RUBIN'S PATHOLOGY:

Clinicopathologic Foundations of Medicine
Fifth edition

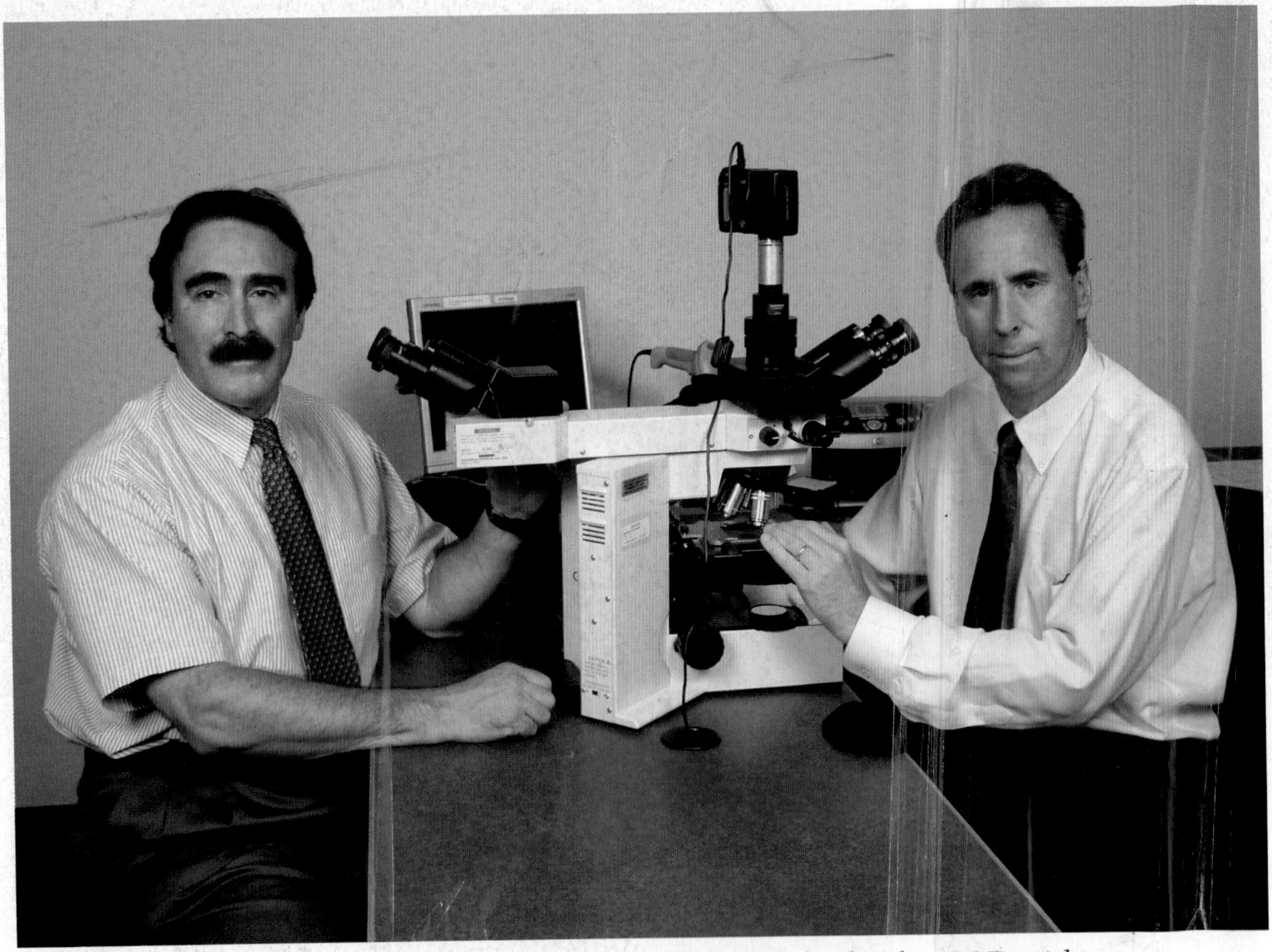

Editors David S. Strayer, M.D., Ph.D., *left* and Raphael Rubin, M.D., *right*.

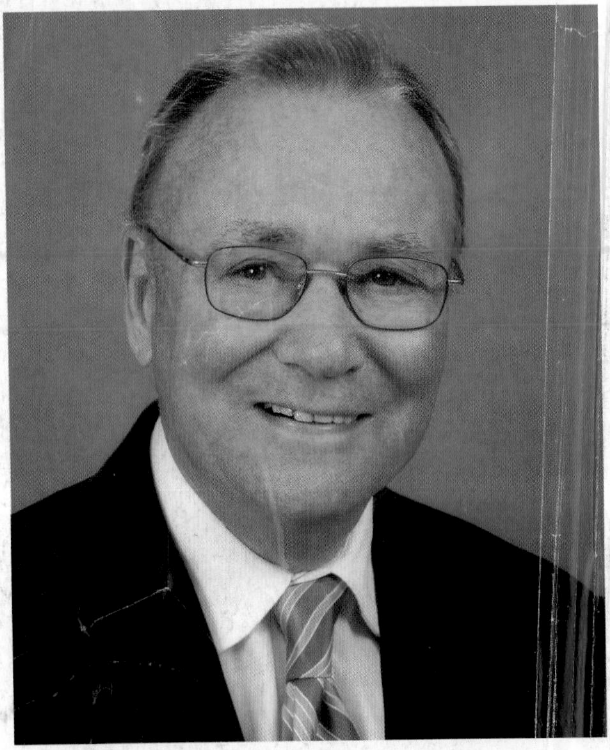

Consulting Editor Emanuel Rubin, M.D.

RUBIN'S PATHOLOGY:

Clinicopathologic Foundations of Medicine

FIFTH EDITION

EDITORS:

Raphael Rubin, M.D.
Professor of Pathology

David S. Strayer, M.D., Ph.D.
Professor of Pathology

Both are in the Department of Pathology, Anatomy, and Cell Biology
Jefferson Medical College of Thomas Jefferson University
Philadelphia, Pennsylvania

CONSULTING EDITOR:

Emanuel Rubin, M.D.
Gonzalo Aponte Distinguished Professor of Pathology
Chairman Emeritus of the Department of Pathology, Anatomy and Cell Biology
Jefferson Medical College
Philadelphia PA.

ASSOCIATE EDITORS:

Jay M. McDonald, M.D.
Professor and Chair, Department of Pathology
Director, Center for Metabolic Bone Disease
Editor-in Chief, American Journal of Pathology
The University of Alabama at Birmingham
Birmingham, Alabama

George K. Michalopoulos, M.D., Ph.D.
Professor and Chairman
Department of Pathology
University of Pittsburgh School of Medicine
Pittsburgh, Pennsylvania

John Q. Trojanowski, M.D., Ph.D.
Professor
Department of Pathology and Laboratory Medicine
University of Pennsylvania School of Medicine
Center for Neurodegenerative Disease Research
Philadelphia, Pennsylvania

Peter A. Ward, M.D.
Godfrey D. Stobbe Professor of Pathology
Department of Pathology
University of Michigan Medical School
Ann Arbor, Michigan

With 44 contributors

Illustrations by Dimitri Karetnikov, George Barile, and Kathy Jaeger

Wolters Kluwer | Lippincott Williams & Wilkins
Health

Philadelphia • Baltimore • New York • London
Buenos Aires • Hong Kong • Sydney • Tokyo

Acquisitions Editor: Betty Sun
Development Editor: Kathleen Scogna
Copy Editor: Dvora Konstant
Marketing Manager: Emilie Linkins
Production Editor: Jennifer P. Ajello and Hearthside Publishing Services
Designer: Risa Clow
Compositor: Maryland Composition, Inc.
Printer: R.R. Donnelley & Sons, Inc.-Willard

351 West Camden Street
Baltimore, MD 21201

530 Walnut Street
Philadelphia, PA 19106

Printed in China

Library of Congress Cataloging-in-Publication Data can be located on the Library of Congress Website: www.libraryof congress.com

ISBN: 0-7817-9516-8 / 978-07817-9516-6

To purchase additional copies of this book, call our customer service department at **(800) 638-3030** or fax orders to **(301) 223-2320**. International customers should call **(301) 223-2300**.

Visit Lippincott Williams & Wilkins on the Internet: http://www.LWW.com. Lippincott Williams & Wilkins customer service representatives are available from 8:30 am to 6:00 pm, EST.

07 08 09 10 11
1 2 3 4 5 6 7 8 9 10

DEDICATION

We dedicate this book to our wives and families, whose love and support throughout this endeavor sustained us; to our colleagues, from whom we have learned so much; and to students everywhere, upon whose curiosity and energy the future of medical science depends.

CONTRIBUTORS

Michael F. Allard, BSc, MD, FRCP(C)
Professor
Department of Pathology & Laboratory Medicine
University of British Columbia
Senior Scientist
The James Hogg iCAPTURE Centre for Cardiovascular and Pulmonary Research
St. Paul's Hospital - Providence Health Care
Vancouver, British Columbia
Canada

Mary Beth Beasley, M.D.
Department of Pathology
Providence Portland Medical Center
Portland, Oregon

Douglas P. Bennett, MD
Clinical Fellow
Division of Infectious Diseases
Department of Medicine
Thomas Jefferson University
Philadelphia, Pennsylvania

Marluce Bibbo, M.D., Sc.D.
Professor of Pathology
Director of Cytopathology
Department of Pathology
Jefferson Medical College
Philadelphia, Pennsylvania

Thomas W. Bouldin, M.D.
Professor and Vice Chair for Faculty & Trainee Development
Department of Pathology and Laboratory Medicine
University of North Carolina at Chapel Hill
Chapel Hill, North Carolina

Mark Curtis, M.D., Ph.D.
Assistant Professor
Department of Pathology, Anatomy, and Cell Biology
Thomas Jefferson University
Philadelphia, Pennsylvania

Ivan Damjanov, M.D., Ph.D
Professor
Department of Pathology
The University of Kansas School of Medicine
Kansas City, Kansas

Giulia De Falco, PhD
Assistant Professor
Department of Human Pathology and Oncology
University of Siena
Siena, Italy

Hormoz Ehya, M.D.
Director of Cytopathology
Department of Pathology
Fox Chase Cancer Center
Philadelphia, Pennsylvania

David Elder, M.D.
Professor
Department of Pathology and Laboratory Medicine
Director of Anatomic Pathology
Hospital of the University of Pennsylvania
Philadelphia, Pennsylvania

Kevin Furlong, D.O.
Clinical Assistant Professor
Division of Endocrinology, Diabetes & Metabolic Diseases
Department of Medicine
Jefferson Medical College
Philadelphia, Pennsylvania

Robert M. Genta, M.D.
Professor of Pathology and Medicine (Gastroenterology)
University of Texas Southwestern Medical Center
Chief, Department of Pathology
Dallas VA Medical Center
Dallas, Texas

Antonio Giordano, M.D., Ph.D
Director
Sbarro Institute for Cancer Research and Molecular Medicine and Center of Biotechnology
College of Science and Technology
Temple University
Philadelphia, PA

Barry Goldstein, M.D., Ph.D.
Director, Division of Endocrinology, Diabetes & Metabolic Diseases
Department of Medicine
Jefferson Medical College
Philadelphia, Pennsylvania

Avrum I. Gotlieb, MDCM, FRCP(C)
Professor and Chair
Department of Laboratory Medicine and Pathobiology
University of Toronto
Toronto, Ontario
Canada

Benjamin Hoch, M.D.
Assistant Professor of Pathology
Director, Orthopaedic Pathology
Director, ENT Pathology
Mount Sinai School of Medicine
New York, New York

Serge Jabbour, MD, FACP, FACE
Associate Professor
Division of Endocrinology, Diabetes & Metabolic Diseases
Department of Medicine
Jefferson Medical College
Philadelphia, Pennsylvania

J. Charles Jennette, M.D.
Kenneth M. Brinkhous Distinguished Professor and Chair
University of North Carolina at Chapel Hill
School of Medicine
Chapel Hill, North Carolina

Lawrence Kenyon, M.D., Ph.D
Assistant Professor
Department of Pathology, Anatomy, and Cell Biology
Jefferson Medical College
Philadelphia, Pennsylvania

Anthony A. Killeen, M.D., Ph.D.
Associate Professor
Director of Clinical Pathology
Department of Laboratory Medicine And Pathology
University of Minnesota
Minneapolis, Minnesota

Robert Kisilevsky MD, PhD, FRCPC
Professor Emeritus
Department of Pathology and Molecular Medicine
Queen's University
Kingston, Ontario
Canada

Gordon K. Klintworth, M.D., Ph.D.
Professor of Pathology and Joseph A.C. Wadsworth Research
Professor of Ophthalmology
Duke University Medical Center
Durham, North Carolina

Gregory Y. Lauwers, M.D.
Director, Gastrointestinal Pathology Service
Massachusetts General Hospital
Associate Professor of Pathology
Harvard Medical School
Boston, Massachussetts

Steven McKenzie, M.D., Ph.D.
Vice President for Research
Thomas Jefferson University
Philadelphia, Pennsylvania

Bruce McManus, M.D., Ph.D, FRSC
Professor
Department of Pathology and Laboratory Medicine
University of British Columbia
Director
The James Hogg iCAPTURE Centre for Cardiovascular and
Pulmonary Research
St. Paul's Hospital-Providence Health Care
Vancouver, British Columbia
Canada

Maria J. Merino-Neumann, M.D.
Senior Principal Investigator
Laboratory of Pathology
National Cancer Institute
National Institutes of Health
Bethesda, Maryland

Mari Mino-Kenudson, M.D.
Assistant in Pathology, Massachusetts General Hospital
Instructor in Pathology, Harvard Medical School
Department of Pathology
Massachusetts General Hospital
Boston, Massachusetts

Michael J. Klein M.D.
Professor of Pathology
Head, Section of Surgical Pathology
University of Alabama School of Medicine
Birmingham, Alabama

Frank A. Mitros, M.D.
Frederic W. Stamler Professor of Anatomical Pathology
Department of Pathology
University of Iowa College of Medicine
Iowa City, Iowa

Hedwig S. Murphy, M.D., Ph.D.
Assistant Professor, Department of Pathology
University of Michigan
Pathologist, Pathology and Laboratory Medicine
Veteran's Affairs Ann Arbor Healthcare System
Ann Arbor, MI

George L. Mutter, M.D.
Associate Professor of Pathology
Harvard Medical School
Department of Pathology
Brigham and Women's Hospital
Boston, Massachusetts

Adeboye O. Osunkoya, M.D.
Clinical and Research Fellow
Division of Genitourinary Pathology
Department of Pathology
The Johns Hopkins Hospital
Baltimore, Maryland

Roger J. Pomerantz, M.D., F.A.C.P.
President, Tibotec
Senior Vice President, World-Wide Therapeutic
Area Head of Virology
Johnson and Johnson Corporation
Yardley, PA

Martha M. Quezado, M.D.
Chief, Neuropathology Unit
Surgical Pathology Section
Laboratory of Pathology
National Cancer Institute
National Institutes of Health
Bethesda, Maryland

Stanley J. Robboy, M.D.
Professor of Pathology
Professor of Obstetrics & Gynecology
Vice Chairman for Diagnostic Services
Duke University Medical Center
Durham, North Carolina

Emanuel Rubin, M.D.
Professor
Department of Pathology, Anatomy, and Cell Biology
Jefferson Medical College of Thomas Jefferson University
Philadelphia, Pennsylvania

Raphael Rubin, M.D.
Professor
Department of Pathology, Anatomy, and Cell Biology
Jefferson Medical College of Thomas Jefferson University
Philadelphia, Pennsylvania

Jeffrey E. Saffitz, M.D., Ph.D
Mallinckrodt Professor of Pathology
Harvard Medical School
Chief, Department of Pathology
Beth Israel Deaconess Medical Center
Boston, Massachusetts

Alan L. Schiller, M.D.
Irene Heinz Given and John LaPorte Given
Professor and Chairman of Pathology
Mount Sinai Medical School
New York, New York

Roland Schwarting, M.D.
Professor & Chair
Cooper University Hospital
Department of Pathology
Camden, New Jersey

David A. Schwartz, M.D., M.S. Hyg.
Associate Clinical Professor
Department of Pathology
Vanderbilt University School of Medicine
Nashville, Tennessee

Gregory C. Sephel, Ph.D.
Associate Professor of Pathology
Vanderbilt University Medical Center
Nashville, Tennessee

Craig A. Storm, M.D.
Assistant Professor
Department of Pathology
Dartmouth-Hitchcock Medical Center
Lebanon, New Hampshire

David S. Strayer, M.D., Ph.D.
Professor
Department of Pathology, Anatomy, and Cell Biology
Jefferson Medical College of Thomas Jefferson University
Philadelphia, Pennsylvania

Ann D. Thor M.D.
Professor and Chair
Department of Pathology
University of Colorado Health Sciences Center at Fitzsimons
Aurora, Colorado

William D. Travis, M.D.
Attending Thoracic Pathologist
Department of Pathology
Memorial Sloan-Kettering Cancer Center
New York, New York

John Q. Trojanowski, M.D., Ph.D.
Professor
Department of Pathology and Laboratory Medicine
University of Pennsylvania School of Medicine
Center for Neurodegenerative Disease Research
Philadelphia, Pennsylvania

Jeffrey S. Warren, M.D.
Warthin/Weller Endowed Professor
and Director, Division of Clinical Pathology
Department of Pathology
University of Michigan Medical School
Ann Arbor, Michigan

Bruce M. Wenig, M.D.
Professor of Pathology
Albert Einstein College of Medicine,
Bronx, NY
Chairman, Department of Pathology and Laboratory Medicine
Beth Israel Medical Center, St. Lukes-Roosevelt Hospitals
New York, New York

Stephen C. Woodward, M.D.
Professor of Pathology, Emeritus
Vanderbilt University Medical Center
Nashville, Tennessee

Robert Yanagawa, Ph.D
Scholar
Faculty of Medicine
University of Toronto
Toronto, Ontario
Canada

Pathology is the study of disease and its effects on the organism. This discipline is a prerequisite for rational medical therapeutics, and has its roots in the early attempts of scholars to understand how human disease begins, manifests and progresses. Celsus (25 BC–50 AD) was the first to describe the cardinal signs of inflammation: *tumor* (swelling), *rubor* (redness), *calor* (heat) and *dolor* (pain). However, deeper understanding of disease awaited several developments that did not occur for one and one half millennia.

The first major advance was the introduction of the necropsy by Antonio Benivieni (1443–1502). The modern approach to autopsy technique was pioneered by Carl Rokitansky (1804–1878) in Vienna. Among the most important applications of postmortem examination is to elucidate the course of a disease in an individual patient, as manifest through its clinical symptoms and signs. Giovanni Morgangni (1682–1771) is credited with developing the concept of clinicopathologic correlation, which remain the foundation of our approach to the study of disease.

The compound microscope was invented in 1595 in Holland by Zacharias Jansen (1588–1631). In 1665, Robert Hooke (1635–1703) in England first coined the term "cell" after examining a piece of cork under a microscope. Nearly 200 years elapsed until the theory of the cell as the building block of all living organisms was enunciated by Matthias Schleiden (1804–1881) and Theodor Schwann (1810–1882). The theory was refined by Rudolf Virchow (1821–1902) to stipulate that all existing cells derive from previously existing cells, and pathologic reactions are, therefore, reactions of cells.

As the techniques used to study the human body in health and disease evolved from structural to mechanistic, diverse scientific disciplines have been at the forefront of medical progress, including physiology, biochemistry, biophysics, immunology, genetics and, more recently, molecular biology, genomics and proteomics. The approaches pioneered by investigators in these areas have been adopted as tools of the pathologist: cellular biochemistry, electron microscopy, immunostaining, flow cytometry, molecular probes and genetic analysis, to name a few. Thus, the coordinate evolution of biological research and pathology continues to provide new opportunities to understand and, hopefully, treat disease. The medical significance of seemingly arcane mutations or signaling pathways is increasingly evident, and with the advent of pharmacologic and genetic manipulation, continues to enter the realm of medical practice.

The basic function of Pathology in the medical curriculum and in medical practice has become less descriptive and more mechanistic and integrative. Pathology, as presented in this text, and as practiced in most medical schools, is in equal measure morphology and pathophysiology. As such, this text seeks to relate clincal and histological manifestations of disease to their basic mechanisms.

The student arrives in the Pathology classroom having mastered the basic sciences of the medical curriculum: physiology, biochemistry, anatomy, molecular biology, etc. It is in the context of Pathology that a framework for future medical training is constructed, by integrating these subjects into the setting of a whole patient. Disease processes may be seen as injuring cells and impairing organ function, altering signaling cascades and cytokine production and upsetting the balance of electrolytes and cells in the blood. But Pathology breathes life into these analyses by focusing on the consequences of these abnormal processes for the human being.

In this context, this 5th edition of *Rubin's Pathology* presents Pathology as the clinicopathologic foundation of medicine, and endeavors to provide medical students and their instructors with a lucid discussion of basic disease processes and their effects on cells, organs and people. Significant advances in the understanding of basic pathophysiologic processes are incorporated into revised chapters on basic disease processes (Chapters 1–9) and specific organ pathology (Chapters 10–30). Notable examples include new sections on proteasomal degradation, stem cells, diabetes and obesity, emerging infections and agents of biowarfare.

This edition also represents a transition in editorship. Emanuel Rubin, the founder and main Editor of this textbook for its first four editions, is now Consulting Editor. With deepest appreciation for Manny's contribution to this work and to our careers, and with the encouragement of the publishers, we have assumed editorial responsibility for this textbook. New contributors from many institutions have joined the distinguished roster of authors. We include for the first time ancillary learning materials: audio questions, on-line text and illustrations and case studies. Self-assessment and review is further available using the companion text *Review of Pathology*.

Pathology is a dynamic discipline. Any textbook such as this is a snapshot of an object in motion. It has been our goal to provide an authoritative instructional and reference text that accurately portrays the field in 2006–2007, both what is known and what remains to be explained. We hope that our students will share the excitement of discovery that we have been privileged to experience in our education and careers.

Raphael Rubin
David S. Strayer
Philadelphia
January, 2007

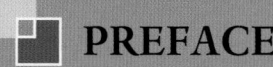

ACKNOWLEDGMENTS

Many dedicated people, too numerous to list, provided insight that made this 5th Edition of *Rubin's Pathology* possible. The editors would like especially to thank the managing and editorial staff at Lippincott, Williams & Wilkins division of Wolters-Kluwer and in particular Betty Sun and Kathleen Scogna, without whose help this volume would not have been possible.

The editors also acknowledge the contributions made by our colleagues who participated in writing previous editions and those who offered suggestions and ideas for the current edition.

Stuart A. Aaronson
Mohammad Alomari
Adam Bagg
Karoly Balogh
Sue Bartow
Hugh Bonner
Patrick J. Buckley
Stephen W. Chensue
Daniel H. Connor
Jeffrey Cossman
John E. Craighead
Mary Cunnane
Joseph C. Fantone
John L. Farber
Gregory N. Fuller
Stanley R. Hamiliton
Terrence J. Harrist
Arthur P. Hays
Robert B. Jennings
Kent J. Johnson
Michael J. Klein
William D. Kocher
Robert J. Kurman
Ernest A. Lack
Antonio Martinez-Hernandez
Wolfgang J. Mergner
Juan Palazzo
Robert O. Peterson
Timothy R. Quinn
Brian Schapiro
Stephen M. Schwartz
Benjamin H. Spargo
Charles Steenbergen, Jr.
Steven L. Teitelbaum
Benjamin F. Trump
Jianzhou Wang
Beverly Y. Wang

TABLE OF CONTENTS

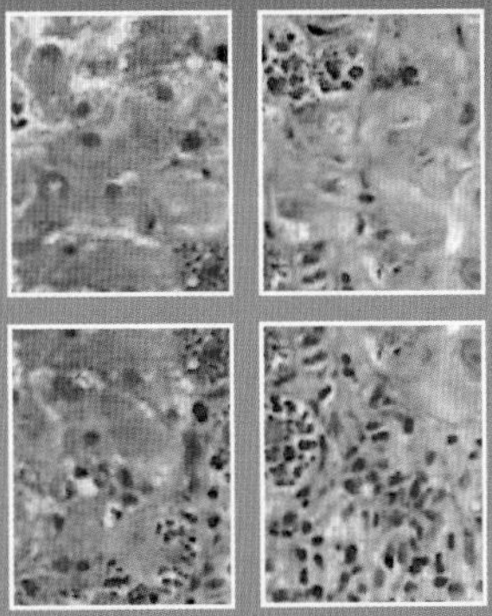

1

Cell Injury

David S. Strayer
Emanuel Rubin

Pathology *is basically the study of structural and functional abnormalities that are expressed as diseases of organs and systems.* Classic theories of disease attributed disease to imbalances or noxious effects of humors on specific organs. In the 19th century, Rudolf Virchow, often referred to as the father of modern pathology, proposed that injury to the smallest living unit of the body, the cell, is the basis of all disease. To this day, clinical and experimental pathology remain rooted in this concept.

Teleology—the study of design or purpose in nature—has long since been discredited as part of scientific investigation. Although facts can only be established by observation, to appreciate the mechanisms of injury to the cell, teleologic thinking can be useful in framing questions. As an analogy, it would be impossible to understand a chess-playing computer without an understanding of the goals of chess and prior knowledge that a particular computer is programmed to play it: it would be futile to search for the sources of defects in the specific program or overall operating system without an appreciation of the goals of the device. In this sense, it is helpful to understand the problems with which the cell is confronted and the strategies that have evolved to cope with them.

A living cell must maintain the ability to produce energy. Thus, the most pressing need for any free living cell, prokaryotic or eukaryotic, is to establish a structural and functional barrier between its internal milieu and a hostile environment. The plasma membrane serves this purpose in several ways:

- It maintains a constant internal ionic composition against very large chemical gradients between the interior and exterior compartments.
- It selectively admits some molecules while excluding or extruding others.
- It provides a structural envelope to contain the informational, synthetic, and catabolic constituents of the cell.
- It provides an environment to house signal transduction molecules that mediate communication between the external and internal milieus.

At the same time, to survive, a cell must be able to adapt to adverse environmental conditions, such as changes in temperature, solute concentrations, or oxygen supply; the presence of noxious agents; and so on. The evolution of multicellular organisms eased the hazardous lot of individual cells by establishing a controlled extracellular environment in which temperature, oxygenation, ionic content, and nutrient supply are relatively constant. It also permitted the luxury of cell differentiation for such widely divergent functions as energy storage (liver cell glycogen and adipocytes), communication (neurons), contractile activity (heart muscle), synthesis of proteins or peptides for export (liver, pancreas, and endocrine cells), absorption (intestine), and defense from foreign invaders (polymorphonuclear leukocytes, lymphocytes, and macrophages).

Cells encounter many stresses as a result of changes in their internal and external environments. *Patterns of response to such stresses is the cellular basis of disease.* If an injury exceeds the adaptive capacity of the cell, the cell dies. A cell exposed to persistent sublethal injury has limited available responses, the expression of which we interpret as evidence of cell injury. In general, mammalian cells adapt to injury by conserving resources: decreasing or ceasing differentiated functions and focusing exclusively on its own survival. *From this perspective, pathology is the study of cell injury and the expression of a cell's preexisting capacity to adapt to such injury.* Such an orientation leaves little room for the concept of parallel—normal and pathologic—biologies.

Reactions to Persistent Stress and Cell Injury

Persistent stress often leads to chronic cell injury. In general, permanent organ injury is associated with the death of individual cells. By contrast, the cellular response to persistent sublethal injury, whether chemical or physical, reflects adaptation of the cell to a hostile environment. Again, these changes are, for the most part, reversible on discontinuation of the stress. In response to persistent stress, a cell dies or adapts. It is thus our view that at the cellular level it is more appropriate to speak of chronic adaptation than of chronic injury. The major adaptive responses are atrophy, hypertrophy, hyperplasia, metaplasia, dysplasia, and intracellular storage. In addition, certain forms of neoplasia may follow adaptive responses.

Proteasomes are Key Participants in Cell Homeostasis, Response to Stress, and Adaptation to Altered Extracellular Environment

Cellular responses to alterations in their milieu were once studied exclusively by analyzing changes in gene expression and protein production. The issue of protein degradation was either ignored or relegated to the nonspecific proteolytic activities of lysosomes. However it has become clear that cellular homeostasis requires mechanisms that allow the cell to destroy certain proteins selectively. Although there is evidence that more than one such pathway may exist, the best understood mechanism by which cells target specific proteins for elimination is the ubiquitin (Ub)-proteasomal apparatus.

Proteasomes

There are two different types of these cellular organelles, 20S and 26S. The degradative unit is the 20S core, to which two additional 19S "caps" may be attached to make a 26S proteasome. There are at least 32 different proteins in the 2.5 MDa proteasomal complex. They are arrayed, as shown in Fig. 1-1, with one 19S subunit at either end of the barrel-like 20S degradative center.

Proteins targeted for destruction are modified as described below, and recognized by one 19S subunit. They are then degraded in an adenosine triphosphate (ATP)-requiring process, by the 20S subunit. The products of this process are peptides that are 3 to 25 amino acids in size, which are released through the lower 19S subunit.

The importance of this structure is underscored by the fact that it may comprise up to 1% of the total protein of the cell. Proteasomes are evolutionarily highly conserved, and are described in all eukaryotic cells. Mutation in key proteins, leading to interference with normal proteasomal function, are lethal.

The 20S proteasomes are important in degradation of oxidized proteins (see below). In 26S proteasomes, ubiquitinated proteins are degraded.

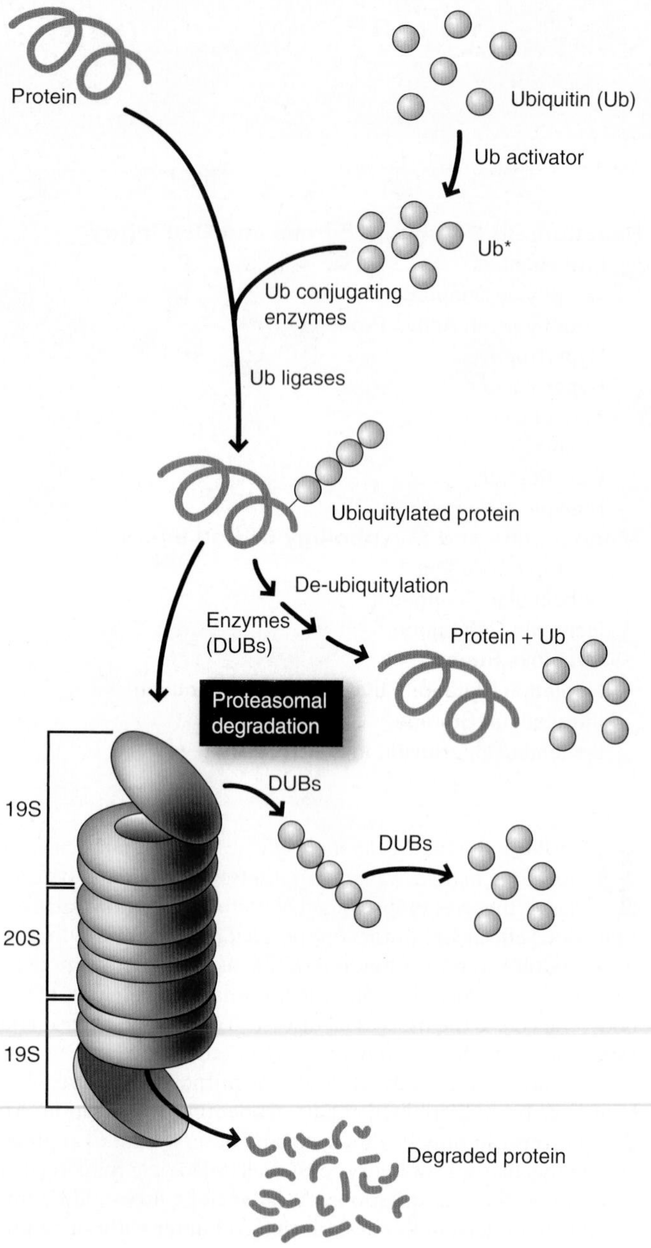

FIGURE 1-1. **Ubiquitin-proteasome pathways.** The mechanisms by which ubiquitin (Ub) targets proteins for specific elimination in proteasomes are shown here. Ub is activated (Ub*) by E1 ubiquitin activating enzyme, then transferred to an E2 (ubiquitin conjugating enzyme). The E2-Ub* complex interacts with an E3 (ubiquitin ligase) to bind a particular protein. The process may be repeated multiple times to append a chain of Ub moieties. These complexes may be deubiquitinated by de-ubiquitinating enzymes (DUBs). If degradation is to proceed, 26S proteasomes recognize the poly-Ub-conjugated protein via their 19S subunit and degrade it into oligopeptides. In the process, Ub moieties are returned to the cell pool of ubiquitin monomers.

Ubiquitin and Ubiquitination

Proteins to be degraded are flagged by attaching small chains of ubiquitin molecules to them. Ub is a 76-amino acid protein that is almost identical in yeast as in humans. It is the key to selective protein elimination: it is conjugated to proteins as a flag to identify those proteins to be destroyed. The process of attaching Ub to proteins is called ubiquitination.

A cascade of enzymes is involved (see Fig. 1-1). Ub activating enzyme, E1, binds Ub then transfers it to one of dozens of Ub conjugating enzymes (E2). These bind one of over 500 Ub ligating enzymes (E3), which add the Ub to an ϵ-amino group of a lysine on the doomed protein. In the multiple cycles of this reaction, subsequent Ub moieties are added to the original, forming a polybuiquitin chain (at least 4 Ubs). The specificity of the process resides in the combinations of E2 and E3 enzymes. Proteins to be degraded have specific structures called degrons, that are recognized by E2-E3 combinations. Degrons are two-part structures with a recognition unit and the site of Ub conjugation.

The system is complex, however. First there are de-ubiquitinating enzymes (DUBs) which can reverse the process. As well, addition of only one or two Ub moieties may occur as part of other cellular functions. Such ubiquitination is important in cell membrane budding, vesicular transport, and protein sorting within cellular compartments.

Further, some modifications of proteins may protect them from ubiquitination. When the tumor suppressor protein, p53, is phosphorylated in response to DNA damage, it is protected from Ub-mediated degradation.

Ubiquitin-like Proteins

There are a number of proteins that resemble, but are structurally distinct from, Ub, and that subserve somewhat different functions. Sentrin/SUMO may be added to proteins similarly to Ub, but is not known to be involved with protein degradation. NEDD8 is a closer homolog of Ub. It may participate in forming some E3 complexes and may substitute for Ub in poly-Ub chains.

How Ubiquitination Matters

The importance of ubiquitination and specific protein elimination is fundamental to cellular adaptation to stress and injury, as the following sections will show. It is also involved in disease processes. Defective ubiquitination may play a role in several important neurodegenerative diseases. Mutations in parkin, a ubiquitin ligase, and a combined E3-DUB enzyme, are implicated in two hereditary forms of Parkinson disease. Manipulation of ubiquitination may be important in tumor development. Thus, human papilloma virus strains that are associated with human cervical cancer (see Chapters 5, 18) produce E6 protein, which inactivates the p53 tumor suppressor. This inactivation is implicated in the genesis of cervical cancer. E6 accomplishes this by binding an E3 (ubiquitin ligase), thereby facilitating its association with p53, leading to increased p53 ubiquitination and accelerating p53 degradation. Finally, there is increasing evidence suggesting that impaired ubiquitination may be involved in some cellular degenerative changes that occur in aging and in some storage diseases.

Ubiquitination also plays a role in gene expression. Nuclear factor-κB (NFκB) is an important transcriptional activator. The inhibitor of NFκB, called IκB, is degraded by ubiquitination. This step appears to be important in NFκB-mediated gene expression since proteasome inhibition greatly decreases NFκB-induced transcriptional activation.

Other Specific Protein Degradation Pathways

There are other mechanisms by which cells may selectively eliminate particular proteins. For example, in chaperone-mediated autophagy (CMA) a chaperone related to heat shock protein-70 (called hsc70) binds particular sequences in proteins and directs them to lysosomes for destruction. CMA is activated as an adaptive response in some stress situations, such as starvation. Defects in this pathway occur during aging and have been related to some lysosomal storage diseases, but the extent to which CMA mechanisms may be involved in other disease processes remains conjectural.

Atrophy Is an Adaptation to Diminished Need or Resources for a Cell's Activities

Clinically, atrophy is often noted as decreased size or function of an organ. It may occur under both pathologic and physiologic circumstances. Thus, atrophy may result from disuse of skeletal muscle or from loss of trophic signals as part of normal aging. Atrophy may be thought of as an adaptive response whereby a cell accommodates to changes in its environment, all the while remaining viable.

One must distinguish atrophy of an organ from cellular atrophy. Reduction in an organ's size may reflect reversible cell atrophy or irreversible loss of cells. For example, atrophy of the brain in Alzheimer disease is secondary to extensive cell death; the size of the organ cannot be restored (Fig. 1-2). Atrophy occurs under a variety of conditions outlined below.

Reduced Functional Demand

The most common form of atrophy follows reduced functional demand. For example, after immobilization of a limb in a cast as treatment for a bone fracture or after prolonged bed rest, the limb's muscle cells atrophy and muscular strength is reduced. When normal activity resumes, the muscle's size and function return.

Inadequate Supply of Oxygen

Interference with blood supply to tissues is called **ischemia**. Total cessation of oxygen perfusion of tissues results in cell death. However, when oxygen deprivation is insufficient to kill cells,

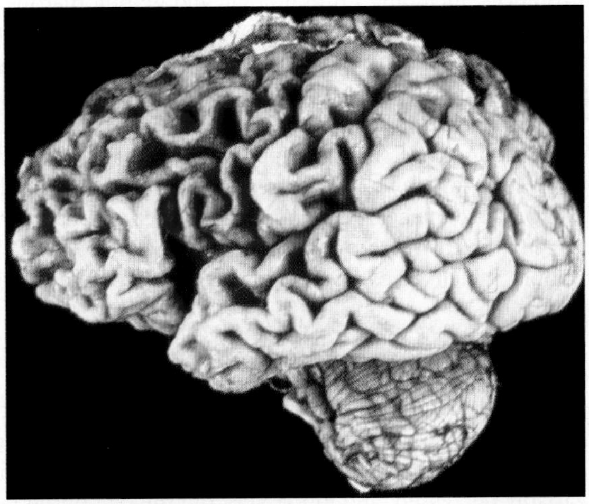

FIGURE 1-2. **Atrophy of the brain.** Marked atrophy of the frontal lobe is noted in this photograph of the brain. The gyri are thinned and the sulci conspicuously widened.

resulting partial ischemia is often compatible with cell viability. Under such circumstances, cell atrophy is common. It is frequently seen around the inadequately perfused margins of ischemic necrosis (infarcts) in the heart, brain, and kidneys following vascular occlusion in these organs.

Insufficient Nutrients

Starvation or inadequate nutrition associated with chronic disease leads to cell atrophy, particularly in skeletal muscle. It is striking that reduction in mass is particularly prominent in cells that are not vital to the survival of the organism. One cannot dismiss the possibility that a portion of the cell atrophy attributed to partial ischemia reflects a lack of nutrients.

Interruption of Trophic Signals

The functions of many cells depend on signals transmitted by chemical mediators. The endocrine system and neuromuscular transmission are the best examples. The actions of hormones or, for skeletal muscle, synaptic transmission, place functional demands on cells. These can be eliminated by removing the source of the signal, e.g., via ablation of an endocrine gland or denervation. If the anterior pituitary is surgically resected, loss of thyroid-stimulating hormone (TSH), adrenocorticotropic hormone (ACTH, also termed corticotropin), and follicle-stimulating hormone (FSH) results in atrophy of the thyroid, adrenal cortex, and ovaries, respectively. Atrophy secondary to endocrine insufficiency is not restricted to pathologic conditions: the endometrium atrophies when estrogen levels decrease after menopause (Fig. 1-3). Even cancer cells may undergo atrophy, to some extent, by hormonal deprivation. Androgen-dependent prostatic cancer partially regresses after administration of testosterone antagonists. Certain types of thyroid cancer may stop growing if one inhibits pituitary TSH secretion by administering thyroxine. If neurologic damage, e.g., from poliomyelitis or traumatic spinal cord injury, leads to denervation of muscle, the neuromuscular transmission necessary for muscle tone is lost and affected muscles atrophy.

Persistent Cell Injury

Persistent cell injury is most commonly caused by chronic inflammation associated with prolonged viral or bacterial infections. Chronic inflammation may be seen in a variety of other circumstances, including immunologic and granulomatous disorders. A good example is the atrophy of the gastric mucosa that occurs in association with chronic gastritis (see Chapter 13). Similarly, villous atrophy of the small intestinal mucosa follows the chronic inflammation of celiac disease. Even physical injury, such as prolonged pressure in inappropriate locations, produces atrophy. Heart failure leads to increased pressure in sinusoids of the liver because the heart cannot pump the venous return from that organ efficiently. Accordingly, the cells in the center of the liver lobule, which are exposed to the greatest pressure, become atrophic.

Aging

One of the hallmarks of aging, particularly in nonreplicating cells such as those of the brain and heart, is cell atrophy. The size of all parenchymal organs decreases with age. The size of the brain is invariably decreased, and in the very old the size of the heart may be so diminished that the term **senile atrophy** has been used.

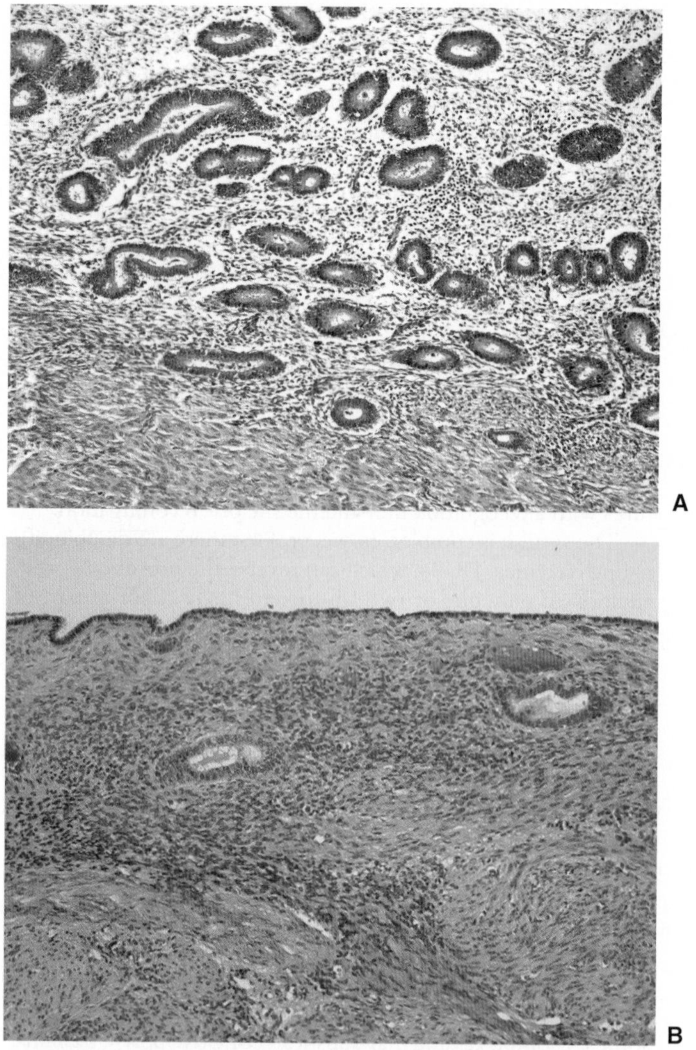

FIGURE 1-3. **Proliferative endometrium. A.** A section of the uterus from a woman of reproductive age reveals a thick endometrium composed of proliferative glands in an abundant stroma. **B.** The endometrium of a 75-year-old woman (shown at the same magnification) is thin and contains only a few atrophic and cystic glands.

Atrophy Is an Active Process

Atrophy involves changes both in production and destruction of cellular constituents. In its most basic sense, atrophy is a cell's reversible restructuring of its activities to facilitate its own survival and adapt to conditions of diminished use.

This process has been most extensively studied in skeletal muscle, which responds rapidly to changes in demand for contractile force. Since striated muscle cells are terminally differentiated, they allow study of atrophy and hypertrophy (see below) without the confounding influence of cell proliferation. This system is used here to illustrate the mechanisms of cell atrophy. When the need for contraction decreases ("unloading," see below), cells institute several selective adaptive mechanisms.

- **Protein synthesis.** Shortly after unloading, protein synthesis decreases. This effect appears mainly to reflect decreased protein elongation at the ribosomes. In the immediate term, RNA levels for contractile proteins are not altered.

- **Protein degradation.** Ubiquitin-related specific protein degradation pathways are activated. These mediate the atrophic response in several ways. They lead to decreases in specific contractile proteins. Ubiquitination of specific transcription factors (e.g., myoD) that increase expression of contractile protein genes further steers the cells adaptive atrophy. The increase in specific protein elimination is transient and if the atrophied state is maintained, the cells reach a new steady state in which mass remains decreased and rates of protein synthesis and degradation re in alignment.
- **Gene expression.** There are selective decreases in transcription of genes for, among other things, contractile activities. Transcription of some genes is upregulated, particularly genes encoding specific E3 enzymes (Ub-ligases) involved in ubiquitinating contractile proteins. Proteasome subunit synthesis is also increased.
- **Signaling.** More complex, and less well understood, changes in intracellular signaling occur. Atrophy-related increased Ub activity causes ubiquitination and elimination of inhibitors of NFκB. This in turn leads to increased NFκB activity. The ramifications of this aspect of the atrophic response are not yet clear.
- **Energy utilization.** A selective decrease in use of free fatty acids as an energy source has been noted during the response to unloading.

Atrophy is thus an active adaptive response, not a passive shutdown of cellular processes, to which the Ub pathway and specific protein elimination by proteasomes are fundamental. The atrophic response is reversible: restoring the pre-atrophy environment allows cells to return to their pre-atrophy functionality.

Hypertrophy Is an Increase in Cell Size and Functional Capacity

When trophic signals or functional demand increase, adaptive changes to satisfy these needs lead to increased cellular size (hypertrophy) and, in some cases, increased cellular number (hyperplasia, see below).

In organs made of terminally differentiated cells (e.g., heart, skeletal muscle), such adaptive responses are accomplished solely by increased cell size (Fig. 1-4). In other organs (e.g., kidney, thyroid) cell numbers and cell size may both increase. This section deals with the mechanisms and consequences when cells enlarge to meet increased functional demands on them. Some mechanisms involved in the hypertrophic response are cell type-specific and some are more general. Also, cells that can divide use some of the same mechanisms to stimulate mitosis that nondividing cells use to increase their size.

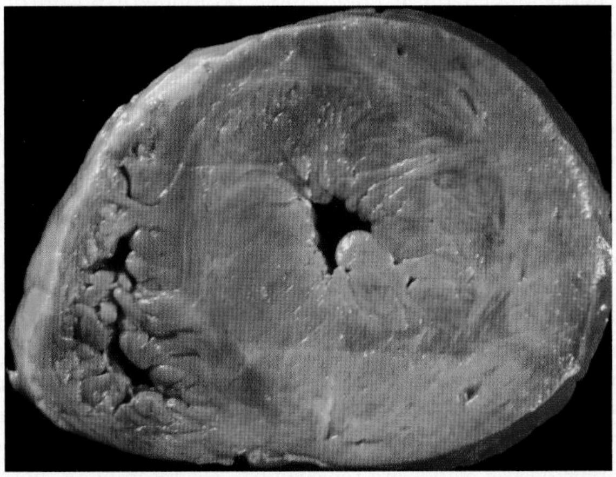

FIGURE 1-4. **Myocardial hypertrophy.** Cross-section of the heart of a patient with long-standing hypertension shows pronounced, concentric left ventricular hypertrophy.

Mechanisms of Cellular Hypertrophy

Whether the stimulus to enlarge is increased work load or increased endocrine or neuroendocrine mediators, there are certain processes that usually contribute to generating cellular hypertrophy.

Cellular Remodeling in Hypertrophy

When cells are stimulated to increase mass one of the first activities is increased proteasomal degradation of selected cellular macromolecular constituents. Thus, proteins that do not contribute to the specific functional need to be expanded are degraded, even as production of proteins that do so contribute increases.

Signaling Mechanisms in Hypertrophy

Although signals that elicit hypertrophic responses vary, depending on the cell type and circumstances, the example of skeletal muscle hypertrophy illustrates some critical general principles. Thus, many types of signaling may lead to cell hypertrophy:

- **Growth factor stimulation.** Each tissue responds to different signals. In many cases certain growth factors appear to be key initiators of hypertrophy. Thus, insulin-like growth factor-I (IGF-I) is increased in load-induced muscle hypertrophy and in experimental settings may elicit hypertrophy even if load does not increase.
- **Neuroendocrine stimulation.** In some tissues, adrenergic or noradrenergic signaling may be important in initiating and/or facilitating hypertrophy.
- **Ion channels.** Ion fluxes may activate adaptation to increased demand. Calcium channel activity, in particular, may stimulate a host of downstream enzymes (e.g., calcineurin) to produce hypertrophy.
- **Other chemical mediators.** Depending on the particular tissue, such factors as nitric oxide (NO•), angiotensin II, and bradykinin may support cell hypertrophic responses.
- **Oxygen supply.** Clearly increased functional demand on cells requires increased energy supply. Angiogenesis is stimulated when a tissue oxygen deficit is sensed and may be an indispensable component of adaptive hypertrophy.
- **Hypertrophy antagonists.** Just as some mechanisms foster cellular hypertrophy, others inhibit it. Atrial and B-type natriuretic factors, high concentrations of NO• and many other factors either brake or prevent cell adaptation by hypertrophy.

Effector Pathways

Whatever mechanisms initiate the signaling process to stimulate hypertrophy, there are a limited number of downstream pathways that mediate the effects of such signaling.

- **Increased protein degradation.** This was discussed above.
- **Increased protein translation.** Shortly after a prohypertrophic signal is received, production of certain proteins increases. This occurs very quickly and without changes in

RNA levels, via increased translational efficiency. Activities of translational initiators and elongation factors are often stimulated in the early phases of hypertrophy, to provide a rapid increase in the proteins needed to meet the increased functional demand.

- **Increased gene expression.** Concentrations of key proteins are also increased by upregulation of transcription of genes that encode those proteins. Many of the signaling pathways activated by cytokines, neurotransmitters, and so forth, activate an array of transcription factors. Thus, for example, calcineurin dephosphorylates the misnamed nuclear factor of activated T lymphocytes (NFAT), facilitating NFAT movement to the nucleus by unmasking its nuclear localization signal and leading to increased transcription of target genes. Hypertrophy may involve increased transcription of genes encoding growth-promoting transcription factors, such as Fos and Myc.
- **Survival.** Among the functions activated during hypertrophy is inhibition of cell death. Thus, stimulation of several receptors increases the activity of several kinases (Akt, PI3K and others) (see below). These in turn promote cell survival, largely by inhibiting programmed cell death (apoptosis, see below).
- **Ancillary functions.** In some situations hypertrophy may involve changes in a cell's relation to its environment, such as remodelling extracellular matrix. It has been suggested that skeletal muscle hypertrophy may include recruiting perimuscular satellite cells to fuse with the muscle syncytia, providing additional nuclei to the expanding muscle.

In sum, the diverse stimuli that lead to cell hypertrophy stimulate adaptive cellular remodeling, increase protein production, facilitate cell function, and promote cell survival.

Hyperplasia Is an Increase in the Number of Cells in an Organ or Tissue

Hypertrophy and hyperplasia are not mutually exclusive and often occur concurrently. The specific stimuli that induce hyperplasia and the mechanisms by which they act vary greatly from one tissue and cell type to the next. Diverse agents that elicit hyperplastic responses in one tissue may do so by entirely different mechanisms. Basically, however it is evoked, hyperplasia involves stimulating resting (G0) cells to enter the cell cycle (G1) and then to multiply. This may be a response to altered endocrine milieu, increased functional demand or chronic injury.

Hormonal Stimulation

Changes in hormone concentrations can elicit proliferation of responsive cells. These changes may reflect developmental, pharmacologic, or pathologic influences. Thus, the normal increase in estrogens at puberty or early in the menstrual cycle leads to increased numbers of endometrial and uterine stromal cells. Estrogen administration to postmenopausal women has the same effect. Enlargement of the male breast, called gynecomastia, may occur in liver failure when the liver's inability to metabolize endogenous estrogens leads to their accumulation, or in men given estrogens as therapy for prostate cancer. Ectopic hormone production, e.g., erythropoietin by renal tumors, may lead to hyperplasia (in this case, of erythrocytes in the bone marrow), and may be a tumor's first presenting symptom.

Increased Functional Demand

Hyperplasia, like hypertrophy, may be a response to increased physiologic demand. At high altitudes low atmospheric oxygen content leads to compensatory hyperplasia of erythrocyte precursors in the bone marrow and increased erythrocytes in the blood (secondary polycythemia) (Fig. 1-5). In this fashion, increased numbers of cells compensate for the decreased oxygen carried by each erythrocyte. The number of erythrocytes promptly falls to normal on return to sea level. Similarly, chronic blood loss, as in excessive menstrual bleeding, also causes hyperplasia of erythrocytic elements.

Immune responsiveness to many antigens may lead to lymphoid hyperplasia, e.g., the enlarged tonsils and swollen lymph nodes that occur with streptococcal pharyngitis. The hypocalcemia that occurs in chronic renal failure leads to increased demand for parathyroid hormone in order to increase blood calcium. The result is hyperplasia of the parathyroid glands.

Chronic Injury

Persistent injury may lead to hyperplasia. Long-standing inflammation or chronic physical or chemical injury often results in a hyperplastic response. For instance, pressure from ill-fitting shoes causes hyperplasia of the skin of the foot, so-called corns or calluses. If one considers that a key function of the skin is to protect underlying structures, such hyperplasia results in thickening of the skin and enhances the skin's functional capacity. Chronic inflammation of the bladder (chronic cystitis) often causes hyperplasia of the bladder epithelium, visible as white plaques on the bladder lining.

Inappropriate hyperplasia can itself be harmful—witness the unpleasant consequences of psoriasis, which is characterized by conspicuous hyperplasia of the skin (see Fig. 1-5D). Excessive estrogen stimulation, whether from endogenous or exogenous sources, may lead to endometrial hyperplasia.

The cellular and molecular mechanisms responsible for hyperplastic responses clearly relate to control of cell proliferation. These topics are discussed in Chapters 3 and 5, and under the heading of liver regeneration in Chapter 14.

Metaplasia Is Conversion of One Differentiated Cell Type to Another

Metaplasia is usually an adaptive response to chronic, persistent injury. That is, a tissue will assume the phenotype that provides it the best protection from the insult. Most commonly, glandular epithelium is replaced by squamous epithelium. Columnar or cuboidal lining cells may be committed to mucus production, but may not be adequately resistant to the effects of chronic irritation or a pernicious chemical. For example, prolonged exposure of the bronchial epithelium to tobacco smoke leads to squamous metaplasia. A similar response occurs in the endocervix, associated with chronic infection (Fig. 1-6). In molecular terms, metaplasia involves replacing the expression of one set of differentiation genes with another.

The process is not restricted to squamous differentiation. When highly acidic gastric contents reflux chronically into the lower esophagus, the squamous epithelium of the esophagus may be replaced by stomach-like glandular mucosa (Barrett epithelium). This can be thought of as an adaption to protect the esophagus from injury by gastric acid and pepsin, to which the normal gastric mucosa is resistant. Metaplasia may also consist of replacement of one glandular epithelium by another. In chronic gastritis, a disorder of the stomach characterized by chronic inflammation, atrophic gastric glands are replaced by cells resembling those of the small intestine. The adaptive value of this condition, known as intestinal metaplasia, is not clear. Metaplasia of transitional epithelium to glandular epithelium occurs when the bladder is chronically inflamed (cystitis glandularis).

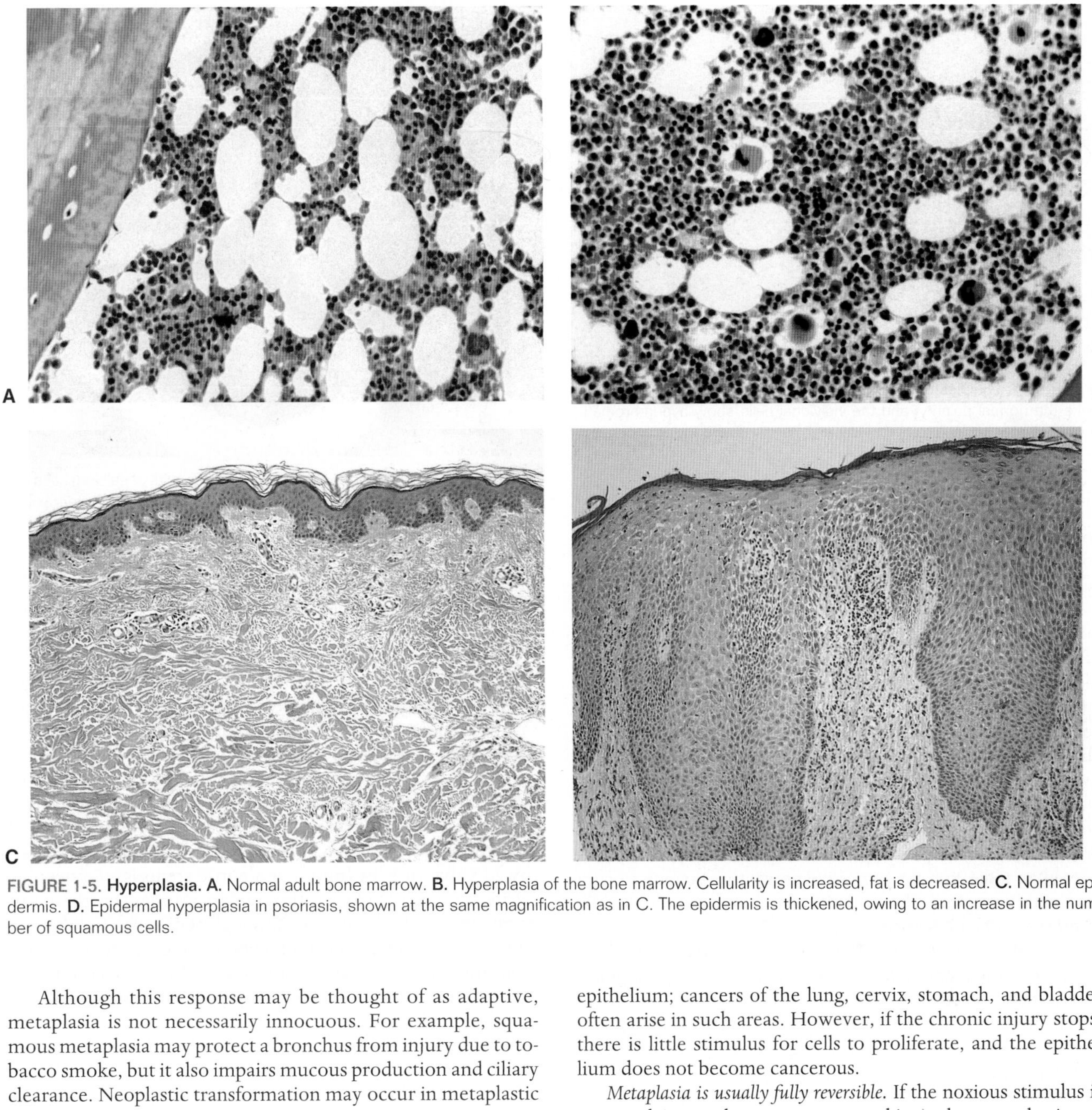

FIGURE 1-5. **Hyperplasia. A.** Normal adult bone marrow. **B.** Hyperplasia of the bone marrow. Cellularity is increased, fat is decreased. **C.** Normal epidermis. **D.** Epidermal hyperplasia in psoriasis, shown at the same magnification as in C. The epidermis is thickened, owing to an increase in the number of squamous cells.

Although this response may be thought of as adaptive, metaplasia is not necessarily innocuous. For example, squamous metaplasia may protect a bronchus from injury due to tobacco smoke, but it also impairs mucous production and ciliary clearance. Neoplastic transformation may occur in metaplastic epithelium; cancers of the lung, cervix, stomach, and bladder often arise in such areas. However, if the chronic injury stops, there is little stimulus for cells to proliferate, and the epithelium does not become cancerous.

Metaplasia is usually fully reversible. If the noxious stimulus is removed (e.g., when one stops smoking), the metaplastic epithelium eventually returns to normal.

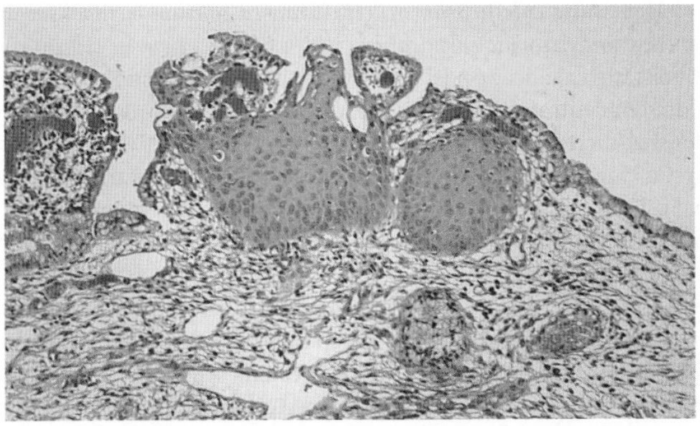

FIGURE 1-6. **Squamous metaplasia.** A section of endocervix shows the normal columnar epithelium at both margins and a focus of squamous metaplasia in the center.

Dysplasia is Disordered Growth and Maturation of the Cellular Components of a Tissue

The cells that compose an epithelium normally exhibit uniformity of size, shape, and nucleus. Moreover, they are arranged in a regular fashion, as, for example, a squamous epithelium progresses from plump basal cells to flat superficial cells. In dysplasia, this monotonous appearance is disturbed by (1) variation in cell size and shape; (2) nuclear enlargement, irregularity, and hyperchromatism; and (3) disarray in the arrangement of cells within the epithelium (Fig. 1-7). Dysplasia occurs most often in hyperplastic squamous epithelium, as seen in epidermal actinic keratosis (caused by sunlight) and in areas of squamous metaplasia, such as in the bronchus or the cervix. It is not, however, exclusive to squamous epithelium. Ulcerative

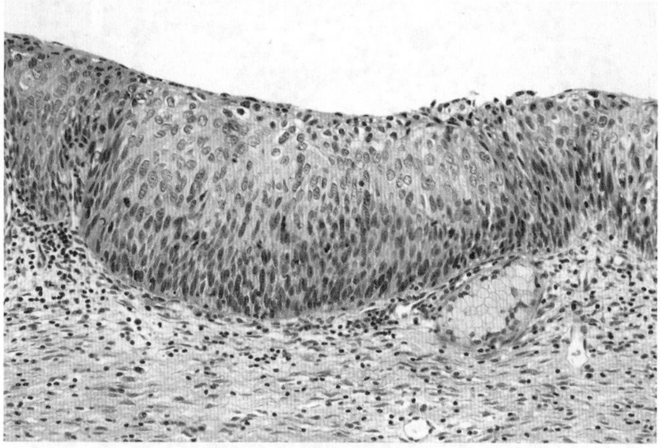

FIGURE 1-7. **Dysplasia.** The dysplastic epithelium of the uterine cervix lacks the normal polarity, and the individual cells show hyperchromatic nuclei, a larger nucleus-to-cytoplasm ratio, and a disorderly arrangement.

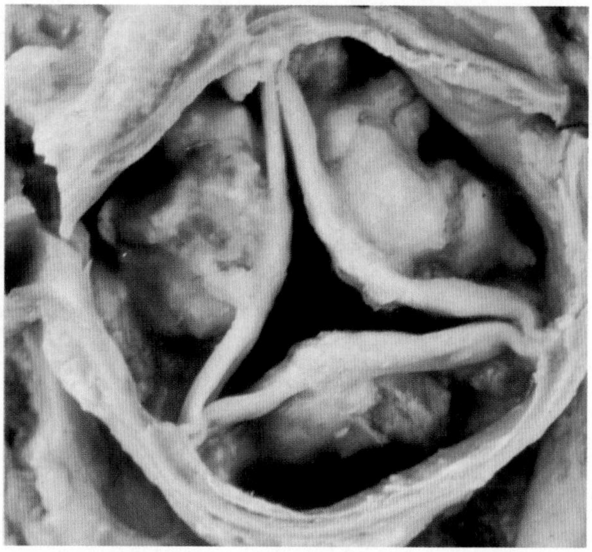

FIGURE 1-8. **Calcific aortic stenosis.** Large deposits of calcium salts are evident in the cusps and the free margins of the thickened aortic valve, as viewed from above.

colitis, an inflammatory disease of the large intestine, is often complicated by dysplastic changes in the columnar mucosal cells.

Like metaplasia, dysplasia is a response to a persistent injurious influence and will usually regress, for example, on cessation of smoking or the disappearance of human papillomavirus from the cervix. However, dysplasia shares many cytologic features with cancer, and the line between the two may be very fine indeed. For example, it may be difficult to distinguish severe dysplasia from early cancer of the cervix. *Dysplasia is a preneoplastic lesion, in that it is a necessary stage in the multistep cellular evolution to cancer.* In fact, dysplasia is included in the morphologic classifications of the stages of intraepithelial neoplasia in a variety of organs (e.g., cervix, prostate, bladder). Severe dysplasia is considered an indication for aggressive preventive therapy to cure the underlying cause, eliminate the noxious agent, or surgically remove the offending tissue.

As in the development of cancer (see Chapter 5), dysplasia results from sequential mutations in a proliferating cell population. The fidelity of DNA replication is imperfect, and occasional mutations are inevitable. When a particular mutation confers a growth or survival advantage, progeny of the affected cell will tend to predominate. In turn, their continued proliferation provides greater opportunity for additional mutations. Accumulation of such mutations progressively distances the cell from normal regulatory constraints. *Dysplasia is the morphologic expression of the disturbance in growth regulation.* However, unlike cancer cells, dysplastic cells are not entirely autonomous, and with intervention, tissue appearance may still revert to normal.

Calcification Is a Normal or Abnormal Process

The deposition of mineral salts of calcium is, of course, a normal process in the formation of bone from cartilage. As we have learned, calcium entry into dead or dying cells is usual, owing to the inability of such cells to maintain a steep calcium gradient. This cellular calcification is not ordinarily visible except as inclusions within mitochondria.

Dystrophic calcification *refers to the macroscopic deposition of calcium salts in injured tissues.* This type of calcification does not simply reflect an accumulation of calcium derived from the bodies of dead cells but rather represents an extracellular deposition of calcium from the circulation or interstitial fluid. Dystrophic calcification apparently requires the persistence of necrotic tissue; it is often visible to the naked eye and ranges from gritty, sandlike grains to firm, rock-hard material. In many locations, such as in cases of tuberculous caseous necrosis in the lung or lymph nodes, calcification has no functional consequences. However, dystrophic calcification may also occur in crucial locations, such as in the mitral or aortic valves (Fig. 1-8). In such instances, calcification leads to impeded blood flow because it produces inflexible valve leaflets and narrowed valve orifices (mitral and aortic stenosis). Dystrophic calcification in atherosclerotic coronary arteries contributes to narrowing of those vessels. Although molecules involved in physiologic calcium deposition in bone—e.g., osteopontin, osteonectin, and osteocalcin—are reported in association with dystrophic calcification, the underlying mechanisms of this process remain obscure.

Dystrophic calcification also plays a role in diagnostic radiography. Mammography is based principally on the detection of calcifications in breast cancers; congenital toxoplasmosis, an infection involving the central nervous system, is suggested by the visualization of calcification in the infant brain.

Metastatic calcification *reflects deranged calcium metabolism, in contrast to dystrophic calcification, which has its origin in cell injury.* Metastatic calcification is associated with an increased serum calcium concentration (hypercalcemia). In general, almost any disorder that increases the serum calcium level can lead to calcification in such inappropriate locations as the alveolar septa of the lung, renal tubules, and blood vessels. Calcification is seen in various disorders, including chronic renal failure, vitamin D intoxication, and hyperparathyroidism.

The formation of stones containing calcium carbonate in sites such as the gallbladder, renal pelvis, bladder, and pancreatic duct is another form of pathologic calcification. Under certain circumstances, the mineral salts precipitate from solution and crystallize about foci of organic material. Those who have suffered the agony of gallbladder or renal colic will attest to the unpleasant consequences of this type of calcification.

Hyaline Refers to Any Material That has a Reddish, Homogeneous Appearance When Stained with Hematoxylin and Eosin

The student will encounter the term **hyaline** in classic descriptions of diverse and unrelated lesions. Standard terminology includes hyaline arteriolosclerosis, alcoholic hyaline in the liver, hyaline membranes in the lung, and hyaline droplets in various cells. The various lesions called hyaline actually have nothing in common. Alcoholic hyaline is composed of cytoskeletal filaments; the hyaline found in arterioles of the kidney is derived from basement membranes; and hyaline membranes consist of plasma proteins deposited in alveoli. The term is anachronistic and of questionable value, although it is still used as a morphologic descriptor.

Mechanisms and Morphology of Cell Injury

All cells have efficient mechanisms to deal with shifts in environmental conditions. Thus, ion channels open or close, harmful chemicals are detoxified, metabolic stores such as fat or glycogen may be mobilized, and catabolic processes lead to the segregation of internal particulate materials. It is when environmental changes exceed the cell's capacity to maintain normal homeostasis that we recognize acute cell injury. If the stress is removed in time or if the cell can withstand the assault, cell injury is reversible, and complete structural and functional integrity is restored. For example, when circulation to the heart is interrupted for less than 30 minutes, all structural and functional alterations prove to be reversible. The cell can also be exposed to persistent sublethal stress, as in mechanical irritation of the skin or exposure of the bronchial mucosa to tobacco smoke. In such instances, the cell has time to adapt to reversible injury in a number of ways, each of which has its morphologic counterpart. On the other hand, if the stress is severe, irreversible injury leads to death of the cell. The precise moment at which reversible injury gives way to irreversible injury, the "point of no return," cannot be identified at present.

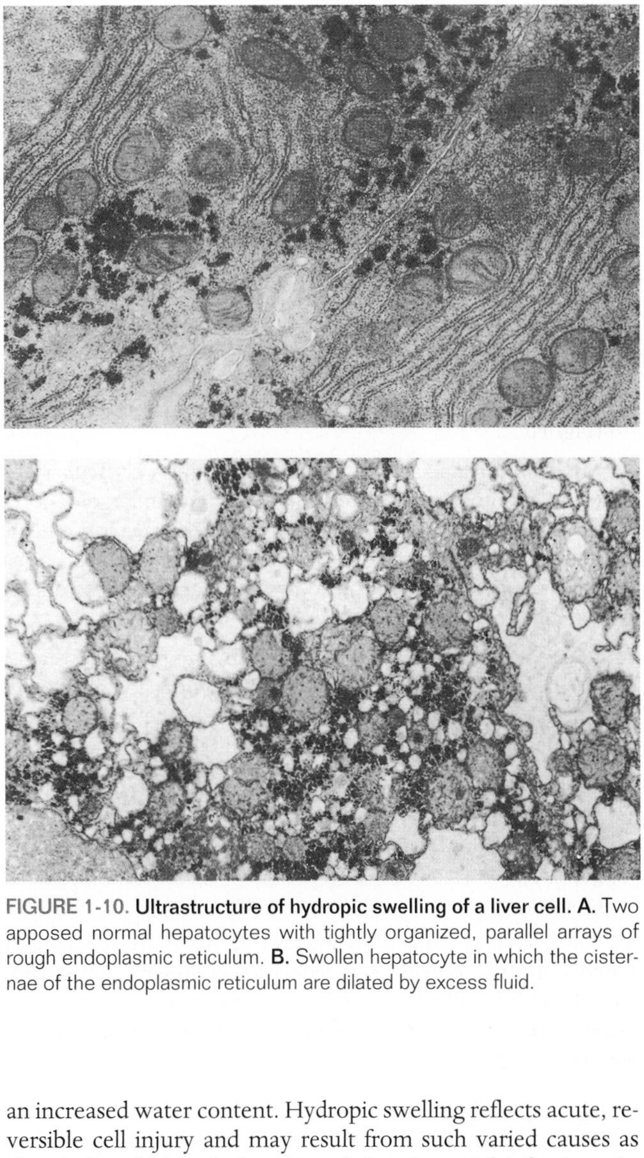

FIGURE 1-10. **Ultrastructure of hydropic swelling of a liver cell. A.** Two apposed normal hepatocytes with tightly organized, parallel arrays of rough endoplasmic reticulum. **B.** Swollen hepatocyte in which the cisternae of the endoplasmic reticulum are dilated by excess fluid.

Hydropic Swelling Is a Reversible Increase in Cell Volume

Hydropic swelling is characterized by a large, pale cytoplasm and a normally located nucleus (Fig. 1-9). The greater volume reflects an increased water content. Hydropic swelling reflects acute, reversible cell injury and may result from such varied causes as chemical and biological toxins, viral or bacterial infections, ischemia, excessive heat or cold, and so on.

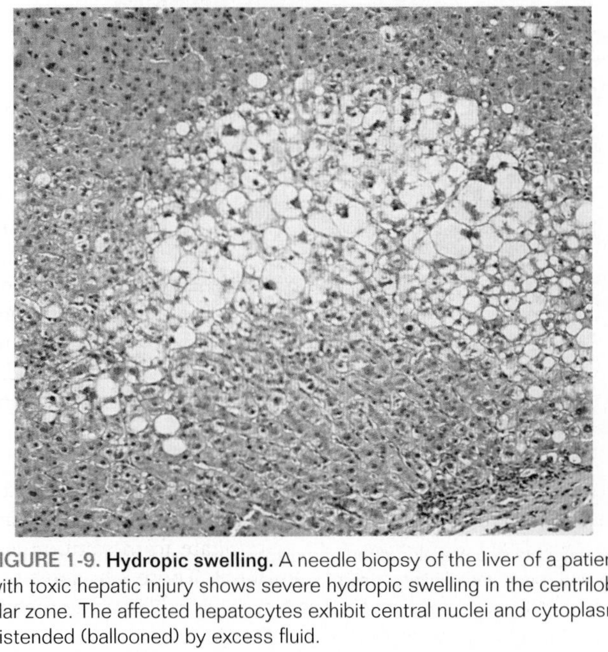

FIGURE 1-9. **Hydropic swelling.** A needle biopsy of the liver of a patient with toxic hepatic injury shows severe hydropic swelling in the centrilobular zone. The affected hepatocytes exhibit central nuclei and cytoplasm distended (ballooned) by excess fluid.

By electron microscopy, the number of organelles is unchanged, although they appear dispersed in a larger volume. The excess fluid accumulates preferentially in the cisternae of the endoplasmic reticulum, which are conspicuously dilated, presumably because of ionic shifts into this compartment (Fig. 1-10). Hydropic swelling is entirely reversible when the cause is removed.

Hydropic swelling results from impairment of cellular volume regulation, a process that controls ionic concentrations in the cytoplasm. This regulation, particularly for sodium, involves three components: (1) the plasma membrane, (2) the plasma membrane sodium pump, and (3) the supply of ATP. The plasma membrane imposes a barrier to the flow of sodium (Na^+) down a concentration gradient into the cell and prevents a similar efflux of potassium (K^+) from the cell. The barrier to sodium is imperfect and the relative leakiness to that ion permits the passive entry of sodium into the cell. To compensate for this intrusion, the energy-dependent plasma membrane sodium pump (Na^+/K^+-ATPase), which is fueled by ATP, extrudes sodium from the cell. Injurious agents may interfere with this membrane-regulated process by (1) increasing the permeability of the plasma membrane to sodium, thereby exceeding the capacity of the pump to extrude sodium; (2) damaging the pump directly; or (3) interfering with the synthesis of ATP, thereby depriving the pump of its fuel. In any event, the accumulation of sodium in the cell leads to an increase in water content to maintain isosmotic conditions, and the cell then swells.

Subcellular Changes Occur in Reversibly Injured Cells

- **Endoplasmic reticulum:** The cisternae of the endoplasmic reticulum are distended by fluid in hydropic swelling (see Fig. 1-10). In other forms of acute, reversible cell injury, membrane-bound polysomes may undergo disaggregation and detach from the surface of the rough endoplasmic reticulum (Fig. 1-11).
- **Mitochondria:** In some forms of acute injury, particularly ischemia, mitochondria swell (Fig. 1-12). This enlargement reflects the dissipation of the energy gradient and consequent impairment of mitochondrial volume control. Amorphous densities rich in phospholipid may appear, but these effects are fully reversible on recovery.
- **Plasma membrane:** Blebs of the plasma membrane—that is, focal extrusions of the cytoplasm—are occasionally noted. These can detach from the membrane into the external environment without the loss of cell viability.
- **Nucleus:** In the nucleus, reversible injury is reflected principally in nucleolar change. The fibrillar and granular components of the nucleolus may segregate. Alternatively, the granular component may be diminished, leaving only a fibrillar core.

These changes in cell organelles (Fig. 1-13) are reflected in functional derangements (e.g., reduced protein synthesis and impaired energy production). *After withdrawal of an acute stress that has led to reversible cell injury, by definition, the cell returns to its normal state.*

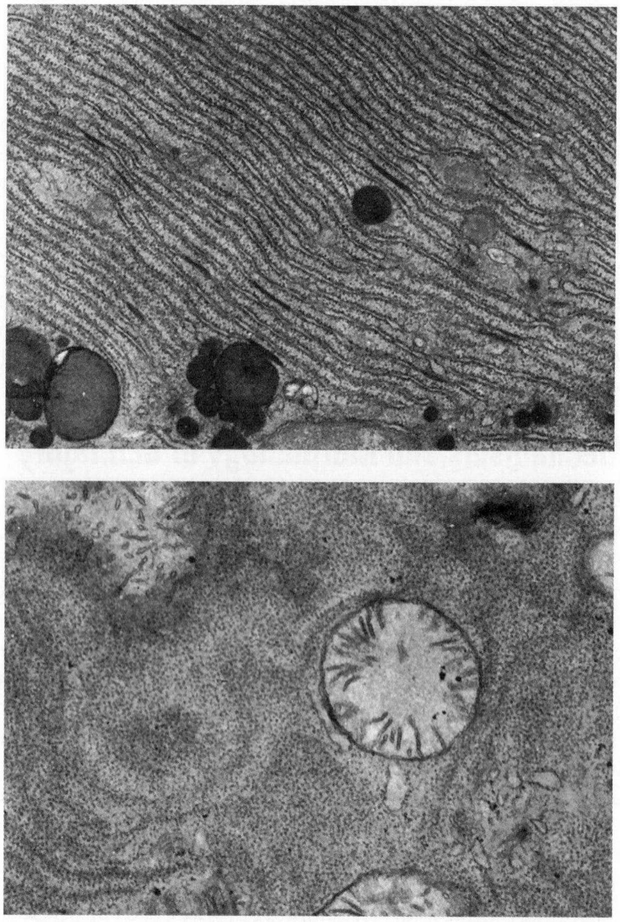

A

B

FIGURE 1-11. **Disaggregation of membrane-bound polyribosomes in acute, reversible liver injury. A.** Normal hepatocyte, in which the profiles of endoplasmic reticulum are studded with ribosomes. **B.** An injured hepatocyte, showing detachment of ribosomes from the membranes of the endoplasmic reticulum and the accumulation of free ribosomes in the cytoplasm.

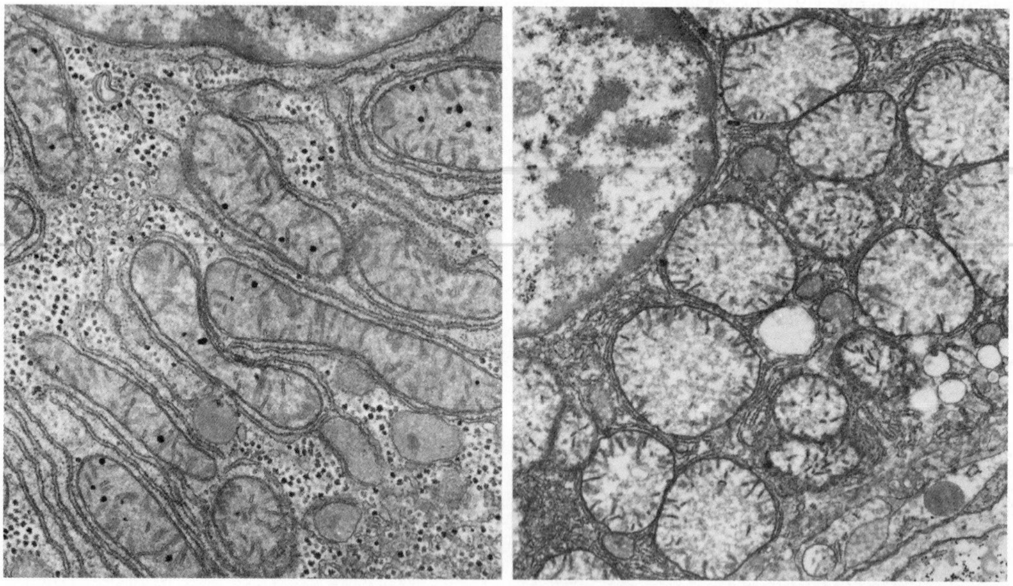

A

B

FIGURE 1-12. **Mitochondrial swelling in acute ischemic cell injury. A.** Normal mitochondria are elongated and display prominent cristae, which traverse the mitochondrial matrix. **B.** Mitochondria from an ischemic cell are swollen and round and exhibit a decreased matrix density. The cristae are less prominent than in the normal organelle.

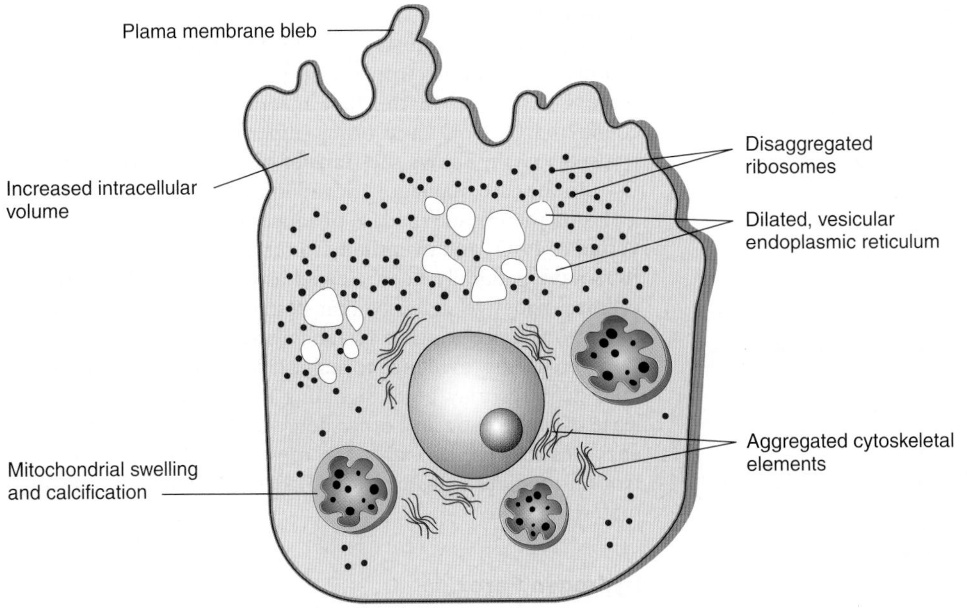

FIGURE 1-13. **Ultrastructural features of reversible cell injury.**

Ischemic Cell Injury Usually Results from Obstruction to the Flow of Blood

When tissues are deprived of oxygen, ATP cannot be produced by aerobic metabolism and is instead generated inefficiently by anaerobic metabolism. Ischemia initiates a series of chemical and pH imbalances, which are accompanied by enhanced generation of injurious free radical species. The damage produced by short periods of ischemia tends to be reversible if the circulation is restored. However, cells subjected to long episodes of ischemia become irreversibly injured and die. The mechanisms of cell damage are discussed below.

Oxidative Stress Leads to Cell Injury in Many Organs

For human life oxygen is both a blessing and a curse. Without it, life is impossible, but its metabolism can produce partially reduced oxygen species that react with virtually any molecule they reach.

Reactive Oxygen Species (ROS)

ROS have been identified as the likely cause of cell injury in many diseases (Fig. 1-14). The inflammatory process, whether acute or chronic, can cause considerable tissue destruction. In such circumstances partially reduced oxygen species produced by phagocytic cells are important mediators of cell injury. Damage to cells resulting from oxygen radicals formed by inflammatory cells has been implicated in diseases of the joints and of many organs, including the kidneys, lungs, and heart. The toxicity of many chemicals may reflect the formation of toxic oxygen species. For example, the killing of cells by ionizing radiation is most likely the result of the direct formation of hydroxyl (•OH) radicals from the radiolysis of water (H_2O). There is also evidence of a role for oxygen species in the formation of mutations during chemical carcinogenesis. Finally, oxidative damage has been implicated in biological aging (see below).

Cells also may be injured when oxygen is present at concentrations greater than normal. In the past, this occurred largely under therapeutic circumstances in which oxygen was given to patients at concentrations greater than the normal 20% of inspired air. The lungs of adults and the eyes of premature newborns were the major targets of such oxygen toxicity.

Oxygen (O_2) has a major metabolic role as the terminal acceptor for mitochondrial electron transport. Cytochrome oxidase catalyzes the four-electron reduction of O_2 to H_2O. The resultant energy is harnessed as an electrochemical potential across the mitochondrial inner membrane.

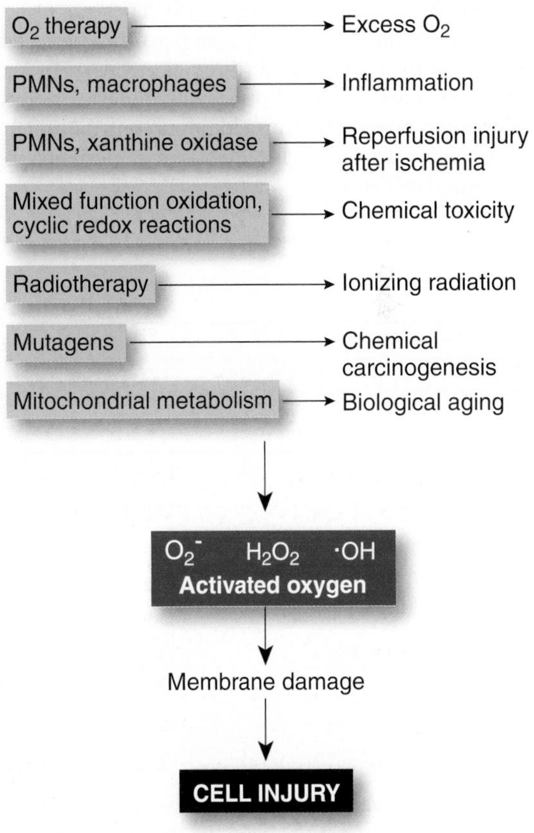

FIGURE 1-14. **The role of activated oxygen species in human disease.** H_2O_2 = hydrogen peroxide; O_2 = oxygen; O_2^- = superoxide; •OH = hydroxyl radical; PMNs = polymorphonuclear neutrophils.

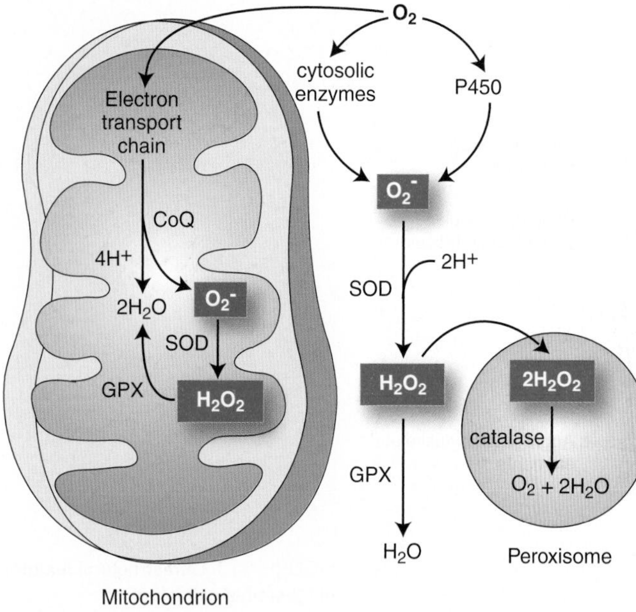

FIGURE 1-15. **Mechanisms by which reactive oxygen radicals are generated from molecular oxygen and then detoxified by cellular enzymes.** CoQ = coenzyme Q; GPX = glutathione peroxidase; H^+ = hydrogen ion; H_2O = water; H_2O_2 = hydrogen peroxide; O_2 = oxygen; O_2^- = superoxide; SOD = superoxide dismutase.

Complete reduction of O_2 to H_2O involves the transfer of four electrons. There are three partially reduced species that are intermediate between O_2 and H_2O, representing transfers of varying numbers of electrons (Fig. 1-15). They are O_2^-, superoxide (one electron); H_2O_2, hydrogen peroxide (two electrons); and •OH, the hydroxyl radical (three electrons). For the most part these ROS are produced principally by leaks in mitochondrial electron transport, with an additional contribution from the mixed-function oxygenase (P450) system. The major forms of ROS are listed in Table 1-1.

Superoxide

The superoxide anion (O_2^-) is produced principally by leaks in mitochondrial electron transport or as part of the inflammatory response. In the first instance, the promiscuity of coenzyme Q (CoQ) and other imperfections in the electron transport chain allows the transfer of electrons to O_2 to yield O_2^-. In the case of phagocytic inflammatory cells, activation of a plasma membrane oxidase produces O_2^-, which is then converted to H_2O_2 and eventually to other ROS (Fig. 1-16). These ROS have generally been viewed as the principal effectors of cellular oxidative defenses that destroy pathogens, fragments of necrotic cells or other phagocytosed material (see Chapter 2). There is now evidence to suggest that their main role in cellular defenses may be as signaling intermediates, to elicit release of proteolytic and other degradative enzymes. It is these enzymes that are probably the most critical effectors of neutrophil-mediated destruction of bacteria and other foreign materials.

Hydrogen Peroxide

O_2^- anions are catabolized by SOD to produce H_2O_2. Hydrogen peroxide is also produced directly by a number of oxidases in cytoplasmic peroxisomes (see Fig. 1-15). By itself, H_2O_2 is not particularly injurious, and it is largely metabolized to H_2O by catalase. However, when produced in excess, it is converted to highly reactive •OH. In neutrophils, myeloperoxidase transforms H_2O_2 to the potent radical hypochlorite (OCl^-), which is lethal for microorganisms and cells.

Most cells have efficient mechanisms for removing H_2O_2. Two different enzymes reduce H_2O_2 to water: (1) catalase within the peroxisomes and (2) glutathione peroxidase (GPX) in both the cytosol and the mitochondria (see Fig. 1-15). GPX uses reduced glutathione (GSH) as a cofactor, producing two molecules of oxidized glutathione (GSSG) for every molecule of H_2O_2 reduced to water. GSSG is re-reduced to GSH by glutathione reductase, with reduced nicotinamide adenine dinucleotide phosphate (NADPH) as the cofactor.

TABLE 1-1

Reactive Oxygen Species (ROS)

Molecule	Attributes
Hydrogen peroxide (H_2O_2)	Forms free radicals via Fe^{2+}-catalyzed Fenton reaction
	Diffuses widely within the cell
Superoxide anion (O_2^-)	Generated by leaks in the electron transport chain and some cytosolic reactions
	Produces other ROS
	Does not readily diffuse far from its origin
Hydroxyl radical (•OH)	Generated from H_2O_2 by Fe^{2+}-catalyzed Fenton reaction
	The intracellular radical most responsible for attack on macromolecules
Peroxynitrite (ONOO•)	Formed from the reaction of nitric oxide (NO) with O_2^- damages macromolecules
Lipid peroxide radicals (RCOO•)	Organic radicals produced during lipid peroxidation
Hypochlorous acid (HOCl)	Produced by macrophages and neutrophils during respiratory burst that accompanies phagocytosis
	Dissociates to yield hypochlorite radical (OCl^-)

Fe^{2+} = ferrous iron

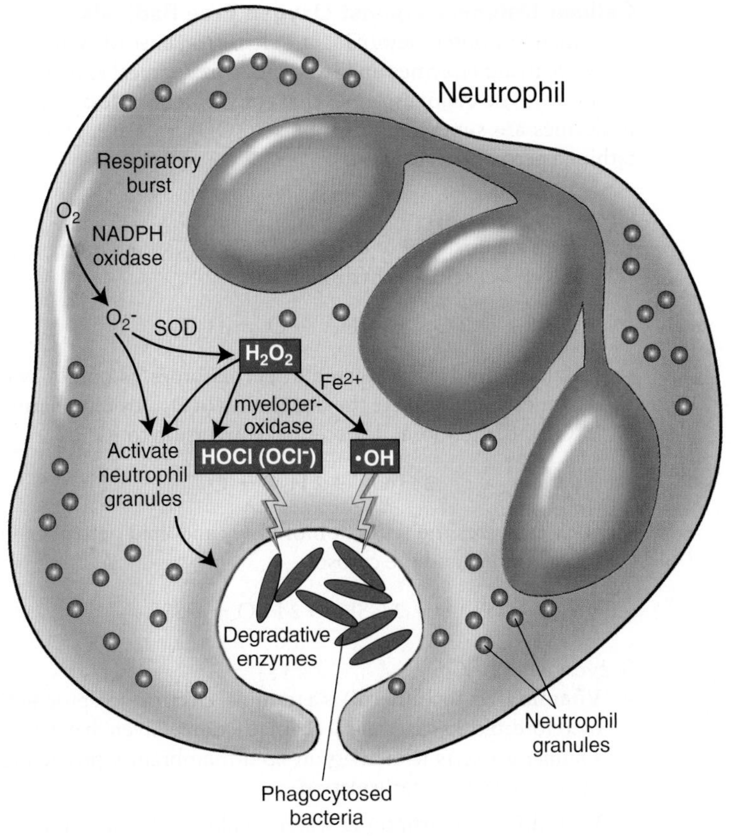

FIGURE 1-16. **Generation of reactive oxygen species in neutrophils as a result of phagocytosis of bacteria.** Fe^{2+} = ferrous iron; H_2O_2 = hydrogen peroxide; HOCl = hypochlorous acid; NADPH = nicotinamide adenine dinucleotide phosphate; OCl^- = hypochlorite radical; •OH = hydroxyl radical; SOD = superoxide dismutase.

Hydroxyl Radical

Hydroxyl radicals (•OH) are formed by (1) the radiolysis of water, (2) the reaction of H_2O_2 with ferrous iron (Fe^{2+}) (the Fenton reaction), and (3) the reaction of O_2^- with H_2O_2 (the Haber-Weiss reaction) (Fig. 1-17). The hydroxyl radical is the most reactive molecule of ROS and there are several mechanisms by which it can damage macromolecules.

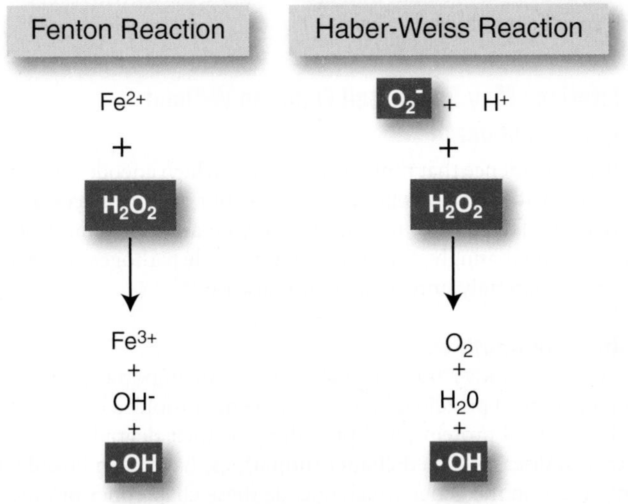

FIGURE 1-17. **Fenton and Haber-Weiss reactions to generate the highly reactive hydroxyl radical.** Reactive species are shown in red. Fe^{2+} = ferrous iron; Fe^{3+} = ferric iron; H^+ = hydrogen ion; H_2O_2 = hydrogen peroxide; OH^- = hydroxide; •OH = hydroxyl radical.

Iron is often an active participant in oxidative damage to cells (see below) by virtue of the Fenton reaction. Many lines of experimental evidence now suggest that in a number of different cell types H_2O_2 stimulates iron uptake and so increases production of hydroxyl radicals.

- **Lipid peroxidation:** The hydroxyl radical removes a hydrogen atom from the unsaturated fatty acids of membrane phospholipids, a process that forms a free lipid radical (Fig. 1-18). The lipid radical, in turn, reacts with molecular oxygen and forms a lipid peroxide radical. This peroxide radical can, in

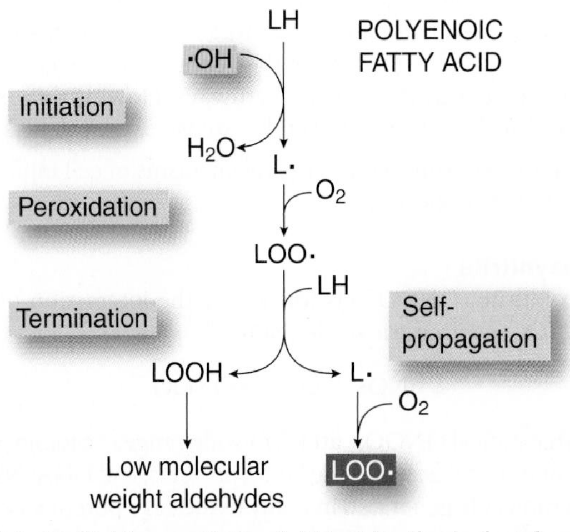

FIGURE 1-18. **Lipid peroxidation initiated by the hydroxyl radical (•OH). H_2O 5 water; O_2 5 oxygen. L•, lipid radical; LOO•, lipid peroxy radical; LOOH, lipid peroxide.**

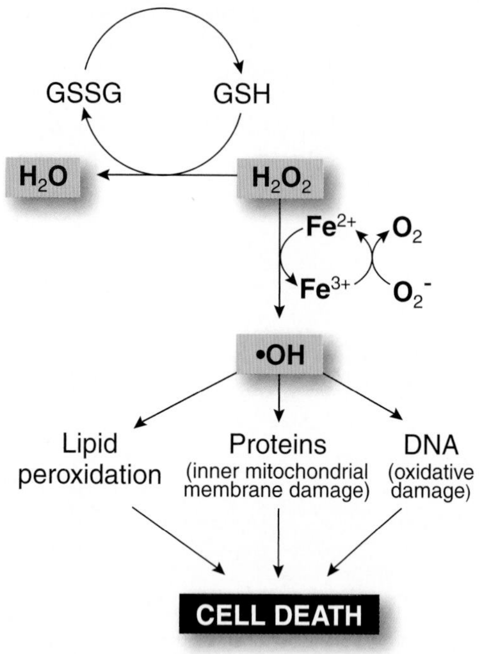

FIGURE 1-19. **Mechanisms of cell injury by activated oxygen species.** Fe^{2+} = ferrous iron; Fe^{3+} = ferric iron; GSH = glutathione; GSSG = glutathione; H_2O_2 = hydrogen peroxide; O_2 = oxygen, O_2^- = superoxide anion; •OH = hydroxyl radical.

turn, function as an initiator, removing another hydrogen atom from a second unsaturated fatty acid. A lipid peroxide and a new lipid radical result and a chain reaction is initiated. Lipid peroxides are unstable and break down into smaller molecules. The destruction of the unsaturated fatty acids of phospholipids results in a loss of membrane integrity.

- **Protein interactions:** Hydroxyl radicals may also attack proteins. The sulfur-containing amino acids cysteine and methionine, as well as arginine, histidine, and proline, are especially vulnerable to attack by •OH. As a result of oxidative damage, proteins undergo fragmentation, cross-linking, aggregation, and eventually degradation.
- **DNA damage:** DNA is an important target of the hydroxyl radical. A variety of structural alterations include strand breaks, modified bases, and cross-links between strands. In most cases, the integrity of the genome can be reconstituted by the various DNA repair pathways. However, if oxidative damage to DNA is sufficiently extensive, the cell dies.

Figure 1-19 summarizes the mechanisms of cell injury by activated oxygen species.

Peroxynitrite

Peroxynitrite ($ONOO^-$) is formed by the interaction of superoxide (O_2^-) with nitric oxide (NO•).

$$NO\bullet + O_2^- \rightarrow ONOO^-$$

The free radical $ONOO^-$ attacks a wide range of biologically important molecules, including lipids, proteins, and DNA. Nitric oxide, a molecule generated in many tissues, is a potent vasodilator and mediator of a number of important biological processes. Thus, the formation of peroxynitrite occupies an important place in free radical toxicology.

Cellular Defenses against Oxygen Free Radicals

Cells manifest potent antioxidant defenses against ROS, including detoxifying enzymes and exogenous free radical scavengers (vitamins). The major enzymes that convert ROS to less reactive molecules are superoxide dismutase (SOD), catalase, and glutathione peroxidase (GPX).

Detoxifying Enzymes

- **SOD** is the first line of defense against O_2^-, converting it to H_2O_2 and O_2. (H^+ = hydrogen ion)

$$2\,O_2^- + 2\,H^+ \rightarrow O_2 + H_2O_2.$$

- **Catalase**, principally located in peroxisomes, is one of two enzymes that complete the dissolution of O_2^- by eliminating H_2O_2 and, therefore, its potential conversion to •OH.

$$2\,H_2O_2 \rightarrow 2\,H_2O + O_2$$

- **GPX** catalyzes the reduction of H_2O_2 and lipid peroxides in mitochondria and the cytosol.

$$H_2O_2 + 2\,GSH \rightarrow 2\,H_2O + GSSG$$

Scavengers of ROS

- **Vitamin E (α-tocopherol)** is a terminal electron acceptor and, therefore, blocks free-radical chain reactions. Given that it is fat soluble, it exerts its activity in lipid membranes, protecting them against lipid peroxidation.
- **Vitamin C (ascorbate)** is water soluble and reacts directly with O_2, •OH, and some products of lipid peroxidation. It also serves to regenerate the reduced form of vitamin E.
- **Retinoids,** the precursors of vitamin A, are lipid soluble and function as chain-breaking antioxidants.
- **NO•** is the product of constitutive or inducible nitric oxide synthases (NOSs). Although it may bind to superoxide to form highly reactive peroxynitrite, nitric oxide is also a major mechanism by which ROS are contained. NO• may accomplish this in several ways. Chelation of iron and scavenging of free radicals have been suggested, but recent studies suggest that the ability of NO• to increase proteasomal activity, and thus decrease cellular iron uptake by the transferrin receptor, may be involved.

Mutations May Impair Cell Function Without Causing Cell Death

There is evidence that mutations in genes which encode proteins that mediate certain cellular activities, but are not necessarily lethal to affected cells, may lead to a wide array of clinical syndromes. Increasingly, such mutations provide pathogenetic links among seemingly unrelated clinical diseases.

Chaperonopathies

As indicated above, molecular chaperones are important in maintaining correct protein folding, recognizing misfolded or improperly modified proteins, and providing for their degradation. An array of diseases, called **chaperonopathies**, have been linked to mutations in the genes which encode these chaperones or other molecules that participate in these processes. The organ systems affected and the presenting symptom complexes of these diseases are diverse. A mutation in a chaperone cofactor is responsible for a form of X-linked retinitis pigmentosa. Hereditary spastic paraplegia is related to a mutation in heat shock protein (hsp)60, a mitochondrial chaperone. In von Hippel-Lindau disease, a mutation in the gene for VHL protein leads to poor chaperone binding to VHL. Consequent VHL protein misfolding inactivates the tumor suppressor activity of the complex of which it is a part and leads to development of tumors of the adrenal, kidney, and brain.

Channelopathies

Ion channels are transmembrane pore-forming proteins that allow ions, principally Na^+, K^+, calcium (Ca^{2+}), and chloride (Cl^-), to flow in or out of the cell. These functions are critical for numerous physiological processes, such as control of the heartbeat, muscular contraction and relaxation, and regulation of insulin secretion in pancreatic beta cells. For example activation and inactivation of sodium and potassium channels are responsible for the action potential in neurons, and calcium channels are important in contraction and relaxation of cardiac and skeletal muscle. Congenital defects caused by mutations in genes that encode ion channel proteins are now termed **channelopathies.** Mutations in over 60 ion channel genes are known to cause a variety of diseases, including cardiac arrhythmias (e.g., short and long QT syndromes) and neuromuscular syndromes (e.g. myotonias, familial periodic paralysis). As an example, a number of inherited human disorders affecting skeletal muscle contraction, heart rhythm, and function of the nervous system are attributable to mutations in genes that encode voltage-gated sodium channels. Channelopathies have also been implicated in certain pediatric epilepsy syndromes. In addition, non-excitable tissues may also be affected. In pancreatic beta cells, ATP-sensitive potassium channels regulate insulin secretion, and mutations in these channel genes lead to certain forms of diabetes.

Intracellular Storage Is Retention of Materials within the Cell

The substance that accumulates may be normal or abnormal, endogenous or exogenous, harmful or innocuous.

- **Nutrients,** such as fat, glycogen, vitamins, and minerals, are stored for later use.
- **Degraded phospholipids,** which result from turnover of endogenous membranes, are stored in lysosomes and may be recycled.
- **Substances that cannot be metabolized** accumulate in cells. These include (1) endogenous substrates that are not further processed because a key enzyme is missing (hereditary storage diseases), (2) insoluble endogenous pigments (e.g., lipofuscin and melanin), (3) aggregates of normal or abnormal proteins, and (4) exogenous particulates, such as inhaled silica and carbon or injected tattoo pigments.
- **Overload of normal body constituents,** including iron, copper, and cholesterol, injures a variety of cells.
- **Abnormal proteins** may be toxic when they are retained within a cell. Examples are Lewy bodies in Parkinson disease and mutant α_1-antitrypsin.

Fat

Bacteria and other unicellular organisms continuously ingest nutrients. By contrast, mammals do not need to eat continuously. They eat periodically and can survive a prolonged fast because they store nutrients in specialized cells for later use—fat in adipocytes and glycogen in the liver, heart, and muscle.

Abnormal accumulation of fat is most conspicuous in the liver, a subject treated in detail in Chapter 14. Briefly, liver cells always contain some fat, because free fatty acids released from adipose tissue are taken up by the liver. There, they are oxidized or converted to triglycerides. Most of newly synthesized triglycerides are secreted by the liver as lipoproteins. When delivery of free fatty acids to the liver is increased, as in diabetes or when intrahepatic lipid metabolism is disturbed, as in alcoholism, triglycerides accumulate in liver cells. Fatty liver is identified morphologically as lipid globules in the cytoplasm. Other organs, including the heart, kidney, and skeletal muscle, also store fat. One must recognize that fat storage is always reversible and there is no evidence that the excess fat in the cytoplasm interferes with cell function.

Glycogen

Glycogen is a long-chain polymer of glucose, formed and largely stored in the liver and to a lesser extent in muscles. It is depolymerized to glucose and liberated as needed. Glycogen is degraded in steps by a series of enzymes, each of which may be deficient as a result of an inborn error of metabolism. Regardless of the specific enzyme deficiency, the result is a glycogen storage disease (see Chapter 6). These inherited disorders affect the liver, heart, and skeletal muscle and range from mild and asymptomatic conditions to inexorably progressive and fatal diseases (see Chapters 11, 14, and 27).

The amount of glycogen stored in cells is normally regulated by the blood glucose concentration, and hyperglycemic states are associated with increased glycogen stores. Thus, in uncontrolled diabetes, hepatocytes and epithelial cells of the renal proximal tubules are enlarged by excess glycogen.

Inherited Lysosomal Storage Diseases

Like glycogen catabolism, breakdown of certain complex lipids and mucopolysaccharides (glycosaminoglycans) takes place by a sequence of enzymatic steps. Since these enzymes are located in the lysosomes, their absence results in lysosomal storage of incompletely degraded lipids, such as cerebrosides (e.g., Gaucher disease) and gangliosides (e.g., Tay-Sachs disease) or products of mucopolysaccharide catabolism (e.g., Hurler and Hunter syndromes). These disorders are all progressive but vary from asymptomatic organomegaly to rapidly fatal brain disease. See Chapter 6 for the metabolic bases of these disorders and Chapters 26 and 28 for specific organ pathology.

Cholesterol

The human body has a love–hate relationship with cholesterol. On the one hand, it is a critical component of all plasma membranes. On the other hand, when stored in excess, it is closely associated with atherosclerosis and cardiovascular disease, the leading cause of death in the Western world (see Chapter 10).

Briefly, the initial lesion of atherosclerosis (fatty streak) reflects accumulation of cholesterol and cholesterol esters in macrophages within the arterial intima. As the disease progresses, smooth muscle cells also store cholesterol. Advanced lesions of atherosclerosis are characterized by extracellular deposition of cholesterol (see Fig 1- 22B).

In a number of disorders characterized by elevated blood levels of cholesterol (e.g., familial hypercholesterolemia or primary biliary cirrhosis), macrophages store cholesterol. When clusters of these cells in subcutaneous tissues become grossly visible, they are termed **xanthomas** (see Fig 1- 22A).

Abnormal Proteins

Several acquired and inherited diseases are characterized by intracellular accumulation of abnormal proteins. The deviant tertiary structure of the protein may result from an inherited mutation that alters the normal primary amino acid sequence or may reflect an acquired defect in protein folding. The following are examples:

- **α_1-Antitrypsin deficiency** is a heritable disorder in which mutations in the coding gene for α_1-antitrypsin yield an insoluble protein. Mutant protein is not easily exported. It accumulates in liver cells (see Fig. 1-22C), causing cell injury and cirrhosis (see Chapter 14).
- **Prion diseases** comprise a group of neurodegenerative disorders (spongiform encephalopathies) caused by the accumulation of abnormally folded prion proteins. The anomaly reflects the conversion of the normal α-helical structure to a β-pleated sheet. Abnormal prion proteins may result from an inherited mutation or from exposure to the aberrant form of the protein (see Chapter 28). The function of normal prion protein is not yet clear. It has been reported to have SOD-like antioxidant activity, a role in T lymphocyte-dendritic cell interactions, the ability to enhance neural progenitor proliferation, and a key role in development of in long- term memory.
- **Lewy bodies** (α-synuclein) are seen in neurons of the substantia nigra in Parkinson disease (Chapter 28).
- **Neurofibrillary tangles** (tau protein) characterize cortical neurons in Alzheimer disease (Chapter 28).
- **Mallory bodies** (intermediate filaments) are hepatocellular inclusions in alcoholic liver injury (Chapter 14).

PATHOGENESIS: After nascent polypeptides emerge from the ribosomes, they fold to assume the tertiary configuration of mature proteins. Correct folding requires proteins to assume one particular structure from a constellation of possible but incorrect conformations. Curiously, it is energetically more favorable for the cell to produce many foldings and then edit the protein repertoire than to produce only a single correct conformation. Molecular chaperones associate with polypeptides in the endoplasmic reticulum and promote correct folding, after which they dissociate from those proteins that have assumed the correct conformation (Fig. 1-20). By contrast, incorrectly folded proteins remain bound to their chaperones and are subsequently degraded by the ubiquitin–proteasome system (see above). Evolutionary preference for energy conservation has dictated that a substantial proportion of newly formed proteins are rogues unsuitable for the society of civilized cells.

Numerous hereditary and acquired diseases are caused by evasion of the quality control system designed to promote correct folding and eliminate faulty proteins. Misfolded proteins can injure the cell in a number of ways.

- **Loss of function:** Certain mutations prevent correct folding of crucial proteins, which then do not function properly or cannot be incorporated into the correct site. For example, some mutations that lead to cystic fibrosis cause misfolding of an ion channel protein, which is then degraded. The protein does not reach its destination at the cell membrane, leading to a defect in chloride transport that produces the disease cystic fibrosis. Other examples of loss of function include mutations of the low-density lipoprotein (LDL) receptor in certain types of hypercholesterolemia and mutations of a copper transport adenosine triphosphatase (ATPase) in Wilson disease.
- **Formation of toxic protein aggregates:** Defects in protein structure may be acquired as well as genetic. Thus, particularly in nondividing cells, age-related impairment of cellular antioxidant defenses leads to protein oxidation, which commonly alters protein tertiary structure, exposing interior hydrophobic amino acids that are normally hidden. In situations of mild to moderate oxidative stress, 20S proteasomes recognize the exposed hydrophobic moieties and degrade these proteins. However if oxidative stress is severe, these proteins aggregate by virtue of a combination of hydrophobic and ionic bonds. Such aggregates are insoluble and tend to sequester Fe^{2+} ions, which in turn help generate additional ROS (see above) and aggregate size increases. Whether or not the proteins contained in the aggregates are ubiquitinated, the aggregates are indigestible (Fig. 1- 21). Any Ub bound to them is lost, which may cause a cellular deficit in Ub and impair protein degradation in general. Both by virtue of their generation of toxic ROS and their inhibition of proteasomal degradation, these aggregates may lead to cell death. Accumulation of amyloid β protein in Alzheimer's disease and α-synuclein in Parkinson's disease may occur by this type of mechanism.
- **Retention of secretory proteins:** Many proteins that are destined to be secreted from the cell require a correctly folded conformation to be transported through cellular compartments and released at the cell membrane. Mutations in genes that encode such proteins (e.g., α_1-antitrypsin) lead to cell injury because of massive accumulation of misfolded proteins within the liver cell. Failure to secrete this antiprotease into the circulation also leads to unregulated proteolysis of connective tissue in the lung and loss of pulmonary elasticity (emphysema).
- **Extracellular deposition of aggregated proteins:** Misfolded proteins tend to exhibit a β-pleated conformation in place of random coils or α helices. These abnormal proteins often form insoluble aggregates, which may be visualized as extracellular deposits, the appearance depending upon the specific disease. These accumulations often assume the forms of various types of amyloid and produce cell injury in systemic amyloidoses (see Chapter 23) and a variety of neurodegenerative diseases (see Chapter 28).

Lipofuscin

Lipofuscin is a mixture of lipids and proteins containing a golden-brown pigment called ceroid. Lipofuscin tends to accumulate by accretion of oxidized, cross-linked proteins (see Fig. 1- 21) *and is indigestible. It occurs mainly in terminally differentiated cells (neurons and cardiac myocytes) or in cells that cycle infrequently (hepatocytes)* (see Fig. 1- 22D). It is often more conspicuous in conditions associated with atrophy of an organ.

Although it was previously thought to be benign, there is increasing evidence that lipofuscin may be both a result and a cause of increasing oxidant stress in cells. It may impair both proteasomal function and lysosomal degradation of senescent or

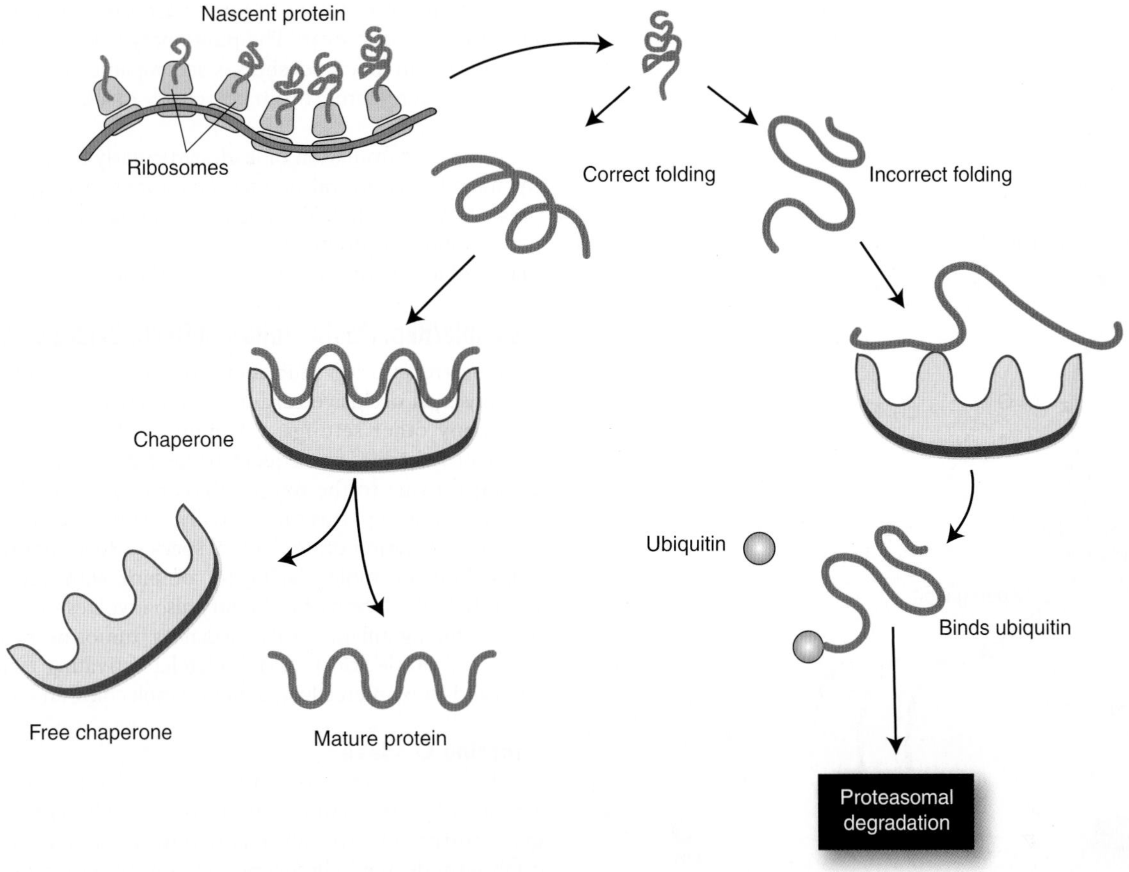

FIGURE 1-20. **Differential handling of protein that is correctly folded *(left arrows)* and protein that is incorrectly folded *(right arrows)*.** Correctly folded proteins are chaperoned from the ribosomes that produce them to their ultimate cellular destination. Incorrectly folded proteins bind to ubiquitin, an association that directs the protein to proteasomes, where the misfolded protein is degraded.

poorly functioning organelles. Consequently, inefficient or poorly functioning mitochondria may accumulate, generate more ROS and perpetuate the cycle.

Melanin

Melanin is an insoluble, brown-black pigment found principally in the epidermal cells of the skin, but also in the eye and other organs (see Fig. 1-22E). It is located in intracellular organelles known as melanosomes and results from the polymerization of certain oxidation products of tyrosine. The amount of melanin is responsible for the differences in skin color among the various races, as well as the color of the eyes. It serves a protective function owing to its ability to absorb ultraviolet light. In white persons, exposure to sunlight increases melanin formation (tanning). The hereditary inability to produce melanin results in the disorder known as **albinism.** The presence of melanin is also a marker of the cancer that arises from melanocytes (melanoma). Melanin is discussed in detail in Chapter 24.

Exogenous Pigments

Anthracosis refers to the storage of carbon particles in the lung and regional lymph nodes (see Fig. 1-22F). Virtually all urban dwellers inhale particulates of organic carbon generated by the burning of fossil fuels. These particles accumulate in alveolar macrophages and are also transported to hilar and mediastinal lymph nodes, where the indigestible material is stored indefinitely within macrophages. Although the gross appearance of the lungs of persons with anthracosis may be alarming, the condition is innocuous.

Tattoos are the result of the introduction of insoluble metallic and vegetable pigments into the skin, where they are engulfed by dermal macrophages and persist for a lifetime.

Iron and Other Metals

About 25% of the body's total iron content is in an intracellular storage pool composed of the iron-storage proteins **ferritin** and **hemosiderin**. The liver and bone marrow are particularly rich in ferritin, although it is present in virtually all cells. Hemosiderin is a partially denatured form of ferritin that aggregates easily and is recognized microscopically as yellow-brown granules in the cytoplasm. Normally, hemosiderin is found mainly in the spleen, bone marrow, and Kupffer cells of the liver.

Total body iron may be increased by enhanced intestinal iron absorption, as in some anemias, or by administration of iron-containing erythrocytes in a transfusion. In either case, the excess iron is stored intracellularly as ferritin and hemosiderin. Increasing the body's total iron content leads to progressive accumulation of hemosiderin, a condition termed **hemosiderosis.** In this condition, iron is present not only in the organs in which it is normally found but also throughout the body, in such places as the skin, pancreas, heart, kidneys, and endocrine organs. Intracellular accumulation of

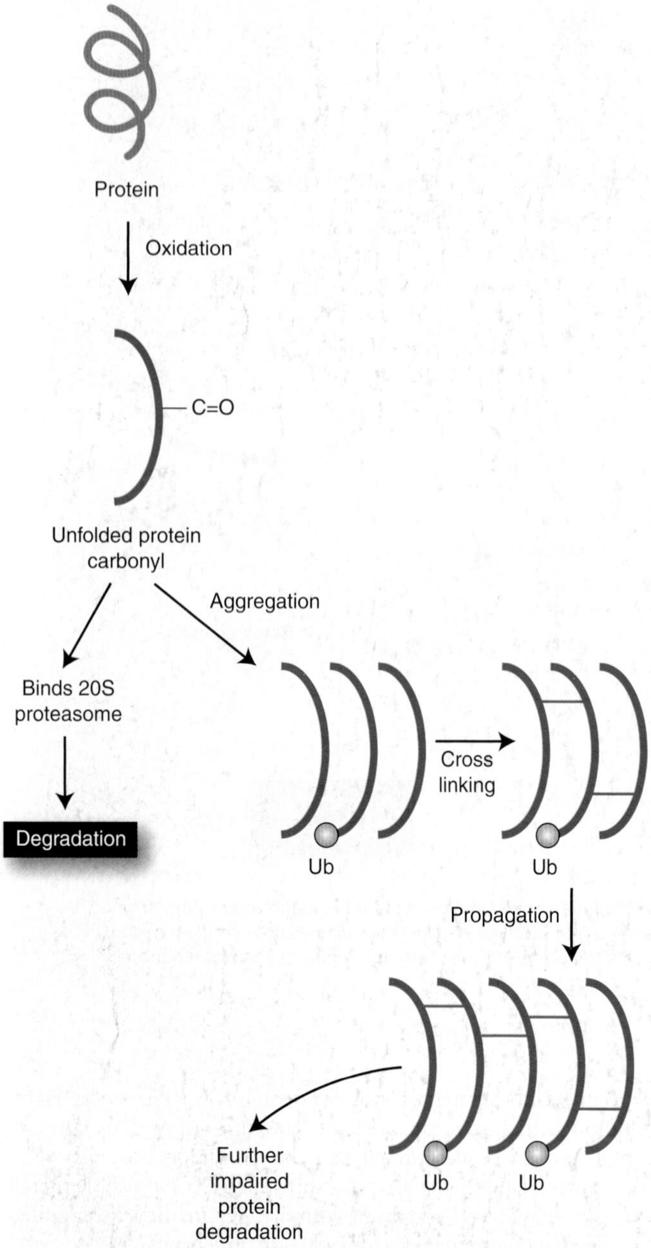

FIGURE 1-21. Mechanism of accumulation and elimination of oxidized proteins. On exposure to reactive oxygen species (ROS), proteins become oxidized to protein carbonyls. This forces a change in protein tertiary structure, exposing hydrophobic residues ordinarily on the protein interior. These protein carbonyls may be eliminated by 20S proteasomes without ubiquitination or, especially if the oxidant stress is heavy, they may aggregate on the basis of hydrophobic interactions. Some aggregated proteins may be ubiquitinated, but such aggregates cannot be degraded. With further accretion, aggregate substituents undergo crosslinking and continue to enlarge. Ub = ubiquitin

iron in hemosiderosis does not usually injure cells. However, if the increase in total body iron is extreme; we speak of **iron overload syndromes** (see Chapter 14), in which iron deposition is so severe that it damages vital organs—the heart, liver, and pancreas. Severe iron overload can result from a genetic abnormality in iron absorption, **hereditary hemochromatosis** (see Fig. 1-22G). Alternatively, severe iron overload may occur after multiple blood transfusions, such as in treating hemophilia or certain hereditary anemias.

Excessive iron storage in some organs is also associated with increased risk of cancer. The pulmonary siderosis encountered among certain metal polishers is accompanied by increased risk of lung cancer. Hemochromatosis leads to a higher incidence of liver cancer.

Excess accumulation of lead, particularly in children, causes mental retardation and anemia. The storage of other metals also presents dangers. In Wilson disease, a hereditary disorder of copper metabolism, storage of excess copper in the liver and brain may lead to severe chronic disease of those organs.

Ischemia/Reperfusion Injury Reflects Oxidative Stress

Ischemia/reperfusion (I/R) injury is a common clinical problem that arises in occlusive cardiovascular disease, infection, shock, and many other settings. I/R injury reflects the interplay of transient ischemia, consequent tissue damage, and exposure of damaged tissue to the oxygen that arrives when blood flow is reestablished (reperfusion). Initially, ischemic cellular damage leads to generation of free radical species. Reperfusion then provides abundant molecular O_2 to combine with free radicals to form ROS. Evolution of I/R injury also involves many other factors, including inflammatory mediators [tumor necrosis factor-α (TNF-α), interleukin-1 (IL-1)], platelet activating factor (PAF), NOS and NO•, intercellular adhesion molecules, and many more.

Xanthine Oxidase

Xanthine dehydrogenase may be converted by proteolysis during a period of ischemia into xanthine oxidase. On reperfusion, oxygen returns and the abundant purines derived from ATP catabolism during ischemia provide substrates for xanthine oxidase. This enzyme requires oxygen to catalyze the formation of uric acid; activated oxygen species are byproducts of this reaction.

The Role of Neutrophils

An additional source of ROS during reperfusion is the neutrophil. Alterations in the cell surface that occur during ischemia and on reperfusion induce the adhesion and activation of circulating neutrophils. These cells release large quantities of activated oxygen species and hydrolytic enzymes, both of which may injure the previously ischemic cells.

Reperfusion also prompts endothelial cells to move preformed P-selectin to the cell surface, allowing neutrophils to bind endothelial membrane intercellular adhesion molecule-1 (ICAM-1) and roll along endothelial cells (see Chapter 2). Recruitment of these inflammatory cells to affected areas increases local production of oxygen free radicals.

The Role of Nitric Oxide

There are two major forms of NOS: a constitutive form, which is common to endothelial cells and parenchymal cells (e.g., hepatocytes, neurons) and an inducible form (iNOS), mostly found in inflammatory cells. Nitric oxide dilates the microvasculature by relaxing smooth muscle, inhibits platelet aggregation, and decreases adhesion between leukocytes and the endothelial surface. These activities are all mediated by the ability of NO• to decrease cytosolic Ca^{2+}, both by extrusion of calcium from the cell and by its sequestration within intracellular stores.

NO• also reacts with O_2^- to form the highly reactive species, $ONOO^-$. Normally, O_2^- is detoxified by SOD and little $ONOO^-$ is produced. However, I/R stimulates iNOS and the NO• produced inactivates SOD, thereby increasing the amount of NO• and favoring production of $ONOO^-$ The free radical

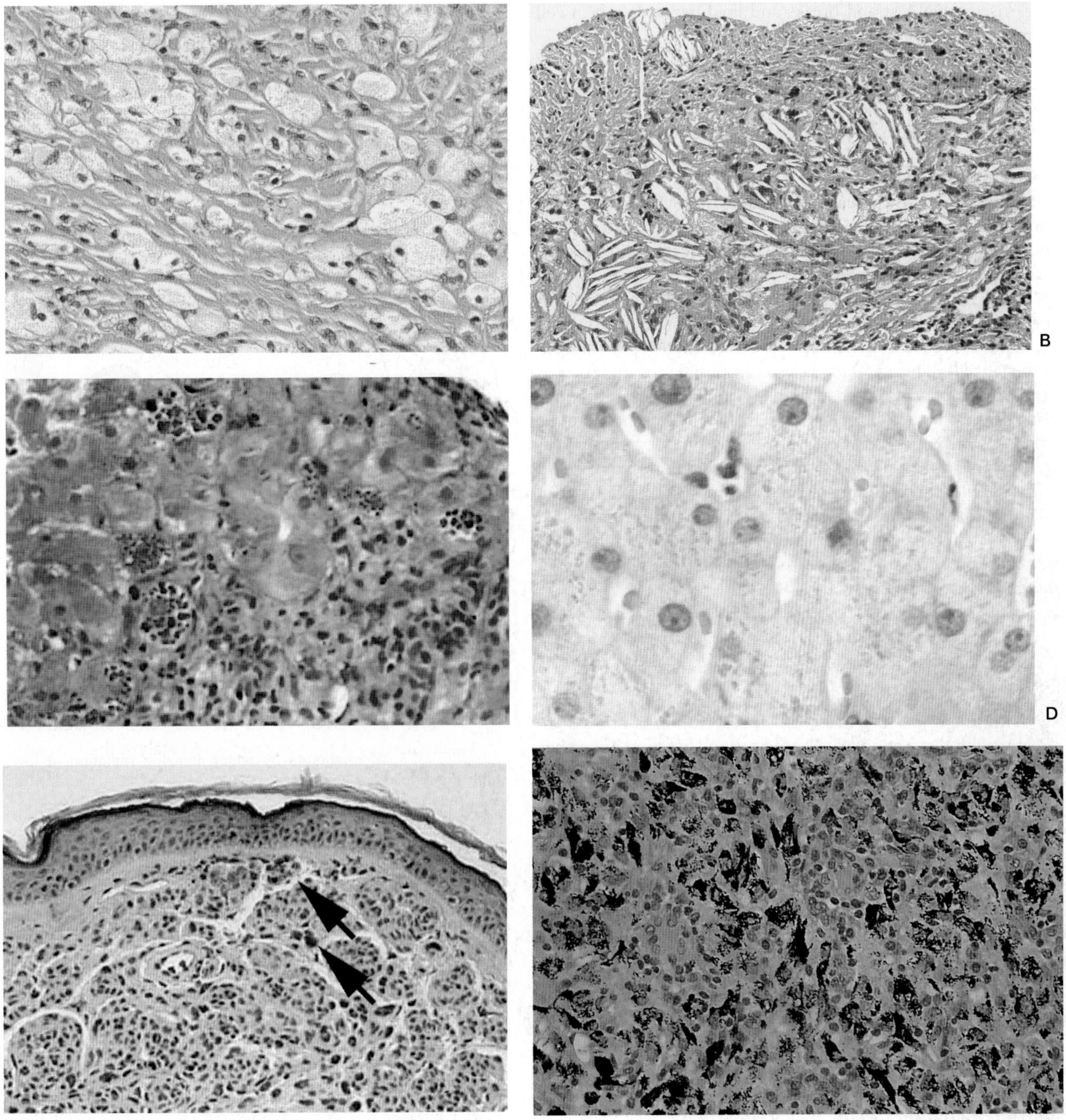

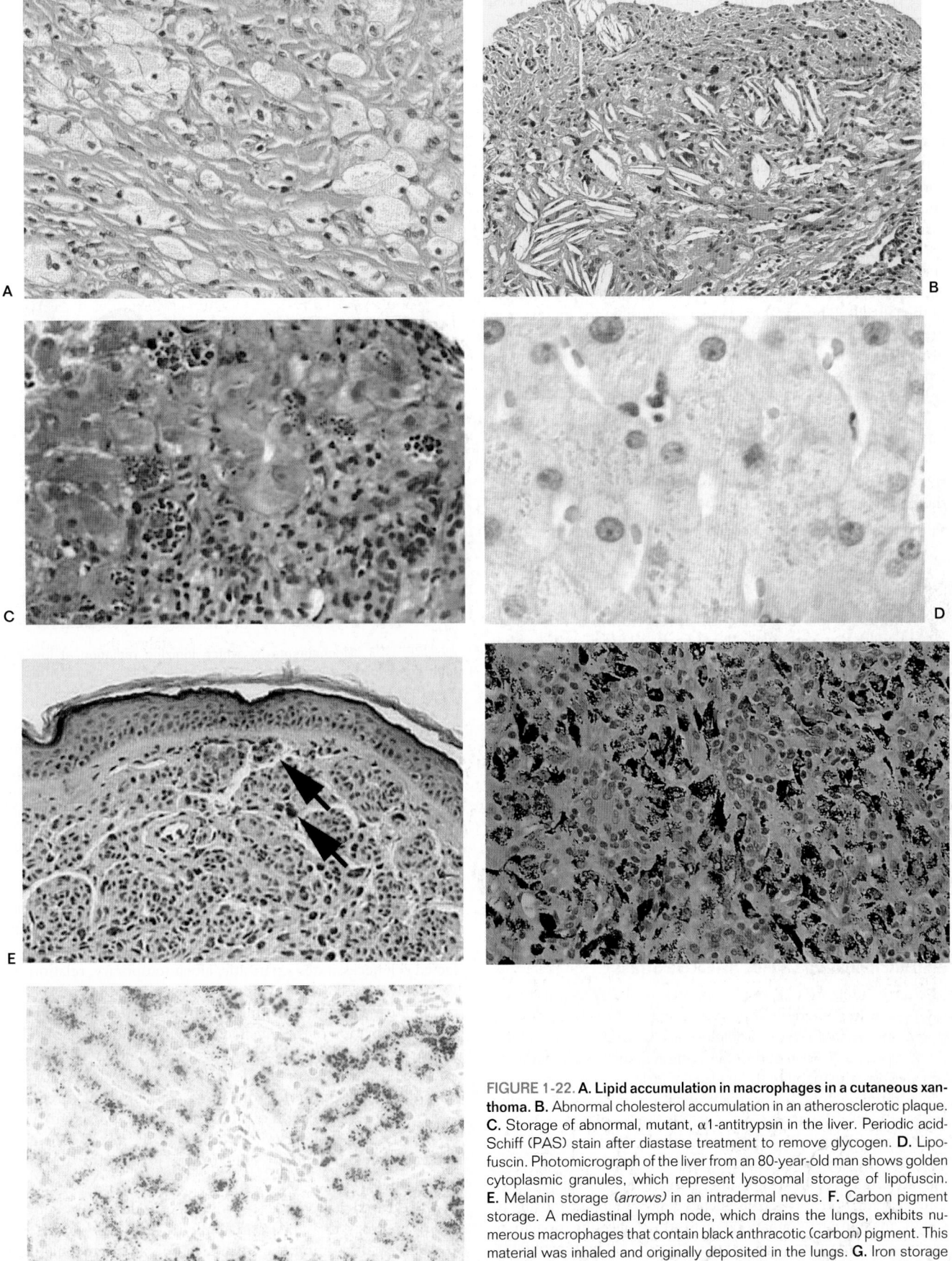

FIGURE 1-22. **A. Lipid accumulation in macrophages in a cutaneous xanthoma. B.** Abnormal cholesterol accumulation in an atherosclerotic plaque. **C.** Storage of abnormal, mutant, α1-antitrypsin in the liver. Periodic acid-Schiff (PAS) stain after diastase treatment to remove glycogen. **D.** Lipofuscin. Photomicrograph of the liver from an 80-year-old man shows golden cytoplasmic granules, which represent lysosomal storage of lipofuscin. **E.** Melanin storage *(arrows)* in an intradermal nevus. **F.** Carbon pigment storage. A mediastinal lymph node, which drains the lungs, exhibits numerous macrophages that contain black anthracotic (carbon) pigment. This material was inhaled and originally deposited in the lungs. **G.** Iron storage in hereditary hemochromatosis. Prussian blue stain of the liver reveals large deposits of iron within hepatocellular lysosomes.

gives rise to DNA strand breaks and lipid peroxidation in cell membranes.

NO• is a double-edged sword in I/R injury, however. Fe^{2+} ion plays an important role in continuing to generate ROS during I/R injury. As noted above, NO• decreases transferrin-mediated iron uptake, and so may also partly protect cells from I/R injury.

Inflammatory Cytokines

I/R injury leads to the release of cytokines that (1) promote vasoconstriction, (2) stimulate the adherence of inflammatory cells and platelets to endothelium, and (3) have effects at sites distant from the ischemic insult itself.

Local release of TNF-α at the site of I/R injury results in chemotaxis and sequestration of neutrophils by upregulating the expression of cell adhesion molecules on both neutrophils and endothelial cells. This cytokine is also responsible for increases in neutrophil trafficking and neutrophil-related damage at locations distant from the site of I/R injury itself, thereby causing systemic effects. By increasing the levels of PAF, I/R injury cripples vascular function both locally and systemically. In addition, augmented release of endothelin during I/R injury promotes the adherence of inflammatory cells and increases vascular tone and permeability.

We can put reperfusion injury in perspective by emphasizing that there are three different degrees of cell injury, depending on the duration of the ischemia:

- With short periods of ischemia, reperfusion (and, therefore, the resupply of oxygen) completely restores the structural and functional integrity of the cell. Cell injury in this case is completely reversible.
- With longer periods of ischemia, reperfusion is not associated with restoration of cell structure and function but rather with deterioration and death of the cells. In this case, lethal cell injury occurs during the period of reperfusion.
- Lethal cell injury may develop during the period of ischemia itself, in which case reperfusion is not a factor. A longer period of ischemia is needed to produce this third type of cell injury. In this case, cell damage does not depend on the formation of activated oxygen species.

Proteasomes and Ischemia/Reperfusion Injury

Many of the cytokines that mediate tissue damage in I/R injury are expressed under the control of NFκB. In a number of experimental models, proteasomal activity is decreased after I/R. This stabilizes the NFκB-IκB complex (see above), and limits tissue damage.

Ionizing Radiation Causes Oxidative Stress

The term "ionizing radiation" connotes an ability to cause radiolysis of water, thereby directly forming hydroxyl radicals. As noted above, hydroxyl radicals interact with DNA and inhibit DNA replication. For a nonproliferating cell, such as a hepatocyte or a neuron, the inability to divide is of little consequence. For a proliferating cell, however, the prevention of mitosis is a catastrophic loss of function. Once a proliferating cell can no longer divide, it dies by **apoptosis,** which rids the body of those cells that have lost their prime function. Direct mutagenic effects of ionizing radiation on DNA are also important. The cytotoxic effects of ionizing radiation are also dose-dependent. Whereas exposure to significant sources of radiation impairs the replicating capacity of cycling cells, massive doses of radiation may kill both proliferating and quiescent cells directly. Figure 1-23 summarizes the mechanisms of cell killing by ionizing radiation.

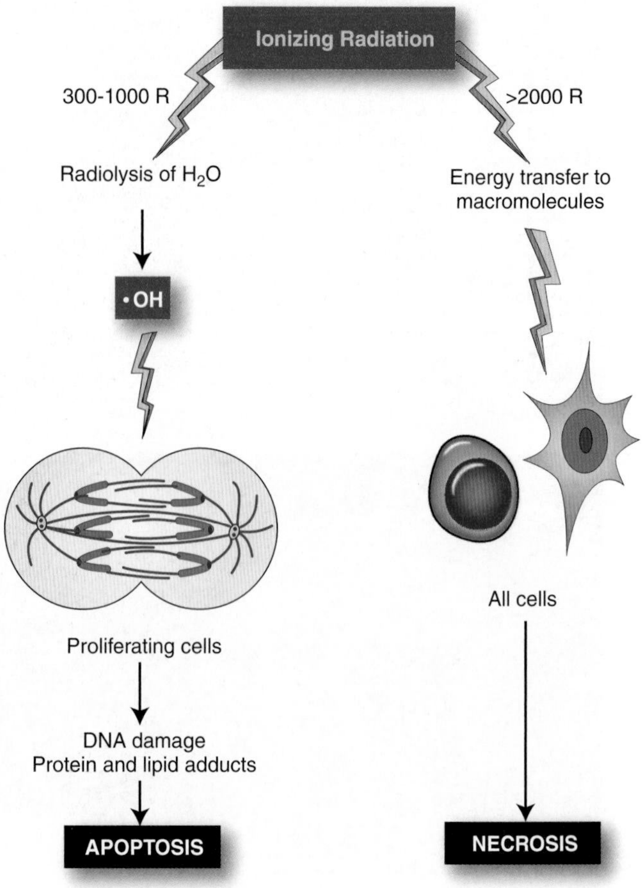

FIGURE 1-23. **Mechanisms by which ionizing radiation at low and high doses causes cell death.** H_2O = water, •OH = hydroxyl radical; R = rads.

Viral Cytotoxicity Is Direct or Immunologically Mediated

The means by which viruses cause cell injury and death are as diverse as viruses themselves. Unlike bacteria, a virus requires a cellular host to (1) house it; (2) provide enzymes, substrates, and other resources for viral replication; and (3) serve as a source for dissemination when mature virions are ready to be spread to other cells. Viruses have evolved mechanisms by which they avoid biting the hand that feeds them (at least until they are ready for other hands). The ability of a virus to persist in an infected cell necessitates a parasitic, albeit temporary, relationship with the host cell. During this vulnerable phase, the virus plays a game of cat and mouse with the immune system as a device to evade elimination of the infected cell. This period is followed by a phase in which the virus disseminates, either by budding (which does not necessarily destroy the cell) or by lysis (which does). In some viral infections (e.g., herpes simplex, measles, zoster-varicella), infection of a host cell may last for many years or a lifetime, in which case the cell is not destroyed. There are patterns of cellular injury related to viral infections that deserve a brief mention:

- **Direct toxicity:** Viruses may injure cells directly by subverting cellular enzymes and depleting the cell's nutrients, thereby disrupting the normal homeostatic mechanisms. The mechanisms underlying virus-induced lysis of cells, however, are probably more complex (Fig. 1-24A).

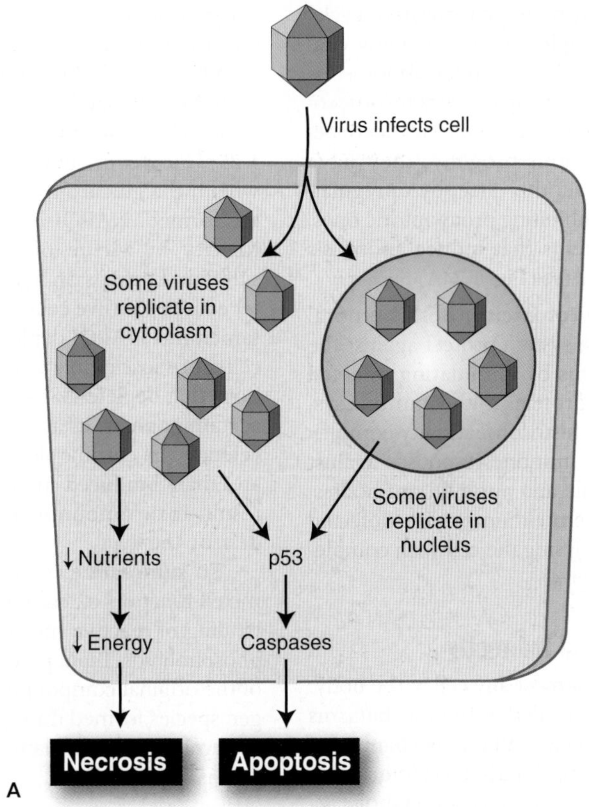

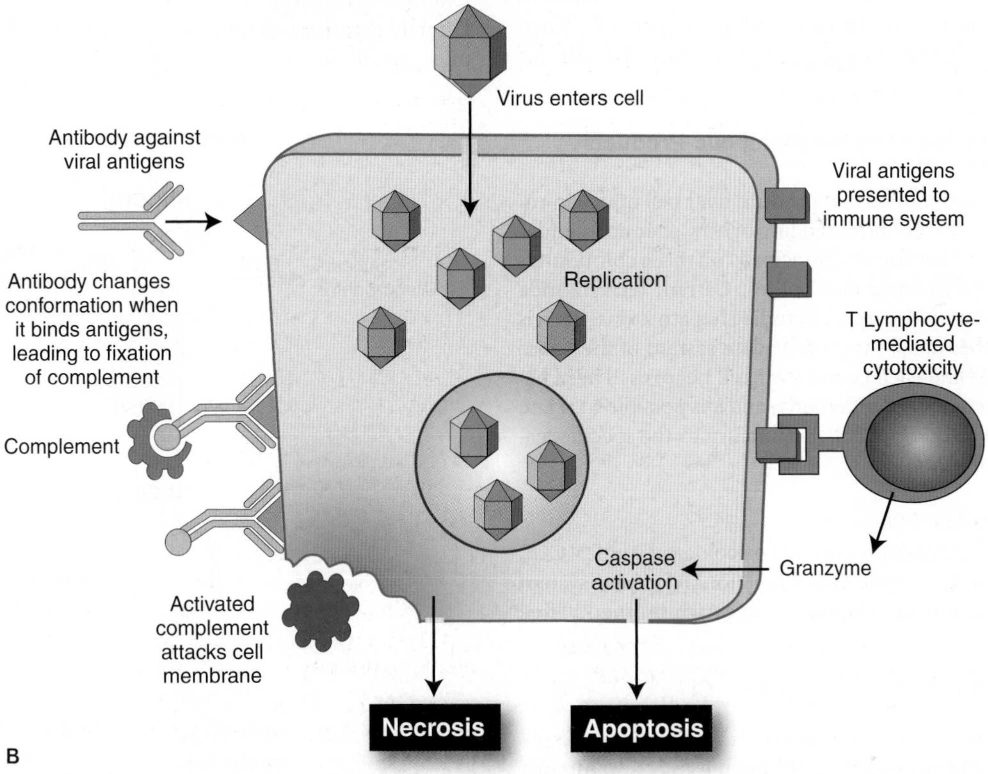

FIGURE 1-24. **Cell injury caused by virus infection. A.** Direct injury caused by virus infection, involving both depletion of cellular resources and activation of apoptotic signaling mechanisms. **B.** Mechanisms that lead to immunologically mediated destruction of virus-infected cells.

- **Manipulation of apoptosis:** During their replicative cycle, and before virion assembly is complete, there are many viral activities that can elicit apoptosis. For example, apoptosis is activated when the cell detects episomal (extrachromosomal) DNA replication. Since viruses must avoid cell death before they have produced infectious progeny, they have evolved mechanisms to counteract this effect by upregulating anti-apoptotic proteins and inhibiting proapoptotic ones. Some viruses also encode proteins that induce apoptosis once daughter virions are mature (see Fig. 1-24A).
- **Immunologically mediated cytotoxicity:** Both humoral and cellular arms of the immune system protect against the harmful effects of viral infections by eliminating infected cells. Thus, presentation of viral proteins to the immune system in the context of a self major histocompatibility complex (MHC) on cell surfaces leads to immune responses against the invader and elicits killer cells and antiviral antibodies. These arms of the immune system eliminate virus-infected cells by inducing apoptosis or by lysing the cell with complement (see Fig. 1-24B) (see Chapter 4).

Chemicals Injure Cells Directly and Indirectly

Innumerable chemicals can damage almost any cell in the body. The science of toxicology attempts to define the mechanisms that determine both target cell specificity and the mechanism of action of such chemicals. Toxic chemicals either: (1) interact directly with cellular constituents without requiring metabolic activation or (2) are themselves not toxic but are metabolized to yield an ultimate toxin that interacts with the target cell. Whatever the mechanism, the result is usually necrotic cell death (see below).

Liver Necrosis Caused by the Metabolic Products of Chemicals

Studies of a few compounds that produce liver cell injury in rodents have enhanced our understanding of how chemicals injure cells. These studies have focused principally on those compounds that are converted to toxic metabolites. Carbon tetrachloride (CCl_4) and acetaminophen are well-studied hepatotoxins. Each is metabolized by the mixed-function oxidase system of the endoplasmic reticulum and each causes liver cell necrosis. These hepatotoxins are metabolized differently, and it is possible to relate the subsequent evolution of lethal cell injury to the specific features of this metabolism.

Carbon Tetrachloride

CCl_4 metabolism is a model system for toxicological studies. CCl_4 is metabolized via the hepatic mixed function oxygenase system (P450) to a chloride ion and a highly reactive trichloromethyl free radical ($CCl_3\bullet$).

$$CCl_4 + e^- \xrightarrow{P450} CCl_3\bullet + Cl^-$$

Like the hydroxyl radical, the trichloromethyl radical is a potent initiator of lipid peroxidation, although it may also interact with other macromolecules. However, in view of the rapidity with which CCl_4 kills cells (hours), peroxidative damage to the plasma membrane is the most likely culprit.

Acetaminophen

Acetaminophen, an important constituent of many analgesics, is innocuous in recommended doses, but when consumed to excess it is highly toxic to the liver. Most acetaminophen is enzymatically converted in the liver to nontoxic glucuronide or sulfate metabolites. Less than 5% of acetaminophen is ordinarily metabolized by isoforms of cytochrome P450 to NAPQI (*N*-acetyl-*p*-benzoquinone imine), a highly reactive quinone (Fig. 1-25). However, when large doses of acetaminophen overwhelm the glucuronidation pathway, toxic amounts of NAPQI are formed. NAPQI is responsible for acetaminophen-related toxicity by virtue of its conjugation with either GSH or sulfhydryl groups on liver proteins to form thiol esters. The latter cause extensive cellular dysfunction and lead to injury. At the same time, NAPQI depletes the antioxidant GSH, rendering the cell more susceptible to free radical-induced injury. Thus, conditions that deplete GSH (e.g., starvation) enhance the toxicity of acetaminophen. In addition, acetaminophen metabolism is accelerated by chronic alcohol consumption, an effect mediated by an ethanol-induced increase in the 3A4 isoform of P450. As a result, toxic amounts of NAPQI rapidly accumulate and may destroy the liver.

To summarize, metabolism of hepatotoxic chemicals by mixed-function oxidation leads to cell injury through covalent binding of reactive metabolites and peroxidation of membrane phospholipids. Lipid peroxidation is initiated by (1) a metabolite of the original compound (as with CCl_4) or (2) by activated oxygen species formed during the metabolism of the toxin (as with acetaminophen), the latter augmented by weakened antioxidant defenses.

Chemicals That Are Not Metabolized

Directly cytotoxic chemicals interact with cellular constituents: prior metabolic conversion is not needed. The critical cellular

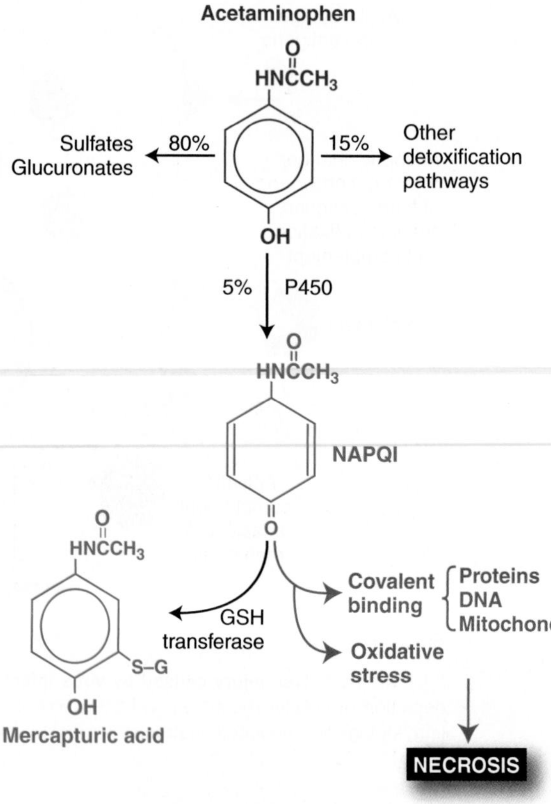

FIGURE 1-25. **Chemical reactions involved in acetaminophen hepatotoxicity.** GSH = glutathione; NAPQI = *N*-acetyl-*p*-benzoquinone imine.

targets are diverse and include, for example, mitochondria (heavy metals and cyanide), cytoskeleton (phalloidin, paclitaxel), and DNA (chemotherapeutic alkylating agents). As well, interaction of directly cytotoxic chemicals with glutathione (alkylating agents) weakens the cell's antioxidant defenses.

Abnormal G Protein Activity Leads to Functional Cell Injury

Normal cell function requires the coordination of numerous activating and regulatory signaling cascades. Hereditary or acquired interference with correct signal transduction can result in significant cellular dysfunction, as illustrated by diseases associated with faulty G proteins. A variety of membrane receptors (e.g., adrenergic or vasopressin receptors) are linked to intracellular G proteins, which activate downstream signaling. Inherited defects in G protein subunits can lead to constitutive activation of the protein. In one such hereditary syndrome, endocrine manifestations predominate, including multiple tumors in the pituitary and thyroid glands. Another G protein mutation appears to predominate in many cases of essential hypertension, in which exaggerated activation of G protein signaling results in increased vascular responsiveness to stimuli that cause vasoconstriction. Certain microorganisms (e.g., *Vibrio cholerae* and *Escherichia coli*) produce their effects by elaborating toxins that activate G proteins.

Decreased responsiveness of G proteins to ligand–receptor interactions may also be caused by certain mutations in G protein subunits. In addition, G protein activity can be inhibited by certain bacterial products, the most important example being pertussis toxin, the cause of whooping cough.

Cell Death

An understanding of the mechanisms underlying cell death is not simply an academic exercise; manipulation of cell viability by biochemical and pharmacologic intervention is currently a major area of research. For example, if we understand the biochemistry of ischemic death of cardiac myocytes, which is responsible for the leading cause of death in the Western world, we may be able to prolong myocyte survival after a coronary occlusion until circulation is restored.

Paradoxically, an organism's survival requires sacrifice of individual cells. Physiologic cell death is integral to the transformation of embryonic anlagen to fully developed organs. It is also crucial for regulation of cell numbers in a variety of tissues, including the epidermis, gastrointestinal tract, and hematopoietic system. Physiological cell death involves activation of an internal suicide program, which results in cell killing by a process termed **apoptosis.**

By contrast, pathologic cell death is not regulated and is invariably injurious to the organism. It may result from a variety of insults to cellular integrity (e.g., ischemia, burns, and toxins). **Necrosis** occurs when an insult interferes with a vital structure or function of an organelle (plasma membrane, mitochondria, etc.) and does not trigger apoptosis. Pathologic cell death, however, can also result from apoptosis, as exemplified by viral infections and ionizing radiation.

Necrosis Results from Exogenous Cell Injury and Is Reflected in Geographic Areas of Cell Death

At the cellular level, necrosis is characterized by cell and organelle swelling, ATP depletion, increased plasma membrane permeability, release of macromolecules, and eventually inflammation. Although the mechanisms responsible for necrosis vary according to the nature of the insult and the organ involved, most instances of necrosis share certain mechanistic similarities. The model of necrotic cell death that has been studied most extensively in mechanistic terms is ischemic injury to cardiac myocytes. The sequence of events is admittedly unique to cardiac myocytes, but most features are pertinent to other cell types and injurious agents.

Necrosis is the Process by Which Exogenous Stress Kills the Cell

Cells exist in a skewed equilibrium with their external environment. The plasma membrane is the barrier that separates the extracellular fluid from the internal cellular milieu. Whatever the nature of the lethal insult, cell necrosis is heralded by disruption of the permeability barrier function of the plasma membrane. Normally, extracellular concentrations of sodium and calcium are orders of magnitude greater than intracellular concentrations. The opposite holds for potassium. The selective ion permeability requires (1) considerable energy, (2) structural integrity of the lipid bilayer, (3) intact ion channel proteins, and (4) normal association of the membrane with cytoskeletal constituents. When one or more of these elements is severely damaged, the resulting disturbance of the internal ionic balance is thought to represent the "point of no return" for the injured cell.

The role of calcium in the pathogenesis of cell death deserves special mention. Ca^{2+} concentration in extracellular fluids is in the millimolar range (10^{-3} M). By contrast, cytosol Ca^{2+} concentration is 10,000-fold lower, on the order of 10^{-7} M. Many crucial cell functions are exquisitely regulated by minute fluctuations in cytosol free calcium concentration. Thus massive influx of Ca^{2+} through a damaged plasma membrane ensures loss of cell viability.

Coagulative Necrosis

Coagulative necrosis refers to light microscopic alterations in a dead or dying cell (Fig. 1-26). Shortly after a cell's death, its outline is maintained. When stained with the usual combination of hematoxylin and eosin, the cytoplasm of a necrotic cell is more deeply eosinophilic than usual. In the nucleus chromatin is initially clumped, and then is redistributed along the nuclear membrane.

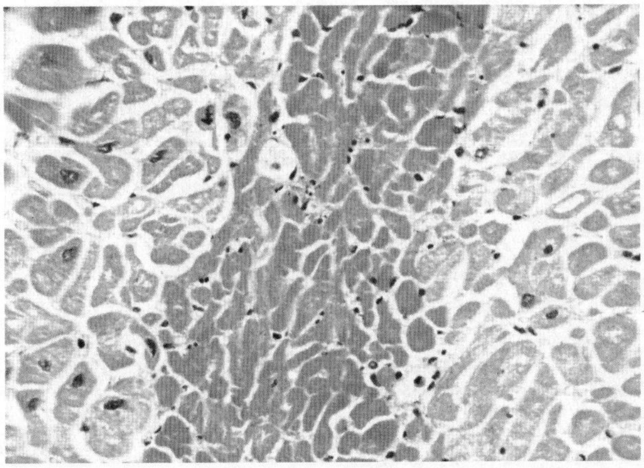

FIGURE 1-26. **Coagulative necrosis.** Photomicrograph of the heart in a patient with an acute myocardial infarction. In the center, the deeply eosinophilic necrotic cells have lost their nuclei. The necrotic focus is surrounded by paler-staining, viable cardiac myocytes.

Three morphologic changes follow:

- **Pyknosis:** The nucleus becomes smaller and stains deeply basophilic as chromatin clumping continues.
- **Karyorrhexis:** The pyknotic nucleus breaks up into many smaller fragments scattered about the cytoplasm.
- **Karyolysis:** The pyknotic nucleus may be extruded from the cell or it may manifest progressive loss of chromatin staining.

Early ultrastructural changes in a dying or dead cell reflect an extension of alterations associated with reversible cell injury (see Fig. 1-11, and Fig. 1-12). In addition to the nuclear changes described above, the dead cell features dilated endoplasmic reticulum, disaggregated ribosomes, swollen and calcified mitochondria, aggregated cytoskeletal elements, and plasma membrane blebs.

After a variable time, depending on the tissue and circumstances, a dead cell is subjected to the lytic activity of intracellular and extracellular enzymes. As a result, the cell disintegrates. This is particularly the case when necrotic cells have elicited an acute inflammatory response.

The appearance of the necrotic cell has traditionally been termed **coagulative necrosis** because of its similarity to coagulation of proteins that occurs upon heating. However, the usefulness of this historical term today is questionable.

Whereas the morphology of individual cell death tends to be uniform across different cell types, the tissue responses are more variable. This diversity is described by a number of terms that reflect specific histologic patterns that depend upon the organ and the circumstances.

Liquefactive Necrosis

When the rate of dissolution of the necrotic cells is considerably faster than the rate of repair, the resulting morphologic appearance is termed **liquefactive necrosis.** The polymorphonuclear leukocytes of the acute inflammatory reaction contain potent hydrolases capable of digesting dead cells. A sharply localized collection of these acute inflammatory cells, generally in response to bacterial infection, produces rapid cell death and tissue dissolution. The result is often an **abscess** (Fig. 1-27), which is a cavity formed by liquefactive necrosis in a solid tissue. Eventually an abscess is walled off by a fibrous capsule that contains its contents.

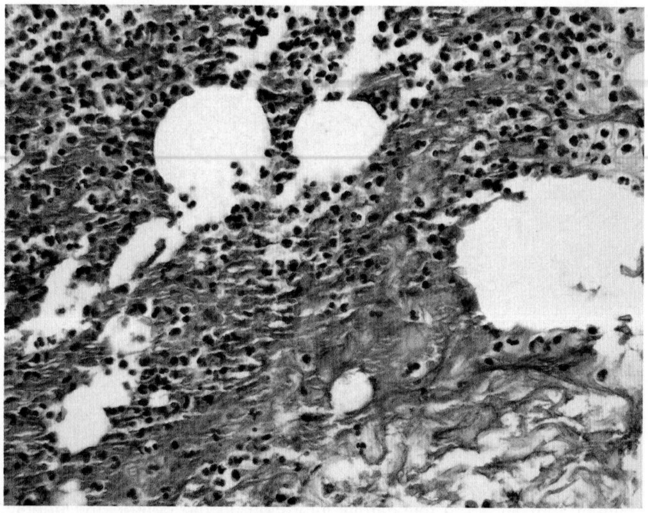

FIGURE 1-27. **Liquefactive necrosis in an abscess of the skin.** The abscess cavity is filled with polymorphonuclear leukocytes.

Coagulative necrosis of the brain may occur after cerebral artery occlusion, and is often followed by rapid dissolution—liquefactive necrosis—of the dead tissue by a mechanism that cannot be attributed to the action of an acute inflammatory response. It is not clear why coagulative necrosis in the brain and not elsewhere, is followed by dissolution of the necrotic cells, but the phenomenon may be related to the presence of more abundant lysosomal enzymes or different hydrolases specific to the cells of the central nervous system. Liquefactive necrosis of large areas of the central nervous system can lead to an actual cavity or cyst that will persist for the life of the person.

Fat Necrosis

Fat necrosis specifically affects adipose tissue and most commonly results from pancreatitis or trauma (Fig. 1-28). The unique feature determining this type of necrosis is the presence of triglycerides in adipose tissue. The process begins when digestive enzymes, normally found only in the pancreatic duct and small intestine, are released from injured pancreatic acinar cells and ducts into the extracellular spaces. On extracellular activation, these enzymes digest the pancreas itself as well as surrounding tissues, including adipose cells:

1. Phospholipases and proteases attack the plasma membrane of fat cells, releasing their stored triglycerides.
2. Pancreatic lipase hydrolyzes the triglycerides, a process to produce free fatty acids.
3. Free fatty acids bind calcium and are precipitated as calcium soaps. These appear as amorphous, basophilic deposits at the edges of irregular islands of necrotic adipocytes.

Grossly, fat necrosis appears as an irregular, chalky white area embedded in otherwise normal adipose tissue. In the case of traumatic fat necrosis, we presume that triglycerides and lipases are released from the injured adipocytes. In the breast, fat

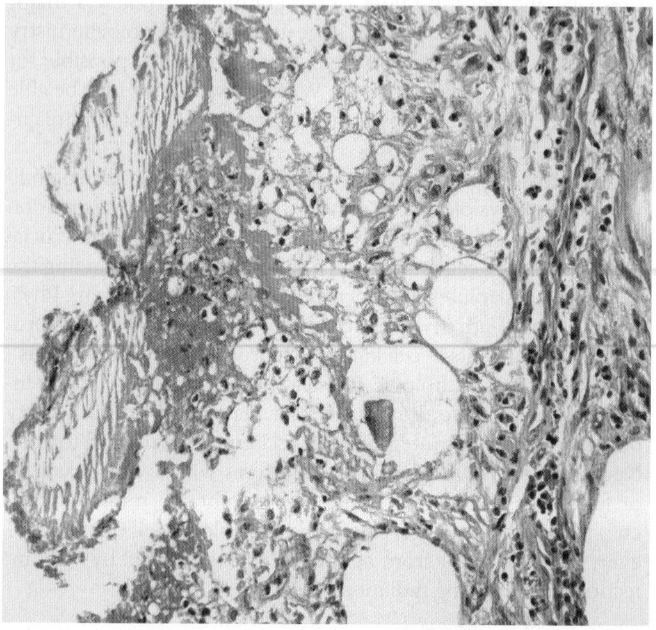

FIGURE 1-28. **Fat necrosis.** Photomicrograph of peripancreatic adipose tissue from a patient with acute pancreatitis shows an island of necrotic adipocytes adjacent to an acutely inflamed area. Fatty acids are precipitated as calcium soaps, which accumulate as amorphous, basophilic deposits at the periphery of the irregular island of necrotic adipocytes.

necrosis secondary to trauma is not uncommon and may mimic a tumor.

Caseous Necrosis

Caseous necrosis is characteristic of tuberculosis (Fig. 1-29). The lesions of tuberculosis are tuberculous granulomas, or tubercles. In the center of such granulomas, the accumulated mononuclear cells that mediate the chronic inflammatory reaction to the offending mycobacteria are killed. In caseous necrosis, unlike coagulative necrosis, the necrotic cells fail to retain their cellular outlines. They do not, however, disappear by lysis, as in liquefactive necrosis. Rather, the dead cells persist indefinitely as amorphous, coarsely granular, eosinophilic debris. Grossly, this debris is grayish white, soft and friable. It resembles clumpy cheese, hence the name **caseous necrosis.** This distinctive type of necrosis is generally attributed to the toxic effects of the mycobacterial cell wall, which contains complex waxes (peptidoglycolipids) that exert potent biological effects.

A

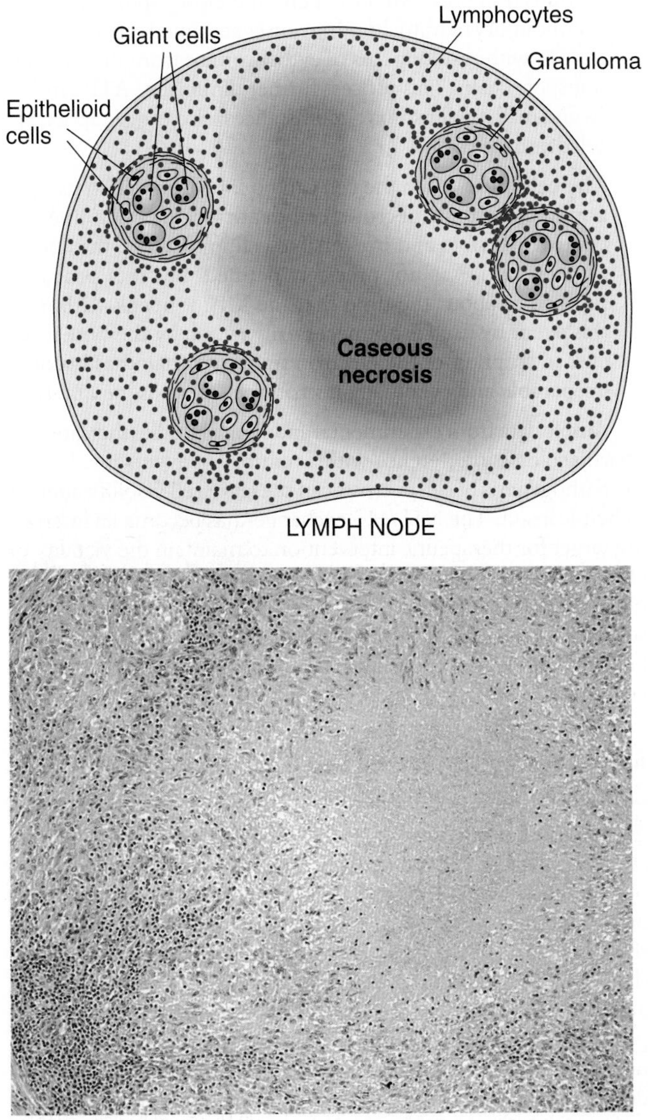

B

FIGURE 1-29. **Caseous necrosis in a tuberculous lymph node. A.** The typical amorphous, granular, eosinophilic, necrotic center is surrounded by granulomatous inflammation. **B.** Photomicrograph showing a tuberculous granuloma with central caseous necrosis.

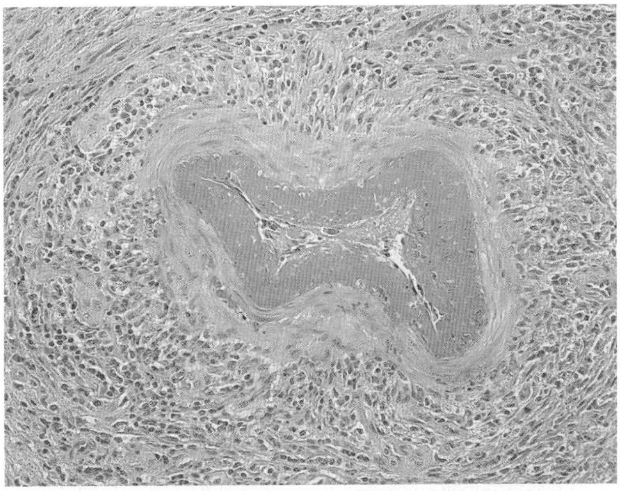

FIGURE 1-30. **Fibrinoid necrosis.** An inflamed muscular artery in a patient with systemic arteritis shows a sharply demarcated, homogeneous, deeply eosinophilic zone of necrosis.

Fibrinoid Necrosis

Fibrinoid necrosis is an alteration of injured blood vessels, in which insudation and accumulation of plasma proteins cause the wall to stain intensely with eosin (Fig. 1-30). The term is something of a misnomer, however, because the eosinophilia of the accumulated plasma proteins obscures the underlying alterations in the blood vessel, making it difficult, if not impossible, to determine whether there truly is necrosis in the vascular wall.

Necrosis Usually Involves Accumulation of a Number of Intracellular Insults

The processes by which cells undergo death by necrosis vary according to the cause, organ, and cell type. The best studied and most clinically important example is ischemic necrosis of cardiac myocytes. The mechanisms underlying the death of cardiac myocytes are in part unique, but the basic processes that are involved are comparable to those in other organs. Some of the unfolding events may occur simultaneously; others may be sequential (Fig. 1-31).

1. **Interruption of blood supply decreases delivery of O_2 and glucose.** Anoxia, whether it arises from ischemia (e.g., atherosclerosis) or other causes (e.g., blood loss from trauma), decreases delivery of both oxygen and glucose to myocytes. For most cells, but especially for cardiac myocytes (which do not store much energy), this combined insult is formidable.
2. **Anaerobic glycolysis leads to overproduction of lactate and decreased intracellular pH.** The lack of O_2 during myocardial ischemia both blocks production of ATP and inhibits mitochondrial oxidation of pyruvate. Instead, pyruvate is reduced to lactate in the cytosol, where its accumulation lowers intracellular pH. The acidification of the cytosol initiates a downward spiral of events that propels the cell towards disaster.
3. **Distortion of the activities of pumps in the plasma membrane skews the ionic balance of the cell.** Na^+ accumulates because the lack of ATP renders the Na^+/K^+ ion exchanger inactive, an effect that leads to activation of the Na^+/H^+ ion exchanger. This pump is normally quiescent, but when intracellular acidosis threatens, it pumps H^+ out of the cell in

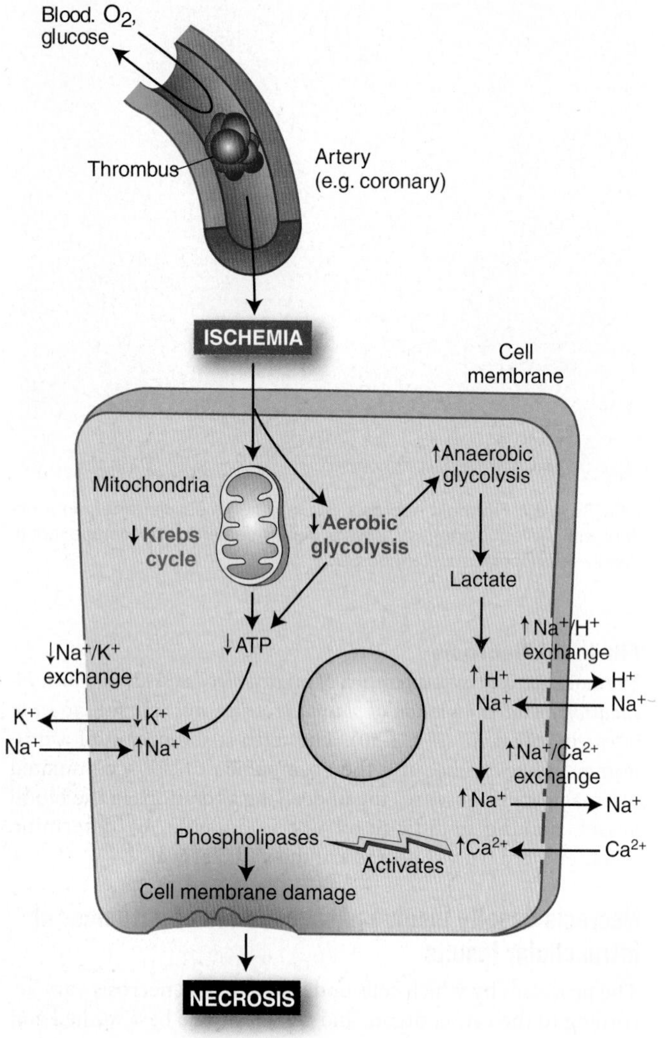

FIGURE 1-31. **Mechanisms by which ischemia leads to cell death.** ATP = adenosine triphosphate; Ca^{2+} = calcium ion; H^+ = hydrogen ion; K^+ = potassium ion; Na^{2+} = sodium ion; O_2 = oxygen.

exchange for Na^+ to maintain proper intracellular pH. The resulting increase in intracellular sodium activates the Na^+/Ca^{2+} ion exchanger, which increases calcium entry. Ordinarily, excess intracellular Ca^{2+} is extruded by an ATP-dependent calcium pump. However, with ATP in very short supply and Ca^{2+} accumulates in the cell.

4. **Activation of phospholipase A_2 (PLA_2) and proteases disrupts the plasma membrane and cytoskeleton.** High calcium concentrations in the cytosol of an ischemic cell activate PLA_2, leading to degradation of membrane phospholipids and consequent release of free fatty acids and lysophospholipids. The latter act as detergents that solubilize cell membranes. Both fatty acids and lysophospholipids are also potent mediators of inflammation (see Chapter 2), an effect that may further disrupt the integrity of the already compromised cell.

   Calcium also activates a series of proteases that attack the cytoskeleton and its attachments to the cell membrane. As the cohesion between cytoskeletal proteins and the plasma membrane is disrupted, membrane blebs form, and the shape of the cell is altered. The combination of electrolyte imbalance and increased cell membrane permeability causes the cell to swell, a frequent morphologic prelude to dissolution of the cell.

5. **The lack of O_2 impairs mitochondrial electron transport, thus decreasing ATP synthesis and facilitating production of ROS.** Under normal circumstances, about 3% of the oxygen entering the mitochondrial electron transport chain is converted to ROS. During ischemia, generation of ROS increases because of (1) decreased availability of favored substrates for the electron transport chain, (2) damage to elements of the chain, and (3) reduced activity of mitochondrial SOD. ROS cause peroxidation of cardiolipin, a membrane phospholipid that is unique to mitochondria and is sensitive to oxidative damage by virtue of its high content of unsaturated fatty acids. This attack inhibits the function of the electron transport chain and decreases its ability to produce ATP.

6. **Mitochondrial damage promotes the release of cytochrome c to the cytosol.** In normal cells the mitochondrial permeability transition pore (MPTP) opens and closes sporadically. Ischemic injury to mitochondria causes sustained opening of the MPTP, with resulting loss of cytochrome c from the electron transport chain. This process further diminishes ATP synthesis and may, under some circumstances, also trigger apoptotic cell death (see below).

7. **The cell dies.** When the cell can no longer maintain itself as a metabolic unit, necrotic cell death occurs. The line between reversible and irreversible cell injury (i.e., the "point of no return,") is not precisely defined, but it is probably reached at about the time that the MPTP opens. Although this event by itself is not necessarily lethal, by the time it occurs, disruption of the electron transport chain has become irreparable and eventually necrotic cell death is inevitable.

Ample data from experimental and clinical studies indicate that pharmacologic interference with a number of events involved in the pathogenesis of cell necrosis can preserve cell viability after an ischemic insult. The Na^+/H^+ exchanger has become an interesting target for therapeutic intervention to maintain the viability of cardiac myocytes during acute ischemia. Treatments that increase glucose uptake and redress some of the ionic imbalances may preserve myocyte viability during ischemia. Indeed, some success has been reported with simple administration of a combination of glucose, insulin, and potassium.

Apoptosis, or Programmed Cell Death, Refers to a Cellular Suicide Mechanism

Apoptosis is a prearranged pathway of cell death triggered by a variety of extracellular and intracellular signals. It is part of the balance between the life and death of cells and determines that a cell dies when it is no longer useful or when it may be harmful to the larger organism. It is also a self-defense mechanism, cells that are infected with pathogens or in which genomic alterations have occurred are destroyed. In this context, many pathogens have evolved mechanisms to inactivate key components of the apoptotic signaling cascades. Apoptosis detects and destroys cells that harbor dangerous mutations, thereby maintaining genetic consistency and preventing the development of cancer. By contrast, as in the case of infectious agents, successful clones of tumor cells often devise mechanisms to circumvent apoptosis.

The Morphology of Apoptosis

Apoptotic cells are recognized by nuclear fragmentation and pyknosis, generally against a background of viable cells. Importantly, individual cells or small groups of cells undergo apoptosis, whereas necrosis characteristically involves larger geographic areas of cell death. Ultrastructural features of apoptotic cells include (1) nuclear condensation and fragmentation; (2) segregation of cytoplasmic organelles into distinct regions; (3) blebs of the plasma membrane; and (4) membrane-bound cellular fragments, which often lack nuclei (Fig. 1-32).

Cells that have undergone necrotic cell death tend to elicit strong inflammatory responses. Inflammation, however, is not generally seen in the vicinity of apoptotic cells (Fig. 1-33). Mononuclear phagocytes may contain cellular debris from apoptotic cells, but recruitment of neutrophils or lymphocytes is uncommon (see Chapter 2). In view of the numerous developmental, physiologic and protective functions of apoptosis, the lack of inflammation is clearly beneficial to the organism.

Apoptosis in Developmental and Physiologic Processes

Fetal development involves the sequential appearance and regression of many anatomical structures: some aortic arches do not persist, the mesonephros regresses in favor of the metanephros, interdigital tissues disappear to allow discrete fingers and toes, and excess neurons are pruned from the developing brain. In the generation of immunologic diversity, clones of cells that recognize normal self antigens are deleted by apoptosis.

Physiologic apoptosis principally involves the progeny of stem cells that are continuously dividing (e.g., stem cells of the hematopoietic system, gastrointestinal mucosa, and epidermis). Apoptosis of mature cells in these organs prevents overpopulation of the respective cell compartments by removing senescent cells and thus maintaining the normal architecture and size of the organ systems.

Apoptosis Eliminates Obsolescent Cells

A normal turnover of cells in many organs is essential to maintain the size and function of that cellular compartment. For example, as cells are continuously supplied to the circulating blood, older and less functional white blood cells must be eliminated to maintain the normal complement of the cells. Indeed, the pathologic accumulation of polymorphonuclear leukocytes in chronic myelogenous leukemia results from a mutation that inhibits apoptosis and therefore allows these cells to persist. In the mucosa of the small intestine, cells migrate from the depths of the crypts to the tips of the villi, where they undergo apoptosis and are sloughed into the lumen.

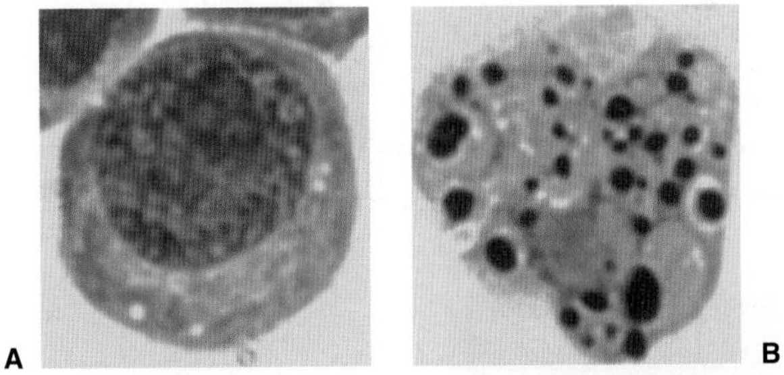

FIGURE 1-32. **Apoptosis.** A viable leukemic cell (**A**) contrasts with an apoptotic cell (**B**) in which the nucleus has undergone condensation and fragmentation.

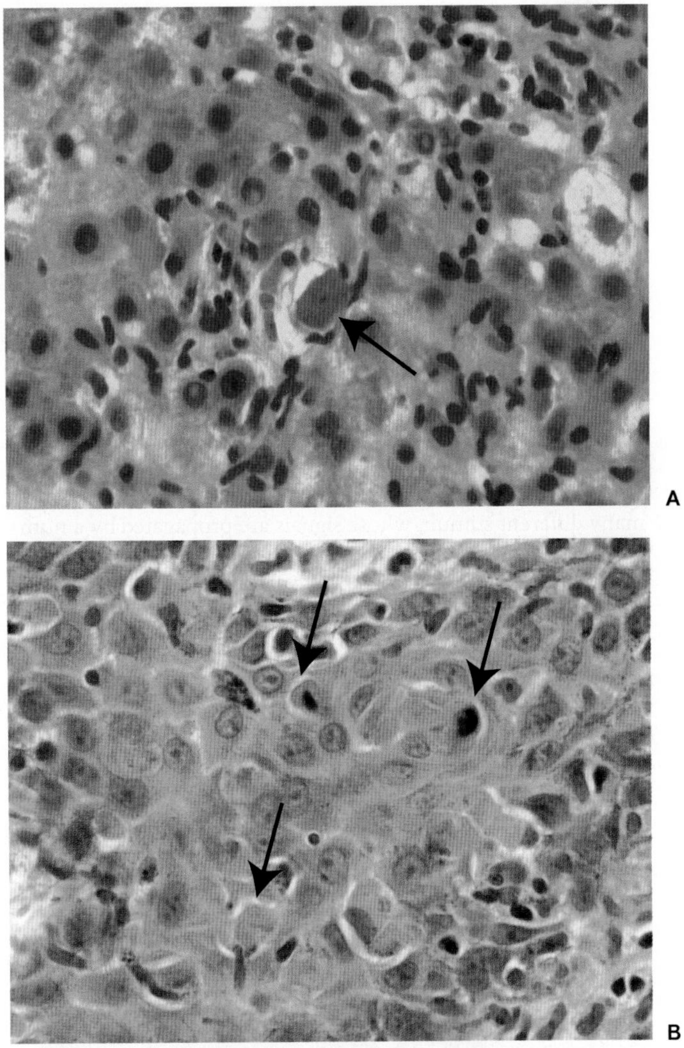

FIGURE 1-33. **Histopathologic illustrations of apoptosis in the liver in viral hepatitis** (**A**) and in the skin in erythema multiforme (**B**). Apoptotic cells are highlighted by *arrows*.

Apoptosis also maintains the balance of cellularity in organs that respond to trophic stimuli, such as hormones. An illustration of such an effect is the regression of lactational hyperplasia of the breast in women who have stopped nursing their infants. On the other side of the reproductive divide, postmenopausal women suffer atrophy of the endometrium after hormonal support has withered.

Apoptosis Deletes Mutant Cells

The integrity of an organism requires that it be able to recognize irreparable damage to DNA, after which the damaged cells must be eliminated by apoptosis. There is a finite error rate in DNA replication, owing to the infidelity of DNA polymerases. In addition, environmental stresses such as ultraviolet (UV) light, ionizing radiation, and DNA-binding chemicals may also alter DNA structure. There are several means, the most important of which is probably p53, by which the cell recognizes genomic abnormalities and "assesses" whether they can be repaired. If the DNA damage is too severe to be repaired, a cascade of events leading to apoptosis is activated and the cell dies. This process protects an organism from the consequences of a nonfunctional cell or one that cannot control its own proliferation (e.g., a cancer cell).

Apoptosis as a Defense against Dissemination of Infection

When a cell "detects" episomal (extrachromosomal) DNA replication, as in a viral infection, it tends to initiate apoptosis. This effect can be viewed as a means to eliminate infected cells before they can spread the virus. Many viruses have evolved protective mechanisms to manipulate cellular apoptosis. Viral gene products that inhibit apoptosis have been identified for many viruses, including human immunodeficiency virus (HIV), human papillomavirus, adenovirus, and many others. In some cases these viral proteins bind and inactivate certain cellular proteins (e.g., p53) that are important in signaling apoptosis. In other instances, they may act at various points in the signaling pathways that activate apoptosis.

Signaling Apoptosis

Apoptosis is a final effector mechanism that can be initiated by many different stimuli, whose signals are propagated by a number of pathways. Unlike necrosis, apoptosis engages the cell's own signaling cascades. That is, a cell that undergoes apoptosis is an active participant in its own death (suicide). Most intermediate enzymes that transduce proapoptotic signals belong to a family of cysteine proteases called **caspases**.

Apoptosis May be Initiated by Receptor–Ligand Interactions at the Cell Membrane

The best understood initiators of apoptosis at the cell membrane are the binding of TNF-α to its receptor (TNFR), and that of the Fas ligand to its receptor (Fas, or Fas receptor). TNF-α is most often a free cytokine, whereas Fas ligand is located at the plasma membrane of certain cells, such as cytotoxic effector lymphocytes.

The receptors for TNF-α and Fas ligand become activated when they bind their ligands. These transmembrane proteins have specific amino acid sequences, termed **death domains,** in their cytoplasmic tails that act as docking sites for death domains of other proteins that participate in the signaling process leading to apoptosis (Fig. 1-34A). After binding to the receptors, the latter proteins activate downstream signaling molecules, especially procaspase-8, which is converted to caspase-8. In turn, caspase-8 initiates an activation cascade of other downstream caspases in

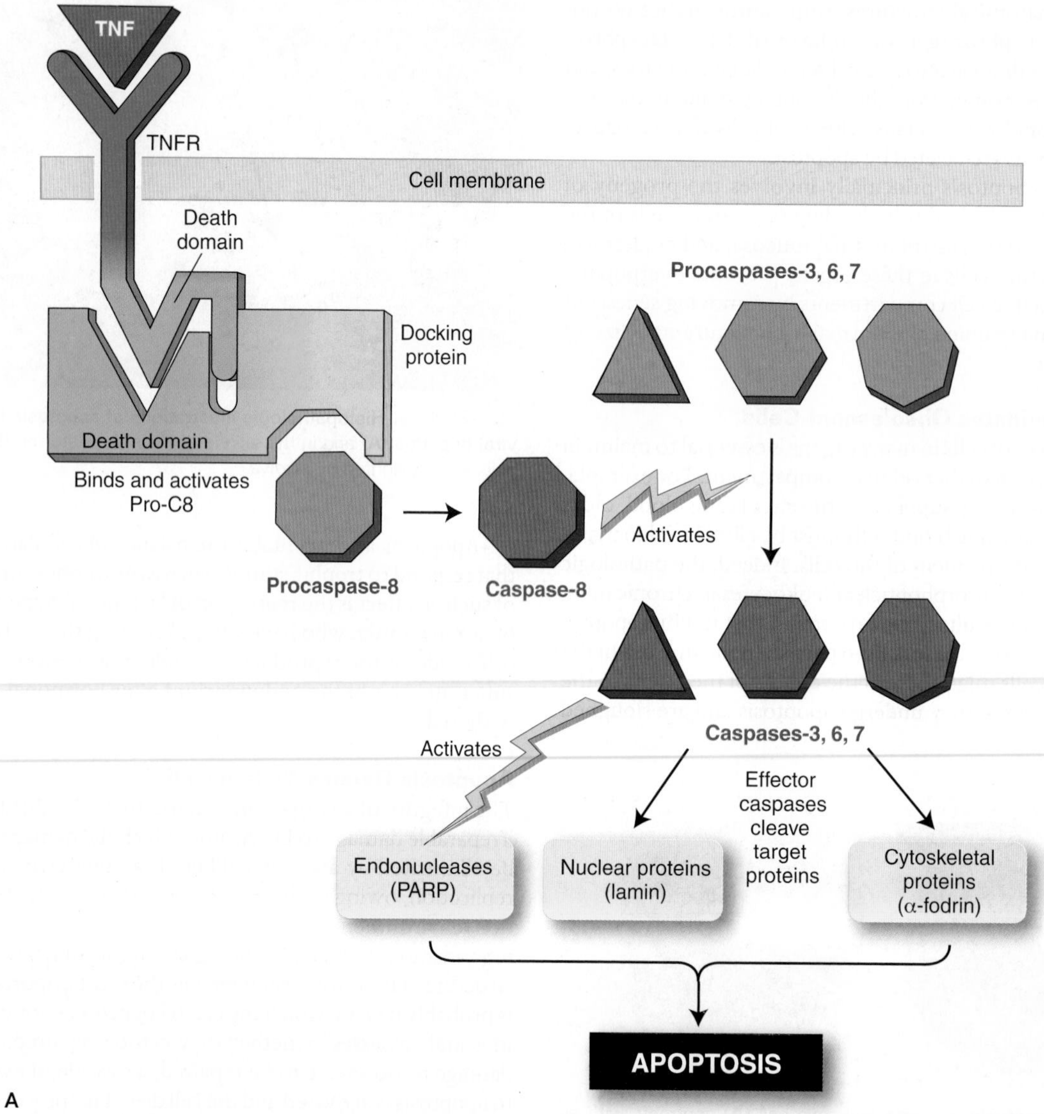

FIGURE 1-34. **Mechanisms by which apoptosis may be initiated, signaled, and executed. A.** Ligand–receptor interactions that lead to caspase activation. TNF = tumor necrosis factor; TNFR = tumor necrosis factor receptor.

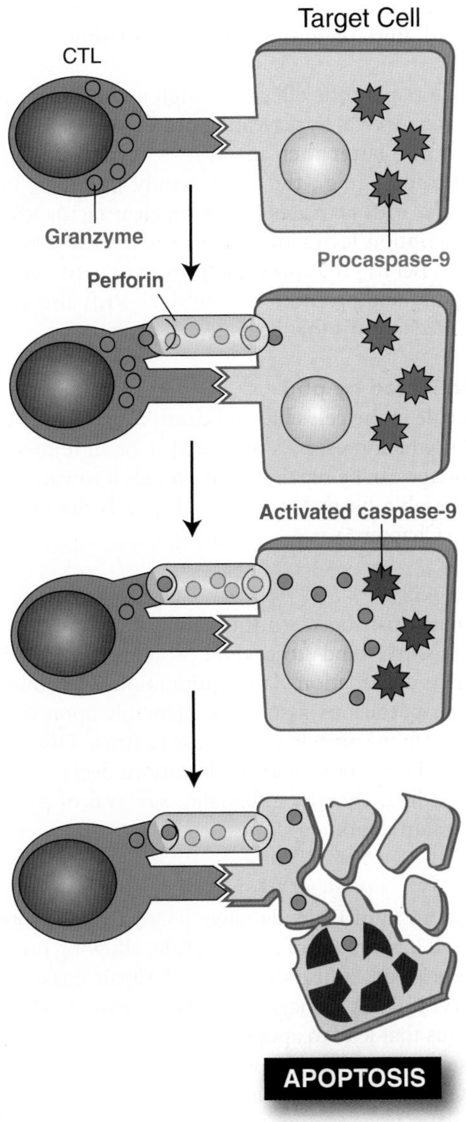

B

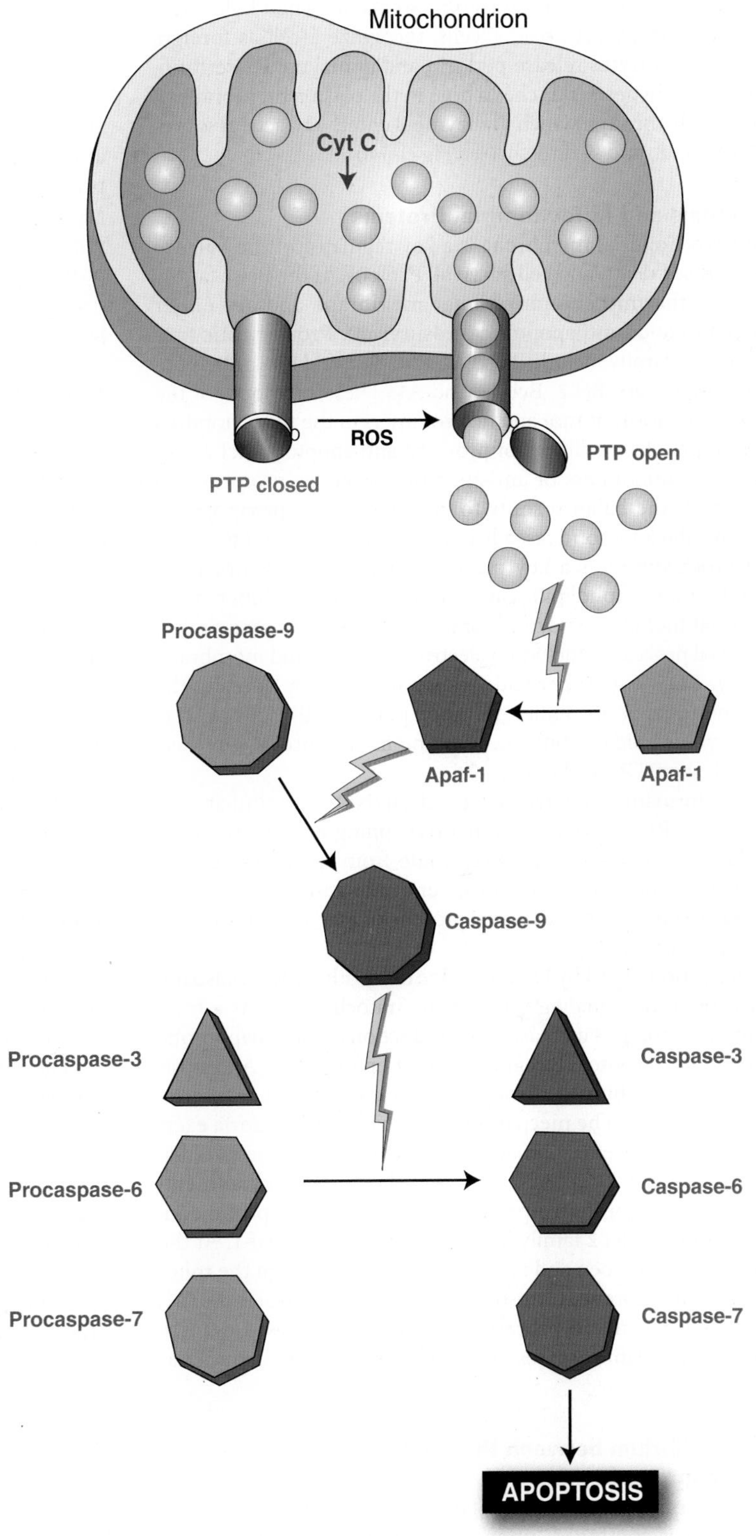

C

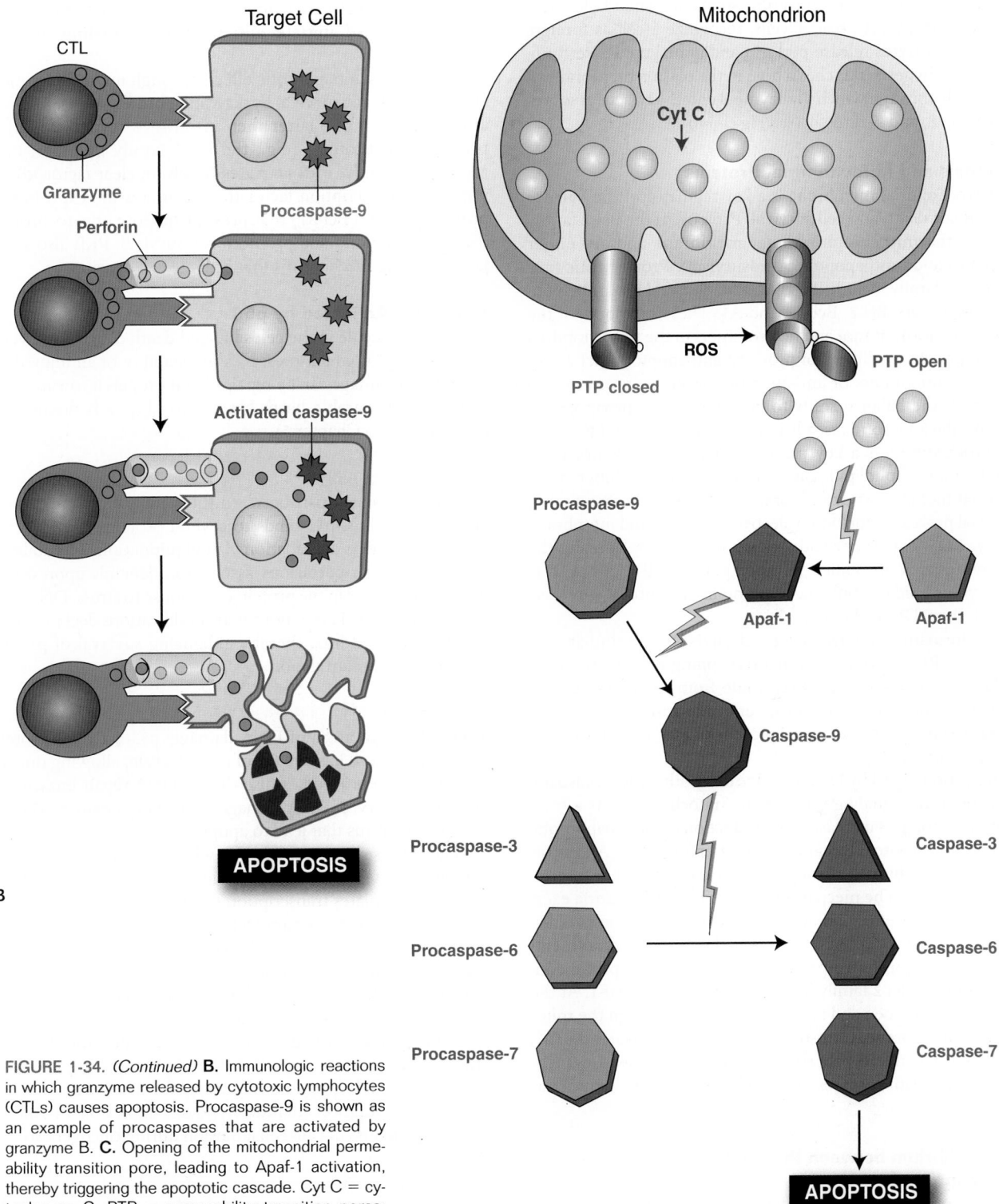

FIGURE 1-34. *(Continued)* **B.** Immunologic reactions in which granzyme released by cytotoxic lymphocytes (CTLs) causes apoptosis. Procaspase-9 is shown as an example of procaspases that are activated by granzyme B. **C.** Opening of the mitochondrial permeability transition pore, leading to Apaf-1 activation, thereby triggering the apoptotic cascade. Cyt C = cytochrome C; PTP = permeability transition pores; ROS = reactive oxygen species.

the apoptosis pathway. These caspases, (3, 6, and 7) activate a number of nuclear enzymes (e.g., poly-adenosine diphosphate [ADP]-ribosyl polymerase [PARP]) that mediate the nuclear fragmentation of apoptotic cell death.

Activation of caspase signaling also occurs when killer lymphocytes, mainly cytotoxic T cells, recognize a cell as foreign. These lymphocytes release perforin and granzyme B. Perforin, as its name suggests, punches a hole in the plasma membrane of a target cell, through which granzyme B enters and activates procaspases-3, -8, and -9 directly (see Fig. 1-34B).

Apoptosis and Mitochondrial Proteins

The mitochondrial membrane is a key regulator of the balance between cell death and cell survival. Proteins of the Bcl-2 family reside in the mitochondrial inner membrane and are either proapoptotic or anti-apoptotic (prosurvival). Proapoptotic proteins in this family include Bax, Bak, Bad, Bid, and Bik; anti-apoptotic proteins are Bcl-2, Bcl-X_L, and A1. These members of the Bcl-2 family form homo- and heterodimers in the mitochondrial membrane. Heterodimers of pro- and anti-apoptotic Bcl-2 proteins, or homodimers of anti-apoptotic proteins, promote cell survival. If the balance shifts to homodimers of proapoptotic proteins, the apoptotic cascade is activated (see Fig. 1-34C).

Cytochrome c is a key player in apoptosis. It is normally bound by a phospholipid, **cardiolipin** (CL), to the inner mitochondrial membrane. Cytochrome c participates in many mitochondrial processes, including electron transport and membrane fluidity. ROS (e.g., superoxide) cause apoptosis by opening the mitochondrial permeability transition pores (PTP). This process may involve oxidation of CL, resulting in cytochrome c release through the PTP (see below).

The formation of nitric oxide radical (NO•) has similar consequences. ROS also activate neutral sphingomyelinase, a cytosolic enzyme that releases ceramide from sphingomyelin in the plasma membrane. In turn, ceramide stimulates cellular stress responses (stress-activated protein kinases), which then activate procaspase-8.

Activation of p53 by DNA damage or by other means also initiates apoptotic signaling through the mitochondria. As a transcription factor, p53 increases the production of the proapoptotic mitochondrial protein Bax and the proapoptotic FasR. Apoptosis is also initiated by p53 through means unrelated to transcriptional activation. The mechanisms by which mitochondria exert such a powerful effect on apoptosis have recently been elucidated (see Fig. 1-34C). Bcl-2 dimers at the mitochondrial membrane bind the protein Apaf-1. A surfeit of proapoptotic constituents of the Bcl-2 family leads to the release of Apaf-1. At the same time, PTP open and cytochrome c leaks through the mitochondrial membrane. Cytosolic cytochrome c activates Apaf-1, which in turn converts procaspase-9 to caspase-9. Caspase-9 activates downstream caspases (3, 6, and 7) in the same manner as caspase-8.

The Equilibrium between Pro- and Anti-apoptotic Signals

Apoptosis can be viewed as a default pathway and the survival of many cells is contingent upon constant anti-apoptotic (prosurvival) signals. In other words, a cell must actively choose life rather than succumbing to the despair of apoptosis. Survival signals are transduced through receptors linked to phosphatidylinositol 3-kinase (PI3K), the enzyme that phosphorylates PIP_2 and PIP_3 (phosphatidyl inositol bis- and triphosphates). By antagonizing apoptosis, PI3K plays a critical role in cell viability. A prototypical receptor that signals via this mechanism is insulin-like growth factor-I receptor (IGF-IR). Paradoxically, PI3K is also activated by TNFR after binding TNF-α.Thus, the same cell membrane receptor that induces apoptosis in some circumstances can also initiate anti-apoptotic signaling in other situations.

PI3K exerts antiapoptotic effects through intracellular mediators, which favor survival by activating protein kinase B (PKB), also called Akt. The latter then inactivates several important proapoptotic proteins (e.g., the Bcl-2 family member, Bad). More importantly, PKB activates NFκB (nuclear factor κB), an important transcription factor that promotes the expression of proteins (A1 and Bcl-X_L) that prevent the loss of cytochrome c from mitochondria and promote cell survival. PKB also stimulates signaling mechanisms that activate cell division.

Apoptosis Activated by p53

A pivotal molecule in the cell's life-and-death dance is the versatile protein p53, which preserves the viability of an injured cell when DNA damage can be repaired, but propels it toward apoptosis after irreparable harm has occurred (p53 is discussed in greater detail in Chapter 5).

Homeostasis of p53

A delicate balance exists between the stabilization and destruction of p53. Thus, p53 binds to several proteins (e.g., Mdm2), which promote its degradation via ubiquitination. The ability of p53 to avoid this pernicious association depends upon certain structural changes in the protein in response to stress, DNA damage, and so forth. These molecular modifications decrease its interaction with Mdm2, thereby enhancing survival of p53 and permitting its accumulation.

Function of p53

After it binds to areas of DNA damage, p53 activates proteins that arrest the cell in stage G1 of the cell cycle, allowing time for DNA repair to proceed. It also directs DNA repair enzymes to the site of injury. If DNA damage cannot be repaired, p53 activates mechanisms that lead to apoptosis.

There are several pathways by which p53 induces apoptosis. It downregulates transcription of the antiapoptotic protein Bcl-2, while it upregulates transcription of the proapoptotic genes *bax* and *bak*. In addition, certain DNA helicases and other enzymes are activated by p53-mediated recognition of DNA damage, an effect that leads to translocation of a number of proapoptotic proteins (e.g., Fas) from the cell membrane to the cytosol.

Stress also leads to accumulation of p53. Activation of certain oncogenes, such as *c-myc,* increases the amount of an Mdm2-binding protein ($p14^{arf}$), thereby protecting p53 from Mdm2-induced destruction. Additional forms of stress that lead to p53 accumulation include hypoxia, depletion of ribonucleotides, and loss of cell–cell adhesion during oncogenesis.

Inactivation of p53

Proteins of a number of oncogenic viruses inactivate p53 by binding to it. In fact, p53 was first identified as a cellular protein that coprecipitated with one such protein (SV40 large T antigen). Inactivating mutations of p53 are the most common DNA alterations in human cancer, which underscores its role as a switch that allows repair of DNA but triggers cellular suicide if that proves to be impossible.

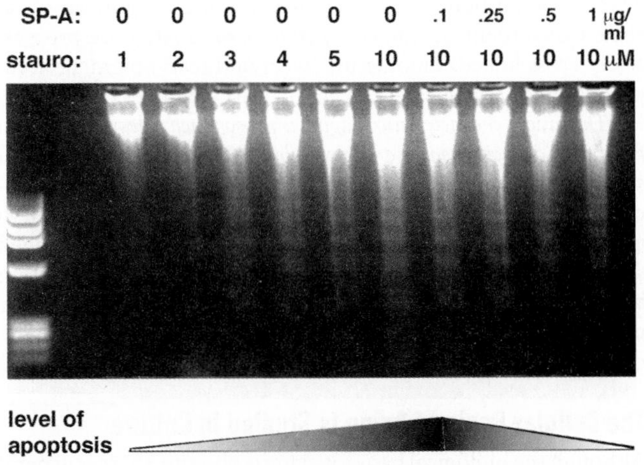

FIGURE 1-35. **DNA fragmentation in apoptosis.** Agarose gel electrophoresis of DNA isolated from lung epithelial cells treated with different amounts of staurosporine, which induces apoptosis, and with different amounts of surfactant protein-A (SP-A), which protects these cells from apoptosis. The schematic at the bottom illustrates the degree of apoptosis observed in these cells as a function of the concentrations of these two agents. At low concentrations of staurosporine or at high concentrations of SP-A, genomic DNA is largely unfragmented and thus remains at the top of the gel. By contrast, internucleosomal cleavage of DNA, such as occurs in apoptosis, is reflected in multiple, regularly spaced genomic DNA fragments, resembling a ladder. This phenomenon is called "laddering."

Quantitative Assays for Apoptosis

Apoptotic cells can be detected by demonstrating fragmented DNA. A popular method involves the demonstration of nucleosomal "laddering." This virtually diagnostic pattern of DNA degradation, which is characteristic of apoptotic cell death, results from cleavage of chromosomal DNA at nucleosomes by activated endonucleases. Since nucleosomes are regularly spaced along the genome, a pattern of regular bands can be seen when fragments of cellular DNA are separated by electrophoresis (Fig. 1-35).

Other assays are also used to detect and quantitate apoptosis. One is the TUNEL assay (terminal deoxyribonucleotidyl transferase [TdT]-mediated deoxyuridine triphosphate [dUTP]-digoxigenin nick end labeling) in which TdT transfers a fluorescent nucleotide to exposed breakpoints in DNA. Apoptotic cells that incorporate the labeled nucleotide are visualized by fluorescence microscopy or flow cytometry. Apoptotic cells that have extruded some of the DNA have less than their normal diploid content. Automated measurement of DNA content in individual cells by flow cytometry thus produces a population distribution according to DNA content (cytofluorography). Other means of detecting apoptosis depend upon quantitating the activated forms of enzymes that signal apoptosis, including the nuclear proteins PARP and lamin A.

In summary, cells are continually poised between survival and apoptosis: their fate rests on the balance of powerful intracellular and extracellular forces, whose signals constantly act upon and counteract each other. Often, apoptosis functions as a self-protective programmed mechanism that leads to a cell's suicide when its survival may be detrimental to the organism. At other times, apoptosis is a pathologic process that contributes to many disorders, especially degenerative diseases. Thus, pharmacologic manipulation of apoptosis is an active frontier of drug development.

Biological Aging

Old age is a consequence of civilization; it is a condition rarely encountered in the animal kingdom or in primitive societies. From an evolutionary perspective, the aging process presents conceptual difficulties. Since animals in the wild do not attain their maximum longevity, how did aging evolve? The consequences of aging arise after the reproductive period and thus should not have an evolutionary impact.

Aging must be distinguished from mortality on the one hand and from disease on the other. Death is a random event; an aged person who does not succumb to the most common cause of death will die from the second, third, or tenth most common cause. Although the increased vulnerability to disease among the elderly is an interesting problem, disease itself is entirely distinct from aging.

Maximal Life Span Has Remained Unchanged

Millennia ago the psalmist sang of a natural life span of 70 years, which with vigor may extend to 80. By contrast, it is estimated that the usual age at death of Neolithic humans was 20 to 25 years, and the average life span today in some regions is often barely 10 years more.

The difference between humans in primitive and in civilized environments is analogous to that observed between animals in their natural habitat and those in a zoo (Fig. 1-36). For animals in the wild, after an initial high mortality during maturation, a progressive linear decline in survival is noted, ending at the maximum life span of the species. This steady decrease in the number of mature animals does not reflect aging but rather sporadic events, such as encounters with beasts of prey, accidental trauma, infection, starvation, and so on. On the other hand, survival in the protected environment of a zoo is characterized by slow attrition until old age, at which time the steep decline in numbers is attributable to the aging process. *Interestingly, the maximum life span attained is not significantly altered by a protected environment.* An analogous situation is seen in studies of human mortality. Less than a century ago, the steep linear slope of mortality in human adults principally reflected random accidents and infections. With improved safety and sanitation, antibiotics and other drugs, and better diagnostic and therapeutic methods, the age-adjusted death rate in the United States has declined by 40% since 1970 and in 2004, life expectancy at

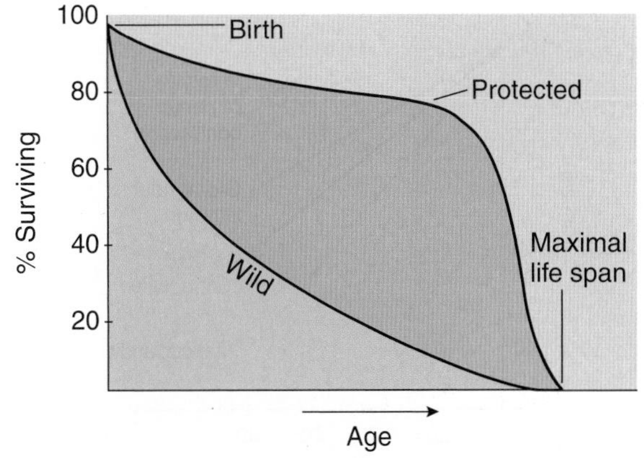

FIGURE 1-36. **Life span of animals in their natural environment compared with that in a protected habitat.** Note that both curves reach the same maximal life span.

the time of birth was 80.4 years for females and 75.2 years for males. At age 60, life expectancy was 20 additional years and 24 additional years, respectively.

Yet the maximum human life span has remained constant at about 110 years. Even if diseases associated with old age, such as cardiovascular disease and cancer, were eliminated, only a modest increase in average life expectancy would be seen. A long period of good health and low mortality rate would be followed by a precipitously increased mortality owing to aging itself; the life span would, for practical purposes, remain on the lower side of 100 years. Given the current life expectancy, the prevention or cure of the causes of premature death would have little impact on mean longevity.

Why do women live longer than men? The male-to-female ratio is 106:100 at birth, but from that time on, more women than men survive at every age, and at age 75 the male-to-female ratio is 2:3. Interestingly, greater female longevity is almost universal in the animal kingdom. At the cellular level, somatic cells with the female genotype are no hardier than those with the male pattern. Factors involved in the difference in average human longevity include the greater male mortality from violent causes and greater susceptibility to cardiovascular disease, cancer, respiratory illness, and cirrhosis in middle and old age. Historical differences between the sexes in cigarette smoking and alcohol consumption are also important in the gender gap in longevity. Indeed, smoking alone has been estimated to account for 4 of the 7 years of sex differential in longevity at birth. Thus, if men escape from these hazards, the gap in longevity between the sexes is progressively reduced with advancing age to just over 1 year beyond age 85.

Functional and Structural Changes Accompany Aging

The insidious effects of aging can be detected in otherwise healthy persons. The great leaps of imagination in theoretical physics and mathematics are almost exclusively made by the young. In many sports, an athlete in his or her 30s may be referred to as "aged." Even in the absence of specific diseases or vascular abnormalities, beginning in the fourth decade of life there is a progressive decline in many physiologic functions (Fig. 1-37), including such easily measurable parameters as muscular strength, cardiac reserve, nerve conduction time, pulmonary vital capacity, glomerular filtration, and vascular elasticity. These functional deteriorations are accompanied by structural changes. Lean body mass decreases and the proportion of fat rises. Constituents of the connective tissue matrix are progressively cross-linked. Lipofuscin ("wear and tear") pigment accumulates in organs such as the brain, heart, and liver.

The salient characteristic of aging is not so much a decrease in basal functional capacity as it is a reduced ability to adapt to environmental stresses. Although resting pulse is unchanged, the maximal increase with exercise is reduced with age and the time required to return to normal heart rate is prolonged. Similarly, the aged show impaired adaptation to ingested carbohydrates: fasting blood glucose levels are often normal compared with younger people, but they rise higher after a carbohydrate meal and decline more slowly.

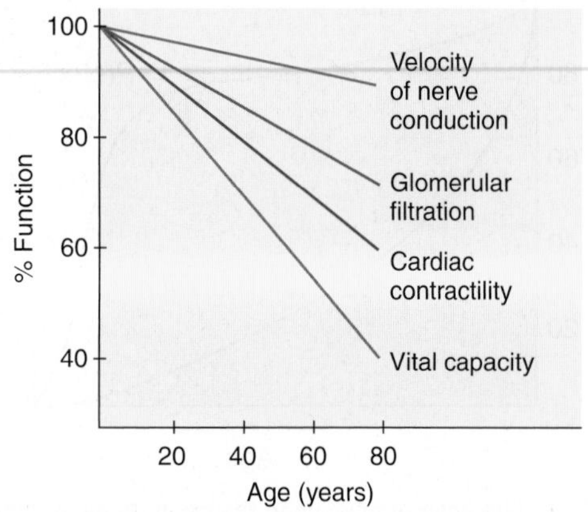

FIGURE 1-37. **Decrease in human physiologic capacities as a function of age.**

The Cellular Basis of Aging Is Studied in Culture

Although the biological basis for aging is obscure, there is general agreement that its elucidation, as in all pathologic conditions, should be sought at the cellular level. Various theories of cellular aging have been proposed, but the evidence adduced for each is at best indirect and is often derived from data obtained in cultured cells. An adequate theory should be parsimonious, compatible with the species-specific differences in life spans and consistent with the fact that most noncycling cells, such as neurons and myocytes, undergo a linear, relatively uniform functional decline with age. Below, we review the major considerations in this controversial field of investigation.

Support for the concept of a genetically programmed life span comes from studies of replicating cells in tissue culture. Unlike cancer cells, normal cells in tissue culture do not exhibit an unrestrained capacity to replicate. Cultured human fibroblasts undergo about 50 population doublings, after which they are irreversibly arrested in the G1 phase of the cell cycle and no longer divide. If they are exposed to an oncogenic virus or a chemical carcinogen, they may continue to replicate; in a sense, they become immortal. A rough correlation between the number of population doublings in fibroblasts and life span has been reported in several species. For example, rat fibroblasts exhibit considerably fewer doublings than do human ones. Moreover, cells obtained from persons afflicted with a syndrome of precocious aging, such as progeria (see below), also display a conspicuously reduced number of population doublings in vitro.

In Vivo Studies

There is no demonstrable age-related change in vivo in the replicative capacity of rapidly cycling cells (e.g., epithelial cells of the intestine). One is, therefore, left with the apparent paradox that replicating cells in culture have a limited life span, whereas aging in vivo seems mainly to affect the functional capacity of postmitotic cells. In other words, persons do not age because cells of the intestinal tract or bone marrow fail to replicate. However, if one considers that a function of cells in vitro is to proliferate, then they indeed display a major failure in functional capacity, and in many studies cells in culture are used as a model for the study of aging.

Just as Greek mythology postulates that the offspring of unions between immortal gods and mortal humans are mortal (e.g., Hercules), cellular senescence in vitro is also a dominant genetic trait. Thus, hybrids between normal human cells in vitro, which exhibit a limited number of cell divisions, and immortalized cells with an indefinite capacity to divide, undergo senescence. This finding shows that senescence is dominant over immortality. Replicative senescence–related genes have been identified on a number of human chromosomes, but the precise function(s) encoded by most of them have not been elucidated.

Telomerase and Senescence

An attractive explanation for cell senescence in vitro centers on the genetic elements at the tips of chromosomes, termed **telomeres.** These are series of short repetitive nucleotide sequences (TTAGGG in vertebrates) that vary in size from 70 in *Tetrahymena* (a protozoan) to 2000 in human chromosomes. Since DNA polymerase cannot copy the linear chromosomes all the way to the tip, the telomeres tend to shorten with each cell division until a critical diminution in size interfered with replication. Moreover, oxidative stress induces single-stranded damage in telomeric DNA, and this defect cannot be repaired in telomeres.

To overcome this "end-replication" problem, most eukaryotic cells use a ribonucleoprotein enzyme termed **telomerase,** which can extend chromosome ends. It has thus been proposed that telomere shortening acts as a molecular clock ("replicometer"), which produces senescence after a defined number of cell divisions in vitro. In this context, ectopic expression of telomerase reverses the senescent phenotype, and after immortalization of cells in vitro, telomerase activity can also be demonstrated.

Senescence also functions as a tumor-suppressing mechanism, limiting cell proliferative capacity in vivo. This idea implies that replicative senescence related to telomere shortening did not evolve to cause aging, but is rather a consequence of a biological device that suppresses tumor formation. Thus, shortening of telomeres to a critical length activates a p53-dependent check point system in the cell cycle. Mice that are mutant for an activated form of p53 display an early onset of phenotypes associated with aging, including a shortened life span, generalized organ atrophy, osteoporosis, and diminished tolerance to a variety of stresses. These data are consistent with the observation that mutant mice that are deficient in telomerase exhibit high levels of activated p53 and also suffer reduced longevity and early senescence-related phenotypes. Other tumor suppressor genes also appear to be activated by telomere shortening and cyclin-dependent kinase inhibitors (p16, p21, and p27) are regarded as the key effectors of replicative senescence. There is also evidence for a telomere-independent pathway for growth arrest in humans. In view of these data, current concepts hold that growth arrest suppresses tumorigenesis but that the functional changes contribute to aging.

Genetic Factors Influence Aging

Experimental Models

Invertebrates, including roundworms and flies, represent a level of biological complexity beyond that afforded by tissue culture. The short generation times of these organisms have been exploited to study genetic influences on aging and longevity.

Caenorhabditis elegans is a worm in which single-gene mutations that extend life span have been identified. A variety of such mutations (*Age* mutations) increase the life spans of these nematode up to fivefold, a greater increase than has been reported for any other model. In addition to prolonging the life span, *Age* mutations in *C. elegans* also confer a complex array of other phenotypes. For example, the so-called clock *(clk)* mutations slow most functions that relate to the overall metabolic rate (cell cycle progression, swimming, food pumping, etc.). *Age* mutations also confer resistance to both environmental (extrinsic) and intrinsic stresses, including oxygen free radicals, heat shock, and ultraviolet radiation. Thus, genes that prolong life in *C. elegans* apparently act to reduce the accumulation of cellular "injuries" that impair homeostatic mechanisms and, thereby, shorten life span.

In experiments with *Drosophila,* strains of long-lived flies can be readily created by using the oldest flies for breeding. In such studies, the better health of the aged flies is associated with a "trade-off" of decreased fitness in the young flies, as evidenced by lesser activity and fertility than in wild-type flies. Thus, the original population must have had a set of alleles that yields greater fitness at a young age and decreased fitness at an older one, a phenomenon termed "antagonistic pleiotropy." This doctrine also applies to the protection against cancer by tumor suppressor mechanisms at the price of promoting the aging process.

Diseases of Premature Aging

In humans, the modest correlation in longevity between related persons and the excellent concordance of life span among identical twins lend credence to the concept that aging is influenced by genetic factors. The existence of heritable diseases associated with accelerated aging buttresses this notion. The entire process of aging, including features such as male-pattern baldness, cataracts, and coronary artery disease, is compressed into a span of less than 10 years in a genetic syndrome termed **Hutchinson-Guilford progeria** (Fig. 1-38). The cause of progeria is apparently a mutation in the LMNA gene, whose product is a protein termed lamin A. The mutant gene codes for a defective precursor of the lamin A protein, which has been termed **progerin.** This abnormal protein accumulates in the nucleus from one cell generation to the next, thereby interfering with the structural

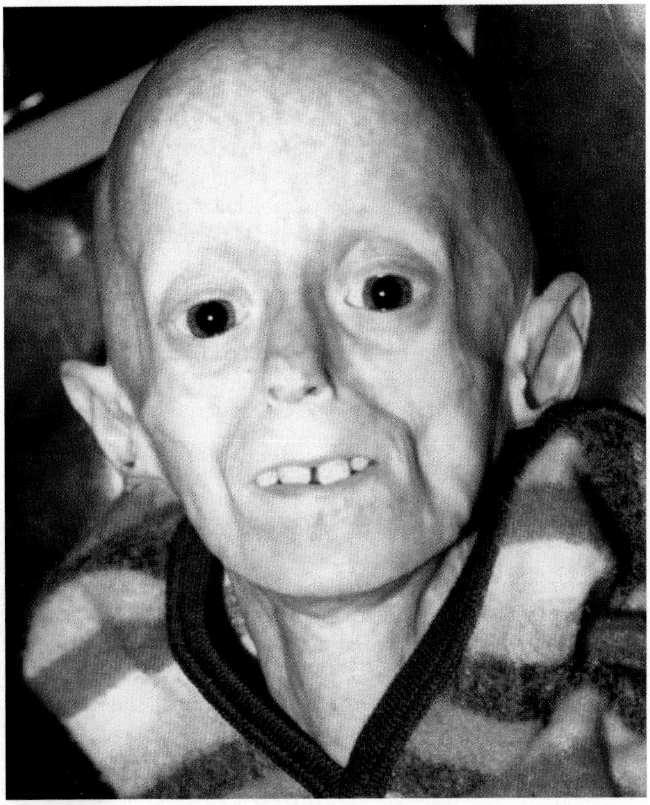

FIGURE 1-38. **Progeria.** A 10-year old girl shows the typical features of premature aging associated with progeria.

integrity of the nucleus and resulting in a lobulated shape. The buildup of progerin also interferes with the organization of nuclear heterochromatin, a component that is thought to regulate the expression of numerous genes. Interestingly, the nuclear changes in cells from patients with progeria were corrected by treating the cells with inhibitors of farnesyltransferase, which prevents progerin from becoming farnesylated. Experimental suppression of the production of progerin has also corrected the nuclear changes in cultured cells from patients with progeria.

Hutchinson-Guilford progeria is now recognized to be one of about 10 disorders associated with mutations in the LMNA gene, comprising a group termed "laminopathies". It is not known whether changes in lamin A contribute to normal aging, but cell nuclei from aged persons have been shown to acquire defects similar to those seen in cells from patients with progeria.

Werner syndrome (WS) is a rare autosomal recessive disease characterized by early cataracts, hair loss, atrophy of the skin, osteoporosis, and atherosclerosis. Affected persons are also at increased risk for the development of a variety of cancers. Patients typically die in the fifth decade from either cancer or cardiovascular disease. This phenotype of patients with WS gives the impression of premature aging. WS is caused by loss of function of the Werner (WRN) gene, which codes for a protein with multiple DNA-dependent enzymatic activities, including ATPase, helicase, exonuclease, and strand annealing. There is experimental evidence that WRN plays a role in the resolution of replication blockage and in telomere maintenance. Its loss leads to defective processing of DNA damage and replication. Experimentally, epigenetic inactivation of WRN by transcriptional silencing associated with promoter hypermethylation results in chromosomal instability and increased apoptosis. It is thought that the increased incidence of cancer in WS may reflect chromosomal changes, whereas accelerated aging probably reflects telomere dysfunction.

Aging May Reflect Accumulated Somatic Damage

Oxidative stress is an invariable consequence of life in an atmosphere rich in oxygen. An important hypothesis holds that the loss of function that is characteristic of aging is caused by progressive and irreversible accrual of molecular oxidative damage. Such lesions would be manifested as (1) peroxidation of membrane lipids, (2) DNA modifications (strand breaks, base alterations, DNA–protein cross-linking), and (3) protein oxidation (loss of sulfhydryl groups, carbonylation). Oxidative stress in normal cells is hardly trivial, since up to 3% of total oxygen consumption generates superoxide anions and hydrogen peroxide. It has been estimated that a single cell undergoes some 100,000 attacks on DNA a day by oxygen free radicals and that at any one time 10% of protein molecules are modified by carbonyl adducts. Thus, antioxidant defenses are not fully efficient and progressive oxidative damage to the cell may be responsible, at least in part, for the aging process.

The rate of generation of ROS correlates with an organism's overall metabolic rate. The theory that aging is related to oxidative stress is based on several observations: (1) larger animals usually live longer than smaller ones, (2) metabolic rate is inversely related to body size (the larger the animal, the lower the metabolic rate), and (3) generation of activated oxygen species correlates inversely with body size.

The role of oxidative stress in aging has been emphasized by experiments in *Drosophila* in which overexpression of genes for SOD or catalase significantly prolongs the fly's life span. Furthermore, as discussed above, virtually all long-lived worms and flies display increased antioxidant defenses. SOD activity in livers of different primates has also been reported to be proportional to maximal life span. The correlation of oxidative damage with aging is further exemplified by the demonstration of increased oxidative damage to lipids, proteins, and DNA in aged animals.

Additional evidence for progressive oxidative damage with aging is the deposition of aggregated proteins and lipofuscin pigment, principally in postmitotic cells of organs such as the brain, heart, and liver (see above). The emerging appreciation of the role of protein and lipid oxidation to the formation of such aggregates and the potential impairment of cell function that results highlight the role of oxidative damage in the decline of cell activities that accompanies aging.

Oxidative damage to mitochondria has also been proposed to play a major role in aging. Aerobic respiration in mitochondria is the richest source of ROS in the cell. Mitochondrial DNA is extremely sensitive to hydroxyl radical damage and progressively develops more than 100 different DNA deletions over the course of a human life. In turn, these DNA defects may lead to further increases in the mitochondrial generation of toxic oxygen species, thereby establishing a vicious circle.

There is increasing evidence that molecular chaperones (see above) decline both in activity and concentration with age, for unknown reasons. Since chaperones such as hsp70 are important in targeting misfolded proteins, loss of chaperone function affects many aspects of organ function and cell repair. Hsp70 influences several facets of the immune response, such as cytokine production and antigen presentation. There are, further, data suggesting that allelic polymorphisms of hsp70 genes may influence longevity in humans. For example, people in whom the amino acid at position #493 in the protein-binding region of HSP70-HOM protein is methionine have been reported to live longer on the average than those in whom this amino acid is threonine. The potential involvement of molecular chaperone function in aging is an active area of investigation.

Caloric restriction in rodents and lower species has long been known to increase longevity. However alluring it may be to extrapolate from lower species to humans, current mathematical models suggest that human life span may not be greatly increased by such severe caloric restriction. There is evidence to indicate that extension of rodent life span by caloric restriction is associated with a hypometabolic state, analogous to the effect of the "clock" mutations in *C. elegans*. Animals subjected to caloric restriction show attenuation of age-related increases in rates of mitochondrial generation of ROS, slower accrual of oxidative damage, and decreased evidence of lipid peroxidation and oxidative alterations of proteins.

Summary Hypothesis of Aging

After the reproductive period, evolution loses interest in an individual and abandons the organism to events against which nature confers no protection. As reviewed above, the doctrine of antagonistic pleiotropy posits the existence of genes that are beneficial during development and the reproductive period but exert baleful influences later in life. The alternative hypothesis of mutation accumulation holds that the evolutionary suppression of genes that are harmful to young individuals of a species creates pressure favoring alleles that defer the attainment of a deleterious phenotype until the postreproductive period. Finally, the major non-

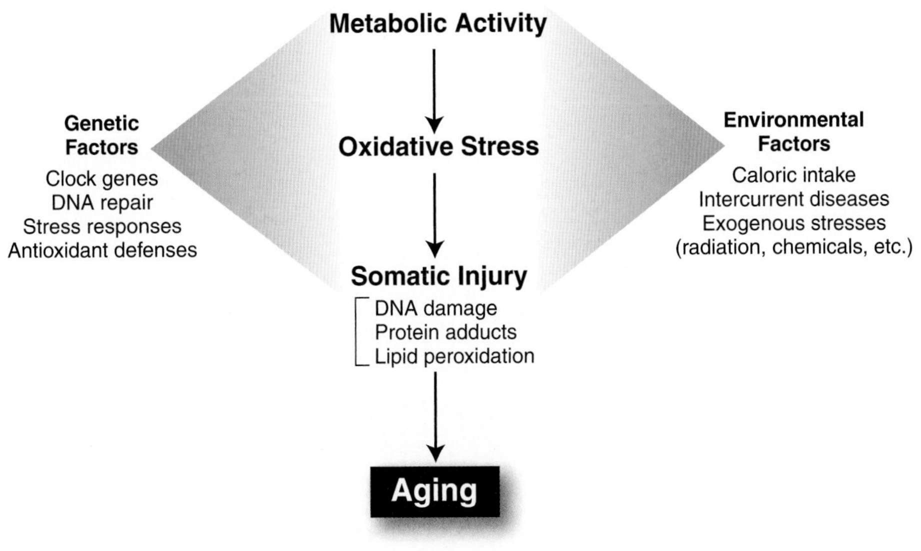

FIGURE 1-39. **Factors that influence the development of biological aging.**

genetic theories postulate that simple accumulation of various cell injuries eventuates in senescence. Current evidence supports the notion that these hypotheses are not mutually contradictory and that all may contribute to aging (Fig. 1-39). *According to this concept, although aging is under some measure of genetic control, it is unlikely that a predetermined genetic program for aging exists.* It is likely that the combined effects of a number of genes eventually lead to the accumulation of somatic mutations, deficiencies in DNA repair, the accretion of oxidative damage to macromolecules, and a variety of other defects in cell function, all culminating in the progressive failure of homeostatic mechanisms characteristic of aging. As Maimonides said, "The same forces that operate in the birth and temporal existence of man also operate in his destruction and death."

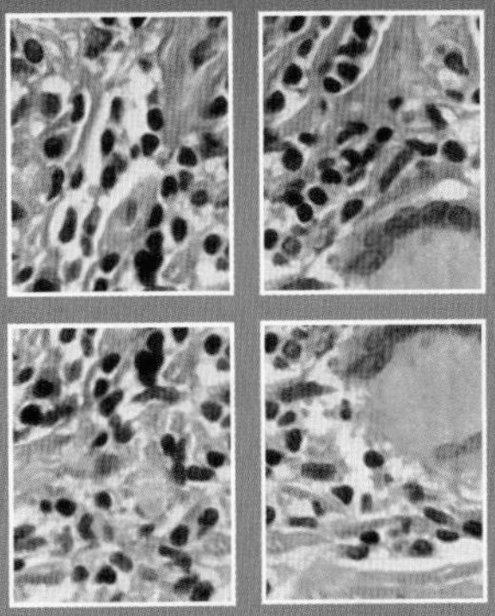

2

Inflammation

Hedwig S. Murphy

Inflammation is the reaction of a tissue and its microcirculation to a pathogenic insult. It is characterized by elaboration of inflammatory mediators and movement of fluid and leukocytes from the blood into extravascular tissues. This response localizes and eliminates altered cells, foreign particles, microorganisms, and antigens and paves the way for the return to normal structure and function.

The clinical signs of inflammation, termed *phlogosis* by the Greeks and *inflammation* in Latin, were described in classical times. In the second century AD, the Roman encyclopedist Aulus Celsus described the four cardinal signs of inflammation, namely, **rubor** (redness), **calor** (heat), **tumor** (swelling), and **dolor** (pain). These features correspond to inflammatory events of vasodilation, edema, and tissue damage. According to medieval concepts, inflammation represented an imbalance of various "humors," including blood, mucus, and bile. Modern appreciation of the vascular basis of inflammation began in the 18th century with John Hunter, who noted dilation of blood vessels and appreciated that pus was accumulated material derived from the blood. Rudolf Virchow first described inflammation as a reaction to prior tissue injury. To the four cardinal signs he added a fifth: **functio laesa** (loss of function). Virchow's pupil Julius Cohnheim was the first to associate inflammation with emigration of leukocytes through the walls of the microvasculature. At the end of the 19th century, the role of phagocytosis in inflammation was emphasized by the eminent Russian zoologist Eli Metchnikoff. Finally, the importance of chemical mediators was described in 1927 by Thomas Lewis, who showed that histamine and other substances increased vascular permeability and caused migration of leukocytes into extravascular spaces. More recent studies have elucidated the molecular and genetic bases of acute and chronic inflammation.

Overview of inflammation

The primary function of the inflammatory response is to eliminate a pathogenic insult and remove injured tissue components, thereby allowing tissue repair to take place. The body attempts to contain

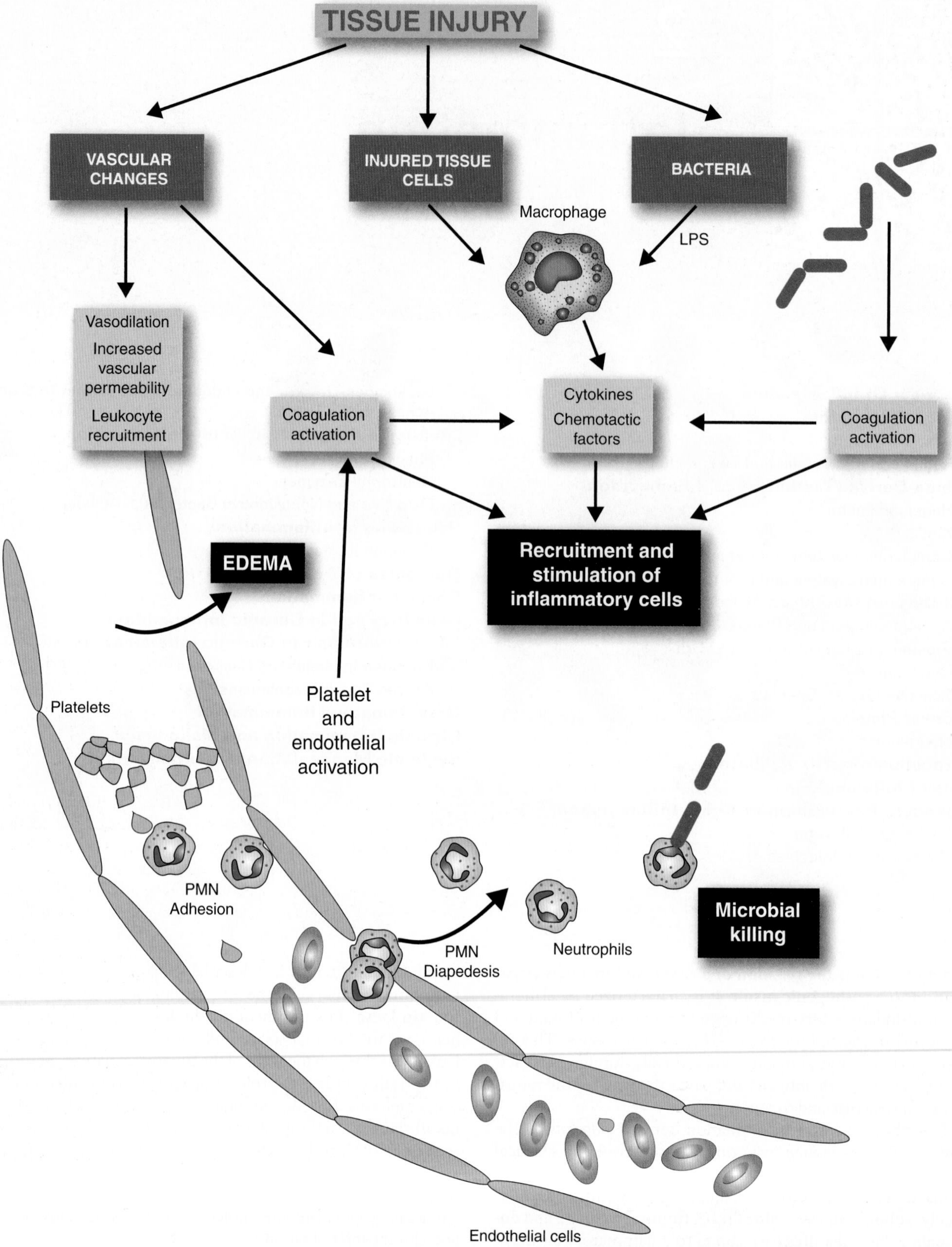

FIGURE 2-1. **The inflammatory response to injury.** Chemical mediators and cells are released from plasma following tissue injury. Vasodilation and vascular injury lead to leakage of fluid into tissues (edema). Platelets are activated to initiate clot formation and hemostasis, and to increase vascular permeability via histamine release. Vascular endothelial cells contribute to clot formation, retract to allow increased vascular permeability, and anchor circulating neutrophils via their adhesion molecules. Microbes initiate activation of the complement cascade, which, along with soluble mediators from macrophages, recruit neutrophils to the site of tissue injury. Neutrophils eliminate microbes and remove damaged tissue so that repair can begin. PMN = polymorphonuclear neutrophil.

or eliminate offending agents, thereby protecting tissues, organs, and ultimately the whole body from damage. Specific cells are imported to attack and destroy injurious agents (e.g., infectious organisms, toxins, or foreign material), enzymatically digest and remove them, or wall them off. During this process, damaged cells and tissues are digested and removed to allow repair to take place. The response to many damaging agents is immediate and stereotypic. The character of the inflammatory response is "modulated" depending upon several factors, including the nature of the offending agent, duration of the insult, extent of tissue damage, and microenvironment.

- **Initiation** of the inflammatory response results in activation of soluble mediators and recruitment of inflammatory cells to the area. Molecules are released from the offending agent, damaged cells, and the extracellular matrix, which alters the permeability of adjacent blood vessels plasma, soluble molecules, and circulating inflammatory cells. This stereotypic, immediate response leads to rapid flooding of the injured tissue with fluid, coagulation factors, cytokines, chemokines, platelets, and inflammatory cells, neutrophils in particular (Figs.2-1 and 2-2). This overall process is termed **acute inflammation.**
- **Amplification** depends upon the extent of injury and activation of mediators such as kinins and complement components. Additional leukocytes and macrophages are recruited to the area.
- **Destruction** of the damaging agent brings the process under control. Enzymatic digestion and phagocytosis reduce or eliminate foreign material or infectious organisms. At the same time, damaged tissue components are also removed, and debris is cleared away, paving the way for repair to begin (see Chapter 3).
- **Termination** of the inflammatory response is mediated by intrinsic anti-inflammatory mechanisms that limit tissue damage and allow for repair and a return to normal physiological function. Alternatively, depending upon the nature of the injury and the specific inflammatory and repair response, a scar may develop in place of normal tissue. Importantly, intrinsic mechanisms are in place to terminate the inflammatory process; to prevent further influx of fluid, mediators, and inflammatory cells; and to avoid digesting normal cells and tissue.

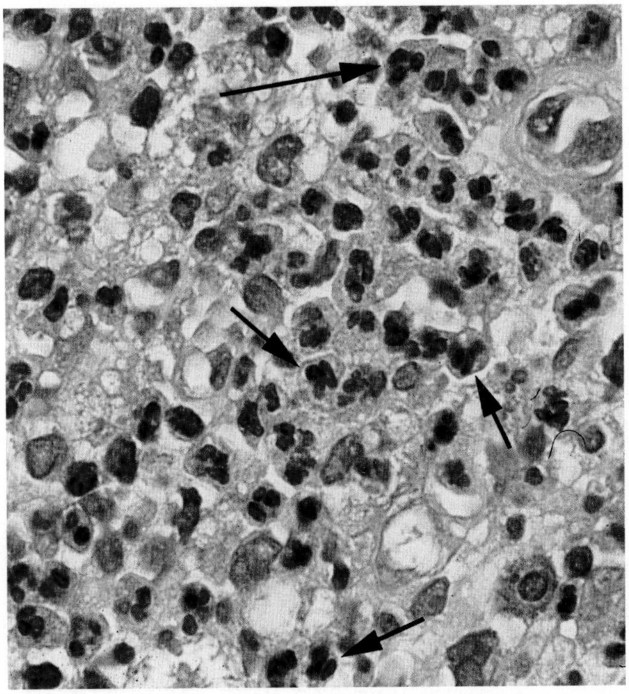

FIGURE 2-2. **Acute inflammation with densely packed polymorphonuclear neutrophils (PMNs) with multilobed nuclei *(arrows).***

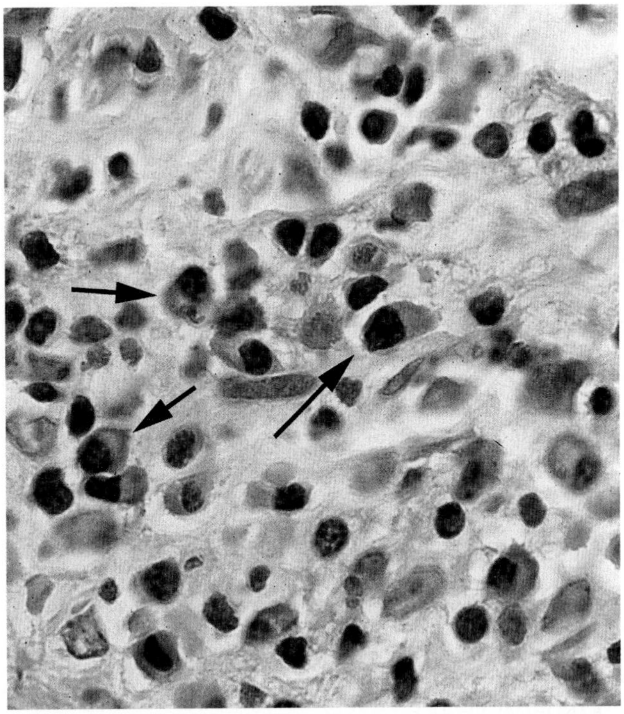

FIGURE 2-3. **Chronic inflammation.** Lymphocytes, plasma cells *(arrows),* and a few macrophages are present.

Certain types of injury trigger a sustained immune and inflammatory response with the inability to clear injured tissue and foreign agents. Such a persistent response is termed **chronic inflammation.** Chronic inflammatory infiltrates are composed largely of lymphocytes, plasma cells, and macrophages (Fig. 2-3). Acute and chronic inflammatory infiltrates often coexist.

Although inflammation usually works to defend the body, inflammation may also be harmful. Acute inflammatory responses may be exaggerated or sustained, with or without clearance of the offending agent. Tissue damage may result: witness the ravages of bacterial pneumonia owing to acute inflammation or joint destruction in septic arthritis. Chronic inflammation may also damage tissue and lead to scarring and loss of function. Indeed, chronic inflammation is the basis for many degenerative diseases.

Impaired inflammatory responses may lead to uncontrolled infection, as in immunocompromised hosts. Several congenital diseases are characterized by deficient inflammatory responses due to defects in inflammatory cell function or immunity.

Acute Inflammation

The acute inflammatory response begins with direct injury or stimulation of cellular or structural components of a tissue, including:

- Parenchymal cells
- Microvasculature

- Tissue macrophages and mast cells
- Mesenchymal cells (e.g., fibroblasts)
- Extracellular matrix (ECM)

Vascular Events After Initiation

A sequence of events occurs following initiation of acute inflammation:

- **Increased vascular permeability leads to accumulation of fluid and plasma components in tissues affected by inflammation.** Fluid exchange occurs normally between intravascular and extravascular spaces, with the endothelium forming a permeability barrier. Endothelial cells are connected to each other by tight junctions and separated from the tissue by a limiting basement membrane (Fig. 2-4). *Disruption of this barrier function is a hallmark of acute inflammation.* One of the earliest responses to tissue injury occurs at the level of capillaries and postcapillary venules. Specific inflammatory mediators are produced at the site of injury and act directly upon blood vessels to increase vascular permeability. Vascular leakage is caused by endothelial cell contraction, endothelial cell retraction, and alterations in transcytosis. Endothelial cells are also damaged, either directly by endothelial injury or indirectly by leukocyte-mediated damage. The loss of the permeability barrier may be extensive and leakage of fluid and cells into the extravascular space, termed **edema** (see Fig. 2-4).
- **Intravascular stimulation of platelets and inflammatory cells, and release of soluble mediators.** Specific inflammatory mediators produced at sites of injury activate platelets and intravascular inflammatory cells. Kinins, complement, and components of the coagulation cascade are activated (see Fig. 2-1 and Fig 2-5), further increasing vascular permeability and edema.
- **Recruitment of neutrophils to the injured site.** Chemotactic factors then recruit leukocytes, especially neutrophils, from the vascular compartment into the injured tissue (see Figs. 2-1 and 2-2). Once present in tissues, recruited leukocytes initiate the process of eliminating the offending agents so damaged components can be removed and tissue repair can commence. These cells secrete additional mediators, which either enhance or inhibit the inflammatory response.

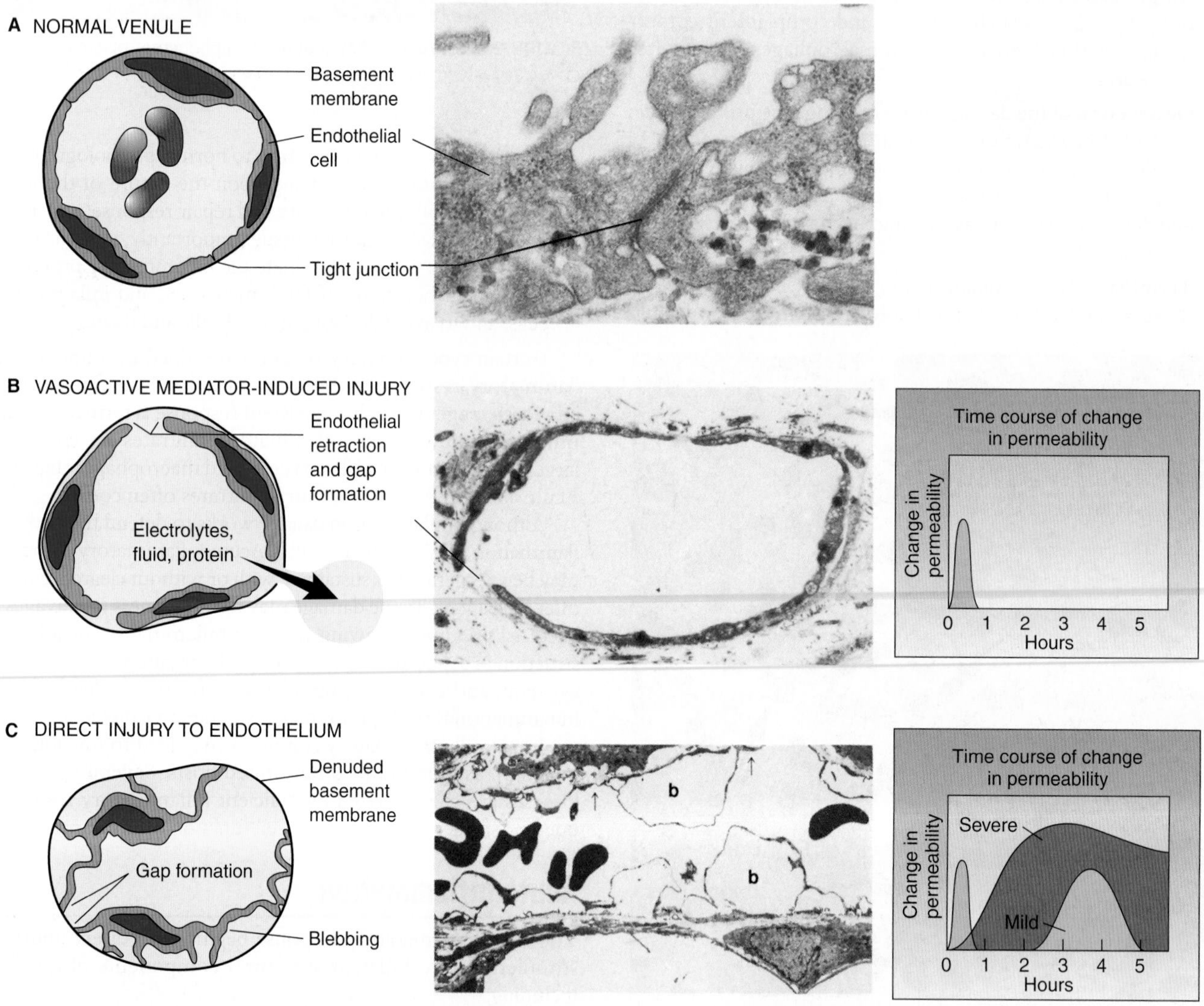

FIGURE 2-4. **Responses of the microvasculature to injury. A.** The wall of the normal venule is sealed by tight junctions between adjacent endothelial cells. **B.** During mild vasoactive mediator-induced injury, the endothelial cells separate and permit the passage of the fluid constituents of the blood. **C.** With severe direct injury, the endothelial cells form blebs *(b)* and separate from the underlying basement membrane. Areas of denuded basement membrane *(arrows)* allow a prolonged escape of fluid elements from the microvasculature.

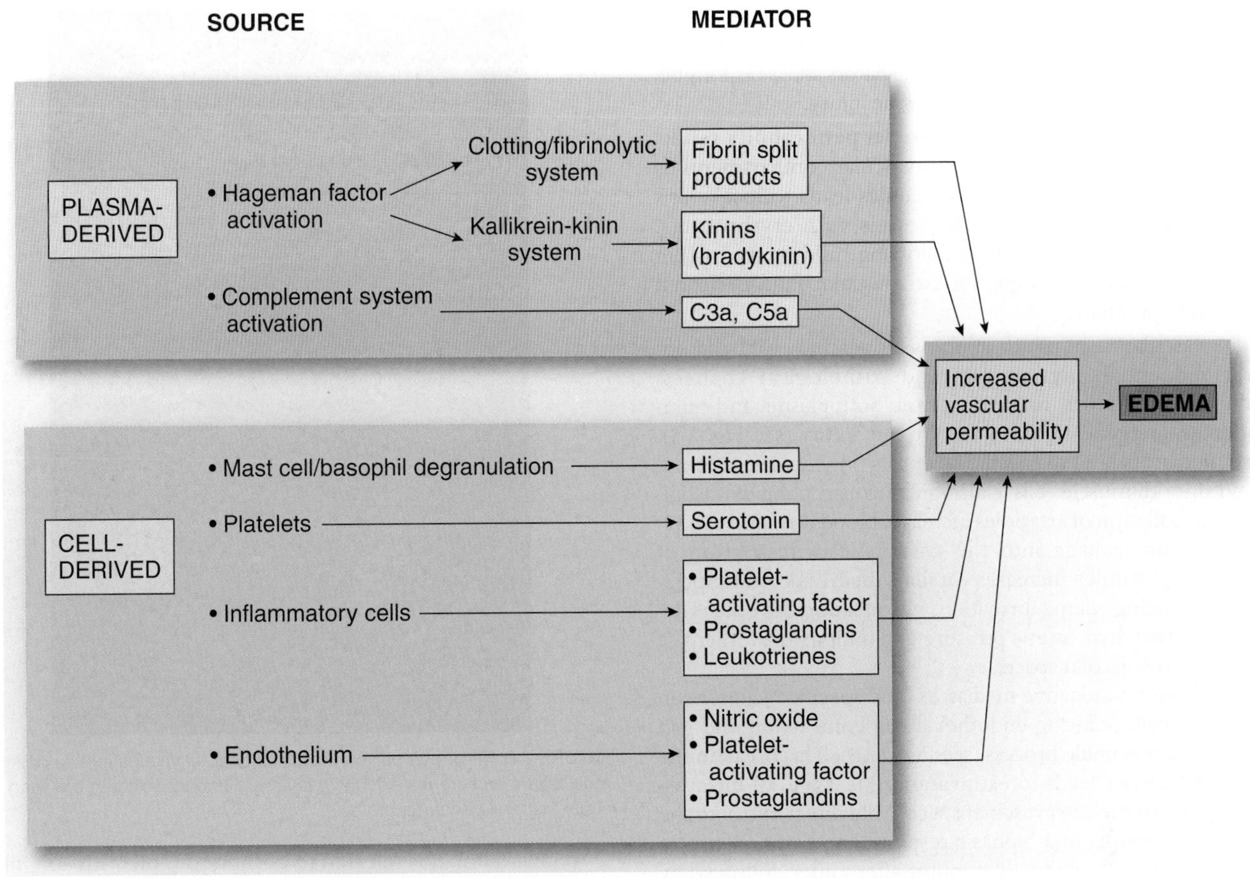

FIGURE 2-5. **Inflammatory mediators of increased vascular permeability.**

Vascular and Tissue Fluids Are Regulated by a Balance of Forces

Under normal circumstances, there is continual movement of fluid from the intravascular compartment to the extravascular space. Fluid that accumulates in the extravascular space is then cleared through lymphatics and returned to the circulation. Regulation of fluid transport across vascular walls is described in part by the **Starling principle**. According to this law, interchange of fluid between vascular and extravascular compartments results from a balance of forces that draw fluid into the vascular space or out into tissues (see also Chapter 7). These forces include:

- **Hydrostatic pressure** results from blood flow and plasma volume. When increased, hydrostatic pressure forces fluid out of the vasculature.
- **Oncotic pressure** reflects the plasma protein concentration, and draws fluid into vessels.
- **Osmotic pressure** is determined by relative amounts of sodium and water in vascular and tissue spaces.
- **Lymph flow**, the passage of fluid through the lymphatic system, continuously drains fluid out of tissues and into lymphatic spaces.

Noninflammatory Edema

When the balance of forces that regulate fluid transport is altered, flow into the extravascular compartment or clearance through lymphatics is disrupted. The net result is fluid accumulation in the interstitial spaces (**edema**). This excess fluid expands the spaces between cells and ECM elements, and leads to tissue swelling. A range of clinical conditions, either systemic or organ specific, are associated with edema. Obstruction of venous outflow (**thrombosis**) or decreased right ventricular function (congestive heart failure) cause back pressure in the vasculature, thereby increasing hydrostatic pressure (see Chapter 7). Loss of albumin (kidney disorders) or decreased synthesis of plasma proteins (liver disease, malnutrition) reduce plasma oncotic pressure. Any abnormality of sodium or water retention will alter the osmotic pressure and the balance of fluid forces. Finally, obstruction of lymphatic flow may occur in various clinical settings but is most commonly due to surgical removal of lymph nodes or tumor obstruction. This fluid accumulation is referred to as **lymphedema**.

Inflammatory Edema

Among the earliest responses to tissue injury are alterations in the anatomy and function of the microvasculature, which may promote fluid accumulation in tissues (see Figs. 2-4 and 2-5). These pathological changes are characteristic of the classic "triple response" first described by Sir Thomas Lewis in 1924. In the original experiments a dull red line developed at the site of mild trauma to skin, followed by a **flare** (red halo), then a **wheal** (swelling). Lewis postulated the presence of a vasoactive mediator that caused vasodilation and increased vascular permeability at the site of injury. The triple response can be explained as follows:

1. **Transient vasoconstriction of arterioles** at the site of injury is the earliest vascular response to mild skin injury. This process is mediated by both neurogenic and chemical mediator systems and usually resolves within seconds to minutes.

2. **Vasodilation of precapillary arterioles** then increases blood flow to the tissue, a condition known as **hyperemia**. Vasodilation is caused by release of specific mediators and is responsible for redness and warmth at sites of tissue injury.
3. **An increase in endothelial cell barrier permeability** results in edema. Loss of fluid from intravascular compartments as blood passes through capillary venules leads to local stasis and plugging of dilated small vessels with erythrocytes. These changes are reversible following mild injury: within several minutes to hours, the extravascular fluid is cleared through lymphatics.

The vascular response to injury is a dynamic event that involves sequential physiological and pathological changes. **Vasoactive mediators,** originating from both plasma and cellular sources, are generated at sites of tissue injury (see Fig. 2-5). These mediators bind to specific receptors on vascular endothelial and smooth muscle cells, causing vasoconstriction or vasodilation. Vasodilation of arterioles increases blood flow and can exacerbate fluid leakage into the tissue. Vasoconstriction of postcapillary venules increases capillary bed hydrostatic pressure, potentiating edema formation. Vasodilation of venules decreases capillary hydrostatic pressure and inhibits movement of fluid into extravascular spaces.

After injury, vasoactive mediators bind specific receptors on endothelial cells, causing endothelial cell contraction and gap formation, a reversible process (see Fig. 2-4B). This break in the endothelial barrier leads to extravasation (leakage) of intravascular fluids into the extravascular space. Mild direct injury to the endothelium results in a biphasic response: an early change in permeability occurs within 30 minutes after injury, followed by a second increase in vascular permeability after 3 to 5 hours. When damage is severe, exudation of intravascular fluid into the extravascular compartment increases progressively peaking 3 to 4 hours after injury.

Severe direct injury to the endothelium, such as is caused by burns or caustic chemicals, may result in irreversible damage. In such cases, the endothelium separates from the basement membrane, resulting in cell blebbing (blisters or bubbles between the endothelium and the basement membrane). This leaves areas of basement membrane naked (see Fig. 2-4C), disrupting the barrier between the intravascular and extravascular spaces.

Several definitions are important for understanding the consequences of inflammation:

- **Edema** is accumulation of fluid within the extravascular compartment and interstitial tissues.
- An **effusion** is excess fluid in body cavities, e.g., peritoneum or pleura.
- A **transudate** is edema fluid with low protein content (specific gravity < 1.015).
- An **exudate** is edema fluid with a high protein concentration (specific gravity > 1.015), which frequently contains inflammatory cells. Exudates are observed early in acute inflammatory reactions and are produced by mild injuries, such as sunburn or traumatic blisters.
- A **serous exudate,** or **effusion,** is characterized by the absence of a prominent cellular response and has a yellow, straw-like color.
- **Serosanguineous** refers to a serous exudate, or effusion, that contains red blood cells and has a red tinge.
- A **fibrinous exudate** contains large amounts of fibrin as a result of activation of the coagulation system. When a fibrinous exudate occurs on a serosal surface, such as the pleura or pericardium, it is referred to as "fibrinous pleuritis" or "fibrinous pericarditis" (Fig. 2-6).

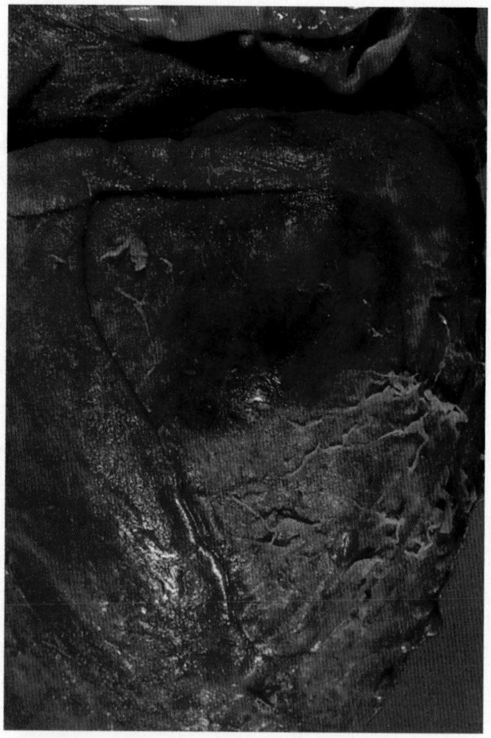

FIGURE 2-6. **Fibrinous pericarditis.** The heart from a patient who died in renal failure and uremia exhibits a shaggy, fibrinous exudate covering the entire visceral pericardium.

- **A purulent exudate or effusion** is one that contains prominent cellular components. Purulent exudates and effusions are frequently associated with pathological conditions such as pyogenic bacterial infections, in which the predominant cell type is the polymorphonuclear neutrophil (PMN) (Fig. 2-7).
- **Suppurative inflammation** describes a condition in which a purulent exudate is accompanied by significant liquefactive necrosis; it is the equivalent of pus.

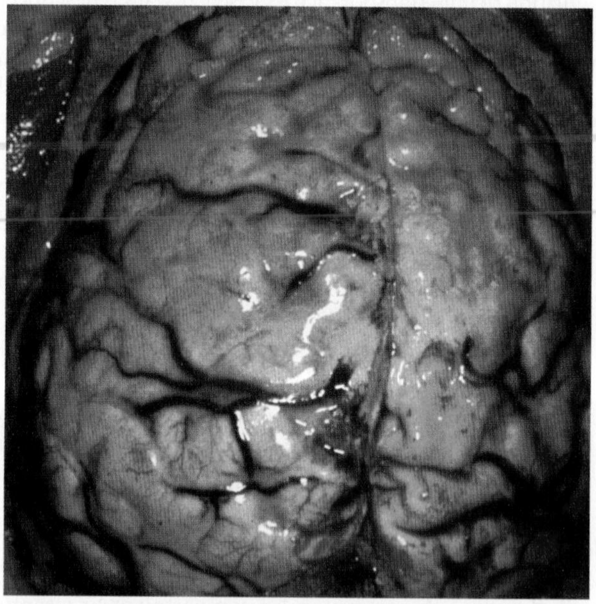

FIGURE 2-7. **Purulent exudate.** In this patient with bacterial meningitis, a viscid, cream-colored, acute inflammatory exudate is present within the subarachnoid space.

Plasma-Derived Mediators Of Inflammation

A large number of chemical mediators are integral to initiation, amplification and termination of inflammatory processes (Fig. 2-8). Cell- and plasma-derived mediators work in concert to activate cells by binding specific receptors, activating cells, recruiting cells to sites of injury, and stimulating of release of additional soluble mediators. These mediators themselves are relatively short-lived, or are inhibited by intrinsic mechanisms, effectively turning off the response and allowing the process to resolve. These are thus important "on" and "off" control mechanisms of inflammation. Cell-derived mediators are considered below.

Plasma contains the elements of three major enzyme cascades, each composed of a series of proteases. Sequential activation of proteases results in release of important chemical mediators. These interrelated systems include (1) the **coagulation cascade**, (2) **kinin generation**, and (3) the **complement system** (Fig. 2-9). The coagulation cascade is discussed in Chapters 10 and 20; the kinin and complement systems are presented here.

Hageman Factor is a Key Source of Vasoactive Mediators

Hageman factor (clotting factor XII), generated within the plasma, is activated by exposure to negatively charged surfaces such as basement membranes, proteolytic enzymes, bacterial lipopolysaccharide, and foreign materials. This key component triggers activation of additional plasma proteases leading to:

- **Conversion of plasminogen to plasmin:** Plasmin generated by activated Hageman factor induces fibrinolysis. Products of fibrin degradation (fibrin-split products) augment vascular permeability in the skin and the lung. Plasmin also cleaves components of the complement system, generating biologically active products, including the anaphylatoxins C3a and C5a.
- **Conversion of prekallikrein to kallikrein:** Plasma kallikrein, also generated by activated Hageman factor, cleaves high-molecular-weight kininogen, thereby producing several vasoactive low molecular weight peptides, collectively termed **kinins**.
- **Activation of the alternative complement pathway.**
- **Activation of the coagulation system** (see Chapters 10 and 20).

Kinins Amplify the Inflammatory Response

Kinins are potent inflammatory agents formed in plasma and tissue by the action of serine protease kallikreins on specific plasma glycoproteins termed **kininogens**. **Bradykinin** and related peptides regulate multiple physiological processes including blood pressure, contraction and relaxation of smooth muscle, plasma

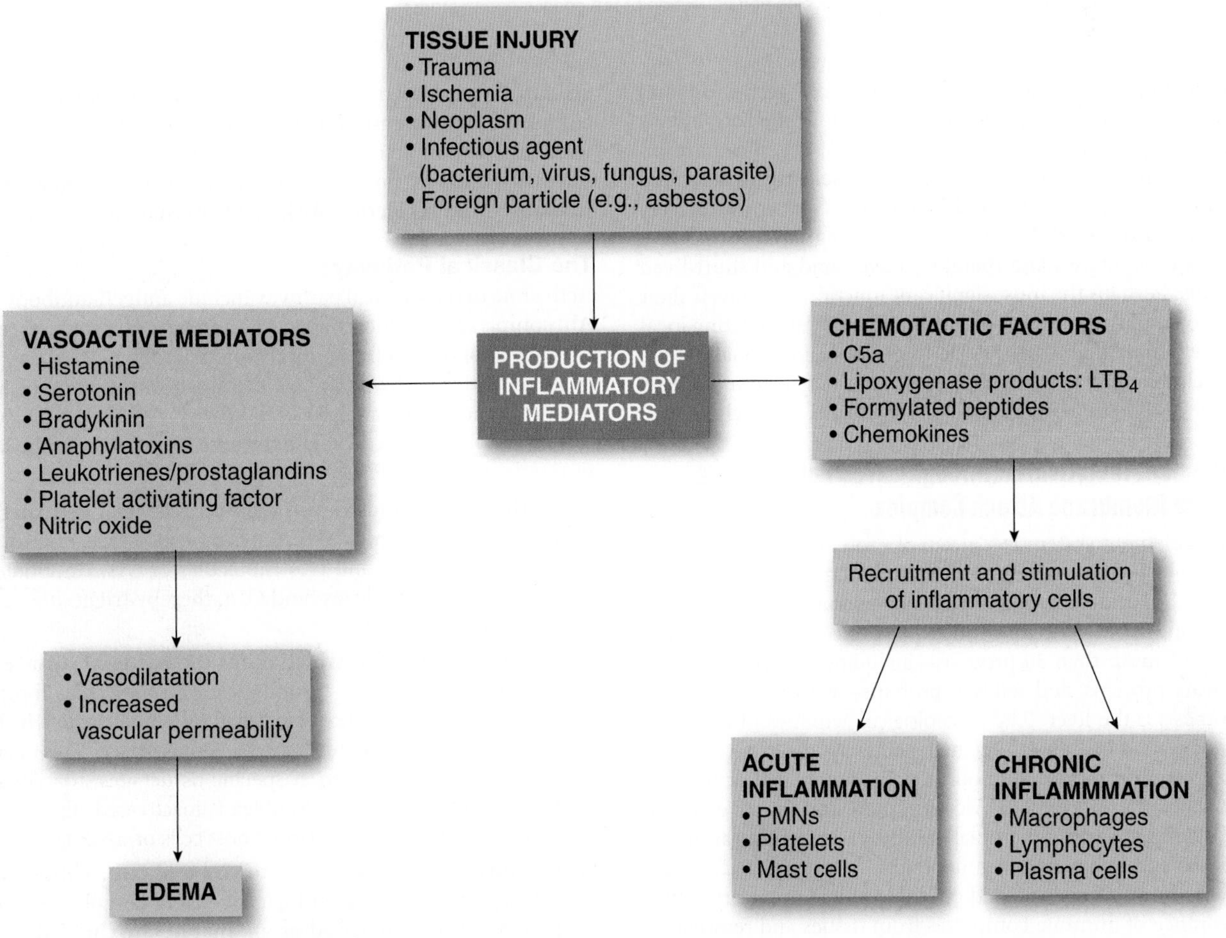

FIGURE 2-8. **Mediators of the inflammatory response.** Tissue injury stimulates the production of inflammatory mediators in plasma and released in the circulation. Additional factors are generated by tissue cells and inflammatory cells. These vasoactive and chemotactic mediators promote edema and recruit inflammatory cells to the site of injury. PMNs = polymorphonuclear neutrophils.

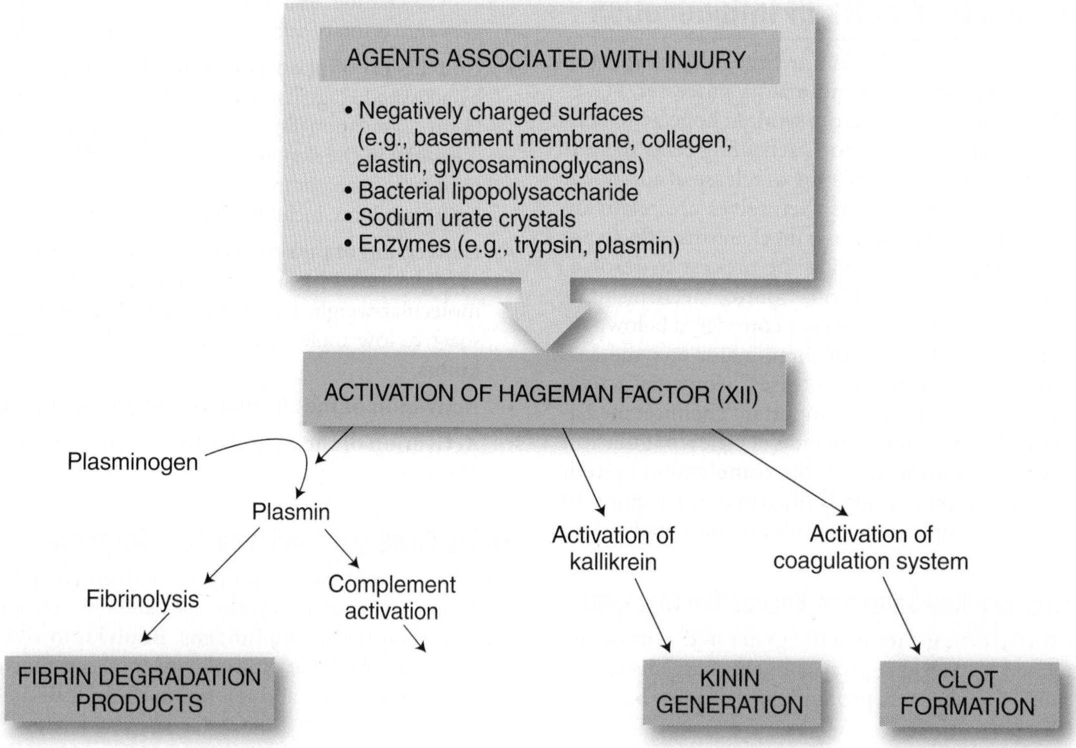

FIGURE 2-9. **Hageman factor activation and inflammatory mediator production.** Hageman factor activation is a key event leading to conversion of plasminogen to plasmin, resulting in generation of fibrin split products and active complement products. Activation of kallikrein produces kinins and activation of the coagulation system results in clot formation.

extravasation, cell migration, inflammatory cell activation, and inflammatory-mediated pain responses. The immediate effects of kinins are mediated by two receptors: B_1 receptors are induced by inflammatory mediators and are selectively activated by bradykinin metabolites, and B_2 receptors are constitutively and widely expressed. Kinins are rapidly degraded to inactive products by kininases and therefore have rapid and short-lived functions. Perhaps the most significant function of kinins is their ability to amplify the inflammatory response by stimulating local tissue cells and inflammatory cells to generate additional mediators, including prostanoids, cytokines (especially tumor necrosis factor-α [TNF-α] and interleukins), nitric oxide, and tachykinins.

Complement Is Activated through Three Pathways To Form The Membrane Attack Complex

The complement system is a group of proteins found in plasma and on cell surfaces, whose primary function is defense against microbes. First identified as a heat-labile serum factor that kills bacteria and "complements" antibodies, the complement system consists of more than 30 proteins—including plasma enzymes, regulatory proteins, and cell lysis proteins—whose principal site of synthesis is the liver. The physiological activities of the complement system include (1) defense against pyogenic bacterial infection by opsonization, chemotaxis, activation of leukocytes and lysis of bacteria and cells; (2) bridging innate and adaptive immunity for defense against microbial agents by augmenting antibody responses and enhancing immunological memory; and (3) disposal of immune products and products of inflammatory injury by clearance of immune complexes from tissues and removal of apoptotic cells. Certain complement components, **anaphylatoxins,** are vasoactive mediators. Other components fix opsonins on cell surfaces and still others induce cell lysis by generating the lytic complex C5b-9 (**membrane attack complex** [**MAC**]). The proteins involved in activating the complement system are themselves activated by three convergent pathways termed **classical, mannose-binding lectin** (**MBL**), and **alternative**.

The Classical Pathway

Activators of the classical pathway include antigen-antibody (Ag-Ab) complexes, products of bacteria and viruses, proteases, urate crystals, apoptotic cells, and polyanions (polynucleotides). The proteins of this pathway are C1 through C9, the nomenclature following the historical order of discovery. Ag-Ab complexes activate C1, initiating a cascade that leads to formation of the MAC proceeds as follows (Fig. 2-10):

1. **Antibodies bound to antigens on bacterial cell surfaces bind the C1 complex.** The C1 complex consists of C1q, two molecules of C1r, and two molecules of C1s. Antibodies in the immune complexes bind C1q, thereby triggering activation of C1r and C1s.
2. **C1s first cleaves C4, which binds the bacterial surface and then cleaves C2.** The resulting cleaved molecules form the C4b2a enzyme complex, also called **C3 convertase,** which remains covalently bound to the bacterial surface. This anchors the complement system at specific tissue sites. If a covalent bond is not formed, the complex is inactivated, aborting the complement cascade in normal host cells or tissues.
3. **C3 convertase cleaves C3 into C3a and C3b.** This is a critical step in generating biologically active complement components. C3a is released as an **anaphylatoxin**. C3b reacts with cell proteins to localize, or "fix" on the cell surface. C3b and its degradation products, especially iC3b, on the surface

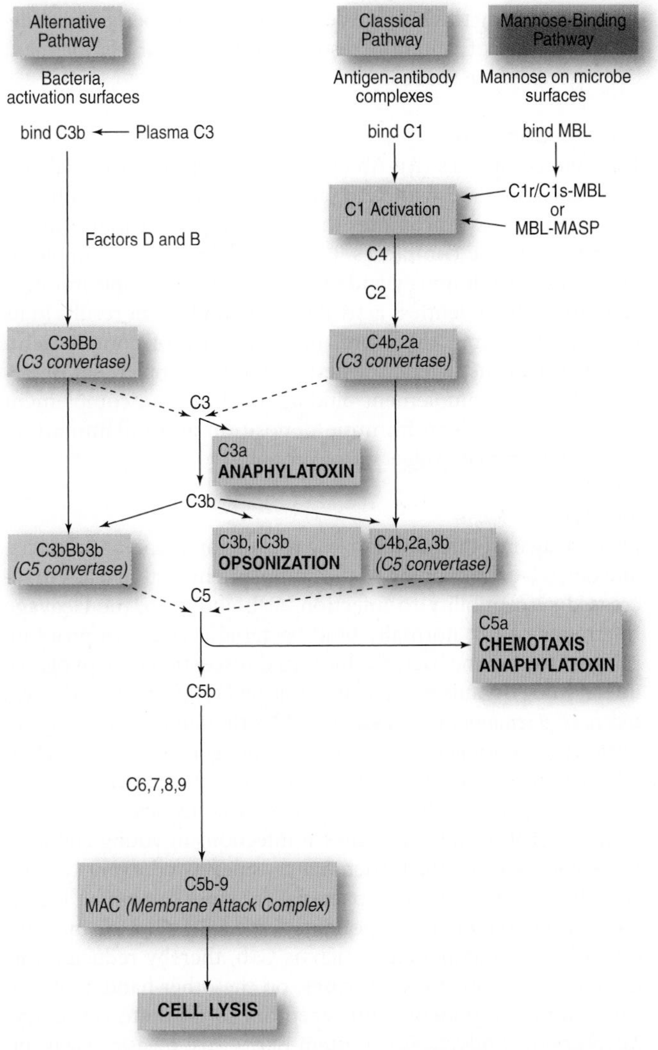

FIGURE 2-10. **Complement activation.** The alternative, classical, and mannose-binding pathways lead to generation of the complement cascade of inflammatory mediators and cell lysis by the membrane attack complex (MAC). MBL = mannose-binding lectin; MBL-MASP = MBL-associated serine protease.

of pathogens, enhance phagocytosis. This process of coating a pathogen with a molecule that enhances phagocytosis is **opsonization**, and the molecule is referred to as an **opsonin**.

4. **The complex of C4b, C2a and C3b (termed C5 convertase) cleaves C5 into C5a and C5b.** C5a also is an anaphylatoxin, and C5b acts as the nidus for the sequential binding of C6, C7, and C8 to form the MAC.
5. **The MAC assembles on target cells**. The MAC directly inserts into the plasma membrane by hydrophobic binding of C7 to the lipid bilayer. The resulting cylindrical transmembrane channel disrupts the barrier function of the plasma membrane and leads to cell lysis.

The Mannose-Binding Pathway

The mannose- or lectin-binding pathway has some components in common with the classical pathway. It is initiated by binding of microbes bearing terminal mannose groups to **MBL**, a member of the family of calcium-dependent lectins, termed the **collectins**. This multifunctional acute phase protein has properties similar to those of immunoglobulin (Ig) M (IgM) antibody (it binds to a wide range of oligosaccharide structures), IgG (it interacts with phagocytic receptors) and C1q. This last property enables it to interact with either C1r-C1s or with a serine protease called MASP (MBL-associated serine protease) to activate complement as follows (see Fig. 2-10):

1. **MBL interacts with C1r and C1s to generate C1 esterase activity.** Alternatively and preferentially, MBL forms a complex with a precursor of the serine protease MASP. MBL and MASP bind to mannose groups on glycoproteins or carbohydrates on bacterial cell surfaces. After MBL binds a substrate, the MASP proenzyme is cleaved into two chains and expresses a C1-esterase activity.
2. **C1-esterase activity, either from C1r/C1s- MBL interaction or MBL-MASP, cleaves C4 and C2, leading to assembly of the classical pathway C3 convertase.** The complement cascade then continues as described for the classical pathway.

Alternative Pathway

The alternative pathway is initiated by derivative products of microorganisms such as endotoxin (from bacterial cell surfaces), zymosan (yeast cell walls), polysaccharides, cobra venom factor, viruses, tumor cells, and foreign materials. Proteins of the alternative pathway are called "factors," followed by a letter. Activation of the alternative pathway proceeds as follows (see Fig. 2-10):

1. **A small amount of C3 in plasma cleaves to C3a and C3b.** This C3b is covalently bound to carbohydrates and proteins on microbial cell surfaces. It binds factor B and factor D to form the alternative pathway C3 convertase, C3bBb. This C3 convertase is stabilized by **properdin**.
2. **C3 convertase generates additional C3b and C3a.** Binding of a second C3b molecule to the C3 convertase converts it to a C5 convertase, C3bBb3b.
3. **As in the classical pathway, cleavage of C5 by C5 convertase generates C5b and C5a and leads to assembly of the MAC.**

The Complement System is Tightly Regulated to Generate Proinflammatory Molecules

Biological Activities of Complement Components

The endpoint of complement activation is formation of the MAC and cell lysis. The cleavage products generated at each step of the way both catalyze the next step in the cascade, and themselves have additional properties that render them important inflammatory molecules:

- **Anaphylatoxins** (C3a, C4a, C5a): These proinflammatory molecules mediate smooth muscle contraction and increase vascular permeability (Fig. 2-11).
- **Opsonins** (C3b, iC3b): Bacterial opsonization is the process by which a specific molecule (e.g., IgG or C3b) binds to the surface of the bacterium. The process enhances phagocytosis by enabling receptors on phagocytic cell membranes (e.g., Fc receptor or C3b receptor) to recognize and bind the opsonized bacterium. Viruses, parasites, and transformed cells also activate complement by similar mechanisms, an effect that leads to their inactivation or death.
- **Proinflammatory molecules** (MAC, C5a): These chemotactic factors also activate leukocytes and tissue cells to generate oxidants and cytokines, induce degranulation of mast cells and basophils.

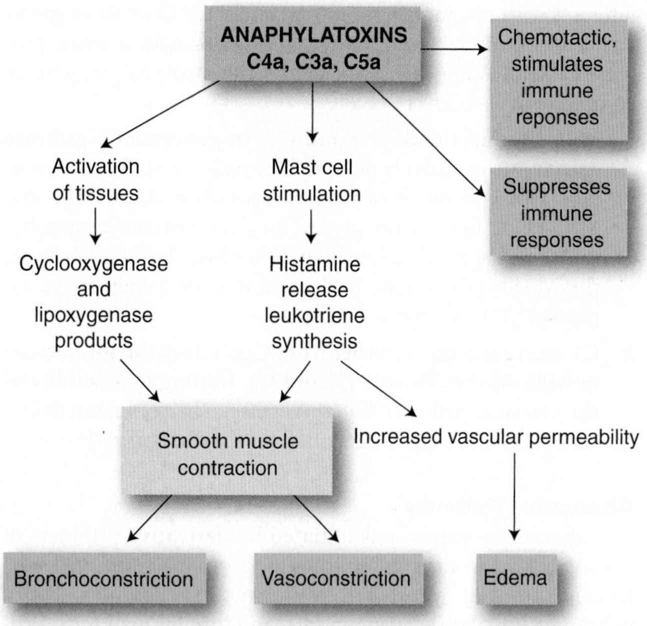

FIGURE 2-11. **Biological activity of the anaphylatoxins.** Complement activation products, generated during activation of the complement cascade, regulate vascular permeability, cell recruitment, and smooth muscle contraction.

- **Lysis (MAC):** C5b binds C6 and C7, and subsequently C8 to the target cell; C9 polymerization is catalyzed to lyse the cell membrane.

Regulation of the Complement System

Proteins in serum and on cell surfaces protect the host from indiscriminate injury by regulating complement activation. There are 4 major mechanisms for this:

- **Spontaneous decay:** C4b2a and C3bBb and their cleavage products, C3b and C4b, decrease by decay.
- **Proteolytic inactivation:** Plasma inhibitors include factor 1 (an inhibitor of C3b and C4b) and serum carboxypeptidase N (SCPN). SCPN cleaves the carboxy-terminal arginine from anaphylatoxins C4a, C3a, and C5a. Removing this single amino acid markedly decreases the biological activity of each of these molecules.
- **Binding of active components:** C1 esterase inhibitor (C1 INA) binds C1r and C1s, forming an irreversibly inactive complex. Additional binding proteins in the plasma include factor H and C4b binding protein. These proteins complex with C3b and C4b, respectively, and enhance their susceptibility to proteolytic cleavage by factor I.
- **Cell membrane-associated molecules:** Two proteins linked to the cell membrane by glycophosphoinositol (GPI) anchors are decay-accelerating factor (DAF) and protectin (CD59). DAF breaks down the alternative pathway C3 convertase, CD59 (membrane cofactor protein, protectin) binds membrane-associated C4b and C3b, promotes its inactivation by factor I and prevents formation of the MAC.

The Complement System and Disease

The complement system is exquisitely regulated so that activation of complement is focused on the surfaces of microorganisms, whereas deposition on normal cells and tissues is limited. When the mechanisms regulating this balance do not function properly, or are deficient because of mutation, resulting imbalances in complement activity can cause tissue injury (Table 2-1).

Immune Complexes

Immune complexes (Ag-Ab complexes) form on bacterial surfaces and associate with C1q, activating the classical pathway. Complement then promotes the physiological clearance of circulating immune complexes. However, when these complexes are formed continuously and in excess (e.g., in chronic immune responses), the relentless activation of complement results in its consumption and, therefore, net depletion of complement. Complement inefficiency, whether due to complement depletion, deficient complement binding, or defects in complement activation, results in immune deposition and inflammation, which in turn may trigger autoimmunity.

Infectious Disease

Defense against infection is a key role of complement products, and defective functioning of the complement system leads to increased susceptibility to infection. C3b and iC3b, the cleavage fragments of C3, normally bind bacterial surfaces to promote phagocytosis of the bacteria. Increased susceptibility to pyogenic infection by organisms such as *Haemophilus influenzae* and *Streptococcus pneumoniae* is associated with defects in antibody production, complement proteins, or phagocyte function. Deficiencies in formation of MAC are associated with increased infections, particularly with meningococci. Deficiency of complement MBL results in recurrent infections in young children. For some bacteria, thick bacterial capsules can prevent lysis by complement. Furthermore bacterial enzymes can inhibit the effects of complement components, especially C5a, or increase catabolism of components, such as C3b, thereby reducing formation of C3 convertase. Viruses, on the other hand, may use cell-bound components and receptors to facilitate cell entry. *Mycobacterium tuberculosis,* Epstein-Barr virus, measles virus, picornaviruses, human immunodeficiency virus (HIV), and flaviviruses use complement components to target inflammatory or epithelial cells.

Inflammation and Necrosis

The complement system amplifies the inflammatory response. Anaphylatoxins C5a and C3a activate leukocytes, and C5a and MAC

TABLE 2-1

Hereditary Complement Deficiencies

Complement Deficiency	Clinical Association
C3b, iC3b, C5, MBL	Pyogenic bacterial infections Membranoproliferative glomerulonephritis
C3, properdin, MAC proteins	Neisserial infection
C1 Inhibitor	Hereditary angioedema
CD59	Hemolysis, thrombosis
C1q, C1r and C1s, C4, C2	Systemic lupus erythematosus
Factor H and Factor I	Hemolytic-uremic syndrome Membranoproliferative glomerulonephritis

MAC = membrane attack complex; MBL = mannose-binding lectin.

activate endothelial cells, inducing generation of oxidants and cytokines that are harmful to tissues when in excess (see Chapter 1). Nonviable or injured tissues cannot regulate complement normally.

Complement Deficiencies

The importance of an intact and appropriately regulated complement system is exemplified in persons who have acquired or congenital deficiencies of specific complement components or regulatory proteins (see Table 2-1). The most common congenital defect is a C2 deficiency, inherited as an autosomal codominant trait. Acquired deficiencies of early complement components occur in patients with some autoimmune diseases, especially those associated with circulating immune complexes. These include certain forms of membranous glomerulonephritis and systemic lupus erythematosus. Deficiencies in early components of complement, e.g., C1q, C1r, C1s, and C4, are strongly associated with susceptibility to systemic lupus erythematosus; patients lacking the middle (C3, C5) components are prone to recurrent pyogenic infections, membranoproliferative glomerulonephritis and rashes; those who lack terminal complement components (C6, C7, or C8) are vulnerable to infections with *Neisseria* species. Such differences in susceptibility further emphasize the importance of individual complement components in host surveillance against bacterial infection. Congenital defects in proteins that regulate the complement system, e.g., C1 inhibitor and SCPN, result in chronic complement activation. C1 inhibitor deficiency is also associated with the syndrome of hereditary angioedema.

Cell-Derived Mediators of Inflammation

Circulating platelets, basophils, PMNs, endothelial cells monocyte/macrophages, tissue mast cells, and the injured tissue itself are all potential cellular sources of vasoactive mediators. In general, these mediators are (1) derived from metabolism of phospholipids and arachidonic acid (e.g., prostaglandins, thromboxanes, leukotrienes, lipoxins, platelet-activating factor [PAF]), (2) preformed and stored in cytoplasmic granules (e.g., histamine, serotonin, lysosomal hydrolases), or (3) derived from altered production of normal regulators of vascular function (e.g., nitric oxide and neurokinins).

Arachidonic Acid and Platelet-Activating Factor Are Derived from Membrane Phospholipids

Phospholipids and fatty acid derivatives released from plasma membranes are metabolized into mediators and homeostatic regulators by inflammatory cells and injured tissues (Fig. 2-12). As part of a complex regulatory network, prostanoids, leukotrienes, and lipoxins, which are derivatives of arachidonic acid, both promote and inhibit inflammation (Table 2-2). The impact depends on several factors, including the level and profile of prostanoid production, both of which change during an inflammatory response.

Arachidonic Acid

Depending on the specific inflammatory cell and the nature of the stimulus, activated cells generate arachidonic acid by one of two pathways (see Fig 2-12). One pathway involves liberation of arachidonic acid from the glycerol backbone of cell membrane phospholipids (in particular, phosphatidylcholine) by stimulus-

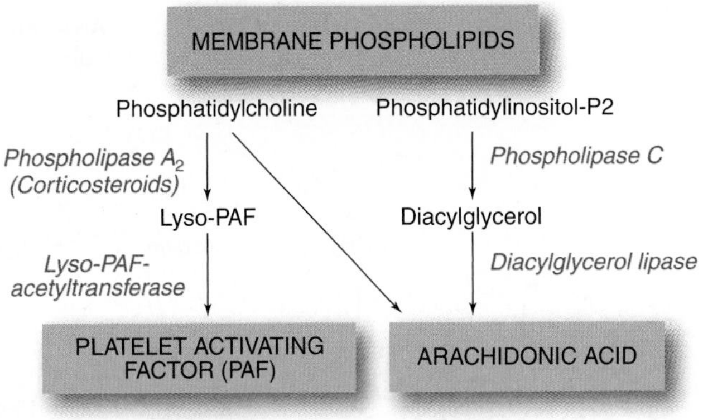

FIGURE 2-12. Cell membrane-derived mediators. Platelet activating factor (PAF) is derived from choline-containing glycerophospholipids in the membrane. Arachidonic acid derives from phosphatidylinositol phosphates and from phosphatidyl choline.

induced activation of phospholipase A_2 (PLA_2). The other is metabolism of phosphatidylinositol phosphates to diacylglycerol and inositol phosphates by phospholipase C. Diacylglycerol lipase then cleaves arachidonic acid from diacylglycerol. Once generated, arachidonic acid is further metabolized through two pathways: (1) **cyclooxygenation**, with subsequent production of prostaglandins and thromboxanes; and (2) **lipoxygenation**, to form leukotrienes and lipoxins (Fig. 2-13).

Corticosteroids are widely used to suppress tissue destruction associated with many inflammatory diseases, including allergic responses, rheumatoid arthritis, and systemic lupus erythematosus. Corticosteroids induce synthesis of an inhibitor of PLA_2 and block release of arachidonic acid in inflammatory cells. Although corticosteroids (e.g., prednisone) are widely used to suppress inflammatory responses, their prolonged administration can have significant harmful effects, including increased risk of infection, damage to connective tissue, and adrenal gland atrophy.

TABLE 2-2

Biological Activities of Arachidonic Acid Metabolites

Metabolite	Biological Activity
PGE_2, PDG_2	Induce vasodilation, bronchodilation; inhibit inflammatory cell function
PGI_2	Induces vasodilation, bronchodilation; inhibits inflammatory cell function
$PGF_{2\alpha}$	Induces vasodilation, bronchoconstriction
TXA_2	Induces vasoconstriction, bronchoconstriction; enhances inflammatory cell functions (esp. platelets
LTB_4	Chemotactic for phagocytic cells; stimulates phagocytic cell adherence; enhances microvascular permeability
LTC_4, LTD_4, LTE_4	Induce smooth muscle contraction; constrict pulmonary airways; increase microvascular permeability

PG . . . = prostaglandin; PD . . . = ; LT . . . = leukotriene; TXA_2 = thromboxane A2

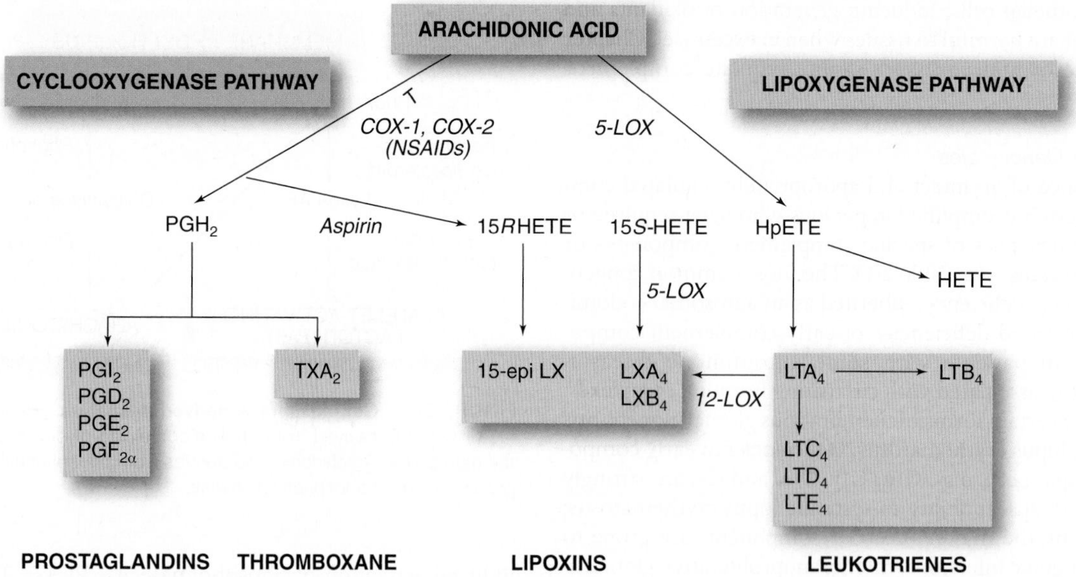

FIGURE 2-13. **Biologically active arachidonic acid metabolites.** The cyclo-oxygenase pathway of arachidonic acid metabolism generates prostaglandins (PG. . .) and thromboxane (TXA_2). The lipoxygenase pathway forms lipoxins (LX. . .) and leukotrienes (LT. . .); COX = cyclooxygenase; HETE = hydroxyicosatetraenoic acid ; HpETE = 5-hydroperoxyeicosatetraenoic acid; NSAIDs = nonsteroidal anti-inflammatory drugs.

Platelet-Activating Factor

Another potent inflammatory mediator derived from membrane phospholipids is PAF, synthesized by virtually all activated inflammatory cells, endothelial cells, and injured tissue cells. During inflammatory and allergic responses, PAF is derived from choline-containing glycerophospholipids in the cell membrane, initially by PLA_2, followed by acetylation by an acetyltransferase (see Fig. 2-12). In plasma, PAF-acetylhydrolase controls PAF activity. PAF has a wide range of activities. PAF stimulates platelets, neutrophils, monocyte/macrophages, endothelial cells, and vascular smooth muscle cells. PAF-induced platelet aggregation and degranulation at sites of tissue injury and enhances release of serotonin, thereby causing changes in vascular permeability. Because PAF primes leukocytes, it enhances functional responses (e.g., O_2 production, degranulation) to a second stimulus and induces adhesion molecule expression, specifically of integrins. PAF is also an extremely potent vasodilator, augmenting permeability of microvasculature at sites of tissue injury. PAF generated by endothelial cells cooperates with P-selectin. When P-selectin lightly tethers a leukocyte to an endothelial cell, PAF from the endothelial cell binds its receptor on the leukocyte and induces intracellular signaling.

Prostanoids, Leukotrienes, and Lipoxins Are Biologically Active Metabolites Of Arachidonic Acid

Prostanoids

Arachidonic acid is further metabolized by cyclooxygenases 1 and 2 (COX-1, COX-2) to generate prostanoids (see Fig. 2-13). **COX-1** is constitutively expressed by most cells and increases upon cell activation. It is a key enzyme in the synthesis of prostaglandins, which in turn (1) protect the gastrointestinal mucosal lining, (2) regulate water/electrolyte balance, (3) stimulate platelet aggregation to maintain normal hemostasis, and (4) maintain resistance to thrombosis on vascular endothelial cell surfaces. **COX-2** expression is generally low or undetectable, but increases substantially upon stimulation, generating metabolites important in inducing pain and inflammation.

The early inflammatory prostanoid response is COX-1-dependent; COX-2 takes over as the major source of prostanoids as inflammation progresses. Both COX isoforms generate prostaglandin H (PGH_2), which is then the substrate for production of prostacyclin (PGI_2), PGD_2, PGE_2, $PGF_{2\alpha}$, and TXA_2 (thromboxane). The profile of prostaglandin production (i.e., the quantity and variety produced during inflammation) depends in part on the cells present and their activation state. Thus, mast cells produce predominantly PGD_2; macrophages generate PGE_2 and TXA_2; platelets are the major source of TXA_2; endothelial cells produce PGI_2. Prostanoids affect immune cell function by binding G protein-coupled cell surface receptors, leading to activation of a range of intracellular signaling pathways in immune cells and resident tissue cells. The repertoire of prostanoid receptors expressed by various immune cells differs, so the functional responses of these cells may be modified differently according to the prostanoids present.

Inhibition of COX is one mechanism by which non-steroidal anti-inflammatory drugs (NSAIDs), including aspirin, indomethacin, and ibuprofen, exert their potent analgesic and antiinflammatory effects. NSAIDS block COX-2–induced formation of prostaglandins, thereby mitigating pain and inflammation. However, they also affect COX-1, lead to decreased homeostatic functions, and so affect the stomach and kidneys adversely. This complication led to development of COX-2–specific inhibitors.

Leukotrienes

Slow-reacting substance of anaphylaxis (SRS-A) has long been recognized as a smooth muscle stimulant and mediator of hypersensitivity reactions. It is, in fact, a mixture of leukotrienes, the second major family of derivatives of arachidonic acid (see Fig. 2-13). The enzyme 5-lipoxygenase (5-LOX) leads to synthesis of 5-hydroperoxyeicosatetraenoic acid (5-HpETE) and leukotriene A_4 (LTA_4) from arachidonic acid; the latter is a precursor for other leukotrienes. In neutrophils and certain macrophage populations, LTA_4 is metabolized to LTB_4, which has potent chemotactic activity for neutrophils, monocytes, and macrophages. In other cell types, especially mast cells, basophils, and macrophages, LTA_4 is converted to LTC_4 and thence to LTD_4 and LTE_4. These three cysteinyl-leukotrienes: (1) stimulate smooth muscle contraction, (2) enhance vascular permeability, and (3) are responsible for development of many of the clinical symptoms associated with allergic-type reactions. They thus play a pivotal role in the development of asthma. Leukotrienes exert their action through high-affinity specific receptors that may prove to be important targets of drug therapy.

Lipoxins

Lipoxins, the third class of products of arachidonic acid, are made within the vascular lumen by cell–cell interactions (see Fig. 2-13). They are proinflammatory, trihydroxytetraene-containing eicosanoids that are generated during inflammation, atherosclerosis, and thrombosis. Several cell types synthesize lipoxins from leukotrienes. LTA_4, released by activated leukocytes, is available for transcellular enzymatic conversion by neighboring cell types. When platelets adhere to neutrophils, LTA_4 from neutrophils is converted by platelet 12-lipoxygenase, forming lipoxin A_4 and B_4 (LXA_4 and LXB_4). Monocytes, eosinophils, and airway epithelial cells generate 15*S*-hydroxyeicosatetraenoic acid (15*S*-HETE), which is taken up by neutrophils and converted to lipoxins via 5-LOX. Activation of this pathway can also inhibit leukotriene biosynthesis, thereby providing a regulatory pathway.

Aspirin initiates transcellular biosynthesis of a group of lipoxins termed "aspirin-triggered lipoxins," or 15-epi-lipoxins (15-epi-LXs). When aspirin is administered in the presence of inflammatory mediators, 15*R*-HETE is generated by COX-2. Activated neutrophils convert 15*R*-HETE to 15 epimeric lipoxins (15-epi-LXs), which are anti-inflammatory lipid mediators. This is another pathway for the beneficial effects of aspirin.

Cytokines Are Cell-Derived Inflammatory Hormones

Cytokines constitute a group of low-molecular-weight proteins secreted by cells. Many cytokines are produced at sites of inflammation, including interleukins, growth factors, colony stimulating factors, interferons and chemokines (Fig. 2-14).

Cytokines

Cytokines produced at sites of tissue injury regulate inflammatory responses, ranging from initial changes in vascular permeability to resolution and restoration of tissue integrity. These molecules are inflammatory hormones that exhibit **autocrine** (affecting themselves), **paracrine** (affecting nearby cells), and **endocrine** (affecting cells in other tissues) functions. While most cells produce cytokines, they differ in their cytokine repertoire. *Through production of cytokines, macrophages are pivotal in orchestrating tissue inflammatory responses.* **Lipopolysaccharide** (LPS), a molecule derived from the outer cell membrane of gram-negative bacteria, is one of the most potent activators of macrophages, as well as endothelial cells and leukocytes (Fig. 2-15). LPS activates cells via specific receptors, either directly or after binding a serum LPS-binding protein (LBP). It is a potent stimulus for production of TNF-α and interleukins (IL-1, IL-6, IL-8, IL-12, and others). Macrophage-derived cytokines modulate endothelial cell–leukocyte adhesion (TNF-α), leukocyte recruitment (IL-8), the acute phase response (IL-6, IL-1), and immune functions (IL-1, IL-6, IL-12).

IL-1 and TNF-α, produced by macrophages as well as other cells, are central to development and amplification of inflammatory responses. These cytokines activate endothelial cells to express adhesion molecules and release cytokines, chemokines, and reactive oxygen species (ROS; see below). TNF-α induces priming and aggregation of neutrophils. IL-1 and TNF-α are also among the mediators of fever, catabolism of muscle, shifts in protein synthesis, and hemodynamic effects associated with inflammatory states (see Fig. 2-15).

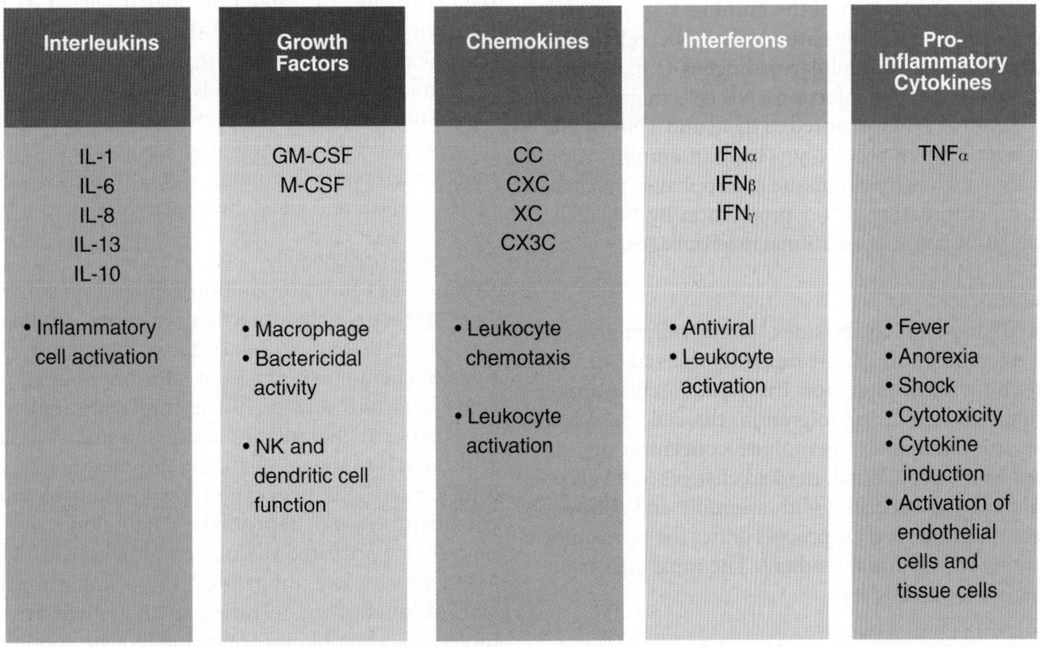

Interleukins
IL-1
IL-6
IL-8
IL-13
IL-10
• Inflammatory cell activation
Growth Factors
GM-CSF
M-CSF
• Macrophage
• Bactericidal activity
• NK and dendritic cell function
Chemokines
CC
CXC
XC
CX3C
• Leukocyte chemotaxis
• Leukocyte activation
Interferons
IFNα
IFNβ
IFNγ
• Antiviral
• Leukocyte activation
Pro-Inflammatory Cytokines
TNFα
• Fever
• Anorexia
• Shock
• Cytotoxicity
• Cytokine induction
• Activation of endothelial cells and tissue cells

FIGURE 2-14. **Cytokines important in inflammation.** GM-CSF = Granulocyte macrophage-colony stimulating factor; IL = interleukin; NK = natural killer; IFN = interferon; TNF = tumor necrosis factor.

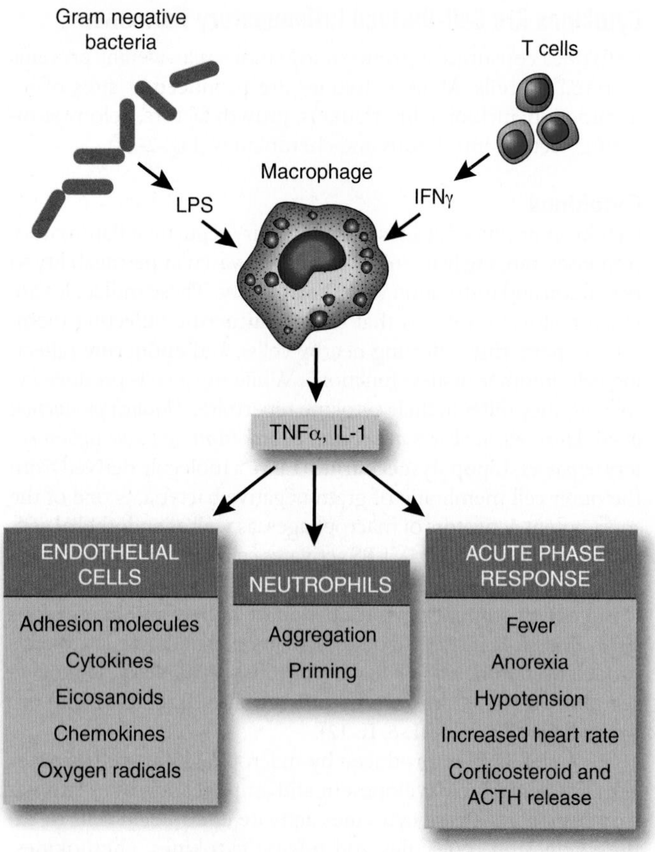

FIGURE 2-15. **Central role of interleukin (IL)-1 and tumor necrosis factor (TNF)-a in inflammation.** Lipopolysaccharide (LPS) and IFN-γ activate macrophages to release inflammatory cytokines, principally IL-1 and TNF-α, responsible for directing local and systemic inflammatory responses. ACTH = adrenocorticotrophic hormone.

Interferon-gamma (IFN-γ), another potent stimulus for macrophage activation and cytokine production, is produced by a subset of T lymphocytes as part of the immune response (see Chapter 4). It is also synthesized by natural killer (NK) cells in the primary host response to intracellular pathogens (e.g., *Listeria monocytogenes*) and certain viral infections. NK cells migrate into tissues at sites of injury. When exposed to IL-12 and TNF-α, NK cells are activated to produce IFN-γ. Thus, an amplification pathway exists by which activated tissue macrophages produce TNF-α and IL-12, stimulating IFN-γ production by NK cells, with subsequent stimulation of additional macrophages.

Chemokines

Chemotactic cytokines, or chemokines, direct cell migration (**chemotaxis**). Accumulation of inflammatory cells at sites of tissue injury requires their migration from the vascular space into extravascular tissue. During migration, the cell extends a pseudopod towards increasing chemokine concentration. At the leading front of the pseudopod, marked changes in levels of intracellular calcium are associated with assembly and contraction of cytoskeleton proteins. This process draws the remaining tail of the cell along the chemical gradient. The most important chemotactic factors for PMNs are

- C5a, derived from complement
- Bacterial and mitochondrial products, particularly low-molecular-weight N-formylated peptides (such as *N*-formyl-methionyl-leucyl-phenylalanine [FMLP])
- Products of arachidonic acid metabolism, especially LTB_4
- Chemokines

Chemokines are a large class of cytokines (over 50 known members) that regulate leukocyte trafficking in inflammation and immunity. Unlike other cytokines, chemokines are small molecules that interact with G-protein–coupled receptors on target cells. These secreted proteins are produced by a variety of cell types, either constitutively or after induction, and differ widely in biological action. This diversity is based on specific cell types targeted, specific receptor activation, and differences in intracellular signaling.

Two functional classes of chemokines have been distinguished: **inflammatory chemokines** and **homing chemokines**. Inflammatory chemokines are produced in response to bacterial toxins and inflammatory cytokines (especially, IL-1, TNF-α, and IFN-γ) by a variety of tissue cells as well as leukocytes themselves. These molecules recruit leukocytes during host inflammatory responses. Homing chemokines are constitutively expressed and upregulated during disease states and direct trafficking and homing of lymphocytes and dendritic cells to lymphoid tissues during an immune response (see Chapter 4).

Structure and Nomenclature

Chemokines are synthesized as secretory proteins consisting of approximately 70 to 130 amino acids, with four conserved cysteines linked by disulfide bonds. The two major subpopulations, termed CXC or CC chemokines (formerly called α and β chemokines)–are distinguished by the position of the first two cysteines, which are either separated by one amino acid (CXC) or are adjacent (CC). Two additional classes of chemokines, each with a single member, have been identified. Lymphotactin has two instead of four conserved cysteines (XC), and fractaline (or neurotactin) has three amino acids between the first two cysteines (CX_3C). Chemokines are named according to their structure, followed by "L" and the number of their gene (CCL1, CXCL1, etc.). However, many of the traditional names for chemokines persist in current usage. Chemokine receptors are named according to their structure, "R," and a number (CCR1, CXCR1, etc.); most receptors recognize more than one chemokine and most chemokines recognize more than one receptor. Receptor binding of chemokines to their ligands may result in an agonistic or antagonistic activity. The same chemokine may act as an agonist for one receptor and an antagonist for another. Leukocyte recruitment or lymphocyte homing is modulated by a combination of these agonistic and antagonistic activities.

Anchoring and Activity

Chemokines function as immobilized or soluble molecules. They generate a chemotactic gradient by binding to proteoglycans of the ECM or to cell surfaces. As a result, high concentrations of chemokines persist at sites of tissue injury. Specific receptors on the surface of the migrating leukocytes bind the matrix-bound chemokines and associated adhesion molecules, which tends to move cells along the chemotactic gradient to the injury site. This process of responding to a matrix-bound chemoattractant is **haptotaxis.** Chemokines are also displayed on cytokine-activated vascular endothelial cells. This process can augment very late antigen-4 (VLA-4) integrin-dependent adhesion of leukocytes, resulting in their firm arrest. As soluble molecules, chemokines control leukocyte motility and localization within extravascular tissues by establishing a chemotactic gradient. The multiplicity and combination of chemokine receptors on cells allows an extensive variety in biological function.

Neutrophils, monocytes, eosinophils, and basophils share some receptors but express other receptors exclusively. Thus specific chemokine combinations can recruit selective cell populations.

Chemokines in Disease

Chemokines are implicated in a variety of acute and chronic diseases. These include disorders with a pronounced inflammatory component, in which case multiple chemokines are expressed in the inflamed tissues. Examples are rheumatoid arthritis, ulcerative colitis, Crohn disease, pulmonary inflammation (chronic bronchitis, asthma), autoimmune diseases (multiple sclerosis, rheumatoid arthritis, systemic lupus erythematosus), and vascular diseases, including atherosclerosis.

Reactive Oxygen Species (ROS) Are Signal-Transducing, Bactericidal, and Cytotoxic Molecules

ROS are chemically reactive molecules derived from oxygen. Normally, they are rapidly inactivated, but when generated inappropriately, they can be toxic to cells (see Chapter 1). ROS activate signal-transduction pathways and combine with proteins, lipids, and DNA, a state termed **oxidative stress**, which can lead to loss of cell function and cell death. Leukocyte-derived ROS, released within phagosomes, are bactericidal. ROS important in inflammation include superoxide (O_2•, O_2^-), nitric oxide (NO•), hydrogen peroxide (H_2O_2) and hydroxyl radical (•OH) (Fig. 2-16) (see below and Chapter 1).

Superoxide

Molecular oxygen is converted to superoxide anion (O_2^-) by several pathways. (1) Within cells, formation of O_2^- occurs spontaneously near the inner mitochondrial membrane; (2) In vascular endothelial cells, O_2^- is generated by flavoenzymes such as xanthine oxidase, as well as lipoxygenase and cyclooxygenase; (3) In the setting of inflammation, leukocytes, as well as endothelial cells, use a reduced nicotinamide adenine dinucleotide phosphate (NADPH) oxidase to produce O_2^-.

In endothelial cells xanthine oxidase, a purine-metabolizing enzyme, converts xanthine and hypoxanthine to uric acid, thereby generating O_2^-. This pathway is a major intracellular source of O_2^- in neutrophil-mediated cell injury. Proinflammatory mediators, including leukocyte elastase and several cytokines, convert xanthine dehydrogenase to the active xanthine oxidase. Intracellular O_2^- interacts with nuclear factor NFκB, activating protein-1 (AP-1), and other molecules to activate signal transduction pathways. It is further metabolized to other free radicals, particularly •OH, which contribute to inflammation-related cell injury.

The NADPH-oxidase of phagocytic cells, neutrophils, and macrophages is a multicomponent enzyme complex, that generates high concentrations of extracellular and intracellular O_2^-, mainly for bactericidal and cytotoxic functions. This oxidase uses NADH and NADPH as substrates for electron transfer to molecular oxygen. A similar enzyme complex is present in vascular endothelial cells, where it generates significant, albeit lower, concentrations of O_2^-.

Nitric Oxide

Nitric oxide (NO•) is synthesized by nitric oxide synthase (NOS), which promotes oxidation of the guanidino nitrogen of L-arginine in the presence of O_2. There are three main NOS isoforms: constitutively expressed neuronal (nNOS) and endothelial (eNOS) forms, and an inducible (iNOS) isoform. Inflammatory cytokines increase expression of iNOS, generating intracellular and extracellular NO•. NO• has diverse roles in the physiology and pathophysiology of the vascular system, including:

- NO• generated by eNOS acts as **endothelium-derived relaxing factor** (EDRF), mediating vascular smooth muscle relaxation.
- In physiological concentrations, NO• alone and in balance with O_2^-, is an intracellular messenger.
- NO• prevents platelet adherence and aggregation at sites of vascular injury, reduces leukocyte recruitment, and scavenges oxygen radicals.
- Excessive production of NO•, especially in parallel with O_2^-, generates the highly reactive and cytotoxic species, peroxynitrite (ONOO•).

Stress Proteins Protect Against Inflammatory Injury

When cells are subjected to stress conditions, many suffer irreversible injury and die, and others are severely damaged. However, mild heat treatment prior to lethal injury provides tolerance to subsequent injury. This phenomenon reflects increased expression of the heat shock family of stress proteins

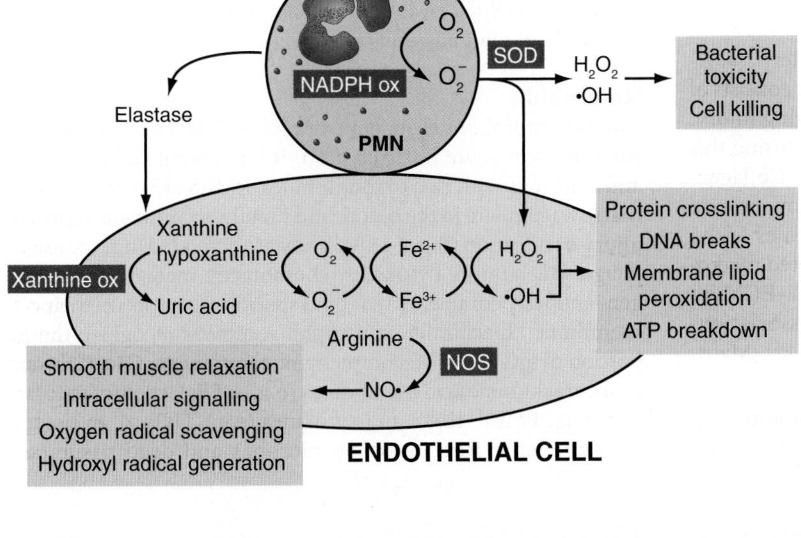

FIGURE 2-16. **Biochemical events in neutrophil-endothelial cell interactions.** When neutrophils are in firm contact with endothelial cells, oxygen radicals and other active molecules generated by both cells interact. Superoxide (O_2^-) generated by the neutrophil NADPH oxidase (NADPH ox) is converted to toxic hydrogen peroxide (H_2O_2) and hydroxyl radical (•OH). Within the endothelial cell, xanthine oxidase oxide (xanthine ox) converts xanthine to uric acid, ultimately generating O_2^- from molecular oxygen. Nitric oxide synthase (NOS) generates nitric oxide (NO•) from arginine. Reactive oxygen species contribute to numerous cellular events. ATP = adenosine triphosphate; Fe^{2+} = ferrous iron; Fe^{3+} = ferric iron; PMN = polymorphonuclear neutrophil.

(HSPs). Stress proteins belong to multigene families and are named according to molecular size, for example, Hsp27, Hsp70, and Hsp90. They are upregulated by diverse stresses, including oxidative/ischemic stress and inflammation, and are associated with protection during sepsis and metabolic stress. Protein damage and misfolded proteins are common denominators in injury and disease. Protection from many kinds of nonlethal stresses is mediated by HSPs, which act as molecular chaperones, increasing protein expression by enhancing folding of nascent proteins and preventing misfolding. Potential functions of stress proteins include suppression of proinflammatory cytokines and NADPH oxidase, increased nitric oxide-mediated cytoprotection, and enhanced collagen synthesis.

Neurokinins Link the Endocrine, Nervous, and Immune Systems

The neurokinin family of peptides includes substance P (SP), neurokinin A (NKA), and neurokinin B (NKB). These peptides are distributed throughout the central and peripheral nervous systems, and represent a link between the endocrine, nervous, and immune systems. A wide range of biological processes is associated with these peptides, including plasma protein extravasation and edema, vasodilation, smooth-muscle contraction and relaxation, salivary secretion, airway contraction, and transmission of nociceptive responses. As early as 1876, Stricker noted an association between sensory afferent nerves and inflammation. *It is now recognized that injury to nerve terminals during inflammation evokes an increase in neurokinins, which in turn influence production of inflammatory mediators, including histamine, NO•, and kinins.* The actions of neurokinins are mediated by activation of at least three classes of receptors—NK1, NK2, and NK3—which are widely distributed throughout the body. The neurokinin system is linked to inflammation in the following settings:

- **Edema formation:** SP, NKA, and NKB induce edema by promoting release of histamine and serotonin from mast cells.
- **Thermal injury:** SP and NKA are produced after thermal injury occurs and mediate early edema.
- **Arthritis:** SP is widely distributed in nerves in joints where it mediates vascular permeability. SP and NKA can modulate the activity of inflammatory and immune cells.
- **Airway inflammation:** SP and NKA have been implicated in bronchoconstriction, mucosal edema, leukocyte adhesion and activation, and increased vascular permeability.

Extracellular Matrix Mediators

The interaction of cells with the extracellular matrix regulates tissue responses to inflammation. The extracellular environment consists of a macromolecular matrix specific to each tissue. During injury, resident inflammatory cells interact with this matrix, using this scaffolding for migration along a chemokine gradient. Collagen, elastic fibers, basement membrane proteins, glycoproteins, and proteoglycans are among the structural macromolecules of the ECM (see Chapter 3). Matricellular proteins are secreted macromolecules that link cells to the ECM or to disrupt cell–ECM interactions. Cytokines and growth factors influence associations among cells, ECM and matricellular proteins (Fig. 2-17). Matricellular proteins include:

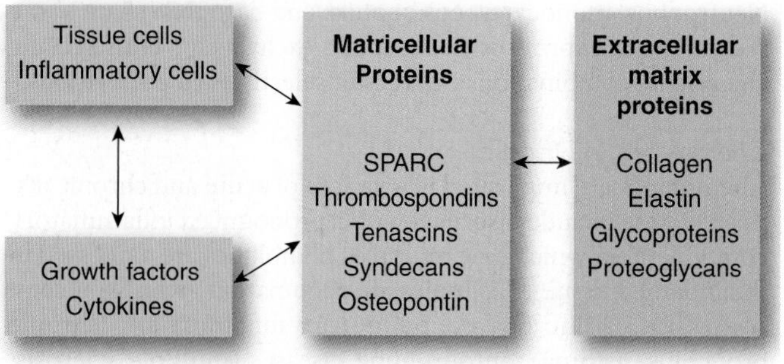

FIGURE 2-17. **Dynamic relationship associates cells, soluble mediators, and matricellular proteins with the extracellular matrix.** SPARC = secreted protein acidic and rich in cysteine.

- **SPARC (secreted protein acidic and rich in cysteine)** is a multifunctional glycoprotein that organizes ECM components and modulates growth factor activity. It affects cell proliferation, migration, and differentiation, and acts as a counter-adhesive protein, especially on endothelial cells.
- **Thrombospondins** are secreted glycoproteins that modulate cell–matrix interactions, influence platelet aggregation and support neutrophil chemotaxis and adhesion.
- **Tenascins C, X, and R** are counter-adhesive proteins expressed during development, tissue injury, and wound healing.
- **Syndecans** are heparan sulfate proteoglycans implicated in coagulation, growth factor signaling, cell adhesion to the ECM, and tumorigenesis.
- **Osteopontin** is a phosphorylated glycoprotein important in bone mineralization. It also (1) mediates cell–matrix interactions, (2) activates cell signaling (particularly in T cells), (3) is chemotactic for and supports adhesion of leukocytes, and (4) has anti-inflammatory effects via regulation of macrophage function.

Cells of Inflammation

Leukocytes are the major cellular components of the inflammatory response and include neutrophils, T and B lymphocytes, monocytes, macrophages, eosinophils, mast cells, and basophils. Specific functions are associated with each of these cell types, but they overlap and vary as inflammation progresses. In addition, local tissue cells interact with one another and with inflammatory cells, in a continuous response to injury and infection. *Inflammatory cells and resident tissue cells interact during inflammation.* They include neutrophils, endothelial cells, monocyte/macrophages, mast cells, eosinophils, and platelets.

Neutrophils

The polymorphonuclear neutrophil, or (PMN), is the cellular participant in acute inflammation. It has granulated cytoplasm and a nucleus with two to four lobules. PMNs are stored in bone marrow, circulate in the blood, and rapidly accumulate at sites of injury or infection (Fig. 2-18A). They are activated in response to phagocytic stimuli, cytokines, chemotactic mediators, or antigen–antibody complexes that bind specific receptors on their cell membrane. Specifically, neutrophil receptors recognize the Fc portion of IgG and IgM; complement components C5a, C3b, and iC3b; arachidonic acid metabolites (e.g., LTB_4); chemotactic factors (e.g., FMLP, IL-8), and cytokines (e.g., TNF-α). In tissues, PMNs phagocytose invading microbes and dead tissue (see

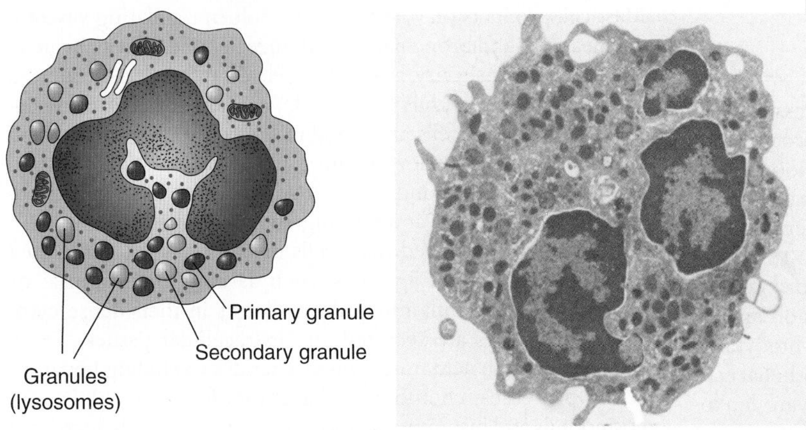

POLYMORPHONUCLEAR LEUKOCYTES

CHARACTERISTICS AND FUNCTIONS
- Central to acute inflammation
- Phagocytosis of microorganisms and tissue debris
- Mediates tissue injury

PRIMARY INFLAMMATORY MEDIATORS
- Reactive oxygen metabolites
- Lysosomal granule contents

Primary granules
Myeloperoxidase
Lysozyme
Defensins
Bactericidal/permeability increasing protein
Elastase
Cathepsins Protease 3
Glucuronidase
Mannosidase
Phospholipase A_2

Secondary granules
Lysozyme
Lactoferrin
Collagenase
Complement activator
Phospholipase A_2
CD11b/CD18
CD11c/CD18
Laminin

Tertiary granules
Gelatinase
Plasminogen activator
Cathepsins
Glucuronidase
Mannosidase

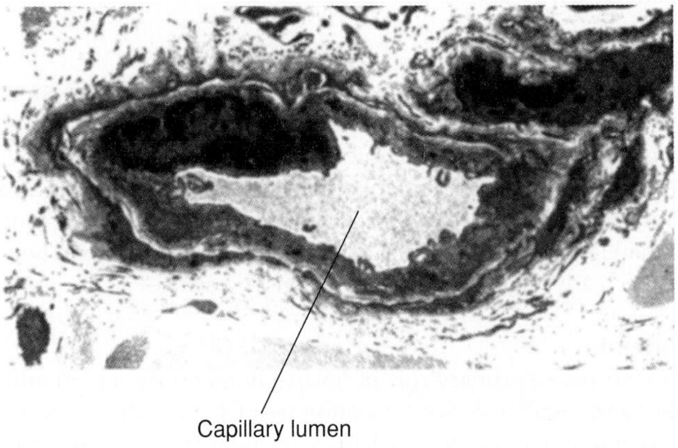

ENDOTHELIAL CELLS

CHARACTERISTICS AND FUNCTIONS
- Maintains vascular integrity
- Regulates platelet aggregation
- Regulates vascular contraction and relaxation
- Mediates leukocyte recruitment in inflammation

PRIMARY INFLAMMATORY MEDIATORS
- von Willebrand factor
- Nitric oxide
- Endothelins
- Prostanoids

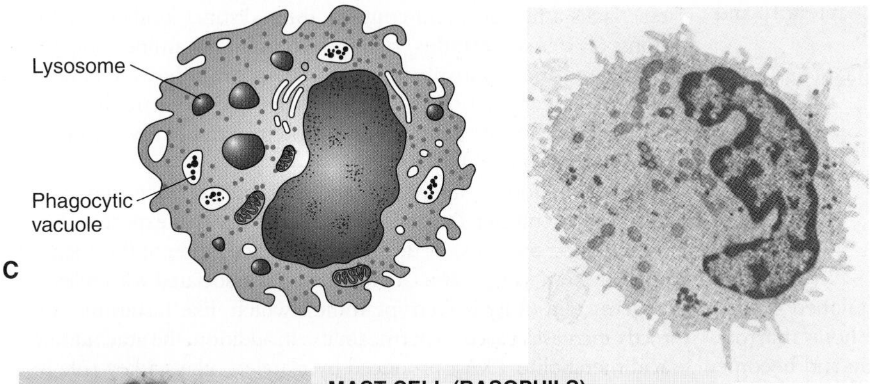

MONOCYTE/MACROPHAGE

CHARACTERISTICS AND FUNCTIONS
- Regulates inflammatory response
- Regulates coagulation/fibrinolytic pathway
- Regulates immune response (see Chapt. 4)

PRIMARY INFLAMMATORY MEDIATORS
- cytokines
  - -IL-1
  - -TNF-α
  - -IL-6
  - -Chemokines (e.g. IL-8, MCP-1)
- lysosomal enzymes
  - -acid hydrolases
  - -serine proteases
  - -metalloproteases (e.g. collagenase)
- cationic proteins
- prostaglandins/leukotrienes
- plasminogen activator
- procoagulant activity
- oxygen metabolite formation

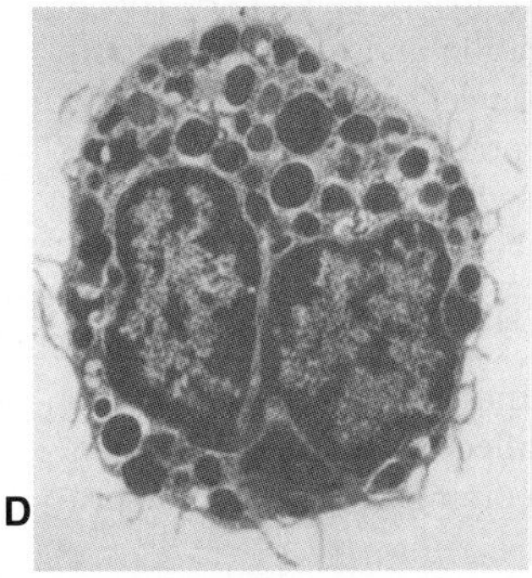

MAST CELL (BASOPHILS)

CHARACTERISTICS AND FUNCTIONS
- Binds IgE molecules
- Contains electron-dense granules

PRIMARY INFLAMMATORY MEDIATORS
- Histamine
- Leukotrienes (LTC, LTD, LTE)
- Platelet activating factor
- Eosinophil chemotactic factors
- Cytokines (e.g., TNF-α IL-4)

FIGURE 2-18. **Cells of inflammation: morphology, and function. A.** Neutrophil. **B.** Endothelial cell. **C.** Monocyte/macrophage. **D.** Mast cell. IL = interleukin; MCP-1 = monocyte chemoattractant protein-1 TNF-α = tumor necrosis factor-α.

below). Once they are recruited into tissue, they do not reenter the circulation.

Endothelial Cells

Endothelial cells, a monolayer of cells lining blood vessels, help to separate intra- and extravascular spaces. They produce antiplatelet and antithrombotic agents that maintain blood vessel patency and also vasodilators and vasoconstrictors that regulate vascular tone. Injury to a vessel wall interrupts the endothelial barrier and exposes a local procoagulant signal (Fig. 2-18B).

Endothelial cells are gatekeepers in inflammatory cell recruitment: they can promote or inhibit tissue perfusion and inflammatory cell influx. Inflammatory agents such as bradykinin and histamine, endotoxin, and cytokines induce endothelial cells to reveal adhesion molecules that anchor and activate leukocytes, present major histocompatibility complex (MHC) class I and II molecules, and generate cytokines and important vasoactive and inflammatory mediators. These mediators include:

- **Nitric oxide (NO•):** Originally identified as EDRF, NO• is a low–molecular-weight vasodilator that inhibits platelet aggregation, regulates vascular tone by stimulating smooth muscle relaxation, and reacts with ROS to create highly reactive radical species (see above).
- **Endothelins:** Endothelins-1, -2, and -3 are low–molecular-weight peptides produced by endothelial cells. They are potent vasoconstrictor and pressor agents, which induce prolonged vasoconstriction of vascular smooth muscle.
- **Arachidonic acid-derived contraction factors:** Oxygen radicals generated by the hydroperoxidase activity of cyclooxygenase and prostanoids such as TXA_2 and PGH_2 induce smooth muscle contraction.
- **Arachidonic acid-derived relaxing factors:** The biological opponent of TXA_2, PGI_2 inhibits platelet aggregation and causes vasodilation.
- **Cytokines:** IL-1, IL-6, TNF-α and other inflammatory cytokines are generated by activated endothelial cells.
- **Anticoagulants:** Heparin-like molecules and thrombomodulin inactivate the coagulation cascade (see Chapters 10 and 20).
- **Fibrinolytic factors:** Tissue-type plasminogen activator (t-PA) promotes fibrinolytic activity.
- **Prothrombotic agents:** von Willebrand factor facilitates adhesion of platelets, and tissue factor activates the extrinsic clotting cascade.

Monocyte/Macrophages

Circulating monocytes (Fig. 2-18C) have a single lobed or kidney-shaped nucleus. They are derived from the bone marrow and can exit the circulation to migrate into tissue and become resident macrophages. In response to inflammatory mediators, they accumulate at sites of acute inflammation and take up and process microbes. These cells can also differentiate into dendritic cells, which are highly efficient antigen-presenting cells. Antigens bind to the **major histocompatibility complex** (MHCII) and are presented to lymphocytes, subsequently activating those cells. Monocyte/macrophages produce potent vasoactive mediators, including prostaglandins and leukotrienes, PAF, and inflammatory cytokines. Macrophages are especially important for maintaining chronic inflammation.

Mast Cells and Basophils

Mast cell products play an important role in regulating vascular permeability and bronchial smooth muscle tone, especially in allergic hypersensitivity reactions (see Chapter 4). Granulated mast cells and basophils (Fig. 2-18D) contain cell surface receptors for IgE. Mast cells are found in the connective tissues, and are especially prevalent along lung and gastrointestinal mucosal surfaces, the dermis, and the microvasculature. Basophils circulate in small numbers and can migrate into tissue.

When IgE-sensitized mast cells or basophils are stimulated by antigen; physical agonists, such as cold and trauma; or cationic proteins, inflammatory mediators in their dense cytoplasmic granules are secreted into extracellular tissues. These granules contain acid mucopolysaccharides (including heparin), serine proteases, chemotactic mediators for neutrophils, and eosinophils and histamine, a primary mediator of early increased vascular permeability. Histamine binds specific H_1 receptors in the vascular wall, inducing endothelial cell contraction, gap formation, and edema, an effect that can be inhibited pharmacologically by H_1-receptor antagonists. Stimulation of mast cells and basophils also leads to the release of products of arachidonic acid metabolism, including LTC_4, LTD_4, and LTE_4, and cytokines, such as TNF-α and IL-4.

Eosinophils

Eosinophils circulate in blood and are recruited to tissue similarly to PMNs. They are characteristic of IgE-mediated reactions, such as hypersensitivity, allergic and asthmatic responses (Fig. 2-19A). Eosinophils contain leukotrienes and PAF, as well as acid phosphatase and peroxidase. They express IgA receptors and contain large granules with eosinophil major basic protein, both of which are involved in defense against parasites.

Platelets

Platelets play a primary role in normal homeostasis and in initiating and regulating clot formation (see Chapter 20). They are sources of inflammatory mediators, including potent vasoactive substances and growth factors that modulate mesenchymal cell proliferation (Fig. 2-19B). The platelet is small (2 mm in diameter), lacks a nucleus, and contains three distinct kinds of inclusions: (1) **dense granules**, rich in serotonin, histamine, calcium and adenosine diphosphate (ADP); (2) ***α* granules**, containing fibrinogen, coagulation proteins, platelet-derived growth factor (PDGF), and other peptides and proteins; and (3) **lysosomes**, which sequester acid hydrolases.

Platelets adhere, aggregate, and degranulate when they contact fibrillar collagen (e.g., after vascular injury that exposes interstitial matrix proteins) or thrombin (after activation of the coagulation system) (Fig. 2-20). Degranulation is associated with release of serotonin (5-hydroxytryptamine), which, like histamine, directly increases vascular permeability. In addition, the arachidonic acid metabolite TXA_2, produced by platelets, plays a key role in the second wave of platelet aggregation and mediates smooth muscle constriction. On activation, platelets, as well as phagocytic cells, secrete cationic proteins that neutralize the negative charges on endothelium and promote increased permeability.

Leukocyte Recruitment in Acute Inflammation

One of the essential features of inflammation is accumulation of leukocytes, particularly PMNs, in affected tissues. Leukocytes adhere to vascular endothelium, becoming activated in the pro-

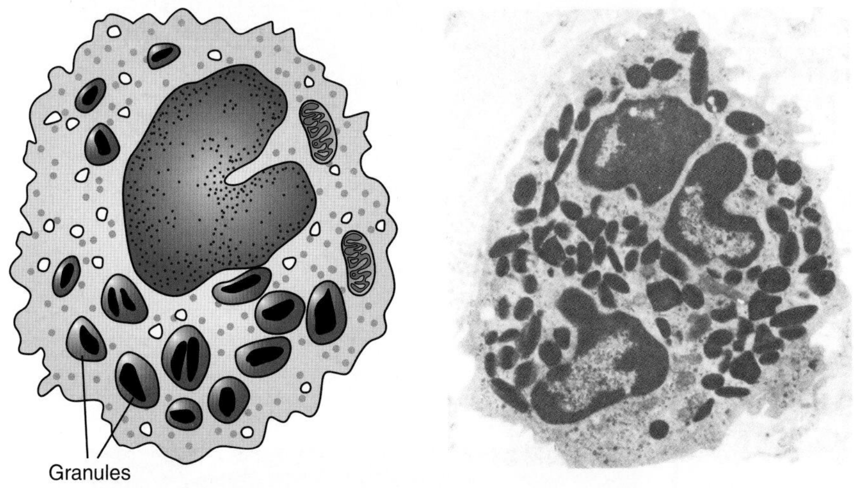

A

EOSINOPHILS

CHARACTERISTICS AND FUNCTIONS
- Associated with:
  - -Allergic reactions
  - -Parasite-associated inflammatory reactions
  - -Chronic inflammation
- Modulates mast cell-mediated reactions

PRIMARY INFLAMMATORY MEDIATORS
- Reactive oxygen metabolites
- Lysosomal granule enzymes (primary crystalloid granules)
  - -Major basic protein
  - -Eosinophil cationic protein
  - -Eosinophil peroxidase
  - -Acid phosphatase
  - -β-glucuronidase
  - -Arylsulfatase B
  - -Histaminase
- Phospholipase D
- Prostaglandins of E series
- Cytokines

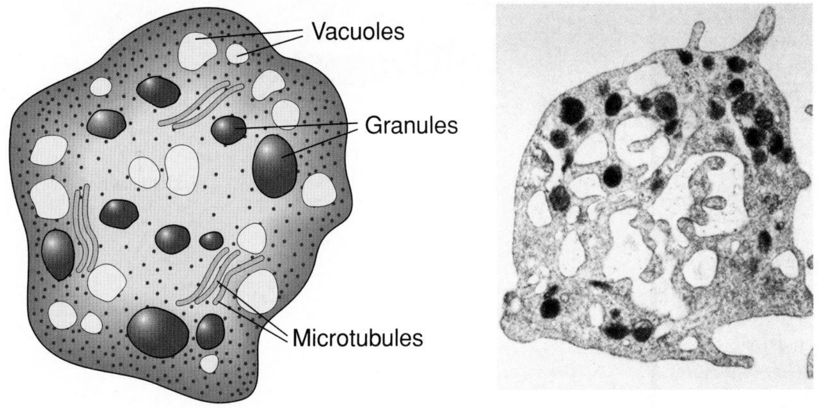

B

PLATELETS

CHARACTERISTICS AND FUNCTIONS
- Thrombosis; promotes clot formation
- Regulates permeability
- Regulates proliferative response of mesenchymal cells

PRIMARY INFLAMMATORY MEDIATORS
- Dense granules
  - -Serotonin
  - -Ca^{2+}
  - -ADP
- α-granules
  - -Cationic proteins
  - -Fibrinogen and coagulation proteins
  - -Platelet-derived growth factor (PDGF)
- Lysosomes
  - -Acid hydrolases
- Thromboxane A_2

FIGURE 2-19. **More cells of inflammation: morphology and function. A.** Eosinophil. **B.** Platelet. ADP = adenosine diphosphate.

cess. They then flatten and migrate from the vasculature, through the endothelial cell layer and into surrounding tissue. In the extravascular tissue, PMNs ingest foreign material, microbes and dead tissue (Fig. 2-21).

Leukocyte Adhesion to Endothelium Results from Interaction of Complementary Adhesion Molecules

Leukocyte recruitment to the postcapillary venules begins with interaction of leukocytes with endothelial cell selectins, which are redistributed to endothelial cell surfaces during activation. This interaction, called **tethering**, slows leukocytes in the blood flow (Fig. 2-22). Leukocytes then move along the vascular endothelial cell surface with a saltatory movement, termed **rolling**. PMNs become activated by proximity to the endothelium and by inflammatory mediators, and adhere strongly to intercellular adhesion molecules (ICAMs) on the endothelium (leukocyte **arrest**). As endothelial cells separate, leukocytes **transmigrate** through the vessel wall and, under the influence of chemotactic factors, leukocytes migrate through extravascular tissue to the site of injury.

The events involved in leukocyte recruitment are regulated by (1) inflammatory mediators, which stimulate resident tissue cells, including vascular endothelial cells; (2) expression of adhesion molecules on vascular endothelial cell surfaces, which bind to reciprocal molecules on the surfaces of circulating leukocytes; and (3) chemotactic factors, which attract leukocytes along a chemical gradient to the site of injury.

Adhesion Molecules

Four molecular families of adhesion molecules are involved in leukocyte recruitment: selectins, addressins, integrins, and immunoglobulins (Fig. 2-23).

Selectins

The selectin family includes P-selectin, E-selectin, and L-selectin, expressed on the surface of platelets, endothelial cells, and leukocytes. Selectins share a similar molecular structure, which includes a chain of transmembrane glycoproteins with an extracellular lectin-binding domain. This calcium-dependent or C-type lectin binds to sialylated oligosaccharides, specifically the sialyl-Lewis X

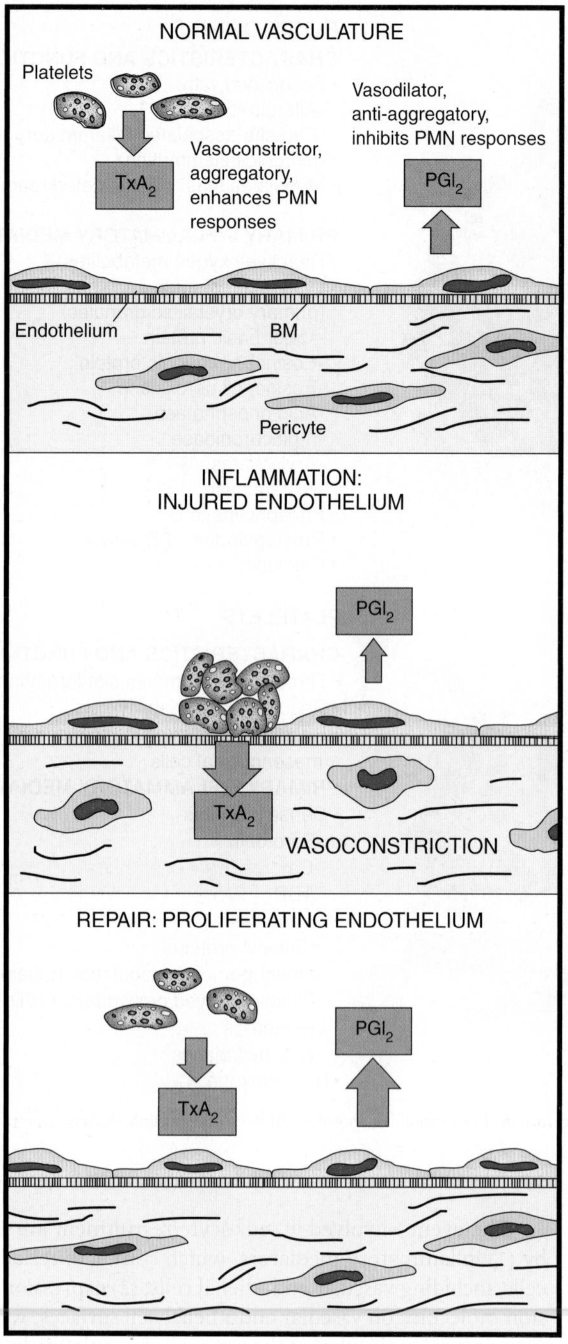

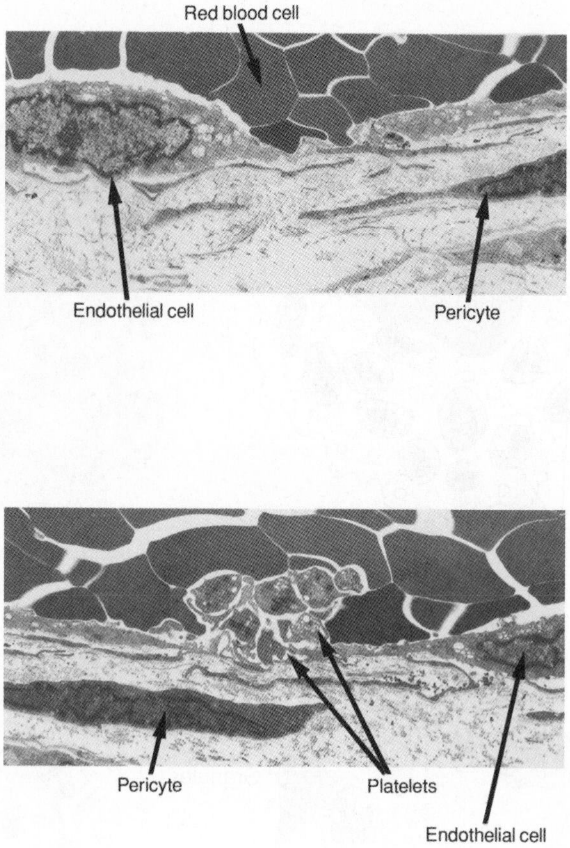

FIGURE 2-20. **Regulation of platelet and endothelial cell interactions by thromboxane A_2 *(TXA_2)* and pro-staglandin I_2 *(PGI_2)*.** During inflammation, the normal balance is shifted to vasoconstriction, platelet aggregation, and polymorphonuclear neutrophil (PMN) responses. During repair, the prostaglandin effects predominate. BM = basement membrane.

moiety on addressins, the binding of which allows rapid attachment and rolling of cells.

P-selectin (CD62P, GMP-140, PADGEM) is preformed and stored within Weibel-Palade bodies of endothelial cells and α-granules of platelets. On stimulation with histamine, thrombin, or specific inflammatory cytokines, P-selectin is rapidly transported to the cell surface, where it binds to sialyl-Lewis X on leukocyte surfaces. Preformed P-selectin can be delivered quickly to the cell surface, allowing rapid adhesive interaction between endothelial cells and leukocytes.

E-selectin (CD62E, ELAM-1) is not normally expressed on endothelial cell surfaces but is induced by inflammatory mediators, such as cytokines or bacterial LPS. E-selectin mediates adhesion of neutrophils, monocytes, and certain lymphocytes via binding to Lewis X or Lewis A

L-selectin (CD62L, LAM-1, Leu-8) is expressed on many types of leukocytes. It was originally defined as the "homing receptor" for lymphocytes. It binds lymphocytes to high endothelial venules (HEV) in lymphoid tissue, thereby regulating their trafficking through this tissue. L-selectin binds glycan-bearing cell adhesion molecule-1 (GlyCAM-1), mucosal addressin cell adhesion molecule-1 (MadCAM-1) and CD34.

Addressins

Vascular addressins are mucin-like glycoproteins including GlyCAM-1, P-selectin glycoprotein-1 (PSGL-1), E-Selection ligand (ESL-1), and CD34. They possess sialyl-Lewis X, which binds the lectin domain of selectins. Addressins are expressed at leukocyte and endothelium surfaces. They regulate localization of subpopulations of leukocytes and are involved in lymphocyte activation.

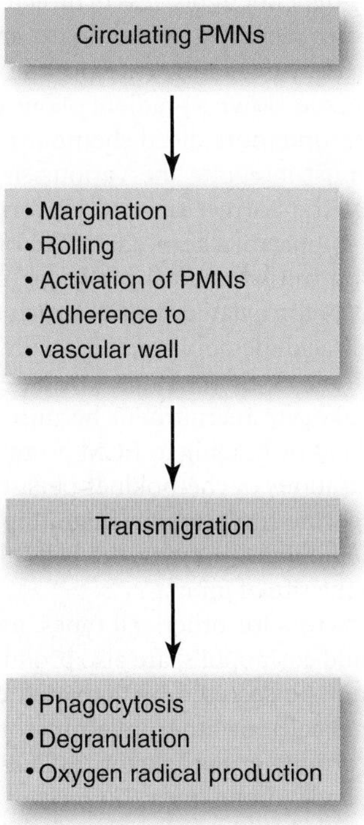

FIGURE 2-21. **Leukocyte recruitment and activation.** PMNs = polymorphonuclear neutrophils.

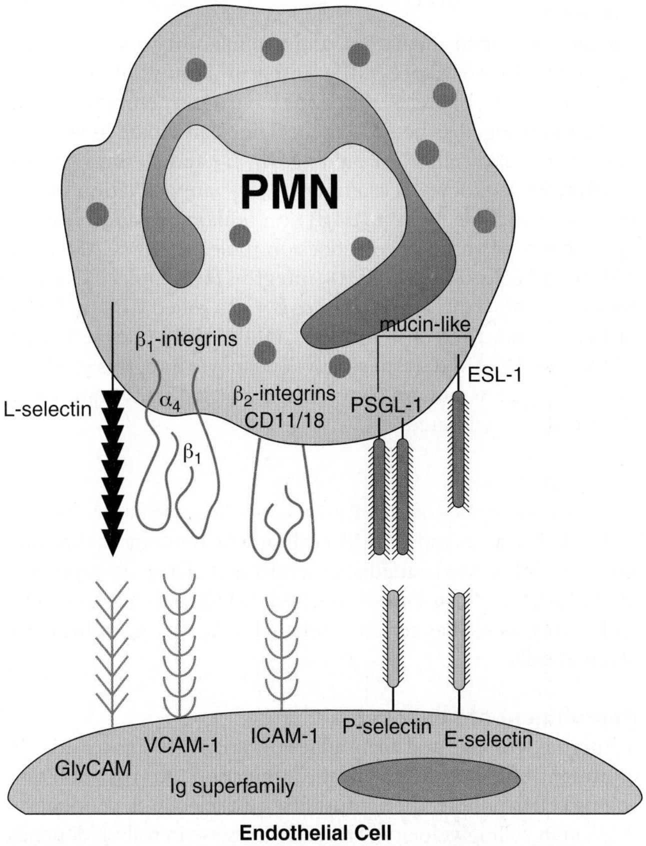

FIGURE 2-23. **Leukocyte and endothelial cell adhesion mole-cules.** GlyCAM = glycan-bearing cell adhesion molecule; ICAM-1 = intercellular adhesion molecule-1; VCAM = vascular cell adhesion molecule.

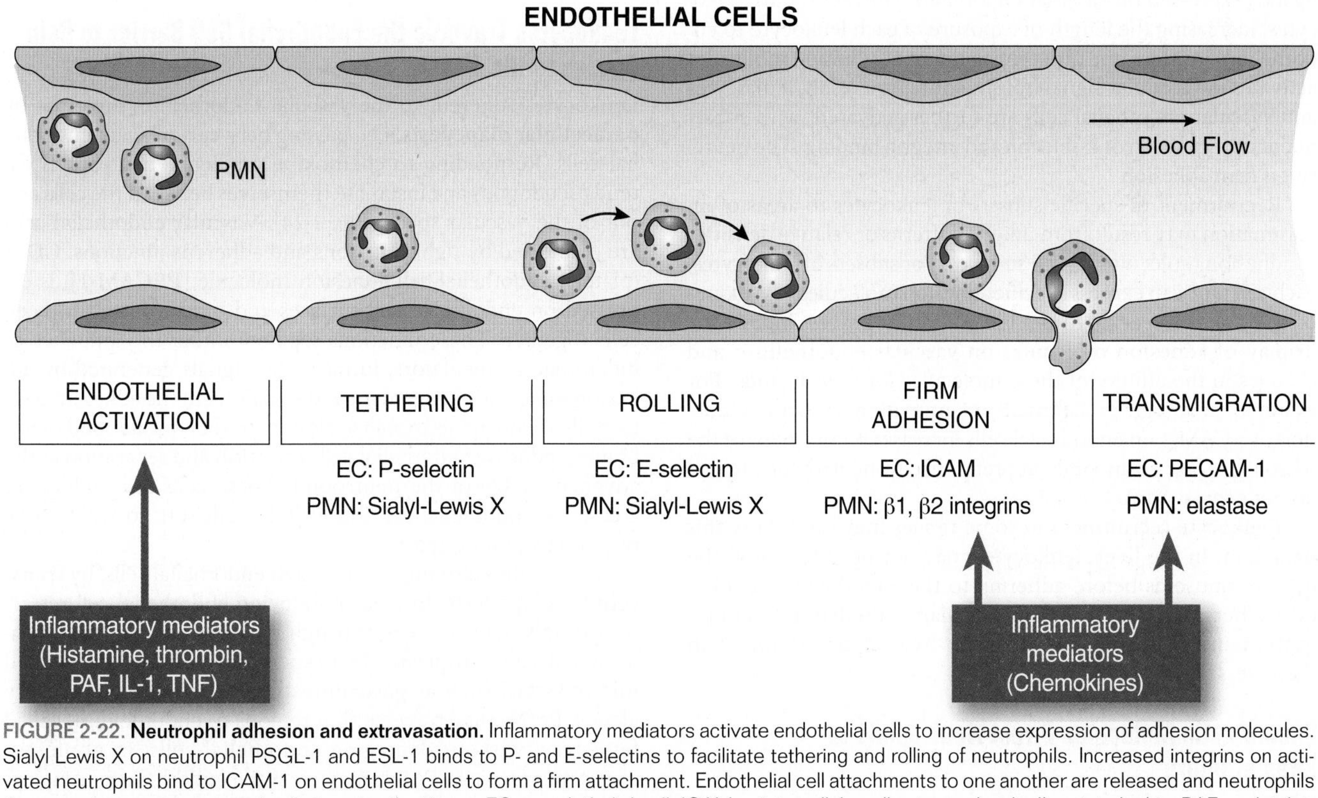

FIGURE 2-22. **Neutrophil adhesion and extravasation.** Inflammatory mediators activate endothelial cells to increase expression of adhesion molecules. Sialyl Lewis X on neutrophil PSGL-1 and ESL-1 binds to P- and E-selectins to facilitate tethering and rolling of neutrophils. Increased integrins on activated neutrophils bind to ICAM-1 on endothelial cells to form a firm attachment. Endothelial cell attachments to one another are released and neutrophils then pass between separated cells to enter the tissue. EC = endothelial cell; ICAM = intercellular adhesion molecule; IL = interleukin; PAF = platelet-activating factor; PMN = polymorphonuclear neutrophil; TNF = tumor necrosis factor.

Integrins

Chemokines, lipid mediators, and proinflammatory molecules activate cells to express the integrin family of adhesion molecules (see Chapter 3). Integrins have transmembrane α and β chains arranged as heterodimers. They participate in cell–cell interactions and cell–ECM binding. β_1, β_2, and β_7 integrins are involved in leukocyte recruitment. Very late activation (VLA) molecules include VLA-4 ($\alpha4\beta1$) on leukocytes and lymphocytes that bind vascular cell adhesion molecule-1 (VCAM-1) on endothelial cells. The $\beta2$ (CD18) integrins form molecules by association with α integrin chains: $\alpha_1\beta_2$ (also called CD11a/CD18 or LFA-1) and $\alpha_m\beta_2$ (also termed CD11b/CD18 or Mac-1) bind ICAM-1 and ICAM-2, respectively. Leukocyte integrins exist in a low affinity state, but are converted to a high affinity state when these cells are activated.

Immunoglobulins

Adhesion molecules of the immunoglobulin superfamily include ICAM-1, ICAM-2, and VCAM-1, all of which interact with integrins on leukocytes to mediate recruitment. They are expressed at the surfaces of cytokine-stimulated endothelial cells and some leukocytes, as well as certain epithelial cells, such as pulmonary alveolar cells.

Recruitment of Leukocytes

Tethering, rolling, and firm adhesion are prerequisites for recruitment of leukocytes from the circulation into tissues. For a rolling cell to adhere, there must first be a selectin-dependent reduction in rolling velocity. The early increase in rolling depends on P-selectin, whereas cytokine-induced E-selectin initiates early adhesion. Integrin family members function cooperatively with selectins to facilitate rolling and subsequent firm adhesion of leukocytes. Leukocyte integrin binding to the Ig superfamily of ligands expressed on vascular endothelium further retard leukocytes, increasing the length of exposure of each leukocyte to endothelium. At the same time, engagement of adhesion molecules activates intracellular signal transduction. As a result, leukocytes and vascular endothelial cells are further activated, with subsequent upregulation of L-selectin and integrin binding. The net result is firm adhesion

Recruitment of specific subsets of leukocytes to areas of inflammation may result from unique patterns or relative densities of adhesion molecules on cell surfaces. For subsets of leukocytes, each cell type can express specific adhesion molecules. Cytokines or chemokines specific to the inflammatory process induce the display of adhesion molecules on vascular endothelium and changes in the affinity of these molecules for their ligands. For example, in allergic or asthmatic inflammation, cytokine induction of VCAM-1 on endothelial cells increases recruitment of the VLA-4–bearing eosinophils in preference to neutrophils, which do not express VLA-4.

Leukocyte recruitment in some tissues may not follow this paradigm. In the liver, leukocytes may not need to roll in the narrow sinusoids before adhering to the endothelium. Leukocyte adherence to arterioles and capillaries also has different requirements, reflecting the different hydrodynamic forces in these vessels.

Chemotactic Molecules Direct Neutrophils to Sites of Injury

Leukocytes must be accurately positioned at sites of inflammatory injury to carry out their biological functions. For specific subsets of leukocytes to arrive in a timely fashion, they must receive very specific directions. *Leukocytes are guided through vascular and extravascular spaces by a complex interaction of attractants, repellants, and adhesion molecules.* **Chemotaxis** is the dynamic and energy-dependent process of directed cell migration. Blood leukocytes are recruited by chemoattractants released by endothelial cells. They then migrate from the endothelium towards the target tissue, down a gradient of one chemoattractant in response to a second more distal chemoattractant gradient.

Neutrophils must integrate the various signals to arrive at the correct site at the correct time to perform their assigned tasks. The most important chemotactic factors for PMNs are C5a, bacterial, and mitochondrial products (particularly low-molecular-weight N-formylated peptides such as FMLP), products of arachidonic acid metabolism, (especially LTB_4), products of ECM degradation and, chemokines. The latter represent a key mechanism of leukocyte recruitment because they generate a chemotactic gradient by binding to ECM proteoglycans. As a result, high concentrations of chemokines persist at sites of tissue injury. In turn, specific receptors on migrating leukocytes bind matrix-bound chemokines, moving the cells along the chemotactic gradient to the site of injury.

Chemotactic factors for other cell types, including lymphocytes, basophils, and eosinophils, are also produced at sites of tissue injury and may be secreted by activated endothelial cells, tissue parenchymal cells, or other inflammatory cells. They include PAF, transforming growth factor-β (TGF-β), neutrophilic cationic proteins, and lymphokines. *The cocktail of chemokines presented within a tissue largely determines the type of leukocyte attracted to the site.* Cells arriving at their destination must then be able to stop in the target tissue. Contact guidance, regulated adhesion, or inhibitory signals may determine the final arrest of specific cells in specific tissue locations.

Leukocytes Traverse the Endothelial Cell Barrier to Gain Access to the Tissue

Leukocytes adherent to the vascular endothelium emigrate by **paracellular diapedesis,** i.e., passing between adjacent endothelial cells. Responding to chemokine gradients, neutrophils extend pseudopods and insinuate themselves between the cells and out of the vascular space (Fig. 2-24). Vascular endothelial cells are connected by tight junctions and adherens junctions. CD31 (platelet endothelial cell adhesion molecule [**PECAM-1**]) is expressed on endothelial cell surfaces and binds to itself to keep cells together. These junctions separate under the influence of inflammatory mediators, intracellular signals generated by adhesion molecule engagement and signals from the adherent neutrophils. Neutrophils mobilize elastase to their pseudopod membranes, inducing endothelial cell retraction and separation at the advancing edge of the neutrophil. These cells also induce increases in endothelial cell intracellular calcium, to which they respond by pulling apart.

Neutrophils also migrate through endothelial cells, by **transcellular diapedesis**. Instead of inducing endothelial cell retraction PMNs may squeeze through small circular pores in endothelial cell cytoplasm. In tissues that contain fenestrated microvessels, such as gastrointestinal mucosa and secretory glands, PMNs may traverse thin regions of endothelium, called **fenestrae**, without damaging endothelial cells. In nonfenestrated microvessels, PMNs may cross the endothelium using endothelial cell caveolae or pinocytotic vesicles, which form small, membrane-bound passageways across the cell.

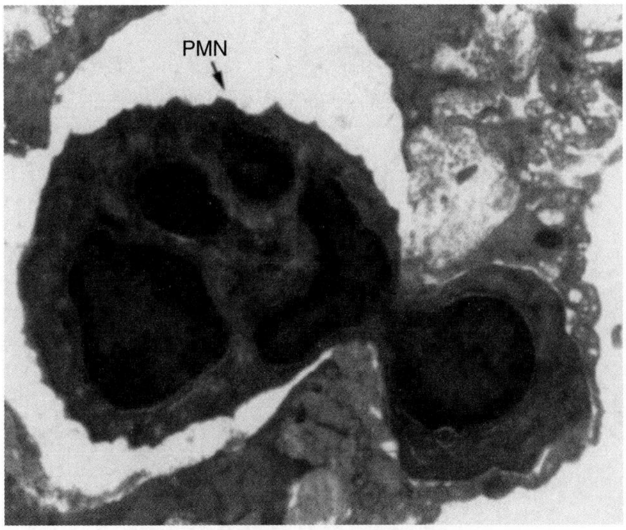

FIGURE 2-24. **Transmission electron micrograph demonstrates neutrophil transmigration.** A neutrophil exits the vascular space by diapedesis across the vascular endothelium. PMN = polymorphonuclear neutrophil.

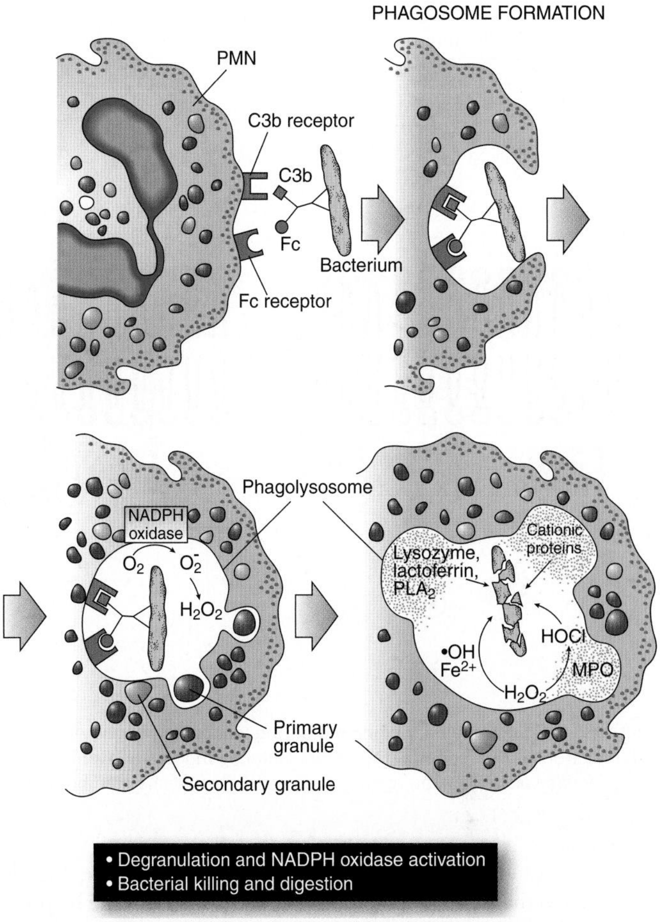

FIGURE 2-25. **Mechanisms of neutrophil bacterial phagocytosis and cell killing.** Opsonins such as C3b coat the surface of microbes allowing recognition by the neutrophil C3b receptor. Receptor clustering triggers intracellular signalling and actin assembly within the neutrophil. Pseudopods form around the microbe to enclose it within a phagosome. Lysosomal granules fuse with the phagosome to form a phagolysosome into which the lysosomal enzymes and oxygen radicals are released to kill and degrade the microbe. Fe^{2+} = ferrous iron; HOCl = hypochlorous acid; MPO = myeloperoxidase; PLA_2 = phospholipase A_2; PMN = polymorphonuclear neutrophil.

Leukocyte Functions in Acute Inflammation

Leukocytes Phagocytose Microorganisms and Tissue Debris

Many inflammatory cells—including monocytes, tissue macrophages, dendritic cells, and neutrophils—recognize, internalize, and digest foreign material, microorganisms, or cellular debris by a process termed **phagocytosis**. This term was first used over a century ago by Elie Metchnikoff and is now defined as ingestion by eukaryotic cells of large (usually $> 0.5\ \mu m$) insoluble particles and microorganisms. The effector cells are **phagocytes**. The complex process involves a sequence of transmembrane and intracellular signaling events.

1. **Recognition:** Phagocytosis is initiated by recognition of particles by specific receptors on the surface of phagocytic cells (Fig. 2-25). Phagocytosis of most biological agents is enhanced by, if not dependent on, their coating (**opsonization**) with plasma components (**opsonins**), particularly immunoglobulins or C3b. Phagocytic cells possess specific opsonic receptors, including those for immunoglobulin Fcγ and complement components. Many pathogens, however, have evolved mechanisms to evade phagocytosis by leukocytes. Polysaccharide capsules, protein A, protein M, or peptidoglycans around bacteria can prevent complement deposition or antigen recognition and receptor binding.
2. **Signaling:** Clumping of opsonins at bacterial surfaces causes phagocyte plasma membrane Fcγ receptors to cluster. Subsequent phosphorylation of immunoreceptor tyrosine-based activation motifs (ITAMs), located in the cytosolic domain or γ subunit of the receptor, trigger intracellular signaling events. Tyrosine kinases that associate with the Fcγ receptor are required for signaling during phagocytosis (Fig. 2-26).
3. **Internalization:** For Fcγ receptor or CR3, actin assembly occurs directly under the phagocytosed target. Polymerized actin filaments push the plasma membrane forward. The plasma membrane remodels to increase surface area and to form pseudopods surrounding the foreign material. The resulting phagocytic cup engulfs the foreign agent. The membrane then "zippers" around the opsonized particle to enclose it in a cytoplasmic vacuole called a **phagosome** (see Figs. 2-25 and 2-26).
4. **Digestion:** The phagosome that contains the foreign material fuses with cytoplasmic lysosomes to form a **phagolysosome**, into which lysosomal enzymes are released. The acid pH within the phagolysosome activates these hydrolytic enzymes, which then degrade the phagocytosed material. Some microorganisms have evolved mechanisms for evading killing by neutrophils by preventing lysosomal degranulation or inhibiting neutrophil enzymes.

Neutrophil Enzymes Are Required for Antimicrobial Defense and Débridement

Although PMNs are critical for degrading microbes and cell debris, they also contribute to tissue injury (Fig. 2-27). PMN release

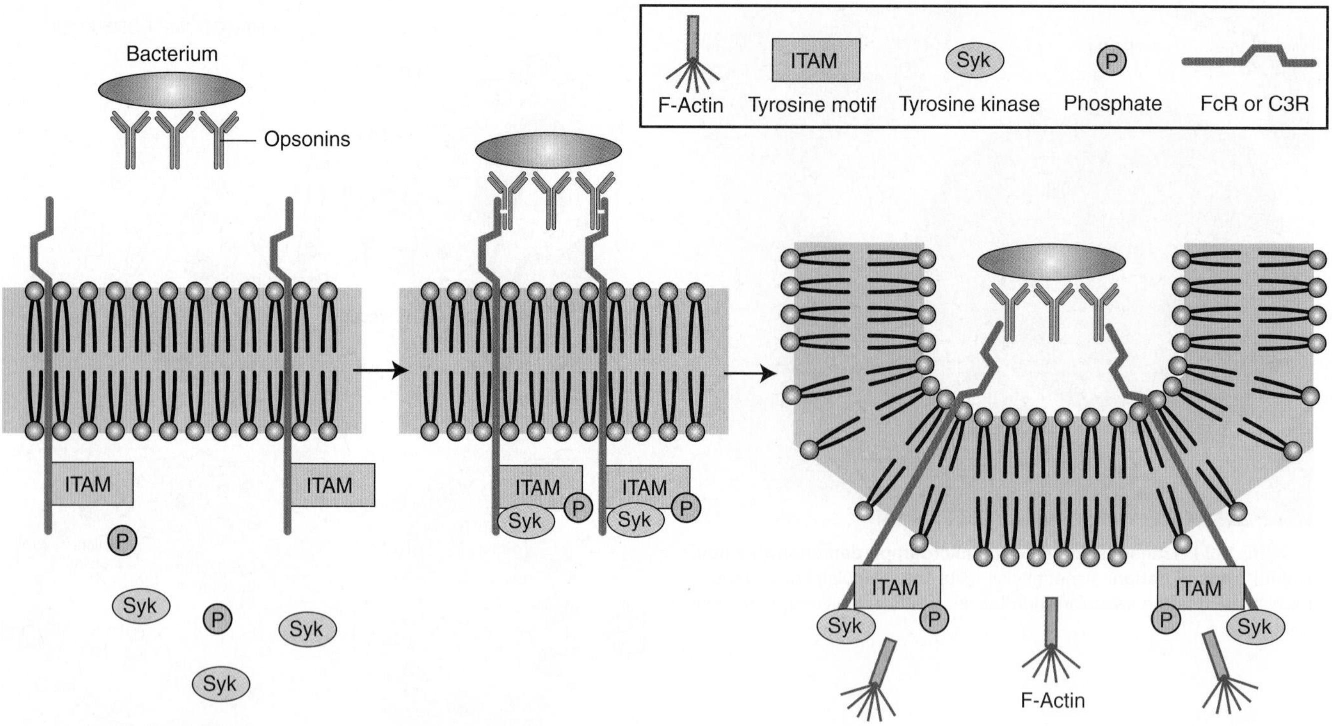

FIGURE 2-26. **Intracellular signaling during leukocyte phagocytosis.** Opsonins coating the surface of microbes or foreign material are recognized by the neutrophil C3b receptor. Receptor clustering triggers phosphorylation of ITAMs on the receptor and tyrosine kinases initiate intracellular signalling. Polymerized actin filament, aggregate beneath the plasma membrane to form a pseudopod to enclose the foreign agent.

of their granule contents at sites of injury is a double-edged sword. On the one hand, débridement of damaged tissue by proteolytic breakdown is beneficial. On the other hand, degradative enzymes can damage endothelial and epithelial cells, as well degrade connective tissue.

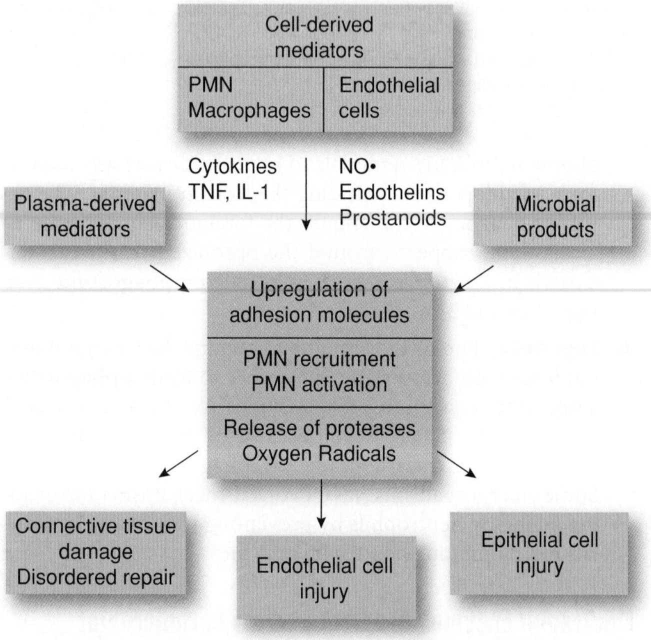

FIGURE 2-27. **Leukocyte-mediated inflammatory injury.** IL = interleukin; LPS = lipopolysaccharide; NO•= nitric oxide; PMN = polymorphonuclear neutrophil; TNF = tumor necrosis factor.

Neutrophil Granules

The armamentarium of enzymes required for degradation of microbes and tissue is generated and contained within PMN cytoplasmic granules. Neutrophil primary, secondary, and tertiary granules are differentiated morphologically and biochemically: each granule has a unique spectrum of enzymes (see Fig. 2-18A).

- **Primary granules (azurophilic granules):** Antimicrobial and proteinase activity of these granules can directly activate other inflammatory cells. Potent acid hydrolases and neutral serine proteases digest a number of macromolecules. Lysozyme and PLA_2 degrade bacterial cell walls and biological membranes and are important in killing bacteria. Myeloperoxidase, a key enzyme in the metabolism of hydrogen peroxide, generates toxic oxygen radicals.
- **Secondary granules (specific granules):** These contain PLA_2, lysozyme, and proteins that initiate killing of specific cells. In addition, their contents include the cationic protein, lactoferrin, a vitamin B_{12}-binding protein and a matrix metalloproteinase (collagenase) specific for type IV collagen.
- **Tertiary granules (small storage granules, C granules):** These granules are released at the leading front of neutrophils during chemotaxis. They are the source of enzymes that promote migration of cells through basement membranes and tissues including proteinases cathepsin, gelatinase, and urokinase-type plasminogen activator (u-PA).

Proteinases

Proteolytic enzymes (proteinases) cleave peptide bonds in polypeptides; they are stored in cytoplasmic granules and secretory vesicles of neutrophils. As these cells emerge from the circulation, they release proteinases that enable them to penetrate the ECM and migrate to sites of injury and there degrade matrix, cell debris, and pathogens. Neutrophils, however, are not the only source of proteinases. These enzymes are also made by most inflammatory cells, including monocytes, eosinophils, basophils, mast cells, and lymphocytes, as well as tissue cells, including vascular endothelial cells.

Proteinases are classified by their catalytic activity into four groups: serine proteinases and metalloproteinases are neutral enzymes that function in extracellular spaces; cysteine proteinases and aspartic proteinases are acidic and act in the acidic milieu of lysosomes (Table 2-3). These enzymes target a variety of intracellular and extracellular proteins, including (1) inflammatory products; (2) debris from damaged cells, microbial proteins, and matrix proteins; (3) microorganisms; (4) plasma proteins, including complement components, clotting factors, immunoglobulins, and cytokines; (5) matrix macromolecules (e.g., collagen, elastin, fibronectin, and laminin); and (6) lymphocytes and platelets.

Serine Proteinases

Serine proteinases degrade extracellular proteins, cell debris and bacteria. Human leukocyte elastase (HLE) is primarily responsible for fibronectin degradation. Cathepsin G (CG) converts angiotensin I to angiotensin II, thereby mediating smooth muscle contraction and vascular permeability. Proteinase 3 (PR3) has antigenic properties related to Wegener granulomatosis. u-PA dissolves fibrin clots to generate plasmin at wound sites, degrades ECM proteins, and activates procollagenases to create a path for leukocyte migration. Although serine proteinases are most important in digesting ECM molecules, they also modify cytokine activity: they solubilize membrane-bound cytokines and receptors by cleaving active cytokines from inactive precursors. They also detach cytokine receptors from cell surfaces, thus regulating cytokine bioactivity.

Metalloproteinases

There are at least 25 members identified (see Chapter 3). Matrix metalloproteinases (**MMPs**, matrixins) degrade all ECM components, including basement membranes. They are subclassified according to substrate specificity into interstitial collagenases, gelatinases, stromelysins, metalloelastases, and matrilysin. Proteins with disintegrin and metalloproteinase domains (ADAMs) regulate neutrophil infiltration by targeting the distintegrins. These molecules are polypeptides that disrupt integrin-mediated binding of cells to each other and to ECM.

TABLE 2-3

Proteinases in Inflammation

Enzyme Class	Examples
Neutral Proteinases	
Serine proteinases	Human leukocyte elastase Cathepsin G Proteinase 3 Urokinase-type plasminogen activator
Metalloproteinase	Collagenases (MMP-1, MMP-8, MMP-13) Gelatinases (MMP-7, MMP-9) Stromelysins (MMP-3, MMP-10, MMP-11) Matrilysin (MMP-7) Metalloelastase (MMP-12) ADAMs-7,-9,-15,-17
Acidic Proteinases	
Cysteine proteinases	Cathepsins, S, L, B, H
Aspartic proteinases	Cathepsin D

MMP: matrix metalloproteinase; ADAM: proteins with *A D*isintegrin and *A M*etalloproteinase domain

Cysteine Proteinases and Aspartic Proteinases

These acid proteinases function primarily within lysosomes of leukocytes to degrade intracellular proteins.

Proteinase Inhibitors

The proteolytic environment is regulated by a battery of inhibitors. During wound healing, these antiproteases protect against damage by limiting protease activity. ECM remodeling occurs in the context of a balance between enzymes and inhibitors. In chronic wounds, continuous influx of neutrophils, with their proteases and ROS, may overwhelm and inactivate these inhibitors, allowing continuation of proteolysis (see Chapter 3). Known proteinase inhibitors include:

- **α_2-Macroglobulin:** Nonspecific inhibitor of all classes of proteinases, primarily found in plasma
- **Serpins:** The major inhibitors of serine proteinases
- **α_1-Antiproteases (α_1-antitrypsin, α_1-antichymotrypsin):** Inhibit human leukocyte elastase and cathepsin G
- **Secretory leukocyte proteinase inhibitor (SLPI), Elafin:** Inhibit proteinase 3
- **Plasminogen activator inhibitors (PAIs):** Inhibit u-PA
- **Tissue inhibitors of metalloproteinases (TIMP-1,-2,-3, -4):** Specific for matrix metalloproteinases in tissue

Inflammatory Cells Have Oxidative and Nonoxidative Bactericidal Activity

The bactericidal activity of PMNs and macrophages is mediated in part by production of ROS and in part by oxygen-independent mechanisms.

Bacterial Killing by Oxygen Species

Phagocytosis is accompanied by metabolic reactions in inflammatory cells that lead to production of several oxygen metabolites (see Chapter 1). These products are more reactive than oxygen itself and contribute to the killing of ingested bacteria (see Fig. 2-25).

- **Superoxide anion** (O_2^-): Phagocytosis activates a NADPH oxidase in PMN cell membranes. NADPH oxidase is a multicomponent electron transport complex that reduces molecular oxygen to O_2^-. Activation of this enzyme is enhanced by prior exposure of cells to a chemotactic stimulus or LPS. NADPH oxidase activation increases oxygen consumption and stimulates the hexose monophosphate shunt. Together, these cell responses are referred to as the **respiratory burst**.
- **Hydrogen peroxide** (H_2O_2): O_2^- is rapidly converted to H_2O_2 by superoxide dismutase at the cell surface and in phagolysosomes. H_2O_2 is stable and serves as a substrate for generating additional reactive oxidants.
- **Hypochlorous acid** (HOCl): Myeloperoxidase (MPO), a neutrophil product with a very strong cationic charge, is secreted from granules during exocytosis and, in the presence

of a halide, usually chlorine, catalyzes conversion of H_2O_2 to HOCl. This powerful oxidant is a major bactericidal agent produced by phagocytic cells. HOCl also participates in activating neutrophil-derived collagenase and gelatinase, both of which are secreted as latent enzymes. HOCl also inactivates α_1-antitrypsin.

- **Hydroxyl radical** (•OH): Reduction of H_2O_2 occurs via the Haber-Weiss reaction to form the highly reactive •OH. This reaction occurs slowly at physiological pH, but in the presence of ferrous iron (Fe^{2+}) the Fenton reaction rapidly converts H_2O_2 to •OH, a radical with potent bactericidal activity. Further reduction of •OH leads to formation of H_2O (see Chapter 1).
- **Nitric oxide** (NO•): Phagocytic cells and vascular endothelial cells produce NO• and its derivatives, which have diverse effects, both physiological and nonphysiological. NO• and other oxygen radical species interact with one another to balance their cytotoxic and cytoprotective effects. NO• can react with oxygen radicals to form toxic molecules such as peroxynitrite and *S*-nitrosothiols, or it can scavenge O_2^-, thereby reducing the amount of toxic radicals.

Monocytes, macrophages and eosinophils also produce oxygen radicals, depending on their state of activation and the stimulus to which they are exposed. Production of ROS by these cells contributes to their bactericidal and fungicidal activity, and their ability to kill certain parasites. The importance of oxygen-dependent mechanisms in bacterial killing is exemplified in **chronic granulomatous disease** of childhood. In this hereditary deficiency of NADPH oxidase, failure to produce O_2^- and H_2O_2 during phagocytosis makes these persons susceptible to recurrent infections, especially with gram-positive cocci. Patients with a related genetic deficiency in MPO cannot produce HOCl, and show increased susceptibility to infections with the fungal pathogen *Candida* (Table 2-4).

TABLE 2-4

Congenital Diseases of Defective Phagocytic Cell Function Characterized by Recurrent Bacterial Infections

Disease	Defect
Leukocyte adhesion deficiency (LAD)	LAD-1 defective β_2-integrin expression or function (CD11/CD18) LAD-2 (defective fucosylation, selectin binding)
Hyper-IgE-recurrent infection, (Job) syndrome	Poor chemotaxis
Chediak-Higashi syndrome	Defective lysosomal granules, poor chemotaxis
Neutrophil-specific granule deficiency	Absent neutrophil granules
Chronic granulomatous disease	Deficient NADPH oxidase, with absent H_2O_2 production
Myeloperoxidase deficiency	Deficient HOCl production

H_2O_2 = hydrogen peroxide; HOCl = hypochlorous acid; Ig = immunoglobulin.

Nonoxidative Bacterial Killing

Phagocytes, particularly PMNs and monocytes/macrophages, have substantial antimicrobial activity which is oxygen-independent. This activity mainly involves preformed bactericidal proteins in cytoplasmic granules. These include lysosomal acid hydrolases and specialized noncatalytic proteins unique to inflammatory cells.

- **Lysosomal hydrolases:** Neutrophil primary and secondary granules, and lysosomes of mononuclear phagocytes contain hydrolases, including sulfatases and phosphatases, and other enzymes capable of digesting polysaccharides and DNA.
- **Bactericidal/permeability-increasing protein (BPI):** This cationic protein in PMN primary granules can kill many gram-negative bacteria but is not toxic to gram-positive bacteria or to eukaryotic cells. BPI inserts into the outer membrane of bacterial envelopes and increases its permeability. Activation of certain phospholipases and enzymes then degrades bacterial peptidylglycans.
- **Defensins:** Primary granules of PMNs and lysosomes of some mononuclear phagocytes contain this family of cationic proteins, which kill a extensive variety of gram-positive and gram-negative bacteria, fungi, and some enveloped viruses. Some of these polypeptides also can also kill host cells. Defensins are chemotactic for phagocytic leukocytes, immature dendritic cells, and lymphocytes, so they help to mobilize and amplify antimicrobial immunity.
- **Lactoferrin:** Lactoferrin is an iron-binding glycoprotein found in the secondary granules of neutrophils, and in most body secretory fluids. Its iron-chelating capacity allows it to compete with bacteria for iron. It may also facilitate oxidative killing of bacteria by enhancing •OH formation.
- **Lysozyme:** This bactericidal enzyme is found in many tissues and body fluids, in primary and secondary granules of neutrophils and in lysosomes of mononuclear phagocytes. Peptidoglycans of gram-positive bacterial cell walls are exquisitely sensitive to degradation by lysozyme; gram-negative bacteria are usually resistant to it.
- **Bactericidal proteins of eosinophils:** Eosinophils contain several granule-bound cationic proteins, the most important of which are major basic protein (MBP) and eosinophilic cationic protein. MBP accounts for about half of the total protein of the eosinophil granule. Both proteins are ineffective against bacteria but are potent cytotoxic agents for many parasites.

Defects in Leukocyte Function

The importance of protection afforded by acute inflammatory cells is emphasized by the frequency and severity of infections when PMNs are greatly decreased or defective. *The most common such deficit is iatrogenic neutropenia resulting from cancer chemotherapy.* Functional impairment of phagocytes may occur at any step in the sequence: adherence, emigration, chemotaxis, or phagocytosis. These disorders may be acquired or congenital. Acquired diseases, such as leukemia, diabetes mellitus, malnutrition, viral infections, and sepsis, are often accompanied by defects in inflammatory cell function. Table 2-4 shows representative examples of congenital diseases linked to defective phagocytic function.

REGULATION OF INFLAMMATION

Plasma- and cell-derived proinflammatory mediators described above amplify tissue responses and represent a positive feedback loop, with progressive amplification of the response and subsequent tissue injury. Left unchecked, this intense inflammatory injury leads to organ failure. Complement factors, proinflammatory cytokines, and in some cases, immune complexes, activate signal transduction pathways that control gene expression of proinflammatory mediators, including TNF-α, IL-1, chemokines, and adhesion molecules. Secreted cytokines then propagate the response by activating other cell types using these and similar pathways.

While the response of cells and tissues is primarily proinflammatory, endogenous mediators control the extent of inflammatory injury by negative feedback inhibition of proinflammatory gene transcription, thereby preventing uncontrolled inflammation. Particularly important endogenous regulators of inflammation include:

- **Cytokines:** IL-6, IL-10, IL-11, IL-12, and IL-13 limit inflammation by reducing production of the powerful proinflammatory cytokine, TNF-α. In some instances, this effect occurs by preventing degradation of IκB (the NFκB inhibitor), thereby inhibiting cell activation and further release of inflammatory mediators.
- **Protease inhibitors:** SLPI and TIMP-2 are particularly important in reducing the responses of a variety of cell types, including macrophages and endothelial cells, and in decreasing connective tissue damage.
- **Lipoxins:** Lipoxins and aspirin-triggered lipoxins are anti-inflammatory lipid mediators that inhibit leukotriene biosynthesis.
- **Glucocorticoids:** Stimulation of the hypothalamic-pituitary-adrenal axis leads to release of immunosuppressive glucocorticoids. These have transcriptional and post-transcriptional suppressive effects on inflammatory response genes.
- **Kininases:** Kininases in plasma and blood degrade the potent proinflammatory mediator bradykinin.
- **Phosphatases:** One of the most common mechanisms used in signal transduction to regulate inflammatory cell signaling is rapid and reversible protein phosphorylation. Phosphatases and associated regulatory proteins provide a balancing, dephosphorylating system.

Common Intracellular Pathways Are Associated with Inflammatory Cell Activation

The process by which diverse stimuli lead to the functional responses of inflammatory cells is referred to as **stimulus–response coupling**. Stimuli can include microbial products and the many plasma- or cell-derived inflammatory mediators described in this chapter. Although intracellular signaling pathways are complex and vary with cell type and stimulus, some common intracellular pathways are associated with inflammatory cell activation, including G protein, TNF receptor (TNFR), and JAK-STAT pathways (Figs. 2-28, 2-29, 2-30, respectively)

G PROTEIN PATHWAYS: Many chemokines, hormones, neurotransmitters, and other inflammatory mediators signal via guanine nucleotide-binding (G) proteins. G proteins vary in their

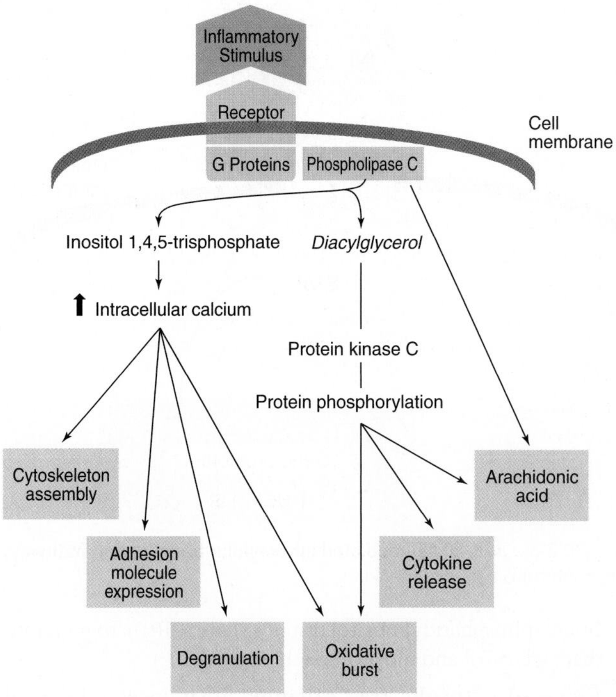

FIGURE 2-28. **G-protein–mediated intracellular signal transduction pathway common to many inflammatory stimuli.**

intracellular connections, but common activities include (see Fig. 2-28):

- **Ligand–receptor binding:** Binding of a stimulatory factor to a specific cell membrane receptor creates a ligand–receptor complex. Exchange of guanosine diphosphate (GDP) for guanosine triphosphate (GTP) activates the G protein, which dissociates into subunits that, in turn, activate phospholipase C and phosphatidylinositol-3-kinase (PI-3-kinase).
- **Phospholipid metabolism of cell membranes:** Phospholipase C hydrolyzes a phosphoinositide in the plasma mem-

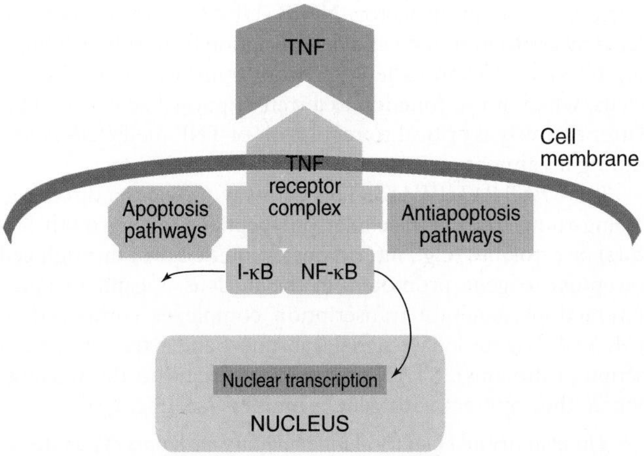

FIGURE 2-29. **TNF receptor-mediated intracellular signal transduction pathway.** TNF = tumor necrosis factor

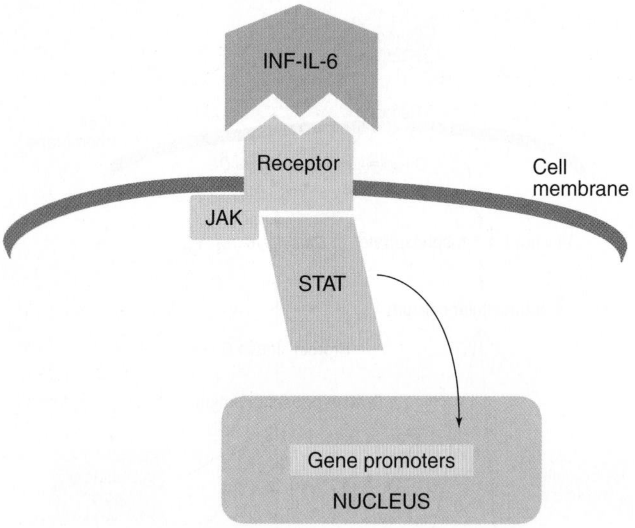

FIGURE 2-30. **JAK-STAT–mediated intracellular transduction pathway.** INF = interferon; IL – interleukin.

brane (phosphatidylinositol bisphosphate [PIP_2]), to generate diacylglycerol and inositol trisphosphate (IP_3).

- **Elevated cytosolic free calcium:** IP_3 induces release of stored intracellular calcium. In conjunction with an influx of calcium ions from the extracellular environment, IP_3 increases cytosolic free calcium, a key event in inflammatory cell activation.
- **Protein phosphorylation and dephosphorylation:** Specific tyrosine kinases bind the ligand–receptor complex and initiate a series of protein phosphorylations.
- **Protein kinase C activation:** Protein kinase C and other protein kinases activate several intracellular signaling pathways, often leading to gene transcription.

TNFR PATHWAYS: TNF is central to the development of inflammation and its symptoms. It also induces tumor cell apoptosis and regulates immune functions (see Fig. 2-29). TNF and related proteins interact with two cell surface receptors to form a multiprotein-signaling complex at the cell membrane. This complex can trigger (1) apoptosis-related enzymes, **caspases** (see Chapter 1) ; (2) inhibitors of apoptosis; or (3) activation of a nuclear transcription factor, **NFκB**. NFκB activation is regulated by association with and disassociation from IκB. IκB binding to NFκB prevents the latter from translocating to the nucleus, where it can function as a transcriptional activator. This latter pathway is critical to regulation of TNF-mediated events during inflammation.

JAK-STAT PATHWAYS: This pathway provides a direct signaling route from extracellular polypeptides (e.g., growth factors) or cytokines (e.g., interferons or interleukins) through cell receptors to gene promoters in the nucleus. Ligand–receptor interactions generate transcription complexes composed of JAK-STAT (Janus kinase-signal transducer and activator of transcription proteins). STAT proteins translocate to the nucleus, where they interact with gene promoters (see Fig. 2-30).

The quantity and quality of inflammatory mediators affects the responses to invading microbes, allergens, or foreign proteins. Regulation occurs at each step of the signal transduction pathways described above, including receptor expression, transcription, and post-transcriptional events.

TRANSCRIPTIONAL CONTROL: Gene promoters for induction of chemokines, adhesion molecules, COX-2, NOS, and collagenase may bind NFκB, AP-1, C/EBP (CAAT/enhancer-binding protein), and ETS transcriptional activators.

POST-TRANSCRIPTIONAL REGULATION: Alterations in mRNA stability have been implicated in suppression of translation of mediators such as TNF-α.

The outcome of these signaling mechanisms and gene transcription is induction or enhancement of specific functional responses, including phagocytosis, degranulation, cell and platelet aggregation, oxidant production, adhesion molecule expression, and cytokine production. Genetics, as well as sex and age of a patient, determines the variable response to injury and in particular, the progression to chronic inflammatory disease. An understanding of inflammatory cell stimulation and regulation provides the basis for new strategies for therapeutic manipulation of both beneficial and harmful inflammatory processes.

Outcomes of Acute Inflammation

As a result of regulatory components and the short life span of neutrophils, acute inflammatory reactions are usually self-limiting and resolve. Resolution involves removal of dead cells, clearance of acute response cells, and reestablishment of the stroma. However inflammatory responses can lead to other outcomes:

- **Resolution:** Under ideal conditions the source of tissue injury is eliminated, inflammation resolves, and normal tissue architecture and physiological function are restored. The progression of inflammation depends on the balance of cell recruitment, cell division, cell emigration, and cell death. For tissue to return to normal, this process must be reversed: the stimulus to injury removed, proinflammatory signals turned off, acute inflammatory cell influx ended, tissue fluid balance restored, cell and tissue debris removed, normal vascular function restored, epithelial barriers repaired, and the ECM regenerated. As signals for acute inflammation wane, PMN apoptosis limits the immune response and resolution begins.
- **Scar:** If a tissue is irreversibly injured, normal architecture is often replaced by a scar, despite elimination of the initial pathological insult (see Chapter 3).
- **Abscess:** If the area of acute inflammation is walled off by inflammatory cells and fibrosis, PMN products destroy the tissue, forming an abscess.
- **Lymphadenitis:** Localized acute inflammation and chronic inflammation may cause secondary inflammation of lymphatic channels (**lymphangitis**) and lymph nodes (**lymphadenitis**). The inflamed lymphatic channels in the skin appear as red streaks, and the lymph nodes are enlarged and painful. Microscopically, the lymph nodes show lymphoid follicle hyperplasias and proliferation of mononuclear phagocytes in the sinuses (sinus histiocytosis).
- **Persistent inflammation:** Failure to eliminate a pathological insult or inability to trigger resolution results in a persistent inflammatory reaction. This may be evident as a prolonged acute response, with continued influx of neutrophils and tissue destruction, or more commonly as chronic inflammation.

Chronic Inflammation

When acute inflammation does not resolve or becomes disordered, chronic inflammation occurs. Inflammatory cells persist, stroma responds by becoming hyperplastic, and tissue destruction and scarring lead to organ dysfunction. This process may be localized, but more commonly progresses to disabling diseases such as chronic lung disease, rheumatoid arthritis, asthma, ulcerative colitis, granulomatous diseases, autoimmune diseases, and chronic dermatitis. Acute and chronic inflammation are ends of a dynamic continuum with overlapping morphological features: (1) inflammation with continued recruitment of chronic inflammatory cells is followed by (2) tissue injury due to prolongation of the inflammatory response, and (3) an often disordered attempt to restore tissue integrity. The events leading to an amplified inflammatory response resemble those of acute inflammation in a number of aspects:

- **Specific triggers,** microbial products or injury, initiate the response.
- **Chemical mediators** direct recruitment, activation, and interaction of inflammatory cells. Activation of coagulation and complement cascades generate small peptides that function to prolong the inflammatory response. Cytokines, specifically IL-6 and RANTES, regulate a switch in chemokines, such that mononuclear cells are directed to the site. Other cytokines (e.g., IFN-γ) then promote macrophage proliferation and activation.
- **Inflammatory cells** are recruited from the blood. Interactions between lymphocytes, macrophages, dendritic cells, and fibroblasts generate antigen-specific responses.
- **Stromal cell activation and extracellular matrix** remodeling occur, both of which affect the cellular immune response. Varying degrees of fibrosis may result, depending on the extent of tissue injury and persistence of the pathological stimulus and inflammatory response.

Chronic inflammation is not synonymous with chronic infection, but if the inflammatory response cannot eliminate an injurious agent, infection may persist. Chronic inflammation does not necessarily require infection: it may follow an acute inflammatory or immune response to a foreign antigen. Signals that result in an extended response include:

- **Bacteria, viruses, and parasites:** These agents can provide signals to support persistence of the inflammatory response, which in this case may be directed towards isolating the invader from the host.
- **Trauma:** Extensive tissue damage releases mediators capable of inducing an extended inflammatory response.
- **Cancer:** Chronic inflammatory cells, especially macrophages and T lymphocytes, may be the morphological expression of an immune response to malignant cells. Chemotherapy may suppress normal inflammatory responses, increasing susceptibility to infection.
- **Immune factors:** Many autoimmune diseases, including rheumatoid arthritis, chronic thyroiditis, and primary biliary cirrhosis, are characterized by chronic inflammatory responses in affected tissues. This may be associated with activation of antibody-dependent and cell-mediated immune mechanisms (see Chapter 4). Such autoimmune responses may account for injury in affected organs.

Cells Involved in Chronic Inflammation

The cellular components of chronic inflammatory responses are recruited from the circulation (macrophages, lymphocytes, plasma cells, dendritic cells, and eosinophils) and affected tissues (fibroblasts, vascular endothelial cells).

Monocyte/Macrophages

Activated macrophages and their cytokines are central to initiating inflammation and prolonging responses that lead to chronic inflammation. (see Fig. 2-18C). Macrophages produce inflammatory and immunological mediators, and regulate reactions leading to chronic inflammation. They also regulate lymphocyte responses to antigens and secrete other mediators that modulate fibroblast and endothelial cell proliferation and activities

The **mononuclear phagocyte system** includes promonocytes and their precursors in the bone marrow, blood monocytes, and different types of histiocytes and macrophages, particularly Kupffer cells. Under the influence of chemotactic stimuli, IFN-γ (interferon-γ) and bacterial endotoxins, resident tissue macrophages are activated and proliferate, while circulating monocytes are recruited and differentiate into tissue macrophages (Fig. 2-31).

Within different tissues, resident macrophages differ in their armamentarium of enzymes and can respond to local inflammatory signals. Blood monocyte granules contain serine proteinases like those found in neutrophils. Circulating monocytes synthesize additional enzymes, particularly MMPs. When monocytes enter tissue and further differentiate into macrophages, they acquire the ability to generate additional MMPs and cysteine proteinases but lose the ability to produce serine proteinases. The activity of these enzymes is central to the tissue destruction in chronic inflammation. In emphysema, for example, resident macrophages generate proteinases, particularly MMPs with elastolytic activity, which destroy alveolar walls and recruit blood monocytes into the lung. Other macrophage products include oxygen metabolites, chemotactic factors, cytokines, and growth factors

Lymphocytes

Naïve lymphocytes home to secondary lymphoid organs, where they encounter antigen-presenting cells and become antigen-specific lymphocytes. Plasma cells and T cells leaving secondary lymphoid organs circulate in the vascular system and are recruited into peripheral tissues.

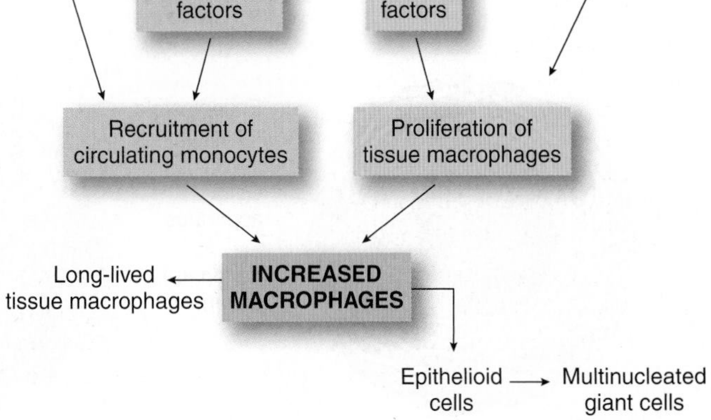

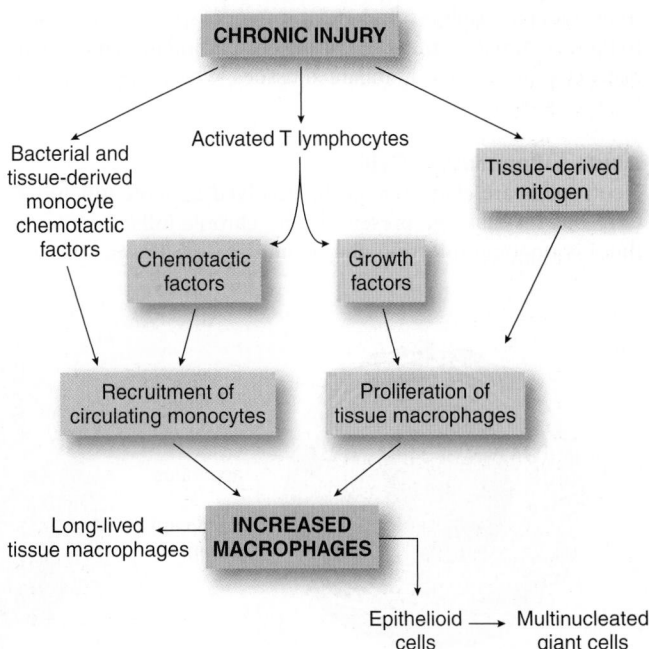

FIGURE 2-31. Accumulation of macrophages in chronic inflammation.

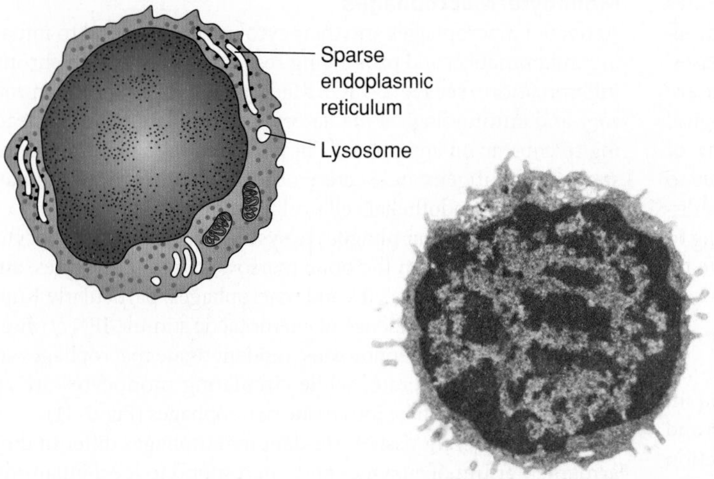

CHARACTERISTICS AND FUNCTIONS

- Associated with chronic inflammation
- Key cells in humoral and cell-mediated immune responses
- Cytokine production
- Multiple subtypes:

B cell ⟶ Plasma cell ⟶ Antibody production

T cell ⟶ Effector cells ⟶ Delayed hypersensitivity; Mixed lymphocyte reactivity; Cytotoxic "killer" cells (K-cells)

T cell ⟶ Regulatory cells ⟶ Helper T cells; Suppressor T cells

Cytotoxic natural killer (NK) cell

Null cell

FIGURE 2-32. **Lymphocyte: Morphology and function.**

T-cells regulate macrophage activation and recruitment by secreting specific mediators (lymphokines), modulate antibody production and cell-mediated cytotoxicity, and maintain immunologic memory (Fig. 2-32). NK cells, as well as other lymphocyte subtypes, help defend against viral and bacterial infections.

Plasma Cells

Plasma cells are rich in rough endoplasmic reticulum and are the primary source of antibodies (Fig. 2-33). The production of antibody to specific antigens at sites of chronic inflammation is important in antigen neutralization, clearance of foreign antigens, and particles and antibody-dependent cell-mediated cytotoxicity (see Chapter 4).

Dendritic Cells

Dendritic cells are professional antigen-presenting cells that trigger immune responses to antigens (see Chapter 4). They phagocytose antigens and migrate to lymph nodes, where they present those antigens. Recognition of antigen and other costimulatory molecules by T cells results in recruitment of specific cell subsets to the inflammatory process. During chronic inflammation, dendritic cells are present in inflamed tissues, where they help prolong responses.

Acute Inflammatory Cells

Neutrophils are characteristically involved in acute inflammation, but may also be present during chronic inflammation, if there is ongoing infection and tissue damage. Eosinophils are particularly prominent in allergic-type reactions and parasitic infestations.

Fibroblasts

Fibroblasts are long-lived, ubiquitous cells whose chief function is to produce components of the ECM (Fig. 2-34). They are derived from mesoderm or neural crest and can differentiate into other connective tissue cells, including chondrocytes, adipocytes, osteocytes, and smooth muscle cells. Fibroblasts are the construction workers of the tissue, rebuilding the scaffolding of ECM upon which tissue is reestablished.

Fibroblasts not only respond to immune signals that induce their proliferation and activation but are also active players in the immune response. They interact with inflammatory cells, particularly lymphocytes, via surface molecules and receptors on both cells. For example, when CD40 on fibroblasts binds its ligand on lymphocytes, both cells are activated. Activated fibroblasts produce cytokines, chemokines, and prostanoids, creating a tissue microenvironment that further regulates the behavior of inflammatory cells in the damaged tissue. (Fibroblast function in wound healing is discussed more fully in Chapter 3.

Injury and Repair in Chronic Inflammation

Chronic inflammation is mediated by both immunological and nonimmunological mechanisms, and is frequently observed in conjunction with reparative responses, namely, granulation tissue and fibrosis.

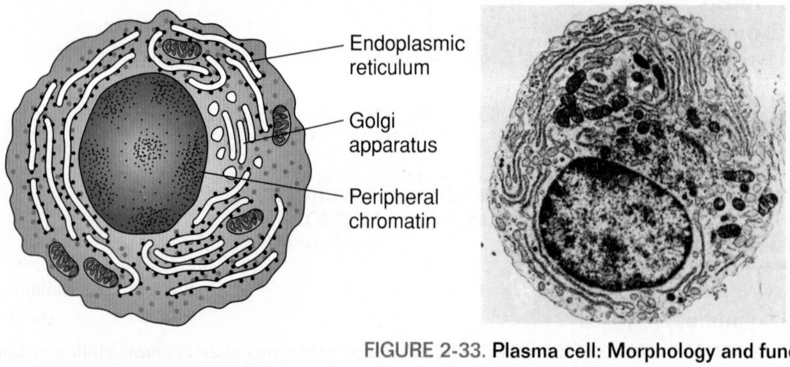

CHARACTERISTICS AND FUNCTIONS

- Associated with:
  - -antibody synthesis and secretion
  - -chronic inflammation
- Derived from B lymphocytes

FIGURE 2-33. **Plasma cell: Morphology and function.**

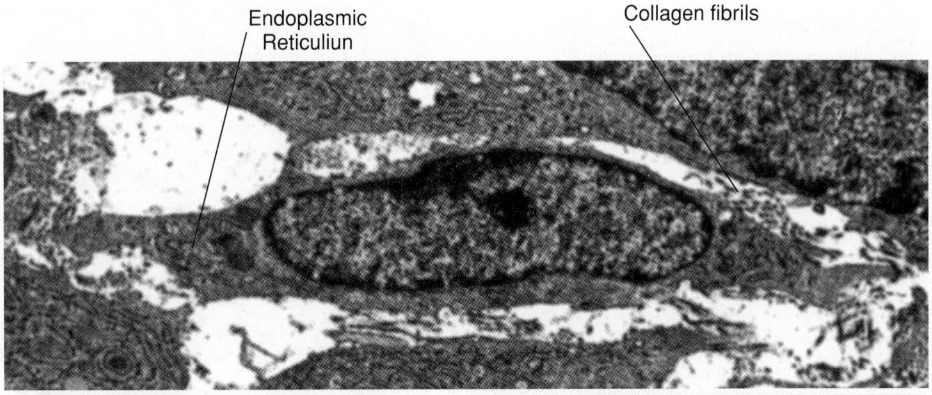

CHARACTERISTICS AND FUNCTIONS	PRIMARY INFLAMMATORY MEDIATORS	
• Produce extracellular matrix proteins	• IL-6	• PGE_2
• Mediate chronic inflammation and wound healing	• IL-8	• CD40 expression
	• Cyclooxygenase-2	• Matricellular proteins
	• Hyaluronan	• Extracellular proteins

FIGURE 2-34. **Fibroblast: Morphology and function.** IL = interleukin.

An Extended Inflammatory Response may Lead to Persistent Injury

The primary role of neutrophils in inflammation is host defense and débridement of damaged tissue. The neutrophil response, however, is a double-edged sword: neutrophil products protect the host by participating in antimicrobial defense and débridement of damaged tissue; however, these same products may prolong tissue damage and promote chronic inflammation if they are not appropriately regulated. Neutrophil enzymes are beneficial when they are digesting phagocytosed organisms intracellularly, but can be destructive if they are released extracellularly. Thus, when neutrophils accumulate connective tissue may be digested by their enzymes.

Persistent tissue injury produced by inflammatory cells is important in the pathogenesis of several diseases, for instance, pulmonary emphysema, rheumatoid arthritis, certain immune complex diseases, gout, and adult respiratory distress syndrome. Phagocytic cell adherence, escape of reactive oxygen metabolites and release of lysosomal enzymes together enhance cytotoxicity and tissue degradation. Proteinase activity is significantly elevated in chronic wounds, creating a proteolytic environment that prevents healing.

Altered Repair Mechanisms Prevent Resolution

Repair processes initiated as part of the inflammation can restore normal architecture and function. Early reparative efforts mimic wound healing. However, when inflammation is prolonged or exaggerated, repair is incompletely effective and altered tissue architecture and tissue dysfunction result. These might include:

- Ongoing proliferation of epithelial cells can result in **metaplasia**. For example, goblet cell metaplasia characterizes the airways of smokers and asthmatics.
- Fibroblast proliferation and activation results in increased ECM. Because ECM components such as collagen now occupy space normally devoted to tissue cells, organ function is altered (see Chapter. 3).
- The ECM may be abnormal. Degradation and production of the matrix change the normal mix of extracellular proteins. For example, elastin degradation plays an important role in development of emphysema.
- Altered ECM (e.g., fibronectin) can be a chemoattractant for inflammatory cells and present an altered scaffolding to cells.

Granulomatous Inflammation

Neutrophils ordinarily remove agents that incite an acute inflammatory response. However, there are circumstances in which reactive neutrophils cannot digest the substances that provoke acute inflammation. Such a situation is potentially dangerous, because it can lead to a vicious circle of (1) phagocytosis, (2) failure of digestion, (3) death of the neutrophil, (4) release of the undigested provoking agent, and (5) re-phagocytosis by a newly recruited neutrophil (Fig. 2-35). *Granuloma formation is a protective response to chronic infection (fungal infections, tuberculosis, leprosy, schistosomiasis) or the presence of foreign material (e.g., suture or talc), preventing dissemination and restricting inflammation, thereby protecting the host tissues.* Some autoimmune diseases are also associated with granulomas, diseases such as rheumatoid arthritis and Crohn's disease In some cases such as sarcoidosis, no inciting agent has yet been identified.

The principal cells involved in granulomatous inflammation are macrophages and lymphocytes (Fig. 2-36). Macrophages are mobile cells that continuously migrate through the extravascular connective tissues. After amassing substances that they cannot digest, macrophages lose their motility, accumulate at the site of injury, and undergo transform themselves into nodular collections of pale, epithelioid cells: the **granuloma**. Multinucleated giant cells are formed by the cytoplasmic fusion of macrophages. When the nuclei of such giant cells are arranged around the periphery of the cell in a horseshoe pattern, the cell is called a **Langhans giant cell** (Fig. 2-37). Frequently, a foreign agent (e.g., silica or a *Histoplasma* spore) or other indigestible material is identified within the cytoplasm of a multinucleated giant cell, in which case the term **foreign body giant cell** is used (Fig. 2-38). Foreign body giant cells tend to have more centrally situated nuclei. Granulomas are further classified histopathologically by the presence or absence of necrosis. Certain infectious

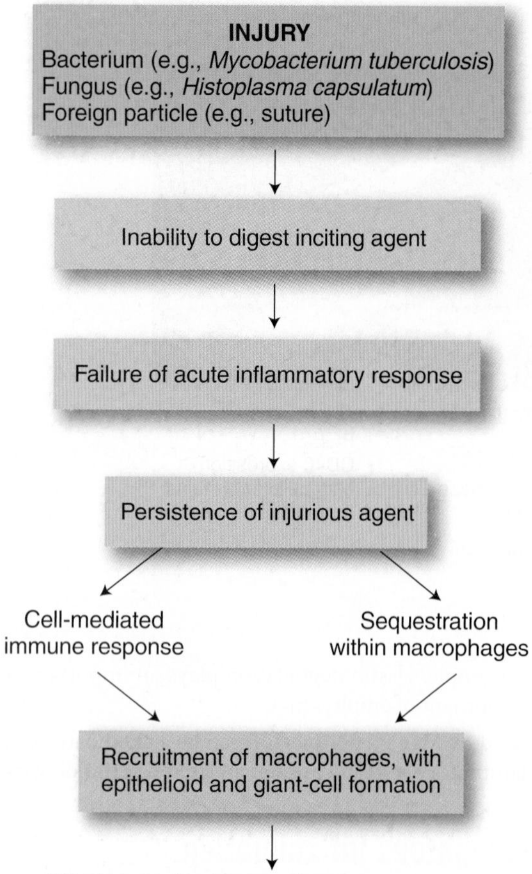

FIGURE 2-35. **Mechanism of granuloma formation.**

agents such as *Mycobacterium tuberculosis* characteristically produce necrotizing granulomas, the centers of which are filled with an amorphous mixture of debris and dead microorganisms and cells. Other diseases such as sarcoidosis are characterized by granulomas that lack necrosis.

Immune granulomas, formed during delayed type hypersensitivity responses contain activated T cells and macrophages, which initiate granuloma formation. CD4+ T cells then recruit and organize cells at the site using CXCL chemokines to develop

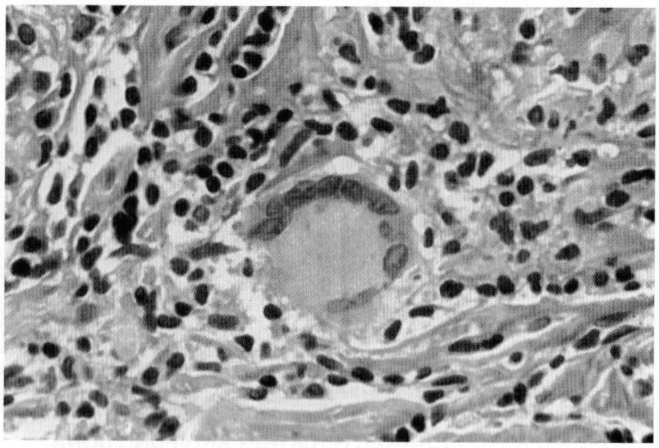

FIGURE 2-37. **A Langhans giant cell shows nuclei arranged on the periphery of an abundant cytoplasm.**

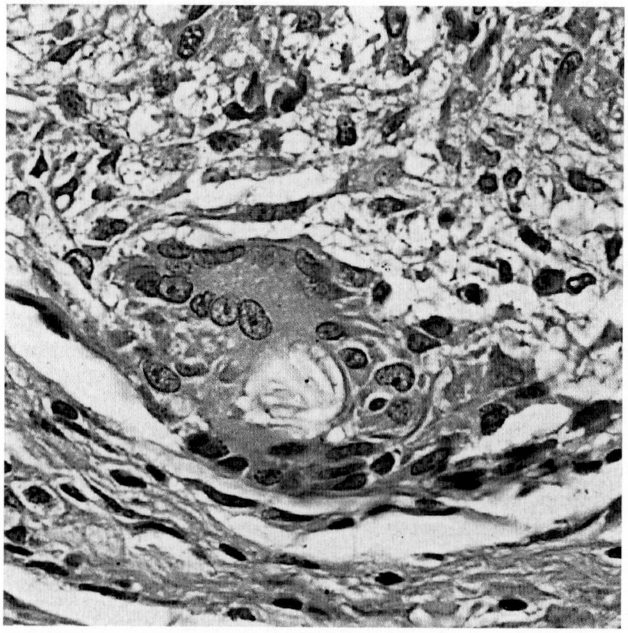

FIGURE 2-38. **A foreign body giant cell has numerous nuclei randomly arranged in the cytoplasm.**

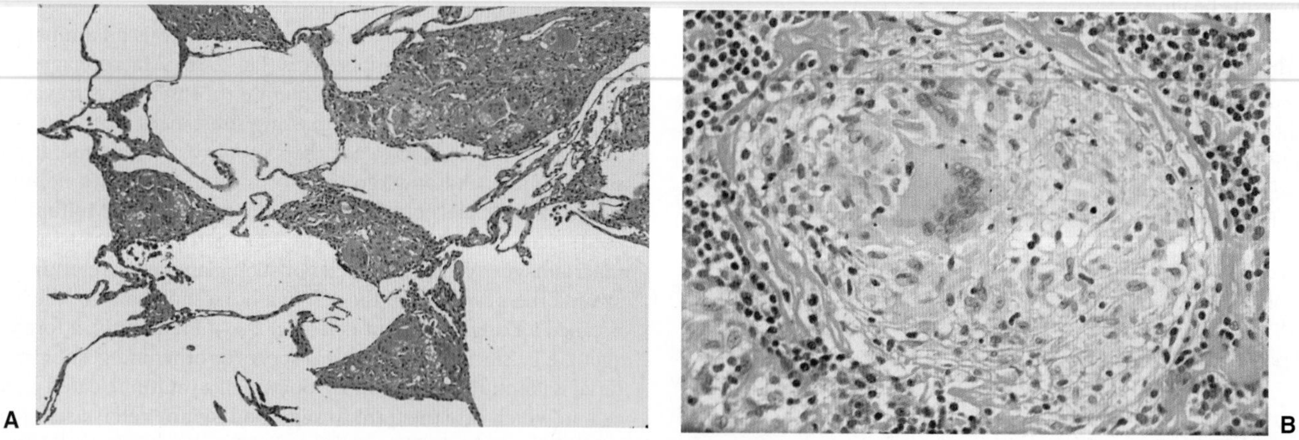

FIGURE 2-36. **Granulomatous inflammation. A.** Section of lung from a patient with sarcoidosis reveals numerous discrete granulomas. **B.** A higher-power photomicrograph of a single granuloma in a lymph node from the same patient depicts a multinucleated giant cell amid numerous pale epithelioid cells. A thin rim of fibrosis separates the granuloma from the lymphoid cells of the node.

Th1 type granulomas and CCL chemokines to develop Th2 type granulomas. Several T cell cytokines stimulate macrophage function (e.g., IFN-γ), whereas others inhibit macrophage activation (e.g., IL-4, IL-10). Thus, lymphocytes are vital for regulating development and resolution of inflammatory responses.

The fate of a granulomatous reaction depends on the toxicity and immunogenicity of the inciting agent. Cell-mediated immune responses to an inciting agent may modify a granulomatous reaction by recruiting and activating more macrophages and lymphocytes. Finally, under the influence of T cell cytokines such as IL-13 and TGFβ, the granuloma burns out and becomes a fibrotic nodule.

Chronic Inflammation and Malignancy

Several chronic infectious diseases are associated with development of malignancies. For example, schistosomiasis of the urinary bladder leads to cancer of that organ. Inflammation that is not specifically linked to infection may also be a risk factor for cancer. Patients with reflux esophagitis or ulcerative colitis are at higher risk for cancer in those organs. The environment created by chronic inflammation promotes malignant transformation by a number of mechanisms (see also Chapter 5):

- **Increased cell proliferation:** Chronically stimulated cell division increases the likelihood of transforming mutations in the proliferating cells
- **Oxygen and NO• metabolites:** Inflammatory metabolites, such as nitrosamines, may cause genomic damage.
- **Chronic immune activation:** Chronic antigen exposure induces an altered cytokine profile, suppressing cell-mediated immune responses and creating an environment permissive for malignant growth.
- **Angiogenesis:** Growth of new vessels is associated with inflammation and wound healing and is required for maintenance of neoplastic lesions.
- **Inhibition of apoptosis:** Chronic inflammation suppresses apoptosis. Increased cell division and decreased apoptosis facilitate survival and expansion of mutated cell populations.

Systemic Manifestations of Inflammation

An effective inflammatory response will: (1) confine the area of injury, (2) clear the inciting pathological agent and damaged tissue, and (3) restore tissue function. However, under certain conditions, local injury may result in prominent systemic effects that can themselves be debilitating. These effects often result when a pathogen enters the bloodstream, a condition known as **sepsis**. Cytokines—including IL-1α, IL-1β, TNF-α, IL-6—and interferons, often acting synergistically, are directly or indirectly responsible for both local and systemic effects of inflammation. The symptoms associated with inflammation, including fever, myalgia, arthralgia, anorexia, and somnolence, are attributable to these cytokines. The most prominent systemic manifestations of inflammation, termed the **systemic inflammatory response syndrome (SIRS)**, are activation of the hypothalamic-pituitary-adrenal axis, leukocytosis, or the acute phase response, fever, and shock.

Hypothalamic-Pituitary-Adrenal Axis

Many of the systemic effects of inflammation are mediated via the hypothalamic-pituitary-adrenal axis, a key component in the response to chronic inflammation and chronic immune disease. Inflammation results in release of anti-inflammatory glucocorticoids from the adrenal cortex. Loss of adrenal function can increase the severity of inflammation.

Leukocytosis

Leukocytosis, defined as an increase in circulating leukocytes, commonly accompanies acute inflammation. Immature PMNs, ("band" forms) may also be seen in the peripheral blood (see Chapter 20). It is most commonly associated with bacterial infections and tissue injury. Leukocytosis is caused by release of specific mediators from macrophages and perhaps other cells. These mediators accelerate release of PMNs, even immature PMNs, from the bone marrow. Subsequently, macrophages and T lymphocytes are stimulated to produce a group of proteins (called "colony-stimulating factors") that induce proliferation of bone marrow hematopoietic precursor cells. On occasion, circulating levels of leukocytes and their precursors may reach very high levels, a situation referred to as a **leukemoid reaction**, which is sometimes difficult to differentiate from leukemia.

In contrast to bacterial infections, viral infections (including infectious mononucleosis) are characterized by **lymphocytosis**, an absolute increase in the number of circulating lymphocytes. Parasitic infestations and certain allergic reactions cause eosinophilia (i.e., increased eosinophils in the peripheral blood).

Leukopenia

Leukopenia is an absolute decrease in circulating white cells. It is occasionally encountered under conditions of chronic inflammation, especially in patients who are malnourished or who suffer from a chronic debilitating disease such as disseminated cancer. Leukopenia may also be caused by typhoid fever and certain viral and rickettsial infections.

Acute Phase Response

The acute phase response is a regulated physiological reaction that occurs in inflammatory conditions. It is characterized clinically by fever, leukocytosis, decreased appetite, and altered sleep patterns, and chemically by changes in plasma levels of acute phase proteins. These proteins (Table 2-5) are synthesized primarily by the liver and released in large numbers into the circulation in response to an acute inflammatory challenge. Changes in plasma levels of acute phase proteins are mediated primarily by IL-1, IL-6 and TNF-α. Increased plasma levels of some acute

TABLE 2-5

Acute Phase Proteins

Protein	Function
Mannose binding protein	Opsonization/ complement activation
C-reactive protein	Opsonization
α_1-Antitrypsin	Serine protease inhibitor
Haptoglobin	Binds hemoglobin
Ceruloplasmin	Antioxidant, binds copper
Fibrinogen	Coagulation
Serum amyloid A protein	Apolipoprotein
α_2-Macroglobulin	Antiprotease
Cysteine protease inhibitor	Antiprotease

phase proteins lead to accelerated **erythrocyte sedimentation rate** (ESR), which is a qualitative index used clinically to monitor the activity of many inflammatory diseases.

Fever

Fever is a clinical hallmark of inflammation. Release of **pyrogens** (molecules that cause fever) by bacteria, viruses or injured cells may directly affect the hypothalamic thermoregulation. More importantly, they stimulate production of endogenous pyrogens, namely cytokines—including IL-1α, IL-1β, TNF-α, IL-6—and interferons, with local and systemic effects. IL-1 stimulates prostaglandin synthesis in hypothalamic thermoregulatory centers, thereby altering the "thermostat" that controls body temperature. Inhibitors of cyclooxygenase (e.g., aspirin) block the fever response by inhibiting IL-1–stimulated PGE_2 synthesis in the hypothalamus. TNF-α and IL-6 also increase body temperature by a direct action on the hypothalamus. Chills (the sensation of cold), rigor (profound chills with shivering and piloerection), and sweats (to allow heat dissipation) are symptoms associated with fever.

Pain

The process of pain is associated with (1) **nociception** (i.e., detection of noxious stimuli and transmission of this information to the brain), (2) pain perception, and (3) suffering and pain behavior. Nociception is primarily a neural response initiated in injured tissues by specific nociceptors, which are high-threshold receptors for thermal, chemical, and mechanical stimuli. Most chemical mediators of inflammation described in this chapter—including ions, kinins, histamine, NO•, prostanoids, cytokines, and growth factors—activate peripheral nociceptors directly or indirectly. Kinins, especially bradykinin, are formed following tissue trauma and in inflammation; they activate primary sensory neurons via B_2 receptors to mediate pain transmission. Another kinin, des-arg bradykinin, activates B_1 receptors to produce pain only during inflammation. Cytokines, particularly TNF-α, IL-1, IL-6 and IL-8, produce pain hypersensitivity to mechanical and thermal stimuli. Prostaglandins and growth factors may directly activate nociceptors but appear to be most important in enhancing nociceptor sensitivity. Pain perception and subsequent behavior arise in response to this enhanced sensitivity to both noxious and normally innocuous stimuli.

Shock

Under conditions of massive tissue injury or infection that spreads to the blood (sepsis), significant quantities of cytokines, especially TNF-α, and other chemical mediators of inflammation may be generated in the circulation. The sustained presence of these mediators induces cardiovascular decompensation through their effects on the heart and on the peripheral vascular system,. Systemic effects include generalized vasodilation, increased vascular permeability, intravascular volume loss, and myocardial depression with decreased cardiac output (SIRS) (see Chapter 7). In severe cases, activation of coagulation pathways may generate microthrombi throughout the body, with consumption of clotting components and subsequent predisposition to bleeding, a condition defined as **disseminated intravascular coagulation** (see Chapter. 20). The net result is **multisystem organ dysfunction** and death.

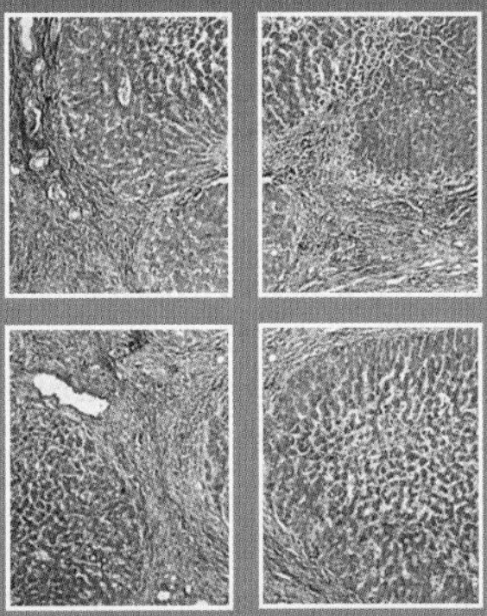

3

Repair, Regeneration, and Fibrosis

Gregory C. Sephel
Stephen C. Woodward

Observations regarding the repair of wounds (i.e., wound healing) date to physicians in ancient Egypt and battle surgeons in classic Greece. The liver's ability to regenerate forms the basis of the Greek myth involving Prometheus. The clotting of blood to prevent exsanguination was recognized as the first necessary event in wound healing. At the time of the American Civil War, the development of "laudable pus" in wounds was thought to be necessary, and its emergence was not appreciated as a symptom of infection but considered a positive sign in the healing process. Later studies of wound infection led to the discovery that inflammatory cells are primary actors in the repair process. Although scurvy (see Chapter 8) was described in the 16th century by the British navy, it was not until the 20th century that vitamin C (ascorbic acid) was found to be necessary for the function of prolyl hydroxylase, an enzyme required for proper folding and stabilization of collagen into a triple helix.

The study of wound healing now encompasses a complex environment containing many cell types, matrix proteins, growth factors, and cytokines, which regulate and modulate the repair process. Nearly every stage in the repair process is redundantly controlled, and there is no single rate-limiting step, with the possible exception of the ingress of inflammatory cells. *Successful healing maintains tissue function and repairs tissue barriers, preventing blood loss and infection, but is usually accomplished through collagen deposition or* ***scarring (fibrosis)***. Advances in our understanding of growth factors, extracellular matrix and stem cell biology are improving healing, and offer the possibility of regenerating tissues to their normal architecture and of engineering replacement tissues.

Successful repair relies upon a crucial balance between the *yin* of matrix deposition and the *yang* of matrix degradation. ***Regenerative processes*** *are favored when the matrix composition and architecture are unaltered.* Thus, wounds that do not heal may reflect excess proteinase activity, decreased matrix accumulation, or altered matrix assembly. Conversely, fibrosis and scarring may result from reduced proteinase activity or increased matrix accumulation. Whereas the formation of new collagen during repair is required for increased strength of the healing site, chronic fibrosis is a major component of diseases that involve chronic injury.

The Basic Processes of Healing

Many of the basic cellular and molecular mechanisms necessary for wound healing are found in other processes involving dynamic tissue changes, such as development and tumor growth. Three key cellular mechanisms are necessary for wound healing:

- **Cellular migration**
- **Extracellular matrix organization and remodeling**
- **Cell proliferation**

Migration of Cells Initiates Repair

Cells That Migrate to the Wound

Ingress of cells into a wound and activation of local cells are initiated by mediators that are either released de novo by resident cells or from reserves stored in the granules of **platelets** and **basophils**. The contents of these granules include cytokines, chemoattractants, proteases, and mediators of inflammation, which together (1) control vascular delivery, (2) degrade damaged tissue, and (3) initiate the repair cascade. Platelets are activated when bound to collagen exposed at sites of endothelial damage, and their ensuing aggregation, in combination with fibrin cross-linking, limits blood loss. Activated platelets release platelet-derived growth factor (PDGF) and other molecules that facilitate adhesion, coagulation, vasoconstriction, repair, and clot resorption. **Mast cells** are bone marrow-derived cells whose granules contain high concentrations of heparin. They reside in connective tissue near small blood vessels and respond to foreign antigens by releasing the contents of their granules, many of which are angiogenic. **Resident macrophages,** tissue-fixed mesenchymal cells, and epithelial cells release mediators that not only contribute to the early response, but also perpetuate it. Their numbers are increased through proliferation and recruitment to the site of injury (Fig. 3-1). *The following are characteristic of skin wounds:*

- **Leukocytes** arrive at the wound site early and migrate rapidly by forming small focal adhesions (focal contacts). A family of small peptide chemoattractants (**chemokines**), are capable of restricted or broad recruitment of particular leukocytes (see Chapter 2).
- **Polymorphonuclear leukocytes** are rapidly recruited from the bone marrow and invade the wound site within the first day. They degrade and destroy nonviable tissue by releasing their granular contents.
- **Macrophages** arrive shortly after neutrophils but persist for days or longer. They phagocytose debris and orchestrate the developing granulation tissue by the release of cytokines and chemoattractants.
- **Fibroblasts, myofibroblasts, pericytes, and smooth muscle cells** are recruited by growth factors and matrix degradation products, arriving in a skin wound by day 3 or 4. These cells are responsible for fibroplasia, synthesis of connective tissue matrix, tissue remodeling, wound contraction, and wound strength.
- **Endothelial cells** form nascent capillaries by responding to growth factors and are visible in a skin wound beyond day 3. The development of capillaries is necessary for the exchange of gases, the delivery of nutrients, and the influx of inflammatory cells.
- **Epithelial cells** in the epidermis move across the surface of a skin wound, penetrate the provisional matrix (see below), and migrate upon stromal collagen, which is coated with plasma glycoproteins, fibrinogen, and fibronectin. The process of reepithelialization is delayed if the migrating epithelial cells must reconstitute a damaged basement membrane. In addition, the phenotype of the epithelial layer is altered in the absence of basement membrane.
- **Stem cells** from bone marrow, the bulb of the hair follicle, and the basal epidermal layer provide a renewable source of epidermal and dermal cells capable of differentiation, proliferation, and migration. Under appropriate conditions, these cells form new blood vessels and new epithelium and regenerate skin structures, such as hair follicles and sebaceous glands.

Mechanisms of Cell Migration

Cell migration uses the most important mechanism of wound healing, namely the response of cells to chemical signals (**cytokines**) and insoluble substrates of the extracellular matrix. Locomotion of the rapidly migrating leukocytes is powered by broad, wavelike, membrane extensions called **lamellipodia**. Slower moving cells, such as fibroblasts, extend narrower, fingerlike membrane protrusions labeled **filopodia**. Cell polarization and membrane extensions are initiated by growth factors or chemokines, which trigger a response by binding to their specific receptors on the cell surface. **Actin fibrils** polymerize and form a network at the membrane's leading edge, thereby propelling lamellipodia and filopodia forward, with traction provided via attachments to the extracellular matrix substrate. Actin-related proteins stimulate actin assembly, and numerous actin-binding proteins act like molecular tinker toys, rapidly constructing, stabilizing and destabilizing actin networks.

The leading edge of the cell membrane impinges upon the extracellular matrix and adheres to it through transmembrane adhesion receptors termed ***integrins*** *(see Chapter 2).* These molecules are highly redundant, and many different integrin heterodimer combinations recognize the same matrix components (e.g., collagen, laminin, fibronectin). Focal contacts develop through the adherence of the integrin extracellular domain to the connective tissue matrix. Focal adhesions form under the cell body, whereas smaller focal contacts form at the leading edge of migrating cells. The focal contact anchors the actin stress fibers, against which myosins pull to extend or contract the cell body. As the cell moves forward, older adhesions at the rear are weakened or destabilized, allowing the trailing edge to retract.

More than 50 proteins have been associated with the formation of adhesion plaques. The cytoplasmic domain of integrins is the foundation of a protein cascade that acts to anchor actin stress fibers. The Rho-family of GTPases (Rho, Rac, and Cdc42) act as molecular switches that interact with surface receptors to regulate matrix assembly, generate focal adhesions, and organize the actin cytoskeleton.

Importantly, the integrins transmit intracellular signals to cells that also regulate cellular survival, proliferation, and differentiation. These functional properties are also affected by other cell activators (e.g., cytokines) by signaling through cytoplasmic tails of integrins from inside the cell to the outside matrix. In this manner, cytokines can also influence the organization and tension in matrix and tissue. Thus, growth factors and integrins share several common signaling pathways, but integrins are unique in their ability to organize and anchor the cytoskeleton. Cytoskeletal connections are involved in cell-cell and cell-matrix connections and determine the shape and differentiation of epithelial, endothelial, and other cells.

Extracellular Matrix Sustains the Repair Process

Three types of extracellular matrix contribute to the organization, physical properties, and function of tissue:

- **Basement membrane**
- **Provisional matrix**
- **Connective tissue (interstitial matrix or stroma)**

Basement Membranes

Basement membranes, also called **basal lamina**, are thin, well-defined layers of specialized extracellular matrix that separate the cells that synthesize it from connective tissue (Fig. 3-2). By light microscopy, a basement membrane appears as a thin lamina that is stained by the periodic acid-Schiff stain (PAS). Epithelium, adipocytes, muscle cells, Schwann cells, and capillary endothelium produce basement membranes.

- Basement membranes are constructed from extracellular matrix molecules, including collagen IV, laminin, entactin/

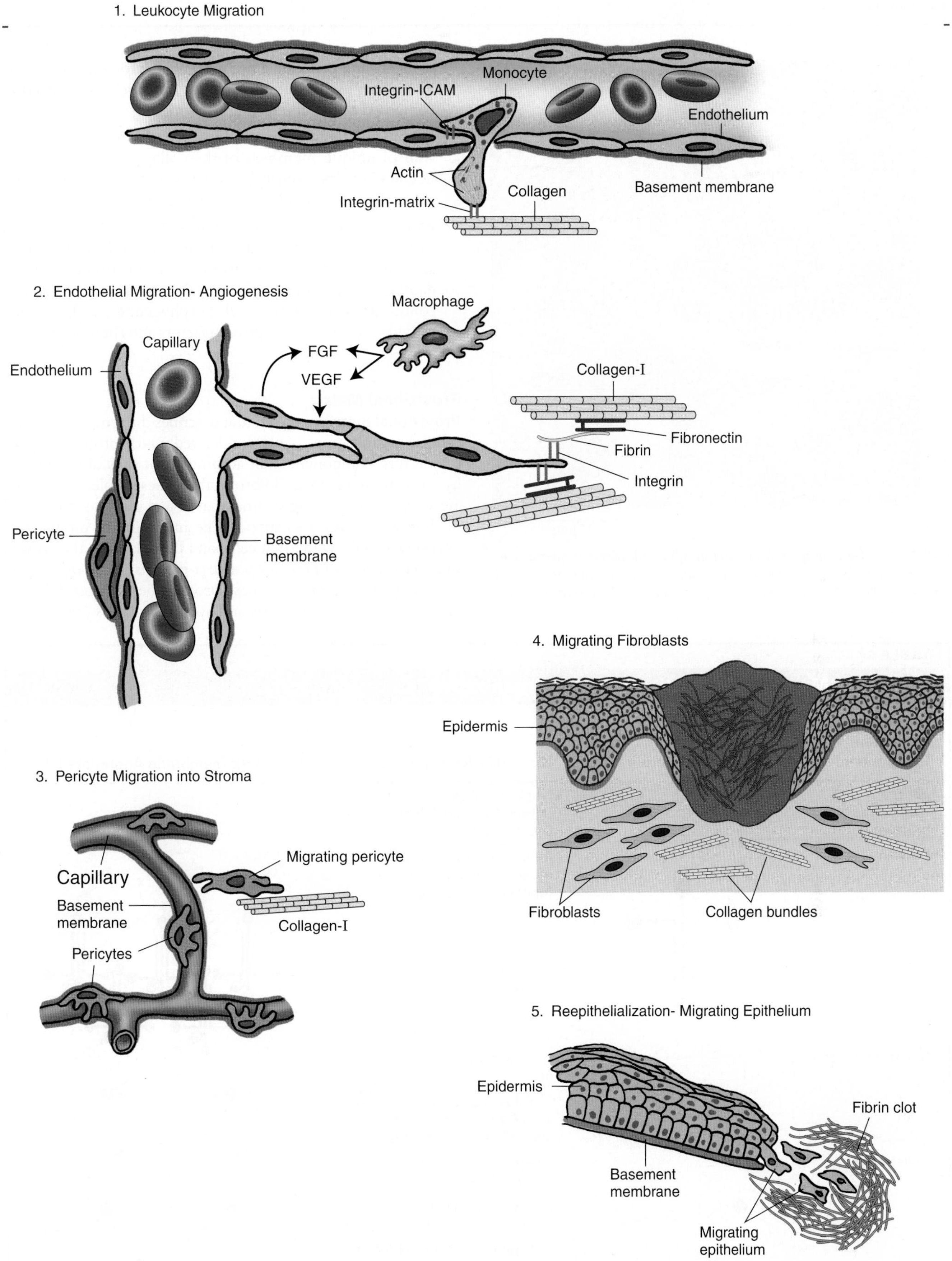

FIGURE 3-1. **Cell migrations during repair.** *(1)* Leukocytes attach to, and migrate between, capillary endothelial cells, penetrate the basement membrane, and enter the matrix. *(2)* Capillary endothelial cells, released from the basement membrane, migrate through the matrix to form new capillaries. *(3)* Pericytes detach from endothelial cells and their basement membranes to migrate into the matrix. *(4)* Fibroblasts become bipolar and migrate through the matrix to the site of injury. *(5)* Epithelial keratinocytes detach from neighboring cells and basement membranes and migrate between the scab and the wound along the provisional matrix of the dermis. FGF = fibroblast growth factor; VEGF = vascular endothelial growth factor.

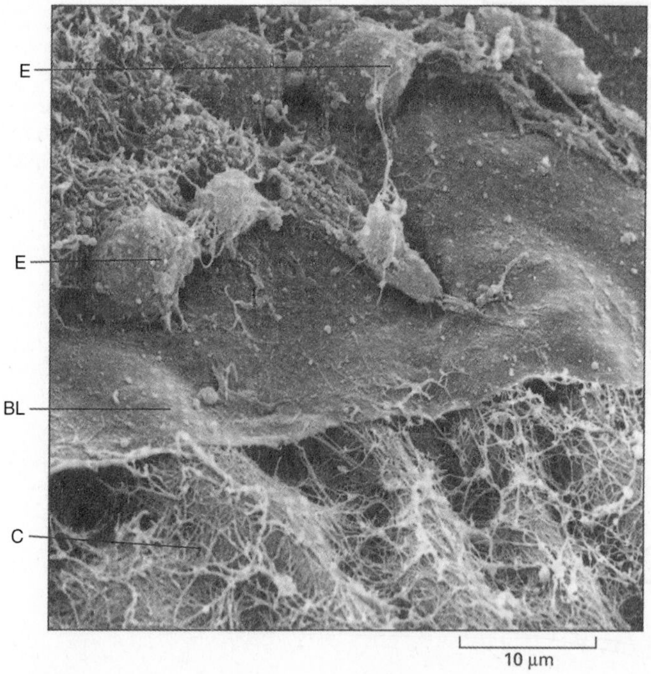

FIGURE 3-2. **Scanning electron micrographs of basement membrane.** Basement membrane (*BL*, basal lamina) separating chick embryo corneal epithelial cells (*E*) from underlying stromal connective tissue with collagen fibrils (*C*).

nidogen, and perlecan, a heparan sulfate proteoglycan (Table 3-1). They self-assemble into a sandwich-like structure composed of two interacting networks.

- Within different tissues and during development, the expression of unique members of the collagen IV and laminin families imparts diversity to the basement membrane and the many structures and functions it supports.
- Basement membranes act as filters, cellular anchors, and a surface for migrating epidermal cells after injury. They also serve to reestablish the neuromuscular junction after nerve damage. Basement membranes also determine cell shape, contribute to developmental morphogenesis, and, notably, provide a repository for growth factors and chemotactic peptides.

Provisional Matrix

Provisional matrix is a term that describes the temporary extracellular organizations of plasma-derived matrix proteins and tissue-derived components that accumulate at sites of injury (e.g. hyaluronan, tenascin, and fibronectin). These molecules associate with the preexisting stromal matrix and serve to stop blood or fluid loss. They also support the migration of monocytes, endothelial cells, epidermal cells, and fibroblasts to the wound site. *Plasma-derived provisional matrix proteins include fibrinogen, fibronectin, and vitronectin.* These proteins become insoluble by binding to the stromal matrix and by forming cross-links.

TABLE 3-1

Basement Membrane Constituents and Organization

Basement Membrane Components	Molecular Structure	Molecular Associations	Basement Membrane Aggregate Form
Perlecan (heparan sulfate proteoglycan)	GAG chains 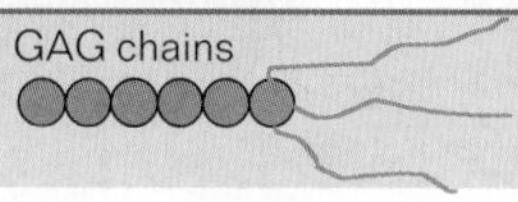	Laminin, collagen IV, fibronectin, growth factors (VEGF, FGF), chemokines	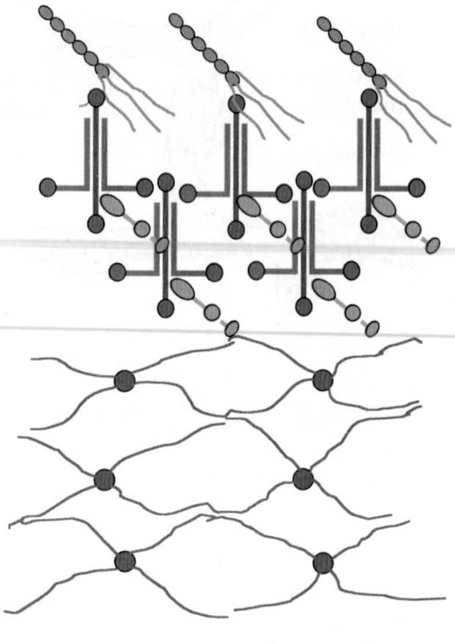
Laminin	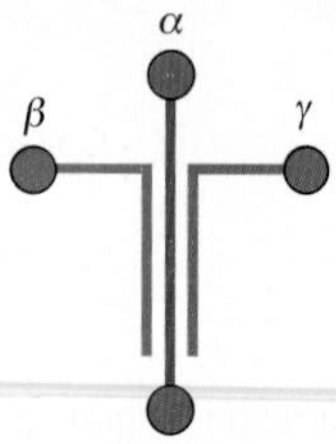 α β γ	Integrin and dystroglycan receptors on variety of cells (epithelium, endothelium, muscle, Schwann cells, adipocytes) Forms self-associated non-covalent network assisted by perlecan Laminin, nidogen/entactin, perlecan, agrin, fibulin	
Nidogen/Entactin	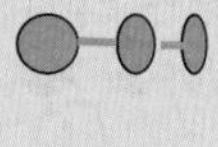	Collagen IV, laminin, perlecan, fibulin Stabilizes basement membrane through association of laminin and collagen IV networks	
Collagen IV	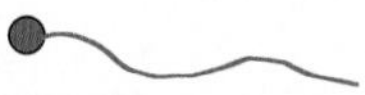	Integrin receptors on many cells Forms covalent self-associated network Collagen IV, perlecan nidogen/entactin, SPARC	
Minor Collagens VIII, XV, XVIII			

FGF = fibroblast growth factor, SPARC = secreted protein acidic and rich in cysteine; VEGF = vascular endothelial growth factor.

Stromal (Connective Tissue) Matrix

Connective tissue forms a continuum between tissue elements such as epithelia, nerves, and blood vessels and provides physical protection by conferring resistance to compression or stretching. The connective tissue stroma is also an important medium for the storage and exchange of bioactive proteins.

Connective tissue contains both extracellular matrix elements and individual cells that synthesize the matrix. The cells are primarily of mesenchymal origin and include fibroblasts, myofibroblasts, adipocytes, chondrocytes, osteocytes, and endothelial cells. Bone marrow-derived cells (e.g., mast cells, macrophages, and transient leukocytes) also populate connective tissue.

The extracellular matrix of connective tissue, commonly referred to as **stroma** or **interstitium**, is defined by fibers formed from a large family of collagen molecules (Table 3-2). Of the fibrillar collagens, type I collagen is the major constituent of bone. Type I and type III collagens are prominent in skin; type II collagen is the predominant form in cartilage. Elastin fibers, which impart elasticity to skin, large blood vessels, and lungs, are decorated by microfibrillar proteins such as fibrillin. The so-called **ground substance** represents a number of molecules, including glycosaminoglycans (GAGs), proteoglycans, and fibronectin, which provide for many important biological functions of connective tissue in addition to the support and modulation of cell attachment.

Collagens

Collagen is the most abundant protein in the animal kingdom; it is essential for the structural integrity of tissues and organs. When collagen synthesis is reduced, delayed, or abnormal, the result is failed wound healing, as seen in scurvy. Excess collagen deposition leads to **fibrosis.** Fibrosis is the basis of connective tissue diseases such as scleroderma and keloids, and also accounts for the compromised tissue function that accompanies chronic damage to many organs, including kidney, lung, and liver.

The collagen superfamily of insoluble extracellular proteins comprises the constituents of connective tissue in all organs, most notably cornea, arteries, dermis, cartilage, tendons, ligaments, and bone. There are more than 20 collagen proteins, assembled from at least 38 different polypeptide chains. Common to all collagen chains are helical segments, largely composed of glycine, proline, hydroxyproline, and hydroxylysine, in which every third amino acid is glycine (Gly-X-Y). The collagen domain that codes for the glycine repeat is important for the formation of the triple helical structure.

Collagen synthesis is complex and is often used as an example of the complexity of post-translational protein modification Each molecule is made by self-association of three α chains that wind around each other to form a triple helix. The triple helix includes members from an α-chain family that is unique for each collagen type. Collagen chains lose stability when errors occur that change the Gly-X-Y sequence, in which case the molecule is more vulnerable to proteinase activity. In general, successful collagen synthesis results from a series of post-translational modifications: (1) alignment of the three chains; (2) formation of the triple helix; (3) cleavage of noncollagenous terminal peptides; (4) molecular alignment and association; and (5) covalent cross-linking, which is mediated by the copper-dependent enzyme lysyl oxidase. Mutational alterations of fibrillar collagen structure are responsible for diseases of bone (osteogenesis imperfecta), cartilage (chondroplasias), skin, joints, and blood vessels (Ehlers-Danlos syndrome) (see Chapters 6 and 26).

Fibrillar collagens include types I, II, and III, V, and XI. Types I, II, and III are the most abundant collagens and appear as long fibrils that are formed from a staggered packing of long, cross-linked collagen molecules, whose triple helix is uninterrupted (see Table 3-2). These fibrillar collagens turn over slowly and are generally resistant to proteinase digestion, except by specific matrix metalloproteinases (MMPs). Type I fibril size and structure can be modified via incorporation of type V molecules or association with type III molecules, while type XI collagen modifies type II fibril size. Mutations in fibrillar collagens, which do not contain nonhelical interruptions, range from lethal to minor and involve skin, blood vessesl, bone, or cartilage. Type I collagen is the most abundant collagen, and mutations in the gene that encodes this molecule, as seen in osteogenesis imperfecta, result in assembly defects in the triple helix, leading to increased bone fractures, thin dermis, and easy bruising (see Chapter 6).

Nonfibrillar collagens (see Table 3-2) contain globular domains that prevent fibril formation. These collagens contain varied numbers of nonhelical domains that interrupt the triple helical segments and confer structural variability and flexibility not possessed by the fibrillar collagens. Nonhelical domains enable small collagens (IX, XII) to associate with fibrillar collagens, modulating fiber packing or a linear collagen. Collagen VI forms beaded filament structures (VI) that encircles fibrillar collagens I and II, is found close to cells, associates with elastin in elastic fibers, and mutations are associated with certain myopathies, as it helps bind muscle cells to basement membrane. Other nonfibrillar collagens act as **transmembrane** proteins (XVII) in the hemidesmosome that attaches epidermal cells to basement membrane and as a **fibrillar anchors** (VII) connecting the hemidesmosome and basement membrane to the underlying stroma. **Network-forming collagens** facilitate the formation of flexible chicken-wire networks of basement membrane collagen (IV) or more ordered hexagonal networks (VIII, X) in other tissues. Mutations in collagen IV cause the abnormal glomerular basement membrane formation seen in Alport's syndrome. Proteolytic fragments of collagen exhibit a different set of biological properties that are also important in tissue remodeling. For example, fragments of basement membrane collagens IV, XV, and XVIII inhibit angiogenesis and tumor growth.

The collagens are called **scleroproteins**, meaning both white and hard; yet in one circumstance, layers of collagen can be translucent, as exemplified by the transparent cornea. The cornea consists of 10 to 20 orthogonally-stacked layers of heterodimeric complexes of Type I and Type V collagens (Fig. 3-3), the fibrils being uniform and smaller sized than Type I collagen fibers in skin. Each layer contains parallel, uniform-sized collagen fibers that are oriented at right angles to the underlying one. In healing, the injured cornea forms disorganized white collagenous scars, which are opaque and interfere with vision. The structure of the cornea surprises those who have seen only dermal collagen, in a loose, random, basket weave-like network. Yet structured orientation of collagen in human skin has long been known. Plastic surgeons use wrinkle lines to promote inconspicuous healing, the wrinkles indicating the primary direction of the underlying dermal collagen. The tensile strength of skin that is broken parallel to creases and wrinkle lines exceeds that which is broken perpendicular to these lines, further suggesting a structured orientation of dermal collagen.

TABLE 3-2

Collagen Molecular Composition and Structure

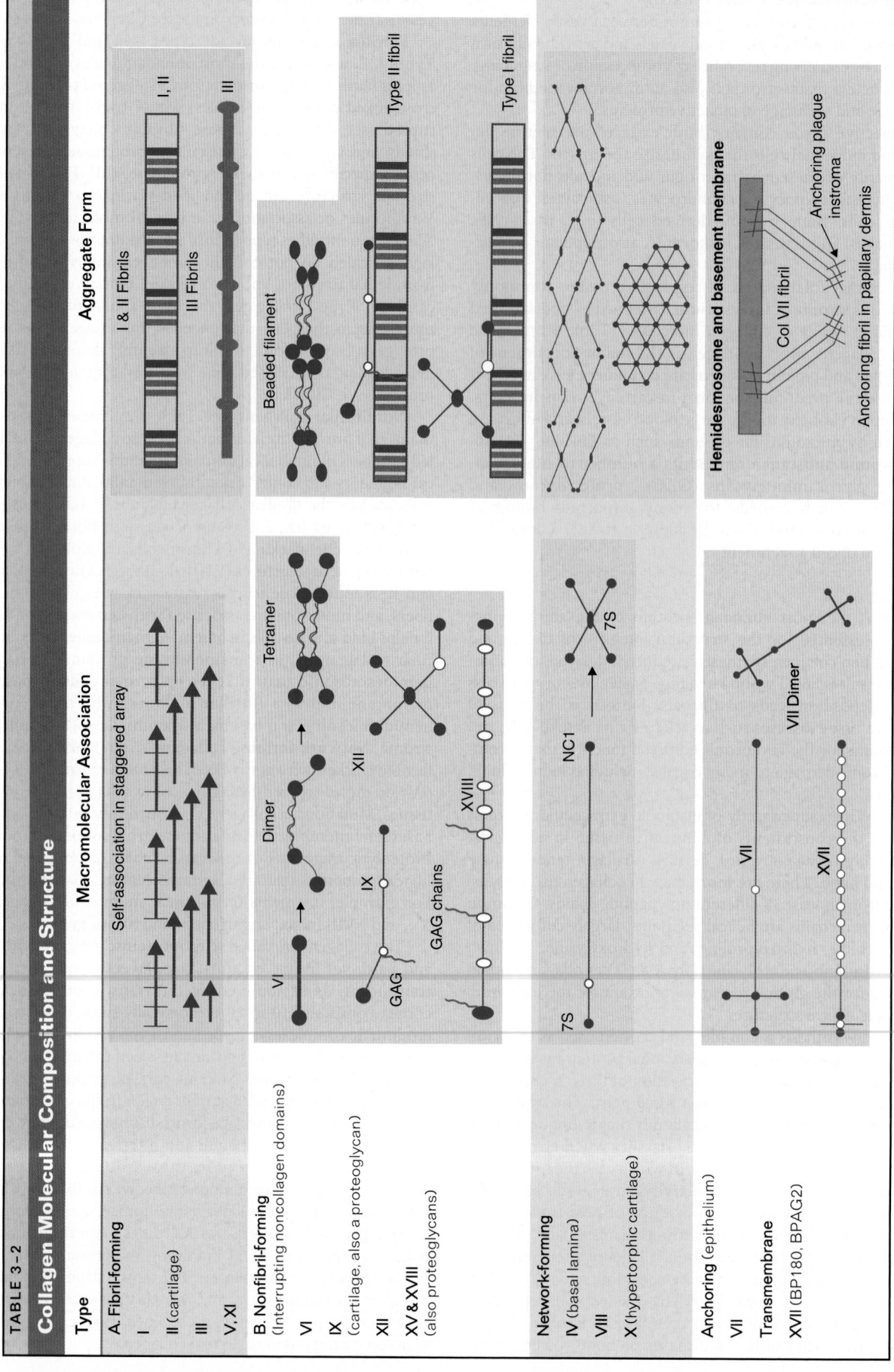

Type	Macromolecular Association	Aggregate Form
A. Fibril-forming I II (cartilage) III V, XI	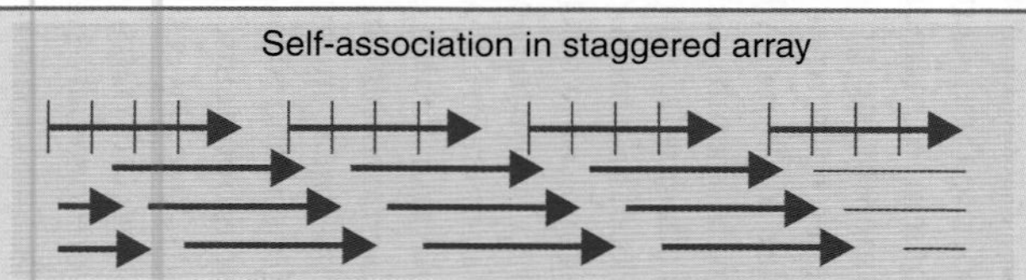	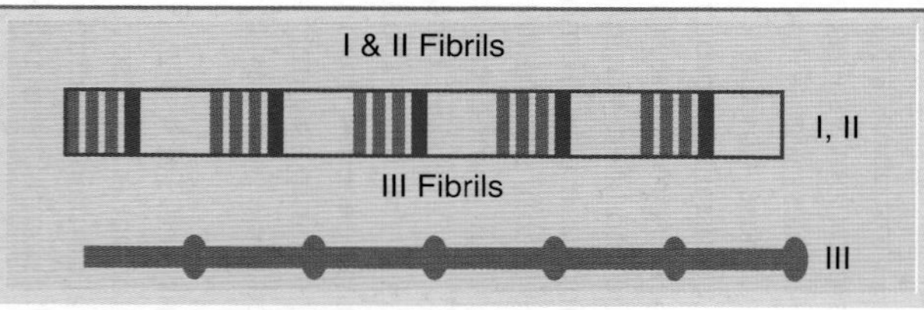
B. Nonfibril-forming (Interrupting noncollagen domains) VI IX (cartilage, also a proteoglycan) XII XV & XVIII (also proteoglycans)	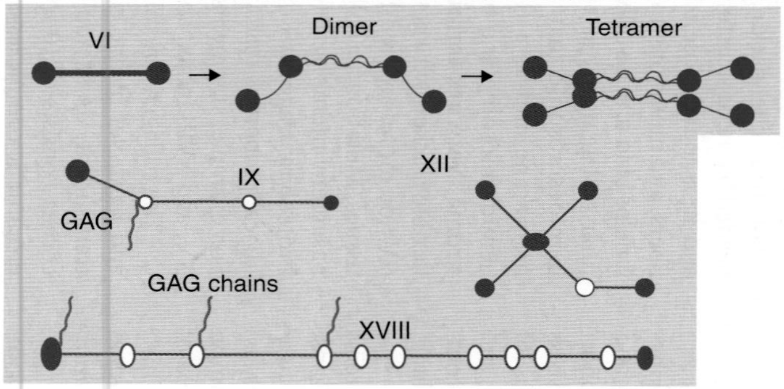	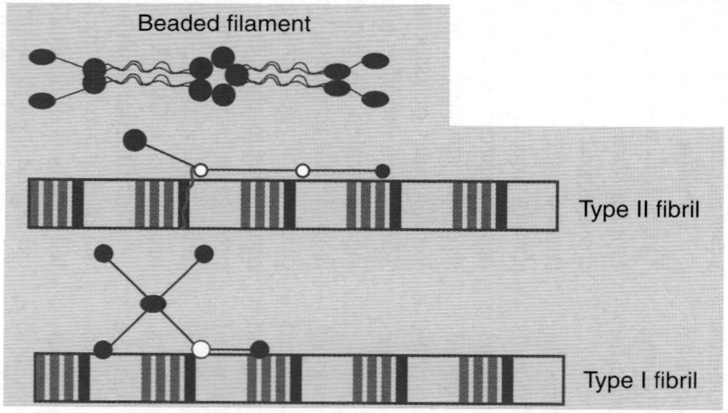
Network-forming IV (basal lamina) VIII X (hypertorphic cartilage)	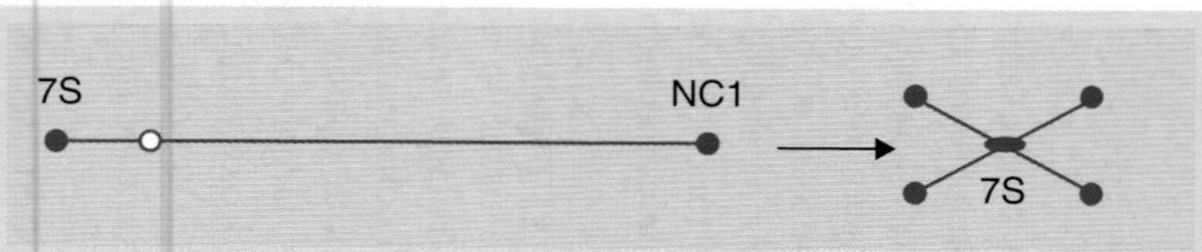	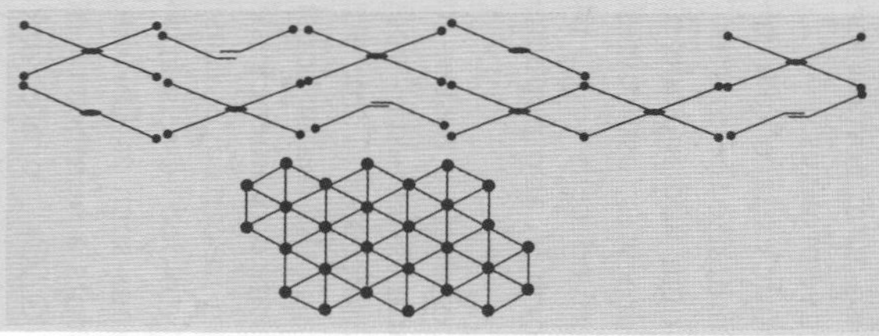
Anchoring (epithelium) VII Transmembrane XVII (BP180, BPAG2)	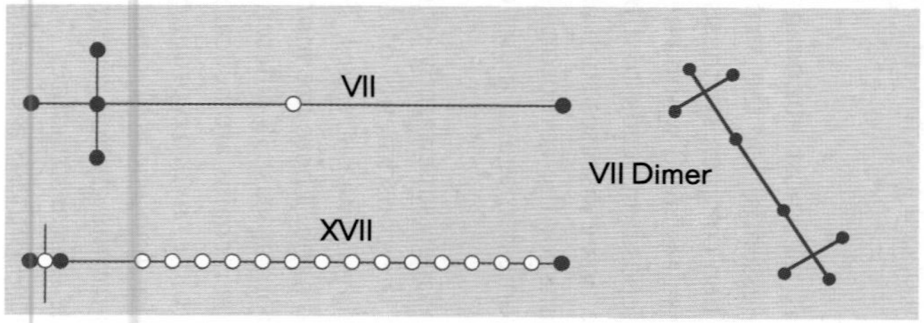	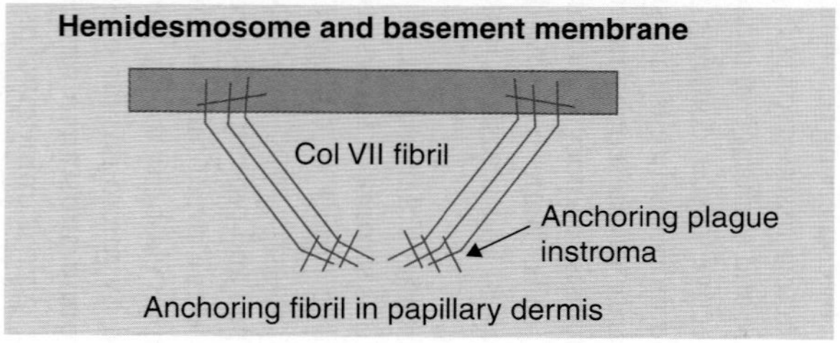

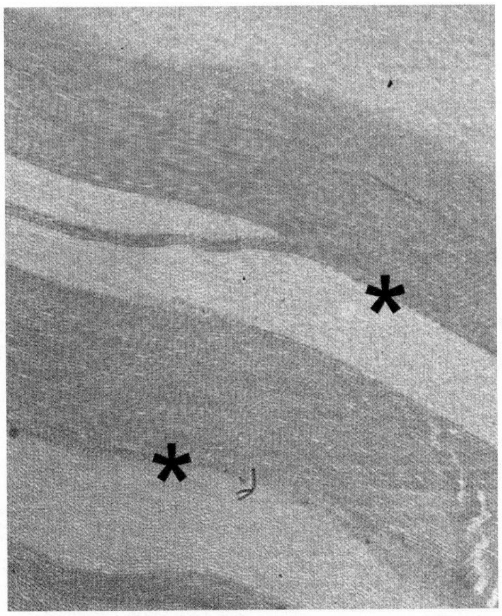

FIGURE 3-3. **Human cornea, near center.** Multiple plywood-like arrays of collagen fibers are of similar width and are sharply demarcated between asterisks (*).

Elastin and Elastic Fibers

Elastin is a secreted matrix protein that, unlike other stromal proteins, is not glycosylated (Table 3-3). Elastin allows deformable tissues such as skin, uterus, ligament, lung, elastic cartilage, and aorta to stretch and bend, and yet recoil. Its lack of carbohydrate and its hydrophobic amino acid sequence make it the most insoluble of all vertebrate proteins. It may seem surprising, therefore, that elastin fibers are damaged by aging and sun exposure, conditions that lead to age-related loss of dermal suppleness. The elastic fiber is crucial for the function of several vital tissues, yet it is not efficiently replaced during repair of skin and lung. The slow accumulation of functional elastin following damage to skin or lung is offset by the fact that it is degraded with difficulty and turns over slowly.

Elastin stability results from its (1) hydrophobicity, (2) extensive covalent cross-linking (mediated by lysyl oxidase, the same enzyme that cross-links collagen), and (3) resistance to most proteolytic enzymes. Arterial wall injury, unlike skin and lung damage, leads to rapid re-formation of the concentric rings of elastic lamellae. This observation illustrates the difference in the elastin synthetic capabilities of the vascular smooth muscle cell and those of dermal or lung fibroblasts.

Elastin is deposited as fibrils, which are complexed with several glycoproteins (microfibrils) that decorate the perimeter of the elastic fiber. The best-characterized microfibrillar protein is **fibrillin** (see Table 3-3). When mutated, abnormal fibrillin causes Marfan syndrome, whose pleomorphic manifestations include dissecting aortic aneurysm (see Chapter 6).

Matrix Glycoproteins

The matrix glycoproteins contribute essential biological functions to basement membrane and stromal connective tissue. In general, these molecules are large (150,000 to 1,000,000 kd) multimeric and multidomain proteins, with long arms that bind other matrix molecules and support or modulate cell attachment. Matrix glycoproteins help to (1) organize tissue topography, (2) support cell migration, (3) orient cells, and (4) induce cell behavior. *The principal matrix glycoprotein of basement membrane is* ***laminin,*** *and that of stromal connective tissue is* ***fibronectin.***

LAMININS: The laminins are a biologically versatile family of basement membrane glycoproteins whose cross-like structure is formed by products of three related gene subfamilies to form α, β, and γ heterotrimers (see Table 3-1). There are 15 known laminin isotypes, which are formed from varying combinations of the 5α, 3β, and 3γ chains. The expression of laminin isotypes in specific tissues contributes to the heterogeneity of tissue morphology and function, in part, by supporting cell attachment. Laminin molecules self-assemble into two-dimensional sheets that associate with type IV collagen sheets and other basement membrane proteins.

The appropriate expression of epidermal laminin is key for both normal epidermal function and reepithelialization of wounds. Epidermal strength is imparted by hemidesmosomes, which develop from the binding of basement membrane laminin to epithelial integrin and collagen VII. The latter is the anchoring fibril that connects the epidermal cell and basement membrane to the dermal connective tissue. Mutations in epidermal laminin, integrin, or collagen VII produce a potentially fatal skin blistering disease, termed **epidermolysis bullosa**

FIBRONECTINS: Fibronectins are versatile, adhesive glycoproteins widely distributed in stromal connective tissue and deposited in wound provisional matrix (see Table 3-3). Fibronectin chains form a V-shaped homo- or heterodimer that is connected at the C terminus by two disulfide bonds. Specific domains within fibronectin bind bacteria, collagen, heparin, fibrin, fibrinogen, and the cell matrix receptor, integrin. Indeed, the integrin receptor family has been partly defined by studies demonstrating its specific binding to fibronectin. The multifunctional dimer is designed to link matrix molecules to one another or to cells. Thrombi support cell migration on the fibronectin that links fibrin strands and are stabilized by cross-linking of factor XIII (transglutaminase) to other provisional and dermal matrix components.

Two classes of fibronectin are formed by a single gene but from different sources: (1) the less soluble cellular form and (2) a hepatocyte-derived, soluble form in plasma. Though they are coded by one gene, as many as 24 variants may be formed by alternative splicing. The plasma-derived thrombus, contains high concentrations of fibronectin, which is cross-linked to fibrin by activated coagulation factor XIII (transglutaminase). Clot-bound fibronectin supports platelet adhesion and promotes reepithelialization of corneal and cutaneous wounds by promoting keratinocyte attachment and migration. Fibronectin synthesized by mesenchymal cells, such as fibroblasts, is polymerized into insoluble fibrils, which are found in granulation tissue and loose connective tissue. Excisional wound clotting and reepithelialization are unaffected by experimentally knocking out plasma fibronectin, suggesting that cellular fibronectin can compensate for its absence.

Glycosaminoglycans (GAGs)

GAGs are long, linear polymers of specific repeating disaccharides arranged in sequence that are also known as mucopolysaccharides. The name of the GAG chain is determined by the disaccharide subunits in the polymer. GAG chains are negatively charged, owing to the presence of carboxylate groups and, with the exception of hyaluronan, the attachment of N- or O-linked sulfate groups to the disaccharide. GAG

TABLE 3–3

Noncollagenous Matrix Constituents of Stroma

Stromal Connective Tissue Components	Molecular Structure	Molecular Associations	Tissue Structures
Fibronectin	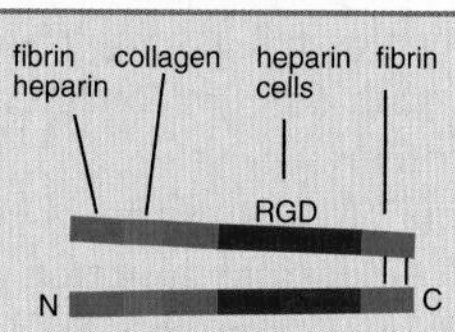 Dimeric protein Chains chosen from ~20 splice variants of one gene	Integrin receptors of many cells (RGD-binding site) Plasma fibronectin is soluble Cellular fibronectin can self-associate into fibrils at cell surface Collagen, heparin, decorin, fibrin, certain bacteria (opsonin), LTBP (latent transforming growth factor-β binding proteins)	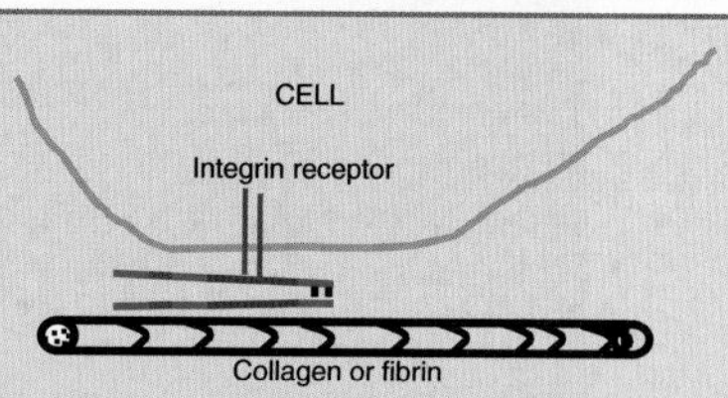
Elastin	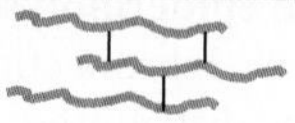 Elastin cross-links to form fiber Monomer with several splice variants, one gene	Self-association to form cross-linked fibers Formed on scaffold of microfibrils	Elastin fiber decorated with microfibrils 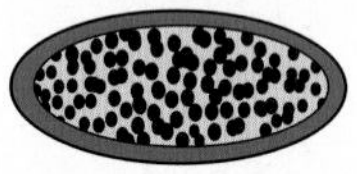
Fibrillin	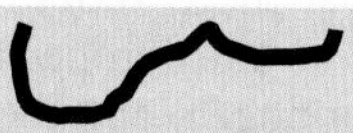 2 members, 2 genes	Other components of microfibrils (LTBP), laminin, versican,	
Versican (hyaluronan-binding proteoglycans)	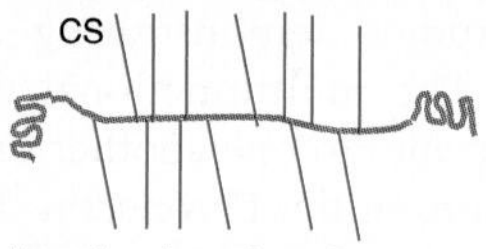 Family of 4 related genes 10–30 chondroitin sulfate and dermatan sulfate GAG chains	Linked to hyaluronan via CD-44 (link protein)	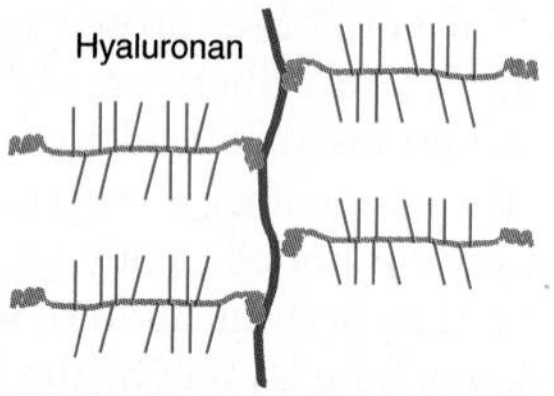
Decorin Small leucine-rich proteoglycans	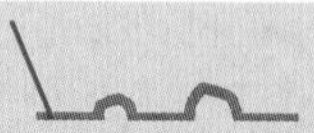 1 protein core, 1 gene One chondroitin sulfate or dermatan sulfate GAG chain Biglycan and fibromodulin structurally related, genetically distinct	Collagen I and II, fibronectin, TGF-β, thrombospondin	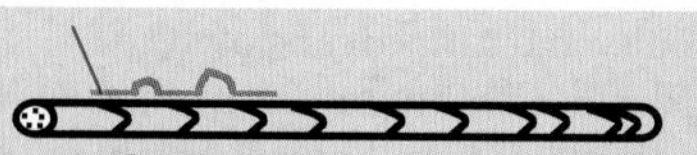 Collagen I or II

GAG = glycosaminoglycan; TGF = transforming growth factor.

sequences have the potential for exceptional diversity owing to epimerization and variability in modifications such as acetylation and sulfation. *When the sulfated GAG chains are O-linked to serine residues of protein cores they are called* ***proteoglycans*** (see below). Glycosaminoglycan storage disorders result from an autosomal recessive (or in one case X-linked) deficiency of one of several lysosomal hydrolases that function to degrade GAGs. The twelve known mucopolysaccharidoses are slowly evolving disorders of connective tissue that significantly decrease life expectancy and affect ossification of cartilage, skeletal structure, and stature facies and may cause psychomotor problems or even mild retardation.

TABLE 3-4

Tissue Expression of Extracellular Matrix Molecules

Tissue or Body Fluid	Primary Mesodermal Cell	Prominent Collagen Types	Noncollagenous Matrix Proteins	Glycosaminolycans Proteoglycans (PGs)
Plasma			Fibronectin, fibrinogen, vitronectin	Hyaluronan
Dermis				
Reticular/ papillary	Fibroblast	I, III, V, VI, XII	Fibronectin, elastin, fibrillin	Hyaluronan, decorin, biglycan, versican
Epidermal junction		VII, VXII (BP 180), anchoring fibrils, hemidesmosome		
Muscle	Muscle cell	I, III, V, VI, VIII, XII	Fibronectin, elastin, fibrillin	Aggrecan, biglycan, decorin, fibromodulin
Peri-, epimysium Aortic media/ adventitia	Fibroblast			
Tendon	Fibroblast	I, III, V, VI, XII	Fibronectin, tenascin (myotendon junction), elastin, fibrillin	Decorin, biglycan, fibromodulin, lumican, versican
Ligament	Fibroblast	I, III, V, VI	Fibronectin, elastin fibrillin	Decorin, biglycan, versican
Cornea	Fibroblast	I, III, V, VI, XII		Lumican, keratocan, mimecan, biglycan, decorin
Cartilage	Chondrocyte	II, IX, VI, VIII, XI X hypertrophic cartilage	Anchorin CII, fibronectin, tenascin	Hyaluronan, aggrecan, biglycan, decorin fibromodulin, lumican, perlecan (minor)
Bone	Osteocyte	I, V	Osteocalcin, osteopontin, bone sialoprotein, SPARC (osteonectin)	Decorin, fibromodulin, biglycan
Basement membrane zones	Epithelial, endothelial adipocytes, Schwann cell, muscle cells (endomysium), pericytes	IV, XV, XVIII	Laminin Nidogen/entactin	Heparan sulfate proteoglycans, perlecan
				Collagen XVIII (vascular), agrin (neuromuscular junctions)

Hyaluronan

Hyaluronan, the only GAG that is not covalently linked to a protein, exists as a random coil of 2,000 to 25,000 disaccharides. Hyaluronan can associate with proteoglycans (defined below) that contain hyaluronan-binding regions. Certain proteoglycans bind ionically via a linking protein along the hyaluronan backbone to form large, hyaluronan/proteoglycan composites, such as **aggrecan** and **versican** (see Table 3-3), molecules that are found in cartilage and stromal tissues. The negatively charged carboxylate backbone of hyaluronan binds large amounts of water, creating a viscous gel that produces turgor in the matrix. The large size and hydrated viscosity of hyaluronan impart resilience and lubrication to joints and connective tissue, and pericellular accumulation of these molecules enables cell migration through the extracellular matrix.

Proteoglycans

Proteoglycans consist of varying numbers of GAGs, heparan, chondroitin sulfate, and keratan sulfate, linked by O-glycosidic bonds to serines or threonines on specific core proteins. They have a higher carbohydrate content than matrix glycoproteins, and though not branched, demonstrate varied modifications such as sulfation, unique linkages, and varying sequences. Individual proteoglycans differ in size, core proteins, choice of GAG chains, and tissue distribution.

Like the matrix glycoproteins, proteoglycans participate in matrix organization, structural integrity, and cell attachment. Though the protein core of proteoglycans often contains biological activity, the properties of several proteoglycans are largely mediated by the GAG chains themselves. Heparan sulfate GAG chains of basement membrane (perlecan and collagen XVIII) and cell-associated proteoglycans modulate the availability and actions of heparin-binding growth factors, such as vascular endothelial growth factor (VEGF), fibroblast growth factor (FGF), and heparin-binding epidermal growth factor (EGF). A group of small proteoglycans, which share a core protein domain of leucine-rich repeats, regulates transforming growth factor-β (TGF-β) activity and fibril formation in collagens I and II (see Table 3-3).

The tissue expressions of extracellular matrix proteins and proteoglycans are summarized in Table 3-4.

Remodeling Is the Long-lasting Phase of Repair

In the later stages of the repair process, inflammatory cells diminish in number, and capillary formation is completed. Remodeling indicates that the equilibrium between collagen deposition and degradation has been restored. The MMPs are the main digestive enzymes in remodeling, but neutrophil protease and serine proteases are also present.

A large family of 25 proteinases, the matrix metalloproteinases (MMPs), are crucial components in wound healing, because they enable cells to migrate through the stroma by degrading matrix proteins (see Table 2-3). They are involved in cell–cell communication, the activation or inactivation of bioactive molecules (e.g., matrix fragments and growth factors), and influence cell growth and apoptosis. The MMPs are synthesized as inactive zymogens and require extracellular activation by already activated MMPs or by serine proteinases. They are classified by the MMP acronym followed by a numerical suffix (e.g., MMP-1, MMP-2) or are called by common names such as collagenase, stromelysin, and gelatinase. MMPs cleave numerous extracellular substrates, many of which are degraded by more than one MMP. As with integrins, such redundancy emphasizes the importance of these molecules in regulatory control. *The list of molecules needed for wound healing is indistinguishable from the list of MMP substrates.* These include:

- Clotting factors
- Extracellular matrix proteins
- Latent growth factors and growth factor-binding proteins
- Receptors for matrix molecules and cell–cell adhesion molecules
- Other MMPs, other proteinases, and proteinase inhibitors
- Chemotactic molecules

Most MMPs are closely regulated at the transcriptional level, the exception being MMP-2 (gelatinase A), which is often constitutively expressed. Transcription is regulated by (1) integrin signaling, (2) growth factor signaling, (3) binding to certain matrix proteins, or (4) tensional force on a cell. As would be predicted by the location of their substrates, MMPs are secreted into the extracellular matrix or are membrane bound. Membrane-bound MMPs are either transmembrane molecules or are linked to glycosylphosphatidylinositol (GPI). MMP-1 and -2 associate with integrins, thereby facilitating cell migration.

In addition to enhancing migration and matrix remodeling, MMPs can disrupt cell–cell adhesions and release, activate, or inactivate bioactive molecules stored in the matrix. These include growth factors, chemokines, growth factor-binding proteins, angiogenic/antiangiogenic factors, and bioactive cryptic fragments released with degradation of matrix molecules.

Once secreted, MMP activity can be minimized by binding to specific proteinase inhibitors. In addition to the important plasma-derived proteinase inhibitor, α_2-macroglobulin, there is a family of endogenous tissue inhibitors of metalloproteinases (TIMPs). Another group of proteolytic enzymes with a metalloproteinase activity that process membrane bound receptors, growth factors, and cytokines are the *ADAM* (a disintegrin and metalloproteinase) family.

Cell Proliferation Is Evoked by Cytokines and Matrix

A prominent early feature in injured tissue is a transient increase in cellularity, which serves to replace damaged cells. Cell proliferation also serves to initiate and perpetuate granulation tissue, which is specialized vascular tissue that is formed transiently during repair (discussed below). Cells of granulation tissue accumulate from labile cell populations, including circulating leukocytes and basal epithelial cells, and from stable cells, such as capillary endothelia and resident mesenchymal cells (fibroblasts, myofibroblasts, pericytes, and smooth muscle cells). Local and marrow-derived stem or progenitor cells may also populate wounds, differentiating into endothelial and fibroblast populations. Cells that are terminally differentiated (e.g., cardiac myocytes, neurons) do not contribute to repair or regeneration (discussed below).

Growth factors and small chemotactic peptides (chemokines) provide soluble autocrine and paracrine signals for cell proliferation, differentiation, and migration. Signals from soluble factors and extracellular matrix also work collectively to influence cell behavior.

The behaviors of cells in healing wounds—proliferation, migration, and altered gene expression—are largely initiated by three receptor systems that share integrated signaling pathways:

- Protein tyrosine kinase receptors for peptide growth factors
- G protein-coupled receptors for chemokines and other factors
- Integrin receptors for extracellular matrix.

Tyrosine kinase receptors, growth factors matrix integrin receptors, and G protein-coupled receptors act in concert to direct cell behavior. These distinct receptor families bind unrelated ligands yet transmit signals within a network of cascading and intersecting intracellular signaling pathways that amplify the messages, often activating similar processes. Even different processes, such as proliferation, differentiation, and migration may share signals, such as those that initiate cytoskeletal changes. A discussion of the myriad intracellular signaling mechanisms that regulate cell growth, survival and proliferation is beyond the scope of the current discussion.

Repair

Outcomes of Injury Include Repair and Regeneration

Repair and regeneration develop following inflammatory responses, inflammation itself being the primary response to tissue injury (see Chapter 2). To understand how inflammation influences repair, it is useful to review the various possible outcomes of acute inflammation. *Transient* acute inflammation may resolve completely, with locally injured parenchymal elements being regenerated without significant scarring. For example, in recovery from a moderate sunburn, small numbers of acute inflammatory cells temporarily accompany transient vasodilation beneath the solar-injured epidermis. By contrast, *progressive* acute inflammation, with emergence of macrophage-predominant inflammation, is intrinsic to the sequence of collagen elaboration and repair. Complete regeneration may be a feature of hepatic injury. For example, normal liver histology is the expected outcome following self-limited toxic drug injury.

Organization represents a pathological outcome of an inflammatory response. It occurs in serous cavities such as the

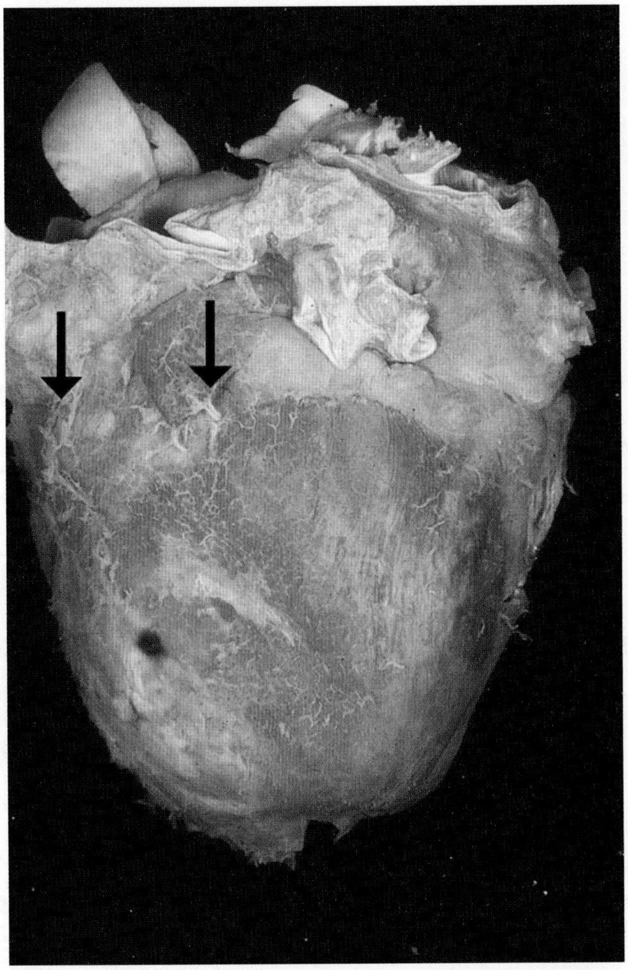

FIGURE 3-4. **Organized strands of collagen in constrictive pericarditis** *(arrows).*

pericardium and peritoneal cavities. In pericarditis, fibroblasts secrete and organize collagen within fibrin strands, thereby binding the visceral and parietal pericardium together (Fig. 3-4). This results in constricted ventricular filling of the heart and may require surgical intervention. Fibrin strands sometimes become organized within the peritoneal cavity following intra-abdominal surgery. Such adhesions (threads of collagen) can trap loops of bowel and cause intestinal obstruction.

Wound Healing Exhibits a Defined Sequence

Wound healing resulting in scar formation remains the predominant mode of repair. Given that wounds in the skin and the extremities are easily accessible, they have been extensively used as models. Though more difficult to study, healing within hollow viscera and body cavities generally parallels the repair sequence in skin (Table 3-5 and Fig. 3-5).

Thrombosis

A thrombus (clot)—referred to as a **scab** or **eschar** after drying out—forms a barrier on the wounded skin to invading surface microorganisms. This barrier also prevents the loss of plasma and tissue fluid. Formed primarily from plasma fibrin, the thrombus is rich in fibronectin. At the site of injury, fibronectin is soon cross-linked by transglutaminase to provide local tensile strength and maintain closure. The thrombus also contains contracting platelets, an initial source of growth factors. Transglutaminase cross-links collagens and fibronectin, which aids in storage of latent growth factors and affects MMP degradation of matrix. Overabundance of transglutaminase may lead to excessive scarring. Much later, the thrombus undergoes proteolysis, after which it is penetrated by regenerating epithelium. The scab then detaches.

Inflammation

Repair sites vary in the amount of local tissue destruction. For example, the surgical excision of a skin lesion leaves little or no devitalized tissue. Demarcated, localized necrosis accompanies medium-sized myocardial infarcts. By contrast, widespread, irregularly defined necrosis is a feature of a large third-degree burn. Initially, an acute, neutrophil-dominated, inflammatory response liquefies the necrotic tissue. Acute inflammation persists as long as necessary, since repair cannot progress until necrotic structures are liquefied and removed. Subsequently, plasma-derived fibronectin binds to collagen and cell membranes to facilitate phagocytosis. Fibronectin and cellular debris are chemotactic for macrophages and fibroblasts (see Fig. 3-5). The appearance of macrophages as the predominant cell at the site of injury signals the onset of the repair process. Macrophages ingest proteolytic products of neutrophils and secrete collage-

TABLE 3-5

Repair in Skin

EARLY	1. Thrombosis: Formation of a growth factor-rich barrier having significant tensile strength
	2. Inflammation: Necrotic debris and microorganisms must be removed by neutrophils; the appearance of macrophages signals and initiates repair
	3. Reepithelialization: Newly formed epithelium establishes a permanent barrier to microorganisms and fluid
MID	4. Granulation tissue formation and function: This specialized organ of repair is the site of extracellular matrix and collagen secretion; it is vascular, edematous, insensitive, and resistant to infection
	5. Contraction: Fibroblasts and possibly other cells also transform to actin-containing myofibroblasts, link to each other and collagen, and contract, stimulated by TGF-β_1 or β_2
LATE	6. Accretion of final tensile strength results primarily from the cross-linking of collagen
	7. Remodeling: The wound site devascularizes and conforms to stress lines in the skin

TGF = transforming growth factor

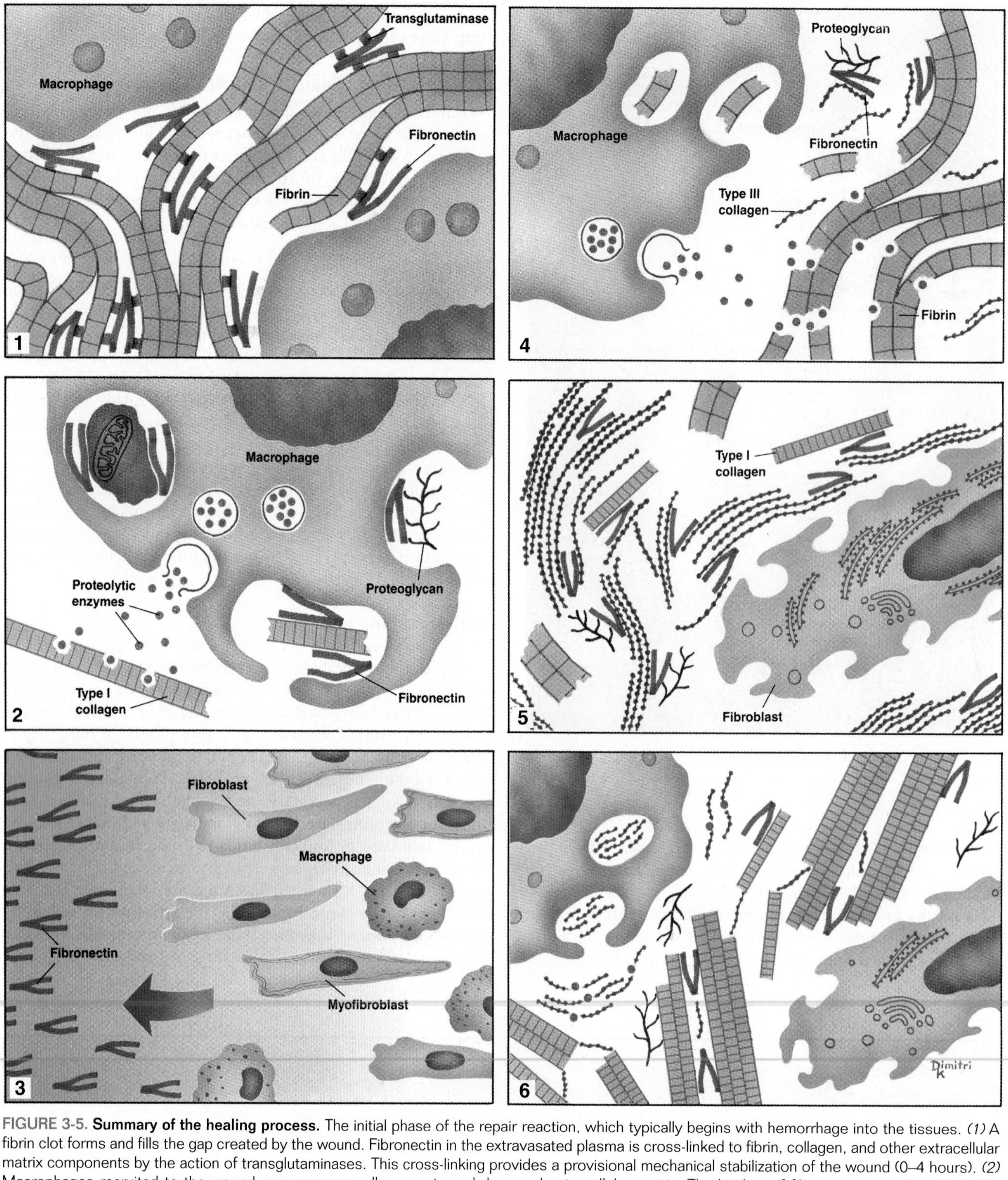

FIGURE 3-5. **Summary of the healing process.** The initial phase of the repair reaction, which typically begins with hemorrhage into the tissues. *(1)* A fibrin clot forms and fills the gap created by the wound. Fibronectin in the extravasated plasma is cross-linked to fibrin, collagen, and other extracellular matrix components by the action of transglutaminases. This cross-linking provides a provisional mechanical stabilization of the wound (0–4 hours). *(2)* Macrophages recruited to the wound area process cell remnants and damaged extracellular matrix. The binding of fibronectin to cell membranes, collagens, proteoglycans, DNA, and bacteria (opsonization) facilitates phagocytosis by these macrophages and contributes to the removal of debris (1–3 days). *(3)* Fibronectin, cell debris, and bacterial products are chemoattractants for a variety of cells that are recruited to the wound site (2–4 days). The intermediate phase of the repair reaction. *(4)* As a new extracellular matrix is deposited at the wound site, the initial fibrin clot is lysed by a combination of extracellular proteolytic enzymes and phagocytosis (2–4 days). *(5)* Concurrent with fibrin removal, there is deposition of a temporary matrix formed by proteoglycans, glycoproteins, and type III collagen (2–5 days). (6) Final phase of the repair reaction. Eventually the temporary matrix is removed by a combination of extracellular and intracellular digestion, and the definitive matrix, rich in type I collagen, is deposited (5 days–weeks).

nase, thereby promoting further liquefaction. They also provide growth factors that stimulate fibroblast proliferation, collagen secretion, and neovascularization.

Fibroblasts are also early responders to injury. These collagen-secreting cells are involved in inflammatory, proliferative, and remodeling phases of wound repair. Fibroblasts are capable of further differentiation to contractile myofibroblasts.

Granulation Tissue

***Granulation tissue** is the transient, specialized organ of repair, which replaces the provisional matrix.* Like the placenta, granulation tissue is only present where and when needed. It is deceptively simple, with a glistening and pebbled appearance (Fig. 3-6). Microscopically, a mixture of fibroblasts and red blood cells first appears, followed by the development of provisional matrix and patent single cell-lined capillaries, which are surrounded by fibroblasts and inflammatory cells.

A key step in the development of granulation tissue is the recruitment of monocytes to the site of injury by chemokines and fragments of damaged matrix. Later, plasma cells are conspicuous, even predominating. Activated macrophages coordinate the development of granulation tissue through the release of growth factors and cytokines (Table 3-6, and see below). These molecules direct angiogenesis, activate fibroblasts to form new stroma, and continue the degradation and removal of the provisional matrix. However, recent studies challenge established concepts regarding the central role of the macrophage in wound repair. Neonatal mice lacking a transcription factor (PU.1) necessary for hematopoietic maturation of macrophages and functioning neutrophils are able to repair skin wounds normally and scar-free.

Granulation tissue is fluid-laden, and its cellular constituents supply antibacterial antibodies and growth factors. It is highly resistant to bacterial infection, allowing the surgeon to create anastomoses at such nonsterile sites as the colon, in which fully one third of the fecal contents consist of bacteria.

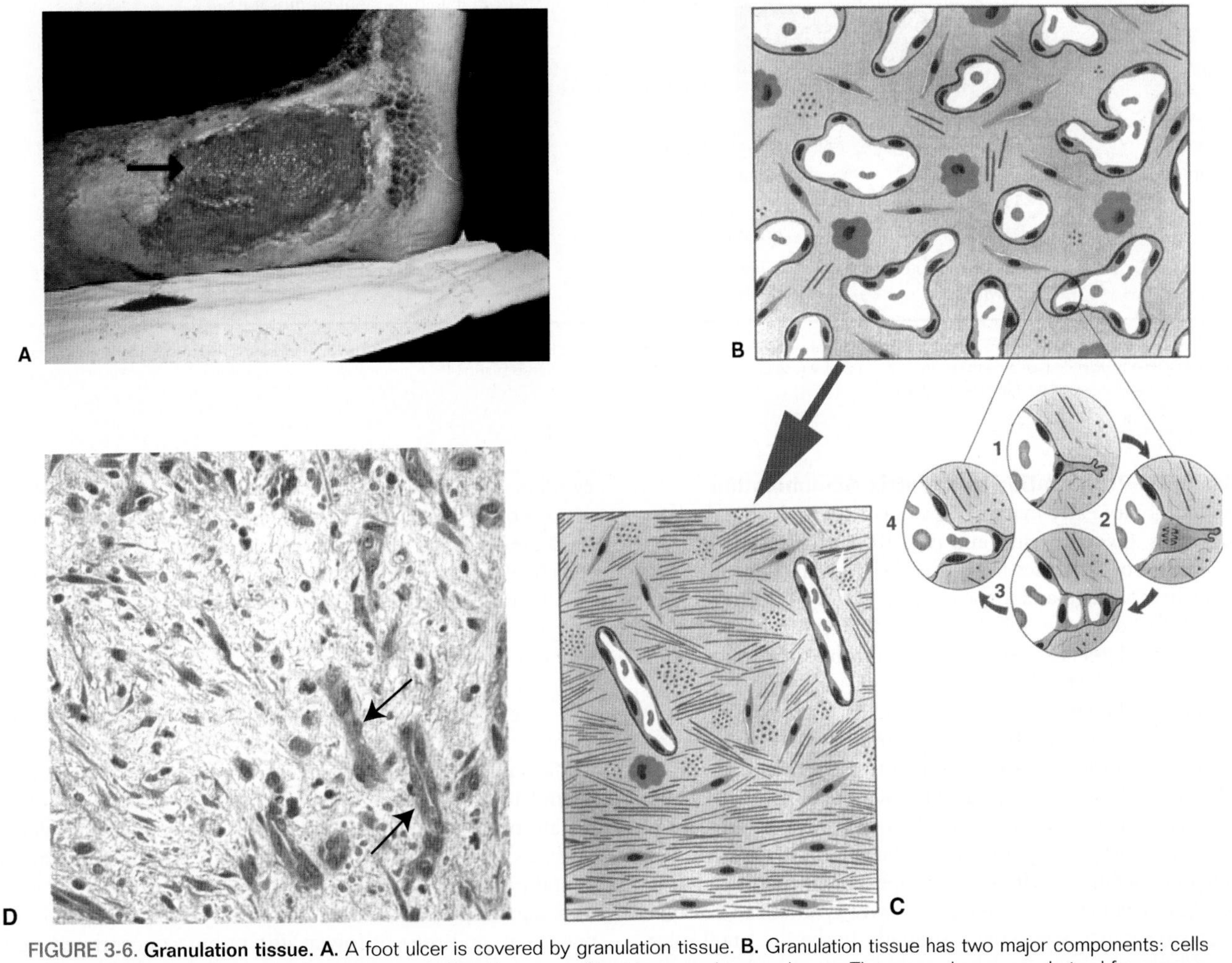

FIGURE 3-6. **Granulation tissue. A.** A foot ulcer is covered by granulation tissue. **B.** Granulation tissue has two major components: cells and proliferating capillaries. The cells are mostly fibroblasts, myofibroblasts, and macrophages. The macrophages are derived from monocytes and macrophages. The fibroblasts and myofibroblasts derive from mesenchymal stem cells, and the capillaries arise from adjacent vessels by division of the lining endothelial cells *(detail)*, in a process termed *angiogenesis*. Endothelial cells put out cell extensions, called *pseudopodia*, that grow toward the wound site. Cytoplasmic growth enlarges the pseudopodia, and eventually the cells divide. Vacuoles formed in the daughter cells eventually fuse to create a new lumen. The entire process continues until the sprout encounters another capillary, with which it will connect. At its peak, granulation tissue is the most richly vascularized tissue in the body. **C.** Once repair has been achieved, most of the newly formed capillaries are obliterated and then reabsorbed, leaving a pale avascular scar. **D.** A photomicrograph of granulation tissue shows thin-walled vessels *(arrows)* embedded in a loose connective tissue matrix containing mesenchymal cells and occasional inflammatory cells.

TABLE 3-6

Extracellular Signals in Wound Repair

Phase	Factor(s)	Source	Effects
Coagulation	XIIIa TGF-α, TGF-β, PDGF, ECGF, FGF	Plasma Platelets	Thrombosis Chemoattraction of subsequently involved cells
Inflammation	TGF-β, Chemokines TNF, IL-1	Neutrophil, macrophages keratinocytes,	Attract monocytes and fibroblasts; differentiates fibroblasts and stem cells
Granulation tissue formation	Basic FGF, TGF-β	Monocytes then fibroblasts	Various factors are bound to proteoglycan matrix
Angiogenesis	VEGFs, FGF	Monocytes, Macrophages, keratinocytes, fibroblasts	Development of blood vessels
Contraction	TGF- β1, β2	Various	Myofibroblasts appear, bind to each other and collagen, and contract
Reepithelialization	EGF, TGF-α	Macrophages, keratinocytes	Epithelial proliferation and migration
Maturation arrest of proliferation	TGF-β1	Platelets, monocytes, fibroblasts	Accumulation of extracellular matrix, fibrosis, tensile strength
	Heparin sulfate proteoglycan (HSPG) Decorin proteoglycan	Endothelium Secretory fibroblasts	HSPG: Capture of TGF-β and of VEFG and basic FGF in basement membrane Decorin: Capture TGF-β, stabilize collagen structure, downregulate migration, proliferation
	Interferon	Plasma monocytes	Suppresses proliferation of fibroblasts and accumulation of collagen
	Increased local oxygen	Repair process	Suppression of release of cytokines
Remodeling	PDGF-FGF	Platelets, fibroblasts	Induction of MMPs
	MMPs, t-PAs, u-PAs	Sprouted capillaries, epithelial cells	Remodeling by permitting in growth of vessels and restructuring of ECM
	Tissue inhibitors of MMPs	Local, not further defined	Balance the effects of MMPs in the evolving repair site

ECGF = endothelial cell growth factor; ECM = extracellular matrix; EGF = epidermal growth factor; FGF = fibroblast growth factor; IL = interleukin; MMPs = matrix metalloproteinases; PDGF = platelet-derived growth factor; TGF = transforming growth factor; TNF = tumor necrosis factor; t-PA = tissue plasminogen activator; u-PA = urokinase-type plasminogen activator; VEGF = vascular endothelial growth factor.

Fibroblast Proliferation and Matrix Accumulation

The temporary early matrix of granulation tissue contains proteoglycans, glycoproteins, and type III collagen (see Fig. 3-5). The release of cytokines from fixed cells in the damaged tissue causes hemorrhage and attracts inflammatory cells to the site. About 2 to 3 days after injury, activated fibroblasts and capillary sprouts are detected. The shape of fibroblasts in the wound changes from oval to bipolar, as they begin to form collagen (Fig. 3-7) and synthesize other matrix proteins, such as fibronectin. The secretion of type III collagen, initially 20% of the total collagen, is transient and a forerunner to the formation of type I collagen, which imparts greater tensile strength. Approaching the peak of matrix accumulation in 5 to 7 days, the release of TGF-β increases the synthesis of collagen and fibronectin and decreases metalloproteinase transcription and matrix degradation. Extracellular cross-linking of newly synthesized collagen progressively increases wound strength. In the PU.1 null mice, which lack macrophages, phagocytic fibroblasts substitute for macrophages engulfing dying cells of skin wounds.

Growth Factors and Fibroplasia

The initial discovery of EGF and the subsequent identification of at least 20 other growth factors have provided explanations for many of the rapidly changing events in repair and regeneration. Redundancy and interaction among growth factors, other cytokines, and MMPs are illustrated in Figures 3-8 and 3-9. The actions of growth factors are not entirely redundant, since each has a predominant function in repair. Specificity derives from (1) selective expression from members of large families, such as FGF and TGF-β; (2) temporal expression of different tyrosine kinase receptors and isotypes in unrelated cell populations; (3) variation in the response pathways or intensity by distinct receptors; and (4) latency or activation of growth factors (Table 3-6). Tables 3-7 and 3-8 exhibit how growth factors control the specific events in repair.

Several growth factor ligands are presented to their receptors bound to extracellular matrix components such as heparan sulfate proteoglycans. Interestingly, certain matrix molecules within the laminin, collagen, tenascin and decorin families contain domains with binding affinity to growth factor receptors. Signals presented in this way are spatially restricted, more persistent, and present lower affinity but concentrated signals that may influence proliferation or migration differently than soluble ligands.

Growth factors expressed as an early wound response (VEGF, FGF, PDGF, EGF, and keratinocyte growth factor [KGF]) support migration, recruitment, and proliferation of cells involved in fibroplasia, re-epithelialization and angiogenesis. Growth factors that peak later (TGF-β, and insulin-like growth factor-I [IGF-I]) sustain the maturation phase and

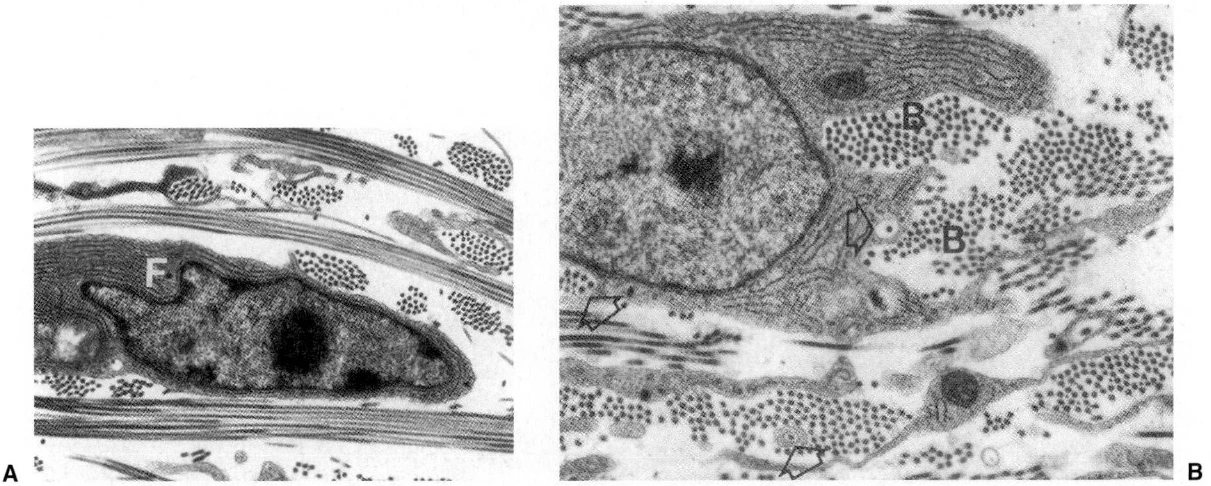

FIGURE 3-7. **Fibroblasts and collagen fibers. Electron micrographs. A.** Chick embryo fibroblast *(F)* lying between collagen fibers and an elastin fiber in lower right corner. The collagen fibers are seen as crosswise strands traversing the field and along the long axis, at a right angle, as dots. **B.** A chick embryo dermal fibroblast with cell surface-associated collagen fibril bundles *(B)*; some bundles are enveloped by fibroblast membrane *(arrows)*. The fibrils are visualized on the long axis as dots.

remodeling of granulation tissue. Tissue regeneration is also driven by signaling networks, which in cooperation with matrix, support self-renewal, maintenance, and differentiation of stem cells.

Wound outcomes vary after exogenous growth factors are added to wounds, depending on the experimental protocol and wound type. PDGF is approved and used to accelerate healing in neuropathic diabetic foot ulcers. In general, however, topical growth factor application does not prevent scars and has not yet been consistently demonstrated to speed or improve healing compared to accepted methods of chronic wound management. Progress in cell culture, matrix, and growth factor biology have advanced in vitro engineering of skin substitutes and improved clinical results for chronic wounds.

Although the roles of growth factors in the initiation and progression of repair are reasonably well understood, the limiting and terminating events are not well defined. Diminishing anoxia as repair progresses may be key to the arrest of the repair process. Repair may also cease because of reduced turnover of extracellular matrix. Finally, increased storage and decreased availability of growth factors may stabilize the matrix, which may then transmit signals that reduce the effects of growth factors. Granulation tissue eventually transitions to scar tissue, as the homeostasis between collagen synthesis and collagen breakdown begins to balance within weeks of injury. Fibroblasts remain active at the wound site, continuing to alter scar appearance over several years.

TABLE 3-7

Growth Factors Control Specific Stages in Repair

Attraction of monocytes/macrophages	PDGFs, FGFs, TGF-β
Attraction of fibroblasts	PDGFs, FGFs, TGF-β, CTGF, EGFs
Proliferation of fibroblasts	PDGFs, FGFs, EGFs, IGF, CTGF, TNFs
Angiogenesis	VEGFs, FGFs
Collagen synthesis	TGF-β, PDGFs, IGF, CTGF, TNFs
Collagen secretion	PDGFs, FGFs, CTGF, TNFs
Migration and proliferation of epithelium-epidermis	KGF, TGF-α, IGF

CTGF = connective tissue growth factor; EGF = epidermal growth factor; FGF = fibroblast growth factor; IGF = insulin-like growth factor; KGF = keratinocyte growth factor; PDGF = platelet-derived growth factor; TGF = transforming growth factor; TNF = tumor necrosis factor.

TABLE 3-8

Growth Factors, Enzymes and Other Factors Regulate Progression of Repair and Fibrosis

Secretion of collagenase	PDGF, EGF, IL-1, TNF, proteases
Movement of surface and stromal cells	t-PA (tissue plasminogen activator) u-Pa (urokinase-type plasminogen activator) MMPs (matrix metalloproteinase) MMP-1 (collagenase 1) MMP-2 (gelatinase A) MMP-3 (stromelysin 1) MMP-13 (collagenase 3)
Maturation or stabilization of blood vessels	Angiopoietins (Ang1, Ang2)
Inhibition of collagen secretion	TGF-β
Reduction in collagen production and turnover	Reduction in anoxia
Collagen cross-linking and maturation	Lysyl oxidase, unknown factor

EGF = epidermal growth factor; IL = interleukin; PDGF = platelet-derived growth factor; TGF = transforming growth factor; TNF = tumor necrosis factor.

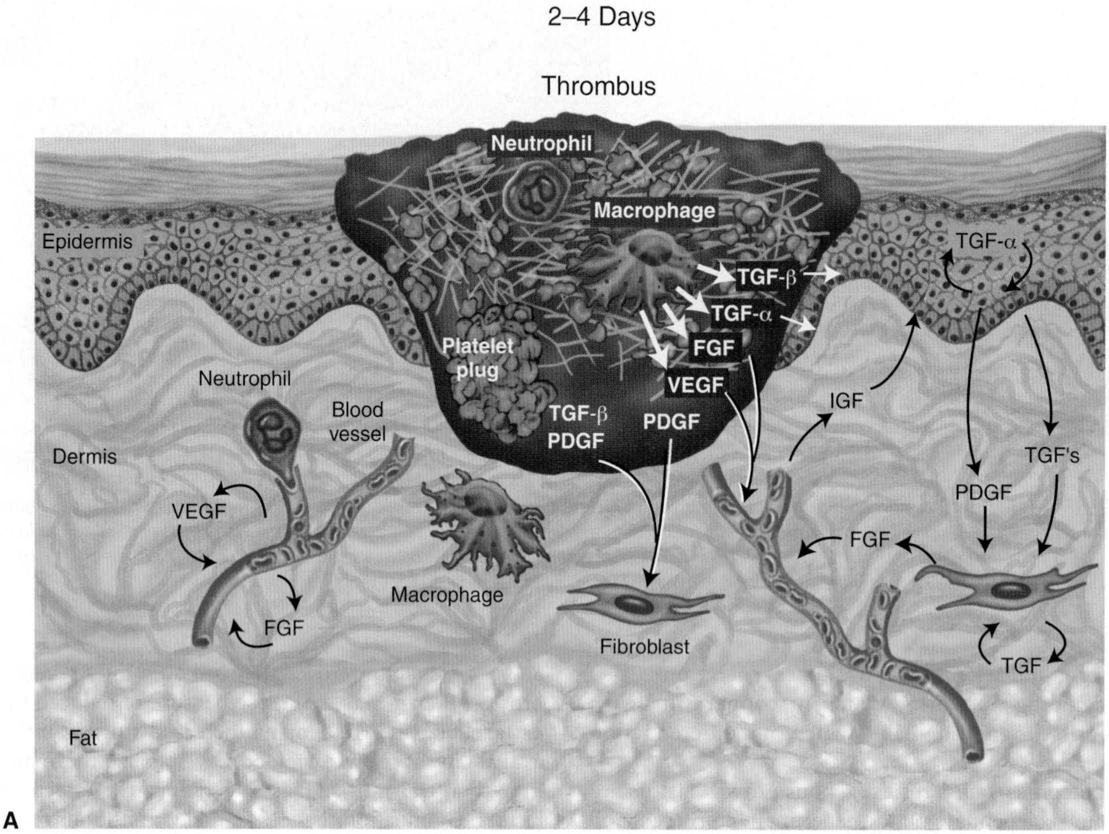

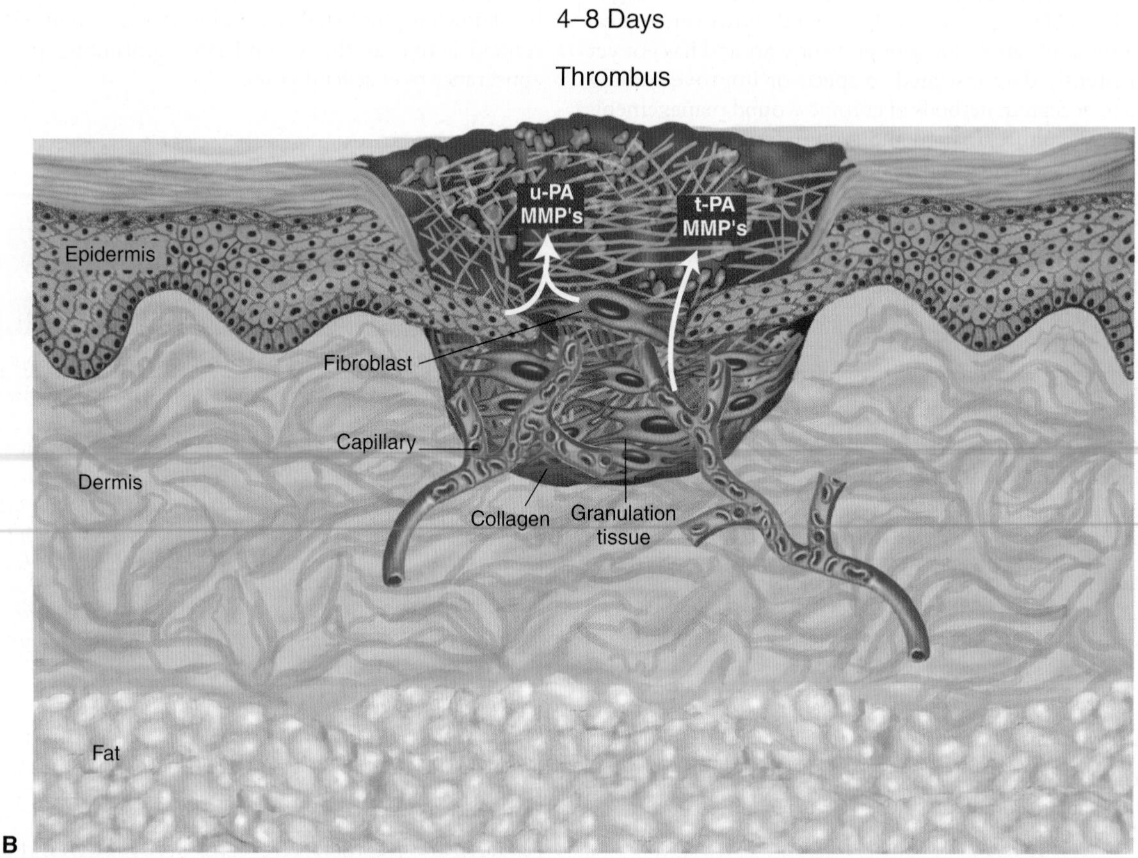

FIGURE 3-8. **Cutaneous wound. A) 2–4 days.** Growth factors controlling migration of cells are illustrated. Extensive redundancy is present, and no growth factor is rate limiting. Most factors have multiple effects, as listed in Table 3-7. **B) 4–8 days.** Blood vessels are proliferating, and the epidermis is penetrating the thrombus, but not at its surface. The upper portion will become an eschar or scab. FGF = fibroblast growth factor; IGF = insulin-like growth factor; TGF = transforming growth factor; PDGF = platelet-derived growth factor; VEGF = vascular endothelial growth factor; MMPs = matrix metalloproteinases; t-PA = tissue plasminogen activator; u-PA = urokinase-type plasminogen activator.

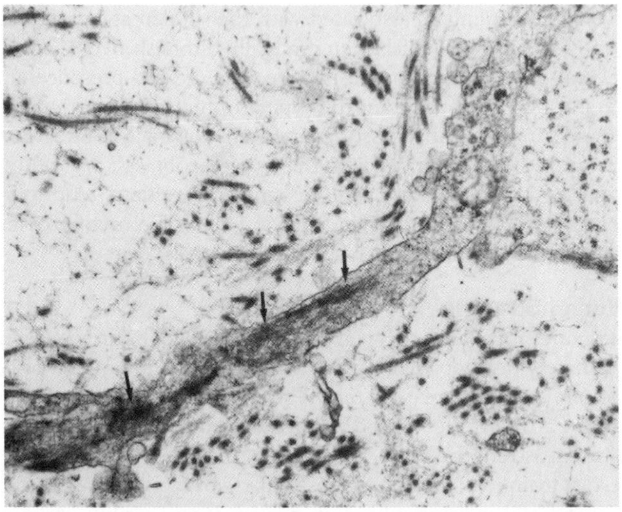

FIGURE 3-9. **Myofibroblast viewed by electron microscopy.** Myofibroblasts have an important role in the repair reaction. These cells, with features intermediate between those of smooth muscle cells and fibroblasts, are characterized by the presence of discrete bundles of myofilaments in the cytoplasm *(arrows)*.

Angiogenesis

The Growth of Capillaries

At its peak, granulation tissue has more capillaries per unit volume than any other tissue. New capillary growth is essential for the delivery of oxygen and nutrients to the cells. New capillaries form by angiogenesis (i.e., sprouting of endothelial cells from preexisting capillary venules) (see Fig. 3-6) and create the granular appearance for which granulation tissue is named. Less often, new blood vessels form de novo from angioblasts. The latter process is known as **vasculogenesis** and is primarily associated with developmental processes.

Angiogenesis in wound repair is tightly regulated. Quiescent capillary endothelial cells are activated by the local release of cytokines and growth factors. The endothelial cells and pericytes are bordered by basement membranes, which must be locally degraded before endothelial cells and pericytes migrate into the provisional matrix. Endothelial passage through the matrix requires the cooperation of plasminogen activators, matrix MMPs, and integrin receptors. The growth of new capillaries is supported by the proliferation and fusion of endothelial cells (see Fig. 3-6), and recent studies suggest that bone marrow-derived endothelial progenitor cells may also be recruited to support the growing vessel.

Migration of cells into the wound site is directed by soluble ligands (by **chemotaxis**) and proceeds along adhesive matrix substrates (by **haptotaxis**). Once capillary endothelial cells are immobilized, cell–cell contacts form, and an organized basement membrane develops on the exterior of the nascent capillary. Association with pericytes and signals from angiopoietin, TGF-β, and PDGF establish a mature vessel phenotype and help form nonleaky capillaries. New capillaries that have not matured may undergo endothelial apoptosis.

Experimentally, stimulation of angiogenesis in cell culture requires extracellular matrix and growth factors. VEGF is the key driver of angiogenesis; the loss of even one allele results in lethal defects in the embryonic vasculature. In vivo angiogenesis is initiated by hypoxia and a redundancy of cytokines, growth factors, and various lipids, which stimulate or regulate VEGF. Activated granulation tissue macrophages and endothelial cells produce beta-FGF and VEGF, and wound epidermal cells release VEGF in response to keratinocyte growth factor (KGF or FGF-7). *Because* the chief target of VEGF is the endothelial cell, this molecule is a critical regulator of embryonic vascular development and angiogenesis, regulating endothelial survival, differentiation, and migration. Splicing variants of VEGF concentrate along both soluble and matrix bound gradients of attraction and help ensure appropriate vessel branching.

The binding of angiogenic growth factors to heparan sulfate-containing GAG chains is a crucial feature of angiogenesis. Association with heparan sulfate chains affects the availability and action of growth factors and vessel pattern formation by (1) creating a storage reservoir of VEGF and beta-FGF in capillary basement membranes and (2) using cell surface proteoglycan receptors to regulate VEGF and beta-FGF receptor congregation, as well as signal delivery and intensity.

Angiogenesis and Receptor Cross-Talk

Surface integrin receptors sense changes in the extracellular matrix and can react by modulating the cellular response to growth factors. This cross-talk is possible because integrin and growth factor signals converge to trigger many of the same signaling cascades that support survival, cell proliferation, differentiation, and migration. Unlike growth factors, integrin receptors drive cell locomotion by organizing cytoskeletal changes at the membrane. When exposed to growth factors or the loss of an organized basement membrane, quiescent endothelial cells express new integrins that modulate endothelial migration on provisional matrix proteins. Capillary sprouting relies principally on β_1-type integrins, although the survival and spatial organization of the capillary network is regulated by different integrins responding to the composition and structure of their extracellular matrix ligands. Without the appropriate matrix or sufficient growth factor signaling, endothelial cells are vulnerable to apoptotic cues.

Reepithelialization

Epidermis constantly renews itself by keratinocyte mitosis at the basal layer. The squamous cells then cornify or keratinize as they mature, move toward the surface, and are shed a few days later. Maturation requires an intact layer of basal cells that are in direct contact with one another and the basement membrane. If cell–cell contact is disrupted, basal epithelial cells reestablish contact with other basal cells through mitosis. In the skin, the hair follicle is the primary source of the regenerating epithelium. Epithelial regeneration is illustrated in Figure 3-8. Once reestablished, the epithelial barrier demarcates the scab from the newly covered wound. When epithelial continuity is reestablished, the epidermis resumes its normal cycle of maturation and shedding.

Epithelialization provides a protective barrier against infection and fluid loss. In addition to epithelial cells, the epidermis includes important immune cells, such as dendritic cells and Langerhans cells. In general, epithelial cells close wounds either by migrating to cover the damaged surface or, less often, by a cinching process called **purse-string closure**. Skin provides the best-studied example of epithelial repair. The basal layer of skin epithelial cells, also called **epidermal cells** or **keratinocytes**, contributes important cytokines (interleukin [IL]-1, VEGF, TGF-α, PDGF, TGF-β) for the initiation of healing and the immune response. To begin migration, keratinocytes must undergo cellular differentiation before forming a new covering over the wound. Normally, these cells are attached to laminin in the underlying basement membrane by hemidesmosome protein complexes containing $\alpha_6\beta_4$ integrin. Among the molecules associated with the hemidesmosome complex are several members of the collagen family, namely, type XVII collagen (BP-180) and collagen type VII, also termed **anchoring fibril** (see Table 3-2). The anchoring fibril connects the hemidesmosome–basement membrane complex to the dermal connective tissue collagen fibers. Mutations in collagen XVII, epidermal laminin, integrin $\alpha_6\beta_4$, or collagen VII produce a potentially fatal skin blistering disease, termed **epidermolysis bullosa,** while autoantibodies against the transmembrane collagen XVII (BP180, BPAG2) causes acquired blistering disorders like **bullous pemphigoid** (see Chapter 24).

Epithelial cells are connected at their lateral edges by **tight junctions** and by **adherens junctions** composed of cadherin receptors. Cadherins are calcium-dependent, integral membrane proteins that form extracellular cell–cell connections and anchor intracellular cytoskeletal connections. Cadherins in the adherens junctions bind stable actin bundles to a cytoplasmic complex of α-, β-, and γ-catenins. The layer of actin that encircles the epithelial cytoplasm creates lateral tension and strength and is referred to as the **adhesion belt.** *The shape and the strength of epithelial sheets result from tension created by cytoskeletal connections to basement membrane and cell-to- cell connections.*

Cellular migration is the predominant means by which the wound surface is reepithelialized. Migrating epidermal cells originate at the margin of the wound and in hair follicles or sweat glands. If the basement membrane is lost, cells come in contact with unfamiliar stromal components, an effect that stimulates cell locomotion and proteinase expression. Experimentally, cells are seen to migrate along a soluble chemical gradient (**chemotaxis**), according to matrix concentration or adhesion (**haptotaxis**), and according to matrix pliability or stiffness (**durotaxis**).

Activation of epithelial motility is driven by the assembly of actin fibers at focal adhesions organized by integrin receptors. Different integrins bind to components of the wound, stromal, or basement membrane matrices and direct the migrating cells along the margin of viable dermis. Movement through cross-linked fibrin apposed to the dermis also requires the activation of plasmin from plasminogen to degrade fibrin. Wound margin epithelial cells of mice lacking plasminogen fail to move through the fibrin matrix. In addition to degrading fibrinogen and fibrin, plasmin aids in the activation of specific MMPs. Proteolytic cleavage of stromal collagens I and III and laminin at focal adhesion contacts can release adhesion or enable keratinocyte migration. Migrating keratinocytes eventually resume their normal phenotype after re-forming a confluent layer and attaching to their newly formed basement membrane.

Wound Contraction

As they heal, open wounds contract and deform. The means by which wounds contract was a mystery until the discovery of a specialized cell of granulation tissue, namely, the **myofibroblast** (Fig. 3-9). This modified fibroblast cannot be distinguished from the collagen-secreting fibroblast by conventional light microscopy. Unlike the fibroblast, the myofibroblast expresses α-smooth muscle actin, desmin, and vimentin, and it responds to pharmacological agents that cause smooth muscle to contract or relax. In short, it is a fibroblast that reacts like a smooth muscle cell. *The myofibroblast is the cell responsible for wound contraction as well as the deforming pathological process termed wound contracture.* The appearance of the myofibroblast, usually about the third day of wound healing, is associated with the sudden appearance of contractile forces, which then gradually diminish over the next several weeks. Myofibroblasts have an increased presence and persistence in fibrosis and in hypertrophic scars, particularly burn scars. Myofibroblasts exert their contractile effects by forming syncytia in which the myofibroblasts are bound together by tight junctions. By contrast, fibroblasts tend to be solitary cells, surrounded by collagen fibers. The myofibroblast may originate as a pericyte, fibroblast, or stem cell.

Wound Strength

Skin incisions and surgical anastomoses in hollow viscera ultimately develop 75% of the strength of the unwounded site. Despite a rapid increase in tensile strength at 7 to 14 days, by the end of 2 weeks the wound has acquired only about 20% of its ultimate strength. Most of the strength of the healed wound results from intermolecular cross-linking of type I collagen. The 2-month-old incision, although healed, is still visibly obvious. The incision line and suture marks are distinct, vascular, and red. By 1 year, the incision is white and avascular but usually still identifiable. As the scar fades further, it is often slowly deformed into an irregular line by stresses in the skin.

Regeneration

Regeneration is the renewal of a damaged tissue or a lost appendage that is identical to the original one. Regeneration requires a population of stem or precursor cells with the potential to differentiate and replicate.

The adult human body is made up of several hundred types of well differentiated cells, yet it maintains the remarkable potential to rebuild itself by replenishing dying cells and to heal itself by recruiting or activating cells that repair or regenerate injured tissue. Some regenerative processes may be thought of as a partial recapitulation of embryonic morphogenesis from pluripotent stem cells. Unlike the newt, humans cannot regenerate limbs, but there are notable examples of regenerative processes. Tissues are adept at healing injury but the regenerative potential is unfortunately restricted to a limited number of adult tissues. Scientists have long recognized that unique cells within bone marrow, epidermis, intestine, and liver maintain sufficient developmental memory to orchestrate tissue specific regeneration. There is a great need to develop similar capabilities in joint cartilage, brain neural tissue, heart myocardium, and pancreatic beta cells. The power to replenish or regenerate tissue is derived from a small number of unspecialized cells, or **stem cells**, unique in their capacity for self-renewal and for producing clonal progeny that differentiate into more specialized cell types.

Embryonic and Adult Stem Cells are Key to Regeneration

Embryonic stem (ES) cells, up to the stage of the pre-implantation blastocyst, are able to differentiate into all cells of the adult organism and preserve small populations of more restricted stem cells. Cells able to divide indefinitely, without terminally differentiating, continue to inhabit many adult tissues and have even been identified in tissues not observed to regenerate. These **adult stem cells** may exist in a specific tissue or be seeded in that tissue from circulating cells of bone marrow origin. Either way, the recently appreciated presence of stem cells within a broader variety of tissues underscores the importance of a permissive and supportive environment for stem cell-driven regeneration (see Table 3-9). Stem cells of adult tissues possess a more restricted

TABLE 3-9

Adult Stem Cells Described in Mammals

	Cell Type	Role in Body
Bone Marrow-Derived Stem Cells	*Hematopoietic stem cells* (HSC) -Multipotent	*Bone marrow* mesenchymal stem cells (MSC) MSC-Multipotent* endothelial progenitors
Tissue Stem Cells (some may be bone-marrow derived)	*Constantly renewing (labile) cells* -Epithelial-like cells (ectoderm- or endoderm-derived)	*Epidermis*: unipotent basal keratinocyte stem cell and multipotent stem cell of hair follicle bulge *Gut:* multipotent crypt cells of small and large intestine *Cornea:* corneal epithelial stem cells are located in the basal layer of the limbus between the cornea and the conjunctiva
	Persistent (stable) cells -Epithelial, parenchyma, neural (endoderm- or ectoderm-derived)	*Liver:* hepatocyte compensatory hyperplasia for maintenance, regeneration, and in response to surgical resection (other liver cells also also divide); Oval cells (bi-potent), canal of Hering, form hepatocytes and biliary epithelial cells in response to severe chemical damage *Kidney:* putative kidney renal epithelial progenitor cell *Lung:* putative lung bronchioalveolar progenitor or stem cells that form bronchiolar Clara cells and alveolar cells *Ear:* pluripotent stem cells residing within and giving rise to hair cell sensory epithelium (neuroepithelium) *Neural stem cells:* (multipotent, thought to be astrocytes); subventricular zone of the lateral ventricle subgranular zone of dentate gyrus
Tissue Mesenchymal (mesoderm-derived) Stem Cells outside bone marrow	Progenitors of connective tissue cells. isolated from several tissues, although bone marrow origin cannot be excluded. *Muscle cells*	*Skeletal:* satellite cells—between sarcolemma and overlying basement membrane of myofiber—originate in bone marrow *Cardiac*: cardiac progenitor cells—cardiomyocytes capable of proliferation; bone marrow mesenchymal stem cells

*These may be the same as mutipotent adult progenitor cells (MAPC), which represent bone marrow stromal cells whose differentiation is influenced by in vitro growth conditions. These cells are capable of seeding tissues outside the bone marrow by one or more of several possible processes: 1) Specific progenitors or multipotent progenitors; 2) Transdifferentiation; 3) Cell Fusion; and 4) Dedifferentiation.

range of cell differentiation than ES cells, yet provide a promising balance between the medical hopes and ethical concerns associated with therapeutic applications using ES stem cells.

Classifying cells by their distinguishing characteristics normally aids our understanding of complex systems. Adult stem cells, however, present challenges in both identification and classification. Their classification typically involves imperfect choices between characteristics such as morphology, developmental tissue of origin, the organ or tissue the cells were isolated from, genetic or immunologic markers, or the capacity to differentiate into multiple or restricted lineages. Exceptions arise for several reasons: (1) any organ or tissue may contain more than one type of stem cell, (2) similar stem cells may be found in different organs, and (3) a stem cell found in tissue may have originated in the bone marrow. Distinguishing between stem cell types using morphology and genetic or phenotypic markers for identification can be difficult and misleading because of the small number of stem cells present in a tissue, shared features between the cells, variance in marker expression through stages of development, and the inherent phenotypic plasticity of stem cells.

Stem cells may be more generally defined by common properties that reflect their exquisite regulation, including:

- The ability to divide without limit and to avoid senescence and maintain genomic integrity
- The ability to intermittently undergo division or to remain quiescent
- The ability to propagate by self-renewal and differentiation
- The absence of lineage markers
- The shared presence of certain growth and transcription markers common to uncommitted cells

Self-Renewal

Self-renewal is the defining in vivo property of adult stem cells and an impermanent property of early ES cells. Relevant stem cells markers based on common traits are experimentally challenging to identify because the populations are small and the cells are difficult to purify. Stem cells may modify their phenotype with changes in cell culture conditions and tissue microenvironments. The presence of stem cells is commonly demonstrated by labeling cellular DNA in the S phase of the cell cycle, while the movement of bone marrow-derived cells to tissue is often studied by observing marker specific transplanted cells in tissues of the irradiated host. Stem cells achieve self-renewal through asymmetric cell division, which produces a new stem cell and a daughter cell able to transiently proliferate and terminally differentiate. In contrast to stem cells, **progenitor** cells have little or no capability for self-renewal. Immortal cancer cells, like stem cells, are capable of self-renewal, however their renewal is unregulated due to their inability to terminally differentiate or revert to quiescence.

This begs the question: Is there a connection between stem cells and cancer cells? Not all cancer cells are capable of regenerating a tumor, suggesting that within a tumor, some cells are more differentiated and do not exhibit stem-like behavior. The cancer cell's capacity for self-renewal may be acquired early in tumorigenesis; or tumors may arise from resident stem cells, multipotent hematopoietic stems cells, or even partially committed progenitor cells that reacquire, through transforming events, stem cell characteristics. Tumors have been likened to wounds that do not heal. Perpetuation of inflammatory processes could provide triggers that release stem or progenitor cells from their normal controls by modifying soluble and matrix based signals of the microenvironment.

Stem Cell Differentiation Potential

The potential of ES cells to differentiate into all lineages diminishes with advancing stages of embryo development. Cells established from the first few divisions of the fertilized egg are **totipotent**, that is, they are capable of forming any of approximately 200 different cell types in the adult body and the cells of the placenta. Nuclei of adult somatic cells can be totipotent, as dramatically proven by nuclear transplantation cloning experiments in amphibians and mammals, but this should not be confused with stem cell potency. ES cells from the inner cell mass of the blastocyst are **pluripotent**, meaning they may differentiate into nearly all cell types. Pluripotent stem cells of the postfertilization zygote, such as neural crest cells, may differentiate into many cell types, but are not totipotent. Many adult stem cells, which must self-renew through the life of the organism, are **multipotent**, or able to differentiate into several cell types within specialized tissues. Hematopoietic stem cells are an example of lineage-restricted multipotent stem cells, capable of forming all the cells found in blood (see Table 3-9). The terms multipotent and pluripotent are often used reciprocally, especially when referring to mesenchymal stem cells from the bone marrow, which appear capable of differentiating into multiple cells types of different tissues.

Progenitor cells are **stable cells** distinguished from stem cells by their lack of significant capacity for self-renewal; however, they maintain the potential for differentiation and rapid proliferation. They are sometimes referred to as unipotent stem cells, as exemplified by the basal keratinocyte of skin, but some may be multipotent or oligopotent.

In addition to normal differentiation pathways within a single tissue, stem cells of one tissue may **transdifferentiate** into cells of another tissue. Transdifferentiation, or **plasticity**, may be induced experimentally using specific *in vitro* culture conditions or by the seeding of transplanted bone marrow stem cells in different tissue microenvironments. Somatic stem or progenitor cells, resident in a several mesenchymal tissues, but of uncertain origin, maintain the capacity to transdifferentiate. Another means of tissue specific differentiation by a circulating cell involves fusion of a circulating stem cell with a resident injured cell, as has been described in animal experiments.

Bone marrow contains hematopoietic, mesenchymal, and endothelial stem cells, providing a multifaceted regenerative capacity. Bone marrow stem cells, which are set aside during embryonic development, replenish the hematopoietic population. Endothelial stem cells from bone marrow have been implicated in tissue angiogenesis and may supplement endothelial hyperplasia during regeneration of blood vessels. Moreover, bone marrow-derived mesenchymal stem cells may populate repairing tissue in other parts of the body (see Table 3-9).

Skin epithelium and hair follicles regenerate from stem cells if the wound does not disrupt the epidermal basement membrane or the hair bulbs. Intestinal epithelium turns over rapidly and is replenished by intestinal stem cells that reside in the crypts of Lieberkuhn. Liver regeneration is partly a misnomer, since the regeneration of liver following partial hepatectomy is a hyperplastic response by mature differentiated hepatocytes and, for the most part, does not involve stem cells. However, there is evidence for stem cell-driven liver regeneration when hepatocytes are damaged by viral hepatitis or toxins. This regenerative potential is thought to arise from "oval cells" in the epithelium of small bile ducts. These putative stem cells have characteristics of both hepatocytes (α-fetoprotein and albumin) and bile duct cells (γ-glutamyl transferase and duct cytokeratins) and may reside in the terminal ductal cells in the canal of Hering.

Influence of Environment on Stem Cells

Stem cells exist in **microenvironments** or **niches** that provide sustaining signals from matrix and neighboring cells to ensure their perpetuation. The mere presence of adult stem cells or progenitor cells is not solely sufficient for tissue regeneration when tissue is damaged. The method of repair is also influenced by the environment of the injury, that is, the growth factors, cytokines, proteinases, and the composition of the extracellular matrix. Whether a wound is repaired by regeneration or scarring and fibrosis is at least partly determined by the concentration, duration, and composition of environmental signals present during inflammation. Epidermal healing during the first or second fetal trimester and maintenance regeneration of adult skin or intestinal epithelium, generally occur without inflammation present and within an innate extracellular matrix. In such instances, normal structures and architecture are regenerated without fibrosis or scarring. Wounds, however, educe physical damage, inflammatory growth factors, and matrix changes that influence the response away from regeneration to scarring. Spinal cord injury, as an example, provides a particularly difficult challenge. Injury-induced cellular reactions lead to the glial scar development, blocking axonal regeneration and complicating the possibility of introducing an appropriately differentiated stem cell that could drive regeneration and reestablish normal tissue function.

Cells Can Be Classified by Their Proliferative Potential

The cells of the body divide at different rates. Some mature cells do not divide at all, whereas others complete a cycle every 16 to 24 hours.

LABILE CELLS: Labile cells are found in tissues that are in a constant state of renewal. Tissues in which more than 1.5% of the cells are in mitosis at any one time are composed of labile cells. However, not all the cells in these tissues are continuously cycling. Stable cells are also constituents of labile tissues that are programmed to divide continuously. Rapidly self-renewing (labile) tissues are typically tissues that form physical barriers between the body and the external environment. These include epithelia of the gut, skin, cornea, respiratory tract, reproductive tract, and urinary tract. Notable in this group are hematopoietic cells of the bone marrow and lymphoid organs involved in immune defense. Polymorphonuclear nucleocytes are the best example of a terminally differentiated cell that is rapidly renewed. *Under appropriate conditions tissues composed of labile cells regenerate after injury, provided that enough stem cells remain.*

STABLE CELLS: Stable cells populate tissues that normally are renewed very slowly but are populated with progenitor cells capable of more rapid renewal after tissue loss. The liver and the proximal renal tubules are examples of stable cell populations. Stable cells populate tissues in which fewer than 1.5% of the cells are in mitosis. Stable tissues (e.g., endocrine glands, endothelium, and liver) do not have conspicuous stem cells. Rather, their cells require an appropriate stimulus to divide. *It is the potential to replicate and not the actual number of steady state mitoses that determines the ability of an organ to regenerate.* For example, the liver, a stable tissue with less than one mitosis for every 15,000 cells, regenerates rapidly after a loss of as much as 75% of its mass.

PERMANENT CELLS: are terminally differentiated, have lost all capacity for regeneration, and do not enter the cell cycle. Traditionally, neurons, cardiac myocytes, and cells of the lens were considered permanent cells, though recent studies are challenging previous dogma. *If lost, permanent cells cannot be replaced.* Although permanent cells do not divide, most of them do renew their organelles. The extreme example of permanent cells is the lens of the eye. Every lens cell generated during embryonic development and postnatal life is preserved in the adult without turnover of its constituents.

Conditions That Modify Repair

Local Factors May Influence Healing

Location of the Wound

In addition to the size and shape of the wound, its location also affects healing. Sites in which skin covers bone with little intervening tissue, such as skin over the anterior tibia, are locations where skin cannot contract. Skin lesions in such areas, particularly burns, often require skin grafts because their edges cannot be apposed. Complications or other treatments, such as infection or ionizing radiation, also slow the repair process.

Blood Supply

Lower extremity wounds of diabetics often heal poorly or even require amputation when it otherwise would not be necessary. In such cases, advanced atherosclerosis in the legs compromises blood supply and impedes repair. Varicose veins of the legs slow the venous return and can also cause ulceration and nonhealing. Bed sores (decubitus ulcers) result from prolonged, localized, dependent pressure, which diminishes both arterial and venous blood flow. Joint (articular) cartilage is largely avascular and has limited diffusion capacity; often it cannot mount a vigorous inflammatory response. As a result, articular cartilage repairs poorly, a phenotype that usually worsens with age.

Systemic Factors

No specific effect of age alone on repair has been found. Although the skin of a 90-year-old person—which exhibits reduced collagen and elastin—may heal slowly, the same person's cataract extraction or colon resection heals normally because the bowel and the eye are practically unaffected by age.

Coagulation defects, thrombocytopenia, and anemia impede repair. Local thrombosis decreases platelet activation, thereby reducing the supply of growth factors and limiting the healing cascade. The decrease in tissue oxygen that accompanies severe anemia also interferes with repair. Exogenous corticosteroids retard wound repair by inhibiting collagen and protein synthesis and by exerting antiinflammatory effects.

Fibrosis and Scarring Contrasted

Successful wound repair that leads to localized scarring is a transient, not chronic, process that leads to rapid resolution of local injury. By contrast, many chronic diseases involve persistent, unresolved inflammation with progression of the repair response culminating in diffuse fibrosis. Inhaled smoke or inhaled silica particles induce persistent inflammation in the lung. Immunologically mediated inflammation of joints initiates rheumatoid arthritis. Inflammatory and noninflammatory factors lead to glomerulosclerosis in the kidney, including infection, hypertension, and diabetes.

Continuing insult or inflammation, mediated through the interplay of monocytes and lymphocytes, results in persistent high levels of cytokines, growth factors, and locally destructive enzymes such as collagenases. Whatever the cause, fibrosis of parenchymal organs such as the lung, kidney, or liver disrupts the normal architecture and reduces or destroys function. The functional unit (alveolus, hepatic lobule, or renal glomerulus or tubule) is replaced by disordered collagen. Fibrosis of parenchymal organs is generally irreversible, calling for measures to prevent exposure to the cause, or therapeutic measures, as in rheumatoid arthritis, to suppress the inflammatory process and so minimize ultimate destruction of joints.

Fibrosis should be viewed as the pathological end result of persistent injury, causing **loss of function.** Often it is the common final result of diverse diseases or injuries the causes of which cannot be ascertained from the end result. As an example, scars of former glomeruli developed following bacterial or immunological injury to the kidney, the specific cause being no longer identifiable. Scarring, however, is often beneficial: the scar resulting from a surgical incision in skin, though cosmetically unattractive, holds the skin together.

Prevention of fibrosis requires either blocking the stimulus of matrix production or increasing the level of matrix degradation. Approaches to controlling fibrotic progression to end-stage kidney disease have therefore targeted profibrotic factors such as TGF-β and plasminogen activator inhibitor (PAI-1). When PAI-1 is inhibited, it fails to activate plasminogen and the resulting plasmin degrades the extracellular matrix either directly or through activating matrix MMPs. Thus matrix deposition in the glomerulus is reduced, protecting the glomerulus from scarring and obliteration. Interestingly, inhibition of PAI could also reduce the incidence of intra-abdominal adhesions, a persistent problem of abdominal surgery and the main cause of intestinal obstruction. The adhesions are initiated by fibrin deposition when mesothelial lining is disrupted. If the fibrin matrix is not dissolved by plasmin within a few days, the fibrinous adhesion is invaded by fibroblasts and eventually transformed into a permanent fibrotic adhesion.

Specific Sites Exhibit Different Repair Patterns

Skin

Healing in the skin involves both repair, primarily dermal scarring, and regeneration, principally of the epidermis and vasculature. The salient features of primary and secondary healing are provided in Figure 3-10.

Primary healing occurs when the surgeon closely approximates the edges of a wound. The actions of myofibroblasts are minimized, and regeneration of the epidermis is optimal, since epidermal cells need migrate only a minimal distance.

Secondary healing proceeds when a large area of hemorrhage and necrosis cannot be completely corrected surgically. In this situation, myofibroblasts contract the wound, and subsequent scarring repairs the defect.

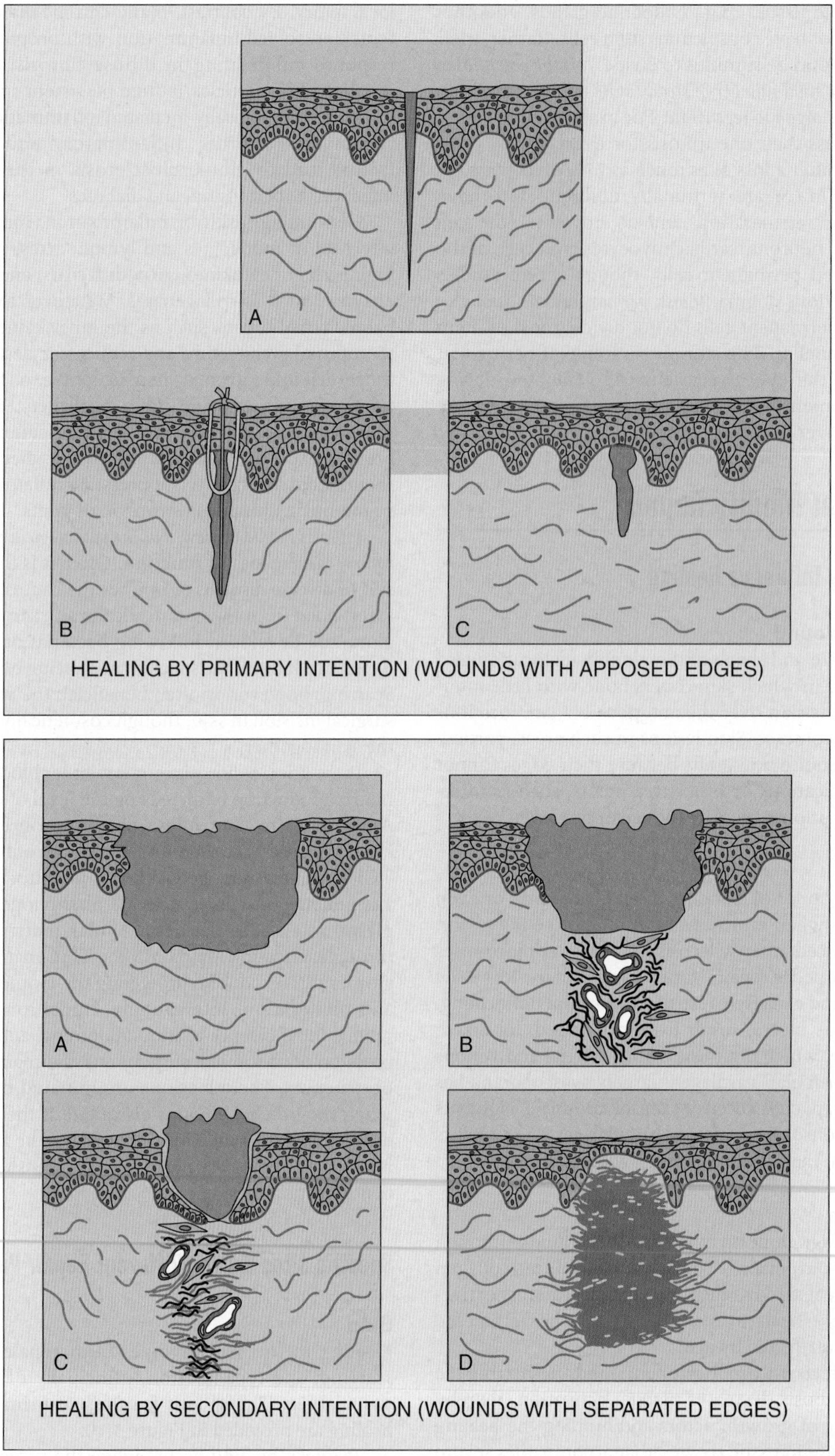

FIGURE 3-10. **Healing by primary intention (top).** (*A*) A wound with closely apposed edges and minimal tissue loss. (*B*) Such a wound requires only minimal cell proliferation and neovascularization to heal. (*C*) The result is a small scar. **Healing by secondary intention (bottom).** (*A*) A gouged wound, in which the edges are far apart and in which there is substantial tissue loss. (*B*) This wound requires wound contraction, extensive cell proliferation, and neovascularization (granulation tissue) to heal. (*C*) The wound is reepithelialized from the margins, and collagen fibers are deposited in the granulation tissue. (*D*) Granulation tissue is eventually resorbed and replaced by a large scar that is functionally and esthetically unsatisfactory.

The success and method of healing following a burn wound depends on the depth of the burn injury. If the burn is superficial or does not extend beyond the upper dermis, stem cells from the sweat glands and hair follicles will regenerate the epidermis. If deep dermis is involved, the regenerative elements are destroyed and surgery and engraftment are necessary to cover or heal the wound site and reduce scaring and severe contractures.

Cornea

The cornea differs from skin in its stromal organization, vascularity, and cellularity. Like skin, the stratified squamous epithelial covering is continually renewed by a stem cell population, which is located in the corneal limbus. Chemical injury to the cornea results in scarring, the white corneal scar effectively blinding the eye. Parenthetically, the cornea, because of its relative avascularity, was the first organ or anatomical structure to be successfully transplanted. Trachoma, an infectious human disease caused by an inflammatory response to *Chlamydia trachomatis*, is the world's most common cause of blindness, resulting from scarring and opacity of the cornea (see Fig 29-1).

Liver

Acute chemical injury or fulminant viral hepatitis causes widespread necrosis of hepatocytes. However, if liver failure is not fatal, and if the connective tissue stroma, vasculature, and bile ducts survive, the parenchyma regenerates and normal form and function are restored. Small cells at the canal of Hering, termed oval cells, are thought to be the stem cell responsible for this method of liver regeneration (see Table 3-9). By contrast, chronic injury in viral hepatitis or alcoholism is associated with the development of broad collagenous scars within the hepatic parenchyma, termed **cirrhosis** of the liver (Fig. 3-11). The hepatocytes form regenerative nodules that lack central veins and expand to obstruct blood vessels and bile flow. Portal hypertension and jaundice ensue despite adequate numbers of regenerated but disconnected hepatocytes.

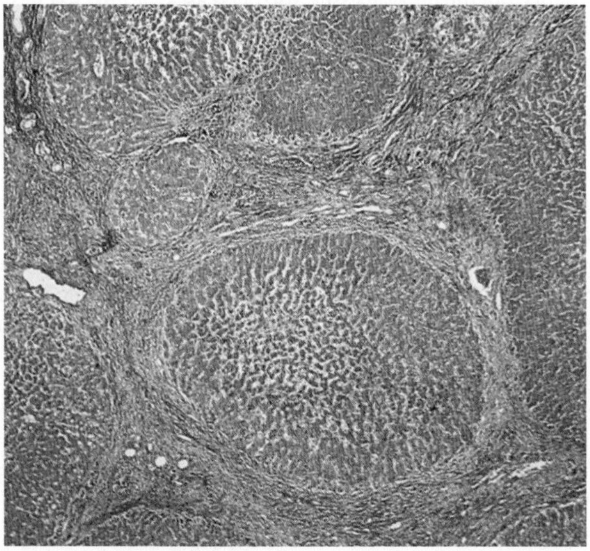

FIGURE 3-11. **Cirrhosis of the liver.** The consequences of chronic hepatic injury is the formation of regenerating nodules separated by fibrous bands. A microscopic section shows regenerating nodules *(red)* surrounded by bands of connective tissue *(blue)*.

In the Greek myth of Prometheus, a vulture tore out his liver every evening, only to have it grow back by morning. It required more than another two millennia for the demonstration that the liver indeed possesses tremendous regenerative capacity, even though the normal hepatic parenchyma is almost devoid of mitoses and virtually all hepatocytes are in cell cycle phase G_0. This method of liver regeneration, after resection, is actually compensatory hyperplasia of hepatocytes. The necessary conditions for hepatic regeneration are complex and beyond the scope of this discussion. Suffice it to say that regeneration is arrested when the normal ratio of liver-to-total body weight is reestablished; the molecular switch that regulates this ratio is obscure. In human liver transplantation, a partial donation of the right lobe of the liver from a living donor is followed by complete regeneration of the normal liver in both the recipient and the donor.

Kidney

Although the kidney has limited regenerative capacity, the removal of one kidney (nephrectomy) is followed by compensatory hypertrophy of the remaining kidney. In the case of renal injury, if it is not extensive and the extracellular matrix framework is not destroyed, the tubular epithelium regenerates. In most renal diseases, however, there is some destruction of the framework. Regeneration is then incomplete, and scar formation is the usual outcome. The regenerative capacity of renal tissue is maximal in cortical tubules, less in medullary tubules, and nonexistent in glomeruli. Recent data suggest tubule repair occurs not from bone-marrow derived cells but due to proliferation of endogenous renal progenitor cells.

Cortical Renal Tubules

Normally, there is some turnover of tubular epithelium, leading to shedding of cells in the urine. No reserve cell has been identified, and simple division accomplishes replacement. The outcome of injury depends on whether the tubular basement membrane is ruptured. If the injury does not produce discontinuities in the basement membrane, the surviving tubular cells in the vicinity of the wound flatten, acquire a squamous appearance, and migrate into the necrotic area along the basement membrane. Mitoses are frequent, and occasional clusters of epithelial cells project into the lumen. Soon, the flattened cells are more cuboidal, and differentiated cytoplasmic elements appear. Tubular morphology and function are normal in 3 to 4 weeks.

Tubulorrhexis

Tubulorrhexis *refers to the rupture of the tubular basement membrane.* The sequence of events resembles that of tubular damage, in which the basement membrane is intact, except that interstitial changes are more prominent. Proliferation of fibroblasts, increased deposition of extracellular matrix, and collapse of the tubular lumen are seen. The final result is regeneration of some tubules and fibrosis of others, usually causing focal losses of functional nephrons.

Medullary Renal Tubules

Medullary diseases of the kidney are often associated with extensive necrosis, which involves tubules, interstitium, and blood vessels. If the lesion is not fatal, the necrotic tissue sloughs into the urine. Healing by fibrosis produces urinary obstruction within the kidney. Although there is some epithelial proliferation, there is no significant regeneration.

Glomeruli

Unlike tubules, glomeruli do not regenerate. Injuries that produce necrosis of glomerular endothelial or epithelial cells, whether focal, segmental, or diffuse, heal by scarring (Fig. 3-12). Mesangial cells are related to smooth muscle cells and seem to have some capacity for regeneration. Following unilateral nephrectomy, the glomeruli in the remaining kidney undergo hypertrophy and hyperplasia to produce greatly enlarged glomeruli.

Lung

The epithelium lining the respiratory tract has an effective regenerative capacity, provided that the underlying extracellular matrix framework is not destroyed. Superficial injuries to tracheal and bronchial epithelia heal by regeneration from the adjacent epithelium. The outcome of alveolar injury ranges from complete regeneration of structure and function to incapacitating fibrosis. As is the case with the liver, the degree of cell necrosis and the extent of the damage to the extracellular matrix framework determine the outcome (Fig. 3-13).

Alveolar Injury with Intact Basement Membranes

Alveolar injury follows a number of insults, for example, infections, shock, and oxygen toxicity. The injury produces a variable degree of alveolar cell necrosis. The alveoli are flooded with an inflammatory exudate particularly rich in plasma proteins. As long as the alveolar basement membrane remains intact, healing is by regeneration, and neutrophils and macrophages clear the alveolar exudate. If these cells fail to liquefy the alveolar exudate, it is organized by granulation tissue, and intra-alveolar fibrosis results. Alveolar type II pneumocytes (the alveolar reserve cells) migrate to denuded areas and undergo mitosis to form cells with features intermediate between those of type I and type II pneumocytes. As these cells cover the alveolar surface, they establish contact with other epithelial cells. Mitosis then stops and the cells differentiate into type I pneumocytes. Regeneration may occur via bone-marrow derived cells or by putative lung bronchioalveolar progenitor or stem cells that differentiate to bronchiolar Clara cells and alveolar cells (see Table 3-9).

Alveolar Injury with Disrupted Basement Membranes

Extensive damage to the alveolar basement membrane evokes scarring and fibrosis. Mesenchymal cells from the alveolar septa proliferate and differentiate into fibroblasts and myofibroblasts. The role of macrophage products in inducing fibroblast proliferation in the lung is well documented. The myofibroblasts and fibroblasts migrate into the alveolar spaces, where they secrete extracellular matrix components, mainly type I collagen and proteoglycans, to produce pulmonary fibrosis. The most common chronic pulmonary disease is emphysema, which involves airspace enlargement and the destruction of alveolar walls. Ineffective replacement of elastin is associated with irreversible loss of tissue resiliency and function.

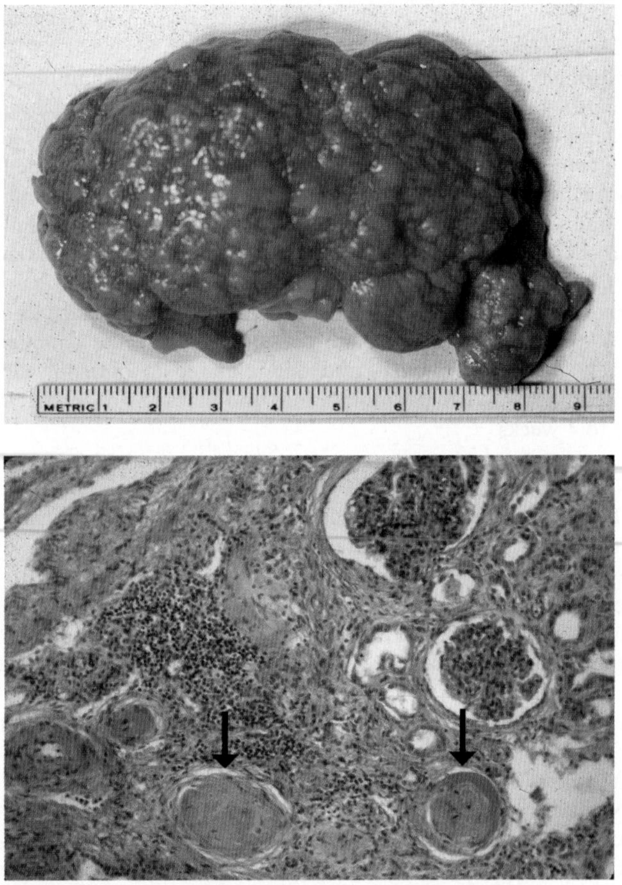

A

B

FIGURE 3-12. **Scarred kidney. A.** Repeated bacterial urinary tract infections have scarred the kidney. **B.** Many glomeruli have been destroyed and appear as circular scars *(arrows).*

Heart

Cardiac myocytes are permanent, nondividing, terminally differentiated cells. Recent studies, however, have provided evidence for minimal regeneration of cardiac myocytes from previously unrecognized stem or reserve cells. The origin of these cells, whether they reside in the myocardium or migrate there following injury from sites unknown, is not resolved. For practical purposes, myocardial necrosis, from whatever cause, heals by the formation of granulation tissue and eventual scarring (Fig. 3-14). Not only does myocardial scarring result in the loss of contractile elements, but the fibrotic tissue also decreases the effectiveness of contraction in the surviving myocardium.

Nervous System

Mature neurons have been described as permanent and postmitotic cells, and recent studies suggesting possible regenerative capacity have not altered well-established observations about injury in the nervous system. Following trauma, only regrowth and reorganization of the surviving neuronal cell processes can reestablish neural connections. Although the peripheral nervous system has the capacity for axonal regeneration, the central nervous system lacks this ability. The olfactory bulb and hippocampal dentate gyrus regions of adult mammalian brain are now known to regenerate via neural precursor or stem cells, although the physiological significance of this finding remains to be determined. Multipotent precursor cells have also been demonstrated in other parts of the brain, raising hope that repair of neural circuitry may eventually be possible (see Table 3-9).

Central Nervous System

Any damage to the brain or spinal cord is followed by the growth of capillaries and gliosis (i.e., the proliferation of astrocytes and

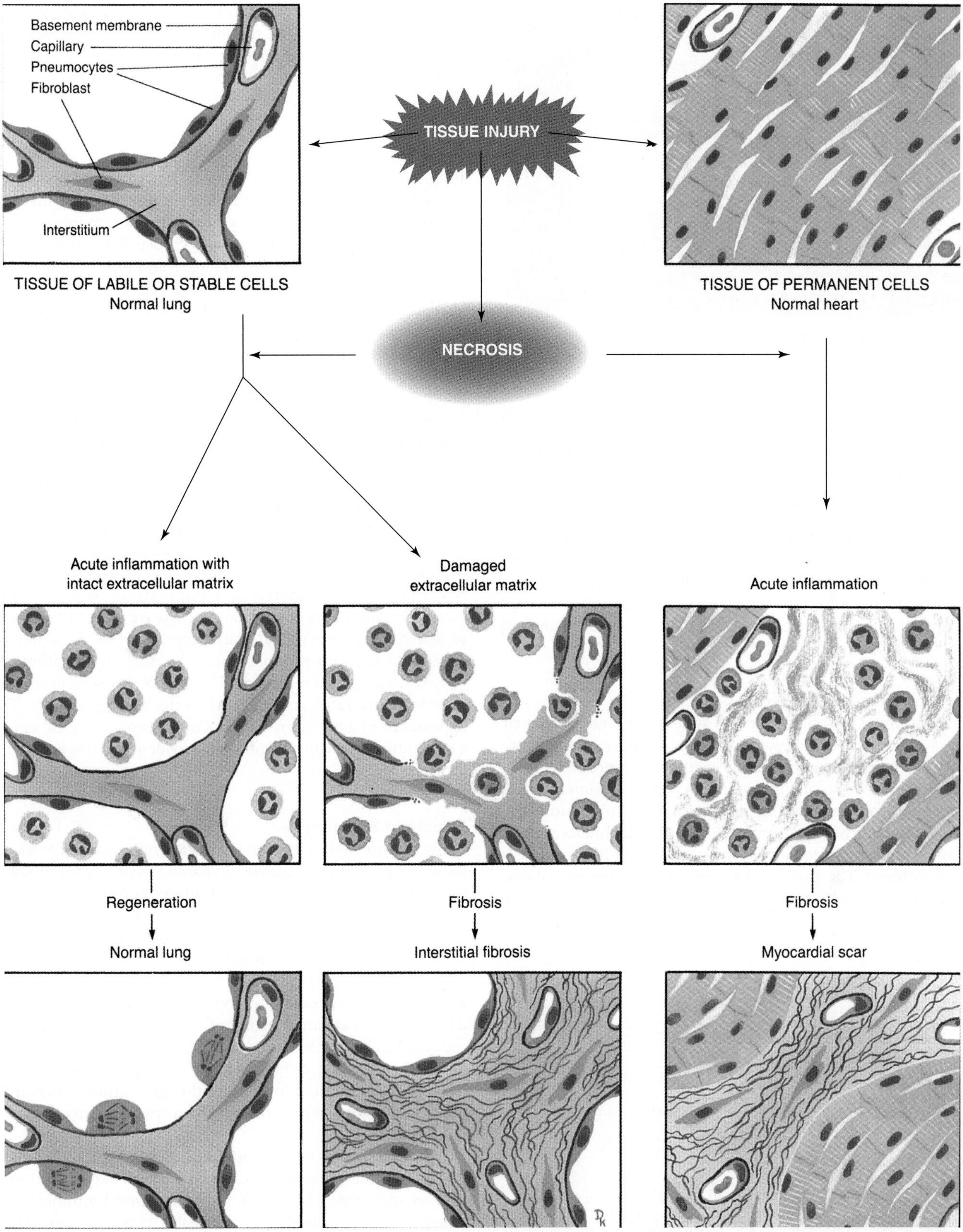

FIGURE 3-13. **Overview of repair.** This figure provides an overview that interrelates the early dynamic events in repair. The time scale in this figure is not linear; initial tensile strength, the first phase, develops almost immediately. Remodeling is ill defined, extending from its early beginning in repair for weeks or months.

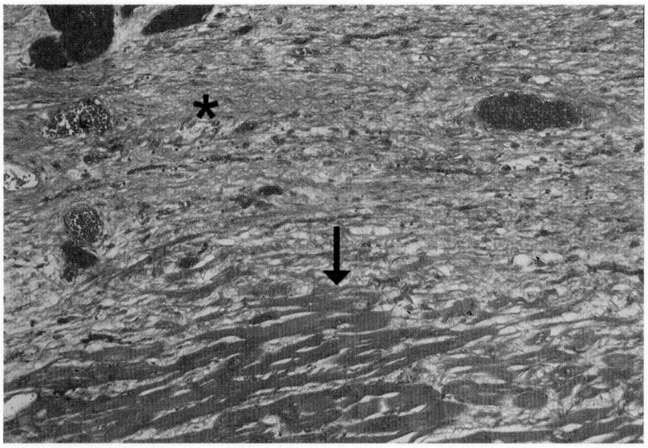

FIGURE 3-14. **Myocardial infarction.** A section through a healed myocardial infarct shows mature fibrosis (*) and disrupted myocardial fibers (*arrow*).

microglia). Gliosis in the central nervous system is the equivalent of scar formation elsewhere; once established, it remains permanently. In spinal cord injuries, axonal regeneration can be seen up to 2 weeks after injury. After 2 weeks, gliosis has taken place and attempts at axonal regeneration end. In the central nervous system, axonal regeneration occurs only in the hypothalamohypophysial region, where glial and capillary barriers do not interfere with axonal regeneration. Axonal regeneration seems to require contact with extracellular fluid containing plasma proteins.

Peripheral Nervous System

Neurons in the peripheral nervous system can regenerate their axons, and under ideal circumstances, interruption in the continuity of a peripheral nerve results in complete functional recovery. However, if the cut ends are not in perfect alignment or are prevented from establishing continuity by inflammation or a scar, a traumatic neuroma results (Fig. 3-15). This bulbous lesion consists of disorganized axons and proliferating Schwann cells and fibroblasts. The regenerative capacity of the peripheral nervous system can be ascribed to (1) the fact that the blood–nerve barrier, which insulates peripheral axons from extracellular fluids, is not restored for 2 to 3 months; and (2) the presence of Schwann cells with basement membranes. Laminin, a basement membrane component, and nerve growth factor (NGF) guide and stimulate neurite growth.

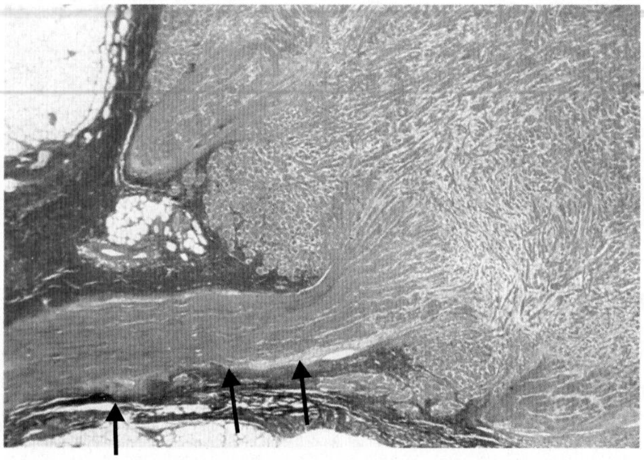

FIGURE 3-15. **Traumatic neuroma.** In this photomicrograph, the original nerve (*arrows*) enters the neuroma. The nerve is surrounded by dense collagenous tissue, which appears dark blue with this trichrome stain.

Fetal Wound Repair

Progress in surgery now permits corrective surgical operations to be performed in utero. Wounds produced in the first and second trimesters of pregnancy heal without scarring; at birth, healed cutaneous incisions are not visible. Fetal wounds also heal more rapidly than adult wounds. Adult-type healing occurs in late pregnancy. Fetal healing is characterized by the virtual absence of acute inflammation, by the regeneration of skin appendages such as hair follicles (not seen in adult healing) and by the absence of TGF-β_1 in fetal skin. Hyaluronan is preserved at higher levels for a longer time in fetal repair as compared with adult repair, apparently inhibiting scarring. MMPs are also increased in fetal skin, promoting scarless healing. The fibroblasts of fetal wounds do not appear to require activation to secrete collagen, in contrast to adult fibroblasts.

The epidermis of the fetal skin is bilayered, as contrasted with the multiple layers of the stratified adult epidermis. Embryonic epidermal cells around the margin of the wound are pulled over the wound via contraction of a thick cable of actin along the leading edge of the cells. Fetal epidermal cells are drawn toward one another as if gathered by a purse-string, whereas adult wound keratinocytes crawl along the matrix using lamellipodia to attach to the provisional matrix glycoproteins. Fetal wound repair continues to provoke study, because to recapture the environment of fetal repair could be extremely useful in circumstances of unwanted scarring, such as the healing of burns. The appearance of a newborn who has undergone a surgical operation in utero, but who has no visible evidence of this at birth, is arresting.

Effects of Scarring

In the absence of the ability to form scars, mammalian life would hardly be possible. Yet scarring in parenchymal organs modifies their complex structure and never improves their function. For example, in the heart, the scar of a myocardial infarction serves to prevent rupture of the heart but reduces the amount of contractile tissue. If extensive enough, it may cause congestive heart failure or the formation of a ventricular aneurysm. Similarly, the aorta that is weakened and scarred by atherosclerosis is prone to dilate as an aneurysm. Scarring of mitral and aortic valves as a result of local inflammation caused by rheumatic fever are often stenotic, regurgitant, or both, leading to congestive heart failure. Persistent inflammation within the pericardium produces fibrous adhesions, which result in constrictive pericarditis and heart failure.

Alveolar fibrosis in the lung causes respiratory failure. Infection within the peritoneum or even surgical exploration may lead to adhesions and intestinal obstruction. Immunological injury to the renal glomerulus eventuates in its replacement by a collagenous scar and, if this process is extensive, renal failure. Scarring in the skin following burns or surgical excision of lesions produces unsatisfactory cosmetic results. An important goal of therapeutic intervention is to create optimum conditions for "constructive" scarring and prevent pathological "overshoot" of this process.

Wound Repair Is Often Suboptimal

Abnormalities in any of three healing processes—repair, contraction, and regeneration—result in unsuccessful or prolonged wound healing. The skill of the surgeon is often of critical importance.

Deficient Scar Formation

Inadequate formation of granulation tissue or an inability to form a suitable extracellular matrix leads to deficient scar formation and its complications.

Wound Dehiscence and Incisional Hernias

Dehiscence (the wound splitting open) is most frequent after abdominal surgery and can be a life-threatening complication. Increased mechanical stress on the wound from vomiting, coughing, or bowel obstruction sometimes causes dehiscence of the abdominal wound. Systemic factors predisposing to dehiscence include metabolic deficiency, hypoproteinemia, and the general inanition that often accompanies metastatic cancer. An **incisional hernia** of the abdominal wall refers to a defect caused by prior surgery. Such hernias resulting from weak scars are often the consequence of insufficient deposition of extracellular matrix or inadequate cross-linking in the collagen matrix. Loops of intestine are sometimes trapped within incisional hernias.

Ulceration

Wounds can ulcerate when there is an inadequate intrinsic blood supply or insufficient vascularization during healing. For example, leg wounds in persons with varicose veins or severe atherosclerosis often ulcerate. Nonhealing wounds also develop in areas devoid of sensation because of persistent trauma. Such **trophic** or **neuropathic** ulcers are commonly seen in diabetic peripheral neuropathy. Occasionally they occur in patients with spinal involvement from tertiary syphilis and leprosy.

Excessive Scar Formation

Excessive deposition of extracellular matrix, mostly excessive collagen, at the wound site results in a hypertrophic scar. **Keloid** is an exuberant scar that tends to progress beyond the site of initial injury and recurs after excision (Fig. 3-16). Histologically, both of these types of scars exhibit broad and irregular collagen bundles, with more capillaries and fibroblasts than expected for a scar of the same age. More clearly defined in keloids than in hypertrophic scars, the rate of collagen synthesis, the ratio of type III to type I collagen, and the number of reducible cross-links, remain high. This situation that indicates a "maturation arrest," or block, in the healing process. Further support for maturation arrest as an explanation for keloid and hypertrophic scars is the overexpression of fibronectin in these lesions. In addition, unlike normal healing tissue, these scar tissues fail to downregulate collagen synthesis when glucocorticoids are administered. Keloids are unsightly, and attempts at surgical repair are always problematic, the outcome likely being a still larger keloid. Dark-skinned persons are more frequently affected by keloids than light-skinned people, and the tendency is sometimes hereditary. By contrast, the occurrence of **hypertrophic scars** is not associated with skin color or heredity.

Excessive Contraction

A decrease in the size of a wound depends on the presence of myofibroblasts, development of cell–cell contacts, and sustained cell contraction. An exaggeration of these processes is termed **contracture** and results in severe deformity of the wound and surrounding tissues. Interestingly, the regions that normally show minimal wound contraction (e.g., the palms, the soles, and the anterior aspect of the thorax) are the ones prone to contractures. Contractures are particularly conspicuous in the healing of serious burns and can be severe enough to compromise the movement of joints. In the alimentary tract, a contracture (stricture) can result in obstruction to the passage of food in the esophagus or a block in the flow of intestinal contents.

Several diseases are characterized by contracture and irreversible fibrosis of the superficial fascia, including Dupuytren contracture (palmar contracture), Lederhosen disease (plantar contracture), and Peyronie disease (contracture of the cavernous tissues of the penis). In these diseases, there is no known precipitating injury, even though the basic process is similar to contracture in wound healing.

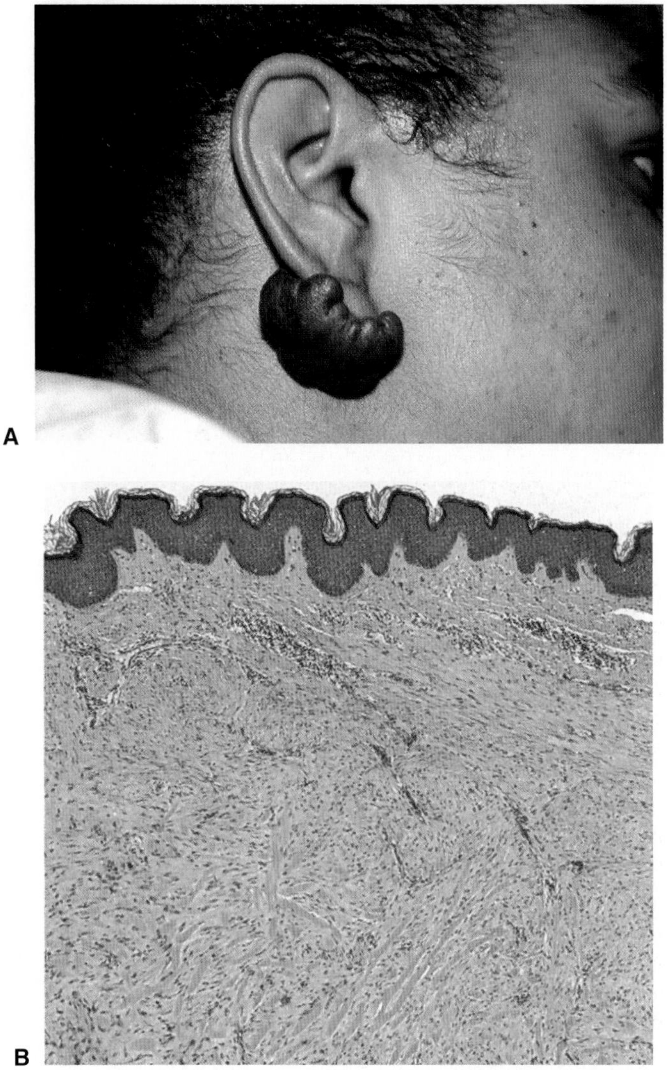

FIGURE 3-16. **Keloid. A.** A light-skinned black woman developed a keloid as a reaction to having her earlobe pierced. **B.** Microscopically, the dermis is markedly thickened by the presence of collagen bundles with random orientation and abundant cells.

Excessive Regeneration and Repair

In addition to the many responses to injury described thus far, an additional lesion merits consideration, namely **pyogenic granuloma**. This lesion is a localized, persistent, exuberant overgrowth of granulation tissue, most commonly seen in gum tissue in pregnant women. It also develops in the squamo-columnar junction of the uterine cervix and at other sites. An injury preceding the development of pyogenic granuloma cannot usually be found. Like injury-induced granulation tissue, it lacks nerves and can be surgically trimmed without anesthesia. Conceptually, pyogenic granuloma is a transitional lesion, resembling granulation tissue but behaving almost as an autonomous benign neoplasm.

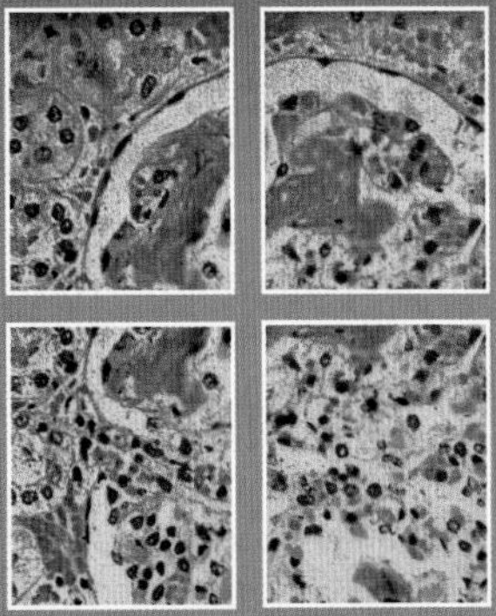

4

Immunopathology

Jeffrey S. Warren
Douglas P. Bennett
Roger J. Pomerantz

The most basic challenge to an organism is to distinguish self from nonself so that it can continue to exist. The chief role of the immune system is to protect the host from invasion by foreign agents. Immune responses can be elicited by a wide range of agents including parasites, bacteria, viruses, chemicals, toxins, drugs, and transplanted tissues. As components of host defense, immune responses are characterized by their ability to distinguish self from nonself, their ability to discriminate among potential invaders (specificity), and immune memory, coupled to the capacity for amplification (i.e., the ability to recall previous exposures and to mount an intensified or anamnestic response).

Humans possess physical barriers such as regionally adapted epithelia (e.g., thick skin, ciliated respiratory epithelium, and a nearly impervious urothelium), chemical–mechanical barriers (e.g., antibacterial lipids and mucus), and indigenous microbial flora that compete with potential pathogens. Patterned hemodynamic responses, cell surface-associated and soluble mediator systems (e.g., complement and coagulation systems), and antigen-nonspecific phagocytes (e.g., resident macrophages, neutrophils) are integral to protective inflammatory responses (see Chapter 2). Host defenses that are not antigen-specific are called the "innate" immune system. Antigen-specific or "adaptive" immune system encompasses lymphocytes, plasma cells, antigen-presenting cells (APCs), specific effector molecules (e.g., immunoglobulins), and a vast array of regulatory mediators.

As noted above, the defining features of adaptive immunity include specificity, memory, and the capacity for amplification. Specificity and immunologic memory are direct results of activation by antigens of lymphocyte clones that bear specific receptors. There are many linkages among the various layers of host defense. For example, an antibody can specifically bind to an epitope on a bacterium, leading to complement fixation, and, in turn, generation of chemotactic peptides that attract phagocytic neutrophils.

It is important to consider the relationships of specific immune system components within the general rubric of acute and chronic inflammation, cell injury, and cell death. For example, immediate (type I) hypersensitivity reactions are immunoglobulin (Ig)E-mediated, depend on generation of vasoactive compounds, and feature inflammatory infiltrates rich in eosinophils. A type III hypersensitivity reaction, which is immune complex-mediated, is characterized by an acute inflammatory infiltrate (mainly neutrophils). Type IV hypersensitivity reactions are triggered by antigen exposure and involve chronic inflammatory infiltrates (mononuclear phagocytes and T lymphocytes). Recognition of these mechanistic and morphologic relationships can be helpful diagnostically and therapeutically.

Biology of the Immune System

The Cells that Comprise the Immune System Derive from Hematopoietic Stem Cells

The cellular components of the immune system are derived from pluripotent hematopoietic stem cells (HSCs). Near the end of the first month of embryogenesis, HSCs appear in the extraembryonic erythropoietic islands adjacent to the yolk sac. At 6 weeks, the primary site of hematopoiesis shifts from extraembryonic blood islands to fetal liver to bone marrow. The process begins at 2 months but by 6 months has completely shifted to bone marrow. Although there are well-defined sequential changes in the primary site of hematopoiesis, there are periods of overlap. By 8 weeks of gestation, lymphoid stem cells derived from HSCs and fated to become T cells circulate to the thymus where they differentiate into mature T lymphocytes. Lymphoid stem cells destined to become B cells differentiate first within fetal liver (8 weeks) and later within bone marrow (12 weeks). In the development of both thymic T lymphocytes and bone marrow B lymphocytes, the microenvironments (e.g., thymic epithelium, bone marrow stromal cells, growth factors) are critical. Mature lymphocytes exit the thymus and bone marrow and "home" to peripheral lymphoid tissues (e.g., lymph nodes, spleen, skin, and mucosa). The population of peripheral lymphoid tissues by mature T and B lymphocytes and the rapid deployment and recirculation of mature lymphocytes to different, often remote, parts of the immune system are anatomically specific. "Lymphocyte homing and recirculation" are orchestrated by a series of leukocyte and endothelial surface molecules called **selectins** and **addressins**. The processes of lymphocyte development and homing/recirculation are important for understanding immune responses, genetic immunodeficiency states, regional host defense, and the underpinnings of modern therapeutics (e.g., HSC transplantation).

The cells of the immune system express a vast array of surface molecules that are important in cellular differentiation and cell-to-cell communication. These surface molecules serve as useful markers of cellular identity. The International Workshop on Human Leukocyte Differentiation Antigens is responsible for nomenclature of these markers and assigns them so-called cluster of differentiation or cluster designation (CD) numbers. Currently, some 300 different molecules have been assigned CD numbers.

Hematopoietic Stem Cells

Pluripotent HSCs account for 1% of bone marrow mononuclear cells. They exhibit characteristic light-scattering properties as assessed by flow cytometry, usually express **CD34** cell surface protein and lack cell surface molecules that characterize more mature lymphocyte subpopulations (e.g., CD2, CD3, CD5, CD7, CD14, CD15, and CD16). Recently, a smaller population of $CD34^-$ HSCs was described. $CD34^+$ HSCs also circulate, and account for 0.01% to 0.1% of mononuclear peripheral blood cells. Bone marrow and blood HSCs are heterogeneous in terms of selected lymphocyte marker expression, myeloid markers, and activation antigens, and in terms of their capacity to engraft bone marrow. Infusion of peripheral blood HSCs in sufficient numbers into transplant recipients leads to faster marrow recovery than occurs in patients who have received marrow-derived HSCs. HSCs are quantified following harvest and before infusion into recipient patients. In clinical HSC transplantation, it is now common practice for donors to receive recombinant growth factors prior to HSC harvest. This practice has led to higher yields of harvested HSCs, decreased time to engraftment, and improved rates of successful engraftment. The proportion of bone marrow transplant recipients who receive harvested peripheral blood HSCs rather than marrow-derived HSCs has increased dramatically in recent years.

Lymphopoiesis and Hematopoiesis

All mature lymphoid and hematopoietic cells are derived from a common population of pluripotential HSCs (Fig. 4-1). Each step in lymphopoiesis and hematopoiesis depends on a microenvironment that encompasses specific structural features and a complex array of growth factors. The primary branch point in differentiation is between lymphoid progenitors and myeloid progenitors. The former ultimately give rise to T lymphocytes, B lymphocytes, and natural killer (NK) cells; whereas the latter develop into granulocytic, erythroid, monocytic–dendritic, and megakaryocytic colony-forming units (GEMM-CFUs). Downstream, CFUs become more lineage-specific. Examples include CFU-GM (granulocyte-monocyte), CFU-Eo (eosinophil), CFU-E (erythrocyte), and so forth. CFU refers to a cell that ultimately gives rise to a specified population of "offspring," such as granulocytes, erythrocytes, monocytes, dendritic cells, and megakaryocytes.

Lymphocytes

There are three major types of lymphocytes—T cells, B cells, and NK cells—which account for 25% of peripheral blood leukocytes. Some 80% of blood lymphocytes are T cells, 10% B cells, and 10% NK cells. The relative proportions of lymphocytes in the peripheral blood and central and peripheral lymphoid tissues vary. In contrast to the blood, only 30% to 40% of splenic and bone marrow lymphocytes are T cells.

T lymphocytes can be subdivided into subpopulations by virtue of their specialized functions, by surface CD molecules, and in some cases, morphologic features. Lymphoid progenitor cells destined to become T cells exit the bone marrow and migrate to the thymus in waves. There, both alpha/beta (α/β) and gamma/delta (γ/δ) T lymphocytes are formed (Fig. 4-2). "Alpha/ beta" and "gamma/delta" are the two major classes of heterodimeric T cell receptors (TCRs) that specifically recognize and bind various antigens. The thymic microenvironment is determined by the epithelial stroma. The early thymus is formed from ectoderm and endoderm derived from the third bronchial cleft and the third and fourth pharyngeal pouches. This thymic anlage is then colonized by HSCs that give rise to T cells, macrophages, and dendritic cells. The thymic cortex is composed of a meshwork of epithelial cell processes that surround groups of immature thymocytes that bear both $CD4^+$ and $CD8^+$ surface molecules (Fig. 4-3). As T lymphocytes mature, they percolate into thymic medulla where, in close proximity to nested groups of epithelial cells, they form more mature cells that are either $CD4^+$ or $CD8^+$.

The thymic corticomedullary junction contains many bone marrow HSC-derived macrophages and dendritic cells. Much of

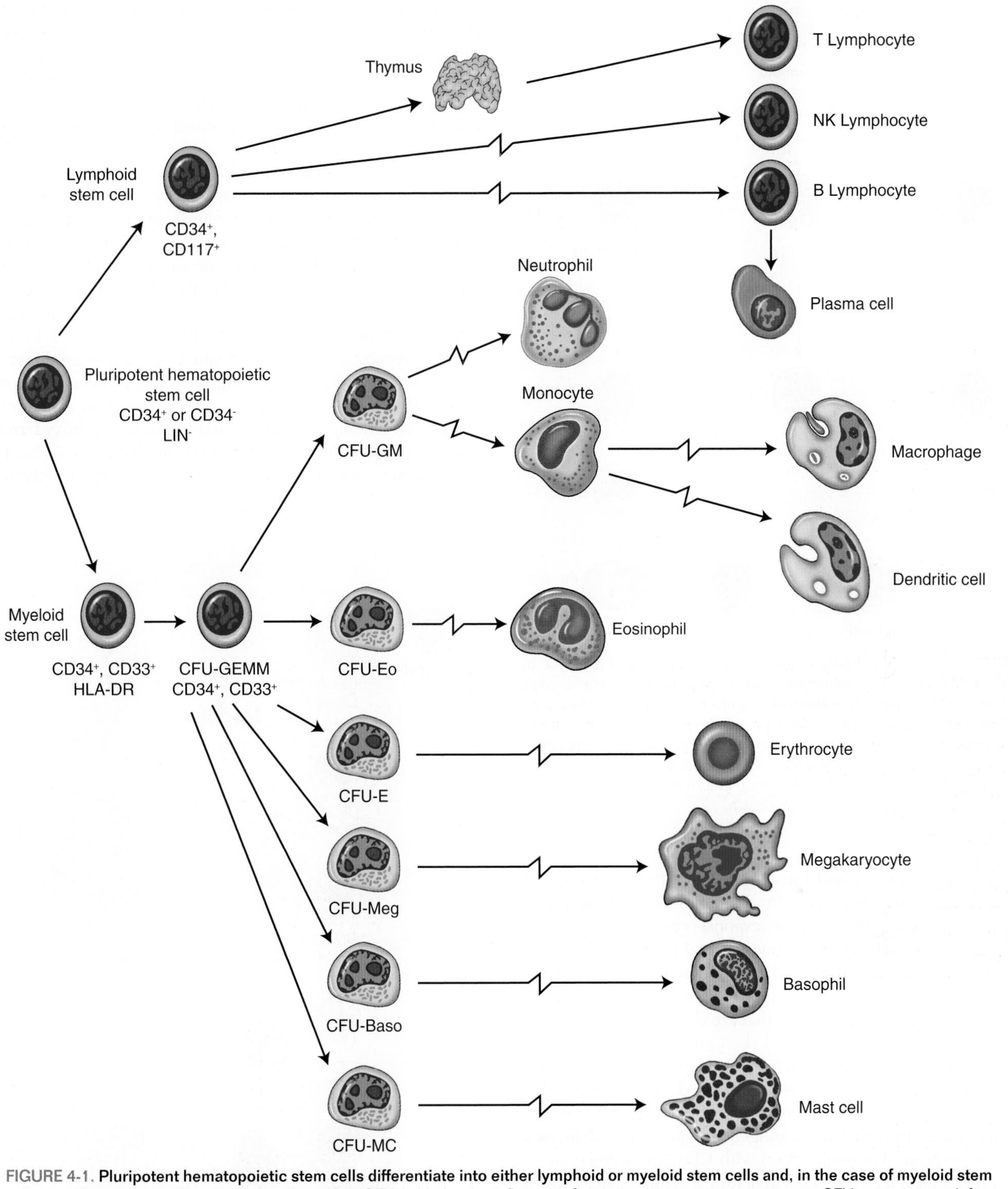

FIGURE 4-1. **Pluripotent hematopoietic stem cells differentiate into either lymphoid or myeloid stem cells and, in the case of myeloid stem cells, into lineage-specific colony-forming units (CFUs).** Under the influence of an appropriate microenvironment, CFUs give rise to definitive cell types. Lymphoid stem cells are precursors of natural killer (NK) cells, T lymphocytes, and B lymphocytes. B lymphocytes give rise to plasma cells. CD = cluster designation; CFU-GEMM = granulocytic, erythroid, monocytic–dendritic, and megakaryocytic colony-forming units; HLA = human leukocyte antigen.

the "positive selection" of thymocytes occurs in the cortex; "negative selection" tends to occur through exposure of developing thymocytes to corticomedullary dendritic cells. In **positive thymic selection** transient binding of cell surface TCRs to a person's own major histocompatibility complex (MHC) class I or II molecules prevents cell death. **Negative thymic selection** is the converse process in which high-affinity TCR-mediated binding to one's own MHC class I or II molecules results in cell death by apoptosis. These complementary thymic selection processes are pivotal to T lymphocyte development, so that T cells can interact with the host's own cells but not in a manner that results in excessive self-reactivity (see below under discussion of autoimmune.)

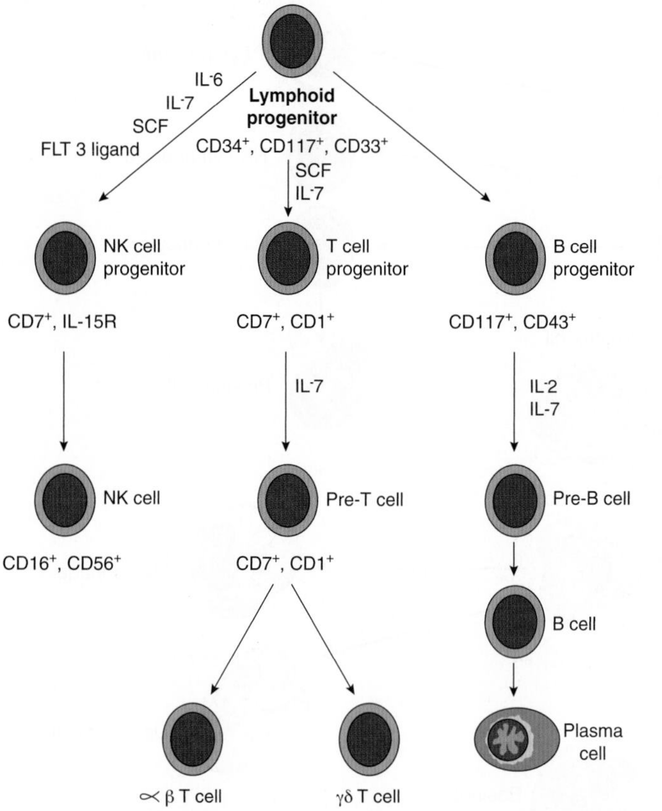

FIGURE 4-2. **Lymphoid progenitors (lymphoid stem cells) give rise to mature but naïve T lymphocytes and B lymphocytes.** Lymphocytes destined to become T lymphocytes migrate to the thymus where they become either α/β or γ/δ T cells. *Type 1* and *type 2* helper cells refer to functional characteristics of T cells (see text). Other lymphocytes differentiate in the bone marrow and give rise to clonal populations of surface immunoglobulin-producing B cells, which in turn can form plasma cells. CD = cluster designation, IL = interleukin.

Thymic selection and lineage-specific differentiation of T lymphocytes are processes fundamental to understanding autoimmunity and the immune response, respectively. Thymic T lymphocyte maturation includes several processes. Developing T cells recombine dispersed gene segments that encode the heterodimeric α/β or γ/δ TCRs. α/β T lymphocytes progress through stages of development that are characterized as $CD4^-$, $CD8^-$, then $CD4^+$, $CD8^+$, and then either $CD4^+$, $CD8^-$ or $CD4^-$, $CD8^+$ (see Fig.4-2 and Fig.4-3). *Most $CD4^+$, $CD8^-$ T cells function as helper cells; most $CD4^-$, $CD8^+$ T cells are cytotoxic cells.*

T lymphocytes exit the thymus and populate peripheral lymphoid tissues. In the thymus, antigen-specific TCRs are formed and are expressed in conjunction with CD3, an essential accessory molecule. Nearly 95% of circulating T lymphocytes express α/β TCRs. In turn, circulating α/β T cells also express either CD4 or CD8. A smaller population (5%) of T cells expresses γ/δ TCRs and CD3 but neither CD4 nor CD8.

B lymphocytes differentiate into antibody-secreting plasma cells in the bone marrow. Similarly to T lymphocyte development, the microenvironment of either the fetal liver or bone marrow, is critical to B lymphocyte development. In both organs, only B lymphocytes that pass through the many stages necessary to produce surface immunoglobulin survive. Conversely, developing B cells in which surface immunoglobulin binds too avidly to self-antigens are negatively selected and eliminated.

Analogous to T cells, B lymphocytes express a surface antigen-binding receptor, namely membrane immunoglobulin (mIg), which bears the same antigen-binding specificity as the soluble immunoglobulin that will ultimately be secreted by the corresponding terminally differentiated plasma cells. Like T cells, B lymphocytes also exhibit a degree of heterogeneity (e.g., $CD5^+$ [B]) and $CD5^-$ [B2]).

TCRs, along with immunoglobulins and MHC class I and class II molecules (see below), confer specificity to the immune system by virtue of their capacity to specifically bind foreign antigens or interact with self-cells, respectively. TCR, immunoglobulin, and a portion of the MHC class I molecule are encoded by members of the immunoglobulin supergene family. The structural variability and, in turn, high specificity of TCRs and immunoglobulins are achieved through genetic recombination of segmented TCR and Ig genes. As noted above, an individual TCR is a heterodimer that forms an antigen-binding site (Fig. 4-4). The proteins that constitute TCRs and immunoglobulins each possesses an amino-terminal antigen-binding variable (V) domain and a carboxy-terminal constant (C) domain. TCRs anchor the antigen to the cell surface, whereas immunoglobulins either anchor the receptor to the B cell

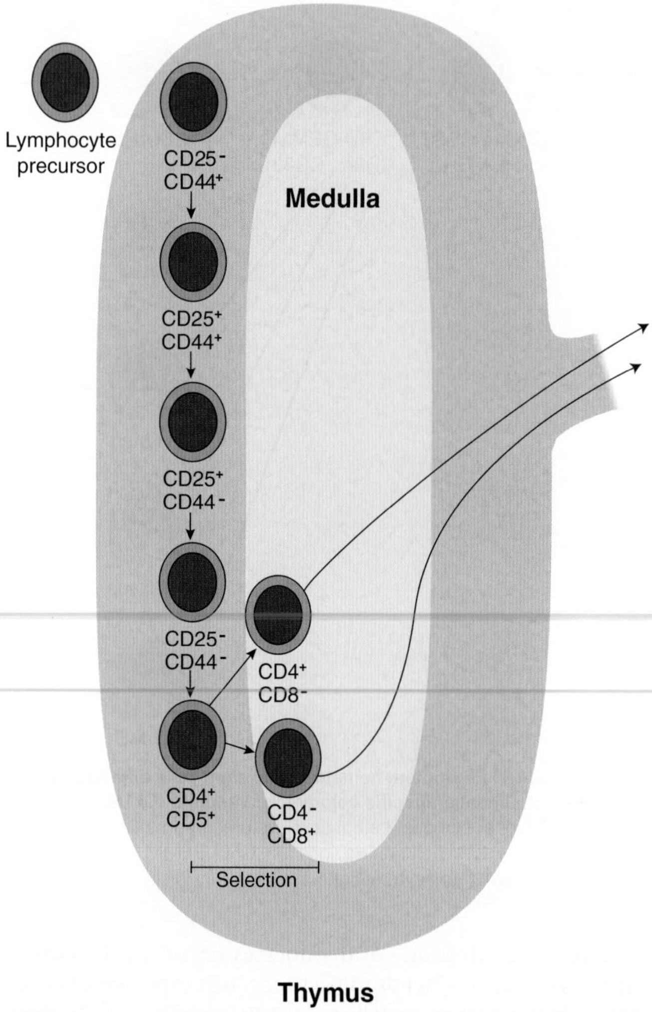

FIGURE 4-3. **Lymphoid progenitors that are destined to become mature, but naïve, T cells differentiate as they percolate through the thymus.** Peripheral $CD4^+$ and $CD8^+$ T cells are derived from thymic precursor cells that are $CD3^+$, $CD4^+$, and $CD8^+$.

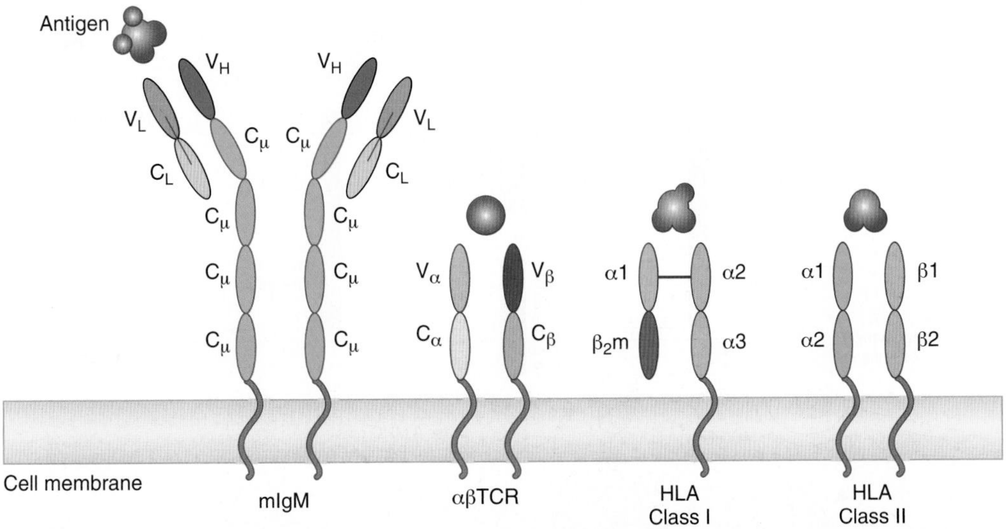

FIGURE 4-4. **The antigen-binding sites of T cell receptors (TCRs) and membrane immunoglobulin (mIg) are formed by the alignment of N-terminal variable domains of two peptide chains.** Each variable (V) domain is derived from a transcript that is the product of a random VJ (TCR) or V(D)J (Ig) gene segment rearrangement. The antigen-binding grooves of major histocompatibility complex (MHC) molecules are formed by the alignment of the $\alpha 1$ and $\alpha 2$ domains of class I and the $\alpha 1$ and $\beta 1$ domains of class II molecules. C indicates a constant domain and $\beta 2m$ represents β_2 microglobulin, which is a component of an intact human leukocyte antigen (HLA) class I molecule.

surface as mIg, or, in the case of soluble immunoglobulin, mediate its biological function (see Fig. 4-4).

NK cells recognize target cells mainly via antigen-independent mechanisms. They are believed to form in both the thymus and bone marrow. NK cells bear several types of class I MHC molecule receptors, which when engaged actually *inhibit* the NK cell's capacity to secrete cytolytic products. Certain tumor cells and virus-infected cells bear reduced numbers of MHC class I molecules and thus do not inhibit NK cells. In this scenario, NK cells engage virus-infected or tumor cells and secrete complement-like cytolytic proteins (perforin), granzymes A and B, and other lytic factors. NK cells also secrete granulysin, a cationic protein that induces target cell apoptosis.

In another example of linkage between different facets of the immune system, NK cells can also lyse target cells via antibody-dependent cellular cytotoxicity (ADCC). In ADCC, NK cells, through their Fc receptors, bind to the Fc domain of IgG that is specifically bound to antigen on surfaces of target cells. As with T and B cells, NK cells exhibit a degree of heterogeneity (e.g., $CD16^+$, $CD16^-$).

Mononuclear Phagocytes, Antigen-Presenting Cells (APCs) and Dendritic Cells

Mononuclear phagocytes, chiefly **monocytes**, account for 10% of circulating white blood cells. Circulating monocytes give rise to resident tissue macrophages including, among others, Kupffer cells, alveolar macrophages, and microglial cells. Monocytes and macrophages express an array of specific cell surface molecules that are important for their host defense functions. These include MHC class II molecules, CD14 (a receptor that binds bacterial lipopolysaccharide and can trigger cell activation), several types of Fc immunoglobulin receptors, toll-like receptors, adhesion molecules, and a variety of cytokine receptors that participate in regulating monocyte/macrophage function. Activated macrophages produce a variety of cytokines and soluble mediators of host defense (e.g., interferon-γ [IFN-γ], interleukin [IL]-1β, tumor necrosis factor-α [TNF-α], and complement components).

APCs, defined by their function and derived from HSCs, acquire the capacity to present antigen to T lymphocytes in the context of histocompatibility, after cytokine-driven upregulation of MHC class II molecules (Fig. 4-5). Monocytes, macrophages, dendritic cells and under certain conditions, B lymphocytes, endothelial cells and epithelial cells, can act as APCs. In some locations, APCs are highly specialized for this function. For instance, in B cell-rich follicles of lymph nodes and spleen, specialized APCs are termed **follicular dendritic cells**. In these sites, through engagement of antibody and complement via Fc and C3b receptors, APCs trap antigen–antibody complexes. In the case of lymph nodes, such complexes arrive via afferent lymphatics, and in spleen, through the blood. Antigen presentation by follicular dendritic cells leads to generation of memory B lymphocytes (Fig. 4-6).

Dendritic cells are specialized APCs that are termed "dendritic" by virtue of their spiderlike morphologic appearance. They are found in B lymphocyte-rich lymphoid follicles, in thymic medulla, and in many peripheral sites, including intestinal lamina propria, lung, genitourinary tract, and skin (Fig. 4-6). Peripherally located dendritic cells are less mature than the APCs found in lymphoid follicles and express lower levels of accessory cell activation molecules (CD80 [B7-1], CD86 [B7-2]) than do mature dendritic cells. An example of a peripheral APC is the **epidermal Langerhans cell**. Upon exposure, the Langerhans cell engulfs antigen, migrates to a regional lymph node through an afferent lymphatic, and differentiates into a more mature dendritic cell. Langerhans cell-derived dendritic cells express high densities of MHC class I and II molecules and costimulatory molecules (CD80, CD86), and present antigen efficiently to T lymphocytes. Again, antigen presentation to T cells occurs through TCRs in the context of histocompatibility determined by MHC class II molecules.

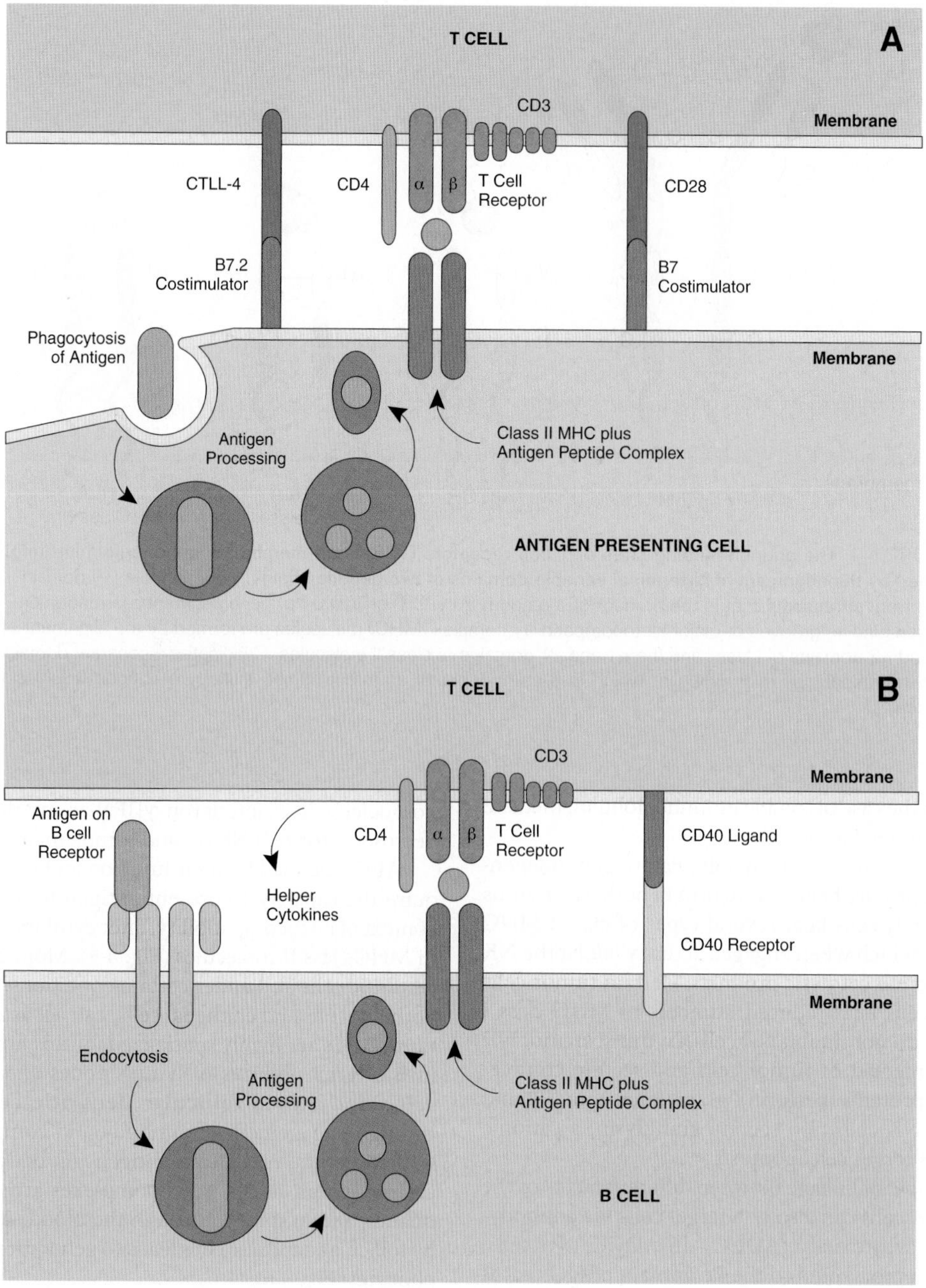

FIGURE 4-5. **A. T lymphocyte activation (by the T cell receptor [TCR]) occurs via peptides cleaved from the phagocytized antigen (antigen processing) and presented to the TCR in the context of a histocompatible class II major histocompatibility complex (MHC) molecule.** T-cell activation also requires accessory or costimulatory signals from cytotoxic lymphoid line (CTLL)-4 or CD28. **B.** A similar process applies to B cell–T cell interactions. The B lymphocyte antigen receptor is membrane immunoglobulin.

Lymphocyte Homing and Recirculation

The segments of DNA that encode the antigen-binding domains of TCRs and immunoglobulin are rearranged in developing T cells and B cells, respectively, to form "new" genes. Through this combinatorial process and a variety of other diversity-generating mechanisms, a large number of different antigen receptors is generated. Adults possesses about 10^{12} lymphocytes, of which only 10% are in the circulation at a given time. Despite the large number of lymphocytes, the number with any specific antigen receptor is relatively small. In addition, the body surfaces that frequently serve as portals of entry for foreign invaders are very large (e.g., skin, 2 m^2; respiratory tract, 100 m^2; gastrointestinal tract, 400 m^2). Lymphocyte trafficking is a necessary aspect of host defense because it allows small numbers of any set of antigen-specific lymphocytes to move to sites of "need." Lymphocyte trafficking, which entails homing and recirculation, has evolved to provide rapid, flexible, and widespread distribution of lymphocytes and a means of focusing specific immunologic processes in anatomically discrete sites (e.g., lymph node cortex).

Following completion of early development, naïve B and T lymphocytes circulate via the vascular system to secondary lym-

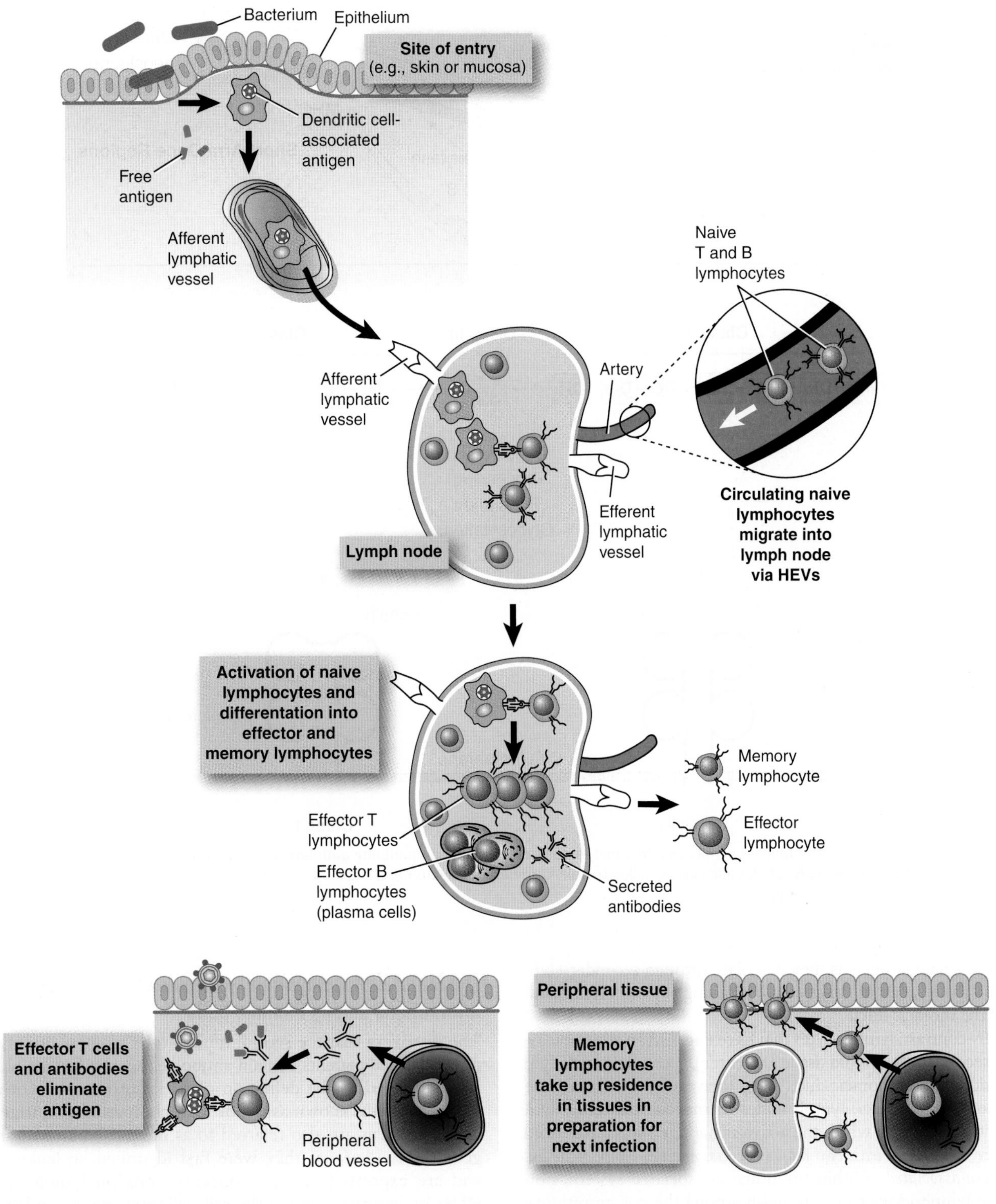

FIGURE 4-6. **In an integrated immune response, antigen is processed and presented by a dendritic cell which migrates via the afferent lymphatics to a regional lymph node.** Within the regional lymph node antigen is presented to lymphocytes, which in turn are activated and may migrate (via homing mechanism) to specific peripheral sites. HEVs = high endothelial venules.

phoid organs and tissues. Included among these tissues are lymph nodes, mucosa-associated lymphoid tissues (e.g., Peyer's patches), and the spleen. Lymphocyte trafficking through lymph nodes occurs through specialized postcapillary venules termed **high endothelial venules** (HEVs) because of the high cuboidal shape of their endothelial cells. HEVs express cellular adhesion molecules (e.g., CD31), which allow lymphocyte binding. The cuboidal shape of HEV cells reduces flow-mediated shear forces and specialized intercellular connections facilitate egress of lymphocytes out of the vascular space. Lymphocytes that do not find

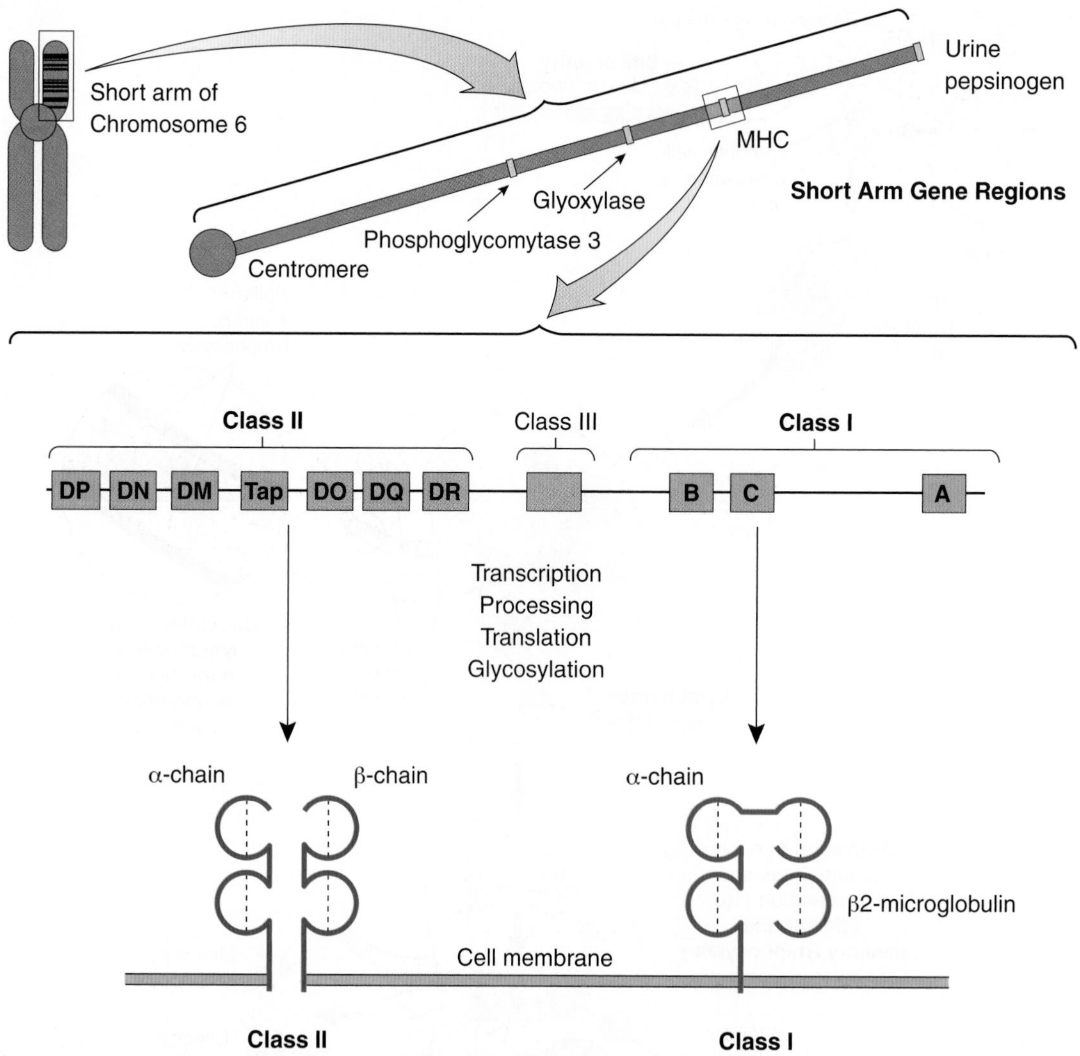

FIGURE 4-7. **The highly polymorphic loci that encode major histocompatibility antigens are located on the short arm of chromosome 6.** Class I and class II molecules exhibit different structures, but each participates in fundamentally important cell-cell interactions.

their cognate antigen as they percolate through secondary lymphoid tissues reenter the circulation through efferent lymphatics and the thoracic duct.

By contrast, lymphocytes that have engaged an antigen leave the secondary lymphoid tissue and enter the circulation via lymphatics and the thoracic duct. They then preferentially bind peripheral tissues (e.g., lymph nodes or mucosa-associated lymphoid tissue) from which the activating antigen was introduced. *Hence there are at least two major circuits, namely, lymph node and mucosa-associated.* Within the mucosa-associated system, non-naïve lymphocytes can distinguish among the gut, respiratory, and genitourinary tracts. Lymphocyte (and neutrophil) homing into sites of inflammation is mediated by different sets of leukocyte and endothelial cell adhesion molecules (see Chapter 2). The best-understood adhesion molecules involved in lymphocyte–lymphoid tissue trafficking include L-selectins (on lymphocytes) and peripheral lymph node addressins, which serve as attachment sites for lymphocytes. Among others, the addressins include CD34, podocalyxin, mucosal addressin cell adhesion molecule-1 (MadCAM-1), and glycosylation-dependent cell adhesion molecule-1 (GlyCAM-1).

The Major Histocompatibility Complex Coordinates Interactions among Immune Cells

The discovery that the sera of multiparous women and multiply-transfused patients contain antibodies against foreign blood leukocytes led to the definition of an intricate system of cell surface proteins known as **major histocompatibility antigens.** These antigens are also referred to as **human leukocyte antigens** (HLAs) because they were first identified on leukocytes and are expressed in high concentrations on lymphocytes. HLAs orchestrate many of the cell–cell interactions fundamental to the immune response. Important interactions between cells of the immune system require histoincompatibility. Conversely, these antigens are major immunogens and are targets in transplant rejection. The MHC includes class I, II, and III antigens. (Class III antigens represent certain complement components and are not histocompatibility antigens *per se.*) Molecules structurally similar to "traditional" MHC class I and II molecules are encoded outside of the more restricted MHC region on the short arm of chromosome 6. Examples include MHC-1b and CD1d which can activate so-called NK T cells. NK

T cells exhibit characteristics of both T lymphocytes and NK cells. Other nontraditional MHC-1 molecules include HLA-E, HLA-F, and HLA-G. These latter molecules are more tissue-restricted than HLA-A, HLA-B, and HLA-C molecules, but their functions are not well understood. These molecules may regulate NK cell activity, and a role in host response to viral infections and tumorigenesis is suspected.

Class I MHC Molecules

Class I molecules are encoded by highly polymorphic genes in the A, B, and C regions of the MHC (see Fig. 4-7). These loci encode similarly structured molecules that are expressed in virtually all tissues. Class I histocompatibility antigens are heterodimeric structures consisting of two chains, a 44-kd polymorphic transmembrane glycoprotein, and a 12-kd nonpolymorphic molecule called β_2-microglobulin. The latter is a superficial surface protein lacking a membrane component and is noncovalently associated with the larger heavy chain. β_2-microglobulin is encoded by a gene on chromosome 15. Structural polymorphism occurs primarily in the extracellular domains of the α-chain. Since the alleles are expressed codominantly, tissues bear class I antigens inherited from each parent. These antigens are recognized by cytotoxic T cells during graft rejection or T lymphocyte-mediated killing of virus-infected cells.

Class II Histocompatibility Molecules

Class II molecules are encoded by multiple loci in the D region: DP, DN, DM, DO, DQ, and DR. The D region loci encode structurally similar molecules that are expressed primarily on accessory cells involved in antigen presentation. As noted above, the chief APCs include monocytes, macrophages, dendritic cells, and B lymphocytes. Class II antigens have also been referred to as "Ia" (immunity-associated) antigens. Class II molecules are heterodimers that consist of two noncovalently linked glycoprotein chains. The 34-kd β-chain possesses a single disulfide bond; its extracellular domain is the major site of class II antigenic variability. The 29-kd α-chain has two disulfide bonds. Both chains are transmembrane proteins. As with class I antigens, D alleles are expressed codominantly and tissues bear antigens from each parent.

Clinical Tissue Typing

"Histocompatibility, HLA, or tissue-typing" laboratories now use several approaches to identify the class I and class II antigens expressed by both potential donor tissues and recipient prior to organ transplantation. Class I antigens have been defined serologically: antisera against various antigens are tested against donor (or recipient) lymphocytes. The system of nomenclature for class I antigens is based on the locus of origin (A1, A2, A3, B4, B6, C1, C2, etc.). Tissue typing reveals the two different antigens codominantly expressed at each locus; one antigen (double dose) when there is homozygosity. Accordingly, a tissue might express A1, A2, B4, B6, DR3, and DR4 antigens. The products of all loci are not universally typed in clinical laboratories. Increasingly, tissue-typing laboratories are using molecular methods including DNA sequence analysis to identify class I and II antigens.

Class II antigens were traditionally defined by serological and functional assays, but these have largely been replaced by molecular techniques, which have demonstrated greater genetic (and structural) variability than was recognized when the standard for typing was serological. The nomenclature for histocompatibility genes and antigens has thus become more complex, a fact reflected in a more detailed system of nomenclature. An example is "HLA-B27" (based on serology) and its sequence based definition B*2701-2725 which encompasses 25 different molecules.

Integrated Cellular and Humoral Immune Responses Protect against Invasion by Foreign Agents

T Lymphocyte Interactions

T lymphocytes recognize specific antigens, usually proteins or haptens bound to proteins. They undergo a series of maturational events when engaged via the TCR in the context of a histocompatible (i.e., MHC-matched) APC. Exogenous signals are delivered by cytokines. $CD4^+$ and $CD8^+$ T cell subsets possess a variety of effector and regulatory functions. Effector functions include secretion of proinflammatory cytokines and killing of cells that express foreign or altered membrane antigens. Regulatory functions include augmenting and suppressing immune responses, usually by secreting specific helper or suppressor cytokines.

$CD4^+$ T cells, and possibly also $CD8^+$ cells, can be further distinguished by the types of cytokines produced. Helper type 1 or Th1, cells produce IFN-γ and IL-2, whereas helper type 2, or Th2, cells secrete IL-4, IL-5, and IL-10. Th1 lymphocytes have been associated with cell-mediated phenomena and Th2 cells with allergic responses. In general, $CD4^+$ T cells promote antibody and inflammatory responses. By contrast, $CD8^+$ cells for the most part exert suppressor and cytotoxic functions. Suppressor cells inhibit the activation phase of immune responses; cytotoxic cells can kill target cells that express specific antigens. However, there is some overlap, as $CD8^+$ cells secrete helper cytokines and $CD4^+$ Th1 and Th2 cells display cross-regulatory suppressive effects.

An important aspect of T cell antigen recognition is the requirement for antigen to be presented on the surface of another cell in association with a histocompatible membrane protein (see Fig. 4-5 and Fig. 4-6). As noted above, T cells bear membrane receptor complexes (α/β TCRs plus CD3 accessory molecules) on their surface. For maximal immune responses, the TCR–CD3 complex must interact with a foreign antigen in the context of cell-to-cell histocompatibility. Thus, antigens are presented to T cells by accessory cells (APCs) that bear appropriate histocompatibility molecules. Antigens may also be presented to T cells by cells that do not "present" antigens but rather express on their surface a foreign or altered self-protein in association with an appropriate histocompatibility molecule.

$CD8^+$ cells (cytotoxic T cells) recognize antigens in conjunction with class I molecules, whereas $CD4^+$ cells (helper T cells) recognize antigens together with class II molecules. The membrane CD4 and CD8 molecules of α/β T cells help to stabilize binding interactions. γ/δ T cells may also acquire CD8 outside the thymus and thereby use class I antigens for binding target cells. *Foreign class I and class II molecules, which are not histocompatible with the host (e.g., transplanted histocompatibility antigens), are themselves potent immunogens and can be recognized by host T cells.* This is why tissue transplantation requires that donor and recipient be HLA-matched. In addition to the binding of foreign peptides presented by MHC molecules to the TCR complex, a number of other receptor–ligand interactions must occur to maximally activate lymphocytes. See Figure 4-5, which summarizes some of the key interactions that occur between $CD4^+$ T helper cells and APCs. A $CD4^+$ T cell becomes an activated effector cell when stimulated via the TCR complex and "accessory" receptors (CD28 and cytotoxic lymphoid line [CTLL]-4), which engage costimulatory molecules (e.g., B7 and B7.2). In turn, an activated T helper cell recognizes an antigen-specific B cell via its receptor. The T helper cell then provides costimulatory and regulatory signals, such as CD40 ligand and "helper" cytokines (e.g., IL-4, IL-5).

B Lymphocyte Interactions

Mature B lymphocytes exist primarily in a resting state, awaiting activation by foreign antigens. Activation requires cross-linking of membrane immunoglobulin receptors by antigens presented by accessory cells and/or interactions with membrane molecules of helper T cells via a mechanism called cognate T cell-B cell help (see Fig. 4-5). The initial stimulus leads to B cell proliferation and clonal expansion, a process amplified by cytokines from both accessory cells and T cells. If no additional signal is provided, proliferating B cells return to a resting state and enter the memory cell pool. These events occur largely in lymphoid tissues and can be seen as germinal centers. Within germinal centers, B cells also undergo further somatic gene rearrangements, leading to generation of cells that produce the various immunoglobulin isotypes and subclasses.

An **isotype** is the class of the defining heavy chain of an immunoglobulin molecule. In turn, each immunoglobulin subtype exhibits a different array of biological activities. In the absence of antigenic stimulation, different B cell clones express a variety of heavy-chain isotypes and subclasses: IgG ($\gamma 1$, $\gamma 2$, $\gamma 3$, $\gamma 4$), IgA ($\alpha 1$, $\alpha 2$) or IgE (ϵ). T cells also influence B cell differentiation. In the presence of antigen, T cells produce helper cytokines that stimulate isotype switching or induce proliferation of previously committed isotype populations. For example, IL-4 induces switching to the IgE isotype.

The final stage of B cell differentiation into antibody-synthesizing plasma cells requires exposure to additional products of T lymphocytes (e.g., IL-5, IL-6), especially in the case of protein antigens. However, some polyvalent agents induce B cell proliferation and differentiation into plasma cells directly, bypassing the requirements for B-cell growth and differentiation factors. Such agents are called **polyclonal B-cell activators** because they do not interact with antigen-binding sites and hence are not specific antigens. Examples of polyclonal B-cell activators are bacterial products (lipopolysaccharide, staphylococcal protein A) and certain viruses (Epstein-Barr virus [EBV], cytomegalovirus [CMV]).

The predominant type of immunoglobulin produced during an immune response changes with age. Newborns tend to produce predominantly IgM. By contrast, older children and adults initially produce IgM following antigenic challenge but rapidly shift toward IgG synthesis.

Mononuclear Phagocyte Activities

Mononuclear phagocyte is a general term applied to phagocytic cell populations in virtually all organs and connective tissues. Among these cells are macrophages, monocytes, Kupffer cells of the liver, and lung alveolar macrophages. The older term "histiocyte" is synonymous with **macrophage**, either a circulating or a fixed tissue macrophage. Subpopulations of macrophages exhibit different functions and phenotypes. Precursor cells (monoblasts and promonocytes) arise in bone marrow, enter the circulation as monocytes, and then migrate into tissues, where they take up residence as tissue macrophages. In the lung, liver, and spleen, numerous macrophages populate sinuses and pericapillary zones to form an effective filtering system that removes effete cells and foreign particulate material from blood. This system, formerly known as the "reticuloendothelial system," is now termed the **mononuclear phagocyte system**. In addition to their "housekeeping" functions, macrophages are critical in inducing immune responses and in maintenance and resolution of inflammatory reactions.

Macrophages are important accessory cells by virtue of their expression of class II histocompatibility antigens. They ingest and process antigens for presentation to T cells in conjunction with class II MHC molecules. The subsequent T cell responses are further amplified by macrophage-derived cytokines. One of the best characterized cytokines is IL-1, which, among a pleiotropic set of activities, promotes expression of IL-2 receptor on T cells, augmenting T cell proliferation, which is driven by IL-2. Among many effects of IL-1 on other tissues is preparation of the body to combat infection. For example, IL-1 induces fever and promotes catabolic metabolism.

Macrophages are dominant participants in subacute and chronic inflammatory reactions. During persistent inflammation, increased numbers of monocytes are recruited from the bone marrow. Under chemotactic influences, they migrate into sites of inflammation, where they mature into macrophages. Both recruited and local tissue macrophages proliferate in these foci, where they secrete proteins, lipids, nucleotides, and reactive oxygen metabolites. Functionally, these molecules are digestive, opsonic, cytotoxic, growth–promoting, and growth-inhibiting.

The functional activities of macrophages and the spectrum of molecules that they produce are regulated by external factors, such as T cell-derived cytokines. Macrophages exposed to such factors become "activated," that is, they acquire a greater capacity to produce reactive oxygen metabolites, kill tumor cells, and eliminate intracellular microorganisms.

If an agent that incites an inflammatory process is difficult to digest, a granulomatous reaction may ensue (see Chapter 2). Under such conditions, macrophages mature further, to become "epithelioid" cells and multinucleated giant cells. Giant cells result from macrophage fusion and are syncytia with multiple nuclei. Different inciting agents elicit different types of giant cells. For example, granulomas caused by mycobacteria often contain Langhans-type giant cells, which have a semicircular arrangement of nuclei. Giant cells of foreign body granulomas exhibit a random distribution of nuclei. Both epithelioid cells and giant cells are poor phagocytes: they mainly sequester and digest foreign material.

Clinical Evaluation of Immune Status

Suspicion of an immune disorder should trigger testing of immune function. For example, patients with chronic, recurrent, or unusual infections, may have an **immune deficiency.** Alternatively, persons who consistently present with localized edema and itching following contact with an object in their environment may be suspected of having a **hypersensitivity response** to an antigen associated with that object.

Defects in the humoral arm usually result in a patient having difficulty clearing encapsulated bacteria from the bloodstream, which may result in life-threatening infections. The bacteria seen in these immunocompromised states are mostly *Streptococcus pneumoniae*, *Haemophilus influenza*, and *Neissera meningitidis*. Defects in humoral immunity may be primary and often present since birth, or they may be acquired. They are quite diverse and include such diseases as selective IgA defiency, common varible immune defiency in which immunoglobin levels are depressed, and the acquired immune defiency state caused by human immunodeficiency virus (HIV)-1 in which immunoglobulin levels are elevated but disordered secondary to immune dysregulation and are therefore ineffective. It is important to realize that patients with asplenia, whether secondary to a functional defect or frank absence, are also at greatly increased risk of overwhelming bacteremia, especially with encapsulated bacteria and subsequent life-threatening sepsis syndrome.

The cellular componet fights viral infections and performs immune surveillance and may prevent or delay malignancy. The best example for the role of T lymphocytes is in advanced HIV-1 disease, acquired immune deficiency syndrome (AIDS), when $CD4^+$ T cells are severely depleted. Such patients develop opportunistic infections with fungi such as cryptococcus, viruses such as CMV and adenovirus, and mycobacteria such as *Mycobacterium tuberculosis* and *Mycobacterium avium-intracellulare* complex.

Immunoglobulin Concentrations are Measured by Electrophoresis

Total aggregate concentrations of IgG, IgA, and IgM can be estimated by serum protein electrophoresis (SPEP). Serum proteins are separated by electrophoresis, stained with dyes that bind to proteins, and quantitated by densitometry. Characteristic electrophoretic patterns of a normal person and a person with hypogammaglobulinemia are compared in Figure 4-8. Immunoglobulins comprise the gammaglobulin fraction, which migrates toward the cathode and is reduced in the patient with hypogammaglobulinemia.

Individual immunoglobulin (i.e., IgG, IgA, IgM) concentrations can be better measured by quantitating individual isotypes using specific antibodies. Quantitation allows identification of selective immunoglobulin subclass deficiencies and, like SPEP, provides a measure of total serum immunoglobulin concentration. There are numerous conditions that involve selective deficiencies of serum IgM, IgG, IgA, or secretory IgA.

Antibody-Dependent Immunity Can be Assessed by Testing for Antibodies Against Specific Antigens

Subtle humoral immune deficiencies are detected by quantitating circulating antibodies to specific antigens to which most people have been exposed via vaccination or common environmental contact (e.g., multivalent pneumococcal vaccine, tetanus toxoid, diphtheria toxoid, rubella virus). These serologic methods may be useful in highlighting deficiencies in specific facets of the humoral immune system, even if total serum immunoglobulin levels may be normal. It may be useful to vaccinate a patient with a "killed" vaccine such as the pneumococcal vaccine, and then recheck levels of antibody to these specific antigens, usually 4 weeks postvaccination. This will allow the clinician to assess the immune system response.

Cell-Mediated Immunity Can Be Measured Using Peripheral Blood T Cells or Skin Sensitivity Testing

Since the large majority (approximately 80%) of blood lymphocytes are T cells, the total lymphocyte count is a crude index of the ability of the body to generate adequate numbers of T cells. Functional screening of T cell function can be done by skin testing for delayed-type hypersensitivity to antigens with which most people are assumed to have come into contact. Subjects receive intradermal injections of small amounts of such antigens (e.g., *Candida albicans*). A normal response is defined by the specific antigen preparation but typically involves development of a specified area of redness and/or induration in a characteristic time frame.

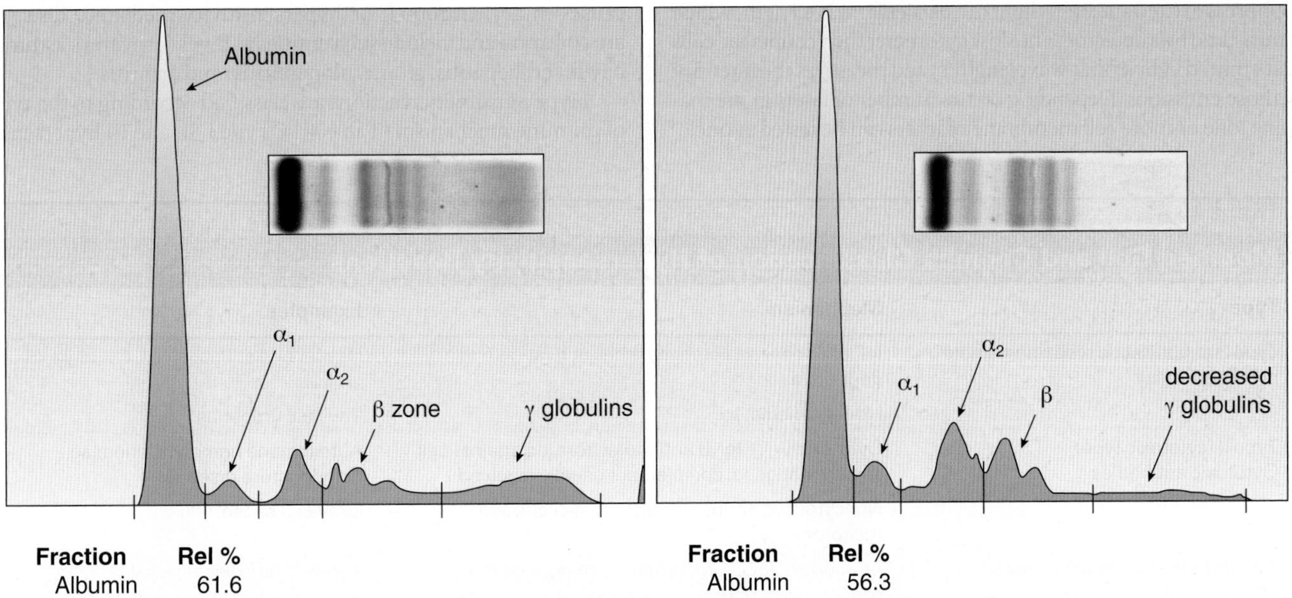

Fraction	Rel %
Albumin	61.6
Alpha 1	4.0
Alpha 2	8.0
Beta	12.5
Gamma	13.9

Fraction	Rel %
Albumin	56.3
Alpha 1	6.7
Alpha 2	16.1
Beta	13.6
Gamma	7.3

FIGURE 4-8. **Normal (*left*) and hypogammaglobulinemic (*right*) serum protein electrophoresis (SPEP).** SPEP provides a rapid means to evaluate the major protein components of serum.

More-sophisticated analyses of T cell function may involve in vitro studies using purified blood lymphocyte preparations. For example, T cell proliferation in response to specific or nonspecific stimuli can provide an indication of T lymphocyte function. Normal T cells (and B cells) proliferate in response to particular mitogenic stimuli. T cell proliferation requires new DNA synthesis, which can be measured by adding labeled nucleotides to the tissue culture medium. Thus, a strong proliferative response to plant lectin phytohemagglutinin (PHA), indicates that the T cell recognition arm of the immune system is likely to be intact. Weak proliferation in response to PHA suggests a qualitative or quantitative defect in T cells or a problem in regulation of T cell proliferation.

Lymphocyte Populations are Commonly Quantitated by Flow Cytometry

Another approach to assessing T and B cell arms of the immune system is quantitating B and T lymphocytes in the blood, usually by flow cytometry (FACS). Peripheral blood lymphocytes are treated with antibodies against specific B or T cell membrane antigens, many of which belong to the system of "cluster designation," or CD, antigens. For example, CD20 is a B cell antigen, whereas a commonly used marker of T cells is CD3. T cells are often further subcategorized by expression of CD4 (helper T cells) or CD8 (effector T cells). CD4 is not unique to T cells; it is also expressed by some mononuclear phagocytes. An example of the clinical utility of lymphocyte subpopulation quantitation is the serial measurement of $CD4^+$ T cells in patients infected with HIV-1.

Monoclonal antibodies against individual antigens, conjugated to fluorescent dyes such as fluorescein or rhodamine (fluorophores), react with the cells in question. A flow cytometer dispenses cells from the whole population in microdroplets that each contain a single cell. As the cell falls, it passes several laser light beams that specifically excite a fluorophore. If the cell bears the antigen recognized by the fluorophore-labeled antibody, the fluorophore is excited and emits light of a particular wavelength, which is measured by a detector. The flow cytometer then counts the cells that emitted light of that wavelength(s) and measures the intensity of those emissions. Depending on the number of lasers in the machine, one or more cell membrane markers can be tested at once.

Such quantitation of T lymphocte populations is routinely used, e.g., to follow the clinical status of patients infected with HIV-1, and to assess the effectiveness of highly active antiretroviral therapy (HAART).

Molecular Evaluation of Immune Status Facilitates Diagnosis of Rare Immune System Defects

A large number of specific, often rare, immunodeficiency disorders have been defined on the basis of mutations within genes that encode various cell membrane-associated, cell-cell communication molecules (e.g., β2-integrins), cytosolic signal-transduction molecules (e.g. Janus kinase 3), cytosolic enzymes (e.g. adenosine deaminase), and transcription factors that are involved in the regulation of host defense gene expression. More than 100 specific genetic defects that can result in impaired immune status have been defined.

Immunologically Mediated Tissue Injury

Immune responses not only protect against invasion by foreign organisms, but may also cause tissue damage. Thus, many inflammatory diseases are examples of "friendly fire" in which the immune system attacks the body's own tissues. A variety of foreign substances (e.g., dust, pollen, bacteria, viruses) may act as antigens and provoke protective immune responses. In certain situations, the protective effects of an immune response give way to deleterious events that elicit a spectrum of lesions. Such lesions can produce manifestations that range from temporary discomfort to substantial injury. For example, in the process of phagocytizing and destroying bacteria, phagocytic cells (neutrophils and macrophages) often cause injury to surrounding tissue. An immune response that leads to tissue injury or disease is broadly called a **hypersensitivity reaction**. Many diseases are categorized as immune disorders or immunologically mediated conditions, in which an immune response to a foreign or self-antigen causes injury. Immune, or hypersensitivity-mediated, diseases are common and include such entities as hives (urticaria), asthma, hay fever, hepatitis, glomerulonephritis, and arthritis.

Hypersensitivity reactions are classified according to the type of immune mechanism (Table 4-1). Type I, II, and III hypersensi-

TABLE 4-1

Modified Gell and Coombs Classification of Hypersensitivity Reactions

Type	Mechanism	Examples
Type I (anaphylactic type): Immediate hypersensitivity	IgE antibody-mediated mast cell activation and degranulation	Hay fever, asthma, hives, anaphylaxis
	Non-IgE-mediated	Physical urticarias
Type II (cytotoxic type): Cytotoxic antibodies	Cytotoxic (IgG, IgM) antibodies formed against cell surface antigens; complement usually involved	Autoimmune hemolytic anemias, Goodpasture disease
	Noncytotoxic antibodies against cell surface receptors	Graves disease
Type III (immune complex type): Immune complex disease	Antibodies (IgG, IgM, IgA) formed against exogenous or endogenous antigens; complement and leukocytes (neutrophils, macrophages) often involved.	Autoimmune diseases (SLE, rheumatoid arthritis), many types of glomerulonephritis
Type IV (cell-mediated type): Delayed-type hypersensitivity	Mononuclear cells (T lymphocytes, macrophages) with interleukin and lymphokine production	Granulomatous disease (tuberculosis) Delayed skin reactions (poison ivy)

Ig = immunoglobulin; SLE = systemic lupus erythematosus.

tivity reactions all require formation of a specific antibody against an exogenous (foreign) or an endogenous (self) antigen. An exception is a subset of type I reactions. The antibody class is a critical determinant of the mechanism by which tissue injury occurs.

In most **type I**, or **immediate-type hypersensitivity reactions,** IgE antibody is formed and binds to high-affinity receptors on mast cells and/or basophils via its Fc domain. Subsequent binding of antigen and crosslinking of IgE triggers rapid (immediate) release of products from these cells, leading to the characteristic symptoms of such diseases as urticaria, asthma, and anaphylaxis.

In **type II hypersensitivity reactions**, IgG or IgM antibody is formed against an antigen, usually a protein on a cell surface. Less commonly, the antigen is an intrinsic structural component of the extracellular matrix (e.g., part of the basement membrane). Such antigen–antibody coupling activates complement, which in turn lyses the cell (cytotoxicity) or damages the extracellular matrix. In some type II reactions, other antibody-mediated effects are operative.

In **type III hypersensitivity reactions**, the antibody responsible for tissue injury is also usually IgM or IgG, but the mechanism of tissue injury differs. The antigen circulates in the vascular compartment until it is bound by antibody. The resulting immune complex is deposited in tissues. Complement activation at sites of antigen–antibody deposition leads to leukocyte recruitment, which is responsible for the subsequent tissue injury. In some type III reactions, antigen is bound by antibody in situ.

Type IV reactions, also known as **cell-mediated**, or **delayed-type, hypersensitivity reactions,** do not involve antibodies. Rather, antigen activation of T lymphocytes, usually with the help of macrophages, causes release of products by these cells, thereby leading to tissue injury.

Many immunologic diseases are mediated by more than one type of hypersensitivity reaction. Thus, in hypersensitivity pneumonitis, lung injury results from hypersensitivity to inhaled fungal antigens. Types I, III, and IV hypersensitivity reactions all appear to be operative in hypersensitivity pneumonitis.

Type I or Immediate Hypersensitivity Reactions Are Triggered by IgE Bound to Mast Cells

Immediate-type hypersensitivity is manifested by a localized or generalized reaction that occurs immediately (within minutes) after exposure to an antigen or "allergen" to which the person has previously been sensitized. The clinical manifestations of a reaction depend on the site of antigen exposure and extent of sensitization. For example, when a reaction involves the skin, the characteristic local reaction is a "wheal and flare," or **urticaria.** When the localized manifestations of immediate hypersensitivity involve the upper respiratory tract and conjunctiva, causing sneezing and conjunctivitis, we speak of **hay fever** (allergic rhinitis). In its generalized and most severe form, immediate hypersensitivity reactions are associated with bronchoconstriction, airway obstruction, and circulatory collapse, as seen in anaphylactic shock. There is a high degree of variability in susceptibility to type I hypersensitivity reactions, which is genetically determined. A variety of linkages and candidate genes have been identified. Particularly susceptible individuals are said to be "atopic."

Type I hypersensitivity reactions usually feature IgE antibodies, which are formed by a $CD4^+$, Th2 T cell–dependent mechanism and which bind avidly to Fc-epsilon (Fcϵ) receptors on mast cells and basophils. The high avidity of binding of IgE accounts for the term **cytophilic** antibody. Once exposed to an specific allergen that elicits IgE, a person is sensitized; subsequent exposures to that allergen or a cross-reacting epitope induce immediate hypersensitivity reactions. After IgE is elicited, repeat exposure to antigen typically induces additional IgE antibody, rather than antibodies of other classes, such as IgM or IgG.

IgE can persist for years bound to Fcϵ receptors on mast cells and basophils, a feature unique to these cells. Upon subsequent reexposure, the soluble antigen or allergen binds the IgE coupled to its surface Fcϵ receptor and activates the mast cell or basophil. This event releases the potent inflammatory mediators that are responsible for the manifestations of this type I hypersensitivity reaction. As shown in Figure 4-9, the antigen (allergen) binds to IgE antibody through its Fab sites. Cross-linking of the antigen to more than one IgE antibody molecule is required to activate the cell. Most cells and basophils can also be activated by agents other than antibodies. For example, some individuals may develop urticaria following exposure to an ice cube (physical urticaria). As also shown in Figure 4-9, the complement-derived anaphylatoxic peptides, C3a and C5a, can directly stimulate mast cells by a different receptor-mediated process. These cell-activating events trigger release of stored granule constituents and rapid synthesis and release of other mediators. Some compounds, such as melittin (from bee venom) and some drugs (e.g., morphine) directly activate mast cells and induce release of granular constituents.

Regardless of how mast cell activation is initiated, cytosolic calcium influx is required. A rise in cytosolic free calcium is associated with increases in cyclic adenosine 3′,5′-monophosphate (cAMP), activation of several metabolic pathways within the mast cell and the subsequent secretion of both preformed and newly synthesized products.

A number of potent mediators are released from granules within minutes. Because they are preformed and stored in granules, they exert immediate biological effects following their release. Of the granule constituents listed in Figure 4-9, the biogenic amine histamine is particularly important. Histamine induces constriction of vascular and nonvascular smooth muscle, causes microvascular dilation, and increases venule permeability. These biological effects are largely mediated through H_1 histamine receptors. Histamine also increases gastric acid secretion through H_2 histamine receptors. In the skin, histamine provokes the wheal-and-flare reaction. In the lung, it is responsible for the early manifestations of immediate hypersensitivity, including bronchospasm, vascular congestion, and edema. Other preformed products released from mast cell granules include heparin, a series of neutral proteases (trypsin, chymotrypsin, carboxypeptidase, and acid hydrolases) and at least two chemotactic factors: a neutrophil chemotactic factor and an eosinophil chemotactic factor. The latter is responsible for the accumulation of eosinophils, a characteristic finding in immediate hypersensitivity. The synthesis and secretion of cytokines by mast cells, by other recruited inflammatory cells and even by indigenous cells (e.g., epithelium) are important in the so-called "late-phase" reaction of immediate hypersensitivity. Late-phase responses typically last for 2 to 24 hours, are marked by a mixed inflammatory infiltrate, and are medicated by many cytokines including IL-1, IL-3, IL-4, IL-5, IL-6, TNF, granulocyte-macrophage colony-stimulating factor (GM-CSF), and macrophage-inflammatory proteins (MIP)-1α and MIP-1β.

Activation of mast cells also results in the synthesis of potent inflammatory mediators. Foremost among these molecules are various products of the arachidonic acid pathway that are

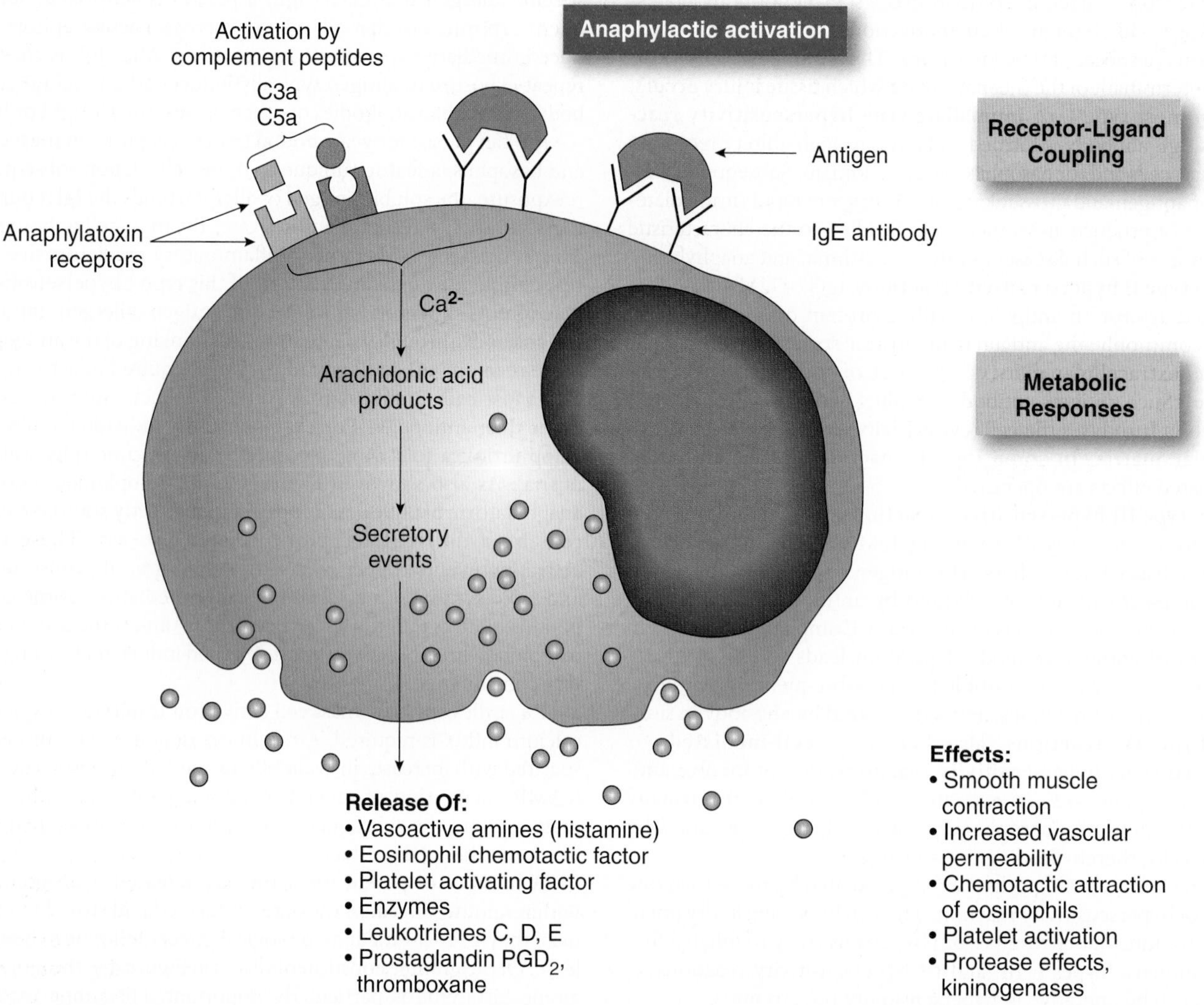

FIGURE 4-9. **In a type I hypersensitivity reaction, allergen binds to cytophilic surface IgE antibody on a mast cell or basophil and triggers cell activation and the release of a cascade of proinflammatory mediators.** These mediators are responsible for smooth muscle contraction, edema formation, and the recruitment of eosinophils. Ca^{2+} = calcium ion; Ig = immunoglobulin; PGD_2 = prostaglandin D_2.

formed following activation of phospholipase A_2. Products derived from the activities of cyclooxygenase (prostaglandins D_2, E_2, F_2 and thromboxane) and lipoxygenase (leukotrienes B_4, C_4, D_4, E_4) are formed. Arachidonic acid products, which are also generated by a variety of other cell types, induce smooth muscle contraction, vasodilation, and edema. Leukotrienes C_4, D_4, and E_4, previously known as the "slow-reacting substances of anaphylaxis" (SRS-As), are important molecules in the delayed bronchoconstriction phase of anaphylaxis. Leukotriene B_4, a potent chemotactic factor for neutrophils, macrophages, and eosinophils, is formed during anaphylaxis and is involved in attracting inflammatory cells into tissues.

Another inflammatory mediator synthesized by mast cells is **platelet activating factor** (PAF), a lipid derived from membrane phospholipids. As its name implies, PAF is a potent inducer of platelet aggregation and release of vasoactive amines from platelets. It is also a potent neutrophil chemotaxin. It has a broad range of biological activities and can activate all types of phagocytic cells.

As mentioned above, activated T cells, specifically Th2 type, produce cytokines that have important roles in allergic responses. Activated Th2 T cell subsets produce IL-4, IL-5, and IL-13, leading to IgE production and increased numbers of mast cells and eosinophils. In allergy-prone persons, a similar response occurs via T cell clones that produce IL-4, IL-6, and IL-2, concentrations of which are also increased in allergic individuals. These persons also have reduced levels of IFN-γ, which suppresses development of Th2 clones and subsequent production of IgE.

To summarize, type I (immediate) hypersensitivity reactions are characterized by a specific cytophilic antibody (IgE), which binds to high-affinity receptors on basophils and mast cells and reacts with a specific antigen. Activated mast cells and basophils release preformed (granule) products and synthesize mediators that cause the classic manifestations of immediate hypersensitivity and the late-phase reaction.

Type II Hypersensitivity Reactions Are Mediated by Antibodies against Fixed Cellular or Extracellular Antigens

IgG and IgM typically mediate type II reactions. An important characteristic of these antibodies is their ability to activate

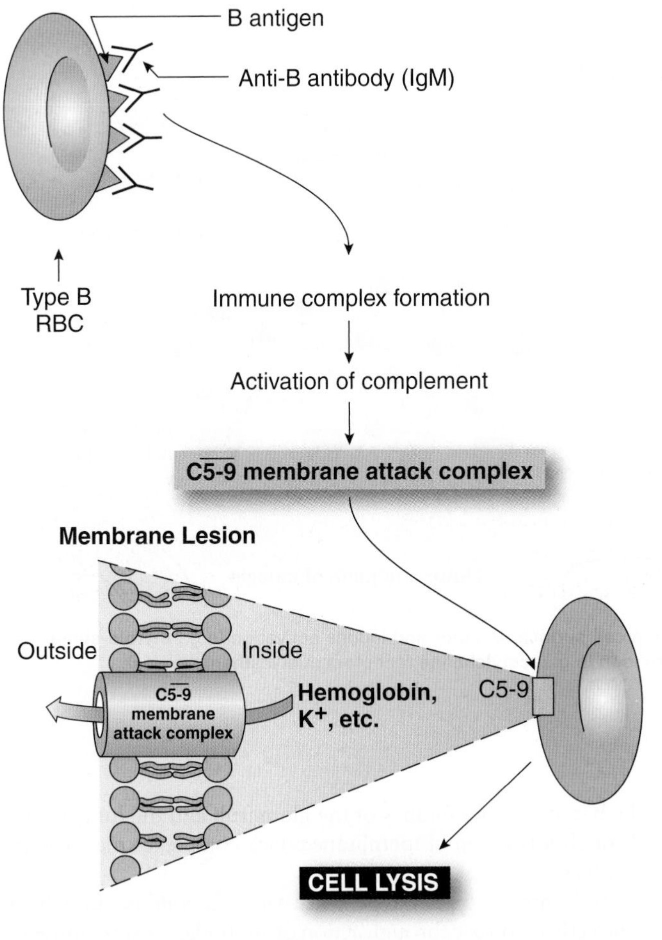

FIGURE 4-10. **In a type II hypersensitivity reaction, binding of IgG or IgM antibody to an immobilized antigen promotes complement fixation.** Activation of complement leads to amplification of the inflammatory response and membrane attack complex (MAC)-mediated cell lysis. Ig = immunoglobulin; K^+ = potassium ion; RBC = red blood cell.

complement through the immunoglobulin Fc domain. There are several antibody-dependent mechanisms of tissue injury.

The prototypic model of antibody-mediated erythrocyte cytotoxicity is illustrated in Figure 4-10. IgM or IgG antibody binds an antigen on the surface of the erythrocyte membrane. At sufficient density, bound immunoglobulin leads to complement fixation via C1q and the classic pathway (see Chapter 2). Once activated, complement can destroy target cells by several distinct mechanisms. Complement products can directly lyse target cells via C5b-9 complement complexes (see Fig. 4-10). This complex is referred to as the **membrane attack complex** because it inserts like the staves of a barrel into the plasma membrane and forms holes or ionic channels, destroying the permeability barrier and inducing cell lysis. This type of complement-mediated cell lysis is exemplified by certain types of autoimmune hemolytic anemias that involve formation of antibodies against blood group antigens on erythrocytes. In transfusion reactions that result from major blood group incompatibilities, hemolysis occurs through activation of complement.

Complement and antibody molecules can also lead to destruction of a target cell by **opsonization**. Target cells coated (opsonized) with immunoglobulin and/or C3b molecules are bound by phagocytes that express Fc or C3b receptors. Complement activation in proximity to a target cell surface leads to formation and covalent bonding of C3b (Fig. 4-11). Many phagocytic cells, including neutrophils and macrophages, have cell membrane Fc and C3b receptors. By binding to its receptor, immunoglobulin or C3b bridges the target cell and the effector (phagocytic) cell, thereby enhancing phagocytosis and the subsequent intracellular destruction of the antibody- or complement-coated cell. Certain types of autoimmune hemolytic anemias and some drug reactions are mediated by antibody- and complement-mediated opsonization.

There is another type of antibody-mediated cytotoxicity that does not require complement. Antibody-dependent cell-mediatal cytotoxicity (**ADCC**) involves cytolytic leukocytes that attack antibody-coated target cells after binding via Fc receptors. Phagocytic cells and NK cells can function as effector cells in ADCC. The mechanisms by which target cells are destroyed in these reactions are not entirely understood. Among

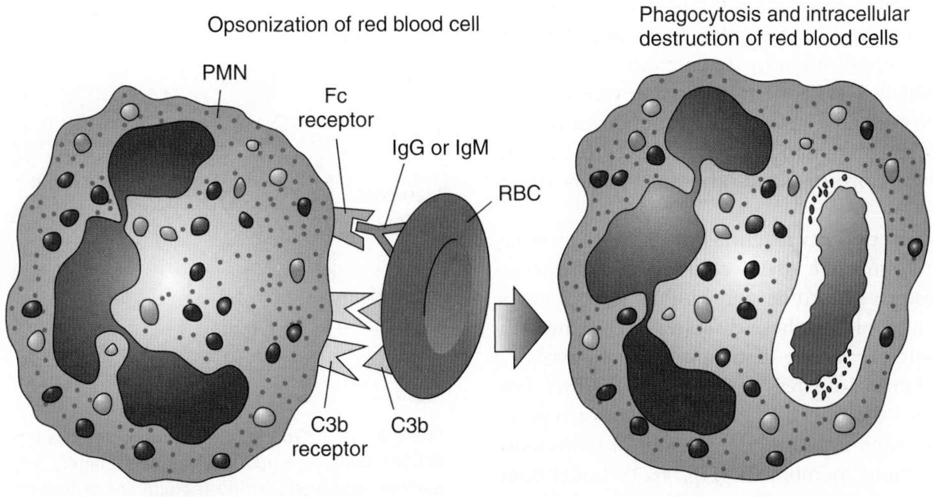

FIGURE 4-11. **In a type II hypersensitivity reaction, opsonization by antibody or complement leads to phagocytosis via either Fc or C3b receptors, respectively.** Ig = immunoglobulin; PMN = polymorphonuclear neutrophil; RBC = red blood cell.

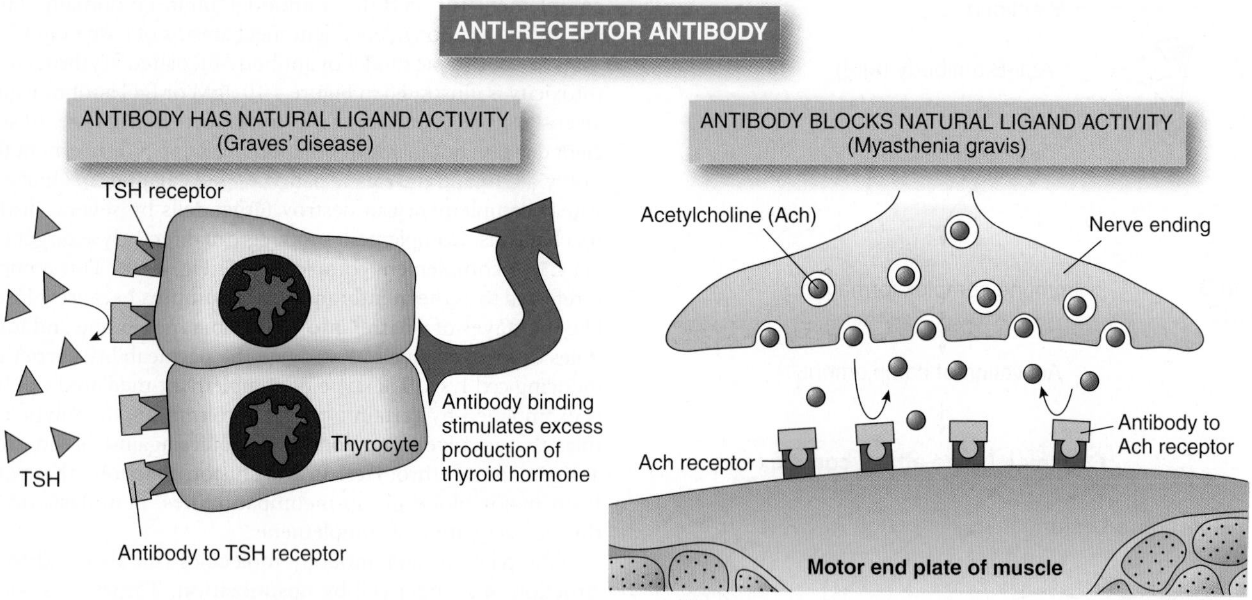

FIGURE 4-12. **In a type II hypersensitivity reaction, antibodies bind to a cell surface receptor and induce activation (e.g., thyroid-stimulating hormone [TSH] receptors in Graves disease) or inhibition/destruction (e.g., acetylcholine receptors in myasthenia gravis).**

an array of mediators, effector cells synthesize homologues of terminal complement proteins (e.g., perforins), which participate in cytotoxic events (see preceding discussion of NK cells). Only rarely is antibody alone directly cytotoxic. In cases involving primarily lymphoid cells, apoptosis is activated. ADCC may also be involved in the pathogenesis of some autoimmune diseases (e.g., autoimmune thyroiditis).

In some type II reactions, antibody binding to a specific target cell receptor does not lead to cell death but rather to a change in function. Autoimmune diseases such as Graves disease and myasthenia gravis feature autoantibodies against cell surface hormone receptors (Fig. 4-12). In Graves disease, autoantibody directed against thyroid-stimulating hormone (TSH) receptor on thyrocytes mimics the effect of TSH, stimulating thyroxine production and leading to hyperthyroidism (see Chapter 21). In contrast, in myasthenia gravis, autoantibodies to acetylcholine receptors in neuromuscular endplates either block acetylcholine binding or mediate internalization or destruction of receptors, thereby inhibiting efficient synaptic transmission (see Chapter 27). Patients with myasthenia gravis thus suffer from muscle weakness. Modulatory autoantibodies against receptors for insulin, prolactin, growth hormone, and other messengers are reported.

Some type II hypersensitivity reactions result from antibody against a structural connective tissue component. Classic examples are Goodpasture syndrome and bullous skin diseases, pemphigus and pemphigoid. In these diseases, circulating antibody binds to intrinsic connective tissue antigens and evokes a destructive local inflammatory response. In Goodpasture syndrome, antibody binds the noncollagenous domain of type IV collagen, which is a major structural component of pulmonary and glomerular basement membranes (Fig. 4-13). Local complement activation results in recruitment of neutrophils into the site, tissue injury, and pulmonary hemorrhage and glomerulonephritis. Direct complement-mediated damage to the basement membranes of the glomeruli and the lung alveoli through formation of membrane attack complexes may also be involved.

In summary, type II hypersensitivity reactions are directly or indirectly cytotoxic through action of antibodies against antigens on cell surfaces or in connective tissues. Complement participates in many of these cytotoxic events. Lysis is mediated directly by complement, indirectly by opsonization and phagocytosis, or via chemotactic attraction of phagocytic cells, which produce a large variety of tissue-damaging products. Complement-independent reactions, such as ADCC, also fall into this category.

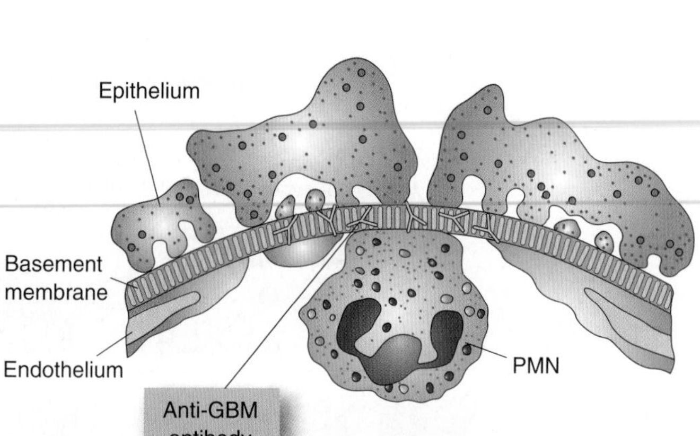

FIGURE 4-13. **Goodpasture syndrome.** In a type II hypersensitivity reaction, antibody binds to a surface antigen, activates the complement system, and leads to the recruitment of tissue-damaging inflammatory cells. Several complement-derived peptides (e.g., C5a) are potent chemotactic factors. GBM = glomerular basement membrane; PMN = polymorphonuclear neutrophil.

In Type III Hypersensitivity Reactions Immune Complex Deposition or Formation in Situ Leads to Complement Fixation and Inflammation

IgG, IgM, and occasionally IgA antibody against either a circulating antigen or an antigen that is deposited or "planted" in a tissue can cause a type III response. Physicochemical characteristics of the immune complexes, such as size, charge, and solubility, in addition to immunoglobulin isotype, determine whether an immune complex can deposit in tissue or fix complement. "Phlogistic" immune complexes elicit inflammatory responses by activating complement, leading to chemotactic recruitment of neutrophils and monocytes to the site. Activated phagocytes release tissue-damaging mediators, such as proteases and reactive oxygen intermediates.

Immune complexes have been implicated in many human diseases (Fig. 4-14). The most compelling cases are those in which demonstration of immune complexes in injured tissue correlates with development of injury. Convincing examples include cryoglobulinemic vasculitis associated with hepatitis C infection, Henoch-Schönlein purpura (in which IgA deposits are found at sites of vasculitis), and systemic lupus erythematosus (SLE) (anti–double-stranded DNA in vasculitic lesions). In many diseases, immune complexes can be detected in plasma without concomitant evidence of tissue injury. The physicochemical properties of circulating immune complexes frequently differ from those of complexes deposited in tissues. In some cases, vasopermeability factors may play a role in the localization of circulating immune complexes. Diseases that seem to be most clearly attributable to immune complex deposition are autoimmune diseases of connective tissue, such as SLE and rheumatoid arthritis, some types of vasculitis, and many varieties of glomerulonephritis.

Serum sickness is an acute, self-limited disease that typically occurs 6 to 8 days after injection of a foreign protein. Human serum sickness is uncommon, but it does occur in patients who have received foreign proteins therapeutically (e.g., antilymphocyte globulin). It is characterized by fever, arthralgias, vasculitis, and acute glomerulonephritis. In experimental acute serum sickness, levels of exogenously injected antigen in the circulation remain constant until about day 6, after which they

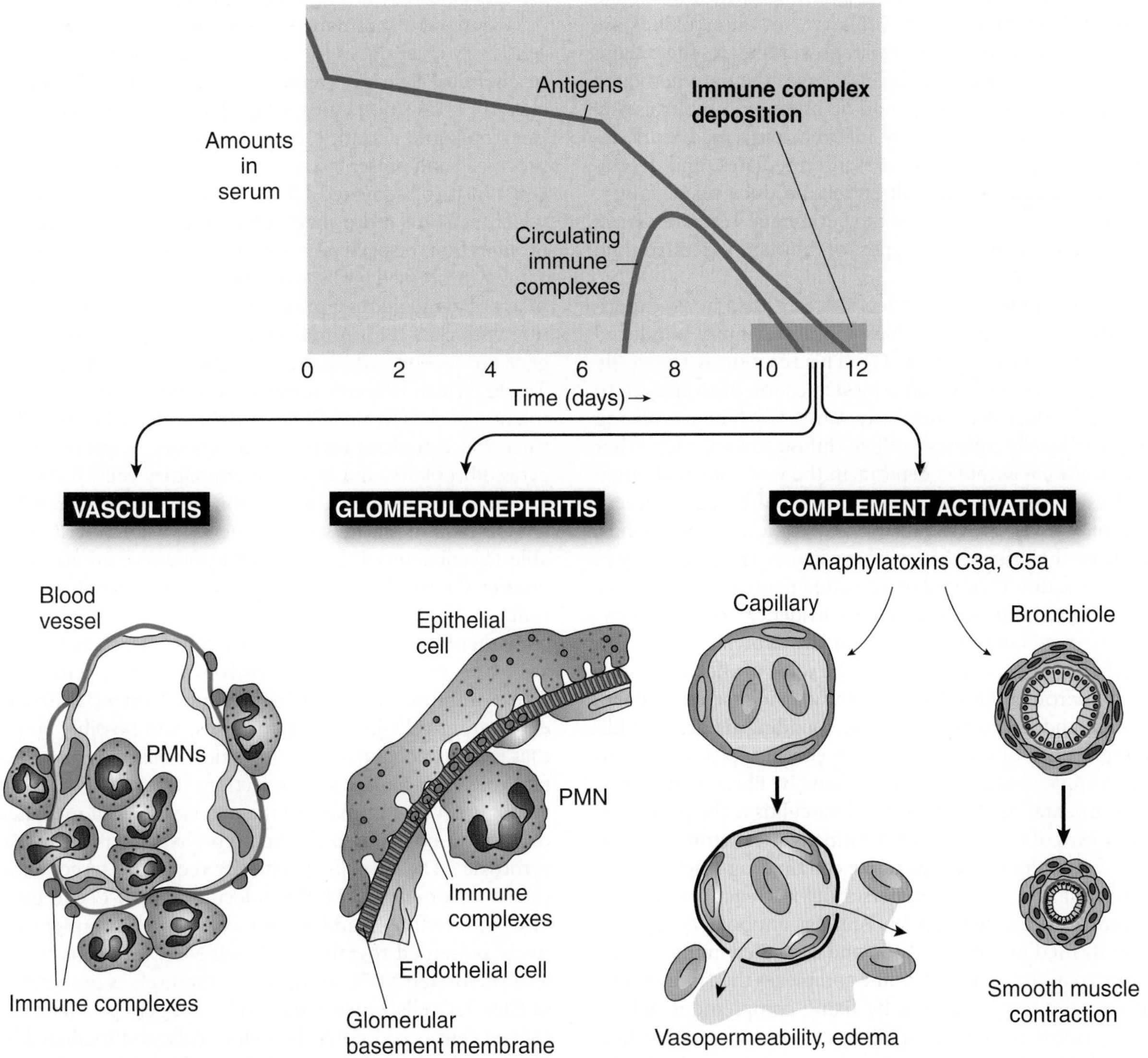

FIGURE 4-14. **In type III hypersensitivity, immune complexes are deposited and can lead to complement activation and the recruitment of tissue-damaging inflammatory cells.** The ability of immune complexes to mediate tissue injury depends on size, solubility, net charge, and ability to fix complement. PMN = polymorphonuclear neutrophil.

fall rapidly (see Fig. 4-14). At the same time, immune complexes (containing IgM or IgG bound to antigen) appear in the circulation. Some of these circulating complexes deposit in tissues such as renal glomeruli and blood vessel walls. They are rendered more soluble by their interaction with the complement system, which enhances tissue deposition. Interaction of immune complexes with complement also generates C3a and C5a, which increase vascular permeability.

Once phlogistic immune complexes are deposited in tissues, they trigger an inflammatory response. Local activation of complement by immune complexes results in formation of C5a, which is a potent neutrophil chemoattractant. Recruitment of inflammatory cells is mediated by chemotactic agents such as C5a, leukotriene B_4, and IL-8. Neutrophil adherence and migration into the sites of immune complex deposition are then mediated by a series of cytokine-mediated adhesive interactions (see Chapter 2). A number of cytokines have been implicated in modulating this response. Early production of IL-1 and TNF-α mediates upregulation of adhesion molecules on endothelial cells and production of other proinflammatory cytokines. These include platelet-derived growth factor (PDGF); transforming growth factor-beta (TGF-β); and IL-4, IL-6, and IL-10; which modulate activation of leukocytes and fibroblasts. Not all cytokines are proinflammatory; IL-10, in particular, downregulates the inflammatory response. Once neutrophils arrive, they are activated through contact with, and ingestion of, immune complexes. Activated leukocytes release many inflammatory mediators, including proteases, reactive oxygen intermediates, and arachidonic acid products, which collectively produce tissue injury. The tissue injury associated with experimental serum sickness mimics that seen in many types of human vasculitis and glomerulonephritis.

The **Arthus reaction** has been characterized in an experimental model of vasculitis in which a localized injury is induced by immune complexes (Fig. 4- 15). This reaction is classically seen in dermal blood vessels after local injection of an antigen to which an individual was previously sensitized. The circulating antibody and locally injected antigen diffuse toward each other and form immune complex deposits in the walls of small blood vessels. Resulting vascular injury is mediated by complement fixation, followed by recruitment and activation of neutrophils, which release their tissue-damaging mediators. Because injury in the Arthus reaction is caused by recruited neutrophils and their products, 2 to 10 hours are required for evidence of tissue injury. This is in marked contrast to more rapidly evolving type I (immediate) hypersensitivity reactions. The walls of affected vessels contain numerous neutrophils and show evidence of damage, with edema and hemorrhage into surrounding tissue. In addition, the presence of fibrin creates the classic appearance of an immune complex-induced vasculitis, namely, fibrinoid necrosis. This experimental model of localized vasculitis is the prototype for many forms of vasculitis seen in humans, for example, the cutaneous vasculitides that characterize certain drug reactions.

To summarize, type III hypersensitivity reactions are immune complex-mediated injuries. Antigen–antibody complexes are either formed in the circulation and deposited in the tissues, or are formed in situ. These immune complexes then induce a localized inflammatory response by fixing complement, which leads to recruitment of neutrophils and monocytes. Activation of these inflammatory cells by immune complexes and complement, accompanied by release of potent inflammatory mediators, is directly responsible for injury (see Fig. 4-15). Many human diseases, including autoimmune diseases such as SLE and many types of glomerulonephritis, are mediated by type III hypersensitivity reactions.

Type IV, or Cell-Mediated, Hypersensitivity Reactions are Cellular Immune Responses That Do Not Involve Antibodies

Included among these reactions are delayed-type cellular inflammatory responses and cell-mediated cytotoxic effects. Type IV reactions often occur together with antibody reactions, which can make it difficult to distinguish these processes. Both clinical observations and experimental studies suggest that the type of tissue response is largely determined by the nature of the inciting agent.

Classically, delayed-type hypersensitivity is a tissue reaction, primarily involving lymphocytes and mononuclear phagocytes, which occurs in response to a soluble protein antigen and reaches greatest intensity 24 to 48 hours after initiation. A classic example of a type IV reaction is the contact sensitivity response to poison ivy. Although chemical ligands in poison ivy are not proteins, they bind covalently to cell proteins, after which the compound molecules are recognized by antigen-specific lymphocytes.

Figure 4-16 summarizes the stages of a delayed-type hypersensitivity reaction. In the initial phase, foreign protein antigens or chemical ligands interact with accessory cells that express class II HLA molecules (Fig. 4-16A). Such accessory cells (macrophages, dendritic cells) secrete IL-12, which along with processed and presented antigen, activates $CD4^+$ T cells (Fig. 4-16B). In turn, activated $CD4^+$ T cells secrete IFN-γ and IL-2, which activate more macrophages and trigger T lymphocyte proliferation, respectively (Fig. 4-16C). The protein antigens are actively processed into short peptides within phagolysosomes of macrophages and then presented on the cell surface in conjunction with class II HLA molecules. Processed and presented antigens are recognized by MHC-restricted, antigen-specific $CD4^+$ T cells, which become activated and synthesize an array of cytokines. Such activated $CD4^+$ cells are referred to as T_H1 cells. In turn, the cytokines recruit and activate lymphocytes, monocytes, fibroblasts, and other inflammatory cells. If the antigenic stimulus is eliminated, the reaction spontaneously resolves after about 48 hours. If the stimulus persists (e.g., poorly biodegradable mycobacterial cell wall components), an attempt to sequester the inciting agent may result in a granulomatous reaction.

Other mechanisms by which T cells (especially $CD8^+$) mediate tissue damage is direct cytolysis of target cells (Fig. 4-17). These immune mechanisms are important in destroying and eliminating cells infected by viruses, and possibly tumor cells that express neoantigens. Cytotoxic T cells also play an important role in transplant graft rejection.

Figure 4-17 summarizes the events in T cell-mediated cytotoxicity. In contrast to delayed-type hypersensitivity reactions, cytotoxic $CD8^+$ T cells specifically recognize target antigens in the context of class I MHC molecules (Fig. 4-17). In the case of virus-infected cells and tumor cells, foreign antigens are actively presented together with self-MHC antigens. In graft rejection, foreign MHC antigens are themselves potent activators of $CD8^+$ T cells. Once activated by antigen, proliferation of cytotoxic cells is promoted by helper cells and mediated by soluble growth factors such as IL-2 (see Fig. 4-17C). An expanded population of antigen-specific cytotoxic cells is thus generated. Actual cell killing involves several mechanisms (see Fig. 4-17D).

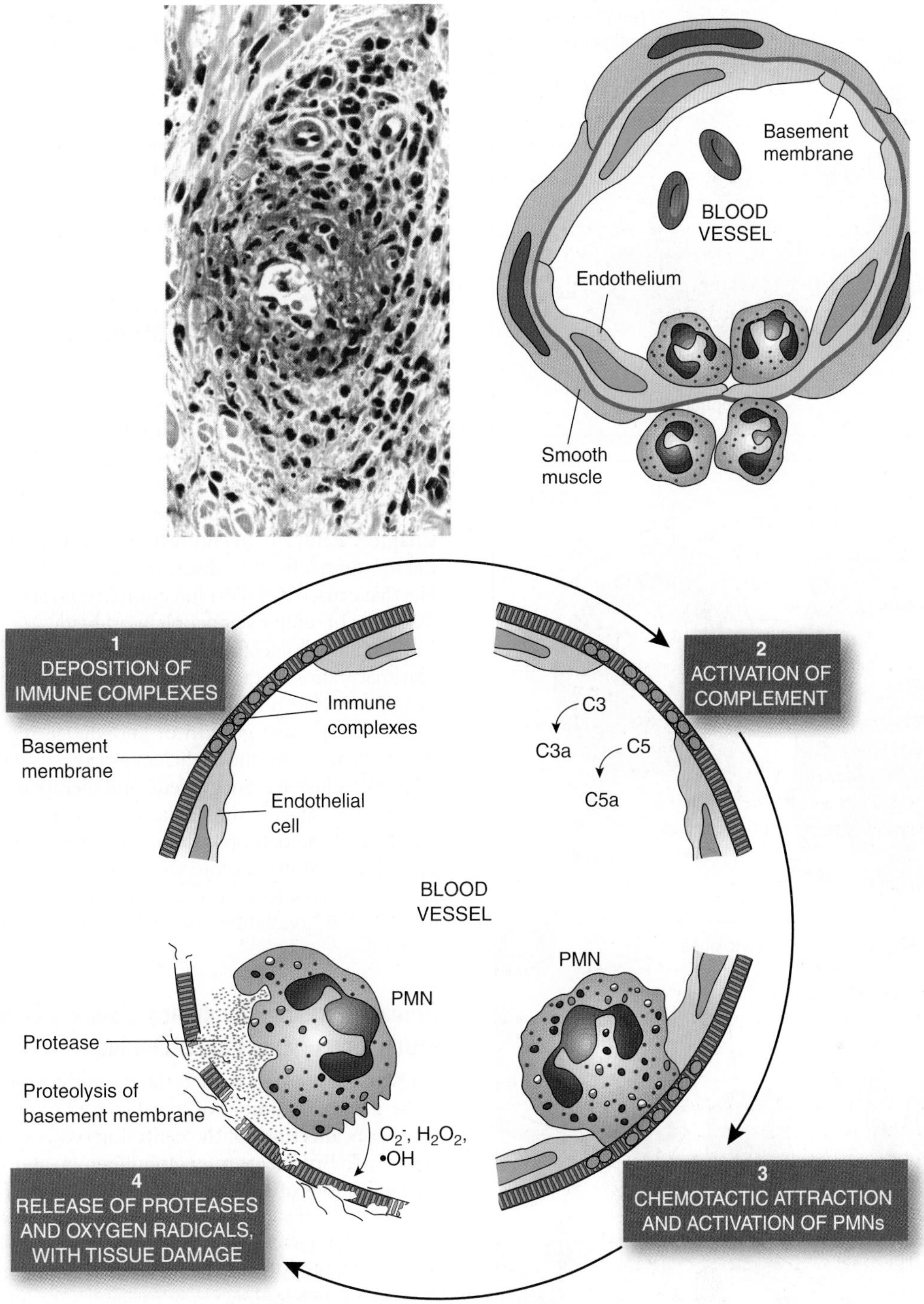

FIGURE 4-15. **The Arthus reaction is a type III hypersensitivity reaction characterized by the deposition of immune complexes and the induction of an acute inflammatory response within blood vessel walls.** Some vasculitic lesions exhibit fibrinoid necrosis. H_2O_2 = hydrogen peroxide; O_2^- = superoxide ion; •OH = hydroxyl radical; PMN = polymorphonuclear neutrophil.

Cytolytic T cells (CTLs) secrete perforins that form pores in target cell membranes and introduce granzymes that activate intracellular caspases, leading to apoptosis. CTLs can also kill targets via engagement of Fas ligand (by the CTL) and Fas (on the target). Fas ligand-Fas interaction triggers apoptosis of the Fas-bearing cell.

The defining characteristics of NK cells have been described, but the extent to which such cells participate in tissue-damaging reactions is unclear. Mounting evidence indicates that NK cells exert both effector and immunoregulatory functions.

Figure 4-18 summarizes target cell killing by NK cells. NK cells can recognize a variety of target cells. Target molecules include membrane glycoproteins expressed by certain virus-infected cells and tumor cells. In a series of events similar to those described for cytotoxic T cells, NK cells bind to target cell through their membrane receptors and then deliver molecular

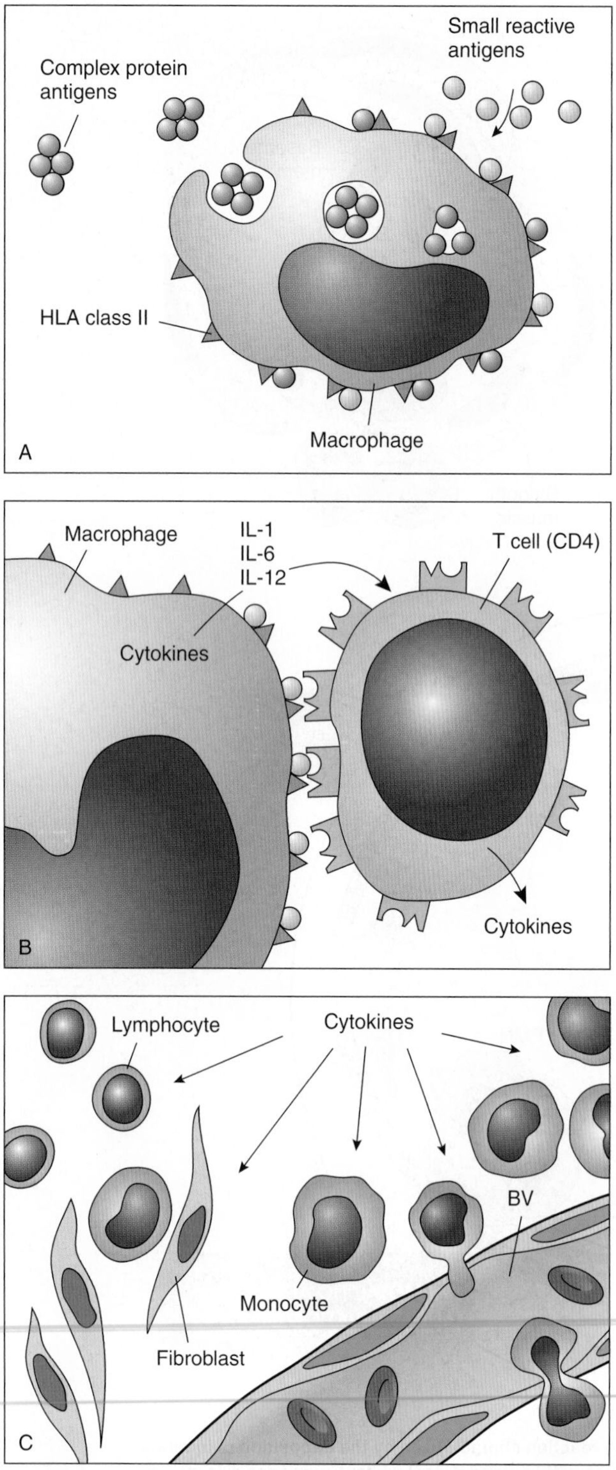

FIGURE 4-16. **In a type IV (delayed type) hypersensitivity reaction, complex antigens are phagocytized, processed, and presented on macrophage cell membranes in conjunction with class II major histocompatibility complex (MHC) antigens.** Antigen-specific, histocompatible, cytotoxic T lymphocytes bind the presented antigens and are activated. Activated cytotoxic T cells secrete cytokines that amplify the response. BV = blood vessel.

signals that result in lysis. NK cells also express membrane Fc receptors, which can bind antibodies that allow cell killing by ADCC. NK cell activity is influenced by a variety of mediators. For example, NK cell activity is increased by IL-2, IL-12, and IFN-γ; and decreased by a variety of prostaglandins.

In sum, in Type IV hypersensitivity reactions, antigens are processed by macrophages and presented to antigen-specific T lymphocytes. These lymphocytes become activated and release a variety of mediators that recruit and activate lymphocytes, macrophages, and fibroblasts. The resulting injury is caused by T lymphocytes themselves, macrophages or both. No antibodies are involved. The chronic inflammation in many autoimmune diseases—including type 1 diabetes, chronic thyroiditis, Sjögren syndrome, and primary biliary cirrhosis—is the result of type IV hypersensitivity.

Immunodeficiency Diseases

Immunodeficiency diseases are classified according to two characteristics: whether the defect is congenital (primary) or acquired (secondary), and the host defense system that is defective. The great majority of primary immunodeficiency disorders are genetically determined. Disorders of the complement system and primary defects of phagocytes are discussed elsewhere (see Chapters 2 and 20). In contrast to the low prevalence of congenital immunodeficiency disorders, acquired immune deficiencies like that caused by HIV-1 infection (AIDS) are common. AIDS affects tens of millions of people worldwide.

Functional defects in lymphocytes can be localized to particular maturational stages in the ontogeny of the immune system or to interruption of discrete immune activation events (Fig. 4-19). The explosive growth of knowledge regarding molecular mechanisms of immunodeficiency disorders has led to improved diagnosis, clinical management, and therapeutic strategies. Identification of specific molecular defects and mechanistic understanding of the pathophysiology of various disorders have also provided great insight into the function of the immune system. A detailed classification scheme for primary immunodeficiency disorders is available via the World Health Organization (WHO).

Primary Antibody Deficiency Diseases Feature Impaired Production of Specific Antibodies

These diseases are characterized by recurrent bacterial infections, a limited number of specific types of viral infections (e.g., echovirus infections of the central nervous system [CNS] in patients with Bruton agammaglobulinemia) and subnormal serum concentrations of either all or specific isotypes of immunoglobulin. There are a variety of immunoglobulin isotype and subclass deficiency states (Table 4-2). These include selective deletions of immunoglobulin heavy chains and selective loss of light-chain expression. In addition, some patients have normal levels of immunoglobulins but fail to produce antibodies against specific antigens, usually polysaccharides. The clinical manifestations of these entities are highly variable; some patients suffer from recurrent mucosal tract infections, whereas others are asymptomatic.

Bruton X-Linked Agammaglobulinemia

The congenital disorder Bruton X-linked agammaglobulinemia typically presents in male infants at 5 to 8 months old, the period during which maternal antibody levels have declined. The infant suffers from recurrent pyogenic infections and severe hypogammaglobulinemia involving all immunoglobulin isotypes. Occasional patients develop chronic enterovirus infections of the CNS. Immunization with live attenuated poliovirus can lead to paralytic poliomyelitis. Approximately a third of Bruton's pa-

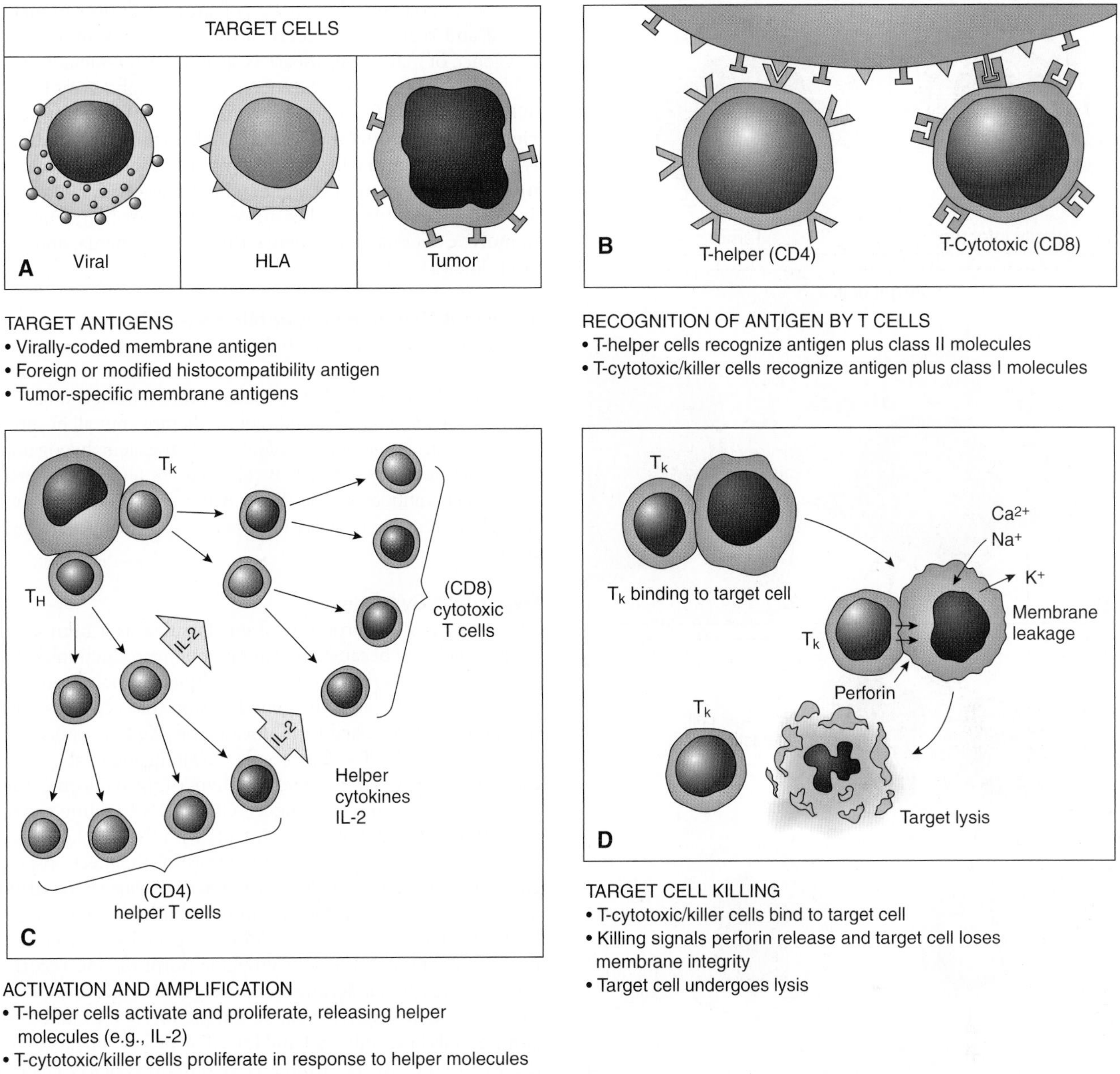
TARGET CELLS
A
Viral
HLA
Tumor
TARGET ANTIGENS
• Virally-coded membrane antigen
• Foreign or modified histocompatibility antigen
• Tumor-specific membrane antigens
B
T-helper (CD4)
T-Cytotoxic (CD8)
RECOGNITION OF ANTIGEN BY T CELLS
• T-helper cells recognize antigen plus class II molecules
• T-cytotoxic/killer cells recognize antigen plus class I molecules
Tk
TH
IL-2
IL-2
(CD8) cytotoxic T cells
Helper cytokines IL-2
(CD4) helper T cells
C
ACTIVATION AND AMPLIFICATION
• T-helper cells activate and proliferate, releasing helper molecules (e.g., IL-2)
• T-cytotoxic/killer cells proliferate in response to helper molecules
Tk
Tk binding to target cell
Ca2+
Na+
K+
Membrane leakage
Tk
Perforin
Tk
Target lysis
D
TARGET CELL KILLING
• T-cytotoxic/killer cells bind to target cell
• Killing signals perforin release and target cell loses membrane integrity
• Target cell undergoes lysis

FIGURE 4-17. **In T cell-mediated cytotoxicity, potential target cells include (A) virus-infected host cells, malignant host cells, and foreign (histoincompatible transplanted) cells. B.** Cytotoxic T lymphocytes recognize foreign antigens in the context of human leukocyte antigen (HLA) class I molecules. **C.** Activated T cells secrete lytic compounds (e.g., perforin and other mediators) and cytokines that amplify the response, that is apoptosis (target cell killing) **(D)**. Ca^{2+} = calcium ion; IL = interleukin; K^+ = potassium ion; Na^+ = sodium ion.

tients have a poorly understood form of arthritis, believed in some cases to be caused by *Mycoplasma*. There are no mature B cells in peripheral blood or plasma cells in lymphoid tissues. Pre-B cells, however, can be detected. The genetic defect, on the long arm of the X chromosome (Xq21.22), inactivates the gene that encodes B-cell tyrosine kinase (Bruton tyrosine kinase [*BTK*]), an enzyme critical to B-lymphocyte maturation (see Table 4-2).

Selective IgA Deficiency

Characterized by low serum and secretory concentrations of IgA, selective IgA deficiency is the most common primary immunodeficiency syndrome. Its incidence ranges from 1:700 among Europeans to 1:18,000 in Japanese. Although patients are often asymptomatic, they occasionally present with respiratory or gastrointestinal infections of varying severity. They also display a strong predilection for allergies and collagen vascular diseases. Patients with IgA deficiency have normal numbers of IgA-bearing B cells; their varied defects result in an inability to synthesize and secrete IgA subclasses (see Table 4-2). Some patients have concomitant IgG subclass deficiencies. Patients with selective IgA deficiency are at risk of allergic, occasionally anaphylactic, reactions to IgA-containing transfused blood products.

Common Variable Immunodeficiency (CVID)

CVID is a heterogenous group of disorders characterized by pronounced hypogammaglobulinemia (see Table 4-2). A variety of defects in either B lymphocyte maturation or T lymphocyte-mediated B lymphocyte maturation appear to be opera-

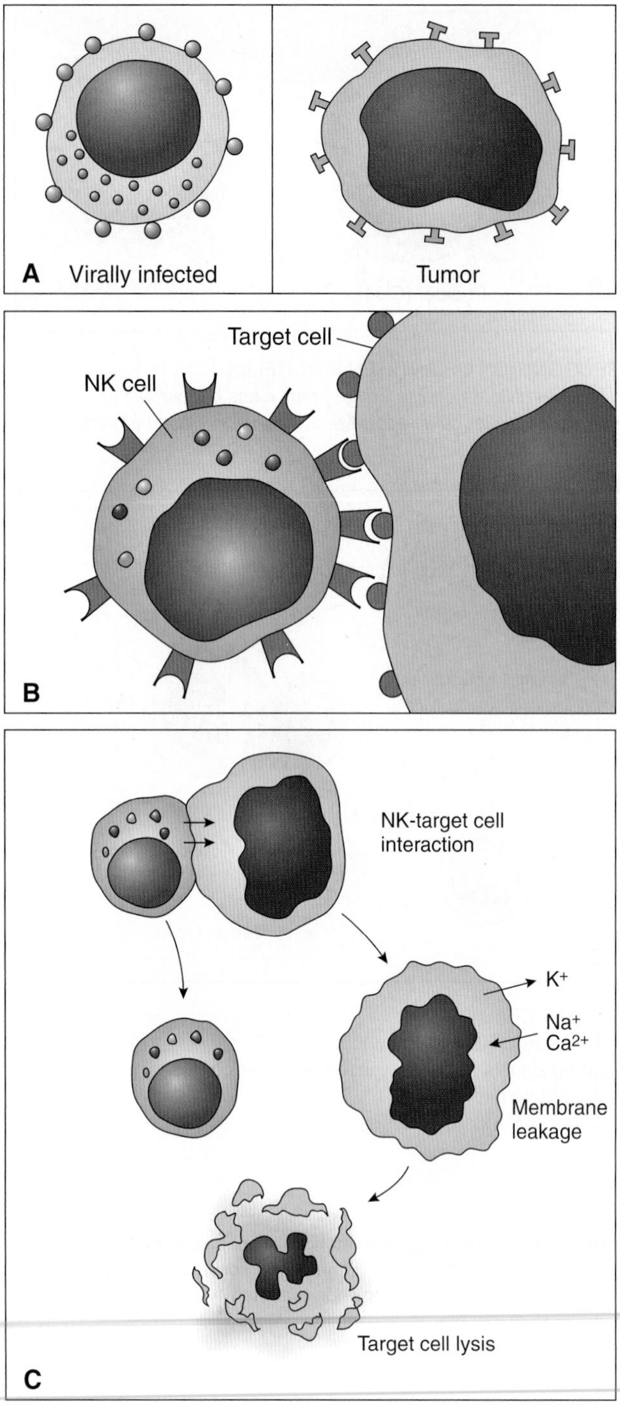

FIGURE 4-18. **In natural killer (NK) cell-mediated cytotoxicity, potential target cells include virus-infected and neoplastic cells (A).** NK cells bind target cells (**B**), are activated, and secrete lytic compounds (**C**). Ca^{2+} = calcium ion; K^+ = potassium ion; Na^+ = sodium ion.

tive. Many relatives of patients with CVID have selective IgA deficiency. Affected patients present with recurrent severe pyogenic infections, especially pneumonia and diarrhea, the latter often due to infestation with *Giardia lamblia*. Recurrent attacks of herpes simplex are common; herpes zoster develops in one fifth of patients. The disease appears years to decades after birth, with a mean age at onset of 30 years. Incidence is estimated to be between 1:50,000 and 1:200,000. The inheritance pattern is variable and the malady features a variety of maturational and regulatory defects of the immune system. A high incidence of malignant disease is seen in CVID, including a 50-fold increase in stomach cancer. Interestingly, lymphoma is 300 times more frequent in women with this immunodeficiency than in affected men. Malabsorption secondary to lymphoid hyperplasia and inflammatory bowel diseases is more frequent than in the general population. CVID patients are also susceptible to other autoimmune disorders, including hemolytic anemia, neutropenia, thrombocytopenia, and pernicious anemia.

Transient Hypogammaglobulinemia of Infancy

Prolonged hypogammaglobulinemia occurs in transient hypogammaglobulinemia of infancy after maternal antibodies in the infant have reached their nadir. Some affected infants develop recurrent infections and require therapy, but all eventually produce immunoglobulins. Infants with transient hypogammaglobulinemia possess mature B cells that are temporarily unable to produce antibodies. The defect is not well understood but is thought to represent a delay in helper T cell signal-generating capacity.

Hyper-IgM Syndrome

The hyper-IgM syndrome is often classified as a humoral immunodeficiency because immunoglobulin production is disordered. It could also be classed as a combined humoral and T lymphocyte defect because the genetic lesion that accounts for the most common X-linked form, located on (Xq26), results in failure to express the T cell molecule, CD40 ligand (Table 4-3). In the remaining 30% of patients with hyper-IgM syndrome, mutations affect the genes that encode CD40, DNA-editing enzyme, activation-induced deaminase. Infants with the X-linked form of the disease exhibit pyogenic and opportunistic infections, especially with *Pneumocystis jiroveci (formerly Pneumocystis carinii)*. They also tend to develop autoimmune diseases involving the formed elements of the blood, especially autoimmune hemolytic anemia, thrombocytopenic purpura, and recurrent, severe neutropenia. Serum levels of IgG and IgA are low, but those of IgM are high normal or conspicuously elevated. Circulating B cells bear only IgM and IgD. The defect appears to be at the level of the "switch" from IgD/IgM to other heavy-chain isotypes. In this context, interaction of the CD40 receptor on the B cell surface with CD40 ligand is required for isotype switching (see Fig. 4-19).

Primary T Cell Immunodeficiency Diseases Typically Result in Recurrent or Protracted Viral and Fungal Infections

DiGeorge Syndrome

In its complete form, the DiGeorge syndrome is one of the most severe T lymphocyte immunodeficiency disorders. It usually appears in an infant with conotruncal congenital heart defects and severe hypocalcemia (due to hypoparathyroidism) and is recognized shortly after birth. Some patients exhibit characteristically abnormal facial features. Infants who survive the neonatal period are subject to recurrent or chronic viral, bacterial, fungal, and protozoal infections. The syndrome is caused by defective embryologic development of the third and fourth pharyngeal pouches, which give rise to the thymus, parathyroid glands, and influence conotruncal cardiac development. Most patients have a point deletion in the long arm of chromosome 22. DiGeorge syndrome is consid-

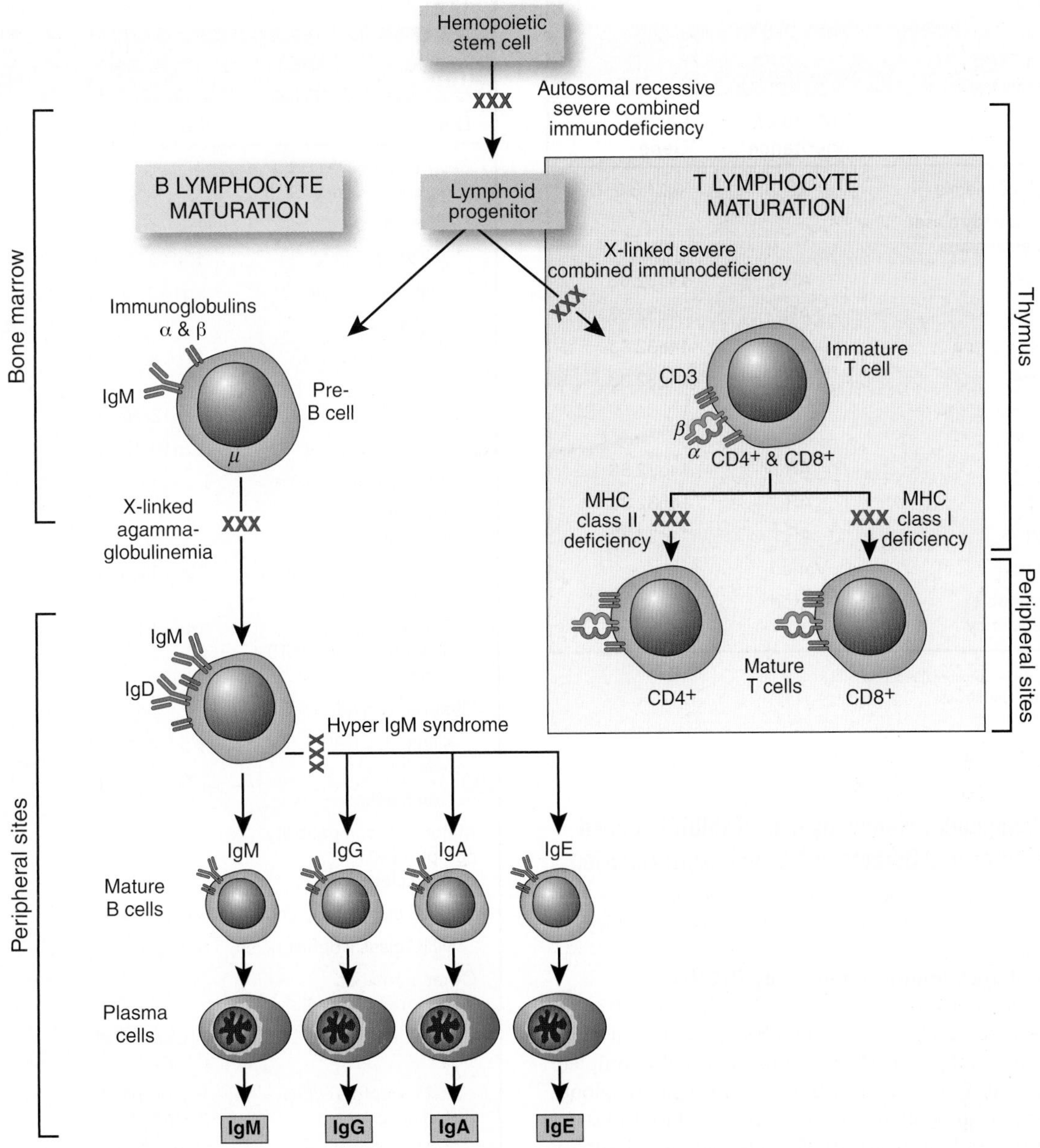

FIGURE 4-19. **Hematopoietic stem cells give rise to lymphoid progenitor cells that, in a predetermined manner, populate either the bone marrow or thymus.** A number of primary immunodeficiency disorders have been characterized at genetic and molecular mechanistic levels. In a number of immunodeficiency disorders, a discrete molecular defect results in a form of "maturational arrest" in the development of fully differentiated and functional lymphocytes. Ig = immunoglobulin.

ered to be a form of so-called 22q11 deletion syndrome. In the absence of a thymus, T cell maturation is interrupted at the pre-T cell stage. The disease has been corrected by transplanting thymic tissue. Most patients have a partial DiGeorge syndrome, in which a small remnant of thymus is present. With time, these persons recover T cell function without treatment. Some patients with the 22q11 mutation are not immunodeficient but suffer only from conotruncal cardiac defects.

Chronic Mucocutaneous Candidiasis

The yeast infection chronic mucocutaneous candidiasis is the result of a congenital defect in T cell function. It is characterized by susceptibility to candidal infections and is associated with an endocrinopathy (hypoparathyroidism, Addison disease, diabetes mellitus). Although most T cell functions are intact, there is an impaired response to *Candida* antigens. The precise cause of the defect in chronic mucocutaneous candidiasis is unknown, but it could occur at any of several points during T cell development. Recent studies suggest that persons with this disorder react to *Candida* antigens differently from normal individuals. In particular, they mount a type 2 (IL-4/IL-6) helper T cell response, which is ineffective in resisting the organism. By contrast, the normal response features type 1 (IL-2/IFN-γ) T cells, which effectively control candidal infections.

TABLE 4-2

Primary Humoral Immunodeficiency Disorders

Disease	Mode of Inheritance*	Locus/ Gene
Agammaglobulinemia	XL	Xq21.3/*BTK*†
Selective antibody class/ subclass deficiencies		
γ1 isotype	AR	14q32.33
γ2 isotype	AR	14q32.33
Partial γ3 isotype	AR	14q32.33
γ4 isotype	AR	14q32.33
IgG subclass ± IgA deficiency	?	-
α1 isotype	AR	14q32.33
α2 isotype	AR	14q32.33
ε isotype	AR	14q32.33
IgA deficiency	Varied	-
Common variable immunodeficiency	Varied	-

* XL = X-linked; AR = autosomal recessive.
†BTK = Bruton tyrosine kinase.
Ig = immunoglobulin.

TABLE 4-3

Combined Humoral and Cellular Immunodeficiencies

Disease	Locus/Gene	Inheritance*
Severe combined immunodeficiency (SCID)		
TB + SCID		
Jak3 deficiency	19p13.1/*JAK3*	AR
X-linked γc-chain	Xq13.1-q13.3	XL
TB- SCID		
Omenn syndrome	11p13/*RAG1*, *RAG2*	AR
RAG1 deficiency	11p13/*RAG1*	AR
RAG2 deficiency	11p13/*RAG2*	AR
Reticular dysgenesis	-	AR
Abnormal purine metabolism		
Adenosine deaminase (ADA) deficiency	20q13.2-q13.11	AR
Purine nucleoside phosphorylase (PNP) deficiency	14q13.1	AR
Hyper-IgM syndrome		
X-linked (CD40L deficiency)	Xq26.3-q27.1	XL
Non-X-linked	-	-
Major histocompatibility complex (MHC) deficiencies		
MHC class I deficiency	6q21.3/*TAP2*	AR
MHC class II deficiencies	Multiple	AR
Other combined immunodeficiencies		
CD3 deficiencies	11q23/*CD3E*, *CD3G*	AR
IL-2 receptor α-chain deficiency	10p14-p15/ *IL2RA*	AR
ZAP-70 deficiency	2q12/*ZAP70*	AR

* XL = X-linked; AR = autosomal recessive.

Combined Immunodeficiency Diseases Exhibit Reduced Immunoglobulins and Defects in T Lymphocyte Function

Severe combined immunodeficiencies are conspicuously heterogenous and represent life-threatening disorders (see Table 4-3).

Severe Combined Immunodeficiency (SCID)

SCID is a group of disorders that ultimately affect both T and B lymphocytes and are characterized by severe recurrent viral, bacterial, fungal, and protozoal infections. A virtually complete absence of T cells is associated with severe hypogammaglobulinemia. Many of these infants have severely reduced mass of lymphoid tissue and an immature thymus that lacks lymphocytes. In some patients, lymphocytes fail to develop beyond pre-B cells and pre-T cells. Because patients with SCID have profound T and B lymphocyte dysfunction, they are susceptible to many pathogens including CMV, varicella, pneumocystic, *Candida,* and many different bacteria.

SCID occurs in both X-linked and autosomal recessive forms and typically appears before 6 months of age (see Table 4-3). In some patients with the autosomal recessive form, B lymphocytes are present but do not function, possibly because of a lack of helper cell activity. In the X-linked form, the most common defect is due to a mutation of the common γ-chain of the IL-2 receptor, which is also used by receptors for other cytokines, namely IL-4, IL-7, IL-9, IL-11, and IL-15. Many patients with the autosomal recessive form have demonstrated mutations of the *Jak-3* gene, which encodes a protein kinase that associates with the γ-chain of cytokine receptors. Thus, abnormalities in the Jak/STAT signaling pathway may account for both of these forms of SCID. Even less common than the so-called T-B positive SCID disorders are the T-B negative SCID diseases, in which neither T nor B lymphocytes are present in appreciable numbers (see Table 4-3). More than a half dozen molecular defects resulting in the SCID phenotype have been described.

Adenosine Deaminase (ADA) deficiency

ADA deficiency is an autosomal recessive form of combined immunodeficiency with mutations in the adenosine deaminase gene (see Table 4-3). ADA participates in purine nucleotide catabolism, converting adenosine to inosine or deoxyadenosine to deoxyinosine. If the enzyme is defective or absent, deoxyadenosine and deoxyadenosine triphosphate accumulate. Deoxyadenosine triphosphate inhibits ribonucleotide reductase, thereby causing depletion of deoxyribonucleoside triphosphates and defective lymphocyte function. The clinical manifestations range from mild to severe dysfunction of T cells and B cells, and include characteristic developmental abnormalities of cartilage.

As noted above, a large number of specific genetic defects that lead to immunodeficiency have been described. Identification of these defects has provided an avenue for specific diagnosis, a basis for fundamental understanding of normal immune function, and rationale for some forms of targeted therapy.

Wiskott-Aldrich Syndrome (WAS) is an X-Linked Defect in Both B- and T-Cell Function

This rare syndrome is characterized by (1) recurrent infections, (2) hemorrhages secondary to thrombocytopenia, and (3) eczema. It typically manifests in boys within the first few months of life as petechiae and recurrent infections (e.g., diarrhea).

WAS is caused by numerous distinct mutations in a gene on the X chromosome (Xp11.22-11.23) that encodes a protein called WASP (Wiskott-Aldrich syndrome protein), which is expressed at high levels in lymphocytes and megakaryocytes. It binds members of the Rho family of guanosine triphosphatases (GTPases), which control many cellular processes, including cell morphology and mitogenesis. WASP itself controls assembly of actin filaments that are required to form microvesicles.

Cellular and humoral immunity are both impaired in WAS. Although levels of most immunoglobulins are normal or elevated, IgM is only about half of normal. Antibody responses to some antigens are normal, but responses to others may be absent. As many polysaccharide antigens, particularly some bacterial polysaccharides, elicit mainly IgM antibody responses, WAS patients are susceptible to infection with encapsulated organisms such as pneumococci.

Boys with WAS also have selective deficiencies in cell-mediated immunity. Numbers of $CD4^+$ and $CD8^+$ T cells are normal, but these children are largely anergic for cutaneous delayed hypersensitivity. Their lymphocytes respond normally to plant lectins that are powerful T-cell mitogens (e.g., PHA), but poorly to specific antigens (e.g., *Candida albicans*). In addition, virus-specific cytotoxic T-cell immunity is usually absent, even though virus-specific antibody responses appear to be normal.

WAS patients typically have recurrent infections with *Streptococcus pneumoniae, Haemophilus influenzae,* and such opportunistic pathogens as *P. jiroveci*. They are also prone to viral infections such as CMV, and not infrequently die of disseminated herpes simplex or varicella. Thrombocytopenia may be severe ($<30{,}000/\mu L$), and the platelets are generally small. One third of these patients typically die of hemorrhage. Rarely, thrombocytopenia alone may be the sole manifestation of mutation in WASP.

A variety of autoimmune diseases may also complicate WAS, including autoimmune hemolytic anemia and thrombocytopenia, polyarthritis and vasculitis of coronary and cerebral arteries. These patients also have a high incidence of lymphoproliferative malignancies. The principal form of thrombocytopenia (nonimmune) is almost always cured by splenectomy. Bone marrow transplantation cures WAS in over 90% of cases.

Autoimmunity and Autoimmune Diseases

Autoimmune Disease Involves an Immune Response Against Self Antigens

Autoimmunity implies that the immune system can no longer differentiate between self- and non–self-antigens effectively. It was classically interpreted as an abnormal immune response that invariably caused disease, but it is now clear that autoimmune responses are common and are necessary in order to regulate the immune system. Anti-idiotype antibodies (antibodies against antigen-binding sites of immunoglobulins), are important in regulating the immune response; their presence is by definition an autoimmune response. When these regulatory mechanisms are in some way disrupted, uncontrolled production of autoantibodies or abnormal cell–cell recognition leads to tissue injury, and autoimmune disease results. While detecting specific autoantibodies is useful to diagnose autoimmune diseases, it is not sufficient for a designation of autoimmune disease. One must demonstrate that the autoimmune reaction (whether cellular or humoral) is directly related to the disease process. Autoimmune diseases may be organ-specific or generalized. At present, only a few diseases (e.g., Hashimoto's thyroiditis, type 1 diabetes, SLE) fit this rigorous criterion.

An abnormal autoimmune response to self-antigens implies a loss of **immune tolerance**. Immune tolerance signifies a situation in which there is no measurable (or clinically consequential) immune response to specific (usually self) antigens. The reasons for loss of tolerance in autoimmune diseases are not understood. Experimental studies suggest that normal tolerance to self-antigens is an active process, and requires contact between self-antigens and immune cells. In the fetus, tolerance is readily established to antigens that cause vigorous immune responses in adults. There is extensive evidence that induction and maintenance of tolerance are active and ongoing immune activities that can be produced through a variety of mechanisms. Thus, tolerance is an active state in which an immune response is blocked or prevented. Induction of tolerance to an antigen is partly related to the dose of antigen to which cells are exposed.

Putative mechanisms of tolerance are divided into two categories: central and peripheral. **Central tolerance** is the processes by which self-reactive T and B lymphocytes are "deleted" during their maturation within the thymus and bone marrow, respectively. Developing self-reactive T cells recognize self peptides in the context of compatible MHC molecules and are induced to undergo apoptosis. These T cells are said to have been "negatively selected." An analogous process occurs to B cells in the bone marrow. **Peripheral tolerance** is important in regulating T cells that escape intrathymic negative selection. These T lymphocytes are held in check in the periphery through anergy, suppression, and/or activation-induced cell death.

Theories of Autoimmunity

Inaccessible Self-Antigens

The simplest hypothesis to explain the loss of tolerance in autoimmune disease states that an immune reaction develops to a self-antigen not normally "accessible" to the immune system. Intracellular antigens are not exposed or released until some type of tissue injury releases them. At that time, an immune response develops. Examples of this type of response are antibody formation against spermatozoa, lens tissue, and myelin. Whether these autoantibodies can induce injury directly is another matter. In the case of antisperm antibodies, aside from a localized orchitis, there is no evidence that they induce generalized injury. Thus, although autoantibodies may form against normally "sequestered" antigens, there is only infrequent evidence that they are pathogenic.

Abnormal T Cell Function

Autoimmune reactions have been suggested to develop as a result of abnormalities in the T lymphocyte system. Most immune responses require T cell participation to activate antigen-specific

B cells. Thus, alterations in the number or functional activities of helper or suppressor T cells would be expected to influence one's ability to mount an immune response. In fact, defects in T cells, particularly suppressor T cells, have been described in many autoimmune diseases. For example, there are reports of defective suppressor cell activity in human and experimental SLE. Lymphocytotropic antibodies have also been described in patients with lupus. Abnormalities in suppressor cell function characterize other autoimmune diseases, including primary biliary cirrhosis, thyroiditis, multiple sclerosis, myasthenia gravis, rheumatoid arthritis, and scleroderma. However, the critical question is whether these alterations in suppressor cell function cause these diseases or whether they merely represent an epiphenomenon. Defects in suppressor cell function have also been described in persons with no evidence of autoimmune disease.

There has also been interest in abnormalities in helper T cell function in autoimmune disease. Helper T cells are defined by their role in antigen-specific B cell activation. It is believed that these cells maintain the helper T cell tolerance induced by low doses of antigen. Recent evidence indicates that these cells become autoreactive in many autoimmune diseases. One key mechanism in autoimmunity is DNA hypomethylation caused by drugs and other agents. This effect leads to upregulation of leukocyte function antigen 1 (LFA-1) and B cell activation independent of antigen. An example of this T cell autoreactivity and loss of antigen specificity is drug-induced lupus. Experimentally, it is also possible to "break" this type of tolerance by altering an antigen so that the helper cell is activated and triggers the B cells. An example is when an antigen is modified by partial degradation or complexing with a carrier protein. Some rheumatic diseases are marked by autoantibodies to partially degraded connective tissue proteins, such as collagen or elastin. In some drug-induced hemolytic anemias, antibody against a drug causes hemolysis when the drug binds to erythrocyte membranes.

Molecular Mimicry

Another mechanism by which the helper T cell tolerance is overcome involves antibodies against foreign antigens that cross-react with self-antigens. Here helper T cells function "correctly" and do not induce autoantibody formation. Rather, the efferent limb of the immune response is abnormal. Thus, in rheumatic heart disease, antibodies against streptococcal bacterial antigens cross-react with antigens from cardiac muscle—a phenomenon known as **molecular mimicry.**

Polyclonal B-Cell Activation

Loss of tolerance may also involve polyclonal B cell activation, in which B lymphocytes are directly activated by complex substances that contain many antigenic sites (e.g., bacterial cell walls and viruses). Development of rheumatoid factor in rheumatoid arthritis, anti-DNA antibodies in lupus erythematosus, and other autoantibodies has been described after bacterial, viral, and parasitic infections.

Tissue Injury in Autoimmune Diseases

Autoimmune diseases have traditionally been considered to be prototypic of immune complex disease, which involves complexes that form either in the circulation or in tissues. Thus, type II (cytotoxic) and type III (immune complex) hypersensitivity reactions are implicated as the cause of tissue injury in most types of autoimmune diseases. Although it is probably true that these hypersensitivity reactions explain most autoimmune tissue injury, the story is more complicated. In some types of autoimmune diseases, T cells sensitized to self-antigens (such as thyroglobulin) may directly cause tissue injury (type IV reaction), but it is not clear to what extent.

Another mechanism of tissue injury is ADCC. Antibodies against an antigen expressed at the cell membrane lead to destruction of that cell. Thus, antibodies against parietal cell H^+/K^+-ATPase are important in the pathogenesis of atrophic gastritis.

However, not all autoantibodies cause disease via cytotoxicity. In antireceptor antibody diseases, such as Graves disease and myasthenia gravis, antibody binds a receptor but the disease process reflects either activation or inactivation of the receptor, rather than cell loss. In Graves disease, autoantibody against TSH receptor acts as an agonist to stimulate thyroid hormone production, whereas in myasthenia gravis the autoantibody prevents acetylcholine binding to its receptor, thereby impairing neuromuscular synaptic transmission. Anti-insulin receptor antibodies have also been described in diseases such as acanthosis nigricans and ataxia telangiectasia, in which some patients exhibit a form of diabetes characterized by extreme insulin resistance.

Type III hypersensitivity reactions (immune complex disease) explain tissue injury in some types of autoimmune diseases. The prototypical disease in this category is SLE. In this disorder, DNA–anti-DNA complexes formed in the circulation (or at local sites) are deposited in tissues, where they induce inflammation and injury, such as occurs in vasculitis and glomerulonephritis. Other examples are rheumatoid arthritis, scleroderma, polymyositis/dermatomyositis, and Sjögren syndrome. All of these disorders are characterized by immune phenomena and are classified under the rubric "collagen vascular" diseases. The clinical manifestations are systemic and many organs and tissues are typically involved. By contrast, cytotoxic (type II-mediated) autoimmune reactions are, for the most part, organ specific.

Systemic Lupus Erythematosus Is a Prototypical Systemic Immune Complex Disease

SLE is a chronic, autoimmune, multisystem, inflammatory disease that may involve almost any organ but characteristically affects kidneys, joints, serous membranes, and skin. Autoantibodies are formed against a variety of self-antigens, including plasma proteins (complement components, clotting factors) and protein-phospholipid complexes cell surface antigens (lymphocytes, neutrophils, platelets, erythrocytes), intracellular cytoplasmic components (microfilaments, microtubules, lysosomes, ribosomes, RNA) and nuclear DNA, ribonucleoproteins, and histones. The most important diagnostic autoantibodies are those against nuclear antigens—in particular, antibody to double-stranded DNA and to a soluble nuclear antigen complex that is part of the spliceosome and termed Sm (Smith) antigen. High titers of these two **antinuclear antibodies** (ANAs) are nearly pathognomonic of SLE but are not directly cytotoxic. Antigen–antibody complexes deposit in tissues, leading to the characteristic vasculitis, synovitis, and glomerulonephritis. For this reason, SLE is a prototype of type III hypersensitivity reactions. Occasionally, directly cytotoxic antibodies are present, particularly antibodies against cell surface antigens of leukocytes and erythrocytes.

The prevalence of SLE varies worldwide and in North America and northern Europe is 40/100,000. In the United States, it appears to be more common and severe in African-Americans and Hispanics, although socioeconomic factors may in part be responsible. Over 80% of cases are in women of childbearing age, and SLE may strike as many as 1 in 700 women in this age group.

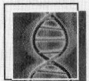

PATHOGENESIS: The etiology of SLE is unknown. The presence of numerous autoantibodies, particularly ANAs, suggests a breakdown in immune surveillance mechanisms that leads to a loss of tolerance. Many manifestations of SLE result from tissue injury caused by immune complex-mediated vasculitis. Other clinical manifestations (e.g., thrombocytopenia or the secondary antiphospholipid syndrome) are caused by autoantibodies against serum components or molecules on cell membranes. However, the diagnostically helpful ANAs are not incriminated in the pathogenesis of SLE. There appear to be many factors that predispose to the development of SLE (Fig. 4-20).

Although there was at one time interest in C-type viral particles in experimental murine models of SLE, most evidence argues against a viral etiology for human SLE. The clear female predisposition for SLE is true for many autoimmune diseases, and sex hormones may in part be the explanation. Immune responses in animals are strongly influenced by sex hormones. In mouse models of SLE, estrogens accelerate disease progression, while androgens have a moderating effect. Whether the course of human SLE is influenced in the same manner is controversial.

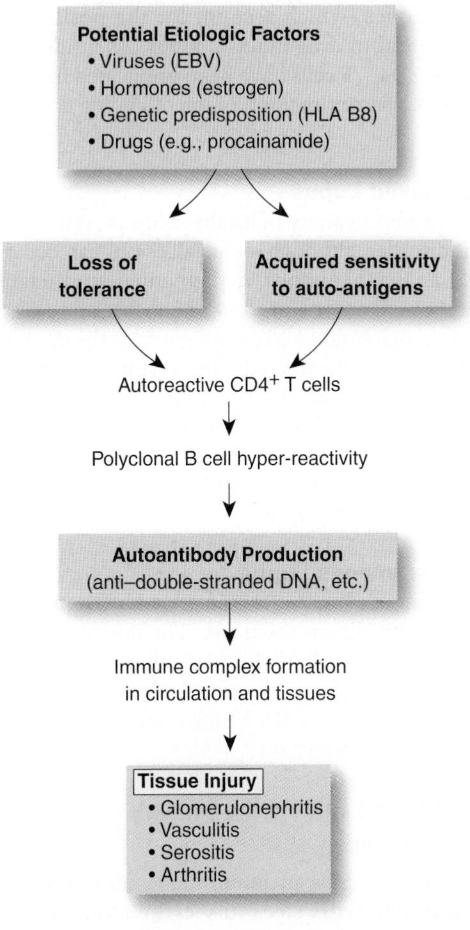

FIGURE 4-20. **The pathogenesis of systemic lupus erythematosus is multifactorial.** EBV = Epstein-Barr virus; HLA = human leukocyte antigen.

Experimentally, estrogens reportedly increase the likelihood of overcoming immune tolerance.

Some genetic predisposition to lupus is suggested by a higher prevalence in some ethic groups, some families, and monozygotic twins. The latter exhibit a concordance of 20% to 30%, suggesting that both genetic and environmental factors play a role. The incidence of SLE (and other autoimmune diseases) is higher among persons who express certain MHC class II DR and DQ antigens. These gene products participate in two unlinked functions, namely, immunoregulation and the effector limb of the immune response. Thus, the HLA-B8 haplotype, which is often found in association with autoimmune diseases, is also associated with the DR antigens in certain immunoregulatory abnormalities. These disorders include abnormal lymphocyte responses to antigens, decreased numbers of circulating suppressor cells, and increased numbers of circulating B cells. Among the effector functions associated with these HLA haplotypes is a decrease in C3b receptors on cells that clear circulating immune complexes. A critical role for the D/DR region in the pathogenesis of SLE is supported by the observation that inherited deficiencies of certain complement components, particularly C2, C4, and C1q are associated with an increased incidence of the disease. The genes that encode these early complement components are within the HLA region, close to the D/DR locus.

Production of autoantibodies against many antigens is characteristic of SLE, but the precise mechanisms underlying B cell hyperreactivity are unknown. Two general hypotheses have been advanced. One attributes the disease to a nonspecific, polyclonal B cell activation, although the nature of the stimulus is speculative. The second hypothesis holds that the antibodies formed in SLE represent a response to specific antigenic stimulation. Support for the latter supposition comes from the observation that with time the antibodies of SLE demonstrate gene rearrangements and mutations that are typical of an antigen-driven response. Moreover, a patient with SLE often has antibodies to more than one epitope on a single antigen, further suggesting a primary role for an antigen-driven process. Although inciting antigens have not been identified, a number of factors render normal body constituents more immunogenic, including infection, ultraviolet light exposure, and other environmental agents that damage cells. Foreign, e.g., viral, antigens might induce molecular mimicry, although direct evidence is lacking.

Whether or not the autoimmune response in SLE is primarily driven by antigens, the variety of autoantibodies strongly suggests a general disturbance of immune tolerance. $CD4^+$ T cells become autoreactive secondary to DNA hypomethylation. These autoreactive $CD4^+$ T cells over-express the cell adhesion molecule LFA-1 (CD11a), which stabilizes the interaction between T cells and APCs such as macrophages. These autoreactive $CD4^+$ T cells have been best described in mouse models; no consistent defect in the T-suppressor cell population has been found in humans. Among other immunologic abnormalities described in SLE is an increase in circulating levels of IL-6, which in these patients is associated with B-cell differentiation.

The evidence for the hypothesis that SLE is predominantly mediated by type III hypersensitivity includes the occurrence of circulating immune complexes, which contain nuclear antigen; the presence of immune complexes in injured tissues, as identified by immunofluorescence; and the observation that immune complexes can be extracted from tissues that contain nuclear antigens. Thus, there is good reason to believe that the bulk of the injury in lupus is due to deposition of circulating immune complexes against self-antigens, particularly against DNA. Additional evidence suggests that under certain conditions immune complex formation also occurs in situ—that is, in tissues rather than in the circulation. Examples include antibody formed against connective tissue components and perhaps the membranous form of lupus glomerulonephritis. Type II hypersensitivity reactions also participate in lupus, since cytotoxic antibodies against leukocytes, erythrocytes, and platelets have been described.

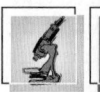

PATHOLOGY AND CLINICAL FEATURES: Because circulating immune complexes deposit in almost all tissues, virtually every organ in the body can be involved.

Skin involvement (see Chapter 24) is common and is manifested by an erythematous rash in sun-exposed sites, a malar "butterfly" rash being the most characteristic. Microscopically, the skin exhibits a perivascular lymphoid infiltrate and liquefactive degeneration of the basal cells. Immunofluorescence studies reveal immunoglobulin and complement deposition at the dermal–epidermal junction ("lupus band").

Joint disease is the most common manifestation of SLE; over 90% of patients have polyarthralgia. An inflammatory synovitis occurs, but unlike rheumatoid arthritis, joint destruction is unusual.

Renal disease, in particular glomerulonephritis, afflicts three fourths of patients with SLE. Immune complexes between DNA and IgG antibodies to double-stranded DNA deposit in glomeruli and lead to glomerulonephritis (see Chapter 16). Although glomerulonephritis is the most common renal manifestation of SLE, interstitial nephritis or (rarely) vasculitis can also be seen. In many of these cases, immunoglobulins and complement are present in the interstitium and blood vessels of the kidney.

Serous membranes are commonly involved in SLE. More than one third of patients have pleuritis and pleural effusion. Pericarditis and peritonitis occur, but less frequently.

Disorders of the respiratory system in SLE occur frequently. The clinical manifestations are diverse, ranging from pleural disease to upper airway involvement and pulmonary parenchymal disease. Pneumonitis is thought to be caused by deposition of immune complexes in alveolar septa and is associated with patchy acute inflammation. Progressive interstitial fibrosis develops in some patients. An increased incidence of pulmonary hypertension has also been reported.

Cardiac involvement (see Chapter 11) is often encountered in SLE, although congestive heart failure is rare and is usually associated with myocarditis. All layers of the heart may be involved, with pericarditis being the most common finding**. Libman-Sacks endocarditis**, which is usually not clinically significant, is characterized by small nonbacterial vegetations on valve leaflets. These lesions should be differentiated from the larger, bulkier vegetations of bacterial endocarditis or the vegetations of rheumatic endocarditis, which are confined to the lines of valve closure.

Disease of the CNS is a life-threatening complication of lupus. Vasculitis is the common underlying lesion, leading to hemorrhage and infarction of the brain, which are often lethal.

Antiphospholipid antibodies are encountered in one third of patients with SLE. This autoimmune phenomenon predisposes patients to thromboembolic complications, including stroke, pulmonary embolism, deep venous thrombosis, portal vein thrombosis, and spontaneous abortions.

Other organ involvement is less frequent and is often due to **vasculitis.** Lesions in the spleen are characterized by thickening and concentric fibrosis of the penicillary arteries, the so-called "onion-skin" pattern.

The clinical course of SLE is highly variable, typically with exacerbations and remissions. Because of immunosuppressive therapies, better recognition of mild forms of the disease and improved antihypertensive medications, overall 10-year survival approaches 90%. The worst prognosis is in patients with severe renal or CNS disease and those with systolic hypertension.

Lupus-like Diseases Feature Immune Complexes

Drug-Induced Lupus

A syndrome that resembles SLE can occur following use of certain drugs, most notably procainamide (for arrhythmias), hydralazine (for hypertension), and isoniazid (for tuberculosis). Drug-induced lupus ranges from asymptomatic laboratory abnormalities (positive ANA test result) to a syndrome that is clinically similar to SLE. Unlike SLE, drug-induced lupus shows no sex predominance and most patients are over 50 years old. Factors that predispose to this syndrome include large daily doses of the offending drug, slow drug-acetylator status and (in hydralazine-induced lupus) HLA-DR4 genotype. As in SLE, deposition of immune complexes is a feature of drug-induced lupus. Patients with drug-induced lupus typically exhibit constitutional signs, polyarthritis, pleuritis, and a positive ANA test result. In addition, they may develop rheumatoid factor, false-positive tests for syphilis, and a positive Coombs test. Unlike in SLE, renal and CNS involvement rarely occurs, and it is unusual to find antibodies to double-stranded DNA and Sm antigen. Autoantibodies to histones (which account for the positive ANA test result) are typical of drug-induced lupus. As in idiopathic SLE, autoreactive $CD4^+$ T cells have been implicated in polyclonal B cell activation. Discontinuation of the offending drug is ordinarily curative.

Chronic Discoid Lupus

The most common variety of localized lupus erythematosus is a cutaneous disorder, although identical lesions can occur in some cases of SLE. Erythematous, depigmented, and telangiectatic plaques are found most commonly on the face and scalp. Deposition of immunoglobulins and complement at the dermal–epidermal interface in chronic discoid lupus is similar to that observed in SLE. However, unlike SLE, uninvolved skin contains no immune deposits. Although ANAs develop in about one third of patients, antibodies to double-stranded DNA and Sm antigen are not encountered. Most patients with discoid lupus are not otherwise ill, but up to 10% eventually manifest features of SLE.

Subacute Cutaneous Lupus

Subacute cutaneous lupus is characterized by papular and annular lesions, principally on the trunk. The disorder is aggravated by exposure to ultraviolet light (via sunlight), although lesions eventually resolve without scarring. Antibodies to a ribonucleoprotein complex (SS-A or Ro antigen) and an association with HLA-DR3 genotype are characteristic.

Sjögren Syndrome Targets the Salivary and Lacrimal Glands

Sjögren syndrome (SS) is an autoimmune disorder characterized by **keratoconjunctivitis sicca** (dry eyes) and **xerostomia** (dry mouth) in the absence of other connective tissue disease. This definition separates primary SS from secondary types that are occasionally associated with other disorders of connective tissue, such as SLE, rheumatoid arthritis, scleroderma, and polymyositis.

The primary type is also frequently associated with involvement of other organs, including the thyroid, lung, and kidney.

Primary SS is the second most common connective tissue disorder after SLE and affects up to 3% of the population. Like most autoimmune diseases, it occurs mostly in women, 30 to 65 years old. There are strong associations between primary SS and certain MHC types, notably HLA-B8, Dw3, HLA-DR3, DRw-52, and HLA-Dw2, as well as MT2, a B cell alloantigen. Familial clustering occurs, and these families also exhibit a high prevalence of other autoimmune diseases.

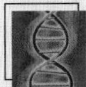

PATHOGENESIS: The cause of SS is unknown. The production of autoantibodies, particularly ANAs against DNA or nonhistone proteins, typically occurs in patients with SS. Autoantibodies to soluble nuclear nonhistone proteins, especially antigens SS-A a (Ro) and SS-B (La), are found in half of patients with primary SS and are associated with more-severe glandular and extraglandular manifestations. Autoantibodies to DNA or histones are rare, and their presence suggests secondary SS associated with lupus. Organ-specific autoantibodies, e.g., against salivary gland antigens, are distinctly uncommon. As in SLE, it remains controversial whether the autoantibodies in SS mainly reflect polyclonal B cell activation or is essentially antigen-driven, although these processes are not mutually exclusive.

SS has become the prototype for investigation of a viral etiology for autoimmune disease. Particular attention has been paid to possible roles of EBV and human T cell leukemia virus-1 (HTLV-1). Although it is still difficult to assign a role for EBV in the pathogenesis of SS, there is evidence that reactivation of this virus may be involved in perpetuating SS, polyclonal B cell activation, and development of lymphoma. In Japan, the seroprevalence of HTLV-1 among patients with SS is 23%, compared with 3.4% among unselected blood donors. Conversely, among HTLV-1 seropositive persons, more than three-quarters demonstrated evidence of SS.

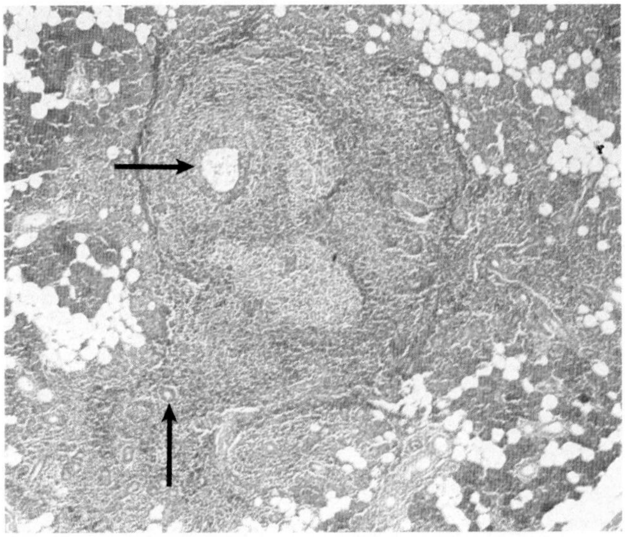

FIGURE 4-21. **Minor gland sialadenitis associated with Sjögren syndrome is characterized by an intense lymphoid infiltrate and acinar destruction.** The salivary ducts *(arrows)* are spared.

PATHOLOGY AND CLINICAL FEATURES: SS is characterized by an intense lymphocytic infiltrate in the salivary and lacrimal glands (Fig. 4-21). Focal lymphocytic infiltrates in these glands are initially observed in a periductal distribution. Most lobules are affected, especially the centers of the lobules. Well-defined germinal centers are rare. The lymphoid infiltrates destroy acini and ducts. The latter often become dilated and filled with cellular debris. The glandular stroma is preserved, which appearance helps to differentiate this disorder from lymphoma. The lymphocytic infiltrates in the glands are predominantly $CD4^+$ T cells, but a few B cells are also present. In the late stage of the disease, the glands atrophy and may be replaced by hyalinized tissue and fibrosis. Owing to the absence of tears, the corneas become dry and fissured and may ulcerate. The lack of saliva causes atrophy, inflammation, and cracking of the oral mucosa. The pathology of the salivary and lacrimal glands is described in greater detail in Chapter 25.

Involvement of extraglandular sites is also common in SS. Pulmonary disease occurs in most patients, particularly bronchial gland atrophy in association with lymphoid infiltration. This causes thick tenacious secretions, focal atelectasis, recurrent infections, and bronchiectasis. The gastrointestinal tract is also affected, and many patients have difficulty swallowing (dysphagia). Esophageal submucosal glands are infiltrated by lymphocytes. In addition, atrophic gastritis occurs secondary to lymphoid infiltration of the gastric mucosa. Liver disease, especially primary biliary cirrhosis, is present in 5% to 10% of patients with SS and is associated with destruction of intrahepatic bile ducts and nodular lymphoid infiltrates. Interstitial nephritis and chronic thyroiditis occasionally accompany SS. SS is associated with a 40-fold increased risk of malignant lymphoma, probably through B-cell clonal expansion.

Scleroderma (Progressive Systemic Sclerosis) Is an Autoimmune Disease of Connective Tissue

Scleroderma is characterized by vasculopathy and excessive collagen deposition in the skin and internal organs, such as the lung, gastrointestinal tract, heart, and kidney. It is four times as common in women as in men, mostly in persons 25 to50 years of age. Familial incidence has been reported. There is an association between HLA-DQB1 and the formation of the autoantibodies characteristic of this disease.

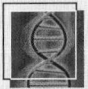

PATHOGENESIS: Patients with scleroderma exhibit abnormalities of the humoral and cellular immune systems. The number of circulating B lymphocytes is normal, but there is evidence of hyperactivity, as manifested by hypergammaglobulinemia and cryoglobulinemia. ANAs are common but are usually at lower titers than in SLE. Antibodies commonly found in scleroderma include nucleolar autoantibodies (primarily against RNA polymerase); antibodies to Scl-70, a nonhistone nuclear protein topoisomerase; and anticentromere antibodies, which are associated with the "CREST" variant of the disease (see below). The Scl-70 autoantibody is the most common and specific for the diffuse form of scleroderma, and is seen in 60% of these patients. However, there is no correlation between ANA titer and disease severity.

Rheumatoid factor is commonly present in scleroderma and autoantibodies are occasionally directed against other issues, such as smooth muscle, thyroid gland, and salivary glands. Antibodies against collagen types I and IV have also been described.

Cellular immune derangements are also seen in patients with progressive systemic sclerosis. Reduced circulating $CD8^+$ T suppressor cells, evidence of T cell activation, alterations in functions mediated by IL-1 and elevated IL-2, and soluble IL-2 receptor occur in active disease. Increased levels of IL-4 and IL-6 have also been described. Tissues exhibit active mononuclear inflammation, which precedes the development of the vasculopathy and fibrosis characteristic of this disease. In these infiltrates, increased numbers of $CD4^+$ and $\gamma\delta+$ T cells (which adhere to fibroblasts) are present, as well as macrophages. Mast cells (degranulated) are also present in skin of these patients. The incidence of other autoimmune disorders, such as thyroiditis and primary biliary cirrhosis, is increased in patients with progressive systemic sclerosis. Circulating male fetal cells have been demonstrated in blood and blood vessel walls of many women with scleroderma who bore male children many years before the disease began. It has been suggested that scleroderma in these patients is similar to graft-versus-host disease (GVHD).

Progressive systemic sclerosis is characterized by widespread excessive collagen deposition. Although the cause remains unclear, there is emerging evidence that there is expansion and activation of fibrogenic clones of fibroblasts. These clones behave autonomously and display augmented procollagen synthesis, including increased circulating levels of type III collagen aminopropeptide. Several factors may be responsible for this fibroblast activation. The $\gamma\delta+$ T cells adhere to fibroblasts and may induce activation via cytokine generation. TGF-β is elevated in tissues of these patients, as are IL-1 and IL-4, all of which stimulate fibroblast proliferation and collagen biosynthesis. IL-6—which is upregulated matrix metalloproteinase and is important in modulation of collagen metabolism—is also elevated. Activated fibroblasts themselves produce cytokines and growth factors, such as IL-1, prostaglandin E (PGE), TGF-β; and PDGF, which may in turn serve to activate other fibroblasts. Finally, activated fibroblasts also express the adhesion molecule ICAM-1 on their surface, which may be important in adherence of T cells and macrophages and their subsequent activation.

PATHOLOGY: The skin in scleroderma initially shows edema and then induration. The thickened skin exhibits a striking increase in collagen fibers in the reticular dermis; thinning of the epidermis with loss of rete pegs; atrophy of dermal appendages; hyalinization and obliteration of arterioles; and variable mononuclear infiltrates, consisting primarily of T cells. The stage of induration may progress to atrophy or revert to normal. Increases in collagen deposition can also occur in synovia, lungs, gastrointestinal tract, heart, and kidneys.

Lesions in the arteries, arterioles, and capillaries are typical, and in some cases may be the first demonstrable pathologic finding in the disease. Initial subintimal edema with fibrin deposition is followed by thickening and fibrosis of the vessel and reduplication or fraying of the internal elastic lamina. The involved vessels can become severely restricted in terms of blood flow and may become occluded by thrombus.

The kidneys are involved in more than half of patients with scleroderma. They show marked vascular changes, often with focal hemorrhage and cortical infarcts (see Chapter 16). Among the most severely affected vessels are the interlobular arteries and afferent arterioles. Early fibromuscular thickening of the subintima causes luminal narrowing, which is followed by fibrosis (Fig. 4-22). Fibrinoid necrosis is commonly seen in afferent arterioles. Glomerular alterations are nonspecific and focal changes range from necrosis extending from the afferent arterioles to fibrosis. There is diffuse deposition of immunoglobulin, complement, and fibrin in affected vessels early in the disease, probably because of increased vascular permeability.

Diffuse interstitial fibrosis is the primary abnormality in lungs. The disease can progress to end-stage pulmonary fibrosis, so-called honeycomb lung.

Most patients with scleroderma have patchy myocardial fibrosis and in about one fourth of cases, more than 10% of the myocardium is involved. These lesions result from focal myocardial necrosis, which may reflect focal ischemia secondary to a Raynaud-like reactivity of coronary microvasculature.

Progressive systemic sclerosis can involve any portion of the gastrointestinal tract. Esophageal dysfunction is the most common and troublesome gastrointestinal complication. Atrophy of smooth muscle and fibrous replacement are seen in the lower esophagus. The small bowel is often involved, with patchy fibrosis, principally of the muscular layers.

CLINICAL FEATURES: Scleroderma presents as two distinct clinical categories, a generalized (progressive systemic) form and a limited variant. Progressive systemic sclerosis (diffuse scleroderma) is characterized by severe and progressive disease of skin and early onset of all or most of the associated abnormalities of visceral organs. Symptoms

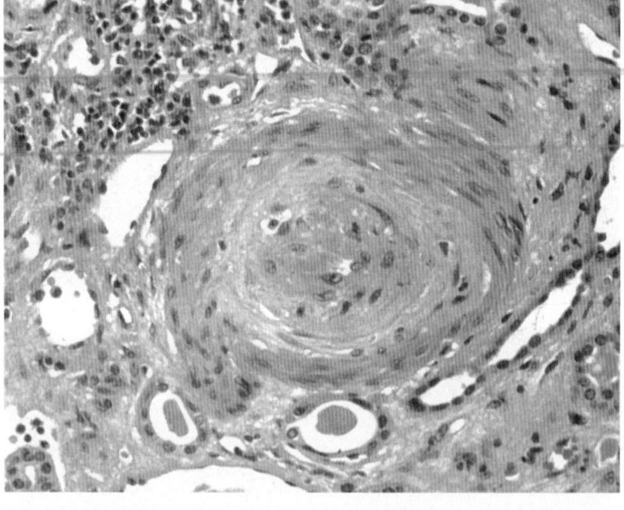

FIGURE 4-22. **Scleroderma that affects the kidney is manifested by vascular involvement.** Here, the interlobular artery exhibits marked luminal narrowing due to pronounced intimal thickening.

usually begin with Raynaud phenomenon, namely, intermittent episodes of ischemia of fingers, marked by pallor, paresthesias, and pain. These symptoms are accompanied or followed by edema of fingers and hands, tightening and thickening of skin, polyarthralgia, and complaints referable to involvement of specific internal organs. The typical patient with generalized scleroderma exhibits "stone facies," owing to tightening of facial skin and restricted motion of the mouth. Progression of vascular lesions in fingers leads to ischemic ulcerations of fingertips, with subsequent shortening and atrophy of digits. Many patients suffer from painful tendinitis and joint pain is common. Esophageal involvement causes hypomotility and dysphagia. Fibrosis in the small bowel interferes with intestinal mobility, with consequent bacterial overgrowth and secondary malabsorption. Dyspnea on exertion is the initial symptom of pulmonary fibrosis in scleroderma, occurring in more than half of patients. The lung disease progresses to dyspnea at rest and eventually to respiratory failure. Patients with long-standing disease are at risk for development of pulmonary hypertension and cor pulmonale. Although most patients with scleroderma have some myocardial fibrosis, congestive heart failure is uncommon. However, ventricular arrhythmias can cause sudden death.

The vascular involvement of the kidneys in generalized scleroderma is responsible for so-called scleroderma renal crisis the sudden onset of malignant hypertension, progressive renal insufficiency, and frequently, microangiopathic hemolytic anemia. The syndrome, which reflects ischemic injury to the kidneys, usually occurs in the first few years of the disease and is marked by conspicuously elevated levels of circulating renin.

The so-called limited form of scleroderma is a milder disease than generalized scleroderma. Typically, such patients exhibit skin involvement, particularly the face and fingers. A variant within the spectrum of limited scleroderma is CREST syndrome. CREST is characterized by calcinosis, Raynaud phenomenon, esophageal dysmotility, sclerodactyly, and telangiectasia. The limited variant usually does not entail severe systemic involvement early in disease but later can progress, primarily in the form of diffuse interstitial lung fibrosis. Patients with limited scleroderma often posses circulating anticentromere antibodies.

Mixed Connective Tissue Disease Combines Features of SLE, Scleroderma, and Dermatomyositis

The incidence of mixed connective tissue disease (MCTD) is unknown. Between 80% and 90% of patients are female, and most are adults (mean age, 37 years). Those symptoms that are characteristic of SLE include rash, Raynaud phenomenon, arthritis, and arthralgias. The characteristics of scleroderma are swollen hands, esophageal hypomotility, and pulmonary interstitial disease. Some patients also develop symptoms suggestive of rheumatoid arthritis. Patients with MCTD have been reported to respond well to corticosteroid therapy, although some studies have challenged this assertion.

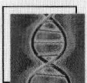

PATHOGENESIS: The etiology and pathogenesis of MCTD are unknown. Patients often have evidence of B cell activation with hypergammaglobulinemia and a positive rheumatoid factor assay result. ANAs are present but, unlike in SLE, they are usually not directed against double-stranded DNA. The most distinctive ANA is directed against an extractable nuclear antigen. Specifically, patients with MCTD have high titers of antibody to uridine-rich ribonucleoprotein (anti-U1-RNP) in the absence of other extractable nuclear antigens, including PM-1 and Jo-1. Anti-RNP antibodies are also occasionally seen in SLE but usually in lower titer than in MCTD.

The cause of the formation and maintenance of the high titer of anti-RNP antibody is unclear. However, there is an association with HLA-DR4 and HLA-DR2 genotypes, suggesting a role for T cells in the autoantibody production. There is no direct evidence that these antibodies induce the characteristic involvement of the various organ systems. There is also controversy over whether MCTD is a separate disease entity or represents a heterogeneous collection of patients with nonclassical presentations of SLE, scleroderma, or polymyositis. For example, in some patients, MCTD seems to evolve into typical scleroderma. Other patients develop evidence of renal disease, consistent with SLE. Still others differentiate into rheumatoid arthritis. Thus, MCTD often seems to be an intermediate stage in a genetically determined progression to a recognized autoimmune disease. Persons whose disease remains undifferentiated may make up a distinct subset. At this time, it is unclear whether MCTD is a distinct entity or simply an overlap of symptoms in patients with other types of collagen vascular diseases.

Immune Reactions to Transplanted Tissues

Antigens encoded by the MHC on chromosome 6 are critical immunogenic molecules that can stimulate rejection of transplanted tissues. Thus, optimal graft survival occurs when recipient and donor are closely matched with regard to histocompatibility antigens. In practice, an exact HLA match is obtained infrequently, except in the case of transplantation between monozygotic twins. Vigilant monitoring of the functional status of the graft and immunosuppressive therapy is thus required after transplantation. In recent years, therapeutic advances (e.g., cyclosporine and tacrolimus) have greatly improved transplant success rates, even when there is a degree of histoincompatibility. When host-versus-graft immune reactions (rejection) occur, any combination of immune responses may injure the graft.

Both T cell-mediated and antibody-mediated reactions are important in the pathophysiology of transplant rejection. Antigen-presenting cells, specifically those bearing foreign MHC molecules in the graft, are recognized by host $CD8^+$ cytotoxic T lymphocytes which mediate tissue injury; and host $CD4^+$ T helper cells which augment antibody production, induce IFN-γ production, and activate macrophages. Induction of IFN-γ leads to enhanced MHC expression with amplification of tissue injury. Host APCs also process foreign donor antigens leading to $CD4^+$-mediated delayed type hypersensitivity and $CD4^+$-mediated antibody production.

Transplant rejection reactions have been traditionally categorized as "hyperacute, acute, and chronic" rejection, based on the clinical tempo of the response and on the pathophysiologic mechanisms involved. However, in practice, there can be overlap of features and ambiguity in diagnosis. The diagnosis of transplant rejection is further complicated by toxic effects of immunosuppressive drugs and by the potential for either mechanical problems (e.g., vascular thrombosis) or recurrence of original disease (e.g., some types of glomerulonephritis). The next sections illustrate rejection in the context of renal transplantation. Similar responses occur in other transplanted tissues, although each transplanted tissue type exhibits its own unique problems.

Hyperacute Rejection Occurs Within Minutes to Hours after Transplantation

Hyperacute rejection is manifested clinically as a sudden cessation of urine output, along with fever and pain in the area of the graft site. This immediate rejection is catastrophic and necessitates prompt surgical removal of the kidney. The histologic features of hyperacute rejection within the transplanted kidney are vascular congestion, fibrin–platelet thrombi within capillaries, neutrophilic vasculitis with fibrinoid necrosis, prominent interstitial edema, and neutrophilic infiltrates (Fig. 4-23A). This form of rejection is mediated by preformed anti-HLA antibodies and complement activation products, including chemotactic and other inflammatory mediators. Fortunately, hyperacute rejection is not common when appropriate pretransplantation antibody screening is performed.

Acute Rejection Is Seen within the First Few Weeks or Months after Transplantation

Acute rejection is characterized by abrupt onset of azotemia and oliguria, which may be associated with fever and graft tenderness. A needle biopsy is often used to differentiate between acute rejection and acute tubular necrosis or toxicity from immunosuppressive agents. Findings vary depending whether the rejection is primarily cellular or humoral. In the former case, microscopic findings include interstitial infiltrates of lymphocytes, and macrophages, edema, lymphocytic tubulitis and tubular necrosis (see Fig. 4-23B). The acute humoral form, sometimes called rejection vasculitis, shows vascular damage manifested as arteritis, fibrinoid necrosis, and thrombosis. Vascular involvement is an ominous sign because it usually means the rejection episode will be refractory to therapy. Acute rejection most typically involves both cell-mediated and humoral mechanisms of tissue damage. If detected in its early stages, acute rejection can be reversed with immunosuppressive therapy.

Chronic Rejection Appears Months to Years after Transplantation

In chronic rejection the patient typically develops progressive azotemia, oliguria, hypertension, and weight gain over a period of months. The dominant histologic features are arterial and arteriolar intimal thickening causing vascular stenosis or obstruction, thickened glomerular capillary walls, tubular atrophy, and interstitial fibrosis (see Fig. 4-23C). The interstitium often exhibits scattered mononuclear infiltrates and tubules contain proteinaceous casts. Chronic rejection may be the end-result of repeated episodes of cellular rejection, either asymptomatic or clinically apparent. This advanced state of damage does not respond to therapy. As in the clinical diagnosis, histologic features of acute and chronic rejection may overlap and vary in degree, so that clear distinction may not be possible on renal biopsy.

Graft-Versus-Host Disease Occurs When Donor Lymphocytes Recognize and React to the Recipient

The advent of transplantation of allogenic (donor) bone marrow or HSCs into patients with hematogenous malignancies or severe connective tissue disorder, has allowed treatment of previously terminal conditions or conditions which were refractory to standard treatment. To allow engraftment of the new bone marrow to the host, the patient's native bone marrow and

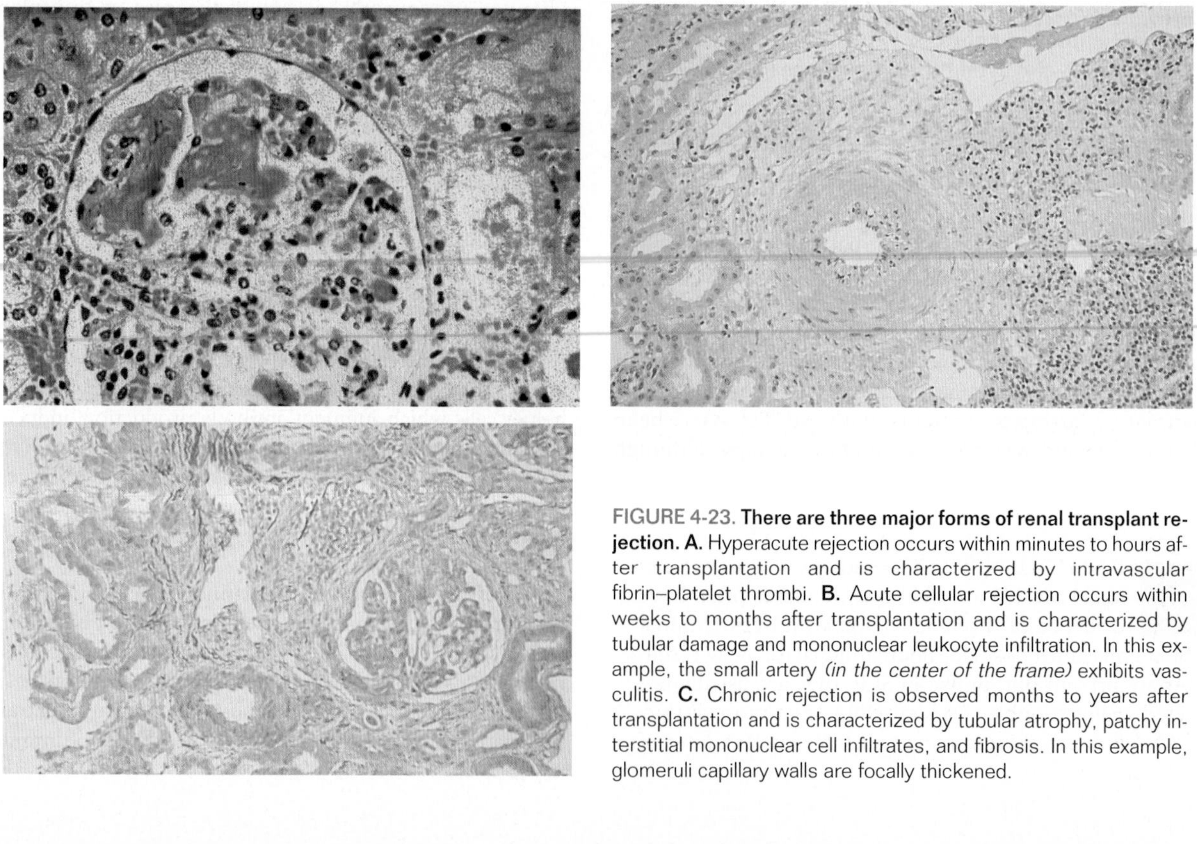

A B C

FIGURE 4-23. **There are three major forms of renal transplant rejection. A.** Hyperacute rejection occurs within minutes to hours after transplantation and is characterized by intravascular fibrin–platelet thrombi. **B.** Acute cellular rejection occurs within weeks to months after transplantation and is characterized by tubular damage and mononuclear leukocyte infiltration. In this example, the small artery *(in the center of the frame)* exhibits vasculitis. **C.** Chronic rejection is observed months to years after transplantation and is characterized by tubular atrophy, patchy interstitial mononuclear cell infiltrates, and fibrosis. In this example, glomeruli capillary walls are focally thickened.

immune system must be "conditioned" (ablated) usually by cytotoxic drugs, sometimes plus radiation. Immunocompetent lymphocytes, if present in the grafted marrow, may react to—"reject"—host tissues, leading to GVHD. GVHD can also occur when a profoundly immunodeficient patient is transfused with blood products containing HLA-incompatible lymphocytes.

The major organs affected in GVHD are skin, gastrointestinal tract, and liver. The skin and intestine exhibit mononuclear cell infiltrates and epithelial cell necrosis. The liver displays periportal inflammation, damaged bile ducts and liver cell injury. Clinically, acute GVHD manifests as rash, diarrhea, abdominal cramps, anemia, and liver dysfunction. The chronic form of GVHD is characterized by dermal sclerosis, sicca syndrome (dry eyes and mouth due to chronic inflammation of lacrimal and salivary glands), and immunodeficiency. Treatment of GVHD requires immunosuppressive therapy. Patients, especially those with chronic GVHD, may be at a higher risk for opportunistic infections, e.g., fungal infection such as invasive aspergillosis are often life-threatening.

Human Immunodeficiency Virus and Acquired Immunodeficiency Syndrome

AIDS is the most common immunodeficiency state worldwide. It is mainly caused by HIV-1, although a small minority of patients are infected with HIV-2, primarily in western Africa. Persons infected with HIV-1 exhibit a variety of immunologic defects, the most devastating of which is a complete eventual loss of cellular immunity, which is progressive if not treated with appropiate HAART. As a result, catastrophic opportunistic infections are virtually inevitable if left untreated. The relentless progression of HIV infection is now recognized as a continuum that extends from an initial asymptomatic state to the immune depletion that characterizes patients with overt AIDS, and the continuum is often referred to as HIV/AIDS. The basic lesion is infection of $CD4^+$ (helper) T lymphocytes by HIV, which leads to depletion of this cell population and consequent impaired immune function and dysregulation. As a result, rather than dying of HIV infection itself, patients with AIDS usually die of opportunistic infections. There is also a high incidence of malignant tumors, principally B-cell lymphomas and Kaposi sarcoma. Finally, infection of the CNS with HIV often leads to an array of syndromes ranging from minor cognitive or motor neuron disorders to frank dementia.

EPIDEMIOLOGY: AIDS was first reported in the United States in 1981, with a report of *Pneumocystis carinii* pneumonia in homosexual men. The starting time for this human epidemic is uncertain: although antibodies to HIV have been found in stored blood from the Congo Republic dating to 1959, sporadic cases of diseases that can retrospectively be attributed to HIV certainly occurred in Africa during the 1960s. By the late 1970s, clusters of strange infectious diseases in New York and Miami among homosexual men, intravenous drug users, and Haitians are now recognized as having been secondary to HIV. By 1982, these unusual infections were associated with Kaposi sarcoma and considered to reflect an underlying immune deficiency. Thus, the acronym "AIDS" was coined. At the same time, it became clear that AIDS was spread by contact with blood of persons suspected of bearing an infectious agent. In addition to homosexual men and intravenous drug users who shared needles, persons at risk were identified among recipients of whole blood and blood products, especially hemophiliacs, heterosexual contacts, and infants born to female drug users. In 1983, the responsible virus, now called *HIV-1*, was identified. Development of a first-generation serologic test to detect antibodies to HIV-1 in 1985 permitted accurate diagnosis and allowed for improved public health measures. Thus, donations of blood and plasma have been screened for HIV-1 antibodies, and clotting factor concentrates used to treat hemophilia are processed to inactivate HIV.

Although AIDS is believed to have originated in sub-Saharan Africa, it is now a worldwide pandemic. The spread of HIV is attributable to the ease of international travel and enhanced population mobility, which in many societies have coincided with a rapid increase in sexual promiscuity and sexually transmitted diseases. Presently, over 40 million people are infected with HIV.

By the mid-1990s more than 1 million HIV-positive persons were reported in the United States. Originally, homosexual men represented two-thirds of these cases, and 30% were accounted for by intravenous drug users and their sexual partners. However, because of behavioral changes, the prevalence of infection among homosexuals has decreased. Men account for the majority of AIDS cases in the United States, although the prevalence in women continues to increase.

Inhabitants of sub-Saharan Africa suffer more from the ravages of AIDS than persons in other regions. Although accurate statistics from this area are not as readily available as in industrialized countries, in parts of sub-Saharan Africa it is estimated that 25% of the population is HIV-positive. The epidemiologic pattern differs from that in the United States, in that African patients rarely report homosexuality or intravenous drug use. The sex ratio for AIDS in Africa shows only a slight male predominance, pointing to a predominance of heterosexual spread of the infection.

Many cases of AIDS have been reported in western Europe. As in the United States, most have been in homosexual men, intravenous drug users and their sexual partners, and prostitutes. AIDS is being reported increasingly in Asia, and some countries on that continent (Thailand, India, and China) have described an exponential increase in the numbers of HIV infections.

HIV is Transmitted by Contact with Blood and Certain Body Fluids, and Through Sexual Activity

Save for intravenous drug users and transfusion recipients, AIDS is transmitted principally as a venereal disease, both homosexually and heterosexually. Transmission to newborns via breast milk is a concern in the developing world. Significant amounts of HIV have been isolated from blood, semen, vaginal secretions, breast milk, and cerebrospinal fluid. Except for the latter, HIV in these fluids is both present in lymphocytes and free virus.

Among homosexual men, the receptive partner in unprotected anal intercourse is at particularly high risk of becoming infected with HIV. The virus is transmitted from semen through tears in the rectal mucosa and it can infect epithelial cells of the rectum directly. In heterosexual contact, transmission from male to female is more likely than the reverse, perhaps reflecting the greater concentration of HIV in semen than in vaginal fluids. The risk of infecting a woman with HIV is evidenced by the demonstration that 8% to 50% of women artificially inseminated with semen from donors later shown to be HIV-positive became infected with the AIDS virus. Additionally, genital lesions, usually caused by other sexually transmitted diseases such as syphilis and human papilloma virus (HPV), facilitate entry of the virus and lead to a particularly high risk of contracting AIDS.

AIDS is not transmissible by nonsexual, casual exposure to infected persons. A particular concern of health care workers is the possibility of HIV infection from accidental exposure to the virus. In prospective studies of hundreds of health care workers who sustained "needle sticks" or other accidental exposures to blood from patients with AIDS, fewer than 1% actually seroconverted and became infected with HIV-1. Immediate postexposure prophalaxis with antiretroviral therapy is indicated in such accidental exposures, with the goal of preventing HIV-1 infection. (Specific recommendations are available online at the Centers for Disease Control and Prevention [CDC].)

The Etiologic Agent of AIDS is HIV-1

HIV-1 is an enveloped member of the retrovirus family, specifically the subfamily of lentiviruses. Animal lentiviruses have been recognized for a century, but human lentiviruses are known for less than 3 decades.

Two identical 9.7-kb single copies of the virus' RNA genome plus some key enzymes needed early in the infectious cycle (see below), such as reverse transcriptase (RNA-dependent DNA polymerase) and integrase, are enclosed within a core of viral proteins. This core is in turn enveloped by a phospholipid bilayer derived from the host cell membrane, in which are found virally encoded glycoproteins (gp120 and gp41). In addition to the *gag, pol,* and *env* genes characteristic of all replication-competent RNA viruses, HIV-1 contains six other genes that code for proteins involved in regulation of viral replication. Specific target cells for HIV-1 are $CD4^+$ helper T lymphocytes and mononuclear phagocytes, although infection of other cells can occur, such as in B lymphocytes, glial cells, and intestinal epithelial cells.

The replicative cycle of HIV-1 is depicted in Figure 4-24.

1. **Binding:** Free HIV or an infected lymphocyte can transmit the virus to an uninfected cell. The HIV envelope glycoprotein gp120, either on the free virus or on the surface of an infected cell, binds the CD4 molecule on the surface of helper T lymphocytes and other cells, as well as one of a family of β-chemokine receptors. The most important of these chemokine receptors are CXCR4 (on T lymphocytes) and CCR-5 (on many phagocytic cells). Binding of both receptors is necessary for HIV entry.

   About 1% of Caucasians are homozygous for major deletions in the CCR-5 gene and remain uninfected with HIV even with extensive exposure to the agent. Even heterozygosity for the mutant CCR-5 allele provides partial protection against HIV infection and if infection does occur they usually progress at a slower pace. Interestingly, the mutant allele is found in up to 20% of Caucasians but is absent in blacks and Asians. Some persons who have been multiply exposed to HIV-1 and who do not seroconvert and possibly some persons with long-term HIV infection who do not progress to AIDS have high levels of chemokines, which may block the coreceptors for HIV.

2. **Internalization:** The binding of gp120 allows gp41 to insert into the target cell's plasma membrane, leading to its fusion with the viral envelope and virus entry.
3. **DNA synthesis:** The virus uncoats in the cytoplasm, and its RNA is copied into double-stranded DNA—complementary DNA (cDNA)—by retroviral reverse transcriptase.
4. **Integration:** Virus cDNA integrates into the host genome using a viral integrase protein, generating the latent proviral form of HIV-1. Viral genes are replicated along with host chromosomes and therefore persist for the life of the cell. As memory T cells have a long life spans, some experts estimate that even if total suppression of HIV-1 replication were achieved, over 60 years would be needed for infected T cells to die off. Also, even with the most effective HAART regiments some replication occurs.
5. **Replication**: Viral RNA is reproduced by transcriptional activation of the integrated HIV provirus, a process that, e.g., for T cells, requires "activation" of the infected cell plus certain inducible host transcription factors.
6. **Dissemination**: To complete its cycle, nascent virus is assembled in the cytoplasm just beneath the cell membrane and disseminated to other target cells. This is accomplished either by fusion of an infected cell with an uninfected one or by the budding of virions from the plasma membrane of the infected cell (Fig. 4-25).

The mechanism by which HIV kills infected T lymphocytes is still incompletely understood. Potential mechanisms for depletion of $CD4^+$ lymphocytes include direct viral cytotoxicity, immune clearance of infected cells, and the actions of secondary mediators such as cytokines. Whatever the mechanism(s), there is a clear association between increasing viral burden and declining $CD4^+$ lymphocyte counts.

The long interval between HIV-1 entry and the appearance of clinical symptoms of AIDS is related to the small number of infected T lymphocytes and viral latency and, it is now becoming clear, extensive virus replication in the gut-associated lymphoid tissue (GALT), away from the circulation. During this asymptomatic period, only 0.01–0.001% of circulation T cells actively transcribe the HIV-1 genome, even though 1% contain integrated proviral DNA. Moreover, virus replication continues apace in the GALT, consuming certain $CD4^+$ T cell populations, particularly memory T cells. When this depletion eventually exceeds the body's ability to replenish these cells, systemic HIV-1 replication supervenes.

In latent infection, the virus can exist in three forms: untranscribed viral RNA in the cytoplasm of resting T cells; unintegrated, and thus untranscribed, viral DNA in the cytoplasm; and integrated proviral DNA, which may remain untranscribed in a resting T cell. The mechanisms underlying latency and conversion of latent to lytic infection are incompletely understood.

Initiation of viral replication in latent HIV-1 infection depends on induction of host proteins during T-cell activation. Viral transcription may be activated by many T-cell mitogens and cytokines produced by monocyte/macrophages, including TNF-α and IL-1, and in addition, by proteins produced by other viruses that infect patients with AIDS, such as herpesvirus, EBV, adenovirus, and CMV. Thus, immune system activation by a variety of infectious agents may promote HIV replication.

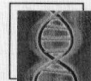

IMMUNOLOGY OF AIDS: The destruction of $CD4^+$ T cells by HIV-1 can essentially disable the entire immune system because this subset of lymphocytes exerts critical regulatory and effector functions that involve both cellular and humoral immunity. Thus, in typical AIDS patients all elements of the immune system are eventually perturbed, including T cells, B cells, NK cells, the monocyte/macrophages lineage of cells, and immunoglobulin production.

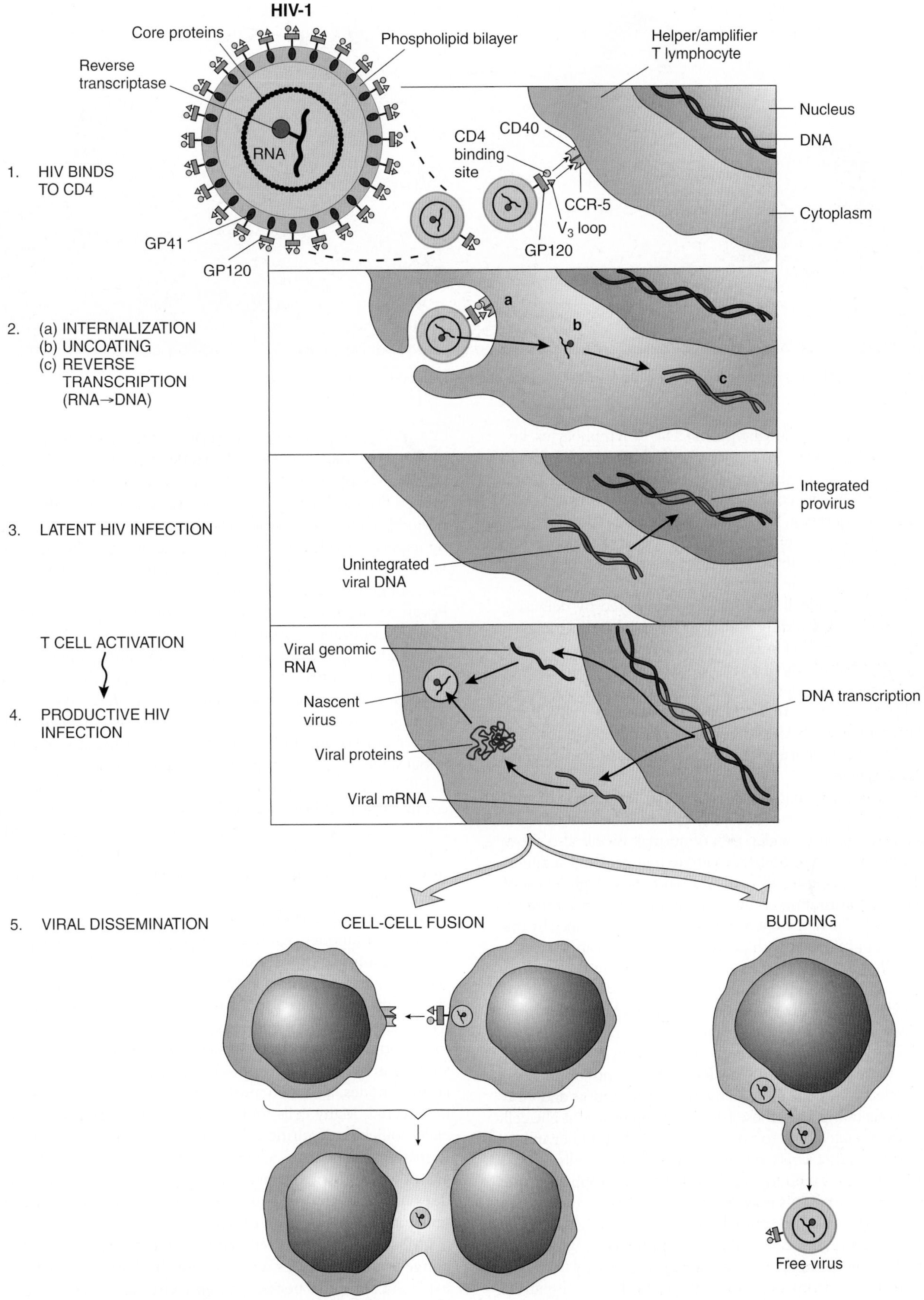

FIGURE 4-24. **The life cycle of human immunodeficiency virus -1 (HIV-1) is a multistep process.** mRNA = messenger RNA.

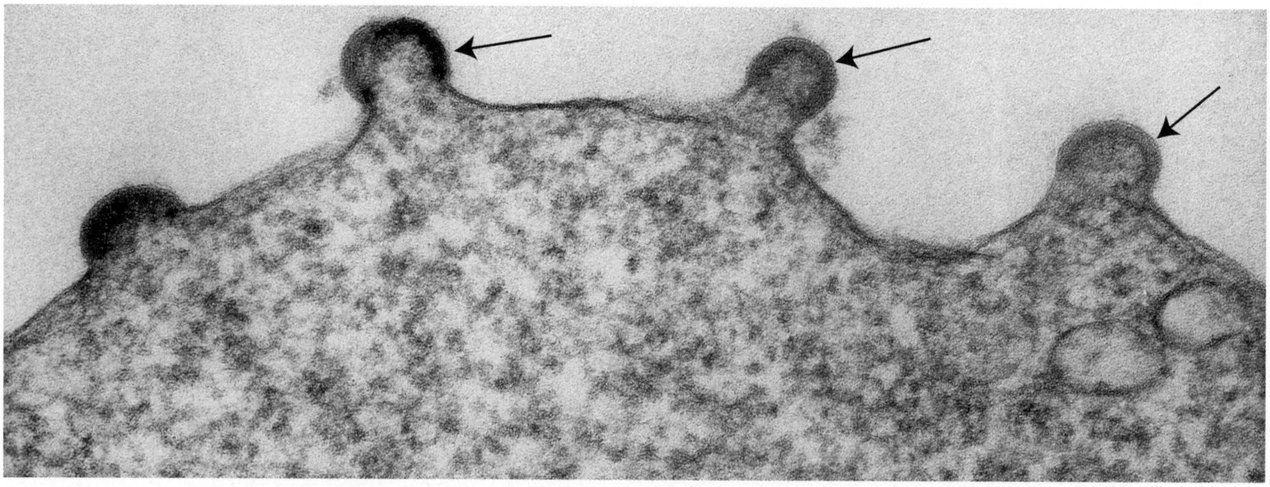

FIGURE 4-25. **Human immunodeficiency virus-1 (HIV-1) virions can be seen budding from an infected cells (*arrows*).**

Of the two functional types of $CD4^+$ T lymphocytes, i.e., helper and amplifier (or inducer) cells, those affected first in HIV infection are the amplifier subset. Eventually, total $CD4^+$ lymphocyte counts fall to less than 500 cells/μL, and helper-to-suppressor T-cell ratios decline from a normal of 2.0 to as little as 0.5. Numbers of $CD8^+$ (cytotoxic/suppressor) cells are variable, although in AIDS, most of these cells seem to be of the cytotoxic variety.

Defects in T-cell function are manifested by defective responses to skin testing with a variety of antigens (delayed hypersensitivity) and impaired proliferative responses to mitogens and antigens in vitro. Moreover, the deficiency of $CD4^+$ cells reduces levels of IL-2, the cytokine produced in response to antigens that stimulate cytotoxic T cell killing. Thus, patients with AIDS cannot generate the antigen-specific cytotoxic T cells that are required to clear viruses and other infectious agents.

Humoral immunity is also abnormal. Production of antibodies in response to specific antigenic stimulation is markedly decreased, often to under 10% of normal. B cells also show poor proliferative responses in vitro to mitogens and antigens. Yet, sera of patients with AIDS usually show high levels of polyclonal immunoglobulins, autoantibodies, and immune complexes. This apparent paradox is probably explained by the concurrent infection with polyclonal B cell-activating viruses (e.g., EBV or CMV) which constantly stimulate B cells nonspecifically to produce immunoglobulins. Lack of $CD4^+$ lymphocytes impairs the cytotoxic T cell proliferation that normally would eliminate B cells infected with EBV.

NK cell activity is severely decreased in AIDS as well. Since these cells kill both virus-infected cells and tumor cells, this defect may contribute to the malignant tumors and viral infections that plague these patients. Suppression of NK cell activity is related both to a decrease in NK cell number and to reduction in IL-2 levels, owing to a loss of $CD4^+$ cells.

Lentiviruses tend to target monocyte/macrophages, and infected macrophages may serve as reservoirs for dissemination of the virus. Interestingly, some macrophages express CD4 on their surfaces. Unlike T lymphocytes, which are killed by HIV, infected macrophages generally survive. Macrophages from patients with AIDS display impaired phagocytosis of immune complexes and opsonized particles, decreased chemotaxis, and impaired responses to antigenic challenges.

PATHOLOGY AND CLINICAL FEATURES OF AIDS: Patients recently infected with HIV-1 may have an acute, usually self-limited flu-like illness called the **acute retroviral syndrome** that resembles infectious mononucleosis. This occurs 2 to 3 weeks after exposure to HIV, before appearance of antibodies against the virus. Less commonly, they present with neurologic symptoms that suggest encephalitis, aseptic meningitis, or a neuropathy. Fever, myalgia, lymphadenopathy, sore throat, and a macular rash are common. Most of these symptoms resolve within 2 to 3 weeks, although lymphadenopathy, fever, and myalgia may persist for a few months. Seroconversion occurs 1 to 10 weeks after the onset of this acute illness. Thus the standard HIV-1 enzyme immunoassay (EIA) and Western Blot testing, which depends on the presence of anti-HIV-1 *gag* antibodies, is negative during the initial stage of the infection. Most patients recover from this initial illness as their immune system mounts a cytotoxic T-cell counterattack, although a small percentage progress rapidely to frank AIDS within a few months. After the initial acute syndrome, most newly infected individuals enter a period of latency and slow immune system decline that averages approximately ten years before they reach a state of serious immune compromise. If unrecognized or untreated, the outcome will eventually be fulminant immunodeficiency and its fatal complications (Fig. 4-26).

Persistent generalized lymphadenopathy is palpable lymph node enlargement at two or more extrainguinal sites, persisting for more than 3 months in a person infected with HIV. The disorder develops either as part of the acute HIV syndrome or within a few months of seroconversion. The most common sites of involvement are the axillary, inguinal, and posterior cervical nodes, although almost any group of lymph nodes can be affected. Many cells within the affected lymph nodes, especially follicular dendritic cells, harbor actively replicating virus. Biopsy reveals reactive changes with follicular hyperplasia, but are not diagnostic. Persistent generalized lymphadenopathy does not have any prognostic significance with respect to progression of HIV infection to AIDS.

Most patients infected with HIV express detectable viral antigens and antibodies within 6 months. Patients will generally experience an initial period of intense viremia with very high viral loads during the acute retroviral syndrome with a corresponding sharp drop in their absolute number of $CD4^+$ T cells. As a patient's immune system begins to recognize the new infection,

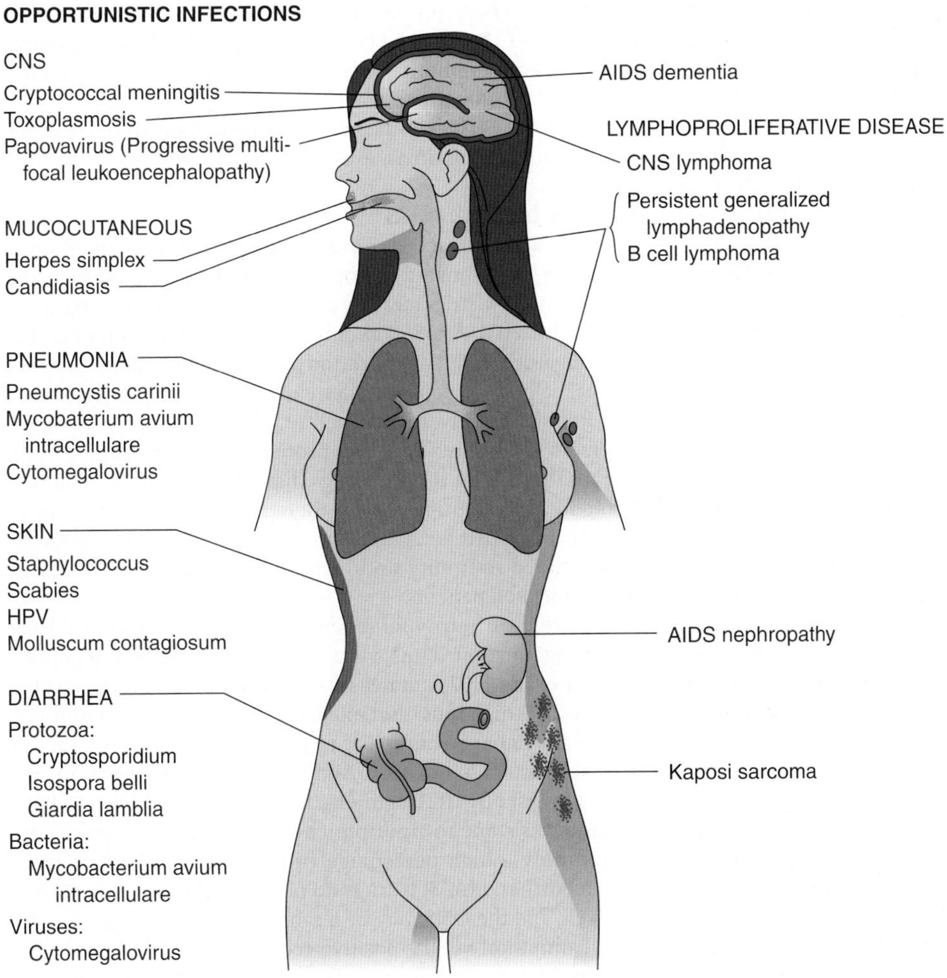

FIGURE 4-26. **Human immunodeficiency virus-1 (HIV-1)–mediated destruction of the cellular immune system results in acquired immunodeficiency syndrome (AIDS).** The infectious and neoplastic complications of AIDS can affect practically every organ system. CNS = central nervous system; HPV = human papilloma virus.

viral load drops and $CD4^+$ T cell count begins to climb. This control of HIV-1 infection occurs via a vigorous cytotoxic T cell response. Viral replication continues but is constrained by the immune response. The immune system and the HIV-1 load eventually enter into a sort of uneasy equilibrium, during which the HIV-1 viral RNA load stays fairly constant at the "viral set point." During this time infected persons are generally asymptomatic. However, virus replication virtually always begins to increase. At some time the number of $CD4^+$ T cells starts to decrease. Patients generally remain asymptomatic until the $CD4^+$ lymphocyte count falls below 500/μL. Then, nonspecific constitutional symptoms may appear, along with opportunistic infections. As $CD4^+$ T cells fall below 350/mL, patients become much more susceptable to primary or reactivation *Mycobacterium tuberculosis,* which may progress rapidly to severe disease or death. Once $CD4^+$ levels are under 150/μL and CD4:CD8 ratios less than 0.8, the disease progresses rapidly. A variety of bacteria, viruses, fungi, and protozoa attack the immunocompromised patient. Kaposi sarcoma and lymphoproliferative disorders may appear, and neurologic disease is common.

Symptoms of CNS dysfunction occur in one-third of AIDS patients and postmortem studies of patients who have died of AIDS reveal CNS pathology in more than three-fourths of the case. HIV is thought to enter the brain via infected blood monocytes and then to reside there in glial cells. Although HIV infection of neurons is not common, HIV gene products cause neuron apoptosis via several mechanisms.

Discussion of the diversity of infectious agents that ravage patients with AIDS is beyond the scope of this chapter, and only a few representative examples are mentioned. It is important to recognize that while most non-immunocompromised patients will have only one infection at a time, HIV-1-infected patients can develop multiple severe infections simultaneously.

Opportunistic Infections, Particularly Polymicrobial Infections are Common in Patients With AIDS

The majority of patients with HIV-1/AIDS suffer from opportunistic pulmonary infections, although this has been greatly reduced through the use of prophylatic antibiotics. *Pneumocystis jiroveci* (formerly *P. carinii*) pneumonia may occur in patients with advanced HIV-1 disease. Lung infection with CMV and *Mycobacterium avium-intracellulare* are less common. Patients with AIDS are also susceptible to *Legionella* infections.

Diarrhea occurs in over 75% of patients, often representing simultaneous infections with more than one organism. The most frequent pathogens are protozoans, including *Cryptosporidium, Isospora belli,* and *Giardia lamblia. M. avium-intracellulare* and *Salmonella* species are the most common bacterial causes of diarrhea in AIDS patients. CMV infection of the gastrointestinal tract can manifest as a colitis associated with watery diarrhea in patients whose CD4 counts are under 50 cells/mm^3.

Cryptococcal meningitis is a devastating complication, and represents 5% to 8% of all opportunistic infections in patients with AIDS. CNS complications include cerebral toxoplasmosis; primary CNS lymphoma; encephalitis caused by herpes siimplex, varicella, or CMV; and progressive multifocal leukoencephalopathy, which is caused by the JC virus

Virtually all patients with AIDS develop some form of skin disease, infections being the most prominent. *Staphylococcus aureus* is the most common, causing bullous impetigo, deeper purulent lesions (ecthyma) and folliculitis. Many of these *S. aureus* isolates carry virulence factors such as the Pantine Valentine leukocidin, which may increase the risk of bacterial invasion and severe disease. Chronic mucocutaneous herpes simplex infection is so characteristic of AIDS that it is considered an index infection in establishing the diagnosis. Skin lesions produced by *Molluscum contagiosum* and HPV are also common, as are scabies and infections with *Candida* species. A varicella zoster outbreak in someone under the age of 50 should raise the question of a possible occult HIV-1 infection.

Among the most common causes of death in patients with HIV/AIDS is hepatitis C virus (HCV) infection (see Chapter 14). In some studies, over a quarter of deaths among HIV-positive individuals are from hepatitis C. A very high percentage of HIV-positive intravenous drug abusers are also infected with HCV. There is evidence suggesting that coinfection with HIV and HCV accelerates the course of disease with both viruses.

Kaposi sarcoma (KS) is an otherwise rare, multicentric, malignant neoplasm. It is characterized by cutaneous and (less commonly) visceral nodules, in which endothelium-lined channels and vascular spaces are admixed with spindle-shaped cells (see Chapter 24). Patients with AIDS, especially homosexual men rather than intravenous drug users, are at very high risk for KS. In fact, occurrence of KS in an otherwise healthy person under 60 years is strong evidence of AIDS. Unlike the classic indolent variety of KS, the tumor in AIDS is usually aggressive, often involving viscera such as the gastrointestinal tract or lungs. Lung involvement frequently leads to death.

A strain of herpesvirus—human herpes virus 8 (HHV8)—is implicated in all forms of KS, including that associated with AIDS. HHV8 is also thought to be the cause of a peculiar lymphoma associated with AIDS (**primary effusion lymphoma**) and of **AIDS-associated Castleman disease**. The virus has been detected in both KS spindle cells and endothelial cells. The finding of HHV8 in the blood strongly predicts later development of KS. In fact, 75% of HIV-infected persons with HHV8 in the blood developed KS within 5 years. It is thought that HHV8 is sexually transmitted, as almost all homosexual HIV carriers are infected, but only a quarter of heterosexual drug users with HIV infection harbor HHV8.

B cell lymphoproliferative diseases are common in patients with AIDS. Congenital and acquired immunodeficiency states are associated with B-cell hyperplasia, usually manifested as generalized lymphadenopathy. This lymphoproliferative syndrome may be followed by appearance of high-grade B-cell lymphomas. In fact, patients who have been subjected to immunosuppressive therapy for renal transplants are at a 35-times-greater risk of developing lymphoma, and in one third of these cases the disease is confined to the CNS. The lymphomas in chronically immunodeficient patients may manifest as an invasive polyclonal B-cell proliferation or as a monoclonal B-cell lymphoma. Many patients exhibit serologic evidence of infection with EBV and the EBV genome has been demonstrated in the lymphoma cells.

B-cell hyperplasia and generalized lymphadenopathy precede malignant lymphoproliferative disease. HIV-associated lymphomas are usually the large cell variety, as in other immunodeficiency conditions, although small cell lymphomas are ometimes seen. A conspicuous feature of lymphomas associated with AIDS is their predilection for extranodal disease, particularly primary lymphomas of the brain. In addition, lymphomas of the gastrointestinal tract, liver, and bone marrow are frequent. The EBV genome has also been demonstrated in many AIDS-related lymphomas, especially in the CNS

Therapy for HIV/AIDS

HIV infection represents a novel challenge in treatment. Human lentivirus infections have not been therapeutic targets in the past. Thus, new strategies have had to be developed to treat patients with HIV/AIDS. Therapy focuses on HIV proteins that are obligatory for HIV replication and sufficiently different from normal cellular proteins to offer clear targets for pharmacotherapy. Initial agents were designed to inhibit the function of HIV reverse transcriptase (RT) and protease (PR). Combining compounds that inhibit RT and drugs that inhibit PR is the mainstay of highly active anti-retroviral therapy (HAART) today. Introduction of HAART revolutionized AIDS treatment, reducing AIDS-related mortality and increasing all indices of health in HIV-1–infected patients.

Unlike most retroviral reverse transcriptases, HIV RT lacks an editing function. Thus, virus genome replication is highly error-prone, and HIV mutates much more often than most other viruses. This high mutation rate facilitates avoidance of immune attack, and enhances its ability to generate functional mutations that are resistent to HAART. Although combining three or more drugs in most HAART regimens depresses viral replication, HIV mutants resistant to multiple chemotherapeutic agents contribute now a high percentage of HIV isolates in the United States. Further, HAART drugs do not cross the blood–brain barrier well, and the CNS may be a sanctuary for the virus.

Quantitation of HIV-positive cells in the body has led to the conclusion that eradication of the virus from the body is not a realistic expectation with the types of chemotherapy currently available. Even HAART patient with no detectable blood HIV-1 continue to deplete their memory $CD4^+$ T cells. Finally, although HAART may eliminate HIV positive cells from the blood, even temporary cessation of therapy leads to rebound, i.e., reactivation of HIV from reservoirs outside the circulation and subsequent viral rebound.

HIV-2 Causes a Clinical Syndrome Similar to that Caused by HIV-1

In 1985, otherwise healthy prostitutes in Senegal were discovered to harbor antibodies that cross-reacted with a monkey retrovirus, now termed *simian immunodeficiency virus* (SIV). A year later, a retrovirus similar to HIV-1 was isolated from West African patients with AIDS who were negative for antibodies against HIV-1. Antibodies to this new retrovirus, now termed *HIV-2,* also cross-reacted with SIV antigens. Frozen sera from West Africa dating to the 1960s have been shown to contain antibodies to HIV-2. In Guinea-Bissau, infection with HIV-2 has been shown in 8% of pregnant women, 10% of male blood donors, and more than one third of prostitutes. The infection has now also been reported from other parts of Africa, Europe, and the United States.

HIV-2 is morphologically similar to HIV-1, and the immunodeficiency state associated with HIV-2 infection is indistinguishable from AIDS caused by HIV-1. The risk factors for infection in both diseases seem to be similar. However, HIV-2 is more difficult to transmit than HIV-1, and persons infected with the former progress at a slower rate to AIDS.

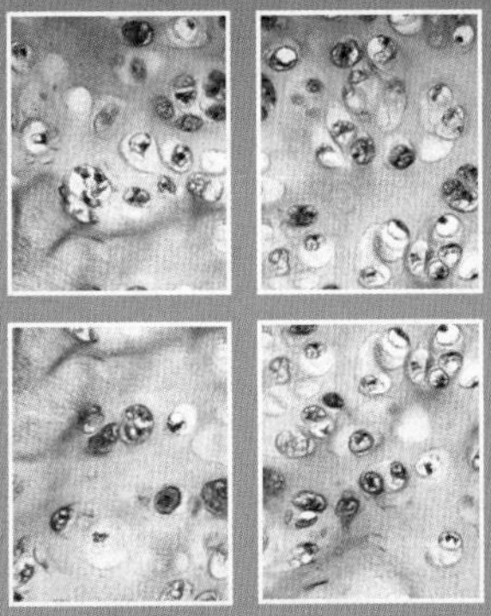

5 Neoplasia

Antonio Giordano
Giulia De Falco
Emanuel Rubin
Raphael Rubin

A **neoplasm** (Greek, *neo,* new + *plasma,* thing formed) is the autonomous growth of tissues that have escaped normal restraints on cell proliferation and exhibit varying degrees of fidelity to their precursors. However, in some instances, for example follicular lymphoma (see Chapter 20), the accumulation of neoplastic cells reflects an aberration in programmed cell death (apoptosis). The structural resemblance of the neoplastic cell to its cell of origin usually enables specific conclusions about its source and potential behavior. In view of their space-occupying properties, solid neoplasms are termed **tumors** (Gr., *swelling*). Tumors that remain localized are considered **benign**, whereas those that spread to distant sites are termed **malignant,** or **cancer.** The neoplastic process entails not only cellular proliferation but also a modification of the differentiation of the involved cell types. Thus, in a sense, cancer may be viewed as a burlesque of normal development.

Cancer is an ancient disease. Evidence of bone tumors has been found in prehistoric remains, and the disease is mentioned in early writings from India, Egypt, Babylonia, and Greece. Hippocrates is reported to have distinguished benign from malignant growths. He also introduced the term *karkinos,* from which our term **carcinoma** is derived. In particular, Hippocrates described cancer of the breast, and in the 2nd century AD, Paul of Aegina commented on its frequency.

The incidence of neoplastic disease increases with age, and greater longevity in modern times necessarily enlarges the population at risk. For this reason alone, the overall incidence of cancer is increasing. In previous generations, on average, humans did not live long enough to develop many cancers that are particularly common in middle and old age, such as those of the prostate, colon, pancreas, and kidney. Despite assertions that contemporary society is or will be subject to an "epidemic" of cancer, the epidemiologic data do not support such a concept. If all deaths from cancers caused by tobacco smoke are removed from the statistics, there has been no increase in the overall age-adjusted cancer death rate in men in the past half-century, and there has been a continually decreasing rate in women. However, the age-adjusted incidence of specific cancers has fluctuated over this time period.

In general, neoplasms are irreversible, and their growth is, for the most part, autonomous. Several observations are important:

- Neoplasms are derived from cells that normally maintain a proliferative capacity. Thus, mature neurons and cardiac myocytes do not give rise to tumors.
- A tumor may express varying degrees of differentiation, from relatively mature structures that mimic normal tissues to a collection of cells so primitive that the cell of origin cannot be identified.
- The stimulus responsible for the uncontrolled proliferation may not be identifiable; in fact, it is not known for most human neoplasms.
- Neoplasia arises from mutations in genes that regulate cell growth, apoptosis, or DNA repair.

Benign versus Malignant Tumors

By definition, benign tumors do not penetrate (invade) adjacent tissue borders, nor do they spread (metastasize) to distant sites. They remain as localized overgrowths in the area in which they arise. As a rule, benign tumors are more differentiated than malignant ones—that is, they more closely resemble their tissue of origin. *By contrast, malignant tumors, or cancers, have the added property of invading contiguous tissues and metastasizing to distant sites, where subpopulations of malignant cells take up residence, grow anew, and again invade.*

In common usage, the terms **benign** and **malignant** refer to the overall biological behavior of a tumor rather than to its morphologic characteristics. In most circumstances, malignant tumors kill, whereas benign ones spare the host. However, so-called benign tumors in critical locations can be deadly. For example, a benign intracranial tumor of the meninges (meningioma) can kill by exerting pressure on the brain. A minute benign tumor of the ependymal cells of the third ventricle (ependymoma) can block the circulation of cerebrospinal fluid, resulting in lethal hydrocephalus. A benign mesenchymal tumor of the left atrium (myxoma) may kill suddenly by blocking the mitral valve orifice. In certain locations, the erosion of a benign tumor of smooth muscle can lead to serious hemorrhage—witness the peptic ulceration of a stromal tumor in the gastric wall. On rare occasions, a functioning, benign endocrine adenoma can be life-threatening, as in the case of the sudden hypoglycemia associated with an insulinoma of the pancreas or the hypertensive crisis produced by a pheochromocytoma of the adrenal medulla. Conversely, certain types of malignant tumors are so indolent that they are curable by surgical resection. In this category are many cancers of breast, and some malignant tumors of connective tissue (e.g., fibrosarcoma).

A number of tumors are difficult to classify because they do not fit all the criteria for either benign or malignant neoplasms. The best-known example is basal cell carcinoma of the skin, which is histologically malignant (i.e., it invades aggressively) but only rarely has been reported to metastasize to distant sites. Similarly, the local growth of a pleomorphic adenoma of a salivary gland, which is classified as benign, may be so aggressive that it defies surgical cure.

Classification of Neoplasms

In any language, the classification of objects and concepts is pragmatic and useful only insofar as its general acceptance permits effective communication. Similarly, the nosology of tumors reflects historical concepts, technical jargon, location, origin, descriptive modifiers, and predictors of biological behavior. Although the language of tumor classification is neither rigidly logical nor consistent, it still serves as a reasonable mode of communication.

Benign Tumors Carry the Suffix "oma"

The primary descriptor of any tumor, benign or malignant, is its cell or tissue of origin. The classification of benign tumors is the basis for the names of their malignant variants. *The suffix "oma" for benign tumors is preceded by reference to the cell or tissue of origin.* For example, a benign tumor that resembles chondrocytes is called a **chondroma** (Fig. 5-1). If the tumor resembles the precursor of the chondrocyte, it is labeled **chondroblastoma.** When a chondroma is located entirely within the bone, it is designated **enchondroma.**

Tumors of epithelial origin are given a variety of names based on what is believed to be their outstanding characteristic. Thus, a benign tumor of the squamous epithelium may be called simply **epithelioma** or, when branched and exophytic, may be termed **papilloma**. Benign tumors arising from glandular epithelium, such as in the colon or the endocrine glands, are named

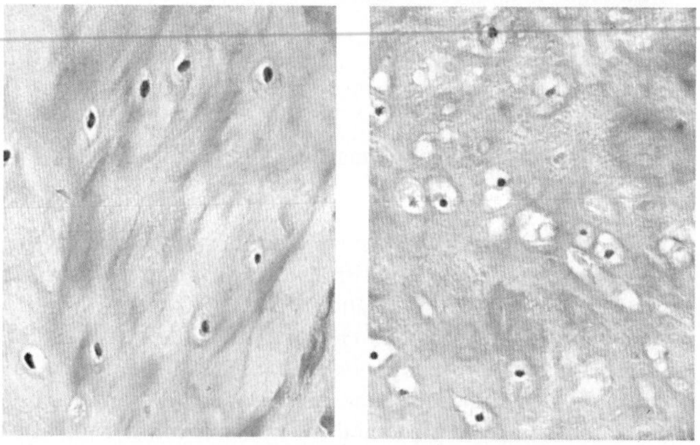

FIGURE 5-1. **Benign chondroma. A.** Normal cartilage. **B.** A benign chondroma closely resembles normal cartilage.

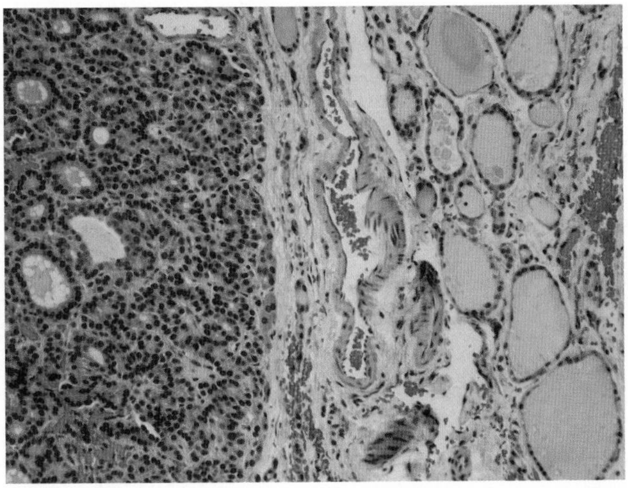

FIGURE 5-2. **Benign thyroid adenoma.** The follicles of a thyroid adenoma *(left)* contain colloid and resemble those of the normal thyroid tissue *(right)*.

adenoma. Accordingly, we refer to a **thyroid adenoma** (Fig. 5-2) or a **pancreatic islet cell adenoma.** In some instances, the predominating feature is the gross appearance, in which case we speak, for example, of an **adenomatous polyp** of the colon.

Benign tumors that arise from germ cells and contain derivatives of different germ layers are labeled **teratoma**. These tumors occur principally in the gonads and occasionally in the mediastinum and may contain a variety of structures, such as skin, neurons and glial cells, thyroid, intestinal epithelium, and cartilage. Localized, disordered differentiation during embryonic development results in a **hamartoma**, a disorganized caricature of normal tissue components (Fig. 5-3). Such tumors, which are not strictly neoplasms, contain varying combinations of cartilage, ducts or bronchi, connective tissue, blood vessels, and lymphoid tissue. Ectopic islands of normal tissue, called **choristoma**, may also be mistaken for true neoplasms. These small lesions are represented by pancreatic tissue in the wall of the stomach or intestine, adrenal rests under the renal capsule, and nodules of splenic tissue in the peritoneal cavity. Certain benign growths, recognized clinically as tumors, are not truly neoplastic but rather represent overgrowth of normal tissue elements. Examples are vocal cord polyps, skin tags, and hyperplastic polyps of the colon.

Malignant Tumors Are Mostly Carcinomas or Sarcomas

*In general, the malignant counterparts of benign tumors usually carry the same name, except that the suffix "**carcinoma**" is applied to epithelial cancers and "**sarcoma**" to those of mesenchymal origin.* For instance, a malignant tumor of the stomach is a **gastric adenocarcinoma** or **adenocarcinoma of the stomach** (Fig. 5-4). **Squamous cell carcinoma** is an invasive tumor of the skin or other organs lined by a squamous epithelium (e.g., the esophagus). In addition, squamous cell carcinoma arises in the metaplastic squamous epithelium of the bronchus or endocervix. **Transitional cell carcinoma** is a malignant neoplasm of the bladder or ureters. By contrast, we speak of **chondrosarcoma** (Fig. 5-5) or **fibrosarcoma.** Sometimes the name of the tumor suggests the tissue type of origin, as in **osteogenic sarcoma** or **bronchogenic carcinoma.** Some tumors display neoplastic elements of different cell types but are not germ cell tumors. For example, **fibroadenoma** of the breast, composed of epithelial and stromal elements, is benign, whereas, as the name implies, **adenosquamous carcinoma** of the uterus or the lung is malignant. A rare malignant tumor that contains intermingled carcinomatous and sarcomatous elements is known as **carcinosarcoma.**

The persistence of certain historical terms adds a note of confusion. **Hepatoma** of the liver, **melanoma** of the skin, **seminoma** of the testis, and the lymphoproliferative tumor, **lymphoma,** are all highly malignant. Tumors of the hematopoietic system are a special case in which the relationship to the blood is

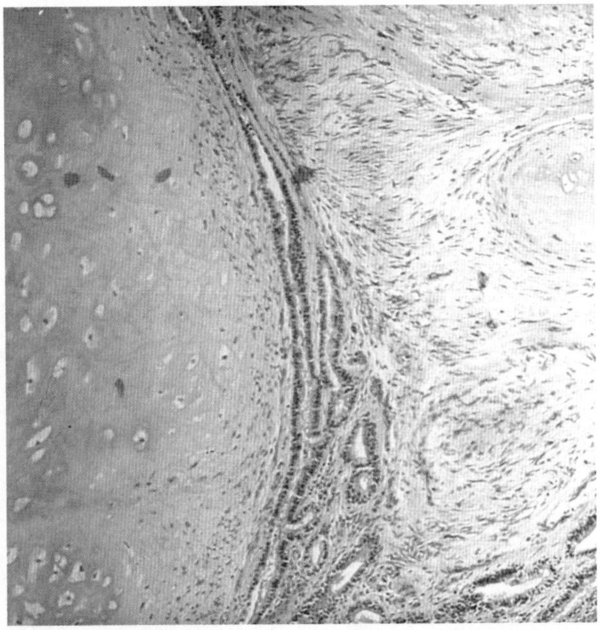

FIGURE 5-3. **Hamartoma of the lung.** The tumor contains islands of hyaline cartilage and clefts lined by cuboidal epithelium embedded in a fibromuscular stroma.

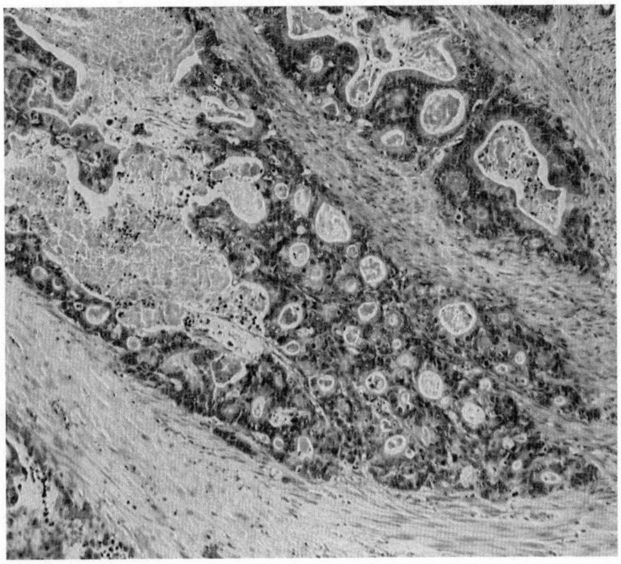

FIGURE 5-4. **Adenocarcinoma of the stomach.** Irregular neoplastic glands infiltrate the gastric wall.

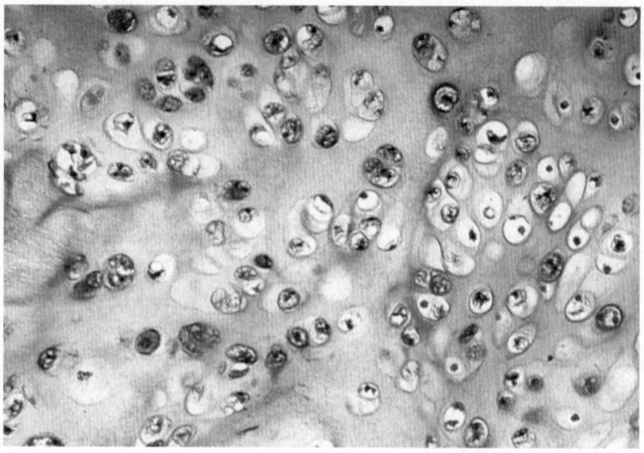

FIGURE 5-5. **Chondrosarcoma of bone.** The tumor is composed of malignant chondrocytes, which have bizarre shapes and irregular hyperchromatic nuclei, embedded in a cartilaginous matrix. Compare with Figure 5-1.

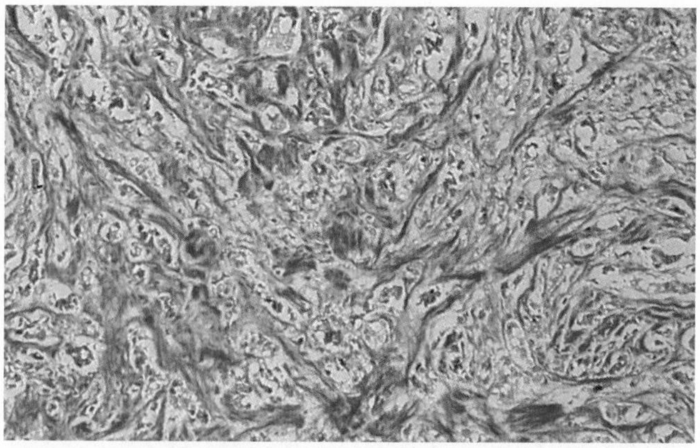

FIGURE 5-7. **Scirrhous adenocarcinoma of the breast.** A trichrome stain shows nests of cancer cells *(red)* embedded in a dense fibrous stroma *(blue)*.

indicated by the suffix "emia." Thus, **leukemia** refers to a malignant proliferation of leukocytes.

Secondary descriptors (again, with some inconsistencies) refer to a tumor's morphologic and functional characteristics. For example, the term **papillary** describes a frondlike structure (Fig. 5-6). **Medullary** signifies a soft, cellular tumor with little connective tissue stroma, whereas **scirrhous** or **desmoplastic** implies a dense fibrous stroma (Fig. 5-7). **Colloid** carcinomas secrete abundant mucus, in which float islands of tumor cells. **Comedocarcinoma** is an intraductal neoplasm in which necrotic material can be expressed from the ducts. Certain visible secretions of the tumor cells lend their characteristics to the classification—for example, production of mucin or serous fluid. A further designation describes the gross appearance of a cystic mass. From all these considerations we derive such common terms as **papillary serous cystadenocarcinoma** of the ovary, **comedocarcinoma** of the breast, **adenoid cystic carcinoma** of the salivary glands, **polypoid adenocarcinoma** of the stomach, and **medullary carcinoma** of the thyroid. Finally, tumors in which the histogenesis is poorly understood are often given an eponym—for example, Hodgkin disease, Ewing sarcoma of bone, or Brenner tumor of the ovary.

Histologic Diagnosis of Malignancy

There are no reliable molecular indicators of malignancy, and the "gold standard" for diagnosis of cancer remains routine microscopy. The distinction between benign and malignant tumors is, from a practical point of view, the most important diagnostic challenge faced by the pathologist. In most cases, the differentiation poses few problems; in a few, careful study is required before an accurate diagnosis is secure. However, there remain tumors that defy the diagnostic skills and experience of any pathologist; in these cases, the correct diagnosis must await the clinical outcome. In effect, the criteria used to assess the true biological nature of any tumor are based not on scientific principles but rather on a historical correlation of histologic and cytologic patterns with clinical outcomes. Although general criteria for malignancy are recognized, they must be used with caution in specific cases. For example, a reactive proliferation of connective cells termed **nodular fasciitis** (Fig. 5-8) has a more alarming histologic appearance than many fibrosarcomas, and misdiagnosis can lead to unnecessary surgery. Conversely, many well-differentiated endocrine adenocarcinomas are histologically indistinguishable from benign adenomas.

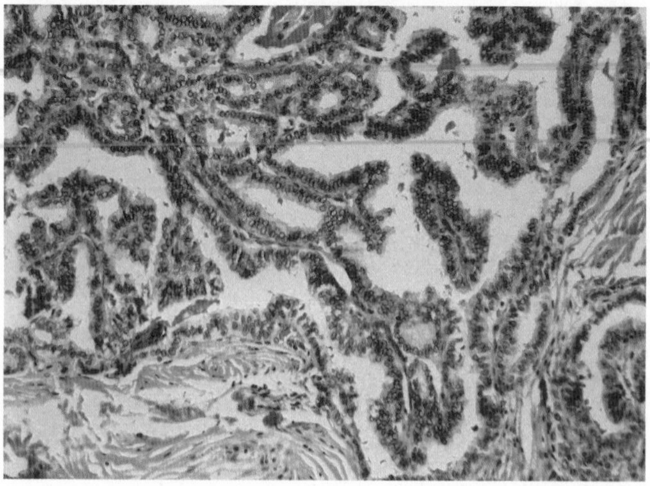

FIGURE 5-6. **Papillary adenocarcinoma of the thyroid.** The tumor exhibits numerous fronds lined by malignant epithelial cells.

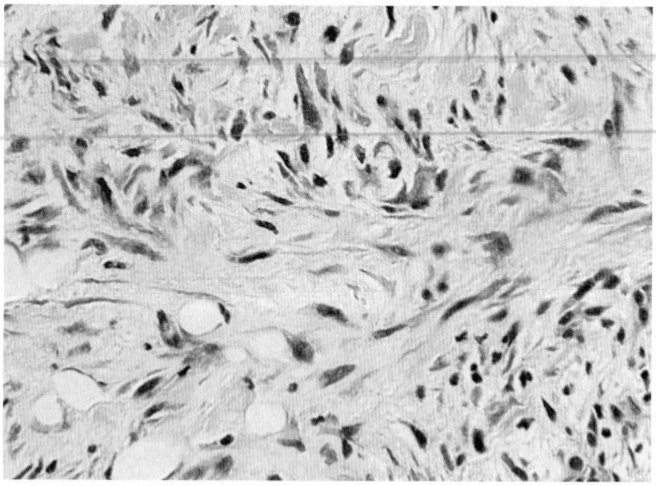

FIGURE 5-8. **Nodular fasciitis.** This cellular reactive lesion contains atypical and bizarre fibroblasts, which may be mistaken for a fibrosarcoma.

Benign Tumors Resemble Their Parent Tissue

Benign tumors tend to be histologically and cytologically similar to their tissues of origin. For example, **lipomas,** despite their often lobulated gross appearance, seem to be composed of normal adipocytes (Fig. 5-9). **Fibromas** are composed of mature fibroblasts and a collagenous stroma. **Chondromas** exhibit chondrocytes dispersed in a cartilaginous matrix. **Thyroid adenomas** form acini and produce thyroglobulin. The gross structure of a benign tumor may depart from the normal and assume papillary or polypoid configurations, as in papillomas of the bladder and skin and adenomatous polyps of the colon. *However, the lining epithelium of a benign tumor resembles that of the normal tissue.* Although many benign tumors are circumscribed by a connective tissue capsule, many equally benign neoplasms are not encapsulated. Unencapsulated benign tumors include papillomas and polyps of the visceral organs, hepatic adenomas, many endocrine adenomas, and hemangiomas. *Remember that the definition of a benign tumor resides above all in its inability to invade adjacent tissue and to metastasize.*

Malignant Tumors Depart from the Parent Tissue Morphologically and Functionally

Despite the histologic divergence of malignant tumors from their tissue of origin, an accurate identification of their source depends not only on the location but also on a morphologic resemblance to a normal tissue. Some of the histologic features that favor malignancy include the following:

- **Anaplasia or cellular atypia:** These terms refer to the lack of differentiated features in a cancer cell. In general, the degree of anaplasia correlates with the aggressiveness of the tumor. Cytologic evidence of anaplasia includes (1) variation in the size and shape of cells and cell nuclei (**pleomorphism**); (2) enlarged and hyperchromatic nuclei with coarsely clumped chromatin and prominent nucleoli; (3) atypical mitoses; and (4) bizarre cells, including tumor giant cells (Fig. 5-10). Many of these features are preceded by a preneoplastic dysplastic epithelium, which may lead to carcinoma in situ (see Chapter 1).

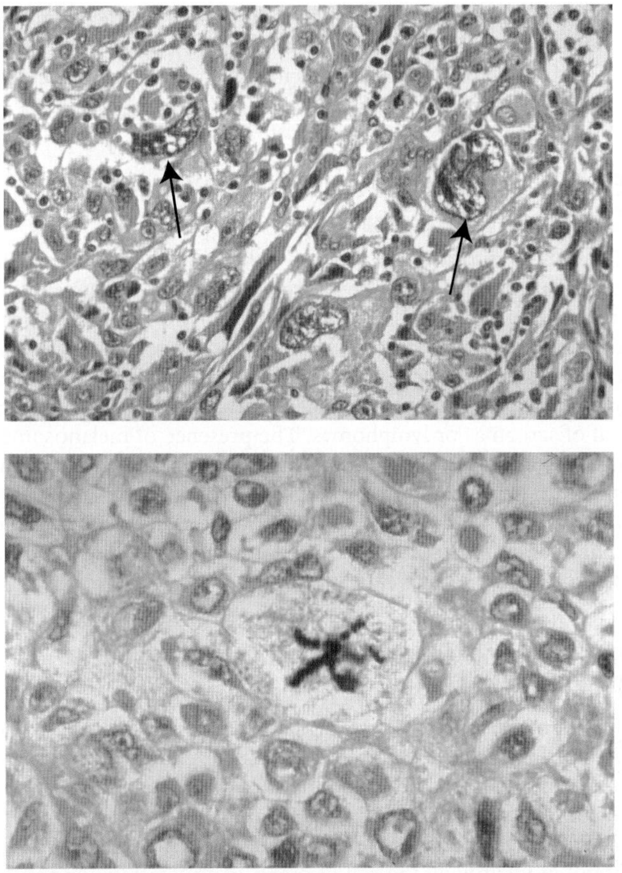

FIGURE 5-10. **Anaplastic features of malignant tumors. A.** The cells of this anaplastic carcinoma are highly pleomorphic (i.e., they vary in size and shape). The nuclei are hyperchromatic and are large relative to the cytoplasm. Multinucleated tumor giant cells are present (*arrows*). **B.** A malignant cell in metaphase exhibits an abnormal mitotic figure.

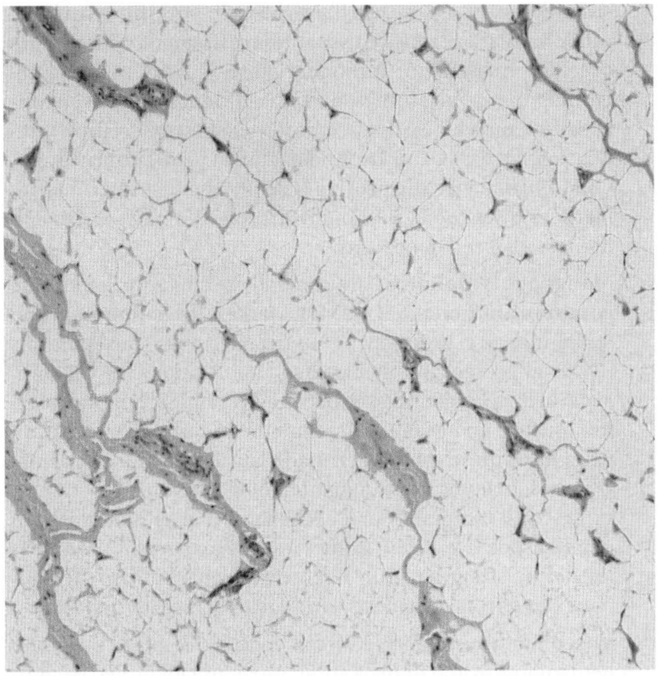

FIGURE 5-9. **Lipoma.** This subcutaneous, nodular tumor of adipocytes is grossly and microscopically indistinguishable from normal fat.

- **Mitotic activity:** Abundant mitoses are characteristic of many malignant tumors but are not a necessary criterion. However, in some cases (e.g., leiomyosarcomas), the diagnosis of malignancy is based on the finding of even a few mitoses.
- **Growth pattern:** In common with many benign tumors, malignant neoplasms often exhibit a disorganized and random growth pattern, which may be expressed as uniform sheets of cells, arrangements around blood vessels, papillary structures, whorls, rosettes, and so forth. Malignant tumors often outgrow their blood supply and display ischemic necrosis.
- **Invasion:** Malignancy is proved by the demonstration of invasion, particularly of blood vessels and lymphatics. In some circumstances (e.g., squamous carcinoma of the cervix or carcinoma arising in an adenomatous polyp), the diagnosis of malignant transformation is made on the basis of local invasion.
- **Metastases:** The presence of metastases identifies a tumor as malignant. In metastatic disease that was not preceded by a clinically diagnosed primary tumor, the site of origin is often

not readily apparent from the morphologic characteristics of the tumor. In such cases, electron microscopic examination and the demonstration of specific tumor markers may establish the correct origin.

Electron Microscopy of Undifferentiated Tumors May Identify the Source

There are no specific determinants of malignancy or even of neoplasia itself that can be detected by electron microscopy. However, this technique may aid in the diagnosis of poorly differentiated cancers, whose classification is problematic by routine light microscopy. For example, carcinomas often exhibit desmosomes and specialized junctional complexes, structures that are not typical of sarcomas or lymphomas. The presence of melanosomes signifies a melanoma, whereas small, membrane-bound granules with dense cores are features of endocrine neoplasms (Fig. 5-11). Another example of a diagnostically useful granule is the characteristic crystal-containing granule of an insulinoma derived from the pancreatic islets.

Immunohistochemical Tumor Markers Are Antigens That Point to the Origin of Neoplasms

Tumor markers are products of malignant neoplasms that can be detected in the cells themselves or in body fluids. The ultimate tumor marker would be one that allows the unequivocal distinction between benign and malignant cells, but unfortunately no such marker exists. Nevertheless, some markers are often useful in identifying the cell of origin of a metastatic or poorly differentiated primary tumor. Metastatic tumors may be so undifferentiated microscopically as to preclude even the distinction between an epithelial and a mesenchymal origin. Tumor markers rely on the preservation of characteristics of the progenitor cell or the synthesis of specialized proteins by the neoplastic cell to make this distinction. The determination of cell lineage of undifferentiated tumors is more than an academic exercise, because therapeutic decisions may be based on their appropriate identification. For example, the treatment of carcinomas usually involves surgery, whereas malignant lymphomas are treated with radiation therapy and chemotherapy. Among these diagnostically useful markers are such diverse products as immunoglobulins, fetal proteins, enzymes, hormones, and cytoskeletal and junctional proteins.

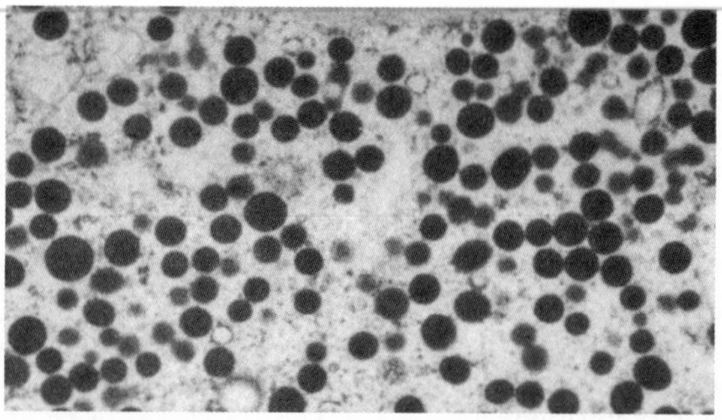

FIGURE 5-11. **Electron micrograph of a metastatic cancer of the adrenal medulla (pheochromocytoma).** The neuroendocrine origin of this poorly differentiated tumor was identified by the presence of characteristic cytoplasmic secretory granules.

- **Carcinomas** uniformly express **cytokeratins,** which are intermediate filaments belonging to a multigene family of proteins. Lineage-associated markers are often useful in establishing the origin of a poorly differentiated carcinoma. For example, prostatic carcinomas consistently express the glycoprotein **prostate-specific antigen** (PSA) and **prostate-specific acid phosphatase** (PSAP). By contrast, colon cancers are negative for these markers, but most of them express **carcinoembryonic antigen** (CEA). Some thyroid carcinomas demonstrate **thyroglobulin,** and breast cancers frequently show nuclear receptors for **estrogen** and **progesterone.** Expression of the sialated form of the **Lewis a antigen** (cancer antigen [CA] 19-9) has been associated with pancreatic and gastrointestinal cancers, whereas **CA 125** is a sensitive marker for ovarian cancers.
- **Neuroendocrine tumors** share the positivity for cytokeratins with other carcinomas. However, they can be identified by their content of **chromogranins,** a family of proteins found in neurosecretory granules. Neuron-specific enolase is another, albeit less specific, marker for neuroendocrine cells. Other markers for neuroendocrine differentiation are **synaptophysin** and Leu-7 (CD57). Specific antibodies exist for a number of peptide hormones, such as gastrin, bombesin, corticotropic hormone (adrenocorticotropic hormone [ACTH]), insulin, glucagon, somatostatin, and serotonin.
- **Malignant melanomas** may be unpigmented and appear similar to other poorly differentiated carcinomas. They can often be distinguished by immunohistochemical studies (Fig. 5-12). Melanomas express HMB-45 and S-100 protein, but unlike most carcinomas, they are not positive for cytokeratins.
- **Soft tissue sarcomas** express the intermediate filament **vimentin.** Since this marker is also present in numerous nonmesenchymal tumors, its expression is meaningful only in concert with other markers and morphologic criteria. **Desmin,** another useful intermediate filament, is present in benign and malignant neoplasms originating from either smooth or striated muscle fibers. **Muscle-specific actin** is another marker for muscle tissue. **Neurofilament proteins** are excellent markers for tumors originating from neurons, including neuroblastomas and ganglioneuroma. **Neuron-specific enolase** (NSE) also shows a strong association with neurogenic tissue and is found in almost all neuroblastomas. **Glial fibrillary acidic protein** (GFAP), the first intermediate filament discovered, is strongly expressed on astrocytes and in most glial cell neoplasms.
- **Malignant lymphomas** are generally positive for **leukocyte common antigen** (LCA, CD45). Markers for lymphomas and leukemias are grouped by so-called cluster designations (CDs), at present numbering over 200. Markers for CD antigens help to discriminate between T and B lymphocytes, monocytes, and granulocytes and the mature and immature variants of these cells. B cell malignancies, including plasmacytomas, manifest immunoglobulin light-chain restriction. A single B cell expresses κ or λ light chains. The presence of both κ- and λ-positive B cells argues against malignancy, whereas the demonstration of only one type of light chain on the lymphocytes strongly suggests a monoclonal B cell lymphoma.
- **Vascular tumors** derived from endothelial cells, including hemangiomas and hemangiosarcomas, are identified by antibodies against **factor VIII-related antigen** or by the binding of certain lectins.

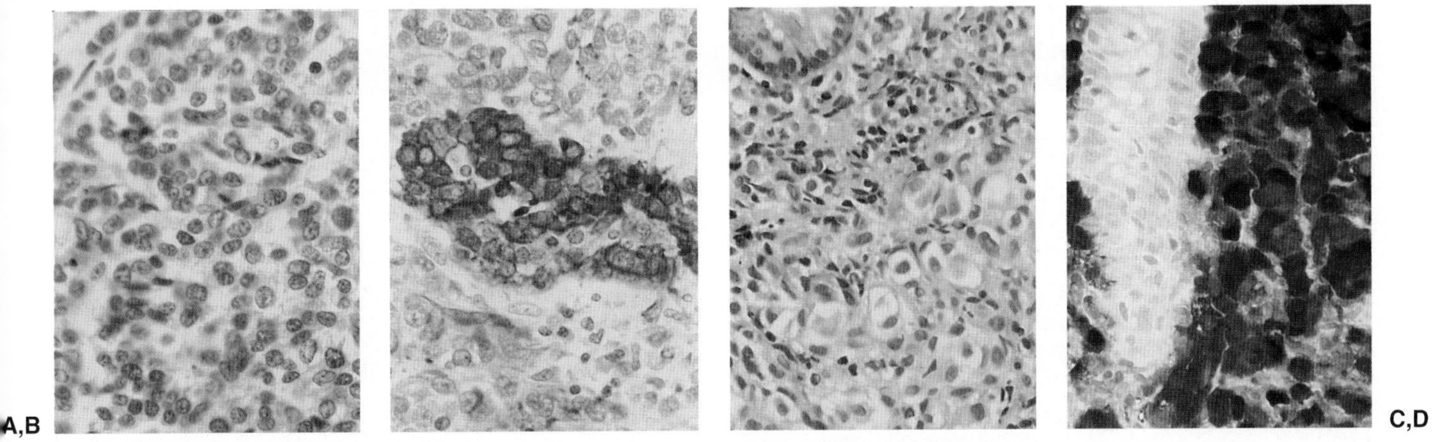

FIGURE 5-12. **Tumor markers in the identification of undifferentiated neoplasms. A.** A poorly differentiated metastatic bladder cancer is difficult to identify as a carcinoma with the hematoxylin and eosin stain. **B.** A section of the tumor depicted in *A* is positive for cytokeratin with an immunoperoxidase stain and is identified as carcinoma. **C.** A metastasis to the colon of an undifferentiated malignant melanoma is not pigmented, and its origin is unclear. **D.** An immunoperoxidase stain of the tumor shown in *C* reveals numerous cells positive for S-100 protein, a commonly used marker for cells of melanocytic origin.

- **Proliferating cells** display **Ki-67** and **proliferating cell nuclear antigen** (PCNA). Although the presence of proliferating cells alone does not establish a diagnosis of malignancy, the presence of cycling cells at sites in which cell growth is normally absent frequently suggests a cancer.

Serum tumor markers are not disease-specific, but they allow monitoring of tumor recurrence after surgery. For example, high serum levels of CEA are associated with carcinomas of the gastrointestinal tract and some carcinomas of the breast. Increased levels of **serum α-fetoprotein** (AFP) suggest liver cancer or a yolk sac tumor. **Human chorionic gonadotropin** (hCG) is used for monitoring the recurrence of malignant trophoblastic tumors. Elevated **CA 19-9** serum titers are found in patients with pancreatic or gastrointestinal cancers, and high **CA 125** levels are associated with ovarian carcinomas. Increased serum levels of PSA accompany prostatic cancers. Elevated titers of human placental alkaline phosphatase (HPAP) occur with seminomas. Table 5-1 lists many of the commonly used tumor markers.

Invasion and Metastasis

The two properties that are unique to cancer cells are the ability to invade locally and the capacity to metastasize to distant sites. These characteristics are responsible for the vast majority of deaths from cancer; the primary tumor itself is generally amenable to surgical extirpation.

Direct Extension Damages the Involved Organ and Adjacent Tissues

Most carcinomas begin as localized growths confined to the epithelium in which they arise. As long as these early cancers do not penetrate the basement membrane on which the epithelium rests, such tumors are termed ***carcinoma in situ*** (Fig. 5-13). In this stage, it is unfortunate that in situ tumors are asymptomatic, because they are invariably curable. When the in situ tumor acquires invasive potential and extends directly through the underlying basement membrane, it can compromise neighboring tissues and metastasize. In situations in which cancer arises from cells that are not confined by a basement membrane—such as connective tissue cells, lymphoid elements, and hepatocytes—an in situ stage is not defined.

Malignant tumors characteristically grow within the tissue of origin, where they enlarge and infiltrate normal structures. They may also extend directly beyond the confines of that organ to involve adjacent tissues. The growth of the cancer is occasionally so extensive that replacement of the normal tissue results in functional insufficiency of the organ. Such a situation is not uncommon in primary liver cancer. Brain tumors, such as astrocytomas, infiltrate the brain until they compromise vital regions. The direct extension of malignant tumors within an organ may also be life-threatening because of their location. A common example is the intestinal obstruction produced by cancer of the colon (Fig. 5-14).

The invasive growth pattern of cancers often leads to their direct extension outside the tissue of origin, in which case the tumor may secondarily impair the function of an adjacent organ. Squamous carcinoma of the cervix frequently grows beyond the genital tract to produce vesicovaginal fistulas and obstruct the ureters. Neglected cases of breast cancer are often complicated by extensive skin ulceration. Even small tumors can produce severe consequences when they invade vital structures. A small lung cancer can cause a bronchopleural fistula when it penetrates the bronchus or exsanguinating hemorrhage when it erodes a blood vessel. The agonizing pain of pancreatic carcinoma results from direct extension of the tumor to the celiac nerve plexus. Tumor cells that reach serous cavities (e.g., those of the peritoneum or pleura) spread easily by direct extension or can be carried by the fluid to new locations on the serous membranes. The most common example is the seeding of the peritoneal cavity by certain types of ovarian cancer (Fig. 5-15).

Metastatic Spread Is the Most Common Cause of Cancer Death

Metastasis refers to the transfer of malignant cells from one site to another not directly connected with it. The invasive properties of malignant tumors bring them into contact with blood and lymphatic vessels. *In the same way that they can invade parenchymal tissue, neoplastic cells can also penetrate vascular and lymphatic channels, through which they are disseminated to distant sites.* In general, metastases resemble the primary tumor histologically, although they are occasionally so anaplastic that their cell of origin is obscure.

TABLE 5–1

Frequently Used Markers to Identify Tumors

Marker	Target Cells
Epithelial Cells	
Cytokeratins (CK)	Carcinomas, mesothelioma
CK7	Many adenocarcinomas
CK20	Gastrointestinal and ovarian carcinomas, urothelial carcinomas, Merkel cell tumor
Epithelial membrane antigen (EMA)	Carcinomas, mesothelioma, some large cell lymphomas
Ber-Ep4	Most adenocarcinomas, but not in mesothelioma
B72.3 (tumor-associated)	Many adenocarcinomas, but not in mesothelioma
Carcinoembryonic antigen (CEA)	Many adenocarcinomas, but not in mesothelioma
CD15	Many adenocarcinomas, but not in mesothelioma
Mesothelial Cells	
Cytokeratins CK5/6	Mesothelioma
Vimentin	Mesothelioma
HBME	Mesothelioma
Calretinin	Mesothelioma
Melanocytes	
HMB-45	Malignant melanoma
S-100 protein	Malignant melanoma
Mel A	Malignant melanoma
Neuroendocrine and Neural Cells	
Chromogranins	Neuroendocrine tumors
Synaptophysin	Neuroendocrine tumors
Neuron-specific enolase	Neuroendocrine tumors
CD57	Neuroendocrine tumors
Glial Cells	
Glial fibrillary acidic protein (GFAP)	Astrocytoma and other glial tumors
Mesenchymal Cells	
Vimentin	Most sarcomas
Desmin	Muscle tumors
Muscle-specific actin	Muscle tumors
CD99	Ewing sarcoma, peripheral neuroectodermal tumors (PNET)
Specific Organs	
Prostate-specific antigen (PSA)	Prostatic cancer
Prostate-specific alkaline phosphatase (PSAP)	Prostatic cancer
Thyroglobulin	Thyroid cancer
α-Fetoprotein (AFP)	Hepatocellular carcinoma, yolk sac tumor
HepPar 1	Hepatocellular carcinoma
CEA	Gastrointestinal cancers
Placental alkaline phosphatase (PLAP)	Seminoma
Human chorionic gonadotropin (hCG)	Trophoblastic tumors
CA19-9	Pancreatic and gastrointestinal carcinomas
CA125	Ovarian carcinoma
Calcitonin	Medullary carcinoma of the thyroid
CD Markers	
CD1	Some T-cell leukemias; Langerhans cell proliferations
CD2	T cells, T-cell malignancies
CD3	T cells, T-cell malignancies
CD4	T cells, T-cell malignancies; Monocytes, monocytic malignancies
CD5	T cells; some B-cell malignancies
CD8	Suppressor T cells; some T-cell malignancies
CD10 (common ALL antigen, CALLA)	Acute lymphoblastic leukemia; some B-cell lymphomas; Renal cell carcinomas
CD15	Hodgkin disease; some myeloid leukemias
CD19	B cells, B-cell malignancies
CD20	B cells, B-cell malignancies
CD30	Hodgkin disease; Anaplastic large cell lymphoma
CD33	Myeloid leukemias
CD34	Acute myeloid or lymphoblastic leukemias; Some spindle cell tumors
Non-CD Leukemia/ Lymphoma Markers	
κ-Light chain	B-cell malignancies
λ-Light chain	B-cell malignancies
TdT	Acute lymphoblastic leukemia
Bcl-1	Mantle cell lymphoma
Bcl-2	Follicular lymphoma
Endothelial Markers	
von Willebrand factor (vWF)	Vascular neoplasms
CD31	Vascular neoplasms
CD34	Vascular neoplasms
Lectins	Vascular neoplasms

CA = cancer antigen; CD = cluster designation; TdT = terminal deoxynucleotidyl transferase.

Hematogenous Metastases

Cancer cells commonly invade capillaries and venules, whereas thicker-walled arterioles and arteries are relatively resistant. Before they can form viable metastases, circulating tumor cells must lodge in the vascular bed of the metastatic site (Fig. 5-16). Here they presumably attach to the walls of blood vessels, either to endothelial cells or to naked basement membranes. For many tumors this sequence of events explains why the liver and the lung are so frequently the sites of metastases. Because abdominal tumors seed the portal system, they lead to hepatic metastases; other tumors penetrate systemic veins that eventually drain into the vena cava and hence to the lungs. In this respect, some tumor cells released into the venous system survive passage through the microcirculation and are thus transported to more distant organs. For instance, tumor cells may traverse the liver and produce pulmonary metastases, and neoplastic cells may also survive passage through the pulmonary microcirculation to reach the brain, bones (Fig. 5-17), and other organs

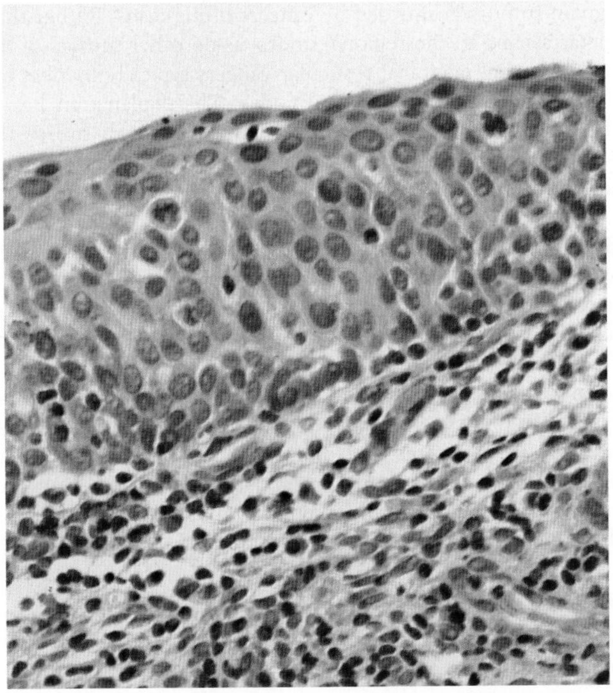

FIGURE 5-13. **Carcinoma in situ.** A section of the uterine cervix shows neoplastic squamous cells occupying the full thickness of the epithelium and confined to the mucosa by the underlying basement membrane.

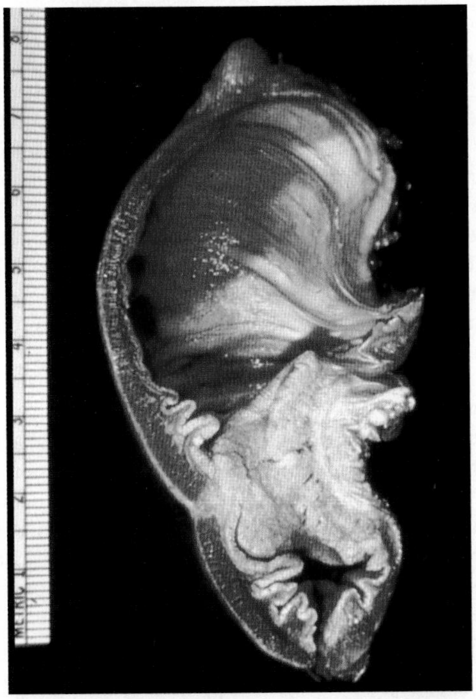

FIGURE 5-14. **Adenocarcinoma of the colon with intestinal obstruction.** The lumen of the colon at the site of the cancer is narrow. The colon above the obstruction is dilated.

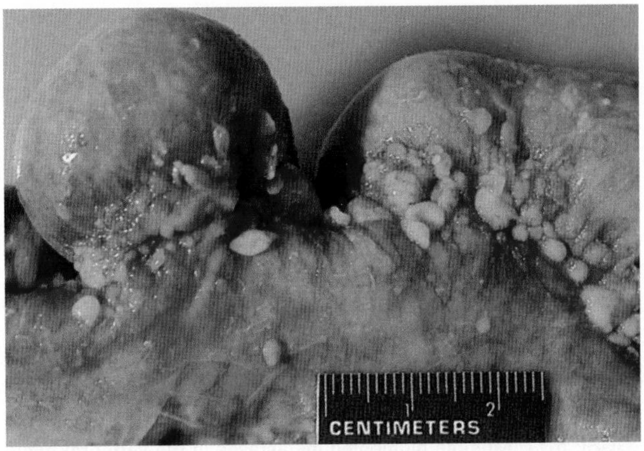

FIGURE 5-15. **Peritoneal carcinomatosis.** The mesentery attached to a loop of small bowel is studded with small nodules of metastatic ovarian carcinoma.

through arterial dissemination. Neoplastic cells arrested in the microcirculation penetrate the vessel walls at the site of metastasis by use of the same mechanisms by which the primary tumor invades.

Lymphatic Metastases

A historical dogma of metastatic spread held that epithelial tumors (carcinomas) preferentially metastasize through lymphatic channels, whereas mesenchymal neoplasms (sarcomas) are distributed hematogenously. This distinction is no longer considered valid because of clinical observations of metastatic patterns and the demonstration of numerous connections between the lymphatic and vascular systems. Tumors arising in tissues that have a rich lymphatic network (e.g., the breast) often metastasize by this route, although the particular properties of specific neoplasms may play a role in the route of spread.

Basement membranes envelop only large lymphatic channels; they are lacking in lymphatic capillaries. Thus, invasive tumor cells may penetrate lymphatic channels more readily than blood vessels. Once in lymphatic vessels, the cells are carried to the regional draining lymph nodes, where they initially lodge in the marginal sinus and then extend throughout the node. Lymph

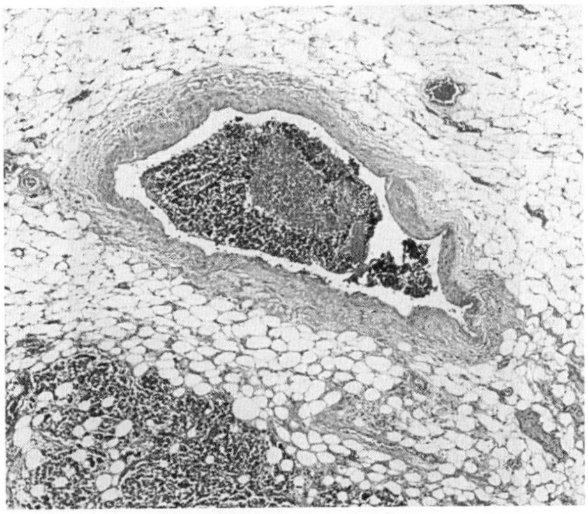

FIGURE 5-16. **Hematogenous spread of cancer.** A malignant tumor *(bottom)* has invaded adipose tissue and penetrated into a small vein.

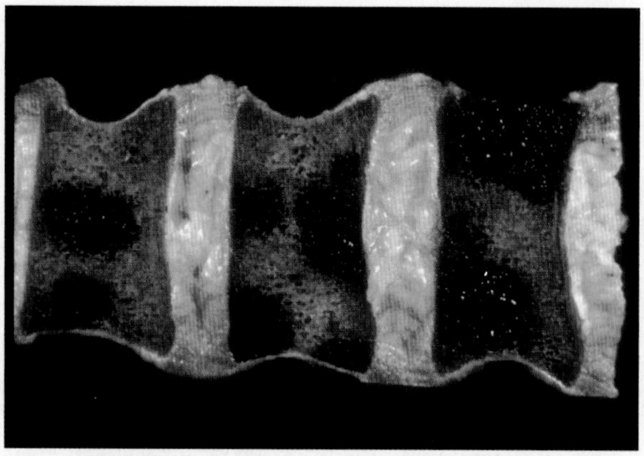

FIGURE 5-17. **Multiple pigmented metastases in the vertebral bodies in a patient who died of malignant melanoma.**

nodes bearing metastatic deposits may be enlarged to many times their normal size, often exceeding the diameter of the primary lesion. The cut surface of the lymph node usually resembles that of the primary tumor in color and consistency and may also exhibit the necrosis and hemorrhage commonly seen in primary cancers (Fig. 5-18).

The regional lymphatic pattern of metastatic spread is most prominently exemplified by breast cancer. The initial metastases are almost always lymphatic, and these regional lymphatic metastases have considerable prognostic significance. Cancers that arise in the lateral aspect of the breast characteristically spread to axillary lymph nodes; those arising in the medial portion drain to the internal mammary thoracic lymph nodes.

Lymphatic metastases are occasionally found in lymph nodes distant from the site of the primary tumor; these are termed **skip metastases**. For example, abdominal cancers may initially be signaled by the appearance of an enlarged supraclavicular node, the so-called **sentinel node**. A graphic example of the relationship of lymphatic anatomy to the spread of malignant tumors is afforded by cancers of the testis. Rather than metastasizing to the regional nodes, as do other tumors of the male external genitalia, testicular cancers typically involve the draining abdominal periaortic nodes. The explanation lies in the descent of the testis from an intra-abdominal site to the scrotum, during which it is accompanied by its own lymphatic supply.

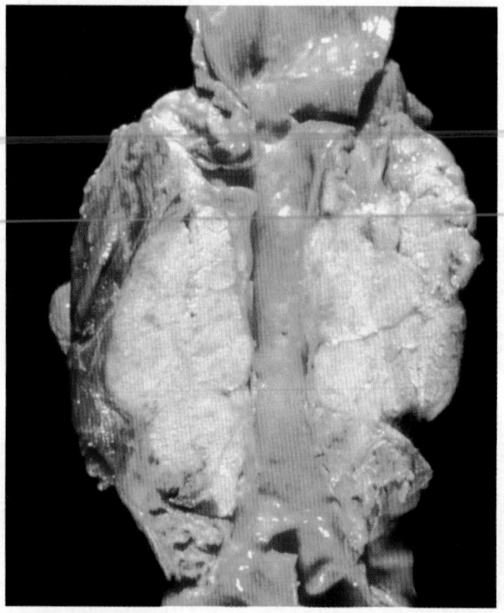

FIGURE 5-18. **Metastatic carcinoma in periaortic lymph nodes.** The aorta has been opened and the nodes bisected.

Seeding of Body Cavities

Malignant tumors that arise in organs adjacent to body cavities (e.g., ovaries, gastrointestinal tract, and lung) may shed malignant cells into these spaces. Such body cavities principally include the peritoneal and pleural cavities, although occasional seeding of the pericardial cavity, joint space, and subarachnoid space, are observed. Similar to tissue culture, tumor in these sites grows in masses and often produces fluid (e.g., ascites, pleural fluid), sometimes in very large quantities. Mucinous adenocarcinoma may also secrete copious amounts of mucin in these locations.

Invasion and Metastasis Are Multistep Events

Several steps are required for malignant cells to establish a metastasis (Fig. 5-19):

1. Invasion of the basement membrane underlying the tumor
2. Movement through extracellular matrix
3. Penetration of vascular or lymphatic channels
4. Survival and arrest within circulating blood or lymph
5. Exit from the circulation into a new tissue site
6. Survival and growth as a metastasis, a process that involves angiogenesis

Most cancers originate from the malignant transformation of a single cell (**monoclonal origin of tumors**). Nevertheless, the inherent genetic instability of the malignant phenotype leads to the appearance of subpopulations with diverse biological characteristics and profound variations in their metastatic potential (**tumor heterogeneity**). The demonstration of tumor heterogeneity has led to the concept that at each step of the metastatic cascade, only the fittest cells survive. Thus, the metastatic process can be viewed as a competition in which a subpopulation of cells within the primary cancer ultimately prevails as a metastasis.

Invasion

Inherent in the definition of a malignant cell is the capacity to invade surrounding tissue. In epithelial tumors, invasion requires disruption of, and penetration through, the underlying basement membrane and passage through the extracellular matrix. Similarly, circulating cells destined to establish metastases must reproduce these same events to exit from the vascular or lymphatic compartment and establish residence at a distant site.

Adhesion Molecules

The entire metastatic sequence, from the initial binding of the tumor cell to the underlying extracellular matrix to the growth in a distant location, depends on the expression of numerous adhesion molecules by the malignant cells. The display of such surface molecules varies with (1) the type of tumor, (2) the individual clone (tumor heterogeneity), (3) the stage of the malignant progression, and (4) the specific step in the metastatic process.

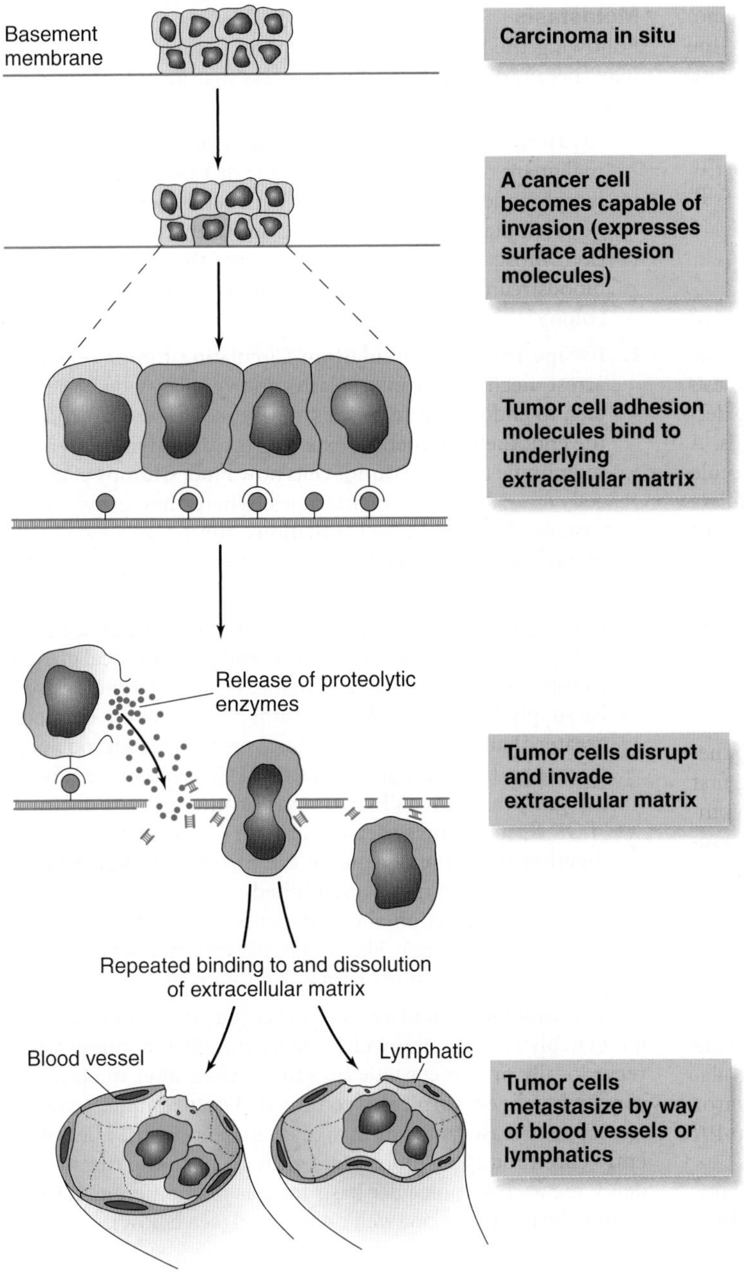
Basement membrane
Carcinoma in situ
A cancer cell becomes capable of invasion (expresses surface adhesion molecules)
Tumor cell adhesion molecules bind to underlying extracellular matrix
Release of proteolytic enzymes
Tumor cells disrupt and invade extracellular matrix
Repeated binding to and dissolution of extracellular matrix
Blood vessel
Lymphatic
Tumor cells metastasize by way of blood vessels or lymphatics

FIGURE 5-19. **Mechanisms of tumor invasion and metastasis.** The mechanism by which a malignant tumor initially penetrates a confining basement membrane and then invades the surrounding extracellular environment involves several steps. The tumor first acquires the ability to bind components of the extracellular matrix. These interactions are mediated by the expression of a number of adhesion molecules. Proteolytic enzymes are then released from the tumor cells, and the extracellular matrix is degraded. After moving through the extracellular environment, the invading cancer penetrates blood vessels and lymphatics by the same mechanisms.

INTEGRINS: Integrins are transmembrane receptors, each consisting of two α and two β subunits, which together confer substrate specificity on the receptor (see Chapter 3). These adhesion receptors mediate cell–matrix and cell–cell attachment. The binding of integrins to their ligands also stimulates intracellular signaling and gene expression, which play a role in cell migration, proliferation, differentiation, and survival. In addition, integrins affect the expression, localization, and activation of collagenases (matrix metalloproteinases [MMPs]; see below) and can guide these enzymes to their targets in the extracellular matrix, where they degrade connective tissue and pave the way for the spread of tumor cells.

IMMUNOGLOBULIN SUPERGENE FAMILY: A number of intercellular adhesion molecules belong to this superfamily, including intercellular adhesion molecule-1 (ICAM-1), MUC18, and vascular cell adhesion molecule-1 (VCAM-1). The expression of ICAM-1 correlates positively with the aggressiveness of a variety of tumor cell types.

CADHERINS AND CATENINS: Cadherins are a family of cell–cell adhesion molecules, which are calcium (Ca^{2+})-dependent transmembrane glycoproteins. The best-characterized of the cadherins, E-cadherin, is expressed on the surface of all epithelia and mediates cell–cell adhesion by mutual **zipper** interactions. Catenins (α, β, and γ) are proteins that interact with the intracellular domain of E-cadherin and create a mechanical linkage between that molecule and the cytoskeleton, which is essential for effective epithelial cell interactions. Overall, cadherins and catenins suppress invasion and metastasis. The expression of both E-cadherin and catenins is reduced or lost in most carcinomas, an effect that permits individual malignant cells to leave the main tumor mass and metastasize. Interestingly, β-catenin also binds to the adenomatous polyposis coli (APC) gene product, an effect that is independent of its interaction with E-cadherin and α-catenin. Mutations in either the APC or β-catenin gene are implicated in the development of colon cancer (see later and Chapter 13).

Growth Factors and Cytokines

Growth factors and cytokines orchestrate cellular responses during development, differentiation, and repair. Aberrant production of growth factors by tumors contributes to neoangiogenesis and attraction of inflammatory cells as well as enhances proliferation, migration, and invasive properties of the tumor cells. A notable example is **autocrine motility factor** (AMF), a molecule that belongs to a family of tumor cell cytokines that stimulate motility via a receptor-mediated signaling pathway. AMF not only regulates motility but also modulates the expression of cell surface integrins. The expression of the AMF receptor (gp78) in normal cells is regulated by cell contact, whereas in many cancer cells, it is constitutively expressed.

Proteolytic Enzymes

A breach of the basement membrane that separates an epithelium from the underlying mesenchymal compartment is the first event in tumor cell invasion. The basement membrane is composed of a number of extracellular matrix components, including type IV collagen, laminin, and proteoglycans (see Chapter 3). Malignant cells and stromal cells associated with cancers elaborate a variety of proteases that degrade one or more of the basement membrane components. Such enzymes include the urokinase-type plasminogen activator (u-PA) and MMPs, including collagenases.

u-PA converts serum plasminogen to plasmin, a serine protease that degrades laminin and activates type IV procollagenase. u-PA activity is balanced by plasminogen activator inhibitor (PAI); changes in the expression of u-PA, the u-PA receptor and PAI have been reported in different cancers.

The MMPs comprise a family of zinc-dependent endopeptidases that are susceptible to tissue inhibitors of MMPs (TIMPs). MMPs include interstitial collagenases, stromelysins, gelatinases, and membrane-type MMPs. These enzymes are synthesized and secreted by normal cells under conditions associated with physiologic tissue remodeling, such as wound healing and placental implantation. Under these circumstances, a balance between MMPs and TIMPs is strictly regulated. By contrast, the invasive and metastatic phenotypes of cancer cells are characterized by dysregulation of this balance.

A direct correlation between increased expression of MMPs and augmented invasive capacity or metastatic potential of tumor cells has been observed in many cancers. In addition, many of these same tumors exhibit decreased TIMP expression. MMPs are present in either tumor cells or surrounding stromal cells or both, depending on the particular neoplasm. In some instances, MMPs secreted by stromal cells are bound to integrins on the surface of the tumor cells, thereby providing a particularly high local concentration of protease activity at the site of tumor invasion. Deregulated MMP activity permits entry of cancer cells into, and their passage through, the extracellular matrix.

Metastasis

Following the invasion of surrounding tissue, malignant cells may spread to distant sites by a process that includes a number of steps:

1. **Invasion of the circulation:** After invading interstitial tissue, malignant cells penetrate lymphatic or vascular channels. In lymph nodes, communications between lymphatics and venous tributaries allow the cells access to the systemic circulation. Most tumor cells do not survive their journey in the bloodstream, and less than 0.1% remain to establish a new colony.
2. **Escape from the circulation:** Circulating tumor cells may arrest mechanically in capillaries and venules, where they attach to endothelial cells. This adherence causes retraction of the endothelium, thereby exposing the underlying basement membrane to which tumor cells now bind. Clumps of tumor cells may also arrest in arterioles, where they grow within vascular lumens. In both situations, tumor cells eventually extravasate by mechanisms similar to those responsible for local invasion.
3. **Local growth:** In a hospitable site, the extravasated cancer cells grow in response to autocrine and possibly local growth factors produced by the host tissue. However, a new vascular supply is necessary for the tumor to grow to a diameter greater than 0.5 mm. Thus, many tumors secrete polypeptides (e.g., fibroblast growth factor [FGF], vascular endothelial growth factor [VEGF], transforming growth factor-β [TGF-β], and platelet-derived growth factor [PDGF]), which together trigger and regulate the process of **angiogenesis** (see below). The newly established metastatic colony must also escape detection and destruction by the host immune defenses (see below). The metastasis can metastasize again, either within the same organ or to distant sites.

The establishment of a metastatic colony does not mean that it inevitably enlarges. It is well known clinically that tumors may recur locally or at metastatic sites many years after the primary cancer has been surgically removed. For example, patients treated for breast cancer or malignant melanoma may be apparently cured for 20 or more years, only to have the tumor suddenly recur. The molecular basis for this phenomenon, termed **tumor dormancy**, is not well understood (see below).

Target Organs in Metastatic Disease

It was recognized more than a century ago that the distribution of metastases in breast cancer is not random. In 1889, Paget proposed that the spread of tumor cells to specific secondary sites depends on compatibility between the tumor cells (the seed) and favorable microenvironment factors in the secondary site (the soil). By contrast, others have argued that metastatic spread depends solely on anatomical factors and the blood flow to an organ. Today, there is evidence that both mechanisms operate, depending on the tumor. For example, cancers of the breast, prostate, and thyroid metastasize to bone, a tropism that suggests a favored "soil." Conversely, despite their size and abundant blood flow, neither the spleen nor skeletal muscle is a common site of metastases. Yet for many cancers, the vascular anatomy unquestionably influences the pattern of metastatic spread. Malignant tumors of the gastrointestinal tract commonly metastasize to the first capillary bed they encounter, namely the liver. Similarly, lung cancers often spread to the brain. An additional factor that regulates homing of malignant cells may be the expression of complementary adhesion molecules, either by the cancer cells or those of the organ to which they home.

The Grading and Staging of Cancers

In an attempt to predict the clinical behavior of a malignant tumor and to establish criteria for therapy, many cancers are classified according to cytologic and histologic grading schemes or by staging protocols that describe the extent of spread.

Cancer Grading Reflects Cellular Characteristics

Low-grade tumors are **well differentiated;** high-grade ones tend to be **anaplastic.** Cytologic and histologic grading, which are necessarily subjective and at best semiquantitative, are based on the degree of anaplasia and on the number of proliferating cells. The degree of anaplasia is determined from the shape and regularity of the cells and from the presence of distinct differentiated features, such as functioning glandlike structures in adenocarcinomas or epithelial pearls in squamous carcinomas. The presence of such characteristics identify a tumor as well differentiated. By contrast, the cells of "poorly differentiated" malignancies bear little resemblance to their normal counterparts. Evidence of rapid or abnormal growth is provided by (1) large numbers of mitoses, (2) atypical mitoses, (3) nuclear pleomorphism, and (4) tumor giant cells. Most grading schemes classify tumors into three or four grades of increasing malignancy (Fig. 5-20). The general correlation between the cytologic grade and the biological behavior of a neoplasm is not invariable: There are many examples of tumors of low cytologic grades that exhibit substantial malignant properties.

Cancer Staging Refers to the Extent of Spread

The choice of a surgical approach or the selection of treatment modalities is influenced more by the stage of a cancer than by its cytologic grade. Moreover, most statistical data related to cancer survival are based on the stage rather than the cytologic grade of the tumor. Clinical staging is independent of cytologic grading. The significant criteria used for staging vary with different organs. Commonly used criteria include:

- Tumor size
- Extent of local growth, whether within or without the organ
- Presence of lymph node metastases
- Presence of distant metastases

These criteria have been codified in the international **TNM cancer staging system,** in which "T" refers to the size of the primary tumor, "N" to regional node metastases, and "M" to the presence and extent of distant metastases. The definitions of numerical scores for T, N, and M (e.g., T1–T4, N1–N3) vary according to specific tumor types.

In some cases, the distinction between benign and malignant tumors is based solely on size. For example, on the basis of clinical experience with papillary renal cancers, tumors smaller than 0.5 cm in diameter are generally considered benign adenomas, whereas those of larger size are labeled renal cell carcinomas. The choice of surgical therapy is often influenced by size alone. For instance, a primary breast cancer smaller than 2 cm in diameter can be treated with local excision and radiation therapy; larger masses often necessitate mastectomy. Local extension can also be used to estimate prognosis, as in the Dukes classification of colorectal cancer. Penetration of the tumor into the muscularis and serosa of the bowel is associated with a poorer prognosis than that of a more superficial tumor. Clearly, the presence of lymph node metastases mandates more aggressive treatment than does their absence, whereas the presence of distant metastases is generally a contraindication to surgical intervention other than for palliation.

The Clonal Origin of Cancer

Studies of human and experimental tumors have provided strong evidence that most cancers arise from a single transformed cell. This theory has been most thoroughly examined in connection with proliferative disorders of the hematopoietic system. The most common piece of clinical evidence in its favor is the production by neoplastic plasma cells of a single immunoglobulin unique to

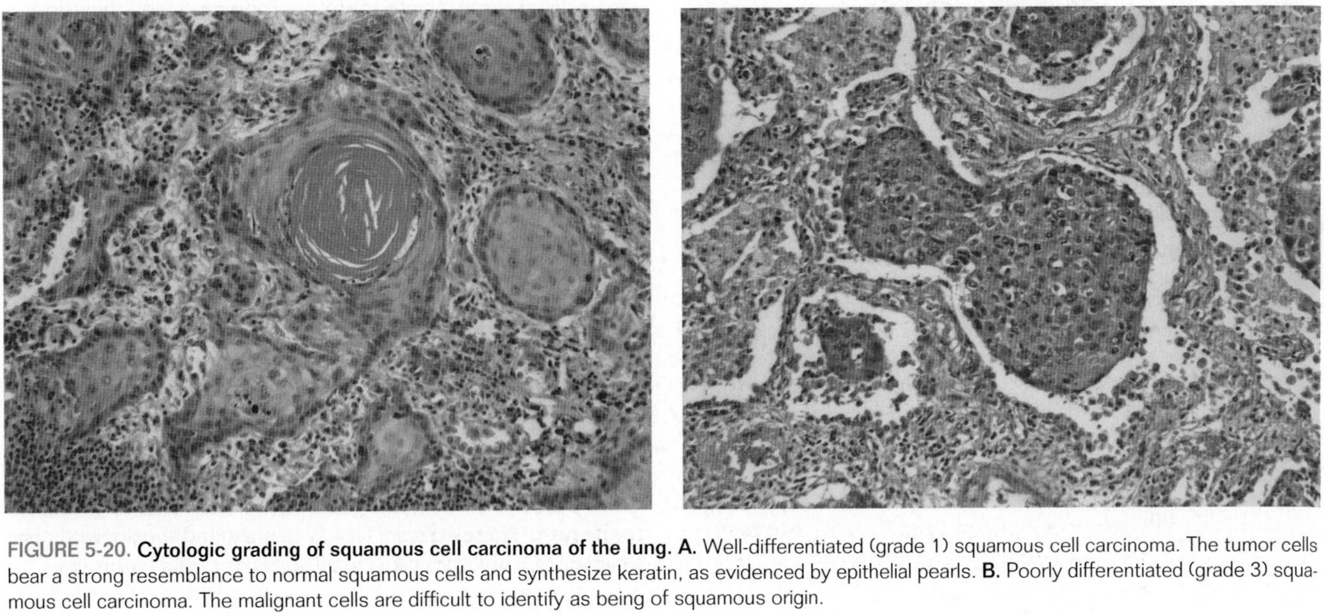

A B

FIGURE 5-20. **Cytologic grading of squamous cell carcinoma of the lung. A.** Well-differentiated (grade 1) squamous cell carcinoma. The tumor cells bear a strong resemblance to normal squamous cells and synthesize keratin, as evidenced by epithelial pearls. **B.** Poorly differentiated (grade 3) squamous cell carcinoma. The malignant cells are difficult to identify as being of squamous origin.

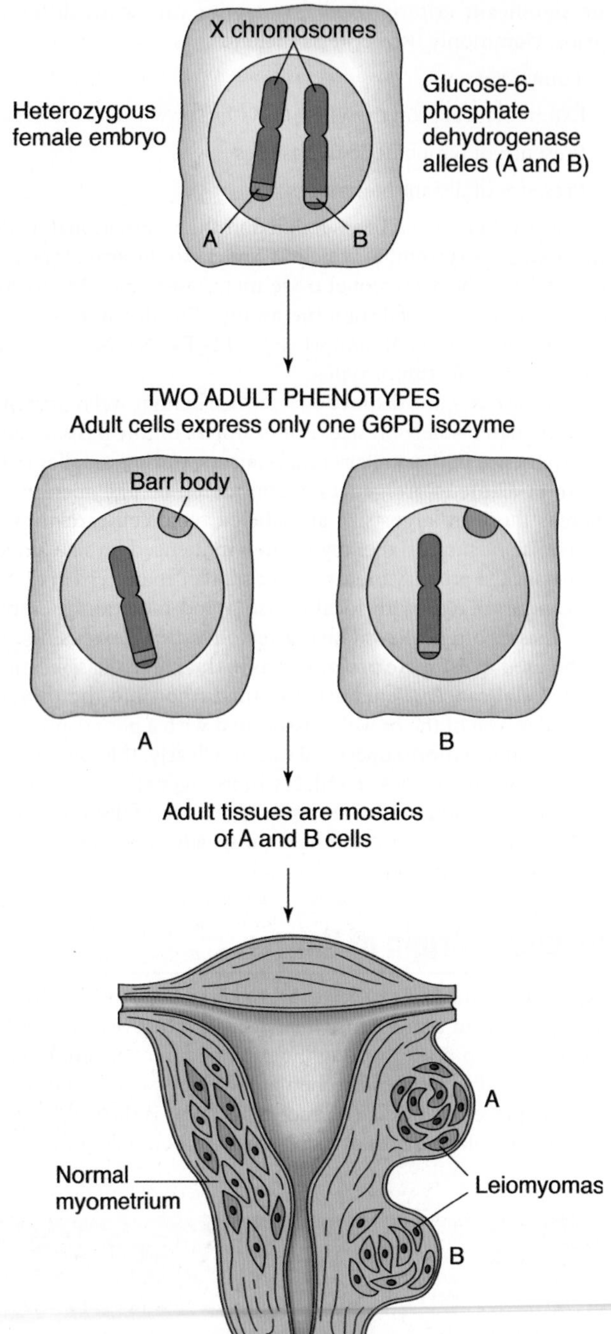

FIGURE 5-21. **Monoclonal origin of human tumors.** Some females are heterozygous for the two alleles of glucose-6-phosphate dehydrogenase (G6PD) on the long arm of the X chromosome. Early in embryogenesis, one of the X chromosomes is randomly inactivated in every somatic cell and appears cytologically as a Barr body attached to the nuclear membrane. As a result, the tissues are a mosaic of cells that express either the A or the B isozyme of G6PD. Leiomyomas of the uterus have been shown to contain one or the other isozyme (A or B) but not both, a finding that demonstrates the monoclonal origin of the tumors.

an individual patient with multiple myeloma. Indeed, such a "monoclonal spike" in the serum electrophoresis from a patient with suspected myeloma is regarded as conclusive evidence of the disease. Similarly, cell surface markers have been used to establish a monoclonal origin for many other hematopoietic malignant disorders. For example, B-cell lymphomas are composed of cells that exclusively display either κ or λ light chains on their surface, whereas polyclonal lymphoid proliferations exhibit both types of cells. Monoclonality has also been demonstrated in the individual metastases of a number of solid tumors.

One of the most important observations in regard to the monoclonal origin of cancer was derived from the study of glucose-6-phosphate dehydrogenase in women who were heterozygous for its two isozymes, A and B (Fig. 5-21). These isozymes are encoded by genes located on the X chromosome. Since one X chromosome is randomly inactivated, only one of these genes is expressed in any given cell. Thus, although the genotypes of all cells are the same, their phenotypes vary with regard to the expression of isozyme A or B. An examination of benign uterine smooth muscle tumors (leiomyomas, or "fibroids") revealed that all the cells in an individual tumor expressed either A or B but not both, indicating that each tumor was derived from a single progenitor cell.

Cancer As Altered Differentiation

In many cancers, the malignant phenotype reflects, at least in part, defects in the normally strict control of cell proliferation. *However, in some cancers, it is thought that the malignant cells result from a maturation arrest in the sequence of development from a stem or progenitor cell to a fully differentiated cell.* According to this theory, tumor cells accumulate because the mechanisms that control the total number of cells in the fully differentiated compartment of some tissues do not apply when less-differentiated precursor cells fail to mature.

SQUAMOUS CELL CARCINOMA: In many tumors most of the neoplastic cells are outside the cell cycle and thus do not contribute to malignancy of the tumor. For example, as noted above, fewer than 3% of the cells in a squamous carcinoma maintain the tumor's malignant potential, and most differentiate and die spontaneously. When such terminally differentiated tumor cells are transplanted into appropriate hosts, they do not grow, whereas their undifferentiated counterparts from the same tumor form typical squamous carcinomas. Such observations support the theory that the initial step in the development of some cancers is a failure of the stem cell to differentiate normally to complete the sequence of cell differentiation.

TERATOCARCINOMA: Further evidence to support the concept of cancer as a failure of differentiation has come from the study of experimental malignant germ cell tumors (teratocarcinomas). A single embryonal carcinoma cell—the stem cell of a teratocarcinoma—when transplanted into a mouse, gives rise to a tumor that contains cells derived from all three germ layers. Clearly, the progeny of the original transplanted tumor cell differentiate into more mature cells that express recognizable phenotypes of more fully differentiated tissues. When these differentiated tissues of the teratocarcinoma are separated from the malignant embryonal cells and transplanted into compatible hosts, they not only survive but also function with no detriment to the host. These cells are clearly benign, and the dogma "once a cancer cell, always a cancer cell" does not hold in this case.

A further refinement of this approach involves the transplantation of a single teratocarcinoma stem cell from a mouse into an early mouse embryo. At term the entirely normal pup is a mosaic composed of cells derived from both the embryo proper and the embryonal carcinoma. The progeny of the malignant cell, under the influence of normal developmental controls, has differentiated into mature tissue elements. Thus, the unregulated growth of the cancer cells may be converted into normal patterns of growth and differentiation.

Clinical analogies to the experimental situation do exist. The best known is the rare spontaneous conversion of a malignant neuroblastoma to its better-differentiated, benign counterpart, ganglioneuroma.

LEUKEMIAS AND LYMPHOMAS: The most comprehensive systematic analysis of human neoplasia from the perspective of developmental biology has come from the study of leukemias and lymphomas. During normal B- and T-lymphocyte maturation, there are well-documented sequential changes of membrane antigens and rearrangements of immunoglobulin and T-cell receptor genes. For example, in acute lymphoblastic leukemia of childhood, the neoplastic cells exhibit only partial assembly of the cell surface receptor molecules that characterize mature lymphocytes. In other words, the leukemic cell phenotype bears a strong resemblance to lymphocytes that appear transiently during the developmental sequence of the normal lymphocyte. Thus, the leukemic cells appear to be "frozen" in the act of receptor gene assembly and expression.

Acute myeloid leukemia is similar to acute lymphoblastic leukemia in that the malignant cells express phenotypes of transient, immature myeloid populations. Likewise, studies of chronic lymphocytic leukemias and lymphomas have revealed that these malignant disorders represent clonal expansions of lymphocyte populations corresponding to subsets found in normal lymphoid tissue.

In normal hematopoietic maturation, differentiation is tightly coupled to proliferation—that is, terminally differentiated cells are continually lost, to be replaced by newly proliferated and differentiated cells. By contrast, the data reviewed above suggest that certain leukemias and lymphomas are not truly proliferative disorders but rather reflect an uncoupling of differentiation from proliferation, with resulting accumulation of cells that have not attained terminal differentiation. According to this theory, leukemia and lymphoma may represent the stabilization of a phenotype that is also expressed, though only transiently, in developing normal cells.

RETINOIDS: The view that certain cancers may reflect impaired differentiation has led to a search for drugs that commit cancer cells to terminal differentiation and, therefore, apoptosis. The interest in the retinoids derives from experiments showing that administration of excess vitamin A or its derivatives inhibits chemically induced carcinogenesis in skin, lung, bladder, colon, and mammary gland.

A dramatic response to all-*trans*-retinoic acid is generated in acute promyelocytic leukemia, in which the administration of this agent induces a complete remission in most patients. In this disease, the reciprocal translocation between chromosomes 15 and 17 results in a fusion gene consisting of the retinoic acid receptor and the promyelocytic leukemia gene (PML) gene. The chimeric protein blocks myeloid differentiation at the promyelocyte stage, a process that is reversed by retinoic acid. Other forms of retinoic acid have shown limited activity against a variety of tumors. In patients with acute promyelocytic leukemia who are refractory to therapy with retinoic acid, arsenic trioxide, a compound that induces partial nonterminal differentiation of leukemic cells, is surprisingly effective.

The Growth of Cancers

Historically, cancer was considered to result from a totally unregulated growth of cells, and a logical corollary was that neoplastic cells divide at a faster rate than normal ones. *It is now clear that tumor cells do not necessarily proliferate more rapidly than their normal counterparts.* Tumor growth depends on other factors, such as the growth fraction (proportion of cycling cells) and the rate of cell death. In normal proliferating tissues (e.g., intestine and bone marrow), an exquisite balance between cell renewal and cell death is strictly maintained. *By contrast, the major determinant of tumor growth is clearly the fact that more cells are produced than die in a given time.* Such an effect can reflect either an excess of cell proliferation over programmed cell death or also normal rates of cell renewal in the face of reduced apoptosis.

Tumor Growth Rates May Be Expressed As Doubling Times

Tumor doubling time is the time taken for the number of cells in the mass to double. Internal cancers are not usually detected before they attain a size of about 1 cm^3 (1 g), which corresponds to 10^8 to 10^9 cells. The origin of most tumors from a single cell implies that the mass has doubled at least 30 times to reach this size. If the cancer is neglected and enlarges to the impressive size of 1 kg, it now contains 10^{12} cells. Yet, the growth from 1 g to 1 kg (assuming no cell death) can be achieved by only 10 population doublings. Thus, when cancers are initially detected clinically, they are already far advanced in their natural history. Because of the variable death rate of tumor cells and differences in cell cycle kinetics, the actual doubling time of human tumors is highly unpredictable.

The doubling time is not necessarily correlated with the growth fraction (i.e., the proportion of cells that are within the cell cycle). Since the duration of mitosis in cancer cells is often prolonged, the increased number of mitoses in a histologic section can be misleading as an indicator of overall growth. For example, a doubling in the time required for mitosis results in twice as many visible mitoses without any real increase in the rate of growth. In most cases, the theoretical tumor doubling time, calculated from the growth fraction and the cell cycle time, bears little relation to the actual clinical situation. To give a particular example, if a tumor weighing 1 g (often the smallest size clinically detectable) produces 2 new cells per 1000 cells in each mitotic cycle, the theoretical net increase would be a staggering 10^6 cells per hour, a figure totally at variance with the experience with most solid tumors. *Because of this difference between the theoretical and observed growth of tumors, it has been estimated that in human skin tumors, as many as 97% of proliferated cells die spontaneously.* The causes of tumor cell death are not precisely defined but probably include such factors as programmed cell death (apoptosis); inadequate blood supply, with consequent ischemia; a paucity of nutrients; and vulnerability to specific and nonspecific host defenses. From a practical point of view, the duration of a malignant tumor cannot be reasonably estimated from its size when it is first discovered.

Tumor Angiogenesis Refers to the Sprouting of New Capillaries

In the absence of new vessels to supply nutrients and remove waste products, malignant tumors do not grow larger than 1 to 2 mm in diameter. In this context, the density of capillaries within the primary tumor (e.g., cancers of the breast, prostate, and colon) correlates directly with metastases and decreased survival. Importantly, tumor angiogenesis occurs in non-neoplastic host tissue and is comparable to that in wound healing and other physiologic circumstances (see Chapter 3). Neovascularization of the evolving cancer may appear at various stages of tumor development and probably is related to phenotypic and genetic changes in the tumors. However, it is still unclear whether tumor angiogenesis is fundamentally a response to tissue hypoxia or to a distinct angiogenic tumor phenotype by which neoplastic cells secrete angiogenic factors. The latter is supported by the observation that neovascularization can begin even in premalignant lesions.

A number of factors can stimulate angiogenesis, including FGF, TGF-α and TGF-β, TNF-α, VEGF, PDGF, and epidermal growth factor (EGF). Some factors act directly on endothelial cells (e.g., VEGF), whereas others stimulate inflammatory cells to promote the formation of new blood vessels (e.g., PDGF). As the new vessels mature, these factors support the recruitment of pericytes and smooth muscle cells, and support the deposition of extracellular matrix. Inactivation of tumor suppressor genes may also play a role in regulating tumor angiogenesis (see below).

VEGF and FGF-2 are thought to be the most important angiogenic factors. Tumor vessels overexpress the tyrosine kinase receptors for VEGFs (VEGFR1 and VEGFR2). The role of such angiogenic factors is underscored by the growth suppression of many solid tumors by both endogenous and synthetic inhibitors of angiogenesis factors, some of which are in clinical use. Tumor angiogenesis may also be influenced by variations in the production of angiogenic inhibitors, such as thrombospondin, TIMPs, platelet factor 4, and interferons α and β. Other factors that have been documented to influence angiogenesis include adhesion molecules, matrix MMPs, and plasmin.

Tumor Dormancy Accounts for the Interval before the Appearance of Metastases

Metastatic disease is often not detectable at the time of the removal of a primary cancer. With some tumors, notably breast cancer and melanoma, metastases may remain dormant for many years, only to become apparent without any obvious cause. It is not clear whether tumor dormancy represents a balance between cell growth and cell death or whether the tumor cells are in cell cycle arrest. Clinically, most patients who have undergone a resection for a primary cancer do not evidence any detectable metastases either radiologically or pathologically. Thus, so-called micrometastases consist of single tumor cells or very small clusters. In the case of dormant tumor cells, it is not known whether they remain in G_0 phase of the cell cycle for prolonged periods of time or whether they do not grow because of interference with angiogenesis, unresponsiveness to growth factors, or the presence of immune growth restraints.

The Molecular Genetics of Cancer

The belief that cancer has a genetic basis, embodied in the concept of "cancer genes," has been prevalent for more than half a century and was rooted in the recognition of four factors: (1) hereditary predisposition, (2) the presence of chromosomal abnormalities in neoplastic cells, (3) a correlation between impaired DNA repair and cancer occurrence, and (4) the close association between carcinogenesis and mutagenesis. *It is now recognized that the unregulated growth of cancer cells results from the sequential acquisition of somatic mutations in genes that control cell growth, differentiation, and apoptosis, or that maintain genomic integrity.* Similar mutations may also be present in the germ line of persons with hereditary cancer predispositions. Mutations can be produced by environmental mutagens such as chemical carcinogens or radiation (see below). They can also arise during normal cellular metabolism, particularly from the formation of activated oxygen species (see Chapter 1).

It is likely that the most common mechanism of mutagenesis relates to spontaneous errors in DNA replication and repair. Considering that 10^{17} mitoses occur during an average human lifetime, corresponding to incorporation of the more than 10^{26} nucleotides into nascent DNA, it is impossible for this much DNA replication to occur without the introduction of unrepaired errors (mutations), particularly with the added burden of environmental mutagenic stresses. Since the body is composed of some 10^{14} cells and the mutation rate is roughly 10^{7} per gene per cell division, it is inevitable that everyone is a somatic mosaic at many genetic loci. Most such mutations are of no consequence, because they either do not affect the function of the cell or are lost as a result of the death of the cell. However, if the mutation involves genes that control growth or stabilize the genome, it may give rise to a clone of cells that possess a growth advantage over their normal neighbors. Successive mutations in similar genes result in increasingly aberrant clones until a malignant phenotype eventually emerges. *In a sense, the emergence of malignancy may be viewed as an evolutionary process wherein we see only the surviving clones.*

Transformed Cells Share Common Attributes

The precise definition of cell transformation is difficult, but it is generally accepted that malignant transformation involves somatic mutations that confer a set of common properties. It is estimated that a minimum of 4 to 7 mutated genes are required for transformation of a normal cell into a malignant phenotype. This **multistep** process takes place over a period of years, an observation that accounts, at least in part, for the fact that the incidence of cancer increases with age. Although mutations in hundreds of genes have been implicated in the pathogenesis of cancer, individual cancers exhibit unique profiles of genetic alterations. Nevertheless, the disruption of a limited number of regulatory pathways in the cell that leads to deregulation of cell proliferation and suppression of apoptosis confers a neoplastic phenotype to diverse cell types. Metazoans must allow cell proliferation upon demand. *Thus, from a teleological perspective, cancer reflects the failure to suppress the deregulated growth of mutated cells.*

Cancer cells are remarkably heterogeneous in appearance, growth rate, invasiveness, and metastatic potential, presumably owing to the interplay between diverse acquired mutations and the inherent gene expression of specific cell lineages. Nevertheless, transformed cells share certain biological features:

- Autonomous generation of mitogenic signals
- Insensitivity to exogenous antigrowth signals
- Resistance to apoptosis
- Limitless replicative potential (immortalization)
- Blocked differentiation

- Ability to sustain angiogenesis
- Capacity to invade surrounding tissues
- Potential to metastasize

Normal genes are mutated in various cancers, including cell cycle regulators, signal transduction factors, transcriptional factors, DNA-binding proteins, growth factor receptors, adhesion molecules, effectors of apoptosis, and telomerase. Thus, the concept of specific "cancer genes" is fanciful. The transforming genes can be grouped into three categories:

- **Oncogenes** are altered versions of normal genes, termed **protooncogenes**, that regulate normal cell growth, differentiation, and survival. Gain-of-function (dominant) mutations activate protooncogenes to become oncogenes and are positive effectors of the neoplastic phenotype.
- **Tumor suppressor genes** are normal genes whose products inhibit cellular proliferation. Loss-of-function (recessive) mutations inactivate inhibitory activities of tumor suppressor genes, thereby permitting unregulated cell growth.
- **Mutator genes (DNA mismatch repair genes)** normally maintain the integrity of the genome and the fidelity of DNA replication. Inactivating mutations of these genes allow the successive accumulation of further mutations.

Cell Cycle Control

The replication of a eukaryotic cell follows a tightly orchestrated program. Myriad intracellular signal transduction pathways connect extracellular signals (growth factors and cytokines) with genes that regulate the cell cycle machinery. Upon growth factor stimulation, a cell leaves the quiescent state (G_0) and enters G1 (Fig. 5-22). DNA replication occurs during S phase, followed by G2 and ultimately mitosis (M phase). Cells progress directly from M phase into G_1 in actively dividing cells.

During G_1, the commitment to enter the S phase occurs at a **restriction (R) point** wherein the cell monitors its internal and external environment and "decides" whether to proceed with replication. The R point is regulated by **cyclins**, so named for their cyclic expression and degradation during the cell cycle. Cyclins complex with and activate a family of related serine/threonine protein kinases, termed **cyclin-dependent kinases** (CDKs). CDK 2, 4, and 6 phosphorylate a family of **retinoblastoma proteins** (pRb). Retinoblastoma (Rb) phosphorylation unleashes transcription factors of the **E2F family**. E2F drives the cell past the R point. Other cyclins and CDKs regulate S to G_2 and G_2 to M transitions.

CDKs are also regulated by **cyclin–dependent kinase inhibitors** (CKIs). The expression of CKIs can be induced by senescence, contact inhibition, extracellular antimitogenic factors (e.g., TGF) and the tumor suppressor protein p53 (see below).

Loss of R point control deregulates progression through the cell cycle. Cancer cells often display loss of R point control through mechanisms such as (1) amplification/overexpression of cyclins/CDKs, (2) loss of CKIs, and (3) mutational inactivation of pRb or p53 proteins. For example, decreased levels of the CKI P27 are associated with a poor prognosis in adenocarcinoma of the colon and certain cancers of the lung. Conversely, a number of malignant tumors overexpress several cyclins and CDKs. Loss of Rb is a feature of many malignancies.

Cell cycle progression depends upon regulatory mechanisms that involve "check points," which ensure that the cell does not progress to mitosis until the S phase has been completed and that any DNA damage has been repaired. Blocks in cell cycle progression in G_1 and G_2 often lead to apoptosis as a default pathway. This phenomenon accounts for induction of tumor cell death in response to various chemotherapeutic agents.

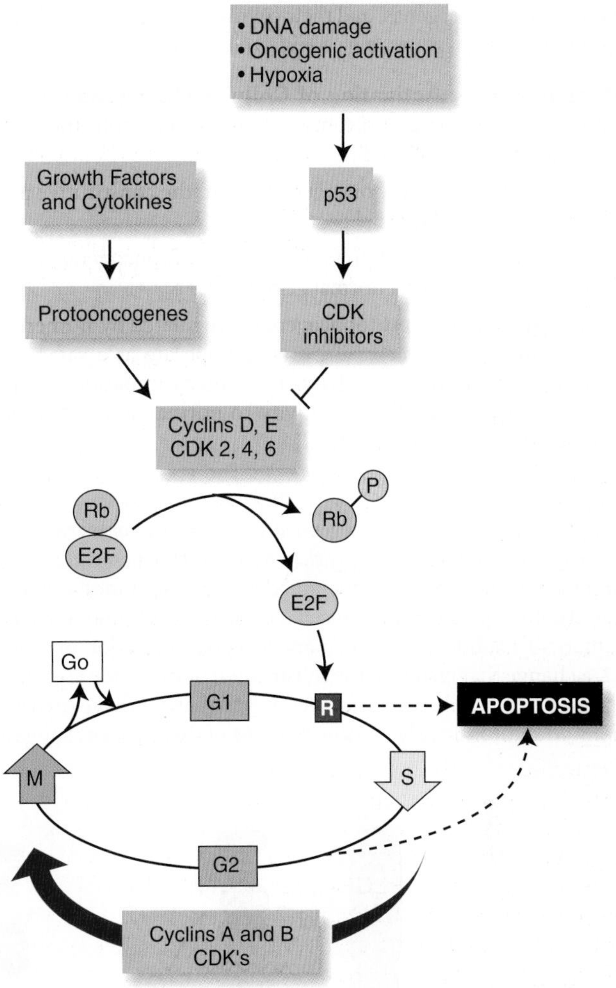

FIGURE 5-22. **Regulation of the cell cycle.** Cells are stimulated to enter G_1 from G_0 by growth factors and cytokines via protooncogene activation. A critical juncture in the transition of cells from G_1 to S phase is the restriction point (R). A major regulatory event in this process is the phosphorylation of retinoblastoma (Rb) by cyclin-dependent kinases (CDKs), which causes the release of the transcriptional activator E2F. CDKs are suppressed by CDK inhibitors (CKIs) that are regulated by p53. Tumor suppressor proteins block cell cycle progression largely within G_1. Interruption of cell cycle progression during G_1 and G_2 may lead to apoptosis as a default pathway. S, G_2, and M phases are also regulated by cyclins, CDKs, and CKIs.

Oncogenes Are Counterparts of Normal Genes

The concept of oncogenes was originally derived from studies of animal tumor viruses. Early research on transforming retroviruses showed that a limited number of viral genes could impart a neoplastic phenotype to virally infected cells. It was subsequently demonstrated that the transfer of specific genes from human tumor cells (**oncogenes**) into rodent cells in vitro could transform the recipient cells. The transforming genes were discovered to be mutant versions of normal genes involved in growth regulation and were termed **protooncogenes**. Transforming viral oncogenes were termed v-*onc* genes, and their cellular counterparts (c-) were individual normal genes (e.g., c-*myc*, c-*jun*, c-*src*).

Mechanisms of Activation of Cellular Oncogenes

There are three general mechanisms by which protooncogene activation is accomplished:

- A mutation of a protooncogene leads to the constitutive production of an abnormal protein.
- An increase in the expression of the protooncogene causes overproduction of a normal gene product.
- The activation of protooncogenes is regulated by numerous auto-inhibitory mechanisms, which operate as a safeguard against inappropriate activity. Thus, many mutations in protooncogenes lead to insensitivity to normal auto-inhibitory and regulatory constraints.

Activation by Mutation

Mutations by which protooncogenes are converted to oncogenes may involve (1) point mutations, (2) deletions, or (3) chromosomal translocations. The first oncogene identified in a human tumor was activated c-*ras* from a bladder cancer. This gene was found to have a remarkably subtle alteration, namely, a point mutation in codon 12, a change that results in the substitution of valine for glycine in the ras protein. Subsequent studies of other cancers have revealed point mutations involving other codons of the *ras* gene, suggesting that these positions are critical for the normal function of the ras protein. Since the discovery of mutations in c-*ras*, alterations in other growth-regulatory genes have been described.

Activating, or gain-of-function, mutations in protooncogenes are usually somatic rather than germ line alterations. Germ line mutations in protooncogenes, which are known to be important regulators of growth during development, are ordinarily lethal in utero. There are several exceptions to this rule. For example, c-*ret* is incriminated in the pathogenesis of certain heritable endocrine cancers, and c-*met,* which encodes the receptor for hepatocyte growth factor, is associated with a hereditary form of renal cancer.

Activation by Chromosomal Translocation

Chromosomal translocations (i.e., the transfer of a portion of one chromosome to another) have been implicated in the pathogenesis of several human leukemias and lymphomas. The first and still the best-known example of an acquired chromosomal translocation in a human cancer is the **Philadelphia chromosome,** which is found in 95% of patients with chronic myelogenous leukemia (Fig. 5-23). The c-*abl* protooncogene on chromosome 9 is translocated to chromosome 22, where it is placed in juxtaposition to a site known as the breakpoint cluster region *(bcr)*. The c-*abl* gene and *bcr* region unite to produce a hybrid oncogene that codes for an aberrant protein with very high tyrosine kinase activity, which generates mitogenic and

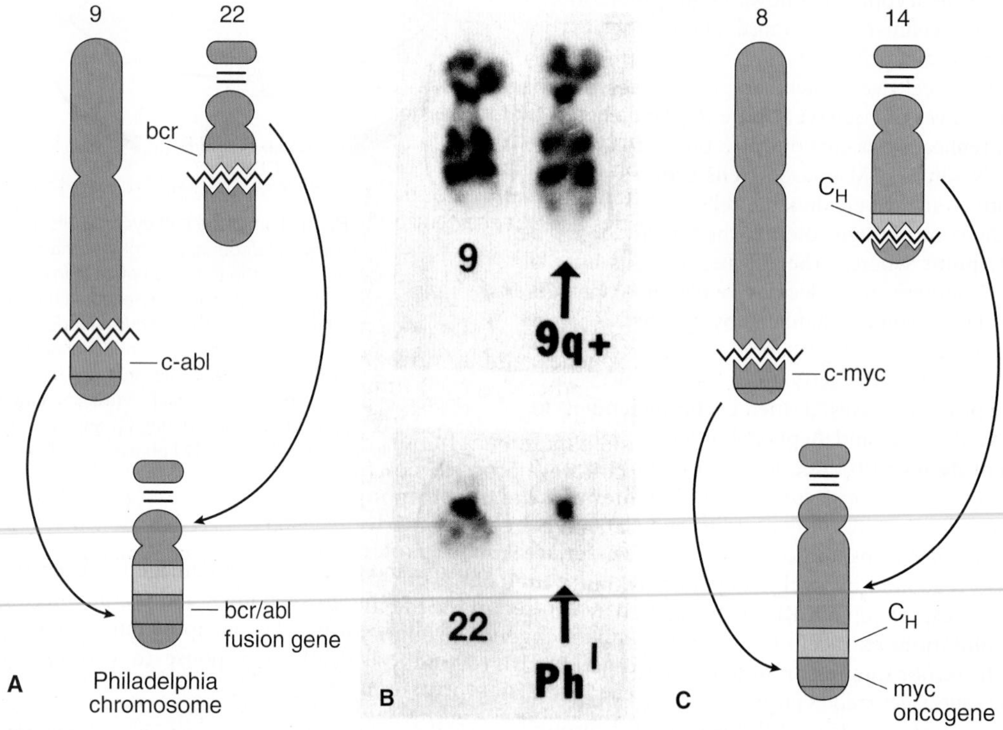

FIGURE 5-23. **Oncogene activation by chromosomal translocation. A.** Chronic myelogenous leukemia. Breaks at the ends of the long arms of chromosomes 9 and 22 allow reciprocal translocations to occur. The c-*abl* protooncogene on chromosome 9 is translocated to the breakpoint region *(bcr)* of chromosome 22. The result is the Philadelphia chromosome, (Ph[1]) which contains a new fusion gene coding for a hybrid oncogenic protein (bcr-abl), presumably involved in the pathogenesis of chronic myelogenous leukemia. **B.** Karyotypes of a patient with chronic myelogenous leukemia showing the results of reciprocal translocations between chromosomes 9 and 22. The Philadelphia chromosome is recognized by a smaller-than-normal chromosome 22 (22q–). One chromosome 9 (9q+) is larger than its normal counterpart. **C.** Burkitt lymphoma. In this disorder, chromosomal breaks involve the long arms of chromosomes 8 and 14. The c-*myc* gene on chromosome 8 is translocated to a region on chromosome 14 adjacent to the gene coding for the constant region of an immunoglobulin heavy chain (C_H). The expression of c-*myc* is enhanced by its association with the promoter/enhancer regions of the actively transcribed immunoglobulin genes.

antiapoptotic signals. The chromosomal translocation that produces the Philadelphia chromosome is an example of oncogene activation by formation of a chimeric (fusion) protein.

In 75% of patients with Burkitt lymphoma (a type of B-cell lymphoma; see Chapter 20), there is a translocation of c-*myc*, a protooncogene involved in cell cycle progression, from its site on chromosome 8 to a position on chromosome 14 (see Fig. 5-23C). This translocation places c-*myc* adjacent to genes that control transcription of the immunoglobulin heavy chains. As a result, the c-*myc* protooncogene is activated by the promoter/enhancer sequences of these immunoglobulin genes and is consequently expressed constitutively rather than in a regulated manner. In 25% of patients with Burkitt lymphoma, the c-*myc* protooncogene remains on chromosome 8 but is activated by translocation of immunoglobulin light-chain genes from chromosome 2 or 22 to the 3′ end of the c-*myc* gene. In either case, a chromosomal translocation does not create a novel chimeric protein but stimulates the overproduction of a normal gene product. In Burkitt lymphoma the excessive amount of the normal c-*myc* product, probably in association with other genetic alterations, leads to the emergence of a dominant clone of B cells, driven relentlessly to proliferate as a monoclonal neoplasm. Many other hematopoietic malignancies, lymphomas, and solid tumors reflect activation of oncogenes by chromosomal translocation. Although some malignant conditions are **initiated** by chromosomal translocations, during the **progression** of many cancers, myriad chromosomal abnormalities take place (translocations, breaks, aneuploidy, etc.).

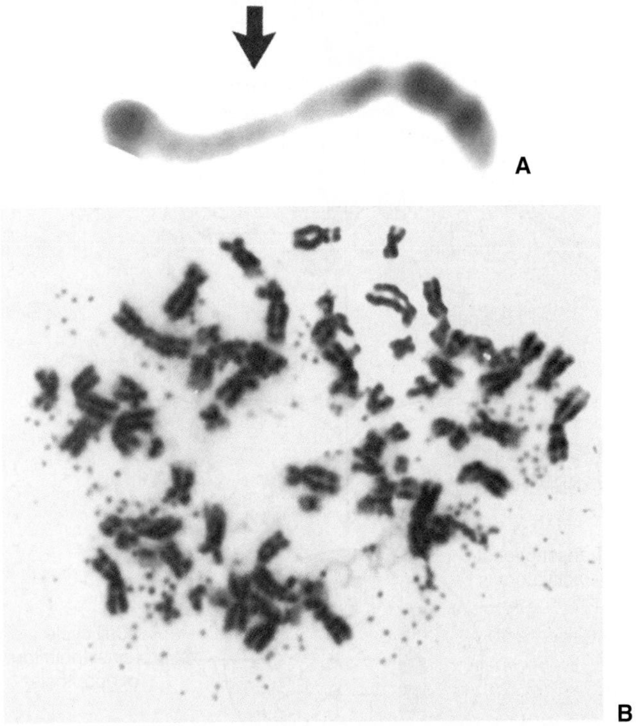

FIGURE 5-24. **Chromosomal alterations in human solid tumors. A.** Homogeneously staining region (HSR; *arrow*) in a chromosome from an ovarian carcinoma. **B.** Double minutes in a karyotype of a soft tissue sarcoma appear as multiple small bodies.

Activation by Gene Amplification

Chromosomal alterations that result in an increased number of gene copies (i.e., gene amplification) have been found primarily in human solid tumors. Such aberrations are recognized as (1) **homogeneous staining regions (HSRs)** (Fig. 5-24A); (2) **abnormal banding regions** on chromosomes; or (3) **double minutes**, which are visualized as multiple, small, paired, cytoplasmic bodies (see Fig. 5-24B). In some cases, gene amplification involves protooncogenes. For example, HSRs derived from the N-*myc* protooncogene may be seen in neuroblastomas. The presence of N-*myc* HSRs is associated with up to a 700-fold amplification of this gene and is a marker of advanced disease with a poor prognosis. Activation of *myc*-family protooncogenes by means of gene amplification has also been demonstrated in small cell carcinoma of the lung, Wilms tumor, and hepatoblastoma.

The *erb B* protooncogene is amplified in up to a third of breast and ovarian cancers. *Erb B2* gene (also designated *HER2/neu*) encodes a receptor-type tyrosine kinase that shows close structural similarity to the EGF receptor. Amplification of *erb B2* in breast and ovarian cancer may be associated with poor overall survival and decreased time to relapse. In this context an antibody targeted against HER2/neu (trastuzumab) is now used as adjunctive therapy for breast cancers that overexpress this protein.

Mechanisms of Oncogene Action

Oncogenes can be classified according to the roles of their normal counterparts (protooncogenes) in the biochemical pathways that regulate growth and differentiation. These include the following (Fig. 5-25 and Fig. 5-26):

- Growth factors
- Cell surface receptors
- Intracellular signal transduction pathways
- DNA-binding nuclear proteins (transcription factors)
- Cell cycle proteins (cyclins and cyclin-dependent protein kinases)
- Inhibitors of apoptosis (bcl-2)

Oncogenes and Growth Factors

The binding of soluble extracellular growth factors to their specific surface receptors initiates signaling cascades that eventuate in entry of the cell into the mitotic cycle. A few protooncogenes encode growth factors that stimulate tumor cell growth. In some instances a growth factor acts upon the same cell that produces it (**autocrine stimulation**). Other growth factors act upon the receptors of neighboring cells (**paracrine stimulation**). Examples of growth factors involved in neoplastic transformation include PDGF and FGF.

PDGF is the protein product of the c-*sis* protooncogene and is a potent mitogen for fibroblasts, smooth muscle cells, and glial cells. Cells derived from human sarcomas and glioblastomas (malignant glial cell tumors) produce PDGF-like polypeptides; their normal counterparts do not. Thus, a normal human gene (c-*sis*) that encodes a growth factor (PDGF) acquires transforming capacity when it is constitutively expressed in a cell that responds to this signal.

An oncogene *(HST)* that codes for a protein with homology to FGF has been identified in human stomach cancer and Kaposi sarcoma. In rodent models, neoplastic cells often express TGF.

Mutational activation of growth factor genes is not well characterized in human cancers. Nevertheless, whether caused by genetic or epigenetic mechanisms, cancer cells generally produce a mixture of growth factors with autocrine or paracrine

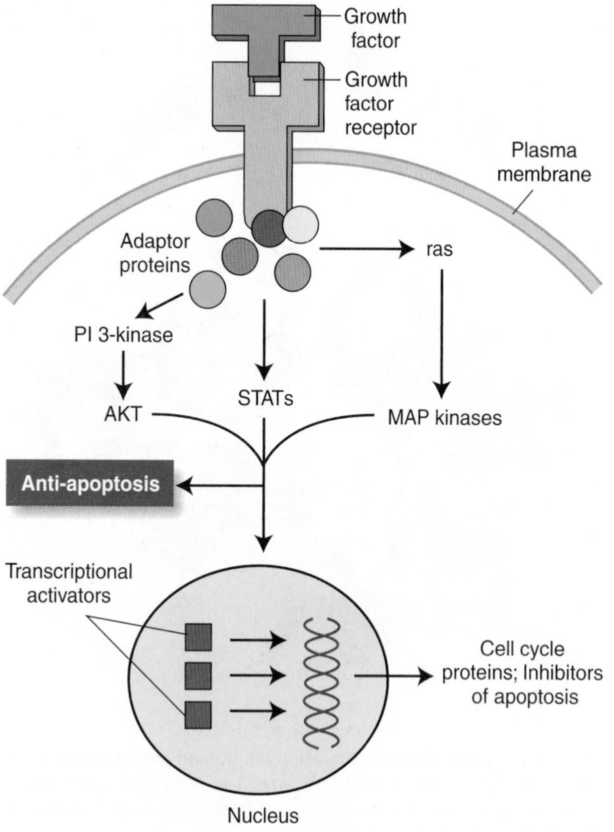

FIGURE 5-25. **Signaling pathways controlling proliferation and apoptosis.** The activation of growth factor receptors by their ligands causes the binding of adaptor proteins and the activation of a series of intracellular signaling molecules leading to transcriptional activation, the induction of cell cycle proteins, and inhibition of apoptosis. Key targets include *ras,* mitogen activated protein (MAP) kinases, signal transducer and activator transcription factors (STATs), phosphatidylinositol 3-kinase (PI 3-kinase), and the serine/threonine kinase AKT.

activity, including insulin-like growth factor-I (IGF-I), PDGF, TGF-α, FGF, colony-stimulating factor-1 (CSF-1), and hepatocyte growth factor (HGF).

Oncogenes and Growth Factor Receptors

Many growth factors stimulate cellular proliferation by interacting with a family of cell surface receptors that are integral membrane proteins with tyrosine kinase activity. In fact, the regulation of the functional responses to growth factors—including cell proliferation, differentiation, and survival—depends principally on the expression of, and relative balance between, various growth factor receptors. Binding of a ligand to the extracellular domain of its receptor stimulates an intrinsic kinase activity in the cytoplasmic domain of the receptor that phosphorylates tyrosine residues on intracellular signaling molecules. *Thus, because growth factor receptors can generate potent mitogenic signals, they harbor a latent oncogenic potential, which when activated, overrides the normal controls of signaling pathways.*

The most common mechanism by which growth factors participate in oncogenesis is overexpression of a normal receptor by enhanced activation of promoters or gene amplification. Under normal circumstances, transient binding of a growth factor to its receptor leads to activation of the cytoplasmic tyrosine kinase domain, after which the receptor reverts to its resting state. Certain mutations of growth factor receptors, including truncation of the extracellular or intracellular domains, point mutations, and deletions, result in unrestrained (constitutive) activation of the receptor, independent of ligand binding. The following examples deserve mention.

- The c-*met* protooncogene encodes a receptor for HGF. Point mutations in the intracellular catalytic domain convert the c-*met* protooncogene to an oncogene that is involved in papillary renal cancers.
- Germline point mutations in c-*ret* lead to constitutive activation of the receptor and are associated with the multiple endocrine neoplasia (MEN) syndromes and familial medullary thyroid carcinoma (see Chapter 21).
- Patients with germ line mutations in the catalytic domain of the c-*kit* tyrosine kinase tend to develop gastrointestinal stromal tumors (GISTs).
- Another abnormality of a growth factor receptor can result from chromosomal translocations that produce hybrid proteins with constitutive tyrosine kinase activity. In the case of the PDGF receptor, a chromosomal translocation [t(5;12)] generates a fusion protein between the cytoplasmic domain of the PDGF receptor and a motif encoded by c-*tel*. The abnormal receptor has been found in patients with myelomonocytic leukemia.

Epigenetic changes that result in increased synthesis of growth factors and their receptors are equally important as mutations and overexpression of growth factor receptors in the pathogenesis of human cancers. In some human malignancies (e.g., breast, ovarian, and stomach cancers), amplification of *HER2/neu* results in autocrine activation that is mediated by overexpression of this growth factor receptor. Of greater importance in human cancers are epigenetic changes that cause increased synthesis of growth factors and receptors.

Oncogenes and Nonreceptor Protein Kinases

A number of proteins that possess tyrosine kinase activity are loosely associated with the inner aspect of the plasma membrane. Although they possess tyrosine kinase activity, they are neither integral membrane proteins nor growth factor receptors. The prototype of a viral oncogene that codes for mutant forms of these protein kinases is v-*src* (see Fig. 5-26). A number of other oncogenes *(abl, lck, yes, fgr, fps, fes)* belong to the *src* family. The homologous c-*src* protooncogene product is expressed in most cells, whereas other members of the *src* family are expressed in specialized cell types, such as hematopoietic cells and epithelia. The src enzymes are activated by most receptor tyrosine kinases and influence cell proliferation, survival, and invasiveness.

The only member of the *src* family that has been implicated in human tumorigenesis is c-*abl*. As discussed above, in chronic myelogenous leukemia this protooncogene, which codes for a cytoplasmic tyrosine kinase, is translocated from chromosome 9 to the breakpoint cluster region *(bcr)* of chromosome 22. The *bcr-abl* fusion gene encodes a mutant protein with conspicuously elevated tyrosine kinase activity, which is necessary for the oncogenic action of the chimeric protein.

Soluble cytoplasmic oncoproteins (*raf, mos, pim*-1) that phosphorylate serine/threonine residues have also been described. The best studied of the soluble cytoplasmic oncoproteins is *raf,* which plays a role in the signal transduction cascade that converts ligand binding by cell surface receptors into nuclear transcriptional activation. Point mutations in c-*raf* occur in up to 10% of human cancers.

Receptor and nonreceptor tyrosine kinases are dephosphorylated and thereby inactivated by a variety of phosphatases. In this context mutations in the phosphatase PTEN (phosphatase and tensin homolog), the product of a tumor suppressor gene (see below), have been linked to a variety of human malignancies.

Ras Oncogenes

Ras is an effector molecule in the signal transduction cascade that couples the activation of growth factor receptors to changes in nuclear gene transcription. The *ras* protooncogene codes for a product, p21, that belongs to a family of small cytoplasmic proteins (G proteins) that bind guanosine triphosphate (GTP) and guanosine diphosphate (GDP). The ras protein, p21, is distinct from the integral membrane G proteins that are involved in receptor-mediated signal transduction (Fig. 5-27). The protein p21 is active when it binds GTP and is inactive when it binds GDP. Bound GTP is converted to GDP by the intrinsic GTPase activity of p21. This enzyme activity is normally very low but is stimulated more than 100-fold by a GTPase-activating protein (GAP). Thus, the inactivating switch for the ras protein is the p21 GTPase.

The discovery of an activated version of the *ras* protooncogene in bladder cancer cells was the first demonstration of a human oncogene. The substitution of valine for glycine at position 12 in p21 was the first mutation characterized in a human oncogene. It is now evident that activation of *ras* genes (Ha-*ras*, Ki-*ras*, or N-*ras*) is the most frequent dominant mutation in human cancers.

The mutant forms of p21 are characterized by persistence of GTP binding, which maintains the protein in its active conformation. Point mutations in the *ras* protooncogene interfere with the hydrolysis of GTP to GDP by rendering p21 resistant to the action of GAP. In addition, some mutations decrease the intrinsic ATPase activity of the ras protein. The persistence of the GTP-bound state results in uncontrolled stimulation of *ras*-related functions, because p21 is locked in the "on" position.

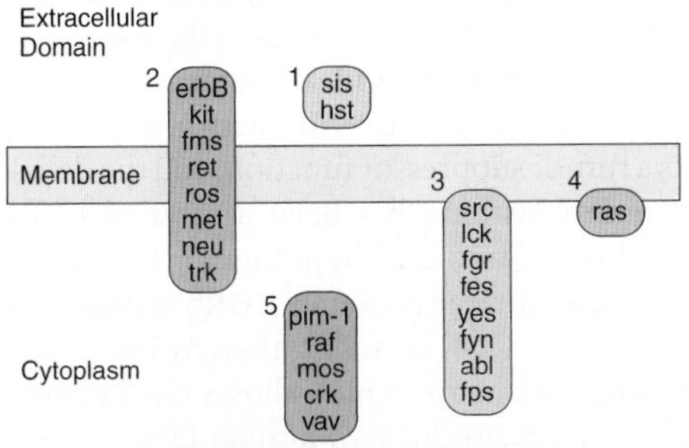

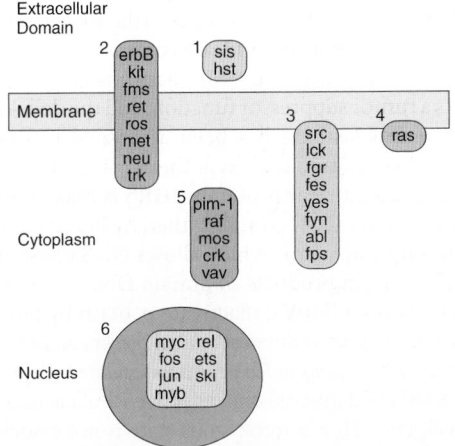

FIGURE 5-26. **Cellular compartments in which oncogene or protooncogene products reside.** *(1)* Growth factors, *(2)* transmembrane growth factor receptors (tyrosine kinase), *(3)* membrane associated kinases, *(4) ras* GTPase family, *(5)* cytoplasmic kinases, *(6)* nuclear transcriptional regulators. GTP = guanosine triphosphate.

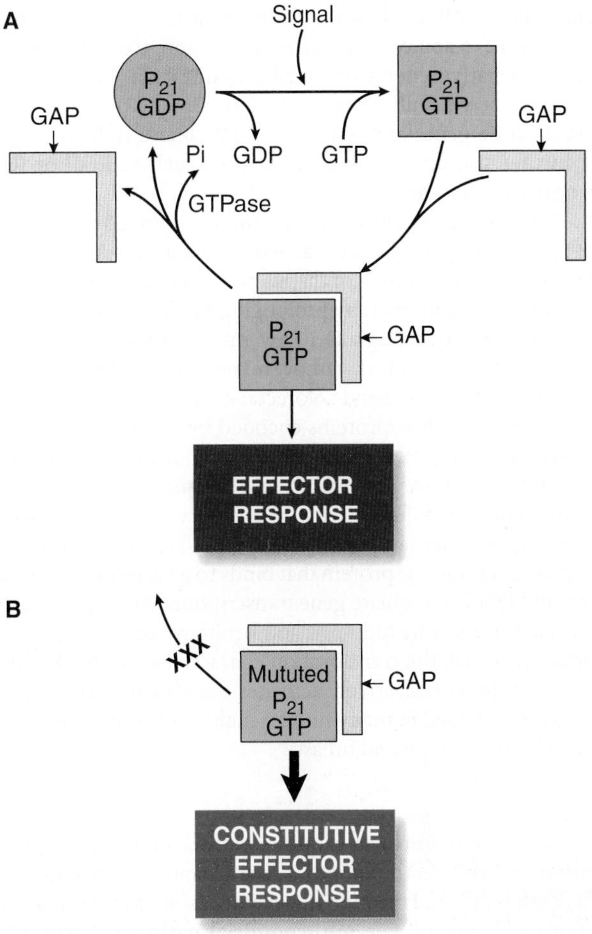

FIGURE 5-27. **Mechanism of action of ras oncogene. A.** Normal. The ras protein p21 exists in two conformational states, determined by the binding of either guanosine diphosphate (GDP) or guanosine triphosphate (GTP). Normally, most of the p21 is in the inactive GDP-bound state. An external stimulus, or signal, triggers the exchange of GTP for GDP, an event that converts p21 to the active state. Activated p21, which is associated with the plasma membrane, binds GTPase-activating protein (GAP) from the cytosol. The binding of GAP has two consequences. In association with other plasma membrane constituents, it initiates the effector response. At the same time, the binding of GAP to p21 GTP stimulates by about 100-fold the intrinsic GTPase activity of p21, thereby promoting the hydrolysis of GTP to GDP and the return of p21 to its inactive state. **B.** Mutated ras protein is locked into the active GTP-bound state because of an insensitivity of its intrinsic GTPase to GAP or because of a lack of the GTPase activity itself. As a result the effector response is exaggerated, and the cell is transformed.

Oncogenes and Nuclear Regulatory Proteins

A number of nuclear proteins encoded by protooncogenes are intimately involved in the sequential expression of genes that regulate cellular proliferation and differentiation. Many of these proteins can bind to DNA, where they regulate the expression of other genes. The transitory expression of several protooncogenes is necessary for the cells to pass through specific points in the cell cycle. For example, the binding of PDGF to cultured fibroblasts causes the cells to leave G_0 and enter the G_1 phase of the cell cycle. Shortly thereafter, several genes, including c-*myc*, c-*fos*, and c-*jun*, are expressed. Protooncogenes that are expressed early in the cell cycle, such as *myc* and *fos*, render the cells competent to receive the final signals for mitosis and are, therefore, termed **competence genes.** In general, competence genes play a role in (1) progression from G_1 to S phase in the cell cycle, (2) stability of the genome, (3) apoptosis, and (4) positive or negative effects on cellular maturation. However, the cells are not yet fully programmed to divide after the expression of these genes and will enter S phase and mitosis only after further stimulation by other factors, such as EGF or IGF-I (**progression factors**).

The proteins encoded by *c-fos* and *c-jun* are components of AP-1, a transcription factor that activates the expression of a variety of genes. Mutations of the *jun* protein eliminate a negative regulatory domain, thereby prolonging its half-life and stimulating progression through G_1. Few mutations of *c-jun* are described in human tumors, but overexpression of the protein has been described in lung and colorectal cancers.

Although nuclear proteins encoded by protooncogenes can promote cellular proliferation, in some circumstances they stimulate differentiation. A rapid increase in *c-fos* expression follows the induction of differentiation in a variety of cells in vitro, including several hematopoietic cell lines and teratocarcinomas.

c-Myc is a nuclear protein that binds to a variety of other proteins and DNA to regulate gene transcription. Among other proteins such targets include p53 and ornithine decarboxylase. As discussed above, the translocation characteristic of Burkitt lymphoma (t8:14) constitutively activates *c-myc* expression. *c-Myc* is also overexpressed in many human malignant tumors (e.g., adenocarcinoma of lung and breast).

Bcl-2 and Apoptosis

Normal tissue requires an exquisite balance between cell proliferation and cell death (apoptosis, see Chapter 1). Programmed cell death is affected through molecular cascades that reflect two major mechanisms. The **mitochondrial pathway** involves the release of cytochrome c, which serves to trigger caspase activation, thereby leading to cell death. A **death receptor pathway** is unleashed by the binding of certain ligands (e.g., Fas, TNF) to cell surface receptors, which results in caspase activation. There is substantial cross-talk between the mitochondrial and the death receptor pathways.

Tumor cells can escape apoptosis by dismantling virtually every aspect of the apoptotic machinery. The most prominent example of suppression of apoptosis in a tumor cell is the upregulation of the antiapoptotic protein bcl-2 in B cell neoplasia. Bcl-2 and its family regulate the permeability of mitochondrial membranes. Bcl-2 itself exerts an antiapoptotic effect by preventing the release of cytochrome c, thereby protecting the cell from the mitochondrial apoptotic pathway.

Follicular B-cell lymphomas (see Chapter 20) display a characteristic chromosomal translocation, t(14;18), in which the *bcl-2* gene on chromosome 18 is brought under the transcriptional control of the immunoglobulin light-chain gene promoter, thereby causing overexpression of *bcl-2*. As a result of the antiapoptotic properties of bcl-2, the neoplastic clone accumulates in the affected lymph nodes. Since its demonstration in follicular lymphomas, *bcl-2* expression has been observed in a variety of other human cancers and nonneoplastic conditions, although the contribution of *bcl-2* to the disease process in these cases is not defined. Many human cancers show other abnormalities in the apoptotic cascades, including the increased expression of endogenous decoys of the death receptors, overexpression of proteins that block caspase activation, inactivating mutations of proapoptotic proteins, and numerous other mechanisms.

Tumor Suppressor Genes Negatively Regulate Cell Growth

The concept of oncogenes postulates a dominant genetic alteration that results in overproduction of a normal gene product or the synthesis of an abnormally active mutant protein (**"gain of function mutations"**). A second general mechanism by which a genetic alteration contributes to carcinogenesis is a mutation that creates a deficiency of a normal gene product (**tumor suppressors** or **"gate keepers"**) that exerts a negative regulatory control of cell growth and thereby suppresses tumor formation (**"loss of function mutations"**). Such genes encode negative transcriptional regulators of the cell cycle, signal-transducing molecules, and cell surface receptors.

Since both alleles of tumor suppressor genes must be inactivated to produce the deficit that allows the development of a tumor, it is inferred that the normal suppressor gene is dominant. In this circumstance, the heterozygous state is sufficient to protect against cancer. The **loss of heterozygosity** (LOH) in a tumor suppressor gene by deletion or somatic mutation of the remaining normal allele predisposes to tumor development.

The Role of Tumor Suppressor Genes in Carcinogenesis

Tumor suppressor genes are increasingly being incriminated in the pathogenesis of both hereditary and spontaneous cancers in humans. Two such genes have been particularly well studied. The Rb and p53 gene products serve to restrain cell division in many tissues, and their absence or inactivation is linked to the development of malignant tumors. In this context, oncogenic DNA viruses encode products that interact with these suppressor proteins, thereby inactivating their functions. *Thus, the mechanisms underlying the development of some tumors associated with germ line and somatic mutations and infections with DNA viruses involve the same cellular gene products.*

Retinoblastoma Gene

Retinoblastoma, a rare childhood cancer, is the prototype of a human tumor whose origin is attributed to the inactivation of a specific tumor suppressor gene. About 40% of cases are associated with a germ line mutation; the remainder are not hereditary. In patients with hereditary retinoblastoma, all somatic cells carry one missing or mutated allele of a gene (the *Rb* gene) located on the long arm of chromosome 13. By contrast, both alleles of the *Rb* gene are inactive in all the retinoblastoma cells. Thus, the *Rb* gene exerts a tumor suppressor function, and the development of hereditary retinoblastoma has been attributed to two genetic events (Knudson's "two-hit" hypothesis) (Fig. 5-28). As mentioned above, the nuclear protein p105Rb is phosphorylated by the activated cyclin/CDK complex, thereby inducing the release of E2F transcription factor, which allows G_1–S phase transition. Additionally, certain products of human DNA viruses (e.g., human papillomavirus [HPV]) inactivate p105Rb by binding to it. *The function of* Rb *genes is the most critical checkpoint in the cell cycle, and inactivating mutations in* Rb *permit unregulated cell proliferation.*

An affected child inherits one defective *Rb* allele together with one normal gene. This heterozygous state is not associated with any observable changes in the retina, presumably because 50% of the *Rb* gene product is sufficient to prevent the development of retinoblastoma. If the remaining normal *Rb* allele is inactivated by deletion or mutation (LOH), the missing suppressor function allows the appearance of a retinoblastoma. Thus, the susceptibil-

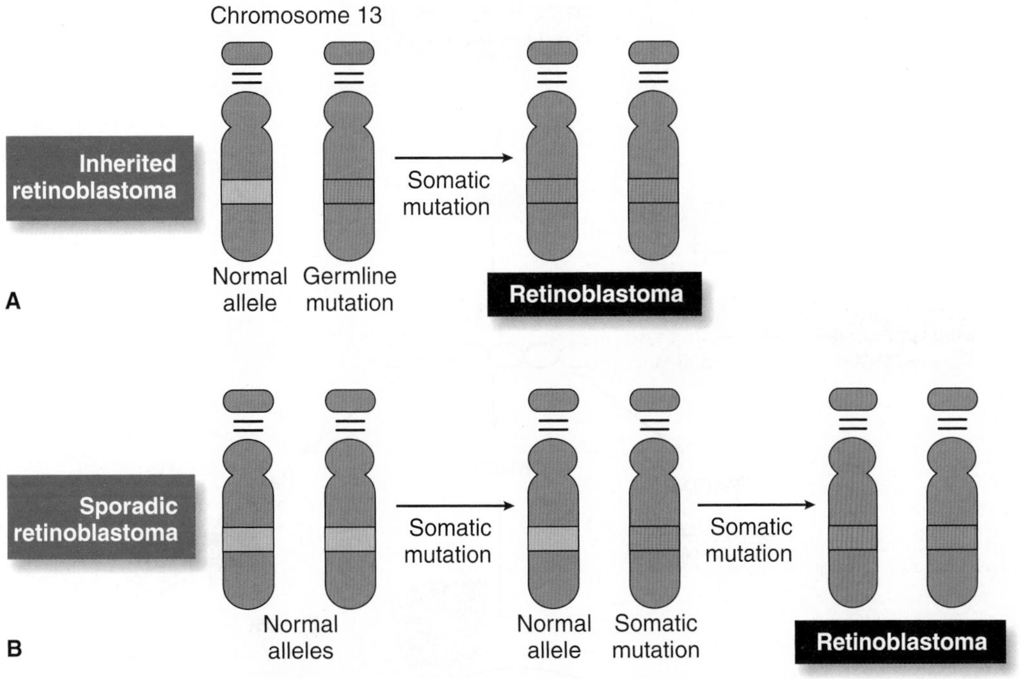

FIGURE 5-28. **The "two-hit" origin of retinoblastoma. A.** A child with the inherited form of retinoblastoma is born with a germ line mutation in one allele of the retinoblastoma gene located on the long arm of chromosome 13. A second somatic mutation in the retina leads to the inactivation of the functioning *Rb* allele and the subsequent development of a retinoblastoma. **B.** In sporadic cases of retinoblastoma, the child is born with two normal *Rb* alleles. It requires two independent somatic mutations to inactivate *Rb* gene function and allow the appearance of a neoplastic clone.

ity to retinoblastoma is inherited in a dominant fashion; that is, the heterozygote develops the disease. Paradoxically, the genetic defect in the tumor itself is recessive. In sporadic cases of retinoblastoma, the child begins life with two normal *Rb* alleles in all somatic cells, but both are inactivated by postzygotic mutations in the retina. Since somatic mutations in the *Rb* gene are uncommon, the incidence of sporadic retinoblastoma is very low (1/30,000).

Children who inherit a mutant *Rb* gene also suffer a 200-fold increased risk of developing mesenchymal tumors in early adult life. More than 20 different cancers have been described, with osteosarcoma being by far the most common. Chromosomal analysis has demonstrated abnormalities of the *Rb* locus in 70% of cases of osteosarcoma and in many instances of small cell lung cancer, carcinomas of the breast, bladder, pancreas, and other human tumors. Many types of *Rb* mutations have been described, including point mutations, insertions, deletions, and translocations. In addition, epigenetic events, such as promoter hypermethylation, may inactivate *Rb*.

The p53 Gene Family

The *p53* tumor suppressor gene is a principal mediator of growth arrest, senescence, and apoptosis (Fig. 5-29). In response to DNA damage, oncogenic activation of other proteins, and other stresses (e.g., hypoxia), p53 levels rise and prevent cells from entering the S phase of the cell cycle, thereby allowing time for DNA repair to take place. In this manner, p53 acts as a "guardian of the genome" by restricting uncontrolled cellular proliferation under circumstances in which cells with abnormal DNA might propagate.

The p53 protein is a transcriptional factor that promotes both the expression of a number of other genes involved in the control of cell cycle progression and apoptosis. DNA damage and other stresses (e.g., hypoxia) upregulate the expression of *p53,* which in turn enhances the synthesis of CKIs. The latter inactivates cyclin/CDK complexes, thereby leading to cell arrest at the G_1/S checkpoint. Cells arrested at this checkpoint may either repair the DNA damage and then reenter the cycle or they may undergo apoptosis. The stimulation of gene transcription by p53 results in the synthesis of proteins (CIP1, GADD45)(see Fig. 5-29) that enhance DNA repair by binding to PCNA. In this manner, the upregulation of p53 has two important and related consequences, namely, arrest of cell cycle progression and promotion of DNA repair.

The *p53* gene is located on the small arm of chromosome 17, and its protein product is present in virtually all normal tissues. This gene is deleted or mutated in 75% of cases of colorectal cancer and frequently in breast cancer, small cell carcinoma of the lung, hepatocellular carcinoma, astrocytoma, and numerous other tumors. *In fact, mutations of p53 seem to be the most common genetic change in human cancer.* Inactivating mutations of *p53* allow cells with damaged DNA to progress through the cell cycle. Many human cancers exhibit deletion of both *p53* alleles, in which case the cell contains no *p53* gene product. By contrast, in some cancers, the malignant cells express one normal *p53* allele and one mutant version. In these cases, the mutant p53 protein forms complexes with the normal p53 protein and thereby inactivates the function of the normal suppressor gene. When a mutant allele inactivates the normal one, the mutant allele is said be a **dominant negative** gene. Theoretically, a cell containing one mutant *p53* allele (i.e., a heterozygote) might have a growth advantage over the normal cells, a situation that would increase the number of cells at risk for a second mutation (loss of heterozygosity) and the development of cancer.

Negative regulation of p53 is principally accomplished by its binding to MDM2 (murine double minute) protein. The formation of the MDM2-p53 complex not only inhibits the function of p53 but also targets it for degradation via the ubiq-

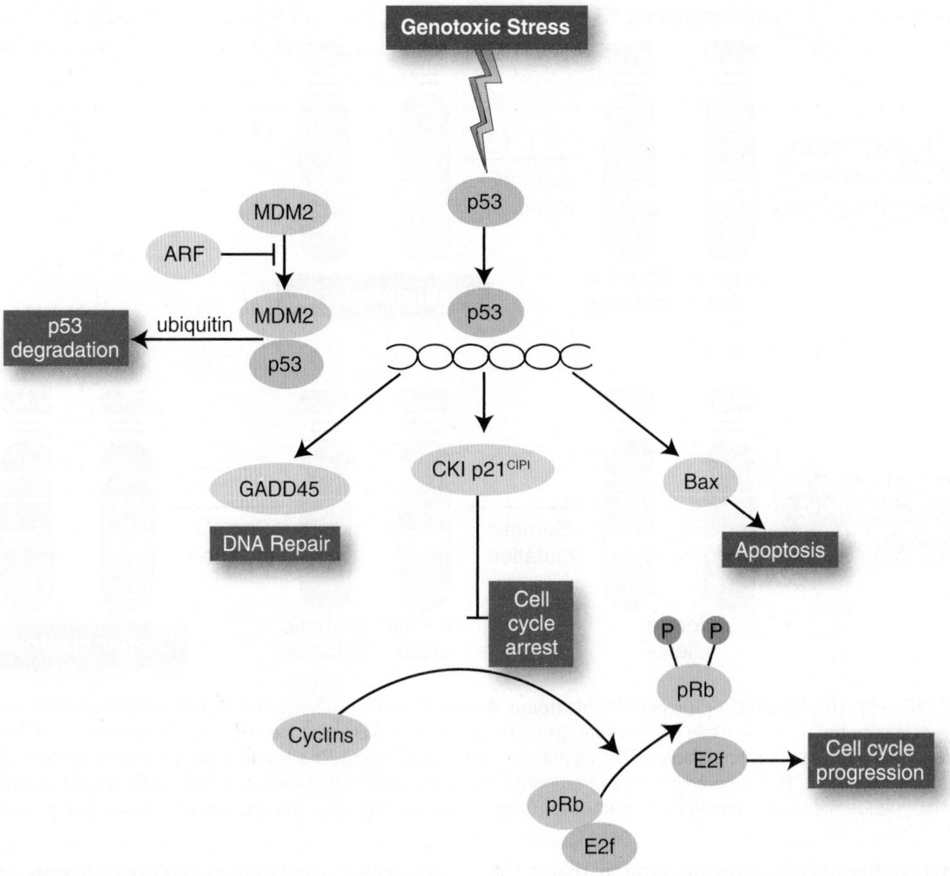

FIGURE 5-29. **P53 regulation of genomic integrity.** In response to genotoxic stress (e.g., ionizing radiation, carcinogens, mutagens), p53 binds to DNA and up-regulates transcription of several genes. Cyclin-dependent kinase inhibitor (CKI) $p21^{CIP1}$ induces cell cycle arrest by preventing the release of E2F from retinoblastoma protein (pRB). GADD45 promotes DNA repair. Bax induces apoptosis, particularly if DNA repair fails. Importantly, cells with loss or mutation of *p53* do not undergo cell cycle arrest and DNA repair, but rather proliferate, generate additional mutations, and increase the risk for the development of malignant tumors. MDM2 (murine double minute) binds to p53 and targets it for ubiquitin-mediated degradation. ARF inhibits MDM2/p53 binding. Reduction in p53 levels in some malignant neoplasms is associated with overexpression of MDM2 or absence of ARF.

uitin pathway. In turn, MDM2 is inhibited by binding to ARF (p14), a protein that is upregulated by any oncogenic stimulus (e.g., *myc, ras*, loss of *Rb*) that induces *Rb* phosphorylation and enhances E2F activity. The function of ARF, which maintains the integrity of p53, establishes *ARF* as another tumor suppressor gene. Some cancers in which both *p53* alleles are normal overexpress MDM2, whereas others do not express functional ARF. As in the case of *Rb*, certain DNA tumor viral products, including HPV E6, promote p53 degradation. Thus, most human cancers display either inactivating mutations of *p53* or abnormalities in the proteins that regulate p53 activity.

Li-Fraumeni syndrome *refers to an inherited predisposition to develop cancers in many organs owing to germ line mutations of* p53. Persons with this condition carry germ line mutations in one *p53* allele, but their tumors display mutations at both alleles. This situation is similar to that determining inherited retinoblastoma and is another example of the two-hit hypothesis (see Fig. 5-28) and LOH.

Other Tumor Suppressor Genes

A number of unrelated syndromes have now been shown to harbor germ line mutations in various tumor suppressor genes:

- ***APC* gene:** This gene is implicated in the pathogenesis of familial adenomatous polyposis coli and most sporadic colorectal cancers (see Chapter 13). The *APC* gene product binds to, and inhibits, the function of β-catenin, an intracellular protein that transmits signals from E-cadherin cell surface adhesion proteins. β-catenin activates certain transcription factors (e.g., tcf/crf-1) that activate several genes, including *myc* and cyclin D, which are involved in cell cycle progression. The products of mutant *APC* genes do not bind to β-catenin and are unable to downregulate its activity. As a result, the expression of *myc* and cyclin D1 is not appropriately repressed, thereby promoting cell proliferation. Further evidence for this mechanism of action comes from the observation that many colorectal tumors in which the *APC* gene is intact exhibit activating mutations in the β-catenin gene. Mutations in both *APC* and β-catenin genes have also been described in other malignant tumors, including malignant melanoma and ovarian cancer.
- ***WT-1* gene:** The tumor suppressor gene *WT-1* is deleted in hereditary Wilms tumor (WT) and is essential for the normal development of the urogenital tract. It encodes a nuclear DNA-binding protein that represses transcription of a variety of genes whose products promote growth and survival, including *PDGF, IGF-I*, and *bcl-2*. Loss of *WT-1* gene expression also occurs in many breast cancers and a few other tumors.
- ***NF-1* gene:** Neurofibromatosis (NF) type 1 is related to germ line mutations of the *NF-1* gene, which encodes *neurofibromin,*

a negative regulator of *ras*. Inactivation of *NF-1* permits unopposed *ras* function and thereby promotes cell growth. Patients with neurofibromatosis-1 are at a substantial risk for the development of neurogenic sarcomas.

- ***VHL* gene:** The inactivation of the von Hippel-Lindau (*VHL*) gene causes the von Hippel-Lindau (VHL) syndrome, which is associated with renal cell carcinoma, hemangioblastoma of the brain, and pheochromocytoma. It is also a major gene involved in the pathogenesis of sporadic renal carcinomas. The normal VHL protein complexes with and inhibits elongin, a molecule that promotes transcriptional elongation of growth-promoting genes by RNA polymerases B and C.
- ***FHIT* gene:** The fragile histidine triad (FHIT) protein is a dinucleoside phosphate hydrolase that is a tumor suppressor. Deletions within the *FHIT* gene, which is found within a fragile chromosome region that is highly susceptible to DNA damage, are associated with cancers of kidney, lung, digestive tract, and other organs. The mechanism by which loss of FHIT activity contributes to tumorigenesis remains to be elucidated, although the normal protein has been shown to be proapoptotic and growth suppressive.
- ***p15* and *p16* genes:** Inactivation of these genes has been identified primarily in breast, pancreas, and prostate tumors, has been detected in many other malignancies. The gene products are CKIs that serve as negative regulators of the cell cycle, and their loss removes a brake on cellular proliferation.
- ***DPC4* gene:** Some 90% of pancreatic carcinomas feature allelic loss or inactivating mutations in the *DPC4* (deleted in pancreatic cancer) gene. The normal DPC4 product is a transcriptional activator that mediates the growth inhibitory response to TGF-β.
- ***BRCA1* and *BRCA2* genes:** These breast (BR) cancer (CA) susceptibility genes, which are also incriminated in some ovarian cancers, are tumor suppressors that are involved in checkpoint functions of the cell cycle related to progression of the cell cycle into S phase, particularly by inducing the CKI p21. BRAC1 and BRAC2 are also thought to promote DNA repair by binding to RAD51, a molecule that mediates DNA double-strand break repairs, thereby functioning as DNA repair genes (see below).
- ***PTEN* gene:** Termed the phosphatase and tensin homologue deleted on chromosome 10, this gene is mutated in most prostate cancers and many gliomas and thyroid cancers, as well as other tumors. The gene product suppresses tumor cell growth by antagonizing tyrosine kinases and may also regulate invasion and metastasis through interactions at focal adhesions. Germ line mutations in *PTEN* are responsible for **Cowden syndrome,** a disorder that includes multiple hamartomas and an increased risk of cancers of the breast, thyroid, and endometrium.

Tumor Suppressor Genes and Oncogenic DNA Viruses

Unlike RNA tumor viruses, whose oncogenes have normal cellular counterparts, the transforming genes of DNA viruses are not homologous with any cellular genes. *The gene products of oncogenic DNA viruses lead to the inactivation of tumor suppressor proteins.* This phenomenon is analogous to the ability of mutant tumor suppressor proteins to inhibit their normal counterparts. Furthermore, the binding of a HPV protein to p53 accelerates the degradation of this suppressor protein. The transforming proteins of polyomaviruses (including SV40), adenoviruses, HPVs, and human herpes virus (HHV)-8 also bind and inactivate Rb protein The interaction of specific viral proteins with Rb releases the E2F family of transcription factors (see Fig. 5-22), which promotes unconstrained cell growth. In addition to activating genes necessary for progression through cell cycle, E2F activates p53 by upregulating the expression of *ARF,* which might provide a defense against aberrant growth. However, DNA tumor viruses have also evolved mechanisms to bind and degrade p53, thereby further "releasing the brake" on cell growth. These observations indicate that oncogenic DNA viruses use common mechanisms for altering growth regulation and, thereby, transforming cells.

DNA Methylation Is an Epigenetic Factor in Cancer

Epigenetics is the alteration in gene expression potential that is unrelated to gene nucleotide sequence. **DNA methylation** represents an important epigenetic regulatory layer for gene transcription. The principal mechanism is the methylation of cytosines within CpG dinucleotides, which occur five times more frequently in so-called CpG islands. DNA methylation patterns are established early in embryogenesis and are finely controlled during development. These regions span the promoter and the first few exons of more than half of all genes. DNA methylation is controlled by a group of enzymes known as the DNA methyltransferases (DNMT) and demethylases. Methylation of these sequences suppresses gene transcription or maintains prior gene silencing by blocking the binding of transcription factors. Another mode of transcriptional repression involves direct binding of specific transcriptional repressors to methylated DNA. DNA methylation can also affect histone modifications and chromatin structure, which, in turn, can alter gene expression. Normal methylation of CpG islands occurs in the case of imprinted genes, inactivated female X chromosomes, germ line genes, and tissue-specific genes. In addition, methylation in the human genome is thought to silence "parasite DNA" such as transposons and endogenous retroviruses, thereby preventing chromosomal instability.

Hypermethylation of many tumor suppressor and DNA repair genes has been demonstrated in human tumors, including the p53 pathway, the APC/β catenin/E-cadherin signaling network, and a number of mismatched DNA repair genes. The pathways controlled by these genes are, therefore, suppressed. For example, about half of human cancers retain unaltered p53. However, the p53 pathway can be inactivated by hypermethylation of *ARF,* thereby preventing inhibition of the MDM2 oncogenic protein and the enhancement of p53 degradation. In this context, aberrant methylation of tumor suppressor genes may be an epigenetic mechanism for a "second hit," thereby leading to LOH. The analysis of gene hypermethylation has promise as a prognostic tool for specific tumors.

The genome of cancer cells also may undergo conspicuous global **hypomethylation**, which may be reflected in up to 60% less DNA methylation than in the normal cell. Hypomethylation usually involves repeated DNA sequences such as long interspersed nuclear elements. Gene hypomethylation may lead to chromosomal instability, derepression of growth regulatory genes, and overexpression of antiapoptotic genes. Unlike genetic changes in cancer, epigenetic changes are potentially reversible, and a search for drugs that influence DNA methylation is under way.

Histone acetylation and deacetylation play important roles in transcriptional regulation by modifying chromatin structure. A high degree of histone acetylation is associated with enhanced transcriptional activity, whereas deacetylation is linked to gene silencing. The yin and yang of acetylation and deacetylation of chromatin are fundamental to the process of cell growth. Experimentally, inhibitors of histone deacetylases arrest tumor growth and prevent the progression of metastases. They also promote apoptosis in animal models of leukemia. Although the precise mechanism of action is not clear, such inhibitors have found a role in the treatment of human acute promyelocytic leukemia and lymphoproliferative diseases.

DNA Repair Genes Protect the Integrity of the Genome

The third class of genes in which mutations contribute to the pathogenesis of cancer are genes involved in DNA mismatch repair, so-called **mutator genes** or **caretaker genes**. The human genome contains roughly 3×10^9 base pairs, distributed evenly among some 10^{14} cells in the body. Considering that DNA is continuously assaulted by mutagenic agents such as radiation, oxidative stress, and chemicals, and that the fidelity of DNA replication is not perfect, it is indeed remarkable that cancer arises in only about one third of the population. In general, the normal versions of the DNA repair genes exercise surveillance over the integrity of genetic information by participating in the cellular response to DNA damage. In this respect, DNA repair genes may be considered "**caretaker genes**." The loss of these gene functions renders the DNA susceptible to the progressive accumulation of mutations; when these affect protooncogenes or tumor suppressor genes, cancer may result.

HEREDITARY NONPOLYPOSIS COLON CANCER (HNPCC): Also known as ***Lynch syndrome****, HNPCC is a familial predisposition to the development of colorectal cancers in persons who do not suffer from APC* (see Chapter 13). It is estimated that some 5% of all colorectal cancers fall into this category. Patients with HNPCC display heterozygous germ line mutations in at least one of five genes involved in the DNA mismatch repair system, whereas the tumors have lost the function of both alleles in the affected gene. After DNA replication is complete, this system leads to the excision and replacement of mismatched nucleotides. Mutations in these error correction genes are associated with up to a 1000-fold general increase in the rate of mutation. Replication errors, termed **microsatellite instability**, are present in the tumor DNA of patients with HNPCC, which arises from uncorrected mispairing of nucleotides and the resulting misalignment of DNA strands. The incidence of cancers of the stomach and small bowel is also increased in patients with HNPCC, and women with this syndrome display an increased risk for endometrial and ovarian cancers.

ATAXIA TELANGIECTASIA: Ataxia telangiectasia (AT) is a rare hereditary syndrome that features cerebellar degeneration; immunologic abnormalities; oculocutaneous telangiectasia; and a predisposition to cancer, including lymphomas, leukemias, stomach cancer, and breast cancer. About 15% of patients with this syndrome eventually die from a malignant disease. The gene responsible for AT (AT mutated [*ATM*]), located on chromosome 11q22-q23, codes for a nuclear phosphoprotein that participates in multiple responses to DNA damage, including control of checkpoints in the cell cycle, activation of DNA repair enzymes, and regulation of apoptosis. There is evidence that heterozygous mutations in *ATM* increase the risk of breast cancer in women. In view of a carrier rate of 1% in the general population, it has been suggested that *ATM* mutations may contribute to a significant number of sporadic breast cancers.

XERODERMA PIGMENTOSUM: Xeroderma pigmentosum is an autosomal recessive disease in which increased sensitivity to sunlight is accompanied by a high incidence of skin cancers, including basal cell carcinoma, squamous cell carcinoma, and malignant melanoma. Several xeroderma pigmentosum genes have been identified that are involved in nucleotide excision of ultraviolet (UV)-damaged DNA.

BLOOM SYNDROME: Bloom syndrome (BS) is an autosomal recessive disorder associated with small size, sun sensitivity, immunodeficiency, and a predisposition to an array of cancers. Cells from patients with BS show a high mutation frequency. The *BS* gene encodes a protein that has helicase activity involved in repair of DNA damage.

Telomerase Is Activated in Most Cancers

As cells in tissue culture continue to divide, the tips of the chromosomes, termed **telomeres**, progressively shorten (see Chapter 1). These structures are thought to protect the integrity of the DNA at the ends of the chromosomes, possibly by preventing exonuclease attack on these regions. Somatic cells do not normally express telomerase, an enzyme that recognizes the end of a chromosome and adds repetitive telomeric sequences to maintain telomere length. Thus, with each round of cell replication, the telomere progressively shortens. It has been proposed that the length of the telomeres acts as a molecular clock that governs the life span of replicating cells. Given that cancer cells have been found to express telomerase, the reactivation of this enzyme is said to be necessary for the immortalization of cancer cells.

Most human cancers show activation of the gene for the catalytic subunit of telomerase: human telomerase reverse transcriptase (hTERT). Although deregulated expression of telomerase might be linked to an increased risk of cancer, telomerase is not classified as an oncogene because it does not lead to growth deregulation. Many immortalized cell lines that express telomerase show no evidence of neoplastic capacity. Thus, despite extensive research in the field, the role of telomerase in oncogenesis remains controversial.

Inherited Cancer Syndromes Encompass a Wide Variety of Tumors

Heritable cancer syndromes attributed to germ line mutations make up only 1% of all cancers. These mutations principally involve tumor suppressor genes and DNA repair genes. As previously discussed for *Rb*, the transmission of a single mutated allele of a tumor suppressor gene results in a heterozygous offspring. Since such persons are at a high risk for LOH (i.e., inactivation of the normal allele), they suffer a conspicuous susceptibility to various types of cancer. Thus, inheritance of cancer susceptibility in such cases is said to be dominant. However, in the tumor cells, both tumor suppressor alleles are inactivated. By contrast, a number of inherited cancer syndromes, mostly involving DNA repair genes, display classical recessive inheritance.

The hereditary tumors can be arbitrarily divided into three categories:

1. Inherited malignant tumors (e.g., Rb, WT, and many endocrine tumors)
2. Inherited tumors that remain benign or have a malignant potential (e.g., APC)
3. Inherited syndromes associated with a high risk of malignant tumors (e.g., Bloom syndrome and ataxia telangiectasia).

TABLE 5-2

Selected Hereditary Conditions Associated with an Increased Risk of Cancer

Syndrome	Gene	Predominant Malignancies	Gene Function	Inheritance*
Chromosomal Instability Syndromes				
Bloom syndrome	*BLM*	Many sites	DNA repair	R
Fanconi anemia	?	Acute myelogenous leukemia	DNA repair	R
Hereditary Skin Cancer				
Familial melanoma	*CDKN2 (p16)*	Malignant melanoma	Cell cycle regulation	D
Xeroderma pigmentosum	*XP group*	Squamous cell carcinoma of skin; malignant melanoma	DNA repair	R
Endocrine System				
Hereditary paraganglioma and pheochromocytoma	*SDHD*	Paraganglioma; pheochromocytoma	Oxygen sensing and signaling	D
Multiple endocrine neoplasia (MEN) type 1	*MEN1*	Pancreatic islet cell tumors	Transcriptional regulation	D
MEN type 2	*RET*	Thyroid medullary carcinoma; Pheochromocytoma (MEN type 2A)	Receptor tyrosine kinase; cell cycle regulation	D
Breast Cancer				
Breast/ovary cancer syndrome	*BRCA1*	Carcinomas of ovary, breast, and prostate	DNA repair	D
Site-specific breast cancer	*BRCA2*	Female and male breast carcinoma; carcinomas of prostate, pancreas and ovary	DNA repair	D
Nervous System				
Retinoblastoma	*Rb*	Retinoblastoma	Cell cycle regulation	D
Phacomatoses				
Neurofibromatosis type 1	*NF1*	Neurofibrosarcomas; astrocytomas; malignant melanomas	Regulator of ras-mediated signaling	D
Neurofibromatosis type 2	*NF2*	Meningiomas; schwannomas	Regulator of cytoskeleton	D
Tuberous sclerosis	*TSC1*	Renal cell carcinoma; astrocytoma	Regulator of cytoskeleton	D
Gastrointestinal System				
Familial adenomatous polyposis	*APC*	Colorectal carcinoma	Cell cycle regulation; migration and adhesion	D
Hereditary nonpolyposis colorectal carcinoma (HNPCC; Lynch syndrome)	*hMSH2, hMSH6, hMLH1, hPMS1, hPMS2*	Carcinomas of colon, endometrium, ovary, and bladder; malignant melanoma	DNA repair	D
Juvenile polyposis coli	*DPC4/SMAD4*	Colorectal carcinoma; endometrial carcinoma	TGF-β signaling	D
Peutz-Jeghers syndrome	*LKB1/STK11*	Stomach, small bowel and colon carcinomas	Serine threonine kinase	D
Kidney				
Hereditary papillary renal cell carcinoma	*MET*	Papillary renal cell carcinoma	Receptor tyrosine kinase; cell cycle regulation	D
Wilms tumor	*WT*	Wilms tumor	Transcriptional regulation	D
Von Hippel-Lindau	*VHL*	Renal cell carcinoma	Regulator of adhesion	D
Multiple Sites				
Carney complex	*PRKARIA*	Testicular neoplasms; thyroid carcinoma	cAMP signaling	D
Cowden syndrome	*PTEN*	Colorectal, breast, and thyroid carcinomas	Protein tyrosine phosphatase	D
Li-Fraumeni syndrome	*TP53*	Breast carcinoma; soft tissue sarcomas; brain tumors; leukemia	Transcriptional regulation	D
Werner syndrome	*WRN*	Soft tissue sarcomas	DNA repair	R
Ataxia-telangiectasia	*ATM*	Lymphoma; leukemia	Cell signaling and DNA repair	R

* D, autosomal dominant; R, autosomal recessive.
ATM = mutated AT (gene); cAMP = cyclic adenosine monophosphate; PTEN = phosphatase and tensin homologue.

Most of these are discussed in detail in the chapters dealing with specific organs, and selected examples are given in Table 5-2. In many cases, the underlying genetic defect responsible for the tumor development has been identified. Some disorders that are difficult to classify, called **phacomatoses** (e.g., tuberous sclerosis, neurofibromatosis), have both developmental and neoplastic features. The tumors associated with these syndromes mostly involve the nervous system.

Although only a small proportion of all cancers show a mendelian pattern of inheritance, certain cancers exhibit an undeniable tendency to run in families. It is estimated that in the case of many tumors, other members of the family of an affected person have a twofold to threefold increase in the risk of developing the same cancer. This predisposition is particularly marked for cancer of the breast and colon. The interplay of heredity and environment is exemplified by the case of lung cancer. Smokers who are closely related to a person with lung cancer have a higher risk of developing lung cancer themselves than smokers without this familial background.

Viruses and Human Cancer

Despite the existence of viral oncogenes, the number of human cancers definitely associated with viral infections is limited. Nevertheless, it is estimated that viral infections are responsible for 15% of all human cancers. The strongest associations between the presence of viruses and the development of cancer in humans are

- Human T-cell leukemia virus type I (HTLV-I) (**RNA retrovirus**) and T-cell leukemia/ lymphoma
- HPV (**DNA**) and carcinoma of the cervix
- Hepatitis B virus (HBV) (**DNA**) and hepatitis C virus (HCV) (**RNA**) and primary hepatocellular carcinoma
- Epstein-Barr virus (EBV) and certain forms of lymphoma and nasopharyngeal carcinoma
- HHV 8 (**DNA**) and Kaposi sarcoma.

Worldwide, infections with hepatitis B and C viruses and HPVs alone account for 80% of all virus-associated cancers.

Human T-Cell Leukemia Virus-I (HTLV-I) Is a Lymphotropic Agent

The one human cancer that has been firmly linked to infection with an RNA retrovirus is the rare adult T cell leukemia, which is endemic in southern Japan and the Caribbean basin and occurs sporadically in other parts of the world. The etiological agent, HTLV-I, is tropic for $CD4^+$ T lymphocytes and has also been incriminated in the pathogenesis of a number of neurologic disorders. It is estimated that leukemia develops in less than 5% of persons infected with HTLV-I and exhibits a latency period on the order of 40 years for the its development. A closely related virus, HTLV-II, has been associated with only a few cases of lymphoproliferative disorders.

The HTLV-I genome contains no known oncogene and does not integrate at specific sites within the host genome. Oncogenic stimulation by HTLV-I is mediated principally by the viral transcriptional activation protein tax. Tax protein not only increases the transcription from its own viral genome, but also promotes the activity of other genes involved in cell proliferation. These include genes that code for interleukin (IL)-2 and its receptor, granulocyte macrophage colony-stimulating factor (GM-CSF), and the protooncogenes *c-fos* and *c-sis*. Lymphocyte transformation in vitro by HTLV-I is initially polyclonal and only later monoclonal. Tax therefore probably initiates transformation, but additional genetic events are required for the appearance of the complete malignant phenotype.

DNA Viruses Encode Proteins That Bind Regulatory Proteins

Four DNA viruses (HPV, EBV, HBV, and HHV 8) are incriminated in the development of human cancers. The transforming genes of oncogenic DNA viruses exhibit virtually no homology with cellular genes, whereas those of RNA retroviruses (oncogenes) are derived from, and are homologous with, their cellular counterparts (protooncogenes). As discussed above, oncogenic DNA viruses have genes that encode protein products that bind to, and inactivate, specific host proteins (the products of tumor suppressor genes, e.g., *Rb, p53*) involved in the regulation of cell proliferation and apoptosis.

Human Papillomaviruses

HPVs induce lesions in humans that progress to squamous cell carcinoma. Papillomaviruses manifest a pronounced tropism for epithelial tissues, and their full productive life cycle occurs only in squamous cells. More than 80 distinct HPVs have been identified, and most are associated with benign lesions of squamous epithelium, including warts, laryngeal papillomas, and condylomata acuminata (genital warts) of the vulva, penis, and perianal region. Occasionally, condylomata acuminata and laryngeal papillomas undergo malignant transformation to squamous cell carcinoma. Although warts of the skin invariably remain benign, in a rare hereditary disease termed **epidermodysplasia verruciformis,** HPV produces flat warts that commonly progress to squamous carcinoma. At least 20 HPV types are associated with cancer of the uterine cervix, especially HPV 16 and 18 (see Chapter 18). A newly available vaccine protects against infection with most oncogenic HPV types and is expected to reduce the incidence of cervical cancer.

The major oncoproteins encoded by HPV are E6 and E7. E6 binds to p53 and targets it for degradation. E7 binds to Rb, thereby releasing its inhibitory effect on cell cycle progression. During the last half century, a cell line derived from cervical cancer, termed *HeLa cells,* has maintained worldwide popularity in the study of cancer. Interestingly, these cells have been found to express HPV-18 E6 and E7, and inactivation of these oncoproteins results in growth arrest. Thus after many years growing in vitro in innumerable laboratories, these cancer cells remain dependent on the expression of HPV proteins.

Epstein-Barr Virus

EBV is a human herpesvirus that is so widely disseminated that 95% of adults in the world have antibodies to it. EBV infects B lymphocytes, transforming them into lymphoblasts with an indefinite lifespan. In a small proportion of primary infections with EBV, this lymphoblastoid transformation is manifested as infectious mononucleosis (see Chapter 9), a short-lived lymphoproliferative disease. However, EBV is also intimately associated with the development of certain human cancers.

When B lymphocytes are infected with EBV, they acquire the ability to proliferate indefinitely in vitro. A number of EBV genes are implicated in this lymphocyte immortalization, including Epstein-Barr nuclear antigens (EBNAs) and latent-infection-associated membrane proteins (LMPs). The EBNAs maintain the EBV genome in its episomal state and activate the transcription of viral and cellular genes. LMP1 interacts with cellular proteins that normally transduce signals from the TNF receptor, a critical pathway in lymphocyte activation and proliferation. *Both EBNAs and LMPs can be demonstrated in most EBV-associated cancers.*

BURKITT LYMPHOMA: EBV was the first virus to be unequivocally linked to the development of a human tumor. In 1958, Burkitt described a form of childhood lymphoma in a geographical belt across equatorial Africa, which he suggested might have a viral etiology. A few years later, Epstein and Barr discovered viral particles in cell lines cultured from patients with Burkitt lymphoma.

African Burkitt lymphoma (BL) is a B cell tumor, in which the neoplastic lymphocytes invariably contain EBV in their DNA and manifest EBV-related antigens (see Chapter 20). The tumor has also been recognized in non-African populations, but in those cases, only about 20% contain the EBV genome. The localization of Burkitt lymphoma to equatorial Africa is not understood, but it has been suggested that prolonged stimulation of the immune system by endemic malaria may be important. Under normal circumstances, the EBV-stimulated B-lymphocyte proliferation is controlled by suppressor T cells. The lack of an adequate T cell response often reported in chronic malarial infections might result in uncontrolled B-cell proliferation, thereby providing the background for further genetic events that lead to the development of lymphoma. As discussed above, one of these is known to be a chromosomal translocation, in which the *c-myc* protooncogene is deregulated by being brought into proximity with an immunoglobulin promoter region. A postulated sequence in the multistep pathogenesis of African Burkitt lymphoma is as follows:

1. Infection and polyclonal lymphoblastoid transformation of B lymphocytes by EBV
2. Proliferation of B cells and inhibition of suppressor T cells induced by malaria
3. Deregulation of the *c-myc* protooncogene by chromosomal translocation in a single transformed B lymphocyte
4. Uncontrolled proliferation of a malignant clone of B lymphocytes

POLYCLONAL LYMPHOPROLIFERATION IN IMMUNODEFICIENT STATES: Congenital or acquired immunodeficiency states can be complicated by the development of EBV-induced B cell proliferative disorders. These lesions may be clinically and pathologically indistinguishable from true malignant lymphomas, but they differ in that most of them are polyclonal. The incidence of lymphoid neoplasia in immunosuppressed renal transplant recipients is 30 to 50 times that of the general population. In virtually all cases of lymphoproliferations associated with organ transplantation, EBNA or EBV genomic material is present in the neoplastic tissue. Similar B cell lymphoproliferative disorders are seen in a number of other acquired immunodeficiencies, notably, acquired immunodeficiency syndrome (AIDS). Occasionally, a true monoclonal lymphoma may develop in the background of an EBV-induced lymphoproliferative disorder. As in the case of Burkitt lymphoma, the deficiency of T cells directed against EBV-infected B cells permits the survival of the latter.

Congenital immunodeficiency states, including X-linked lymphoproliferative syndrome (XLP), Wiskott-Aldrich syndrome, and AT, are associated with EBV infections and aggressive lymphoproliferations. In the familial disorder XLP, clinical immunodeficiency is commonly inapparent until the onset of a particularly severe, and often fatal, form of infectious mononucleosis. In many of these patients who survive infectious mononucleosis, lymphoproliferative disorders and lymphomas ensue. Patients with XLP lack EBV-specific immune responses, including the formation of cytotoxic T cells that normally eliminate EBV-infected B cells.

NASOPHARYNGEAL CARCINOMA: Nasopharyngeal carcinoma is a variant of squamous cell carcinoma that has a worldwide distribution and is particularly common in certain parts of Africa and Asia. EBV DNA and EBNA are present in virtually all of these cancers. It is thought that epithelial cells are exposed to EBV by lysis of infected lymphocytes traveling through lymphoid-rich epithelium. The pathogenesis of nasopharyngeal carcinoma may be related to infection with EBV in early childhood, with reactivation at 40 to 50 years of age and the appearance of tumors 1 to 2 years thereafter. Fortunately, 70% of patients with this disease are cured by radiation therapy alone.

Hepatitis B and C Viruses

Epidemiologic studies have established a strong association between chronic infection with HBV and HCV (chronic hepatitis and cirrhosis) and the development of primary hepatocellular carcinoma (see Chapter 14). Two mechanisms have been invoked to explain the mechanism of carcinogenesis in virus-related liver cancer. One theory holds that the continued liver cell proliferation that accompanies chronic liver injury eventually leads to malignant transformation. However, a small subset of patients with HBV infection develop hepatocellular carcinoma in noncirrhotic livers. A second theory implicates a virally encoded protein in the pathogenesis of HBV-induced liver cancer. Transgenic mice expressing HBx, a small viral regulatory protein, also develop liver cancer, but without evident preexisting liver cell injury and inflammation. The *HBx* gene product has been shown in vitro to upregulate a number of cellular genes. In addition, like other DNA viral oncoproteins, HBx binds to and inactivates p53. The underlying mechanisms in HBV-induced carcinogenesis are still controversial and require further investigation.

Human Herpesvirus 8 (HHV 8)

Kaposi sarcoma is a vascular neoplasm that was originally described in eastern European elderly men and later in central African blacks (see Chapter 10). Kaposi sarcoma is today the most common neoplasm associated with AIDS. The neoplastic cells contain sequences of a novel herpesvirus, HHV 8. Interestingly, HHV 8 has also been demonstrated in specimens of Kaposi sarcoma from HIV-negative patients. In addition to infecting the spindle cells of Kaposi sarcoma, HHV 8 is lymphotropic and has been implicated in two uncommon B-cell lymphoid malignancies, namely, **primary effusion lymphoma** and **multicentric Castleman disease.**

Like other DNA viruses, the viral genome encodes proteins that interfere with the p53 and RB tumor suppressor pathways. HHV 8 also encodes gene products that downregulate class I major histocompatibility complex (MHC) expression, a mechanism by which the infected cells may evade recognition by cytotoxic T lymphocytes.

Chemical Carcinogenesis

The field of chemical carcinogenesis originated some 2 centuries ago in descriptions of an occupational disease (this was not the first recognition of an occupation-related cancer, since a peculiar predisposition of nuns to breast cancer was appreciated even earlier). The English physician Sir Percival Pott gets credit for relating cancer of the scrotum in chimney sweeps to a specific chemical exposure, namely, soot. Today we realize that other products of the combustion of organic materials are responsible for a man-made epidemic of cancer, namely, lung cancer in cigarette smokers.

The experimental production of cancer by chemicals dates to 1915, when Japanese investigators produced skin cancers in rabbits with coal tar. Since that time, the list of organic and inorganic carcinogens has grown exponentially. Yet a curious paradox existed for many years. Many compounds known to be potent carcinogens are relatively inert in terms of chemical reactivity. *The solution to this riddle became apparent in the early 1960s, when it was shown that most, although not all, chemical carcinogens require metabolic activation before they can react with cell constituents.* On the basis of those observations and the close correlation between mutagenicity and carcinogenicity, an in vitro assay using *Salmonella* organisms for screening potential chemical carcinogens—the Ames test—was developed a decade later. Subsequently, a variety of genotoxicity assays have been developed and are still used to screen chemicals and new drugs for potential carcinogenicity.

Chemical Carcinogens Are Mostly Mutagens

Associations between exposure to a specific chemical and human cancers have historically been established on the basis of epidemiologic investigations. These studies have numerous inherent disadvantages, including uncertainties in estimated doses, variability of the population, long and variable latency, and dependence on clinical and public health records of questionable accuracy. As an alternative to epidemiologic studies, investigators turned to the use of studies involving animals. Indeed, such studies are legally required before the introduction of a new drug. Yet the logarithmic increase in the number of chemicals synthesized every year makes even this method prohibitively cumbersome and expensive. The search for rapid, reproducible, and reliable screening assays for potential carcinogenic activity has centered on the relationship between carcinogenicity and mutagenicity.

*A **mutagen** is an agent that can permanently alter the genetic constitution of a cell.* The Ames test uses the appearance of frameshift mutations and base-pair substitutions in a culture of bacteria of a *Salmonella* species. Mutations, unscheduled DNA synthesis, and DNA strand breaks are also detected in rat hepatocytes, mouse lymphoma cells, and Chinese hamster ovary cells. Cultured human cells are now used increasingly for assays of mutagenicity. About 90% of known carcinogens are mutagenic in these systems. Moreover, most, but not all, mutagens are carcinogenic. This close correlation between carcinogenicity and mutagenicity presumably occurs because both reflect damage to DNA. Although not infallible, in vitro mutagenicity assays have proved to be valuable tools in screening for the carcinogenic potential of chemicals.

Chemical Carcinogenesis Is a Multistep Process

Studies of chemical carcinogenesis in experimental animals have shed light on the distinct stages in the progression of normal cells to cancer. Long before the genetic basis of cancer was appreciated, it was demonstrated that a single application of a carcinogen to the skin of a mouse was not, by itself, sufficient to produce cancer. However, when a proliferative stimulus was then applied locally, in the form of a second, noncarcinogenic, irritating chemical (e.g., a phorbol ester), tumors appeared. The first effect was termed **initiation.** The action of the second, noncarcinogenic chemical was called **promotion.** Subsequently, further experiments in rodent models of a variety of organ-specific cancers (liver, skin, lung, pancreas, colon, etc.) expanded the concept of a two-stage mechanism to our present understanding of *carcinogenesis as a multistep process that involves numerous mutations.*

From these studies, one can abstract four stages of chemical carcinogenesis:

1. **Initiation** likely represents a mutation in a single cell.
2. **Promotion** reflects the clonal expansion of the initiated cell, in which the mutation has conferred a growth advantage. During promotion the altered cells remain dependent on the continued presence of the promoting stimulus. This stimulus may be an exogenous chemical or physical agent or may reflect an endogenous mechanism (e.g., hormonal stimulation [breast, prostate] or the effect of bile salts [colon]).
3. **Progression** is the stage in which growth becomes autonomous (i.e., independent of the carcinogen or the promoter). By this time, sufficient mutations have accumulated to immortalize cells.
4. **Cancer,** the end result of the entire sequence, is established when the cells acquire the capacity to invade and metastasize.

The morphologic changes that reflect multistep carcinogenesis in humans are best exemplified in epithelia, such as those of the skin, cervix, and colon. Although initiation has no morphologic counterpart, *promotion and progression are represented by the sequence of hyperplasia, dysplasia, and carcinoma in situ.*

Chemical Carcinogens Usually Undergo Metabolic Activation

The International Agency for Research in Cancer (IARC) has listed about 75 chemicals as human carcinogens. Chemicals cause cancer either directly or, more often, after metabolic activation. The direct-acting carcinogens are inherently reactive enough to bind covalently to cellular macromolecules. A number of organic compounds, such as nitrogen mustard, *bis*(chloromethyl)ether, and benzyl chloride, as well as certain metals are included in this category. Most organic carcinogens, however, require conversion to an ultimate, more reactive compound. This conversion is enzymatic and, for the most part, is effected by the cellular systems involved in drug metabolism and detoxification. Many cells in the body, particularly liver cells, possess enzyme systems that can convert procarcinogens to their active forms. Yet each carcinogen has its own spectrum of target tissues, often limited to a single organ. The basis for organ specificity in chemical carcinogenesis is not well understood.

POLYCYCLIC AROMATIC HYDROCARBONS: The polycyclic aromatic hydrocarbons, originally derived from coal tar, are among the most extensively studied carcinogens. In this class are such model compounds as benzo(a)pyrene, 3-methylcholanthrene, and dibenzanthracene. These compounds have a broad range of target organs and generally produce cancers at the site of application. The specific type of cancer produced varies with the route of administration and includes tumors of the skin, soft tissues, and breast. Polycyclic hydrocarbons have been identified in cigarette smoke, and so it has been suggested, but not proved, that they are involved in the production of lung cancer.

Polycyclic hydrocarbons are metabolized by cytochrome P450-dependent mixed function oxidases to electrophilic epoxides, which in turn react with proteins and nucleic acids. The formation of the epoxide depends on the presence of an unsaturated carbon–carbon bond. For example, vinyl chloride, the simple two-carbon molecule from which the widely used plastic polyvinyl chloride is synthesized, is metabolized to an epoxide, which is responsible for its carcinogenic properties. Workers exposed to the vinyl chloride monomer in the ambient atmosphere later developed hepatic angiosarcomas.

ALKYLATING AGENTS: Many chemotherapeutic drugs (e.g., cyclophosphamide, cisplatin, busulfan) are alkylating agents that transfer alkyl groups (methyl, ethyl, etc.) to macromolecules, including guanines within DNA. Although such drugs destroy cancer cells by damaging DNA, they also injure normal cells. Thus, alkylating chemotherapy carries a significant risk of solid and hematological malignancies at a later time.

AFLATOXIN: In contrast to the polycyclic hydrocarbons, which are for the most part formed either by the combustion of organic material or synthetically, a heterocyclic hydrocarbon, aflatoxin B_1, is a natural product of the fungus *Aspergillus flavus*. Like the polycyclic aromatic hydrocarbons, aflatoxin B_1 is metabolized to an epoxide, which can bind covalently to DNA. Aflatoxin B_1 is among the most potent liver carcinogens recognized, producing tumors in fish, birds, rodents, and primates. Since *Aspergillus* species are ubiquitous, contamination of vegetable foods exposed to the warm moist conditions, particularly peanuts and grains, may result in the formation of significant amounts of aflatoxin B_1. It has been suggested that in addition to hepatitis B and C, aflatoxin-rich foods may contribute to the high incidence of cancer of the liver in parts of Africa and Asia. In rodents exposed to aflatoxin B_1, the resulting liver tumors exhibit a specific inactivating mutation in the *p53* gene (G:C → T:A transversion at codon 249). Interestingly, human liver cancers in areas of high dietary concentrations of aflatoxin carry the same *p53* mutation.

AROMATIC AMINES AND AZO DYES: Aromatic amines and azo dyes, in contrast to the polycyclic aromatic hydrocarbons, are not ordinarily carcinogenic at the point of application. However, they commonly produce bladder and liver tumors, respectively, when fed to experimental animals. Both aromatic amines and azo dyes are primarily metabolized in the liver. The activation reaction undergone by aromatic amines is N-hydroxylation to form the hydroxylamino derivatives, which are then detoxified by conjugation with glucuronic acid. In the bladder, hydrolysis of the glucuronide releases the reactive hydroxylamine. Occupational exposure to aromatic amines in the form of aniline dyes has resulted in bladder cancer.

NITROSAMINES: Carcinogenic nitrosamines are a subject of considerable study because it is suspected that they may play a role in human gastrointestinal neoplasms and possibly other cancers. The simplest nitrosamine, dimethylnitrosamine, produces kidney and liver tumors in rodents. Nitrosamines are also potent carcinogens in primates, although unambiguous evidence of cancer induction in humans is lacking. However, the extremely high incidence of esophageal carcinoma in the Hunan province of China (100 times higher than in other areas) has been correlated with the high nitrosamine content of the diet. There is concern that nitrosamines may also be implicated in other gastrointestinal cancers because nitrites, commonly added to preserve processed meats and other foods, may react with other dietary components to form nitrosamines. In addition, tobacco-specific nitrosamines have been identified, although a contribution to carcinogenesis has not been proved. Nitrosamines are activated by hydroxylation, followed by formation of a reactive alkyl carbonium ion.

METALS: A number of metals or metal compounds can induce cancer, but the carcinogenic mechanisms are unknown. Divalent metal cations, such as nickel (Ni^{2+}), lead (Pb^{2+}), cadmium (Cd^{2+}), cobalt (Co^{2+}), and beryllium (Be^{2+}), are electrophilic and can, therefore, react with macromolecules. In addition, metal ions react with guanine and phosphate groups of DNA. A metal ion such as Ni^{2+} can depolymerize polynucleotides. Some metals can bind to purine and pyrimidine bases through covalent bonds or pi electrons of the bases. These reactions all occur in vitro, and the extent to which they occur in vivo is not known. Most metal-induced cancers occur in an occupational setting (see Chapter 9).

Endogenous and Environmental Factors Influence Chemical Carcinogenesis

Chemical carcinogenesis in experimental animals involves consideration of genetic aspects (species and strain, age and sex of the animal), hormonal status, diet, and the presence or absence of inducers of drug-metabolizing systems and tumor promoters. A similar role for such factors in humans has been postulated on the basis of epidemiologic studies.

METABOLISM OF CARCINOGENS: **Mixed-function oxidases** are enzymes whose activities are genetically determined, and a correlation has been observed between the levels of these enzymes in various strains of mice and their sensitivity to chemical carcinogens. Since most chemical carcinogens require metabolic activation, agents that enhance the activation of procarcinogens to ultimate carcinogens should lead to greater carcinogenicity, whereas those that augment the detoxification pathways should reduce the incidence of cancer. In general, this is the case experimentally. Since humans are exposed to many chemicals in the diet and environment, such interactions are potentially significant.

SEX AND HORMONAL STATUS: These factors are important determinants of susceptibility to chemical carcinogens but are highly variable and in many instances not readily predictable. In experimental animals, there is sex-linked susceptibility to the carcinogenicity of certain chemicals. However, the effects of sex and hormonal status on chemical carcinogenesis in humans are not clear.

DIET: The composition of the diet can affect the level of drug-metabolizing enzymes. Experimentally, a low-protein diet, which reduces the hepatic activity of mixed-function oxidases, is associated with decreased sensitivity to hepatocarcinogens. In the case of dimethylnitrosamine, the decreased incidence of liver tumors is accompanied by an increased incidence of kidney tumors, an observation that emphasizes the fact that the metabolism of carcinogens may be regulated differently in different tissues.

Physical Carcinogenesis

The physical agents of carcinogenesis discussed here are UV light, asbestos, and foreign bodies. Radiation carcinogenesis is discussed in Chapter 9.

Ultraviolet Radiation Causes Skin Cancers

Among fair-skinned persons, a glowing tan is commonly considered the mark of a successful holiday. However, this overt manifestation of the alleged healthful effects of the sun conceals underlying tissue damage. The harmful effects of solar radiation were recognized by ladies of a bygone era, who shielded themselves from the sun with parasols to maintain a "roses-and-milk" complexion and to prevent wrinkles. The more recent fad for a tanned complexion has been accompanied not only by cosmetic deterioration of facial skin but also by an increased incidence of the major skin cancers.

Cancers attributed to sun exposure, namely, basal cell carcinoma, squamous carcinoma, and melanoma, occur predominantly in persons of the white race. The skin of persons of the darker races is protected by the increased concentration of melanin pigment, which absorbs UV radiation. In fair-skinned people, the areas exposed to the sun are most prone to develop skin cancer. Moreover, there is a direct correlation between total exposure to sunlight and the incidence of skin cancer.

UV radiation is the short-wavelength portion of the electromagnetic spectrum adjacent to the violet region of visible light. It appears that only certain portions of the UV spectrum are associated with tissue damage, and a carcinogenic effect occurs at wavelengths between 290 and 320 nm. *The effects of UV radiation on cells include enzyme inactivation, inhibition of cell division, mutagenesis, cell death, and cancer.*

The most important biochemical effect of UV radiation is the formation of **pyrimidine dimers** in DNA, a type of DNA damage that is not seen with any other carcinogen. Pyrimidine dimers may form between thymine and thymine, between thymine and cytosine, or between cytosine pairs alone. Dimer formation leads to a cyclobutane ring, which distorts the phosphodiester backbone of the double helix in the region of each dimer. Unless efficiently eliminated by the nucleotide excision repair pathway, genomic injury produced by UV radiation is mutagenic and carcinogenic.

Xeroderma pigmentosum, an autosomal recessive disease, exemplifies the importance of DNA repair in protecting against the harmful effects of UV radiation. In this rare disorder, sensitivity to sunlight is accompanied by a high incidence of skin cancers, including basal cell carcinoma, squamous cell carcinoma, and melanoma. Both the neoplastic and non-neoplastic disorders of the skin in xeroderma pigmentosum are attributed to an impairment in the excision of UV-damaged DNA.

Asbestos Causes Mesothelioma

Pulmonary asbestosis and asbestosis-associated neoplasms are discussed in Chapter 12. Here we review possible mechanisms of carcinogenesis attributed to asbestos. In this context, it is not conclusively established whether the cancers related to asbestos exposure should be considered examples of chemical carcinogenesis or of physically induced tumors, or both.

Asbestos, a material widely used in construction, insulation, and manufacturing, is a family of related fibrous silicates, which are classed as "serpentines" or "amphiboles." Serpentines, of which chrysotile is the only example of commercial importance, occur as flexible fibers; the amphiboles, represented principally by crocidolite and amosite, are firm narrow rods.

*The characteristic tumor associated with asbestos exposure is **malignant mesothelioma** of the pleural and peritoneal cavities.* This cancer, which is exceedingly rare in the general population, has been reported to occur in 2% to 3% (in some studies even more) of heavily exposed workers. The latent period (i.e., the interval between exposure and the appearance of a tumor) is usually about 20 years but may be twice that figure. It is reasonable to surmise that mesotheliomas of both pleura and peritoneum reflect the close contact of these membranes with asbestos fibers transported to them by lymphatic channels.

The pathogenesis of asbestos-associated mesotheliomas is obscure. Thin crocidolite fibers are associated with a considerably greater risk of mesothelioma than shorter and thicker amosite fibers or flexible chrysotile fibers. However, the distinction between these fibers in the causation of human disease should not be taken as absolute, particularly since mixtures of these fibers are characteristically found in human lungs.

An association between cancer of the lung and asbestos exposure is clearly established in smokers. A slight increase in the prevalence of lung cancer has been reported in nonsmokers exposed to asbestos, but the small number of cases renders an association questionable. Claims that exposure to asbestos increases the risk of gastrointestinal cancer have not withstood statistical analysis of the collected data. In any case, the widespread adoption of strict safety standards will undoubtedly relegate the hazards of asbestos to historical interest.

Foreign Bodies Produce Experimental Cancer

In implantation of inert materials induces sarcomas in certain experimental animals. However, *humans are resistant to foreign body carcinogenesis, as evidenced by the lack of cancers following the implantation of prostheses constructed of plastics and metals.* A few reports of cancer developing in the vicinity of foreign bodies in humans probably reflect scar formation, which in some organs seems to be associated with an increased incidence of cancers. Despite numerous contrary claims in lawsuits, there is no evidence that a single traumatic injury can lead to any form of cancer.

The genomic mechanisms underlying the development of neoplasia are summarized in Figure 5-30.

Tumor Immunology

It has long been recognized that malignant tumors elicit a chronic inflammatory response that is unrelated to necrosis or infection of the tumor. This observation led early investigators to postulate a host immune reaction to the neoplastic cells, but a refined understanding awaited the development of modern immunology. The inflammatory reaction is correlated with a better prognosis in some tumors, such as medullary carcinoma of the breast and seminoma, but in general no clear correlation exists. Although the infiltrate is composed principally of T cells and macrophages, suggesting a cell-mediated immune response, the antigens to which the cells respond have not been identified. Despite the paucity of direct evidence in human cancers, it is clear from animal experiments that immune defenses against malignant tumors exist.

Immunologic Defenses against Cancer Have Been Demonstrated in Experimental Animals and Humans

To invoke a role for an immune defense against cancer, it is necessary to postulate that tumor cells express antigens that differ from those of normal cells and that are recognized as foreign by the host. Such a condition has been indirectly demonstrated in experiments with inbred mice. When cells from a chemically induced or virally induced tumor are transplanted into a syngeneic mouse, the cells form a tumor. When cells from this tumor are passed into a second mouse, they again form a tumor. *However, if the first transplanted tumor is removed before it metastasizes (i.e., the mouse is cured of its tumor), reinjection of the tumor cells back into the cured mouse will not produce a tumor.* The transplanted tumor is **rejected** because of immunity acquired as a result of the first tumor transplant. Moreover, irradiated tumor cells or preparations of tumor cell membranes, when injected experimentally, aug-

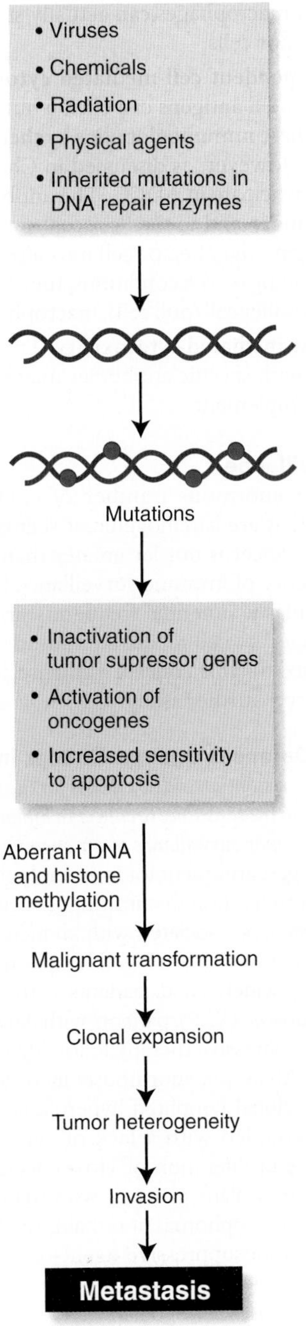

FIGURE 5-30. **Summary of the genomic mechanisms of cancer.**

ment resistance to tumor growth. Why the original tumor is not destroyed by the immunologic reaction remains unexplained.

An important observation is that tumors induced by the same chemical in different mice are antigenically distinct, whereas those induced by the same virus express the same virally determined antigens. Accordingly, mice sensitized to one chemically induced tumor do not reject a second tumor induced by the same chemical. By contrast, mice that have received a virus-induced tumor reject another similar tumor. These experiments provide compelling evidence that immunologic mechanisms can play a role in host defenses against tumors, at least against experimental tumors in animals.

Further evidence for the existence of immune mechanisms in the defense against cancer comes from studies in nude mice. These animals are devoid of T-cell-mediated immunity and thus accept grafts from different species. Similarly, tumors from different species grow in an unrestrained fashion when transplanted into nude mice.

The effectiveness of immune mechanisms to limit the growth of malignant cells can be demonstrated by mixing mouse tumor cells with immune effector cells from a syngeneic mouse that has been sensitized to the tumor. The mixture is then injected into a normal (unsensitized) syngeneic recipient. In many instances, the growth of the tumor cells in the recipient is inhibited, compared with that of tumor cells mixed with unsensitized lymphoid cells. Similar approaches have been tested in cases of human melanoma. However, it has not proved possible to cure human melanomas by reinjecting tumor-sensitized lymphocytes into the patient.

Tumor Antigens

The immune response to experimental tumors must necessarily be directed against tumor antigens on the surface of malignant cells. Such antigens can be tumor-specific; that is, they are uniquely expressed by the cancer cells but not by their normal cellular counterparts. Alternatively, other tumor antigens represent proteins that are expressed by some normal cells, such as those in developing embryos. Such antigens are tumor-associated, rather than tumor-specific.

In experimental animals, tumors produced by chemicals and viruses display tumor-specific antigens. As noted above, each chemically induced cancer expresses unique tumor antigens; that is, no two tumors are antigenically alike. The precise nature of these antigens is obscure, although some may be altered histocompatibility antigens. By contrast, all tumors induced by the same virus express the same tumor-specific antigens, presumably because they are products encoded by the viral genome.

It is much more difficult to document the presence of tumor-specific antigens in human cancers, because patients cannot be subjected to an immunization challenge with tumor cells, as is used in experimental animals. Yet despite this experimental limitation, candidate human tumor-specific antigens have begun to emerge, for example, virally encoded antigens in tumors whose pathogenesis is linked to viruses (e.g., HPV). Neoantigens encoded by altered gene sequences have also been detected in malignant cells resulting from mutations or translocations. The tumor-specific antigens identified to date are peptides complexed to human leukocyte antigen (HLA) molecules on tumor cell surfaces.

There has been even more progress in identifying tumor-associated antigens for both human and experimental animal tumors. Early studies on melanoma showed that certain HLA-associated peptide antigens correspond to proteins that are present in small amounts in the adult but are abundant during development. Such tumor-associated oncodevelopmental antigens are not specific for a given patient's tumor per se but instead are shared by cancers in different persons and sometimes of varying histologic type. Although, there is no reason to believe that immune responses to these fetal antigens play any role in the host defense against cancer, their presence in the blood or the tumor (e.g., CEA, AFP) is useful in clinical diagnosis and treatment.

Inroads into the identification of tumor antigens have created new opportunities for developing immunotherapies against human cancers, at least in theory. Passive immunotherapies can draw upon tumor-infiltrating lymphocytes with specificity for

HLA-associated tumor peptide antigens and antibodies directed against various tumor surface proteins. Alternatively, active immunotherapeutic strategies can invoke tumor antigens as vaccines to elicit systemic antitumor immune responses.

Mechanisms of Immunologic Cytotoxicity

The contribution of any specific immunologic mechanism to tumor cell destruction in vivo has not been clearly defined. A number of possible mechanisms are recognized (Fig. 5-31):

- **T cell-mediated cytotoxicity:** The capacity of cytotoxic T cells to mediate the specific rejection of transplanted tumors is evidenced by the demonstration that lymphocytes from tumor-bearing hosts can transfer tumor immunity when injected into normal animals. Moreover, the transferred immunity is eliminated by the administration of antibodies directed against T-cell antigens. The mechanisms of T cell-mediated immunological cell killing are discussed in Chapter 4.
- **Natural killer cell-mediated cytotoxicity:** Another set of lymphocytes, the natural killer (NK) cells, have tumoricidal activity that does not depend on prior sensitization. These lymphocytes are generally more effective than untransformed cells in killing tumor cells. Tumor cells that are resistant to the action of NK cells may be lysed by NK cells that have been activated by IL-2. Such activated NK cells are referred to as **lymphokine-activated killer (LAK) cells.**
- **Macrophage-mediated cytotoxicity:** Macrophages are capable of killing tumor cells in a nonspecific manner. However, their role in the control of malignant tumors is far from clear, since under some circumstances in vitro factors derived from macrophages can actually stimulate the proliferation of tumor cells.
- **Antibody-dependent cell-mediated cytotoxicity (ADCC):** Tumor-associated antigens can elicit a humoral antibody response, but these immunoglobulins by themselves do not kill tumor cells. However, as discussed in Chapter 4, such antibodies can participate in ADCC. The antibody binds both to the tumor antigen and to the Fc receptor of the effector cell, thereby bringing the effector cell into direct contact with its target. Depending on the conditions, the effector cells may be a lymphocyte killer cell (null cell), macrophage, or neutrophil.
- **Complement-mediated cytotoxicity:** Tumor cells that have been coated with specific antibodies may be lysed by the activation of complement.

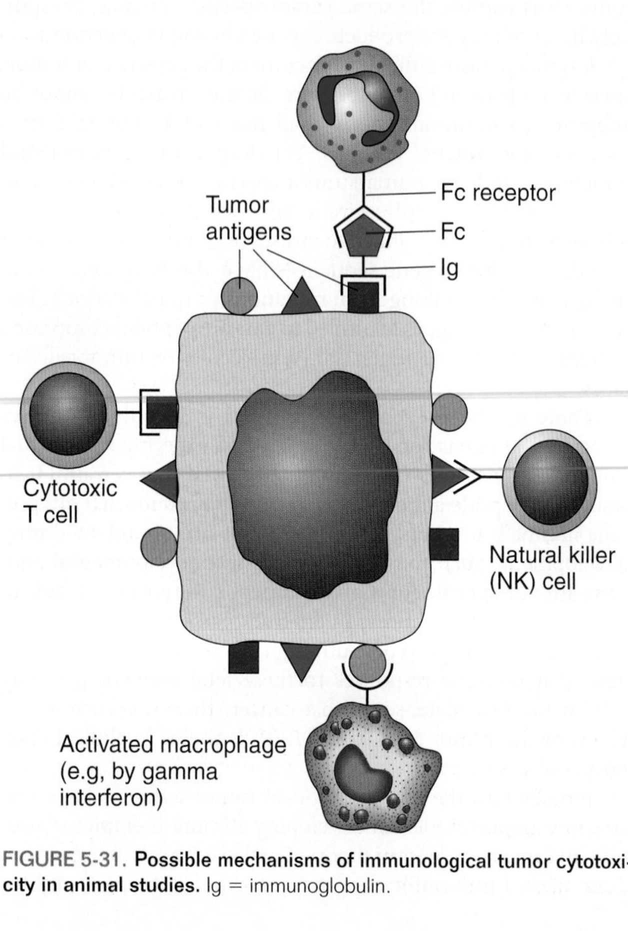

FIGURE 5-31. **Possible mechanisms of immunological tumor cytotoxicity in animal studies.** Ig = immunoglobulin.

Immune Surveillance

Considering the enormous number of chemical, viral, and physical agents that are carcinogenic, it seems remarkable that the incidence of cancer is not far greater than current statistics indicate. The theory of immune surveillance holds that mutant clones with neoplastic potential frequently arise but are recognized and expunged by cell-mediated immune responses. However, the evidence for this concept is highly controversial, and the subject deserves further study.

Immunologic Defenses against Cancer in Humans

Although some circumstantial evidence exists for the participation of immunologic defenses in the resistance to cancer in humans, conclusive proof that immunologic tumor surveillance is an ongoing process is lacking. Perhaps the strongest argument for immunologic tumor rejection in humans is the observation that immunodeficiency, whether acquired or congenital, is associated with an increased incidence of cancers, almost all of which are B-cell lymphomas. Three prominent examples are widely cited: patients with X-linked lymphoproliferative syndrome (XLP), patients with AIDS, and those who receive immunosuppressive therapy following organ transplantation. In XLP and AIDS, the enormously increased risk can be attributed to a polyclonal lymphoid hyperplasia induced by infection with EBV, coupled with a lack of cytotoxic T cells that normally limit the proliferation of virus-infected B cells. In immunosuppressed transplant patients, who manifest a 75-fold increased incidence of lymphomas, it remains unclear whether a direct effect of immunosuppressive agents on the regulation of lymphocyte proliferation and maturation or a nonspecific depression of immune defenses is responsible.

Additional arguments for the effectiveness of immunologic defenses against cancer in humans are also far from definitive. Rare instances of the regression of primary and metastatic tumors have been attributed to immunologic mechanisms, but many other factors may have been responsible (e.g., hormonal, nutritional, or vascular). Similarly, as noted above, the phenomenon of tumor dormancy may be related to comparable nonimmunologic circumstances. The presence of lymphoid cells and macrophages in the stroma of many cancers may represent a reaction to tumor antigens, but their effectiveness in limiting growth is problematic.

Tumor Cells May Be Able to Evade Immunologic Cytotoxicity

The fact that cancer is alive and well despite the presence of potential immunologic defenses implies that such mechanisms are either ineffective or that tumor cells can evade immunologic cytotoxicity. A number of factors have been proposed to account for the failure of immune responses to limit tumor growth. These explanations remain theoretical and even controversial.

It is intuitively clear that an absence of tumor-specific antigens or a lack of immunogenicity by such antigens will permit unhampered growth of the neoplasm. *In this respect, tumor antigens are sometimes found to be expressed at low levels on human tumors, in conjunction with deficient HLA expression or antigenic peptide processing*. The concept of tumor heterogeneity predicts that even in strongly antigenic tumors, clones will arise that do not express tumor antigens or histocompatibility antigens and thus will be selected for survival. Besides antigenic variation, tumor cells tend to lack surface molecules such as co-stimulators that are needed for T cell activation. Additionally, malignant cells can express a variety of immunosuppressive factors that enable them to blunt anti-tumor immunologic responses. Defining and tackling these immune evasion mechanisms will be essential for developing effective immunotherapies for cancer.

Systemic Effects of Cancer on the Host

The symptoms of cancer are, for the most part, referable to the local effects of either the primary tumor or its metastases. However, in a minority of patients, cancer produces remote effects that are not attributable to tumor invasion or to metastasis, which are collectively termed **paraneoplastic syndromes**. Although such effects are rarely lethal, in some cases they dominate the clinical course. It is important to recognize these syndromes for several reasons. First, the signs and symptoms of the paraneoplastic syndrome may be the first clinical manifestation of a malignant tumor. When they are recognized, the cancer may be detected early enough to permit a cure. Second, the syndromes may be mistaken for those produced by advanced metastatic disease and may, therefore, lead to inappropriate therapy. Third, when the paraneoplastic syndrome itself is disabling, treatment directed toward alleviating those symptoms may have important palliative effects. Finally, certain tumor products that result in paraneoplastic syndromes provide a means of monitoring recurrence of the cancer in patients who have had surgical resections or are undergoing chemotherapy or radiation therapy.

Fever

It is not uncommon for cancer patients to present initially with fever of unknown origin that cannot be explained by an infectious disease. Fever attributed to cancer correlates with tumor growth, disappears after treatment, and reappears on recurrence. The cancers in which this most commonly occurs are Hodgkin disease, renal cell carcinoma, and osteogenic sarcoma, although many other tumors are occasionally complicated by fever. Tumor cells may themselves release pyrogens or the inflammatory cells in the tumor stroma can produce IL-1.

Anorexia and Weight Loss

A paraneoplastic syndrome of anorexia, weight loss, and cachexia is very common in patients with cancer, often appearing before its malignant cause becomes apparent. For example, a small asymptomatic pancreatic cancer may be suspected only on the basis of progressive and unexplained weight loss. Although cancer patients often have a decreased caloric intake because of anorexia and abnormalities of taste, restricted food intake does not explain the profound wasting so common among them. The mechanisms responsible for this phenomenon are poorly understood. It is known, however, that unlike starvation, which is associated with a lowered metabolic rate, cancer is often accompanied by an elevated metabolic rate. It has been demonstrated that TNF-α and other cytokines (interferons, IL-6) can produce a wasting syndrome in experimental animals.

Endocrine Syndromes

Malignant tumors may produce a number of peptide hormones whose secretion is not under normal regulatory control. Most of these hormones are normally present in the brain, gastrointestinal tract, or endocrine organs. Their inappropriate secretion can cause a variety of effects.

CUSHING SYNDROME: Ectopic secretion of ACTH by a tumor leads to features of Cushing syndrome, including hypokalemia, hyperglycemia, hypertension, and muscle weakness (see Chapter 21). ACTH production is most commonly seen with cancers of the lung, particularly small cell carcinoma. It also complicates carcinoid tumors and other neuroendocrine tumors, such as pheochromocytoma, neuroblastoma, and medullary thyroid carcinoma.

INAPPROPRIATE ANTIDIURESIS: The production of arginine vasopressin (antidiuretic hormone [ADH]) by a tumor may cause sodium and water retention to such an extent that it is manifested as water intoxication, resulting in altered mental status, seizures, coma, and sometimes death. The tumor that most often produces this syndrome is small cell lung carcinoma. It is also reported with carcinomas of the prostate, gastrointestinal tract, and pancreas and with thymomas, lymphomas, and Hodgkin disease.

HYPERCALCEMIA: A paraneoplastic complication that afflicts 10% of all cancer patients, hypercalcemia, is usually caused by metastatic disease of bone. However, in about one tenth of cases it occurs in the absence of bony metastases. The most common cause of paraneoplastic hypercalcemia is the secretion of a parathormone-like peptide by an epithelial tumor, usually squamous cell lung carcinoma or breast adenocarcinoma. In multiple myeloma and lymphomas, hypercalcemia is attributed to the secretion of osteoclast activating factor. Other mechanisms of hypercalcemia involve the production of prostaglandins, active metabolites of vitamin D, TGF-α, and TGF-β.

HYPOCALCEMIA: Cancer-induced hypocalcemia is actually more common than hypercalcemia and complicates osteoblastic metastases from cancers of the lung, breast, and prostate. The cause of hypocalcemia is not known. Low calcium levels have been reported in association with calcitonin-secreting medullary carcinoma of the thyroid.

GONADOTROPIC SYNDROMES: Gonadotropins may be secreted by germ cell tumors, gestational trophoblastic tumors (choriocarcinoma, hydatidiform mole), and pituitary tumors. Less commonly, gonadotropin secretion is observed with hepatoblastomas in children and cancers of the lung, colon, breast, and pancreas in adults. High gonadotropin levels lead to precocious puberty in children, gynecomastia in men, and oligomenorrhea in premenopausal women.

HYPOGLYCEMIA: The best-understood cause of hypoglycemia associated with tumors is excessive insulin production by pancreatic islet cell tumors. Other tumors, especially large mesotheliomas, fibrosarcomas, and primary hepatocellular carcinoma, are associated with hypoglycemia. The cause of hypoglycemia in nonendocrine tumors is not established, but the most likely candidate is production of somatomedins (IGFs), a family of peptides normally produced by the liver under regulation by growth hormone.

Neurologic Syndromes

Neurologic disorders are common in cancer patients, usually resulting from metastases or from endocrine or electrolyte disturbances. Vascular, hemorrhagic, and infectious conditions affecting the nervous system are also common. However, there remains a small group of cancer patients who suffer from a variety of neurologic complaints without any demonstrable cause. Most of these cases reflect an autoimmune etiology mediated by circulating antibodies directed against neural antigens or by reactive T cells. Cerebral complications include dementia, subacute cerebellar degeneration, limbic encephalitis, and optic neuritis.

Spinal Cord

Subacute motor neuropathy, a disorder of the spinal cord, is characterized by slowly developing lower motor neuron weakness without sensory changes. It is so strongly associated with cancer that an intensive search for an occult neoplasm, often a lymphoma, should be made in patients who present with these symptoms.

Amyotrophic lateral sclerosis is well described among cancer patients. Conversely, as many as 10% of patients with this neurologic disease are found to have cancer.

Peripheral Nerves

Sensorimotor peripheral neuropathy, characterized by distal weakness and wasting and sensory loss, is common in cancer patients and when not associated with an overt neoplasm suggests the possibility of an occult tumor. Interestingly, the removal of the primary tumor usually does not reverse the neuropathy.

Purely sensory neuropathy, resulting from degenerative changes in the dorsal root ganglia, may also develop in persons with cancer.

Autonomic and gastrointestinal neuropathies, manifested as orthostatic hypotension, neurogenic bladder, and intestinal pseudoobstruction, are associated with small cell carcinoma of the lung.

Skeletal Muscle Syndromes

Patients with dermatomyositis or polymyositis have an incidence of cancer five to seven times higher than that in the general population. The association is most conspicuous in affected men older than 50 years; in this group more than 70% have cancer. In most cases, the muscle disorder and cancer present within a year of each other.

Eaton-Lambert syndrome is an uncommon myasthenic disorder that is strongly associated with small cell lung carcinoma. Although the symptoms superficially resemble those of true myasthenia gravis, muscle strength improves with exercise, and there is a poor response to an anticholinesterase. Thymoma has a well-recognized association with **myasthenia gravis,** but a wide variety of other tumors have on occasion been linked to this disorder of the neuromuscular junction.

Hematologic Syndromes

The most common hematologic complications of neoplastic diseases result either from direct infiltration of the marrow or from treatment. However, hematologic paraneoplastic syndromes, which antedate the modern era of chemotherapy and radiation therapy, are well described.

Erythrocytosis

Cancer-associated erythrocytosis (polycythemia) is a complication of some tumors, particularly renal cell carcinoma, hepatocellular carcinoma, and cerebellar hemangioblastoma. Interestingly, benign kidney disease, such as cystic disease or hydronephrosis, and uterine myomas can lead to erythrocytosis. Elevated erythropoietin levels are found in the tumor and in the serum in about half of patients with erythrocytosis.

Anemia

One of the most common findings in patients with cancer is anemia, but the mechanism underlying this disorder is not clear. The anemia is usually normocytic and normochromic, although **iron deficiency anemia** is common in cancers that bleed into the gastrointestinal tract, such as colorectal cancers. **Pure red cell aplasia,** often associated with thymomas, and megaloblastic anemia are sometimes encountered.

Autoimmune hemolytic anemia may be associated with B cell neoplasms and with solid tumors, particularly in the elderly. In fact, autoimmune hemolytic anemia in an older person suggests the possibility of an underlying neoplasm. **Microangiopathic hemolytic anemia** is occasionally seen, often in association with disseminated intravascular coagulation and thrombotic thrombocytopenic purpura.

Leukocytes and Platelets

Paraneoplastic granulocytosis, characterized by a peripheral granulocyte count over 20,000/μL, is a finding that may lead to an erroneous diagnosis of leukemia. This condition is usually caused by the secretion of a colony-stimulating factor by the tumor.

Eosinophilia is occasionally noted in association with cancer, particularly in Hodgkin disease, in which it may occur in one fifth of cases.

Thrombocytosis, with platelet counts above 400,000/μL, occurs in one third of cancer patients. The platelet count usually returns to normal with successful treatment of the malignant disease.

The Hypercoagulable State

The association between cancer and venous thrombosis was noted more than a century ago. Since then, other abnormalities resulting from a hypercoagulable state (e.g., disseminated intravascular coagulation and nonbacterial thrombotic endocarditis) have been recognized. The cause of this hypercoagulable state is still debated.

VENOUS THROMBOSIS: This condition is most distinctly associated with carcinoma of the pancreas, in which there is a 50-fold increased incidence of this complication. Venous thrombosis, commonly in the deep veins of the legs, is also particularly frequent in association with other mucin-secreting adenocarcinomas of the gastrointestinal tract and with lung cancer. Tumors of the breast, ovary, prostate, and other organs are occasionally complicated by venous thrombosis.

DISSEMINATED INTRAVASCULAR COAGULATION: The widespread appearance of thrombi in small vessels in association with cancer may come to attention because of the chronic occurrence of thrombotic phenomena or an acute hemorrhagic diathesis. Sometimes a coagulation disorder is detected by laboratory tests alone. This complication is most commonly found with acute promyelocytic leukemia and adenocarcinomas.

NONBACTERIAL THROMBOTIC ENDOCARDITIS: The presence of noninfected verrucous deposits of fibrin and platelets on the left-sided heart valves occurs in cancer patients, particularly in debilitated persons (see Chapter 11). Although the effects on the heart are not of clinical importance, emboli to the brain and rarely the coronary arteries present a great danger. Paraneoplastic endocarditis may develop early in the course of a cancer and signal its presence long before the tumor would otherwise become symptomatic. This cardiac complication is most common with solid tumors but may occasionally be noted with leukemias and lymphomas.

Gastrointestinal Syndromes

Malabsorption of a variety of dietary components is an occasional paraneoplastic symptom, and half of cancer patients develop some histologic abnormalities of the small intestine, even though the tumor may not directly involve the bowel.

Hypoalbuminemia may result from a paraneoplastic depression of albumin synthesis by the liver or, in rare cases, a protein-losing enteropathy.

Nephrotic Syndrome

Nephrotic syndrome, as a consequence of renal vein thrombosis or amyloidosis, is a well-known complication of cancer. The nephrotic syndrome may also represent a paraneoplastic complication in the form of minimal-change disease (lipoid nephrosis) or glomerulonephritis produced by the deposition of immune complexes.

Cutaneous Syndromes

Pigmented lesions and keratoses are well-recognized paraneoplastic effects.

- **Acanthosis nigricans** is a cutaneous disorder marked by hyperkeratosis and pigmentation of the axilla, neck, flexures, and anogenital region. *It is of particular interest because more than half of patients with acanthosis nigricans have cancer.* The development of the disease may precede, accompany, or follow, the detection of the cancer. Over 90% of cases occur in association with gastrointestinal carcinomas, with tumors of the stomach accounting for one half to two thirds.
- **Exfoliative dermatitis** occasionally complicates certain lymphomas and Hodgkin disease, without any cutaneous involvement by tumor.
- **Erythema gyratum repens** is an unusual skin disorder, which presents with scaling and itching and is seen almost exclusively in cancer patients.

Amyloidosis

About 15% of cases of amyloidosis occur in association with cancers, particularly with multiple myeloma and renal cell carcinoma but also with other solid tumors and lymphomas (see Chapter 23). The presence of amyloidosis implies a poor prognosis; in patients with myeloma, amyloidosis is associated with a median survival of 14 months or less.

Epidemiology of Cancer

The mere compilation of raw epidemiologic data is of little use unless they are subjected to careful analysis. In evaluating the relevance of epidemiologic observations to cancer causation, the Hill criteria are germane:

- Strength of the association
- Consistency under different circumstances
- Specificity
- Temporality (i.e., the cause must precede the effect)
- Biological gradient (i.e., there is a dose–response relationship)
- Plausibility
- Coherence (i.e., a cause-and-effect relationship does not violate basic biological principles)
- Analogy to other known associations

It is not mandatory that a valid epidemiologic study satisfy all these criteria, nor does adherence to them guarantee that the hypothesis derived from the data is necessarily true. However, as a guideline they remain useful.

Cancer accounts for one-fifth of the total mortality in the United States and is the second leading cause of death after cardiovascular diseases and stroke. For most cancers, death rates in the United States have largely remained flat for more than half a century, with some notable exceptions (Fig. 5-32). The death rate from cancer of the lung among men has risen dramatically from 1930, when it was an uncommon tumor, to the present, when it is by far the most common cause of death from cancer in men. As discussed in Chapter 8, the entire epidemic of lung cancer deaths is attributable to smoking. Among women, smoking did not become fashionable until World War II. Considering the time lag needed between starting to smoke and the development of cancer of the lung, it is not surprising that the increased death rate from lung cancer in women did not become significant until after 1965. In the United States, the death rate from lung cancer in women now exceeds that for breast cancer, and it is now, as in men, the most common fatal cancer. By contrast, for reasons difficult to fathom, cancer of the stomach, which in 1930 was by far the most common cancer in men and was more common than breast cancer in women, has shown a remarkable and sustained decline in frequency. Similarly, there has been a conspicuous decline in the death rate from cancer of the uterus corpus and cervix, possibly explained by better screening, diagnostic techniques, and therapeutic methods. Overall, after decades of steady increases, the age-adjusted mortality due to all cancers has now reached a plateau. The ranking of the incidence of tumors in men and women in the United States is shown in Table 5-3.

Individual cancers have their own age-related profiles, but for most, increased age is associated with an increased incidence. The most striking example of the dependency on age is carcinoma of the prostate, in which the incidence increases 30-fold between men ages 50 and 85 years. Certain neoplastic diseases, such as acute lymphoblastic leukemia in children and testicular cancer in young adults, show different age-related peaks of incidence (Fig. 5-33).

Geographic and Ethnic Differences Influence Cancer Incidence

NASOPHARYNGEAL CANCER: Nasopharyngeal cancer is rare in most of the world except for certain regions of China, Hong Kong, and Singapore.

ESOPHAGEAL CARCINOMA: The range in incidence of esophageal carcinoma varies from extremely low in Mormon

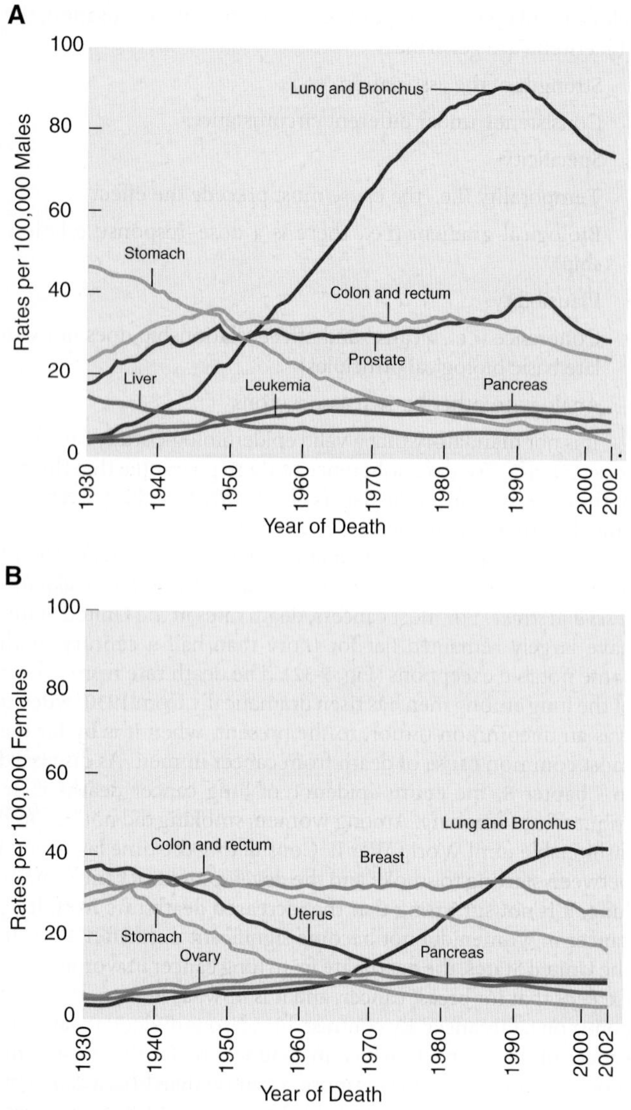

FIGURE 5-32. **Cancer death rates in the United States,** 1930 to 2002, among men (**A**) and women (**B**).

TABLE 5-3

Most Common Tumor Types in Men and Women

Tumor Type	%	Tumor Type	%
Men		**Women**	
Prostate	33	Breast	32
Lung and bronchus	14	Lung and bronchus	12
Colon and rectum	11	Colon and rectum	11
Urinary bladder	6	Uterine corpus	6
Melanoma	4	Ovary	4
Non-Hodgkin lymphoma	4	Non-Hodgkin lymphoma lymphoma	4
Kidney	3	Melanoma	3
Oral cavity	3	Thyroid	3
Leukemia	3	Pancreas	2
Pancreas	2	Urinary bladder	2
All other sites	17	All other sites	20

women in Utah to a value some 300 times higher in the female population of northern Iran. Particularly high rates of esophageal cancer are noted in a so-called Asian esophageal cancer belt, which includes the great land mass stretching from Turkey to eastern China. Interestingly, throughout this region, as the incidence rises, the proportional excess in males decreases; in some of the areas of highest incidence there is even a female excess. The disease is also more common in certain regions of sub-Saharan Africa and among blacks in the United States. The causes of esophageal cancer are obscure, but it is known that it disproportionately affects the poor in many areas of the world, and the combination of alcohol abuse and smoking is associated with a particularly high risk.

STOMACH CANCER: The highest incidence of stomach cancer occurs in Japan, where the disease is almost 10 times as frequent as it is among American whites. A high incidence has also been observed in Latin American countries, particularly Chile. Stomach cancer is also common in Iceland and eastern Europe.

COLORECTAL CANCER: The highest incidence of colorectal cancer is found in the United States, where it is three or four times more common than in Japan, India, Africa, and Latin America. It has been theorized that the high fiber content of the diet in low-risk areas and the high fat content in the United States are related to this difference, although this concept has been seriously questioned.

LIVER CANCER: There is a strong correlation between the incidence of primary hepatocellular carcinoma and the prevalence of hepatitis B and C. Endemic regions for both diseases include large parts of sub-Saharan Africa and most of Asia, Indonesia, and the Philippines. It must be remembered that levels of aflatoxin B_1 are high in the staple diets of many of the high-risk areas.

SKIN CANCER: As noted above, the rates for skin cancers vary with skin color and exposure to the sun. Thus, particularly high rates have been reported in northern Australia, where the population is principally of English origin and sun exposure is intense. Increased rates of skin cancer have also been noted among the white population of the American Southwest. The lowest rates are found among persons with pigmented skin (e.g., Japanese, Chinese, and Indians). The rates for African blacks, despite their heavily pigmented skin, are occasionally higher than those for Asians because of the higher incidence of melanomas of the soles and palms in blacks.

BREAST CANCER: Adenocarcinoma of the breast, the most common female cancer in many parts of Europe and North America, shows considerable geographic variation. The rates in African and Asian populations are only one-fifth to one-sixth of those prevailing in Europe and the United States. Epidemiological studies have contributed little to our understanding of the etiology of breast cancer. Although hormonal factors are clearly involved, except for a good correlation with age at first pregnancy, few confirmed hormonal correlations have surfaced. The role of dietary fat in the pathogenesis of breast cancer is still debated.

CERVICAL CARCINOMA: Striking differences in the incidence of squamous carcinoma of the cervix exist between ethnic groups and different socioeconomic levels. For instance, the very low rate in Ashkenazi Jews of Israel contrasts with a 25 times greater rate in the Hispanic population of Texas. In general, groups of low socioeconomic status have a higher incidence

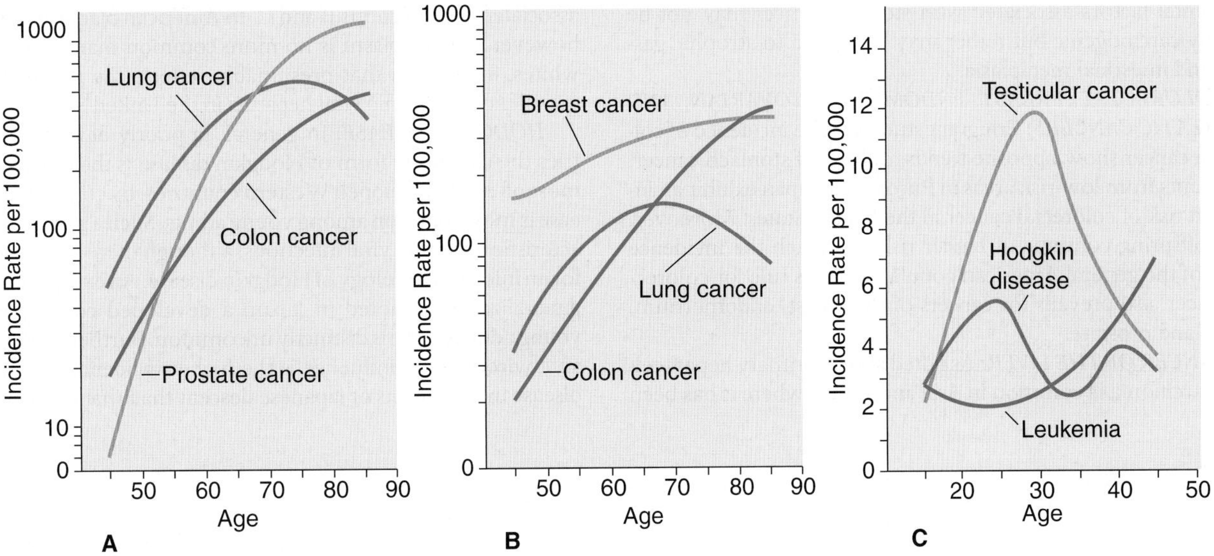

FIGURE 5-33. **Incidence of specific cancers as a function of age.** (A) Men. (B) Women. (C) Testicular cancer in men and Hodgkin disease and leukemia in both sexes. The incidence of these cancers in *C* peaks at younger ages than do those in *A* and *B*.

of cervical cancer than the more prosperous and better educated. This cancer is also directly correlated with early sexual activity and multiparity, and is rare among women who are not sexually active, such as nuns. It is also uncommon among women whose husbands are circumcised. A strong association with infection by HPVs has been demonstrated, and cervical cancer should be classed as a venereal disease.

CHORIOCARCINOMA: Choriocarcinoma, an uncommon cancer of trophoblastic differentiation, is found principally in women, following a pregnancy, although it can present as a testicular tumor. The rates of this disease are particularly high in the Pacific rim of Asia (Singapore, Hong Kong, Japan, and the Philippines).

PROSTATIC CANCER: Very low incidences of prostatic cancer are reported for Asian populations, particularly Japanese, whereas the highest rates described are in American blacks, in whom the disease occurs some 25 times more often. The incidence in American and European whites is intermediate.

TESTICULAR CANCER: An unusual aspect of testicular cancer is its universal rarity among black populations. Interestingly, although the rate in American blacks is only about one-fourth that in whites, it is still considerably higher than the rate among African blacks.

CANCER OF THE PENIS: This squamous carcinoma is virtually nonexistent among circumcised men of any race but is common in many parts of Africa and Asia. It is usually associated with HPV infection.

CANCER OF THE URINARY BLADDER: The rates for transitional cell carcinoma of the bladder are fairly uniform. Squamous carcinoma of the bladder, however, is a special case. Ordinarily far less common than transitional cell carcinoma, it has a high incidence in areas where schistosomal infestation of the bladder (bilharziasis) is endemic.

BURKITT LYMPHOMA: Burkitt lymphoma, a disease of children, was first described in Uganda, where it accounts for half of all childhood tumors. Since then, a high frequency has been observed in other African countries, particularly in hot, humid lowlands. It has been noted that these are areas where malaria is also endemic. High rates have been recorded in other tropical areas, such as Malaysia and New Guinea, but European and American cases are encountered only sporadically.

MULTIPLE MYELOMA: This malignant tumor of plasma cells is uncommon among American whites but displays a three to four times higher incidence in American and South African blacks.

CHRONIC LYMPHOCYTIC LEUKEMIA: Chronic lymphocytic leukemia is common among elderly persons in Europe and North America but is considerably less common in Japan.

Studies of Migrant Populations Give Clues to Cancer Development

Although planned experiments on the etiology of human cancer are hardly feasible, certain populations have unwittingly performed such experiments by migrating from one environment to another. Initially at least, the genetic characteristics of such persons remained the same, but the new environment differed in climate, diet, infectious agents, occupations, and so on. *Consequently, epidemiologic studies of migrant populations have provided many intriguing clues to the factors that may influence the pathogenesis of cancer.* The United States, which has been the destination of one of the greatest population movements of all time, is the source of most of the important data in this field.

CANCER OF THE STOMACH: A study of Japanese residents of Hawaii found that emigrants from Japanese regions with the highest risk of stomach cancer continued to exhibit an excess risk in Hawaii. By contrast, their offspring who were born in Hawaii had the same incidence of this cancer as American whites. Although dietary factors, such as pickled vegetables and salted fish, have been postulated to account for the higher incidence in Japan and the lower incidence in Hawaii, no firm evidence has been adduced to support this contention. More recently it has been shown in Japan that the population in regions at high risk for stomach cancer also display a high prevalence of chronic atrophic gastritis with intestinal metaplasia, lesions that are considered precursors of gastric cancer. Interestingly, when persons from these regions move to low-risk areas, they carry the high prevalence of intestinal metaplasia with them. Thus, the environmental factors associated with stomach cancer may not be directly carcinogenic but rather may be related to atrophic gastritis and intestinal metaplasia.

COLORECTAL, BREAST, ENDOMETRIAL, OVARIAN, AND PROSTATIC CANCERS: Emigrant studies of the incidence of colorectal cancer show opposite trends to those of stomach cancer. Emigrants from low-risk areas in Europe and Japan exhibit an increased risk of colorectal cancer in the United States. Moreover, their offspring continue at higher risk and reach the incidence levels of the general American population. This rule for colorectal cancer also prevails for cancers of the breast, endometrium, ovary, and prostate.

CANCER OF THE LIVER: As noted above, primary hepatocellular carcinoma is common in Asia and Africa, where it has been associated with hepatitis B and C. In American blacks and Asians, however, the neoplasm is no more common than in American whites, a situation that presumably reflects the relatively low prevalence of chronic viral hepatitis in the United States.

HODGKIN DISEASE: In general, in poorly developed countries the childhood form of Hodgkin disease is the one reported most often. In developed Western countries, by contrast, the disease is most common among young adults. Such a pattern is characteristic of certain viral infections, although there is no evidence for an infectious etiology of Hodgkin disease. An exception to this generalization is noted in Japan, a developed country where young adult disease is distinctly uncommon. Further evidence for an environmental influence is the higher incidence of Hodgkin disease in Americans of Japanese descent than that in Japan.

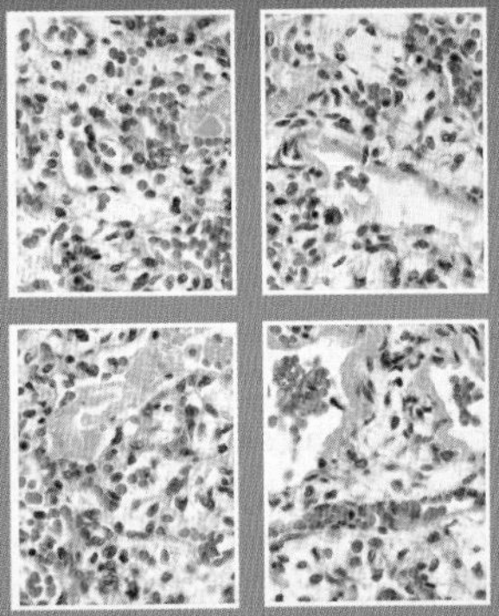

6

Developmental and Genetic Diseases

Anthony A. Killeen
Emanuel Rubin
David S. Strayer

Glossary

The following terms are used in the text or figures of this chapter:

Allele–An alternative form of a gene.

Alternative splicing–A regulatory mechanism by which variations in the incorporation of a gene's exons, or coding regions, into messenger RNA (mRNA) lead to the production of more than one related protein, or isoform.

Autosomes–All of the nuclear chromosomes except for the sex chromosomes.

Centromere–The constricted region near the center of a chromosome, which has a critical role in cell division.

Codon–A three-base sequence of DNA or RNA that specifies a single amino acid.

Conservative mutation–A change in a DNA or RNA sequence that leads to the replacement of one amino acid with a biochemically similar one.

Epigenetic–A term describing nonmutational phenomena, such as methylation and histone modification, that alter the expression of a gene.

Exon–A region of a gene that codes for a protein.

Frame-shift mutation–The addition or deletion of a number of DNA bases that is not a multiple of three, thus causing a shift in the reading frame of the gene. This shift leads to a change in the reading frame of all parts of the gene that are downstream from the mutation, often creating a premature stop codon and ultimately, a truncated protein.

Gain-of-function mutation–A mutation that produces a protein that takes on a new or enhanced function.

Genomics–The study of the functions and interactions of all the genes in the genome, including their interactions with environmental factors.

Genotype–A person's genetic makeup, as reflected by his or her DNA sequence.

Haplotype–A group of nearby alleles that are inherited together.

Hemizygous–Having a gene on one chromosome for which there is no counterpart on the opposite chromosome.

Heterozygous–Having two different alleles at a specific autosomal (or X chromosomal in a female) gene locus.

Homozygous–Having two identical alleles at a specific autosomal (or X chromosomal in a female) gene locus.

Intron–A region of a gene that does not code for a protein.

Linkage disequilibrium–The nonrandom association in a population of alleles at nearby loci.

Loss-of-function mutation–A mutation that decreases the production or function of a protein (or both).

Missense mutation–A mutation that decreases the production or function of a protein (or both).

Monogenic–Caused by a mutation in a single gene.

Motif–A DNA-sequence pattern within a gene that, because of its similarity to sequences in other known genes, suggests a possible function of the gene, its protein product, or both.

Multifactorial–Caused by the interaction of multiple genetic and environmental factors.

Nonconservative mutation–A change in the DNA or RNA sequence that leads to the replacement of one amino acid with a very dissimilar one.

Nonsense mutation–Substitution of a single DNA base that results in a stop codon, thereby leading to the truncation of a protein.

Penetrance–The likelihood that a person carrying a particular mutant gene will have an altered phenotype.

Phenotype–The clinical presentation or expression of a specific gene or genes, environmental factors, or both.

Point mutation–The substitution of a single DNA base in the normal DNA sequence.

Regulatory mutation–A mutation in a region of the genome in multiple identical or closely related copies.

Repeat sequence–A stretch of bases that occurs in the genome in multiple identical or closely related copies.

Silent mutation–Substitution of single DNA base that produces no change in the amino acid sequence of the encoded protein.

Single-nucleotide polymorphism (SNP)–A common variant in the genome sequence; the human genome contains about 10 million SNPs.

Stop codon–A codon that leads to the termination of a protein rather than the addition of an amino acid. The three stop codons are TGA, TAA, and TAG.

It has been known since biblical times that certain disorders are inherited or related to disturbances in intrauterine development. The earliest sanitary codices contain guidelines on how to choose a healthy spouse, how to conceive healthy children, and what to do or not do during pregnancy. Nevertheless, most of our scientific understanding of developmental and genetic disorders is from only the past 3 decades, and the exponential growth of molecular genetics has provided tools for unraveling the etiology and pathogenesis of these disorders. In fact, the molecular basis of most inherited disorders caused by single-gene mutations are either known today or likely to be known within the next few years.

Diseases that present during the perinatal period may be caused solely by factors in the fetal environment, solely by genomic abnormalities, or by interaction between genetic defects and environmental influences. An example is phenylketonuria, in which a genetic deficiency of phenylalanine hydroxylase causes mental retardation only if an infant is exposed to dietary phenylalanine.

Developmental and genetic disorders are classified as follows:

- Errors of morphogenesis
- Chromosomal abnormalities
- Single-gene defects
- Polygenic inherited diseases

The fetus may also be injured by adverse transplacental influences or deformities and injuries caused by intrauterine trauma or during parturition. After birth, acquired diseases of infancy and childhood are also important causes of morbidity and mortality.

Magnitude of the Problem

Each year, about one quarter of a million babies in the United States are born with a birth defect. Worldwide, at least 1 in 50 newborns has a major congenital anomaly, 1 in 100 has a single-gene abnormality, and 1 in 200 has a major chromosomal abnormality.

In more than two thirds of all birth defects, the cause is not apparent (Fig. 6-1). No more than 6% of total birth defects can be attributed to uterine factors; maternal disorders such as metabolic imbalances or infections during pregnancy; and other environmental hazards, including exposure to drugs, chemicals, and radiation. Most of the remainder are accounted for by genomic defects, either hereditary traits or spontaneous mutations, and a smaller number by chromosomal abnormalities.

Although chromosomal abnormalities account for only a small fraction of birth defects in newborns, cytogenetic analyses of fetuses spontaneously aborted early in pregnancy show that up to 50% have chromosomal abnormalities. *The incidence of specific numerical chromosomal abnormalities in abortuses is several times higher than in term infants, indicating that most such chromosomal defects are lethal.* Thus only a small number of children with cytogenetic abnormalities are born alive.

In Western countries, developmental and genetic birth defects account for half of the deaths in infancy and childhood.

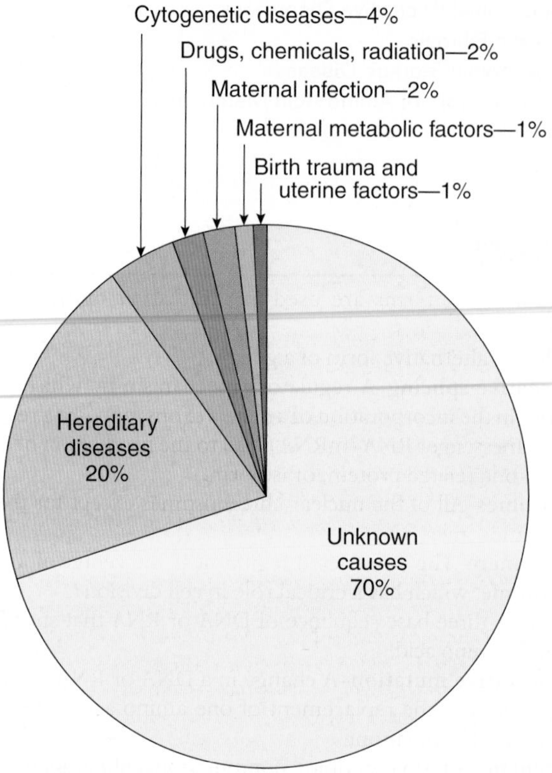

FIGURE 6-1. **Causes of birth defects in humans.** Most birth defects have unknown causes.

In less-developed countries, in contrast, 95% of infant mortality reflects environmental causes such as infectious diseases and malnutrition. Further reduction in the incidence of birth anomalies in industrialized societies will require genetic counseling, early prenatal diagnosis, identification of high-risk pregnancies, and avoidance of possible exogenous teratogens. Thus, prenatal dietary folic acid supplements have reduced the incidence of congenital neural tube defects.

Principles of Teratology

Teratology is the study of developmental anomalies (Greek. *teraton,* monster). **Teratogens** are chemical, physical, and biological agents that cause developmental anomalies. There are few proven teratogens in humans. However, many drugs and chemicals are teratogenic in animals and should, thus, be treated as potentially dangerous for humans.

***Malformations** are morphologic defects or abnormalities of an organ, part of an organ, or anatomical region due to perturbed morphogenesis.* Exposure to a teratogen may result in a malformation, but this is not invariably the case. Such observations have led to the formulation of general principles of teratology:

- **Susceptibility to teratogens is variable.** Presumably the principal determinants of this variability are the genotypes of the fetus and the mother. Experimental evidence for this concept comes from the demonstration that certain strains of inbred mice are susceptible to some teratogens whereas others are not. An example of human variability in the vulnerability to teratogens is the fetal alcohol syndrome, which affects some children of alcoholic mothers, but not others.
- **Susceptibility to teratogens is specific for each embryologic stage.** Most agents are teratogenic only at particular times in development (Fig. 6-2). For example, maternal rubella infection only causes fetal abnormalities if it occurs during the first trimester of pregnancy.
- **The mechanism of is specific for each teratogen.** Teratogenic drugs inhibit crucial enzymes or receptors, interfere with formation of mitotic spindles or block energy production, thereby inhibiting metabolic steps critical for normal morphogenesis. Many drugs and viruses affect specific tissues (e.g., neurotropism, cardiotropism) and so damage some developing organs more than others.
- **Teratogenesis is dose-dependent.** Theoretically, this means that each teratogen should have a "safe" dose, below which no teratogenesis occurs. In practice, however, because of the multiple determinants of teratogenesis, all established

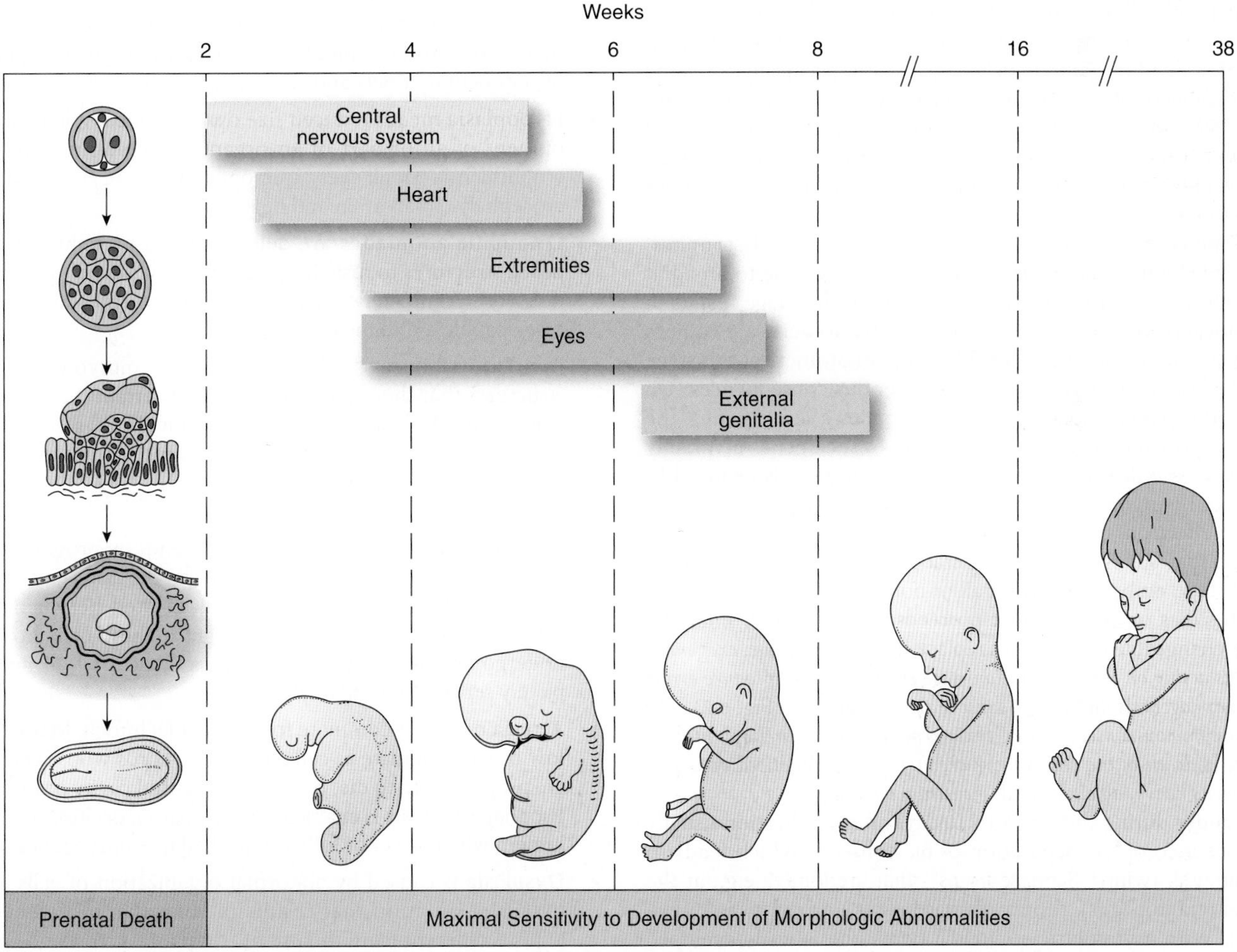

FIGURE 6-2. **Sensitivity of specific organs to teratogenic agents at critical stages of human embryogenesis.** Exposure to adverse influences in the preimplantation and early postimplantation stages of development *(far left)* leads to prenatal death. Periods of maximal sensitivity to teratogens *(horizontal bars)* vary for different organ systems but overall are limited to the first 8 weeks of pregnancy.

teratogens should be avoided during pregnancy; an absolutely safe dose cannot be predicted for every woman.

- **Teratogens produce death, growth retardation, malformation, or functional impairment.** The outcome depends on the interaction between the teratogenic influences, the maternal organism and the fetal–placental unit.

The search for human teratogens requires (1) population surveys, (2) prospective and retrospective studies of single malformations, and (3) investigation of reported adverse effects of drugs or other chemicals. The list of proven teratogens is long and includes most cytotoxic drugs, alcohol, some antiepileptic drugs, heavy metals, and thalidomide. Many drugs and chemicals have been declared safe for use during pregnancy because they were not teratogenic in laboratory animals. However, the fact that a drug is not teratogenic for mice or rabbits does not necessarily mean that it is innocuous for humans: thalidomide was found not to be teratogenic in mice and rats but caused complex human malformations when many pregnant women ingested it in their first trimester of pregnancy. Interestingly, long after thalidomide was known to be teratogenic in humans, its teratogenicity in rabbits and monkeys was also demonstrated.

Errors of Morphogenesis

Normal intrauterine and postnatal development depends on sequential activation and repression of genes. A fertilized ovum (zygote) has all the genes of an adult organism, but most of them are inactive. As the zygote enters cleavage stages of development, individual genes or sets of genes are specifically activated according to the stage of embryogenesis at which they are needed. Initially, only genes essential for cell replication and growth, cell-cell interaction, and morphogenetic movements are activated. *Abnormal gene activation or structure in early embryonic cells can cause early death.*

The cells that form 2-cell and 4-cell embryos (blastomeres) are developmentally equipotent: each can give rise to an adult organism. Separation of embryonic cells at this stage results in identical twins or quadruplets. Since the blastomeres are equipotent and interchangeable, loss of a single blastomere at this stage of development may occur without serious consequences. On the other hand, if one blastomere contains a lethal genes, the others probably do as well. Activation of such genes invariably leads to the death. Furthermore, if a conceptus is exposed to harmful exogenous influences, the noxious agent exerts the same effect on all blastomeres and also causes death. We conclude that adverse environmental influences on preimplantation-stage embryos exert an all-or-nothing effect: either a conceptus dies or development proceeds uninterrupted, since the interchangeable blastomeres replace the loss. *As a rule, exogenous toxins acting on preimplantation-stage embryos do not produce errors of morphogenesis and do not cause malformations* (see Fig. 6-2). *The most common consequence of toxic exposure at the preimplantation stage is death of the embryo, which often passes unnoticed or is perceived as heavy, albeit delayed, menstrual bleeding.*

Injury during the first 8 to 10 days after fertilization usually causes incomplete separation of blastomeres, which leads to conjoined, twins ("Siamese twins") that are joined, e.g., at the head (craniopagus), thorax (thoracopagus), or rump (ischiopagus). With asymmetric conjoined twins one is well-developed and one rudimentary or hypoplastic. The latter is always abnormal and is externally attached to, or internally included in, the body of the better-developed sibling (fetus in fetu). Some congenital teratomas, especially in the sacrococcygeal area, are actually asymmetric monsters.

Most complex developmental abnormalities affecting several organ systems are due to injuries that occur between implantation of the blastocyst and early organogenesis. This period is characterized by rapid cell division, cell differentiation, and formation of so-called **developmental fields,** in which cells interact and determine each other's developmental fate. This process leads to irreversible differentiation of groups of cells. Complex morphologic movements form organ primordia (anlage), and organs are then interconnected in functionally active systems. *Formation of primordial organ systems is the stage of embryonic development most susceptible to teratogenesis, and many major developmental abnormalities are probably due to faulty gene activity or the effects of exogenous toxins* (see Fig. 6-2). Disorganized or disrupted morphogenesis may have minor or major consequences at the level of (1) cells and tissues, (2) organs or organ systems, and (3) anatomical regions.

- **Agenesis** is the complete absence of an organ primordium. It may manifest as (1) total lack of an organ, as in unilateral or bilateral renal agenesis; (2) absence of part of an organ, as in agenesis of the corpus callosum of the brain; or (3) lack of tissue or cells within an organ, as in the absence of testicular germ cells in congenital infertility ("Sertoli cell only" syndrome).
- **Aplasia** is the persistence of an organ anlage or rudiment, without the mature organ. Thus, in aplasia of the lung the main bronchus ends blindly in nondescript tissue composed of rudimentary ducts and connective tissue.
- **Hypoplasia** means reduced size owing to incomplete development of all or part of an organ. Examples include microphthalmia (small eyes), micrognathia (small jaw), and microcephaly (small brain and head).
- **Dysraphic anomalies** are defects caused by failure of apposed structures to fuse. In spina bifida, the spinal canal does not close completely, and overlying bone and skin do not fuse, leaving a midline defect.
- **Involution failures** denote persistence of embryonic or fetal structures that should have involuted at certain stages of development. A persistent thyroglossal duct is the result of incomplete involution of the tract that connects the base of the tongue with the developing thyroid.
- **Division failures** are caused by incomplete cleavage of embryonic tissues, when that process depends on programmed cell death. Fingers and toes are formed at the distal end of the limb bud through the loss of cells located between the primordia that contain the cartilage. If these cells do not undergo apoptosis, the fingers will be conjoined or incompletely separated (syndactyly).
- **Atresia** reflects incomplete formation of a lumen. Many hollow organs originate as cell strands and cords whose centers are programmed to die, producing a central cavity or lumen. Esophageal atresia is characterized by partial occlusion of the lumen, which was not fully established in embryogenesis.
- **Dysplasia** is caused by abnormal organization of cells into tissues, a situation that results in abnormal histogenesis. (This is different from the use of "dysplasia" to describe precancerous epithelial lesions [see Chapters 1 and 5].) Tuberous sclerosis is a striking example of dysplasia, being characterized by abnormal development of the brain, which contains

aggregates of normally developed cells arranged into grossly visible "tubers."

- **Ectopia, or heterotopia,** is an anomaly in which an organ is situated outside its normal anatomic site. Thus, an ectopic heart is not in the thorax. Heterotopic parathyroid glands can be within the thymus in the anterior mediastinum.
- **Dystopia** refers to inadequate migration of an organ that remains where it was during development, rather than migrating to its proper site. For example, the kidneys are first in the pelvis, and then move cephalad out of the pelvis. Dystopic kidneys remain in the pelvis. Dystopic testes are retained in the inguinal canal, and do not descend into the scrotum (cryptorchidism).

Developmental anomalies caused by interference with morphogenesis are often multiple:

- ***A polytopic effect** occurs when a noxious stimulus affects several organs that are simultaneously in critical stages of development.*
- ***A monotopic effect** refers to a single localized anomaly that results in a cascade of pathogenetic events.*
- ***A developmental sequence anomaly** (anomalad or complex anomaly) is a pattern of defects related to a single anomaly or pathogenetic mechanism:* different factors lead to the same consequences through a common pathway. In the Potter complex (Fig. 6-3), pulmonary hypoplasia, external signs of intrauterine fetal compression, and morphologic changes of the amnion are all related to oligohydramnios (a severely reduced amount of amniotic fluid). A fetus in an amniotic sac with insufficient fluid develops the distinctive features of Potter complex irrespective of the cause of oligohydramnios.

A **developmental syndrome** *refers to multiple anomalies that are pathogenetically related.* The term **syndrome** implies a single cause for anomalies in diverse organs that have been damaged by the same polytopic effect during a critical develop mental period. Many developmental syndromes are related to chromosomal abnormalities or single-gene defects. By contrast, **developmental association,** or **syntropy,** refers to multiple anomalies that are associated statistically but that do not necessarily share the same pathogenetic mechanisms. Many of the anomalies that now seem unrelated may one day prove to have the same cause. However, until such associations are proved, it is important to bear in mind that not all congenital anomalies in a child with multiple defects are necessarily interrelated. Thus, the birth of a child with multiple anomalies does not prove that the mother was exposed to an exogenous teratogen or that all the diverse anomalies were caused by the same genetic defect. The recognition of specific syndromes, and their distinction from random associations, is essential to assess the risk of recurrence of similar anomalies in subsequent children of the same family.

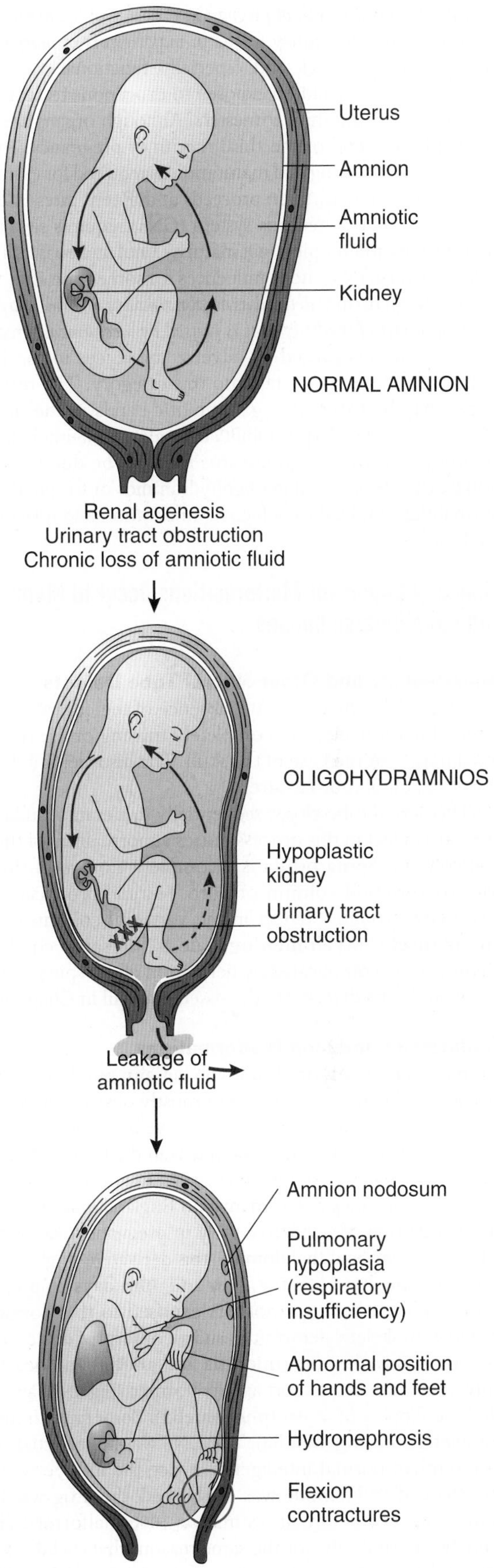

FIGURE 6-3. **Potter complex.** The fetus normally swallows amniotic fluid and, in turn, excretes urine, thereby maintaining its normal volume of amniotic fluid. In the face of urinary tract disease (e.g., renal agenesis or urinary tract obstruction) or leakage of amniotic fluid, the volume of amniotic fluid decreases, a situation termed **oligohydramnios.** Oligohydramnios results in a number of congenital abnormalities termed **Potter complex,** which includes pulmonary hypoplasia and contractures of the limbs. The amnion has a nodular appearance. In cases of urinary tract obstruction, congenital hydronephrosis is also seen, although this abnormality is not considered part of Potter complex.

After the third month of pregnancy, exposure of the human fetus to teratogenic influences rarely results in major errors of morphogenesis. However, morphologic and, especially, functional consequences may still occur in children exposed to exogenous teratogens during the second and third trimesters. Although organs are already formed by the end of the third month of pregnancy, most still undergo restructuring and maturation as required for extrauterine life. Functional maturation proceeds at different rates in different organs: the central nervous system (CNS) requires several years after birth to attain functional maturity until and so is still susceptible to adverse exogenous influences for some time after birth.

A **deformation** *is defined as an abnormality of form, shape, or position of a part of the body that is caused by mechanical forces.* Most anatomic defects caused by adverse influences in the last two trimesters of pregnancy fall into this category. The responsible forces may be external (e.g., amniotic bands in the uterus) or intrinsic (e.g., fetal hypomobility caused by CNS injury). Thus, a deformity known as equinovarus foot can be due to compression by the uterine wall in oligohydramnios or to spinal cord abnormalities that lead to defective innervation and movement of the foot.

Clinically Important Malformations Occur in Many Organs and Have Diverse Causes

Anencephaly and Other Neural Tube Defects

Anencephaly is the congenital absence of the cranial vault. The cerebral hemispheres are completely missing or are reduced to small masses at the base of the skull. The disorder is a dysraphic defect of neural tube closure.

The neural tube closes sequentially in a craniocaudad direction, so a defect in this process causes abnormalities of the vertebral column. **Spina bifida** is incomplete closure of the spinal cord or vertebral column or both. Hernial protrusion of the meninges through a defect in the vertebral column is termed **meningocele. Myelomeningocele** is the same condition as meningocele, complicated by herniation of the spinal cord itself

Neural tube defects are discussed in detail in Chapter 28.

Thalidomide-Induced Malformations

Limb-reduction deformities, involving any number of extremities, are rare congenital defects of mostly obscure origin that affect 1 in 5000 liveborn infants. They have been known for ages: a Goya depiction of a typical example is in the Louvre Museum in Paris. In the 1960s, a sudden increase in the incidence of limb-reduction deformities in Germany and England was linked to maternal ingestion of a sedative early in pregnancy. Known under the generic name of thalidomide, this derivative of glutamic acid is teratogenic between the 28th and 50th days of pregnancy. Many children born to mothers exposed to thalidomide presented with skeletal deformities and pleomorphic defects in other organs, mostly the ears (**microtia** and **anotia**) and heart. Typically, their arms were short and malformed (Fig. 6-4), and resembled the flippers of a seal (**phocomelia).** Sometimes limbs were completely missing (**amelia).** The CNS was not affected, and the children had normal intelligence. Once the link between phocomelia and thalidomide was established, the drug was banned (1962), but not before an estimated 3000 malformed children were born. Ironically, for the same reasons that thalidomide hinders limb growth–its anti-angiogenic properties and, perhaps, its ability to induce caspase-8-dependent apoptosis– the drug also has recently been reintroduced to treat certain malignancies.

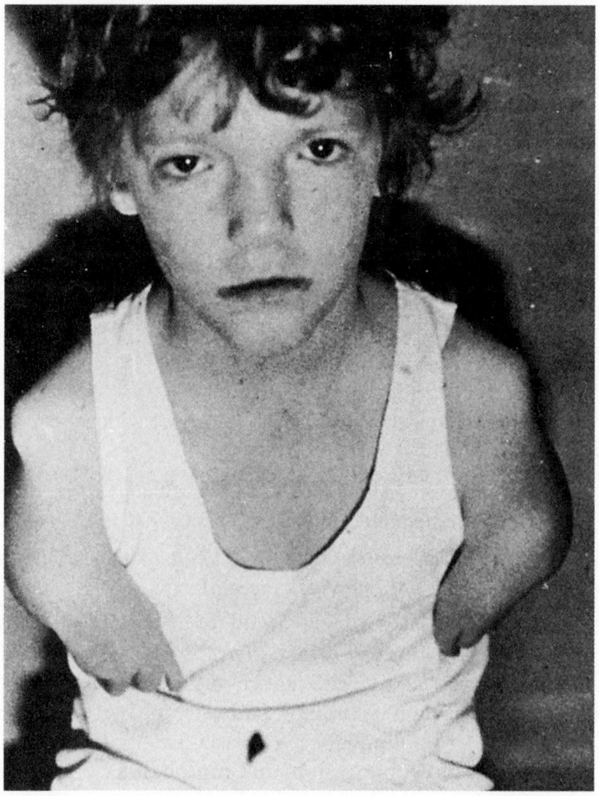

FIGURE 6-4. **Thalidomide-induced deformity of the arms.**

Fetal Hydantoin Syndrome

Ten percent of children born to epileptic mothers who were treated with antiepileptic drugs such as hydantoin during pregnancy show characteristic facial features, hypoplasia of nails and digits, and various congenital heart defects. Since this syndrome occurs only two to three times more often in treated epileptics than in untreated ones, it is uncertain whether the defects all reflect adverse effects of the drug. Nevertheless, it appears that fetal susceptibility to this disorder correlates with the fetal level of the microsomal detoxifying enzyme epoxide hydrolase. Presumably, accumulation of poorly detoxified reactive intermediates of hydantoin metabolism promotes teratogenesis.

Fetal Alcohol Syndrome

Fetal alcohol syndrome is caused by maternal consumption of alcoholic beverages during pregnancy. It is a complex of abnormalities including: (1) growth retardation, (2) CNS dysfunction, and (3) characteristic facial dysmorphology. Because not all children adversely affected by maternal alcohol abuse show all these abnormalities, the term **fetal alcohol effect** is also used.

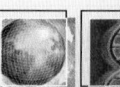

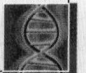

EPIDEMIOLOGY AND PATHOGENESIS: An injurious effect of intrauterine exposure to alcohol was noted in biblical times and was reported during the historic London gin epidemic (1720 to 1750). However, it was only in 1968 that a specific syndrome was identified. The prevalence of fetal alcohol syndrome in the United States and Europe is 1 to 3 per 1000 live births. However, in populations with extremely high rates of alcoholism, such as some tribes of Native Americans, incidence may reach 20 to 150 per 1000. *It is thought that abnormalities related to fetal alcohol effect, particularly mild mental deficiency and emotional disorders, are far more common than the full-blown fetal alcohol syndrome.*

The minimum amount of alcohol that results in fetal injury is not well established, but children with the entire spectrum of fetal alcohol syndrome are usually born to mothers who are chronic alcoholics. Heavy alcohol consumption during the first trimester of pregnancy is particularly dangerous. The mechanism by which alcohol damages the developing fetus remains unknown despite a large body of research.

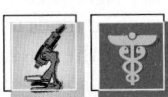

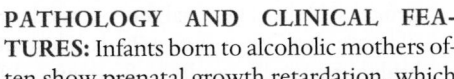

PATHOLOGY AND CLINICAL FEATURES: Infants born to alcoholic mothers often show prenatal growth retardation, which continues after birth. These infants also may show microcephaly, epicanthal folds, short palpebral fissures, maxillary hypoplasia, a thin upper lip, a small jaw (micrognathia), and a poorly developed philtrum. Cardiac septal defects may affect up to one third of patients, although these often close spontaneously. Minor abnormalities of joints and limbs may occur.

Fetal alcohol syndrome is the most common cause of acquired mental retardation. One fifth of children with fetal alcohol syndrome have intelligence quotients (IQs) below 70, and 40% are between 70 and 85. Even if their IQ is normal, these children tend to have short memory spans, and to exhibit impulsive behavior and emotional instability (see Chapter 8).

TORCH Complex

The acronym, TORCH, refers to a complex of similar signs and symptoms produced by fetal or neonatal infection with: Toxoplasma *(T), rubella (R), cytomegalovirus (C), and herpes simplex virus (H). In the acronym TORCH, the letter "O" represents "others."* The term was coined to alert pediatricians to the fact that fetal and newborn infections by TORCH agents are usually indistinguishable from each other and that assessment should include testing for all TORCH agents, and for some possible others as well (Fig. 6-5). "Other" infections include syphilis, tuberculosis, listeriosis, leptospirosis, varicella-zoster virus infection, and Epstein-Barr virus infection. Human immunodeficiency virus (HIV) and human parvovirus (B19) have been suggested as additions to the list.

Infections with TORCH agents occur in 1% to 5% of all liveborn infants in the United States and are major causes of neonatal morbidity and mortality. The severe damage inflicted by these organisms is mostly irreparable, and prevention (if possible) is the only alternative. Unfortunately, titers of serum antibodies against TORCH agents in infants or mothers are usually not diagnostic, and the precise etiology is often unclear.

- **Toxoplasmosis:** Asymptomatic toxoplasmosis is common, and 25% of women in their reproductive years have antibodies to this organism. On the other hand, intrauterine *Toxoplasma* infection occurs in only 0.1% of all pregnancies.
- **Rubella:** Vaccination against rubella in the United States has virtually eliminated congenital rubella. Fewer than 10 cases are reported each year.
- **Cytomegalovirus (CMV):** In the United States, 2/3 of women of childbearing age have antibody to CMV, and up to 2% of newborns are congenitally infected. Most normal infants have maternally derived antibodies, so CMV is diagnosed by urine culture.
- **Herpesvirus:** Intrauterine infection with herpes simplex virus type 2 (HSV-2) is uncommon. The neonatal infection is usually acquired during passage through the birth canal of a mother with active genital herpes. Clinical examination of the mother, the appearance of typical skin lesions in the newborn, and serologic testing and culture for HSV-2 establish the diagnosis. Congenital herpes infection can be prevented by cesarean section of mothers who have active genital lesions.

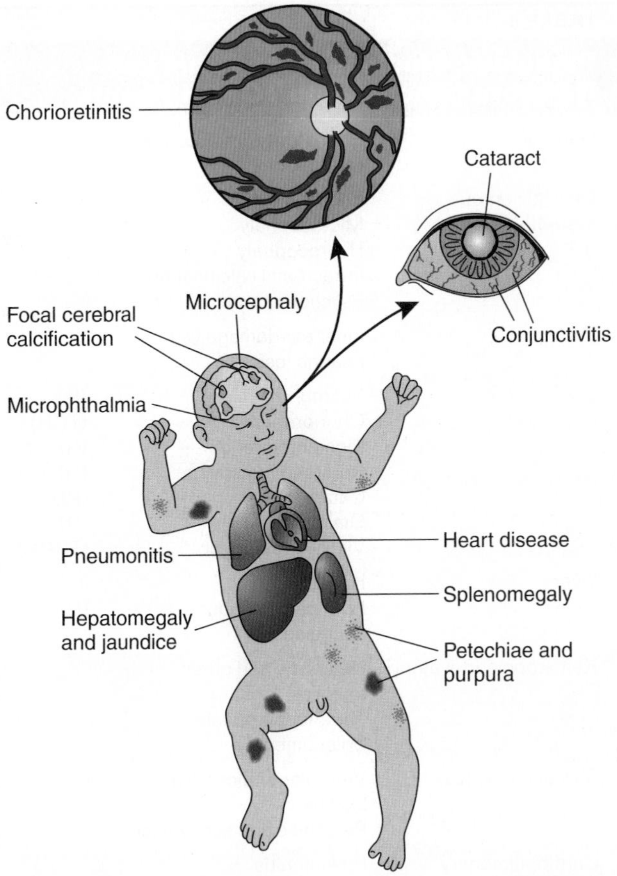

FIGURE 6-5. **TORCH complex.** Children infected in utero with *Toxoplasma*, rubella virus, cytomegalovirus, or herpes simplex virus show remarkably similar effects.

The specific organisms of the TORCH complex are discussed in detail in Chapter 9.

PATHOLOGY: The clinical and pathologic findings in the symptomatic newborn vary. Only a minority present with multisystem disease and the entire spectrum of abnormalities (Table 6-1). Growth retardation and abnormalities of the brain, eyes, liver, hematopoietic system, and heart are common.

Lesions of the brain are the most serious pathologic changes in TORCH-infected children. In acute encephalitis, foci of necrosis are initially surrounded by inflammatory cells. Later these lesions calcify, most prominently in congenital toxoplasmosis. Microcephaly, hydrocephalus, and abnormally shaped gyri and sulci (microgyria) are frequent. Radiologically, defects of cerebral matter (porencephaly), missing olfactory bulbs, and other major brain

TABLE 6-1

Pathologic Findings in the Fetus and Newborn Infected with TORCH Agents

General	Prematurity, intrauterine retardation	
Central nervous system	Encephalitis Microcephaly Hydrocephaly Intracranial calcifications Psychomotor retardation	
Ear	Inner ear damage with hearing loss	
Eye	Microphthalmia Chorioretinitis Pigmented retina Keratoconjunctivitis Cataracts Glaucoma Visual impairment	(R) (TCH) (R) (H) (RH) (R) (TRCH)
Liver	Hepatomegaly Liver calcifications Jaundice	 (R)
Hematopoietic system	Hemolytic and other anemias Thrombocytopenia Splenomegaly	
Skin and mucosae	Vesicular or ulcerative lesions Petechiae and ecchymoses	(H)
Cardiopulmonary system	Pneumonitis Myocarditis Congenital heart disease	
Skeleton	Various bone lesions	

T - *Toxoplasma;* R = rubella virus; C = cytomegalovirus; H = herpesvirus.

defects may be identified. Severe brain damage is reflected in psychomotor retardation, neurologic defects, and seizures.

Ocular defects are prominent in the TORCH complex, particularly with rubella infection, in which over 2/3 of patients have cataracts and microphthalmia. Glaucoma and retinal malformations (coloboma) may occur. Choroidoretinitis is common in with rubella, *Toxoplasma,* and CMV, is usually bilateral and on funduscopy appears as pale, mottled areas surrounded by a pigmented rim. Keratoconjunctivitis is the most common ocular lesion in newborns afflicted with herpes simplex.

Cardiac anomalies occur in many children with the TORCH complex, mostly in congenital rubella. Patent ductus arteriosus and various septal defects are the most common cardiac abnormalities. Pulmonary artery stenosis and complex cardiac anomalies are occasionally seen.

Congenital Syphilis

The organism that causes syphilis, *Treponema pallidum,* is transmitted to the fetus by a mother who has acquired syphilis during pregnancy. The fetus may possibly develop syphilis if the mother became infected in the 2 years before the pregnancy, although the actual risk cannot be accurately assessed. Congenital syphilis affects about 1 in 2000 liveborn infants in the United States. In pregnant syphilitic women, stillbirth occurs in 1/3, and 2/3 of infants carried to term manifest congenital syphilis.

T. pallidum may invade the fetus at any point in pregnancy. Early infections most likely induce abortions, and grossly visible signs of congenital syphilis appear only in fetuses infected after the 16th week of pregnancy. Spirochetes grow in all fetal tissues, and the clinical presentation is thus variable.

Children with congenital syphilis are normal at first, or show changes like those of the TORCH complex. Early lesions in various organs teem with spirochetes. They show perivascular infiltrates of lymphocytes and plasma cells, and granuloma-like lesions termed **gummas.** Many infants are asymptomatic, only to develop the typical stigmata of congenital syphilis in the first few years of life. Late symptoms of congenital syphilis appear many years later and reflect slowly evolving tissue destruction and repair:

- **Rhinitis:** A conspicuous mucopurulent nasal discharge, "snuffles," is almost always present as an early sign of congenital syphilis. The nasal mucosa is edematous and tends to ulcerate, leading to nosebleeds. Destruction of the nasal bridge eventually results in flattening of the nose, so-called **saddle nose.**
- **Skin:** A maculopapular rash is common early in congenital syphilis. Palms and soles are usually affected (as in secondary syphilis of adults), although it may involve the entire body or any part. Cracks and fissures (**rhagades**) occur around the mouth, anus, and vulva. Flat raised plaques (**condylomata lata**) around the anus and female genitalia may develop early or after a few years.
- **Visceral organs:** A distinctive pneumonitis, characterized by pale hypocrepitant lungs (**pneumonia alba),** may develop in the neonatal period. Hepatosplenomegaly, anemia, and lymphadenopathy may also be observed in early congenital syphilis.
- **Teeth:** The buds of incisors and 6th-year molars develop early in postnatal life, the time when congenital syphilis is particularly aggressive. Thus, the permanent incisors may be notched (**Hutchinson teeth**) and the molars malformed (**mulberry molars).**
- **Bones:** The most common osseous lesion is an inflammation of the periosteum together with new bone formation (periostitis). This complication is particularly evident in the anterior tibia, resulting in a distinctive outward curving (**saber shins).**
- **Eye:** A progressive corneal vascularization (**interstitial keratitis**) is an especially vexing complication of congenital syphilis, occurring as early as 4 years of age and as late as 20 years. The cornea eventually scars and becomes opaque.
- **Nervous system:** The nervous system is commonly involved, with symptoms starting in infancy or after 1 year. **Meningitis** predominates in early congenital syphilis, leading to convulsions, mild hydrocephalus, and mental retardation. **Meningovascular syphilis** is a common lesion in later syphilis, which may result in deafness, mental retardation, paresis and other manifestations of neurosyphilis. **Hutchinson triad** refers to the combination of deafness, interstitial keratitis, and notched incisor teeth.

The diagnosis of congenital syphilis is suggested by clinical findings plus a history of maternal infection. Serologic confirmation of syphilis may be difficult in newborns because transplacental transfer of maternal immunoglobulin (Ig)G gives false-positive results. Penicillin is the drug of choice for intrauterine and postnatal syphilis. If penicillin is given during intrauterine life or during the first 2 years of postnatal life, the prognosis is excellent, and most symptoms of early and late congenital syphilis will be prevented.

Chromosomal Abnormalities

Cytogenetics is the study of chromosomes and their abnormalities. The current system of classification is the International System for Human Cytogenetic Nomenclature (ISCN).

The Normal Chromosomal Complement Is 44 Autosomes and 2 Sex Chromosomes

Cytogenetic analysis can be done on any dividing cell but most studies use circulating lymphocytes, which are easily stimulated to undergo mitosis. The dividing cells are treated with colchicine to arrest them in metaphase. Cells are then spread on glass slides to disperse the chromosomes, which are stained to faciitate more precise identification of chromosomes and their distinct bands.

Chromosome Structure

Using a stain such as Giemsa, chromosomes are classified according to their **length** and the positions of their constrictions, or **centromeres.** The centromere is the point at which the two identical strands of chromosomal DNA, called **sister chromatids,** attach to each other during mitosis. The location of the centromere is used to classify chromosomes as **metacentric, submetacentric,** or **acrocentric.** In **metacentric chromosomes** (1, 3, 19, and 20) the centromere is exactly in the middle. In **submetacentric chromosomes** (2, 4–12, 16–18, and X), it divides the chromosome into a short arm (p, from French, *petit*) and a long arm (q, the next letter in the alphabet). **Acrocentric chromosomes** (13, 14, 15, 21, 22, and Y) display very short arms or stalks and satellites attached to an eccentrically located centromere (Fig. 6-6).

Stains are used to classify chromosomes into seven groups, A to G. Thus, group A contains 2 large metacentric and a large submetacentric chromosome, group B has 2 large submetacentric chromosomes, group C includes 6 submetacentric chromosomes, etc.

Fluorescence In Situ Hybridization (FISH)

FISH uses fluorophore-labeled DNA probes to identify DNA sequences, varying in size from individual genes or small regions of chromosomes (Figs. 6-6 and 6-7). It is also used to identify genetic material lost or gained. Using probes with different fluorophores, one can demonstrate chromosomal translocations. More-recent applications, termed **multicolor FISH,** or **spectral karyotyping,** utilize probes that hybridize to whole chromosomes, which facilitates detection of gross chromosomal abnormalities (Figs. 6-6 and 6-7).

Chromosomal Banding

To identify each chromosome individually, special stains delineate specific bands of different staining intensity on each chromosome. *The pattern of bands is unique to each chromosome and makes possible to (1) pair two homologous chromosomes, (2) recognize each chromosome, and (3) identify defects on each segment of a chromosome.*

Chromosome bands are labeled as follows:

- **G bands:** These segments are highlighted using Giemsa stain (hence "G").
- **Q bands:** These stain with Giemsa and fluoresce when treated with quinacrine (thus, "Q").
- **R bands:** On appropriate staining, R bands present as reverse (hence "R") images of G and Q bands; that is, dark G bands are light R bands and vice versa.
- **C banding:** This is a method for staining centromeres (hence "C") and other portions of chromosomes containing constitutive heterochromatin. By contrast, facultative heterochromatin forms the inactive X chromosome (Barr body).

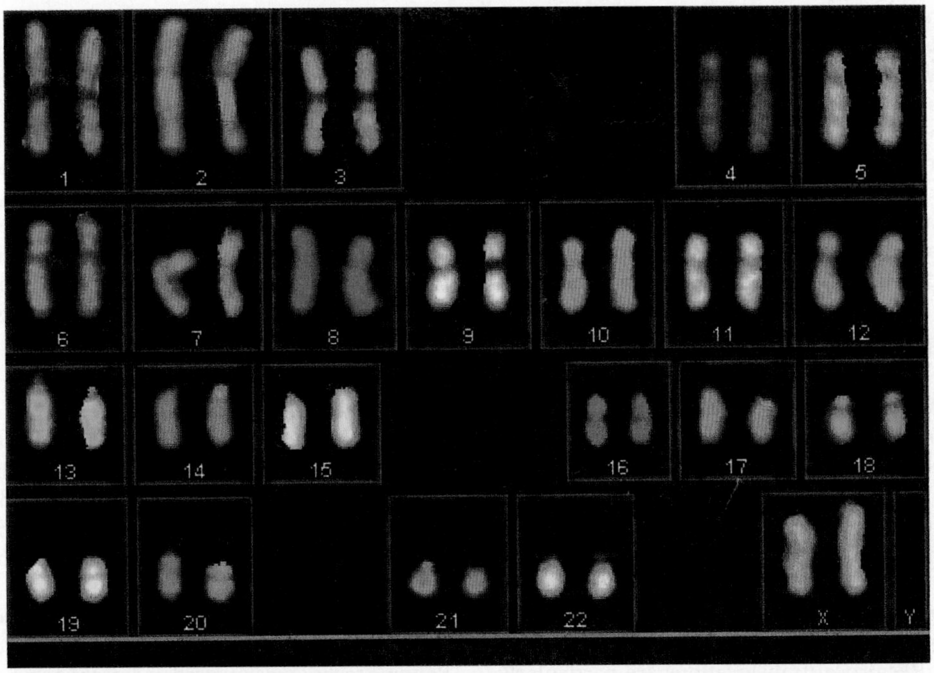

FIGURE 6-6. Spectral karyotype of human chromosomes.

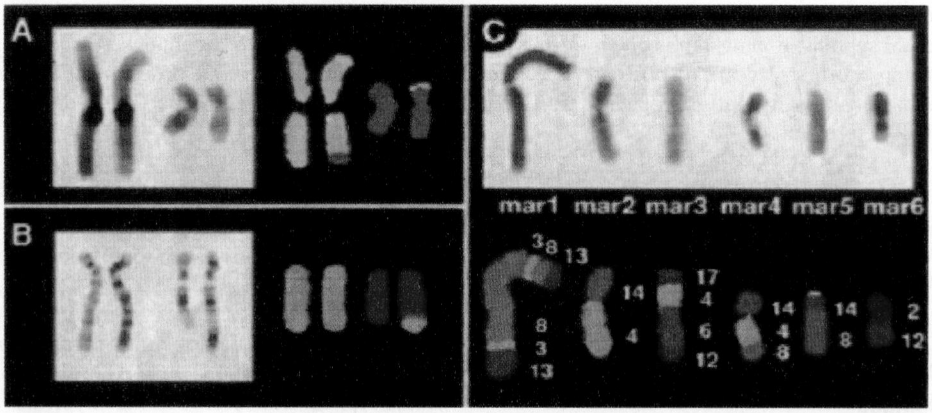

FIGURE 6-7. **Translocations in human chromosomes demonstrated by spectral karyotyping. A.** Balanced translocation: t (1; 11). **B.** Unbalanced karyotype: Derivative chromosome 12 with chromosome 4 material attached (partial trisomy for 4q and partial monosomy for 12q). **C.** Characterization of marker chromosomes from an aneuploid breast cancer showing multiple translocations.

- **Nucleolar organizing region (NOR) staining:** Secondary constrictions (stalks) of chromosomes with satellites are demonstrated by NOR staining.
- **T banding:** This technique stains the terminal (hence "T") ends of chromosomes.

Structural Chromosomal Abnormalities May Arise during Somatic Cell Division (Mitosis) or during Gametogenesis (Meiosis)

Changes in chromosome structure that occur in somatic cells during mitosis may: (1) not affect a cell's basic functions and thus be silent, (2) interfere with one or more key cellular activities and lead to cell death, or (3) change a key cell function (e.g., increase mitotic activity) so as to lead to dysfunction without cell death (see Chapter 5).

The structural chromosomal abnormalities that arise during gametogenesis are important in a different context, because they are transmitted to all somatic cells of the individual's offspring and may result in heritable diseases. During normal meiosis, homologous chromosomes (e.g., two chromosomes 1) form pairs, termed **bivalents.** By a normal process known as crossing-over, parts of these chromosomes are exchanged, thus rearranging the genetic constituents of each chromosome.

By an abnormal process termed **translocation,** such exchanges may also involve nonhomologous chromosomes (e.g., chromosomes 3 and 21). Two major types of chromosomal translocations are recognized: reciprocal and robertsonian.

Reciprocal Translocations

Reciprocal translocation refers to exchange of acentric chromosomal segments between different (nonhomologous) chromosomes (Fig. 6-8). A reciprocal translocation is **balanced** if there is no loss of genetic material, so that each chromosomal segment is translocated in its entirety. When such translocations are present in the gametes (sperm or ova), progeny maintain the abnormal chromosomal structure in all somatic cells. *Balanced translocations are not generally associated with loss of genes or disruption of vital gene loci, so most carriers of balanced translocations are phenotypically normal.* Balanced reciprocal translocations can be inherited for many generations. Reciprocal translocations are particularly well demonstrated by current banding techniques.

Offspring of carriers of balanced translocations, however, are at risk because they will have unbalanced karyotypes and may show severe phenotypic abnormalities (Fig. 6-9). The abnormal positions of the exchanged chromosomal segments may disturb meiosis and lead to abnormal segregation of chromosomes. In a translocation carrier, formation of bivalents may be disturbed. To achieve complete pairing of translocated segments, a cross-like structure (quadriradial) is formed from the two chromosomes with the translocations plus their two normal homologues. Unlike the normal bivalent, which typically resolves by orderly migration each chromosome to the opposite pole, a quadriradial can divide along several different planes. Some resulting gametes carry unbalanced chromosomes and on fertilization yield zygotes with various combinations of partial trisomy and monosomy for segments of the translocated chromosomes.

Robertsonian Translocations

Robertsonian translocation (centric fusion) involves the centromere of acrocentric chromosomes. When two nonhomologous chromosomes are broken near the centromere, they may exchange two arms to form one large metacentric chromosome and a small chromosomal fragment. The latter lacks a centromere and is usually lost in subsequent divisions. As in reciprocal translocation, robertsonian translocation is balanced if there is no significant loss of genetic material. The carrier is also usually phenotypically normal, but may be infertile. *If the carrier is fertile, however, their gametes may produce unbalanced translocations (see Figs. 6-7 and 6-8), in which case the offspring may have congenital malformations.*

Chromosomal Deletions

A deletion is loss of a portion of a chromosome and involves either a terminal or an intercalary (middle) segment. Disturbances during meiosis in germ cells or breaks of chromatids during mitosis in somatic cells may result in formation of chromosomal fragments that are not incorporated into any chromosome and are thus lost in subsequent cell divisions.

The shortening of a chromosome because of a deletion may be apparent in routinely stained chromosome preparations. Banding techniques are used to determine whether the arm of the chromosome is shortened because of a deletion of the terminal

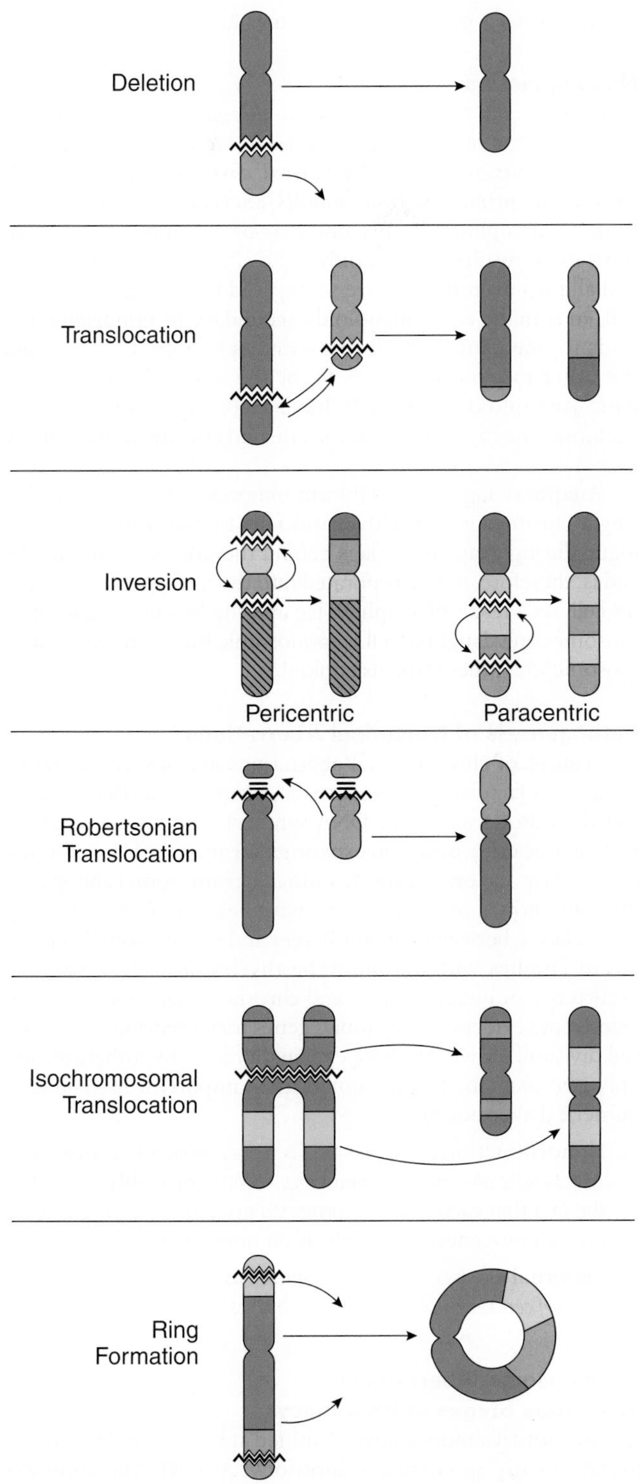

FIGURE 6-8. **Structural abnormalities of human chromosomes.** The deletion of a portion of a chromosome leads to the loss of genetic material and a shortened chromosome. A reciprocal translocation involves breaks on two nonhomologous chromosomes, with exchange of the acentric segments. An inversion requires two breaks in a single chromosome. If the breaks are on opposite sides of the centromere, the inversion is **pericentric;** it is **paracentric** if the breaks are on the same arm. A Robertsonian translocation occurs when two nonhomologous acrocentric chromosomes break near their centromeres, after which the long arms fuse to form one large metacentric chromosome. Isochromosomes arise from faulty centromere division, which leads to duplication of the long arm (iso q) and deletion of the short arm, or the reverse (iso p). Ring chromosomes involve breaks of both telomeric portions of a chromosome, deletion of the acentric fragments, and fusion of the remaining centric portion.

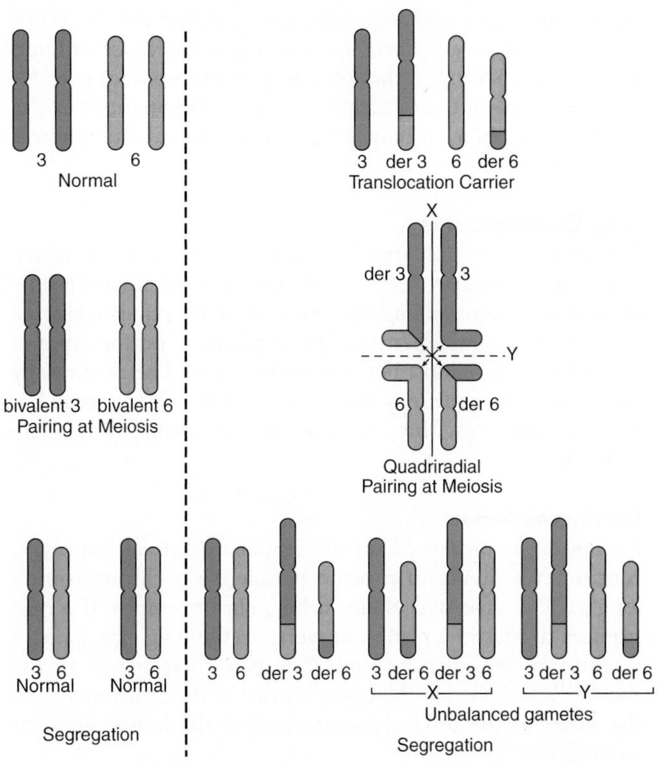

FIGURE 6-9. **Meiotic segregation in a reciprocal balanced translocation involving chromosomes 3 and 6.** The pairing of homologous chromosomes 3 and 6 in normal meiosis forms bivalents, which then segregate uniformly to create two gametes, each of which bears a single chromosome 3 and chromosome 6. Here the translocation carrier carries a balanced exchange of portions of the long arms of chromosomes 3 and 6. The chromosomes that carry the translocated genetic material are termed **derivative chromosomes** (der 3 and der 6). Diploid germ cells contain pairs of homologous chromosomes 3 and 6, each of which consists of one normal chromosome and one that carries a translocation. During meiosis, instead of the normal pairing into two bivalents, a quadriradial structure, containing all four chromosomes, is formed. In this circumstance, the chromosomes can segregate along several different planes of cleavage, shown as *X* and *Y*. In addition, the chromosomes can segregate diagonally *(arrows)*. As a result, six different gametes can be produced, four of which are unbalanced and can result in congenital abnormalities.

portion or because of a double break in the more central portions. The latter event leads to intercalary deletion and subsequent fusion of adjoining residual fragments.

Gametic deletion can be associated with either normal or abnormal development. An example of the latter is the **cri du chat syndrome,** in which the short arm of chromosome 5 is deleted. Deletions may be related to several human cancers, including some hereditary forms of cancer. For example, some familial **retinoblastomas** are associated with deletions in the long arm of chromosome 13 (see Chapter 5). **Wilms tumor aniridia syndrome** is associated with deletions in the short arm of chromosome 11.

Chromosomal Inversions

Chromosomal inversion refers to a process in which a chromosome breaks at two points, the affected segment inverts and then reattaches. **Pericentric inversions** result from breaks on opposite sides of the centromere, whereas **paracentric inversions** involve breaks on the same arm of the chromosome (see Fig. 6-8). During meiosis, homologous chromosomes that carry inversions do not exchange segments of chromatids by crossing over as readily as normal chromosomes, because of interference with pairing. Although this is of little consequence for the phenotype of the offspring, it may be important in evolutionary terms, since it may lead to clustering of certain hereditary features.

Ring Chromosomes

Ring chromosomes are formed by a break involving both telomericends of a chromosome, deletion of the acentric fragments and end-to-end fusion of the remaining centric portion of the chromosome (see Fig. 6-8). The consequences depend primarily on the amount of genetic material lost because of the break. The abnormally shaped chromosome may impede normal meiotic division, but in most instances, this chromosomal abnormality is of no consequence.

Isochromosomes

Isochromosomes are formed by faulty centromere division. Normally, centromeres divide in a plane parallel to a chromosome's long axis, to give two identical hemichromosomes. If a centromere divides in a plane transverse to the long axis, pairs of isochromosomes are formed. One pair corresponds to the short arms attached to the upper portion of the centromere and the other to the long arms attached to the lower segment (see Fig. 6-8).

The most important clinical condition involving isochromosomes is **Turner syndrome,** in which 15% of those affected have an isochromosome of the X chromosome. Thus, a woman with a normal X chromosome and an isochromosome composed of long arms of the X chromosome is monosomic for all the genes located on the missing short arm (i.e., the other isochromosome, which is lost during the meiotic division). She also has three sets of the genes located on the long arm. The absence of the genes from the short arm accounts for the abnormal development in these persons.

The Causes of Abnormal Chromosome Numbers Are Largely Unknown

A number of terms are important in understanding developmental defects associated with abnormal chromosome numbers.

- **Haploid:** A single set of each chromosome (23 in humans). Only germ cells have a haploid number (n) of chromosomes.
- **Diploid:** A double set (2n) of each of the chromosomes (46 in humans). Most somatic cells are diploid.
- **Euploid:** Any multiple (from n to 8n) of the haploid number of chromosomes. For example, many normal liver cells have twice (4n) the diploid DNA of somatic cells and are, therefore, euploid or, more specifically, tetraploid. If the multiple is greater than 2 (i.e., greater than diploid), the karyotype is **polyploid.**
- **Aneuploid:** Karyotypes that are not exact multiples of the haploid number. Many cancer cells are aneuploid, a characteristic often associated with aggressive behavior.
- **Monosomy:** The absence in a somatic cell of one chromosome of a homologous pair. For example, in Turner syndrome there is a single X chromosome.
- **Trisomy:** The presence of an extra copy of a normally paired chromosome. For example, Down syndrome is caused by the presence of three chromosomes 21.

Nondisjunction

Nondisjunction is a failure of paired chromosomes or chromatids to separate and move to opposite poles of the spindle at anaphase, during mitosis or meiosis. ***Numerical chromosomal abnormalities arise primarily from nondisjunction.*** Nondisjunction leads to aneuploidy if only one pair of chromosomes fails to separate. It results in polyploidy if the entire set does not divide and all the chromosomes are segregated into a single daughter cell. In somatic cells, aneuploidy secondary to nondisjunction leads to one daughter cell that exhibits trisomy ($2n + 1$) and the other monosomy ($2n - 1$) for the affected chromosome pair. Aneuploid germ cells have two copies of the same chromosome ($n + 1$) or lack the affected chromosome entirely ($n - 1$).

Anaphase lag is a special form of nondisjunction in which a single chromosome or chromatid fails to pair with its homologue during anaphase. It lags behind the others on the spindle and is, therefore, not incorporated into the nucleus of the daughter cell. As a result of anaphase lag and the loss of a single chromosome, one daughter cell is monosomic for the missing chromosome; the other remains euploid.

Pathogenesis of Numerical Aberrations

The causes of chromosomal aberrations are obscure. Putative exogenous factors, such as radiation, viruses, and chemicals, affect the mitotic spindle or DNA synthesis and produce mitotic and meiotic disturbances in experimental animals. However, the role of these factors in causing human chromosomal abnormalities is unknown. Immune factors have been invoked, as there is a correlation between autoantibodies and chromosomal anomalies in families with autoimmune thyroid disorders. Familial occurrence of meiotic failure and chromosomal anomalies provides some evidence that human genes may predispose to faulty cell division. However, these explanations are hypothetical, and only two phenomena are known to be important in genesis of numerical aberrations.

- **Nondisjunction** *during meiosis is more common in persons with structurally abnormal chromosomes.* This is probably related to the fact that such chromosomes do not pair or segregate during gametogenesis as readily as do normal ones.
- **Maternal age** *has long been recognized as a major factor in the etiology of certain nondisjunction syndromes, particularly trisomy 21.*

Chromosomal Aberrations at Various Stages of Pregnancy

Chromosomal abnormalities identified at birth differ from those found in early spontaneous abortions. At birth, the common chromosomal abnormalities are trisomies 21 (most frequent), 18, 13, and X or Y (47,XXX; 47,XXY; and 47,XYY). Approximately 0.3% of all liveborn infants have a chromosomal abnormality. Among spontaneous abortions, the most common chromosomal abnormalities are 45,X (most frequent), then trisomies 16, 21, and 22. However, trisomy of almost any chromosome can be observed in spontaneous abortions. *Up to 35% of spontaneous abortions have a chromosomal abnormality.* The reason for these differences is presumably related to survival in utero. Very few fetuses with 45,X survive to term, and trisomy 16 is nearly always lethal in utero; a fetus with trisomy 21 has a better chance of surviving to birth.

Effects of Chromosomal Aberrations

Most major chromosomal abnormalities are incompatible with life. The defects are usually lethal to a developing conceptus, and cause early death and spontaneous abortion. Loss of genetic material (e.g., autosomal monosomies) results in embryos that generally do not survive pregnancy. Monosomy of the X chromosome (45,X) may be compatible with life, although over 95% of such embryos are lost during pregnancy. Absence of an X chromosome (i.e., 45,Y) invariably leads to early abortion.

Autosomal trisomies lead to several developmental abnormalities. Affected fetuses usually die during pregnancy or shortly after birth. Trisomy 21, which defines Down syndrome, is an exception, and people with Down syndrome may survive for years. Trisomy of the X chromosome may result in abnormal development but is not lethal.

Mitotic nondisjunction may involve embryonic cells during early stages of development and result in chromosomal aberrations that are transmitted through some cell lineages but not others. *This is called* **mosaicism:** *the body contains two or more karyotypically different cell lines.* Mosaicism may involve autosomes or sex chromosomes, and the phenotype depends on the chromosome involved and the extent of mosaicism. Autosomal mosaicism is rare, probably because this condition is usually lethal. On the other hand, mosaicism involving sex chromosomes is common and is found in patients with gonadal dysgenesis who present with Turner or Klinefelter syndrome.

Nomenclature of Chromosomal Aberrations

Structural and numerical chromosomal abnormalities are classified by:

1. Total number of chromosomes
2. Designation (number) of affected chromosomes
3. Nature and location of the defect on the chromosome (Table 6-2).

Karyotypes are described sequentially by:

1. Total number of chromosomes
2. Sex chromosome complement
3. Any abnormality.

The short arm of a chromosome is designated **p,** and the long arm, **q.** The addition of chromosomal material, whether an entire chromosome or a part of one, is indicated by a plus sign (+) before the number of the affected chromosome. A minus sign (−) denotes loss of part or all of a chromosome. Alternatively, loss (deletion) of part of a chromosome may be designated by **del,** followed by the location of the deleted material on the affected chromosome. A translocation is written as a **t,** followed by brackets containing the involved chromosomes. Structural or numerical chromosomal aberrations are seen in 5 to 7 per 1000 liveborn infants, although most are balanced translocations and are asymptomatic.

Numerical Autosomal Aberrations in Liveborn Infants are Virtually All Trisomies

Structural aberrations that may result in clinical disorders include translocations, deletions and chromosomal breakage (Table 6-3).

Trisomy 21 (Down Syndrome)

Trisomy 21 is the most common cause of mental retardation. Furthermore, liveborn infants are only a fraction of all conceptuses with this defect. Two thirds abort spontaneously or die in utero. Life expectancy is also reduced. Advances in treating infections, congenital heart defects, and leukemia—the leading causes of death in patients with Down syndrome—have increased life expectancy.

TABLE 6-2

Chromosomal Nomenclature

Numerical designation of autosomes	1–22
Sex chromosomes	X, Y
Addition of a whole or part of a chromosome	+
Loss of a whole or part of a chromosome	−
Numerical mosaicism (e.g., 46/47)	/
Short arm of chromosome (petite)	p
Long arm of chromosome	q
Isochromosome	i
Ring chromosome	r
Deletion	del
Insertion	ins
Translocation	t
Derivative chromosome (carrying translocation)	der
Terminal	ter
Representative Karyotypes	
Male with trisomy 21 (Down syndrome)	47, XY, +21
Female carrier of fusion-type translocation between chromosomes 14 and 21	45,XX,−14, −21, + t(14q21q)
Cri du chat syndrome (male) with deletion of a portion of the short arm of chromosome 5	46,XY,del(5p)
Male with ring chromosome 19	46,XY,r(19)
Turner syndrome with monosomy X	45,X
Mosaic Klinefelter syndrome	46,XY/47,XXY

PATHOGENESIS: There are three mechanisms by which three copies of the genes on chromosome 21 that cause Down syndrome may be present in somatic cells:

- **Nondisjunction** in the first meiotic division of gametogenesis accounts for most (92%–95%) patients with trisomy 21. The extra chromosome 21 is of maternal origin in about 95% of Down syndrome children. Virtually all maternal nondisjunction seems to result from events in the first meiotic division (meiosis I).
- **Translocation** of an extra long arm of chromosome 21 to another acrocentric chromosome causes about 5% of cases of Down syndrome.
- **Mosaicism** for trisomy 21 is caused by nondisjunction during mitosis of a somatic cell early in embryogenesis and accounts for 2% of children born with Down syndrome.

TABLE 6-3

Clinical Features of the Autosomal Chromosomal Syndromes

Syndromes	Features
Trisomic Syndromes	
Chromosome 21 (Down syndrome 47,XX or XY,+21:1/800)	Epicanthic folds, speckled irides, flat nasal bridge, congenital heart disease, simian crease of palms, Hirschsprung disease, increased risk of leukemia
Chromosome 18 (47,XX or XY, +18: 1/8000)	Female preponderance, micrognathia, congenital heart disease, horseshoe kidney, deformed fingers
Chromosome 13 (47,XX or XY, +13: 1/20,000)	Persistent fetal hemoglobin, microcephaly, congenital heart disease, polycystic kidneys, polydactyly, simian crease
Deletion Syndromes	
5p - syndrome (Cri du chat 46,XX or XY,5p −)	Catlike cry, low birth weight, microcephaly, epicanthic folds, congenital heart disease, short hands and feet, simian crease
11p - syndrome (46,XX or XY, 11p −)	Aniridia, Wilms tumor, gonadoblastoma, male genital ambiguity
13q - syndrome (46,XX or XY,13q −)	Low birth weight, microcephaly, retinoblastoma, congenital heart disease

All of these syndromes are associated with mental retardation.

EPIDEMIOLOGY: *The incidence of trisomy 21 correlates strongly with increasing maternal age: children of older mothers have much greater risk of having Down syndrome* (Fig. 6-10). Up to their mid-30s, women have a constant risk of giving birth to a trisomic child of about 1 per 1000 liveborn infants. Incidence then increases sharply, to 1 in 30 at age 45 years. The risk of a mother having a second child with Down syndrome is 1%, regardless of maternal age, unless the syndrome is associated with translocation of chromosome 21.

PATHOGENESIS: The mechanism by which increasing maternal age increases the risk of bearing a child with trisomy 21 is poorly understood. Molecular studies have shown that the maternal age effect is related to maternal nondisjunction events, which implies that the defect lies in meiosis in oocytes. Down syndrome associated with translocation or mosaicism is not related to maternal age.

Down syndrome caused by translocation of an extra portion of chromosome 21 occurs in two situations. Either parent may be a phenotypically normal carrier of a balanced translocation, or a translocation may arise de novo during gametogenesis. These translocations are typically robertsonian, tending to involve only acrocentric chromosomes, with short arms consisting of a satellite and stalk (chromosomes 13, 14, 15, 21, and 22). Translocations between these chromosomes are particularly common since they cluster during meiosis and so are subjected to breakage and recombination more than other chromosomes. The most common translocation in Down syndrome (50%) is fusion of the long arms of chromosomes 21 and 14, t(14q;21q), followed in frequency (40%) by similar fusion involving two chromosomes 21, t(21q;21q).

If the translocation is inherited from a parent, a balanced translocation has been converted to an unbalanced one (see Figure 6-7B). By this scheme, one would expect a one in three chance of Down syndrome among offspring of a carrier of a balanced robertsonian translocation. However, if the mother carries the translocation, the actual incidence is only 10% to 15% and it is less than 5% if the father is the carrier. This reduced incidence probably relates to the early loss of most embryos with trisomy 21.

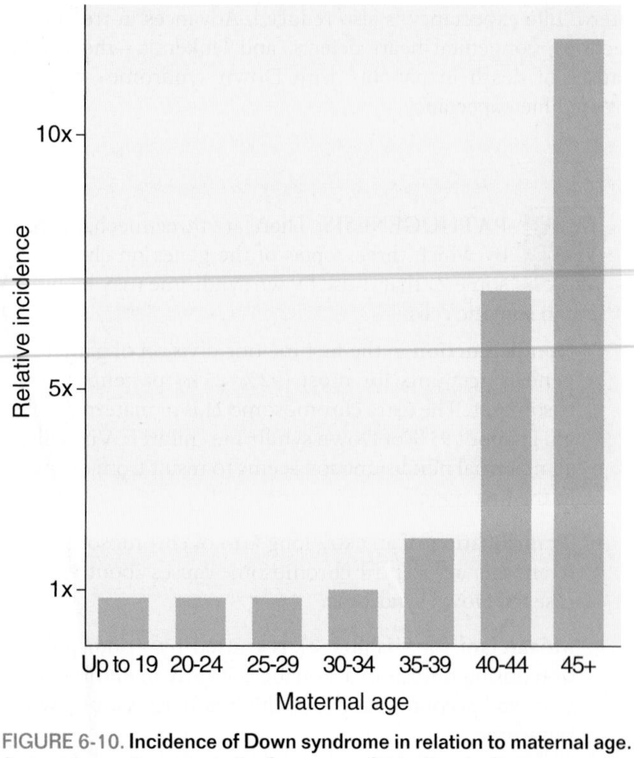

FIGURE 6-10. **Incidence of Down syndrome in relation to maternal age.** A conspicuous increase in the frequency of this disorder is seen over the age of 35 years.

Molecular Genetics of Down Syndrome

Chromosome 21 is the smallest human autosome, with less than 2% of all human DNA. It has an acrocentric structure, and all genes of known function (except for ribosomal RNA) are on the long arm (21q). Based on studies of inherited translocations, in which only a portion of chromosome 21 is duplicated, the region on chromosome 21 responsible for the full Down syndrome phenotype is in band 21q22.2, a 4-Mb region of DNA termed the **Down syndrome critical region** (DSCR). Genes in the DSCR that might be involved in Down syndrome have recently been identified. They encode transcription factors of the nuclear factor of activated T cells (NFAT) family, which are known to influence somatic development.

PATHOLOGY AND CLINICAL FEATURES: Diagnosis of Down syndrome is ordinarily made at the time of birth by virtue of the infant's flaccid state and characteristic appearance. The diagnosis is then confirmed by cytogenetic analysis. As the child develops, a typical constellation of abnormalities appears (Fig. 6-11).

- **Mental status:** Children with Down syndrome are invariably mentally retarded. Their IQs decline relentlessly and progressively with age. Mean IQs are 70 below the age of 1 year, declining during the first decade of life to a mean of 30. The major defect seems to be an inability to develop more-advanced cognitive strategies and processes, problems that become more apparent as the child grows older. These children were traditionally described as particularly gentle and affectionate, newer studies have cast serious doubt on the validity of these personality stereotypes.
- **Craniofacial features:** Face and occiput tend to be flat, with a low-bridged nose, reduced interpupillary distance, and oblique palpebral fissures. Epicanthal folds of the eyes impart an Oriental appearance, which accounts for the obsolete term **mongolism.** A speckled appearance of the iris is referred to as **Brushfield spots.** Ears are enlarged and malformed. A prominent tongue, which typically lacks a central fissure, protrudes through an open mouth.
- **Heart:** One third of children with Down syndrome have cardiac malformations. The incidence is even higher in aborted fetuses. Anomalies include atrioventricular canal, ventricular and atrial septal defects, tetralogy of Fallot, and patent ductus arteriosus. Most cardiac defects seem to reflect a problem in formation of the heart's venous inflow tract.
- **Skeleton:** These children tend to be small, owing to shorter than normal bones of the ribs, pelvis, and extremities. The hands are broad and short and exhibit a "simian crease," that is, a single transverse crease across the palm. The middle phalanx of the fifth finger is hypoplastic, an abnormality that leads to inward curvature of this digit.
- **Gastrointestinal tract:** Duodenal stenosis or atresia, imperforate anus and Hirschsprung disease (megacolon) occur in 2% to 3% of children with Down syndrome.
- **Reproductive system:** Men with trisomy 21 are invariably sterile, due to arrested spermatogenesis. A few women with Down syndrome have given birth to children, 40% of which had trisomy 21.
- **Immune system:** The immune system in Down syndrome has been the subject of numerous studies, but no clear pattern of defects has emerged. Still, affected children are unusually susceptible to respiratory and other infections.
- **Hematologic disorders:** Persons with Down syndrome are at a particularly high risk of developing leukemia at all ages. *The risk of leukemia in Down syndrome children younger than the age of 15 years is about 15-fold greater than normal.* In children younger under 3 years, acute nonlymphocytic leukemia predominates. After that, when most of the leukemias in Down syndrome occur, most cases are acute lymphoblastic leukemias. The basis for the high incidence of leukemia is unknown, but leukemoid reactions (transient pronounced neutrophilia) are frequent in the newborn with Down syndrome. Interestingly, leukemias that develop in patients who are mosaic for Down syndrome, are invariably trisomic for chromosome 21.
- **Neurologic disorders:** There is no clear pattern of neuropathology associated with Down syndrome, nor are there characteristic changes in the electroencephalogram. Nevertheless, the neurons in trisomy 21 may in fact differ from normal. Virtually all electrical parameters and a number of physiologic ones are altered in cultured neurons from infants with Down syndrome. *One of the most intriguing neurologic features of Down syndrome is its association with Alzheimer disease,* a relationship that has been appreciated for more than half a

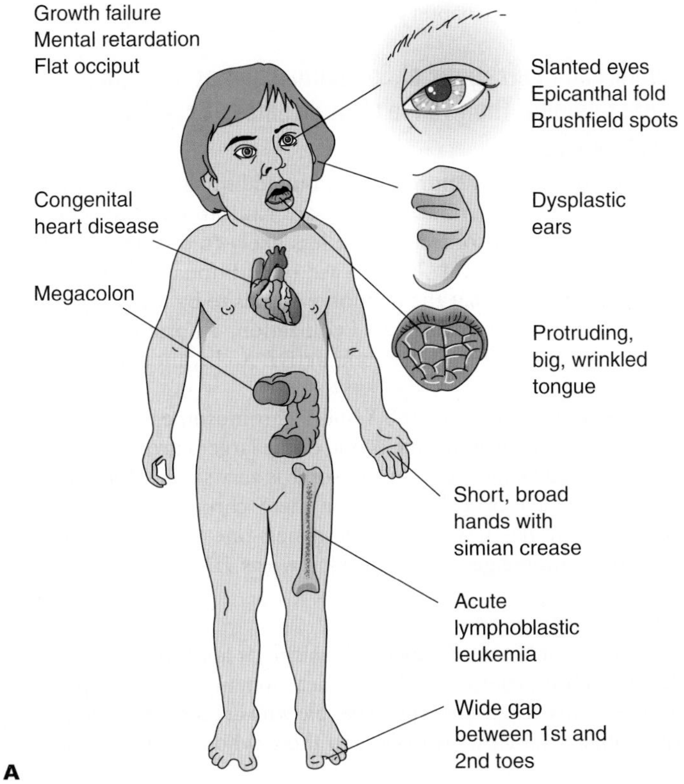

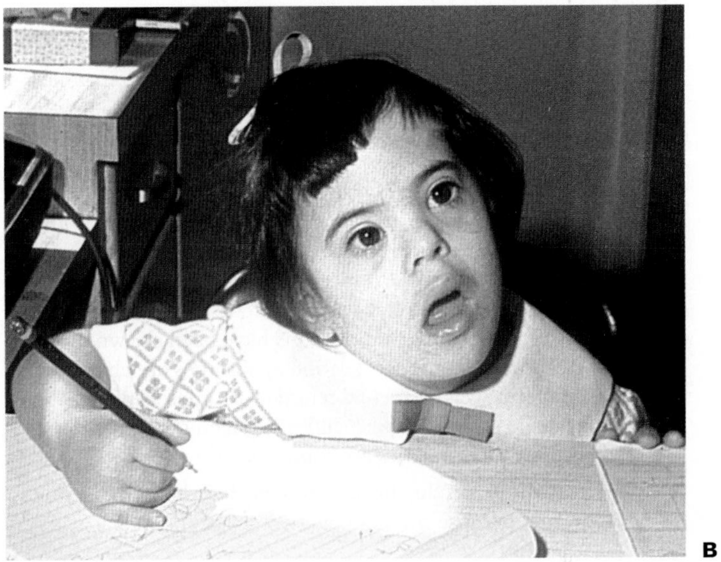

FIGURE 6-11. **A.** Clinical features of Down syndrome. **B.** A young girl with the facial features of Down syndrome.

century. The lesions characteristic of Alzheimer disease are universally demonstrable by age 35, including: (1) granulovacuolar degeneration, (2) neurofibrillary tangles, (3) senile plaques, and (4) loss of neurons (see Chapter 28). The senile plaques and cerebral blood vessels of both Alzheimer disease and Down syndrome always contain an amyloid composed of the same fibrillar protein (β-amyloid protein). The similarity between the neuropathology of Down syndrome and that of Alzheimer disease is also reflected in the appearance of dementia in one-fourth to one-half of older patients with Down syndrome and progressive loss of many intellectual functions that cannot be attributed to mental retardation alone.

- **Life expectancy:** During the first decade of life, the presence or absence of congenital heart disease is the major determinant of survival in Down syndrome. Of those whose hearts are normal, only about 5% die before age 10, while about 25% with heart disease die by then. For those who reach age 10, the estimated age at death is 55, which is 20 years or more lower that of the general population. Only 10% reach age 70.

Trisomies of Chromosomes 18, 13 and 22

Trisomy 18 is the second most common autosomal syndrome, occurring about once in 8000 live births, an order of magnitude less frequent than Down syndrome. The disorder results in mental retardation and affects females four times as often as males. Virtually all infants with trisomy 18 have congenital heart disease and die in the first 3 months of life.

Trisomies 13 and 22 are rare and both are associated with mental retardation, congenital heart disease, and other abnormalities. Syndromes associated with trisomies of chromosomes 8 and 9 have also been described.

Translocation Syndromes

The prototypical translocation that causes partial trisomy is Down syndrome. Many other partial trisomies are reported, the best documented of which is 9p-trisomy. In this disorder, the short arm of chromosome 9 may be translocated to one of several autosomes. Many kindreds with this syndrome have been described. Carriers of a balanced chromosome 9 translocation are asymptomatic but may pass an unbalanced translocation on to their offspring. The clinical disorder is characterized by mental retardation, microcephaly, and other craniofacial abnormalities. A reciprocal translocation between the long arms of chromosomes 22 and 11 is also well known. Offspring of carriers may have an extra chromosome with parts of both 11 and 22, in which case they have partial trisomy of both chromosomes, leading to microcephaly and other anomalies.

Chromosomal Deletion Syndromes

Deletion of an entire autosomal chromosome (i.e., monosomy) is usually not compatible with life. However, several syndromes arise from deletions of parts of several chromosomes (see Table 6-3). In most cases, the congenital syndromes are sporadic, but in a few instances, reciprocal translocations have been shown in the parents. Virtually all of these deletion syndromes are characterized by low birth weight, mental retardation, microcephaly, and craniofacial and skeletal abnormalities. Congenital heart disease and urogenital abnormalities are common.

- **5p–syndrome (cri du chat):** This is the best-known deletion syndrome, because the high-pitched cry of the infant is like that of a kitten and calls attention to the disorder. Most cases are sporadic, but reciprocal translocations have been reported in some parents.
- **11p–syndrome:** Deletion of the short arm of chromosome 11, specifically band 11p13, leads absence of the iris (aniridia), and is often accompanied by Wilms tumor.
- **13q–syndrome:** Loss of the long arm of chromosome 13 is associated with retinoblastoma, owing to the loss of the *Rb* tumor suppressor gene (see Chapter 5).
- **Other deletion syndromes:** Deletions of both short and long arms of chromosome 18 are documented, producing varying patterns of mental retardation and craniofacial anomalies. Loss of material from chromosomes 19, 20, 21, and 22 is usually associated with ring chromosomes. Syndromes associated with 21q–and 22q–are the most common and often resemble Down syndrome.
- **Deletions and rearrangements of subtelomeric sequences:** Telomeres are a repetitive sequence $(TTAGGG)_n$ at the ends of chromosomes. Subtelomeric regions of chromosomes are rich in genes. Deletions and rearrangements of these regions can only be demonstrated by FISH, and are major causes of mild to severe mental retardation and dysmorphic features, and are found in about 5% of such patients.

Chromosomal Breakage Syndromes

Several recessive syndromes associated with frequent chromosomal breakage and rearrangements are accompanied by significant risk of leukemia and other cancers. These disorders include xeroderma pigmentosum, Bloom syndrome (congenital telangiectatic erythema with dwarfism), Fanconi anemia (constitutional aplastic pancytopenia), and ataxia telangiectasia. Acquired chromosome breaks and translocations are associated with leukemias and lymphomas, the best documented of which are chronic myelogenous leukemia, t(9;22) and Burkitt lymphoma, mostly t(8;14) (see Chapters 5, 20).

Numerical Aberrations of Sex Chromosomes Are Much More Common Than Those of Autosomes, Save for Trisomy 21

The reasons are not entirely clear, but additional sex chromosomes (Fig. 6-12) produce less severe clinical manifestations than do extra autosomes and are less likely to disturb critical stages of development. In the case of additional X chromosomes, the reason that the phenotype tends to be less severely affected is probably related to Lyonization, a normal process in which each cell only has one active X-chromosome (see below).

The contrast between the X and Y chromosomes is striking. Whereas the X chromosome is one of the larger chromosomes, with 6% of all DNA, the Y chromosome is very small. More than 1300 genes have been identified on the X chromosome; the Y chromosome has fewer than 400 genes, one of which is the testis-determining gene (*SRY,* also known as *TDF*).

The Y Chromosome

In humans, unlike some lower organisms, it appears that genes on the Y chromosome are the key determinants of gender phenotype. Thus, the phenotype of people who are XXY (Klinefelter syndrome; see below) is male, and those who are XO (Turner

Gametes: Ovum \ Sperm	X	Y	XY	O
X	46,XX Normal ♀	46,XY Normal ♂	47,XXY Klinefelter ♂	45,X Turner ♀
XX	47,XXX ♀	47,XXY Klinefelter ♂	48,XXXY Klinefelter ♂	46,XX Normal ♀
XXX	48,XXXX ♀	48,XXXY Klinefelter ♂	49,XXXXY Klinefelter ♂	47,XXX Triple X ♀
O	45,X Turner ♀	45,Y LETHAL	46,XY LETHAL	44 LETHAL

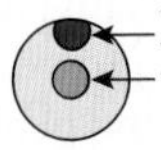

FIGURE 6-12. **Numerical aberrations of sex chromosomes.** Nondisjunction in either the male or female gamete is the principal cause of these abnormalities.

syndrome) are female. The testis-determining gene (*SRY,* sex-determining region, Y) is an intron-less gene near the end of the short arm of the Y chromosome. The *SRY* gene encodes a small nuclear protein with a DNA-binding domain. This protein binds another protein (SIP-1) to form a complex that is a transcriptional activator of autosomal genes that control development of a male phenotype. Mutations in this gene lead to XY females, while translocations that introduce this gene into an X chromosome produce XX males.

A small proportion of infertile men with azoospermia or severe oligospermia have small deletions in regions of the Y chromosome. However, the size and location of these deletions are variable and do not correlate with the severity of spermatogenic failure.

The X Chromosome

Males carry only one X chromosome but the same amounts of X chromosome gene products as do females. This seeming discrepancy isexplained by the **Lyon effect:**

- In females, one X chromosome is irreversibly inactivated early in embryogenesis. The inactivated X chromosome is detectable in interphase nuclei as a heterochromatic clump of chromatin attached to the inner nuclear membrane, termed the **Barr body.** The inactive X chromosome is extensively methylated at gene control regions and transcriptionally repressed. Nevertheless, a significant minority of X-linked genes escape inactivation and continue to be expressed by both X chromosomes. The probability that an X chromosome is rendered inactive seems to correlate with the level of expression of another X-linked gene, *XIST,* which is expressed only by the inactive partner.
- Either the paternal or maternal X chromosome is inactivated randomly.
- Inactivation of the X chromosome is virtually complete.
- Inactivation of the X chromosome is permanent and transmitted to progeny cells: paternally or maternally derived X chromosomes are propagated clonally. *All females are therefore mosaic for paternally and maternally derived X chromosomes.* Mosaicism for glucose-6-phosphate dehydrogenase in females was important in demonstrating the monoclonal origin of neoplasms (see Chapter 5).

The issue is not quite so simple, however. If one X chromosome is entirely nonfunctional, persons with XXY (Klinefelter) or XO (Turner) karyotypes should be phenotypically normal. They are not, and the fact that they show phenotypic abnormalities indicates that the inactivated X chromosome still functions, at least in part. Indeed, a part of the short arm of the X chromosome is known to escape X-inactivation. This region, which can pair with a homologous region on the short arm of the Y chromosome and undergo meiotic recombination between the two, is known as the **pseudoautosomal region.** Genes in this location are present in two functional copies in both males and females. Thus patients with Turner syndrome (45,X) are haploinsufficient for these genes, and those with more than two X chromosomes (e.g., Klinefelter patients) have more than two functional copies. One gene in this region, *SHOX,* is associated with height, and its haploinsufficiency in Turner syndrome may explain the short stature of Turner patients. Several other genes outside the pseudoautosomal region also escape X inactivation. *In both phenotypically male and female children with extra X chromosomes, the degree of mental retardation correlates roughly with the number of X chromosomes.*

Klinefelter Syndrome (47,XXY)

In Klinefelter syndrome, or testicular dysgenesis, there are one or more X chromosomes beyond the normal male XY complement. This is the most important clinical condition involving trisomy of sex chromosomes (Fig. 6-13). This syndrome is a prominent cause of male hypogonadism and infertility.

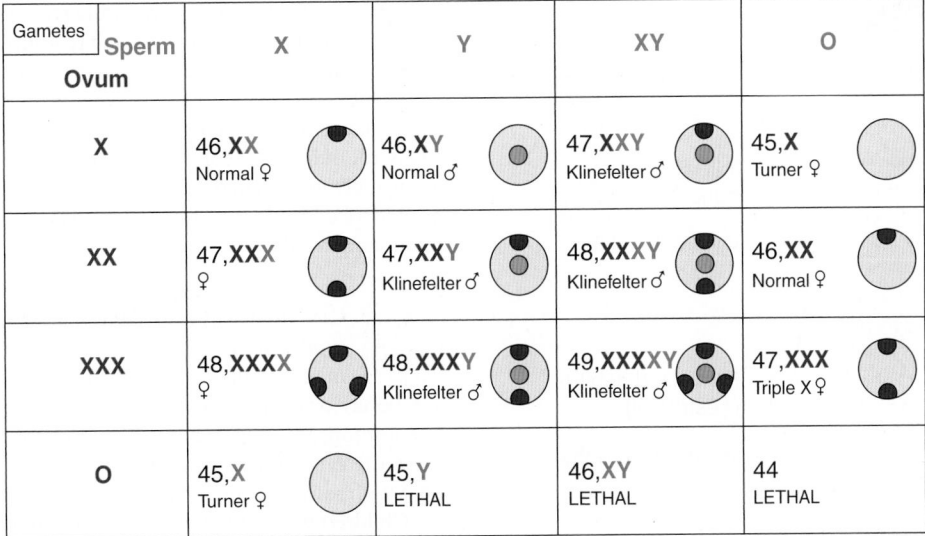

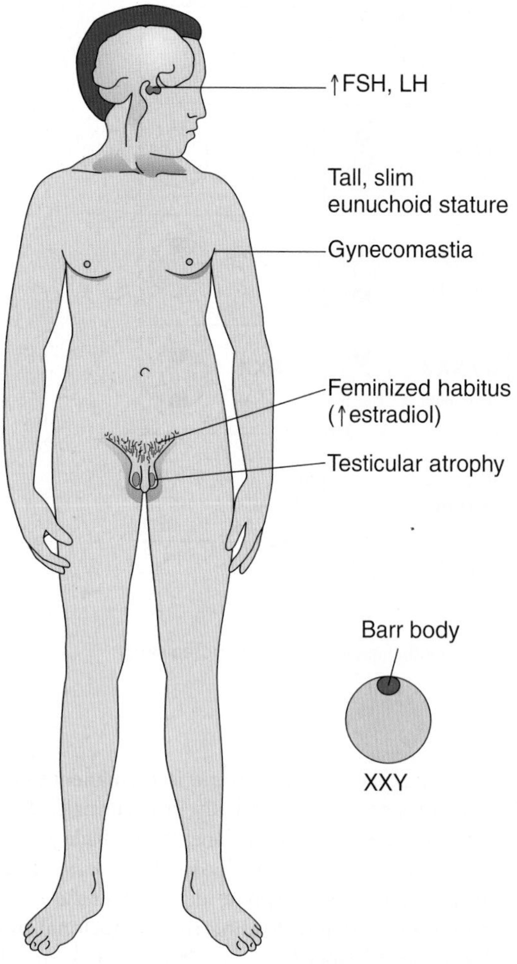

FIGURE 6-13. **Clinical features of Klinefelter syndrome.** FSH = follicle-stimulating hormone; LH = leuteinizing hormone

PATHOGENESIS: Most people with Klinefelter syndrome (80%) have a single extra X chromosome, that is, a 47,XXY karyotype. A minority are mosaics (e.g., 46,XY/47,XXY) or have more than two X chromosomes (e.g., 48,XXXY). *Interestingly, regardless of the number of supernumerary X chromosomes (even up to 4), the Y chromosome ensures a male phenotype.* The additional X chromosomes correlate with a more abnormal phenotype, despite the inactivation of the extra X chromosomes. Presumably, the same genes that escape inactivation in normal females are still functional in Klinefelter syndrome.

Klinefelter syndrome occurs in 1 per 1000 male newborns, roughly comparable to the incidence of Down syndrome. Interestingly, half of all 47,XXY conceptuses are lost due to spontaneous abortion. The additional X chromosome(s) arises as a result of meiotic nondisjunction during gametogenesis. In half of cases, nondisjunction occurs during paternal meiosis I, leading to a sperm containing both an X and a Y chromosome. Fertilization of a normal oocyte by such a sperm produces a 47,XXY karyotype.

PATHOLOGY: After puberty, the intrinsically abnormal testes do not respond to gonadotropin stimulation and show sequentially regressive alterations. Seminiferous tubules display atrophy, hyalinization, and peritubular fibrosis. Germ cells and Sertoli cells are usually absent and eventually the tubules become dense cords of collagen. Leydig cells are usually increased in number, but their function is impaired, as evidenced by low testosterone levels in the face of elevated luteinizing hormone (LH) levels.

CLINICAL FEATURES: The diagnosis of Klinefelter syndrome is usually made after puberty, because the main manifestations of the disorder during childhood are behavioral and psychiatric. Gross mental retardation is uncommon, although average IQ is probably somewhat reduced. Since the syndrome is so common, it should be suspected in all boys with some mental deficiency or severe behavioral problems.

Children with Klinefelter syndrome tend to be tall and thin, with relatively long legs (eunuchoid body habitus). Normal testicular growth and masculinization do not occur at puberty, and testes and penis remain small. Feminine characteristics include a high-pitched voice, gynecomastia, and a female pattern of pubic hair (female escutcheon). Azoospermia results in infertility. All of these changes are due to hypogonadism and a resulting lack of androgens. Serum testosterone is low to normal, but LH and follicle-stimulating hormone are remarkably high, indicating normal pituitary function. High circulating estradiol levels increase the estradiol-to-testosterone ratio, which determines the degree of feminization. Treatment with testosterone will virilize these patients but does not restore fertility.

The XYY Male

Interest in the XYY phenotype (1 per 1000 male newborns) comes from studies in penal institutions suggesting that the prevalence of this karyotype was significantly higher than in the general population. However, the idea that these "supermales" manifest aggressive antisocial behavior because of an extra Y chromosome has not been substantiated in other studies and the topic remains controversial. The only features of the XYY phenotype that are agreed on are tall stature, a tendency toward cystic acne, and some problems in motor and language development. Aneuploidy of the Y chromosome is a consequence of meiotic nondisjunction in the father.

Turner Syndrome

Turner syndrome refers to the spectrum of abnormalities that results from complete or partial X chromosome monosomy in a phenotypic female. It occurs in about 1 liveborn female infant in 5000. In 3/4 of cases, the single X chromosome of Turner syndrome is of maternal origin, suggesting that the meiotic error tends to be paternal. The incidence of the syndrome does not correlate with maternal age, and the risk of producing a second affected female infant is not increased.

The 45,X karyotype is actually one of the most common aneuploid abnormalities in human conceptuses, but almost all are aborted spontaneously. In fact, up to 2% of abortuses show this aberration. Since patients with Turner syndrome survive normally after birth, why is the missing X chromosome lethal during fetal development? Perhaps the inactivated X chromosome in normal females (or the Y chromosome in males) protects against early demise of the embryo. It is believed that homologues of Y genes in the pseudoautosomal region of the X chromosome escape inactivation and are critical to the survival of a female conceptus.

Only about half of women with Turner syndrome lack an entire X chromosome (monosomy X). The remainder are mosaics or have structural X chromosome aberrations, such as isochromosome of the long arm, translocations, and deletions. Mosaics with a 45,X/46,XX karyotype (15%) tend to have milder phenotypic manifestations of Turner syndrome and may even be fertile. In about 5% of patients, the mosaic karyotype is 45,X/46,XY, in which case an original male zygote was subsequently modified by a mitotic nondisjunction. Such persons are at a 20% risk of developing a germ cell cancer and should have prophylactic removal of the abnormal gonads.

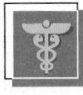

PATHOLOGY AND CLINICAL FEATURES: The clinical hallmark of Turner syndrome is sexual infantilism with primary amenorrhea and sterility (Fig. 6-14). In most cases, the disorder is not discovered until the absence of menarche brings the child to medical attention. Virtually all of these women are less than 5 ft (152 cm) tall. Other clinical features include a short, webbed neck (pterygium coli), low posterior hairline, wide carrying angle of the arms (cubitus valgus), broad chest with widely spaced nipples, and hyperconvex fingernails. Half of patients have anomalies on urograms, the most common being horseshoe kidney and malrotation. Many have facial abnormalities, including a small mandible, prominent ears, and epicanthal folds. Defective hearing and vision are common, and as many as 20% are noted to be mentally defective. Pigmented nevi become prominent as the patient ages. For unknown reasons, women with Turner syndrome are at a greater risk for chronic autoimmune thyroiditis and goiter.

Cardiovascular anomalies occur in almost half the patients in Turner syndrome. Coarctation of the aorta is seen in 15%, and a bicuspid aortic valve in as many as a third. Essential hypertension occurs in some patients, and dissecting aneurysm of the aorta is occasionally a cause of death.

The ovaries of women with Turner syndrome show a curious acceleration of normal aging. Ovaries of a normal female fetus initially contain 7 million oocytes each. Fewer than half of these survive to the time of birth. Relentless loss of oocytes continues, so that at menarche only about 5% (400,000) of the original remain, and at menopause a mere 0.1% have survived. Ovaries of fetuses with Turner syndrome contain oocytes at first, but they lose them rapidly, so that none remain by 2 years of age. The ovaries are converted to fibrous streaks, whereas the uterus, fallopian tubes, and vagina develop normally. It may be said that the child with Turner syndrome has undergone menopause long before reaching menarche.

Interestingly, families are known in which several women have premature menopause and show deletions of portions of the long arm of one X chromosome. Such data, together with observations of Turner syndrome, further support the concept that the genes controlling ovarian development and function in the inactivated X chromosome continue to be expressed in the normal female.

Children with Turner syndrome are treated with growth hormone and estrogens and enjoy an excellent prognosis for a normal life, albeit infertile.

Syndromes in Females with Multiple X Chromosomes

One extra X chromosome in a phenotypic female (i.e., a 47,XXX karyotype) is the most frequent abnormality of sex chromosomes in women, occurring at about the same rate as Klinefelter syndrome. Most of these women are of normal intelligence, although they may have some difficulty in speech, learning, and emotional responses. Minor physical anomalies are encountered, including epicanthal folds and clinodactyly (inward curvature of the fifth finger). Fertility is the rule, but incidence of congenital defects may be increased in the children of 47,XXX women.

Women with 4 and 5 X chromosomes are reported. Virtually all have been mentally retarded. They superficially resemble women with Down syndrome and do not mature sexually. Women with supernumerary X chromosomes have additional Barr bodies, indicating inactivation of all but one X chromosome. Clearly, some genes on the inactivated X chromosomes continue to be expressed.

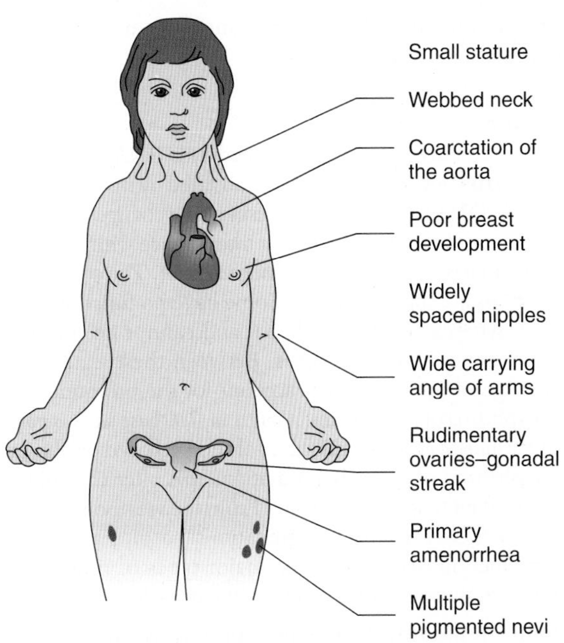

FIGURE 6-14. **Clinical features of Turner syndrome.**

Single Gene Abnormalities Confer Traits That Segregate Sharply Within Families

The classic laws of mendelian inheritance, named in honor of Gregor Mendel, are:

- **A mendelian trait** is determined by two copies of the same gene, called alleles, located at the same locus on two homologous chromosomes. In the case of the X and Y chromosomes in males, a trait is determined by just one allele.
- **Autosomal genes** refer to those located on one of the 22 autosomes.
- **Sex-linked traits** are encoded by loci on the X chromosome.
- **A dominant phenotypic trait** requires the presence of only one allele of a homologous gene pair. In other words, the dominant phenotype is present whether the allelic genes are homozygous or heterozygous.
- **A recessive phenotypic trait** demands that both alleles be identical, that is homozygous.
- **Codominance** refers to a situation in which both alleles in a heterozygous gene pair are fully expressed (e.g., the AB blood group genes).

Mendelian traits are classified as:

1. **Autosomal dominant**
2. **Autosomal recessive**
3. **Sex-linked dominant**
4. **Sex-linked recessive.**

Diseases due to sex-linked dominant genes are rare and of little practical significance.

Mutations

To make proteins, DNA is transcribed into RNA, which is processed into mRNA, which in turn is translated by ribosomes. Thus, a change in DNA can lead to a corresponding change in the amino acid sequence of a specific protein or interference with its synthesis.

A mutation is a stable heritable change in DNA. The consequences of mutations are highly variable. Some have no functional consequences, whereas others are lethal and cannot be transmitted from one generation to another. Between these extremes is a broad range of mutations that account for the profound genetic polymorphisms of any species. *About 1 in 1000 base pairs is polymorphic in the human genome.* Indeed, evolution is based on the occurrence over time of nonlethal mutations that alter the abiity of a species to adapt to its environment. From the viewpoint of human disease, we focus principally on mutations that alter protein structure or function detectably. The major types of mutations encountered in the study of human genetic disorders (Fig. 6-15) are

- **Point mutations:** Replacement of one base by another is a **point mutation.** If it is in the coding region (the part of the gene that is translated into a protein), a point mutation has three possible consequences.
  - In a **synonymous mutation** the new codon with the mutation still codes for the same amino acid. For example, CGA and CGC both code for arginine.
  - A **missense mutation** (three fourths of base changes in the coding region) occurs when the new codon codes for a different amino acid. In sickle cell anemia, an adenine to thymine change in the β-globin gene replaces glutamic acid (GAG) with valine (GUG).
  - A **nonsense mutation** (4%) is one in which a base substitution stops translation. A codon for an amino acid is changed to a termination codon, yielding a truncated protein. For example, UAU codes for tyrosine, but UAA is a stop codon.
- **Frameshift mutations:** Amino acids are encoded by trinucleotide sequences. If the number of nucleotides in a gene is changed by insertion or deletion, and if the number of bases added or deleted is not a multiple of 3, *the reading frame of the message is changed.* Then, even though the downstream sequence is the same, it will code for a different amino acid sequence and probably a termination signal. Frameshift mutations can also alter transcription, splicing or processing of mRNA.
- **Large deletions:** When a large segment of DNA is deleted, the coding region of a gene may be entirely removed, in which case the protein product is absent. On the other hand, a large deletion may result in the apposition of coding regions of nearby genes, giving rise to a fused gene that codes for a hybrid protein, one in which part or all of one protein is followed by part or all of another.
- **Expansion of unstable trinucleotide repeat sequences:** The human genome contains frequent tandem trinucleotide repeat sequences, some of which are associated with disease. The number of copies of certain repetitive trinucleotide sequences varies among individuals, representing allelic polymorphism of the genes in which they are found. In general, the number of repeats below a particular threshold does not change during mitosis or meiosis, whereas above this threshold, the number of repeats can expand or contract, expansion being far more common. A number of distinct trinucleotide expansions have been identified in human disease (Table 6-4).

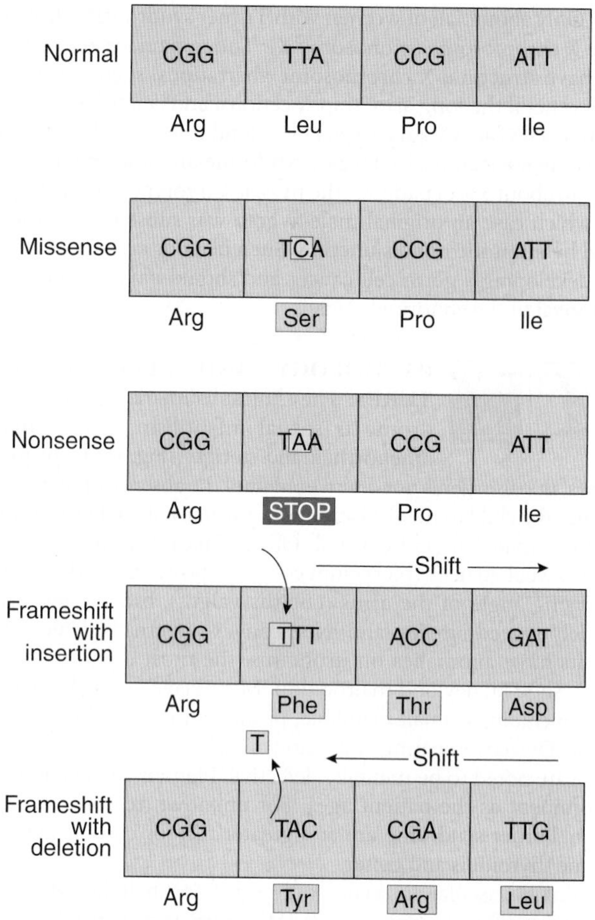

FIGURE 6-15. **Point mutations that alter the reading frame of DNA.** A variety of mutations in the second codon of a normal sequence of four amino acids is depicted. With a missense mutation, a change from T to C substitutes serine (Ser) for leucine (Leu). With a nonsense mutation, a change from T to A converts the leucine codon to a stop codon. A shift in the reading frame to the right results from insertion of a T, thus changing the sequence of all subsequent amino acids. Conversely, deletion of a T shifts the reading frame one base to the left and also changes the sequence of subsequent amino acids. Arg = arginine; Asp = aspartate; Ile = isoleucine; Phe = phenylalanine; Pro = proline; Thr = threonine; Tyr = tyrosine.

Huntington disease (HD): HD is an inherited neurodegenerative disease caused by expansion of a CAG repeat within the coding sequence of the gene, IT15, that codes for the protein **huntingtin.** In HD, the stable alleles contain 10 to 30 repeats, while persons affected by the disease have 40 to 100 repeats. CAG codes for glutamine, and abnormal expansion of the polyglutamine tract in HD confers a toxic gain-of-function to huntingtin. Although the precise mechanism by which mutant huntingtin causes selective neuronal loss is not understood, there is evidence to suggest that altered protein–protein interactions are responsible. In addition to HD, expanded CAG repeats are involved in a number of other neurodegenerative disorders (see Table 6-4).

Fragile X syndrome: This genetic disorder, the most common cause of inherited mental retardation (see below), is due to expansion of a CGG repeat in a noncoding region immediately adjacent to the *FMR1* gene on the X chromosome. The expanded CGG repeat somehow silences the *FMR1* gene by methylation of its pro-

TABLE 6-4

Representative Diseases Associated with Trinucleotide Repeats

Disease	Location	Sequence	Normal Length	Premutation	Full Mutation
Huntington disease	4p16.3	CAG	10–30	-	40–100
Kennedy disease	Xq21	CAG	15–25	-	40–55
Spinocerebellar ataxia	6p23	CAG	20–35	-	45–80
Fragile X syndrome	Xq27.3	CGG	5–55	50–200	200– >1000
Myotonic dystrophy	19q13	CTG	5–35	37–50	50–2000
Friedreich ataxia	9q13	GAA	7–30	-	120–1700

moter. The abnormal repeat is also associated with an inducible "fragile site" on the X chromosome, which appears in cytogenetic studies as a nonstaining gap or an apparent chromosomal break.

Myotonic dystrophy (MD): MD, the most common form of autosomal muscular dystrophy (see Chapter 27), is caused by expansion of a CTG repeat in the 3′-untranslated region of the MD gene. Normal persons have up to 35 CTG repeats, but patients with MD may have up to 2000 repeats. The structure of the protein product of the gene, a protein kinase, is unchanged but it is suspected that other nearby genes are rendered dysfunctional.

Friedreich ataxia (FA): FA is an autosomal recessive degenerative disease affecting the CNS and the heart that is associated with expansion of a GAA repeat in the *frataxin* gene (see Chapter 28), which encodes a mitochondrial protein. Affected persons have 120 to 1700 repeats in the first intron (noncoding) of the frataxin gene.

Functional Consequences of Mutations

A biochemical pathway represents the sequential actions of a series of enzymes, which are coded for by specific genes. A typical pathway can be represented by the conversion of a substrate (A) through intermediate metabolites (B and C) to the final product (D).

A	→	B → C	→	D
initial substrate		intermediary metabolites		end-products

A single gene defect can have several consequences:

- **Failure to complete a metabolic pathway:** In this situation, the end-product (D) is not formed because an enzyme that is essential for the completion of a metabolic sequence is missing:

  $$A \rightarrow B \rightarrow C -/ /\rightarrow (D)\,(\downarrow)$$

  An example of the failure to complete a metabolic pathway is **albinism**, a pigment disorder caused by a deficiency of tyrosinase. This enzyme catalyzes the conversion of tyrosine to melanin (through the intermediate formation of dihydroxyphenylalanine (DOPA)). Without tyrosinase, the end-product, melanin, is not formed, and an affected person (an "albino") has no pigment in all organs that normally contain it, primarily the eyes and skin.

- **Accumulation of unmetabolized substrate:** The enzyme that converts the initial substrate into the first intermediary metabolite may be missing, a situation that results in excessive accumulation of the initial substrate.

  $$A\,(\uparrow)^{\sim} / /\rightarrow B\,(\downarrow)\,C\,(\downarrow)\,D\,(\downarrow)$$

  In phenylketonuria, dietary phenylalanine accumulates because of an inborn deficiency of phenylalanine hydroxylase. The resulting toxic concentration of phenylalanine interferes with postnatal development of the brain and causes severe mental retardation.

- **Storage of an intermediary metabolite:** An intermediary metabolite, which is readily processed into the final product and is normally present only in minute amounts, accumulates in large quantities if the enzyme responsible for its metabolism is deficient.

  $$A \rightarrow B\,(\uparrow)^{\sim} \rightarrow / /\rightarrow C\,(\downarrow)\,D\,(\downarrow)$$

  This type of genetic disorder is exemplified by von Gierke disease, a glycogen storage disease that results from a deficiency of glucose-6-phosphatase. The inability to convert glucose-6-phosphate into glucose leads to its alternative conversion to glycogen.

- **Formation of an abnormal end-product:** In this situation, a mutant gene codes for an abnormal protein. Sickle cell anemia results from substitution of valine for glutamic acid in the β globin part of hemoglobin.

Mutation Hotspots

Certain regions of the genome mutate at a much higher rate than average. The best-characterized hotspot is the dinucleotide pair CG, which is prone to undergo mutation to form TG. The reason is that methylation of cytosine in CG dinucleotides is a common occurrence that is implicated in regulating gene expression. Generally, the methylation product, 5-methylcytosine, represses gene transcription. Importantly, 5-methylcytosine can undergo spontaneous deamination to thymine (Fig. 6-16). If this occurs in a gamete, it can become a fixed, heritable trait in the offspring.

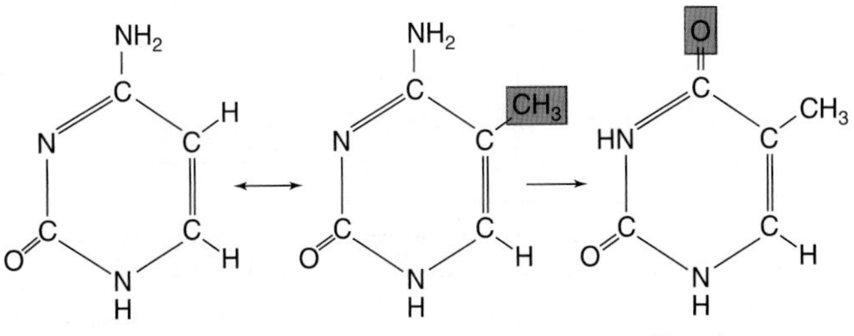

FIGURE 6-16. **5-Methylcytosine is formed from cytosine.** Spontaneous deamination of 5-methylcytosine produces thymine.

Autosomal Dominant Disorders Are Expressed in Heterozygotes

A dominant disease occurs when only one defective gene (i.e., mutant allele) is present, whereas its paired allele on the homologous chromosome is normal. The salient features of autosomal dominant traits are (Fig. 6-17):

- Males and females are equally affected, since by definition, the mutant gene resides on one of the 22 autosomal chromosomes. As a consequence, there can be father-to-son transmission (which is absent in X-linked dominant disorders).
- The trait encoded by the mutant gene can be transmitted to successive generations (unless the disease interferes with reproductive capacity).
- Unaffected members of a family do not transmit the trait to their offspring. Unless the disease represents a new mutation, everyone with the disease has an affected parent.
- The proportions of normal and diseased offspring of patients with the disorder are on average equal, because most affected persons are heterozygous, whereas their normal mates do not harbor the defective gene.

New Mutations versus Inherited Mutations

As noted above, an autosomal dominant disease may result from a new mutation rather than transmission from an affected parent. Nevertheless, the offspring of persons with a new dominant mutation are at a 50% risk for the disease. *The ratio of new mutations to transmitted ones among persons with dominant autosomal disorders varies with the effect of the disease on reproductive capacity.* Greater impairment of reproductive capacity, means a greater proportion will be new mutations. A dominant mutation that leads to complete infertility would have to be a new mutation. If reproductive capacity is only partially impaired, the proportion of new mutations is correspondingly lower. Thus, **tuberous sclerosis** is an autosomal dominant condition in which mental retardation limits reproductive potential. In this disease, new mutations account for 80% of cases. If a dominant disease has little effect on reproductive activity (e.g., familial hypercholesterolemia), virtually all affected persons will have pedigrees showing classic vertical transmission of the disorder.

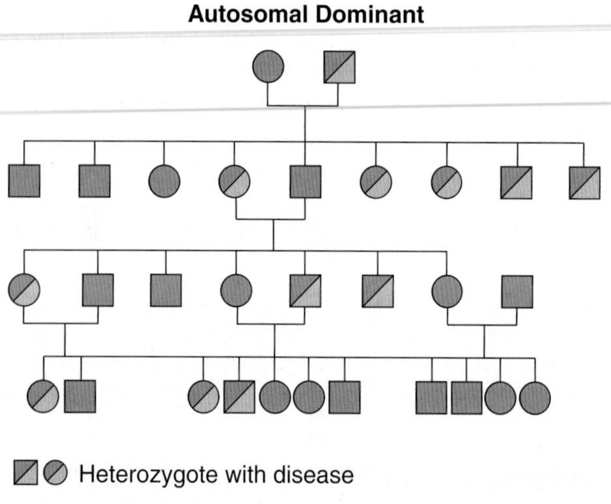

FIGURE 6-17. **Autosomal dominant inheritance.** Only symptomatic persons transmit the trait to the next generation, and heterozygotes are symptomatic. Both males and females are affected.

Biochemical Basis of Autosomal Dominant Disorders

There are several major mechanisms by which the presence of one mutant allele and one normal allele is responsible for clinical disease.

- When the gene product is a rate-limiting component of a complex metabolic network (e.g., a receptor or an enzyme), half of the normal amount of gene product may be insufficient to maintain the normal state. This is known as **haploinsufficiency.** Examples of this mechanism include βthalassemia and familial hypercholesterolemia caused by defects in the low-density lipoprotein (LDL) uptake receptor by hepatocytes.
- In some diseases, the presence of an extra copy of an allele gives rise to a phenotype. An example of this is Charcot-Marie-Tooth disease, type IA, which is caused by duplication of the peripheral myelin protein-22 gene.
- Constitutive activation of a gene is seen in some familial cancer syndromes. For example, mutations in the *RET* protooncogene are found in families with multiple endocrine neoplasia, type 2. These cause abnormally increased activity of a tyrosine kinase that stimulates cell proliferation.
- Mutations in genes that encode structural proteins (e.g., collagens, cytoskeletal constituents) result in abnormal molecular interactions and disruption of normal morphologic patterns. Such a situation is exemplified by osteogenesis imperfecta and hereditary spherocytosis.

More than 1000 human diseases are inherited as autosomal dominant traits, although most are rare. Examples of human autosomal dominant diseases are given in Table 6-5.

TABLE 6-5

Representative Autosomal Dominant Disorders

Disease	Frequency	Chromosome
Familial hypercholesterolemia	1/500	19p
von Willebrand disease	1/8000	12p
Hereditary spherocytosis (major forms)	1/5000	14,8
Hereditary elliptocytosis (all forms)	1/2500	1,1p,2q,14
Osteogenesis imperfecta (types I–IV)	1/10,000	17q,7q
Ehlers-Danlos syndrome, type III	1/5000	?
Marfan syndrome	1/10,000	15q
Neurofibromatosis type 1	1/3500	17q
Huntington chorea	1/15,000	4p
Retinoblastoma	1/14,000	13q
Wilms tumor	1/10,000	11p
Familial adenomatous polyposis	1/10,000	5q
Acute intermittent porphyria	1/15,000	11q
Hereditary amyloidosis	1/100,000	18q
Adult polycystic kidney disease	1/1000	16p

Heritable Diseases of Connective Tissue Are Heterogeneous and Often Inherited As Autosomal Dominant Traits

This discussion is limited to three of the most common and best-studied entities that affect connective tissue: Marfan syndrome, Ehlers-Danlos syndrome, and osteogenesis imperfecta. Even in these well-delineated disorders, clinical symptomatology often overlaps. For instance, some patients exhibit the joint dislocations typical of the Ehlers-Danlos syndrome, but other members of the same family suffer from multiple fractures characteristic of osteogenesis imperfecta. Yet others in the family, with the same genetic defect, may have no symptoms. Thus current classifications based on clinical criteria, will eventually be replaced by references to specific gene defects, as with the hemoglobinopathies.

Marfan Syndrome

Marfan syndrome is an autosomal dominant, inherited disorder of connective tissue characterized by a variety of abnormalities in many organs, including the heart, aorta, skeleton, eyes, and skin. One third of cases represent sporadic mutations. The incidence in the United States is 1 per 10,000.

PATHOGENESIS: The cause of Marfan syndrome is a missense mutation in the gene for *fibrillin-1 (FBN1),* on the long arm of chromosome 15 (15q21.1). Fibrillin is a family of connective tissue proteins analogous to the collagens, of which there are now about a dozen genetically distinct forms. It is widely distributed in many tissues in the form of a fiber system termed **microfibrils.** By electron microscopy, microfibrils are threadlike filaments that form larger fibers, which are organized into rods, sheets, and interlaced networks. **Microfibrillar fibers** are scaffolds for elastin deposition during embryonic development, after which they constitute part of elastic tissues. For example, the deposition of elastin on lamellae of microfibrillar fibers produces the concentric rings of elastin in the aortic wall. By use of immunofluorescent microscopy, abnormal microfibrillar fibers have been visualized in all the tissues affected in Marfan syndrome.

Fibrillin-1 is a large, cysteine-rich glycoprotein that forms 10-nm microfibrils in the extracellular matrix of many tissues. Interestingly, the ciliary zonules that suspend the lens of the eye are devoid of elastin but consist almost exclusively of microfibrillar fibers (fibrillin). Dislocation of the lens is a characteristic feature of Marfan syndrome. Deficiencies in the amount and distribution of microfibrillar fibers have been shown in the skin and fibroblast cultures of patients with Marfan syndrome, which renders the elastic fibers incompetent to resist normal stress.

PATHOLOGY AND CLINICAL FEATURES: People with Marfan syndrome are usually (but not invariably) tall, and the lower body segment (pubis-to-sole) is longer than the upper body segment. A slender habitus, which reflects a paucity of subcutaneous fat, is complemented by long, thin extremities and fingers, which accounts for the term **arachnodactyly** (spider fingers) (Fig. 6-18). Overall, the affected persons resemble figures in paintings by El Greco.

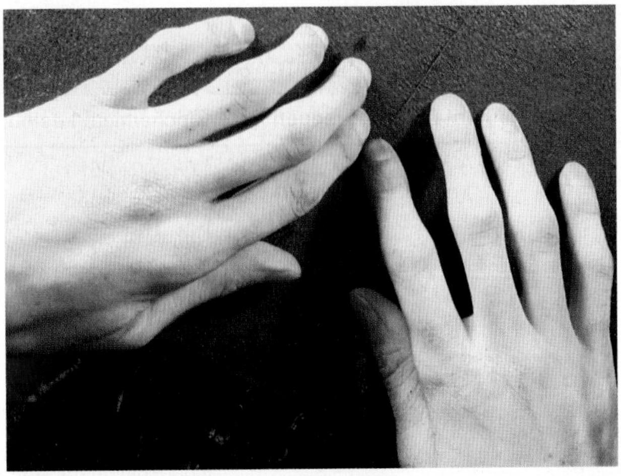

FIGURE 6-18. **Long, slender fingers (arachnodactyly) in a patient with Marfan syndrome.**

- **Skeletal system:** The skull in Marfan syndrome is characteristically long (dolichocephalic), with prominent frontal eminences. Disorders of the ribs are conspicuous and produce pectus excavatum (concave sternum) and pectus carinatum (pigeon breast). The tendons, ligaments and joint capsules are weak, a condition that leads to hyperextensibility of the joints (double-jointedness), dislocations, hernias, and kyphoscoliosis; the last is often severe.
- **Cardiovascular system:** *The most important vascular defect is in the aorta, in which the principal lesion is a weal tunica media.* Weakness of the media leads to variable dilation of the ascending aorta and a high incidence of dissecting aneurysms. The dissecting aneurysm, usually of the ascending aorta, may rupture into the pericardial cavity or make its way down the aorta and rupture into the retroperitoneal space. Dilation of the aortic ring results in aortic regurgitation, which may be severe enough to produce angina pectoris and congestive heart failure. The mitral valve may have redundant leaflets and chordae tendineae—leading to mitral valve prolapse syndrome. Cardiovascular disorders are the most common causes of death in Marfan syndrome.

  Microscopic examination of the aorta reveals conspicuous fragmentation and loss of elastic fibers, accompanied by an increase in metachromatic mucopolysaccharide. Focally, the defect in the elastic tissue results in discrete pools of amorphous metachromatic material, reminiscent of that seen in Erdheim (idiopathic) cystic medial necrosis of the aorta. Smooth muscle cells are enlarged and lose their orderly circumferential arrangement.
- **Eyes:** Ocular changes are common in Marfan syndrome and reflect the intrinsic lesion in connective tissue. These include dislocation of the lens (ectopia lentis), severe myopia owing to elongation of the eye and retinal detachment.

Untreated men with Marfan syndrome usually die in their 30s, and untreated women often die in their 40s. However, with antihypertensive therapy and replacement of the aorta with prosthetic grafts, life expectancy approaches normal.

Ehlers-Danlos Syndromes

The Ehlers-Danlos syndromes (EDS) are rare, autosomal dominant, inherited disorders of connective tissue that feature remarkable hyperelasticity and fragility of the skin, joint hypermobility, and often a bleeding diathesis. The disorder is clinically and genetically hete-

TABLE 6-6

Ehlers-Danlos Syndromes

Type	Inheritance	Frequency	Biochemical Lesion	Clinical Features
I	AD	1/30,000	Type V collagen	Hyperextensible skin; hypermobile joints
II	AD	1/30,000	Type V collagen	Similar to, but less severe than, type I
III	AD	1/5000	Unknown	Hypermobile joints
IV	AD	1/100,000	Type III collagen	Thin skin, easy bruising, rupture of arteries, intestine and gravid uterus
V	XLR	Rare	Unknown	Similar to type II
VI	AR	Rare	Lysyl hydoxylase	Ocular lesions and blindness, hyperextensible, hypermobile joints
VII	AD	Rare	Type I collagen	Congenital hip dislocation, hypermobile joints
VIII	AD	Rare	Unknown	Periodontal disease, hyperextensible skin
IX	XLR	Rare	Lysyl oxidase (copper metabolism)	Lax skin, bladder diverticula and rupture, skeletal deformities
X	AR	Rare	Fibronectin	Similar to type II

AD = autosomal dominant; AR = autosomal recessive; XLR = X-linked recessive.

rogeneous (Table 6-6). More than 10 varieties of EDS have been distinguished, and the molecular lesions have been identified in several.

PATHOGENESIS: The genetic and biochemical lesions in 7 of the 10 types of EDS have been established. *The common feature of all is a generalized defect in collagen, including abnormalities in its molecular structure, synthesis, secretion, and degradation.* In EDS I through IV, VI, and X, electron microscopic studies of the skin have shown an increased size of collagen fibrils, with unusually small bundles, features that are consistent with the presence of abnormal collagen. Such changes involve type III collagen in EDS IV and type I collagen in EDS VII. EDS VII arises from mutations that alter the amino-terminal cleavage sites of either the 1 or 2 procollagen chains of type I collagen. Deficiencies of specific collagen-processing enzymes, including lysyl hydroxylase and lysyl oxidase, have been identified in EDS VI and IX, respectively. Whatever the underlying biochemical defect may be, the end result is deficient or defective collagen. Depending on the type of EDS, these molecular lesions are associated with conspicuous weakness of the supporting structures of the skin, joints, arteries, and visceral organs.

PATHOLOGY AND CLINICAL FEATURES: All types of EDS are characterized by soft, fragile, hyperextensible skin. Patients typically can stretch their skin many centimeters and trivial injuries can lead to serious wounds. Sutures do not hold well, so dehiscence of surgical incisions is common. Hypermobility of the joints allows unusual extension and flexion, e.g., as in the "human pretzel" and other contortionists. EDS IV is the most dangerous variety, owing to a tendency to spontaneous rupture of the large arteries, bowel, and gravid uterus. Death from such complications is common in the third and fourth decades of life.

Ehlers-Danlos syndrome VI also has major complications, including severe kyphoscoliosis, blindness from retinal hemorrhage, or rupture of the globe and death from aortic rupture. Severe periodontal disease, with loss of teeth by the third decade, characterizes EDS VIII. EDS IX features the development of bladder diverticula during childhood, with a danger of bladder rupture and skeletal deformities.

Many persons who exhibit clinical abnormalities suggesting EDS do not conform to any of the documented types of this disorder. Further genetic and biochemical characterization of such cases is likely to expand the classification of EDS.

Osteogenesis Imperfecta

Osteogenesis imperfecta (OI), or brittle bone disease, is a group of inherited disorders in which a generalized abnormality of connective tissue is expressed principally as fragility of bone. OI is inherited in an autosomal dominant pattern, although there are rare cases that are autosomal recessive.

PATHOGENESIS: The genetic defects in the 4 types of OI are heterogeneous, but all affect type I collagen synthesis. In 90% of cases, mutations in pro-$\alpha 1$(I) and pro-$\alpha 2$(I) collagen genes mostly cause substitution of other amino acids for the obligate glycine at every third residue.

PATHOLOGY AND CLINICAL FEATURES: Type I OI is characterized by a normal appearance at birth, but fractures of many bones occur during infancy and at the time the child learns to walk. Such patients have been described as being as "fragile as a china doll." Children with type I OI typically have blue sclerae as the deficiency in collagen fibers, which imparts translucence to the sclera. A high incidence of hearing loss occurs because fractures and fusion of the bones of the middle ear restrict their mobility.

Type II OI is usually fatal in utero or shortly after birth. The infants have a characteristic facial appearance and skeletal abnormalities. Those who are born alive usually die of respiratory failure within the first month of life.

Type III OI is the progressively deforming variant, which is ordinarily detected at birth by the presence of short stature and deformities caused by fractures in utero. Dental defects and hearing loss are common. Unlike other types of OI, type III is often inherited as an autosomal recessive trait.

Type IV OI is similar to type I, except that sclerae are normal and the phenotype is more variable.

Osteogenesis imperfecta is discussed in further detail in Chapter 26.

Neurofibromatosis

The neurofibromatoses include two distinct autosomal dominant disorders characterized by the development of multiple neurofibromas, which are benign tumors of peripheral nerves of Schwann cell origin.

Neurofibromatosis Type I (von Recklinghausen Disease)

Neurofibromatosis type I (NF1) is characterized by (1) disfiguring neurofibromas, (2) areas of dark pigmentation of the skin (café au lait spots), and (3) pigmented lesions of the iris (Lisch nodules). It is one of the more common autosomal dominant disorders, affecting 1 in 3500 persons of all races. The *NF1* gene has an unusually high rate of mutation and half of cases are sporadic rather than familial. NF1 was first described in 1882 by von Recklinghausen, but references to this disorder can be found as early as the 13th century.

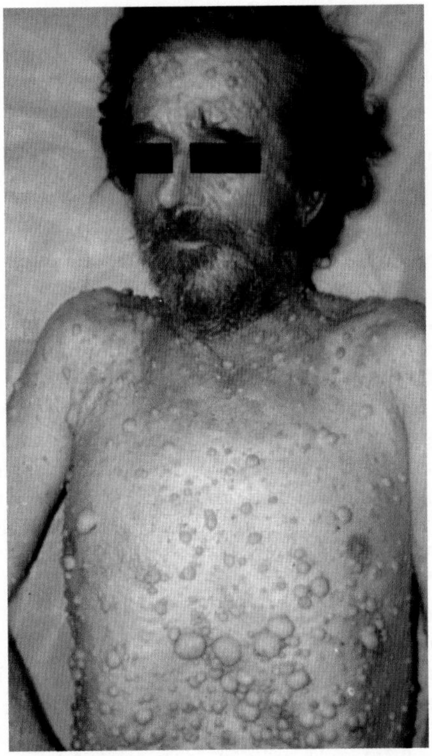

FIGURE 6-19. **Neurofibromatosis, type I.** Multiple cutaneous neurofibromas are noted on the face and trunk.

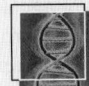

PATHOGENESIS: Germline mutations in the NF1 gene, on the long arm of chromosome 17 (17q11.2), include deletions, missense mutations, and nonsense mutations. The gene product, *neurofibromin,* belongs to a family of GTPase-activating protein (GAP), which inactivate the ras protein (see Chapter 5). In this sense, NF1 is a classic tumor suppressor. The loss of GAP activity permits uncontrolled ras activation, which presumably predisposes to formation of neurofibromas.

PATHOLOGY AND CLINICAL FEATURES: The clinical manifestations of NF1 are highly variable and difficult to explain entirely on the basis of a single gene defect. The typical features of NF1 include:

- **Neurofibromas:** More than 90% of patients with NF1 develop cutaneous and subcutaneous neurofibromas in late childhood or adolescence. These cutaneous tumors, which may total more than 500, appear as soft, pedunculated masses, usually about 1 cm in diameter (Fig. 6-19). However, on occasion they may reach alarming proportions and dominate the physical appearance of a patient, attaining 25 cm in dimeter. Subcutaneous neurofibromas present as soft nodules along the course of peripheral nerves. **Plexiform neurofibromas** occur only within the context of NF1 and are diagnostic of that condition. These tumors usually involve the larger peripheral nerves but on occasion may arise from cranial or intraspinal nerves. Plexiform neurofibromas are often large, infiltrative tumors that cause severe disfigurement of the face or an extremity. The microscopic appearance of neurofibromas is discussed in Chapter 28. *A major complication of NF1, occurring in 3% to 5% of patients, is the appearance of a neurofibrosarcoma in a neurofibroma, usually a larger one of the plexiform type.* NF1 is also associated with an increased incidence of other neurogenic tumors, including meningioma, optic glioma and pheochromocytoma.
- **Café au lait spots:** Although normal persons may exhibit occasional light brown patches on the skin, more than 95% of persons affected by NF1 display six or more such lesions. These are over 5 mm before puberty and greater than 1.5 cm thereafter. Café au lait spots tend to be ovoid, with the longer axis oriented in the direction of a cutaneous nerve. Numerous freckles, particularly in the axilla, are also common.
- **Lisch nodules:** Over 90% of patients with NF1 have pigmented nodules of the iris, which are masses of melanocytes. These lesions are thought to be hamartomas.
- **Skeletal lesions:** A number of bone lesions occur frequently in NF1. These include malformations of the sphenoid bone and thinning of the cortex of the long bones, with bowing and pseudarthrosis of the tibia, bone cysts, and scoliosis.
- **Mental status:** Mild intellectual impairment is frequent in patients with NF1, but severe retardation is not part of the syndrome.
- **Leukemia:** The risk of malignant myeloid disorders in children with NF1 is 200 to 500 times the normal risk. In some patients, both alleles of the NF1 gene are inactivated in leukemic cells.

Neurofibromatosis Type II (Central Neurofibromatosis)

Neurofibromatosis type II (NF2) refers to a syndrome defined by bilateral tumors of the eighth cranial nerve (acoustic neuromas) and, commonly, by meningiomas and gliomas. The disorder is considerably less common than NF1, occurring in 1 in 50,000 persons. Most patients suffer from bilateral acoustic neuromas, but the condition can be diagnosed in the presence of a unilateral eighth nerve tumor if two of the following are present: neurofibroma, meningioma, glioma, schwannoma, or juvenile posterior lenticular opacity.

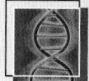

PATHOGENESIS: Despite the superficial similarities between NF1 and NF2, they are not variants of the same disease and, indeed, have separate genetic origins. The *NF2* gene resides in the middle of the long arm of chromosome 22 (22q,11.1-13.1). In contrast to NF1, the tumors in NF2 frequently show deletions or loss of heterozygous DNA markers in the affected chromosome. The *NF2* gene encodes a tumor-suppressor protein termed **merlin,** or **schwannomin,** which is a member of a superfamily of proteins that link the cytoskeleton to the cell membrane. Other members of this family include ezrin, moesin, radixin, talin, and protein 4.1. Merlin is detectable in most differentiated tissues, including Schwann cells.

Achondroplastic Dwarfism

Achondroplastic dwarfism is an autosomal dominant, hereditary disturbance of epiphyseal chondroblastic development that leads to inadequate enchondral bone formation. This abnormality causes a distinctive form of dwarfism characterized by short limbs with a normal head and trunk. The affected person has a small face, a bulging forehead, and a deeply indented bridge of the nose. Achondroplastic dwarfism is not infrequent, occurring in 1 per 3000 live births. Achondroplasia is discussed in Chapter 26.

Familial Hypercholesterolemia

Familial hypercholesterolemia is an autosomal dominant disorder characterized by high levels of LDLs in the blood, and deposition of cholesterol in arteries, tendons, and skin. It is one of the most common autosomal dominant disorders, and affecting 1 in 500 adults in the United States in its heterozygous form. Only 1 person in 1 million is homozygous for the disease. *Interest in this disease stems from the striking acceleration of atherosclerosis and its complications.* (see Chapter 10).

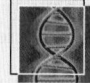

PATHOGENESIS: Familial hypercholesterolemia results from abnormalities in the gene that codes for the cell surface receptor that removes LDL from the blood. This gene is on the short arm of chromosome 19. Over 150 different mutations of all kinds in the LDL receptor gene are known.

The LDL receptor is (1) synthesized in the endoplasmic reticulum (ER), (2) transferred to the Golgi complex, (3) transported to the cell surface, and (4) internalized by receptor-mediated endocytosis in coated pits after binding LDL. Genetic defects in each of these steps have been described:

- **Class 1:** This is the most common type of defect and leads to failure of synthesis of nascent LDL-receptor protein in the ER. Most such defects reflect large deletions in the gene (null alleles).
- **Class 2:** These mutations prevent transfer of the nascent receptor from the ER to the Golgi apparatus (transport-defective alleles). Thus, mutant receptor never appears at the cell surface.
- **Class 3:** LDL receptors of class 3 mutations are expressed on the cell surface but are defective in the ligand-binding domain (binding-defective alleles).
- **Class 4:** In this rare class of mutations, LDL binding to the receptor is normal, but the defect prevents receptor clustering in coated pits, thus blocking their internalization by endocytosis (internalization-defective alleles).
- **Class 5:** In this case, internalized LDL–receptor complexes are not discharged from the endosome, and the receptor does not recycle to the plasma membrane (recycling-defective alleles).

Hepatocytes are the main cell type expressing LDL receptor. After LDL bind the receptor, they are internalized and degraded in lysosomes, freeing cholesterol for further metabolism. Lacking LDL receptor function, high levels of LDL circulate, are taken up by tissue macrophages, and accumulate to form occlusive arterial plaques (atheromas) and papules or nodules of lipid-laden macrophages (xanthomas) (see Chapter 10).

CLINICAL FEATURES: Heterozygous and homozygous familial hypercholesterolemia are two distinct clinical syndromes, reflecting a clear gene-dosage effect. In heterozygotes, elevated blood cholesterol (mean, 350 mg/dL; normal, < 200 mg/dL) are seen at birth. Tendon xanthomas develop in half the patients before the age of 30, and symptoms of coronary heart disease often occur before age 40. In homozygotes, blood cholesterol content reaches astronomic levels (600 to 1200 mg/dL) and virtually all patients have tendon xanthomas and generalized atherosclerosis in childhood. Untreated homozygotes typically die of myocardial infarction before they reach 30 years of age.

Autosomal Recessive Disorders Cause Symptoms in People who have Defective Alleles on both Homologous Chromosomes

Most genetic metabolic diseases exhibit an autosomal recessive mode of inheritance (Fig. 6-20) (Table 6-7). The fact that recessive genes are uncommon and the need for two mutant alleles to produce

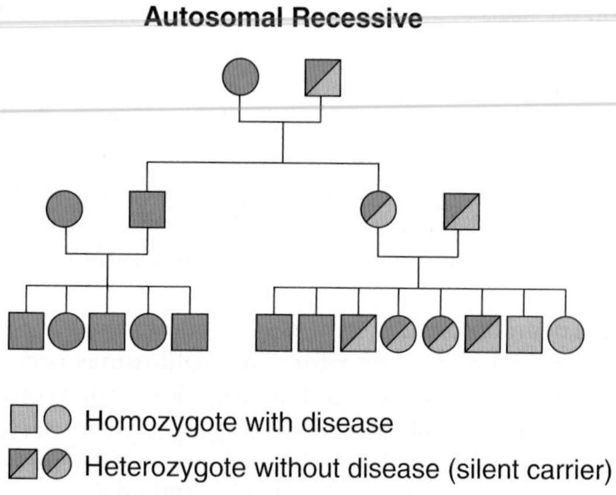

FIGURE 6-20. **Autosomal recessive inheritance.** Symptoms of the disease appear only in homozygotes, male or female. Heterozygotes are asymptomatic carriers. Symptomatic homozygotes result from the mating of asymptomatic heterozygotes.

TABLE 6–7

Representative Autosomal Recessive Disorders

Disease	Frequency	Chromosome
Cystic fibrosis	1/2500	7q
α-Thalassemia	High	16p
β-Thalassemia	High	11p
Sickle cell anemia	High	11p
Myeloperoxidase deficiency	1/2000	17q
Phenylketonuria	1/10,000	12q
Gaucher disease	1/1000	1q
Tay-Sachs disease	1/4000	15q
Hurler syndrome	1/100,000	22p
Glycogen storage disease Ia (von Gierke disease)	1/100,000	17
Wilson disease	1/50,000	13q
Hereditary hemochromatosis	1/1000	6p
α_1-Antitrypsin deficiency	1/7000	14q
Oculocutaneous albinism	1/20,000	11q
Alkaptonuria	<1/100,000	3q
Metachromatic leukodystrophy	1/100,000	22q

clinical disease determine the key characteristics of autosomal recessive inheritance. Some of the salient features of such disorders are

- The more infrequent the mutant gene in the general population, the lower the chance that unrelated parents carry the trait. *Rare autosomal recessive disorders often derive from consanguineous marriages.*
- Both parents are usually heterozygous for the trait and are clinically normal.
- Symptoms appear on average in 1 of 4 of their offspring. Half of all offspring are heterozygous for the trait and are asymptomatic. Thus, 2/3 of unaffected offspring are heterozygous carriers.
- As in autosomal dominant disorders, autosomal recessive traits are transmitted equally to males and females.
- Symptomatology of autosomal recessive disorders is ordinarily less variable than with dominant diseases. Recessive traits therefore present more commonly in childhood, while dominant disorders may initially appear in adults.
- The variability in clinical expression of many autosomal recessive diseases is a function of the residual functionality of the affected enzyme. This variability is manifested in (1) different degrees of clinical severity, (2) age at onset, or (3) the existence of acute and chronic forms of the specific disease.

Most mutant genes responsible for autosomal recessive disorders are rare in the general population, because those homozygous for the trait tend to die before reaching reproductive age. Paradoxically, a few lethal autosomal recessive diseases are common. Sickle cell anemia may confer a biological advantage in increasing resistance of heterozygotes to malarial parasitization, and thus compensates for the loss of homozygotes. Almost all males with cystic fibrosis (CF) are sterile because of congenital bilateral absence of the vas deferens, and females have decreased fertility; any enhanced biological fitness of the heterozygote remains obscure.

New mutations for recessive diseases are difficult to identify clinically because resulting heterozygotes are asymptomatic. Nonconsanguineous mating of two such heterozygotes would occur by chance, and many generations later, if at all.

Biochemical Basis of Autosomal Recessive Disorders

Autosomal recessive diseases characteristically are caused by deficiencies in enzymes rather than in structural proteins. A mutation that inactivates an enzyme does not usually cause an abnormal phenotype in heterozygotes. For instance, since most cellular enzymes operate at substrate concentrations well below saturation, an enzyme deficiency is easily corrected simply by increasing the amount of substrate. Diseases caused by impaired catabolism of dietary substances (e.g., phenylketonuria, galactosemia) or cellular constituents (e.g., Tay-Sachs, Hurler) are autosomal recessive, in heterozygotes, increased substrate concentrations overcome the partial lack of enzyme. By contrast, loss of both alleles in a homozygote results in complete loss of enzyme activity, which situation cannot be corrected by such mechanisms.

Cystic Fibrosis Is the Most Common Lethal Autosomal Recessive Disorder in the White Population

CF is characterized by (1) chronic pulmonary disease; (2) deficient exocrine pancreatic function; and (3) other complications of inspissated mucus in several organs, including the small intestine, liver, and reproductive tract. The disease results from a defective chloride channel, the **cystic fibrosis transmembrane conductance regulator** (CFTR).

EPIDEMIOLOGY: More than 95% of cases have been reported in whites; the disease is only exceptionally found in blacks and almost never in Asians. About 1 in 25 whites is a heterozygous carrier of the gene and the incidence of the disease is 1 in 2,500 newborns. Within the white population, the incidence of CF varies widely by geographic location. It is highest in the northern European Celtic populations such as Ireland and Scotland, and much lower among southern Europeans.

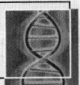

PATHOGENESIS: The CFTR gene is on the long arm of chromosome 7 (7q31.2). (see Table 6-7) It encodes a protein of 1480 amino acids that is a member of the adenosine triphosphate (ATP)-binding family of membrane transporter proteins. It is a chloride channel in most epithelia, with two membrane-spanning domains, two domains that bind ATP and an "R" domain that contains phosphorylation sites.

CFTR activity is regulated by the balance between kinase and phosphatase activities (i.e., phosphorylation and dephosphorylation). Phosphorylation of the R domain, mostly by cyclic adenosine monophosphate (cAMP)-dependent protein kinase A stimulates chloride channel activity by enhancing ATP binding. Secretion of chloride anions by mucus-secreting epithelial cells controls the parallel secretion of fluid and, consequently, the viscosity of the mucus. In normal mucus-secreting epithelia, cAMP activates protein kinase A, which phosphorylates the regulatory domain of CFTR and permits channel opening. The most common mutation in the white population is a deletion of 3 base pairs that delets a phenylalanine residue (ΔF_{508}). This mutation accounts for 70% of mutations in the white population. The next most common mutation accounts for only 2% of all mutations.

Mutations in the *CFTR* gene that disturb chloride channel function fall into several functional groupings (Fig. 6-21):

- **Failure of CFTR synthesis:** Mutations that result in premature termination signals interfere with synthesis of the full-length CFTR protein. As a result there is no CFTR-mediated chloride secretion in the involved epithelia.
- **Failure of CFTR transport to the plasma membrane:** Certain mutations prevent proper folding of the nascent protein, so it is then targeted for proteasomal degradation rather than for transport to the plasma membrane (see Chapter 1). The ΔF_{508} mutation is of this class. However, the role of the ΔF_{508} mutation in CF varies significantly by geography and ethnicity. In Denmark, it accounts for almost 90% of all CF cases; among Ashkenazi Jews, the figure is only 30%. An analysis of haplotypes suggested that the ΔF_{508} mutation originated 50,000 years ago in the Middle East, from where it progressively spread throughout the European land mass.
- **Defective ATP binding to CFTR:** Certain mutations allow CFTR proteins to reach the plasma membrane but affect ATP-binding domains, thus interfering with regulation of the channel and decreasing, but not abolishing, chloride secretion.
- **Defective chloride secretion by mutant CFTR:** Mutations in the channel pore inhibit chloride secretion.

The relationship between these genotypes (more than 1000 mutations are known) and the clinical severity of CF is complicated and not always consistent. The best correlation seems to be between children with or without pancreatic insufficiency. Severe symptoms are generally found in those with pancreatic insufficiency (85% of all cases of CF), whereas milder cases are associated with preservation of pancreatic function. Class I and class II mutations are generally found among severely affected patients. By contrast, milder forms of CF feature class III and class IV mutations.

All pathologic consequences of CF can be attributed to the abnormally thick mucus, which obstructs lumina of airways, pancreatic, and biliary ducts, and the fetal intestine, and impairs airway mucociliary function. CF was once called **mucoviscidosis.** Normal CFTR corrects the defect in chloride secretion in cultured cells from CF patients.

PATHOLOGY: CF affects many organs that produce exocrine secretions.

RESPIRATORY TRACT: Pulmonary disease is responsible for most of the morbidity and mortality associated with CF. The earliest lesion is obstruction of bronchioles by mucus, with secondary infection and inflammation of bronchiolar walls. Recurrent cycles of obstruction and infection result in **chronic bronchiolitis** and **bronchitis,** which increase in severity as the disease progresses. Bronchial mucous glands undergo hypertrophy and hyperplasia, and airways are distended by thick and tenacious secretions. Widespread **bronchiectasis** becomes apparent by age 10 and often earlier. In late stages of the disease, large bronchiectatic cysts and lung abscesses are common. Secondary pulmonary hypertension may complicate the chronic bronchitis.

PANCREAS: Most (85%) of patients with CF have a form of **chronic pancreatitis,** and in long-standing cases, little or no functional exocrine pancreas remains. Inspissated secretions in the

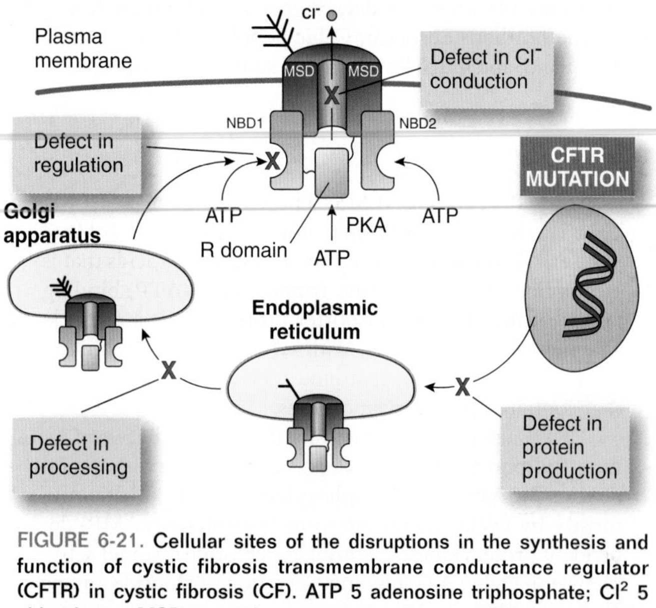

FIGURE 6-21. **Cellular sites of the disruptions in the synthesis and function of cystic fibrosis transmembrane conductance regulator (CFTR) in cystic fibrosis (CF). ATP 5 adenosine triphosphate; Cl² 5 chloride ion; MSD 5 membrane-spanning domain; NBD 5 nucleotide-binding domain; PKA 5 protein kinase A.**

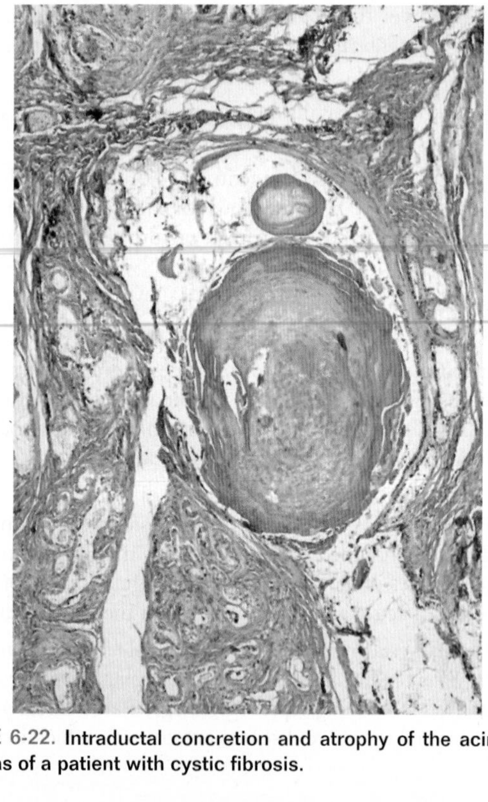

FIGURE 6-22. **Intraductal concretion and atrophy of the acini in the pancreas of a patient with cystic fibrosis.**

pancreatic ducts produce secondary dilation and cystic change of the distal ducts (Fig. 6-22). Recurrent pancreatitis leads to loss of acinar cells and extensive fibrosis. At autopsy, the pancreas is often simply cystic fibroadipose tissue containing islets of Langerhans.

LIVER: Inspissated mucous secretions in the intrahepatic biliary system obstruct the flow of bile in the drainage areas of the affected ducts and lead to focal **secondary biliary cirrhosis,** which is seen in one fourth of patients at autopsy. Microscopically, the liver shows inspissated concretions in bile ducts and ductules, chronic portal inflammation and septal fibrosis. On occasion (2%5%), the hepatic lesions are sufficiently widespread to lead to the clinical manifestations of biliary cirrhosis.

GASTROINTESTINAL TRACT: Shortly after birth, a normal newborn passes the intestinal contents that have accumulated in utero (meconium). The most important lesion of the gut in CF is small bowel obstruction in the newborn, **meconium ileus,** which is caused by failure to pass meconium in the immediate postpartum period. This complication occurs in 5% to 10% of newborns with CF and has been attributed to the failure of pancreatic secretions to digest meconium, possibly augmented by the greater viscosity of small bowel secretions.

REPRODUCTIVE TRACT: Almost all boys with CF have atrophy or fibrosis of the reproductive duct system, including the vas deferens, epididymis, and seminal vesicles. The pathogenesis of these lesions relates to obstruction of the lumen by inspissated secretions early in life and even in utero. As a result, only 2% to 3% of males become fertile, most demonstrating an absence of spermatozoa in the semen.

Only a minority of women with CF are fertile, and many of them suffer from anovulatory cycles as a result of poor nutrition and chronic infections. Moreover, the cervical mucous plug is abnormally thick and tenacious.

CLINICAL FEATURES: *The diagnosis of CF is most reliably made by detecting increased concentrations of electrolytes in the sweat and by genetic studies that demonstrate the disease-causing mutations.* The decreased chloride conductance characteristic of CF results in a failure of chloride reabsorption by the cells of the sweat gland ducts and hence to the accumulation of sodium chloride in the sweat (Fig. 6-23). Children with CF have been described as "tasting salty" and may even display salt crystals on their skin after vigorous sweating.

The clinical course of CF is highly variable. At one extreme, death may result from meconium ileus in the neonatal period, whereas some patients have reportedly survived to age 50. Improved medical care and recognition of milder cases of CF have served to prolong the average life span which is now about 30 years of age.

The pulmonary symptoms of CF begin with cough, which eventually becomes productive of large amounts of tenacious and purulent sputum. Episodes of infectious bronchitis and bronchopneumonia become progressively more frequent, and eventually shortness of breath develops. Respiratory failure and the cardiac complications of pulmonary hypertension (cor pulmonale) are late sequelae.

The most common organisms that infect the respiratory tract in CF are *Staphylococcus* and *Pseudomonas* species. As the disease advances, *Pseudomonas* may be the only organism cultured from the lung. *In fact, the recovery of* Pseudomonas *species, particularly the mucoid variety, from the lungs of a child with chronic pulmonary disease is virtually diagnostic of CF.* Infection with *Burkholderia cepacia* is associated with **cepacia syndrome,** a very severe pulmonary infection that is highly resistant to treatment with antibiotics and is commonly fatal.

The failure of pancreatic exocrine secretion leads to malabsorption of fat and protein, an effect that is reflected in bulky, foul-smelling stools (steatorrhea), nutritional deficiencies, and growth retardation.

Postural drainage of the airways, antibiotic therapy, and pancreatic enzyme supplementation are the mainstays of treatment. Molecular prenatal diagnosis of CF is now accurate in 95% of cases.

Lysosomal Storage Diseases Are Characterized by Accumulation of Unmetabolized Normal Substrates in Lysosomes Because of Deficiencies of Specific Acid Hydrolases

Lysosomes are membrane-bound collections of hydrolytic enzymes that are used for the controlled intracellular digestion of macromolecules. Lysosomal digestive enzymes are called "acid hydrolases" since their optimal pH is in the acidic range (pH 3.5–5.5). This environment is maintained by an ATP-dependent proton pump in the lysosomal membrane. These enzymes de-

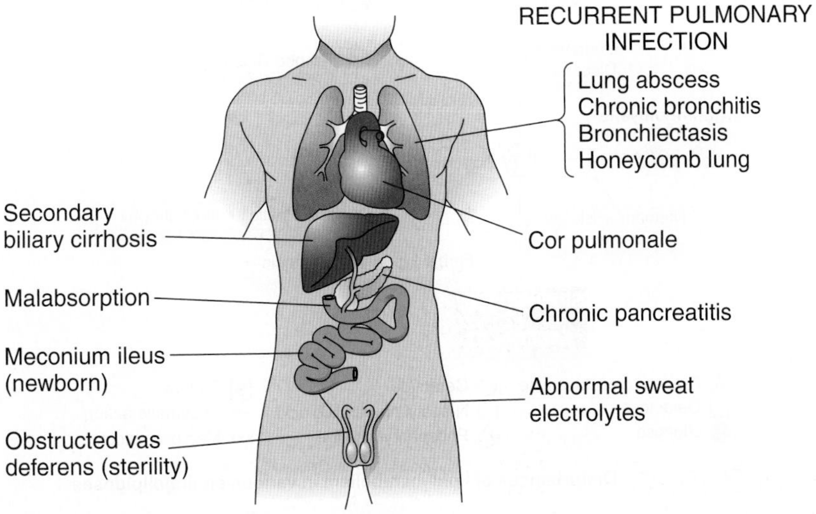

FIGURE 6-23. **Clinical features of cystic fibrosis.**

grade virtually all types of biological macromolecules. Extracellular macromolecules that are incorporated by endocytosis or phagocytosis and intracellular constituents that are subjected to autophagy are digested in lysosomes to their basic components. End-products may be transported across the lysosomal membrane into the cytosol, where they are reused in the synthesis of new macromolecules.

Virtually all lysosomal storage diseases result from mutations in genes that encode lysosomal hydrolases. A deficiency in one of the more than 40 acid hydrolases can result in an inability to catabolize the normal macromolecular substrate of that enzyme. As a result, undigested substrate accumulates in and engorges lysosomes, expanding the lysosomal compartment of the cell. The resulting lysosomal distention is often at the expense of other critical cellular components, particularly in the brain and heart, and can lead to a failure of cell function.

Lysosomal storage diseases are classified according to the material retained within the lysosomes. Thus, when the substrates that accumulate are sphingolipids, they are **sphingolipidoses.** Storage of mucopolysaccharides (glycosaminoglycans) leads to the **mucopolysaccharidoses.** More than 30 distinct lysosomal storage diseases are known, but we restrict our discussion to the more important examples.

Sphingolipidoses are lysosomal storage diseases characterized by accumulation of lipids derived from the turnover of obsolete cell membranes. Cerebrosides, gangliosides, sphingomyelin, and sulfatides are sphingolipid components of the membranes of a variety of cells. These substances are degraded within lysosomes by complex pathways to sphingosine and fatty acids (Fig. 6-24). Deficiencies of many of the acid hydrolases that mediate specific steps in these pathways lead to accumulation of undigested intermediate substrates in the lysosomes.

Gaucher Disease

Gaucher disease is characterized by accumulation of glucosylceramide, primarily in macrophage lysosomes. The disorder was first described in 1882 in a doctoral thesis by Gaucher, but its familial occurrence was not recognized for some 20 years.

PATHOGENESIS: The abnormality in Gaucher disease is a deficiency in glucocerebrosidase, a lysosomal acid β-glucosidase. The enzyme deficiency can be traced to a variety of single base mutations in the β-glucosidase gene, on the long arm of chromosome 1 (1q21) (see Table 6-7). Each of the three clinical types of the disease (see below) exhibits heterogeneous mutations in the β-glucosidase gene, although the molecular basis for the phenotypic differences remains to be firmly established.

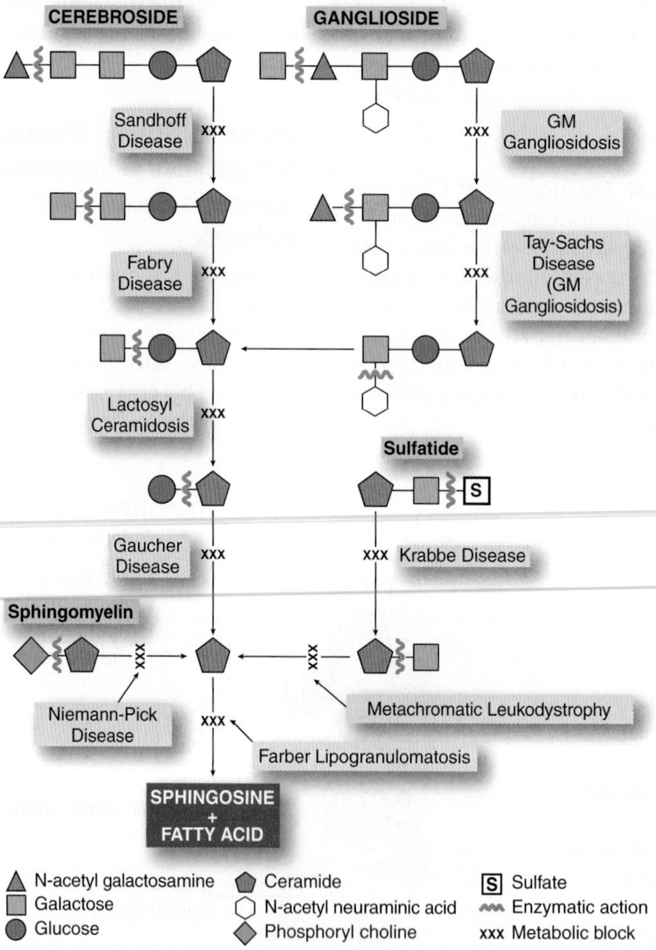

FIGURE 6-24. **Disturbances of lipid metabolism in various sphingolipidoses.**

The glucosylceramide that accumulates in Gaucher cells of the spleen, liver, bone marrow, and lymph nodes derives principally from catabolism of senescent leukocytes. The membranes of these cells are rich in cerebrosides, and when their degradation is blocked by the deficiency of glucocerebrosidase, the intermediate metabolite, glucosylceramide, accumulates. The glucosylceramide of Gaucher cells in the brain is believed to originate from turnover of plasma membrane gangliosides of cells in the CNS.

PATHOLOGY: The hallmark of this disorder is the **Gaucher cells,** which are lipid-laden macrophages characteristically present in the red pulp of the spleen, liver sinusoids, lymph nodes, lungs, and bone marrow, although they may be found in virtually any organ. These cells are derived from resident macrophages in the respective organs, for example, Kupffer cells in the liver and alveolar macrophages in the lung. In the uncommon variants of Gaucher disease with involvement of the CNS, Gaucher cells originate from periadventitial cells in Virchow-Robin spaces.

Gaucher cells are large (20–100 μm) with clear cytoplasm and eccentric nuclei (Fig. 6-25). By light microscopy, the cytoplasm has a characteristic fibrillar appearance, which has been likened to "wrinkled tissue paper" and is intensely positive with periodic acid-Schiff (PAS) stain. By electron microscopy, the storage material is found within enlarged lysosomes and appears as parallel layers of tubular structures.

Enlargement of the spleen is virtually universal in Gaucher disease. In the adult form of the disorder, splenomegaly may be massive, with spleen weights up to 10 kg. The cut surface of the enlarged spleen is firm and pale and often contains sharply demarcated infarcts. Microscopically, the red pulp shows nodular and diffuse infiltrates of Gaucher cells, and moderate fibrosis.

The liver is usually enlarged by Gaucher cells within sinusoids, but hepatocytes are unaffected. In severe cases, hepatic fibrosis and even cirrhosis may ensue. The extent of bone marrow involvement is variable but leads to radiological abnormalities in 50% to 75% of cases (see Chapter 26).

Gaucher cells may also be found in many other organs, including lymph nodes, lungs, endocrine glands, skin, gastrointestinal tract, and kidneys, although symptoms referable to these organs are uncommon.

When the brain is affected, Gaucher cells are present in Virchow-Robin spaces around blood vessels. In the infantile (neuronopathic) form of Gaucher disease, these cells have also been found in the parenchyma, where they may stimulate gliosis and formation of microglial nodules.

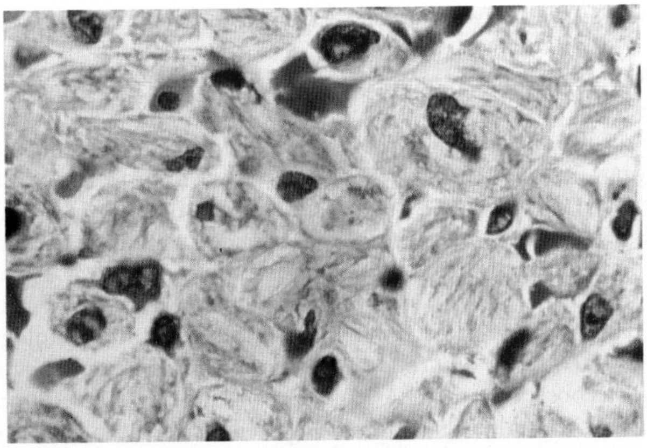

FIGURE 6-25. **The spleen in Gaucher disease.** Typical Gaucher cells have foamy cytoplasm and eccentrically located nuclei.

CLINICAL FEATURES: Gaucher disease is classified into three distinct forms, based on the age at onset and degree of neurologic involvement.

- **Type 1 (chronic non-neuronopathic):** This variant is the most common of all lysosomal storage diseases and is found principally in adult Ashkenazi Jews, among whom the incidence is 1 in 600 to 1 in 2500. The age at onset is highly variable, some cases being diagnosed in infants and others in persons 70 years old. Similarly, the severity of clinical manifestations varies widely. Most cases are diagnosed as adults and present initially as painless splenomegaly and the complications of hypersplenism (i.e., anemia, leukopenia, and thrombocytopenia). Whereas hepatomegaly is common, clinical liver disease is infrequent. Bone involvement, in the form of pain and pathologic fractures, is the leading cause of disability and may be severe enough to confine the patient to a wheelchair. The life expectancy of most persons with type 1 Gaucher disease is normal. This type of Gaucher disease is now successfully treated by intravenous administration of modified acid glucose cerebrosidase, although the extremely high cost limits its use. Marrow transplantation is also effective but is little used because of the risks associated with this therapy. Prenatal diagnosis, based on β-glucosidase activity in amniotic fluid or chorionic villi or on DNA technology, is now routinely available.
- **Type 2 (acute neuronopathic):** Type 2 Gaucher disease is rare and distinctly different from type 1 in the age at onset and clinical presentation. It usually presents by age 3 months with hepatosplenomegaly and has no ethnic predilection. Within a few months, the infant shows neurologic signs, with the classic triad of trismus, strabismus, and backward flexion of the neck. Further neurologic deterioration rapidly follows, and most patients die before the age of 1 year.
- **Type 3 (subacute neuronopathic):** This form is also rare and combines features of type 1 and type 2. Neurologic deterioration presents at an older age than in type 2 and progresses more slowly.

Tay-Sachs Disease (GM_2 Gangliosidosis, Type 1)

Tay-Sachs disease is the catastrophic infantile variant of a class of lysosomal storage diseases known as the GM_2 gangliosidoses, in which this ganglioside is deposited in neurons of the CNS, owing to a failure of lysosomal degradation. The association of a "cherry-red spot" in the retina and profound mental and physical retardation was first pointed out in 1881 by Warren Tay, a British ophthalmologist. Fifteen years later, Bernard Sachs, an American neurologist, described the histologic features of the disorder and coined the term "amaurotic (blind) family idiocy." Tay-Sachs disease is inherited as an autosomal recessive trait and is predominantly a disorder of Ashkenazi Jews, in whom the carrier rate is 1 in 30, and the natural incidence of homozygotes is 1 in 4000 live newborns. By contrast, the incidence of Tay-Sachs disease in non-Jewish American populations is less than 1 in 100,000 live births. Screening programs for heterozygotes among Ashkenazi Jews have now reduced the disease incidence by 90%. The other GM_2 gangliosidoses are exceedingly rare.

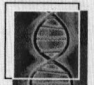

PATHOGENESIS: Gangliosides are glycosphingolipids consisting of a ceramide and an oligosaccharide chain that contains *N*-acetylneuraminic acid (see Fig. 6-24). They are present in the outer leaflet of the plasma membrane of animal cells, particularly in brain neurons.

Lysosomal catabolism of 1 of the 12 known gangliosides in the brain, namely ganglioside GM_2, is through the activity of the β-hexosaminidases (A and B), which have α and β subunits and require GM_2-activator protein. A deficiency in any of these components results in clinical disease.

Tay-Sachs disease (also known as hexosaminidase α-subunit deficiency) results from about 50 different mutations in the gene on chromosome 15q23-24 that codes for the α subunit of hexosaminidase A, with a resulting defect in the synthesis of this enzyme (see Table 6-7). An insertion of four nucleotides in exon 11 is the most common mutation among Ashkenazi Jews, accounting for over two thirds of the carriers, or about 2% of that population. The β subunits are synthesized normally and associate to form the dimer known as hexosaminidase B, levels of which are normal or even increased in Tay-Sachs disease.

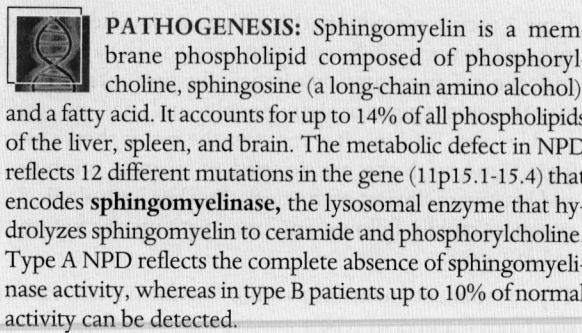

PATHOGENESIS: Sphingomyelin is a membrane phospholipid composed of phosphorylcholine, sphingosine (a long-chain amino alcohol), and a fatty acid. It accounts for up to 14% of all phospholipids of the liver, spleen, and brain. The metabolic defect in NPD reflects 12 different mutations in the gene (11p15.1-15.4) that encodes **sphingomyelinase,** the lysosomal enzyme that hydrolyzes sphingomyelin to ceramide and phosphorylcholine. Type A NPD reflects the complete absence of sphingomyelinase activity, whereas in type B patients up to 10% of normal activity can be detected.

Sandhoff disease is caused by a mutation in the gene for the β subunit on chromosome 5, and leads to deficiencies of both hexosaminidase A and B.

A third, rare variant is the result of a defect in the synthesis of the GM_2-activator protein (chromosome 5) in the face of normal activities of the hexosaminidases.

PATHOLOGY: GM_2 ganglioside accumulates in lysosomes of all organs in Tay-Sachs disease, but it is most prominent in brain neurons and cells of the retina. The size of the brain varies with the length of survival of the affected infant. Early cases are marked by brain atrophy, whereas the brain may be as much as doubled in weight in those who survive beyond a year. Microscopic examination reveals neurons markedly distended with storage material that stains positively for lipids. By electron microscopy, the neurons are stuffed with "membranous cytoplasmic bodies," composed of concentric whorls of lamellar structures (Fig. 6-26). As the disease progresses, neurons are lost, and many lipid-laden macrophages are conspicuous in the cortical gray matter. Eventually, gliosis becomes prominent and myelin and axons in the white matter are lost. The pathologies of the other forms of GM_2 gangliosidosis are similar to those of Tay-Sachs disease, although usually less severe.

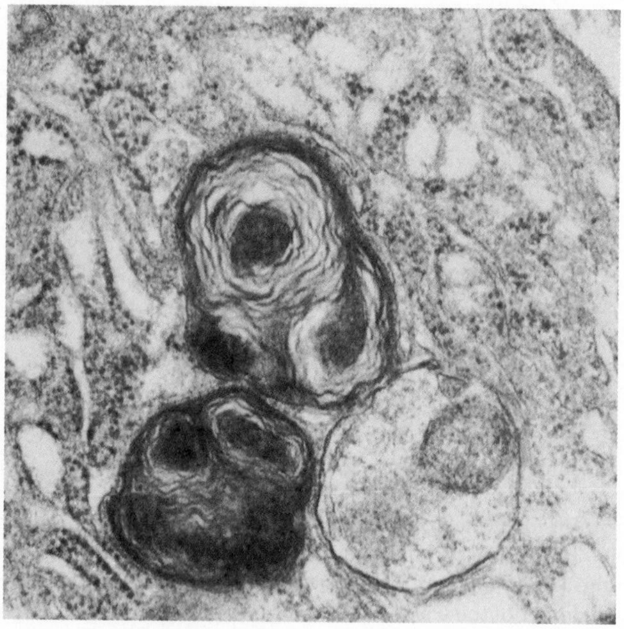

FIGURE 6-26. **Tay-Sachs disease.** The cytoplasm of the nerve cell contains lysosomes filled with whorled membranes.

CLINICAL FEATURES: Tay-Sachs disease presents between 6 and 10 months of age and is characterized by progressive weakness, hypotonia, and decreased attentiveness. Progressive motor and mental deterioration, often with generalized seizures, follow rapidly. Vision is seriously impaired. Involvement of retinal ganglion cells is detected by ophthalmoscopy as a **cherry-red spot** in the macula. This feature reflects the pallor of the affected cells, which enhances the prominence of blood vessels underlying the central fovea. Most children with Tay-Sachs disease die before 4 years of age.

Niemann-Pick Disease

Niemann-Pick disease (NPD) refers to lipidoses that are characterized by the lysosomal storage of sphingomyelin in macrophages of many organs, in hepatocytes, and in the brain. These disorders are classified into two categories, termed **types A and B.** Type A NPD appears in infancy and is characterized by hepatosplenomegaly and progressive neurodegeneration, with death occurring by 3 years of age. Type B NPD is more variable and features principally hepatosplenomegaly and minimal neurologic symptomatology, with survival to adulthood. A particularly high frequency of NPD is observed among Ashkenazi Jews, but the disorder is present in other ethnic groups. Among the former, the incidence of type A NPD is 1 in 40,000 and of type B 1 in 80,000, with a combined heterozygote prevalence of 1 in 100.

PATHOLOGY: The characteristic storage cell in NPD is a foam cell, that is, an enlarged (20–90 μm) macrophage in which the cytoplasm is distended by uniform vacuoles that contain sphingomyelin and cholesterol. By electron microscopy, whorls of concentrically arranged lamellar structures distend the lysosomes.

Foam cells are particularly numerous in the spleen, lymph nodes, and bone marrow but are also found in the liver, lungs, and gastrointestinal tract. The spleen is enlarged, often to massive size, and microscopically, foam cells are diffusely distributed throughout the red pulp. Lymph nodes enlarged by foam cells are seen in many locations. The hematopoietic tissues in the bone marrow may be displaced by aggregates of foam cells. The liver is enlarged by the stored sphingomyelin and cholesterol in lysosomes of both Kupffer cells and hepatocytes.

The brain is the most important organ involved in type A NPD, and neurologic damage is the usual cause of death. At autopsy, the brain is atrophic and in severe cases may be as little as half the normal weight. Neurons are distended by vacuoles containing the same stored lipids found elsewhere in the body. Advanced cases are characterized by a severe loss of neurons and sometimes by demyelination. Foam cells are noted in many locations. Half of children affected by type A disease demonstrate a cherry-red spot in the retina, similar to that seen in Tay-Sachs disease.

CLINICAL FEATURES: Type A NPD manifests in early infancy with conspicuous spleen and liver enlargement, and psychomotor retardation. There is a progressive loss of motor and intellectual function, and the child typically dies between the ages of 2 and 3 years. Most type B patients present in childhood with marked hepatosplenomegaly. Pulmonary infiltration with sphingomyelin-laden macrophages eventually leads to compromised respiratory function in many patients with type B disease. However, these patients have little in the way of neurological symptoms and may survive for many years.

Mucopolysaccharidoses

The mucopolysaccharidoses (MPS) are an assortment of lysosomal storage diseases characterized by accumulation of glycosaminoglycans (mucopolysaccharides) in many organs. All types of MPS are inherited as autosomal recessive traits, except for Hunter syndrome, which is X-linked recessive. These rare diseases are caused by deficiencies in any one of the 10 lysosomal enzymes that catabolize glycosaminoglycans (Fig. 6-27). Six abnormal phenotypes are described, each varying with the specific enzyme deficiency (Table 6-8).

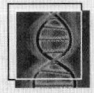

PATHOGENESIS: Glycosaminoglycans (GAGs) are large polymers of repeating disaccharide units containing *N*-acetylhexosamine and a hexose or hexuronic acid. Either disaccharide may be sulfated. The accumulated GAGs (dermatan sulfate, heparan sulfate, keratan sulfate, and chondroitin sulfates) in MPS are all derived from cleavage of proteoglycans, which are important extracellular matrix constituents. GAGs are degraded stepwise by removing sugar residues or sulfate groups. Thus, a deficiency in any one of the glycosidases or sulfatases results in the accumulation of undegraded GAGs. A special case is a deficiency of an *N*-acetyltransferase, which leads to deposition of heparan sulfate in Sanfilippo C disease.

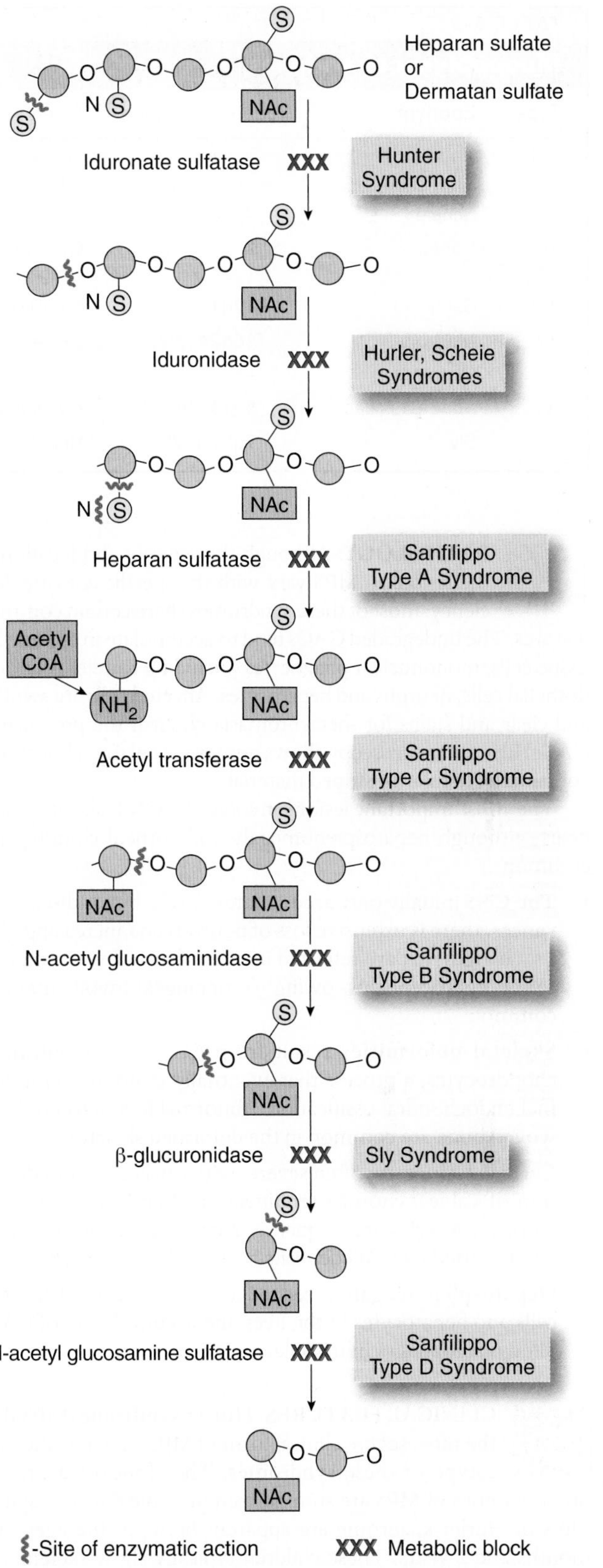

FIGURE 6-27. **Metabolic blocks in various mucopolysaccharidoses that affect the degradation of heparan sulfate and dermatan sulfate. Acetyl CoA 5 acetyl coenzyme A; NAc 5 *N*- acetyl moiety.**

TABLE 6-8

Mucopolysaccharidoses

Type	Eponym	Location of Gene	Clinical Features
I H	Hurler	4p16.3	Organomegaly, cardiac lesions, dysostosis multiplex, corneal clouding, death in childhood
I S	Scheie	4p16.3	Stiff joints, corneal clouding, normal intelligence, longevity
II	Hunter	X	Organomegaly, dysostosis multiplex, mental retardation, death earlier than 15 years of age
III	Sanfillipo	12q14	Mental retardation
IV	Morquio	16q24	Skeletal deformities, corneal clouding
V	Obsolete	–	–
VI	Maroteaux Lamy	5q13–14	Dysostosis multiplex, corneal clouding, death in second decade
VII	Sly	7q21.1–22	Hepatosplenomegaly, dysostosis multiplex

PATHOLOGY: Although the severity and location of the lesions in MPS vary with the specific enzyme deficiency, most ot these syndromes share certain common features. The undegraded GAGs tend to accumulate in connective tissue cells, mononuclear phagocytes (including Kupffer cells), endothelial cells, neurons and hepatocytes. Affected cells are swollen and clear and stains for metachromasia confirm the presence of GAGs. Electron microscopy shows numerous enlarged lysosomes containing granular or striped material.

The most important lesions involve the CNS, skeleton, and heart, although hepatosplenomegaly and corneal clouding are common.

- **The CNS** initially only accumulates GAGs, but as disease advances, there is extensive loss of neurons and increasing gliosis, changes that are reflected in cortical atrophy. Communicating hydrocephalus, owing to meningeal involvement, is common.
- **Skeletal deformities** result from CAG accumulation in chondrocytes, a process that eventually interferes with normal endochondral ossification. Abnormal foci of osteoid and woven bone are common in the deformed skeleton.
- **Cardiac lesions** are often severe, with thickening and distortion of valves, chordae tendineae, and endocardium. The coronary arteries are frequently narrowed by intimal thickening caused by GAG deposits in smooth muscle cells.
- **Hepatosplenomegaly** is secondary to distention of Kupffer cells and hepatocytes in the liver and accumulation of CAG-filled macrophages in the spleen.

CLINICAL FEATURES: Hurler syndrome (MPS IH), the most severe clinical form of MPS, remains the prototype of these syndromes. The clinical features of other varieties of MPS are summarized in Table 6-8. The symptoms of Hurler syndrome are apparent between the ages of 6 months and 2 years. These children typically show skeletal deformities, enlarged livers and spleens, a characteristic facies, and joint stiffness. The combination of coarse facial features and dwarfism is reminiscent of gargoyle figures that decorate Gothic cathedrals and accounts for the term **gargoylism** previously appended to this syndrome.

Children with Hurler syndrome suffer developmental delay, hearing loss, corneal clouding, and progressive mental deterioration. Increased intracranial pressure, due to communicating hydrocephalus, can be troublesome. Most patients die from recurrent pulmonary infections and cardiac complications before they reach 10 years.

Detection of heterozygotes is difficult, because of the overlap in enzyme activity of cultured cells with the normal population. Prenatal diagnosis is possible for all the MPS and is routine for Hurler and Hunter syndromes.

Glycogenoses (Glycogen Storage Diseases)

The glycogenoses are a group at least 10 distinct inherited disorders characterized by glycogen accumulation, principally in the liver, skeletal muscle, and heart. Each entity reflects a deficiency of one of the specific enzymes involved in glycogen metabolism (Fig. 6-28). With one rare exception (X-linked phosphorylase kinase deficiency), all types of glycogen storage disease are autosomal recessive traits. The glycogenoses are rare, varying in frequency from 1 in 100,000 to 1 in 1 million.

Glycogen is a large glucose polymer (20,000–30,000 glucose units per molecule), that is stored in most cells to provide a ready source of energy during the fasting state. Liver and muscle are particularly rich in glycogen, although its function is different in each organ. The liver stores glycogen not for its own use but rather for rapid supply of glucose to the blood, particularly for the benefit of the brain. By contrast, glycogen in skeletal muscle is used as a local fuel when oxygen or glucose supply falls. Glycogen is synthesized and degraded sequentially by a number of enzymes, a deficiency in any of which leads to accumulation of glycogen.

Although each of the glycogen storage diseases causes glycogen accumulation, the significant organ involvement varies with the specific enzyme defect. Some mainly affect the liver, whereas others principally cause cardiac or skeletal muscle dysfunction. *Importantly, the symptoms of a glycogenosis can reflect either accumulation of glycogen itself* (**Pompe disease, Andersen disease**) *or the lack of the glucose that is normally derived from glycogen degradation* (**von Gierke disease, McArdle disease**). We discuss only several representative examples of the known glycogenoses.

von GIERKE DISEASE (TYPE IA GLYCOGENOSIS): *von Gierke disease is a result of a deficiency in glucose-6-phosphatase and is characterized by accumulation of glycogen in the liver.* Symptoms reflect the inability of the liver to convert glycogen to glucose, a defect that results in hepatomegaly and hypoglycemia. The

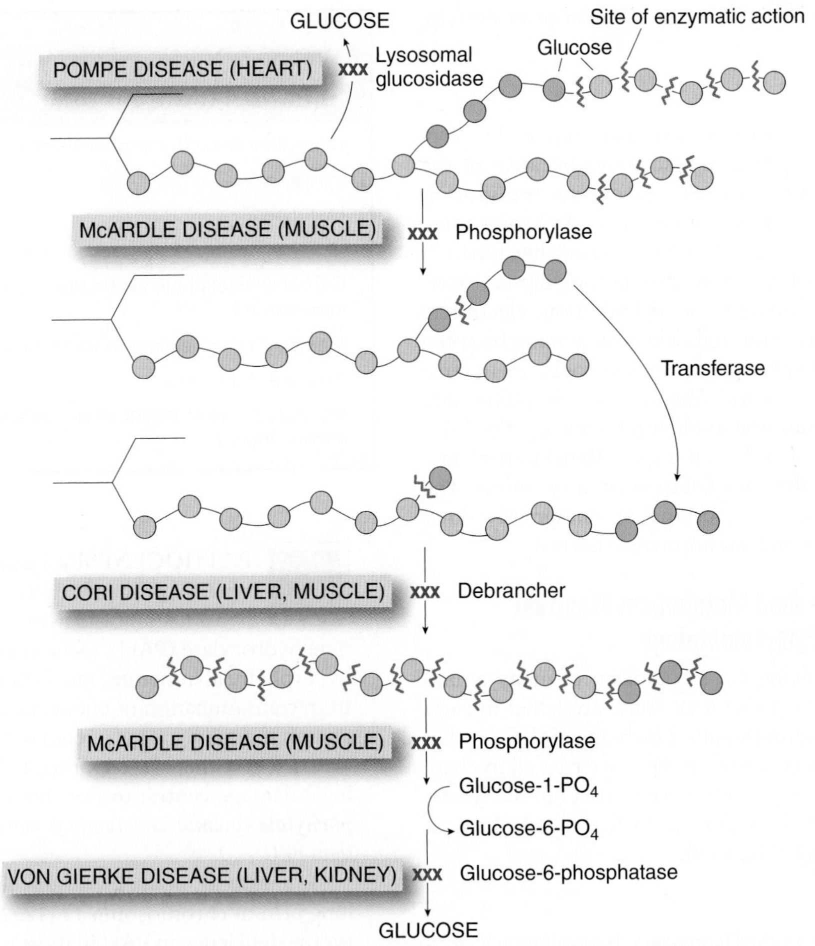

FIGURE 6-28. **Sequential catabolism of glycogen and the enzymes that are deficient in various glycogenoses.** Glycogen is a long-chain branched polymer of glucose residues, which are connected by α-1,4 linkages, except at branch points, where an α-1,6 linkage is present. Phosphorylase hydrolyzes α-1,4 linkages to a point three glucose residues distal to an α-1,6-linked sugar. These three glucose residues are transferred to the chain linked by α-1,4 bonds, by the bifunctional debrancher enzyme amylo-1,6-glucosidase. Subsequently the same enzyme removes the α-1,6 linked sugar at the original branch point. This creates a linear α-1,4 chain, which is degraded by phosphorylase to glucose-1-phosphate. Following the conversion to glucose-6-phosphate, glucose is released by the action of glucose-6-phosphatase. A small proportion of glycogen is totally degraded within lysosomes by acid α-glucosidase. Red x's-metabolic block.

disorder is usually evident in infancy or early childhood. Growth is commonly stunted, but with treatment, the prognosis for normal mental development and longevity are generally good.

POMPE DISEASE (TYPE II GLYCOGENOSIS): *Pompe disease is a lysosomal storage disease that involves virtually all organs and results in death from heart failure before the age of 2.* The juvenile and adult variants are less common and have a better prognosis. Normally, a small proportion of cytoplasmic glycogen is degraded within lysosomes after an autophagic sequence. Type II glycogenosis is caused by a deficiency in the lysosomal enzyme acid α-glucosidase (17q23), which leads to inexorable accumulation of undegraded glycogen in lysosomes of many different cells. Interestingly, patients do not suffer from hypoglycemia, because the major metabolic pathways of glycogen synthesis and degradation in the cytoplasm are intact.

ANDERSEN DISEASE (TYPE IV GLYCOGENOSIS): *Andersen disease is a very rare condition in which an abnormal form of glycogen, termed* **amylopectin**, *is deposited principally in the liver but also in the heart, muscles, and nervous system.* Children with type IV glycogenosis typically die between the ages of 2 and 4 years from **cirrhosis of the liver.** The disorder results from a deficiency in the branching enzyme (amyloglucantransferase) (3p12) that creates the branch points in normal glycogen molecules. The absence of brancher enzyme leads to formation and accumulation of an insoluble and toxic form of glycogen that is normally not present in animal cells and resembles plant starch. Liver transplantation cures Andersen disease. Remarkably, the deposits of amylopectin in the heart and other extrahepatic tissues are greatly reduced following liver transplantation, although the mechanism for this effect is obscure.

McARDLE DISEASE (TYPE V GLYCOGENOSIS): *McArdle disease is characterized by accumulation of glycogen in skeletal muscles, due to a deficiency of muscle phosphorylase (11q13), the enzyme that releases glucose-1-phosphate from glycogen.* Symptoms usually appear in adolescence or early adulthood and consist of muscle cramps and spasms during exercise and sometimes myocytolysis and resulting myoglobinuria. Avoidance of exercise prevents the symptoms.

Cystinosis

Cystinosis is a lysosomal storage disease characterized by accumulation of crystalline cystine in lysosomes because of the absence of **cystinosin,** a transmembrane cystine transporter. The gene that is affected by this mutation is at chromosome 17p13. Cystinosis occurs in 1 per 100,000 to 200,000 live births. It is characterized by renal Fanconi syndrome (polydipsia, excretion of large amounts of dilute urine, dehydration, electrolyte imbalances, growth retardation, and rickets) beginning between 6 and 12 months of age. Untreated, cystinosis progresses to renal failure, often before adolescence. Abnormalities in pulmonary and brain function are common in older patients. Cystine crystals are present in almost all cells and organs. Renal transplantation can be used to treat the renal failure seen in cystinosis. The use of cysteamine to decrease lysosomal cystine greatly slows progression of the disease and has improved survival.

Inborn Errors of Amino Acid Metabolism Manifest with Variably Severe Symptomatology

Heritable disorders involving the metabolism of many amino acids have been described (Table 6-9). Some are lethal in early childhood; others are asymptomatic biochemical defects that have no clinical significance. Some of these are treated in chapters dealing with specific organs. Here we restrict our discussion to the examples provided by defects in the metabolism of phenylalanine and tyrosine (Fig. 6-29).

Phenylketonuria

Phenylketonuria (PKU, hyperphenylalaninemia) is an autosomal recessive deficiency of the hepatic enzyme phenylalanine hydroxylase. The disorder is characterized by high levels of circulating phenylalanine, leading to progressive mental deterioration in the first few years of life. The overall incidence of PKU is 1 per 10,000 in white and Asian populations, but it varies widely across different geographic areas. Its frequency is highest (1 in 5000) in Ireland and western Scotland and among Yemenite Jews.

TABLE 6-9

Representative Inherited Disorders of Amino Acid Metabolism

Phenylketonuria (hyperphenylalaninemia)
Tyrosinemia
Histidinemia
Ornithine transcarbamylase deficiency (ammonia intoxication)
Carbamyl phosphate synthetase deficiency (ammonia intoxication)
Maple syrup urine disease (branched chain ketoacidemia)
Arginase deficiency
Arginosuccinic acid synthetase deficiency (citrulline accumulation)

PATHOGENESIS: Phenylalanine is an essential amino acid derived exclusively from the diet. It is oxidized in the liver to tyrosine by phenylalanine hydroxylase (PAH). Deficiency in PAH results in both hyperphenylalaninemia and formation of phenylketones from transamination of phenylalanine. Phenylpyruvic acid and its derivatives are excreted in the urine, but phenylalanine itself, rather than its metabolites, causes the neurologic damage central to this disease. *Thus, the term **hyperphenylalaninemia** is actually a more appropriate designation than PKU.*

A variety of point mutations in the *PAH* gene, on the long arm of chromosome 12 (12q22-24.1), are responsible for the deficiency in PAH in most patients of European origin. By contrast, PKU among Yemenite Jews reflects a single deletion in the *PAH* gene. An analysis of family histories of the Yemenite Jewish community has traced the origin of this defect to a common ancestor from Sanà, Yemen, before the 18th century. A different *PAH* gene deletion causes the disease in the affected Scottish population.

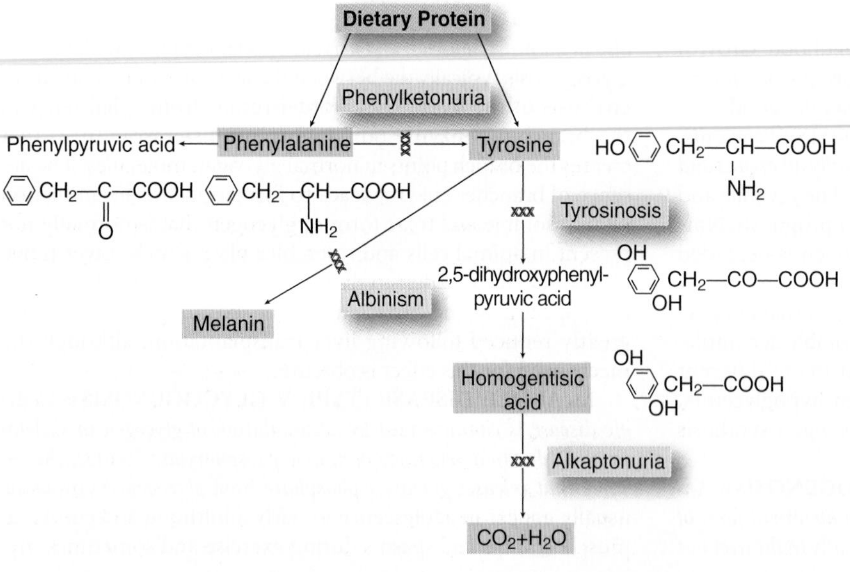

FIGURE 6-29. **Diseases caused by disturbances of phenylalanine and tyrosine metabolism.**

The mechanism of the neurotoxicity associated with hyperphenylalaninemia during infancy has not been precisely established, but several processes have been implicated: (1) competitive interference with amino acid transport systems in the brain, (2) inhibition of the synthesis of neurotransmitters, and (3) disturbance of other metabolic processes. These effects presumably lead to inadequate development of neurons and defective synthesis of myelin.

The lack in PAH activity is not always absolute: hyperphenylalaninemia milder than occurs in classic PKU is described. In such cases, phenylpyruvic acid is not excreted in the urine. Patients with $<1\%$ of the normal activity of PAH generally have a PKU phenotype, whereas those with more than 5% are considered to exhibit non-PKU hyperphenylalaninemia, do not suffer neurologic damage, and develop normally. It is presumed that non-PKU hyperphenylalaninemia is caused by mutations different from those in classic PKU.

Malignant hyperphenylalaninemia occurs in a few ($<$ 5%) infants with hyperphenylalaninemia. In this condition, dietary restriction of phenylalanine does not arrest neurologic deterioration. These patients have a deficiency in tetrahydrobiopterin (BH_4), a cofactor required for hydroxylation of phenylalanine by PAH. In some instances, this defect results from a failure to regenerate BH_4, owing to an inherited lack of dihydropteridine reductase (DHPR), the enzyme that reduces dihydrobiopterin (BH_2) to the tetrahydro form (BH_4). The mutant *DHPR* gene is on the short arm of chromosome 4, and so is distinct from the *PAH* gene. Alternatively, in some cases synthesis of BH_4 is impaired. Although infants with malignant hyperphenylalaninemia are initially indistinguishable phenotypically from those with classic PKU, BH_4 deficiency also interferes with synthesis of the neurotransmitters dopamine (tyrosine hydroxylase-dependent) and serotonin (tryptophan hydroxylase-dependent). Thus, the mechanism underlying brain damage in malignant hyperphenylalaninemia likely involves more than a simple elevation in the levels of phenylalanine.

CLINICAL FEATURES: Phenylketonuria illustrates the interaction between "nature and nurture" in the pathogenesis of disease. The disorder is based on a genetic defect, but its expression depends on the provision of a dietary constituent. *The affected infant appears normal at birth, but mental retardation is evident within a few months.* By the age of 12 months, the untreated infant has lost about 50 IQ points, which means that a child with normal intelligence has been reduced to an imbecile who requires institutionalization. Infants with PKU tend to have fair skin, blond hair, and blue eyes, because the inability to convert phenylalanine to tyrosine leads to reduced melanin synthesis. They exude a "mousy" odor, due to the phenylacetic acid they make.

Treatment of PKU involves restriction of dietary phenylalanine to 250 to 500 mg/day, which usually requires a semisynthetic formula. How long such dietary therapy is necessary is controversial. At one time it was believed that the dietary regimen could be relaxed after the brain has in large part matured, i.e., by 6 years of age. Newer evidence suggests that many older patients suffer some harm when phenylalanine is reintroduced into the diet. Thus, how long phenylalanine restriction should be maintained is not certain.

In developed countries, the clinical phenotype of classical PKU is now more of historical interest than of significant public health concern. About 10 million newborns worldwide are screened annually for hyperphenylalaninemia by a simple blood test, and most of the estimated 1000 new cases are promptly treated.

The success of newborn screening programs in detecting PKU, and the prompt institution of a low-phenylalanine diet allows many PKU homozygotes to live a normal life and to reproduce. Expectant mothers who are homozygous for PKU (maternal PKU) must consume a low-phenylalanine diet during pregnancy if the fetus is to avoid complications associated with maternal hyperphenylalaninemia. Infants exposed to high levels of phenylalanine in utero show microcephaly, mental and growth retardation, and cardiac anomalies. In other words, high levels of phenylalanine are teratogenic.

Tyrosinemia

Hereditary tyrosinemia (hepatorenal tyrosinemia, tyrosinemia type I) is a rare (1 in 100,000) autosomal recessive inborn error of tyrosine catabolism that manifests as acute liver disease in early infancy or as a more chronic disease of the liver, kidneys, and brain in children. Elevated levels of tyrosine and its metabolites are found in the blood. Both forms of the disease are caused by a deficiency of fumarylacetoacetate hydrolase (15q23-25), the last enzyme in the catabolic pathway that converts tyrosine to fumarate and acetoacetate. In the acute form there is no enzyme activity, whereas children with chronic disease have variable residual activity. Cell injury in hereditary tyrosinemia is attributed to abnormal toxic metabolites, succinylacetone, and succinylacetoacetate.

Acute tyrosinemia manifests in the first few months of life as hepatomegaly, edema, failure to thrive, and a cabbagelike odor. Within a few months, infants die of hepatic failure.

Chronic tyrosinemia is characterized by cirrhosis of the liver, renal tubular dysfunction (Fanconi syndrome), and neurologic abnormalities. **Hepatocellular carcinoma** *supervenes in more than a third of patients.* Most children die before the age of 10 years. Liver transplantation corrects the hepatic metabolic abnormalities and prevents the neurologic crises. Combined liver–kidney transplants have also been done to treat chronic tyrosinemia. Prenatal diagnosis is accomplished by demonstrating succinylacetone in amniotic fluid or fumarylacetoacetate hydrolase deficiency in cells obtained by amniocentesis or chorionic villus sampling.

Alkaptonuria (Ochronosis)

Alkaptonuria is a rare autosomal recessive deficiency of hepatic and renal homogentisic acid oxidase. It features excretion of homogentisic acid in the urine, generalized pigmentation and arthritis. The enzyme deficiency prevents catabolism of homogentisic acid, an intermediate gene product in phenylalanine and tyrosine metabolism. Alkaptonuria is of greater historical significance than of clinical importance. Studies almost a century ago by Garrod and others described the inheritance of alkaptonuria and were among the first to define the concept of hereditary inborn errors of metabolism.

Patients with alkaptonuria excrete urine that darkens rapidly on standing, due to formation of a pigment on the nonenzymatic oxidation of homogentisic acid (Fig. 6-30). In longstanding alkaptonuria, a similar pigment is deposited in numerous tissues, particularly the sclera, cartilage in many areas (ribs, larynx, trachea), tendons, and synovial membranes. Although the pigment appears bluish black on gross examination, it is brown under the

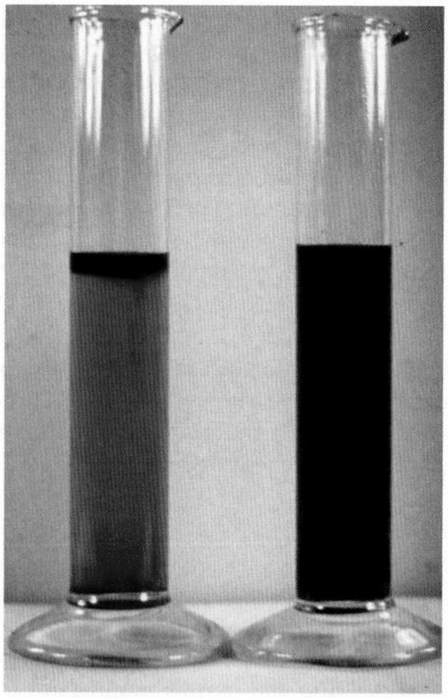

FIGURE 6-30. **Urine from a patient with alkaptonuria.** The specimen on the left, which has been standing for 15 minutes, shows some darkening at the surface, owing to the oxidation of homogentisic acid. After 2 hours *(right)*, the urine is entirely black.

microscope, accounting for the term **ochronosis** (color of ocher) coined by Virchow. A degenerative and frequently disabling **arthropathy** ("ochronotic arthritis") often develops after years of alkaptonuria. It is tempting to ascribe the joint disease to the pigment deposition, but this has not been proved. Despite the involvement of many organs, alkaptonuria does not reduce the longevity of affected persons.

Albinism

Albinism refers to a heterogeneous group of at least 10 inherited disorders in which absent or reduced biosynthesis of melanin causes hypopigmentation. This condition is found throughout the animal kingdom (from insects to humans). The most common type is oculocutaneous albinism (OCA), a family of closely related diseases that (with a single rare exception) represent autosomal recessive traits (see Table 6-7). OCA is characterized by a deficiency or complete absence of melanin pigment in the skin, hair follicles, and eyes. The frequency of OCA in whites is 1 per 18,000 in the United States and is 1 in 10,000 in Ireland. American blacks have the same high frequency of OCA as the Irish.

Two major forms of OCA are distinguished by the presence or absence of tyrosinase, the first enzyme in the biosynthetic pathway that converts tyrosine to melanin (see Fig. 6-29).

Tyrosinase-positive OCA is the most common type of albinism in whites and blacks. Patients typically begin life with complete albinism, but with age, a small amount of clinically detectable pigment accumulates. A defect in the *P* gene (15q11.2-13) prevents melanin synthesis. The *P* gene has been postulated to code for a tyrosine-transport protein.

Tyrosinase-negative OCA is the second most common type of albinism and is characterized by complete absence of tyrosinase (11q14-21) and melanin: melanocytes are present but contain unpigmented melanosomes. Affected people have snow-white hair, pale pink skin, blue irides, and prominent red pupils, owing to an absence of retinal pigment. They typically have severe ophthalmic problems, including photophobia, strabismus, nystagmus, and decreased visual acuity.

The skin of all types of albinos is strikingly sensitive to sunlight. Exposed skin areas require strong sunscreen lotions. These patients are at a greatly increased risk for squamous cell carcinomas of sun-exposed skin. In fact, among a group of more than 500 albinos in equatorial Africa, not one survived beyond the age of 40 years, nearly all having succumbed to cancer. Interestingly, albinos seem to have a lower than normal frequency of malignant melanoma.

An X-Linked Disorder Features an Abnormal Gene on the X Chromosome

Expression of an X-linked disorder (Fig. 6-31) is different in males and females. Females, having two X chromosomes, may be homozygous or heterozygous for a given trait. It follows that clinical expression of the trait in a female is variable, depending on whether it is dominant or recessive. By contrast, males have only one X chromosome and are said to be **hemizygous** for the same trait. *Thus, regardless of whether the trait is dominant or recessive, it is invariably expressed in the male.*

A cardinal attribute of all X-linked inheritance, is lack of transmission from father to son: a symptomatic father donates only a normal Y chromosome to his male offspring. By contrast, he always donates his abnormal X chromosome to his daughters, who are therefore obligate carriers of the trait. As a consequence, the disease classically skips a generation in the male, the female carrier transmitting it to grandsons of the original symptomatic male.

X-Linked Dominant Traits

X-linked dominance refers to expression of a trait only in the female, since the hemizygous state in the male precludes a distinction between dominant and recessive inheritance (Fig. 6-32).

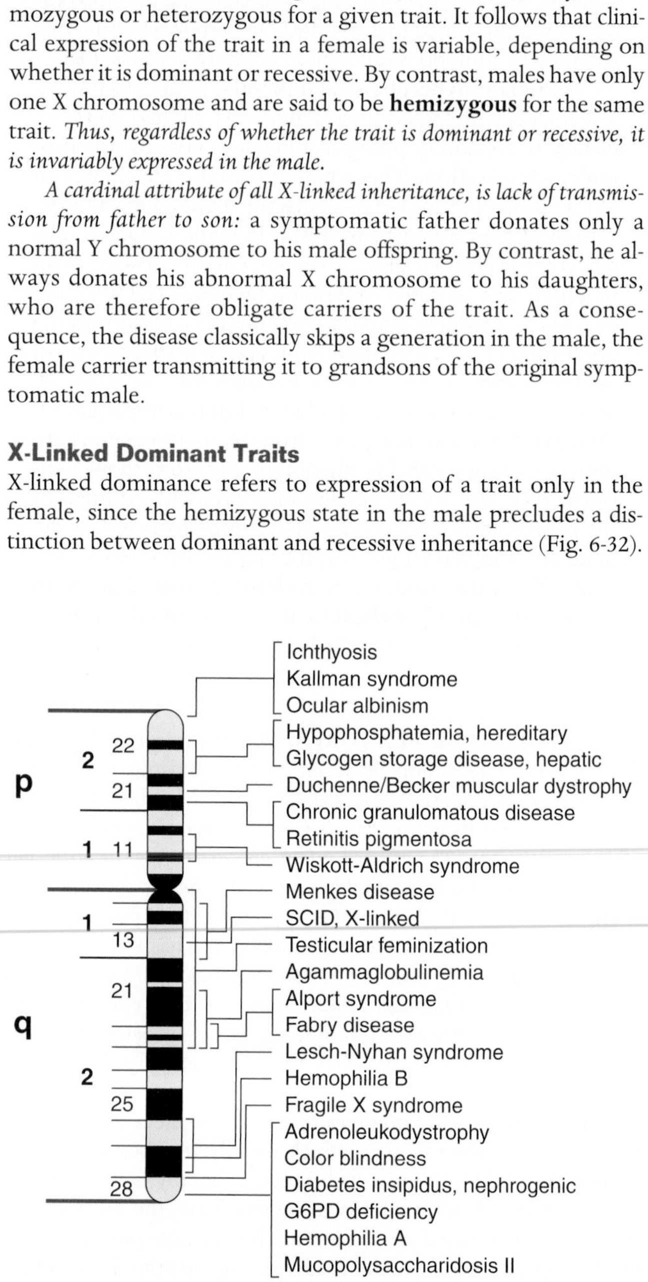

FIGURE 6-31. **Localization of representative inherited diseases on the X chromosome. G6PD 5 glucose-6-phosphate dehydrogenase; SCID 5 severe comvbined immunodeficiency (syndrome).**

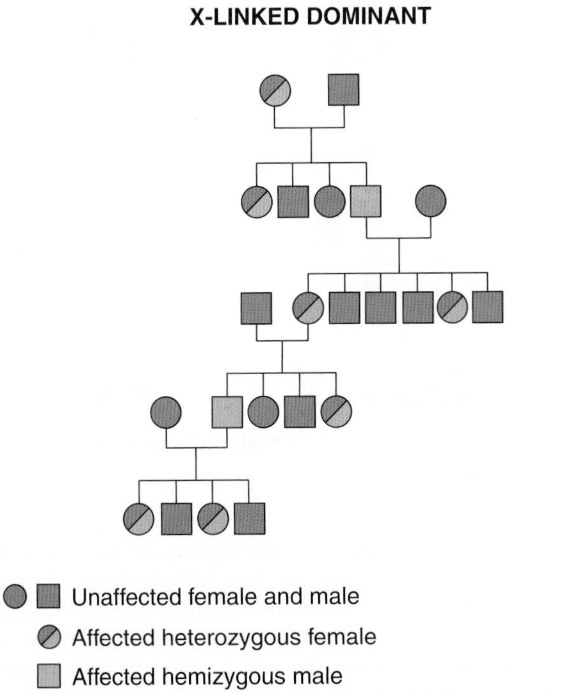

FIGURE 6-32. **X-linked dominant inheritance.** A heterozygous woman transmits the trait equally to males and females; men transmit the trait only to their daughters. Asymptomatic males and females do not carry the trait.

The distinctive features of X-linked dominant disorders are:

- Females are affected twice as frequently as males.
- A heterozygous woman transmits the disorder to half her children, whether male or female.
- A man with a dominant X-linked disorder transmits the disease only to his daughters.
- Clinical expression of the disease tends to be less severe and more variable in heterozygous females than in hemizygous males.

Only a few X-linked dominant disorders are described, among which are familial hypophosphatemic rickets and ornithine transcarbamylase deficiency. In such diseases, variations in the phenotype of the trait in the female may be explained, at least in part, by the Lyon effect (i.e., inactivation of one X chromosome). This random inactivation results in mosaicism for the mutant allele, leading to inconstant expression of the trait.

X-Linked Recessive Traits

Most X-linked traits are recessive; that is, heterozygous females do not have clinical disease (Fig. 6-33). The characteristics of this mode of inheritance are

- Sons of women who are carriers have a 50% chance of inheriting the disease; daughters are not symptomatic. However, 50% of daughters will also be carriers.
- All daughters of affected men are asymptomatic carriers, but the sons of these men do not have the trait and cannot transmit it to their children.
- Symptomatic homozygous females can result from the rare mating of an affected man and an asymptomatic, heterozygous woman. Alternatively, Lyonization may preferentially inactivate the normal X chromosome, which in extreme cases may lead to a heterozygous female expressing an X-linked recessive trait.
- The trait tends to occur in maternal uncles and in male cousins descended from the mother's sisters.

Table 6-10 presents a list of representative X-linked recessive disorders.

X-Linked Muscular Dystrophies (Duchenne and Becker Muscular Dystrophies)

The muscular dystrophies are devastating muscle diseases. Most are X-linked, although a few are autosomal recessive. The X-linked muscular dystrophies are among the most frequent human genetic diseases, occurring in 1 per 3500 boys, an incidence approaching that of CF. ***Duchenne muscular dystrophy (DMD),*** the most common variant, is a fatal progressive degeneration of muscle that appears before the age of 4 years. ***Becker muscular dystrophy (BMD)*** is allelic with DMD but is less common and milder.

Muscular dystrophy is discussed in Chapter 27.

Hemophilia A (Factor VIII Deficiency)

Hemophilia A is an X-linked recessive disorder of blood clotting that results in spontaneous bleeding, particularly into joints, muscles, and internal organs. The disease is discussed in Chapter 20.

Fragile X Syndrome

Fragile X syndrome is the most common form of inherited mental retardation and is caused by expansion of a CGG repeat at the Xq27 fragile site. It is second only to Down syndrome as an identifiable cause of mental retardation. The disease afflicts 1 in 1250 males and 1 in 2500 females.

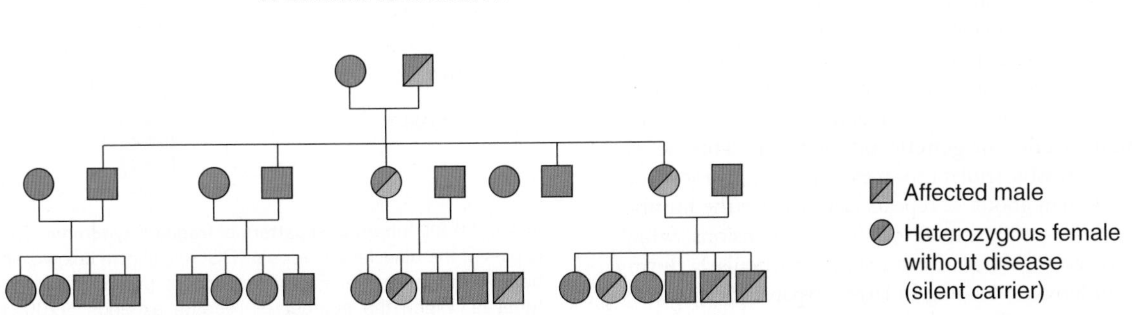

FIGURE 6-33. **X-linked recessive inheritance.** Only males are affected; daughters of affected men are all asymptomatic carriers. Asymptomatic men do not transmit the trait. Clinical expression of the disease skips a generation.

TABLE 6-10

Representative X-Linked Recessive Diseases

Disease	Frequency in Males
Fragile X syndrome	1/2000
Hemophilia A (factor VIII deficiency)	1/10,000
Hemophilia B (factor IX deficiency)	1/70,000
Duchenne-Becker muscular dystrophy	1/3500
Glucose-6-phosphate dehydrogenase deficiency	Up to 30%
Lesch-Nyhan syndrome (HPRT deficiency)	1/10,000
Chronic granulomatous disease	Not rare
X-linked agammaglobulinemia	Not rare
X-linked severe combined immunodeficiency	Rare
Fabry disease	1/40,000
Hunter syndrome	1/70,000
Adrenoleukodystrophy	1/100,000
Menke disease	1/100,000

HPRT = hypoxanthine-guanine phosphoribosyltransferase

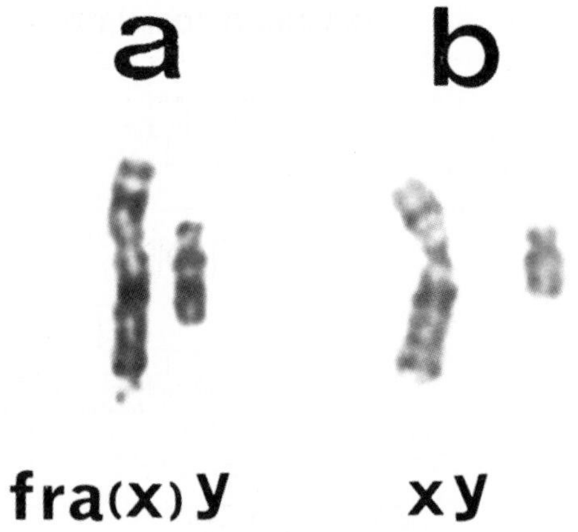

FIGURE 6-34. **Fragile X chromosome.**

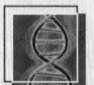

PATHOGENESIS: The well-known fact that more males than females are institutionalized for mental retardation was traditionally ascribed to societal factors. However, it was recognized in the early 1970s that X-linked inheritance of mental retardation accounted for most of this excess of males. Whereas fully 20% of all cases of heritable mental retardation are X-linked disorders, one-fifth of these are associated with a single genetic defect, namely, an inducible fragile site on the X chromosome (Xq27).

A **fragile site** represents a specific locus, or band, on a chromosome that breaks easily. It is usually detected in cytogenetic preparations as a nonstaining gap or constriction (Fig. 6-34). Importantly, under the routine conditions of preparing cells for karyotypic analysis, most fragile sites are not detected. However, when the same cells in culture are treat so as to impair DNA synthesis (e.g., with methotrexate, floxuridine), fragile sites are revealed. At least 11, and possibly as many as 50, fragile sites occur in the genomes of most persons, both on autosomes and on the X chromosome. *However, the locus at Xq27 is associated with mental retardation and other clinical findings that characterize fragile X syndrome.* As discussed, the fragile site at Xq27 is a distinct kind of mutation characterized by amplification of a CGG repeat.

Within fragile X families, the probability of being affected is related to position in the pedigree; that is, later generations are more likely than earlier ones to be affected (**Sherman paradox or genetic anticipation**). This fact relates to progressive triplet repeat expansion. Chromosomes with more than about 52 repeats can increase the number of repeats—so-called expansion. Small expansions, which tend to be asymptomatic, can enlarge, particularly during meiosis in females, leading to larger expansions in successive generations. These are known as **premutations.** Expansions with more than 200 repeats are associated with mental retardation and represent full mutations. Expansion of a premutation to a full mutation during gametogenesis only occurs in females. Thus, daughters of men with premutations (carriers) are never clinically symptomatic, whereas the sisters of the transmitting males occasionally produce affected daughters. However, the daughters of carrier males always harbor the premutation. The frequency of conversion of a premutation to a full mutation in such women (i.e., the probability that their sons will have fragile X syndrome) varies with the length of the expanded tract. Premutations with more than 90 repeats are almost always converted to full mutations. As fragile X syndrome is recessive, most daughters of carrier males transmit mental retardation to 50% of their sons. These considerations explain the greater risk of the disorder in succeeding generations of fragile X families (Fig. 6-35).

CLINICAL FEATURES: A male newborn with fragile X syndrome appears normal, but during childhood, typical features appear, including increased head circumference, facial coarsening, joint hyperextensibility, enlarged

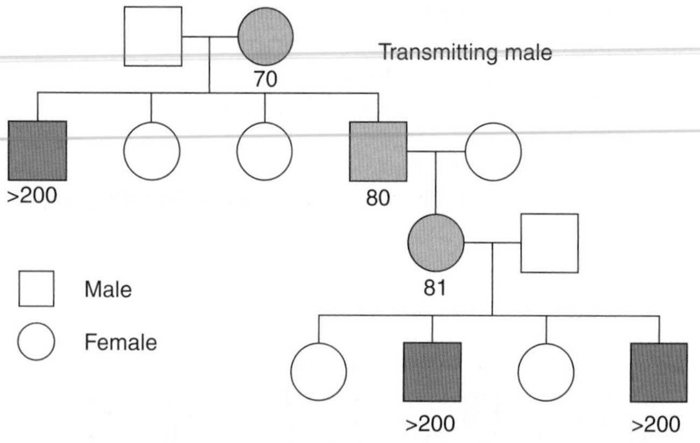

FIGURE 6-35. **Inheritance pattern of fragile X syndrome.** The number of copies of the trinucleotide repeat (CGG) is shown below selected members in this pedigree. Expansion occurs primarily during meiosis in females. When the number of repeats exceeds ~200, the clinical syndrome is manifested. Individuals shaded orange carry a premutation and are asymptomatic.

testes, and heart valve abnormalities. Mental retardation is profound: IQ scores vary from 20 to 60. *Interestingly, a significant proportion of autistic male children carry a fragile X chromosome.* Among female carriers who are mentally handicapped, the severity of the impairment varies from a learning disability with normal IQ to serious retardation.

Only 80% of males with the Xq27 fragile site are mentally retarded; the others are clinically normal, but can transmit the trait. They have expansions in less than 200 copies of the trinucleotide repeat. Recently, a new syndrome characterized by tremors, ataxia, and declining congitive abilities was described in elderly men with fragile X premutations. This disorder has some clinical similarities to Parkinson disease and Alzheimer disease, and has been called fragile X tremor ataxia syndrome (FTAXS). Among females who are known to bear a fragile X chromosome (obligate carriers), two thirds are intellectually normal, and the fragile site on the X chromosome cannot be demonstrated. By contrast, of the 1/3 of female carriers who are mentally retarded, virtually all display a fragile Xq27 locus. It has been suggested that this variability in phenotypic expression in females may relate to the pattern of X inactivation.

Fabry Disease

Fabry disease is a deficiency of lysosomal α-galactosidase A. This X-linked syndrome leads to accumulation of globotriaosylceramide and other glycosphingolipids in the endothelium of the brain, heart, skin, kidneys, and other organs. A particular type of tumor, angiokeratoma, is a characteristic cutaneous manifestation of Fabry disease. The functionally affected microvasculature is increasingly compromised, leading to progressive vascular insufficiency, then cerebral, renal, and cardiac infarcts. Affected people die in early adulthood from complications of their vascular disease. Recent treatments using recombinant α-D-galactosidase A show promise in arresting the disease.

Mitochondrial Diseases

Mitochondrial proteins are encoded by both nuclear and mitochondrial genes. Most mitochondrial respiratory chain proteins are encoded by nuclear genes, although several are products of the mitochondrial genome. A few rare, autosomal recessive (mendelian) disorders that represent defects in nuclear encoded mitochondrial proteins have been described. However, most inherited defects in mitochondrial function result from mutations in the mitochondrial genome itself. To understand these conditions an explanation of the unique genetics of the mitochondria is needed. These features include:

- **Maternal inheritance:** All vertebrate mitochondria are inherited from the mother via the ovum, which possesses up to 300,000 copies of mitochondrial DNA (mtDNA).
- **Variability of mtDNA copies:** The number of mitochondria and the number of copies of mtDNA per mitochondrion vary in different tissues. Each mitochondrion carries 2 to 10 mtDNA copies, and the need of various cell types for ATP correlates with the DNA content per mitochondrion.
- **Threshold effect:** Since any given cell has many mitochondria and thus hundreds or thousands of mtDNA copies, mutations in mtDNA lead to mixed populations of mutant and normal mitochondrial genomes, a situation is called **heteroplasmy.** The phenotype associated with mtDNA mutations reflects the severity of the mutation, the proportion of mutant genomes, and the demand of the tissue for ATP. In this context, different tissues require different minimum rates (or thresholds) of ATP production to sustain their characteristic metabolic activity; the brain, heart, and skeletal muscle have particularly great energy demands.
- **High mutation rate:** The rate of mutation of mtDNA is considerably higher than that of nuclear DNA, owing (at least in part) to less DNA repair capacity.

Diseases caused by mutations in the mitochondrial genome principally affect the nervous system, heart, and skeletal muscle. The functional deficits in all of these disorders can be traced to inadequate oxidative phosphorylation (OXPHOS). **OXPHOS diseases** have been divided into the following classes: I, nuclear mutations; II, mtDNA point mutations; III, mtDNA deletions; and IV, as yet undefined defects.

All inherited mitochondrial diseases are rare and have variable clinical presentations based on the considerations discussed above. The first human mtDNA disease to be discovered was **Leber hereditary optic neuropathy,** which is characterized by progressive loss of vision. Various mitochondrial myopathies and encephalomyopathies are known; they are discussed in Chapter 27. Hypertrophic cardiomyopathy (see Chapter 11) is also a common manifestation of OXPHOS diseases.

Genetic Imprinting

Genetic imprinting refers to the observation that the phenotype associated with some genes differs, depending on whether the allele is inherited from the mother or the father. In the case of imprinted genes, either the maternal or paternal allele is maintained in an inactive state. This normal physiologic process results from methylation of DNA cytosine residues in regulatory elements in the imprinted allele. The nonimprinted allele provides the biological function for that locus. If the nonimprinted allele is disrupted through mutation, the imprinted allele remains inactivated: it cannot compensate for the missing function. Imprinting occurs in meiosis during gametogenesis, and the pattern of imprinting is maintained to variable degrees in different tissues. It is reset during meiosis in the next generation, so the selection of a given allele for imprinting can vary from one generation to the next.

In the extreme case, experimental embryos that obtain both sets of chromosomes exclusively from either the mother or the father never survive to term. A less severe manifestation of genetic imprinting is seen in **uniparental disomy,** in which both members of a single chromosome pair are inherited from the same parent. The pair of chromosomes may be copies of one parental chromosome (uniparental isodisomy) or may be the same pair found in one parent (uniparental heterodisomy). Uniparental disomy is rare, but has been implicated in unexpected patterns of inheritance of genetic traits. For instance, a child with uniparental isodisomy may manifest a recessive disease when only one parent carries the trait, as has been observed in a few cases of cystic fibrosis and hemophilia A. Loss of a chromosome from a trisomy or duplication of a chromosome in the case of a monosomy can lead to uniparental disomy. Interestingly, as many as 1% of viable pregnancies carry uniparental disomy for at least one chromosome.

Genetic imprinting is well illustrated by certain hereditary diseases whose phenotype is determined by the parental source of the mutant allele. Deletion of the 15q11-13 locus results in **Prader-Willi syndrome** when the affected chromosome is inherited maternally and in **Angelman syndrome** when it is of paternal origin. The phenotypes of these disorders are remarkably different. Prader-Willi syndrome features hypotonia, obesity, hypogonadism, mental retardation, and a specific facies. By contrast, Angelman syndrome patients are hyperactive, display inappropriate laughter, have a facies different from that of Prader-Willi syndrome, and suffer from seizures. Prader-Willi syndrome develops because the maternal locus is imprinted (silenced), and the same region on the paternal chromosome is deleted. The converse obtains in Angelman syndrome: the paternal gene is imprinted and the maternal locus is inactivated by mutation, e.g., deletion. This pattern is similar to loss of heterozygosity in tumor-suppressor genes by aberrant methylation in some cases of cancer (see Chapter 5). The gene responsible for Angelman syndrome appears to be *UBE3A*. The gene(s) responsible for Prader-Willi syndrome have not been definitively identified.

Genetic imprinting is implicated in a number of other situations relevant to human disease. For example, in some childhood cancers, including Wilms tumor, osteosarcoma, bilateral retinoblastoma, and embryonal rhabdomyosarcoma, the maternal allele of a putative tumor-suppressor gene is lost and the remaining allele is on a chromosome of paternal origin. In the case of familial glomus tumor, an adult neoplasm, both males and females may carry the trait, but it is transmitted only through the male. Thus, the responsible gene is active only when it is located on the paternal autosome. Finally, as noted above, the premutation of fragile X syndrome is expanded to the full mutation only during female gametogenesis, implying that the trinucleotide repeat is treated differently on passage through the female than in the male.

Multifactorial Inheritance

Multifactorial inheritance *describes a process by which a disease results from the effects of a number of abnormal genes and environmental factors.* Most normal human traits reflect such complexities, and are not inherited as simple dominant nor as recessive mendelian attributes. For example, multifactorial inheritance determines height, skin color, and body habitus. Similarly, most of the common chronic disorders of adults–diabetes, atherosclerosis, and many forms of cancer and arthritis and hypertension–represent multifactorial genetic diseases and are well known to "run in families." The inheritance of many birth defects is also multifactorial (e.g., cleft lip and palate, pyloric stenosis, and congenital heart disease) (Table 6-11).

TABLE 6-11

Representative Diseases Associated with Multifactorial Inheritance

Adults	Children
Hypertension	Pyloric stenosis
Atherosclerosis	Cleft lip and palate
Diabetes, type II	Congenital heart disease
Allergic diathesis	Meningomyelocele
Psoriasis	Anencephaly
Schizophrenia	Hypospadias
Ankylosing spondylitis	Congenital hip dislocation
Gout	Hirschprung disease

The concept of multifactorial inheritance is based on the notion that multiple genes interact with each other and with environmental factors to produce disease in an individual patient. Such inheritance leads to familial aggregation that does not obey simple mendelian rules. Thus, inheritance of polygenic diseases is studied by population genetics, rather than by analysis of individual families.

The number of involved genes for any polygenic disease is not known. Thus, it is not possible to ascertain accurately the risk of a particular disorder in an individual case. The probability of disease can only be predicted from the numbers of relatives affected, the severity of their disease and statistical projections based on population analyses. Whereas monogenic inheritance implies a specific risk of disease (e.g., 25% or 50%), the probability of symptoms in first-degree relatives of a person affected with a polygenic disease is usually about 5% to 10%.

The biological basis of polygenic inheritance rests on the evidence that more than one fourth of all genetic loci in normal humans contain polymorphic alleles. Such genetic heterogeneity provides a background for wide variability in susceptibility to many diseases, which is compounded by the many interactions with environmental factors.

- **Expression of symptoms is proportional to the number of mutant genes.** Close relatives of an affected person have more mutant genes than the population at large and a greater chance of expressing the disease. The probability of expressing the same number of mutant genes is highest in identical twins.
- **Environmental factors influence expression of the trait.** Thus, concordance for the disease may occur in only one third of monozygotic twins.
- **The risk in first-degree relatives (parents, siblings, children) is the same (5%–10%).** The probability of disease is much lower in second-degree relatives.
- **The probability of a trait's expression in later offspring is influenced by its expression in earlier siblings.** If one or more children are born with a multifactorial defect, the chance of its recurrence in later offspring is doubled. For simple mendelian traits, in contrast, the probability is independent of the number of affected siblings.
- **The more severe a defect, the greater the risk of transmitting it to offspring.** Patients with more-severe polygenic defects presumably have more mutant genes and their children thus have a greater chance of inheriting the abnormal genes than the offspring of less severely affected persons.
- **Some abnormalities characterized by multifactorial inheritance show a sex predilection.** For example, pyloric stenosis is more common in males, while congenital dislocation of the hip is more common in females. Such differential susceptibility is believed to represent a difference in the threshold for expression of mutant genes in the two sexes. For example, if the number of mutant genes required for pyloric stenosis in males is A, it may require 4A in the female. Then, a woman who had pyloric stenosis as an infant has more mutant genes to transmit to her children than does a similarly afflicted man. Indeed, the son of such a woman actually has a 25% chance of being born with pyloric stenosis, compared with a 4% risk for the son of an affected man. *As a general rule, if there is an altered sex ratio in the incidence of a polygenic defect, a member of the less commonly affected sex has a much greater probability of transmitting the defect.*

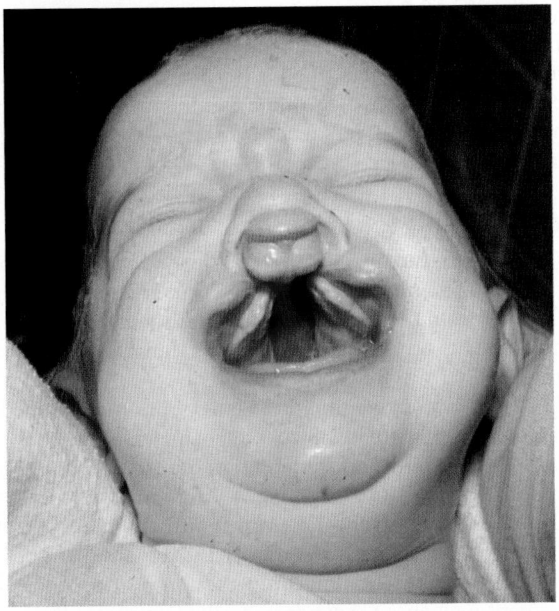

FIGURE 6-36. **Cleft lip and palate in an infant.**

Cleft Lip and Cleft Palate Exemplify Multifactorial Inheritance

At the 35th day of gestation, the frontal prominence fuses with the maxillary process to form the upper lip. This process is under the control of many genes, and disturbances in gene expression (hereditary or environmental) at this time lead to interference with proper fusion and result in cleft lip, with or without cleft palate (Fig. 6-36). This anomaly may also be part of a systemic malformation syndrome caused by teratogens (rubella, anticonvulsants) and is often encountered in children with chromosomal abnormalities.

The incidence of cleft lip, with or without cleft palate, is 1 in 1000, and the incidence of cleft palate alone is 1 in 2500. If one child is born with a cleft lip, the chances are 4% that the second child will exhibit the same defect. If the first two children are affected, the risk of cleft lip increases to 9% for the third child. The more severe the anatomical defect, the greater the probability of transmitting cleft lip will be. Whereas 75% of cases of cleft lip occur in boys, the sons of women with cleft lip have a four times higher risk of acquiring the defect than the sons of affected fathers.

Screening for Carriers of Genetic Disorders

Until recently, screening for carriers of genetic diseases was not uncommon. Among Ashkenazi Jews, screening to identify carriers of Tay-Sachs disease, an autosomal recessive disease, has been done because of the relatively high frequency of the disease in that group. A number of other inherited conditions are also included in a so-called "Ashkenazi screen." The objective is to identify couples in which both members are heterozygous carriers and who thus have a 25% risk of having an affected offspring with each pregnancy. These couples can be offered prenatal diagnosis to determine the genetic status of the fetus. In vitro fertilization combined with preimplantation genetic diagnosis is available in some centers to ensure that an implanted embryo will not have this disease.

Prenatal screening for carriers of CF has been recommended by national professional organizations for several years. This represents the first large-scale adoption of testing for carriers of genetic diseases. Guidelines recommend that screening for CF be offered to all white and Ashkenazi Jewish women because of the relatively high frequency of CF in these groups. A panel of 25 CF mutations has been chosen for this DNA-based testing. If a woman is a carrier of a CF mutation, then her partner should be tested to see if the couple is at risk of having an affected offspring. Because of the distribution of CF mutations, the recommended panel will detect only about 80% of known CF mutations in whites, but over 97% among Ashkenazi Jews. Among other ethnic groups, detection rates are lower.

Prenatal Diagnosis of Genetic Disorders

Amniocentesis and chorionic villus biopsy are the most important methods for diagnosis of a developmental or genetic disorder. Both procedures are safe, reliable, and easily performed. The indications for chorionic villus biopsy or amniocentesis are:

- **Age 35 years old and over:** The risk of having a child with Down syndrome is about 1 in 300 for a 40-year-old woman, compared with 1 in 1200 at age 25. This risk rises even higher with advanced maternal age.
- **Previous chromosomal abnormality:** The overall risk of recurrence of Down syndrome in a succeeding child of a woman who has already borne an infant with trisomy 21 is 1%.
- **Translocation carrier:** Estimates of risks to the offspring of translocation carriers vary from 3% to 15%. Carriers of balanced translocations are at increased risk for producing children with unbalanced karyotypes and resulting phenotypic abnormalities.
- **History of familial inborn error of metabolism:** Recessive inborn errors of metabolism have a 25% risk for each child if each parent is heterozygous for the trait. Prenatal diagnosis can identify disorders for which a biochemical diagnosis can be made.
- **Identified heterozygotes:** Carrier detection programs, such as Tay-Sachs Disease Prevention Program, identify couples in which both spouses are carriers of the same recessive gene. Each pregnancy in such couples has a 25% risk of an affected child and prenatal diagnosis can be made routinely.
- **Family history of X-linked disorders:** Fetal sex determination, using amniotic cells, can be offered to women known to be carriers of X-linked disorders. The diagnosis of some of these conditions can be established biochemically by amniotic fluid analysis.

New molecular techniques for carrier detection and early prenatal diagnosis are of ever-increasing utility. Gene-specific DNA probes have been developed for many genetic diseases, including hemophilia A and B, the hemoglobinopathies, phenylketonuria, and α_1-antitrypsin deficiency. Most heterozygous carriers for Duchenne and Becker muscular dystrophies, Huntington chorea, and CF can be identified by such techniques.

Diseases of Infancy and Childhood

The period from birth to puberty has been traditionally subdivided into several stages.

- Neonatal age (the first 4 weeks)
- Infancy (the first year)

- Early childhood (1 to 4 years)
- Late childhood (5 to 14 years)

Each of these periods has its own distinct anatomical, physiologic, and immunologic characteristics, which determine the nature and form of various pathologic processes. Morbidity and mortality rates in the neonatal period differ considerably from those in infancy and childhood. Infants and children are not simply "small adults," and they may be afflicted by diseases unique to their particular age group.

Prematurity and Intrauterine Growth Retardation

Human pregnancy normally lasts 40 ± 2 weeks, and most newborns weigh 3300 ± 600 g. The World Health Organization defines prematurity as a gestational age of less than 37 weeks (timed from the first day of the last menstrual period). Traditionally prematurity was defined as a birth weight below 2500 g, regardless of gestational age. However, it is now appreciated that full-term infants may weigh under 2500 g because of intrauterine growth retardation rather than prematurity. Thus, **low-birth-weight infants** (<2500 g) are termed (1) appropriate for gestational age (AGA) or (2) small for gestational age (SGA).

In the United States, the frequency of low-birth-weight infants is less than 6% among whites. Two thirds of these infants are premature (AGA). By contrast, when the frequency of low-birth-weight infants exceeds 10%, as it does for blacks (>12%), most of these newborns suffer from intrauterine growth retardation and are considered SGA.

About 1% of all infants born in the United States weigh less than 1500 g and are classified as **very-low-birth-weight infants.** Such babies account for half of neonatal deaths, and their survival is determined by their birth weight. If premature newborns are cared for in neonatal intensive care units, 90% of infants over 750 g survive. Between 500 g and 750 g, 45% survive, of whom more than half develop normally.

- **Etiology:** The factors that predispose to premature birth of an infant (AGA) are (1) maternal illness, (2) uterine incompetence, (3) fetal disorders, and (4) placental abnormalities. When the life of a fetus is threatened by such conditions, it may be necessary to induce premature delivery to save the infant. In a substantial proportion of AGA infants, the cause of premature birth is unknown. Intrauterine growth retardation and the resulting birth of SGA infants are associated with disorders that (1) impair maternal health and nutrition, (2) interfere with placental circulation or function, or (3) disturb the growth or development of the fetus.

CLINICAL FEATURES: There is a substantial overlap between the complications of prematurity itself (AGA) and intrauterine growth retardation (SGA). However, certain general principles apply. Prematurity is often associated with severe respiratory distress, metabolic disturbances (e.g., hyperbilirubinemia, hypoglycemia, hypocalcemia), circulatory problems (anemia, hypothermia, hypotension), and bacterial sepsis. By contrast, SGA infants are a much more heterogeneous group, including many infants with congenital anomalies and infections acquired in utero. Even when these causes of intrauterine growth retardation are excluded, neonatal complications in SGA infants reflect gestational age more than birth weight. In addition to the many problems associated with prematurity, SGA infants often suffer from perinatal asphyxia, meconium aspiration, necrotizing enterocolitis, pulmonary hemorrhage, and disorders related to birth defects or inherited metabolic diseases.

Organ Immaturity is a Cause of Neonatal Problems

The maturity of the newborn can be defined in both anatomic and physiologic terms. Maturing organs in infants born prematurely differ from those in term infants, although complete maturation of many organs may require days (lungs) to years (brain) after birth.

LUNGS: Pulmonary immaturity is a common and immediate threat to the viability of low-birth-weight infants. The lining cells of the fetal alveoli do not differentiate into type I and type II pneumocytes until late in pregnancy. Amniotic fluid fills the fetal alveoli and drains from the lungs at birth. Sometimes immature infants show sluggish respiratory movement that does not fully expel the amniotic fluid from the lungs. Respiratory embarassment may ensue, a syndrome called **amniotic fluid aspiration,** but that actually represents retained amniotic fluid. Air passages contain desquamated squamous cells (**squames**) and lanugo hair from the fetal skin and protein-rich amniotic fluid (Fig. 6-37).

The ability of the alveoli to remain expanded during the respiratory cycle, i.e., not to collapse when the individual exhales, is largely due to **pulmonary surfactant,** which reduces intraalveolar surface tension. Surfactant is produced by type II pneumocytes, and is a complex mixture of several phospholipids, 75% phosphatidylcholine (lecithin), and 10% phosphatidylglycerol. The

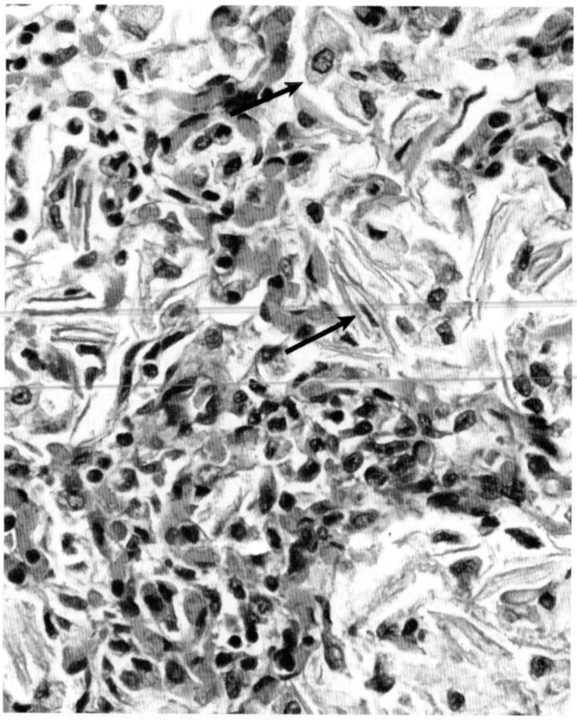

FIGURE 6-37. **Retention of amniotic fluid in the lung of a premature newborn.** The incompletely expanded lung contains squames *(arrows)*, consisting of squamous epithelial cells shed into the amniotic fluid from the fetal skin.

composition of lung surfactant changes as the fetus matures: (1) The concentration of lecithin increases rapidly at the beginning of the third trimester and thereafter rises rapidly to reach a peak near term (Fig. 6-38). (2) Whereas most of the lecithin in the mature lung is dipalmitate, in the immature lung it is the less-surface-active α-palmitate, α-myristate species. (3) Phosphatidylglycerol is not present in the lungs before the 36th week of pregnancy. (4) Before the 35th week, the immature surfactant contains a higher proportion of sphingomyelin than adult surfactant.

Pulmonary surfactant is released into the amniotic fluid, which can be sampled by amniocentesis to assess the maturity of the fetal lung. A lecithin-to-sphingomyelin ratio above 2:1 implies that the fetus should survive without developing respiratory distress syndrome. After the 35th week, the appearance of phosphatidylglycerol in the amniotic fluid is the best proof of the maturity of the fetal lungs.

LIVER: The liver of premature infants is morphologically similar to that of the adult organ, with the exception of conspicuous extramedullary hematopoiesis. However, the hepatocytes tend to be functionally immature. The fetal liver is deficient in glucuronyl transferase and the resulting inability of the organ to conjugate bilirubin often leads to neonatal jaundice. This enzyme deficiency is aggravated by the rapid destruction of fetal erythrocytes, a process that results in an increased supply of bilirubin.

BRAIN: Although the brain of the immature newborn differs from that of the adult, both morphologically and functionally, this difference is rarely fatal. On the other hand, the incomplete development of the CNS is often reflected in poor vasomotor control, hypothermia, feeding difficulties, and recurrent apnea.

The Apgar Score

Clinical assessments of neonatal maturity in general are usually performed 1 minute and 5 minutes after delivery, and certain parameters are scored according to the criteria recommended by Virginia Apgar (Table 6-12). In general, the higher the **Apgar score,** the better the clinical condition of the infant. The score taken at 1 minute is an index of asphyxia and of the need for assisted ventilation. The 5-minute score is a more accurate indication of impending death or the likelihood of persistent neurologic damage. For example, in newborns weighing less than 2000 g who have a 5-minute Apgar score of 9 or 10, the mortality during the first month is less than 5%; it is almost 80% when the Apgar score is reduced to 3 or less.

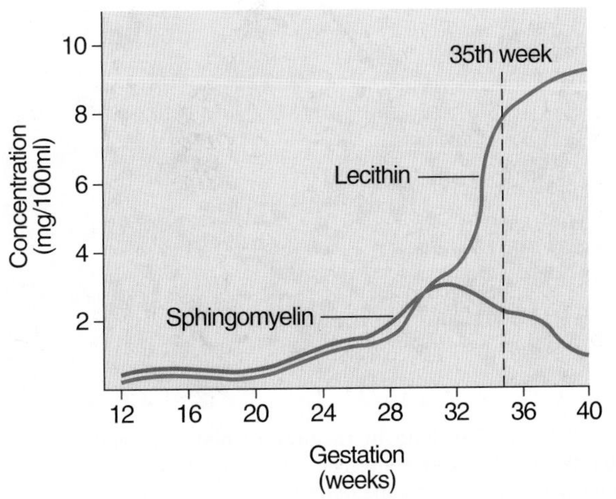

FIGURE 6-38. **Changes in amniotic fluid composition during pregnancy.**

TABLE 6-12

Apgar Score*

Sign	0	1	2
Heart rate	Not detectable	Below 100/min	Over 100/min
Respiratory effort	None	Slow, irregular	Good, crying
Muscle tone	Poor	Some flexion of extremities	Active motion
Response to catheter in nostril	No response	Grimace	Cough or sneeze
Color	Blue, pale	Body pink, extremities blue	Completely pink

*Sixty seconds after the completion of birth, these five objective signs are evaluated, and each is given a score of 0, 1, or 2. A maximum score of 10 is assigned to infants in the best possible condition.

Neonatal Respiratory Distress Syndrome (RDS) is due to Deficiency of Surfactant

Neonatal RDS is the leading cause of morbidity and mortality among premature infants. It accounts for half of all neonatal deaths in the United States. Its incidence varies inversely with gestational age and birth weight. Thus, more than half of newborns younger than 28 weeks gestational age have RDS, whereas only one fifth of infants between 32 and 36 weeks do. In addition to prematurity, other risk factors for RDS include (1) neonatal asphyxia, (2) maternal diabetes, (3) delivery by cesarean section, (4) precipitous delivery, and (5) twin pregnancies.

PATHOGENESIS: *The pathogenesis of RDS of the newborn is intimately linked to a deficiency of surfactant* (Fig. 6-39). When a newborn starts breathing, type II cells release their surfactant stores. The biophysical role of surfactant is to reduce surface tension, i.e., to decrease the affinity of alveolar surfaces for each other. This allows alveoli to remain open when the baby exhales and reduces resistance to reinflating the lungs with the second breath. If surfactant function is inadequate, as it is in many premature infants with immature lungs, alveoli collapse when the baby exhales and resist expansion when the child tries to take its second breath. The energy required for the second breath must then overcome the cell-cell affinity within the alveoli and inspiration therefore requires considerable effort and damages the alveolar lining. The injured alveoli leak plasma into airspaces. Plasma constituents, including fibrinogen and albumin, bind surfactant and impair its function, thus further exacerbating the respiraptory insufficiency. Many alveoli are perfused with blood, but not ventilated by air, which leads to hypoxia and acidosis and further compromise in the ability of type II pneumocytes to produce surfactant. Moreover, hypoxia produces pulmonary arterial vasoconstriction, thereby increasing right-to-left shunting through the ductus arteriosus and foramen

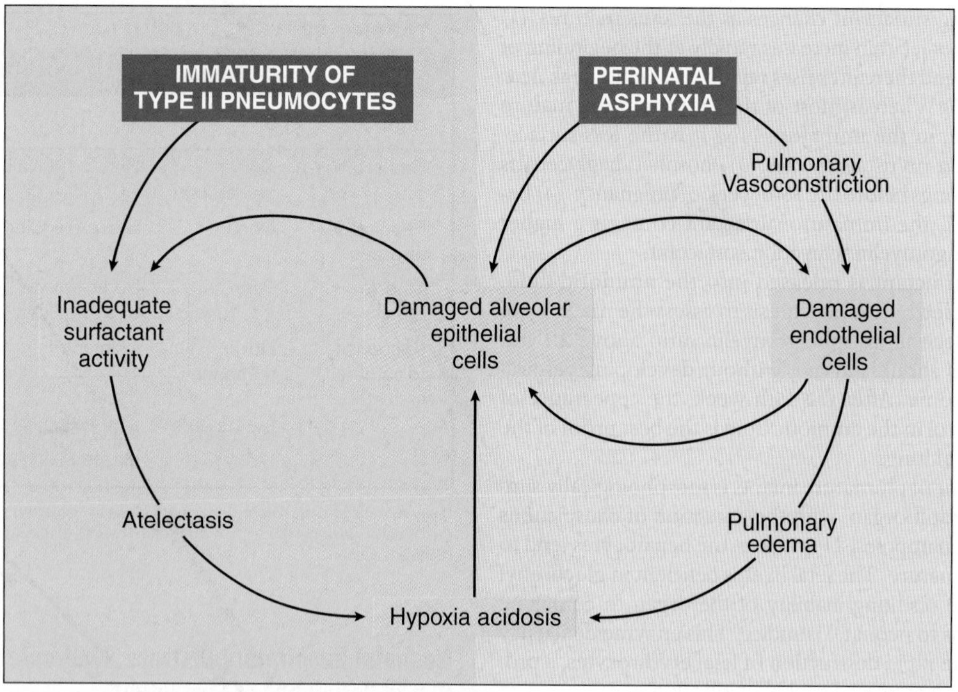

FIGURE 6-39. **Pathogenesis of the respiratory distress syndrome of the neonate.** Immaturity of the lungs and perinatal asphyxia are the major pathogenetic factors.

ovale and within the lung itself. The resulting pulmonary ischemia further aggravates alveolar epithelial damage and injures the endothelium of the pulmonary capillaries. The leak of protein-rich fluid into the alveoli from the injured vascular bed contributes to the typical clinical and pathologic features of RDS.

PATHOLOGY: On gross examination, the lungs are dark red and airless. Alveoli are collapsed. Alveolar ducts and respiratory bronchioles are dilated and contain cellular debris, proteinaceous edema fluid and erythrocytes. The alveolar ducts are lined by conspicuous, eosinophilic, fibrin-rich, amorphous structures, called **hyaline membranes,** hence the original term for neonatal RDS, **hyaline membrane disease** (Fig. 6-40). Walls of collapsed alveoli are thick, capillaries are congested and lymphatics are filled with proteinaceous material.

CLINICAL FEATURES: Most newborns destined to develop RDS appear normal at birth and have high Apgar scores. The first symptom, usually appearing within an hour of birth, is increased respiratory effort, with forceful intercostal retraction and the use of accessory neck muscles. Respiratory rate increases to more than 100 breaths per minute, and the baby becomes cyanotic. Chest radiographs show a characteristic "ground-glass" granularity and in terminal stages the fluid-filled alveoli appear as complete "white out" of the lungs. In severe cases, the infant becomes progressively obtunded and flaccid. Long periods of apnea ensue and the infant

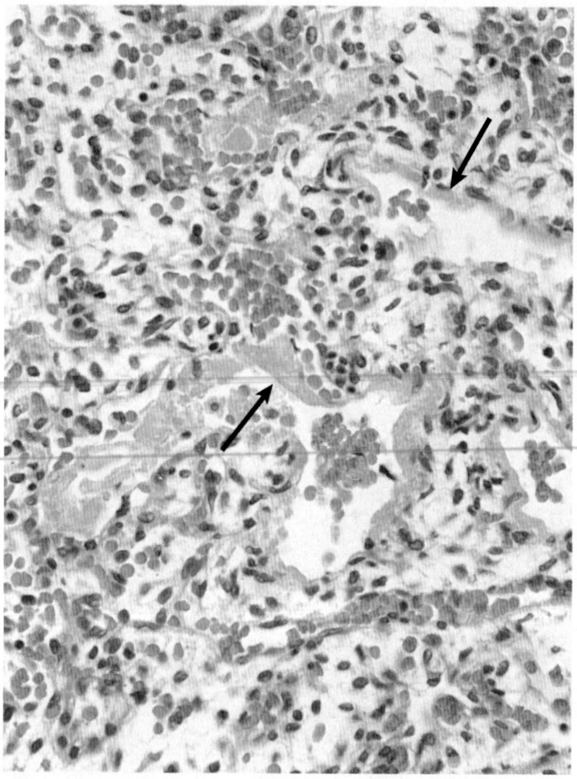

FIGURE 6-40. **The lung in respiratory distress syndrome of the neonate.** The alveoli are atelectatic, and a dilated alveolar duct is lined by a fibrin-rich hyaline membrane *(arrows)*.

eventually dies of asphyxia. Despite advances in neonatal intensive care, the overall mortality of RDS is about 15%, and one third of infants born before 30 weeks of gestational age die of this disorder. In milder cases, the disorder peaks within 3 days, after which gradual improvement takes place.

The major complications of RDS relate to anoxia and acidosis and include:

- **Intraventricular cerebral hemorrhage:** The periventricular germinal matrix in the newborn brain is particularly vulnerable to hemorrhage because the dilated, thin-walled veins in this area rupture easily (Fig. 6-41). The pathogenesis of this complication is not fully understood but is believed to reflect anoxic injury to the periventricular capillaries, venous sludging and thrombosis and impaired vascular autoregulation.
- **Persistent patent ductus arteriosus:** In almost 1/3 of newborns who survive RDS, the ductus arteriosus remains patent. With recovery from the pulmonary disease, pulmonary arterial pressure declines, and the higher pressure in the aorta reverses the direction of blood flow in the ductus, thereby creating a persistent left-to-right shunt. Congestive heart failure may ensue and necessitate correction of the patent ductus.
- **Necrotizing enterocolitis:** This intestinal complication of RDS is the most common acquired gastrointestinal emergency in newborns. It is thought to be related to ischemia of the intestinal mucosa, which leads to bacterial colonization, usually with *Clostridium difficile*. The lesions vary from those of typical pseudomembranous enterocolitis to gangrene and perforation of the bowel.
- **Bronchopulmonary dysplasia (BPD):** BPD is a late complication of RDS usually in infants who weigh less than 1500 g and were maintained on a positive-pressure respirator with high oxygen tensions. It is thought that the disorder results from oxygen toxicity superimposed on RDS. In such patients, respiratory distress persists after the third or fourth day and is reflected in hypoxia, acidosis, oxygen dependency, and the onset of right-sided heart failure. Radiographs of the lungs show a change from almost complete opacification to a spongelike appearance, with small lucent areas alternating with denser foci. The bronchiolar epithelium is hyperplastic, with squamous metaplasia in the bronchi and bronchioles. There are atelectasis, interstitial edema, and thickening of alveolar basement membranes. BPD is a chronic disease; affected infants may continue to require oxygen supplementation into their second or third years of life. Some studies also suggest that a degree of respiratory impairment may persist, even into adolescence and beyond.

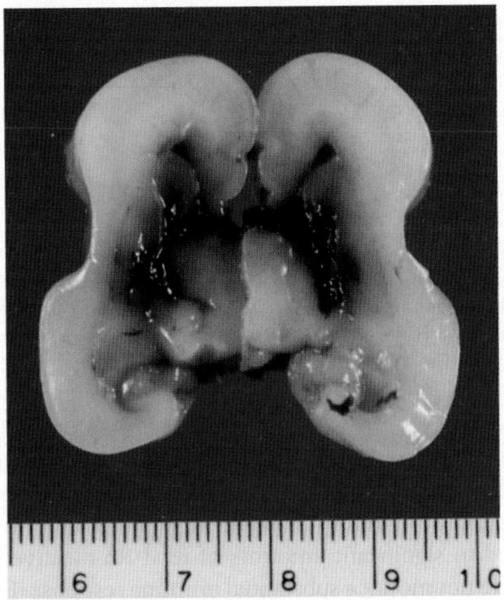

FIGURE 6-41. **Intraventricular hemorrhage in a premature infant suffering from respiratory distress syndrome of the neonate.**

Advances in treatment of neonatal RDS have dramatically improved the prognosis for preterm infants. Antenatal glucocorticoids are often administered to women experiencing preterm labor to accelerate pulmonary maturation. Surfactant preparations, the most effective of which are derived from natural surfactants, have greatly increased survival. Improvements in ventilatory support have, as well, been instrumental in the improved survival of these infants.

Erythroblastosis Fetalis Is a Hemolytic Disease Caused by Maternal Antibodies Against Fetal Erythrocytes

The disorder was first recognized by Hippocrates but was not fully understood until 1940, when the Rh (Rhesus) antigen on erythrocytes was identified. More than 60 antigens on red blood cell membranes can elicit antibody responses, but only antibodies against Rh D antigen and the ABO system cause a significant incidence of hemolytic disease.

Rh Incompatibility

The distribution of Rh antigens among ethnic groups varies. In American whites, 15% are Rh-negative (Rh D−), whereas only 8% of blacks are Rh D−. Japanese, Chinese, and Native American Indian populations contain essentially no Rh D− persons. By contrast, in the Basque population, among whom the mutation that causes the Rh D− phenotype may have arisen, the prevalence of Rh D− persons is 35%.

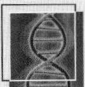

PATHOGENESIS: The Rh blood group system consists of some 25 components, of which only the alleles cde/CDE need be considered in this discussion. Among infants with erythroblastosis fetalis caused by Rh incompatibility, 90% are due to antibodies against D, the remaining cases involving C or E. Rh-positive fetal erythrocytes (>1 mL) enter the circulation of an Rh-negative mother at the time of delivery, eliciting antibodies in her to the D antigen (Fig. 6-42). Because the quantity of fetal blood necessary to sensitize the mother is introduced into her circulation only at the time of delivery, erythroblastosis fetalis does not ordinarily affect the first baby. However, when a sensitized mother again carries an Rh-positive fetus, much smaller quantities of fetal D antigen elicit an increase in antibody titer. In contrast to IgM, IgG antibodies are small enough to cross the placenta and thus produce hemolysis in the fetus. This cycle is exaggerated in multiparous women and the severity of erythroblastosis tends to increase progressively with each succeeding pregnancy.

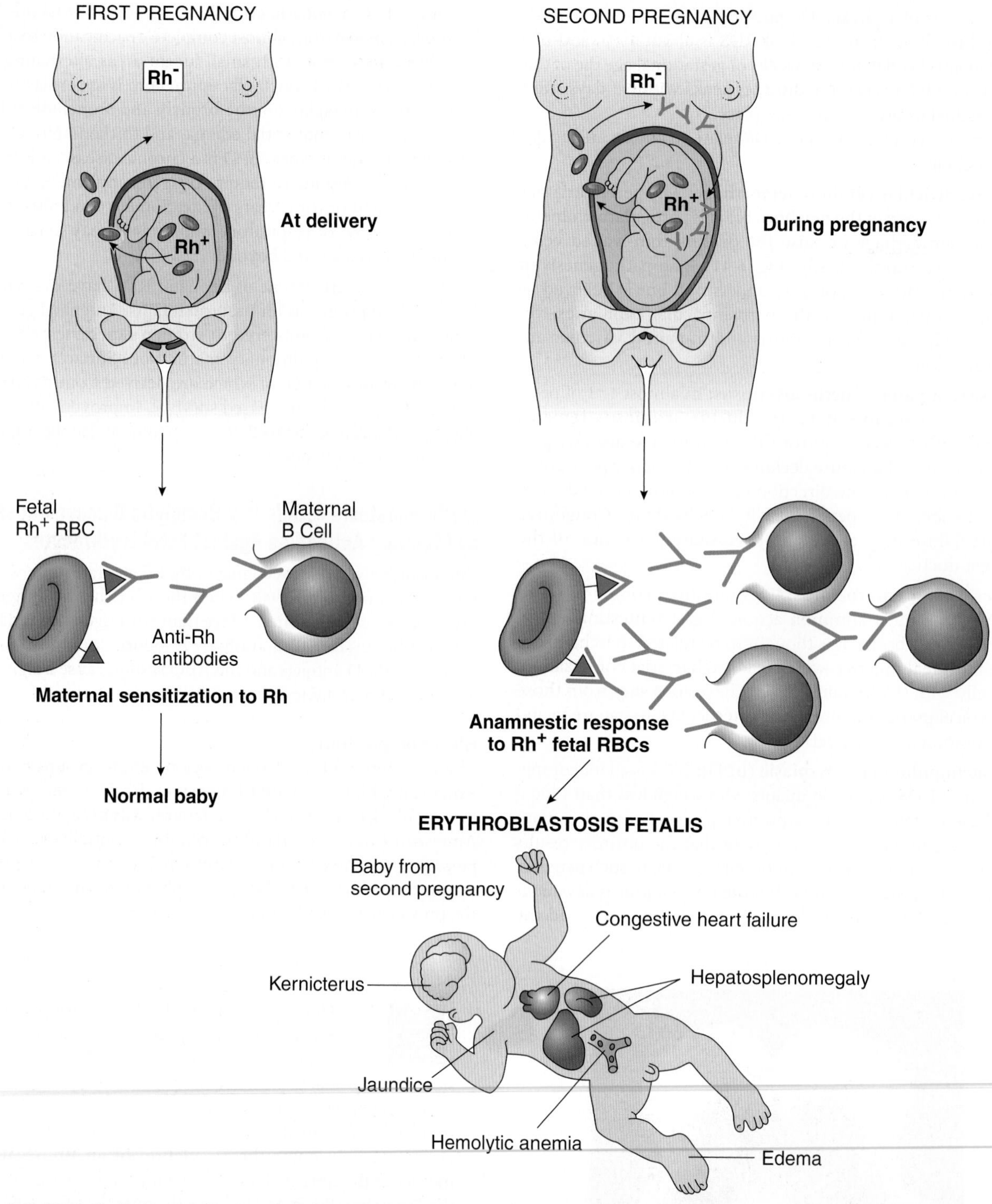

FIGURE 6-42. **Pathogenesis of erythroblastosis fetalis due to maternal–fetal Rh incompatibility.** Immunization of the Rh-negative mother with Rh-positive erythrocytes in the first pregnancy leads to the formation of anti-Rh antibodies of the immunoglobulin (Ig)G type. These antibodies cross the placenta and damage the Rh-positive fetus in subsequent pregnancies.

Since 15% of white women are Rh D−, and since they have an 85% chance of marrying an Rh D+ man, 13% of all marriages are theoretically at risk for maternal–fetal Rh incompatibility. The actual incidence of erythroblastosis fetalis is, however, much lower. This apparent discrepancy is explained by several factors: (1) More than half of Rh-positive men are heterozygous (D/d), and thus only half of their offspring express the D antigen. (2) Only half of all pregnancies have large enough fetal-to-maternal transfusions to sensitize the mother. (3) Even in those Rh-negative women who are exposed to significant amounts of fetal Rh-positive blood, many do not mount a substantial immune response. Even after multiple pregnancies, only 5% of Rh-negative women are ever delivered of infants with erythroblastosis fetalis.

PATHOLOGY AND CLINICAL FEATURES: The severity of erythroblastosis fetalis varies from a mild hemolysis to fatal anemia, and the pathologic findings are determined by the extent of the hemolytic disease.

- **Death in utero** occurs in the most extreme form of the disease, in which case severe maceration is evident on delivery. Numerous erythroblasts are demonstrable in visceral organs that are not extensively autolyzed.
- **Hydrops fetalis** *is the most serious form of erythroblastosis fetalis* (Fig. 6-43) *in liveborn infants. It is characterized by severe edema secondary to congestive heart failure caused by the severe anemia.* Affected infants generally die, unless adequate exchange transfusions with Rh-negative cells correct the anemia and ameliorate the hemolytic disease. Infants are not jaundiced at birth, but develop progressive hyperbilirubinemia rapidly. Those who die have hepatosplenomegaly and bile-stained organs, erythroblastic hyperplasia in the bone marrow, and extramedullary hematopoiesis in the liver, spleen, lymph nodes, and other sites.
- **Kernicterus,** *also termed* **bilirubin encephalopathy,** *is defined as a neurologic condition associated with severe jaundice and characterized by bile staining of the brain, particularly of the basal ganglia, pontine nuclei, and dentate nuclei in the cerebellum.* Although brain damage in jaundiced newborns was first mentioned in the 15th century, the association of kernicterus with high levels of unconjugated bilirubin was not appreciated until 1952. Kernicterus (from the German, *kern,* nucleus) is essentially confined to newborns with severe unconjugated hyperbilirubinemia, usually related to erythroblastosis. The bilirubin derived from the destruction of erythrocytes and the catabolism of the released heme is not easily conjugated by the immature liver, which is deficient in glucuronyl transferase.

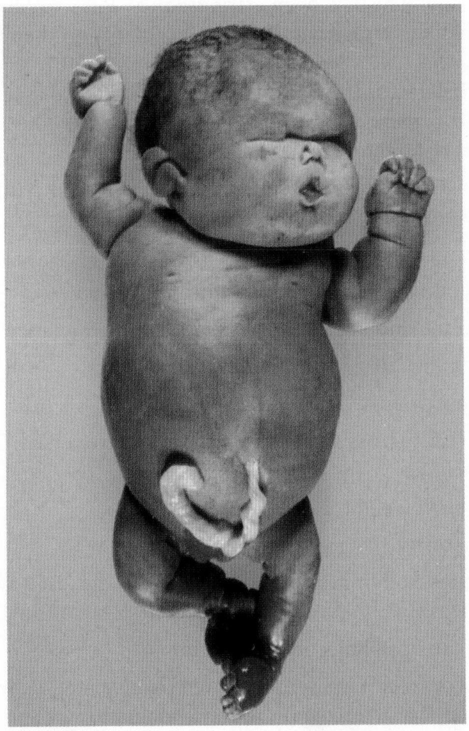

FIGURE 6-43. **Hydrops fetalis.** The infant shows severe anasarca.

The development of kernicterus is directly related to the level of unconjugated bilirubin and is rare in term infants when serum bilirubin levels are below 20 mg/dL. Premature infants are more vulnerable to hyperbilirubinemia and may develop kernicterus at levels as low as 12 mg/dL. Bilirubin is thought to injure the cells of the brain by interfering with mitochondrial function. Severe kernicterus leads initially to loss of the startle reflex and athetoid movements, which in 75% progresses to lethargy and death. Most surviving infants have severe choreoathetosis and mental retardation; a minority have varying degrees of intellectual and motor retardation.

PREVENTION AND TREATMENT: Exchange transfusions may keep the maximum serum bilirubin at an acceptable level. However, phototherapy, which converts the toxic unconjugated bilirubin into isomers that are nontoxic and excreted in the urine, has greatly reduced the need for exchange transfusions.

The incidence of erythroblastosis fetalis secondary to Rh incompatibility has been greatly reduced (to $<$1% of women at risk) by the use of human anti-D globulin (RhoGAM) within 72 hours of delivery. The quantity of RhoGAM administered to the mother suffices to neutralize 10 mL of antigenic fetal cells that may have entered the maternal circulation during delivery.

ABO Incompatibility

The availability of RhoGAM for Rh-negative mothers has drastically decreased the incidence of Rh-incompatible erythroblastosis. Today ABO incompatibility is the main cause of hemolytic disease of the newborn. Although 25% of pregnancies result in ABO incompatibility between mother and offspring, hemolytic disease develops in only 10% of such children, usually infants with blood type A. The low antigenicity of the ABO factors in the fetus accounts for the mildness of ABO hemolytic disease. Natural anti-A and anti-B antibodies are IgM, which does not cross the placenta. However, certain incomplete antibodies to A antigen may be IgG, which does cross the placenta, so ABO isoimmune disease may be seen in firstborn infants. However, most cases of hemolytic anemia from ABO incompatibility are seen after a previous incompatible pregnancy.

Most infants with ABO incompatibility have mild disease, jaundice being the only clinical feature. The complications of erythroblastosis associated with Rh incompatibility are unusual with ABO disease. Nevertheless, kernicterus has occasionally been reported.

Birth Injury Spans the Spectrum from Mechanical Trauma to Anoxic Damage

Some birth injuries relate to poor obstetric manipulation, whereas many are unavoidable sequelae of routine delivery. Birth injuries occur in about 5 per 1000 live births. Factors that predispose to birth injury include cephalopelvic disproportion, dystocia (difficult labor), prematurity, and breech presentation.

Cranial Injury

- **Caput succedaneum** refers to edema of the scalp caused by trauma to the head incurred during the passage through the birth canal. The swelling rapidly disappears and is more a source of parental anxiety than of clinical concern.
- **Cephalohematoma** is defined as a subperiosteal hemorrhage that is confined to a single cranial bone and becomes apparent within the first few hours after birth. It may or may not be associated with a linear fracture of the underlying bone.

Most cephalohematomas resolve without complication and require no treatment.

- **Skull fractures** during birth result from the impact of the head on the pelvic bones or pressure from obstetric forceps. Linear fractures, the most common variety, are asymptomatic and do not require any treatment. Depressed fractures are usually caused by trauma from forceps. Although many depressed fractures do not initially produce symptoms, they usually require mechanical elevation because of the risk of underlying cranial trauma from persistent pressure. In contrast to most fractures, those of the occipital bone often extend through the underlying venous sinuses and produce fatal hemorrhage.
- **Intracranial hemorrhage** is one of the most dangerous birth injuries and may be traumatic, secondary to asphyxia, or a result of an underlying bleeding diathesis. Traumatic intracranial hemorrhage occurs in the setting of (1) significant cephalopelvic disproportion, (2) precipitous delivery, (3) breech presentation, (4) prolonged labor, or (5) the inappropriate use of forceps. These traumas can result in **subdural or subarachnoid hemorrhage,** which are commonly secondary to lacerations of the falx cerebri or tentorium cerebelli that involve the vein of Galen or the venous sinuses. As noted above, anoxic injury from asphyxia, particularly in the premature infant, is often associated with intraventricular hemorrhage.

The prognosis for newborns with intracranial hemorrhage depends on its extent. Massive hemorrhage is often rapidly fatal. A surviving infant may recover completely or may have long-term impairment, usually in the form of cerebral palsy or hydrocephalus. However, many cases of cerebral palsy have been shown by ultrasound studies to relate to brain damage acquired 2 weeks or more prior to birth rather than from birth trauma.

Peripheral Nerve Injury

Brachial palsy, with varying degrees of paralysis of the upper extremity, is caused by excessive traction on the head and neck or shoulders during delivery. The injury may be permanent if the nerves are severed. Function may return within a few months if the palsy results from edema and hemorrhage.

Phrenic nerve paralysis and associated paralysis of a hemidiaphragm may be associated with brachial palsy and result in breathing difficulties. The condition generally resolves spontaneously within a few months.

Facial nerve palsy usually presents as a unilateral flaccid paralysis of the face caused by injury to the seventh cranial nerve during labor or delivery, especially with forceps. When severe, the entire affected side of the face is paralyzed and even the eyelid cannot be closed. The prognosis again depends on whether the nerve was lacerated or simply injured by pressure.

Fractures

The **clavicle** is more vulnerable to fracture during delivery than any other bone and may be associated with fracture of the **humerus.** Immobilization of the arm and shoulder usually provides for complete healing. Fractures of other long bones and the nose occasionally occur during birth but heal easily.

Rupture of the Liver

The only internal organ other than the brain that is injured with any frequency during labor and delivery is the liver. This organ is injured by mechanical pressure during difficult or premature births. Rupture of the liver may lead to the formation of a hematoma large enough to cause a palpable abdominal mass and anemia; surgical repair of the laceration may be required.

Sudden Infant Death Syndrome Does Not Have a Known Cause

The sudden infant death syndrome (SIDS), also known as "crib death," is defined as "the sudden death of an infant or young child which is unexpected by history and in which a thorough postmortem examination fails to demonstrate an adequate cause of death." Although the diagnosis of SIDS is arrived at solely by excluding other specific causes of sudden death, this catastrophe is nevertheless considered a distinct clinicopathologic entity. SIDS actually was first described in the American colonies in 1686, but modern attention to the disorder dates only a few decades.

Typically, the victim of SIDS is an apparently healthy young infant who has been asleep without any hint of impending calamity. Clinically, the infant does not awaken from an otherwise normal sleep period. Postmortem examination does not identify a cause of death, such as pneumonia, food aspiration, sepsis, or cerebral hemorrhage. This tragic sequence has aroused great public concern, because it must be separated from homicide, which has been demonstrated in a number of cases to be the true cause of mysterious death in children.

EPIDEMIOLOGY: After the neonatal period, SIDS is the leading cause of death in the first year of life, accounting for more than one third of all deaths in this period. Incidence in the United States is 2 per 1000 live births. Most (90%) cases occur before 6 months of age. Most deaths from SIDS are during the winter months, but no association between particular respiratory infections and infant death has been established. Most deaths occur at night or during periods associated with sleep. The reported death rates for SIDS have declined dramatically. This has been attributed to "Back to Sleep" campaigns that encourage parents to place infants on their backs for sleeping.

The risk factors for SIDS have been difficult to ascertain and are based principally on retrospective studies. The strongest **maternal risk factors** appear to be:

- Low socioeconomic status (poor education, unmarried mother, poor prenatal care)
- Black race
- Age younger than 20 years at first pregnancy
- Cigarette smoking during and following pregnancy
- Use of illicit drugs during pregnancy
- Increased parity

The risk factors for the infant are controversial. The consensus includes:

- Low birth weight
- Prematurity
- An illness, often gastrointestinal, within the last 2 weeks before death
- Subsequent siblings of SIDS victims
- Survivors of an apparent life-threatening event, defined as an episode characterized by some combination of apnea, color change, marked alteration in muscle tone, and choking or

gagging. A definite cause, such as seizures or aspiration after vomiting, is established in only half the cases of an apparent life-threatening event.

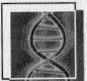

PATHOGENESIS: The pathogenesis of SIDS is elusive and controversial. No clear answers are available at this time. It is also unclear whether SIDS is a single entity or the common end-point of several different conditions. The most popular hypothesis relates SIDS to a prolonged spell of apnea, followed by cardiac arrhythmia or shock, in sleeping infants who cannot arouse themselves and prevent the process from progressing to a fatal outcome. However, fewer than 10% of parents of SIDS victims report episodes of apnea or an apparent life-threatening event at any time prior to the fatal event. *Thus, sleep apnea may contribute to the sequence of events leading to SIDS, but available data do not support a strong and predictable relationship between the two conditions.*

Numerous other causes for SIDS have found various champions, but the evidence for any one of these is indeed weak. They include cardiovascular abnormalities triggering fatal arrhythmias, abnormal brainstem sensitivity to respiratory stimuli, gastroesophageal reflux, various infections, inborn errors of metabolism, and bronchopulmonary dysplasia.

PATHOLOGY: At autopsy, several morphologic alterations are described in victims of SIDS, but their relevance to the etiology and pathogenesis of this disorder remains unclear. Chronic hypoxia brainstem gliosis, medial hypertrophy of small pulmonary arteries, persistence of extramedullary hematopoiesis in the liver, retention of periadrenal brown fat, and right ventricular hypertrophy may suggest a degree of chronic hypoxia. However, except for brainstem gliosis, none of these changes occurs with any regularity. Petechiae on the surfaces of the lungs, heart, pleura, and thymus, which have been reported in most infants dying of SIDS, are probably terminal events and have been attributed to negative intrathoracic pressure produced by respiratory efforts.

Neoplasms of Infancy and Childhood

Malignant tumors between the ages of 1 and 15 years are distinctly uncommon, but cancer remains the leading cause of death from disease in this age group. In children, 10% of all deaths are due to malignancies, and only accidental trauma kills a larger number. *Unlike adults, in whom most cancers are of epithelial origin (e.g., carcinomas of the lung, breast, and gastrointestinal tract), most malignant tumors in children arise from hematopoietic, nervous and soft tissues* (Fig. 6-44). Another feature that distinguishes childhood tumors from those of adults is the fact that many of the former are part of developmental complexes. Examples include Wilms tumor associated with aniridia, genitourinary malformations, and mental retardation (WAGR complex); hemihypertro-

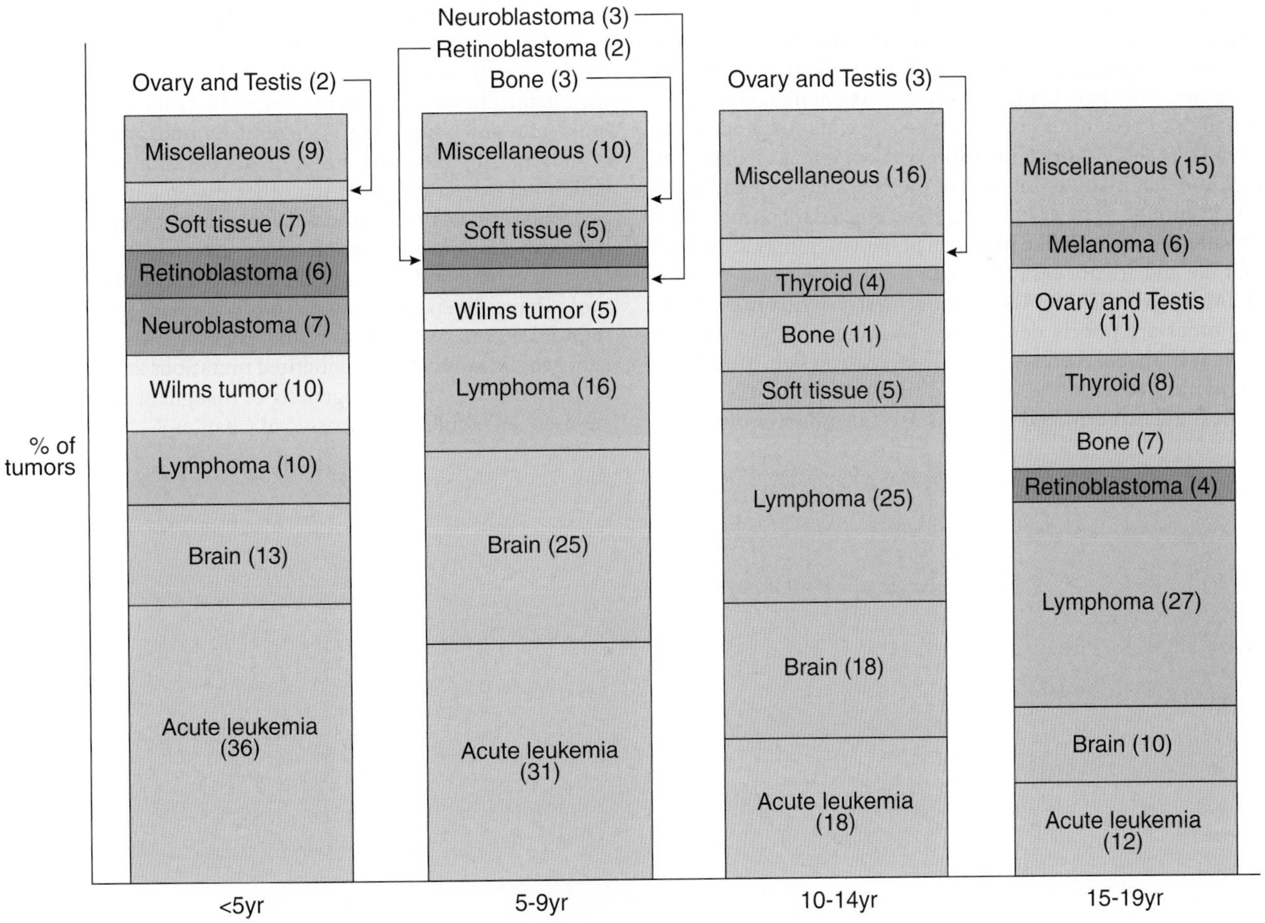

FIGURE 6-44. Distribution of childhood tumors according to age and primary site.

phy of the body associated with Wilms tumor, hepatoblastoma, and adrenal carcinoma; and tuberous sclerosis in association with renal tumors and rhabdomyomas of the heart. Some neoplasms are apparent at birth and are obviously developmental tumors that have evolved in utero. In addition, abnormally developed organs, persistent organ primordia, and displaced organ rests are all vulnerable to neoplastic transformation.

The individual cancers of childhood, including disorders such as the leukemias, neuroblastoma, Wilms tumor, various sarcomas, and germ cell neoplasms, are discussed in detail in the chapters dealing with the respective organs. The basic principles of neoplasia and carcinogenesis, including those applicable to pediatric cancers, are discussed in Chapter 5.

Benign Tumors and Tumorlike Conditions Encompass a Wide Range of Abnormalities

HAMARTOMAS: These lesions represent focal, benign overgrowths of one or more of the mature cellular elements of a normal tissue, often with one element predominating. Although the cells of a hamartoma are often arranged in a highly irregular fashion, the distinction between this developmental abnormality and a true benign neoplasm is often conjectural.

CHORISTOMAS: Also called **heterotopias,** choristomas are similar to hamartomas but are minute or microscopic aggregates of normal tissue components in aberrant locations. Choristomas are represented by rests of pancreatic tissue in the wall of the gastrointestinal tract or of adrenal tissue in the renal cortex.

HEMANGIOMAS: These lesions, of varying size and in diverse locations, are the most frequently encountered tumors in childhood. Whether hemangiomas are true neoplasms or hamartomas is unclear, although half are present at birth and most regress with age. Large, rapidly growing hemangiomas occasionally can be serious lesions, especially when they occur on the head or neck. A **port wine stain** is a congenital capillary hemangioma that involves the skin of the face and scalp and is often large enough to be disfiguring, imparting a dark purple color to the affected area. Unlike many small hemangiomas, they persist for life and are not easily treated.

LYMPHANGIOMAS: Also termed **cystic hygromas,** lymphangiomas are poorly demarcated swellings that are usually present at birth and thereafter rapidly increase in size. Most lymphangiomas occur on the head and neck, but the floor of the mouth, mediastinum, and buttocks are not uncommon sites. The classification of these tumors is imprecise; some researchers consider them developmental malformations or hamartomas and others call them neoplasms. Lymphangiomas appear as unilocular or multilocular cysts with thin, transparent walls and straw-colored fluid. Microscopically, myriad dilated lymphatic channels are separated by fibrous septa. Unlike hemangiomas, these lesions do not regress spontaneously and should be resected.

SACROCOCCYGEAL TERATOMAS: Although rare, these germ cell neoplasms are the most common solid tumors in the newborn, with an incidence of 1 in 40,000 live births. At least 75% of sacrococcygeal teratomas occur in girls, and a substantial number have been encountered in twins. The tumors are usually noticed at birth as a mass in the region of the sacrum and buttocks. They are commonly large, lobulated masses, often as large as the infant's head. One half of tumors grow externally and may be connected to the body by a small stalk. Some have both external and intrapelvic components, whereas a few grow entirely in the pelvis. Microscopically, sacrococcygeal teratomas are composed of numerous tissues, particularly of neural origin. Most (90%) sacrococcygeal teratomas detected before the age of 2 months are benign, but up to half of those diagnosed later in life are malignant. Associated congenital anomalies of the vertebrae, genitourinary system and anorectum are common. The lesion should be resected promptly.

Cancers in the Pediatric Age Group Are Uncommon

The incidence of childhood malignancies is 1.3 per 10,000 per year in children under the age of 15 years. The mortality clearly varies with the intrinsic behavior of the tumor and the response to therapy, but as an overall figure, the death rate for childhood cancer is only about one-third the incidence. Almost half of all malignant diseases in patients under 15 years of age are acute leukemias and lymphomas. Leukemias alone, particularly acute lymphoblastic leukemia, account for one third of all cases of childhood cancer. Most of the other malignant neoplasms are neuroblastomas, brain tumors, Wilms tumors, retinoblastomas, bone cancers, and various soft tissue sarcomas.

The genetic influences in the development of childhood tumors have been particularly well studied in the case of retinoblastoma, Wilms tumor and osteosarcoma. The issues relating to the interaction of inherited mutations and environmental influences in the pathogenesis of malignant tumors in both children and adults are discussed in Chapter 5.

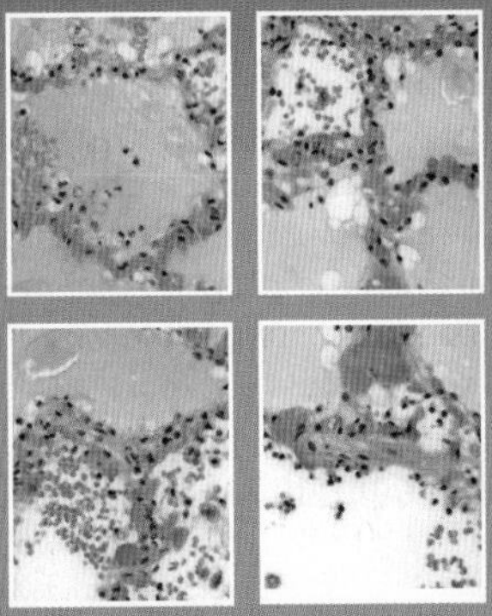

7 Hemodynamic Disorders

Bruce M. McManus
Michael F. Allard
Robert Yanagawa

Normal Circulation

Normal function and metabolism of organs and cells depends on an intact circulatory system for continuous delivery of oxygen, nutrients, hormones, electrolytes, and water, as well as for removal of metabolic waste and carbon dioxide. The circulatory system is a vascular conduit made of a muscular pump connected to tubes (or blood vessels) that deliver blood to organs and tissues and return it to the heart to complete the circuit. Delivery and elimination at the cellular level are controlled by exchanges between the intravascular space, interstitial space, cellular space, and lymphatic space, which occur via the smallest-diameter blood vessels in the body (the microcirculation).

The Heart Is a Two-Sided Pump With Vascular Circuits in Series

The amount of blood handled by the right ventricle-which pumps blood to the lungs (pulmonary circulation)–must, over time, exactly equal the amount of blood going through the left ventricle–which distributes blood to the body (systemic circulation). The hemodynamically important parameters are cardiac output, perfusion pressure, and peripheral vascular resistance.

- **Cardiac output** is the volume of blood pumped by each ventricle per minute and represents the total blood flow in pulmonary and systemic circuits. Cardiac output depends on heart rate and stroke volume, and, as the **cardiac index**, is often adjusted for body surface area (in square meters) as an indicator of ventricular function.
- **Perfusion pressure** (also called **driving pressure**) is the difference in dynamic pressure between two points along a blood vessel. Blood flow to any segment of the circulation ultimately depends on arterial driving pressure. However, each organ can autoregulate flow and so determine the amount of blood it receives from the circulation. Such local control of perfusion depends on continuous modulation of microvascular beds by hormonal, neural, metabolic, and hemodynamic factors.
- **Peripheral vascular resistance** refers to the sum of the factors that determine regional blood flow in each organ. Two-thirds of the resistance in the systemic vasculature is determined by the arterioles.

The sum of all regional flows equals the venous return, which in turn determines the cardiac output. Determination of the cardiac response to inflow (preload) and outflow (afterload) relies on cardiac reflexes as well as cardiac muscle integrity and neurohormonal regulation.

The Aorta and Arteries Are Conducting Vessels

The major functions of the aorta and arteries are transport of blood to the organs and conversion of pulsatile flow into sustained regular flow. The latter function derives from the elastic properties of the aorta and the resistance produced by the arteriolar sphincters.

The Microcirculation Includes Arterioles, Capillaries, and Venules

The blood vessels of the microcirculation are less than 100 μM in diameter. Blood from an arteriole enters the capillaries, which freely anastomose with each other (Fig. 7-1), either directly or through metarterioles. Capillary length, measured from terminal arteriole to collecting venule, ranges from 0.1 to 3 mm, averaging 1 mm. However, the path length by which blood cells traverse the capillaries may actually be longer because of their extensive anastomoses. This fact is likely an important factor with respect to microvascular exchange of substances such as oxygen because it will increase the time available for exchange to take place. The large aggregate surface area of capillaries determines that velocity of blood is low, which further enhances microvascular exchange. The density of capillaries in a tissue also influences microvascular exchange by affecting the diffusion distance. For example, in tissues with high oxygen demands, such as the heart, capillary density is very high. Entry into the capillary system is guarded by precapillary sphincters, except for **thoroughfare channels**, which bypass capillaries and are always open. Since not all capillaries are always open, blood flow can be increased by recruiting additional capillaries. The sum of blood flow through the capillary bed, the thoroughfare channels, and the arteriovenous anastomoses determines the regional blood flow.

The exact means by which an organ regulates blood flow according to its metabolic needs are still debated, but there is a link between oxygen demand and blood flow. In the heart, blood flow is adjusted on a second-to-second basis. Factors that mediate and link metabolic vasodilation to cellular metabolism include adenosine, other nucleotides, nitric oxide, certain prostaglandins, carbon dioxide, and pH. The microcirculation is an important contributor to all forms of hyperemia and edema, and is a target in septic shock (see below). Vasoregulation in conducting arteries, resistance arteries, and veins relies on delicate interactions between blood, endothelium, smooth muscle cells, and surrounding stroma.

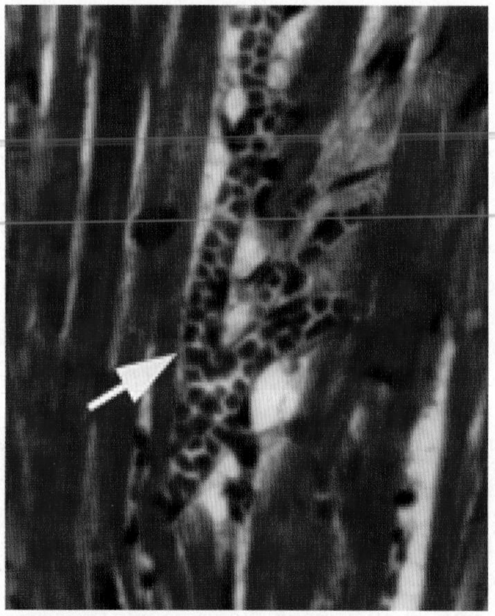

FIGURE 7-1. **Microcirculation.** Photomicrographs of myocardium show anastomosing capillaries *(arrow)*.

The Normal Endothelium Provides a Continuous Partition between Blood and Tissues

Endothelial cells play important roles in anticoagulation, facilitation of migration of substances from blood to tissue and back, regulation of vessel tone (particularly that of resistance arteries), and regulation of vasopermeability (also see Chapters 2 and 10).

Veins and Venules Return Blood to the Heart

Blood from the capillaries enters venules and eventually veins on its route back to the heart. Veins not only serve as a conduits for blood, but also act as a blood reservoir; 64% of the total blood volume resides in the venous system.

The Interstitium Represents 15% of Total Body Volume

The interstitial fluid between cells provides a means for the delivery of nutrients and the elimination of waste. Most of the interstitial water is bound to a dense network of glycosaminoglycans.

Lymphatics Reabsorb Interstitial Fluid

Interstitial fluid is reabsorbed into the circulation at the venous end of the capillary, and a small portion is drained through lymphatics. Lymphatic capillaries conduct lymph from the periphery to the central venous system via the thoracic duct. Normal oscillatory constrictions and relaxations of lymphatic vessels contribute to steady return of lymph fluid to the central circulation. Lymph is a solvent for large molecules that cannot return to the circulation through blood capillaries.

Disorders of Perfusion

Hemodynamic disorders are characterized by disturbed perfusion that may result in organ and cellular injury.

Hyperemia Is an Excess of Blood in an Organ

Hyperemia may be caused either by an increased supply of blood from the arterial system (**active hyperemia**) or by impaired exit of blood through venous pathways (**passive hyperemia** or **congestion**).

Active Hyperemia

Active hyperemia is augmented supply of blood to an organ. It is usually a physiologic response to increased functional demand, as in the heart and skeletal muscle during exercise. Neurogenic and hormonal influences play a role in active hyperemia, e.g., the blushing bride and the menopausal flush. Although the utility of vasodilation in these examples is not clear, cutaneous hyperemia in febrile states serves to dissipate heat. In addition, skeletal muscle may increase its blood flow (and thus oxygen delivery) 20-fold during exercise. The increased blood supply occurs by arteriolar dilation and recruitment of unperfused capillaries.

The most striking active hyperemia occurs in association with inflammation. Vasoactive materials released by inflammatory cells (see Chapter 2) cause dilation of blood vessels; in the skin this contributes to classic "tumor, rubor, and calor" of inflammation. In pneumonia, for example, alveolar capillaries are engorged with erythrocytes as a hyperemic response to inflammation. Because inflammation can also damage endothelial cells and increase capillary permeability, inflammatory hyperemia is often accompanied by edema and local extravasation of erythrocytes.

Reactive hyperemia occurs after temporary interruption of blood supply (ischemia). The release of the obstruction is followed by active hyperemia, probably due to ischemic tissue injury and release of inflammatory agents such as histamine. The degree and duration of hyperemia is proportional to the period of occlusion until a plateau of hyperemic response is reached.

Passive Hyperemia (Congestion)

Passive hyperemia, or congestion, is engorgement of an organ with venous blood. Acute passive congestion is clinically a consequence of acute left or right ventricular failure. Regarding the former, resultant venous engorgement of the lung leads to accumulation of a transudate in the alveoli, a condition termed **pulmonary edema**. With acute failure of the right ventricle, the liver can become severely congested.

A generalized increase in venous pressure, typically from chronic heart failure, results in slower blood flow and consequent increase in blood volume in many organs, including liver, spleen, and kidneys. In the past, heart failure from rheumatic mitral stenosis was a common cause of generalized venous congestion, but with the decline in the prevalence of rheumatic fever and the advent of surgical valve replacement, such cases are unusual. Congestive heart failure secondary to coronary artery disease and hypertension, and right-sided failure due to pulmonary disease is now more common.

Passive congestion may also be confined to a limb or an organ as a result of more-localized obstruction to venous drainage. Examples include deep venous thrombosis of the leg veins, with resulting edema of the lower extremity and thrombosis of hepatic veins (Budd-Chiari syndrome) with secondary chronic passive congestion of the liver.

LUNGS: Chronic left ventricle failure impedes blood flow out of the lungs, and leads to chronic passive pulmonary congestion. As a result, pressure in the alveolar capillaries increases and these vessels become engorged with blood. Increased pressure in the alveolar capillaries has four major consequences:

- Microhemorrhages release erythrocytes into alveolar spaces, where they are phagocytosed and degraded by alveolar macrophages. The released iron, in the form of hemosiderin, remains in the macrophages, which are then called "heart failure cells" (Fig. 7-2).
- Fluid is forced from the blood into the alveolar spaces, resulting in pulmonary edema (Fig. 7-3), which interferes with gas exchange in the lung.
- Fibrosis increases in the interstitium of the lung. The presence of fibrosis and iron is viewed grossly as a firm, brown lung (**brown induration**).
- **Pulmonary hypertension** occurs when the pressure is transmitted to the pulmonary arterial system. This may lead to right-sided heart failure and consequent generalized systemic venous congestion.

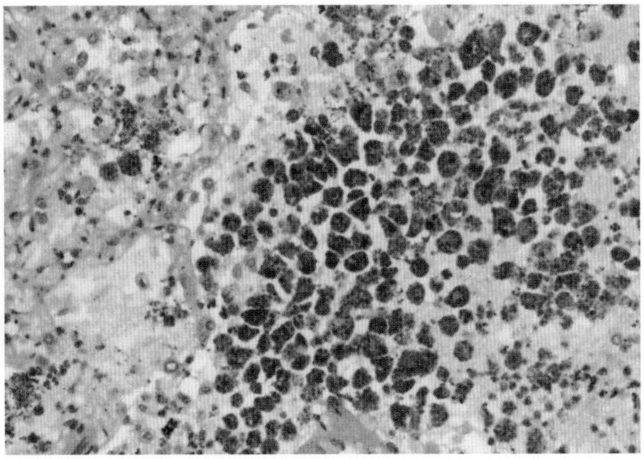

FIGURE 7-2. **Passive congestion of lung.** Hemosiderin-laden macrophages in the lung of a patient with congestive heart failure.

In Chapter 12 the morphologic changes associated with chronic passive congestion of the lungs are discussed.

LIVER: The hepatic veins empty into the vena cava immediately inferior to the heart, so the liver is particularly vulnerable to acute or chronic passive congestion (see Chapter 14). The central veins of hepatic lobules become dilated. The increased venous pressure is transmitted to the sinusoids, which dilate, and centrilobular hepatocytes undergo pressure atrophy (Fig. 7-4). Grossly, the cut surface of the chronically congested liver exhibits dark foci of centrilobular congestion surrounded by paler zones of unaffected peripheral portions of the lobules. The result is a reticulated appearance that resembles a cross-section of a nutmeg ("nutmeg liver") (see Fig. 7-4). In extreme cases associated with acute right ventricular failure, frank hemorrhagic necrosis of hepatocytes in the centrilobular zones is conspicuous. Prolonged hepatic venous congestion eventually leads to thickening of central veins and centrilobular fibrosis. Only in the most extreme cases of venous congestion (e.g., constrictive pericarditis or tricuspid stenosis) is the fibrosis sufficiently generalized and severe to justify the label **cardiac cirrhosis**.

SPLEEN: Increased intravascular pressure in the liver, from cardiac failure or an intrahepatic obstruction to blood flow (e.g., cirrhosis), leads to higher pressure in the splenic vein, and congestion of the spleen. The organ becomes enlarged and tense,

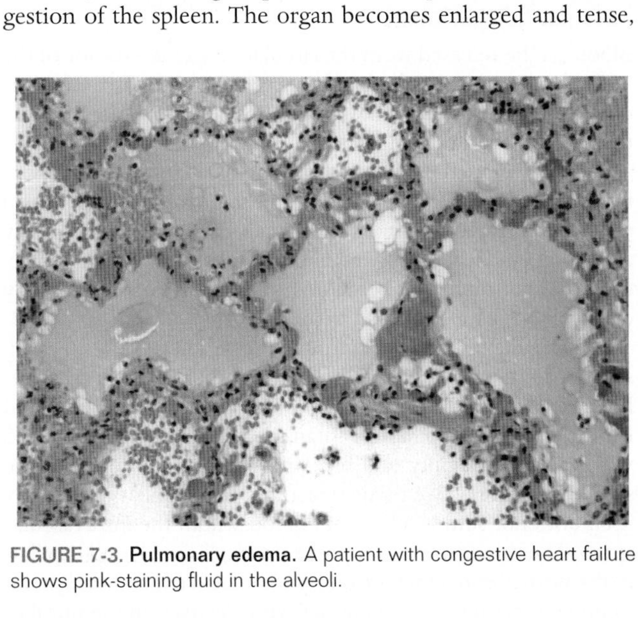

FIGURE 7-3. **Pulmonary edema.** A patient with congestive heart failure shows pink-staining fluid in the alveoli.

A

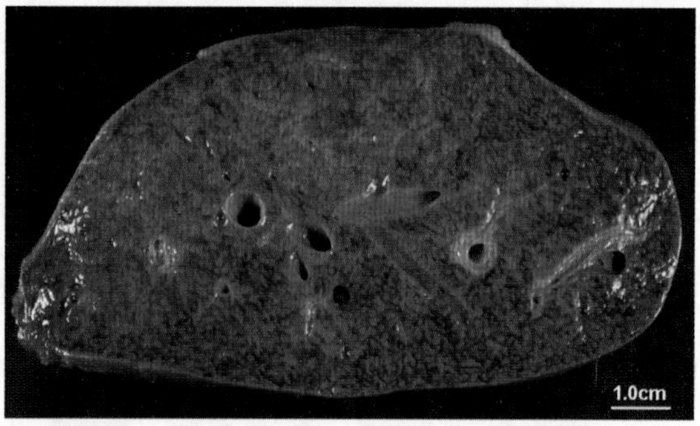

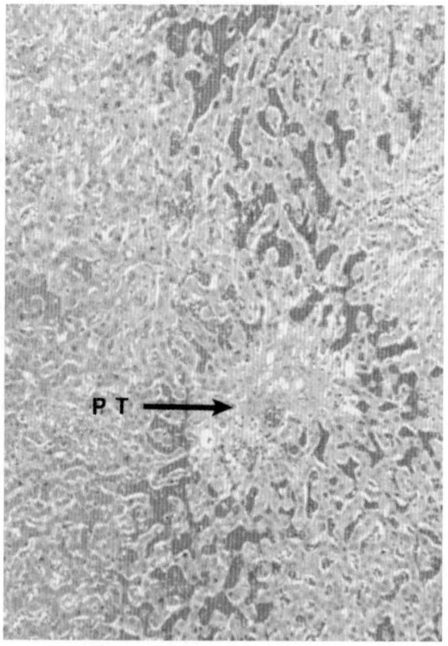

B

FIGURE 7-4. **Passive congestion of liver. A.** A gross photograph of liver shows nutmeg appearance, reflecting congestive failure of the right ventricle. **B.** A photomicrograph of liver shows centrilobular sinusoids dilated with blood. The intervening plates of hepatocytes exhibit pressure atrophy. *PT*, portal tract.

and the cut section oozes dark blood. In long-standing congestion, diffuse splenic fibrosis develops, as do iron-containing, fibrotic, and calcified foci of old hemorrhage (Gamna-Gandy bodies). Such a spleen may weigh 250 to 750 g, compared with a normal weight of 150 g. The enlarged spleen sometimes displays excessive functional activity—termed **hypersplenism**—which leads to hematologic abnormalities (e.g., thrombocytopenia).

EDEMA AND ASCITES: Venous congestion impedes blood flow through the capillaries, thereby increasing hydrostatic pressure and promoting edema formation (see below for a discussion of the mechanisms of edema formation). Accumulation of edema fluid in heart failure is particularly noticeable in dependent tissues—the legs and feet in ambulatory patients and the back in bedridden persons. **Ascites** is accumulation of fluid in the peritoneal space and reflects (among other factors) lack of tissue rigor, a condition in which there is no countervailing external pressure to oppose hydrostatic pressure within the blood vessels.

Hemorrhage Is a Discharge of Blood out of the Vascular Compartment

Blood can be released from the circulation to the exterior of the body or into nonvascular body spaces. The most common and obvious cause is trauma. Severe atherosclerosis may so weaken the wall of the abdominal aorta that it balloons to form an aneurysm, which then may rupture and bleed into the retroperitoneal space (see Chapter 10). In the same way, an aneurysm may complicate a congenitally weak cerebral artery (berry aneurysm) and lead to subarachnoid hemorrhage. Certain infections (e.g., pulmonary tuberculosis) and invasive neoplasms may erode blood vessels and lead to hemorrhage.

Hemorrhage also results from damage to capillaries. For instance, rupture of capillaries by blunt trauma leads to a bruise. Increased venous pressure also causes extravasation of blood from pulmonary capillaries. Vitamin C deficiency is associated with capillary fragility and bleeding, owing to a defect in the supporting connective tissue structures. The capillary barrier by itself does not suffice to contain blood within the intravascular space. The minor trauma imposed on small vessels and capillaries by normal movement requires an intact coagulation system to prevent hemorrhage. Thus, a severe decrease in the number of platelets (thrombocytopenia) or deficiency of a coagulation factor (e.g., factor VIII in hemophilia A) is associated with spontaneous hemorrhage without apparent trauma (see Chapter 10).

A person may exsanguinate into an internal cavity, as in gastrointestinal hemorrhage from a peptic ulcer (arterial hemorrhage) or esophageal varices (venous hemorrhage). In such cases, large amounts of fresh blood fill the entire gastrointestinal tract. Bleeding into a serous cavity can result in accumulation of a large amount of blood, even to the point of exsanguination.

A few definitions are in order:

- **Hematoma:** Hemorrhage into soft tissue. Such collections of blood can be merely painful, as in a muscle bruise, or fatal, if located in the brain.
- **Hemothorax:** Hemorrhage into the pleural cavity.
- **Hemopericardium:** Hemorrhage into the pericardial space.
- **Hemoperitoneum:** Bleeding into the peritoneal cavity.
- **Hemarthrosis:** Bleeding into a joint space.
- **Purpura:** Diffuse superficial hemorrhages in the skin, up to 1 cm in diameter.
- **Ecchymosis:** A larger superficial hemorrhage in the skin (Fig. 7-5). The initially purple discoloration turns green and

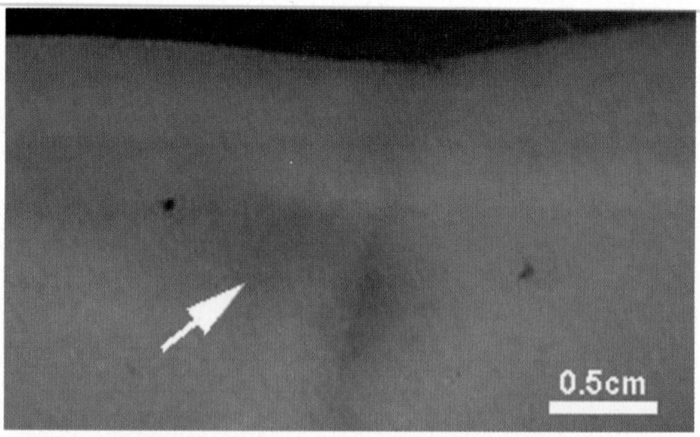

FIGURE 7-5. **Ecchymosis.** Superficial diffuse hemorrhage *(arrow)* in a forearm caused by a needle puncture.

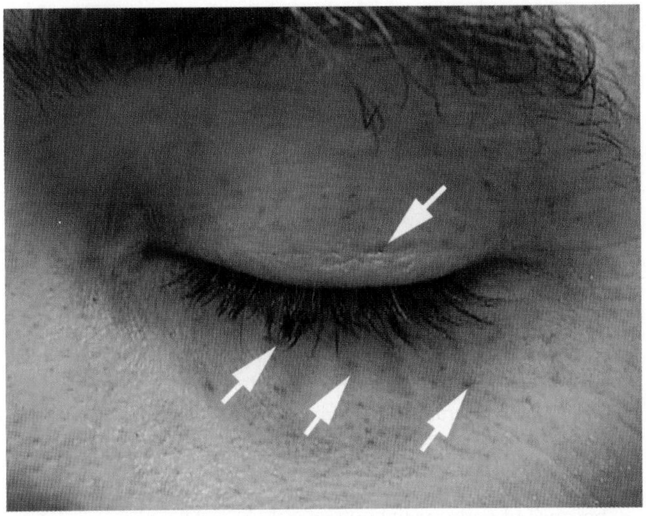

FIGURE 7-6. **Petechiae.** Periorbital microhemorrhages *(arrows)* appear as punctate red foci.

then yellow before resolving. This sequence of events reflects progressive oxidation of bilirubin released from the hemoglobin of degraded erythrocytes. A good example of an ecchymosis is a "black eye."

- **Petechiae:** Pinpoint hemorrhages, usually in the skin or conjunctiva (Fig. 7-6). This lesion represents the rupture of a capillary or arteriole and occurs in conjunction with coagulopathies or vasculitis. Petechiae may also be produced by microemboli from infected heart valves (bacterial endocarditis).

Thrombosis

Thrombosis refers to the formation of a thrombus, defined as an aggregate of coagulated blood containing platelets, fibrin, and entrapped cellular elements, within a vascular lumen. A **thrombus** by definition adheres to vascular endothelium and should be distinguished from a simple blood clot, which reflects only activation of the coagulation cascade and can form in vitro or even postmortem. Similarly, a thrombus differs from a hematoma, which results from hemorrhage and subsequent clotting outside the vascular system. Thrombus formation and the coagulation cascade are discussed in more detail in Chapters 10 and 20. Here we present the causes and consequences of thrombosis in different sites.

Thrombosis in the Arterial System Is Usually Due to Atherosclerosis

PATHOGENESIS: The vessels most commonly involved in arterial thrombosis are coronary, cerebral, mesenteric, and renal arteries, and arteries of the lower extremities. Less commonly, arterial thrombosis occurs in other disorders, including inflammation of arteries (arteritis), trauma, and blood diseases. Thrombi are common in aneurysms (localized dilations of the lumen) of the aorta and its major branches, in which the distortion of blood flow, combined with intrinsic vascular disease, promotes thrombosis.

A major risk factor for thrombosis is immobilization after surgery or after leg casting. Other risk factors include obesity, advanced age, previous thrombosis, and cancer. The pathogenesis of arterial thrombosis involves principally three factors:

- **Damage to endothelium,** usually by atherosclerosis, disturbs the anticoagulant properties of the vessel wall and serves as a nidus for platelet aggregation and fibrin formation.
- **Alterations in blood flow,** whether from turbulence in an aneurysm or at sites of arterial bifurcation is conducive to thrombosis. Slowing of blood flow in narrowed arteries favors thrombosis.
- **Increased coagulability of the blood,** as seen in polycythemia vera or in association with some cancers, leads to an increased risk of thrombosis.

PATHOLOGY: An arterial thrombus attached to a vessel wall is initially soft, friable, and dark red, with fine alternating bands of yellowish platelets and fibrin, the lines of Zahn (Fig. 7-7). Once formed, arterial thrombi have several possible outcomes.

- **Lysis,** owing to the potent thrombolytic activity of the blood.
- **Propagation** (i.e., an increase in its size), because a thrombus serves as a focus for further thrombosis.
- **Organization**, the eventual invasion of connective tissue elements, which causes a thrombus to become firm and grayish white.
- **Canalization**, by which new lumina lined by endothelial cells form in an organized thrombus (Fig. 7-8). The functional significance of this change is often questionable.
- **Embolization**, when part or all of the thrombus becomes dislodged, travels through the circulation, and lodges in a blood vessel some distance from the site of thrombus formation (see below for further discussion).

The organized structure of a thrombus reflects a tight interaction between platelets and fibrin and differs in appearance from a postmortem clot or one formed in a test tube. Determination of

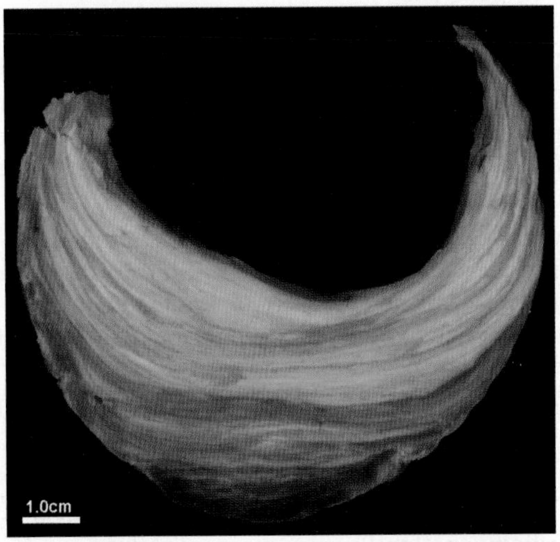

FIGURE 7-7. **Arterial thrombus.** Gross photograph of a thrombus from an aortic aneurysm shows the laminations of fibrin and platelets known as the lines of Zahn.

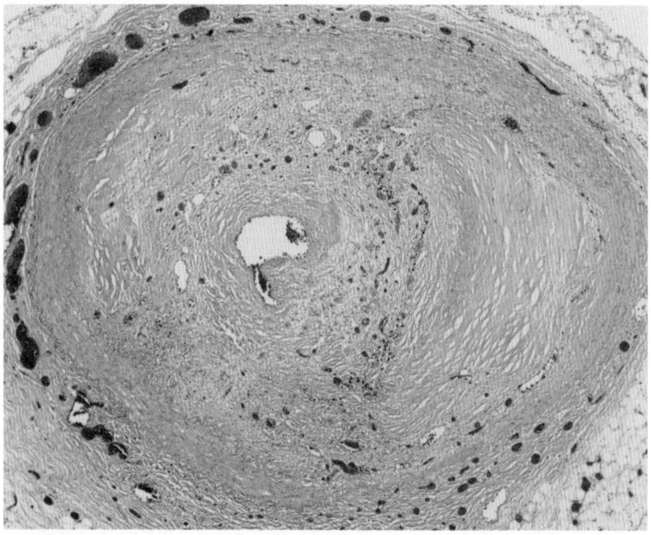

FIGURE 7-8. **Canalization of thrombus.** Photomicrograph of the left anterior descending coronary artery shows severe atherosclerosis and canalization.

whether or not a clot formed during life (antemortem clot) or after death (postmortem clot) is often important in a medical autopsy and in forensic pathology. Lines of Zahn stabilize a thrombus formed during life, while a postmortem clot has a more gelatinous structure. Postmortem clots occur in stagnant blood in which gravity fractionates the blood. The part of the clot containing many red blood cells has a reddish, gelatinous appearance, and is referred to as "currant jelly." The overlying clot is firmer and yellow-white, representing coagulated plasma without red blood cells. It is called "chicken fat" because of its color and consistency.

CLINICAL FEATURES: *Arterial thrombosis due to atherosclerosis is the most common cause of death in Western industrialized countries.* Since most arterial thrombi occlude the vessel, they often lead to ischemic necrosis of tissue supplied by that artery (i.e., an **infarct**). Thus, thrombosis of a coronary or cerebral artery results in **myocardial infarct** (heart attack) or **cerebral infarct** (stroke), respectively. Other end-arteries that are affected by atherosclerosis and often suffer thrombosis include mesenteric arteries (intestinal infarction), renal arteries (kidney infarcts), and arteries of the leg (gangrene).

Thrombosis in the Heart Develops on the Endocardium

As in the arterial system, endocardial injury and changes in blood flow in the heart may lead to mural thrombosis, i.e., a thrombus adhering to the underlying wall of the heart. The disorders in which mural thrombosis occurs include:

- **Myocardial infarction:** Adherent mural thrombi form in the left ventricular cavity over areas of myocardial infarction, owing to damaged endocardium and alterations in blood flow associated with a poorly functional or adynamic segment of the myocardium.
- **Atrial fibrillation:** Disordered atrial rhythm (atrial fibrillation) leads to slower blood flow and impaired left atrial contractility a situation that predisposes to formation of mural thrombi in atria.
- **Cardiomyopathy:** Primary myocardial diseases are associated with mural thrombi in the left ventricle, presumably because of endocardial injury and altered hemodynamics associated with poor myocardial contractility.
- **Endocarditis:** Small thrombi, **vegetations,** may also develop on cardiac valves, usually mitral or aortic, that are damaged by a bacterial infection (bacterial endocarditis) (Fig. 7-9). Occasionally, vegetations form in the absence of valve infection, on a mitral or tricuspid valve injured by systemic lupus erythematosus (Libman-Sacks endocarditis). In chronic wasting states, as in terminal cancer, large, friable vegetations may appear on cardiac valves (marantic endocarditis), possibly reflecting a hypercoagulable state.

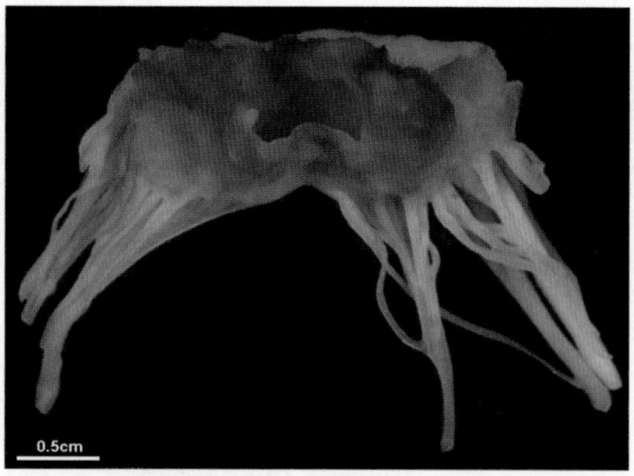

FIGURE 7-9. **Endocarditis.** The anterior leaflet of the mitral valve is damaged by a friable bacterial vegetation.

The major complication of thrombi in any location in the heart is detachment of fragments and their lodging in blood vessels at distant sites (**embolization**).

Thrombosis in the Venous System Is Multifactorial

At one time, venous thrombosis was widely referred to as **thrombophlebitis**, implying that an inflammatory or infectious process had injured the vein, thereby causing thrombosis. However, with recognition that there is no evidence of inflammation in most cases, the term **phlebothrombosis** is more accurate. Nevertheless, both terms have been replaced for the most part by the expression **deep venous thrombosis**. This last term is particularly appropriate for the most common manifestation of the disorder, namely, thrombosis of the deep venous system of the legs.

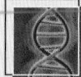

PATHOGENESIS: Deep venous thrombosis is caused by the same factors that favor arterial and cardiac thrombosis—endothelial injury, stasis, and a hypercoagulable state. Conditions that favor the development of deep venous thrombosis include:

- **Stasis** (heart failure, chronic venous insufficiency, postoperative immobilization, prolonged bed rest)
- **Injury** (trauma, surgery, childbirth)
- **Hypercoagulability** (oral contraceptives, late pregnancy, cancer, inherited thrombophilic disorders (see Chapter 20))
- **Advanced age** (venous varicosities, phlebosclerosis)
- **Sickle cell disease** (see Chapter 20)

PATHOLOGY: Most (>90%) venous thromboses occur in deep veins of the legs; the rest usually involve pelvic veins. Most venous thrombi begin in the calf veins, frequently in the sinuses above the venous valves. In this location, venous thrombi have several potential fates:

- **Lysis:** They may remain small and are eventually lysed, posing no further threat to health.
- **Organization:** Many undergo organization similar to those of arterial origin. Small, organized venous thrombi may be incorporated into the vessel wall; larger ones may undergo canalization, with partial restoration of venous drainage.
- **Propagation:** Venous thrombi often serve as a nidus for further thrombosis and thereby propagate proximally to involve the larger iliofemoral veins (Fig. 7-10).
- **Embolization:** Large venous thrombi or those that have propagated proximally represent a significant hazard to life, since they may dislodge and be carried to the lungs as pulmonary emboli.

CLINICAL FEATURES: Small thrombi in the calf veins are ordinarily asymptomatic, and even larger thrombi in the iliofemoral system may cause no symptoms. Some patients have calf tenderness, often associated with forced dorsiflexion of the foot (**Homan sign**). Occlusive thrombosis of femoral or iliac veins leads to severe congestion, edema, and cyanosis of the lower extremity. Symptomatic deep venous thrombosis is treated with systemic anticoagulants, and thrombolytic therapy may be useful in selected cases. In some cases, a filter is inserted into the vena cava to prevent pulmonary embolization.

The function of venous valves is always impaired in a vein subjected to thrombosis and organization. As a result, chronic deep venous insufficiency (i.e., impaired venous drainage) is virtually inevitable. If a lesion is restricted to a small segment of the deep venous system, the condition may remain asymptomatic. However, more extensive involvement leads to pigmentation, edema, and induration of leg skin. Ulceration above the medial malleolus can occur and is often difficult to treat.

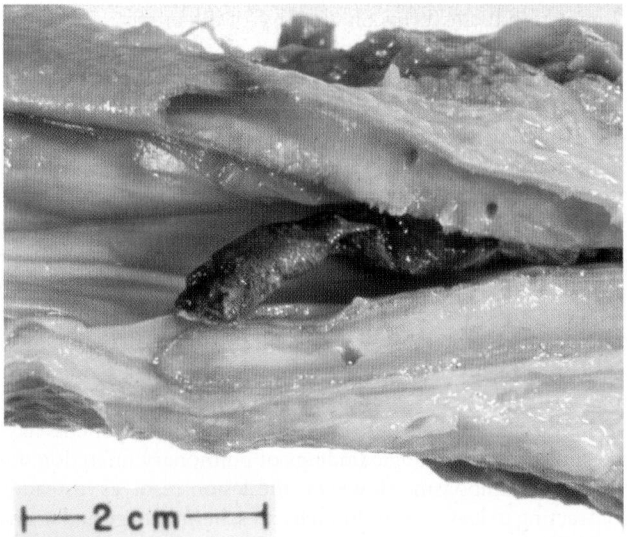

FIGURE 7-10. **Venous thrombosis.** The femoral vein has been opened to reveal a large thrombus within the lumen.

Venous thrombi elsewhere may also be dangerous. Thrombosis of mesenteric veins can cause hemorrhagic small bowel infarction; thrombosis of cerebral veins may be fatal; hepatic vein thrombosis (Budd-Chiari syndrome) may destroy the liver.

Inherited disorders of blood clotting may lead to susceptibility to these types of events. These diseases are covered in detail in Chapter 20.

Embolism

Embolism is passage through venous or arterial circulations of any material that can lodge in a blood vessel and obstruct its lumen. The most common embolus is a thromboembolus—that is, a thrombus formed in one location that detaches from a vessel wall at its point of origin and travels to a distant site.

Pulmonary Arterial Embolism Is Potentially Fatal

Pulmonary embolism is an important diagnostic and therapeutic challenge. In fact, pulmonary thromboemboli are reported in more than half of all autopsies. Furthermore, this complication occurs in 1% to 2% of postoperative patients over the age of 40. The risk after surgery increases with advancing age, obesity, length of operative procedure, postoperative infection, cancer, and preexisting venous disease.

Most pulmonary emboli (90%) arise from deep veins of the lower extremities; most fatal ones form in iliofemoral veins (Fig. 7-11). Only half of patients with pulmonary thromboembolism have signs of deep vein thrombosis. Some thromboemboli arise from the pelvic venous plexus and others from the right side of the heart. Emboli are also derived from thrombi around indwelling lines in the systemic venous system or pulmonary artery. The upper extremities are a rare source of thromboemboli.

The clinical features of pulmonary embolism are determined by the size of the embolus, the health of the patient, and whether embolization occurs acutely or chronically. Acute pulmonary embolism is divided into the following syndromes:

- Asymptomatic small pulmonary emboli
- Transient dyspnea and tachypnea without other symptoms
- Pulmonary infarction, with pleuritic chest pain, hemoptysis, and pleural effusion
- Cardiovascular collapse with sudden death

Chronic pulmonary embolism, with numerous (usually asymptomatic) emboli lodged in small arteries of the lung, can lead to pulmonary hypertension and right-sided heart failure (see below).

Massive Pulmonary Embolism

One of the most dramatic calamities complicating hospitalization is the sudden collapse and death of a patient who appeared to be well on the way to an uneventful recovery. The cause of this catastrophe is often massive pulmonary embolism due to release of a large deep venous thrombus from a lower extremity. Classically, a postoperative patient succumbs upon getting out of bed for the first time. The muscular activity dislodges a thrombus that formed as a result of the stasis from prolonged bed rest. Excluding deaths related to surgery itself, pulmonary embolism is the most common cause of death after major orthopedic surgery and is the most frequent nonobstetric cause of postpartum death. It also is an especially common cause of death in patients who suffer from chronic heart and lung diseases and in

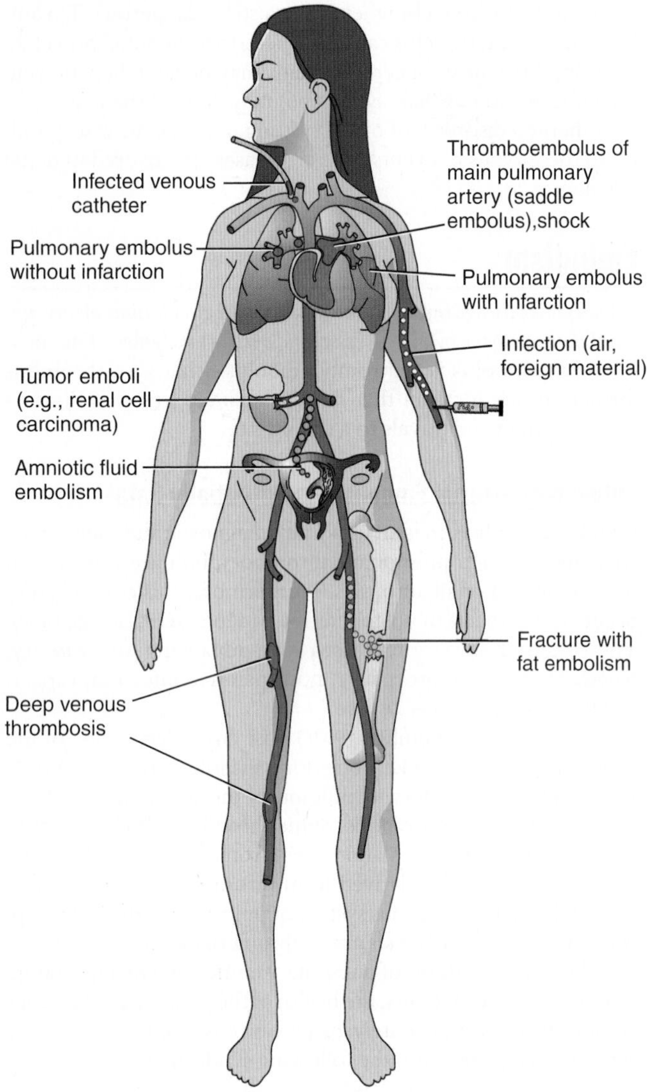

FIGURE 7-11. **Sources and effects of venous emboli.**

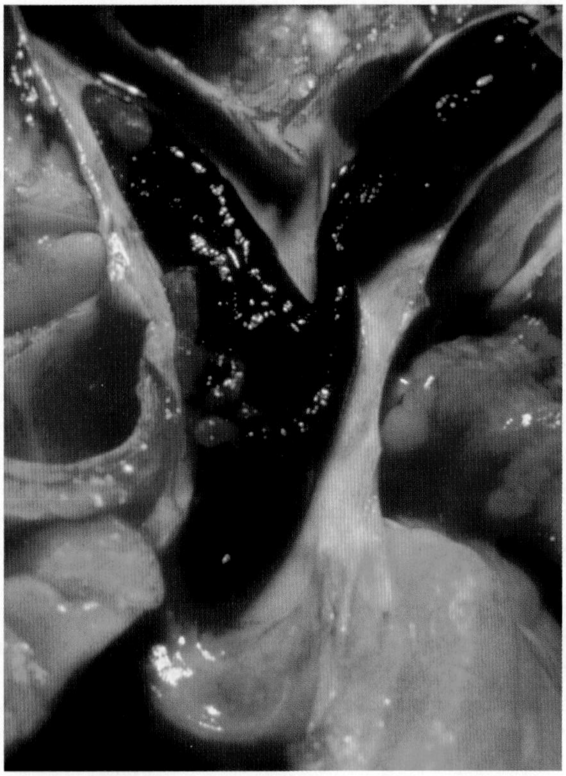

FIGURE 7-12. **Pulmonary embolism.** The main pulmonary artery and its bifurcation have been opened to reveal a large saddle embolus.

those who are subjected to prolonged immobilization for any reason. Prolonged immobilization associated with air travel can also lead to venous thrombosis and, occasionally, sudden death from a pulmonary embolus.

A large pulmonary embolus may lodge at the bifurcation of the main pulmonary artery (**saddle embolus**), obstructing blood flow to both lungs (Fig. 7-12). Large lethal emboli may also be found in the first branching of the right or left pulmonary arteries. Multiple smaller emboli may lodge in secondary branches and prove fatal. With acute obstruction of more than half of the pulmonary arterial tree, the patient often experiences immediate severe hypotension (or shock) and may die within minutes.

The hemodynamic consequences of such massive pulmonary embolism are acute right ventricular failure from sudden obstruction of outflow and pronounced reduction in left ventricular cardiac output, secondary to the loss of right ventricular function. The low cardiac output is responsible for the sudden appearance of severe hypotension.

Pulmonary Infarction

Small pulmonary emboli are not ordinarily lethal. They tend to lodge in peripheral pulmonary arteries. Sometimes (15%–20% of all pulmonary emboli) they produce lung infarcts. Clinically, pulmonary infarction is usually seen in the context of congestive heart failure or chronic lung disease, because the normal dual circulation of the lung ordinarily protects against ischemic necrosis; since the bronchial artery pumps blood into the necrotic area, pulmonary infarcts are typically hemorrhagic. They tend to be pyramidal, with the base of the pyramid on the pleural surface. Patients experience cough, stabbing pleuritic pain, shortness of breath, and occasional hemoptysis. Pleural effusion is common and often bloody. With time, the blood in the infarct is resorbed, and the center of the infarct becomes pale. Granulation tissue forms on the edge of the infarct, after which it is organized to form a fibrous scar.

Pulmonary Embolism without Infarction

Since the lung is supplied by both the bronchial arteries and the pulmonary artery, most (75%) small pulmonary emboli do not produce infarcts. Although most small emboli do not attract clinical attention, a few lead to a syndrome characterized by dyspnea, cough, chest pain, and hypotension. Rarely (3%), recurrent pulmonary emboli cause pulmonary hypertension by mechanical blockage of the arterial bed. In this circumstance, reflex vasoconstriction and bronchial constriction, owing to release of vasoactive substances, may contribute to a reduction in size of the functional pulmonary vascular bed.

In the clinical syndrome of "partial infarction," patients have the clinical and radiologic findings of pulmonary infarction due to thromboembolism. However, the lesion resolves instead of contracting to leave a scar. In such cases, hemorrhage and necrosis of the lung tissue in the affected area occur, but the tissue framework remains. Collateral circulation maintains tissue viability and enables its regeneration.

Fate of Pulmonary Thromboemboli

Small pulmonary emboli may completely resolve, depending on (1) the embolic load, (2) the adequacy of the pulmonary vascular reserve, (3) the state of the bronchial collateral circulation, and (4) the thrombolytic process. Alternatively, thromboemboli may become organized and leave strings of fibrous tissue attached to a vessel wall in the lumen of pulmonary arteries. Radiologic studies have indicated that half of all pulmonary thromboemboli are resorbed and organized within 8 weeks, with little narrowing of the vessels.

Paradoxical Embolism

Paradoxical embolism refers to emboli that arise in the venous circulation and bypass the lungs by traveling through an incompletely closed foramen ovale, subsequently entering the left side of the heart and blocking flow to the systemic arteries. Since left atrial pressure usually exceeds that in the right, most of these cases occur in the context of a right-to-left shunt (see Chapter 11).

Systemic Arterial Embolism Often Causes Infarcts

Thromboembolism

The heart is the most common source of arterial thromboemboli (Fig. 7-13), which usually arise from mural thrombi (Fig. 7-14) or diseased valves. These emboli tend to lodge at points where the vessel lumen narrows abruptly (e.g., at bifurcations or in the area of an atherosclerotic plaque). The viability of tissue supplied by the vessel depends on the availability of collateral circulation and on the fate of the embolus itself. The thromboembolus may propagate locally and lead to a more severe obstruction or it may fragment and lyse. Organs that suffer the most from arterial thromboembolism include:

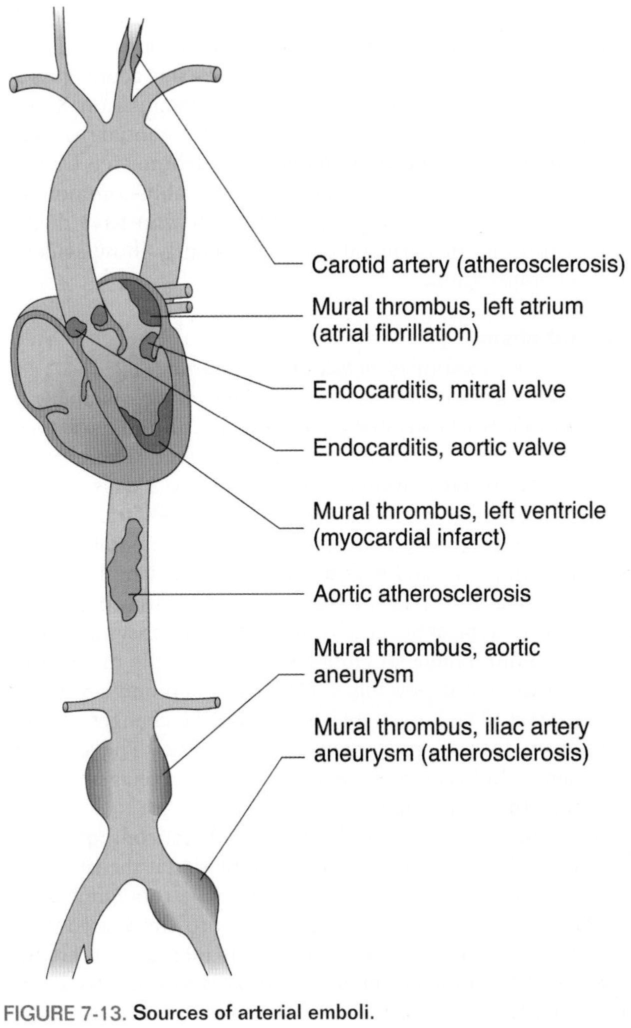

FIGURE 7-13. **Sources of arterial emboli.**

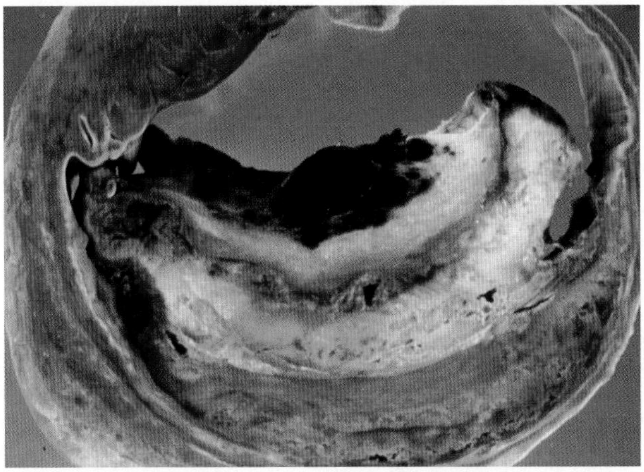

FIGURE 7-14. **Mural thrombus of the left ventricle.** A laminated thrombus adheres to the endocardium overlying a healed aneurysmal myocardial infarct.

- **Brain:** Arterial emboli to the brain cause ischemic necrosis (strokes).
- **Intestine:** In the mesenteric circulation, emboli cause bowel infarction, which manifests as an acute abdomen and requires immediate surgery.
- **Lower extremity:** Embolism to an artery of the leg leads to sudden pain, absence of pulses, and a cold limb. In some cases, the limb must be amputated.
- **Kidney:** Renal artery embolism may infarct an entire kidney but more commonly causes small peripheral infarcts.
- **Heart:** Coronary artery embolism and resulting myocardial infarcts occur but are rare.

The more common sites of infarction from arterial emboli are summarized in Figure 7-15.

Air Embolism

Air may enter the venous circulation through neck wounds, thoracocentesis, or punctures of the great veins during invasive procedures or hemodialysis. Small amounts of circulating air in the form of bubbles are of little consequence, but quantities of 100 mL or more can lead to sudden death. Air bubbles tend to coalesce and physically obstruct blood flow in the right side of the heart, the pulmonary circulation, and the brain. Histologically, air bubbles appear as empty spaces in capillaries and small vessels of the lung.

Persons exposed to increased atmospheric pressure, such as scuba divers and workers in underwater occupations (e.g., tunnels, drilling platform construction) are subject to **decompression sickness**, a unique form of gas embolism. During descent, large amounts of inert gas (nitrogen or helium) are dissolved in bodily fluids. When the diver ascends, the gas is released from solution and exhaled. However, if ascent is too rapid, gas bubbles form in the circulation and within tissues, obstructing blood flow and directly injuring cells. Air embolism is the second most common cause of death in sport diving (drowning is the first).

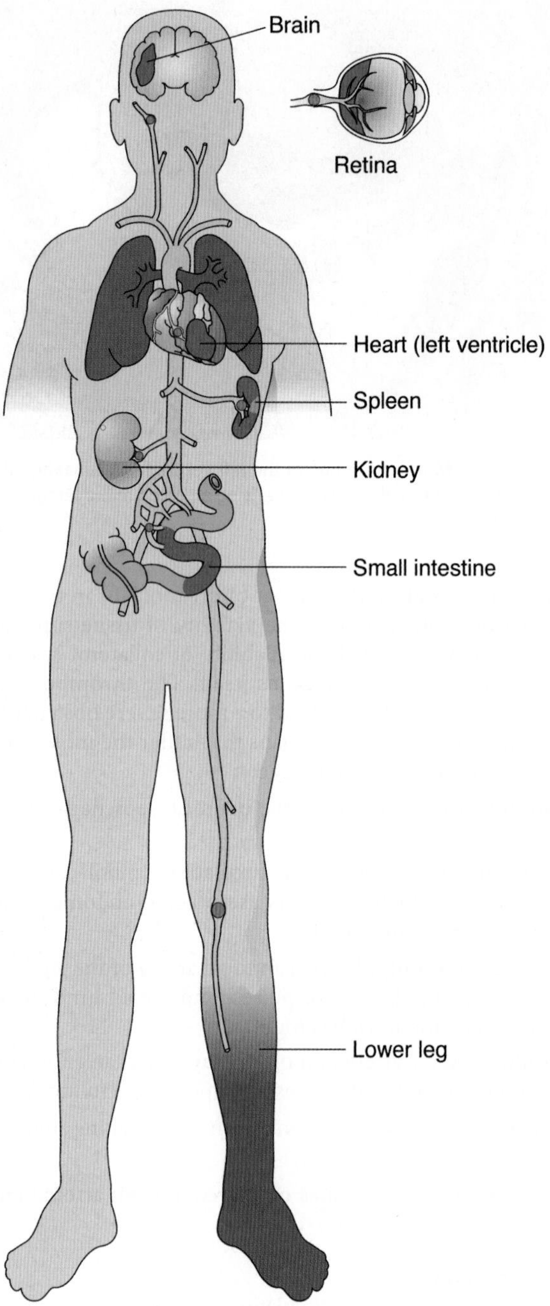

FIGURE 7-15. Common sites of infarction from arterial emboli.

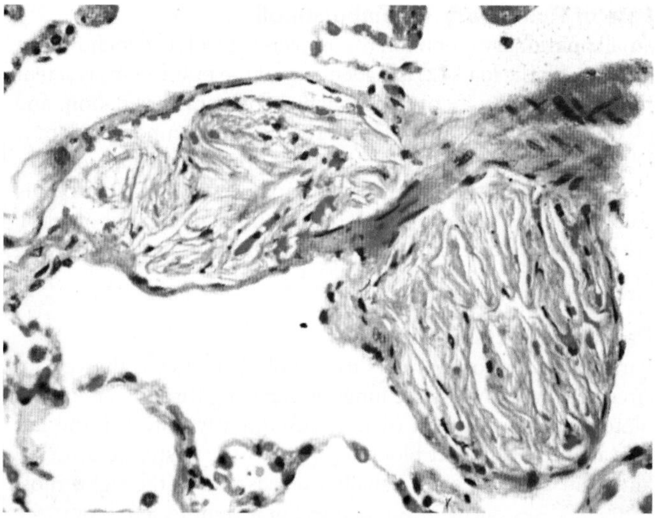

FIGURE 7-16. **Amniotic fluid embolism.** A section of lung shows pulmonary capillaries distended by epithelial squames.

Acute decompression sickness, "the bends," is characterized by temporary muscular and joint pain, owing to small vessel obstruction in these tissues. However, severe involvement of cerebral blood vessels may cause coma or even death.

Caisson disease refers to decompression sickness in which vascular obstruction causes multiple foci of ischemic (avascular) necrosis of bone, particularly affecting the head of the femur, tibia, and humerus. This complication was originally described in construction workers in diving bells (or caissons).

Amniotic Fluid Embolism

In amniotic fluid embolism, amniotic fluid containing fetal cells and debris enter the maternal circulation through open uterine and cervical veins. It is a rare maternal complication of childbirth, but can be catastrophic when it occurs. This disorder usually occurs at the end of labor when the pulmonary emboli are composed of the solid epithelial constituents (squames) contained in the amniotic fluid (Fig. 7-16). Of greater importance is the initiation of a potentially fatal consumptive coagulopathy caused by the high thromboplastin activity of amniotic fluid.

The clinical presentation of amniotic fluid embolism can be dramatic, with sudden onset of cyanosis and shock, followed by coma and death. If the mother survives this acute episode, she may die of disseminated intravascular coagulation. Should she overcome this complication, she is at substantial risk of developing **acute respiratory distress syndrome** (see Chapter 12). Minor amniotic fluid embolism is probably common and asymptomatic, since autopsies of mothers who have died of other causes in the perinatal period frequently show evidence of this complication.

Fat Embolism

Fat embolism is release of emboli of fatty marrow (Fig. 7-17) *into damaged blood vessels following severe trauma to fat-containing tissue, particularly accompanying bone fractures.* In most instances, fat embolism is clinically inapparent. However, severe fat embolism leads to **fat embolism syndrome** 1 to 3 days after the injury. In its most severe form, which may be fatal, this syndrome is characterized by respiratory failure, mental changes, thrombocytopenia, and widespread petechiae. Chest radiography reveals diffuse opacity of the lungs, which may progress to a "whiteout" typical of acute respiratory distress syndrome. At autopsy, innumerable fat globules are seen in the microvasculature of the lungs (see Fig. 7-17B) and brain and sometimes other organs. The lungs typically exhibit the changes of acute respiratory distress syndrome (see Chapter 12). The lesions in the brain include cerebral edema, small hemorrhages, and occasionally microinfarcts.

Fat embolism is usually considered a direct consequence of trauma, with fat entering ruptured capillaries at the site of the fracture. However, this explanation may be too simplistic. It has been suggested that hemorrhage into the marrow and perhaps also into the subcutaneous fat increases interstitial pressure above capillary pressure, so fat is forced into the circulation. Moreover, there is more fat in the pulmonary vascular system than can be accounted for by simple transfer of fat

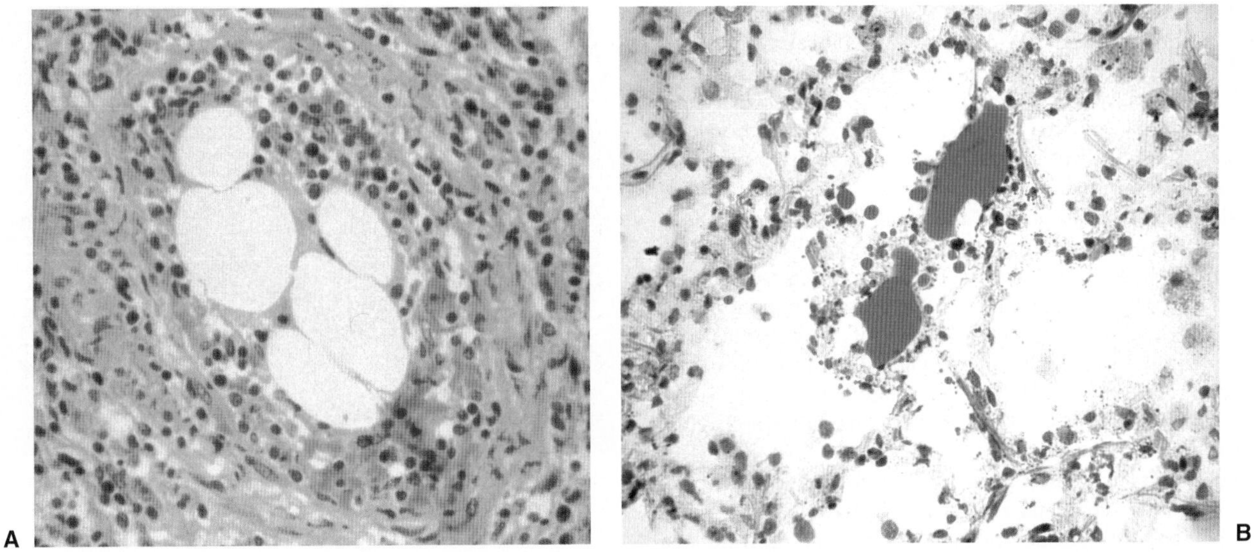

FIGURE 7-17. **Fat embolism. A.** The lumen of a small pulmonary artery is occluded by a fragment of bone marrow consisting of fat cells and hematopoietic elements. **B.** A frozen section of lung stained with Sudan red shows capillaries occluded by red-staining fat emboli.

from peripheral depots and the chemical composition of the fat in the lung differs from that in tissue. Finally, there is a discrepancy between the frequency of fat embolism and bone marrow embolism.

Bone Marrow Embolism

Bone marrow emboli to the lungs, complete with hematopoietic cells and fat, are often encountered at autopsy after cardiac resuscitation, a procedure in which fractures of the sternum and ribs commonly occur. They also occasionally occur after fractures of long bones. In most cases no symptoms are attributed to bone marrow embolism.

Miscellaneous Pulmonary Emboli

Intravenous drug abusers who use talc as a carrier for illicit drugs may introduce it into the lung via the bloodstream. **Talc emboli** produce a granulomatous response in the lungs (Fig. 7-18). **Cotton emboli** are surprisingly common and are due to cleansing of the skin prior to venipuncture. **Schistosomiasis** may be associated with the embolization of ova to the lungs from bladder or gut, in which case they incite a foreign body granulomatous reaction. **Tumor emboli** are occasionally seen in the lung during hematogenous dissemination of cancer.

Infarction

Infarction is the process by which coagulative necrosis develops in an area distal to the occlusion of an end-artery. The necrotic zone is an **infarct**. Infarcts of vital organs such as heart, brain, and intestine are serious medical conditions and are major causes of morbidity and mortality. If the victim survives, the infarct heals with a scar. Partial arterial occlusion (i.e., stenosis) occasionally causes necrosis, but it more commonly leads to atrophic changes associated with chronic ischemia. For example, in the heart these changes include vacuolization of cardiac myocytes, atrophy, loss of muscle cell myofibrils, and interstitial fibrosis.

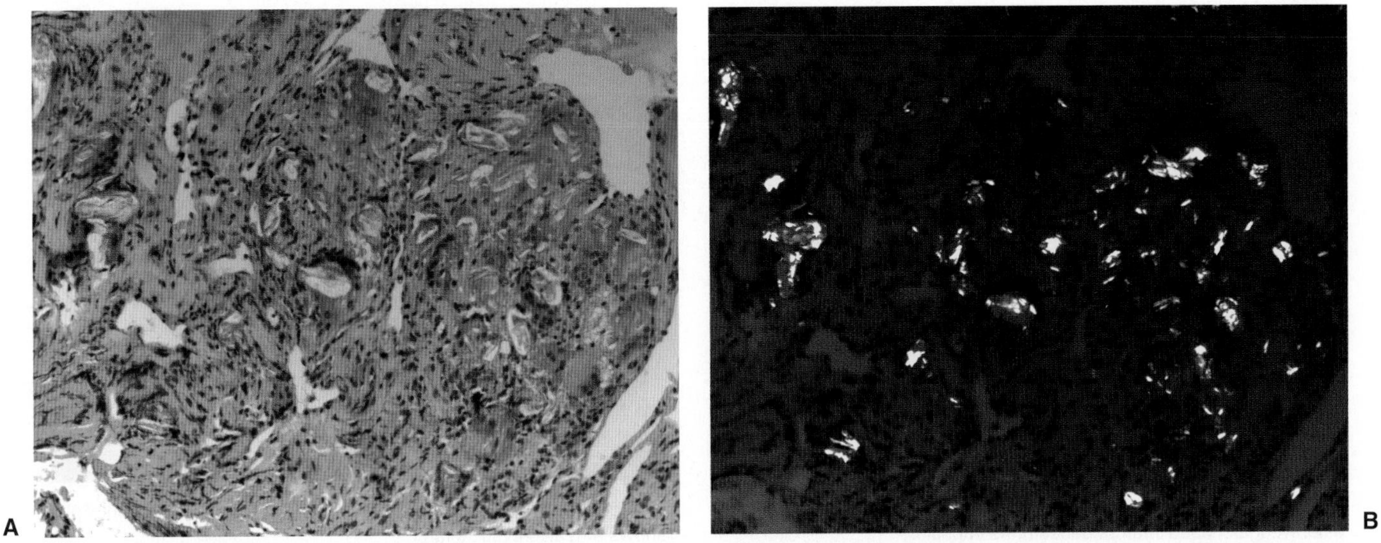

FIGURE 7-18. **Talc emboli.** A section of lung from an intravenous drug abuser shows talc particles before (**A**) and after (**B**) polarization of light.

PATHOLOGY: The gross and microscopic appearance of an infarct depends on its location and age. Upon arterial occlusion, the area supplied by the vessel rapidly becomes swollen and deep red. Microscopically, vascular dilation and congestion and occasionally interstitial hemorrhage are noted. Subsequently, several types of infarcts are distinguishable by gross examination.

Pale infarcts are typical in the heart, kidneys, and spleen (Fig. 7-19), although certain renal infarcts may be cystic. **Dry gangrene** of the leg due to arterial occlusion (often noted in diabetes) is actually a large pale infarct. On gross examination, 1 or 2 days after the initial hyperemia, the infarct becomes soft, sharply delineated, and light yellow (Fig. 7-20). The border tends to be dark red, reflecting hemorrhage into surrounding viable tissue. Microscopically, a pale infarct exhibits uniform coagulative necrosis.

Red infarcts may result from either arterial or venous occlusion and are also characterized by coagulative necrosis. However, they are distinguished by bleeding into the necrotic area from adjacent arteries and veins. *Red infarcts occur principally in organs with a dual blood supply*, such as the lung, or those with extensive collateral circulation, such as the small intestine and brain. In the heart, a red infarct occurs when the infarcted area is reperfused, as may occur following spontaneous or therapeutically induced lysis of the occluding thrombus. Grossly, red infarcts are sharply circumscribed, firm and dark red to purple (Fig. 7-21). Over a period of several days, acute inflammatory cells infiltrate the necrotic area from the viable border. The cellular debris is phagocytosed and digested by polymorphonuclear leukocytes and later by macrophages. Granulation tissue eventually forms, to be replaced ultimately by a scar. In a large infarct of an organ such as the heart or kidney, the necrotic center remains inaccessible to the inflammatory exudate and may persist for months. In the brain, an infarct typically undergoes liquefactive necrosis and may become a fluid-filled cyst, which is referred to as a **cystic infarct** (Fig. 7-22).

Septic infarct results when the necrotic tissue of an infarct is seeded by pyogenic bacteria and becomes infected. Pulmonary infarcts are not uncommonly infected, presumably because the necrotic tissue offers little resistance to inhaled bacteria. In the case of bacterial endocarditis, the emboli themselves are infected and the resulting infarcts are often septic. A septic infarct may become a frank abscess (Fig. 7-23).

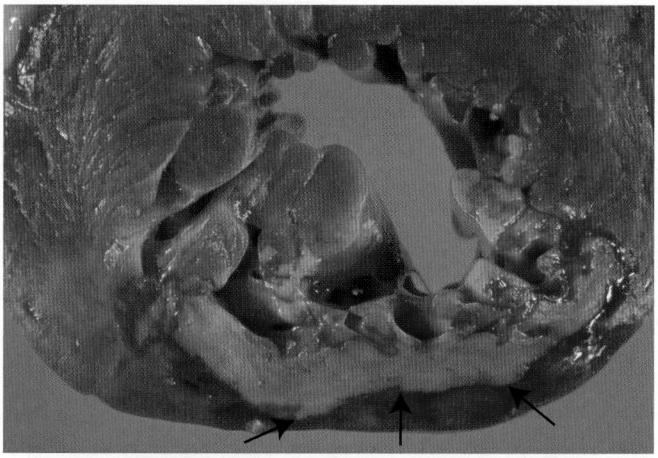

FIGURE 7-20. **Acute myocardial infarct.** A cross-section of the left ventricle reveals a sharply circumscribed, soft, yellow area of necrosis in the posterior free wal (*arrows*).

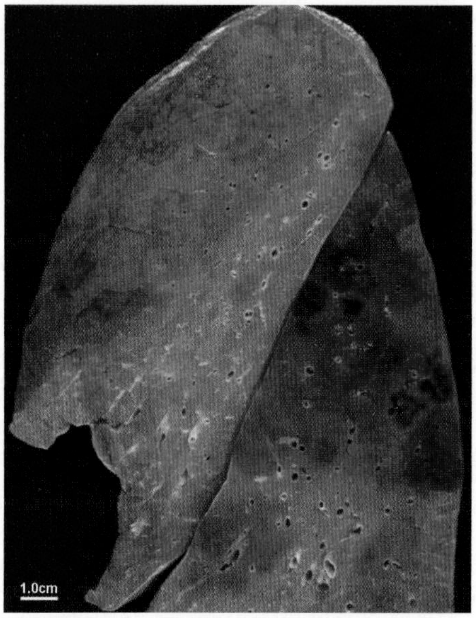

FIGURE 7-21. **Red infarct.** A sagittal slice of lung shows a hemorrhagic infarct in upper segments of the lower lobe.

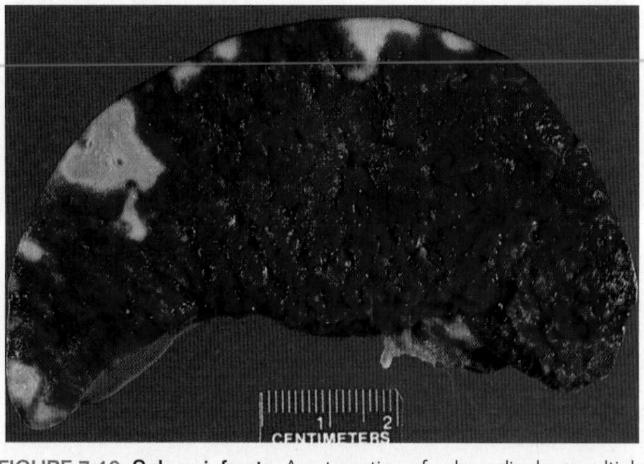

FIGURE 7-19. **Spleen infarcts.** A cut section of spleen displays multiple pale, wedge-shaped infarcts beneath the capsule.

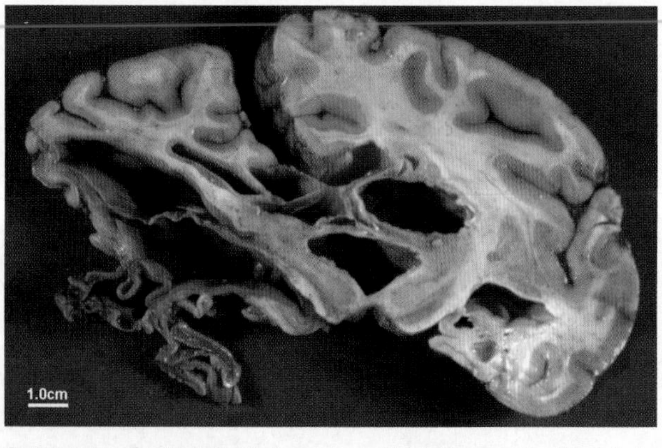

FIGURE 7-22. **Cystic infarct.** A cross-section of brain in the frontal plane shows a healed cystic infarct.

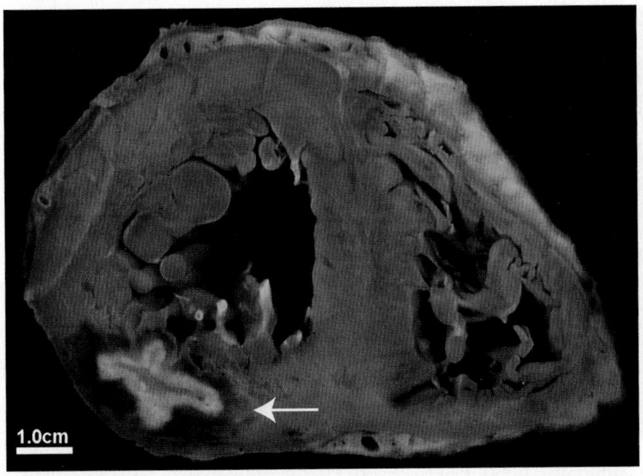

FIGURE 7-23. **Septic infarct.** A myocardial abscess (*arrow*) within the left ventricular free wall was due to infection with *Staphylococcus aureus*.

Infarction in Specific Locations Is Often Fatal

Myocardial Infarcts

Myocardial infarcts are transmural (through the entire wall) or subendocardial. A transmural infarct results from complete occlusion of a major extramural coronary artery. Subendocardial infarction reflects prolonged ischemia caused by partially occluding, atherosclerotic, stenotic lesions of the coronary arteries when the requirement for oxygen exceeds the supply. Such a situation prevails in disorders such as shock, anoxia, or severe tachycardia (rapid pulse). A myocardial infarct may be pale or red, depending upon the extent of reflow of blood into the infarcted area (Fig. 7-24).

Pulmonary Infarcts

Only about 10% of pulmonary emboli elicit clinical symptoms referable to pulmonary infarction, usually after occlusion of a middle-sized pulmonary artery. Infarction occurs only if circulation from bronchial arteries inadequately compensates for supply lost from the pulmonary arteries. This circumstance is often found in congestive heart failure, although stasis in the pulmonary circulation may contribute. Hemorrhage into the alveolar spaces of the necrotic lining tissue occurs within 48 hours.

Cerebral Infarcts

Infarction of the brain may result from local ischemia or a generalized reduction in blood flow. The latter often results from systemic hypotension, as in shock, and produces infarction in the border zones between the distributions of the major cerebral arteries (**watershed infarct**). If prolonged, severe hypotension can cause widespread brain necrosis. The occlusion of a single vessel in the brain (e.g., after an embolus has lodged) causes ischemia and necrosis in a well-defined area. This type of cerebral infarct may be pale or red, the latter being common with embolic occlusions. The occlusion of a large artery produces a wide area of necrosis, which may ultimately resolve as a large fluid-filled cavity in the brain.

Intestinal Infarcts

The earliest tissue changes in intestinal ischemia are necrosis of the tips of the villi in the small intestine and necrosis of the superficial mucosa in the large intestine. In either case, more severe ischemia leads to hemorrhagic necrosis of the submucosa and muscularis but not the serosa. Small mucosal infarcts heal in a few days, but more severe injury leads to ulceration. These ulcers can eventually reepithelialize. However, if ulcers are large, they are repaired by scarring, a process that may lead to strictures. Severe transmural necrosis is associated with massive bleeding or bowel perforation, complications that often result in irreversible shock, sepsis, and death.

Edema

Edema is excess fluid in interstitial spaces of the body. It may be local or generalized. **Local edema** in most instances occurs with inflammation, the "tumor" of "tumor, rubor, and calor." Local

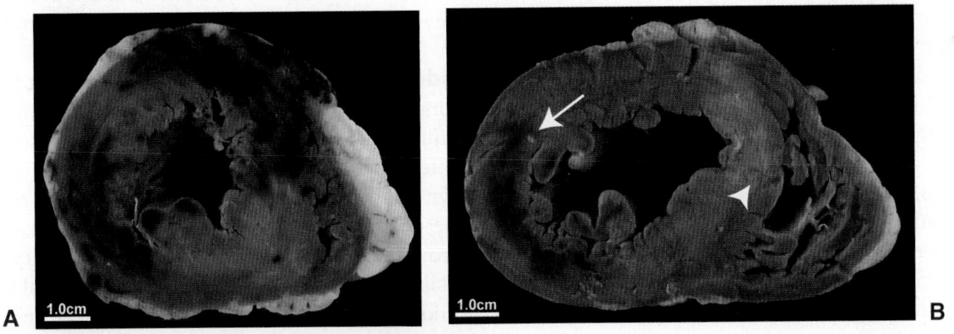

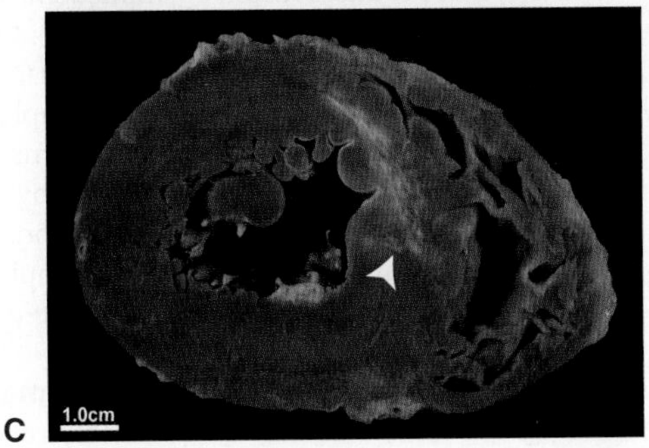

FIGURE 7-24. **Myocardial infarct.** Transverse sections of ventricular myocardium show (**A**) reperfused, (**B**) acute (*arrow*) and healed (*arrowhead*) together, and (**C**) healed infarct. Reperfusion is typically associated with hemorrhage as in (A) and (B). In (C), a white scar (*arrowhead*) is evident in the anterior (*arrowhead*) ventricular septum.

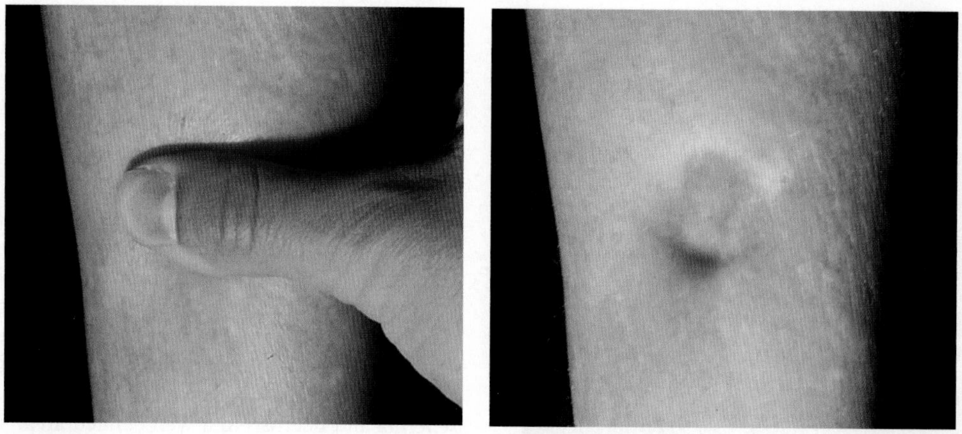

A B

FIGURE 7-25. **Pitting edema of the leg. A.** In a patient with congestive heart failure, severe edema of the leg is demonstrated by applying pressure with a finger. **B.** The resulting "pitting" reflects the inelasticity of the fluid-filled tissue.

edema of a limb, usually the leg, results from venous or lymphatic obstruction. Burns cause prominent local edema by disrupting the permeability of the local vasculature. Local edema may be a prominent component of an immune reaction, for example, urticaria (hives), or edema of the epiglottis or larynx (angioneurotic edema).

Generalized edema, affecting visceral organs and the skin of the trunk and lower extremities (Fig. 7-25), reflects a global disorder of fluid and electrolyte metabolism, most often occasioned by heart failure. Generalized edema is also seen in certain renal diseases associated with loss of serum proteins into the urine (nephrotic syndrome) and in cirrhosis of the liver. **Anasarca** is extreme generalized edema, a condition evidenced by conspicuous fluid accumulation in subcutaneous tissues, visceral organs, and body cavities. Edema fluid may accumulate in body spaces, such as the pleural cavity (**hydrothorax**), peritoneal cavity (**ascites**), or pericardial cavity (**hydropericardium**).

Normal Capillary Filtration

Normal formation and retention of interstitial fluid depends on filtration and reabsorption at the level of the capillaries (Starling forces). The internal or hydrostatic pressure in the arteriolar segment of the capillary is 32 mm Hg. At the middle of the capillary, it is 20 mm Hg. Since the interstitial hydrostatic pressure is only 3 mm Hg, there is an outward fluid filtration of 14 mL/min. Hydrostatic pressure is opposed by plasma oncotic pressure (26 mm Hg), which results in osmotic reabsorption of 12 mL/min at the venous end of the capillary. Thus, interstitial fluid is formed at the rate of 2 mL/min and is reabsorbed by the lymphatics, so that in equilibrium there is no net fluid gain or loss in the interstitium.

Sodium and Water Metabolism

Water represents 50% to 70% of body weight and is divided between the extracellular and the intracellular fluid spaces. Extracellular fluid is further divided into interstitial and vascular compartments. Interstitial fluid constitutes about 75% of the latter.

Total body sodium is the principal determinant of extracellular fluid volume because it is the major cation in the extracellular fluid. In other words, increased total body sodium must be balanced by more extracellular water to maintain constant osmolality. Control of extracellular fluid volume depends to a large extent on regulation of renal sodium excretion, which is influenced by (1) atrial natriuretic factor, (2) the renin–angiotensin system of the juxtaglomerular apparatus, and (3) sympathetic nervous system activity (see Chapter 10).

Edema Caused by Increased Hydrostatic Pressure

Unopposed increases in hydrostatic pressure result in greater filtration of fluid into the interstitial space and its retention as edema. Such a situation is particularly prominent in decompensated heart disease, in which back-pressure in the lungs secondary to left ventricle failure leads to acute pulmonary edema and right sided heart failure, and contributes to systemic edema. Similarly, back-pressure caused by venous obstruction in the lower extremity causes edema of the leg. Obstruction to portal blood flow in cirrhosis of the liver contributes to formation of abdominal fluid (ascites).

Edema Caused by Decreased Oncotic Pressure

The difference in pressure between intravascular and interstitial compartments is largely determined by the concentration of plasma proteins, especially albumin. Any condition that lowers plasma albumin levels, whether it is albuminuria in the nephrotic syndrome or reduced albumin synthesis in chronic liver disease or severe malnutrition, tends to promote generalized edema.

Edema Caused by Lymphatic Obstruction

Under normal circumstances, more fluid is filtered into the interstitial spaces than is reabsorbed into the vascular bed. This excess interstitial fluid is removed by lymphatics. Thus, obstruction to lymphatic flow leads to localized edema. Lymphatic channels can be obstructed by (1) malignant neoplasms, (2) fibrosis resulting from inflammation or irradiation, and (3) surgical ablation. For instance, the inflammatory response to filarial worms (Bancroftian and Malayan filariasis; see Chapter 9) can result in lymphatic obstruction that produces massive lymphedema of the scrotum and lower extremities (**elephantiasis**) (Fig. 7-26). Lymphedema of the arm often complicates radical mastectomies for breast cancer, due to removal of axillary lymph nodes and lymphatics.

Lymphatic edema differs from other forms of edema in its high protein content, since lymph is the vehicle by which proteins and interstitial cells are returned to the circulation. The increased protein concentration may be a fibrogenic stimulus in the formation of dermal fibrosis in chronic edema (indurated edema).

The Role of Sodium Retention in Edema

Generalized edema and ascites invariably reflect increased total body sodium, as a consequence of renal sodium retention. When

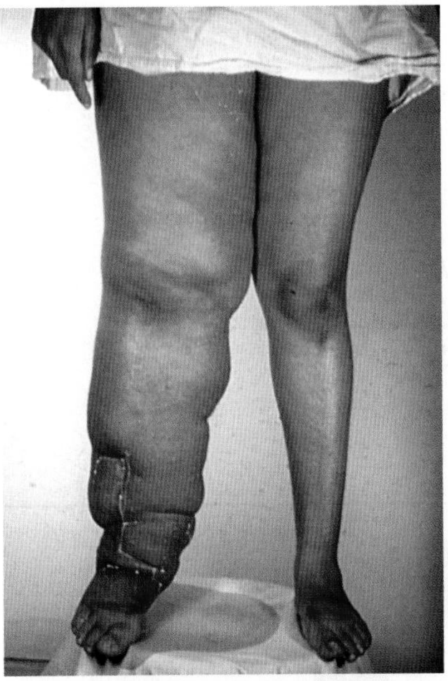

FIGURE 7-26. **Edema secondary to lymphatic obstruction.** Massive edema of the right lower extremity (elephantiasis) in a patient with obstruction of lymphatic drainage.

peripheral edema is first detectable clinically, extracellular fluid volume has already expanded by at least 5 L. The most common conditions in which generalized edema is found include congestive heart failure, cirrhosis of the liver, nephrotic syndrome, and some cases of chronic renal insufficiency. The mechanisms of edema formation and representative disorders associated with them are summarized in Figure 7-27 and Table 7-1.

Congestive Heart Failure Is the Consequence of Inadequate Cardiac Output

It is estimated that two to three million people in the United States have congestive heart failure, of whom 15% die annually. Half of all patients with congestive heart failure who require admission to the hospital will die within 1 year. In the United States, this disorder is most commonly associated with ischemic heart disease, although virtually any chronic cardiac disorder may eventuate in congestive heart failure (see Chapter 11).

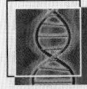

PATHOGENESIS: The argument regarding the relative contributions of "forward failure" (low cardiac output) versus "backward failure" (venous congestion) in the pathogenesis of edema in congestive heart failure is no longer a burning issue. Both systolic and diastolic dysfunction contribute to the low cardiac output and high ventricular filling pressure characteristic of congestive heart failure, although systolic dysfunction is more important in most patients.

Inadequate cardiac output in congestive heart failure leads to decreased glomerular filtration and increased renin secretion. The latter activates angiotensin, leading to release of aldosterone, subsequent sodium reabsorption, and fluid retention. Furthermore, reduced hepatic blood flow impairs catabolism of aldosterone, thereby further raising its concentration in the blood. As a compensatory mechanism, increased fluid volume preserves an adequate intracardiac pressure. In addition, increased sympathetic discharge leads to augmented levels of catecholamines, which stimulate cardiac contractility and further counteract the impairment in cardiac performance. At the same time, distention of the atria by the increased blood volume promotes release of atrial natriuretic peptide, which stimulates renal sodium excretion.

After long-standing heart failure, these compensatory mechanisms fail, in which case renal sodium retention again becomes important. The further expansion of plasma volume leads to increased pulmonary and systemic venous pressure, which produces increased hydrostatic pressure in the respective capillary beds. The increased capillary pressure, together with decreased plasma oncotic pressure, results in the edema of congestive heart failure.

PATHOLOGY: Failure of the left ventricle is associated principally with passive congestion of the lungs and pulmonary edema (Fig. 7-28). When chronic, these conditions lead to pulmonary hypertension and eventual failure of the right ventricle. Right ventricular failure is characterized by generalized subcutaneous edema (most prominent in the dependent portions of the body), ascites, and pleural effusions. The liver, spleen, and other splanchnic organs are typically congested. At autopsy, the heart is enlarged and its chambers dilated

CLINICAL FEATURES: The effects of heart failure depend upon which ventricle is failing, recognizing that both may be failing simultaneously. Patients in left-sided heart failure complain of shortness of breath (**dyspnea**) on exertion and when recumbent (**orthopnea**). They may be awakened from sleep by sudden episodes of shortness of breath (**paroxysmal nocturnal dyspnea**). Physical examination usually reveals distended jugular veins. Persons with right-sided failure have pitting edema of the legs and an enlarged and tender liver. When ascites is present, the abdomen is distended. Patients in congestive heart failure with pulmonary edema have crackling breath sounds (**rales**) caused by expansion of fluid-filled alveoli.

Pulmonary Edema Features Increased Fluid in the Alveolar Spaces and Interstitium of the Lung

This condition leads to decreased gas exchange in the lung, causing hypoxia and retention of carbon dioxide (**hypercapnia**).

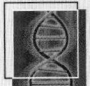

PATHOGENESIS AND PATHOLOGY: The lung is a loose tissue without much connective tissue support and, therefore, requires certain conditions to prevent the development of edema. Among these protective devices are

- Low perfusion pressure in lung capillaries, owing to low right ventricular pressure
- Effective drainage of the interstitial space of the lung by lymphatics, which are under a slightly negative pressure and can accommodate up to 10 times the regular lymph flow
- Tight cellular junctions between endothelial cells, which control capillary permeability

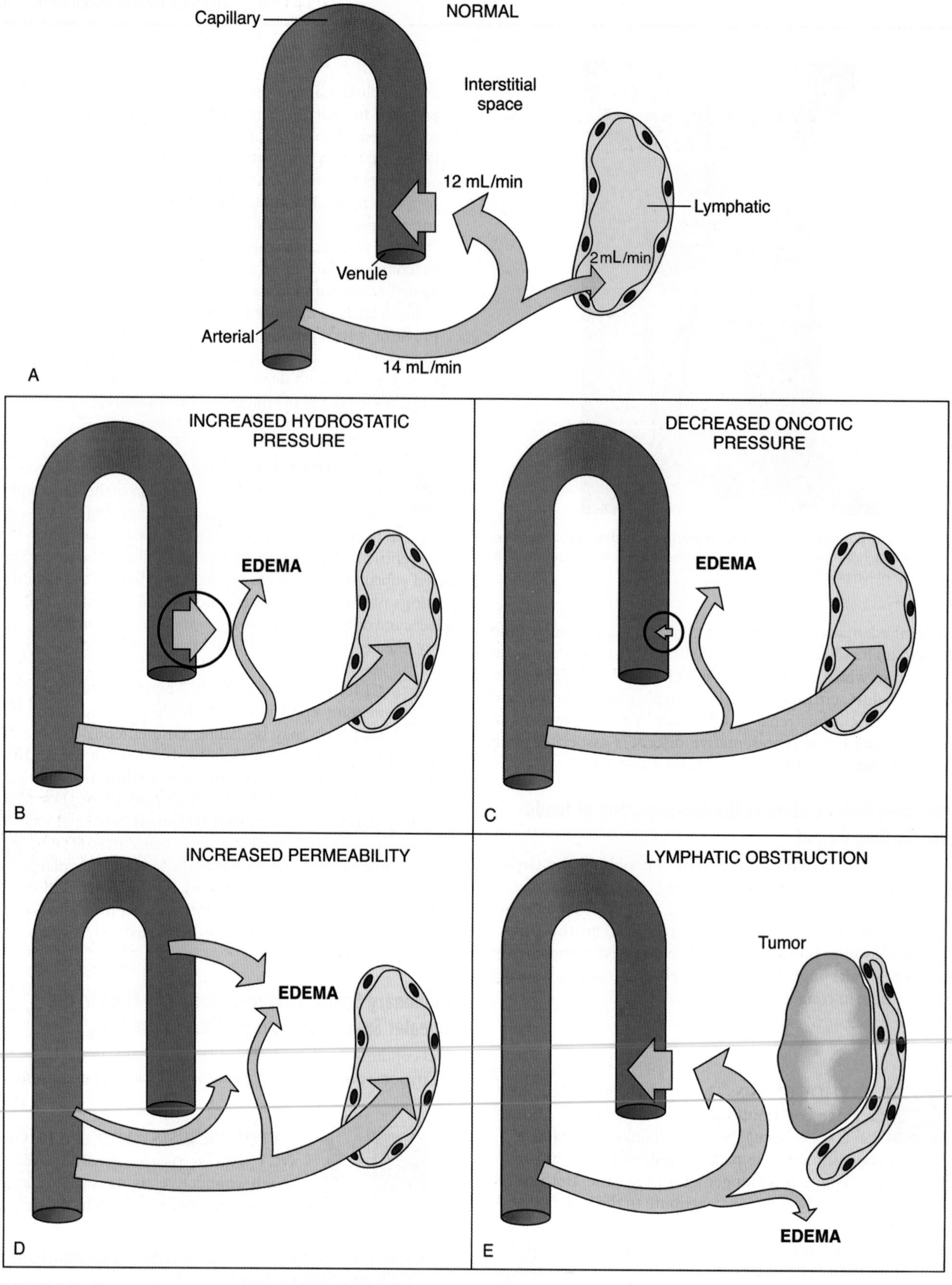

FIGURE 7-27. **The capillary system and mechanisms of edema formation. A. Normal.** The differential between the hydrostatic and oncotic pressures at the arterial end of the capillary system is responsible for the filtration into the interstitial space of approximately 14 mL of fluid per minute. This fluid is reabsorbed at the venous end at the rate of 12 mL/min. It is also drained through the lymphatic capillaries at a rate of 2 mL/min. Proteins are removed by the lymphatics from the interstitial space. **B. Hydrostatic edema.** If the hydrostatic pressure at the venous end of the capillary system is elevated, reabsorption decreases. As long as the lymphatics can drain the surplus fluid, no edema results. If their capacity is exceeded, however, edema fluid accumulates. **C. Oncotic edema.** Edema fluid also accumulates if reabsorption is diminished by decreased oncotic pressure of the vascular bed, owing to a loss of albumin. **D. Inflammatory and traumatic edema.** Edema, either local or systemic, results if the vascular bed becomes leaky following injury to the endothelium. **E. Lymphedema.** Lymphatic obstruction causes the accumulation of interstitial fluid because of insufficient reabsorption and deficient removal of proteins, the latter increasing the oncotic pressure of the fluid in the interstitial space.

TABLE 7-1

Disorders Associated with Edema

Increased hydrostatic pressure	
Arteriolar dilation	Inflammation Heat
Increased venous pressure	Venous thrombosis Congestive heart failure Cirrhosis (ascites) Postural inactivity (e.g., prolonged standing)
Hypervolemia	Sodium retention (e.g., decreased renal function)
Decreased oncotic pressure	
Hypoproteinemia	Nephrotic syndrome Cirrhosis Protein-losing gastroenteropathy Malnutrition
Increased capillary permeability	Inflammation Burns Adult respiratory distress syndrome
Lymphatic obstruction	Cancer Postsurgical lymphedema Inflammation

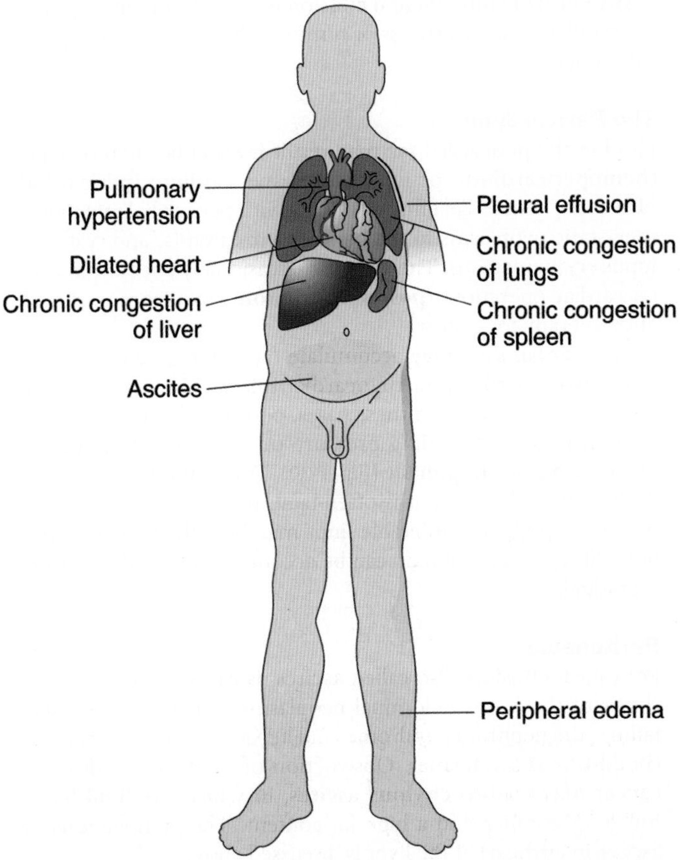

FIGURE 7-28. **Pathologic consequences of chronic congestive heart failure.**

Pulmonary edema results if the above-mentioned protective mechanisms are disturbed. The most common causes of pulmonary edema relate to hemodynamic alterations in the heart that increase perfusion pressure in pulmonary capillaries and block effective lymphatic drainage. These conditions include left ventricular failure (the most common cause), mitral stenosis, and mitral insufficiency. Disruption of capillary permeability is the cause of pulmonary edema in acute lung injury associated with adult respiratory distress syndrome, inhalation of toxic gases, aspiration of gastric contents, viral infections, and uremia. Acute lung injury is reflected in destruction of endothelial cells or disruption of their tight junctions (see Chapter 12).

Pulmonary edema may be interstitial or alveolar. Interstitial edema is the earliest phase and is an exaggeration of normal fluid filtration. Lymphatics become distended and fluid accumulates in the interstitium of lobular septa and around veins and bronchovascular bundles. Radiologic examination reveals a reticulonodular pattern, more marked at lung bases. Lobular septa become edematous and produce linear shadows ("Kerley B lines") on chest radiographs. Edema results in shunting of blood flow from the bases to the upper lobes and increased airflow resistance occurs because of edema of the bronchovascular tree. Patients are often asymptomatic in this early stage.

When the fluid can no longer be accommodated in the interstitial space, it spills into the alveoli, a condition termed **alveolar edema**. At this stage, a radiologic alveolar pattern is seen, usually worse in central portions of the lung and in lower zones. The patient becomes acutely short of breath and bubbly rales are heard. In extreme cases, frothy fluid is coughed up or wells up out of the trachea.

Microscopic examination of the edematous lung reveals severely congested alveolar capillaries and alveoli filled with a homogeneous, pink-staining fluid permeated by air bubbles (see Fig. 7-3). If pulmonary edema is caused by alveolar damage, cell debris, fibrin, and proteins form films of proteinaceous material, called **hyaline membranes**, in the alveoli (Fig. 7-29).

CLINICAL FEATURES: Pulmonary fluid accumulation may go unnoticed initially, but eventually dyspnea and coughing become prominent. If edema is severe, large amounts of frothy pink sputum are expectorated. Hypoxemia is manifested as cyanosis.

Pulmonary function is restricted in severe congestion and in interstitial pulmonary edema because accumulation of fluid in the interstitial space causes reduced compliance (i.e., stiffening of the lung tissue). Thus, increased respiratory work is required to maintain ventilation. Since alveolar walls are thickened, there is a greater barrier to oxygen and carbon dioxide exchange. The latter is less affected than the former, resulting in hypoxia with near-normal carbon dioxide levels. Mismatch between ventilation (which is reduced) and perfusion (which persists) contributes to development of hypoxemia in patients with pulmonary edema.

Edema in Cirrhosis of the Liver Is Commonly an End-Stage Condition

Cirrhosis of the liver is often accompanied by ascites and peripheral edema (see Chapter 14). Liver scarring obstructs portal blood flow and leads to portal hypertension, and increased hydrostatic pressure in the splanchnic circulation. This situation

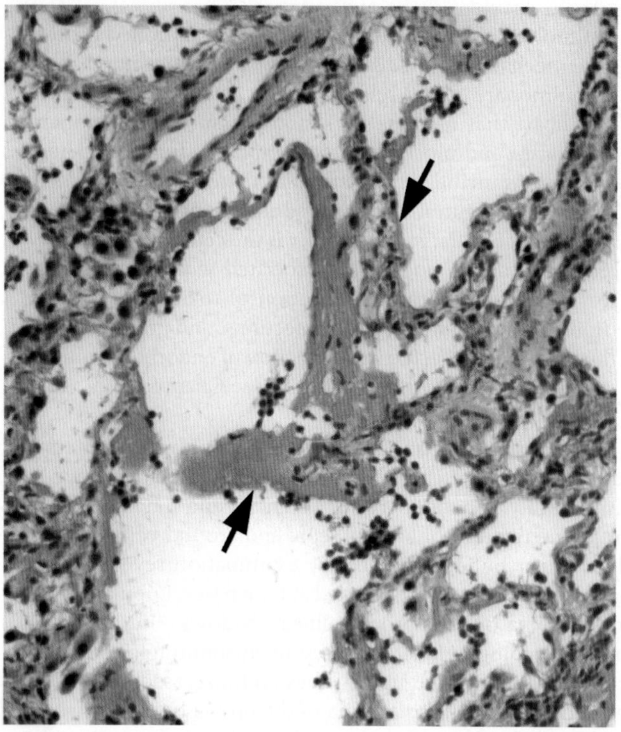

FIGURE 7-29. **Pulmonary edema due to diffuse alveolar damage.** A section of lung shows hyaline membranes *(arrows)* in alveoli.

is compounded by decreased hepatic synthesis of albumin as a result of liver dysfunction. Consequent accumulation of peritoneal fluid leads to a lower effective blood volume, which results in renal retention of sodium by mechanisms similar to those operative in congestive heart failure. Alternatively, chronic liver disease itself causes renal retention of sodium. Subsequent expansion of extracellular fluid volume further promotes ascites and edema, thus establishing a vicious circle. In addition, increased transudation of lymph from the liver capsule adds to the accumulation of fluid in the abdomen.

The Nephrotic Syndrome Reflects Massive Proteinuria

In the nephrotic syndrome, the magnitude of protein loss in the urine exceeds the rate at which it is replaced by the liver (see Chapter 16). The resulting decline in the concentration of plasma proteins, particularly albumin, reduces plasma oncotic pressure and promotes edema. The ensuing decrease in blood volume stimulates the renin–angiotensin–aldosterone mechanism, leading to sodium retention. The edema is generalized but appears preferentially in soft connective tissues, the eyes, the eyelids, and subcutaneous tissues. Ascites and pleural effusions also occur.

Cerebral Edema Often Causes a Fatal Increase in Intracranial Pressure

Edema of the brain is dangerous because the rigidity of the cranium allows little room for expansion. Increased intracranial pressure from edema compromises cerebral blood supply, distorts the gross structure of the brain and interferes with central nervous system function (see Chapter 28). Cerebral edema is divided into vasogenic, cytotoxic, and interstitial forms.

- **Vasogenic edema,** the most common variety of edema, is excess fluid in the extracellular space of the brain. It results from increased vascular permeability, mainly in white matter. The tight endothelial junctions of the blood–brain barrier are disrupted and fluid filters into the interstitial space. Disorders associated with cerebral vasogenic edema include trauma, neoplasms, encephalitis, abscesses, infarcts, hemorrhage, and toxic brain injury (e.g., lead poisoning).
- **Cytotoxic edema** is equivalent to hydropic cell swelling (i.e., accumulation of intracellular water). It is usually a response to cell injury, such as that produced by ischemia. Cytotoxic cerebral edema preferentially affects the gray matter.
- **Interstitial edema** is a consequence of hydrocephalus, in which fluid accumulates in the cerebral ventricles and periventricular white matter.

At autopsy, an edematous brain is soft and heavy. Gyri are flattened and sulci narrowed. Because of alterations in brain function, patients with cerebral edema suffer vomiting, disorientation, and convulsions. Severe cerebral edema leads to herniation of the cerebral tonsils, ordinarily a lethal event.

Fluid Accumulates in Body Cavities as Extensions of the Interstitial Space

The Pleural Space

Pleural effusion (fluid in the pleural space) is a straw-colored transudate of low specific gravity that contains few cells (mainly exfoliated mesothelial cells). Fluid commonly accumulates as an expression of a generalized tendency to form edema in diseases such as the nephrotic syndrome, cirrhosis of the liver, and congestive heart failure. Pleural effusion is also a frequent response to an inflammatory process or tumor in the lung or on the pleural surface.

The Pericardium

Fluid in the pericardial sac may result from either hemorrhage (**hemopericardium**) or injury to the pericardium (**pericardial effusion**). Pericardial effusions occur with pericardial infections, metastatic neoplasms to the pericardium, uremia, and systemic lupus erythematosus. They are also occasionally encountered after cardiac operations (**postpericardiotomy syndrome**) or radiation therapy for cancer.

Pericardial fluid may accumulate rapidly, e.g., with hemorrhage from a ruptured myocardial infarct, dissecting aortic aneurysm or trauma. In these cases, pericardial cavity pressure rises to exceed the filling pressure of the heart, a condition termed **cardiac tamponade** (Fig. 7-30). The resulting precipitous decline in cardiac output is often fatal. If pericardial fluid accumulates rapidly, the tolerable limit may be only 90 to 120 mL, but a liter or more of fluid can be accommodated if the process is gradual.

Peritoneum

Peritoneal effusion, also called **ascites**, is caused mainly by cirrhosis of the liver, abdominal neoplasms, pancreatitis, cardiac failure, the nephrotic syndrome, and hepatic venous obstruction (Budd-Chiari syndrome). Obstruction of the thoracic duct by cancer may lead to **chylous ascites**, in which the fluid has a milky appearance and a high fat content. The pathogenesis of ascites in cirrhosis of the liver is discussed above.

Patients with severe ascites accumulate many liters of fluid and have hugely distended abdomens. The complications of as-

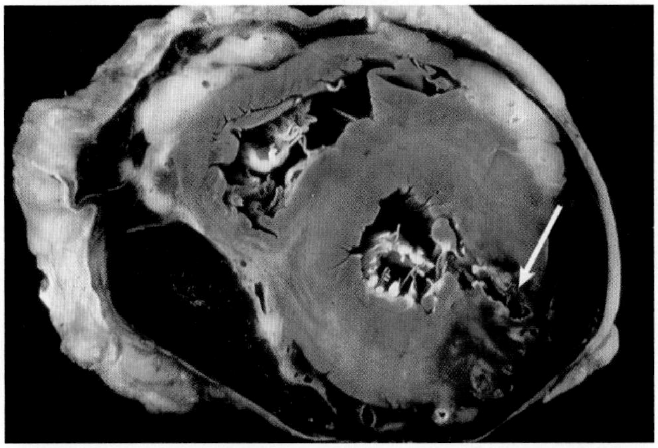

FIGURE 7-30. **Cardiac tamponade.** A cross-section of the heart shows rupture of a myocardial infarct *(arrow)* with the accumulation of a large quantity of blood in the pericardial cavity.

cites derive from increased abdominal pressure and include anorexia and vomiting, reflux esophagitis, dyspnea, ventral hernia, and leakage of fluid into the pleural space.

Fluid Loss and Overload

Excessive fluid loss (dehydration) and fluid overload are clinical situations that have potentially grave consequences. Fluid imbalance causes hemodynamic disorders; alterations in osmolality, and quantity of fluid in intravascular, interstitial, and cellular spaces may affect perfusion or the delivery of substrates, electrolytes or fluids.

Dehydration Features Inadequate Fluid to Fill the Fluid Compartments

Dehydration results from insufficient fluid intake, excessive fluid loss, or both. Water loss may exceed intake in cases of vomiting, diarrhea, burns, excessive sweating, and diabetes insipidus. When excessive fluid loss occurs, fluid is recruited from the interstitial space to the plasma space. fluids in the cell and within the interstitial and vascular compartments become more concentrated, particularly if there is a preferential loss of water, such as during inappropriate secretion of antidiuretic hormones in diabetes insipidus. When patients suffer from burns, vomiting, excessive sweating, or diarrhea, they not only lose fluid but also suffer electrolyte disturbances.

Clinically, only dryness of the skin and mucous membranes are noted initially, but as dehydration progresses, skin turgor is lost. If dehydration persists, **oliguria** (reduced urine output) occurs as a compensation for the fluid loss. More severe fluid loss is accompanied by a shift of water from the intracellular space to the extracellular space, leading to severe cell dysfunction, particularly in the brain. Shrinkage of brain tissue may result in the rupture of small vessels and subsequent bleeding. Systemic blood pressure falls with continuous dehydration and declining perfusion eventually leads to death.

In Overhydration, Fluid Intake Exceeds Renal Excretory Capacity

Overhydration is rare, unless injury to the kidneys limits their excretory function or they are prevented from proper counter-regulation (e.g., via excessive secretion of antidiuretic hormone). Fluid overload today is mostly caused by administration of excessive amounts of intravenous fluids. The most serious effect of such fluid overload is induction of cerebral edema or congestive heart failure in patients with cardiac dysfunction.

Shock

Shock is a condition of profound hemodynamic and metabolic disturbance characterized by failure of the circulatory system to maintain an appropriate blood supply to the microcirculation, with consequent inadequate perfusion of vital organs. In this often catastrophic circumstance, tissue perfusion and oxygen delivery fall below levels required to meet normal demands, including failure to remove metabolites adequately. The term **shock** encompasses all the reactions that occur in response to such disturbances. In the course of uncompensated shock, a rapid circulatory collapse leads to impaired cellular metabolism and death. However, in many cases, compensatory mechanisms sustain the patient, at least for a while. When these adaptations fail, shock becomes irreversible. Shock has been a major cause of morbidity and mortality in intensive care units and despite endeavors to suppress portions of the immune response, the outcome of shock has been unchanged in the past 50 years.

Shock is not synonymous with low blood pressure, although hypotension is often part of the shock syndrome. Hypotension is actually a late sign in shock and indicates a failure of compensation. At the same time that peripheral blood flow falls below critical levels, extreme vasoconstriction can maintain arterial blood pressure. The distinction between shock and hypotension is important clinically because rapid restoration of systemic blood flow is the primary goal in treating shock. When blood pressure alone is raised with vasopressive drugs, systemic blood flow may actually be diminished.

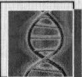

PATHOGENESIS: Decreased perfusion in shock most commonly results from decreased cardiac output, either due to the inability of the heart to pump the normal venous return or to decreased effective blood volume that leads to decreased venous return. These two mechanisms underlie two of the major types of shock: **cardiogenic** and **hypovolemic** shock. Systemic vasodilation, with or without increases in vascular permeability, is responsible for the other categories of shock: septic shock, anaphylactic shock, and neurogenic shock (Fig. 7-31).

- **Cardiogenic shock** is caused by myocardial pump failure. It usually arises after massive myocardial infarction, but myocarditis may also be responsible. Conditions that prevent left or right heart filling reduce cardiac output, resulting in "obstructive" shock. Such conditions include pulmonary embolism, cardiac tamponade, (see Fig. 7-30), and (rarely) atrial myxoma.
- **Hypovolemic shock** is secondary to a pronounced decrease in blood or plasma volume, caused by loss of fluid from the vascular compartment. Hemorrhage, fluid loss from severe burns, diarrhea, excessive urine formation, perspiration, and trauma are the major mechanisms of fluid loss that can lead to hypovolemic shock. In the case of burns or trauma, direct damage to the microcirculation increases vascular permeability.

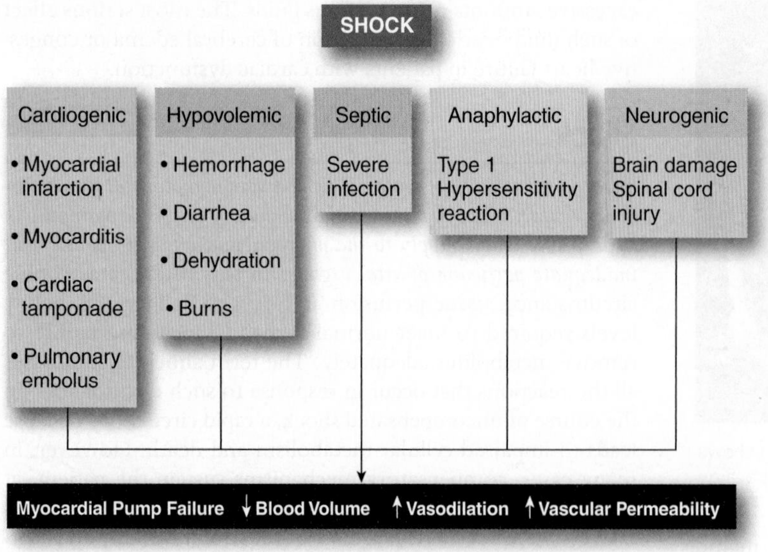

FIGURE 7-31. **Classification of shock.** Shock results from (1) an inability of the heart to pump adequately (cardiogenic shock), (2) decreased effective blood volume as a consequence of severely reduced blood or plasma volume (hypovolemic shock), or (3) widespread vasodilation (septic, anaphylactic or neurogenic shock). Increased vascular permeability may complicate vasodilation by contributing to reduced effective blood volume.

- **Septic shock** is caused by severe systemic microbial infections. The pathogenesis of septic shock is complex and is discussed in detail below.
- **Anaphylactic shock** is a consequence of a systemic type I hypersensitivity reaction, which leads to widespread vasodilation and increased vascular permeability.
- **Neurogenic shock** can follow acute injury to the brain or spinal cord, which impairs the neural control of vasomotor tone, causing generalized vasodilation. In the case of both anaphylactic and neurogenic shock, the subsequent redistribution of blood to the periphery, with or without increased vascular permeability, reduces the effective circulating blood and plasma volume. This effect ultimately leads to the same consequences as in hypovolemic shock.

In hypovolemic and cardiogenic shock, lower cardiac output and resultant decreased tissue perfusion are the key steps in the progression from reversible to irreversible shock. Cellular hypoxia is the common consequence of the initial decrease in tissue perfusion. Although such changes do not initially result in irreversible injury, a vicious circle of decreasing tissue perfusion and further cell injury is perpetuated by several mechanisms:

- Injury to endothelial cells, secondary to the hypoxia caused by decreased tissue perfusion and increased vascular permeability, leads to escape of fluid from the vascular compartment.
- Increased exudation of fluid from the circulation reduces (1) blood volume; (2) venous return; and (3) cardiac output, thereby aggravating hypoxic cell injury.
- Decreased perfusion of the kidneys and skeletal muscles results in metabolic acidosis, which in turn further decreases cardiac output and tissue perfusion.
- Decreased perfusion of the heart injures the myocardial cells and decreases their ability to pump blood, further reducing cardiac output and tissue perfusion.

Systemic Inflammatory Response Syndrome Characterizes Septic Shock

Systemic inflammatory response syndrome (SIRS) is an exaggerated and generalized manifestation of a local immune or inflammatory reaction, and is often fatal. SIRS is a hypermetabolic state that features two or more signs of systemic inflammation—such as fever, tachycardia, tachypnea, leukocytosis, or leukopenia—in the setting of a known cause of inflammation. **Septic shock** is defined as clinical SIRS so severe that it leads to organ dysfunction and hypotension. The mechanisms responsible for the development of septic shock are illustrated in Figure 7-32. These processes often progress to **multiple organ dysfunction syndrome** (MODS), a term used to describe otherwise unexplained abnormalities of organ function in critically ill patients (see below).

The massive inflammatory reaction defined by SIRS results from systemic release of cytokines, the most important being tumor necrosis factor (TNF), interleukin-1 (IL-1), IL-6, and platelet-activating factor (PAF). Over 30 endogenous mediators are described in this condition. Their interactions may be important in the pathogenesis of SIRS.

Septicemia with gram-negative organisms is the most common cause of septic shock. The invading bacteria release **endotoxin,** a lipopolysaccharide (LPS), whose toxic activity resides in the lipid A component. On entry into the circulation, LPS, via lipid A binds to LPS-binding protein, after which the complex binds to the CD14 receptor on the surface of monocyte/macrophages. The recognition complex resides on the plasma membrane and includes the toll-like receptor (TLR) family of proteins and CD14. TLRs represent the primary sensors of the innate immune system, which collectively recognize bacteria, fungi, and protozoa. Immediately downstream of TLR binding are the myeloid differentiation protein 88 (MyD 88), toll-interleukin-1 (TIR) domain-containing adaptor protein, TIR receptor domain-containing adaptor protein inducing interferon β (TRIF), and TRIF-related adaptor molecule. They mediate signaling through activation of the transcription factor, nuclear factor-kappaB (NF-κB) and upregulate TNF expression. LPS binding to TLR-4 causes mononuclear phagocytes to secrete large quantities of cytokines, such as TNF, IL-1, IL-6, IL-8, IL-12, and others, that mediate a variety of responses. These cytokines,

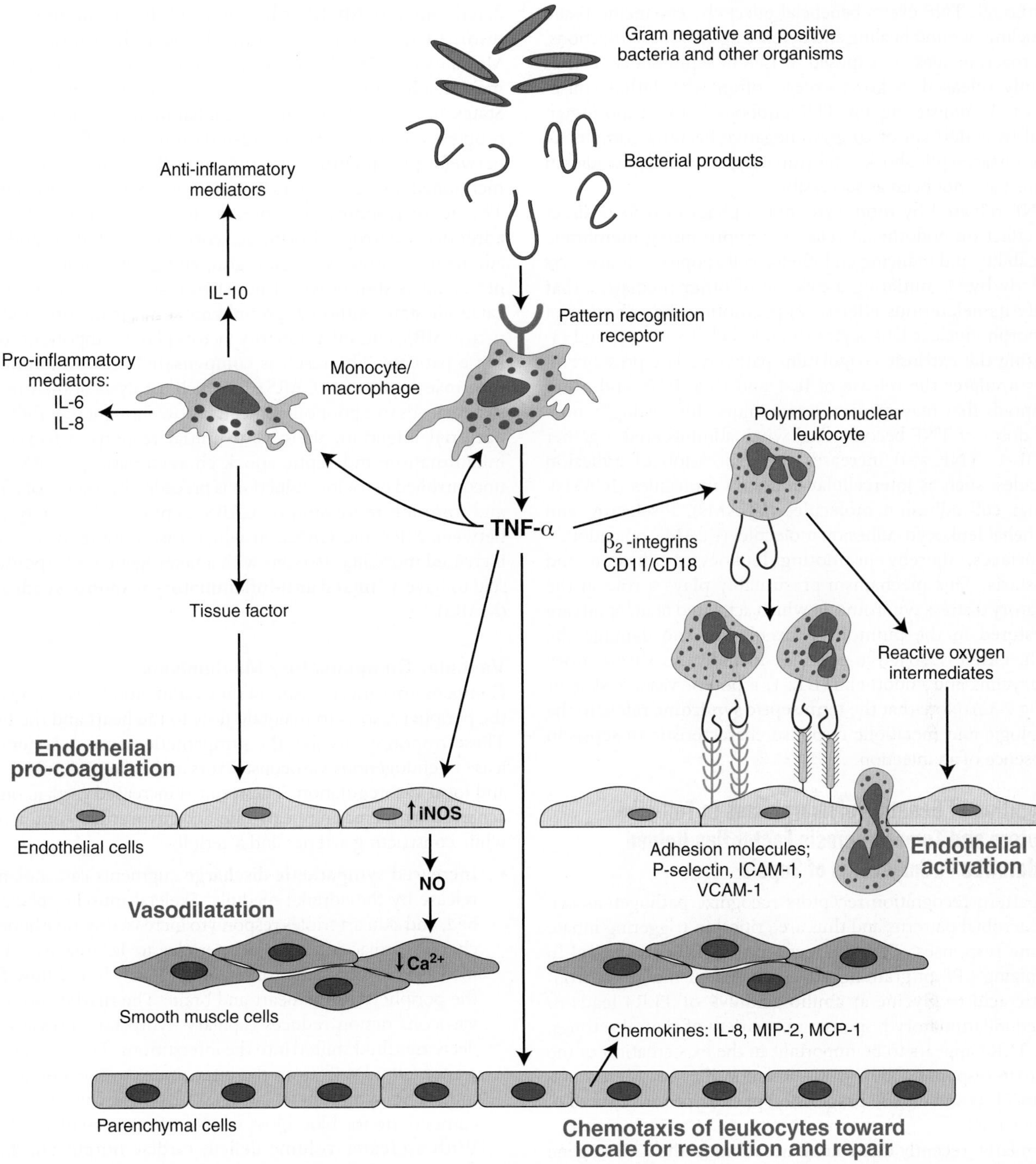

FIGURE 7-32. **Pathogenesis of endotoxic shock.** Sepsis is caused primarily by gram-negative bacteria and bacterial products such as endotoxin (lipopolysaccharide [LPS]) which is released into the circulation, where it binds to a pattern recognition receptor on the surface of monocyte/ macrophages. Such binding stimulates the secretion of substantial quantities of tumor necrosis factor-alpha (TNF-α). TNF-α mediates septic shock by a number of mechanisms: (1) stimulation of the release of various pro- and anti-inflammatory mediators; (2) induction of endothelial procoagulation by tissue factor, thereby leading to thrombosis and local ischemia; (3) direct cytotoxic damage to endothelial cells; (4) endothelial activation, which enhances the adherence of polymorphonuclear leukocytes; (5) stimulation of endothelial cell nitric oxide production and vasodilation; and (6) release of chemokines to attract leukocytes for resolution and repair of tissue injury. Ca^{2+} = calcium ion; ICAM = intercellular adhesion molecule; IL = interleukin; iNOS = inducible nitric oxide synthetase; MCP-1 = monocyte chemotactic protein-1; MIP-2 = macrophage-inflammatory protein-2; NO = nitric oxide; VCAM -1 = vascular cell adhesion molecule-1.

and subsequent production of nitric oxide (NO) and procoagulant proteins, ultimately cause the overwhelming cardiovascular collapse characteristic of septic shock. In this context activation of inducible NO synthase (iNOS) by TNF upregulates NO synthesis from L-arginine, an effect that is primarily responsible for the drop in blood pressure during sepsis. TNF is also involved in the pathogenesis of shock unassociated with endotoxemia (e.g., cardiogenic shock). LPS is the most potent stimulus for TNF release, but other antigens also promote its secretion. These include toxin-1 of the toxic shock syndrome; enterotoxin; antigens of mycobacteria, fungi, parasites, and viruses; and products of complement activation.

Although TNF exerts beneficial effects by enhancing tissue remodeling, wound healing and defense against local infections, when macrophages are exposed to LPS in septic shock TNF is suddenly released in great excess, often with lethal consequences. Administering anti-TNF antibody before exposing an animal to endotoxin or to gram-negative bacteria completely protects from septic shock. Unfortunately, comparable studies in humans have not been as successful.

TNF released by monocyte/macrophages exerts a direct toxic effect on endothelial cells by compromising membrane permeability and inducing endothelial cell apoptosis. It also acts indirectly by (1) initiating a cascade of other mediators that amplify its deleterious effects, (2) promoting the adhesion of polymorphonuclear leukocytes to endothelial surfaces, and (3) activating the extrinsic coagulation pathway. The presence of TNF stimulates the release of IL-1 and IL-6, PAF, and other eicosanoids that may mediate tissue injury. Interestingly, nonlethal doses of TNF become fatal when administered together with IL-1. TNF also increases the expression of adhesion molecules, such as intercellular adhesion molecules (ICAMs), vascular cell adhesion molecules (VCAMs), P-selectin, and endothelial-leukocyte adhesion molecules (ELAMs) on endothelial surfaces, thereby promoting leukocyte adhesion and leukostasis. This mechanism presumably plays a role in the respiratory distress syndrome, in which activated neutrophils are sequestered in the pulmonary circulation and damage the alveoli. Other vasoactive peptides include the vasodilatory prostacyclins and endothelin (ET)-1, a potent vasoconstrictor (see Fig 7-32). Note that the term **septic syndrome** refers to the physiologic and metabolic response characteristic of sepsis in the absence of an infection.

Recognition of Genetic Polymorphisms in Toll-Like Receptors and Tumor Necrosis Factor Has Helped Elucidate the Pathogenesis of Sepsis

TLR-pattern recognition receptors recognize pathogen-associated microbial patterns and thus are critical in triggering innate immune responses. Toll-like receptor-4 (TLR4) is critical in recognizing LPS of gram-negative bacteria. A mutation, from aspartic acid to glycine at amino acid 299 of TLR4 leads to reduced inflammatory responses in a variety of clinical settings. Thus, TLR4 appears to be important in the exacerbation of the endotoxin response and in sepsis. Relationships between mutations in TLRs and disease progression phenotypes are an area of intense study.

Similarly, recently discovered mutations in the TNF-α gene have improved understanding of the role of TNF-α in sepsis. For example a G to A base change at base 308 of the TNF-α promoter leads to enhanced promoter activity and increased expression of TNF-α and is associated with an increased risk of sepsis and shock.

Multiple Organ Dysfunction Syndrome (MODS) Is the End-Result of Shock

Improvements in the early treatment of shock and sepsis have allowed patients to survive long enough to manifest a new problem, progressive deterioration of organ function. Almost all septic shock patients suffer from dysfunction of at least one organ. However multiple organ dysfunction occurs in one third of patients with septic shock, trauma, or burns, and a quarter of those with acute pancreatitis. Whatever the cause, the clinical deterioration of MODS is held to result from common mechanisms of tissue injury subsumed under the rubric of SIRS. Mortality of SIRS/MODS exceeds 50%, making it responsible for most deaths in noncoronary intensive care units in the United States. In most circumstances the inflammatory reaction and the progression from sepsis to organ dysfunction reflects a balance between proinflammatory and antiinflammatory factors. As mentioned above, TNF-α, IL-1, and NO have systemic effects. The acute response to sepsis is characterized by release of adrenocorticotropic hormone, cortisol, adrenaline and noradrenaline, vasopressin, glucagon, and growth hormone. The net result is shut-down of noncritical systems and an overall catabolic state. Although proinflammatory mediators predominate in SIRS, anti-inflammatory factors play an important role in some patients. The result is **compensated anti-inflammatory response syndrome** (CARS), in which paralysis of the immune system leads to a poor outcome. It is now thought that following bacterial infection, there is an initial response of excessive inflammation and septic shock characteristic of SIRS. Such uncontrolled cytokine induction is preceded by a stage of anergy and immune repression or CARS. Septic patients may cycle between SIRS and CARS, in which case they tend to exhibit increased mortality. Persons with a heterogeneous response are said to have a **"mixed anti-inflammatory response syndrome"** (MARS).

Vascular Compensatory Mechanisms

Compensatory mechanisms in shock shift blood flow away from the periphery, so as to maintain flow to the heart and the brain. These responses involve the sympathetic nervous system, release of endogenous vasoconstrictors and hormonal substances, and local vasoregulation. The result is increased cardiac output achieved by increasing heart rate and myocardial contractility, while constricting arteries and arterioles.

- **Increased sympathetic discharge** augments catecholamine release by the adrenal medulla. Skeletal muscle, splanchnic bed, and skin arterioles respond to increased sympathetic discharge; cardiac and cerebral arterioles are less reactive. Thus, increased sympathetic tone works to shift blood flow from the periphery to the heart and brain. The marked arteriolar vasoconstriction reduces capillary hydrostatic pressure and decreases fluid shifted into the interstitium. This facilitates an osmotic fluid shift from the interstitium to the vascular system. The sympathetic–adrenal response can completely compensate for blood loss of 10% of intravascular volume. With a greater volume deficit, cardiac output and blood pressure are affected and blood flow to tissues is reduced.
- **The renin–angiotensin–aldosterone system** also helps compensate, by stimulating sodium and water reabsorption, thereby helping to maintain intravascular volume. A similar water-preserving action is provided by pituitary antidiuretic hormone.
- **Vascular autoregulation** preserves regional blood flow to vital organs, particularly the heart and brain, by vasodilation in the coronary and cerebral circulations in response to hypoxia and acidosis. Vasoconstriction mediated largely by α-adrenergic receptors in mesenteric venules and veins helps maintain cardiac filling and arterial pressure. Circulation to organs such as skin and skeletal muscles, which are less sensitive to hypoxia, does not display such tightly controlled autoregulation.

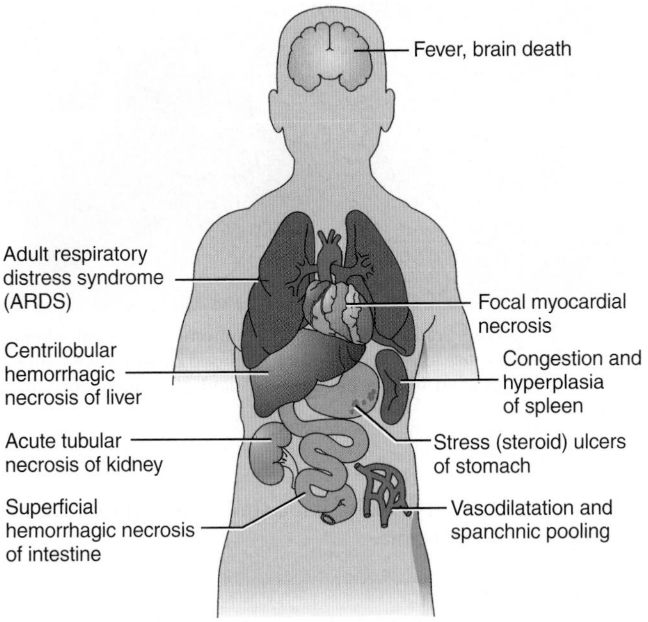

FIGURE 7-33. **Complications of shock.**

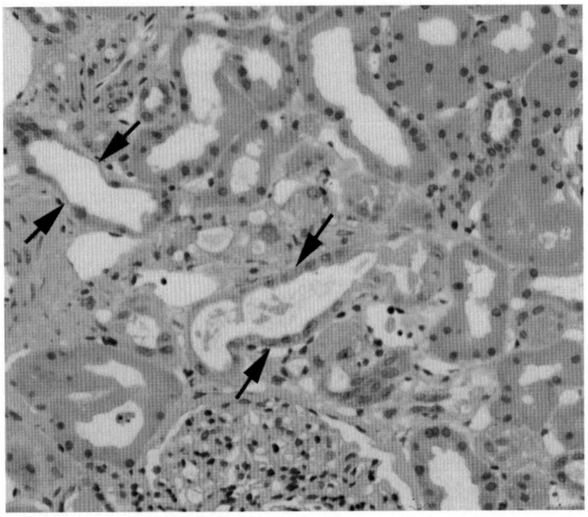

FIGURE 7-34. **Acute tubular necrosis.** A section of kidney shows swelling and degeneration of tubular epithelium. *Arrows* indicate the thinned and damaged epithelium.

PATHOLOGY: Shock is associated with specific changes in a number of organs (Fig. 7-33), including acute renal tubular necrosis, acute respiratory distress syndrome, liver failure, depression of host defense mechanisms, and heart failure.

Heart

The heart shows petechial hemorrhages of the epicardium and endocardium. Microscopically, necrotic foci in the myocardium range from loss of single fibers to large areas of necrosis. Prominent contraction bands are visible by light microscopy but are better seen by electron microscopy. Ultrastructurally, flattened areas of the intercalated disk are a sign of cell swelling, and invagination of adjacent cells is considered to be a catecholamine-induced lesion.

Kidney

Acute tubular necrosis (acute renal failure), a major complication of shock, has been divided into three phases: (1) **initiation**, from the onset of injury to the beginning of renal failure; (2) **maintenance**, from the onset of renal failure to a stable, reduced renal function; and (3) **recovery**. In those who survive an episode of shock, the recovery phase begins about 10 days after its onset and may last up to 8 weeks.

Renal blood flow is restricted to one-third of normal following the acute ischemic phase. This effect is even more severe in the outer cortex. The constriction of arterioles reduces the filtration pressure, thereby reducing the amount of filtrate and contributing to oliguria. Interstitial edema occurs, possibly through a process termed **backflow.** Excessive vasoconstriction is also related to stimulation of the renin–angiotensin system.

During acute renal failure, the kidney is large, swollen, and congested, although the cortex may be pale. A cross-section reveals blood pooling in the outer stripe of the medulla. Microscopically, fully developed acute tubular necrosis is evidenced by dilation of the proximal tubules and focal necrosis of cells (Fig. 7-34). Frequently, pigmented casts in tubular lumina indicate leakage of hemoglobin or myoglobin. Coarse, "ropy" casts are seen in the distal nephron and distal convoluted tubules. Interstitial edema is prominent in the cortex and mononuclear cells accumulate within tubules and surrounding interstitium. Acute tubular necrosis is discussed in more detail in Chapter 16.

Lung

After the onset of severe and prolonged shock, injury to alveolar walls can result in **shock lung**, which is a cause of **acute respiratory distress syndrome** (ARDS) (see Chapter 12). The sequence of changes is mediated by polymorphonuclear leukocytes and includes interstitial edema, necrosis of endothelial and alveolar epithelial cells, and formation of intravascular microthrombi and hyaline membranes lining the alveolar surface.

Macroscopically, the lung is firm and congested and a frothy fluid often exudes from the cut surface. Interstitial edema is first seen around peribronchial connective tissue and lymphatics, subsequently filling the interstitial connective tissue. In this initial period, a large fluid volume drains into the pulmonary lymphatics. If removal of this fluid becomes inadequate, or if the balance of forces that keep the fluid in the interstitial space is disturbed, alveolar edema develops.

Shock-induced lung injury leads to alveolar hyaline membranes (see Fig. 7-29), which also frequently line alveolar ducts and terminal bronchioles. These lung changes may heal entirely, but in half of patients, the repair processes cause a thickening of the alveolar wall. Type II pneumocytes proliferate to replace damaged type I pneumocytes and line the alveoli. Fibrous tissue proliferation may lead to organization of the alveolar exudate. These chronic changes may result in persistent respiratory distress and even death. Shock lung and ARDS are more fully discussed in Chapter 12.

Gastrointestinal Tract

Shock often results in diffuse gastrointestinal hemorrhage. Erosions of the gastric mucosa and superficial ischemic necrosis in the intestines are the usual sources of this bleeding. Interruption of the barrier function of the intestine may lead to septicemia. More-severe necrotizing lesions contribute to deterioration in the final phase of shock.

Liver

In patients who die in shock, the liver is enlarged and has a mottled cut surface that reflects marked centrilobular pooling of blood. The most prominent histologic lesion is centrilobular congestion and necrosis. The basis for the apparent increased sensitivity of centrilobular hepatocytes to shock may not simply represent their greater distance from the source of blood delivered via the portal tracts, a matter that is not settled (see Chapter 14).

Pancreas

The splanchnic vascular bed, which supplies the pancreas, is particularly affected by impaired circulation during shock. Resulting ischemic damage to the exocrine pancreas unleashes activated catalytic enzymes and causes acute pancreatitis, a complication that further promotes shock.

Brain

Brain lesions are rare in shock. Microscopic hemorrhages may be seen, but patients who recover do not ordinarily have neurologic deficits. In severe cases, particularly in persons with cerebral atherosclerosis, hemorrhage and necrosis may appear in the overlapping region between the terminal distributions of major arteries, so-called **watershed infarcts** (see Chapter 28).

Adrenals

In severe shock, adrenal glands exhibit conspicuous hemorrhage in the inner cortex. The hemorrhage is often focal. However, it can be massive and accompanied by hemorrhagic necrosis of the entire gland, as seen in the **Waterhouse-Friderichsen syndrome** (Fig. 7-35), typically associated with overwhelming meningococcal septicemia.

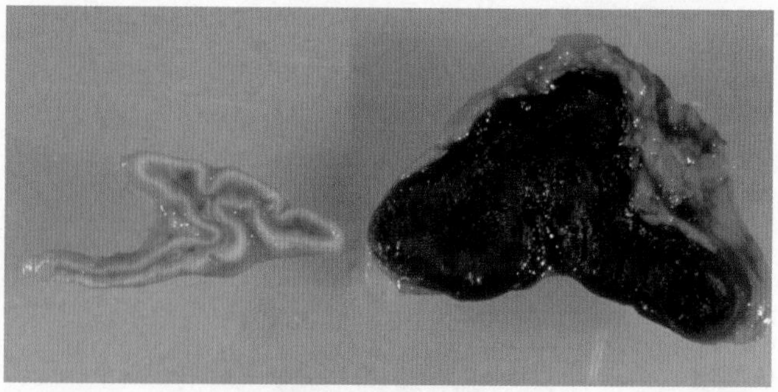

FIGURE 7-35. **Waterhouse-Friedrickson syndrome.** A normal adrenal gland *(left)* in contrast to an adrenal gland enlarged by extensive hemorrhage *(right)*, obtained from a patient who died of meningococcemic shock.

Host Defenses

The alterations of the immunologic system and host defenses in shock are not well understood, although it is common for patients who survive the acute phase of shock to succumb to subsequent overwhelming infection. It may well be that several factors interact, namely, ischemic colitis, tissue trauma, and immune and metabolic suppression of host defenses. Humoral immunity and phagocytic activity by leukocytes and macrophages are both depressed, but the mechanisms underlying these effects are not clear.

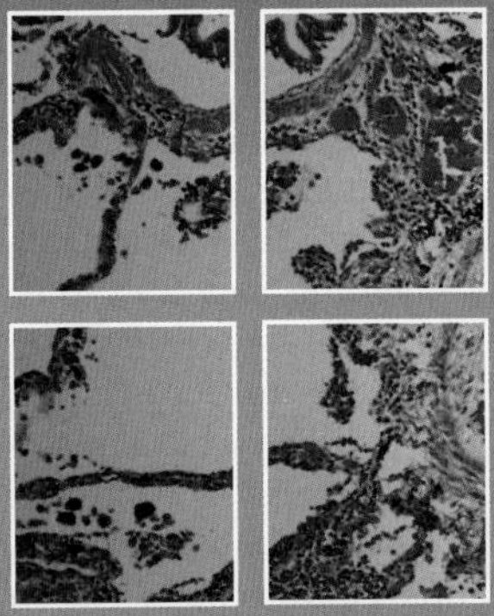

8 Environmental and Nutritional Pathology

David S. Strayer
Emanuel Rubin

Environmental pathology is the study of diseases caused by exposure to harmful external agents and deficiencies of vital substances. In a sense it encompasses all nutritional, infectious, chemical, and physical causes of illness. With heightened awareness of the fact that chemical agents may mediate tissue changes and recognition that many of these are environmental contaminants, "occupational pathology" has developed. In this chapter we concentrate on diseases caused by (1) exposure to toxic agents, (2) physical damage, and (3) nutritional deficiencies.

Smoking

Smoking tobacco is the single largest preventable cause of death in the United States, with direct health costs to the economy of tens of billions of dollars a year. *Over 400,000 deaths per year—about one sixth of the total deaths in the United States—occur prematurely because of smoking.* Estimates have incriminated tobacco in 11% to 30% of cancer deaths, 17% to 30% of cardiovascular deaths, 30% of deaths from lung diseases, and 20% to 30% of the incidence of low–birth-weight infants. Life expectancy is shortened, and overall mortality is proportional to the amount and duration of cigarette smoking, commonly quantitated as "pack-years" (Fig. 8-1). For example, a person who smokes two packs of cigarettes a day at the age of 30 years will live an average of 8 years less than a nonsmoker. The increasing adoption of smoking by many women has led to their being afflicted with the same epidemic of smoking-related disease that assaulted men more than a generation earlier. The characteristics of smoking-related illnesses reflect the amount smoked, not the gender of the smoker. In fact, mortality from lung cancer, almost all of which is related to cigarette smoking, exceeds that from cancers of the breast and prostate, the most common cancers in the United States. The excess mortality associated with cigarette smoking declines after one quits smoking: after 15 years of abstinence from cigarettes, the mortality of ex-smokers approaches that of people who have never smoked. Overall mortality among those who smoke only cigars or pipes is only slightly higher than that in the nonsmoking population.

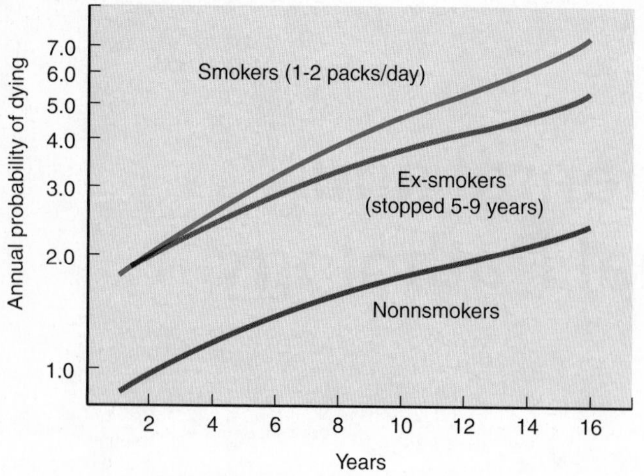

FIGURE 8-1. **The risk of dying in smokers and nonsmokers.** Note that the annual probability of an individual dying, indicated on the ordinate, is a logarithmic scale. Individuals who have smoked for 1 year have a twofold greater probability of dying than a nonsmoker, whereas those who have smoked for more than 15 years have more than a threefold greater probability of dying.

The major diseases responsible for excess mortality reported in cigarette smokers are, in order of frequency, coronary heart disease, lung cancer, and chronic obstructive pulmonary disease. Cancers of the oral cavity, larynx, esophagus, pancreas, bladder, kidney, colon, and cervix are all more common in smokers than in nonsmokers. Also, smokers show excess mortality from atherosclerotic aortic aneurysms and peptic ulcer disease.

Cardiovascular Disease Is a Major Complication of Smoking

Cigarette smoking is a major independent risk factor for myocardial infarction. It acts synergistically with other risk factors, such as elevated blood pressure and blood cholesterol levels (Fig. 8-2). Smoking precipitates initial myocardial infarction, increases risk for second heart attacks, and diminishes survival after a heart attack among those who continue to smoke. Smoking also increases the incidence of sudden cardiac death: it contributes to instability and erosion of atherosclerotic plaques and may lead to ischemia and rhythm disturbances as well.

Cigarette smoking is an independent risk factor for ischemic stroke. The risk correlates with the number of cigarettes smoked and is reduced after cessation of smoking. Tobacco use also increases risk of certain forms of intracranial hemorrhage. The combination of smoking and oral contraceptive use in women older than 35 years of age increases the likelihood of myocardial infarction. Similarly, use of cigarettes by women who are using oral contraceptives significantly increases their risk of stroke.

Atherosclerosis of the coronary arteries and aorta is more severe and extensive among cigarette smokers than among nonsmokers, and the effect is dose-related. As a consequence, cigarette smoking is a strong risk factor for atherosclerotic aortic aneurysms. The incidence and severity of atherosclerotic peripheral vascular disease are also remarkably increased by smoking. Smoking is also a major risk factor for coronary vasospasm. It disturbs regional coronary blood flow in patients with coronary artery disease and lowers the threshold for ventricular fibrillation and cardiac arrest in patients with established ischemic heart disease. The pharmacologic actions of nicotine itself, carbon monoxide (CO) inhalation, reduced plasma high-density lipoprotein levels, increased plasma fibrinogen levels, and higher leukocyte counts are all consequences of smoking that may predispose to myocardial infarction.

Buerger disease, a peculiar inflammatory and occlusive disease of the lower leg vasculature occurs almost only in heavy smokers, mainly Eastern European Jews (see Chapter 10). Although Buerger disease is unquestionably related to smoking, it is rare today.

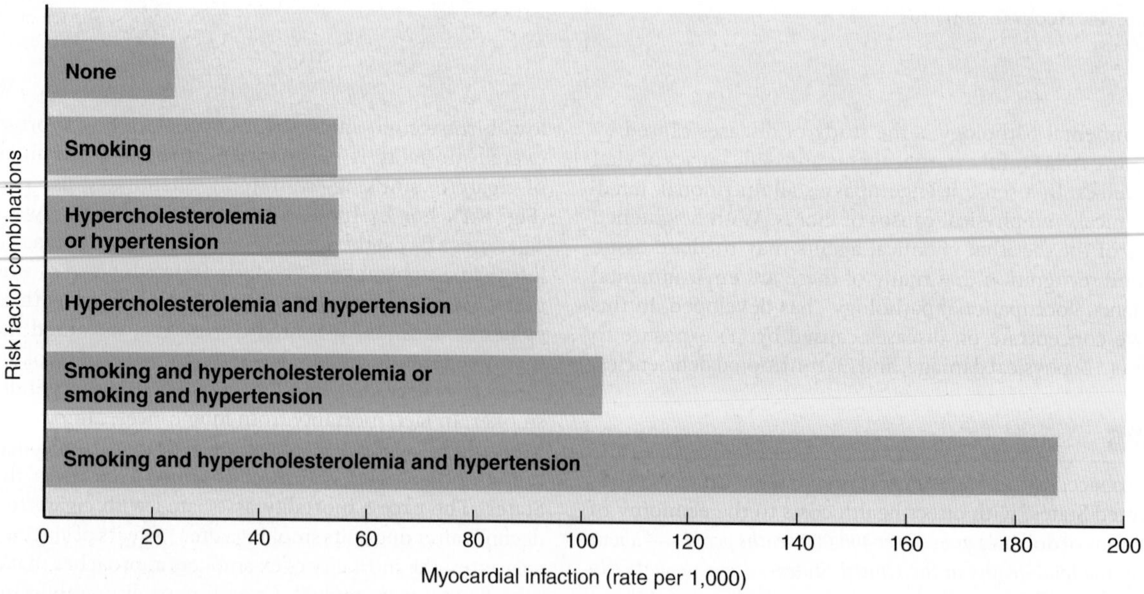

FIGURE 8-2. **The risk of myocardial infarction in cigarette smokers.** Smoking is an independent risk factor and increases the risk of a myocardial infarction to about the same extent as does hypertension or hypercholesterolemia alone. The effects of smoking are additive to those of these other two risk factors.

Cancer of the Lung Is Largely a Disease of Cigarette Smokers

More than 85% of deaths from lung cancer, the single most common cancer death in both men and women in the United States today, are attributed to cigarette smoking (Fig. 8-3). Although the precise offenders in cigarette smoke have not been identified, clearly cigarette smoke is toxic and carcinogenic to the bronchial mucosa. When cigarette smoke is passed through a filter, it is separated into gas and particulate phases. Cigarette tar, the material that is deposited on the filter, contains more than 3000 compounds, many of which have been identified as carcinogens, tumor promoters, and ciliotoxic agents. Compounds with similar toxic properties are found in the gas phase, but they are fewer. The risk of developing lung cancer is directly related to the number of cigarettes smoked.

Cigarette smoking is also an important factor in the induction of lung cancer that is associated with certain occupational exposures. For instance, uranium miners have an increased rate of lung cancer, presumably because of inhalation of radon daughters. However, the rate of lung cancer among miners who smoke is considerably higher than for non-miners with similar smoking habits. Another example is the case of asbestos workers. Whereas heavy smokers in the general population have a risk of lung cancer some 20 times greater than nonsmokers, asbestos workers who manifest pulmonary fibrosis and smoke heavily have a risk that is more than 60 times that of nonsmokers.

- **Cancers of the lip, tongue, and buccal mucosa** occur principally (>90%) in tobacco users. All forms of tobacco use—cigarette, cigar and pipe smoking, as well as tobacco chewing—expose the oral cavity to the compounds found in raw tobacco or tobacco smoke.

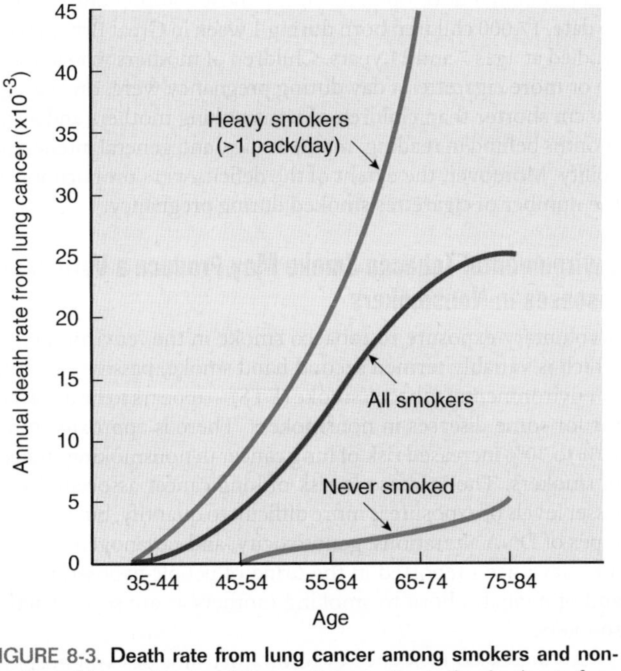

FIGURE 8-3. **Death rate from lung cancer among smokers and nonsmokers.** Nonsmokers exhibit a small, linear rise in the death rate from lung cancer from the age of 50 onward. By contrast, those who smoke more than one pack per day show an exponential rise in the annual death rate from lung cancer starting at about age 35. By age 70, heavy smokers have about a 20-fold greater death rate from lung cancer than nonsmokers.

- **Cancer of the larynx,** is similarly related to cigarette smoking. In some large studies, white male smokers have from 6 to 13 greater death rate from laryngeal cancer as nonsmokers.
- **Cancer of the esophagus** in the United States and Great Britain is estimated to result from smoking in 80% of cases.
- **Cancer of the bladder** is twice as frequent a cause of death in cigarette smokers as in nonsmokers. In fact, 30% to 40% of all bladder cancers are attributable to smoking. As with most tobacco-related disorders, there is a clear dose-response relationship between incidence of bladder cancer, numbers of cigarettes smoked per day, and duration of cigarette smoking.
- **Carcinoma of the kidney** is increased 50% to 100% among smokers. A modest increase in cancer of the renal pelvis has also been documented.
- **Cancer of the pancreas** has shown a steady increase in incidence, which is, at least in part, related to cigarette smoking. The risk ratio in male smokers for adenocarcinoma of the pancreas is 2 to 3 and a dose-response relationship exists. Men who smoke over two packs a day have five times greater risk of developing pancreatic cancer than nonsmokers.
- **Cancer of the uterine cervix** is significantly increased in women smokers. It has been estimated that about 30% of cervical cancer mortality is attributable to this habit.
- **Acute myelogenous leukemia** has been reported by some as associated with smoking, but the issue is controversial.

Smokers Are At Higher Risk for Certain Nonneoplastic Diseases

- **Chronic bronchitis and emphysema** occur primarily in cigarette smokers. The incidence of these diseases is a function of the amount of cigarettes smoked (Fig. 8-4) (see Chapter 12).
- **Peptic ulcer disease** is 70% more common in male cigarette smokers than in nonsmokers.
- **Osteoporosis** in women is exacerbated by tobacco use. Women who smoke one pack of cigarettes per day during their reproductive period will exhibit a 5% to 10% deficit in bone density at menopause. This deficit is enough to increase the risk of bone fractures.
- **Thyroid diseases** are linked to cigarette smoking. The most conspicuous association is with Graves disease, especially when hyperthyroidism is complicated by exophthalmos.
- **Ocular diseases,** particularly macular degeneration and cataracts are reportedly more frequent in smokers.

Smoking Impairs Female Reproductive Function

Women who smoke experience an **earlier menopause** than nonsmokers, possibly because of the effects of tobacco on estrogen metabolism.

In the liver, estradiol is hydroxylated to estrone, which then enters one of two irreversible metabolic pathways. In one, 16-hydroxylation leads to production of estriol, a potent estrogen. In the other, 2-hydroxylation yields methoxyestrone, which has no estrogenic activity. *In female smokers, the latter pathway, i.e., the one that leads to the inactive metabolite, is stimulated. Consequently circulating levels of estriol, the active estrogen, are reduced.* The increased incidence of postmenopausal osteoporosis mentioned above has been attributed to decreased estriol levels.

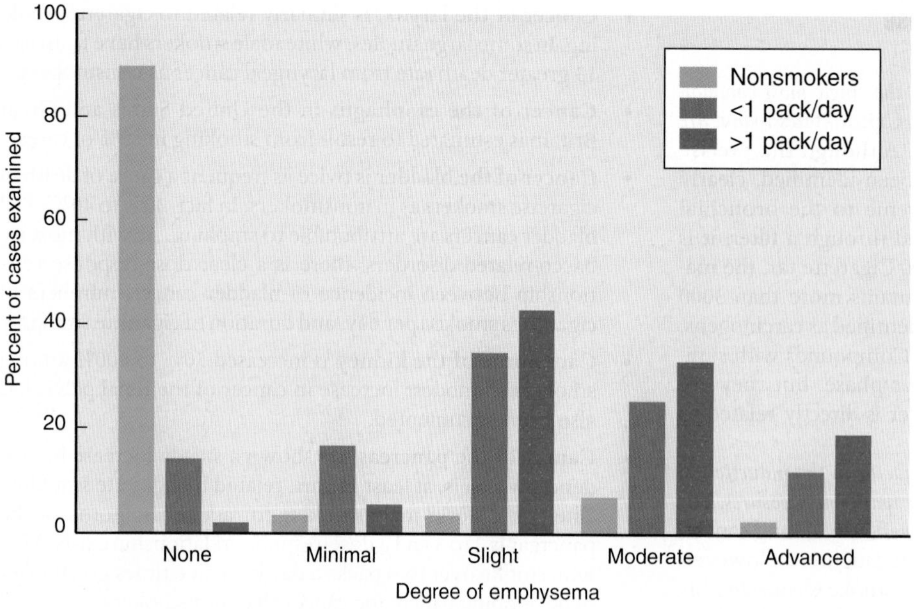

FIGURE 8-4. **The association between cigarette smoking and pulmonary emphysema.** Some 90% of nonsmokers have no detectable emphysema at autopsy. In contrast, virtually all those who smoke more than one pack per day have morphologic evidence of emphysema at autopsy. Emphysema shows a slight dose dependence on the number of cigarettes smoked. Those who smoke less than one pack per day tend to have less severe emphysema, but 85% to 90% of such smokers have some emphysema at autopsy.

Fetal Tobacco Syndrome Produces Smaller Infants

Maternal cigarette smoking impairs the development of the fetus. Infants born to women who smoke during pregnancy are, on average, 200 g lighter than infants born to comparable women who do not smoke. *These infants are not born preterm but rather are small for gestational age at every stage of pregnancy.* In fact, 20% to 40% of the incidence of low birth weight can be attributed to maternal cigarette smoking (Fig. 8-5). Thus, this effect of smoking is not idiosyncratic but reflects a direct retardation of fetal growth.

The harmful consequences of maternal cigarette smoking on the fetus are illustrated by its effect on the uteroplacental unit. Perinatal mortality is higher among offspring of smokers, the increases ranging from 20% among progeny of women who smoke less than a pack per day to almost 40% among offspring of those who smoke over one pack per day, with the excess mortality reflecting problems related to the uteroplacental system. *Incidences of abruptio placentae, placenta previa, uterine bleeding, and premature rupture of membranes are all increased* (Fig. 8-6). These complications of smoking tend to occur at times when the fetus is not viable or is at great risk, i.e., from 20 to 32 weeks' of gestation.

Children born of cigarette-smoking mothers have been reported to be more susceptible to several respiratory diseases, including respiratory infections and otitis media.

Substantial evidence indicates that maternal cigarette smoking inflicts lasting harm on children, and impairs physical, cognitive, and emotional development. Thus, these children showed measurable deficits in physical growth, intellectual maturation, and emotional development. In the most comprehensive study to date, 17,000 children born during 1 week in Great Britain were studied at ages 7 and 11 years. Children of mothers who smoked 10 or more cigarettes a day during pregnancy were, on average, 1.0 cm shorter than children of nonsmoking mothers and 3 to 5 months behind in reading, mathematics, and general intellectual ability. Moreover, the extent of the deficits were proportional to the number of cigarettes smoked during pregnancy.

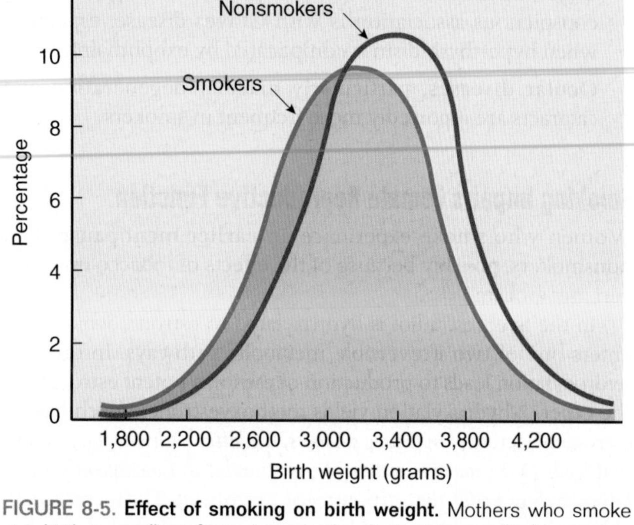

FIGURE 8-5. **Effect of smoking on birth weight.** Mothers who smoke give birth to smaller infants. In particular, the incidence of babies weighing less than 3000 g is increased significantly by smoking.

Environmental Tobacco Smoke May Produce a Variety of Diseases in Nonsmokers

Involuntary exposure to tobacco smoke in the environment—which is variably termed second-hand smoke, passive smoking, or environmental tobacco smoke (ETS)—appears to be a risk factor for some diseases in nonsmokers. There is approximately a 20% to 30% increased risk of lung cancer in nonsmoking spouses of smokers. The increase in risk of lung cancer associated with lesser levels of exposure is more difficult to quantify, but the same types of DNA alterations, genotoxicity, and carcinogen metabolites have been reported in the urine of people exposed to ETS and of neonates born to smoking mothers as are seen in active smokers.

An increased incidence of respiratory illnesses and hospitalizations has been reported among infants whose parents smoke, and several studies have reported mild impairment of pulmonary function among children of smokers and exacerbation of preexisting asthma. Reduced indices of pulmonary function are also seen in children of smokers.

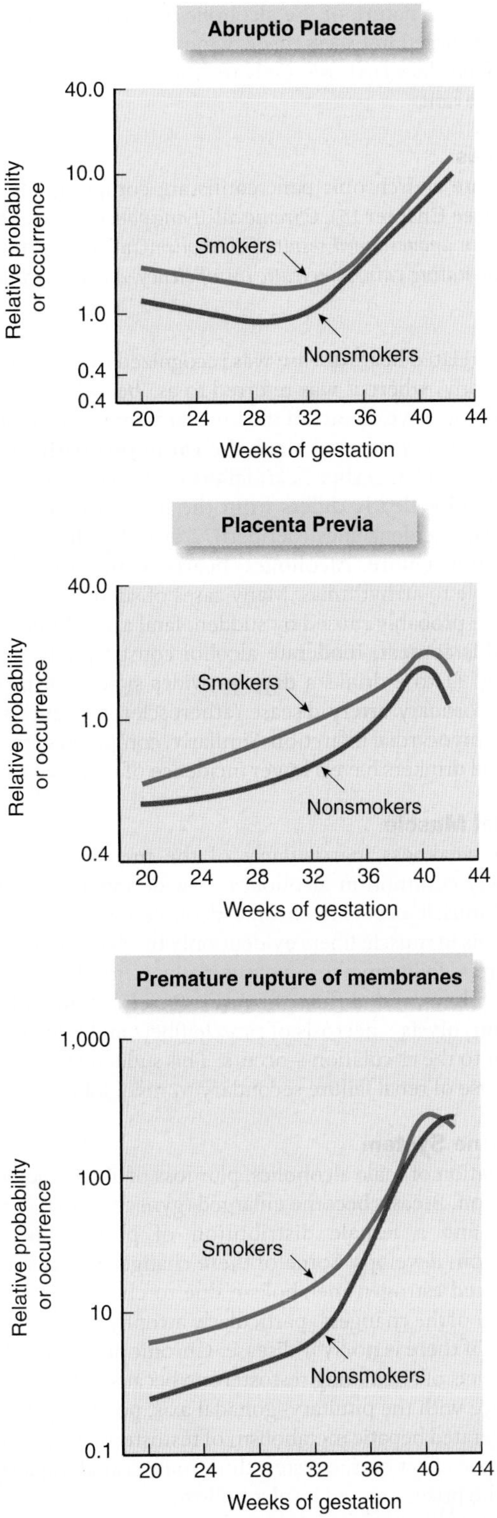

FIGURE 8-6. **Effect of smoking on the incidence of abruptio placentae (*top*), placenta previa (*middle*), and the premature rupture of amniotic membranes (*bottom*).** In each, the ordinate shows the probability of one of three complications of the third trimester of pregnancy. Note that it is a logarithmic scale. Smoking increases the probability of abruptio placentae and premature rupture of the amniotic membranes prior to 34 weeks' of gestation, at which time the fetus is still premature. Smoking increases the risk of placenta previa up to 40 weeks' of gestation.

ETS has been linked to an increased risk of both coronary artery disease and sudden death. The magnitude of the risk is dose-dependent and disproportionate to the level of smoke exposure as compared to smokers. Nonsmokers are highly sensitive to certain effects of ETS, including increased platelet aggregation, endothelial cell damage, impaired vasodilation, lower blood levels of high-density lipoprotein (HDL), oxidative stress, and impaired responsiveness to oxidative stress. In one study, the city of Helena, Montana banned cigarette smoking in workplaces and public places. This ban was overturned by court order 6 months later. During the interval when the ban was in effect, the number of acute cardiac events leading to hospital admission decreased by about 50%. When the ban on smoking was removed, hospital admissions for acute cardiac events rebounded almost to the levels seen before the ban was instituted.

Alcoholism

Alcoholism is addiction to ethanol that features dependence and withdrawal symptoms and results in acute and chronic toxic effects of alcohol on the body. It is estimated that there are about 12 million alcoholics in the United States, about one-tenth of the population at risk. The proportion has been estimated to be even higher in other countries. Certain ethnic groups, such as Native Americans and Eskimos, have high rates of alcoholism, while others, such as Chinese and Jews, are less afflicted. Although alcoholism is more common in men, the number of female alcoholics has been increasing.

Chronic alcoholism has been defined as regular intake of sufficient alcohol to injure a person socially, psychologically, or physically. Although there are no firm rules, for most persons, daily consumption of more than 45 g alcohol should probably be discouraged, and 100 g or more a day may be dangerous (10 g alcohol = 1 oz, or 30 mL, of 86 proof [43%] spirits).

The short-term effects of alcohol on the brain are familiar to most people, but the mechanism of inebriation is not understood. Like other anesthetic agents, alcohol is a central nervous system (CNS) depressant. However, it is such a weak anesthetic that it must be drunk by the glassful to exert any significant effect. In a normal person, characteristic behavioral changes can be detected at low alcohol concentrations (below 50 mg/dL). Levels above 80 to 100 mg/dL are usually associated with gross incoordination, and in American jurisdictions are considered legal evidence of intoxication while driving a motor vehicle. At levels above 300 mg/dL, most people become comatose and at concentrations above 400 mg/dL, death from respiratory failure is common. In humans, the LD_{50} (median lethal dose) is about 5 g of alcohol per kilogram of body weight.

The situation is somewhat different in chronic alcoholics, who develop CNS tolerance to alcohol. Such persons may easily tolerate blood alcohol levels of 100 to 200 mg/dL; and in fatal automobile accidents, blood levels of 500 to 600 mg/dL or more have been found by medical examiners. The mechanism underlying tolerance has not been established.

Acute alcohol intoxication is hardly a benign condition. Some 40% of all fatalities from motor vehicle accidents involve alcohol—about 16,600 deaths in 2004 in the United States. Alcoholism is also a major contributor to fatal home accidents, death in fires, and suicide.

Many chronic diseases associated with alcoholism were once attributed to malnutrition, and some alcoholics do suffer from nutritional deficiencies, such as thiamine deficiency (Wernicke

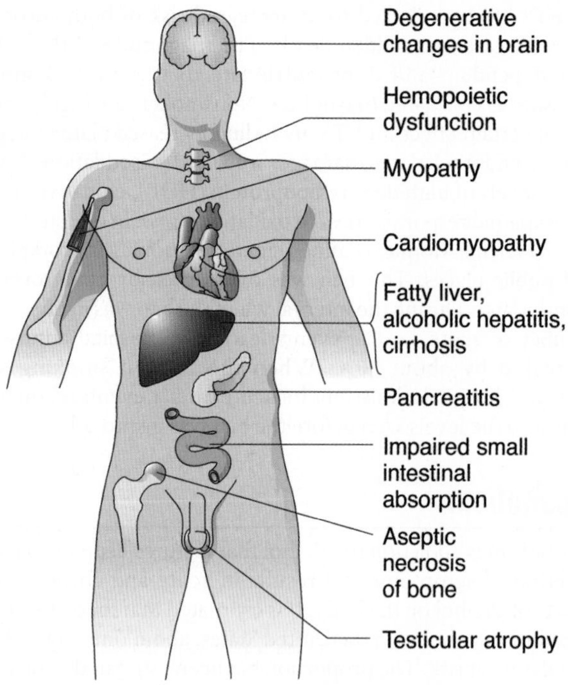

FIGURE 8-7. **Complications of chronic alcohol abuse.**

encephalopathy) or folic acid deficiency (megaloblastic anemia). *However, most alcoholics have adequate diets, and the great majority of alcohol-related disorders should be attributed to the toxic effects of alcohol.* The diseases associated with alcoholism are discussed in detail in chapters dealing with individual organs, and we restrict this discussion to the spectrum of disease (Fig. 8-7).

Alcohol Ingestion Affects Organs and Tissues

Liver

Alcoholic liver disease, the most common medical complication of alcoholism, has been known for thousands of years and accounts for a large proportion of cases of cirrhosis of the liver (Fig. 8-8) *in industrialized countries.* The nature of the alcoholic beverage is largely irrelevant; consumed in excess, beer, wine, whiskey, hard cider, and so on all produce cirrhosis. Only the total daily dose of alcohol itself is relevant.

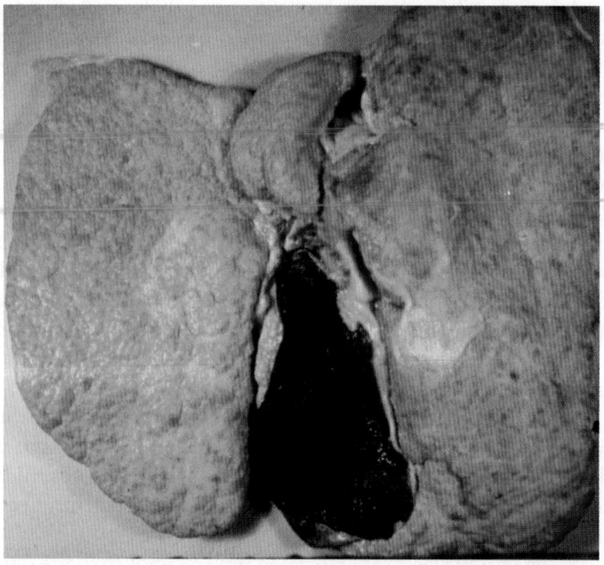

FIGURE 8-8. **Cirrhosis of the liver in a chronic alcoholic.** The surface displays innumerable small nodules of hepatocytes separated by interconnecting bands of fibrous tissue. The dark structure is the gallbladder.

Pancreas

Both acute and chronic pancreatitis are complications of alcoholism (see Chapter 15). *Chronic calcifying pancreatitis, on the other hand, is an unquestioned result of alcoholism and an important cause of incapacitating pain, pancreatic insufficiency, and pancreatic stones.*

Heart

Alcohol-related heart disease was recognized over a century ago in Germany, where it was referred to as "beer-drinker's heart." This degenerative disease of the myocardium is a form of dilated cardiomyopathy, termed **alcoholic cardiomyopathy** and leads to low-output congestive heart failure (see Chapter 11). This cardiomyopathy clearly differs from the heart disease associated with thiamine deficiency (beriberi), a disorder characterized by high-output failure. Alcoholics' hearts seem also to be more susceptible to arrhythmias. Many cases of sudden death in alcoholics are probably caused by sudden, fatal arrhythmias.

In this context, moderate alcohol consumption, or "social drinking" (1 to 2 drinks a day), provides significant protection against coronary artery disease (atherosclerosis) and its consequence, myocardial infarction. Similarly, compared with abstainers, social drinkers have a lower incidence of ischemic stroke.

Skeletal Muscle

Muscle weakness, particularly of the proximal muscles, is extremely common in alcoholics. A wide range of changes in skeletal muscle occurs in chronic alcoholics, varying from mild alterations in muscle fibers evident only by electron microscopy to severe, debilitating chronic myopathy, with degeneration of muscle fibers and diffuse fibrosis. Rarely, **acute alcoholic rhabdomyolysis**—necrosis of muscle fibers and release of myoglobin into the circulation—occurs. This sudden event can be fatal because of renal failure secondary to myoglobinuria.

Endocrine System

Feminization of male alcoholics, plus loss of libido and potency, is common. Breasts become enlarged (gynecomastia), body hair is lost, and a female distribution of pubic hair (female escutcheon) develops. Some of these changes can be attributed to impaired estrogen metabolism due to chronic liver disease, but many of the changes—particularly atrophy of the testes—occur even if there is no liver disease. Chronic alcoholism leads to lower levels of circulating testosterone because of a complex interference with the pituitary–gonadal axis, possibly complicated by accelerated hepatic metabolism of testosterone. Alcohol has a direct toxic effect on the testes; thus, male sexual impairment is one of the prices exacted by alcoholism.

Gastrointestinal Tract

Since the esophagus and stomach may be exposed to 10 M ethanol, it is not surprising that a direct toxic effect on the mucosa of these organs is common. Injury to the mucosa of both organs is potentiated by hypersecretion of gastric hydrochloric acid stimulated by ethanol. **Reflux esophagitis** may be particularly painful, and peptic ulcers are also more common in alcoholics. Violent retching may lead to tears at the esophageal-gastric junction (**Mallory-Weiss syndrome**), sometimes severe enough to cause exsanguinating hemorrhage (see Chapter 13). Small intestine mucosal cells are also exposed to circulating alcohol, and a variety of absorptive abnormalities and ultrastructural changes have been demonstrated. Alcohol inhibits active transport of amino acids, thiamine, and vitamin B_{12}.

Blood

Megaloblastic anemia is not uncommon in alcoholics, and reflects a combination of dietary deficiency of folic acid and the fact that alcohol is a weak folic acidantagonist in humans. Moreover, folate absorption by the small intestine may be decreased in alcoholics. In addition, chronic ethanol intoxication leads directly to an **increase in mean corpuscular volume erythrocytes.** In the presence of alcoholic cirrhosis, the spleen is often enlarged by portal hypertension; in such cases, **hypersplenism** often causes **hemolytic anemia.** Acute transient **thrombocytopenia** is common after acute alcohol intoxication and may result in bleeding. Alcohol also interferes with platelet aggregation, thereby contributing to bleeding.

Bone

Chronic alcoholics, particularly postmenopausal women, are at increased risk for **osteoporosis.** Although it is well established that alcohol, at least in vitro, inhibits osteoblast function, the precise mechanism responsible for accelerated bone loss is not understood. Interestingly, moderate alcohol intake seems to exert a protective effect against osteoporosis. Male alcoholics exhibit an unusually high incidence of **aseptic necrosis of the head of the femur.** The mechanism for this complication is also obscure.

Immune System

Alcoholics seem to be prone to many infections (particularly pneumonias) with organisms that are unusual in the general population, such as *Haemophilus influenzae*. Experimentally, a number of alcohol-induced effects on immune function have been reported.

Nervous System

General cortical atrophy of the brain is common in alcoholics and may reflect a toxic effect of alcohol (see Chapter 28). By contrast, most of the characteristic brain diseases in alcoholics are probably a result of nutritional deficiency.

- **Wernicke encephalopathy** is caused by thiamine deficiency and is characterized by mental confusion, ataxia, abnormal ocular motility, and polyneuropathy, reflecting pathologic changes in the diencephalon and brainstem.
- **Korsakoff psychosis** is characterized by retrograde amnesia and confabulatory symptoms. It was once believed to be pathognomonic of chronic alcoholism but has also been seen in several organic mental syndromes and is considered nonspecific.
- **Alcoholic cerebellar degeneration** is differentiated from other acquired or familial cerebellar degeneration by the uniformity of its manifestations. Progressive unsteadiness of gait, ataxia, incoordination, and reduced deep tendon reflex activity are present.
- **Central pontine myelinolysis** is another characteristic change in the brain of alcoholics, apparently caused by electrolyte imbalance—usually after electrolyte therapy, after an alcoholic binge, or during withdrawal. In this complication, a progressive weakness of bulbar muscles terminates in respiratory paralysis.
- **Amblyopia** (impaired vision) is occasionally seen in alcoholics. It may reflect alcohol-related decreases in tissue vitamin A, although other vitamin deficiencies may also be involved.
- **Polyneuropathy** is common in chronic alcoholics. It is usually associated with deficiencies of thiamine and other B vitamins, but a direct neurotoxic effect of ethanol may play a role. The most common complaints include numbness, paresthesias, pain, weakness, and ataxia.

Fetal Alcohol Syndrome Results from Alcohol Abuse in Pregnancy

Infants born to mothers who consume excess alcohol during pregnancy may show a cluster of abnormalities that together constitute the fetal alcohol syndrome. These include growth retardation, microcephaly, facial dysmorphology, neurologic dysfunction, and other congenital anomalies. About 6% of the offspring of alcoholic mothers are afflicted by the full syndrome. More often, exposure of the fetus to high concentrations of ethanol leads to less severe abnormalities, prominent among which are mental retardation, intrauterine growth retardation, and minor dysmorphic features. Animal models of fetal alcohol syndrome have demonstrated that ethanol exposure at certain phases of gestation causes apoptosis of some cell populations. Fetal alcohol syndrome is discussed in greater detail in Chapter 6.

Alcohol Increases the Risk of Some Cancers

Cancers of the oral cavity, larynx, and esophagus occur more often in alcoholics than in the general population. As most alcoholics are also smokers, the differential contributions of ethanol and cigarette smoke to these observed increases are not defined.

The Mechanisms by Which Alcohol Injures Tissues Are Not Understood

The pathogenesis of ethanol-induced organ damage remains obscure. In the liver, the change in the redox potential occasioned by the metabolism of ethanol has been proposed as a major factor. During the oxidation of ethanol to acetaldehyde, NAD is reduced to NADH, thereby greatly increasing the reducing power of the cell. However, although certain metabolic abnormalities may be attributed to this change in the NAD/NADH ratio, no tissue injury has been directly shown to be caused by it. Moreover, other organs that also exhibit alcohol-induced injury, such as the heart and the pancreas, do not metabolize ethanol to any appreciable extent.

Acetaldehyde is the highly toxic product of alcohol metabolism. In the liver, acetaldehyde is rapidly converted by aldehyde dehydrogenase to acetate, but measurable levels of acetaldehyde can be found in the liver. However, circulating levels of acetaldehyde are extremely low, and it is difficult to attribute all of the changes associated with alcoholism to this metabolite. Other metabolites that have been proposed as causes of tissue injury include fatty acid ethyl esters, phosphatidyl ethanol, and hydroxyethanol.

An effect of ethanol common to all cells, regardless of their origin or location, is disordering of cell membranes. Like all anesthetics, ethanol intercalates within the lipid bilayer and decreases the molecular order of the acyl chains of phospholipids (a process known as fluidization). As an adaptive response, the composition of the membranes is changed, so that they become resistant to this fluidizing effect of ethanol. The relationship of this effect to cell injury requires further study.

Drug Abuse

Drug abuse has been defined as "the use of any substance in a manner that deviates from the accepted medical, social, or legal patterns within a given society." For the most part, drug abuse involves agents that are used to alter mood and perception. These include (1) derivatives of opium (heroin, morphine); (2) depressants (barbiturates, tranquilizers, alcohol); (3) stimulants (cocaine, amphetamines), marijuana, psychedelic drugs (PCP, lysergic acid diethylamide [LSD]), and (4) inhalants (amyl nitrite, organic solvents such as those in glue). Use of illicit drugs is estimated to cause about 17,000 deaths a year in the United States.

Illicit Drugs Are Responsible for Many Pathologic Syndromes

Heroin

Heroin is a common illicit opiate used to induce euphoria. It is usually taken subcutaneously or intravenously and in the usual dosage is effective for about 5 hours. Overdoses are characterized by hypothermia, bradycardia, and respiratory depression. Other opiates that are subject to abuse include morphine, Dilaudid, and oxycodone.

Cocaine

Cocaine is an alkaloid derived from South American coca leaves. The more potent freebase form of cocaine is hard and is "cracked" into smaller pieces that are smoked ("crack"). The half-life of cocaine in the blood is about 1 hour.

Cocaine users report extreme euphoria and heightened sensitivity to a variety of stimuli. However, with addiction, paranoid states and conspicuous emotional lability occur. The mechanism of action of cocaine is related to its interference with the reuptake of the neurotransmitter dopamine.

Cocaine overdose leads to anxiety and delirium and occasionally to seizures. Cardiac arrhythmias and other effects on the heart may cause sudden death in otherwise apparently healthy persons. Chronic abuse of cocaine is associated with the occasional development of a characteristic dilated cardiomyopathy, which may be fatal.

Amphetamines

Amphetamines, mainly metamphetamine, are sympathomimetic and resemble cocaine in their effects, although they have longer duration of action. The most serious complications of the abuse of amphetamines are seizures, cardiac arrhythmias, and hyperthermia. Amphetamine use has been reported to lead to vasculitis of the CNS and both subarachnoid and intracerebral hemorrhages have been described.

Hallucinogens

Hallucinogens are a group of chemically unrelated drugs that alter perception and sensory experience.

Phencyclidine (PCP) is an anesthetic agent that has psychedelic or hallucinogenic effects. As a recreational drug, it is known as "angel dust" and is taken orally, intranasally or by smoking. The anesthetic properties of phencyclidine lead to a diminished capacity to perceive pain and, therefore, to self-injury and trauma. Other than the behavioral effects, PCP commonly produces tachycardia and hypertension. High doses result in deep coma, seizures, and even decerebrate posturing.

LSD (lysergic acid diethylamide) is a hallucinogenic drug whose popularity peaked in the late 1960s, and is little used today. It causes perceptual distortion of the senses, interference with logical thought, alteration of time perception, and a sense of depersonalization. "Bad trips" are characterized by anxiety and panic and objectively by sympathomimetic effects that include tachycardia, hypertension, and hyperthermia. Large overdoses cause coma, convulsions, and respiratory arrest.

Organic Solvents

The recreational inhalation of organic solvents is widespread, particularly among adolescents. Various commercial preparations such as fingernail polish, glues, plastic cements, and lighter fluid are all sniffed. Among the active ingredients are benzene, carbon tetrachloride, acetone, xylene, and toluene. However, many of these compounds are also industrial solvents and reagents, and so chronic low-level occupational exposure occurs. These compounds are all CNS depressants, although early effects (e.g., with xylene) may be excitatory. Acute intoxication with organic solvents resembles inebriation with alcohol. Large doses produce nausea and vomiting, hallucinations, and eventually coma. Respiratory depression and death may follow. Chronic exposure to, or abuse of, organic solvents may result in damage to the brain, kidneys, liver, lungs, and hematopoietic system. Benzene, for example is a bone marrow toxin and has been associated with the development of acute myelogenous leukemia. Unfortunately, for many such chemicals, occupational exposures are to solvents and solvent vapors, which are usually mixtures of different chemical species.

Intravenous Drug Abuse Has Many Medical Complications

Apart from reactions related to pharmacologic or physiological effects of substance abuse, the most common complications (15% of directly drug-related deaths) are caused by introducing infectious organisms by a parenteral route. Most occur at the site of injection: cutaneous abscesses, cellulitis, and ulcers (Fig. 8-9). When these heal, "track marks" persist and these areas may be hypopigmented or hyperpigmented. Thrombophlebitis of the veins draining sites of injection is common. Intravenous introduction of bacteria may lead to septic complications in internal

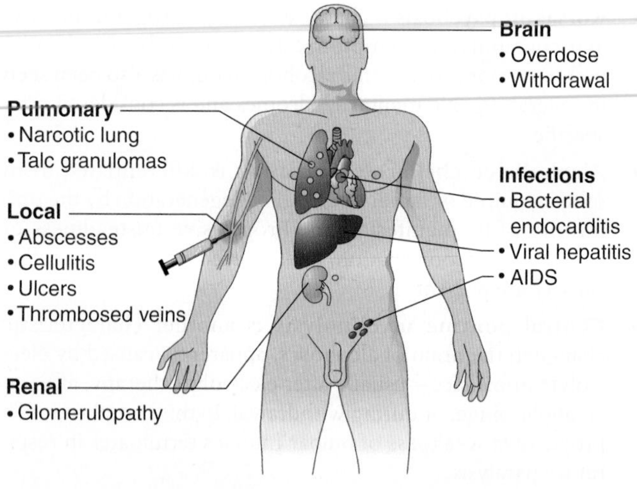

FIGURE 8-9. Complications of intravenous drug abuse. AIDS 5 acquired immunodeficiency syndrome.

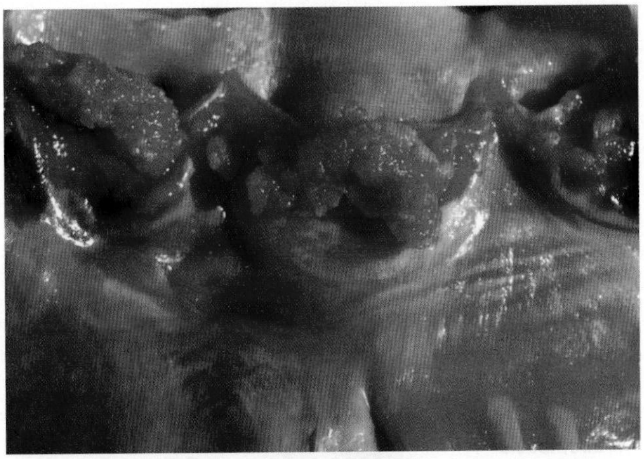

FIGURE 8-10. **Bacterial endocarditis.** The aortic valve of an intravenous drug abuser displays adherent vegetations.

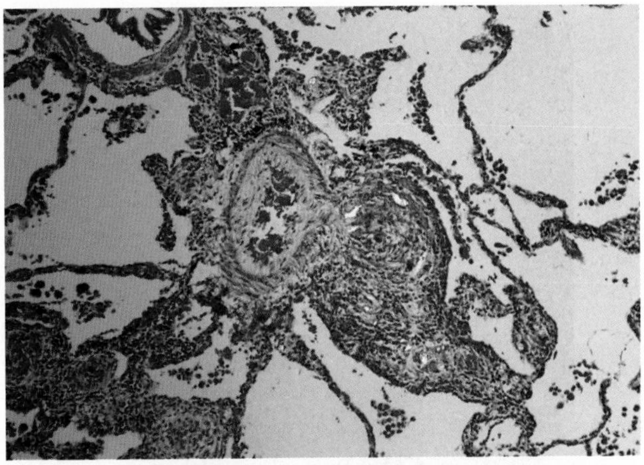

FIGURE 8-12. **Talc granulomas in the lung.** A section of lung from an intravenous drug abuser viewed under polarized light reveals a granuloma adjacent to a pulmonary artery. The refractile material is talc that was used to dilute the drug prior to its intravenous injection.

organs. Bacterial endocarditis, often involving *Staphylococcus aureus,* occurs on both sides of the heart (Fig. 8-10) and may lead to pulmonary, renal, and intracranial abscesses; meningitis; osteomyelitis, and mycotic aneurysms (Fig. 8-11).

Intravenous drug abusers are at very high risk for acquired immunodeficiency syndrome (AIDS), as well as hepatitis B and C. These people may also suffer from the complications of viral hepatitis, such as chronic active hepatitis, necrotizing angiitis, and glomerulonephritis. A focal glomerulosclerosis ("heroin nephropathy") is characterized by immune complexes and has been ascribed to an immune reaction to impurities that contaminate illicit drugs.

Intravenous injection of talc, which is used to dilute pure drug, is associated with the appearance of foreign body granulomas in the lung (Fig. 8-12). These may be severe enough to lead to interstitial pulmonary fibrosis.

Drug Addiction in Pregnant Women Poses Risks for the Fetus

Maternal drug use may lead to addiction of newborn infants, who often exhibit a full-blown withdrawal syndrome. Moreover, the appearance of the drug withdrawal syndrome in the fetus during labor may result in excessive fetal movements and increased oxygen demand, a situation that increases the risk of intrapartum hypoxia and meconium aspiration. If labor occurs when maternal drug levels are high, the infant is often born with respiratory depression. Mothers who are addicted to drugs experience higher rates of toxemia of pregnancy and premature labor.

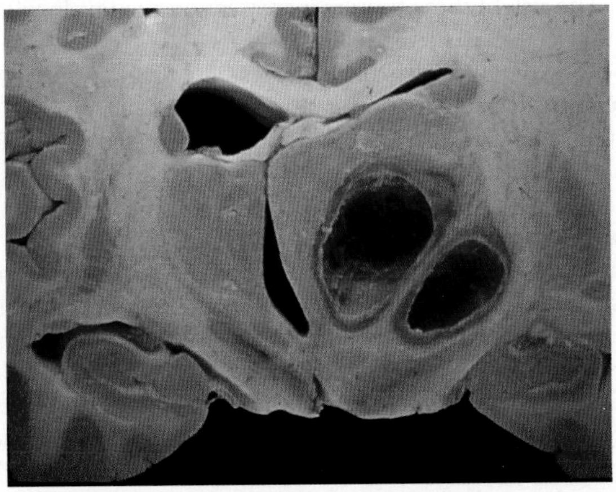

FIGURE 8-11. **Brain abscess.** Cross-section of the brain from an intravenous drug abuser shows two encapsulated cavities.

Maternal use of illicit drugs during pregnancy may injure the developing fetus in other ways. Thus, pregnant women who use cocaine more commonly experience placental abruption and premature labor. Infants born to such mothers are prone to be low birth weight, to have one of an array of CNS and other anomalies, and to show impaired brain function after birth. Maternal addiction to heroin carries a number of risks of abnormalities of pregnancy and premature birth. It is also associated with a large number of postnatal problems (in addition to heroin withdrawal), including sudden infant death syndrome (SIDS), neonatal respiratory distress syndrome, and developmental retardation. Maternal abuse of other substances, e.g., amphetamines and hallucinogens, also leads to variably severe fetal and postnatal disorders.

Iatrogenic Drug Injury

Iatrogenic drug injury refers to the unintended side effects of therapeutic or diagnostic drugs prescribed by physicians. Adverse reactions to pharmaceuticals are surprisingly common. They are seen in 2% to 5% of patients hospitalized on medical services; of these reactions, 2% to 12% are fatal. The typical hospitalized patient is given about 10 different medications, and some receive five times as many. The risk of an adverse reaction increases proportionately with the number of different drugs; for example, the risk of injury is at least 40% when more than 15 drugs are administered. Because they are so ubiquitously prescribed, drugs represent a significant environmental hazard. Untoward effects of drugs result from (1) overdose, (2) exaggerated physiological responses, (3) a genetic predisposition, (4) hypersensitivity, (5) interactions with other drugs, and (6) other unknown factors. The characteristic pathologic changes associated with drug reactions are treated in chapters dealing with specific organs. An example of a drug reaction is illustrated in Figure 8-13.

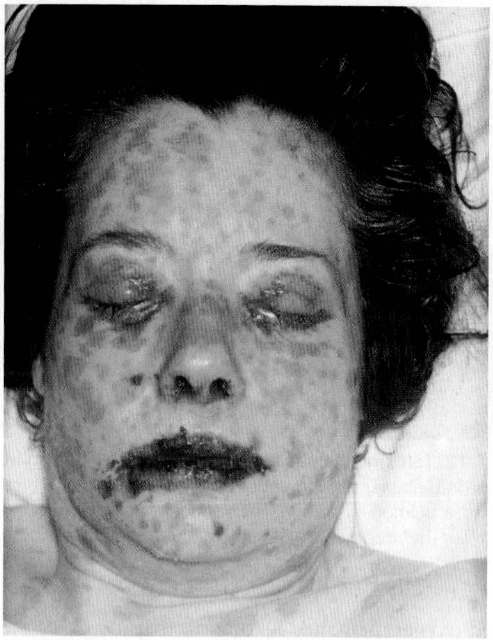

FIGURE 8-13. Erythema multiforme secondary to sulfonamide therapy.

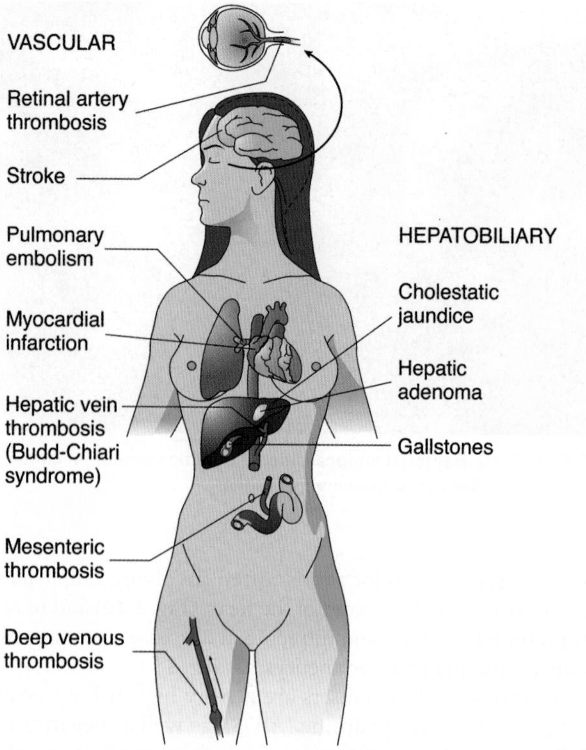

FIGURE 8-14. Complications of oral contraceptives.

Sex Hormones

Oral Contraceptives Carry a Small Risk of Complications

Orally administered hormonal contraceptives (OCs) are now the most commonly used method of birth control in industrialized countries. Current formulations are combinations of synthetic estrogens and steroids with progesterone-like activity. They act either by inhibiting the gonadotropin surge at midcycle, thereby preventing ovulation, or by preventing implantation by altering the phase of the endometrium. Data available to date include studies focusing on second- and third-generation OCs, which contain lower doses of both estrogens and progestogens than did earlier oral contraceptives. There are as yet little data available on longer-acting formulations, designed to decrease the numbers of menstrual periods as well as protect against conception. Most complications of oral contraceptives involve either the vasculature or reproductive organs (Fig. 8-14).

Vascular Complications

Deep vein thrombosis is a recognized complication of oral contraceptive use, the risk being increased three to four times. As a consequence, the risk of thromboembolism is correspondingly increased, especially in women who are already at high risk for this condition. Obesity and smoking magnify the risk of venous thrombosis attendant to OCs, as do coexisting disorders that increase clotting (thrombophilia).

The risk of arterial thrombotic events in women taking oral contraceptives is also increased, although different studies give conflicting results. Thus, both myocardial infarction and thrombotic stroke are reported to be increased in some, but not all, studies.

Neoplastic Complications

Tumors of several of the female reproductive organs, especially ovary, endometrium, and breast, are strongly influenced by female hormones. Repeated epidemiologic studies indicate that OC use decreases the risk of ovarian and endometrial cancers by about half, presumably because of suppression of the production of pituitary gonadotropins. Interestingly, there have been suggestions that OCs also decrease risk of colorectal cancers in women.

There is a small increase in the frequency of breast cancers in OC users. This observation applies mainly to nonfamilial breast cancers and to individuals currently taking OCs. The increased risk appears to endure for about 10 years following cessation of OC administration. Interestingly, this increased risk is not associated with increased mortality as tumors tend to be more localized to the breast at the time of discovery.

Squamous carcinoma of the cervix in women positive for human papilloma virus (HPV) may be somewhat increased in association with long-term (more than 5 years) OC use.

Benign liver adenomas are rare hepatic neoplasms that are significantly increased in incidence among women who use OCs. The risk of these tumors increases conspicuously with the duration of use, particularly after 5 years.

Several small studies have suggested a small increased risk of **hepatocellular carcinoma** among women using OCs. Fortunately, this cancer is rare in young women without chronic viral hepatitis.

Other Complications

For reasons unknown, oral contraceptives may induce an increased pigmentation of the malar eminences, called **chloasma,** which is accentuated by sunlight and persists for a long time after the contraceptives are discontinued.

Cholelithiasis is more frequent (twofold increase) in women who have used OCs for 4 years or less, but its incidence becomes lower than normal after that period of time. Thus, OCs accelerate the process of cholelithiasis but do not increase its overall incidence.

Benefits of Oral Contraceptives

In considering the potential side effects of the use of oral contraceptive agents, it is important to recognize that certain benefits accrue. In addition to a significant reduction in the risk of ovarian and endometrial cancers, the use of these agents decreases the risk of pelvic inflammatory disease, uterine leiomyomas, endometriosis, and fibrocystic disease of the breast.

Postmenopausal Hormone Replacement Therapy Increases the Risk of Some Cancers

Hormone replacement preparations containing either estrogen or estrogen plus progestin are given to postmenopausal women in an effort to alleviate menopausal symptoms and decrease risk of myocardial infarction and osteoporosis. These agents have proved effective in the treatment of postmenopausal symptoms. However, recent studies have cast doubt on their effectiveness in preventing myocardial infarction and osteoporosis.

Women who take these preparations have increased risk for cancers of the breast and endometrium. Hormone replacement regimens involving estrogens with or without added progestins increase risk of both cancers. However increased breast cancer incidence is somewhat greater for hormone replacements that contain both progestin and estrogen, compared to estrogen only, but is significant for both types of formulation.

It has been reported that postmenopausal women taking hormone replacements have a slightly increased risk of deep venous thrombotic events. This increase declines once treatment stops.

Environmental Chemicals

Awareness of potential hazards posed by harmful chemicals in the environment is not new. In the 12th century Maimonides wrote:

> Comparing the air of cities to the air of deserts is like comparing waters that are befouled and turbid to waters that are fine and pure. In the city, because of the height of its buildings, the narrowness of its streets and all that pours forth from its inhabitants, the air becomes stagnant, turbid, thick, misty and foggy. . . . Wherever the air is altered . . . men develop dullness of understanding, failure of intelligence and defects of memory.

Humans are surrounded by, breathe in, and consume many chemicals that are added to, or appear as contaminants in, foods, water, and air. Several important mechanisms govern the effect of toxic agents, including the toxin's absorption, distribution, metabolism, and excretion. Absorption (whether through pulmonary, gastrointestinal, or cutaneous routes) depends largely on the chemical in question. For example, because of their solubility in lipids, the insecticides chlordane and heptachlor are rapidly absorbed and stored in body fat. By contrast, the water-soluble herbicide paraquat is readily eliminated.

The storage, distribution, and excretion of chemicals control their concentrations in the organism at any given time. Agents stored in adipose tissue may exert prolonged low-level effects, while more water-soluble materials that are easily excreted by the kidney usually have a shorter duration of action.

Among the most important chemical hazards to which humans are exposed are environmental dusts and carcinogens. Inhalation of mineral and organic dusts occurs primarily in occupational settings (e.g., mining, industrial manufacturing, farming) and occasionally as a result of unusual situations (e.g., bird fanciers, pituitary snuff inhalation). Inhaling mineral dusts leads to pulmonary diseases known as **pneumoconioses**, whereas organic dusts may produce **hypersensitivity pneumonitis**. Pneumoconioses were formerly common, but control of dust exposure in the workplace by modifying manufacturing techniques, improvements in air handling, and use of masks has substantially reduced the incidence of these diseases. Because of their importance, pneumoconioses and hypersensitivity pneumonitis are discussed in detail in Chapter 12.

Chemical carcinogens are ubiquitous in the environment. Their potential for causing disease has elicited widespread concern. In particular, exposure to carcinogens in the workplace has been associated epidemiologically with a number of cancers (Table 8-1), which are reviewed in Chapter 5.

Toxic Effects Differ from Hypersensitivity Responses

Many substances elicit disease in a variety of animal species in a dose-dependent manner, with a regular time delay and a predictable target organ response. Furthermore, the morphologic changes in injured tissues are constant and reproducible. By contrast, other agents show great variability in their ability to produce disease, irregular lag times before injury is apparent, no dose dependency, and lack of reproducibility. Generally, predictable dose-response reactions reflect direct actions of a compound or its metabolite on a tissue—a "toxic" effect. The second, unpredictable type of reaction is believed to reflect "hypersensitivity," or an immunologic response or idiosyncratic side effect.

Chemical Toxicity May Follow Occupational or Environmental Exposure

Beginning with the industrial revolution, there has been an exponential rise in the number of chemicals manufactured and a corresponding increase in the risk of human exposure. In any consideration of this topic, one must differentiate between acute

TABLE 8-1

Cancers Associated with Exposure to Occupational Carcinogens

Agent or Occupation	Site of Cancer
Arsenic	Lung cancer
Asbestos	Mesothelioma (pleura and peritoneum) Lung cancer (in smokers)
Aromatic amines	Bladder cancer
Benzene	Leukemia, multiple myeloma
bis-(Chloromethyl)ether	Lung cancer
Chromium	Lung cancer
Furniture and shoe manufacturing	Nasal carcinoma
Hematite mining	Lung cancer
Nickel	Lung cancer, paranasal sinus cancer
Tars and oils	Cancers of lung, gastrointestinal tract, bladder, and skin
Vinyl chloride	Angiosarcoma of liver

poisoning and chronic toxicity. One must also distinguish industrial and accidental exposure from that which is likely to occur in the general environment. The lack of adequate quantitative exposure data in humans and the difficulties involved in assessing long-term risks of low-level exposures have led to use of data derived from animal studies to assess toxicities and risks in humans. Such projections can be hazardous because of (1) species differences in sensitivity, (2) differing routes of administration, (3) species-to-species variations in metabolic pathways by which some compounds are modified and, (4) extrapolation from very high levels needed to show an effect in a short experimental time frame in animals to low-level exposures over years in humans. These considerations necessarily complicate the need to understand and quantify the potential for human toxicity of a plethora of chemicals.

Except for certain hypersensitivity reactions in susceptible persons, acute poisoning by environmental chemicals does not pose a significant threat to the general population. Concentrations necessary to cause acute functional disorders or structural damage are ordinarily encountered only in the workplace or as a consequence of uncommon accidents.

Accidental mass poisonings with the pesticides endrin and parathion have led to as many as 100 deaths in a single event, but long-term sequelae among the survivors have been difficult to document. The experimental literature dealing with the short- and long-term toxicity of industrial chemicals is voluminous and complicated and often contradictory. For this reason we largely restrict the following discussion to documented effects in humans.

Volatile Organic Solvents and Vapors

Volatile organic solvents and vapors are widely used in industry in many capacities. With few exceptions, exposures to these compounds are industrial or accidental, and represent short-term dangers rather than long-term toxicity. For the most part, exposure to solvents is by inhalation rather than by ingestion.

- **Chloroform (CHCl3) and carbon tetrachloride (CCl_4):** These solvents exert anesthetic (depressant) effects on the CNS, and on the heart and blood vessels, but are better known as hepatotoxins. With both, but classically with carbon tetrachloride, large doses lead to acute hepatic necrosis, fatty liver, and liver failure. Long-term exposure to carbon tetrachloride does not pertain to humans, as each exposure to it causes recognizable clinical liver injury, so that continued exposure would not be permitted.
- **Trichloroethylene (C_2HCl_3):** A ubiquitous industrial solvent, trichloroethylene in high concentrations depresses the CNS, but hepatotoxicity is minimal. There is no evidence for chronic sequelae in humans following ordinary long-term industrial exposure.
- **Methanol (CH_3OH):** Because methanol, unlike ethanol, is not taxed, it is used by some impoverished alcoholics as a substitute for ethanol or by unscrupulous merchants as an adulterant of alcoholic beverages. In methanol poisoning, inebriation similar to that produced by ethanol is succeeded by gastrointestinal symptoms, visual dysfunction, seizures, coma, and death. The major toxicity of methanol is believed to arise from its metabolism, first to formaldehyde and then to formic acid. Metabolic acidosis is common after methanol ingestion.

  The most characteristic lesion of methanol toxicity is necrosis of retinal ganglion cells and subsequent degeneration of the optic nerve. Severe poisoning may lead to lesions in the putamen and globus pallidus.
- **Ethylene glycol ($HOCH_2CH_2OH$):** Because of its low vapor pressure, toxicity of ethylene glycol chiefly results from ingestion. It is commonly used in antifreeze, and has been drunk by chronic alcoholics as a substitute for ethanol for many years. Poisoning with this compound has come into prominence because it has been used to adulterate wines in Austria and Italy, owing to its sweet taste and solubility. The toxicity of ethylene glycol is chiefly due to its metabolites, particularly oxalic acid, and occurs within minutes of ingestion. Metabolic acidosis, CNS depression, nausea and vomiting, and hypocalcemia-related cardiotoxicity are seen. Oxalate crystals in the tubules and oxaluria are often noted and may cause renal failure.
- **Gasoline and kerosene:** These fuels are mixtures of aliphatic hydrocarbons and branched, unsaturated and aromatic hydrocarbons. Chronic exposure is by inhalation. Despite prolonged exposure to gasoline by gas station attendants, auto mechanics, etc., there is no evidence that inhalation of gasoline over the long term is particularly injurious. Acutely, gasoline is an irritant, but really only causes systemic problems if inhaled in very high concentrations. Increased use of kerosene for home heating has led to accidental poisoning of children.
- **Benzene (C_6H_6):** The prototypic aromatic hydrocarbon is benzene, which must be distinguished from benzine, a mixture of aliphatic hydrocarbons. Benzene is one of the most widely used chemicals in industrial processes, being a starting point for innumerable syntheses and a solvent. It is also a constituent of fuels, accounting for as much as 3% of gasoline. Virtually all cases of acute and chronic benzene toxicity have occurred as industrial exposures, e.g., in shoemakers and workers in shoe manufacturing, occupations that at one time were associated with heavy exposure to benzene-based glues.

  Acute benzene poisoning primarily affects the CNS, and death results from respiratory failure. However, it is the long-term effects of benzene exposure that have attracted the most attention. In these cases, the bone marrow is the principal target. Patients who develop hematologic abnormalities characteristically exhibit **hypoplasia or aplasia of the bone marrow and pancytopenia.** Aplastic anemia usually is seen while the workers are still exposed to high concentrations of benzene. In a substantial proportion of cases of benzene-induced anemias, **acute myeloblastic leukemia, erythroleukemia, or multiple myeloma** develops during continuing exposure to benzene, or after a variable latent period following removal of the worker from the hazardous environment. Some cases of acute leukemia have occurred without a prior history of aplastic anemia. Although instances of chronic myeloid and chronic lymphocytic leukemia have been reported, a cause-and-effect relationship with benzene exposure is less convincing than that with cases of acute leukemia. Overall, the risk of leukemia is increased 60-fold in workers exposed to the highest atmospheric concentrations of benzene. The closely related compounds toluene and xylenes, also widely used as solvents, have not been incriminated as a cause of hematologic abnormalities, possibly because they are metabolized via different pathways.

Agricultural Chemicals

Pesticides, fungicides, herbicides, fumigants, and organic fertilizers are crucial to the success of modern agriculture. Without pesticides, agricultural productivity would be severely compromised. However, many of these chemicals persist in soil and water and may pose a potential long-term hazards. Acute poisoning with very large concentrations of any of these chemicals has already been mentioned above. It is clear that exposure to industrial concentrations or inadvertently contaminated food can cause severe acute illness. Children are particularly susceptible and may ingest home gardening preparations.

Symptoms of acute toxicity are often related to the mode of action of the toxin. For example, organophosphate insecticides are acetylcholinesterase inhibitors that are readily absorbed through the skin. Thus acute toxicity in humans mainly involves neuromuscular disorders such as visual disturbances, dyspnea, mucous hypersecretion, and bronchoconstriction. Death may come from respiratory failure. In the United States, 30 to 40 persons die annually of acute pesticide poisoning. Long-term exposure produces symptoms similar to acute exposure.

Organochlorine pesticides, such as DDT (dichlorodiphenyltrichloroethane), chlordane, and others, have caused concern because they accumulate in soils and in human tissues, and break down very slowly. High levels of any such pesticide can be harmful to humans in acute exposures, but the side effects of chronic contact with the materials and their buildup are of greatest interest. Many of these compounds function as weak estrogens, but no harmful effects related to this activity have been documented. Some of these compounds, such as aldrin and dieldrin, have been associated with tumor development, but the toxicity of most organochlorine insecticides relates to inhibition of CNS GABA responses.

Human exposure to herbicides is not infrequent. Among the best known of these is paraquat. Occupational paraquat exposure is usually via the skin, although toxicity from ingestion and inhalation are documented. The compound is very corrosive, and causes burns or ulcers of whatever it contacts. It is transported actively to the lung, where it can damage to the pulmonary epithelium, causing edema and even respiratory failure. High level exposures may lead to death from cardiovascular collapse, while when lower doses are involved, pulmonary fibrosis may ultimately lead to death.

Aromatic Halogenated Hydrocarbons

The halogenated aromatic hydrocarbons that have received considerable attention include (1) the polychlorinated biphenyls (PCBs); (2) chlorophenols (pentachlorophenol, used as a wood preservative); (3) hexachlorophene, used as an antibacterial agent in soaps); and (4) the dioxin TCDD (2,3,7,8-tetrachlorodibenzo-p-dioxin) a byproduct of the synthesis of herbicides and hexachlorophene and, therefore, a contaminant of these preparations. Chronic exposure to TCDD does not appear to produce demonstrable toxicity. Serious questions have been raised regarding the danger of long-term exposure to dioxin, and there is now a consensus that at the very least this compound is far more carcinogenic in rodents than in humans. The problem of the presence of PCBs in the environment resembles that of agricultural chemicals: long-term animal toxicity is well documented, but there are no significant increases in the incidence of cancer or other diseases in workers exposed to PCBs. The same situation pertains to hexachlorophene and pentachlorophenol.

Cyanide

Prussic acid (HCN) is the classic murderer's tool in detective fiction, where the smell of bitter almonds (*Prunus amygdalus*) betrays the crime. A more contemporary homicidal application of cyanide is its surreptitious addition to a number of commercially available medicinal capsules. Amygdalin, a glycoside found in the pits of several fruits (including apricots, peaches, and wild cherries) and in the seeds of almonds and hydrangeas, is a combination of glucose, benzaldehyde, and cyanide. Although humans do not possess the β-glucosidase needed to liberate the cyanide, intestinal flora can perform this function, thereby leading to cyanide intoxication. Amygdalin is, therefore, far more toxic when ingested than when injected intravenously. These considerations may appear esoteric, except for the fact that extracts of apricot pits were used in the formulation of fraudulent anticancer nostrums and resulted in cases of cyanide poisoning.

Cyanide blocks cellular respiration by reversibly binding to mitochondrial cytochrome oxidase, the terminal acceptor in the electron transport chain, which is responsible for reducing molecular oxygen to water. The pathologic consequences are similar to those produced by any acute global anoxia.

Air Pollutants

A precise definition of air pollution is elusive, since the meaning of "pure air" is not established. However, for the purposes of this discussion, the most important pollutants are those generated by the combustion of fossil fuels, industrial and agricultural processes, and so forth. The most important air pollutants that are implicated as factors in human disease are the irritants sulfur dioxide (SO_2), oxides of nitrogen, CO, and ozone, as well as suspended particulates and acid aerosols.

Most common chemical constituents of air pollution are mainly irritants and have been suggested as contributing to development or predisposition to several respiratory illnesses, but are not usually implicated directly as increasing mortality in the developed world. Dissecting the specific effects of these chemicals from the effects of other air pollutants, especially particulates (see below) is difficult. **SO_2** is highly irritative and may be oxidized to sulfuric acid. SO_2 mainly derives from burning fossil fuels. Acute exposure leads to bronchoconstriction and respiratory tract inflammation. Chronic experimental exposure to high levels of SO_2 may lead to a chronic bronchitis-like syndrome, but it is not clear that there are significant sequelae of human exposure to the concentrations of SO_2 normally found in smog.

CO is a colorless, odorless gas that has a very high affinity for hemoglobin. It is problematic when indoor combustion is used for heating (see below), but atmospheric CO is more an indicator of fossil fuel combustion than an environmental hazard.

Nitrogen oxides are generally written NOx, because they are a mixture of several compounds. They, as well, are derived from burning fossil fuels, especially in generating electricity. These gasses are oxidants and respiratory irritants that induce airway hyperreactivity in acute exposure settings. Adverse effects attributable to chronic atmospheric levels of NOx have not been demonstrated. Trophospheric **ozone** (i.e., ozone near the ground as opposed to in the upper atmosphere) is largely produced by the action of sunlight on NO_2, especially on warm, sunny days. It is a strong oxidant that causes both respiratory (cough, dyspnea) and nonrespiratory (nausea, headache) symptoms on acute exposure. Chronic exposure to ozone in smog is reported to lead to deterioration in pulmonary function and is associated with a slight but significant increase in mortality.

Particulates in the air include solid particles and liquid droplets. These vary in size, composition and origin, and are generally divided into those between 2.5 μm and 10μm in aerodynamic diameter, and those under 2.5 μm. The former (coarse particulates) are mostly deposited in the tracheobronchial tree and are largely derived from natural sources, e.g., windblown soil, dusts. Bioaerosols (e.g., spores, pollens) are included in this group. The fine particulates are mostly from combustion processes. Because of their small size, they penetrate more deeply into the lungs. Even finer particles, ($<$100 nm) have recently attracted interest as they penetrate very deeply, have a high ratio of surface area:mass ratio (which allows for greater potential delivery of noxious components) and have been found to pass through the alveolar capillaries into the bloodstream.

Most studies of the effects of air pollution on health have focused on particulates. Many large short-term and long-term epidemiologic studies have shown that particulate air pollution is associated with increased mortality, both overall and from cardiovascular disease and cancer. Thus, the American Cancer Society estimated that overall, cardiopulmonary and lung tumor deaths were greater respectively by 4%, 6%, and 8% for every 10 $\mu g/m^3$ increase in average annual exposure to fine particulates. Shorter term studies showed significant increases in acute myocardial infarction as a consequence of exposure to higher levels of fine particulates. It has been suggested that residence within 100 meters of a freeway greatly increases the likelihood of cardiovascular death. Furthermore, experimental studies have shown that particulate exposure may lead to greater atherosclerosis, blood pressure, heart rate, coagulability, and levels of inflammatory mediators.

There is experimental evidence to support a suggestion that inflammation and oxidative stress are responsible for at least part of the harmful effects of pollutants. Thus, the frequency of exacerbations of asthma is related to levels of fine particulates, especially derived from diesel exhaust, and ozone in the air. A cohort of asthmatic children in Mexico City was found to have mutations in glutathione S-transferase, an enzyme that metabolizes a variety of toxins and that can detoxify reactive oxygen species. Treating these children with antioxidant vitamins C and E resulted in clinical improvement.

Carbon Monoxide

CO is an odorless and nonirritating gas that results from the incomplete combustion of organic substances. It combines with hemoglobin with an affinity 240 times greater than that of oxygen to form carboxyhemoglobin. CO binding to hemoglobin also increases the affinity of the remaining heme moieties for oxygen. Oxygen does not dissociate from such hemoglobin in the tissues as readily as it should. The hypoxia that results from CO poisoning is thus far greater than can be attributed to loss of oxygen-carrying capacity alone.

Atmospheric CO is derived principally from automobile exhaust, and does not pose a health problem. Carboxyhemoglobin concentrations under 10% are common in smokers and ordinarily do not produce symptoms. Indoor combustion, particularly from space heaters, however can generate much higher concentrations of CO, which can be hazardous. Concentrations up to 30% usually cause only headache and mild exertional dyspnea. Higher levels of carboxyhemoglobin lead to confusion and lethargy. Above 50%, coma and convulsions ensue. Levels greater than 60% are usually fatal. In fatal CO poisoning, a characteristic cherry-red color is imparted to the skin by the carboxyhemoglobin in the superficial capillaries. Recovery from severe CO poisoning may be associated with brain damage, which may be manifested as subtle intellectual deficits, memory loss, or extrapyramidal symptoms (e.g., parkinsonism). Treatment of acute CO poisoning, as in persons who attempt suicide or are trapped in fires, consists principally of the administration of 100% oxygen.

Deleterious effects of long-term exposure to low levels of CO have been difficult to substantiate. However, in patients with ischemic heart disease concentrations of carboxyhemoglobin below 5% to 8% (often found in smokers) may accelerate onset of exertional angina and cause changes in electrocardiograms. Thus, carboxyhemoglobin saturation levels even as low as 2.5% are considered undesirable in such patients.

Metals

Metals are an important group of environmental chemicals that have caused disease in humans from ancient times to the present.

Lead

Lead is a ubiquitous heavy metal that is common in the environment of industrialized countries. Before widespread awareness of chronic exposure to lead in the 1950s and 1960s, the classic symptoms of lead poisoning were commonly encountered in children and adults. In the United States, lead poisoning was primarily a pediatric problem related to pica—the habit of chewing on cribs, toys, furniture, and woodwork—and eating painted plaster and fallen paint flakes. Most dwellings built before 1940 had lead-containing paint (up to 40% of dry weight) on interior and exterior walls. Children living in dilapidated older homes heavily coated with flaking paint were at significant risk for chronic lead poisoning. To these sources of lead was added a heavy burden of atmospheric lead in the form of dust derived from the combustion of lead-containing gasoline. Children and adults living near point sources of environmental lead contamination, such as smelters, were exposed to even higher levels of lead.

In adults, occupational exposure to lead occurred primarily among those engaged in lead smelting, which releases metal fumes and deposits lead oxide dust in the area. Lead oxide is a constituent of battery grids and an occupational exposure to lead is a hazard in the manufacture and recycling of automobile batteries. Accidental poisonings occasionally occurred from pottery that had been improperly fired with a lead glaze, renovation of old residences heavily coated with lead paint, "moonshine" whiskey made in lead stills, or "sniffing" lead-containing gasoline.

METABOLISM: Lead is absorbed through the lungs or, less often, the gastrointestinal tract. Once in the blood, it rapidly equilibrates with the plasma and erythrocytes and is excreted by the kidneys. A portion of blood lead remains freely diffusible. Lead crosses the blood-brain barrier readily and concentrations in the brain, liver, kidneys, and bone marrow are directly related to its toxic effects. It binds sulfhydryl groups and interferes with the activities of zinc (Zn)-dependent enzymes. As well, it interferes with enzymes involved in synthesis of steroids and cell membranes.

By contrast, bones, teeth, nails, and hair represent a tightly bound pool of lead that is not generally regarded as harmful. With chronic exposure, 90% of the total body lead burden is in the bones. During metaphyseal bone formation in children, lead and calcium are deposited to produce the increased bone densities ("lead lines") seen radiographically at the metaphysis, thereby providing a simple method of detecting increased body stores of lead in children.

TOXICITY: Classic lead overexposure, which is rarely seen in the United States today, affects many organs but its major toxicity involves dysfunction in: (1) the nervous system, (2) the kidneys, and (3) hematopoiesis (Fig. 8-15).

The brain is the target of lead toxicity in children; adults usually present with manifestation of peripheral neuropathy. Children with lead encephalopathy are typically irritable and ataxic. They may convulse or display altered states of consciousness, from drowsiness to frank coma. Children with blood lead levels above 80 μg/dL, but with concentrations lower than those in children with frank encephalopathy (120 μg/dL), exhibit mild CNS symptoms such as clumsiness, irritability, and hyperactivity.

Lead encephalopathy is a condition in which the brain is edematous and displays flattened gyri and compressed ventricles. There may be herniation of the uncus and cerebellar tonsils. Microscopically, congestion, petechial hemorrhages and foci of neuronal necrosis are seen. A diffuse astrocytic proliferation in both the gray and white matter may accompany these changes. Vascular lesions in the brain are particularly prominent, with capillary dilation and proliferation.

Peripheral motor neuropathy is the most common manifestation of lead neurotoxicity in the adult, typically affecting the radial and peroneal nerves and resulting in **wristdrop** and **footdrop,** respectively. Lead-induced neuropathy is probably also the basis of the paroxysms of gastrointestinal pain known as lead colic.

Anemia is a cardinal sign of lead intoxication. Lead disrupts heme synthesis in bone marrow erythroblasts by inhibiting δ-aminolevulinic acid dehydratase, the second enzyme in de novo synthesis of heme. It also inhibits ferrochelatase, which catalyzes the incorporation of ferrous iron into the porphyrin ring. The resulting inability to produce heme adequately is expressed as a microcytic and hypochromic anemia resembling that seen in iron deficiency, in which heme synthesis is also impaired. The anemia of lead intoxication is also characterized by prominent basophilic stippling of erythrocytes, related to clustering of ribosomes. Erythrocyte life span is decreased; thus, the anemia of lead intoxication is due to both ineffective hematopoiesis and accelerated erythrocyte turnover.

Lead nephropathy reflects the toxic effect of the metal on the proximal tubular cells of the kidney. The resulting dysfunction is characterized by aminoaciduria, glycosuria, and hyperphosphaturia (Fanconi syndrome). Such functional alterations are accompanied by the formation of inclusion bodies in the nuclei of the proximal tubular cells. These inclusions are characteristic of lead nephropathy and are composed of a lead–protein complex containing more than 100 times the concentration of lead in the whole kidney.

Lead poisoning is treated with chelating agents such as calcium ethylene diamine tetra-acetic acid (EDTA), either alone or in combination with dimercaprol (BAL). Both the hematologic and renal manifestations of lead intoxication are usually reversible; alterations in the CNS are generally irreversible.

Laboratory diagnosis is made by demonstrating high blood levels of lead and increased free erythrocyte protoporphyrin. Elevated urinary excretion of δ-aminolevulinic acid and decreased levels of aminolevulinic acid dehydratase in erythrocytes are confirmatory.

EFFECTS OF CHRONIC EXPOSURE TO LOW LEAD LEVELS: Due to the removal of lead from gasoline, improvements in housing, substitution of titanium for lead in paints, and control of industrial point sources, ambient levels of lead have fallen significantly: blood levels in the general population of the United States decreased from an average of 16 μg/dL in 1976 to 1.0 μg/dL in 2000. The dramatic fall in mean blood lead levels was accompanied by the near elimination of lead-related childhood fatalities and encephalopathy. However, low lead exposure in children, while not producing recognizable symptoms, may permanently decrease cognitive performance. The regulatory safe threshold for blood levels of lead in children has been progressively reduced and is now thought to be below 10 μg/dL.

The evidence is compelling that low level lead exposure in children, while not producing recognizable symptoms, creates deficits in intellectual and motor functions that persist into adult life. Efforts to reduce environmental lead have led to decreases in the percentage of children in the United States with blood levels of 10 μg/dL of lead or more from 88% in the 1970s to 4.4% in the

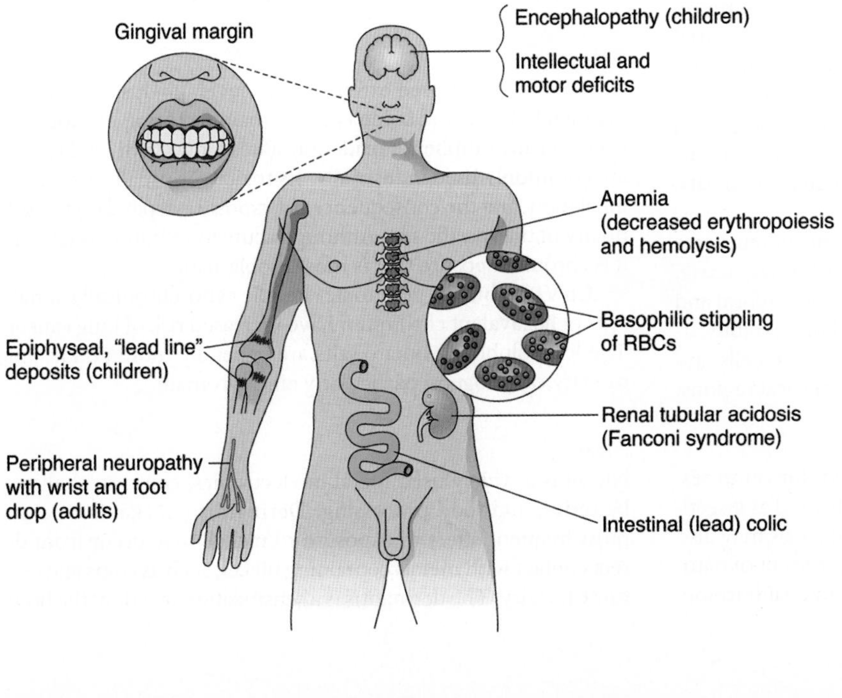

FIGURE 8-15. **Complications of lead intoxication. RBCs 5 red blood cells.**

1990s. However, high blood lead concentrations remain a problem among poor, mainly urban, children and more vigorous campaigns to address this situation are justified.

Mercury

Inorganic mercury has been used since prehistoric times and has been known to be an occupation-related hazard at least since the Middle Ages. Although mercury poisoning still occurs in some occupations, there has been increasing concern over the potential health hazards brought about by the contamination of many ecosystems following several well-known outbreaks of methylmercury poisoning. The most widely publicized episodes occurred in Japan, first in Minamata Bay in the 1950s and then in Niigata. In both cases, local inhabitants developed severe, chronic organic mercury intoxication. This poisoning was traced to the consumption of fish contaminated with mercury that had been discharged into the environment in the effluents from a fertilizer and a plastics factory. Children exposed in utero showed delayed developmental milestones and abnormal reflexes, despite the fact that fetal exposure was estimated to be 1/5 to 1/10 times that in adults.

Mercury released into the environment may be bioconcentrated and enter the food chain. Bacteria in bays and oceans can convert inorganic mercury compounds from industrial wastes into highly neurotoxic organomercurials. These compounds are then transferred up the food chain and are eventually concentrated in the large predatory fish (e.g., tuna, pike) that make up a substantial part of the diet in many countries.

Although inorganic mercury is not efficiently absorbed in the gastrointestinal tract, organic mercurial compounds are readily absorbed because of their lipid solubility. Both inorganic and organic mercury are preferentially concentrated in the kidney, and methylmercury also distributes to the brain. *The kidney is the principal target of the toxicity of inorganic mercury, but the brain is damaged by organic mercurials.*

NEPHROTOXICITY: At one time, mercuric chloride was widely used as an antiseptic, and acute mercuric chloride poisoning was much more common; the compound was ingested by accident or for suicidal purposes. Under such circumstances, **proximal tubular necrosis** was accompanied by oliguric renal failure. Mercurial diuretics were also widely prescribed in the past, and chronic mercury nephrotoxicity was a not uncommon complication of their long-term use. Today, chronic mercurial nephrotoxicity is almost always a consequence of long-term industrial exposure. Proteinuria is common in chronic mercurial nephrotoxicity, and there may be a nephrotic syndrome with more severe intoxication. Pathologically, there is a membranous glomerulonephritis with subepithelial electron-dense deposits, suggesting immune complex deposition.

NEUROTOXICITY: The neurologic effects of mercury are manifested as a constriction of visual fields, paresthesias, ataxia, dysarthria, and hearing loss. Pathologically, there is cerebral and cerebellar atrophy. Microscopically, the cerebellum exhibits atrophy of the granular layer, without loss of Purkinje cells and spongy softenings in the visual cortex and other cortical regions.

Arsenic

The toxic properties of arsenic have been known for centuries. Arsenic-containing compounds have been widely used as insecticides, weed killers, and wood preservatives. Arsenicals may also contaminate soil and leach into ground water as a result of naturally occurring arsenic-rich rock formations, from coal burning, or use of arsenical pesticides. As with mercury, there is evidence for the bioaccumulation of arsenic along the food chain.

Acute arsenic poisoning is almost always the result of accidental or homicidal ingestion. Death is due to **CNS toxicity.** Chronic arsenic intoxication affects many organ systems. It is characterized initially by such nonspecific symptoms as malaise and fatigue. Eventually, gastrointestinal, cardiovascular, and hematologic dysfunction become evident. Both encephalopathy and peripheral neuropathy develop. The latter is characterized by paresthesias, motor palsies, and painful neuritis. On epidemiological grounds, **cancers of the skin, respiratory tract, and gastrointestinal tract** have been attributed to industrial and agricultural exposure to arsenic. In some parts of the world, exposure of workers in rice paddies to arsenic in the ground water has been associated with skin cancers.

Cadmium

Cadmium is used in ever-increasing quantities in the manufacture of alloys, in the production of rechargeable batteries, in electroplating of other metals (e.g., automobile parts and musical instruments), as a plasticizer, and as a pigment. Fumes of cadmium oxide are released in the course of welding steel parts previously plated with a cadmium anticorrosive. It accumulates in the human body, with a half life of over 20 years, and, since it is rarely recycled, the increase in industrial use of the metal is of concern.

The main routes of exposure for the general population are ingestion and inhalation. Both plant- and animal-derived foodstuffs may contain substantial levels of cadmium.

Short-term cadmium inhalation irritates the respiratory tract, with pulmonary edema the most dangerous result. The lungs and the kidneys, and to a lesser extent, the skeletal and vascular systems, are the principal target organs of chronic cadmium intoxication. Emphysema has been the major finding in the fatal cases of chronic cadmium pneumonitis that have been studied. A number of studies report increased lung cancer in people chronically exposed to cadmium by inhalation. Although the confounding effects of smoking complicate interpretation of some of these studies, cadmium does appear to lead to some lung cancers. Proteinuria, which reflects tubular rather than glomerular damage, has been the most consistent finding in cadmium workers with renal damage.

Chromium

Chromium (Cr) is used extensively in several industries, including metal plating and some types of manufacturing. Although it occurs in any number of oxidation states, only Cr(III) and Cr(VI) are commonly used industrially. Its toxicity is usually a result of inhalation, and the consequences of exposure depend on the solubility of the specific salt. Although acute intoxication is known, it is chronic exposure that is most problematic.

Cr(VI) is highly genotoxic. People who chronically inhale salts of hexavalent chromium have increased risk of lung cancer. The less soluble chromate salts are generally more potent pulmonary carcinogens, particularly zinc chromate.

Nickel

Nickel is a widely used metal in electronics, coins, steel alloys, batteries, and food processing. Dermatitis ("nickel itch"), the most frequent effect of exposure to nickel, may occur from direct contact with metals containing nickel, such as coins and costume jewelry. The dermatitis is a sensitization reaction; the body reacts to nickel-conjugated proteins formed following the penetration of the epidermis by nickel ions. Exposure to nickel, as to arsenic, increases the risk of development of specific types of cancer. Epidemiologic studies have demonstrated that workers who were occupationally exposed to nickel compounds have an increased incidence of lung cancer and cancer of the nasal cavities.

Iron

Iron deficiency anemia is a common disease, particularly in premenopausal women. Oral iron preparations contain largely ferrous sulfate, the form absorbed by the gastrointestinal mucosa and then converted to the trivalent form. Acute ferrous sulfate poisoning from accidental ingestion, mainly by little children. As little as 1 to 2 g of ferrous sulfate may be lethal, but most fatal cases follow ingestion of 3 to 10 g. Hemorrhagic gastritis and acute liver necrosis have been the most prominent findings at autopsy.

Long-term, excessive dietary intake of iron does not ordinarily lead to abnormal iron accumulation. South African Bantus, however, have a diet very high in iron, largely derived from iron drums used to prepare fermented alcoholic beverages. The acidic pH of these brews readily solubilizes the iron, and their low alcohol content allows large volumes to be consumed. A large proportion of the excess iron is in the liver, and there is a correlation between the degree of siderosis and the presence of cirrhosis. There is also a high incidence of diabetes and heart disease in this "Bantu siderosis."

Miscellaneous Metals

COBALT: In the 1960s, an epidemic of an unusual cardiomyopathy, clinically characterized by fulminant congestive heart failure, appeared in drinkers of a particular brand of beer, first in the Canadian province of Quebec and subsequently in the United States and Europe. The heart disease was traced to an excessive intake of cobalt, which had been added to the beer to enhance foaming qualities. When the cobalt was removed from the beer, no further cases of heart disease were reported.

ALUMINUM: "Dialysis encephalopathy" was first reported in patients with uremia undergoing chronic renal dialysis. The subsequent finding of high concentrations of aluminum in the gray matter of the brains of patients who died led to the suggestion that the encephalopathy resulted from aluminum intoxication. Epidemiologic studies implicated the aluminum in the tap water used to prepare the dialysates, and the disease could be eliminated by removing aluminum from the water. Aluminum intoxication with encephalopathy and osteomalacia can occur in patients (generally children) with uremia who are not dialyzed but who are given oral phosphate-binding gels that contain aluminum.

Radioactive Elements

Elements whose radioactive isotopes are potentially hazardous include radium, strontium, uranium, plutonium, thorium, and iodine. Chronic toxicities relate principally to radiation-induced carcinogenesis. The individual tumors reflect the organ localization of the elements and are discussed in the chapters that address specific organ pathology.

Biological Toxins are Organisms and Their Nonviable Components

These toxins are mostly of microbial, algal, plant, protozoan, arthropod, or mammalian origin. They include whole organisms, intact particulate or soluble products of those organisms (e.g., exotoxins, pollens), and fragments of organisms. Adverse reactions may result from inhalation, ingestion, or other contact; and they may reflect infectious, hypersensitivity, and toxic effects of those materials. This discussion addresses the latter. Infectious and hypersensitivity reactions to foreign matter are considered in Chapters 9 and 4 respectively, as well as individual organ-specific discussions (e.g., hypersensitivity pneumonitis in Chapter 12.).

The toxic effects of microbial products are the best characterized of biological toxicities. **Organic dust toxic syndrome** (ODTS) is a systemic reaction to the direct toxicities of many, mainly fungal, toxins. It consists of flu-like symptoms (fever, malaise, etc.), often with a respiratory component (dyspnea, cough). Unlike hypersensitivity pneumonitis, ODTS appears to reflect cell death and the consequent acute inflammatory reaction. It is usually associated with fungal toxins produced by many common fungi.

Aspergillus, Stachybotrys, Penicillium, and *Fusarium* species are the most common culprits. These fungi are particularly abundant in water-damaged buildings and moist warm environments. Their mycotoxins include trichothecenes and β-1,3-glucans, which may elicit disease by ingestion and inhalational routes.

One particular toxin produced by *Aspergillus flavus* and *Aspergillus parasiticus,* called **aflatoxin**, is highly hepatotoxic and is recognized as a potent hepatocarcinogen. There are several known varieties of aflatoxin.

Bacterial endotoxins are lipopolysaccharides derived from gram-negative bacterial cell walls. They are often complexed with proteins and phospholipids. Injected endotoxins are used experimentally to elicit inflammatory and febrile responses characterized by local or systemic macrophage activation. Inhaled, these compounds elicit profuse pulmonary inflammatory responses, involving release of inflammatory mediators (tumor necrosis factor [TNF]-α, interleukin [IL]-1, etc.), causing fever, pneumonitis, and pulmonary edema.

Thermal Regulatory Dysfunction

Hypothermia is a Decrease in Body Temperature Below 35°C (95°F)

Hypothermia can result in systemic or focal injury, the latter exemplified by **trench foot** or **immersion foot.** In localized hypothermia of these types, actual tissue freezing does not occur. **Frostbite,** by contrast, involves the crystallization of tissue water.

Generalized Hypothermia

Acute immersion in water at 4°C to 10°C (39.2° to 50°F) reduces central blood flow. Coupled with decreased core body temperature and cooling of the blood perfusing the brain, this results in mental confusion. Tetany makes swimming impossible. Furthermore, increased vagal discharge leads to premature ventricular contractions, ventricular arrhythmias, and even fibrillation.

Attempting to increase heat production, the immersed body immediately responds by increasing muscle activity and oxygen consumption. However, there are limits to the sources of energy available for sustained warming. Within 30 minutes, heat loss exceeds heat production because of the combination of high direct conduction of heat from the whole skin surface and altered muscle tone caused by decreased arterial carbon dioxide and exhaustion. Core temperature then begins to fall. Peripheral vasoconstriction is another response to conserve heat. In addition, there is an increased sympathetic neural discharge, resulting in increased heart and basal metabolic rates and shivering. When the core temperature approaches 35°C, this activity may be three to six times above normal. Below 35°C respiratory rate, heart rate, and blood pressure decline because the functional reserve is reduced.

With prolonged cooling, a "cold-induced" diuresis results in increased blood viscosity. As a result, blood flow decreases and oxygen–hemoglobin association is less effective. Cardiac stroke volume decreases and peripheral vascular resistance increases as a direct result of both blood "sludging" and loss of plasma. The most important factor in causing death is cardiac arrhythmia or sudden cardiac arrest. These observations have been confirmed and extended, largely because of the need to induce hypothermia in some patients undergoing open-heart surgery. In fact, with careful pharmacologic control, prolonged periods of lower body temperature can be achieved with no residual harm.

If hypothermia is prolonged, decreased body temperature alters cerebrovascular function. When body core temperature reaches 32°C (89.6°F), the person becomes lethargic, apathetic and withdrawn. A characteristic response is inappropriate behavior, including disrobing, even when cold. If temperature falls further, intermittent "stupor" and eventually coma supervene. If core temperature goes below 28°C (82.4°F) pulse and breathing weaken.

Although there are no specific morphologic changes in those who die from hypothermia, the skin shows red and purple discolorations, ears and hands swell, and there is irregular vasoconstriction and vasodilation. Areas of cardiac myocytolysis are seen. Lungs may display pulmonary edema and intra-alveolar, intrabronchial, and interstitial hemorrhage.

Focal Thermal Alterations

As discussed above, local reduction in tissue temperature, particularly in the skin, is associated with local vasoconstriction. Tissue water crystallizes if blood circulation is insufficient to counter persistent thermal loss. When freezing occurs slowly, ice crystals form within tissue cells and in the interstitial space. Concomitantly, electrolyte-rich gels are excluded. Injury to cellular organelles reflects the drastic changes in ion concentrations in the excluded volume. Denaturation of macromolecules, and physical disruption of cellular membranes by the ice, ensue. When freezing is rapid, a gel-like structure forms within the cell that lacks water crystalloids. This water-solid reduces the extent of mechanical and chemical injury. The most significant cellular damage apparently occurs on thawing, when mechanical disruption of membrane structures occurs, perhaps the result of transformation from a gel to a crystal.

The most biologically significant cell injury appears in the endothelial lining of the capillaries and venules, which alters small vessel permeability. This injury initiates extravasation of plasma, formation of localized edema and blisters and an inflammatory reaction. Whereas frostbite results from the actual freezing of water, immersion foot (trench foot) is caused by a prolonged reduction in tissue temperature to a point not low enough to freeze tissue. This cooling causes cellular disruption. Endothelial cell damage leads to local thrombosis and changes caused by altered permeability are prominent. Vascular occlusion often leads to gangrene.

Hyperthermia Means an Increase in Body Temperature

Tissue responses to hyperthermia are similar in some respects to those caused by freezing injuries. In both instances, injury to the vascular endothelium results in altered vascular permeability, edema, and blisters. The degree of injury depends on the extent of temperature elevation and how quickly it is reached. Small increases in body temperature increase the metabolic rate. However, above a certain limit enzymes denature and other proteins precipitate and "melting" of lipid bilayers of cell membranes takes place.

Systemic Hyperthermia

Systemic hyperthermia, or **fever**, is an elevation of body core temperature. It occurs because of (1) increased heat production, (2) decreased elimination of heat from the body (reflecting an aberrant response of the thermal regulatory center), or (3) a disturbance of the thermal regulatory center itself. Hyperthermia can also occur because heat is conducted into the body faster than the system can clear it.

A body temperature above 42.5°C (108.5°F) leads to profound functional disturbances, including general vasodilation, inefficient cardiac function, and altered respiration. Isolated heart–lung preparations fail at about the same temperature, suggesting an inherent limitation in the cardiovascular system and perhaps in the myocardial cells themselves. *In general, systemic temperature elevations above 41° to 42°C (105° to 107.6°F) are not compatible with life.*

During infectious and inflammatory responses, several cytokines including IL-1, IL-6, and TNF -α, interact with a portion of the hypothalamus at the roof of the third ventricle, the organum vasculosum laminae terminalis, and apparently reset the body's "thermostat" to permit a higher body core temperature. There is also evidence that for mild pyrogens, parasympathetic activation may be involved.

Few, if any, defined pathologic changes are associated with fever alone. Physical findings include increased heart and respiratory rates, peripheral vasodilation, and diaphoresis, all recognized mechanisms for thermal regulation. The CNS may respond with irritability, restlessness, and (particularly in children) convulsions. Nocturnal temperature elevations with "night sweats" are a feature of pulmonary granulomatous infection (especially tuberculosis) and are also observed in lymphoproliferative diseases. Prolonged temperature elevation can produce wasting, principally because of an increased metabolic rate.

Malignant hyperthermia is a thermal alteration, accompanied by a hypermetabolic state and often by rhabdomyolysis (muscle necrosis), that occurs after anesthesia in susceptible persons. This autosomal dominant disorder is associated with mutations in the gene for the sarcoplasmic reticulum ryanodine receptor. Muscle damage is caused by an abnormally high calcium concentration produced by accelerated release of Ca^{2+} through the mutant calcium release channel.

Heat stroke is a form of hyperthermia that occurs under conditions of very high ambient temperatures and is not mediated by endogenous pyrogens. It reflects impaired thermal regulatory cooling responses and characteristically occurs in infants, young children, and the very aged. Often the disorder is associated with an underlying chronic illness and use of diuretics, tranquilizers that may affect the hypothalamic thermal regulatory center, or drugs that inhibit perspiration. Another form of heat stroke is seen in healthy men during unusually vigorous exercise. Lactic acidosis, hypocalcemia, and rhabdomyolysis may be severe problems and almost one third of patients with exertional heat stroke develop myoglobinuric acute renal failure. Heat stroke is not amenable to treatment with standard antipyretics and only external cooling and fluid and electrolyte replacement are effective therapy.

Cutaneous Burns

Cutaneous burns are the most common form of localized hyperthermia. Both the elevated temperature and rate of temperature change are important in determining the tissue response. A temperature of 50°C (120°F) may be sustained for 10 minutes or more without cell death, while a temperature 70°C (158°F) or higher for even several seconds causes necrosis of the entire epidermis.

Cutaneous burns have been separated into three categories of severity: first-, second-, and third-degree burns (Fig. 8-16). A more contemporary classification refers to full-thickness (third-degree) and partial thickness (first- and second-degree) burns.

- **First-degree burns,** such as a mild sunburn, are recognized by congestion and pain but are not associated with necrosis. Mild endothelial injury produces vasodilation, increased vascular permeability, and slight edema.
- **Second-degree burns** cause epidermal necrosis, but spare the dermis. Clinically, these burns are recognized by blisters, in which the epithelium separates from the dermis.
- **Third-degree burns** char both epidermis and dermis. Histologically, they are carbonized and cellular structure is lost.

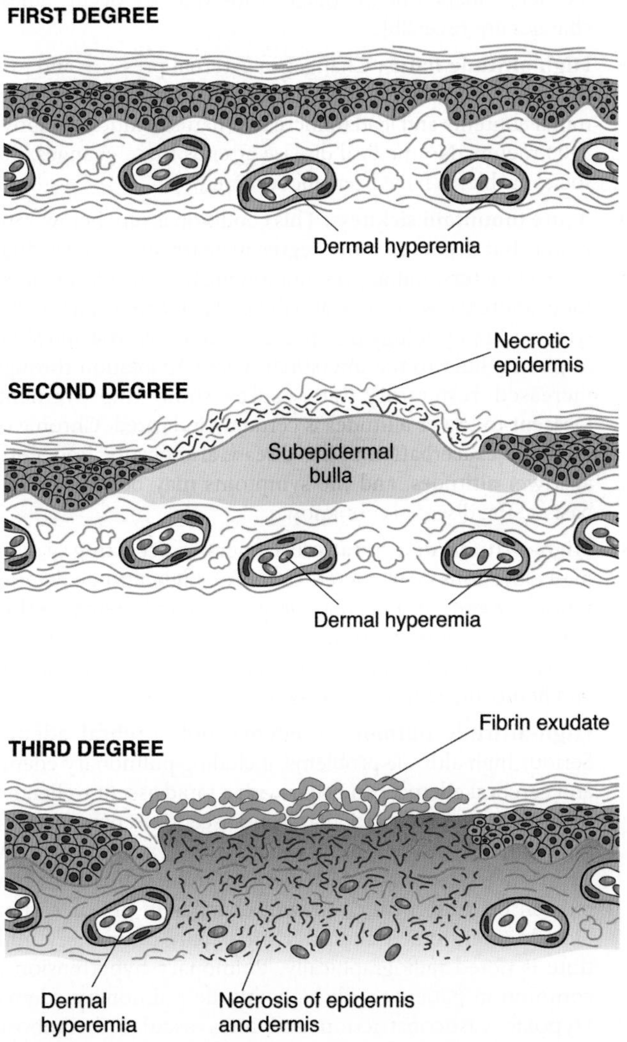

FIGURE 8-16. **The pathology of cutaneous burns.** A first-degree skin burn exhibits only dilation of the dermal blood vessels. In a second-degree burn, there is necrosis of the epidermis, and subepidermal edema collects under the necrotic epidermis to form a bulla. In a third-degree burn, both the epidermis and dermis are necrotic.

Among the most important functions of the skin are fluid retention and protection from infectious agents. Not surprisingly, then, when skin is severely damaged its ability to subserve these functions is compromised. One of the most serious systemic disturbances caused by extensive cutaneous burns is fluid loss. Persons with third-degree burns can lose about 0.3 mL of body water/cm^2 of burned area per day. Resulting hemoconcentration and poor vascular perfusion of the skin and other viscera complicate the recovery of these patients. Many severely burned persons, particularly those with more than 70% of their body surface involved with third-degree burns, develop shock and acute tubular necrosis of the kidneys, and mortality is very high. Severely burned patients who survive longer are at great risk of lethal surface infections and sepsis. Even normal skin saprophytes may cause infection of charred tissue and pose another difficulty for healing.

Healing of cutaneous burns is related to the extent of tissue destruction. First-degree burns, by definition, have little if any cell loss, and healing requires only repair or replacement of injured endothelial cells. Second-degree burns also heal without a scar because epidermal basal cells remain, and are a source of regenerating cells for the epithelium. Third-degree burns, in which the entire thickness of the epidermis is destroyed, pose a separate set of problems. If the skin appendages are spared, reepithelialization can arise from them. Initially, islands of proliferation at the orifices of these glands grow and coalesce to cover the surface. Deeper burns that destroy the skin appendages require new epidermis to be grafted to the débrided area to establish a functional covering. Burned skin that is not replaced by a graft heals with dense scarring. Since this scar tissue lacks the elasticity of normal skin, contractures that limit motion may eventually result. In severe burns, epithelial layers have been produced in vitro from cultured keratinocytes derived from the patient's own surviving skin. This approach has permitted some severely injured patients to survive, who previously would surely have died.

Inhalation Burns

Persons trapped in burning buildings and vehicles are exposed to air and aerosolized flammable materials heated to very high temperatures. Inhalation of these noxious fumes injures or destroys respiratory tract epithelium from the oral cavity to the alveoli. If a patient survives the acute episode, acute respiratory distress syndrome (ARDS), which itself may be fatal (see Chapter 12), may develop.

Electrical Burns

Electrical injury produces damage through: (1) electrical dysfunction of cardiovascular conduction and the nervous system, and (2) conversion of electrical energy to heat energy when the current encounters the resistance of the tissues. *Because electrical energy can potentially disrupt the electrical system within the heart, it frequently causes death through ventricular fibrillation.* The amount of current necessary for such a disruption depends in part on its

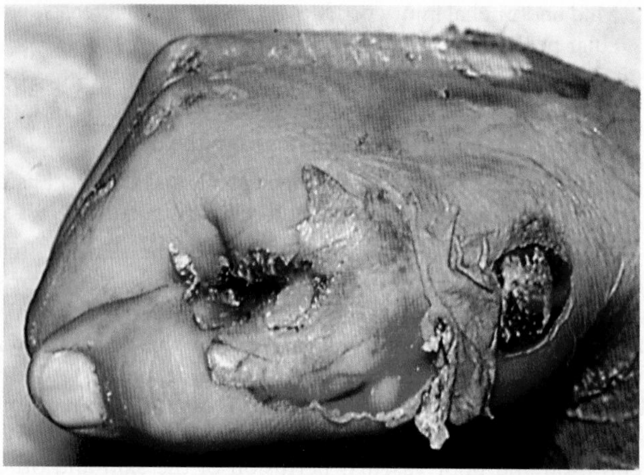

FIGURE 8-17. **Electrical burn of the skin.** The victim was electrocuted after attempting to stop a fall from a ladder by grasping a high-voltage electrical line.

pathway through the body and its ease in penetrating the skin. Someone who inadvertently touches a 120-V line in a living room may suffer burns on the hand because the skin that contacts the wire has substantial resistance to the flow of electrical current. If that resistance is decreased, as when a person inadvertently touches the same line in a bathtub, the lower resistance increases transmitted current, leading to disordered cardiac electrical activity.

Electrical burns of the skin reflect the voltage, the area of electrical conductance, and the duration of current flow (Fig. 8-17). Very high-voltage current chars tissue and produces a third-degree burn. On the other hand, broad, moist surfaces exposed to the same flow exhibit less-severe change. With exposure to very high-voltage currents, the force may be almost "explosive," in which case vaporization of tissue water produces extensive damage.

Altitude-related Illnesses

High-altitude illness is rare, in large part because mountain climbers tend to acclimate before extreme altitudes are achieved. However, there is an altitude limit beyond which human life cannot be sustained for prolonged periods. Communities in the Andes succeed at 4000 to 4300 meters (13,124 to 14,108 ft). Inhabitants adapt to the decreased pressure and availability of oxygen by developing elevated hematocrits and large "barrel" chests with increased lung volume. Even those who live in this zone do not survive at elevations above 5500 to 6000 meters (18,045 to 19,686 ft). Prolonged stays at this altitude result in weight loss, difficulty in sleeping, and lethargy, perhaps because of the redirection of cellular energy simply for survival. For example, 75% to 90% of the oxygen available at 6000 meters is used simply for the effort of inspiration.

The modifications induced by high altitude are related to decreased atmospheric pressure and consequent decreased oxygen availability. Unlike sea level, where activity does not change oxygen saturation, physical activity at these elevations leads to decreased partial pressure of arterial oxygen. At sea level, cardiac output limits exercise; at high altitudes, the diffusing capacity of the lung for oxygen seems to be the determinant.

Acclimation to chronic hypoxia at high altitudes results in a reduced ventilatory drive. Acclimated persons exhibit increases in: (1) capillaries per unit volume of brain, muscle, and myocardium; (2) myoglobin within tissues; (3) mitochondria per cell; and (4) hematocrit. An increase in erythrocyte levels of 2′3′-diphosphoglycerate, which enhances oxygen delivery to tissues, occurs within hours, but polycythemia takes months. Some of the minor effects of high altitude are systemic edema, retinal hemorrhages, and flatulence. The more serious nonfatal diseases are acute and chronic mountain sickness and high-altitude deterioration. Fatal **high-altitude pulmonary edema** and **high-altitude encephalopathy** may ensue.

- **High-altitude systemic edema:** This condition results from asymptomatic increases in vascular permeability, particularly in hands, face, and feet, and most often at elevations over 3000 meters. It is reflected only in weight gain; on return to lower altitude, diuresis causes the edema to disappear. This disorder may in part reflect endothelial cell responses to hypoxia and is twice as common in women as in men.
- **High-altitude retinal hemorrhage:** A critical analysis by funduscopic examination revealed that 30% to 60% of those sleeping above 5000 meters had retinal hemorrhages. The initial effect includes retinal vascular engorgement and tortuousness. Optic disc hyperemia is also noted, and multiple flame-shaped hemorrhages subsequently occur. These changes are reversible.
- **High-altitude flatus:** Changes in external pressure and production of intestinal gas provide for expansion of intestinal luminal contents and lead to increased flatus at altitudes above 3500 meters. No medical disease attends these changes, but social problems have been encountered.
- **Acute mountain sickness:** This condition is rare below 2500 meters but occurs to some degree in nearly everyone at 3000 to 3600 meters. Initial presentation includes headache, lassitude, anorexia, weakness, and difficulty sleeping. The underlying pathophysiology is in part related to hypoxia and shifts in plasma fluid to the interstitial space. Adaptation through increased respiratory rate causes some improvement. Descent to lower altitudes is certainly indicated. Chronic or subacute exacerbation of this disease also occurs, frequently at lower altitudes, and the symptoms may be severe. The basis of the disease is not known.
- **High-altitude deterioration:** Generally occurring at very high elevations (5500 meters or more), high-altitude deterioration presents as a decrease in physical and mental performance. The combination of chronic hypoxia, inadequate fluid intake, inadequate nutrition, decreased plasma volume, and hemoconcentration are aggravating factors.
- **High-altitude pulmonary edema and cerebral edema:** Serious high-altitude problems, including pulmonary edema and cerebral edema, can occur with a rapid ascent to heights over 2500 meters, particularly in susceptible persons who have difficulty sleeping at higher altitudes. Tachycardia, right ventricular overload, and marked reduction in arterial oxygen pressure occur, without changes in pH or carbon dioxide retention. A characteristic patchy pulmonary infiltrate is noted radiographically. Pulmonary hypertension is common in patients with high-altitude pulmonary edema. Hypoxic vasoconstriction and intravascular thrombosis have been proposed as causes of pulmonary hypertension. Eventually, cardiac output is decreased and systemic blood pressure falls. The precapillary arterioles become dilated, increasing capillary bed pressure and inducing interstitial and

alveolar edema. Autopsy findings include severe confluent pulmonary edema, proteinaceous alveolar exudates, and hyaline membrane formation. Capillary obstruction by thrombi has been noted. A dilated heart and enlarged pulmonary arteries are commonly found.

- **High-altitude encephalopathy** is characterized by confusion, stupor, and coma. Autopsies reveal cerebral edema and vascular congestion. A proposed mechanism is severe cerebral hypoxia, with inhibition of the sodium pump and resultant intracellular edema.

Physical Injuries

The effect of mechanical trauma is related to (1) the force transmitted to the tissue, (2) the rate at which the transfer occurs, (3) the surface area to which the force is transferred, and (4) the area of the body involved. The compressibility of the tissue adjacent to the transmitted force in part determines its effect. However, transmission of absorbed energy can produce alterations elsewhere in the body. Blows over a hollow viscus can rupture the organ because of compression of the fluid or gas it contains; organs nestled beneath the skin, such as the liver, can be easily ruptured. An impact directly over the heart can even disturb its electrical systems. However, a blow over a large muscle mass, such as the thigh or upper arm, is often less injurious than a direct blow to a poorly shielded bone, such as the anterior tibia. Furthermore, the distribution of the force is important.

A Contusion Is a Localized Mechanical Injury with Focal Hemorrhage

A force with sufficient energy may disrupt capillaries and venules within an organ by physical means alone. The result may be so limited that the only histologic change is hemorrhage in tissue spaces outside the vascular compartment. A discrete extravascular blood pool within the tissue is called a **hematoma.** Initially, the deoxygenated blood renders the area blue to blue-black, as in the classic "black eye." Macrophages ingest the erythrocytes, convert their hemoglobin to bilirubin and so change the color from blue to yellow. Both mobilization of the pigment by macrophages and further metabolism of bilirubin cause the yellow to fade to yellowish green and then to disappear.

An Abrasion Is a Skin Defect Caused by Crushes or Scrapes

The disruptive force may provide a portal of entry for microorganisms. The impact of the agent and its configuration are frequently seen in these wounds and are of special interest to the forensic pathologist.

A Laceration Is a Split or Tear of the Skin

Lacerations result from an impact stronger than that causing an abrasion and are usually the result of unidirectional displacement. When they have crushed margins, they are termed abraded lacerations.

Wounds Are Mechanical Disruptions of Tissue Integrity

An incision is a deliberate opening in the skin by a cutting instrument, e.g., a surgeon's scalpel. Incisions have sharp edges and, importantly, spare no tissue to the depth of the wound. **Deep penetrating wounds** made by high-velocity projectiles, such as bullets, are often deceptive, because the energy of the missile as it passes through the body may be released at sites distant from the entrance itself. Bullets, because they rotate, produce a well-defined and usually round entrance wound (Fig. 8-18). Once the projectile enters the flesh, however, it may fragment, tumble, or actually explode, resulting in considerable tissue damage and a large, ragged exit wound.

Radiation

We can define radiation simply as emission of energy by one body, its transmission through an intervening medium, and its absorption by another body. By this definition, radiation encompasses the entire electromagnetic spectrum and certain charged particles emitted by radioactive elements. Alpha particles, and the beta particles of elements such as tritium (^3H) and carbon 14 (^{14}C), are of immense use scientifically and diagnostically but pose few hazards for humans. High-energy radiation, in the form of gamma or x-rays, mediates most of the biological effects discussed here. We do not consider the effects of ultraviolet radiation here; they are discussed in Chapters 5 and 24.

A

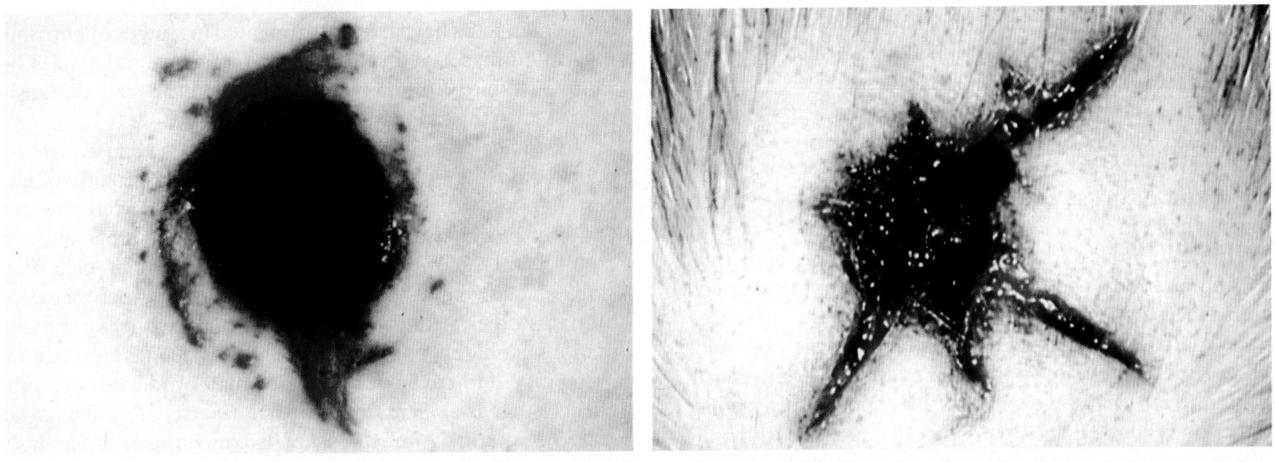

B

FIGURE 8-18. **Bullet wounds. A**. The entrance wound is sharply punched out. **B**. The exit wound is irregular with characteristic stellate lacerations.

Radiation is quantitated in a number of ways:

- **A roentgen** is a measure of the emission of radiant energy from a source. This unit refers to the amount of ionization produced in air.
- **A rad** measures absorption of radiant energy, which is biologically the more important parameter. A rad defines the energy, expressed as ergs, absorbed by a tissue. One rad equals 100 ergs per gram of tissue.
- **A gray** (Gy) corresponds to 100 rads (1 joule/kg of tissue), and a centigray (cGy) is equivalent to 1 rad.
- **The rem** was introduced to describe the biological effect caused by a rad of high-energy radiation, since low-energy particles produce more biological damage than gamma or x-rays.
- **A sievert** (Sv) is the dose in gray multiplied by an appropriate quality factor Q, so that 1 Sv of radiation is roughly equivalent in biological effectiveness to 1 Gy of gamma rays.

For the purposes of this discussion of radiation-induced pathology, the rad, gray, rem, and sievert are considered comparable.

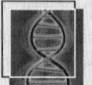

PATHOGENESIS: At the cellular level, radiation essentially has two effects: (1) a somatic effect, associated with acute cell killing; and (2) genetic damage. Radiation-induced cell death is believed to be caused by the acute effects of the radiolysis of water (see Chapter 1). The production of activated oxygen species may result in lipid peroxidation, membrane injury, and possibly an interaction with macromolecules of the cell. Genetic damage to the cell—whether caused by direct absorption of energy by DNA (the target theory) or caused indirectly by a reaction of DNA with oxygen radicals—is expressed either as mutation or as reproductive failure. Both mutation and reproductive failure may lead to delayed cell death and mutation is incriminated in the development of radiation-induced neoplasia.

Different tissues are differently sensitive to radiation. The vulnerability of a tissue to radiation-induced damage depends on its proliferative rate, which in turn correlates with the natural life span of the constituent cells. For example, the intestine and the hematopoietic bone marrow are far more vulnerable than tissues such as bone and brain. Damage to the DNA of a long-lived, nonproliferating cell does not necessarily impair its function or viability because its reproductive and metabolic functions are separate properties. By contrast, a short-lived, proliferating cell, such as an intestinal crypt cell or a hematopoietic precursor, must be rapidly replaced by division of precursor cells. If radiation-induced DNA damage precludes mitosis of these cells, the mature elements are not replaced and the tissue can no longer function.

It is important to distinguish between whole-body irradiation and localized irradiation. Except for unusual circumstances, as in the high-dose irradiation that precedes bone marrow transplantation, significant levels of whole-body irradiation result only from industrial accidents or from nuclear weapons explosions. By contrast, localized irradiation is an inevitable byproduct of any diagnostic radiologic procedure, and it is the intended result of radiation therapy. Rapid somatic cell death occurs only with extremely high doses of radiation, well in excess of 1000 rads. It is morphologically indistinguishable from coagulative necrosis produced by other causes (see Chapter 1). By contrast, irreversible damage to the replicative capacity of cells requires far lower doses, possibly as few as 50 rads.

Whole-Body Irradiation Injures Many Organs

Fortunately, there have been few instances of human disease caused by whole-body irradiation, and most of our information has been derived from studies of Japanese atom bomb survivors. Further information is now available from the study of the survivors of the much smaller sample of persons exposed in the accident at the Chernobyl nuclear power plant in Ukraine in 1986.

Since comparable doses of radiant energy are transmitted to all organs in whole-body irradiation, development of the different acute radiation syndromes reflects the dissimilarities in vulnerability of the target tissues (Fig. 8-19).

- **300 cGy:** At this dose, a syndrome characterized by **hematopoietic failure** develops within 2 weeks. Following an initial depletion of circulating lymphocytes, a progressive decrease in formed elements of the blood eventually leads to bleeding, anemia, and infection. The last is often the cause of death.
- **10 Gy:** In the vicinity of this dose, the main cause of death is related to the **gastrointestinal system**. Although gastrointestinal symptoms occur through the entire dose range of whole-body exposure, at higher levels, the entire epithelium of the gastrointestinal tract is destroyed within 3 days, i.e., the time of the normal life span of villous and crypt cells. As a result, fluid homeostasis of the bowel is disrupted and severe diarrhea and dehydration ensue. Moreover, the epithelial barrier to intestinal bacteria is breached; gut organisms invade and disseminate throughout the body. Septicemia and shock kill the victim.
- **20 Gy:** With whole-body doses of 20 Gy and above, CNS damage causes death within hours. In most cases, cerebral edema and loss of the integrity of the blood–brain barrier, owing to endothelial injury, predominate. With extreme doses, radiation necrosis of neurons can be expected. Convulsions, coma, and death follow.

FETAL EFFECTS: The effects of whole-body irradiation on the human fetus have been documented in studies of Hiroshima nuclear bomb survivors. Pregnant women exposed to 25 cGy or more gave birth to infants with reduced head size, diminished overall growth, and mental retardation.

In studies of the clinical status of children exposed to therapeutic doses of radiation between the 3rd and 20th week of gestation, growth retardation and microcephaly were observed. Other effects of irradiation in utero include hydrocephaly, microphthalmia, chorioretinitis, blindness, spina bifida, cleft palate, clubfeet, and genital abnormalities. Data from experimental and human studies strongly suggest that major congenital malformations are highly unlikely at doses below 20 rads after day 14 of pregnancy. However, lower doses may produce more-subtle effects, such as a decrease in mental capacity. *To protect against such a possibility, the established maximum permissible dose of radiation to the fetus from exposure of the expectant mother is far below the known teratogenic dose.*

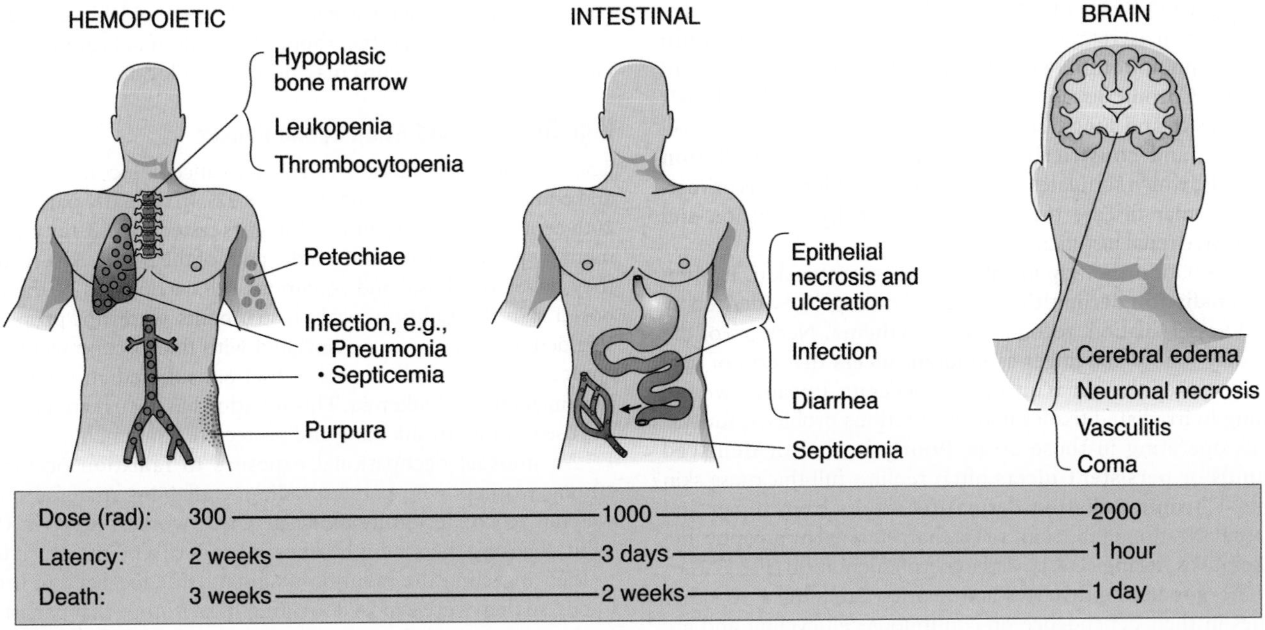

FIGURE 8-19. **Acute radiation syndromes.** At a dose of approximately 300 rads of whole body radiation, a syndrome characterized by hematopoietic failure develops within 2 weeks. In the vicinity of 1000 rads, a gastrointestinal syndrome with a latency of only 3 days is seen. With doses of 2000 rads or more, disease of the central nervous system appears within 1 hour, and death ensues rapidly.

GENETIC EFFECTS: Most data on which predictions of human genetic effects are based are derived from experimental data and analysis of nuclear bomb survivors. *After long-term follow-up, even survivors of Hiroshima and Nagasaki have showed no evidence of genetic damage in the form of either congenital abnormalities or hereditable diseases in subsequent offspring or their descendants.* In experimental animals, the risk of induced mutation per rad is at most 0.5% to 5% of the risk of spontaneous mutation (the spontaneous risk of mutation in humans is estimated to be 10% of live births). By extension, 20 to 200 rads of radiation is necessary to double the spontaneous mutation rate. Consequently, the risk of genetic damage to future generations from radiation appears to be small.

AGING: There is to date no evidence that radiation exposure leads to premature aging. A mortality study of survivors of the nuclear bomb explosions in Japan did not show excess mortality beyond that attributable to neoplasia. Nor is there any evidence of acceleration in disease among the survivors in any part of the age range.

Localized Radiation Injury Complicates Radiation Therapy for Tumors

In the course of radiation therapy for malignant neoplasms, some normal tissue is inevitably irradiated. Although almost any organ can be damaged by radiation, the skin, lungs, heart, kidney, bladder, and intestine are both susceptible and difficult to shield (Fig. 8-20). Localized damage to the bone marrow is clearly of little functional consequence because of the immense reserve capacity of the hematopoietic system.

PATHOLOGY: Persistent damage to radiation-exposed tissue can be attributed to: (1) compromise of the vascular supply and (2) a fibrotic repair reaction to acute necrosis and chronic ischemia. Radiation-induced tissue injury predominantly affects small arteries and arterioles. The endothelial cells are the most sensitive elements in the blood vessels and in the short term exhibit swelling and necrosis. With time, vascular walls become thickened by endothelial cell proliferation and subintimal deposition of collagen and other connective tissue elements. Striking vacuolization of intimal cells, so-called foam cells, is typical. Fragmentation of the internal elastic lamina, loss of smooth muscle cells, scarring in the media, and fibrosis of the adventitia are seen in the small arteries. Bizarre fibroblasts with large hyperchromatic nuclei are common and probably reflect radiation-induced DNA damage.

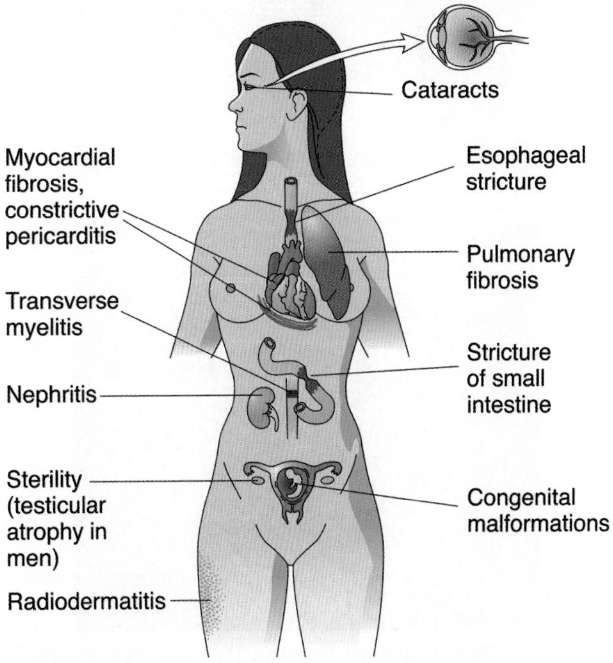

FIGURE 8-20. **The nonneoplastic complications of radiation.**

CLINICAL FEATURES: Acute necrosis from radiation is represented by such disorders as **radiation pneumonitis, cystitis, dermatitis,** and diarrhea from **enteritis.** Chronic disease is characterized by **interstitial fibrosis** in the heart and lungs, strictures in the esophagus and small intestine, and **constrictive pericarditis.** Chronic **radiation nephritis,** which simulates malignant nephrosclerosis, is primarily a vascular disease that leads to severe hypertension and progressive renal insufficiency.

As radiation therapy inevitably traverses the skin, it often causes **radiation dermatitis.** The initial damage is evidenced by blood vessel dilation, recognized as **erythema.** Necrosis of the skin may follow and linger as **indolent ulcers** that do not heal because the epithelium is unable to regenerate. Impaired wound healing in irradiated tissues may pose serious problems for surgeons operating in those areas. **Poorly healed** or **dehisced wounds** or **persistent ulcers** often require full-thickness skin grafts. **Chronic radiation dermatitis** results from repair and revascularization of the skin, and is characterized by atrophy, hyperkeratosis, telangiectasia, and hyperpigmentation (Fig. 8-21).

The gonads, both testes and ovaries, are similar to other tissues in their dependence on continuous cell cycling and are exquisitely radiosensitive. Acute inhibition of mitosis in the testis results in necrosis of the germinal stem cells, the spermatogonia. The combination of radiation-induced vascular injury and direct damage to the germ cells leads to progressive atrophy of seminiferous tubules, peritubular fibrosis, and loss of reproductive function. Interstitial and Sertoli cells do not cycle rapidly, and so persist, thereby preserving normal hormonal status. Comparable injury is seen in the irradiated ovary; the follicles become atretic and the organ eventually becomes fibrous and atrophic.

Cataracts (lenticular opacities) may be produced if the eye lies in the path of the radiation beam. **Transverse myelitis** and paraplegia occur when the spinal cord is unavoidably irradiated during treatment of certain thoracic or abdominal tumors. **Vascular damage in the cord** may bring about localized ischemia.

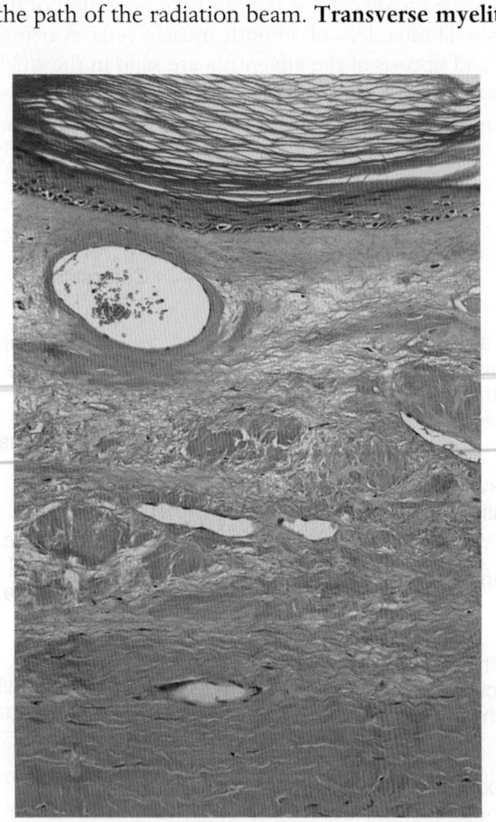

FIGURE 8-21. **Chronic radiation dermatitis.** The epidermis is atrophic. The dermis is densely fibrotic and contains dilated superficial blood vessels.

High Doses of Radiation Cause Cancer

The evidence that radiation can lead to cancer is incontrovertible and comes from many sources (Fig. 8-22). In the early part of the 20th century, scientists and radiologists tested their X-ray equipment by placing their hands in the path of the beam. As a result, they developed basal and squamous cell carcinomas of the exposed skin. In addition, early instruments were not properly shielded and the hazards associated with fluoroscopy were not appreciated. The radiologists of that era suffered an unusually high incidence of leukemia. This situation has been rectified with the use of modern shielding and protective equipment.

An unusual occupational exposure to radiation occurred among workers who painted radium-containing material onto watches to create luminous dials. These workers were in the habit of licking their paint brushes to produce a point, which led to their ingesting the radium. It subsequently localized in their bones, so they were exposed to a long-lived isotope that persisted in their bones indefinitely. These people experienced a high incidence of cancer of the bone and of the paranasal sinuses. Another example of occupational exposure to a radioactive element is the high rate of lung cancer in uranium miners who inhaled

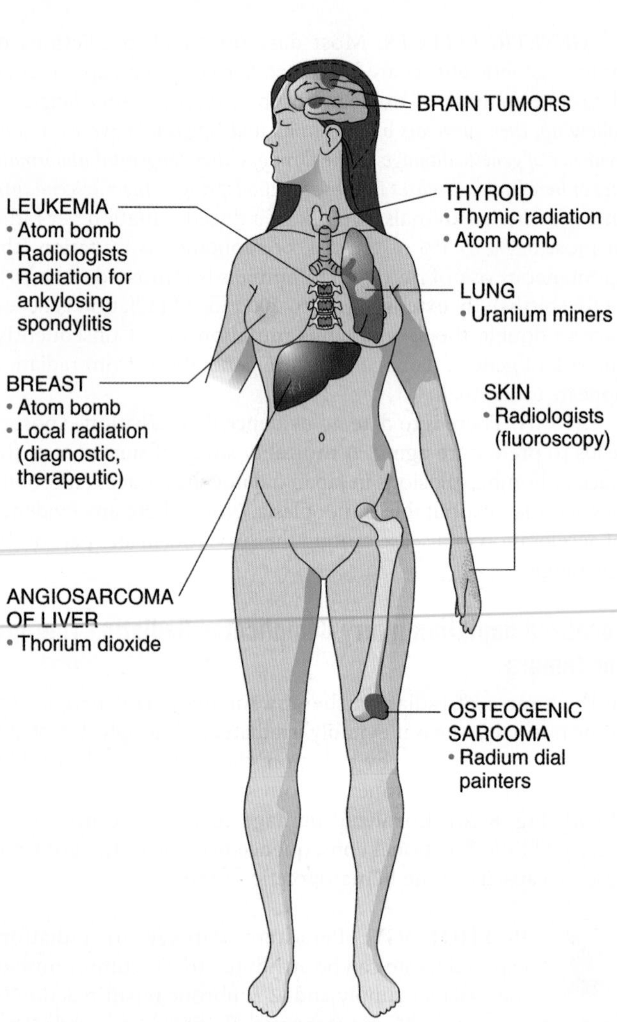

FIGURE 8-22. **Radiation-induced cancers.**

radioactive dust. Most of these workers also smoked, and evidence strongly favors a synergistic effect in lung carcinogenesis.

Iodine is concentrated by the thyroid. If radioactive iodine isotopes are inhaled or ingested, that gland will experience highly concentrated exposure to radioactivity. An explosive increase in the incidence of thyroid cancer among children in geographical areas contaminated by the nuclear catastrophe at Chernobyl in Ukraine in 1986 has been linked to release of radioactive iodine isotopes in that incident.

The risk of **solid tumors,** especially breast cancer, is particularly high among adult women who were treated with thoracic radiation for Hodgkin disease as children. Long-term survivors of childhood Hodgkin disease, who were treated with radiation therapy, have almost 20-fold increased risk of developing a second neoplasm owing to the radiation. Another example of iatrogenic cancer resulted in Great Britain from widespread use of low-dose spinal irradiation to treat ankylosing spondylitis. These patients later developed aplastic anemia, myelogenous leukemia, and other tumors with high frequency. An increase in brain tumors was found in persons who had received cranial irradiation for tinea capitis infection of the scalp in childhood. Thorium dioxide (Thorotrast), a material avidly ingested by phagocytic cells, was used a few decades ago for radionuclide imaging. The persistence in the liver of a long-lived radioisotope resulted in the development of a number of tumors, particularly angiosarcomas of the liver.

The survivors of the nuclear bomb explosions in Japan suffered from a number of cancers. They exhibited a more than 10-fold increase in the incidence of leukemia, which peaked from 5 to 10 years after exposure, then declined to background rates. Two thirds were of cases were acute leukemia; the remainder were of chronic myelogenous leukemia. Chronic lymphocytic leukemia, an uncommon disease in Japan, showed no increase in incidence. The risk of multiple myeloma increased fivefold, and there was a small increment in the incidence of lymphoma. The frequency of solid tumors, although not as great as that for leukemia, was clearly increased for the breast, lung, thyroid, gastrointestinal tract, and urinary tract. The development of malignant tumors, including leukemia, showed a dose-response relationship.

LOW-LEVEL RADIATION AND CANCER: Few debates have engendered as much heat and as little light as that concerning the potential carcinogenic effect of low levels of radiation. All assumptions are based on extrapolations to zero of the risk of cancer at higher doses or from epidemiologic studies to which valid exception may be taken. *The key question that needs to be answered is whether there is a threshold dose of radiation below which there is no increase in the incidence of cancer, or whether any exposure carries a significant risk.*

Data currently available from studies of cancer induction in animals, chromosomal damage in human cell cultures, malignant transformation of mammalian cells in vitro, and populations exposed to radiation show that the estimates of risk at low radiation doses is very low. The data do not show that the risk of cancer from low-level radiation is zero. *When data from atomic bomb survivors are subjected to a conservative analysis, the lifetime risk from 1 cGy of whole-body x- or gamma irradiation is 1 excess cancer death per 10,000 persons.*

RADON: The finding that some homes in the United States are contaminated with radon has elicited considerable public concern. Radon is a radioactive noble gas formed from the decay of uranium 238 (^{238}U), which is found in soil and rock formations. Radon is itself inert. Concern about the environmental hazards of radon focus on its radioactive decay products, which are called radon daughters. These include radioactive isotopes of bismuth, lead, and polonium, which are chemically active and which bind to particulates and lung tissues. The half-life of the α-emitting isotope, ^{218}Po, is 103 years.

Previously, studies of the risk of radon gas were done in uranium miners and were not well controlled for smoking as an independent risk factor. More recent large-scale studies indicate that people who dwell in homes containing high concentrations of radon gas have increased risk of developing lung cancer. The relative risk is by far the greatest for smokers and ex-smokers. However, recent studies also indicate that people who never smoked also have increased risk of lung cancer. The additional risk of radon exposure for developing lung cancer is proportionate to the concentration of radon in the air (measured in Becquerel [Bq]/m^3) and numbers of years spent in that environment.

Microwave Radiation, Electromagnetic Fields, and Ultrasound Are Not Ionizing

Microwaves, produced by ovens, radar, and diathermy, are electromagnetic waves that penetrate tissue but do not produce ionization. Unlike x- and gamma radiation, absorption of microwave energy produces only heat. The activation energy of radiofrequency and microwave radiation is too low to modify chemical bonds or alter DNA. Thus, exposure to microwave radiation under ordinary circumstances is highly unlikely to produce any injury. Moreover, a study of 20,000 radar technicians in the Navy who were chronically exposed to high levels of microwave radiation failed to detect any increased incidence of cancer.

Controversy also surrounds possible carcinogenic—especially leukemogenic—effects of exposure to nonionizing electromagnetic fields, such as those encountered in the vicinity of high-voltage electric lines. Recent epidemiologic evidence has led to a consensus that exposure to electromagnetic fields does not raise the incidence of leukemia or other cancers.

Ultrasound, the vibrational waves in air above the audible range, produces mechanical compression but, again, no ionization. Highly focused and energetic ultrasound devices are used to disrupt tissue in vitro for chemical analysis and to clean various surfaces, including teeth. However, there is no reason to believe that diagnostic ultrasound or accidental exposure to any industrial device results in any measurable damage.

Nutritional Disorders

Protein-Calorie Malnutrition Reflects Starvation or Specific Deficiencies

Marasmus is the term used to denote a deficiency of calories from all sources. **Kwashiorkor** is a form of malnutrition in children caused by a diet deficient in protein alone.

Marasmus

Global starvation—that is, a deficiency of all elements of the diet—leads to marasmus. The condition is common throughout the nonindustrialized world, particularly when breast feeding is stopped, and a child must subsist on a calorically inadequate diet. Pathologic changes are similar to those in starving adults and include decreased body weight, diminished subcutaneous fat, a protuberant abdomen, muscle wasting, and a wrinkled face. In general, the child is a "shrunken old person." Wasting and increased lipofuscin pigment are seen in most visceral organs, especially the heart and the liver. No edema is present. Pulse, blood pressure, and temperature are low; diarrhea is common. Since immune responses are impaired, the child suffers from numerous infections. An important consequence of marasmus is growth failure. If these children are not provided with adequate food in childhood, they will not reach their full potential stature as adults. The effects on ultimate intelligence are controversial.

Kwashiorkor

Kwashiorkor (Fig. 8-23) results from a deficiency of protein in diets relatively high in carbohydrates. It is one of the most common diseases of infancy and childhood in the nonindustrialized world. Like marasmus, it usually occurs after an infant is weaned, when a protein-poor diet, consisting principally of staple carbohydrates, replaces mother's milk. There is generalized growth failure and muscle wasting, as in marasmus, but subcutaneous fat is normal, since caloric intake is adequate. Extreme apathy is notable, in contrast to children with marasmus, who may be alert. Also in contrast to marasmus, severe edema, hepatomegaly, depigmentation of the skin, and dermatoses are usual. "Flaky paint" lesions of the skin on the face, extremities, and perineum, are dry and hyperkeratotic. Hair becomes a sandy or reddish color; a characteristic linear depigmentation of the hair ("flag sign") provides evidence of particularly severe periods of protein deficiency. The abdomen is distended because of flaccid abdominal muscles, hepatomegaly, and ascites due to hypoalbuminemia. Along with general atrophy of the viscera, villous atrophy of the intestine may interfere with nutrient absorption. Diarrhea is common. Anemia is the rule, but it is not generally life-threatening. The nonspecific effects on growth, pulse, temperature, and the immune system are similar to those in marasmus. Although it has been claimed that kwashiorkor not only impairs physical development but also stunts later intellectual growth, the subject requires further study.

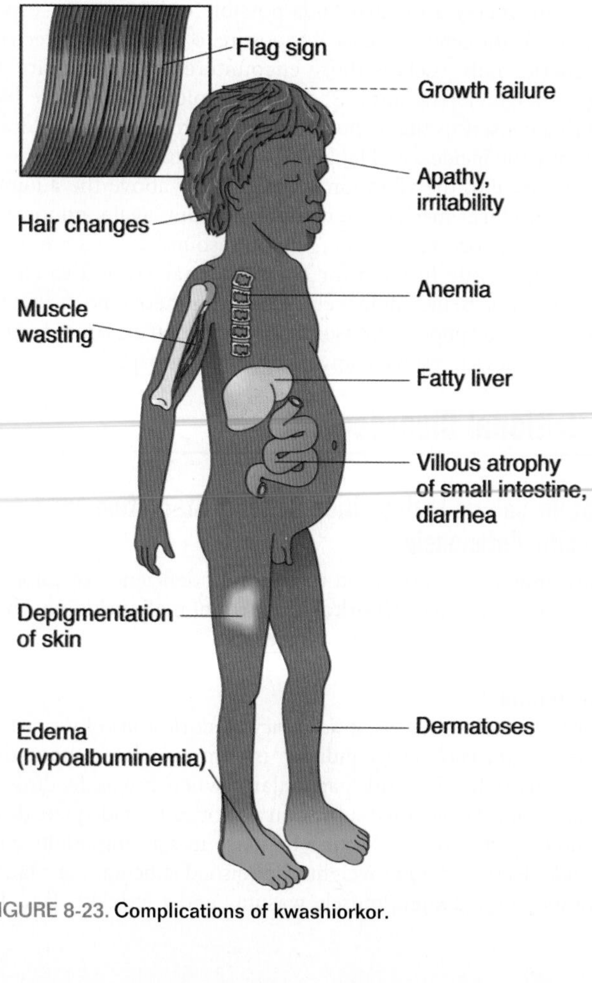

FIGURE 8-23. Complications of kwashiorkor.

PATHOLOGY: Microscopically, the liver in kwashiorkor is conspicuously fatty. Accumulation of lipid within the cytoplasm of the hepatocyte displaces the nucleus to the periphery of the cell. The adequacy of dietary carbohydrate provides lipid for the hepatocyte, but the inadequate protein stores do not permit synthesis of enough apoprotein carrier to transport the lipid from the liver cell. The changes, with the possible exception of mental retardation, are fully reversible when sufficient protein is made available. In fact, the fatty liver reverts to normal after early childhood, even if the diet remains deficient in protein. In any event, hepatic changes are not progressive and do not lead to chronic liver disease.

Vitamins Are Organic Catalysts That are Both Required for Normal Metabolism and Available Only From Dietary Sources

Thus, vitamins in one species are not necessarily vitamins in another. For example, humans cannot synthesize ascorbic acid (vitamin C) and so require dietary ascorbate to prevent scurvy, but most lower animals can produce their own vitamin C and do not require it as a vitamin.

Vitamin A

Vitamin A is a fat-soluble substance that is important for skeletal maturation, maintenance of specialized epithelial linings, and cell membrane structure. In addition, it is an important constituent of the photosensitive pigments in the retina. Vitamin A occurs naturally as retinoids or as a precursor, β-carotene. The source of the precursor—carotene—is in plants, principally leafy, green vegetables. Fish livers are a particularly rich source of vitamin A itself.

Metabolism

β-Carotene is modified in the intestinal mucosa to retinoids, which are absorbed with chylomicrons. It is stored in the liver, where 90% of the body's vitamin A is located. At times when fat absorption is impaired (e.g., diarrhea), vitamin A absorption decreases.

Vitamin A Deficiency

Although vitamin A deficiency is uncommon in developed countries, it is a significant health problem in poorer regions of the world, including much of Africa, China and Southeast Asia.

PATHOLOGY: *Deficiency of vitamin A results principally in squamous metaplasia, especially in glandular epithelium* (Fig. 8-24). Thus, keratin debris blocks sweat and tear glands. Squamous metaplasia is common in the trachea and bronchi, and bronchopneumonia is a frequent cause of death. The epithelia lining the renal pelvis, pancreatic ducts, uterus, and salivary glands are also commonly affected. Epithelial changes in the renal pelvis may be associated with kidney

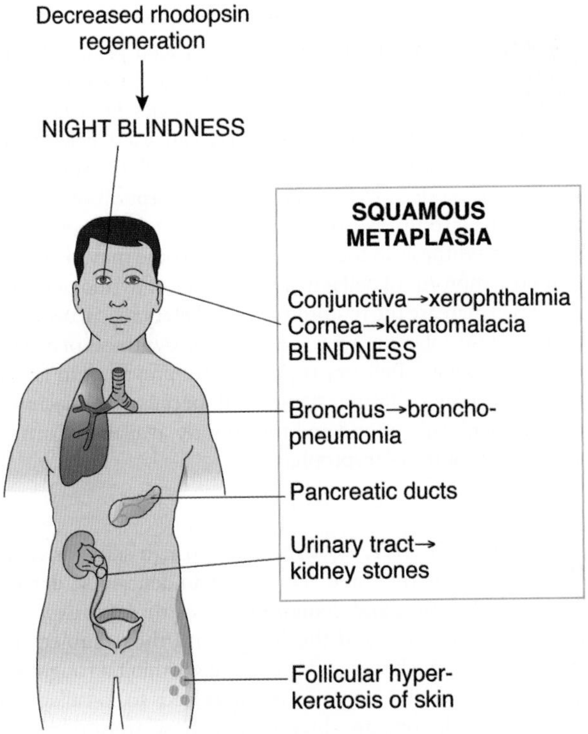

FIGURE 8-24. **Complications of vitamin A deficiency.**

stones. With further diminution of vitamin A stores, squamous metaplasia of conjunctival and tear duct epithelial cells occurs, which leads to **xerophthalmia,** dryness of the cornea, and conjunctiva. The cornea becomes softened (**keratomalacia**) and vulnerable to ulceration and bacterial infection, which may lead to blindness. **Follicular hyperkeratosis,** a skin disorder caused by occluded sebaceous, is also a feature of this disease.

CLINICAL FEATURES: The earliest sign of vitamin A deficiency often is diminished vision in dim light. Vitamin A is a necessary component in retinal rod pigment, and is active in light transduction. Because vitamin A aldehyde, retinal, is constantly degraded in generating the light signal, a continuous supply of vitamin A is necessary for night vision.

Vitamin A Toxicity

Vitamin A poisoning is usually caused by overenthusiastic administration of vitamin supplements to children. Early Arctic explorers were said to have experienced vitamin A toxicity because they ate polar bear livers, which are particularly rich in the vitamin. Enlargement of the liver and spleen are common; microscopically these organs show lipid-laden macrophages. In the liver, vitamin A is also present in hepatocytes, and prolonged hypervitaminosis A has been incriminated cirrhosis. Bone pain and neurological symptoms, such as hyperexcitability and headache, may be the presenting symptoms. Discontinuing the excess vitamin A consumption reverses all or most of the lesions. Excessive carotene intake is benign and simply stains the skin yellow, which may be mistaken for jaundice.

Synthetic derivatives of retinoic acid are now increasingly pharmacologically to alleviate severe acne. Both retinoic acid and a high dietary intake of preformed vitamin A are particularly dangerous in pregnancy because they are potent teratogens.

Vitamin B Complex

Vitamins in the B group of water-soluble vitamins are numbered 1 through 12, but most are not distinct vitamins. The members of the complex currently recognized as true vitamins are vitamins B_1 (thiamine), B_3 (niacin), B_2 (riboflavin), B_6 (pyridoxine), and B_{12} (cyanocobalamin). With the exception of vitamin B_{12}, which is derived only from animal sources, B complex vitamins are found principally in leafy green vegetables, milk, and liver.

Thiamine

Thiamine was the active ingredient in the original description of vitamin B, which was defined as a water-soluble extract in rice polishings that cured beriberi (clinical thiamine deficiency). This disease was classically seen in the Orient, where the staple food was polished rice that had been deprived of its thiamine content by processing. With increased awareness of the disease and improved nutrition in some areas of Asia, the disorder is less common now than in previous generations. In Western countries, the disease occurs in alcoholics, neglected persons with poor overall nutrition, and food faddists. *The cardinal symptoms of thiamine deficiency are polyneuropathy, edema, and cardiac failure* (Fig. 8-25). The deficiency syndrome is classically divided into **dry beriberi,** with symptoms referable to the neuromuscular system and **wet beriberi,** in which manifestations of cardiac failure predominate.

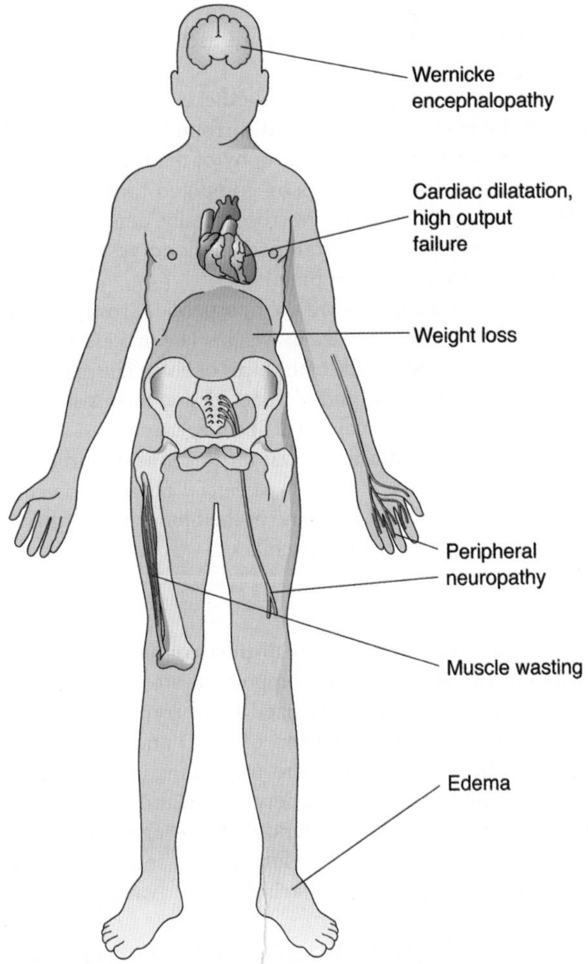

FIGURE 8-25. **Complications of thiamine deficiency (beriberi).**

CLINICAL FEATURES: Patients with dry beriberi present with paresthesias, depressed reflexes and weakness, and muscle atrophy in the extremities. Wet beriberi is characterized by generalized edema, a reflection of severe congestive failure. The basic lesion is uncontrolled, generalized vasodilation and significant peripheral arteriovenous shunting. This combination leads to a compensatory increases in cardiac output, and eventually to a large dilated heart and congestive heart failure. In a patient without documented metabolic disease (e.g., hyperthyroidism), high output failure, and generalized edema strongly suggest thiamine deficiency. The biochemical basis for the symptoms of thiamine deficiency is not understood.

Thiamine deficiency in chronic alcoholics may be manifested by CNS involvement, in the form of Wernicke syndrome, in which progressive **dementia, ataxia, and ophthalmoplegia** (paralysis of the extraocular muscles) are prominent. Korsakoff syndrome, in which a thought disorder is conspicuous, at one time was attributed solely to thiamine deficiency, but is now understood to be seen both in chronic alcoholics and in patients with other organic mental syndromes.

PATHOLOGY: Pathologic examination of the nervous system in thiamine deficiency has not defined a pathognomonic change in the peripheral nerves, given that similar or identical changes can be seen other peripheral neuropathies. A characteristic alteration is myelin sheath degeneration, which often begins in the sciatic nerve, then involves other peripheral nerves and sometimes the spinal cord itself. In advanced cases, axon fragmentation may be seen.

The most striking lesions in Wernicke encephalopathy are found in the mamillary bodies and surrounding areas that abut on the third ventricle. Indeed, atrophy of the mamillary bodies can be visualized in alcoholics by computed tomography and magnetic resonance imaging. Microscopically, degeneration and loss of ganglion cells, rupture of small blood vessels and ring hemorrhages are seen in the brain.

The changes in the heart are also nonspecific. Grossly, the heart is flabby, dilated, and increased in weight. The process may affect either the right or the left side of the heart or both. The microscopic changes are nondescript and include edema, inconsistent fiber hypertrophy, and occasional foci of fiber degeneration.

The most reliable diagnostic test for thiamine deficiency is an immediate and dramatic response to parenteral administration of thiamine. Measurements of thiamine in the blood and erythrocyte transketolase activity are also useful.

Niacin

Niacin refers to two chemically distinct compounds: nicotinic acid and nicotinamide. These components are derived from dietary niacin or are biosynthesized from tryptophan. Niacin plays a major role in formation of NAD and its phosphate (NADP). These compounds are important in intermediary metabolism and a extensive variety of oxidation–reduction reactions. Animal protein, as found in meat, eggs, and milk, is high in tryptophan and is therefore a good source of endogenously synthesized niacin. Niacin itself is available in many types of grain.

Pellagra is the term for clinical niacin deficiency. It is uncommon today.

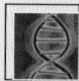

PATHOGENESIS: Pellagra is seen principally in patients who have been weakened by other diseases, and in malnourished alcoholics. Food faddists who do not eat sufficient protein may suffer a deficiency of tryptophan, which in combination with a lack of exogenous niacin may result in mild pellagra. Malabsorption of tryptophan, as in Hartnup disease, or excessive use of tryptophan for serotonin synthesis in the carcinoid syndrome may also lead to mild symptoms of pellagra. Deficiencies of pyridoxine and riboflavin increase the requirement for dietary niacin because both of these cofactors are required for biosynthesis of niacin from tryptophan. Pellagra is particularly prevalent in areas where corn (maize) is the staple food, because the niacin in corn is chemically bound and thus poorly available. Corn is also a poor source of tryptophan.

PATHOLOGY: Pellagra (Ital., "rough skin") is characterized by the three "Ds" of niacin deficiency: **dermatitis, diarrhea, and dementia** (Fig. 8-26). Areas exposed to light, such as the face and the hands, and those subjected to pressure, such as the knees and the elbows, exhibit a rough, scaly dermatitis. The involvement of the hands leads to so-called glove dermatitis. The lesions are discrete and show areas of pigmentation and of depigmentation. Microscopically, hyperkeratosis, vascularization, and chronic inflammation of the skin are characteristic. Subcutaneous fibrosis and scarring may be seen in late stages. Similar lesions are found in the mucous membranes of the mouth and vagina. In the mouth, inflammation and edema lead to a large, red tongue, which in the chronic stage is fissured and is likened to raw meat. Chronic, watery diarrhea is typical for the disease, presumably due to mucosal atrophy and ulceration in the entire gastrointestinal tract, particularly in the colon. The dementia, characterized by aberrant ideation bordering on psychosis, is represented in the brain by degeneration of ganglion cells in the cortex. Myelin degeneration of tracts in the spinal cord resembles the subacute combined degeneration of vitamin B_{12} deficiency. Severe long-standing pellagra adds another "**D**," namely death.

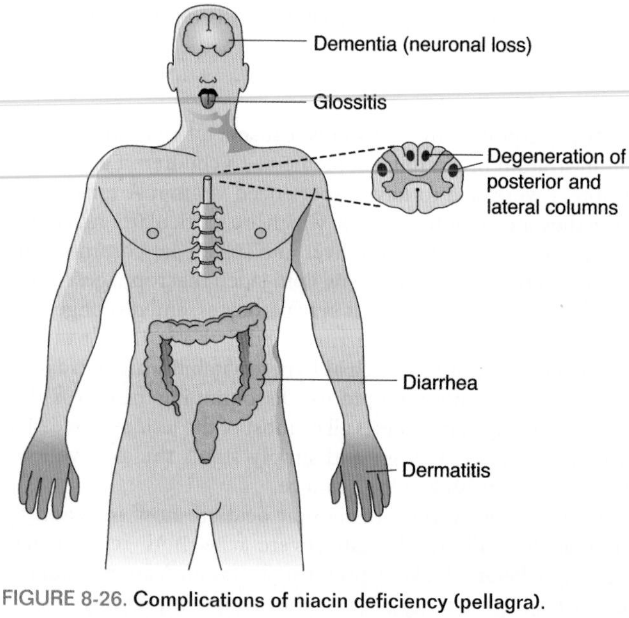

FIGURE 8-26. **Complications of niacin deficiency (pellagra).**

Riboflavin

Riboflavin, a vitamin derived from many plant and animal sources, is important for synthesis of flavin nucleotides, which are important in electron transport and other reactions in which energy transfer is crucial. Riboflavin is converted within the body to flavin mononucleotides and dinucleotides. Clinical symptoms of riboflavin deficiency are uncommon; they are usually seen only in debilitated patients with a variety of diseases and in poorly nourished alcoholics.

Deficiencies of thiamine, riboflavin, and niacin are unusual in industrialized countries because bread and cereals are fortified with these vitamins. Occasionally, a mild riboflavin deficiency is seen during pregnancy and lactation, or during a phase of rapid growth in childhood and adolescence, when increased demands are combined with moderate nutritional deprivation.

PATHOLOGY: Riboflavin deficiency is manifested principally by lesions of the facial skin and corneal epithelium. **Cheilosis,** a term used for fissures in the skin at the angles of the mouth, is a characteristic feature (Fig. 8-27). These cracks in the skin may be painful and often become infected. Microscopically, hyperkeratosis and a mild mononuclear infiltrate of the skin are noted. **Seborrheic dermatitis,** an inflammation of the skin that exhibits a greasy, scaling appearance, typically involves the cheeks and the areas behind the ears. The tongue is smooth and purplish (magenta), owing to mucosal atrophy. The most troubling lesion may be **corneal interstitial keratitis,** which is followed by opacification of the cornea and eventual ulceration. The localization of the lesions in riboflavin deficiency is not explained biochemically.

Pyridoxine

Vitamin B_6 activity is found in three related, naturally occurring compounds: pyridoxine, pyridoxal, and pyridoxamine. For convenience, they are grouped under the heading pyridoxine. These compounds are widely distributed in vegetable and animal foods.

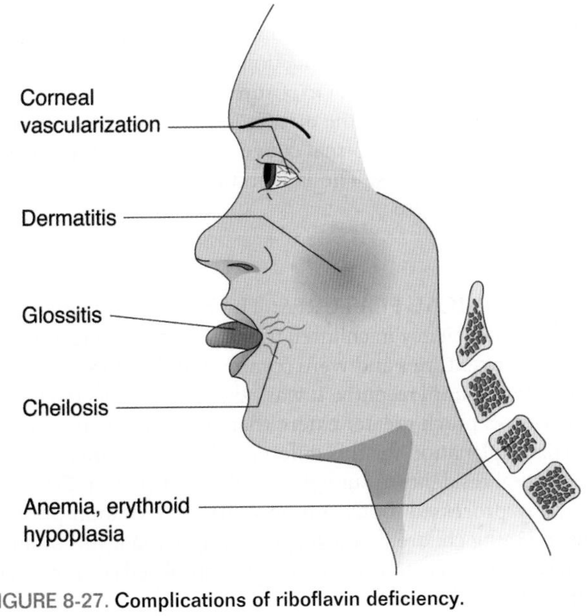

FIGURE 8-27. **Complications of riboflavin deficiency.**

PATHOGENESIS: Pyridoxine is converted to pyridoxal phosphate, a coenzyme for many enzymes, including transaminases and carboxylases. Pyridoxine deficiency is rarely caused by an inadequate diet, although infants who have been fed poorly prepared powdered formula in which pyridoxine was destroyed during preparation have suffered convulsions. A higher demand for the vitamin, as may occur in pregnancy, may lead to a secondary deficiency state. Of particular concern is the deficiency of pyridoxine that follows prolonged medication with a number of drugs, particularly isoniazid, cycloserine, and penicillamine. A deficiency state is also occasionally reported in alcoholics.

CLINICAL FEATURES: There are no clinical manifestations of pyridoxine deficiency that can be considered characteristic or pathognomonic. The usual dermatologic complications of other B vitamin deficiencies occur with pyridoxine deficiency. *The primary expression of the disease is in the CNS, a feature consistent with the role of this vitamin in the formation of pyridoxal-dependent decarboxylase of the neurotransmitter GABA.* In infants and children, diarrhea, anemia, and seizures have occurred.

Conditions are encountered in which there is no clinical or biochemical evidence of pyridoxine deficiency, yet large (pharmacologic) doses of the vitamin are useful in treating the disorder. Such diseases are termed pyridoxine-dependency syndromes and include anemia, convulsions, and homocystinuria caused by cystathionine synthetase deficiency.

Pyridoxine-responsive anemia is hypochromic and microcytic and therefore can be confused with iron deficiency anemia. Unlike iron deficiency anemia, however, pyridoxine-responsive anemia is characterized by saturation of iron stores and increased saturation of transferrin. Thus, administration of iron may simply make pyridoxine-responsive anemia worse. By definition, the anemia responds well to massive doses of pyridoxine.

Vitamin B_{12} and Folic Acid Deficiencies

Deficiency of vitamin B_{12} is almost always seen in cases of pernicious anemia and result from the lack of secretion of intrinsic factor in the stomach, which prevents absorption of the vitamin in the ileum.

PATHOGENESIS: Since vitamin B_{12} is found in almost all animal protein, including meat, milk, and eggs, dietary deficiency is seen only in rare cases of extreme vegetarianism and then only after many years of a restricted diet. Parasitization of the small intestine by the fish tapeworm *Diphyllobothrium latum* (from undercooked fish) may lead to vitamin B_{12} deficiency because the parasite absorbs the vitamin in the gut lumen.

Deficiency of folic acid is commonly of dietary origin. Leafy vegetables, liver, kidney, and yeast are rich sources of folic acid. However, excessive cooking destroys much of the folic acid in foods. Dietary folic acid deficiency is usually accompanied by multiple vitamin deficiencies. Pregnancy increases the requirement for folic acid 5- to 10-fold. *It has been estimated that two thirds of anemic pregnant women are folate deficient,* although this may be combined with iron deficiency. Folic acid is absorbed principally in the upper third of the small intestine and thus folate deficiency is common in certain diseases of malabsorption, notably nontropical and tropical celiac disease. The latter condition responds to treatment with folic acid.

CLINICAL FEATURES: Deficiencies of both vitamin B_{12} and folic acid are associated with megaloblastic anemia. In addition, pernicious anemia is complicated by a neurologic condition called subacute combined degeneration of the spinal cord. Comprehensive discussions of vitamin B_{12} and folic acid deficiencies are found in Chapters 20 and 28. In pregnant women, deficiency of folate may lead to spina bifida and other dysraphic anomalies in the fetus, which are in turn prevented by folate supplementation (see Chapter 6).

Vitamin C (Ascorbic Acid)

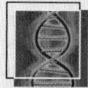

PATHOGENESIS: Ascorbic acid is a powerful biological reducing agent involved in many oxidation–reduction reactions and in proton transfer. This vitamin is important for chondroitin sulfate synthesis and for proline hydroxylation to form the hydroxyproline of collagen. It serves many other important functions: it prevents oxidation of tetrahydrofolate and augments absorption of iron from the gut. Without vitamin C, biosynthesis of certain neurotransmitters is impaired because dopamine β-hydroxylase activity is reduced. Wound healing and immune functions also involve ascorbic acid. The best dietary sources of vitamin C are citrus fruits, green vegetables, and tomatoes.

Scurvy *is the clinical vitamin C deficiency state.* The first demonstration of the need for this vitamin was the remarkable effect of lime in preventing scurvy among 18th century British sailors. The distribution of limes in the British navy led to the name "limey" for the seamen. Scurvy is uncommon in the Western world, but is often noted in nonindustrialized countries in which other forms of malnutrition are prevalent. In industrialized countries, scurvy is now a disease of persons afflicted with chronic diseases who do not eat well, the neglected aged, and malnourished alcoholics. The stress of cold, heat, fever, or trauma (accidental or surgical) leads to an increased requirement for vitamin C. Children who are fed only milk for the first year of life develop scurvy, as do alcoholics. Mild depression of ascorbic acid levels also occurs in other conditions, including cigarette smoking, tuberculosis, rheumatic fever, and many debilitating disorders. Some women who use oral contraceptives may have mildly decreased serum vitamin C levels. About 3% of the body's ascorbic acid is catabolized per day.

PATHOLOGY: *Most of the events associated with vitamin C deficiency are caused by formation of abnormal collagen that lacks tensile strength* (Fig. 8-28). Within 1 to 3 months, subperiosteal hemorrhages lead to pain in bones and joints. Petechial hemorrhages, ecchymoses, and purpura are common, particularly after mild trauma or at pressure points. Perifollicular hemorrhages in the skin are particularly typical of scurvy. In advanced cases, swollen, bleeding gums are a classic finding. Alveolar bone resorption results in loss of teeth. Wound healing is poor and dehiscence of previously healed wounds occurs. Anemia may result from prolonged bleeding, impaired iron absorption, or associated folic acid deficiency.

In children, vitamin C deficiency leads to growth failure and collagen-rich structures such as teeth, bones, and blood vessels develop abnormally. Effects on developing bone are conspicuous and relate principally to impaired function of osteoblasts (see Chapter 26).In addition to poor wound healing, scorbutic patients have difficulty walling off infections to form abscesses, so that infections spread more easily. The diagnosis of scurvy is confirmed by finding low levels of ascorbic acid in the serum.

While the claims that ascorbic acid may help to prevent upper respiratory infections lack substantiation, ingestion of large amounts of vitamin C is not known to be harmful.

Vitamin D

Vitamin D is a fat-soluble steroid hormone found in two forms: vitamin D_3 (cholecalciferol) and vitamin D_2 (ergocalciferol), both of which have equal biological potency in humans. Vitamin D_3 is produced in the skin and vitamin D_2 is derived from plant ergosterol. The vitamin is absorbed in the jejunum along with fats and is transported in the blood bound to an α-globulin (vitamin D-binding protein). *To achieve biological potency, vitamin D must be hydroxylated to active metabolites in the liver and kidney. The active form of the vitamin promotes calcium and phosphate absorption from the small intestine and may directly influence mineralization of bone.*

Vitamin D Deficiency

PATHOGENESIS: *In children, vitamin D deficiency causes rickets; in adults, osteomalacia occurs.* Vitamin D deficiency results from (1) insufficient dietary vitamin D, (2) insufficient production of vitamin D in the skin because of limited sunlight exposure, (3) inadequate absorption of vitamin D from the diet (as in the fat malabsorption syndromes), or (4) abnormal conversion of vitamin D to its bioactive metabolites. The last occurs in liver disease and chronic renal failure.

CLINICAL FEATURES: The bone lesions of vitamin D deficiency in children (rickets) have been recognized for centuries and were common in the Western industrialized world until recently. It was a disease that affected the urban poor to a much greater extent than their rural counterparts. A partial explanation for this difference lies in the greater exposure of rural residents to sunlight. Addition of vitamin D to milk and many processed foods, administration of vitamin preparations to young children, and generally improved levels of nutrition have made rickets a curiosity in industrialized countries. See Chapter 26 for more details.

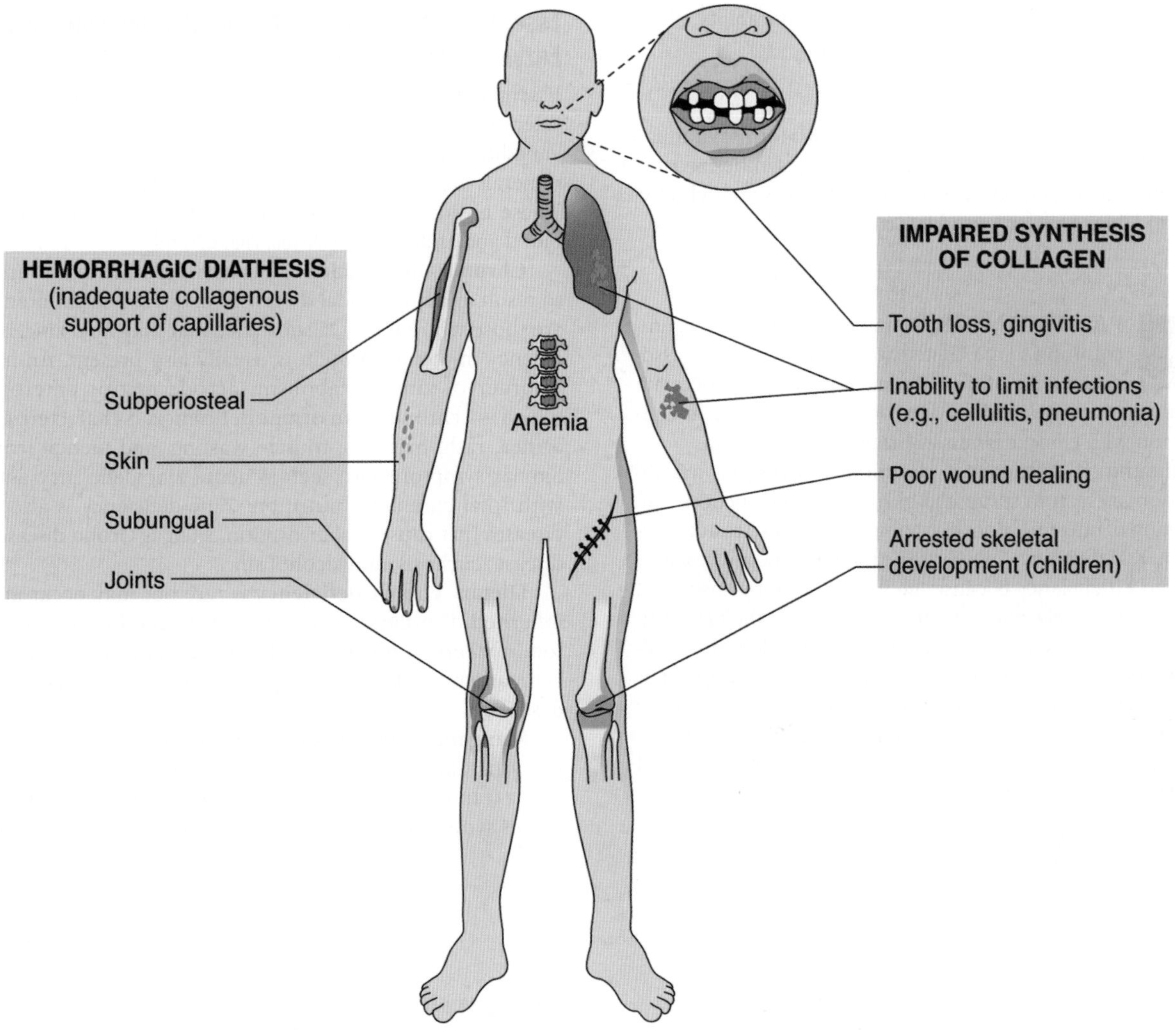

FIGURE 8-28. **Complications of vitamin C deficiency (scurvy).**

Hypervitaminosis D

The most common cause of excess vitamin D is the inordinate consumption of vitamin preparations. Abnormal conversion of vitamin D to biologically active metabolites is occasionally seen in granulomatous diseases such as sarcoidosis. In cases of calcium malabsorption, when the underlying disease is corrected, the sensitivity of target tissues to vitamin D may be increased.

PATHOLOGY: The initial response to excess vitamin D is **hypercalcemia,** which leads to nonspecific symptoms such as weakness and headaches. Increased renal calcium excretion results in **nephrolithiasis** or **nephrocalcinosis. Ectopic calcification** in other organs, such as blood vessels, heart, and lungs, may be seen. Infants are particularly susceptible to excess vitamin D and if the condition is not corrected, they may develop premature arteriosclerosis, supravalvular aortic stenosis, and renal acidosis.

Vitamin E

Vitamin E is an antioxidant that (experimentally at least) protects membrane phospholipids against lipid peroxidation by free radicals formed by cellular metabolism. The activity of this fat-soluble vitamin is found in a number of dietary constituents, principally in α-tocopherol. Corn and soy beans are particularly rich in vitamin E.

Dietary deficiency of vitamin E is rare, except among patients receiving total parenteral nutrition. Low vitamin E levels have also been found in patients with disorders of fat absorption from the intestine. No clearly definable syndrome associated with vitamin E deficiency has been identified in adults. Inconsistent reports of abnormalities of the posterior columns of the spinal cord, together with functional disturbances of gait, proprioception, and vibration have been recorded. Although erythrocyte life span may be shortened, clinical anemia is not attributable to vitamin E deficiency alone.

In premature infants, hemolytic anemia, thrombocytosis, and edema have been associated with vitamin E deficiency. Vitamin E therapy has been reported to improve hemolytic anemia in premature newborns, and may reduce the severity but not the incidence of retrolental fibroplasia. Vitamin E is reported to retard development of cirrhosis in infants with congenital biliary atresia. A number of interesting experimental effects are produced by vitamin E, such as inhibition of (1) platelet aggregation, (2) conversion of dietary nitrites to carcinogenic nitrosamines, and (3) prostaglandin synthesis. Protection against toxins that exert their activity through production of free radical oxygen species has also been shown. The applicability of these results to humans requires further study.

Vitamin K

Vitamin K, a fat-soluble material, occurs in two forms: vitamin K_1, from plants and vitamin K_2, which is principally synthesized by the normal intestinal bacteria. Green leafy vegetables are rich in vitamin K, and liver and dairy products contain smaller amounts.

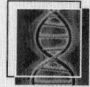

PATHOGENESIS: Dietary deficiency is very uncommon in the United States; most cases are associated with other disorders. However, inadequate dietary intake of vitamin K does occasionally occur in conjunction with chronic illness associated with anorexia.

Vitamin K deficiency is common in severe fat malabsorption, as seen in sprue and biliary tract obstruction. Destruction of intestinal flora by antibiotics may also result in vitamin K deficiency. Newborn infants frequently exhibit vitamin K deficiency because the vitamin is not transported well across the placenta, and the sterile gut of the newborn does not have bacteria to produce it. Vitamin K confers calcium-binding properties to certain proteins and is important for the activity of four clotting factors: prothrombin, factor VII, factor IX, and factor X. Deficiency of vitamin K can be serious, because it can lead to catastrophic bleeding. Parenteral vitamin K therapy is rapidly effective.

Essential Trace Minerals Are Mostly Components of Enzymes and Cofactors

Essential trace minerals include iron, copper, iodine, zinc, cobalt, selenium, manganese, nickel, chromium, tin, molybdenum, vanadium, silicon, and fluorine. Dietary deficiencies of these minerals are clinically important in the case of iron and iodine. These are discussed in Chapters 20 and 21, which deal with blood and endocrine diseases, respectively.

Chronic zinc deficiency has been reported in Iran and Egypt to result in hypogonadal dwarfism in boys. The children usually are those who eat clay, a substance that may bind zinc, but a deficiency in dietary protein is usually also present. An inherited disorder of zinc metabolism, acrodermatitis enteropathica, which is a chronic form of zinc deficiency, is characterized by diarrhea, rash, hair loss, muscle wasting, and mental irritability. Similar symptoms are seen in acute zinc deficiency associated with total parenteral nutrition. Zinc deficiency is also seen in diseases that cause malabsorption, such as Crohn disease, celiac disease, cirrhosis, and alcoholism.

Dietary copper deficiency is rare but may occur in certain inherited disorders, in malabsorption syndromes, and during total parenteral nutrition. The most common result is microcytic anemia, although megaloblastic changes have also been described.

Manganese deficiency has been described and causes poor growth, skeletal abnormalities, reproductive impairment, ataxia/ and convulsions. **Industrial exposure to manganese** causes symptoms closely related to those of parkinsonism.

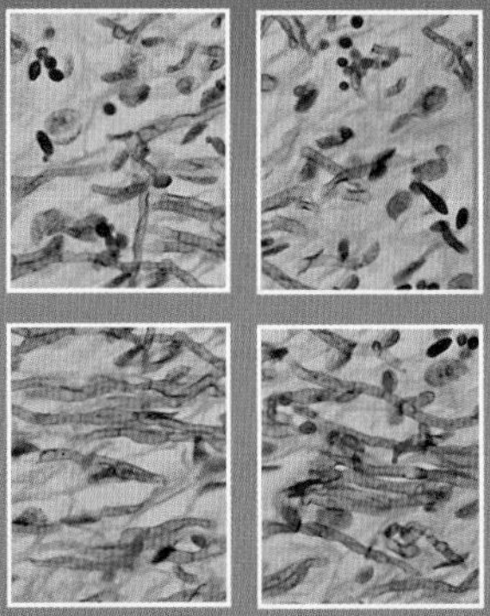

9

Infectious and Parasitic Diseases

David A. Schwartz
Robert M. Genta
Douglas P. Bennett
Roger J. Pomerantz

- Brucellosis
- Plague
- Tularemia
- Anthrax
- Listeriosis
- Cat-Scratch Disease
- Glanders
- Bartonellosis

Infections Caused by Branching Filamentous Organisms

- Actinomycosis
- Nocardiosis

SPIROCHETAL INFECTIONS

Syphilis

- Primary Syphilis
- Secondary Syphilis
- Tertiary Syphilis
- Congenital Syphilis

Nonvenereal Treponematoses

- Yaws
- Bejel
- Pinta

Lyme Disease

Leptospirosis

Relapsing Fever

Fusospirochetal Infections

- Tropical Phagedenic Ulcer
- Noma

CHLAMYDIAL INFECTIONS

Chlamydia trachomatis

- Genital and Neonatal Infections
- Lymphogranuloma Venereum
- Trachoma

Psittacosis (Ornithosis)

Chlamydia pneumoniae

RICKETTSIAL INFECTIONS

Rocky Mountain Spotted Fever

Epidemic (Louse-Borne) Typhus

Endemic (Murine) Typhus

Scrub Typhus

Q Fever

MYCOPLASMAL INFECTIONS

MYCOBACTERIAL INFECTIONS

Tuberculosis

- Primary Tuberculosis
- Secondary (Cavitary) Tuberculosis

Leprosy

- Tuberculoid Leprosy
- Lepromatous Leprosy

***Mycobacterium avium-intracellulare* Complex**

- Granulomatous Pulmonary Disease
- Disseminated Infection in AIDS

Atypical Mycobacteria

FUNGAL INFECTIONS

***Pneumocystis jiroveci* Pneumonia**

Candida

Aspergillosis

- Allergic Bronchopulmonary Aspergillosis
- Aspergilloma
- Invasive Aspergillosis

Mucormycosis (Zygomycosis)

Cryptococcosis

Histoplasmosis

Coccidioidomycosis

Blastomycosis

Paracoccidioidomycosis (South American Blastomycosis)

Sporotrichosis

Chromomycosis

Dermatophyte Infections

Mycetoma

PROTOZOAL INFECTIONS

Malaria

Babesiosis

Toxoplasmosis

- *Toxoplasma* Lymphadenopathy Syndrome
- Congenital *Toxoplasma* Infections
- Toxoplasmosis in Immunocompromised Hosts

Amebiasis

- Intestinal Amebiasis
- Amebic Liver Abscess

Cryptosporidiosis

Giardiasis

Leishmaniasis

- Localized Cutaneous Leishmaniasis
- Mucocutaneous Leishmaniasis
- Visceral Leishmaniasis (Kala Azar)

Chagas Disease (American Trypanosomiasis)

- Acute Chagas Disease
- Chronic Chagas Disease

African Trypanosomiasis

Primary Amebic Meningoencephalitis

HELMINTHIC INFECTION

Filarial Nematodes

- Lymphatic Filariasis
- Onchocerciasis
- Loiasis

Intestinal Nematodes

- Ascariasis
- Trichuriasis
- Hookworms
- Strongyloidiasis
- Pinworm Infection (Enterobiasis)

Tissue Nematodes

- Trichinosis
- Visceral Larva Migrans (Toxocariasis)
- Cutaneous Larva Migrans
- Dracunculiasis

Trematodes (Flukes)

- Schistosomiasis
- Clonorchiasis
- Paragonimiasis
- Fascioliasis
- Fasciolopsiasis

Cestodes: Intestinal Tapeworms

- Cysticercosis
- Echinococcosis

EMERGING AND RE-EMERGING INFECTIONS

AGENTS OF BIOWARFARE

THE TOLL OF INFECTIOUS DISEASES

Perhaps the greatest scourge to humankind, the diverse group of disorders collectively known as the infectious diseases have caused more pain, suffering, disability, and premature death than any other group of diseases in history. Bacterial and viral diarrheas, bacterial pneumonias, tuberculosis, measles, malaria, hepatitis B, pertussis, and tetanus kill more people each year than all cancers and cardiovascular diseases (Table 9-1). The impact of infectious diseases is greatest in less-developed countries, where millions of people, mostly children younger than 5 years of age, die of treatable or preventable infectious diseases. Even in the developed countries of Europe and North America, the mortality, morbidity, and loss of economic productivity from infectious diseases is enormous. In the United States each year, infectious diseases cause over 200,000 deaths, more than 50 million days of hospitalization, and almost 2 billion days lost from work or school. It is estimated that smallpox claimed between 300 and 500 million human lives during the 20th century alone. Although smallpox has been eradicated from the natural environment, a multitude of other infectious agents continue to claim millions of lives each year. Infectious diseases such as tuberculosis, malaria, childhood diarrhea and human immunodeficiency virus (HIV)/acquired immunodeficiency disease (AIDS) continue to ravage the developing world, taking millions of lives each year. Even in industrialized nations, the morbidity and mortality from infectious disease is still substantial. In the United States alone sepsis is responsible for an estimated 200,000 deaths per year.

Despite the untold past and present (and, undoubtedly, future) misery for which these diseases are responsible, past accomplishments of individuals great and small illustrate the contributions that can be made in this area to the alleviation of human suffering: Edward Jenner's use of the cowpox (vaccinia) virus in 1798 to immunize against smallpox; John Snow's removal of the Broad Street pump handle which ended the 1854 choleria outbreak in London; the discovery in 1843 by Oliver Wendell Holmes, Sr., that simply washing hands between patients could dramatically reduce the incidence of puerperal fever. All these discoveries were made before an intelligible theory of causation of these illnesses existed. That theory was to come only with the work of Koch, Pasteur, and Lister, who established the field of microbiology which led directly to identification of agents responsible for many infectious diseases, establishment of effective standards of antisepsis, and, eventually, the discovery and development of antibiotics to treat common bacterial, fungal, helminthic, and protozoal diseases.

By the 1970s it seemed that infectious diseases would become medical curiosities due to the advanced antibiotics, improved sanitation, and vaccination. It is instructive that in 1970, the Surgeon General of the United States declared, "the time has come for us to close the book on infectious disease." The fact that we had not conquered infectious diseases and, in fact, that tremendous problems were lurking was illustrated by the discovery of Legionnaires' disease in 1976. The end of our naive expectations that infectious diseases were conquered came in 1981, with the first reports of HIV-1/AIDS. Since then, many other infections have emerged, for which we currently have little treatment and no cures: Ebola virus, severe acute respiratory syndrome (SARS), drug-resistant tuberculosis, and others. The recent concern over these and other infectious diseases underscores the facts that the potential for future infectious threats to human existence is real, animal reservoirs of microbes that can be transmitted to humans are bottomless, and vigilence should never be relaxed. Finally, the possibly that people may seek to use infectious agents as weapons of warfare should dispel any complacency we have developed that we are safe from these pathogens.

TABLE 9-1
Sources of Global Deaths

Illness	Annual Deaths
Cardiovascular disease	12×10^6
Diarrheal diseases (Rotavirus, Norwalk-like viruses, *Salmonella*, *Shigella*, diarrheogenic *Escherichia coli*)	5×10^6
Cancer	4.8×10^6
Pneumonia	4.8×10^6
Tuberculosis	3×10^6
Chronic obstructive lung disease	2.7×10^6
Measles	1.5×10^6
Malaria	$1\text{–}2 \times 10^6$
Hepatitis B	$1\text{–}2 \times 10^6$
Tetanus (neonatal)	775×10^3
Pertussis (whooping cough)	500×10^3
Maternal mortality	500×10^3
AIDS	200×10^3
Schistosomiasis	200×10^3
Amebiasis	$40\text{–}110 \times 10^3$
Hookworm	$50\text{–}60 \times 10^3$
Rabies	35×10^3
Typhoid	25×10^3
Yellow fever	25×10^3
African trypanosomiasis (sleeping sickness)	20×10^3
Ascariasis	20×10^3

AIDS = acquired immunodeficiency virus.

Infectious Diseases are Disorders in Which Tissue Damage or Dysfunction Results from an Invading Transmissable Agent

These diseases represent many of the familiar taxa: bacteria, fungi, protozoa, and various parasitic worms. Yet some infectious agents do not qualify as completely independent organisms. Viruses cannot replicate by themselves and are obligate intracellular parasites that hijack the replicative machinery of susceptable cells. Likewise, the class of proteinaceous infectious agents, prions, lack nucleic acids and clearly represent a different infectious disease paradigm.

There is great diversity in how various infectious diseases are acquired. Many of these diseases, such as influenza, syphilis, and tuberculosis, are contagious, that is, transmissible from person to person. Yet many infectious diseases, such as legionellosis, histoplasmosis, and toxoplasmosis, are not contagious but are rather acquired from the enviroment. *Legionella* species bacteria normally replicate in aquatic amebas but can infect humans via aerosolized water or through microaspiration of contaminated water. Other infectious agents come from many diverse sources, including animals, insects, soil, air, inanimate objects, and the endogenous microbial flora of the human body.

Perhaps the greatest paradox is that certain retroviruses have actually been incorporated into the human genome and are passed from generation to generation. Their function is unclear but their possible activation during placentation has lead to speculation that such endogenous retroviruses may have allowed placental mammals to evolve.

Infectivity and Virulence

Virulence refers to the complex of properties that allows an organism to achieve infection and cause disease of different degrees of severity. The organism must (1) gain access to the body, (2) avoid multiple host defenses, (3) accommodate to growth in the human milieu, and (4) parasitize human resources. Virulence reflects both the structures inherent to the offending microbe and the interplay of those factors with host defense mechanisms.

Host Defense Mechanisms

The means by which the body prevents or contains infections are known as defense mechanisms (Table 9-2). There are major anatomical barriers to infection—the skin and the aerodynamic filtration system of the upper airway—that prevent most organisms from ever penetrating the body. The mucociliary blanket of the airways is also an essential defense, providing a means of expelling organisms that gain access to the respiratory system. The microbial flora normally resident in the gastrointestinal tract and in various body orifices compete with outside organisms, preventing them from gaining sufficient nutrients or binding sites in the host. The body's orifices are also protected by secretions that possess antimicrobial properties, both nonspecific (e.g., lysozyme and interferon) and specific (usually IgA immunoglobulins). In addition, gastric acid and bile chemically destroy many ingested organisms.

TABLE 9–2

Host Defenses Against Infection
Skin
Tears
Normal bacterial flora
Gastric acid
Bile
Salivary and pancreatic secretions
Filtration system of nasopharynx
Mucociliary blanket
Bronchial, cervical, urethral, and prostatic secretions
Neutrophils
Monocytes
Complement
Stationary mononuclear phagocyte system
Immunoglobulins
Cell-mediated immunity

Heritable Differences

The first step in infection is often a highly specific interaction of a binding molecule on the infecting organism with a receptor molecule on the host. If the host lacks a suitable receptor, the organism cannot attach to the target. An example is *Plasmodium vivax,* one of the organisms that cause human malaria. It infects human erythrocytes by using Duffy blood group determinants on the cell surface as receptors. Many persons, particularly blacks, lack these determinants and are not susceptible to infection with *P. vivax*. As a result, *P. vivax* malaria is absent from much of Africa. Similar racial or geographic differences in susceptibility are apparent for many infectious agents, including *Coccidioides immitis* and *Coccidioides. posadasii,* which are 14 times more common in blacks and 175 times more frequent in persons of Filipino ancestry than in whites.

Age

The effect of age on the outcome of exposure to many infectious agents is well illustrated by fetal infections. Some organisms produce more-severe disease in utero than in children or adults. Infections of the fetus with cytomegalovirus (CMV), rubellavirus, parvovirus B19, and *Toxoplasma gondii* interfere with fetal development. Normally, the fetus is protected by maternal immunoglobulin [Ig]G (generated by a specific previous infection) that passively crosses the placenta. In acute infection of a pregnant women without neutralizing antibody, certain pathogens may cross the placenta. These infections are usually subclinical or produce minimal disease in the mother. Depending on the organism and time of exposure, fetal infection can produce minimal damage, major congenital abnormalities, or death.

Age also affects the course of common illnesses, such as the diverse viral and bacterial diarrheas. In older children and adults, these infections cause discomfort and inconvenience, but rarely severe disease. The outcome can be different in children uner 3 years, who cannot compensate for rapid volume loss resulting from profuse diarrhea. In 2000, the World Health Organization (WHO) estimated that acute diarrheal diseases kill 2.2 million children yearly.

Other examples include infection with *Mycobacterium tuberculosis,* which produces severe, disseminated tuberculosis in children younger than 3 years, probably because of the immaturity of the cell-mediated immune system. By contrast, older persons fare much better. Maturity, however, is not always an advantage in infections. Epstein-Barr virus (EBV) is more likely to cause symptomatic infections in adolescents and adults than in younger children. Varicella-zoster virus, the cause of chickenpox, produces more severe disease in adults, who are more likely to develop viral pneumonia.

The elderly fare more poorly with almost all infections than younger persons. Common respiratory illnesses such as influenza and pneumococcal pneumonia are more often fatal in those older than 65 years of age.

Human Behavior Plays a Large Role in Exposure to Infectious Agents

The link between behavior and infection is probably most obvious for sexually transmitted diseases. Syphilis, gonorrhea, urogenital chlamydial infections, AIDS, and a number of other infectious diseases are transmitted primarily by sexual contact. The type and number of sexual encounters profoundly influence the risk of acquiring sexually transmitted diseases.

Other aspects of behavior also influence the risk of acquiring infections. Humans contract brucellosis and Q fever, which are primarily bacterial diseases of domesticated farm animals, by close contact with infected animals or their secretions. These infections occur in farmers, herders, meat processors, and, in the case of brucellosis, in persons who drink unpasteurized milk. Transmission of a number of parasitic diseases is strongly affected by behavior. Schistosomiasis, acquired when water-borne infective parasite larvae penetrate the skin of a susceptible host, is primarily a disease of farmers who work in fields irrigated by infected water. In addition, children who swim in lakes and ponds containing these organisms become infected. The larvae of hookworm and *Strongyloides stercoralis* live in humid soil and penetrate the skin of the lower extremities in people who walk barefoot. The introduction of shoes has probably been the single most important factor in reducing the prevalence of infection with soil-transmitted nematodes. Anisakiasis and diphyllobothriasis are helminthic diseases acquired by eating incompletely cooked fish. Toxoplasmosis is a protozoan infection transmitted from animals to humans by ingestion of incompletely cooked, infected meat or by exposure to infected cat feces. Botulism, a food poisoning caused by a bacterial toxin, is contracted by ingestion of improperly canned food, which contains the toxin; ingestion of spores often via honey by infants; or from inoculation of wounds by spores which then germinate in devitalized tissue.

As humans change their behavior, they open up new possibilities for infectious diseases. Although the agent of Legionnaires disease is common in the environment, aerosols generated by cooling plants, faucets, and humidifiers have provided the means for causing human infections. Traditional behaviors are not necessarily health promoting. Hundreds of thousands of cases of neonatal tetanus in less-developed countries are linked to coating umbilical stumps with dirt, dung, or home-made cheese to stop bleeding. These materials do arrest the bleeding but often contain *Clostridium tetani* spores, which germinate and release the toxin that causes tetanus. In parts of Africa, numerous cases of cysticercosis are caused by the ingestion of locally prepared potions containing, among other ingredients, the stools of persons infected with *Taenia solium*.

People with Compromised Defenses are More Likely to Contract Infections and to Have More Severe Infections

Disruption or absence of any of the complex host defenses results in increased numbers and severity of infections. Disruption of epithelial surfaces by trauma or burns frequently leads to invasive bacterial or fungal infections. Injury to the mucociliary apparatus of the airways, as in smoking or influenza, impairs clearance of inhaled microorganisms and leads to increased incidence of bacterial pneumonia. Congenital absence of complement components C5, C6, C7, and C8 prevents formation of a fully functional membrane attack complex and permits disseminated, and often recurrent, *Neisseria* infections (see Chapt. 2). Diseases such as diabetes mellitus and chemotherapeutic drugs that interfere with neutrophil production or function increase the likelihood of bacterial infection or invasive fungal infections (see Chapter 20).

Immunologically compromised states create diagnostic and therapeutic challenges, and are the consequence of cytotoxic and immunosuppressive therapies, our ability to prolong the lives of debilitated persons, and the explosion of the AIDS epidemic. In addition, burn and trauma units, transplantation centers, and medical and surgical intensive care facilities are filled with patients whose primary conditions have left them unable, or insufficiently able, to protect themselves from infections, either by lacking the capacity to mount inflammatory or immune responses. Compromised hosts become infected more easily and they are often attacked by organisms that are innocuous to normal persons. For example, patients deficient in neutrophils frequently develop life-threatening bloodstream infections with commensal microorganisms that normally populate the skin and gastrointestinal tract.

Such organisms, that cause disease mainly in hosts with impaired immunity, are **opportunistic pathogens**. These organisms, many of which are part of the normal endogenous human or environmental microbial flora, take advantage of a host's inadequate defenses to stage a more violent and sustained attack.

VIRAL INFECTIONS: INTRODUCTION

Viruses range from 20 to 300 nm and consist of RNA or DNA contained in a protein shell. Some are also enveloped in lipid membranes. *Viruses do not engage in metabolism or reproduction independently, and thus are obligate intracellular parasites: they require living cells in order to replicate.* After invading cells, they divert the cells' biosynthetic and metabolic capacities to synthesizing virus-encoded nucleic acids and proteins.

Viruses often cause disease by killing infected cells, but many do not. For example, rotavirus, a common cause of diarrhea, interferes with the function of infected enterocytes without immediately killing them. It prevents enterocytes from synthesizing proteins that transport molecules from the intestinal lumen and thereby causes diarrhea.

Viruses may also promote the release of chemical mediators that elicit inflammatory or immunologic responses. The symptoms of the common cold are due to the release of bradykinin from infected cells. Other viruses cause cells to proliferate and form tumors. Human papillomaviruses (HPVs), for instance, cause squamous cell proliferative lesions, which include common warts and anogenital warts.

Some viruses infect and persist in cells without interfering with cellular functions, a process known as **latency**. Latent viruses can emerge to produce disease years after the primary infection. Opportunistic infections are frequently caused by viruses that have established latent infections. CMV and herpes simplex viruses are among the most frequent opportunistic pathogens because they are commonly present as latent agents and emerge in persons with impaired cell-mediated immunity.

Finally, some viruses may reside within cells, either by integrating into their genomes or by remaining episomal, and cause those cells to generate tumors. Examples of this are EBV, which causes endemic Burkitt's lymphoma in Africa, and other tumors in different settings, and human T cell leukemia virus-1 (HTLV-1, see Chapter 5), which causes a form of T-cell lymphoma.

This section is divided into diseases caused by RNA viruses and those caused by DNA viruses. This division reflects fundamental differences in the biology of these agents. Some viruses with highly organ-specific tropisms are not described here in detail, but are addressed in those chapters that deal with the organs that are principally affected: thus, HIV (Chapter 4, Immunopathology), hepatitis B and C (Chapter 14, Liver), etc.

VIRAL INFECTIONS: RNA VIRUSES

RNA viruses generally follow different paths to causing disease than do most DNA viruses: the enzymes needed for their infectious cycles may be vastly different, and important aspects of their biology do not have correlates among DNA viruses. Therefore, RNA viruses are treated as a separate category of disease-causing agent.

One of the important differences between some of these viruses and many DNA viruses is that the polymerases of a number of important pathogenic RNA viruses (e.g., HIV-1, hepatitis C virus [HCV]) do not proofread the strand being synthesized. This has two important consequences. First, the mutation rate—and therefore the plasticity of these viruses in circumvening therapies—is very high. Second, a greater percentage of daughter virions are inactive.

Respiratory Viruses

The Common Cold Is the Most Common Viral Disease

The common cold (coryza) is an acute, self-limited upper respiratory tract disorder caused by infection with a variety of RNA viruses, including over 100 distinct rhinoviruses and several coronaviruses. Colds are frequent and worldwide in distribution, spreading from person to person by contact with infected secretions. Infection is more likely during the winter months in temperate areas and during the rainy seasons in the tropics, when spread is facilitated by indoor crowding. In the United States, children usually suffer six to eight colds per year and adults two to three.

The viruses infect the nasal respiratory epithelial cells, causing increased mucus production and edema. Rhinoviruses and coronaviruses have a tropism for respiratory epithelium and optimally reproduce at temperatures well below 37°C (98.6°F). Thus, infection remains confined to the cooler passages of the upper airway. Infected cells release chemical mediators, such as bradykinin, which produce most of the symptoms associated with the common cold: increased mucus production, together with nasal congestion and eustachian tube obstruction. Resulting stasis may predispose to secondary bacterial infection and lead to bacterial sinusitis and otitis media. Rhinoviruses and coronaviruses do not destroy the respiratory epithelium and produce no visible alterations. Clinically, the common cold is characterized by rhinorrhea, pharyngitis, cough, and low-grade fever. Symptoms last about a week.

Influenza May Predispose to Bacterial Pneumonia

Influenza is an acute, usually self-limited, infection of upper and lower airways, caused by influenza virus. These viruses are enveloped and contain single-stranded RNA.

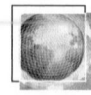

EPIDEMIOLOGY: There are three distinct types of influenza virus—types A, B, and C—that cause human disease, but influenza A is by far the most common and causes the most severe disease. Ten to 40 million cases of influenza occur annually in the United States, accounting for over 35,000 deaths. Influenza is highly contagious, and epidemics often spread around the world. New strains emerge regularly, often from animal hosts, infect humans in parts of the world where humans and animals live in close contact, and then disseminate rapidly. Influenza strains are identified by their type (A, B, C) and the serotype of their hemagglutinin (H) and neuraminidase. Thus, the avian influenza virus that emerged in 2003 and continues to spread around the globe is designated A(H5N1). Because epidemic influenza virus antigens change so often, host immunity that develops in one epidemic rarely protects against the next one.

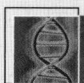

PATHOGENESIS: Influenza spreads from person to person by virus-containing respiratory droplets and secretions. Upon reaching the respiratory epithelial cell surface, the virus binds and enters the cell by fusion with the cell membrane, a process mediated by a viral glycoprotein (hemagglutinin) that binds to sialic acid residues on human respiratory epithelium. Once inside the cell, the virus directs it to produce progeny viruses and causes cell death. The infection usually involves both the upper and the lower airways. Destruction of the ciliated epithelium cripples the mucociliary blanket, predisposing to bacterial pneumonia, especially with *Staphylococcus aureus* and *Streptococcus pneumoniae*.

PATHOLOGY: Influenza virus causes necrosis and desquamation of the ciliated respiratory tract epithelium, associated with a predominantly lymphocytic inflammatory infiltrate. Extension of the infection to the lungs leads to necrosis and sloughing of alveolar lining cells and the histologic appearance of viral pneumonitis.

CLINICAL FEATURES: Influenza manifests with a rapid onset of fever, chills, myalgia, headaches, weakness, and nonproductive cough. Symptoms may be primarily those of an upper respiratory infection or those of tracheitis, bronchitis, and pneumonia. Epidemics are accompanied by deaths from both the disease and its complications, particularly in the elderly and persons with underlying cardiopulmonary disease. Killed viral vaccines specific to epidemic strains are 75% effective in preventing influenza.

Parainfluenza Virus Is Associated with Croup

The parainfluenza viruses cause acute upper and lower respiratory tract infections, particularly in young children. These enveloped, single-stranded negative-sense RNA viruses are the most common cause of croup (laryngotracheobronchitis), which is characterized by stridor on inspiration and a barking cough.

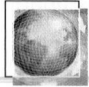

EPIDEMIOLOGY: This condition is common in children younger than the age of 3 years and is characterized by subglottic swelling, airway compression, and respiratory distress. These viruses spread from person to person through infectious respiratory aerosols and secretions. Infection is highly contagious, and disease is present worldwide. The parainfluenza viruses are isolated from 10% of young children with acute respiratory tract illnesses.

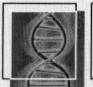

PATHOGENESIS AND PATHOLOGY: Parainfluenza viruses infect and kill ciliated respiratory epithelial cells and elicit an inflammatory response. In very young children, this process frequently extends into the lower respiratory tract, causing bronchiolitis and pneumonitis. In young children, the trachea is narrow, and the larynx is small. When laryngotracheitis occurs, the local edema compresses the upper airway enough to obstruct breathing and cause croup. Parainfluenza infection is associated with fever, hoarseness, and cough. Croup is evidenced by a characteristic barking cough and inspiratory stridor. In older children and adults symptoms are usually mild.

Respiratory Syncytial Virus (RSV) Causes Bronchiolitis in Infants

EPIDEMIOLOGY: RSV belongs to the same family, Paramyxoviridae, as parainfluenza virus. It spreads rapidly from child to child in respiratory aerosols and secretions, and is commonly disseminated in daycare centers, hospitals, and other settings when small children are confined. The virus, which is present worldwide, is highly contagious, and most children have been infected with RSV by school age.

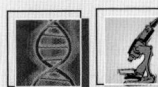

PATHOGENESIS AND PATHOLOGY: Viral surface proteins interact with specific receptors on host respiratory epithelium to cause viral binding and fusion. RSV produces necrosis and sloughing of bronchial, bronchiolar, and alveolar epithelium, associated with a predominantly lymphocytic inflammatory infiltrate. Multinucleated syncytial cells are sometimes seen in infected tissues.

CLINICAL FEATURES: Infants and young children with RSV bronchiolitis or pneumonitis present with wheezing, cough, and respiratory distress, sometimes accompanied by fever. The illness is usually self-limited, resolving in 1 to 2 weeks. In older children and adults, RSV produces much milder disease. Among otherwise healthy young children, the mortality from RSV infection is very low, but it rises dramatically, up to 20% to 40%, among hospitalized children with congenital heart disease or immunosuppression.

Severe Acute Respiratory Syndrome (SARS) is an Emergent Viral Disease Causing Outbreaks of Pneumonia

In early 2002 an epidemic of severe pneumonia was traced to Guangdong Province of China. As outbreaks occurred in Hong Kong, Viet Nam, and Singapore, the disease swept around the globe via routes of international air travel. This emerging clinical disease, termed SARS, eventually spread to the United States, Canada, and Europe. The causative agent is a novel coronavirus, termed the SARS-associated cornonavirus (SARS-CoV), which derived from a nonhuman host, now felt most likely to be bats. SARS is a potentially fatal viral respiratory illness with an incubation period of 2 to 7 days, with cases ranging up to 10 days.

PATHOLOGY: The lungs of patients who died from SARS disclose diffuse alveolar damage (see Chapter 12). Multinucleated syncytial cells without viral inclusions have also been observed.

CLINICAL FEATURES: Clinically, SARS begins with fever and headache, followed shortly by cough and dyspnea. Coryza is often absent and diarrhea is quite common. Lymphopenia is common, and the aminotransferase levels are modestly increased. Some patients develop adult respiratory distress syndrome (ARDS, see Chapter 12) and are at high risk of complications and death. Most patients recover, but the mortality rate is as high as 15% in the elderly and in patients who suffer from other respiratory disorders. No specific treatment is available although corticosteroids may offer some benefit. Unfortunately, no data from controlled clinical trials is available.

Viral Exanthems

Measles (Rubeola) is a Highly Contagious Virus That May Cause Fatal Infection

Measles virus is an enveloped, single-stranded RNA virus that causes an acute illness, characterized by upper respiratory tract symptoms, fever, and rash.

EPIDEMIOLOGY: The measles virus is transmitted to humans in respiratory aerosols and secretions. In nonimmunized populations, measles is primarily a disease of children. Currently available live, attenuated vaccines are highly effective in preventing measles and in eliminating the spread of the virus. Recent efforts at nationwide immunization have made measles uncommon in the United States. Similar efforts are under way worldwide to immunize all children.

Measles is a particularly severe disease in the very young, the sick, or the malnourished. In impoverished countries, the disease has a high mortality rate (10%–25%). In recent years, measles has been estimated to kill 1.5 million children each year and remains a major vaccine-preventable cause of death worldwide. When measles was first introduced to previously unexposed populations (e.g., Native Americans, Pacific Islanders), the resulting widespread infections had devastatingly high mortality rates.

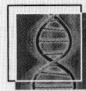

PATHOGENESIS: The initial site of infection is the mucous membranes of the nasopharynx and bronchi. Two surface glycoproteins, designated the "H" and "F" proteins, mediate viral attachment and fusion with respiratory epithelium. From these cells, the virus extends to the regional lymph nodes and then to the bloodstream, leading to widespread dissemination with prominent involvement of the skin and lymphoid tissues. The rash results from the action of T lymphocytes on virally infected vascular endothelium.

PATHOLOGY: Measles virus produces necrosis of infected respiratory epithelium, associated with a predominantly lymphocytic inflammatory infiltrate. The virus produces a vasculitis of small blood vessels in the skin.

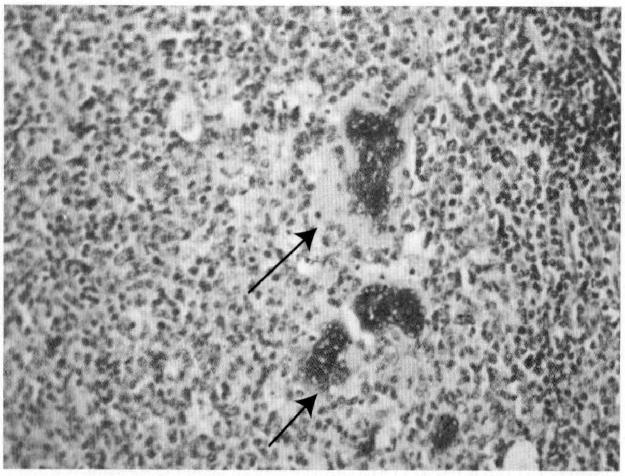

FIGURE 9-1. **Warthin-Finkeldey giant cells in measles.** A hyperplastic lymph node from a patient with measles shows several multinucleated giant cells *(arrows).*

Lymphoid hyperplasia is often prominent in the cervical and mesenteric lymph nodes, spleen, and appendix. In lymphoid tissues, the virus sometimes causes fusion of infected cells, producing multinucleated giant cells containing up to 100 nuclei, with both intracytoplasmic and intranuclear inclusions. These cells, named **Warthin-Finkeldey giant cells** (Fig. 9-1), are pathognomonic for measles.

CLINICAL FEATURES: Measles first manifests with fever, rhinorrhea, cough, and conjunctivitis and progresses to the characteristic mucosal and skin lesions. The mucosal lesions, known as "Koplik spots," appear on the posterior buccal mucosa and consist of minute gray-white dots on a red base. The skin lesions begin on the face as an erythematous maculopapular rash, which usually spreads to involve the trunk and extremities. The rash fades in 3 to 5 days, and the symptoms gradually resolve. The clinical course of measles may be much more severe in very young children, malnourished persons, or immunocompromised patients. Measles often leads to secondary bacterial infections, especially otitis media and pneumonia. Central nervous system (CNS) invasion is probably a common event as suggested by changes in electroencepahlograph (EEG) readings. Acute encephalitis is rare but does occur. Uncommonly, patients can develop subacute sclerosing panencephalitis (SSPE), a slow, chronic neurodegenerative disorder that occurs years after a measles infection. The exact pathophsiology of SSPE is unclear, as there is no animal model. Wild type measles virus is the cause of SSPE, and prophylactic vaccination against measles has greatly reduced the incidence of SSPE.

Rubella Infection in Utero Is Associated with Congenital Anomalies

Rubellavirus is an enveloped, single-stranded RNA virus that causes a mild, self-limited systemic disease, usually associated with a rash (also known as "German measles"). Many infections are so mild that they go unnoticed. However, in pregnant women, rubella is a destructive fetal pathogen. Infection early in gestation can produce fetal death, premature delivery, and congenital anomalies, including deafness, cataracts, glaucoma, heart defects, and mental retardation.

EPIDEMIOLOGY: The agent spreads from person to person primarily by the respiratory route. Infection occurs worldwide. Rubella is not highly contagious, and in unvaccinated populations, 10% to 15% of young women remain susceptible to infection into their reproductive years. The live attenuated viral vaccine currently available prevents rubella and has largely eliminated the disease from developed countries.

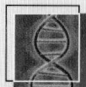

PATHOGENESIS: Rubella infects respiratory epithelium and then disseminates to various organs through the bloodstream and lymphatics. The rubella rash is believed to result from an immunologic response to the disseminated virus. Fetal infection occurs through the placenta during the viremic phase of maternal illness. A congenitally infected fetus remains persistently infected and sheds large amounts of virus in body fluids, even after birth. Maternal infection after 20 weeks' gestation usually does not cause significant fetal disease.

PATHOLOGY: In most patients, rubella is a mild, acute febrile illness, with rhinorrhea, conjunctivitis, postauricular lymphadenopathy, and a rash that spreads from face to trunk and extremities. The rash resolves within 3 days, and complications are rare. As many as 30% of infections are completely asymptomatic.

In the fetus, the heart, eye, and brain are the organs most frequently affected. Cardiac lesions include pulmonary valvular stenosis, pulmonary artery hypoplasia, ventricular septal defects, and patent ductus arteriosus. Cataracts, glaucoma, and retinal defects may occur. Deafness is a common complication of fetal rubella. Severe brain involvement can produce microcephaly and mental retardation.

MUMPS

Mumps virus is an enveloped, single-stranded RNA virus that causes an acute, self-limited systemic illness, characterized by parotid gland swelling and meningoencephalitis.

EPIDEMIOLOGY: Mumps is present worldwide and is primarily a disease of childhood. It spreads from person to person via the respiratory route. The virus is highly contagious, and 90% of exposed, susceptible persons become infected, although only 60% to 70% develop symptoms. A live attenuated mumps vaccine prevents mumps, and the disease has been largely eliminated from most developed countries.

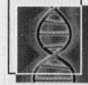

PATHOGENESIS: Mumps begins with viral infection of respiratory tract epithelium. The virus then disseminates through the blood and lymphatic systems to infect other sites, most commonly the salivary glands (especially parotids), CNS, pancreas, and testes. The CNS is involved in more than half of cases, producing symptomatic disease in 10%. Epididymoorchitis occurs in 30% of males infected after puberty.

PATHOLOGY: Mumps virus causes necrosis of infected cells, which is associated with a predominantly lymphocytic inflammatory infiltrate. The affected salivary glands are swollen, the ducts lined by necrotic epithelium, and the interstitium infiltrated with lymphocytes. In mumps epididymoorchitis, the testis can be swollen to three times the normal size. The swelling of testicular parenchyma, confined within the tunica albuginea, produces focal infarctions. Mumps orchitis is usually unilateral and, thus, rarely causes sterility.

CLINICAL FEATURES: Mumps begins with fever and malaise, followed by painful swelling of the salivary glands, usually one or both parotids. Symptomatic meningeal involvement most often manifests as headache, stiff neck, and vomiting. Prior to widespread vaccination, mumps was a leading cause of viral meningitis and encephalitis in the United States. Although severe disease of the pancreas is rare in mumps, most patients exhibit elevated serum amylase activity.

Intestinal Virus Infections

Rotavirus Infection Is the Most Common Cause of Severe Diarrhea Worldwide

Rotavirus produces profuse watery diarrhea that can lead to dehydration and death if untreated. This double-stranded RNA virus usually infects young children.

EPIDEMIOLOGY: Rotavirus infection spreads from person to person by the oral–fecal route. Infection is most common among children, who shed huge amounts of virus in the stool. Siblings, playmates, parents, as well as food, water, and environmental surfaces are readily contaminated with virus. The peak age of infection is 6 months to 2 years, and virtually all children have been infected by the age of 4 years. In the United States, rotavirus causes about 100 deaths in young children and worldwide leads to over 1 million deaths.

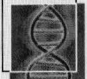

PATHOGENESIS: Rotavirus infects the enterocytes of the upper small intestine, disrupting the absorption of sugars, fats, and various ions. The resulting osmotic load causes a net loss of fluid into the bowel lumen, producing diarrhea and dehydration. Infected cells are shed from intestinal villi, and the regenerating epithelium initially lacks full absorptive capabilities.

PATHOLOGY: Pathologic changes in rotavirus infection are largely confined to the duodenum and jejunum, where there is shortening of the intestinal villi associated with a mild infiltrate of neutrophils and lymphocytes.

CLINICAL FEATURES: Rotavirus infection manifests as vomiting, fever, abdominal pain, and profuse, watery diarrhea. The vomiting usually persists for 2 to 3 days, whereas diarrhea continues for 5 to 8 days. Without adequate fluid replacement, diarrhea can produce fatal dehydration in young children.

Norwalk Virus and Other Gastrointestinal Viruses Often Cause Outbreaks of Diarrhea

In addition to rotavirus, there are numerous other viral causes of diarrhea, including adenoviruses, caliciviruses, and astroviruses. The best understood are the Norwalk family of nonenveloped RNA viruses, a group of caliciviruses that carry a host of individual names (e.g., Norwalk virus, Snow Mountain virus, Sapporo virus) associated with the locations of particular outbreaks. Norwalk viruses are responsible for one third of all outbreaks of diarrheal disease. They produce gastroenteritis in children and adults, with self-limited vomiting and diarrhea, similar to that caused by rotavirus. The Norwalk viruses infect cells of the upper small bowel and produce changes similar to those that occur with rotavirus.

Viral Hemorrhagic Fevers

Viral hemorrhagic fevers are a group of at least 20 distinct viral infections that cause varying degrees of hemorrhage and shock and sometimes death. There are many similar viral hemorrhagic fevers in different parts of the world, for the most part named for the area where they were first described. The viral hemorrhagic fevers encompass members of four virus families—the Bunyaviridae, Flaviviridae, Arenaviridae, and Filoviridae. On the basis of differences in routes of transmission, vectors, and other epidemiologic characteristics, the viral hemorrhagic fevers have been divided into four groups (Table 9-3): mosquito-borne; tick-borne; zoonotic; and the filoviruses, Marburg and Ebola virus, in which the route of transmission is unknown.

TABLE 9-3
Viral Hemorrhagic Fevers

Vector	Viral Fever
Mosquitoes	Yellow fever Rift valley fever Dengue hemorrhagic fever Chikungunya hemorrhagic fever
Ticks	Omsk hemorrhagic fever Crimean hemorrhagic fever Kyasanuf forest disease
Rodents	Lassa fever Bolivian hemorrhagic fever Argentine hemorrhagic fever Korean hemorrhagic fever
Undefined	Ebola virus disease Marburg virus disease

Yellow Fever May Lead to Fulminant Hepatic Failure

Yellow fever is an acute hemorrhagic fever, sometimes associated with extensive hepatic necrosis and jaundice. The illness is caused by an insect-borne flavivirus, an enveloped, single-stranded RNA virus. Other pathogenic flaviviruses cause Omsk hemorrhagic fever and Kyasanur Forest disease.

EPIDEMIOLOGY: Yellow fever was first recognized as a nosological entity in the New World in the 17th century, but its origins probably were in Africa. Today, the virus is restricted to certain regions of Africa and South America, including both jungle and urban settings. The usual reservoir for the virus is tree-dwelling monkeys, the agent being passed among them in the forest canopy by mosquitoes. These monkeys serve as a reservoir because the virus neither kills them nor makes them ill. Humans acquire jungle yellow fever by entering the forest and being bitten by infected *Aedes* mosquitoes. Felling trees increases the risk of infection, because mosquitoes are brought down with the tree. On returning to the village or city, the human victim becomes the reservoir for epidemic yellow fever in the urban setting, where *Aedes aegyptii* is the vector.

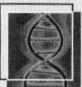

PATHOGENESIS: On inoculation by the mosquito, the virus multiplies within tissue and vascular endothelium and then disseminates through the bloodstream. The virus has a tropism for liver cells, where it sometimes produces extensive acute hepatocellular destruction. Extensive damage to the endothelium of small blood vessels may lead to the loss of vascular integrity, hemorrhages, and shock.

PATHOLOGY: Yellow fever virus causes coagulative necrosis of hepatocytes, which begins among cells in the middle of hepatic lobules and spreads toward the central veins and portal tracts. The infection sometimes produces confluent areas of necrosis in the middle of the hepatic lobules (i.e., midzonal necrosis). In the most severe cases, the entire lobule may be necrotic. Some necrotic hepatocytes lose their nuclei and become intensely eosinophilic. They often dislodge from adjacent hepatocytes, in which case they are known as Councilman bodies (recognized today as apoptotic bodies). Hepatocytes also show microvesicular fatty change.

CLINICAL FEATURES: Yellow fever is characterized by the abrupt onset of fever, chills, headache, myalgias, nausea, and vomiting. After 3 to 5 days, some patients develop manifestations of hepatic failure, with jaundice (hence the term "yellow" fever), deficiencies of clotting factors, and diffuse hemorrhages. Vomiting of clotted blood ("black vomit") is a classic feature of severe cases of yellow fever. Patients with massive hepatic failure lapse into coma and die, usually within 10 days of onset of illness. Overall mortality of yellow fever is 5%, but among those with jaundice, it rises to 30%.

Ebola Hemorrhagic Fever Is a Fatal African Disease

Ebola hemorrhagic fever is a severe viral disease caused by the Ebola virus, an RNA virus belonging to the Filoviridae. It causes a hemorrhagic disease with a high mortality rate in humans in several regions of Africa. The only other filovirus pathogenic to humans is the Marburg virus, which produces Marburg hemorrhagic fever.

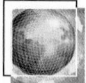

EPIDEMIOLOGY: Ebola virus first emerged in Africa with two major disease outbreaks that occurred almost simultaneously in Zaire and Sudan in 1976. Outbreaks of Ebola hemorrhagic fever have occurred in Africa through 2005. In Uganda, the virus infected 425 persons with a 53% mortality rate, and in the border area of the Republic of the Congo and Gabon, there were 122 persons infected, with an 80% fatality rate.

In the wild, the virus infects humans, gorillas, chimpanzees, and monkeys. Recent field evidence from Gabon and the Republic of the Congo area of western Africa has implicated several species of fruit bats as the natural reservoir of Ebola virus. Healthcare workers and family members have become infected as a result of viral exposure while treating patients with Ebola hemorrhagic fever or during funerary preparation of the bodies of deceased victims. The virus can be transmitted via bodily secretions, blood, and used needles.

PATHOGENESIS AND PATHOLOGY: *Ebola virus results in the most widespread destructive tissue lesions of all viral hemorrhagic fever agents.* The virus undergoes massive replication in endothelial cells, mononuclear phagocytes, and hepatocytes. Necrosis is most severe in the liver, kidneys, gonads, spleen, and lymph nodes. Characteristic findings in the liver include hepatocellular necrosis, Kupffer cell hyperplasia, Councilman bodies, and microsteatosis. The lungs are usually hemorrhagic, and petechial hemorrhages are present in the skin, mucous membranes, and internal organs. Injury to the microvasculature and increased endothelial permeability are important causes of shock.

CLINICAL FEATURES: The incubation period varies from 2 to 21 days. The initial symptoms include headache, weakness, and fever followed by diarrhea, nausea, and vomiting. Some patients develop overt hemorrhage including bleeding from injection sites, petechia, gastrointestinal bleeding, and gingival hemorrhage.

West Nile Virus is Spread by Mosquito Vectors and Birds

EPIDEMIOLOGY: The virus, a member of the family Flaviviridae, is increasing its geographic distribution as a result of spread by infected migratory birds and among arthropods transported between continents in pooled water in cargo ships. West Nile virus (WNV) was isolated in 1937 from the blood of a febrile woman in the West Nile region of Uganda. Since then it has spread rapidly through the

Mediterranean and temperate parts of Europe. In 1999, WNV was identified in the Western Hemisphere for the first time when it caused an outbreak of meningoencephalitis (West Nile fever) in New York City and the surrounding metropolitan area. By 2003, the infection had been identified in 4000 persons from 40 states, and resulted in 263 fatalities.

PATHOGENESIS AND PATHOLOGY: The virus can be recovered from blood for up to 10 days in immunocompetent febrile patients, as late as 22 to 28 days after infection in immunocompromised patients. Laboratory findings include a slightly increased sedimentation rate and a mild leukocytosis; cerebrospinal fluid in patients with CNS involvement is clear, with moderate pleiocytosis and elevated protein. Brains show mononuclear meningoencephalitis or encephalitis. The brainstem, particularly the medulla, can be extensively involved, and in some cases the cranial nerve roots had endoneural mononuclear inflammation. There are varying degrees of neuronal necrosis in gray matter, neuronal degeneration, and neuronophagia.

CLINICAL FEATURES: Most WNV infections among humans are subclinical, with overt disease occurring in only 1 of 100 infections. The incubation period ranges from 3 to 15 days. When symptoms occur, they usually consist of fever, often accompanied by rash, lymphadenopathy, and polyarthropathy. Patients with severe illness can develop acute aseptic meningitis or encephalitis, and develop convulsions and coma. Anterior myelitis, hepatosplenomegaly, hepatitis, pancreatitis, and myocarditis occur. The probability of developing severe illness increases with increasing age. CNS infection is associated with a 4% to 13% mortality rate and is highest among elderly persons.

VIRAL INFECTIONS: DNA VIRUSES

Adenovirus

Adenoviruses are nonenveloped DNA viruses that are isolated from the respiratory and intestinal tract of humans and animals. Certain serotypes are common causes of acute respiratory disease and adenovirus pneumonia in military recruits. Some adenoviruses are important causes of chronic pulmonary disease in infants and young children.

PATHOLOGY: Pathologic changes include necrotizing bronchitis and bronchiolitis, in which the sloughed epithelial cells and inflammatory infiltrate may fill the damaged bronchioles. Interstitial pneumonitis is characterized by areas of consolidation with extensive necrosis, hemorrhage, and a mononuclear inflammatory infiltrate. Two distinctive types of intranuclear inclusions—smudge cells and Cowdry type A inclusions—involve bronchiolar epithelial cells and alveolar lining cells. Adenoviruses types 40 and 41 infect colonic and small intestinal epithelial cells and may cause diarrhea in both immunocompetent and immunocompromised hosts. Patients with AIDS are particularly susceptible to urinary tract infections caused by adenovirus type 35.

Human Parvovirus B19

Human parvovirus B19 is a single-stranded DNA virus that causes a benign self-limited febrile illness in children known as erythema infectiosum. It also causes systemic infections characterized by rash, arthralgias, and transient interruption in erythrocyte production in nonimmune adults.

PATHOGENESIS: Human parvovirus B19 spreads from person to person by the respiratory route. Infection is common and occurs in outbreaks, mostly among children. It is not known which cells, other than erythroid precursors, support parvovirus B19 replication, but replication at some respiratory site prior to dissemination to erythropoietic cells seems likely.

PATHOLOGY: Human parvovirus B19 produces characteristic cytopathic effects in erythroid precursor cells and gains entry to this cell via the erythrocyte P antigen. The nucleus of an affected cell is enlarged, and the chromatin is displaced peripherally by central glassy eosinophilic material that represents nuclear inclusion bodies. These enlarged cells are called giant pronormoblasts.

CLINICAL FEATURES: Most persons suffer a mild exanthematous illness, known as **erythema infectiosum ("fifth disease")**, accompanied by an asymptomatic interruption in erythropoiesis. In persons with chronic hemolytic anemias, however, the interruption in erythrocyte production causes profound, potentially fatal anemia, known as **transient aplastic crisis** (see Chapter 20). When the fetus is infected by human parvovirus B19, a transient cessation of erythropoiesis can lead to severe anemia, hydrops fetalis, and death in utero, an outcome that occurs in about 10% of maternal infections.

Smallpox (Variola)

Smallpox is a highly contagious exanthematous viral infection produced by the variola virus, a member of the family Poxviridae.

EPIDEMIOLOGY: Smallpox is an ancient disease: a rash resembling smallpox was found in the mummified remains of Egyptian pharaoh Ramses V, who died in 1160 BC. In the 6th century, a Swiss bishop named the etiologc agent of smallpox "variola" from the Latin *varius*, meaning pimple or spot. The infection was common in Europe, and arrived in the New World with the Spanish colonists. Native populations were often decimated by it. In 1796, Edward Jenner performed the first successful vaccination when he inoculated a child with lymph from the hand of a milkmaid infected with cowpox. Once the cowpox pustule had regressed, Jenner challenged that child with smallpox and demonstrated that he was protected from the disease. In 1967, the WHO began its uniquely successful campaign to eradicate smallpox. The last occurrence of endemic smallpox was in Somalia in 1977, and the last reported human cases were laboratory-acquired infections in 1978. On May 8, 1980, the WHO declared that smallpox had been eradicated. Two known repositories of variola virus remain: one at the Centers for Disease Control and Prevention (CDC) in the United States, and one at the Institute for Virus Preparation in Russia. There has been considerable vigilance to its reemergence, either naturally or as a bioweapon.

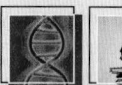

PATHOGENESIS AND PATHOLOGY: Smallpox was transmitted between smallpox victims and susceptible persons via droplets or aerosol of infected saliva. Viral titers in the saliva were highest during the first week of infection. The virus is highly stable and retains its infectivity for long periods outside its human host. Two distinctive types of smallpox have been recognized. *Variola major* was prevalent in Asia and parts of Africa and represented the prototypical form of the infection. *Variola minor* (or alastrim) was found in Africa, South America, and Europe and was distinguished by its milder systemic toxicity and smaller pox lesions.

Microscopic features of the skin vesicle of variola include reticular degeneration and scarce areas of ballooning degeneration. The eosinophilic, intracytoplasmic inclusion bodies (Guarnieri bodies) are of limited diagnostic value as they are not specific for smallpox but occur in most poxviral infections. Vesicles could also occur in the palate, pharynx, trachea, and esophagus. In severe cases of smallpox there were gastric and intestinal involvement, hepatitis, and interstitial nephritis.

CLINICAL FEATURES: The incubation period of smallpox is approximately 12 days (range, 7 to 17 days) following exposure. On exposure to the aerosolized virus, variola travels from the upper and lower respiratory tract to regional lymph nodes, where replication occurs and results in viremia. Clinical manifestations begin abruptly with malaise, fever, vomiting, and headache. The characteristic rash, most prominent on the face but also involving the hands and forearms, follows in 2 to 3 days. Following subsequent eruptions on the lower extremities, the rash spreads centrally during the next week to the trunk. Lesions are more abundant in a centrifugal distribution, that is, on the face and extremities. Lesions progress quickly from macules to papules and then to pustular vesicles (Fig. 9-2). Smallpox lesions generally remain synchronous in their stage of development. In 8 to 14 days after onset, the pustules form scabs, which leave depressed scars on healing after 3 to 4 weeks. The case fatality rate is 30% in unvaccinated persons.

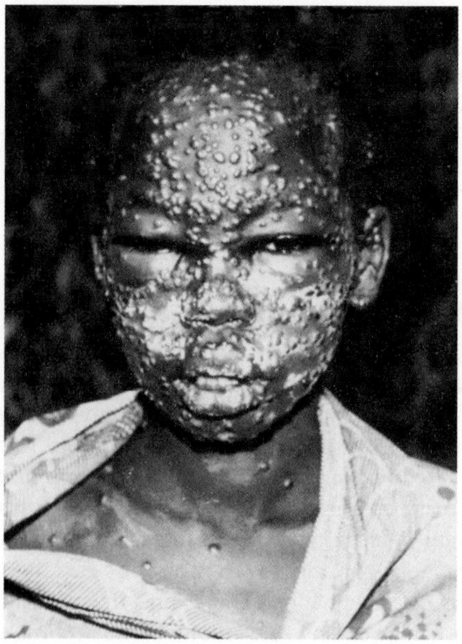

FIGURE 9-2. Child with smallpox, eastern Congo, 1968.

Herpesviruses

The virus family Herpesviridae includes a large number of enveloped, DNA viruses, many of which infect humans. Almost all herpesviruses express some common antigenic determinants, and many produce type A nuclear inclusions (acidophilic bodies surrounded by a halo). The most important human pathogens among the herpesviruses are varicella-zoster, herpes simplex, EBV, human herpesvirus 6 (HHV6, the cause of roseola), and cytomegalovirus. Recently, human herpesvirus 8 (HHV8) was implicated in the pathogenesis of Kaposi sarcoma in HIV-infected patients. These viruses are also distinguished by their capacity to remain latent for long periods of time.

Varicella-Zoster Infection Causes Chickenpox and Herpes Zoster

The first exposure to varicella-zoster virus (VZV) produces chickenpox, an acute systemic illness whose dominant feature is a generalized vesicular skin eruption (Fig. 9-3). The virus then becomes latent, and its reactivation causes herpes zoster ("shingles"), a localized vesicular skin eruption.

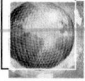

EPIDEMIOLOGY: VZV is restricted to human hosts and spreads from person to person primarily by the respiratory route. It can also be spread by contact with secretions from skin lesions. The virus is present worldwide and is highly contagious. Most children in the United States are infected by early school age, but an effective vaccine has reduced this incidence.

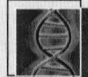

PATHOGENESIS: VZV initially infects cells of the respiratory tract or conjunctival epithelium. There it reproduces and spreads through the blood and lymphatic systems. Many organs are infected during this viremic stage, but skin involvement usually

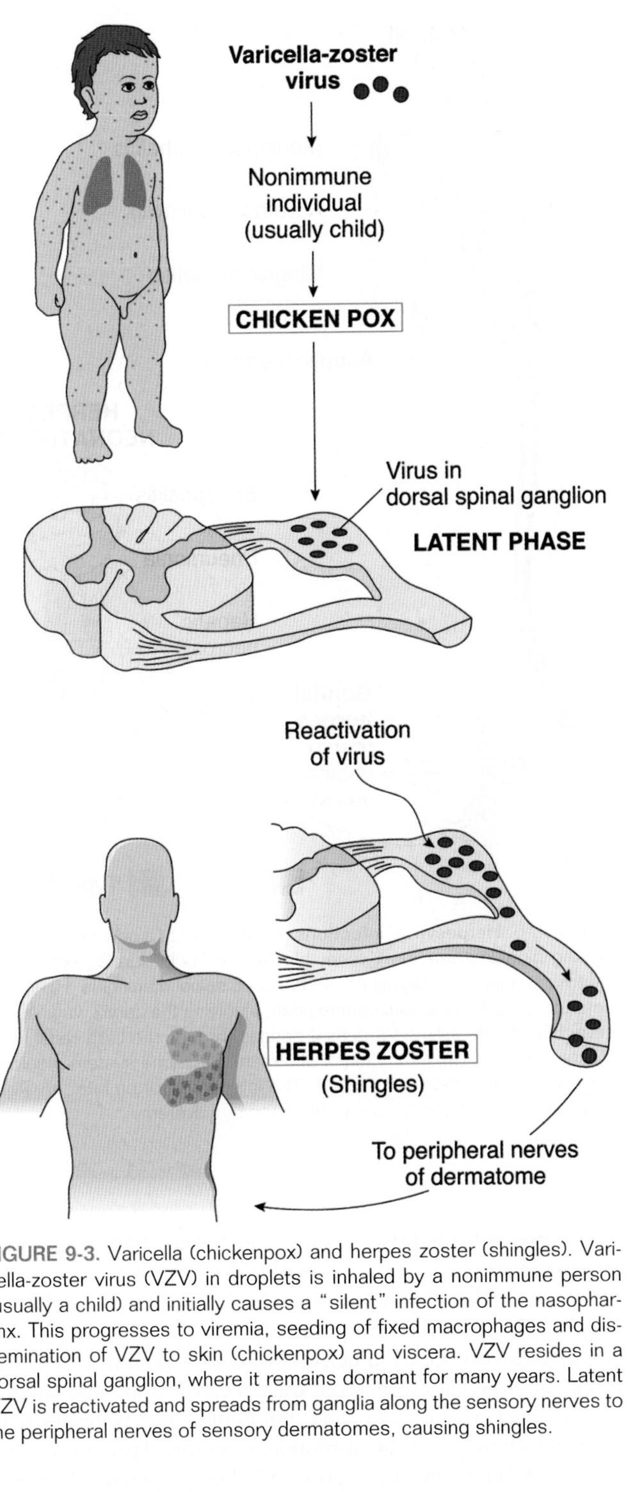

FIGURE 9-3. Varicella (chickenpox) and herpes zoster (shingles). Varicella-zoster virus (VZV) in droplets is inhaled by a nonimmune person (usually a child) and initially causes a "silent" infection of the nasopharynx. This progresses to viremia, seeding of fixed macrophages and dissemination of VZV to skin (chickenpox) and viscera. VZV resides in a dorsal spinal ganglion, where it remains dormant for many years. Latent VZV is reactivated and spreads from ganglia along the sensory nerves to the peripheral nerves of sensory dermatomes, causing shingles.

dominates the clinical picture. The virus spreads from the capillary endothelium to the epidermis, where its replication destroys the basal cells. As a result, the upper layers of the epidermis separate from the basal layer to form vesicles.

During primary infection, VZV establishes latent infection in perineuronal satellite cells of the dorsal nerve root ganglia. Transcription of viral genes continues during latency, and viral DNA can be demonstrated years after the initial infection.

Shingles occurs when full virus replication occurs in ganglion cells and the agent travels down the sensory nerve for a single dermatome. It then infects the corresponding epidermis, producing a localized, painful vesicular eruption. The risk of shingles in an infected person increases with age, and most cases occur among the elderly. Impaired cell-mediated immunity also increases the risk of herpes zoster reactivation.

PATHOLOGY: The skin lesions of chickenpox and shingles are indentical to each other and also to the lesions of herpes simplex virus (HSV). Vesicles fill with neutrophils and soon erode to become shallow ulcers. In infected cells, VZV produces a characteristic cytopathic effect, consisting of nuclear homogenization, intranuclear inclusions (Cowdry type A). The inclusion is large and eosinophilic and is separated from the nuclear membrane by a clear zone (halo). Multinucleated cells are common (Fig. 9-4). Over several days, vesicles become pustules, then rupture and heal.

CLINICAL FEATURES: Chickenpox causes fever, malaise, and a distinctive pruritic rash, that starts on the head and spreads to the trunk and extremities. Skin lesions begin as maculopapules that rapidly evolve into vesicles, then pustules that soon ulcerate and crust. Vesicles may also appear on mucous membranes, especially the mouth. Fever and systemic symptoms resolve in 3 to 5 days; skin lesions heal in several weeks.

Shingles presents with a unilateral, painful, vesicular eruption, similar in appearance to chickenpox, but in a dermatomal pattern, usually localized to a single dermatome. Pain can persist for months after resolution of the skin lesions.

Herpes Simplex Virus Produces Necrotizing Infections at Diverse Body Sites

Herpes simplex viruses (HSVs) are common human viral pathogens, which most frequently produce recurrent painful vesicular eruptions of the skin and mucous membranes (Table 9-4). Two antigenically and epidemiologically distinct HSVs cause human disease (Fig. 9-5):

- **HSV-1** is transmitted in oral secretions and typically causes disease "above the waist," including oral, facial, and ocular lesions.

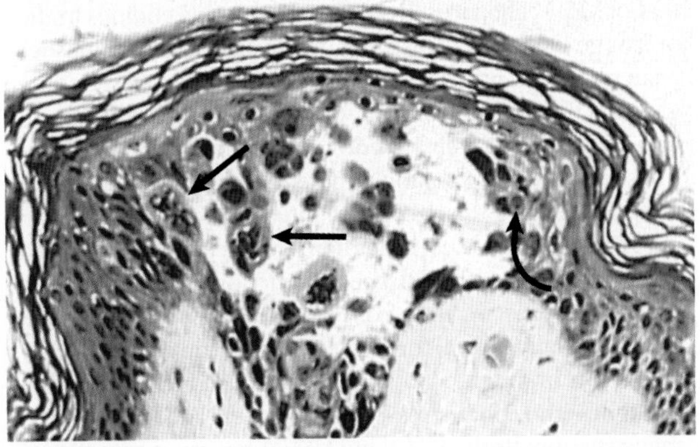

FIGURE 9-4. **Varicella.** Photomicrograph of the skin from a patient with chickenpox shows an intraepidermal vesicle. Multinucleated giant cells *(straight arrows)* and nuclear inclusions *(curved arrow)* are present.

TABLE 9-4

Herpes Simplex Viral Diseases

Viral Type	Common Presentations	Infrequent Presentations
HSV-1	Oral-labial herpes	Conjunctivitis, keratitis Encephalitis Herpetic whitlow Esophagitis* Pneumonia* Disseminated infection*
HSV-2	Genital herpes	Perinatal infection Disseminated infection*

* These conditions usually occur in immunocompromised hosts.

- **HSV-2** is transmitted in genital secretions and typically produces disease "below the waist," including genital ulcers and neonatal herpes infection.

EPIDEMIOLOGY: HSV spreads from person to person, primarily through direct contact with infected secretions or open lesions. HSV-1 spreads in oral secretions, and infection frequently occurs in childhood, most persons (50% to90%) being infected by adulthood. HSV-2 spreads by contact with genital lesions and is primarily a venereally transmitted pathogen. Neonatal herpes is acquired during passage of the newborn through an infected birth canal.

PATHOGENESIS: Primary HSV disease occurs at a site of initial viral inoculation, such as the oropharynx, genital mucosa, or skin. The virus infects epithelial cells, producing progeny viruses and destroying basal cells in the squamous epithelium, with resulting formation of vesicles. Cell necrosis also elicits an inflammatory response, initially dominated by neutrophils and then followed by lymphocytes. Primary infection resolves with the development of humoral and cell-mediated immunity to the virus.

Latent infection is established in a manner analogous to that of VZV. The virus invades sensory nerve endings in the oral or genital mucosa, ascends within axons, and establishes a latent infection in sensory neurons within corresponding ganglia. From time to time, the latent infection is reactivated, and HSV travels back down the nerve to the epithelial site served by the ganglion, where it again infects epithelial cells. Sometimes this secondary infection produces ulcerating vesicular lesions. At other times, the secondary infection does not cause visible tissue destruction, but contagious progeny viruses are shed from the site of infection. Various factors, usually typical for a given person, can induce the reactivation of latent HSV infection. These include intense sunlight, emotional stress, febrile illness, and, in women, menstruation. Both HSV-1 and HSV-2 can cause severe protracted and disseminated disease in immunocompromised persons.

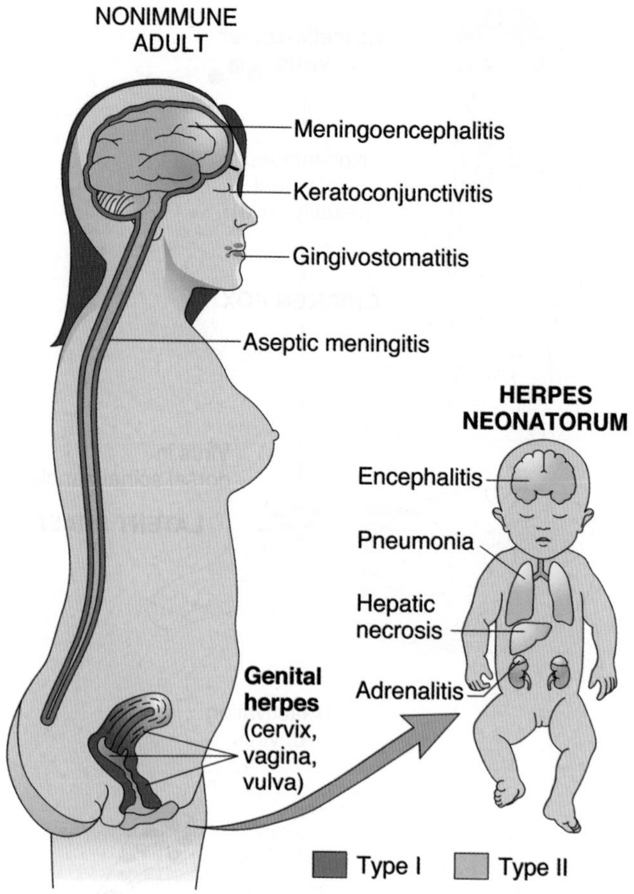

FIGURE 9-5. **Herpesvirus infections.** HSV-1 infects a nonimmune adult, causing gingivostomatitis ("fever blister" or "cold sore"), keratoconjunctivitis, meningoencephalitis, and aseptic spinal meningitis. HSV-2 infects the genitalia of a nonimmune adult, involving the cervix, vagina, and vulva. HSV-2 infects the fetus as it passes through the birth canal of an infected mother. The infant's lack of a mature immune system results in disseminated infection with HSV-1. The infection is often fatal, involving lung, liver, adrenal glands, and central nervous system.

Herpes encephalitis is a rare (1 in 100,000 HSV infections), but devastating, manifestation of HSV-1 infection. In some instances, it occurs when virus, latent in the trigeminal ganglion, is reactivated and travels retrograde to the brain. However, herpes encephalitis also occurs in persons who have no history of "cold sores," and the pathogenesis of the encephalitis in these cases is poorly understood (see Chapter 28). Equally rare is **herpes hepatitis,** which may occur in immunocompromised patients but has been also reported in young, previously healthy pregnant women.

Neonatal herpes is a serious complication of maternal genital herpes. The virus is transmitted to the fetus from the infected birth canal, often the uterine cervix, and readily disseminates in the unprotected newborn child.

Aseptic meningitis without genital involvement may be a manifestation of HSV-2 infection.

PATHOLOGY: The skin and mucous membranes are the usual sites of HSV infection, but the disease sometimes involves the brain, eye, liver, lungs, and other organs. In any location, both HSV-1 and HSV-2 cause necrosis of infected cells, accompanied by a vigorous inflammatory response. Clusters of painful ulcerating vesicular lesions on the skin or mu-

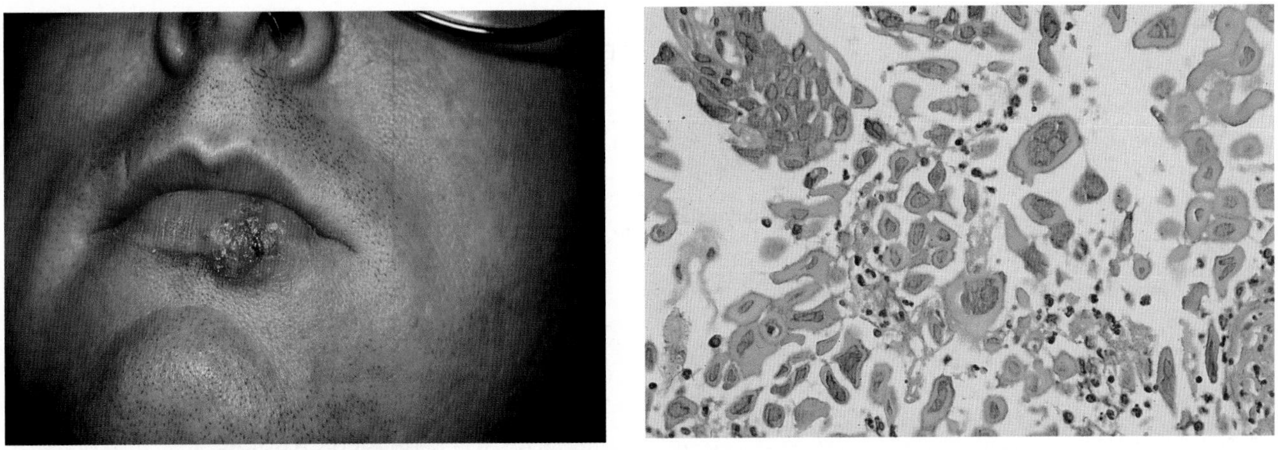

A B

FIGURE 9-6. **Herpes simplex,** type 1. **A.** Herpetic vesicles are seen on the surface of the lower lip. **B.** Epithelial cells infected with HSV-1 demonstrate Cowdry type A intranuclear inclusions and multinucleated giant cells.

cous membranes are the most frequent manifestation of HSV infection (Fig. 9-6A). These lesions persist for 1 to 2 weeks and then resolve. The cellular alterations include (1) nuclear homogenization, (2) Cowdry type A intranuclear inclusions, and (3) multinucleated giant cells (see Fig. 9-6B).

CLINICAL FEATURES: The clinical features of HSV infections vary according to host susceptibility (e.g., neonate, normal host, compromised host), viral type, and site of infection. A prodromal "tingling" sensation at the site often precedes the appearance of skin lesions. Recurrent lesions appear weeks, months, or years later, at the initial site or at a site subserved by the same nerve ganglion. Recurrent herpetic lesions in the mouth or on the lip are commonly called "cold sores" or "fever blisters" and frequently appear following sun exposure, trauma, or a febrile illness.

Patients with AIDS and other immunocompromised persons are prone to develop herpes esophagitis. Early lesions consist of rounded 1- to 3-mm vesicles located predominantly in the mid to distal esophagus. As the HSV-infected squamous cells slough from the lesions, sharply demarcated ulcers with elevated margins form and coalesce. This process may result in denudation of the esophageal mucosa. Superimposed *Candida* infection is common at this stage. In immunocompromised patients, HSV may also infect the anal mucosa, where it causes painful blisters and ulcers.

Neonatal herpes begins 5 to 7 days after delivery, with irritability, lethargy, and a mucocutaneous vesicular eruption. The infection rapidly spreads to involve multiple organs, including the brain. The infected newborn develops jaundice, bleeding problems, respiratory distress, seizures, and coma. Treatment of severe HSV infections with acyclovir is often effective, but neonatal herpes still carries a high mortality.

Epstein-Barr Virus

Infectious mononucleosis is a viral disease characterized by fever, pharyngitis, lymphadenopathy, and increased circulating lymphocytes. By adulthood, most persons have been infected with EBV. In most instances, infection is asymptomatic, but in some persons, EBV causes infectious mononucleosis. EBV has also been associated with several cancers, including African Burkitt lymphoma, B-cell lymphoma in immunosuppressed persons, and nasopharyngeal carcinoma. These neoplastic complications are discussed in Chapters 20 and 25.

EPIDEMIOLOGY: In areas of the world where children often live in crowded conditions, infection with EBV usually occurs before the age of 3 years and infectious mononucleosis is not encountered. In developed countries, many persons remain uninfected into adolescence or early adulthood. Two thirds of those newly infected after childhood develop clinically evident infectious mononucleosis.

EBV spreads from person to person primarily through contact with infected oral secretions (Fig. 9-7). EBV, once it enters the body, remains for life, analogous to latent infections with other herpesviruses. A few people (10% to 20%) intermittently shed the virus. Transmission requires close contact with infected persons. Thus, EBV spreads readily among young children in crowded conditions, where there is considerable "sharing" of oral secretions. Kissing is also an effective mode of transmission, hence the term "kissing disease" attached for youngsters.

PATHOGENESIS: The virus first binds to and infects nasopharyngeal cells and then B lymphocytes, which carry the virus throughout the body, producing a generalized infection of lymphoid tissues.

EBV is a polyclonal activator of B cells. In turn, activated B cells stimulate proliferation of specific killer T lymphocytes and suppressor T cells. The former destroy virally infected B cells, whereas suppressor cells inhibit production of immunoglobulins by B cells. The virus is also implicated in Burkitt lymphoma (see Chapters 5 and 20).

PATHOLOGY: The pathology of infectious mononucleosis involves the lymph nodes and spleen prominently. In most patients, lymphadenopathy is symmetric and most striking in the neck. The nodes are movable, discrete, and tender. Microscopically, the general architecture is preserved. The germinal centers are enlarged and have indistinct margins, because of a proliferation of immunoblasts. The nodes contain occasional large hyperchromatic cells with polylobular nuclei that resemble Reed-Sternberg cells. Lymph node histology may be difficult to distinguish from Hodgkin disease or other lymphomas (see Chapter 20).

The spleen is large and soft, owing to hyperplasia of the red pulp, and is susceptible to rupture. Immunoblasts are abundant throughout the pulp and infiltrate the walls of vessels, the trabeculae, and the capsule. The liver is almost always involved, and the sinusoids and portal tracts contain atypical lymphocytes.

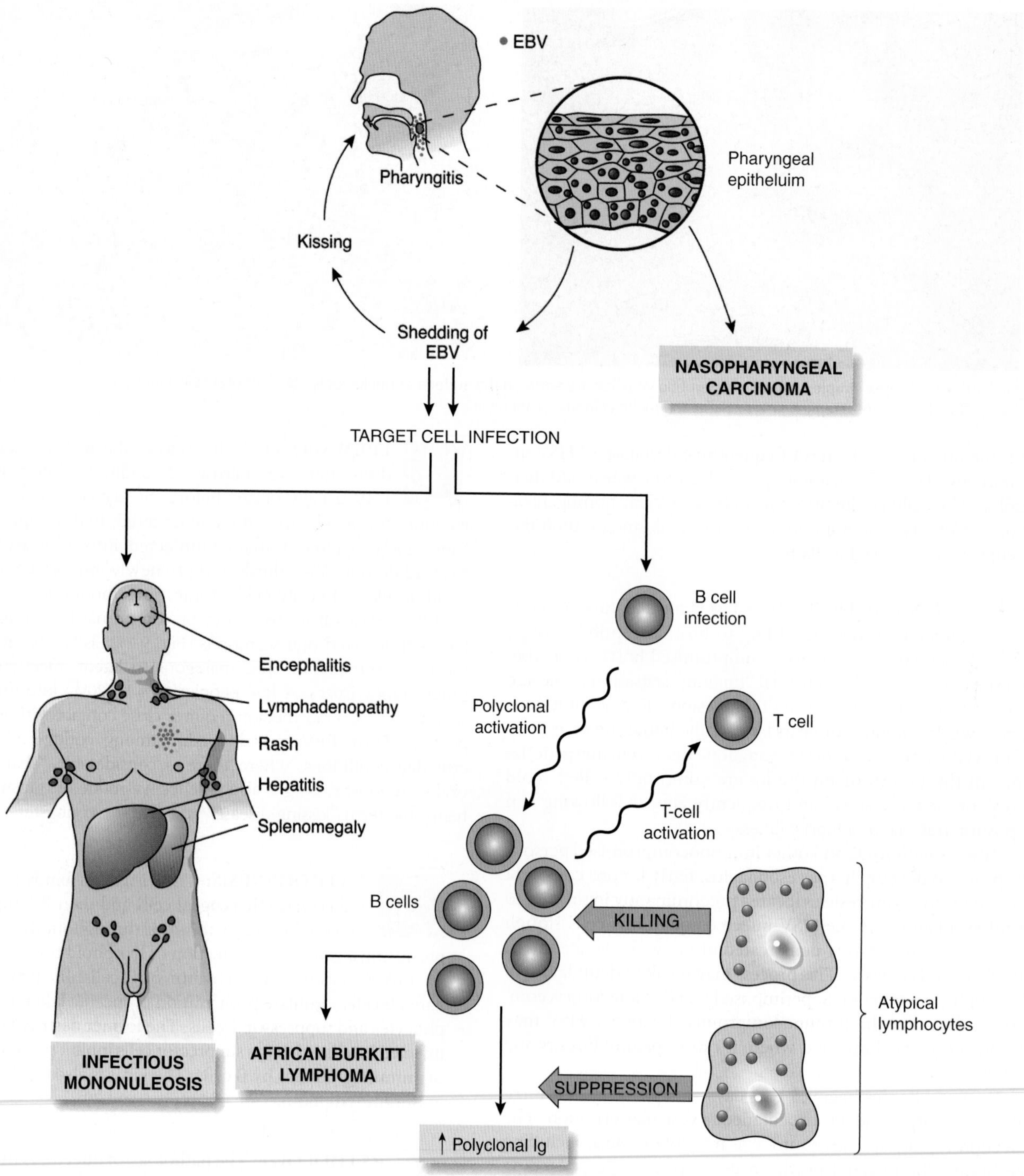

FIGURE 9-7. Role of Epstein-Barr virus (EBV) in infectious mononucleosis, nasopharyngeal carcinoma, and Burkitt lymphoma. EBV invades and replicates within the salivary glands or pharyngeal epithelium and is shed into the saliva and respiratory secretions. In some persons, the virus transforms pharyngeal epithelial cells, leading to nasopharyngeal carcinoma. In persons who are not immune from childhood exposure, EBV causes infectious mononucleosis. EBV infects B lymphocytes, which undergo polyclonal activation. These B cells stimulate the production of atypical lymphocytes, which kill virally infected B cells and suppress the production of immunoglobulins. Some infected B cells are transformed into immature malignant lymphocytes of Burkitt lymphoma.

CLINICAL FEATURES: One of the features of infectious mononucleosis is a lymphocytosis with atypical lymphocytes. These are activated T cells with lobulated, eccentric nuclei and vacuolated cytoplasm, and are involved in suppression and killing of EBV-infected B lymphocytes. Another distinguishing feature of infectious mononucleosis is the development of a specific heterophile antibody—an immunoglobulin produced in one species that reacts with antigens of another species—known as Paul Bunnell antibody. Paul Bunnell antibodies in persons with infectious mononucleosis are detected by their affinity for sheep erythrocytes. This heterophile reaction is a standard diagnostic test for infectious mononucleosis. Specific serologic tests for antibodies against EBV and for EBV antigens are also available.

Infectious mononucleosis manifests as fever, malaise, lymphadenopathy, pharyngitis, and splenomegaly. Patients usually have an elevated leukocyte count, with a predominance of lymphocytes and monocytes. Treatment is supportive, and symptoms usually resolve in 3 to 4 weeks.

Cytomegalovirus I

Cytomegalovirus (CMV) is a congenital and opportunistic pathogen that usually produces an asymptomatic infection. However, the fetus and immunocompromised persons are particularly vulnerable to the destructive effects of the virus. CMV infects 0.5% to 2.0% of all fetuses and injures 10% to 20% of those infected, making it the most common congenital pathogen.

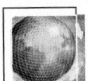

EPIDEMIOLOGY: CMV spreads from person to person by contact with infected secretions and bodily fluids, and is transmitted to the fetus across the placenta. Children spread virus in saliva or urine, whereas among adolescents and adults, transmission occurs primarily through sexual contact.

PATHOGENESIS: CMV infects various human cells, including epithelial cells, lymphocytes, and monocytes, and establishes latency in white blood cells. The normal immune response rapidly controls CMV infection: infected persons rarely show ill effects, although they shed virus periodically in body secretions. Like other herpesviruses, CMV may remain latent for life.

When an infected pregnant woman passes CMV to her fetus, the fetus is not protected by maternally derived antibodies and the virus invades fetal cells with little initial immunologic response, causing widespread necrosis and inflammation. The virus produces similar lesions in persons with suppressed cell-mediated immunity.

CMV infection is often symptomatic in immunosuppressed persons such as organ transplant recipients. In that setting, the CMV infection usually represents reactivation of endogenous latent infection, whether the source is the graft or the recipient. Subsequent dissemination may lead to severe systemic disease.

PATHOLOGY: In the fetus with CMV disease, the most common sites of involvement are the brain, inner ears, eyes, liver, and bone marrow. The most severely affected fetuses may have microcephaly, hydrocephalus, cerebral calcifications, hepatosplenomegaly, and jaundice. Microscopically, the lesions of fetal CMV disease show cellular necrosis and a characteristic cytopathic effect, consisting of marked cellular and nuclear enlargement, with nuclear and cytoplasmic inclusions. The giant nucleus, which is usually solitary, contains a large central inclusion surrounded by a clear zone (Fig. 9-8). The cytoplasmic inclusions are less prominent.

CLINICAL FEATURES: Congenitally acquired CMV has a wide range of clinical presentations. Severe disease causes fetal death in utero, conspicuous lesions of the CNS, liver disease, and bleeding problems. However, most congenital CMV infections do not produce gross abnormalities, but manifest as subtle neurologic or hearing defects, which may not be detected until later in life.

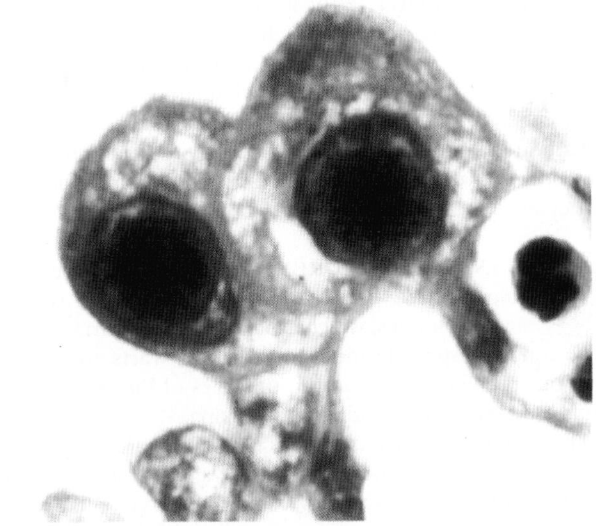

FIGURE 9-8. **Cytomegalovirus pneumonitis.** Type II pneumocytes display enlarged nuclei containing solitary inclusions surrounded by a clear zone.

CMV disease in immunosuppressed patients has diverse clinical manifestations. It can manifest as decreased visual acuity (chorioretinitis), diarrhea or gastrointestinal hemorrhage (colonic ulcerations), change in mental status (encephalitis), shortness of breath (pneumonitis), or a wide range of other symptoms.

Human Papillomavirus

Human papillomaviruses (HPVs) cause proliferative lesions of squamous epithelium, including common warts, flat warts, plantar warts, anogenital warts (condyloma acuminatum) as well as laryngeal papillomatosis. Some HPV serotypes cause squamous cell dysplasias and squamous cell carcinomas of the genital tract (see Chapter 18).

HPVs are nonenveloped, double-stranded DNA viruses. Over 100 types of HPV are known, different ones being associated with different lesions. Thus, HPV types 1, 2, and 4 produce common warts and plantar warts. Types 6, 10, 11, and 40 through 45 cause anogenital warts. Types 16, 18, and 31 are associated with squamous carcinoma of the female genital tract.

HPV infection is widespread. It is transmitted from person to person by direct contact. Most children develop common warts. The viruses that cause genital lesions are transmitted sexually.

PATHOGENESIS: HPV infection begins with viral inoculation into a stratified squamous epithelium, where the virus enters the nuclei of basal cells. Infection stimulates replication of the squamous epithelium, producing the various HPV-associated proliferative lesions. The rapidly growing squamous epithelium replicates innumerable progeny viruses, which are shed in the degenerating superficial cells. Many HPV lesions resolve spontaneously, although depressed cell-mediated immunity is associated with the persistence and spread of HPV lesions. The mechanism by which HPV infections participate in malignant change is discussed in Chapter 5.

PATHOLOGY: HPV infection produces squamous proliferative lesions, which vary in appearance and biological behavior. Most lesions show thickening of the affected epithelium, owing to enhanced squamous cell proliferation. Some HPV-infected cells display a characteristic cytopathic effect, termed **koilocytosis**, which features large squamous cells with shrunken nuclei enveloped in large cytoplasmic vacuoles (koilocytes).

CLINICAL FEATURES: Common warts (verruca vulgaris) are firm, circumscribed, raised, rough-surfaced lesions, which usually appear on surfaces subject to trauma, especially the hands. **Plantar warts** are similar squamous proliferative lesions on the soles of the feet but are compressed inward by standing and walking.

Anogenital warts (condyloma acuminatum) are soft, raised, fleshy lesions found on the penis, vulva, vaginal wall, cervix, or perianal region. When caused by certain HPV types, flat warts can develop into malignant squamous cell proliferations. The relationship between HPV, cervical intraepithelial neoplasia (CIN), and invasive squamous carcinoma of the cervix is discussed in Chapter 18.

PRIONS: A NEW DISEASE PARADIGM

In the last several decades it has become clear that infection can be transmitted and propagated solely by proteins and without nucleic acids. Despite considerable resistance to this disease paradigm, it is clear that filterable particles that lack nucleic acids can transmit disease. To date, these particles, prions, are only known to cause CNS disease. Prions are essentialy missfolded proteins that aggregate in the CNS and cause progressive neurodegeneration that leads to death. The prion protein (PrP) exists in a normal isoform and in a pathogenic form that may be transmissible. These pathogenic isoforms aggregate into prion rods which are one diagnostic characteristic of these rare disorders. Of particular importance is the uncommon persistence of these infectious agents which are highly resistent to the normal methods of sterilization and which may be transmitted via surgical instruments or electrodes which are implanted in nervous tissue, unless special protocols are followed.

- **Kuru:** The prototypical prion disease for humans is Kuru, a progressive neurodegenerative disease that was only found in the Fore tribe in the remote highlands of Papa New Guinea. Kuru was transmitted via cannibalism. Experimental transmission of Kuru has been accomplished using tissue from Kuru victims and to pass the infection to non-human primates.
- **Sporadic, Familial, and Iatrogenic Creutzfeldt-Jakob Disease** (sCJD, fCJD and iCJD): CJD is a rapidely progressive neurodegenerative disorder characterized by myoclonus, behavior changes and dementia (see Chapter 28). With a frequency of 1/1,000,000, sCJD is probably the most common human prion disease. Rarely, CJD has resulted from transmission through transplanting such tissues as cornea and dural matter. Before the advent of recombinant protein therapeutics, CJD was also transmitted from human growth hormone isolated from human cadaver pituitaries.
- **New Variant Creutzfeld-Jakob Disease** (vCJD): One of the more infamous emerging infectious diseases of the last few decades, both vCJD and the associated bovine spongiform encephalopathy (BSE), also known as "mad cow "disease, underscore the interrelatedness of animal and human infectious agents. The use of certain animal products in feeds for domestic ungulates led to and amplified a prion disease epidemic in cattle herds of the United Kingdom. Nearly 150 persons have been infected with this relentless terminal disease. All patients to date have the uncommon genetic arrangement of being homozygous, having methionine-methionine at codon 129 of the gene (PRNP) that encodes for the prion protein. Presentations have varied from the previously recognized forms of CJD in a number of important ways with age of onset being most notable. While the mean onset of CJD has been 65 years of age, vCJD has mainly occurred in young adults,with a mean age of 26 years. Psychiatric signs and symptoms has also been predominant in vCJD. Pathologic changes in vCJD are strikingly similar to those seen in BSE and differ somewhat from changes seen in the sporadic form.
- **Fatal Familial Insomnia:** This is rare inherited prion disorder that has as its hallmark a progressive course of insomnia that worsenes over time until the patient barely sleeps or not at all. There is also autonomic instability that usually manifests as what appears to be increased sympathetic tone. Altered sensorium may also be present, and signs of motor system degeneration follow. Spongiform changes like those seen in other transmissable spongiform encephalopathies are also seen later in the disease.
- **Gerstmann-Straussler-Scheinker Syndrome:** This is another rare transmissable spongiform encephalopathy that is usually familial, although rare sporadic cases have been described. Patients may present with a variety of symptoms but signs and symptoms of cerebellar degeneration usually predominate. Later in the course dementia may and often becomes a common feature.

BACTERIAL INFECTIONS

Bacteria, at 0.1 to 10 μm, are the smallest living cells. They have three basic structural components: nuclear body, cytosol, and envelope. The **nuclear body** consists of a single, coiled circular molecule of double-stranded DNA with associated RNA, and proteins. It is not separated from the cytoplasm by a special membrane, which feature distinguishes bacteria, as prokaryotes, from eukaryotes. The **cytosol** is densely packed with ribosomes, proteins, and carbohydrates and lacks structured organelles, such as mitochondria and Golgi apparatus, of eukaryotic cells. The **bacterial envelope** serves as a permeability barrier and is also actively involved in transport, protein synthesis, energy generation, DNA synthesis, and cell division.

Bacteria are classified according to the structural features of their envelope. The simplest envelope is only a phospholipid–protein bilayer membrane. Mycoplasmas have such an envelope. Most bacteria, however, have a rigid cell wall that surrounds the cell membrane. Two types of bacterial cell walls are identified by their Gram stain properties:

- **Gram-positive bacteria** retain iodine-crystal violet complexes when decolorized and appear dark blue. Their cell walls contain teichoic acids and a thick peptidoglycan layer.
- **Gram-negative bacteria** lose the iodine-crystal violet stain when decolorized and appear red with a counterstain. The outer membrane of gram-negative bacteria contains a

lipopolysaccharide component, known as endotoxin, which is a potent mediator of the shock that complicates infections with these organisms.

Both gram-positive and gram-negative cell walls may be surrounded by an additional layer of polysaccharide or protein gel, a **capsule.** Capsules aid in bacterial attachment and colonization, and may protect bacteria from phagocytosis. Because capsules are important in many infections, bacteria may be divided into those that are **encapsulated** and those that are **unencapsulated**.

The cell wall confers rigidity to bacteria and allows them to be distinguished on the basis of shape and pattern of growth in cultures. Round or oval bacteria are **cocci**. Those that grow in clusters are called **staphylococci**, while those that grow in chains are called **streptococci.** Elongate bacteria are **rods** or **bacilli**, and curved ones are **vibrios**. Some spiral-shaped bacteria are called **spirochetes**.

Most bacteria can be cultured on chemical media, and so are frequently described according to their growth requirements on these media. Bacteria that need high levels of oxygen are called **aerobic**, those that grow best without oxygen are **anaerobic,** and those that thrive with limited amounts of oxygen are **microaerophilic**. Bacteria that grow well with or without oxygen are **facultative anaerobes**.

BACTERIAL EXOTOXINS: Many bacteria secrete toxins (exotoxins) that damage human cells either at the site of bacterial growth or at a distant site. These toxins are often named for the site or mechanism of their activity. Thus, those that act on the nervous system are called **neurotoxins;** those that affect intestinal cells are termed **enterotoxins**. Some toxins, such as diphtheria toxin or some of the *Clostridium perfringens* toxins, that kill target cells are called **cytotoxins**. Others, such as the diarrheagenic toxin of *Vibrio cholerae* or the potent neurotoxin of *Clostridium botulinum*, disturb the normal functions of their target cells damaging or killing them. *Clostirdium perfringens* produces over 20 different toxins that damage the human body in diverse ways.

BACTERIAL ENDOTOXINS: As mentioned above, gram-negative bacteria contain in their outer membranes a structural element called **lipopolysaccharide**. Also known as **endotoxin**, lipopolysaccharide activates complement, coagulation, fibrinolysis, and bradykinin systems. It also causes release of primary inflammatory mediators, including tumor necrosis factor (TNF) and interleukin-1 (IL-1), and various colony-stimulating factors. Endotoxin may cause shock, complement depletion, and disseminated intravascular coagulation.

Many bacteria damage tissues through the inflammatory or immune responses they elicit. The capsule of *Streptococcus pneumoniae* protects it from phagocytosis while activating the host's inflammatory response. Within the lung, the encapsulated organism causes exudation of fluid and cells that fills the alveoli. This inflammation impairs breathing but does not, at least initially, limit proliferation of the organism. *Treponema pallidum,* the spirochete that causes syphilis, persists in the body for years and elicits inflammatory and immune responses that continuously damage host tissues.

Many common bacterial infections (e.g., *Staphylococcus aureus* skin infections) are characterized by purulent exudates, but tissue responses to bacteria are highly variable. In some cases, such as cholera, botulism, and tetanus, there is no inflammatory response at critical sites of cellular injury. Other bacterial infections, including syphilis and Lyme disease, lead to a predominantly lymphocytic and plasma cellular response. Still others (e.g., brucellosis) are characterized by granuloma formation.

Many bacterial diseases are caused by organisms that normally inhabit the human body. There is an extensive endogenous bacterial flora of the gastrointestinal tract, upper respiratory tract, skin, and vagina. Normally, these microorganisms are commensal and cause no harm. However, if they gain access to usually sterile sites or if host defenses are impaired, they can cause extensive destruction. *Staphylococcus aureus, Streptococcus pneumoniae,* and *Escherichia coli* are normal flora that are also major human pathogens.

Pyogenic Gram-Positive Cocci

Staphylococcus aureus Produces Suppurative Infections

S. aureus is a gram-positive coccus that typically grows in clusters and is one of the most common bacterial pathogens. It normally resides on the skin and is readily inoculated into deeper tissues, where it causes suppurative infections. *In fact, it is the most common cause of suppurative infections of the skin, joints, and bones, and it is a leading cause of infective endocarditis. S. aureus* is commonly distinguished from other, less virulent staphylococci by the coagulase test. *S. aureus* is coagulase-positive; the other staphylococci are coagulase-negative.

S. aureus spreads by direct contact with colonized surfaces or persons. Most people are intermittently colonized with *S. aureus*, carrying the organism on the skin, nares, or clothing. The organism also survives on inanimate surfaces for long periods.

PATHOGENESIS: Many *S. aureus* infections begin as localized infections of the skin and skin appendages, producing cellulites and abscesses. The organism, equipped with destructive enzymes and toxins, sometimes invades beyond the initial site, spreading by the blood or lymphatics to almost any location in the body. The bones, joints, and heart valves are the most common sites of metastatic *S. aureus* infections. *S. aureus* also causes several distinct diseases by elaborating toxins that are carried to distant sites.

PATHOLOGY: When *S. aureus* is introduced into a previously sterile site, the infection usually produces suppuration and abscess formation. Abscesses range from microscopic foci to lesions several centimeters in diameter and are filled with pus and bacteria.

CLINICAL FEATURES: The clinical manifestations of *S. aureus* disease vary according to the sites and types of infection.

- **Furuncles (boils) and styes:** Deep-seated *S. aureus* infections occur in and around hair follicles, often in a nasal carrier. They localize on hairy surfaces, such as the neck, thighs and buttocks of men; and the axillae, pubic area, and eyelids of both sexes. The boil begins as a nodule at the base of a hair follicle, followed by a pimple that remains painful and red for a few days. A yellow apex forms and the central core becomes necrotic and fluctuant. Rupture or incision of the boil relieves the pain. **Styes** are boils that involve the sebaceous glands around the eyelid. **Paronychia** are staphylococcal

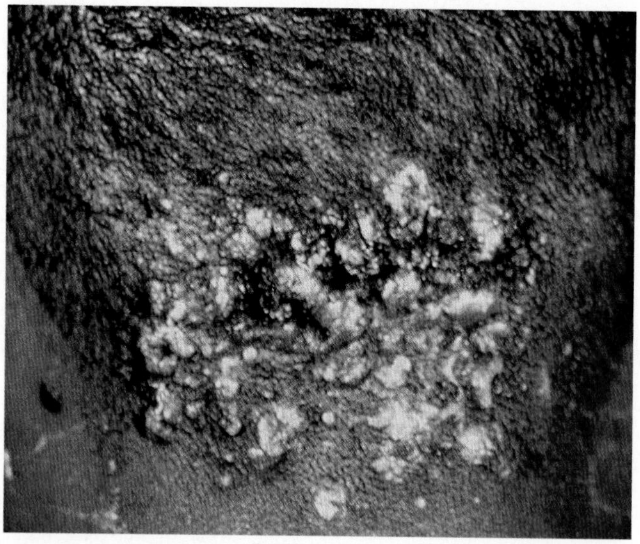

FIGURE 9-9. **Staphylococcal carbuncle.** The posterior neck is indurated and shows multiple follicular abscesses discharging purulent material.

infections of nail beds and **felons** are the same infections on the palmar side of the fingertips.

- **Carbuncles:** These lesions, mostly on the neck, result from coalescing infections with *S. aureus* around hair follicles and produce draining sinuses (Fig. 9-9).
- **Scalded skin syndrome:** This disease affects infants and children under 3 years who present with a sunburnlike rash that begins on the face and spreads over the body. Bullae begin to form and even gentle rubbing causes the skin to desquamate. The disease begins to resolve in 1 to 2 weeks, as the skin regenerates. Desquamation is due to systemic effects of a specific exotoxin and the site of *S. aureus* proliferation is often occult.
- **Osteomyelitis:** Acute staphylococcal osteomyelitis, usually in the bones of the legs, most commonly afflicts boys between 3 and 10 years old, most of whom have a history of infection or trauma. Osteomyelitis may become chronic if not properly treated. Adults older than 50 are more frequently afflicted with vertebral osteomyelitis, which may follow staphylococcal infections of the skin or urinary tract, prostatic surgery, or pinning of a fracture.
- **Infections of burns or surgical wounds:** These sites often become infected with *S. aureus* from the patient's own nasal carriage or from medical personnel. Newborns and elderly, malnourished, diabetic, and obese persons all have increased susceptibility.
- **Respiratory tract infections:** Staphylococcal respiratory tract infections are most common in infants under 2 years, and especially under 2 months. The infection is characterized by ulcers of the upper airway, scattered foci of pneumonia, pleural effusion, empyema, and pneumothorax. In adults, staphylococcal pneumonia may follow viral influenza, which destroys the ciliated surface epithelium and leaves the bronchial surface vulnerable to secondary infection.
- **Bacterial arthritis:** *S. aureus* is the causative organism in half of all cases of septic arthritis, mostly in patients 50 to 70 years old. Rheumatoid arthritis and corticosteroid therapy are common predisposing conditions.
- **Septicemia:** Septicemia with *S. aureus* afflicts patients with lowered resistance who are in the hospital for other diseases. Some have underlying staphylococcal infections (e.g., osteomyelitis, septic arthritis), some have had surgery (e.g., transurethral resection of the prostate), and some have infections from an indwelling intravenous catheter. Miliary abscesses and endocarditis are serious complications.
- **Bacterial endocarditis:** Bacterial endocarditis is a common complication of *S. aureus* septicemia. It may develop spontaneously on normal valves, valves damaged by rheumatic fever, or prosthetic valves. Intravenous drug abuse is a predisposing factor to staphylococcal endocarditis.
- **Toxic shock syndrome:** This disorder most commonly afflicts menstruating women, who present with high fever, nausea, vomiting, diarrhea, and myalgias. Subsequently, they develop shock and within several days a sunburnlike rash. The disease is associated with use of tampons, particularly hyperabsorbent tampons, which provide a site for *S. aureus* replication and toxin elaboration. Toxic shock syndrome occurs rarely in children and men and is then usually associated with an occult *S. aureus* infection.
- **Staphylococcal food poisoning:** Staphylococcal food poisoning typically begins less than 6 hours after a meal. Nausea and vomiting begin abruptly and usually resolve within 12 hours. This disease is caused by preformed toxin, rather than by secretion of toxin by ingested bacteria.
- **Antibiotic-resistant *S. aureus*.** One of the most important clinical issues concerning *S. aureus* is the relentless increase in antibiotic resistence that has occurred over the last 6 decades since the introduction of penicillin in the early 1940s. *S. aureus* was one of the first important pathogens to become completely resistant to penicillin and, subsequently, to each subsequent generation of penicillin derivatives. Today, methicillin-resistant *S. aureus* (MRSA) infections are usually acquired in the hospital, in an environment that selects for antibiotic-resistant bacteria. MRSA represents one of the most dreaded of nosocomial infections. According to the CDC, between 1995 and 2004 the percentage of *S. aureus* infections in patients in intensive care units that were due to MRSA almost doubled, from slightly over one-third, to almost two-thirds, of all *S. aureus* infections. The most worrisome feature of MRSA infection is the difficulty in treatment when it becomes invasive and imperils health. The recent increase in community-acquired MRSA raises concerns of dissemination of antibiotic resistance among *Staphyloccocus* and other bacteria.

Coagulase-Negative Staphylococci Infect Prosthetic Devices

Coagulase-negative staphylococci are the major cause of infections associated with the introduction of medical devices, including intravenous catheters, prosthetic heart valves, heart pacemakers, orthopedic prostheses, cerebrospinal fluid shunts, and peritoneal catheters.

Disease caused by coagulase-negative staphylococci usually derives from the normal bacterial flora. Of the more than 20 known species of coagulase-negative staphylococci, 10 are normal residents of human skin and mucosal surfaces. Staphylococcus epidermidis *is the most frequent cause of infections associated with medical devices.* Another species, *Staphylococcus saprophyticus*, causes 10% to 20% of acute urinary tract infections in young women.

PATHOGENESIS: Coagulase-negative staphylococci readily contaminate foreign bodies. The organisms slowly proliferate on implanted devices, inducing an inflammatory response that damages adjacent tissue. If the bacteria are present on an intravascular surface, such as the tip of an intravascular catheter, they can spread through the bloodstream to cause metastatic infections. Coagulase-negative staphylococci lack the enzymes and toxins that permit *S. aureus* to cause extensive local tissue destruction. Some strains of coagulase-negative staphylococci produce a polysaccharide gel, called a biofilm, which enhances adherence of the bacteria to foreign objects and protects them from host antimicrobial defenses and from many antibiotics.

PATHOLOGY: Medical devices infected with coagulase-negative staphylococci are usually thinly coated with tan, fibrinous material. In contrast to infections caused by *S. aureus*, coagulase-negative staphylococcal infections usually do not produce extensive local tissue necrosis or large quantities of pus. Microscopic examination of infected devices shows clusters of gram-positive bacteria embedded in fibrin and cellular debris, with an associated acute inflammatory infiltrate.

CLINICAL FEATURES: Coagulase-negative staphylococcal infections usually have subtle clinical presentations, and the only symptom of infection may be persistent low-grade fever. Infection of orthopedic prostheses frequently causes progressive loosening and dysfunction of the devices. In most persons, these infections are indolent, but in neutropenic or otherwise severely compromised persons, the infections can be fatal. Treatment usually requires replacement of any infected foreign object and appropriate antibiotic therapy. Nosocomial strains of coagulase-negative *Staphylococcus* are often multi-drug resistent and close to 80% of such hospital acquired isolates have the *mecA* gene, which encodes resistence to the all classes of β-lactam antibiotics. If a β-lactam antibiotic is used, clinical failure is almost guaranteed.

Streptococcus pyogenes Causes Suppurative, Toxin-Related, and Immunologic Reactions

S. pyogenes, *also known as group A streptococcus, is one of the most common human bacterial pathogens, causing many diseases of diverse organ systems, from acute self-limited pharyngitis to major illnesses such as rheumatic fever* (Fig. 9-10). *S. pyogenes* is a gram-positive coccus that is frequently part of the endogenous flora of the skin and oropharynx.

Diseases caused by *S. pyogenes* fall into two categories: suppurative and nonsuppurative. Suppurative diseases occur at sites where the bacteria invade and cause tissue necrosis, usually inducing an acute inflammatory response. Suppurative *S. pyogenes* infections include pharyngitis, impetigo, cellulitis, myositis, pneumonia, and puerperal sepsis. By contrast, nonsuppurative diseases occur at sites remote from the site of bacterial invasion. *S. pyogenes* causes two major nonsuppurative complications: rheumatic fever and acute poststreptococcal glomerulonephritis. These (1) involve organ systems far from the sites of streptococcal invasion, (2) usually occur some time after the acute infection, and (3) are probably caused by an immune responses. Rheumatic fever is discussed in Chapter 11 and poststreptococcal glomerulonephritis in Chapter 16.

S. pyogenes *elaborates several exotoxins, including erythrogenic toxins and cytolytic toxins (streptolysins S and O).* Erythrogenic toxins are responsible for the rash of scarlet fever. Streptolysin S lyses bacterial protoplasts (L forms) and probably destroys neutrophils after they ingest *S. pyogenes*. Streptolysin O induces a persistently high antibody titer, an effect that provides a useful marker for the diagnosis of *S. pyogenes* infections and their nonsuppurative complications.

Streptococcal Pharyngitis ("Strep Throat")

S. pyogenes, the common bacterial cause of pharyngitis, spreads from person to person by direct contact with oral or respiratory secretions. "Strep throat" occurs worldwide, predominantly affecting children and adolescents.

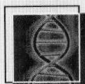

PATHOGENESIS: *S. pyogenes* attaches to epithelial cells by binding to fibronectin on their surface. The bacterium produces hemolysins, DNAase, hyaluronidase, and streptokinase, which allow it to damage and invade human tissues. *S. pyogenes* also has cell wall components that protect it from the inflammatory response. One of these, designated **M protein**, protrudes from the cell wall of virulent strains and prevents complement deposition, thereby protecting bacteria from phagocytosis. Another surface protein destroys C5a, blocking its opsonizing effect and inhibiting phagocytosis. The invading organism elicits an acute inflammatory response, often producing an exudate of neutrophils in the tonsillar fossae.

CLINICAL FEATURES: "Strep throat" is a sore throat, with fever, malaise, headache, and elevated leukocyte count. It usually lasts 3 to 5 days. *In a few cases, streptococcal pharyngitis leads to rheumatic fever or acute poststreptococcal glomerulonephritis.* Penicillin treatment shortens the course of "**strep throat**" and, more importantly, prevents the major nonsuppurative sequelae.

Scarlet Fever

Scarlet fever (scarlatina) describes a punctate red rash on skin and mucous membranes in some suppurative S. pyogenes *infections, most commonly pharyngitis.* It usually begins on the chest and spreads to the extremities. The tongue may develop a yellow-white coating, which sheds to reveal a "beefy-red" surface. Scarlet fever is caused by an erythrogenic toxin.

Erysipelas

Erysipelas is an erythematous swelling of the skin caused chiefly by S. pyogenes (Fig. 9-11). The rash usually begins on the face and spreads rapidly. Erysipelas is common in warm climates but is not often seen before the age of 20 years. A diffuse, edematous, acute inflammatory reaction in the epidermis and dermis extends into subcutaneous tissues. The inflammatory infiltrate is principally composed of neutrophils and is most intense around vessels and adnexa of the skin. Cutaneous microabscesses and small foci of necrosis are not uncommon.

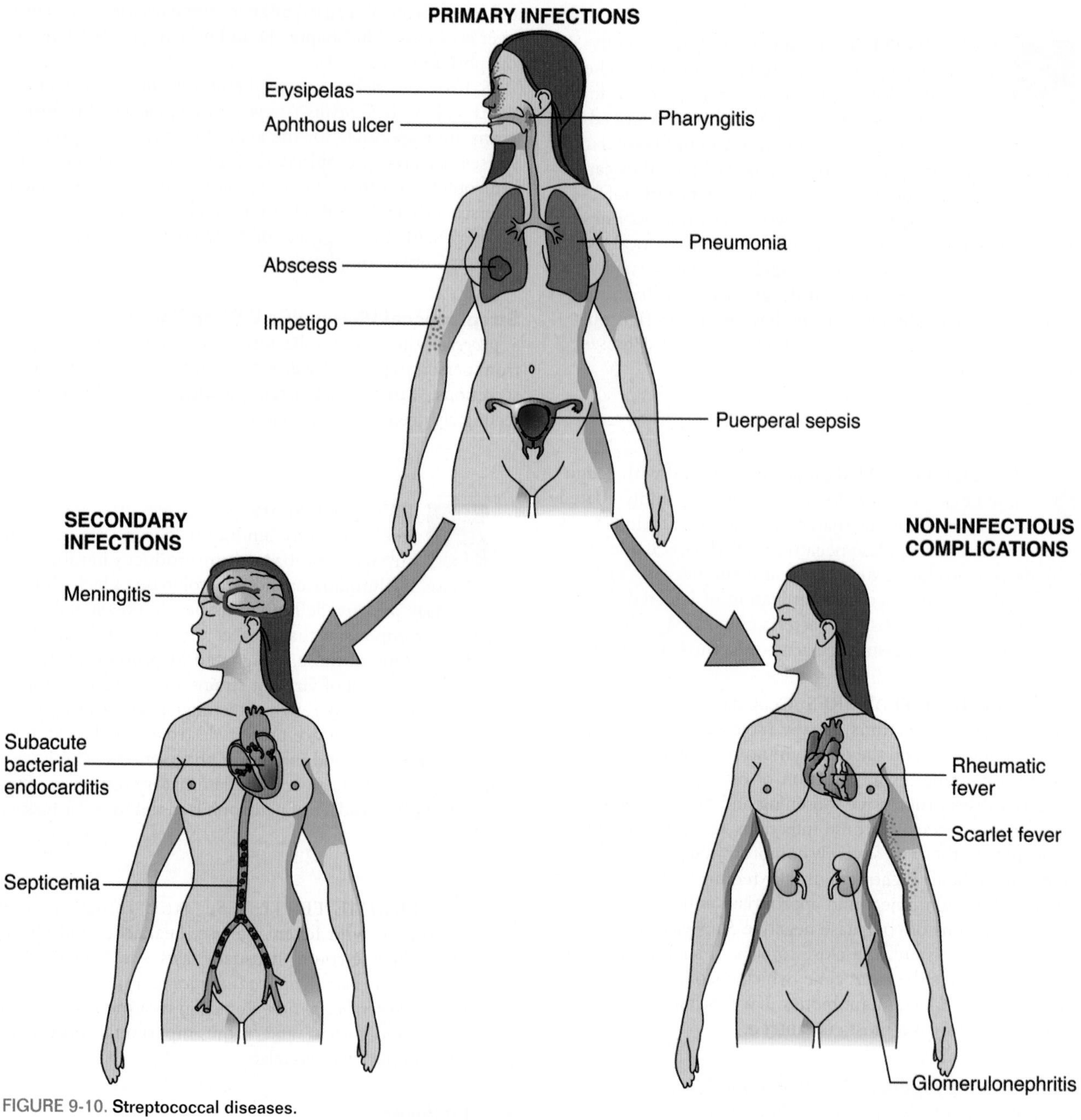

FIGURE 9-10. **Streptococcal diseases.**

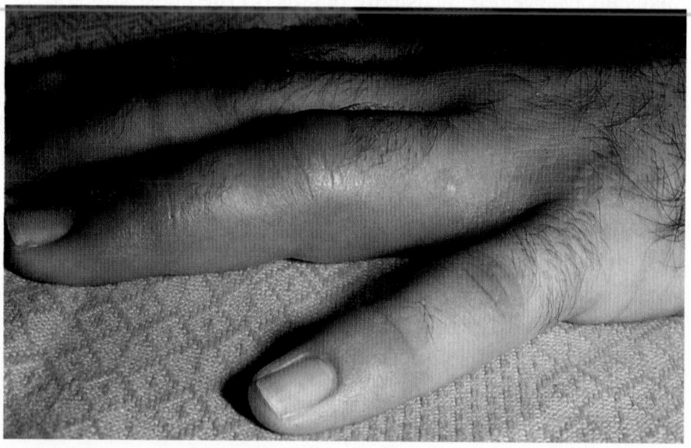

FIGURE 9-11. **Erysipelas.** Streptococcal infection of the skin has resulted in an erythematous and swollen finger.

Impetigo

Impetigo (pyoderma) is a localized, intraepidermal infection of the skin that is caused by S. pyogenes *or* S. aureus. The strains of *S. pyogenes* that cause impetigo are antigenically and epidemiologically distinct from those that cause pharyngitis.

Impetigo spreads from person to person by direct contact. The disease most commonly affects children aged 2 to 5 years. A person, usually a child, first develops skin colonization with the causative organism. Minor trauma or an insect bite then inoculates the bacteria into the skin, where they form an intraepidermal pustule, which ruptures and leaks a purulent exudate.

Lesions begin on exposed body surfaces as localized erythematous papules (Fig. 9-12). These become pustules, which erode within a few days to form a thick honey-colored crust. Impetigo sometimes leads to poststreptococcal glomerulonephritis but not to rheumatic fever.

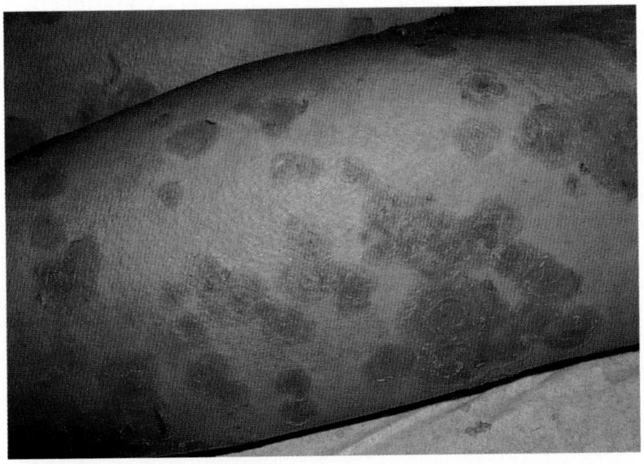

FIGURE 9-12. **Streptococcal impetigo.** The lower extremities exhibit numerous erythematous papules, with central ulceration and the formation of crusts.

Streptococcal Cellulitis

S. pyogenes *causes an acute spreading infection of the loose connective tissue of the deeper layers of the dermis.* This suppurative infection results from traumatic inoculation of microorganisms into the skin and frequently occurs on the extremities in the context of impaired lymphatic drainage. Cellulitis usually begins at sites of unnoticed injury and appears as spreading areas of redness, warmth, and swelling.

Puerperal Sepsis

Puerperal sepsis refers to postpartum infection of the uterine cavity by S. pyogenes. The disease was formerly common but is now rare in developed countries. The infection originates from the contaminated hands of attendants at delivery.

Streptococcus pneumoniae Infection Is a Major Cause of Lobar Pneumonia

Streptococcus pneumoniae, often simply called **pneumococcus**, causes pyogenic infections, primarily involving the lungs (pneumonia), middle ear (otitis media), sinuses (sinusitis), and meninges (meningitis). *It is one of the most common bacterial pathogens of humans, and by age 5, most children in the world have suffered at least one episode of pneumococcal disease (usually otitis media).*

S. pneumoniae is an aerobic, gram-positive diplococcus. Most *S. pneumonia* that cause clinical disease posses a capsule although nonserotypeable isolates are a known cause of epidemic conjunctivitis. There are over 80 antigenically distinct serotypes of pneumococcus; antibody to one does not protect from infection with another. *S. pneumoniae* is a commensal organism in the oropharynx and virtually all persons are colonized at some time.

PATHOGENESIS AND PATHOLOGY: Pneumococcal disease begins when the organism gains access to sterile sites, usually those in proximity to its normal residence in the oropharynx. Pneumococcal sinusitis and otitis media are usually preceded by a viral illness, such as the common cold, which injures the protective ciliated epithelium and fills affected air spaces with fluid. Pneumococci then thrive in the nutrient-rich tissue fluid. Infection of the sinuses or middle ear can spread to the adjacent meninges.

Pneumococcal pneumonia arises in a similar fashion. The lower respiratory tract is protected by the mucociliary blanket and cough response, which normally expel organisms that are inhaled into the lower airway. Insults that interfere with respiratory defenses, including influenza, other viral respiratory illness, smoking, and alcoholism, allow access to *S. pneumoniae.* Once in the alveoli, the organisms proliferate and elicit an acute inflammatory response. As the bacteria multiply and fill the alveoli they gain access to other alveoli via the pores of Kohn. The polysaccharide capsule of *S. pneumoniae* prevents activation of the alternate complement pathway, thereby blocking the production of the opsonin C3b. Thus, before a specific IgG antibody is produced, the organism can proliferate and spread unimpeded by phagocytes. In the lungs, *S. pneumoniae* spreads rapidly to involve an entire lobe or several lobes (lobar pneumonia). Alveoli fill with proteinaceous fluid, neutrophils, and bacteria. The clinical features of pneumococcal infections are discussed in Chapter 12. Unlike pneumonia caused by *Staphylococcus aureus,* which can cause permanent lung damage, pneumonia caused by *S. pneumoniae* often resolves completely. If pneumococcal disease is invasive, there is usually an underlying problem such as chronic aspiration, diabetes, alcohol abuse, or other diseases that compromises bacterial opsonization, like multiple myeloma, hypogammaglobemia, patients with sickle cell disease, or previous splenectomy. Splenectomized patients are at a greatly increased risk of rapid, fulminant septic shock, and death.

Group B Streptococci Are the Leading Cause of Neonatal Pneumonia, Meningitis, and Sepsis

These organisms are also an infrequent cause of pyogenic infections in adults. Group B streptococci are gram-positive bacteria that grow in short chains. Several thousand neonatal infections with group B streptococci occur in the United States each year, and about 30% of infected infants die. Group B streptococci are part of the normal vaginal flora and are found in 10% to 30% of women. Most newborns born to colonized women acquire the organisms as they pass through the birth canal.

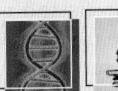

PATHOGENESIS AND PATHOLOGY: Particular risk factors associated with the development of neonatal group B streptococcal infections include premature delivery and low levels of maternally derived IgG antibodies against the organism. Newborns have little functional reserve for granulocyte production, and once established, the bacterial infection rapidly overwhelms the body's defense capacity. Group B streptococcal infection may be limited to the lungs or CNS or may be widely disseminated. Histopathologically, the involved tissues show a pyogenic response, often with overwhelming numbers of gram-positive cocci.

Bacterial Infections of Childhood

Diphtheria Is a Necrotizing Upper Respiratory Tract Infection

Infection with *Corynebacterium diphtheriae*—an aerobic, pleomorphic, gram-positive rod—may lead to cardiac and neurologic disturbances due to toxin production. The disease is preventable by vaccination with inactivated *C. diphtheriae* toxin (toxoid).

EPIDEMIOLOGY: Humans are the only known reservoir for *C. diphtheriae*, and most persons are asymptomatic carriers. The organism spreads from person to person in respiratory droplets or oral secretions. At one time, diphtheria was a leading cause of death in children 2 to 15 years of age, but in Western countries, immunization programs have largely eliminated the disease. However, diphtheria persists as a major health problem in less-developed countries.

PATHOGENESIS: *C. diphtheriae* enters the pharynx and proliferates, often on the tonsils. Diphtheria toxin is absorbed systemically and acts on tissues throughout the body, with the heart, nerves, and kidneys being most susceptible to damage. Diphtheria toxin is composed of *A* and *B* subunits.The B subunit binds to glycolipid receptors on target cells, and the A subunit acts within the cytoplasm on elongation factor 2 to interrupt protein synthesis. The toxin is one of the most potent known, and one molecule suffices to kill a cell. Not all strains of C. *dipheriae* produce exotoxin. The gene encoding the exotoxin is carried by a bacteriphage, lysogenic beta phage.

PATHOLOGY: The characteristic lesions of diphtheria are the thick, gray, leathery membranes composed of sloughed epithelium, necrotic debris, neutrophils, fibrin, and bacteria that line affected respiratory passages (from the Greek, *diphtheria*, "leather"). The epithelial surface beneath the membranes is denuded, and the submucosa is acutely inflamed and hemorrhagic. The inflammatory process often produces swelling in the surrounding soft tissues, which can be severe enough to cause respiratory compromise. When the heart is affected, the myocardium displays fat droplets in the myocytes and focal necrosis (Fig. 9-13). In the case of neural involvement, the affected peripheral nerves exhibit demyelination.

CLINICAL FEATURES: Diphtheria begins with fever, sore throat, and malaise. The dirty gray membrane usually develops first on the tonsils and may spread throughout the posterior oropharynx. The membrane is firmly adherent, and an attempt to strip it from the underlying mucosa produces bleeding. Cardiac and neurologic symptoms develop in a minority of infected persons, usually those with the most severe local disease.

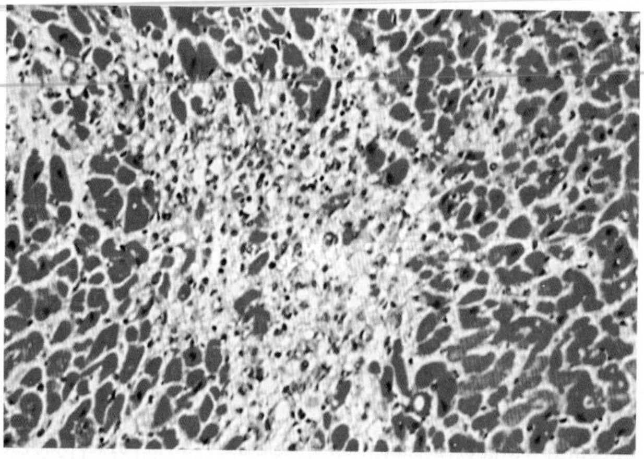

FIGURE 9-13. **Diphtheric myocarditis.** Focal degeneration of cardiac myocytes is evident.

Cutaneous diphtheria, which results from inoculation of the organism into a break in the skin, manifests as a pustule or ulcer; it rarely leads to cardiac or neurologic complications. Diphtheria is treated by prompt administration of antitoxin and antibiotics.

Pertussis Is Characterized by Debilitating Paroxysmal Coughing

The paroxysm is followed by a long, high-pitched inspiration, the "whoop," which gives the disease its name, "whooping cough." The causative organism is *Bordetella pertussis*, a small, gram-negative coccobacillus.

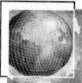

EPIDEMIOLOGY: *B. pertussis* is highly contagious and spreads from person to person, primarily by infected respiratory aerosols. Humans are the only reservoir of infection. In susceptible populations, pertussis is primarily a disease of children younger than the age of 5 years although infection incidence is increasing among adults. Vaccination protects against *B. pertussis*, but worldwide, there are some 50 million cases of pertussis each year, resulting in almost 1 million deaths, particularly in infants.

PATHOGENESIS AND PATHOLOGY: *B. pertussis* initiates infection by attaching to the cilia of respiratory epithelial cells. The organism then elaborates a cytotoxin that kills ciliated cells. The progressive destruction of ciliated respiratory epithelium and the ensuing inflammatory response cause the local respiratory symptoms. Several other toxins include "pertussis toxin," an agent that causes the pronounced lymphocytosis often associated with whooping cough. Another toxin inhibits adenylyl cyclase, an effect that blocks bacterial phagocytosis.

B. pertussis causes an extensive tracheobronchitis, with necrosis of the ciliated respiratory epithelium and an acute inflammatory response. With the loss of the protective mucociliary blanket, there is an increased risk of pneumonia from aspirated oral bacteria. Coughing paroxysms and vomiting make aspiration likely. Secondary bacterial pneumonia commonly causes death.

CLINICAL FEATURES: Whooping cough is a prolonged upper respiratory tract illness, lasting 4 to 5 weeks and passing through three stages:

- The **catarrhal stage** resembles a common viral upper respiratory tract illness, with low-grade fever, runny nose, conjunctivitis, and cough.
- The **paroxysmal stage** occurs one week into the illness. Cough worsens and becomes paroxysmal, with 5 to 15 consecutive coughs, often followed by an inspiratory whoop. The patient develops a marked lymphocytosis: total leukocyte counts often exceed 40,000 cells/μL. The paroxysms persist for 2 to 3 weeks.
- The **convalescent phase** usually lasts for several weeks.

Haemophilus influenzae Causes Pyogenic Infections in Young Children

Haemophilus influenzae *infections involve the middle ear, sinuses, facial skin, epiglottis, meninges, lungs, and joints.* The organism is a major pediatric bacterial pathogen and a leading cause of bacterial meningitis worldwide. It is an aerobic, pleomorphic gram-negative coccobacillus that may be either encapsulated or not. Nonencapsulated strains (type a) usually produce localized infections; encapsulated strains, designated type b, are more virulent and cause over 95% of the invasive bacteremic infections.

EPIDEMIOLOGY: *H. influenzae* is a strict parasite of humans and spreads from person to person, primarily in respiratory droplets and secretions. The organism is normally resident in the human nasopharynx, colonizing 20% to 50% of healthy adults. Most colonizing strains are nonencapsulated, but 3% to 5% are *H. influenzae* type b.

Most severe *H. influenzae* type b infections occur in children younger than the age of 6 years. The incidence of serious disease peaks at 6 to 18 months of age, corresponding to the period between the loss of maternally acquired immunity and the acquisition of native immunity. Complications can be prevented by inoculating infants with *H. influenzae* type b vaccine. This vaccine has been credited with greatly reducing invasive H. influenzae type b disease, particularly meningitis, in children. However, because vaccination also reduces *H. influenzae* type b carriage and the repeated immunologic boosting effect that carriage provides, continued vigilance is important.

PATHOGENESIS: Unencapsulated *H. influenzae* strains produce disease by spreading locally from their normal sites of residence to adjoining sterile locations, such as the sinuses or middle ear. This is facilitated by injury to normal defense mechanisms, as occurs with a viral upper respiratory tract illness. Within these previously sterile sites, unencapsulated organisms proliferate and elicit an acute inflammatory response, which injures local tissue but eventually contains the infection. Under most circumstances, unencapsulated strains do not produce bacteremia.

H. influenzae type b is capable of tissue invasion. The capsular polysaccharide of type b organisms allows them to evade phagocytosis and bacteremic infections are common. Epiglottitis, facial cellulitis, septic arthritis, and meningitis result from invasive bacteremic infections. *H. influenzae* type b also elaborates an IgA protease, which facilitates local survival of the organism in the respiratory tract.

PATHOLOGY: *H. influenzae* elicits strong acute inflammatory responses. Specific pathologic features vary according to the sites affected. *H. influenzae* meningitis resembles other acute bacterial meningitides, with a predominantly acute inflammatory leptomeningeal infiltrate, sometimes involving the subarachnoid space.

H. influenzae pneumonia usually complicates chronic lung disease. In half of patients it follows a viral infection of the respiratory tract. The alveoli are filled with neutrophils, macrophages containing bacilli, and fibrin. The bronchiolar epithelium is necrotic and infiltrated by macrophages.

Epiglottitis is swelling and acute inflammation of the epiglottis, aryepiglottic folds, and pyriform sinuses. It may sometimes completely obstruct the upper airway. In facial cellulitis, the site of infection and inflammation is the dermis, usually of the cheek or periorbital region.

CLINICAL FEATURES: Most bacteremic *H. influenzae* infections afflict young children. H. influenzae *is the most common cause of meningitis in children younger than the age of 2 years,* although vaccination has reduced its frequency. Onset is insidious and may follow an otherwise unremarkable upper respiratory tract infection or otitis media.

- **Bronchopneumonia or lobar pneumonia** is characterized by fever, cough, purulent sputum, and dyspnea.
- **Epiglottitis** affects primarily children aged 2 to 7 years but also occurs in adults. Death may occur from obstruction of the upper respiratory tract.
- **Septic arthritis** is secondary to bacteremic seeding of large weight-bearing joints. Symptoms include fever, heat, erythema, swelling, and pain on movement.
- **Facial cellulitis** or periorbital cellulitis is another severe bacteremic infection affecting primarily young children. Patients present with fever; profound malaise; and a raised, hot, red-blue discolored area of the face, usually involving the cheek or an area about the eye. There is often concomitant meningitis or septic arthritis.

Neisseria meningitides Causes Pyogenic Meningitis and Overwhelming Shock

Neisseria meningitidis, *commonly termed* ***meningococcus,*** *produces disseminated blood-borne infections, often accompanied by shock and profound disturbances in coagulation* (Fig. 9-14). The organism is

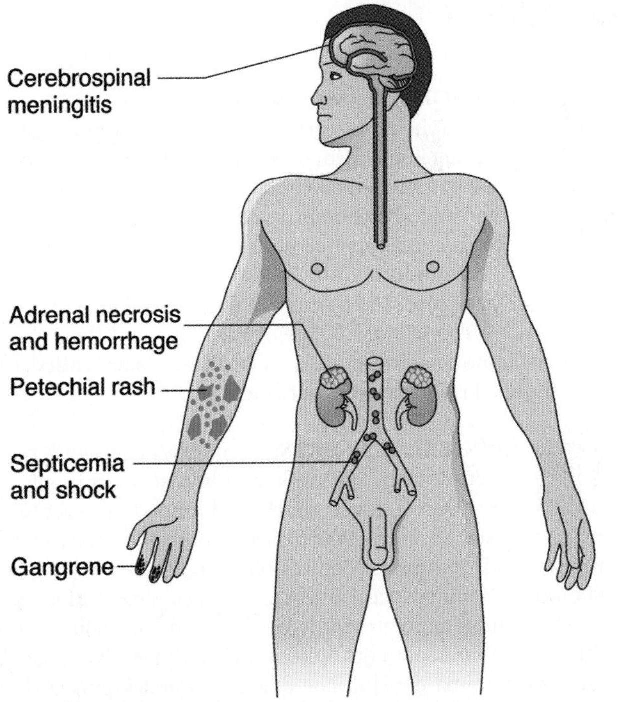

FIGURE 9-14. **Meningococcemia.** Meningococcal infections have a variety of clinical manifestations including meningitis, septicemia, shock, and associated complications.

aerobic and appears as paired, bean-shaped, gram-negative cocci. There are eight major serogroups, of which A, B, and C are most important.

EPIDEMIOLOGY: Meningococci spread from person to person, primarily by respiratory droplets. About 5% to 15% of the population carries the organism as a commensal in the nasopharynx. Carriers develop antibodies to their colonizing strain of *N. meningitidis* and are not susceptible to disease caused by that strain.

Meningococcal diseases appear as sporadic cases, clusters of cases and epidemics. Most infections in industrialized countries are sporadic and afflict children under the age of 5. Epidemic disease occurs most frequently in crowded quarters, such as among military recruits in barracks. There are over 6000 cases of meningococcal meningitis each year in the United States, and over 600 deaths. Fatalities from meningococcal disease are more common in less-developed countries.

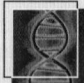

PATHOGENESIS: On colonizing the upper respiratory tract, *N. meningitidis* attaches to nonciliated respiratory epithelium by means of its pili. Most exposed persons then develop protective bactericidal antibodies over the following weeks, and some become carriers. If the organism spreads to the bloodstream before the development of protective immunity, it can proliferate rapidly in unprotected human tissue, resulting in fulminant meningococcal disease.

Many of the systemic effects of meningococcal disease are due to the endotoxin of the outer membrane lipopolysaccharide of the bacterium. Endotoxin promotes a conspicuous increase in the production of TNF and the simultaneous activation of the complement and coagulation cascades. Disseminated intravascular coagulation, fibrinolysis, and shock follow.

PATHOLOGY: Meningococcal disease can be confined to the CNS or may be disseminated throughout the body in the form of septicemia. In the former case, the leptomeninges and subarachnoid space are infiltrated with neutrophils and underlying brain parenchyma is swollen and congested. Meningococcal septicemia is characterized by diffuse damage to the endothelium of small blood vessels, with widespread petechiae, and purpura in the skin and viscera.

Rarely (3% to 4% of all cases), vasculitis and thrombosis produce hemorrhagic necrosis of both adrenals, called the **Waterhouse-Friderichsen syndrome.**

CLINICAL FEATURES: Meningitis begins with rapid onset of fever, stiff neck, and headache. In meningococcal sepsis, fever, shock, and mucocutaneous hemorrhages appear abruptly. Patients can progress to shock within minutes, and treatment requires blood pressure support and antibiotics. Meningococcal disease was once almost invariably fatal, but antibiotic treatment has reduced the mortality to less than 15%. Some patients who survive the early phase of meningococcemia develop late allergic complications such as polyarthritis, cutaneous vasculitis, and pericarditis. Severe vasculitis may be associated with extensive cutaneous ulceration and even gangrene of the distal extremities.

Sexually Transmitted Bacterial Diseases

Gonorrhea Remains a Common Infection That Causes Sterility

Neisseria gonorrhoeae, *also termed* ***gonococcus,*** *causes gonorrhea, an acute suppurative genital tract infection, which is reflected in urethritis in men and endocervicitis in women.* It is one of the oldest and still one of the most common sexually transmitted diseases. *N. gonorrhoeae* is an aerobic, bean-shaped, gram-negative diplococcus.

Gonococcal pharyngitis and proctitis are not uncommon, and are also sexually transmitted. In women, infection often ascends the genital tract, producing endometritis, salpingitis, and pelvic inflammatory disease. Ascending spread in men is less common, but if it occurs, epididymitis results. Gonococcal infection may rarely be bacteremic, in which case septic arthritis and skin lesions develop. Neonatal infections derived from the birth canal of a mother with gonorrhea usually manifest as conjunctivitis, although disseminated infections are occasionally seen. Neonatal gonococcal conjunctivitis it is still a major cause of blindness in much of Africa and Asia but is largely eliminated in developed countries by routine instillation of antibiotics into the conjunctiva at birth.

EPIDEMIOLOGY: This common infection is spread directly from person to person. Except for perinatal transmission, spread is almost always by sexual intercourse. Infected persons who are asymptomatic are a significant reservoir of infection.

PATHOGENESIS: Gonorrhea begins in the mucous membranes of the urogenital tract (Fig. 9-15). Bacteria attach to surface cells, after which they invade superficially and provoke acute inflammation. Gonococcus lacks a true polysaccharide capsule, but hair-like extensions, termed "pili," project from the cell wall. The pili contain a protease that digests IgA on the mucous membrane, thereby facilitating the attachment of the bacterium to the columnar and transitional epithelium of the urogenital tract.

PATHOLOGY: Gonorrhea is a suppurative infection, characterized by a vigorous acute inflammatory response, producing copious pus and often forming submucosal abscesses. Stained smears of pus reveal numerous neutrophils, often containing phagocytosed bacteria. If untreated, the inflammatory response becomes chronic, with macrophages and lymphocytes predominant.

CLINICAL FEATURES: Men exposed to *N. gonorrhoeae* present with purulent urethral discharge and dysuria. If treatment is not instituted promptly, urethral stricture is a common complication. The organisms may also extend to the prostate, epididymis, and accessory glands, where they cause epididymitis and orchitis, and may result in infertility.

In about one half of infected women, gonorrhea remains asymptomatic. The other infected women initially exhibit endocervicitis, with a vaginal discharge or bleeding. Urethritis presents as dysuria rather than as a urethral discharge. Infection

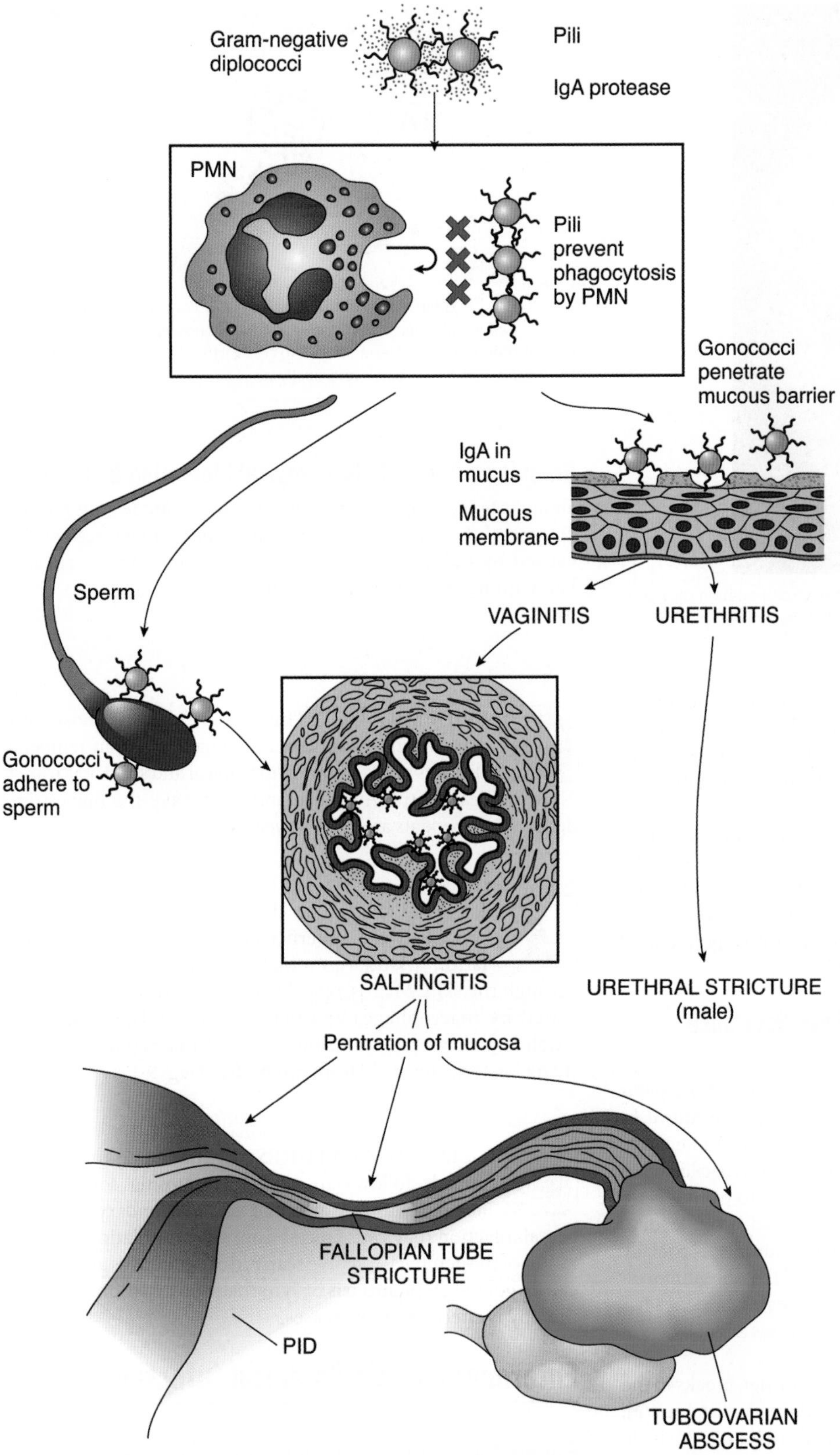

FIGURE 9-15. Pathogenesis of gonococcal infections. *Neisseria gonorrhoeae* is a gram-negative diplococcus whose surface pili form a barrier against phagocytosis by neutrophils. The pili contain an IgA protease that digests IgA on the luminal surface of the mucous membranes of the urethra, endocervix, and fallopian tube, thereby facilitating attachment of gonococci. Gonococci cause endocervicitis, vaginitis, and salpingitis. In men, gonococci attached to the mucous membrane of the urethra cause urethritis and, sometimes, urethral stricture. Gonococci may also attach to sperm heads and be carried into the fallopian tube. Penetration of the mucous membrane by gonococci leads to stricture of the fallopian tube, pelvic inflammatory disease (PID), or tuboovarian abscess. IgA = immunoglobulin A; PMN = polymorphonuclear neutrophil.

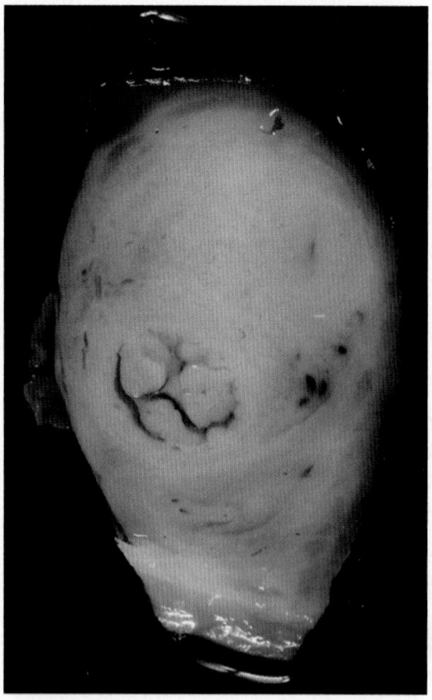

FIGURE 9-16. **Gonorrhea of the fallopian tube.** Cross-section of a "pus tube" shows thickening of the wall and a lumen swollen with pus.

often extends to the fallopian tubes, where it produces acute and chronic salpingitis and eventually pelvic inflammatory disease. The fallopian tubes swell with pus (Fig. 9-16), causing acute abdominal pain. Infertility occurs when inflammatory adhesions block the tubes.

From the fallopian tubes, gonorrhea spreads to the peritoneum, healing as fine "violin string" adhesions between the liver and the parietal peritoneum (Fitz-Hugh-Curtis syndrome). Chronic endometritis is a persistent complication of gonococcal infection and is usually the consequence of chronic gonococcal salpingitis.

Chancroid Causes Genital Ulcers in Less-Developed Geographic Regions

Chancroid, sometimes called "the third venereal disease" (after syphilis and gonorrhea), is an acute sexually transmitted infection caused by Haemophilus ducreyi. The organism is a small, gram-negative bacillus, which appears in tissue as clusters of parallel bacilli and as chains, resembling schools of fish. Infections lead to painful genital ulcerations and lymphadenopathy. Chancroid is the leading cause of genital ulcers in many less-developed countries, especially in Africa and parts of Asia. It has been suggested that the genital ulcers facilitate the spread of HIV. In the United States incidence has risen in the past decade: there are about 5000 cases annually.

PATHOLOGY: *H. ducreyi* enters through breaks in the skin, where it multiplies and produces a raised lesion, which then ulcerates. Ulcers vary from 0.1 to 2 cm in diameter. Organisms are carried within macrophages to regional lymph nodes, which may suppurate. Seven to 10 days after the appearance of the primary lesion, half of patients develop unilateral, painful, suppurative, inguinal lymphadenitis (bubo). Overlying skin becomes inflamed, breaks down, and drains pus from the underlying node. The diagnosis is made by identifying the bacillus in tissue sections or gram-stained smears from the ulcers. Treatment with erythromycin is usually effective.

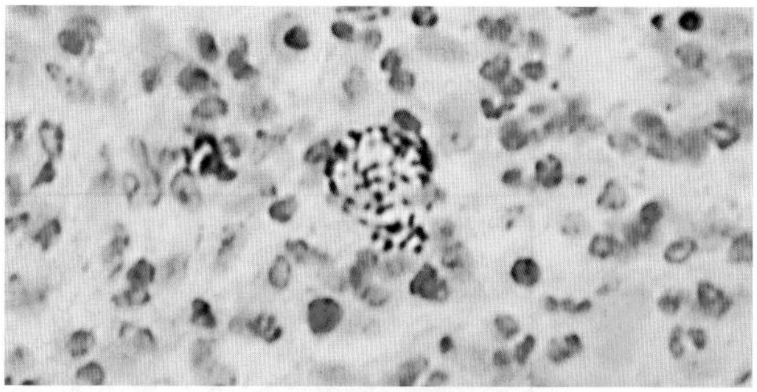

FIGURE 9-17. **Granuloma inguinale.** A photomicrograph of a skin lesion shows *Calymmatobacterium granulomatis* (Donovan bodies) clustered in a large macrophage. Intense silvering by Warthin-Starry technique makes the organisms large, black and easily seen.

Granuloma Inguinale Is a Tropical Ulcerating Disease

Granuloma inguinale is a sexually transmitted, chronic, superficial ulceration of the genitalia and the inguinal and perianal regions. It is caused by *Calymmatobacterium granulomatis,* a small, encapsulated, nonmotile, gram-negative bacillus.

EPIDEMIOLOGY: Humans are the only hosts of *C. granulomatis*. Granuloma inguinale is rare in temperate climates but is common in tropical and subtropical areas. New Guinea, central Australia, and India have the highest incidence. Most patients are 15 to 40 years of age.

PATHOLOGY: The characteristic lesion is a raised, soft, beefy-red, superficial ulcer. The exuberant granulation tissue resembles a fleshy mass herniating through the skin. Microscopically, dermis and subcutis are infiltrated by macrophages and plasma cells and by fewer neutrophils and lymphocytes. Interspersed macrophages contain many bacteria, termed **Donovan bodies** (Fig. 9-17).

CLINICAL FEATURES: Untreated granuloma inguinale follows an indolent, relapsing course, often healing with an atrophic scar. Secondary fusospirochetal infection may cause ulceration, with mutilation or amputation of the genitalia. Massive scarring of the dermis and subcutis causes genital **elephantiasis** by lymphatic obstruction. Antibiotic therapy is effective in early cases.

Enteropathogenic Bacterial Infections

Escherichia coli is a Common Cause of Diarrhea and Urinary Tract Infections

E. coli *is among the most frequent and important human bacterial pathogens, causing over 90% of all urinary tract infections and many cases of diarrheal illness worldwide.* It is also a major opportunistic pathogen, frequently causes pneumonia and sepsis in immunocompromised hosts, and meningitis and sepsis in newborns.

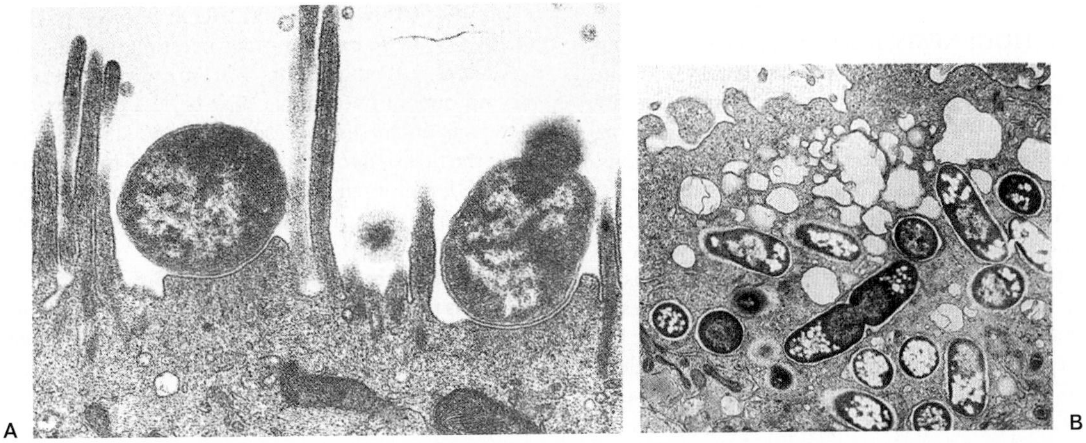

FIGURE 9-18. **A.** Enteropathogenic *E. coli* infection. An electron micrograph shows adherence of the bacteria to the intestinal mucosal cells and localized destruction of microvilli. **B.** Enteroinvasive *E. coli* infection. An electron micrograph shows organisms within a cell.

E. coli are a group of antigenically and biologically diverse, aerobic (facultatively anaerobic), gram-negative bacteria. Most strains are intestinal commensals, well adapted grow in the human colon without harming the host. However, *E. coli* can be aggressive when it gains access to usually sterile body sites, such as the urinary tract, meninges, or peritoneum. Strains of *E. coli* that produce diarrhea possess specialized virulence properties, usually plasmid-borne, which confer the capacity to cause intestinal disease.

E. coli Diarrhea

There are four distinct strains of *E. coli* that cause diarrhea.

ENTEROTOXIGENIC E. **coli:** *Enterotoxigenic* E. coli *is a major cause of diarrhea in poor tropical areas and probably causes most "traveler's diarrhea" among visitors to such regions.* It is acquired from contaminated water and food. Many persons in Latin America, Africa, and Asia are asymptomatic carriers of the infection.

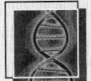

PATHOGENESIS: Nonimmune persons (local children or travelers from abroad), develop diarrhea when they encounter the organism. Enterotoxigenic strains produce diarrhea by adhering to the intestinal mucosa and elaborating one or more of at least three enterotoxins that cause secretory dysfunction of the small bowel. One of the enterotoxins is structurally and functionally similar to cholera toxin, and another acts on guanylyl cyclase. Enterotoxigenic *E. coli* produces no distinctive macroscopic or light-microscopic alterations in the intestine.

Enterotoxigenic *E. coli* causes an acute, self-limited diarrheal illness with watery stools lacking neutrophils and erythrocytes. In severe cases, fluid and electrolyte loss can cause extreme dehydration and even death.

ENTEROPATHOGENIC E. **coli:** *Historically, enteropathogenic* E. coli *was the first group of this genus to be identified as a causal agent of diarrhea.* The organism is a major cause of diarrheal illness in poor tropical areas, especially in infants and young children. Although it has virtually disappeared from developed countries, it still causes sporadic outbreaks of diarrhea, particularly among hospitalized infants younger than 2 years. Enteropathogenic *E. coli* is acquired by ingesting contaminated food or water. The organism is not invasive, and causes disease by adhering to and deforming the microvilli of the intestinal epithelial cells (Fig. 9-18A). Enteropathogenic *E. coli* produces diarrhea, vomiting, fever, and malaise.

ENTEROHEMORRHAGIC E. **coli:** *Enterohemorrhagic* E. coli *(**serotype 0157:H7**) causes a bloody diarrhea, which occasionally is followed by the hemolytic–uremic syndrome* (see Chapter 16). The source of infection is usually the ingestion of contaminated meat or milk. Enterohemorrhagic *E. coli* adheres to the colonic mucosa and elaborates an enterotoxin, virtually identical to Shigatoxin (see below), that destroys the epithelial cells. Patients infected with *E. coli* 0157:H7 present with cramping abdominal pain, low-grade fever, and sometimes bloody diarrhea. Microscopic examination of the stool shows both leukocytes and erythrocytes.

ENTEROINVASIVE E. **coli:** *Enteroinvasive* E. coli *causes foodborne dysentery which is clinically and pathologically indistinguishable from that caused by* Shigella. The agent shares extensive DNA homology and antigenic and biochemical characteristics with *Shigella*. It invades and destroys mucosal cells of the distal ileum and colon (see Fig. 9-18B). As in shigellosis, the mucosa of the distal ileum and colon are acutely inflamed and focally eroded and are sometimes covered by an inflammatory pseudomembrane. Patients exhibit abdominal pain, fever, tenesmus, and bloody diarrhea. Symptoms persist for about a week. Antibiotic treatment is similar to that for shigellosis.

E. coli Urinary Tract Infection

EPIDEMIOLOGY: Urinary tract infections with *E. coli* are most common in sexually active women and in persons of both sexes who have structural or functional abnormalities of the urinary tract. Such infections are extremely common, afflicting more than 10% of the human population, often repeatedly. *E. coli* in the urinary tract usually derives from the resident flora of the perineum and periurethral -areas, reflecting fecal contamination of these regions.

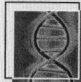

PATHOGENESIS: *E. coli* gains access to the sterile proximal urinary tract by ascending from the distal urethra. Because the shorter female urethra provides a less effective mechanical barrier to infection, women are much more prone to urinary tract infections. Sexual intercourse can suffice to propel organisms into the female urethra. Uropathogenic *E. coli* organisms have specialized adherence factors (Gal-Gal) on the pili, which enable them to bind to galactopyranosyl-galactopyranoside residues on the uroepithelium. Structural abnormalities of the urinary tract (e.g., congenital deformities, prostatic hyperplasia, strictures) and instrumentation (catheterization) overwhelm normal host defenses and facilitate the establishment of urinary tract infections. These conditions account for most urinary tract infections in men.

PATHOLOGY AND CLINICAL FEATURES: *E. coli* urinary tract infections initially produce an acute inflammatory infiltrate at the site of infection, usually the bladder mucosa. Urinary tract infections involving the bladder or urethra manifest as urinary urgency, burning on urination (**dysuria**) and leukocytes in the urine. If infection ascends to involve the kidney (**pyelonephritis**), patients develop acute flank pain, fever, and elevated leukocyte counts. An infiltrate of neutrophils spills from the mucosa into the urine, and the blood vessels of the submucosa are dilated and congested. Chronic infections exhibit an inflammatory infiltrate of neutrophils and mononuclear cells. Chronic infection of the kidneys may lead to chronic pyelonephritis and renal failure (see Chapter 16).

E. coli Pneumonia

Pneumonia caused by enteric gram-negative bacteria is considered opportunistic, mostly occurring in debilitated persons. *E. coli* is the most common cause, but other normal bowel flora, such as *Klebsiella*, *Serratia*, and *Enterobacter* species, produce similar disease. *The discussion below applies to all opportunistic gram-negative pneumonias.*

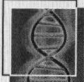

PATHOGENESIS AND PATHOLOGY: Enteric gram-negative bacteria are transiently introduced into the oral cavity of healthy persons but cannot compete successfully with the predominant gram-positive flora, which adhere to the fibronectin that coats the surface of mucosal cells. Chronically ill or severely stressed persons elaborate a salivary protease that degrades fibronectin, allowing gram-negative enteric bacteria to overcome the normal gram-positive flora and colonize the oropharynx.

Inevitably, droplets of the resident oral flora are aspirated into the respiratory tract. Debilitated patients often have markedly diminished local defenses and cannot destroy these organisms. Decreased gag and cough reflexes; abnormal neutrophil chemotaxis; injured respiratory epithelium; and foreign bodies, such as endotracheal tubes, all facilitate entry and survival of the aspirated organisms.

E. coli pneumonia results from proliferation of aspirated organisms in terminal airways, usually at multiple sites in the lung. Multifocal areas of consolidation result and terminal airways and alveoli are filled with proteinaceous fluid, fibrin, neutrophils, and macrophages.

CLINICAL FEATURES: Because pneumonia caused by *E. coli* and other enteric gram-negative organisms afflicts patients who are often already severely ill, symptoms of pneumonia may be less obvious than in healthy persons. Increased malaise, fever, and labored breathing are often the first signs of pneumonia. If *E. coli* pneumonia remains untreated, the organisms may invade the blood to produce a fatal septicemia. Treatment requires parenteral antibiotics.

E. coli Sepsis (Gram-Negative Sepsis)

E. coli is the most common cause of enteric gram-negative sepsis, but other gram-negative rods, including *Pseudomonas*, *Klebsiella*, and *Enterobacter* species, produce identical disease. *The discussion below relates to gram-negative sepsis in general.*

PATHOGENESIS: *E. coli* sepsis is usually an opportunistic infection, occurring in persons with predisposing conditions, such as neutropenia, pyelonephritis, or cirrhosis, and in hospitalized patients. Together with other enteric gram-negative rods that normally reside in human colon, *E. coli* occasionally seeds the bloodstream. In healthy persons, mononuclear macrophages and circulating neutrophils phagocytose these bacteria. Patients with neutropenia or cirrhosis develop *E. coli* sepsis because of an impaired capacity to eliminate even low-level bacteremias. Persons with ruptured abdominal organs or acute pyelonephritis suffer gram-negative sepsis because the large numbers of organisms that gain access to the circulation overwhelm the normal defenses.

The presence of *E. coli* in the bloodstream causes septic shock through the effects of TNF, whose release from macrophages is stimulated by bacterial endotoxin. Septic shock is discussed in Chapters 7 and 20.

Neonatal *E. coli* Meningitis and Sepsis

E. coli and group B streptococci are the main causes of meningitis and sepsis in the first month after birth. Both colonize the vagina, and the newborn acquires them on passage through the birth canal. *E. coli* then colonizes the infant's gastrointestinal tract. It is postulated that the organisms spread to the bloodstream from the gastrointestinal tract, then seed the meninges. The pathology of *E. coli* meningitis is identical to that of other bacterial meningitides. Although antibiotic treatment for neonatal *E. coli* meningitis and sepsis is often effective, the mortality rate is still 15% to 50%. Almost half of survivors suffer neurologic sequelae.

Salmonella Enterocolitis and Typhoid Fever Are Both Intestinal Infections

The bacterial genus *Salmonella* comprises over 1500 antigenically distinct but biochemically and genetically related gram-negative rods, which cause two important human diseases: *Salmonella* enterocolitis and typhoid fever.

Salmonella Enterocolitis

Salmonella *enterocolitis is an acute self-limited (1 to 3 days) gastrointestinal illness that manifests as nausea, vomiting, diarrhea, and fever.* Infection is typically acquired by eating food contaminated with nontyphoidal *Salmonella* strains and is commonly called *Salmonella food poisoning.*

EPIDEMIOLOGY: Nontyphoidal *Salmonella* infect diverse animal species, including amphibians, reptiles, birds, and mammals. They also readily contaminate foodstuffs derived from infected animals (e.g., meat, poultry, eggs, dairy products). If these foods are not cooked, pasteurized, or irradiated, the bacteria persist and proliferate, particularly at warm temperatures. Once a person is infected, the organism can spread from person to person by the fecal–oral route, which is infrequent among adults but common among small children in day-care settings or within families. *Salmonella* enterocolitis remains a major cause of childhood mortality in less-developed countries.

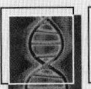

PATHOGENESIS AND PATHOLOGY: *Salmonella* proliferate in the small intestine and invade enterocytes in the distal small bowel and colon. The nontyphoidal *Salmonella* species elaborate several toxins that contribute to the dysfunction of intestinal cells. The mucosa of the ileum and colon is acutely inflamed and sometimes superficially ulcerated.

CLINICAL FEATURES: *Salmonella* enterocolitis characteristically manifests as diarrhea, beginning 12 to 48 hours after consuming contaminated food. This contrasts with staphylococcal food poisoning, which is caused by a preformed toxin and begins 1 to 6 hours after eating. The diarrhea of *Salmonella* food poisoning is self-limited. It lasts 1 to 3 days and is often accompanied by nausea, vomiting, cramping abdominal pain, and fever. Treatment is supportive: antibiotics rarely improve the clinical course.

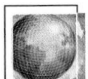

Typhoid Fever

Typhoid fever is an acute systemic illness caused by infection with Salmonella typhi. **Paratyphoid fever** is a clinically similar but milder disease that results from infection with other species of *Salmonella,* including *Salmonella paratyphi.* The term **enteric fever** includes both typhoid and paratyphoid fever.

EPIDEMIOLOGY: Humans are the only natural reservoir for *S. typhi* and typhoid fever is acquired from infected patients or chronic carriers. The latter tend to be older women with gallstones or biliary scarring: *S. typhi* colonizes their gallbladder or biliary tree. The disease is spread primarily by ingestion of contaminated water and food, especially dairy products and shellfish. Less commonly, the organisms are disseminated by direct finger-to-mouth contact with feces, urine, or other secretions. Infected food handlers with poor personal hygiene and urine from patients with typhoid pyelonephritis can be a significant source of infection. Typhoid fever accounts for over 25,000 annual deaths worldwide but is uncommon in the United States.

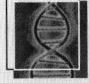

PATHOGENESIS: *S. typhi* attaches to and invades small bowel mucosa without causing clinical enterocolitis. Invasion tends to be most prominent in the ileum in areas overlying Peyer patches, where the organisms are engulfed by macrophages. The organisms block the respiratory burst of the phagocytes and multiply within these cells. They spread first to regional lymph nodes and then throughout the body through the lymphatics and bloodstream, infecting mononuclear macrophages in lymph nodes, bone marrow, liver, and spleen. Infection of macrophages stimulates IL-1 and TNF production, thereby causing the prolonged fever, malaise, and wasting characteristic of typhoid fever.

PATHOLOGY: The earliest pathologic change in typhoid fever is degeneration of the intestinal epithelium brush border. As bacteria invade, Peyer patches become hypertrophic. In some cases, intestinal lymphoid hyperplasia progresses to capillary thrombosis, causing necrosis of overlying mucosa and the characteristic ulcers oriented along the long axis of the bowel (Fig. 9-19). These ulcers frequently bleed and occasionally perforate, producing infectious peritonitis. Systemic dissemination of the organisms leads to focal granulomas in the liver, spleen, and other organs, termed **typhoid nodules.** These are composed of aggregates of macrophages ("typhoid cells") containing ingested bacteria, erythrocytes, and degenerated lymphocytes.

CLINICAL FEATURES: Prior to the antibiotic era, untreated typhoid fever was classically divided into five stages (Fig. 9-20):

- **Incubation:** (10 to 14 days)
- **Active invasion/bacteremia:** the patient suffers for about a week with a variety of nonspecific symptoms, including daily stepwise elevation in temperature (up to 41°C [105.8°F]), malaise, headache, arthralgias, and abdominal pain.
- **Fastigium:** Fever and malaise increase over several days until the infected person is prostrate. Patients may become toxic from the release of endotoxins from dead bacteria. Hepatomegaly is accompanied by derangements in liver function. The spleen is conspicuously enlarged.
- **Lysis:** Patients destined to survive exhibit a gradual reduction in fever, and toxic symptoms recede. Although gastrointestinal bleeding and perforation of the intestine at sites of ulceration may occur in any stage, they are most common during lysis, which commonly lasts a week;
- **Convalescence:** Fever abates and patients gradually recover over several weeks to months. Some relapse or have metastatic foci of infection.

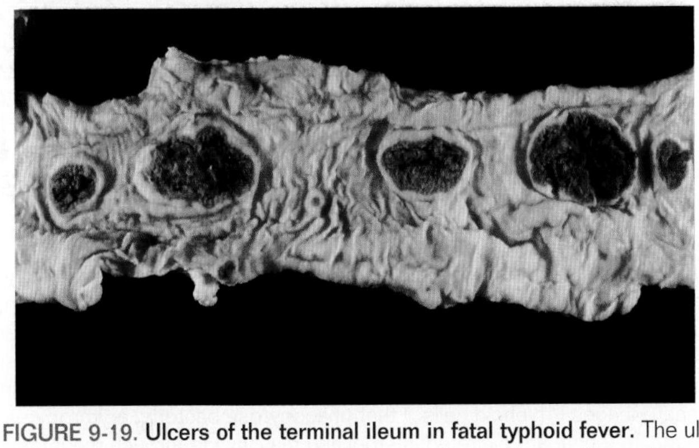

FIGURE 9-19. **Ulcers of the terminal ileum in fatal typhoid fever.** The ulcers have a longitudinal orientation because they are located over hyperplastic and necrotic Peyer patches.

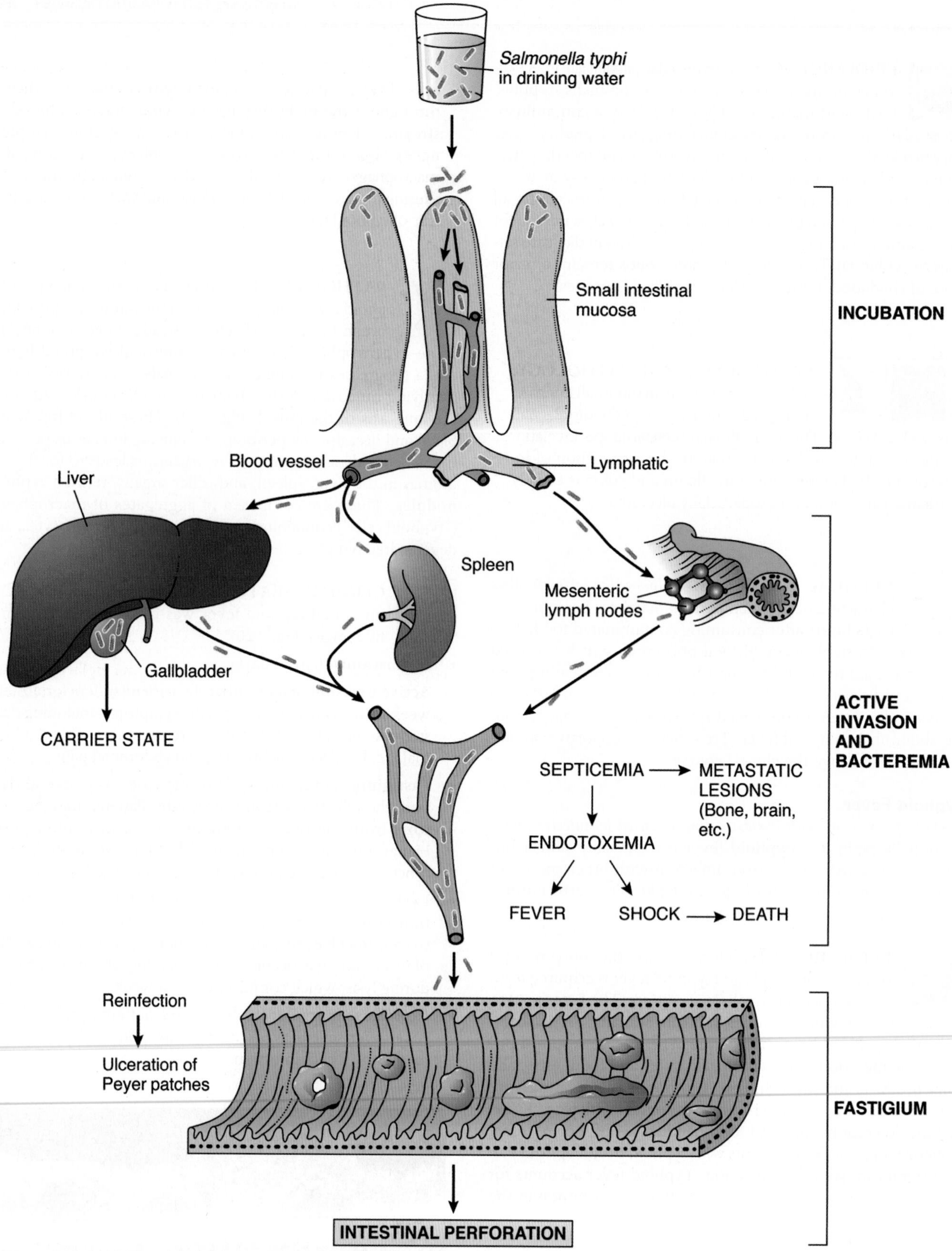

FIGURE 9-20. Stages of typhoid fever.

Incubation (10–14 days). Water or food contaminated with *Salmonella typhi* is ingested. Bacilli attach to the villi in the small intestine, invade the mucosa and pass to the intestinal lymphoid follicles and draining mesenteric lymph nodes. The organisms proliferate further within mononuclear phagocytic cells of the lymphoid follicles, lymph nodes, liver, and spleen. Bacilli are sequestered intracellularly in the intestinal and mesenteric lymphatic system.

Active invasion/bacteremia (1 week). Organisms are released and produce a transient bacteremia. The intestinal mucosa becomes enlarged and necrotic, forming characteristic mucosal lesions. The intestinal lymphoid tissues become hyperplastic and contain "typhoid nodules"—aggregates of macrophages ("typhoid cells") that phagocytose bacteria, erythrocytes, and degenerated lymphocytes. Bacilli proliferate in several organs, reappear in the intestine, are excreted in stool and may invade through the intestinal wall.

Fastigium (1 week). Dying bacilli release endotoxins that cause systemic toxemia.

Lysis (1 week). Necrotic intestinal mucosa sloughs, producing ulcers, which hemorrhage or perforate into the peritoneal cavity.

The treatment of typhoid fever entails antibiotics and supportive care. Ten to 20% of untreated patients die, usually of secondary complications, such as pneumonia. However, treatment within 3 days of the onset of fever is generally curative.

Shigellosis Is an Acute Bacterial Dysentery

Shigellosis is characterized by a necrotizing infection of the distal small bowel and colon. It is caused by any of four species of *Shigella (Shigella boydii, Shigella dysenteriae, Shigella flexneri* and *Shigella sonnei),* which are aerobic, gram-negative rods. Of these species, *S. dysenteriae* is the most virulent. Shigellosis is a self-limited disease that typically presents with abdominal pain and bloody, mucoid stools.

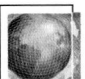

EPIDEMIOLOGY: *Shigella* organisms are spread from person to person by the fecal–oral route. Shigellae have no animal reservoir and do not survive well outside the stool. Therefore, infection usually occurs through ingestion of fecally contaminated food or water, but it can be acquired by oral contact with any contaminated surface (e.g., clothing, towels, or skin surfaces). As a result, endemic shigellosis is more common in populations with poor standards of hygiene and sanitation. Shigellosis is also spread in closed communities, such as hospitals, barracks, and households. In developed countries, *S. flexneri* and *S. sonnei* are more common, and infection tends to be sporadic.

In the United States, there are estimated to be 300,000 cases of shigellosis annually, but the incidence of the disease is much higher in countries lacking sanitary systems for human waste disposal. Like the other diarrheal illnesses, shigellosis is a significant cause of childhood mortality in developing countries.

PATHOGENESIS: Shigellae are among the most virulent enteropathogens known. Disease is produced by ingestion of as few as 10 to 100 organisms, and there are few asymptomatic carriers. The agent proliferates rapidly in the small bowel and attaches to enterocytes, where it replicates within the cytoplasm. Endocytosis is essential for virulence and the factor that induces it is encoded by a plasmid. Replicating shigellae kill infected cells then spread to adjacent cells and into the lamina propria.

Shigellae also produce a potent exotoxin, known as **Shiga toxin**. This toxin interfers with 60S ribosomal subunits and inhibits protein synthesis. It also causes watery diarrhea, probably by interfering with fluid absorption in the colon. Although shigellae extensively damage the epithelium of the ileum and colon, they rarely invade beyond the intestinal lamina propria, and bacteremia is uncommon.

PATHOLOGY: The distal colon is almost always affected, although the entire colon and distal ileum can be involved. The affected mucosa is edematous, acutely inflamed, and focally eroded. Ulcers appear first on the edges of mucosal folds, perpendicular to the long axis of the colon. A patchy inflammatory **pseudomembrane**, composed of neutrophils, fibrin, and necrotic epithelium, is commonly found on the most severely affected areas. Regeneration of infected colonic epithelium occurs rapidly, and healing is usually complete within 10 to 14 days.

CLINICAL FEATURES: Shigellosis often begins with watery diarrhea, which changes in character within 1 to 2 days to the classic dysenteric stools. These are small-volume stools that contain gross blood, sloughed pseudomembranes, and mucus. Cramping abdominal pain, tenesmus, and urgency at stool typically accompany the diarrhea. Symptoms persist for 3 to 8 days, if the disease is untreated. Treatment with antibiotics shortens the course of the illness.

Cholera Is an Epidemic Enteritis Usually Acquired from Contaminated Water

Cholera is a severe diarrheal illness caused by the enterotoxin of Vibrio cholerae, *an aerobic, curved gram-negative rod.* The organism proliferates in the lumen of the small intestine and causes profuse watery diarrhea, rapid dehydration, and (if fluids are not restored) shock and death within 24 hours of the onset of symptoms.

EPIDEMIOLOGY: Cholera is common in most parts of the world, but it periodically "disappears" spontaneously. A major pandemic occurred between 1961 and 1974, extending throughout Asia, the Middle East, southern Russia, the Mediterranean basin, and parts of Africa. Cholera remains endemic in the river deltas of India and Bangladesh, where it may cause up to a half-million deaths annually.

It is acquired by ingesting *V. cholerae,* primarily in contaminated food or water. Epidemics spread readily in areas where human feces pollute the water supply. Shellfish and plankton may serve as a natural reservoir for the organism, and shellfish ingestion accounts for most of the sporadic cases seen in the United States.

PATHOGENESIS AND PATHOLOGY: Bacteria that survive passage through the stomach thrive and multiply in the mucous layer of the small bowel. *They do not themselves invade the mucosa but cause diarrhea by elaborating a potent exotoxin,* ***cholera toxin***. The toxin is composed of A and B subunits. The latter binds to GM_1 ganglioside in the enterocyte cell membrane. The A subunit then enters the cell, where it activates adenylyl cyclase. The consequent rise in cell cyclic adenosine monophosphate (cAMP) content results in massive secretion of sodium and water by the enterocyte into the intestinal lumen (Fig. 9-21). The greatest fluid secretion occurs in the small bowel, where there is a net loss of water and electrolytes. *V. cholerae* causes little visible alteration in the affected intestine, which appears grossly normal or only slightly hyperemic. Microscopically, the intestinal epithelium is intact but depleted of mucus.

CLINICAL FEATURES: Cholera begins with a few loose stools, usually evolving within hours into severe watery diarrhea. The stools are often flecked with mucus, imparting a "rice water" appearance. The volume of diarrhea is highly variable, but the rapidity and volume loss in severe cases can be staggering. With adequate volume replacement, infected adults can lose up to 20 L of fluid in a day. Fluid and electrolyte loss can lead to shock and death within hours if fluid volume is not replaced. Untreated cholera has a 50% mortality rate. Replacing lost salts and water is a simple, effective treatment, which can often be accomplished by oral rehydration with preparations

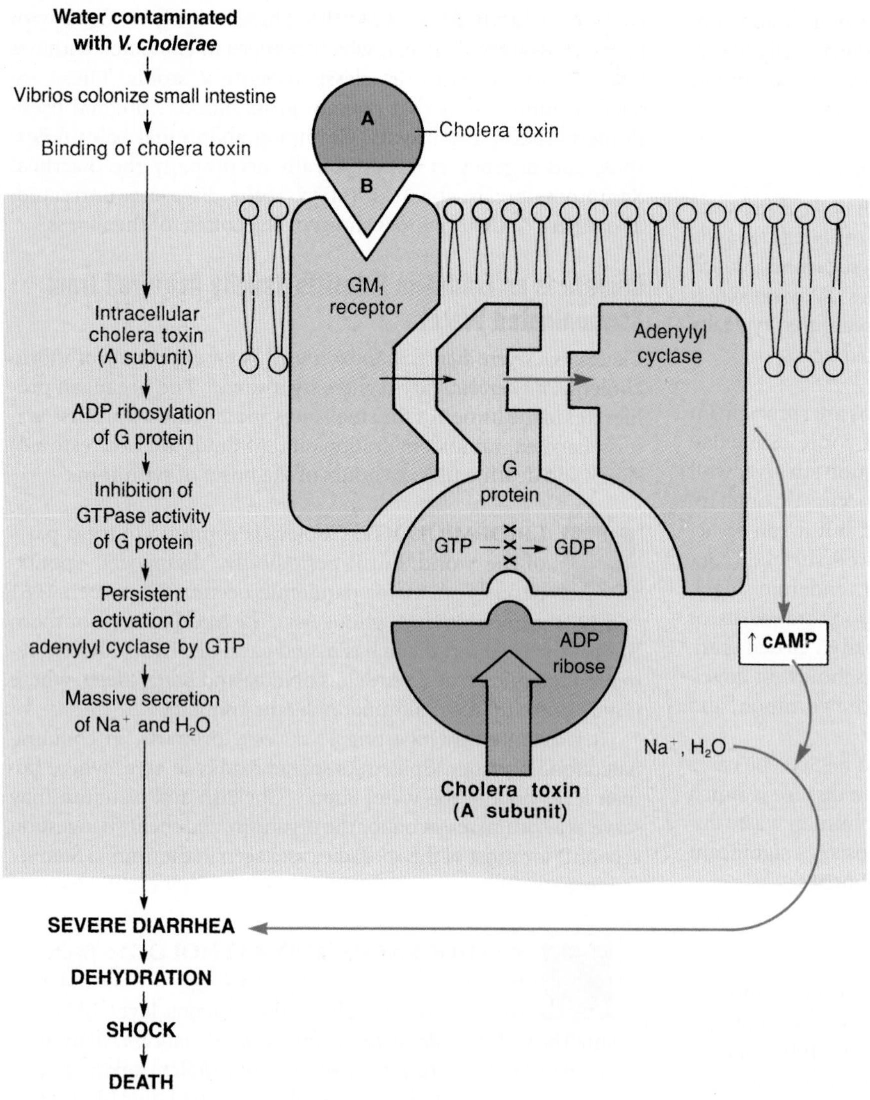

FIGURE 9-21. **Cholera.** Infection comes from water contaminated with *Vibrio cholerae* or food prepared with contaminated water. Vibrios traverse the stomach, enter the small intestine, and propagate. Although they do not invade the intestinal mucosa, vibrios elaborate a potent toxin that induces a massive outpouring of water and electrolytes. Severe diarrhea ("ricewater stool") leads to dehydration and hypovolemic shock.

of salt, glucose, and water. The illness subsides spontaneously in 3 to 6 days, which can be shortened by antibiotic therapy. Infection with *V. cholerae* confers long-term protection from recurrent illness, but available vaccines have limited effectiveness.

Vibrio parahaemolyticus

There are a number of so-called "noncholera" vibrios, of which *V. parahaemolyticus* is the most common. This organism is a gram-negative bacillus that causes acute gastroenteritis. It is found in marine life and coastal waters around the world in temperate climates, causing outbreaks in the summer. Its range maybe expanding, whether due to global warming or other factors, as confirmed cases have occurred in Alaska, more than 1,000 miles north of any previous outbreaks. Gastroenteritis is associated with consumption of inadequately cooked or poorly refrigerated seafood. The clinical syndrome resembles *Salmonella* enteritis. No deaths have been reported.

Campylobacter jejuni Is the Most Common Cause of Bacterial Diarrhea in the Developed World

C. jejuni *is the major human pathogen in the genus Campylobacter. It causes an acute, self-limited inflammatory diarrheal illness.* The organism is distributed worldwide and is responsible for over 2 million cases annually in the United States. *C. jejuni* is a microaerophilic, curved gram-negative rod, morphologically similar to the vibrios.

EPIDEMIOLOGY: *C. jejuni* infection is acquired through contaminated food or water. These bacteria inhabit gastrointestinal tracts of diverse animal species, including cows, sheep, chickens, and dogs, which are a significant animal reservoir for infection. In fact, *Campylobacter* infections cause serious economic losses to farmers because of abortions and infertility of infected cattle and sheep. Raw milk and inadequately cooked poultry and meat are frequent sources of disease. *C. jejuni* can also spread from person to person by fecal–oral contact. The organism is a major cause of childhood mortality in developing countries and is responsible for many cases of "travelers' diarrhea."

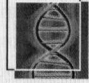

PATHOGENESIS: Ingested *C. jejuni* that survive gastric acidity multiply in the alkaline environment of the upper small intestine. The agent elaborates several toxic proteins that correlate with the severity of the symptoms.

PATHOLOGY: *C. jejuni* causes a superficial enterocolitis, primarily involving the terminal ileum and colon, with focal necrosis of the intestinal epithelium, accompanied by an acute inflammatory infiltrate. In severe cases, it progresses to small ulcers and patchy inflammatory exudates (pseudomembranes) composed of necrotic cells, neutrophils, fibrin, and debris. The crypts of the colonic epithelium often fill with neutrophils, forming so-called crypt abscesses. These pathologic changes resolve in 7 to 14 days.

CLINICAL FEATURES: Patients with *C. jejuni* usually produce more than 10 stools per day, varying from profuse watery stools to small-volume stools containing gross blood and mucus. Symptoms resolve in 5 to 7 days. Treatment with antibiotics is probably of marginal benefit. A few patients develop a more severe, protracted illness resembling acute ulcerative colitis. Gastrointestinal infections with *C. jejuni* have been associated with Guillain-Barré syndrome.

Yersinia Infections Produce Painful Diarrhea

Yesinia enterocolitica and *Yersinia pseudotuberculosis* are gram-negative coccoid or rod-shaped bacteria.

EPIDEMIOLOGY: These organisms are facultative anaerobes found in feces of wild and domestic animals, including rodents, sheep, cattle, dogs, cats and horses. *Y. pseudotuberculosis* is also often encountered in domestic birds, including turkeys, ducks, geese, and canaries. Both organisms have been isolated from drinking water and milk. *Y. enterocolitica* is more likely to be acquired from contaminated meat, and *Y. pseudotuberculosis* from contact with infected animals.

PATHOLOGY AND CLINICAL FEATURES: *Y. enterocolitica* proliferates in the ileum, invades the mucosa, produces ulceration and necrosis of Peyer patches, and migrates by way of lymphatics to mesenteric lymph nodes. Fever, diarrhea (sometimes bloody), and abdominal pain begin 4 to 10 days after mucosal penetration. Abdominal pain in the right lower quadrant has led to an incorrect diagnosis of appendicitis. Arthralgia, arthritis, and erythema nodosum are complications. Septicemia is uncommon, but kills about one half of those affected.

Y. pseudotuberculosis penetrates ileal mucosa, localizes in ileal–cecal lymph nodes, and produces abscesses and granulomas in the lymph nodes, spleen, and liver. Fever, diarrhea, and abdominal pain may also suggest appendicitis.

Pulmonary Infections with Gram-Negative Bacteria

Klebsiella and Enterobacter Produce Nosocomial Infections That Cause Necrotizing Lobar Pneumonia

Klebsiella *and* Enterobacter *species are short, encapsulated, gram-negative bacilli.*

EPIDEMIOLOGY: These organisms cause 10% of all hospital-acquired (nosocomial) infections, including pneumonia and infections of the urinary tract, biliary tract, and surgical wounds. Person-to-person transmission by hospital personnel is a special hazard. Predisposing factors are obstructive pulmonary disease in endotracheal tubes, indwelling catheters, debilitating conditions, and immunosuppression. Secondary pneumonia caused by these bacteria may complicate influenza or other respiratory viral infections.

PATHOLOGY: *Klebsiella* and *Enterobacter* are inhaled and multiply within the alveolar spaces. The pulmonary parenchyma becomes consolidated, and the mucoid exudate that fills the alveoli is dominated by macrophages, fibrin, and edema fluid. As the exudate accumulates, alveolar walls become compressed and then necrotic. Numerous small abscesses may coalesce and lead to cavitation.

CLINICAL FEATURES: The onset of pneumonia is sudden, with fever, pleuritic pain, cough, and a **characteristic thick mucoid sputum.** When infection is severe, these symptoms progress to dyspnea, cyanosis, and death in 2 to 3 days. *Klebsiella* and *Enterobacter* infections may be complicated by fulminating, often fatal, septicemia, and aggressive antibiotic therapy is required.

Legionnaires Disease (Legionellosis) Is a Noncontagious Environmental Hazard

Legionella *species cause pneumonia that ranges from relatively mild to severe, life-threatening necrotizing disease, called Legionnaires disease.* *Legionella pneumophila* is a minute aerobic bacillus that has the cell wall structure of a gram-negative organism but reacts poorly with Gram stains. *L. pneumophila* was first identified 6 months after an outbreak of a severe respiratory disease of unknown cause at the 1976 American Legion convention in Philadelphia. Subsequently, retrospective studies demonstrated antibodies in sera from previously unexplained epidemics, dating to 1957.

EPIDEMIOLOGY: *Legionella* is present in small numbers in natural bodies of fresh water. It survives chlorination and proliferates in devices such as cooling towers, water heaters, humidifiers, and evaporative condensers. Infection occurs when people inhale aerosols from contaminated sources. The disease is not contagious, and the organism is not normal human oropharyngeal flora. There are an estimated 75,000 cases of *Legionella* infection in the United States annually.

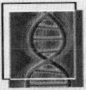

PATHOGENESIS: *Legionella* causes two distinct diseases, namely, pneumonia and **Pontiac fever.** The pathogenesis of *Legionella* pneumonia (Legionnaires disease) is understood in some detail, whereas that of Pontiac fever remains largely a mystery. *Legionella* pneumonia begins with the arrival of the organisms in the terminal bronchioles or alveoli, where they are phagocytosed by alveolar macrophages. The bacteria replicate within the phagosomes and protect themselves by blocking fusion of lysosomes with the phagosomes. The multiplying *Legionella* are released and infect freshly arriving macrophages. When immunity develops, macrophages are activated and cease to support intracellular growth of the organisms.

The native respiratory tract defenses, such as the mucociliary blanket of the airway, provide a first line of defense against *Legionella* infection in the lower respiratory tract. Smoking, alcoholism, and chronic lung diseases, which interfere with respiratory defenses, increase the risks of developing *Legionella* pneumonia.

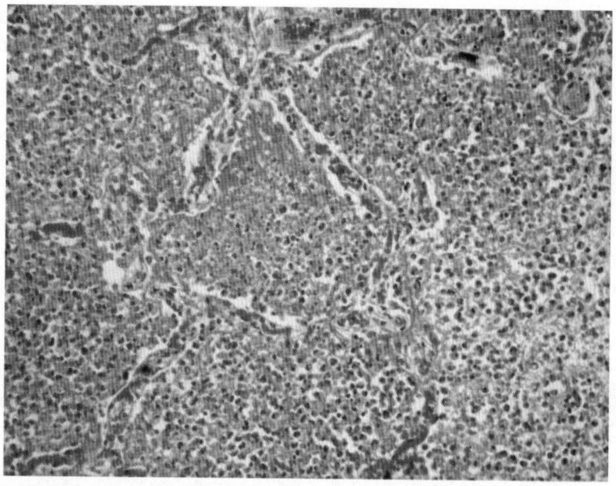

FIGURE 9-22. **Legionnaires pneumonia.** The alveoli are packed with an exudate composed of fibrin, macrophages, and neutrophils.

PATHOLOGY: Legionnaires disease is an acute bronchopneumonia, usually patchy but sometimes with a lobar pattern of infiltration. Affected alveoli and bronchioles are filled with an exudate composed of proteinaceous fluid, fibrin, macrophages and neutrophils (Fig. 9-22), and microabscesses. Alveolar walls become necrotic and are destroyed. Many macrophages show eccentric nuclei, pushed aside by cytoplasmic vacuoles containing *L. pneumophila*. As the pneumonia resolves, the lungs heal with little permanent damage.

CLINICAL FEATURES: After incubating 2 to 10 days, clinical onset is characterized by a rapidly progressive pneumonia, fever, nonproductive cough, and myalgia. Chest radiographs reveal unilateral, diffuse, patchy consolidation, progressing to widespread nodular consolidation. Toxic symptoms, hypoxia, and obtundation may be prominent, and death may follow within a few days. In those who survive, convalescence is prolonged. The mortality rate among hospitalized patients averages 15%, although there is a much greater risk of death if there is a serious underlying illness. Erythromycin was the antibiotic of choice for many years, but has beeen supplanted by newer macrolides such as azithromycin and fluoroquinolones such as levofloxacin.

Pontiac fever is a self-limited, flulike illness with fever, malaise, myalgias, and headache. It differs from Legionnaires disease in showing no evidence of pulmonary consolidation. The disease resolves spontaneously in 3 to 5 days.

Pseudomonas aeruginosa is a Highly Antibiotic-Resistant Opportunsitic Pathogen

The organism only infrequently infects humans. However it causes disease, particularly in hospital environments, where it is associated with pneumonia, wound infections, urinary tract disease, and sepsis in debilitated or immunosuppressed persons. Burns, urinary catheterization, cystic fibrosis, diabetes, and neutropenia all predispose to infection with *P. aeruginosa*.

It is a ubiquitous aerobic, gram-negative rod that requires moisture and only minimal nutrients. It thrives in soil and water, on animals, and on moist environmental surfaces. *Antibiotic use selects for* P. aeruginosa *infection, as the organism is resistant to most antibiotics.*

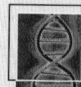

PATHOGENESIS: *P. aeruginosa* elaborates an array of proteins that allow it to attach to, invade, and destroy host tissues, while avoiding host inflammatory and immune defenses. Injury to epithelial cells uncovers surface molecules that serve as binding sites for the pili of *P. aeruginosa*. Many strains of *P. aeruginosa* produce a proteoglycan that surrounds the bacteria and protects them from mucociliary action, complement, and phagocytes. The organism releases extracellular enzymes—including an elastase, an alkaline protease, and a cytotoxin—which facilitate tissue invasion and are partially responsible for the necrotizing lesions of *Pseudomonas* infections. The elastase is probably responsible for the distinctive ability of *P. aeruginosa* to invade blood vessel walls. The organism also produces systemic pathologic effects through endotoxin and several systemically active exotoxins.

PATHOLOGY: *Pseudomonas* infection produces an acute inflammatory response. The organism often invades small arteries and veins, producing vascular thrombosis and hemorrhagic necrosis, particularly in the lungs and skin. Blood vessel invasion predisposes to dissemination and sepsis, and leads to the development of multiple nodular lesions in the lungs. Gram stains of necrotic tissue infected with *Pseudomonas* commonly show blood vessel walls densely infiltrated with organisms. Sometimes disseminated infections are marked by the development of typical skin lesions called **ecthyma gangrenosum.** These nodular, necrotic lesions represent sites where the organism has disseminated to the skin, invaded blood vessels, and produced localized hemorrhagic infarctions.

CLINICAL FEATURES: *Pseudomonas* infections are among the most aggressive human bacterial diseases, often progressing rapidly to sepsis. They require immediate medical intervention and are associated with high mortality.

Melioidosis Features Abscesses in Many Organs

Melioidosis (Rangoon beggars disease) is an uncommon disease caused by Pseudomonas pseudomallei, *a small gram-negative bacillus in the soil and surface water of Southeast Asia and other tropical areas.* During the conflict in Vietnam, several hundred American servicemen acquired melioidosis. The organism flourishes in wet environments, such as rice paddies and marshes. The skin is the usual portal of entry, and organisms enter through preexisting lesions, including penetrating wounds and burns. Humans may also be infected by inhaling contaminated dust or aerosolized droplets. The incubation period may last months to years, and the clinical course is variable.

PATHOLOGY AND CLINICAL FEATURES: ***Acute melioidosis*** *is a pulmonary infection, ranging from a mild tracheobronchitis to an overwhelming cavitary pneumonia* (Fig. 9-23). Patients with severe cases present with the sudden onset of high fever, constitutional symptoms, and a cough that may produce blood-stained sputum. Splenomegaly, hepatomegaly, and jaundice are sometimes present. Diarrhea may be as severe as in cholera. Fulminating septicemia, shock, coma, and death may develop in spite of antibiotic therapy. Acute

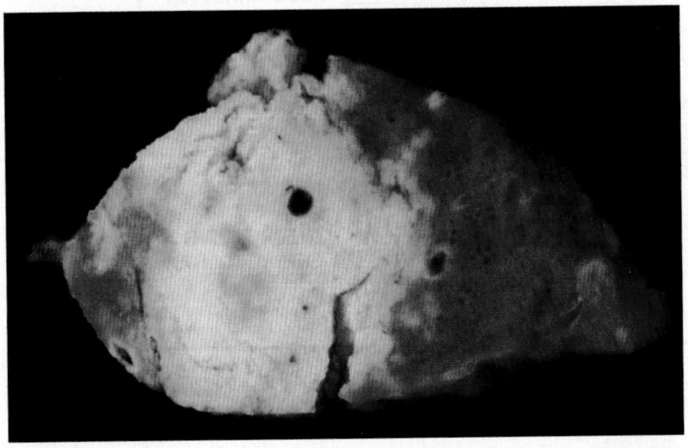

FIGURE 9-23. **Acute melioidosis.** The lung is consolidated and necrotic.

septicemic melioidosis causes discrete abscesses throughout the body, especially in the lungs, liver, spleen, and lymph nodes.

Chronic melioidosis *is a persistent localized infection involving the lungs, skin, bones, or other organs.* The lesions are suppurative or granulomatous abscesses and in the lung may be mistaken for tuberculosis. Chronic melioidosis may lie dormant for months or years, only to appear suddenly.

Clostridial Diseases

Clostridia are gram-positive, spore-forming, obligate anaerobic bacilli. The vegetative bacilli are found in the gastrointestinal tract of herbivorous animals and humans. Anaerobic conditions promote vegetative division, whereas aerobic ones lead to sporulation. Spores pass in animal feces and contaminate soil and plants, where they can survive unfavorable environmental circumstances. Under anaerobic conditions, the spores revert to vegetative cells, thereby completing the cycle. During sporulation, vegetative cells degenerate and their plasmids produce a variety of specific toxins that cause widely differing diseases, depending on the species (Fig. 9-24).

- **Food poisoning and necrotizing enteritis (pigbel)** are caused by the enterotoxins of *Clostridium perfringens*.
- **Gas gangrene** is produced by the myotoxins of *C. perfringens*, *Clostridium novyi*, *Clostridium septicum*, and other species.
- **Tetanus** is due to the neurotoxin of *Clostridium tetani*.
- **Botulism** results from the action of the neurotoxins of *Clostridium. botulinum*.
- **Pseudomembranous enterocolitis** is caused by the exotoxins of *Clostridium difficile*.

Clostridial Food Poisoning Is Common and is Self-Limited

C. perfringens is one of the most common causes of bacterial food poisoning in the world, characterized by an acute, generally benign, diarrheal disease, usually lasting less than 24 hours. It is omnipresent in the environment, contaminating soil, water, air samples, clothing, dust, and meat.

Its spores survive cooking temperatures and germinate to yield vegetative forms, which proliferate when food is allowed to stand without refrigeration. Cooking drives out enough air to make the food anaerobic, a condition that is conducive to growth but not to sporulation. As a result, the contaminated food contains the vegetative clostridia but little preformed enterotoxin. The vegetative bacteria sporulate in the small bowel, where they elaborate a variety of exotoxins, which are cytotoxic to enterocytes and cause the loss of intracellular ions and fluid. Certain types of food, including meats, gravies, and sauces, are ideal substrates for *C. perfringens*. Clostridial food poisoning presents as abdominal cramping and watery diarrhea. Symptoms begin 8 to 24 hours after the ingestion of contaminated food and usually resolve within 24 hours.

Necrotizing Enteritis Is a Catastrophic Childhood Infection in New Guinea

C. perfringens *type C also produces an enterotoxin that causes necrotizing enterocolitis.* The illness is rare in the industrialized world but remains endemic in parts of New Guinea, especially in children who have participated in pig feasts (hence the pidgin term *pigbel*). Adults, because they have circulating antibodies, tend not to develop the disease, which is segmental and may be restricted to a few centimeters, or may involve the entire small intestine. Green, necrotic pseudomembranes are seen in areas of necrosis and peritonitis. More-advanced lesions perforate the bowel wall. Histologic sections reveal infarction of intestinal mucosa, with edema, hemorrhage, and a suppurative transmural infiltrate.

Gas Gangrene May Complicate Penetrating Wounds

Gas gangrene (clostridial myonecrosis) is a necrotizing, gas-forming infection that begins in contaminated wounds and spreads rapidly to adjacent tissues. The disease can be fatal within hours of onset. *C. perfringens* is the most common cause of gas gangrene, but other clostridial species occasionally produce the disease.

PATHOGENESIS: Gas gangrene follows anaerobic deposition of *C. perfringens* into tissue. Clostridial growth requires extensive devitalized tissue, as in severe penetrating trauma, wartime injuries, and septic abortions. Clostridial myonecrosis is rare if wounds are débrided promptly.

Necrosis of previously healthy muscle is caused by myotoxins elaborated by a few species of clostridia. *C. perfringens* type A is the source of myotoxin in 80% to 90% of cases, but *C. novyi* and *C. septicum* may also produce myotoxin. Clostridial myotoxin is a phospholipase that destroys the membranes of muscle cells, leukocytes, and erythrocytes.

PATHOLOGY: Affected tissues rapidly become mottled and then frankly necrotic. Tissues such as muscle may even liquefy. The overlying skin becomes tense, as edema and gas expand underlying soft tissues. Microscopic examination shows extensive tissue necrosis with dissolution of the cells. A striking feature is the paucity of neutrophils, which are apparently destroyed by the myotoxin. Gram stain of affected tissues often shows typical, lozenge-shaped, gram-positive rods.

CLINICAL FEATURES: The incubation period of gas gangrene is commonly 2 to 4 days after injury. Sudden, severe pain occurs at the site of the wound, which is tender and edematous. Skin darkens, because of hemorrhage and cutaneous necrosis. The lesion develops a thick, serosanguineous discharge, which has a fragrant odor and may contain gas bubbles. Hemolytic anemia, hypotension, and renal failure may develop; and in the terminal stages, coma, jaundice, and shock supervene.

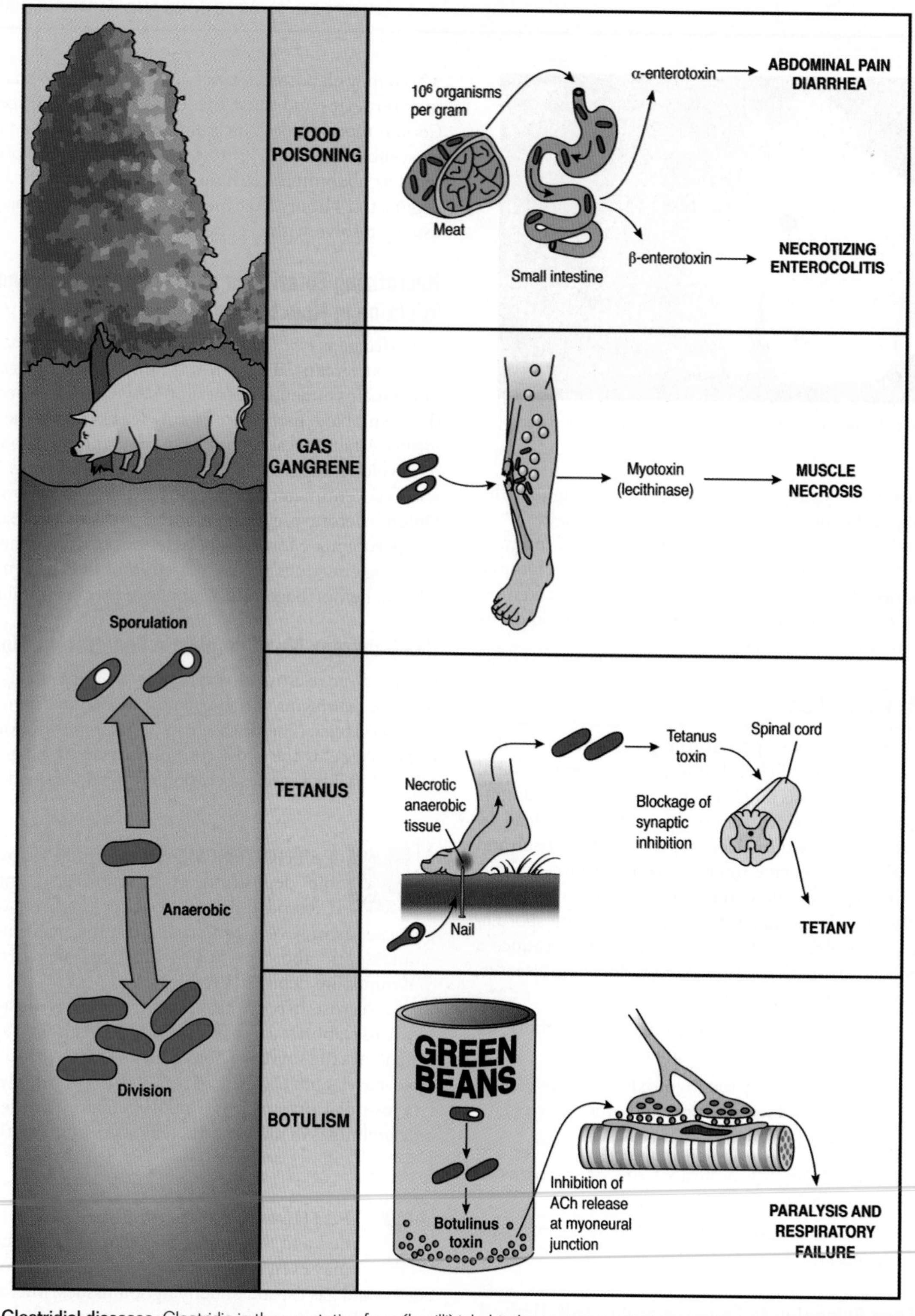

FIGURE 9-24. **Clostridial diseases.** Clostridia in the vegetative form (bacilli) inhabit the gastrointestinal tract of humans and animals. Spores pass in the feces, contaminate soil and plant materials, and are ingested or enter sites of penetrating wounds. Under anaerobic conditions they revert to vegetative forms. Plasmids in the vegetative forms elaborate toxins that cause several clostridial diseases.

Food poisoning and necrotizing enteritis. Meat dishes left to cool at room temperature grow large numbers of clostridia ($>10^6$ organisms per gram). When contaminated meat is ingested, *Clostridum perfringens* types A and C produce α enterotoxin in the small intestine during sporulation, causing abdominal pain and diarrhea. Type C also produces β enterotoxin.

Gas gangrene. Clostridia are widespread and may contaminate a traumatic wound or surgical operation. *C. perfringens* type A elaborates a myotoxin (α toxin), >α lecithinase that destroys cell membranes, alters capillary permeability, and causes severe hemolysis following intravenous injection. The toxin causes necrosis of previously healthy skeletal muscle.

Tetanus. Spores of *Clostridium tetani* are in soil and enter the site of an accidental wound. Necrotic tissue at the wound site causes spores to revert to the vegetative form (bacilli). Autolysis of vegetative forms releases tetanus toxin. The toxin is transported in peripheral nerves and (retrograde) through axons to the anterior horn cells of the spinal cord. The toxin blocks synaptic inhibition and the accumulation of acetylcholine in damaged synapses leads to rigidity and spasms of the skeletal musculature (tetany).

Botulism. Improperly canned food is contaminated by the vegetative form of *Clostridium botulinum,* which proliferates under aerobic conditions and elaborates a neurotoxin. After the food is ingested, the neurotoxin is absorbed from the small intestine and eventually reaches the myoneural junction, where it inhibits the release of acetylcholine (ACh). The result is a symmetric descending paralysis of cranial nerves, trunk and limbs, with eventual respiratory paralysis and death.

Tetanus is Spastic Skeletal Muscle Contractions Caused by C. tetani Neurotoxin

It is also known as "lockjaw" because of early involvement of the muscles of mastication.

EPIDEMIOLOGY: *C. tetani* is present in the soil and lower intestine of many animals. Tetanus occurs when the organism contaminates wounds and proliferates in tissue, releasing its exotoxin. Using a vaccine composed of inactivated tetanus toxin, immunization programs have largely eliminated the disease from developed countries. Nonetheless, tetanus remains a frequent and lethal disease in developing countries. Many deaths occur in newborns in primitive societies, due to the custom of coating umbilical stumps with dirt or dung to prevent bleeding.

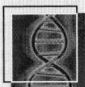

PATHOGENESIS: Necrotic tissue and suppuration create a fertile anaerobic environment for the spores to revert to vegetative bacteria. Tetanus toxin is released from autolyzed vegetative cells. Although the infection remains localized, the potent neurotoxin (**tetanospasmin**) undergoes retrograde transport through the ventral roots of peripheral nerves to the anterior horn cells of the spinal cord. It crosses the synapse and binds to ganglioside receptors on presynaptic terminals of motor neurons in the ventral horns. Following internalization, its endopeptidase activity selectively cleaves a protein responsible for exocytosis of synaptic vesicles. Thus, release of inhibitory neurotransmitters is blocked, permitting unopposed neural stimulation and sustained contraction of skeletal muscles (**tetany**). The loss of inhibitory neurotransmitters also accelerates heart rate and leads to hypertension and cardiovascular instability.

CLINICAL FEATURES: The incubation period of tetanus is 1 to 3 weeks. The disease begins subtly with fatigue, weakness, and muscle cramping that progresses to rigidity. Spastic rigidity often begins in the muscles of the face, giving rise to lockjaw, which extends to several facial muscles, causing a fixed grin *(risus sardonicus)*. Rigidity of the muscles of the back produces a backward arching *(opisthotonos)* (Fig. 9-25). Abrupt stimuli, including noise, light, or touch, can precipitate painful generalized muscle spasms. Prolonged spasm of respiratory and laryngeal musculature may lead to death. Infants and persons older than 50 years of age have the highest mortality.

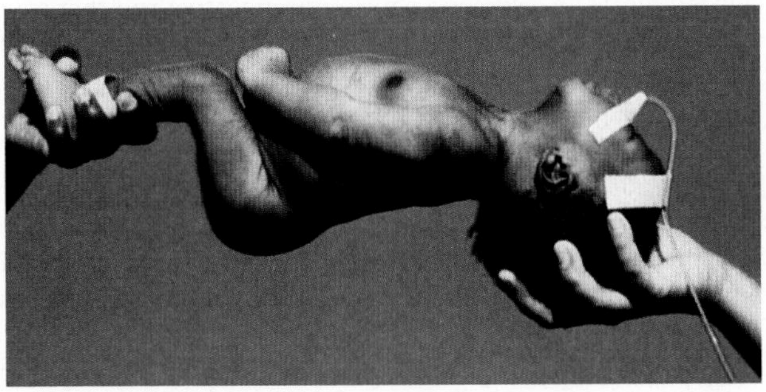

FIGURE 9-25. **Tetanus.** Opisthotonus (backward arching) in an infant due to intense contraction of the paravertebral muscles.

Botulism Is a Paralyzing Disease Due to *C. botulinum* Neurotoxin

The disease is characterized by a symmetric descending paralysis of cranial nerves, limbs, and trunk.

EPIDEMIOLOGY: *C. botulinum* spores are widely distributed and are especially resistant to drying and boiling. *In the United States, the toxin is most often present in foods that have been improperly home canned and stored without refrigeration. These circumstances provide suitable anaerobic conditions for growth of the vegetative cells that elaborate the neurotoxin.* Botulism can also be contracted from home-cured ham and other meats that have been left unrefrigerated for several days and from raw, smoked, and fermented fish products. The disease is also caused by absorption of toxin from organisms proliferating in infants' intestines (**infantile botulism**) or rarely by absorption of toxin from organisms growing in contaminated wounds (**wound botulism**).

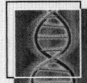

PATHOGENESIS: Ingested botulinum neurotoxin resists gastric digestion and is readily absorbed into the blood from the proximal small intestine. Circulating toxin reaches the cholinergic nerve endings at the myoneural junction. There are 7 serotypes of neurotoxin (A–G), with diverse mechanisms of action. The most common serotype, A, binds gangliosides at presynaptic nerve terminals and inhibits acetylcholine release.

CLINICAL FEATURES: Botulism is characterized by a descending paralysis, first affecting cranial nerves and causing blurred vision, photophobia, dry mouth, and dysarthria. Weakness progresses to involve neck muscles, extremities, diaphragm, and accessory muscles of breathing. Respiratory weakness can progress rapidly to complete respiratory arrest and death. Untreated botulism is usually lethal, but treatment with antitoxin reduces the mortality to 25%. Botulinum toxin is often used as treatment for many forms of dystonia, and has recently found popularity as a cosmetic vehicle to transiently erase frown lines (Botox).

Clostridium difficile Colitis Follows Antibiotic Treatment

C. difficile *colitis is an acute necrotizing infection of the terminal small bowel and colon.* It is responsible for a large fraction (25% to 50%) of the antibiotic-associated diarrheas and is potentially lethal.

EPIDEMIOLOGY: *C. difficile* resides in the colon in some healthy persons. A change in intestinal flora, often due to antibiotic administration (e.g., clindamycin), allows the organism to flourish, produce toxin, and damage the colonic mucosa. Such colitis can also be precipitated by other insults to the colonic flora, such as bowel surgery, dietary changes, and antineoplastic chemotherapeutic agents. In hospitals where many patients receive antibiotics, fecal shedding of the organism results in person-to-person spread.

PATHOGENESIS: As mentioned above, colonic bacteria ordinarily limit the growth of *C. difficile,* but alterations in normal flora permit the organism to proliferate, elaborate toxins, and destroy mucosal cells. The bacterium does not invade the colonic mucosa but rather produces two exotoxins. Toxin A causes fluid secretion; toxin B is directly cytopathic.

PATHOLOGY: *C. difficile* destroys colonic mucosal cells and incites an acute inflammatory infiltrate. Lesions range from focal colitis limited to a few crypts and only detectable on biopsy, to massive confluent mucosal ulceration. Inflammation initially involves only the mucosa, but if the disease progresses, it can extend into the submucosa and muscularis propria. An inflammatory exudate, called a "pseudomembrane," of cellular debris, neutrophils, and fibrin often forms over affected areas of the colon. *C. difficile* colitis is often called **pseudomembranous colitis**, even though that condition may have many etiologies.

CLINICAL FEATURES: *C. difficile* colitis may present with very mild symptoms or with diarrhea, fever, and abdominal pain. Stools may be profuse and often contain neutrophils. The symptoms and signs are not specific and do not distinguish *C. difficile* colitis from other acute inflammatory diarrheal illnesses. Mild cases of *C. difficile* diarrhea can often be treated simply by discontinuing the precipitating antibiotic. More-severe cases require treatment with an antibiotic effective against *C. difficile.*

Bacterial Infections with Animal Reservoirs or Insect Vectors

Brucellosis Is a Chronic Febrile Disease Acquired from Domestic Animals

Brucellosis is a zoonotic disease caused by one of four Brucella *species. Human brucellosis may manifest as an acute systemic disease or as a chronic infection characterized by waxing and waning febrile episodes, weight loss, and fatigue. Brucella* species are small, aerobic, gram-negative rods that in humans primarily infect monocytes/macrophages.

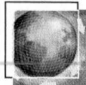

EPIDEMIOLOGY: Each species of *Brucella* has its own animal reservoir:

- *Brucella melitensis:* sheep and goats
- *Brucella abortus:* cattle
- *Brucella suis:* swine
- *Brucella canis:* dogs

Brucellosis is encountered worldwide, Virtually every type of domesticated animal and many wild ones are affected. The organisms reside in the genitourinary systems of animals, and infection is often endemic in animal herds. Humans acquire the bacteria by several mechanisms, including (1) contact with infected blood or tissue, (2) ingestion of contaminated meat or milk, or (3) inhalation of contaminated aerosols. Brucellosis is an occupational hazard among ranchers, herders, veterinarians, and slaughterhouse workers.

Elimination of infected animals and vaccination of herds have reduced the incidence of brucellosis in many countries, including the United States, where only about 200 cases are reported annually. Yet, the disease remains prevalent throughout Central and South America, Africa, Asia, and Southern Europe. Unpasteurized milk and cheese remain a major source of infection in these areas. In the arctic and subarctic regions, humans acquire brucellosis by eating raw bone marrow of infected reindeer.

PATHOLOGY: Bacteria enter the circulation through skin abrasions, the conjunctiva, oropharynx, or lungs. They then spread in the bloodstream to the liver, spleen, lymph nodes, and bone marrow, where they multiply in macrophages. Generalized hyperplasia of these cells may ensue, causing lymphadenopathy and hepatosplenomegaly in 15% of patients infected with *B. melitensis,* and in 40% of those infected with *B. abortus.* Patients infected with *B. abortus* develop conspicuous noncaseating granulomas in the liver, spleen, lymph nodes, and bone marrow. By contrast, classic granulomas are not present in patients infected with *B. melitensis,* who may have only small aggregates of mononuclear inflammatory cells scattered throughout the liver. *B. suis* infection may cause suppurative liver abscesses rather than granulomas. The organisms usually cannot be demonstrated histologically. Periodic release of organisms from infected phagocytic cells may be responsible for the febrile episodes of the illness.

CLINICAL FEATURES: Brucellosis is a systemic infection that can involve any organ or organ system of the body, with an insidious onset in half of cases. The disease is characterized by a multitude of somatic complaints, such as fever, sweats, anorexia, fatigue, weight loss, and depression. Fever occurs in all patients at some time during the illness, but it can wax and wane (hence the term **undulant fever**) over a period of weeks to months when untreated. The mortality rate from brucellosis is less than 1%; death is usually caused by endocarditis.

The most common complications of brucellosis involve the bones and joints and include spondylitis of the lumbar spine and suppuration in large joints. Peripheral neuritis, meningitis, orchitis, endocarditis, myocarditis, and pulmonary lesions are described. Prolonged treatment with tetracycline is usually effective; the relapse rate is dramatically reduced if rifampin or an aminoglycoside is added.

Yersinia pestis Causes Bubonic Plague, the Medieval "Black Death"

Plague is a bacteremic, often fatal, infection that is usually accompanied by enlarged, painful regional lymph nodes (buboes). Historically, plague caused massive epidemics that killed much of the then civilized world. *Y. pestis* is a short gram-negative rod that stains more heavily at the ends (i.e., bipolar staining), particularly with Giemsa stains.

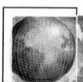

EPIDEMIOLOGY: *Y. pestis* infection is an endemic zoonosis in many parts of the world, including the Americas, Africa, and Asia. The organisms are found in wild rodents, such as rats, squirrels, and prairie dogs. Fleas transmit it from animal to animal, and most human infections result from bites of infected fleas. Some infected humans develop plague pneumonia, and shed large numbers of organisms in aerosolized respiratory secretions, which allow disease transmission from person to person.

Major plague epidemics have occurred when *Y. pestis* was introduced into large urban rat populations in crowded, squalid cities. Infection spread first among rats; then, as they died, infected fleas fed on the human population, causing widespread disease. The Black Death pandemic that struck Europe in the mid-14th century (1347–1350) killed about a third of Europe's population, perhaps 34 million people. In the United States, 30 to 40 cases of plague occur annually, mostly in the desert Southwest.

PATHOGENESIS AND PATHOLOGY: After inoculation into the skin, *Y. pestis* is phagocytosed by neutrophils and macrophages. Organisms ingested by neutrophils are killed, but those engulfed by macrophages survive and replicate intracellularly. The bacteria are carried to regional lymph nodes, where they continue to multiply, producing extensive hemorrhagic necrosis. From the regional lymph nodes, they disseminate throughout the body through the bloodstream and lymphatics. In the lungs, *Y. pestis* produces a necrotizing pneumonitis that releases organisms into the alveoli and airways. These are expelled by coughing, enabling pneumonic spread of the disease. Affected lymph nodes, known as "buboes," are frequently enlarged and fluctuant, owing to extensive hemorrhagic necrosis. Infected patients often develop necrotic, hemorrhagic skin lesions, hence the name "black death" for this disease.

CLINICAL FEATURES: There are three clinical presentations of *Y. pestis* infection, although they often overlap.

- **Bubonic plague** begins within 2 to 8 days of the flea bite, with headache, fever, and myalgias, and with painful enlargement of regional lymph nodes, mostly in the groin, because flea bites usually occur in the lower extremities. Disease progresses to septic shock within hours to days after appearance of the bubo.
- **Septicemic plague** (10% of cases) occurs when bacteria are inoculated directly into the blood and do not produce buboes. Patients die of overwhelming bacterial growth in the bloodstream. Fever, prostration, and meningitis occur suddenly, and death ensues within 48 hours. All blood vessels contain bacilli, and fibrin casts surround the organisms in renal glomeruli and dermal vessels.
- **Pneumonic plague** results from inhalation of airborne particles from carcasses of animals or the cough of infected persons. Within 2 to 5 days after infection, high fever, cough, and dyspnea begin suddenly. The sputum teems with bacilli. Respiratory insufficiency and endotoxic shock kill the patient within 1 to 2 days.

All types of plague carry a high mortality rate (50% to 75%) if untreated. Tetracycline combined with streptomycin is the recommended therapy.

Tularemia Is an Acute Febrile, Disease Usually Acquired from Rabbits

Tularemia is caused by Francisella tularensis, *a small, gram-negative coccobacillus.*

EPIDEMIOLOGY: Tularemia is a zoonosis whose most important reservoirs are rabbits and rodents, although other wild and domestic animals may harbor the organisms. Human infection with *F. tularensis* results from contact with infected animals or from the bites of infected insects, including ticks, deerflies, and mosquitoes. Ticks and rabbits are responsible for most human infections. The blood-sucking insects inoculate the organism into the skin. Bacteria may also enter via unnoticed breaks in the skin if there is direct contact with an infected animal. In addition, tularemia can result from the inhalation of infected aerosols, ingestion of contaminated food and water, or inoculation into the eye. Tularemia is found in temperate zones of the Northern Hemisphere. The incidence of the infection has fallen dramatically in the United States in the past 5 decades, to about 250 cases annually, presumably related to a decline in hunting and trapping.

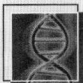

PATHOGENESIS: *F. tularensis* multiplies at the site of inoculation, where it produces a focal ulceration. The bacteria then spread to regional lymph nodes. Dissemination in the bloodstream leads to metastatic infections that involve the monocyte/macrophage system and sometimes the lungs, heart, and kidneys. *F. tularensis* survives within macrophages until these cells are activated by a cell-mediated immune response to the infection.

PATHOLOGY: Lesions of tularemia occur at the inoculation site and in lymph nodes, spleen, liver, bone marrow, lungs (Fig. 9-26), heart, and kidneys. The initial skin lesion is an exudative, pyogenic ulcer. Later, disseminated lesions undergo central necrosis and are surrounded by a perimeter of granulomatous reaction resembling the lesions of tuberculosis. Hyperemia and the presence of numerous macrophages in the sinuses make lymph nodes large and firm; they subsequently soften as necrosis and suppuration develop. The spleen tends to be enlarged but shows only nonspecific changes. The pulmonary lesions resemble those of primary tuberculosis.

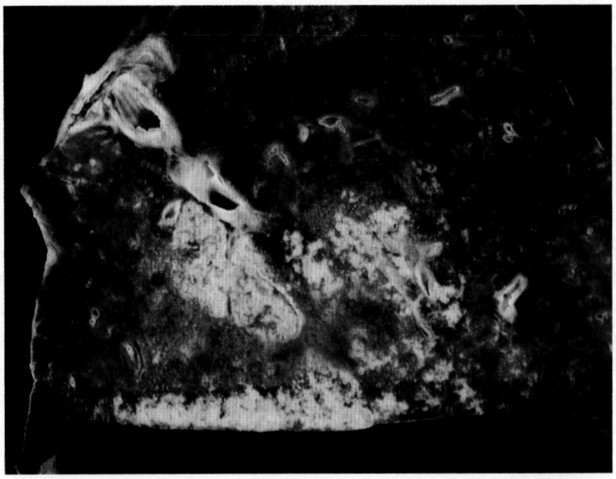

FIGURE 9-26. **Tularemia.** The lung shows firm, consolidated and necrotic areas.

CLINICAL FEATURES: The incubation period of tularemia ranges from 1 to 14 days, depending on the dose and route of transmission, with a mean of 3 to 4 days. There are four distinct clinical presentations.

- **Ulceroglandular tularemia** is the most common form of the disease (80% to 90% of cases) and begins as a tender, erythematous papule at the site of inoculation, usually on a limb. This develops into a pustule, which then ulcerates. Regional lymph nodes become large and tender and may suppurate and drain through sinus tracts. In some instances, generalized lymphadenopathy (glandular tularemia) is the first manifestation of infection.

  Initial bacteremia is accompanied by fever, headache, myalgias, and occasionally prostration. Within a week, generalized lymphadenopathy and splenomegaly are evident. The most serious infections are complicated by secondary pneumonia and endotoxic shock, in which case the prognosis is grave. Some patients develop meningitis, endocarditis, pericarditis, or osteomyelitis.
- **Oculoglandular tularemia** is rare (<2% of cases) and is characterized by a primary conjunctival papule, which forms a pustule and ulcerates. Lymphadenopathy of the head and neck become prominent. Severe ulceration may cause blindness, if infection penetrates the sclera and reaches the optic nerve.
- **Typhoidal tularemia** is diagnosed when fever, hepatosplenomegaly, and toxemia are the presenting signs and symptoms.
- **Pneumonic tularemia**, in which pneumonia is a major feature, may complicate any of the other types.

The duration of illness is 1 week to 3 months, but this may be shortened by prompt treatment with streptomycin.

Anthrax Is Rapidly Fatal When It Disseminates

Anthrax is a necrotizing disease caused by Bacillus anthracis, *which is a large spore-forming, gram-positive rod.*

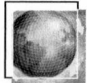

EPIDEMIOLOGY: Anthrax has been recognized for centuries, and descriptions of disease consistent with anthrax were reported in early Hebrew, Roman, and Greek records. The major reservoirs are goats, sheep, cattle, horses, pigs, and dogs. Spores form in the soil and dead animals, resisting heat, desiccation, and chemical disinfection for years. Humans are infected when spores enter the body through breaks in the skin, by inhalation, or by ingestion. Human disease may also result from exposure to contaminated animal byproducts, such as hides, wool, brushes, or bone meal.

Anthrax has been a persistent problem in Iran, Turkey, Pakistan, and Sudan. One of the largest recorded naturally occurring outbreaks of anthrax occurred in Zimbabwe, when an estimated 10,000 persons became infected in 1978 to 1980. In North America, human infection is extremely rare (one case per year for the past few years) and usually results from exposure to imported animal products. However, increased vigilance for anthrax has emerged following a recent bioterrorism epidose involving transport of organisms by the postal system (see below).

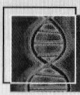

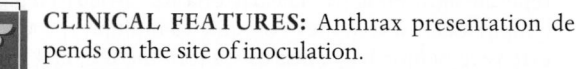

PATHOGENESIS: The spores of *B. anthracis* germinate in the human body to yield vegetative bacteria that multiply and release a potent necrotizing toxin. In 80% of cases of cutaneous anthrax, the infection remains localized, and the host immunologic response eventually eliminates the organism. If the infection disseminates, as occurs when the organisms are inhaled or ingested, the resulting widespread tissue destruction is usually fatal.

PATHOLOGY: *B. anthracis* produces extensive tissue necrosis at the sites of infection, associated with only a mild infiltrate of neutrophils. Cutaneous lesions are ulcerated, contain numerous organisms, and are covered by a black scab. Pulmonary infection produces a necrotizing, hemorrhagic pneumonia, associated with hemorrhagic necrosis of mediastinal lymph nodes and widespread dissemination of the organism.

CLINICAL FEATURES: Anthrax presentation depends on the site of inoculation.

- **Malignant pustule** is the cutaneous form of the disease and accounts for 95% of all anthrax. The infected person presents with an elevated skin papule that enlarges and erodes into an ulcer. Bloody purulent exudate accumulates and gradually darkens to purple or black. The ulcer is often surrounded by a zone of brawny edema, which is disproportionately large for the size of the ulcer. Regional lymphadenitis portends a poor prognosis, as lymphatic invasion precedes septicemia. If infection does not disseminate, cutaneous lesions heal without sequelae.
- **Pulmonary, or inhalational, anthrax,** sometimes called "woolsorters' disease," is a hazard of handling raw wool and develops after the inhalation of the spores of *B. anthracis*. Pulmonary anthrax presents as a flulike illness that rapidly progresses to respiratory failure and shock. Death often ensues within 24 to 48 hours of onset. Only 18 cases of inhalational anthrax were reported in the United States from 1900 to 1980. As a result of the anthrax bioterror attack in the United States in 2001, 11 cases of inhalational anthrax occurred. The only hope is early antibiotic therapy.
- **Septicemic anthrax** more commonly follows pulmonary anthrax than malignant pustule. Disseminated intravascular coagulation is a common complication. Moreover, a bacterial toxin depresses the respiratory center, which explains why death can occur even when antibiotic therapy has cured the infection.
- **Gastrointestinal anthrax** is rare and is acquired by eating contaminated meat. Ulceration of the stomach or bowel and invasion of the regional lymphatics are common. Death is caused by fulminant diarrhea and massive ascites.

Listeriosis Is a Systemic Multiorgan Infection That Carries a High Mortality

It is caused by Listeria monocytogenes, *a small, motile, gram-positive coccobacillus.*

EPIDEMIOLOGY: Listeriosis is usually sporadic but may be epidemic. The organism has been isolated worldwide from surface water, soil, vegetation, feces of healthy persons, many species of wild and domestic mammals, and several species of birds. However, spread of infection from animals to humans is rare. Most human infections are in urban rather than rural environments and, in the Northern

Hemisphere, occur during July and August. *L. monocytogenes* grows at refrigerator temperatures, and outbreaks have been traced to unpasteurized milk, cheese, and dairy products.

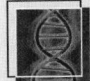

PATHOGENESIS: *L. monocytogenes* has an unusual life cycle, which accounts for its ability to evade intracellular and extracellular antibacterial defense mechanisms. After phagocytosis by host cells, the organism enters a phagolysosome, where the acidic pH activates *listeriolysin O*, an exotoxin that disrupts the vesicular membrane and permits the bacterium to escape into the cytoplasm. After replicating, bacteria usurp the contractile elements of the host cytoskeleton to form elongated protrusions that are engulfed by adjacent cells. Thus, *Listeria* spread from one cell to another without exposure to the extracellular environment.

PATHOLOGY AND CLINICAL FEATURES: **Listeriosis of pregnancy** includes prenatal and postnatal infections. Listeriosis of the adult population is most commonly characterized by meningoencephalitis and septicemia, but may be localized to skin, eyes, lymph nodes, endocardium, or bones.

Maternal infection early in pregnancy may lead to abortion or premature delivery. Infected infants rapidly develop respiratory distress, hepatosplenomegaly, cutaneous and mucosal papules, leukopenia, and thrombocytopenia. Intrauterine infections involve many organs and tissues, including amniotic fluid, placenta, and the umbilical cord. Abscesses are found in many organs. Microscopically, foci of necrosis and suppuration contain many bacteria. Older lesions tend to be granulomatous. Neurologic sequelae are common, and the mortality of neonatal listeriosis is high even with prompt antibiotic therapy. Neonatal listeriosis may also be acquired during delivery, in which case the onset of clinical disease is 3 days to 2 weeks after birth.

Chronic alcoholics, patients with cancer, those receiving immunosuppressive therapy, and patients with AIDS are far more susceptible to infection than is the general population. Meningitis is the most common form of the disease in adults and resembles other bacterial meningitides.

Septicemic listeriosis is a severe febrile illness most common in immunodeficient patients. It may lead to shock and disseminated intravascular coagulation, a situation that may be misdiagnosed as gram-negative sepsis. Prolonged treatment with antimicrobials is usually required because patients tend to experience relapse if therapy is administered for less than 3 weeks. The mortality from systemic listeriosis remains at 25%.

Cat-Scratch Disease Is a Self-Limited Granulomatous Lymphadenitis

Cat-scratch disease is a self-limited infection usually caused by Bartonella henselae *and more rarely by* Bartonella quintana. The bacteria are small (0.2 to 0.6 μm) gram-negative rods. They are difficult to culture but are easily seen in tissue sections of the skin, lymph nodes and conjunctiva, when stained with a silver impregnation technique (Fig. 9-27).

EPIDEMIOLOGY: The reservoir is thought to be cats; various surveys have shown that up to 30% of cats are bacteremic. Infection begins when the bacillus is inoculated into the skin by the claws of cats (and rarely, other animals) or by thorns or splinters. Sometimes the conjunctiva is contaminated by close contact with a cat, possibly by licking around the eye. Infections are more common in children (80%) than in adults, and there may be clustering of cases when a stray cat joins a family.

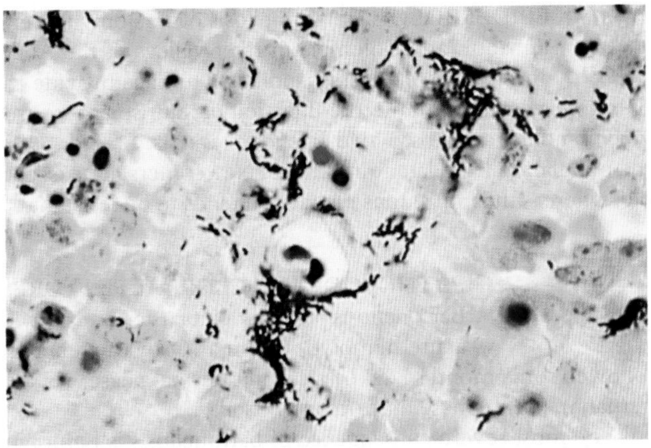

FIGURE 9-27. **Cat-scratch disease.** Section of a lymph node shows the bacilli, which are gram-negative but difficult to visualize with tissue gram stains. They are blackened by the Warthin-Starry silver impregnation technique.

PATHOLOGY AND CLINICAL FEATURES: Bacteria multiply in the walls of small vessels and about collagen fibers at the site of inoculation. The organisms are then carried to regional lymph nodes, where they cause a suppurative and granulomatous lymphadenitis. In early lesions, clusters of bacteria fill and expand lumina of small blood vessels. However, bacteria are rare in late lesions. After a papule develops at the site of inoculation, tenderness and enlargement of regional lymph nodes ensue. Nodes remain enlarged for 3 to 4 months and may drain through the skin. About half of patients have other symptoms, including fever and malaise, rash, a brief encephalitis, and erythema nodosum. **Parinaud oculoglandular syndrome** (preauricular adenopathy secondary to conjunctival infection) is common. Antibiotics are not known to help.

Glanders Is a Granulomatous Infection Acquired From Horses

Glanders is an infection of equine species (horses, mules, donkeys) that is only rarely transmitted to humans, in whom it causes acute or chronic granulomatous disease. The cause is *Pseudomonas mallei*, a small gram-negative, nonmotile bacillus. Although uncommon, the infection remains endemic in South America, Asia, and Africa. Humans acquire the disease by contact with infected equines through broken skin or by inhalation of contaminated aerosols.

- **Acute glanders** is characterized by bacteremia, with severe prostration and fever. Granulomatous abscesses may form in subcutaneous tissues and many other organs, including the lung, liver, spleen, muscles, and joints. Acute glanders is almost always fatal.
- **Chronic glanders** features low-grade fever, draining abscesses of the skin, lymphadenopathy, and hepatosplenomegaly. Granulomas in many organs mimic tuberculosis. The mortality in chronic glanders exceeds 50%.

Bartonellosis Causes Acute Anemia and Chronic Skin Disease

Bartonellosis is an infection by Bartonella bacilliformis, *a small, multiflagellated, gram- negative coccobacillus (Oroya fever) (verruga peruana).*

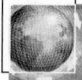

EPIDEMIOLOGY: Bartonellosis occurs only in Peru, Ecuador, and Colombia in river valleys of the Andes and is transmitted by sandflies. Humans provide the only reservoir and acquire the infection at sunrise and sunset, when sandflies are most active. In endemic areas, 10% to 15% of the population have latent infections. Newcomers are susceptible, whereas the indigenous population tends to be resistant.

PATHOLOGY AND CLINICAL FEATURES: Bartonellosis presents a biphasic pattern, with acute hemolytic anemia (Oroya fever) first, followed some months later by a chronic dermal phase (verruga peruana). Either phase may occur by itself.

The most severe consequence of bartonellosis is hemolytic anemia. After *B. bacilliformis* is inoculated into the skin by a sandfly, bacteria proliferate in the vascular endothelium and then invade erythrocytes, thereby producing profound hemolysis.

The **acute anemic phase** follows a 3 week incubation period and is characterized by abrupt onset of fever, skeletal pains, and severe, hemolytic anemia. In untreated bartonellosis, 40% of patients in the anemic phase die. Secondary *Salmonella* sepsis is frequent and contributes to the high mortality.

The **dermal eruptive phase** of bartonellosis may coexist with the anemic phase but is usually separated by an interval of 3 to 6 months. Many small hemangioma-like lesions stud the dermis, and bacteria may be identified in endothelial cells. Nodular lesions may be prominent on the extensor surfaces of the arms and legs. Large deep-seated lesions, which tend to ulcerate, develop near joints and limit motion. The dermal eruptive phase is often prolonged but eventually heals spontaneously. The mortality in this phase is less than 5%.

Infections Caused by Branching Filamentous Organisms

Actinomycosis Is Characterized by Abscesses and Sinus Tracts

Actinomycosis is a slowly progressive, suppurative, fibrosing infection involving the jaw, thorax, or abdomen. The disease is caused by a number of anaerobic and microaerophilic bacteria termed *Actinomyces*. These organisms are branching, filamentous, gram-positive rods that normally reside in the oropharynx, gastrointestinal tract, and vagina. Although *Actinomyces* are bacteria with filamentous morphology. Several *Actinomyces* species cause human disease, the most common being *Actinomyces israelii*.

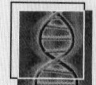

PATHOGENESIS AND PATHOLOGY: *Actinomyces* is not ordinarily virulent: the organisms reside as saprophytes in the body without producing disease. Two uncommon conditions must occur for *Actinomyces* to cause disease. First, the organism must be inoculated into deeper tissues, since it cannot invade. Second, an anaerobic atmosphere is necessary for bacterial proliferation. Trauma can produce tissue necrosis, providing an excellent anaerobic medium for growth of *Actinomyces,* and can inoculate the organism into normally sterile tissue. Actinomycosis occurs at four distinct sites:

- **Cervicofacial actinomycosis** results from jaw injury, dental extraction, or dental manipulation.
- **Thoracic actinomycosis** is caused by the aspiration of organisms contaminating dental debris.
- **Abdominal actinomycosis** follows traumatic or surgical disruption of the bowel, especially the appendix.
- **Pelvic actinomycosis** is associated with the prolonged use of intrauterine devices (IUDs).

Actinomycosis begins as a nidus of proliferating organisms that attracts an acute inflammatory infiltrate. The small abscess grows slowly, becoming a series of abscesses connected by sinus tracts. Tracts burrow across normal tissue boundaries and into adjacent organs. Eventually, a tract may penetrate onto an external surface or mucosal membrane, producing a draining sinus. The walls of the abscess and tracts are composed of granulation tissue, often thick, densely fibrotic, and chronically inflamed. Within the abscesses and sinuses are pus and colonies of organisms.

The colonies of *Actinomyces* within these lesions can grow to several millimeters in diameter and be visible to the naked eye. They appear as hard, yellow grains known as **sulfur granules**, because of their resemblance to elemental sulfur. Sulfur granules consist of tangled masses of narrow, branching filaments, embedded in a polysaccharide–protein matrix (**Splendore-Hoeppli material**). Histologically, the colonies appear as rounded, basophilic grains with scalloped eosinophilic borders (Fig. 9-28A). Individual filaments of *Actinomyces* cannot be discerned with the

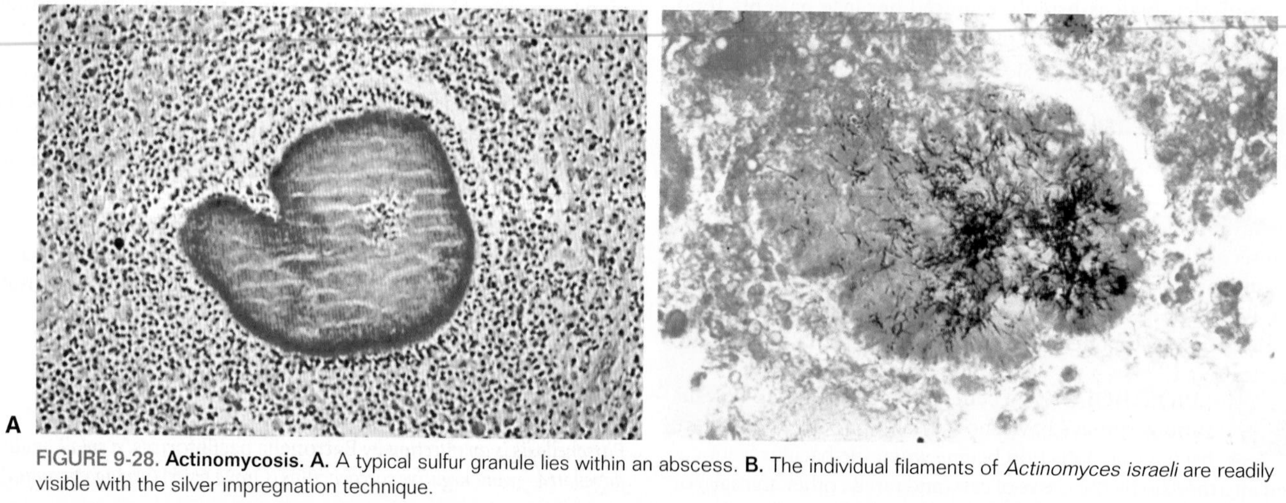

FIGURE 9-28. **Actinomycosis. A.** A typical sulfur granule lies within an abscess. **B.** The individual filaments of *Actinomyces israeli* are readily visible with the silver impregnation technique.

hematoxylin and eosin stain but are readily visible on Gram staining or silver impregnation (see Fig. 9-28B).

CLINICAL FEATURES: The signs and symptoms of actinomycosis depend on the site of infection. If infection originates in a tooth socket or the tonsils it is characterized by swelling of the jaw ("lumpy jaw"), face, and neck, at first painless and fluctuant but later painful. In pulmonary infections, sinus tracts may penetrate from lobe to lobe, through the pleura, and into ribs and vertebrae. Abdominal or pelvic disease may be encountered as an expanding mass, suggesting a locally spreading tumor. Actinomycosis responds to prolonged antibiotic therapy, and penicillin is highly effective.

Nocardiosis Is a Suppurative Respiratory Infection in Immunocompromised Hosts

From the lung it often spreads to the brain and skin. *Nocardia* are aerobic, gram-positive filamentous, branching bacteria. They are weakly acid-fast, a characteristic used to distinguish them from the morphologically similar actinomycetes.

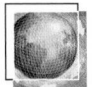

EPIDEMIOLOGY: *Nocardia* species are widely distributed in soil. Human disease is caused by inhaling or inoculating soil-borne organisms. It is not transmitted from person to person. *Nocardia asteroides* is the species most often involved in human disease. Nocardiosis is most common in persons with impaired immunity, particularly cell-mediated immunity. Organ transplantation, long-term corticosteroid therapy, lymphomas, leukemias, and other debilitating diseases predispose to *Nocardia* infections.

Two other pathogenic species of *Nocardia*, *Nocardia brasiliensis* and *Nocardia caviae*, may cause pulmonary nocardiosis resembling that produced by *N. asteroides*. However, they are usually encountered in underdeveloped countries as a cause of mycetomas.

PATHOLOGY AND CLINICAL FEATURES: The respiratory tract is the usual portal of entry for Nocardia. The organism elicits a brisk infiltrate of neutrophils, and disease begins as a slowly progressive, pyogenic pneumonia. If the infected person mounts a vigorous cell-mediated immune response, the infection may be eliminated. In immunocompromised persons, however, Nocardia produces pulmonary abscesses, which are frequently multiple and confluent. Direct extension to the pleura, trachea, and heart, and metastases to the brain or skin through the circulation carry a grave prognosis. Nocardial abscesses are filled with neutrophils, necrotic debris, and scattered organisms. Bacteria can be demonstrated by silver impregnation (Fig. 9-29). With the Gram stain, they appear as beaded, filamentous, gram-positive rods. Untreated nocardiosis is usually fatal. Sulfonamides or related antibiotics for several months are often effective therapy.

SPIROCHETAL INFECTIONS

Spirochetes are long, slender, helical bacteria with specialized cell envelopes that permit them to move by flexion and rotation. The thinner organisms are below the resolving power of routine light microscopy. Specialized techniques, such as darkfield microscopy or silver impregnation, are needed for their demonstration. Although spirochetes have the basic cell wall structure of gram-negative bacteria, they stain poorly with the Gram stain.

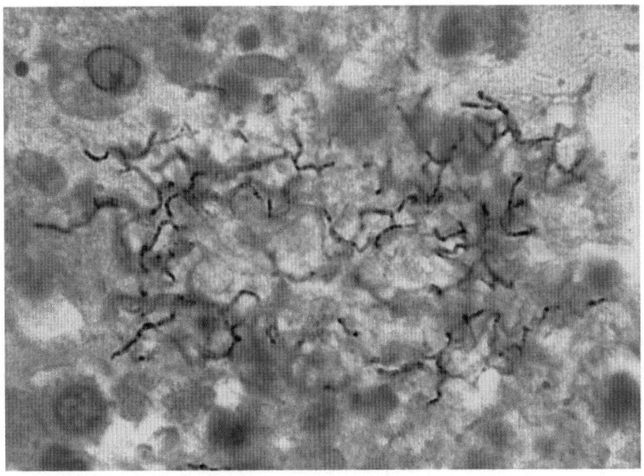

FIGURE 9-29. **Nocardiosis.** A silver stain of a necrotic exudate reveals the branching, filamentous rods of *Nocardia asteroides*.

Three genera of spirochetes, *Treponema, Borrelia,* and *Leptospira,* cause human disease (Table 9-5). They are adept at evading host inflammatory and immunological defenses, and diseases caused by these organisms are all chronic or relapsing.

Syphilis

Syphilis (lues) is a chronic, sexually transmitted, systemic infection caused by Treponema pallidum. *T. pallidum* is a thin, long spirochete (Fig. 9-30) that cannot be grown in artificial media. The disease was first recognized in Europe in the 1490s and has been related to Columbus'return from the New World. Urbanization and mass movements of people caused by war contributed to its rapid spread. Originally, syphilis was an acute disease that caused destructive skin lesions and early death, but it has become milder, with a more protracted and insidious clinical course.

EPIDEMIOLOGY: Syphilis is a worldwide disease that is transmitted almost exclusively by sexual contact. Infection is also spread from an infected mother to her fetus (**congenital syphilis**). The incidence of primary and secondary syphilis has declined since the introduction of penicillin therapy at the end of World War II.

PATHOGENESIS: *T. pallidum* is very fragile and is killed by soap, antiseptics, drying, and cold. Person-to-person transmission requires direct contact between a rich source of spirochetes (e.g., an open lesion) and mucous membranes or abraded skin of the genital organs, rectum, mouth, fingers, or nipples. The organisms reproduce at the site of inoculation, pass to regional lymph nodes, gain access to systemic circulation, and disseminate throughout the body. Although *T. pallidum* induces an inflammatory response and is taken up by phagocytic cells, it persists and proliferates. Chronic infection and inflammation cause tissue destruction, sometimes for decades. The course of syphilis is classically divided into three stages (Fig. 9-31).

TABLE 9-5

Spirochete Infections

Disease	Organism	Clinical Manifestation	Distribution	Mode of Transmission
	Treponemes			
Syphilis	*Treponema pallidum*	See text	Common worldwide	Sexual contact, congenital
Bejel	*Treponema endenicum (Treponema pallidum,* subspecies *endenicum)*	Mucosal, skin, and bone lesions	Middle East	Mouth-to-mouth contact
Yaws	*Treponema pertenue (Treponema pallidum* subspecies *pertenue)*	Skin and bone	Tropics	Skin-to-skin contact
Pinta	*Treponemacarateum*	Skin lesions	Latin America	Skin-to-skin contact
	Borrelia			
Lyme disease	*Borrelia burgdorferi*	See text	North America, Europe, Russia, Asia, Africa, Australia	Tick bite
Relapsing fever	*Borrelia recurrentis* and related species	Relapsing flulike illness	Worldwide	Tick bite, louse bite
	Leptospira			
Leptospirosis	*Leptospira interrogans*	Flulike illness, meningitis	Worldwide	Contact with animal urine

Primary Syphilis Features a Chancre

The classic lesion of primary syphilis is the chancre (Fig. 9-32), a characteristic ulcer at the site of *T. pallidum* entry, usually the penis, vulva, anus, or mouth. It appears 1 week to 3 months after exposure, with an average incubation period of 3 weeks. It tends to be solitary and has a firm, raised border. Spirochetes tend to concentrate in vessel walls and in the epidermis around the ulcer. *Chancres, as well as the lesions of the other stages of syphilis, display a characteristic "luetic vasculitis," in which endothelial cells proliferate and swell, and vessel walls become thickened by lymphocytes and fibrous tissue.*

The chancre quickly erodes to a characteristic ulcer. Chancres are painless and can go unnoticed in some locations, such as the uterine cervix, anal canal, and mouth. They last 3 to 12 weeks, are frequently accompanied by inguinal lymphadenopathy and heal without scarring.

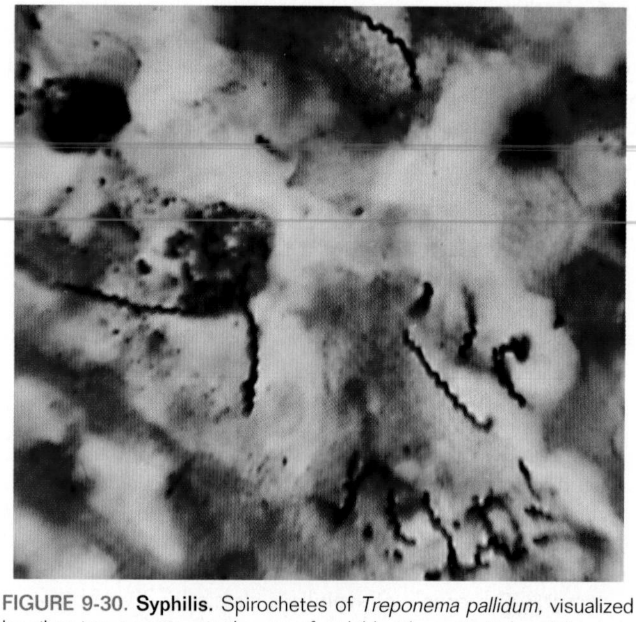

FIGURE 9-30. **Syphilis.** Spirochetes of *Treponema pallidum*, visualized by silver impregnation, in the eye of a child with congenital syphilis.

Secondary Syphilis Reflects Dissemination of Spirochetes

In secondary syphilis *T. pallidum* spreads systemically and proliferates to cause lesions in the skin, mucous membranes, lymph nodes, meninges, stomach, and liver. Lesions show perivascular lymphocytic infiltration and endarteritis obliterans.

- **Skin:** The most common presentation of secondary syphilis is an erythematous and maculopapular rash, involving the trunk and extremities, and often including the palms (Fig. 9-33) and soles. The rash appears 2 weeks to 3 months after the chancre heals. A variety of other skin lesions in secondary syphilis includes **condylomata lata** (exudative plaques in the perineum, vulva, or scrotum, which abound in spirochetes) (Fig. 9-34), **follicular syphilids** (small papular lesions around hair follicles that cause loss of hair), and **nummular syphilids** (coinlike lesions involving the face and perineum).
- **Mucous membranes:** Lesions on mucosal surfaces of the mouth and genital organs, called **mucous patches**, teem with organisms and are highly infectious.
- **Lymph nodes:** Characteristic changes in lymph nodes, especially epitrochlear nodes, include a thickened capsule, follicular hyperplasia, increased numbers of plasma cells, and macrophages and luetic vasculitis. Numerous spirochetes are present in the lymph nodes of secondary syphilis.
- **Meninges:** Although the meninges are commonly seeded with *T. pallidum,* this involvement is frequently asymptomatic.

Tertiary Syphilis Causes Neurologic and Vascular Diseases

After lesions of secondary syphilis have subsided, an asymptomatic period lasts for years or decades. However, spirochetes

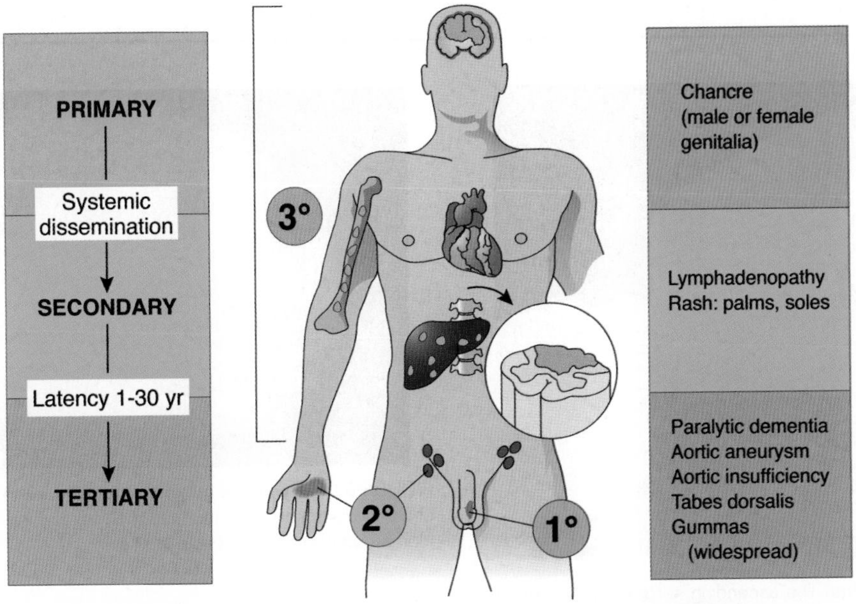

FIGURE 9-31. **Clinical characteristics of the various stages of syphilis.**

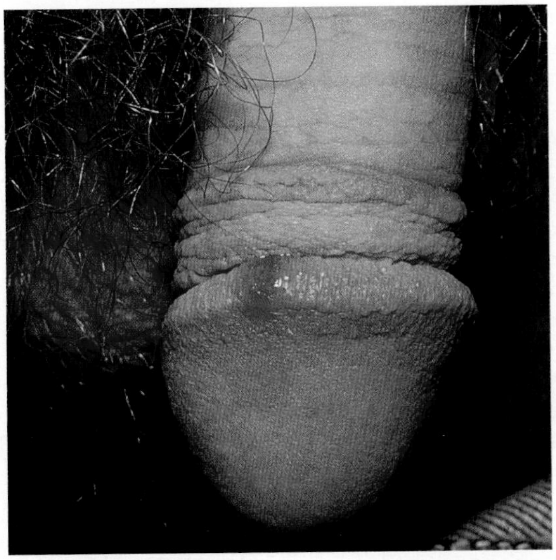

FIGURE 9-32. **Syphilitic chancre.** A patient with primary syphilis displays a raised, erythematous penile lesion.

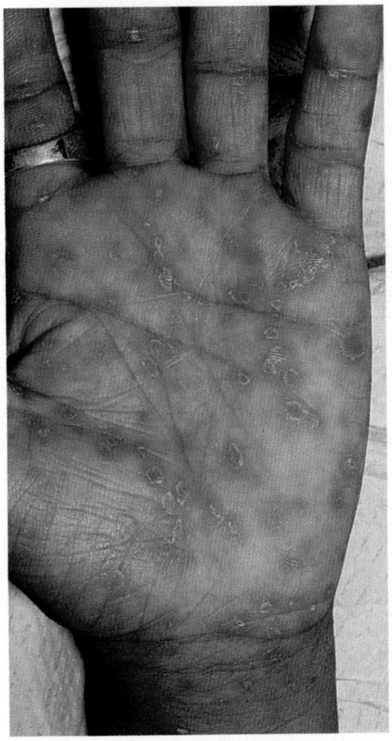

FIGURE 9-33. **Secondary syphilis.** A maculopapular rash is present on the palm.

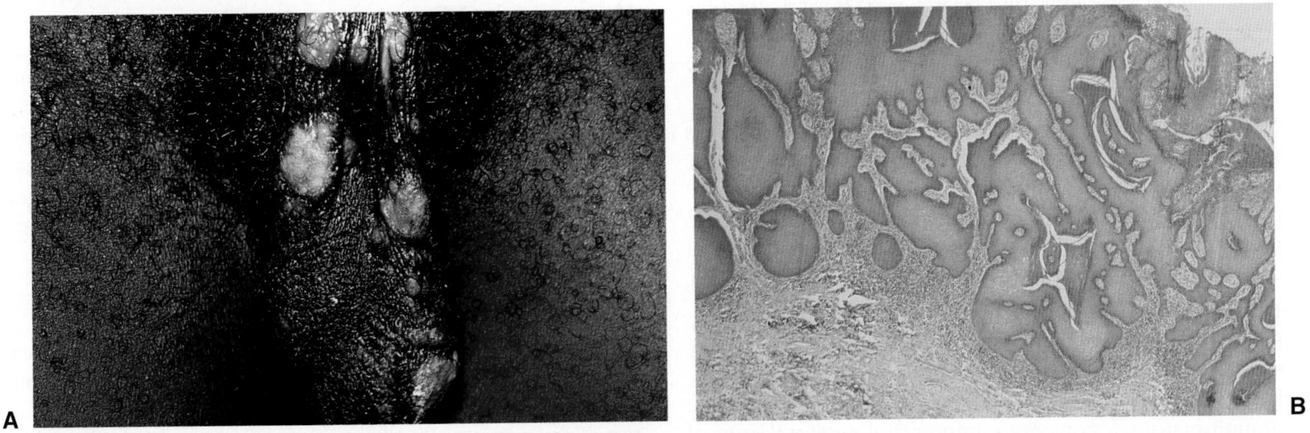

FIGURE 9-34. **Condylomata lata in secondary syphilis. A.** Whitish plaques are seen on the vulva and perineum. **B.** A photomicrograph shows papillomatous hyperplasia of the epidermis with underlying chronic inflammation.

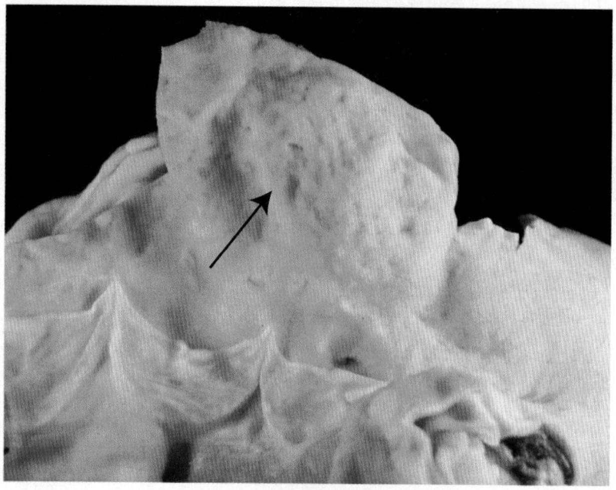

FIGURE 9-35. **Syphilitic aortitis.** The ascending aorta exhibits a roughened intima (*arrow*, "tree bark" appearance), owing to destruction of the media.

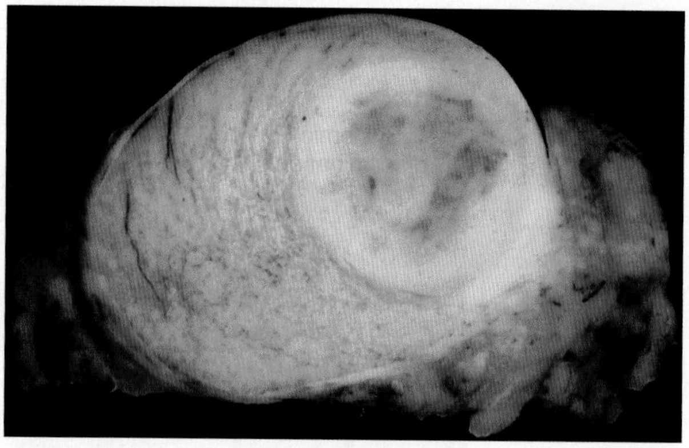

FIGURE 9-36. **Syphilitic gumma.** A patient with tertiary syphilis shows a sharply circumscribed gumma in the testis, characterized by a fibrogranulomatous wall and a necrotic center.

continue to multiply and the deep-seated lesions of tertiary syphilis gradually develop in one third of untreated patients. *Focal ischemic necrosis secondary to obliterative endarteritis is the underlying mechanism for many of the processes associated with tertiary syphilis.* *T. pallidum* induces a mononuclear inflammatory infiltrate predominantly composed of lymphocytes and plasma cells. These cells infiltrate small arteries and arterioles, producing a characteristic obstructive vascular lesion (**endarteritis obliterans**). The small arteries are inflamed and their endothelial cells are swollen. They are surrounded by concentric layers of proliferating fibroblasts, which confer an "onion skin" appearance to the vascular lesions.

- **Syphilitic aortitis:** This lesion results from a slowly progressive endarteritis obliterans of vasa vasorum that eventually leads to necrosis of the aortic media, gradual weakening and stretching of the aortic wall, and aortic aneurysm. Syphilitic aneurysms are saccular and involve the ascending aorta, an unusual site for the much more common atherosclerotic aneurysms. On gross examination, the aortic intima is rough and pitted (**tree-bark appearance**) (Fig. 9-35) (see Chapter 10). The aortic media is gradually replaced by scar tissue, after which the aorta loses its strength and resilience. The aorta gradually stretches, becoming progressively thinner to the point of rupture, massive hemorrhage, and sudden death. *Damage to, and scarring of, the ascending aorta also commonly lead to dilation of the aortic ring, separation of the valve cusps, and regurgitation of blood through the aortic valve (aortic insufficiency).* Luetic vasculitis may narrow or occlude the coronary arteries and cause myocardial infarction.
- **Neurosyphilis:** The slowly progressive infection damages the meninges, cerebral cortex, spinal cord, cranial nerves, or eyes. Tertiary syphilis involving the CNS is subclassified according to the predominant tissue affected. Thus, there are **meningovascular syphilis** (meninges), **tabes dorsalis** (spinal cord), and **general paresis** (cerebral cortex) (see Chapter 28).
- **Benign tertiary syphilis:** The appearance of a gumma (Fig. 9-36) in any organ or tissue is the hallmark of benign tertiary syphilis. Gummas are most commonly found in the skin, bone, and joints, although they can occur anywhere. These granulomatous lesions are composed of a central area of coagulative necrosis, epithelioid macrophages, occasional giant cells, and peripheral fibrous tissue. Gummas are usually localized lesions that do not significantly damage the patient.

Congenital Syphilis is Transmitted from an Infected Mother to the Fetus

In this setting, the organism disseminates in fetal tissues, which are injured by the proliferating organisms and accompanying inflammatory response. Fetal infection produces stillbirth, neonatal illness or death, or progressive postnatal disease.

PATHOLOGY: Histopathologically, the lesions of congenital syphilis are identical to those of adult disease. Infected tissues show a chronic inflammatory infiltrate, composed of lymphocytes and plasma cells, and endarteritis obliterans. Virtually any tissue can be affected, but skin, bones, teeth, joints, liver, and CNS are characteristically involved (see Chapter 6).

CLINICAL FEATURES: The presentation of congenital syphilis is variable, and infected newborns are often asymptomatic. Early signs of infection include a rhinitis (**snuffles**) and a desquamative rash. Infection of periosteum, bone, cartilage, and dental pulp produce deformities of bones and teeth, including **saddle nose,** anterior bowing of the legs (**saber shins**), and peg-shaped upper incisor teeth (**Hutchinson teeth**). Progression of congenital syphilis can be arrested by penicillin.

Nonvenereal Treponematoses

In tropical and subtropical countries, there is a group of nonvenereal, chronic diseases that are caused by treponemes indistinguishable from *T. pallidum*. Like syphilis, they result from the inoculation of the organism into mucocutaneous surfaces. They also pass through clearly defined clinical and pathologic stages, including a primary lesion at the site of inoculation; secondary skin eruptions; a latent period; and a tertiary, late stage.

Yaws is a Tropical Disease Caused by T. pertenue

Yaws occurs among poor rural populations in warm, humid areas of tropical Africa, South America, Southeast Asia, and Oceania. Children and adolescents living in deprived tropical regions are at risk. Transmission is by skin-to-skin contact and is facilitated by breaks or abrasions. Two to 5 weeks after exposure, a single "mother yaw" appears at the site of inoculation, usually on an exposed part. The lesion begins as a papule and becomes a 2- to 5-cm "raspberry-like" papilloma. The secondary or disseminated stage begins with the eruption of similar, but smaller, yaws on other parts of the skin. Microscopically, the mother yaw and the disseminated lesions show hyperkeratosis, papillary acanthosis, and an intense neutrophilic infiltrate of the epidermis. The epidermis at the apex of the papilloma lyses to form a shallow ulcer, and plasma cells invade the upper dermis. Spirochetes are numerous in the dermal papillae.

Painful papillomas on the soles of the feet lead patients to walk on the side of their feet like a crab, a condition called *"crab yaw."* The treponemes are borne by the blood to bones, lymph nodes, and skin. There they grow during a latent period of 5 or more years. The lesions in the late stage include gummas of the skin, which are destructive to the face and upper airway. Periostitis of the tibia causes "saber shins" or "boomerang legs." A single dose of long-acting penicillin cures yaws.

Bejel Is Characterized by Gummas of the Skin, Airways, and Bone

Bejel (also known as "endemic syphilis") has a focal distribution in Africa, western Asia, and Australia. Bejel is transmitted by nonvenereal routes, such as from an infected infant to the breast of the mother, from mouth to mouth, or from utensils to the mouth and is caused by *T. pallidum* subspecies *endemicum*. Other than on the nursing breast, primary lesions are rare. Secondary lesions in the mouth are identical to the mucosal lesions of syphilis and may spread from the upper airway to the larynx. Lesions of the perineum and bone are encountered, and gummas of the breast occur.

Pinta Is a Tropical Skin Disease

Pinta (from the Spanishfor "painted" or "blemish") is a treponematosis characterized by variably colored spots on the skin. It is caused by *Treponema carateum* and prevails in remote, arid, inland regions and river valleys of the American tropics. The lesions of the three stages of pinta are limited to the skin and tend to merge. Transmission is by skin-to-skin inoculation, usually after long intimate contact with an infected person.

Lyme Disease

Lyme disease is a chronic systemic infection, which begins with a characteristic skin lesion and later manifests as cardiac, neurologic, or joint disturbances. The causative agent is *Borrelia burgdorferi,* a large, microaerophilic spirochete.

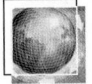

EPIDEMIOLOGY: Lyme disease was first described in patients from Lyme, Connecticut, but was later recognized in many other areas. *B. burgdorferi* is transmitted from its animal reservoir to humans by the bite of the minute *Ixodes* tick. The insect is found in wooded areas, where it usually feeds on mice and deer. Transmission to humans is most likely to occur from May through July, when nymph forms of the tick feed.

Lyme disease is a growing problem in the United States, where it has become the most common tick-borne illness, causing an estimated 15,000 to 20,000 cases annually. It is concentrated along the eastern seaboard from Maryland to Massachusetts, in the Midwest in Minnesota and Wisconsin, and in the West in California and Oregon. The disease is also present in Europe, Australia, and Asia.

PATHOLOGY AND CLINICAL FEATURES: *B. burgdorferi* reproduces locally at the site of inoculation, spreads to regional lymph nodes, and is disseminated throughout the body in the bloodstream. Like other spirochetal diseases, Lyme disease is chronic, occurring in stages, with remissions and exacerbations. Studies of skin and synovium have shown that *B. burgdorferi* elicits a chronic inflammatory infiltrate, composed of lymphocytes and plasma cells. In patients who died of the disease, organisms have been seen at autopsy in virtually every organ affected, including skin, myocardium, liver, CNS, and the musculoskeletal system.

Lyme disease is a prolonged illness in which three clinical stages are described.

- **Stage 1:** The characteristic skin lesion, **erythema chronicum migrans,** appears at the site of the tick bite. It begins 3 to 35 days after the bite as an erythematous macule or papule, which grows into an erythematous patch 3 to 7 cm in diameter. It often is intensely red at its periphery, with some central clearing, imparting an annular appearance. Erythema chronicum migrans is accompanied by fever, fatigue, headache, arthralgias, and regional lymphadenopathy. Secondary annular skin lesions develop in about half of patients and may persist for long periods. During this phase, patients experience constant malaise and fatigue, headache, and fever. Intermittent manifestations may also include meningeal irritation, migratory myalgia, cough, generalized lymphadenopathy, and testicular swelling.
- **Stage 2:** The second stage begins within several weeks to months of the skin lesion and is characterized by exacerbation of migratory musculoskeletal pains and cardiac and neurologic abnormalities. In 10% of cases, conduction abnormalities, particularly atrioventricular block, result from myocarditis. Neurologic abnormalities, most commonly meningitis and facial nerve palsies, occur in 15% of patients.
- **Stage 3:** The third stage of Lyme disease begins months to years afterwards, and is manifested by joint, skin, and neurologic abnormalities. Joint abnormalities develop in over half of infected persons and include severe arthritis of the large joints, especially the knee. The histopathology of affected joints is virtually indistinguishable from that of rheumatoid arthritis, with villous hypertrophy and a conspicuous mononuclear infiltrate in the subsynovial lining area.

It is now recognized that neurologic manifestations may begin months to years after the disease begins. They range from intermittent tingling paresthesias without demonstrable neurologic deficits to slowly progressive encephalomyelitis, transverse myelitis, organic brain syndromes, and dementia. There is a distinctive late skin manifestation of Lyme disease, acrodermatitis chronica atrophicans, which occurs years after erythema chronicum migrans and presents as patchy atrophy and sclerosis of the skin.

The diagnosis of Lyme disease is established by culturing *B. burgdorferi* from infected patients, but the yield is low. Therefore, the determination of antibody titers (initially IgM and later IgG) against the organism remains the most practical way to establish the diagnosis. Treatment with tetracycline or erythromycin is effective in eliminating early Lyme disease. In later stages and when there are extensive extracutaneous manifestations, high doses of intravenous penicillin G and other combinations of antibiotic regimens for long periods are necessary.

LEPTOSPIROSIS

Leptospirosis is an infection with spirochetes of the genus Leptospira, *which is for the most part (90% of patients) a mild, self-limited, febrile disease. In persons with more severe infections, hepatic and renal failure may prove fatal.*

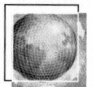

EPIDEMIOLOGY: Leptospirosis is a zoonosis of worldwide distribution. Leptospires penetrate abraded skin or mucous membranes following contact with infected rats, contaminated water, or mud. Since warm, moist environments favor survival of the spirochetes, the incidence is higher in the tropics. Between 30 and 100 cases of leptospirosis are reported annually in the United States, some of them in slaughterhouse workers and trappers, but recently some cases were reported among destitute persons in urban areas.

PATHOLOGY AND CLINICAL FEATURES: The symptoms of leptospirosis begin 4 days to 3 weeks after exposure to *Leptospira interrogans*. In most cases, the disease resolves within a week without sequelae. In more severe infections, leptospirosis is a biphasic disease.

- The **leptospiremic phase** is characterized by the presence of leptospires in the blood and cerebrospinal fluid. There is an abrupt onset of fever, shaking chills, headache, and myalgias. After 1 to 2 weeks, the symptoms abate as the leptospires disappear from the blood and bodily fluids.
- The **immune phase,** which begins within 3 days of the end of the leptospiremic phase, is accompanied by the production of IgM antibodies. The earlier symptoms recur, and signs of meningeal irritation become apparent. At this time, the cerebrospinal fluid shows a prominent pleiocytosis. In severe cases, jaundice appears and may be followed by hepatic and renal failure and the appearance of widespread hemorrhages and shock. This severe form of leptospirosis has historically been referred to as **Weil disease**.

Untreated Weil disease carries a mortality rate of 5% to 30%. At autopsy the tissues are bile-stained, and hemorrhages are observed in many organs. Microscopically, the principal lesion is a diffuse vasculitis with capillary injury. The liver shows dissociation of the liver cell plates, erythrophagocytosis by Kupffer cells, minimal necrosis of hepatocytes, neutrophils in the sinusoids, and a mixed inflammatory cell infiltrate in the portal tracts. The kidneys display swollen and necrotic tubules. Spirochetes are numerous in the lumina of the tubules and particularly in bile-stained casts (Fig. 9-37).

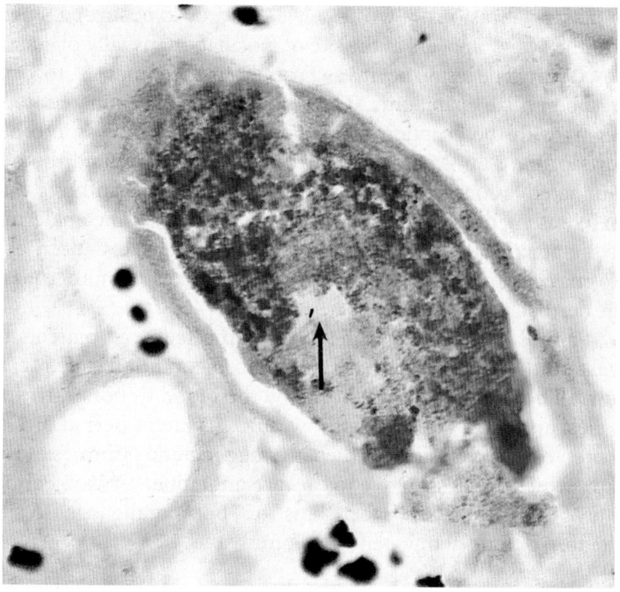

FIGURE 9-37. **Leptospirosis.** A distal renal tubule is obstructed by a bile-stained mass of hemoglobin and cellular debris. A leptospire *(arrow)* is in the center of this mass.

Relapsing Fever

Relapsing fever is an acute, febrile, septicemic illness caused by spirochetes of the genus Borrelia. There are two main types of relapsing fever:

- **Epidemic relapsing fever** is caused by *Borrelia recurrentis* and is transmitted by the bite of an infected louse. Humans are the only reservoir.
- **Endemic relapsing fever** is produced by a number of *Borrelia* species and is transmitted from rodents and other animals by the bite of an infected tick.

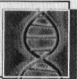

EPIDEMIOLOGY AND PATHOGENESIS: The human body louse, *Pediculus humanus humanus,* becomes infected with *B. recurrentis* when it feeds on an infected person. The spirochetes cross the gut wall of the louse into the hemolymph, where they multiply. Here they remain, unless the louse is crushed when feeding. If this occurs, the borrelliae escape and penetrate at the site of the bite or even through the intact skin. War, crowded migrant worker camps, and heavy clothing during cold weather all favor mobilization of lice and the spread of relapsing fever. Furthermore, lice dislike the higher temperatures of the feverish victims and seek new hosts, another factor in the rapid spread of relapsing fever during epidemics. Louse-borne relapsing fever is currently encountered in a number of African countries, especially Ethiopia and Sudan, and is also seen in the South American Andes.

In endemic, tick-borne relapsing fever, ticks are infected while biting rats and other hosts. The borrelliae grow in the hemocoelom of the tick and invade other tissues, including the salivary glands. Humans are infected by saliva or coxal fluid of the tick. Ticks have a considerably longer life span than lice and may harbor spirochetes for 12 to 15 years without a blood meal. Tick-borne relapsing fever occurs sporadically worldwide.

PATHOLOGY: In fatal infections, the spleen is enlarged and contains miliary microabscesses. Spirochetes form tangled aggregates around the necrotic centers. Lymphocytes and neutrophils infiltrate central and midzonal areas of the liver, where spirochetes lie free in the sinusoids. Focal hemorrhages involve many organs.

CLINICAL FEATURES: Following the bite of an infected arthropod, fever, headache, myalgias, arthralgias, and lethargy appear within 1 to 2 weeks. The liver and spleen enlarge, and there are petechiae of the skin, conjunctival hemorrhages, and abdominal tenderness. Within 3 to 9 days after the onset of symptoms, the fever ends abruptly, only to begin 7 to 10 days later. During the afebrile period, the spirochetes disappear from the blood and change their antigenic coats. With each relapse, the symptoms are milder and the duration of illness is shorter. In severe cases, the initial episode may be characterized by a rash, meningitis, myocarditis, liver failure, and coma. Tetracycline is an effective treatment for both types of relapsing fever.

Fusospirochetal Infections

Tropical Phagedenic Ulcer Is a Painful Lesion of the Leg

Tropical phagedenic (rapid spreading and sloughing) ulcer, also known as **tropical foot,** is a painful, necrotizing lesion of the skin and subcutaneous tissues of the leg that afflicts persons in tropical climates. Although flora in the ulcers are often mixed, bacteriologic studies indicate *Bacillus fusiformis* and *Treponema vincentii* to be causal. Malnutrition may predispose to infection.

PATHOLOGY AND CLINICAL FEATURES: The lesion usually starts on the skin at a point of trauma and develops rapidly. The surface sloughs to form an ulcer with raised borders and a cup-shaped crater, which contains a gray, putrid exudates (Fig. 9-38). The ulcer may be so deep that the underlying bone and tendons are exposed. The margin becomes fibrotic, but complete healing may be delayed for years. In addition to secondary infection, tibial osteomyelitis and squamous cell carcinoma may be late complications. Antibiotics may be effective, but reconstructive plastic surgery is often necessary to close the defect.

Noma Is a Destructive Lesion of the Face

Noma (gangrenous stomatitis, cancrum oris) is a rapidly progressive necrosis of soft tissues and bones of the mouth and face and, less commonly, of such other sites as the chest, limbs, and genitalia. It afflicts malnourished children in the tropics, many of whom are further debilitated by recent infections (e.g., measles, malaria, leishmaniasis). A variety of bacteria may be recovered from these lesions, but *Treponema vincentii,*

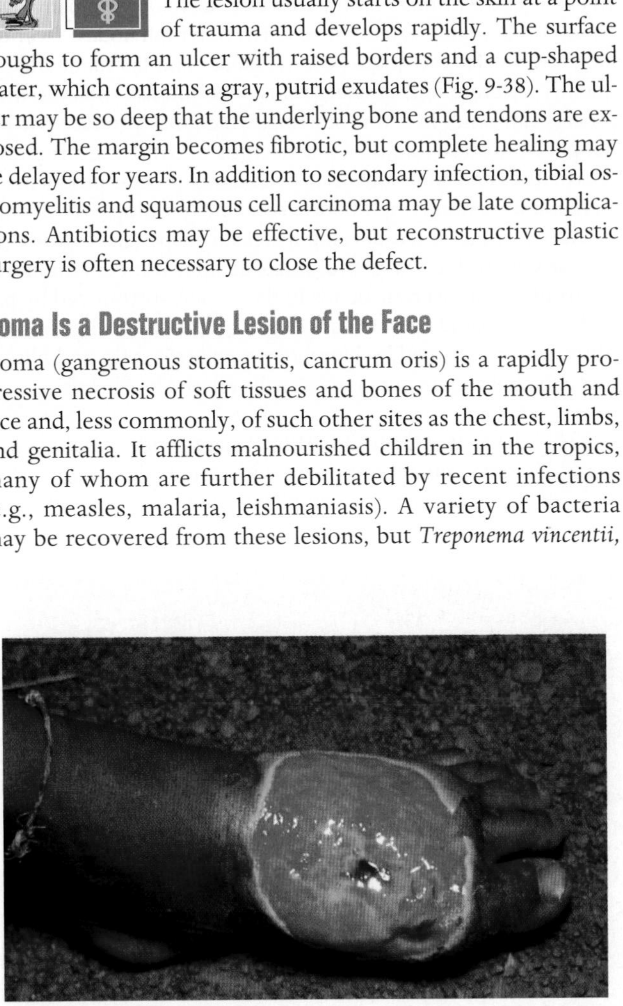

FIGURE 9-38. Tropical phagedenic ulcer caused by infection by fusospirochetal organisms, following penetrating trauma.

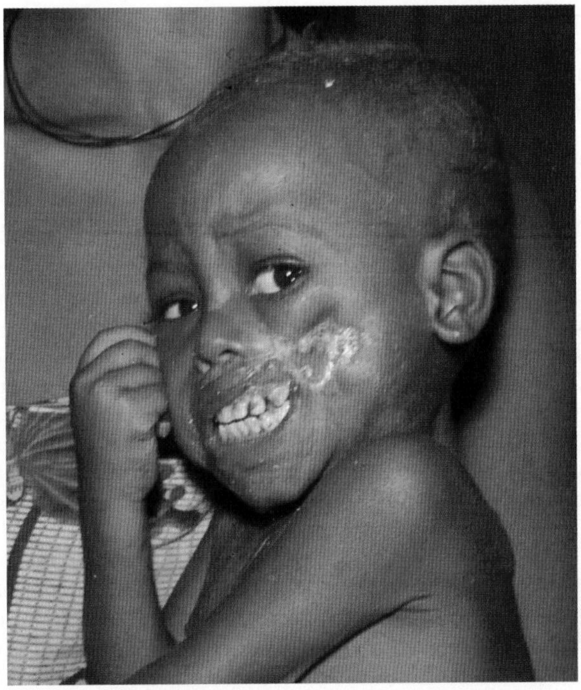

FIGURE 9-39. **Noma.** There is massive destruction of the soft tissues and bones of the mouth and cheek.

Bacillus fusiformis, Bacteroides spp., and *Corynebacterium* spp. tend to predominate.

PATHOLOGY AND CLINICAL FEATURES: The ulcer is destructive, disfiguring and usually unilateral (Fig. 9-39). Initially it is a small papule, often on the cheek opposite the molars or premolars. Large malodorous defects quickly develop. The lesions are painful and advanced lesions reveal necrosis of skin, muscle, and adipose tissue, with exposure of underlying bone. Without treatment, patients usually die. Antibiotics are helpful, but reconstructive surgery is often required.

CHLAMYDIAL INFECTIONS

Chlamydiae are obligate intracellular parasites that are smaller than most other bacteria. They lack the enzymatic capacity to generate adenosine triphosphate (ATP) and must parasitize the metabolic machinery of a host cell to reproduce. The chlamydial life cycle involves two distinct morphologic forms. The **elementary body** is the smaller, metabolically inactive form, which survives extracellularly. It attaches to the appropriate host cell and induces endocytosis, forming a vacuole. It then transforms into the larger, metabolically active form, the **reticulate body,** which commandeers host cell metabolism to fuel chlamydial replication. The reticulate body divides repeatedly, forming daughter elementary bodies and destroying the host cell. Necrotic debris elicits inflammatory and immunologic responses that further damage infected tissue.

Chlamydial infections are widespread among birds and mammals and as many as 20% of humans are infected. Three species of chlamydiae (Chlamydia *trachomatis,* Chlamydia *psittaci,* and Chlamydia *pneumoniae*) cause human infection.

Chlamydia Trachomatis Infection

The species *C. trachomatis* contains a variety of strains (serovars), which cause three distinct types of disease: (1) genital and neonatal disease, (2) lymphogranuloma venereum, and (3) trachoma.

Genital and Neonatal Infections with C. trachomatis Are among the Most Common Sexually Transmitted Diseases

C. trachomatis *serovars D through K cause genital epithelial infection* that is the most common sexually contracted disease in North America. In men, it produces urethritis and sometimes epididymitis or proctitis. In women, it usually begins with cervicitis, which can progress to endometritis, salpingitis, and generalized infection of the pelvic adnexal organs (pelvic inflammatory disease). Repeated episodes of salpingitis are associated with scarring, which cause scarring and lead to infertility or ectopic pregnancy. Perinatal transmission of *C. trachomatis* causes neonatal conjunctivitis and pneumonia.

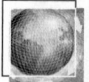

EPIDEMIOLOGY: The organism spreads from person to person in genital secretions. Infection is chronic and frequently asymptomatic, providing an enormous reservoir for transmission. As with all sexually transmitted diseases, persons with the largest number of sexual partners are at greatest risk of infection. Newborns acquire the organism by contact with infected endocervical secretions on passage through an infected birth canal. Two thirds of exposed newborns develop *C. trachomatis* conjunctivitis.

PATHOLOGY: Chlamydial infection elicits an infiltrate of neutrophils and lymphocytes. Lymphoid aggregates, with or without germinal centers, may appear at the site of infection. In newborns, the conjunctival epithelium often contains characteristic vacuolar cytoplasmic inclusions, and the disease is frequently called **inclusion conjunctivitis**. Most genital infections are asymptomatic. In men, clinically apparent infection presents as a purulent penile discharge, with dysuria and urinary urgency. Chlamydial cervicitis causes a mucopurulent drainage from the cervical os.

CLINICAL FEATURES: Chlamydial disease in the newborn presents as reddened conjunctivae with a watery or purulent discharge. Untreated neonatal conjunctivitis is potentially serious, although it may resolve without sequelae. Chlamydial pneumonia manifests in the second or third month with tachypnea and paroxysmal cough, usually without fever. Inclusion conjunctivitis is treated with systemic or topical antibiotics.

Lymphogranuloma Venereum is a Sexually Transmitted Disease that Causes Necrotizing Lymphadenitis

Lymphogranuloma venereum begins as a genital ulcer, spreads lymph nodes (Fig. 9-40A), *and may cause local scarring.* It is caused by *C. trachomatis* serovars L1 to L3.

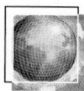

EPIDEMIOLOGY: Lymphogranuloma venereum is uncommon in developed countries, but is endemic in the tropics and subtropics. It accounts for 5% of sexually transmitted disease in Africa, India, parts of southeast Asia, South America, and the Caribbean. In North America and Europe, it is primarily a disease of homosexual men.

PATHOLOGY: The organism is introduced through a break in the skin. After an incubation period of 4 to 21 days, an ulcer appears, usually on the penis, vagina, or cervix, although lips, tongue, and fingers may also be primary sites. The organisms are transported by lymphatics to regional lymph nodes, where a necrotizing lymphadenitis erupts 1 to 3 weeks after the primary lesion. Abscesses develop within involved lymph nodes, often extending to adjacent lymph nodes. Over the next few weeks, the nodes become tender and fluctuant and frequently ulcerate and discharge pus. The intense inflammatory process can result in severe scarring, which may produce chronic lymphatic obstruction, ischemic necrosis of overlying structures, or strictures and adhesions. The necrotizing process produces enlarged and matted lymph nodes, containing multiple, coalescing abscesses, which often develop a stellate shape (see Fig. 9-40B). The abscesses have a granulomatous appearance, containing neutrophils and necrotic debris in the center, surrounded by palisading epithelioid cells, macrophages, and occasional giant cells. Abscesses are rimmed by lymphocytes, plasma cells, and fibrous tissue. Nodal architecture is eventually effaced by fibrosis.

CLINICAL FEATURES: Patients with lymphogranuloma venereum present with lymphadenopathy. Most infections resolve completely, even without antimicro-

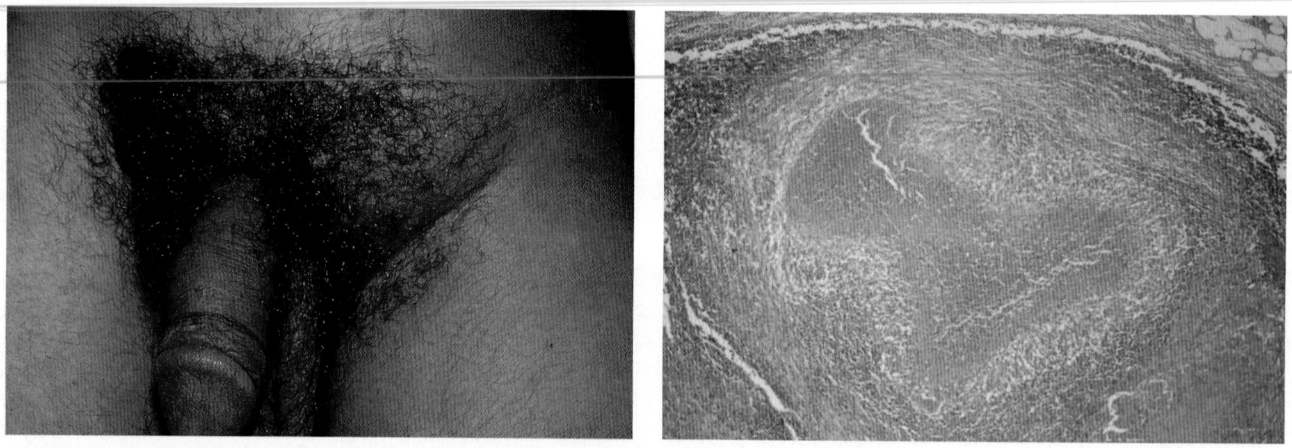

A B

FIGURE 9-40. **Lymphogranuloma venereum. A.** Painful inguinal lymphadenopathy in a man infected with *C. trachomatis*. **B.** Microscopic section of a lymph node shows a necrotic central area surrounded by a granulomatous zone.

bial therapy. However, progressive ulceration of the penis, urethra, or scrotum, with fistulas and urethral stricture, develop in 5% of men. Women and homosexual men often present with hemorrhagic proctitis, and most late complications, such as rectal stricture, rectovaginal fistulas, and genital elephantiasis, occur in women.

Trachoma Is a Leading Cause of Blindness in Many Developing Countries

Trachoma is a chronic infection that causes progressive scars of the conjunctiva and cornea. C. trachomatis serovars A, B, Ba and C cause the disease.

EPIDEMIOLOGY: Trachoma is worldwide, associated with poverty, and most prevalent in dry or sandy regions. Only humans are naturally infected, and poor personal hygiene and inadequate public sanitation are common factors. Trachoma remains a major problem in parts of Africa, India, and the Middle East. The infection is spread mostly by direct contact, but may also be transmitted by fomites, contaminated water, and probably flies. Subclinical infections are an important reservoir. In endemic areas, infection is acquired early in childhood, becomes chronic, and eventually progresses to blindness.

PATHOLOGY: When *C. trachomatis* is inoculated into the eye, it reproduces in the conjunctival epithelium, inciting a mixed acute and chronic inflammatory infiltrate. Histologic examination of early lesions shows chronic inflammation, lymphoid aggregates, focal degeneration, and chlamydial inclusions in the conjunctiva. As trachoma progresses, lymphoid aggregates enlarge and the conjunctiva becomes scarred and focally hypertrophic. The cornea is invaded by blood vessels and fibroblasts, forming a scar reminiscent of a cloth ("pannus" in Latin), and is eventually opacified.

CLINICAL FEATURES: Early trachoma is characterized by abrupt onset of palpebral and conjunctival inflammation, which leads to tearing, purulent conjunctivitis, and photophobia. The lymphoid aggregates appear as small yellow grains beneath the palpebral conjunctivae within 3 to 4 weeks of infection. After months or years, eyelid deformities eventually interfere with normal ocular function and secondary bacterial infections and corneal ulcerations are common. Blindness is a common end point.

Psittacosis (Ornithosis)

Psittacosis is a self-limited pneumonia transmitted to humans from birds. The causative agent, *Chlamydia psittaci,* is spread by infected birds, and the resulting disease is known as both psittacosis (association with parrots) or ornithosis (contact with birds in general).

EPIDEMIOLOGY: *C. psittaci* is present in the blood, tissues, excreta, and feathers of infected birds. Humans inhale infectious excreta or dust from feathers. Although infection is endemic in tropical birds, *C. psittaci* can infect almost any species. Human disease has resulted from exposure to various bird species, including parrots, parakeets, canaries, pigeons, sea gulls, ducks, chickens, and turkeys. Use of tetracycline-containing bird feeds and quarantine of imported tropical birds limits the spread of disease, and fewer than 50 cases of psittacosis are reported annually in the United States.

PATHOLOGY: *C. psittaci* first infects pulmonary macrophages, which carry the organism to the phagocytic cells of the liver and spleen, where it reproduces. The organism is then distributed by the bloodstream, producing systemic infection, particularly diffuse involvement of the lungs. *C. psittaci* reproduces in alveolar lining cells, whose destruction elicits an inflammatory response.

The pneumonia is predominantly interstitial, with an interstitial lymphocytic inflammatory infiltrate. Type II pneumocytes are hyperplastic and may show characteristic chlamydial cytoplasmic inclusions. In severe pulmonary disease, hemorrhage and fibrin fill the alveoli and bacterial superinfection may produce multiple abscesses. Dissemination of the infection is characterized by foci of necrosis in the liver and spleen and diffuse mononuclear cell infiltrates in the heart, kidneys, and brain.

CLINICAL FEATURES: The spectrum of clinical illness varies widely. There is usually a persistent dry cough, with constitutional symptoms of high fever, headache, malaise, myalgias, and arthralgias. Untreated, fever persists for 2 to 3 weeks and then subsides as the pulmonary disease regresses. With tetracycline therapy, the disease is rarely fatal.

Chlamydia Pneumoniae

Chlamydia pneumoniae *is a causes acute, self-limited, usually mild respiratory tract infections, including pneumonia.* It is transmitted from person to person, and infection appears to be very common. In the developed world, half of all adults show evidence of past exposure, but only 10% of infections cause clinical pneumonia. Symptomatic persons complain of fever, sore throat, and cough. Severe pneumonia occurs only if there is an underlying pulmonary condition. Untreated disease usually resolves in 2 to 4 weeks.

RICKETTSIAL INFECTIONS

The rickettsiae are small, gram-negative coccobacillary bacteria that are obligate intracellular pathogens and cannot replicate outside a host. Rickettsiae can synthesize their own ATP via a proton-translocating ATPase and can also obtain ATP from the host through the ATP/adenosine diphosphate (ADP) translocase. The organisms induce endocytosis by target cells and replicate within the cytoplasm of the host cell. They have the cell wall structure of gram-negative bacteria but, unlike chlamydiae, replicate by binary fission. Although structurally gram-negative, the rickettsiae do not stain well with the Gram stain and are best demonstrated by the Gimenez method or with acridine orange.

Humans are accidental hosts for most species of *Rickettsia.* The organisms reside in animals and insects and do not require humans for perpetuation. Human rickettsial infection results from insect bites. Several species of *Rickettsia* cause different human diseases (Table 9-6), but rickettsial infections have many features in common. *The human target cell for all rickettsiae is the endothelial cell of capillaries and other small blood vessels.* The organisms reproduce within these cells, killing them in the process and producing a necrotizing vasculitis. Human rickettsial infections are traditionally divided into the "spotted fever group" and the "typhus group."

TABLE 9-6

Rickettsial Infections

Disease	Organism	Distribution	Transmission
	Spotted-fever group (genus *Rickettsia*)		
Rocky Mountain spotted fever	*R. rickettsii*	Americas	Ticks
Queensland tick fever	*R. australis*	Australia	Ticks
Boutonneuse fever, Kenya tick fever	*R. conorii*	Mediterranean, Africa, India	Ticks
Siberian tick fever	*R. sibirica*	Siberia, Mongolia	Ticks
Rickettsialpox	*R. akari*	United States, Russia, Central Asia, Korea, Africa	Mites
	Typhus group		
Louse-borne typhus (epidemic typhus)	*R. prowazekii*	Latin America, Africa, Asia	Lice
Murine typhus (endemic typhus)	*R. typhi*	Worldwide	Fleas
Scrub typhus	*R. tsutsugamushi*	South Pacific, Asia	Mites
Q fever	*Coxiella burnetti*	Worldwide	Inhalation

Rocky Mountain Spotted Fever

Rocky Mountain spotted fever is an acute, potentially fatal, systemic vasculitis, usually manifested by headache, fever, and rash. The causative organism, *Rickettsia rickettsii*, is transmitted to humans by tick bites.

EPIDEMIOLOGY: Rocky Mountain spotted fever is acquired by bites of infected ticks, which are the vectors for *R. rickettsii*. The organism passes from mother to progeny ticks without killing them, thereby maintaining a natural reservoir for human infection. Rocky Mountain spotted fever occurs in various areas throughout North, Central, and South America. About 500 cases occur annually in the United State, mostly from the eastern seaboard (Georgia to New York) westward to Texas, Oklahoma, and Kansas. Its name derives from its discovery in Idaho, but the disease is uncommon in the Rocky Mountain region.

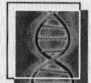

PATHOGENESIS: *R. rickettsii* in salivary glands of ticks is introduced into the skin while the ticks feed. The organisms spread via lymphatics and small blood vessels to the systemic and pulmonary circulation. Here they attach to vascular endothelial cells, are engulfed, and reproduce within the cytoplasm. They are then shed into the vascular and lymphatic systems. Further infection and destruction of vascular endothelium causes a systemic vasculitis. The rash, produced by inflammatory damage to cutaneous vessels, is the most visible manifestation of the generalized phenomenon of vascular injury. Whereas other rickettsiae infect only capillary endothelial cells, *R. rickettsii* spreads to vascular smooth muscle and endothelium of larger vessels. Extensive damage to blood vessel walls causes loss of vascular integrity, exudation of fluid, and disseminated intravascular coagulation. Fluid loss can be so extensive that it leads to shock. Damage to pulmonary capillaries can produce pulmonary edema and acute alveolar injury.

PATHOLOGY: The vascular lesions of Rocky Mountain spotted fever are seen throughout the body, affecting capillaries, venules, arterioles, and sometimes larger vessels. Necrosis and reactive hyperplasia of vascular endothelium are often associated with thrombosis of the smaller-caliber vessels. Vessel walls are infiltrated, initially with neutrophils and macrophages, and later with lymphocytes and plasma cells. Microscopic infarctions and extravasation of blood into surrounding tissues are common. The orientation of the intracellular bacilli in parallel rows and in an end-to-end pattern gives them the appearance of a "flotilla at anchor facing the wind."

CLINICAL FEATURES: Rocky Mountain spotted fever manifests with fever, headache and myalgias, followed by a rash. Skin lesions begin as a maculopapular eruption but rapidly become petechial, spreading centripetally from the distal extremities to the trunk (Fig. 9-41). Cutaneous lesions usually appear on the palms and soles, a distinctive feature of the disease. If untreated, more than 20% to 50% of infected persons die within 8 to 15 days. Prompt diagnosis and antibiotic treatment (chloramphenicol and tetracycline) is life saving: mortality in the United States is less than 5%.

Epidemic (Louse-Borne) Typhus

Epidemic typhus is a severe systemic vasculitis transmitted by the bite of infected lice. The disease is caused by *Rickettsia prowazekii*, an organism that has a human-louse-human life cycle (Fig. 9-42).

EPIDEMIOLOGY: *R. prowazekii* is transmitted from one infected person to another by the bite of an infected body louse. The disease is widely distributed in some regions of Africa, Asia, Europe, and the Western Hemisphere. Devastating epidemics of typhus were associated with cold climates, poor sanitation, and crowding during natural disasters, famine, or war. Infrequent bathing and lack of changes of clothing lead to louse infestation of human populations and consequently epidemics of typhus. With the mass displacements of populations in Eastern Europe in World War I, epidemic typhus affected over 30 million persons, killing over 3 million. Epidemic louse-borne typhus last occurred in the United States in 1921.

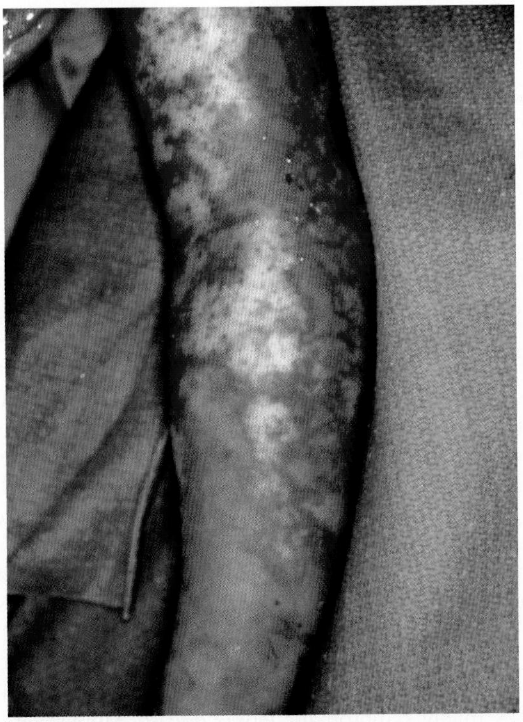

FIGURE 9-41. **Rocky mountain spotted fever.** A severe petechial and purpuric eruption is noted on the arm in this fatal case.

PATHOGENESIS: After a louse takes a blood meal from a person infected with *R. prowazekii*, the organisms enter the epithelial cells of the midgut, multiply and rupture the cells within 3 to 5 days. Large numbers of rickettsiae are released into the lumen of the louse intestine. The louse deposits its contaminated feces on the skin or clothing of a second host, where they may remain infectious for more than 3 months. A person becomes infected when the contaminated louse feces penetrate an abrasion or scratch or when the person inhales airborne rickettsiae from clothing containing louse feces. Epidemic typhus begins with localized infection of capillary endothelium and progresses to a systemic vasculitis. Louse-borne typhus differs from the other rickettsial diseases in that *R. prowazekii* can establish latent infection and produce recrudescent disease (Brill-Zinsser disease) many years after primary infection.

PATHOLOGY: The pathology produced by *R. prowazekii* is similar to Rocky Mountain spotted fever and other rickettsial diseases. At autopsy, there are few gross findings except for splenomegaly and occasional areas of necrosis. Microscopically, collections of mononuclear cells are found in various organs (e.g., skin, brain, and heart). The infiltrate includes mast cells, lymphocytes, plasma cells, and macrophages, frequently arranged as **typhus nodules** around arterioles and capillaries. Throughout the body, the endothelium of small blood vessels is focally necrotic and hyperplastic and the walls contain inflammatory cells. Rickettsiae can be demonstrated within the endothelial cells.

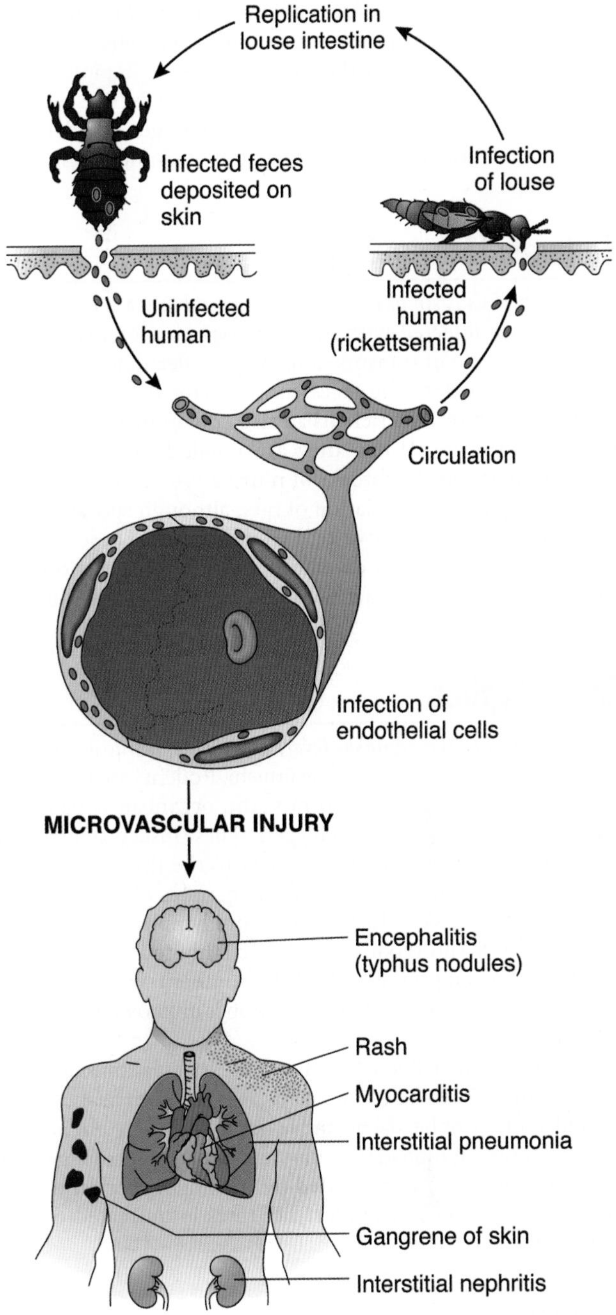

FIGURE 9-42. **Epidemic typhus (louse-borne typhus).** *Rickettsia prowazekii* has a man-louse-man life cycle. The organism multiplies in endothelial cells, which detach, rupture and release organisms into the circulation (rickettsemia). A louse taking a blood meal becomes infected with rickettsiae, which enter the epithelial cells of its midgut, multiply, and rupture the cells, thereby releasing rickettsiae into the lumen of the louse intestine. Contaminated feces are deposited on the skin or clothing of a second host, penetrate an abrasion or are inhaled. The rickettsiae then enter endothelial cells, multiply and rupture the cells, thus completing the cycle.

CLINICAL FEATURES: Louse-borne typhus is characterized by fever, headache, and myalgias, followed by a rash. Macular lesions, which become petechial, appear on the upper trunk and axillary folds and spread centrifugally to the extremities. In fatal cases, the rash commonly becomes confluent and purpuric. Mild rickettsial pneumonia is followed by a superimposed bacterial pneumonia. Dying patients may exhibit the symptoms of encephalitis, myocarditis, interstitial pneumonia, interstitial nephritis, and shock. Fatalities usually occur during the second or third week of illness. In patients who recover, the symptoms abate after about 3 weeks.

Epidemic typhus can be controlled by large-scale delousing of the population, by steam sterilization of clothing, and use of insecticides.

Endemic (Murine) Typhus

Endemic typhus is similar to epidemic typhus but tends to be milder. Humans are infected with *Rickettsia typhi* by interrupting the rat-flea-rat cycle of transmission. When a flea defecates on the surface of the skin, the feces contaminate the small wound made by the bite. The rickettsiae also contaminate clothes and become airborne. When they are inhaled, they cause pulmonary infection. Outbreaks of murine typhus are associated with an exploding population of rats, although sporadic infections occur in the southwestern United States. These are associated with rat-infested dwellings and with occupations that bring humans into contact with rats, such as the handling and storage of grain.

Scrub Typhus

*Scrub typhus (**Tsutsugamushi fever**) is an acute, febrile illness of humans caused by* Rickettsia tsutsugamushi. Rodents are the natural mammalian reservoir. From rats, the organism is passed to trombiculid mites known as chiggers. These insects transmit the infection to their larvae, which crawl to the tips of vegetation and attach to passers-by. While feeding, mites inoculate the organisms into the skin. Rickettsemia and lymphadenopathy follow shortly. Scrub typhus is widely distributed in eastern and southern Asia and the islands of the southern and western Pacific, including Japan. Endemic infection is unknown in the western world.

A multiloculated vesicle forms at the inoculation site and ulcerates, after which an eschar forms. As the lesion heals, there is a sudden onset of headache and fever, followed by pneumonia, a macular rash, lymphadenopathy, and hepatosplenomegaly. Severe infections are complicated by meningoencephalitis, myocarditis, and shock. The mortality rates in untreated patients have ranged up to 30%.

Q Fever

Q fever is a self-limited, systemic infection, usually manifesting as headache, fever, and myalgias. The disease is caused by *Coxiella burnetii*, a small pleomorphic coccobacillus with a gram-negative cell wall. Unlike true rickettsiae, *C. burnetii* enters cells by a passive mechanism, being phagocytized by macrophages. *C. burnetii* infection does not produce a vasculitis, and thus there is no associated rash.

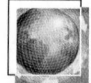

EPIDEMIOLOGY: Humans acquire Q fever by exposure to infected animals or animal products. Infection is endemic in many wild and domesticated animals, but cattle, sheep, and goats are the usual sources of human infection. These animals shed large numbers of organisms in urine, feces, milk, bodily fluids, and birth products. Q fever is most often seen in herders, slaughterhouse workers, veterinarians, dairy workers, and other persons with occupational exposure to infected domesticated animals. Aerosol droplets may spread the infection from person to person. Q fever is rare in the United States.

PATHOLOGY: Q fever begins with inhalation of organisms, which are phagocytosed by alveolar macrophages and replicate in phagolysosomes. Recruitment of neutrophils and macrophages produces a focal bronchopneumonia. The nonactivated phagocytes fail to kill *C. burnetii*, and the organism disseminates through the body, primarily infecting monocytes and/macrophages. Most infections resolve with the onset of specific cell-mediated immunity, but occasional cases persist as chronic infections.

The lungs and liver are the organs most prominently involved in Q fever. The lungs demonstrate single or multiple irregular areas of consolidation, in which the pulmonary parenchyma is infiltrated by neutrophils and macrophages. Organisms may be demonstrated in macrophages by the Giemsa stain. Hepatic involvement in Q fever is usually characterized by multiple microscopic granulomas, which have a distinctive "fibrin ring" or "doughnut ring" configuration. In these granulomas, epithelioid macrophages encircle a ring of fibrin, sometimes containing a lipid vacuole.

CLINICAL FEATURES: Q fever is usually a self-limited mildly symptomatic febrile disease. More-severe cases may present with headache, fever, fatigue, and myalgias, with no rash. Pulmonary infection is virtually always present, but it may appear as an atypical pneumonia with dry cough, a rapidly progressive pneumonia or chest roentgenographic abnormalities without significant respiratory symptoms. Many patients have some hepatosplenomegaly. The disease resolves spontaneously in 2 to 14 days.

MYCOPLASMAL INFECTIONS

At less than 0.3 μm in greatest dimension, mycoplasmas are the smallest free-living **prokaryotes**. They lack the rigid cell walls of more complex bacteria. Mycoplasmas are widespread, both geographically and ecologically, as saprophytes and as parasites of many animals and plants. Numerous *Mycoplasma* species inhabit the human body, but only three are pathogenic: *Mycoplasma pneumoniae, Mycoplasma hominis,* and *Ureaplasma urealyticum*. The diseases associated with these organisms are shown in Table 9-7.

TABLE 9-7
Mycoplasmal Infections

Organism	Disease
Mycoplasma pneumoniae	Tracheobronchitis Pneumonia Pharyngitis Otitis media
Ureaplasma urealyticum	Urethritis Chorioamnionitis Postpartum fever
Mycoplasma hominis	Postpartum fever

M. pneumoniae *produces acute, self-limited lower respiratory tract infections, affecting mostly children and young adults.* It can also cause pharyngitis and otitis media.

EPIDEMIOLOGY: Most infections occur in small groups of persons who have frequent close contact (e.g., families, college fraternities, military units, and residents of closed institutions). The organism is spread by aerosol transmission from person to person over a period of several months, with an attack rate exceeding 50% within the group. *M. pneumoniae* infection occurs worldwide, and in developed countries, the organism causes 15% to 20% of all pneumonias.

PATHOGENESIS: *M. pneumoniae* initiates infection by attaching to a glycolipid on the surface of the respiratory epithelium. The organism remains outside the cells, where it reproduces and causes progressive dysfunction and eventual death of the host cells. Because *M. pneumoniae* infection rarely produces symptomatic disease in children younger than the age of 5 years, it is thought that the host immune response plays a role in tissue injury.

PATHOLOGY: Pneumonia caused by *M. pneumoniae* usually shows patchy consolidation of a single segment of a lower lung lobe, although the process can be more widespread. The mucosa of affected airways is edematous and infiltrated by a mostly mononuclear inflammatory infiltrate. The alveoli show a largely interstitial process, with reactive alveolar lining cells and mononuclear infiltration. Pulmonary changes are often complicated by bacterial superinfection. The organism itself is too small to be seen by routine light microscopy.

CLINICAL FEATURES: *Mycoplasma* pneumonia tends to be milder than other bacterial pneumonias, and is sometimes called "walking pneumonia." Fever rarely lasts more than 2 weeks, although cough may linger for 6 weeks or more. Death from *M. pneumoniae* infection is rare. However, life-threatening cases of Stevens-Johnson syndrome have been linked to mycoplasma infection.

MYCOBACTERIAL INFECTIONS

Mycobacteria are distinctive organisms, 2 to 10 μm in length, which share the cell wall architecture of gram-positive bacteria but also contain large amounts of lipid. The high lipid content interferes with staining by aniline dyes, including crystal violet used in the Gram stain. Thus, although mycobacteria are structurally gram-positive, this property is difficult to demonstrate by routine staining. *The waxy lipids of the cell wall make the mycobacteria "acid fast" (i.e., they retain carbolfuchsin after rinsing with acid alcohol).*

The mycobacteria grow more slowly than other pathogenic bacteria, and their diseases are chronic, slowly progressive illnesses. The organisms produce no known toxins. They damage human tissues by inducing inflammatory and immune responses. Most mycobacterial pathogens replicate within cells of the monocyte/macrophage lineage and elicit granulomatous inflammation. The outcome of mycobacterial infection is largely determined by the host's capacity to contain the organism through delayed-type hypersensitivity mechanisms and cell-mediated immune responses.

The two main mycobacterial pathogens, *Mycobacetrium tuberculosis* and *Mycobacterium leprae,* only infect humans and have no environmental reservoir. Other pathogenic mycobacteria are environmental organisms that only occasionally cause human disease.

Tuberculosis

Tuberculosis is a chronic, communicable disease in which the lungs are the prime target, although any organ may be infected. disease is mainly caused by M. tuberculosis hominis *(Koch bacillus) but also occasionally by* M. tuberculosis bovis. *The characteristic lesion is a spherical granuloma with central caseous necrosis.*

M. tuberculosis is an obligate aerobe, a slender, beaded, nonmotile, acid-fast bacillus (Fig. 9-43). The organism grows slowly in culture, with a doubling time of 24 hours, and 3 to 6 weeks are commonly required to produce visible growth in culture.

EPIDEMIOLOGY: Tuberculosis is worldwide and is one of the most important humanbacterial diseases. Although the rate of infection is now low in developed countries, HIV-infected persons, homeless, and malnourished persons in impoverished areas are highly susceptible, as are immigrants from areas where the disease is endemic. In the United States, the annual incidence of tuberculosis is 12 per 100,000 and mortality is 1 to 2 per 100,000. In some developing countries, the incidence reaches 450 per 100,000, with a high fatality rate. There are also racial and ethnic differences—Africans, Native Americans, and Eskimos are the more susceptible than are white people. In the United States, tuberculosis is commonest in the elderly, possibly reflecting reactivation of infections acquired early in life before the decline in the prevalence of the disease.

M. tuberculosis is transmitted from person to person by aerosolized droplets. Coughing, sneezing, and talking all create aerosolized respiratory droplets; usually, droplets evaporate, leaving an organism (droplet nucleus) that is readily carried in the air. Tuberculosis can also be caused by the closely related *M. tuberculosis bovis,* which is acquired by drinking nonpasteurized milk from infected cows.

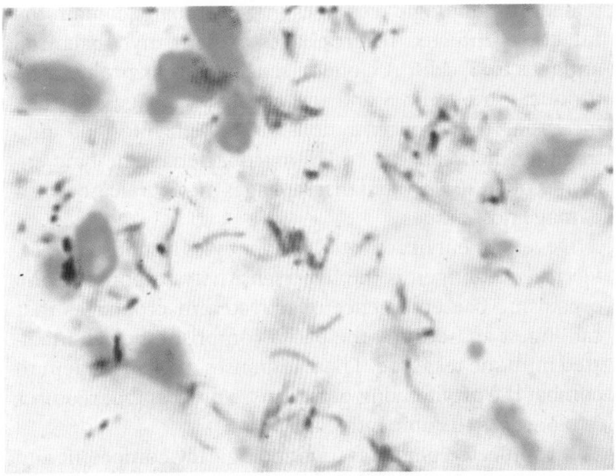

FIGURE 9-43. ***Mycobacterium tuberculosis.*** A smear of a pulmonary lesion shows slender, beaded, acid-fast bacilli.

PATHOGENESIS: The course of tuberculosis depends on age and immune competence, as well as total burden of organisms. Some patients have only an indolent, asymptomatic infection, while in others, tuberculosis is a destructive, disseminated disease. Many more persons are infected with *M. tuberculosis* than develop clinical symptoms. Thus, one must distinguish between infection and active tuberculosis. **Tuberculous infection** refers to growth of the organism in a person, whether there is symptomatic disease or not. **Active tuberculosis** denotes the subset of tuberculous infections manifested by destructive, symptomatic disease.

Primary tuberculosis occurs on first exposure to the organism, and can pursue either an indolent or aggressive course (Fig. 9-44). **Secondary tuberculosis** is disease that develops long after a primary infection, mostly as a result of reactivation of a primary infection. Secondary tuberculosis can also be produced by exposure to exogenous organisms and is always an active disease.

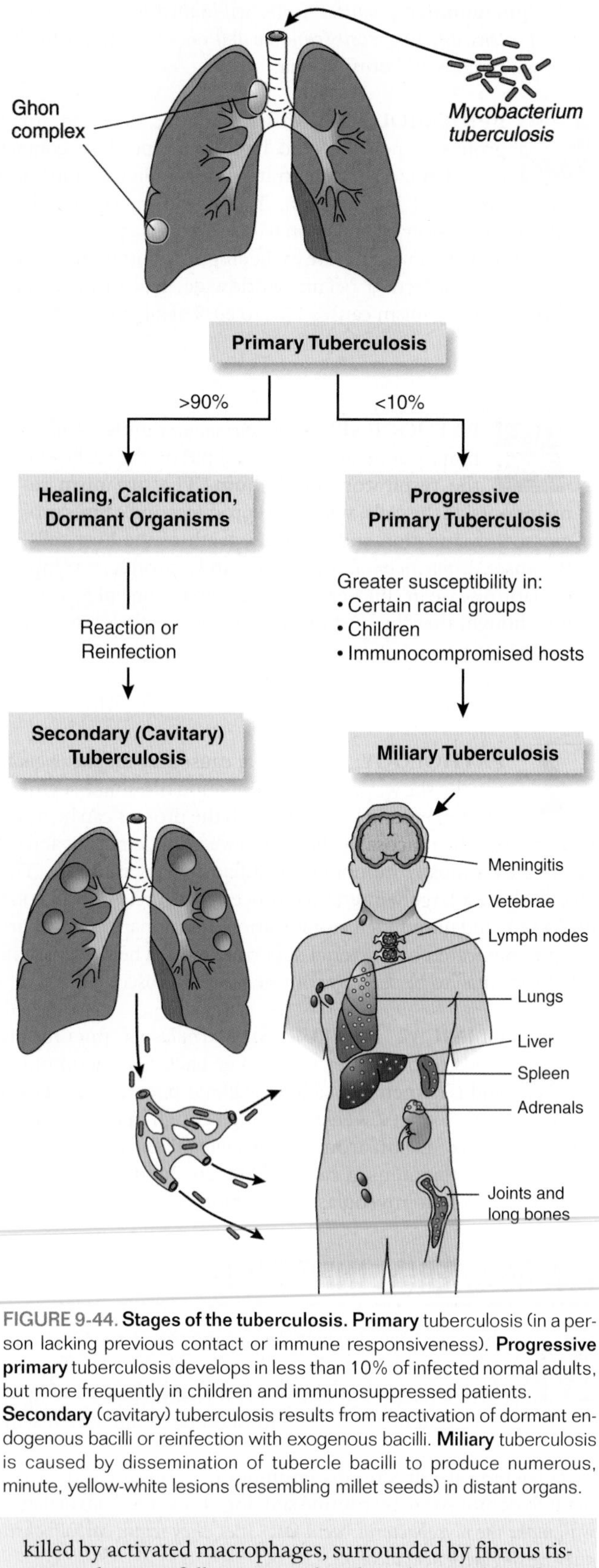

FIGURE 9-44. **Stages of the tuberculosis. Primary** tuberculosis (in a person lacking previous contact or immune responsiveness). **Progressive primary** tuberculosis develops in less than 10% of infected normal adults, but more frequently in children and immunosuppressed patients. **Secondary** (cavitary) tuberculosis results from reactivation of dormant endogenous bacilli or reinfection with exogenous bacilli. **Miliary** tuberculosis is caused by dissemination of tubercle bacilli to produce numerous, minute, yellow-white lesions (resembling millet seeds) in distant organs.

Primary Tuberculosis Is a First Exposure to the Tubercle Bacillus

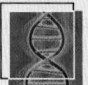

PATHOGENESIS: Inhaled *M. tuberculosis* is deposited in alveoli, usually in the lower segments of lower and middle lobes and anterior segments of upper lobes. The organisms are phagocytosed by alveolar macrophages but resist killing; cell wall lipids of *M. tuberculosis* apparently block fusion of phagosomes and lysosomes and allow the bacilli to proliferate within macrophages. As the bacilli multiply, macrophages degrade some, and present antigens to T lymphocytes. Some macrophages carry organisms from the lung to regional (hilar and mediastinal) lymph nodes, from which they may be disseminated by the bloodstream to other areas in the body. Bacilli continue to proliferate at the primary site in the lungs, and elsewhere including lymph nodes, kidneys, meninges, epiphyseal plates of long bones and vertebrae, and apical areas of the lungs.

Although the macrophages that first ingest *M. tuberculosis* cannot kill it, they initiate hypersensitivity and cell-mediated immunologic responses that eventually contain the infection. Infected macrophages present mycobacterial antigens to T cells. A clone of sensitized cells proliferates, produces interferon γ and activates macrophages, thereby increasing their concentrations of lytic enzymes and augmenting their capacity to kill mycobacteria. The lytic enzymes of these activated macrophages may, if released, also damage host tissues.

Development of activated lymphocytes responsive to *M. tuberculosis* antigen is the hypersensitivity response to the organism. The emergence of activated macrophages that can ingest and destroy the bacilli comprises the cell-mediated immune response. These responses work in tandem to combat the proliferating organisms, a process that requires 3 to 6 weeks to come into play.

If an infected person is immunologically competent and the burden of organisms is small, a vigorous granulomatous reaction is produced. Tubercle bacilli are ingested and killed by activated macrophages, surrounded by fibrous tissue, and successfully contained. When the number of organisms is high, the hypersensitivity reaction produces significant tissue necrosis, which has a characteristic cheeselike (caseous) consistency. Although not invariably caused by *M. tuberculosis*, caseous necrosis is so strongly associated with tuberculosis, that its discovery in tissue must raise a suspicion of this disease.

In immunologically immature subjects (a young child or immunosuppressed patient) granulomas are poorly formed or not formed at all, and infection progresses at the primary site in the lung, in the regional lymph nodes, or in multiple sites of dissemination. This process produces **progressive primary tuberculosis**.

PATHOLOGY: The lung lesion of primary tuberculosis is known as a **Ghon focus**. It is found in the subpleural area of the upper segments of the lower lobes or in the lower segments of the upper lobes. Initially, it is a small, ill-defined area of inflammatory consolidation, which then drains to hilar lymph nodes. The combination of a peripheral Ghon focus and involved mediastinal or hilar lymph nodes is called the **Ghon complex**.

Microscopically, the classic lesion of tuberculosis is a caseous granuloma (Fig. 9-45), which has a soft, semisolid core surrounded by epithelioid macrophages, Langhans giant cells, lymphocytes, and peripheral fibrous tissue. If the infected person lacks an appropriate immunologic response, the granuloma formed in response to *M. tuberculosis* is less organized and may consist of only an aggregate of macrophages, lacking the architecture and Langhans giant cells of the classic granuloma.

In over 90% of normal adults, tuberculous infection is self-limited. In both lungs and lymph nodes, the Ghon complex heals, undergoing shrinkage, fibrous scarring, and calcification, the latter visible radiographically. Small numbers of organisms may remain viable for years. Later, if immune mechanisms wane or fail, resting bacilli may proliferate and break out, causing serious secondary tuberculosis.

Progressive primary tuberculosis is an alternative course in which the immune response fails to control the tubercle bacilli. Infection takes this course in less than 10% of normal adults, but it is common in children younger than 5 and in patients with suppressed or defective immunity. The Ghon focus enlarges and may even erode into the bronchial tree. Affected hilar and mediastinal lymph nodes also enlarge, sometimes compressing the bronchi to produce atelectasis of the distal lung; collapse of the middle lobe (**middle lobe syndrome**) is a common result of this compression. In some instances, the infected lymph nodes erode into an airway to spread organisms throughout the lungs.

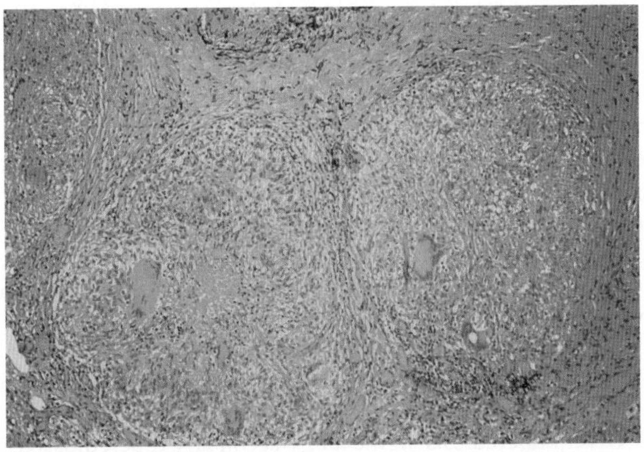

FIGURE 9-45. **Primary tuberculosis.** Photomicrograph of a hilar lymph node shows a tuberculous granuloma with central caseation.

***Miliary tuberculosis** occurs when infection disseminates to produce multiple, small, yellow, nodular lesions in several organs* (Fig. 9-46). The term "miliary" refers to the resemblance of these lesions to millet seeds. The lungs, lymph nodes, kidneys, adrenals, bone marrow, spleen, and liver are common sites of miliary lesions. Progressive disease may involve the meninges and cause tuberculous meningitis.

CLINICAL FEATURES: Most people successfully contain primary infection, and primary tuberculosis is generally asymptomatic. In those who develop progressive primary disease, symptoms are usually insidious and nonspecific, with fever, weight loss, fatigue, and night sweats. Sometimes onset of symptoms is abrupt, with high fever, pleurisy, pleural effusion, and lymphadenitis. Cough and hemoptysis develop only when active pulmonary disease is well established. In miliary tuberculosis, symptoms vary according to the organs affected and tend to occur late in the course of disease.

A

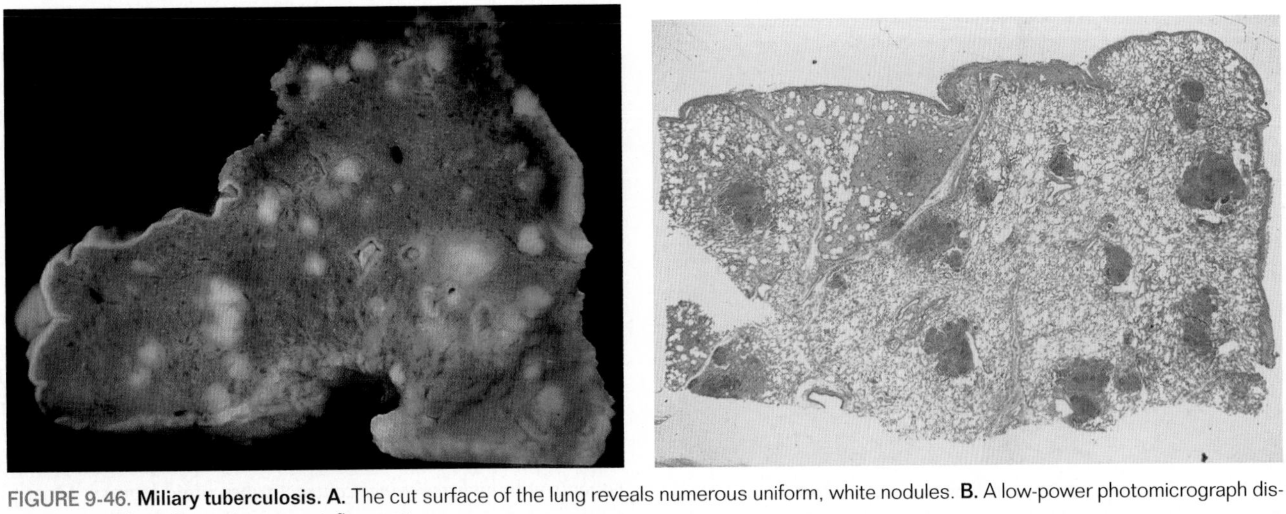

B

FIGURE 9-46. **Miliary tuberculosis. A.** The cut surface of the lung reveals numerous uniform, white nodules. **B.** A low-power photomicrograph discloses many foci of granulomatous inflammation.

Secondary (Cavitary) Tuberculosis Results from Proliferation of M. tuberculosis in Someone Who Has Previously Contained the Infection

The mycobacteria in secondary tuberculosis may be either dormant organisms from old granulomas (which is usually the case) or newly acquired bacilli. Various conditions, including cancer, antineoplastic chemotherapy, immunosuppressive therapy, AIDS, and old age, predispose to reemergence of endogenous dormant *M. tuberculosis*. Secondary tuberculosis may develop even decades after primary infection.

PATHOLOGY: Any location may be involved but the lungs are by far the most common site for secondary tuberculosis. In the lungs, secondary tuberculosis usually begins in apical–posterior segments of the upper lobes, where organisms are commonly seeded during primary infection. There, the bacilli proliferate and elicit an inflammatory response, causing localized consolidation. *Ensuing T cell-mediated immune responses to the now familiar tuberculous antigens lead to tissue necrosis and production of tuberculous cavities* (Fig. 9-47). Apical cavities are optimal sites for multiplication of *M. tuberculosis*, and large numbers of organisms are produced in this environment. Cavities are typically 2 to 4 cm in diameter when first detected clinically but can exceed 10 cm. These cavities contain necrotic material teeming with mycobacteria, and are surrounded by a granulomatous response.

The pulmonary lesions of secondary tuberculosis may be complicated by a variety of secondary effects: (1) scarring and calcification; (2) spread to other areas; (3) pleural fibrosis and adhesions; (4) rupture of a caseous lesion, spilling bacilli into the pleural cavity; (5) erosion into a bronchus, which seeds bronchioles, bronchi, and trachea; and (6) implantation of bacilli in the larynx, causing hoarseness and pain on swallowing. Tubercle bacilli may also spread throughout the body through the lymphatics and bloodstream to cause miliary tuberculosis.

CLINICAL FEATURES: Cough (which may be mistakenly attributed to smoking or a cold), low-grade fever, general malaise, fatigue, anorexia, weight loss, and often night sweats are the usual manifestations. Cavitation may be accompanied by hemoptysis, on occasion severe enough to cause exsanguination. Chest radiographs showing unilateral or bilateral apical cavities suggest the diagnosis of secondary tuberculosis. If disease is disseminated, the signs and symptoms reflect the particular organs involved.

Untreated secondary tuberculosis is a wasting disease that is eventually fatal, and at one time chronic cavitary tuberculosis was a most common cause of secondary amyloidosis. Tuberculosis is now treated with prolonged courses of antituberculous antibiotics, including isoniazid, pyrazinamide, rifampin, and ethambutol. Strains of *M. tuberculosis* resistant to these antibiotics have recently emerged, usually as a result of failure to take prescribed medications consistently and for the full time.

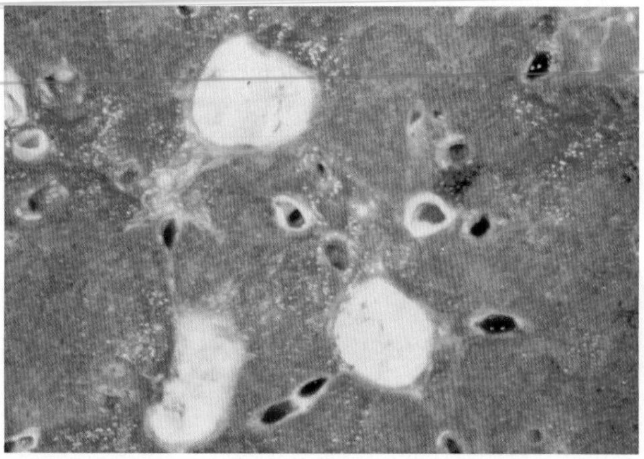

FIGURE 9-47. Secondary pulmonary tuberculosis. A cross-section of lung shows several tuberculous cavities filled with necrotic, caseous material.

LEPROSY

Leprosy (Hansen disease) is a chronic, slowly progressive, destructive process involving peripheral nerves, skin, and mucous membranes, caused by Mycobacterium leprae. This agent is a slender, weakly acid-fast rod, which cannot be cultured on artificial media or in cell culture.

EPIDEMIOLOGY: Leprosy is one of the oldest recognized human diseases. Lepers were isolated from the community in the Old Testament, although some of those segregated persons may have suffered from psoriasis and other skin conditions. For centuries, leprosy was widespread in Europe, including England. In 1873, Hansen first documented the causative agent.

Lepra bacilli multiply in experimental animals at sites with temperatures below that of the internal organs, such as foot pads of mice and ear lobes of hamsters, rats, and other rodents. Naturally acquired leprosy has been recognized in armadillos in Louisiana and Texas. Lepra bacilli have been experimentally transmitted to armadillos, whose susceptibility is related, at least in part, to their low body temperature (32° to 35°C [89.6° to 95°F]).

Leprosy is transmitted from person to person, usually as a result of years of intimate contact. *M. leprae* is present in nasal secretions or ulcerated lesions of infected persons. The mode of infection is unclear, but probably involves inoculation of bacilli into the respiratory tract or open wounds. Although leprosy is now rare in developed countries, 15 million persons are infected worldwide, primarily in tropical areas, including India, Papua-New Guinea, Southeast Asia, and tropical Africa. Fewer than 400 cases are diagnosed yearly in the United States; most in immigrants from endemic areas.

PATHOGENESIS: *M. leprae* multiplies best at temperatures below core human body temperature and lesions tend to occur in cooler parts of the body (e.g., hands and face). Leprosy exhibits a bewildering variety of clinical and pathologic features. Lesions vary from the small, insignificant, and self-healing macules of tuberculoid leprosy to the diffuse, disfiguring, and sometimes fatal lesions of lepromatous leprosy (Fig. 9-48). This extreme variation in disease presentation probably reflects differences in immune reactivity.

Most (95%) persons have a natural protective immunity to *M. leprae* and are not infected, despite intimate and prolonged exposure. Susceptible individuals (5%) span a broad immunologic spectrum from anergy to hyperergy and may develop symptomatic infection. *At one end of the spectrum, anergic patients have little or no resistance and develop* ***lepromatous leprosy****, while hyperergic patients with high resistance contract* ***tuberculoid leprosy****.* Most patients, in between these extremes, have **borderline leprosy.**

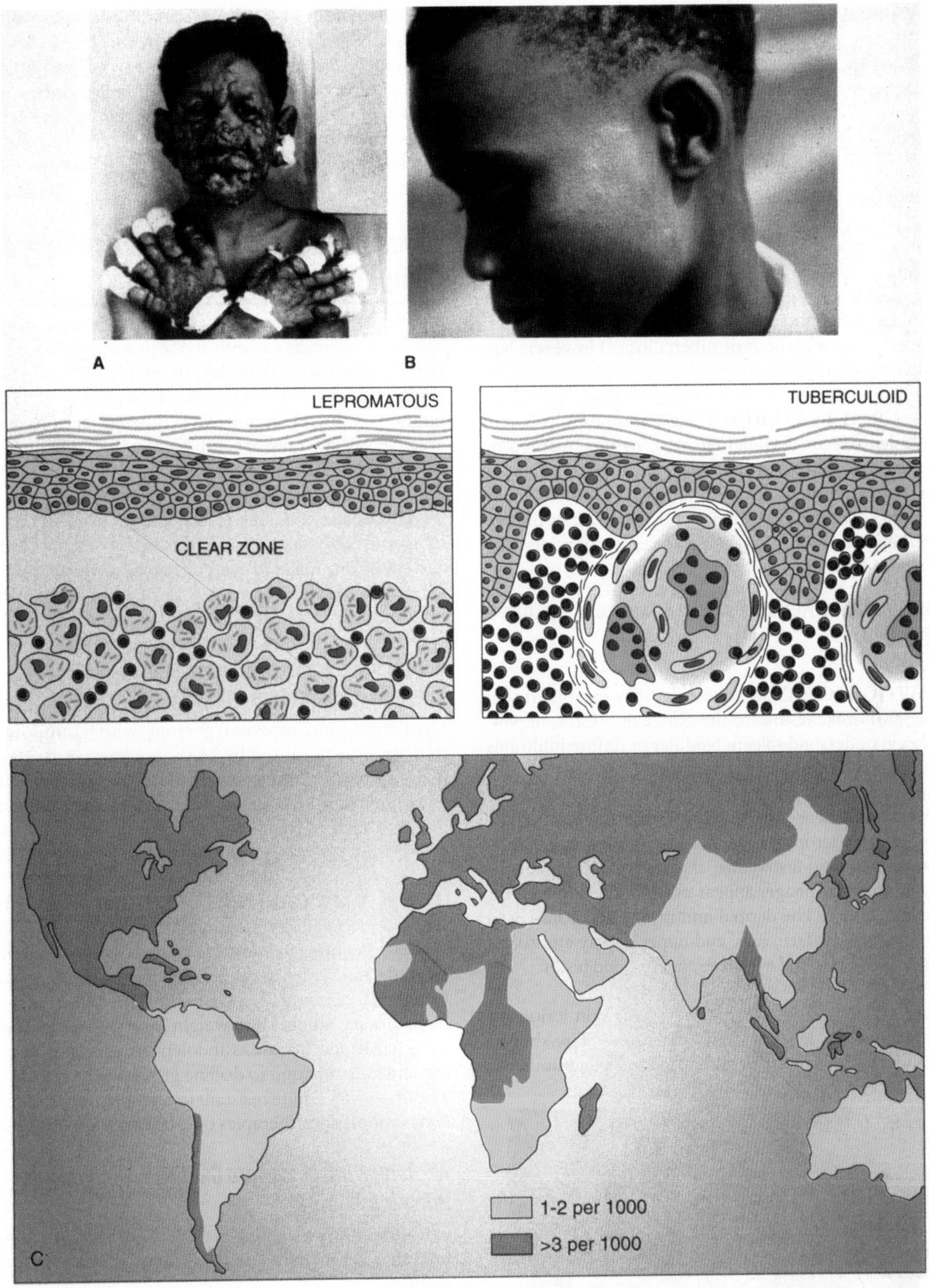

FIGURE 9-48. **A.** *(Top)* Lepromatous leprosy. There is diffuse involvement, including a leonine face, loss of eyebrows and eyelashes, and nodular distortions, especially on the face, ears, forearms and hands—the exposed (cool) parts of the body. *(Bottom)* The nodular skin lesions of advanced lepromatous leprosy. Swelling has flattened the epidermis (loss of Rete ridges). A characteristic "clear zone" of uninvolved dermis separates the epidermis from tumorlike accumulations of macrophages, each containing numerous lepra bacilli *(M. leprae)*. **B.** *(Top)* Tuberculoid leprosy on the cheek, showing a hypopigmented macule with a raised, infiltrated border. The central portion may be hypesthetic or anesthetic. *(Bottom)* Macular skin lesion of tuberculoid leprosy. Skin from the raised "infiltrated" margin of the plaque contains discrete granulomas that extend to the basal layer of the epidermis (without a clear zone). The granulomas are composed of epithelioid cells and Langhans giant cells and are associated with lymphocytes and plasma cells. Lepra bacilli are rare. **C.** Distribution of leprosy. Prevalence is greatest in tropical regions of Africa, Asia, and Latin America.

Tuberculoid Leprosy Occurs in Infected Persons Who Mount an Effective Granulomatous Response

PATHOLOGY: Tuberculoid leprosy is characterized by a single lesion or very few lesions of the skin, usually on the face, extremities, or trunk. Microscopically lesions show well-formed, circumscribed dermal granulomas with epithelioid macrophages, Langhans giant cells, and lymphocytes. Nerve fibers are almost invariably swollen and infiltrated with lymphocytes. Destruction of small dermal nerve twigs accounts for the sensory deficit associated with tuberculoid leprosy. Bacilli are rare and often not found with acid-fast stains. The term "tuberculoid leprosy" is used because the granulomas vaguely resemble those of tuberculosis. However, leprous granulomas lack caseation.

CLINICAL FEATURES: The skin lesions of tuberculoid leprosy are well-demarcated, hypopigmented or erythematous, dry, hairless patches, with raised outer edges. Nerve involvement leads to decreased sensation or numbness within the patch. As the lesion expands at its periphery, it often heals centrally. The lesions of tuberculoid leprosy cause minimal disfigurement and are not infectious.

Lepromatous Leprosy Reflects a Poor Immune Response to Lepra Bacilli

PATHOLOGY: Lepromatous leprosy exhibits multiple, tumorlike lesions of the skin, eyes, testes, nerves, lymph nodes, and spleen. Nodular or diffuse infiltrates of foamy macrophages contain myriad bacilli (Fig. 9-49). The epidermis is stretched thinly over the nodules, and beneath it is a narrow, uninvolved "clear zone" of the dermis. Rather than destroying the bacilli, macrophages seem to act as microincubators. When subjected to acid-fast stains, the numerous organisms within the foamy macrophages appear as aggregates of acid-fast material, called "globi." The dermal infiltrates expand slowly to distort and disfigure the face, ears, and upper airway and to destroy the eyes, eyebrows and eyelashes, nerves, and testes.

CLINICAL FEATURES: The nodular skin lesions of lepromatous leprosy may ulcerate. Claw-shaped hands, hammertoes, saddle nose, and pendulous ear lobes are common. Nodular lesions of the face may coalesce to produce a lionlike appearance ("leonine facies"). Involvement of the upper airways leads to chronic nasal discharge and voice change. Infection of the eyes may cause blindness.

The most commonly used drug, dapsone, effectively eliminates lepra bacilli in 4 to 5 years, but it must be continued indefinitely. Dapsone-resistant strains of *M. leprae* have appeared, and multidrug regimens are often used.

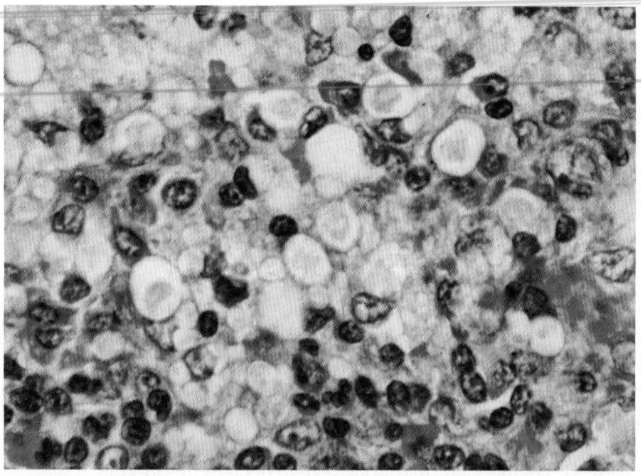

FIGURE 9-49. **Lepromatous leprosy.** A section of skin shows a tumorlike mass of foamy macrophages. The faint masses within the vacuolated macrophages are enormous numbers of lepra bacilli.

Mycobacterium Avium-Intracellulare Complex

Mycobacterium avium and *Mycobacterium intracellulare* are similar species, which cause identical diseases and grouped as *M. avium-intracellulare* (MAI) complex, or simply MAI. MAI causes two types of disease: (1) a rare, slowly progressive granulomatous pulmonary disease in immunocompetent persons and (2) a progressive systemic disease in patients with AIDS. Because of the AIDS epidemic, infection with MAI is the third most common opportunistic infection in AIDS patients in the United States.

MAI is found in soil, water, and foodstuffs worldwide. Humans probably acquire it from the environment by inhaling aerosols from infected water sources. Colonization by the organisms is common. As many as 70% of healthy persons show immunologic responsiveness to MAI, indicating prior exposure.

Granulomatous MAI Disease Occurs in Immunocompetent Persons

Most immunocompetent persons with granulomatous pulmonary disease caused by MAI are older (50 to 70 years), and many suffer from preexisting pulmonary disease. Clinically and pathologically MAI disease resembles tuberculosis but progresses much more slowly. It causes pulmonary nodules and cavities and caseating granulomas.

CLINICAL FEATURES: The most common antecedent illnesses predisposing to pulmonary MAI infection are chronic obstructive pulmonary disease, treated tuberculosis, pneumoconioses, and bronchiectasis. Cough is a common symptom, but the disease lacks the fever, night sweats, fatigue, and weight loss that characterize tuberculosis. MAI lung disease is indolent or only slowly progressive, causing lung function to decline gradually over years or decades. The organism is quite resistant to first-line antituberculous drugs, and combinations therapies often yield disappointing results.

M. Avium-Intracellulare Causes Disseminated Infection in AIDS

One third of AIDS patients in the United States develop overt MAI infection; as many as one half have evidence of infection at autopsy.

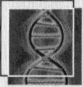

PATHOGENESIS: In patients with AIDS, progressive depletion of helper T cells cripples immune responses that normally prevent MAI disease. Although macrophages phagocytose the organisms, they cannot kill them. The bacilli replicate, fill the cells, spread to other macrophages, and spread throughout the body via the lymphatics and bloodstream.

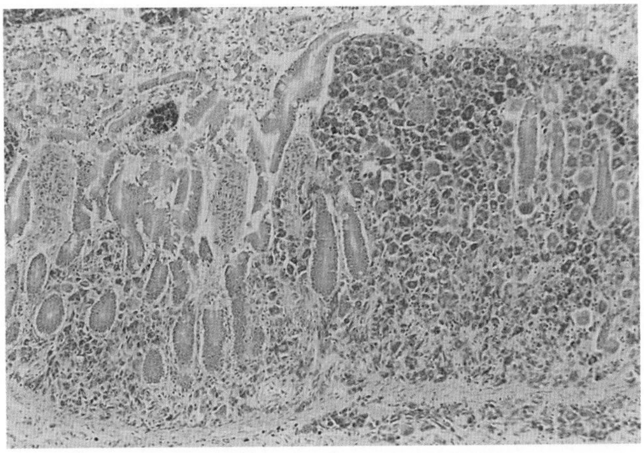

FIGURE 9-50. ***Mycobacterium avium-intracellulare* (MAI).** A section of small bowel from a patient with acquired immunodeficieny syndrome (AIDS) reveals the presence of numerous macrophages stuffed with acid-fast bacilli in the lamina propria.

PATHOLOGY: Infected macrophages are found in many organs. Proliferation of the organisms leads to recruitment of additional macrophages, causing expanding nodular lesions that range from structured epithelioid granulomas with few organisms, to loose aggregates of foamy macrophages packed with acid-fast bacilli (Fig. 9-50). Eventually, lymph nodes, spleen, and bone marrow may be almost completely replaced by aggregates of macrophages and lesions in the bowel erode into the lumen of the gut.

CLINICAL FEATURES: Early, constitutional symptoms of MAI disease in AIDS resemble those of tuberculosis: fever, night sweats, fatigue, and weight loss. Progressive small bowel involvement produces malabsorption and diarrhea, often accompanied by abdominal pain. Although the lungs are commonly involved, pulmonary disease is not usually symptomatic. Combinations of five or more different antibiotics, including clarithromycin, may control, but rarely cure, widespread MAI infection in AIDS patients.

Atypical Mycobacteria

Several other species of environmental mycobacteria occasionally produce human disease. These organisms are also present in surface waters, dust, and dirt and people acquire infection by inhalation, inoculation, or ingestion of environmental material.

These bacteria, including MAI, are often lumped together as the "atypical mycobacteria" (in contrast to *M. tuberculosis*, regarded as the "typical" mycobacterium). The atypical mycobacteria are biologically diverse and the uncommon diseases that they produce in humans differ in circumstances of acquisition, pathology, clinical presentations, and therapies. The features of these diseases are compared in Table 9-8.

- *Mycobacterium* ***kansasii*** causes a chronic, slowly progressive granulomatous pulmonary disease in older persons (over age 50 years), similar to that produced by MAI in immunocompetent patients.
- *Mycobacterium* ***scrofulaceum,*** a common soil inhabitant, causes a draining, granulomatous, cervical lymphadenitis in young children (aged 1 to 5 years). The infection affects the submandibular lymph nodes and probably results from inoculation or ingestion of organisms by toddlers playing in soil. The disease is localized, and surgical excision of the affected lymph nodes is curative.
- *Mycobacterium* ***marinum,*** commonly found on underwater surfaces, produces a localized nodular skin lesion ("swimming pool granuloma"), sometimes with lymphatic involvement. Infection is acquired by traumatic inoculation, such as abrading an elbow on a swimming pool ladder or cutting a finger on a fish spine. The tissue reaction can be pyogenic or granulomatous.
- *Mycobacterium* ***ulcerans*** leads to a severe ulcerating skin disease in Australia, Africa, and New Guinea. Infection presents as a solitary, undermining, deep ulcer of the skin and subcutaneous fat of the extremities.
- *Mycobacterium* ***chelonae*** **and** *Mycobacterium* ***fortuitum*** are closely related organisms that are present throughout the en-

TABLE 9-8

Atypical Mycobacterial Infections

Organism	Disease	Ages Affected	Pathology	Source	Distribution
Mycobacterium kansasii	Chronic granulomatous pulmonary disease (similar to that caused by *M. avium-intracellulare*)	50–70	Granulomatous inflammation	Inhaled organisms from soil, dust, or water	Worldwide
Mycobacterium scrofulaceum	Cervical lymphadenitis	1–5	Granulomatous inflammation	Probably ingested organisms from soil or dust	Worldwide
Mycobacterium marinum	Localized skin lesions	All	Granulomatous inflammation	Direct inoculation of organisms from fish or underwater surfaces (swimming pools, fish tanks)	Worldwide
Mycobacterium ulcerans	Large, solitary, severe ulcer of skin and subcutaneous tissue	Usually 5–25	Coagulative necrosis	Probably inoculation of environmental organisms	Australia, Africa
Mycobacterium fortuitum and *Mycobacterium chelonei*	Infections associated with traumatic or iatrogenic inoculations	All	Pyogenic inflammation	Inoculation of environmental organisms	Worldwide

vironment. Infection is associated with traumatic or iatrogenic inoculation of material contaminated with organisms. Painless, fluctuant abscesses appear at the site of inoculation, ulcerate, and gradually heal spontaneously. The tissue reaction can be pyogenic or granulomatous.

FUNGAL INFECTIONS

Of more than 100,000 known fungi, only a few cause human disease. Of these, most are "opportunists": they only infect people with impaired immune mechanisms. *Thus, corticosteroid administration, antineoplastic therapy, and congenital or acquired T-cell deficiencies all predispose to mycotic infections.*

Fungi are larger and more complex than bacteria. They vary from 2 to 100 μm and are eukaryotes. Thus, they possess nuclear membranes and cytoplasmic organelles, such as mitochondria and endoplasmic reticulum.

There are two basic morphologic types of fungi: yeasts and molds.

- **Yeasts** are unicellular forms of fungi. They are round or oval cells that reproduce by budding, by which process daughter organisms pinche off from a parent. Some yeasts produce buds that do not detach but instead produce a chain of elongated yeast cells that resemble hyphae and are termed **pseudohyphae**.
- **Molds** are multicellular filamentous fungal colonies with branching tubules, or **hyphae**, 2 to 10 μm in diameter. The mass of tangled hyphae in the mold form is called a **mycelium**. Some hyphae are separated by septa that are located at regular intervals; others are nonseptate.
- **Dimorphic fungi** may grow as yeasts or molds, depending on their environment.

Most fungi are visible on tissue sections stained with hematoxylin and eosin. The periodic acid–Schiff (PAS) reaction and Gomori methenamine silver (GMS) stain outline fungal cell walls and are commonly used to detect fungal infection in tissues.

Pneumocystis Jiroveci Pneumonia

Pneumocystis jiroveci *(formerly,* carinii) *causes progressive, often fatal, pneumonia in persons with impaired cell-mediated immunity and is a common opportunistic pathogen in persons with AIDS.* The organism has recently been reclassified with the fungi.

EPIDEMIOLOGY: *P. jiroveci* is distributed worldwide and since 75% of the population have acquired antibodies by 5 years of age, it is likely that the organisms are inhaled by all. In persons with intact cell-mediated immunity, infection is rapidly contained without producing symptoms.

In the 1960s and 1970s, 100 to 200 cases of active *Pneumocystis* disease were reported annually in the United States, mainly in people with hematologic malignancies, transplant recipients, or those treated with corticosteroids or cytotoxic therapy. Pneumocystis became a common pathogen with the AIDS pandemic: before the introduction of highly active antiretroviral therapy (see Chapter 4), *80% of AIDS patients developed* Pneumocystis *pneumonia.*

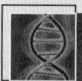

PATHOGENESIS: *P. jiroveci* reproduces in association with alveolar type 1 lining cells and active disease is confined to the lungs. Infection begins with attachment of *Pneumocystis* trophozoites to alveolar lining cells. The trophozoites feed on host cells, enlarge, and transforms into the cyst form, which contains daughter organisms. The cyst ruptures to release new trophozoites, which attach to additional alveolar lining cells. If the process is not checked by the host immune system or antibiotic therapy, the infected alveoli eventually fill with organisms and proteinaceous fluid. The progressive filling of alveoli prevents adequate gas exchange and the patient slowly suffocates.

It is assumed, but not proven, that most cases of pneumocystosis derive from latent endogenous infection. Outbreaks of *Pneumocystis* pneumonia have also occurred among severely malnourished (and thus immunosuppressed) infants in nurseries; these are believed to represent primary infection with the organism.

PATHOLOGY: *P. jiroveci* causes progressive consolidation of the lungs. Microscopically, alveoli contain a frothy eosinophilic material, composed of alveolar macrophages and cysts and trophozoites of *P. carinii* (Fig. 9-51). There are hyaline membranes and prominent type 2 pneumocytes. In newborns, alveolar septa are thickened by lymphoid cells and macrophages. The prominence of plasma cells in the infantile disease led to the now obsolete term *plasma cell pneumonia.*

The various forms of *P. carinii* are best visualized with methenamine silver stains. The cyst form measures about 60 μm in diameter (see Fig. 9-51B); extracellular trophozoites and intracystic forms of the organism appear as irregularly shaped cells, 1 to 3 μm across, with punctate violet nuclei by Giemsa staining.

CLINICAL FEATURES: *P. jiroveci* pneumonia features fever and progressive shortness of breath, often exacerbated by exertion and accompanied by a nonproductive cough. Dyspnea may be subtle in onset and slowly progressive over many weeks. Chest radiographs show a diffuse pulmonary process. The diagnosis requires recovery of alveolar material (by bronchoscopy, endobronchial washing or sputum induction) for staining. *The disease is fatal if untreated.* Therapy is with trimethoprim-sulfamethoxazole or pentamidine.

Candida

The genus *Candida,* comprising over 20 species of yeasts, includes the most common opportunistic pathogens. Many *Candida* species are endogenous human flora, well adapted to life on or in the human body. However, they can cause disease when host defenses are compromised. Although the various forms of candidiasis vary in clinical severity, most are localized, superficial diseases, limited to a particular mucocutaneous site, including:

- **Intertrigo:** infection of opposed skin surfaces
- **Paronychia:** infection of the nail bed
- **Diaper rash**
- **Vulvovaginitis**
- **Thrush:** oral infection
- **Esophagitis**

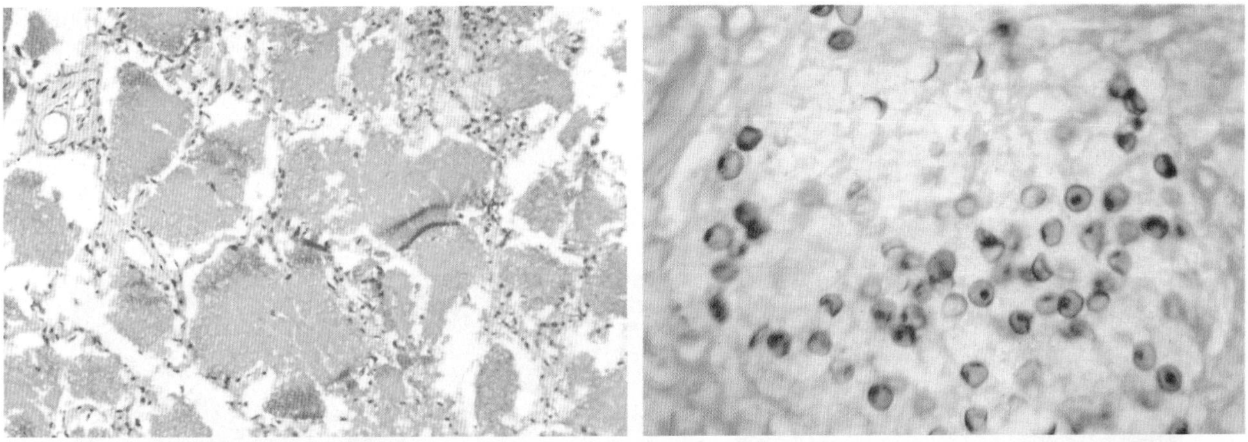

A B

FIGURE 9-51. ***Pneumocystis carinii* pneumonia. A.** The alveoli contain a frothy eosinophilic material that is composed of alveolar macrophages and cysts and trophozoites of *P. carinii*. **B.** A silver stain shows crescent-shaped organisms, which are collapsed and degenerated. Some have a characteristic dark spot in their walls.

Candidal infections of deep tissues are much less common than superficial infections but can be life-threatening. The most common deep sites affected are the brain, eye, kidney, and heart. Deep infections, with candidal sepsis and disseminated candidiasis, occur only in immunologically compromised persons and are often fatal.

Most candidal infections derive from endogenous flora. *Candida albicans* resides in small numbers in the oropharynx, gastrointestinal tract, and vagina and is the most frequent candidal pathogen, being responsible for more than 95% of these infections.

PATHOGENESIS: Mechanical barriers, inflammatory cells, humoral immunity, and cell-mediated immunity relegate *Candida* to superficial, nonsterile sites. In turn, the resident bacterial flora normally limits the number of fungal organisms. Bacteria (1) block candidal attachment to epithelial cells, (2) compete with the organisms for nutrients, and (3) prevent conversion of the fungus to its tissue-invasive forms. When any of the above defenses is compromised, candidal infections can occur (Table 9-9). *Antibiotic use results in the suppression of the competing bacterial flora and is the most common precipitating factor for candidiasis.* Under conditions of unopposed growth, the yeast converts to its invasive form (hyphae or pseudohyphae), invades superficially and elicits an inflammatory or immunologic response.

Even though *Candida* inhabits skin surfaces, it does not cause cutaneous disease without a predisposing skin lesion. The most common such factor is maceration, or softening and destruction of the skin. Chronically warm and moist areas, such as between fingers and toes, between skinfolds, and under diapers, are prone to maceration and thus superficial candidal disease.

The incidence of invasive candidal infections is increasing. Frequent use of potent broad-spectrum antibiotics eliminates bacteria that otherwise limit *Candida* colonization. Expanded use of medical devices, such as intravascular catheters, monitoring devices, endotracheal tubes, and urinary catheters, provides access to sterile sites. AIDS and iatrogenic neutropenias render individuals less capable of defending themselves from even weak pathogens, such as *Candida*. Finally, intravenous drug users develop deep candidal infections because of inoculation of the fungi into the bloodstream.

PATHOLOGY AND CLINICAL FEATURES: Superficial infections of the skin, oropharynx (Fig. 9-52A) and esophagus show invasive organisms in the most superficial layers of the epithelium and are associated with acute inflammatory infiltrates. Yeasts, pseudohyphae, and hyphae are present (see Fig. 9-52B). The yeast are round and 3 to 4 μm in diameter and the hyphae are septate. Candidal vaginitis is characterized by superficial invasion of the squamous epithelium, but inflammation is usually scanty. Deep candidal infections consist of multiple microscopic abscesses with yeasts, hyphae, necrotic debris, and neutrophils. Rarely, the organism elicits a granulomatous response.

The various superficial cutaneous infections manifest as tender, erythematous papules, which expand to form confluent erythematous areas.

- **Thrush:** This lesion involves the tongue and mucous membranes of the mouth. Early in life, it is the most common form of mucocutaneous candidiasis. Candidal vaginitis

TABLE 9–9

Candidal Infections

Disease	Predisposing Conditions
Superficial Infections	
Intertrigo (opposed skin surfaces)	Maceration
Paronychia (nail beds)	Maceration
Diaper rash	Maceration
Vulvovaginitis	Alteration in normal flora
Thrush (oral)	Decreased cell-mediated immunity
Esophagitis	Decreased cell-mediated immunity
Deep Infections	
Urinary tract infections	Indwelling urinary catheters
Sepsis and disseminated infection	Neutropenia, indwelling vascular catheters, and change in normal flora

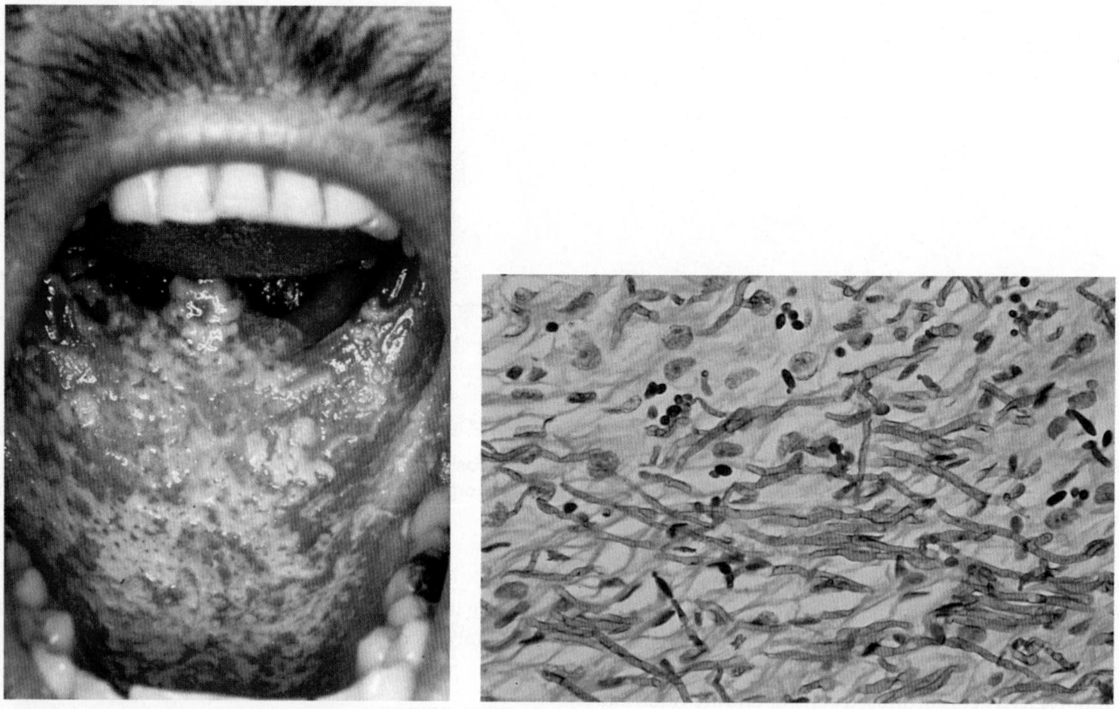

A B

FIGURE 9-52. **Candidiasis. A.** The oral cavity of a patient with acquired immunodeficieny syndrome (AIDS) is covered by a white, curdlike exudate containing numerous fungal organisms. **B.** A periodic acid-Schiff (PAS) stain shows numerous septate hyphae and yeast forms.

during pregnancy predisposes newborns to infection. Thrush consists of friable, white, curdlike membranes adherent to affected surfaces. These patches contain fungi, necrotic debris, neutrophils, and bacteria and can be dislodged by scraping. Removal of the membranes leaves a painful, bleeding surface.

- **Candidal vulvovaginitis:** This condition causes a thick, white vaginal discharge with vaginal and vulvar itching. Involved areas of the vulva are erythematous and tender. Candidal vaginitis is most intense when vaginal pH is low. Antibiotics, pregnancy, diabetes, and corticosteroids predispose to this form of vaginitis.
- **Candidal sepsis and disseminated candidiasis:** Systemic candidiasis is rare, and it is ordinarily a terminal event of an underlying disorder involving altered immunity or neutropenia. Several candidal species can produce invasive disease in this context. Organisms may enter through ulcerated skin or mucous membrane lesions or may be introduced iatrogenically (e.g., peritoneal dialysis, intravenous lines, or urinary catheters). The urinary tract is most commonly involved, and the incidence in women is four times that in men. Renal lesions may be blood-borne or may arise from an ascending pyelonephritis.
- **Candidal endocarditis:** This infection is characterized by large vegetations on the heart valves and a high incidence of embolization to large arteries. In most patients with candidal endocarditis, the cause is not immunosuppression but unusual vulnerability. Drug addicts who use unsterilized needles and persons with preexisting valvular disease who have had prolonged antibacterial therapy or indwelling vascular catheters are at risk for endocarditis. One of the most serious complications of invasive candidiasis is septic embolism to the brain.

ASPERGILLOSIS

Aspergillus species are common environmental fungi that cause opportunistic infections, usually involving the lungs. There are three types of pulmonary aspergillosis: (1) allergic bronchopulmonary aspergillosis, (2) colonization of a preexisting pulmonary cavity (aspergilloma or fungus ball), and (3) invasive aspergillosis (see Chapter 12). Of the over 200 identified species of *Aspergillus,* approximately 20 cause human disease. *Aspergillus fumigatus,* is by far the most frequent human pathogen.

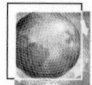

EPIDEMIOLOGY: *Aspergillus* is a saprophyte found worldwide in soil, decaying plant matter, and dung. Pulmonary aspergillosis is acquired by inhaling small (2 to 3 μm) spores, known as *conidia,* that are in the air in almost every human environment. The spores are small enough to reach the alveoli when inhaled. Exposure is greatest when the fungus' habitat is disturbed, as during soil excavations or handling decaying organic matter.

In tissues, *Aspergillus* shows septate hyphae, 2 to 7 μm in diameter, branching progressively at acute angles. The multiple dichotomous branching led to the name *Aspergillus* (from the Latin *aspergere,* "to sprinkle"). It derived from a fancied resemblance to the aspergillum, a device used to sprinkle holy water during Catholic religious ceremonies.

Allergic Bronchopulmonary Aspergillosis Complicates Asthma

Inhalation of *Aspergillus* spores exposes airways and alveoli to fungal antigens; contact subsequently initiates an allergic response in susceptible persons. The situation is aggravated if spores can germinate and grow in the airways, thereby causing long-term exposure to the antigen. Allergic bronchopulmonary aspergillosis is virtually restricted to asthmatics, 20% of whom eventually develop this disorder (see Chapter 12).

Bronchi and bronchioles show infiltrates of lymphocytes, plasma cells, and variable numbers of eosinophils. Sometimes airways are impacted with mucus and fungal hyphae. Patients experience exacerbations of asthma, often accompanied by pulmonary infiltrates and eosinophilia.

Aspergilloma Occurs in Persons with Pulmonary Cavities or Bronchiectasis

Inhaled spores germinate in the warm humid atmosphere provided by these hollows and fill them with masses of hyphae. The organisms do not invade (see Chapter 12).

PATHOLOGY: An aspergilloma is a dense, roundish mass of tangled hyphae, 1 to 7 cm in diameter, within a fibrous cavity. The cavity wall is collagenous connective tissue, with lymphocytes and plasma cells. The hyphae do not invade adjacent tissues.

CLINICAL FEATURES: Aspergillomas occur most commonly older tuberculous cavities. Symptoms reflect the underlying disease. The radiologic appearance of a dense round ball in a cavity is characteristic. Aspergillomas are usually best left untreated, but surgical excision may be indicated in some cases.

Invasive Aspergillosis Afflicts Neutropenic Patients

Whenever neutrophil number or activity is compromised, invasive aspergillosis may occur. The most common settings are high-dose steroid or cytotoxic therapy, or acute leukemia. In profoundly neutropenic patients, inhaled spores germinate to produce hyphae, which invade through bronchi into the lung parenchyma, from where the fungi may spread widely.

PATHOLOGY: *Aspergillus* readily invades blood vessels and produces thrombosis (Fig. 9-53). As a result, multiple nodular infarcts are seen throughout both lungs. Involvement of larger pulmonary arteries results in large, wedge-shaped, pleural-based infarcts. Vascular invasion by the fungi also leads to their dissemination to other organs. Microscopically, *Aspergillus* hyphae are arranged radially around blood vessels and extend through their walls. Acute aspergillosis may also start in a nasal sinus and spread to the face, orbit, and brain.

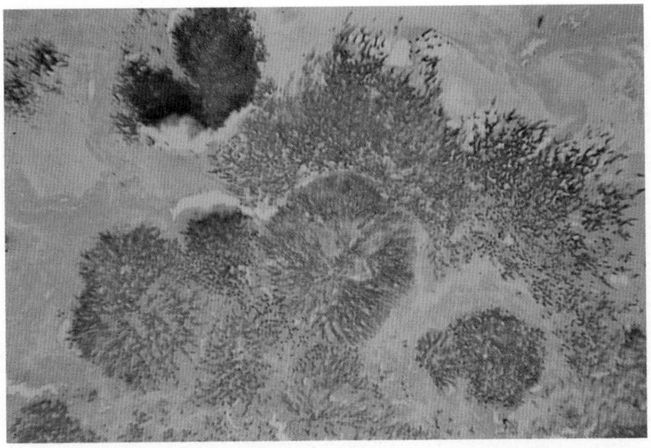

FIGURE 9-53. **Invasive aspergillosis.** A section of lung impregnated with silver shows branching fungal hyphae surrounding blood vessels and invading the adjacent parenchyma.

CLINICAL FEATURES: Invasive aspergillosis presents as fever and multifocal pulmonary infiltrates in a compromised patient. Because of frequent thrombosis and bloodstream dissemination, the disease is often fatal. Antifungal therapy with amphotericin B may be successful but must be initiated early and given in high doses.

Mucormycosis (Zygomycosis)

Several related environmental fungi, members of the class Zygomycetes—namely, *Rhizopus, Mucor, Rhizomucor, and Absidia*—produce severe, necrotizing, invasive, opportunistic infections that begin in the nasal sinuses or lungs. The infections they produce are usually called mucormycoses or zygomycoses.

In tissues, zygomycetes have large (8–15 μm across) hyphae that branch at right angles, have thin walls, and lack septa. In tissue sections, they appear as hollow tubes. Lacking cross walls, their liquid contents flow, leaving long empty segments. They also may resemble "twisted ribbons," which represent collapsed hyphae.

EPIDEMIOLOGY: *Rhizopus, Rhizomucor, Mucor, and Absidia* are ubiquitous in the environment, inhabiting soil, food, and decaying vegetable matter. The spores are inhaled and in susceptible persons, disease begins in the lungs. Mucormycosis occurs almost exclusively in the context of compromised defenses. Common causes include severe neutropenia (e.g., following treatment for leukemia), high-dose glucocorticoid therapy, and particularly severe diabetes.

PATHOLOGY AND CLINICAL FEATURES: The three predominant forms of mucormycosis are rhinocerebral, pulmonary, and subcutaneous.

- **Rhinocerebral mucormycosis:** Fungi proliferate in nasal sinuses and invade surrounding tissues, extending into facial soft tissues, nerves, blood vessels, and the brain. The palate or nasal turbinates are covered by a black crust and underlying tissue is friable and hemorrhagic. Fungal hyphae grow into the arteries and cause devastating, rapidly progressive, septic infarction of he affected tissues. Extension into the brain leads to fatal, necrotizing, hemorrhagic encephalitis. Therapy requires surgical excision of involved tissues, amphotericin B, and correction of the predisposing abnormality.
- **Pulmonary mucormycosis:** This infection resembles invasive pulmonary aspergillosis, including vascular invasion and multiple areas of septic infarction (Fig. 9-54). Both rhinocerebral and pulmonary mucormycosis are usually fatal.
- **Subcutaneous zygomycosis:** This infection is limited to the tropics and is caused by *Basidiobolus haptosporus*. The fungus grows slowly in the panniculus, producing a gradually enlarging, hard inflammatory mass, usually on the shoulder, trunk, buttock, or thigh.

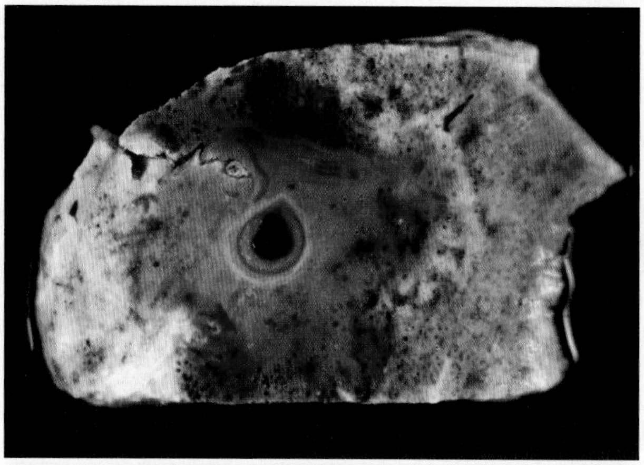

FIGURE 9-54. **Pulmonary mucormycosis.** A cross-section of the lung shows the vessel in the center of the field to be invaded by mucormycetes and occluded by a septic thrombus. The surrounding tissue is infarcted.

Cryptococcosis

Cryptococcosis is a systemic mycosis caused by Cryptococcus neoformans, *which principally affects the meninges and lungs* (Fig. 9-55). *C. neoformans* has a worldwide distribution. Its main reservoir is pigeon droppings, which are alkaline and hyperosmolar. These conditions keep cryptococci small, allowing inhaled organisms to reach the terminal bronchioles. *C. neoformans* is unique among pathogenic fungi in having a proteoglycan capsule, which is essential for their pathogenicity. The organisms appear as faintly stained, basophilic yeasts with a clear 3- to 5-μm thick mucinous capsule.

EPIDEMIOLOGY: Cryptococcus *almost exclusively affects persons with impaired cell-mediated immunity.* Although the organism is ubiquitous and exposure is common, cryptococcosis is rare in the absence of predisposing illness. Disease is uncommon even among persons such as pigeon fanciers, who are exposed to high concentrations of the organism. Cryptococcosis occurs in patients with AIDS, lymphomas (particularly Hodgkin disease), leukemias, and sarcoidosis, and in those treated with high doses of corticosteroids.

PATHOGENESIS: In immunologically intact persons, neutrophils and alveolar macrophages kill *C. neoformans* and no clinical disease develops. By contrast, in a patient with defective cell-mediated immunity, the cryptococci survive, reproduce locally, and then disseminate. Although the lung is the site of entry the CNS is the most common site of disease, owing to the excellent environment provided by the cerebrospinal fluid.

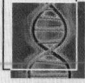

PATHOLOGY: Over 95% of cryptococcal infections involve the meninges and brain. Lesions in the lungs can be demonstrated in half of patients. In a small minority skin, liver and other involvement occurs. In cryptococcal meningoencephalitis, the entire brain is swollen and soft and leptomeninges are thickened and gelatinous, from infiltration by the thickly encapsulated organisms. Inflammatory responses are variable but are often minimal, with large numbers of cryptococci infiltrating tissue with no inflammatory response. If present, inflammation may be neutrophilic, lymphocytic, or granulomatous.

Cryptococcosis in the lung may appear as diffuse disease or as isolated areas of consolidation. Affected alveoli are distended by clusters of organisms, usually with minimal associated inflammation.

Because of its thick capsule, *C. neoformans* stains poorly with routine hematoxylin and eosin and appears as bubbles or holes in tissue sections (Fig. 9-56A). Fungal stains (PAS and GMS) demonstrate the yeasts well but do not stain the polysaccharide capsule. The organism thus appears to be surrounded by a halo. The capsule can be highlighted using a mucicarmine stain (see Fig. 9-56B).

CLINICAL FEATURES: Cryptococcal CNS disease often begins insidiously with nonfocal symptoms, including headache, dizziness, sleepiness, and loss of coordination. Untreated cryptococcal meningitis is invariably fatal. Therapy requires prolonged systemic administration of antifungal agents. Cryptococcal pneumonia presents as diffuse progressive pulmonary disease.

Histoplasmosis

Histoplasmosis is caused by Histoplasma capsulatum. *The disease is usually self-limited but may lead to a systemic granulomatous disease.* Although most cases histoplasmosis are asymptomatic, progressive disseminated infections occur in persons with impaired cell-mediated immunity. *H. capsulatum* is a dimorphic fungus of worldwide distribution that grows as a mold at ambient temperatures and as a yeast in the body (37°C [98.6°F]). The yeast cell is round and has a central basophilic body surrounded by a clear zone or halo, which in turn is encircled by a rigid cell wall 2 to 4 μm in diameter. In caseous lesions, silver impregnation identifies the remains of degenerating yeast forms.

EPIDEMIOLOGY: Histoplasmosis is acquired by inhalation of infectious spores of *H. capsulatum* (see Fig. 9-55). The reservoir for the fungus is bird droppings and soil. In the Americas, hyperendemic areas are the eastern and central United States, western Mexico, Central America, the northern countries of South America and Argentina. In the tropics, bat nests, caves and soil beneath trees are foci of exposure.

PATHOGENESIS: The disease resembles tuberculosis in many ways. Primary infection begins with phagocytosis of microconidia by alveolar macrophages. Like *M. tuberculosis, H. capsulatum* reproduces in immunologically naïve macrophages. As organisms grow, additional macrophages are recruited to the site of infection, producing an area of pulmonary consolidation. A few macrophages carry organisms first to hilar and mediastinal lymph nodes and then throughout the body, where fungi further infect monocytes/macrophages. The organisms proliferate within these cells until the onset of hypersensitivity and cell-mediated immune responses, usually within 1 to 3 weeks. Normal immune responses usually limit the infection. Activated macrophages destroy the phagocytosed yeasts, forming necrotizing granulomas at sites of infection.

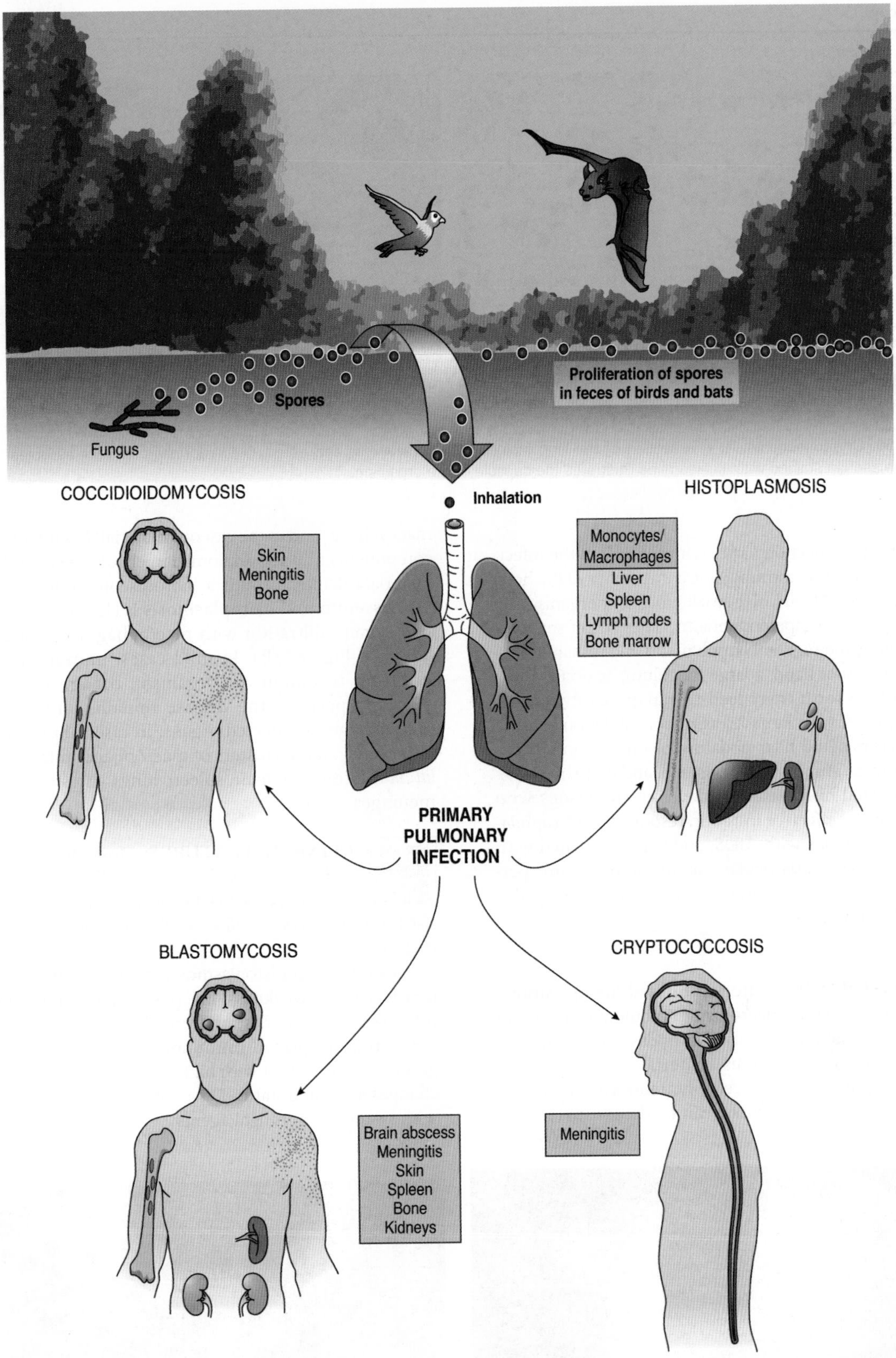

FIGURE 9-55. **Pulmonary and disseminated fungal infection.** Fungi grow in soil, air, and in the feces of birds and bats; they produce spores, some of which are infectious. When inhaled, spores cause primary pulmonary infection. In a few patients, the infection disseminates.

Histoplasmosis. Primary infection is in the lung. In susceptible patients, the fungus disseminates to target organs, namely, the monocyte/macrophage system (liver, spleen, lymph nodes, and bone marrow) and the tongue, mucous membranes of mouth, and the adrenals.

Cryptococcosis. Primary infection of the lung disseminates to the meninges.

Blastomycosis. Primary infection of the lung disseminates widely. The principal targets are the brain, meninges, skin, spleen, bone, and kidney.

Coccidioidomycosis. Primary infection of the lung may disseminate widely. The skin, meninges, and bone are common targets.

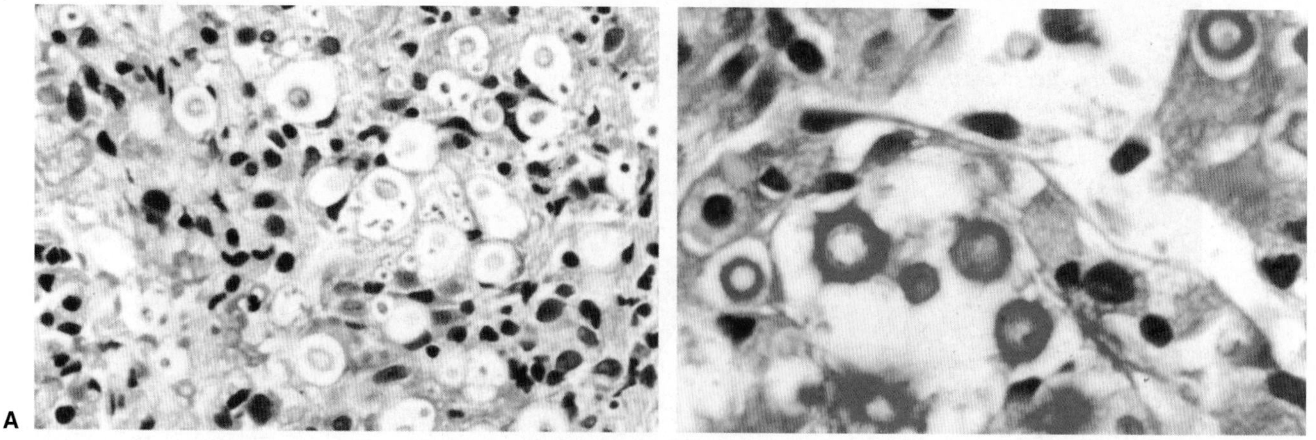

FIGURE 9-56. **Cryptococcosis. A.** In a section of the lung stained with hematoxylin and eosin, *C. neoformans* appears as holes or bubbles. **B.** The same section stained with mucicarmine illustrates the capsule of the organism.

The course of infection varies with the size of the infecting inoculum and the immunologic competence of the host. Most infections (95%) involve small inocula of organisms in immunologically competent persons. They affect small areas of the lung and regional lymph nodes and remain unnoticed. On the other hand, a large inoculum, as occurs in an excavated bird roost, may lead to rapidly evolving pulmonary disease, with large areas of consolidation, prominent mediastinal and hilar nodal involvement, and extension of the infection to the liver, spleen, and bone marrow.

Disseminated histoplasmosis develops in persons who fail to mount an effective immune response to *H. capsulatum*. Infants, persons with AIDS, and patients treated with corticosteroids are at particular risk. In addition, some persons with no known underlying illness also develop disseminated histoplasmosis.

PATHOLOGY: Acute self-limited histoplasmosis is characterized by necrotizing granulomas in the lung, mediastinal and hilar lymph nodes, spleen, and liver. Early in infection, the caseous material is surrounded by macrophages, Langhans giant cells, lymphocytes, and plasma cells. Yeast forms of *H. capsulatum* can be demonstrated within macrophages and in the caseous material. Eventually, the cellular components of the granuloma largely disappear and the caseous material calcifies, forming a "fibrocaseous nodule" (Fig. 9-57A).

Disseminated histoplasmosis is characterized by progressive organ infiltration with macrophages carrying *H. capsulatum* (see Fig. 9-57B). In mild cases, immune responses are sufficient to inhibit the organism, though not eliminate it. For long periods, the disease remains largely confined to macrophages in infected organs. In cases of profound immunodeficiency, large clusters of macrophages filled with *H. capsulatum* infiltrate the liver, spleen, lungs, intestine, adrenals, and meninges.

CLINICAL FEATURES: Most infections are asymptomatic, but with extensive disease, patients present with fever, headache, and cough. The symptoms persist for a few days to a few weeks, but the disease requires no therapy.

Disseminated histoplasmosis features weight loss, intermittent fever, and weakness. In cases of subtle immunodeficiency, the disease may persist and progress for years, even decades. With more-profound immunodeficiency, dissemination progresses rapidly, often with high fever, cough, pancytopenia, and changes in mental status. Disseminated histoplasmosis is treated with systemic antifungal agents.

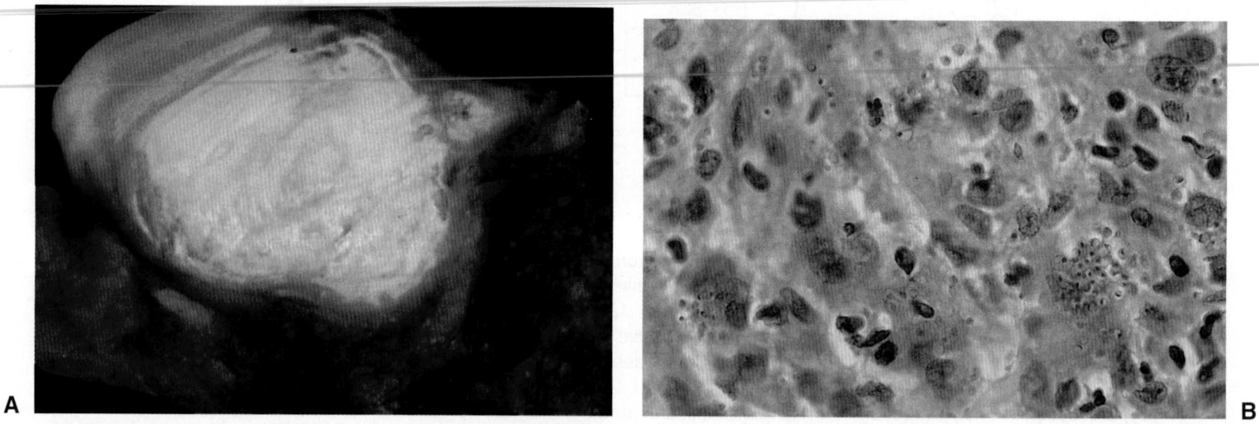

FIGURE 9-57. **Histoplasmosis. A.** A section of lung shows an encapsulated, subpleural, fibrocaseous nodule. **B.** A section of liver from a patient with disseminated histoplasmosis reveals Kupffer cells containing numerous yeasts of *H. capsulatum* (perodic acid-Schiff [PAS] stain).

Coccidioidomycosis

Coccidioidomycosis is a chronic, necrotizing mycotic infection that clinically and pathologically resembles tuberculosis. The disease, caused by *Coccidioides immitis,* includes a spectrum of infections that begin as focal pneumonitis. Most are mild and asymptomatic and are limited to the lungs and regional lymph nodes. Occasionally, *C. immitis* infections spread outside the lungs to produce life-threatening disease.

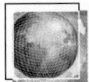

EPIDEMIOLOGY: *C. immitis* is a dimorphic fungus that grows as a mold in the soil, where it forms spores. The spores are inhaled into alveoli and terminal bronchioles (see Fig. 9-55), enlarge into spherules and then mature to form sporangia, which are 30 to 60 μm across. These gradually fill with 1 to 5 μm endospores, which accumulate by endosporulation, a process unique among the pathogenic fungi. The sporangia eventually rupture and release endospores, that then repeat the cycle.

C. immitis is present in the soil in restricted climatic regions, particularly the Lower Sonoran life zones of the Western hemisphere. These are areas with sparse rainfall, hot summers, and mild winters. In the United States, large portions of California, Arizona, New Mexico, and Texas are a natural habitat for *C. immitis*. The disease is particularly common in the San Joaquin Valley of California, where it is called "valley fever." Coccidioidomycosis also occurs in Mexico and parts of South America.

Long-term residents of endemic regions are almost always infected with *C. immitis*. Even brief visits to these areas can cause infection (usually asymptomatic). Dry, windy weather, which lifts spores into the air, favors infection. The disease is not contagious.

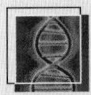

PATHOGENESIS: Coccidioidomycosis begins with focal bronchopneumonia where the spores are deposited. These elicit mixed inflammatory infiltrates of neutrophils and macrophages, but the spores survive these immunologically naïve inflammatory cells. As in tuberculosis and histoplasmosis, the host controls *C. immitis* infection only when inflammatory cells become immunologically activated. Necrotizing granulomas form with the onset of specific hypersensitivity and cell-mediated immune responses, which kills or contains the fungi.

The course of coccidioidomycosis varies from acute, self-limited disease to disseminated infection, depending on the size of the infecting dose and the immune status of the host. Coccidioidomycosis begins with focal bronchopneumonia. *Most infections are produced by small inocula of organisms in immunologically competent hosts and are acute and self-limited.* Extensive pulmonary involvement and fulminant disease may occur in persons from a nonendemic region exposed to large numbers of organisms.

Disseminated coccidioidomycosis occurs in immunocompromised persons, from a primary infection or reactivation of old disease. Immunologically compromised patients are at greatest risk. Certain racial groups, including Filipinos, other Asians, and blacks, are particularly susceptible to dissemination of coccidioidomycosis, probably because of a specific immunologic defect. The risk of dissemination in Filipinos is 175 times that in whites. Pregnant women are also unusually susceptible to spread of the disease if they develop primary infection during the latter half of pregnancy.

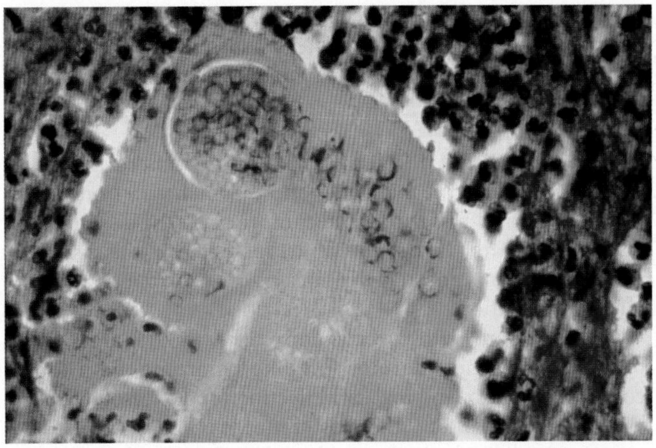

FIGURE 9-58. **Coccidioidomycosis.** A photomicrograph of the lung from a patient with acute coccidioidal pneumonia shows an acute inflammatory infiltrate surrounding spherules and endospores of *Coccidioides immitis*.

PATHOLOGY: Acute self-limited coccidioidomycosis causes solitary lesions or patchy pulmonary consolidation, in which affected alveoli are infiltrated by neutrophils and macrophages (Fig. 9-58). *C. immitis* spherules elicit an infiltrate of macrophages, whereas endospores predominantly attract neutrophils. Once an immune reaction begins, necrotizing, caseous granulomas develop. Successful immune responses cause the granuloma to heal, sometimes leaving a fibrocaseous nodule composed of caseous material and rimmed by residual macrophages and a thin capsule. In contrast to histoplasmosis, old granulomas of coccidioidomycosis rarely calcify.

The spherules and endospores of *C. immitis* stain with hematoxylin and eosin. Spherules in various stages of development appear as basophilic rings. Mature spherules (sporangia) contain endospores that appear as smaller basophilic rings. As in other fungal infections, PAS and GMS stains can be used to enhance the staining of *C. immitis*.

Disseminated coccidioidomycosis may involve almost any body site and may manifest as a single extrathoracic site or as widespread disease, including lesions of the skin (Fig. 9-59),

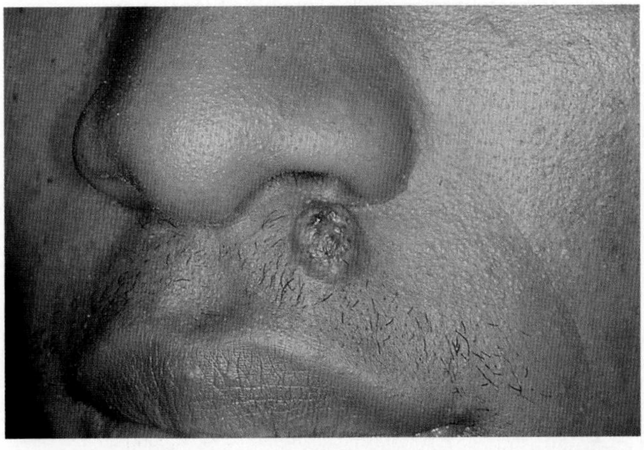

FIGURE 9-59. **Disseminated coccidioidomycosis.** A single raised, central ulcerated lesion is present on the face.

bones, meninges, liver, spleen, and genitourinary tract. The inflammatory response at the sites of dissemination is highly variable, ranging from an infiltrate of neutrophils to a granulomatous response.

CLINICAL FEATURES: Coccidioidomycosis is a disease of protean manifestations, which vary from a subclinical respiratory infection to one that disseminates and is rapidly fatal. Like syphilis and typhoid fever, this disease is a great imitator: almost any complaint or syndrome may be its initial presentation.

Most persons with coccidioidomycosis (>60%) are asymptomatic. The others develop a flulike syndrome, with fever, cough, chest pain, and malaise. Infection usually resolves spontaneously. Cavitation is the most frequent complication of pulmonary coccidioidomycosis, although it fortunately occurs in only few patients (<5%). The cavity, which may be mistaken for tuberculosis, is usually solitary and may persist for years. Progression or reactivation may lead to destructive lesions in the lungs, or more seriously, to disseminated lesions.

The signs and symptoms of disseminated coccidioidomycosis vary according to the site affected. Coccidioidal meningitis manifests with headache, fever, alteration in mental statis or seizures, and is fatal if untreated. Skin lesions in disseminated disease often have a warty appearance (see Fig. 9-59). Even with prolonged amphotericin B therapy, the prognosis is poor in acute disseminated coccidioidomycosis although the response rate can be quite good with some of the newer azole antifungal agents.

Blastomycosis

Blastomycosis is a chronic granulomatous and suppurative pulmonary disease, which is often followed by dissemination to other body sites, principally the skin and bone. The causative organism, *Blastomyces dermatitidis,* is a dimorphic fungus that grows as a mold in warm moist soil, rich in decaying vegetable matter.

EPIDEMIOLOGY: Blastomycosis is acquired by inhalation of infectious spores from the soil (see Fig. 9-55). The infection occurs within restricted geographic regions of the Americas, Africa, and possibly the Middle East. In North America, the fungus is endemic along the distributions of the Mississippi and Ohio Rivers, the Great Lakes, and the St. Lawrence River. Disturbance of the soil, either by construction or by leisure activities such as hunting or camping, leads to formation of aerosols containing fungal spores.

PATHOGENESIS: Inhaled spores of *B. dermatitidis* germinate to form yeasts, which reproduce by budding. The host responds to the proliferating organisms with neutrophils and macrophages, producing a focal bronchopneumonia. However, organisms persist until the onset of specific hypersensitivity and cell-mediated immunity, when activated neutrophils and macrophages kill them.

PATHOLOGY: Blastomycosis is usually confined to the lungs, where infection mostly produces small areas of consolidation. *B. dermatitidis* incites a mixed suppurative and granulomatous inflammatory response and even in the same patient, lesions may range from neutrophilic abscesses to epithelioid granulomas. Pulmonary disease usually resolves by scarring, but some patients develop progressive miliary lesions or cavities. The skin (>50%) and bones (>10%), are the most common sites of extrapulmonary involvement. Skin infection often elicits a marked pseudoepitheliomatous hyperplasia, imparting a warty appearance to the lesions.

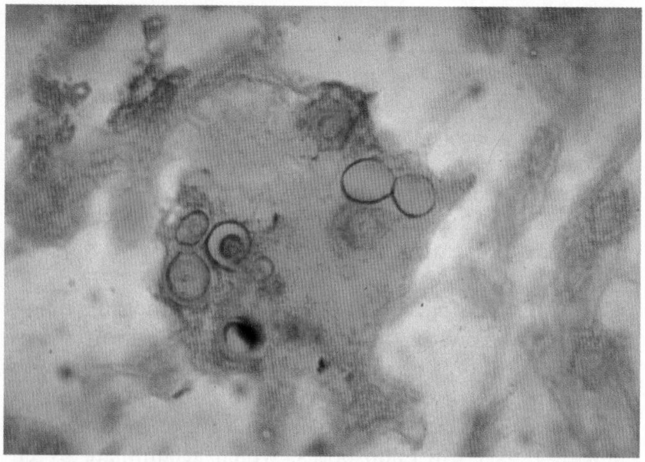

FIGURE 9-60. Blastomycosis. The yeasts of *Blastomyces dermatitidis* have a doubly contoured wall and nuclei in the central body. The buds have broad-based attachments.

Infected areas contain numerous yeasts of *B. dermatitidis,* which are spherical and 8 to 14 μm across, with broad-based buds and multiple nuclei in a central body (Fig. 9-60). With hematoxylin and eosin stains, the yeast are rings with thick, sharply defined cell walls. They may be found in epithelioid cells, macrophages, or giant cells, or they may lie free in microabscesses.

CLINICAL FEATURES: Pulmonary blastomycosis is self-limited in one third of cases. Symptomatic acute infection presents as a flulike illness, with fever, arthralgias, and myalgias. Progressive pulmonary disease is characterized by low-grade fever, weight loss, cough, and predominantly upper lobe infiltrates on the chest radiograph. Skin lesions often resemble squamous cell carcinomas of the skin, and are the most common signs of extrapulmonary dissemination. Although the lung infection may appear to resolve totally, in some patients, blastomycosis may appear at distant sites months to years later.

Paracoccidioidomycosis (South American Blastomycosis)

Paracoccidioidomycosis is a chronic granulomatous infection that begins with lung involvement and disseminates to involve skin, oropharynx, adrenals, and the macrophages of the liver, spleen, and lymph nodes. The causative organism is *Paracoccidioides brasiliensis,* a dimorphic fungus, whose mold form is thought to reside in the soil.

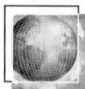

EPIDEMIOLOGY: Paracoccidioidomycosis is acquired by inhalation of spores from the environment in restricted regions of Central and South America. Most infections are asymptomatic. Reactivation of latent infection occurs and persons can develop active disease many years after moving from an endemic region. Interestingly, men develop

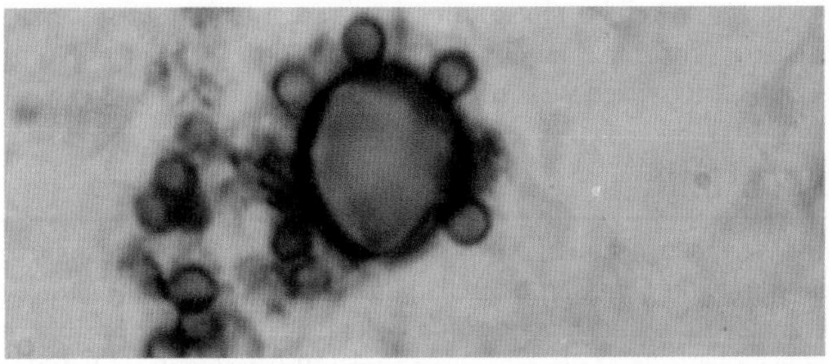

FIGURE 9-61. **Paracoccidioidomycosis.** The lung contains *Paracoccidioides braziliensis,* which displays many external buds arising circumferentially from the mother organism.

symptomatic infections 15 times more often than women, perhaps because of hormonal influences on conversion of the organism to its yeast phase.

PATHOLOGY: Paracoccidioidomycosis can involve the lungs alone (Fig. 9-61) or multiple extrapulmonary sites, most commonly skin, mucosal surfaces and lymph nodes. *P. brasiliensis* elicits a mixed suppurative and granulomatous response, producing lesions similar to those seen in blastomycosis and coccidioidomycosis.

CLINICAL FEATURES: Paracoccidioidomycosis is usually an acute, self-limited, and minimally symptomatic disease. The symptoms of progressive pulmonary involvement resemble those of tuberculosis. Chronic mucocutaneous ulcers are a frequent manifestation of extrapulmonary disease.

Sporotrichosis

Sporotrichosis is a chronic infection of the skin, subcutaneous tissues, and regional lymph nodes caused by Sporothrix schenckii. This dimorphic fungus grows as a mold in soil and decaying plant matter, and as yeast in the body.

EPIDEMIOLOGY: Sporotrichosis is endemic in parts of the Americas and southern Africa. Most cases are cutaneous, resulting from accidental inoculation of the fungus from thorns (especially rose thorns) or splinters or by handling reeds or grasses. Cutaneous sporotrichosis is particularly common among gardeners, botanical nursery workers, and other persons who suffer abrasions while working with soil, moss, hay, or timbers. Infected animals, particularly cats, can also transmit the disease.

PATHOLOGY: On entry into the skin, *S. schenckii* proliferates locally, eliciting an inflammatory response that produces an ulceronodular lesion. The infection frequently spreads along subcutaneous lymphatic channels, resulting in a chain of similar nodular skin lesions (Fig. 9-62A). Extracutaneous disease is much less common than skin disease. Joint and bone involvement is the commonest form of extracutaneous disease and infections of the wrist, elbow, ankle, or knee account for most (80%) of the cases.

The lesions of cutaneous sporotrichosis are usually in the dermis or subcutaneous tissue. The periphery of the nodules is granulomatous and the center is suppurative. Surrounding skin shows exuberant pseudoepitheliomatous hyperplasia. Some yeasts are surrounded by an eosinophilic, spiculated zone and are termed "asteroid bodies" (see Fig. 9-62B). The material surrounding the yeasts ("Splendore-Hoeppli substance") probably consists of antigen–antibody complexes.

CLINICAL FEATURES: Cutaneous sporotrichosis begins as a solitary nodular lesion at the site of inoculation, typically on a hand, arm, or leg. Weeks afterwards, additional nodules may appear along the lymphatic drainage of the primary lesion. Nodules often ulcerate and drain serosanguineous fluid. Joint involvement appears as pain and swelling of the affected joint, without involving overlying skin. Untreated cutaneous sporotrichosis continues to spread along the skin. The skin infection responds to systemic iodine therapy, but extracutaneous sporotrichosis requires systemic antifungal therapy.

A

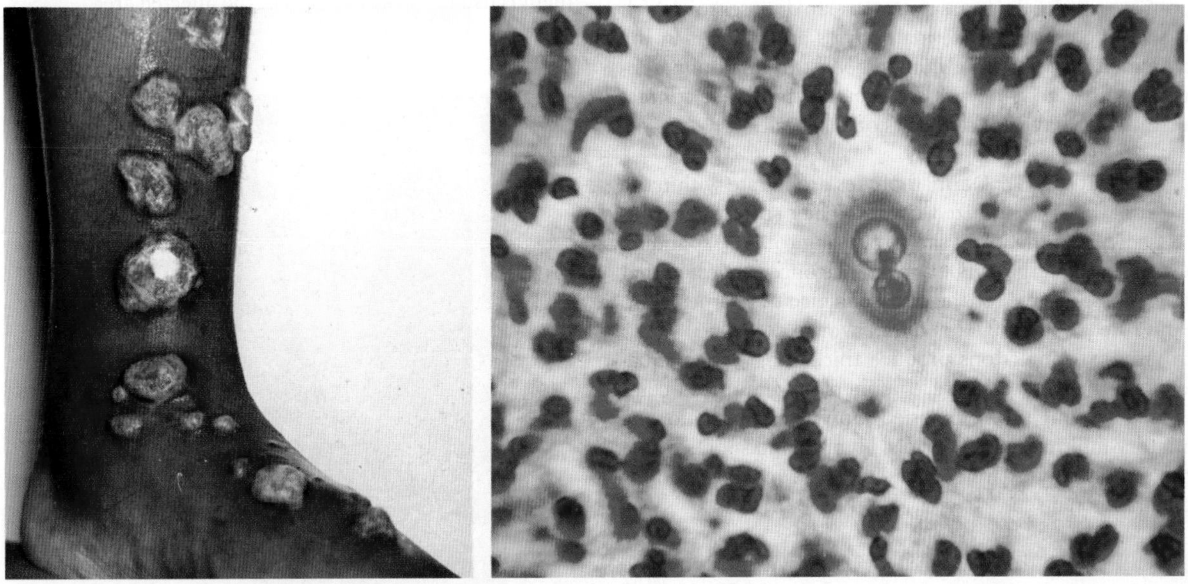

B

FIGURE 9-62. **Sporotrichosis. A.** The leg shows typical lymphocutaneous spread. **B.** A section of the lesion in (A) shows an asteroid body, composed of a pair of budding yeasts of *Sporothrix schenckii* surrounded by a layer of Splendore-Hoeppli substance, with radiating projections.

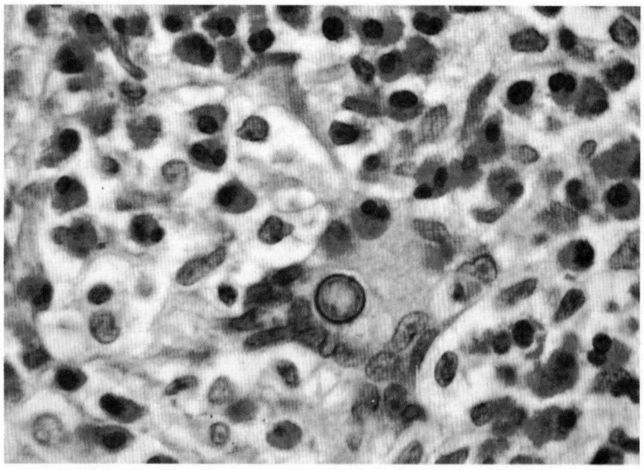

FIGURE 9-63. **Chromomycosis.** A section of skin shows a giant cell in the center, which contains a thick-walled, brown, sclerotic body (copper penny), representing the fungus.

Chromomycosis

Chromomycosis is a chronic skin infection caused by several species of fungi that live as saprophytes in soil and decaying vegetable matter. The fungi are brown, round, thick walled, and 8 μm across and have been likened to "copper pennies" (Fig. 9-63). The infection is most common in barefooted agricultural workers in the tropics, in whom the fungus is implanted by trauma, usually below the knee. The lesions begin as papules and over the years become verrucous, crusted, and sometimes ulcerated. The infection spreads by contiguous growth and through lymphatics and eventually may involve an entire limb.

Dermatophyte Infections

Dermatophytes are fungi that cause localized superficial infections of keratinized tissues, including skin, hair, and nails. There are about 40 species of dermatophytes in 3 genera: *Trichophyton, Microsporum,* and *Epidermophyton.* Dermatophyte infections are minor illnesses, but are among the most common skin diseases for which persons seek medical help. Dermatophytes are resident in the soil, on animals, and on other humans. Most dermatophyte infections in temperate countries are acquired by direct contact with persons who have infected hairs or skin scales.

PATHOLOGY: Dermatophytes proliferate within the superficial keratinized tissues. They spread centrifugally from the initial site, producing round, expanding lesions with sharp margins. The appearance once suggested that a worm was responsible for the disease, hence the names **ringworm** and **tinea** (from the Latin *tinea*, "worm").

Dermatophyte infections produce thickening of the squamous epithelium, with increased numbers of keratinized cells. Lesions severe enough to be biopsied show a mild lymphocytic inflammatory infiltrate in the dermis. Hyphae and spores of the infecting dermatophytes are confined to the nonviable portions of skin, hair, and nails.

CLINICAL FEATURES: Dermatophyte infections are named according to the sites of involvement (e.g., scalp, tinea capitis; feet, tinea pedis, "athlete's foot"; nails, tinea unguium; intertriginous areas of the groin, tinea cruris, "jock itch"). These infections range from asymptomatic disease to chronic, fiercely pruritic eruptions. Dermatophyte infections are treated with topical antifungal agents.

Mycetoma

A mycetoma is a slowly progressive, localized, and often disfiguring infection of the skin, soft tissues, and bone produced by inoculation of various soil-dwelling fungi and filamentous bacteria. Responsible organisms include *Madurella mycetomatis, Petrilidium boydii, Actinomadura madurae,* and *Nocardia brasiliensis.*

EPIDEMIOLOGY: Mycetoma usually occurs in the tropics among farmers and outdoor laborers whose skin is exposed to trauma. The foot is a common site of infection in locales where persons walk barefoot on soggy ground, and the disease is also known as **Madura foot.** Frequent immersion of the foot macerates the skin and facilitates deep inoculation with soil organisms.

PATHOLOGY: In the subcutaneous tissue, the organisms proliferate and spread to adjacent tissues, including bone. This incites a mixed suppurative and granulomatous inflammatory infiltrate which fails to eliminate the infecting organism. Surrounding granulation tissue and scarring produce progressive disfigurement of the affected sites.

A mycetoma begins as a solitary subcutaneous abscess, which slowly expands to form multiple abscesses interconnected by sinus tracts (Fig. 9-64). Sinus tracts eventually drain to the skin surface. Abscesses contain colonies of compact bacteria or fungi surrounded by neutrophils and an outer layer of granulomatous inflammation. The colonies of organisms, called "grains," resemble the "sulfur granules" of actinomycosis.

CLINICAL FEATURES: A mycetoma initially manifests as a painless, localized swelling at a site of penetrating injury. The lesion slowly expands, and produces sinus tracts that tend to follow fascial planes in their lateral and deep spread through connective tissue, muscle, and bone. Treatment is usually wide excision of the affected area.

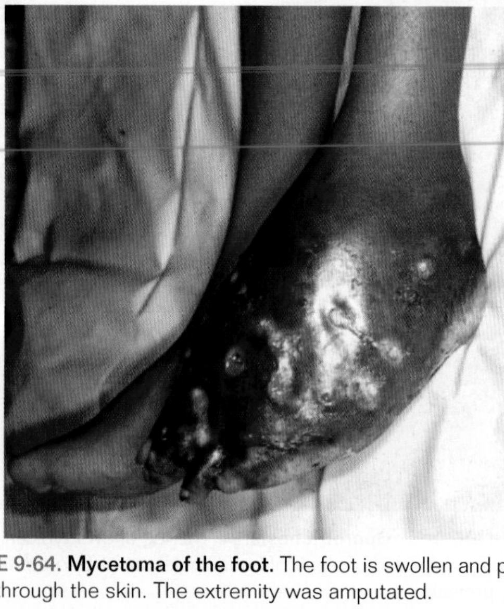

FIGURE 9-64. **Mycetoma of the foot.** The foot is swollen and painful and drains through the skin. The extremity was amputated.

PROTOZOAL INFECTIONS

The protozoa are single-celled eukaryotes that fall into three general classes: **amebae, flagellates,** and **sporozoites**. Amebae move by projection of cytoplasmic extensions termed **pseudopods**. Flagellates move through threadlike structures, flagella, which extend out from the cell membrane. Sporozoites do not have organelles of locomotion and also differ from amebae and flagellates in their mode of replication.

Protozoa cause human disease by diverse mechanisms. Some, such as *Entamoeba histolytica,* are extracellular parasites that digesting and invading human tissues. Others, such as plasmodia, are obligate intracellular parasites that replicate in, and kill, human cells. Still others, such as trypanosomes, damage human tissue largely by inflammatory and immunologic responses they elicit. Some protozoa (e.g., *Toxoplasma gondii*) can establish latent infections and cause reactivation disease in immunocompromised hosts.

Malaria

Malaria is a mosquito-borne, hemolytic, febrile illness. Malaria infects over 200 million persons and yearly kills more than 1 million. Four species of *Plasmodium* cause malaria: *Plasmodium falciparum, Plasmodium vivax, Plasmodium ovale,* and *Plasmodium malariae*. All these plasmodia infect and destroy human erythrocytes, producing chills, fever, anemia, and splenomegaly. *P. falciparum* causes more severe disease than the others and accounts for most malarial deaths.

EPIDEMIOLOGY: Malaria has been eradicated in developed countries but continues to afflict people tropical and subtropical areas, especially Africa, South and Central America, India, and Southeast Asia (Fig. 9-65). The rural poor, infants, children, malnourished persons and pregnant women are all especially susceptible to infection.

Malaria is transmitted by the bite of the female *Anopheles* mosquito. *P. falciparum* and *P. vivax* are the most common pathogens, but there is considerable geographic variation in species distribution. *P. vivax* is rare in Africa, where much of the black population lacks the erythrocyte cell surface receptors required for infection. *P. falciparum* and *P. ovale* are the predominant species in Africa. *P. malariae* is the least common and mildest form of malaria, although it has a broad geographic distribution.

PATHOGENESIS: The life cycle of the *Plasmodium* species responsible for human malaria requires both human and mosquito hosts (Fig. 9-66). Infected humans produce forms of the organism (gametocytes) that mosquitoes acquire on feeding. Within these insects, the organism reproduces sexually, producing plasmodial forms (sporozoites), which the mosquito transmits to humans when it feeds.

The anopheline mosquito inoculates the sporozoites into a human's bloodstream. There, they undergo asexual division ("schizogony"). Circulating sporozoites rapidly invade hepatocytes and reproduce in the liver, yielding numerous daughter organisms, "merozoites" (exoerythrocytic phase). Within 2 to 3 weeks of hepatic infection, these rupture host hepatocytes exit into the bloodstream and invade erythrocytes.

Merozoites feed on hemoglobin, grow and reproduce inside erythrocytes. Within 2 to 4 days, mature progeny merozoites are produced. These merozoites burst from infected erythrocytes, invade naïve red cells, and so initiate another cycle of erythrocytic parasitism. The erythrocytic cycle is repeated many times. Eventually, subpopulations of merozoites differentiate into sexual forms called gametocytes, which are ingested when a mosquito feedsing on an infected host, thus completing the parasite's life cycle.

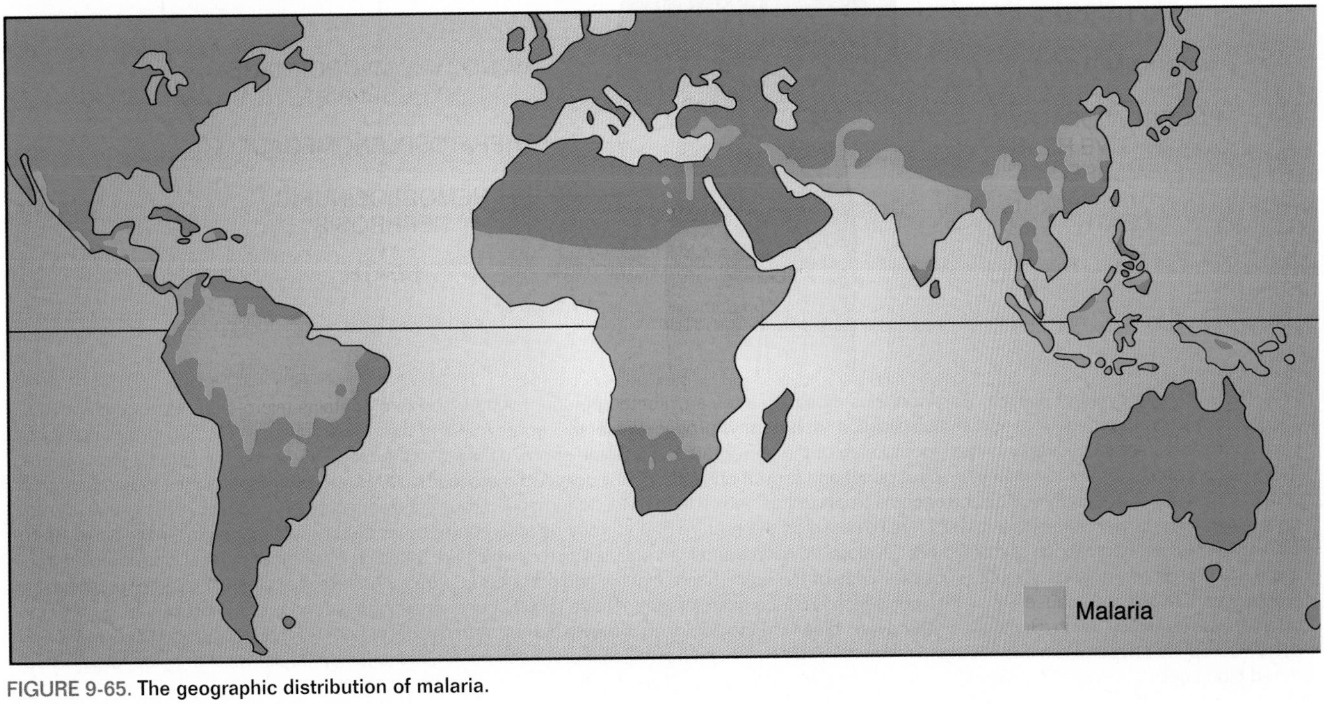

FIGURE 9-65. The geographic distribution of malaria.

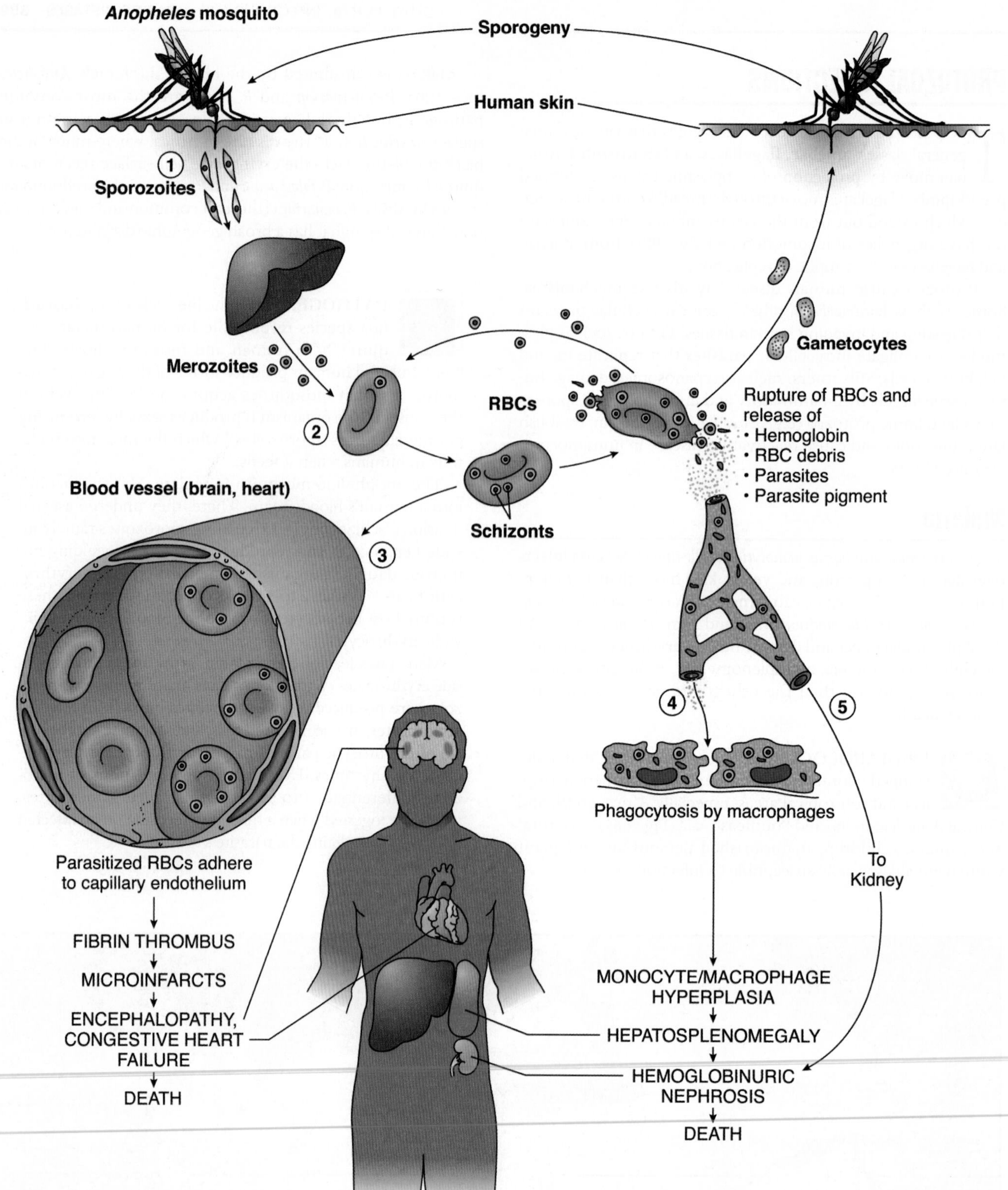

FIGURE 9-66. **Life cycle of malaria.** An *Anopheles* mosquito bites an infected person, taking blood that contains micro- and macrogametocytes (sexual forms). In the mosquito, sexual multiplication (sporogony) produces infective sporozoites in the salivary glands. ***(1)*** During the mosquito bite, sporozoites are inoculated into the bloodstream of the vertebrate host. Some sporozoites leave the blood and enter the hepatocytes, where they multiply asexually (exoerythrocytic schizogony) and form thousands of uninucleated merozoites. ***(2)*** Rupture of hepatocytes releases merozoites, which penetrate erythrocytes and become trophozoites, which then divide to form numerous schizonts (intraerythrocytic schizogony). Schizonts divide to form more merozoites, which are released on the rupture of erythrocytes and reenter other erythrocytes to begin a new cycle. After several cycles, subpopulations of merozoites develop into micro- and macrogametocytes, which are taken up by another mosquito to complete the cycle. ***(3)*** Parasitized erythrocytes obstruct capillaries of the brain, heart, kidney, and other deep organs. Adherence of parasitized erythrocytes to capillary endothelial cells causes fibrin thrombi, which produce microinfarcts. These result in encephalopathy, congestive heart failure, pulmonary edema, and frequently death. Ruptured erythrocytes release hemoglobin, erythrocyte debris, and malarial pigment. ***(4)*** Phagocytosis leads to monocyte/macrophage hyperplasia and hepatosplenomegaly. ***(5)*** Released hemoglobin produces hemoglobinuric nephrosis, which may be fatal. RBCs = red blood cells.

The rupture of infected erythrocytesreleases pyrogens and causes the chills and fever of malaria. Anemia results both from loss of circulating infected erythrocytes and sequestration of cells in the enlarging spleen. The fixed mononuclear phagocytes of the liver and spleen respond to the infestation by causing enlargement of the liver and spleen.

P. falciparum, causes malignant malaria, a much more aggressive disease than the other plasmodia. It is distinguished from other malarial parasites in four respects:

- It has no secondary exoerythrocytic (hepatic) stage.
- It parasitizes erythrocytes of any age, causing marked parasitemia and anemia. In other types of malaria, only subpopulations of erythrocytes (e.g., only young or old forms) are parasitized, and thus low-level parasitemias and more modest anemias occur.
- There may be several parasites in a single red cell.
- *P. falciparum* alters flow characteristics and adhesive properties of infected erythrocytes, so they adhere to the endothelial cells of small blood vessels. Obstruction of small blood vessels frequently produces severe tissue ischemia, which is probably the most important factor in the virulence of *P. falciparum.*

PATHOLOGY: All forms of malaria display hepatosplenomegaly as red blood cells are sequestered by fixed mononuclear phagocytes. The organs of this system (liver, spleen, lymph nodes) are darkened ("slate gray") by macrophages filled with hemosiderin and malarial pigment, the end-product of parasitic digestion of hemoglobin.

Adherence of infected red cells to microvascular endothelium in falciparum malaria has two consequences. First, parasitized erythrocytes attached to endothelial cells do not circulate, so patients with severe falciparum malaria have few circulating parasites. Second, capillaries of deep organs, especially the brain, become obstructed, leading to ischemia of the brain, kidneys, and lungs. Brains of persons who die of cerebral malaria show congestion and thrombosis of small blood vessels in the white matter, which are rimmed with edema and hemorrhage ("ring hemorrhages") (Fig. 9-67). Obstruction of renal blood flow produces acute renal failure, whereas intravascular hemolysis leads to hemoglobinuric nephrosis (**blackwater fever**). In the lung, damage to alveolar capillaries produces pulmonary edema and acute alveolar damage.

CLINICAL FEATURES: Recurrent **paroxysms** of chills and high fever are characteristic of malaria. They begin with chills and sometimes headache, followed by a high, spiking fever with tachycardia, often accompanied by nausea, vomiting, and abdominal pain. The high fever produces marked vasodilation and often associated orthostatic hypotension. The patient defervesces after several hours, and is usually exhausted and drenched in sweat.

A period of 2 to 3 days follows, during which the patient feels well, only to be followed by a new paroxysm. Paroxysms recur for weeks, eventually subsiding as an immunologic response is mounted. Each paroxysm reflects the rupture of infected erythrocytes and release of daughter merozoites. As the mononuclear macrophage system responds to the infection, patients develop hepatosplenomegaly. Splenic enlargement can be dramatic. Indeed, some of the largest spleens on record represent the effects of chronic malaria. Hypersplenism can exacer-

A
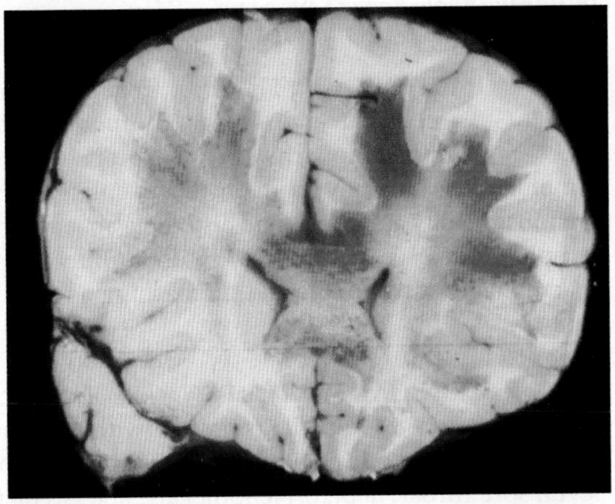

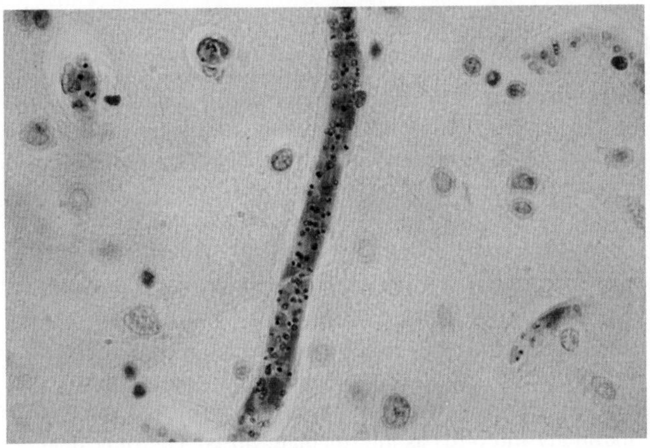
B

C
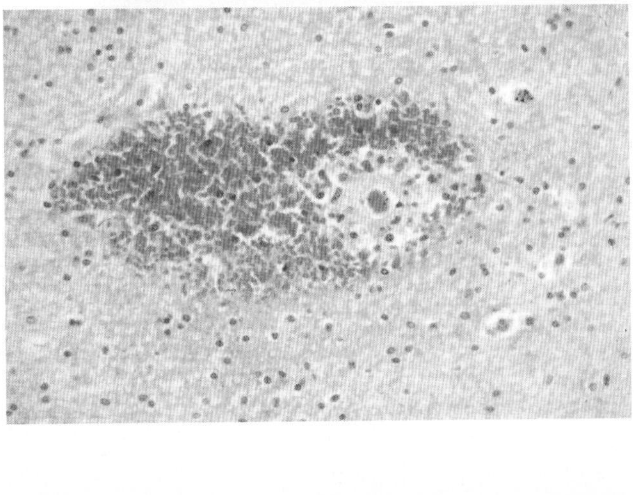

FIGURE 9-67. **Acute falciparum malaria of the brain. A.** There is severe diffuse congestion of the white matter and focal hemorrhages. **B.** A section of *(A)* shows a capillary packed with parasitized erythrocytes. **C.** Another section of *(A)* displays a ring hemorrhage around a thrombosed capillary, which contains parasitized erythrocytes in a fibrin thrombus.

bate the anemia of malarial infection. *P. falciparum* infection produces a graver disease than the other forms of malaria. As the level of parasitemia grows, fever may become virtually continuous. Ischemic brain injury causes symptoms from somnolence, hallucinations, and behavioral changes, to seizures and coma. CNS disease has a mortality of 20% to 50%.

Malaria is diagnosed by demonstrating the organisms on Giemsa-stained blood smears. The several species are distinguished by their appearance in infected erythrocytes. Malarias other than falciparum malaria are treated with oral chloroquine, sometimes with primaquine. Therapy for falciparum malaria varies, as new treatments are constantly being developed to meet the challenge of widespread chloroquine resistance.

Babesiosis

Babesiosis is a malaria-like infection caused by protozoa of the genus Babesia, *which is transmitted by hard-bodied ticks.*

EPIDEMIOLOGY: *Babesia* infections are common in animals and in some locations are responsible for serious economic losses to the livestock industry. By contrast, human babesiosis is almost a medical curiosity, with the parasites infecting humans only when they intrude into the zoonotic cycle between the tick vector and its vertebrate host. Human babesiosis has been reported only in Europe and North America. Infections in the United States have been concentrated in islands off the New England coast. The organisms invade and destroy erythrocytes, causing hemoglobinemia, hemoglobinuria, and renal failure. The disease is usually self-limited, but uncontrolled infections can be fatal. *Babesia* spp. are resistant to most antiprotozoal drugs.

Toxoplasmosis

Toxoplasmosis is a worldwide infectious disease caused by a protozoan, Toxoplasma gondii. *Most infections are asymptomatic, but if they occur in a fetus or immunocompromised host, devastating necrotizing disease may result.*

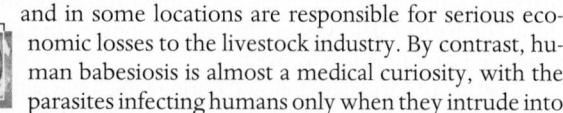

EPIDEMIOLOGY AND PATHOGENESIS: In some areas (e.g., France), the prevalence of *T. gondii* infection exceeds 80% of adults; in other regions (e.g., the southwestern United States), few people are affected. *T. gondii* infects many mammals and birds as intermediate hosts. The only final host is the cat, which becomes infected by ingesting cysts of the organism in tissues of an infected mouse or other intermediate host. Within the cat's intestinal epithelium, five multiplicative stages end with the shedding of oocysts. Oocysts sporulate in feces and soil and differentiate into sporocysts, which contain sporozoites. These are ingested by intermediate hosts, such as birds, mice, or humans and develop in the intermediate host to complete the life cycle.

T. gondii has two stages in tissue, tachyzoites and bradyzoites, both crescent-shaped and measuring 2 × 6 μm. During acute infection, tachyzoites multiply rapidly to form "groups" within intracellular vacuoles of the parasitized cells, eventually causing the cells to rupture. Tachyzoites spread from the gut through the lymphatics to regional lymph nodes and through the blood to the liver, lungs, heart, brain, and other organs. During chronic infection, the organisms, now called "bradyzoites," multiply slowly. The bradyzoites store PAS-positive material and hundreds of organisms are tightly packed in "cysts." The cysts originate in intracellular vacuoles, enlarge beyond the usual size of the cell, and push the nucleus to the periphery.

Except for congenital infection, toxoplasmosis is acquired by eating infectious forms of the organism. In the tropics, where infection is generally acquired in childhood, oocysts in contaminated soil are the main source of infection. In developed countries, the major mechanism of infection is eating incompletely cooked meat (lamb and pork) that carries *Toxoplasma* tissue cysts. Another source of infection is cat feces: oocysts contaminate the hands and food of people who live in close proximity to cats. Congenital infection is acquired by transplacental transmission of infectious forms from an acutely infected (usually asymptomatic) mother to the fetus.

The active infection is usually terminated by cell-mediated immunologic responses. *In most* T. gondii *infections, little significant tissue destruction occurs before the immune response brings the active phase of the infection under control and infected persons suffer few clinical effects. T. gondii* establishes latent infection, however, by forming dormant tissue cysts in some infected cells. These survive for decades in host cells. If an infected person loses cell-mediated immunity, the organism can emerge from its encysted form and reestablish a destructive infection.

Toxoplasma Lymphadenopathy Occurs in Immunocompetent Persons

PATHOLOGY: The most frequent manifestation of *T. gondii* infection in the immunocompetent host is lymphadenopathy (see Chapter 20). Virtually any lymph node group may be involved, but enlarged cervical nodes are most readily apparent. The histologic appearance of affected lymph nodes is distinctive, with numerous epithelioid macrophages surrounding and encroaching on reactive germinal centers.

CLINICAL FEATURES: In *Toxoplasma* lymphadenitis (Fig. 9-68A), patients present with nontender regional lymph node enlargement, sometimes accompanied by fever, sore throat, hepatosplenomegaly, and circulating atypical lymphocytes. Hepatitis, myocarditis (see Fig. 9-68B) and myositis have been documented. Lymphadenopathy usually resolves spontaneously in several weeks to several months and therapy is seldom required.

Congenital Toxoplasma Infections Principally Affect the Brain

T. gondii infection in a fetus is far more destructive than is postnatal infection (see Chapter 6).

PATHOLOGY: The developing brain and eye are readily infected, and the fetus lacks the immunologic capacity to contain the infection. CNS infection causes a necrotizing meningoencephalitis, which in the most severe cases leads to

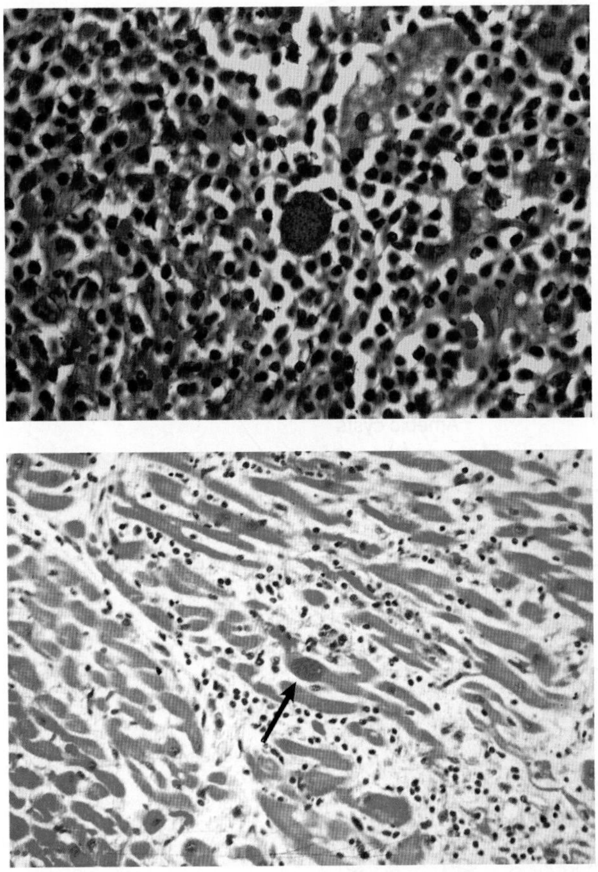

FIGURE 9-68. **Toxoplasmosis. A.** A photomicrograph of an enlarged lymph node reveals bradyzoites of *Toxoplasma gondii* within a cyst. **B.** A section of heart shows a cyst of bradyzoites of *T. gondii* within a myofiber *(arrow)*, with edema and inflammatory cells in the adjacent tissue.

loss of brain parenchyma, cerebral calcifications, and marked hydrocephalus (Fig. 9-69). Ocular infection causes chorioretinitis (i.e., necrosis and inflammation of the choroid and retina).

CLINICAL FEATURES: The most severe fetal disease is produced by infection early in pregnancy and often terminates in spontaneous abortion. In infants born with congenital toxoplasmosis, the effects of brain involvement range from severe mental retardation and seizures to subtle psychomotor defects. Ocular involvement may cause congenital visual impairment. Latent ocular infection established in utero may also recrudesce later in life to produce visual loss. Some newborns have *Toxoplasma* hepatitis, with large areas of necrosis and giant cells. Adrenal necrosis is also occasionally observed. Congenital toxoplasmosis requires therapy with antiprotozoal agents.

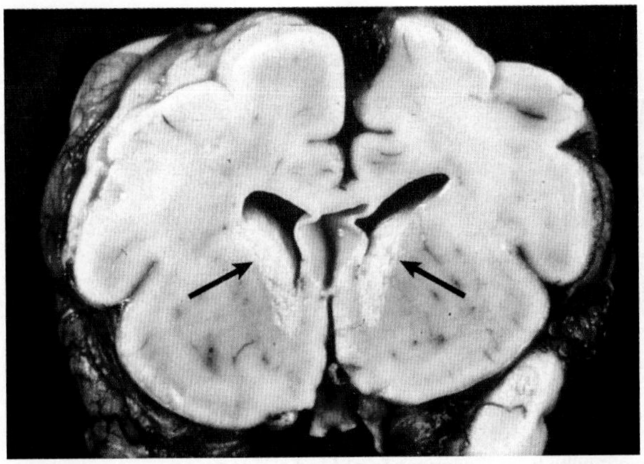

FIGURE 9-69. **Congenital toxoplasmosis.** The brain of a premature infant reveals subependymal necrosis with calcification appearing as bilaterally symmetric areas of whitish discoloration *(arrows)*.

Toxoplasmosis in Immunocompromised Hosts Produces Encephalitis

Devastating *T. gondii* infections occur in persons with decreased cell-mediated immunity (e.g., patients with AIDS or those receiving immunosuppressive therapy). In most cases, the disease represents reactivation of a latent infection. The brain is the most commonly affected organ, where infection with *T. gondii* produces a multifocal necrotizing encephalitis. Patients with encephalitis present with paresis, seizures, alterations in visual acuity, and changes in mentation. *Toxoplasma* encephalitis in immunocompromised patients is fatal if not treated with effective antiprotozoal agents.

Amebiasis

Amebiasis is infection with Entamoeba histolytica, *which principally involves the colon and occasionally the liver. E. histolytica* is named for its lytic actions on tissue. Intestinal infection ranges from asymptomatic colonization to severe invasive infections with bloody diarrhea. On occasion, parasites spread beyond the colon to involve other organs. The most common site of extraintestinal disease is the liver, where *E. histolytica* causes slowly expanding, necrotizing abscesses.

EPIDEMIOLOGY: Humans are the only known reservoir for *E. histolytica,* which reproduces in the colon and passes in the feces. Although amebiasis is found worldwide, it is more common and more severe in tropical and subtropical areas, where poor sanitation prevails. *Amebiasis is acquired by ingestion of materials contaminated with human feces.*

PATHOGENESIS: *E. histolytica* has three distinct stages: the trophozoite, the precyst, and the cyst.

Amebic trophozoites, 10 to 60 μm across, are found in the stools of patients with acute symptoms. They are spherical or oval and have a thin cell membrane, a single nucleus, condensed chromatin on the interior of the nuclear membrane, and a central karyosome. The trophozoites sometimes contain phagocytosed erythrocytes. PAS stains the cytoplasm of the trophozoites and makes them stand out in tissue sections. In the colon, the trophozoite develops into a cyst through an intermediate form termed the precyst, during which process the trophozoite stops feeding, becomes round and nonmotile, loses some of its digestive vacuoles, and forms a glycogen mass and chromatoidal bodies.

Amebic cysts are the infecting stage and are found only in stools, since they do not invade tissue. They are spherical, have thick walls, measure 5 to 25 μm across and usually have four nuclei. From the stools, the cysts contaminate water, food, or fingers. (Fig. 9-70). On ingestion, cysts traverse the stomach and excyst in the lower ileum. A metacystic ameba containing four nuclei divides to form four small, immature trophozoites, which then grow to full size.

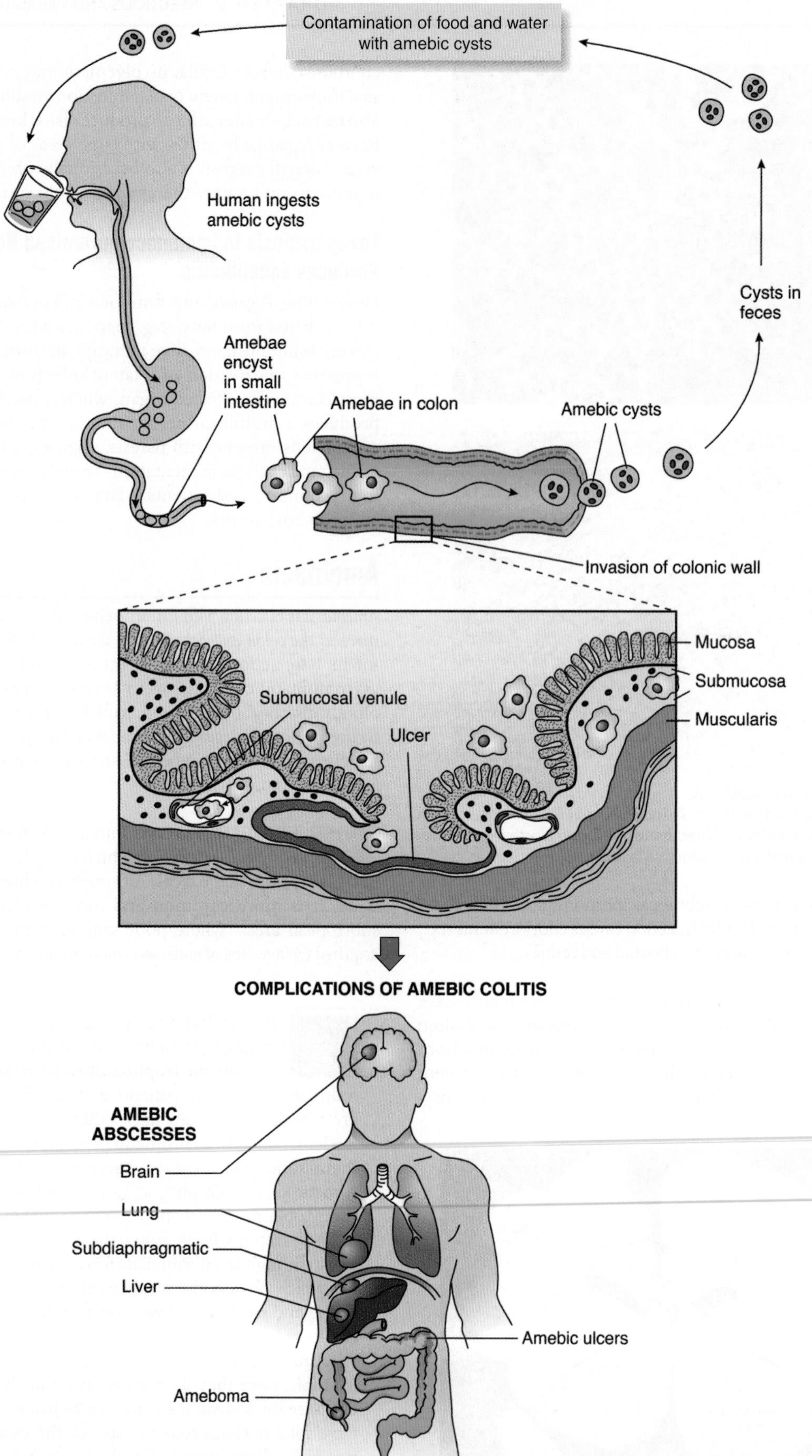

FIGURE 9-70. **Amebic colitis and its complications.** Amebiasis results from the ingestion of food or water contaminated with amebic cysts. In the colon, the amebae penetrate the mucosa and produce flask-shaped ulcers of the mucosa and submucosa. The organisms may invade submucosal venules, thereby disseminating the infection to the liver and other organs. The liver abscess can expand to involve adjacent structures.

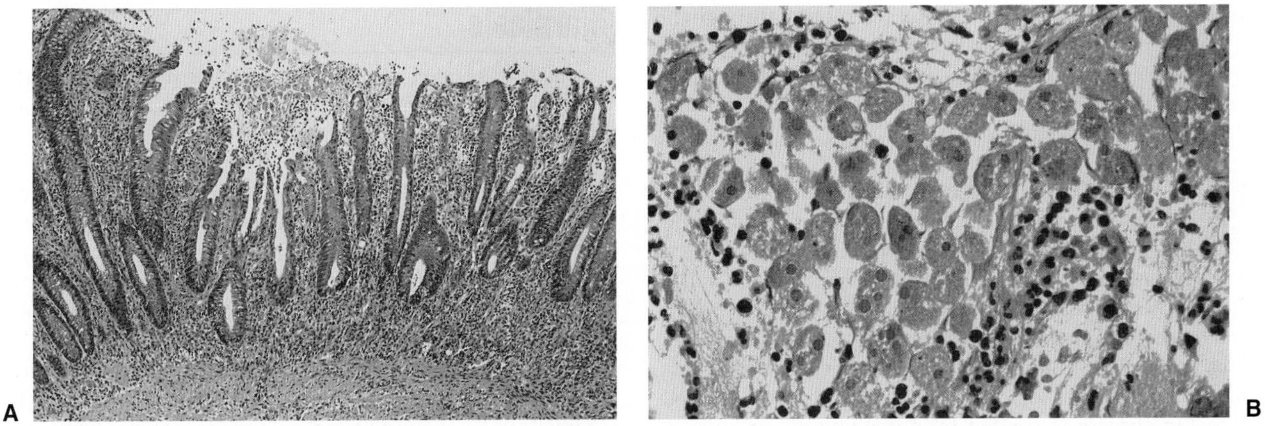

FIGURE 9-71. **Intestinal amebiasis. A.** The colonic mucosa shows superficial ulceration beneath a cluster of trophozoites of *Entamoeba histolytica.* The lamina propria contains excess acute and chronic inflammatory cells, including eosinophils. **B.** Higher-power view shows numerous trophozoites in the luminal exudate.

These thrive in the colon and feed on bacteria and human cells. They may colonize any part of the large bowel, but the cecum is most affected. Patients with symptomatic amebic colitis pass both cysts and trophozoites. The latter survive only briefly outside the body and are also destroyed by gastric secretions. Host factors, such as nutritional status, coexistent colonic flora, and immunologic status, also affect the course of *E. histolytica* infection. Invasion begins with attachment of a trophozoite to a colonic epithelial cell. The organism kills the target cell by elaborating a lytic protein that breaches the cell membrane. Progressive death of mucosal cells produces a superficial ulcer.

Intestinal Amebiasis Is an Ulcerating Disease of the Colon

PATHOLOGY: Amebic lesions begin as small foci of necrosis that progress to ulcers (Fig. 9-71A). Undermining of the ulcer margin and confluence of expanding ulcers lead to irregular sloughing of the mucosa. The ulcer bed is gray and necrotic, with fibrin and cellular debris. The exudate raises the undermined mucosa, producing chronic amebic ulcers whose shape has been described as resembling a flask or a bottle neck.

Trophozoites are found on the surface of the ulcer, in the exudate and in the crater (see Fig. 9-71B). They are also frequent in the submucosa, muscularis propria, serosa, and small veins of the submucosa. There is little inflammatory response in early amebic ulcers. However, as the ulcer enlarges, acute and chronic inflammatory cells accumulate.

An **ameboma** is an infrequent complication of amebiasis, occurring when amebae invade through the intestinal wall. It is an inflammatory thickening of the bowel wall that resembles colon cancer and tends to form a "napkin-ring constriction." It consists of granulation tissue, fibrosis and clusters of trophozoites.

CLINICAL FEATURES: Intestinal amebiasis ranges from completely asymptomatic to a severe dysenteric disease. The incubation period for acute amebic colitis is 8 to 10 days. Gradually increasing abdominal discomfort, tenderness, and cramps are accompanied by chills and fever. Nausea, vomiting, malodorous flatus and intermittent constipation are typical features. Liquid stools (up to 25 a day) contain bloody mucus, but diarrhea is rarely prolonged enough to cause dehydration. Amebic colitis often persists for months or years and patients may become emaciated and anemic. Clinical features may be bizarre and sometimes must be differentiated from those of appendicitis, cholecystitis, intestinal obstruction, or diverticulitis. In severe amebic colitis, massive destruction of colonic mucosa may lead to fatal hemorrhage, perforation, or peritonitis. Therapy for intestinal amebiasis includes metronidazole, which acts against trophozoites and diloxanide, which is effective against cysts.

Amebic Liver Abscess Is a Major Complication of Intestinal Amebiasis

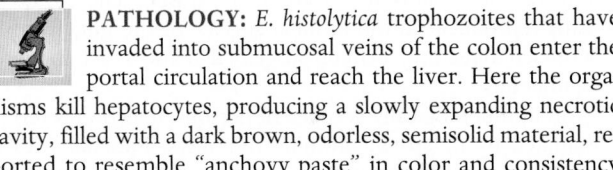

PATHOLOGY: *E. histolytica* trophozoites that have invaded into submucosal veins of the colon enter the portal circulation and reach the liver. Here the organisms kill hepatocytes, producing a slowly expanding necrotic cavity, filled with a dark brown, odorless, semisolid material, reported to resemble "anchovy paste" in color and consistency (Fig. 9-72). Neutrophils are rare within the cavity and trophozoites are found along the edges adjacent to hepatocytes.

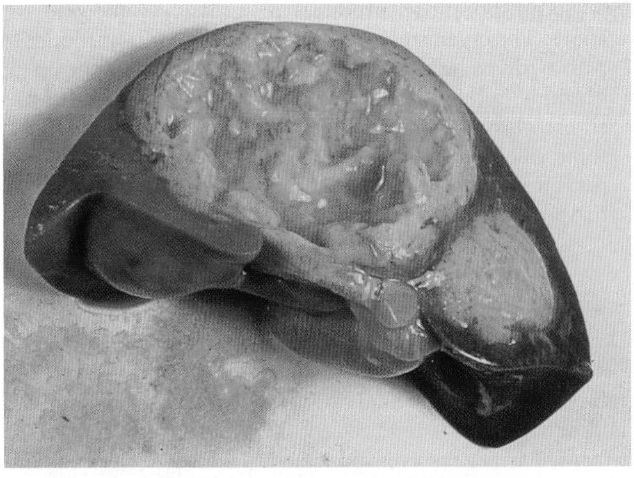

FIGURE 9-72. **Amebic abscesses of the liver.** The cut surface of the liver shows multiple abscesses containing "anchovy paste" material.

An amebic liver abscess may expand and rupture through the capsule, extending into the peritoneum, diaphragm, pleural cavity, lungs, or pericardium. Rarely, a liver abscess, or even a lesion in the colon, may spread amebae to the brain by a hematogenous route to form large necrotic lesions.

CLINICAL FEATURES: Patients with amebic liver abscess present with severe right upper quadrant pain, low-grade fever, and weight loss. Only a minority of patients give a history of an antecedent diarrheal illness and *E. histolytica* is demonstrated in the feces of less than one-third of patients with extraintestinal disease. The diagnosis is usually made by radiologic or ultrasound demonstration of the abscess, in conjunction with serologic testing for antibodies to *E. histolytica*. Amebic abscess is treated by percutaneous or surgical drainage and antiamebic drugs.

Cryptosporidiosis

Cryptosporidiosis is an enteric infection with protozoa of the genus Cryptosporidium *that cause diarrhea in persons with compromised immunity.* The infection varies from a self-limited gastrointestinal infection to a potentially life-threatening illness. It is acquired by ingesting *Cryptosporidium* oocysts, which are shed in feces of infected humans and animals. Most infections probably result from person-to-person transmission, but many domesticated animals harbor the parasite, and are a large reservoir for human infection.

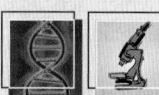

PATHOGENESIS AND PATHOLOGY: *Cryptosporidium* oocysts survives passage through the stomach and release forms that attach to the microvillous surface of the small bowel. Unlike *Toxoplasma* and other coccidia, *Cryptosporidium* remains an extracellular parasite. The organisms reproduce on the luminal surface of the gut, from stomach to rectum, forming progeny that also attach to the epithelium.

In immunologically competent persons, infection is terminated by unknown immune responses. Patients with AIDS and some congenital immunodeficiencies cannot contain the parasite and develop chronic infections, which sometimes spread from the bowel to involve the gallbladder and intrahepatic bile ducts.

Cryptosporidiosis produces no grossly visible alterations. The organisms are visible microscopically as round, 2- to 4-μm blebs attached to the luminal surface of the epithelium. In the small intestine, there may be moderate or severe chronic inflammation in the lamina propria and some villous atrophy directly related to the density of the parasites. The colon has a chronic active colitis, with minimal architectural disruption.

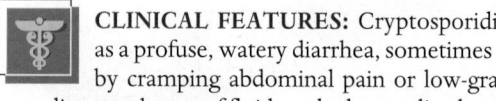

CLINICAL FEATURES: Cryptosporidiosis presents as a profuse, watery diarrhea, sometimes accompanied by cramping abdominal pain or low-grade fever. Extraordinary volumes of fluid can be lost as diarrhea and intensive fluid replacement is required. In immunologically competent persons, diarrhea resolves spontaneously in 1 to 2 weeks. In immunocompromised patients, diarrhea persists indefinitely and may contribute to death.

Giardiasis

Giardiasis is an infection of the small intestine caused by the flagellated protozoan Giardia lamblia *and characterized by abdominal cramping and diarrhea.*

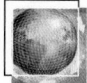

EPIDEMIOLOGY: *G. lamblia* has a worldwide distribution, with a prevalence of infection from less than 1% to more than 25% in some areas with warmer climates and crowded, unsanitary environments. Children are more susceptible than adults. Giardiasis is acquired by ingesting infectious cyst forms of the organism, which are shed in the feces of infected humans and animals. Infection spreads directly from person to person and also in contaminated water or food. *Giardia* can be acquired from wilderness water sources, where infected animals, such as beavers and bears, serve as the reservoir of infection. The infection may be epidemic and outbreaks have occurred in orphanages and institutions.

PATHOGENESIS AND PATHOLOGY: *G. lamblia* has two stages: trophozoites and cysts. The former are flat, pear-shaped, binucleate organisms with 4 pairs of flagella. They are most numerous in the duodenum and proximal small intestine. A curved, disklike "sucker plate" on their ventral surface aids mucosal attachment. Ingested cysts contain 2 or 4 nuclei and revert to trophozoites on reaching the intestine. The stools usually contain only cysts, but trophozoites may also be present in patients with diarrhea.

Giardia cysts survive gastric acidity and rupture within the duodenum and jejunum to release trophozoites. The latter attach to the small bowel epithelial microvilli and reproduce. Giardiasis produces no grossly visible alterations. Microscopic examination shows *Giardia* trophozoites on the surface of villi and within crypts, with minimal associated mucosal changes.

CLINICAL FEATURES: *G. lamblia* is a harmless commensal in most persons, but can cause acute or chronic symptoms. Acute giardiasis occurs with abrupt onset of abdominal cramping and frequent, foul-smelling stools. The infection is highly variable. In some patients, symptoms resolve spontaneously in 1 to 4 weeks. Others complain of persistent abdominal cramping and poorly formed stools for months. In children, chronic giardiasis may cause malabsorption, weight loss, and retarded growth. The infection is treated effectively with various antibiotics, including metronidazole.

Leishmaniasis

Leishmaniae are protozoans that are transmitted to humans by insect bites and cause a spectrum of clinical syndromes, ranging from indolent, self-resolving cutaneous ulcers to fatal disseminated disease. There are numerous species of *Leishmania,* which differ in their natural habitats and the types of disease that they produce.

EPIDEMIOLOGY: Leishmaniasis is transmitted by *Phlebotomus* sandflies, which acquire the infection by feeding on infected animals. In many subtropical and tropical areas, leishmanial infection is endemic in animal populations; thus, dogs, ground squirrels, foxes, and jackals are reservoirs and potential sources for transmission to humans. It is mainly a disease of less-developed countries where humans live in close proximity to animal hosts and the fly vector. There are estimated to be 20 million persons infected worldwide.

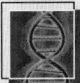

PATHOGENESIS: Infection begins when the organisms are inoculated into human skin by the bite of the sandfly. Shortly thereafter, leishmaniae are phagocytosed by mononuclear phagocytes and transformed into amastigotes, which reproduce within the macrophage. Daughter amastigotes eventually rupture from the cell and spread to other macrophages. Reproduction continues in this way and eventually a cluster of infected macrophages forms at the site of inoculation.

From this initial local infection, the disease may take widely divergent courses depending on two factors: the immunologic capabilities of the host and the infecting species of *Leishmania*. Three distinct clinical entities are recognized: (1) localized cutaneous leishmaniasis, (2) mucocutaneous leishmaniasis, and (3) visceral leishmaniasis.

Localized Cutaneous Leishmaniasis Is an Ulcerating Disorder

Several *Leishmania* species in Central and South America, Northern Africa, the Middle East, India, and China produce localized cutaneous disease, also known as "oriental sore" or "tropical sore."

PATHOLOGY: Localized cutaneous leishmaniasis begins as a collection of amastigote-filled macrophages that ulcerates the overlying epidermis. In tissue sections, the oval amastigotes measure 2 μm and contain two internal structures, a nucleus and a kinetoplast. Under low power, amastigotes in macrophages appear as multiple regular cytoplasmic dots, **Leishman-Donovan bodies.** With progressive development of cell-mediated immunity, macrophages become activated and kill the intracellular parasites. The lesion slowly assumes a more mature granulomatous appearance, with epithelioid macrophages, Langhans giant cells, plasma cells, and lymphocytes. Over the course of months, the cutaneous ulcer heals spontaneously.

CLINICAL FEATURES: Cutaneous leishmaniasis begins as an itching, solitary papule, which erodes to form a shallow ulcer with a sharp, raised border. This ulcer can grow to 6 to 8 cm in diameter. Satellite lesions develop along draining lymphatics. The ulcers begin to resolve at 3 to 6 months, but healing may take a year or longer.

Diffuse cutaneous leishmaniasis develops in some patients who lack specific cell-mediated immune responses to leishmaniae. The disease begins as a single nodule, but adjacent satellite nodules slowly form, eventually involving much of the skin. These lesions so closely resemble lepromatous leprosy that some patients have been cared for in leprosaria. The nodule of anergic leishmaniasis is caused by enormous numbers of macrophages replete with leishmaniae.

Mucocutaneous Leishmaniasis Is a Late Complication of Cutaneous Leishmaniasis

Mucocutaneous leishmaniasis is caused by infection with *Leishmania braziliensis*. Most cases occur in Central and South America, where rodents and sloths are reservoirs.

PATHOLOGY AND CLINICAL FEATURES: The early course and pathologic changes of mucocutaneous leishmaniasis are similar to those of localized cutaneous leishmaniasis. A solitary ulcer appears, expands and resolves spontaneously. Years after a primary lesion has healed, an ulcer develops at a mucocutaneous junction, such as the larynx, nasal septum, anus, or vulva. The mucosal lesion is slowly progressive, highly destructive and disfiguring, eroding mucosal surfaces and cartilage. Destruction of the nasal septum sometimes produces a "tapir nose" deformity. The ulcers may also kill the patient by obstructing the airways. Mucocutaneous leishmaniasis requires treatment with systemic antiprotozoal agents.

Visceral Leishmaniasis (Kala Azar) Is a Potentially Fatal Infection of the Monocyte/Macrophage System

EPIDEMIOLOGY: *Kala azar is produced by several subspecies of* Leishmania donovani. Reservoirs of the agent and susceptible age groups vary in different parts of the world. Humans are the reservoir in India, and foxes in, for instance, southern France and central Italy. Other canine and rodent species serve as reservoirs elsewhere in the world.

PATHOLOGY: Infection with *L. donovani* begins with a localized collection of infected macrophages at the site of a sandfly bite (Fig. 9-73); these spread the organisms throughout the mononuclear phagocyte system. Most persons destroy *L. donovani* by cell-mediated immune responses, but 5% develop visceral leishmaniasis. Young children and malnourished persons are especially susceptible. The liver (Fig. 9-74A), spleen, and lymph nodes become massively enlarged, as macrophages in these organs fill with proliferating leishmanial amastigotes. Normal organ architecture is gradually replaced by sheets of parasitized macrophages (see Fig. 9-74B). Eventually, these cells accumulate in other organs, including the heart and kidney.

CLINICAL FEATURES: Patients with visceral leishmaniasis have persistent fever, progressive weight loss, hepatosplenomegaly, anemia, thrombocytopenia, and leukopenia. Light-skinned persons develop darkening of the skin; the Hindi name for leishmaniasis, *kala azar,* means "black sickness." Over the course of months, a patient with visceral leishmaniasis becomes profoundly cachectic with massive splenomegaly. The untreated disease is invariably fatal. Treatment entails systemic antiprotozoal therapy.

Chagas Disease (American Trypanosomiasis)

Chagas disease is an insect-borne, zoonotic infection by the protozoan Trypanosoma cruzi, *which causes a systemic infection of humans. Acute manifestations and long-term sequelae occur in the heart and gastrointestinal tract.*

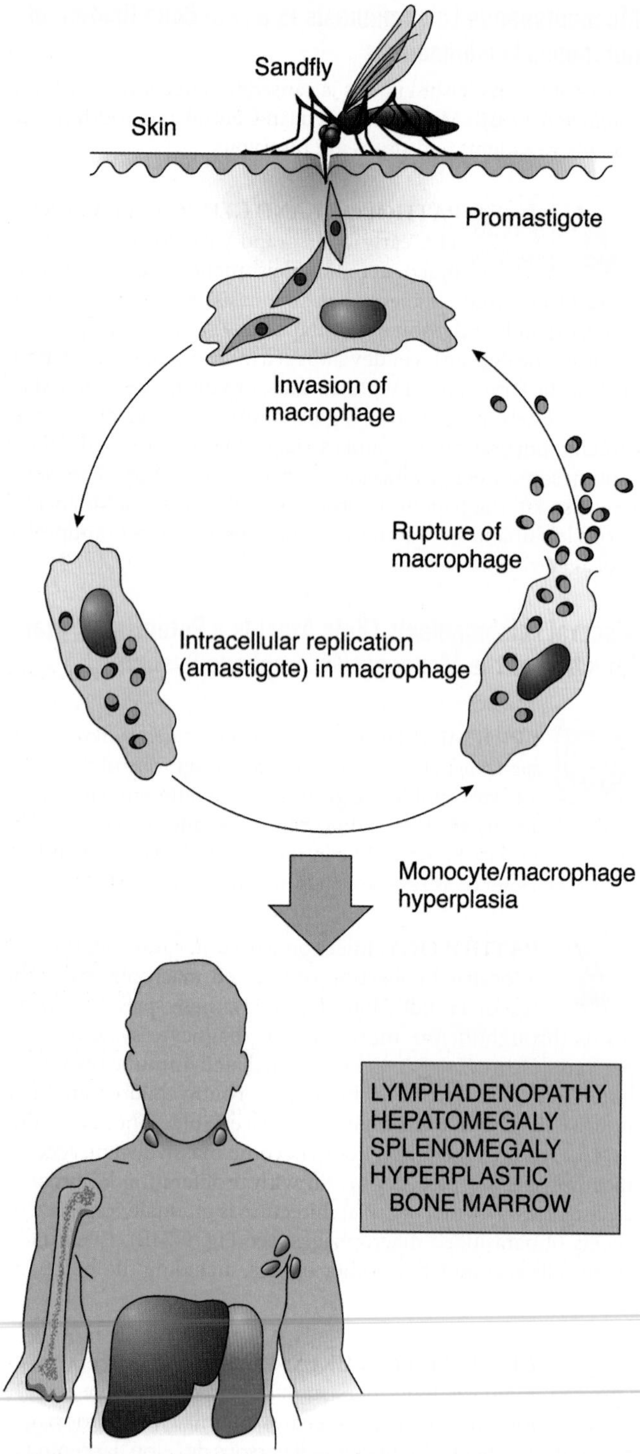

FIGURE 9-73. **Leishmaniasis.** Blood-sucking sandflies ingest amastigotes from an infected host. These are transformed in the sandfly gut into promastigotes, which multiply and are injected into the next vertebrate host. There they invade macrophages, revert to the amastigote form and multiply, eventually rupturing the cell. They then invade other macrophages, thus completing the cycle.

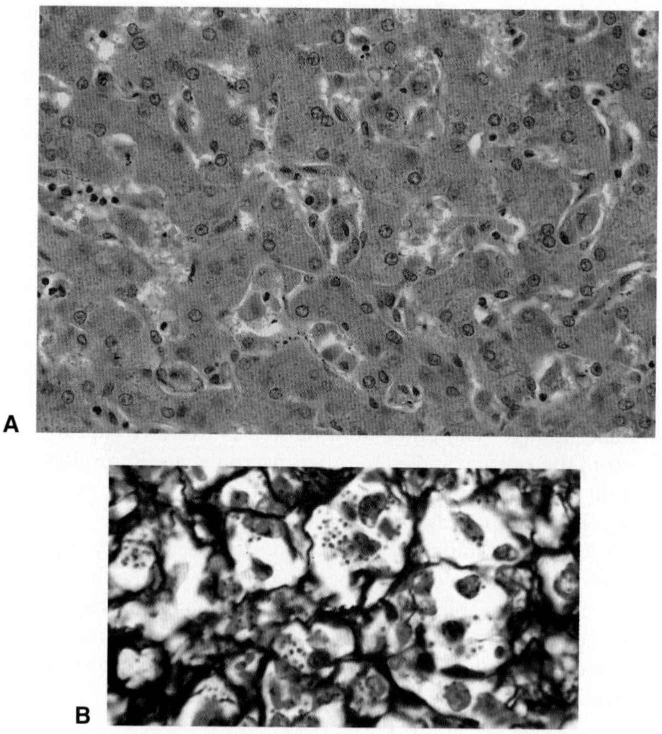

FIGURE 9-74. **Visceral leishmaniasis. A.** A photomicrograph of an enlarged liver shows prominent Kupffer cells distended by leishmanial amastigotes. **B.** A section of bone marrow subjected to silver impregnation shows macrophages filled with proliferating leishmanial amastigotes.

EPIDEMIOLOGY: *T. cruzi* infection is endemic in wild and domesticated animals (e.g., rats, dogs, goats, cats, armadillos) in Central and South America, where the parasite is transmitted by the reduviid ("kissing") bug. Infection with *T. cruzi* is promoted by contact between humans and infected bugs, usually in mud or thatched dwellings of the rural and suburban poor. The bugs hide in cracks of rickety houses and in vegetal roofing, emerge at night and feed on sleeping victims. Congenital infection occurs upon passage of the parasite from mother to fetus. It is estimated that some 20 million persons in Latin America are infected with *T. cruzi,* more than half of whom live in Brazil. An annual total of 50,000 deaths are attributable to Chagas disease.

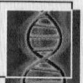

PATHOGENESIS: Infective forms of *T. cruzi* are discharged in the feces of the reduviid bug as it takes its blood meal. Itching and scratching promote contamination of the wound. The trypomastigotes penetrate at the site of the bite or other abrasions, or may penetrate the mucosa of the eyes or lips. Once in the body, they lose their flagella and undulating membranes, round up to become amastigotes, and enter macrophages, where they undergo repeated divisions. Amastigotes also invade other sites, including cardiac myocytes and brain. Within host cells, amastigotes differentiate into trypomastigotes, which break out and enter the bloodstream (Fig. 9-75). Ingested in a subsequent bite of a reduviid bug, trypomastigotes multiply in the insect's alimentary tract and differentiate into metacyclic trypomastigotes, which congregate in the rectum of the bug and are discharged in the feces.

T. cruzi infects and reproduces in cells at the site of inoculation, to form a localized nodular inflammatory lesion, a **chagoma**. The organism then disseminates in the bloodstream, infecting cells throughout the body. Strains of *T. cruzi* differ in their predominant target cells; infections of

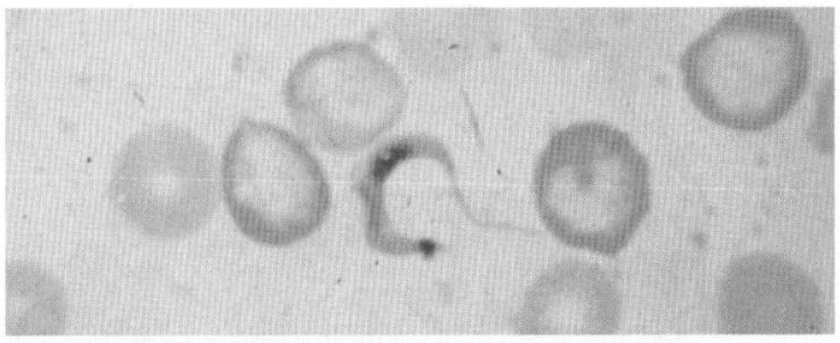

FIGURE 9-75. **Chagas disease.** A blood smear demonstrates a trypomastigote of *Trypanosoma cruzi* with its characteristic "C" shape, flagellum, nucleus, and terminal kinetoplast.

cardiac myocytes, gastrointestinal ganglion cells, and meninges produce the most significant disease. Parasitemia and widespread cellular infection are responsible for the systemic symptoms of acute Chagas disease. The onset of cell-mediated immunity eliminates the acute manifestations, but chronic tissue damage may continue. Progressive destruction of cells at sites of infection—particularly the heart, esophagus, and colon—causes organ dysfunction, manifested decades after the acute infection.

Acute Chagas Disease May Cause Fatal Myocarditis

PATHOLOGY: *T. cruzi* circulates in the blood as a 20-μm long, curved, flagellate that is easily recognized on blood films. Within infected cells, it reproduces as a nonflagellated amastigote, 2 to 4 μm in diameter. In fatal cases, the heart is enlarged and dilated, with a pale, focally hemorrhagic myocardium. Microscopically, numerous parasites are seen in the heart and amastigotes are evident within pseudocysts in myofibers (Fig. 9-76). There is extensive chronic inflammation and phagocytosis of parasites is conspicuous.

CLINICAL FEATURES: Acute symptoms develop 1 to 2 weeks after inoculation with *T. cruzi*. A chagoma (see above), develops at the site. Parasitemia appears 2 to 3 weeks after inoculation and is usually associated with a mild illness characterized by fever, malaise, lymphadenopathy, and hepatosplenomegaly. However, the disease can be lethal when there is extensive myocardial or meningeal involvement.

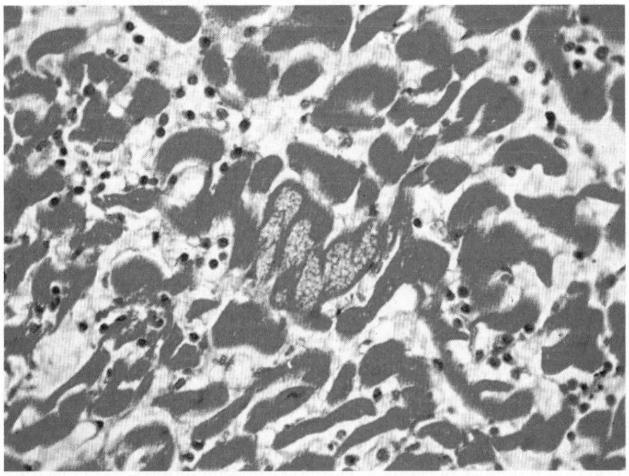

FIGURE 9-76. **Acute Chagas myocarditis.** The myofibers in the center contain numerous amastigotes of *T. cruzi* and are surrounded by edema and chronic inflammation.

Chronic Chagas Disease Is Associated with Cardiac Failure and Gastrointestinal Disease

The most frequent and most serious consequences of infection with *T. cruzi* develop years or decades after the acute infection. It is estimated that 10% to 40% of acutely infected persons eventually develop chronic disease. In this phase of the illness, *T. cruzi* is no longer present in blood or tissue. Infected organs have been damaged, however, by a chronic, progressive inflammatory process.

PATHOLOGY AND CLINICAL FEATURES: Chronic myocarditis is characterized by a dilated heart, prominent right ventricular outflow tract, and dilation of the valve rings. The interventricular septum is often deviated to the right and may immobilize the adjacent tricuspid leaflet. Microscopically, there is extensive interstitial fibrosis, hypertrophied myofibers, and focal lymphocytic inflammation, often involving the cardiac conduction system. Progressive cardiac fibrosis causes dysrhythmia or congestive heart failure. In endemic regions, chronic Chagas disease is a leading cause of heart failure in young adults.

Megaesophagus, dilation of the esophagus caused by failure of the lower esophageal sphincter (achalasia), is a common complication of chronic Chagas disease. It results from destruction of parasympathetic ganglia in the wall of the lower esophagus, and leads to difficulty in swallowing, which may be so severe that the patient can consume only liquids.

Megacolon, massive dilation of the large bowel, is similar to megaesophagus in that the myenteric plexus of the colon is destroyed. The progressive aganglionosis of the colon causes severe constipation.

Congenital Chagas disease occurs in some pregnant women with parasitemia. Infection of the placenta and fetus leads to spontaneous abortion. In the infrequent live births, the infants die of encephalitis within a few days or weeks.

Antiprotozoal chemotherapy is effective for acute Chagas disease but not for its chronic sequelae. Cardiac transplantation has been effective in a number of patients.

African Trypanosomiasis

African trypanosomiasis, popularly termed ***sleeping sickness****, is an infection with* Trypanosoma brucei gambiense *or* Trypanosoma brucei rhodesiense, *which produces a life-threatening meningoencephalitis.* Gambian trypanosomiasis is a chronic infection often lasting more than a year. By contrast, East African (Rhodesian) trypanosomiasis is a rapidly progressive infection that kills the patient in 3 to 6 months. The organisms are curved flagellates, 15 to 30 μm in length. Although they can be demonstrated in blood or cerebrospinal fluid, they are difficult to find in infected tissues.

EPIDEMIOLOGY: *T. brucei gambiense* and *T. brucei rhodesiense* are hemoflagellate protozoa are transmitted by several species of blood-sucking tsetse flies of the genus *Glossina*. The patchy distribution of African trypanosomiasis is related to the habitats of these flies. In Gambian trypanosomiasis, *T. brucei gambiense* is transmitted by tsetse flies of the riverine bush, mainly in endemic pockets of West and Central Africa. *Humans are the only important reservoir for this trypanosome.*

In East African trypanosomiasis, *T. brucei rhodesiense* is spread by tsetse flies of the woodland savanna of East Africa. Antelope, other game animals, and domestic cattle are natural reservoirs of *T. brucei rhodesiense*. *Infection of humans is an occupational hazard of game wardens, fishermen, and cattle herders.*

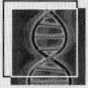

PATHOGENESIS: While biting an infected animal or human, the tsetse fly ingests trypomastigotes with the blood (Fig. 9-77). These (1) lose their coat of surface antigen, (2) multiply in the midgut of the fly, (3) migrate to the salivary gland, (4) develop for 3 weeks through the epimastigote stage, and (5) multiply in the fly's saliva as infective metacyclic trypomastigotes. During another bite, metacyclic trypomastigotes are injected into the lymphatics and blood vessels of a new host. The organisms disseminate to the bone marrow and tissue fluids and some eventually invade the CNS. After replicating by binary fission in blood, lymph, and spinal fluid, trypomastigotes are ingested by another fly to complete the cycle.

African trypanosomiasis involves immune complex formation by variable trypanosomal antigens and antibodies. Autoantibodies to antigens of erythrocytes, brain, and heart may participate in the pathogenesis of this disease. The trypanosome evades immune attack in mammalian hosts by periodically altering its glycoprotein antigen coat. The alterations take place in a genetically determined pattern, not by mutation. Thus, each wave of circulating trypomastigotes includes immunologically distinct antigenic variants that are a step ahead of the immune response.

PATHOLOGY: *T. brucei* multiplies at sites of inoculation, occasionally producing localized nodular lesions: "primary chancres." Generalized involvement of lymph nodes and spleen is prominent early in the disease. Microscopic changes in affected nodes and spleen include foci of lymphocyte and macrophage hyperplasia. Infection eventually localizes to small blood vessels of the CNS, where replicating organisms elicit a destructive vasculitis, producing the progressive decrease in mentation characteristic of sleeping sickness. In *T. brucei rhodesiense* infection, the organisms also localize to blood vessels in the heart, sometimes causing a fulminant myocarditis.

Lesions in the lymph nodes, brain, heart, and various other sites (including the inoculation site) show vasculitis of small blood vessels, with endothelial cell hyperplasia and dense perivascular infiltrates of lymphocytes, macrophages, and plasma cells. The CNS vasculitis causes destruction of neurons, demyelination, and gliosis. The perivascular infiltrate thickens the leptomeninges and involves the Virchow-Robin spaces (Fig. 9-78).

CLINICAL FEATURES: African trypanosomiasis is divided into 3 clinical stages:

1. **Primary chancre:** After 5 to 15 days, a 3- to 4-cm papillary swelling topped by a central red spot appears at the inoculation site. It subsides spontaneously within 3 weeks.
2. **Systemic infection:** Shortly after the appearance of the chancre (if any) and within 3 weeks of the bite, bloodstream invasion is marked by intermittent fever, for up to a week, often accompanied by splenomegaly and local and generalized

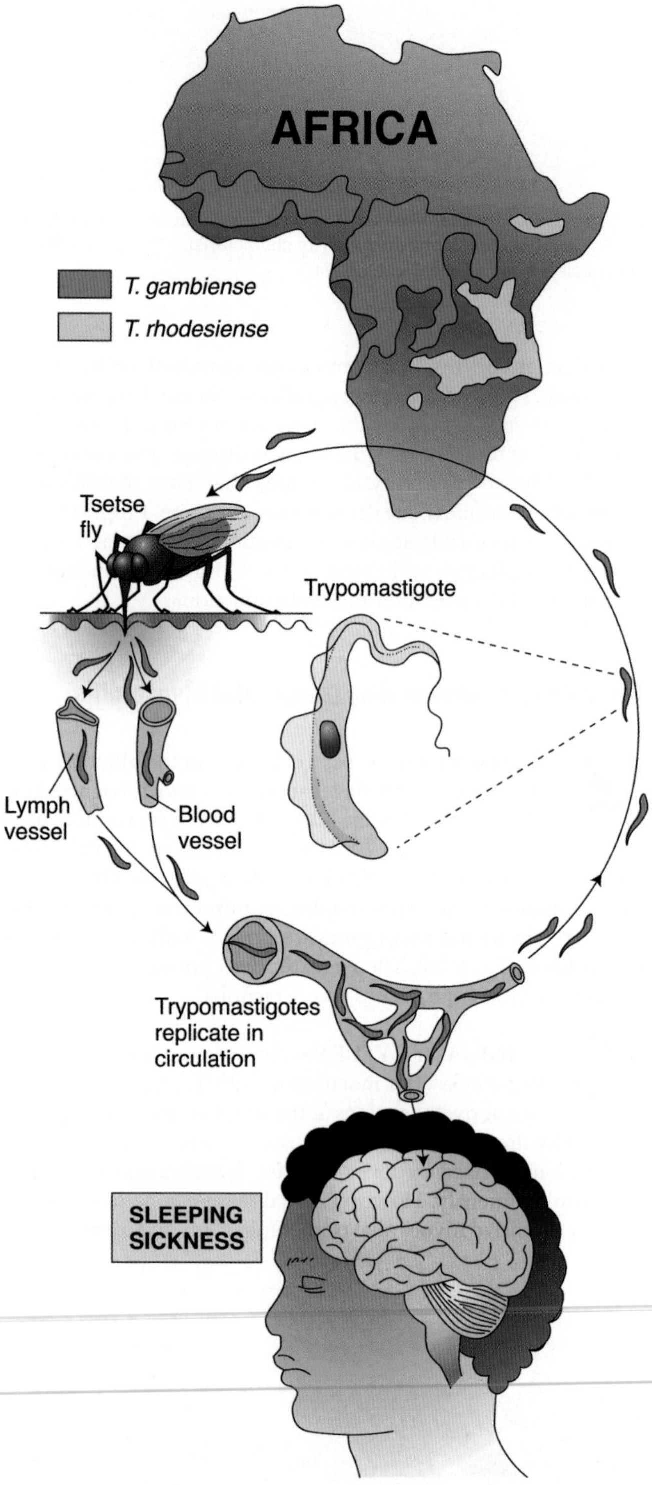

FIGURE 9-77. **African trypanosomiasis (sleeping sickness).** The distribution of Gambian and Rhodesian trypanosomiasis is related to the habitats of the vector tsetse flies (*Glossina* spp.). A tsetse fly bites an infected animal or human and ingests trypomastigotes, which multiply into infective, metacyclic trypomastigotes. During another fly bite, these are injected into lymphatic and blood vessels of a new host. A primary chancre develops at the site of the bite (stage 1a). Trypomastigotes replicate further in the blood and lymph, causing a systemic infection (stage 1b). Another fly ingests hypomastigotes to complete the cycle. In stage 2, invasion of the central nervous system by trypomastigotes leads to meningoencephalomyelitis and associated symptoms, including lethargy and daytime somnolence. Patients with Rhodesian trypanosomiasis may die within a few months. *T. gambiense* = *Trypanosoma brucei gambiense* *T. rhodeseince* = *Trypanosoma* brucei rhodesiense.

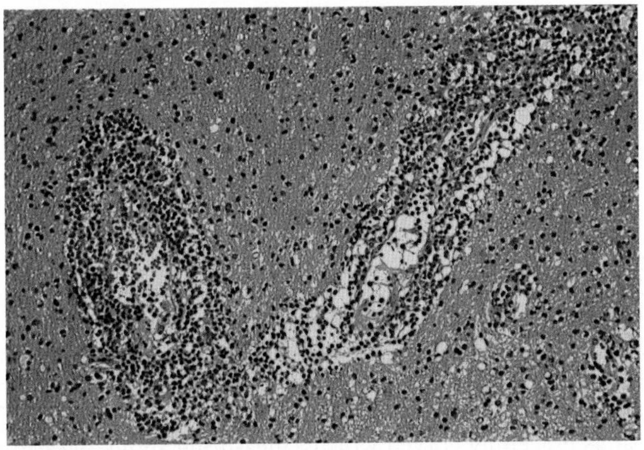

FIGURE 9-78. **African trypanosomiasis.** A section of brain from a patient who died from infection with *T. brucei rhodesiense* shows a perivascular mononuclear cell infiltrate.

lymphadenopathy. Enlargement of posterior cervical lymph nodes, "Winterbottom sign," is characteristic of Gambian trypanosomiasis. The evolving illness is marked by remitting irregular fevers, headache, joint pains, lethargy, and muscle wasting. Myocarditis may be a complication and is more common and severe in Rhodesian trypanosomiasis. Dysfunction of the lungs, kidneys, liver, and endocrine system is frequently observed in both forms of the disease.

3. **Brain invasion:** Differences between the forms of sleeping sickness are primarily a matter of time scale, especially with regard to invasion of the brain. This feature develops early (weeks or months) in Rhodesian trypanosomiasis and late (months or years) in the Gambian form. Brain invasion is marked by apathy, daytime somnolence, and sometimes coma. A diffuse meningoencephalitis is characterized by tremors of the tongue and fingers; fasciculations of the muscles of the limbs, face, lips, and tongue; oscillatory movements of the arms, head, neck, and trunk; indistinct speech; and cerebellar ataxia, causing problems in walking.

Primary Amebic Meningoencephalitis

Amebic meningoencephalitis is fatal and is caused by Naegleria fowleri.

EPIDEMIOLOGY: *N. fowleri* is a free-living, soil ameba that inhabits ponds and lakes throughout tropical and subtropical regions but has been reported in temperate areas, including the United States. Primary amebic meningoencephalitis is a rare disease (fewer than 300 reported cases) affecting persons who swim or bathe in these waters.

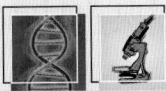

PATHOGENESIS AND PATHOLOGY: *N. fowleri* is inoculated into nasal mucosa near the cribriform plate when a person swims in or dives into water containing high concentrations of the organism. Amebae invade the olfactory nerves, migrate into the olfactory bulbs, then proliferate in the meninges and brain.

In tissue sections, the trophozoites are 8 to 15 μm across, with sharply outlined nuclei that stain deeply with hematoxylin. Grossly, the brain is swollen and soft, with vascular congestion and a purulent exudate on the meningeal surface, most prominent over the lateral and basal areas. There is massive destruction of the brain by amebae, which invade the brain along the Virchow-Robin spaces. Thrombosis and destruction of blood vessels are associated with extensive hemorrhage. The olfactory tract and bulbs are enveloped and destroyed, and there is an exudate between the bulb and the inferior surface of the temporal lobe. Proliferation of *Naegleria* in the brain may produce solid masses of amebae (amebomas). Meningitis can extend the full length of the cord.

CLINICAL FEATURES: Primary amebic meningoencephalitis due to *N. fowleri* begins suddenly with fever, nausea, vomiting, and headache. Disease progresses rapidly. Within hours the patient suffers profound deterioration in mental status. Cerebrospinal fluid contains numerous neutrophils, blood, and amebae. The disease is rapidly fatal.

HELMINTHIC INFECTION

Helminths, or worms, are among the most common human pathogens. At any given time, 25% to 50% of the world's population carries at least one helminth species. Although most such infections cause little harm, some produce significant disease. Schistosomiasis, for instance, ranks among the leading global causes of morbidity and mortality.

Helminths are the largest and most complex organisms capable of living within the human body. Their adult forms range from 0.5 mm over 1 m in length. Most are visible to the naked eye. Helminths are multicellular animals with differentiated tissues, including specialized nervous tissues, digestive tissues, and reproductive systems. Their maturation from eggs or larvae to adult worms is complex, often involving multiple morphologic transformations (molts). Some undergo these metamorphoses in different hosts before attaining adulthood, and the human host may be only one in a series that supports this maturation process. Within the human body, the helminths frequently migrate from the port of entry through several organs to a site of final infection.

Most helminths that infect humans are well adapted to human parasitism, causing limited or no host tissue damage. Helminths gain entry by ingestion, skin penetration, or insect bites. With two excetions, helminths cannot multiply within the human body; thus a single organism cannot become an overwhelming infection. The exceptions are *Strongyloides stercoralis* and *Capillaria philippinensis*, which can complete their life cycle and multiply within the human body.

Helminths cause disease in various ways. A few compete with their human host for certain nutrients. Some grow to block vital structures, producing disease by mass effect. Most, however, cause dysfunction through the destructive inflammatory and immunologic responses that they elicit. For example, morbidity in schistosomiasis, the most destructive helminthic infection, results from the granulomatous response to the schistosome eggs deposited in tissue.

Eosinophils contain basic proteins toxic to some helminths and are a major component of inflammatory responses to these organisms. Parasitic helminths are categorized based on overall morphology and the structure of digestive tissues:

- **Roundworms** (**nematodes**) are elongate cylindrical organisms with tubular digestive tracts.

- **Flatworms (trematodes)** are dorsoventrally flattened organisms with digestive tracts that end in blind loops.
- **Tapeworms (cestodes)** are segmented organisms with separate head and body parts; they lack a digestive tract and absorb nutrients through their outer walls.

Filarial Nematodes

Lymphatic Filariasis Results in Massive Lymphedema (Elephantiasis)

Lymphatic filariasis (bancroftian and Malayan filariasis) is an inflammatory parasitic infection of lymphatic vessels caused by the roundworms *Wuchereria bancrofti* and *Brugia malayi*. Adult worms inhabit the lymphatics, most frequently in inguinal, epitrochlear and axillary lymph nodes, testis, and epididymis. There they cause acute lymphangitis and, in a minority of infected subjects, lymphatic obstruction, leading to severe lymphedema (Fig. 9-79). These and similar organisms are known as filarial worms, because of their threadlike appearance (from the Latin *filum*, meaning thread).

EPIDEMIOLOGY: The elephantiasis characteristic of lymphatic filariasis was familiar to Hindi and Persian physicians as early as 600 BC. Humans, the only definitive host of these filarial nematodes, acquire infection from the bites of at least 80 species of mosquitoes of the genera *Culex, Aedes, Anopheles, and Mansonia*. *W. bancrofti* infection is widespread in southern Asia, the Pacific, Africa, and portions of South America. *B. malayi* is localized to coastal southern Asia and western Pacific islands. Worldwide, 100 to 200 million persons are estimated to be infected.

PATHOGENESIS: Mosquito bites transmit infectious larvae that migrate to lymphatics and lymph nodes. After maturing into adult forms over several months, worms mate and the female releases microfilariae into lymphatics and the bloodstream. The manifestations of filariasis result from inflammatory responses to degenerating adult worms in the lymphatics. Repeated infections are common in endemic regions and produce numerous bouts of lymphangitis (filarial fevers), that cause extensive scarring and obstruction of lymphatics over years. This blockage causes localized dependent edema, most commonly affecting legs, arms, genitalia, and breasts. In its most severe form (less than 5% of the infected population), this is known as **elephantiasis.**

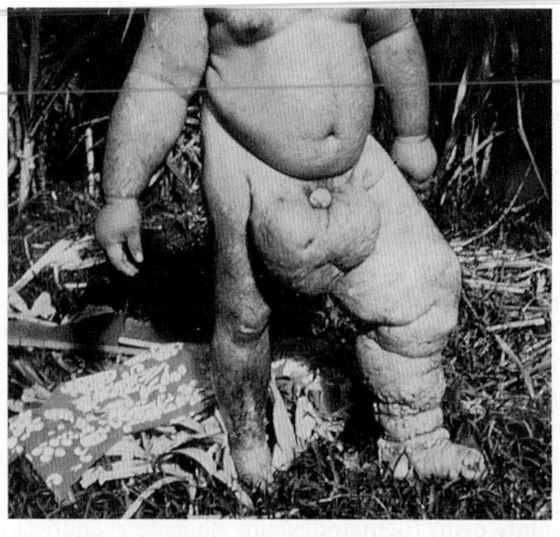

FIGURE 9-79. **Bancroftian filariasis.** Massive lymphedema (elephantiasis) of the scrotum and left lower extremity are present.

PATHOLOGY: The adult nematode is a white, threadlike worm that is much convoluted within the lymph nodes. The female measures 80 to 100 mm in length and 0.20 to 0.3 mm in width, twice the size of the male. In blood films stained with Giemsa, the microfilariae appear as gracefully curved worms, measuring about 300 μm in length.

Lymphatic vessels harboring adult worms are dilated, and their endothelial lining is thickened. In adjacent tissue, a chronic inflammatory infiltrate, including eosinophils, surrounds the worms. A granulomatous reaction may develop and degenerating worms can provoke acute inflammation. Microfilariae are seen in blood vessels and lymphatics and degenerating microfilariae also provoke a chronic inflammatory reaction. After repeated bouts of lymphangitis, lymph nodes and lymphatics become densely fibrotic, often containing calcified remnants of the worms.

CLINICAL FEATURES: In endemic areas, most of the infected population displays either antifilarial antibodies with no detectable infection or asymptomatic microfilaremia. A smaller number develop recurrent episodes of filarial fevers, with malaise, lymphadenopathy, and lymphangitis, which persist for 1 to 2 weeks and then resolve spontaneously. In a small subset of these patients, late manifestations of disease appear after two to three decades of recurrent bouts of filarial fevers. Lymphatic obstruction leads to chronic edema of dependent tissues. The overlying skin becomes thickened and warty. The diagnosis is made by identifying microfilariae in blood samples. Diethylcarbamazine and ivermectin are the agents effective against lymphatic filariasis.

Occult filariasis, a condition characterized by indirect evidence of filarial infection (circulating antifilarial antibodies), is the cause of **tropical pulmonary eosinophilia**. This condition is virtually restricted to southern India and some Pacific Islands. Patients present with cough, wheezing diffuse pulmonary infiltrates, and peripheral eosinophilia. The severity ranges from mild asthma to fatal pneumonia.

Onchocerciasis Causes Blindness

Onchocerciasis ("river blindness") is a chronic inflammatory disease of the skin, eyes and lymphatics caused by the filarial nematode *Onchocerca volvulus*.

EPIDEMIOLOGY: Onchocerciasis is one of the world's major endemic diseases, afflicting an estimated 40 million persons, of whom 2 million are blind. Humans are the only definitive host. On biting, *Simulium damnosum* blackflies transmit infectious larvae to humans. These insects require rapidly running water for breeding. Onchocerciasis is thus endemic along rivers and streams (hence, "**river blindness**") in parts of tropical Africa, southern Mexico, Central America, and South America.

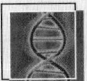

PATHOGENESIS: Adult worms live as coiled tangled masses in the deep fasciae and subcutaneous tissues. They do not cause tissue damage and or elicit inflammatory responses, but gravid females release millions of microfilariae, which migrate into the skin, eyes, lymph nodes, and deep organs, producing corresponding onchocercal lesions. Ocular onchocerciasis results from migration of microfilariae into all regions of the eye, from the cornea to the optic nerve head.

When microfilariae die, they incite vigorous inflammatory and immune responses. Inflammatory damage to the cornea, choroids, or retina leads to partial or total loss of vision. Cutaneous inflammation causes microabscess formation and chronic degenerative changes in the epidermis and dermis. In the lymph nodes and lymphatics, the response to dying microfilariae causes chronic lymphatic obstruction and localized dependent edema.

PATHOLOGY: *Onchocerca volvulus* is a thin, very long nematode, the female is 400 × 0.3 mm and the male 30 × 0.2 mm. Masses of adult worms become encapsulated by a fibrous scar, forming discrete, 1- to 3-cm, **onchocercal nodules** in the deep dermis and subcutis. Nodules form over bony prominences of the skull, scapula, ribs, iliac crest, trochanter, sacrum, and knee. Microscopically, these nodules have an outer fibrous layer and a central inflammatory infiltrate, which varies from suppurative to granulomatous. Active lesions in the eyes and lymphatics all show degenerating microfilariae surrounded by chronic inflammation, including eosinophils. Involvement of the eye leads to sclerosing keratitis, iridocyclitis, chorioretinitis, and optic atrophy. The femoral inguinal nodes become enlarged and then fibrotic.

CLINICAL FEATURES: Symptoms of onchocerciasis result from inflammatory responses to degenerating microfilariae. Skin manifestations begin with generalized pruritus that becomes so intense that it can interfere with sleeping. Continuing damage produces areas of depigmentation, hypertrophy, or atrophy of the skin. Progressive destruction of the cornea, choroid, or uvea leads to loss of vision. Chronic lymphadenitis results in localized edema that may cause chronic swelling (elephantiasis) of the legs, scrotum, or other dependent portions of the body. Systemic antihelminthic therapy, particularly with ivermectin, is effective.

Loiasis Principally Affects the Eyes and Skin

Loiasis is infection by the filarial nematode Loa loa, *the African "eyeworm."*

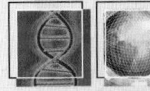

EPIDEMIOLOGY AND PATHOGENESIS: Loiasis is prevalent in the rain forests of Central and West Africa. Humans and baboons are the definitive hosts and infection is transmitted by mango flies. Adult worms (4 cm long) migrate in the skin and occasionally cross the eye beneath the conjunctiva, making the patient acutely aware of this infection (Fig. 9-80). Gravid worms discharge microfilariae, which circulate in the blood during the day but reside in capillaries of the skin, lungs, and other organs at night.

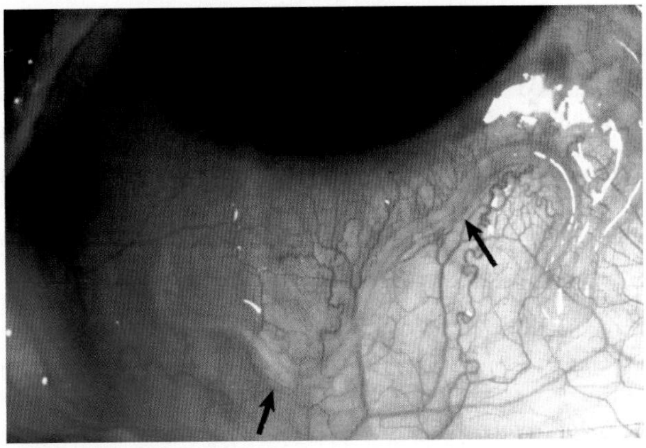

FIGURE 9-80. **Loiasis.** A threadlike *Loa loa (arrows)* is migrating in the subconjunctival tissues.

PATHOLOGY: Migrating worms cause no inflammation, but static ones are surrounded by eosinophils, other inflammatory cells, and a foreign body giant cell reaction. Rarely, infected subjects may develop acute generalized loiasis. At autopsy, these patients have obstructive fibrin thrombi in small vessels of most organs, which contain degenerating microfilariae. When the brain is involved, obstruction of vessels by filarial thrombi kills the patient through sudden and diffuse ischemia.

CLINICAL FEATURES: Most infections are asymptomatic but persist for years. Some patients have pruritic, red, subcutaneous "Calabar" swellings, which may be a reaction to migrating adult worms or to microfilariae in the skin. Ocular symptoms include swelling of the eyelids, itching, and pain. Worms may be extracted during their migration beneath the conjunctiva. Systemic reactions include fever, pain, itching, urticaria, and eosinophilia. Dead worms in or near major nerves may cause paresthesia or paralysis. Treatment with microfilariacides may cause massive death of microfilariae and provoke fever, meningoencephalitis, and death.

Intestinal Nematodes

The adult forms of several nematode species (Table 9-10) reside in the human bowel but rarely cause symptomatic disease. Clinical symptoms occur almost exclusively in persons who carry very large numbers of worms or who are immunocompromised. Humans are the exclusive or primary host for all of intestinal nematodes and infection spreads from person to person via eggs or larvae passed in the stool or deposited in the perianal region. Infection is most prevalent in settings where hand washing and hygienic disposal of feces are lacking (e.g., less-developed countries, day-care centers). Warm, moist climates are required for survival of the infectious forms of many of the intestinal nematodes outside the body. These worms are, therefore, endemic in tropical and subtropical environments.

Ascariasis Is Usually an Asymptomatic Infestation of the Small Bowel

Ascariasis refers to infection by the large roundworm Ascaris lumbricoides. It is the most common helminth infection of humans, affecting at least one billion people, usually without causing symptoms. It is found worldwide, but infection is most common in areas with warm climates and poor sanitation.

TABLE 9–10

Intestinal Nematodes

Species	Common Name	Site of Adult Worm	Clinical Manifestations
Ascaris lumbricoides	Roundworm	Small bowel	Allergic reactions to lung migration; intestinal obstruction
Ancylostoma duodenale	Hookworm	Small bowel	Allergic reactions to cutaneous inoculation and lung migration; intestinal blood loss
Necator americanus	Hookworm	Small bowel	Allergic reactions to cutaneous inoculation and lung migration; intestinal blood loss
Trichuris trichiura	Whipworm	Large bowel	Abdominal pain and diarrhea; rectal prolapse (rare)
Strongyloides stercoralis	Threadworm	Small bowel	Abdominal pain and diarrhea; dissemination to extraintestinal sites in immunocompromised persons
Enterobius vermicularis	Pinworm	Cecum, appendix	Perianal and perineal itching

PATHOGENESIS: Adult worms live in the small intestine, where gravid females discharge eggs that pass in the feces. These eggs hatch when ingested. *Ascaris* larvae emerge in the small intestine, penetrate the bowel wall, and reach the lungs through the venous circulation. From the pulmonary capillaries they enter alveolar spaces and migrate up the trachea to the glottis, where they are swallowed and again reach the small bowel. There, they mature and live as adult worms within the lumen for 1 to 2 years.

PATHOLOGY AND CLINICAL FEATURES: Adult worms (15 to 35 cm long) usually cause no pathologic changes. Heavy infections may cause vomiting, malnutrition, and sometimes intestinal obstruction (Fig. 9-81). On rare occasions, worms migrate into the ampulla of Vater or pancreatic or biliary ducts, where they may cause obstruction, acute pancreatitis, suppurative cholangitis, and liver abscesses. Eggs deposited in the liver or other tissues may produce necrosis, granulomatous inflammation, and fibrosis. *Ascaris* pneumonia, which may be fatal, develops when large numbers of larvae migrate within the air spaces.

The diagnosis of ascariasis is made by identifying eggs in the feces. Occasionally, adult worms may pass with the stools or even emerge from the nose or mouth. Ascaricidal drugs are effective.

Trichuriasis Is a Superficially Invasive Infection of the Large Bowel

Trichuriasis is caused by the intestinal nematode Trichuris trichiura *("whipworm").*

EPIDEMIOLOGY: Whipworm infection is found worldwide, affecting over 800 million people. Parasitism is most common in warm, moist places with poor sanitation, but over 2 million persons in the United States are infected. Children are especially susceptible. Adult worms live in the cecum and upper colon, where female worms produce eggs that pass in the feces. Eggs embryonate in moist soil and become infective in 3 weeks. Humans are infected by ingesting eggs in contaminated soil, food, or drink.

PATHOGENESIS AND PATHOLOGY: Larvae emerge from ingested eggs in the small bowel and migrate to the cecum and colon, where the adult worms burrow their anterior portions into the superficial mucosa (Fig. 9-82). This invasion causes small erosions, focal active inflammation, and continuous loss of small quantities of blood. *T. trichiura* measures 3 to 5 cm in length, with a long, slender anterior portion and a short, blunt posterior.

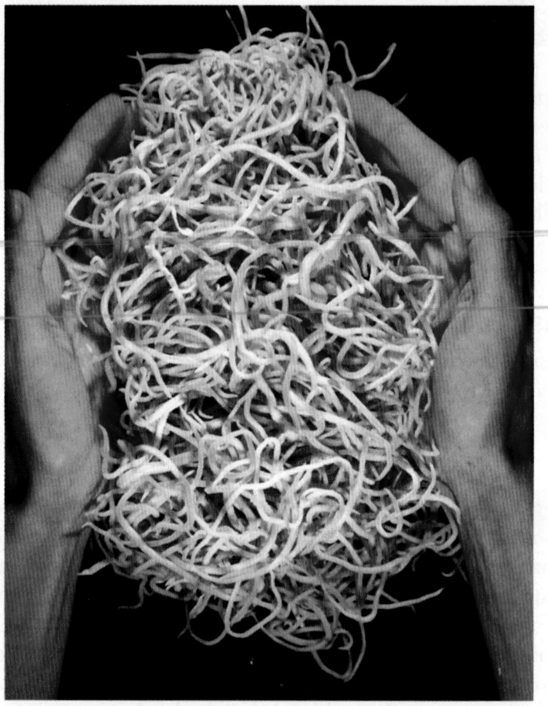

FIGURE 9-81. **Ascariasis.** This mass of over 800 worms of *Ascaris lumbricoides* obstructed and infarcted the ileum of a 2-year-old girl in South Africa.

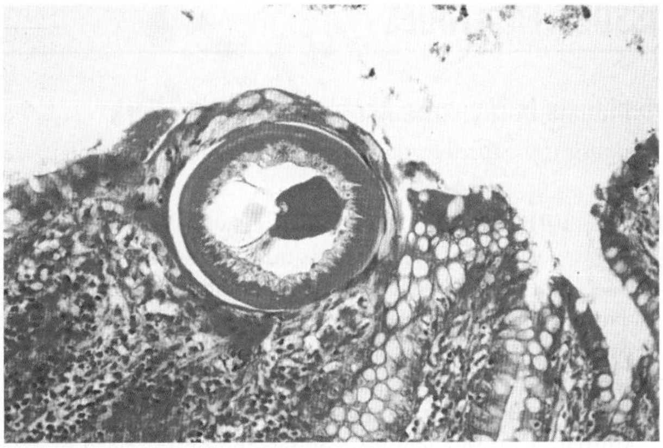

FIGURE 9-82. **Trichuriasis.** The anterior "whip" end of *Trichuris trichiura* is threaded into the mucosa of the colon.

CLINICAL FEATURES: Most *T. trichiura* infections are asymptomatic. Heavy infestation of worms may produce cramping abdominal pain, bloody diarrhea, weight loss, and anemia. The diagnosis is made by finding the characteristic eggs in the stool. Mebendazole is effective therapy.

Hookworms Cause Intestinal Blood Loss and Anemia

Necator americanus *and* Ancylostoma duodenale *("hookworms") are intestinal nematodes that infect the human small bowel. They lacerate the bowel mucosa, causing intestinal blood loss, which can produce symptomatic disease in heavy infestations.*

EPIDEMIOLOGY: Hookworm infections are found in moist, warm, temperate and tropical areas and cause serious public health problems worldwide. In fact, both *A. duodenale* ("Old World" hookworm) and *N. americanus* ("American" hookworm) prevail on most continents and have overlapping epidemiologic boundaries. More than 700 million persons are infected with hookworms. It is estimated that a half-million persons in the United States harbor the parasite.

PATHOGENESIS AND PATHOLOGY: On contact with human skin, filariform larvae directly penetrate the epidermis and enter the venous circulation. They travel to the lungs, where they lodge in alveolar capillaries. After rupturing into the alveoli, larvae migrate up the trachea to the glottis and are then swallowed. They molt in the duodenum, attach to the mucosal wall with toothlike buckle plates, and clamp off a section of the villus and ingest it (Fig. 9-83). With extensive worm infections, particularly with *A. duodenale,* blood loss can be sufficient to cause anemia. Hookworms are about 1 cm in length. They are grossly visible attached to the small bowel mucosa alongside punctate areas of hemorrhages. There is no associated inflammation.

CLINICAL FEATURES: *Although most persons with hookworm infection are not symptomatic, infection with this parasite is the most important cause of chronic anemia worldwide.* In persons with heavy worm burdens (particularly women who consume a diet low in iron) and in populations with inadequate iron intake, chronic intestinal blood loss can produce severe iron deficiency anemia. Skin penetration is sometimes associated with a pruritic eruption ("ground itch"), and the phase of larval migration through the lungs occasionally causes asthmalike symptoms.

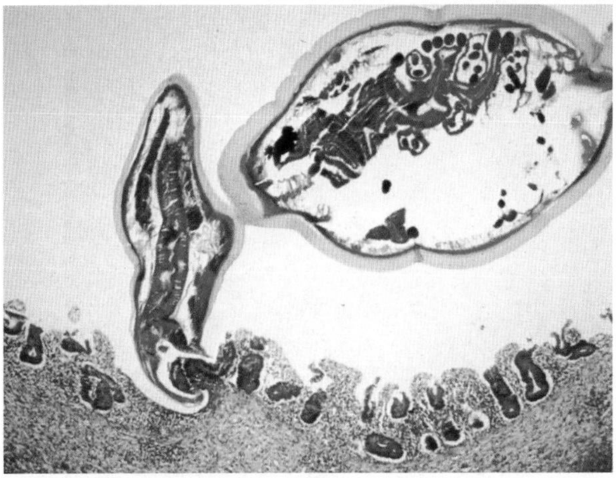

FIGURE 9-83. **Ancylostomiasis.** Section of the ileum shows two portions of a single adult worm, *Ancylostoma duodenale.* A plug of mucosa is in the buccal cavity of the hookworm.

Strongyloidiasis Is Disseminated in Immunocompromised Hosts

Strongyloidiasis is a small intestinal infection with a nematode, Strongyloides stercoralis *("threadworm"). Although most cases are asymptomatic, the infection can progress to lethal disseminated disease in immunocompromised persons.* Infection is most frequent in areas with warm, moist climates and poor sanitation. However, endemic pockets of strongyloidiasis still exist in the United States, particularly in the Appalachian region and in institutions where personal hygiene is poor, such as hospitals for the mentally ill.

PATHOGENESIS AND PATHOLOGY: *S. stercoralis* is the smallest of the intestinal nematodes, measuring 0.2 to 0.3 cm in length. Adult females are buried in the crypts of the duodenum or jejunum but produce no visible alterations. Microscopic examination shows the coiled females, along with eggs and developing larvae, within the mucosa, usually with no associated inflammation (Fig. 9-84).

Parasitic females live within the mucosa of the small intestine, where they lay eggs that hatch quickly and release rhabditiform larvae. The larvae are passed in the feces, and in the soil become filariform, the infective stage that penetrates human skin. On entering the skin, *S. stercoralis* larvae pass in the bloodstream to the lungs and then to the small bowel, in a manner similar to that of hookworms. The worms mature in the small bowel. Unlike other intestinal nematodes, *S. stercoralis* may reproduce in human hosts by a mechanism known as **autoinfection**. This occurs when rhabditiform larvae become infective (filariform) within a host's intestine and repenetrate either the intestinal wall or the perianal skin, thereby starting a new parasitic cycle within a single host.

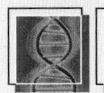

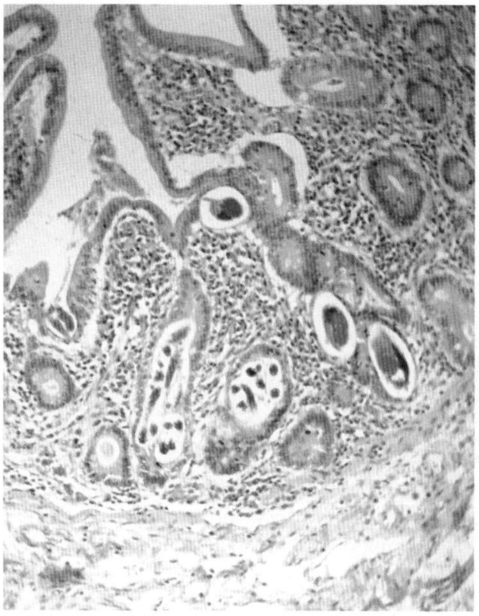

FIGURE 9-84. **Strongyloidiasis.** A section of jejunum shows adult worms, larvae and eggs of *Strongyloides stercoralis* in the mucosal crypts. The lamina propria is infiltrated with lymphocytes, plasma cells, and eosinophils. The patient had a hyperinfected syndrome and presented with malabsorption.

CLINICAL FEATURES: Most infected persons are completely asymptomatic, but moderate eosinophilia is common. **Disseminated strongyloidiasis or hyperinfection syndrome** occurs in patients with suppressed immunity, particularly those receiving corticosteroids. In such patients, the rate of internal autoinfection is greatly increased, and extraordinary numbers of filariform larvae penetrate intestinal walls and disseminate to distant organs. In disseminated strongyloidiasis, the gut may exhibit ulceration, edema, and severe inflammation. Sepsis, usually with gram-negative organisms and infection of parenchymal organs eventuate. Untreated, disseminated strongyloidiasis is fatal; even with prompt treatment with thiabendazole or ivermectin, only one-third survive.

Pinworm Infection (Enterobiasis) Leads to Perianal Itching

Enterobius vermicularis *("pinworm") is an intestinal nematode that is encountered worldwide but is more frequent in temperate zones.* Although people can be infected at any age, parasitism is most common among young children. It is estimated that more than 200 million persons are infected with *E. vermicularis* worldwide; some 5 million school-age children harbor the worm in the United States.

The adult female worm resides in the cecum and appendix but migrates to the perianal and perineal skin to deposit eggs. The eggs stick to fingers, bed linens, towels, and clothing and are readily transmitted from person to person. Ingested eggs hatch in the small bowel to yield larvae that mature into adult worms. Some infected persons are asymptomatic, but most complain of perineal pruritus, caused by the migrating worms depositing eggs. Several agents, including mebendazole, are effective against pinworms.

TISSUE NEMATODES

Trichinosis Is Myositis Acquired by Eating Pork

Trichinosis is produced by the roundworm Trichinella spiralis.

EPIDEMIOLOGY: Infection with *T. spiralis* occurs worldwide. Humans acquire trichinosis by ingesting inadequately cooked meat containing encysted *T. spiralis* larvae. The larvae are found in the skeletal muscles of various carnivorous or omnivorous wild and domesticated animals, including pigs, rats, bears, and walruses. Pork is the most common source of human trichinosis (Fig. 9-85).

Animals acquire trichinosis by feeding on the flesh of other infected animals. Infection is common among some wild animal populations and can be readily introduced into domesticated animals, such as pigs, when they feed on garbage or uncooked meat. Meat inspection programs and restriction of feeding practices have largely eliminated *T. spiralis* from domesticated pigs in many developed countries. Although only about 100 cases of trichinosis are reported in the United States annually, these represent only the most severely symptomatic cases and infection is probably much more common.

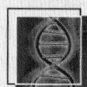

PATHOGENESIS: In the small bowel, *T. spiralis* larvae emerge from the ingested tissue cysts and burrow into the intestinal mucosa, where they develop into adult worms. The adults mate, and the female worm liberates larvae that invade the intestinal wall and enter the circulation. Production of larvae may continue for 1 to 4 months, until the worms are finally expelled from the intestine. The larvae can invade nearly any tissue but can survive only in striated skeletal muscle, where they encyst and remain viable for years. The resulting myositis is especially prominent in the diaphragm, extrinsic ocular muscles, tongue, intercostal muscles, gastrocnemius, and deltoids. Sometimes the CNS or heart is also involved in the inflammatory response, producing a meningoencephalitis or myocarditis.

PATHOLOGY: Skeletal muscle is the major sites of tissue damage in trichinosis. When a larva infects a myocyte, the cell undergoes basophilic degeneration and swelling. Early myocyte infection elicits an intense inflammatory infiltrate rich in eosinophils and macrophages. The larva grows to 10 times its initial size, folds on itself, and develops a capsule. With encapsulation, the inflammatory infiltrate subsides. Several years later, the larva dies and the cyst calcifies. In *T. spiralis* infections, the small bowel is grossly unremarkable. In heavy infestations, adult worms may be found on microscopic examination at the base of villi and may be associated with an inflammatory infiltrate.

CLINICAL FEATURES: Most human infections with *T. spiralis* involve small numbers of cysts and are asymptomatic. Symptomatic trichinosis is usually self-limited and patients recover in a few months. If

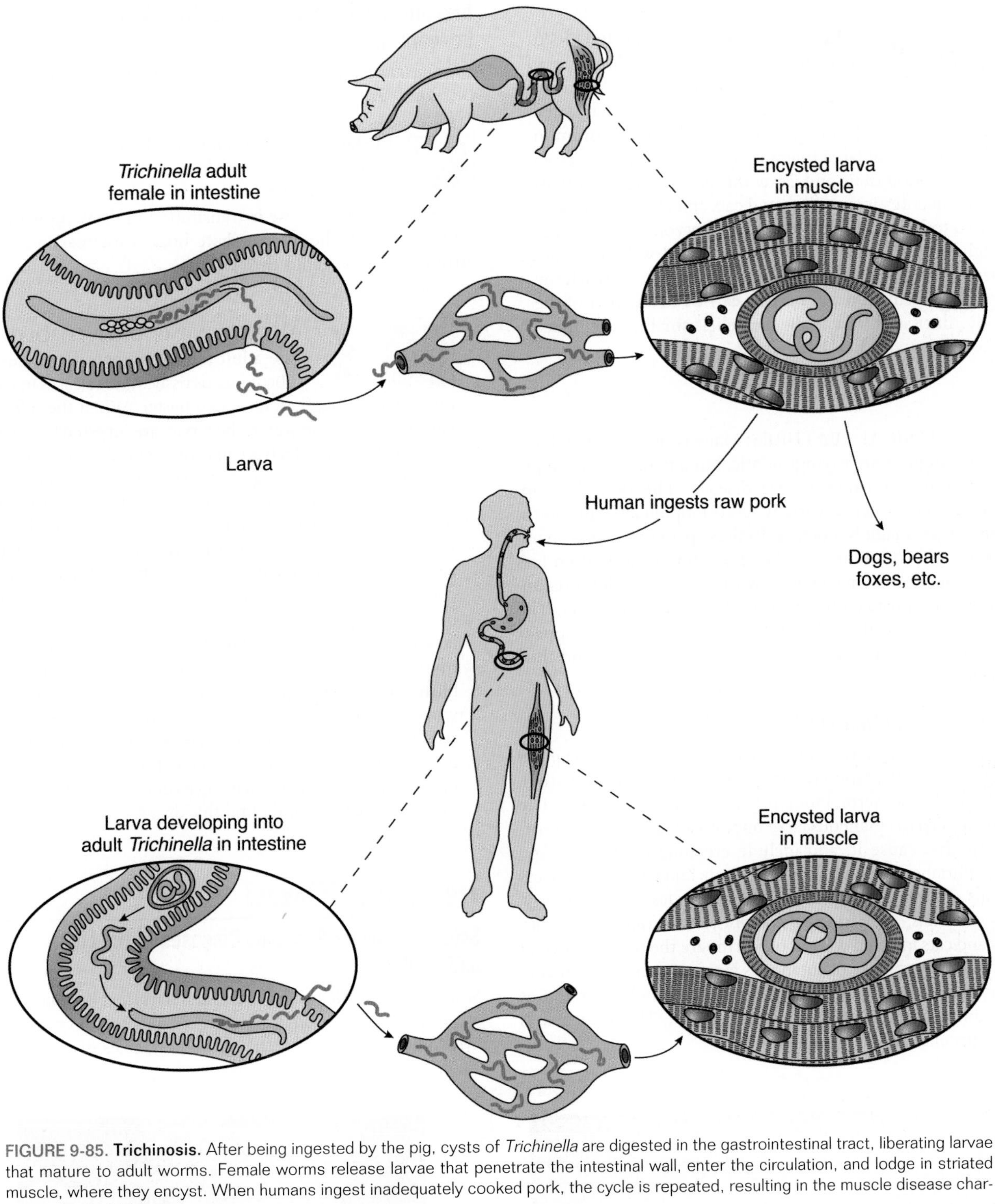

FIGURE 9-85. **Trichinosis.** After being ingested by the pig, cysts of *Trichinella* are digested in the gastrointestinal tract, liberating larvae that mature to adult worms. Female worms release larvae that penetrate the intestinal wall, enter the circulation, and lodge in striated muscle, where they encyst. When humans ingest inadequately cooked pork, the cycle is repeated, resulting in the muscle disease characteristic of trichinosis.

large numbers of cysts are eaten, abdominal pain and diarrhea may result from small bowel invasion by the worms. Major symptoms usually develop several days later when skeletal muscles are invaded. Patients suffer severe pain and tenderness of affected muscles, fever, and weakness. *Eosinophilia may be extreme (over 50% of all leukocytes).* Involvement of the extraocular muscles produces periorbital edema. Infection of the brain or myocardium can be fatal. Severe trichinosis is treated with corticosteroids to attenuate the inflammation. Antihelminthic drugs are required to remove adult worms from the intestine.

Visceral Larva Migrans (Toxocariasis) Is Transmitted by Cats and Dogs

Visceral larva migrans is an infection of deep organs by helminthic larvae migrating in aberrant hosts.

PATHOGENESIS AND PATHOLOGY: The infestation is a sporadic disease, primarily of young children, which characteristically occurs in areas where there are overcrowded dwellings, as well as dogs and cats. The most common causes of visceral larva migrans are *Toxocara* species, especially *Toxocara canis* and *Toxocara cati.* The roundworms live in the intestines of dogs and cats and infection is transmitted to humans by ingestion of embryonated ova. Eggs hatch and the larvae invade the intestinal wall. They are carried to the liver, from where a few emerge to reach the systemic circulation and may be carried to any part of the body. In tissues, larvae die and elicit small granulomas, which eventually heal by scarring.

CLINICAL FEATURES: Many cases of visceral larva migrans are asymptomatic, but any infection can potentially cause severe disease. The typical symptomatic patient is a child with hypereosinophilia, pneumonitis, and hypergammaglobulinemia. In these patients, ocular manifestations are common, and the chief complaint is often loss of vision in one eye. In fact, eyes with toxocaral endophthalmitis have been mistakenly enucleated for retinoblastoma. The infection is generally self-limited and symptoms disappear within a year. It is treated with diethylcarbamazine and thiabendazole.

Cutaneous Larva Migrans Is a Pruritic Eruption

Cutaneous larva migrans is caused by migration of larval nematodes through the skin. Migrating worms provoke severe inflammation, which appears as serpiginous urticarial trails (Fig. 9-86). The names applied to cutaneous larva migrans are as varied as the organisms that cause it, and include creeping eruptions, sand worm, plumber's itch, duck hunter's itch, and epidermis linearis migrans. The more common larval nematodes include *Strongyloides stercoralis, Ancylostoma braziliensis, and Necator americanus.* Dogs and cats infected with hookworms are the major source of the disease. Outbreaks of cutaneous larva migrans occur at subtropical and tropical beaches. Plumbers who crawl under houses and animal caretakers are frequently infected. Thiabendazole is the treatment of choice.

Dracunculiasis Features Long Adult Worms beneath the Skin

Dracunculiasis (guinea worm) is an infection of the connective and subcutaneous tissues with the guinea worm, Dracunculus medinensis.

EPIDEMIOLOGY: Dracunculiasis is common in rural areas of sub-Saharan Africa, the Middle East, India, and Pakistan, where it is estimated that 10 million persons are infected. The disease is transmitted in drinking water contaminated with the intermediate host, a microscopic aquatic crustacean of the genus *Cyclops.*

PATHOGENESIS AND PATHOLOGY: The adult female nematode resides in subcutaneous tissues and releases numerous larvae through an ulcerated blister. When the infected part is immersed in water, the larvae are ingested by the *Cyclops* crustaceans, which are in turn ingested by humans.

About a year after ingestion of infected crustaceans, systemic allergic symptoms appear, including a pruritic urticarial rash. A reddish papule, often around the ankles, develops and vesiculates. Beneath this sterile blister is the anterior end of the female worm. The blister bursts when it comes into contact with water and the female worm, now measuring up to 120 cm in length and containing 3 million larvae, partially emerges (Fig. 9-87). The worm then spews myriad larvae into the water. Secondary infection of the blister, often with spreading cellulitis, is common. Dead worms provoke an intense inflammatory response, accounting for the debilitation seen in many patients with dracunculosis. The worm is often extracted by local practitioners by progressively twisting it onto a small stick. Treatment also includes anthelminthic drugs.

Trematodes (Flukes)

Schistosomiasis Produces Diseases of the Liver and Bladder

Schistosomiasis (bilharziasis) is the most important helminthic disease of humans. Intense inflammatory and immune responses damage the liver, intestine, or urinary bladder. Three species of schistosomes,

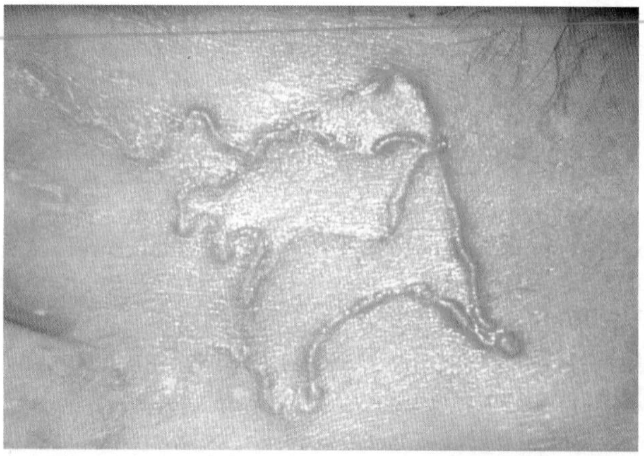

FIGURE 9-86. **Cutaneous larva migrans.** The skin shows a creeping eruption with the characteristic serpiginous, raised lesion.

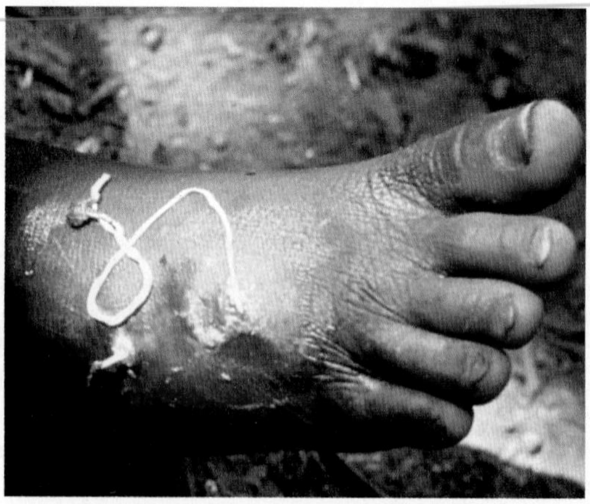

FIGURE 9-87. **Dracunculiasis.** A female guinea worm is seen emerging from the foot, which is swollen because of secondary bacterial infection.

Schistosoma mansoni, Schistosoma haematobium, and *Schistosoma japonicum,* are the causative agents.

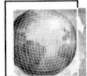

EPIDEMIOLOGY: *Schistosomiasis causes greater morbidity and mortality than all other worm infections.* The disease affects about 10% of the world's population and ranks second only to malaria as a cause of disabling disease. The three schistosomal pathogens inhabit distinct geographic regions, dictated by the distribution of their specific host snail species (Fig. 9-88). *S. mansoni* is found in much of tropical Africa, parts of southwest Asia, South America, and the Caribbean islands. *S. haematobium* is endemic in large regions of tropical Africa and parts of the Middle East. *S. japonicum* occurs in parts of China, the Philippines, Southeast Asia, and India.

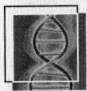

PATHOGENESIS: The schistosomes have complicated life cycles, alternating between asexual generations in the invertebrate host (snail) and sexual generations in the vertebrate host (Fig. 9-89). A schistosome egg hatches in fresh water, liberating a motile form (miracidium) that penetrates a snail, where it develops into the final larval stage, the cercaria. Cercariae escape into the water and penetrate the skin of the human host, during which process they lose their forked tails and become "schistosomula." These migrate through tissues, penetrate blood vessels and thence to the lung and liver. In the intestinal venules of the portal drainage, schistosomula mature, forming pairs of male and female worms. The females of *S. mansoni* and *S. japonicum* deposit eggs in intestinal venules, whereas *S. haematobium* lays eggs in those of the urinary bladder. Embryos develop during the passage of eggs through these tissues. The larvae are mature when eggs pass through the wall of the intestine or the bladder and are discharged in feces or urine. They hatch in fresh water, liberating miracidia and completing the life cycle.

PATHOLOGY: *The basic lesion is a circumscribed granuloma or a cellular infiltrate of eosinophils and neutrophils around an egg.* Adult schistosomes provoke no inflammation while alive in the veins. Granulomas that form about the eggs also obstruct the microvascular blood supply and produce ischemic damage to adjacent tissue. The result is progressive scarring and dysfunction in the affected organs.

The female worm deposits hundreds or thousands of eggs daily for 5 to 35 years. Most infected persons harbor fewer than 10 adult females. However, when the worm burden is large, the granulomatous response to the enormous number of eggs poses significant problems. The site of involvement is determined by the tropism of the particular schistosome species.

- *S. mansoni* inhabits the branches of the inferior mesenteric vein, thereby affecting the distal colon and liver.
- *S. haematobium* winds its way to the veins serving the rectum, bladder, and pelvic organs.
- *S. japonicum* deposits eggs predominantly in the branches of the superior mesenteric vein, thereby damaging the small bowel, ascending colon, and liver.

Liver disease caused by *S. mansoni* or *S. japonicum* begins as periportal granulomatous inflammation (Fig. 9-90) and progresses to dense periportal fibrosis (**pipestem fibrosis**) (Fig. 9-91). In severe cases of hepatic schistosomiasis, this effect results in obstruction of portal blood flow and portal hypertension. *S. mansoni* and *S. japonicum* also damage the intestine, where the granulomatous response produces inflammatory polyps and foci of mucosal and submucosal fibrosis.

Urogenital schistosomiasis, caused by *S. haematobium*, features eggs that are most numerous in the bladder, ureter, and seminal vesicles, although they may also reach lungs, colon, and appendix. Eggs in the bladder and ureters lead to a granulomatous reaction, inflammatory protuberances, and patches of mucosal and mural fibrosis. These can obstruct urine flow, thus producing secondary inflammatory damage to the bladder,

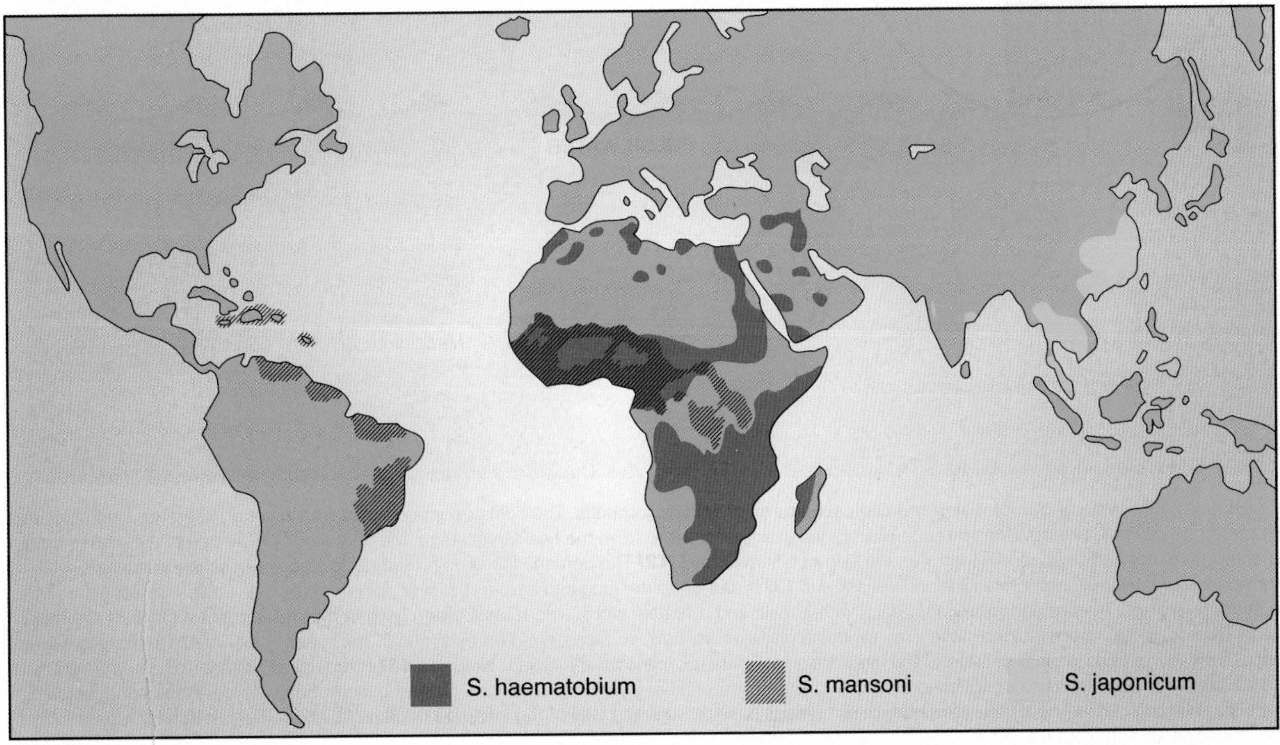

FIGURE 9-88. Distribution of schistosomiasis caused by *Schistosoma mansoni, Schistosoma haematobium,* and *Schistosoma japonicum.*

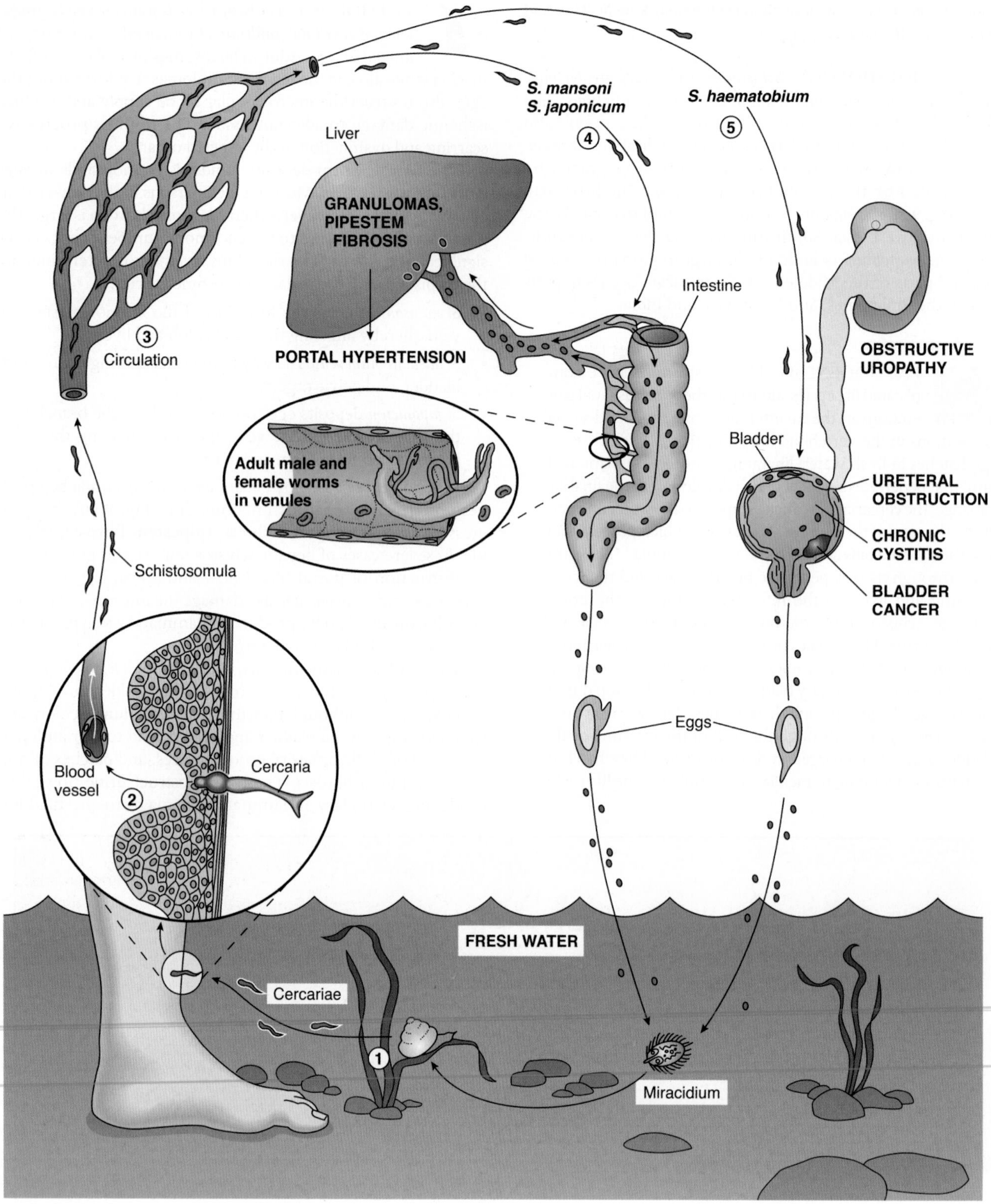

FIGURE 9-89. **Life cycle of *Schistosoma* and clinical features of schistosomiasis.** The schistosome egg hatches in water, liberates a miracidium that penetrates a snail, and develops through two stages to a sporocyst to form the final larval stage, the cercaria. ***(1)*** The cercaria escapes from the snail into water, "swims," and penetrates the skin of a human host. ***(2)*** The cercaria loses its forked tail to become a schistosomulum, which migrates through tissues, penetrates a blood vessel, and ***(3)*** is carried to the lung and later to the liver. In hepatic portal venules, the schistosomula become sexually mature and form pairs, each with a male and a female worm, the female worm lying in the gynecophoral canal of the male worm. The organism causes lesions in the liver, including granulomas, portal ("pipestem") fibrosis, and portal hypertension. ***(4)*** The female worm deposits immature eggs in small venules of the intestine and rectum (*S. mansoni* and *S. japonicum*) or ***(5)*** of the urinary bladder (*S. haematobium*). The bladder infestation leads to obstructive uropathy, ureteral obstruction, chronic cystitis, and bladder cancer. Embryos develop during passage of the eggs through tissues and larvae are mature when eggs pass through the wall of the intestine or urinary bladder. Eggs hatch in water and liberate miracidia to complete the cycle.

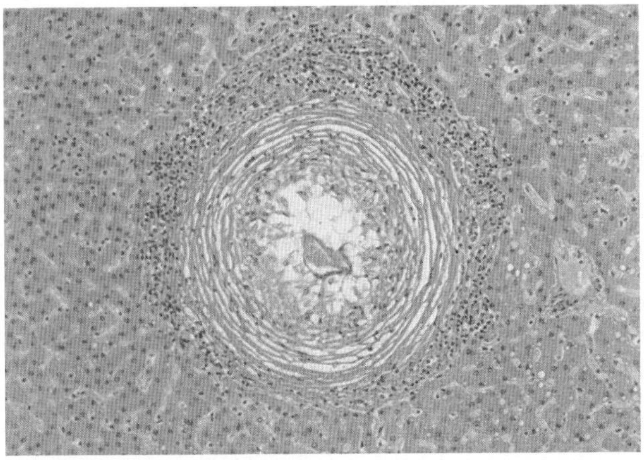

FIGURE 9-90. **Hepatic schistosomiasis.** A hepatic granuloma surrounds a degenerating egg of *S. mansoni.*

ureters, and kidneys. *The bladder disease produced by* S. haematobium *may lead to squamous cell carcinoma of the bladder.*

The granulomas of schistosomiasis surround schistosome eggs. Eosinophils often predominate in early granulomas. In older granulomas, epithelioid macrophages and giant cells are conspicuous and the oldest granulomas are densely fibrotic. Eggs of the various schistosomal species are identified on the basis of their size and shape.

CLINICAL FEATURES: Skin penetration by the schistosome larvae is sometimes associated with a self-limited, intensely pruritic rash. Most cases are dominated by the manifestations of chronic granulomatous tissue damage. Hepatic involvement leads to portal hypertension, splenomegaly, ascites, and bleeding esophageal varices. Intestinal disease is usually only minimally symptomatic, but some patients experience abdominal pain and blood in the stools. Schistosomiasis of the bladder causes hematuria, recurrent urinary tract infections, and sometimes progressive obstruction leading to renal failure. The diagnosis is made by identifying schistosome eggs in the urine or feces. Although schistosomes are effectively killed by systemic antihelminthic agents, the structural changes resulting from extensive fibrosis and scarring are irreversible.

Clonorchiasis Leads To Biliary Obstruction

Clonorchiasis is an infection of the hepatic biliary system by the Chinese liver fluke, Clonorchis sinensis. Although the fluke usually causes only mild symptoms, it is sometimes associated with bile duct stones, cholangitis, and bile duct cancer.

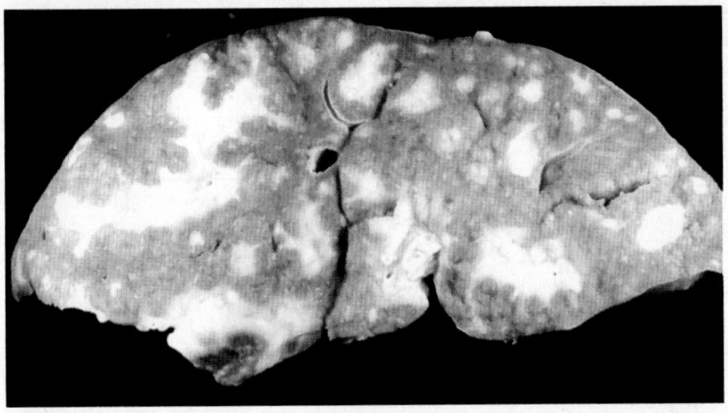

FIGURE 9-91. **Hepatic schistosomiasis.** Chronic infection of the liver with *S. japonicum* has led to the characteristic "pipestem" fibrosis.

EPIDEMIOLOGY: Clonorchiasis is endemic in east Asia, from Vietnam to Korea, where uncooked freshwater fish is common fare. In parts of Vietnam, China, and Japan, over 50% of the adult population is infected. Human infection is acquired by the ingestion of inadequately cooked freshwater fish containing *C. sinensis* larvae.

Adult worms are flat and transparent, live in human bile ducts, and pass eggs to the intestine and feces. After ingestion by a specific snail, the egg hatches into a miracidium. Cercariae escape from the snail and seek out certain fish, which they penetrate and in which they encyst. When humans eat the fish, the cercariae emerge in the duodenum, enter the common bile duct through the ampulla of Vater, and mature in the distal bile ducts to an adult fluke.

PATHOGENESIS AND PATHOLOGY: The presence of *Clonorchis* in the bile ducts elicits an inflammatory response, which fails to eliminate the worm but causes dilation and fibrosis of the ducts. Sometimes the worms cause calculus formation within the hepatic bile ducts, leading to ductal obstruction. The adult *Clonorchis* persists in the ducts for decades, and long-standing infection is associated with an increased incidence of carcinoma of the bile duct epithelium (cholangiocarcinoma).

In heavy *Clonorchis* infections, the liver may be up to three times normal size. Dilated bile ducts are seen through the capsule, and the cut surface is punctuated with thick-walled dilated bile ducts (Fig. 9-92). The flukes (up to 2.5 cm in length), sometimes in the thousands, can be expressed from the bile ducts. Microscopically, the epithelial ductlining is initially hyperplastic and then becomes metaplastic. Surrounding stroma is fibrotic. Secondary bacterial infection is common and may be associated with suppurative cholangitis. Eggs deposited in the hepatic parenchyma are surrounded by a fibrous and granulomatous reaction. Masses of eggs may become lodged in the bile ducts and cause cholangitis. The pancreatic ducts may also be invaded and become dilated, thickened, lined by metaplastic epithelium, and eventually surrounded by scar tissue.

CLINICAL FEATURES: Migration of *C. sinensis* into the bile ducts results in transient fever and chills, although most infected persons are completely asymptomatic. Patients with clonorchiasis may die of a variety of complications, including biliary obstruction, bacterial cholangitis, pancreatitis, and cholangiocarcinoma. The diagnosis of clonorchiasis is made by identifying eggs of *C. sinensis* in stools or duodenal aspirates. The infestation is treated effectively with systemic antihelminthic agents.

Paragonimiasis Is a Lung Disease

Paragonimiasis refers to a pulmonary infection by several species of the genus *Paragonimus,* the oriental lung fluke. The most common human pathogen is *Paragonimus westermani*. The infestation is common in Asian countries (Korea, the Philippines, Taiwan,

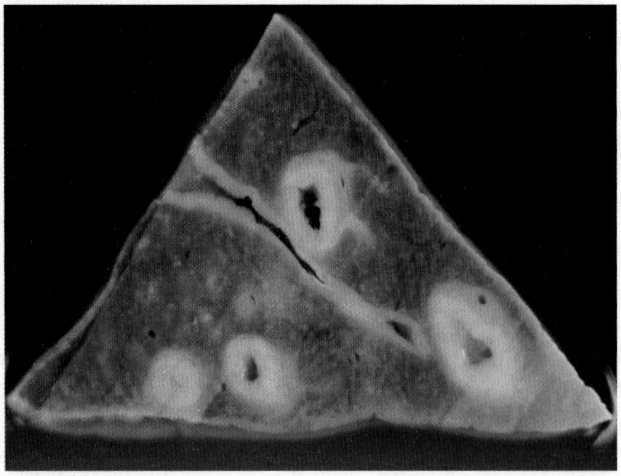

FIGURE 9-92. **Clonorchiasis of the liver**. The bile ducts are greatly thickened and dilated because of the presence of adult flukes *(Clonorchis sinensis)*.

and China), where uncooked, lightly salted, or wine-soaked fresh crabs are considered delicacies. The use of raw crab juices as medicinal beverages or seasonings also has been associated with the infection.

CLINICAL FEATURES: Pulmonary paragonimiasis is frequently misdiagnosed as tuberculosis. The disease manifests as fever, malaise, night sweats, chest pain, and cough. However, unlike tuberculosis, peripheral eosinophilia is common. The sputum is sometimes blood-tinged and chest radiographs reveal transient diffuse pulmonary infiltrates. The prognosis in pulmonary paragonimiasis is good, but ectopic lesions of the brain may be fatal. Eggs in the sputum or stools provide the definitive diagnosis.

Fascioliasis Is a Biliary Disease Acquired from Sheep

Fascioliasis is an infection of the liver by the sheep liver fluke, Fasciola hepatica. Humans may acquire the infection wherever sheep are raised. People become infected by eating vegetation, such as watercress, that is contaminated with the cysts passed by sheep.

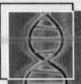

PATHOGENESIS: After reaching the duodenum, cysts liberate metacercariae that pass into the peritoneal cavity, penetrate the liver, and migrate through the hepatic parenchyma into the bile ducts. The larvae mature to adults and live in both the intrahepatic and extrahepatic bile ducts. Later, the adult flukes penetrate the wall of the bile ducts and wander back into the liver parenchyma, where they feed on liver cells and deposit their eggs.

PATHOLOGY AND CLINICAL FEATURES: The eggs of *F. hepatica* lead to hepatic abscesses and granulomas. The worms induce hyperplasia of the lining epithelium of the bile ducts, portal and periductal fibrosis, proliferation of bile ductules, and varying degrees of biliary obstruction. Eosinophilia, vomiting, and acute gastric pain are characteristic features. Severe untreated infections may be fatal. The diagnosis is made by recovering eggs from the stools or biliary tract.

Fasciolopsiasis Is an Infestation of the Small Intestine

Fasciolopsiasis is caused by the giant intestinal fluke, Fasciolopsis buski. The disease is common in the Orient. Humans are infected by eating aquatic vegetables contaminated with the encysted cercariae. The worm is large (3 × 7 cm) and attaches to the duodenal or jejunal wall. The point of attachment may ulcerate and become infected, causing pain like that of a peptic ulcer. Acute symptoms may also be caused by intestinal obstruction or by toxins released by large numbers of worms. The diagnosis is made by identifying the eggs of *F. buski* in the stool. Treatment is with systemic antihelminthic agents.

CESTODES: Intestinal Tapeworms

Taenia saginata, Taenia solium, and Diphyllobothrium latum are tapeworms that infect humans, growing to their adult forms within the intestine (Table 9-11). The presence of these adult worms rarely damages the human host.

EPIDEMIOLOGY: Intestinal tapeworm infections are acquired by eating inadequately cooked beef *(T. saginata),* pork *(T. solium),* or fish *(D. latum)* containing larval forms of these organisms. Tapeworm life cycles involve cystic larval stages in animals and worm stages in the human. The life cycles of the beef and pork tapeworms require that the animals ingest material tainted with infected human feces. The cystic larval forms develop in the muscles of the animals. Modern cattle and pig farming practices, plus meat inspection, have largely eliminated beef and pork tapeworms in industrialized countries, but infection remains common in the underdeveloped world. Fish tapeworm infection is prevalent in regions where raw, pickled, or partly cooked freshwater fish are common fare. Tapeworm infections are usually asymptomatic, although it may be distressing when an infected person passes portions of the worm in the stool. The fish tapeworm *(D. latum)* competes for vitamin B_{12} and a small number (<2%) of infected persons develop pernicious anemia (see Chapter 20).

Cysticercosis Is a Systemic Infection by the Larvae of the Pork Tapeworm

The adult *T. solium* is acquired by eating undercooked pork infected with cysticerci (measly pork).

TABLE 9-11

Tapeworm Infections

Species	Human Disease	Source of Human Infection
Taenia saginata	Adult tapeworm in intestine	Beef
Taenia solium	Adult tapeworm in intestine; cysticercosis	Pork; human feces
Diphyllobothrium latum	Adult tapeworm in intestine	Fish
Echinococcus granulosus	Hydatid cyst disease	Dog feces

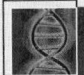

PATHOGENESIS: Pigs acquire cysticerci by ingesting eggs of *T. solium* in human feces. This cycle, although a public health concern, is essentially benign for both humans and pigs. *However, when humans accidentally ingest tapeworm eggs from human feces and become infected with cysticerci, the consequences may be catastrophic.* The eggs release oncospheres, which penetrate the wall of the gut, enter the bloodstream, lodge in tissue, encyst, and differentiate to cysticerci.

PATHOLOGY: The cysticercus is a spherical, milky white cyst about 1 cm in diameter that contains fluid and an invaginated scolex (head of the worm) with birefringent hooklets. Viable cysts can be shelled out from the infected tissue. They remain viable for an indefinite period and provoke no inflammation; rather, as they grow they compress adjacent tissues. Degenerating cysts, the ones usually responsible for symptoms, are attached to the tissue and are densely inflamed with eosinophils, neutrophils, lymphocytes, and plasma cells. Multiple cysticerci in the brain sometimes impart a "Swiss cheese" appearance to the tissue (Fig. 9-93).

CLINICAL FEATURES: Cysticercosis of the brain manifests as headaches or seizures and symptoms vary according to the sites affected. Massive cysticercosis of the brain causes convulsions and death. Cysticerci in the retina blind the patient. In the heart, cysticerci may cause arrhythmias and sudden death. Depending on the involved site, cysticercosis is treated with surgery or antihelminthic therapy.

Echinococcosis Features Cysts of the Liver and Lungs

Echinococcosis (hydatid disease) is a zoonotic infection caused by larval cestodes of the genus *Echinococcus*. The most common offender is *Echinococcus granulosus,* which causes cystic hydatid disease. Rarely, *Echinococcus multilocularis* and *Echinococcus vogeli* infect humans.

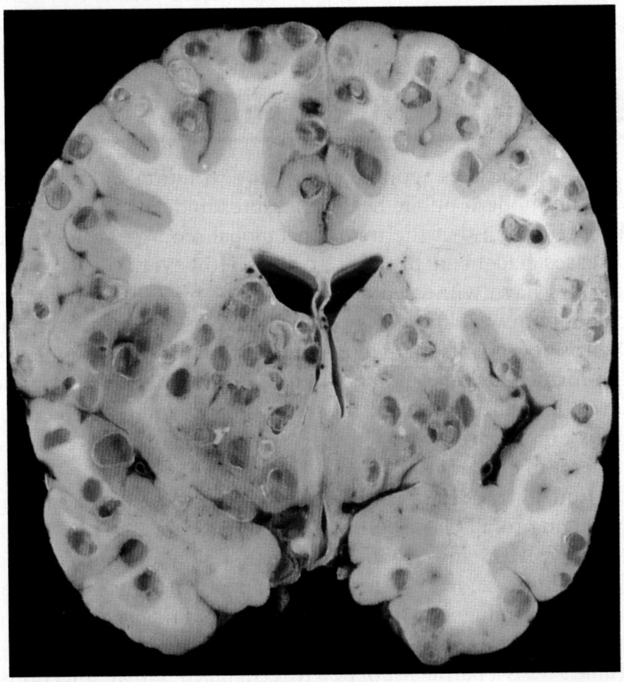

FIGURE 9-93. **Cysticercosis.** A cross-section of the brain from a patient infected with the larvae of *Taenia solium* shows many cysticerci in the gray matter, imparting a "Swiss cheese" appearance.

EPIDEMIOLOGY: Infestation with the tapeworm *E. granulosus* is endemic in sheep, goats, and cattle as well as their attendant dogs. Dogs contaminate their habitats (and their human keepers) with infectious eggs. Humans become infected when they inadvertently ingest the tapeworm eggs. The resulting hydatid disease is present worldwide among herding populations who live in close proximity to dogs and herd animals, especially Australia, New Zealand, Argentina, Greece, and herding countries of Africa and the Middle East. In the United States, hydatid cyst disease is seen among immigrants and among the indigenous sheep-herding populations of the southwest.

E. multilocularis causes the alveolar hydatid disease in humans. Dogs and cats are domestic definitive hosts and the domestic intermediate host is the house mouse. Rare infections by *E. multilocularis* have been reported in Germany, Switzerland, China, and the republics of the former Soviet Union.

Dogs are definitive hosts for *E. vogeli*. Humans may become accidental intermediate hosts for *E. vogeli* by ingesting eggs shed by domestic dogs. Polycystic hydatid disease caused by *E. vogeli* has been reported in Central and South America.

PATHOGENESIS: The adult tapeworms (2 to 6 mm long) live in the small intestine of carnivorous hosts, for example,wolves, foxes, and so forth. (Fig. 9-94). *E. granulosus* has a scolex with suckers and numerous hooklets for attachment to the intestinal mucosa. A short neck is followed by three segments (proglottids). The terminal gravid proglottid breaks off and releases eggs, which are eliminated in the feces. Contaminated herbage is then eaten by herbivorous intermediate hosts, such as cattle and sheep. Humans are also infected by ingesting plant material contaminated by the cestode eggs. Larvae released from the eggs penetrate the wall of the gut, enter the bloodstream, and disseminate to deep organs, where they grow to form large cysts containing brood capsules and scolices. If the flesh of the herbivore is eaten by a carnivore, scolices develop into sexually mature worms in the latter, thereby completing the cycle.

PATHOLOGY AND CLINICAL FEATURES: The slowly growing hydatid cyst is found by chance or becomes obvious when its size and position interferes with normal functions. A hepatic cyst may manifest as a palpable right upper quadrant mass. Compression of intrahepatic bile ducts by the cyst may lead to obstructive jaundice. Pulmonary cysts (Fig. 9-95) are often asymptomatic and discovered incidentally on a chest radiograph.

A major complication of cyst rupture is seeding of adjacent tissues with brood capsules and scolices. When these "seeds" germinate, they produce many additional cysts, each with the growth potential of the original cyst. Traumatic rupture of a hydatid cyst of the liver or other abdominal organ results in severe diffuse pain, resembling that of peritonitis. Rupture of a pulmonary cyst may cause pneumothorax and empyema. Moreover, when a hydatid cyst ruptures into a body cavity, release of cyst contents can cause fatal allergic reactions. Treatment of

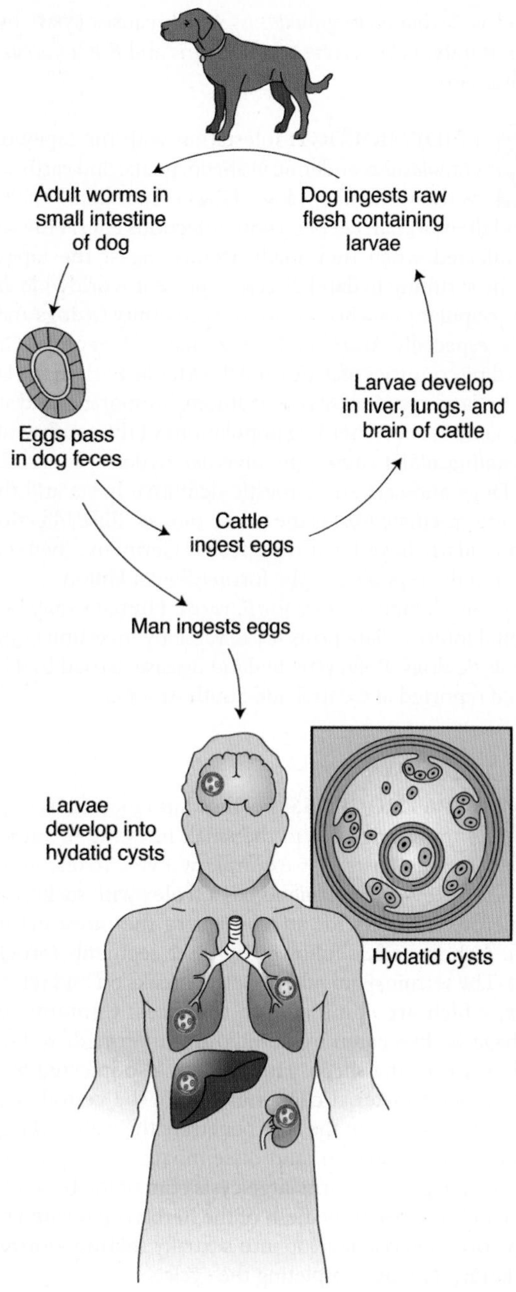

FIGURE 9-94. **Life cycle of *Echinococcus granulosus* and cystic hydatid disease.** The adult cestode lives in the small intestine of a dog (the definitive host). A gravid proglottid ruptures, releasing cestode eggs into the dog's feces. Cestode eggs are ingested by cattle or sheep (the intermediate hosts), hatch in the intestine and release oncospheres that penetrate the wall of the gut, enter the bloodstream, disseminate to various deep organs, and grow to form hydatid cysts, containing brood capsules and scolices. When another dog ingests raw flesh from the cattle or sheep, the scolices are ingested and develop into mature worms in the dog's intestine to complete the cycle. A person who ingests cestode eggs in contaminated plant material becomes an accidental intermediate host. The larvae increase in size, but the parasite reaches a "dead end" without developing into an adult tapeworm. Hydatid cysts in humans occur predominantly in the liver but may also involve lung, kidney, brain, and other organs.

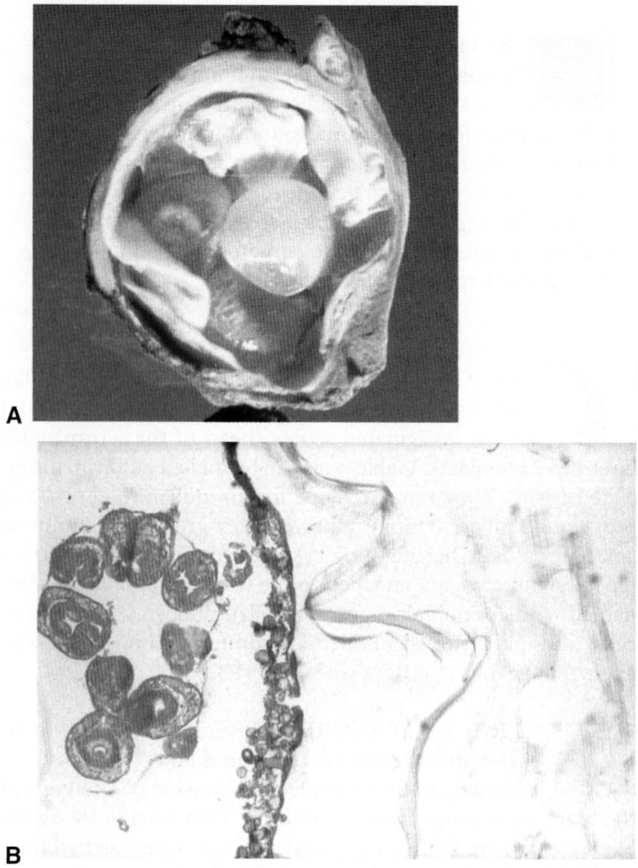

FIGURE 9-95. **Echinococcal cyst. A.** An echinococcal cyst showing daughter cysts was resected from the liver of a patient infected with *E. granulosus*. **B.** A photomicrograph of the cyst wall shows *(from right to left)* a laminated, non-nuclear layer, a nucleated germinal layer with brood capsules attached, and numerous scolices in the cyst cavity.

echinococcal cysts frequently requires careful surgical removal. Cysts must be sterilized with formalin before drainage or extirpation to prevent intraoperative anaphylactic shock.

EMERGING AND RE-EMERGING INFECTIONS

Several decades ago, the antibiotic revolution, vaccinations, and modern public health measures understandably led to the notion that the traditional global scourge of infectious diseases had been brought to bay. However, the last few decades have witnessed a resurgence of microbial threats includes both well-known agents that have become resurgent, as well as new agents that were previously unknown. Examples of the former include cholera, yellow fever, diphtheria, dengue fever, influenza, measles, tuberculosis, and anthrax. The ominous emergence of antibiotic-resistant organisms presents a new set of challenges.

Equally important has been the discovery of new pathogens belonging to all classes: viruses, bacterial, parasites, and fungi. Notably, AIDS and hepatitis C infection alone have accounted for millions of deaths, despite therapeutic advances. The resilience of influenza virus as a pathogen is underscored by the possibility of a global avian influenza pandemic (e.g., H5N1). Table 9-12 is a partial list of newly recognized human infections. It should serve as a reminder that the equilibrium between hu-

TABLE 9-12

Examples of recently discovered and emerging infections

Year	Agent	Human Disease/Association
2006	*Rickettsia massiliae*	Rickettsial spotted fever
2006	*Mycobacterium tilburgii*	Multiorgan disease
2005	Coronavirus HCoV-HKU-1	Pneumonia
2005	*Rickettsia mongolotimonae*	Lymphangitis
2004	H5N1 "Avian" influenza	Pneumonia
2004	Arcobacter species	Intestinal infection
2004	*Rickettsia parkeri*	Rickettsial spotted fever
2002	SARS-associated coronavirus	Severe atypical pneumonia (SARS-CoV)
2002	*Rickettsia aeschlimannii*	Rickettsial spotted fever
2000	*Rickettsia felis*	Rickettsial spotted fever
2000	Human metapneumovirus (hMPV)	Respiratory tract infection
1999	Nipah virus	Acute respiratory syndrome
1997	Alkhurma hemorrhagic fever virus	Saudi Arabian hemorrhagic fever
1997	*Rickettsia slovaca* (tickborne lymphadenopathy); TIBOLA	Lymph node enlargement
1996	*Rickettsia africae*	African tick bite fever
1995	New variant Creutzfeldt-Jakob Disease	Spongiform encephalopathy ("mad cow")
1994	Hendra virus	Acute respiratory syndrome
1994	Sabiá virus	Brazilian hemorrhagic fever
1994	Human herpesvirus 8 (HHV8)	Kaposi's sarcoma, body cavity lymphomas
1994	*Ehrlichia phagocytophilia*-like agent	Human granulocytic ehrlichiosis
1993	*Balamuthia mandrillaris*	Amebic meningoencephalitis
1993	*Cyclospora cayetanensis*	Coccidan diarrhea
1993	Sin nombre virus	Hantavirus pulmonary syndrome
1993	*Septata intestinalis* (now *Encephalitozoon intestinalis*)	Intestinal and disseminated microsporidiosis
1992	Vibrio cholerae O139	Epidemic cholera
1992	*Bartonella henselae*	Bacillary angiomatosis, cat scratch fever
1991	*Ehrlichia chaffeensis*	Human ehrlichiosis
1991	Guanarito virus	Venezuelan hemorrhagic fever
1991	*Encephalitozoon hellem*	Disseminated microsporidiosis
1990	*Anaplasma phagocytophilum*	Human granulocytic anaplasmosis
1990	*Hemophilus influenzae* biotype *aegyptius*	Brazilian purpuric fever
1990	Human herpesvirus 7 (HHV7)	Aseptic meningitis
1989	*Pythium insidiosum*	Cutaneous & deep fungal infections
1989	*Chlamydia pneumoniae* (TWAR)	Respiratory infection
1989	Hepatitis C virus	Chronic hepatitis, cirrhosis, liver cancer
1989	Barmah Forest virus	Polyarthritis
1986	Human herpesvirus 6 (HHV6)	Roseola (Exanthema subitum)
1986	Porogia virus	Hemorrhagic fever/renal syndrome (HFRS)
1986	HIV-2	AIDS-like illness
1985	*Enterocytozoon bieneusi*	Intestinal and hepatobiliary microsporidiosis
1983	HIV-1	AIDS
1983	*Helicobacter pylori*	Gastric and duodenal infection, ulcers
1983	Hepatitis E virus	"Epidemic" non-A non-B hepatitis
1983	*Borrelia burgdorferi*	Lyme disease

AIDS = acquired immunodeficiency syndrome; HIV = human immunodeficiency virus; SARS = severe acute respiratory syndrome; SARS-CoV = severe acute respiratory syndrome-associated corona virus

TABLE 9-13

Potential Biological Agents of Warfare and Bioterror

Bacteria
Bacillus anthracis
Brucella abortus, B. suis, B. melitensis
Pseudomonas mallei, P. pseudomallei
Rickettsia prowazekii, R. rickettsii
Pseudomonas mallei, P. pseudomallei
Coxiella burnetii, Francisella tularensis, Yersinia pestis
Clostridium botulinum and Botulinum neurotoxin-producing species of *Clostridium*
Viruses
Arenaviruses - Lassa, Machupo, Sabia, Junin, Guanarito
Bunyaviruses - Rift Valley Fever virus, Congo-Crimean hemorrhagic fever virus
Filoviruses - Ebolavirus, Marburgvirus
Flaviviruses - Kyasanur Forest Disease,
Influenza
Kumlinge, Omsk hemorrhagic fever, Russian Spring-Summer encephalitis, Tick-borne encephalitis
Poxviruses - Smallpox (Variola) and Monkeypox
Togaviruses - Eastern Equine Encephalitis Virus
Venezuelan Equine Encephalitis Virus
Biological Toxins
Botulinum, *Clostridium perfringens* epsilon toxin
Staphylococcal enterotoxin B
Shigatoxin
Conotoxins
Abrin
Ricin
Tetrodotoxin
Saxitoxin
T-2 toxin
Diacetoxyscirpenol
Microcystins
Aflatoxins
Satratoxin H
Palytoxin
Anatoxin A

mans and the pathogens that confront them is a dynamic one: continuous vigilance is in order and complacency is an invitation to disaster. The reader is referred to other sources for those infections not discussed above.

AGENTS OF BIOWARFARE

Biological agents have been used as weapons since ancient times. Perhaps the first resort to a bioweapon was in 184 BC by Hannibal, the great leader of Carthage. In preparation for a naval battle against King Eumenes of Pergamum, his army filled earthenware pots with serpents and hurled them to the decks of the Pergamene ships. In 1346, the Tatars lay siege to the Genoese-controlled seaport of Caffa (modern-day Feodosiya, Ukraine). During the siege, the Tatars were ravaged by plague. The Tatar leader catapulted his own dead soldiers, victims of the disease, into the besieged town to spread the epidemic, and forced the Genoese army to flee to Italy. Similar tactics were used at Karlstein in Bohemia in 1422 and by Russian troops in fighting Swedish forces in Reval in 1710.

Smallpox was used as a biological weapon by Francisco Pizarro in his conquest of South America in the 15th century when he gave variola-contaminated clothing as gifts. The English used a similar tactic during the French-Indian War in 1763, when Sir Jeffrey Amherst presented smallpox-laden blankets to the Delaware Indians loyal to the French. The deliberate delivery of smallpox was later used by American colonists against their adversaries during the Revolutionary War. The colonists were immune to smallpox, as General George Washington had ordered mandatory vaccination.

Allegations of biowarfare surfaced in World War I. The Germans were reported to spread cholera to Italy, plague to St. Petersburg, and anthrax and glanders to the United States and elsewhere Although no definite evidence of any of these actions by Germany was identified by the League of Nations following the war, the psychological impact of the potential use of biological weaponry in inducing terror was firmly established in modern times. The United States established Camp Detrick in Maryland in 1942–1943 to investigate biological weapons. The 20th century has seen many national bioweapons research programs, mainly covert, and a few notorious for human experimentation. Accidental contamination has occurred. In 1942, Gruinard Island off the northwest coast of Scotland was rendered uninhabitable for almost 50 years following field trials of anthrax by the British. An outbreak of inhalational anthrax in 1979 in Sverdlovsk (former Soviet Union) killed over 60 people. Prior to the Persion Gulf War of 1990, Iraq had prepared an arsenal of biological weapon delivery systems using botulinum toxin, aflatoxin, and anthrax.

There is legitimate fear in modern times over the use of bioweapons as a terrorist tool. In September 1984, an outbreak of salmonella gastroenteritis was caused by followers of the Indian guru Bagwan Shree Rajneesh in Oregon, infecting over 700 persons. In 1993 an apocalyptic Japanese cult group sprayed anthrax spores from a high-rise building in Tokyo, but no one was injured. The same cult group was found to be preparing vast quantities of *Clostridium difficile* spores for terrorist use. In 1995, the American Type Culture Collection (ATCC), a nonprofit organization that supplies biological specimens to scientists, shipped a package containing three vials of *Yersinia pestis* to the home of a political extremist in Ohio. A search of his home revealed a variety of explosive devices, detonating fuses, and triggers. Most recently, dried anthrax was mailed in letters through the United States postal system, resulting in five deaths.

Only a few biological agents have been considered or proven to be effective as weapons of biowarfare or bioterrorism (Table 9-13). The important factors which make an infectious agent suitable for large-scale biowarfare include (1) ease of large-scale production; (2) ability to cause death or incapacity of humans at doses which are deliverable; (3) appropriate particle size as an aerosol; (4) ease of dissemination; (5) stability of the agent during storage, in the environment, or placement into a delivery system; and (6) susceptibility of intended victims, but nonsusceptibility of friendly forces.

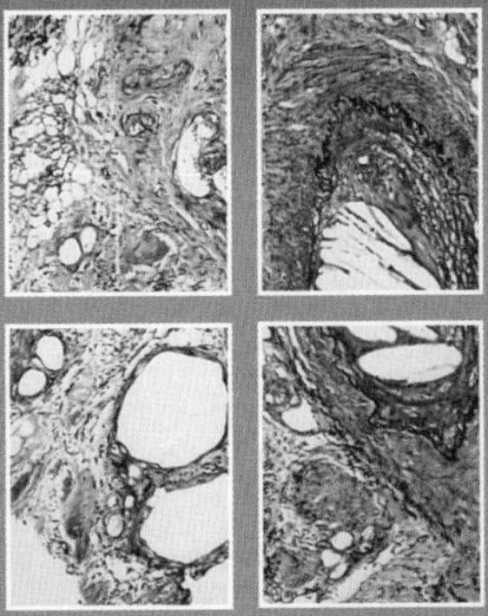

10 Blood Vessels

Avrum I. Gotlieb

Embryonic Development and Structure of Blood Vessels

Vascular smooth muscle cells are derived from local mesoderm after endothelial tubes are formed. However, smooth muscle cells that populate major arteries in the upper part of the body are derived from neural crest (Fig. 10-1). Thus, vascular smooth muscle cell diversity, both structural and functional, has a developmental basis and may have implications in the development of pathological lesions in the adult vascular system.

The Vessel Wall Comprises Endothelial Cells and Smooth Muscle Cells

Most vascular diseases result from dysfunction of endothelial and smooth muscle cells.

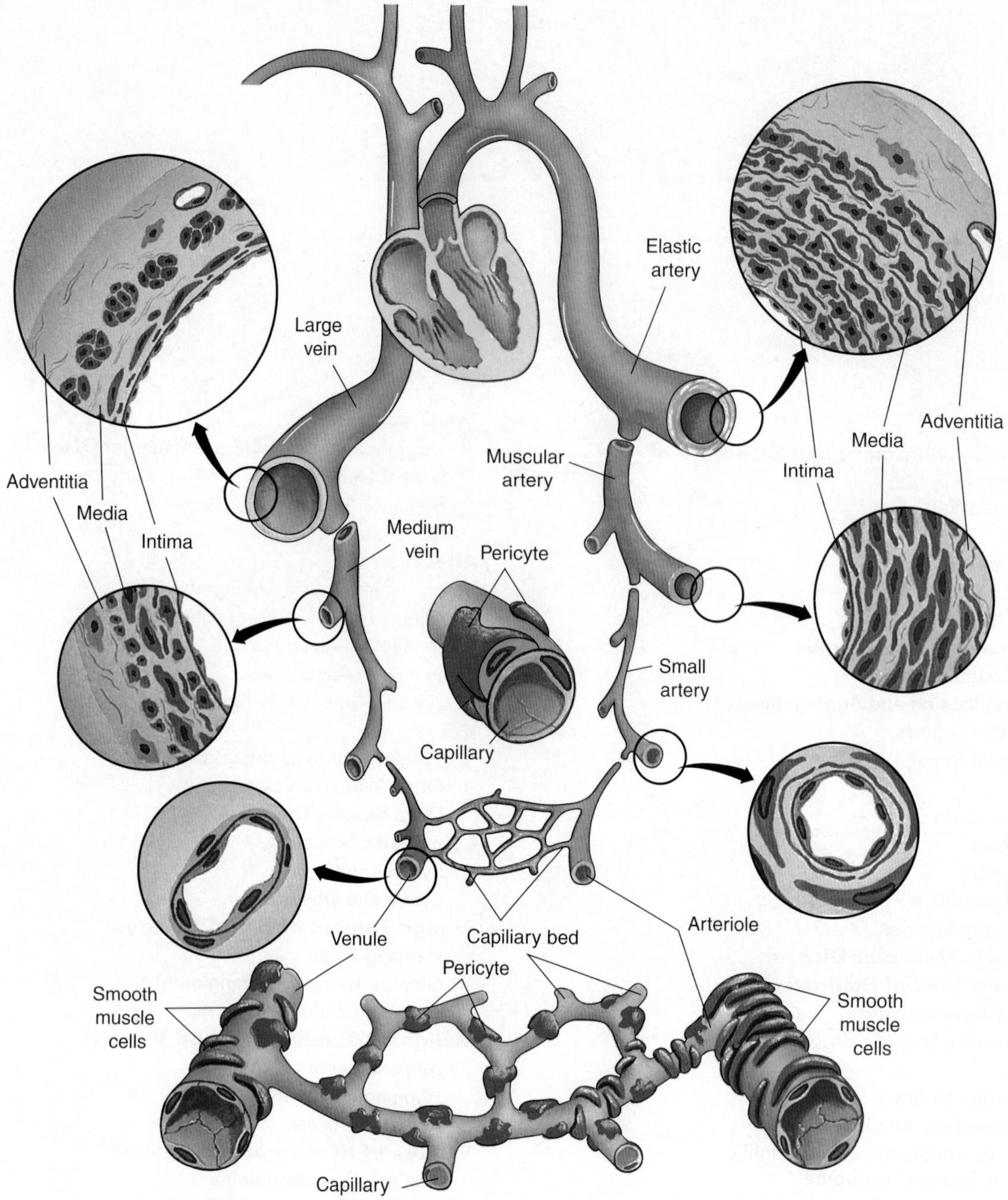

FIGURE 10-1. **Differentiation of vessels in early embryos.** The course of events from the development of blood islands on the chorioallantoic membrane starts with differentiation of endothelium and proceeds to fully developed arteries and veins.

Endothelial Cells

The endothelium forms (1) a macromolecular barrier, (2) a thromboresistant surface, (3) a cell layer that modulates vascular smooth muscle cell function, and (4) a single row of highly metabolic endothelial cells intimately involved in several biological functions, including coagulation, platelet regulation, fibrinolysis, inflammation, immunoregulation, and repair. The endothelium also forms a unique mechanotransduction structure that modulates endothelial morphology and function in response to shear stress. By virtue of mechanical sensing, endothelial cell membranes may deform, biochemical and signaling responses may be activated, leading to expression of vasoactive compounds, growth factors, coagulation/fibrinolytic/complement factors, matrix degradation enzymes, inflammatory mediators, and adhesion molecules.

A single row of endothelial cells lines the tunica intima, the innermost layer of the blood vessel wall, and form the interface with the flowing blood (Figs. 10-1, 10-2 and 10-3). The integrity of the endothelium depends on several types of adhesion complexes which promote cell-substratum, cell-cell, and endothelial cell-leukocyte adhesion (see Chapter 2).

- **Cell-substrate adhesion molecules** attach endothelial cells to their substratum (e.g., basal lamina). They complex with intracellular cytoskeleton, which participates in intracellular signal transduction. For example, integrins are heterodimeric transmembrane molecules which bind endothelial cells to extracellular matrix adhesive molecules, including laminin, fibronectin, fibrinogen, von Willebrand factor, and thrombospondin. The cytoplasmic tails of the integrins bind the complex of proteins that regulate adhesion at focal contact sites and associate with actin microfilaments and microtubules of the cytoskeleton (Fig. 10-4).

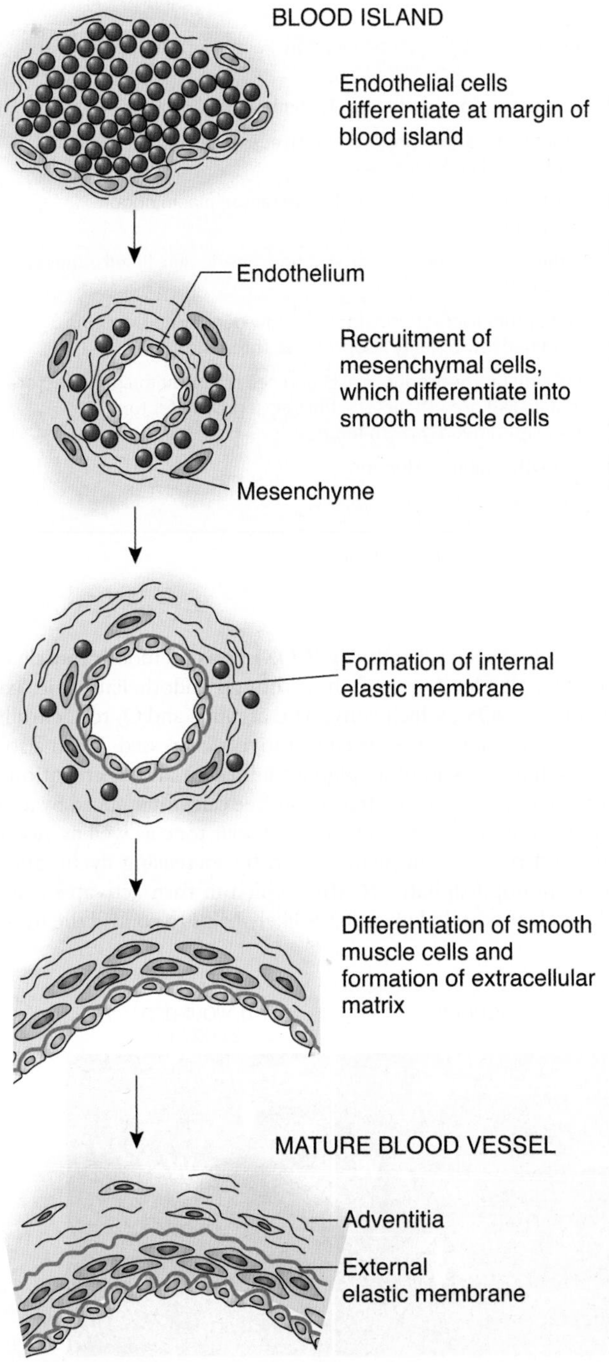

FIGURE 10-2. **Subdivisions and histologic structure of the vascular system.** Each subdivision is subject to a set of pathologic changes conditioned by the structure–function relationship of that part of the system. For example, the aorta, an elastic artery subject to great pressure, frequently shows a pathologic dilation (aneurysm) if the supporting elastic media is damaged. Muscular arteries are the most significant sites of atherosclerosis. Small arteries, particularly arterioles, are sites of hypertensive changes. Capillary beds, venules, and veins each display their own types of pathologic changes.

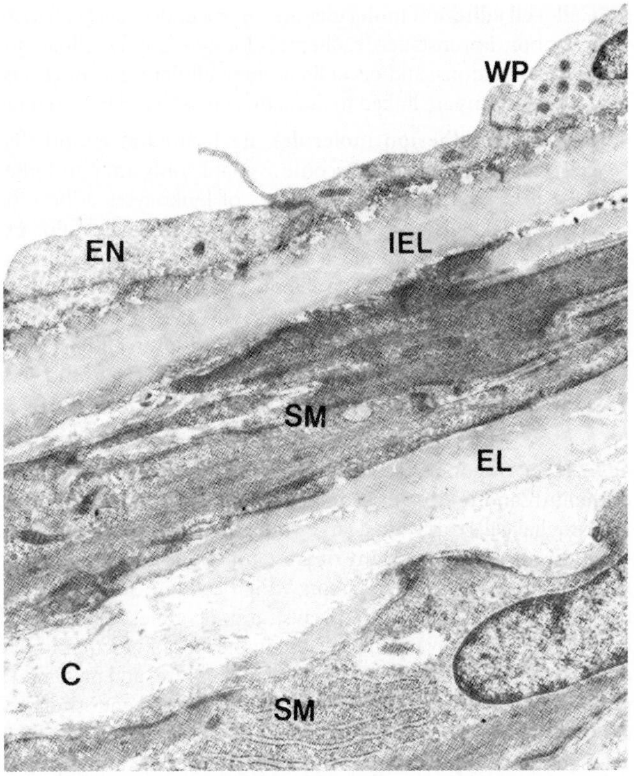

FIGURE 10-3. **Luminal side of the rat aorta.** An electron micrograph shows endothelial cells *(EN)* with Weibel-Palade bodies *(WP)*, internal elastic lamina *(IEL)*, smooth muscle cells *(SM)*, collagen *(C)*, and elastic lamellae *(EL)*.

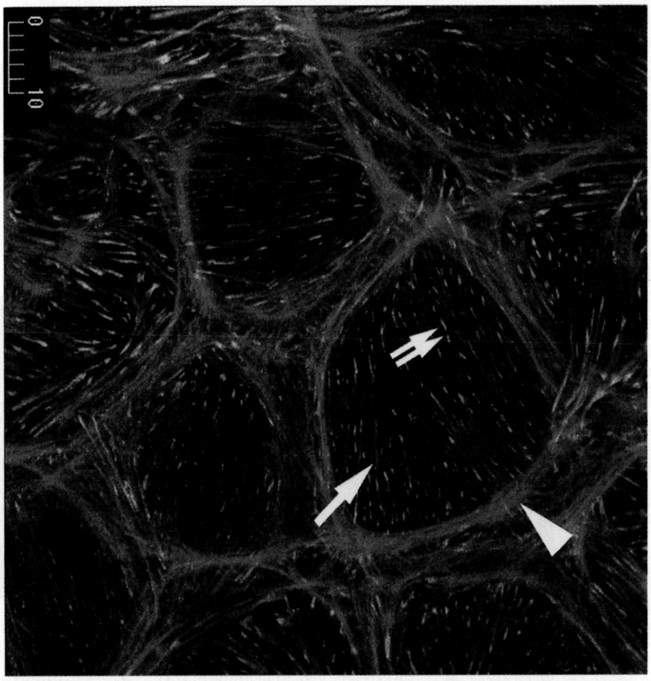

FIGURE 10-4. **Focal adhesion protein, vinculin.** Porcine aortic endothelial cells were grown to confluency and double-stained for actin/vinculin. Endothelial cells in confluent monolayers contain a *dense peripheral band* (DPB) of actin microfilament bundles *(arrow head)* and central microfilament or "stress fibers" *(single arrow)*. Vinculin in confluent monolayer localizes to the tips of stress fibers *(double arrow)*.

- **Cell–cell adhesion molecules** attach one endothelial cell to its neighbor. For instance, cadherin is located at intercellular adhesion junctions, and occludin at intercellular tight junctions. The cadherins are linked to the actin cytoskeleton by catenins.
- **Leukocyte adhesion molecules** are located at endothelial cell surfaces and several become available only after endothelial cell activation. Different types of leukocytes adhere to endothelial cells through these adhesion molecules. For example E-selectin and P-selectin at endothelial surfaces bind to ligands on leukocytes. P-selectin binds counter-receptors such as P-selectin glycoprotein ligand-1 (PSGL-1). Vascular cell adhesion molecule 1 (VCAM-1) and intercellular adhesion molecule 1 (ICAM-1) on the endothelial surface bind very late antigen 4 (VLA-4) and leukocyte function antigen-1 (LFA-1) present on leukocytes.

A layer of connective tissue is interposed between the endothelium and underlying smooth muscle of the tunica media. Endothelial cells carry out a large variety of important metabolic functions (Table 10-1). Many of these functions are regulated by serum and hemodynamic factors which activate surface receptors, signal transduction pathways, and/or genes. Endothelial cells do not normally proliferate, but in the face of vascular injury and loss of endothelial cells, they spread, migrate, and proliferate rapidly to reestablish the structural integrity of the endothelium, and thus protect the wall from disease (Fig. 10-5).

Endothelial dysfunction plays a significant role in the pathogenesis of vascular disease. It may be associated with subendothelial accumulation of blood-borne materials. For example, accretion of lipid beneath the endothelium in atherosclerotic lesions reflects, in part, failure of the endothelium to serve as an effective barrier between tissue and plasma, and adhesion and subsequent transmigration of monocytes across the endothelium to become subendothelial lipid-laden macrophages, which release lipids into the matrix.

Endothelial cells synthesize a number of biologically active factors that are released upon activation of the endothelial cell. Some are potent bioactive molecules that are released locally, act at short distances, and are rapidly inactivated. For example, prostacyclin (PGI_2), a product of arachidonic metabolism derived from the cyclooxygenase pathway (COX), relaxes smooth muscle and inhibits platelet aggregation. Although endothelial nitric oxide synthase (NOS), which converts L-arginine and O_2 to L-citrulline and nitric oxide (NO•), is constitutively expressed, it can also be regulated. NO• inhibits platelet adhesion and aggregation by attenuating the rise in intracellular free calcium induced by a variety of agonists. NO• modulates vascular tone as well as vascular smooth muscle cell proliferation by increasing cyclic guanosine monophosphate (cGMP), which in turn activates cGMP-dependent protein kinase. NO• likely helps to control the muscu-

TABLE 10-1

Functions of Endothelial Cells of the Blood Vessels

Permeability barrier
Vasoactive factors: Nitric oxide (EDRF), endothelin
Antithrombotic agent production: Prostacyclin (PGI_2), adenine metabolites
Prothrombotic agent production: Factor VIIIa (von Willebrand factor)
Anticoagulant production: Thrombomodulin, other proteins
Fibrinolytic agent production: Tissue plasminogen activator, urokinase-like factor
Procoagulant production: Tissue factor, plasminogen activator/inhibitor, factor V
Inflammatory mediator production: Interleukin-1, cell adhesion molecules
Receptors for factor IX, factor X, low-density lipoproteins, modified low-density lipoproteins, thrombin
Growth factor production: Blood cell colony-stimulating factors, insulin-like growth factors, fibroblast growth factor, platelet-derived growth factor
Growth inhibitor: Heparin
Replication

EDRF = endothelium-derived relaxing factor

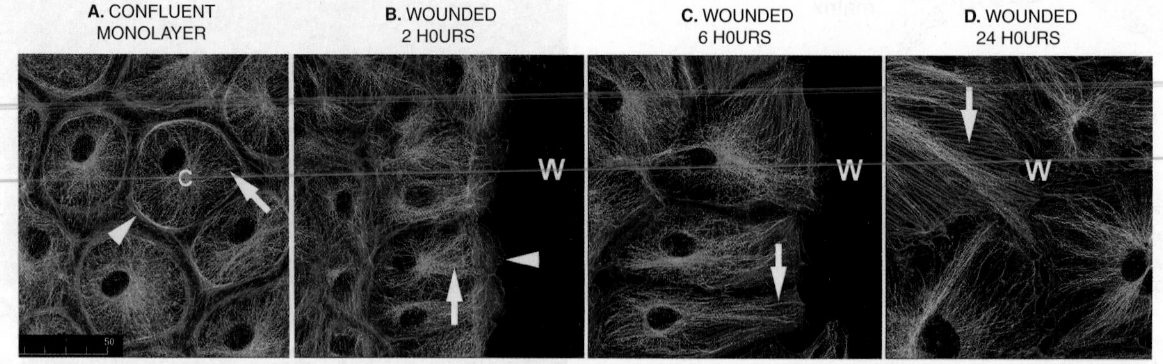

FIGURE 10-5. **Remodeling in response to loss of endothelial integrity.** Porcine aortic endothelial cells were grown to confluency, and a 1-mm wound was created using a scraper. Cells were fixed and double-stained for actin/tublin at 2, 6, and 24 hours after wounding. **A.** Endothelial cells in confluent monolayers contain a dense peripheral band (DPB) of actin microfilament bundles *(arrow head)* and centrosomes *(c)* toward the cell periphery. **B.** Two hours after wounding, there is formation of lamellipodia *(arrow head)*, and stress fibers *(arrow)* rearrange to become parallel to the wound edge *(w)*. Centrosomes migrate around the nucleus toward the wound edge, and the microtubules begin emanating toward the wound *(w)*. **C.** By 6 hours, changes in microtubules and microfilaments are more prominent, the microtubule/microfilaments are more prominent, and the microtubule–microfilament networks *(arrow)* begin to reorganize perpendicular to the wound edge *(w)* as the cells begin to spread. **D.** 24 hours after wounding, the microtubule–microfilament networks *(arrow)* are aligned perpendicular to the wound edge *(w)* as the cells migrate into the wound.

lar tone of large arteries and resistance vessels. After stimulation of endothelial receptors by agonists, prostacyclin and NO• are released and together inhibit platelet aggregation. Compounds that promote NO• release include acetylcholine, bradykinin, and adenosine diphosphate (ADP). NO• is even more labile than prostacyclin, with a half-life of 6 seconds.

Vascular tone is also affected by a number of bioactive peptides. The endothelins are a family of potent vasoconstrictive proteins synthesized by endothelial cells. Their functional effects are mediated by two distinct receptor subtypes; both are found on smooth muscle cells, but only one on endothelial cells. The endothelial enzyme angiotensin-converting enzyme (ACE) converts angiotensin I to angiotensin II, a potent vasoconstrictor which is is important in the pathogenesis of hypertension.

Endothelial cell-derived factors also control some immune responses. Like macrophages, endothelial cells express class II histocompatibility antigens when they are stimulated. They may thus participate with monocytes—or even replace them—in activating lymphocytes. Immune responses to endothelial cells are a major part of organ rejection following transplantation and play a role in the pathogenesis of graft arteriosclerosis.

Smooth Muscle Cells

Smooth muscle cells maintain blood vessel integrity and provide support for the endothelium. They control blood flow by contracting or dilating in response to specific stimuli. Smooth muscle cells synthesize the connective tissue matrix of the vessel wall, which includes elastin, collagen, and proteoglycans. In normal arteries, smooth muscle cells rarely divide, but, like endothelial cells, proliferate in response to injury, an important event in the pathogenesis of the atherosclerotic plaque.

Leukocytes that enter the vessel wall, especially macrophages and lymphocytes, also promote vascular disease. T cells play a role in atherosclerosis and in vasculitis, and polymorphonuclear leukocytes are important in acute vasculitis. Fibroblasts of the adventitia of blood vessels, and the pericytes of capillaries and venules (see Fig. 10-1), may also contribute to the pathogenesis of vascular diseases. Pericytes influence endothelial cell function and the fibroblasts of the adventitia proliferate and migrate in reaction to medial disruption, as in severe vasculitis and following angioplasty.

Arteries Include Conducting and Resistance Vessels

The simple two-cell structure of blood vessels is made more complex by the organization of the wall into layers called "tunicae" (see Fig. 10-1).

Elastic Arteries

The largest blood vessels in the body, the aorta and the elastic arteries, are conduits for blood flow to smaller arterial branches and are composed of three layers:

- **Tunica intima:** This layer consists of endothelium, a few smooth muscle cells, and connective tissue on the luminal side of the internal elastic lamina. The aortic intima is thick and contains a matrix of collagen, proteoglycans, and small amounts of elastin. Occasional resident lymphocytes, macrophages, and other blood-derived inflammatory cells are also present.
- **Tunica media:** The next layer outward, the tunica media, is bounded by internal and external elastic laminae, and displays layers of smooth muscle cells. In elastic arteries, elastic fibers are interposed between smooth muscle cells and minimize energy loss during the pressure changes between systole and diastole. A breakdown of the media, particularly of its elastic layers, leads to dilation of the artery, called an **aneurysm**. Much arterial disease (e.g., atherosclerosis) involves proliferation of medial smooth muscle cells. Alternatively, during normal aging and in hypertension, smooth muscle cells replicate their DNA without cell division. As a result, they become tetraploid, octaploid, or of even higher ploidy.

  Medial smooth muscle cells may also undergo atrophy or cell death if they do not receive adequate nutrients or cannot effectively exchange wastes with the blood. In smaller elastic arteries nutrition for the media is provided by diffusion from the blood vessel lumen. Nutrients traverse the endothelium and the layers of smooth muscle. However, blood vessels with more than 28 layers of smooth muscle cells have a vasculature of their own, the **vasa vasorum**. These small vessels penetrate the exterior of the artery and provide blood for the tunica media. The rich blood supply of atherosclerotic plaques is derived from vasa vasorum. The tunica media also contains autonomic nerve fibers that influence vascular contractility.
- **Tunica adventitia:** The most external vessel wall layer contains fibroblasts, connective tissue, and small vessels that give rise to the vasa vasorum and nerves. Occasional inflammatory cells may also be present in the adventitia.

Muscular Arteries

The blood conducted by the elastic arteries is distributed to individual organs through large muscular arteries (Fig. 10-6). The tunica media of a muscular artery consists of layers of smooth muscle cells without prominent bands of elastin, although a prominent internal elastic lamina and usually an external elastic lamina are seen. Fenestrae interrupt the continuity of the internal elastic lamina, permitting smooth muscle cells to migrate from the media into the intima. The absence of the heavy elastin layers allows muscular arteries to contract more efficiently. The intima of muscular arteries, like that of the aorta, also contains smooth muscle cells, connective tissue, and occasional inflammatory cells. Vasa vasorum penetrate the walls of the thicker muscular arteries but are not seen in the smaller ones. As the vascular tree branches further, the tunica media becomes thinner, and except for the endothelium, the tunica intima disappears.

The small muscular arteries are important regulators of blood flow. Their narrow lumens increase resistance, thereby reducing blood pressure to levels appropriate for exchange of water and plasma constituents across the thin-walled capillaries. The small muscular arteries, sometimes called **resistance vessels**, also maintain systemic pressure by regulating total peripheral resistance.

Arterioles

Arterioles are the smallest elements of the arterial system. They have an endothelial lining surrounded by one or two layers of smooth muscle cells. No elastic layers are evident. The smallest arterioles provide dynamic regulation of blood flow by controlling the distribution of blood in the capillary tree.

Capillaries Permit Transport from the Blood to the Interstitium

In these smallest blood vessels, the endothelium is supported only by sparse smooth muscle cells. The capillary endothelium provides for exchange of solutes and cells between the blood and the extracellular fluid. A necessary feature of this exchange is a

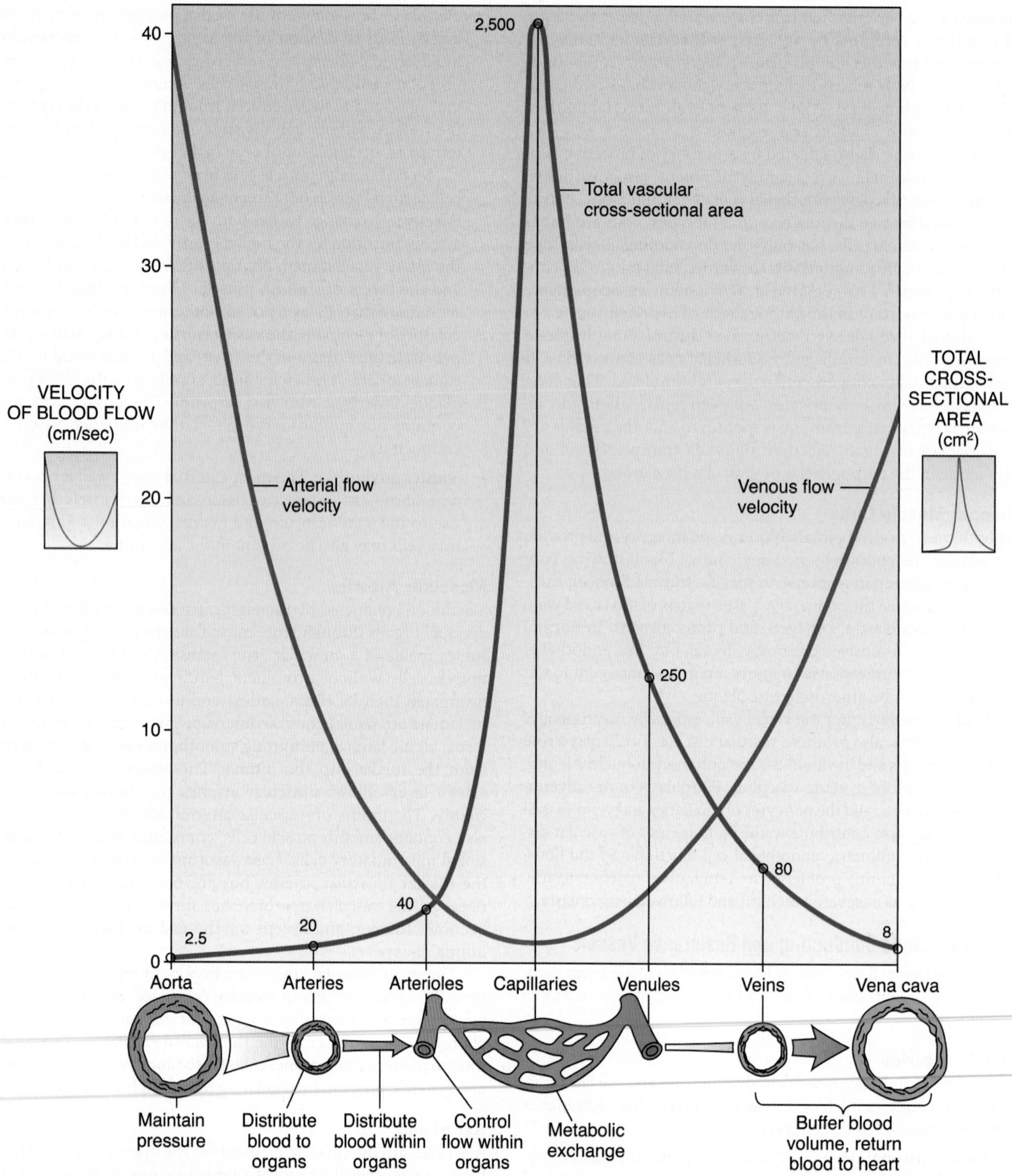

FIGURE 10-6. **Relationship between velocity of blood flow and cross-sectional area in the vasculature.** The vascular tree is a circuit that conducts blood from the heart through large-diameter, low-resistance conducting vessels to small arteries and arterioles, which lower blood pressure and protect the capillaries. The capillaries are thin-walled and allow the exchange of nutrients and waste products between tissue and blood, a process that requires a very large surface area. The circuit back to the heart is completed by the veins, which are distensible and provide a volume buffer that acts as a capacitance for the vascular circuit.

marked lowering of pressure, which prevents the vascular fluid from shifting into the extracellular space.

The capillary endothelium is a semipermeable membrane, in which exchange of plasma solutes with extracellular fluid is controlled by molecular size and charge. It also synthesizes cytokines that influence the surrounding tissues, modifies molecules in transit across the endothelium, and synthesizes inflammatory mediators.

Pericytes are modified smooth muscle cells that surround the capillaries. They are in close contact with endothelial cells, as both share the same basement membrane (see Fig. 10-1). The functions of pericytes are largely unknown. They may have a contractile function and may regulate the function of adjacent endothelial cells, especially their rate of proliferation. The capillary adventitia merges with, and is indistinguishable from, the surrounding connective tissue.

The permeability of capillaries depends on their endothelial cells. Brain capillaries are highly impermeable because junctions between endothelial cells are tightly sealed junctions, preventing exchange of proteins across the vessel wall. Transport in other capillary beds is mediated either by the passage of molecules through incomplete cell junctions or by pinocytosis, a process by which molecules traverse the cytoplasm through vesicular transport. Some investigators have suggested that vesicles are connected with each other to provide a channel for direct transport of plasma proteins across the cytoplasm. In some locations, the capillary endothelium itself may have permanent channels through endothelial cells or discontinuous gaps between them. Fenestrated capillaries in the renal glomerulus are specifically adapted to filter plasma. The liver sinusoids, which are not true capillaries, also show a fenestrated endothelium, which permits free access of plasma to liver cells.

Veins Return Blood to the Heart

The venules are the first vessels to collect blood from capillaries. Their thin media is appropriate for a vessel that does not face high intraluminal pressures. Venules merge into small and medium-sized veins, which in turn converge into large veins. The walls of large veins do not display the characteristic elastic lamellae of elastic arteries, and even the internal elastic lamina is well developed only in the largest veins. The media is thin and is virtually absent in the smaller tributaries. Many veins, particularly those in the extremities, have valves formed by endothelial-lined folds of the tunica intima. These structures prevent backflow and assist in moving blood under the low pressure of the venous circulation. The postcapillary venules are the site of leukocyte transmigration into tissue in inflammatory reactions (see Chapter 2).

Lymphatics Drain Interstitial Fluid

Lymphatic circulation is composed of blind-ended lymphatic capillaries, consisting of (1) endothelium with no pericytes; (2) precollecting lymphatics; and (3) collecting lymphatics, which pump lymph towards the lymph nodes, lymphatic trunks, and finally to thoracic and right lymphatic ducts, which return lymph back to the blood. Filtrate from capillaries and venules enters the lymphatics, which act as a pathway to regional lymph nodes for cells, foreign material, and microorganisms. The collecting lymphatics have an intrinsically contractile layer of smooth muscle cells that propel lymph forward. Intraluminal valves, as in veins, prevent back flow. Embryonic development and postnatal growth of lymphatics are regulated by vascular endothelial growth factors (VEGFs), platelet-derived growth factors (PDGFs), and angiopoietin 1 and 2.

Hemostasis and Thrombosis

***Hemostasis** is the arrest of hemorrhage, and is a response to vascular injury.* This process involves vasoconstriction, tissue swelling, coagulation, platelet aggregation, and thrombosis.

The hemostatic system is an exquisitely controlled mechanism that prevents blood loss following injury. The complex system comprises (1) a network of activating and inactivating enzymes, and (2) cofactors derived from different cells and tissues, some circulating and some locally produced (Table 10-2). Disorders of hemostasis are discussed in detail in Chapter 20.

TABLE 10-2

Coagulation Factor Designations

Factor	Standard Name
I	Fibrinogen
II	Prothrombin
III	Tissue factor
IV	Calcium ions
V	Proaccelerin
VII	Proconvertin
VIII	Antihemophilic factor (AHF)
IX	Plasma thromboplastin (PTC)
X	Stuart factor
XI	Plasma thromboplastin antecedent (PTA)
XII	Hageman factor
XIII	Fibrin stabilizing factor (FSF)
–	Prekallikrein
–	High-molecular-weight kininogen

The hemostatic complex can be divided into several functional areas that combine coagulation of blood proteins and aggregation of platelets to form a hemostatic "plug." ***Thrombosis** is formation of a blood clot in the circulation.* A thrombus is an aggregate of coagulated blood that contains platelets, fibrin, leukocytes, and red blood cells. Its formation involves a "tug of war" between those factors that favor clotting and those that inhibit it. *Thrombosis occurs when antithrombotic systems fail to balance prothrombotic processes.*

One must understand the difference between **coagulation** and **thrombosis**. Coagulation can occur in vitro by activation of the clotting cascade. By contrast, thrombosis also involves (1) adherence and aggregation of platelets, (2) participation of cellular elements of the monocyte/macrophage system, and (3) active participation of endothelial cells.

Blood Coagulation Occurs When Fibrinogen Is Converted to Fibrin

Coagulation of blood entails conversion of soluble plasma fibrinogen to an insoluble fibrillar polymer–fibrin; a reaction catalyzed by the proteolytic enzyme thrombin. This event cannot represent a sudden process, since the entire circulation might be converted into a massive clot. Instead, a series of finely tuned steps is mediated by a number of coagulation factors (see Table 10-2), many of which are restricted by specific inhibitors This coagulation cascade amplifies an initial signal into the eventual generation of thrombin, the production of which is probably the most important factor in progression and stabilization of a thrombus.

Historically, the coagulation cascade was divided into "intrinsic" and "extrinsic" pathways. The former could be initiated without an extrinsic trigger, and required only contact of factor XII with a thrombogenic surface. By contrast, the extrinsic pathway required exposure of blood to an extravascular tissue factor. However, dividing coagulation into two distinct arms does not accurately reflect the underlying mechanisms of clotting.

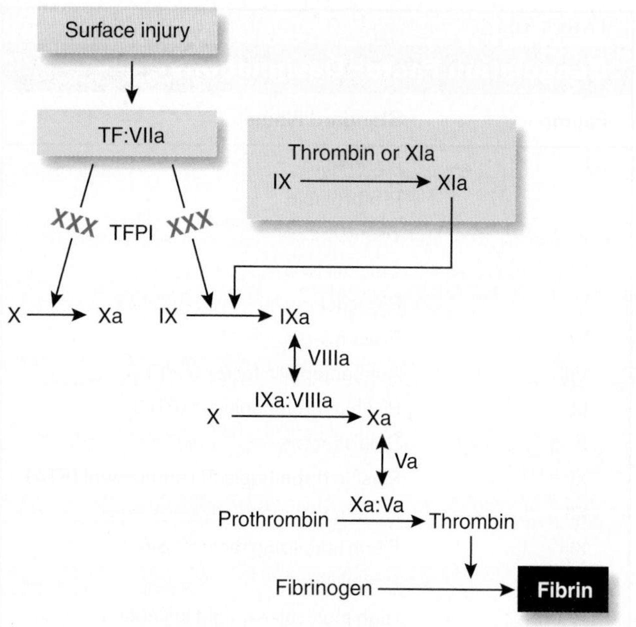

FIGURE 10-7. **Coagulation cascade.** The coagulation cascade is initiated by endothelial injury, which releases tissue factor (TF). The latter combines with activated factor VII (VIIa) to form a complex that activates small amounts of X to Xa and IX to IXa. The complex of IXa with VIIIa further activates X. The complex of Xa with Va then catalyzes the conversion of prothrombin to thrombin, after which fibrin is formed from fibrinogen. TFPI = tissue factor pathway inhibitor.

The current view of coagulation (Fig. 10-7) highlights the importance of **tissue factor** (TF), a membrane-bound glycoprotein. The dynamic association of factor VIIa–TF complexes with TF pathway inhibitor (TFPI) is crucial to thrombosis. TFPI inhibits initiation of coagulation by binding the TF–FXa–FVIIa complex. A major pool of TFPI on the surface of endothelial cells thus probably regulates coagulation. Initiation of hemostasis takes place when activated factor VII (VIIa) encounters TF at a site of injury. Small amounts of factors X and IX are activated to Xa and IXa. Activation of larger amounts of X to Xa is promoted by factors VIIIa and IXa. Traces of thrombin catalyze activation of factor XI, which in turn augments conversion of factor IX to IXa. The IXa and VIIIa complex converts more factor X to Xa, which then binds Va to form the **prothrombinase complex**. This complex then converts prothrombin to thrombin, which is a serine protease.

Besides its important role in coagulation and platelet aggregation, thrombin participates in production of fibrinolytic molecules and regulation of growth factors and leukocyte adhesion molecules. It also mediates the protein C anticoagulant pathway by binding thrombomodulin at the surface of endothelial cells. Factor V, an essential coagulation factor, also exhibits anticoagulant activity by exerting a cofactor function in the activated protein C system, which then down-regulates factor VIIIa activity. Thrombin also increases endothelial permeability by promoting alterations in endothelial cell shape and disruption of endothelial cell–cell adhesion junctions.

Platelet Adhesion and Aggregation Occur after Injury to a Blood Vessel

Under normal circumstances circulating platelets are in a nonadherent state. However, injury up-regulates platelet adhesiveness, after which platelets interact with one another to form a platelet thrombus, that is, an aggregate of activated platelets (Fig. 10-8).

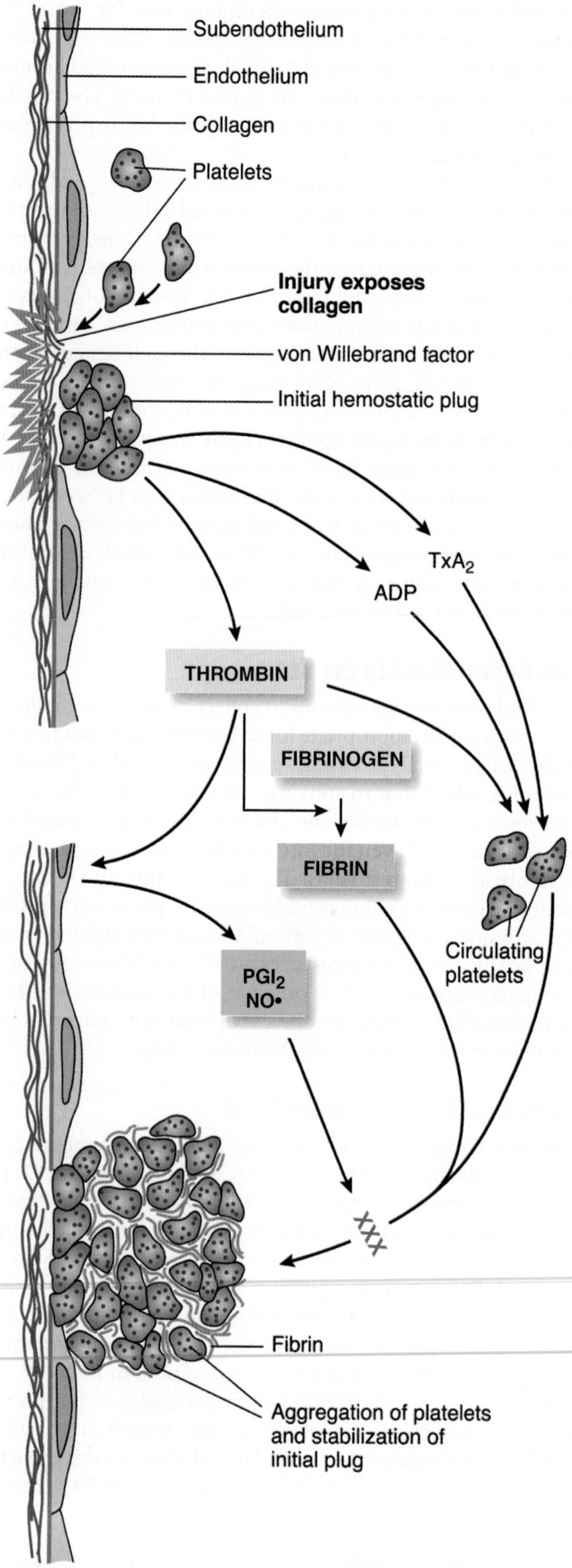

FIGURE 10-8. **The role of platelets in thrombosis.** Following vessel wall injury and alteration in flow, platelets adhere and then aggregate. Adenosine diphosphate (ADP) and thromboxane A_2 (TxA_2) are released and, along with locally generated thrombin, recruit additional platelets, causing the mass to enlarge. The growing platelet thrombus is stabilized by fibrin. Other elements, including leukocytes and red blood cells, are also incorporated into the thrombus. The release of prostacyclin (PGI_2) and nitric oxide (NO•) by endothelial cells regulates the process by inhibiting platelet aggregation.

Changes in platelet shape that reflect reorganization of actin microfilaments are essential to enable platelets to aggregate. Several molecules may promote platelet aggregation including thrombin, collagen, ADP, epinephrine, thromboxame A_2, platelet-activating factor (PAF), and vasopression. Platelet aggregates occlude injured small vessels and prevent leakage of blood.

Once platelets are stimulated to adhere to the vessel wall, their granular contents are released, in part by contraction of the platelet cytoskeleton. In turn, these granules promote aggregation of other platelets. Platelet adhesion is enhanced by release of subendothelial von Willebrand factor, which is adhesive for Gp1b platelet membrane protein and for fibrinogen. Activated platelets also release ADP and thromboxane A_2, a product of arachidonic acid metabolism, which recruit additional platelets to the process. The platelet membrane protein complex GpIIb–IIIa binds to fibrinogen, thereby forming fibrinogen bridges between platelets, enhancing aggregation, and stabilizing the nascent thrombus. Activated platelets, in turn, release factors that initiate coagulation, thus forming a complex thrombus on the vessel wall. Thrombin itself stimulates further release of platelet granules and subsequent recruitment of new platelets.

Endothelial Factors Regulate Both Anticoagulant and Procoagulant Processes

The endothelium plays an active role in the control of thrombosis (Table 10-3). A major antithrombotic mechanism of the endothelium is the secretion of **PGI_2**, which inhibits platelet aggregation. Endothelial NO is also a potent inhibitor of platelet aggregation and adhesion to the vessel wall. Endothelial cells metabolize ADP, a strong promoter of thrombogenesis, to metabolites that are antithrombogenic. The luminal surface of the endothelium is coated with heparan sulfate, a molecule that binds a number of clotting factors, including the antiprotease β_2-macroglobulin. Endothelial cells may also lyse some clots as they form through the **plasminogen/plasminogen activator/plasmin system**.

Endothelial cells have several other anticoagulant activities. A cofactor on the endothelial cell surface inactivates thrombin by forming a complex with thrombin and antithrombin 3 (a plasma antiprotease). Thrombin itself activates protein C by interacting with its receptor, **thrombomodulin**, which is located at endothelial cell surfaces. Both protein C and thrombomodulin are synthesized by endothelial cells. Activated protein C destroys coagulation factors V and VIII. TFPI generated during coagulation is bound to endothelium, where it inhibits the TF–VIIa complex (see Fig. 10-7). TF and TFPI are synthesized and secreted by endothelial cells as well as other vascular cells.

The endothelium is also intimately involved in initiation and propagation of thrombosis. The major event that triggers most thrombosis is endothelial injury, which imparts a prothrombotic property to endothelium (see Fig. 10-8).

Endothelial cells synthesize von Willebrand factor, which promotes platelet adherence and activates clotting factor V. Endothelial cells also bind factors IX and X, a process that favors coagulation on the endothelial surface. Finally, inflammatory agents, including cytokines released from monocytes, activate procoagulant activities on the surface of intact endothelium. Endothelial cells treated with interleukin-1 or tumor necrosis factor present thromboplastin to the plasma, thereby potentially initiating coagulation through the extrinsic pathway. Thus thrombi may form when endothelial function is altered, when endothelial continuity is lost, or when flow in a blood vessel becomes abnormal, such as when. turbulent or static. Simple loss of endothelial cells or injury to a vessel with good flow produces platelet pavementing but not thrombosis (Fig. 10-9).

TABLE 10-3

Regulation of Coagulation at the Endothelial Cell Surface

Down-Regulation
1. Thrombin inactivators
a. Antithrombin III
b. Thrombomodulin
2. Activated protein C pathway
a. Synthesis and expression of thrombomodulin
b. Synthesis and expression of protein S
c. Thrombomodulin-mediated activation of protein C
d. Inactivation of factor V_a and factor VIII_a by APC-protein S complex
3. Tissue factor pathway inhibition
4. Fibrinolysis
a. Synthesis of tissue plasminogen activator, urokinase plasminogen activator, and plasminogen activator inhibitor 1
b. Conversion of Glu-plasminogen to Lys-plasminogen
c. APC-mediated potentiation
5. Synthesis of unsaturated fatty acid metabolites
a. Lipoxygenase metabolites-13-HODE
b. Cyclooxygenase metabolites-PGI_2 and PGE_2
Procoagulant Pathways
1. Synthesis and expression of:
a. Tissue factor (thromboplastin)
b. Factor V
c. Platelet activating factor (PAF)
2. Binding of clotting factors IX/IX_a, X (prothrombinase complex)
3. Down-regulation of APC pathway
4. Increased synthesis of plasminogen activator inhibitor
5. Synthesis of 15-HPETE

APC = adenomatous polyposis coli; 13-HODE = 13-hydroxy-octadeca-dienoic acid HPETE = hydroperoxy eicosatetraenoic acid; PGE_2 = prostaglandin E_2, PGI_2 = prostacyclin

Endothelial Cells Repair Defects by Spreading and Migrating into Areas of Denudation

The most common denuding injury is progressive endothelial disruption by atherosclerotic plaque. Denuding endothelial injury has also been described in homocystinuria, hypoxia, and endotoxemia, as well as during construction of saphenous vein bypass grafts, angioplasty, insertion of intravascular stents, and atherectomy. Interactions of a thrombus with underlying adjacent endothelial cells may further disturb endothelial integrity. Both fibrin and thrombin affect the endothelial cytoskeleton and initiate endothelial shape changes with gaps forming between cells, and so promote disruption of endothelial integrity.

Disrupted endothelium can reestablish a thromboresistant barrier by rapidly spreading and migrating into an area of denudation (see Figure 10-5). This is followed by endothelial cell proliferation to restore normal cell density. However, these mechanisms may become dysfunctional at sites of persistent endothelial cell damage.

Another hypothesized mechanism of repair is migration of endothelial precursor cells (EPCs) derived from the bone marrow

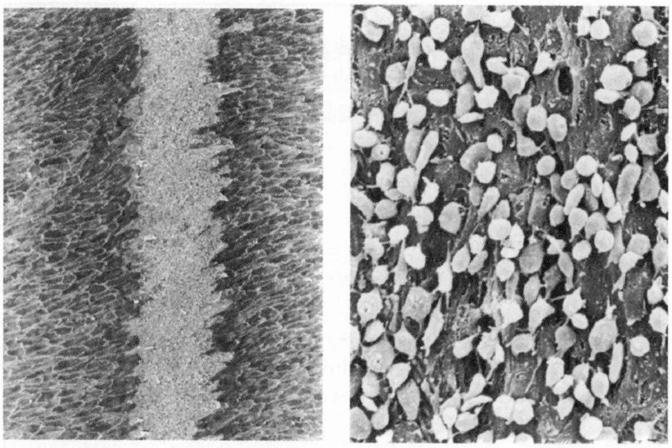

FIGURE 10-9. **Scanning electron micrograph of the endothelial surface of a rat aorta 1 hour after the endothelial cells were removed by scraping with a nylon filament. A.** Intact endothelium and scratched portion. **B.** Higher-power view of the scratched area shows a pavement of intact platelets that adheres to the underlying connective tissue in the high-velocity arterial stream.

(see Chapter 3). EPCs are thought to proliferate after vascular injury and physiologic stress. They then are released into the peripheral circulation, where they target injured vessel walls, attach to the denuded surface, and differentiate to reestablish endothelial integrity.

Clot Lysis Is a Regulatory Mechanism

A thrombus may undergo several fates, including (1) lysis, (2) growth and propagation, (3) embolization, or (4) organization and canalization. The combination of aggregated platelets and clotted blood is made unstable by activation of the fibrinolytic enzyme plasmin (Fig. 10-10). During clot formation, plasminogen is bound to fibrin and therefore is an integral part of the forming platelet mass. Endothelial cells synthesize plasminogen activator, but in larger thrombi, circulating plasminogen may also be converted to plasmin by products of the coagulation cascade. Plasminogen activator bound to fibrin activates plasmin. In turn, by digesting fibrin, plasmin lyses clots and disrupts the thrombus. The clearance of fibrin also prevents its accumulation in atherosclerotic plaque, where it tends to promote plaque growth and attract inflammatory cells. Endothelial cells also synthesize plasminogen activator inhibitor-1 (PAI-1) and plasmin is inhibited by α_2 antiplasmin. Thus, the regional fibrinolytic balance depends on the balance between plasminogen activation and inhibition.

Thrombi may undergo organization and become incorporated into the vessel wall. This occurs when arterial smooth muscle cells or venous fibroblasts migrate into the thrombus meshwork of cross-linked fibrin and produce matrix. The matrix proteolytic enzymes remodel the thrombus, digest the fibrin, and form a fibrous structure with its own new blood vessels. This revascularization process is called **recanalization**. Macrophages also likely participate in this remodeling.

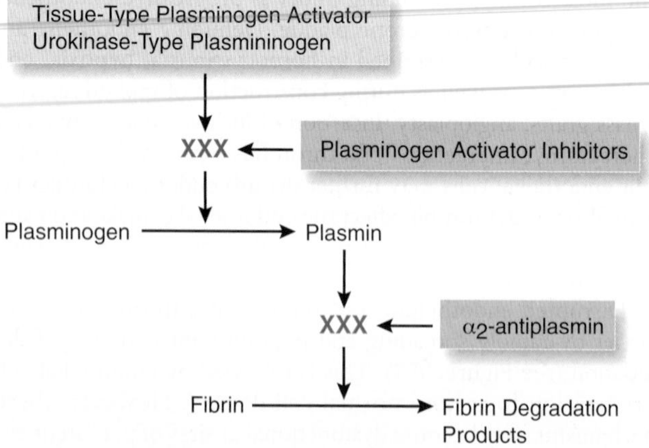

FIGURE 10-10. **Mechanisms of fibrinolysis.** Plasmin formed from plasminogen lyses fibrin. The conversion of plasminogen to plasmin and the activity of plasmin itself are suppressed by specific inhibitors.

TABLE 10-4

Atherogenesis

- Initiation and growth of fibro-inflammatory lipid atheroma is a slowly evolving dynamic process with superimposed acute events
- Risk factors accelerate progression
- The pathogenesis is multifactorial and thus the relative importance of specific genetic and environmental factors may vary in individuals.
- Interactions between cellular and matrix components of the vessel wall, and serum constituents, leukocytes, platelets, and physical forces regulate the formation of the fibro-inflammatory lipid atheroma.

Atherosclerosis

In atherosclerosis, inflammatory cells, smooth muscle cells, lipid, and connective tissue progressively accumulate in the intima of large and medium-sized elastic and muscular arteries. The classical atherosclerotic lesion is best described as a fibroinflammatory lipid plaque (**atheroma**). These plaques develop over several decades (Table 10-4, Table 10-5). Their continued growth encroaches on the media of the arterial wall and into the lumen of the vessel, resulting in narrowing (stenosis) of the lumen. Atherosclerotic lesions are also called atherosclerotic plaques, atheromas, fibrous plaques, or fibrofatty lesions.

TABLE 10-5

Important Components of Fibroinflammatory Lipid Atheroma

Cells	- Endothelial cells	Lipids and lipoproteins
	- Foam cells	Serum proteins
	- Giant Cells	Platelet and leukocyte products
	- Lymphocytes	Necrotic debris
	- Mast cells	New microvessels
	- Macrophages	Hydroxyapatite crystals
Matrix	- Collagen	Growth factors
	- Elastin	Oxidants/Antioxidants
	- Glycoproteins	Proteolytic enzymes
	- Proteoglycans	Procoagulant factors

EPIDEMIOLOGY: The major complications of atherosclerosis, including ischemic heart disease, myocardial infarction, stroke, and gangrene of the extremities, account for more than half of the annual mortality in the United States. Ischemic heart disease itself is the leading cause of death. The incidence of ischemic heart disease in Western countries rose progressively to a peak in the late 1960s. Subsequently it has declined by more than 30%. There are wide geographic and racial variations in the incidence of ischemic heart disease.of the lesions or their progression to clinically significant disease

PATHOGENESIS: Several hypotheses have been proposed to explain the origins of atherosclerotic plaques. These hypotheses are not mutually exclusive and numerous experimental and clinical observations have shown how processes highlighted in one theory may be linked to those in another. Viewed in this light, most of the controversies lie in opinions about which process is most important in initiation .

INSUDATION HYPOTHESIS: Conventional wisdom holds that the critical events in atherosclerosis center on focal accumulation of fat in a vessel wall. The insudation hypothesis states that the lipid in these lesions derives from plasma lipoproteins, a view consistent with the role of blood lipids as risk factors for myocardial infarction. Although there is still controversy over how the lipid enters the vessel wall, this hypothesis is now widely accepted. Whereas it explains the source of plaque lipid, it does not completely explain the pathogenesis of atherosclerotic lesions, since it does not explain other clinically important features of the plaque, such as smooth muscle proliferation and thrombosis. Thus lipid deposition appears to be necessary but not sufficient to explain atherosclerosis.

Low-density lipoprotein (LDL) is the form of lipid in the plasma most closely associated with accelerated atherosclerosis. LDL particles are far too large (20 nm in diameter) to penetrate the tightly closed endothelial cell junctions. However, endothelial cells have receptors for both LDL and modified forms of LDL. Transport across an intact endothelium can occur either by receptor-mediated uptake of lipoprotein or by nonspecific uptake into micropinocytic channels. Alternatively, lipid may be engulfed by macrophages in blood and then transported into the vascular wall as these cells transmigrate between dysfunctional endothelial cells.

ENCRUSTATION HYPOTHESIS: A theory first suggested in the 19th century asserted that material from the blood is deposited on the inner surface of arteries and leads to thickening of the inner lining. At the time this suggestion was made, the details of clotting and platelet function in thrombosis were unknown. A modern version of this idea holds that small mural thrombi are the initial events in atherosclerosis. Organization of these thrombi leads to plaque formation, and expansion of these lesions reflects repeated episodes of thrombosis and organization.

We now know from experimental studies of hyperlipidemic animals and autopsy studies of children that mural thrombi do not initiate atherogenesis. However, mural thrombosis is a critical part of later progression of atherosclerotic lesions and is a major event leading to vascular occlusion, especially in coronary arteries.

REACTION TO INJURY HYPOTHESIS: This theory attempts to explain how smooth muscle cells accumulate in atherosclerotic lesions. This hypothesis suggests that smooth muscle proliferation depends on release of polypeptide growth factors by endothelial cells, macrophages, and smooth muscle cells themselves that accumulate at sites of injury. This theory has been broadened to focus on the roles of all cell types present in artery walls in initiation and growth of atherosclerotic lesions: dysfunctional endothelial cells, inflammatory cells, macrophages, and lymphocytes. It has recently been modified to suggest that cellular responses that occur during atherosclerogenesis constitute an inflammatory and fibroproliferative response to injury. In this theory, endothelial dysfunction compromises the integrity of the endothelial barrier to macromolecules and activates leukocyte adhesion molecules to promote infiltration of macrophages in the subendothelium.

The "reaction to injury" hypothesis evolved from the discovery that growth of smooth muscle cells in culture requires one or more platelet-derived polypeptides. The best known of these is PDGF, which is secreted by macrophages and vascular wall cells. PDGF is not only mitogenic for smooth muscle cells in vitro, but is also chemotactic for them. Thus, in addition to stimulating proliferation of cells already in the intima, it may recruit smooth muscle cells from the media. The number of growth factors that can potentially induce proliferation of cells in culture has multiplied and now includes fibroblast growth factor (FGF), transforming growth factor-β (TGF-β), thrombin, LDL, endothelin, and others. There are also growth inhibitors, such as heparin and NO.

MONOCLONAL HYPOTHESIS: The monoclonal concept is focused on smooth muscle proliferation and comes from the observation that the smooth muscle cells that form the fibrous caps of atherosclerotic plaques (see below) appear to migrate from the underlying media, then proliferate. Can the lesion arise as an aberration of growth control in one cell, or at most a few cells, similarly to the process in a benign smooth muscle tumor such as a leiomyoma? On the other hand, might it not arise from polyclonal proliferation of many cells, as in a healing wound?

Based on studies of women who are mosaic for X-linked markers, it has been established that many plaques are monoclonal; that is, they originate from one or very few smooth muscle cells. The monoclonality of the fibrous cap suggests that some unknown etiologic factor might induce cap formation by altering growth control in the smooth muscle cells of the arterial wall. Although research has been done on the possible pathogenetic role of viruses in atherosclerosis, particularly herpesvirus and cytomegalovirus, a cause-and-effect relationship has not been established.

A Unifying Hypothesis

The sequence of events in atherogenesis (Figs. 10-11 to 10-14) may begin as early as fetal life, with the formation of intimal cell masses, or perhaps shortly after birth, when fatty streaks begin to evolve. However, the characteristic lesion, which is not initially clinically significant, requires as long as 20 to 30 years to form. Once formed, serious acute complications may occur or complicated lesions may emerge after several more years of development.

To tie the foregoing concepts together, we can construct a hypothetical sequence divided into three stages: (1) initiation and formation, (2) adaptation, and (3) clinical. Biologically active molecules regulate a number of dynamic cellular functions. At present, identification of a single "master" atherogenic gene is unlikely. Rather, one should consider that the products of multiple genes interact with the environment and with each other. The imbalance between proatherogenic and antiatherogenic factors and processes most likely leads to initiation and growth of atherosclerotic plaques.

Initiation and Formation Stage

1. Intimal lesions initially occur at sites that appear to be predisposed to lesion formation. In humans, atherosclerotic lesions tend to arise at sites where shear stresses are low but fluctuate rapidly, such as at branch points and bifurcations. Endothelial dysfunction or accumulation of subendothelial smooth muscle cells occurs in an intimal cell mass at branch and at other points in certain vessels. This cell mass is considered a predisposing condition for plaque formation. The coronary arteries are particularly affected in this regard. The distribution of atherosclerotic lesions in large vessels, and differences in location and frequency of lesions in different vascular beds, encourage a belief in the role of hemodynamic factors. The fact that hypertension enhances the severity of atherosclerotic lesions, e.g., in the pulmonary artery in pulmonary hypertension, further supports a role for hemodynamic factors in the development of atherosclerosis.

   It has been demonstrated that hemodynamic forces induce gene expression of several factors in endothelial cells that are likely to promote atherosclerosis, including FGF-2, TF, plasminogen activator, and endothelin. However, shear stress also induces gene expression of agents that may be antiatherogenic, including NOS and PAI-1. In persons at increased risk of atherosclerosis, lesions also occur in areas that are not predisposed to the disease.

2. Lipid accumulation depends on disruption of the integrity of the endothelial barrier through cell loss and/or cell dysfunction. LDLs carry lipids into the intima. Macrophages adhere to activated endothelial cells and transmigrate into the intima bringing lipids with them. Some of these "foamy" macrophages undergo necrosis and release lipids. The types of connective tissue (e.g., proteoglycans) synthesized by the smooth muscle cells in the intima also render these sites prone to lipid accumulation by trapping lipids in the intima. Oxidative stress in endothelial cells and macrophages leads to cellular dysfunction and damage.

3. As proposed in the "reaction to injury" hypothesis, mononuclear macrophages, in addition to playing a central atherogenic role by participating in lipid accumulation, release growth factors, thereby stimulating further accumulation of smooth muscle cells. **Oxidized lipoproteins** induce tissue damage and further macrophage accumulation. Monocyte/macrophages synthesize PDGF, FGF, TNF, interleukin (IL)-1, interferon-α (IFN-α), and TGF-β, each of which can stimulate or inhibit growth of smooth muscle or endothelial cells. For example, IFN-γ and TGF-γ limit cell proliferation and could account for the failure of endothelial cells to maintain continuity over the lesion. Alternatively, they could inhibit growth-stimulatory peptides. Of particular interest is the discovery that IL-1 and TNF stimulate endothelial cells to produce PAF, TF, and PAI. Thus, the combination of macrophages and endothelial cells may transform the normal anticoagulant vascular surface to a procoagulant one.

4. As a lesion progresses, mural thrombi may form on the damaged intimal surface. This stimulates PDGF release, which accelerates smooth muscle proliferation and secretion of matrix components. The thrombus may grow, lyse, or become organized, and incorporate into the plaque.

5. The deeper parts of the thickened intima are poorly nourished and undergo necrosis, which is augmented by proteolytic enzymes released by macrophages and tissue damage caused by oxidized LDL, reactive oxygen species, and other agents. This initiates angiogenesis, with new vasa vasorum forming in the plaque.

6. The fibroinflammatory lipid plaque is formed, with a central necrotic core and a fibrous cap, which separates the core from the blood in the lumen. The plaque becomes heterogeneous with respect to inflammatory cell infiltration, lipid deposition, and matrix organization. TGF-β is an important regulator of extracellular matrix deposition. It induces formation of several types of collagen, fibronectin, and proteoglycans. TGF-β enhances expression of protease inhibitors and inhibits proteolytic enzymes that promote matrix degradation.

Adaptation Stage

7. As the plaque protrudes into the lumen (e.g., in coronary arteries), the wall of the artery remodels to maintain lumen size. When a plaque occupies half the lumen, compensatory remodeling can no longer compensate, and the arterial lumen becomes narrowed (stenosis). Hemodynamic shear stress, an important regulator of vessel wall remodeling, acts through the mechanotransduction properties of endothelial cells. It is likely that smooth muscle cell turnover, proliferation, apoptosis, and matrix synthesis and degradation modulate remodeling of the vessel and the plaque in the face of atherosclerosis. Matrix metalloproteinases (MMPs) and their inhibitors (TIMP) are important in this remodeling (see Chapter 3). Although remodeling maintains vessel patency, it may delay clinical diagnosis of atherosclerosis as a plaque may be "clinically silent." Even though a plaque may be small, even at this stage, it can rupture with catastrophic results, as noted below.

Clinical Stage

8. As a plaque encroaches on the lumen, hemorrhage into it may increase its size without rupture. Expression of human leukocyte antigen (HLA)-DR antigens on endothelial and smooth muscle cells in plaques implies that these cells may have undergone some type of immunologic activation, perhaps in response to IFN-γ released by activated T cells in the plaque. In this scenario, the presence of T cells reflects an autoimmune response, e.g., against oxidized LDL, that is important for progression of atherosclerotic lesions.
9. Complications develop in the plaque, including surface ulceration, fissure formation, calcification, and aneurysm formation. Activated mast cells at sites of erosion may release proinflammatory mediators and cytokines. Continued plaque growth leads to severe stenosis or occlusion of the lumen. Plaque rupture, involving the fibrous cap, and ensuing thrombosis and occlusion may precipitate catastrophic events in these advanced plaques (e.g., acute myocardial infarction). However, recent angiographic studies suggest that even plaques causing less than 50% stenosis may suddenly rupture.

Figure 10-11 shows how these hypothetical mechanisms may operate in the pathogenesis of atherosclerosis.

The Initial Lesion of Atherosclerosis

PATHOLOGY: Two distinct lesions have been seen as precursors of atherosclerotic plaques.

FATTY STREAK: Fatty streaks are flat or slightly elevated lesions in the intima that contain accumulations of intracellular and extracellular lipid. They are found in young children as well as in adults. Cells filled with lipid droplets ("foam cells") accumulate (see Figs. 10-11 and Fig. 10-12). Macrophages contain the greatest amounts of lipid, but smooth muscle cells also contain fat.

In children who die accidentally, significant numbers of fatty streaks may be evident in many parts of the arterial tree. However, they do not correspond to the distribution of atherosclerotic lesions in adults. For example, fatty spots are common in the thoracic aorta in children, but atherosclerosis in adults is more prominent in the abdominal aorta. Nonetheless, many believe that fatty infiltration is the precursor lesion of atherosclerosis and that other factors control the transition from fatty streak to clinically significant atherosclerotic plaque.

INTIMAL CELL MASS: The intimal cell mass is another candidate for the initial lesion of atherosclerosis. Intimal cell masses are white, thickened areas at branch points in the arterial tree. Microscopically, they contain smooth muscle cells and connective tissue but no lipid. The location of these lesions, also known as "cushions," at arterial branch sites correlates well with the locations of later atherosclerotic lesions.

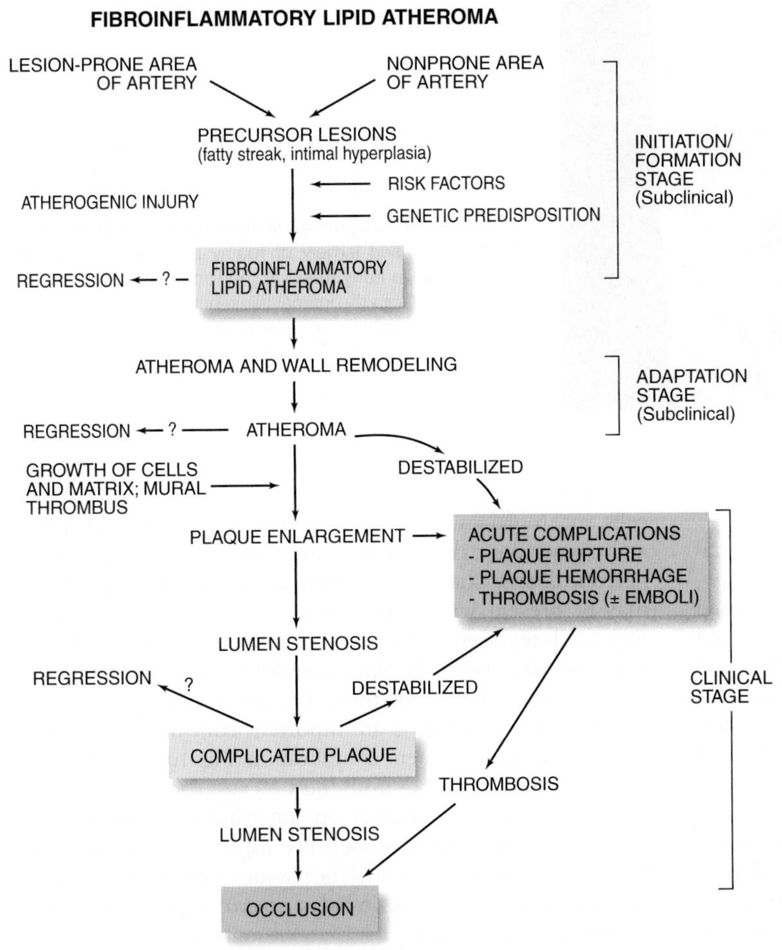

FIGURE 10-11. **A unifying hypothesis for the pathogenesis of atherosclerosis.**

A

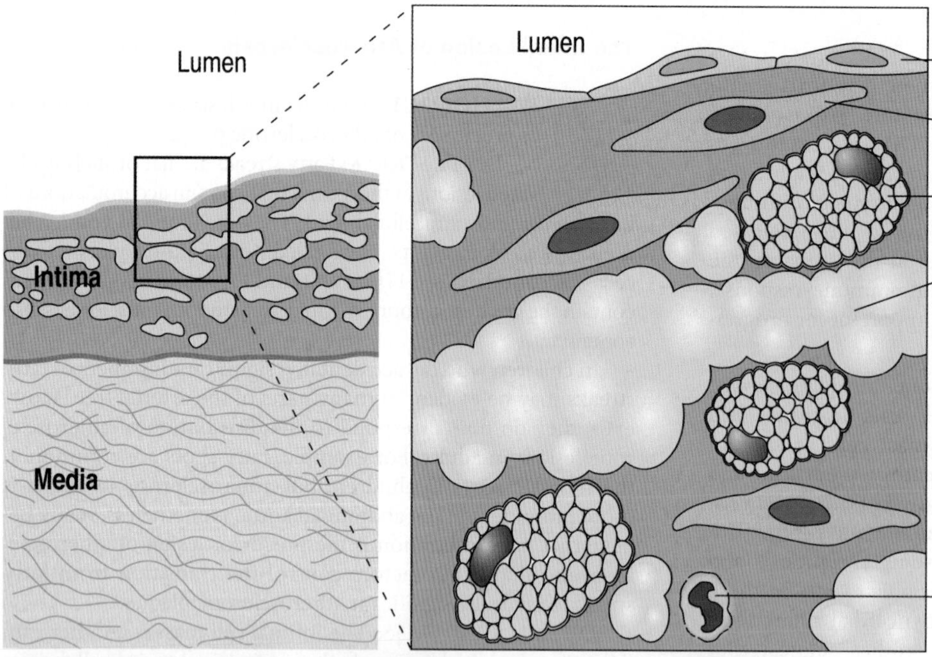

B

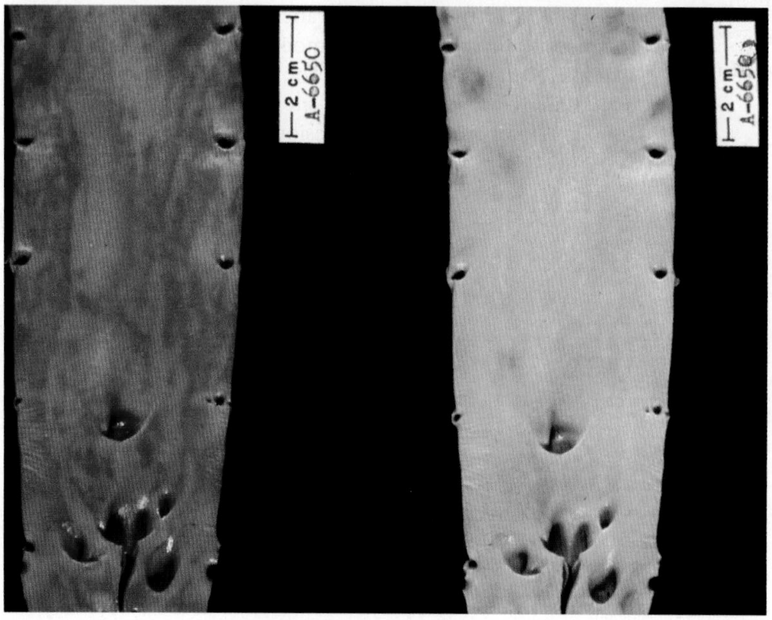

FIGURE 10-12. **Fatty streak of atherosclerosis. A.** The fatty streak, composed largely of foamy macrophages, is presumed to be an early stage in the formation of atherosclerotic lesions. Note the intimal thickening in the *left panel* and the infiltrating cells in the enlargement on the *right*. **B.** The aorta of a young man shows numerous fatty streaks on the luminal surface when stained with Sudan red. The unstained specimen is shown on the *right*.

The Characteristic Lesion of Atherosclerosis

The characteristic lesion of atherosclerosis is the fibroinflammatory lipid plaque. Simple plaques are focal, elevated, pale yellow, smooth-surfaced lesions, irregular in shape but with well-defined borders. Fibrofatty plaques (Fig. 10-13) represent more-advanced lesions and tend to be oval, with diameters of 8 to 12 cm. In smaller vessels, such as the coronary or cerebral arteries, a plaque is often eccentric; that is, it occupies only part of the circumference of the lumen. In later stages, fusion of plaques in muscular arteries can give rise to larger lesions, which occupy several square centimeters.

Microscopically, atherosclerotic plaques are initially covered by endothelium and tend to involve the intima and very little of the upper media (see Fig. 10-13). The area between the lumen and the necrotic core –the **fibrous cap**–contains smooth muscle cells, macrophages, lymphocytes, lipid-laden cells (foam cells), and connective tissue components. The central core contains necrotic debris. Cholesterol crystals and foreign body giant cells may be present within the fibrous tissue and necrotic areas. Foam cells represent both macrophages and smooth muscle cells that have taken up lipids. Numerous inflammatory and immune cells, especially T cells, are present within a plaque.

Neovascularization is an important contributor to plaque growth and its subsequent complication (Fig. 10-14). It is postulated that vessels grow in from the vasa vasorum. They are rare in healthy coronary arteries but plentiful in atherosclerotic plaques. Newly formed vessels are fragile and may rupture, resulting in acute expansion of the plaque from intraplaque hemorrhage. Foci of hemosiderin-laden macrophages are often present in plaques, indicating a remote intraplaque hemorrhage.

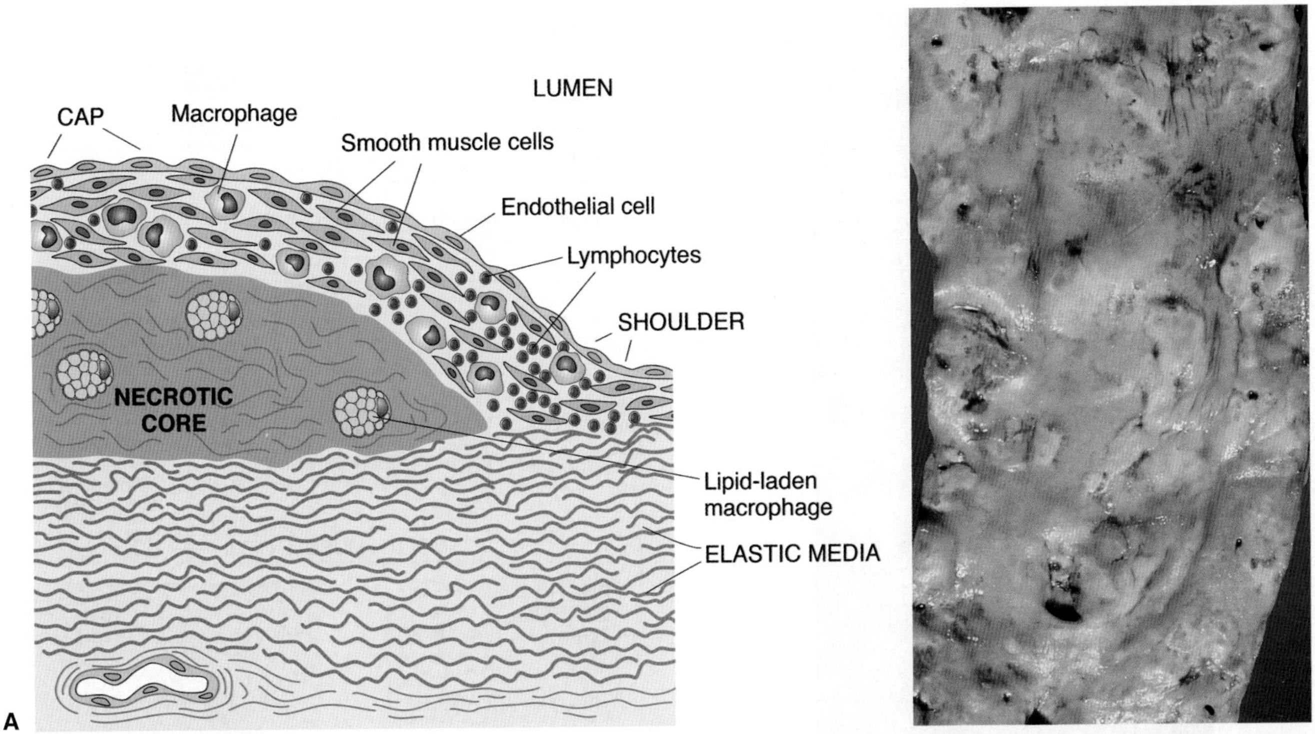

FIGURE 10-13. **Fibrofatty plaque of atherosclerosis. A.** In this fully developed fibrous plaque, the core contains lipid-filled macrophages and necrotic smooth muscle cell debris. The "fibrous" cap is composed largely of smooth muscle cells, which produce collagen, small amounts of elastin, and glycosaminoglycans. Also shown are infiltrating macrophages and lymphocytes. Note that the endothelium over the surface of the fibrous cap frequently appears intact. **B.** The aorta shows discrete, raised, tan plaques. Focal plaque ulcerations are also evident.

Complicated Atherosclerotic Plaques

The term **complicated** plaque describes several conditions: erosion, ulceration or fissuring of the plaque surface; plaque hemorrhage; mural thrombosis; calcification; and aneurysm (see Fig. 10-14 and Fig. 10-15). Progression from a simple fibrofatty atherosclerotic plaque to a complicated lesion may occur while some persons are still in their 20s, but most affected people are 50 or 60 years of age. Cellular interactions involved in progression of atherosclerotic lesions are summarized in Fig. 10-16.

- **Calcification** occurs in areas of necrosis and elsewhere in the plaque. Calcification in the artery is thought to depend on mineral deposition and resorption, which are regulated by osteoblast-like and osteoclast-like cells in the vessel wall.
- **Mural thrombosis** results from turbulent blood flow around the plaque, where it protrudes into the lumen. The disturbance in flow also causes damage to the endothelial lining, which may become dysfunctional or locally denuded and no longer present a thromboresistant surface. Thrombi often form at sites of erosion and fissuring on the surface of the fibrous cap. Mural thrombi in the proximal region of a coronary artery may embolize to more distal sites.

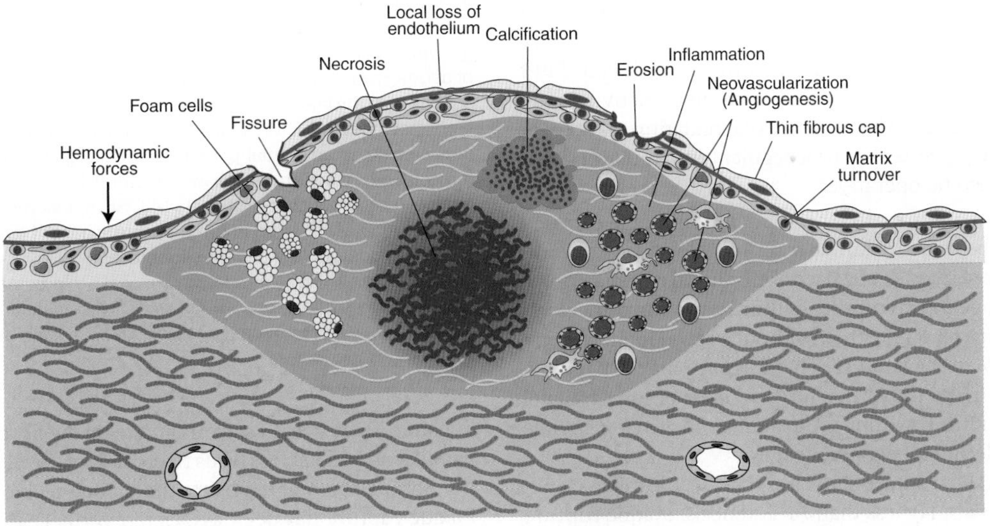

FIGURE 10-14. **Factors involved in the pathogenesis of complicated atherosclerotic plaques.**

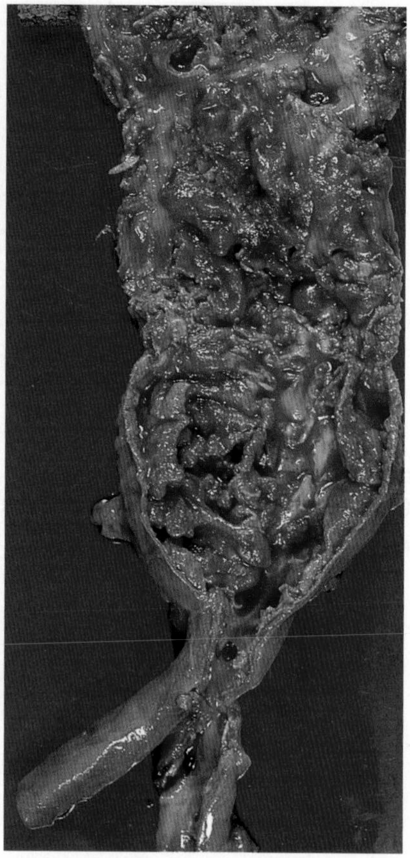

FIGURE 10-15. **Complicated lesions of atherosclerosis.** The luminal surface of the abdominal aorta and the common iliac arteries shows numerous fibrous plaques and raised, ulcerated lesions containing friable, atheromatous debris. The distal portion of the aorta displays a small aneurysmal dilation.

- **The vulnerable atheroma** has structural and functional alterations that predispose to plaque destabilization
- **Atheroma destabilization**, often resulting in acute coronary syndromes, may occur at any time when the dynamic balance of opposing biological and physical processes is disrupted, leading to mural thrombosis, fibrous cap rupture, or intraplaque hemorrhage. Clinically silent ruptures occur and can heal. In a ruptured plaque, the necrotic material that comes in contact with the blood contains TF and is very thrombogenic. Adjacent endothelium has reduced TFPI levels and lower antiplatelet and fibrinolytic activities, all favoring coagulation. The presence of circulating markers of inflammation suggests that procoagulant inflammatory mediators may also be operative.

Once a plaque ruptures, the thrombogenic material exposed promotes thrombosis in the lumen, causing an occlusive thrombus. Plaque rupture may also heal without clinical complications. Plaque hemorrhage due to rupture of thin, newly formed vessels may occur within a plaque with or without a subsequent rupture of the fibrous cap. In the latter case hemorrhage may expand the plaque, and so narrow the lumen further. The hemorrhage will be resorbed over time within the plaque, and leaving telltale residual hemosiderin-laden macrophages.

Most plaques that rupture show less than 50% luminal stenosis, and over 95% display less than 70% stenosis. Plaque rupture often occurs at the shoulder of the plaque, suggesting that hemodynamic shear stress weakens and tears the fibrous cap. If not repaired, endothelial loss leads to erosion of the plaque, weakening the fibrous cap and exposing the plaque to blood constituents. Plaque rupture has been associated with (1) areas of inflammation, (2) large lipid core size, (3) thin fibrous cap ($<65\ \mu M$),

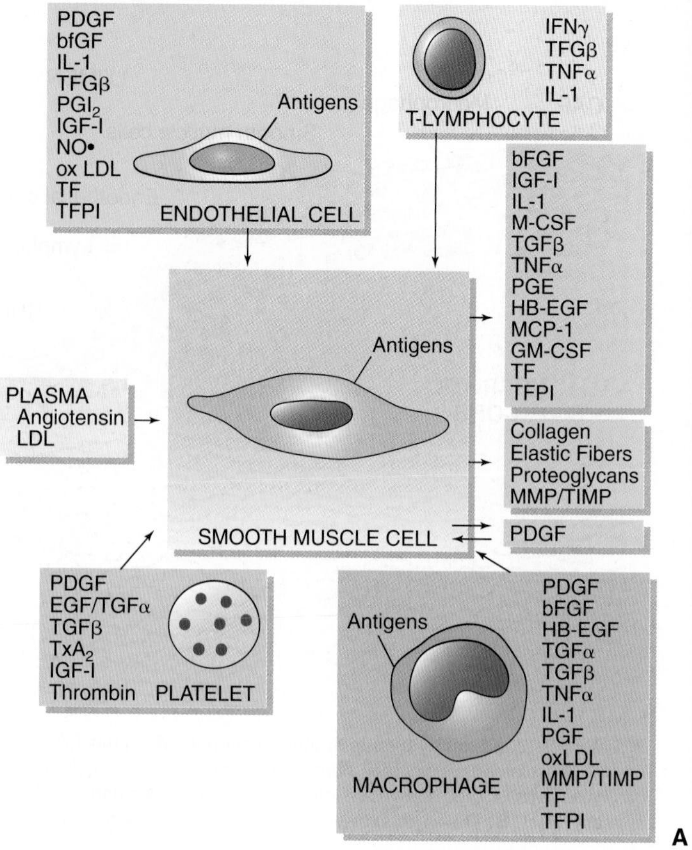

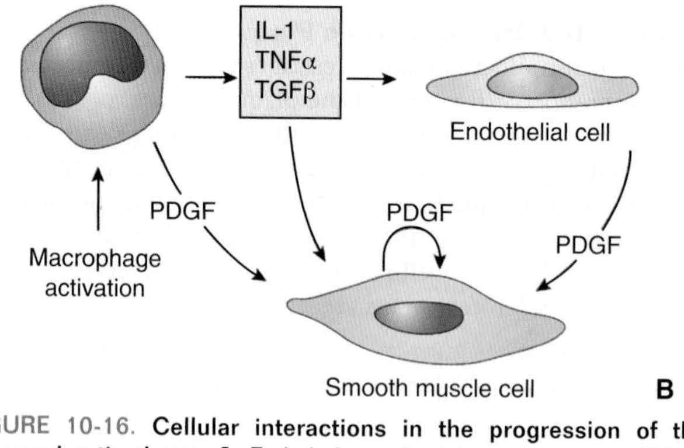

FIGURE 10-16. **Cellular interactions in the progression of the atherosclerotic plaque. A.** Endothelium, platelets, macrophages, T lymphocytes, and smooth muscle cells elaborate a variety of cytokines, growth factors, and other substances. The scheme illustrated here emphasizes their influence on smooth muscle cells. **B.** The cellular interactions that promote the proliferation of smooth cells. bfGF = basic fibroblast growth factor; EGF = endothelial growth factor; HB-EGF = heparin-binding epidermal growth factor-like growth factor; IFN = interferon; IGF-I = insulin-like growth factor-I; IL = interleukin; MCP-1 = monocyte chemotactic protein-1; M-CSF = macrophage colony-stimulating factor; MMP = matrix metalloproteinase; NO = nitric oxide; ox LDL = oxidated low-density lipoprotein; PDGF = platelet-derived growth factor; PGE = prostaglandin; PGI_2 = prostacyclin; TF = tissue factor; TFG = tumor growth factor; TFPI = tissue factor pathway inhibitor; TNF = tumor necrosis factor; TMIP = inhibitors of MMPs; TxA_2 = thromboxane A_2.

(4) decreased smooth muscle cells owing to apoptosis, (5) imbalance of proteolytic enzymes and their inhibitors in the fibrous cap, (6) calcification in the plaque, and (7) intraplaque hemorrhage leading to inside-out rupture of the fibrous cap.

Several circulating markers have been associated with plaque burden, including C-reactive protein (CRP), fibrinogen, soluble VCAM, IL-1, IL-6, and TNF.

Complications of Atherosclerosis

The complications of atherosclerosis vary with the location and the size of the affected vessel and the chronicity of the process (Fig. 10-17).

- **Acute occlusion:** Thrombosis on an atherosclerotic plaque, may abruptly occlude the lumen of a muscular artery (Fig. 10-18). The result is ischemic necrosis (infarction) of the tissue supplied by that vessel, manifested clinically as myocardial infarction, stroke, or gangrene of the intestine or lower extremities. Some occlusive thrombi can be dissolved by enzymes that activate plasma fibrinolytic activity, including streptokinase and tissue plasminogen activator.
- **Chronic narrowing of the vessel lumen:** As an atherosclerotic plaque grows, it often impinges on the lumen, thereby progressively reducing blood flow to the tissue in the distribution of the artery. Chronic ischemia of the affected tissue is evidenced by atrophy of the organ, as exemplified by (1) unilateral renal artery stenosis with renal atrophy, (2) intestinal stricture in mesenteric artery atherosclerosis, or (3) ischemic atrophy of the skin in a diabetic with severe peripheral vascular disease.
- **Aneurysm formation:** The complicated lesions of atherosclerosis may extend into the media of an elastic artery and weaken the wall so as to allow formation of an aneurysm, typically in the abdominal aorta. These aneurysms may suddenly rupture and precipitate a vascular catastrophe.
- **Embolism:** A thrombus formed over an atherosclerotic plaque may detach and lodge in a distal vessel. For example, embolization from a thrombus in an abdominal aortic aneurysm may acutely occlude the popliteal artery, with subsequent gangrene of the leg. Ulceration of an atherosclerotic plaque may also dislodge atheromatous debris and produce so-called "cholesterol crystal emboli," which appear as needle-shaped spaces in affected tissues (Fig. 10-19), most commonly in the kidney.

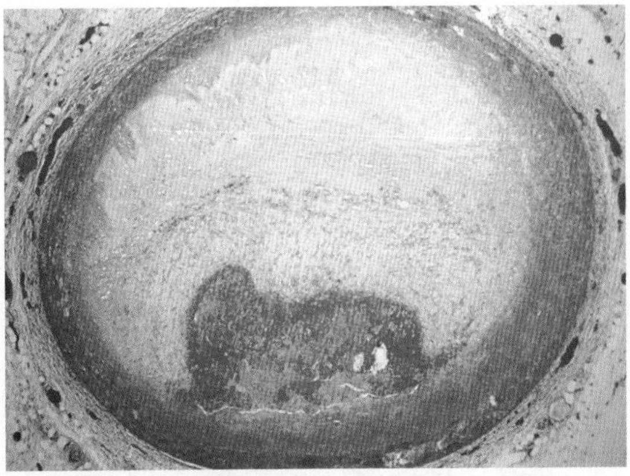

FIGURE 10-18. **Coronary artery thrombosis.** A microscopic section of a coronary artery shows severe atherosclerosis and a recent thrombus in the narrowed lumen.

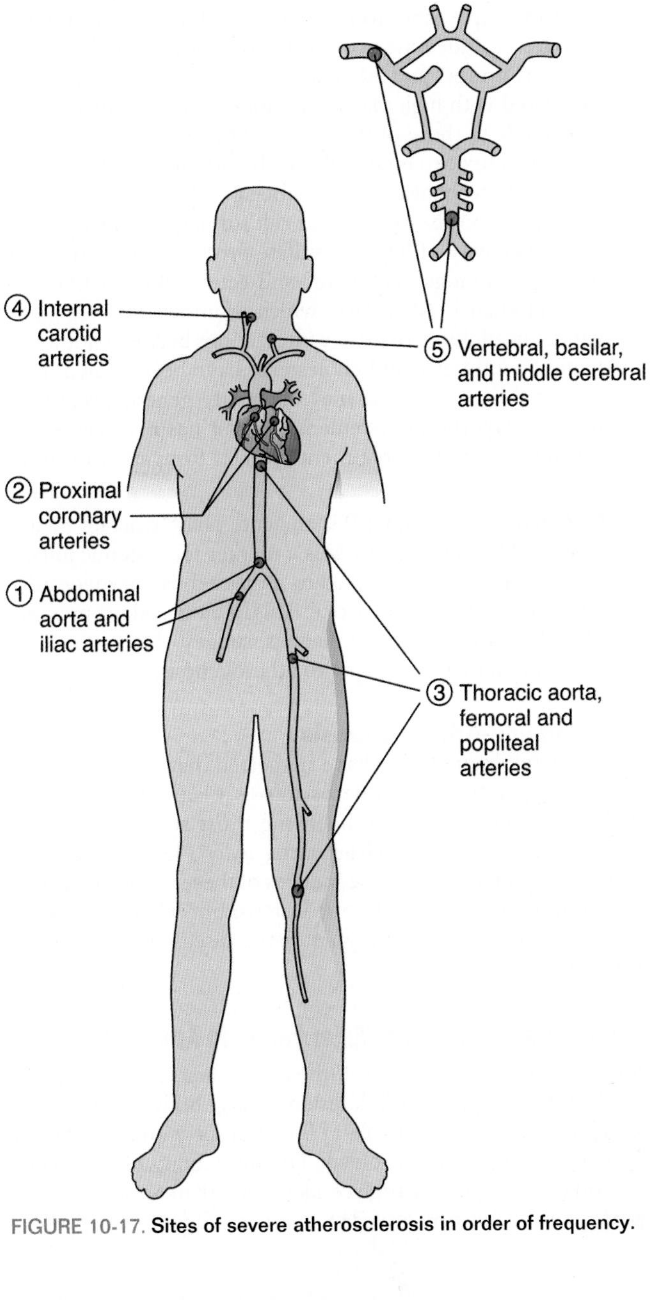

FIGURE 10-17. **Sites of severe atherosclerosis in order of frequency.**

Restenosis Occurs After Interventional Therapy

Percutaneous transluminal coronary angioplasty is an important form of interventional therapy for stenotic atherosclerotic vascular disease, especially that of the epicardial coronary arteries. A balloon catheter is inserted into the coronary arteries, where it is inflated to dilate the stenotic artery. The balloon causes endothelial damage and tears in the plaque and the media. In 30% to 40% of cases in which the vessel lumen is satisfactorily dilated, restenosis takes place over a period of 3 to 6 months.

Intimal hyperplasia due to smooth muscle cell proliferation and matrix deposition, with or without an organized mural thrombus on the luminal surface, leads to restenosis. In addition, vascular wall remodeling, induced in part by trauma to the vessel wall and involving the adventitia, also results in luminal narrowing through contraction of the vessel wall. The use of stents coated with certain biocompatible polymers and biologically active agents began in 2002 and has resulted in less restenosis. For

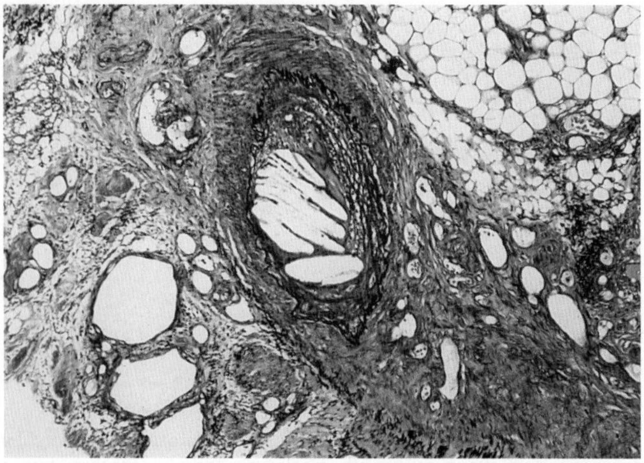

FIGURE 10-19. **Cholesterol crystal embolus.** Needle-shaped clefts are seen in an atherosclerotic embolus that has occluded a small artery.

example, drug-eluting stents with anti-proliferative agents block cell cycle progression and thus inhibit the overgrowth of smooth muscle cells in the vessel wall. However short-term and long-term complications are not fully known, especially as they relate to thrombosis.

Transplanted saphenous veins used as autografts in coronary artery bypass operations undergo a series of adaptive and reparative changes. These include (1) intimal thickening associated with phlebosclerosis, (2) occasional medial calcification, (3) focal muscle cell hypertrophy, and eventually, (4) scarring of the adventitia. However, venous grafts in place for a few years exhibit atherosclerotic plaques indistinguishable from those found in native coronary arteries. Half of these grafts occlude within 5 to 10 years, owing to neointimal hyperplasia and atherosclerosis.

Risk Factors for Atherosclerosis Are Predictors of Ischemic Events

Factors associated with a two-fold or greater risk of ischemic heart disease include:

- **Hypertension:** High blood pressure is consistently associated with greater risk of myocardial infarction. This increased risk had previously been associated solely with the diastolic component, but recent evidence suggests that the systolic hypertension is equally important. Men with systolic blood pressures over 160 mm Hg have almost three times the incidence of myocardial infarction as those with systolic pressures under 120 mm Hg. Control of hypertension has significantly decreased the incidence of myocardial infarction and stroke.
- **Blood cholesterol level:** Serum cholesterol have been directly correlated with ischemic heart disease. *Indeed, serum cholesterol seems to be the most important determinant of the geographic differences in incidence of atherosclerotic coronary artery disease.* In the absence of genetic disorders of lipid metabolism (see below), the amount of cholesterol in the blood is strongly related to the dietary intake of saturated fat. The incidence of myocardial infarction is reduced by treatment with cholesterol-lowering drugs.
- **Cigarette smoking:** Coronary and aortic atherosclerosis is more severe and extensive among cigarette smokers than nonsmokers, and the effect is dose-related (see Chapter 8). Thus, smoking markedly increases the risk of myocardial infarction, ischemic stroke, and abdominal aortic aneurysms.
- **Diabetes:** Diabetics are at greater risk for occlusive atherosclerotic vascular disease in many organs, but the relative contributions of carbohydrate intolerance itself, advanced glycation end-products, and secondary changes in blood lipids are not well defined (see Chapter 22).
- **Increasing age and male sex:** These factors are strong determinants of the risk for myocardial infarction, but both are probably secondary to the accumulated effects of other risk factors.
- **Physical inactivity and stressful life patterns:** Both of these factors correlate with increased risk of ischemic heart disease, although their precise relationship to the evolution of atherosclerosis is not established.
- **Homocysteine:** Homocystinuria is a rare autosomal recessive disease caused by mutations in the gene encoding cystathionine synthase. The disorder causes premature and severe atherosclerosis. Mild elevations of plasma homocysteine in people who do not have this disease are common, and are an independent risk factor for atherosclerosis of coronary arteries and other large vessels. This increase in risk associated with high plasma homocysteine is comparable in magnitude to those of smoking and hyperlipidemia. Homocysteine is toxic to endothelial cells and impairs several anticoagulant mechanisms in endothelial cells. It inhibits thrombomodulin on the endothelial cell surface, antithrombin III binding activity of heparan sulfate proteoglycan, binding of tissue plasminogen activator, and ecto-ADPase activity on the endothelial cell surface, which promotes platelet aggregation. In addition, oxidative interactions between homocysteine, lipoproteins, and cholesterol have been shown. Low dietary folic acid intake may aggravate genetic predispositions to hyperhomocysteinemia, but it has not been established that folic acid treatment protects from atherosclerotic vascular disease.
- **C-Reactive Protein:** CRP is an acute phase reactant mainly produced by hepatocytes. It is a marker for systemic inflammation, and has been linked to increased risk of myocardial infarction and ischemic stroke. This finding, and the presence of CRP in atherosclerotic plaques, suggest that systemic inflammation may contribute to atherogenesis.

Infection and Atherosclerosis

Seroepidemiologic studies have suggested that some infectious agents may contribute to atherosclerosis. *Chlamydia pneumoniae* and cytomegalovirus have been the most studied, although there is also interest in *Helicobacter pylori,* herpesvirus, and other organisms. Genomic sequences of these agents have been found in human atherosclerotic lesions, but whether they are causally associated or simply enter the diseased artery wall is not known.

Lipid Metabolism Is the Major Factor in Atherosclerosis

Since Rudolf Virchow in the 19th century first identified cholesterol crystals in atherosclerotic lesions, a large body of information on lipoproteins and their role in lipid transport and metabolism and atherosclerosis has evolved. The insolubility of cholesterol and other lipids (mainly triglycerides) necessitates a special transport system, a function served by a system of lipoprotein particles

TABLE 10-6
The Apolipoproteins

Apolipoprotein	Approximate Molecular Weight	Major Density Class	Major Sites of Synthesis in Humans	Major Function in Lipoprotein Metabolism
AI	28,000	HDL	Liver, intestine	Activates lecithin: cholesterol acyltransferase
AII	18,000	HDL	Liver, intestine	
AIV	45,000	Chylomicrons	Intestine	
B-100	250,000	VLDL, IDL, LDL	Liver	Binds to LDL receptor
B-48	125,000	Chylomicrons, VLDL IDL	Intestine	
CI	6500	Chylomicrons, VLDL, HDL	Liver	Activates lecithin: cholesterol acyltransferase
CII	10,000	Chylomicrons, VLDL, HDL	Liver	Activates lipoprotein lipase
CIII	10,000	Chylomicrons	Liver	Inhibits lipoprotein uptake by the liver
D	20,000	HDL		Cholesteryl ester exchange protein
E	40,000	Chylomicrons, VLDL, HDL	Liver, macrophage	Binds to E receptor system

HDL = high-density lipoprotein; IDL = intermediate-density lipoprotein; LDL = low-density lipoprotein; VLDL = very low-density lipoprotein.

(Table 10-6; Fig. 10-20). These are categorized according to density:

- Chylomicrons
- Very-low-density lipoproteins (VLDLs)
- LDLs
- High-density lipoproteins (HDLs)

Each of these particles consists of a lipid core with associated proteins (apolipoproteins), as indicated in Table 10-6. The metabolic pathways for lipoproteins containing the B apolipoproteins (apoB) are two major lipoprotein cascades, one from the intestine and the other from the liver (Fig. 10-21).

EXOGENOUS PATHWAY: This metabolic route involves chylomicrons containing apoB-48 secreted by the intestine. Following secretion, chylomicrons rapidly acquire apoCII and apoE from HDL. These triglyceride-rich lipoproteins primarily transport lipid from intestine to liver. The triglycerides in chylomicrons are hydrolyzed by lipoprotein lipase, which is at the surface of capillary endothelial cells. ApoCII activates lipoprotein lipase and causes removal of triglycerides, converting chylomicrons to "remnants," and finally to intermediate-density lipoproteins (IDLs). The chylomicron remnants are removed by hepatocytes through an apoE-mediated (remnant) receptor process.

ENDOGENOUS PATHWAY: This network of reactions involves triglyceride-rich lipoproteins containing apoB-100 secreted by the liver. Liver VLDL particles acquire apoCII and apoE from HDL shortly after their secretion. The triglycerides on VLDL are hydrolyzed by lipoprotein lipase. The lipoproteins containing apoB-100 are initially converted to IDLs and finally to LDLs. Hepatic lipoprotein lipase converts, at least in part, IDL to LDL, at which point most apoCII and apoE dissociates from the particles and reassociates with HDL. Lipoprotein lipase acts both as a triglyceride hydrolase and, more importantly, as a phospholipase. LDL, which contains apoB-100, interacts with high-affinity receptors on hepatocytes and on peripheral cells, including smooth muscle cells, fibroblasts, and adrenal cells (see Fig. 10-21). The interaction of LDL with its receptor initiates receptor-mediated endocytosis, which is followed by catabolism of LDL.

HIGH-DENSITY LIPOPROTEIN: HDL containing apoAI and apoAII is synthesized by several pathways. These include direct

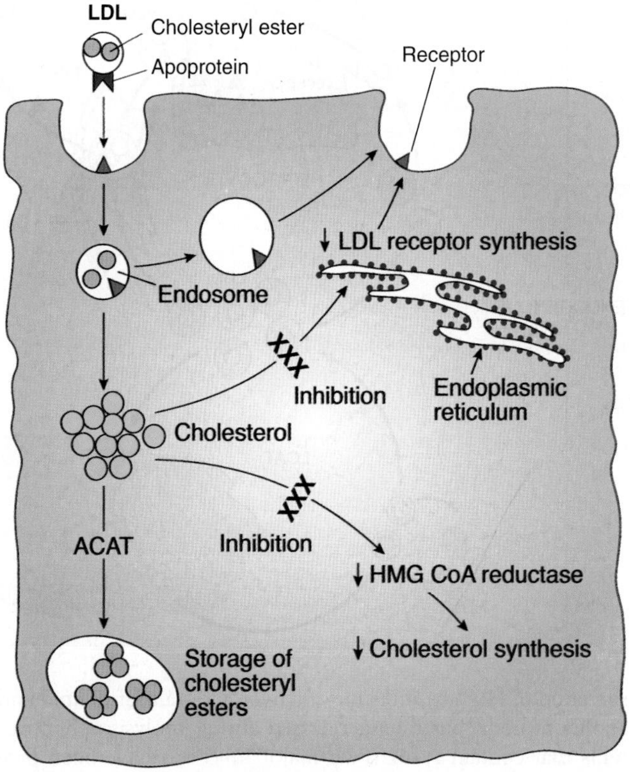

FIGURE 10-20. **The relationship between circulating low-density lipoprotein (LDL)-cholesterol, LDL receptors, and the synthesis of cholesterol.** LDL, which contains cholesteryl esters, is taken up by cells into vesicles by a receptor-mediated pathway to form an endosome. The receptor and lipids are dissociated, and the receptor is returned to the cell surface. The exogenous cholesterol, now in the cytoplasm, causes a reduction in receptor synthesis in the endoplasmic reticulum and inhibits the activity of hydroxy methylglutaryl coenzyme A (HMG–CoA) reductase in the cholesterol synthesizing pathway. Excess cholesterol in the cell is esterified to cholesteryl esters and stored in vacuoles. ACAT = acyl-CoA:cholesterol acyltransferase.

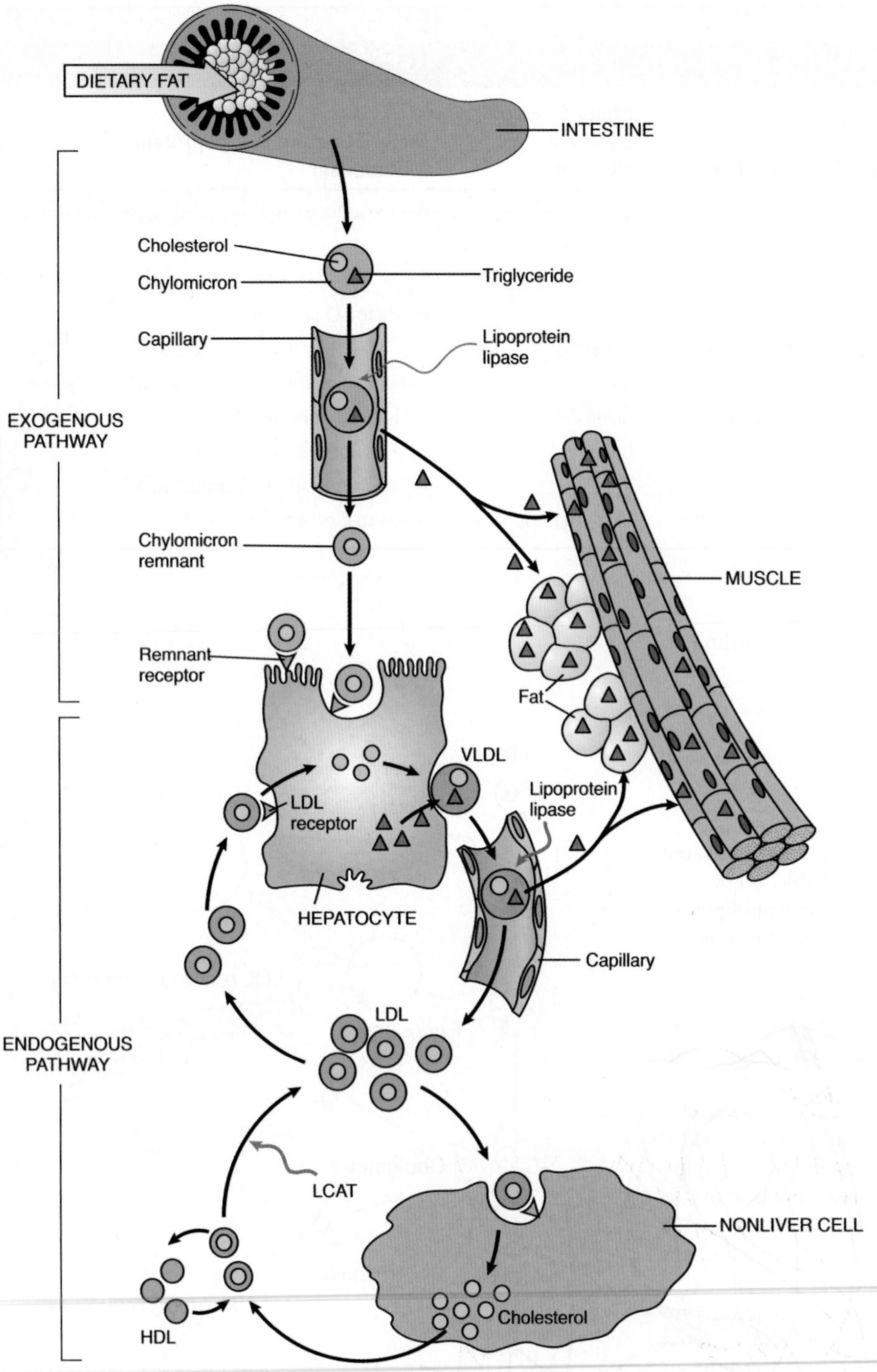

FIGURE 10-21. **Exogenous and endogenous cholesterol transport pathway.** In the exogenous pathway, cholesterol and fatty acids from food are absorbed through the intestinal mucosa. Fatty acid chains are linked to glycerol to form triglycerides. Triglycerides and cholesterol are packaged into chylomicrons that are returned via the lymph to the blood. The lipids are coupled to proteins by enzymes such as the microsomal transfer protein complex. In the capillaries (mainly of fat tissue and muscle, but also other tissues), the ester bonds holding the fatty acids in triglycerides are split by lipoprotein lipase. Fatty acids are removed, leaving cholesterol-rich lipoprotein remnants. These bind to special remnant receptors and are taken up by liver cells. The cholesterol of the remnant is either secreted into the intestine, largely as bile acids, or packaged as very low-density lipoprotein (VLDL) particles, which are then secreted into the circulation. This is the first step in the endogenous cycle. In fat or muscle tissue the triglyceride is removed from the VLDL with the aid of lipoprotein lipase. The intermediate-density lipoprotein (IDL) particles (not shown) remain in the circulation. Some IDL is immediately taken up by the liver via the mediation of LDL receptors for ApoB/E. The remaining IDL in the circulation is either taken up by nonliver cells or converted to LDL. Most of the LDL in the circulation binds to hepatocytes or other cells and is removed from the circulation. High-density lipoproteins (HDLs) take up cholesterol from cells. This cholesterol is esterified by the enzyme lecithin:cholesterol acyltransferase (LCAT), after which the esters are transferred to LDL and taken up by cells.

secretion of HDL by intestine and liver and transfer of lipid and apolipoprotein constituents released during lipolysis of lipoproteins that contain apoB. Two major functions have been proposed for HDL: (1) a reservoir for apolipoproteins, particularly apoCII and apoE; and (2) interaction with cells in the transport system to carry extrahepatic cholesterol, including that in the arterial wall, to the liver for ultimate removal from the body. The latter function has been termed **reverse cholesterol transport**. The cholesterol removed from cells is principally free cholesterol, which rapidly undergoes esterification to cholesteryl esters. Cholesteryl esters are transferred to the core of the lipoprotein particle or are exchanged to VLDL and LDL. Transfer of cholesteryl esters between lipoprotein particles is mediated by specific transfer proteins such as cholesterol ester transfer protein. Defects in cholesteryl ester transfer and exchange lead to dyslipoproteinemia, increased intracellular cholesteryl ester concentrations, and premature atherosclerosis.

LOW-DENSITY LIPOPROTEIN: LDL cholesterol has numerous effects on endothelial cells, smooth muscle cells, and monocyte/macrophages. For example, it regulates cyclooxygenase-2–dependent prostacyclin formation in vitro.

Each of the cell types in atherosclerotic lesions (macrophages, endothelial cells, smooth muscle cells) can oxidize LDL. This change facilitates LDL recognition by the macrophage scavenger receptor and causes massive uptake of cholesterol by macrophages. Oxidized lipoproteins also affect other processes that may contribute to atherogenesis, including regulation of vascular tone, activation of inflammatory and immune responses, and coagulation. Autoantibodies to oxidized LDL are present in patients with atherosclerosis in both plasma and plaques and may be important in the pathogenesis of plaques. Oxidized LDL are toxic to vascular wall cells, may disrupt endothelial integrity, and lead to accumulation of cell debris within the atheroma. Oxidized LDL is also chemotactic for macrophages, thereby further promoting their accumulation in atheromas. Epidemiologic studies suggest that dietary intake of antioxidants is inversely associated with risk of atherosclerosis, implying that oxidized LDL may be an important mediator of vascular disease. Further investigation is, however, necessary to establish this point.

Several Heritable Dyslipoproteinemias are Now Recognized

Familial clustering of ischemic heart diseases is well documented (Table 10-7).

FAMILIAL HYPERCHOLESTEROLEMIA: The LDL receptor is a cell surface glycoprotein that regulates plasma cholesterol by mediating endocytosis and recycling of apoE, the major plasma cholesterol transport protein. Mutations in the LDL receptor gene, located on the short arm of chromosome 19, lead to familial hypercholesterolemia, an autosomal dominant disease in which the prevalence of heterozygotes is about 1 in 500 persons. However, among persons who have had myocardial infarctions associated with hyperlipidemia, the prevalence of familial hypercholesterolemia may approach 6%.

More than 400 mutant alleles for familial hypercholesterolemia have been described, including point mutations, insertions, and deletions. The mutations fall into five main classes, based on their effects on the functions of the receptor protein (Fig. 10-22). Genetic issues in familial hypercholesterolemia are discussed more fully in Chapter 6.

The early onset and malignant course of ischemic heart disease in patients with homozygous familial hypercholesterolemia may be the most compelling arguments for a relationship between circulating cholesterol and atherosclerosis. Homozygotes have plasma cholesterol levels between 600 and 1000 mg/dL, 4- to 6-fold higher than the mean values in most whites. Most untreated homozygotes die from coronary artery disease before the age of 20. In heterozygotes, LDL cholesterol levels vary from 250 to 500 mg/dL, roughly twice normal. These patients also suffer from premature myocardial infarction but at a later age than do the homozygotes (40 to 45 years in men).

In addition to accelerated accumulation of cholesterol in arteries (premature atherosclerosis), LDL cholesterol also deposits in skin and tendons to form xanthomas (Fig. 10-23). In some cases (before age 10 in homozygotes), an arcus lipoides is present in the cornea.

APOLIPOPROTEIN E (APOE): Genetic variations in various apoproteins are also known to be accompanied by alterations in LDL levels. Polymorphisms in apoE and variants of apolipoprotein AI and AII have been observed. Apolipoprotein E is one of the main protein constituents of VLDL and of a subclass of HDL. The gene locus that codes for apoE is polymorphic; three common alleles, E2, E3, and E4, code for three major apoE isoforms, respectively, and determine the six apoE phenotypes. Some 20% of the variability in serum cholesterol has been attributed to apoE polymorphism. In men, the apoE 3/2 phenotype is associated with a 20% lower LDL level than the most common phenotype, apoE 3/3. By contrast, the E4 allele is associated with elevated serum cholesterol. Interestingly, E2 allele is increased and E4 decreased among male octogenarians.

TABLE 10-7

Molecular Defects in Dyslipoproteinemias

Disease	Genetic Defect	Clinical Features
Apolipoprotein Defects		
ApoA1 deficiency	ApoA1 truncations or rearrangements (11q23)	Absent HDL, severe atherosclerosis
ApoA1 variants	ApoA1 point mutations (11q23)	Reduced HDL, variable atherosclerosis
Abetalipoproteinemia (absence of both ApoB-100 and ApoB-48)	Microsomal triglyceride protein mutations (4q22–24)	Ataxia, malabsorption, hemolytic anemia, visual defects, absence of atherosclerosis
ApoB-100 absence	Unknown (2p24)	Mild ataxia, malabsorption, absence of atherosclerosis
ApoCII deficiency	ApoCII mutations (19q13.2)	Type I hyperlipidemia: severe hypertriglyceridemia, variable atherosclerosis
ApoE variants	ApoE mutations (19q13.2)	Type III hyperlipidemia: elevated triglycerides, premature atherosclerosis
Enzyme Defects		
Lipoprotein lipase deficiency	Lipoprotein lipase mutations (8p22)	Type I hyperlipidemia: hypertriglyceridemia; minimal atherosclerosis
Hepatic lipase deficiency	Hepatic lipase mutations (15q21–23)	Elevations of IDL and HDL; severe atherosclerosis
Lecithin:cholesterol acyltransferase (LCAT) deficiency	LCAT mutations (16q22.1)	Mild hypertriglyceridemia; reduced HDL; corneal opacities; variable atherosclerosis
Receptor Defect		
Familial hypercholesterolemia	LDL receptor mutations (19p13.2)	Type II hyperlipidemia: severe elevation of LDL; premature atherosclerosis

Apo = apoprotein; HDL = high-density lipoprotein; IDL = intermediate-density lipoprotein; LDL = low-density lipoprotein.

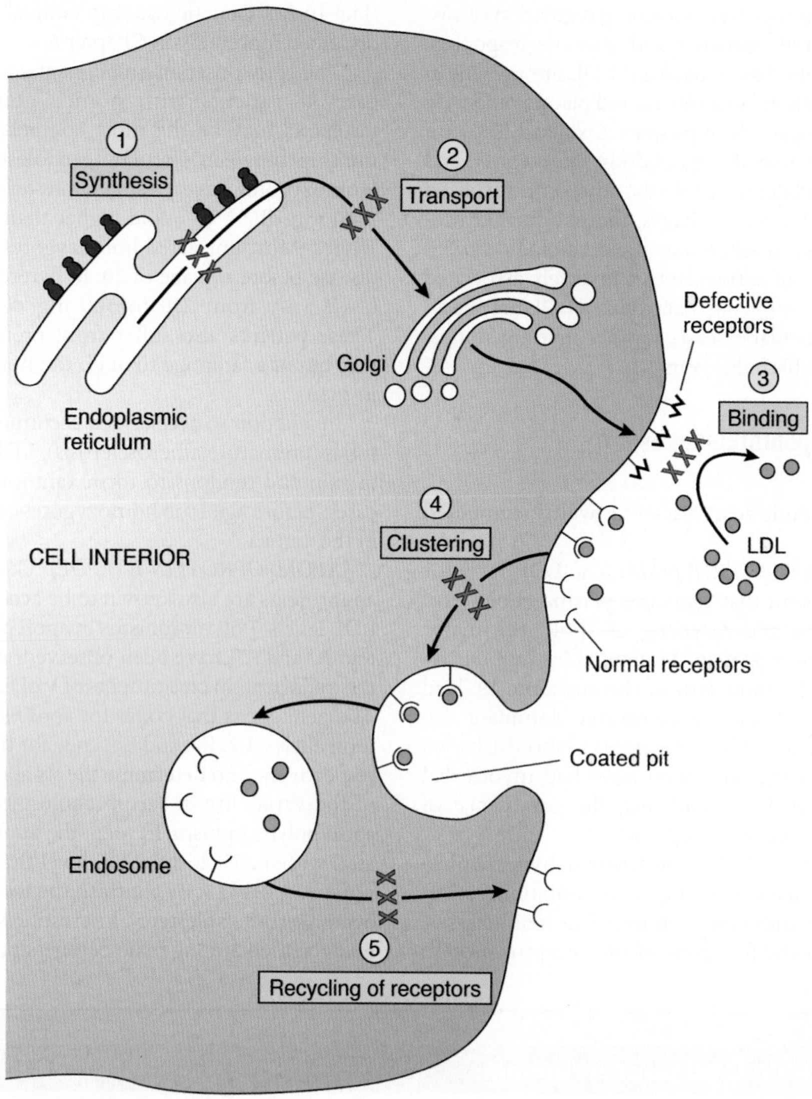

FIGURE 10-22. **Mutations of the low-density lipoprotein (LDL) receptor in familial hypercholesterolemia.**

HIGH-DENSITY LIPOPROTEIN: An inverse correlation between ischemic heart disease and HDL cholesterol levels has been established. The genes for apolipoproteins AI and CIII are on chromosome 11 and are physically linked, whereas the gene for A-II is on chromosome 1. Polymorphisms of apoAI are associated with premature atherosclerosis, as are rare cases of hereditary apoAI deficiency. Factors that increase HDL levels include female gender, estrogens, vigorous exercise, and moderate alcohol consumption. Decreased HDL occurs with low-fat diets, diets high in polyunsaturated fats, truncal obesity, diabetes, smoking, and androgen administration. Hypertriglyceridemia is often associated with low HDL cholesterol.

LIPOPROTEIN (a) (LP[A]): High circulating levels of Lp(a) are associated with an augmented risk of atherosclerotic disease of the coronary arteries and larger cerebral vessels. Plasma levels of this cholesterol-rich lipoprotein vary greatly (<1 to >140 mg/dL) and appear to be independent of LDL levels. The Lp(a)-specific protein, apo(a), has been detected in atherosclerotic lesions and high Lp(a) levels correlate with target organ damage in hypertensive patients.

Lp(a) is an LDL-like particle to which the glycoprotein apo(a) is attached through a disulfide bridge with apoB-100. Apo(a) is encoded by a gene on chromosome 6 (6q2.7), close to the gene for plasminogen, with which apo(a) is highly homologous. Both apo(a) and plasminogen display similar domains that mediate an interaction with fibrin and cell surface receptors. Lp(a) enhances cholesterol delivery to injured blood vessels, suppresses generation of plasmin, and promotes smooth muscle proliferation. Thus, it may be an important link between atherosclerosis and thrombosis.

Lp(a) plasma levels are heritable and not altered by most cholesterol-lowering drugs, although they are reduced by nicotinic acid. Taken together, this information distinguishes a risk factor that appears superficially to be related to serum cholesterol, but the effect of which may actually be linked to an alteration in clot lysis.

Hypertensive Vascular Disease

Hypertension affects up to 20% of the population in industrial countries and is seen in more than half of cases of myocardial infarction, stroke, and chronic renal disease. Blacks are particularly plagued by hypertension, and are more likely than whites to experience severe complications. Three-fourths of patients with

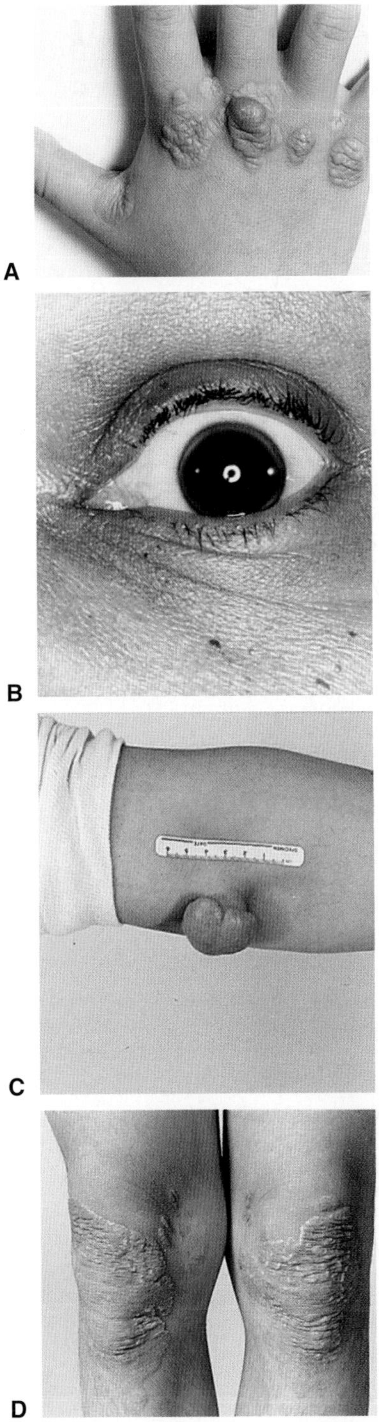

FIGURE 10-23. **Xanthomas in familial hypercholesterolemia. A.** Dorsum of hand. **B.** Arcus lipoides represents the deposition of lipids in the peripheral cornea. **C.** Extensor surface of elbow. **D.** Knees

dissecting aortic aneurysm, intracerebral hemorrhage, or myocardial wall rupture also have elevated blood pressure. In 95% of patients hypertension occurs without a clearly identifiable cause. Thus, most hypertensive persons are said to have **essential** or **primary** hypertension. Whatever the etiology, treatment of hypertension prolongs life.

The definition of hypertension depends on a statistical estimate of the distribution of systolic and diastolic blood pressures in the general population. Over the course of the day, blood pressure varies widely, depending on exertion, emotional state, and other poorly understood factors. Blood pressure also varies with age. The mean systolic blood pressure in 20-year-old men is about 130 mm Hg, but the 95% confidence limits range from 105 to 150 mm Hg. With age, average systolic blood pressure increases, so that in 80-year-olds, it reaches 170 mm Hg, with 95% confidence limits from 125 to 220. The World Health Organization defines hypertension as systolic pressure above 160 mm Hg and/or diastolic pressure above 90.

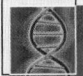

PATHOGENESIS: Blood pressure is the product of cardiac output and systemic vascular resistance to blood flow. However, both of these functions are critically influenced by renal function and sodium homeostasis. The most widespread hypothesis holds that primary hypertension results from an imbalance in the interactions between these mechanisms (Fig. 10-24).

A complex endocrine axis centers on the renin–angiotensin system. Renal artery occlusion or dietary salt restriction leads to increased renal secretion of renin. Renin is a protease that cleaves angiotensinogen to a decapeptide, angiotensin I. In turn, angiotensin I is converted to angiotensin II by the endothelial surface protein, ACE. Angiotensin II causes vasoconstriction and also affects centers in the CNS that control sympathetic outflow and stimulate adrenal aldosterone release. Aldosterone acts on renal tubules to increase sodium reabsorption. The net effect of all these actions is increased total body fluid volume. Thus, the **renin–angiotensin** system elevates blood pressure by three mechanisms:

- Increased sympathetic output
- Increased mineralocorticoid secretion
- Direct vasoconstriction

This axis is antagonized by atrial natriuretic factor (ANF), a hormone secreted by specialized cells in the cardiac atria. ANF binds specific receptors in kidney and increases urinary sodium excretion, thus opposing angiotensin II-induced vasoconstriction. Secretion of ANF may be controlled by atrial distention, a consequence of increased volume, or by as-yet undefined endocrine interactions.

The importance of this hormonal axis in regulating blood pressure in hypertension is demonstrated by the therapeutic success of sympathetic antagonists (β-adrenergic blockers), diuretics, and inhibitors of ACE. Nonetheless, it has proved difficult to identify a central defect in the renin–angiotensin axis, because the vasculature responds quickly to hemodynamic changes in the tissues by autoregulation (Fig. 10-25).

In the case of hypertension, the end-result of autoregulation is always increased peripheral resistance. For example, hypertension can be induced experimentally by surgically removing large amounts of renal tissue, followed by administering excess sodium and water. Cardiac output, and therefore blood pressure, increase rapidly as a result of the rapid change in blood volume. However, within a few days, pressure-induced diuresis restores near-normal cardiac output and plasma volume. At this point, blood pressure is maintained by increased peripheral resistance. Although the blood pressure elevation was initially due to increased volume, compensatory mechanisms successfully masked the volume changes and caused apparent essential

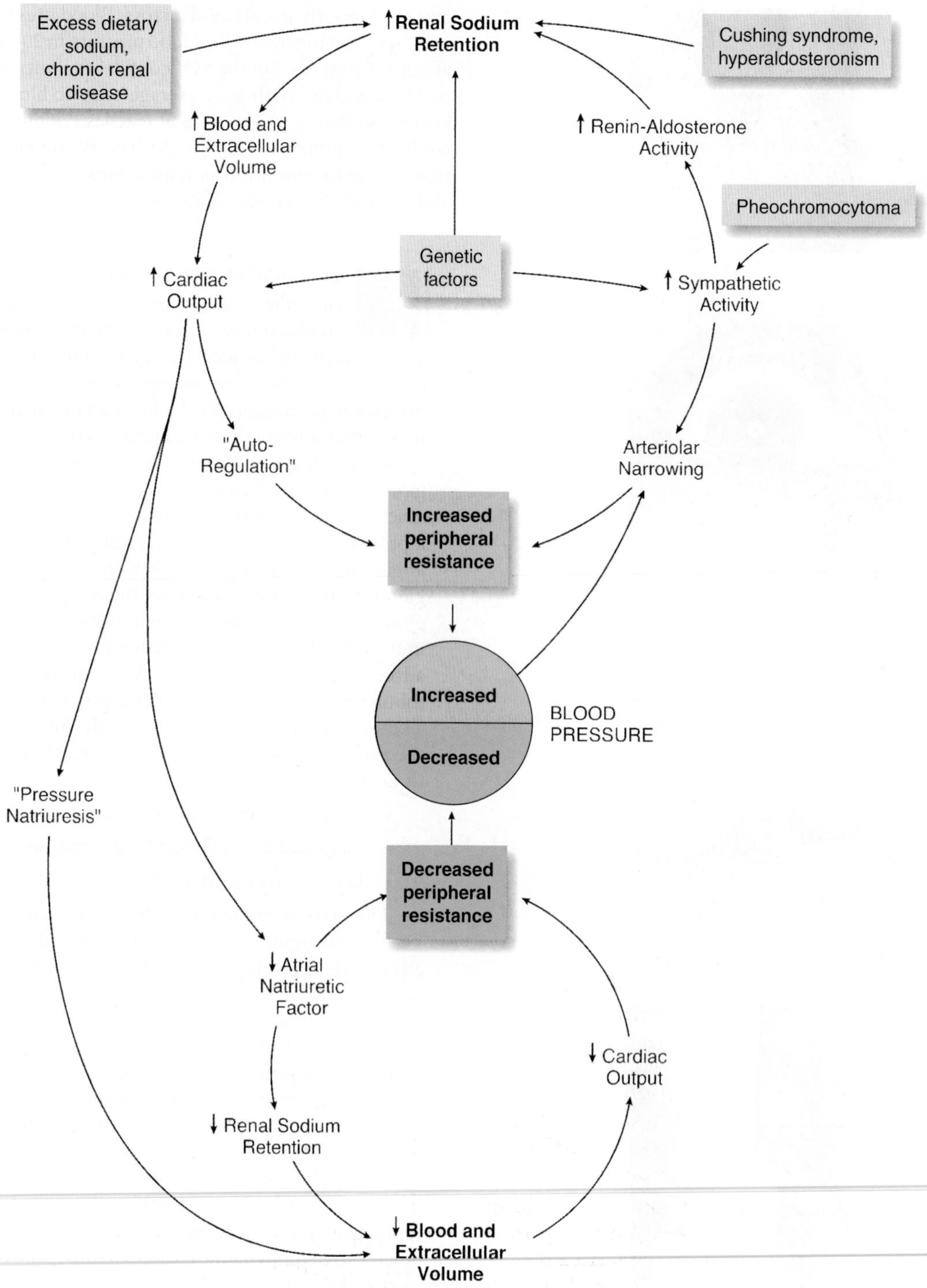

FIGURE 10-24. **Factors contributing to hypertension and the counterregulatory factors that lower blood pressure.** An imbalance in these factors results in the increased peripheral resistance that is responsible for most cases of essential (primary) hypertension. Note the central role of peripheral resistance.

hypertension. Many cases of human hypertension may also result from a process that begins with alterations in cardiac output, salt metabolism, or ANF release.

Molecular Genetics of Hypertension

We know from family and twin studies that genetic factors are likely to be important in the pathogenesis of essential hypertension. For example, there is a familial association of hypertension with alterations in membrane transport of sodium (measured as lithium transport). Interestingly, spontaneous hypertension can be produced in rats in as few as six generations of inbreeding for elevated blood pressure. However, no specific genetic defect has been shown to be causal in rats or humans. Inheritance of essential hypertension is most likely polygenic and not due to single-gene conditions.

Although essential hypertension likely involves interactions of a number of gene products, the study of rare inherited forms

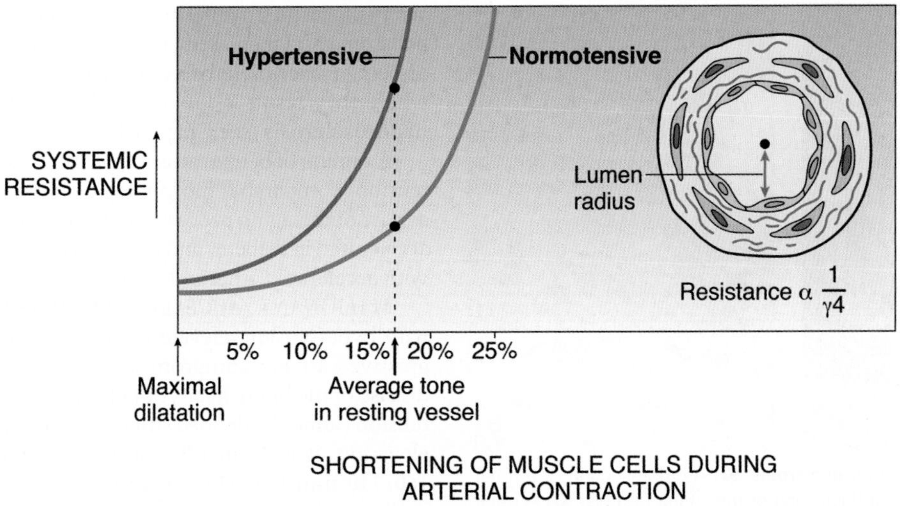

FIGURE 10-25. **Structural autoregulation of blood pressure.** Hypertension, regardless of its primary cause, increases the ability of the resistance vessel walls to respond to vasoactive stimuli. Resistance is increased even in maximally dilated vessels because the lumen size is decreased in the hypertensive vascular bed. As the smooth muscle cells contract, the increase in vessel wall thickness increases the resistance, which is inversely proportional to the fourth power of the radius of the lumen. Note that at the average resting muscular tone, the resistance in hypertensive persons is considerably higher than normal.

of hypertension has helped identify genes that may contribute to control of blood pressure. Three inherited monogenic forms of hypertension have been defined:

- **Glucocorticoid-remediable aldosteronism (GRA):** GRA is an autosomal dominant trait in which congenital hypertension is mediated by the mineralocorticoid receptor in the kidney. Here, excess aldosterone production is prompted by corticotropin (or adrenocorticotropic hormone [ACTH]) rather than by the normal secretagogue for aldosterone, angiotensin II. The aldosterone synthase gene on chromosome 8 is normally expressed in the adrenal glomerulosa, where its product catalyzes the biosynthesis of aldosterone. This gene is 95% homologous with the steroid 11 β-hydroxylase gene, which regulates adrenal cortisol biosynthesis. Nearby on the same chromosome, mutations in aldosterone synthase and 11 β-hydroxylase genes create a hybrid gene, with ectopic production of aldosterone in the zona fasciculata under the control of ACTH. In turn, the unrestrained secretion of mineralocorticoids leads to prolonged volume expansion and hypertension.
- **Syndrome of apparent mineralocorticoid excess (AME):** In this autosomal recessive form of early-onset hypertension, the mineralocorticoid receptor is stimulated despite very low levels of aldosterone. Under normal circumstances, the mineralocorticoid receptor responds not only to aldosterone but also, albeit much more weakly, to cortisol. Cortisol's aldosterone-like activity is suppressed when 11 β-hydroxysteroid dehydrogenase in renal tubular epithelial cells converts it to cortisone. In AME, inactivating mutations in the gene for this enzyme allow cortisol to accumulate and constitutively stimulate the mineralocorticoid receptor. Interestingly, the consumption of large quantities of licorice can produce a syndrome similar to AME, because licorice contains glycyrrhetinic acid, which inhibits 11 β-hydroxysteroid dehydrogenase.
- **Liddle syndrome:** This autosomal dominant form of hypertension stems from a "gain-of-function" mutation in the gene on chromosome 16 that codes for the amiloride-sensitive epithelial sodium channel. Patients have constitutively activated renal tubule sodium channels but low levels of mineralocorticoids. Sustained channel activation leads to excessive renal reabsorption of salt and water, independent of mineralocorticoids, causing volume expansion and hypertension.

All mutations that cause hereditary hypertension result in constitutively increased renal sodium reabsorption. Conversely, mutations that result in sodium wastage (pseudohypoaldosteronism type I and Gitelman syndrome) are associated with profound hypotension. *Thus, these Mendelian disorders illustrate the central role for sodium homeostasis in determining blood pressure.*

Increasing evidence indicates that common polymorphisms of the angiotensinogen gene contribute to essential hypertension. Three findings buttress the potential importance of angiotensinogen variants: (1) the angiotensinogen locus is linked to elevated blood pressure in sibling pairs, (2) specific angiotensinogen variants have been tied to hypertension in case-control studies, and (3) the same variants are associated with increased plasma angiotensinogen.

Acquired Causes of Hypertension

Causes of hypertension are identifiable in a small proportion of cases. These include renal artery stenosis, most forms of chronic renal disease, including diabetes mellitus, primary elevation of aldosterone levels (Conn syndrome), Cushing syndrome, pheochromocytoma, hyperthyroidism, coarctation of the aorta, and renin-secreting tumors. In addition, persons with severe atherosclerosis may have high systolic pressure, because a sclerotic aorta cannot properly absorb the kinetic energy of the pulse wave, and renovascular hypertension is more common.

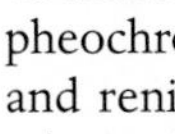

PATHOLOGY: The central lesion in most cases of hypertension is compromised lumens of small muscular arteries and arterioles (see Fig. 10-25). These resistance vessels control blood flow through the capillary beds. The lumen may be restricted by active contraction of the vessel wall, in-

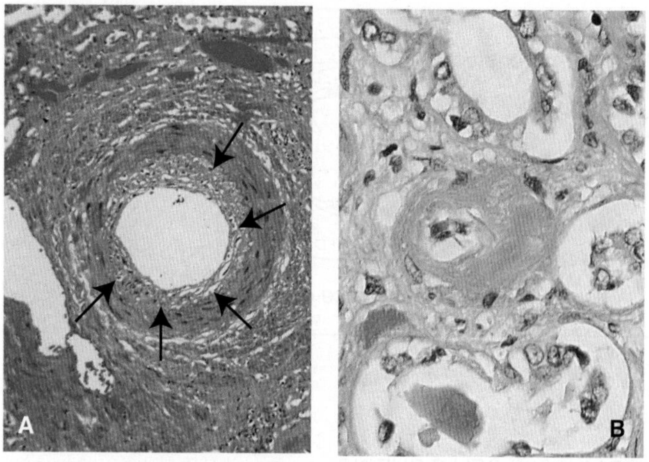

FIGURE 10-26. **Benign arteriosclerosis. A.** A cross-section of a renal intralobular shows irregular thickening of the intima *(arrows)*. **B.** A renal arteriole exhibits hyaline arteriolosclerosis.

creased mass of the vessel wall or both. Structural changes in hypertension have been shown by morphometric analysis of arterial walls. Structurally thicker vessel walls would be expected to narrow vascular lumens more than would normal, thinner walls. The rapid drop in blood pressure after treatment of hypertensive animals or persons with smooth muscle relaxants suggests that active constriction is very important.

Arteriosclerosis

Chronic hypertension leads to reactive changes in smaller arteries and arterioles throughout the body, collectively termed **arteriosclerosis**. In the arterioles, the alterations are termed *arteriolosclerosis*.

BENIGN ARTERIOSCLEROSIS: This condition reflects mild chronic hypertension, and the major change is a variable increased arterial wall thickness (Fig. 10-26A). In the smallest arteries and arterioles, these lesions are referred to as **hyaline arteriosclerosis** and **arteriolosclerosis**. "Hyaline" refers to the glassy, scarred appearance of the blood vessel walls as seen by light microscopy. Arteriolar walls are thickened by deposition of basement membrane material and accumulation of plasma proteins (see Fig. 10-26B). The small muscular arteries display new layers of elastin, manifesting as reduplication of the intimal elastic lamina and increased connective tissue. The vascular lesions of benign arteriosclerosis are particularly evident in the kidney, where they result in loss of renal parenchyma, termed **benign nephrosclerosis** (see Chapter 17).

A finding of benign arteriosclerosis is not diagnostic of hypertension: comparable morphologic alterations commonly occur as part of the aging process. However, hyaline arteriosclerosis is accelerated in diabetes and hypertension, diseases also associated with accelerated atherosclerosis.

MALIGNANT (ACCELERATED) HYPERTENSION: In malignant hypertension, elevated blood pressure causes rapidly progressive vascular compromise, with the onset of symptomatic disease of the brain, heart, or kidney. Although malignant hypertension cannot be defined strictly by the degree of blood pressure elevation, it is ordinarily not associated with pressures below 160/110 mm Hg. Modern antihypertensive therapy has made malignant hypertension a rare disorder.

Malignant hypertension produces dramatic microvascular pathologic changes. Segmental constriction and dilation of retinal arterioles in severely hypertensive persons are sufficiently prominent to allow one to make the diagnosis by ophthalmoscopy. If blood pressure rises rapidly, retinal arterioles show microaneurysms, focal hemorrhages, and scarring of the retina. Ischemic necrosis and edema of the retina are visible with the ophthalmoscope as "cotton wool spots" (see Chapter 29). These retinal changes are typical of those in other resistance vessels when the pressure rises rapidly.

In malignant hypertension, small muscular arteries show segmental dilation due to necrosis of smooth muscle cells. Endothelial integrity is lost in these regions, and increased vascular permeability leads to entry of plasma proteins into the vessel wall, deposition of fibrin, and an appearance termed **fibrinoid necrosis**. The period of acute injury is rapidly followed by smooth muscle proliferation and a striking concentric increase in the number of layers of smooth muscle cells, which yields the so-called onion-skin appearance (Fig. 10-27). This form of smooth muscle proliferation may be a response to the release of growth factors derived from platelets and other cells at sites of vascular injury. Together, these changes are labeled **malignant arteriosclerosis** or **arteriolosclerosis**, depending on the size of the vessels affected. In the kidney, lesions of malignant hypertension are known as **malignant nephrosclerosis**.

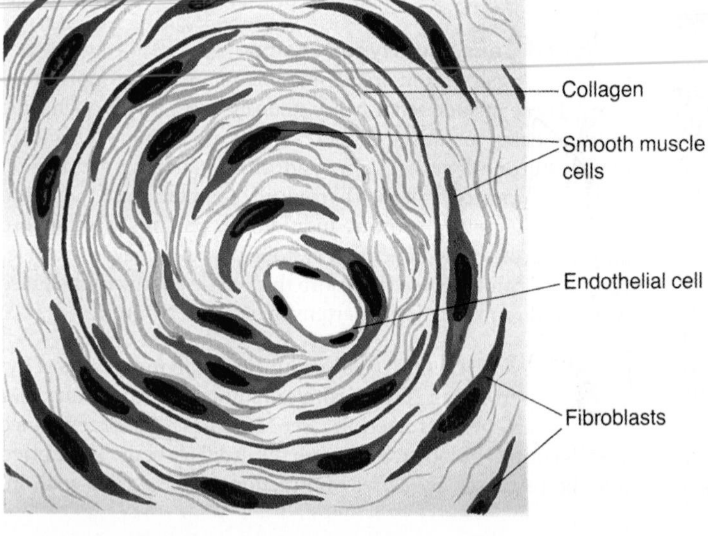

FIGURE 10-27. **Arteriolosclerosis.** In cases of hypertension, the arterioles exhibit smooth muscle cell proliferation and increased amounts of intercellular collagen and glycosaminoglycans, resulting in an "onion-skin" appearance. The mass of smooth muscle and associated elements tends to fix the size of the lumen and restrict the arteriole's capacity to dilate.

Mönckeberg Medial Sclerosis

Mönckeberg medial sclerosis refers to degenerative calcification of the media of large and medium-sized muscular arteries. The disorder occurs principally in older persons and most often involves arteries of the upper and lower extremities.

PATHOLOGY: Involved arteries are hard and dilated. Microscopically, the smooth muscle of the media is focally replaced by pale-staining, acellular, hyalinized fibrous tissue, with concentric dystrophic calcification. Osseous metaplasia in calcified areas is occasionally observed. Mönckeberg medial sclerosis is distinct from atherosclerosis and ordinarily does not lead to any clinical disorder.

Raynaud Phenomenon

Raynaud phenomenon refers to intermittent, bilateral attacks of ischemia of the fingers or toes, and sometimes ears or nose. It is characterized by severe pallor (Fig. 10-28) and often accompanied by paresthesias and pain. Symptoms are precipitated by cold or emotional stimuli and relieved by heat.

Raynaud phenomenon may occur as an isolated disorder or as a part of a number of systemic diseases of connective tissue (collagen vascular disorders), particularly scleroderma and systemic lupus erythematosus. The entity includes primary and secondary cold sensitivity, livedo reticularis, and acrocyanosis. Whatever the cause, Raynaud phenomenon reflects arterial vasospasm in the skin.

Primary cold sensitivity of the Raynaud type is more common in women, often starting in the late teens. It is bilateral and symmetric and, on rare occasions, may lead to ulcers or gangrene of the tips of digits. The hands are more commonly affected than feet.

Fibromuscular Dysplasia

Fibromuscular dysplasia is a rare, noninflammatory thickening of large and medium-sized muscular arteries, which is distinct from atherosclerosis and arteriosclerosis. The cause is unknown. In renal arteries, stenosis produced by this condition is an important cause of renovascular hypertension, although fibromuscular dysplasia may affect almost any other vessel, including carotid, vertebral, and splanchnic arteries. It is typically a disease of women during their reproductive years, but it can appear at any age, even in childhood.

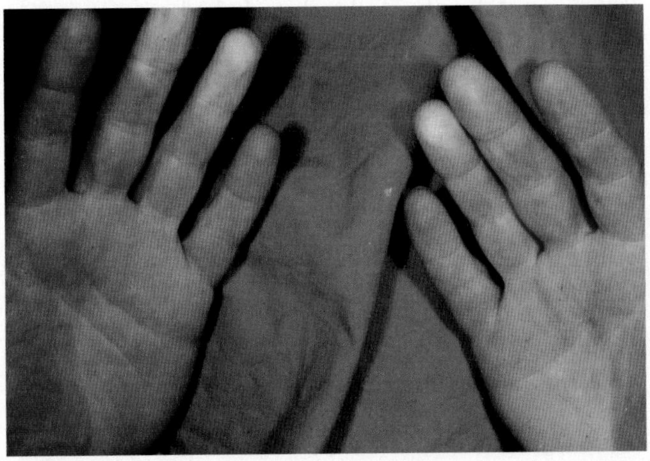

FIGURE 10-28. **Raynaud phenomenon.** The tips of the fingers show marked pallor.

TABLE 10-8

Inflammatory Disorders of Blood Vessels

Polyarteritis nodosa group of systemic necrotizing vasculitis	
	Classic polyarteritis nodosa
	Allergic angiitis and granulomatosis (Churg-Strauss variant)
	"Overlap syndrome" of systemic angiitis
Hypersensitivity vasculitis	
	Serum sickness and similar reactions
	Henoch-Schönlein purpura
	Vasculitis associated with connective tissue disorders
	Vasculitis in cases of essential mixed cryoglobulinemia
	Vasculitis associated with other primary disorders
Wegener granulomatosis	
Lymphomatoid granulomatosis	
Giant cell arteritis	
	Temporal arteritis
	Takayasu arteritis
Central nervous system vasculitis	
Vasculitis associated with cancer	
Mucocutaneous lymph node syndrome (Kawasaki disease)	
Thromboangiitis obliterans (Buerger disease)	
Behçet disease	
Miscellaneous vasculitis syndromes	

PATHOLOGY: In most cases, the distal two-thirds of the renal artery and its primary branches display several segmental stenoses, which represent fibrous and muscular ridges that project into the lumen. Microscopically, these segments exhibit a disorderly arrangement and proliferation of the cellular elements of the vessel wall, without necrosis or inflammation. Smooth muscle is replaced by fibrous tissue and myofibroblasts. In some cases, intimal fibroplasia predominates and in unusual instances, connective tissue encircles the adventitia. Other than renal hypertension, the major complication of fibromuscular dysplasia is dissecting aneurysm of the affected arteries.

Vasculitis

Vasculitis is inflammation and necrosis of blood vessels, and may affect arteries, veins, and capillaries (Table 10-8). Arteries or veins may be damaged by immune mechanisms, infectious agents, mechanical trauma, radiation, or toxins. However, in many cases, no specific cause is determined.

PATHOGENESIS: Vasculitic syndromes are thought to involve immune mechanisms, including (1) deposition of immune complexes, (2) direct attack on vessels by circulating antibodies, and (3) various forms of cell-mediated immunity. Although the agents responsible for inciting these reactions are largely unknown, there is evidence that in some instances it is associated with viral infection.

Serum sickness was one of the first human immunologic disorders to be linked with vasculitis. In animal models of serum sickness, immune complexes and complement are found in local tissue reaction (see Chapter 4). However, in most human cases, immune complexes are only sometimes present, and firm evidence for them in most cases of vasculitis is lacking.

Viral antigens may cause vasculitis in experimental animals and in humans, e.g., chronic infection with hepatitis B virus is associated with some cases of polyarteritis nodosa. In this case, viral antigen–antibody complexes circulate and are deposited in the vascular lesions. Human vasculitis has also been associated with other viral infections, including herpes simplex, cytomegalovirus, and parvovirus, and with several bacterial antigens as well.

Small vessel vasculitides (e.g., Wegener granulomatosis and microscopic polyarteritis; see below) are associated with antineutrophil cytoplasmic antibodies (ANCA), but the contributions of these autoantibodies to the pathogenesis of the vasculitis is not understood. ANCA may cause endothelial damage by activating neutrophils, and antibody titers correlate with disease activity in some cases. ANCA is detected by indirect immunofluorescence assays using the patient's serum and ethanol-fixed neutrophils. Common patterns include a perinuclear immunofluorescence (P-ANCA, mainly against myeloperoxidase) and a more general cytoplasmic immunofluorescence (C-ANCA, mainly against proteinase 3). Although the significance of ANCA requires further study, myeloperoxidase and proteinase 3 are expressed on the surface of neutrophils activated by cytokines in vitro, which then leads to degranulation.

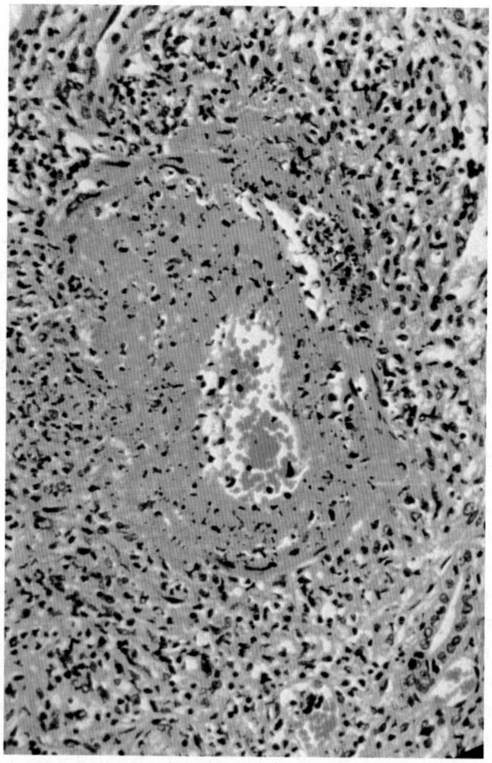

FIGURE 10-29. **Polyarteritis nodosa.** The intense inflammatory cell infiltrate in the arterial wall and surrounding connective tissue is associated with fibrinoid necrosis and disruption of the vessel wall.

Polyarteritis Nodosa Is an Acute, Necrotizing Vasculitis

Polyarteritis nodosa affects medium-sized and smaller muscular arteries, and occasionally larger arteries. It is somewhat more common in men than in women. The disease was regarded as a rarity until the 1940s, when there was a striking rise in its incidence. The increased frequency of polyarteritis nodosa at that time seemed to be associated with the widespread use of antisera to bacteria and toxins produced in animals and with use of sulfonamides. The incidence of polyarteritis nodosa now seems to be subsiding.

PATHOLOGY: The characteristic lesions of polyarteritis nodosa are found in small to medium-sized muscular arteries and are distributed in patchily. However, on occasion they extend into larger arteries, such as the renal, splenic, or coronary arteries. Each lesion is no more than a millimeter long and may involve the entire circumference of the vessel or only a part of it. The most prominent morphologic feature of the affected artery is an area of fibrinoid necrosis, in which the medial muscle and adjacent tissues are fused into a structureless eosinophilic mass that stains for fibrin. A vigorous acute inflammatory response envelops the area of necrosis, usually involving the entire adventitia (periarteritis), and extends through the other coats of the vessel (Fig. 10-29). Neutrophils, lymphocytes, plasma cells, and macrophages are present in varying proportions, and eosinophils are often conspicuous. Polyarteritis nodosa affecting small vessels is often associated with P-ANCA (see below).

As a result of thrombosis in affected segment of an artery, infarcts are commonly found in involved organs. Injury to larger arteries causes small aneurysms (<0.5 cm in diameter), particularly in branches of the renal, coronary, and cerebral arteries. An aneurysm may rupture and, if located in a critical area, may result in fatal hemorrhage.

If the patient survives for some months, many vascular lesions will show evidence of healing, especially if corticosteroids have been administered. The necrotic tissue and inflammatory exudate are resorbed, and the vessel is left with fibrosis of the media and conspicuous gaps in the elastic laminae.

CLINICAL FEATURES: Clinical manifestations of polyarteritis nodosa are highly variable, and depend on the chance locations of lesions in different organs. Kidneys, heart, skeletal muscle, skin, and mesentery are most frequently involved, but lesions may occur in almost any organ, including the bowel, pancreas, lungs, liver, and brain. Constitutional symptoms such as fever and weight loss are common.

Without treatment, polyarteritis nodosa is usually fatal, but antiinflammatory and immunosuppressive therapy, in the form of corticosteroids and cyclophosphamide, leads to remissions or cures in most patients.

Hypersensitivity Angiitis Is a Response to Exogenous Substances

Hypersensitivity angiitis refers to a broad category of inflammatory vascular lesions that are thought to represent a reaction to foreign materials (e.g., bacterial products or drugs). In the case of vascular lesions confined predominantly to skin, the terms **leukocytoclastic vasculitis** (referring to the nuclear debris from disintegrating neutrophils), **cutaneous vasculitis** *or* **cutaneous necrotizing venulitis** (emphasizing the predominant involvement of the venules) are applied. **Systemic hypersensitivity angiitis**, also referred to as **microscopic polyarteritis**, affects many of the same organs as polyarteritis nodosa but is restricted to the smallest arteries and arterioles.

CLINICAL FEATURES: Cutaneous vasculitis may follow administration of many drugs, including aspirin, penicillin, and thiazide diuretics. It is also commonly related to disparate infections such as streptococcal and staphylococcal illnesses, viral hepatitis, tuberculosis, and bacterial endocarditis. The disease typically presents as palpable purpura, principally on the lower extremities. Microscopically, superficial cutaneous venules display fibrinoid necrosis with acute inflammatory reaction. Cutaneous vasculitis is generally self-limited. A detailed description of this disease is found in Chapter 24.

Systemic hypersensitivity angiitis may be an isolated entity or a feature of other conditions, including collagen vascular diseases (lupus erythematosus, rheumatoid arthritis, Sjögren syndrome), Henoch-Schönlein purpura, dysproteinemias, and a variety of malignant neoplasms. Patients with systemic hypersensitivity angiitis may also have purpuric lesions in the skin. The most feared complication of microscopic polyarteritis is renal involvement, characterized by rapidly progressive glomerulonephritis and renal failure (see Chapter 16). Microscopic polyarteritis is strongly associated with the presence of ANCA (60% P-ANCA and 40% C-ANCA).

Allergic Granulomatosis and Angiitis (Churg-Strauss Syndrome) is a Systemic Vasculitis that Occurs in Young Persons with Asthma

Two thirds of patients have C-ANCA or P-ANCA.

PATHOLOGY: Widespread necrotizing lesions of the small and medium-sized arteries (Fig. 10-30), arterioles, and veins are found in the lungs, spleen, kidney, heart, liver, CNS, and other organs. These lesions are granulomas and an intense eosinophilic infiltrates in and around blood vessels. The resulting fibrinoid necrosis, thrombosis and aneurysm formation may simulate polyarteritis nodosa, although Churg-Strauss syndrome seems to be a distinct entity. It must also be distinguished from other eosinophilic syndromes, such as parasitic and fungal infestations, Wegener granulomatosis, eosinophilic pneumonia (Loeffler syndrome), and drug vasculitis.

Untreated persons with allergic granulomatosis and angiitis have a poor prognosis, but corticosteroids are now almost always successful in treating the disease.

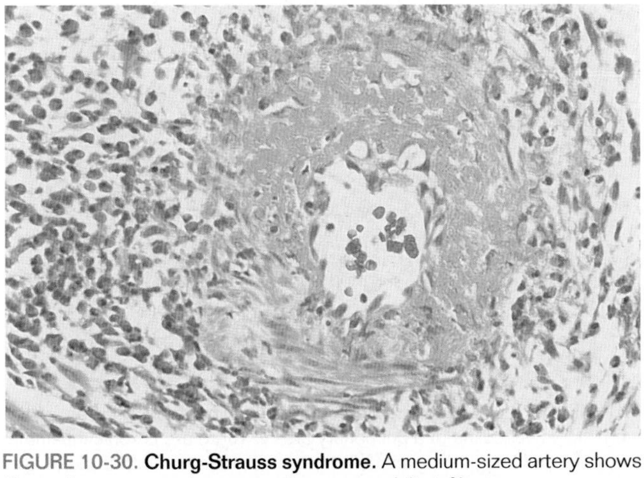

FIGURE 10-30. **Churg-Strauss syndrome.** A medium-sized artery shows fibrinoid necrosis and a surrounding eosinophilic infiltrate.

Giant Cell Arteritis (Temporal Arteritis, Granulomatous Arteritis) Is the Most Common Vasculitis

Giant cell arteritis is focal, chronic, granulomatous inflammation of the temporal arteries. Although it most often affects the temporal artery, it may also involve additional cranial arteries, the aorta (giant cell aortitis) and its branches and occasionally other arteries. Aortic aneurysm and dissection occur. The average age at onset is 70 years, and it is rare before age 50. Incidence rises with age and may reach 1% by 80 years of age. Women are slightly more often affected than men. The age at onset helps differentiate this entity from other vasculitides that may involve the same vessels, such as Takayasu disease, which occurs in much younger persons.

PATHOGENESIS: The etiology of giant cell arteritis is obscure. Its association with HLA-DR4 and its occurrence in first-degree relatives support a genetic component in its pathogenesis. The morphologic alterations, including the presence of activated CD4+ T-helper cells and macrophages, and association of giant cell arteritis with a specific polymorphism of the leukocyte adhesion molecule ICAM-1, suggest an immunologic reaction. B-lymphocytes are lacking. Macrophages at the border of the intima and media produce MMPs which digest matrix. ANCA is not detected in giant cell arteritis. Generalized muscle aching and widespread distribution of its manifestations are consistent with a relationship to rheumatoid diseases.

PATHOLOGY: In giant cell arteritis, affected vessels are cordlike and show nodular thickening. The lumen is reduced to a slit or may be obliterated by a thrombus (Fig. 10-31A). Microscopically, there is granulomatous inflammation of the media and intima, consisting of aggregates of macrophages, lymphocytes, and plasma cells, with varying admixtures of eosinophils and neutrophils. Giant cells tend to be distributed at the internal elastic lamina (see Fig. 10-31B) but vary widely in number. Both foreign-body giant cells and Langhans giant cells may be found. Foci of necrosis are characterized by changes in the internal elastica, which becomes swollen, irregular, and fragmented, and in advanced lesions may completely disappear. Fragments of the elastica occasionally appear in the giant cells. In the late stages, the intima is conspicuously thickened, and the media is fibrotic. Thrombosis may obliterate the lumen, after which organization and canalization occur.

CLINICAL FEATURES: Giant cell arteritis tends to be benign and self-limited, and symptoms subside in 6 to 12 months. Patients present with headache and throbbing temporal pain. In some instances, there are early constitutional symptoms, including malaise, fever, and weight loss, plus generalized muscular aching or stiffness in shoulders and hips. Throbbing and pain over the temporal artery are accompanied by swelling, tenderness, and redness in overlying skin. Visual symptoms occur in almost half of patients and may proceed from transient to permanent blindness in one or both eyes, sometimes rapidly. Occasionally, the disease causes infarcts in the myocardium, brain, or gastrointestinal tract, which may be fatal. Because the inflammatory process is not continuous, but

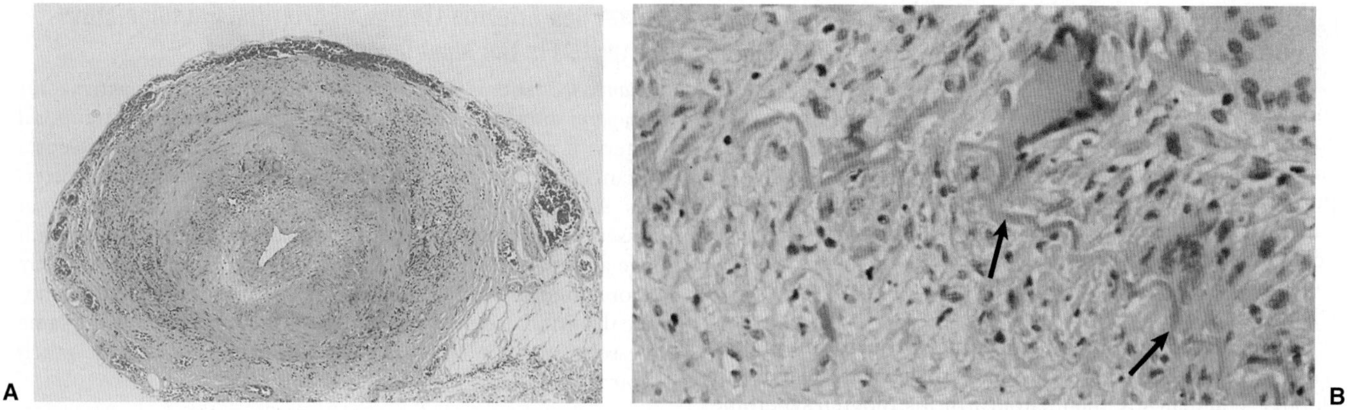

FIGURE 10-31. **Temporal arteritis. A.** A photomicrograph of a temporal artery shows chronic inflammation throughout the wall, giant cells, and a lumen severely narrowed by intimal thickening. **B.** A high-power view shows giant cells adjacent to the fragmented internal elastic lamina *(arrows)*.

rather skips areas of the temporal artery, biopsy of temporal artery may not be diagnostic in as many as 40% of patients with otherwise classic manifestations. The response to corticosteroid therapy is usually dramatic, and symptoms subside within days.

Wegener Granulomatosis Is a Vasculitis of the Respiratory Tract and Kidney

Wegener granulomatosis is a systemic necrotizing vasculitis of unknown etiology characterized by granulomatous lesions of the nose, sinuses, and lungs and renal glomerular disease. Men are affected more often than women, usually in the fifth and sixth decades of life. The etiology of the disease is unknown. More than 90% of patients with Wegener granulomatosis exhibit ANCA, of whom 75% have C-ANCA. It has been suggested that these antibodies activate circulating neutrophils to attack blood vessels. The response to immunosuppressive therapy supports an immunologic basis for the disease.

PATHOLOGY: The lesions of Wegener granulomatosis feature parenchymal necrosis, vasculitis and a granulomatous inflammation composed of neutrophils, lymphocytes, plasma cells, macrophages, and eosinophils. Individual lesions in the lung may be as large as 5 cm across and must be distinguished from tuberculosis. Vasculitis involving small arteries and veins may be seen anywhere but occurs most frequently in the respiratory tract (Fig. 10-32), kidney and spleen. Arteritis is characterized principally by chronic inflammation, although acute inflammation, necrotizing and nonnecrotizing granulomatous inflammation, and fibrinoid necrosis are frequently present. Medial thickening and intimal proliferation are common and often lead to narrowing or obliteration of the lumen.

The most prominent pulmonary feature is persistent bilateral pneumonitis, with nodular infiltrates that undergo cavitation similarly to tuberculous lesions (although the mechanisms are clearly different). Chronic sinusitis and ulcers of the nasopharyngeal mucosa are common. The kidney at first shows focal necrotizing glomerulonephritis, which progresses to crescentic glomerulonephritis (see Chapter 17).

CLINICAL FEATURES: Most patients present with symptoms referable to the respiratory tract, particularly pneumonitis and sinusitis. In fact, the lung is eventually involved in over 90% of patients. Radiologically, multiple pulmonary infiltrates are prominent, which are often cavitary. Hematuria and proteinuria are common, and glomerular disease can progress to renal failure. Rash, muscular pains, joint involvement, and neurologic symptoms occur. In untreated Wegener granulomatosis, most persons (80%) die within a year of onset, with a mean survival of 5 to 6 months. Treatment with cyclophosphamide produces both complete remissions and substantial disease-free intervals in most patients. Interestingly, administration of antimicrobial sulfa drugs significantly reduces the incidence of relapses, suggesting a relationship of the disease to bacterial infections.

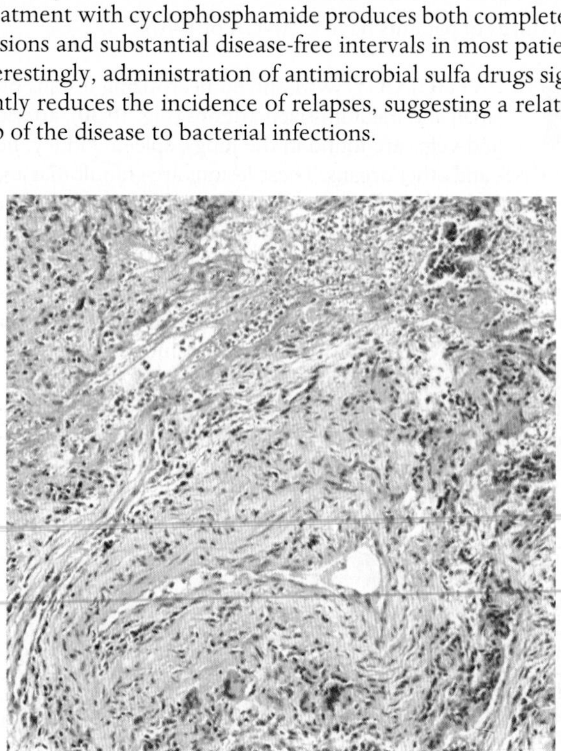

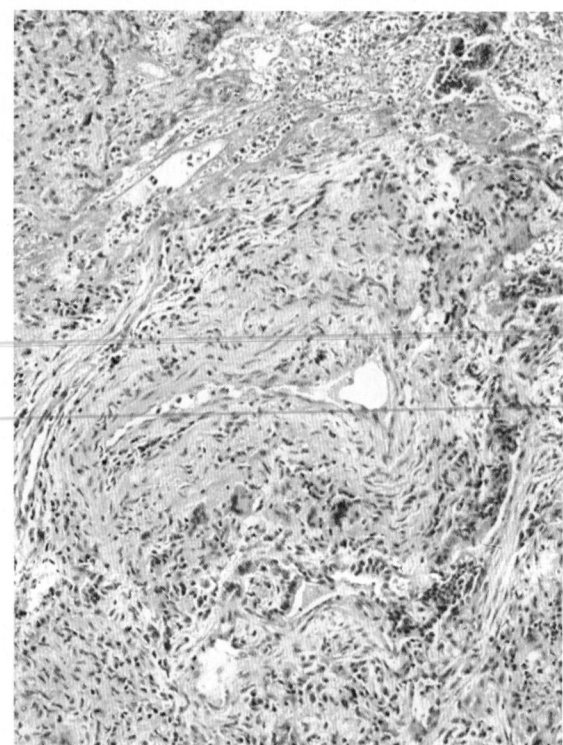

FIGURE 10-32. **Wegener granulomatosis.** A photomicrograph of the lung shows vasculitis of a pulmonary artery. There are chronic inflammatory cells and Langhans giant cells in the wall, together with thickening of the intima.

Takayasu Arteritis is an Inflammatory Disease Affecting the Aorta and its Major Branches

This form of arteritis is seen worldwide, and mainly affects women (90%), most of whom are under 30 years of age. The cause of Takayasu arteritis is unknown, but an autoimmune basis has been proposed.

PATHOLOGY: Takayasu arteritis is classified according to the extent of aortic involvement: (1) disease restricted to the aortic arch and its branches, (2) arteritis involving only the descending thoracic and abdominal aorta and its branches, and (3) combined involvement of the arch and descending aorta. The pulmonary artery is also occasionally affected and involvement of the retinal vasculature is often a prominent feature.

On gross examination, the aorta is thickened, and the intima exhibits focal, raised plaques. The branches of the aorta often display localized stenosis or occlusion, which interferes with blood flow and accounts for the synonym "**pulseless disease**" when the subclavian arteries are affected. The aorta, particularly the distal thoracic and abdominal segments, commonly shows variably sized aneurysms. The early lesions of the aorta and its main branches consist of an acute panarteritis, with infiltrates of neutrophils, mononuclear cells, and occasional Langhans giant cells. Inflammation of the vasa vasorum in Takayasu arteritis requires differentiation from syphilitic aortitis. Late lesions display fibrosis and severe intimal proliferation. Secondary atherosclerotic changes may obscure the basic disease.

CLINICAL FEATURES: Patients with early Takayasu arteritis complain of constitutional symptoms, dizziness, visual disturbances, dyspnea, and occasionally syncope. As the disease progresses, cardiac symptoms become more severe with intermittent claudication of the arms or legs. Asymmetric differences in blood pressure may develop and the pulse in one extremity may actually disappear. Hypertension may reflect coarctation of the aorta or renal artery stenosis. Most patients eventually show congestive heart failure. They may lose visual acuity, ranging from field defects to total blindness. Early Takayasu arteritis responds to corticosteroids, but the later lesions require surgical reconstruction.

Kawasaki Disease (Mucocutaneous Lymph Node Syndrome) Is a Childhood Vasculitis That Targets Coronary Arteries

Kawasaki disease is an acute necrotizing vasculitis of infancy and early childhood characterized by high fever, rash, conjunctival and oral lesions, and lymphadenitis. In 70% of patients, the vasculitis affects the coronary arteries and leads to coronary artery aneurysms (Fig. 10-33), which may cause death in 1% to 2% of cases.

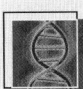

PATHOGENESIS: Kawasaki disease is usually self-limited. Although an infectious cause has been sought, none has been conclusively proved. Infection with *parvovirus B19* or with *New Haven coronavirus* has been implicated in some cases, and there is evidence for various bacterial infections including staphylococcus, streptococcus, and chlamydia, in others. The common theme seems to be viral or bacterial production of superantigens, i.e., molecules that bind to major histocompatability complex (MHC) class II receptors and the V-beta region of the T cell receptor, thereby massively the immune system in an antigen-nonspecific manner. Autoantibodies to endothelial and smooth muscle cells have been identified in some patients.

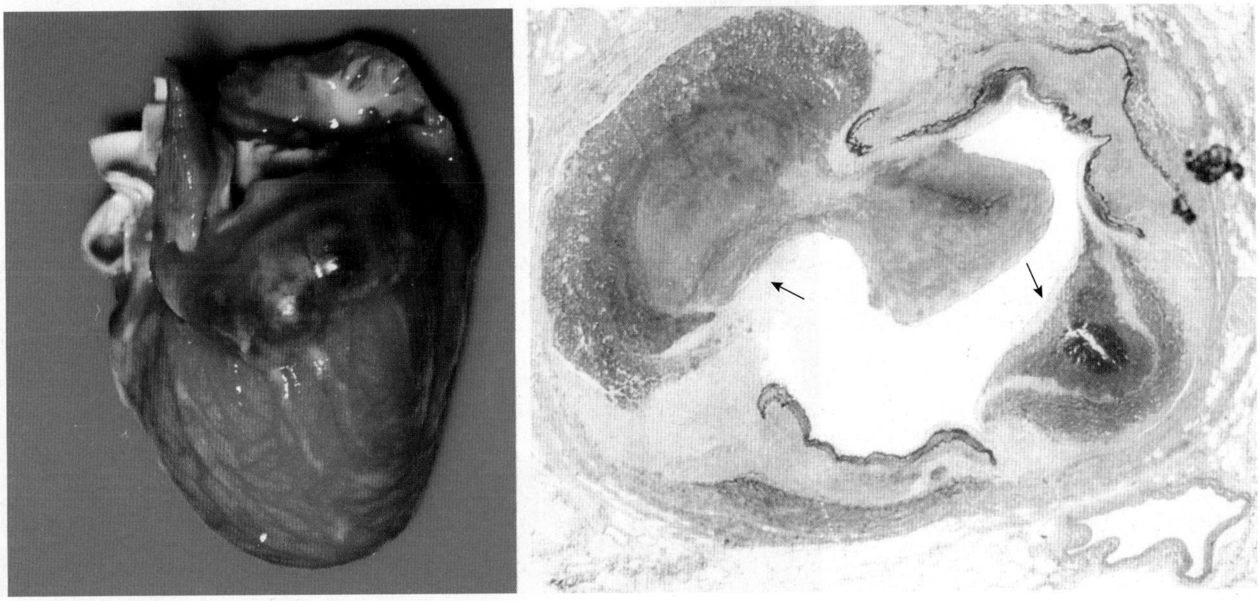

A B

FIGURE 10-33. **Kawasaki disease. A.** The heart of a child who died from Kawasaki disease shows conspicuous coronary artery aneurysms. **B.** A microscopic section of a coronary artery from the same patient shows two large defects *(arrows)* in the internal elastic lamina, with two small aneurysms filled with thrombus.

Thromboangiitis Obliterans (Buerger Disease) is a Peripheral Vascular Disease of Smokers

It is an occlusive inflammatory disease of medium and small arteries in the distal arms and legs. At one time Buerger disease occurred almost exclusively in young and middle-aged men who smoked heavily, but it is now described in women as well. It is more prevalent in the Mediterranean area, Middle East, and Asia.

PATHOGENESIS: The etiologic role of smoking in Buerger disease is underscored by the fact that cessation of smoking may lead to remission, and resumption of smoking to exacerbation. Yet, how tobacco smoke produces Buerger disease is obscure. Certain polyphenols from tobacco elicit antibodies and can induce inflammation. Smokers show a higher incidence of such sensitivity to tobacco than do nonsmokers. Cell-mediated hypersensitivity to collagen types II and III has also been observed. Endothelium-dependent vasodilatory responses in nondiseased blood vessels are dysfunctional in some patients, suggesting that there may be a generalized impairment of endothelial function. HLA-A9 and HLA-B5 haplotypes are more common among patients with the disease, further suggesting that a genetically controlled hypersensitivity to tobacco is involved in the pathogenesis of disease.

PATHOLOGY: The earliest change in Buerger disease is an acute inflammation of medium-sized and small arteries. The neutrophilic infiltrate extends to involve neighboring veins and nerves. The involvement of the endothelium in inflamed areas leads to thrombosis and obliteration of the lumen (Fig. 10-34A). Small microabscesses of the vessel wall, featuring a central area of neutrophils surrounded by fibroblasts and Langhans giant cells, distinguish the process from thrombosis associated with atherosclerosis. The early lesions often become severe enough to result in gangrene of the extremity, for which the only treatment is amputation. Late in the course of the disease, the thrombi are completely organized and partly canalized.

CLINICAL FEATURES: Symptoms of Buerger disease usually start between the ages of 25 and 40 and take the form of intermittent claudication (cramping pains in muscles after exercise, quickly relieved by rest). Patients often present with painful ulceration of a digit, which progresses to destruction of the tips of the involved digits (see Fig. 10-34B). Persons with Buerger disease who continue to smoke may slowly lose both hands and feet.

Behçet Disease Is a Vasculitis Mainly Involving Mucous Membranes of Many Organs

Behçet disease *is a systemic vasculitis characterized by oral aphthous ulcers, genital ulceration, and ocular inflammation and occasionally lesions in the CNS, gastrointestinal tract, and cardiovascular system.* Both large and small vessels display vasculitis. The mucocutaneous lesions show a nonspecific vasculitis of arterioles, capillaries, and venules, with infiltration of vessel walls and perivascular tissue by lymphocytes and plasma cells. Occasional endothelial cells are proliferated and swollen. Medium and large arteries show destructive arteritis, with fibrinoid necrosis, mononuclear infiltration, thrombosis, aneurysms, and hemorrhage. The cause is unknown, but an association with specific HLA subtypes suggests an immune basis. The disease often responds to corticosteroids.

Radiation Vasculitis Has Acute and Chronic Phases

The acute phase of radiation vasculitis shows endothelial injury and denudation, ballooning degeneration of intimal smooth muscle cells and macrophages, and medial smooth muscle cell necrosis, which may be fibrinoid. Thrombosis may be present

A
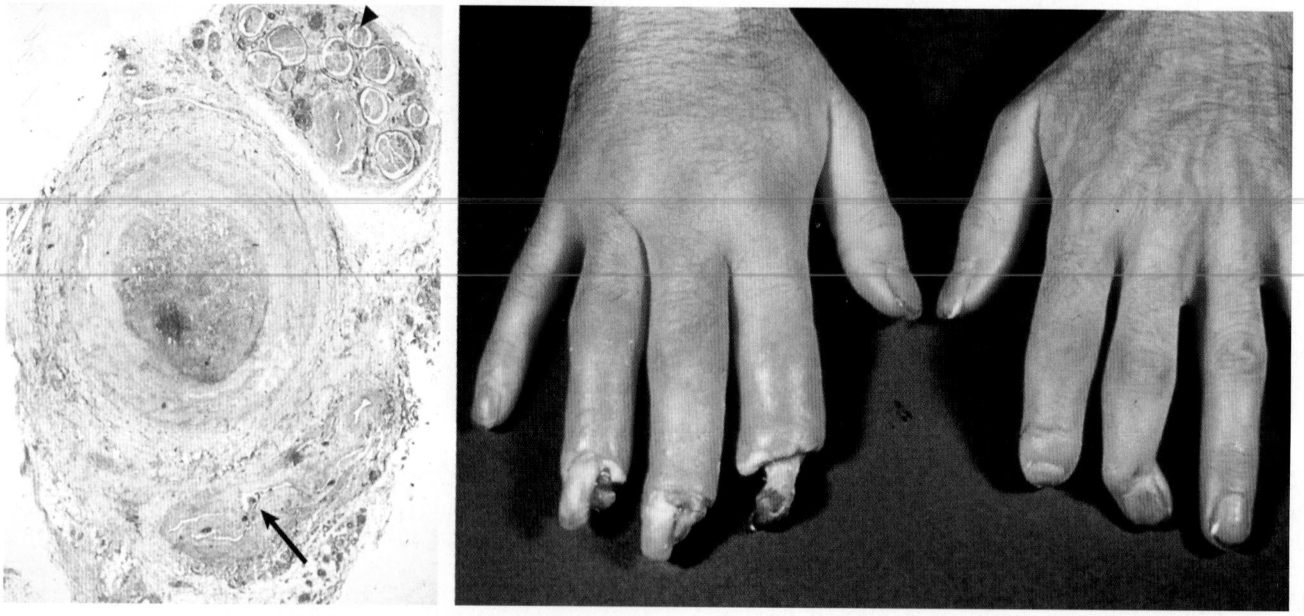
B

FIGURE 10-34. **Buerger disease. A.** Section of the upper extremity shows an organized arterial thrombus that has occluded the lumen. Some inflammatory cells are evident in the adventitial fat. In this instance, the vein *(arrow)* and the adjacent nerve *(arrowhead)* show foci of chronic inflammation. **B.** The hand shows necrosis of the tips of the fingers.

in small arteries and arterioles. In the chronic phase, intimal hyperplasia and fibrosis of the vessel wall are noted. Occasionally the vessel shows complete fibrous occlusion. Radiation damage predisposes to accelerated atherosclerosis.

Rickettsial Vasculitis Is Caused by Intracellular Parasites

Rickettsiae are obligate intracellular parasites that produce a characteristic vasculitis. The vasculitis in each of the different rickettsial diseases affects different types of small vessels and its extent and severity varies. In general, the organisms disseminate from the entry site into the bloodstream and invade endothelial cells, smooth muscle cells of the media of small vessels and capillaries. These infections are discussed in detail in Chapter 9.

Aneurysms

Arterial aneurysms are localized dilations of blood vessels caused by a congenital or acquired weakness of the media. They are not rare, and their incidence tends to rise with age. Aneurysms of the aorta and other arteries are found in as many as 10% of autopsies. The wall of an aneurysm is formed by the stretched remnants of the arterial wall.

Aneurysms are classified by location, configuration, and etiology (Fig. 10-35). The location refers to the type of vessel involved—artery or vein—and the specific vessel affected, such as the aorta or popliteal artery. The gross morphology of aneurysms reveals several different pathologic features.

- **Fusiform aneurysm** is an ovoid swelling parallel to the long axis of the vessel.
- **Saccular aneurysm** is a bubble-like arterial wall outpouching at a site of weakened media.
- **Dissecting aneurysm** is actually a dissecting hematoma, in which blood from hemorrhage into the media separates the layers of the vascular wall.
- **Arteriovenous aneurysm** is a direct communication between an artery and a vein.

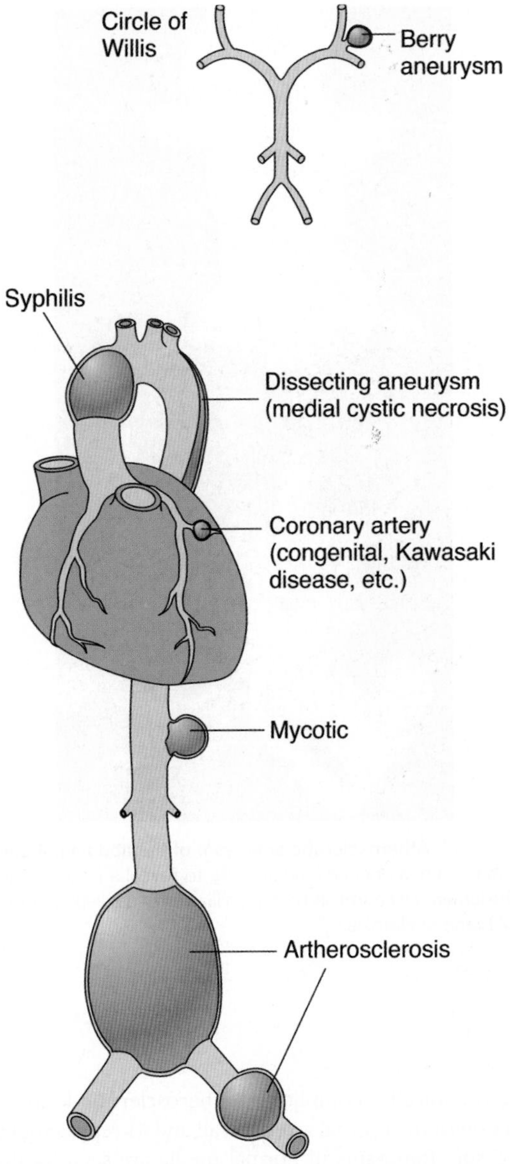

FIGURE 10-35. **The locations of aneurysms.** Syphilitic aneurysms are the common variety in the ascending aorta, which is usually spared by the atherosclerotic process. Atherosclerotic aneurysms can occur in the abdominal aorta or muscular arteries, including the coronary and popliteal arteries and other vessels. Berry aneurysms are seen in the circle of Willis, mainly at branch points; their rupture leads to subarachnoid hemorrhage. Mycotic aneurysms occur almost anywhere that bacteria can deposit on vessel walls.

Abdominal Aortic Aneurysms Are Complications of Atherosclerosis

Abdominal aortic aneurysms are dilations that increase vessel wall diameter by at least 50%. They are the most frequent aneurysms, usually developing after the age of 50, and are associated with severe atherosclerosis of the artery. Prevalence rises to 6% after age 80. Aortic aneurysms occur much more often in men than in women, and half of patients are hypertensive. Occasionally, aneurysms are found in ascending, arch, and descending parts of the thoracic aorta, and in iliac and popliteal arteries.

Although abdominal aortic aneurysms invariably occur in the context of atherosclerosis, it is thought that the disease is actually multifactorial. Familial clustering suggests a genetic predisposition. A variety of changes in the extracellular matrix of the aortic wall have been described, including local dysfunction of elastolytic and collagenlytic activity in the wall. Inflammation or alterations in cell mediated immune responses have also been implicated in pathogenesis as have hemodynamic factors, especially hypertension.

PATHOLOGY: Most abdominal aortic aneurysms are distal to the renal arteries and proximal to the bifurcation (Fig. 10-36). They are usually fusiform, although saccular varieties are occasionally encountered. The lesions may be of almost any size, but most of the symptomatic ones are more than 5 to 6 cm in diameter. Some extend into the iliac arteries, which occasionally exhibit distinct aneurysms distal to the one in the aorta. Aneurysms that extend above the renal arteries may occlude the origin of the superior mesenteric artery and the celiac axis.

Most abdominal aortic aneurysms are lined by raised, ulcerated, and calcified (complicated) atherosclerotic lesions. Most contain mural thrombi of varying degrees of organization. portions of which may embolize to peripheral arteries. Infrequently, the thrombus itself may enlarge enough to compromise the lumen of the aorta.

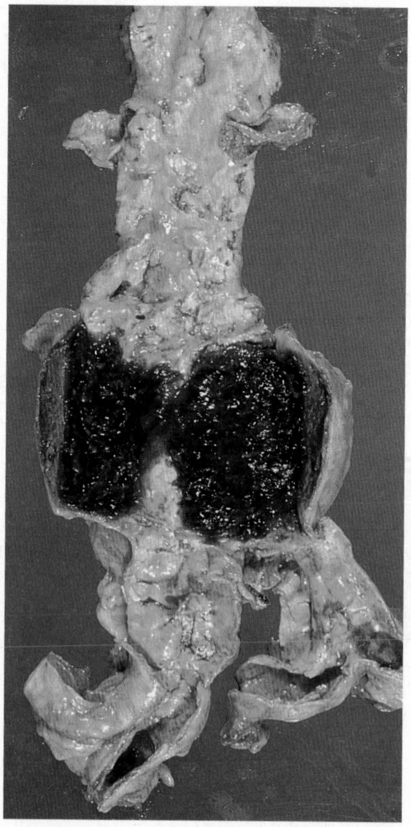

FIGURE 10-36. **Atherosclerotic aneurysm of the abdominal aorta.** The aneurysm has been opened longitudinally to reveal a large mural thrombus in the lumen. The aorta and common iliac arteries display complicated lesions of atherosclerosis.

Microscopically, complicated atherosclerotic lesions show destruction of the normal arterial wall and its replacement by fibrous tissue. Remnants of normal media are seen focally, and atheromatous lesions extend to variable depths. The adventitia is thickened and focally inflamed, as a response to severe atherosclerosis.

CLINICAL FEATURES: Many abdominal aortic aneurysms are asymptomatic and are discovered only by palpation of a mass in the abdomen or on radiologic examination for some other reason. In some cases the condition is brought to medical attention by the onset of abdominal pain, which often reflects aneurysmal expansion. Abrupt occlusion of a peripheral artery by an embolus from the mural thrombus presents as sudden ischemia of a lower limb. The most dreaded complication of aortic aneurysms is rupture and exsanguinating retroperitoneal (or thoracic) hemorrhage, in which case the patient presents with pain, shock, and a pulsatile mass in the abdomen. Such a situation is an acute emergency and even with prompt surgical intervention, half of patients die. Therefore, large aneurysms, even if entirely asymptomatic, are often replaced by or bypassed with prosthetic grafts.

The risk of rupture of an abdominal aortic aneurysm is a function of its size. Aneurysms under 4 cm in diameter rarely rupture (2%), while 25% to 40% of those larger than 5 cm rupture within 5 years of their discovery.

Aneurysms of Cerebral Arteries Lead to Subarachnoid Hemorrhage

The most common type of cerebral aneurysm is saccular and is called a **berry aneurysm**, because it resembles a berry attached to a twig of the arterial tree. It results from a congenital defect in a branch point of the arterial wall. Berry aneurysms tend to arise at branching angles in the circle of Willis or in one of the arterial branches. The most common sites are (1) between the anterior cerebral artery and the anterior communicating artery, (2) between the internal carotid artery and the posterior communicating artery, and (3) between the first main divisions of the middle cerebral artery and the bifurcation of the internal carotid artery. Berry aneurysms are discussed in detail in Chapter 28.

Dissecting Aneurysm Is a Hematoma of the Aortic Wall

Blood enters into the arterial wall and separates the layers of the wall as it dissects a path along the length of the vessel (Fig. 10-37). The dissection is essentially a false lumen within the wall of the artery. Although this lesion is conventionally termed an aneurysm, it is actually a form of hematoma. Dissecting aneurysms most often affect the aorta and its major branches. Their frequency has been estimated to be as high as 1 in 400 autopsies, with men affected three times as frequently as women. They may occur at almost any age, but are most common in the sixth and seventh decades. Most patients have histories of hypertension.

PATHOGENESIS: The basis of dissecting aneurysms is usually weakening of the aortic media. The changes were originally described as **cystic medial necrosis (of Erdheim)**, because focal loss of elastic and muscle fibers in the media leads to "cystic" spaces filled with a metachromatic myxoid material. These spaces are not true cysts but are rather pools of matrix collected between the cells and tissues of the media. The cause of medial degeneration is not known. Some cases are complications of Marfan syndrome, a systemic connective tissue disorder caused by mutations in the gene encoding the extracelluar matrix protein, fibrillin (see Chapter 6). Aging also results in mild degenerative changes in the aorta, characterized by focal elastin loss and medial fibrosis. Patients with dissection of the thoracic aorta show decreased expression of fibulin-5 and extracellular protein that regulates elastic fiber assembly. Disruption in the release of MMP-2 and its inhibitor by smooth muscle cells have been implicated in aortic aneurysms. In animals, defective cross-linking of collagen induced by a copper-deficient diet (lysyl oxidase is a copper-dependent enzyme) causes dissecting aneurysm of the aorta. The same lesion is produced by feeding β-aminopropionitrile, an inhibitor of lysyl oxidase. Persons with Wilson disease who are treated with penicillamine, a copper chelator, also may develop medial necrosis of the aorta. Taken together, these data suggest that the common factor in these several situations is a defect that leads to weakness of aortic connective tissue.

The initial event that triggers medial dissection is controversial. Over 95% of cases have a transverse tear in the intima and internal media, and it is widely held that spontaneous laceration of the intima allows blood from the lumen to enter and dissect the media. Alternatively, it has been proposed that hemorrhage from vasa vasorum into a

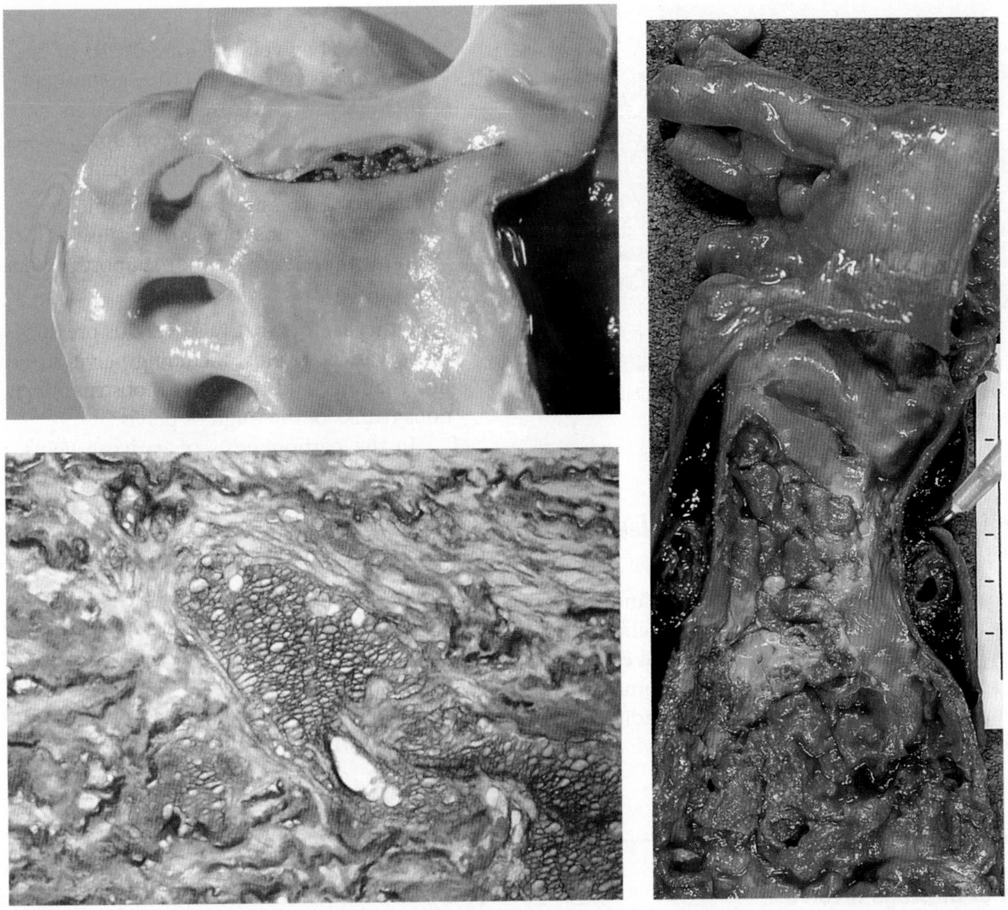

FIGURE 10-37. **Dissecting aneurysm of the aorta. A.** A transverse tear is present in the aortic arch. The orifices of the great vessels are on the *left*. **B.** The thoracic aorta has been open longitudinally and reveals clotted blood dissecting the media of the vessel. The luminal surface shows extensive complicated lesions of atherosclerosis. **C.** A section of the aortic wall stained with aldehyde fuchsin shows pools of metachromatic material characteristic of the degenerative process known as cystic medial necrosis.

media weakened by cystic medial necrosis initiates stress on the intima, which in turn leads to the ubiquitous intimal tear.

PATHOLOGY: Most intimal tears are in the ascending aorta, 1 or 2 cm above the aortic ring. Dissection in the media, occurs within seconds, and separates the inner two-thirds of the aorta from the outer third. It can also involve coronary arteries, great vessels of the neck, and renal, mesenteric, or iliac arteries. Since the outer wall of the false channel of the dissecting aneurysm is thin, hemorrhage into the extravascular space—including the pericardium, mediastinum, pleural space, and retroperitoneum—frequently causes death. In 5% to 10% of cases, the blood within the dissection reenters the lumen via a second distal tear to form a "double-barreled aorta." In a comparable proportion, a reentry site leads to communication of the aorta with a major artery, most often the iliac artery.

CLINICAL FEATURES: The typical patient with an aortic dissection presents with acute onset of severe, "tearing" pain in the anterior chest, which is sometimes misdiagnosed as myocardial infarction. Loss of one or more arterial pulses is common and a murmur of aortic regurgitation is often present. Whereas hypertension is a frequent finding, hypotension is an ominous sign, suggesting aortic rupture. Cardiac tamponade or congestive heart failure is diagnosed by the usual criteria.

Before antihypertensive and surgical treatment became available, more than a third of patients with aortic dissection died within 24 hours, and 80% succumbed by 2 weeks. Half of the survivors died within 3 months. Surgical intervention and control of hypertension have now reduced overall mortality to less than 20%.

Syphilitic Aneurysms are Due to Inflammation of Aortic Vasa Vasorum

Syphilis was once the most common cause of aortic aneurysms, but as this infection has become less common, so has syphilitic vascular disease, including aortitis and aneurysms. Syphilitic aneurysms mainly affect the ascending aorta, where microscopic examination shows endarteritis and periarteritis of vasa vasorum. These vessels ramify in the adventitia and penetrate the outer and middle thirds of the aorta, where they become encircled by lymphocytes, plasma cells, and macrophages. Obliterative changes in the vasa vasorum cause focal necrosis and scarring of the media, with disruption and disorganization of elastic lamellae. The depressed medial scars lead to a roughened intimal surface, which imparts a "tree bark" appearance (Fig. 10-38). The weakened wall of the ascending aorta and aortic arch eventually yields to the relentless pressure of the blood and balloons to form a fusiform aneurysm.

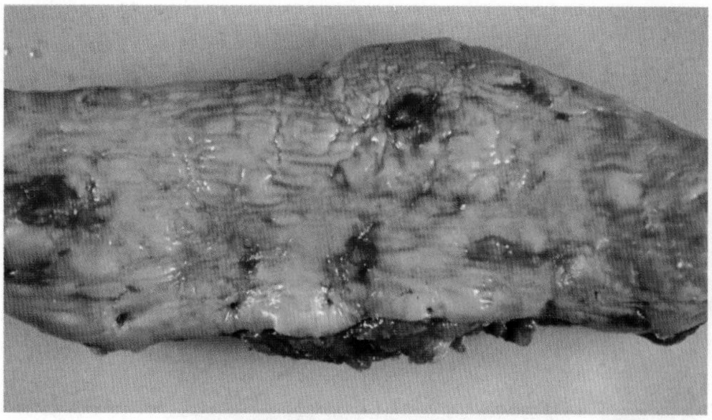

FIGURE 10-38. **Syphilitic aortitis.** The thoracic aorta is dilated, and its inner surface shows the typical "tree bark" appearance.

Mycotic (Infectious) Aneurysms Result from Weakening of the Vessel Wall by a Microbial Infection

Mycotic aneurysms have a tendency to rupture and hemorrhage. They may develop in the aortic wall or in cerebral vessels during septicemia, most commonly due to bacterial endocarditis. Mesenteric, splenic, or renal arteries are also commonly affected. In addition, mycotic aneurysms may occur adjacent to a tuberculous infection or a bacterial abscess.

Veins

Varicose Veins of the Legs Involve the Superficial Saphenous System

A varicose vein is an enlarged and tortuous vein. Superficial varicosities of leg veins are usually in the saphenous system, and are very common. They vary from a trivial knot of dilated veins to disabling distention of the whole venous system of the leg, with secondary trophic disturbances. It is estimated that as much as 10% to 20% of the population has some varicosities in the leg veins, but only a fraction of these persons develop symptoms.

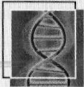

PATHOGENESIS: There are a number of risk factor for varicose veins:

- **Age:** Varicose veins increase in frequency with age and may reach 50% in persons over 50. This upswing in incidence may reflect age-related degenerative changes in the connective tissues of the vein walls, and loss of supporting fat and connective tissues, a more flaccid muscle tone, and inactivity.
- **Sex:** Among 30- to 50-year-olds, women are more often affected by varicose veins than men, particularly women who have experienced increased venous pressure from the pressure of a pregnant uterus on the iliac veins.
- **Heredity:** There is a strong familial predisposition to varicose veins, possibly owing to inherited configurations or structural weaknesses of the walls or valves of the veins.
- **Posture:** Leg vein pressure is 5 to 10 times higher when someone is erect, rather than recumbent. As a result, the incidence of varicose veins and its complications are greater in people whose occupations require them to stand in one place for long periods.
- **Obesity:** Excessive body weight increases the incidence of varicose veins, possibly because of increased intraabdominal pressure or poor support provided by subcutaneous fat to vessel walls.

Other factors that raise venous pressure in the legs can cause varicose veins, including pelvic tumors, congestive heart failure, and thrombotic obstruction of the main venous trunks of the thigh or pelvis.

In the pathogenesis of varicose veins, it is not clear whether incompetence of the valves or dilation of the vessels comes first. Whatever the case, the two reinforce each other. The vein increases in length and diameter, so that tortuousities develop. Once the process begins, the varicosity extends progressively throughout the length of the affected vein. As each valve becomes incompetent, increasing strain is put on the vessel and valve below. The role of inflammation is not well studied, although elevated expression of leukocyte-endothelial adhesion molecules is reported in affected veins.

PATHOLOGY: Microscopically, varicose veins show variations in wall thickness. Thinning due to dilation is present in some areas, whereas others are thickened by smooth muscle hypertrophy, subintimal fibrosis, and incorporation of mural thrombi into the wall. Patchy calcification is frequently seen. Valvular deformities consist of thickening, shortening, and rolling of the cusps.

CLINICAL FEATURES: The diagnosis of varicose veins of the leg is easily made by inspection. Most varicose veins are without clinical effects and are mainly cosmetic problems. The principal symptoms are aching in the legs, aggravated by standing and relieved by elevation. Severe varicosities (Fig. 10-39) may lead to trophic alterations in the skin drained by the affected veins, termed **stasis dermatitis**. Surgical intervention is mandated if the overlying skin has ulcerated, or if the patient has spontaneous bleeding or extensive thrombosis (which may lead to pulmonary embolism).

Varicose Veins Also Occur at Other Sites

HEMORRHOIDS: These are dilations of the veins of the rectum and anal canal, and may occur inside or outside the anal sphincter (see Chapter 13). Although there may be a hereditary predisposition, the condition is aggravated by factors that increase intra-abdominal pressure, such as constipation and pregnancy, or venous obstruction by rectal tumors. Hemorrhoids often bleed, which may be confused with bleeding rectal cancers. Thrombosed hemorrhoids are exquisitely painful.

ESOPHAGEAL VARICES: This complication of portal hypertension is caused mainly by cirrhosis of the liver (see Chapter 14). High portal pressure leads to distention of the anastomoses between portal and systemic venous systems at the lower end of the esophagus. Although they may be prominent radiologically,

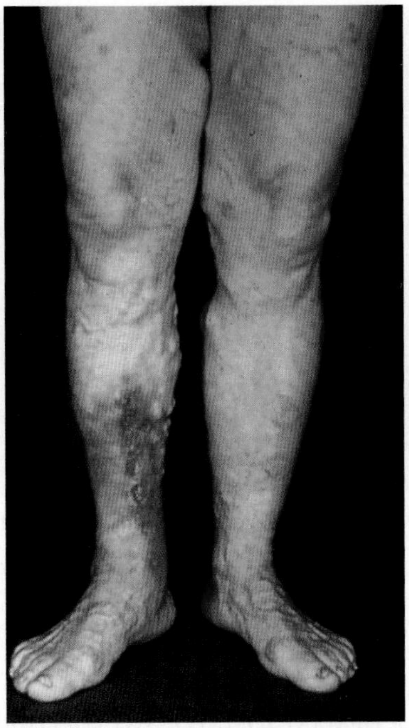

FIGURE 10-39. **Varicose veins of the legs.** Severe varicosities of the superficial leg veins have led to stasis dermatitis and secondary ulcerations.

esophageal varices are usually unimpressive at autopsy. After their collapse at death, often all that is evident on gross examination are bluish streaks in the esophageal mucosa. Hemorrhage from esophageal varices is one of the most common causes of death in cirrhosis.

VARICOCELE: This palpable scrotal mass represents varicosities of the pampiniform plexus (see Chapter 17).

Deep Venous Thrombosis Principally Affects Leg Veins

- **Thrombophlebitis** is inflammation and secondary thrombosis of small veins and sometimes larger ones, commonly as part of a local reaction to bacterial infection.
- **Phlebothrombosis** is the term for venous thrombosis that occurs without an initiating infection or inflammation.
- **Deep venous thrombosis** now refers to both phlebothrombosis and thrombophlebitis. Since most cases of venous thrombosis are not associated with inflammation or infection, the condition is currently associated with prolonged bed rest or reduced cardiac output. It is most frequent in deep leg veins and can be a major threat to life because of pulmonary embolization (witness the well-known phenomenon of sudden death with ambulation after surgery). Deficiencies of anticoagulants, such as protein C and antithrombin, increase the incidence of venous thromboembolism. Deep venous thrombosis is discussed more fully in Chapter 7.

Lymphatic Vessels

The lymphatic vessels are thin-walled low-pressure channels that are important for normal tissue fluid balance; provide drainage of plasma filtrates, cells, and foreign material from the interstitial spaces; and are important in fat digestion and in immune surveillance. Lymphatic vessels are more permeable than blood vessels, in part because the former have fewer tight junctions. NO• may act as mediator of several growth factors that are lymphangiogenic and may be important in lymphatic function. For example, NO• release may inhibit pumping in collecting lymphatics. Lymphatic pathways for spread of inflammation and neoplasia, may be modulated in disease.

Lymphangitis Reflects Infection and Inflammation in Lymphatic Vessels

Transport of infectious material to regional lymph nodes incites **lymphadenitis**. The periphery of a focus of inflammation reveals dilated lymphatics filled with fluid exudate, cells, cellular debris, and bacteria. When tissues are expanded by exudate, there is comparable distention of lymphatic channels and an opening of intercellular channels between endothelial cells.

Almost any virulent pathogen can cause acute lymphangitis, but β-hemolytic streptococci (pyogenes) are particularly notorious offenders. The process may extend beyond these channels into surrounding tissues. Draining lymph nodes are regularly enlarged and inflamed. Painful subcutaneous red streaks, often accompanied by painful regional lymph nodes, characterize acute lymphangitis.

Lymphatic Obstruction Causes Lymphedema

Lymphatics may be obstructed by scar tissue, intraluminal tumor cells, pressure from surrounding tumor tissue, or plugging with parasites. As collateral lymphatic routes are abundant, lymphedema (distention of tissue by lymph) usually occurs only when major trunks are obstructed, especially in the axilla or groin. For example, when radical mastectomy for breast cancer was routine, axillary lymph node dissection frequently disrupted lymphatic channels and led to lymphedema of the arm. Prolonged lymphatic obstruction causes progressive dilation of lymphatic vessels, termed **lymphangiectasia**, and overgrowth of fibrous tissue. The term **elephantiasis** describes a lymphedematous limb that has become grossly enlarged. An important cause of elephantiasis in the tropics is filariasis, in which a parasitic worm invades lymphatics (see Chapter 9).

Milroy disease *is an inherited type of lymphedema that is present at birth.* It usually affects only one limb, but it may be more extensive and involve the eyelids and lips. Affected tissues show hugely dilated lymphatic channels, and the entire area appears honeycombed or spongy. This lesion is more properly considered lymphangiectasia rather than simply lymphedema.

Benign Tumors of Blood Vessels

Tumors of the vascular system are common. Many are hamartomas, that is, masses of mature but disorganized cells and tissues characteristic of the particular organ, rather than true neoplasms. Some mutations have been linked to vascular anomalies. For example, endoglin and ALK-1 mutations have been identified in hereditary hemorrhagic telangiectasia and several gene mutations have been identified in familial cerebral cavernous malformation.

Hemangiomas Are Common Benign Tumors of Vascular Channels

Hemangiomas usually occur in the skin but may also be found in internal organs.

PATHOGENESIS: Although hemangiomas are clearly benign, their origin is uncertain; they represent either true neoplasms or hamartomas. The evidence favoring hamartoma (i.e., a malformation) includes: (1) the lesion is present at birth; (2) it grows only as the rest of the body grows, and remains limited in size; and (3) after growth ceases, it usually remains unchanged indefinitely absent trauma, thrombosis, or hemorrhage.

The development of these vascular malformations recalls the embryology of the vascular system. A network of endothelial channels undergoes remodeling, acquiring a muscular coat and adventitia. In this view, vascular malformations reflect the persistence of the original or modified channels and mixtures of connective tissue elements derived from the mesenchyme. At present, hemangiomas are classified by histologic type and location although molecular characterization will likely lead to new classifications and better understanding of the prognosis of given lesions.

PATHOLOGY:

CAPILLARY HEMANGIOMA: This lesion is composed of vascular channels with the size and structure of normal capillaries. Capillary hemangiomas may be located in any tissue. The most common sites are skin; subcutaneous tissues; mucous membranes of lips and the mouth; and internal viscera, including spleen, kidneys, and liver. Capillary hemangiomas vary from a few millimeters to several centimeters in diameter. They are bright red to blue, depending on the degree of oxygenation of the blood. In the skin, capillary hemangiomas are known as **birthmarks** or **ruby spots**. The only disability is cosmetic disfiguration.

JUVENILE HEMANGIOMA: Also called **strawberry hemangiomas**, these lesions are found on the skin of newborns. They grow rapidly in the first months of life, begin to fade at 1 to 3 years of age and completely regress in most (80%) cases by 5 years of age. Juvenile hemangiomas contain packed masses of capillaries separated by connective tissue stroma. The endothelium-lined channels are usually filled with blood. Thromboses, sometimes organized, are common. Occasionally, the vascular channels rupture, causing scarring and accumulation of hemosiderin. Juvenile hemangiomas are usually well demarcated despite lacking capsules, although fingerlike projections of the vascular tissue may give the impression of invasion. However, these growths are benign. They do not invade or metastasize.

CAVERNOUS HEMANGIOMA: This designation is reserved for lesions consisting of large vascular channels, frequently interspersed with small, capillary-type vessels. Cavernous hemangiomas occur in the skin (Fig. 10-40), where they are termed **port wine stains**. They also appear on mucosal surfaces and visceral organs, including the spleen, liver, and pancreas. Occasionally, they occur in the brain, where they may slowly enlarge and cause neurologic symptoms after long quiescent periods.

A cavernous hemangioma is a red-blue, soft, spongy mass, with a diameter of up to several centimeters. Unlike the capillary hemangioma, a cavernous hemangioma does not regress spontaneously. Although the lesion is demarcated by a sharp border, it is not encapsulated. Large endothelial-lined, blood-containing spaces are separated by sparse connective tissue.

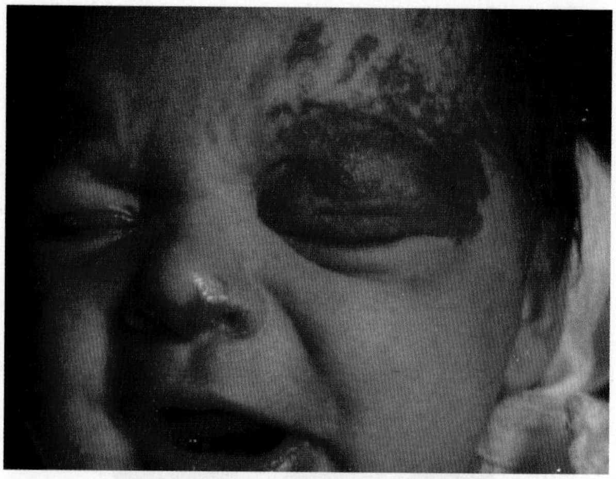

FIGURE 10-40. **Congenital cavernous hemangioma of the skin.**

Cavernous hemangiomas can undergo a variety of changes, including thrombosis and fibrosis, cystic cavitation, and intracystic hemorrhage.

MULTIPLE HEMANGIOMATOUS SYNDROMES: More than one hemangioma may occur in a single tissue. Two or more tissues may be involved, such as skin and nervous system or spleen and liver. Eponym enthusiasts have defined various combinations of sites. **von Hippel-Lindau syndrome** is a rare entity in which cavernous hemangiomas occur in the cerebellum or brainstem and the retina. **Sturge-Weber syndrome** involves a developmental disturbance of blood vessels in the brain and skin. Other closely related lesions are plexiform or racemose angiomas, cirsoid aneurysms, and angiomatous dilation of vessels of the brain and elsewhere.

Glomus Tumor (Glomangioma) Is a Painful Arteriolar–Venous Anastomosis

A glomus tumor is a benign neoplasm of the glomus body. Glomus bodies are normal neuromyoarterial receptors that are sensitive to temperature and regulate arteriolar flow. They are widely distributed in the skin, mostly in the distal regions of fingers and toes. This pattern is reflected in the location of glomus tumors at these sites, typically in a subungual location.

PATHOLOGY: The lesions are small, usually under 1 cm in diameter; many are smaller than a few millimeters. In the skin, they are slightly elevated, rounded, red-blue, and firm (Fig. 10-41). The two main histologic components are branching vascular channels in a connective tissue stroma and aggregates or nests of the specialized glomus cells. The latter are regular, round to cuboidal cells that reveal typical smooth muscle cell features by electron microscopy.

Hemangioendothelioma May Metastasize to Distant Sites

Hemangioendothelioma is a vascular tumor of endothelial cells that is intermediate between benign hemangiomas and frankly malignant angiosarcomas. The epithelioid or histiocytoid, variant displays endothelial cells with considerable eosinophilic, often vacuolated, cytoplasm. Vascular lumina are evident and there are few mitoses. These tumors occur in almost all locations. Surgical removal is generally curative, but about one fifth of patients develop metastases.

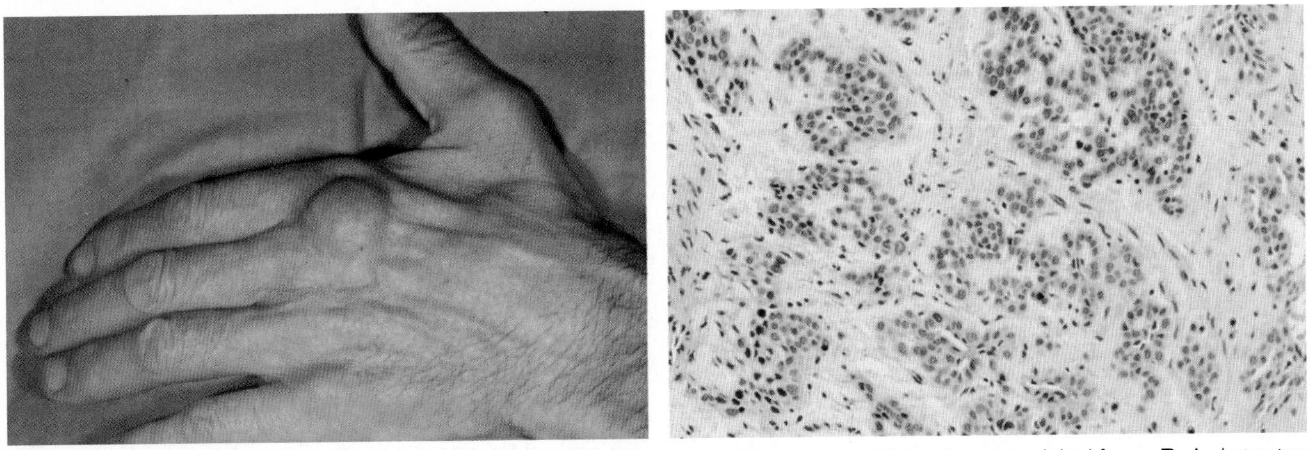

A B

FIGURE 10-41. **Glomus tumor. A.** The dorsal surface of the hand displays a prominent tumor nodule on the proximal third finger. **B.** A photomicrograph of *(A)* reveals nests of glomus tumor cells embedded in a fibrovascular stroma.

Spindle cell hemangioendothelioma occurs principally in males of any age, usually in the dermis and subcutaneous tissue of distal extremities. It features vascular, endothelial-lined spaces into which papillary projections extend. Although the lesion may recur locally after excision, it rarely metastasizes.

Malignant Tumors of Blood Vessels

Malignant vascular neoplasms are rare, and only a few arise in preexisting benign tumors.

Angiosarcoma is a Rare, Highly Malignant Tumor of Endothelial Cells

The lesions occur in either sex and at any age, and begin as small, painless, sharply demarcated, red nodules. The most common locations are skin, soft tissue, breast, bone, liver, and spleen. Eventually, most enlarge to become pale gray, fleshy masses without a capsule. Often these tumors undergo central necrosis, with softening and hemorrhage.

PATHOLOGY: Angiosarcomas exhibit varying degrees of differentiation, ranging from those composed mainly of distinct vascular elements to undifferentiated tumors with few recognizable blood channels. The latter display frequent mitoses, pleomorphism, and giant cells and tend to be more malignant. Almost half of patients with angiosarcoma die of the disease.

Angiosarcoma of the liver is of special interest because of its association with environmental carcinogens, particularly arsenic (a component of pesticides) and vinyl chloride (used in the production of plastics). Hepatic angiosarcoma is also associated with administration of thorium dioxide, radioactive contrast medium (Thorotrast), a material used by radiologists prior to 1950. The Thoratrast is engulfed by macrophages of the liver sinusoids, where it remains for life.

There is a long latent period between exposure to the chemicals or radionuclide and development of hepatic angiosarcoma. The earliest detectable changes are atypism and diffuse hyperplasia of the cells lining the hepatic sinusoids. The tumors are frequently multicentric and may arise in the spleen as well. Hepatic angiosarcomas are highly malignant and show both local invasion and metastatic spread.

Hemangiopericytoma

Hemangiopericytoma is a rare neoplasm previously thought to arise from pericytes, modified smooth muscle cells outside the walls of capillaries and arterioles. However, there is no convincing evidence that the neoplasm actually derives from these cells. These tumors present as small masses of capillary-like channels surrounded by, and frequently enclosed within, nests and masses of round to spindle-shaped cells. The tumor cells are characteristically invested by a basement membrane.

Hemangiopericytomas can occur anywhere, but are most common in the retroperitoneum and lower extremities. Most are removed surgically without having invaded or metastasized. Malignant hemangiopericytomas metastasize to lungs, bone, liver, and lymph nodes.

Kaposi Sarcoma Is a Complication of Acquired Immunodeficiency Syndrome (AIDS)

Kaposi sarcoma is a malignant angioproliferative tumor derived from endothelial cells.

EPIDEMIOLOGY: Kaposi sarcoma was originally described in the 19th century by Moritz Kaposi as a sporadic tumor endemic in parts of central Africa but otherwise an oddity that occurred mainly in men in the sixth and seventh decades. However, Kaposi sarcoma now appears in epidemic form in association with AIDS and in immunosuppressed patients. A member of the herpesvirus family, human herpesvirus 8 (HHV8) (Kaposi sarcoma-associated herpes virus [KSHV]), is thought to be responsible for this tumor. Only a small faction of KSHV-infected individuals develop Kaposi sarcoma. Cofactors that influence risk of Kaposi sarcoma among individuals who are not infected with human immunodeficiency virus (HIV) are not well understood.

PATHOLOGY: Kaposi sarcoma begins as painful purple or brown cutaneous nodules, 1 mm to 1 cm in diameter. They appear most often on the hands or feet but may occur anywhere. The histologic appearance is highly variable. One form resembles a simple hemangioma, with tightly packed clusters of capillaries and scattered hemosiderin-laden macrophages. Other forms are highly cellular and the vascular spaces are less prominent (Fig. 10-42).

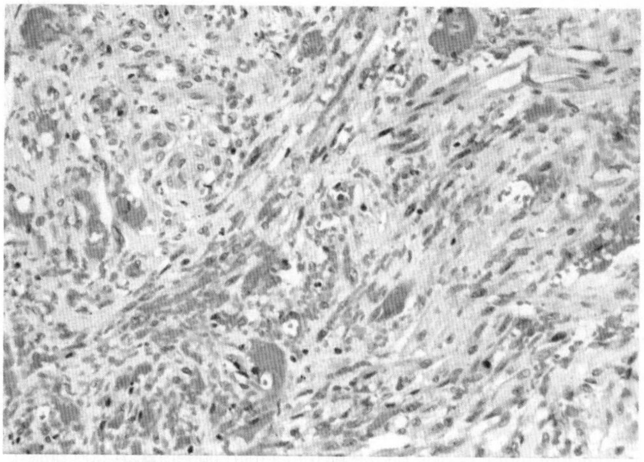

FIGURE 10-42. **Kaposi sarcoma.** A photomicrograph of a vascular lesion from a patient with acquired immune deficiency syndrome shows numerous poorly differentiated, spindle-shape neoplastic cells and a vascular lesion filled with red blood cells.

These lesions may be difficult to distinguish from fibrosarcomas, but the characteristic features of endothelial cells can be demonstrated immunochemically and by electron microscopy. Although Kaposi sarcoma is considered a malignant lesion and may be widely disseminated in the body, it is only exceptionally a cause of death.

Tumors of the Lymphatic System

Many histologic and clinical variants of local enlargements of the lymphatics have been described. It is difficult to distinguish among anomalies, proliferations due to stasis, and true neoplasms. In general, lymphatic tumors are distinguished by their size and location. The spaces may be small, as in capillary lymphangiomas, or large and dilated, as in cystic or cavernous lesions. Lymphangiomatous lesions can arise at almost any site, including skin, mediastinum, retroperitoneum, spleen, and elsewhere.

Capillary Lymphangioma

Sometimes called "simple lymphangiomas," these benign tumors are small, circumscribed, grayish pink, fleshy nodules, which can be single or multiple. They are subcutaneous and found in the skin of the face, lips, chest, genitalia, or extremities. Capillary lymphangiomas are composed of variably sized, thin-walled spaces that are lined by endothelial cells and contain lymph and occasional leukocytes.

Cystic Lymphangioma (Cystic Hygroma, Cavernous Lymphangioma) Cystic Hygromas, and Cavernous Lymphangioma

These benign lesions are most common in the neck and axilla, but also occur in the mediastinum and occasionally in the retroperitoneum. They may reach 10 to 15 cm or more in diameter and fill the axilla or distort structures of the neck.

PATHOLOGY: Cystic lymphangiomas are soft, spongy, and pink, and watery fluid exudes from their cut surface. Microscopically, they contain endothelial lined spaces with a protein-rich fluid. These spaces are distinguished from blood vessels by their lack of erythrocytes and leukocytes. An abundance of irregularly distributed smooth muscle and connective tissue cells may be present.

Lymphangiosarcoma May Follow Lymphedema or Radiation

A rare malignant tumor develops in 0.1% to 0.5% of patients with lymphedema of the arm after radical mastectomy. A distinction between this tumor and angiosarcoma is difficult, and some authors equate the two cancers. Lymphangiosarcoma may also occur in other regions, for example, in the leg following radiation therapy for uterine cervical carcinoma.

PATHOLOGY: Lymphangiosarcomas present as purplish, frequently multiple, nodules in edematous skin. Histologically, the nodules are composed of cells resembling capillary endothelial cells and showing zonulae adherentes between cells. The walls of tumor vessels have a rudimentary form of basal basement membrane. Lymphangiosarcomas are highly malignant and, despite radical surgery, carry a poor prognosis.

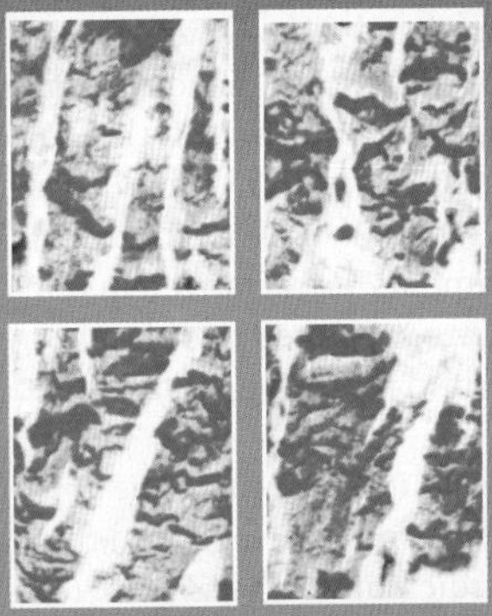

11 The Heart

Jeffrey E. Saffitz

The heart is a fist-sized muscular pump that has a remarkable capacity to work unceasingly for the 80 or more years of a human lifetime. As demand requires, it can increase its output manyfold, in part because the coronary circulation can augment its blood flow to over 10 times normal. The ventricles also respond to short-term increases in workload by dilating, in accordance with Starling law of the heart. When an increased workload is imposed for a longer period (e.g., in cases of essential hypertension) the left ventricle hypertrophies, an adaptation that increases its work capacity. However, when this compensatory mechanism reaches its limits, the heart no longer provides an adequate supply of blood to peripheral tissues, and the result is congestive heart failure. Damage to the myocardium, caused mostly by ischemic heart disease, also limits the capacity of the left ventricle to pump blood and similarly results in heart failure.

Anatomy of the Heart

The heart of an adult man weighs 280 to 340 g, and that of a woman, 230 to 280 g. The organ is a two-sided pump. Blood enters each side through a thin-walled atrium, from which it is propelled forward by thicker muscular ventricles. The right ventricle is considerably thinner (<0.5 cm) than the left ventricle (1.3 to 1.5 cm) owing to the low venous pressure and relatively low afterload on the right side. Blood enters the ventricles across the atrioventricular valves, the mitral valve on the left and the tricuspid valve on the right. The leaflets of these valves are held in place by chordae tendineae, strong fibrous cords attached via papillary muscles to the inner surface of the ventricular wall. The aorta and pulmonary arteries are guarded respectively by aortic and pulmonary valves, each consisting of three semilunar cusps. The heart wall has three layers: outer epicardium, middle myocardium, and inner endocardium. The heart is surrounded and enclosed by visceral and parietal pericardia, which are separated by the pericardial cavity.

Cardiac Myocytes Generate Contractile Force

The myocardium is composed of a network of individual myocytes, each of which normally has a single nucleus and is separated from adjacent cells by intercalated disks which contain cell–cell mechanical and electrical junctions. Electron microscopy reveals the structure and distribution of the sarcolemma, sarcoplasmic reticulum (SR), T system of tubules, nucleus, and numerous mitochondria (Fig. 11-1). The contractile elements of the myocyte, the myofilaments, are arranged in bundles, referred to as myofibrils, which are separated by mitochondria and SR. Myofibrils are organized into repeating units termed **sarcomeres.**

The sarcomere is the basic functional unit of the contractile apparatus. It consists of a Z disk on each end and interdigitated thick and thin filaments, oriented perpendicular to the Z disk (see Fig. 11-1). The thick filaments contain myosin heavy chains, myosin binding protein C, and myosin light chains. The thick

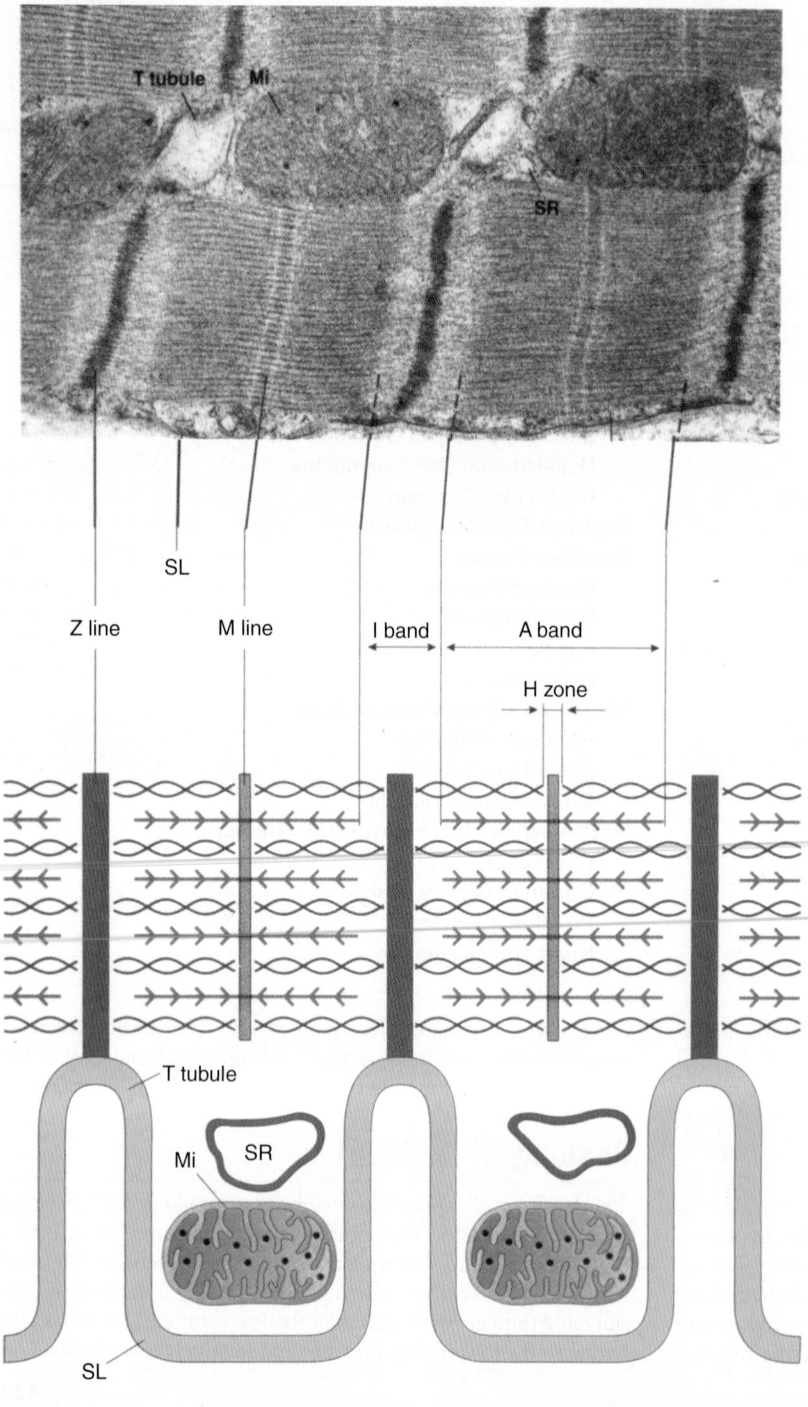

FIGURE 11-1. **Ultrastructure of the myocardium. (Top)** Electron micrograph of left ventricle in the longitudinal plane, showing the sarcolemma (SL); the sarcomeres of the myofibrils, delimited by Z lines; A bands; I bands; H zones; and M lines. Also present are mitochondria (Mi), sarcoplasmic reticulum (SR), and T tubules. The I bands and H zones are absent when the myofibrils are shortened. **(Bottom)** The structural basis for the banding shown in the electron micrograph. The fine threads that extend at right angles to the thick (myosin) filaments are the cross bridges that form the force-generating cross-links with actin. The amount of force that can be generated is proportional to the length of the adjoining myofilaments and is at a maximum when the sarcomeres are between 2 and 2.2 μm in length. When the sarcomeres are less than 2 μm in length, the thin filaments slide across each other and overlap, decreasing the potential for force-generating cross-links; similarly, when the sarcomeres are stretched beyond 2.2 μm, there is a decrease in force that is proportional to the widening of the H zone. This mechanism can be invoked as the basis for Starling law of the heart.

filaments, which are limited to the A band, interact with the giant sarcomeric protein, titin (~27,000 amino acids long), which spans from the Z disk to the M line, thereby forming a third filament system of the sarcomere. Titin helps maintain precise assembly of myofibrillar proteins and contributes to the viscoelastic properties of cardiac muscle. The thin filaments contain actin and regulatory proteins, including **tropomyosin** and the **troponin complex** (troponins I, C, and T), and extend from the Z disk through the I band and into the A band. The interaction of these myofilaments generates the force for contraction. The amount of force that can be generated is proportional to the extent of overlap between adjoining thick and thin filaments and is maximum when sarcomeres are 2.0 to 2.2 μm in length.

When sarcomere length is under 2 μm, the thin filaments slide across each other and overlap, decreasing the potential for force-generating cross-links. When it is stretched beyond 2.2 μm, force decreases in proportion to the widening of the H zone. *This mechanism is the basis for Starling law of the heart, which states that the contractile force of the heart is a function of diastolic fiber length.* Average sarcomere length is about 2.2 μm when left ventricular end-diastolic pressure is at the upper limit of normal.

Contraction of cardiac muscle is initiated by increases in cytosol free calcium. In a normal myocyte, an action potential triggers entry of calcium ions into the myocyte through voltage-gated L-type calcium channels in the sarcolemma. In turn, the entering calcium stimulates release of calcium (Ca^{2+}) sequestered in the SR (Ca^{2+}-induced Ca^{2+} release) via the cardiac ryanodine receptor (RyR2). The increase in cytosolic free calcium produces a conformational change in the regulatory myofilament proteins, in particular troponin, which permits cross-bridges between actin and myosin to break and reform repetitively. As a result, the filaments slide over one another, causing myocardial contraction. *The number of contractile sites activated, and the resulting force generated, are directly proportional to the concentration of calcium nearby the myofibrils.*

The myocardium relaxes when cytosolic calcium returns to its normal low concentration of 10^{-7} M. This process depends on calcium ATPase of the SR, which pumps Ca^{2+} from the cytosol into the SR. Cytosolic Ca^{2+} also is lowered by its outward transport through sodium–calcium exchange and sarcolemmal calcium pumps. *Thus, myocardial relaxation is an active, energy-requiring event.*

The Conduction System Consists of Specialized Myocytes

These myocytes have two major functions: (1) they initiate heartbeats by generating electric current through their automatic rhythmicity, which is more rapid in the sinoatrial node than in the more distal parts of the system; and (2) they distribute electric current to activate atrial and ventricular myocardium in an appropriate temporal–spatial pattern. Fibers of the atrioventricular conduction system generally conduct impulses at a faster rate (~1–2 m/sec) than do working (contractile) atrial and ventricular fibers (~0.5–1 m/sec). By contrast, conduction through the atrioventricular node is exceptionally slow (~0.1 m/sec). Slow conduction through the atrioventricular junction delays ventricular activation, and thereby facilitates their filling.

The heartbeat normally originates in the sinoatrial node. If the node is diseased or otherwise prevented from functioning as the pacemaker, more-distal components of the conduction system or even the ventricular muscle itself assume the role of pacemaker. *As a rule, the more distal the pacemaker site, the slower the heart rate.* On leaving the sinoatrial node, an electrical impulse activates the atria. Atrial wavefronts converge on the atrioventricular node, which conducts the impulse through the common bundle (bundle of His) to the left and right bundle branches of the Purkinje system. Purkinje fibers run within the endocardium on either side of the interventricular septum and distribute current to the overlying ventricular muscle. During each cycle, ventricular contraction begins along the interventricular septum and at the apex. It progresses from apex to base, resulting in smooth and efficient ejection of blood into the great vessels.

The His bundle in the normal adult heart is the only electrical connection between the atria and ventricles. However, additional abnormal connections may occasionally arise as small bundles or tracts of cardiac myocytes. Such "bypass tracts" can activate ventricular muscle before the normal impulse arrives via the conduction system and are found in patients with the **Wolff-Parkinson-White syndrome** and in various forms of **supraventricular tachycardia**. Congenital discontinuities in the conduction system may be caused by placentally transmitted autoantibodies in mothers with connective tissue disease such as systemic lupus erythematosus (SLE). Acquired defects may arise because of infarction, inflammatory or infiltrative disease, cardiac surgery, or cardiac catheterization.

Coronary Arteries Supply Blood Flow to the Heart

The right and left main coronary arteries originate in, or immediately above, the sinuses of Valsalva of the aortic valve. The left main coronary artery bifurcates within 1 cm of its origin into the left anterior descending (LAD) and left circumflex coronary arteries. The left circumflex coronary artery rests in the left atrioventricular groove and supplies the lateral wall of the left ventricle (Fig. 11-2). The LAD coronary artery lies in the anterior interventricular groove and provides blood to the (1) anterior left ventricle, (2) adjacent anterior right ventricle, and (3) anterior half-to-two thirds of the interventricular septum. In the apical region, the LAD artery supplies the ventricles circumferentially (see Fig. 11-2).

The right coronary artery travels along the right atrioventricular groove and nourishes the bulk of the right ventricle and posteroseptal left ventricle (see Fig. 11-2), including the posterior third-to-half of the interventricular septum at the base of the heart (also referred to as the "inferior" or "diaphragmatic" wall). From these distributions, one can predict the location of infarcts that result from occlusion of any of the three major epicardial coronary arteries.

The epicardial coronary arteries are usually arranged in a so-called right coronary-dominant distribution. The pattern of dominance is determined by the coronary artery that contributes most of the blood to the posterior descending coronary artery. Ten percent of human hearts display a left-dominant pattern, with the left circumflex coronary artery supplying the posterior descending coronary artery.

Blood flow in the myocardium occurs inward from epicardium to endocardium. Thus, as a general rule, endocardium is most vulnerable to ischemia when flow through a major epicardial coronary artery is compromised. Some of the small intramyocardial coronary arteries branch as they course through the ventricular wall; others maintain a large diameter and pass to the endocardial surface without branching (Fig. 11-3). Because capillary networks arising from penetrating arteries do not interconnect, the borders be-

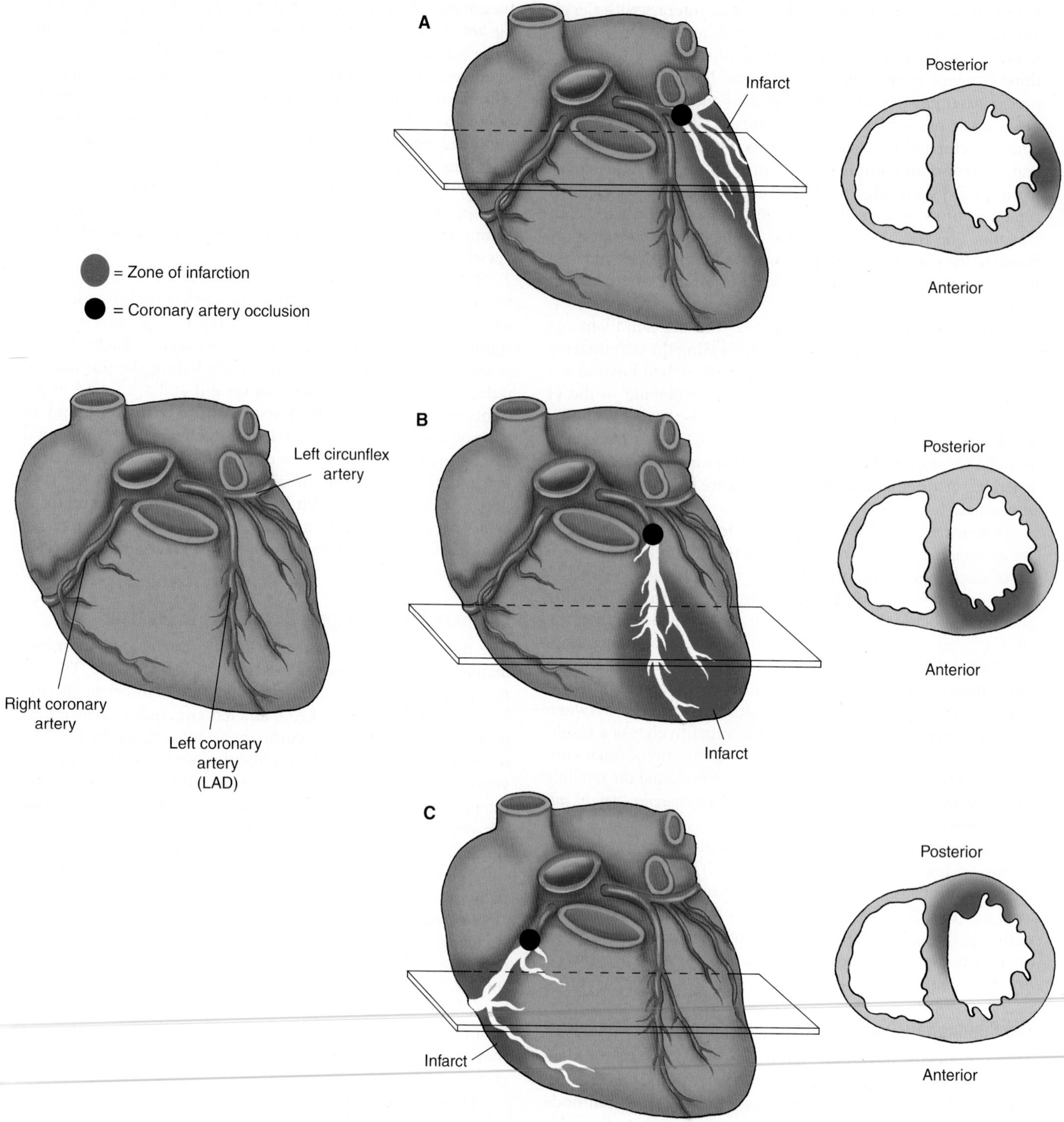

FIGURE 11-2. **Position of left ventricular infarcts resulting from occlusion of each of the three main coronary arteries. A.** Posterolateral infarct, which follows occlusion of the left circumflex artery and is present in the posterolateral wall. **B**. Anterior infarct, which follows occlusion of the anterior descending branch (left anterior descending, LAD) of the left coronary artery. The infarct is located in the anterior wall and adjacent two-thirds of the septum. It involves the entire circumference of the wall near the apex. **C.** A posterior ("inferior" or "diaphragmatic") infarct results from occlusion of the right coronary artery and involves the posterior wall, including the posterior third of the interventricular septum and the posterior papillary muscle in the basal half of the ventricle.

tween viable and infarcted myocardium after coronary artery occlusion are distinct.

The epicardial portion of each coronary artery fills and expands during systole and empties and narrows during diastole. The intramyocardial arteries have the opposite action and are narrowed by the systolic muscular pressure. As a result, blood flow within myocardium, especially in the subendocardial ventricular regions, is decreased or absent during systole. Nevertheless, blood flow is roughly equal throughout the myocardium because of autoregulation.

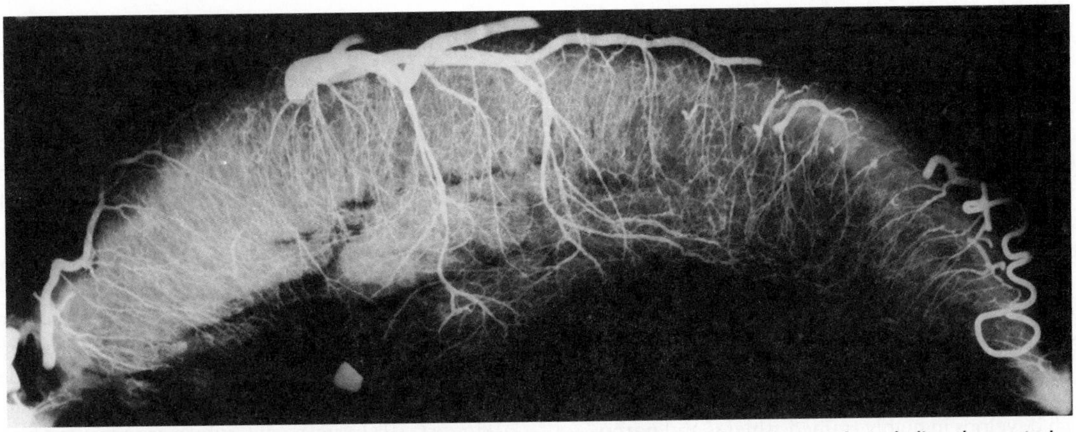

FIGURE 11-3. **Arteriogram of a longitudinal segment of the posterior wall of the left ventricle including the posterior papillary muscle.** Note the two types of branches passing into the myocardium at right angles to the epicardial artery *(top)*: class A, which quickly divide into a fine network, and class B, which maintain a large diameter and pass with little branching into the subendocardial region and the papillary muscle.

Myocardial Hypertrophy and Heart Failure

The ventricles are compliant in a normal heart, and diastolic filling occurs at low atrial pressures. During systole, ventricles contract vigorously and eject about 60% of the blood present in the ventricle at the end of diastole (ejection fraction). When a heart is injured, the clinical consequences are similar, regardless of the cause of cardiac dysfunction. *If the initial impairment is severe, cardiac output is not maintained despite compensatory changes and the result is acute, life-threatening,* ***cardiogenic shock***. When the functional impairment is less, compensatory mechanisms (see below) maintain cardiac output by increasing diastolic ventricular filling pressure and end-diastolic volume. This situation results in the characteristic signs and symptoms of congestive heart failure. Because of the heart's capacity to compensate, congestive heart failure is often tolerated for years.

The ability of the heart to adapt to injury is based on the same mechanisms that allow cardiac output to increase in response to stress. *The fundamental compensatory mechanism is the Frank-Starling mechanism: the cardiac stroke volume is a function of diastolic fiber length and, within certain limits, a normal heart will pump whatever volume is brought to it by the venous circulation* (Fig. 11-4). Stroke volume, a measure of ventricular function, is enhanced by increasing ventricular end-diastolic volume secondary to an increase in atrial filling pressure.

The increased contractile force in response to ventricular dilation is a result of myofibrillar organization, in which stretching of the sarcomeres results in a greater potential for overlap of thick and thin filaments during contraction. This allows enhanced force generation, provided the sarcomere is not stretched beyond 2.2 μm. When there is a sudden need to increase cardiac output in a normal heart, such as during exercise, catecholamine stimulation increases both heart rate and contractility. The latter is mainly mediated by modulating the activities of key proteins that regulate calcium transients during excitation–contraction coupling. As a result, the normal relationship between end-diastolic volume and stroke volume is shifted upward (from curve A to curve X in Fig. 11-4). End-diastolic volume may also increase, causing a large increase in cardiac output.

If the heart is injured, overall cardiac function tends to be depressed in the basal state. Then, higher than normal filling pressures are required to maintain cardiac output (curve Y in Fig. 11-4). Moreover, catecholamine stimulation is often present in the basal state in cardiac failure, so a comparable increase in cardiac output requires a larger increase in atrial pressure in a failing heart than in a normal one. *The most prominent feature of heart failure is the abnormally high atrial filling pressure relative to stroke volume.* However, the absolute values of stroke volume and cardiac output are generally well maintained.

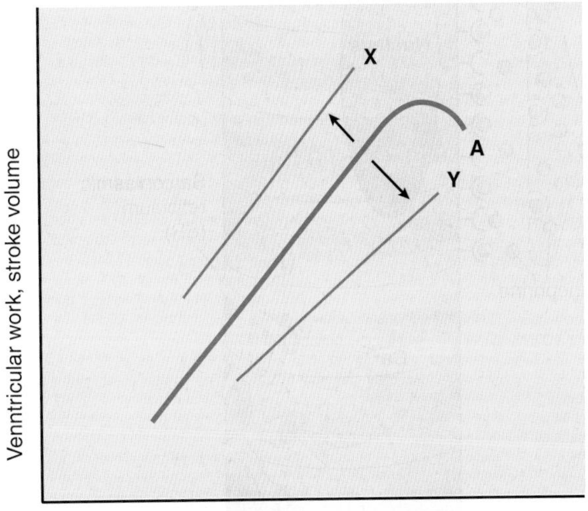

FIGURE 11-4. **Relation between the work of the heart (or stroke volume) and the level of venous inflow, as measured by atrial pressure, ventricular end-diastolic volume (EDV), or end-diastolic pressure (EDP).** *Curve A* indicates that as ventricular EDV, EDP, or left atrial pressure increases, the amount of work done by the heart increases linearly up to a point. Beyond this point, the work done decreases, and the heart fails. However, the downslope of this curve is reached only at very high left atrial pressures. The curve may shift upward to position *X* or downward to position *Y*, depending on whether contractility has increased (e.g., because of the action of norepinephrine) or decreased (i.e., in failure), respectively. The failing heart usually functions on the ascending limb of a depressed curve.

PATHOGENESIS: Myocardial hypertrophy is an adaptive response that augments myocyte contractile strength. It develops as a compensatory response to hemodynamic overload, which occurs in association with chronic hypertension or valvular stenosis (pressure overload), myocardial injury, valvular insufficiency (volume overload) and other stresses that increase heart workload. The importance of this adaptive mechanism was noted more than a century ago by Austin Flint, who suggested that like the enlargement of skeletal muscle in athletes, cardiac hypertrophy compensates for hemodynamic overloading of the heart. A distinction must be made, however, between **physiologic hypertrophy** of a heart, which develops in highly trained athletes and **pathologic hypertrophy**, which occurs in response to injury or overload. Hypertrophic responses feature enlargement of cardiac myocytes and accumulation of sarcomeric proteins, without an increase in the number of cardiac myocytes. Hypertrophy initially reflects a compensatory and potentially reversible mechanism, but faced with persistent stress, the myocardium becomes irreversibly enlarged and dilated (Fig. 11-5).

Receptor-mediated myocardial events that are triggered by a stimulus promote the hypertrophic response by autocrine and paracrine mechanisms. Contractile cells respond to mechanical stimuli, such as stretching, by activating receptor-mediated signaling pathways that produce hypertrophy. Among the most important ligands that activate these pathways are (1) angiotensin II (ANG-II), (2) endothelin-1 (Et-1), and (3) various growth factors, including insulin-like growth factor-I (IGF-I) and transforming growth factor-β (TGF-β). Some of these mediators may also act on interstitial fibroblasts in the heart to promote synthesis and deposition of extracellular matrix. The most important signaling cascades involve (1) mitogen-activated protein kinase (MAPK) and protein kinase C (PKC) pathways, which are activated by G protein-coupled receptors; and (2) calcineurin A and calcium/calmodulin-dependent protein kinase (CamK) pathways, which are regulated by calcium. Events mediated by the adrenergic receptor are implicated in the transition from compensatory hypertrophy to heart failure.

ANGIOTENSIN II: All components of the renin–angiotensin system (renin, angiotensinogen, angiotensin-converting enzyme [ACE], and Ang II receptors) are pre-

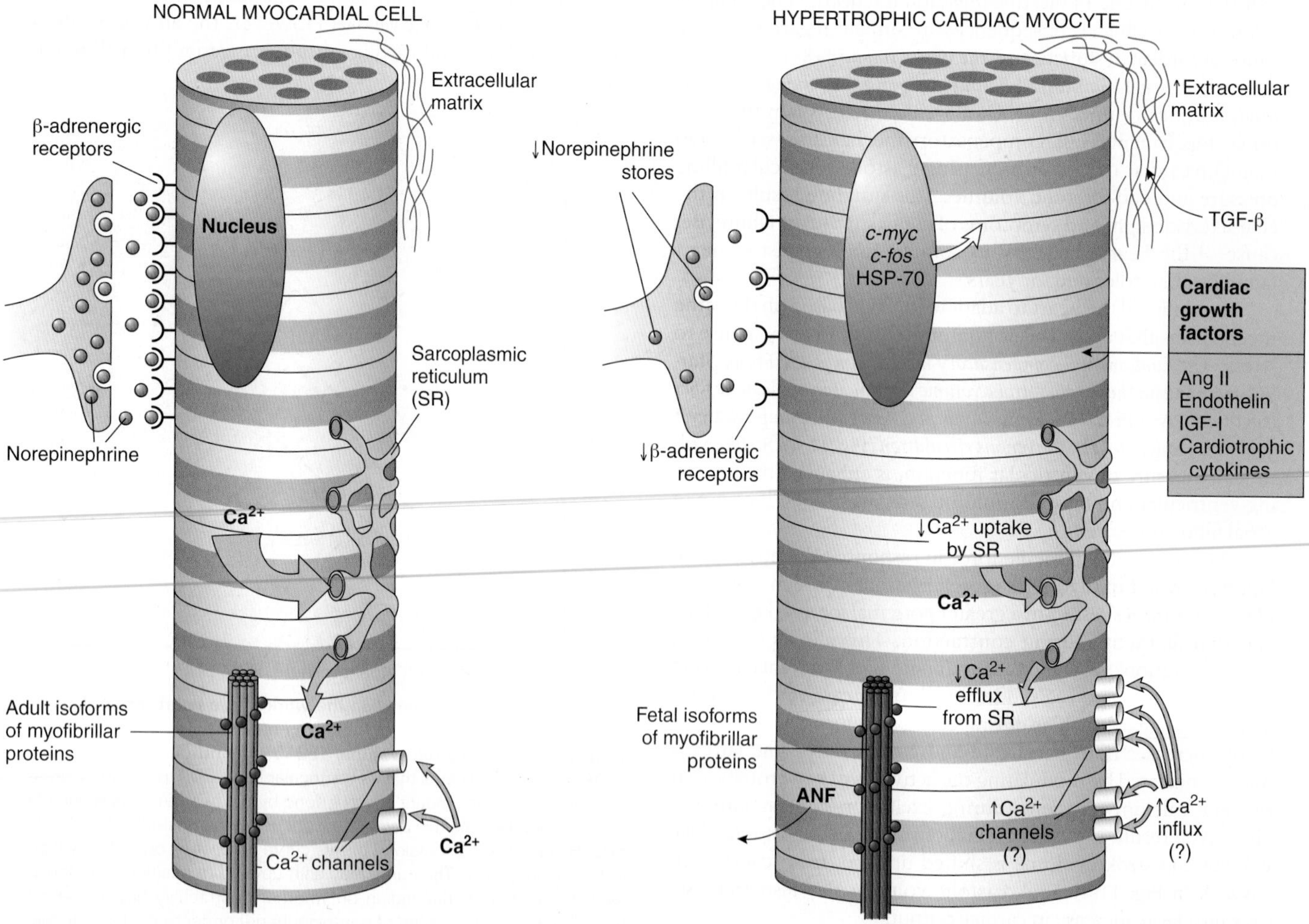

FIGURE 11-5. **Biochemical characteristics of myocardial hypertrophy and congestive heart failure.** ANF = atrial natriuretic factor; ANG II = angiotensin II; HSP-70 = heat shock protein 70; IGF = insulin-like growth factor; TGF = transforming growth factor.

sent in both cardiac myocytes and interstitial fibroblasts of the myocardium. Ang II is released locally in response to load or stress stimuli and acts by autocrine and paracrine mechanisms to promote myocyte hypertrophy and produce extracellular matrix. In this context, treatment with an ACE inhibitor tends to reverse cardiac hypertrophy and to normalize heart size. ACE inhibitors also prevent cardiac hypertrophy induced by experimental hypertension, without reducing the elevated arterial pressure.

ENDOTHELIN-I): ET-1 is a powerful vasoconstrictor produced by many cells, including endothelial cells and cardiac myocytes. It is also a potent growth factor for cardiac myocytes. Like Ang II, ET-1 activates MAPK cascades on binding to its receptor to promote cardiac hypertrophy.

INSULIN-LIKE GROWTH FACTOR-1: IGF-I is a growth-promoting peptide synthesized locally in most tissues. As a growth factor for cardiac myocytes, IGF-I probably contributes to the development of cardiac hypertrophy.

EXTRACELLULAR MATRIX: Short-term heart overload leads to a prompt increase in collagen synthesis. Interstitial fibrosis, which occurs in virtually all forms of heart failure, is an obligatory feature of the hypertrophic response. Deposition of matrix proteins results, at least in part, from stimulation of cardiac fibroblasts by TGF-β and Ang II. After myocardial infarction, fibrosis is important in replacing necrotic myocytes and preventing cardiac rupture. As with many adaptive responses of the heart, however, myocardial fibrosis eventually interferes with diastolic relaxation and impairs diffusion of oxygen and nutrients.

β-ADRENERGIC DESENSITIZATION: The chronically failing heart responds poorly to catecholamines, which is presumably an adaptive response to elevated circulating levels of autonomic neurotransmitters in heart failure. Desensitization of β-adrenergic receptors contributes to sluggish responses of a failing heart to exercise. Chronic overstimulation of these myocyte receptors by endogenous catecholamines leads to a decrease in both the number and responsiveness of receptors. In addition, there appears to be a defect in the coupling of the β-adrenergic receptor to adenylyl cyclase through G proteins. The failing heart also stores less norepinephrine in autonomic nerve endings. Although β_1-adrenergic receptors are desensitized in heart failure, treatment with blockers of this receptor class have been shown in clinical trials to reduce mortality and improve contractile function in patients with advanced heart failure. Seemingly paradoxical, this response is consistent with abundant evidence that β_1-adrenergic receptors mediate cardiotoxic effects of norepinephrine in the failing heart including maladaptive cardiac myocyte hypertrophy and apoptosis, interstitial fibrosis, contractile dysfunction, and sudden death

CALCIUM HOMEOSTASIS: A variety of defects in calcium homeostasis occurs in hypertrophy and heart failure. The expression and function of important calcium-regulating proteins in cardiac myocytes are altered, including (1) RyR2, (2) SR Ca^{2+}-dependent ATPase (SERCA), and (3) phospholamban.

- **RyR2,** the major calcium release channel in the SR, is activated during the action potential by influx of extracellular Ca^{2+} through voltage-gated calcium channels in the sarcolemma. A decrease in the number of RyR2 channels impairs contractile function by reducing the rate of Ca^{2+} release from SR.
- **SERCA** is the pump responsible for Ca^{2+} reuptake into SR after contraction. Decreased Ca^{2+} uptake by the SR is mediated by a reduced amount and abnormal regulation of SERCA. As a result, interference with Ca^{2+} sequestration during diastole leads to impaired relaxation.
- **Phospholamban** is a key regulator of cardiac contractility that inhibits SERCA. Enhanced phospholamban—SERCA interactions lead to chronically elevated Ca^{2+} levels during diastole and have been implicated in chronic heart failure.
- **Calcineurin A and CamK pathways,** both of which are regulated by Ca^{2+}, have also been implicated in the hypertrophic response.

PROTOONCOGENES AND MYOCARDIAL HYPERTROPHY: Within an hour of the stress produced by acute pressure overload, myocardial cells respond by expressing protooncogenes *c-jun* and *c-fos* and heat shock protein 70 (HSP 70). It is likely that transcription of protooncogenes helps orchestrate the reexpression of fetal protein isoforms in the hypertrophic heart.

EXPRESSION OF FETAL GENES: A number of protein isoforms are expressed in the fetal heart but not after birth. In cardiac hypertrophy induced by hemodynamic overload, many of these genes are reexpressed. For example, atrial natriuretic factor (ANF) is expressed in the fetal ventricle and atrium, but after birth, its production is restricted to the atrium. In a hypertrophic ventricle, however, ANF and brain natriuretic protein (BNP) are abundantly reexpressed and reduce hemodynamic overload through their effects on salt and water metabolism (see Chapter 7).

Cardiac hypertrophy is also accompanied by reexpression of fetal isoforms of several contractile proteins. In the rat, the normal adult isoform is β-myosin that has high ATPase activity and a rapid shortening velocity. By contrast, the fetal type is β-myosin that has lower ATPase activity and a slower shortening velocity. In experimental cardiac hypertrophy, "fast" β-myosin is replaced by "slow" β-myosin, leading to impaired myocardial contractility. However, this change in myosin gene expression is also adaptive, since it increases the tension generated during systole and improves contraction efficiency, thus conserving energy. Hypertrophied hearts exhibit similar, but not identical, changes in myosin isoforms. The ventricle contains only slow myosin, and the hypertrophic heart changes from fast to slow myosin only in the atrium. However, fetal isoforms of other myofibrillar proteins appear in ventricular myocardium, including fetal forms of actin and tropomyosin. The hypertrophied heart also contains abnormal varieties of lactic dehydrogenase (LDH), creatine kinase (CK) and the sarcolemmal sodium pump.

Another adaptive gene switch occurs in expression of proteins involved in energy metabolism. The fetal heart relies primarily on maternally derived glucose for adenosine triphosphate (ATP) production. After birth, however, the heart downregulates genes encoding glycolytic enzymes and increases expression of genes that encode proteins involved in β-oxidation of fatty acids. The failing heart reverts to using glucose by reexpressing the fetal pattern of genes regulating energy metabolism. Although a mole of glucose yields less ATP than a mole of fatty acid, glycolytic metabolism uses less oxygen. In the case of the failing heart, this switch is, therefore, advantageous.

Recent advances in understanding the molecular pathogenesis of heart failure have identified a role for histone acetylases and deacetylases in stress-activated myocyte signaling pathways. DNA-binding histone proteins control gene expression by modulating chromatin structure and controlling access of transcriptional activitors and repressors to critical regulatory DNA sequences. Activation of stress-related signaling pathways involving G-protein coupled receptors for adrenergic agonists, endothelin, angiotensin. and others ultimately shifts patterns of histone acetylation and gene expression patterns, which is mediated by changes in subcellular location and activites of histone acetylases and deacetylases. Manipulation of histone-modifying enzymes may, therefore, be an attractive new therapeutic approach to prevent heart failure.

Apoptosis of cardiac myocytes may be important in heart failure. A 5-fold increase in the number of cardiac myocytes undergoing apoptosis has been observed in animal models of heart disease, and senescent rats have 30% fewer cardiac myocytes than young ones. Pathologic hypertrophy is generally associated with greater cardiac myocyte apoptosis, which may contribute to the transition from compensated hypertrophy to heart failure. Signaling by agonists such as angiotensin and endothelin increases expression of pro-apoptotic genes, and signaling by adrenergic agonists increases the sensitivity of cardiac myocytes to apoptotic stimuli. In contrast, signaling via IGF-1 may enhance survival. Thus, various signaling pathways in cardiac hypertrophy may exert both pro- and anti-apoptotic influences with the final outcome dependent on the intricate balance of opposing actions.

CARDIAC STEM CELLS AND MYOCARDIAL REGENERATION: The heart has traditionally been thought of as a static organ incapable of growing new myocytes to regenerate or repair damage due to a lack of cardiac stem cells. In this view, cardiac myocytes must last a lifetime and can respond to injury only by hypertrophy or death. Many controversies remain, but there is now compelling evidence that cardiac stem cells exist in adults. For example, male transplant recipients who have received female hearts exhibit fully differentiated cardiac myocytes bearing the Y chromosome. Moreover, embryonic stem cells and adult bone-marrow-derived cells can experimentally repopulate areas of myocardial injury and differentiate into cardiac myocytes. Thus, the failing heart is a candidate for potential stem cell therapy (see Chapter 3).

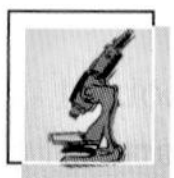

PATHOLOGY: Anything that increases cardiac workload for a prolonged period or produces structural damage may eventuate in myocardial failure. *Ischemic heart disease is by far the most common condition responsible for cardiac failure, accounting for more than 80% of deaths from heart disease.* Most of the remaining deaths are caused by nonischemic forms of heart muscle disease (cardiomyopathies) and congenital heart disease. Virtually all body organs suffer when the heart fails. The subject is discussed in detail in Chapter 7, and only the salient features are reviewed here.

Other than changes characteristic of specific disease entities (e.g., ischemic heart disease or cardiac amyloidosis) the morphology of the failing heart is nonspecific. *Ventricular hypertrophy is observed in virtually all conditions associated with chronic heart failure.* Initially, only the left ventricle may be hypertrophied, as in compensated hypertensive heart disease. But when the left ventricle fails, some right ventricular hypertrophy usually follows, owing to the increased work load imposed on the right ventricle by the failing left ventricle. *In most cases of clinically apparent heart failure, the ventricles are conspicuously dilated.* The distribution of end-organ involvement depends on whether the heart failure is predominantly left-sided or right-sided.

Left-sided heart failure is more common, because the most frequent causes of cardiac injury (e.g., ischemic heart disease and hypertension) primarily affect the left ventricle. To compensate for left ventricular failure, left atrial and pulmonary venous pressures increase, resulting in passive pulmonary congestion. The capillaries in the alveolar septa fill with blood and small ruptures allow erythrocytes to escape. As a result, alveoli contain many hemosiderin-laden macrophages (so-called heart failure cells). Moreover, if capillary hydrostatic pressure exceeds plasma osmotic pressure, fluid leaks from capillaries into alveoli. Resultant **pulmonary edema** (see Chapter 10) may be massive, with alveoli being "drowned" in a transudate. Interstitial pulmonary fibrosis results when congestion is present over an extended period.

Right-sided heart failure commonly complicates left-sided failure, or it can develop independently secondary to intrinsic pulmonary disease or pulmonary hypertension, which create resistance to blood flow through the lungs. As a consequence, right atrial pressure and systemic venous pressure both increase, resulting in jugular venous distention, edema of lower extremities, and congestion of liver and spleen. Hepatic congestion in heart failure is characterized by distended central veins, which stand out on the cut surface of the liver as dark red foci against the yellow of the cells in the lobular periphery. This gives the liver a gross appearance that has been compared to the cut surface of a nutmeg (hence, **nutmeg liver;** see Chapter 14).

Chronically injured cardiac myocytes exhibit loss of myofibrils. Regardless of the type of injury, dysfunctional myocytes lose sarcomeres and correspondingly increase cytosol and glycogen, which causes the cells to appear vacuolated (**myocytolysis**) (Fig. 11-6). These changes are apparently reversible and likely result

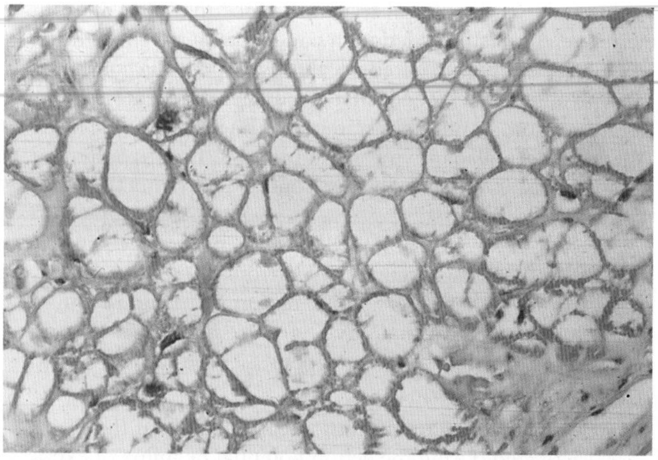

FIGURE 11-6. **Severe myocytolysis in a patient with end-stage heart failure.** Chronically injured myocytes show dramatic loss of myofibrils, giving the cells a marked vacuolated appearance. Only a thin rim of contractile cytoplasm is present, immediately beneath the sarcolemma.

from perturbations in myocyte metabolism. Myofibrillar loss may be an adaptive response to enhance myocyte survival in the face of chronic injury. Such histopathology is especially prominent in "**hibernating myocardium**," a condition in which contractile function is impaired at rest in the setting of reduced coronary blood flow.

Diastolic heart failure is often seen in elderly patients. As a heart ages, the ventricles become progressively stiffer and require greater filling (diastolic) pressures. Some patients exhibit signs and symptoms of heart failure even though their hearts are normal in size and have normal systolic contractile function. These patients do not easily tolerate increases in blood volume and are susceptible to developing pulmonary edema in response to a fluid challenge. Microscopically, these hearts typically exhibit intersitial fibrosis, which may contribute to the decreased compliance of ventricular myocardium.

CLINICAL FEATURES: Symptoms of left-sided failure include **dyspnea on exertion, orthopnea** (dyspnea when lying down), and **paroxysmal nocturnal dyspnea.** Dyspnea on exertion reflects the increasing pulmonary congestion that accompanies a higher end-diastolic pressure in the left atrium and ventricle. Orthopnea and paroxysmal nocturnal dyspnea result when thoracic blood volume increases, owing to reduced blood volume in the lower extremities during recumbency.

Although much of the clinical presentation of heart failure can be explained by venous congestion (**backward failure**), two aspects of congestive failure involve inadequate arterial perfusion of vital organs (**forward failure**). Most patients with left-sided heart failure retain sodium and water (edema), owing to decreased renal perfusion, decreased glomerular filtration rate, and activation of the renin–angiotensin–aldosterone system (see Chapter 7). Inadequate cerebral perfusion can lead to confusion, memory loss, and disorientation. Reduced perfusion of skeletal muscle leads to fatigue and weakness.

Congenital Heart Disease

Congenital heart disease (CHD) results from faulty embryonic development, expressed either as misplaced structures (e.g., transposition of the great vessels) or an arrest in the progression of a normal structure from an early stage to a more advanced one (e.g., atrial septal defect).

Significant CHD occurs in almost 1% of all live births. This does not include certain common defects that are not functionally important, e.g., an anatomically patent foramen ovale that is functionally closed by the left atrial flap that covers it. In this circumstance, the foramen ovale remains closed as long as left atrial pressure exceeds that in the right atrium. A bicuspid aortic valve is also common and is usually asymptomatic until adulthood. Estimates of the incidence of particular cardiovascular anomalies vary, depending on many factors. A range derived from several sources is shown in Table 11-1.

TABLE 11-1

Relative Incidence of Specific Anomalies in Patients with Congenital Heart Disease

Ventricular septal defects—25% to 30%
Atrial septal defects—10% to 15%
Patent ductus arteriosus—10% to 20%
Tetralogy of Fallot—4% to 9%
Pulmonary stenosis—5% to 7%
Coarctation of the aorta—5% to 7%
Aortic stenosis—4% to 6%
Complete transposition of the great arteries—4% to 10%
Truncus arteriosus—2%
Tricuspid atresia—1%

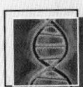

PATHOGENESIS: The cause(s) of CHD is usually not ascertained. However, it is worthwhile to determine whether a defect in any one case can be recognized as being mainly of genetic origin or primarily acquired, as this issue is important to parents in planning future pregnancies. Most congenital heart defects reflect both multifactorial genetic and environmental influences. As in other diseases with multifactorial inheritance (see Chapter 6), the risk of recurrence is increased among siblings of an affected child: the incidence of CHD in the general population is 1%, but it increases to 2% to 15% for a second pregnancy after the birth of a child with a heart defect. The risk for a third affected child may be as high as 30%. Moreover, an infant born to a mother with CHD also has an increased risk of cardiac defects.

Single-gene syndromes are rare causes of CHD. Chromosomal abnormalities associated with increased incidence of congenital heart anomalies include, most prominently Down syndrome (trisomy 21), other trisomies, Turner syndrome, and DiGeorge syndrome. Together, these account for no more than 5% of all cases of CHD.

Much has been learned recently about genes encoding transcription factors that regulate cardiogenesis. The best studied is *Csx/Mkx2-5*, a member of the evolutionarily conserved *NK* homeobox gene family. *Csx/Mkx2-5* is a mammalian homolog of the *Drosophila* gene *NK4*, also known as *tinman* (from the Wizard of Oz) because deletion of this gene leads to failure of cardiac myocyte fate specification and lack of formation of a heart. The cardiac myocyte lineage is formed when *Csx/Mkx2-5* is deleted in mammals, but certain features of morphogenesis are arrested and growth of the heart tube is retarded. Expression of several cardiac genes is also reduced including genes encoding myosin light chain 2v, atrial natriuretic peptide, cardiac ankyrin repeat protein, and various transcription factors such as dHAND and eHAND which are expressed in chamber-specific patterns and exert important regulatory influences over development of the right and left ventricles. Various mutations in *Csx/Mkx2-5* in humans have been associated with a spectrum of congenital cardiac malformations including atrial and ventricular septal defects, Tetralogy of Fallot, double-outlet right ventricle, tricuspid valve abnormalities, and hypoplastic left heart syndrome.

The best evidence for intrauterine influence in the occurrence of congenital cardiac defects relates to maternal rubella infection during the first trimester, especially during the first 4 weeks of gestation. An association with other viral infections is suspected but is not as well documented. Maternal use of certain drugs in early pregnancy is also associated with increased numbers of cardiac defects in offspring. For example, in the thalidomide syndrome (phocomelia) there was a 10% incidence of CHD. Other drugs implicated in CHD include alcohol, phenytoin, amphetamines, lithium, and estrogenic steroids. Maternal diabetes is also associated with an increased incidence of CHD.

Classifications of Congenital Heart Disease Reflect Cyanosis and Shunting

There are several ways to categorize congenital heart defects. One of the earliest clinically useful schemes was proposed by Maude Abbott, who grouped cases into 3 groups based on the presence or absence of cyanosis:

- **The acyanotic group** does not have an abnormal communication between the two circulations. Examples of the acyanotic group include coarctation of the aorta, right-sided aortic arch, and Ebstein malformation.
- **The cyanose tardive** group is defined as an initial left-to-right shunt with late reversal of flow, including patent ductus arteriosus (PDA), patent foramen ovale, and ventricular septal defect. In patients with these anomalies, cyanosis supervenes later (i.e., tardive). Although the shunt is initially left to right, it later becomes right-to-left (Eisenmenger complex) because progressive increases in pulmonary vascular resistance cause right ventricular pressure to exceed that in the left ventricle.
- **The cyanotic group** describes a permanent right-to-left shunt. This category of CHD includes tetralogy of Fallot, truncus arteriosus, tricuspid atresia, and complete transposition of the great vessels.

Additional classification schemes have been developed to provide the detail necessary to meet clinical requirements, especially those of the cardiac surgeon. A more contemporary classification divides the cases into the groups shown in Table 11-2.

TABLE 11-2

Classification of Congenital Heart Disease

Initial left-to-right shunt
Ventricular septal defect
Atrial septal defect
Patent ductus arteriosus
Persistent truncus arteriosus
Anomalous pulmonary venous drainage
Hypoplastic left heart syndrome
Right-to-left shunt
Tetralogy of Fallot
Tricuspid atresia
No shunt
Complete transposition of the great vessels
Coarctation of the aorta
Pulmonary stenosis
Aortic stenosis
Coronary artery origin from pulmonary artery
Ebstein malformation
Complete heart block
Endocardial fibroelastosis

Early Left-to-Right Shunt Reflects Higher Pressure on the Left Side of the Heart

Ventricular Septal Defect

Ventricular septal defects are the most common congenital heart lesion (see Table 11-1). They occur as isolated lesions or in combination with other malformations.

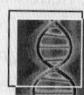

PATHOGENESIS: The fetal heart consists of a single chamber until the fifth week of gestation, after which it is divided by the development of interatrial and interventricular septa and by formation of atrioventricular valves from endocardial cushions. A muscular interventricular septum grows upward from the apex toward the base of the heart (Fig. 11-7). It is joined by the down-growing membranous septum, separating right and left ventricles. *The most common ventricular septal defect is related to failure of the membranous portion of the septum to form in whole or in part.*

PATHOLOGY: Ventricular septal defects occur as (1) a small hole in the membranous septum; (2) a large defect involving more than the membranous region (perimembranous defects); (3) defects in the muscular portion, which are more common anteriorly but can occur anywhere in the muscular septum; or (4) complete absence of the muscular septum (leaving a single ventricle).

Ventricular septal defects are most common in the superior portion of the septum below the pulmonary artery outflow tract (below the crista supraventricularis, i.e., infracristal) and behind the septal leaflet of the tricuspid valve. The common bundle (bundle of His) is located immediately below the defect (inlet type). Less commonly, the defect is above the crista supraventricularis (supracristal) and just below the pulmonary valve (infra-arterial). The supracristal variety of septal defect is often associated with other defects, such as an overriding pulmonary artery (the **Taussig-Bing** type of double-outlet right ventricle), transposition of the great vessels, or persistent truncus arteriosus.

CLINICAL FEATURES: *A small septal defect may have little functional significance and may actually close spontaneously as the child matures.* Closure is accomplished by either hypertrophy of adjacent muscle or adherence of tricuspid valve leaflets to the margins of the defect. In infants with large septal defects, higher left ventricular pressure creates initially a left-to-right shunt. Left ventricular dilation and congestive heart failure are common complications of such shunts. If a defect is small enough to permit prolonged survival, augmented pulmonary blood flow caused by shunting of blood into the right ventricle eventually results in thickening of pulmonary arteries and increased pulmonary vascular resistance. This increased vascular resistance may be so great that the direction of the shunt is reversed and goes from right to left (**Eisenmenger complex**). A patient with this condition displays late onset of cyanosis (i.e., tardive cyanosis), right ventricular hypertrophy, and right-sided heart failure.

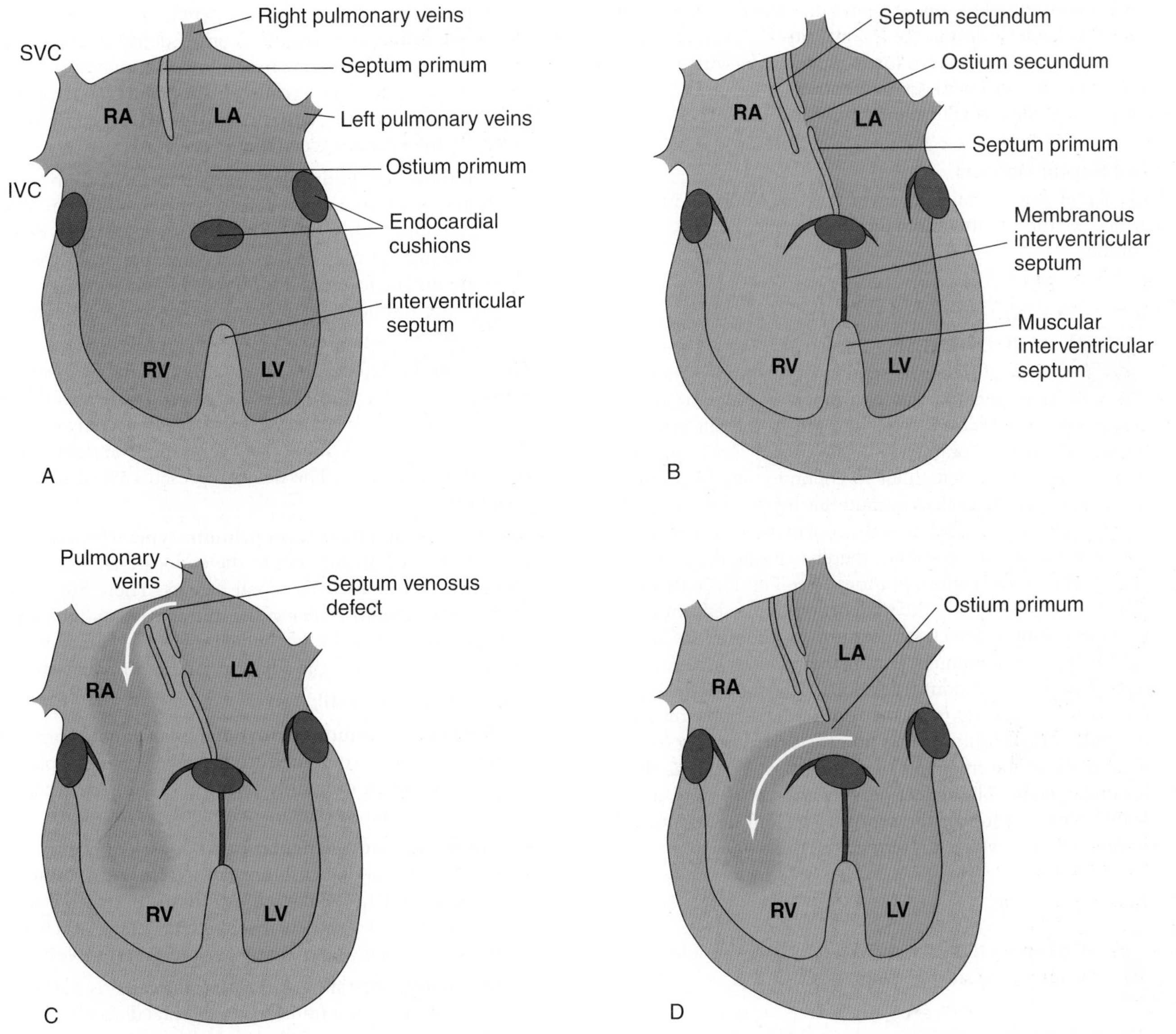

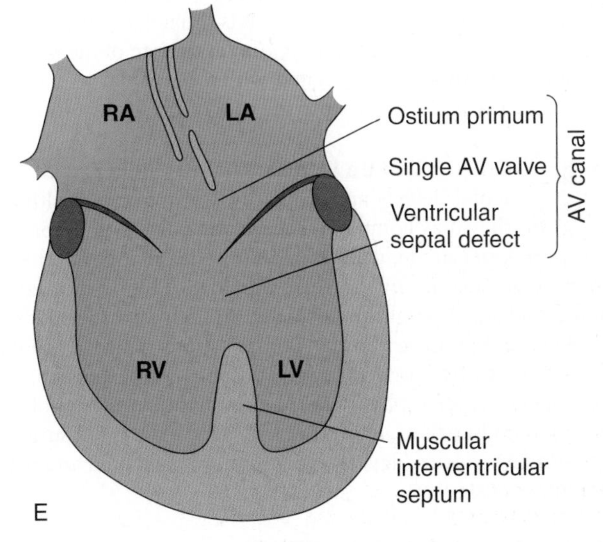

FIGURE 11-7. **Pathogenesis of ventricular and atrial septal defects.** **A.** The common atrial chamber is being separated into the right and left atria (RA and LA) by the septum primum. Because the septum primum has not yet joined the endocardial cushions, there is an open ostium primum. The ventricular cavity is being divided by a muscular interventricular septum into right and left chambers (right and left ventrilces, RV and LV). SVC = superior vena cava; IVC = inferior vena cava. **B.** The septum primum has joined the endocardial cushions but at the same time has developed an opening in its midportion (the ostium secundum). This opening is partly overlaid by the septum secundum, which has grown down to cover, in part, the foramen ovale. Simultaneously, the membranous septum joins the muscular interventricular septum to the base of the heart, completely separating the ventricles. **C.** The sinus venosus type of atrial septal defect is located in the most cephalad region and is adjacent to the inflow of the right pulmonary veins, which thus tend to open into the RA. **D.** The ostium primum defect occurs just above the atrioventricular (AV) valve ring, sometimes in the presence of an intact valve ring. It may also, in conjunction with a defect of the valve ring and ventricular septum, form an AV canal, as shown in (**E**). This common opening allows free communication between the atria and the ventricles.

Additional complications of ventricular septal defects include (1) infective endocarditis at the lesional site, (2) paradoxical emboli, and (3) prolapse of an aortic valve cusp (with resulting aortic valve insufficiency). Large ventricular septal defects are repaired surgically, usually in infancy.

Atrial Septal Defects

Atrial septal defects range in severity from clinically insignificant and asymptomatic anomalies to chronic, life-threatening conditions.

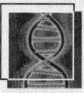

PATHOGENESIS: The embryologic development of the atrial septum occurs in a sequence that permits the continued passage of oxygenated placental blood from the right to the left atrium through the patent foramen. The developing atrial septum permits this right-to-left shunt to continue until birth. Beginning at the fifth week of intrauterine life, the septum primum extends downward from the roof of the atrium to join with the endocardial cushions, thereby closing the incomplete segment, or "ostium primum" (see Fig. 11-7). Before this closure is complete, the midportion of the septum primum develops a defect, or "ostium secundum," so that right-to-left flow continues. During the sixth week, a second septum (septum secundum) develops to the right of the septum primum, passing from the roof of the atrium toward the endocardial cushions. This process leaves a patent foramen at about the midpoint of the septum, known as the **foramen ovale**. The defect persists after birth until it is sealed off by fusion of the septum primum and septum secundum, after which it is termed the **fossa ovalis**.

PATHOLOGY: The atrial septum may be defective at a number of sites (see Fig 11-7).

- **Patent foramen ovale:** Tissue derived from the septum primum situated on the left side of the foramen ovale functions as a flap valve that normally fuses with the margins of the foramen ovale, thereby sealing the opening. An incomplete seal of the foramen ovale, which can be detected with a probe (**probe patent foramen ovale**), is found in 25% of normal adults and is not normally functional. However, it may become a true shunt if circumstances increase right atrial pressure, as can occur with recurrent pulmonary thromboemboli. If this situation develops, a right-to-left shunt will be produced, and thromboemboli from the right-sided circulation will pass directly into the systemic circulation. These **paradoxical emboli** can produce infarcts in many parts of the arterial circulation, most commonly in the brain, heart, spleen, intestines, kidneys, and lower extremities. A widely patent foramen ovale is occasionally encountered and is actually an acquired atrial septal defect caused by a disproportion between the size of the foramen ovale and the length of the valve covering it.
- **Atrial septal defect, ostium secundum type:** This is by far the most common of atrial septal defect, accounting for 90% of all cases. It is a true deficiency of the atrial septum and should not be confused with a patent foramen ovale. An ostium secundum defect occurs in the middle portion of the septum and varies from a trivial opening to a large defect of the entire fossa ovalis region. A small defect is usually not functional, but a larger one may allow shunting of sufficient blood from left to right to cause dilation and hypertrophy of the right atrium and ventricle. In this setting, pulmonary artery diameter may exceed that of the aorta.
  - **Lutembacher syndrome**, a variant of the ostium secundum type of atrial septal defect, is the combination of mitral stenosis and an ostium secundum atrial septal defect. Mitral stenosis may be due to a congenital malformation or rheumatic fever. It is thought that increased left atrial pressure secondary to mitral valve obstruction influences the continued patency of the atrial septum.
- **Sinus venosus defect:** This anomaly occurs in the upper portion of the atrial septum, above the fossa ovalis, near the entry of the superior vena cava. It is usually accompanied by drainage of the right pulmonary veins into the right atrium or superior vena cava. This defect represents 5% of atrial septal defects.
- **Atrial septal defect, ostium primum type:** This condition involves the region adjacent to the endocardial cushion and comprises 7% of all atrial septal defects. There are usually clefts in the anterior leaflet of the mitral valve and the septal leaflet of the tricuspid valve, which may be accompanied by an associated defect in the adjacent interventricular septum.
- **Atrioventricular canal:**
  - **Persistent common atrioventricular canal** represents fully developed combined atrial and ventricular septal defects. Although ordinarily uncommon, this defect is encountered often in patients with Down syndrome.
  - **Complete atrioventricular canal** occurs when atrioventricular endocardial cushions fail to fuse. As a result, the defect includes (1) enlarged ostium primum atrial septal defect, (2) inlet ventricular septal defect, and (3) clefts in the septal leaflets of the tricuspid and mitral valves.
  - **Incomplete (partial) atrioventricular canal** is a situation in which an ostium primum atrial septal defect is adjacent to the atrioventricular valves, which are often abnormal.
- **Coronary sinus atrial septal defect:** This abnormality is the rarest of the atrial septal defects. It is situated in the posteroinferior part of the interatrial septum at the site of the coronary sinus ostium and is associated with a persistent left superior vena cava, which drains into the roof of the left atrium.

CLINICAL FEATURES: Young children with atrial septal defects are ordinarily asymptomatic, although they may complain of easy fatigability and dyspnea on exertion. Later in life, usually in adulthood, changes in the pulmonary vasculature may reverse the flow of blood through the defect and create a right-to-left shunt. In such cases, cyanosis and clubbing of the fingers ensue. Complications of atrial septal defects include atrial arrhythmias, pulmonary hypertension, right ventricular hypertrophy, heart failure, paradoxical emboli, and bacterial endocarditis. Symptomatic cases are treated surgically or with new closure devices, which can be delivered and placed percutaneously.

Patent Ductus Arteriosus (PDA)

The early embryo supposedly recapitulates an ancestral evolutionary stage, with six aortic arches connecting the ventral and dorsal aortas as part of the branchial cleft system (Fig. 11-8). The left sixth aortic arch is partly preserved as the pulmonary arteries, and the arterial continuation on the left to the descending thoracic aorta is retained as the **ductus arteriosus**. The ductus conveys most of the pulmonary outflow into the aorta. After birth, the ductus constricts in response to the increased arterial oxygen content and becomes occluded by fibrosis (ligamentum arteriosus).

PATHOGENESIS: Persistent PDA is one of the most common congenital cardiac defects and is especially common in infants whose mothers were infected with rubellavirus early in pregnancy. It is also common in premature infants, in whom prematurity precluded closure. In these patients, the ductus usually closes spontaneously. In full-term infants with PDA, however, the ductus has an abnormal endothelium and media and only rarely closes spontaneously.

CLINICAL FEATURES: The lumenal diameter of a PDA varies greatly. A small shunt has little effect on the heart, whereas a large one leads to considerable diversion of blood from the aorta to the low-pressure pulmonary artery. In severe cases, more than half of the left ventricular output may be shunted into the pulmonary circulation. Left ventricular hypertrophy and heart failure ensue as due to increased demand for cardiac output. In patients with a large PDA, the increased volume and pressure of blood in the pulmonary circulation eventually lead to pulmonary hypertension and its cardiac complications. Infective endarteritis is a frequent complication of untreated PDA.

PDA can be corrected surgically or by cardiac catheterization. It can be caused to contract and then close by instillation of prostaglandin synthesis inhibitors (e.g., indomethacin). Conversely, it can be kept open after birth by administering prostaglandins (PGE_2). This effect is used to treat patients born with a cardiac defect whose survival requires a left-to-right or right-to-left shunt. Examples include patients with isolated pulmonary stenosis, complete transposition of the great vessels, or hypoplastic left heart syndrome.

Aortopulmonary window is a defect between the base of the aorta and the pulmonary artery. It is a rare condition that is functionally similar to PDA and is clinically difficult to differentiate from it.

Other abnormalities of the aortic arch system can be predicted by visualizing the variations that could occur in the development of the complete aortic arch system (see Fig. 11-8). For example, the right side of the aortic arch system rather than the left may be retained, resulting in the condition known as a **right aortic arch**. This variant is seen in about 25% of patients with tetralogy of Fallot and in 50% of patients with truncus arteriosus. A right aortic arch is innocuous unless it creates a vascular ring that compresses the esophagus and trachea.

Truncus Arteriosus

Persistent truncus arteriosus refers to a common trunk for the origin of the aorta, pulmonary arteries, and coronary arteries. It results from absent or incomplete partitioning of the truncus arteriosus by the spiral septum.

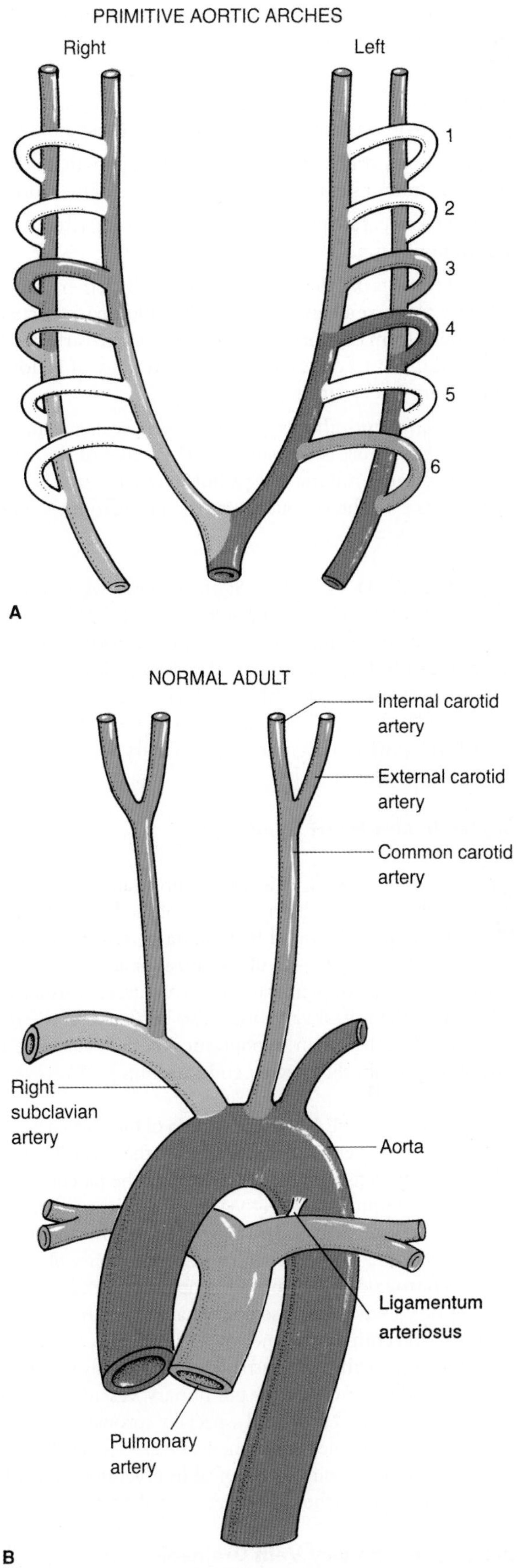

FIGURE 11-8. **Derivatives of the aortic arches. A.** Complete primitive aortic arch system. **B.** In the normal adult, the left fourth aortic arch is preserved as the arch of the adult aorta, and the left sixth arch gives rise to the pulmonary artery and ligamentum arteriosus (closed ductus arteriosus).

PATHOLOGY: There are several variants of truncus arteriosus:

- **Type 1** is most common, and consists of a single trunk that gives rise to a common pulmonary artery and ascending aorta.
- **Type 2** displays right and left pulmonary arteries that originate from a common site in the posterior midline of the truncus.
- **Type 3** has separate pulmonary arteries arising laterally from a common trunk.
- **Type 4** consists of other rare variants in which there is no pulmonary trunk at all and in which the pulmonary circulation is supplied from the aorta by enlarged bronchial arteries. This type is difficult to differentiate from tetralogy of Fallot with pulmonary artery atresia.

Truncus arteriosus always overrides a ventricular septal defect and receives blood from both ventricles. The valve of the truncus usually has three semilunar cusps but may have as few as two or as many as six. The coronary arteries arise from the base of the valve.

CLINICAL FEATURES: Most infants with truncus arteriosus have torrential pulmonary blood flow, causing heart failure, recurrent respiratory tract infections, and often early death. Pulmonary vascular disease develops in children with prolonged survival, in which case cyanosis, polycythemia, and clubbing of the fingers appear. Open-heart surgery prior to development of significant pulmonary vascular changes is an effective treatment.

Hypoplastic Left Heart Syndrome

PATHOLOGY: This usually profound malformation is characterized by hypoplasia of the left ventricle and ascending aorta and hypoplasia or atresia of the left-sided valves. Severe aortic valvular stenosis or aortic atresia is often the main defect. Some mitral valve structures are usually present, although the mitral valve may also be atretic. If the mitral valve is atretic rather than hypoplastic, the left ventricle may consist of only a thin slit lined by endocardium.

CLINICAL FEATURES: Atresia of the aortic valve precludes left ventricular outflow into the aorta. There is an obligate left-to-right shunt through the patent foramen ovale. Cardiac output is entirely via the right ventricle and pulmonary artery. Systemic blood flow depends on flow from the pulmonary trunk to the aorta through a PDA. Coronary blood flow depends on retrograde flow from a hypoplastic ascending aorta to the sinuses of Valsalva. Because pulmonary vascular resistance is high at birth, and both the foramen ovale and ductus arteriosus are patent, newborns with hypoplastic left heart syndrome may appear well initially. However, as pulmonary vascular resistance falls, and systemic blood flow (and especially coronary blood flow) decreases, infants become symptomatic. Over 95% will die within the first month of life without surgical intervention. Treatment includes surgical approaches or cardiac transplantation.

Anomalous Pulmonary Vein Drainage

The pulmonary veins form a network in the dorsal mesoderm. A bud from the region of the atrium joins the pulmonary venous confluence, and eventually all four pulmonary veins drain into the left atrium. Failure of these tissues to join correctly results in various venous anomalies.

PATHOLOGY: Total anomalous pulmonary vein drainage may occur as an isolated defect, or it may be part of the asplenia syndrome (splenic agenesis, congenital heart defects, and situs inversus of abdominal organs). Most commonly, the pulmonary veins drain into a common pulmonary venous chamber, and then through a persistent left superior vena cava (the persistent left pericardial vein) into the innominate vein or the right superior vena cava. A second route for common pulmonary vein drainage leads into the coronary sinus. A third drainage route consists of persistent posterior and subcardinal veins, which form a middorsal trunk that crosses the diaphragm and enters the portal vein or ductus venosus. The third type of drainage is often associated with some pulmonary venous obstruction.

CLINICAL FEATURES: In total anomalous pulmonary drainage, there is no direct venous return to the left side of the heart and life is sustained only by an atrial septal defect or patent foramen ovale. Heart failure, severe hypoxemia, and pulmonary venous obstruction result from total anomalous pulmonary vein drainage. Good results have been obtained with surgical correction.

Partial anomalous pulmonary venous drainage may result from less severe circulatory impairment. This anomaly may involve one or two pulmonary veins, especially in association with a sinus venosus type of atrial septal defect. The prognosis is excellent, similar to that for atrial septal defects.

Right-to-Left Shunt Is the Most Common Cyanotic Congential Heart Disease

Tetrology of Fallot

Tetralogy of Fallot represents 10% of all cases of CHD.

PATHOLOGY

The four anatomical changes that define the tetralogy of Fallot are (Fig. 11-9):

- **Pulmonary stenosis**
- **Ventricular septal defect**
- **Dextroposition of the aorta so that it overrides the ventricular septal defect**
- **Right ventricular hypertrophy**

The ventricular septal defect, which may be as large as the aortic orifice, is the result of incomplete closure of the membranous septum and involves both the muscular septum and the endocardial cushions. In addition, the development of the spiral septum, which normally divides the common truncus region into an aorta and pulmonary artery, is abnormal. As a result, the aorta is displaced into a more dextral position overlying the septal defect. The ventricular septal defect is immediately below the overriding aorta. Pulmonary stenosis is often due to subpulmonary muscular hypertrophy, with an enlarged infundibular muscle obstructing blood flow into the pulmonary artery. In about one third of these hearts, the valve itself is the main cause of stenosis; in such cases, the valve is usually funnel shaped, with the narrow part more distal.

The heart is hypertrophied so as to give it a boot shape. Almost half of patients with tetralogy of Fallot have other cardiac anomalies, including ostium secundum atrial septal defects, PDA, left superior vena cava, and endocardial cushion defects. The aortic arch is on the right side in about 25% of cases of tetralogy of Fallot. The surgeon must remember that a large branch of the right coronary artery may cross the pulmonary conus

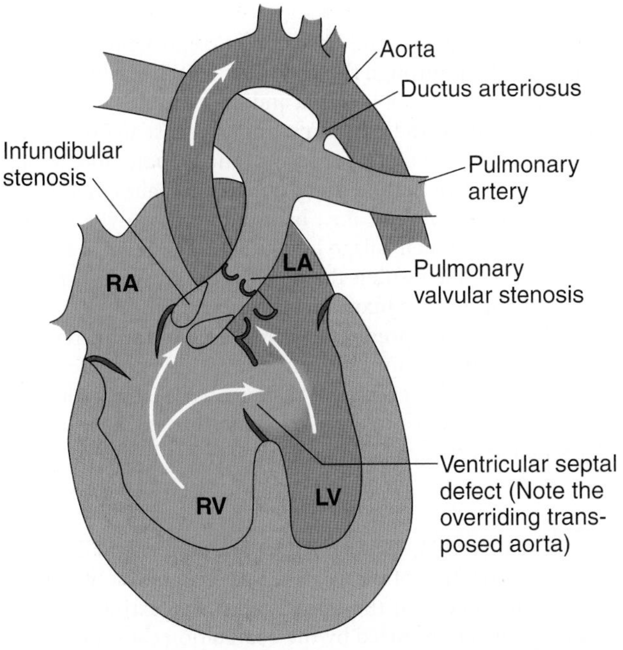

FIGURE 11-9. **Tetralogy of Fallot.** Note the pulmonary stenosis, which is due to infundibular hypertrophy as well as pulmonary valvular stenosis. The ventricular septal defect involves the membranous septum region. Dextroposition of the aorta and right ventricular hypertrophy are shown. Because of the pulmonary obstruction, the shunt is from right to left, and the patient is cyanotic. LA = left atrium; LV = left ventricle; RA = right atrium; RV = right ventricle.

region, which is the site of the cardiotomy made to enlarge the outflow tract. Patency of the ductus arteriosus is actually protective, because it provides a source of blood to the otherwise deprived pulmonary vascular bed.

CLINICAL FEATURES: In the face of severe pulmonary stenosis, right ventricular blood is shunted through the ventricular septal defect into the aorta, resulting in arterial desaturation and cyanosis. Surgical correction is typically performed in the first 2 years of life. In children who are unrepaired, dyspnea on exertion is particularly noticeable, and the affected child often assumes a squatting position to relieve the shortness of breath. Physical development is characteristically retarded. Cerebral thromboses may complicate the disease owing to marked polycythemia. Patients are also at risk for bacterial endocarditis and brain abscesses. Increasing cyanosis and shortness of breath may indicate that a beneficial PDA has closed spontaneously. Left-sided heart failure is not common.

Without surgical intervention, tetralogy of Fallot has a dismal prognosis. However, total correction is now possible with open-heart surgery, which carries less than 10% mortality. After successful surgery, patients are asymptomatic and have an excellent long-term prognosis.

Tricuspid Atresia

PATHOLOGY: *Tricuspid atresia, a congenital absence of the tricuspid valve, results in an obligate right-to-left shunt through the patent foramen ovale.* This defect usually occurs with a ventricular septal defect through which blood gains access to the pulmonary artery. Type I tricuspid atresia, (75% of patients with tricuspid atresia) is associated with normally related great arteries. Type II is associated with D-transposition of the great arteries, and type III (rare) features L-malposition.

CLINICAL FEATURES: Infants with tricuspid atresia present with cyanosis due to the atrial right-to-left shunt. If the ventricular septal defect is small, the limitation of pulmonary blood flow can result in even more significant cyanosis. In this scenario, a prominent cardiac murmur is typically noted. Surgical intervention is aimed at bypassing the atretic tricuspid valve and small right ventricle. Staged surgical palliation is the goal of current therapy.

Congenital Heart Diseases Without Shunts Involve Various Cardiovascular Sites

Transposition of the Great Arteries

In transposition of the great arteries (TGA), the aorta arises from the right ventricle and the pulmonary artery from the left ventricle. The condition shows a male predominance and is more common in offspring of mothers with diabetes. TGA is responsible for more than half of deaths in infants younger than 1 year with cyanotic heart disease.

PATHOGENESIS: The normal division of the embryonic truncus arteriosus into the aorta and pulmonary artery depends on the spiral septum. Its abnormal development can produce aberrant positioning of the great arteries, such that the aorta is anterior to the pulmonary artery and connects with the right ventricle. Then, the pulmonary artery receives the left ventricular outflow (Fig. 11-10). Because the venous blood from the right side of the heart flows to the aorta, and the oxygenated blood from the lungs returns to the pulmonary artery, there are in effect two independent and parallel blood circuits for the systemic and pulmonary circulations.

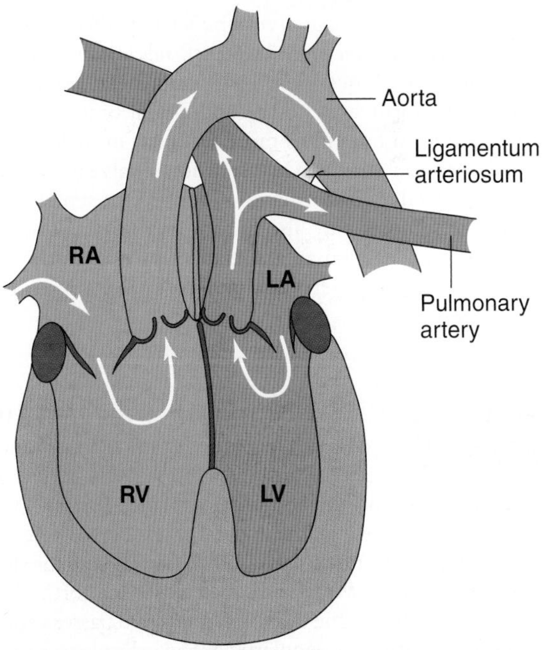

FIGURE 11-10. **Complete transposition of great arteries, regular type.** The aorta is anterior to, and to the right of, the pulmonary artery ("D-transposition") and arises from the right ventricle. In the absence of interatrial or interventricular connections or patent ductus arteriosus, this anomaly is incompatible with life. LA = left atrium; LV = left ventricle; RA = right atrium; RV = right ventricle.

Survival is possible only if there is a communication between the circuits. Virtually all infants with TGA have an atrial septal defect. One half of patients exhibit a ventricular septal defect, and two thirds have a PDA.

PATHOLOGY: The aorta normally arises posterior and to the left of the pulmonary artery. In its ascending portion, it courses behind and to the right of the pulmonary artery. In TGA, the aorta is anterior to the pulmonary artery and to its right ("D" or dextrotransposition) all the way from its origin.

CLINICAL FEATURES: Before cardiac surgery, the outlook for infants with TGA was hopeless: 90% died in their first year. It is now possible to correct the malformation within the first 2 weeks of life using an arterial-switch operation, with overall survival of 90%.

Congenitally corrected transposition is a condition in which the aorta is anterior to, but passes to the left of, the pulmonary artery ("L" transposition). Although the great arteries are thus abnormally related to each other and arise from discordant ventricles, the circulatory pattern is functionally corrected because of coexistent atrioventricular discordance. Patients in whom corrected TGA is the only malformation are clinically entirely normal. Unfortunately, many cases are complicated by other cardiac anomalies, which require their own specific interventions.

The **Taussig-Bing malformation** is a double-outlet right ventricle (both great vessels arise from the right ventricle) in which a ventricular septal defect is above the crista supraventricularis and directly beneath an overriding pulmonary artery. This condition is functionally and clinically similar to TGA with a ventricular septal defect and pulmonary hypertension.

Coarctation of the Aorta

Coarctation of the aorta is a local constriction that almost always occurs immediately below the origin of the left subclavian artery at the site of the ductus arteriosus. Rare coarctations can occur at any point from the aortic arch to the abdominal bifurcation. The condition is two to five times more frequent in males than females and is associated with a bicuspid aortic valve in two-thirds of cases. Mitral valve malformations, ventricular septal defects, and subaortic stenosis may also accompany coarctation of the aorta. There is a particular association of coarctation with Turner syndrome, and berry aneurysms in the brain are also more common.

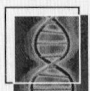

PATHOGENESIS AND PATHOLOGY: The pathogenesis of coarctation of the aorta is related to the pattern of flow in the ductus arteriosus during fetal life (Fig. 11-11). In utero blood flow through the ductus is considerably greater than that across the aortic valve. The blood leaving the ductus is diverted into two streams by a posterior aortic shelf opposite the orifice of the ductus. One stream passes cephalad into the relatively hypoplastic aortic isthmus to supply the head and upper extremities; the other enters the descending thoracic aorta. In late fetal life, increasing left ventricular output dilates the isthmus, and the increased blood flow bypasses the obstruction (represented by the posterior shelf) through the wide ductal orifice. After birth, the ductal orifice is obliterated and the posterior shelf normally involutes, thereby removing the obstruction. The shelf may not involute because of inadequate antegrade flow in the aortic arch in utero due to anomalies that limit left ventricular output (e.g., bicuspid aortic valve). Often the obstructing shelf fails to involute for unknown reasons. In any event, the result is the most common type of coarctation of the aorta, a **juxtaductal constriction**.

The **infantile (preductal) type of coarctation** results when the aortic isthmus remains narrow (hypoplastic) into late fetal life and after birth. This lesion is usually accompanied by a PDA and a right-to-left shunt through a ventricular septal defect.

CLINICAL FEATURES: The clinical hallmark of coarctation of the aorta is a discrepancy in blood pressure between the upper and lower extremities. The pressure gradient produced by the coarctation causes hypertension proximal to the narrowed segment and, occasionally, dilation of that portion of the aorta.

Hypertension in the upper part of the body results in left ventricular hypertrophy and may produce dizziness, headaches, and nosebleeds. The increased pressure may also increase the risk of rupture of a berry aneurysm and consequent subarachnoid hemorrhage. Hypotension below the coarctation leads to weakness, pallor, and coldness of lower extremities. In an attempt to bridge the obstruction between the upper and lower aortic segments, collateral vessels enlarge. Radiologic examination of the chest shows *notching of the inner surfaces of the ribs*, produced by increased pressure in markedly dilated intercostal arteries.

Most patients with coarctation of the aorta die by age 40 unless they are treated. Complications include (1) heart failure, (2) rupture of a dissecting aneurysm (secondary to cystic medial necrosis of the aorta), (3) infective endarteritis at the point of narrowing or at the site of jet-stream impingement on the wall immediately distal to the coarctation, (4) cerebral hemorrhage, and (5) stenosis or infective endocarditis of a bicuspid aortic valve. Coarctation of the aorta is successfully treated by surgical excision of the narrowed segment, preferably between 1 and 2 years of age for asymptomatic patients. Balloon dilation of the narrowed area by cardiac catheterization has also been performed.

Pulmonary Stenosis

Pulmonary stenosis results from (1) developmental deformities arising from the endocardial cushion region of the heart (with involvement of the pulmonary valves); (2) an abnormality of the right ventricular infundibular muscle (subvalvular or infundibular stenosis, especially as part of tetralogy of Fallot); or (3) abnormal development of the more distal parts of the pulmonary artery tree (peripheral pulmonary stenosis). Peripheral pulmonary stenosis, which is much less common than the other two, may produce "coarctation" of the pulmonary arteries at one or several sites. This anomaly is more frequent in newborns with **Williams syndrome**, a disorder often associated with deletion mutations in the gene encoding elastin.

Isolated pulmonary stenosis ordinarily involves the valve cusps, which are fused to form an inverted cone or funnel type

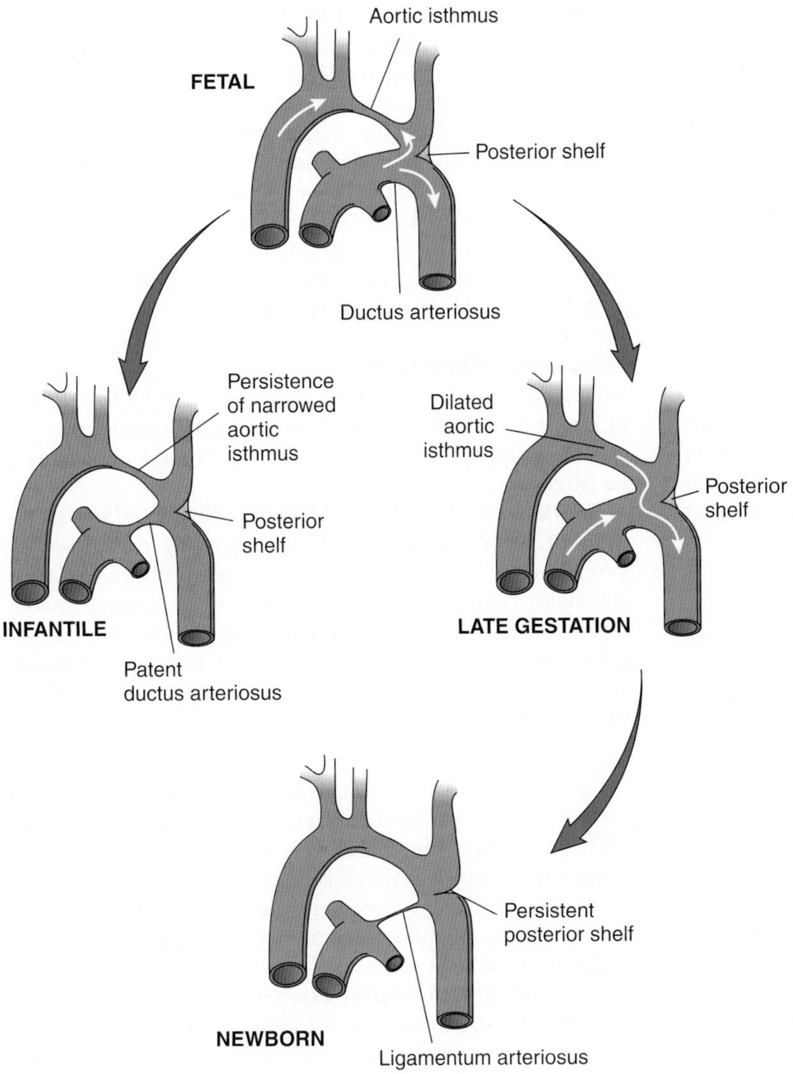

FIGURE 11-11. **Pathogenesis of coarctation of the aorta.** In the fetus, ductal blood is diverted into cephalad and descending streams by the posterior aortic shelf. In late fetal life, the isthmus dilates and the increased descending blood flow is accommodated by the ductal orifice. After birth, if the shelf does not undergo the normal involution, obliteration of the ductal orifice does not permit free flow around the persistent posterior shelf, thereby creating a juxtaductal obstruction of blood flow to the distal aorta. If the aortic isthmus does not dilate during late fetal life, it remains narrow, resulting in an infantile or preductal coarctation. In this circumstance, the ductus arteriosus usually remains patent.

of constriction. The artery distal to the valve may develop poststenotic dilation after several years. In severe cases, infants exhibit right ventricular and atrial hypertrophy. If the foramen ovale is patent, there is a right-to-left shunt with cyanosis, secondary polycythemia, and clubbing of the fingers. Good results have been obtained with balloon dilation of the stenotic valve by cardiac catheterization.

Congenital Aortic Stenosis

Three types of congenital aortic stenosis are recognized: valvular, subvalvular, and supravalvular.

VALVULAR AORTIC STENOSIS: The most common congenital aortic stenosis, bicuspid valve, arises through abnormal development of the endocardial cushions. A congenitally bicuspid aortic valve is considerably more frequent (4:1) in males than females and is associated with other cardiac anomalies (e.g., coarctation of the aorta) in 20% of cases. A bicuspid valve typically features fusion of two of the three semilunar cusps (the right coronary cusp with one of the adjacent two cusps).

CLINICAL FEATURES: Many children with bicuspid aortic stenosis are asymptomatic. Over the years, the resulting bicuspid valve tends to become thickened and calcified, generally leading to symptoms in adulthood. More severe forms of congenital aortic stenosis result in a unicommissural valve or one without any commissures. These malformations cause symptoms in early life. Exertional dyspnea and angina pectoris may be prominent. Sudden death, principally owing to ventricular arrhythmias, is a distinct threat for patients with severe obstruction. Bacterial endocarditis sometimes complicates the disease. In symptomatic cases, aortic valvulotomy has had a high degree of success, although valve replacement is occasionally indicated.

SUBVALVULAR AORTIC STENOSIS: This defect accounts for 10% of all cases of congenital aortic stenosis and is caused by abnormal development of a band of subvalvular fibroelastic tissue or a muscular ridge. Stenosis results from a membranous diaphragm or fibrous ring that surrounds the left ventricular outflow tract immediately below the aortic valve. It is twice as common in males as in females.

In many persons with subvalvular aortic stenosis, thickening and immobility of the aortic cusps develops, with mild aortic regurgitation. Bacterial endocarditis carries its own risks and may also aggravate the regurgitation. Surgical treatment of subvalvular aortic stenosis involves excising the membrane or fibrous ridge.

SUPRAVALVULAR AORTIC STENOSIS: This type of stenosis is much less common than the other two, and is often associated with idiopathic infantile hypercalcemia (**Williams syndrome**), characterized by mental retardation and multiple system disorders.

Origin of a Coronary Artery from the Pulmonary Artery

A single coronary artery or, rarely, both may originate from the pulmonary artery rather than the aorta. When one coronary artery has an anomalous origin (most commonly the left coronary), anastomoses develop between the right and left coronary arteries. This produces an arteriovenous shunt through which blood flows from the artery originating from the aorta to that arising from the pulmonary artery. As a result, the myocardium supplied by the anomalous artery is vulnerable to episodes of ischemia. The result may be myocardial infarction, fibrosis and calcification, and endocardial fibroelastosis.

Ebstein Malformation

Ebstein malformation results from downward displacement of an abnormal tricuspid valve into an underdeveloped right ventricle. One or more tricuspid valve leaflets is plastered to the right ventricular wall for a variable distance below the right atrioventricular annulus.

PATHOLOGY: Septal and posterior tricuspid valve leaflets are usually affected. They are irregularly elongated and adherent to the right ventricular wall, so that the upper part of the right ventricular cavity (inflow region) functions separately from the distal chamber. The anterior leaflet is usually the least involved, and may be normal. The valve ring may or may not be displaced downward from its usual position. In any event, the effective tricuspid valve orifice is displaced downward into the ventricle, thereby dividing it into two separate parts: the "atrialized" ventricle (proximal ventricle) and the functional right ventricle (distal ventricle). In two thirds of cases, conspicuous dilation of the functional ventricle hinders its ability to pump blood efficiently through the pulmonary arteries. The degree of insufficiency of the tricuspid valve depends on the severity and configuration of the defect in the leaflets.

CLINICAL FEATURES: Ebstein malformation leads to heart failure, massive right atrial dilation, arrhythmias with palpitations and tachycardia, and sudden death. Surgical treatment has met with variable success.

Congenital Heart Block

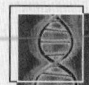

PATHOGENESIS: Congenital complete heart block is usually associated with other cardiac anomalies. In such cases, disruption in the continuity of the conduction system is probably caused by the accompanying cardiac abnormality. However, in cases of isolated complete heart block, failure of the atrioventricular conduction system is believed to result from lack of regression of the sulcus tissue, which entirely encloses the conducting tissue during early development. Congenital heart block in the absence of structural heart disease has been linked to maternal connective tissue disease, especially SLE. If maternal SS-A/Ro or SS-B/La autoantibodies are trans-placentally transmitted to the fetus, the incidence of congenital complete heart block approaches 100%.

PATHOLOGY AND CLINICAL FEATURES: The hearts of patients with congenital heart block tend to show a lack of continuity between the atrial myocardium and the atrioventricular node. Alternatively, the defect may consist of a fibrous separation of the atrioventricular node from the ventricular conducting tissue. Although the heart rate is abnormally slow, patients with isolated heart block often have little functional difficulty. Later in life, cardiac hypertrophy, attacks of Stokes–Adams syncope (dizziness and unexpected fainting), arrhythmias, and heart failure may develop.

Endocardial Fibroelastosis

Endocardial fibroelastosis (EFE) is characterized by fibroelastotic thickening of the endocardium of the left ventricle, which may also affect the valves. The disorder is classified as primary or secondary, the latter being far more common.

SECONDARY ENDOCARDIAL FIBROELASTOSIS: This disorder occurs in association with underlying cardiovascular anomalies that lead to left ventricular hypertrophy in the face of an inability to meet the increased myocardial oxygen demands. Thus secondary EFE is a frequent complication of congenital aortic stenosis (including hypoplastic left ventricle syndrome) and coarctation of the aorta. Presumably, some type of endocardial injury is involved in its pathogenesis.

PATHOLOGY: On gross examination, the left ventricle endocardium displays irregular, opaque, grey-white patches, which also may be present on the cardiac valves. Microscopically, these plaques are areas of endocardial fibroelastotic thickening, frequently accompanied by degeneration of adjacent subendocardial myocytes. The valves may show collagenous thickening.

PRIMARY ENDOCARDIAL FIBROELASTOSIS: Defined as fibroelastosis in the absence of any associated lesion, this disorder is now quite rare. It afflicts infants, usually 4 to 10 months of age. Although it has occurred in siblings, no specific mode of inheritance has been established. Recent evidence links primary EFE to mumps infection, which may explain why this condition is now so rarely encountered.

PATHOLOGY: The left ventricle is usually conspicuously dilated but occasionally contracted and hypertrophic. Diffuse endocardial thickening involves most of the left ventricle (Fig. 11-12) and aortic and mitral valve leaflets. The thickened endocardium tends to obscure the trabecular pattern of the underlying myocardium, and papillary muscles and chordae tendineae are thick and short. Mural thrombi may complicate the situation.

Infants with primary EFE develop progressive heart failure. The prognosis is dismal, and cardiac transplantation offers the only hope for a cure.

Dextrocardia

Dextrocardia is rightward orientation of the base–apex axis of the heart. It is often associated with a mirror image of the normal left-sided location and configuration. The position of the ventricles is determined by the direction of the embryonic cardiac loop. If the loop protrudes to the right, the future right ventricle develops on the right and the left ventricle comes to occupy its proper position. If the loop protrudes to the left, the opposite occurs.

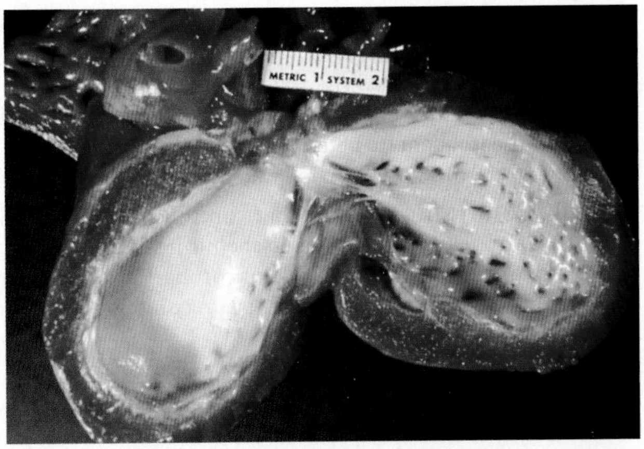

FIGURE 11-12. **Endocardial fibroelastosis.** The left ventricle of an infant who died of endocardial fibroelastosis has been opened to reveal a thickened endocardium lining most of the cavity and virtually obliterating the trabeculae carneae.

PATHOLOGY: When dextrocardia occurs without abnormal positioning of the visceral organs (situs inversus), the condition is invariably associated with severe cardiovascular anomalies. These include transposition of the great arteries, a variety of atrial and ventricular septal defects, anomalous pulmonary venous drainage and many others. In dextrocardia that occurs with situs inversus, the heart is functionally normal, although minor anomalies are not uncommon.

Ischemic Heart Disease

Ischemic heart disease is, in most cases, a consequence of coronary artery atherosclerosis. It develops when blood flow is inadequate to meet the oxygen demands of the heart. *Ischemic heart disease is by far the most common type of heart disease in the United States and other industrialized nations, where it remains the leading cause of death. It is responsible for at least 80% of all deaths attributable to heart disease.* By contrast, atherosclerotic heart disease is far less frequent in underdeveloped countries. The principal effects of ischemic heart disease are angina pectoris, myocardial infarction, chronic congestive heart failure, and sudden death.

ANGINA PECTORIS: This term refers to the pain of myocardial ischemia. It typically occurs in the substernal portion of the chest and may radiate to the left arm, jaw, and epigastrium. It is the most common symptom of ischemic heart disease. Coronary atherosclerosis usually becomes symptomatic only when the luminal cross-sectional area of the affected vessel is reduced by more than 75%. A patient with typical angina pectoris exhibits recurrent episodes of chest pain, usually brought on by increased physical activity or emotional excitement. The pain is of limited duration (1 to 15 minutes) and is relieved by reducing physical activity or by treatment with sublingual nitroglycerin (a potent vasodilator).

Although the most common cause of angina pectoris is severe coronary atherosclerosis, decreased coronary blood flow can result from other conditions, including coronary vasospasm, aortic stenosis, or aortic insufficiency. Angina pectoris is not associated with anatomic changes in the myocardium as long as the duration and severity of ischemic episodes are insufficient to cause myocardial necrosis.

Prinzmetal angina (variant angina) *is an atypical form of angina that occurs at rest and is caused by coronary artery spasm.* The responsible mechanisms are not fully understood. Spasm can occur in structurally normal coronary arteries and may be part of a systemic syndrome of abnormal arterial vasomotor reactivity, which includes migraine headache and Raynaud phenomenon. Usually, however, it develops in atherosclerotic coronary arteries, often in a portion of a vessel nearby an atherosclerotic plaque. Whereas coronary artery spasm may contribute to the pathogenesis of an acute myocardial infarction or to the size of the infarct, it is generally not the principal cause of infarction.

Unstable angina, *a variety of chest pain that has a less predictable relationship to exercise than does stable angina and may occur during rest or sleep, is associated with development of nonocclusive thrombi over atherosclerotic plaques.* In some cases of unstable angina, episodes of chest pain become progressively more frequent and longer in duration over a 3- to 4-day period. Electrocardiographic changes are not characteristic of infarction and serum levels of cardiac-specific intracellular proteins, such as MB isoform of CK (MB-CK) or cardiac troponins T or I, (evidence of myocardial necrosis), remain normal. Unstable angina is also termed **preinfarction angina, accelerated angina** or **"crescendo" angina**. Without pharmacologic or mechanical intervention to "open up" the coronary narrowing, many patients with unstable angina progress to myocardial infarction.

MYOCARDIAL INFARCT: A *myocardial infarct is a discrete focus of ischemic muscle necrosis in the heart.* This definition excludes patchy foci of necrosis caused by drugs, toxins, or viruses. The development of an infarct is related to the duration of ischemia and the metabolic rate of the ischemic tissue. In experimental coronary artery ligation, foci of necrosis form after 20 minutes of ischemia and become more extensive as the period of ischemia lengthens.

CHRONIC CONGESTIVE HEART FAILURE: Because early mortality associated with acute myocardial infarction has fallen to less than 5%, many patients with ischemic heart disease survive longer and eventually develop chronic congestive heart failure. In more than 75% of all patients with heart failure, coronary artery disease is the major cause of their heart failure. Contractile impairment in these patients is due to irreversible loss of myocardium (previous infarcts) and hypoperfusion of surviving muscle, which leads to chronic ventricular dysfunction ("hibernating" myocardium). Many of these patients die suddenly, especially those in whom contractile impairment is not severe. Others develop progressive pump failure and die of multi-organ failure. Because coronary artery disease is often so extensive in these patients and many have already undergone coronary artery bypass surgery, the only treatments available are cardiac transplantation or the use of artificial pumps (ventricular assist devices).

SUDDEN DEATH: In some patients, the first and only clinical manifestation of ischemic heart disease is sudden death due to spontaneous ventricular fibrillation. Some authorities consider death to be sudden only if it occurs within 1 hour of the onset of symptoms. Others regard death within 24 hours after the onset of symptoms to be sudden or require that sudden death be diagnosed only if it is unexpected. *In any event, coronary atherosclerosis underlies most cases of cardiac death occurring during the first hour after the onset of symptoms.*

Experimental animals subjected to acute coronary occlusion show a high incidence of ventricular fibrillation during the first hour of ischemia. Sudden cardiac death due to ventricular fibrillation also occurs in humans as a result of acute coronary artery thrombosis. On the other hand, such an arrhythmia also appears in patients with marked coronary artery disease and no detectable thrombosis. Clinical studies of patients who have been defibrillated and survived an arrhythmia have shown that most have not had acute myocardial infarction. No serum markers of myocardial necrosis can be found, and electrocardiographic changes indicating infarction do not develop. *Thus, in many cases, lethal arrhythmia is likely triggered by acute ischemia without overt myocardial infarction.* The presence of a healed infarct or ventricular hypertrophy increases the risk that an episode of acute ischemia will initiate a life-threatening ventricular arrhythmia.

EPIDEMIOLOGY: *The major risk factors that predispose to coronary artery disease are (1) systemic hypertension, (2) cigarette smoking, (3) diabetes mellitus, and (4) elevated blood cholesterol level.* Any one of these factors significantly increases risk of myocardial infarction, but a combination of multiple factors augments risk more than sevenfold (see Chapter 8).

During the 20th century, the United States experienced first a dramatic increase and then a dramatic reversal in mortality from ischemic heart disease. In 1950, the age-adjusted death rate from myocardial infarction was 226 per 100,000 cases; 40 years later it was 108. This shift reflects many factors, including reduced smoking; lower dietary saturated fat; and new drugs that control hypertension, reduce cholesterol, and dissolve coronary thrombi. Important advances in medical technology include construction of coronary care units, coronary revascularization procedures, and use of defibrillators and ventricular assist devices. Concurrently, the role of hyperlipidemia in the pathogenesis of coronary artery atherosclerosis attracted much more attention. This was driven initially by epidemiologic evidence showing that populations in which men have high mean serum cholesterol values had higher rates of coronary artery disease. Since then, multiple studies established that elevated serum low-density lipoproteins (LDLs) increase risk of myocardial infarction, whereas high levels of high-density lipoproteins (HDLs) decrease risk. The total cholesterol/HDL cholesterol ratio appears to be a better predictor of coronary artery disease than serum cholesterol level alone.

Although blood lipid profile is an important indicator of the risk of atherogenesis, other risk factors exert powerful independent effects. A person with a blood pressure of 160/95 mm Hg has twice the risk of ischemic heart disease as one whose blood pressure is 140/75 mm Hg or less. The risk of ischemic heart disease increases in proportion to the number of cigarettes smoked. Serum factors involved in thrombosis or thrombolysis or which contribute to endothelial injury have also been implicated in atherogenesis. For example, plasma fibrinogen levels directly correlate with risk of ischemic heart disease, presumably because of the role of fibrinogen in atherogenesis and coronary artery thrombosis. Other factors reported to contribute to increased risk of myocardial infarction include factor VII, plasminogen activator inhibitor-1 (PAI-1), homocysteine, and decreased fibrinolytic activity. Levels of selected serum markers of inflammation such as C-reactive protein also predict ischemic heart disease risk.

During the past several years, there has been a remarkable increase in the incidence of type II diabetes in the United States, which mirrors a similar increase in obesity (see Chapter 22). Ischemic heart disease is a consequence of both type 1 and type 2 diabetes, the risk being twofold to threefold greater than in nondiabetic persons. Conversely, atherosclerotic cardiovascular disease (myocardial infarction, stroke, peripheral vascular disease) accounts for 80% of all deaths in patients with diabetes.

Other risk factors for ischemic heart disease include:

- **Obesity:** In a major, longitudinal study of one population (Framingham Heart Study), obesity was an independent risk factor for cardiovascular disease, with an increased risk for obese persons over lean ones of 2 to 2.5.
- **Age:** The risk of infarction is greater with increasing age, up to age 80 years.
- **Sex:** Men have increased risk of ischemic heart disease: 60% of coronary events occur in men. Angina pectoris is considerably more frequent in men than in women; the ratio at ages younger than 50 years is 4:1 and that at age 60 years is 2:1.
- **Family history:** In one study that controlled for other risk factors, relatives of patients with ischemic heart disease had a twofold to fourfold increased risk for coronary artery disease. The genetic basis for this familial risk may interact with the other risk factors.
- **Use of oral contraceptives:** Women over 35 years who smoke cigarettes and use oral contraceptives have a modestly increased incidence of myocardial infarction.
- **Sedentary life habits:** Regular exercise reduces risk of myocardial infarction, perhaps by increasing HDL levels. In one study, the least-fit quartile of persons subjected to exercise testing had 6 times the risk of myocardial infarction than persons in the fittest quartile.
- **Personality features:** Early studies suggested that aggressive, time-conscious, executive-type individuals ("type A" personality) have more heart disease than do easygoing, relaxed persons ("type B" personality). "Coronary-prone" subjects, those of the type A behavior pattern, differ from type B individuals in having higher plasma triglyceride and cholesterol levels and greater urinary catecholamine excretion. However, the relationship between coronary artery disease and type A personality is controversial, and recent studies have failed to show the strong association previously reported.

Many Conditions Limit the Supply of Blood to the Heart

The heart is an aerobic organ, requiring oxidative phosphorylation to provide energy for contraction. The anaerobic glycolysis used by skeletal muscle under conditions of extreme physical exertion is insufficient to sustain cardiac contraction. Ischemic heart disease is caused by an imbalance between the oxygen demands of the myocardium and the supply of oxygenated blood (Table 11-3).

Atherosclerosis and Thrombosis

The pathogenesis of atherosclerosis is detailed in Chapter 10. Here we discuss only briefly the features of special importance to ischemic heart disease. The coronary arteries are conductance vessels, small muscular arteries with a prominent internal elastic lamina. Their principal role is to deliver blood to the regulatory vasculature (small intramural arteries and arterioles), which controls nutritive myocardial blood flow. A healthy person has substantial coronary flow reserve and myocardial perfusion can be increased to 4 to 8 times the resting blood flow. In a normal heart, the large coronary arteries provide almost no resistance to blood flow; and myocardial circulation is mainly controlled by constriction and dilation of small, intramyocardial branches less than 400 μm in diameter. In advanced atherosclerosis of the main epicardial coronary arteries, luminal stenosis decreases blood pressure distal to the narrowed zone. To compensate for the reduced perfusion pressure, microvessels dilate, thereby maintaining normal resting blood flow. Thus, most patients with coronary atherosclerosis do not have ischemia or angina at rest. However, with exercise, the capacity of the microcirculation to dilate further is limiting, and myocardial oxygen demand exceeds the supply. The result is ischemia and angina.

TABLE 11-3

Causes of Ischemic Heart Disease

Decreased supply of oxygen	
Conditions that influence the supply of blood	
	Atherosclerosis and thrombosis
	Thromboemboli
	Coronary artery spasm
	Collateral blood vessels
	Blood pressure, cardiac output, and heart rate
	Miscellaneous: arteritis (e.g., periarteritis nodosa), dissecting aneurysm, luetic aortitis, anomalous origin of coronary artery, muscular bridging of coronary artery
Conditions that influence the availability of oxygen in the blood	
	Anemia
	Shift in the hemoglobin-oxygen dissociation curve
	Carbon monoxide
	Cyanide
Increased oxygen demand (i.e., increased cardiac work)	
	Hypertension
	Valvular stenosis or insufficiency
	Hyperthyroidism
	Fever
	Thiamine deficiency
	Catecholamines

Maximal blood flow to the myocardium is not impaired until about 75% of the cross-sectional area of coronary artery (~50% of the diameter as assessed during coronary angiography) is compromised by atherosclerosis. However, resting blood flow is not reduced until more than 90% of the lumen is occluded. In patients with long-standing angina pectoris, the extent and distribution of collateral circulation exerts an important influence on the risk of acute myocardial infarction. In some conditions (e.g., hypotension or tachycardia) demand for oxygen and perfusion pressure may so out of imbalance that myocardial infarction ensues even when a coronary artery is not ordinarily sufficiently narrowed to produce ischemia.

Although myocardial infarction often occurs during physically demanding activities such as running or shoveling snow, many infarcts occur at rest or even during sleep. Thus, for most persons, conversion of the clinically silent disease of coronary atherosclerosis to the catastrophic event of myocardial infarction involves a sudden, marked decrease in myocardial blood flow, with or without an increase in myocardial oxygen demand. *It is now well established that coronary artery thrombosis is the event that usually precipitates an acute myocardial infarction. Thrombosis typically results from spontaneous rupture of an atherosclerotic plaque, usually in a region that contains numerous inflammatory cells and a thin fibrous cap.* The initiating event may be hemorrhage into or beneath the plaque.

Thromboemboli

Thromboembolism is a rare cause of myocardial infarction. The coronary embolus is usually traced to the heart itself, usually valvular vegetations caused by infective or nonbacterial endocarditis. Coronary emboli occur in patients with atrial fibrillation and mitral valve disease who have mural thrombi in the left atrial appendage (Fig. 11-13). Thromboembolic occlusion of a coronary artery is also seen in patients with mural thrombi in the left ventricle secondary to infarction, aneurysm or dilated cardiomyopathy.

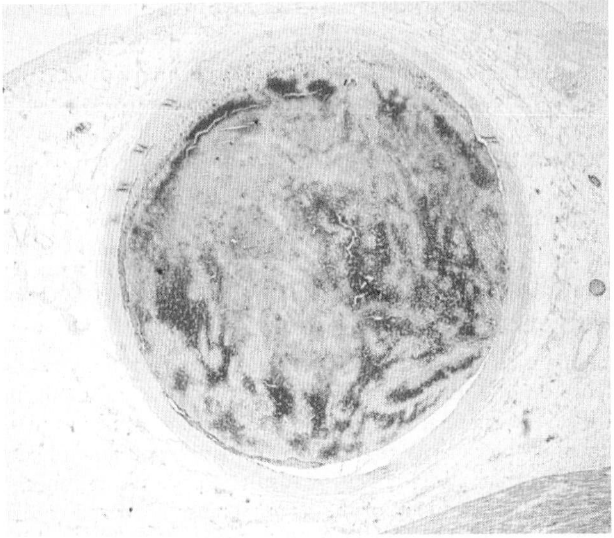

FIGURE 11-13. **Thromboembolus** in the left anterior descending coronary artery of a man who had old rheumatic heart disease, mitral stenosis, and a mural thrombus in the left atrial appendage.

Coronary Collateral Circulation

Normal coronary arteries function as end-arteries. Although most normal hearts have anastomoses 20 to 200 μm in diameter between coronary vessels, these collateral vessels do not function under normal circumstances because there is no pressure gradient between the arteries that they connect. However, after abrupt occlusion of a coronary artery, the resulting pressure differential allows blood to flow from the patent coronary artery to the ischemic area. Extensive collateral connections develop in hearts with severe coronary atherosclerosis. These collaterals may actually provide enough arterial flow to prevent infarction completely or to limit its size when a major epicardial coronary artery undergoes acute thrombotic occlusion

Well-developed coronary collaterals can explain certain unusual situations, such as anterior infarction after recent thrombotic occlusion of the right coronary artery (so-called infarction at a distance). This circumstance reflects the presence of coronary collaterals between the LAD and right coronary arteries that formed in response to gradual atherosclerotic narrowing of the LAD. As a result, myocardium normally supplied by the LAD distal to the occlusion now depends on blood flow from the right coronary artery via collaterals. Under these conditions, acute thrombosis of the right coronary artery causes paradoxical infarction of the anterior left ventricle.

Other Conditions That Limit Coronary Blood Flow

- **Coronary arteritis** is caused by various vasculitides such as polyarteritis nodosa or Kawasaki disease. It may produce luminal narrowing due to vessel wall thickening. It can also create local aneurysms that become occluded by thrombus.
- **Dissecting aneurysm of the aorta** occasionally extends into and obstructs the coronary arteries. Occasionally, medial necrosis and dissecting aneurysms are confined to the coronary artery.
- **Syphilitic aortitis** characteristically involves the ascending aorta, where it may obliterate a coronary artery orifice.
- **Congenital anomalous origin of a coronary artery** (origin of a coronary artery from the pulmonary trunk or passage of

an anomalous coronary artery between the aorta and pulmonary artery) has been associated with sudden death.

- **An intramural course of the LAD coronary artery** may cause myocardial ischemia and sudden death. The artery normally runs in the epicardial fat but in some hearts, it dips into the myocardium for a short distance. The muscular bridge over the LAD coronary artery may compress the vessel during systole or predispose to coronary spasm.

In Settings When Oxygen Availability is Limited, the Myocardium is At Risk for Ischemia

Anemia is a common cause of decreased oxygen supply to the myocardium. Although a heart with normal circulation can survive severe anemia, the presence of coronary atherosclerosis may limit the capacity to increase coronary blood flow to such an extent that cardiac necrosis results. Furthermore, anemia increases the workload of the heart because increased cardiac output is required to oxygenate vital organs adequately.

Carbon monoxide (CO) poisoning decreases oxygen delivery to the tissues. The high affinity of hemoglobin for CO displaces oxygen, thereby depriving tissues of oxygen. It should be noted, in this regard, that cigarette smoking produces significant levels of carboxyhemoglobin (a measure of CO) in the blood.

Increased Oxygen Demand May Cause Cardiac Ischemia

Any increase in cardiac workload increases the heart's need for oxygen. Conditions that raise blood pressure or cardiac output, such as exercise or pregnancy, augment oxygen demand by the myocardium, which may lead to angina pectoris or myocardial infarction. Disorders in this category include valvular disease (mitral or aortic insufficiency, aortic stenosis), infection, and conditions such as hypertension, coarctation of the aorta, and hypertrophic cardiomyopathy (HCM) (see Table 11-3). The increased metabolic rate and tachycardia in patients with hyperthyroidism are accompanied by increased oxygen demand as well as an increase in the workload of the heart. In fact, treatment of the underlying thyroid disease is the best therapy for a hyperthyroid patient with symptoms of ischemic heart disease. Fever also increases basal metabolic rate, cardiac output, and heart rate.

Myocardial Infarcts May be Mainly Subendocardial or Transmural

PATHOLOGY

Location of Infarcts

There are important differences between these two types of infarction (Table 11-4).

*A **subendocardial infarct** affects the inner one- third to one-half of the left ventricle.* It may arise within the territory of one of the major epicardial coronary arteries or it may be circumferential, involving subendocardial territories of multiple coronary arteries. Subendocardial infarction generally occurs as a consequence of hypoperfusion of the heart. It may result from atherosclerosis in a specific coronary artery or develop in disorders that limit myocardial blood flow globally, such as aortic stenosis, hemorrhagic shock, or hypoperfusion during cardiopulmonary bypass. Most subendocardial infarcts do not involve occlusive coronary thrombi, although small particles of platelet–fibrin thrombus may be seen in the epicardial coronary artery that supplies the region of infarction. In the case of circumferential subendocardial infarction caused by global hypoperfusion of the myocardium, coronary artery stenosis need not be present. Because necrosis is limited to the inner layers of the heart, complications arising in transmural infarcts (e.g., pericarditis and ventricular rupture) are not seen in subendocardial infarcts.

TABLE 11-4

Differences between Subendocardial and Transmural Infarcts

Subendocardial Infarcts	Transmural Infarcts
Multifocal	Unifocal
Patchy	Solid
Circumferential	In distribution of a specific coronary artery
Coronary thrombosis rare	Coronary thrombosis common
Often result from hypotension or shock	Often causes shock
No epicarditis	Epicarditis common
Do not form aneurysms	May result in aneurysm

*A **transmural infarct** involves the full left ventricular wall thickness and usually follows occlusion of a coronary artery.* As a result, transmural infarcts typically conform to the distribution of one of the three major coronary arteries (see Fig. 11-2).

- **Right coronary artery:** Occlusion of the proximal portion of this vessel results in an infarct of the posterior basal region of the left ventricle and the posterior third to half of the interventricular septum ("inferior" infarct).
- **LAD coronary artery:** Blockage of this artery produces an infarct of the apical, anterior, and anteroseptal walls of the left ventricle.
- **Left circumflex coronary artery:** Obstruction of this vessel is the least common cause of myocardial infarction and leads to an infarct of the lateral wall of the left ventricle.

Myocardial infarction does not occur instantaneously. Rather, it first develops in the subendocardium and progresses as a wave front of necrosis from subendocardium to subepicardium over the course of several hours. Transient coronary occlusion may cause only subendocardial necrosis, whereas persistent occlusion eventually leads to transmural necrosis. The goal of acute coronary interventions (pharmacologic or mechanical thrombolysis) is to interrupt this wave front and limit myocardial necrosis.

The volume of arterial collateral flow is the chief factor in the transmural progression of an infarct. In chronic cardiac ischemia, extensive collateral circulation, which preferentially supplies the outer or subepicardial layer, often limits the infarct to subendocardial myocardium. However, in fatal cases of acute myocardial infarction, transmural infarcts are more common than those restricted to the subendocardium.

Infarcts involve the left ventricle much more commonly and extensively than the right ventricle. This difference may be partly explained by the greater workload imposed on the left ventricle by systemic vascular resistance and the greater thickness of the left ventricular wall. Right ventricular hypertrophy (e.g., in pulmonary hypertension) increases the incidence of right ventricular infarction. Infarction of the posterior right ventricle occurs in about a third of left ventricular posteroseptal infarcts (right coronary artery territory), but infarcts limited to the right ventricle are rare.

Macroscopic Characteristics of Myocardial Infarcts

The early stages in the evolution of a myocardial infarct have been characterized most thoroughly in experimental animals. About 10 seconds after ligation of a coronary artery, the affected myocardium becomes cyanotic and, rather than contracting, bulges outward during systole. If the obstruction is promptly relieved, myocardial contractions resume and no anatomical damage ensues, although contractility may be depressed in the postischemic tissue for many hours (**stunned myocardium**). This reversible stage continues for 20 to 30 minutes of total ischemia, beyond which time damaged myocytes progressively die.

On gross examination, an acute myocardial infarct is not identifiable within the first 12 hours. By 24 hours, it can be recognized on the cut surface of the involved ventricle by its pallor. After 3 to 5 days, it becomes mottled and more sharply outlined, with a central pale, yellowish, necrotic region bordered by a hyperemic zone (Fig. 11-14). By 2 to 3 weeks, the infarcted region is depressed and soft, with a refractile, gelatinous appearance. Older, healed infarcts are firm and contracted and have the pale gray appearance of scar tissue (Fig. 11-15).

Microscopic Characteristics of Myocardial Infarcts

THE FIRST 24 HOURS: Electron microscopy is required to discern the earliest morphologic features of ischemic injury (Fig. 11-16). Reversibly injured myocytes show subtle changes of sarcoplasmic edema, mild mitochondrial swelling, and loss of glycogen. After 30 to 60 minutes of ischemia, when myocyte injury has become irreversible, mitochondria are greatly swollen with disorganized cristae and amorphous matrix densities. The nucleus shows clumping and margination of chromatin, and the sarcolemma is focally disrupted.

Loss of sarcolemmal integrity leads to release of intracellular proteins, such as myoglobin, LDH, CK, and troponins I and T. Ion gradients are also dissipated, and tissue potassium decreases as sodium and chloride increase.

The noncontractile ischemic myocytes are stretched with each systole and become "**wavy fibers**." By 24 hours, myocytes are deeply eosinophilic (Fig. 11-17) and show the characteristic

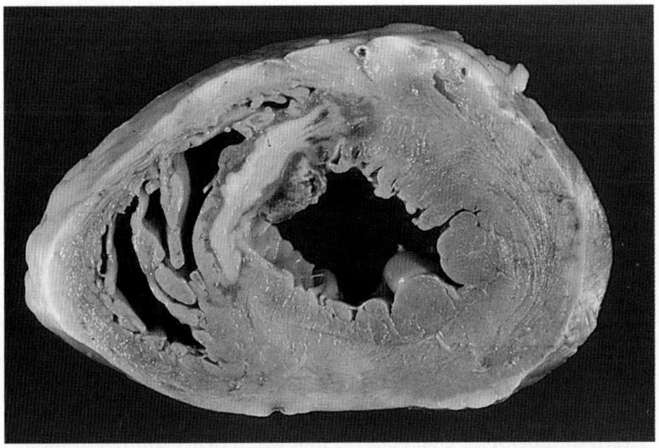

FIGURE 11-14. **Acute myocardial infarct.** A transverse section of the heart of a patient who died a few days after the onset of severe chest pain shows a transmural infarct in the anteroseptal region of the left ventricle (left anterior descending [LAD] coronary artery territory). The necrotic myocardium is soft, yellowish, and sharply demarcated.

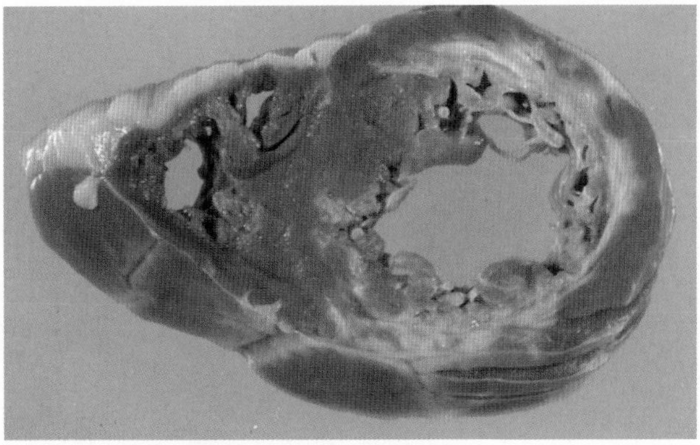

FIGURE 11-15. **Healed myocardial infarct.** A cross-section of the heart from a man who died after a long history of angina pectoris and several myocardial infarctions shows circumferential scarring of the left ventricle.

changes of coagulation necrosis (see Chapter 1). However, it takes several days for the myocyte nucleus to disappear totally.

TWO TO 3 DAYS: Polymorphonuclear leukocytes are attracted to necrotic myocytes, but they gain access only at the periphery of the infarct, where blood flow is maintained. Hence they accumulate at infarct borders and reach maximal concentration after 2 to 3 days (see Fig. 11-17 and Fig. 11-18). Interstitial edema and microscopic areas of hemorrhage may also appear. By 2 to 3 days, muscle cells are more clearly necrotic, nuclei disappear, and striations become less prominent. Some of the polymorphonuclear leukocytes that were attracted to the area begin to undergo karyorrhexis.

FIVE TO 7 DAYS: By this time, few, if any, polymorphonuclear leukocytes remain. The periphery of the infarcted region shows phagocytosis of dead muscle by macrophages. Fibroblasts begin to proliferate, and new collagen deposited. Lymphocytes and pigment-laden macrophages are prominent. The process of replacing necrotic muscle with scar tissue is initiated at about 5 days, beginning at the periphery of the infarct and gradually extending toward the center.

ONE TO 3 WEEKS: Collagen deposition proceeds, the inflammatory infiltrate gradually recedes, and the newly sprouted capillaries are progressively obliterated.

MORE THAN 4 WEEKS: Considerable dense fibrous tissue is present. The debris is progressively removed, and the scar becomes more solid and less cellular as it matures (Fig. 11-19).

This sequence of inflammatory and reparative events can be altered by local or systemic factors. For example, the immediate extension of an infarct into a region that previously displayed patchy necrosis may not show the expected changes. A large infarct tends not to mature in its center as rapidly as a smaller one. In estimating the age of a large infarct, it is more accurate to base the interpretation on the outer border where repair begins, rather than on changes in the central region. In fact, in some large infarcts, rather than being removed, dead myocytes remain indefinitely "mummified."

Reperfusion of Ischemic Myocardium

The foregoing descriptions pertain to healing of infarcts caused by persistent coronary occlusion, such as those arising from thrombotic occlusion of an epicardial coronary artery. However, blood flow may be restored to regions of evolving infarcts either because of spontaneous thrombolysis or in response to pharmacologic or mechanical means of opening up occluded

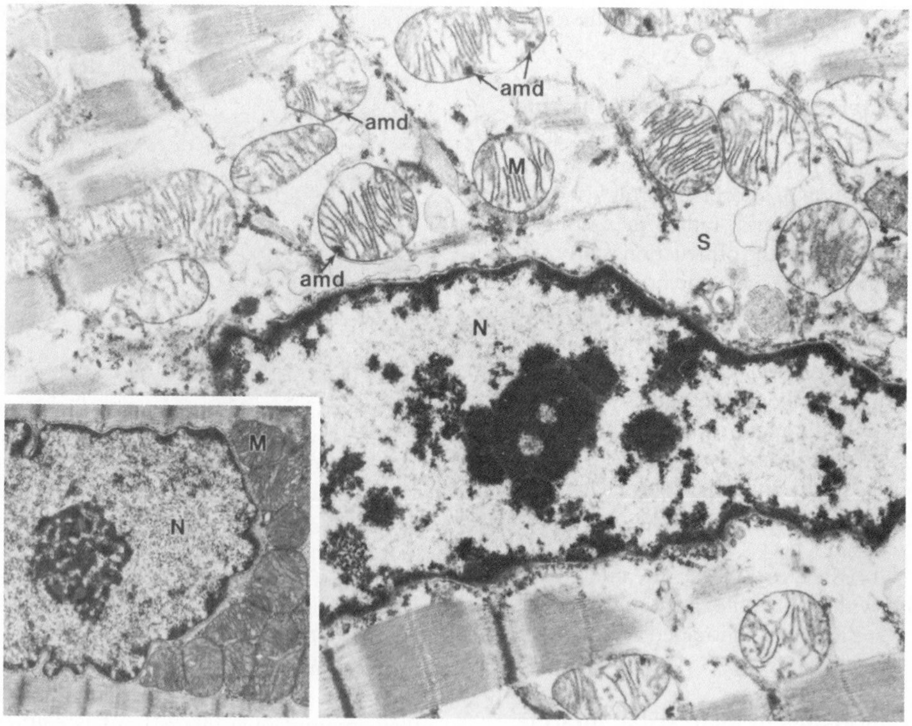

FIGURE 11-16. **Ultrastructure of myocardial ischemia.** Electron micrograph of an irreversibly injured myocyte from a canine heart subjected to 40 minutes of low-flow ischemia induced by proximal occlusion of the circumflex branch of the left coronary artery. (**Inset** shows a nonischemic control myocyte from the same heart, N-nucleus.) The affected myocyte is swollen and has abundant clear sarcoplasm (S). The mitochondria (M) are also swollen and contain amorphous matrix densities (amd), which are characteristic of lethal cell injury. The sarcolemma of this myocyte *(not shown)* exhibited small areas of disruption. The chromatin of the nucleus (N) is aggregated peripherally, in contrast to the uniformly distributed chromatin in normal tissue.

coronary arteries. When that happens, the infarct's gross and microscopic appearances change. Reperfused infarcts are typically hemorrhagic, the result of blood flow through a damaged microvasculature. Thus, while infarcts following persistent occlusion become grossly apparent only after about 12 hours and are pale, the presence of hemorrhage immediatly highlights reperfused infarcts. Reperfusion also accelerates acute inflammatory responses. Neutrophils can gain access throughout the infarct rather than only at the periphery. They accumulate more rapidly but also disappear more rapidly. In general, replacement of necrotic muscle by fibrous scar also proceeds more quickly, at least in areas of the infarct in which perfusion persists.

One of the most characteristic features of reperfused infarcts is **contraction band necrosis.** Contraction bands are thick, irregular, transverse eosinophilic bands in necrotic myocytes (Fig. 11-20). By electron microscopy, these bands are small groups of hypercontracted and disorganized sarcomeres with thickened Z lines. The sarcolemma is disrupted and mitochondria located between the contraction bands swell. They may contain deposits of calcium phosphate in the matrix, as well as amorphous matrix densities. Contraction bands occur whenever there is a massive influx of Ca^{2+} into cardiac myocytes. Reperfusion of ischemic myocardium causes extensive sarcolemmal damage mediated largely by reactive oxygen species, which permits unrestrained entry of extracellular Ca^{2+} into myocytes. The massive Ca^{2+} influx leads to hypercontraction in cells still able to contract. Contraction band necrosis is most prominent when necrotic myocardium is reperfused (e.g., after thrombolytic therapy or following prolonged cardiopulmonary bypass in which the myocardium has sustained irreversible injury). In infarcts arising from persistent coronary occlusion, microscopic foci of contraction band necrosis are often seen at the margins, where dynamic ebb and flow of blood creates conditions that favor Ca^{2+} influx. Other conditions associated with contraction band injury include massive catecholamine release in patients with pheochromocytoma or head injuries or patients in shock treated with large doses of pressors.

CLINICAL FEATURES:

Clinical Diagnosis

The onset of acute myocardial infarction is often sudden and associated with severe, crushing substernal, or precordial pain. The pain may be experienced as epigastric burning (simulating indigestion) or it may extend into the jaw or down the inside of either arm. It is often accompanied by sweating, nausea, vomiting, and shortness of breath. In some cases an acute myocardial infarction is preceded by unstable angina of several days duration. *One-fourth to one-half of all nonfatal myocardial infarctions occur without any symptoms and infarcts are identified only later by electrocardiographic changes or at autopsy.* These "clinically silent" infarcts are particularly common among diabetic patients with autonomic dysfunction and also in cardiac transplant patients whose hearts are denervated.

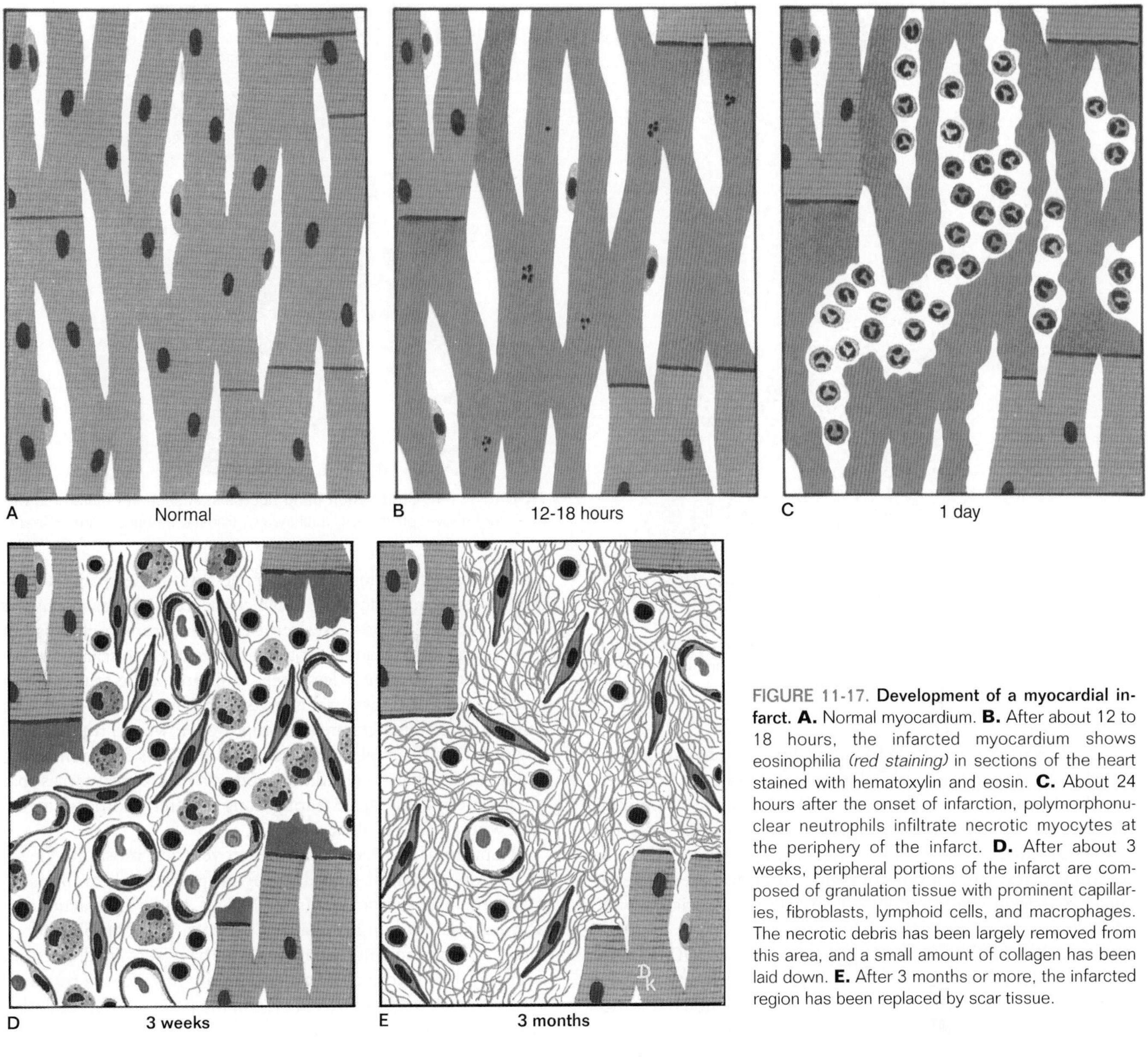

FIGURE 11-17. **Development of a myocardial infarct. A.** Normal myocardium. **B.** After about 12 to 18 hours, the infarcted myocardium shows eosinophilia *(red staining)* in sections of the heart stained with hematoxylin and eosin. **C.** About 24 hours after the onset of infarction, polymorphonuclear neutrophils infiltrate necrotic myocytes at the periphery of the infarct. **D.** After about 3 weeks, peripheral portions of the infarct are composed of granulation tissue with prominent capillaries, fibroblasts, lymphoid cells, and macrophages. The necrotic debris has been largely removed from this area, and a small amount of collagen has been laid down. **E.** After 3 months or more, the infarcted region has been replaced by scar tissue.

The diagnosis of acute myocardial infarction is confirmed by electrocardiography and the appearance of increased levels of certain enzymes or proteins in the serum. The electrocardiogram exhibits new Q waves and changes in the ST segment and the conformation of the T wave. Identification in serum of cardiac proteins such as MB- CK or cardiac troponins T and I is evidence of myocardial necrosis.

Complications of Myocardial Infarction

Early mortality in acute myocardial infarction (within 30 days) has dropped from 30% in the 1950s to less than 5% today. Nevertheless, the clinical course after acute infarction may be dominated by functional or mechanical complications of the infarct.

ARRHYTHMIAS: Virtually all patients who have a myocardial infarct have abnormal cardiac rhythm at some time during their illness. Arrhythmias still account for half of all deaths caused by ischemic heart disease, although the advent of coronary care units and defibrillators has greatly reduced early mortality. Acute infarction is often associated with premature ventricular beats, sinus bradycardia, ventricular tachycardia, ventricular fibrillation, and paroxysmal atrial tachycardia. Partial or complete heart block can also occur. The causes of these arrhythmias are often multifactorial. Acute ischemia alters conduction, increases automaticity and promotes triggered activity related to after-depolarizations. Enhanced sympathetic activity mediated by increased levels of local or circulating catecholamines plays an important role.

LEFT VENTRICULAR FAILURE AND CARDIOGENIC SHOCK: Development of left ventricular failure soon after myocardial infarction is an ominous sign that generally indicates massive loss of muscle. Fortunately, cardiogenic shock occurs in less than 5% of cases, owing to the development of techniques that limit the extent of infarction (thrombolytic therapy, angioplasty) or assist damaged myocardium (intraaortic balloon pump). Cardiogenic shock tends to develop early after infarction when 40% or more of the left ventricle has been lost; mortality is as high as 90%.

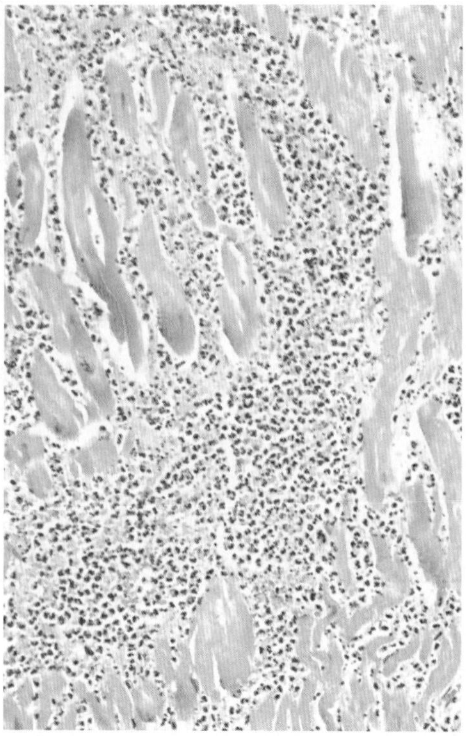

FIGURE 11-18. **Acute myocardial infarct.** The necrotic myocardial fibers, which are eosinophilic and devoid of cross striations and nuclei, are immersed in a sea of acute inflammatory cells.

EXTENSION OF THE INFARCT: Clinically recognizable extension of an acute myocardial infarct occurs in the first 1 to 2 weeks in up to 10% of patients. In careful echocardiographic studies, half of all patients with anterior myocardial infarction showed some extension of the infarct during the first 2 weeks, indicating that many episodes of infarct extension are not recognized. Clinically significant infarct extension is associated with a doubling of mortality.

RUPTURE OF THE FREE WALL OF THE MYOCARDIUM: Myocardial rupture (Fig. 11-21) may occur at almost any time during the 3 weeks following acute myocardial infarction but is most common between the first and fourth days, when the infarcted wall is weakest. During this vulnerable period, the infarct is composed of soft, necrotic tissue in which the extracellular matrix has been degraded by proteases released by inflammatory cells but new matrix deposition has not yet occurred. Once scar tissue begins to form, rupture is less likely. Rupture of the free wall is a complication of transmural infarcts; surviving muscle overlying subendocardial infarcts prevents rupture. However, rupture usually occurs in relatively small transmural infarcts. The remaining viable, contractile myocardium produces mechanical forces that can initiate and propagate tearing along the lateral border of the infarct where neutrophils accumulate.

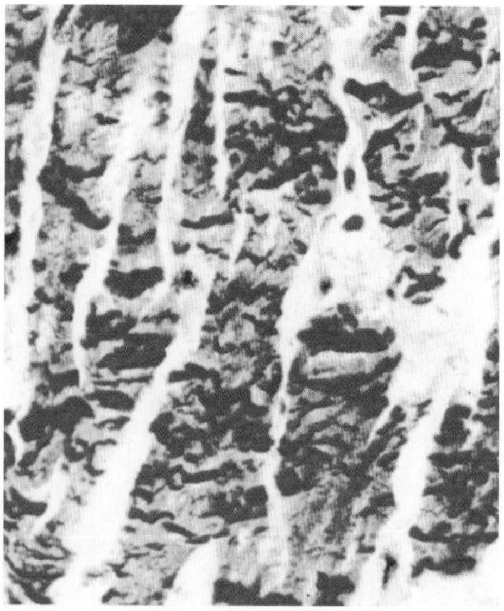

FIGURE 11-20. **Contraction band necrosis.** A section of infarcted myocardium shows prominent, thick, wavy, transverse bands in myofibers.

Rupture of the free wall of the left ventricle most often leads to hemopericardium and death from pericardial tamponade. Myocardial rupture accounts for 10% of deaths after acute myocardial infarction in hospitalized patients. This complication is more common in elderly patients who have sustained a first infarct (most of whom are women). In rare instances, a ruptured ventricle may become walled off and the patient survives with a false aneurysm (Fig. 11-22).

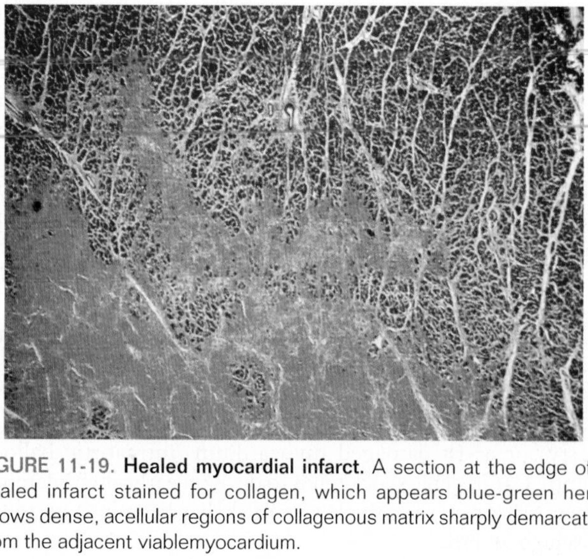

FIGURE 11-19. **Healed myocardial infarct.** A section at the edge of a healed infarct stained for collagen, which appears blue-green here, shows dense, acellular regions of collagenous matrix sharply demarcated from the adjacent viablemyocardium.

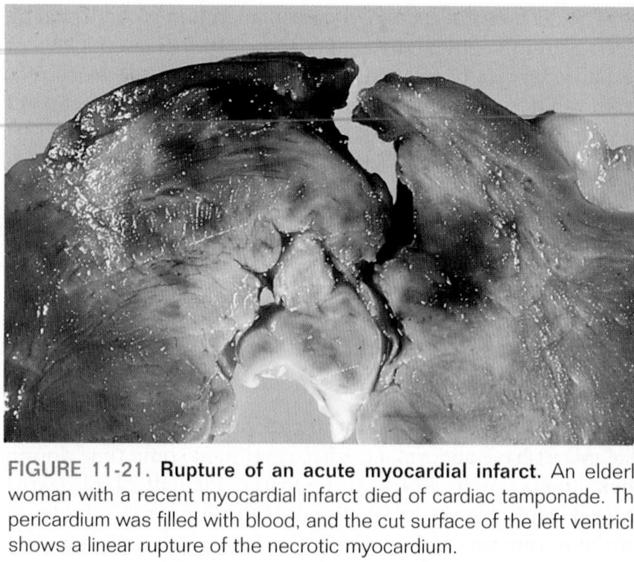

FIGURE 11-21. **Rupture of an acute myocardial infarct.** An elderly woman with a recent myocardial infarct died of cardiac tamponade. The pericardium was filled with blood, and the cut surface of the left ventricle shows a linear rupture of the necrotic myocardium.

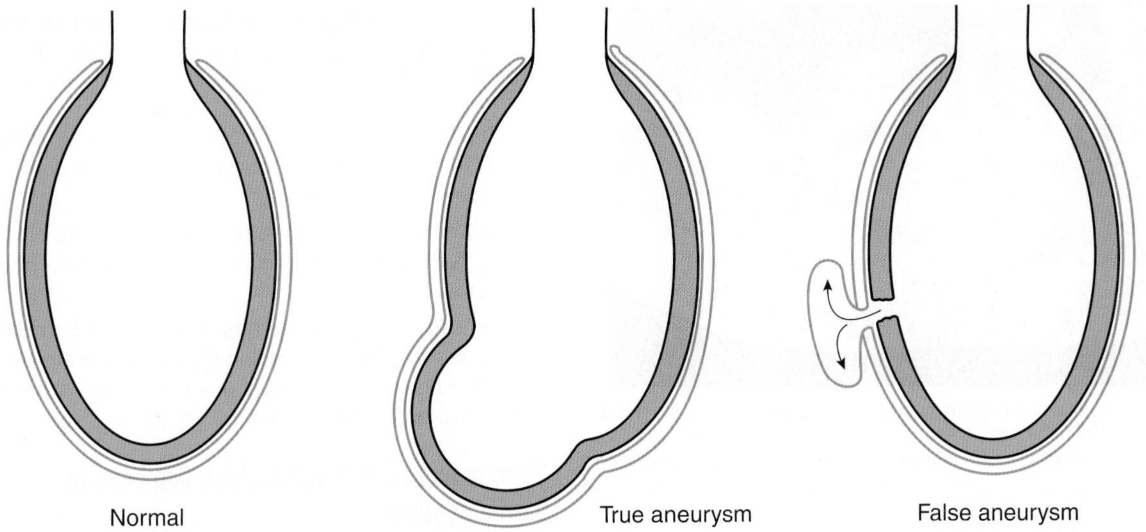

FIGURE 11-22. **True and false aneurysms of the left ventricle. (Left)** Normal heart. The left ventricular wall *(shaded)* is enclosed by the pericardial sac. **(Center)** True aneurysm shows an intact wall *(black)*, which bulges outward. **(Right)** False aneurysm shows a ruptured infarct that is walled off externally by adherent pericardium. Note that the mouth of the true aneurysm is wider than that of the false aneurysm.

OTHER FORMS OF MYOCARDIAL RUPTURE: A few patients in whom a myocardial infarct involves the interventricular septum develop **septal perforation,** varying in length from 1 cm or more. The magnitude of the resulting left-to-right shunt and, therefore, the prognosis vary with the size of the rupture.

Rupture of a portion of a papillary muscle results in mitral regurgitation. In some cases, an entire papillary muscle is transected, in which case, massive mitral valve incompetence may be fatal.

ANEURYSMS: Left ventricular aneurysms complicate 10% to 15% of transmural myocardial infarcts. After acute transmural infarction, the affected ventricular wall tends to bulge outward during systole in one third of patients. As the infarct heals, the newly deposited collagenous matrix is susceptible to further stretching, although eventually the scar tissue becomes nondistensible. Localized thinning and stretching of the ventricular wall in the region of a healing myocardial infarct has been termed "infarct expansion" but is actually an early aneurysm. Such an aneurysm is composed of a thin layer of necrotic myocardium and collagenous tissue, which expands with each contraction of the heart. As the evolving aneurysm becomes more fibrotic, its tensile strength increases. However, the aneurysm continues to dilate with each beat, thereby "stealing" some of the left ventricular output and increasing the workload of the heart. Patients with left ventricular aneurysms are at increased risk of developing ventricular tachycardia, owing to increased opportunities for reentry along the periphery of the aneurysm. Mural thrombi often develop within aneurysms and are a source of systemic emboli.

A distinction should be made between "**true**" and "**false**" **aneurysms** (see Fig. 11-22). True aneurysms are much more common than false aneurysms and are caused by bulging of the weakened, but intact, left ventricular wall (Fig. 11-23). By contrast, false aneurysms result from rupture of a portion of the left ventricle that has been walled off by pericardial scar tissue. Thus, the wall of a false aneurysm is composed of pericardium and scar tissue but not left ventricular myocardium.

MURAL THROMBOSIS AND EMBOLISM: Half of all patients who die after myocardial infarction have mural thrombi overlying the infarct at autopsy (Fig. 11-24). This occurs particularly often when the infarct involves the apex of the heart. In turn, half of these patients have some evidence of systemic embolization.

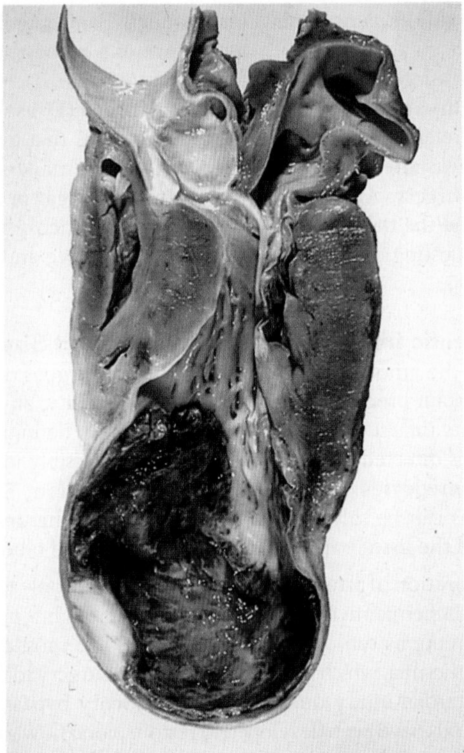

FIGURE 11-23. **Ventricular aneurysm.** The heart of a patient with a history of an anteroapical myocardial infarct who developed a massive ventricular aneurysm. The apex of the heart shows marked thinning and aneurysmal dilation.

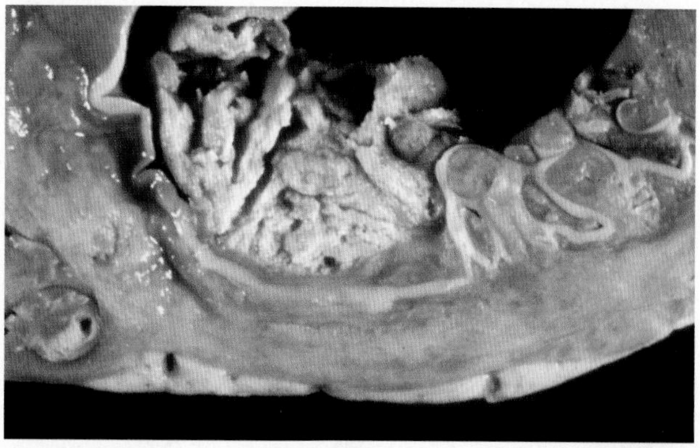

FIGURE 11-24. **Mural thrombus overlying a healed myocardial infarct.** In this cross-section of a fixed heart, an organized, friable, grayish white mural thrombus overlies a thickened endocardium situated over a scarred myocardium.

Inflammation of the endocardium lining an infarct promotes platelet adhesion and fibrin deposition. Also, the poor contractile function of the underlying myocardium allows the fibrin–platelet mural thrombus to grow. Particles of thrombus can detach and be swept along with the arterial blood, potentially causing strokes or myocardial or visceral infarcts. Documented mural thrombosis justifies anticoagulant therapy and antiplatelet medications.

PERICARDITIS: A transmural myocardial infarct involves the epicardium and leads to inflammation of the pericardium in 10% to 20% of patients. Pericarditis is manifested clinically as chest pain and may produce a pericardial friction rub. A fourth of patients with acute myocardial infarction, particularly those with larger infarcts and congestive heart failure, develop a pericardial effusion, with or without pericarditis. Less frequently, anticoagulant therapy has been associated with appearance of a hemorrhagic pericardial effusion and even with cardiac tamponade.

Postmyocardial infarction syndrome (Dressler syndrome) refers to a delayed form of pericarditis that develops 2 to 10 weeks after infarction. A similar disorder may occur after cardiac surgery. Antibodies to heart muscle appear in these patients, and the the condition improves with corticosteroid therapy, suggesting that Dressler syndrome may have an immunologic basis.

Therapeutic Interventions Can Limit Infarct Size

Because the amount of myocardium that undergoes necrosis is an important predictor of morbidity and mortality, any therapy that limits infarct size should be beneficial. By definition, such therapy is directed at preventing death of reversibly injured, ischemic myocytes and limiting infarct extension. Damaged myocytes can be salvaged for some time after the onset of ischemia if the tissue can be reperfused with arterial blood.

- **Restoration of arterial blood flow** remains the only way to salvage ischemic myocytes permanently, although a number of interventions can delay ischemic injury. The most notable is hypothermia, which is used during cardiac surgery to minimize myocardial injury during cardiopulmonary bypass. Several methods have been developed to restore blood flow to the area of myocardium supplied by an obstructed coronary artery.
- **Thrombolytic enzymes** such as tissue plasminogen activator or streptokinase can be infused intravenously to dissolve the clot causing the obstruction.
- **Percutaneous transluminal coronary angioplasty (PTCA)** is dilation of a narrowed coronary artery by inflation with a balloon catheter. This can be done as a primary procedure immediately after onset of ischemia or as a rescue procedure when thrombolytic agents fail to restore arterial blood flow. PTCA also allows placement of a stent in the coronary artery to maintain its patency.
- **Coronary artery bypass grafting** can restore blood flow to the distal segment of a coronary artery with a proximal occlusion.

Procedures that restore blood flow must be performed as quickly as possible, preferably in the first few hours after the onset of symptoms. Beyond 6 hours, it is unlikely that much salvageable ischemic myocardium remains.

Chronic Ischemic Heart Disease Can Lead to Cardiomyopathy

In a minority of patients with severe coronary atherosclerosis, myocardial contractility is impaired globally without discrete infarcts, as in dilated cardiomyopathy. This situation usually reflects a combination of ischemic myocardial dysfunction, diffuse fibrosis, and multiple small healed infarcts. However, there is a group of patients with left ventricular failure in whom cardiac dysfunction occurs without obvious infarction. These patients are said to have **ischemic cardiomyopathy**. In some patients, the dysfunctional myocardium has been subjected to repetitive episodes of ischemic injury, which causes degenerative changes in myocytes, characterized principally by loss of myofibrils (hibernating myocardium) (see Fig. 11-6). The contractile function of hibernating myocardium is restored when affected tissue is revascularized. Thus, to the extent that hibernation plays a role in ischemic cardiomyopathy, surgical revascularization is potentially beneficial.

Hypertensive Heart Disease

Effects of Hypertension on the Heart

Hypertension has been defined by the World Health Organization as a persistent increase of systemic blood pressure above 140 mm Hg systolic or 90 mm Hg diastolic, or both (see Chapter 10). Systemic hypertension is one of the most prevalent and serious causes of coronary artery and myocardial disease in the United States. Chronic hypertension leads to pressure overload resulting first in compensatory left ventricular hypertrophy and, eventually, cardiac failure. The term **hypertensive heart disease** is used when the heart is enlarged in the absence of a cause other than hypertension.

PATHOLOGY: Hypertension causes compensatory left ventricular hypertrophy as a result of the increased cardiac workload. The left ventricular free walls and interventricular septum become thickened uniformly and concentrically (Fig. 11-25), and heart weight increases, exceeding 375 g in men and 350 g in women. Microscopically, hypertrophic myocardial cells have an increased diameter, with enlarged, hyperchromatic, and rectangular ("boxcar") nuclei (Fig. 11-26).

CLINICAL FEATURES: Myocardial hypertrophy clearly adds to the ability of the heart to handle an increased workload. However, there is a limit beyond which additional hypertrophy no longer compensates. This upper

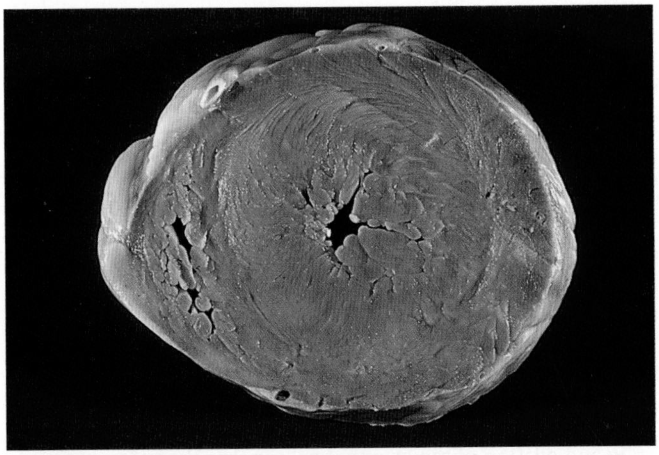

FIGURE 11-25. **Hypertensive heart disease.** A transverse section of the heart shows marked hypertrophy of the left ventricular myocardium without dilation of the chamber. The right ventricle is of normal dimensions.

limit to useful hypertrophy may reflect increasing diffusion distance between the interstitium and the center of each myofiber; if the distance becomes too great, the oxygen supply to the myofiber will be deficient.

Diastolic dysfunction is the most common functional abnormality caused by hypertension and by itself can lead to congestive heart failure. Some interstitial fibrosis typically develops as part of hypertrophy, which further contributes to left ventricular stiffness. *Hypertension also is associated with increased severity of coronary artery atherosclerosis. The combination of increased cardiac workload (systolic dysfunction), diastolic dysfunction, and narrowed coronary arteries leads to greater risk of myocardial ischemia, infarction and heart failure.*

Congestive Heart Failure is the Major Cause of Death in Patients with Untreated Hypertension

Fatal intracerebral hemorrhage is also common. Death may also result from coronary atherosclerosis and myocardial infarction, dissecting aneurysm of the aorta, or ruptured berry aneurysm of the cerebral circulation. Renal failure may supervene when nephrosclerosis induced by hypertension becomes severe.

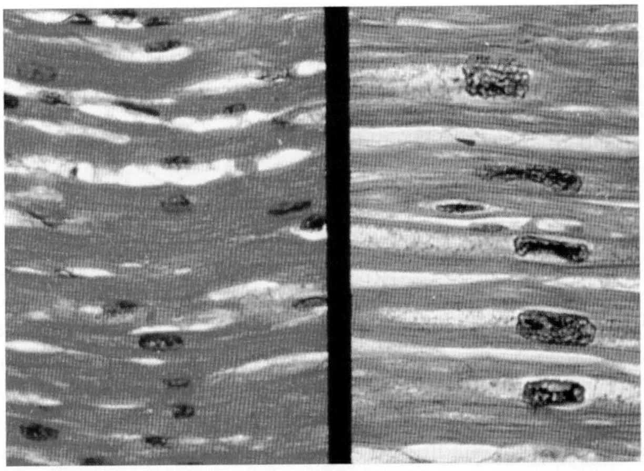

FIGURE 11-26. **Hypertensive heart disease with myocardial hypertrophy. (Left)** Normal myocardium. **(Right)** Hypertrophic myocardium shows thicker fibers and enlarged, hyperchromatic, rectangular nuclei.

Cor Pulmonale

Cor pulmonale is right ventricular hypertrophy and dilation due to pulmonary hypertension. Increased pressure in the pulmonary circulation may reflect a disorder of lung parenchyma or, more rarely, a primary disease of the vasculature (e.g., primary pulmonary hypertension, recurrent small pulmonary emboli).

Acute cor pulmonale is the sudden occurrence of pulmonary hypertension, most commonly as a result of sudden, massive pulmonary embolization. This condition causes acute right-sided heart failure and is a medical emergency. At autopsy, the only cardiac findings are severe dilation of the right ventricle and sometimes the right atrium.

Chronic cor pulmonale is a common heart disease, accounting for 30% to 40% of all cases of heart failure in an English study and 10% to 30% in a series in the United States. This frequency reflects the prevalence of chronic pulmonary disease in these countries, especially chronic bronchitis and emphysema. In many cases of chronic lung disease, the severity of pulmonary hypertension correlates more closely with survival than any other variable. In fact, fewer than 10% of patients with a pulmonary artery pressure greater than 45 mm Hg survive 5 years.

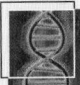

PATHOGENESIS: Chronic cor pulmonale may be caused by any pulmonary disease that interferes with ventilatory mechanics or gas exchange or obstructs the pulmonary vasculature (Table 11-5). *The most common causes of chronic cor pulmonale are chronic obstructive pulmonary disease and pulmonary fibrosis.* Severe kyphoscoliosis may deform the chest wall and interfere with its function as a bellows, resulting in hypoxemia and pulmonary vasoconstriction. A few cases of cor pulmonale are attributed to **primary pulmonary hypertension**, a disorder of unknown etiology. As discussed above, some congenital heart diseases associated with increased pulmonary blood flow are complicated by pulmonary hypertension and cor pulmonale.

The pathogenesis of pulmonary hypertension secondary to recurrent pulmonary emboli is related clearly to progressive mechanical obstruction of blood flow. However, mechanisms of pulmonary hypertension in chronic parenchymal diseases of the lungs are more complicated. In addition to the obliteration of blood vessels in the lung, these disorders also lead to pulmonary arteriolar vasoconstriction, which reduces the effective cross-sectional area of the pulmonary vascular bed without destroying the vessels. Hypoxia, acidosis, and hypercapnia directly cause pulmonary vasoconstriction. Hypoxia also increases pulmonary vascular resistance indirectly by leading to polycythemia, which causes hyperviscosity of the blood. Persons living at very high altitude, for instance, natives of the Andes mountain range, often develop cor pulmonale secondary to the effects of chronic hypoxemia.

TABLE 11-5

Causes of Cor Pulmonale

Parenchymal diseases of the lung
Chronic bronchitis and emphysema
Pulmonary fibrosis (from any cause)
Cystic fibrosis
Pulmonary Vascular Diseases
Recurrent pulmonary emboli
Primary pulmonary hypertension
Peripheral pulmonary stenosis
Intravenous drug abuse
Residence at high altitude
Schistosomiasis
Congenital heart diseases
Impaired movement of the thoracic cage
Kyphoscoliosis
Pickwickian syndrome
Pleural fibrosis
Neuromuscular disorders
Idiopathic hypoventilation

PATHOLOGY: Chronic cor pulmonale is characterized by conspicuous right ventricular hypertrophy (Fig. 11-27), to the extent of exceeding 1.0 cm in thickness (normal range, 0.3 to 0.5 cm). Dilation of the right ventricle and right atrium are often present. Normally, the interventricular septum is concave to the left (i.e., it is part of the left ventricle). With development of severe right ventricular hypertrophy, the interventricular septum remodels by straightening or even becoming concave to the right.

Acquired Valvular and Endocardial Diseases

A variety of inflammatory, infectious, and degenerative diseases damage cardiac valves and impair their function. The valves normally consist of thin flexible membranes, which close tightly to prevent backward blood flow. When they become damaged, leaflets or cusps may be thickened and fused enough to narrow the aperture and obstruct blood flow, a condition labeled **valvular stenosis**. Diseases that destroy valve tissue may also allow retrograde blood flow, termed **valvular regurgitation** or **insufficiency**. In many cases, diseases of the cardiac valves produce both stenosis and insufficiency, but generally one or the other predominates.

Stenosis of a cardiac valve results in hypertrophy of the myocardium proximal (in terms of blood flow) to the obstruction. Once compensatory mechanisms are exhausted **pressure overload** eventually causes myocardial dilation and failure of the chamber proximal to the valve. Thus, mitral stenosis leads to left atrial hypertrophy and dilation. As the left atrium decompensates and can no longer force the venous return through the stenotic mitral valve, signs of pulmonary congestion develop, followed by right ventricular hypertrophy and even cor pulmonale. Similarly, aortic stenosis causes left ventricular hypertrophy and eventually left heart failure.

Valvular regurgitation or insufficiency also results in hypertrophy and dilation of the chamber proximal to the valve, owing to **volume overload.** In aortic insufficiency, the left ventricle first hypertrophies and then dilates when it can no longer accommodate the regurgitant volume and provide adequate cardiac output. On the other hand, an incompetent mitral valve leads to hypertrophy and dilation of both the left atrium and left ventricle, because both are subjected to volume overload. Marked left ventricular dilation from any condition in which cardiac contractility is inadequate (e.g., congestive failure after a large myocardial infarct) also may widen the mitral valve ring. This effect may be so severe that the valve leaflets do not close properly, leading to mitral regurgitation.

The semilunar valves are structurally and functionally simple compared with the atrioventricular valves. The latter consist of the valve leaflets, muscular valve annuli, and the subvalvular apparatus (chordae tendineae and papillary muscles). In general, valvular stenosis involves pathological changes of leaflets themselves, but regurgitation can be caused by abnormalities of valve leaflets, annulus, or subvalvular apparatus.

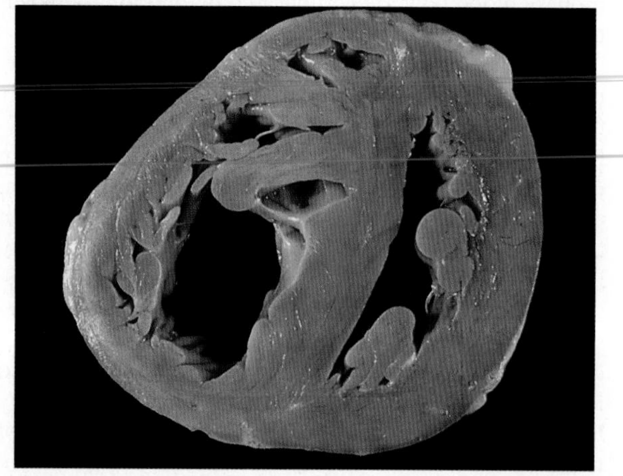

FIGURE 11-27. **Cor pulmonale.** A transverse section of the heart from a patient with primary (idiopathic) pulmonary hypertension shows a markedly hypertrophied right ventricle (on the left). The right ventricular free wall has a thickness equal to the left ventricular wall. The right ventricle is dilated. The straightened interventricular septum has lost its normal curvature toward the left ventricle as part of the remodeling process in cor pulmonale.

Rheumatic Heart Disease Encompasses Acute Myocarditis and Residual Valvular Deformities

Acute Rheumatic Fever

Rheumatic fever (RF) is a multisystem childhood disease that follows a streptococcal infection and is characterized by an inflammatory reaction involving the heart, joints, and central nervous system.

EPIDEMIOLOGY: RF is a complication of an acute streptococcal infection, almost always pharyngitis (i.e., "strep" throat) (see Chapter 9). The offending agent is *Streptococcus pyogenes*, also known as group A β-hemolytic *Streptococcus*. In some epidemics of streptococcal pharyngitis, the incidence of RF has been as high as 3%. RF is principally a disease of childhood, the median age being 9 to 11 years, although it can occur in adults.

In the first half of the 20th century, RF reached almost epidemic proportions in the United States, but its incidence has decreased dramatically. Between 1950 and 1972, the death rate fell from 14.5 to 6.8 per 100,000, and it has decreased further since then. Although this decline may have been partly the result of widespread antibiotic treatment, such therapy cannot account for the entire reduction, because the death rate had begun to decrease well before antibiotics were generally available. Improved socioeconomic conditions, in particular less crowded living circumstances, probably contributed to the decrease. *Despite its declining importance in industrialized countries, RF is a leading cause of death of heart disease in persons 5 to 25 years old in less-developed regions.*

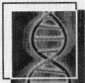

PATHOGENESIS: The pathogenesis of RF remains unclear, and with the exception of the link to streptococcal infection, no theory has been proven unequivocally. Most hypotheses relate rheumatic carditis to antibodies against streptococcal antigens that cross-react with heart antigens, an observation that raises the possibility of an autoimmune etiology related to so-called molecular mimicry (Fig. 11-28).

Streptococcal antigens structurally similar to those in the heart include hyaluronate in the bacterial capsule, cell wall polysaccharides similar to the carbohydrate moiety of heart valve glycoproteins, and bacterial membrane antigens that share epitopes with sarcolemma and smooth muscle constituents. Although antibodies to these antigens are found in patients with RF, it has not been proved that they are cytotoxic or that they are directly involved in the pathogenesis of the disease. A direct toxic effect of some streptococcal product on the myocardium has not yet been excluded.

PATHOLOGY: Acute rheumatic heart disease is a pancarditis, involving all three layers of the heart (endocardium, myocardium, and pericardium).

MYOCARDITIS: In severe cases of RF, a few patients may die during the earliest acute phase of the illness before the characteristic granulomatous inflammation has developed. At this early stage, the heart tends to be dilated and exhibits a nonspecific myocarditis, in which lymphocytes and macrophages predominate, although a few neutrophils and eosinophils may be evident. Fibrinoid degeneration of collagen, in which fibers become swollen, fragmented, and eosinophilic, is characteristic of this early phase.

The **Aschoff body** is the characteristic granulomatous lesion of rheumatic myocarditis (Fig. 11-29), developing several weeks after symptoms begin. This structure initially consists of a perivascular focus of swollen eosinophilic collagen surrounded by lymphocytes, plasma cells, and macrophages. With time, the Aschoff body assumes a granulomatous appearance, with a central fibrinoid focus associated with a perimeter of lymphocytes, plasma cells, macrophages, and giant cells. Eventually, the Aschoff body is replaced by a nodule of scar tissue.

Anitschkow cells are unusual cells within the Aschoff body, whose nuclei contain a central band of chromatin. These nuclei have an "owl eye" appearance in cross-section, and they resemble a caterpillar when cut longitudinally (see Fig 11-29). These cells are macrophages that are normally present in small numbers but accumulate and become prominent in certain types of inflammatory diseases of the heart. Anitschkow cells may become multinucleated, in which case they are termed **Aschoff giant cells.**

PERICARDITIS: Tenacious irregular fibrin deposits are found on both visceral and parietal surfaces of the pericardium during the acute inflammatory phase of RF. These deposits resemble the shaggy surfaces of two slices of buttered bread that have been pulled apart ("bread-and-butter pericarditis"). The pericarditis may be recognized clinically by hearing a friction rub, but it has little functional effect and ordinarily does not lead to constrictive pericarditis.

ENDOCARDITIS: During the acute stage of rheumatic carditis, valve leaflets become inflamed and edematous. All four valves are affected, but left-sided valves are most injured because they close under greater pressures than do right-sided valves. The result is damage and focal loss of endothelium along the lines of closure of the valve leaflets. This leads to deposition of tiny nodules of fibrin, which can be recognized grossly as "verrucae" along the leaflets (so-called verrucous endocarditis of acute RF).

CLINICAL FEATURES: There is no specific test for RF. The clinical diagnosis is made when two major—or one major and two minor—criteria (the Jones criteria) are met. If the diagnosis is supported by evidence of a recent streptococcal infection, the probability of RF is high.

The **major criteria** of acute RF include carditis (murmurs, cardiomegaly, pericarditis, and congestive heart failure), polyarthritis, chorea, erythema marginatum, and subcutaneous nodules.

The minor criteria are previous history of RF, arthralgia, fever, certain laboratory tests indicating an inflammatory process (e.g., increased sedimentation rate, positive test result for C-reactive protein, leukocytosis), and electrocardiographic changes.

The symptoms of RF occur 2 to 3 weeks after an infection with *S. pyogenes*. By that time, throat cultures are usually negative. Increasing titers of serum antibodies to group A streptococcal antigens, such as antistreptolysin O, anti-DNAase B, and antihyaluronidase, provide concrete evidence of a recent infection with group A *Streptococcus*. Acute symptoms of RF usually subside within 3 months, but with severe carditis, clinical activity may continue for 6 months or more. The mortality from acute rheumatic carditis is low. The main cause of death is heart failure due to myocarditis, although valvular dysfunction may also play a role.

Recurrent attacks of RF are associated with types of group A β-hemolytic streptococci to which the patient has not been previously exposed and, therefore, to which immunity has not developed. The rate of recurrence of RF is related to the elapsed interval between the initial episode and a subsequent streptococcal infection. In patients with a history of a recent attack of RF, the recurrence rate is as high as 65%, whereas after 10 years, a streptococcal infection is followed by an acute relapse in only 5%.

Prompt treatment of streptococcal pharyngitis with antibiotics prevents an initial attack of RF and, less often, a recurrence of the disease. There is no specific treatment for acute RF, but corticosteroids and salicylates are helpful in managing the symptoms.

Chronic Rheumatic Heart Disease

PATHOLOGY: The myocardial and pericardial components of rheumatic pancarditis typically resolve without permanent sequelae. By contrast, the acute valvulitis of RF often results in long-term structural and functional alterations. During the healing phase, valve leaflets develop diffuse fibrosis and become thickened, shrunken, and less pliable. At the same time, healing of the verrucous lesions along the lines of closure often leads to formation of fibrous "adhesions" between leaflets, especially at the commissures (commissural fusion). The result is a stenotic valve that does not open freely because the leaflets are rigid and partially fused. Blood flow across such a valve is turbulent, which can cause even more scarring and deformation of the leaflets because of chronic "wear and tear" on the valve. Severe valvular scarring may develop months or years after a single bout of acute RF. On the other

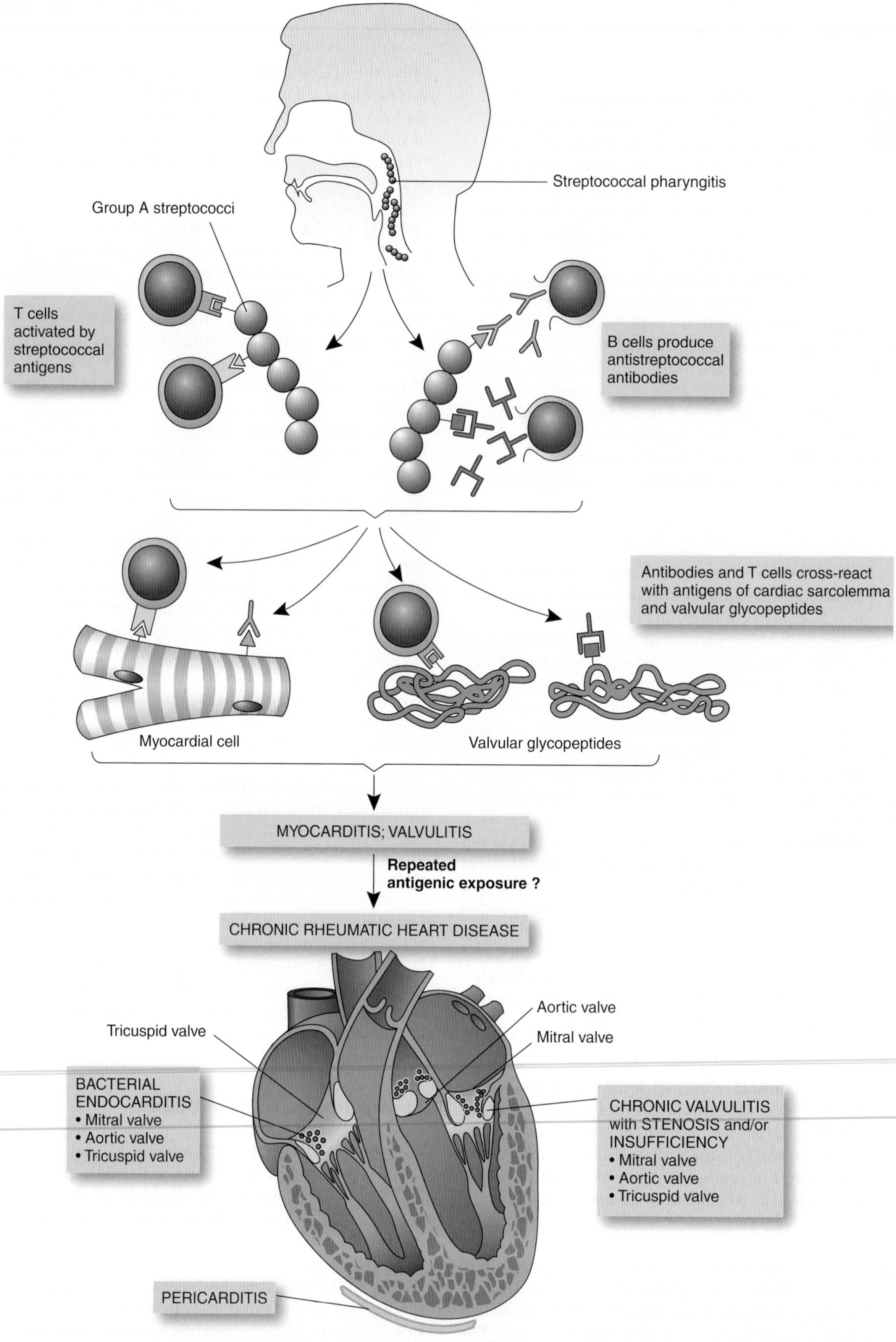

FIGURE 11-28. **Biological factors in rheumatic heart disease.** The upper portion illustrates the initiating β-hemolytic streptococcal infection of the throat, which introduces the streptococcal antigens into the body and may also activate cytotoxic T cells. These antigens lead to the production of antibodies against various antigenic components of the streptococcus, which can cross-react with certain cardiac antigens, including those from the myocyte sarcolemma and glycoproteins of the valves. This may be the mechanism for inflammation of the heart in acute rheumatic fever, which involves all cardiac layers (endocarditis, myocarditis, and pericarditis). This inflammation becomes apparent after a latent period of 2 to 3 weeks. Active inflammation of the valves may eventually lead to chronic valvular stenosis or insufficiency. These lesions involve the mitral, aortic, tricuspid, and pulmonary valves, in that order of frequency.

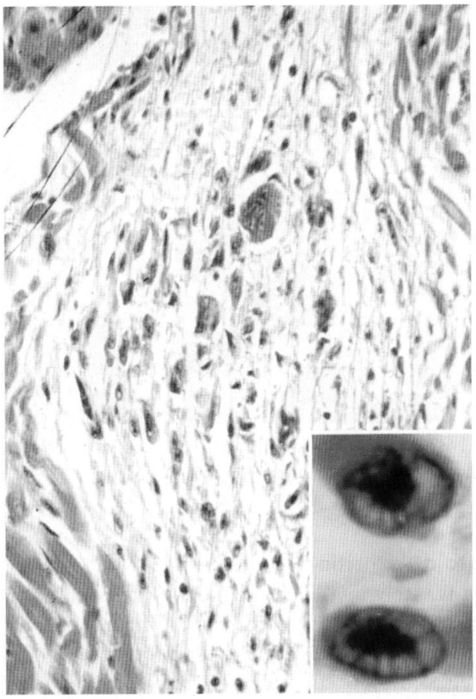

FIGURE 11-29. **Acute rheumatic heart disease.** An Aschoff body is located interstitially in the myocardium. Note collagen degeneration, lymphocytes, and a multinucleated Aschoff giant cell. **(Inset)** Nuclei of Anitschkow myocytes, showing "owl-eye" appearance in cross-section and "caterpillar" shape longitudinally.

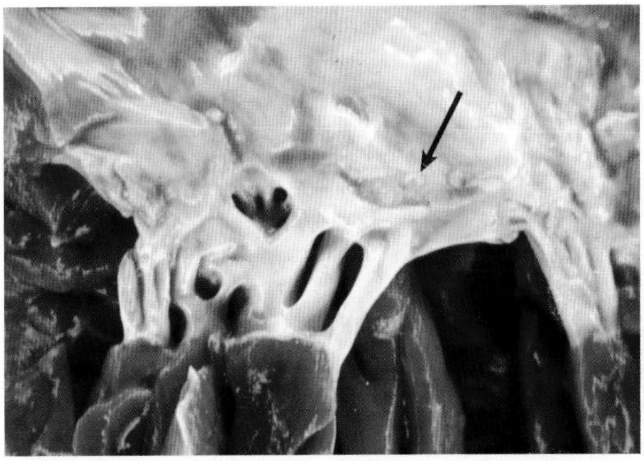

FIGURE 11-30. **Chronic rheumatic valvulitis.** The mitral valve leaflets are thickened and focally calcified *(arrow)*, and the commissures are partially fused. The chordae tendineae are also short, thick, and fused.

hand, recurrent episodes of acute RF are common and result in repeated and progressively increasing damage to the heart valves.

The mitral valve is the most commonly and severely affected valve in chronic rheumatic disease. It snaps shut under systolic pressure and, thus, bears the greatest mechanical burden of all cardiac valves. Chronic mitral valvulitis is characterized by conspicuous, irregular thickening and calcification of the leaflets, often with fusion of the commissures and chordae tendineae (Fig. 11-30). In severe chronic rheumatic mitral valve disease, the valve orifice becomes reduced to a fixed narrow opening that has the appearance of a "fish mouth" when viewed from the ventricular aspect (Fig. 11-31). Mitral stenosis is the predominant functional lesion, but such a valve is also regurgitant. Chronic regurgitation produces a "jet" of blood directed at the posterior aspect of the left atrium, which damages the atrial endocardium and produces a discrete focus of rough, wrinkled endocardium referred to as a "MacCallum patch."

The aortic valve, which snaps shut under diastolic pressure, is the second most commonly involved valve in rheumatic heart disease. Diffuse fibrous thickening of the cusps and fusion of the commissures cause aortic stenosis, which may be mild initially but which progresses because of the chronic effects of turbulent blood flow across the valve. Often, cusps become rigidly calcified as the patient ages, resulting in stenosis and insufficiency, although either lesion may predominate (Fig. 11-32). The lower pressures experienced by the right-sided valves are usually protective. In cases of recurrent RF, however, the tricuspid valve may become deformed, virtually always in association with mitral and aortic lesions. The pulmonic valve is rarely affected.

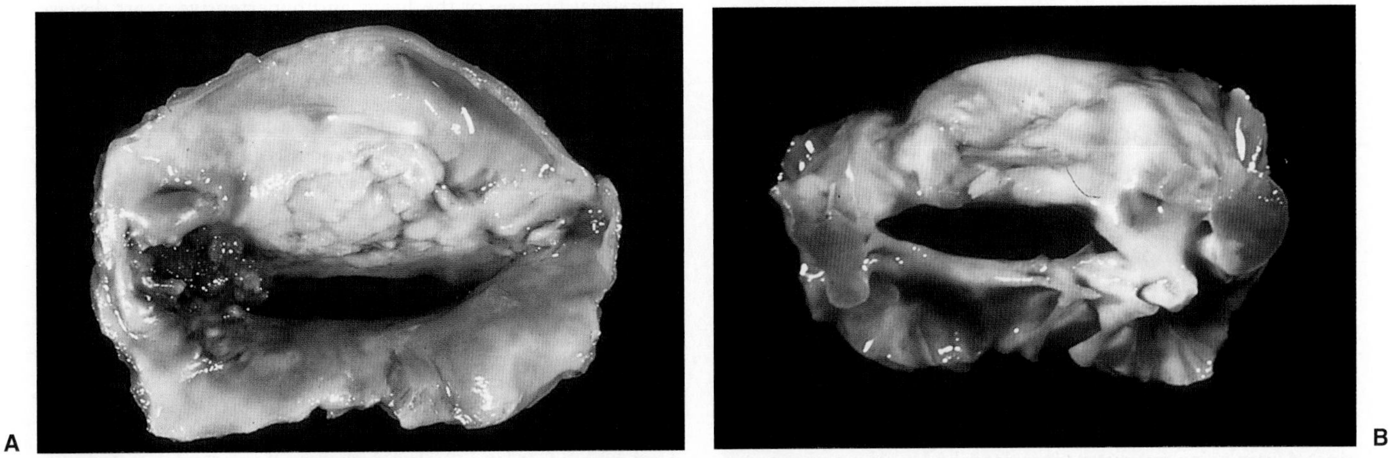

FIGURE 11-31. **Chronic rheumatic valvulitis.** A view of a surgically excised rheumatic mitral valve from the left atrium (**A**) and left ventricle (**B**) shows rigid, thickened, and fused leaflets with a narrow orifice, creating the characteristic "fish mouth" appearance of rheumatic mitral stenosis. Note that the tips of the papillary muscles *(shown in B)* are directly attached to the underside of the valve leaflets, reflecting marked shortening and fusion of the chordae tendineae.

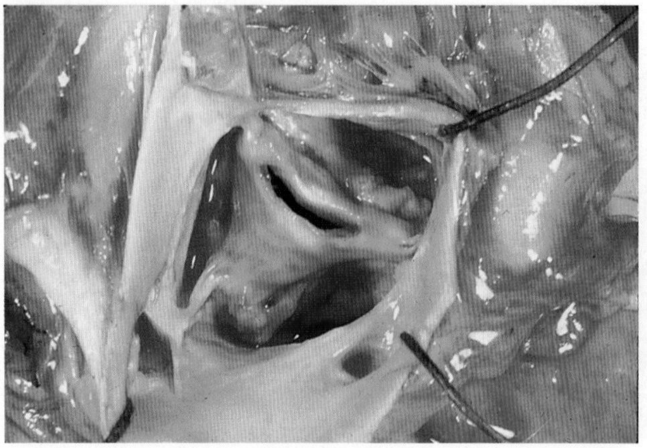

FIGURE 11-32. **Chronic rheumatic valvulitis.** An example of severe rheumatic aortic stenosis. Three sinuses of Valsalva are recognizable, but the cusps are rigidly fibrotic and calcified, and extensive fusion of the commissures has narrowed the orifice into a fixed slitlike configuration that does not change during the cardiac cycle.

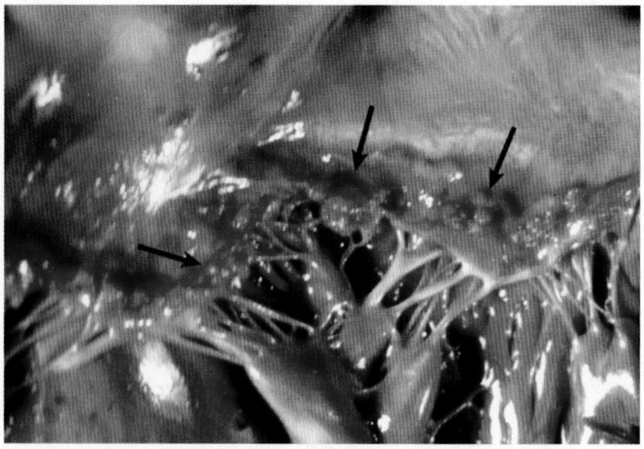

FIGURE 11-33. **Libman-Sacks endocarditis.** The heart of a patient who died of complications of systemic lupus erythematosus displays verrucous vegetations *(arrows)* on the leaflets of the mitral valve.

Complications of Chronic Rheumatic Heart Disease

- **Bacterial endocarditis** follows episodes of bacteremia, e.g., during dental procedures. The scarred valves of rheumatic heart disease provide an attractive environment for bacteria that would bypass a normal valve.
- **Mural thrombi** form in atrial or ventricular chambers in 40% of patients with rheumatic valvular disease. They give rise to thromboemboli, which can produce infarcts in various organs. Rarely, a large thrombus in the left atrial appendage develops a stalk and acts as a ball valve that obstructs the mitral valve orifice.
- **Congestive heart failure** is associated with rheumatic disease of both mitral and aortic valves.
- **Adhesive pericarditis** commonly follows the fibrinous pericarditis of the acute attack, but almost never results in constrictive pericarditis.

Collagen Vascular Diseases Affect Both Cardiac Valves and Myocardium

Systemic Lupus Erythematosus

The heart is often involved in SLE, but cardiac symptoms are usually less prominent than other manifestations of the disease.

PATHOLOGY: The most common cardiac lesion is **fibrinous pericarditis,** usually with an effusion. **Myocarditis** in SLE, at least in the form of subclinical left ventricular dysfunction, is also common and reflects the severity of the disease in other organs. Microscopically, fibrinoid necrosis of small vessels and focal degeneration of interstitial tissue are seen.

Endocarditis is the most striking cardiac lesion of SLE. Verrucous vegetations, up to 4 mm across, occur on endocardial surfaces and are termed **Libman-Sacks endocarditis**. They are most common on the mitral valve (Fig. 11-33), characteristically the undersurface, close to the origin of the leaflets from the valve ring. Aortic valve involvement is described rarely, and the verrucae may extend onto the chordae tendineae and the papillary muscles. Ordinarily, Libman-Sacks endocarditis heals without scarring and does not produce a functional deficit.

Rheumatoid Arthritis

The heart is rarely involved in patients with rheumatoid arthritis. Characteristic rheumatoid granulomatous inflammation, with fibrinoid necrosis and palisaded lymphocytes and macrophages, may occur in the pericardium, myocardium, or valves. Involvement of the heart in rheumatoid arthritis does not compromise function.

Ankylosing Spondylitis

A characteristic aortic valve lesion develops in as many as 10% of patients with long-standing ankylosing spondylitis. The aortic valve ring is dilated and its cusps are scarred and shortened. Focal inflammatory lesions occur in all layers of the aortic wall, particularly near the valve ring. Aortic regurgitation is the principal functional consequence.

Scleroderma (Progressive Systemic Sclerosis)

Cardiac involvement is second only to renal disease as a cause of death in scleroderma. The myocardium exhibits intimal sclerosis of small arteries, which leads to small infarcts and patchy fibrosis. As a result, congestive heart failure and arrhythmias are common. In fact, electrocardiographic studies have revealed ventricular ectopy in two thirds of patients with scleroderma and serious arrhythmias in one fourth. Cor pulmonale secondary to interstitial fibrosis of the lungs and hypertensive heart disease (caused by renal involvement) are also seen.

Polyarteritis Nodosa

The heart is involved in up to 75% of cases of polyarteritis nodosa. Necrotizing lesions in branches of the coronary arteries result in myocardial infarction, arrhythmias or heart block. Cardiac hypertrophy and failure secondary to renal vascular hypertension are common.

Bacterial Endocarditis is Infection of the Cardiac Valves

Fungi, chlamydia, and rickettsiae may also cause infective endocarditis, but such cases are uncommon. Before the antibiotic era, bacterial endocarditis was untreatable and almost invariably fatal. The infection was classified according to its clinical course as either acute or subacute endocarditis.

Acute bacterial endocarditis was described as an infection of a normal cardiac valve by highly virulent suppurative organisms, typically *Staphylococcus aureus* and *S. pyogenes*. The affected valve was rapidly destroyed, and the patient died within 6 weeks in acute heart failure or of overwhelming sepsis.

Subacute bacterial endocarditis was a less fulminant disease in which less-virulent organisms (e.g., *Streptococcus viridans* or *Staphylococcus epidermidis*) infected a structurally abnormal valve, which typically had been deformed by rheumatic heart disease. In these cases, patients typically survived for 6 months or more, and infectious complications were uncommon.

Antimicrobial therapy changed the clinical patterns of bacterial endocarditis, and classical presentations described earlier are today unusual. The disease is now classified according to the anatomical location and the offending organism (Table 11-6).

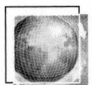

EPIDEMIOLOGY: Most children with bacterial endocarditis have an underlying cardiac lesion. In the past, rheumatic heart disease accounted for a third of such cases. However, as incidence of RF has declined, under 10% of cases of bacterial endocarditis in children are today attributable to this disease. *The most common predisposing condition for bacterial endocarditis in children now is congenital heart disease.*

The epidemiology of bacterial endocarditis has also changed in adults. Rheumatic heart disease once comprised three fourths of the cases, but now underlies only a few. More than half of adults with bacterial endocarditis have no predisposing cardiac lesion. *Mitral valve prolapse (MVP) and congenital heart disease are today the most frequent bases for bacterial endocarditis in adults.*

- In **rheumatic heart disease,** the mitral valve is affected in over 85% of cases of bacterial endocarditis, and the aortic valve is involved in 50%. Involvement of a single valve occurs more often in women (2:1) in the case of mitral valve disease, whereas the male-to-female ratio in isolated aortic endocarditis is 4:1.
- **Intravenous drug abusers** inject pathogenic organisms along with their illicit drugs, and bacterial endocarditis is a notorious complication. In such patients, 80% have no underlying cardiac lesion, and the tricuspid valve is infected in half of cases. The most common source of bacteria in intravenous drug abusers is the skin, with *S. aureus* causing more than half of the infections.
- **Prosthetic valves** are sites of infection in 15% of all cases of endocarditis in adults, and 4% of patients with prosthetic valves have this complication. Staphylococci are again responsible for half of these infections, and most of the rest are caused by gram-negative aerobic organisms, streptococci and enterococci, and fungi. Another iatrogenic form of endocarditis originates from bacterial colonization of indwelling vascular catheters.
- **Transient bacteremia** from any procedure may lead to infective endocarditis. Examples include dental procedures, urinary catheterization, gastrointestinal endoscopy, and obstetric procedures. Antibiotic prophylaxis is recommended during such maneuvers for patients at increased risk for bacterial endocarditis (e.g., those with a history of RF or a cardiac murmur).
- **The elderly** also have an increasing tendency to develop endocarditis. A number of degenerative changes in heart valves, including calcific aortic stenosis and calcification of the mitral annulus, predispose to endocarditis.
- **Diabetes** and **pregnancy** are also associated with increased incidence of bacterial endocarditis.

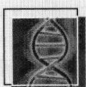

PATHOGENESIS: Virulent organisms, such as *S. aureus*, can infect apparently normal valves, but the mechanism of such bacterial colonization is poorly understood. The pathogenesis of the infection of a damaged valve by less-virulent organisms has been related to (1) hemodynamic factors, (2) the formation of an initially sterile platelet–fibrin thrombus, and (3) the adherence properties of the microorganisms. A key feature is abnormal blood flow across a damaged valve. The pressure gradient formed across a narrow orifice (valve or congenital defect) produces turbulent flow at the periphery and a high-velocity jet stream at the center, both of which

TABLE 11-6

Etiologic Factors in Bacterial Endocarditis

	Children (%)		Adults (%)	
	Newborns	<15 years	15–60 years	>60 years
Underlying disease				
Congenital heart disease	30	80	10	2
Rheumatic heart disease	–	5	25	8
Mitral valve prolapse	–	10	10	10
Valvular calcification	–	–	5	30
Intravenous drug abuse	–	–	15	10
Other	–	–	10	10
None	70	5	25	30
Microorganisms*				
Staphylococcus aureus	45	25	35	30
Coagulase-negative staphylococci	10	5	5	10
Streptococci	15	45	45	35
Enterococci	–	5	5	15
Gram-negative bacteria	10	5	5	5
Fungi	10	Rare	Rare	Rare
Negative culture	5	10	5	5

* 5% of neonatal infections are polymicrobial

tend to denude endothelial surfaces of valves on the low-pressure side of the orifice. This leads to focal deposition of platelets and fibrin, creating small sterile vegetations that are hospitable sites for bacterial colonization and growth. Microorganisms that gain access to the circulation, as a result of a dental procedure for example, can be deposited within the vegetations. In this protected environment, colony counts upon culture may reach 10^{10} organisms per gram of tissue.

Factors that promote bacterial adherence to the sterile vegetations are believed to be important in the pathogenesis of endocarditis. Cell-associated and circulating fibronectin both bind to surface molecules of the bacteria, facilitating adhesion of fibrin, collagen, and cells. Some microorganisms produce extracellular polysaccharides, which also function as adhesion factors.

PATHOLOGY: Bacterial endocarditis most commonly involves the left-sided heart valves (mitral or aortic valves or both).

The most common congenital heart lesions that underlie bacterial endocarditis are PDA, tetralogy of Fallot, ventricular septal defect, and bicuspid aortic valve, which is an increasingly recognized risk factor, especially in men over 60 years. *As a rule, vegetations in bacterial endocarditis form on the atrial side of the atrioventricular valves and the ventricular side of the semilunar valves, often at points of closure of the leaflets or cusps* (Fig. 11-34). Vegetations are composed of platelets, fibrin, cell debris, and masses of organisms. Underlying valve tissue is edematous and inflamed and may eventually become so damaged that a leaflet perforates, causing regurgitation. Lesions vary in size from a small, superficial deposit to bulky, exuberant vegetations. The infective process may spread locally to involve the valve ring or adjacent mural endocardium and chordae tendineae.

Infected thromboemboli travel to multiple systemic sites, causing infarcts or abscesses in many organs, including the brain, kidneys, intestine, and spleen.

Focal segmental glomerulonephritis may complicate infective endocarditis (see Chapter 16). It is the result of immune-complex deposition in glomeruli, producing a patchy hemorrhagic appearance of the kidneys referred to as "flea-bitten kidneys."

CLINICAL FEATURES: Many patients show early symptoms of bacterial endocarditis within a week of the bacteremic episode, and almost all are symptomatic within 2 weeks. The disease begins with nonspecific symptoms of low-grade fever, fatigue, anorexia, and weight loss. Heart murmurs develop almost invariably, often with a changing pattern, during the course of the disease. In cases of more than 6 weeks duration, splenomegaly, petechiae, and clubbing of the fingers are frequent. In a third of patients, systemic emboli are recognized at some time during the illness. Pulmonary emboli characterize tricuspid valve endocarditis in drug addicts. One third of the victims of bacterial endocarditis manifest some evidence of neurologic dysfunction, owing to the frequency of embolization to the brain. Mycotic aneurysms of cerebral vessels, brain abscesses, and intracerebral bleeding are observed.

Antibacterial therapy is effective in limiting the morbidity and mortality of bacterial endocarditis. Most patients defervesce within a week of instituting such therapy. However, the prognosis depends to some extent on the offending organism and the stage at which the infection is treated. *A third of cases of S. aureus endocarditis are still fatal.* Surgical replacement of a valve destroyed by endocarditis is risky and carries high surgical mortality unless the infection is fully cleared. *The most common serious complication of bacterial endocarditis is congestive heart failure, usually due to destruction of a valve.* Myocardial abscesses and infarction secondary to coronary artery emboli occasionally contribute to heart failure. At this stage the prognosis is grim.

Nonbacterial Thrombotic Endocarditis Is a Complication of Wasting Diseases

Nonbacterial thrombotic endocarditis (NBTE), also known as marantic endocarditis, refers to sterile vegetations on apparently normal cardiac valves, almost always in association with cancer or some other wasting disease. NBTE affects mitral (Fig. 11-35) and aortic valves with equal frequency. Its gross appearance is similar to that of infective endocarditis, but it does not destroy the affected valve, and on microscopic examination, neither inflammation nor microorganisms can be demonstrated.

The cause of NBTE is poorly understood. It has been attributed to increased blood coagulability or immune-complex deposition. It is seen commonly as a paraneoplastic condition, usually complicating adenocarcinomas (particularly of pancreas

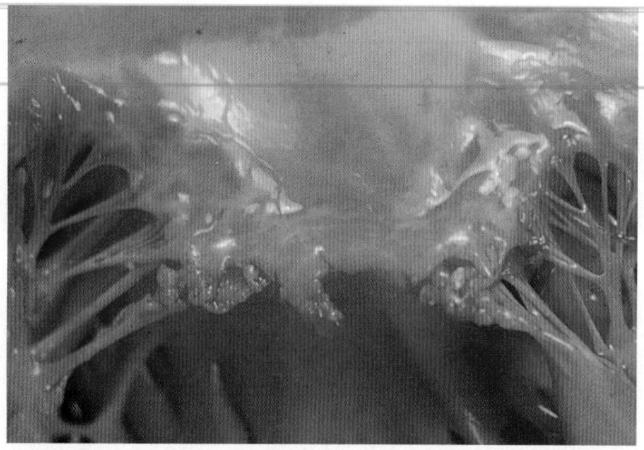

FIGURE 11-34. **Bacterial endocarditis.** The mitral valve shows destructive vegetations, which have eroded through the free margins of the valve leaflets.

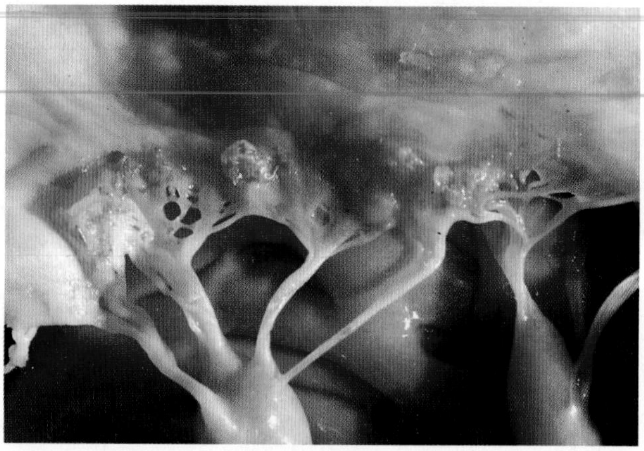

FIGURE 11-35. **Marantic endocarditis.** Sterile platelet–fibrin vegetations are seen on the leaflets of a structurally normal mitral valve.

and lung) and hematologic malignancies. It may also occur in disseminated intravascular coagulation or accompany a variety of debilitating non-neoplastic diseases, accounting for the term "marantic endocarditis" (from the Greek, *marantikos,* "wasting away"). The main danger posed by NBTE is embolization to distant organs, clinically manifested as infarcts of many organs.

Calcific Aortic Stenosis Reflects Chronic Damage to the Valve

Calcific aortic stenosis refers to a narrowing of the aortic valve orifice as a result of calcium deposition in the cusps and valve ring.

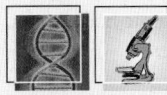

PATHOGENESIS AND PATHOLOGY: Calcific aortic stenosis has three main causes.

- **Rheumatic aortic valve disease** is characterized by diffuse fibrous thickening and scarring of the cusps, commissural fusion, and deposition of calcium, all of which reduce the valve orifice and limit valve mobility (see Fig. 11-32). Rheumatic aortic stenosis virtually never occurs in isolation; there is nearly always evidence of rheumatic mitral valve disease as well. Now that acute RF has become so rare in the United States and most elderly patients with rheumatic valve disease have either undergone valve replacement or died, calcific aortic stenosis is usually attributed to other causes.
- **Degenerative (senile) calcific stenosis** develops in elderly patients as a degenerative process involving a symmetric tricuspid aortic valve. Valve cusps become rigidly calcified, but there is no commissural fusion (Fig. 11-36), which is a hallmark of the rheumatic aortic valve. The mitral valve is usually normal in patients with senile calcific aortic stenosis, although the mitral annulus may also be calcified.
- **Congenital bicuspid aortic stenosis** often develops with age (Fig. 11-37).
- **Calcific aortic stenosis** in both congenitally malformed valves and normal ones is probably related to the cumulative effect of years of trauma, owing to turbulent blood flow around the valve. For example, although a bicuspid valve is not inherently stenotic, its orifice is elliptical rather than round, and flow across the valve is somewhat turbulent. Increasing rigidity of the cusps eventually produces functional derangements, typically in patients beyond the age of 60.

In any of the forms of calcific aortic stenosis, calcification produces nodules restricted to the base and lower half of the cusps, rarely involving free margins. Without rheumatic scarring, the commissures are not fused, and three distinct cusps are evident.

Aortic valve calcification is not a purely passive process in which devitalized tissue becomes mineralized, as the term "dystrophic calcification" seems to imply. In fact, valvular calcification is an active process involving modulation of valvular interstitial cells to an osteoblastic phenotype and new gene expression resulting in cell-mediated mineralization of the extracellular matrix. For example, expression of bone morphogenetic protein-2 (BMP-2) has been implicated in both vascular and valvular calcification.

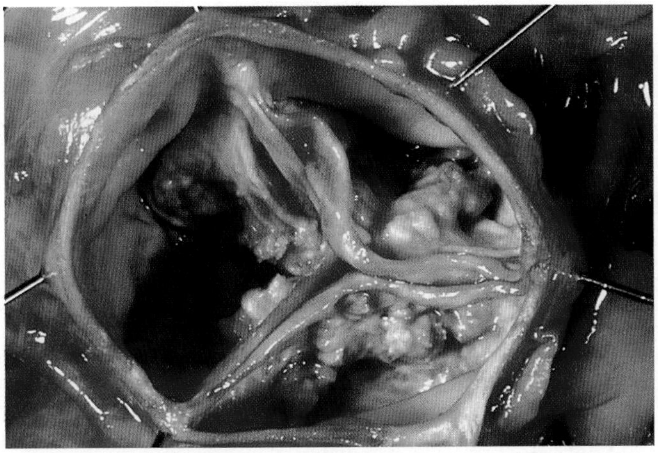

FIGURE 11-36. **Calcific aortic stenosis in a three-cuspid aortic valve in an elderly person.** The leaflets are heavily calcified, but there is no commissural fusion (compare with Fig. 11-32).

CLINICAL FEATURES: Severe aortic stenosis results in striking concentric left ventricular hypertrophy. Eventually, the heart dilates and fails. The disease is treated with great success (5-year survival rate of 85%) with surgical valve replacement, provided the operation is performed before ventricular dysfunction becomes irreversible. The hypertrophic left ventricle is then restored to normal size.

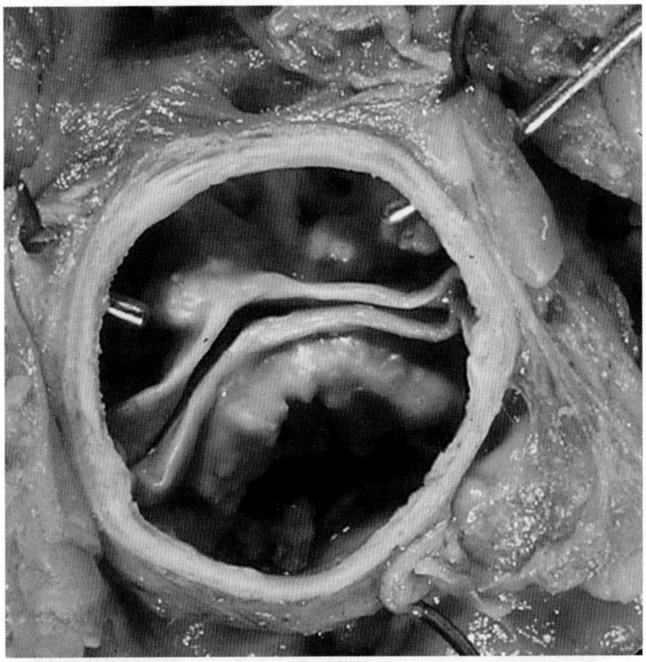

FIGURE 11-37. **Calcific aortic stenosis of a congenitally bicuspid aortic valve.** The two leaflets are heavily calcified, but there is no commissural fusion.

Calcification of the Mitral Valve Annulus Is Usually Asymptomatic

Calcification of the mitral valve annulus occurs commonly in the elderly and is usually without functional significance, although it often produces a murmur. However, if it is severe enough to interfere with mitral leaflet closure during systole, mitral regurgitation occurs. Calcification of the mitral valve annulus in the elderly differs from that in rheumatic mitral valve disease. The former features little or no deformation of the valve leaflets, and calcification is most prominent in the annulus rather than the leaflets. About 40% of women older than 90 years exhibit this lesion, whereas the incidence is only 15% in men. Calcification of the mitral valve annulus is aggravated by the presence of aortic stenosis, hypertension, and diabetes.

Calcific deposits transform the mitral ring into a rigid, curved bar up to 2 cm in diameter, which may be evident radiologically. The posterior mitral leaflet is often distorted and displaced upward. Amorphous masses of calcified material first develop in the connective tissue of the valve ring. However, with time, the calcification extends into the base of the leaflets and eventually to the ventricular septum.

Mitral Valve Prolapse Is the Most Common Indication for Valve Replacement

MVP is a condition in which mitral valve leaflets become enlarged and redundant, and chordae tendineae become thinned and elongated, such that the billowed leaflets prolapse into the left atrium during systole (Fig. 11-38A). Also referred to as "floppy mitral valve syndrome," MVP is the most frequent cause of mitral regurgitation that requires surgical valve replacement. As much as 5% of the adult population may show echocardiographic evidence of MVP, although most will not have regurgitation severe enough to warrant surgical intervention.

PATHOGENESIS: MVP has an important hereditary component and many cases appear to be transmitted as an autosomal dominant trait. Patients with primary MVP exhibit a striking accumulation of myxomatous connective tissue in the center of the valve leaflet (see Fig. 11-38B). This abnormality is believed to be related to an undefined defect in the metabolism of extracellular matrix. The amount of proteoglycans in the valve is increased, and by electron microscopy, collagen fibrils are fragmented. Presumably, the extracellular matrix defect allows the leaflets and chordae to enlarge and stretch under the high-pressure conditions they experience during the cardiac cycle. MVP is usually an isolated finding, although it may occur in the context of a variety of other conditions, including Marfan syndrome, inherited disorders of collagen metabolism, and myotonic muscular dystrophy. It is also seen in hyperthyroidism, certain congenital heart lesions, and von Willebrand disease. MVP is unusually common in persons with an asthenic habitus and a number of congenital thoracic deformities.

PATHOLOGY: On gross examination, mitral valve leaflets are redundant and deformed (see Fig. 11-38A). On cross-section they have a gelatinous appearance and slippery texture, owing to accumulation of acid mucopolysaccharides (proteoglycans). The myxomatous degenerative process also affects the annulus and chordae tendineae, which increases the degree of prolapse and regurgitation. Damage to the chordae may be so severe that they rupture, producing a flail mitral valve that is totally incompetent. Although the mitral valve is usually the only valve affected, myxomatous degeneration can develop in the other cardiac valves, especially in patients with Marfan syndrome, 90% of whom have some clinical evidence of MVP.

CLINICAL FEATURES: Most patients with MVP are asymptomatic. Clinical recognition of MVP is based on recognition of the classical auscultatory findings of a mid-to-late systolic click, caused by the snap of the redundant leaflets as they prolapse into the left atrium. A late systolic murmur is present if mitral regurgitation is significant. Endocarditis, both infective and nonbacterial, is sometimes a serious complication, and cerebral emboli are common. Significant mitral regurgitation develops in 15% of patients after 10 to 15 years of MVP, after which mitral valve replacement is indicated.

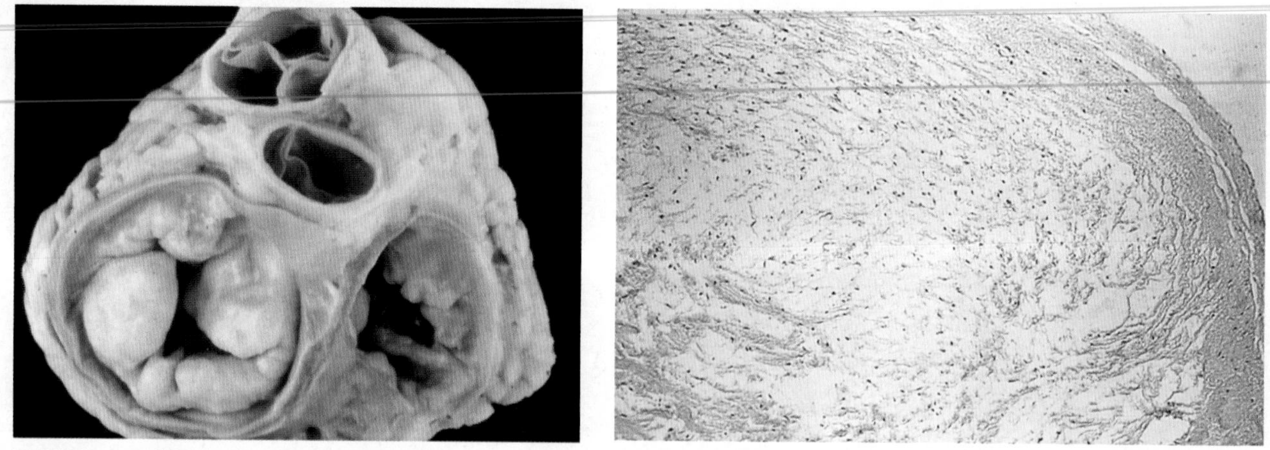

A B

FIGURE 11-38. **Mitral valve prolapse. A.** A view of the mitral valve *(left)* from the left atrium shows redundant and deformed leaflets, which billow into the left atrial cavity. **B.** A microscopic section of one of the mitral valve leaflets reveals conspicuous myxomatous connective tissue in the center of the leaflet.

Papillary Muscle Dysfunction May Produce Mitral Regurgitation

Dysfunction of the left ventricular papillary muscles is most often caused by ischemia. The papillary muscles are especially vulnerable to ischemic injury because they are supplied by the terminal branches of the intramyocardial coronary arteries. Thus, any reduction in coronary blood flow may preferentially interfere with papillary muscle function. Brief periods of ischemia (e.g., during episodes of angina pectoris) can result in transient papillary muscle dysfunction (stunning) and temporary mitral regurgitation. By contrast, severe myocardial infarction and subsequent scarring of papillary muscles can lead to permanent mitral regurgitation. In fact, one third of all patients being evaluated for coronary artery bypass surgery have some evidence of "ischemic mitral regurgitation." Papillary muscle dysfunction may also be associated with a healed myocardial infarct, in which impaired myocardial contractility at the base of the papillary muscle interferes with its function. Rarely, patients may suddenly develop life-threatening mitral regurgitation after rupture of an acutely infarcted papillary muscle.

Carcinoid Heart Disease Affects Right-Sided Valves

Carcinoid heart disease is an unusual condition that uniquely affects the right side of the heart and produces tricuspid regurgitation and pulmonary stenosis. It arises in patients with carcinoid tumors, usually of the small intestine, that have metastasized to the liver.

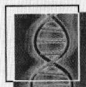

PATHOGENESIS: The pathogenesis of carcinoid heart disease is not fully understood. The valvular and endocardial lesions are thought to be caused by high concentrations of serotonin or other vasoactive amines and peptides produced by the tumor in the liver. Because these moieties are metabolized in the lung, carcinoid heart disease affects the right side of the heart almost exclusively. There are rare reports of left-sided involvement in patients with atrial or ventricular septal defects.

During the 1990s, reports surfaced of mitral and aortic valve disease in patients taking the appetite-suppressing drugs fenfluramine–phentermine ("fen-phen"). Gross and microscopic features of the valve lesions are strikingly similar to those seen in carcinoid heart disease, except that they develop on the left-sided valves. Since then, other anorexogenic drugs and ergot alkaloid drugs such as methysergide and ergotamine used to treat migraine headaches have also been linked to this type of valve disease. Because these drugs interfere with serotonin metabolism and signaling, it has been suggested that the pathogenesis of drug-related and carcinoid valve disease is similar.

PATHOLOGY: The cardiac lesions are plaquelike deposits of dense, pearly gray, fibrous tissue on the tricuspid (Fig. 11-39) and pulmonary valves and on the endocardial surface of the right ventricle. Microscopically, these patches appear "tacked on" to valve leaflets and are not associated with inflammation or apparent damage to underlying valve structures. However, leaflets become deformed, and their surface area reduced. As a result, the tricuspid leaflets become "stuck down" onto adjacent right ventricular mural endocardium, resulting in tricuspid insufficiency or stenosis. Shrinkage of the pulmonary valve and its annulus leads to pulmonary stenosis.

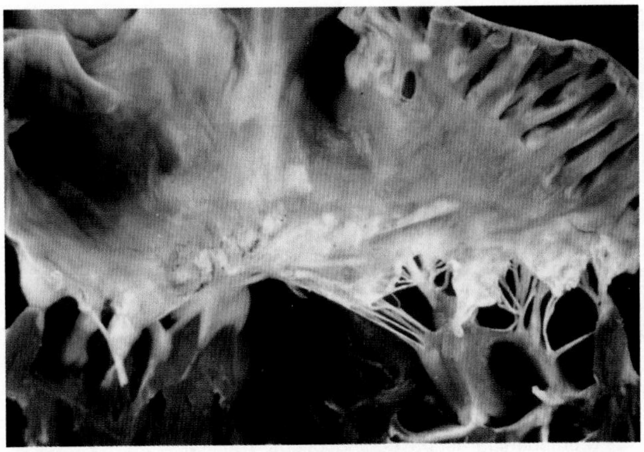

FIGURE 11-39. **Carcinoid heart disease.** Pearly white deposits are seen on the tricuspid valve leaflets and adjacent endocardium. Although the valve leaflets have not been destroyed, they have become deformed and "stuck down" on the ventricular endocardium, which usually produces tricuspid regurgitation.

Myocarditis

Myocarditis is inflammation of the myocardium associated with myocyte necrosis and degeneration. This definition specifically excludes ischemic heart disease. The true incidence of myocarditis is difficult to establish because many cases are asymptomatic. It can occur at any age but is most common in children between the ages of 1 and 10. It is one of the few heart diseases that can produce acute heart failure in previously healthy children, adolescents, or young adults. Severe myocarditis can cause arrhythmias and even sudden cardiac death.

Viral Myocarditis

Most cases of myocarditis in North America occur without an easily demonstrable cause. Most are believed to be viral, although the evidence is usually circumstantial unless polymerase chain reaction (PCR) studies are performed to identify viral nucleic acids in heart biopsies. The most common viruses that cause myocarditis are listed in Table 11-7.

PATHOGENESIS: The pathogenesis of viral myocarditis is believed to involve direct viral cytotoxicity and/or cell-mediated immune reactions directed against infected myocytes. There is

TABLE 11-7

Causes of Myocarditis

Idiopathic

Infectious

- Viral: Coxsackievirus, adenovirus, echovirus, influenza virus, human immunodeficiency virus, and many others
- Rickettsial: Typhus, Rocky Mountain spotted fever
- Bacterial: Diphtheria, staphylococcal, streptococcal, meningococcal, borrelial (Lyme disease), and leptospiral infection
- Fungi and protozoan parasites: Chagas disease, toxoplasmosis, aspergillosis, cryptococcal, and candidal infection
- Metazoan parasites: *Echinococcus, Trichina*

Noninfectious

- Hypersensitivity and immunologically related diseases: Rheumatic fever, systemic lupus erythematosus, scleroderma, drug reaction (e.g., to penicillin or sulfonamide), and rheumatoid arthritis
- Radiation
- Miscellaneous: Sarcoidosis, uremia

substantial evidence for both mechanisms. In animal models, inoculation of a cardiotropic virus is followed shortly by replication of the virus in the myocardium. Microscopically, there are only small isolated foci of acute myocyte necrosis with little if any inflammatory cell infiltration, and there is little evidence of functional impairment. Over the next few days, mononuclear cells, principally T lymphocytes and macrophages, infiltrate the myocardium extensively. At the point of maximum inflammation, the animals show signs of heart failure, although viral cultures of both blood and myocardium are negative. This finding is consistent with the observation that patients with symptomatic myocarditis generally have negative viral cultures. Nevertheless, it may still be possible to identify viral nucleic acid sequences by PCR. Furthermore, viral proteins may degrade some components of the myocyte cytoskeleton and thereby contribute to contractile dysfunction. In some models of experimental viral myocarditis, it is clear that T lymphocytes cause much or all of the myocyte injury. The stimulus for the immune attack on myocytes is not established but appears to involve major histocompatibility antigens.

PATHOLOGY: The hearts of patients with myocarditis who develop clinical heart failure during the active inflammatory phase show biventricular dilation and generalized myocardial hypokinesis. At autopsy, these hearts are flabby and dilated. The histologic changes of viral myocarditis vary with the clinical severity of the disease, but with few exceptions, microscopic features are nonspecific and indistinguishable from toxic myocarditis. Most cases show a patchy or diffuse interstitial, predominantly mononuclear, inflammatory infiltrate composed principally of T lymphocytes and macrophages (Fig. 11-40). Multinucleated giant cells may also be present. The inflammatory cells often surround individual myocytes, and focal myocyte necrosis is seen. During the resolving phase, fibroblast proliferation and interstitial collagen deposition predominate. Ordinarily, neutrophils are not seen in viral myocarditis. However, if necrosis is extensive, the histologic features may resemble those seen in an infarct, namely a neutrophilic infiltrate followed by organization and repair. Most viruses that cause myocarditis also cause pericarditis.

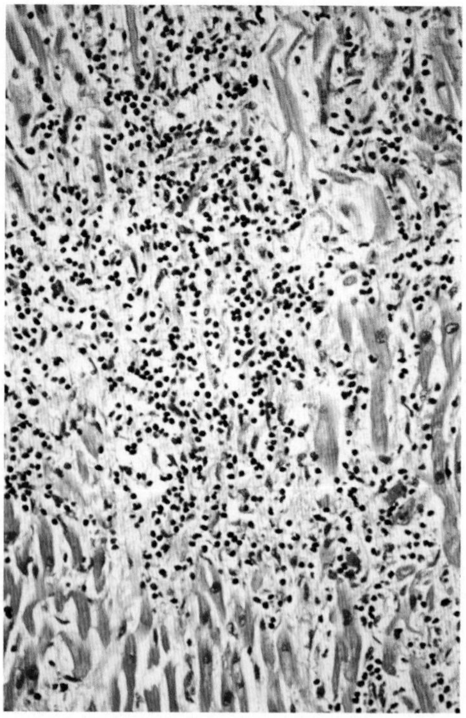

FIGURE 11-40. **Viral myocarditis.** The myocardial fibers are disrupted by a prominent interstitial infiltrate of lymphocytes and macrophages.

CLINICAL FEATURES: Many persons who develop viral myocarditis may be asymptomatic. When symptoms do occur, they usually begin a few weeks after infection. Most patients recover from acute myocarditis, although a few die of congestive heart failure or arrhythmias. The disease may be unusually severe in infants and pregnant women. Despite resolution of the active inflammatory phase of viral myocarditis, subtle functional impairment may persist for years and progression to overt cardiomyopathy is well documented. There is no specific treatment for viral myocarditis, and supportive measures are the rule.

MYOCARDITIS IN ACQUIRED IMMUNODEFICIENCY SYNDROME (AIDS): A significant proportion of symptomatic patients with AIDS have some clinical or pathologic evidence of cardiac disease (pericardial effusions, myocarditis, endocarditis, or cardiomyopathy). An unusually high incidence of viral myocarditis due to cardiotropic viruses, such as Coxsackie B and adenovirus, is documented in AIDS. Human immunodeficiency virus (HIV) infection of cardiac myocytes appears to play a minor role.

Other Transmissible Agents May Cause Infectious Myocarditis

In addition to viruses, other microorganisms that gain access to the bloodstream can infect the heart. For example, brucellosis, meningococcemia, and psittacosis are often associated with an infectious myocarditis. Moreover, some bacteria (e.g., diphtheria organisms) produce cardiotoxins, which may produce a fatal myocarditis. The most common cause of myocarditis in South America the protozoan *Trypanosoma cruzi,* the agent of Chagas disease (see Chapter 9).

- **Bacterial infection** of the myocardium is characterized by multiple foci of a mixed inflammatory cell infiltrate, with neutrophils as the major component. Microabscesses can occur when septic emboli lodge in the coronary circulation, often as a consequence of infective endocarditis.
- **Rickettsial diseases** commonly cause widespread vasculitis, which affects small coronary blood vessels.
- **Fungal infection** of the myocardium typically occurs in immunocompromised patients, although the heart is relatively resistant to fungal infection.
- **Toxoplasmosis** can involve the myocardium in immunosuppressed patients; the intracellular parasites proliferate within cardiac myocytes and elicit a focal mixed inflammatory response, with neutrophils and eosinophils.
- **Chagas disease** is associated with proliferation of parasites within cardiac myocytes and a mixed inflammatory cell infiltrate, composed principally of lymphocytes, plasma cells and macrophages.

Hypersensitivity Myocarditis is a Reaction to Drugs

PATHOLOGY: The inflammation consists of an interstitial and perivascular infiltrate, which is often confined to the myocardium and does not affect other organs. The inflammatory infiltrate in hypersensitivity myocarditis resembles that seen in viral myocarditis, but the former displays numerous eosinophils, as well as lymphocytes and plasma cells. Another typical feature is the virtual absence of myocyte necrosis, even when the infiltrate is intense.

CLINICAL FEATURES: Hypersensitivity myocarditis is usually clinically silent, and the diagnosis is often made as an incidental finding at autopsy. However, it may produce chest pain and electrocardiographic changes that resemble acute myocardial ischemia. Occasionally, it is responsible for fatal ventricular arrhythmias. When the disease causes symptoms, treatment consists of discontinuing the offending drug and administering corticosteroids or immunosuppressive agents.

Giant Cell Myocarditis is Usually Fatal

Giant cell myocarditis is a rare, highly aggressive disease of the heart characterized by intense inflammation, extensive areas of myocyte necrosis, and numerous multinucleated giant cells of macrophage origin. The cause is unknown, but it sometimes occurs in patients with SLE, hyperthyroidism, or thymoma. An autoimmune etiology has been suggested, but there is no persuasive evidence for this theory.

Giant cell myocarditis is usually a rapidly fatal disease of adults in the third to fifth decades of life, although it can also occur in adolescents. Patients die of congestive heart failure or sudden death from arrhythmias. At autopsy, the heart is flabby and dilated and may contain mural thrombi. Microscopically, prominent giant cells, together with lymphoid cells and macrophages, are seen at the margins of serpiginous areas of myocardial necrosis. The only effective treatment for giant cell myocarditis is cardiac transplantation. However, the disease recurs in the transplanted heart in one fourth of cases. Aside from cardiac transplantation, there is no effective therapy.

Metabolic Diseases of the Heart

Hyperthyroidism Causes High-Output Failure

Thyroid hormone has direct inotropic and chronotropic effects on the heart: (1) it increases the activity of the sarcolemmal sodium pump; (2) it enhances the synthesis of a myosin isoform with rapid ATPase activity and reduces production of a slower isoform; and (3) it upregulates expression of slow calcium channels in the sarcolemma, thereby facilitating contractility. ***Hyper*thyroidism** thus causes conspicuous tachycardia and an increased cardiac workload, owing to decreased peripheral resistance and increased cardiac output. It may eventually lead to angina pectoris and high-output failure.

Hypothyroid Heart Disease Diminishes Cardiac Output

Patients with severe ***hypo*thyroidism** (**myxedema**) have decreased cardiac output, reduced heart rate, and impaired myocardial contractility—changes that are the reverse of those seen in hyperthyroidism. There may be a pericardial effusion created by increased capillary permeability and leakage of fluid and protein into the pericardial cavity. Pulse pressure is decreased because of higher peripheral resistance and lower blood volume.

The hearts of patients with myxedema are flabby and dilated, and the myocardium exhibits myofiber swelling. Basophilic (mucinous) degeneration is common. Interstitial fibrosis may also be present. Despite these changes, myxedema does not produce congestive heart failure in the absence of other cardiac disorders.

Thiamine Deficiency (Beriberi) Heart Disease is Similar to Hyperthyroidism

Beriberi heart disease develops in patients who consume a diet inadequate in vitamin B_1 (thiamine) for at least 3 months (see Chapter 8). It is seen in parts of Asia where the diet consists largely of shelled rice. In the United States, thiamine deficiency is occasionally seen in alcoholics or neglected persons. Beriberi heart disease results in decreased peripheral vascular resistance and increased cardiac output, a combination similar to that produced by hyperthyroidism. The result is high-output failure. Interestingly, heart failure may develop so suddenly that patients die within 2 days of the onset of symptoms. At autopsy, the heart is dilated and shows only nonspecific microscopic changes.

Cardiomyopathy

Cardiomyopathy refers to a primary disease of the myocardium and excludes damage caused by extrinsic factors. Dilated cardiomyopathy (DCM) is the most common type of cardiomyopathy and is characterized by biventricular dilation, impaired contractility, and eventually congestive heart failure. DCM can develop in response to a large number of known insults that directly injure cardiac myocytes ("secondary DCM"), or it may be idiopathic (primary).

Idiopathic Dilated Cardiomyopathy Is Characterized by Impaired Contractility

PATHOGENESIS: Numerous etiologies have been implicated in idiopathic DCM but the pathogenesis is unresolved.

Genetic factors now appear to be more important than previously believed. Among patients with idiopathic DCM, a third have a familial disease. The proportion may be even greater because incomplete penetrance often makes it difficult to identify early or latent disease in family members. Most familial cases seem to be transmitted as an autosomal dominant trait, but autosomal recessive, X-linked recessive, and mitochondrial inheritance patterns have all been described.

Mutations in several known genes including those encoding dystrophin, δ-sarcoglycan, troponin T, β-myosin heavy chain, actin, lamin A/C, and desmin have been identified as causing a phenotype (Table 11-8). *A current hypothesis holds that defects in force transmission lead to development of a dilated, poorly contracting heart* (Fig 11-41). Stabilization of sarcomeres by attachments of the actin cytoskeleton to the extracellular matrix via dystrophin and δ-sarcoglycan may be perturbed by mutations in genes encoding these proteins. Mutations in the cytoskeletal protein desmin may act similarly. Interestingly, mutations in proteins such as actin, troponin T, and β-myosin heavy chain may produce either dilated or hypertrophic cardiomyopathy phenotypes, perhaps depending on whether they produce a defect in force generation (hypertrophic cardiomyopathy) or force transmission. For example, actin mutations associated with hypertrophic cardiomyopathy have been localized to a portion of the molecule near a myosin-binding site, which could impair sarcomeric function. By contrast, DCM-associated mutations in actin are located within the region that binds to the dystrophin–sarcoglycan complex (see Fig. 11-41). Defects in lamin A/C, filamentous proteins associated with the inner surface of the nuclear envelope, could make the nucleus more vulnerable to mechanical stress and thereby cause myocyte death.

Viral myocarditis may eventually lead to DCM, but how this would develop has not been clear. Interestingly, a protease expressed by cardiotropic enteroviruses, has been shown to cleave dystrophin, thus providing a potential mechanistic link between viral infection and development of a dilated cardiomyopathy phenotype. As noted above, in some instances the acute inflammatory phase of viral myocarditis may be followed by an autoimmune attack on the myocardium, which injures cardiac myocytes and eventually causes DCM. Indeed, persistance of viral genomes in the heart detected by PCR is associated with progressive impairment of left ventricular function, whereas spontaneous viral elimination is associated with improved function.

Immunologic abnormalities involving both cellular and humoral effects have been recognized in both myocarditis and idiopathic DCM. Autoantibodies to cardiac antigens that have been identified include those directed against a variety of mitochondrial antigens, cardiac myosin, and β-adrenergic receptors. However, as in many cases of autoimmune disease, a pathogenic role for immune mechanisms remains to be proved, and circulating autoantibodies may simply result from rather than cause long-standing myocardial injury.

PATHOLOGY: The pathologic changes in patients with DCM are generally nonspecific and are similar whether the disorder is idiopathic or secondary to a known injurious agent. At autopsy, the heart is invariably enlarged, reflecting conspicuous left and right ventricular hypertrophy. The weight of the heart may be as much as tripled (>900 g). As a rule, all chambers of the heart are dilated, though the ventricles are more severely affected than are the atria (Fig. 11-42). At end-stage, left ventricular dilation is usually so severe that the left ventricular wall appears to be of normal thickness or even thinned. The myocardium is flabby and pale, and small subendocardial scars are occasionally evident. The left ventricle endocardium, especially at the apex, tends to be thickened. Adherent mural thrombi are often present in this area.

Microscopically, DCM is characterized by atrophic and hypertrophic myocardial fibers. Cardiac myocytes, especially in the subendocardium, often show advanced degenerative changes characterized by myofibrillar loss, an effect that gives cells a vacant, vacuolated appearance. Interstitial and perivascular fibrosis of myocardium is evident, also most prominently in the subendocardial zone. Scattered chronic inflammatory cells may be present, but are not conspicuous. Electron microscopy typically shows loss of sarcomeres and an apparent increase mitochondria.

CLINICAL FEATURES: The clinical courses of idiopathic and secondary DCM are comparable. The disease begins insidiously with compensatory ventricular hypertrophy and asymptomatic left ventricular dilation. Commonly, exercise intolerance progresses relentlessly to frank congestive heart failure and 75% of patients die within 5 years of the onset of symptoms. Half of all deaths in DCM patients are sudden and are attributed to ventricular arrhythmias Abnormalities in intracellular Ca^{2+} handling and certain repolarizing (potassium, K^+) currents are common features in all forms of heart failure. They tend to prolong the QT interval and increase the likelihood of arrhythmias initiated by triggered activity. Although supportive treatment is useful, cardiac transplantation or use of a ventricular assist device eventually becomes the only option.

Secondary Dilated Cardiomyopathy Has Many Causes

Almost 100 distinct myocardial diseases can result in the clinical features of DCM. Thus, secondary DCM is best viewed as a final common pathway for the effects of virtually any toxic, metabolic, or infectious disorder that directly injures cardiac myocytes. In this context, alcohol abuse, hypertension, pregnancy, and viral myocarditis predispose to secondary DCM. Diabetes mellitus and cigarette smoking are also associated with increased incidence of this disorder.

Toxic Cardiomyopathy

Numerous chemicals and drugs cause myocardial injury but only a few of the more important chemicals are discussed here.

ETHANOL: Alcoholic cardiomyopathy is the single most common identifiable cause of DCM in the United States and Europe. Ethanol abuse can lead to chronic, progressive cardiac

TABLE 11-8

Gene Defects Associated with Dilated Cardiomyopathy (DCM)

Gene Product	Chromosome and Inheritance*		Skeletal Involvement	High Risk of SD or HF†	Remarks	Mutations in the Same Gene Can Cause MD or HCM‡
Dystrophin	Xp21	X	Mild	HF	Rapid progression to end-stage heart failure	Becker and Duchenne MD
Troponin T	1q3	AD	Not reported	SD, HF	Early-onset ventricular dilation	HCM
δ-Sarcoglycan	5q33–q34	AD	None to subclinical	SD, HF	Early-onset ventricular dilation	Limb girdle MD
β-Myosin heavy chain	14q11.2–12	AD	None	HF	Early-onset ventricular dilation	HCM
Actin	15q14	AD	Not reported		Defect located in dystrophin-binding region	HCM
Lamin A/C	1q21.3	AD	None to mild	SD	Occurs in DCM associated with conduction abnormalities	Emerey-Dreifuss MD, Limb girdle MD
Desmin	2q35	AD	None to severe	Can develop severe skeletal weakness	Desmin skeletal myopathy	
Titin	2q31	AD	None	Two mutations in Z-line binding domain	HCM in one case	

* X = X-linked; AD = autosomal dominant.
† SD = sudden death; HF = rapid progression to heart failure.
‡ MD = primary muscular dystrophy; HCM = hypertrophic cardiomyopathy.

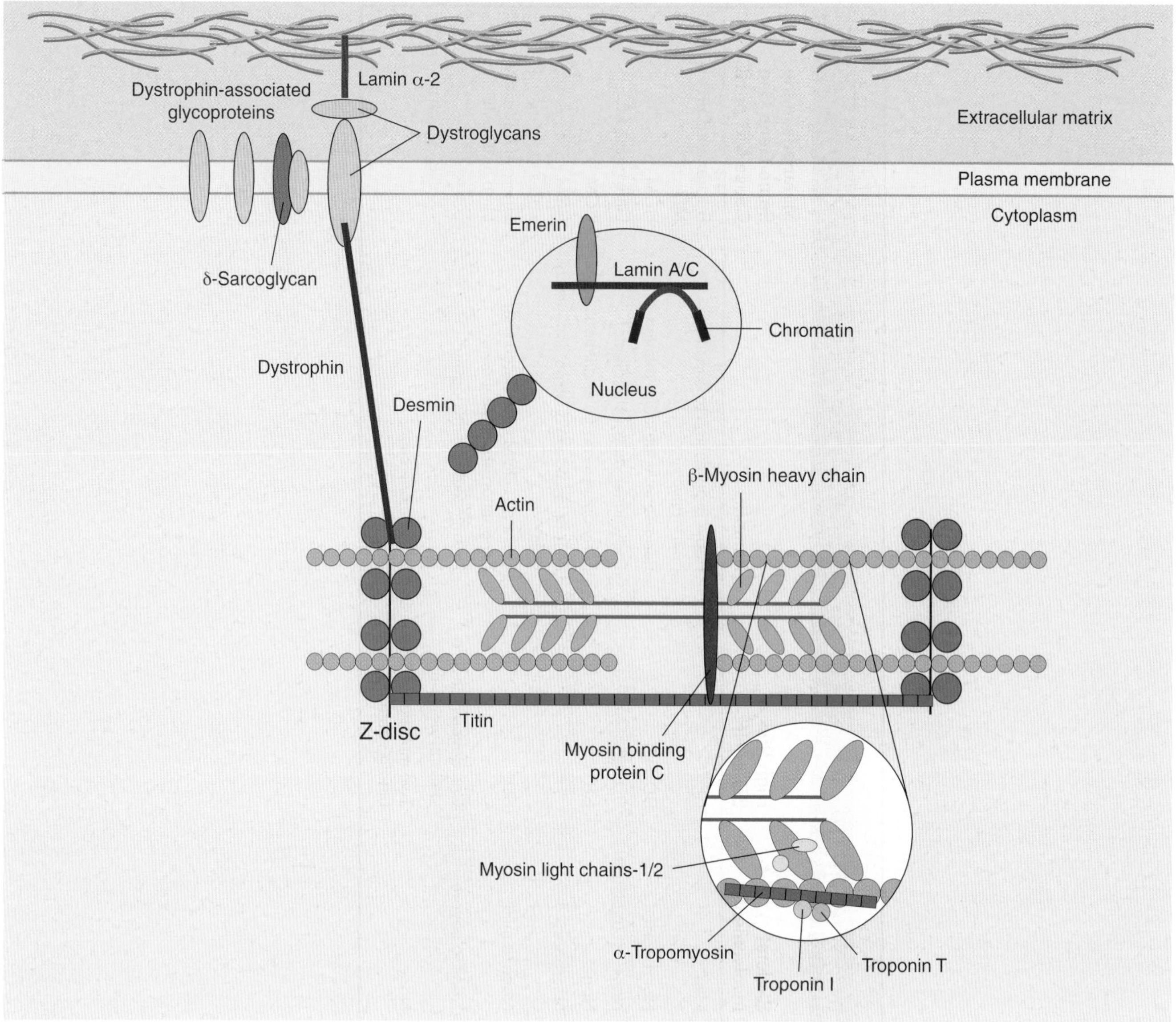

FIGURE 11-41. **Subcellular distribution and molecular interactions of mutant proteins implicated in the pathogenesis of dilated and hypertrophic cardiomyopathy.** The specific mutations responsible for each type are provided in Tables 11-8 and 11-9.

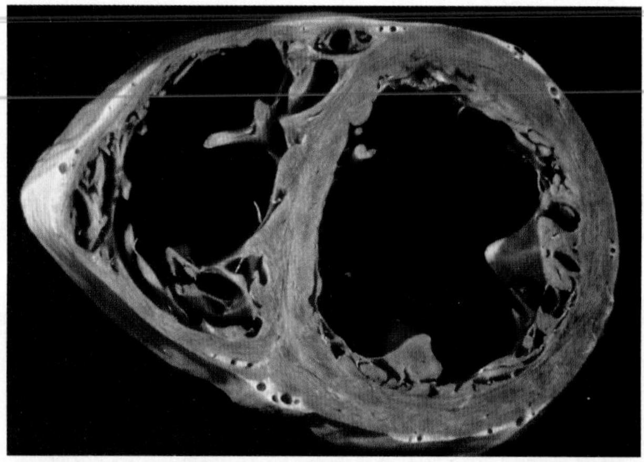

FIGURE 11-42. **Idiopathic dilated cardiomyopathy.** A transverse section of the enlarged heart reveals conspicuous dilation of both ventricles. Although the ventricular wall appears thinned, the increased mass of the heart indicates considerable hypertrophy.

dysfunction, which may be fatal. The disorder is more common in men, because alcoholism is more frequent in men than in women. The typical patient is between 30 and 55 years of age and has been drinking heavily for at least 10 years.

PATHOGENESIS: The mechanism by which alcohol injures the heart is obscure, but the degree of myocardial damage correlates with the total lifetime dose of ethanol. Ethanol has an immediate negative inotropic effect on the heart. Although the short-term action of alcohol on cardiac myocytes is reversible, the cumulative injury eventually becomes irreversible. Abstinence ameliorates or even reverses early stages of alcoholic cardiomyopathy but may be too late in advanced stages.

COBALT: The cardiac toxicity of cobalt is discussed in Chapter 8.

CATECHOLAMINES: In high concentrations, catecholamines can cause focal myocyte necrosis. Toxic myocarditis may occur in patients with pheochromocytomas or who require high doses of inotropic drugs to maintain blood pressure and in accident victims who sustain massive head trauma. Multiple mechanisms contribute to myocardial injury, but the most important is enhanced calcium flux into myocytes. Focal ischemia caused by platelet aggregation and microvascular constriction may also contribute.

ANTHRACYCLINES: Doxorubicin (adriamycin) and other anthracycline drugs are potent chemotherapeutic agents whose usefulness is limited by cumulative, dose-dependent, cardiac toxicity. The clinical major effect is poor myocyte contractility due to chronic, irreversible degeneration of cardiac myocytes. The histopathology of this disorder includes vacuolization and loss of myofibrils. Myocyte necrosis is rare, but once severe degeneration occurs, intractable congestive heart failure develops and the prognosis is grim.

PATHOGENESIS: DCM begins to appear in patients who receive a cumulative dose of more than 500 mg doxorubicin per m^2, and those who are treated with more than 550 mg/m^2 have a 35% incidence of cardiomyopathy. The mechanism by which anthracyclines damage the heart appears related to diminished capacity to handle reactive oxygen species. Although the heart is relatively resistant to radiation injury, anthracyclines and radiation act synergistically. Thus, a patient who has received radiotherapy to the mediastinum is at risk of developing anthracycline cardiac toxicity at a lower dose than someone who was not irradiated.

CYCLOPHOSPHAMIDE: This potent chemotherapeutic drug is often used in high doses before bone marrow transplantation. Although it does not cause classical DCM, it can cause pericarditis and occasionally massive hemorrhagic myocarditis. The latter is thought to be secondary to endothelial injury and thrombocytopenia.

COCAINE: Cocaine use is frequently associated with chest pain and palpitations. True DCM is an unusual complication of cocaine abuse, but myocarditis, focal necrosis, and thickening of intramyocardial coronary arteries have been reported. Myocardial ischemia or infarction associated with cocaine use has been attributed to coronary vasoconstriction in the face of increased myocardial oxygen demand. Sudden death due to spontaneous ventricular tachyarrhythmias is well documented. Mechanisms underlying arrhythmogenic effects of cocaine include vasoconstriction, sympathomimetic activity, hypersensitivity responses, and direct toxicity.

Cardiomyopathy of Pregnancy

A unique form of DCM develops in the last trimester of pregnancy or the first 6 months after delivery. The disorder is relatively uncommon in the United States, but in some regions of Africa, it is encountered in as many as 1% of pregnant women. The risk of cardiomyopathy of pregnancy is greatest in black, multiparous women, older than 30 years. The cause of this form of DCM is unknown. Some patients exhibit inflammatory cells in heart biopsies taken during the symptomatic phase of the illness, consistent with the hypothesis that disordered immunity may underlie development of DCM in this setting.

Unlike most other varieties of DCM, half of women with cardiomyopathy of pregnancy spontaneously recover normal cardiac function. The other half is left with persistent left ventricular dysfunction or proceed to overt congestive heart failure and early death. In patients who survive, subsequent pregnancies pose a high risk of recurrence and maternal mortality.

In Hypertrophic Cardiomyopathy Cardiac Hypertrophy is out of Proportion to the Hemodynamic Load

HCM develops for no apparent physiologic reason, is probably genetically determined in most patients, and is identified as an autosomal dominant trait in half of patients. Many people without a family history probably have spontaneous mutations or a mild form of disease that is difficult to detect. HCM is now known to be far more common than previously appreciated: its prevalence in the United States is about 1 in 500.

PATHOGENESIS: The clinical picture of HCM is caused by more than 100 mutations in at least nine genes encoding proteins of the sarcomere (Table 11-9 and see Fig.11-41).The mutated genes most commonly involved encode (1) β-myosin heavy chain (35%), (2) myosin-binding protein C (20%), and (3) troponin T (15%). Mutations in other genes such as titin and myosin light chains are rare. The mutant protein is incorporated into the sarcomere, where it acts in a dominant-negative fashion to alter sarcomeric function. *This proposed mechanism has led to the hypothesis that HCM is related to defects in force generation owing to altered sarcomeric function.* In turn, hypertrophy is a compensatory response. Other mutations, such as those involving myosin light chain and α-tropomyosin genes, may actually enhance contractility and, thereby, lead to hypertrophy. Still others (e.g., mutations in the myosin-binding protein C gene) may produce proteins that do not become incorporated into sarcomeres. These might lead to hypertrophy through a lack of the functional protein, rather than by a dominant-negative effect.

Specific mutations are associated with certain clinical features of HCM (see Table 11-9). For example, selected mutations in β-myosin heavy chain and troponin T genes involve a high likelihood of sudden death. In the case of the β-myosin heavy chain mutations, the risk of sudden death correlates with the amount of hypertrophy, whereas troponin T mutations, which are also linked to sudden death, produce minimal or no hypertrophy. HCM in patients with myosin-binding protein C mutations is usually benign clinically and is associated with slowly progressive hypertrophy developing late in life.

PATHOLOGY: The heart in HCM is always enlarged, but the degree of hypertrophy is different in different genetic forms. The left ventricle wall is thick, and its cavity is small, sometimes being reduced to a slit. Papillary muscles and trabeculae carneae are prominent and encroach on the ventricular lumen. More than half of cases exhibit asymmetric hypertrophy of the interventricular septum, with a ratio of the thickness of the septum to that of the left ventricular free wall greater than 1.5 (Fig. 11-43A). There are some rare genetic forms of HCM in which only the apical portion of the left ventricle or papillary muscles are selectively hypertrophied. Often, the thickened, hypertrophied interventricular septum bulges into the left ventricular outflow tract early in ventricular systole, causing subvalvular obstruction of the aortic outflow tract. In

TABLE 11-9

Gene Defects Associated with Hypertrophic Cardiomyopathy (HCM)

Gene Product	Chromosome	Risk of Sudden Death	Mutations	Remarks
β-Myosin heavy chain	14q11-2-12	High*	Missense	Degree of hypertrophy correlates with risk of sudden death
Myosin-binding protein C	11p11.2	Low	Missense, deletions, splice defects	Benign clinical course, progressive hypertrophy with late onset
Troponin T	1q3	High	Missense, deletions, splice defects	High risk of sudden death; mild or absent hypertrophy
Troponin 1	19q13.4	High	Missense	Apical variant of HCM, occasionally DCM-like features in elderly patients
α-Tropomyosin	15q22	High	Missense	Usually favorable prognosis, high phenotypic variability
Myosin light chain-1	3p21	Low	Missense	Papillary muscle thickening, only rare cases
Myosin light chain-2	12q23-24.3	Low	Missense	Papillary muscle thickening, only rare cases
Actin	15q14	Low	Missense	Some mutations also cause DCM
α-Myosin heavy chain	Spontaneous	Low	Missense	Late onset; rare
Titin	Spontaneous	–	Missense	Only one patient reported

* For selected mutations.

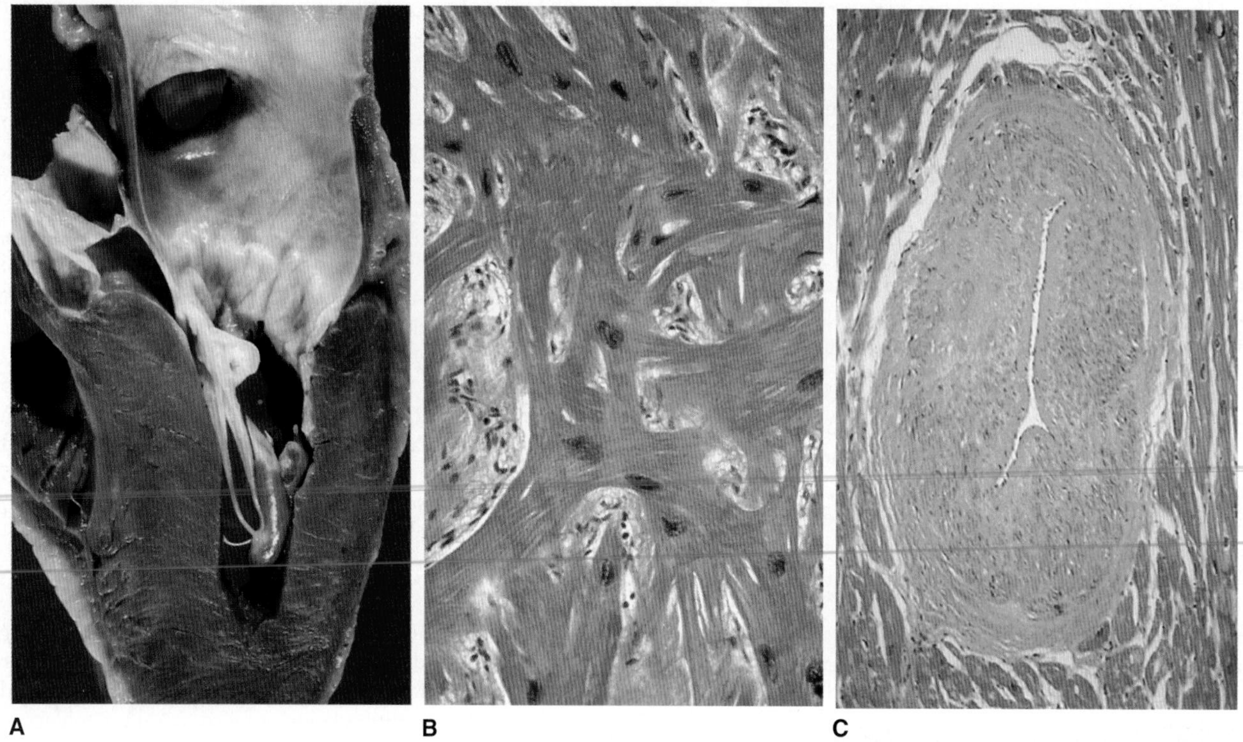

FIGURE 11-43. **Hypertrophic cardiomyopathy (HCM). A**. The heart has been opened to show striking asymmetric left ventricular hypertrophy. The interventricular septum is thicker than the free wall of the left ventricle and impinges on the outflow tract such that it contacts the underside of the anterior mitral valve leaflet. **B.** A section of the myocardium shows the characteristic myofiber disarray and hyperplasia of interstitial cells. **C.** A small intramural coronary artery shows a thickened, hypercellular media. This type of remodeling of coronary vessels could contribute to development of angina-like symptoms in some patients with HCM.

this situation, an endocardial mural plaque is typically seen in the outflow tract, corresponding to the contact point where the anterior mitral valve leaflet impinges on the septal wall of the outflow tract during systole. Both atria are commonly dilated.

The most notable histologic feature of HCM is ***myofiber disarray****, which is most extensive in the interventricular septum.* Instead of the usual parallel arrangement of myocytes into muscle bundles, myofiber disarray is characterized by an oblique and often perpendicular orientation of adjacent hypertrophic myocytes (see Fig. 11-43B). By electron microscopy, myofibrils and myofilaments within individual myocytes are also disorganized. Such structural disarrangements are also frequently present in infants with congenital heart defects and can be observed under a variety of circumstances. However, they are always extensive in HCM and are not as widespread in other situations. There is usually hyperplasia of interstitial cells, and intramural coronary arteries may become thick and cellular (see Fig. 11-43C).

CLINICAL FEATURES: Most patients with HCM have few if any symptoms, and the diagnosis is commonly made during screening of the family with an affected member. Despite a lack of symptoms, such persons may be at risk for sudden death, particularly during severe exertion. In fact, unsuspected HCM is a commonly found at autopsy in young competitive athletes who die suddenly. Clinical recognition of HCM can occur at any age, often in the third, fourth, or fifth decade of life, but the disorder also is encountered in the elderly. Some patients with HCM become incapacitated by cardiac symptoms, of which dyspnea, angina pectoris, and syncope are most common. The clinical course tends to remain stable for many years, although eventually the disease can progress to congestive heart failure. In 10% of patients, DCM supervenes.

Despite the fact that mutant proteins impair the sarcomere, contractile function in HCM tends to be hyperdynamic. Ejection fractions are typically very high and most of the stroke volume is ejected during early systole. The most prominent dysfunctional aspect of HCM is decreased left ventricular compliance (diastolic dysfunction), which results in increased end-diastolic pressure. Mitral regurgitation is also seen in many HCM patients. These features contribute to the atrial dilation commonly seen in HCM. In one fourth of patients, functional obstruction of the left ventricular outflow tract occurs near the end of systole, resulting in a pressure gradient between the apex and the subvalvular region of the left ventricle.

HCM responds paradoxically to pharmacologic interventions. Heart failure from other causes is typically treated with cardiac glycosides to increase myocardial contractility and with diuretics to reduce intravascular volume. In HCM, these drugs aggravate symptoms. The most efficacious treatment of HCM is β-adrenergic blockers and calcium channel blockers, which reduce contractility, decrease outflow-tract obstruction, and may improve left ventricular relaxation during diastole. Surgical removal of a portion of the hypertrophic septum or injection of ethanol into a septal artery to cause localized infarction has been successful in relieving symptoms of obstruction but seems to have no impact on the risk of sudden death.

Restrictive Cardiomyopathy Impairs Diastolic Function

Restrictive cardiomyopathy describes a group of diseases in which myocardial or endocardial abnormalities limit diastolic filling, while contractile function remains normal. It is the least common category of cardiomyopathy in Western countries, although in some less-developed regions (e.g., parts of equatorial Africa, South America, and Asia), endomyocardial disease related to parasitic infections leads to many cases of restrictive cardiomyopathy.

PATHOGENESIS AND PATHOLOGY: Restrictive cardiomyopathy is caused by (1) interstitial infiltration of amyloid, metastatic carcinoma, or sarcoid granulomas; (2) endomyocardial disease characterized by marked fibrotic thickening of the endocardium; (3) storage diseases, including hemochromatosis; and (4) markedly increased interstitial fibrous tissue. The pathophysiologic consequence is a pre-load-dependent state, characterized by defective diastolic compliance, restricted ventricular filling, increased end-diastolic pressure, atrial dilation, and venous congestion. In many respects, these hemodynamic changes are similar to the consequences of constrictive pericarditis. Many cases of restrictive cardiomyopathy are classified as idiopathic, with interstitial fibrosis as the only histologic abnormality.

The disease almost invariably progresses to congestive heart failure, and only 10% of the patients survive for 10 years.

Amyloidosis

The heart is affected in most forms of generalized amyloidosis (see Chapter 23). In fact, restrictive cardiomyopathy is the most common cause of death in AL amyloidosis of plasma cell dyscrasias.

PATHOLOGY: Amyloid infiltration of the heart results in cardiac enlargement without ventricular dilation, and the gross appearance of the heart may resemble that of hypertrophic cardiomyopathy. Ventricular walls are typically thickened, firm, and rubbery. Microscopically, amyloid accumulation is most prominent in interstitial, perivascular, and endocardial regions (Fig. 11-44). Endocardial involvement is common in the atria, where nodular endocardial deposits often impart a granular

A

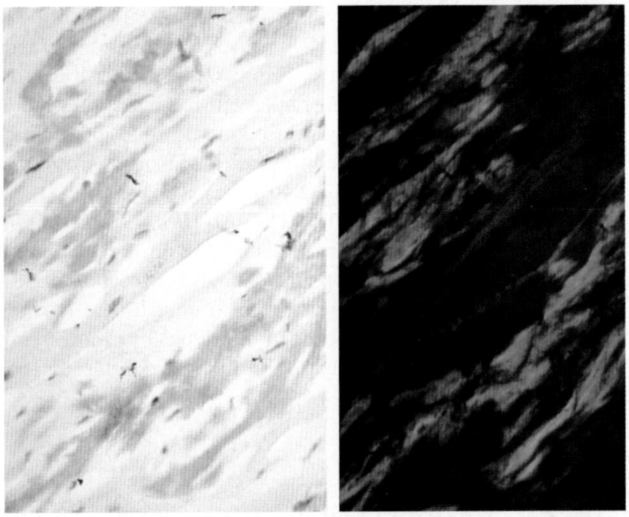

B

FIGURE 11-44. **Cardiac amyloidosis. A.** A section of myocardium stained with Congo red shows interstitial, pink-staining deposits of amyloid. **B.** Under polarized light, the same section displays the characteristic green birefringence of amyloid fibrils.

appearance and gritty texture to the endocardial surface. Amyloid deposits also can cause thickening of cardiac valves. In rare cases, amyloid deposition within the walls of intramural coronary arteries narrows the lumens and causes ischemic injury.

CLINICAL FEATURES: Cardiac amyloidosis is most often a restrictive cardiomyopathy, with symptoms mainly referable to right-sided heart failure. Infiltration of the conduction system can result in arrhythmias, and sudden cardiac death is not unusual. Cardiomegaly is characteristically prominent. Echocardiography shows marked wall thickening and decreased wall motion. Low voltage of the QRS complex is a characteristic feature of the electrocardiogram.

Some patients with cardiac amyloidosis initially present with congestive heart failure secondary to impaired systolic or contractile function. In these patients, diastolic dysfunction is often inconspicuous. As in patients with a restrictive presentation, the prognosis is grim: most survive less than 1 year once the disease becomes symptomatic.

SENILE CARDIAC AMYLOIDOSIS: Senile cardiac amyloidosis refers to the deposition of a protein closely related to prealbumin (transthyretin) in the hearts of elderly persons (see Chapter 23). The disorder may be present to some extent in up to 25% of patients who are 80 years old or older. It not only involves the heart (atria and ventricles) but, in many cases, the lungs and rectum as well. Amyloid deposits also may be found in blood vessel walls in many organs, but virtually never in the renal glomeruli. The functional significance of senile cardiac amyloidosis is often minimal, and it is usually an incidental finding at autopsy. Even when amyloid deposition is extensive and is associated with symptoms of congestive heart failure, progression of the disease is much slower than that in AL amyloidosis.

Two additional forms of isolated cardiovascular amyloidosis are common in the elderly: **senile aortic amyloidosis** and **isolated atrial amyloidosis**. Neither of these forms of amyloid contains prealbumin or closely related proteins.

Endomyocardial Disease

Endomyocardial disease (EMD) comprises two geographically separate disorders.

ENDOMYOCARDIAL FIBROSIS: This disorder is particularly common in equatorial Africa, where it accounts for 10% to 20% of all deaths from heart disease. The malady is also occasionally seen in other tropical and subtropical regions of the world. It is most common is children and young adults but has been reported to occur in persons up to age 70 years. Endomyocardial fibrosis leads to progressive myocardial failure and has a poor prognosis, although survival for as long as 12 years has been reported.

EOSINOPHILIC ENDOMYOCARDIAL DISEASE (LÖFFLER ENDOCARDITIS): This is a cardiac disorder of temperate regions characterized by hypereosinophilia (as high as 50,000/μL). It is usually encountered in men in the fifth decade and is often accompanied by rash. Löffler endocarditis typically progresses to congestive heart failure and death, although corticosteroids may improve survival.

PATHOGENESIS: Endomyocardial fibrosis and Löffler endocarditis were once considered distinct entities, but there is a growing consensus that they represent variants of the same underlying disease.

EMD is suspected to result from myocardial injury produced by eosinophils, possibly mediated by cardiotoxic granule components. In the tropics, transient high blood eosinophil counts often result from parasitic infestations; in temperate climates, idiopathic hypereosinophilia is often persistent.

EMD can be divided into three stages:

1. The necrotic stage occurs within the first few months of the illness and is characterized by an intense eosinophilic infiltrate involving the inner layers of the myocardium, usually of both ventricles. The infiltrate is perivascular and interstitial, and there is evidence of vascular injury and myocyte necrosis. The necrotic stage lasts for several months, but significant functional impairment is rare.
2. The thrombotic stage develops about a year later and features mural thrombi attached to the injured and slightly thickened endocardium. At this time, the myocardium is no longer inflamed but shows early hypertrophy. Embolization is a common complication.
3. The fibrotic stage is the chronic phase of EMD and features conspicuous fibrotic thickening of the endocardium. Marked endocardial fibrosis results in decreased compliance and abnormal diastolic function. Adherence of the posterior mitral valve leaflet to the endocardium results in mitral regurgitation or, in the case of the right side, tricuspid regurgitation.

PATHOLOGY: At autopsy, a grayish white layer of thickened endocardium extends from the apex of the left ventricle over the posterior papillary muscle to the posterior leaflet of the mitral valve and for a short distance into the left outflow tract. On cut section of the ventricle, endocardial fibrosis spreads into the inner one-third to one-half of the wall. Mural thrombi in various stages of organization may be present. When the right ventricle is involved, the entire cavity may exhibit endocardial thickening, which may penetrate as far as the epicardium. Microscopically, the fibrotic endocardium contains only a few elastic fibers. Myofibers trapped within the collagenous tissue display nonspecific degenerative changes.

Storage Diseases

The various lysosomal storage diseases are discussed in detail in Chapter 6. Only the cardiac manifestations are reviewed here.

GLYCOGEN STORAGE DISEASES: Of the various forms of glycogen storage disease, types II (Pompe disease), III (Cori disease), and IV (Andersen disease) affect the heart. The most common and severe involvement is with Pompe disease. In infants with this condition, the heart is markedly enlarged (up to seven times normal), and endocardial fibroelastosis is seen in 20% of patients. The myocytes are vacuolated as a result of the large amounts of stored glycogen. The functional changes are those of a restrictive type of cardiomyopathy, and the usual cause of death is cardiac failure.

MUCOPOLYSACCHARIDOSES: Several of the mucopolysaccharidoses involve the heart. Cardiac disease results from lysosomal accumulation of mucopolysaccharides (glycosaminoglycans) in various cells. In general, pseudohypertrophy of the ventricles develops and contractility gradually diminishes. The coronary arteries may be narrowed by thickening of the intima and media, and in Hurler and Hunter syndromes, myocardial infarction is common. Valve leaflets may be thickened, thereby producing progressive valvular dysfunction, manifested as aortic stenosis (Scheie syndrome) or mitral regurgitation (Hurler and Morquio syndromes). Cor pulmonale may result from pulmonary hypertension related to narrowing of the airways.

SPHINGOLIPIDOSES: **Fabry disease** may result in accumulation of glycosphingolipids in the heart, with functional and pathologic changes similar to those that complicate the mucopolysaccharidoses. Fabry disease typically produces gross and microscopic changes that mimic HCM, but the characteristic vacuolated appearance of cardiac myocytes is an important clue of an underlying storage disease. **Gaucher disease**, which only rarely involves the heart, may feature interstitial infiltration of the left ventricle by cerebroside-laden macrophages, leading to impairment of left ventricular compliance and cardiac output.

HEMOCHROMATOSIS: This multiorgan disease is associated with excessive iron deposition in many tissues (see Chapter 14). The degree of iron deposition in the heart varies and only roughly correlates with that in other organs. Cardiac involvement has features of both dilated and restrictive cardiomyopathy, with systolic and diastolic impairment. *Congestive heart failure occurs in as many as one third of patients with hemochromatosis.*

At autopsy, the heart is dilated, and ventricular walls are thickened. The brown color seen on gross examination correlates with iron deposition in cardiac myocytes. Interstitial fibrosis is invariable, but its extent does not correlate well with the degree of iron accumulation. The severity of myocardial dysfunction seems to be proportional to the quantity of iron deposited.

Sarcoidosis

Sarcoidosis is a generalized granulomatous disease that may involve the heart (see Chapter 12). A quarter of sarcoidosis cases that come to autopsy show some granulomas in the heart, but fewer than 5% of patients with this condition have clinical symptoms. Sarcoid heart disease is seen clinically as a mixed pattern of dilated and restrictive cardiomyopathy. Sarcoid granulomas are highly necrotizing and often produce large areas of myocardial damage. The base of the interventricular septum is preferentially involved. Because this region contains major components of the atrioventricular conduction system, bundle branch blocks or complete heart block are often seen. More serious life-threatening arrhythmias are also common, and sudden death is common. Microscopic examination of the heart in severe cases of sarcoid heart disease reveals infiltration of the myocardium by noncaseating granulomas, massive destruction of myocytes and replacement by interstitial fibrosis (Fig. 11-45).

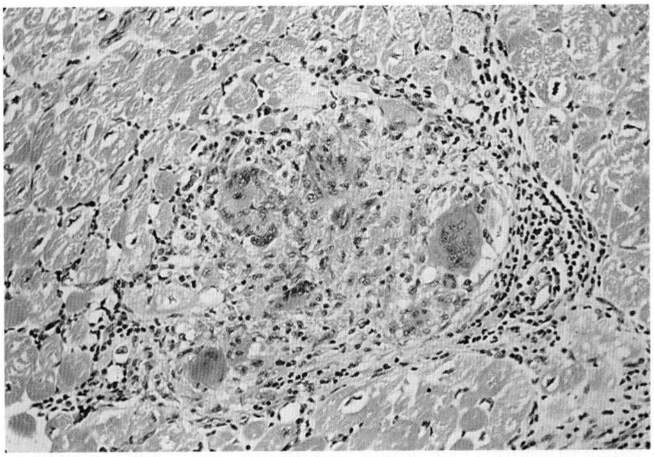

FIGURE 11-45. **Cardiac sarcoidosis.** The myocardium is infiltrated by noncaseating granulomas, with prominent giant cells. There is considerable destruction of cardiac myocytes with fibrosis.

Sudden Cardiac Death

More than 300,000 people in the United States die suddenly each year. Most of these deaths are caused by spontaneous lethal ventricular tachyarrhythmias—ventricular tachycardia and ventricular fibrillation—in patients with some type of heart disease. Many sudden deaths occur out-of-hospital in apparently healthy individuals who exhibit coronary artery disease at autopsy but may have shown little clinical evidence of heart disease during life. Common causes of sudden cardiac death differ in young and old individuals. This has been studied most thoroughly in competitive atheletes (Fig. 11-46). In subjects under 35 years of age,

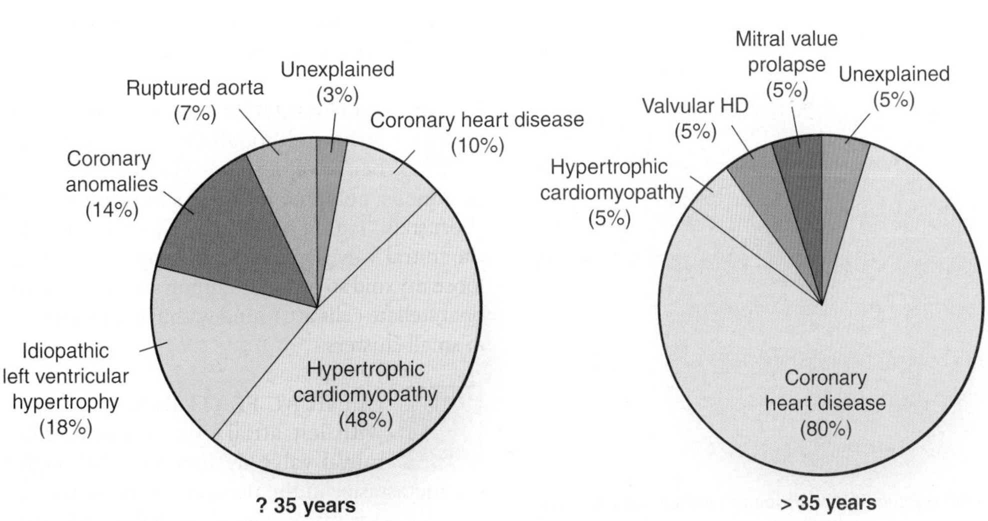

FIGURE 11-46. **Different causes of sudden cardiac death in young and older adult competitive atheletes.** Cm/CM = cardiomyopathy; Hd/HD = heart disease; LVH = left ventricular hypertrophy (Adapted with permission from Zipes DP, Wellens HJ. Sudden Cardiac Death. *Circulation* 1998;98:2334–2351).

HCM, idiopathic left ventricular hypertrophy (presumably reflecting genetic forms of heart muscle disease in at least some), and congenital coronary anomalies account for more than 75% of sudden deaths. In Italy and other Mediterranean countries, arrhythmogenic right ventricular cardiomyopathy is a leading cause of sudden death in young people. This familial cardiomyopathy, uncommon in non-Mediterranean populations, is characterized by replacement of right ventricular myocardium by fat and fibrous tissue (Fig. 11-47) and a high incidence of tachyarrhythmias of right ventricular origin. *However, in virtually all economically developed nations, coronary artery disease is responsible for most sudden deaths in middle-aged and older adults.*

Sudden cardiac death can occur in patients with structurally normal hearts at autopsy, but this is rare. Some (perhaps many) of these patients have "channelopathies," genetic diseases in which mutations in genes for sodium (Na^+), K^+, and Ca^{2+} channel proteins are responsible for sudden death syndromes such as long QT syndrome, Brugada syndrome, and catecholaminergic polymorphic ventricular tachycardia. For example, in long QT syndrome, loss-of-function mutations in K^+ channels prolong repolarization (and so prolong the QT interval on the surface electrocardiogram [ECG]), thereby favoring arrhythmias triggered by after-depolarizations. In the case of catecholaminergic polymorphic ventricular tachycardia, mutations in the cardiac ryanodine receptor, RyR2, cause diastolic Ca^{2+} leakage from the SR which also promotes after-depolarizations.

Spontaneous lethal arrhythmias are also important causes of death in patients with dilated and hypertrophic cardiomyopathies, primary diseases of cardiac myocytes which typically lead to marked changes in cardiac structure and electrophysiology.

PATHOLOGY: The surface ECG may occasionally indicate the presence of a specific pathologic structure that can be implicated in causing sudden death such as an accessory atrioventricular connection in Wolff-Parkinson-White syndrome or a lesion that disrupts a discrete component of the ventricular conduction system causing new bundle branch block. *However, lethal arrhythmias usually arise from pathologic changes affecting conduction properties of the working ventricular myocardium.* At autopsy, the heart of a sudden death victim typically exhibits structural alterations of myocardium that create "anatomic substrates of arrhythmias." These structural changes may be localized (e.g., discrete healed myocardial infarcts or left ventricular aneurysms) or diffuse (e.g., variable degrees of cardiac myocyte hypertrophy and interstitial fibrosis). Spontaneous development of a lethal cardiac arrhythmia may be regarded as a stochastic event arising from complex interactions between relatively fixed anatomic substrates and acute, transient triggering events such as acute ischemia, neurohormonal activation, changes in electrolytes, or other transient stresses. The most frequent clinicopathologic scenario in which sudden death occurs involves acute ischemia (a transient triggering event) in an area of the heart containing a healed infarct (a common anatomic substrate).

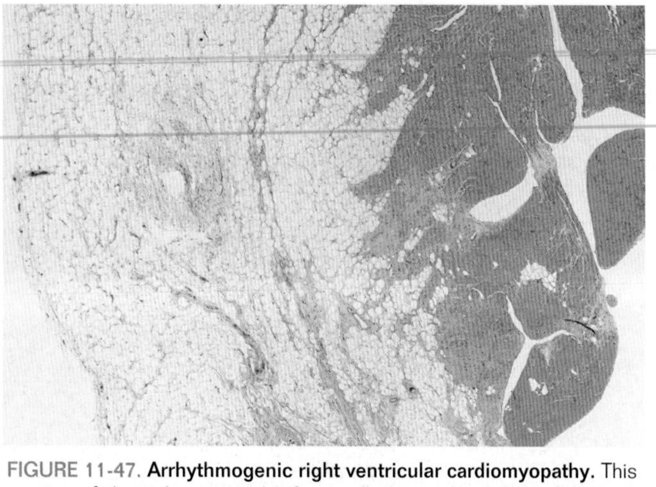

FIGURE 11-47. **Arrhythmogenic right ventricular cardiomyopathy.** This section of the right ventricular free wall shows that much of the myocardium has been replaced by mature adipose tissue and fibrosis such that only subendocardial muscle bundles remain.

The pathologic features of anatomic substrates of recurrent ventricular tachycardia were elucidated in the late 1970s when reentrant ventricular arrhythmia circuits were mapped in patients, and discrete subendocardial areas adjacent to healed infarcts or surrounding ventricular aneurysms were found to exhibit conduction abnormalities. This led to surgical procedures to interrupt arrhythmia circuits by excision of these tissues. Microscopic analysis revealed bundles of viable myocardial fibers embedded in dense fibrous tissue. Subsequent electrophysiologic studies demonstrated highly discontinuous conduction through these tissues with frequent areas of conduction block. These observations, therefore, identified the structural abnormalities responsible for conduction derangements known to underlie many ventricular tachyarrhythmias. They also led to the recognition that many patients have potential arrhythmia substrates in their hearts that, in most cases, may be necessary, but are not sufficient for arrhythmogenesis. Indeed, an arrhythmia is most likely when acute electrophysiological changes caused, for example, by transient ischemia, are superimposed on an existing substrate of remodeled myocardium with characteristic conduction abnormalities.

Cardiac Tumors

Primary cardiac tumors are rare, but can result in serious problems when they occur.

Cardiac Myxoma Is the Most Common Primary Tumor of the Heart

Cardiac myxoma accounts for 3% to 50% of all primary cardiac tumors. It is usually sporadic, but it is occasionally associated with familial autosomal dominant syndromes.

PATHOLOGY: Most myxomas (75%) arise in the left atrium, although they can occur in any cardiac chamber or on a valve. The tumor appears as a glistening, gelatinous, polypoid mass, usually 5 to 6 cm in diameter, with a short stalk (Fig. 11-48). It may be sufficiently mobile to obstruct the mitral valve orifice. Microscopically, cardiac myxoma has a loose myxoid stroma containing abundant proteoglycans. Polygonal stellate cells are found within the matrix, occurring singly or in small clusters.

CLINICAL FEATURES: More than half of patients with left atrial myxoma have clinical evidence of mitral valve dysfunction. Although the tumor does not metastasize in the usual sense, it often embolizes. A third of patients with myxomas of the left atrium or left ventricle die from tumor embolization to the brain. Surgical removal of the tumor is successful in most cases.

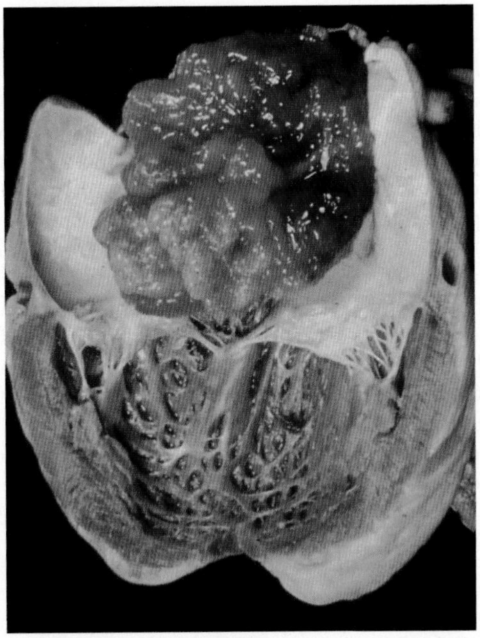

FIGURE 11-48. **Cardiac myxoma.** The left atrium contains a large, polypoid tumor that protrudes into the mitral valve orifice.

Rhabdomyoma Is a Childhood Tumor

Rhabdomyoma is the most common primary cardiac tumor in infants and children and forms nodular masses in the myocardium. It may actually be a hamartoma (see below) rather than a true neoplasm, although the issue is still debated. Almost all are multiple and involve both ventricles and, in one third of cases, the atria as well. In half of cases, the tumor projects into a cardiac chamber and obstructs the lumen or valve orifices.

PATHOLOGY: On gross examination, cardiac rhabdomyomas are pale masses, from 1 mm to several centimeters in diameter. Microscopically, tumor cells show small central nuclei and abundant glycogen-rich clear cytoplasm, in which fibrillar processes containing sarcomeres radiate to the margin of the cell ("spider cell"). Rhabdomyomas often occur in association with tuberous sclerosis (one third to one half of cases). A few cardiac rhabdomyomas have been successfully excised.

Papillary Fibroelastoma Involves the Valves

Papillary fronds resembling a sea anemone and measuring up to 3 to 4 cm in diameter may grow on the heart valves. These tumors are not neoplasms and are more appropriately termed **hamartomas**. The fronds have a central dense core of collagen and elastic fibers surrounded by looser connective tissue. They are covered by a continuation of valvular endothelial cells on which the tumor originates. In most instances, papillary fibroelastomas pose no clinical problem, but they can fragment and embolize to other organs or occlude a coronary artery orifice and produce myocardial ischemia.

Other Tumors are Rare

Other primary tumors of the heart are even rarer than those above. These include angiomas, fibromas, lymphangiomas, neurofibromas, and their sarcomatous counterparts. Lipomatous hypertrophy of the interatrial septum and encapsulated lipomas have been reported.

Metastatic tumors to the heart are seen most frequently in patients with the most prevalent forms of carcinomas—those of lung, breast, and gastrointestinal tract. Still, only a minority of patients with these tumors will show cardiac metastases. Lymphomas and leukemia also may involve the heart. Of all tumors, the one most likely to metastasize to the heart is malignant melanoma (Fig. 11-49). Metastatic cancer of the myocardium can result in clinical manifestations of restrictive cardiomyopathy, particularly if the cardiac tumors are associated with extensive fibrosis.

Diseases of the Pericardium

Pericardial Effusion Can Cause Cardiac Tamponade

Pericardial effusion is accumulation of excess fluid within the pericardial cavity, either as a transudate or an exudate. The pericardial sac normally contains no more than 50 mL of lubricating fluid. If the pericardium is slowly distended, it can accommodate up to 2 L of fluid without notable hemodynamic consequences. However, rapid accumulation of as little as 150 to 200 mL of pericardial fluid or blood may significantly increase intrapericardial pressure and restrict diastolic filling, especially of the right ventricle.

- **Serous pericardial effusion** is often a complication of an increase in extracellular fluid volume, as occurs in congestive heart failure or the nephrotic syndrome. The fluid has a low protein content and few cellular elements.
- **Chylous effusion** (fluid containing chylomicrons) results from a communication of the thoracic duct with the pericardial space secondary to lymphatic obstruction by tumor or infection.
- **Serosanguineous pericardial effusion** may develop after chest trauma, either accidentally or caused by cardiopulmonary resuscitation.
- **Hemopericardium** is bleeding directly into the pericardial cavity (Fig. 11-50). The most common cause is ventricular free wall rupture at a myocardial infarct. Less frequent causes are penetrating cardiac trauma, rupture of a dissecting aneurysm of the aorta, infiltration of a vessel by tumor, or a bleeding diathesis.

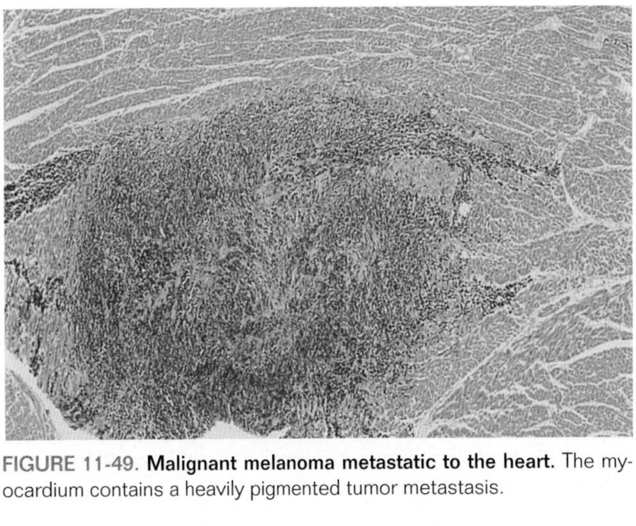

FIGURE 11-49. **Malignant melanoma metastatic to the heart.** The myocardium contains a heavily pigmented tumor metastasis.

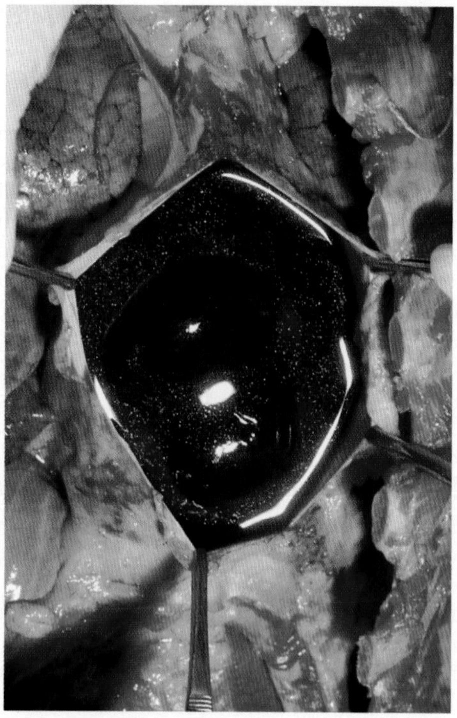

FIGURE 11-50. **Hemopericardium.** The parietal pericardium has been opened to reveal the pericardial cavity distended with fresh blood. The patient sustained a rupture of a myocardial infarct.

***Cardiac tamponade** is the syndrome produced by rapid accumulation of pericardial fluid, which restricts the filling of the heart.* The hemodynamic consequences range from a minimally symptomatic condition to abrupt cardiovascular collapse and death. As the pericardial pressure increases, it reaches and then exceeds central venous pressure, thereby limiting return of blood to the heart. Cardiac output and blood pressure decrease, and **pulsus paradoxus** (an abnormal decrease in systolic pressure with inspiration) occurs in almost all patients. Acute cardiac tamponade is almost invariably fatal unless the pressure is relieved by removing pericardial fluid, by either needle pericardiocentesis or surgical procedures.

Acute Pericarditis May Follow Viral Infections

Pericarditis refers to inflammation of the visceral or parietal pericardium.

PATHOGENESIS: The causes of pericarditis are similar to those for myocarditis (see Table 11-7). In most cases, the cause of acute pericarditis is obscure and (as in myocarditis) is attributed to undiagnosed viral infection. Bacterial pericarditis is distinctly unusual in the antibiotic era. Metastatic tumors may induce serofibrinous or hemorrhagic exudative and inflammatory reactions when they involve the pericardium. The most common tumors to involve the pericardium and cause a malignant pericardial effusion are breast and lung carcinomas. Pericarditis associated with myocardial infarction and rheumatic fever is discussed above.

PATHOLOGY: Acute pericarditis can be classified as **fibrinous, purulent,** or **hemorrhagic,** depending on the gross and microscopic characteristics of the pericardial surfaces and fluid. The most common form is fibrinous pericarditis, in which the normal smooth, glistening appearance of the pericardial surfaces becomes replaced by a dull, granular fibrin-rich exudate (Fig. 11-51). The rough texture of the inflamed pericardial surfaces produces the characteristic friction rub heard by auscultation. The effusion fluid in fibrinous pericarditis is usually rich in protein, and the pericardium contains primarily mononuclear inflammatory cells. Uremia can cause fibrinous pericarditis (Fig. 11-52), although with the widespread availability of renal dialysis, uremic pericarditis is now unusual in the United States. The most common causes are viral infection and pericarditis following myocardial infarcts.

Bacterial infection leads to a purulent pericarditis, in which the pericardial exudate resembles pus and contains many neutrophils. Bleeding into the pericardial space caused by aggressive infectious or neoplastic processes or coagulation defects leads to hemorrhagic pericarditis.

CLINICAL FEATURES: The initial manifestation of acute pericarditis is sudden, severe, substernal chest pain, sometimes referred to the back, shoulder, or neck. It is distinguished from the pain of angina pectoris or myocardial infarction by its failure to radiate down the left arm. A characteristic pericardial friction rub is easily heard. Electrocardiographic changes reflect repolarization abnormalities of the myocardium.

Idiopathic or viral pericarditis is a self-limited disorder, although it may infrequently lead to constrictive pericarditis. Corticosteroids are the treatment of choice. The therapy for other specific forms of acute pericarditis varies with the cause.

Constrictive Pericarditis May Mimic Right Heart Failure

Constrictive pericarditis is a chronic fibrosing disease of the pericardium that compresses the heart and restricts inflow.

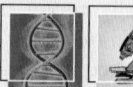

PATHOGENESIS AND PATHOLOGY: Constrictive pericarditis is not an active inflammatory condition. Rather, it results from an exuberant healing response after acute

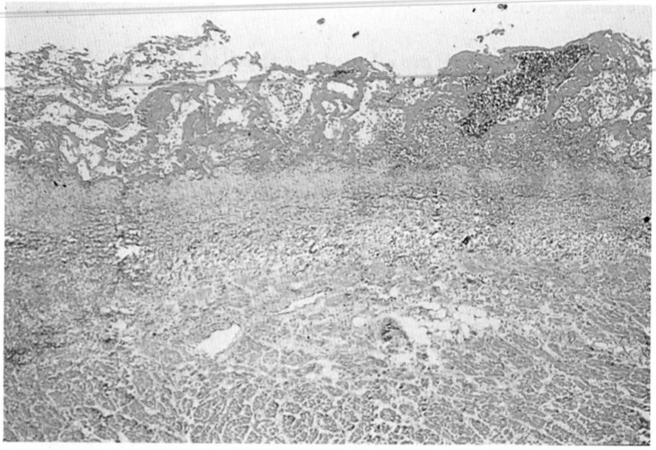

FIGURE 11-51. **Fibrinous pericardial exudate.** The epicardial surface is edematous, inflamed, and covered with tentacles of fibrin.

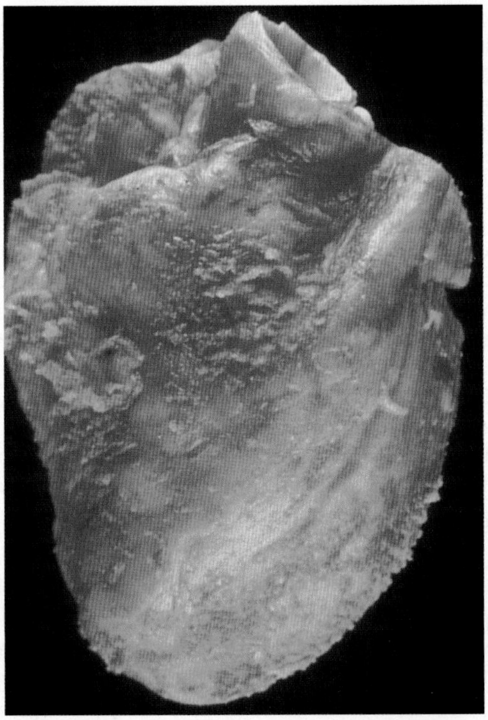

FIGURE 11-52. **Fibrinous pericarditis.** The heart of a patient who died in uremia displays a shaggy, fibrinous exudate covering the visceral pericardium.

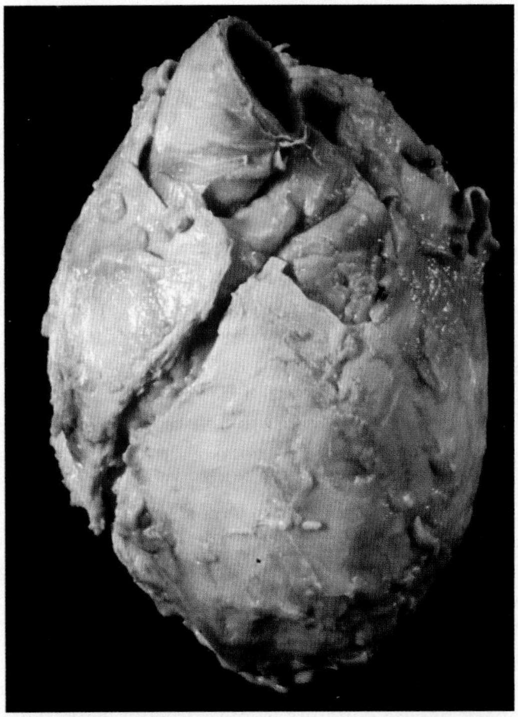

FIGURE 11-53. **Constrictive pericarditis.** The pericardial space has been obliterated, and the heart is encased in a fibrotic, thickened pericardium.

pericardial injury, in which the pericardial space becomes obliterated and visceral and parietal layers become fused in a dense, rigid mass of fibrous tissue. The scarred pericardium may be so thick (up to 3 cm) that it narrows the orifices of the venae cavae (Fig. 11-53). The fibrous envelope may contain calcium deposits. The condition is infrequent today and, in developed countries, is predominantly idiopathic. Prior radiation therapy to the mediastinum and cardiac surgery account for more than one third of cases. In others, constrictive pericarditis follows a purulent or tuberculous infection. Although tuberculosis today accounts for under 15% of cases of constrictive pericarditis in industrialized countries, it is still the major cause in underdeveloped regions.

CLINICAL FEATURES: Patients with constrictive pericarditis have a small, quiet heart in which venous inflow is restricted, and the rigid pericardium determines the diastolic volume of the heart. These patients have high venous pressure, low cardiac output, small pulse pressure, and fluid retention with ascites and peripheral edema. Total pericardiectomy is the treatment of choice.

Adhesive pericarditis is a much milder form of healing of an inflamed pericardium. Commonly seen as an incidental finding at autopsy, it is the outcome of many different types of pericarditis that have healed and left only minor fibrous adhesions between the visceral and parietal surfaces.

Pathology of Interventional Therapies

Coronary Angioplasty and Stenting are Used to Treat Atherosclerotic Coronary Disease

PTCA and stenting are used to mechanically dilate an artery narrowed by an atherosclerotic plaque and keep the lumen open. A catheter with a deflated balloon covered by a collapsed cylindrical metallic mesh (**stent**) is positioned in the stenotic segment. Inflating the balloon fractures the plaque and stretches the vessel wall. As the stent deploys, it holds the fragmented wall open and keeps the lumen patent. Acute complications of PTCA such as coronary artery dissection, acute thrombotic occlusion, and perforation are uncommon. However, restenosis occurs within 4 to 6 months after PTCA (with or without placement of a bare metal stent) in up to 40% of patients. Restenosis reflects a fibroproliferative response of intimal smooth muscle cells to injury sustained during the procedure, resulting in variable intimal thickening and hyperplasia. Recent use of drug-eluting stents which slowly release immunosuppressive agents such as rapamycin or tacrolimus (FK 506), or antiproliferative agents has dramatically reduced the incidence of restenosis.

Coronary Bypass Grafts Circumvent Obstructed Segments

Coronary bypass grafting, using a saphenous vein or left internal mammary artery to direct blood around a blockage, is a common procedure for treatment of proximal coronary stenosis. Although operative mortality is low and early symptomatic relief occurs in most patients, improvement in myocardial perfusion is not permanent, owing to several complications: (1) early thrombosis,

(2) intimal hyperplasia, and (3) atherosclerosis of vein grafts. Moreover, progressive atherosclerosis of the native coronary arteries is not affected by the grafting procedure.

Internal mammary artery grafts develop fewer pathologic changes and, thus, last longer than vein grafts. Excised saphenous vein segments used as grafts are subjected to unavoidable surgical manipulation and an interval of ischemia during harvesting, which results in endothelial cell injury. Also, the grafted vein is exposed to blood pressures much higher than those in its native location. Finally, the caliber of the vein, which is expanded by arterial blood pressure, is usually much greater than that of the distal coronary artery at the graft anastomosis, which mismatch promotes blood stasis. In the immediate postoperative period, these factors enhance the probability of thrombosis and probably play a role in the eventual development of intimal hyperplasia. Intimal hyperplasia is characterized by a concentric proliferation of smooth muscle cells and fibroblasts and collagen deposition in the intima of the vein. After several years, lipids may deposit and atherosclerotic plaques may form in the thickened intima of vein grafts. Atherosclerosis is the most frequent cause of vein graft failure in patients who have had good graft function for several years after surgery.

Because arteries are better suited than veins to serve as aortocoronary bypass conduits, some surgeons have developed total arterial bypass procedures that use the internal mammary, radial, and selected abdominal arteries, which can be harvested without causing significant end-organ damage.

There are Two Types of Valve Replacements: Tissue Xenografts and Mechanical Valves

In most patients with severe valve dysfunction, valve replacement is the best prospect for long-term symptomatic improvement. Operative mortality is low, especially for patients with good preoperative myocardial function. Half of all patients with prosthetic valves are free of complications after 10 years.

TISSUE VALVES: The most commonly used tissue-valve prostheses use a mechanical frame to which glutaraldehyde-fixed porcine aortic valve cusps or pieces of bovine pericardium are attached. These valves have good hemodynamic characteristics, cause little obstruction, and resist thromboembolic complications. Unfortunately, they are not very durable. The most common cause of failure of tissue-valve prostheses is tissue degeneration with severe calcification and fragmentation of the prosthetic valve cusps. This complication affects virtually all porcine aortic valves within 5 years of implantation and leads to valve failure in 20% to 30% of patients within 10 years. However, improved understanding of prosthetic tissue valve calcification have led to development of anti-calcification treatments that improve valve longevity and performance. For example, extraction of tissue lipids with ethanol prior to glutaraldehyde fixation renders the collagenous matrix less susceptible to calcification.

MECHANICAL VALVES: The most widely used mechanical prostheses involve single or bileaflet tilting disk designs that do not obstruct blood flow across the valve and have excellent durability. However, the risk of thromboembolism makes long-term anticoagulant therapy imperative.

Heart Transplantation Cures End-Stage Heart Disease

Development of effective immunosuppressive drugs and institution of surveillance endomyocardial biopsy protocols has made cardiac transplantation an effective treatment for end-stage heart disease. Allograft rejection, however, is a major complication of cardiac transplantation.

Hyperacute rejection occurs if there are blood-group incompatibility or major histocompatibility differences. In these situations, preformed antibodies cause immediate vascular injury to the donor heart, with diffuse hemorrhage, edema, intracapillary platelet–fibrin thrombi, vascular necrosis, and infiltration of neutrophils. Screening for blood-group incompatibility has rendered this complication rare.

Acute humoral rejection is characterized by vascular deposition of antibody and complement, endothelial cell swelling, and edema. This unusual form of rejection has a worse prognosis than acute cellular rejection.

Acute cellular rejection, the most common form of allograft rejection, usually occurs in the first few months after transplantation. It begins as perivascular T-cell infiltration, which is focal and

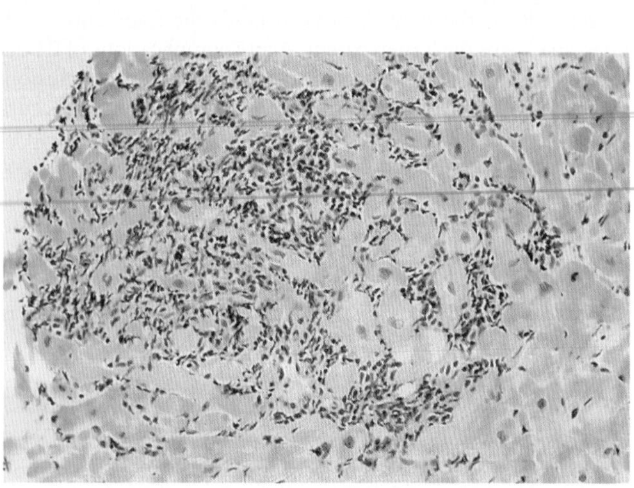

FIGURE 11-54. **Cardiac transplant rejection.** An endomyocardial biopsy shows lymphocytes surrounding individual myocytes and expanding the interstitium.

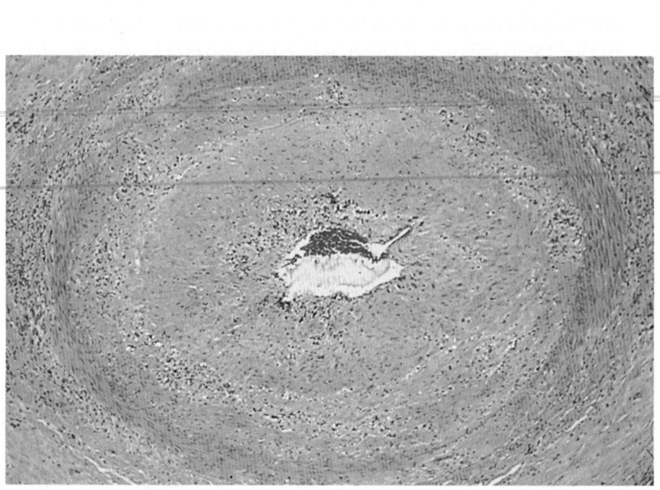

FIGURE 11-55. **Chronic cardiac transplant rejection.** An intramyocardial branch of a coronary artery shows prominent intimal proliferation and inflammation with narrowing of the lumen.

is not associated with acute myocyte necrosis. This reaction often resolves spontaneously and, therefore, does not necessitate a change in the immunosuppressive regimen. Moderate cellular rejection is characterized by T-cell infiltration into adjacent interstitial spaces, where lymphocytes surround individual myocytes and expand the interstitium (Fig. 11-54). In this instance, focal acute myocyte necrosis is also present. Moderate cellular rejection usually does not produce detectable functional impairment and tends to resolve within a few days to a week after treatment. However, additional immunosuppressive therapy is instituted because moderate cellular rejection can progress to severe rejection. The latter is characterized by vascular damage, widespread myocyte necrosis, neutrophil infiltration, interstitial hemorrhage, and functional impairment, which is difficult to reverse.

The early stage of cellular allograft rejection is typically asymptomatic. Once symptoms develop, rejection is usually much more advanced and has caused irrecoverable loss of cardiac myocytes. The most reliable screening procedure is endomyocardial biopsy of the right side of the interventricular septum, performed by cardiac catheterization.

Chronic vascular rejection, also referred to as **accelerated coronary artery disease**, is the most common cause of death in heart transplant patients beyond the first year after transplantation. It affects proximal and distal epicardial coronary arteries, the penetrating coronary artery branches and even the arterioles. Microscopically, accelerated coronary artery disease is characterized by concentric intimal proliferation (Fig. 11-55),which can lead to coronary occlusion and myocardial infarction. This complication is silent because the transplanted heart is denervated. Thus extensive myocardial damage can develop before the transplant patient is aware that ischemic injury has occurred.

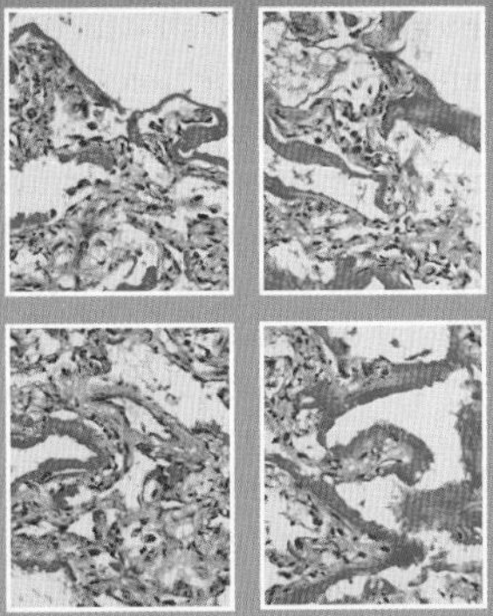

12

The Respiratory System

Mary Beth Beasley
William D. Travis
Emanuel Rubin

THE NORMAL RESPIRATORY SYSTEM

Embryology

The respiratory system comprises the larynx, trachea, bronchi, bronchioles, and alveoli. During the fourth week of gestation, the laryngotracheal groove develops as a ventral outpouching of the foregut.

The embryonic period of lung development occurs between 4 and 6 weeks' gestation. During this period, the tracheobronchial bud divides to form the proximal airways to the level of the segmental bronchi.

The pseudoglandular period occupies weeks 6 to 16 of gestation, after which time the distal airways are formed up to the level of the terminal bronchioles.

The acinar or canalicular period encompasses weeks 17 to 28 of gestation. This is the time when (1) the framework of the gas-exchanging unit of the lung develops, (2) the acinus is formed, (3) the vascular system develops, (4) capillaries reach the epithelium, and (5) gas exchange becomes possible. At this point extrauterine life becomes possible.

The saccular period extends from 28 to 34 weeks of gestation. The primary saccules become subdivided by secondary crests, a process that results in greater complexity of the gas-exchanging surface and thinning of air-space walls.

The alveolar period corresponds to 34 to 36 weeks of gestation and is the last step in lung development when alveoli begin developing. At birth, the number of alveoli is highly variable, ranging from 20–150 million. Most alveoli develop in the first 2 years of life.

Anatomy

TRACHEA AND BRONCHI: The trachea is a hollow tube up to 25 cm in length and up to 2.5 cm in diameter. The right bronchus diverges at a lesser angle from the trachea than does the left, which is why foreign material is more frequently aspirated on the right side. On entering the lung, the bronchi divide into lobar bronchi, then into segmental bronchi, which supply the 19 lung segments. Because the segments are individual units with their own bronchovascular supply, they can be resected individually.

The tracheobronchial tree contains cartilage and submucosal mucous glands in the wall (Fig. 12-1). The latter are compound tubular glands with mucous cells (pale) and serous cells (granular, more basophilic). The lining is pseudostratified epithelium, which appears as layers, although all cells reach the basement membrane. Most cells are ciliated, but there are also mucus-secreting (goblet) cells, and basal cells. The basal cells, which do not reach the surface, are thought to be precursor cells that differentiate to form the more specialized cells of the tracheobronchial epithelium. There are also nonciliated columnar cells, or **Clara cells**, which accumulate and detoxify many inhaled toxic agents (e.g., nitrogen dioxide [NO_2]). Scattered in the tracheobronchial mucosa are **Kulchitsky cells**, neuroendocrine cells that contain a variety of hormonally active polypeptides and vasoactive amines.

BRONCHIOLES: Distal to the bronchi are bronchioles, which differ from bronchi in that they lack cartilage and mucus-secreting glands (see Fig. 12-1). Bronchiolar epithelium becomes thinner with progressive branching, until only one cell layer is present. The last purely conducting structure free of alveoli is the **terminal bronchiole,** which has a circumferential layer of pseudostratified ciliated respiratory epithelium and a smooth muscle wall. Mucous cells gradually disappear from the lining of the bronchioles until they are entirely replaced in the small bronchioles by the nonciliated, columnar Clara cells. The terminal bronchioles divide into **respiratory bronchioles,** which merge into **alveolar ducts** and **alveoli**. The **acinus**, which is the unit of gas exchange in the lung, consists of respiratory bronchioles, alveolar ducts, and alveoli.

ALVEOLI: The alveoli are lined by two types of epithelium (see Fig. 12-1). ***Type I cells*** *cover 95% of the alveolar surface, but comprise only 40% of alveolar epithelial cells.* They are thin and have a large surface area, a combination that facilitates gas exchange. ***Type II cells*** *produce surfactant and are 60% of the alveolar lining cells.* However, as they are more cuboidal, they constitute only 5% of the alveolar surface. Type I cells are particularly vulnerable to injury. When they are lost, type II pneumocytes multiply and differentiate to form new type I cells, reconstituting the alveolar surface.

Alveolar epithelial and endothelial cells are arranged ideally for gas exchange. The cytoplasm of epithelial and endothelial cells is spread very thinly on either side of a fused basement membrane, allowing efficient exchange of oxygen and carbon dioxide. An abundant capillary network covers 85% to 95% of the alveolar surface. Away from the site of gas exchange, there is more abundant interstitial connective tissue consisting of collagen, elastin, and proteoglycans. Fibroblasts and myofibroblasts may also be present. This expanded region forms the interstitial space of the alveolar wall, where significant fluid and molecular exchange occurs.

PULMONARY VASCULATURE: The lung has a dual blood supply: the pulmonary circulation and the bronchial system. Pulmonary arteries accompany the airways in a sheath of connective tissue, the **bronchovascular bundle**. The more proximal arteries are elastic. They are succeeded by muscular arteries, the pulmonary arterioles and eventually the pulmonary capillaries.

The smallest veins, which resemble the smallest arteries, join other veins and drain into the lobular septa, connective tissue partitions that subdivide the lung into small respiratory units. The veins then continue in the lobular septa, joining other veins to form a network that is separate from the bronchovascular bundles.

The bronchial arteries arise from the thoracic aorta and nourish the bronchial tree as far as the respiratory bronchioles. These arteries are accompanied by their respective veins, which drain into the azygous or hemiazygous veins.

There are no lymphatics in most alveolar walls. The lymphatics commence in alveoli at the periphery of the acinus, which lies along a lobular septum, a bronchovascular bundle, or the pleura. The lymphatics of the lobular septa and bronchovascular bundle accompany these structures, and the pleural lymphatics drain toward the hilus through the bronchovascular lymphatics.

Defense Mechanisms

The respiratory system has effective defense mechanisms to cope with the numerous particulates and infectious agents inhaled on inspiration.

The **nose and trachea** warm and humidify the air entering the lung. The nose traps almost all particles over 10 μm in diameter and about half of all particles of 3 μm aerodynamic diameter (Fig. 12-2). (Aerodynamic diameter refers to the way particles behave in air rather than to their actual size.)

The **mucociliary blanket** of the airway epithelium disposes of particles 2 to 10 μm in diameter. The ciliary beat drives the

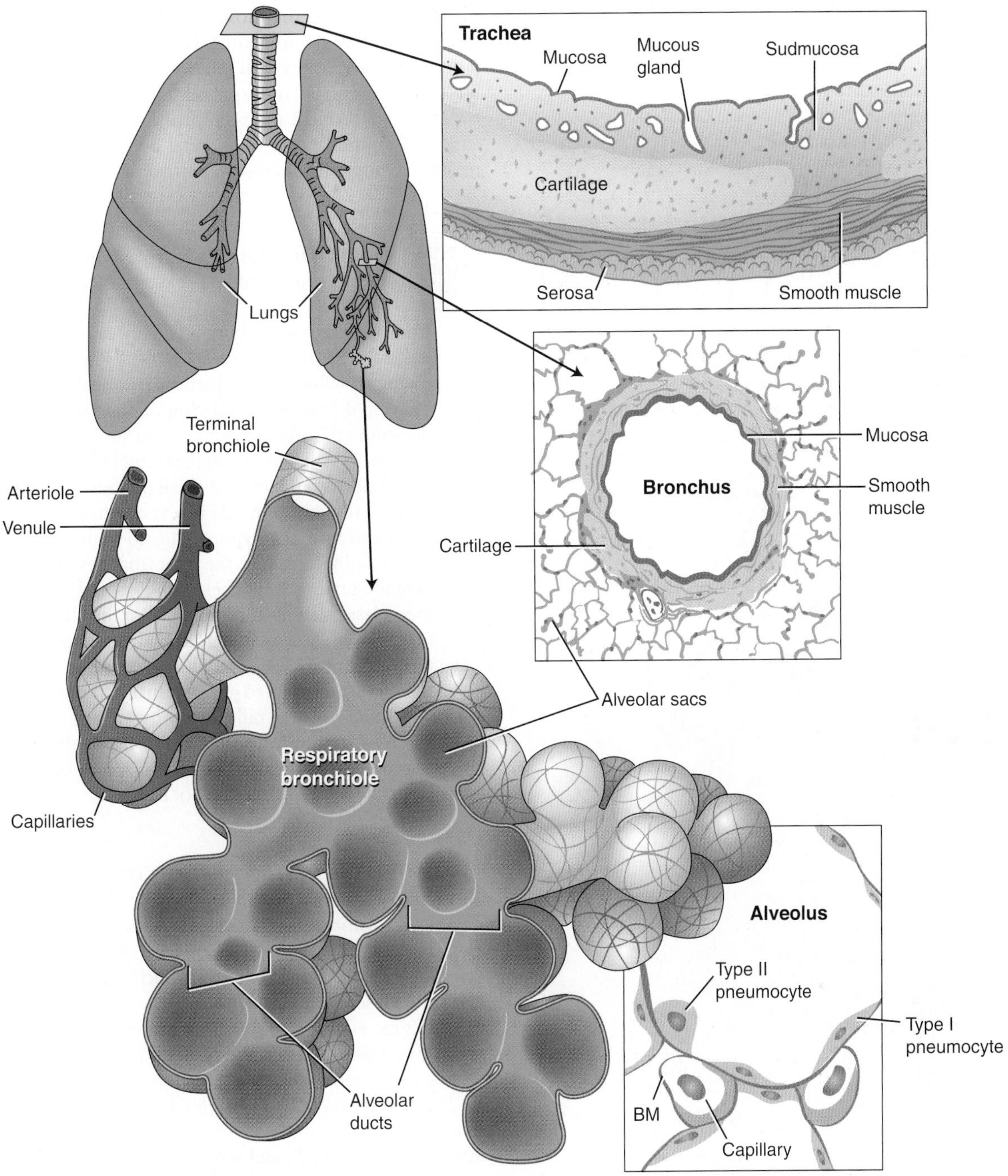

FIGURE 12-1. **Anatomy of the lung.** The conducting structures of the lung include (1) the trachea, which has horseshoe-shaped cartilages; (2) the bronchi, which have plates of cartilage in their walls (both the trachea and bronchi have mucus-secreting glands in their walls); and (3) the bronchioles, which do not have cartilage in their walls and terminate in the terminal bronchioles. The gas-exchanging components compose the unit distal to the terminal bronchiole, namely, the acinus. Alveoli are lined by type I cells, which are large, flat cells that cover most of the alveolar wall, and by type II cells, which secrete surfactant and are the progenitor cells of the alveolar epithelium. Gas exchange occurs at the level of the alveolar wall.

mucous blanket toward the trachea. Particles that land on it are thus removed from the lungs and swallowed or coughed up.

Alveolar macrophages protect the alveolar space. These cells are derived from the bone marrow, probably undergo a maturation division in the interstitium of the lung, and then enter the alveolar space. They are particularly effective in dealing with particles with aerodynamic diameters under 2 μm. Very small particles are not phagocytosed and are exhaled.

THE LUNGS

Congenital Anomalies

BRONCHIAL ATRESIA: This abnormality most often involves the bronchus to the apical posterior segment of the left upper lobe. In infants, the lesion may result in an overexpanded part of

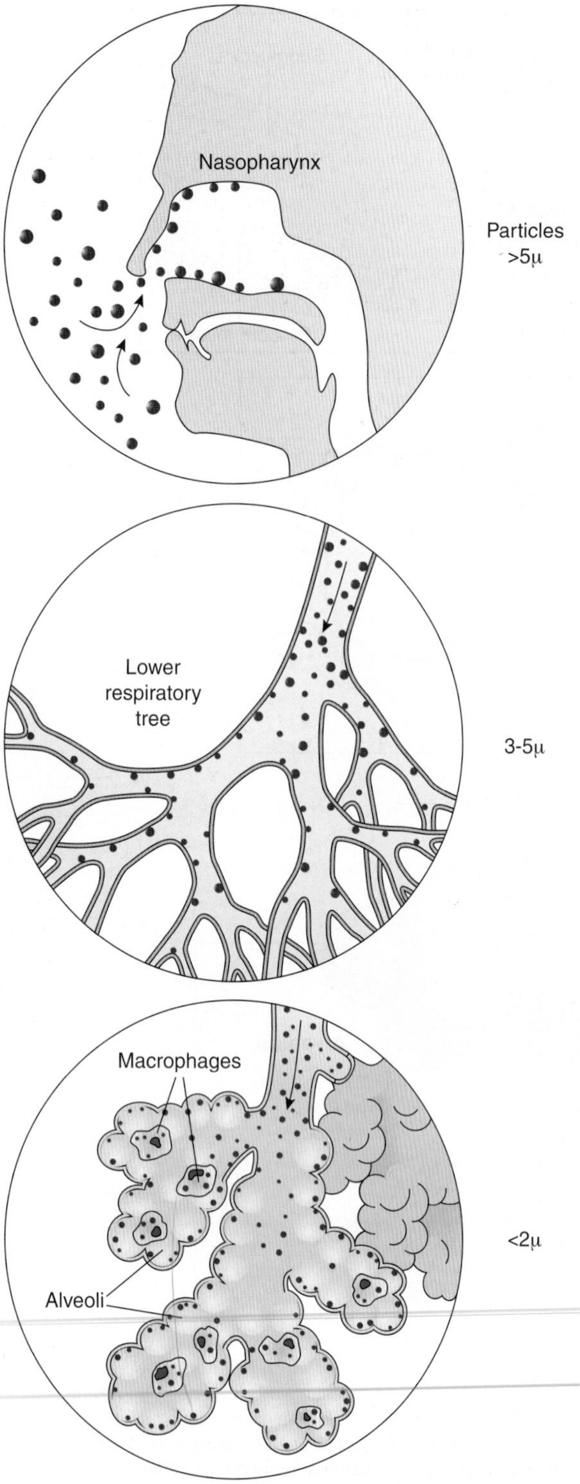

FIGURE 12-2. **Deposition of particles in the respiratory tract.** Large particles are trapped in the nose. Intermediate-sized particles deposit on the bronchi and bronchioles and are removed by the mucociliary blanket. Smaller particles terminate in the air spaces and are removed by macrophages. Very small particles behave as a gas and are breathed out.

the lung. In later life, the overexpanded lobe may also be emphysematous. Bronchial mucus accumulating distal to the atretic region may appear on radiologic examination as a mass.

PULMONARY HYPOPLASIA: This condition reflects incomplete or defective development of the lung. The lung is smaller than normal, owing to fewer acini or a decrease in their size. Pulmonary hypoplasia, the most common congenital lesion of the lung, is found in 10% of neonatal autopsies. In most cases (90%), it occurs in association with other congenital anomalies, most of which impinge on the thorax. The lesion may be accompanied by hypoplasia of bronchi and pulmonary vessels if the insult occurs early in gestation, as in congenital diaphragmatic hernia. Pulmonary hypoplasia also is seen in trisomies 13, 18, and 21.

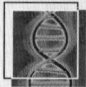

PATHOGENESIS: Three major factors have been implicated as causes of pulmonary hypoplasia:

- **Compression of the lung** is usually caused by a congenital diaphragmatic hernia, typically on the left side, owing to failure of the pleuroperitoneal canal to close. Varying degrees of herniation of abdominal viscera are present in the affected hemithorax, and the degree of hypoplasia is variable. At one extreme, the lung on the affected side is reduced to a small nubbin of tissue and the lung on the opposite side is severely hypoplastic. At the other extreme, the hypoplasia is so slight that the infant has no symptoms and the abnormalities are noted incidentally on a routine chest radiograph. Other causes of hypoplasia include abnormalities of the chest wall, pleural effusions, and ascites, as in hydrops fetalis.
- **Oligohydramnios** (inadequate volume of amniotic fluid) is usually due to genitourinary anomalies and is an important cause of pulmonary hypoplasia.
- **Decreased respiration** has been shown experimentally to produce hypoplastic lungs, which may be caused by a lack of repetitive stretching of the lung.

CONGENITAL CYSTIC ADENOMATOID MALFORMATION: This common anomaly consists of abnormal bronchiolar structures of varying sizes or distribution. Most cases are seen in the first 2 years of life. The lesion usually affects one lobe of the lung and consists of multiple cystlike spaces lined by bronchiolar epithelium and separated by loose fibrous tissue (Fig. 12-3). Some patients with congenital cystic adenomatoid malformation have other congenital anomalies. The most common presenting symptom is respiratory distress and cyanosis. Surgical resection is the treatment of choice.

BRONCHOGENIC CYST: This lesion is a discrete, extrapulmonary, fluid-filled mass lined by respiratory epithelium and limited by walls that contain muscle and cartilage. It is most commonly found in the middle mediastinum. In the newborn, a bronchogenic cyst may compress a major airway and cause respiratory distress. Secondary infection of the cyst in older patients may lead to hemorrhage and perforation. Many bronchogenic cysts are asymptomatic and are found on routine chest radiographs.

EXTRALOBAR SEQUESTRATION: Extralobar sequestration is a mass of lung tissue that is not connected to the bronchial tree and is located outside the visceral pleura. An abnormal artery, usually arising from the aorta, supplies the sequestered tissue (Fig. 12-4).

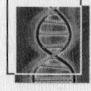

PATHOGENESIS: This lesion is thought to originate from an outpouching of the foregut, distinct from the pulmonary anlage but later loses its connection to the original foregut. It is 3 to 4 times as common in males as in females, and is associated with other anomalies in two thirds of patients.

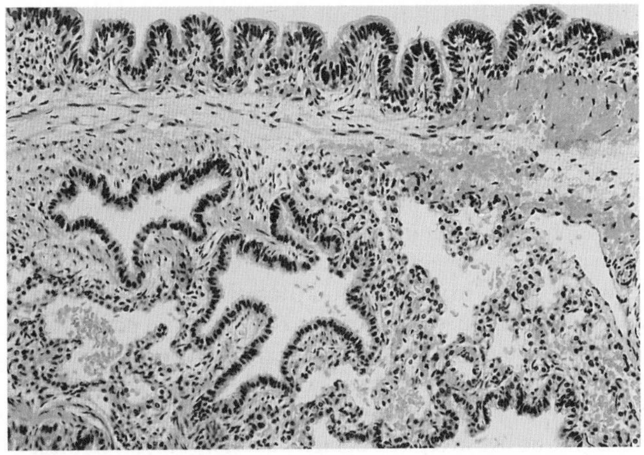

FIGURE 12-3. **Congenital cystic adenomatoid malformation.** Multiple glandlike spaces are lined by bronchiolar epithelium.

PATHOLOGY: On gross examination, extralobar sequestration is a pyramidal or round mass covered by pleura, from 1 to 15 cm in greatest dimension. Microscopically, dilated bronchioles, alveolar ducts and alveoli are noted. Infection or infarction may alter the histologic appearance.

CLINICAL FEATURES: In half of cases, extralobar sequestration is recognized in the first month of life. By age 2 years, the diagnosis has been made in 75% of patients. In the neonatal period, often during the first day of life, the disorder may manifest as dyspnea and cyanosis. In older children, it may come to medical attention because of recurrent bronchopulmonary infections. Surgical excision is curative.

INTRALOBAR SEQUESTRATION: Intralobar sequestration is a mass of lung tissue within the visceral pleura, isolated from the tracheobronchial tree and supplied by a systemic artery (Fig. 12-5). For many years, it was considered a congenital malformation, but it is now thought to be acquired.

PATHOLOGY: Intralobar sequestration is found in a lower lobe in almost all cases. Bilateral involvement is distinctly unusual. On gross examination, the sequestered pulmonary tissue shows the result of chronic recurrent

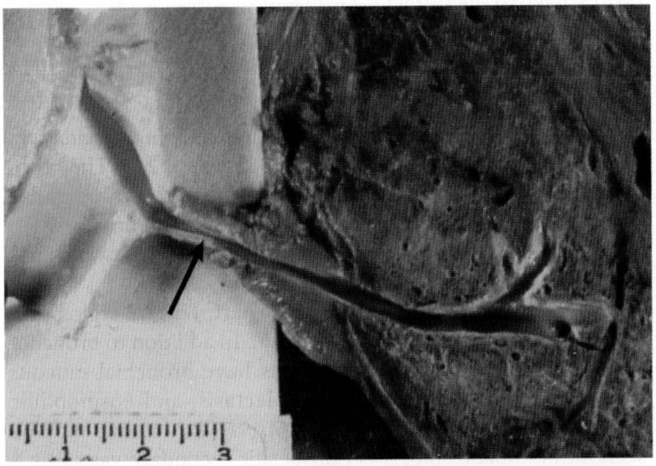

FIGURE 12-4. **Extralobar sequestration.** The sequestered pulmonary tissue is situated outside the lung parenchyma. It is supplied by an aberrant artery *(arrow)* from the aorta and is not connected to the bronchial tree.

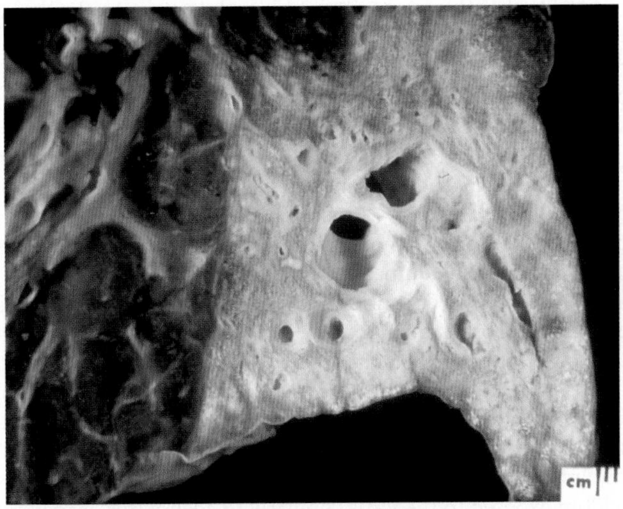

FIGURE 12-5. **Intralobar sequestration.** The sequestered tissue lies within the visceral pleura and exhibits cystic change and dense fibrosis. An aberrant arterial supply to this lesion was identified (not shown).

pneumonia, with end-stage fibrosis and honeycomb cystic changes. The cysts range up to 5 cm in diameter and lie in a dense fibrous stroma. Microscopically, the cystic spaces are mostly lined by cuboidal or columnar epithelium and the lumen contains foamy macrophages and eosinophilic material. Interstitial chronic inflammation and hyperplasia of lymphoid follicles is often prominent. Acute and organizing pneumonia may be seen.

CLINICAL FEATURES: Cough, sputum production, and recurrent pneumonia are noted in almost all patients. Most cases are discovered in adolescents or young adults. Only one fourth of patients are in the first decade of life, and the lesion is rarely identified in infants. Surgical resection is often indicated.

Diseases of the Bronchi and Bronchioles

Most bronchial and bronchiolar diseases deal with acute conditions and their sequelae. We reserve the discussion of chronic bronchitis for the section devoted to chronic obstructive pulmonary disease (COPD).

Airway Infections Are Caused by Diverse Organisms

In this section, we distinguish between infections of the airways and parenchyma for reasons of classification and convenience, but this division should not be thought of as rigid. The agents causing these infections are discussed in detail in Chapter 9.

Many infectious agents that involve the intrapulmonary airways tend to affect the more peripheral airways (**bronchiolitis**). The classic examples are adenovirus, respiratory syncytial virus (RSV) and measles. All are more serious in malnourished children and populations not ordinarily exposed to these agents. Severe symptomatic illnesses with these agents are more commonly encountered in infants and children, and recovery is the rule. Symptoms include cough, a feeling of tightness in the chest, and, in extreme cases, shortness of breath and even cyanosis.

INFLUENZA: This is a characteristic example of tracheobronchitis, and in the occasional patient who dies with this infection, the appearance of the bronchi is dramatic. The surface of the airway is fiery red, reflecting acute inflammation and congestion of the mucosa.

ADENOVIRUS: Infection with this adenovirus produces the most serious sequelae, including extensive inflammation of bronchioles (Fig. 12-6) and subsequent healing by fibrosis. Bronchioles may become obliterated or occluded by loose fibrous tissue (**obliterative bronchiolitis**).

RESPIRATORY SYNCYTIAL VIRUS (RSV): RSV infection tends to occur in epidemics in nurseries. It is usually self-limited, but rare fatal cases occur. It can cause nosocomial infection in children and (rarely) in adults. Histologically, one encounters peribronchiolar inflammation and disorganization of the epithelium. Severe overdistention may be found without obvious bronchiolar obstruction, possibly due to displacement of surfactant from the bronchiolar surface.

MEASLES: At one time a major cause of bronchiolitis, measles is rarely a problem in developed countries since the advent of the measles vaccine. However, measles-induced bronchiolitis remains a serious problem, particularly in populations seldom exposed to the virus. Similarly to adenovirus, it may result in bronchiolar obliteration and bronchiectasis.

BORDETELLA PERTUSSIS: This bacterium commonly infects the airways and is the cause of whooping cough. After widespread use of a pertussis vaccine, the disease became rare in the United States. Unfortunately, in England, where vaccination is no longer compulsory, the incidence of pertussis is increasing. Clinically, whooping cough is typified by fever and severe prolonged bouts of coughing, followed by a characteristic deep whooping inspiration. Severe bronchial and bronchiolar inflammation has been found in fatal cases. Before immunization was available, whooping cough commonly led to development of bronchiectasis.

HAEMOPHILUS INFLUENZAE AND STREPTOCOCCUS PNEUMONIAE: These organisms have been implicated in exacerbations of chronic bronchitis. Such episodes contribute to the morbidity of chronic bronchitis and are treated with antibiotics.

CANDIDA ALBICANS: This fungus is a normal commensal organism in the oral cavity, gut, and vagina, and is best known for its infection of those regions. It may also affect the lungs, usually as a noninvasive growth on the airwaysurface epithelium, where it may produce mucosal ulceration. Predisposing factors for invasive growth include trauma, burns, gastrointestinal surgery and indwelling catheters, as well as neutropenia associated with acute leukemia and cytotoxic chemotherapy.

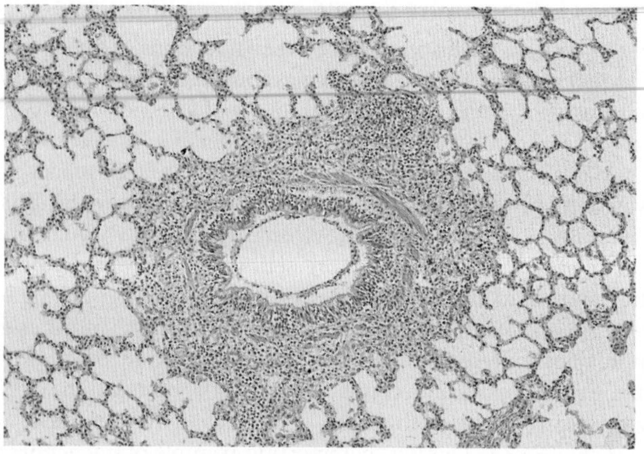

FIGURE 12-6. Bronchiolitis due to adenovirus. The wall of this bronchiole shows an intense chronic inflammatory infiltrate with local extension into the surrounding peribronchial tissue.

Irritant Gases Derive from Air Pollution and Accidents

The most important irritant gases in the atmosphere are oxidants (ozone, nitrogen oxides) and sulfur dioxide (SO_2). Oxidants are particularly related to the action of sunlight on automobile exhaust fumes and are important in major urban areas that have temperature inversions. SO_2 is derived mainly from burning fossil fuels. Although the precise effects of these agents in low concentration is not certain, it seems unlikely that they are a major cause of serious respiratory disease, despite their nuisance value. However, they may compound adverse effects of tobacco smoke. Indeed, persons living in urban and more polluted areas have worse pulmonary function, as expressed by reduced expiratory flow rates, than do those who reside in cleaner environments. Respiratory infections are also more common in young children who live in regions of high pollution. However, these effects are small in the healthy population.

In persons with chronic pulmonary disease, the situation is different: experimentally, ozone makes airways more reactive, an effect related to airway inflammation. Thus, air pollution may exacerbate symptoms of asthmatic persons and those with established respiratory disease. In high concentrations, irritant gases produce serious morphologic and functional effects.

NO_2: Exposure to NO_2 is often encountered in industrial settings, including welding, electroplating, metal cleaning, and blasting. The gas is also produced by decaying grain stored in silos. Because NO_2 is heavier than air, it accumulates immediately above the surface of the grain. A worker entering the silo inhales high concentrations of the gas, with resulting injury to the lung, a condition known as **silo-filler disease**. The onset of respiratory symptoms is delayed for up to 30 hours, after which the patient develops cough and dyspnea. Most patients recover but some develop progressive bronchiolitis obliterans and may die of respiratory failure.

SO_2: This highly soluble gas, when inhaled chronically by experimental animals, produces lesions in the more central airways that resemble chronic bronchitis and that may progress to squamous metaplasia. In humans, exposure to very high concentrations of SO_2 has been associated with severe inflammation and bronchiolitis.

CHLORINE AND AMMONIA: These gases are released in high concentrations in industrial accidents. On inhalation, they produce extensive bronchial and bronchiolar mucosal injury. Secondary inflammation may culminate in extensive bronchiectasis, in part from bronchiolar obliteration and in part from direct damage to the bronchi.

Bronchocentric Granulomatosis Usually Reflects Allergic Responses to Infection

Bronchocentric granulomatosis refers to nonspecific granulomatous inflammation centered on bronchi or bronchioles (Fig. 12-7). The histologic pattern can be seen in a number of clinical settings and is not a distinct clinical entity. Bronchocentric granulomatosis can be the predominant pulmonary pathologic finding in two groups of patients, asthmatics and nonasthmatics.

Asthmatic patients, for the most part, have allergic bronchopulmonary aspergillosis (see below). In addition to bronchocentric granulomatosis, such patients have bronchial mucous plugs, bronchiectasis and bronchiolectasis, and eosinophilic pneumonia. Irregular, fragmented *Aspergillus* hyphae may be seen in the mucous plugs. A nonspecific secondary vasculitis is centered on the airways rather than the vessels.

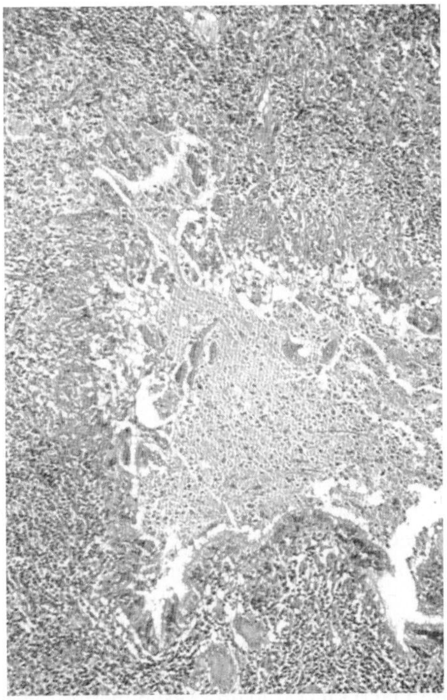

FIGURE 12-7. **Bronchocentric granulomatosis.** The wall of a bronchiole is destroyed by necrotizing granulomatous inflammation. The lumen is filled with necrotic debris.

Nonasthmatic patients with bronchocentric granulomatosis are likely to have an infection, especially tuberculosis or fungi such as *Histoplasma capsulatum*. Bronchocentric granulomatosis can also be a manifestation of rheumatoid arthritis, ankylosing spondylitis, and Wegener granulomatosis. Patients with bronchocentric granulomatosis of either allergic or nonallergic type generally respond well to corticosteroid therapy.

Constrictive Bronchiolitis May Obliterate the Airway

Constrictive bronchiolitis is an uncommon disorder in which an initial inflammatory bronchiolitis is followed by bronchiolar scarring and fibrosis, resulting in constrictive narrowing and eventually complete obliteration of the airway lumen (Fig. 12-8). **Obliterative bronchiolitis** is a synonym.

PATHOLOGY: Bronchioles show chronic mural inflammation and varying amounts of submucosal fibrosis. These lesions are often focal and may be difficult to identify. Elastic stains may assist in recognizing the scarred bronchioles. Bronchiolectasis and mucous plugs may be seen in adjacent airways. The surrounding lung is usually normal.

CLINICAL FEATURES: Patients may have dyspnea and wheezing owing to severe obstructive pulmonary function. The chest radiograph and computed tomography (CT) scan may be normal, or they may show overinflation, caused by air trapping distal to the obliterated bronchioles. This pattern of fibrosis is seen in a number of situations, including: (1) bone marrow transplantation (graft-versus-host disease), (2) lung transplantation (chronic rejection), (3) collagen vascular diseases (especially rheumatoid arthritis), (4) postinfectious disorders (especially viral infections), (5) after inhalation of toxins (SO_2, ammonia, phosgene), and (6) intake of certain drugs (penicillamine).

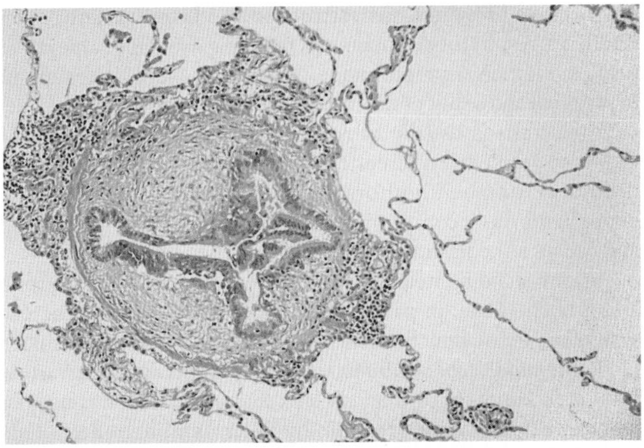

FIGURE 12-8. **Constrictive bronchiolitis.** The lumen of a bronchiole is markedly narrowed, owing to marked submucosal fibrosis.

It also may occur as an idiopathic entity. Most patients have a relentless progressive clinical course. Many are treated with steroids, but no therapy is effective for this disease.

Bronchial Obstruction Leads to Atelectasis

Bronchial obstruction in adults is most often the consequence of the endobronchial extension of primary lung tumors, although mucous plugs from aspirated gastric contents or foreign bodies may be responsible, especially in children. In the case of partial obstruction, the trapped air may lead to overdistention of the distal affected segment; complete obstruction results in atelectasis. Areas distal to the obstruction are also susceptible to pneumonia, pulmonary abscess, and bronchiectasis (see below).

Atelectasis *refers to the collapse of expanded lung tissue* (Fig. 12-9). If the supply of air is obstructed, the loss of gas from the alveoli to the blood causes collapse of the affected region. Atelectasis is an important postoperative complication of abdominal surgery, occur-

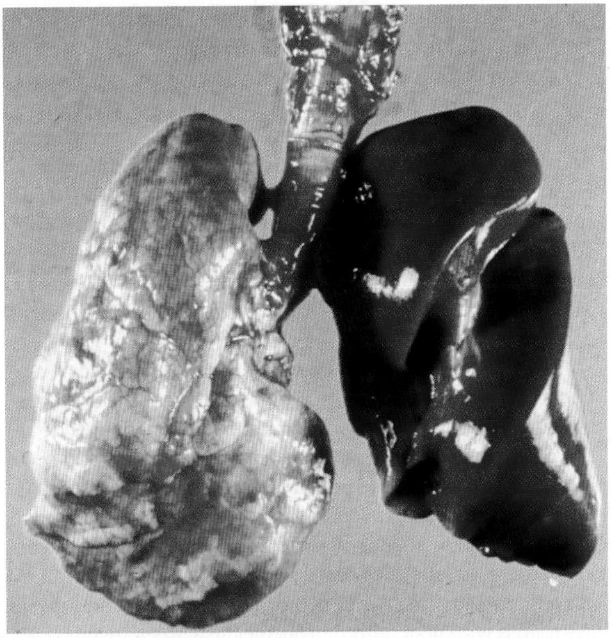

FIGURE 12-9. **Atelectasis.** The right lung of an infant is pale and expanded by air; the left lung is collapsed.

ring because of (1) mucous obstruction of a bronchus and (2) diminished respiratory movement resulting from postoperative pain. It is often asymptomatic, but when severe, it results in hypoxemia and a shift of the mediastinum *toward* the affected side.

Atelectasis is usually caused by bronchial obstruction, but may also result from direct compression of the lung (e.g., hydrothorax or pneumothorax). Such compression, if severe enough, seriously compromises the function of the affected lung and causes a mediastinal shift *away* from the affected side.

In long-standing atelectasis, the collapsed lung becomes fibrotic and bronchi dilate, in part because of infection distal to the obstructeion. Permanent bronchial dilation (bronchiectasis) results.

Right middle lobe syndrome *refers to atelectasis due to obstruction of the bronchus to the right middle lobe.* Such obstruction is usually due to external compression by hilar lymph nodes. This bronchus is particularly susceptible to external compression because it is long and slender and surrounded by lymph nodes. Histologically, the lung shows bronchiectasis, chronic bronchitis and bronchiolitis, lymphoid hyperplasia, abscess formation, and dense fibrosis. Both acute and organizing pneumonia may be present. The lymph node enlargement can be due to tuberculous lymphadenitis or metastatic lung cancer. Often, however, the cause of the obstruction remains undetermined.

Bronchiectasis Is Irreversible Dilation of Bronchi Caused by Destruction of Bronchial Wall Muscle and Elastic Elements

PATHOGENESIS: Bronchiectasis may be obstructive or nonobstructive.

Obstructive bronchiectasis is localized to a segment of the lung distal to a mechanical obstruction of a central bronchus by a variety of lesions, including tumors, inhaled foreign bodies, mucous plugs in asthma, and compressive lymphadenopathy. **Nonobstructive bronchiectasis** is usually a complication of respiratory infections or defects in the defense mechanisms that protect the airways from infection. It may be localized or generalized.

Localized nonobstructive bronchiectasis was once common, usually resulting from childhood bronchopulmonary infections such as measles, pertussis, or other bacterial infections. Although vaccines and antibiotics have reduced the frequency of bronchiectasis, one-half to two-thirds of all cases still follow a bronchopulmonary infection. At present, adenovirus and RSV infections are frequent causes of bronchiectasis in children. Childhood respiratory infections remain important causes of bronchiectasis in less-developed parts of the world.

Generalized bronchiectasis is, for the most part, secondary to inherited impairment in host defense mechanisms or acquired conditions that permit introduction of infectious organisms into the airways. The acquired disorders that predispose to bronchiectasis include (1) neurologic diseases that impair consciousness, swallowing, respiratory excursions, and the cough reflex; (2) incompetence of the lower esophageal sphincter; (3) nasogastric intubation; and (4) chronic bronchitis. The principal inherited conditions associated with generalized bronchiectasis are cystic fibrosis, the dyskinetic ciliary syndromes, hypogammaglobulinemias, and deficiencies of specific immunoglobulin (Ig)G subclasses.

Kartagener syndrome *is one of the immotile cilia (ciliary dyskinesia) syndromes and comprises the triad of dextrocardia (with or without situs inversus), bronchiectasis, and sinusitis.* It is caused by absence of inner or outer dynein arms of cilia. Other dyskinetic ciliary syndromes include radial spoke deficiency ("Sturgess syndrome") and an absence of the central doublet of the cilium. In these diseases cilia are deficient throughout the body. Both men and women are sterile, because of impaired ciliary mobility in the vas deferens and the fallopian tube. In the respiratory tract, ciliary defects lead to repeated upper and lower respiratory tract infections in the lung and, thus, to bronchiectasis.

Immunodeficiency diseases similarly predispose to repeated pulmonary infections and are associated with bronchiectasis. Hypogammaglobulinemia can result in recurrent pulmonary infections owing to the absence of IgAs or IgGs that protect against viruses or bacteria. Acquired and inherited disorders of neutrophils also lead to a greater risk of respiratory infections and bronchiectasis.

PATHOLOGY: On gross examination, bronchial dilation is saccular, varicose, or cylindrical.

- **Saccular bronchiectasis** affects the proximal third to fourth branches of the bronchi (Fig. 12-10). These bronchi are severely dilated and end blindly in dilated sacs, with collapse and fibrosis of the distal lung parenchyma.

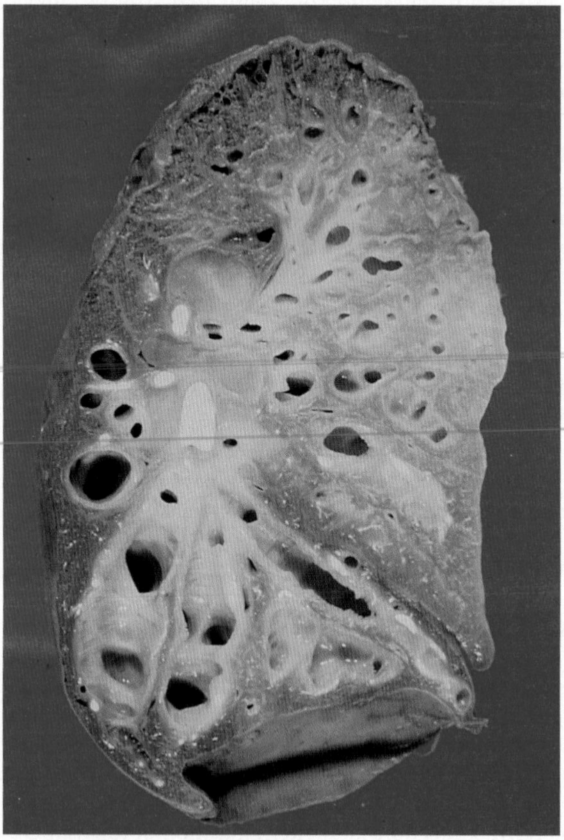

FIGURE 12-10. **Bronchiectasis.** The resected upper lobe shows widely dilated bronchi, with thickening of the bronchial walls and collapse and fibrosis of the pulmonary parenchyma.

- **Cylindrical bronchiectasis** involves the sixth to eighth bronchial branchings, which show uniform, moderate dilation. It is a milder disease than saccular bronchiectasis and leads to fewer clinical symptoms.
- **Varicose bronchiectasis** results in bronchi that resemble varicose veins when visualized by radiologic bronchography, with irregular dilations and constrictions. Two to eight branchings of bronchi are recognized grossly. Bronchiolar obliteration is not as severe, and parenchymal abnormalities are variable.

Generalized bronchiectasis is usually bilateral and is most common in the lower lobes, the left more commonly involved than the right. Localized bronchiectasis may occur wherever there was obstruction or infection. Bronchi are dilated and have white or yellow thickened walls. Bronchial lumens frequently contain thick, mucopurulent secretions. Microscopically, severe inflammation of bronchi and bronchioles results in destruction of all components of the bronchial wall. With the consequent collapse of distal lung parenchyma, the damaged bronchi dilate. Inflammation of the central airways leads to hypersecretion of mucus and abnormalities of the surface epithelium, including squamous metaplasia and increased goblet cells. Lymphoid follicles are often seen in the bronchial walls. The distal bronchi and bronchioles are scarred and often obliterated. The bronchial arteries increase in size to supply the inflamed bronchial wall and fibrous tissue. A vicious circle may be established, because a pool of mucus is liable to further infection, which leads to progressive destruction of the bronchial walls.

CLINICAL FEATURES: Patients with bronchiectasis have chronic productive cough, often with several hundred milliliters of mucopurulent sputum a day. Hemoptysis is common, as bronchial inflammation erodes through the walls of adjacent bronchial arteries. Dyspnea and wheezing are variable, depending on the extent of the disease. Pneumonia is a common complication, and patients with longstanding cases are at risk of chronic hypoxia and pulmonary hypertension. Radiologically, the bronchi appear dilated and have thickened walls. The definitive diagnosis is made by CT scans of the lung. Surgical treatment of localized bronchiectasis may be necessary, especially if complications such as severe hemoptysis or pneumonia arise. However, in the generalized disease, surgical resection is more palliative than curative.

Acute, reversible dilation of bronchi may occur as a consequence of bacterial or viral bronchopulmonary infection, and it may take months before the bronchi return to normal size.

Infections

Pulmonary infections are discussed in detail in Chapter 9. The major pulmonary entities are described below, with particular emphasis on pathologic features.

Bacterial Pneumonia is Inflammation and Consolidation of the Lung Parenchyma

Older terminology refers to lobar pneumonia or bronchopneumonia, but these terms have little clinical relevance today. In general, **lobar pneumonia** refers to consolidation of an entire lobe (Fig. 12-11) while **bronchopneumonia** is scattered solid foci in the same or several lobes (Fig. 12-12).

Streptococcus pneumoniae was the classic cause of lobar pneumonia, but today, largely due to antibiotic therapy, the involvement of a lobe tends to be incomplete, and more than one lobe is usually affected. By contrast, bronchopneumonia is still a common cause of death. It typically develops in terminally ill patients, usually in the dependent and posterior portions of the lung. Scattered irregular foci of pneumonia are centered on terminal bronchioles and respiratory bronchioles. Bronchiolitis is present, with exudation of polymorphonuclear leukocytes into the adjacent alveoli. Large continuous areas of alveolar involvement do not occur in bronchopneumonia.

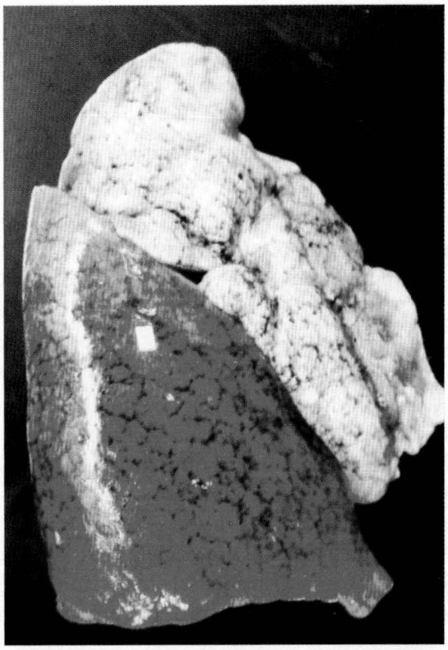

FIGURE 12-11. **Lobar pneumonia.** The entire left lower lobe is consolidated and in the stage of red hepatization. The upper lobe is normally expanded.

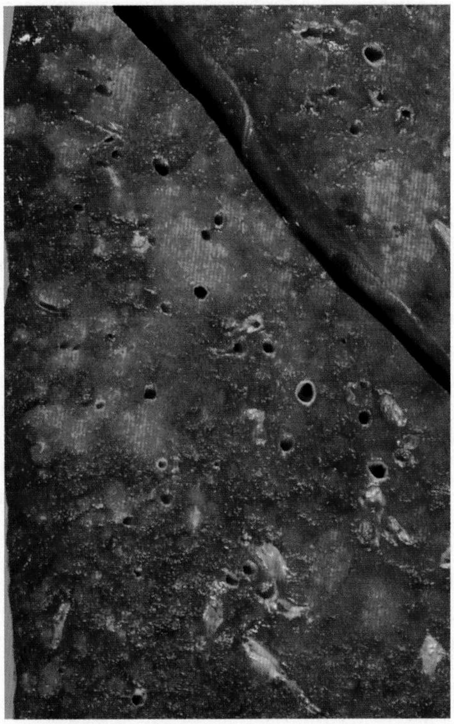

FIGURE 12-12. **Bronchopneumonia.** Scattered foci of consolidation are centered on bronchi and bronchioles.

Bacterial pneumonias occur in three settings:

- **Community-acquired pneumonia** arises outside the hospital in persons with no primary disorder of the immune system.
- **Nosocomial pneumonia** represents an infection spread by organisms in the hospital environment to particularly susceptible patients.
- **Opportunistic pneumonia** afflicts persons whose immune status is compromised.

PATHOGENESIS: Most bacteria that cause pneumonia are normal inhabitants of the oropharynx and nasopharynx and reach alveoli by aspiration of secretions. Other routes of infection include inhalation from the environment, hematogenous dissemination from an infectious focus elsewhere and (rarely) spread of bacteria from an adjacent site. A change in oropharyngeal flora from the normal commensals to a virulent organism often precedes the development of pneumonia. A number of conditions predispose to infection by depressing the host defenses, including cigarette smoking, chronic bronchitis, alcoholism, severe malnutrition, wasting diseases and poorly controlled diabetes. Alterations in oropharyngeal flora commonly occur in debilitated or immunosuppressed patients in the hospital, in whom nosocomial pneumonia can occur in as many as 25%.

Bacterial pneumonias should be classified on the basis of the etiologic agent, because clinical and morphologic features, and thus therapies, often vary with the causative organism.

Pneumococcal Pneumonia

Despite the impact of antibiotic therapy, pneumonia caused by *Streptococcus pneumoniae* (pneumococcus) remains a significant problem. Pneumococcal pneumonia is principally a disease of young to middle-aged adults. It is rare in infants, less common in the elderly, and considerably more frequent in men than in women.

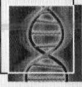

PATHOGENESIS: Pneumococcal pneumonia is mostly a consequence of altered defense barriers in the respiratory tract. Frequently this pneumonia follows a viral infection of the upper respiratory tract (e.g., influenza). The bronchial secretions stimulated by a viral infection provide a hospitable environment for proliferation of *S. pneumoniae*, which are normal flora of the nasopharynx. The thin, watery secretions carry the organisms into the alveoli, thereby initiating an inflammatory response. The remarkably severe acute inflammation with spreading edema suggests that immunologic mechanisms may be involved. The aspiration of pneumococci is also promoted by factors that impair the epiglottic reflex, including exposure to cold, anesthesia, and alcohol intoxication. Lung injury caused by factors such as congestive heart failure and irritant gases also renders the lung more susceptible to pneumococcal pneumonia.

The capsule of the pneumococcus provides a defense against phagocytosis by the alveolar macrophages, and the organisms must, therefore, be opsonized before they can be ingested and killed. In an immune-competent person, antipneumococcal antibodies function as opsonins, but a host not previously exposed to the specific infecting strain of *S. pneumoniae* must use the alternative complement pathway to opsonize the bacteria.

PATHOLOGY: In the earliest stage of pneumococcal pneumonia, protein-rich edema fluid containing numerous organisms fills the alveoli (Fig. 12-13). Marked capillary congestion leads to massive outpouring of polymorphonuclear leukocytes and intra-alveolar hemorrhage (Fig. 12-14). Because the firm consistency of the affected lung is reminiscent of the liver, this stage has been aptly named "red hepatization" (see Fig. 12-13).

The next phase, occurring after 2 or more days, depending on the success of treatment, involves lysis of polymorphonuclear leukocytes and appearance of macrophages, which phagocytose the fragmented neutrophils and other inflammatory debris. At this stage, the congestion has diminished, but the lung is still firm ("grey hepatization") (see Fig. 12-13). The alveolar exudate is then removed and the lung gradually returns to normal.

A number of complications may follow pneumococcal pneumonia:

- **Pleuritis,** often painful, is common, because the pneumonia readily extends to the pleura.
- **Pleural effusion** occurs frequently, but usually resolves.
- **Pyothorax** results from an infection of a pleural effusion and may heal with extensive fibrosis.
- **Empyema** (a loculated collection of pus with fibrous walls) results from the persistence of pyothorax.
- **Bacteremia** is present in more than 25% of patients in the early stages of pneumococcal pneumonia and may lead to endocarditis or meningitis. Patients whose spleens have been removed often die of this bacteremia.
- **Pulmonary fibrosis** is a rare complication in which the intraalveolar exudate becomes organized and forms intraalveolar plugs of granulation tissue, also known as **organizing pneumonia**. Gradually, increasing alveolar fibrosis leads to a shrunken and firm lobe, a rare complication known as **carnification**.
- **Lung abscess** is an unusual complication of pneumococcal pneumonia.

CLINICAL FEATURES: The onset of pneumococcal pneumonia is acute, with fever and chills. Chest pain secondary to pleural involvement is common. Hemoptysis is frequent and is characteristically "rusty," because it is derived from altered blood in alveolar spaces. Radiologic examination shows alveolar filling in large areas of lung, producing a solid appearance that extends to entire lobes or segments. Before antibiotic therapy, the clinical course was characterized by severe fever, dyspnea, debility, and even loss of consciousness. The dramatic event was the **crisis**, 5 to 10 days after the onset of respiratory symptoms, when a moribund patient would suddenly become afebrile and return from Death's door. Satisfactory resolution of a crisis was the result of the immune response to the infection. Unfortunately, the outcome was often not favorable, and in one third of cases, the patient

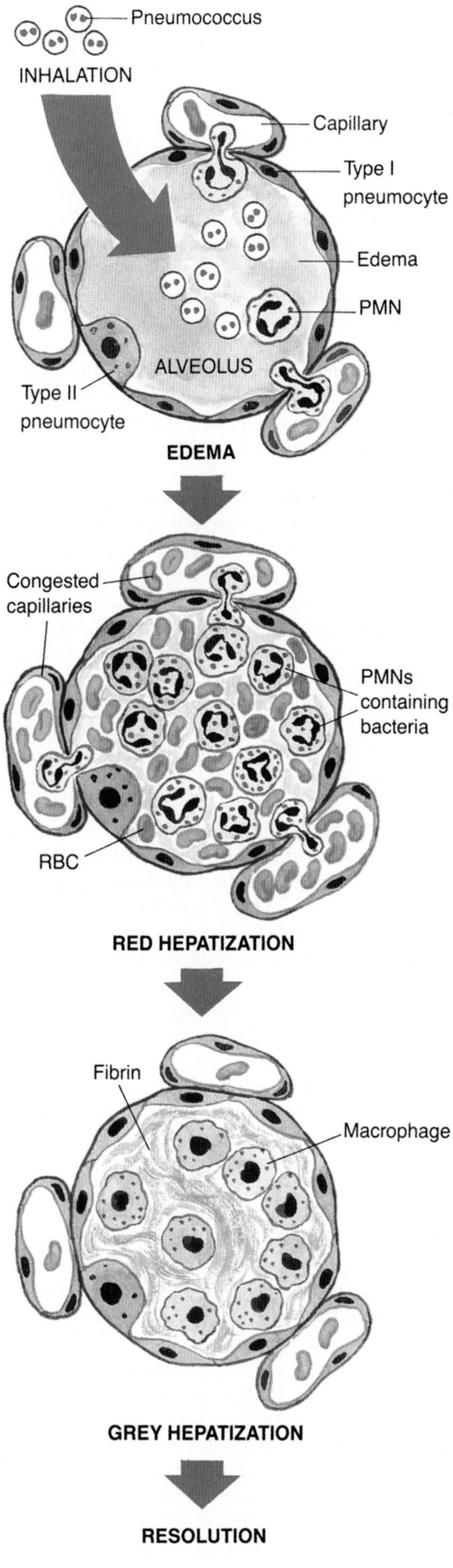

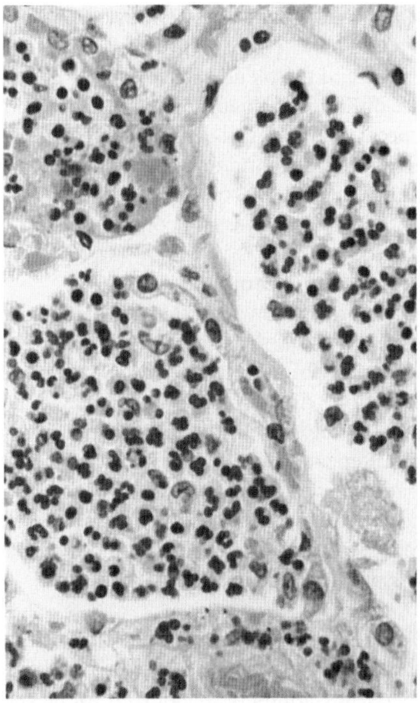

FIGURE 12-14. **Pneumococcal pneumonia.** The alveoli are packed with an exudate composed of polymorphonuclear leukocytes and occasional macrophages.

died. In the modern era, pneumococcal pneumonia is treated effectively with antibiotics. Although symptoms of pneumonia respond rapidly to antibiotics, radiologically, the lesion still takes several days to resolve.

Klebsiella Pneumonia

Other than *S. pneumoniae, Klebsiella pneumoniae* is the only organism that causes lobar pneumonia with any frequency. However, it accounts for no more than 1% of all cases of community-acquired pneumonia. The disease is commonly associated with alcoholism and is seen most frequently in middle-aged men, although persons with diabetes and chronic pulmonary disease are also at risk.

PATHOLOGY: The stages in *Klebsiella* pneumonia are not so well described as those in pneumococcal pneumonia, but the congestion and hemorrhage in the acute phase are less pronounced. *K. pneumoniae* has a thick, gelatinous capsule, which feature is responsible for the characteristic mucoid appearance of the cut surface of the lung. Another distinctive characteristic of *Klebsiella* pneumonia is that the affected lobe increases in size, so that the fissure "bulges" toward the unaffected region. There is a tendency toward tissue

FIGURE 12-13. **Pathogenesis of pneumococcal lobar pneumonia.** Pneumococci, characteristically in pairs (diplococci), multiply rapidly in the alveolar spaces and produce extensive edema. They incite an acute inflammatory response in which polymorphonuclear leukocytes and congestion are prominent (red hepatization). As the inflammatory process progresses, macrophages replace the polymorphonuclear leukocytes and ingest debris (grey hepatization). The process usually resolves, but complications may ensue. PMN =polymorphonuclearneutrophil; RBC = red blood cell.

necrosis and abscess formation. A serious complication is **bronchopleural fistula**, (i.e., a communication between the bronchial airway and the pleural space).

The onset of *Klebsiella* pneumonia is less dramatic than that of pneumococcal pneumonia, but the disease may be more dangerous. Before the antibiotic era, mortality rates in *Klebsiella* pneumonia ranged from 50% to 80%. Even with prompt antibiotic treatment, the mortality is still considerable.

Staphylococcal Pneumonia

Community-acquired staphylococcal pneumonia is uncommon, accounting for only 1% of these bacterial pneumonias. However, pulmonary infection with *Staphylococcus aureus* is a common superinfection after influenza and other viral respiratory tract infections. In the 1918 influenza pandemic, it was a major cause of death. Repeated episodes of staphylococcal pneumonia are seen in patients with cystic fibrosis, owing to colonization of the bronchiectatic airways. Nosocomial staphylococcal pneumonia typically occurs in weakened, chronically ill patients, who are prone to aspiration, and in intubated persons.

PATHOLOGY: Like staphylococcal infection elsewhere, staphylococcal pneumonia is characterized by abscess development. In contrast to the classic solitary lung abscess, the multiple foci of staphylococcal pneumonia produce many small abscesses. In infants and, to a lesser extent, in adults, these may lead to **pneumatoceles**, thin-walled cystic spaces lined primarily by respiratory tissue. Pneumatoceles may expand rapidly and compress surrounding lung or rupture into the pleural cavity and cause a tension pneumothorax. A pneumatocele develops when an abscess breaks into an airway, allowing expansion of the former by the pressure of inspired air. Cavitation and pleural effusions are common complications of staphylococcal pneumonia, but empyema is infrequent.

Staphylococcal pneumonia requires aggressive therapy, particularly because *S. aureus* is often antibiotic-resistant.

Other Streptococcal Pneumonias

Pulmonary infection with group A *Streptococcus pyogenes* was identified among soldiers as early as the 19th century, and its pathologic features were described during World War I. Streptococcal pneumonia typically follows viral respiratory tract infections and is thought to have been a common superinfection in the 1918–1919 influenza pandemic. It is distinctly unusual in a community setting but is occasionally encountered in debilitated persons.

PATHOLOGY: On gross examination, the lungs of patients who die of streptococcal pneumonia are heavy and display bloody edema. Dry consolidation (hepatization) is not a feature of the disease. Microscopically, the alveoli are filled with fibrin-containing fluid, but neutrophils are few. After prolonged pneumonia, alveolar necrosis may be encountered. Empyema is a common complication.

CLINICAL FEATURES: Patients with streptococcal pneumonia have abrupt fever, dyspnea, cough, chest pain, hemoptysis, and often cyanosis. Radiologically, a pattern of bronchopneumonia is observed; lobar consolidation is not seen. Intensive antibiotic therapy is indicated.

Streptococcal pneumonia in the newborn is usually caused by group B streptococci *(Streptococcus agalactiae)*, a normal resident of the female genital tract. Symptoms are similar to those of the infantile respiratory distress syndrome. The infants, however, are often full term, have severe toxemia, and may die within a few hours.

Legionella Pneumonia

In 1976, a mysterious respiratory ailment that carried a high mortality broke out at an American Legion convention in Philadelphia. The responsible organism, *Legionella pneumophila*, was soon identified as a fastidious bacterium, with special requirements to grow in culture. Serologic and histologic studies revealed that several previously unrecognized epidemics of the same disease had occurred.

Legionella organisms thrive in aquatic environments and outbreaks of pneumonia have been traced to contaminated water in air-conditioning cooling towers, evaporative condensers, and construction sites. Person-to-person spread does not occur, and there is no animal or human reservoir.

PATHOLOGY: In fatal cases of *Legionella* pneumonia, multiple lobes exhibit a bronchopneumonia, with large confluent areas. Microscopically, alveoli contain fibrin and inflammatory cells, with either neutrophils or macrophages predominating. Necrosis of inflammatory cells (leukocytoclasis) may be extensive. If the patient survives for several weeks, the exudate may show fibrous organization. One third of cases have been complicated by empyema. *Legionella* organisms are usually abundant within and outside the phagocytic cells. They are gram-negative but are difficult to visualize with conventional stains. Silver impregnation and immunofluorescent stains show them well.

CLINICAL FEATURES: The onset of *Legionella* pneumonia tends to be abrupt, with malaise, fever, muscle aches and pains and, curiously, abdominal pain. A productive cough is usual, and chest pain due to pleuritis occasionally occurs. The chest radiograph is variable, but the most common pattern shows focal alveolar infiltrates, which may be bilateral. Symptoms are usually less severe than chest radiographs suggest. Mortality has been high (10%–20%), especially in immunocompromised patients. Erythromycin is the antibiotic of choice.

Pontiac fever, also caused by *Legionella* species, is mainly a febrile illness with slight respiratory symptoms, radiologic abnormalities, and a good prognosis. It has occurred in epidemics in office buildings and affects apparently healthy persons.

Opportunistic Pneumonia Caused by Gram-Negative Bacteria

Pneumonias caused by gram-negative organisms have become more common with the advent of immunosuppressive and cytotoxic therapies, treatment with broad-spectrum antibiotics, and acquired immunodeficiency syndrome (AIDS). The most common bacteria are *Escherichia coli* and *Pseudomonas aeruginosa*.

ESCHERICHIA COLI: Pneumonia caused by *E. coli* is a recognized complication of bacteremia after gastrointestinal and urogenital surgery, even in patients who are not immunosuppressed. It also is encountered in cancer patients given chemotherapy and in persons with chronic lung or heart disease. It occurs as a bronchopneumonia and responds poorly to treatment.

PSEUDOMONAS AERUGINOSA: *Pseudomonas* pneumonia is most often seen in immunocompromised persons, in patients with burns, and in those with cystic fibrosis. A history of antibiotic treatment of another infection is common. Often an infectious vasculitis, in which large numbers of organisms can be seen in the wall of a blood vessel, results in pulmonary infarction. *Pseudomonas* infection is common in people with cystic fibrosis. Antibiotic treatment of *Pseudomonas* pneumonia is often unsatisfactory.

Pneumonia Caused by Anaerobic Organisms

Many anaerobic organisms are normal commensals of the oral cavity, especially in patients with poor dental hygiene. These include certain streptococci, fusobacteria, and *Bacteroides* species. Aspiration of these organisms commonly occurs with swallowing disorders, as in stuporous alcoholics, anesthetized patients, and persons subject to seizures. Pulmonary infection with anaerobic organisms leads to necrotizing pneumonias, which are frequently complicated by lung abscesses. The most dramatic complication is gangrene of the lung, a result of thrombosis of a branch of the pulmonary artery and consequent infarction. This is a medical emergency and requires resection of the affected lung.

Psittacosis

Psittacosis is a pulmonary infection that results from the inhalation of **Chlamydia psittaci** *in dust contaminated with excreta from birds, usually pets and often parrots.* It is characterized by severe systemic symptoms, with fever, malaise, and muscle aches, but surprisingly few respiratory symptoms other than cough. Chest radiographs may be negative, and when abnormal, they show irregular consolidation and an interstitial pattern. The morphologic patterns in most cases are unknown, but the disease is likely to be an interstitial pneumonia. In fatal cases, varying degrees of diffuse alveolar damage are present, together with edema, intra-alveolar pneumonia, and necrosis.

Anthrax Pneumonia and Pneumonic Plague

Recent world events have refocused a great deal of attention toward infectious agents that may be used as potential weapons of bioterrorism. Chief among these are *Bacillus anthracis* and *Yersinia pestis*.

B. anthracis, the causative agent of anthrax, is a gram-positive, spore-forming bacillus. Anthrax occurs in many species of domestic animals, and infection of humans is seen infrequently or in sporadic outbreaks. Transmission is via direct contact with the spores. Person-to-person transmission is uncommon. Cutaneous anthrax is rarely fatal, whereas inhalational anthrax has a high mortality. Anthrax spores are highly resistant to drying, and when inhaled they are transported to mediastinal lymph nodes. From there, bacilli emerge and rapidly disseminate through the bloodstream to other organs, including the lungs. Hemorrhagic necrosis of infected organs ensues, the most pronounced of which is a hemorrhagic mediastinal mass. In the lungs, the disease is manifested by hemorrhagic bronchitis and confluent areas of hemorrhagic pneumonia.

Y. pestis, the causative agent of *plague,* produces two forms of infection, a bubonic form and a pneumonic form. In pneumonic plague the organisms are inhaled directly without transmission by an arthropod vector, and the disease may be spread from person to person. The lungs typically show extensive hemorrhagic bronchopneumonia, pleuritis and enlargement of mediastinal lymph nodes. The untreated disease progresses rapidly and is highly fatal.

Mycoplasma Pneumoniae Causes Atypical Pneumonia

In contrast to lobar pneumonia, the onset of atypical pneumonia is insidious, leukocytosis is absent or slight and the course is prolonged. Respiratory symptoms may be minimal or severe, and the chest radiograph shows a patchy intra-alveolar pneumonia or an interstitial infiltrate. The infection characteristically causes a bronchiolitis with a neutrophilic intraluminal exudate and an intense lymphoplasmacytic infiltrate in the bronchiolar wall (Fig. 12-15). *Mycoplasma* lack the rigid cell wall characteristic of most bacteria and are thus slow growing and often difficult to isolate by traditional culture methods. The diagnosis is often established clinically on the basis of serologic studies detecting *M. pneumoniae* antibodies or cold agglutinins. Erythromycin is effective, and the infection is only rarely fatal.

Tuberculosis Is the Classic Granulomatous Infection

Known since ancient Egypt, tuberculosis became the scourge of 19th century Europe and North America. There was an exponential decline in its prevalence in the 20th century, and the advent of antituberculosis drugs has further diminished the impact of the disease. However, there has been a recent resurgence of tuberculosis and the emergence of drug-resistant strains, particularly among patients with AIDS. The infection is discussed in detail in Chapter 9, and here we consider only the pulmonary pathology.

Tuberculosis represents infection with *Mycobacterium tuberculosis,* although atypical mycobacterial infections may mimic tuberculosis. The disease is divided into primary and secondary (or reactivation) tuberculosis.

PRIMARY TUBERCULOSIS: The disease is acquired from the initial exposure to *M. tuberculosis,* most commonly as a result of inhaling infected aerosols generated when a person with cavitary tuberculosis coughs. The inhaled organisms multiply in the alveoli because the alveolar macrophages cannot readily kill the bacteria.

PATHOLOGY: The **Ghon complex** is the first lesion of primary tuberculosis and consists of a peripheral parenchymal granuloma, often in the upper lobes. When it is associated with an enlarged mediastinal lymph node a **Ranke complex** is formed (Fig. 12-16). On gross examination, the healed, subpleural Ghon nodule is 1 to 2 cm in diameter, well

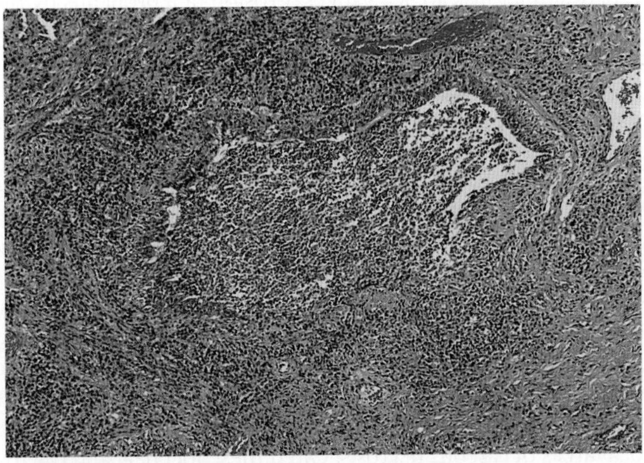

FIGURE 12-15. **Mycoplasma pneumonia.** Chronic bronchiolitis with a neutrophilic luminal exudate.

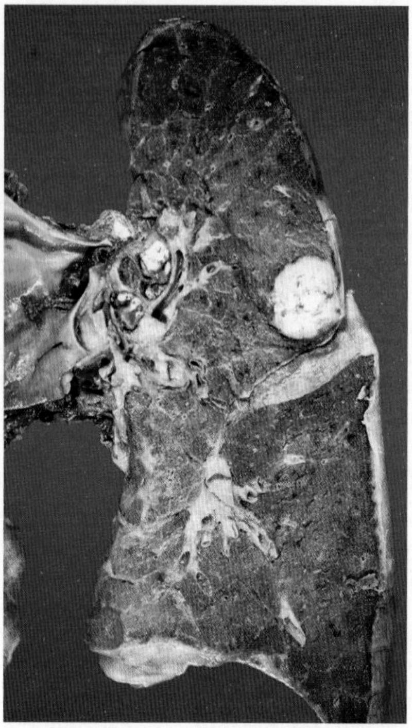

FIGURE 12-16. **Primary tuberculosis.** A healed Ranke complex is represented by a subpleural nodule and involved hilar lymph nodes.

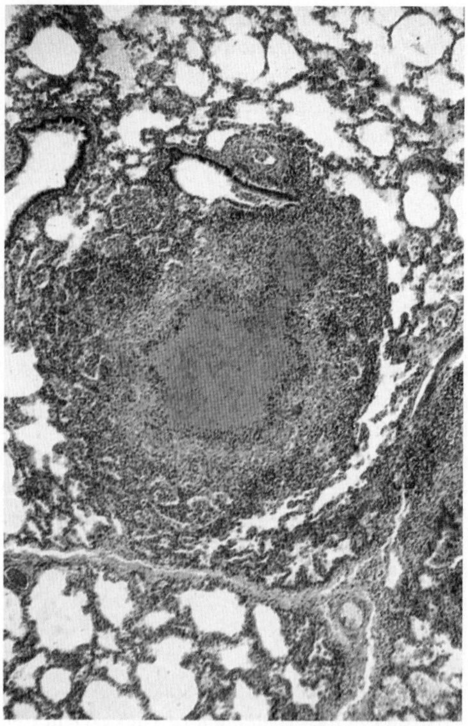

FIGURE 12-17. **Necrotizing granuloma due to *Mycobacterium tuberculosis*.** A small tuberculous granuloma with conspicuous central caseation is present in the pulmonary parenchyma. The necrotic center is surrounded by histiocytes, giant cells. and fibrous tissue.

circumscribed, and centrally necrotic. In later stages, it is fibrotic and calcified. Microscopically, a granuloma with central caseous necrosis (Fig. 12-17) shows varying degrees of fibrosis. The microscopic features of draining hilar lymph nodes are similar to those of the peripheral parenchymal lesion.

Most (90% or more) primary infections are asymptomatic, and lesions remain localized and heal. In some instances there is self-limited extension to the pleura, with secondary pleural effusion. Less commonly, primary tuberculosis does not remain limited but spreads to other parts of the lung (**progressive primary tuberculosis**). This usually happens in young children or immunosuppressed adults. The initial lesion enlarges, producing necrotic areas up to 6 cm or more in greatest dimension. Central liquefaction results in cavities, which may expand to occupy most of the lower lobe. At the same time, draining lymph nodes display similar histologic changes. Erosion of a bronchus by the necrotizing process leads to further pulmonary dissemination of the disease.

SECONDARY TUBERCULOSIS: This stage represents either reactivation of primary pulmonary tuberculosis or a new infection in a host previously sensitized by primary tuberculosis.

PATHOLOGY: The initial reaction to *M. tuberculosis* is different in secondary tuberculosis. A cellular immune response occurs after a latent interval and leads to formation of many granulomas and extensive tissue necrosis. The apical and posterior segments of the upper lobes are most commonly involved, but the superior segment of the lower lobe is also often affected, and no part of the lung can be excluded. A diffuse, fibrotic, poorly defined lesion develops, which displays focal areas of caseous necrosis. Often these foci heal and calcify, but some erode into a bronchus, after which drainage of infectious material creates a tuberculous cavity.

Tuberculous cavities range in size from under 1 cm in diameter to large, cystic areas occupying almost the entire lung. Most measure 3 to 10 cm in diameter and tend to be situated in the apices of the upper lobes (Fig. 12-18), although they may occur anywhere in the lung. The wall of the cavity is an inner, thin, gray membrane encompassing soft necrotic nodules; a middle zone of granulation tissue; and an outer collagenous border. The lumen is filled with caseous material containing acid-fast bacilli. The tuberculous cavity often communicates freely with a bronchus, and release of the infectious material into the airways spreads the infection within the lung. The walls of healed tuberculous cavities eventually become fibrotic and calcified.

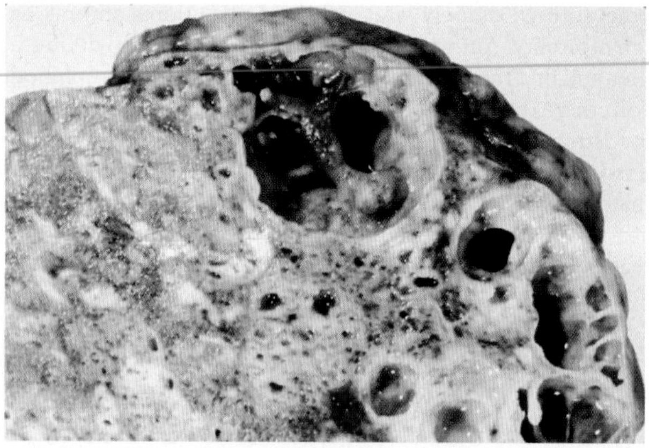

FIGURE 12-18. **Cavitary tuberculosis.** The apex of the left upper lobe shows tuberculous cavities surrounded by consolidated and fibrotic pulmonary parenchyma that contains small tubercles.

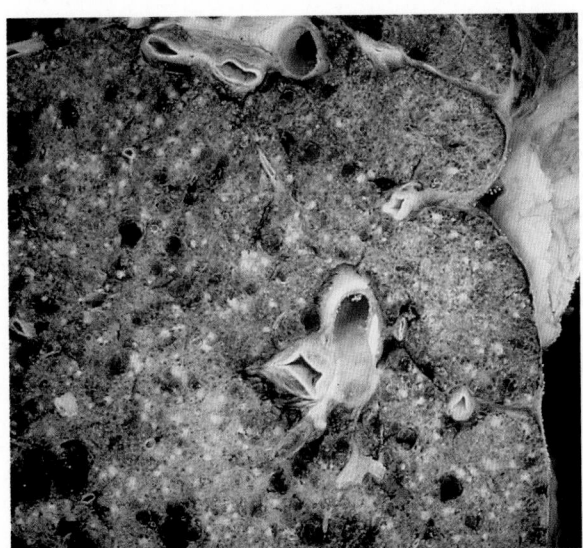

FIGURE 12-19. **Miliary tuberculosis.** Multiple millimeter-sized nodules are scattered throughout the lung parenchyma.

Secondary tuberculosis is associated with a number of complications:

- **Miliary tuberculosis** refers to the presence of multiple, small (size of millet seeds), tuberculous granulomas (Fig. 12-19) in many organs. It results from hematogenous dissemination of the organisms, usually from secondary pulmonary tuberculosis, but occasionally from primary pulmonary tuberculosis or from other sites.
- **Hemoptysis** is caused by erosion of small pulmonary arteries in the wall of a cavity. It may be severe enough to drown patients in their own blood.
- **Bronchopleural fistula** occurs when a subpleural cavity ruptures into the pleural space. In turn, tuberculous empyema and pneumothorax result.
- **Tuberculous laryngitis** is a consequence of coughing up infectious material.
- **Intestinal tuberculosis** may follow swallowing of the same tuberculous material.
- **Aspergilloma** is a fungal mass that follows superinfection of a persistent open cavity with *Aspergillus;* it may fill the entire cavity.

MYCOBACTERIUM AVIUM-INTRACELLULARE (MAI): In patients who have AIDS, the ability to mount a granulomatous reaction may be impaired, and MAI pneumonia is characterized by an extensive infiltrate of macrophages and innumerable acid-fast organisms (Fig. 12-20). MAI may colonize the airways of older, immunocompetent individuals with underlying pulmonary disorders such as bronchiectasis, or it may produce granulomatous inflammation with or without cavitation. *Mycobacterium kansasii* produces a spectrum of disease similar to MAI but is not as frequently encountered due to a more restricted geographic distribution.

Actinomycosis Features Multiple Lung Abscesses

Actinomycosis is caused by infection with actinomycetes, and the usual pulmonary organism is *Actinomyces israelii.* Although actinomycetes resemble fungi in appearance, they are anaerobic filamentous bacteria. These gram-positive organisms normally inhabit the mouth and nose, and infect the lung by aspiration of oropharyngeal contents or by extension from an actinomycotic subdiaphragmatic abscess or liver abscess.

PATHOLOGY: Lung lesions consist of multiple, interconnecting, small lung abscesses. The margin of an abscess is granulomatous, but the central necrotic area is purulent and contains colonies of organisms, which form "sulfur granules." The colonies consist of thin, branching, filamentous gram-positive bacteria. Clubbed basophilic filaments are noted at the margins of the colonies, which are visible to the naked eye as small yellow particles (sulfur granules). The abscesses invade the pleura and produce bronchopulmonary fistulas and empyema. They may also invade the chest wall.

Nocardia Is Usually an Opportunistic Organism

Nocardia is a gram-positive filamentous bacteria that causes an acute progressive or chronic bacterial pneumonia. It is frequently encountered in immunocompromised persons, particularly patients with lymphomas, neutropenia, chronic granulomatous disease of childhood and pulmonary alveolar proteinosis. *Nocardia asteroides* is the most common *Nocardia* species to cause pneumonia.

A

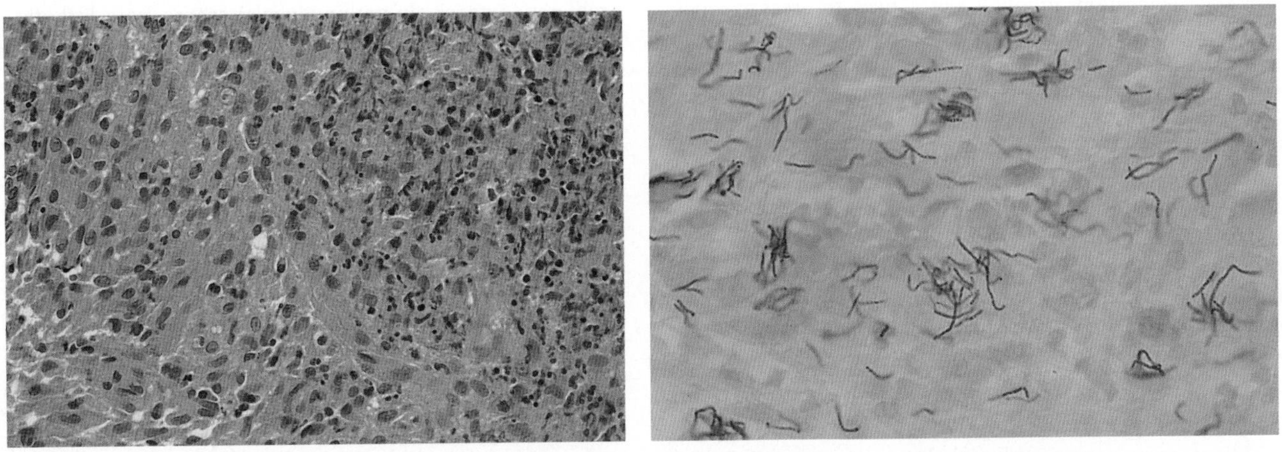

B

FIGURE 12-20. ***Mycobacterium avium-intracellulare* pneumonia in acquired immunodeficiency syndrome (AIDS). A.** The pneumonia is characterized by an extensive infiltrate of macrophages. **B.** The Ziehl-Neelsen stain shows numerous acid-fast organisms.

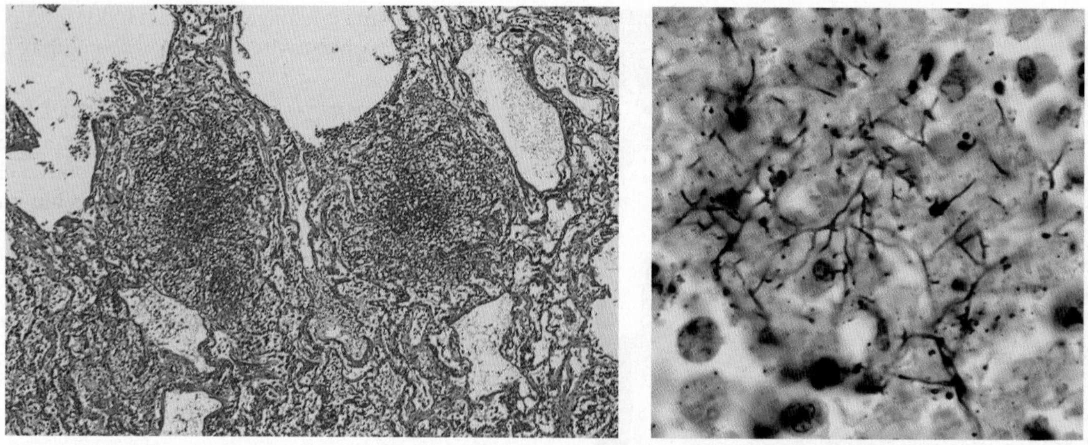

A B

FIGURE 12-21. **Nocardiosis. A.** This lung shows abscesses consisting of focal collections of acute inflammation. **B**. The organisms are thin, filamentous, branching bacteria (Gomori methenamine silver).

PATHOLOGY: Histologically, lungs show abscesses (Fig. 12-21A), which may have granulomatous features in chronic infections. The organisms are delicate, beaded, thin filaments, which branch mostly at right angles (see Fig. 12-21B). In tissue sections, the organisms are best seen with a Gram stain or Gomori methenamine silver stain (see Fig. 12-21B). They are also weakly acid fast.

Fungal Infections may be Geographic or Opportunistic

Histoplasmosis

Histoplasmosis is a disease of the midwestern and southeastern United States., particularly the Mississippi and Ohio river valleys. It is caused by inhalation of *Histoplasma capsulatum* in infected dust, commonly from bird droppings.

PATHOLOGY: Histoplasmosis has many clinical and pathologic similarities to tuberculosis. Most infections are asymptomatic and result in lesions comparable to the Ghon complex, including a parenchymal granuloma and similar lesions in the draining lymph nodes. The granulomas are particularly prone to calcify, often with a concentric laminar pattern. The acute phase, in which numerous organisms are seen within macrophages, is followed by granulomatous inflammation, with central areas of necrosis. The granulomas heal by fibrosis and calcification, although central necrotic areas may persist. The organisms are generally not visible on routine stains and are best seen with a silver stain. They are 2-4 μm in diameter, spherical in shape and exhibit narrow-based budding.

In a few cases, pulmonary lesions progress or reactivate, leading to a progressive fibrotic and necrotic lesion that closely resembles reactivation tuberculosis. However, the lesion of histoplasmosis is more fibrotic than that of tuberculosis and cavitation is less common. The reason for progression is not known, although a large infective dose and a poor host response are usually considered to be responsible. Immunocompromised persons are at particular risk for dissemination of *Histoplasma* within the lungs and spread to other organs.

Coccidioidomycosis

Coccidioidomycosis, caused by inhalation of spores of *Coccidioides immitis,* was originally known as San Joaquin Valley fever, after the location where the disease has been endemic for many years. However, the infection is widespread throughout the southwestern part of the United States and shares many of the clinical and pathologic features of histoplasmosis and tuberculosis. In histologic sections the organism is a spherule, 30-100 μm in diamter, and exhibits a thick refractile wall. The spherules contain innumerable endospores 2–5μm in diameter. Empty spherules or endospores which have been released into the tissue may also be visible.

PATHOLOGY: In most instances, lesions are limited to a peripheral parenchymal granuloma, with or without lymph node granulomas. In a few instances, the lesion may be slowly progressive. Immunocompromised persons may experience rapid progression of the disease, with release of endospores into the lung, in which case the tissue reaction may be purulent as well as granulomatous.

Cryptococcosis

Cryptococcosis results from inhalation of spores of *Cryptococcus neoformans,* which is often found in pigeon droppings. Lung lesions range from small parenchymal granulomas to several large granulomatous nodules, pneumonic consolidation, and even cavitation. Most serious cases of pulmonary cryptococcosis occur in immunocompromised persons, in whom the organisms proliferate extensively within alveolar spaces, with little tissue reaction. *Cryptococcus* organisms are typically 4–6 μm in diameter, but may be larger, and show narrow-based budding and a thick mucoid capsule.

North American Blastomycosis

Blastomycosis is an uncommon condition caused by *Blastomyces dermatitidis*. It is concentrated in the basins of the Missouri, Mississippi, and Ohio rivers in the United States and in southern Manitoba and northwestern Ontario in Canada. The clinical and pathologic features resemble those associated with the fungi mentioned earlier. The infection manifests as a lesion resembling a Ghon complex or as a progressive pneumonitis. Unlike the tuberculous Ghon complex, the focal lesion of blastomycosis exhibits central necrosis with a purulent reaction, surrounded by granulomatous inflammation. *Blastomyces* organisms are 8–15 μm in diameter, have a thick refractile wall and are characterized by broad-based budding.

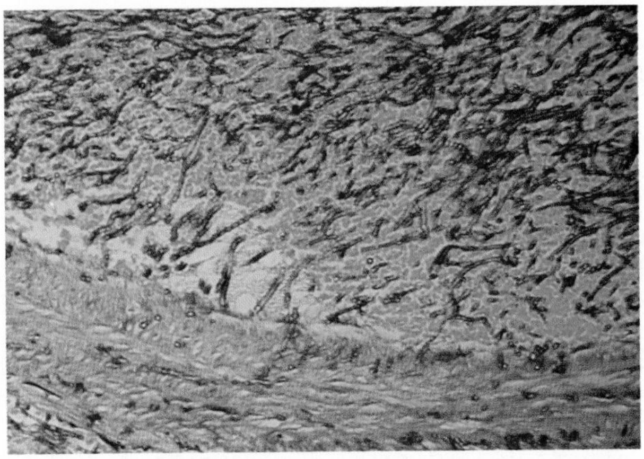

FIGURE 12-22. **Invasive pulmonary aspergillosis.** A branch of the pulmonary artery shows fungal hyphae in the wall and within the lumen.

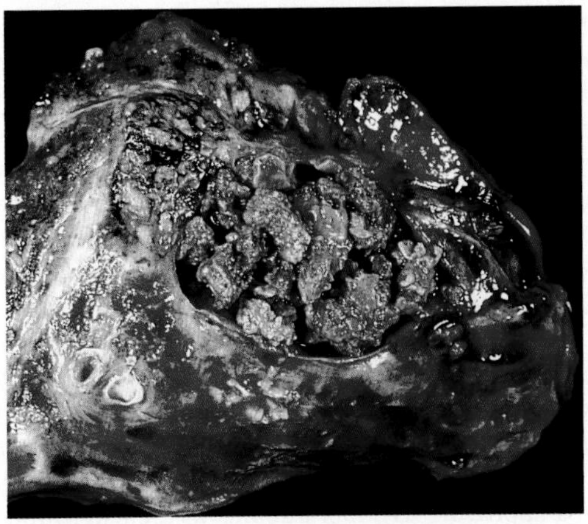

FIGURE 12-23. ***Aspergillus* fungus ball.** The lung contains a cavity filled with a fungus ball.

Aspergillosis

Infection of the lungs by *Aspergillus* species, usually *Aspergillus niger* or *Aspergillus fumigatus,* can occur under a number of circumstances.

- **Invasive aspergillosis:** This is the most serious form of *Aspergillus* infection, occurring almost exclusively as an opportunistic infection in persons with compromised immunity, usually due to cytotoxic therapy or AIDS. The lungs exhibit patchy, multifocal areas of consolidation and occasionally cavities. Extensive blood vessel invasion (usually arterial [Fig. 12-22]) results in occlusion, thrombosis, and infarction of lung tissue. Invasive aspergillosis is a fulminant pulmonary infection that is not amenable to therapy.
- **Aspergilloma ("fungus ball" or mycetoma):** *Aspergillus* species may grow in preexisting cavities, such as those caused by tuberculosis or bronchiectasis. They proliferate to form a fungus ball within these cavities (Fig. 12-23). Radiologic examination shows a large mass within a cavity that is separated from the wall by air. In most instances, the fungus ball is clinically unrecognized and represents merely an interesting radiologic finding. However, sometimes it becomes clinically evident, the most important symptom being hemoptysis, owing either to the underlying condition, or less commonly, to fungal infection of the cavity wall.
- **Allergic bronchopulmonary aspergillosis (ABPA):** Certain asthmatic persons demonstrate an unusual immunologic reaction to *Aspergillus* characterized by (1) transient pulmonary infiltrates on chest radiographs, (2) eosinophilia of blood and sputum, (3) skin sensitivity and serum precipitins to *A. fumigatus,* and (4) increased serum IgE. Roentgenograms show thickened bronchial walls and mucous plugs in the bronchi.

PATHOLOGY: ABPA is invariably associated with proximal (central) bronchiectasis, involving segmental bronchi and the next two to four orders of subsegmental bronchi. Histologically, the lungs show bronchial and bronchiolar mucous plugs, infiltrates of eosinophils and Charcot-Leyden crystals (Fig. 12-24 A,B). Bronchocentric granulomatosis and eosinophilic pneumonia may be present. The bronchial mucus may contain septate, branching fungal hyphae, with 45° branching. Interestingly, the peripheral bronchial tree is spared.

CLINICAL FEATURES: Patients with ABPA have wheezing, chest pain, cough, and often produce thick mucous plugs. Administration of systemic corticosteroids usually controls the acute episode.

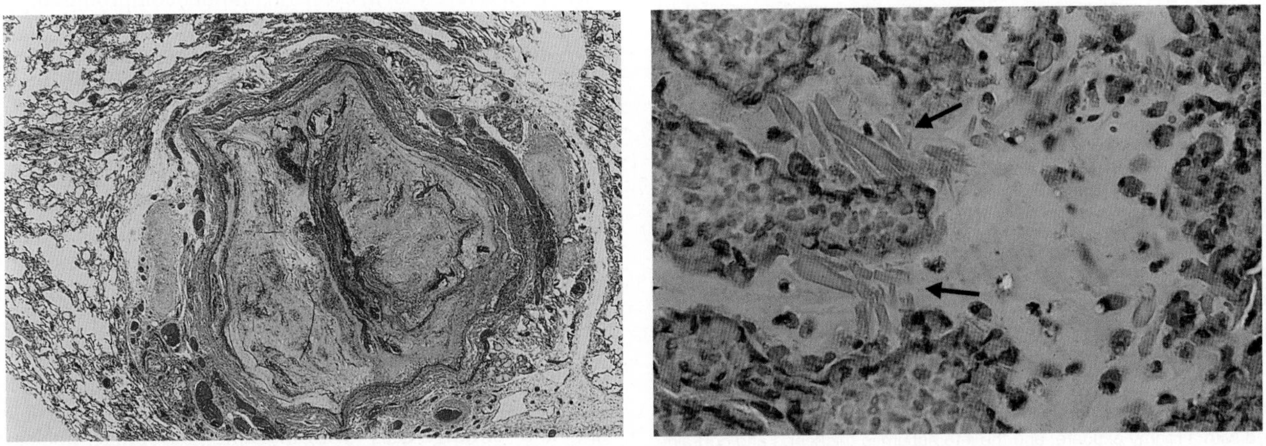

A B

FIGURE 12-24. **Allergic bronchopulmonary aspergillosis. A.** A dilated bronchus is filled with a mucous plug that has dense layers of eosinophilic infiltrates. **B.** Higher magnification shows numerous eosinophils and Charcot-Leyden crystals *(arrows).*

Pneumocystis jiroveci

First described as "plasma cell pneumonia," pulmonary infection with *Pneumocystis jiroveci* (formerly *Pneumocystis carinii*) was identified in malnourished infants at the end of World War II. It was increasingly recognized as the use of immunosuppression for renal transplantation and in the chemotherapy for malignant disease became common. *It is also a frequent cause of infectious pneumonia in patients with AIDS.* Once considered a protozoan, *Pneumocystis* has been reclassified as a fungus.

PATHOLOGY: The classic lesion of *Pneumocystis* pneumonia is an interstitial infiltrate of plasma cells and lymphocytes and hyperplasia of type II pneumocytes. Alveoli are filled with a characteristic foamy exudate, the organisms appearing as small bubbles in a background of proteinaceous exudate (Fig. 12-25A). With silver impregnation, cysts appear as round or indented ("crescent moon") bodies, 5 μm in diameter (see Fig. 12-25B). A darkly stained focus represents focal thickening of the capsule. After sporozoites develop within the cyst, it ruptures and assumes an indented shape. Sporozoites develop into trophozoites, which may be seen with stains such as Giemsa in cytology specimens; they are very difficult to see in routine histologic sections. Granulomatous inflammation in *Pneumocystis* pneumonia is rare but may be seen in up to 5% of lung biopsies from human immunodeficiency virus (HIV)-infected patients. Pneumocystis may also produce diffuse alveolar damage (see below) in some cases.

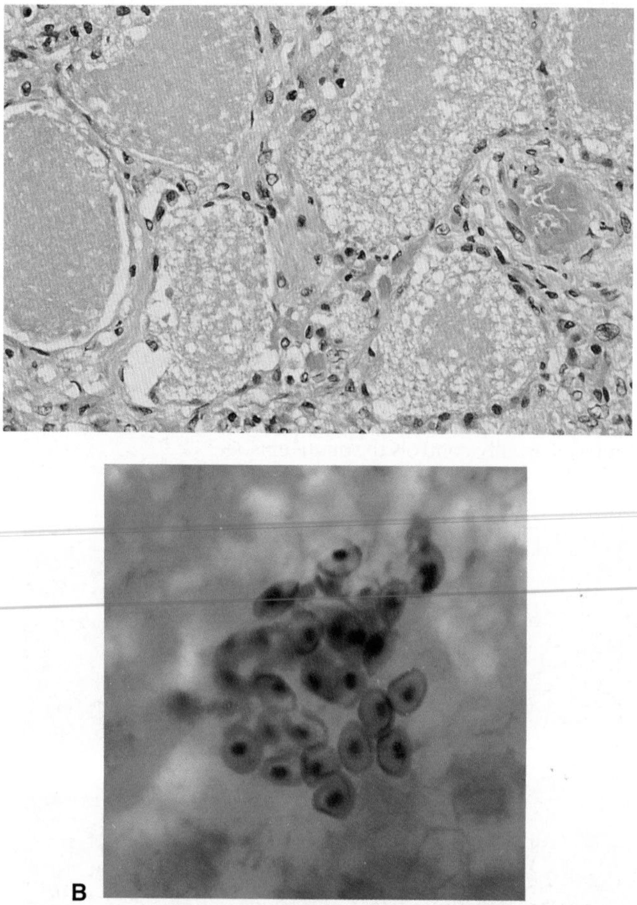

FIGURE 12-25. ***Pneumocystis jiroveci* pneumonia. A.** The alveoli are filled with a foamy exudate, and the interstitium is thickened and contains a chronic inflammatory infiltrate. **B.** A centrifuged bronchoalveolar lavage specimen impregnated with silver shows a cluster of *Pneumocystis* cysts.

CLINICAL FEATURES: Clinically and radiologically, the presentation of *Pneumocystis* pneumonia is variable. At one extreme, the symptoms are minimal; at the other, there is rapidly progressive respiratory failure. In HIV-infected patients, thin-walled cysts may develop and predispose to pneumothorax. The diagnosis is made by identifying the organism with a variety of procedures including sputum examination, bronchoalveolar lavage, transbronchial biopsy, needle aspiration of the lung, and open-lung biopsy. Treatment is with trimethoprim–sulfamethoxazole or pentamidine.

Viral Infections of the Lung Produce Diffuse Alveolar Damage or Interstitial Pneumonia

PATHOLOGY: Viral infections initially affect the alveolar epithelium and result in a mononuclear infiltrate in the interstitium of the lung (Fig. 12-26). Necrosis of type I epithelial cells and the formation of hyaline membranes result in an appearance that is indistinguishable from diffuse alveolar damage from other causes. In some instances, alveolar damage may be indolent, and the disease is characterized by hyperplasia of type II pneumocytes and interstitial inflammation. This appearance contrasts with that of most bacterial infections, in which an intra-alveolar exudates predominate and the interstitium is only incidentally involved (Fig. 12-27).

Cytomegalovirus produces a characteristic interstitial pneumonia that features an intense interstitial lymphocytic infiltrate. The alveoli are lined by type II cells that have regenerated to cover the epithelial defect left by necrosis of type I cells. The infected alveolar cells are very large (cytomegaly) with a single, dark, basophilic nuclear inclusion with a peripheral halo and multiple indistinct cytoplasmic, basophilic inclusions (Fig. 12-28).

Measles infection, which involves both the airways and the parenchyma, is characterized by very large (100 μm across) multinucleated giant cells that have nuclear inclusions and large eosinophilic cytoplasmic inclusions (Fig. 12-29). Although interstitial pneumonia is a well-characterized complication of measles, it is rarely fatal, except in immunocompromised, previously unexposed persons.

Varicella infection (both chickenpox and herpes zoster) produces disseminated, focally necrotic lesions in the lung, as well as interstitial pneumonia. Pulmonary involvement is usually asymptomatic, except in immunocompromised hosts, in whom it may be fatal. The viral inclusions are nuclear, eosinophilic, and refractile and are surrounded by a clear halo. Multinucleation can occur.

Herpes simplex can cause a necrotizing tracheobronchitis as well as diffuse alveolar damage. The viral inclusions are identical to those seen in varicella infection.

Adenovirus pneumonia results in a necrotizing bronchiolitis and bronchopneumonia. It can cause two types of nuclear inclusions: eosinophilic nuclear inclusions surrounded by a clear halo and "smudge cells" with indistinct, basophilic, nuclear inclusions that fill the entire nucleus and are surrounded by only a thin rim of chromatin (Fig. 12-30).

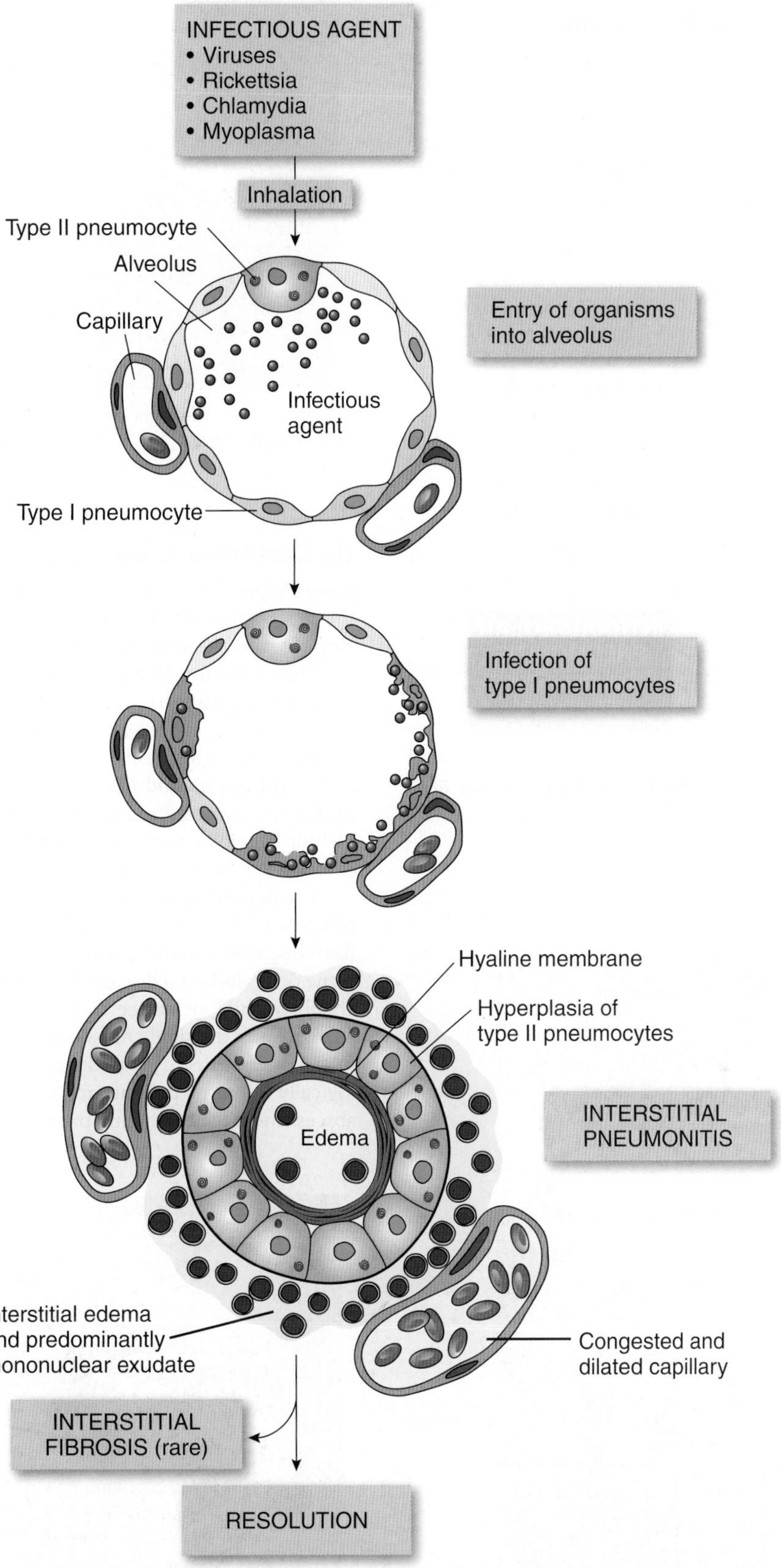

FIGURE 12-26. **Pathogenesis of interstitial pneumonia.** Although interstitial pneumonia is most commonly caused by viruses, other organisms also may cause significant interstitial inflammation. Type I cells are the most sensitive to damage, and loss of their integrity leads to intraalveolar edema. The proteinaceous exudate and cell debris form hyaline membranes, and type II cells multiply to line the alveoli. Interstitial inflammation is characterized mainly by mononuclear cells. The disease generally resolves completely but occasionally progresses to interstitial fibrosis.

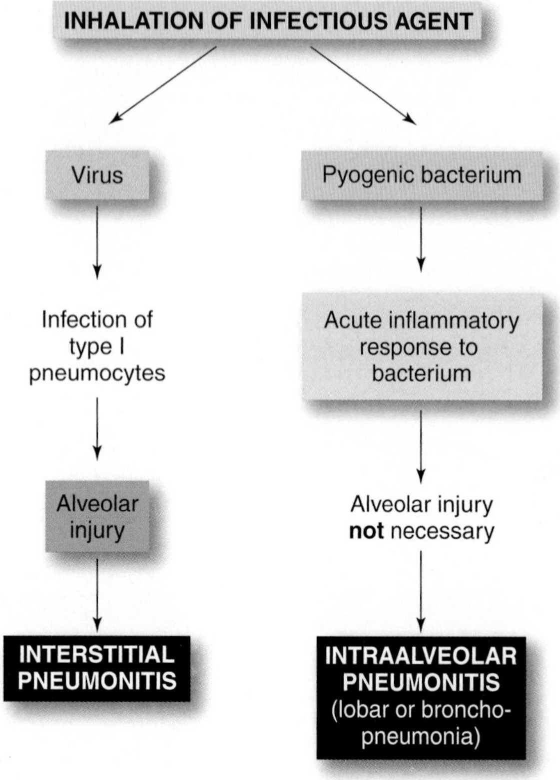

FIGURE 12-27. **Pathogenesis of interstitial and intraalveolar pneumonitis.**

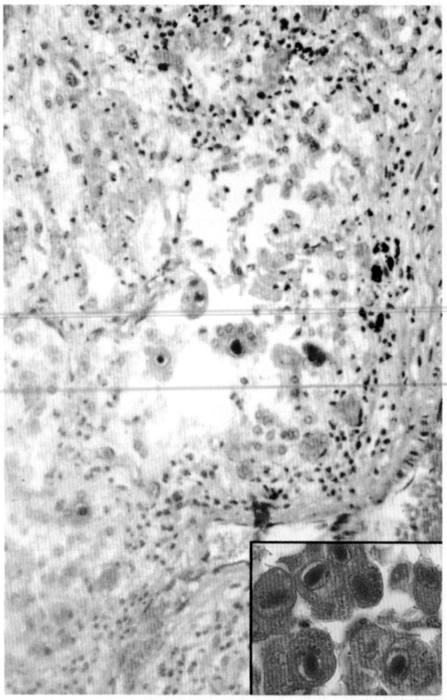

FIGURE 12-28. **Cytomegalovirus pneumonitis.** The infected alveolar cells are enlarged and display the typical dark-blue nuclear inclusions. *Inset:* A higher-power view shows infected alveolar cells that display a single basophilic nuclear inclusion with a perinuclear halo and multiple, indistinct, basophilic, cytoplasmic inclusions.

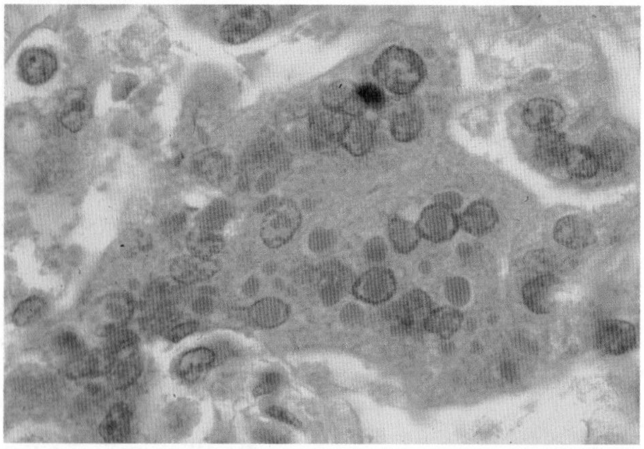

FIGURE 12-29. **Measles pneumonitis.** This multinucleated giant cell shows single, eosinophilic, refractile inclusions within each of the nuclei, as well as multiple, irregular, eosinophilic, cytoplasmic inclusions.

The Most Common Cause of Lung Abscess is Aspiration

Lung abscess is a localized accumulation of pus accompanied by the destruction of pulmonary parenchyma, including alveoli, airways, and blood vessels.

The aspiration that leads to pulmonary abscesses often occurs in the setting of depressed consciousness. Over 90% of lung abscesses reflect aspiration of anaerobic bacteria from the oropharynx. Infections are typically polymicrobial, with fusiform bacteria and *Bacteroides* species often isolated. Other organisms encountered in lung abscesses caused by aspiration include *Staphylococcus aureus, Klebsiella pneumoniae, Streptococcus pneumoniae,* and *Nocardia*.

The deposition of enough bacteria to produce a lung abscess requires two conditions. A large number of anaerobic bacteria must be present in the oral flora, as in persons with poor oral hygiene or periodontal disease. In addition, the cough reflex or tracheobronchial clearance must be impaired. Not surprisingly, alcoholism is the single most common condition predisposing to lung abscess. Persons with drug overdose, epileptics, and neurologically impaired patients are also at risk. Other causes of lung abscess include necrotizing pneumonias, bronchial obstruction,

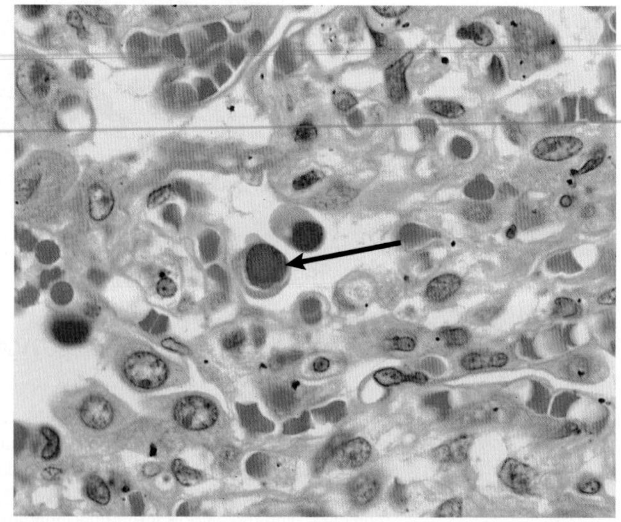

FIGURE 12-30. **Adenovirus pneumonia.** The "smudge" cell in the center (*arrow*) consists of a smudgy basophilic nuclear inclusion.

infected pulmonary emboli, penetrating trauma, and extension of infection from tissues adjacent to the lung.

PATHOLOGY: Lung abscesses mostly range from 2 to 6 cm in diameter, and 10% to 20% have multiple cavities, usually after a necrotizing pneumonia or a shower of septic pulmonary emboli. The right side of the lung is more often involved than the left, because the right main bronchus follows the direction of the trachea more closely at its bifurcation. Acute lung abscesses are not well separated from the surrounding pulmonary parenchyma. They exhibit abundant polymorphonuclear leukocytes and, depending on the age of the lesion, variable numbers of macrophages. Debris from necrotic tissue may be evident. The abscess is surrounded by hemorrhage, fibrin, and inflammatory cells. As the abscess ages, a fibrous wall forms around the margin. Lung abscesses differ from those elsewhere in their capacity for spontaneous drainage. The cavity thus formed contains air, necrotic debris, and inflammatory exudate (Fig. 12-31), creating a fluid level that is easily seen radiographically. The cavity lining becomes covered with regenerating squamous epithelium. Walls of old abscesses may be lined by ciliated respiratory epithelium, making distinction from bronchiectasis difficult.

CLINICAL FEATURES: Almost all patients with lung abscess are first seen with cough and fever. One of the most characteristic symptoms is production of large amounts of foul-smelling sputum. Many patients complain of pleuritic chest pain, and 20% develop hemoptysis.

The differential diagnosis of lung abscess includes lung cancer and cavitary tuberculosis. Indeed, cancer is now a more common cause of cavitation than is lung abscess. About half of all cavitation due to cancer reflects necrosis of the tumor; the others follow obstruction of the bronchi and subsequent infection. A tuberculous cavity only rarely displays the air–fluid level characteristic of a lung abscess.

Complications of lung abscess include rupture into the pleural space, with resulting empyema and severe hemoptysis. The abscess may drain into a bronchus, with subsequent dissemination of the infection to other parts of the lung. Despite vigorous antimicrobial therapy, principally directed against anaerobic bacteria, the mortality of lung abscess remains 5% to 10%.

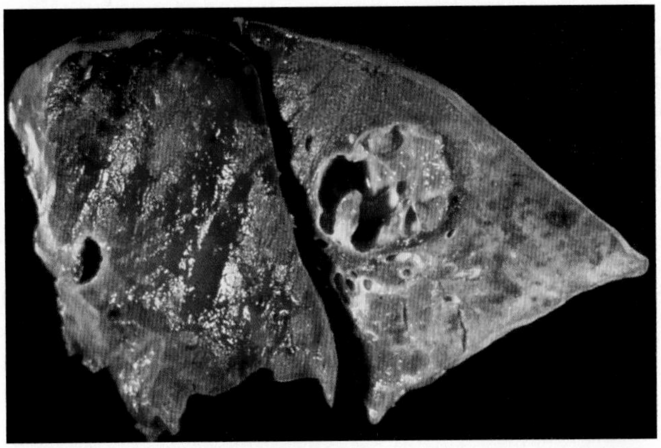

FIGURE 12-31. **Pulmonary abscess.** A large cystic abscess contains a purulent exudate and is contained by a fibrous wall. Pneumonia is present in the surrounding pulmonary parenchyma.

Diffuse Alveolar Damage (Acute Respiratory Distress Syndrome)

Diffuse alveolar damage (DAD) refers to a pattern of reaction to injury of alveolar epithelial and endothelial cells from a variety of acute insults (Table 12-1). The clinical counterpart of severe DAD is the acute respiratory distress syndrome (ARDS). In this disorder, a patient with apparently normal lungs sustains pulmonary damage and then develops rapidly progressive respiratory failure. The condition reflects decreased lung compliance (usually requiring mechanical ventilation) and hypoxemia and features extensive radiologic opacities in both lungs ("white-out"). The overall mortality of ARDS is more than 50%, and in patients older than 60 years, it is as high as 90%.

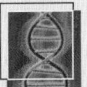

PATHOGENESIS: DAD is a final common pathology caused by a large variety of insults (see Table 12-1). These include respiratory tract infections, sepsis, shock, aspiration of gastric contents, inhalation of toxic gases, near-drowning, radiation pneumonitis, and a large assortment of drugs and other chemicals. Although these conditions are quite diverse, they can all injure the epithelial and endothelial cells of the alveoli, thereby producing DAD. *Importantly, the precise cause of DAD cannot be determined from the morphologic appearance of the lung alone, unless a specific infectious agent is identified.* Some patients have an idiopathic form of DAD, in which no cause can be found. Idiopathic DAD is referred to clinically as **acute interstitial pneumonia** (AIP) and also includes cases historically referred to as **Hamman-Rich disease**.

TABLE 12-1

Important Causes of the Acute Respiratory Distress Syndrome

Nonthoracic Trauma	Infection	Aspiration	Drugs and Therapeutic Agents
Shock due to any cause	Gram-negative septicemia	Near-drowning	Heroin
Fat embolism	Other bacterial infections	Aspiration of gastric contents	Oxygen
	Viral infections		Radiation
			Paraquat
			Cytotoxic drugs

Injury to endothelial cells allows leakage of protein-rich fluid from alveolar capillaries into the interstitial space (Fig. 12-32). Destruction of type I pneumocytes permits exudation of fluid into alveolar spaces, where deposition of plasma proteins results in formation of fibrin-containing precipitates (hyaline membranes) on the injured alveolar walls (Fig. 12-33). Although it is denuded of type I pneumocytes, the alveolar basement membrane remains intact and functions as a scaffold for type II pneumocytes, whose proliferation replaces the normal epithelial lining of the alveoli. In response to the cell injury of DAD, inflammatory cells accumulate in the interstitial space.

If the patient survives the acute phase of ARDS, fibroblasts proliferate in the interstitial space and deposit collagen in the alveolar walls (Fig. 12-34). In patients who recover completely, lesions may heal, with resorption of the alveolar exudate and hyaline membranes and restitution of normal alveolar epithelium. Fibroblastic proliferation ceases, and the extra collagen is metabolized. It is well documented that patients with ARDS who recover do regain normal pulmonary function. In patients who do not recover, DAD can progress to end-stage fibrosis; remodeling of the lung architecture produces multiple cystlike spaces throughout the lung (**honeycomb lung**). These spaces

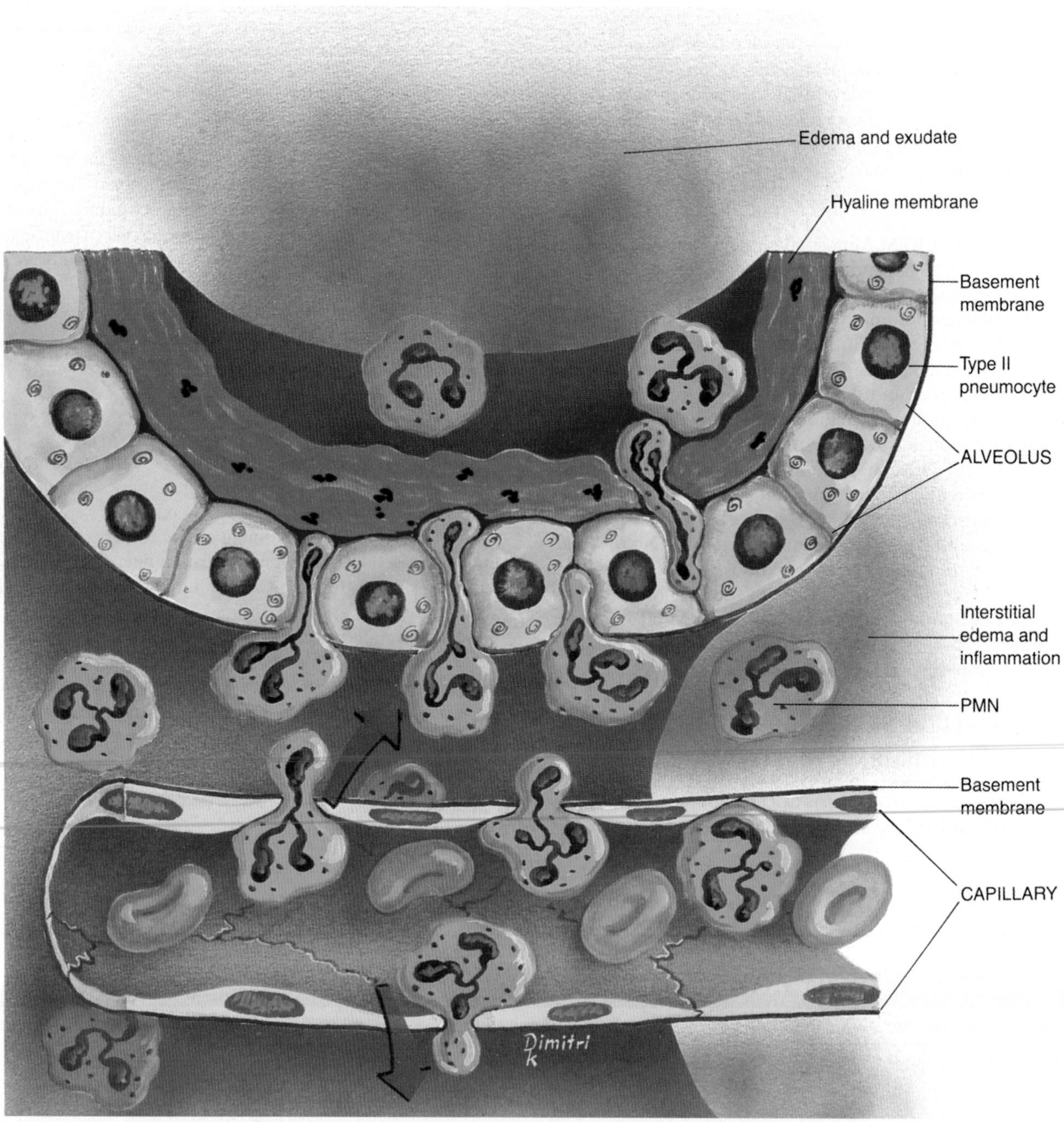

FIGURE 12-32. **Diffuse alveolar damage (adult respiratory distress syndrome, ARDS).** In ARDS, type I cells die as a result of diffuse alveolar damage. Intraalveolar edema follows, after which there is formation of hyaline membranes composed of proteinaceous exudate and cell debris. In the acute phase, the lungs are markedly congested and heavy. Type II cells multiply to line the alveolar surface. Interstitial inflammation is characteristic. The lesion may heal completely or progress to interstitial fibrosis. PMN = polymorphonuclear neutrophil.

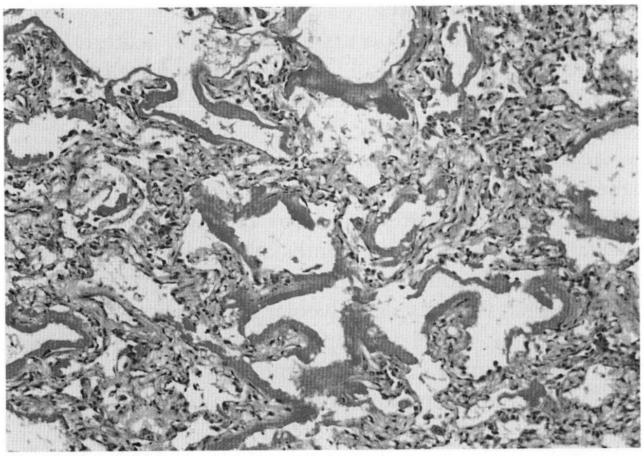

FIGURE 12-33. **Diffuse alveolar damage, acute (exudative) phase.** The alveolar septa are thickened by edema and a sparse inflammatory infiltrate. The alveoli are lined by eosinophilic hyaline membranes.

are separated from each other by fibrous tissue and lined by type II pneumocytes, bronchiolar epithelium, or squamous cells.

PATHOGENESIS: The pathogenesis of DAD is not entirely clear. It is thought that activation of complement (e.g., by endotoxin in the case of gram-negative septicemia) results in sequestration of neutrophils in the marginating pool. Only a small proportion, perhaps one third, of neutrophils actively circulate in the blood; most of the remainder are found in the lung. Normally, the neutrophils cause no damage, but after activation by complement, they release oxygen radicals and hydrolytic enzymes, which damage the capillary endothelium of the lung. The role of polymorphonuclear leukocytes in the pathogenesis of DAD is still debated because ARDS has been reported in severely neutropenic patients.

In DAD produced by inhalation of toxic gases or near-drowning, the damage occurs primarily at the alveolar epithelial surface. The alveolar epithelial junctions are usually very tight; damage to the epithelium disrupts these junctions, permitting exudation of fluid and proteins from the interstitium into the alveolar spaces.

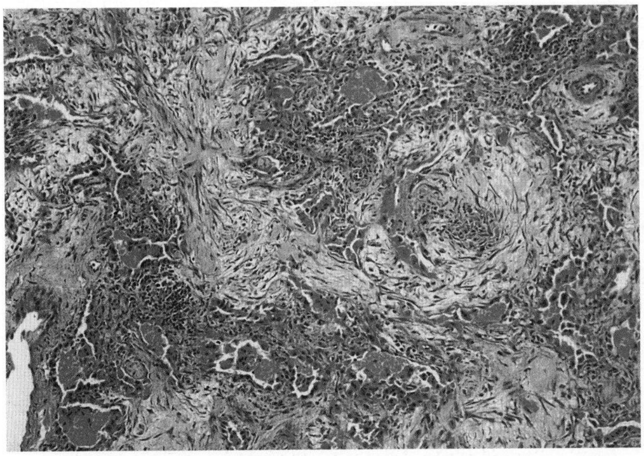

FIGURE 12-34. **Diffuse alveolar damage, acute and organizing phase.** In addition to hyaline membranes, the alveolar walls are thickened by fibroblasts and loose connective tissue.

PATHOLOGY: As DAD evolves, the initial exudative phase is followed by an organizing phase.

The exudative phase of DAD develops during the first week after pulmonary insult and features edema, leakage of plasma proteins, accumulation of inflammatory cells, and hyaline membranes (see Fig. 12-33). The earliest alveolar injury is detected by electron microscopy, which reveals degenerative changes in endothelial cells and type I pneumocytes. This is followed by sloughing of type I cells, leaving basement membranes denuded. Interstitial and alveolar edema is prominent by the first day but soon recedes. "Hyaline membranes" begin to appear by the second day and are the most conspicuous morphologic feature of the exudative phase after 4 to 5 days. These eosinophilic, glassy "membranes" consist of precipitated plasma proteins and cytoplasmic and nuclear debris from sloughed epithelial cells. Interstitial inflammation, consisting of lymphocytes, plasma cells, and macrophages, is apparent early and reaches its maximum in about a week. Toward the end of the first week and persisting during the subsequent organizing stage, regularly spaced, cuboidal type II pneumocytes become arrayed along the denuded alveolar septa. The alveolar capillaries and pulmonary arterioles may exhibit fibrin thrombi. In fatal cases of DAD, the lungs are heavy, edematous, and virtually airless.

The organizing phase of DAD, beginning about a week after the initial injury, is marked by proliferation of fibroblasts within alveolar walls (see Fig. 12-34). Interstitial inflammation and proliferated type II pneumocytes persist, but hyaline membranes are no longer formed. Alveolar macrophages digest the remnants of hyaline membranes and other cellular debris. Loose fibrosis thickens the alveolar septa. This fibrosis resolves in mild cases; in severe ones, it progresses to restructuring of the pulmonary parenchyma and cyst formation.

CLINICAL FEATURES: Patients destined to develop ARDS have a symptom-free interval for a few hours after the initial insult, after which tachypnea and dyspnea mark the onset of the syndrome. Blood gas analyses show arterial hypoxemia and decreased $P\text{CO}_2$. As ARDS progresses, dyspnea worsens and the patient becomes cyanotic. Diffuse, bilateral interstitial, and alveolar infiltrates are noted radiologically. Arterial hypoxemia at this stage cannot be reversed simply by increasing oxygen tension in the inspired air, and mechanical ventilation becomes necessary. In fatal cases the combination of increasing tachypnea and decreasing tidal volume eventuates in alveolar hypoventilation, progressive hypoxemia, and increasing $P\text{CO}_2$.

Patients who survive ARDS may recover normal pulmonary function but, in severe cases, are left with scarred lungs, respiratory dysfunction and, in some instances, pulmonary hypertension.

Diffuse Alveolar Damage May Have Specific Causes

Oxygen

During World War II, aviators were required to breathe increased concentrations of oxygen at high altitude. Animal experiments had demonstrated harmful effects of oxygen on the lung. Later observations with patients who received high levels of oxygen for respiratory problems documented the development of DAD. Pulmonary lesions have developed in patients with long-term exposure to as little as 28% oxygen, but it is usually safe to breathe 40% to 60% oxygen for long periods. Oxygen toxicity is thought to be caused by increased production of activated oxygen species in the lung (see Chapter 1).

Shock

ARDS often follows shock from any cause, including gram-negative sepsis, trauma, or blood loss, in which case the pulmonary condition is colloquially referred to as "shock lung." The pathogenesis of DAD associated with shock is poorly understood, but is likely multifactorial. Tissue necrosis in organs damaged by trauma or by ischemia may lead to release of vasoactive peptides into the circulation. These enhance vascular permeability in the lung. Disseminated intravascular coagulation may damage alveolar capillaries, and fat emboli from bone fractures may obstruct the distal capillary bed of the lung. The pathogenesis of endothelial cell injury in endotoxic shock is discussed in Chapter 7.

Aspiration

Aspiration of gastric contents introduces acid with a pH less than 3.0 into the alveoli. The severe chemical injury to the alveolar lining cells leads to DAD. In near-drowning, aspiration of water leads to pulmonary injury and ARDS.

Drug-Induced Diffuse Alveolar Damage

Many drugs cause DAD, especially cytotoxic chemotherapeutic agents. The best known is bleomycin. Other known causes include 1,3-bis-(2-chloroethyl)-1-nitrosourea (BCNU), methotrexate, 5-fluorouracil, busulfan, and cyclophosphamide. With bleomycin, an imprecise dose-dependent relation has been demonstrated, but such an effect is not apparent with most other drugs.

Bizarre, atypical, hyperchromatic nuclei in type II cells are particularly common in cases of alveolar damage from chemotherapy (Fig. 12-35). Damage progresses despite discontinuation of the offending agent, although it may be modified by the administration of corticosteroids. Progressive interstitial fibrosis occurs, usually with retention of lung structure. Methotrexate differs from the other chemotherapeutic agents in that it may sometimes cause a hypersensitivity reaction in the lung. Under these circumstances, DAD is reversible after the drug is discontinued. The lesions that reflect hypersensitivity are characterized by granulomatous inflammation and occasionally vasculitis.

Drugs other than chemotherapeutic agents also cause DAD. Examples are nitrofurantoin, amiodarone, and penicillamine.

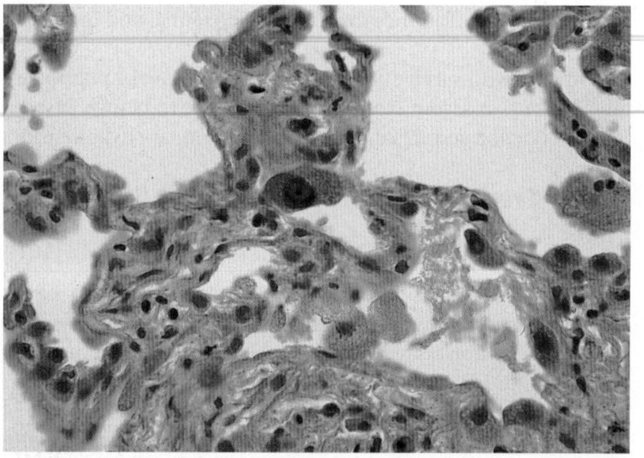

FIGURE 12-35. **Diffuse alveolar damage (DAD) associated with busulfan treatment.** An atypical pneumocyte was encountered in a case of organizing DAD associated with busulfan therapy.

Radiation Pneumonitis

Radiation pneumonitis occurs in two forms, acute DAD and chronic pulmonary fibrosis. Alveolar injury is believed to be caused by oxygen radicals generated by the radiolysis of water (see Chapter 1).

Acute radiation pneumonitis occurs in as many as 10% of patients irradiated for cancer of the lung or breast or for mediastinal lymphoma. DAD caused by radiation is mostly dose-related and appears 1 to 6 months after radiation therapy. Patients have fever, cough, and dyspnea. Microscopic examination of the lungs reveals atypical alveolar lining cells, with enlarged hyperchromatic nuclei and multinucleated cells. Most patients recover from acute radiation pneumonitis.

Chronic radiation pneumonitis is characterized by interstitial fibrosis and may follow acute DAD or may develop insidiously. Lung biopsy demonstrates interstitial fibrosis, radiation-induced vascular changes, and atypical type II pneumocytes. The disease remains asymptomatic unless a substantial volume of the lung is affected.

Paraquat

The ingestion of the widely used herbicide paraquat is associated with DAD. Pulmonary disease becomes apparent 4 to 7 days after ingestion, as ARDS develops. Patients rarely recover once pulmonary complications have evolved. A curious intraalveolar exudate and organization occur, as well as the more usual interstitial fibrosis. The intra-alveolar exudate organizes in such a way that the alveolar framework persists and the airspaces are filled with loose granulation tissue.

Respiratory Distress Syndrome of the Newborn is a Counterpart of ARDS

The counterpart of ARDS in newborns is termed respiratory distress syndrome of the newborn (NRDS). NRDS, also called **hyaline membrane disease**, is a result of immaturity in the surfactant system at birth, usually as a consequence of severe prematurity. The advent of surfactant replacement therapy and improvements in ventilatory techniques have improved survival and decreased the frequency of complications of NRDS in older premature infants, but very premature infants may still develop **bronchopulmonary dysplasia (BPD).** This infantile disorder was caused initially by damage to pulmonary acini and later by repair, which led to atelectasis, fibrosis, and destruction of clusters of acini. Since the advent of surfactant replacement therapy, the necrotizing bronchiolitis and alveolar septal fibrosis of bronchopulmonary dysplasia have largely disappeared, and the major change now encountered is one of decreased alveolarization in infants following birth. NRDS and BPD are discussed in further detail in Chapter 6.

Rare Alveolar Diseases

Alveolar Proteinosis Features Excess Intraalveolar Lipid-Rich Material

Alveolar proteinosis, also termed lipoproteinosis, *is a rare condition in which the alveoli are filled with a granular eosinophilic material, which has a very high surfactant content.* The disease was initially described as idiopathic, but recent studies have associated alveolar proteinosis with (1) compromised immunity; (2) a number of cancers, particularly leukemia and lymphoma; (3) respiratory infections; and (4) exposure to environmental inorganic dusts.

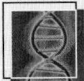

PATHOGENESIS: The origin of alveolar proteinosis is obscure, but impaired activity of alveolar macrophages and overproduction of lipid (surfactant) by type II pneumocytes may be responsible. However, the large amount of protein in the material indicates an additional (although unknown) mechanism. In most cases, no etiologic agent is identifiable. However, recent studies suggest that a deficiency in granulocyte-monocyte colony stimulating factor (GM-CSF) may be involved.

PATHOLOGY: On gross examination, the lungs are very heavy and viscid, and yellow fluid leaks from the cut surface. Scattered, firm, yellow-white nodules vary in size from a few millimeters to 2 cm in diameter. Microscopically, the granular material is noted in the alveoli, respiratory bronchioles and alveolar ducts (Fig. 12-36). Within the eosinophilic material may be found cellular debris, foamy macrophages, ghosts of degenerated cells, and detached type II pneumocytes. High concentrations of surfactant are demonstrated by immunostaining and electron microscopy shows characteristic surfactant tubular myelin structures. Importantly, the interstitial architecture of the lung is intact, and little inflammation is present.

CLINICAL FEATURES: Alveolar proteinosis is a disease of adults, although a few cases have been reported in infants and children. Patients have fever, a productive cough, and dyspnea. The most common finding on the chest radiograph is diffuse, bilateral, symmetric, alveolar infiltrates, which may radiate from the hilar regions. Repeated respiratory tract infections, often with fungi or *Nocardia,* are common. Before treatment became available, alveolar proteinosis gradually progressed to respiratory failure in one-third of patients. Today, bronchoalveolar lavage is used to remove the alveolar material, and repeated lavage (sometimes for years) cures or halts the progress of the disease.

Diffuse Pulmonary Hemorrhage Syndromes Are Mainly Immunologic Disorders

Diffuse alveolar hemorrhage can occur in diverse clinical settings (Table 12-2). Histologically, the diseases are characterized by acute hemorrhage (numerous intra-alveolar red blood cells) or chronic hemorrhage (hemosiderosis). In virtually all of these disorders, a neutrophilic infiltrate of the alveolar wall (**neutrophilic capillaritis**) is present and is reminiscent of leukocytoclastic vasculitis seen in other organs such as the skin. This lesion tends to be most prominent in hemorrhagic syndromes associated with Wegener granulomatosis or systemic lupus erythematosus.

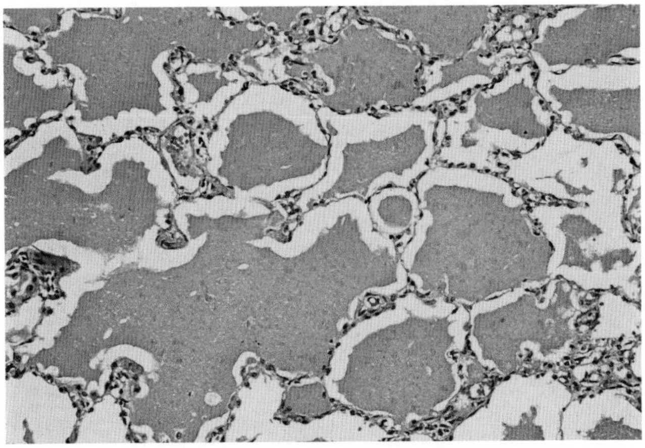

FIGURE 12-36. **Alveolar proteinosis.** The alveoli and alveolar ducts contain a granular, eosinophilic material.

Diffuse pulmonary hemorrhage syndromes can be classified according to the associated immunofluorescence patterns. A linear pattern of fluorescence is seen in antibasement membrane antibody disease or Goodpasture syndrome. A granular pattern is present in immune complex–associated diseases, such as systemic lupus erythematosus. Pauciimmune disorders consist of antineutrophil cytoplasm antibody (ANCA)-associated diseases (e.g., Wegener granulomatosis or idiopathic pulmonary hemorrhage syndromes), in which no etiology or immunologic mechanism can be determined (see Table 12-2).

Goodpasture Syndrome (AntiGlomerular Basement Membrane Antibody Disease)

Goodpasture syndrome refers to a triad of diffuse alveolar hemorrhage, glomerulonephritis, and a circulating cytotoxic autoantibody to a component of basement membranes. Cross-reactivity between alveolar and glomerular basement membranes accounts for the simultaneous attack on the lung and kidney. The pathogenesis of Goodpasture syndrome is discussed in greater detail in Chapter 16.

TABLE 12-2

Conditions of Pulmonary Hemorrhage

Disease	Immunological Mechanism	Immunofluorescence Pattern
Goodpasture syndrome	Antibasement membrane antibody	Linear
Systemic lupus erythematosus	Immune complexes	Granular
Mixed cryoglobulinemia		
Henoch-Schönlein purpura		
IgA disease		
Wegener granulomatosis	Antineutrophil cytoplasmic antibody (ANCA)	Negative or pauciimmune
Idiopathic glomerulonephritis		
Idiopathic pulmonary hemorrhage	No immunological marker	

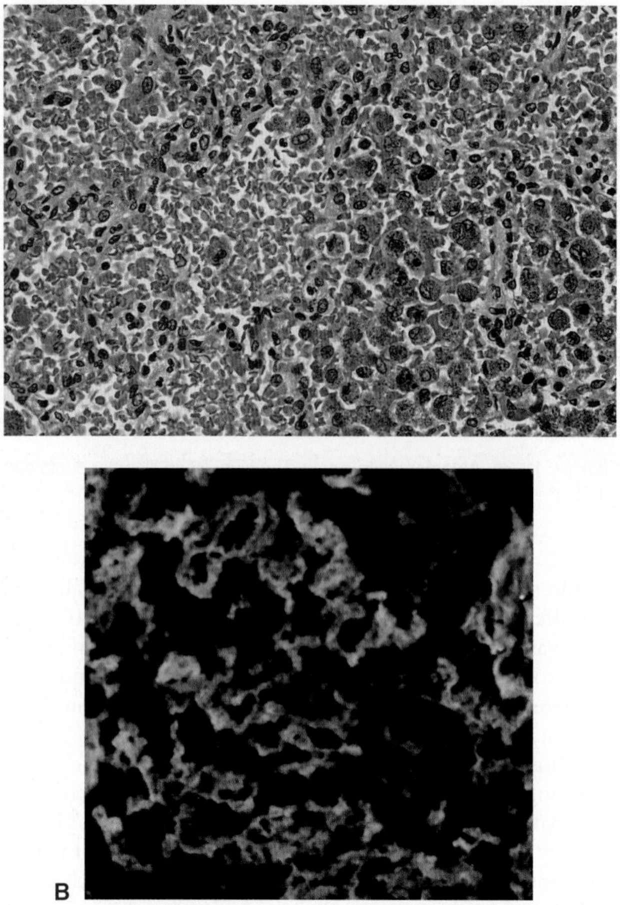

FIGURE 12-37. **Goodpasture syndrome. A.** A section of lung shows extensive intra-alveolar hemorrhage. The alveolar septa are thickened, and the alveoli are lined by hyperplastic type II pneumocytes. **B.** Linear deposition of IgG within the alveolar septa is demonstrated by immunofluorescence.

PATHOLOGY: Patients with Goodpasture syndrome suffer extensive intra-alveolar hemorrhage (Fig. 12-37A). Grossly, the lungs are dark red and heavy in the acute phase and rusty brown later, when the erythrocytes have been phagocytosed. Histologically, erythrocytes and hemosiderin-laden macrophages fill the airspaces. The presence of neutrophils in and around alveolar capillaries may suggest an "alveolitis," although this reaction may be transient. The alveolar septa are mildly thickened by interstitial fibrosis and hyperplasia of type II pneumocytes. Immunofluorescence shows linear deposition of IgG and complement in basement membranes of alveoli and glomeruli (see Fig. 12-37B).

CLINICAL FEATURES: Patients with Goodpasture syndrome are typically young men, although the disease may affect adults of either sex and of any age. Most (95%) patients are seen initially with hemoptysis, often accompanied by dyspnea, weakness, and mild anemia. Evidence of glomerulonephritis follows the pulmonary manifestations in about 3 months (1 week to 1 year), although some patients do not develop renal disease. Radiographic examination reveals diffuse, bilateral alveolar infiltrates, which may resolve rapidly in a matter of days as erythrocytes lyse and are phagocytosed. Hypoxemia and respiratory alkalosis are common, but respiratory function returns to normal as the hemorrhage resolves. The diagnosis is made on the basis of a renal or pulmonary biopsy.

Goodpasture syndrome is treated with corticosteroids and cytotoxic drugs, and plasmapheresis. Before such aggressive treatment was instituted, the mortality of Goodpasture syndrome was 80%. Even with current treatment, 2-year survival is only 50%, and the outlook is worse if renal failure is present.

Idiopathic Pulmonary Hemorrhage

Idiopathic pulmonary hemorrhage (also known as idiopathic pulmonary hemosiderosis) is a rare disease characterized by diffuse alveolar bleeding similar to that of Goodpasture syndrome but lacking renal involvement or antibasement membrane antibodies. Microscopically, it is indistinguishable from the lung of Goodpasture syndrome.

CLINICAL FEATURES: The malady primarily affects children, but 20% of patients are adults, usually younger than 30 years. There is a 2:1 male predominance in adults, but an equal sex distribution in children. The patients are first seen with cough (with or without hemoptysis), dyspnea, substernal chest pain, fatigue, and iron-deficiency anemia. Pulmonary hemorrhages are recurrent and intermittent, and the course is more protracted than that of Goodpasture syndrome.

The response to corticosteroids is variable, and mean survival is 3 to 5 years. One fourth of patients die rapidly of massive hemorrhage. Another fourth have persistent, active disease; repeated episodes of hemoptysis result in interstitial fibrosis and cor pulmonale. In another fourth of patients, the disease remains inactive, but persistent dyspnea and anemia are troublesome. The remaining patients recover completely without recurrence.

Hypersensitivity to cow's milk in infants and children generally younger than 2 years can result in diffuse pulmonary hemorrhage similar to that seen in idiopathic pulmonary hemorrhage. Removal of milk from the diet ameliorates the condition.

Eosinophilic Pneumonia Is Principally an Allergic Disorder

Eosinophilic pneumonia refers to the accumulation of eosinophils in alveolar spaces. Eosinophilic pneumonia is classified as **idiopathic** or **secondary** to an underlying illness (Table 12-3).

Idiopathic Eosinophilic Pneumonia

SIMPLE EOSINOPHILIC PNEUMONIA: Simple eosinophilic pneumonia (Löffler syndrome) is a mild condition characterized by fleeting pulmonary infiltrates, which usually resolve within a month. Patients typically have peripheral blood eosinophilia but are often asymptomatic. Histologically, the lung shows eosinophilic pneumonia, but the diagnosis is usually established clinically, and lung biopsy is rarely performed.

ACUTE EOSINOPHILIC PNEUMONIA: In this disorder, patients are first seen with fewer than 7 days of symptoms, which include fever, hypoxemia, and diffuse interstitial and alveolar infiltrates on chest radiograph. The etiology of acute eosinophilic pneumonia is not known, but it is thought to be a type of hypersensitivity reaction. Although peripheral blood eosinophilia is frequently absent, bronchoalveolar lavage consistently demonstrates increased eosinophils. Leukocytosis is usually present. Histologically, the lung shows eosinophilic pneumonia accompanied by features of diffuse alveolar damage (i.e., hyaline membranes). Patients respond dramatically to corticosteroids, and in contrast to chronic eosinophilic pneumonia, acute eosinophilic pneumonia does not recur.

TABLE 12-3

Types of Eosinophilic Pneumonia

- Idiopathic
  - Chronic eosinophilic pneumonia
  - Acute eosinophilic pneumonia
  - Simple eosinophilic pneumonia (Löffler syndrome)
- Secondary eosinophilic pneumonia
  - Infection
    - Parasitic
      - Tropical eosinophilic pneumonia
      - *Ascaris lumbricoides, Toxocara canis*, filaria
      - Dirofilaria
    - Fungal
      - *Aspergillus*
  - Drug-induced
    - Antibiotics
    - Cytotoxic drugs
    - Anti-inflammatory agents
    - Antihypertensive drugs
    - L-Tryptophan (eosinophilic fasciitis)
  - Immunological or systemic diseases
    - Allergic bronchopulmonary aspergillosis
    - Churg-Strauss syndrome
    - Hypereosinophilic syndrome

CHRONIC EOSINOPHILIC PNEUMONIA: The etiology of chronic eosinophilic pneumonia is unknown, but an allergic diathesis is noted in some patients.

PATHOLOGY: The alveolar spaces are flooded with eosinophils, alveolar macrophages, and a proteinaceous exudate (Fig. 12-38). Some cases may also show an eosinophilic interstitial pneumonia. Hyperplasia of type II pneumocytes may be prominent. Eosinophilic abscesses, with central masses of necrotic eosinophils surrounded by palisaded macrophages, are sometimes encountered. A mild eosinophilic vasculitis may be seen. An organizing pneumonia pattern is also occasionally described (see below).

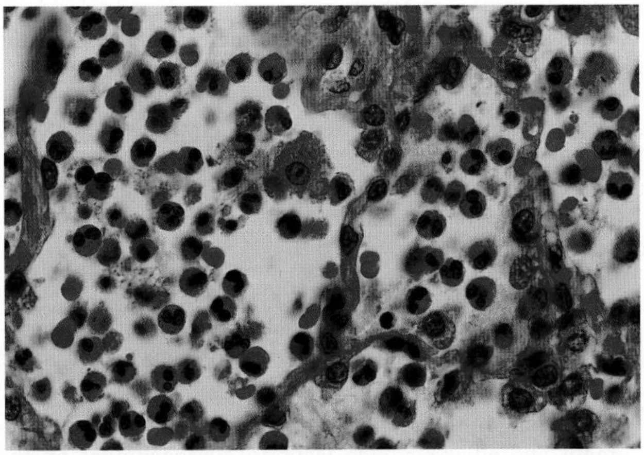

FIGURE 12-38. **Eosinophilic pneumonia.** The alveolar spaces are filled with an inflammatory exudate composed of eosinophils and macrophages. The alveolar septa are thickened by the presence of numerous eosinophils.

CLINICAL FEATURES: Patients have fever, night sweats, weight loss, cough productive of eosinophils, and dyspnea. Asthma is present in many patients, and circulating eosinophilia may be conspicuous. The chest radiograph is diagnostic and has been described as "the photographic negative of pulmonary edema," characterized by peripheral alveolar infiltrates with sparing of the hilum. The response to corticosteroids is dramatic and helps to confirm the diagnosis.

Secondary Eosinophilic Pneumonia

Eosinophilic pneumonia can occur in a variety of known clinical settings, including parasitic or fungal infection, drug toxicity, and systemic disorders such as Churg-Strauss syndrome (see Table 12-3) In industrialized countries, the most frequent cause of eosinophilic pneumonia is drug hypersensitivity, including reactions to antibiotics, anti-inflammatory agents, cytotoxic drugs, and antihypertensive agents. The pulmonary disease resolves without long-term sequelae. The clinical presentations and histologic findings are the same as described above.

The classic form of **infectious eosinophilic pneumonia** associated with parasitic infection is **tropical eosinophilic pneumonia**. The migration of parasites through the lung is often accompanied by an acute, self-limited, respiratory illness, characterized clinically by (1) fever, (2) a cough productive of sputum containing eosinophils, and (3) transient pulmonary infiltrates.

In temperate zones, *Ascaris lumbricoides* is the usual inciting organism. Hypersensitivity to *Toxocara canis* is also occasionally encountered. However, the most distinctive infection associated with eosinophilic pneumonia is allergic bronchopulmonary aspergillosis (see discussion above on aspergillosis).

In tropical regions, eosinophilic pneumonia is most commonly a response to infestation with the filarial nematodes *Wuchereria bancrofti* and *Brugia malayi,* although other parasites may also produce this syndrome.

Endogenous Lipid Pneumonia Reflects Bronchial Obstruction

Endogenous lipid pneumonia, also termed "golden pneumonia," *is a localized condition distal to an obstructed airway, characterized by lipid-laden macrophages in the alveolar spaces.* The size of the affected area corresponds to the caliber of the involved bronchus. Bronchial obstruction results in the retention of secretions and breakdown products of inflammatory and epithelial cells. Whereas the protein component is readily digested, lipids are phagocytosed by macrophages, which fill the alveoli distal to the obstruction.

PATHOLOGY: Endogenous lipid pneumonia has a characteristic golden-yellow color owing to accumulation of fine lipid droplets within alveolar macrophages. Microscopically, alveoli are flooded by foamy macrophages with needle-shaped clefts characteristic of cholesterol crystals. Alveolar walls typically remain intact. The pneumonia is accompanied by mild chronic inflammation and fibrosis. If the obstruction is relieved, the affected parenchyma can return to its normal state unless bronchiectasis and chronic recurrent bronchopneumonia have led to irreversible parenchymal changes.

Exogenous Lipid Pneumonia Is a Response to Aspirated Oils

Causes of exogenous pneumonia include mineral oil (a laxative and a carrier for medications in nose drops), vegetable oils used in cooking, and animal oils ingested in the form of cod-liver oil and other vitamin preparations. Oil-based contrast media used for radiologic bronchography has also been associated with the disorder. Exogenous lipid pneumonia is most common in older persons who take nose drops or laxatives at bedtime and aspirate during sleep. Children may aspirate oily medications while vigorously resisting the dosing.

PATHOLOGY: On gross examination, exogenous lipid pneumonia is gray, greasy, and poorly demarcated. Microscopically, foamy macrophages are seen in the alveolar and interstitial spaces (Fig. 12-39). Large oil droplets in both locations are surrounded by a foreign-body granulomatous response. Because most of the oil dissolves out in paraffin processing, empty vacuolar spaces are noted in histologic sections. In chronic cases, the affected areas may become densely fibrotic.

Patients with exogenous lipid pneumonia are usually asymptomatic, and the condition is brought to medical attention when a mass simulating an infectious process or a tumor is noted on a chest radiograph.

Obstructive Pulmonary Diseases

Several different diseases, including chronic bronchitis, emphysema, asthma, and in some classifications bronchiectasis and cystic fibrosis, are grouped together because they have in common an obstruction to air flow in the lungs.

COPD applies to chronic bronchitis and emphysema, in which forced expiratory volume, measured by spirometriy, is decreased.

Air flow has a hydraulic basis and can be reduced by increasing resistance to air flow or reducing outflow pressure. In the lung, narrowed airways produce increased resistance, whereas loss of elastic recoil results in diminished pressure. Airway narrowing occurs in chronic bronchitis or asthma, and emphysema causes loss of recoil.

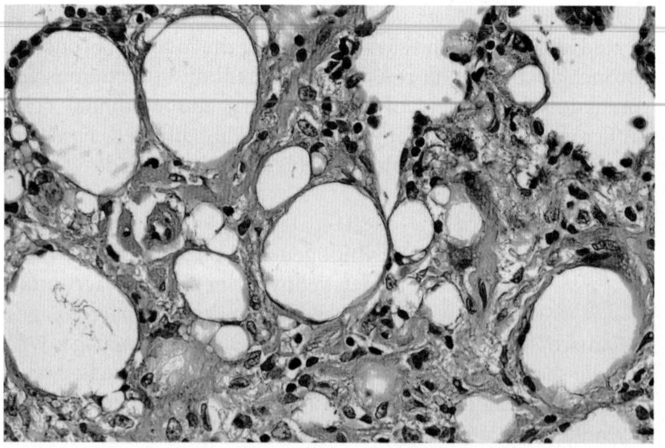

FIGURE 12-39. **Exogenous lipoid pneumonia (mineral oil aspiration).** The cystic spaces are empty because the lipid was washed out during paraffin processing. A giant-cell reaction is also present.

Chronic Bronchitis Is Defined as the Presence of a Chronic Productive Cough without a Discernible Cause for More Than Half of the Time Over 2 Years

The pathologic definition of the disease is less satisfactory, because its morphologic alterations are a continuum; in milder chronic bronchitis, they overlap with those seen in ostensibly normal persons.

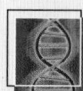

PATHOGENESIS: *Chronic bronchitis is primarily a disease of cigarette smokers (see Chapter 8): 90% of cases occur in smokers.* Chronic bronchitis occurs in less than 5% of nonsmokers, 10% to 15% of moderate smokers, and more than 25% of heavy smokers. The frequency and severity of acute respiratory tract infections are increased in patients with chronic bronchitis; conversely, infections have been incriminated in its etiology and progression. Chronic bronchitis is more common among urban dwellers in areas of substantial air pollution and in workers exposed to toxic industrial inhalants, but the effects of cigarette smoking far outweigh other contributing factors.

How cigarette smoke and other pollutants injure bronchi is not well understood. Experimentally, rodents that inhale cigarette smoke or SO_2, or are given dilute acids by instillation, exhibit squamous metaplasia of the bronchial epithelium. A similar change is produced by introducing certain proteases into the bronchi, whose effect is prevented by pretreating with anti-proteases. Bronchial epithelial metaplasia also occurs in rodents given adrenergic and cholinergic agonists, suggesting that autonomic stimulation may play a role in the pathogenesis of chronic bronchitis.

PATHOLOGY: The main morphologic finding in chronic bronchitis is an increase in size of the bronchial mucus-secreting apparatus (Fig. 12-40). Two types of cells line the mucous glands: pale mucous cells, which are more common, and serous cells, which are more basophilic and contain granules. *Chronic bronchitis is characterized by hyperplasia and hypertrophy of the mucous cells and an increased ratio of mucous to serous cells.* Thus, both the individual acini and the glands enlarge (Fig. 12-41).

The Reid index is a measure of the increase in the size of the mucous glands (see Fig. 12-40). The area occupied by the glands in the plane vertical to the cartilage and epithelium is expressed as a proportion of the thickness of the entire bronchial wall (basement membrane to inner perichondrium). A normal Reid index is 0.4 or less; in chronic bronchitis it is more than 0.5.

Other morphologic changes in chronic bronchitis are variable and include:

- Excess mucus in central and peripheral airways
- "Pits" on the surface of the bronchial epithelium, which represent dilated bronchial gland ducts into which several glands open
- Thickening of the bronchial wall by mucous gland enlargement and edema, which leads to encroachment on the bronchial lumen
- An increase in the number of goblet cells (hyperplasia) in the bronchial epithelium

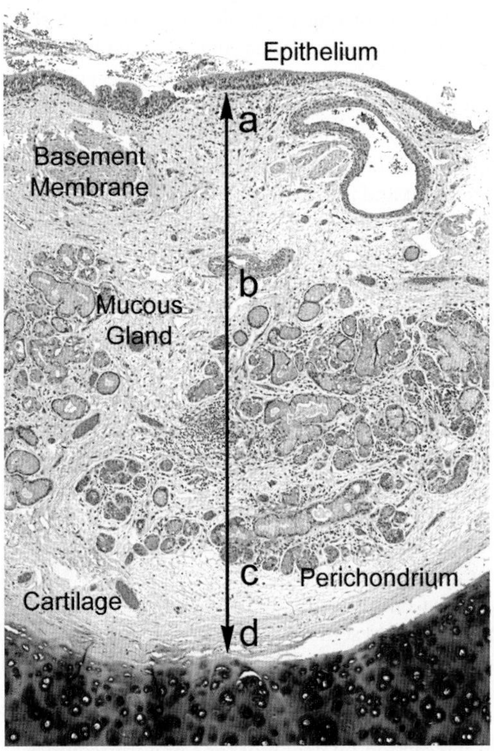

FIGURE 12-40. **Chronic bronchitis.** The bronchial submucosa is greatly expanded by hyperplastic submucosal glands that compose well over 50% of the thickness of the bronchial wall. The Reid index equals the maximum thickness of the bronchial mucous glands internal to the cartilage *(b to c)* divided by the bronchial wall thickness *(a to d)*.

- Increased smooth muscle, which may indicate bronchial hyperreactivity
- Squamous metaplasia of the bronchial epithelium, reflecting epithelial damage from tobacco smoke, which effect is probably independent of the other changes seen in chronic bronchitis

CLINICAL FEATURES: Chronic bronchitis is often accompanied by emphysema (see below); it is often difficult to separate the relative contribution of each disease to the clinical presentation. In general, patients with predominantly chronic bronchitis have had a productive cough for many years. Cough and sputum production are initially more severe in the winter months, but as the malady becomes more chronic, it progresses from hibernal to perennial. Exertional dyspnea and cyanosis supervene, and cor pulmonale may ensue. The combination of cyanosis and edema secondary to cor pulmonale has led to the label "blue bloater" for such patients.

Acute respiratory failure in patients with advanced chronic bronchitis, consisting of progressive hypoxemia and hypercapnia, may be precipitated by pulmonary infections, thromboembolism and left ventricular failure, and by major episodes of air pollution. Because of retained mucous secretions, patients with chronic bronchitis have increased risk for bacterial infections of the lung, particularly with *Haemophilus influenzae* and *Streptococcus pneumoniae.*

Persons with chronic bronchitis must be admonished to stop smoking. Prompt antibiotic treatment of pulmonary infections, administration of bronchodilator drugs, and occasionally bronchopulmonary drainage are the mainstays of treatment.

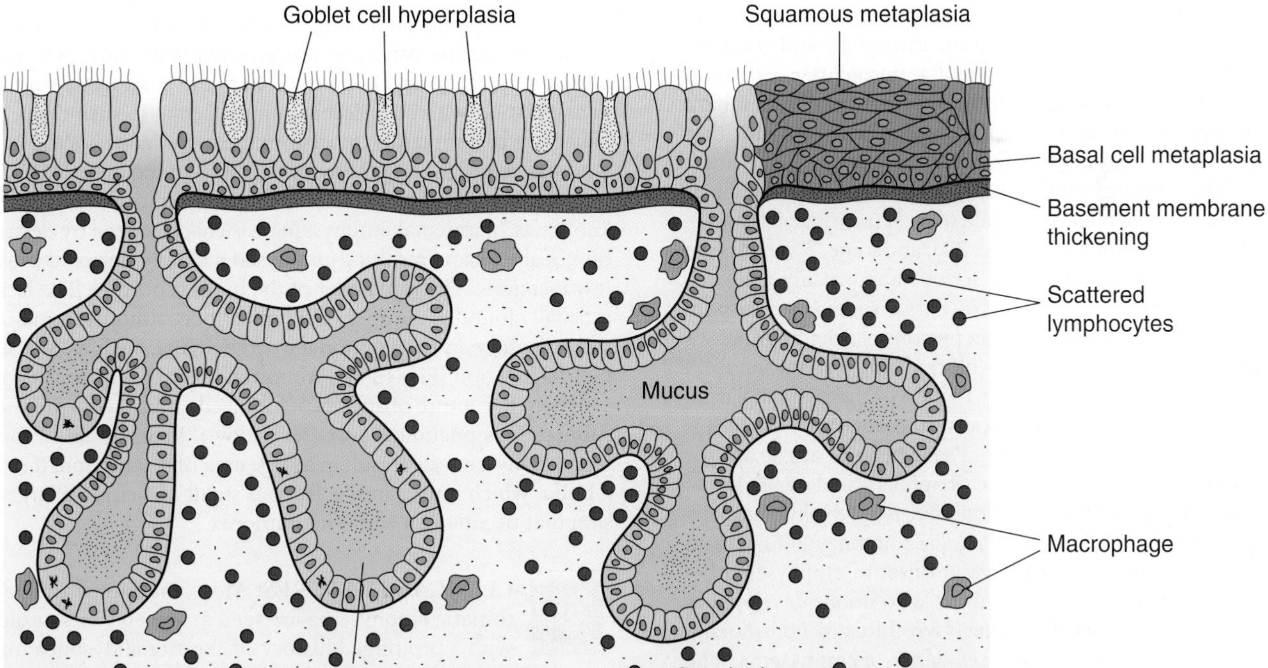

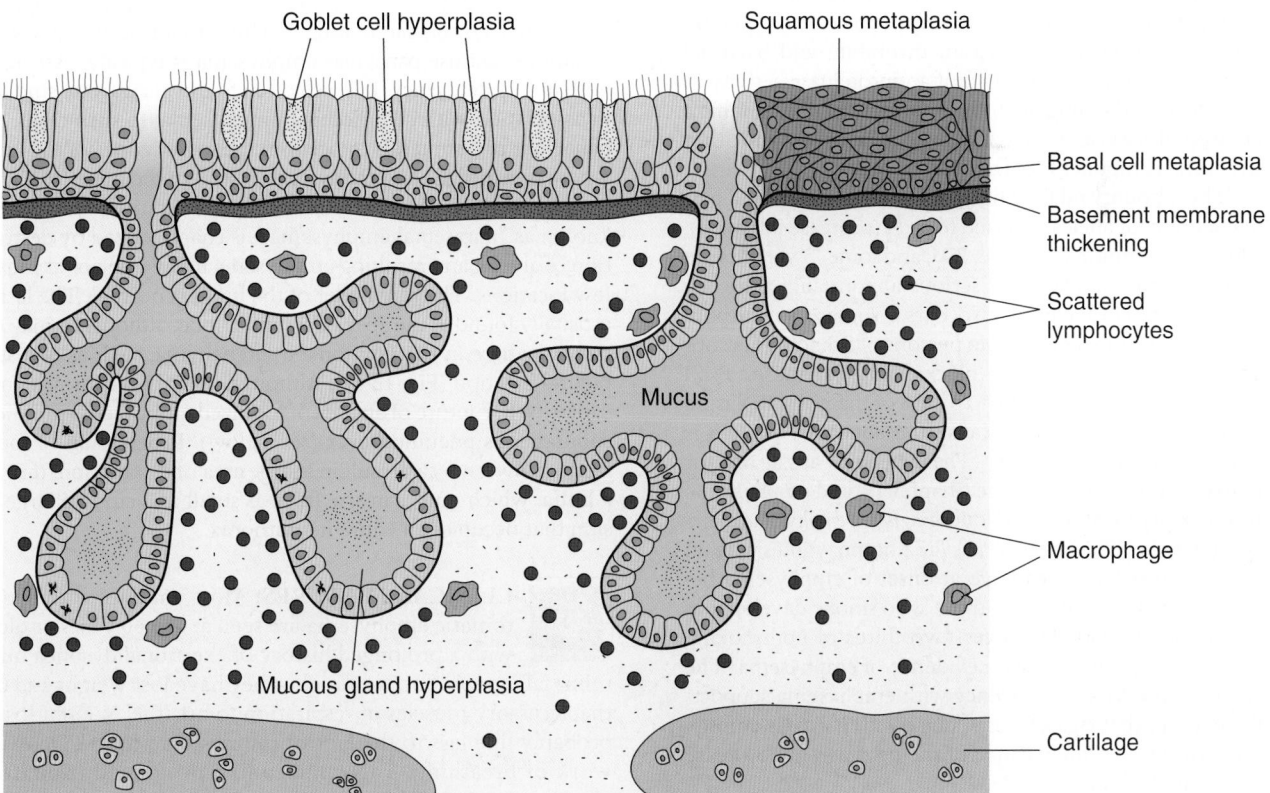

FIGURE 12-41. **Chronic bronchitis.** Morphological changes in chronic bronchitis.

Emphysema Causes Overinflation of the Lungs in Smokers

Emphysema is a chronic lung disease characterized by enlargement of airspaces distal to the terminal bronchioles, with destruction of their walls but without fibrosis. Although emphysema is classified in anatomical terms, *the severity of emphysema is more important than the type.* In practical terms, as emphysema becomes more severe, it becomes more difficult to classify. Moreover, several anatomical patterns may be present in the same lung.

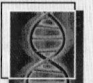

PATHOGENESIS: *The major cause of emphysema is cigarette smoking. Moderate-to-severe emphysema is rare in nonsmokers (see Chapter 8).* In considering the pathogenesis of emphysema, it is thought that a balance exists between elastin synthesis and catabolism in the lung (Fig. 12-42). In other words, emphysema results when elastolytic activity increases or antielastolytic activity is reduced.

Increased numbers of neutrophils, which contain serine elastase and other proteases, are found in the bronchoalveolar lavage fluid of smokers. Smoking also interferes with α_1-antitrypsin (α_1-AT) activity, by oxidizing methionine residues in α_1-antitrypsin. In this way, unopposed and increased elastolytic activity leads to destruction of elastic tissue in the walls of distal airspaces, thereby impairing elastic recoil. At the same time, other cellular proteases may be involved in injury to the airspace walls. This theory awaits further confirmation.

α_1-AT DEFICIENCY: A hereditary deficiency in α_1-AT accounts for about 1% of all patients with COPD and is considerably more common in young persons with severe emphysema. α_1-AT–a circulating glycoprotein produced in the liver–is a major inhibitor of a variety of proteases, including elastase, trypsin, chymotrypsin, thrombin, and bacterial proteases. It accounts for 90% of antiproteinase activity in the blood. In the lung, its most important action to inhibit neutrophil elastase, an enzyme that digests elastin and other structural components of the alveolar septa.

The amount and type of α_1-AT is determined by a pair of codominant alleles, referred to as *Pi* (protease inhibitor). The most common genotype, *PiM,* and some 75 variants are now recognized. The most serious abnormality is associated with the *PiZ* allele, which occurs in some 5% of the population. It is more common in persons of Scandinavian origin and is rare in Jews, blacks, and Japanese. *PiZZ* homozygotes have only 15% to 20% of the normal plasma concentration of α_1-AT because the abnormal protein is poorly secreted by the liver. These persons are at risk for both cirrhosis of the liver (see Chapter 14) and emphysema. *In fact, most patients with clinically diagnosed emphysema under age 40 have α_1-AT deficiency (PiZ). PiZZ* homozygotes who do not smoke show a mean age at onset of emphysema between ages 45 and 50 years; those who smoke develop it at about age 35 years. However, two thirds of nonsmoking *PiZZ* homozygotes show no evidence of emphysema. The association of α_1-AT deficiency with emphysema supports the concept that cigarette smoking by itself causes emphysema by altering the balance of the protease–antiprotease system in the lung.

PATHOLOGY: Emphysema is morphologically classified according to the location of the lesions within the pulmonary acinus (Fig. 12-43). Only the proximal part of the acinus (respiratory bronchiole) is selectively involved in centrilobular emphysema, whereas the entire acinus is destroyed in panacinar emphysema.

CENTRILOBULAR EMPHYSEMA: This form of emphysema is most frequent and is usually associated with cigarette smoking and with clinical symptoms. Centrilobular emphysema is characterized by destruction of the cluster of terminal bronchioles near the end of the bronchiolar tree in the central part of the pulmonary lobule (Fig. 12-44A). The lobule is the smallest portion of the lung bounded by septa, and includes several acini. Dilated respiratory bronchioles form enlarged airspaces that are separated from each other and from the lobular septa by normal alveolar ducts and alveoli. As centrilobular emphysema progresses, these distal structures also may be involved (Fig. 12-44B). Bronchioles proximal to the emphysematous spaces are inflamed and narrowed. Centrilobular emphysema is most severe in the upper zones of the lung, the upper lobe, and the superior segment of the lower lobe.

Focal dust emphysema, a disease of coal miners, resembles centrilobular emphysema but differs in that the enlarged spaces are smaller and more regular and inflammation of the bronchioles is not apparent. Importantly, the lesion is primarily distensive rather than destructive. Focal dust emphysema is discussed below in the section on coal worker's pneumoconiosis.

PANACINAR EMPHYSEMA: In panacinar emphysema, the acinus is uniformly involved, with destruction of the alveolar septa from the center to the periphery of the acinus (Fig. 12-45A,B). The loss of alveolar septa is illustrated in the histologic comparison of lung affected by α_1-AT deficiency with normal lung at the same magnification (Fig. 12-46). In the final stage, panacinar emphysema leaves behind a lacy network of supporting tissue ("cotton-candy lung"). This variant occurs in several situations. Diffuse panacinar emphysema is typically associated with α_1-AT deficiency. It is also often found in cigarette smokers in association with centrilobular emphysema. In such cases, the panacinar pattern tends to occur in the lower zones of the lung, whereas centrilobular emphysema is seen in the upper regions.

LOCALIZED EMPHYSEMA: This condition, previously known as "paraseptal emphysema," is characterized by destruction of alveoli and resulting emphysema in only one or at most a few locations. The remainder of the lungs is normal. The lesion is usually found at the apex of an upper lobe, although it may occur anywhere in the pulmonary parenchyma, such as in a subpleural location (Fig. 12-47). Although it is of no clinical significance itself, rupture of an area of localized emphysema produces spontaneous pneumothorax (see below). Progression of localized emphysema can result in a large area of destruction, termed a **bulla**, which ranges in size from as small as 2 cm to a large lesion that occupies an entire hemothorax.

CLINICAL FEATURES: Most patients with symptomatic emphysema are seen at age 60 years or older with a prolonged history of exertional dyspnea but a minimal, nonproductive cough. They have lost weight and use the accessory muscles of respiration to breathe. Weight loss is probably due less to the lack of calories than to the increased work of breathing. Tachypnea and a prolonged expiratory phase are typical. The most prominent radiologic abnormality is overinflation of the lung, as evidenced by enlarged lungs,

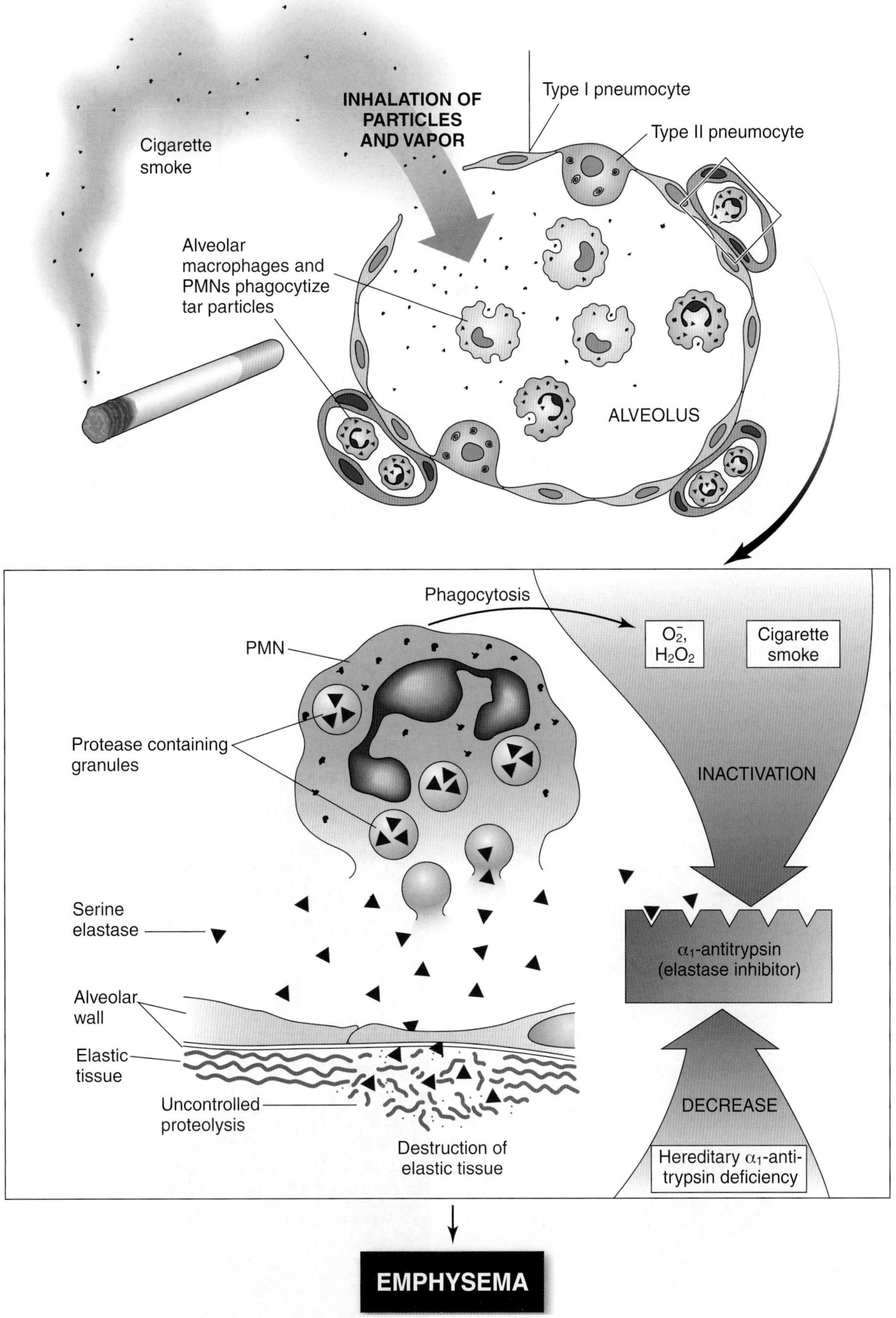

FIGURE 12-42. **The proteolysis–antiproteolysis theory of the pathogenesis of emphysema.** Cigarette (tobacco) smoking is closely related to the development of emphysema. Some product in tobacco smoke induces an inflammatory reaction. The serine elastase in polymorphonuclear leukocytes, which is a particularly potent elastolytic agent, injures the elastic tissue of the lung. Normally, this enzyme activity is inhibited by α_1-antitrypsin, but tobacco smoke, directly or through the generation of free radicals, inactivates α_1-antitrypsin (protease inhibitor). H_2O_2 = hydrogen peroxide; O_2^- = superoxide ion; PMN = polymorphonuclear neutrophil.

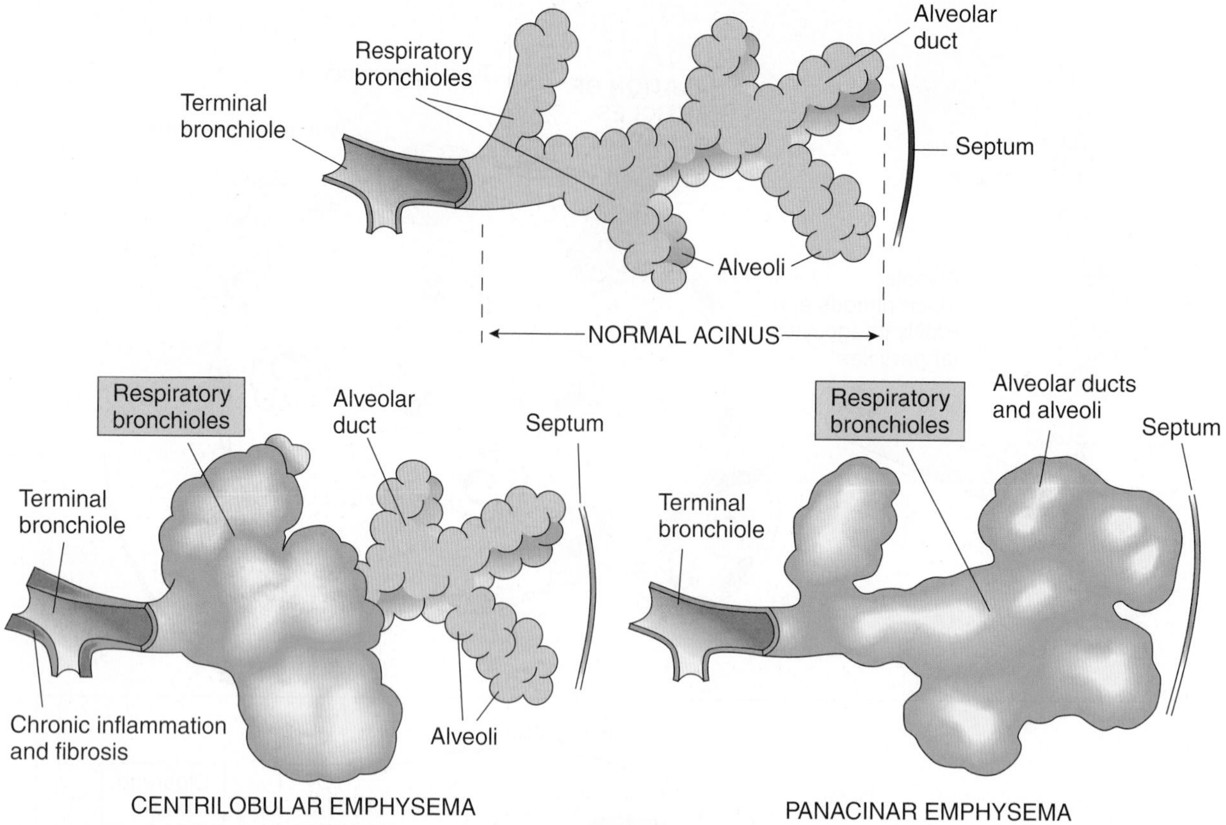

FIGURE 12-43. **Types of emphysema.** The acinus is the unit gas-exchanging structure of the lung distal to the terminal bronchiole. It consists of (in order) respiratory bronchioles, alveolar ducts, alveolar sacs, and alveoli. In centrilobular (proximal acinar) emphysema, the respiratory bronchioles are predominantly involved. In paraseptal (distal acinar) emphysema, the alveolar ducts are particularly affected. In panacinar (panlobular) emphysema, the acinus is uniformly damaged.

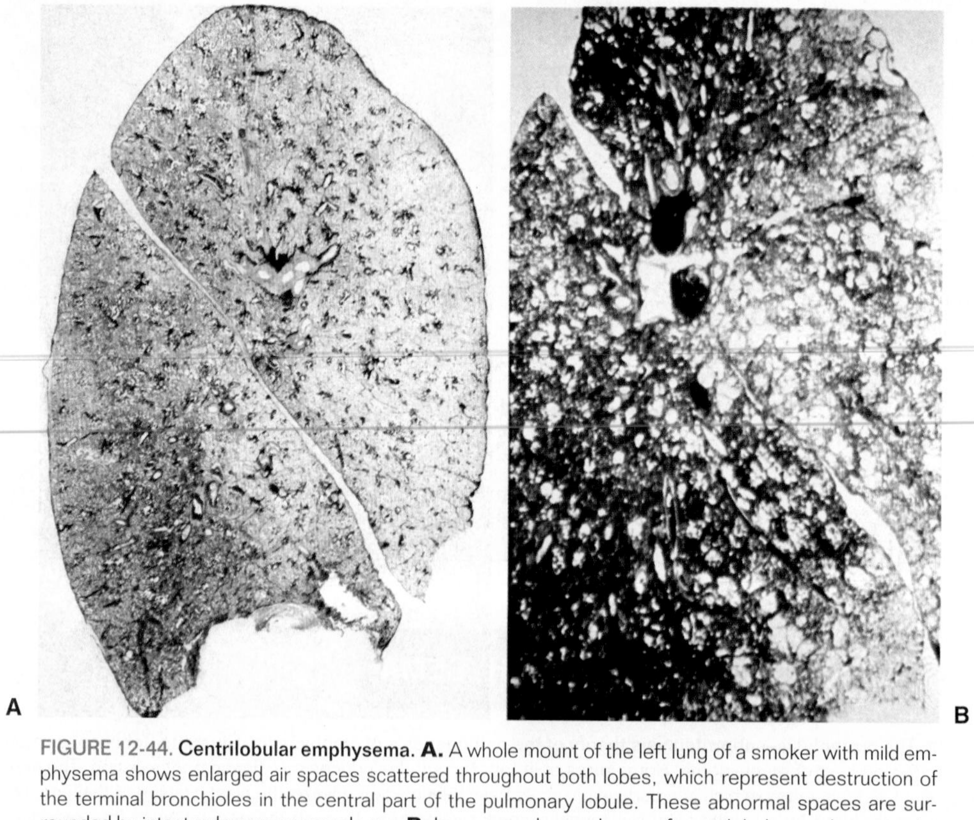

FIGURE 12-44. **Centrilobular emphysema. A.** A whole mount of the left lung of a smoker with mild emphysema shows enlarged air spaces scattered throughout both lobes, which represent destruction of the terminal bronchioles in the central part of the pulmonary lobule. These abnormal spaces are surrounded by intact pulmonary parenchyma. **B.** In a more advanced case of centrilobular emphysema, the destruction of the lung has progressed to produce large, irregular air spaces.

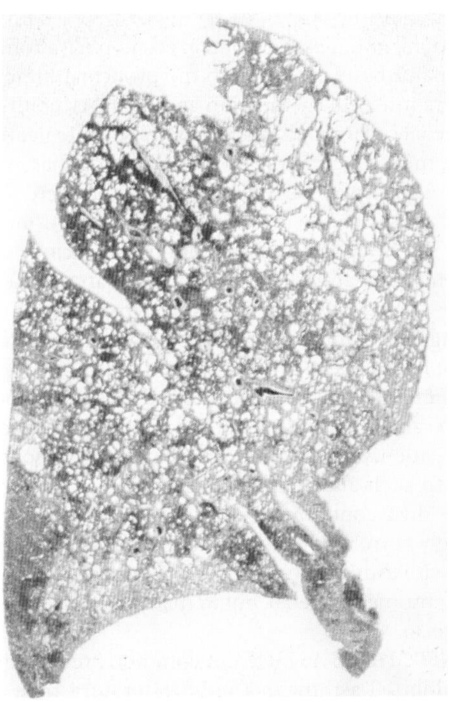
A

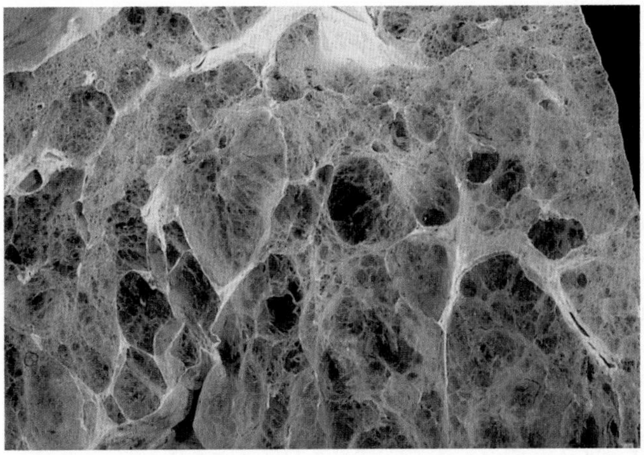
B

FIGURE 12-45. **Panacinar emphysema. A.** A whole mount of the left lung from a patient with severe emphysema reveals widespread destruction of the pulmonary parenchyma, which in some areas leaves behind only a lacy network of supporting tissue. **B**. The lung from this patient with α_1-antitrypsin deficiency shows a panacinar pattern of emphysema. The loss of alveolar walls has resulted in markedly enlarged air spaces.

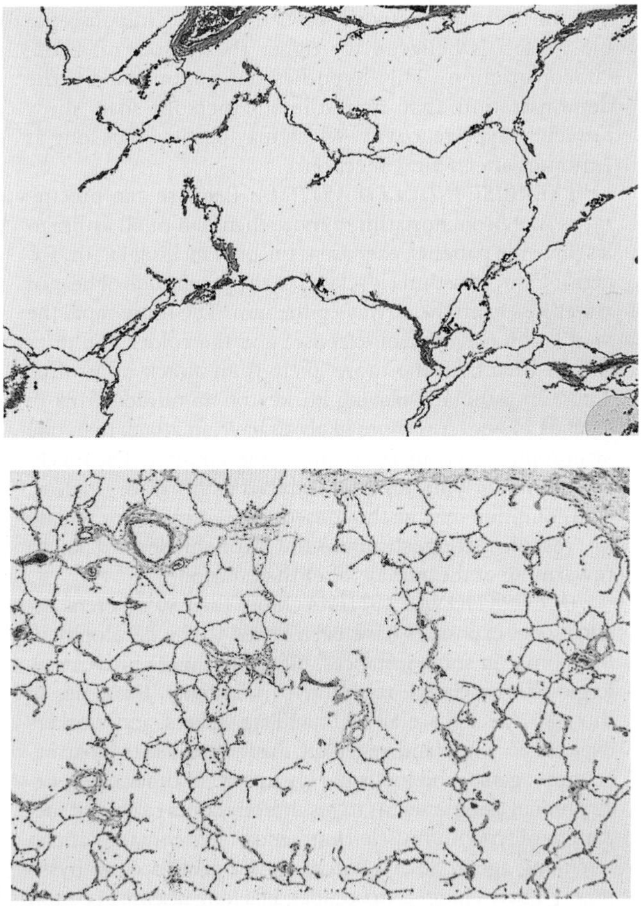
A
B

FIGURE 12-46. **Panacinar emphysema. A.** This lung, from a patient with α_1-antitrypsin deficiency, shows large, irregular air spaces and a markedly reduced number of alveolar walls. **B.** The extensive loss of alveolar walls in A is emphasized by comparison with this section of normal lung at the same magnification.

depressed diaphragms and an increased posteroanterior diameter (barrel chest). The bronchovascular markings do not extend to the peripheral lung fields. Because these patients have a higher respiratory rate and an increased minute volume, they can maintain arterial hemoglobin saturation at near-normal levels and so are called "pink puffers." In contrast to patients with predominantly chronic bronchitis, those with emphysema are at lower risk of recurrent pulmonary infections and are not so prone to develop cor pulmonale. The clinical course of emphysema is marked by inexorable decline in respiratory function and progressive dyspnea, for which no treatment is adequate.

Asthma Is Characterized by Episodic Air-Flow Obstruction in Response to a Number of Stimuli

Patients typically have paroxysms of wheezing, dyspnea and cough. Acute episodes of asthma may alternate with asymp-

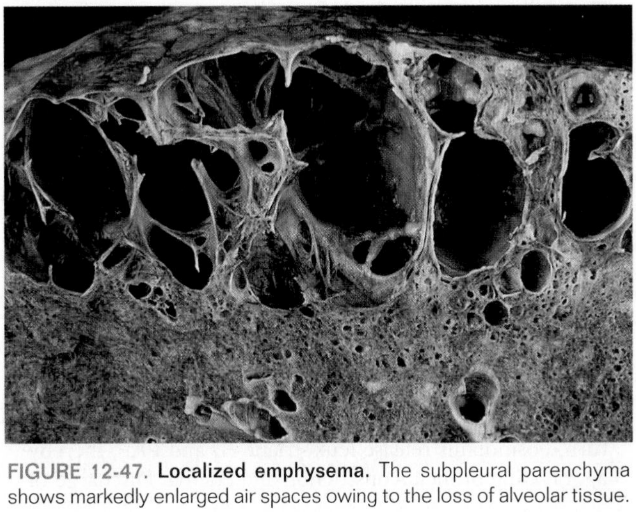

FIGURE 12-47. **Localized emphysema.** The subpleural parenchyma shows markedly enlarged air spaces owing to the loss of alveolar tissue.

tomatic periods or be superimposed on a background of chronic airway obstruction. Severe acute asthma unresponsive to therapy is termed **status asthmaticus**. Most asthmatic patients, even when apparently well, have some persistent air-flow obstruction and morphologic lesions.

In the United States, bronchial asthma affects up to 10% of children and 5% of adults. For reasons unknown, since 1980, the prevalence of asthma in the United States has doubled. Although the initial attack of the disease can occur at any age, half of cases appear in patients younger than 10 years, and the incidence is twice as high in boys as in girls. By age 30, both sexes are affected equally.

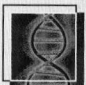

PATHOGENESIS: Asthma was classically divided into extrinsic (allergic) and intrinsic (idiosyncratic) categories depending on inciting factors. In the former, bronchospasm is induced by inhaled antigens, usually in children with a personal or family history of allergic disease (e.g., eczema, urticaria, or hay fever). Intrinsic asthma was a disease of adults in which bronchial hyperreactivity was precipitated by a variety of factors unrelated to immune mechanisms. It now seems more appropriate simply to discuss asthma in terms of the different inciting factors and the common effector pathways.

The consensus hypothesis attributes bronchial hyperresponsiveness in asthma to an inflammatory reaction to diverse stimuli. After exposure to an inciting factor (e.g., allergens, drugs, cold, exercise), inflammatory mediators released by activated macrophages, mast cells, eosinophils, and basophils induce bronchoconstriction, increased vascular permeability, and mucous secretion. Moreover, resident inflammatory cells may be activated to release chemotactic factors that in turn recruit more effector cells and amplify the response of the airways. Inflammation of the bronchial walls also may injure the epithelium, stimulating nerve endings and initiating neural reflexes that further aggravate and propagate the bronchospasm.

Many inflammatory mediators and chemotactic factors have been implicated in leading to the bronchospasm and mucous hypersecretion of asthma. The relative contributions of the different substances probably vary with the inciting stimulus. The best-studied situation associated with the induction of asthma is inhaled allergens.

In a sensitized person, an inhaled allergen interacts with T_H2 cells and IgE antibody bound to the surface of mast cells that are interspersed among the epithelial cells of the bronchial mucosa (Fig. 12-48). As a result, T_H2 cells and mast cells release mediators of type I (immediate) hypersensitivity, including histamine, bradykinin, leukotrienes, prostaglandins, thromboxane A_2, and platelet-activating factor (PAF), as well as cytokines such as interleukin (IL)-4 and IL-5. The inflammatory mediators lead to (1) smooth muscle contraction, (2) mucous secretion, and (3) increased vascular permeability and edema. Each of these effects is a potent, albeit reversible, cause of airway obstruction. IL-5 causes terminal differentiation of eosinophils in the bone marrow. Chemotactic factors–including leukotriene B_4 and neutrophil–and eosinophil chemotactic factors attract neutrophils, eosinophils, and platelets to the bronchial wall. In turn, eosinophils release leukotriene B_4 and PAF, thereby aggravating bronchoconstriction and edema. Discharge of eosinophil granules that contain eosinophil cationic protein and major basic protein into the bronchial lumen further impairs mucociliary function and damages epithelial cells. Epithelial cell injury is suspected to stimulate nerve endings in the mucosa, initiating an autonomic discharge that contributes to airway narrowing and mucous secretion. Moreover, leukotriene B_4 and PAF recruit more eosinophils and other effector cells, and so continue the vicious circle that prolongs and amplifies the asthmatic attack. Recent evidence suggests that activated T lymphocytes also help propagate the inflammatory response through various cytokine networks.

ALLERGIC ASTHMA: This is the most common form of asthma and is usually seen in children. One third to one half of all patients with asthma have known or suspected reactions to such allergens as pollens, animal hair or fur, and house dust contaminated with mites. Allergic asthma is strongly correlated with skin-test reactivity. Half of all children with asthma have a substantial or complete remission of symptoms by age 20, but in many, asthma may recur after age 30.

INFECTIOUS ASTHMA: A common precipitating factor in childhood asthma is a viral respiratory tract infection rather than an allergic stimulus. In children under 2 years, RSV is the usual agent; in older children, rhinovirus, influenza, and parainfluenza are common inciting organisms. The inflammatory response to viral infection in a susceptible person is believed to trigger the episode of bronchoconstriction. This hypothesis is supported by the demonstration that nonasthmatic persons also show bronchial hyperreactivity, which may persist for as long as 2 months after a viral infection.

EXERCISE-INDUCED ASTHMA: Exercise can precipitate some bronchospasm in more than half of all asthmatics. In some patients, exercise is the only inciting factor. Exercise-induced asthma is related to the magnitude of heat or water loss from the airway epithelium. The more rapid the ventilation (severity of exercise) and the colder and drier the air breathed, the more likely is an attack of asthma. Thus, an asthmatic playing hockey on an outdoor rink in Canada in winter is more likely to have an attack than one swimming slowly in Texas during the summer. The mechanisms underlying exercise-induced asthma are unclear. The condition may be the consequence of mediator release or vascular congestion in the bronchi secondary to rewarming of the airways after the exertion.

OCCUPATIONAL ASTHMA: More than 80 different occupational exposures have been linked to the development of asthma. In some instances, these substances provoke allergic asthma via IgE-related hypersensitivity. Examples of those so affected are animal handlers, bakers, and workers exposed to wood and vegetable dusts, metal salts, pharmaceutical agents, and industrial chemicals. In other cases, occupational asthma seems to result from direct release of mediators of smooth muscle contraction after contact with an offending agent. Such a mechanism is postulated in byssinosis ("brown lung"), an occupational lung disease in cotton workers. Some occupational exposures affect the autonomic nervous system directly. For instance, organic phosphorus insecticides act as anticholinesterases and produce overactivity of the parasympathetic nervous system. Substances such

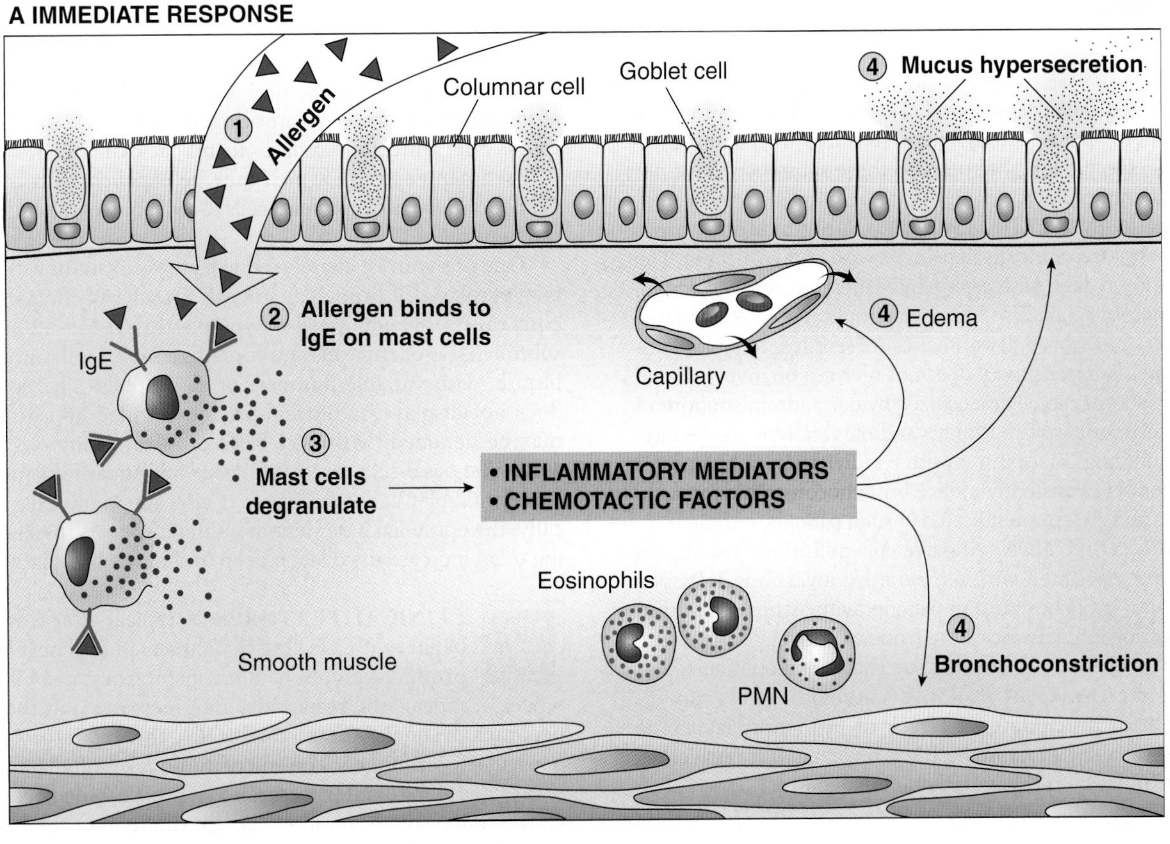

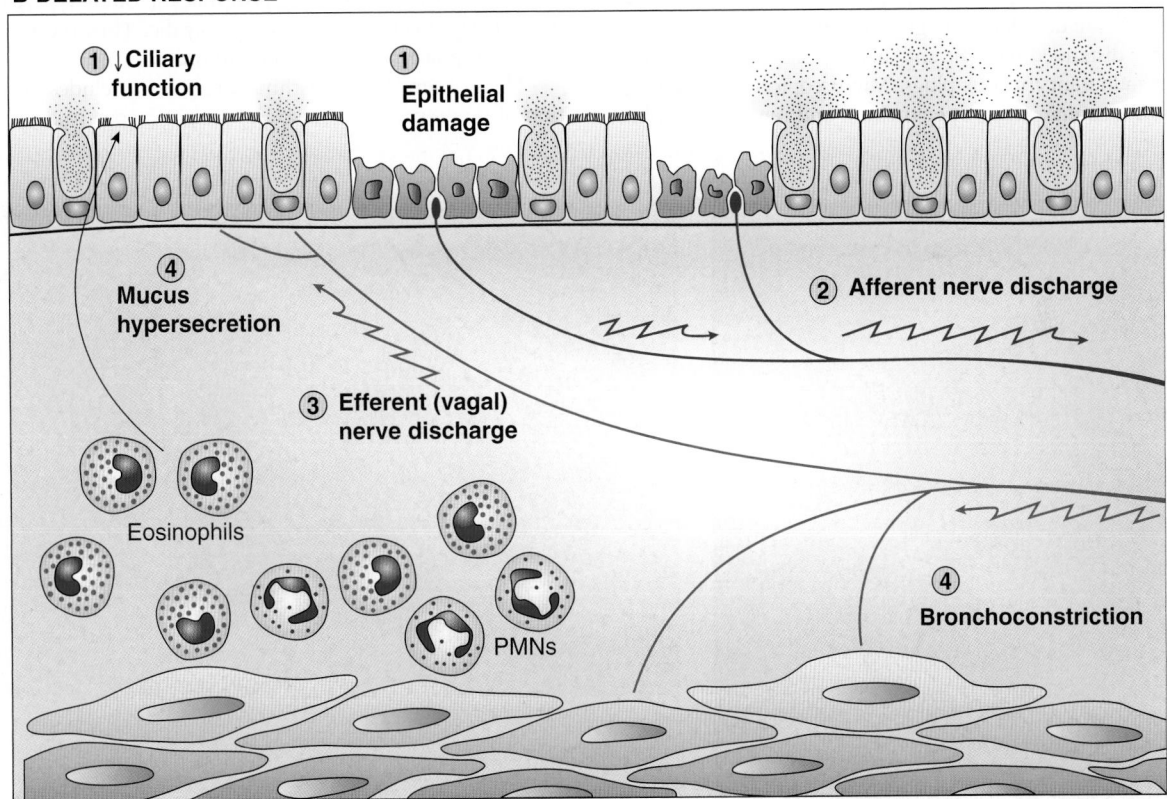

FIGURE 12-48. **Pathogenesis of asthma. A.** Immunologically mediated asthma. Allergens interact with immunoglobulin E (IgE) on mast cells, either on the surface of the epithelium or, when there is abnormal permeability of the epithelium, in the submucosa. Mediators are released and may react locally or by reflexes mediated through the vagus. **B.** The discharge of eosinophilic granules further impairs mucociliary function and damages epithelial cells. Epithelial cell injury stimulates nerve endings in the mucosa, thereby initiating an autonomic discharge that contributes to airway narrowing and mucous secretion. PMNs = polymorphonuclear neutrophils.

as toluene diisocyanate and western red cedar dust are thought to operate through hypersensitivity mechanisms, although specific IgE antibodies to these substances have not been identified.

DRUG-INDUCED ASTHMA: Drug-induced bronchospasm occurs mostly in patients with known asthma. The best-known offender is aspirin but other nonsteroidal anti-inflammatory agents also have been implicated. It is estimated that up to 10% of adult asthmatics are sensitive to aspirin. Immediate hypersensitivity does not seem to be involved, and these patients can be desensitized by daily administrations of small doses of aspirin. Rhinitis and nasal polyps are also frequent findings in aspirin-sensitive individuals. β-Adrenergic antagonists consistently induce bronchoconstriction in asthmatics and are contraindicated in such patients.

AIR POLLUTION: Massive air pollution, usually in episodes associated with temperature inversions, is associated with bronchospasm in patients with asthma and other preexisting lung diseases. SO_2, oxides of nitrogen, and ozone are the commonly implicated environmental pollutants.

EMOTIONAL FACTORS: Psychological stress can aggravate or precipitate an attack of bronchospasm in as many as half of all asthmatics. It is believed that vagal efferent stimulation is the underlying mechanism.

PATHOLOGY: Most information on the pathology of asthma has been derived from autopsies on patients who have died in status asthmaticus, and thus the most severe lesions are described. On gross examination, the lungs are remarkably distended with air and airways are filled with thick, tenacious, adherent mucous plugs. Microscopically, these plugs (Fig. 12-49A) contain strips of epithelium and many eosinophils. Charcot-Leyden crystals, derived from phospholipids of the eosinophil cell membrane, are also seen (see Fig. 12-24B). In some cases, the mucoid exudate forms a cast of the airways (Curschmann spirals), which may be expelled with coughing. Compact clusters of epithelial cells (Creola bodies) also are seen in the sputum.

One of the most characteristic features of status asthmaticus is hyperplasia of bronchial smooth muscle. Bronchial submucosal mucous glands are also hyperplastic (see Fig. 12-49A). The submucosa is edematous and contains a mixed inflammatory infiltrate, with variable numbers of eosinophils. The epithelium does not display the normal pseudostratified appearance and may be denuded, with only basal cells remaining (see Fig. 12-49B). The basal cells are hyperplastic and squamous metaplasia is seen. Goblet cell hyperplasia is also apparent. Characteristically, the epithelial basement membrane appears thickened, owing to an increase in collagen deep to the true basal lamina.

CLINICAL FEATURES: A typical attack of asthma begins with a feeling of tightness in the chest and nonproductive cough. Both inspiratory and expiratory wheezes appear, the respiratory rate increases and the patient becomes dyspneic. Characteristically, the expiratory phase is particularly prolonged. The end of the attack is often heralded by severe coughing and expectoration of thick, mucus containing Curschmann spirals, eosinophils, and Charcot–Leyden crystals.

***Status asthmaticus** refers to severe bronchoconstriction that does not respond to the drugs that usually abort the acute attack.* This situation is potentially serious and requires hospitalization. Patients in status asthmaticus have hypoxemia and often hypercapnia. In particularly severe episodes, they may die. They require oxygen and other pharmacologic interventions.

The cornerstone of asthma treatment includes administration of β-adrenergic agonists, inhaled corticosteroids, cromolyn

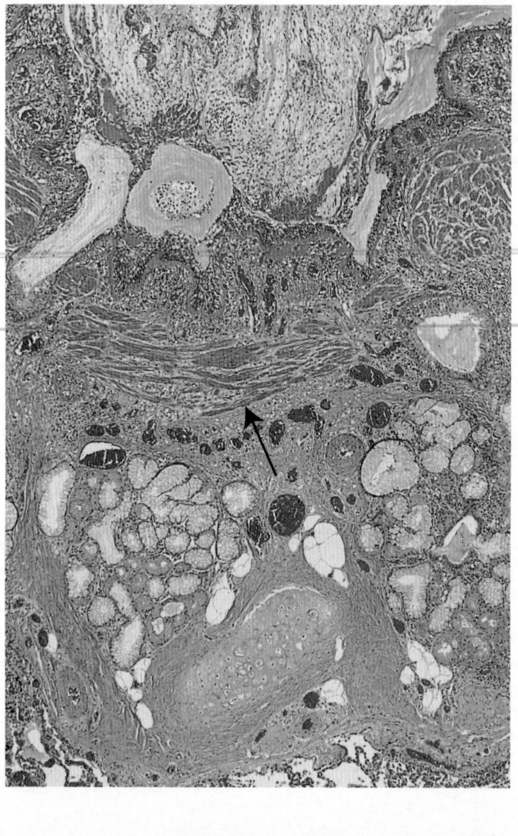
A

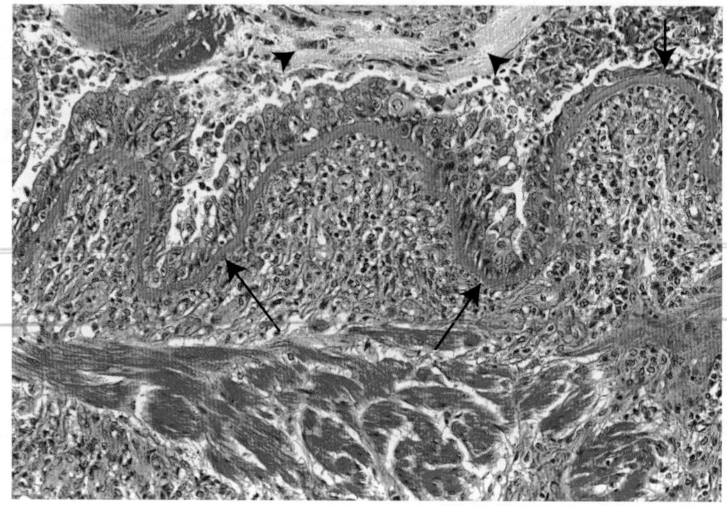
B

FIGURE 12-49. **Asthma. A.** A section of lung from a patient who died in status asthmaticus reveals a bronchus containing a luminal mucous plug, submucosal gland hyperplasia, and smooth muscle hyperplasia *(arrow)*. **B.** Higher magnification shows hyaline thickening of the subepithelial basement membrane *(long arrows)* and marked inflammation of the bronchiolar wall, with numerous eosinophils. The mucosa exhibits an inflamed and metaplastic epithelium *(arrowheads)*. The epithelium is focally denuded *(short arrow)* sodium, methylxanthines, and anticholinergic agents. Systemic corticosteroids are reserved for status asthmaticus or resistant chronic asthma. The inhalation of bronchodilators often provides dramatic relief.

Pneumoconioses

The pneumoconioses are pulmonary diseases caused by dust inhalation. More than 40 inhaled minerals cause lung lesions and radiographic abnormalities. Most, such as tin, barium, and iron, are innocuous and simply accumulate in the lung. However, some lead to crippling pulmonary diseases. The specific types of pneumoconioses are named according to the substance inhaled (e.g., silicosis, asbestosis, talcosis). Sometimes, the offending agent is uncertain, and often the occupation is simply cited (e.g., "arc welder's lung"). Historically, occupations were recognized as predisposing to lung disease before an etiology was recognized. Thus, "knife grinder's lung" was used before the disease was recognized as silicosis.

PATHOGENESIS: *The most important factor in the production of symptomatic pneumoconioses is the capacity of inhaled dusts to stimulate fibrosis* (Fig. 12-50). Thus, small amounts of silica or asbestos may produce extensive fibrosis, whereas coal and iron are only weakly fibrogenic.

In general, lung lesions produced by inorganic dusts reflect the dose and size of the particles that reach the lung. The dose is a function of the amount of dust in the ambient air and the time spent in that environment. As inhaled particles are often irregular, it is important to express their size as aerodynamic particle diameter, a parameter that describes the motion of the particle in inspired air. The aerodynamic particle diameter determines where inhaled dusts deposit in the lung (see Fig. 12-2). The most dangerous particles are those that reach the peripheral zones (i.e., the smallest bronchioles and the acini). Particles over 10 μm in diameter deposit on bronchi and bronchioles and are removed by the mucociliary escalator. Smaller particles reach the acinus, and the smallest ones behave as a gas and are exhaled.

Alveolar macrophages ingest the inhaled particles and are the primary defenders of the alveolar space. Most phagocytosed particles ascend to the mucociliary carpet and are expectorated or swallowed. Others migrate into the interstitium of the lung, then into the lymphatics. A significant number of ingested particles accumulate in and about respiratory bronchioles and terminal bronchioles. Others are not phagocytosed but migrate through epithelial cells into the interstitium.

Silicosis Is Caused by Inhalation of Silicon Dioxide (Silica)

The earth's crust is composed largely of silicon and its oxides, and silicosis is one of the oldest recorded diseases, possibly having begun in the Paleolithic period when humans began to fashion flint instruments. Dyspnea in metal diggers was reported by Hippocrates and early Dutch pathologists wrote that the lungs of stone cutters sectioned like a mass of sand. The 19th-century English literature provided numerous descriptions of silicosis, and the disease remained the major cause of death in workers exposed to silica dust for the first half of the 20th century.

Silicosis was described historically as a disease of sandblasters. Mining also involves exposure to silica, as do numerous other occupations, including stone cutting, polishing and sharpening of metals, ceramic manufacturing, foundry work, and the cleaning of boilers. The use of air-handling equipment and face masks has substantially reduced the incidence of silicosis.

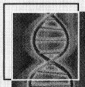

PATHOGENESIS: The biological effects of silica particles depend on a number of factors, some involving the particle itself and others related to the host response. Crystalline silica (quartz) is more toxic than amorphous forms, and its biological activity is related to its surface properties. Particles of 0.2 to 2.0 μm are the most dangerous. Removal of the soluble surface layer by acid washing or the creation of new surfaces by sandblasting enhances the biological activity of silica particles.

After their inhalation, silica particles are ingested by alveolar macrophages. Silicon hydroxide groups on the surface of the particles form hydrogen bonds with phospholipids and proteins, an interaction that is presumed to damage cellular membranes and thereby kill the macrophages. The dead cells release free silica particles and fibrogenic factors. The released silica is then reingested by macrophages and the process is amplified.

PATHOLOGY: *SIMPLE NODULAR SILICOSIS:* This is the most common form of silicosis and is almost inevitable in any worker with long-term exposure to silica. Twenty to 40 years after the initial exposure to silica (but sometimes after only 10 years), the lungs contain silicotic nodules, which are less than 1 cm in diameter (usually 2 to 4 mm). On histologic examination, they have a characteristic whorled appearance, with concentrically arranged collagen that forms the largest part of the nodule (Fig. 12-51). At the periphery, there are aggregates of mononuclear cells, mostly lymphocytes and fibroblasts. Polarized light reveals doubly refractile needle-shaped silicates within the nodule.

Hilar nodes may become enlarged and calcified, often at the periphery of the node ("eggshell calcification"). Simple silicosis is not ordinarily associated with significant respiratory dysfunction.

PROGRESSIVE MASSIVE FIBROSIS: Progressive massive fibrosis is defined radiologically as nodular masses of more than 2 cm diameter in a background of simple silicosis. These larger lesions represent the coalescence of smaller nodules. Most of these lesions are 5 to 10 cm across and are usually in the upper zones of the lungs bilaterally (Fig. 12-52). Morphologically, they often exhibit central cavitation. Progressive massive fibrosis is related to the amount of silica in the lung. Disability is caused by destruction of lung tissue that has been incorporated into the nodules.

ACUTE SILICOSIS: Now uncommon, acute silicosis results from heavy exposure to finely particulate silica during sandblasting or boiler scaling. It is associated with diffuse fibrosis of the lung. Silicotic nodules are not found. Dense eosinophilic material accumulates in alveolar spaces to produce an appearance that resembles alveolar lipoproteinosis (**silicoproteinosis**). The disease progresses rapidly over a few years, in contrast to other forms of silicosis in which progression is measured in decades. On radiologic examination, acute silicosis shows diffuse linear fibrosis and reduced lung volume. Clinically, there is a severe restrictive defect.

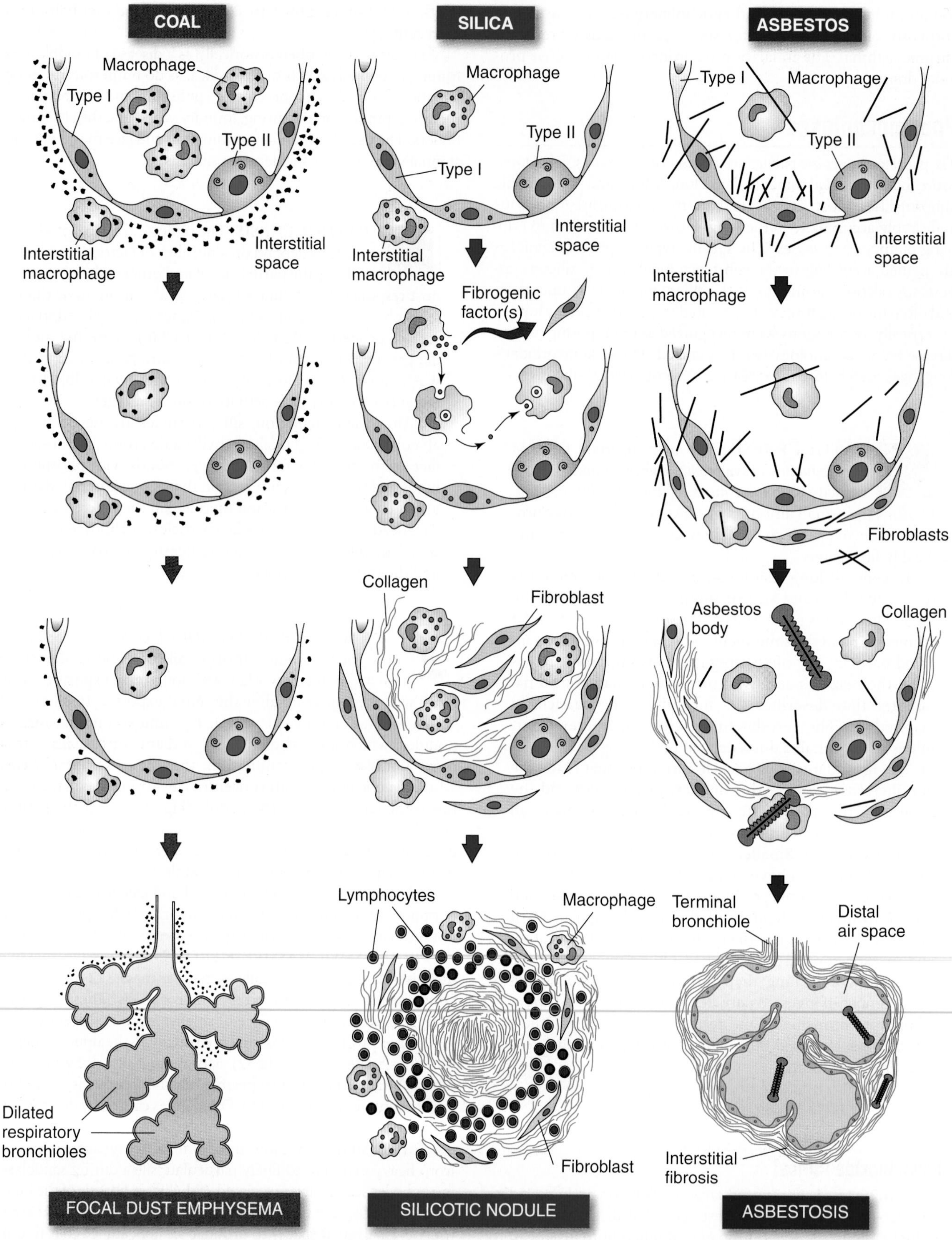

FIGURE 12-50. **Pathogenesis of pneumoconioses.** The three most important pneumoconioses are illustrated. In simple coal workers' pneumoconiosis, massive amounts of dust are inhaled and engulfed by macrophages. The macrophages pass into the interstitium of the lung and aggregate around the respiratory bronchioles. Subsequently, the bronchioles dilate. In silicosis, the silica particles are toxic to macrophages, which die and release a fibrogenic factor. In turn the released silica is again phagocytosed by other macrophages. The result is a dense fibrotic nodule, the silicotic nodule. Asbestosis is characterized by little dust and much interstitial fibrosis. Asbestos bodies are the classic features.

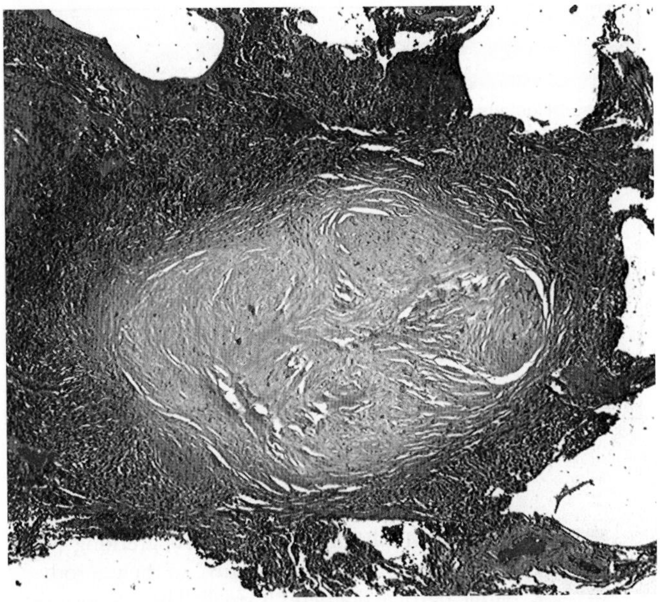

FIGURE 12-51. **Silicosis.** A silicotic nodule is composed of concentric whorls of dense, sparsely cellular collagen. At the edge of the nodule are dust deposits that contain carbon pigment and silica particles.

CLINICAL FEATURES: Simple silicosis is usually a radiologic diagnosis without significant symptoms. Dyspnea on exertion and later at rest suggests progressive massive fibrosis or other complications of silicosis. In acute silicosis, dyspnea may become rapidly disabling, after which respiratory failure ensues.

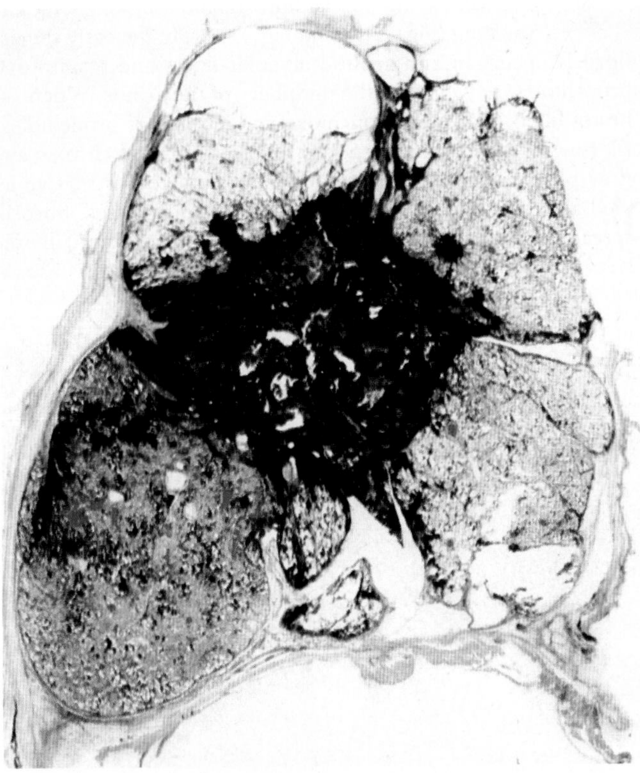

FIGURE 12-52. **Progressive massive fibrosis.** A whole mount of a silicotic lung from a coal miner shows a large area of dense fibrosis containing entrapped carbon particles.

It is well recognized that tuberculosis is much more common in patients with silicosis than in the general population. The incidence of tuberculosis in patients with silicosis is higher in acute silicosis and among populations with a high prevalence of tuberculosis. Despite a decline in the incidence of tuberculosis in the general population, the association with silicosis has persisted. Silicosis does not predispose to lung cancers.

Coal Workers' Pneumoconiosis (CWP) Reflects Inhalation of Carbon Particles

PATHOGENESIS: Coal dust is composed of amorphous carbon and other constituents of the earth's surface, including variable amounts of silica. Anthracite (hard) coal contains significantly more quartz than does bituminous (soft) coal. Workers in certain occupations, such as those who work within mines, inhale more quartz particles than those working above ground or loading coal for transport. In this context, one must recognize that amorphous carbon by itself is not fibrogenic, owing to its inability to kill alveolar macrophages. It is simply a nuisance dust that causes an innocuous anthracosis. By contrast, silica is highly fibrogenic, and inhaled anthracotic particles may thus lead to **anthracosilicosis**. (see Fig. 12-53)

PATHOLOGY: CWP is typically divided into **simple CWP** and **complicated CWP** (a.k.a. progressive massive fibrosis). The characteristic lung lesions of simple CWP include nonpalpable **coal-dust macules** and palpable **coal-dust nodule**. Both are typically multiple and scattered throughout the lung as 1- to 4-mm black foci. Microscopically, a coal-dust macule exhibits numerous carbon-laden macrophages which surround distal respiratory bronchioles, extend to fill adjacent alveolar spaces and infiltrate peribronchiolar interstitial spaces. There is an accompanying mild dilation of respiratory bronchioles (focal dust emphysema), which probably results from atrophy of smooth muscle.

Nodules are round or irregular, may or may not be associated with bronchioles and consist of dust-laden macrophages associated with a fibrotic stroma. They occur when coal is admixed with fibrogenic dusts such as silica and are more properly classified as anthracosilicosis (Fig. 12-53). Coal-dust macules and nodules appear on a chest radiograph as small nodular densities. Although simple CWP was once thought to cause severe disability, it is now clear that at worst it causes a minor impairment of pulmonary function. When coal miners have severe air-flow obstruction, it is usually due to smoking. **Complicated CWP** occurs on a background of simple CWP and is defined as a lesion 2.0 cm or greater in size. Patients with complicated CWP may have significant respiratory impairment.

Caplan syndrome was originally described as the presence of rheumatoid nodules (**Caplan nodules**) in the lungs of coal miners with rheumatoid arthritis. However, the term is now also used for the association of pulmonary rheumatoid nodules

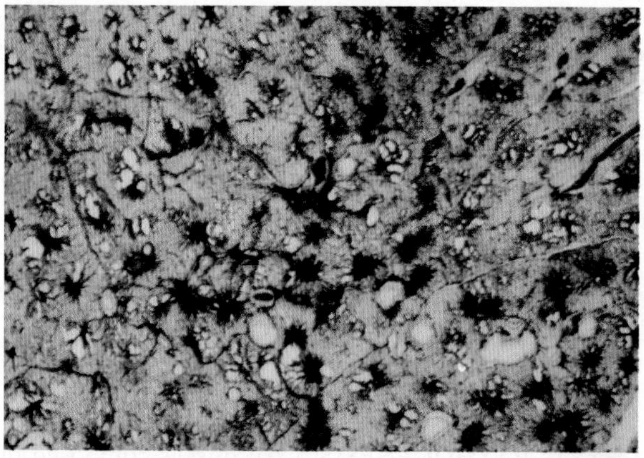

FIGURE 12-53. **Anthracosilicosis.** A whole mount of the lung of a coal miner demonstrates scattered, irregular, pigmented nodules throughout the parenchyma.

with other pneumoconioses, such as silicosis or asbestosis. These nodular lesions are large (1–10 cm in diameter), multiple, bilateral, and usually peripheral. Microscopically, a Caplan nodule has the appearance of a rheumatoid nodule associated with inhaled dust deposits. Rheumatoid nodules consist of large, central, necrotic areas surrounded by a border of chronic inflammation and palisading macrophages. Caplan nodules are similar but not identical to rheumatoid nodules and may represent a combination of silicotic and rheumatoid nodules.

Asbestos-Related Diseases may be Reactive or Neoplastic

Asbestos (Greek, *unquenchable*) includes a group of fibrous silicate minerals that occur as long, thin fibers. It has been used for a variety of purposes for more than 4000 years, since early Finns fashioned pottery from it. The Roman vestal virgins used asbestos to manufacture oil-lamp wicks, and Marco Polo remarked on the asbestos-containing Chinese cloth that resisted fire. More recently, asbestos has been used in a variety of products including insulation, construction materials. and automative brake linings. Asbestos mining proceeded exponentially in the 20th century until its deleterious effects eventually elicited alarm.

There are six natural types of asbestos, which can be divided into two mineralogic groups. **Chrysotile** accounts for the bulk of commercially used asbestos. The **amphiboles** include amosite, crocidolite, tremolite, actinolite, and anthophyllite. Of the amphiboles, only amosite and crocidolite have been used commercially to any extent. If coal is the classic example of much dust and little fibrosis, asbestos is the prototype of little dust and much fibrosis (see Fig. 12-50). Exposure to asbestos can cause a number of thoracic complications including asbestosis, benign pleural effusion, pleural plaques, diffuse pleural fibrosis, rounded atelectasis, and mesothelioma (Table 12-4). All commercially used forms of asbestos have been associated with asbestos-related lung diseases. However, the amphiboles, and crocidolite in particular, have a much greater propensity to produce disease than does chrysotile.

ASBESTOSIS: Asbestosis is diffuse interstitial fibrosis resulting from inhalation of asbestos fibers. The development of asbestosis requires heavy exposure to asbestos of the type historically seen in asbestos miners, millers, and insulators.

TABLE 12-4

Asbestos-Related Lung Disease

Pleural lesions
Benign pleural effusion
Parietal pleural plaques
Diffuse pleural fibrosis
Rounded atelectasis
Interstitial lung disease
Asbestosis
Malignant mesothelioma
Carcinoma of the lung (in smokers)

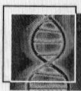

PATHOGENESIS: Asbestos fibers are long (up to 100 μm) but thin (0.5–1 μm), so their aerodynamic particle diameter is small. They deposit in distal airways and alveoli, particularly at bifurcations of alveolar ducts. The smallest particles are engulfed by macrophages, but many larger fibers penetrate into the interstitial space. The first lesion is an alveolitis that is directly related to asbestos exposure. Release of inflammatory mediators by activated macrophages and the fibrogenic character of the free asbestos fibers in the interstitium promote interstitial pulmonary fibrosis.

PATHOLOGY: Asbestosis is characterized by bilateral, diffuse interstitial fibrosis, and asbestos bodies in the lung (Fig. 12-54 and Fig. 12-55). In the early stages, fibrosis occurs in and around alveolar ducts and respiratory bronchioles, as well as in the periphery of the acinus. When asbestos fibers deposit in bronchioles and respiratory bronchioles, they incite a fibrogenic response that leads to mild chronic airflow obstruction. Thus, asbestos may produce obstructive as well as restrictive defects. As the disease progresses, fibrosis spreads beyond the peribronchiolar location and eventually results in an end-stage or ("honeycomb") lung. Asbestosis is usually more severe in the lower zones of the lung.

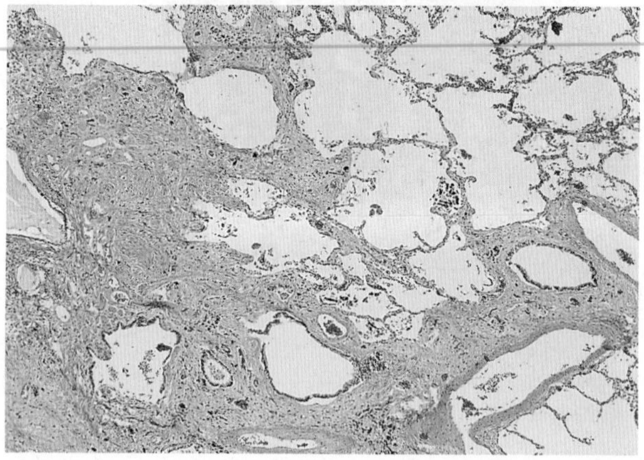

FIGURE 12-54. **Asbestosis.** The lung shows patchy, dense, interstitial fibrosis.

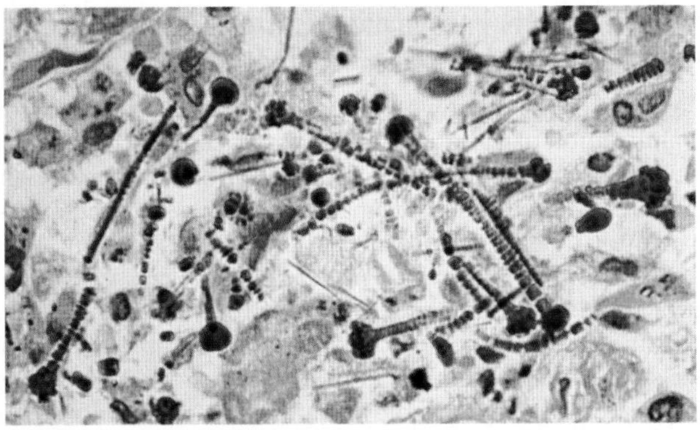

FIGURE 12-55. **Asbestos bodies.** These ferruginous bodies are golden brown and beaded, with a central, colorless, nonbirefringent core fiber. Asbestos bodies are encrusted with protein and iron.

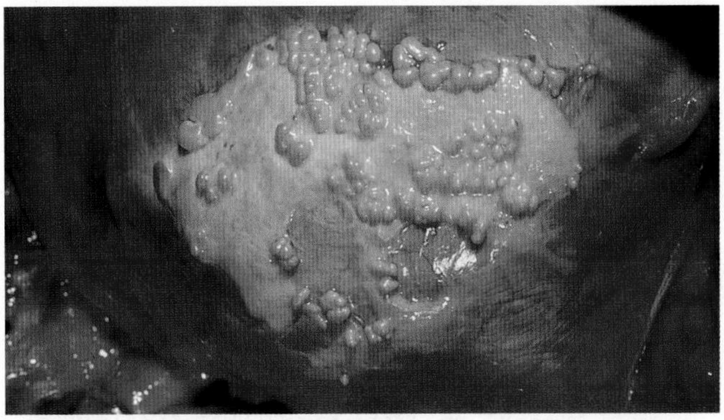

FIGURE 12-56. **Pleural plaque.** The dome of the diaphragm is covered by a smooth, pearly white, nodular plaque.

Asbestos bodies are found in the walls of bronchioles or within alveolar spaces, often engulfed by alveolar macrophages. The particle has distinctive morphologic features, consisting of a clear, thin asbestos fiber (10–50 μm long) surrounded by a beaded iron–protein coat. By light microscopy, it is golden brown (see Fig. 12-55) and stains strongly with the Prussian blue stain for iron. The fibers are only partly engulfed by macrophages because they are too large for a single cell. The macrophages coat the asbestos fiber with protein, proteoglycans and ferritin.

An incidental finding of asbestos bodies in autopsies does not warrant a diagnosis of asbestosis; the lungs must also show diffuse interstitial fibrosis. Digests and concentrates of lung tissue show that asbestos bodies occur to varying degrees in the lungs of virtually all patients who come to autopsy.

BENIGN PLEURAL EFFUSION: Benign pleural effusion associated with asbestos inhalation is diagnosed by: (1) a history of asbestos exposure, (2) identification of a pleural effusion with radiographs or thoracentesis, (3) absence of other diseases that could cause effusion, and (4) no malignant tumor after 3 years of follow-up. Pleural effusions often occur within 10 years of initial exposure and have been observed in about 3% of workers exposed to asbestos.

PLEURAL PLAQUES: Pleural plaques typically occur on parietal and diaphragmatic pleura, often 10 to 20 years after exposure to asbestos. Plaques may be found in up to 15% of the general population and half of all patients with plaques at autopsy may not have a history of asbestos exposure. Plaques occur most often on the parietal pleura, in the posterolateral regions of the lower thorax and on the domes of the diaphragm.

On gross examination, pleural plaques are pearly white and have a smooth or nodular surface (Fig. 12-56). They are usually bilateral, although not necessarily symmetric. Plaques may measure over 10 cm in diameter and become calcified. Histologically, they consist of acellular, dense, hyalinized fibrous tissue, with numerous slitlike spaces in a parallel fashion ("basketweave pattern"). Pleural plaques are not predictors of asbestosis, nor do they evolve into mesotheliomas.

DIFFUSE PLEURAL FIBROSIS: Fibrosis limited to the pleura is usually detected at least 10 years after initial exposure to asbestos. It must be distinguished from asbestosis, in which fibrosis diffusely affects the interstitium of the underlying lung. Plaques and pleural fibrosis can occur in association with all types of asbestos.

ROUNDED ATELECTASIS: Asbestosis exposure occasionally leads to a condition in which pleural fibrosis and adhesions are associated with atelectasis, which has a rounded appearance on chest radiograph. Radiographically, rounded atelectasis is characterized by a pleural-based, rounded or oval, 2.5- to 5.0-cm shadow, which usually lies along the posterior surface of a lower lobe. Pathologically, the lung shows pleural fibrosis or plaques, with curved pleural invaginations extending several centimeters into the underlying parenchyma. The condition is clinically benign.

MESOTHELIOMA: The relation between asbestos exposure and malignant mesothelioma is firmly established. Sometimes exposure is indirect and slight, e.g., wives of asbestos workers who wash their husbands' clothes. More often, mesothelioma is seen in workers heavily exposed to asbestos, mainly crocidolite. This disease are discussed below with diseases of the pleura.

CARCINOMA OF THE LUNG: Lung cancer has been reported to be 3- to 5- times more common in nonsmoking asbestos workers than in similar workers not exposed to asbestos, but this figure is based on small numbers and remains to be firmly established. However, in asbestos workers who smoke, the incidence of carcinoma of the lung is vastly increased: up to 60 times that of the general population. The link between asbestos and lung cancer is most convincingly supported in the presence of asbestosis (diffuse interstitial fibrosis).

Berylliosis Displays Noncaseating Granulomas

Berylliosis refers to the pulmonary disease that follows inhalation of beryllium. Today this metal is used principally in structural materials in aerospace industries, in the manufacture of industrial ceramics, and in nuclear reactors. Exposure to beryllium may also occur in those who mine and extract beryllium ores.

PATHOLOGY: Berylliosis occurs as an acute chemical pneumonitis or a chronic pneumoconiosis. In the acute form, symptoms begin within hours or days after inhalation of metal particles and mainfest pathologically as diffuse alveolar damage. Of all persons with acute beryllium pneumonitis, 10% progress to chronic disease, although chronic berylliosis is often encountered in workers without any history of an acute illness.

Chronic berylliosis differs from other pneumoconioses in that the amount and duration of exposure may be small. The lesion is thus suspected to be a hypersensitivity reaction. Pathologically, the pulmonary lesions are indistinguishable from those of sarcoidosis (see below). Multiple noncaseating granulomas are distributed along the pleura, septa, and bronchovascular bundles (Fig. 12-57). The beryllium lymphocyte proliferation

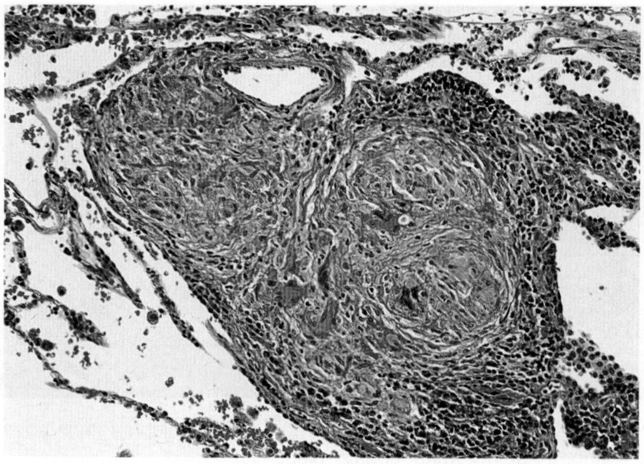

FIGURE 12-57. **Berylliosis.** A noncaseating granuloma consists of a nodular collection of epithelioid macrophages and multinucleated giant cells.

test may aid in separating these two entities. Disease progression can lead to end-stage fibrosis and **honeycomb lung.** Patients with chronic berylliosis have an insidious onset of dyspnea 15 or more years after the initial exposure. The disease appears to be associated with an increased risk of lung cancer.

Talcosis Results From Prolonged and Heavy Exposure to Talc Dust

Talc consists of magnesium silicates that are used in a number of industries for their lubricant properties, and in cosmetics and pharmaceuticals. Occupational exposure to talc occurs among workers engaged in mining and milling the mineral and in the leather, rubber, paper, and textile industries. Industrial talc is usually mixed with other minerals such as asbestos or silica. Cosmetic talc is more than 90% pure and rarely causes lung disease.

PATHOLOGY: On gross examination, talcosis lesions vary from minute nodules to severe fibrosis. Microscopically, foreign-body granulomas associated with birefringent platelike talc particles are scattered throughout the parenchyma, which displays fibrotic nodules and interstitial fibrosis. Associated minerals, such as silica or asbestos, may contribute to the fibrotic changes.

Intravenous drug abusers who use talc as a carrier for illicit drugs may develop vascular and interstitial granulomas in the lung and variable degrees of fibrosis. Arterial changes of pulmonary hypertension are common. Persons with these changes may initially present with cor pulmonale.

Interstitial Lung Disease

A large number of pulmonary disorders are grouped as interstitial, infiltrative, or restrictive diseases because they are characterized by inflammatory infiltrates in the interstitial space and have similar clinical and radiologic presentations. These diverse maladies (1) are acute or chronic, (2) are of known or unknown etiology, and (3) vary from minimally symptomatic conditions to severely incapacitating and lethal interstitial fibrosis. Restrictive lung diseases are typically characterized by decreased lung volume and decreased oxygen-diffusing capacity on pulmonary function studies.

Hypersensitivity Pneumonitis (Extrinsic Allergic Alveolitis) Is a Response to Inhaled Antigens

Many antigens are known to cause hypersensitivity pneumonitis. Inhalation of these antigens leads to acute or chronic interstitial inflammation in the lung. Most of the responsible antigens are encountered in occupational settings, and the diseases are often labeled according to a specific vocation. Thus, **farmer's lung** occurs in farmers exposed to *Micropolyspora faeni* from moldy hay, **bagassosis** results from exposure to *Thermoactinomyces sacchari* in moldy sugar cane, **maple bark–stripper's disease** is seen in persons exposed to the fungus *Cryptostroma corticale* from moldy maple bark, and **bird fancier's lung** affects bird keepers with long-term exposure to proteins from bird feathers, blood, and excrement. Other causes of hypersensitivity pneumonitis include inhalation of pituitary snuff (**pituitary snuff taker's disease**), moldy cork (**suberosis**), and moldy compost (**mushroom worker's disease**). Hypersensitivity pneumonitis may also be caused by fungi growing in stagnant water in air conditioners, swimming pools, hot tubs, and central heating units. Skin tests and serum precipitating antibodies are often used to confirm the diagnosis. In many cases, especially in the chronic form of hypersensitivity pneumonitis, the inciting antigen is never identified.

PATHOGENESIS: Acute hypersensitivity pneumonitis is characterized by a neutrophilic infiltrate in alveoli and respiratory bronchioles; chronic lesions display mononuclear cells and granulomas, typical of delayed hypersensitivity. Most cases have serum IgG precipitating antibodies against the offending agent. Hypersensitivity pneumonitis represents a combination of immune complex-mediated (type III) and cell-mediated (type IV) hypersensitivity reactions, although the precise contribution of each is still debated (Fig. 12-58). Importantly, most persons with serum precipitins to inhaled antigens do not develop hypersensitivity pneumonitis on exposure, a fact that suggests a genetic component in host susceptibility.

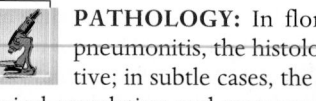

PATHOLOGY: In florid cases of hypersensitivity pneumonitis, the histologic picture is strongly suggestive; in subtle cases, the diagnosis may require careful clinical correlation and may remain tentative even then. The main microscopic features of chronic hypersensitivity pneumonitis include bronchiolocentric cellular interstitial pneumonia, noncaseating granulomas, and organizing pneumonia (Fig. 12-59A,B). The bronchiolocentric cellular interstitial infiltrate varies from severe to subtle and consists of lymphocytes, plasma cells, and macrophages; eosinophils are distinctly uncommon. Poorly formed noncaseating granulomas are present in two thirds of cases (see Fig. 12-59B). Organizing pneumonia is found in two thirds of cases and may form the lesion of bronchiolitis obliterans (see Fig. 12-59A). In the end stage, interstitial inflammation recedes, leaving pulmonary fibrosis, which may resemble usual interstitial pneumonia.

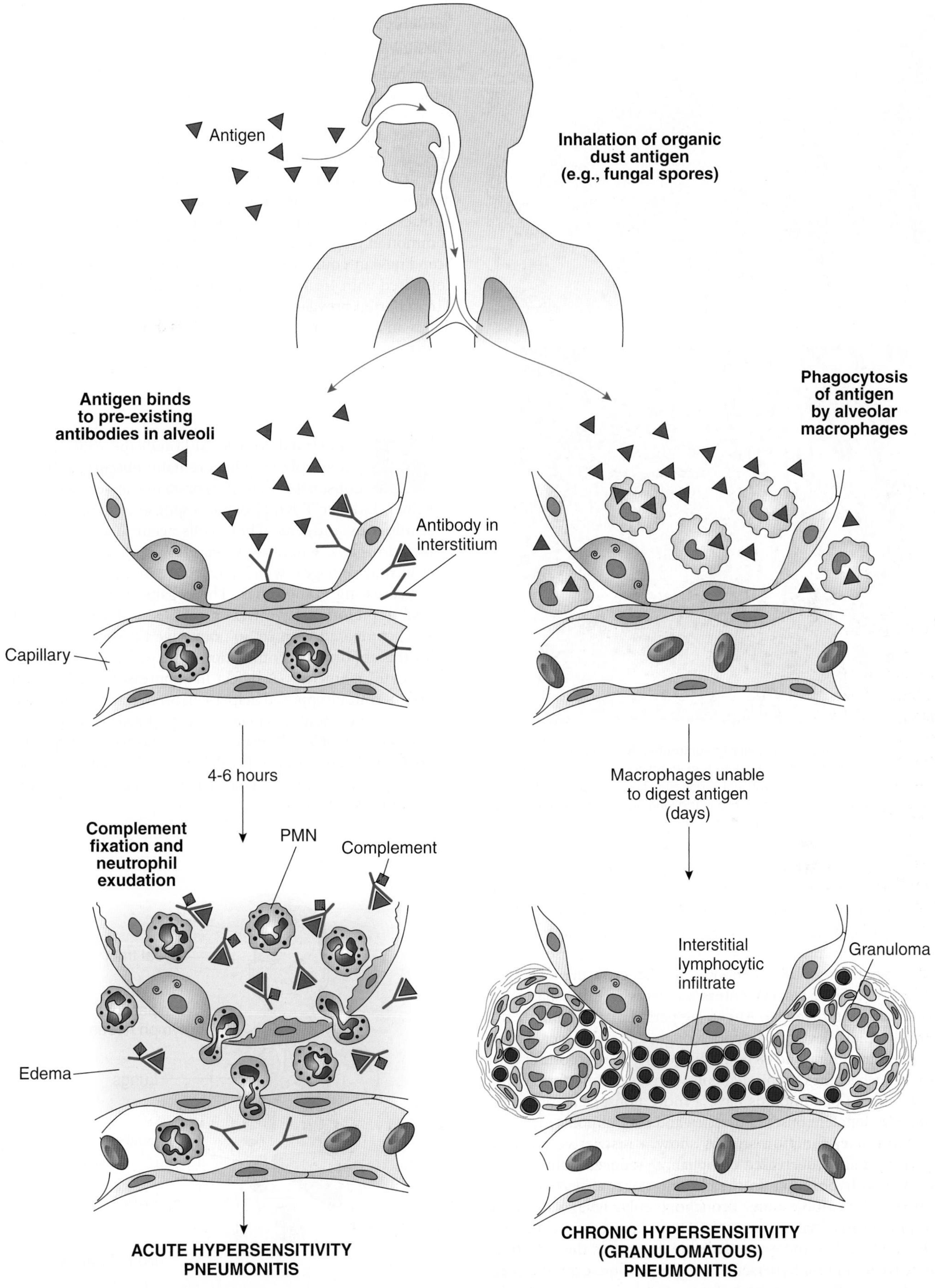

FIGURE 12-58. **Hypersensitivity pneumonitis.** An antigen–antibody reaction occurs in the acute phase and leads to acute hypersensitivity pneumonitis. If exposure is continued, this is followed by a cellular or subacute phase, with the formation of granulomas and chronic interstitial pneumonitis. PMN = polymorphonuclear neutrophil.

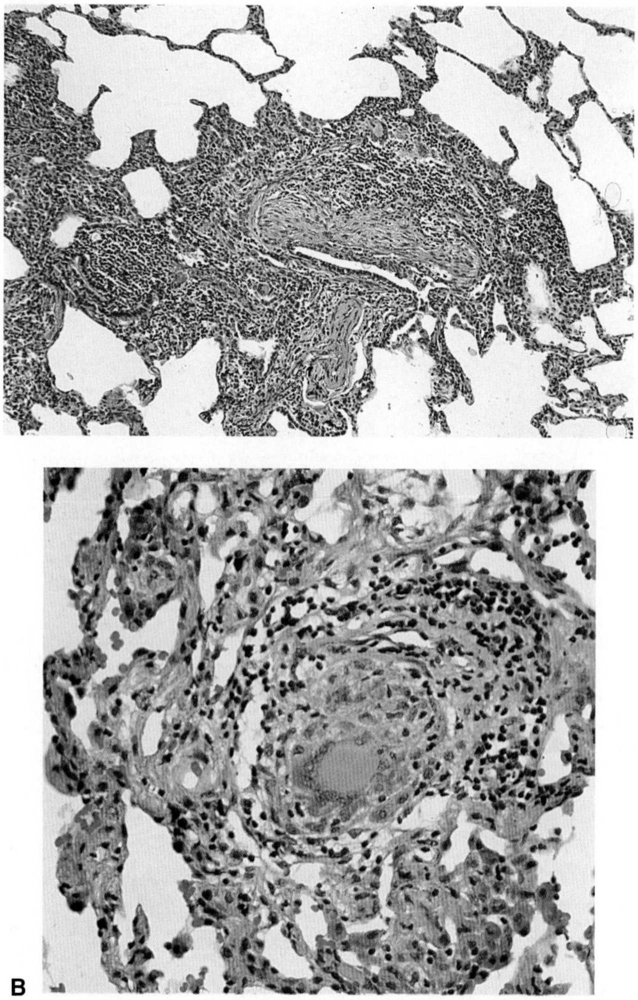
A
B

FIGURE 12-59. **Hypersensitivity pneumonitis. A**. A lung biopsy specimen shows a mild peribronchiolar chronic inflammatory interstitial infiltrate, with a focus of intraluminal organizing fibrosis. **B**. Focal poorly formed granulomas were scattered in the lung biopsy specimen.

CLINICAL FEATURES: Hypersensitivity pneumonitis may be first seen as acute, subacute, or chronic pulmonary disease, depending on the frequency and intensity of exposure to the offending antigen. The prototype of hypersensitivity pneumonitis is "farmer's lung," caused by inhalation of thermophilic actinomycetes that grow in moldy hay. Typically, a farm worker enters a barn where hay has been stored for winter feeding. After a lag period of 4 to 6 hours, the worker rapidly develops dyspnea, cough, and mild fever. Symptoms remit within 24 to 48 hours but return on reexposure; with time, they become chronic. Patients with the chronic form of hypersensitivity pneumonitis have a more nonspecific presentation, with indolent onset of dyspnea and cor pulmonale.

Pulmonary-function studies show a restrictive pattern, characterized by decreased compliance, reduced diffusion capacity, and hypoxemia. In the chronic stage, airway obstruction may be troublesome. Bronchoalveolar lavage shows T lymphocytosis, predominantly CD8+ suppressor/cytotoxic cells. Removal of the environmental antigen is the only adequate treatment for hypersensitivity pneumonitis. Steroid therapy may be effective in acute forms and for some chronically affected patients.

Sarcoidosis Is a Granulomatous Disease of Unknown Etiology

In sarcoidosis the lung is the organ most frequently involved but lymph nodes, skin, and eye are also common targets (Fig. 12-60).

EPIDEMIOLOGY: Sarcoidosis is a worldwide disease, affecting all races and both sexes. The differences in prevalence among racial and ethnic groups are remarkable. In North America, sarcoidosis is much more common in blacks than in whites, the ratio being about 15:1, but is uncommon in tropical Africa. The disease is often encountered in Scandinavian countries, where the prevalence is 64/100,000, compared with 10/100,000 in France, and 3/100,000 in Poland. The reported prevalence of sarcoidosis in Irish women in London is an astonishing 200/100,000. It is distinctly uncommon in China.

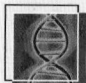

PATHOGENESIS: Although the exact pathogenesis of sarcoidosis remains obscure, there is a consensus that it represents an exaggerated helper/inducer T lymphocyte response to exogenous or autologous antigens. These cells accumulate in the affected organs, where they secrete lymphokines and recruit macrophages, which participate in the formation of noncaseating granulomas. The organs that contain sarcoid granulomas have CD4+ to CD8+ T cell ratios of 10:1, compared with 2:1 in uninvolved tissues. The basis for this abnormal accumulation of helper/inducer T lymphocytes is unclear. A defect in suppressor-cell function may permit unopposed helper-cell proliferation. Inherited or acquired differences in immune-response genes may favor one type of T cell response over another. Nonspecific polyclonal activation of B cells by T-helper cells leads to hyperglobulinemia, a characteristic feature of active sarcoidosis.

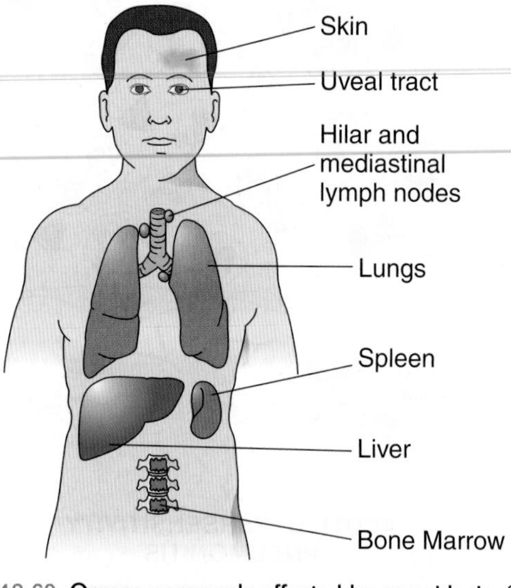

FIGURE 12-60. **Organs commonly affected by sarcoidosis.** Sarcoidosis involves many organs, most commonly the lymph nodes and lung.

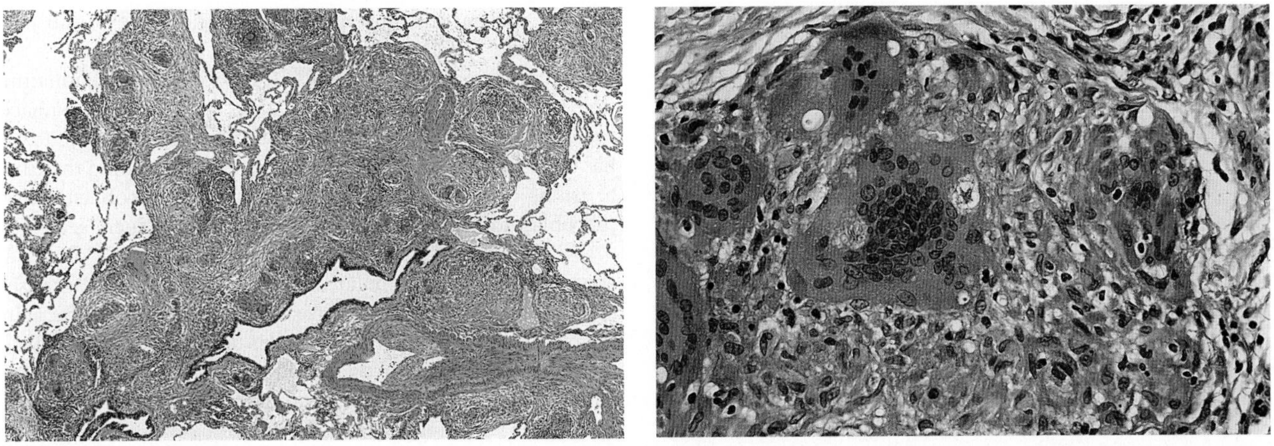

FIGURE 12-61. **Sarcoidosis. A.** Multiple noncaseating granulomas are present along the bronchovascular interstitium. **B.** Noncaseating granulomas consist of tight clusters of epithelioid macrophages and multinucleated giant cells. Several asteroid bodies are present.

PATHOLOGY: Pulmonary sarcoidosis most commonly affects the lung and hilar lymph nodes, although either involvement may occur separately. Radiologically, a diffuse reticulonodular infiltrate is typical, but in occasional cases, larger nodules are present. Histologically, multiple sarcoid granulomas are scattered in the interstitium of the lung (Fig. 12-61). The distribution is distinctive—along the pleura and interlobular septa and around bronchovascular bundles (see Fig. 12-61A). Frequent bronchial or bronchiolar submucosal infiltration by sarcoid granulomas accounts for the high diagnostic yield (<90%) on bronchoscopic biopsy. Granulomas in the airways may occasionally be so prominent as to lead to airway obstruction (endobronchial sarcoid).

The cellular granulomatous phase of sarcoidosis can progress to a fibrotic phase. Fibrosis often begins at the periphery of the granuloma and may show an onion-skin pattern of lamellar fibrosis around the giant cells. Although significant necrosis is usually absent, small foci of necrosis are seen in one third of open lung biopsies. Interstitial chronic inflammation tends to be inconspicuous. Vasculitis can be demonstrated in two thirds of open lung biopsy specimens from patients with sarcoidosis. **Asteroid bodies** (star-shaped crystals) may be seen in the granulomas (see Fig. 12-61B). **Schaumann bodies** (small calcifications with a lamellar structure) may also be present. Although asteroid and Schaumann bodies are commonly encountered, they are not specific for sarcoid and may be seen in most granulomatous process.

In most cases of pulmonary sarcoidosis, interstitial fibrosis is not prominent. However, in rare instances, progressive pulmonary fibrosis leads to a honeycomb lung, respiratory insufficiency, and cor pulmonale.

CLINICAL FEATURES: Sarcoidosis most often occurs in young adults of both sexes. **Acute sarcoidosis** has an abrupt onset, usually followed by spontaneous remission within 2 years and an excellent response to steroids. **Chronic sarcoidosis** has an insidious onset, and patients are more likely to have persistent or progressive disease. Sarcoidosis causes several chest radiographic patterns, the most classic of which is bilateral hilar adenopathy, with or without interstitial pulmonary infiltrates. The malady may also affect the skin (erythema nodosum and lupus pernio), more commonly in women. Black patients tend to have more severe uveitis, skin disease, and lacrimal gland involvement. Cough and dyspnea are the major respiratory complaints. However, the disease can be mild and may be discovered as an incidental finding on a chest radiograph in an asymptomatic patient.

No laboratory test is specific for the diagnosis of sarcoidosis. Transbronchial lung biopsy via a fiberoptic bronchoscope often reveals granulomas. Occasionally, the diagnosis is based on finding multiple noncaseating granulomas in the biopsy of a mediastinal lymph node by mediastinoscopy. Bronchoalveolar lavage often demonstrates an increase in the proportion of T lymphocytes that show a predominance of CD4+ cells. Increased uptake of gallium-67, a material phagocytosed by activated macrophages, can demonstrate granulomatous areas. Serum levels of angiotensin-converting enzyme (ACE) are elevated in two-thirds of patients with active sarcoidosis, and 24-hour urine calcium is frequently increased. The laboratory data, together with the clinical and radiologic findings, allow the diagnosis of sarcoidosis to be established with a high probability.

Other organs commonly involved include the skin, eye (uveal tract), heart, central nervous system, extrathoracic lymph nodes, spleen, and liver (see Fig. 12–60). These are discussed separately in individual chapters.

The prognosis in pulmonary sarcoidosis is favorable and most patients do not develop clinically significant sequelae. Resolution occurs in 60% of patients with pulmonary sarcoidosis but is less likely in older patients and those with extrathoracic lesions, particularly in the bone and skin. In up to 20% of cases, the disorder does not remit or recurs at intervals, but sarcoidosis directly accounts for the death of the patient in only 10% of cases. Corticosteroid therapy is effective for active sarcoidosis.

Usual Interstitial Pneumonia (UIP) Refers Clinically to Idiopathic Pulmonary Fibrosis

UIP is one of the most common types of interstitial pneumonia, with an annual incidence of 6 to 14.6 cases per 100,000 persons. It has a slight male predominance and a mean age at onset of 50 to 60 years. The clinical terms ***idiopathic pulmonary fibrosis*** *(IPF)* or ***cryptogenic fibrosing alveolitis*** *(CFA),* are often applied.

PATHOGENESIS: The etiology of UIP is unknown, but viral, genetic, and immunologic factors are thought to play a role. A viral etiology is favored by a history of flu-like illness in some patients. A genetic role is suggested by cases of familial UIP and the association of UIP-like diseases in patients with inherited disorders such as neurofibromatosis and Hermansky-Pudlak syndrome. An immunologic component has been proposed because collagen vascular disease may be associated in about 20% of cases, including rheumatoid arthritis, systemic lupus erythematosus, and progressive systemic sclerosis. UIP also occurs in the context of other autoimmune disorders (e.g., Hashimoto thyroiditis, primary biliary cirrhosis, chronic hepatitis, idiopathic thrombocytopenic purpura, and myasthenia gravis). In addition, patients with UIP frequently exhibit circulating autoantibodies (e.g., antinuclear antibodies and rheumatoid factor). Immune complexes have been demonstrated in the circulation, the inflamed alveolar walls, and bronchoalveolar-lavage specimens, although the antigen has not been identified. It has been postulated that alveolar macrophages become activated on phagocytosis of immune complexes, after which they release cytokines that recruit neutrophils. These in turn damage alveolar walls, setting in motion a series of events that culminates in interstitial fibrosis.

PATHOLOGY: *UIP demonstrates a histologic pattern that occurs in a variety of clinical settings, including collagen vascular disease, chronic hypersensitivity pneumonitis, drug toxicity, and asbestosis.* The lungs are small in UIP, and fibrosis tends to be worse in the lower lobes, subpleural regions, and along interlobular septa. Retraction of the scars, especially of lobular septa, gives the external surface of the lung a hobnail appearance, reminiscent of cirrhosis of the liver. Fibrosis is often patchy, with areas of dense scarring and honeycomb cystic change (Fig. 12-62A).

The histologic hallmark of UIP is patchy chronic inflammation and interstitial fibrosis, with areas of normal lung adjacent to fibrotic areas (see Fig. 12-62B). The fibrosis itself exhibits what has been termed "temporal heterogeneity," meaning that the fibrosis is of different ages. Areas of loose fibroblastic tissue (fibroblast foci) are found adjacent to dense collagen (see Fig. 12-62C). The fibrosis is most pronounced beneath the pleura and adjacent to the interlobular septa (see Fig. 12-62B). Because of alveolitis and subsequent fibrosis, the distal part of the acinus shrinks and the proximal bronchioles dilate. The bronchiolar epithelium grows into the dilated air spaces, which may represent damaged proximal respiratory bronchioles but are no longer recognized as such (Fig. 12-63). The areas of dense scarring fibrosis cause remodeling of the lung architecture, resulting in collapse of alveolar walls and formation of cystic spaces (see Fig. 12-62A). The cystic spaces are typically lined by bronchiolar or cuboidal epithelium and contain mucus, macrophages, or neutrophils. Interstitial chronic inflammation is mild or moderate. Lymphoid aggregates, sometimes containing germinal centers, are occasionally noted, particularly in UIP associated with rheumatoid arthritis. Extensive vascular changes, particularly intimal fibrosis and thickening of the media, may be associated with pulmonary hypertension.

CLINICAL FEATURES: UIP begins insidiously, with the gradual onset of dyspnea on exertion and dry cough, usually over a period of 1 to 3 years. Patients have restrictive lung disease. Chest radiographs show diffuse bilateral infiltrates, predominantly in the lower lobes, and a reticular pattern. Clubbing of the fingers is common, especially late in the disease. In approximately 50% of patients, high-resolution CT shows distinctive findings, consisting of peripheral, subpleu-

A

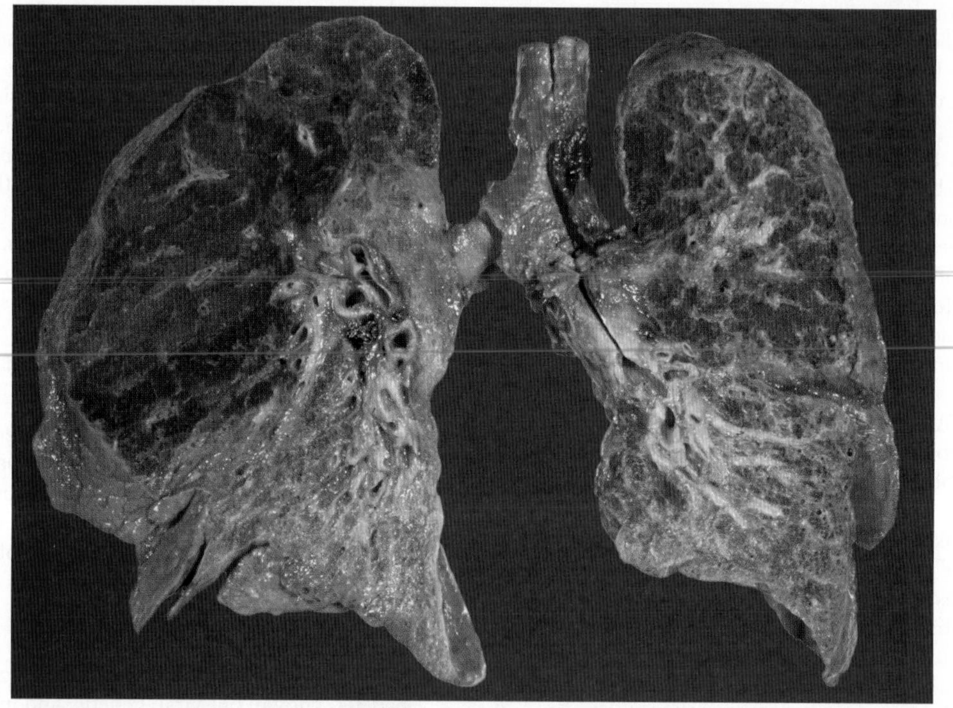

FIGURE 12-62. **Usual interstitial pneumonitis. A.** A gross specimen of the lung shows patchy dense scarring with extensive areas of honeycomb cystic change, predominantly affecting the lower lobes. This patient also had polymyositis.

B

C

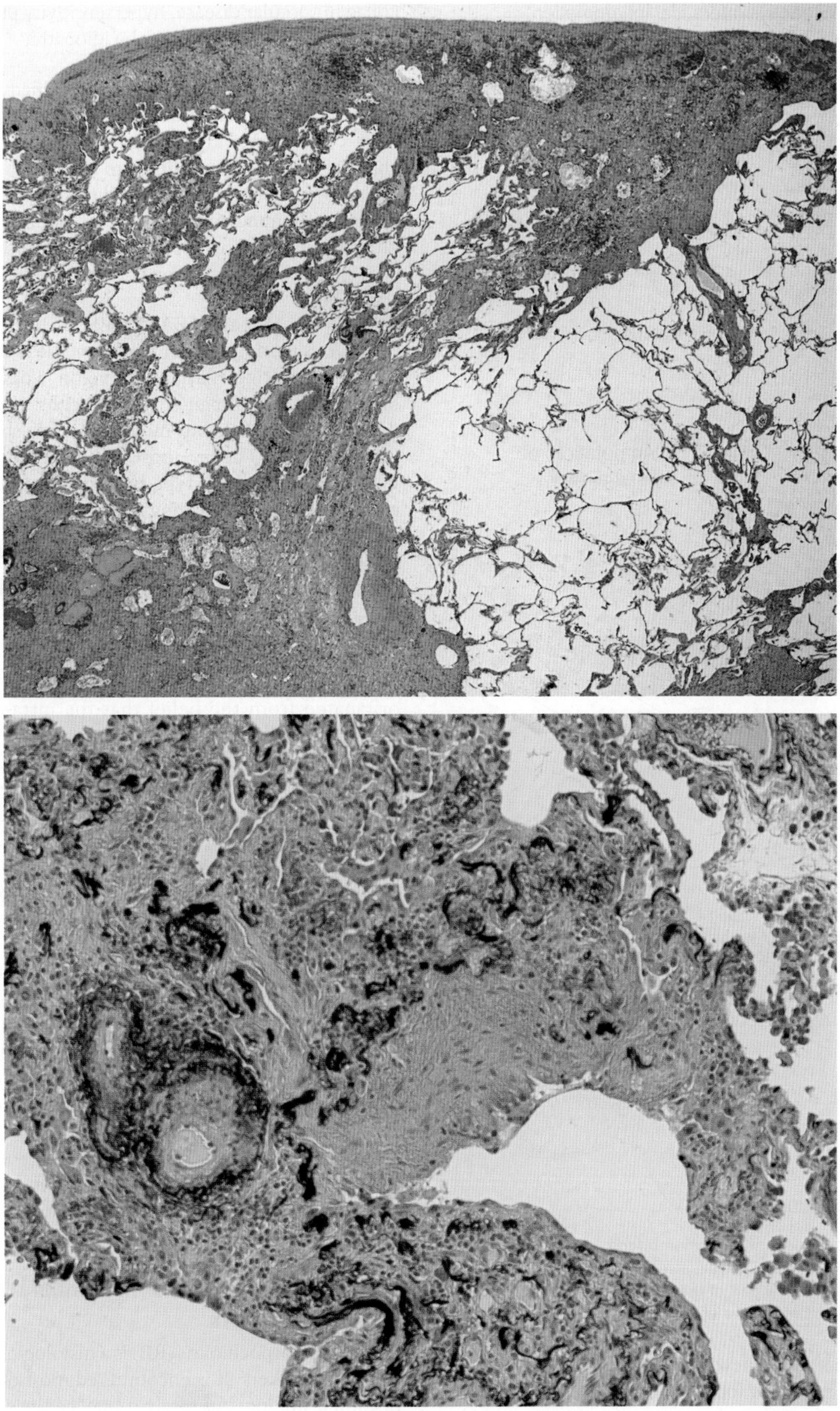

FIGURE 12-62. *(continued)* **B.** A microscopic view shows patchy subpleural fibrosis with microscopic honeycomb fibrosis. The areas of dense fibrosis display remodeling, with loss of the normal lung architecture. **C.** Movat stain highlights the fibroblastic focus in green, which contrasts with the adjacent area of yellow staining of dense collagen and black staining of collapsed elastic fibers.

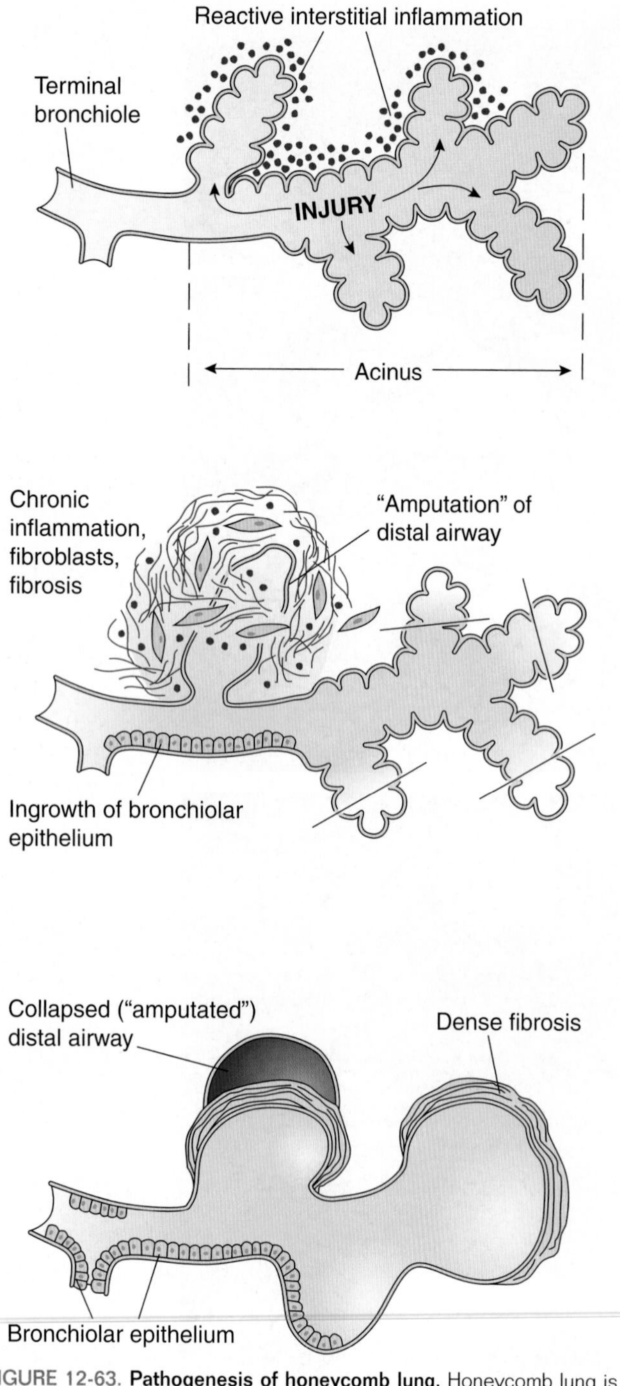

FIGURE 12-63. **Pathogenesis of honeycomb lung.** Honeycomb lung is the result of a variety of injuries. Interstitial and alveolar inflammation destroys ("amputates") the distal part of the acinus. The proximal parts dilate and become lined by bronchiolar epithelium.

ral reticular opacitie,s and honeycombing, predominantly in the posterior aspects of the lower lobes.

The classic auscultatory finding is late inspiratory crackles and fine ("Velcro") rales at the lung bases. Tachypnea at rest, cyanosis, and cor pulmonale eventually ensue. The prognosis is bleak, with a mean survival of 4 to 6 years. Patients are treated with corticosteroids and sometimes cyclophosphamide, but lung transplantation generally offers the only hope of a cure.

Nonspecific Interstitial Pneumonia Has Multiple Etiologies

Nonspecific interstitial pneumonia (NSIP) is a histologic pattern of disease that may reflect diverse potential etiologies (infection, collagen vascular disease, hypersensitivity pneumonitis, drug reaction, and others) or it may be idiopathic.

PATHOLOGY: NSIP is classified into two subtypes—**cellular** and **fibrosing**. In contrast to the patchy distribution and temporal heterogeneity of UIP, NSIP is characterized by diffuse uniform changes in the lung. In the cellular form, alveolar septa are diffusely involved by a mild to moderate lymphcytic infiltrate. In the fibrosing form, septa are diffusely involved by fibrosis, with or without significant associated inflammation.

CLINICAL FEATURES: NSIP typically presents at a slightly younger age than UIP although there is considerable overlap. Patients develop worsening shortness of breath and cough over several months to years. Radiographic findings are variable but most frequently show diffuse "ground glass" changes. The prognosis of NSIP is favorable compared to UIP, with the cellular type having a near 100% 5-year survival and the fibrotic type having a 10-year survival of 35%.

Desquamative Interstitial Pneumonia (DIP) is a Diffuse Lung Disease Characterized by Marked Accumulation of Intraalveolar Mcrophages

There is minimal associated interstitial fibrosis in DIP (Fig. 12-64A,B). The term "desquamative" is actually a misnomer that originated from the belief that the intra-alveolar cells were desquamated epithelial cells, whereas they are now recognized as macrophages. DIP is distinguished from UIP by preservation of alveolar architecture in the former and the lack of patchy scarring and remodeling of lung parenchyma characteristic of UIP. The macrophages contain a fine golden-brown pigment. Alveolar walls in DIP may, however, show mild thickening by chronic inflammation and interstitial fibrosis (see Fig. 12-64B). Scattered lymphoid aggregates also may be present. Hyperplasia of type II pneumocytes is often prominent.

DIP is seen almost exclusively in cigarette smokers, typically in the fourth or fifth decade and occurs twice as often in males as females. The prevailing opinion is that DIP and respiratory bronchiolitis–interstitial lung disease (RB-ILD; below) represent a spectrum of disease related to cigarette smoking, although the mechanism is unclear. The radiographic picture of DIP is not specific but is most frequently described as bilateral ground glass infiltrates with a lower lobe predominance. DIP has a much better prognosis than UIP, with an overall 10-year survival between 70% and 100%. Most patients respond well to steroid therapy and smoking cessation.

Respiratory Bronchiolitis–Interstitial Lung Disease is a Malady of Smokers

Respiratory bronchiolitis (RB) is a histologic lesion that occurs in cigarette smokers. It is encountered most often as an incidental histologic finding, but rarely it may be the sole cause of interstitial lung disease (ILD), and the clinical term **respiratory bronchiolitis–interstitial lung disease** (RB-ILD) is appropriate.

PATHOLOGY: Histologically, the process is patchy and consists of prominent accumulation of pigmented macrophages in the air spaces, centered on bronchioles (Fig. 12-65). The macrophages are present within the lumina of bronchioles and the adjacent alveolar spaces. Bronchiolar walls show mild chronic inflammation and fibrosis. However, interstitial fibrosis does not extend into the surrounding lung.

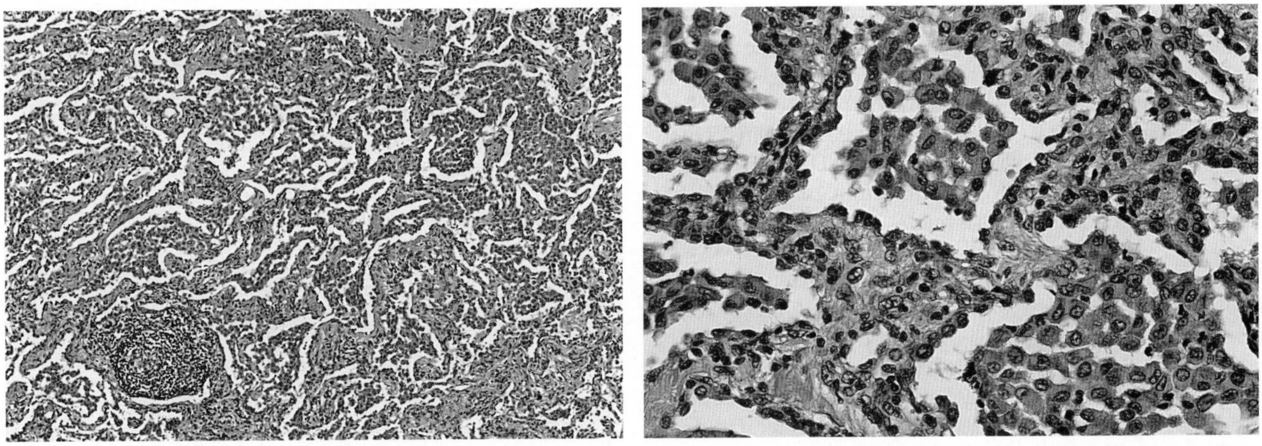

A B

FIGURE 12-64. **Desquamative interstitial pneumonia (DIP). A.** A diffuse process in the lungs is characterized by the accumulation of alveolar macrophages, preservation of the alveolar architecture, and a lymphoid aggregate. **B.** In addition to alveolar macrophage accumulation, there is mild alveolar septal fibrosis, type II pneumocyte hyperplasia, and mild interstitial chronic inflammation.

The pigment within the macrophages is usually brown and finely granular. In contrast to DIP, in which the process is diffuse, in RB the lesion is bronchiolocentric and patchy.

CLINICAL FEATURES: Patients have mild respiratory dysfunction. Radiographically, there is an upper lobe predominance, with thickening of the peripheral bronchioles. Patients with RB–ILD have an excellent prognosis, and the symptoms usually resolve after cessation of smoking.

Organizing Pneumonia Pattern (Cryptogenic Organizing Pneumonia) Features Polypoid Plugs of Tissue that Fill the Bronchiolar Lumen and Surrounding Alveolar Spaces

Organizing pneumonia pattern was previously referred to as "bronchiolitis obliterans–organizing pneumonia" *(BOOP)*. Organizing pneumonia pattern is not specific for any particular etiologic agent, and the cause cannot be determined from the morphologic appearance. It is observed in many settings, including respiratory tract infections (particularly viral bronchiolitis), inhalation of toxic materials, administration of a number of drugs, and several inflammatory processes (e.g., collagen vascular diseases). Importantly, a substantial number of cases remain idiopathic and are referred to as cryptogenic organizing pneumonia (or idiopathic BOOP).

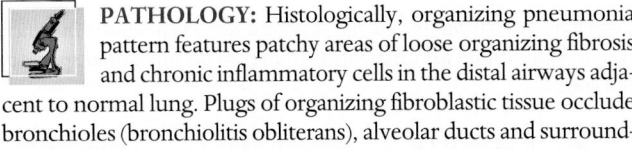

PATHOLOGY: Histologically, organizing pneumonia pattern features patchy areas of loose organizing fibrosis and chronic inflammatory cells in the distal airways adjacent to normal lung. Plugs of organizing fibroblastic tissue occlude bronchioles (bronchiolitis obliterans), alveolar ducts and surrounding alveoli (organizing pneumonia; Fig. 12-66). The pattern is

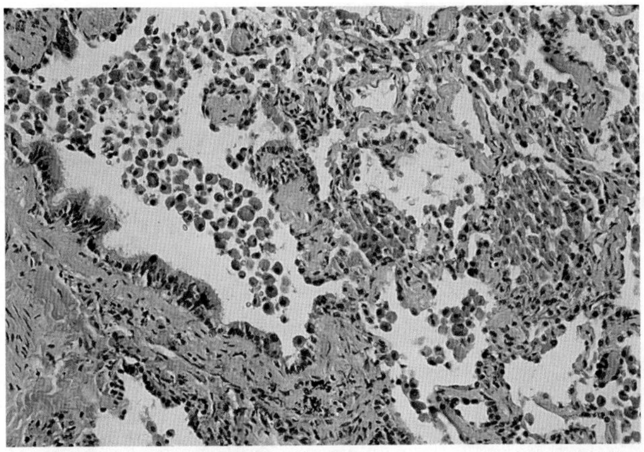

FIGURE 12-65. **Respiratory bronchiolitis.** There is marked accumulation of macrophages within the bronchioles and surrounding air spaces. Mild fibrotic thickening and chronic inflammation of the bronchiolar wall are present.

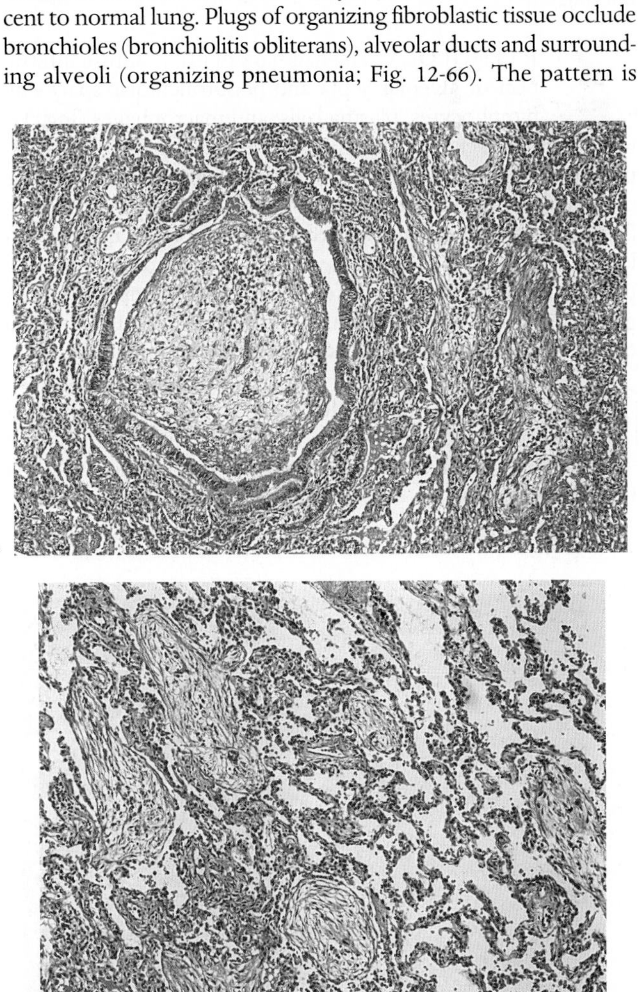

A B

FIGURE 12-66. **Organizing pneumonia pattern. A.** Polypoid plugs of loose fibrous tissue are present in a bronchiole and the adjacent alveolar ducts and alveoli. **B.** The alveolar spaces contain similar plugs of loose organizing connective tissue.

predominantly one of patchy alveolar organizing pneumonia, and bronchiolitis obliterans may not be seen in all cases. The architecture of the lung is preserved, with none of the remodeling or honeycomb changes seen in UIP. An obstructive or endogenous lipid pneumonia may develop if there is significant bronchiolitis obliterans owing to the occlusion of the distal airways. The alveolar septa are only slightly thickened with chronic inflammatory cells, and hyperplasia of type II pneumocytes is mild.

CLINICAL FEATURES: Organizing pneumonia pattern presents at age 55 on the average. Onset is acute, with fever, cough, and dyspnea. Many patients have a history of a flu-like illness 4 to 6 weeks before the onset of symptoms. As noted above, some may have predisposing conditions. Chest radiographs reveal localized opacities or bilateral interstitial infiltrates, which may migrate over time. Pulmonary function studies demonstrate a restrictive ventilatory pattern. Corticosteroid therapy is effective, and some patients recover within weeks to months even without therapy.

Lymphoid Interstitial Pneumonia Occurs in the Setting of Autoimmune Diseases

Lymphoid interstitial pneumonia (LIP) is a rare pneumonitis in which lymphoid infiltrates are distributed diffusely in the interstitial spaces of the lung.

PATHOLOGY: The hallmark of LIP is diffuse infiltration of alveolar septa and peribronchiolar spaces by lymphocytes, plasma cells, and macrophages (Fig. 12-67). Alveolar architecture is preserved without scarring or remodeling of the lung. Hyperplasia of type II pneumocytes may be conspicuous, and inconspicuous foci of organizing interstitial fibrosis are occasionally present. Sarcoidlike, noncaseating granulomas are often seen. The alveolar spaces tend to contain a proteinaceous exudate. Occasionally, scattered lymphoid aggregates are present, some containing germinal centers. Hyperplasia of peribronchiolar lymphoid tissue may be prominent.

CLINICAL FEATURES: LIP may be idiopathic, but often occurs in patients with dysproteinemia, collagen vascular disease (especially Sjögren syndrome), and HIV infection (Table 12-5). It is principally encountered in adults, but cases in children are recorded. In children, LIP is one of the defining criteria for the diagnosis of AIDS. Associated autoimmune manifestations include increased or reduced serum gamma globulins, a variety of dysproteinemias, and increased circulating autoantibodies, such as rheumatoid factor and antinuclear antibodies. Rarely, lymphoma can develop in patients with LIP, particularly in those with Sjögren syndrome and AIDS.

Patients with LIP have cough and progressive dyspnea. The disease varies from an indolent condition to one that progresses to end-stage lung and respiratory failure. Corticosteroids and cytotoxic agents have been of some benefit.

TABLE 12-5

Conditions Associated with Lymphocytic Interstitial Pneumonia (LIP)

Idiopathic
Dysproteinemia
Polyclonal gammopathy
Macroglobulinemia
Hypogammaglobulinemia
Pernicious anemia
Collagen vascular disease
Sjögren syndrome
Systemic lupus erythematosus
Rheumatoid arthritis
Immunodeficiency
HIV infection
Severe combined immunodeficiency syndrome
Infection
Pneumocystis jirovecii pneumonia;
Epstein-Barr virus (lymphoproliferative disorder)
Chronic hepatitis
Iatrogenic
Bone marrow transplantation
Phenytoin (Dilantin)

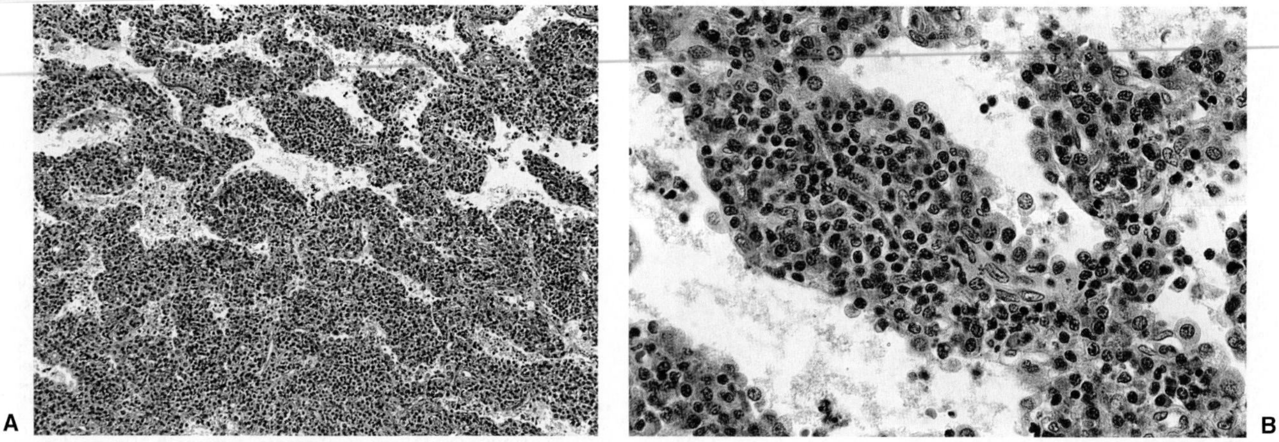

FIGURE 12-67. **Lymphocytic interstitial pneumonia (LIP). A.** The walls of the alveolar septa are diffusely infiltrated by chronic inflammation. **B.** The inflammatory infiltrate is composed of lymphocytes and plasma cells.

Langerhans Cell Histiocytosis (Histiocytosis X) Encompasses a Spectrum of Localized and Systemic Cell Proliferations

Different presentations of Langerhans cell histiocytosis (LCH) have been called eosinophilic granuloma, Hand-Schüller-Christian disease, and Letterer-Siwe disease (see Chapter 20). LCH can affect the lung as a distinctive form of ILD. In adults the disorder occurs most often as an isolated form (also known as **pulmonary eosinophilic granuloma**), with extrapulmonary manifestations such as bone lesions or diabetes insipidus occurring in 10% to 15% of cases. *Virtually all of these patients are cigarette smokers.* In children, lung involvement may occur in association with Letterer-Siwe disease or Hand-Schüller-Christian disease.

PATHOLOGY: Histologically, pulmonary LCH appears as scattered nodular infiltrates with a stellate border extending into the surrounding interstitium (Fig. 12-68A). These lesions are frequently centered on bronchioles or subpleurally. The cellular lesions contain varying proportions of Langerhans cells admixed with lymphocytes, eosinophils, and macrophages. Langerhans cells are round to oval, with a moderate amount of eosinophilic cytoplasm and prominently grooved nuclei with small inconspicuous nucleoli (see Fig. 12-68B). As the disease progresses, lesions cavitate and become fibrotic, and honeycomb fibrosis may result. Lung parenchyma adjacent to the nodular lesions may show marked accumulation of intraalveolar macrophages, due to respiratory bronchiolitis caused by smoking.

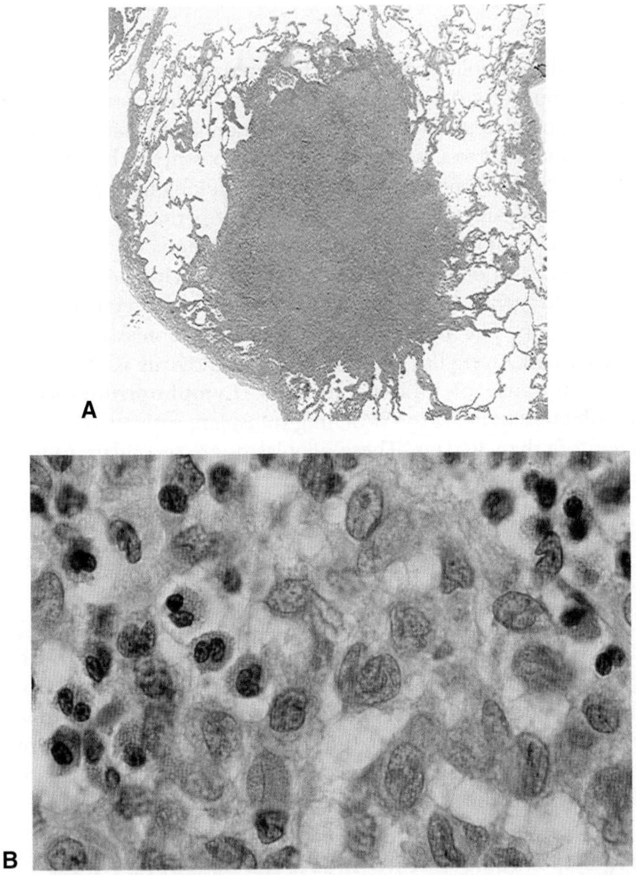

FIGURE 12-68. **Langerhans cell histiocytosis. A.** The interstitial nodular infiltrate has a stellate shape, with extension of the cells into the adjacent alveolar septa **B.** Higher power view shows Langerhans cells with moderate amount of eosinophilic cytoplasm and prominently grooved nuclei. Eosinophils are present

Langerhans cells have distinctive characteristics, including (1) cytoplasmic Birbeck granules (detected by electron microscopy); (2) C3, $IgG\text{-}F_c$ receptors, CD1a, and human leukocyte antigen (HLA)-DR expression; and (3) S-100 protein expression. Whether pulmonary LCH represents a neoplastic proliferation or an abnormal immunologic response to antigens within cigarette smoke remains to be determined.

CLINICAL FEATURES: Pulmonary LCH usually affects patients in their third and fourth decades. The most common presenting symptoms are a nonproductive cough, dyspnea on exertion, and spontaneous pneumothorax. Some 25% of patients are asymptomatic at the time of diagnosis. Chest radiographs show diffuse bilateral reticulonodular lesions, usually in the upper lobes. The lesions frequently undergo cavitation. Although most patients have a good prognosis, some develop chronic pulmonary dysfunction. In a small subset of cases, progressive pulmonary fibrosis can lead to death. Cessation of smoking is beneficial in the early stages of the disease.

Lymphangioleiomyomatosis (LAM) Features Abnormal Smooth Muscle Proliferation in the Lung and Lymphatics

LAM is a rare ILD that occurs in women of childbearing age and is characterized by the widespread abnormal proliferation of smooth muscle in lung, mediastinal and retroperitoneal lymph nodes, and major lymphatic ducts. Its etiology is unknown, but clinical responses to oophorectomy and progesterone therapy suggest that the smooth muscle proliferation is under hormonal control. The facts that LAM occurs in patients with tuberous sclerosis and that it may be associated with renal angiomyolipomas suggest that LAM may be a forme fruste of tuberous sclerosis.

PATHOLOGY: Grossly, the lungs show bilateral, diffuse enlargement, with extensive cystic changes resembling those of emphysema (Fig. 12-69A). Histologically, numerous cystic spaces are lined by focal nodules or bundles of abnormal smooth muscle cells. These round or spindle-shaped cells (LAM cells) resemble immature smooth muscle cells but lack the parallel orientation of normal smooth muscle around airways and blood vessels (see Fig. 12-69B). The smooth muscle proliferation typically follows a lymphatic distribution in the lung, around blood vessels and bronchioles, and along the pleura and interlobular septa. Blood vessel walls, especially in small pulmonary veins, also may be infiltrated, resulting in microscopic hemorrhage and hemosiderin accumulation in alveolar macrophages. Immunostaining for HMB-45 (a melanoma antigen) specifically decorates LAM cells but not other smooth muscle cells in the lung. LAM cells are sometimes positive for estrogen or progesterone receptors.

CLINICAL FEATURES: Patients with LAM have shortness of breath, spontaneous pneumothorax, hemoptysis, cough, and chylous effusions. In early stages, the chest radiograph may appear normal. However, as the disease progresses it may show a diffuse interstitial reticular or cystic pattern. Pleural effusions, marked hyperinflation of the lungs and pneumothorax may ensue. Pulmonary function tests show markedly increased total lung capacity, decreased diffusing capacity and obstructive or restrictive features. Although some

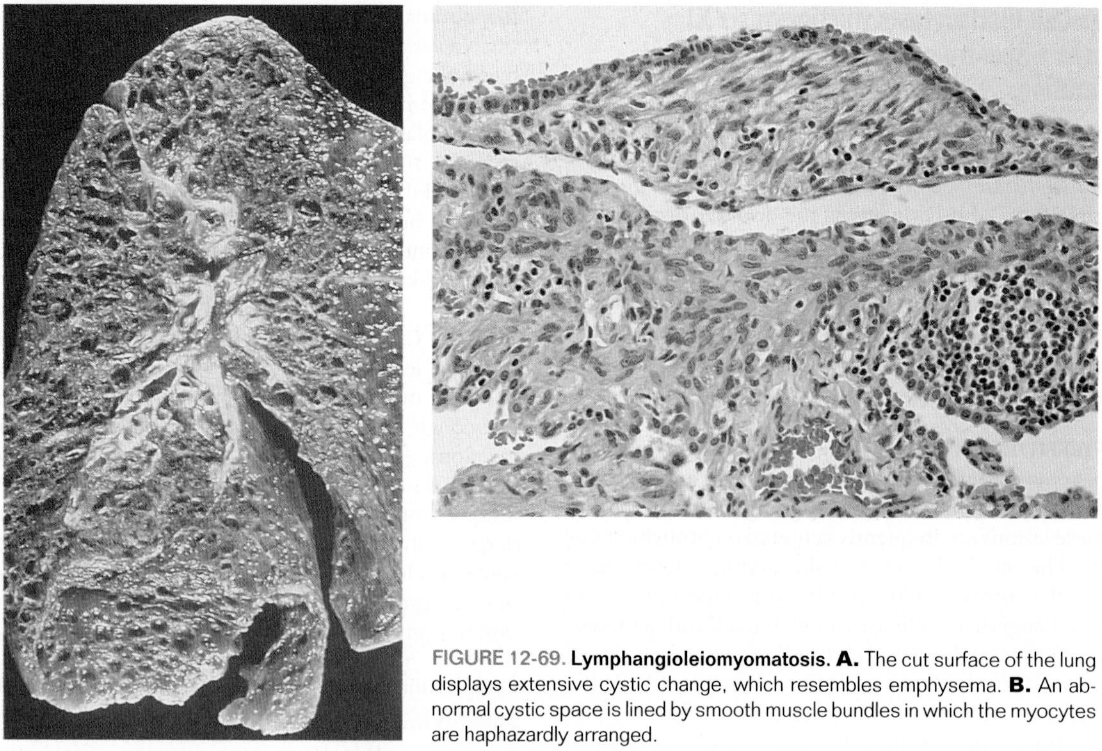

A

B

FIGURE 12-69. **Lymphangioleiomyomatosis. A.** The cut surface of the lung displays extensive cystic change, which resembles emphysema. **B.** An abnormal cystic space is lined by smooth muscle bundles in which the myocytes are haphazardly arranged.

patients have an indolent clinical course, many die of progressive respiratory failure. Hormonal ablation through oophorectomy, as well as antiestrogen (tamoxifen) and progesterone therapy, have shown some promise.

Lung Transplantation

Patients who undergo lung transplantation are prone to acute and chronic rejection, and infection. Histologic clues to acute rejection include perivascular infiltrates of small round lymphocytes, plasmacytoid lymphocytes, macrophages, and eosinophils. In severe cases, the inflammation may spill over into adjacent alveoli, and hyaline membranes may be seen. The major pattern of chronic rejection is bronchiolitis obliterans, characterized by bronchiolar inflammation and varying degrees of fibrosis. The latter can take the form of polypoid plugs of intraluminal granulation tissue or concentric mural fibrosis, with the pattern of constrictive bronchiolitis (Fig. 12-70). Bronchiectasis is common in long-term survivors of lung transplants, which may reflect poor perfusion of the airways, denervation, and recurrent airway infection.

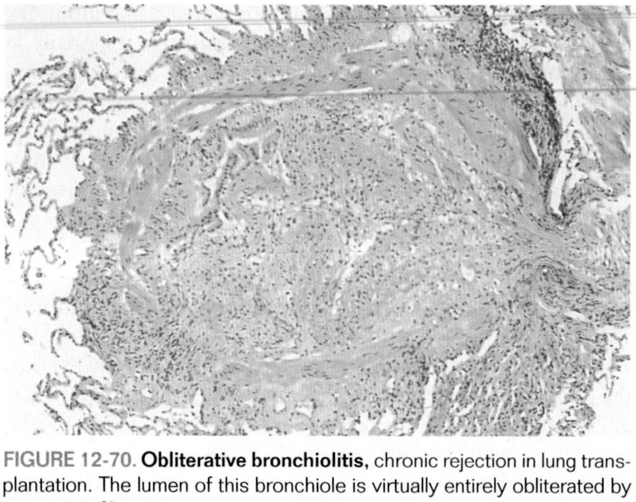

FIGURE 12-70. **Obliterative bronchiolitis,** chronic rejection in lung transplantation. The lumen of this bronchiole is virtually entirely obliterated by concentric fibrosis.

A spectrum of opportunistic infections, including bacteria, fungi, viral agents, and *Pneumocystis jirovecii*, can be seen in transplant patients. The most common fungal pneumonias are due to *Candida* and *Aspergillus* species. Cytomegalovirus is the most common cause of viral pneumonia. **Lymphoproliferative disorders** occur in 3% to 8% of lung-transplant patients who survive more than 30 days. These neoplasms are secondary to uncontrolled proliferation of B lymphocytes infected with the Epstein-Barr virus (EBV) as a result of immunosuppression by cyclosporine.

Vasculitis and Granulomatosis

Many pulmonary conditions result in vasculitis, most of which are secondary to other inflammatory processes, such as necrotizing granulomatous infections. Only a few primary idiopathic vasculitis syndromes affect the lung, the most important of which are Wegener granulomatosis (WG), Churg-Strauss granulomatosis, and necrotizing sarcoid granulomatosis.

Wegener Granulomatosis Affects the Respiratory Tract and Kidneys

WG is a disease of unknown cause characterized by aseptic, necrotizing, granulomatous inflammation, and vasculitis that affect both upper and lower respiratory tracts, and the kidneys. The disease is

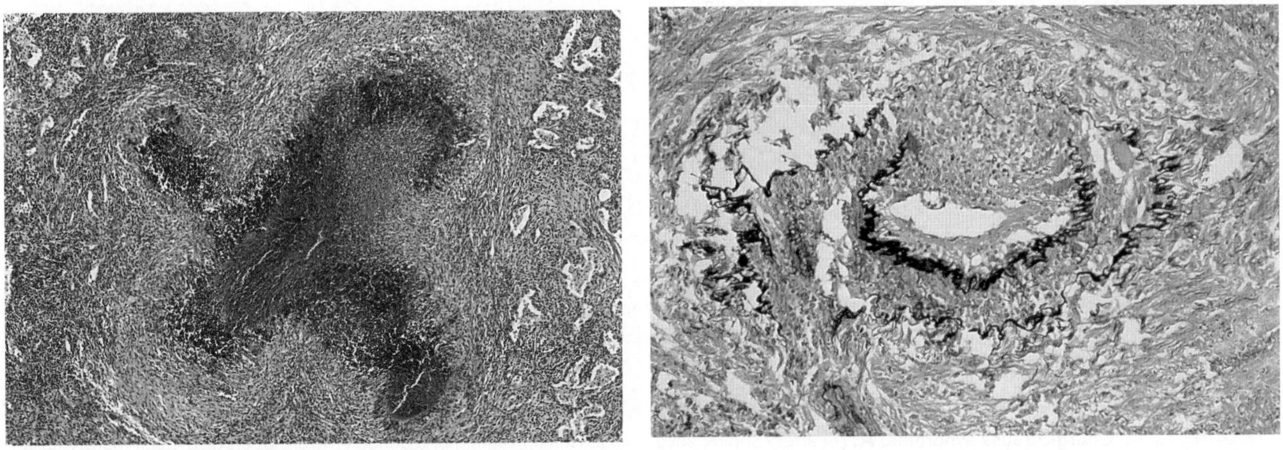
A B

FIGURE 12-71. **Wegener granulomatosis. A.** This large area of necrosis has a "geographical" pattern with serpiginous borders and a basophilic center. **B.** Vasculitis in this artery is characterized by a focal, eccentric, transmural chronic inflammatory infiltrate that destroys the inner and outer elastic laminae (elastic stain).

described in Chapter 10. The glomerulonephritis associated with WG is discussed in Chapter 16, and the lesions of the upper respiratory tract are described in Chapter 25. Here, we deal only with the pulmonary manifestations of WG.

PATHOLOGY: In the lung WG shows necrotizing granulomatous inflammation, parenchymal necrosis, and vasculitis. In most cases of pulmonary WG, multiple bilateral nodules, averaging 2 to 3 cm in diameter, are seen. The nodules have irregular edges, tan-brown or hemorrhagic cut surfaces and frequent central cavitation.

Nodules of parenchymal consolidation consist of (1) tissue necrosis; (2) granulomatous inflammation with a mixed inflammatory infiltrate composed of lymphocytes, plasma cells, neutrophils, eosinophils, macrophages, and giant cells; and (3) fibrosis. Necrosis can take the form of neutrophilic microabscesses or large basophilic zones of "geographical" necrosis with irregular serpiginous borders (Fig. 12-71A). The granulomas may show several patterns, including palisading macrophages along the border of the large necrotic zones, loosely clustered multinucleated giant cells, and scattered giant cells. Vasculitis may affect arteries (see Fig. 12-71B), veins, or capillaries, and the vascular lesions may show acute, chronic, or granulomatous inflammation. The most common pattern of fibrosis consists of a nonspecific organizing pneumonia at the edges of the nodules of inflammatory consolidation. The lungs often show acute or chronic intra-alveolar hemorrhage. "Neutrophilic capillaritis," consisting of neutrophilic infiltration of alveolar walls, is often present.

CLINICAL FEATURES: WG most commonly affects the head and neck, followed by the lung, kidney, and eye. Respiratory manifestations include cough, hemoptysis, and pleuritis. Chest radiographs commonly show multiple intrapulmonary nodules, although single nodules may also be encountered. Head and neck manifestations consist of sinusitis, nasal disease, otitis media, hearing loss, subglottic stenosis, ear pain, cough, and oral lesions. Other systemic manifestations are arthralgias, fever, skin lesions, weight loss, peripheral neuropathy, central nervous system abnormalities, and pericarditis.

Diffuse pulmonary hemorrhage,an important complication of WG, is a fulminant life-threatening crisis characterized by severe respiratory failure. It is usually accompanied by acute renal failure.

The serum ANCA test is a useful marker for WG and other vasculitis syndromes. When these antibodies react with ethanol-fixed neutrophils, there are two major immunofluorescence patterns: cytoplasmic or classical (C-ANCA) and perinuclear (P-ANCA). C-ANCAs react with proteinase 3 and occur in more than 85% of patients with active generalized WG. Most P-ANCAs are specific for myeloperoxidase and are found in patients with idiopathic necrotizing and crescentic glomerulonephritis, and in patients with polyarteritis nodosa or Churg-Strauss syndrome.

Most patients with WG are treated effectively with corticosteroids and cyclophosphamide. Some respond to trimethoprim-sulfamethoxazole, suggesting the possibility of a bacterial infection.

Churg-Strauss Syndrome (Allergic Angiitis and Granulomatosis) Is Defined by Asthma, Eosinophilia and Vasculitis

Churg-Strauss syndrome is a disorder of unknown etiology.

PATHOLOGY: The lungs of patients with Churg-Strauss syndrome show changes of asthmatic bronchitis or bronchiolitis (see above discussion of asthma). Histologic features include eosinophilic pneumonia, vasculitis (Fig. 12-72A), parenchymal necrosis (see Fig. 12-72B), and granulomatous inflammation. Infiltrates of eosinophils may be seen in any anatomical compartment of the lung. Involvement of blood vessel walls causes vasculitis and damage to airway walls, and results in bronchitis or bronchiolitis. The vasculitis includes diverse inflammatory cells: eosinophils, lymphocytes, plasma cells, macrophages, giant cells, and neutrophils (see Fig. 12-72A). Necrotic foci have eosinophilic centers owing to the accumulation of dead eosinophils (see Fig. 12-72B).

CLINICAL FEATURES: Churg-Strauss syndrome passes through three clinical phases.

- **Prodrome:** Patients have one or more of: allergic rhinitis, asthma, peripheral eosinophilia, and eosinophilic infiltrative disease (eosinophilic pneumonia or eosinophilic enteritis).
- **Systemic vasculitic phase:** Extrapulmonary vasculitic manifestations are present, such as cutaneous leukocytoclastic vasculitis or peripheral neuropathy.
- **Postvasculitic phase:** Patients may continue to have asthma and allergic rhinitis, and complications of neuropathy and

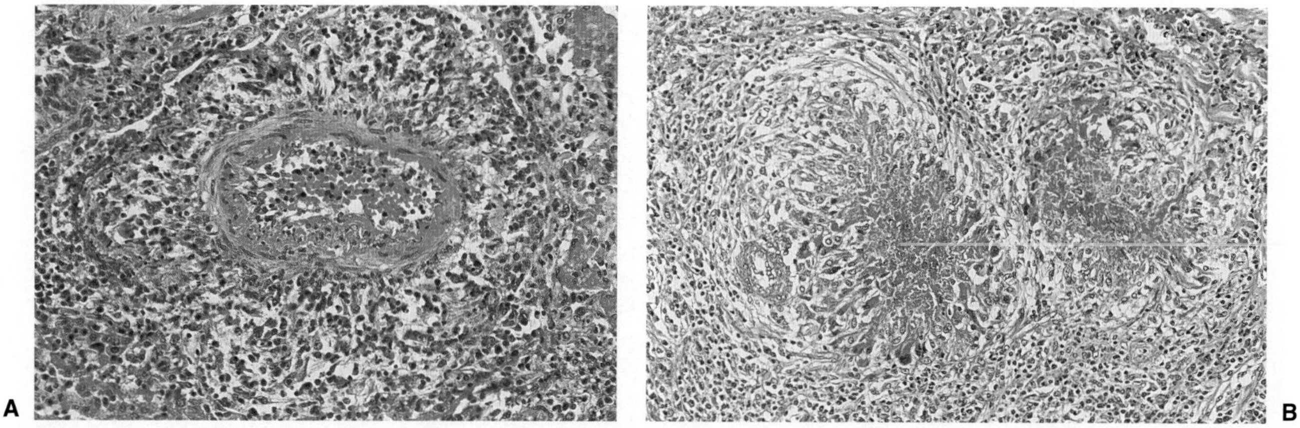

FIGURE 12-72. **Churg-Strauss syndrome. A.** An artery shows severe vasculitis consisting of a dense infiltrate of chronic inflammatory cells and eosinophils. **B.** A necrotic ("allergic") granuloma has a central eosinophilic area of necrosis surrounded by palisading macrophages and giant cells.

hypertension may persist. Cardiovascular manifestations are common and often consist of pericarditis, hypertension, and cardiac failure. Renal disease and sinus involvement are usually less severe than those in WG.

Patients with Churg-Strauss usually are positive for P-ANCA during the vasculitic phase. Most patients respond to corticosteroid therapy, but cyclophosphamide may be needed in severe cases.

Necrotizing Sarcoid Granulomatosis Demonstrates Large Zones of Necrosis and Vasculitis

Necrotizing sarcoid granulomatosis is a rare condition that features nodular confluent sarcoidal granulomas (Fig. 12-73). This disorder is not a systemic vasculitis, but a disorder usually limited to the lung. The vasculitis displays giant cells, necrotizing granulomas (see Fig. 12-73B), and chronic inflammation consisting of lymphocytes and plasma cells. Most patients are asymptomatic, and chest radiographs typically show multiple, well-circumscribed, pulmonary nodules. Extrapulmonary disease is uncommon, and localized lesions may be treated effectively by surgical removal. Corticosteroids are usually effective for patients with multiple lesions. The prognosis is excellent.

Pulmonary Hypertension

In fetal life, pulmonary arterial walls are thick and pulmonary arterial pressure is correspondingly high. Blood is oxygenated through the placenta, not the lungs. Thus, the high fetal pulmonary arterial pressure serves to shunt the output of the right ventricle through the ductus arteriosus into the systemic circulation, effectively bypassing the lungs. After birth, the lungs are responsible for oxygenating venous blood, and the ductus arteriosus closes. The lungs must thus adapt to accept the entire cardiac output, a situation that demands the high-volume and low-pressure system of the mature lung. Accordingly, by the third day of life, pulmonary arteries dilate, their walls become thin, and pulmonary arterial pressure declines.

Increased pulmonary arterial pressure is defined as a mean pressure exceeding 25 mm Hg at rest. Increases in either pulmonary blood flow or vascular resistance may lead to higher pulmonary arterial pressure. Whatever the cause, characteristic morphologic abnormalities result from increased pulmonary artery pressure (Fig. 12-74). The grading system for the arterial changes of pulmonary hypertension was devised to determine if corrective cardiac surgery would reverse the hypertensive changes. Grades 1, 2, and 3 are generally reversible; grades 4 and above are generally not.

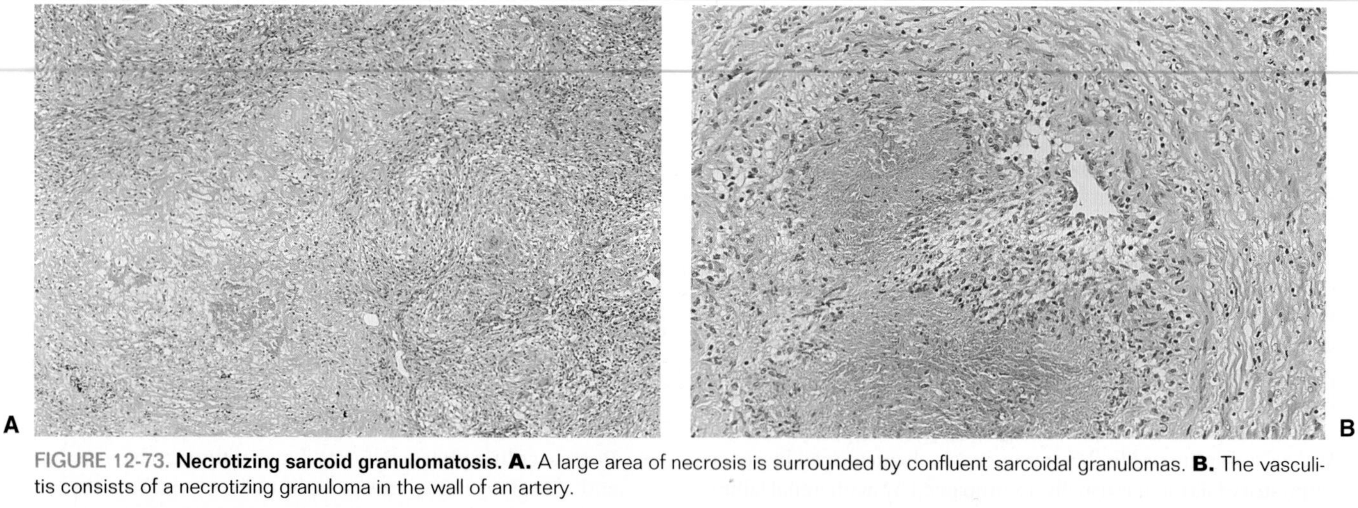

FIGURE 12-73. **Necrotizing sarcoid granulomatosis. A.** A large area of necrosis is surrounded by confluent sarcoidal granulomas. **B.** The vasculitis consists of a necrotizing granuloma in the wall of an artery.

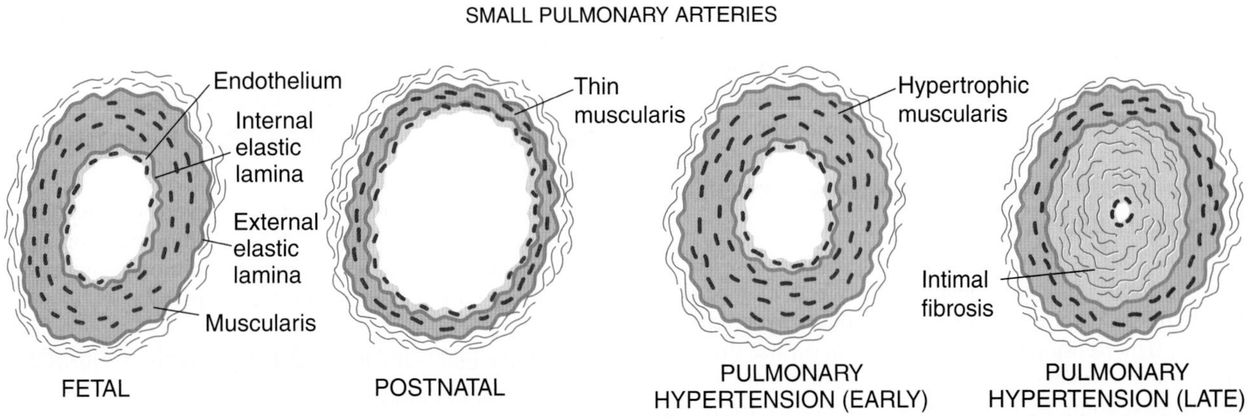

FIGURE 12-74. **Histopathology of pulmonary hypertension.** In late gestation, the pulmonary arteries have thick walls. After birth, the vessels dilate, and the walls become thin. Mild pulmonary hypertension is characterized by thickening of the media. As pulmonary hypertension becomes more severe, there is extensive intimal fibrosis and muscle thickening.

- **Grade 1:** Medial hypertrophy of muscular pulmonary arteries and appearance of smooth muscle in pulmonary arterioles
- **Grade 2:** Intimal proliferation with increasing medial hypertrophy
- **Grade 3:** Intimal fibrosis of muscular pulmonary arteries and arterioles, which may be occlusive (Fig. 12-75A)
- **Grade 4:** Formation of plexiform lesions together with dilation and thinning of pulmonary arteries. These nodular lesions are composed of irregular interlacing blood channels and impose a further obstruction in the pulmonary circulation (see Fig. 12-75B).
- **Grade 5:** Plexiform lesions in combination with dilation or angiomatoid lesions. Rupture of dilated thin walled vessel, with parenchymal hemorrhage and hemosiderosis, is also present.
- **Grade 6:** Fibrinoid necrosis of arteries and arterioles

A

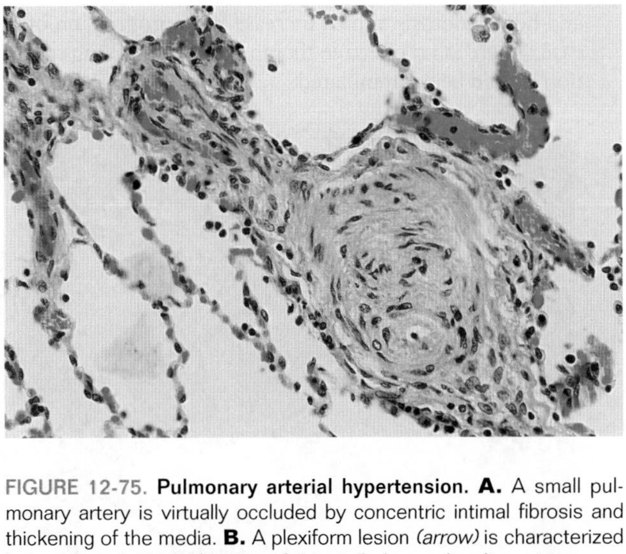

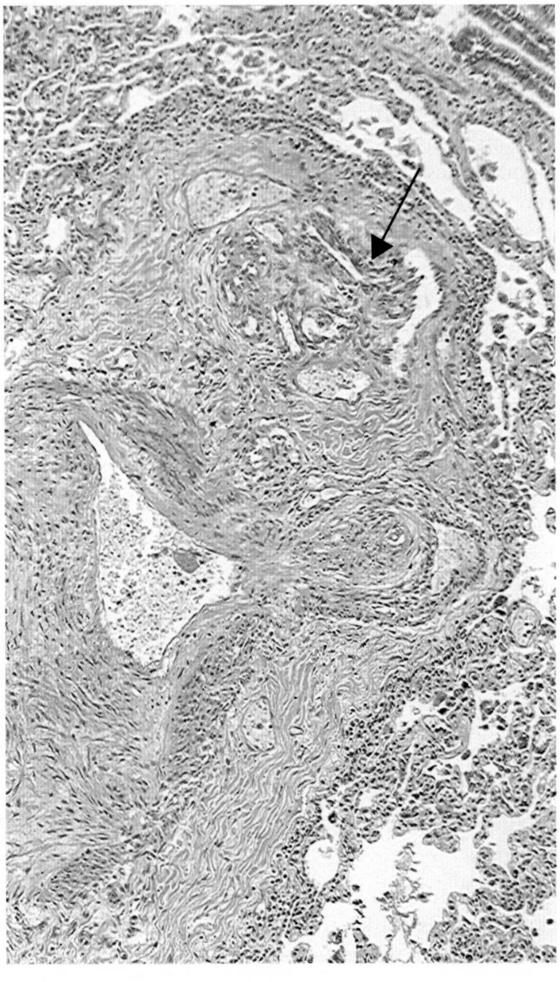

B

FIGURE 12-75. **Pulmonary arterial hypertension. A.** A small pulmonary artery is virtually occluded by concentric intimal fibrosis and thickening of the media. **B.** A plexiform lesion *(arrow)* is characterized by a glomeruloid proliferation of thin-walled vessels adjacent to a parent artery, which shows marked hypertensive changes of intimal fibrosis and medial thickening.

Even mild atherosclerosis is uncommon when pulmonary arterial pressure is normal. However, with all grades of pulmonary hypertension, atherosclerosis is seen in the largest pulmonary arteries. Increased pressure in the lesser circulation leads to hypertrophy of the right ventricle (**cor pulmonale**).

Pulmonary Hypertension May be Considered Precapillary or Postcapillary in Origin

The primary source of increased flow or resistance, whether proximal or distal to the pulmonary capillary bed, may be used to understand the pathophysiology of pulmonary hypertension. Precapillary hypertension includes left-to-right cardiac shunts as well as primary pulmonary hypertension, thromboembolic pulmonary hypertension, and hypertension secondary to fibrotic lung disease and hypoxia. Postcapillary hypertension includes pulmonary veno-occlusive disease as well as hypertension secondary to left-sided cardiac disorders such as mitral stenosis and aortic coarctation.

Left-to-Right Shunts

A shunt from the systemic circulation to the pulmonary circulation results in increased flow to the lungs. Most cases represent congenital left-to-right shunts (see Chapter 11). An additional lesion is present when hypertension exists from birth. At this time, the pulmonary artery and the aorta have about the same number of elastic lamellae in their media. In normal infants, there is a loss of elastic lamellae in the pulmonary artery after birth, but when pulmonary hypertension is present, the fetal pattern persists.

Primary Pulmonary Hypertension

Primary pulmonary hypertension is a rare condition caused by increased tone within the pulmonary arteries. It occurs at all ages, but is most common in young women in their 20s and 30s. The disorder is seen as an insidious onset of dyspnea. Physical signs and radiologic abnormalities are initially slight, but become more apparent with time. Severe pulmonary hypertension (i.e., plexiform lesions) eventually ensues, and patients die of cor pulmonale. Medical treatment is ineffective, and heart–lung transplantation is indicated. Although primary pulmonary hypertension is typically idiopathic, some patients with collagen vascular diseases have identical clinical and morphologic findings.

Recurrent Pulmonary Emboli

Multiple thromboemboli in the smaller pulmonary vessels often result from asymptomatic, episodic showers of small emboli from the periphery. They gradually restrict pulmonary circulation, and lead to pulmonary hypertension. Some patients have evidence of peripheral venous thrombosis, usually in the leg veins, or a history of circumstances predisposing to venous thrombosis. In addition to the vascular lesions of pulmonary hypertension, organized thromboemboli are evidenced by fibrous bands ("webs") that extend across the lumina of small pulmonary arteries. If the condition is diagnosed during life, placement of a filter in the inferior vena cava prevents further embolization.

Any Disorder That Produces Hypoxemia Can Result in Constriction of Small Pulmonary Arteries and Pulmonary Hypertension

Predisposing conditions include chronic air-flow obstruction (chronic bronchitis), ILD, and living at high altitude. Severe kyphoscoliosis or extreme obesity (**Pickwickian syndrome**) may interfere with the mechanics of ventilation and lead to hypoxemia and pulmonary hypertension.

Left Ventricular Failure Increases Pulmonary Venous Pressure and, to Some Extent, Pulmonary Arterial Pressure

By contrast, mitral stenosis produces severe venous hypertension and significant pulmonary artery hypertension. In such cases, the lungs exhibit lesions of both pulmonary hypertension and chronic passive congestion (see Chapter 7).

Pulmonary Veno-occlusive Disease Involves Fibrotic Obstruction of Small Veins

Pulmonary veno-occlusive disease is a rare condition of uncertain etiology characterized by extensive occlusion of small pulmonary veins and venules by loose, sparsely cellular, intimal fibrosis (Fig. 12-76). Some large veins may also be involved, and in half of cases, similar but less severe lesions involve the pulmonary arteries. Canalization of the obstructive lesions suggests that they represent organized thrombi. The disease has been reported to follow viral infections, exposure to toxic agents and chemotherapy. More than half of cases are encountered in the first 3 decades of life. In children, girls and boys are affected similarly, but after age 15, it is more common in men.

PATHOLOGY: Pulmonary veno-occlusive disease produces severe pulmonary hypertension. Gross examination reveals brown induration of the lung and atherosclerosis of large pulmonary arteries. Microscopic examination shows partial or total occlusion of small veins and venules and eccentric intimal thickening of larger veins. Moderate fibrosis of alveolar walls is usually noted, and foci of hemosiderosis are common. The pulmonary arterial tree exhibits severe lesions of pulmonary hypertension. Recent thrombi are regularly observed.

CLINICAL FEATURES: The clinical presentation of progressive dyspnea is similar to that of primary pulmonary hypertension, but pulmonary veno-occlusive disease has a more fulminant course. Radiologic examination reveals scattered infiltrates in the lung, representing hemorrhage and hemosiderosis, which increase with progression of the disease. There is no effective therapy, and heart–lung transplantation should be contemplated.

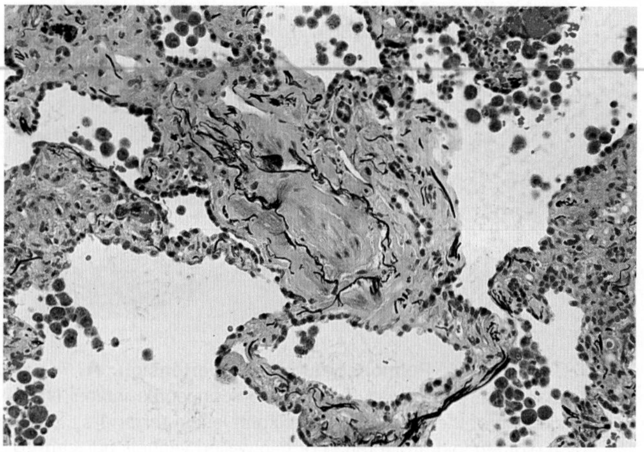

FIGURE 12-76. **Veno-occlusive disease of the lung.** This pulmonary vein is occluded by intimal fibrosis (Movat stain).

Pulmonary Hamartoma

Although the term *hamartoma* implies a malformation, hamartomas are true tumors. They typically occur in adults, with a peak in the sixth decade of life. They are the cause of some 10% of "coin" lesions discovered incidentally on chest radiographs. A characteristic ("popcorn") pattern of calcification is often seen by x-ray.

PATHOLOGY: Grossly, pulmonary hamartomas are solitary, circumscribed, lobulated masses, averaging 2 cm in diameter, with a white or gray, cartilaginous cut surface (Fig. 12-77A). The tumor consists of elements usually present in the lung, including cartilage, fibromyxoid connective tissue, fat, bone, and occasionally smooth muscle (see Fig. 12-77B). These components are interspersed with clefts lined by respiratory epithelium. The tumor is benign and well circumscribed and shells out from the surrounding lung parenchyma. Most are seen in the peripheral parenchyma, but 10% occur in a central endobronchial location. The latter may cause symptoms due to bronchial obstruction.

Carcinoma of the Lung

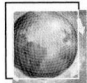

EPIDEMIOLOGY: Regarded as a rare tumor as late as 1945, carcinoma of the lung is the most common cause of cancer death worldwide, including the United States, where it is the most common cause of cancer death in both men and women. Some 85% of lung cancers occur in cigarette smokers (see Chapter 8). Most types are linked to cigarette smoking, but the strongest association is with squamous cell carcinoma and small cell carcinoma. The nonsmoker who develops cancer of the lung usually has an adenocarcinoma. The peak age for lung cancer is between 60 and 70 years, and most patients are between 50 and 80 years old. The former male predominance is decreasing, owing to increased smoking among women.

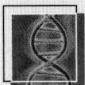

PATHOGENESIS: Mutations in the K-*ras* oncogene, particularly codons 12 and 13, are seen in 25% of adenocarcinomas, 20% of large cell carcinomas, and 5% of squamous cell carcinomas, but rarely in small cell tumors. These mutations correlate with cigarette smoking and with a poor prognosis in patients with adenocarcinoma. *Myc* oncogene overexpression occurs in 10% to 40% of small cell carcinomas but is rare in other types. Two important tumor-suppressor genes in lung cancer are the *p53* and retinoblastoma *(Rb)* genes. Mutations in *p53* are found in more than 80% of small cell carcinomas and 50% of non-small cell tumors. *Rb* mutations occur in over 80% of small cell carcinomas and 25% of non-small cell cancers. Deletions in the short arm of chromosome 3 (3p) are frequently found in all types of lung cancers. The protooncogene *bcl-2,* which encodes a protein that inhibits programmed cell death (apoptosis), is expressed in 25% of squamous cell carcinomas and 10% of adenocarcinomas.

PATHOLOGY: In the past, the term **bronchogenic** carcinoma was often used for primary lung cancer, but it is perhaps too specific, implying an origin from the bronchi. A substantial proportion, perhaps one-fourth, of primary lung cancers do not have an obvious bronchial origin. The most important issue in the histological subclassification of lung cancer is separating small cell carcinoma from the other types (non-small cell carcinoma), because small cell carcinoma responds to chemotherapy, whereas other histological types do not.

Histologic subtyping of lung cancer is based on the best-differentiated component, unless an area of small cell carcinoma is present. However, the degree of differentiation is graded according to the worst-differentiated component. For example, if a tumor is mostly poorly differentiated large cells but has foci of squamous cells or adenocarcinoma, it is classified as a poorly differentiated squamous cell carcinoma or adenocarcinoma, respectively. Any cancer with a component of small cell carcinoma is regarded as a subtype of that tumor (see below).

CLINICAL FEATURES: Overall 5-year survival for all patients with lung cancer has remained 15% for the past 2 decades. The 5-year survival at all stages is 42% for bronchioloalveolar carcinoma, 17% for adenocarcinoma, 15% for squamous cell carcinoma, 11% for large cell carcinoma,

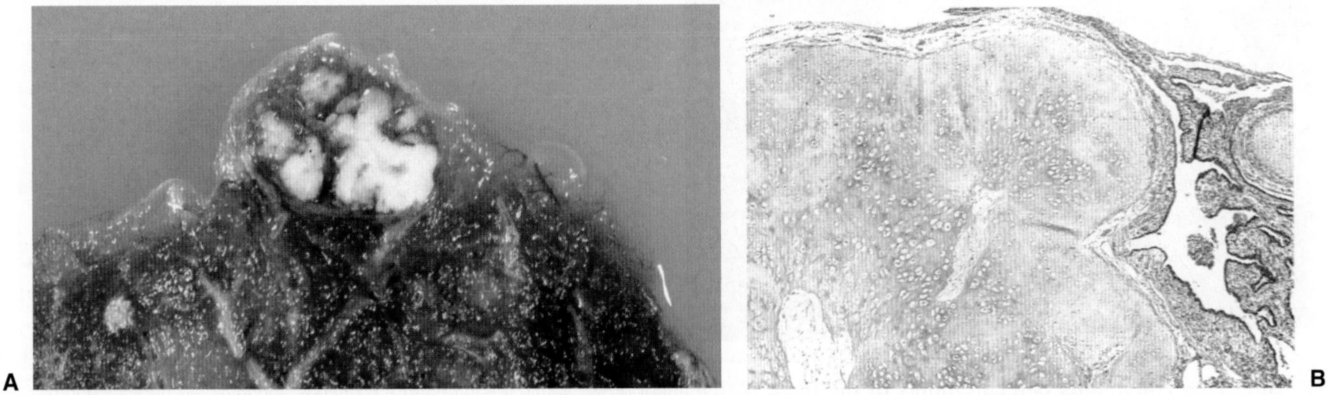

FIGURE 12-77. **Pulmonary hamartoma. A.** The cut surface of a sharply circumscribed, peripheral pulmonary nodule shows a lobulated structure. **B.** A photomicrograph reveals nodules of hyaline cartilage separated by connective tissue lined by respiratory epithelium.

and 5% for small cell carcinoma. Tumor stage remains the single most important predictor of prognosis.

General Features of Lung Cancer

LOCAL EFFECTS: Lung cancer can produce cough, dyspnea, hemoptysis, chest pain, obstructive pneumonia, and pleural effusion. Growth of a lung cancer (usually squamous) in the apex of the lung (**Pancoast tumor**) may extend to involve the eighth cervical and first and second thoracic nerves, leading to shoulder pain that radiates down the arm in an ulnar distribution (**Pancoast syndrome**). A Pancoast tumor also may paralyze cervical sympathetic nerves and cause **Horner syndrome**, characterized on the affected side by (1) depression of the eyeball (enophthalmos), (2) ptosis of the upper eyelid, (3) constriction of the pupil (miosis), and (4) absence of sweating (anhidrosis).

Most central endobronchial tumors produce symptoms related to bronchial obstruction: persistent cough, hemoptysis and obstructive pneumonia, or atelectasis. Effusions can result from extension of the tumor into the pleura or pericardium. Lymphangitic spread of the tumor within the lung may interfere with oxygenation. Tumors arising peripherally are more likely to be discovered either on routine chest radiographs or after they have become advanced. The latter circumstance features invasion of the chest wall with resulting chest pain, superior vena cava syndrome, and nerve-entrapment syndromes.

MEDIASTINAL SPREAD: Growth of the tumor within the mediastinum can cause the superior vena cava syndrome (owing to tumorous obstruction of this vein) and nerve-entrapment syndromes.

METASTASES: Carcinomas of the lung metastasize most frequently to regional lymph nodes, particularly the hilar and mediastinal nodes, but also to the brain, bone, and liver. The most frequent site of extranodal metastases is the adrenal gland, although adrenal insufficiency is distinctly uncommon.

PARANEOPLASTIC SYNDROMES: Disorders associated with lung cancer include acanthosis nigricans, dermatomyositis/polymyositis, clubbing of the fingers, and myasthenic syndromes, such as Eaton-Lambert syndrome and progressive multifocal encephalopathy. Endocrine syndromes are also encountered, for example, Cushing syndrome or inappropriate release of antidiuretic hormone (SIADH) by small cell carcinoma, and hypercalcemia (secretion of a parathormone-like substance by squamous cell carcinoma).

Histologic Subtypes of Lung Carcinoma

Squamous Cell Carcinoma

Squamous cell carcinoma accounts for 30% of all invasive lung cancers in the United States. After injury to the bronchial epithelium, such as occurs with cigarette smoking, regeneration from the pluripotent basal layer commonly occurs in the form of squamous metaplasia. The metaplastic mucosa follows the same sequence of dysplasia, carcinoma in situ, and invasive tumor as that observed in sites that are normally lined by squamous epithelium, such as the cervix or skin.

PATHOLOGY: Most squamous cell carcinomas arise in the central portion of the lung from the major or segmental bronchi, although 10% arise in the periphery. They tend to be firm, grey-white, 3- to 5-cm ulcerated lesions that extend through the bronchial wall into the adjacent parenchyma (Fig. 12-78A). The appearance of the cut surface is variable, depending on the degree of necrosis and hemorrhage. Central cavitation is frequent. On occasion, a central squamous carcinoma occurs as an endobronchial tumor.

The microscopic appearance of squamous cell carcinoma is highly variable. Well-differentiated squamous cell carcinomas display keratin "pearls," which are small round nests of brightly eosinophilic aggregates of keratin surrounded by concentric ("onion skin") layers of squamous cells (see Fig. 12-78B). Individual cell keratinization also occurs, in which a cell's cytoplasm assumes a glassy, intensely eosinophilic appearance. Intercellular bridges are identified in some well-differentiated squamous cancers as slender gaps between adjacent cells, which are traversed by fine strands of cytoplasm. By contrast, some squamous tumors are so poorly differentiated that they show no foci of keratinization and are difficult to distinguish from large cell, small cell, or spindle cell carcinomas. Tumor cells may be readily

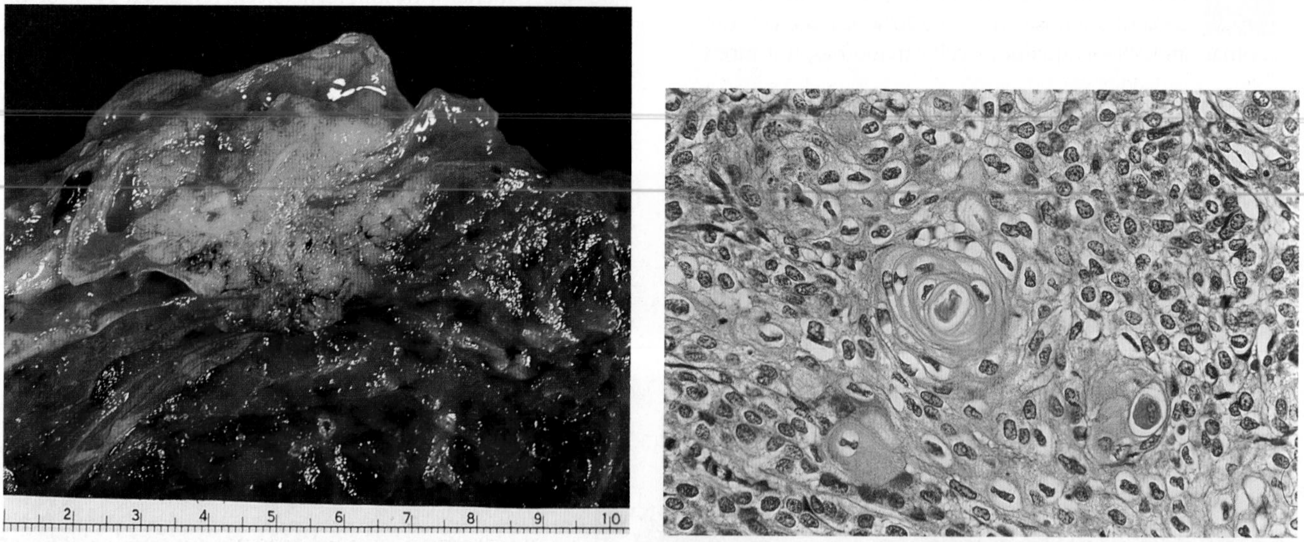

A B

FIGURE 12-78. **Squamous cell carcinoma of the lung. A.** The tumor grows within the lumen of a bronchus and invades the adjacent intrapulmonary lymph node. **B.** A photomicrograph shows well-differentiated squamous cell carcinoma with a keratin pearl composed of cells with brightly eosinophilic cytoplasm.

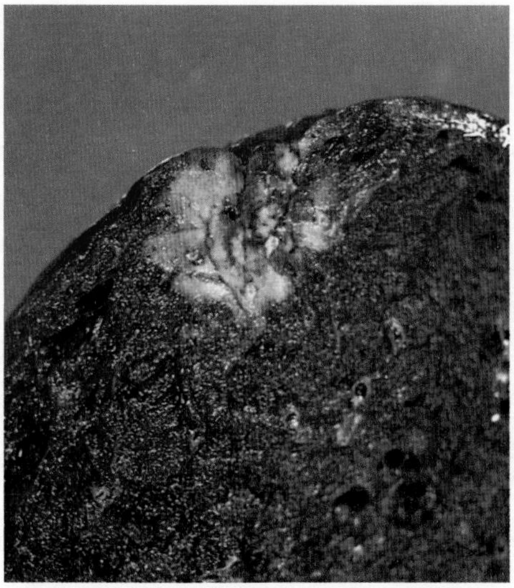

FIGURE 12-79. **Adenocarcinoma of the lung.** A peripheral tumor of the right upper lobe has an irregular border and a tan or grey cut surface and causes puckering of the overlying pleura.

found in the sputum, in which case the diagnosis is made by exfoliative cytology.

Adenocarcinoma

Adenocarcinoma of the lung comprises a third of all invasive lung cancers. In the United States and many other countries it has overtaken squamous cell carcinoma as the most common subtype of lung cancer and is the most common type in women. It tends to arise in the periphery and is often associated with pleural fibrosis and subpleural scars, which can result in pleural puckering (Fig. 12-79). In the past, these cancers were thought to arise in scars secondary to old tuberculosis or healed infarcts but it is now recognized that most of these scars represent a desmoplastic response to the tumor.

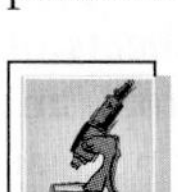

PATHOLOGY: At initial presentation, adenocarcinomas of the lung most often appear as irregular masses 2 to 5 cm in diameter, although they may be so large as to replace an entire lobe. On cut section, the tumor is grayish white and often glistening, depending on the amount of mucus production. Central adenocarcinomas may have predominantly endobronchial growth and invade bronchial cartilage.

There are four major subtypes of adenocarcinoma, as defined by the World Health Organization (Fig. 12-80, and see Fig. 12-81, and Fig. 12-82): (1) acinar, (2) papillary, (3) solid with mucus formation, and (4) bronchioloalveolar. Although some adenocarcinomas consist purely of one of these patterns, it is common to encounter a mixture of these histologic subtypes. Bronchioloalveolar carcinoma is distinctive enough to merit special attention (see below).

Pulmonary adenocarcinoma may reflect the architecture and cell population of any part of the respiratory mucosa, from the large bronchi to the smallest bronchioles. The neoplastic cells may resemble ciliated or nonciliated columnar epithelial cells, goblet cells, cells of bronchial glands, or Clara cells. The most common histologic type of adenocarcinoma features the acinar pattern, which is distinguished by regular glands lined by cuboidal or columnar cells, (see Fig. 12-80A). Papillary adenocarcinomas exhibit a single cell layer on a core of fibrovascular

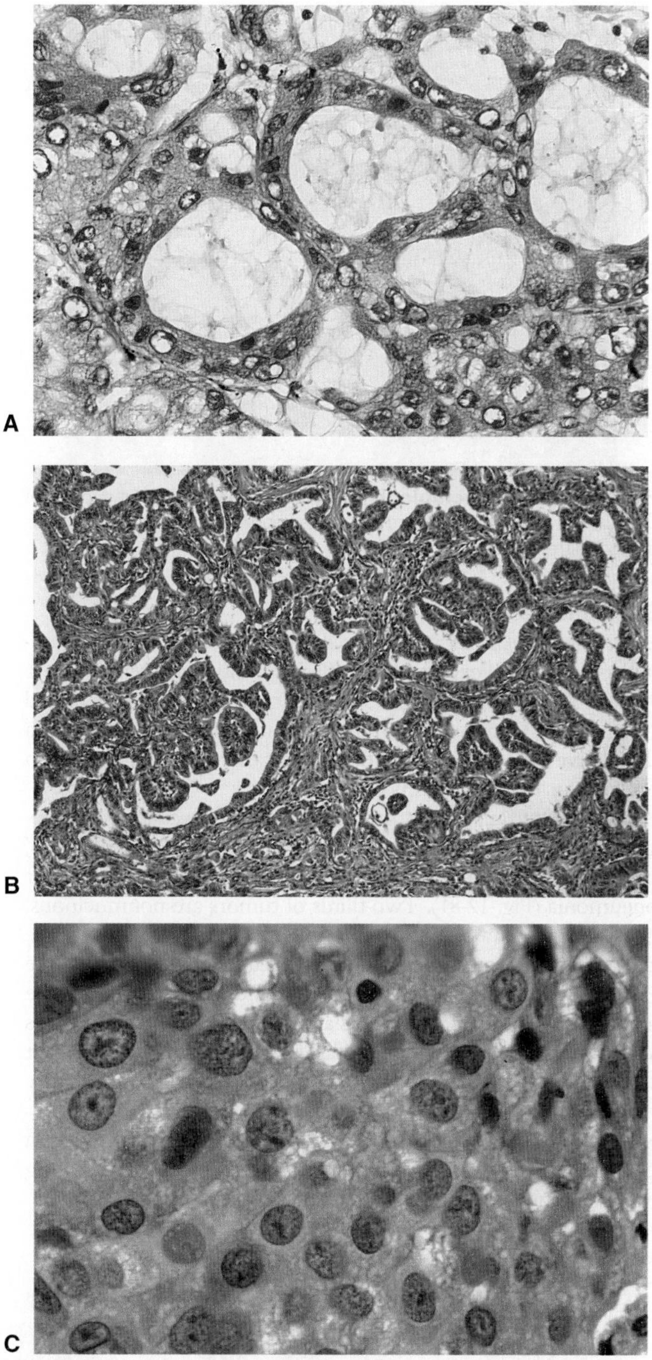

FIGURE 12-80. **Adenocarcinoma of the lung. A.** The malignant epithelial cells of an acinar adenocarcinoma form glands. **B.** A papillary adenocarcinoma consists of malignant epithelial cells growing along thin fibrovascular cores. **C.** A tumor grows in the pattern of solid adenocarcinoma with mucin formation. Several intracytoplasmic mucin droplets stain positively with the mucicarmine stain.

connective tissue (see Fig. 12-80B). Solid adenocarcinomas with mucus formation are poorly differentiated tumors, distinguishable from large cell carcinomas by demonstrating mucin with mucicarmine or periodic acid-Schiff (PAS) stains (see Fig. 12-80C).

Patients with stage I adenocarcinomas (localized to the lung) who undergo complete surgical removal have a 5-year survival of 50% to 80%.

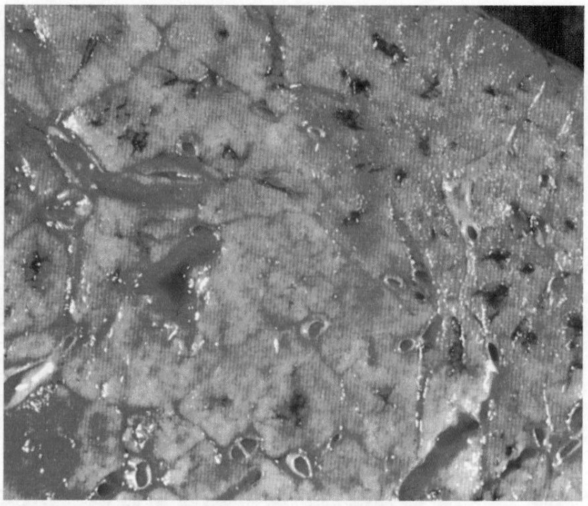

FIGURE 12-81. **Bronchioloalveolar carcinoma.** The cut surface of the lung is solid, glistening, and mucoid, an appearance that reflects a diffusely infiltrating tumor.

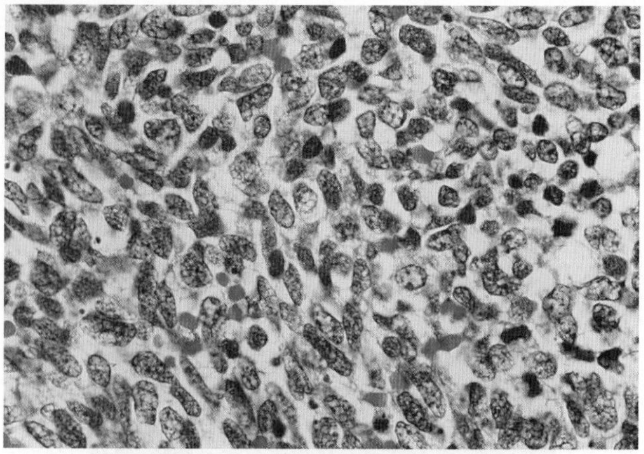

FIGURE 12-83. **Small cell carcinoma of the lung.** This tumor consists of small oval to spindle-shaped cells with scant cytoplasm, finely granular nuclear chromatin, and conspicuous mitoses.

Bronchioloalveolar Carcinoma

Bronchioloalveolar carcinoma is a distinctive subtype of adenocarcinoma that grows along preexisting alveolar walls and accounts for 1% to 5% of all invasive lung tumors. It has not been definitively linked to smoking. Copious mucin in the sputum (bronchorrhea) is a distinctive sign of bronchioloalveolar carcinoma but is seen in fewer than 10% of patients.

On gross examination, bronchioloalveolar carcinoma may appear as a single peripheral nodule or coin lesion (>50% of cases), multiple nodules, or a diffuse infiltrate indistinguishable from lobar pneumonia (Fig. 12-81). Two-thirds of tumors are nonmucinous, consisting of Clara cells and type II pneumocytes (Fig. 12-82A); the remaining third are mucinous tumors featuring goblet cells (see Fig. 12-82B). In nonmucinous tumors cuboidal cells grow along the alveolar walls. Mucinous tumors are composed of columnar cells with abundant apical cytoplasm filled with mucus. It is important to exclude the possibility that the tumor is actually a pulmonary metastasis, particularly for mucinous tumors.

Patients with stage I bronchioloalveolar carcinomas have a good prognosis; those who have multiple nodules or diffuse lung involvement are more likely to have a poor outcome.

Small Cell Carcinoma

Small cell carcinoma (previously "oat cell" carcinoma) is a highly malignant epithelial tumor of the lung that exhibits neuroendocrine features. It accounts for 20% of all lung cancers and is strongly associated with cigarette smoking. The male-to-female ratio is 2:1. The tumor grows and metastasizes rapidly, and 70% of patients are first seen in an advanced stage. A variety of paraneoplastic syndromes are distinctive for small cell carcinoma, including diabetes insipidus, ectopic ACTH (corticotropin) syndrome, and the Eaton-Lambert syndrome.

PATHOLOGY: Small cell carcinoma usually appears as a perihilar mass, frequently with extensive lymph node metastases. On cut section, it is soft and white but often shows extensive hemorrhage and necrosis. The tumor typically spreads along bronchi in a submucosal and circumferential fashion.

Histologically, small cell carcinoma consists of sheets of small, round, oval or spindle-shaped cells with scant cytoplasm. Their nuclei are distinctive, featuring finely granular nuclear chromatin and absent or inconspicuous nucleoli (Fig. 12-83). By

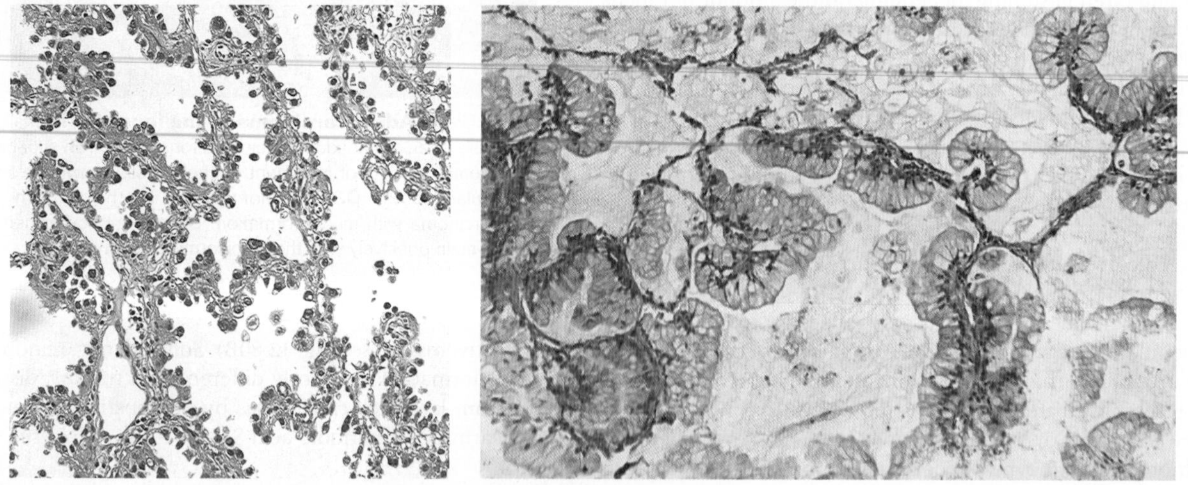

A B

FIGURE 12-82. **Bronchioloalveolar carcinoma. A.** Nonmucinous bronchioloalveolar carcinomas consist of atypical cuboidal to low columnar cells proliferating along the existing alveolar walls. **B.** Mucinous bronchioloalveolar carcinoma consists of tall columnar cells filled with apical cytoplasmic mucin that grow along the existing alveolar walls.

electron microscopy, many of the cells contain secretory neuroendocrine granules. A high mitotic rate is characteristic, with an average of 60 to 70 mitoses per 10 high-power fields. Necrosis is frequent and extensive. Although there is no absolute measure for the size of the tumor cells, a useful rule of thumb in small cell carcinoma is the diameter of three small lymphocytes.

Unlike other lung cancers small cell carcinomas show marked sensitivity to chemotherapy. From an oncologist's standpoint, then, all other lung cancers are grouped together as "non-small cell carcinoma."

Large Cell Carcinoma

Large cell carcinoma is a diagnosis of exclusion in a poorly differentiated tumor that does not show features of squamous or glandular differentiation and has been shown not to be a small cell carcinoma (Fig. 12-84). This tumor type accounts for 10% of all invasive lung tumors. The cells are large and exhibit ample cytoplasm. The nuclei frequently show prominent nucleoli and vesicular chromatin. Some large cell carcinomas exhibit pleomorphic giant cells or spindle cells.

Carcinoid Tumors

Carcinoid tumors of the lung comprise two subtypes of neuroendocrine neoplasms and are thought to arise from the resident neuroendocrine cells normally found in the bronchial epithelium. These neoplasms account for 2% of all primary lung cancers, show no sex predilection, and are not related to cigarette smoking. Although neuropeptides are readily demonstrated in the tumor cells, most are endocrinologically silent. A small subset of cases is associated with an endocrinopathy, such as Cushing syndrome with ectopic ACTH production by tumor cells. The carcinoid syndrome (see Chapter 13) occurs in 1% of cases, usually in the setting of hepatic metastases.

PATHOLOGY: Onethird of carcinoid tumors are central, one-third are peripheral (subpleural), and one-third are in the midportion of the lung. Central carcinoid tumors tend to have a large endobronchial component, with a fleshy, smooth, polypoid mass protruding into the bronchial lumen (Fig. 12-85A). The tumors average 3.0 cm in diameter, but range from 0.5 to 10 cm.

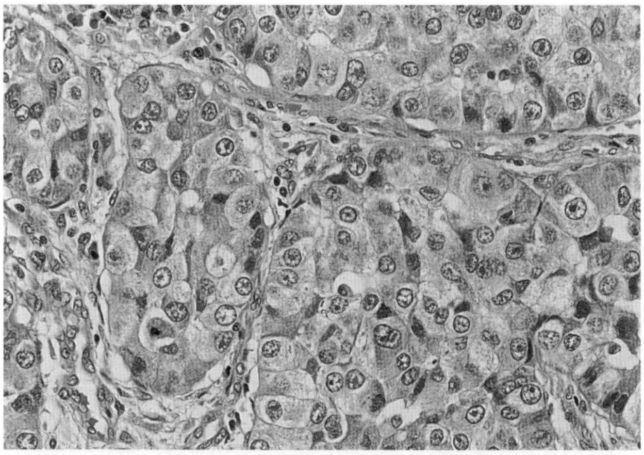

FIGURE 12-84. **Large cell carcinoma of the lung.** This poorly differentiated tumor is growing in sheets. The tumor cells are large and contain ample cytoplasm and prominent nucleoli.

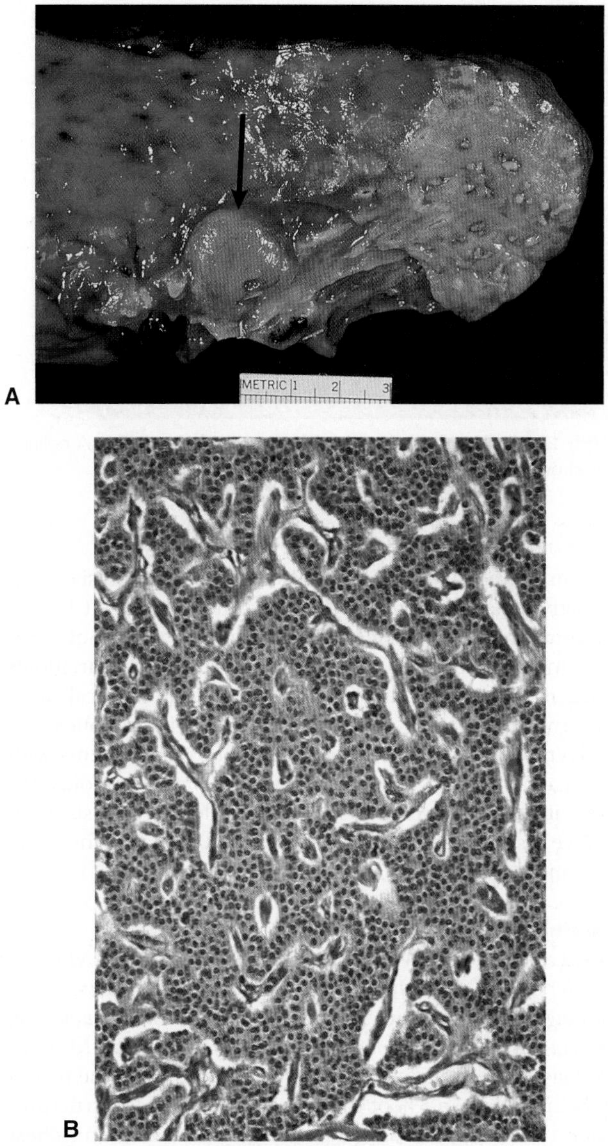

FIGURE 12-85. **Carcinoid tumor of the lung. A.** A central carcinoid tumor (arrow) is circumscribed and protrudes into the lumen of the main bronchus. The compression of the bronchus by the tumor caused the postobstructive pneumonia seen in the distal lung parenchyma *(right)*. **B.** A microscopic view shows ribbons of tumor cells embedded in a vascular stroma.

Carcinoid tumors are characterized histologically by an organoid growth pattern and uniform cytologic features: eosinophilic, finely granular cytoplasm and nuclei with finely granular chromatin (see Fig. 12-85B). A variety of neuroendocrine patterns may be seen, including trabecular growth, peripheral palisading, and rosettes.

Atypical carcinoid tumors differ from typical carcinoids by: (1) increased mitoses, with 2 to 10 mitoses per 2 mm^2 of tumor; (2) tumor necrosis (Fig. 12-86); (3) areas of increased cellularity and disorganization of the architecture; and (4) nuclear pleomorphism, hyperchromatism and high nuclear:cytoplasmic ratio.

CLINICAL FEATURES: Carcinoid tumors grow so slowly that half of patients are asymptomatic at presentation. Such tumors are often discovered as a mass in a chest radiograph. In symptomatic patients, the most

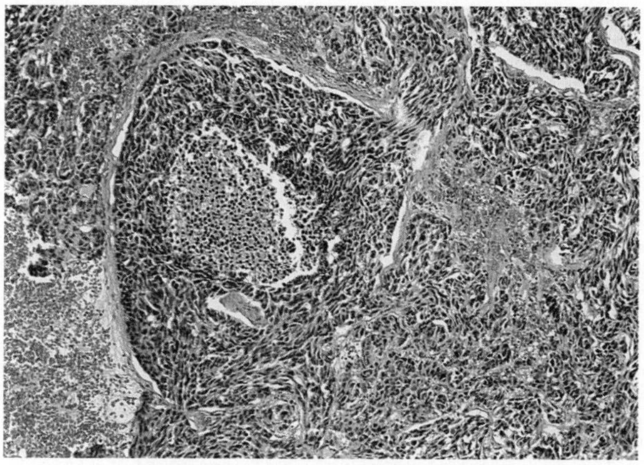

FIGURE 12-86. **Atypical carcinoid tumor of the lung.** A cellular tumor shows central necrosis and a disorganized architecture.

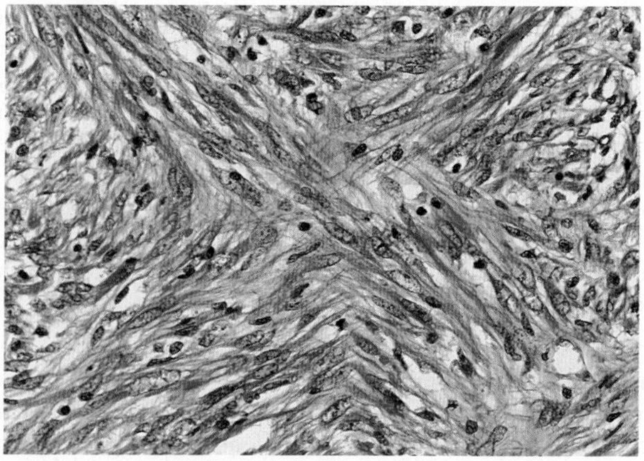

FIGURE 12-87. **Inflammatory pseudotumor.** A photomicrograph shows intersecting spindle cells and scattered lymphocytes and macrophages.

common pulmonary manifestations include hemoptysis, postobstructive pneumonitis, and dyspnea. There is a slight female predominance. The mean age at diagnosis is 55 years, but carcinoid tumors can occur at any age. In fact, bronchial carcinoids are the most common lung tumor in childhood. Atypical carcinoid tumors tend to be more aggressive than typical ones. Regional lymph node metastases are found in 20% of patients with typical carcinoids and 50% of those with atypical carcinoids. Patients with typical carcinoids have an excellent prognosis, with 90% 5-year survival after surgery, compared with 60% for atypical carcinoids.

Rare Pulmonary Tumors

INFLAMMATORY MYOFIBROBLASTIC TUMOR (INFLAMMATORY PSEUDOTUMOR): Inflammatory myofibroblastic tumor of the lung is an uncommon lesion that consists of variable amounts of inflammatory cells, foamy macrophages, and fibroblasts. Most of these masses are contained within the lung, although the pleura may be involved. In 5% of cases, the tumor invades structures outside the lung, such as the esophagus, mediastinum, chest wall, diaphragm, or pericardium.

Inflammatory myofibroblastic tumor had been regarded as an inflammatory, non-neoplastic process. However, genetic studies suggest that at least some of these may represent true neoplasms. A previous history of a pulmonary infection can be elicited in one third of patients.

PATHOLOGY: The tumors are solitary circumscribed, with a mean size of 4 cm. Virtually any inflammatory cells may be present, including lymphocytes, plasma cells, macrophages, giant cells, mast cells, and eosinophils. Inflammatory pseudotumor causes consolidation of the lung parenchyma and loss of architecture. Two major histologic patterns are fibrohistiocytic (Fig. 12-87) and plasma cell granuloma, depending on the predominant component. In some cases, foamy macrophages impart a xanthomatous pattern.

CLINICAL FEATURES: Most patients are younger than 40 years, although inflammatory pseudotumor can occur at any age and is one of the most common lung tumors of childhood. Half of patients are asymptomatic at presentation. Most inflammatory pseudotumors are cured by surgical excision, but 5% recur within the chest.

PULMONARY EPITHELIOID HEMANGIOENDOTHELIOMA: Pulmonary epithelioid hemangioendotheliomas are rare low- to intermediate-grade vascular sarcomas. Most patients are young adults and 80% are women. The course tends to be indolent, and half of patients are asymptomatic.

PATHOLOGY: Most patients are first seen with multiple pulmonary nodules. Histologically, the tumor consists of oval-shaped nodules that have a central, sclerotic, hypocellular zone and a cellular peripheral zone. The tumor spreads within alveolar spaces (Fig. 12-88). Tumor cells have abundant cytoplasm, with frequent intracytoplasmic vascular lumina, which may contain red blood cells. The intercellular stroma consists of an abundant eosinophilic matrix. The tumors express vascular markers, such as factor VIII. Epithelioid hemangioendotheliomas with a histological pattern similar to that seen in the lung may occur in the liver, bone, and soft tissue. Pulmonary epithelioid hemangioendothelioma has a variable clinical course, with a mean survival of 5 years.

CARCINOSARCOMA: Occasionally, a cancer of the lung appears like both a carcinoma and a sarcoma in different parts of the tumor, with the two patterns intimately mingled. In most cases, the epithelial component is a squamous carcinoma. The sarcomatous portion is usually spindle cells but may also exhibit heterologous elements, such as osteosarcoma, chondrosarcoma,

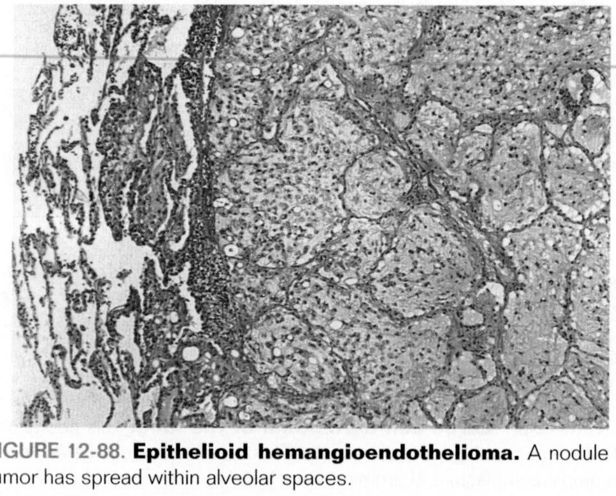

FIGURE 12-88. **Epithelioid hemangioendothelioma.** A nodule of tumor has spread within alveolar spaces.

and rhabdomyosarcoma. Metastases can contain both histologic components. The primary approach to therapy for carcinosarcoma is surgery, but the prognosis is poor, with a median survival of 9 to 12 months.

PULMONARY BLASTOMA: This malignant tumor resembles embryonal lung, with a glandular component consisting of poorly differentiated columnar cells arranged in tubules, without mucous secretion. The intervening tumor is formed by spindle cells that resemble embryonal mesoderm. There is a histologic overlap between pulmonary blastoma and carcinosarcoma, including heterologous elements, and the clinical features are similar.

Despite the embryonal appearance of pulmonary blastoma, the tumor occurs primarily in adults (median age range, 35–43 years), and most patients are cigarette smokers. The prognosis for patients with biphasic tumors is poor and comparable to that for carcinoma of the lung.

MUCOEPIDERMOID CARCINOMA AND ADENOID CYSTIC CARCINOMA: These neoplasms resemble their namesakes in the salivary glands. They are derived from the tracheobronchial mucous glands and are seen in the trachea or proximal bronchus as a luminal mass, often associated with obstructive symptoms. Adenoid cystic carcinomas are difficult to resect locally and often metastasize.

PULMONARY ARTERY SARCOMA: Pulmonary artery sarcoma is a rare tumor of connective tissue (Fig. 12-89), which has a broad histologic spectrum, including fibrosarcoma, leiomyosarcoma, osteosarcoma, rhabdomyosarcoma, angiosarcoma, or unclassifiable sarcoma. These tumors are rarely diagnosed during life and may be discovered because of pulmonary hypertension. The tumor often grows in an intraluminal fashion within proximal arteries and may extend in a wormlike fashion to peripheral pulmonary artery branches, resulting in peripheral infarcts.

Lymphomatoid Granulomatosis

Lymphomatoid granulomatosis is a lymphoproliferative disorder characterized by pulmonary nodular lymphoid infiltrates with frequent central necrosis and vascular permeation (Fig. 12-90). It affects middle-aged persons and is more common in immunosuppressed people. The lung is the major location, but kidney, skin and upper respiratory tract may also be involved. The lymphoid infiltrate is angiocentric and angioinvasive and consists of polymorphous, small to medium-sized lymphocytes, which are mainly T cells, admixed with variable numbers of large atypical B cells. The latter typically express EBV, which is thought to drive the proliferative process.

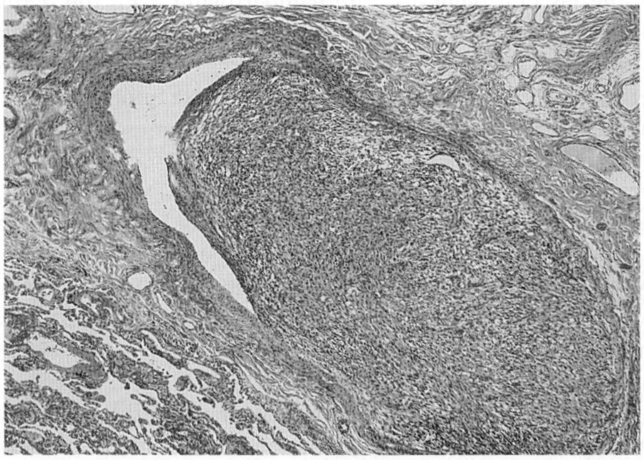

FIGURE 12-89. **Pulmonary artery sarcoma.** A polypoid mass of malignant spindle cells is spreading within the lumen of this pulmonary artery.

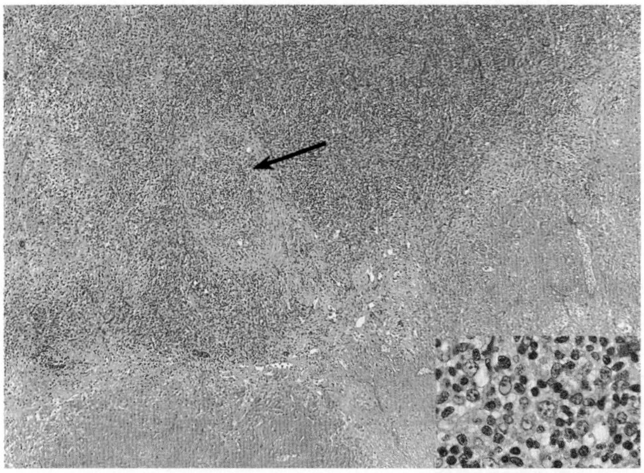

FIGURE 12-90. **Lymphomatoid granulomatosis.** This extensively necrotic nodular mass consists of a cellular lymphoid infiltrate that penetrates a blood vessel *(arrow)* at the edge of the lesion. *Inset:* The lymphoid infiltrate is composed of a polymorphous population of small, medium-sized, and large atypical lymphoid cells.

Despite remissions induced by chemotherapy, half of all patients eventually develop large cell lymphoma. Even with aggressive treatment, the prognosis of lymphomatoid granulomatosis is poor.

Pulmonary Metastases are More Common than Primary Lung Tumors

In one-third of all fatal cancers, pulmonary metastases are evident at autopsy. Metastatic tumors in the lung are typically multiple and circumscribed. When large nodules are seen in the lungs radiologically, they are called "cannon ball" metastases (Fig. 12-91).

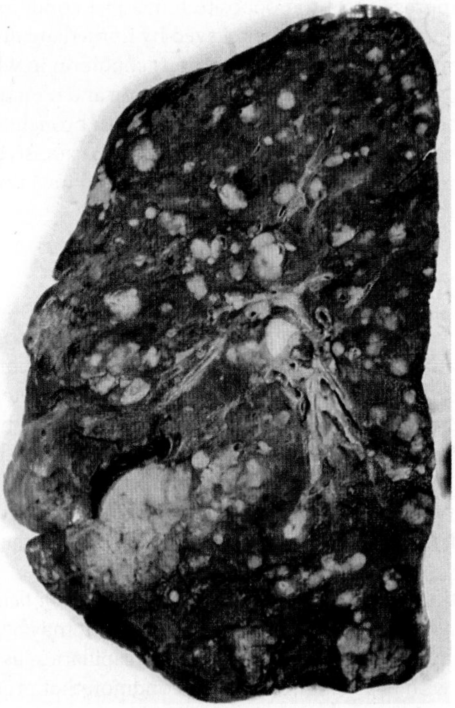

FIGURE 12-91. **Metastatic carcinoma of the lung.** A section through the lung shows numerous nodules of metastatic carcinoma corresponding to "cannon ball" metastases seen radiologically.

The histologic appearance of most metastases resembles that of the primary tumor. Uncommonly, metastatic tumors may mimic bronchioloalveolar carcinoma, in which cases the usual primary site is the pancreas or stomach.

In **lymphangitic carcinoma** a metastatic tumor spreads widely through pulmonary lymphatic channels to form a sheath of tumor around the bronchovascular tree and veins. Clinically, patients suffer from cough and shortness of breath and display a diffuse reticulonodular pattern on the chest radiograph. The common primary sites are the breast, stomach, pancreas, and colon.

THE PLEURA

Pneumothorax

Pneumothorax is defined as the presence of air in the pleural cavity. It may occur with traumatic perforation of the pleura or may be "spontaneous." Traumatic causes include penetrating wounds of the chest wall (e.g., a stab wound or a rib fracture). Traumatic pneumothorax is most commonly iatrogenic and is seen after aspiration of fluid from the pleura (thoracentesis), pleural or lung biopsies, transbronchial biopsies, and positive pressure-assisted ventilation.

Spontaneous pneumothorax is typically encountered in young adults. For example, while exercising vigorously, a tall young man develops acute chest pain and shortness of breath. A chest radiograph shows collapse of the lung on the side of the pain and a large collection of air in the pleural space. The condition is due to rupture, usually of a subpleural emphysematous bleb. In most cases, spontaneous pneumothorax subsides by itself, but some patients required withdrawal of the air.

Tension pneumothorax refers to unilateral pneumothorax extensive enough to shift the mediastinum to the opposite side, with compression of the opposite lung. The condition may be life-threatening and must be relieved by immediate drainage.

Bronchopleural fistula is a serious condition in which there is free communication between the airway and pleura. It is usually iatrogenic, caused by the interruption of bronchial continuity by biopsy or surgery. It may also be due to extensive infection and necrosis of lung tissue, in which case the infection is more important than the air.

Pleural Effusion

Pleural effusion is accumulation of excess fluid in the pleural cavity. Only a small amount of fluid in the pleural cavity lubricates the space between the lungs and chest wall. Fluid secreted into the pleural space from the parietal pleura is absorbed by the visceral pleura. The severity of a pleural effusion varies from a few milliliters of fluid, which is detected only radiologically as obliteration of the costophrenic angle, to a massive accumulation that shifts the mediastinum and the trachea to the opposite side.

HYDROTHORAX: This term refers to an effusion that resembles water and would be regarded as edema elsewhere. It may be due to increased hydrostatic pressure within the capillaries, as occurs in patients with heart failure or in any condition that produces systemic or pulmonary edema. Hydrothorax also occurs in patients with low serum osmotic pressure, as in nephrotic syndrome, cirrhosis of the liver, or severe starvation. Other important causes of hydrothorax are the collagen vascular diseases (notably systemic lupus erythematosus and rheumatoid arthritis) and asbestos exposure.

PYOTHORAX: A turbid effusion containing many polymorphonuclear leukocytes (pyothorax) results from infections of the pleura. This may occasionally be caused by an external penetrating wound that introduces pyogenic organisms into the pleural space. More commonly, it is a complication of bacterial pneumonia that extends to the pleural surface, the classic example of which is pneumococcal pneumonia. Pyothorax is a rare complication of medical procedures involving the pleural cavity.

EMPYEMA: This disorder is a variant of pyothorax in which thick pus accumulates within the pleural cavity, often with loculation and fibrosis.

HEMOTHORAX: This term refers to blood in the pleural cavity as a result of trauma or rupture of a vessel (e.g., dissecting aneurysm of the aorta). A pleural effusion may be blood-stained in tuberculosis, cancers involving the pleura, and pulmonary infarction.

CHYLOTHORAX: Chylothorax is accumulation milky, lipid-rich fluid (chyle) in the pleural cavity as a result of lymphatic obstruction. It has an ominous portent, because lymphaticobstruction suggests disease of the lymph nodes in the posterior mediastinum. Chylothorax is thus a rare complication of malignant tumors in the mediastinum, such as lymphoma. In tropical countries, it results from nematode infestations. Chylothorax can also be seen in pulmonary lymphangioleiomyomatosis.

Pleuritis

Pleuritis, or inflammation of the pleura, may result from the extension of any pulmonary infection to the visceral pleura, bacterial infections within the pleural cavity, viral infections, collagen vascular disease, or pulmonary infarction that involves the surface of the lung. The most striking symptom is sharp, stabbing chest pain on inspiration. It is frequently associated with a pleural effusion.

Tumors of the Pleura

Localized (Solitary) Fibrous Tumor of the Pleura Are Usually Benign

Solitary fibrous tumor of the pleura is an uncommon localized neoplasm arising in association with the pleura. Most are benign, but a small percentage are malignant. Some 80% of these tumors arise on the visceral pleura, the remainder being from the parietal pleura. Similar tumors can develop in any location with a mesothelial surface, including the mediastinum, peritoneum, pericardium, liver, and tunica vaginalis. These tumors arise from submesothelial connective tissue, rather than mesothelium, and are unrelated to asbestos exposure.

PATHOLOGY: The tumors may be pedunculated. More than 60% are over 10 cm in diameter and some reach 40 cm and may weigh up to 3800 g. The cut surface is grey-white, with a nodular, whorled or lobulated appearance (Fig. 12-92A). Cysts are occasionally present, especially at the base near the pleural attachment.

The most common histological apperance is the "patternless pattern." disorderly or randomly arranged mixtures of fibroblast-like cells and connective tissue. Other arrangements include he-

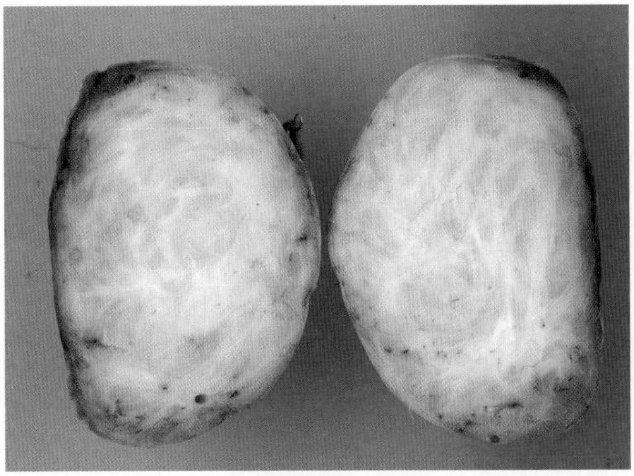

A

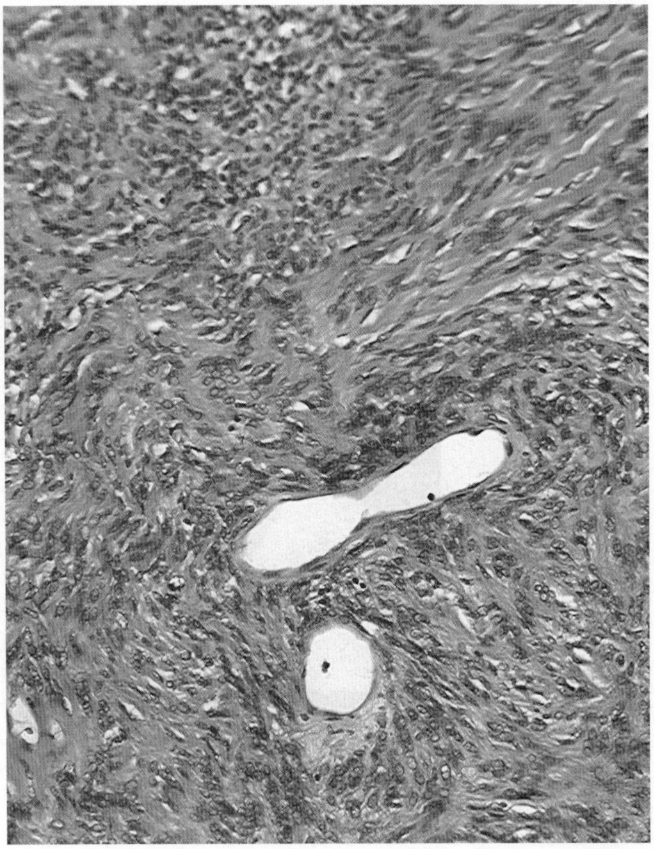

B

FIGURE 12-92. **Pleural localized (solitary) fibrous tumor. A.** The tumor is circumscribed with a whorled, tan, cut surface. **B.** The tumor cells are round to oval and spindle shaped, with a dense eosinophilic or "ropy" collagen stroma and slitlike blood vessels.

mangiopericytoma-like, storiform, herringbone, leiomyoma-like, or neurofibroma-like arrangements (Fig. 12-92B). The tumor cells are spindle- to oval-shaped, often with a fibroblast-like appearance. The collagen is compressed between the cells in a lacy network or it may form dense, wirelike bands. Histologic features suggesting malignancy include increased cellularity, pleomorphism, necrosis, and more than four mitoses per 10 high-power fields. Most tumors are immunopositive for CD34 and *bcl*-2.

CLINICAL FEATURES: The median age of patients diagnosed with localized fibrous tumor of the pleura is 55 years (range, 9–86 years) without any sex predominance. They present most often with chest pain, followed by shortness of breath, cough, hypoglycemia, weight loss, hemoptysis, fever, and night sweats. Patients with benign fibrous tumors of pleura have an excellent prognosis. Half of histologically malignant tumors are cured if completely resected.

Malignant Mesothelioma is a Complication of Asbestos Exposure

Malignant mesothelioma is a neoplasm of mesothelial cells that is most common in the pleura but also occurs in the peritoneum, pericardium, and the tunica vaginalis of the testis.

EPIDEMIOLOGY: Some 2000 new persons develop these tumors yearly in the United States. *In the United States, Great Britain, and South Africa, 80% of patients report exposure to asbestos.* The latency period between asbestos exposure and the appearance of malignant mesothelioma is usually to 40 years, with a range of 12 to 60 years.

PATHOLOGY: Grossly, pleural mesotheliomas often encase and compress the lung, extending into fissures and interlobar septa, a distribution often referred to as a "pleural rind" (Fig. 12-93A). Invasion of pulmonary parenchyma is generally limited to the periphery adjacent to the tumor, and lymph nodes tend to be spared. Microscopically, classic mesotheliomas show a biphasic appearance, with epithelial and sarcomatous patterns (see Fig. 12-93B). Glands and tubules that resemble adenocarcinoma are admixed with sheets of spindle cells that are similar to a fibrosarcoma. In some instances, only one or the other component: if it is epithelial, the tumor may be difficult to distinguish from adenocarcinoma. Less commonly, only a sarcomatous component is present. Useful criteria for diagnosing mesothelioma include absence of mucin, presence of hyaluronic acid (positive Alcian blue staining), and demonstration of long, slender microvilli by electron microscopy.

Immunohistochemistry provides more-refined criteria for differentiating mesothelioma from adenocarcinoma (see Chapter 5). Adenocarcinomas often, but not always, express carcinoembryonic antigen, Leu-M1, B72.3, and BER-EP4. Mesotheliomas are negative for these markers. Both mesothelioma and adenocarcinoma are positive for cytokeratins. Calretinin, a recently developed marker, usually stains mesotheliomas, whereas adenocarcinoma is typically negative. Wilms tumor-1 (WT-1),

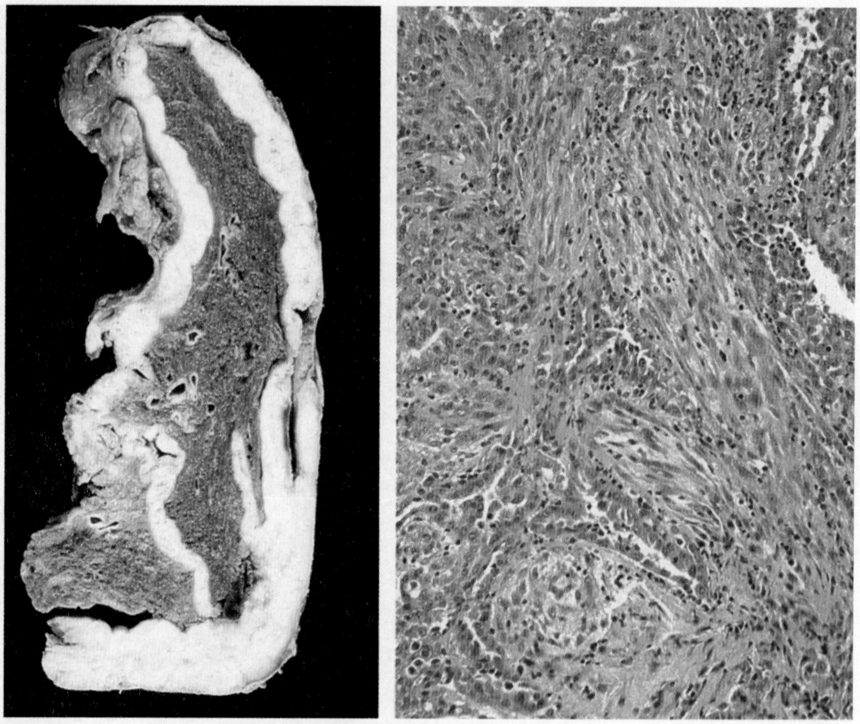

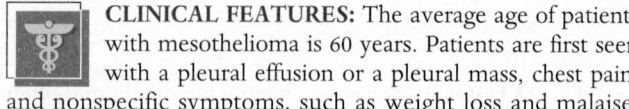

FIGURE 12-93. **Pleural malignant mesothelioma. A.** The lung is encased by a dense pleural tumor that extends along the interlobar fissures but does not involve the underlying lung parenchyma. **B**. This mesothelioma is composed of a biphasic pattern of epithelial and sarcomatous elements.

thrombomodulin, and podoplanin are other markers typically expressed in mesotheliomas but not pulmonary adenocarcinomas.

CLINICAL FEATURES: The average age of patients with mesothelioma is 60 years. Patients are first seen with a pleural effusion or a pleural mass, chest pain, and nonspecific symptoms, such as weight loss and malaise. Pleural mesotheliomas tend to spread locally within the chest cavity, invading and compressing major structures. Metastases can occur to the lung parenchyma and mediastinal lymph nodes, as well as to extrathoracic sites such as the liver, bones, peritoneum,and adrenals. Treatment is largely ineffective and prognosis is poor: few patients survivie longer than 18 months after diagnosis.

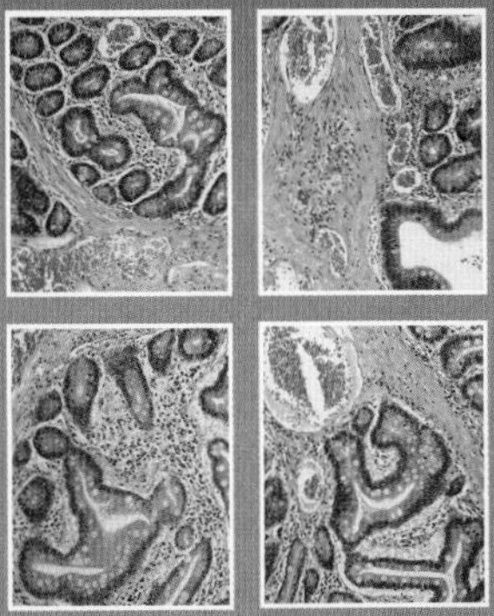

13

The Gastrointestinal Tract

Frank A. Mitros
Emanuel Rubin

THE ESOPHAGUS

Anatomy

Embryologically, the gut and respiratory tract arise from the same anlage and constitute a single tube. This structure divides into two separate tubes, the esophagus being dorsal and the future respiratory tract, ventral. Initially, columnar epithelium lines the esophagus in its early embryonic development, but it is replaced by a stratified squamous epithelium.

The adult esophagus is a 25-cm tube that is a conduit for the passage of food and liquid into the stomach. It contains striated and smooth muscle in its upper portion and smooth muscle alone in its lower portion. The organ is fixed superiorly at the cricopharyngeus muscle, which is considered the upper esophageal sphincter. It courses inferiorly through the posterior mediastinum behind the trachea and heart, and exits the thorax through the hiatus of the diaphragm. Tonic muscular contraction at its lower end creates an action like that of a one-way flutter valve. The so-called **lower esophageal sphincter** is not a true anatomical sphincter but rather a functional one.

The esophagus has a mucosa, submucosa, muscularis propria, and adventitia. The transition from the squamous mucosa of the esophagus to the gastric mucosa at the esophagogastric junction occurs abruptly at the level of the diaphragm. The esophageal submucosa contains mucous glands and a rich lymphatic plexus. The lymphatics of the upper third of the esophagus drain to cervical lymph nodes, those of the middle third to the mediastinal nodes, and those of the lower third to the celiac and gastric lymph nodes. These anatomic features are significant in the spread of esophageal cancer.

The venous drainage of the esophagus is important in portal hypertension, in which esophageal varices occur. These varices are invariably found in the lower third of the esophagus, because the veins of the upper third drain into the superior vena cava and those of the middle third drain into the azygous system. Only the veins of the lower third of the esophagus drain into the portal vein via the gastric veins.

Congenital Disorders

Tracheoesophageal Fistula Leads to Aspiration Pneumonia

Tracheoesophageal fistula is the most common esophageal anomaly (Fig. 13-1). It is frequently combined with some form of **esophageal atresia.** In some cases, it is associated with a complex of anomalies identified by the acronym Vater syndrome (vertebral defects, anal atresia, tracheoesophageal fistula, and renal dysplasia). Maternal hydramnios has been recorded in some cases of esophageal atresia and, less commonly, in cases of tracheoesophageal fistula. Esophageal atresia and fistulas are often associated with congenital heart disease.

PATHOLOGY: In 90% of tracheoesophageal fistulas, the upper portion of the esophagus ends in a blind pouch and the superior end of the lower segment communicates with the trachea. *In this type of atresia, the upper blind sac soon fills with mucus, which the infant then aspirates.* Surgical correction is feasible albeit difficult.

Among the remaining 10% of fistulas, the most common is a communication between the proximal esophagus and the

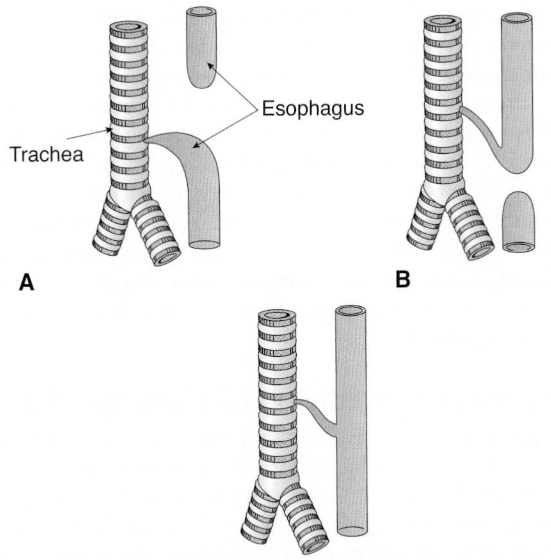

FIGURE 13-1. **Congenital tracheoesophageal fistulas. A.** The most common type is a communication between the trachea and the lower portion of the esophagus. The upper segment of the esophagus ends in a blind sac. **B.** In a few cases, the proximal esophagus communicates with the trachea. **C.** The least common anomaly, the H type, is a fistula between a continuous esophagus and the trachea.

trachea; the lower esophageal pouch communicates with the stomach. *Infants with this condition develop aspiration immediately after birth.* In another variant, termed an *H-type fistula,* a communication exists between an intact esophagus and an intact trachea. In some cases, (see Fig. 13-1C) the lesion becomes symptomatic only in adulthood, when repeated pulmonary infections call attention to it.

Rings and Webs Cause Dysphagia

ESOPHAGEAL WEBS: Occasionally, a thin mucosal membrane projects into the esophageal lumen. Webs are usually single, but may be multiple, and can occur anywhere in the esophagus. They are often successfully treated by dilation with large rubber bougies; occasionally, they can be excised with biopsy forceps during endoscopy.

PLUMMER-VINSON (PATERSON-KELLY) SYNDROME: This disorder is characterized by (1) a cervical esophageal web, (2) mucosal lesions of the mouth and pharynx, and (3) iron-deficiency anemia. Dysphagia, often associated with aspiration of swallowed food, is the most common clinical manifestation. Ninety percent of cases occur in women. *Carcinoma of the oropharynx and upper esophagus is a recognized complication of the Plummer-Vinson syndrome.*

SCHATZKI RING: This lower esophageal narrowing is usually seen at the gastroesophageal junction (Fig. 13-2). The upper surface of the mucosal ring has stratified squamous epithelium; the lower, columnar epithelium. Although it has been noted in up to 14% of barium meal examinations, Schatzki ring is usually asymptomatic. Patients with narrow Schatzki rings however, may complain of intermittent dysphagia.

Esophageal Diverticula Often Reflect Motor Dysfunction

A **true esophageal diverticulum** is an outpouching of the wall that contains all layers of the esophagus. If a sac has no muscular layer, it is a **false** diverticulum. Esophageal diverticula occur in the hypopharyngeal area above the upper esophageal sphincter, in the middle esophagus, and immediately proximal to the lower esophageal sphincter.

ZENKER DIVERTICULUM: Zenker diverticulum is an uncommon lesion that appears high in the esophagus and affects men more than women. It was once believed to result from luminal pressure exerted in a structurally weak area and was therefore classed as a **pulsion diverticulum.** The cause is probably more complicated, but disordered function of cricopharyngeal musculature is still generally thought to be involved in the pathogenesis of this false diverticulum. Most affected persons who come to medical attention are older than 60, suggesting that this diverticulum is acquired.

Zenker diverticula can enlarge conspicuously and accumulate a large amount of food. The typical symptom is regurgitation of food eaten some time previously (occasionally days), in the absence of dysphagia. Recurrent aspiration pneumonia may be a serious complication. When symptoms are severe, surgical intervention is the rule.

TRACTION DIVERTICULA: Traction diverticula are outpouchings that occur principally in the midportion of the esophagus. They were so named because of their attachment to adjacent mediastinal lymph nodes, usually associated with tuberculous lymphadenitis. However, such adhesions are today uncommon and it is believed that these pouches often reflect a disturbance in the motor function of the esophagus. A diverticulum in the midesophagus ordinarily has a wide stoma and the pouch is usually higher than its orifice. Thus, it does not retain food or secretions and remains asymptomatic, with only rare complications.

EPIPHRENIC DIVERTICULA: These diverticula are located immediately above the diaphragm. Motor disturbances of the esophagus (e.g., achalasia, diffuse esophageal spasm) are found in two thirds of patients with this true diverticulum. In addition, reflux esophagitis may play a role in the pathogenesis of epiphrenic diverticula.

Unlike other diverticula, epiphrenic diverticula are encountered in young persons. Nocturnal regurgitation of large amounts of fluid stored in the diverticulum during the day is

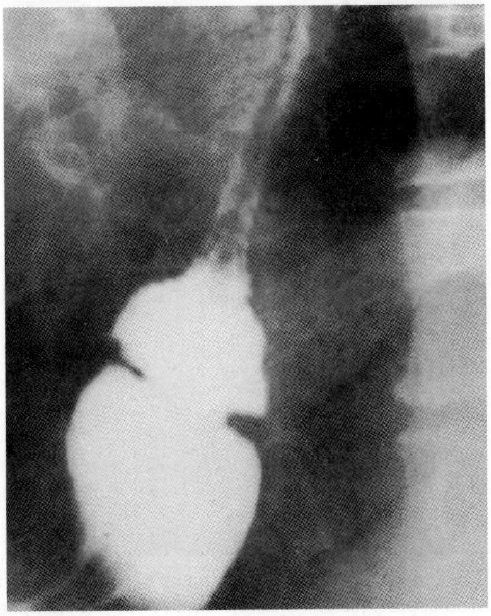

FIGURE 13-2. **Schatzki mucosal ring.** A contrast radiograph illustrates the lower esophageal narrowing.

typical. When symptoms are severe, surgical intervention directed toward correcting the motor abnormality (e.g., myotomy) is appropriate.

Motor Disorders

The automatic coordination of muscular movement during swallowing is termed a **motor function** and results in free passage of food through the esophagus. The hallmark of motor disorders is difficulty in swallowing, termed **dysphagia.** Dysphagia is often an awareness that a bolus of food is not moving downwards, and in itself is not painful. Pain on swallowing is **odynophagia.** Motor disorders can be caused by:

- **Dysfunction of striated muscle** in the upper esophagus
- **Systemic diseases of skeletal muscle** such as myasthenia gravis, dermatomyositis, amyloidosis, hyperthyroidism, and myxedema
- **Neurologic diseases** that affect nerves to skeletal muscle (e.g., cerebrovascular accidents, amyotrophic lateral sclerosis)
- **Peripheral neuropathy** associated with diabetes or alcoholism

Achalasia Features Impaired Function of the Lower Esophageal Sphincter

Achalasia, at one time termed ***cardiospasm,*** *is characterized by failure of the lower esophageal sphincter to relax in response to swallowing and absence of peristalsis in the body of the esophagus.* As a result of these defects in both the outflow tract and the pumping mechanisms of the esophagus, food is retained within the esophagus and the organ hypertrophies and dilates conspicuously (Fig. 13-3).

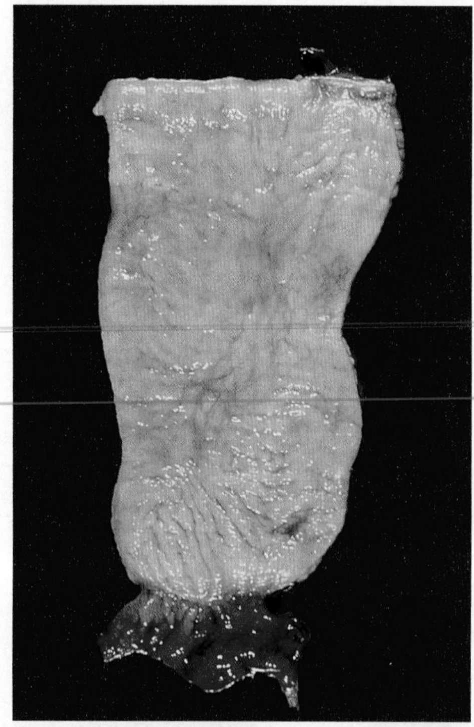

FIGURE 13-3. **Esophagus and upper stomach of a patient with advanced achalasia.** The esophagus is markedly dilated above the esophagogastric junction, where the lower esophageal sphincter is located. The esophageal mucosa is redundant and has hyperplastic squamous epithelium.

Achalasia is associated with loss or absence of ganglion cells in the esophageal myenteric plexus. Degenerative changes in the dorsal motor nucleus of the vagus and extraesophageal vagus nerves have also been described. Ganglion cell loss may be accompanied by chronic inflammation. In Latin America, achalasia is a common complication of **Chagas disease,** in which the ganglion cells are destroyed by the protozoa *Trypanosoma cruzi.*

Dysphagia, occasionally odynophagia, and regurgitation of material retained in the esophagus are common symptoms of achalasia. Squamous carcinoma is also a complication. Treatment is by dilation or surgical myotomy, which can lead to gastroesophageal reflux.

Scleroderma Causes Fibrosis of the Esophageal Wall

Scleroderma (progressive systemic sclerosis) causes fibrosis in many organs and produces a severe abnormality of esophageal muscle function. The disease mainly affects the lower esophageal sphincter, which may become so impaired that the lower esophagus and upper stomach are no longer distinct functional entities and are visualized as a common cavity. In addition, there may be a lack of peristalsis in the entire esophagus.

Microscopically, fibrosis of esophageal smooth muscle (especially the inner layer of the muscularis propria) and nonspecific inflammatory changes are seen. Intimal fibrosis of small arteries and arterioles is common and may play a role in the pathogenesis of the fibrosis. Clinically, patients have dysphagia and heartburn caused by peptic esophagitis, owing to reflux of acid from the stomach. Severe reflux changes may occur (see below).

Hiatal Hernia

Hiatal hernia is a herniation of the stomach through an enlarged esophageal hiatus in the diaphragm. Two basic types of hiatal hernia are observed (Fig. 13-4).

SLIDING HERNIA: An enlargement of the diaphragmatic hiatus and laxity of the circumferential connective tissue allows a cap of gastric mucosa to move upward to a position above the diaphragm. This condition is common. Sliding hiatal hernia is asymptomatic in most patients: only 5% of patients diagnosed radiologically complain of symptoms referable to gastroesophageal reflux.

PARAESOPHAGEAL HERNIA: This uncommon form of hiatal hernia is characterized by herniation of a portion of gastric fundus alongside the esophagus through a defect in the diaphragmatic connective tissue membrane that defines the esophageal hiatus. The hernia progressively enlarges, and the hiatus grows increasingly wide. In extreme cases, most of the stomach herniates into the thorax.

CLINICAL FEATURES: Symptoms of hiatal hernia, particularly heartburn and regurgitation, are attributed to gastroesophageal reflux of gastric contents, primarily related to incompetence of the lower esophageal sphincter. Classically, symptoms are exacerbated when the affected person is recumbent, which facilitates acid reflux. Dysphagia, painful swallowing, and occasionally bleeding may also be troublesome. Large herniations carry a risk of gastric volvulus or intrathoracic gastric dilation.

Sliding hiatal hernias generally do not require surgical repair; symptoms are often treated medically. By contrast, an enlarging paraesophageal hernia should be surgically treated, even in the absence of symptoms.

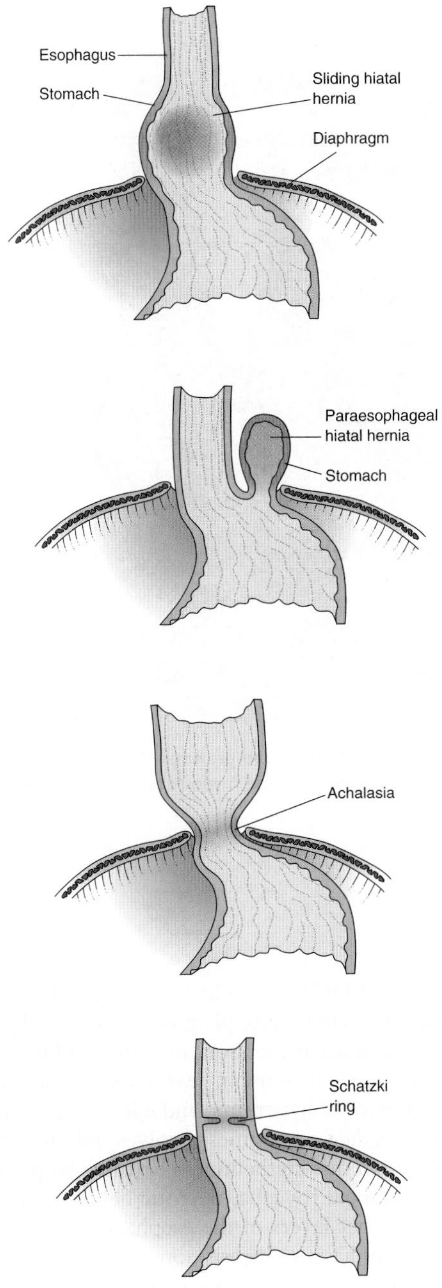

FIGURE 13-4. **Disorders of the esophageal outlet.**

Esophagitis

Reflux Esophagitis Is Caused by Regurgitation of Gastric Contents

By far the most common type of esophagitis, reflux esophagitis is often found in conjunction with a sliding hiatal hernia, although it may occur through an incompetent lower esophageal sphincter without any demonstrable anatomical lesion.

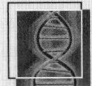

PATHOGENESIS: The principal barrier to reflux of gastric contents into the esophagus is the lower esophageal sphincter. Transient reflux is a normal event, particularly after a meal. When these episodes become more frequent and are prolonged, esophagitis results. Agents that decrease the pressure of the lower esophageal sphincter (e.g., alcohol, chocolate, fatty foods, cigarette smoking) are also associated with reflux. Certain central nervous system depressants (e.g., morphine, diazepam), pregnancy, estrogen therapy, and the presence of a nasogastric tube may lead to reflux esophagitis. Although acid is damaging to the esophageal mucosa, the combination of acid and pepsin may be particularly injurious. Moreover, gastric fluid often contains refluxed bile from the duodenum, which is harmful to the esophageal mucosa. Alcohol, hot beverages, and spicy foods also may damage the mucosa directly.

PATHOLOGY: The first grossly evident change caused by gastroesophageal reflux is hyperemia. Areas affected by reflux are susceptible to superficial mucosal erosions and ulcers, which often appear as vertical linear streaks. Microscopically, mild injury to the squamous epithelium is manifested by cell swelling (hydropic change). The basal region of the epithelium is thickened, and the papillae of the lamina propria are elongated and extend toward the surface because of reactive proliferation. Capillary vessels within the papillae are often dilated. An increase in lymphocytes is seen in the squamous epithelium and eosinophils and neutrophils may be present. Esophageal stricture may eventuate in those patients in whom the ulcer persists and damages the esophageal wall deep to the lamina propria. In this circumstance, reactive fibrosis can narrow the esophageal lumen.

Barrett Esophagus Is Replacement of Esophageal Squamous Epithelium by Columnar Epithelium

Barrett esophagus is a result of chronic gastroesophageal reflux. Its incidence has been increasing in recent years, particularly among white men. This disorder occurs in the lower third of the esophagus but may extend higher.

There is a slight male predominance and a more than twofold increased risk for Barrett esophagus among smokers. Patients with Barrett esophagus are placed in a regular surveillance program to detect early microscopic evidence of dysplastic mucosa.

PATHOLOGY: Metaplastic Barrett epithelium may partially involve the circumference of short segments or may line the entire lower esophagus (Fig. 13-5A). Microscopically, the sine qua non of Barrett esophagus is the presence of a distinctive type of epithelium, referred to as "specialized epithelium." It consists of an admixture of intestine-like epithelium characterized by well-formed goblet cells interspersed with gastric foveolar cells (see Fig. 13-5B). Complete intestinal metaplasia, with Paneth cells and absorptive cells, occurs occasionally. Inflammatory changes are often superimposed on the epithelial alterations. *Barrett esophagus may transform into adenocarcinoma, the risk correlating with the length of the involved esophagus and the degree of dysplasia* (see below). The dysplastic change occurs in the "specialized epithelium."

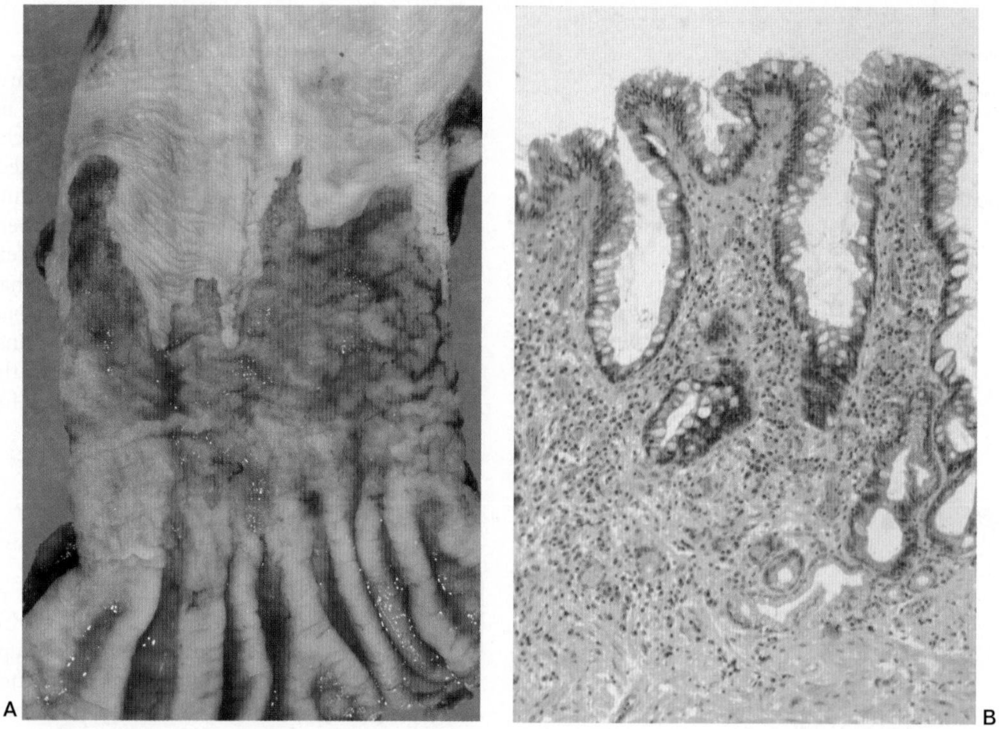

FIGURE 13-5. **Barrett esophagus A.** The presence of the tan tongues of epithelium interdigitating with the more proximal squamous epithelium is typical of Barrett esophagus. **B.** The specialized epithelium has a villiform architecture and is lined by cells that are foveolar gastric type cells and intestinal goblet type cells.

Eosinophilic Esophagitis is Distinct from Reflux Esophagitis

Eosinophilic esophagitis appears is likely allergic in etiology. Patients often complain of the sensation of food "sticking" upon swallowing and may relate the sensation to specific foodstuffs. Affected individuals are often first identified after they fail to improve on standard anti-reflux therapy. There is often a mild peripheral eosinophilia.

PATHOLOGY: The endoscopic appearance of eosinophilic esophagitis is often characteristic with the presence of transverse ridges (which can mimic the appearance of the trachea) and small white plaques. Intra-epithelial esopinophils are abundant, typically 20 or more per high power field, and tend to cluster superficially.

Infective Esophagitis Is Associated with Immunosuppression

CANDIDA ESOPHAGITIS: This fungal infection has become commonplace because of an increasing number of immunocompromised persons who (1) receive chemotherapy for malignant disease, (2) are treated with immunosuppressive drugs after organ transplantation, or (3) have contracted acquired immunodeficiency syndrome (AIDS). Esophageal candidiasis also occurs in patients with diabetes, those receiving antibiotic therapy, and uncommonly in persons with no known predisposing factors. Dysphagia and severe pain on swallowing are usual.

PATHOLOGY: In mild cases of candidiasis, a few small, elevated white plaques surrounded by a hyperemic zone are present on the mucosa of the middle or lower third of the esophagus. In severe cases, confluent pseudomembranes lie on a hyperemic and edematous mucosa. Microscopically, *Candida* sometimes involves only the superficial layers of the squamous epithelium. The candidal pseudomembrane contains fungal mycelia, necrotic debris, and fibrin. Involvement of deeper layers of the esophageal wall can lead to disseminated candidiasis or fibrosis, sometimes severe enough to create a stricture.

HERPETIC ESOPHAGITIS: Esophageal infection with herpesvirus type I is most frequently associated with lymphomas and leukemias and is often manifested by odynophagia. However, it may occur in otherwise healthy individuals on occasion.

PATHOLOGY: The well-developed lesions of herpetic esophagitis grossly resemble those of candidiasis. In early cases, vesicles, small erosions or plaques are seen; as infection progresses, these may coalesce to form larger lesions. Microscopically, lesions are superficial and epithelial cells exhibit typical nuclear herpetic inclusions and occasional multinucleation (see Fig. 9-6). Necrosis of infected cells leads to ulceration and candidal and bacterial superinfection results in the formation of pseudomembranes.

CYTOMEGALOVIRUS ESOPHAGITIS: Esophageal involvement with cytomegalovirus usually reflects systemic viral disease in patients with AIDS. Mucosal ulceration, like that in herpetic esophagitis, is common. Characteristic inclusion bodies of cytomegalovirus are present in endothelial cells and granulation tissue fibroblasts.

Chemical Esophagitis Results from Ingestion of Corrosive Agents

Chemical injury to the esophagus usually reflects accidental poisoning in children, attempted suicide in adults, or contact with medication. Ingestion of strong alkaline agents (e.g., lye) or strong acids (e.g., sulfuric or hydrochloric acid), both of which are used in various cleaning solutions, can produce chemical esophagitis. The alkaline solutions are particularly insidious, because they are generally odorless and tasteless and so easily swallowed before protective reflexes come into play.

PATHOLOGY: Microscopically, alkali-induced liquefactive necrosis is accompanied by conspicuous inflammation and saponification of membrane lipids in the epithelium, submucosa, and muscularis propria of the esophagus and stomach. Thrombosis of small vessels adds ischemic necrosis to the injury. Severe injury is the rule with liquid alkali, but less than 25% of those who ingest granular preparations have severe complications.

Strong acids produce immediate coagulation necrosis, which results in a protective eschar that limits injury and penetration. Nevertheless, half of patients who ingest concentrated hydrochloric or sulfuric acid have severe esophageal injury.

Drug-related esophagitis is most often caused by direct chemical effects on the squamous-lined mucosa, especially with capsules; esophageal dysmotility and cardiac enlargement (which impinges on the esophagus) may be contributing factors.

Esophagitis May Complicate Systemic Illnesses

Esophageal squamous mucosa resembles, and shares some reactions with, the epidermis.

The **dystrophic form of epidermolysis bullosa** involves all organs lined by, or derived from, squamous epithelium, including skin, nails, teeth, and esophagus. Bullae, which occur episodically, evolve from fluid-filled vesicles to weeping ulcers. Dysphagia and painful swallowing are the rule. Stricture, usually in the upper esophagus, may occur.

Pemphigoid produces subepithelial bullae in the skin and esophagus, but does not lead to scarring. Other dermatologic disorders associated with esophagitis include pemphigus, dermatitis herpetiformis, Behçet syndrome, and erythema multiforme.

Graft-versus-host disease in recipients of bone marrow transplants can cause esophageal lesions and dysphagia, odynophagia, and gastroesophageal reflux. The upper and middle thirds of the esophageal mucosa appear friable and esophageal motor function of the esophagus.

Esophagitis May be Iatrogenic

External irradiation for treatment of thoracic cancers may include portions of the esophagus and lead to esophagitis and even stricture. **Nasogastric tubes** may cause pressure ulcers when they are in place for prolonged periods, although acid reflux also plays a role in these cases.

Esophageal Varices

Esophageal varices are dilated veins immediately beneath the mucosa (Fig. 13-6) *that are prone to rupture and hemorrhage* (also see Chapter 14). They arise in the lower third of the esophagus, virtually always in patients with cirrhosis and portal hypertension. The lower esophageal veins are linked to the portal system through gastroesophageal anastomoses. If portal system pressure exceeds a critical level, these anastomoses become prominent in the upper stomach and lower esophagus. When varices are greater than 5 mm in diameter, they are prone to rupture, leading to life-threatening hemorrhage. Reflux injury or infective esophagitis can contribute to variceal bleeding.

A B

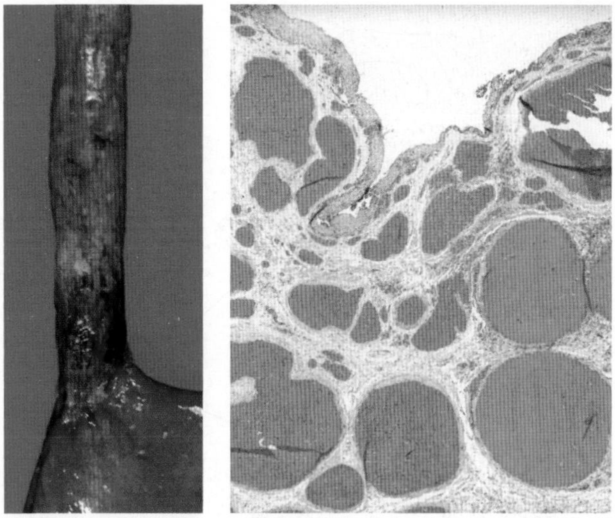

FIGURE 13-6. **Esophageal varices. A.** Numerous prominent blue venous channels are seen beneath the mucosa of the everted esophagus, particularly above the gastroesophageal junction. **B.** Section of the esophagus reveals numerous dilated submucosal veins.

Lacerations and Perforations

Lacerations of the esophagus result from external trauma, such as automobile accidents and falls from great heights as well as from medical instrumentation. However, the most common cause is severe vomiting, during which intraesophageal pressure may reach 300 mm Hg. The diaphragm descends rapidly, and a portion of the upper stomach is forced up through the hiatus. As a result, forceful retching may cause mucosal tears, beginning in the gastric epithelium and extending into the esophagus.

Mallory-Weiss syndrome *refers to severe retching, often associated with alcoholism, that leads to mucosal lacerations of upper stomach and lower esophagus.* These tears result in the vomiting of bright red blood and bleeding may be severe enough to require transfusion of many units of blood. The lacerations may also cause perforation into the mediastinum. Esophageal rupture due to vomiting is **Boerhaave syndrome.**

Esophageal perforation, whether from trauma or vomiting, can be catastrophic. It is a well-known occurrence in newborns, in whom it is caused occasionally by suctioning or feeding with a nasogastric tube. However, it may also occur spontaneously.

The major non-neoplastic disorders of the esophagus are summarized in Figure 13-7.

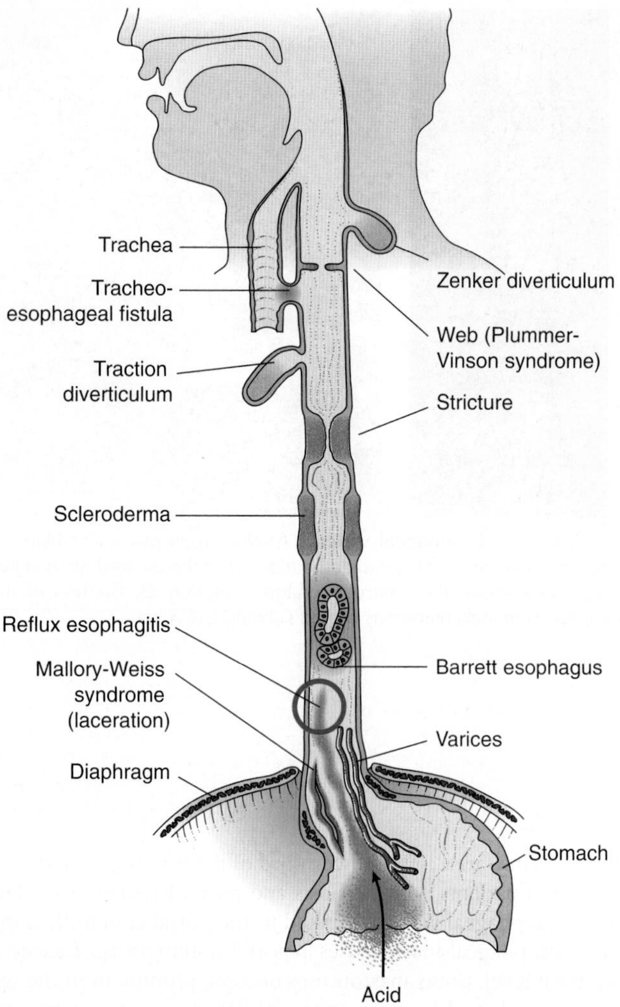

FIGURE 13-7. **Nonneoplastic disorders of the esophagus.**

Neoplasms

Benign Tumors of the Esophagus are Uncommon

Unlike the remainder of the gastrointestinal tract, most spindle cell submucosal tumors of the esophagus derive from smooth muscle (**leiomyoma**) rather than from interstitial cells of Cajal (gastrointestinal stromal tumors [GIST tumors]; see below). They are almost always benign. Squamous papilloma of the esophagus is rare.

Esophageal Carcinoma Varies Geographically and Histologically

EPIDEMIOLOGY: Worldwide, most esophageal cancers are squamous cell carcinomas but adenocarcinoma is now more common in the United States (see below). Esophageal cancer is uncommon and accounts for about 2% of cancer deaths in the United States.

Worldwide geographic variations in the incidence of esophageal carcinoma are striking, and areas of high incidence are located adjacent to areas of low incidence. There is an esophageal cancer belt extending across Asia from the Caspian Sea region of northern Iran and the former Soviet Union through Central Asia and Mongolia to northern China. In parts of China, the mortality rate from esophageal cancer in men may be 70 times that in the United States. American blacks have a much higher incidence than whites, and in the United States, urban dwellers are at greater risk than those in rural areas. Cancer of the esophagus is also common in certain regions of France, Finland, Switzerland, Chile, Japan, India, and Africa.

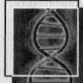

PATHOGENESIS: Geographic variations in esophageal cancer, even in relatively homogeneous populations, suggest that environmental factors contribute strongly to its development. However, no single factor has been incriminated.

- **Cigarette smoking** increases risk of esophageal cancer 5- to 10-fold. The number of cigarettes smoked correlates with the presence of esophageal dysplasia.
- **Excessive consumption of alcohol** is a major risk factor in the United States, even when cigarette smoking is taken into account.
- **Nitrosamines** and aniline dyes produce esophageal cancer in animals. Although high levels of nitrosamines and other potentially carcinogenic compounds have been found in the diets of persons living in high-incidence areas, direct evidence for their contribution to esophageal cancer is lacking. Moreover, such chemical agents have not been detected in many high-risk areas, such as northern Iran.
- **Diets low in fresh fruits, vegetables, animal protein, and trace metals** are described in areas with endemic esophageal cancer, and in some hyperendemic areas, as are deficiencies of various vitamins and minerals. However, the close proximity of endemic and nonendemic areas renders a causative role for these dietary factors unlikely.
- **Plummer-Vinson syndrome, celiac sprue, and achalasia** are associated with an increased incidence of esophageal cancer, for obscure reasons.
- **Chronic esophagitis** has been related to esophageal cancer in areas in which this tumor is endemic.
- **Chemical injury with esophageal stricture** is a risk factor. Of persons who have an esophageal stricture after ingestion of lye, 5% develop cancer 20 to 40 years later.
- **Webs, rings and diverticula** are sometimes associated with esophageal cancer.

PATHOLOGY: About half of cases of esophageal cancer involve the lower third of the esophagus; the middle and upper thirds account for the remainder. Grossly, the tumors are of three types: (1) polypoid, which projects into the lumen (Fig. 13-8B); (2) ulcerating, which is usually smaller than polypoid (Fig. 13-8A); and (3) infiltrating, in which the principal plane of growth is in the wall. The bulky polypoid tumors tend to obstruct early, whereas ulcerated ones are more likely to bleed. Infiltrating tumors gradually narrow the lumen by circumferential compression. Local extension of tumor into mediastinal structures is commonly a major problem.

Microscopically, neoplastic squamous cells range from well differentiated, with epithelial "pearls," to poorly differentiated

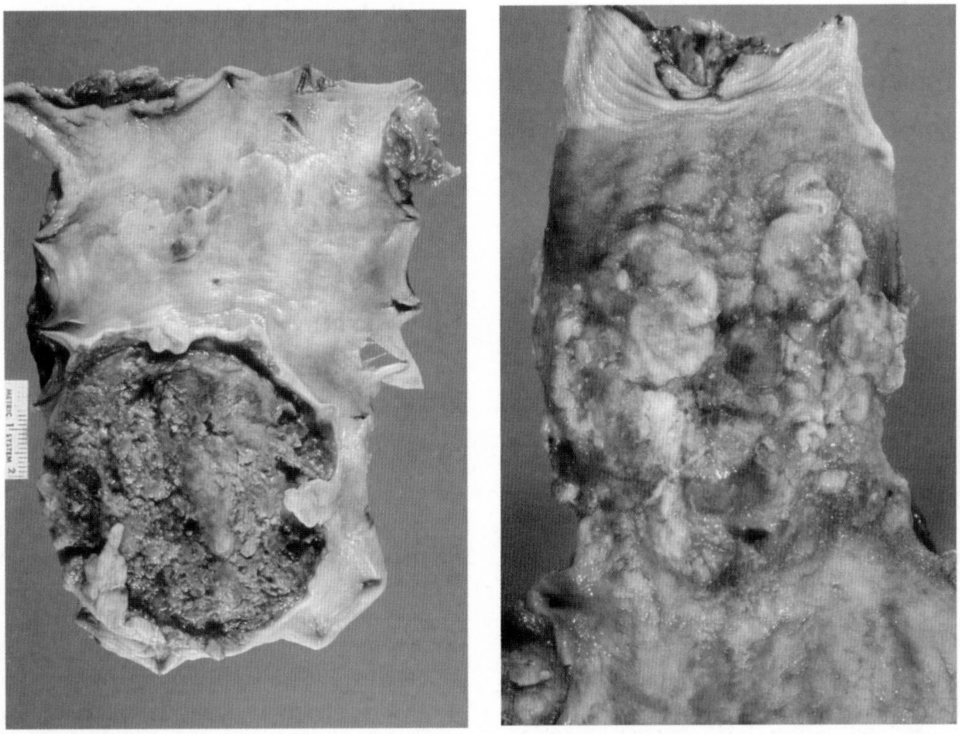

A B

FIGURE 13-8. **Esophageal carcinoma. A.** Squamous cell carcinoma. There is a large ulcerated mass present in the squamous mucosa with normal squamous mucosa intervening between the carcinoma and the stomach. **B.** Adenocarcinoma. There is a large exophytic ulcerated mass lesion just proximal to the gastroesophageal junction. The well-differentiated adenocarcinoma was separated from the most proximal squamous epithelium by a tan area representing Barrett esophagus.

tumors that lack evidence of squamous differentiation. Occasional tumors have a predominant spindle cell population of tumors cells (metaplastic carcinoma).

The rich lymphatic drainage of the esophagus provides a route for most metastases. Accordingly, tumors of the upper third metastasize to cervical, internal jugular, and supraclavicular nodes. Cancer of the middle third metastasizes to the paratracheal and hilar lymph nodes and to nodes in the aortic, cardiac, and paraesophageal regions. As the lower third of the esophagus is fed by the left gastric artery, lower esophageal tumors spread via accompanying lymphatics to retroperitoneal, celiac, and left gastric nodes. Metastases to liver and lung are common, but almost any organ may be involved.

CLINICAL FEATURES: The most common presenting complaint is dysphagia, but by this time most tumors are unresectable. Patients with esophageal cancer are almost invariably cachectic, owing to anorexia, difficulty in swallowing, and the remote effects of a malignant tumor. Odynophagia occurs in half of patients and persistent pain suggests mediastinal extension of the tumor or involvement of spinal nerves. Compression of the recurrent laryngeal nerve produces hoarseness and tracheoesophageal fistula is manifested clinically by a chronic cough. Surgery and radiation therapy are useful for palliation, but the prognosis remains dismal. Many patients are inoperable and of those who undergo surgery, only 20% survive for 5 years.

Adenocarcinoma of the Esophagus

As its incidence has recently increased, adenocarcinoma of the esophagus is now more common (60%) in the United States than squamous carcinoma. *Virtually all adenocarcinomas arise in the background of Barrett esophagus,* although a rare case originates in submucosal mucous glands. Endoscopic surveillance for adenocarcinoma is now commonly done in patients with Barrett esophagus, particularly in those with dysplasia. The symptoms and clinical course of esophageal adenocarcinoma are similar to those of squamous cell carcinoma.

THE STOMACH

Anatomy

The stomach, a J-shaped saccular organ with a volume of 1200 to 1500 mL, arises as a dilation of the primitive foregut. It is continuous with the esophagus superiorly and the duodenum inferiorly. Situated in the upper abdomen, the stomach extends from the left hypochondrium across the epigastrium. The convexity of the stomach, extending leftward from the gastroesophageal junction, is termed the **greater curvature.** The concavity of the right side of the stomach, called the **lesser curvature,** is only about one fourth as long as the greater curvature. The entire stomach is invested in peritoneum, which descends from the greater curvature as the **greater omentum.**

The stomach is divided into 5 regions, superiorly to inferiorly (Fig. 13-9):

1. The **cardia** is a small, grossly indistinct zone that extends a short distance from the gastroesophageal junction.
2. The **fundus** is the dome-shaped part of the stomach located to the left of the cardia and extends superiorly above the level of the gastroesophageal junction.

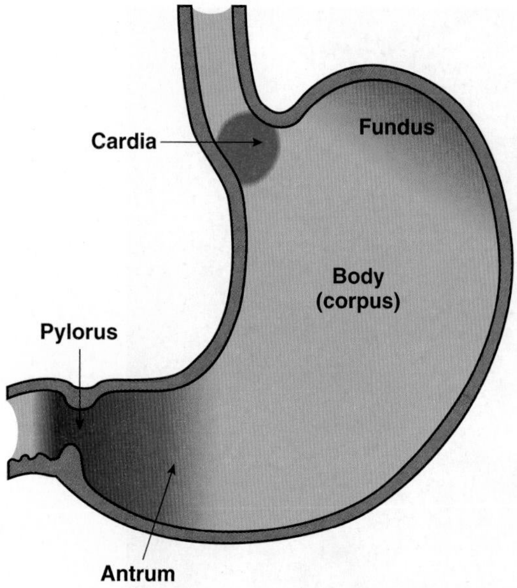

FIGURE 13-9. **Anatomical regions of the stomach.**

3. **The body, or corpus,** is two-thirds of the stomach and descends from the fundus to the most inferior region, where the organ turns right to form the bottom of the J.
4. **The antrum** is the distal third of the stomach. It is positioned horizontally and extends from the body to the pyloric sphincter.
5. **The pyloric sphincter** is the most distal tubular segment of the stomach. It is entirely surrounded by the thick muscular layer that controls passage of food into the duodenum.

The wall of the stomach is composed of a mucosa, submucosa, muscularis, and serosa. The lining of the fundus and body has prominent folds, the gastric rugae.

Branches of the celiac, hepatic, and splenic arteries supply blood to the stomach. Gastric veins drain either directly into the portal system or indirectly through splenic and superior mesenteric veins. A rich plexus of lymphatic channels empties into gastric and other regional lymph nodes. Both vagal nerves supply parasympathetic innervation to the stomach and the celiac plexus provides sympathetic innervation.

The histology of the gastric mucosa varies with the anatomic region. Surface mucus-secreting, columnar epithelium extends into numerous foveolae, or pits. These are the orifices of millions of branched, tubular glands. There are three types of glands:

- **Cardiac glands** are located in the cardia.
- **Parietal** (**oxyntic**) **glands** are found in the body and fundus of the stomach.
- **Pyloric glands** are situated in the antrum and the pyloric canal.

The gastric glands, the principal secretory elements of the stomach, are densely arranged perpendicular to the mucosa and enter the base of the foveola through a narrowed segment called the **neck of the gland.** Gastric glands contain 5 cell types:

- **Zymogen, or chief, cells:** These are primarily in the lower half of gastric glands. They are pyramidal, basophilic cells with zymogen granules that contain pepsinogen.
- **Parietal, or oxyntic, cells:** These cells occupy the upper half of the gastric gland. They are oval or pyramidal eosinophilic cells that secrete hydrochloric acid. They contain numerous mitochondria to provide energy for the ion transport needed for acid secretion. Ultrastructurally, parietal cells have many surface membrane invaginations, **secretory canaliculi,** which vastly expand the surface area for acid secretion. Parietal cells also produce intrinsic factor, which is necessary for intestinal absorption of vitamin B_{12}.
- **Mucous neck cells:** These mucus-secreting, basophilic components are interspersed among the parietal cells in the neck of the gastric gland.
- **Endocrine cells:** These cells are scattered in the gastric glands, mostly between the zymogen cells and the basement membrane. They are small, round, or pyramidal cells filled with granules. Endocrine cells are scattered among the pyloric glands and contain biogenic amines such as serotonin and polypeptide hormones (e.g., gastrin and somatostatin). The endocrine cells include gastrin-secreting cells (G cells). Vasoactive intestinal peptide (VIP) is found in neural elements of the mucosa but not within endocrine cells. These cells are best visualized by immunoperoxidase techniques, either with more generic markers such as chromogranin or synaptophysin or with antibodies directed against specific peptides, such as gastrin.
- **Pyloric glands** are branched and conspicuously coiled structures, emptying into foveolae that are substantially deeper than those elsewhere in the stomach. The glands are lined by pale cells similar in appearance to mucous neck cells and cells of Brunner glands in the duodenum. The endocrine cells include G cells.
- **Cardiac glands** are lined by cells that are similar to mucous neck cells and those of the pyloric glands but lack G cells.

Congenital Disorders

Congenital Pyloric Stenosis Causes Projectile Vomiting in Infancy

Congenital pyloric stenosis is concentric enlargement of the pyloric sphincter and narrowing of the pyloric canal that obstructs the gastric outlet. This disorder is the most common indication for abdominal surgery in the initial 6 months of life. It is four times more common in boys than in girls and affects first-born children more than subsequent ones. It occurs in 1 in 250 white infants but is rare in blacks and Asians.

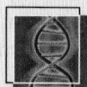

PATHOGENESIS: Congenital pyloric stenosis may have a genetic basis; there is a familial tendency, and the condition is more common in identical twins than in fraternal ones. It also has been seen together with other developmental abnormalities, such as Turner syndrome, trisomy 18, and esophageal atresia. Embryopathies associated with rubella infection and maternal intake of thalidomide have also been associated with congenital pyloric stenosis. In some cases, congenital pyloric stenosis is associated with a deficiency of nitric oxide synthase in the nerves of pyloric smooth muscle (nitric oxide mediates relaxation of smooth muscle).

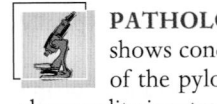

PATHOLOGY: Gross examination of the stomach shows concentric pyloric enlargement, and narrowing of the pyloric canal. The only consistent microscopic abnormality is extreme hypertrophy of the circular muscle coat. After pyloromyotomy, the lesion disappears, although occasionally a small mass remains.

CLINICAL FEATURES: Projectile vomiting is the main symptom and is usually seen within the first month of life. Consequent loss of hydrochloric acid leads to hypochloremic alkalosis in one third of infants. A palpable pyloric lesion and visible peristalsis are common. Surgical incision of hypertrophied pyloric muscle is curative.

Congenital Diaphragmatic Hernia

Congenital diaphragmatic hernias of variable size and location are associated with defective closure of embryological foramina or abnormalities of the esophageal hiatus. These hernias are often associated with congenital malrotations of the intestine. The stomach, together with other abdominal organs, may eventrate into the thoracic cavity.

Congenital Abnormalities Are Rare

DUPLICATIONS, DIVERTICULA, AND CYSTS: These lesions are usually lined by normal gastric mucosa and are distinctly uncommon. Whereas all layers of the stomach wall tend to be present in congenital duplications, muscle coats are often deficient in diverticula and cysts. Patients with these disorders are generally asymptomatic.

SITUS INVERSUS: This causes the stomach to be located to the right of the midline, as is the esophageal hiatus. Correspondingly, the duodenum is on the left.

ECTOPIC PANCREATIC TISSUE: Nodules of pancreatic tissue are common in the wall of the antrum and pylorus. Histologically, these embryonic rests are identical to normal pancreatic tissue, except that islets are rare. Heterotopic pancreatic tissue is usually asymptomatic, but pyloric obstruction and epigastric pain have been reported.

PARTIAL GASTRIC ATRESIAS: Lack of development of the body, antrum, and pylorus have been described, as have cases in which the stomach ends blindly.

CONGENITAL PYLORIC AND ANTRAL MEMBRANES: These lesions are presumably caused by failure of the stomach to canalize during embryogenesis. They may cause symptoms of obstruction in the neonatal period but more commonly become symptomatic in adults.

Gastritis

Acute Hemorrhagic Gastritis Is Associated with Drugs and Stress

Acute hemorrhagic erosive gastritis is characterized by mucosal necrosis. Erosion of the mucosa may extend into the deeper tissues to form an ulcer. The necrosis is accompanied by an acute inflammatory response and hemorrhage, which may be severe enough to result in exsanguination.

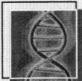

PATHOGENESIS: Acute hemorrhagic gastritis is most commonly associated with the intake of aspirin, other nonsteroidal anti-inflammatory agents, or excess alcohol, or with ischemic injury. These agents injure the gastric mucosa directly and exert their effects topically. Oral administration of corticosteroids also may be complicated by acute hemorrhagic gastritis. Uncommonly, accidental or suicidal ingestion of corrosive substances, such as those that produce erosive esophagitis, causes acute gastric injury. Any serious illness that is accompanied by profound physiologic alterations that require substantial medical or surgical intervention renders the gastric mucosa more vulnerable to acute hemorrhagic gastritis because of mucosal ischemia. The factor common to all forms of acute hemorrhagic gastritis is thought to be the breakdown of the mucosal barrier, permitting acid-induced injury.

Stress ulcers and erosions are occur in severely burned persons (**Curling ulcer**) and commonly result in bleeding. Ulceration may be deep enough to cause perforation of the stomach. Patients occasionally exhibit both gastric and duodenal ulcers.

Central nervous system trauma, accidental or surgical (**Cushing ulcer**), may also cause stress ulcers. These ulcers, which also may occur in the esophagus or duodenum, are characteristically deep and carry a substantial risk of perforation. Injury to the brain, particularly if it results in a decerebrate state, often leads to increased acid secretion in the stomach, presumably as a result of increased vagal tone. **Severe trauma,** especially if accompanied by **shock, prolonged sepsis, and incapacitation** from many debilitating chronic diseases also predisposes to development of acute hemorrhagic gastritis.

Hypersecretion of gastric acid has been incriminated in the pathogenesis of acute hemorrhagic gastritis, but its role is not clear. Acid secretion is often increased in some circumstances, such as neurologic trauma, but the development of stress ulcers is not generally accompanied by any such increase. Nevertheless, gastric acid plays a permissive role, because inhibition of gastric acid secretion (e.g., with histamine-receptor antagonists) protects against the development of stress ulcers.

Microcirculatory changes in the stomach induced by shock or sepsis suggest that ischemic injury may contribute to the development of acute hemorrhagic gastritis.

Each of these defensive factors of the gastric mucosa has been individually investigated:

- **Corticosteroids and aspirin** lead to decreased mucus production and gastric ulcers after experimental administration.
- **Prostaglandin deficiency,** caused by nonsteroidal anti-inflammatory agents that inhibit prostaglandin synthesis, has been postulated to decrease mucosal resistance to gastric contents. By contrast, certain prostaglandins that stimulate mucus secretion also protect against gastric erosions.
- **Renewal of gastric epithelial cells** is clearly necessary for healing erosions of any etiology.
- **Decreased intramural pH of the gastric mucosa** has been shown to protect from gastric erosions in hemorrhagic shock. Thus, acid-induced damage to the gastric mucosa is important in the pathogenesis of certain erosions.

PATHOLOGY: Acute hemorrhagic gastritis is characterized grossly by widespread petechial hemorrhages in any portion of the stomach or regions of confluent mucosal or submucosal bleeding (Fig. 13-10). Lesions vary from 1 to 25 mm across and appear occasionally as sharply punched-out ulcers. Microscopically, patchy mucosal necrosis, which can extend to the submucosa, is visualized adjacent to normal mucosa. Fibrinous exudate, edema and hemorrhage in the lamina propria are present in early lesions. Necrotic epithelium is eventually sloughed, but deeper erosions and hemorrhage may be present. In extreme cases, penetrating ulcers may reach the serosa.

CLINICAL FEATURES: Symptoms of acute hemorrhagic gastritis range from vague abdominal discomfort to massive, life-threatening hemorrhage, or clinical manifestations of gastric perforation. Patients with gastritis induced by aspirin and other nonsteroidal anti-inflammatory agents may be seen with hypochromic, microcytic anemia caused by undetected chronic bleeding. However, in patients with a severe underlying illness, the first sign of stress ulcers may be exsanguinating hemorrhage. Treatment with antacids and histamine-receptor antagonists has proved useful.

Chronic Gastritis is Autoimmune or Environmental

Chronic gastritis refers to chronic inflammatory diseases of stomach, which range from mild superficial involvement of gastric mucosa to severe atrophy. This is a heterogeneous group of disorders with distinct anatomical distributions within the stomach, varying etiologies, and characteristic complications. The predominant symptom is dyspepsia. The diseases are also commonly discovered in asymptomatic persons undergoing routine endoscopic screening.

Autoimmune Atrophic Gastritis and Pernicious Anemia

Autoimmune atrophic gastritis is a chronic, diffuse inflammatory disease of the stomach that is restricted to the body and fundus and is associated with autoimmune phenomena. This disorder typically exhibits:

- Diffuse atrophic gastritis in the body and fundus of the stomach, with lack of, or minimal involvement of, the antrum
- Antibodies to parietal cells and intrinsic factor
- Significant reduction in or absence of gastric secretion, including acid
- Increased serum gastrin, owing to G-cell hyperplasia of the antral mucosa
- Enterochromaffin-like (ECL) cell hyperplasia in atrophic oxyntic mucosa, secondary to gastrin stimulation

Pernicious anemia *is a megaloblastic anemia caused by malabsorption of vitamin B_{12}, due to a deficiency of intrinsic factor. In most cases, pernicious anemia is a complication of autoimmune gastritis.* The latter disorder is also associated with extragastric autoimmune diseases such as chronic thyroiditis, Graves disease, Addison disease, vitiligo, diabetes mellitus type I, and myasthenia gravis.

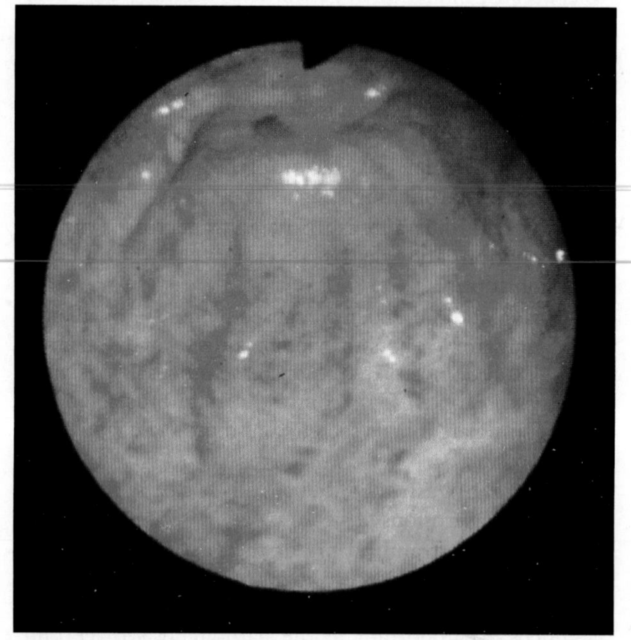

FIGURE 13-10. **Erosive gastritis.** This endoscopic view of the stomach in a patient who was ingesting aspirin reveals acute hemorrhagic lesions.

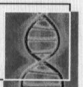

PATHOGENESIS: Autoimmune gastritis is so named because of the presence of autoantibodies and the association with other diseases that have a similar pathogenesis.

CYTOTOXIC ANTIBODIES: Circulating antibodies to parietal cells, some of which are cytotoxic in the presence of complement, occur in 90% of patients with pernicious anemia. Parietal cell autoantibodies react with α and β subunits of the proton pump (H^+/K^+ ATPase). This enzyme is the major protein of the secretory canaliculi of parietal cells and mediates secretion of H^+ in exchange for K^+. Importantly, some 20% of persons over 60 years have parietal cell antibodies, but few have pernicious anemia.

INTRINSIC FACTOR ANTIBODIES: In addition to the postulated immunologicl destruction of parietal cells, two types of autoantibodies to intrinsic factor are common in pernicious anemia. Two thirds of patients have an antibody to intrinsic factor that impedes its binding to vitamin B_{12}, preventing formation of the complex that is absorbed in the ileum. About half of patients with this antibody also have an antibody against the intrinsic factor–vitamin B_{12} complex that interferes with its absorption.

OTHER ANTIBODIES: Half of patients with pernicious anemia have circulating antibodies to thyroid tissue. Conversely, about one third of patients with chronic thyroiditis possess gastric autoantibodies.

Multifocal Atrophic Gastritis (Environmental Metaplastic Atrophic Gastritis)

Multifocal atrophic gastritis is a disease of uncertain etiology that typically involves the antrum and adjacent areas of the body. This form of chronic gastritis has these features:

- It is considerably more common than the autoimmune variety of atrophic gastritis and is four times as frequent among whites as in other races.
- It is not linked to autoimmune phenomena.

- Like autoimmune gastritis, it is often associated with reduced acid secretion (hypochlorhydria).
- Complete absence of gastric secretion (achlorhydria) and pernicious anemia are uncommon.

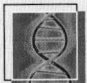

EPIDEMIOLOGY AND PATHOGENESIS: The age and geographic distribution of environmental metaplastic atrophic gastritis parallel those of gastric carcinoma, and this type of gastritis seems to be a precursor of this cancer. The disease exhibits a striking localization to certain populations, being particularly common in Asia, Scandinavia, and parts of Europe and Latin America. It also increases in incidence with age in all populations in which it is prevalent. Offspring of emigrants from areas of high risk for stomach cancer to those of low risk lose their predisposition to this tumor. Environmental etiologic factors include *Helicobacter pylori* (see below) and diet.

PATHOLOGY: The pathologic features of autoimmune and multifocal atrophic gastritis are similar, except for the localization of the autoimmune type to the fundus and body and the multifocal variety mainly to the antrum.

ATROPHIC GASTRITIS: This condition is characterized by prominent chronic inflammation in the lamina propria. Occasionally, lymphoid cells are arranged as follicles, an appearance that has led to an erroneous diagnosis of lymphoma, especially in patients with *H. pylori* infection (see below). Involvement of gastric glands leads to degenerative changes in their epithelial cells and ultimately to a conspicuous reduction in the number of glands (thus the name **atrophic gastritis**; Fig. 13-11). Eventually, inflammation may abate, leaving only a thin atrophic mucosa, in which case the term **gastric atrophy** is applied.

INTESTINAL METAPLASIA: This lesion is a common and important histopathologic feature of both autoimmune and multifocal types of atrophic gastritis. In response to injury of the gastric mucosa, the normal epithelium is replaced by one composed of cells of the intestinal type (see Fig. 13-11C). Numerous mucin-containing goblet cells and enterocytes line cryptlike glands. Paneth cells, which are not normal inhabitants of the gastric mu-

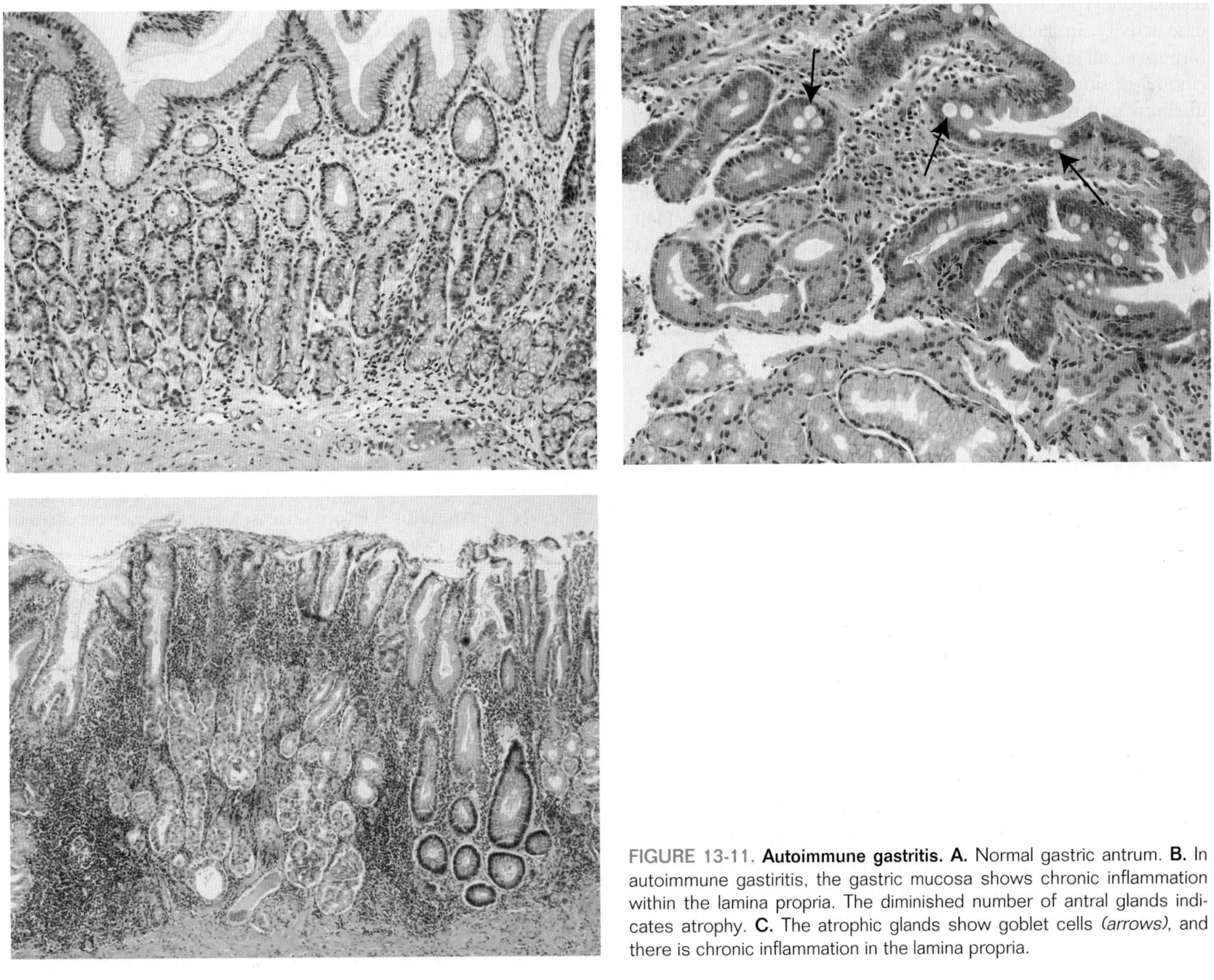

FIGURE 13-11. **Autoimmune gastritis. A.** Normal gastric antrum. **B.** In autoimmune gastiritis, the gastric mucosa shows chronic inflammation within the lamina propria. The diminished number of antral glands indicates atrophy. **C.** The atrophic glands show goblet cells *(arrows)*, and there is chronic inflammation in the lamina propria.

cosa, are present. Intestinal-type villi may occasionally form. The metaplastic cells also contain enzymes characteristic of the intestine but not of the stomach (e.g., alkaline phosphatase, aminopeptidase).

In the fundus of the stomach with autoimmune atrophic gastritis, the normal parietal and zymogen cells may be replaced by clear mucous glands similar to those of the cardia or antrum, a change termed **pseudopyloric metaplasia.** Therefore, the pathologist must know the precise location from which a biopsy specimen was taken, because fundal pseudopyloric metaplasia may be mistaken for gastritis of the antrum.

Atrophic Gastritis and Stomach Cancer

Persons with autoimmune or multifocal atrophic gastritis have greater risk of carcinoma of the stomach. Atrophic gastritis is usually asymptomatic and so does not ordinarily come under medical scrutiny so this relationship is hard to quantify. However, patients with pernicious anemia, who invariably have atrophic gastritis, have a 3-fold greater risk for gastric adenocarcinoma and 13-fold higher risk of carcinoid (neuroendocrine) tumors.

Cancer arises in the antrum several times more frequently than in the body of the stomach, suggesting that antral gastritis is related to gastric carcinogenesis.

Intestinal metaplasia of the stomach has been identified as a preneoplastic lesion for several reasons: (1) gastric cancer arises in areas of metaplastic epithelium, (2) half of all stomach cancers are of the intestinal cell type, and (3) many gastric cancers show aminopeptidase activity similar to that seen in areas of intestinal metaplasia. Moreover, all grades of dysplasia, from low-grade dysplasia to carcinoma in situ, have been observed in metaplastic intestinal epithelium and are felt to be precursors of invasive gastric cancer.

Helicobacter pylori Gastritis

H. pylori *gastritis is a chronic inflammatory disease of the antrum and body of the stomach caused by* H. pylori *and occasionally by* Helicobacter heilmannii. It is the most common type of chronic gastritis in the United States. The organism causes one of the most frequent chronic infections. *H. pylori* infection is also strongly associated with peptic ulcer disease of the stomach and duodenum (see below).

PATHOGENESIS: *Helicobacter* species are small, curved, gram-negative rods (Proteobacteria) with polar flagella and display a corkscrew-like motion. *H. pylori* has been isolated from diverse populations throughout the world. The prevalence of infection with this organism increases with age: by age 60 years, half the population has serologic evidence of infection. Twin studies have shown genetic influences in susceptibility to infection with *H. pylori*. Intrafamilial clustering of *H. pylori* infection suggests that these bacteria may spread from person to person. Two thirds of those who have been infected with *H. pylori* show histologic evidence of chronic gastritis.

H. pylori is considered to be the pathogen responsible for chronic antral gastritis rather than as a commensal that colonizes injured gastric mucosa because: (1) gastritis develops in healthy persons after ingesting the organism, (2) *H. pylori* attaches to the epithelium in areas of chronic gastritis and is absent from uninvolved areas of the gastric mucosa, (3) eradicating the infection with bismuth or antibiotics cures the gastritis, (4) antibodies against *H. pylori* are routinely found in persons with chronic gastritis, and (5) the increasing prevalence of *H. pylori* infection with age parallels that of chronic gastritis.

H. pylori is found only on the epithelial surface and does not invade. Its pathogenicity is related to the *cag* pathogenicity island in its genome—a horizontally acquired locus of 40 kb that contains 31 genes. This virulence marker is putatively associated with duodenal ulcer and gastric cancer. A separate region of the genome contains the gene for vacuolating cytotoxin *(vac A),* which is also associated with duodenal ulcer disease. Chronic infection with *H. pylori* also predisposes to the development of mucosa-associated lymphoid tissue (MALT) lymphoma of the stomach.

PATHOLOGY: The curved rods of *H. pylori* are found in the surface mucus of epithelial cells and in gastric foveolae (Fig. 13-12). The uncommon bacterium *H. heilmannii* is long and has tight spirals, an appearance similar to that of spirochetes. Active gastritis features polymorphonuclear leukocytes in glands and their lumina and increased numbers of plasma cells and lymphocytes in the lamina propria (see Fig. 13-12A). Lymphoid hyperplasia with germinal centers is frequent.

Reactive (Chemical) Gastropathy

Reactive (chemical) gastropathy is being recognized with increasing frequency. It was first recognized in patients with bile reflux, but is currently most commonly seen in association with chronic nonsteroidal anti-inflammatory drug (NSAID) use. Reflux of bile is commonly occurs after a gastroduodenostomy or gastrojejunostomy, but can be seen in intact stomachs.

PATHOLOGY: The normal flat mucosal surface is replaced by villiform projections in which the lamina propria shows fibromuscular proliferation. Surface foveolar cells show prominent reactive nuclear atypia out of proportion to the sparse inflammatory infiltrate. Unlike *H. pylori* gastritis, inflammatory infiltrates are minimal.

Granulomatous Gastritis

Granulomatous gastritis may be secondary to infection (e.g., *Mycobacterium tuberculosis;* fungus) or as a manifestation of systemic illness (e.g., sarcoidosis, Crohn disease). However, most cases of granulomatous gastritis are idiopathic.

Miscellaneous Forms of Chronic Gastritis

Eosinophilic gastritis, *often in association with eosinophilic enteritis, is disease in which eosinophils involve all layers of the stomach wall or are selectively localized in a single layer.* In classic cases, the antrum and pylorus are mainly affected: diffuse thickening of the wall, presumably by muscular hypertrophy, may narrow the pylorus and cause symptoms of obstruction. These are occasionally severe enough to require surgical relief. In some cases, ulceration in an affected area leads to chronic blood loss and anemia. Peripheral eosinophilia and a history of food allergies are common, but many patients have neither. Corticosteroid therapy is often effective.

Lymphocytic gastritis is characterized by prominent intraepithelial lymphocytes (>20 per 100 epithelial nuclei). It can

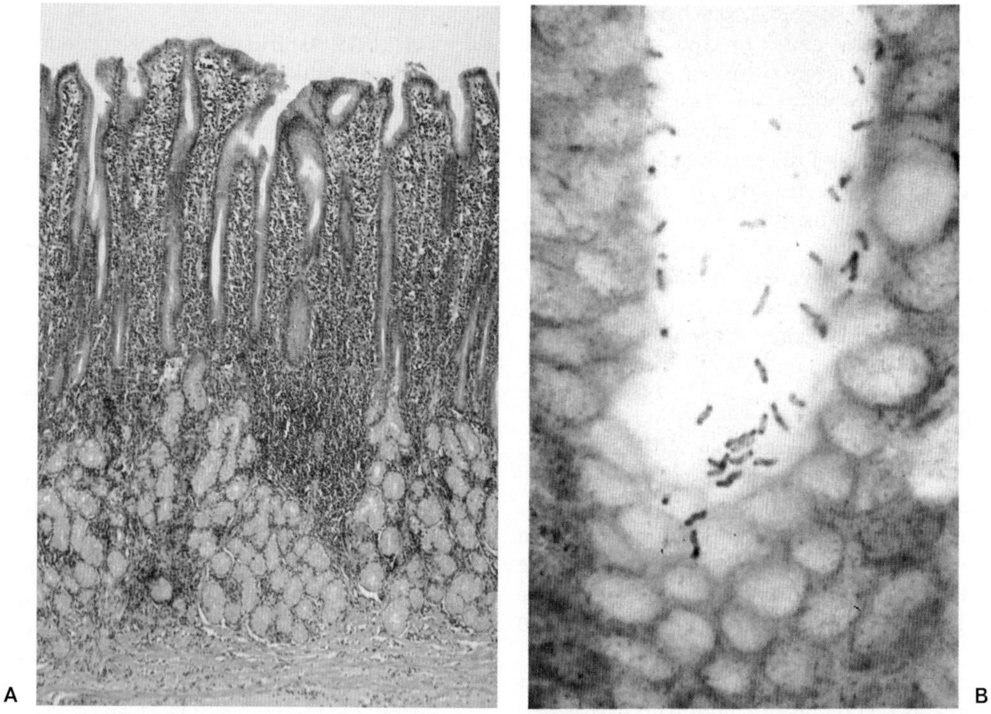

FIGURE 13-12. ***Helicobacter pylori*-associated gastritis. A.** The antrum shows an intense lymphocytic and plasma cell infiltrate which tends to be heaviest in the superficial portions of the lamina propria. **B.** The microorganisms appear on silver staining as small, curved rods on the surface of the gastric mucosa.

be associated with celiac disease, although in most cases the etiology is unknown. Some cases may be related to prior *H. pylori* infection.

Vascular gastropathies include gastric antral vascular ectasia (GAVE) and portal hypertensive gastropathy (see Chapter 14). GAVE is characterized by prominent lamina propria vessels with focal thrombosis. It has a characteristic endoscopic appearance termed "watermelon stomach". GAVE mostly occurs in elderly patients, and may be associated with significant blood loss.

Ménétrier Disease Causes Protein Loss

Ménétrier disease (hyperplastic hypersecretory gastropathy) is an uncommon gastric disorder characterized by enlarged rugae. It is often accompanied by a severe loss of plasma proteins (including albumin) from the altered gastric mucosa. A childhood form is due to cytomegalovirus infection; an adult form is attributed to overexpression of transforming growth factor-α (TGF-α).

PATHOLOGY: The stomach is enlarged. The folds of the greater curvature in the fundus and body of the stomach, and occasionally in the antrum, are increased in height and thickness, forming a convoluted brainlike surface (Fig. 13-13). Microscopically, Ménétrierdisease is restricted to the oxyntic mucosa. Hyperplasia of the gastric pits results in a conspicuous increase in their depth and a tortuous (corkscrew) structure. Mucus-secreting cells of the surface or neck type line the foveolae. The glands are elongated, and many appear cystic. These dilated glands, which are lined by superficial-type, mucus-secreting epithelial cells rather than parietal and chief cells, may penetrate the muscularis mucosae, and in so doing resemble the sinuses of Rokitansky-Aschoff in the gallbladder. Pseudopyloric metaplasia may be seen, but intestinal metaplasia does not occur. Lymphocytes, plasma cells, and occasional neutrophils are seen in the lamina propria. Concurrent lymphocytic gastritis is often present.

CLINICAL FEATURES: Ménétrier disease is four times more common in men than women and affects persons of all ages. The presenting symptom is usually postprandial pain, relieved by antacids. Weight loss, sometimes of rapid onset, occasionally occurs. Peripheral edema is com-

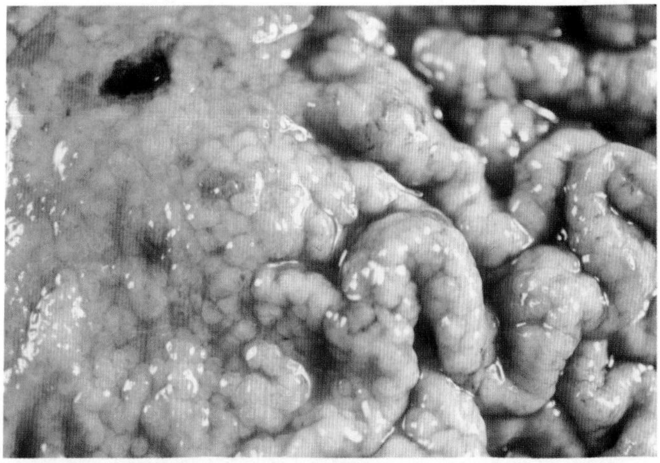

FIGURE 13-13. **Ménétrier disease.** The folds of the stomach are increased in height and thickness, forming a convoluted surface that has been likened to those of the cerebrum.

mon. In some cases, ascites and cachexia, which are related to a loss of plasma proteins from the gastric mucosa, may suggest a malignancy. The cause of the enormous protein loss into the lumen of the stomach is obscure, but treatment with anticholinergic agents or an inhibitor of acid secretion may be successful. Although gastric acidity is usually low, severe peptic ulceration associated with hyperacidity has occasionally been observed.

Ménétrier disease does not usually resolve spontaneously in adults, and in intractable cases, partial gastrectomy is necessary. *The disorder is considered a precancerous condition, and periodic endoscopic surveillance is recommended.* Cytomegalovirus-associated Ménétrier disease in children is often self-limited.

Peptic Ulcer Disease

"Peptic ulcer disease" refers to focal destruction of gastric mucosa and small intestine, principally the proximal duodenum, caused by the action of gastric secretions. About 10% of the population of Western industrialized countries may develop such ulcers at some time during their lives. However, both the incidence and prevalence of duodenal ulcers have declined substantially during the past 30 years.

Although peptic ulceration can occur as high as Barrett esophagus and as low as Meckel diverticulum with gastric heterotopia, *for practical purposes, peptic ulcer disease affects the distal stomach and proximal duodenum.* Many clinical and epidemiologic features distinguish gastric from duodenal ulcers; *the common factor that unites them is the gastric secretion of hydrochloric acid.*

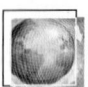

EPIDEMIOLOGY: The peak age for peptic ulcer disease has progressively increased in the past 50 years, and for duodenal ulcer disease it is now between 30 and 60 years of age, although the disorder may occur in persons of any age and even in infants. Gastric ulcers afflict the middle-aged and elderly more than the young. For duodenal ulcers there is a male predominance. By contrast, the incidence of gastric ulcers is similar in men and women.

Racial differences in the incidence of peptic ulcers have been noted, but studies of different ethnic populations are confounded by variations in many other environmental factors. For example, in Africa, duodenal ulcers are rare among blacks, whereas in the United States, the incidence is the same in blacks and whites. The preponderance of evidence suggests that in an urban Western setting, all ethnic groups are susceptible.

Surveys in the United States and Great Britain suggest a trend towards an inverse relation between duodenal ulcers and socioeconomic status and education.

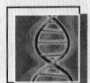

PATHOGENESIS: Numerous etiologic factors have been implicated in the pathogenesis of peptic ulcers, but no single agent seems to be responsible.

Environmental Factors

DIET: Despite the folk wisdom that spicy food and caffeine are ulcerogenic, little evidence actually supports the contention that any food or beverage, including coffee and alcohol, contributes to the development or persistence of peptic ulcers. However, cirrhosis from any cause is associated with increased incidence of peptic ulcers.

DRUGS: **Aspirin** is an important contributing factor for duodenal, and especially gastric, ulcers. **Other nonsteroidal anti-inflammatory agents and analgesics** have been incriminated in production of peptic ulcers. Prolonged treatment with high doses of corticosteroids may also increase the risk of peptic ulceration slightly.

CIGARETTE SMOKING: Smoking is a definite risk factor for duodenal and gastric ulcers, particularly gastric ulcers.

Genetic Factors

First-degree relatives of people with duodenal or gastric ulcers have a threefold increased risk of developing an ulcer, but only at the same site. These data are confirmed by a considerably higher concordance for these ulcers in monozygotic than in dizygotic twins. Identical twins show only a 50% concordance indicating that environmental factors must also be involved.

Blood-group antigens provide further evidence for the role of genetic factors. The risk of duodenal ulcer is 30% higher in persons with type O blood than in those with other types. Interestingly, patients with gastric ulcers do not exhibit a greater frequency of blood group O. People who do not secrete blood-group antigens in saliva or gastric juice carry a 50% increased risk for duodenal ulcers. Those who are both blood group O and nonsecretors (10% of white people) have a 2.5-fold increase in duodenal ulcers.

Pepsinogen I is secreted by gastric chief and mucous neck cells, and appears in gastric juice, blood, and urine. Serum levels of this proenzyme correlate with the capacity for gastric acid secretion and are considered a measure of parietal cell mass. *A person with a high circulating level of pepsinogen I has 5 times the normal risk of developing a duodenal ulcer.* Hyperpepsinogenemia I occurs in half of children of ulcer patients with hyperpepsinogenemia and has been attributed to autosomal dominant inheritance. Thus, hyperpepsinogenemia may reflect an inherited tendency to increased parietal cell mass.

Familial tendencies for other features are reported in ulcer patients. Many patients with peptic ulcer have normal pepsinogen I secretion and familial aggregation has also been shown among such persons. Familial clustering of duodenal ulcers and rapid gastric emptying have been noted, and familial hyperfunction of antral G cells is also reported. Patients with a childhood duodenal ulcer are much more likely to have a family history of ulcers than persons in whom the disease begins when they are adults.

Hydrochloric acid secretion is necessary for *formation and persistence of peptic ulcers in the stomach and duodenum.* This is evidenced principally by: (1) all patients with duodenal ulcers and almost all with gastric ulcers are gastric acid secretors; (2) experimental ulcer production in animals requires acid; (3) hypersecretion of acid is present in many, but not all, patients with duodenal ulcers (there is no evidence that acid overproduction alone is explains duodenal ulceration); and (4) surgical or medical treatment that reduces acid production results in the healing of peptic ulcers. Gastric secretion of pepsin, which may also play a role in peptic ulceration, parallels that of hydrochloric acid.

Physiologic Factors in Duodenal Ulcers

The maximal capacity for gastric acid production reflects total parietal cell mass. Patients with duodenal ulcers may have up to double normal parietal cell mass and maximal acid secretion. *However, there is a large overlap with normal values, and only one third of these patients secrete excess acid.* Increased chief cell mass often accompanies increased parietal cells, a situation that is consistent with the increased prevalence of hyperpepsinogenemia in patients with ulcers.

Gastric secretion of acid stimulated by food is increased in magnitude and duration in those with duodenal ulcers, although here, too, there is significant overlap with normal values. In a few patients this may involve, at least in part, altered G cell responses to meals. Such persons exhibit postprandial hypergastrinemia and increased numbers of antral G cells. Most patients with duodenal ulcers, however, show no evidence of G-cell hyperfunction.

Acid secretion in people with duodenal ulcers may also be more sensitive than normal to gastric secretagogues such as gastrin, possibly as due to increased vagal tone or increased affinity of parietal cells for gastrin. It is further possible that brisk secretion of acid after a meal is stimulated by increased vagal tone.

Accelerated gastric emptying has been noted in patients with duodenal ulcers. This condition might lead to excessive acidification of the duodenum. However, as with other factors, there is overlap with normal rates. Normally, duodenal bulb acidification inhibits further gastric emptying. In most patients with duodenal ulcer, this inhibitory mechanism is absent: duodenal acidification leads to continued, rather than delayed, gastric emptying. Rapid gastric emptying may in some cases be an inherited trait.

The pH of the duodenal bulb reflects the balance between delivery of gastric juice and its neutralization by biliary, pancreatic, and duodenal secretions. Duodenal ulceration requires an acidic pH in the bulb, that is, an excess of acid over-neutralizing secretions. In ulcer patients, duodenal pH after a meal decreases to a lower level and remains depressed for a longer time than in normal persons. Such duodenal hyperacidity certainly reflects the gastric factors discussed above. The role of neutralizing factors, particularly secretin-stimulated bicarbonate secretion by the pancreas and production of bicarbonate by the duodenal mucosa, is uncertain.

Impaired mucosal defenses have been invoked as contributing to peptic ulceration. These mucosal factors, including prostaglandin function, may or may not be similar to those protecting the gastric mucosa (see above).

Physiologic Factors in Gastric Ulcers

Gastric ulcers almost invariably arise in the setting of epithelial injury by H. pylori *or chemical gastritis.* The mechanisms by which chronic gastritis predisposes to gastric ulceration are obscure. *Most patients with gastric ulcers secrete less acid than do those with duodenal ulcers and even less than normal persons.* Factors implicated include (1) back-diffusion of acid into the mucosa, (2) decreased parietal cell mass, and (3) abnormalities of the parietal cells themselves. A minority of patients with gastric ulcers show acid hypersecretion. The ulcers in these persons are usually near the pylorus, and are considered variants of duodenal ulcers. Interestingly, the intense gastric hypersecretion that occurs in the Zollinger-Ellison syndrome is associated with severe ulceration of the duodenum and even the jejunum but rarely of the stomach.

The concurrence of gastric ulcers and gastric hyposecretion implies: (1) the gastric mucosa may in some way be particularly sensitive to low concentrations of acid; (2) something other than acid may damage the mucosa, e.g., NSAIDs; or (3) the gastric mucosa may be exposed to potentially injurious agents for unusually long periods. As discussed above, the mucosal barrier to the action of acid and perhaps to other contents of the stomach, may be impaired in some patients with gastric ulcers, although the evidence is far from conclusive. Bile reflux (particularly deoxycholic acid and lysolecithin) and pancreatic secretions have been suggested as causes of gastric ulcers.

The Role of *Helicobacter pylori*

H. pylori *is isolated from the gastric antrum of virtually all patients with duodenal ulcers.* The converse is not true; that is, only a small minority of persons infected with this bacterium have duodenal ulcer disease. Thus, *H. pylori* infection may be a necessary, but not sufficient, condition for development of peptic ulcers in the duodenum.

Just how *H. pylori* infection predisposes to duodenal ulcers are not completely known, but several mechanisms have been proposed. Cytokines produced by inflammatory cells that respond to *H. pylori* infection stimulate gastrin release and suppress somatostatin secretion. Interleukin (IL)-1β, an acid inhibitor, has also emerged as an important mediator of inflammation in *H. pylori*-infected gastric mucosa. These effects, together with release of histamine metabolites from the organism itself, may stimulate basal gastric acid secretion. In addition, luminal cytokines from the stomach may enter and injure duodenal epithelium. There is some evidence that *H. pylori* infection blocks inhibitory signals from the antrum to both the G cells and the parietal cell region, resulting in increased gastrin release and impaired inhibition of gastric acid secretion. Such an effect might lead to increased acid load in the duodenum, thereby contributing to duodenal ulceration. Acidification of the duodenal bulb leads to islands of metaplastic gastric mucosa in the duodenum in many patients with a peptic ulcer. This gastric epithelium in the duodenum is sometimes colonized with *H. pylori*, like the gastric mucosa. It has been postulated that infection of the metaplastic epithelium by *H. pylori* renders the mucosa more susceptible to peptic injury (Fig. 13-14).

Infection with H. pylori *is probably also important in the pathogenesis of gastric ulcers,* because this organism is responsible for most cases of the chronic gastritis that underlies this disease. About 75% of patients with gastric ulcers harbor *H. pylori*. The remaining 25% of cases may represent an association with other types of chronic gastritis. The various gastric and duodenal factors that have been implicated as possible mechanisms in the pathogenesis of duodenal ulcers are summarized in Figure 13-15.

Diseases Associated with Peptic Ulcers

CIRRHOSIS: The incidence of duodenal ulcers in patients with cirrhosis is 10 times that in normal persons.

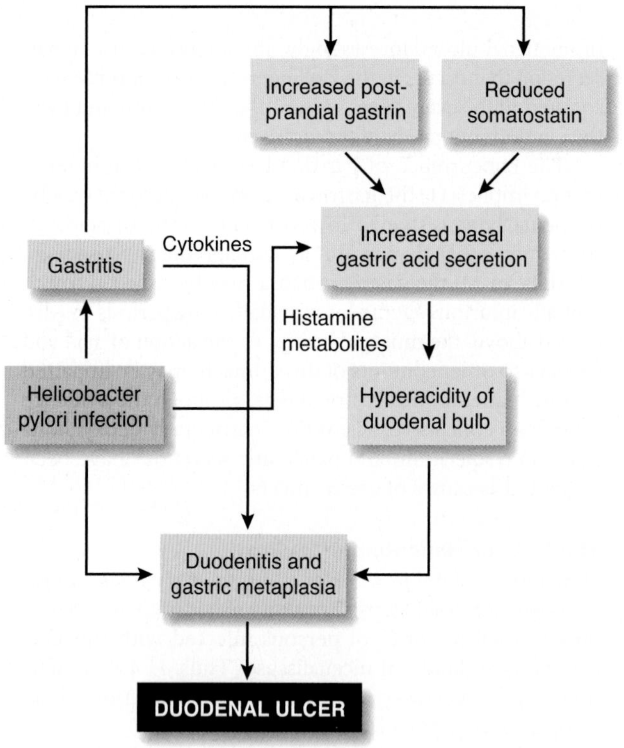

FIGURE 13-14. **Possible mechanisms in the pathogenesis of duodenal ulcer disease associated with *Helicobacter pylori* infection.**

CHRONIC RENAL FAILURE: End-stage renal disease with hemodialysis increases the risk of peptic ulceration. Patients subjected to renal transplantation also show a substantially increased incidence of peptic ulceration and its complications, such as bleeding and perforation.

HEREDITARY ENDOCRINE SYNDROMES: There is an increased incidence of peptic ulcers in persons with **multiple endocrine neoplasia, type I** (see Chapter 21). Zollinger-Ellison syndrome, a cause of severe peptic ulceration, is characterized by gastric hypersecretion caused by a gastrin-producing islet cell adenoma of the pancreas.

α_1-ANTITRYPSIN DEFICIENCY: Almost one third of patients with this disease have peptic ulcers, which incidence is even higher if patients also have lung disease. Moreover, peptic ulcer is increased in people heterozygous for mutant α_1-antitrypsin.

CHRONIC PULMONARY DISEASE: Long-standing pulmonary dysfunction significantly increases the risk of ulcers, and it is estimated that fully one fourth of those with such disorders have peptic ulcer disease. Conversely, chronic lung disease is increased 2- to 3-fold in persons who have peptic ulcers.

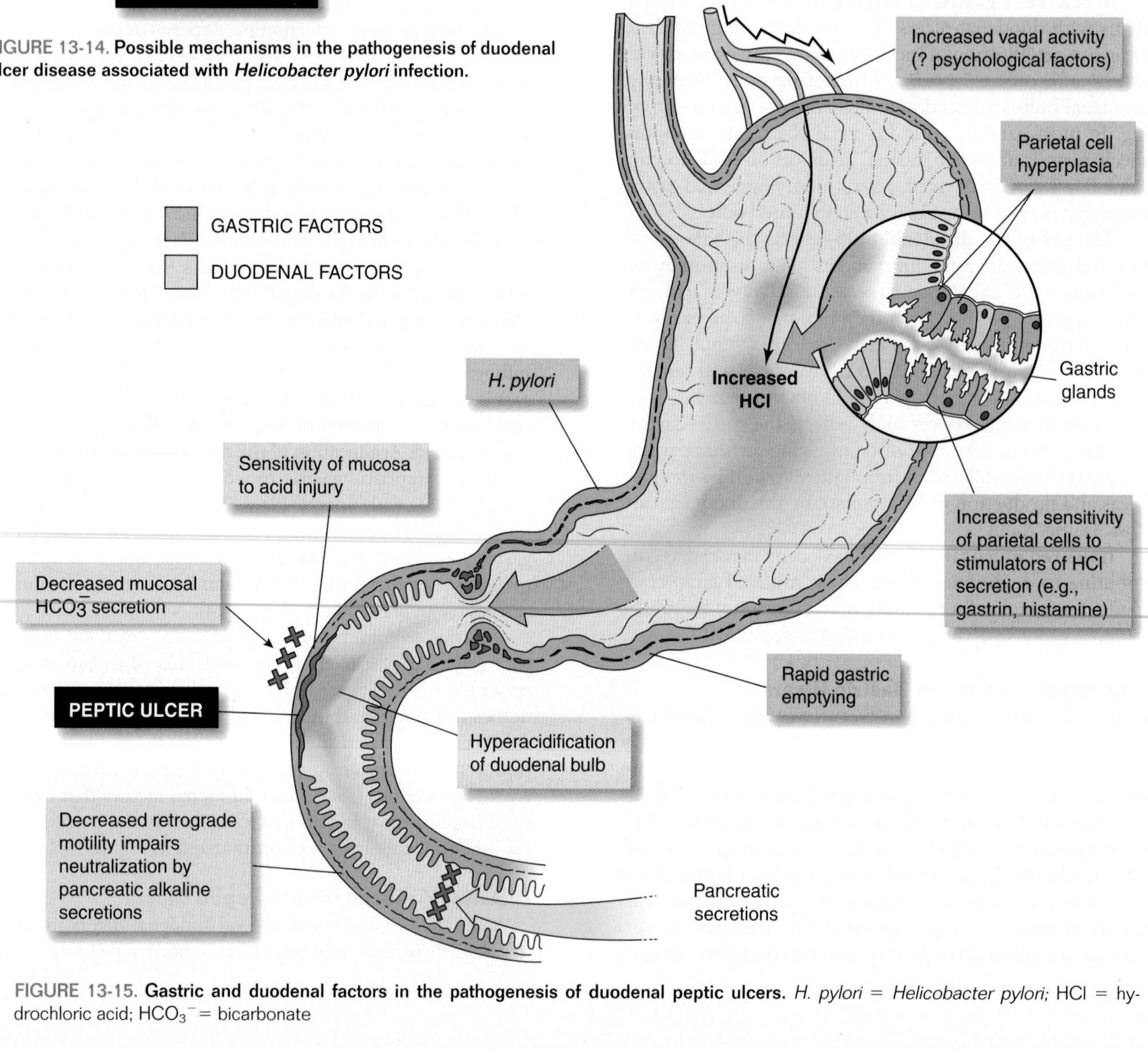

FIGURE 13-15. **Gastric and duodenal factors in the pathogenesis of duodenal peptic ulcers.** *H. pylori* = *Helicobacter pylori;* HCl = hydrochloric acid; HCO_3^- = bicarbonate

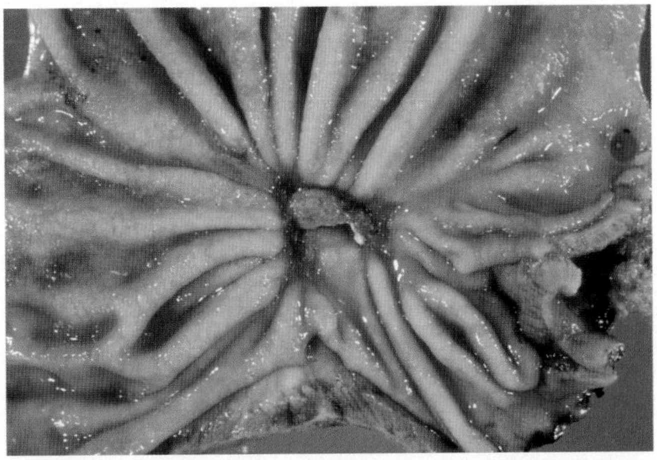

FIGURE 13-16. **Gastric ulcer.** There is a characteristic sharp demarcation from the surrounding mucosa, with radiating gastric folds. The base of the ulcer is gray owing to fibrin deposition.

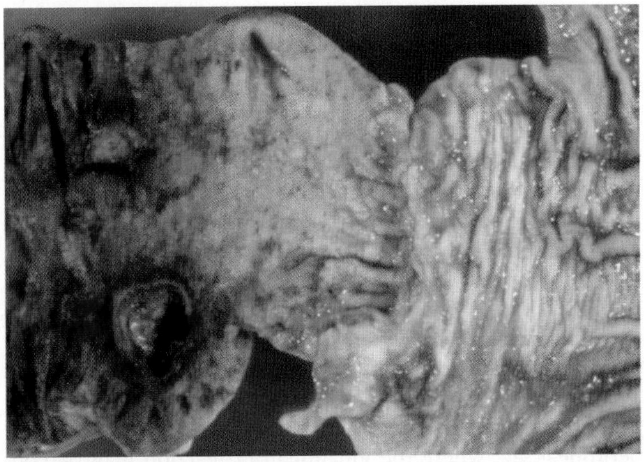

FIGURE 13-17. **Duodenal ulcer.** There are two sharply demarcated duodenal ulcers surrounded by inflamed duodenal mucosa. The gastroduodenal junction is in the mid portion of the photograph.

PATHOLOGY: Most peptic ulcers arise in the lesser gastric curvature, in the antral and prepyloric regions and in the first part of the duodenum.

Gastric ulcers (Fig. 13-16) are usually single and smaller than 2 cm in diameter. Ulcers on the lesser curvature are commonly associated with chronic gastritis, whereas those on the greater curvature are often related to NSAIDs. Edges tend to be sharply punched out, with overhanging margins. Deeply penetrating ulcers produce a serosal exudate that may cause adherence of the stomach to surrounding structures. Scarring of ulcers in the prepyloric region may be severe enough to produce pyloric stenosis. *Grossly, chronic peptic ulcers may closely resemble ulcerated gastric carcinomas.* Thus, the endoscopist must take multiple biopsies from the edges and bed of any gastric ulcer.

Duodenal ulcers (Fig. 13-17) are ordinarily on the anterior or posterior wall of the first part of the duodenum, close to the pylorus. Lesions are usually solitary, but it is not uncommon to find paired ulcers on both walls, so-called kissing ulcers.

Microscopically, gastric and duodenal ulcers are similar (Fig. 13-18). From the lumen outward, the following are noted: (1) a superficial zone of fibrinopurulent exudate; (2) necrotic tissue; (3) granulation tissue; and (4) fibrotic tissue at the base of the ulcer, which exhibits variable degrees of chronic inflammation. Ulceration may penetrate the muscle layers, causing them to be interrupted by scar tissue after healing. Blood vessels on the margins of the ulcer are often thrombosed. The mucosa at the margins tends to be hyperplastic, and with healing grows over the ulcerated area as a single layer of epithelium. Duodenal ulcers are usually accompanied by peptic duodenitis, with Brunner gland hyperplasia and gastric mucin cell metaplasia.

CLINICAL FEATURES: The symptoms of gastric and duodenal ulcers are sufficiently similar that the two conditions are generally not distinguishable by history or physical examination. The classic case of duodenal ulcer is characterized by epigastric pain 1 to 3 hours after a meal, or that awakens the patient at night. Both alkali and food relieve the symptoms. Dyspeptic symptoms commonly associated with gallbladder disease, including fatty food intolerance, distention, and belching, occur in half of patients with peptic ulcers. The major complications of peptic ulcer disease are hemorrhage, perforation with peritonitis and obstruction.

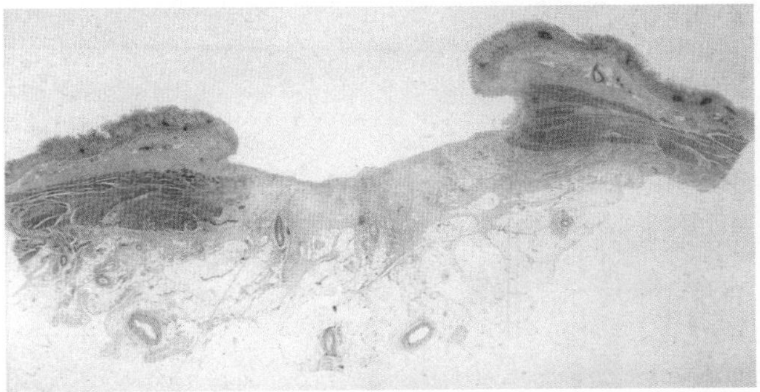

A

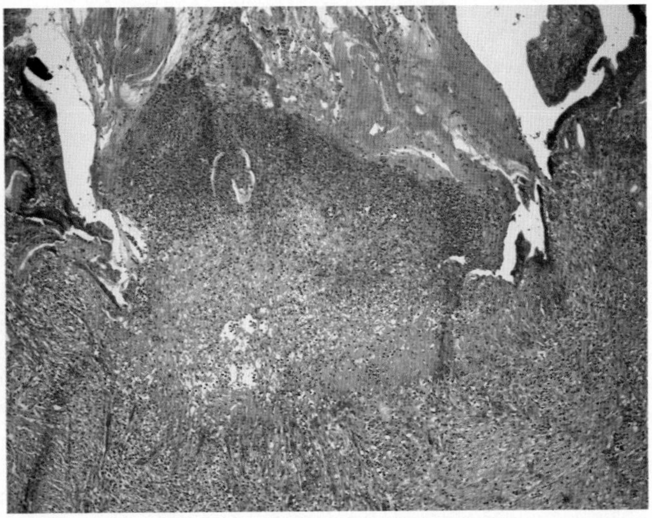

B

FIGURE 13-18. **Gastric ulcer. A.** There is full thickness replacement of the gastric muscularis with connective tissue. **B.** Photomicrograph of a peptic ulcer with superficial exudate over necrosis, granulation tissue and fibrosis.

HEMORRHAGE: The most common complication of peptic ulcers is bleeding, which occurs in up to 20% of patients. Bleeding is often occult and, in the absence of other symptoms, may manifest as iron-deficiency anemia or occult blood in stools. *Massive life-threatening bleeding is a well-known complication of active peptic ulcers.*

PERFORATION: Perforation is a serious complication of peptic ulcers that occurs in 5% of patients; in one third of cases, there are no antecedent symptoms of a peptic ulcer. Perforations occur more often with duodenal than with gastric ulcers, mostly on the anterior wall of the duodenum. Because the anterior walls of the stomach and duodenum are undefended by contiguous tissue, ulcers in these locations are more likely to be complicated by free perforation, which leads to generalized peritonitis and accumulation of air in the abdominal cavity, called **pneumoperitoneum.** Posterior gastric ulcers perforate into the lesser peritoneal sac, where the inflammatory reaction may be contained. When ulcers penetrate into the pancreas, liver or greater omentum, they cause intractable symptoms. They may also penetrate the biliary tract and fill it with air.

Perforation carries a high mortality rate. The risk of death for perforated gastric ulcers is 10% to 40%, two to four times more than for duodenal ulcers (10%). Perforations are occasionally complicated by hemorrhage. Although shock, abdominal distention, and pain are common symptoms, perforations are occasionally diagnosed for the first time at autopsy, particularly in institutionalized, elderly patients.

PYLORIC OBSTRUCTION (GASTRIC OUTLET OBSTRUCTION): Pyloric obstruction occurs in up to 10% of ulcer patients and peptic ulcer disease is its most common cause in adults. Narrowing of the pyloric lumen by an adjacent peptic ulcer may be caused by muscular spasm, edema, muscular hypertrophy, or contraction of scar tissue; most commonly it is due to a combination of these. Eventually obstruction may ensue.

DEVELOPMENT OF COMBINED ULCERS: Gastric and duodenal ulcers may occur together in the same patient far more often than can be accounted for by chance alone. Patients with either one have a much greater risk of developing the other later.

MALIGNANT TRANSFORMATION OF BENIGN GASTRIC ULCERS: It is extremely difficult to distinguish a cancer arising in a preexisting gastric ulcer from an ulcerated primary carcinoma. In contrast, *malignant transformation of a duodenal ulcer is very uncommon.* However, although cancers originating in benign peptic ulcers probably account for under 1% of all malignant tumors in the stomach, such tumors have been well documented.

TREATMENT: In the past, peptic ulcers were treated by subtotal gastrectomy. However, the disease is now cured using antibiotics to eliminate *H. pylori,* blocking gastric acid secretion, with histamine receptor blockers and proton pump inhibitors.

Benign Neoplasms

Stromal Tumors in the Stomach Tend to Be NonAggressive

Nearly all gastrointestinal stromal tumors (GISTs) are derived from the pacemaker cells of Cajal and include the vast majority of mesenchymal derived stromal tumors of the entire gastrointestinal tract. The pacemaker cells and the tumor cells express the c-*kit* oncogene (CD117) that encodes a tyrosine kinase that regulates cell proliferation and apoptosis. The criteria to evaluate aggressive behavior in all GISTs include size, necrosis, and the number of mitotic figures. Interestingly, many of gastric GISTs, independently of size, tend to behave in a nonaggressive fashion, as opposed to small and large bowel tumors, which more commonly behave in a malignant manner.

Gastric GISTs are usually submucosal (Fig. 13-19) and covered by intact mucosa or, when they project externally, by peritoneum. The cut surface is whorled. Microscopically, the tumors are variably cellular, and are composed of spindle-shaped cells with cytoplasmic vacuoles embedded in a collagenous stroma. The cells are disposed in whorls and interlacing bundles. Bizarre and giant nuclei do not necessarily suggest malignancy. GISTs

A

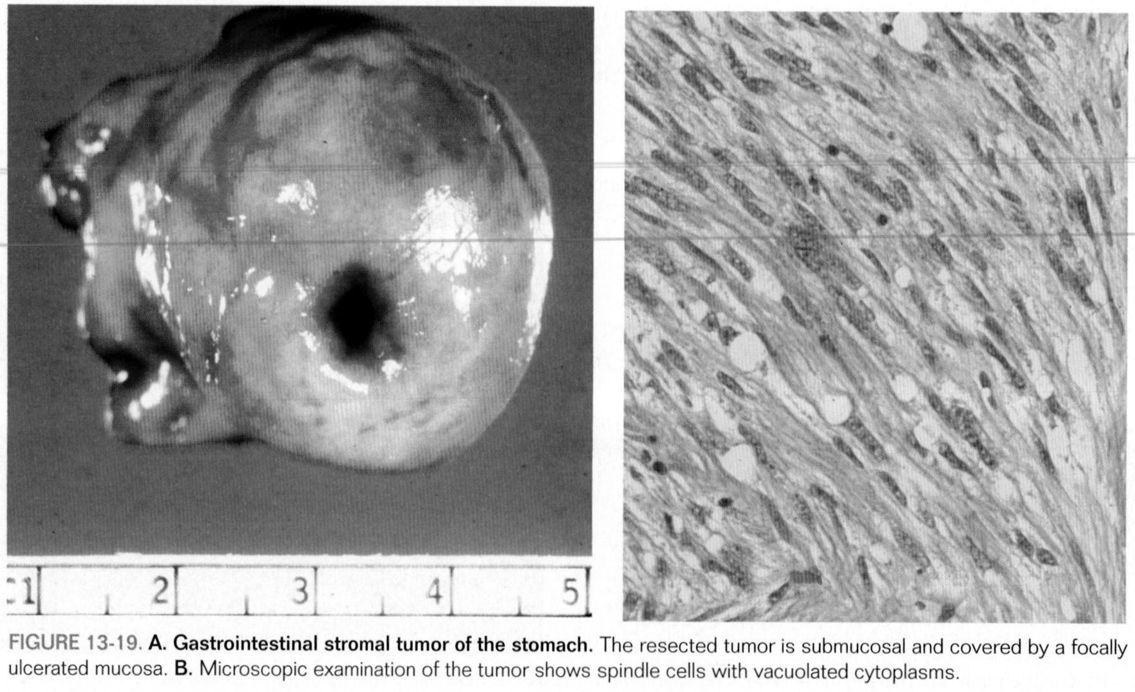

B

FIGURE 13-19. **A. Gastrointestinal stromal tumor of the stomach.** The resected tumor is submucosal and covered by a focally ulcerated mucosa. **B.** Microscopic examination of the tumor shows spindle cells with vacuolated cytoplasms.

can also appear more epithelioid, with cells that are polygonal and have eosinophilic cytoplasm.

With few exceptions, GISTs are considered tumors of low malignant potential. Treatment of GISTs consists mainly of surgical resection.

Epithelial Polyps

HYPERPLASTIC POLYPS: These lesions are by far the most common of the gastric polyps. They may be single or multiple, and are seen as pedunculated or sessile lesions of variable sizes. Hyperplastic polyps are common in the atrophic oxyntic mucosa of the body and fundus of patients with autoimmune metaplastic atrophic gastritis, but they also occur in the antrum of patients with *H. pylori* gastritis. Microscopically, the polyps consist of elongated, branched crypts lined by foveolar epithelium, beneath which pyloric or gastric glands are present. They appear to represent a response to injury and their epithelium is not dysplastic. *Hyperplastic polyps have no malignant potential.*

TUBULAR ADENOMAS (ADENOMATOUS POLYPS): These are true neoplasms that occur most commonly in the antrum. They range from smaller than 1 cm in diameter to a considerable size. Many are about 4 cm. Most adenomatous polyps are sessile, and are usually solitary. Microscopically, adenomas show tubular structures or a combination of tubular and villous structures. The glands are usually lined by dysplastic epithelium, which is sometimes intestinalized. *Adenomatous polyps manifest a malignant potential, variably reported at 5% to 75%.* This risk increases with the size of the polyp and is greatest for lesions over 2 cm. Dysplasia can also occur in flat gastric mucosa. The presence of multiple tubular adenomas in patients with familial adenomatous polyposis greatly increases the risk of developing adenocarcinoma.

FUNDIC GLAND POLYPS: Fundic gland polyps are characterized by dilated oxyntic glands lined by parietal and chief cells and by mucous cell metaplasia. They were originally described in patients with familial adenomatous polyposis. Currently they are mostly seen in patients treated with proton pump inhibitors. These polyps are not considered preneoplastic, and patients have no increased risk of gastric carcinoma.

Malignant Tumors

Carcinoma of the Stomach Relates to Many Environmental Factors

EPIDEMIOLOGY: As recently as the mid-20th century, gastric carcinoma was the most common cause of cancer death in men in the United States. For reasons that are unclear, the incidence of gastric carcinoma has decreased steadily. It now accounts for only about 3% of cancer deaths in the United States. The incidence of stomach cancer remains exceedingly high in such countries as Japan and Chile, where rates are seven to eight times that in the United States. Emigrants from high-risk to low-risk areas show a decline in the incidence of cancer of the stomach (see Chapter 5), which observation strongly implicates environmental factors in its gastric carcinogenesis.

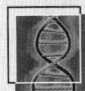

PATHOGENESIS: Although correlations have been demonstrated with a number of factors, the cause of gastric cancer remains elusive.

DIETARY FACTORS: Ingredients in the diet have been invoked to account for geographic variations in the incidence of gastric cancer. The tumor is more common among persons who eat large amounts of starch, smoked fish and meat, and pickled vegetables. Benzpyrene, a potent carcinogen, has been detected in smoked foods.

NITROSAMINES: Attention has focused on a possible role of nitrosamines, which are powerful carcinogens in animals. Secondary amines are nonenzymatically converted to nitrosamines in the presence of nitrates or nitrites. High concentrations of nitrate have been found in the soil and water in certain areas where incidence of gastric cancer is high, and processed meats and vegetables are high in nitrates and nitrites.

The decrease in gastric cancer in the United States parallels increased use of refrigeration, which inhibits conversion of nitrates to nitrites and also obviates the need for such food preservatives. Consumption of whole milk and fresh vegetables rich in vitamin C is inversely related to the occurrence of stomach cancer. Vitamin C inhibits the nitrosation of secondary amines in vivo.

GENETIC FACTORS: Although a few familial clusters and several cases in twins have been reported heredity is not thought to play a role in most cases of gastric carcinoma. Gastric cancer occurs with higher frequency in hereditary nonpolyposis colorectal cancer (HNPCC) syndrome, a disorder caused by germline mutations of genes responsible for DNA nucleotide mismatch repair. Blood type A is found in 38% of the general population, whereas half of patients with gastric cancer display this blood type.

AGE AND SEX: Gastric cancer is uncommon in persons younger than 30 years and shows a sharp peak in incidence in persons over 50. However, the age at onset is somewhat lower in Japan, where the disease is endemic. In the United States, there is only a slight male predominance, but in countries with a high incidence of this tumor, the male-to-female ratio is about 2:1.

HELICOBACTER PYLORI: *Serologic studies have shown a high prevalence of gastric infection with* H. pylori *many years before the appearance of stomach cancer.* Persons seropositive for *H. pylori* were three times more likely than seronegative persons to develop gastric adenocarcinoma in the ensuing 1 to 24 years of follow-up. In view of the observation that risk of stomach cancer is determined largely by environmental factors in the first decades of life, it is noteworthy that populations at high risk for this tumor show a high prevalence of childhood infection with *H. pylori,* while those at low risk do not. Since gastric adenocarcinoma develops in only a small proportion of persons infected with *H. pylori,* and since some stomach cancers are found in uninfected persons, *H. pylori* alone is neither sufficient nor necessary for gastric carcinogenesis.

LOW SOCIOECONOMIC SETTINGS: These situations pose an increased risk of gastric cancer, an observation that has been used to explain the higher frequency of the tumor among American blacks and the fact that the incidence of the disease in that population has not declined as rapidly as it has among whites.

Atrophic gastritis, pernicious anemia, subtotal gastrectomy, and **gastric adenomatous polyps** are discussed above as factors associated with a high risk of stomach cancer.

PATHOLOGY: Gastric adenocarcinoma accounts for over 95% of malignant gastric tumors. It occurs in two major but overlapping types: diffuse and intestinal. Cancers are most common in the distal stomach, the lesser curvature of the antrum and the prepyloric region. Adenocarcinoma may occur anywhere, but is rare in the fundus.

ADVANCED GASTRIC CANCER: By the time most gastric cancers in the Western world are detected, they are advanced; that is, they have penetrated beyond the submucosa into the muscularis propria and may extend through the serosa. The macroscopic appearance of these advanced cancers is of great importance not only to the pathologist but also to the radiologist and the endoscopist, who may be called on to distinguish carcinomas from benign lesions and to assess the degree of spread.

Advanced gastric cancers are divided into three major macroscopic types:

- **Polypoid (fungating) adenocarcinoma** accounts for one third of advanced cancers. It is a solid mass, often several centimeters in diameter, that projects into the stomach lumen. The surface may be partly ulcerated, and deeper tissues may or may not be infiltrated.
- **Ulcerating adenocarcinomas** comprise another third of all gastric cancers. They have shallow ulcers of variable size (Fig. 13-20). Surrounding tissues are firm, raised and nodular. Characteristically, the lateral margins of the ulcer are irregular and the base is ragged. This appearance stands in contrast to that of the usual benign peptic ulcer, which exhibits punched-out margins and a smooth base. Despite these differences, radiologic differentiation of ulcerating cancer from peptic ulcer is occasionally difficult.
- **Diffuse or infiltrating adenocarcinoma** accounts for one tenth of all stomach cancers. No true tumor mass is seen; instead, the wall of the stomach is thickened and firm (Fig. 13-21). If the entire stomach is involved, it is called a **linitis plastica** tumor. In the diffuse type of gastric carcinoma, invading tumor cells induce extensive fibrosis in the submucosa and muscularis. Thus, the wall is stiff and may be more than 2 cm thick.

Microscopically, the histologic pattern of advanced gastric cancer varies from a well-differentiated adenocarcinoma with gland formation (intestinal type) to a poorly differentiated carcinoma without glands. The polypoid variant typically contains well-differentiated glands, whereas linitis plastica is characteristically poorly differentiated. Particularly in the ulcerated type of cancer, tumor cells may be arranged in cords or small foci. Tumor cells may contain cytoplasmic mucin that displaces the nucleus to the periphery of the cell, resulting in the so-called signet ring cell (Fig. 13-22). Extracellular mucinous material may be so prominent that the malignant cells seem to float in a gelatinous matrix, in which case it is called a **mucinous (colloid) carcinoma.**

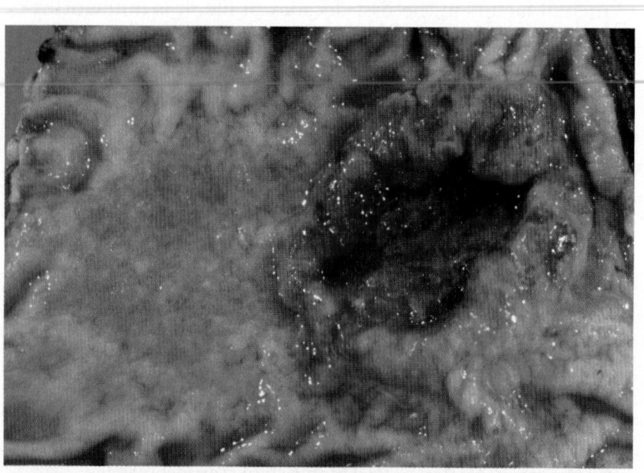

FIGURE 13-20. **Ulcerating gastric carcinoma.** In contrast to the benign peptic ulcer the edges of this lesion are raised and firm. Note the atrophy of the surrounding mucosa.

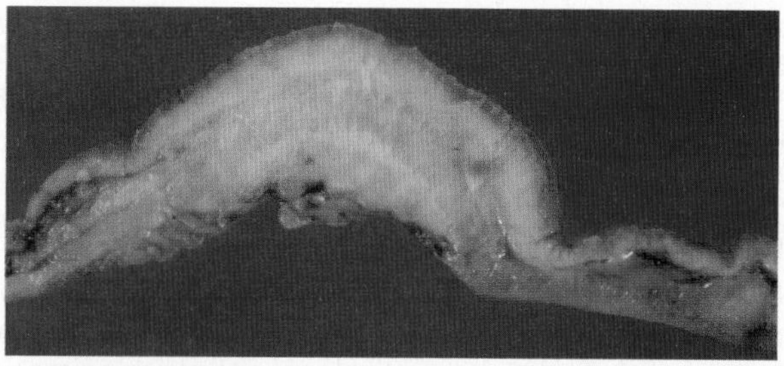

FIGURE 13-21. **Infiltrating gastric carcinoma (linitis plastica).** Cross section of gastric wall thickened by tumor and fibrosis.

EARLY GASTRIC CANCER: Early gastric cancer is defined as a tumor limited to the mucosa or submucosa (Fig. 13-23). The older term, **superficial spreading carcinoma,** is synonymous with early gastric cancer. In Japan, early gastric cancer accounts for one third of all stomach cancers, but only 5% in the United States and Europe.

Early gastric cancer is strictly a pathologic diagnosis based on depth of invasion; the term does not refer to the duration of the disease, its size, presence of symptoms, absence of metastases or curability. Up to 20% of early gastric cancers have already metastasized to lymph nodes at the time of detection.

Like advanced cancer, most early gastric cancers are in the distal stomach and are classified according to their macroscopic appearance:

- **Type I** protrudes into the lumen as a polypoid or nodular mass.
- **Type II** is a superficial, flat lesion that may be slightly elevated or depressed.
- **Type III** is an excavated malignant ulcer that does not ordinarily occur alone but rather represents ulceration of type I or type II tumors.

The polypoid and superficial elevated varieties of early gastric cancer are typically well-differentiated intestinal-type adenocarcinomas. In flattened or depressed superficial early cancers, patterns range from well differentiated to poorly differentiated. The excavated lesions have the highest proportion of undifferentiated tumors.

Most intestinal type gastric cancers originate from areas of ***intestinal metaplasia.*** By contrast, less-differentiated and anaplastic tumors of the diffuse type are more likely to derive from the necks of gastric glands without intestinal metaplasia.

Intuitively, one would suppose that early gastric cancer would be the precursor of advanced gastric cancer. However, this is not always the case. Early gastric cancer may sometimes be a different disease from advanced cancer, with a more benign course and greater curability because it has an inherently lower biological potential for invasion. This difference in biology may reflect differences between intestinal and gastric cell types. For example, even if there are lymph node metastases, early gastric cancer has a much better prognosis than does advanced cancer. The 10-year survival rate for surgically treated advanced gastric cancer is about 20%, compared with 95% for early gastric

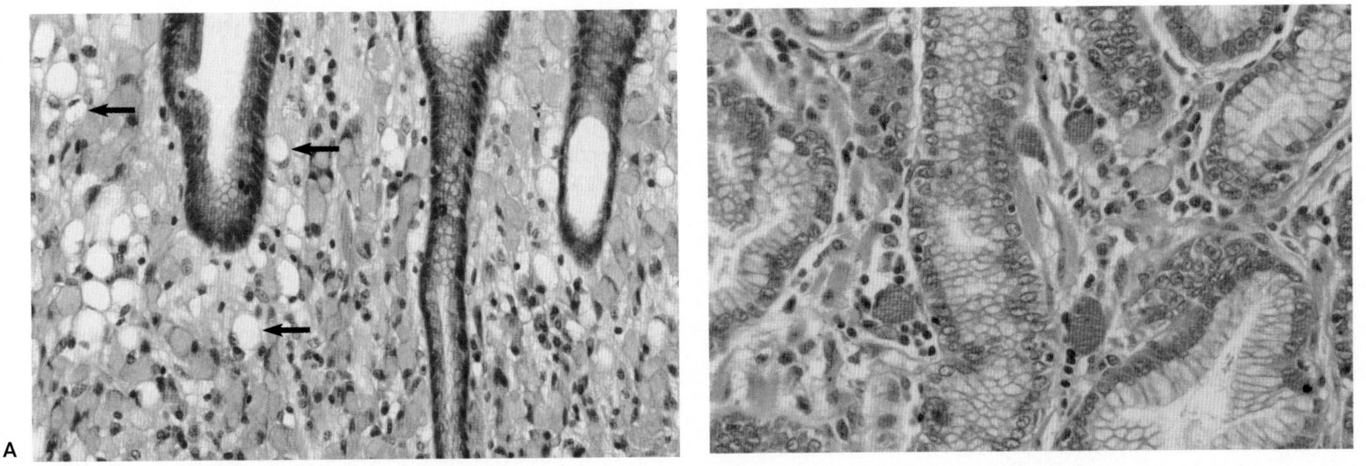

FIGURE 13-22. **Infiltrating gastric carcinoma. A.** Numerous signet ring cells (arrows) infiltrate the lamina propria between intact crypts. **B.** Mucin stains highlight the presence of mucin within the neoplastic cells.

cancer. Moreover, the mean age at onset of early gastric cancer is uniformly younger than that of advanced cancer, and the early variety shows a striking geographic distribution.

Gastric cancer metastasizes mainly via lymphatics to regional lymph nodes of the lesser and greater curvature, porta hepatis, and subpyloric region. Distant lymphatic metastases also occur, the most common being an enlarged supraclavicular node, called **Virchow node.** Hematogenous spread may seed any organ, including liver, lung, or brain. Direct extension to nearby organs is often seen. It can also spread to ovary, where it commonly elicits a desmoplastic response, which is termed a **Krukenberg tumor.**

Figure 13-24 schematically depicts the major types of gastric cancer.

CLINICAL FEATURES: In the United States and Europe, most patients with gastric cancer have metastases when they are first seen for examination. Thus, the symptoms and course are usually those of advanced cancer. The most frequent initial symptom is weight loss, usually with anorexia and nausea. Most patients complain of epigastric or back pain, a symptom that mimics benign gastric ulcer and is often relieved by antacids or H_2-receptor antagonists. However, as the disease advances, symptomatic amelioration with medical therapy disappears.

Gastric outlet obstruction may occur with large tumors of the antrum or prepyloric region. Massive bleeding is uncommon, but chronic bleeding often leads to anemia and finding occult blood in the stools. Tumors involving the esophagogastric junction cause dysphagia and may mimic achalasia and esophageal adenocarcinoma.

Patients with early gastric cancer may be asymptomatic but usually complain of dyspepsia or epigastric pain. Weight loss, melena and anemia are present in a minority.

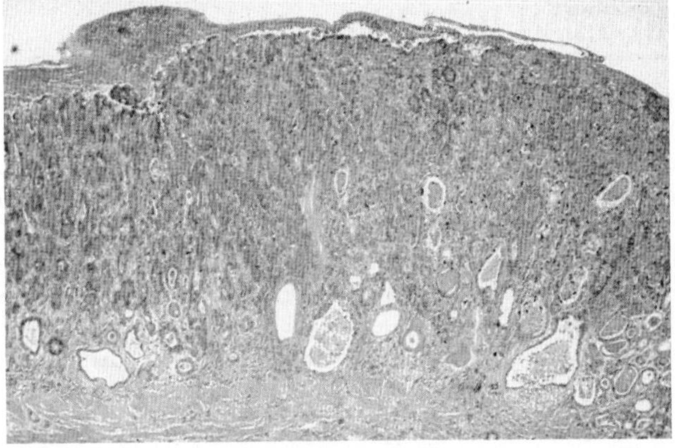

FIGURE 13-23. **Early gastric cancer.** Gastric adenocarcinoma showing malignant glands infiltrating into the submucosa.

Gastric Neuroendocrine (Carcinoid) Tumors are Low-Grade Malignancies

Various endocrine cells in the gastric mucosa may give rise to neoplasms, collectively termed carcinoid tumor (neuroendocrine tumors; NETs). These tumors may recur locally and metastasize. The probability of metastases depends more on tumor size than on histopathologic characteristics. Most gastric NETs are not hormonally functional but may occasionally secrete serotonin and metastases can cause **carcinoid syndrome.**

Gastric NETs arise in the setting of hypergastrinemia associated with autoimmune gastritis. In this context, NETs derive from hyperplastic neuroendocrine cells in the proximal stomach (ECL cells) in response to hypergastrinemia that follows loss of parietal cells. Sporadic gastric NETstend to be more aggressive.

Gastric Lymphoma Is the Most Common Extranodal Lymphoma

Primary lymphoma of the stomach accounts for about 5% of all gastric malignancies, and 20% of all extranodal lymphomas. Clinically and radiologically, it mimics gastric adenocarcinoma. Presenting symptoms, as with gastric adenocarcinoma, are usually weight loss, dyspepsia, and abdominal pain. The age at diagnosis is usually 40 to 65 years and there is no sex predominance. The tumors grossly resemble carcinomas, because they may be polypoid, ulcerating or diffuse (Fig. 13-25). Most gastric lymphomas are low-grade B-cell neoplasms of the MALToma type and arise in the setting of chronic *H. pylori* gastritis with lymphoid hyperplasia. Some of actually regress after eradication of the *H. pylori* infection. Other histopathologic varieties are similar to those in primary nodal lymphomas.

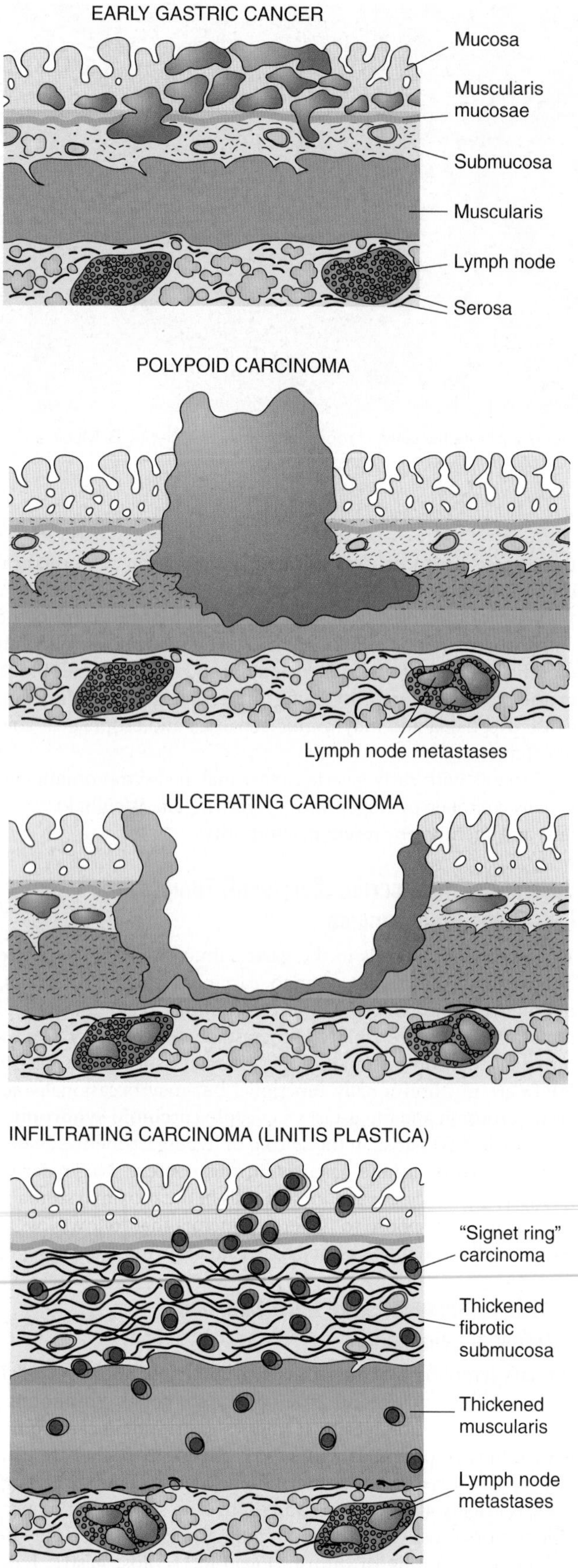

FIGURE 13-24. **The major types of gastric cancer.**

Gastrointestinal Stromal Tumors Have Low Malignant Potential

These spindle cell tumors almost always arise from the interstitial cells of Cajal (pacemaker cells) in the muscularis propria. GISTs constitute about 1% of gastric cancers. They are seen as palpable masses in up to half of patients with this tumor. It is often difficult to predict the biological behavior of a GIST from its morphologic appearance in the absence of infiltration or metastases. Macroscopically malignant GISTs are larger than their benign counterparts. Cellular pleomorphism and hyperchromasia may be present in both benign and malignant tumors, but the size and number of mitoses are greater in malignant GISTs. In some cases, the biology of a tumor is apparent only after long-term follow-up. Metastases are usually to the liver and peritoneal surfaces. Direct spread to adjacent tissues may occur. Treatment is surgical excision. A drug that specifically inhibits the *c-kit* signal transduction pathway (imatinib) is an effective treatment in many patients with advanced metastatic GISTs.

Bezoars

Bezoars are foreign bodies made of food or hair altered by the digestive process.

PHYTOBEZOAR: These vegetable concretions are unusual, except in persons who eat many persimmons or swallow unchewed bubble gum. Phytobezoars are usually seen in persons with delayed gastric emptying, as in the peripheral neuropathy of diabetes or gastric cancer, and in people undergoing therapy with anticholinergic agents.

Recently, phytobezoars have been found principally in patients who display delayed gastric emptying and hypochlorhydria after partial gastrectomy, particularly when surgery includes vagotomy. Plant bezoars contain vegetable or fruit fibers. Most patients with persimmon bezoars have bleeding from an associated gastric ulcer.

The preferred treatment of phytobezoars is chemical attack with cellulase; in some cases, manual disruption by endoscopic techniques, including jets of water, has been successful. However, enzymatic therapy is usually not effective for persimmon bezoars, and surgery is required.

TRICHOBEZOAR: This mass is a hairball within a gelatinous matrix, usually seen in long-haired girls or young women who eat their own hair as a nervous habit. Trichobezoars may grow by accretion to form a complete cast of the stomach, potentially reaching 3 kg (Fig. 13-26).

THE SMALL INTESTINE

Anatomy

Early in development, the intestinal tract begins as a tube that joins the stomach to the cloaca. This tube progressively elongates and its cephalic portion becomes the segment that extends from the distal duodenum to the proximal ileum. The more caudal portion develops into distal ileum and the proximal two thirds of transverse colon. The vitelline duct, which connects the primitive duct with the yolk sac, may persist as a Meckel diverticulum. To achieve the final position of the intestine, the fetal gut undergoes a complex series of rotations.

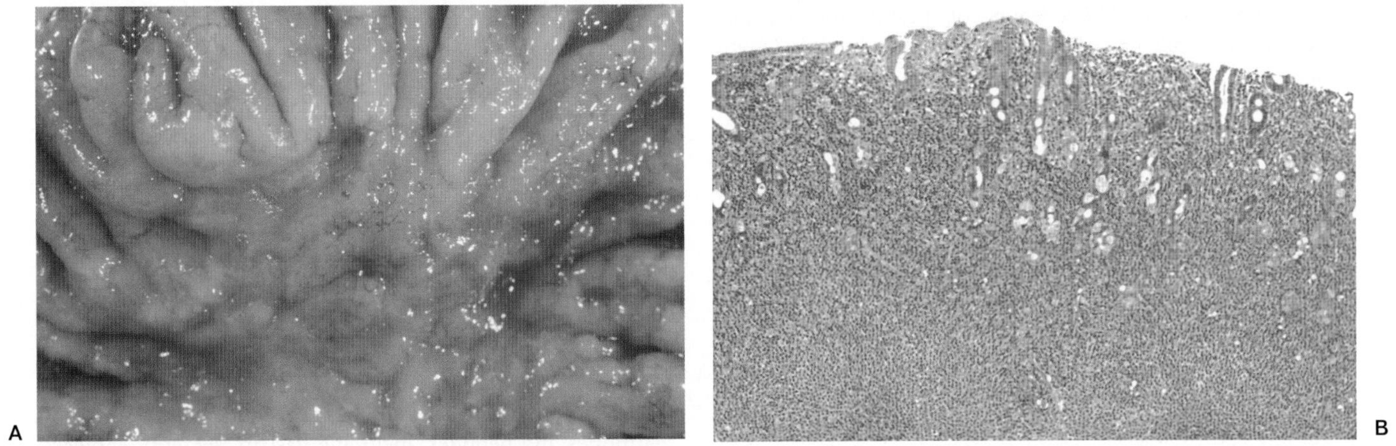

FIGURE 13-25. **Mucosa-associated lymphoid tissue (MALT) lymphoma. A.** There is loss of detail within the gastric mucosa as a MALT lymphoma infiltrates the mucosa over a large surface area, although a discrete mass was not formed. **B.** Microscopically, there is a monotonous population of lymphoid cells expands the lamina propria.

The small intestine extends from the pylorus to the ileocecal valve and, depending on its muscle tone, is from 3.5 to 6.5 m long. It is divided into three regions:

1. **The duodenum** extends to the ligament of Treitz.
2. **The jejunum** is the proximal 40% of the remainder of the small intestine.
3. **The ileum** is the distal 60%.

The duodenum is almost entirely retroperitoneal and therefore fixed. The remainder of small intestine, which is disposed in redundant loops, is movable.

The C-shaped duodenum surrounds the head of the pancreas. It receives biliary drainage of the liver and the pancreatic secretions through the common bile duct at the ampulla of Vater. The distal duodenum becomes invested by mesentery and merges with the jejunum at the ligament of Treitz. The proximity of the duodenum to its neighbors means that it may be affected by disorders such as cancer of the pancreas and cholecystoduodenal fistulas. Conversely, duodenal ulcers may penetrate into the pancreas or liver. There is no demarcation between jejunum and ileum, which merge gradually. The wall of the jejunum is thicker and its lumen wider than that of the ileum.

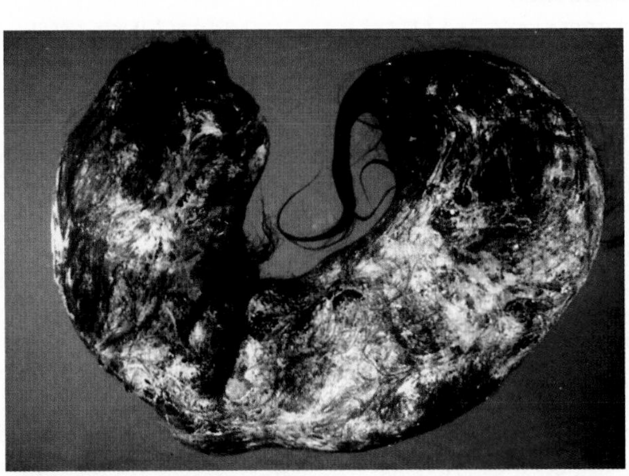

FIGURE 13-26. **Trichobezoar (hairball).** A mass of hair in a gelatinous matrix forms a cast of the stomach.

The plicae circularis, the spiral folds that consist of mucosa and submucosa, are most prominent in the distal duodenum and proximal jejunum, usually disappearing in the terminal ileum. **Peyer patches** are lymphoid aggregates in the submucosa measuring up to 3 cm in diameter. They are located in the antimesenteric aspect of the distal half of the ileum. The ileocecal valve is not a true valve but rather a muscular sphincter that regulates the flow of intestinal contents into the cecum.

The duodenum is served by the pancreaticoduodenal branch of the hepatic artery, which arises from the celiac artery. The jejunum and ileum are supplied by the superior mesenteric artery (a branch of the aorta), which is arranged in arcades in the mesentery, thereby providing abundant collateral circulation in its distal reaches. The veins draining the small intestine empty into the portal venous system. Duodenal lymphatic channels drain into portal and pyloric lymph nodes; those of the jejunum and ileum communicate with mesenteric lymph nodes. The lymphatics of terminal ileum empty into ileocolic nodes. The small intestine is innervated by sympathetic fibers from the celiac plexus and ganglia and by parasympathetic fibers from the vagus nerve. The small intestinal wall has four layers: mucosa, submucosa, muscularis, and serosa. In the retroperitoneal duodenum, however, only the anterior wall is covered by a serosa.

SEROSA AND MUSCULARIS PROPRIA: The serosa contains loose connective tissue bounded by a single layer of mesothelial cells. The muscularis propria has an outer longitudinal layer and an inner circular layer, both of which function in a coordinated manner to propel the intestinal contents by peristalsis.

SUBMUCOSA: This region consists of vascularized connective tissue and a few scattered lymphocytes, plasma cells, and macrophages, with occasional mast cells and eosinophils. In the proximal duodenum, the submucosa is occupied by Brunner glands, branched structures that contain mucous and serous cells. These secrete mucus and bicarbonate, which protect the duodenal mucosa from peptic ulceration. The lymphatic and venous capillaries of the mucosa drain into a highly developed system of lymphatic and venous plexuses in the submucosa. The **myenteric nerve plexus of Auerbach,** which lies between the two layers of the muscularis, and **Meissner plexus** in the submucosa are interconnected.

MUCOSA: The distinctive feature of intestinal mucosa is its arrangement in villi, fingerlike projections 0.5 to 1 mm in length that expand the absorptive area enormously. The macroscopic structure of the villi varies in different regions of the small intestine. In the proximal duodenum, villi tend to be broad and blunted, whereas in the distal duodenum and proximal jejunum, they are more slender, leaf-shaped. Shorter, finger-shaped villi are the rule in distal jejunum and ileum.

Villi are composed of columnar epithelium resting on a basement membrane, a lamina propria, and a muscularis mucosae, which separates the mucosa from the submucosa. The connective tissue of the lamina propria forms the core of the villus and surrounds the crypts of Lieberkuhn at the base of the villi. The normal lamina propria contains lymphocytes, plasma cells and macrophages. Plasma cells in this location principally secrete immunoglobulin A (IgA) into the intestinal lumen or the lamina propria itself. Occasional eosinophils and mast cells are scattered throughout. A few smooth muscle cells and fibroblasts are also present. The cellular composition of the lamina propria reflects its role in protecting against invasion by bacteria that may penetrate the mucosa and segregating foreign material that breaches the mucosa.

Some IgA is produced by plasma cells in the lamina propria as a dimer that diffuses through the basement membrane of the crypt. IgA then reaches the basal or lateral surface of epithelial cells, where it combines with a secretory component produced by that cell. Resulting **secretory IgA** is taken up by epithelial cells and secreted into the lumen. Secretory IgA is more resistant to proteolysis than is serum IgA. It binds food antigens and prevents bacterial adherence to the intestinal epithelium. Moreover, it can neutralize bacterial toxins and inhibit viral replication and mucosal penetration.

Lymphoid nodules (MALT) are scattered throughout the mucosa and aggregate into visible Peyer patches. The villous columnar epithelial cells are mainly absorptive, whereas those lining the crypts are the source of cell renewal and secretion. There are normally a moderate number of intraepithelial T lymphocytes.

Absorptive cells, or enterocytes (Fig. 13-27), are the principal lining cells of intestinal villi. The villi also exhibit a few goblet and endocrine cells. Enterocytes are tall and display basally situated nuclei. Numerous microvilli extend from the surface of these cells into the lumen, thereby hugely increasing the absorptive surface. The plasma membrane of the microvilli is covered by a glycocalyx (fuzzy coat) produced by the absorptive cells. Disaccharidases and peptidases reside in this glycocalyx. Certain receptors, such as that for the intrinsic factor–vitamin B_{12} complex in the ileum, are also present in the membrane–glycocalyx complex. The cytoplasm just under the microvilli contains a network of actin microfilaments, termed the **terminal web.** These filaments, which are also associated with myosin and other contractile proteins, insert into the core of the microvilli and presumably serve as a contractile apparatus. The lateral borders of adjacent plasma membranes form tight junctions that are impermeable to macromolecules but permit passive transport of small molecules by the paracellular route. Absorbed material is transported from epithelial cells to the intercellular space between absorptive cells, through lateral or basal plasma membranes. It then penetrates the basement membrane, traverses the lamina propria and enters a capillary or a lymphatic channel.

Four cell types are recognized in the crypts:

- **Paneth cells** at the base of the crypts are similar to the zymogen cells of the pancreas and salivary glands that are actively engaged in exocrine secretion. Within Paneth cells, eosinophilic secretory granules fill a basophilic cytoplasm. These cells play a role in **mucosal defense,** as evidenced by the presence of lysozyme, antimicrobial products, including peptides called **crypt defensins** (cryptdins) and CD95 ligand, which is a member of the tumor necrosis factor (TNF) family of cytokines.
- **Goblet cells** of the lateral walls of the crypts are flask-shaped and filled with mucus granules. They are similar in structure and function to goblet cells elsewhere and contain neutral and acid mucins.
- **Endocrine cells** appear inverted, with an apical nucleus and basal granules. The granules are most likely secreted into the lamina propria. These cells make several gastrointestinal hormones and peptides, including gastrin, secretin, cholecystokinin, glucagon, VIP, and serotonin. These hormones are felt to regulate many gastrointestinal functions, and tumors derived from these cells often exhibit striking hormone secretion.
- **Undifferentiated cells** are located in the lateral crypt walls and are interspersed between the Paneth cells at their bases. They are the most numerous cells of the crypts. Small glycoprotein secretory granules are grouped in the apical cytoplasm of some of the undifferentiated cells. These cells function as reserve cells from which all other mucosal cells are renewed, and thus mitoses are numerous among them.

Cell renewal in the small intestine is limited to the crypts, where undifferentiated cells divide. The newly formed cells migrate up the villus, where they terminally differentiate into absorptive cells and goblet cells and eventually undergo apoptosis or slough into the lumen at the tip of the villus. Their absorptive capacity is maximal when they reach the upper third of the villus. The mucosal epithelium of the small intestine is replaced within a period of 4 to 7 days. This rapid cell proliferation explains why the intestinal epithelium is particularly sensitive to radiation and chemotherapeutic agents.

Congenital Disorders

Atresia and Stenosis Cause Neonatal Intestinal Obstruction

ATRESIA: Atresia is defined as a complete occlusion of the intestinal lumen, which may manifest as (1) a thin intraluminal diaphragm, (2) blind proximal and distal sacs joined by a cord, or (3) disconnected blind ends. One fourth of atresias are associated with meconium ileus and cystic fibrosis is involved in one tenth of the cases.

STENOSIS: This is an incomplete stricture, which narrows but does not occlude, the lumen. Stenosis may also be caused by an incomplete diaphragm. It is usually symptomatic in infancy, but cases presenting in middle-aged adults have been recorded.

One fourth of mothers of fetuses with high intestinal atresia develop polyhydramnios in their last trimester of pregnanacy, presumably because the fetus does not swallow amniotic fluid. Intestinal atresia or stenosis is diagnosed on the basis of persistent vomiting of bile-containing fluid within the first day of life. Meconium is not passed. The obstructed fetal intestine is dilated and filled with fluid, which can be detected radiologically. Surgi-

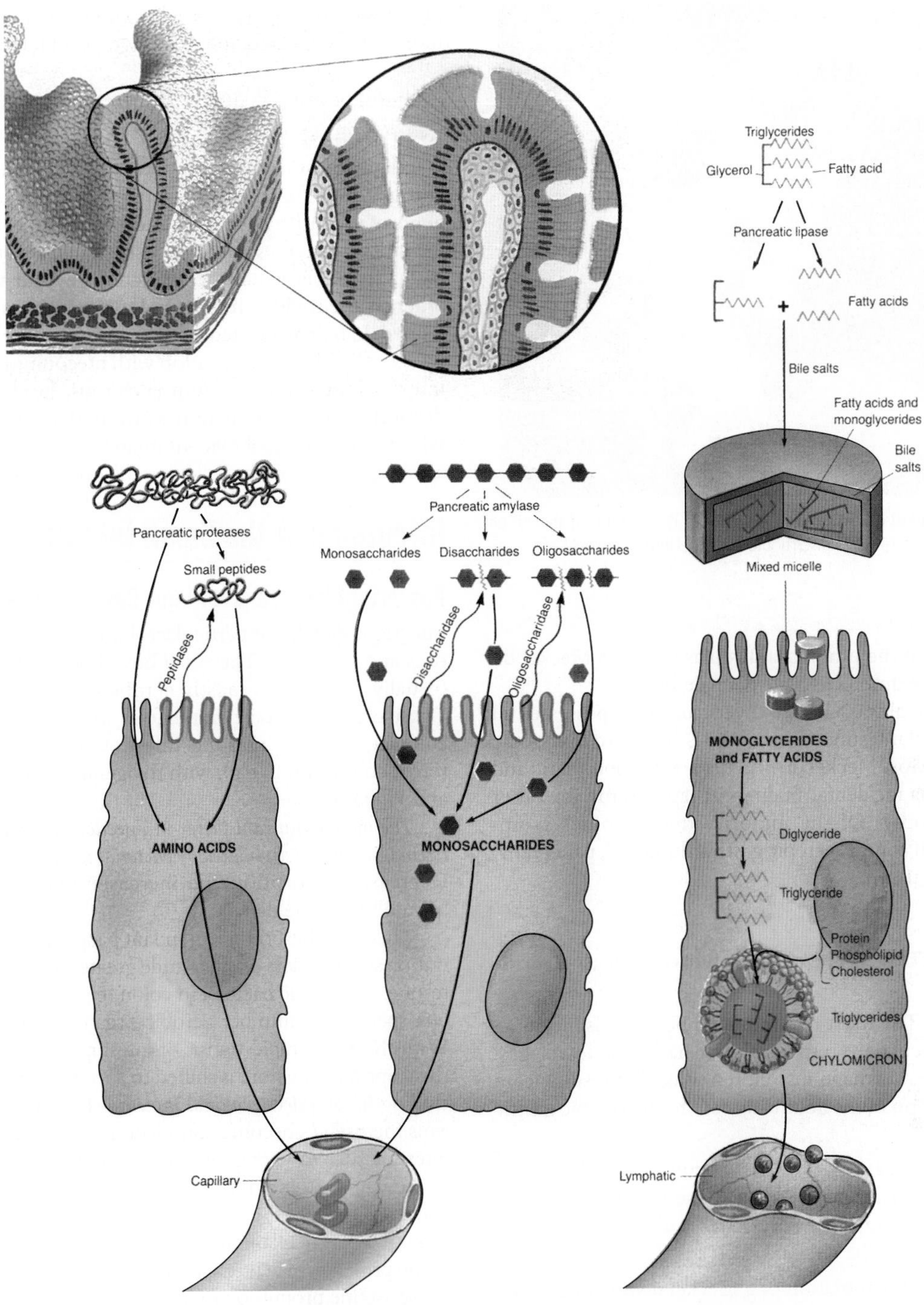

FIGURE 13-27. **Mechanisms of nutrient absorption in the small intestine.**

cal correction is usually successful, but there are often other complicating anomalies.

Duplications (Enteric Cysts) May Occur From the Esophagus to the Anus

These cysts are spherical or tubular structures attached to the alimentary tract. They may be seen as cystic structures or may communicate with the gut lumen. Intestinal duplications are most common in the ileum and less so in the jejunum. They have a smooth muscle wall and gastrointestinal type epithelium. Communicating duplications are often lined by gastric mucosa, a situation that may lead to peptic ulceration, bleeding, or perforation.

Meckel Diverticulum Causes Bleeding, Obstruction, and Perforation

Meckel diverticulum, caused by persistence of the vitelline duct, is an outpouching of the gut on the antimesenteric ileal border, 60 to 100 cm from the ileocecal valve in adults. It is the most common and the most clinically significant congenital anomaly of the small intestine (Fig. 13-28). Two thirds of patients are younger than 2 years.

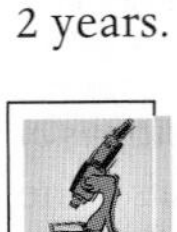

PATHOLOGY: Meckel diverticulum is about 5 cm long, slightly narrower than the ileum. A fibrous cord may hang freely from the apex of the diverticulum or

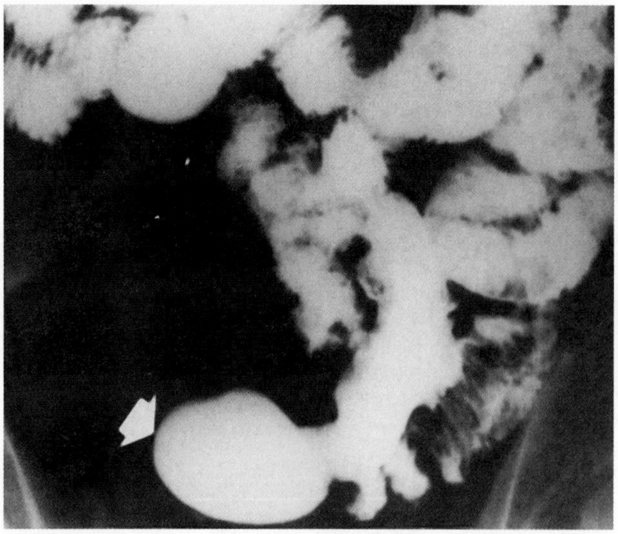

FIGURE 13-28. **Meckel diverticulum.** A contrast radiograph of the small intestine shows a barium-filled diverticulum of the ileum *(arrow)*.

may be attached to the umbilicus. Fistulas between Meckel diverticulum and the umbilicus have been described.

Meckel diverticulum is a true diverticulum. It possesses all the coats of normal intestine; the mucosa is similar to that of the adjoining ileum. Most Meckel diverticula are asymptomatic and discovered only as incidental findings at laparotomy for other causes or at autopsy. Of the minority that becomes symptomatic, about half contain ectopic gastric, duodenal, pancreatic, biliary, or colonic tissue.

CLINICAL FEATURES: The complications of Meckel diverticulum are several.

- **Hemorrhage:** The most common complication is bleeding. Meckel diverticula are responsible for half of all lower gastrointestinal hemorrhage in children. Bleeding results from **peptic ulceration** of the ileum adjacent to the ectopic gastric mucosa.
- **Intestinal obstruction:** The diverticulum may be a lead point for **intussusception** and so cause intestinal obstruction. Obstruction can also be caused by **volvulus** around the fibrotic remnant of the vitelline duct.
- **Diverticulitis:** Inflammation of a Meckel diverticulum (i.e., diverticulitis) leads to symptoms indistinguishable from those of appendicitis. Thus, a surgeon suspecting acute appendicitis who encounters a normal appendix, is well advised to search for a Meckel diverticulum.
- **Perforation:** Peptic ulceration, either in the diverticulum or in the ileum, may cause perforation, and lead to rapidly spreading peritonitis.
- **Fistula:** A fecal discharge from the umbilicus may be observed.

Malrotation May Lead to Bowel Obstruction

Defective intestinal rotation in fetal life leads to abnormal positions of small intestine and colon, anomalous attachments, and bands. The clinical importance of such rotational anomalies lies in their propensity to cause catastrophic volvulus of the small and large intestine and incarceration of bowel in an internal hernia.

Meconium Ileus is an Early Complication of Cystic Fibrosis

Neonatal intestinal obstruction in cystic fibrosis is caused by accumulation of tenacious meconium in the small intestine. The abnormal consistency of the meconium reflects a deficiency in pancreatic enzymes and high viscosity of intestinal mucus. The distal ileum is usually contracted beyond the obstruction, whereas the midileum proximal to the inspissated meconium is dilated. In half of affected infants, meconium ileus is complicated by (1) volvulus, (2) perforation with meconium peritonitis, or (3) intestinal atresia. Meconium ileus must be differentiated from distal intestinal obstruction associated with cystic fibrosis, in which a small plug of meconium in the distal colon may eventually be passed, thereby relieving the obstruction.

Infections of the Small Intestine

Bacterial Diarrhea is a Major Cause of Death Worldwide

Infectious diarrhea is particularly lethal in underdeveloped countries and in infants. The small bowel normally has few bacteria (usually $<10^4$/mL), mostly aerobic bacilli such as lactobacilli. These organisms travel in the food stream and ordinarily do not colonize the small intestine. Infectious diarrhea is caused by bacteroa; colonization, e.g., with toxigenic strains of *Escherichia coli* and *Vibrio cholerae*.

The most significant factor in infectious diarrhea is increased intestinal secretion, stimulated by bacterial toxins and enteric hormones. Decreased absorption and increased peristaltic activity contribute less to the diarrhea.

The colon harbors an abundant bacterial flora, with a concentration seven orders of magnitude greater than that of the small intestine. Anaerobic bacteria in colon (e.g., *Bacteroides* and *Clostridium* species) outnumber aerobic organisms by a factor of 1000. With the more rapid transit of intestinal contents during a diarrheal episode, the flora is shifted to a more aerobic population, including *E. coli, Klebsiella,* and *Proteus*. Moreover, offending organisms themselves become conspicuous and pathogens of the small intestine such as *V. cholerae* may be the major isolate in the stools.

Several factors limit the numbers of bacteria in the stomach and small bowel: (1) gastric acid production is inimical to bacterial growth, which explains the overgrowth of bacteria in the stomach in the presence of achlorhydria; (2) bile has antimicrobial activity; (3) peristaltic propulsion of intestinal contents limits bacterial accumulation; (4) normal flora secrete their own antimicrobial substances to maintain an ecological balance (indeed, treatment with broad-spectrum antibiotics alters the natural flora and allows overgrowth of ordinarily harmless organisms); and (5) plasma cells of the lamina propria secrete IgA into the intestinal lumen.

Individual agents responsible for infectious diarrhea are discussed in Chapter 9. Here we only briefly review the major entities. The agents of infectious diarrhea are conveniently classified into toxigenic organisms, which produce diarrhea by elaborating toxins, adherent bacteria, and invasive bacteria.

Toxigenic Diarrhea

The prototypic organisms that produce diarrhea by secreting toxins are V. cholerae *and toxigenic strains of* E. coli. Toxigenic diarrhea is characterized by:

- Damage to the intestinal mucosa is minimal or absent.
- The organism remains on the mucosal surface, where it secretes its toxin.
- Fluid secreted into the small intestine causes watery diarrhea, which can lead to dehydration, particularly in the case of cholera.

Although many organisms have been isolated in so-called travelers' diarrhea, the most common pathogen in almost all studies is toxigenic *E. coli.*

Diarrhea Caused by Invasive Bacteria

Invasive bacteria, as their name implies, cause diarrhea by directly injuring the intestinal mucosa. Among these organisms, *Shigella, Salmonella,* and certain strains of *E. coli, Yersinia,* and *Campylobacter* are the most widely recognized. Invasive organisms tend to infect distal ileum and colon, while toxigenic bacteria mainly involve the upper intestinal tract. The mechanism by which they produce diarrhea is uncertain. Enterotoxins have been identified, but their role in causing diarrhea has not been established. Invasion of the mucosa by bacteria increases the synthesis of prostaglandins in the affected tissue and inhibitors of prostaglandin synthesis seem to block fluid secretion. It is also possible that the damaged mucosa is unable to resorb fluid from the lumen.

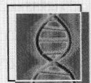

PATHOGENESIS AND PATHOLOGY: *SHIGELLOSIS:* Shigellosis principally affects the colon, although the terminal ileum is occasionally involved. Microscopically, a granular and hemorrhagic mucosa exhibits numerous shallow serpiginous ulcers. The inflammation, which is especially severe in the sigmoid colon and rectum, is usually superficial. In the early stage, the accumulation of neutrophils in damaged crypts (crypt abscesses) is similar to that in ulcerative colitis and the lymphoid follicles of the mucosa break down to form ulcers. As the infection recedes, the ulcers heal and the mucosa returns to normal.

TYPHOID FEVER: Typhoid fever (*Salmonella* enteritis) is today uncommon in the industrialized world but is still a problem in underdeveloped countries. Necrosis of lymphoid tissue, principally in the terminal ileum, leads to scattered ulcers. Infection of Peyer patches results in oval ulcers, in which the longer dimension is in the long axis of the intestine. Occasionally, lymphoid follicles in the large bowel or the appendix are ulcerated. The base of the ulcer is composed of black necrotic tissue mixed with fibrin.

The early lesions of typhoid fever contain large basophilic macrophages filled with typhoid bacilli, erythrocytes, and necrotic debris. Necrosis of lymphoid follicles becomes confluent and mucosal ulceration follows. Similar lymphoid hyperplasia and necrosis are seen in regional lymph nodes. Within a week of the acute symptoms ulcers heal completely, leaving little fibrosis or other sequelae. **Intestinal hemorrhage and perforation,** principally in the ileum, are the most feared complications of typhoid fever and tend to occur in the third week and during convalescence.

NONTYPHOIDAL SALMONELLOSIS: Formerly known as **paratyphoid fever,** this enteritis is caused by *Salmonella* strains other than *Salmonella typhi* and is generally far less serious than typhoid fever. The principal target is the ileum, although minor involvement of the colon may also occur. Organisms invade the mucosa, which shows mild ulceration, edema, and infiltration with neutrophils. Hematogenous dissemination from the intestine may carry infection to bones, joints, and meninges. Interestingly, people with sickle cell anemia tend to develop *Salmonella* osteomyelitis, presumably because phagocytosis of the products of hemolysis prevents further cellular ingestion of the *Salmonella* organisms and allows their dissemination through the bloodstream.

ENTEROINVASIVE AND ENTEROHEMORRHAGIC STRAINS OF E. COLI: These organisms may uncommonly cause bloody diarrhea similar to shigellosis. Certain strains of *E. coli,* particularly serotype 0157:H7, produce *Shigella*-like toxins, but the role of these proteins in the pathogenesis of the enterocolitis is not understood. Serotype 0157:H7 has also been implicated in the hemolytic–uremic syndrome in children.

YERSINIA *ENTEROCOLITIS: Yersinia enterocolitica* and *Yersinia pseudotuberculosis* are transmitted by pets or contaminated food and infection is most common in young children. *Yersinia* infection causes diarrhea, cramps, and fever and lasts 1 to 3 weeks. Disease is characterized by hyperplasia of Peyer patches, with acute ulceration of overlying mucosa. A fibrinopurulent exudate covers the ulcers and often contains many organisms.

In addition to causing enterocolitis, *Yersinia* causes acute mesenteric adenitis and pain in the right lower quadrant. Infected children have undergone laparotomy because the disease was mistaken for appendicitis. Microscopically the lymph nodes show epithelioid granulomas with central necrotic zones in the case of infection with *Y. pseudotuberculosis.* The ileum and appendix may contain similar granulomas, causing an appearance that has been mistaken for Crohn disease.

Adults, who are less susceptible to infection with *Yersinia* than are children, have an acute diarrhea, often followed within a few weeks by erythema nodosum, erythema multiforme, or polyarthritis. Patients with chronic debilitating diseases may develop a fatal *Yersinia* bacteremia that is resistant to antibiotic treatment. Interestingly, persons with thalassemia have a propensity for *Y. enterocolitica* infection.

CAMPYLOBACTER JEJUNI: C. jejuni is one of the most common causes of bacterial diarrhea. Some investigators report a higher incidence of *Campylobacter* than of nontyphoidal *Salmonella* and *Shigella* infections in the United States. In one study from Great Britain, half of all bacterial diarrhea was caused by *Campylobacter.* Humans contract the disease mainly by contact with infected domestic animals or ingestion of poorly cooked or contaminated food. Adults usually recover in less than 1 week.

Food Poisoning

Infectious agents can produce diarrhea by elaborating enterotoxins in contaminated food that is then ingested.

STAPHYLOCOCCUS AUREUS: This bacterium is a common cause of food poisoning. Symptoms result from ingesting food contaminated with *Staphylococcus* strains that produce an exotoxin that damages the gastrointestinal epithelium. Within 6 hours, severe vomiting and abdominal cramps occur, often followed by diarrhea. Most patients recover in 1 to 2 days.

CLOSTRIDIUM PERFRINGENS: This bacterium elaborates an enterotoxin that causes vomiting and diarrhea. Although the organism is anaerobic, it tolerates exposure to air for up to 3 days. Enterotoxin activity is maximal in the ileum. In most cases, watery diarrhea and severe abdominal pain begin 8 to 24 hours after ingestion of contaminated food, and last only about 1 day.

Rotavirus and Norwalk Virus are the Most Common Causes of Viral Gastroenteritis in the United States

ROTAVIRUS: Rotavirus infection is a common cause of infantile diarrhea. It accounts for about half of acute diarrhea in hospitalized children under 2 years. Rotavirus has been demonstrated in duodenal biopsy specimens and is associated with injury to the surface epithelium and impaired intestinal absorption for periods of up to 2 months.

NORWALK VIRUSES: These agents account for one third of the epidemics of viral gastroenteritis in the United States. The virus targets the upper small intestine, where it causes patchy mucosal lesions and malabsorption. Vomiting and diarrhea are usual, but the symptoms resolve within 2 days.

Other viruses implicated as etiological agents of infective diarrhea include echovirus, coxsackievirus, cytomegalovirus, adenovirus, and coronavirus.

Intestinal Tuberculosis Occurs After Ingesting *Mycobacterium Bovis*

Historically an important disease, gastrointestinal tuberculosis is now uncommon in industrialized countries, although it is still a problem in underdeveloped areas of the world. Intestinal tuberculosis usually involves infection with *M. bovis,* which was mainly transmitted by contaminated milk. However, the control of tuberculosis in dairy herds and pasteurization of milk have made infection with this organism a curiosity.

Most cases of intestinal tuberculosis are caused either by ingesting bacteria in food or by swallowing infectious sputum. The tubercle bacillus is protected from digestion by its waxy capsule, and passes into the small bowel. It then establishes a locus of infection, usually (90% of patients) in the ileocecal region, where lymphoid tissue is abundant. Infection also occurs in the colon, jejunum, appendix, rectum, and duodenum, in that order of frequency.

PATHOLOGY: Intestinal tuberculosis may present with circular ulcers of varying size in the transverse plane of the bowel. As the ulcers heal, reactive fibrosis may cause a circumferential ("napkin ring") stricture of the bowel lumen. Mesenteric lymph nodes are typically enlarged and display caseous necrosis.

Granulomas may also be found in all layers of the bowel wall, particularly in Peyer patches and lymphoid follicles. Tuberculous strictures are difficult to distinguish from other causes of stricture, such as ischemic enterocolitis or Crohn disease.

CLINICAL FEATURES: Almost all patients with intestinal tuberculosis complain of chronic abdominal pain and about two thirds have a palpable abdominal mass, usually in the right lower quadrant. Malnutrition, weight loss, fever, and weakness are common. Complications include obstruction, fistulas, perforation, and abscess.

Intestinal Fungal Infections Occur Mainly in Immunocompromised Patients

Since the gastrointestinal tract is not a hospitable environment for fungi and the number of commensal organisms is miniscule (mostly yeasts and anaerobic actinomycetes), *gastrointestinal fungal infections are usually opportunistic.* Suppression of normal bacterial flora by antibiotics also favors fungal growth. Under these circumstances, the most common mycosis is caused by *Candida.* Other fungi, including *Histoplasma* and *Mucor,* are occasionally found.

PATHOLOGY: Candidiasis and mucormycosis typically cause mucosal erosions; these may progress to larger ulcers that are surrounded by hemorrhage and necrosis. The inflammation is characteristically neutrophilic and there may be remarkably little reaction to the fungi because of immunosuppression. Mucormycosis often invades blood vessels, with thrombosis and infarction, but hematogenous dissemination from the intestine is rare. Disseminated histoplasmosis may involve the bowel, where it causes elevated plaques that ulcerate and may even perforate.

Small Intestinal Parasites Include Both Protozoan and Metazoan Species

Parasitic diseases of the small bowel are discussed in detail in Chapter 9. These parasites include (1) **protozoa,** such as *Giardia lamblia, Coccidia* species, and cryptosporidia; (2) **nematodes (roundworms)** such as *Ascaris, Strongyloides,* and hookworms; and (3) **flatworms.** The latter are divided into tapeworms (cestodes), such as *Diphyllobothrium latum, Taenia solium, Taenia saginata,* and *Hymenolepis nana.* Flukes (trematodes) include various schistosomes and the giant intestinal fluke *Fasciolopsis buski.* In addition, trichinosis has an intestinal phase during which vomiting, diarrhea, and colic mimic acute food poisoning or bacterial enteritis.

Vascular Diseases of the Small Intestine

Decreased intestinal blood flow from any cause can lead to **ischemic bowel disease.** Analogous to coronary heart disease, there is a spectrum of manifestations. The most common type of ischemic bowel disease is acute intestinal ischemia, which is associated with injury ranging from mucosal necrosis to transmural bowel infarction. Chronic intestinal ischemic syndromes are less common and generally require the severe compromise of two or more major arteries, usually by atherosclerosis.

Superior Mesenteric Artery Occlusion is the Most Common Cause of Acute Intestinal Ischemia

PATHOGENESIS:

ARTERIAL OCCLUSION: Sudden occlusion of a large artery by thrombosis or embolization leads to small bowel infarction before collateral circulation comes into play. Depending on the size of the artery, infarction may be segmental or may lead to gangrene of virtually the entire small bowel (Fig. 13-29). Occlusive intestinal infarction is most often caused by embolic or thrombotic occlusion of the superior mesenteric artery. A lesser number are the result of vasculitis, which often involves small arteries.

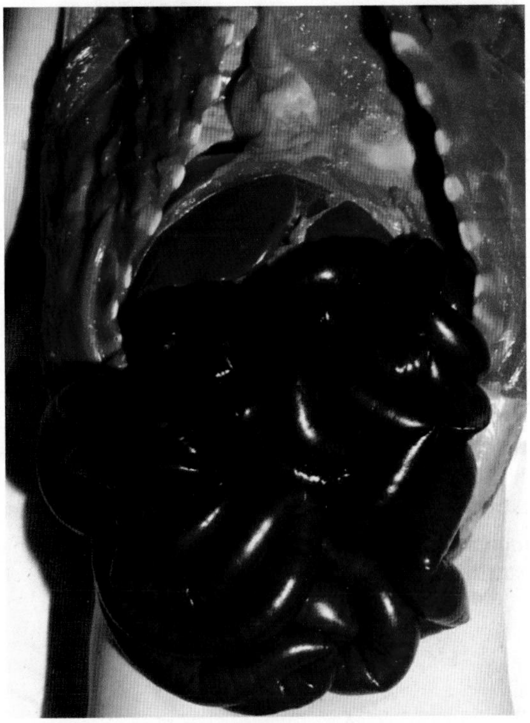

FIGURE 13-29. **Infarct of the small bowel.** This infant died after an episode of intense abdominal pain and shock. Autopsy demonstrated volvulus of the small bowel that had occluded the superior mesenteric artery. The entire small bowel is dilated, gangrenous, and hemorrhagic.

In addition to intrinsic vascular lesions, volvulus, intussusception and incarceration of the intestine in a hernial sac may all lead to arterial as well as venous occlusion.

NONOCCLUSIVE INTESTINAL ISCHEMIA: Intestinal ischemic necrosis in which no acute vascular occlusion is evident is more common than the occlusive type. Nonocclusive intestinal infarction may be extensive and is seen in hypoxic patients with reduced cardiac output from shock of a variety of causes including hemorrhage, sepsis, and acute myocardial infarction. Shock leads to redistribution of blood flow to the brain and other vital organs. In addition, patients in shock often receive α-adrenergic agents, which may further shunt blood away from the intestine. The drastically lowered perfusion pressure in the arterioles leads to their collapse, thereby aggravating the ischemia.

THROMBOSIS OF MESENTERIC VEINS: Causes of mesenteric vein thrombosis include hypercoagulable states, stasis, and inflammation (pylephlebitis). Almost all thromboses affect the superior mesenteric vein; only 5% involve the inferior mesenteric vein. The collateral flow in the distribution of the superior mesenteric vein usually suffices to preclude infarction of the intestine.

PATHOLOGY: Infarcted bowel is edematous and diffusely purple. The demarcation between infarcted bowel and normal tissue is usually sharp, although venous occlusion may lead to a more diffuse appearance. Extensive hemorrhage is seen in the mucosa and submucosa. Hemorrhage is prominent especially in venous occlusion (e.g., mesenteric vein thrombosis). The mucosal surface shows irregular white sloughs, the wall becomes thin and distended and bubbles of gas (pneumatosis) may be present in the bowel wall and mesenteric veins. The serosal surface is cloudy and covered by an inflammatory exudate.

Dysfunction of smooth muscle interferes with peristalsis and leads to **adynamic ileus,** in which the bowel proximal to the lesion is dilated and filled with fluid. Intestinal organisms may pass through the damaged wall and cause **peritonitis** or **septicemia.**

In nonocclusive intestinal ischemia, the principal lesion is restricted initially to the mucosa. Mucosal changes range from foci of dilated capillaries with a few extravasated erythrocytes to severe hemorrhagic necrosis and bleeding into the lumen. If the patient survives the episode of hypoperfusion, the bowel may be completely repaired, or it may heal with granulation tissue and fibrosis, with eventual **stricture formation.**

CLINICAL FEATURES: Mesenteric artery occlusion is heralded by abrupt onset of abdominal pain. Bloody diarrhea, hematemesis, and shock are common. In untreated cases, perforation is frequent. *As infarction progresses, systemic manifestations become more severe (multiple organ dysfunction syndrome).* In extensive infarction, as a result of occlusion in the proximal portion of the superior mesenteric artery, almost the entire small bowel must be resected, a situation not compatible with ultimate survival.

Chronic Intestinal Ischemia Leads to Recurrent Abdominal Pain

Atherosclerotic narrowing of major splanchnic arteries leads to chronic intestinal ischemia. As in the heart, it causes intermittent abdominal pain, termed **intestinal (abdominal) angina.** Characteristically, the pain begins within a half hour of eating and lasts for a few hours. Many cases of frank infarction of the intestine are preceded by abdominal angina. Recurrent abdominal pain may also reflect pressure on the celiac axis from surrounding structures and has been labeled the **celiac compression syndrome.**

PATHOLOGY: Chronic small bowel ischemia may lead to fibrosis and stricture formation. Ischemic strictures of the small bowel may be single or multiple, and produce intestinal obstruction or, occasionally, malabsorption due to stasis and bacterial overgrowth. These strictures are concentric, and the mucosa of this region is atrophic and often exhibits one or more small ulcers. The submucosa is thickened and fibrotic and displays granulation tissue, which may extend into the muscular layers Hemosiderin deposition may be prominent, particularly near the muscularis mucosae.

Malabsorption

Malabsorption is a general term that describes a number of clinical conditions in which important nutrients are inadequately absorbed by the gastrointestinal tract. Although some nutrient absorption occurs in the stomach and colon, only absorption from the small intestine, mainly in the proximal portion, is clinically important. Two substances are preferentially absorbed by the distal small intestine: bile salts and vitamin B_{12}.

Normal intestinal absorption is characterized by a luminal phase and an intestinal phase (Fig. 13-30). The **luminal phase,** consisting of those processes that occur within the lumen of the small intestine, alters the physicochemical state of the various nutrients so that they can be taken up by the small bowel absorptive cells. The **intestinal phase** includes those processes that occur in the cells and transport channels of the intestinal wall. Each phase includes several critical components; derangement of one or more leads to impaired absorption.

In the luminal phase of intestinal absorption, **pancreatic enzymes** and **bile acids** must be secreted into the duodenal lumen in adequate amounts and in a normal physicochemical condition. Two additional factors are important for optimal activity of both pancreatic enzymes and bile salts: a normal and regulated flow of gastric contents into the duodenum and an appropriately high pH of the duodenal contents. Normal pancreatic enzyme excretion into the duodenum requires adequate pancreatic exocrine function and an unobstructed flow of pancreatic juice.

Supply of a normal quantity and quality of bile to the duodenum requires (1) adequate hepatocellular function, (2) unobstructed flow of bile, and (3) intact enterohepatic circulation of bile salts. The enterohepatic circulation of bile begins with absorption of most intestinal bile salts from the distal ileum and ends with their excretion into the duodenum through the bile ducts. Normally, 95% of intestinal bile salts are recycled through the enterohepatic circulation; 5% are excreted in the stools. Normal functioning of the enterohepatic circulation requires (1) normal intestinal microflora, (2) normal ileal absorptive function, and (3) an unobstructed biliary system.

Luminal-Phase Malabsorption Often Reflects Insufficient Bile Acids

- **Interruption of the normal continuity of the distal stomach and duodenum** occurs after gastroduodenal surgery (gastrectomy, antrectomy, pyloroplasty).
- **Pancreatic dysfunction** can occur as a result of chronic pancreatitis, pancreatic carcinoma, or cystic fibrosis.

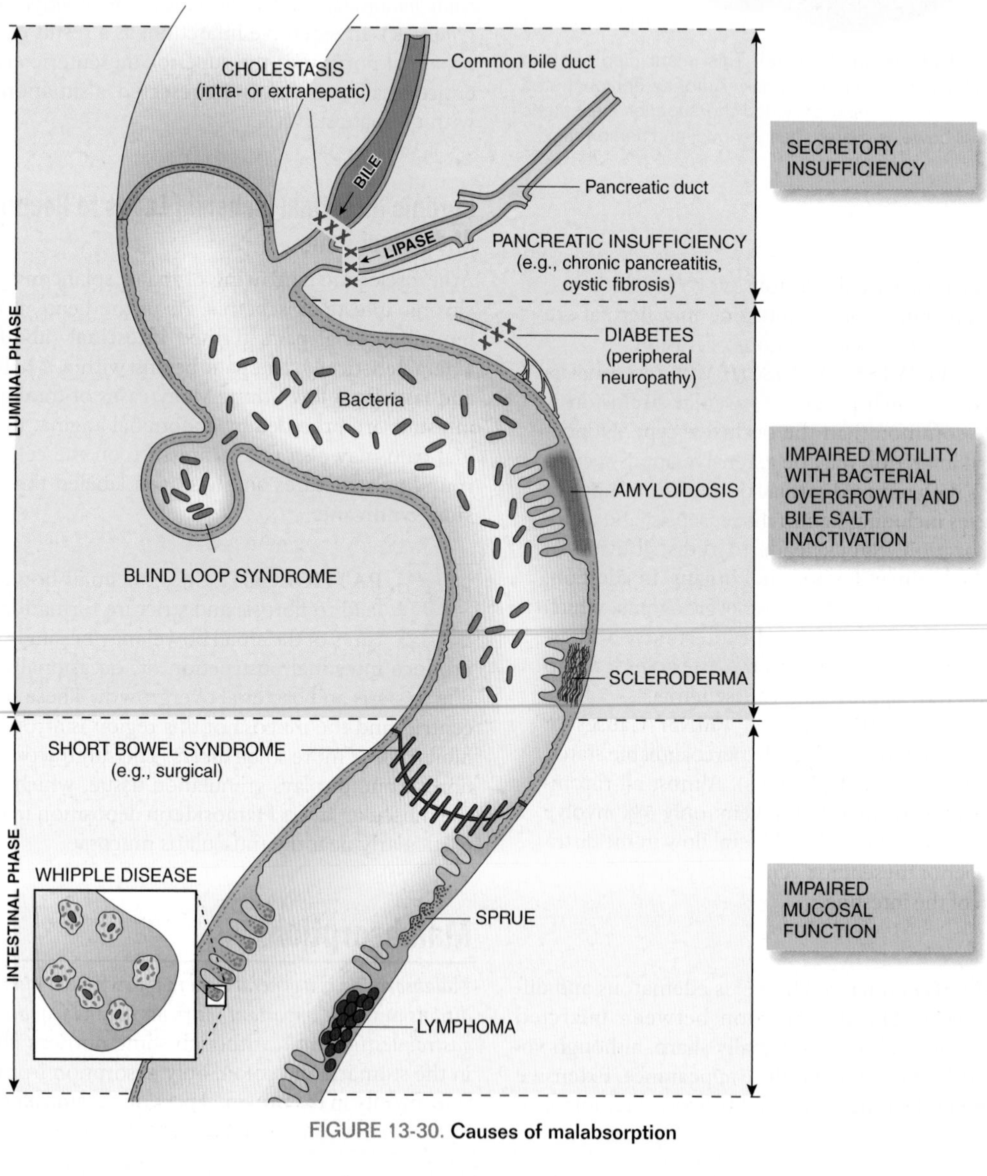

FIGURE 13-30. **Causes of malabsorption**

- **Deficient or ineffective bile salts** may result from three possible causes:
  1. **Impaired excretion of bile** resulting from liver disease.
  2. **Bacterial overgrowth** from a disturbance in gut motility. This is seen in such conditions as blind-loop syndrome, multiple diverticula of the small bowel, and muscular or neurogenic defects of the intestinal wall (e.g., amyloidosis, scleroderma, diabetic enteropathy). When gastrointestinal motility is defective, bile salts are deconjugated by the excess bacterial flora, after which they cannot form micelles, which are essential for normal absorption of monoglycerides and free fatty acids.
  3. **Deficient bile salts** due to the absence or bypass of the distal ileum caused by surgical excision, surgical anastomoses, fistulas, or ileal disease (e.g., Crohn disease, lymphoma).

Intestinal-Phase Malabsorption Frequently Reflects Specific Enzyme Defects or Impaired Transport

Although abnormalities in any one of the four components of the intestinal phase may cause malabsorption, some diseases affect more than one of these components. Figure 13-30 summarizes the major causes of malabsorption.

PATHOGENESIS:
MICROVILLI: The intestinal disaccharidases and oligopeptidases are integrally bound to the microvillous membranes. Disaccharidases are essential for sugar absorption, because only monosaccharides can be absorbed by intestinal epithelial cells. Oligopeptides and dipeptides may be absorbed by alternate mechanisms that do not require peptidases. Abnormal function of the microvilli may be primary, as in primary disaccharidase deficiencies; or secondary, when there is damage to the villi, as in celiac disease (sprue). The various enzyme deficiencies (e.g., of lactase) are characterized by intolerance for the corresponding disaccharides.

ABSORPTIVE AREA: The considerable length of the small bowel and the amplification of its surface wall by the intestinal folds (valves of Kerkring) provide a large absorptive surface. Severe diminution in this area may result in malabsorption. The surface area may be diminished by (1) small bowel resection (short bowel syndrome), (2) gastrocolic fistula (bypassing the small intestine), or (3) mucosal damage due to a number of small intestinal diseases (celiac disease, tropical sprue, and Whipple disease).

METABOLIC FUNCTION OF THE ABSORPTIVE CELLS: For their subsequent transport to the circulation, nutrients within the absorptive cells depend on their metabolism within these cells. Monoglycerides and free fatty acids are reassembled into triglycerides and coated with proteins (apoproteins) to form chylomicrons and lipoprotein particles. Specific metabolic dysfunction is seen in abetalipoproteinemia (associated with erythrocyte acanthocytosis), a disorder in which the absorptive cells cannot synthesize the apoprotein required for the assembly of lipoproteins and chylomicrons. Nonspecific damage to small intestinal epithelial cells occurs in celiac disease, tropical sprue, Whipple disease, and hyperacidity due to gastrinoma.

TRANSPORT: Nutrients are transported from the intestinal epithelium through the intestinal wall by way of blood capillaries and lymphatic vessels. Impaired transport of nutrients through these conduits is probably an important factor in the malabsorption associated with Whipple disease, intestinal lymphoma, and congenital lymphangiectasia.

CLINICAL FEATURES: Malabsorption may be either specific or generalized.

- ***Specific or isolated malabsorption*** *refers to an identifiable molecular defect that causes malabsorption of a single nutrient.* Examples of this group are the disaccharidase deficiencies (notably lactase deficiency) and deficiency of gastric intrinsic factor, which causes malabsorption of vitamin B_{12} and consequently pernicious anemia. Specific deficiency states may present with anemia due to deficiency of iron, folic acid, or vitamin B_{12} or a combination of these three. Patients may have a bleeding diathesis due to vitamin K deficiency or malabsorption of vitamin D and calcium may lead to tetany, osteomalacia (in adults), or rickets (in children). In some persons, a deficiency of water-soluble vitamins of the B group may occur.
- ***Generalized malabsorption*** *describes a condition in which absorption of several or all major nutrient classes is impaired.* It leads to generalized malnutrition. In adults, this appears as weight loss and sometimes cachexia; in children, it is expressed as "failure to thrive" with poor growth and weight gain.

Secondary effects of nonabsorbed or partially absorbed substances may lead to diarrhea. In disaccharidase deficiency, unhydrolyzed sugars in the gut are metabolized by colonic bacteria to lactic acid, carbon dioxide (CO_2), and water, causing explosive fermentative diarrhea. In patients with ileal dysfunction, bile salts that are not absorbed enter the colon and cause choleretic diarrhea because of they stimulate colonic secretion.

Laboratory Evaluation Detects Specific Forms of Malabsorption

Diverse laboratory tests are used to assess malabsorption. For example, disaccharidase deficiency is diagnosed by measuring blood sugar after oral administration of a standard amount of disaccharide, as in the **lactose-tolerance test,** or by quantitating disaccharidase activity in small bowel biopsy specimens. Vitamin B_{12} absorption is assessed by the **Schilling test,** in which isotopically labeled vitamin B_{12} is given orally and its blood level then determined. This test helps to distinguish between malabsorption resulting from intrinsic-factor deficiency and other causes of vitamin B_{12} malabsorption.

In generalized malabsorption, there is almost always impaired absorption of dietary fat. Quantitative fecal fat analysis is the most reliable and sensitive test of overall digestive and absorptive function and is a standard for all other tests for malabsorption. Steatorrhea (fat in the stools) is the hallmark of generalized malabsorption, and the two terms are often used interchangeably.

A few of the tests currently in use for the evaluation of various causes of malabsorption merit mention.

- **D-Xylose Absorption:** Xylose is a 5-carbon sugar whose absorption does not require any of the components of the luminal phase. Blood levels and urinary excretion of this compound after ingestion of a defined amount thus serve as useful tests for the intestinal phase of absorption.

- **$^{14}CO_2$-cholyl-glycine breath test:** Measurement of $^{14}CO_2$ in exhaled air after oral administration of $^{14}CO_2$-cholylglycine is a test of bile salt absorption by the ileum. It is used in the diagnosis of the blind- or stagnant-loop syndrome (caused by bacterial overgrowth) and of ileal absorptive function. A newer test to detect bacterial overgrowth is the ^{14}C-xylose breath test.
- **Schilling test:** Originally devised to diagnose pernicious anemia, this test has been modified to test ileal absorption, bacterial overgrowth, and pancreatic function.

Lactase Deficiency Causes Intolerance to Milk Products

The intestinal brush border contains disaccharidases that are important for the absorption of carbohydrates. As a prominent constituent of milk and many other dairy products, lactose is one of the most common disaccharides in the diet. Acquired lactase deficiency is a widespread disorder of carbohydrate absorption. Typically, symptoms of the disease begin in adolescence. Patients complain of abdominal distention, flatulence, and diarrhea after the ingestion of dairy products. Eliminating milk and its products from the diet relieves these symptoms. Diseases that injure the intestinal mucosa (e.g., celiac disease or radiation enteritis) may also lead to acquired lactase deficiency. Congenital lactase deficiency is rare but may be lethal if not recognized.

Celiac Disease Reflects an Immune Response to Gluten in Cereals

Celiac disease (celiac sprue, gluten-sensitive enteropathy) is characterized by (1) generalized malabsorption, (2) small intestinal mucosal lesion,s and (3) prompt clinical and histopathologic response to withdrawal of gluten-containing foods from the diet.

EPIDEMIOLOGY: Celiac disease is worldwide and affects all ethnic groups. There is a slight female predominance, 1.3:1. It may be seen any time after cereals are introduced into the diet. Most cases are diagnosed during childhood, although the disease may become clinically apparent for the first time as late as the seventh decade of life.

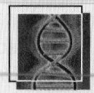

PATHOGENESIS: Genetic predisposition and gliadin exposure are crucial factors in the development of celiac disease.

ROLE OF CEREAL PROTEINS: Experiments on successfully treated, asymptomatic patients with celiac disease have shown that ingestion or instillation of wheat, barley, or rye flour into the small intestine is followed by the clinical and histopathologic features of celiac sprue. Other grains, such as rice and corn flour, do not have such an effect. Both the water-insoluble portion of wheat flour, **gluten** and an alcoholic extract called **gliadin** have the same effect.

GENETIC FACTORS: Celiac sprue is caused by an interplay of complex genetic factors plus an abnormal immune response to ingested cereal antigens. Overt and latent celiac disease run in families. Concordance for celiac disease in first-degree relatives ranges between 8% and 18% and reaches 70% in monozygotic twins. About 90% of patients with celiac disease carry the histocompatibility antigen human leukocyte antigen (HLA)-B8 and a comparable frequency has been reported for HLA DR8 and DQ2.

IMMUNOLOGIC FACTORS: The intestinal lesion in celiac disease is characterized by damage to the epithelial cells and a marked increase in the number of T lymphocytes within the epithelium and of plasma cells in the lamina propria. Gliadin challenge of persons with treated celiac sprue stimulates local immunoglobulin synthesis.

A region of amino acid sequence homology has been found between α-gliadin and a protein of an adenovirus (serotype 12) that infects the human gastrointestinal tract. Most (90%) untreated patients with celiac disease have serologic evidence of prior infection with this virus. Exposure of a genetically susceptible person to gluten-containing cereals might then stimulate an immune reaction to gliadin at the intestinal epithelial cell surface.

Serum antigliadin and anti-endomysial antibodies are present in almost all patients, but their role in the pathogenesis of the disease remains to be established.

ASSOCIATION WITH DERMATITIS HERPETIFORMIS: Celiac disease is occasionally associated with dermatitis herpetiformis (DH), a vesicular skin disease that typically affects extensor surfaces and exposed parts of the body. In DH, subepidermal neutrophil infiltration leads to local edema and blister formation. Basement membrane IgA deposits are detected. Almost all patients with DH have a small bowel mucosal lesion similar to that of celiac disease, although only 10% have overt malabsorption. Treatment with a strict gluten-free diet leads to improvement in both gastrointestinal symptoms and skin lesions. The histocompatibility antigen HLA-B8 is much more frequent in patients with dermatitis herpetiformis than in normal persons.

Malabsorption in celiac disease probably results from multiple factors, including reduced intestinal mucosa surface area (due to blunting of villi and microvilli) and impaired intracellular metabolism within damaged epithelial cells. A probable aggravating factor is secondary disaccharidase deficiency, related to damage to microvilli. A hypothetical mechanism for the pathogenesis of celiac disease is presented in Figure 13-31.

PATHOLOGY: A microscopic finding in small bowel biopsies that can precede the more characteristic findings is an intraepithelial lymphocytic infiltrate involving crypts and surface epithelium in normal appearing villi. The hallmark of fully developed celiac disease is a flat mucosa, with (1) blunting or total disappearance of villi, (2) damaged mucosal surface epithelial cells with numerous intraepithelial lymphocytes (T cells), and (3) increased plasma cells in the lamina propria but not in deeper layers (Fig. 13-32). The most severe histologic abnormalities in untreated celiac disease usually occur in the duodenum and proximal jejunum. There is a progressive decrease in severity distally and in some cases the ileal mucosa appears virtually normal. The clinical severity of the disease is related to the length of the affected intestine.

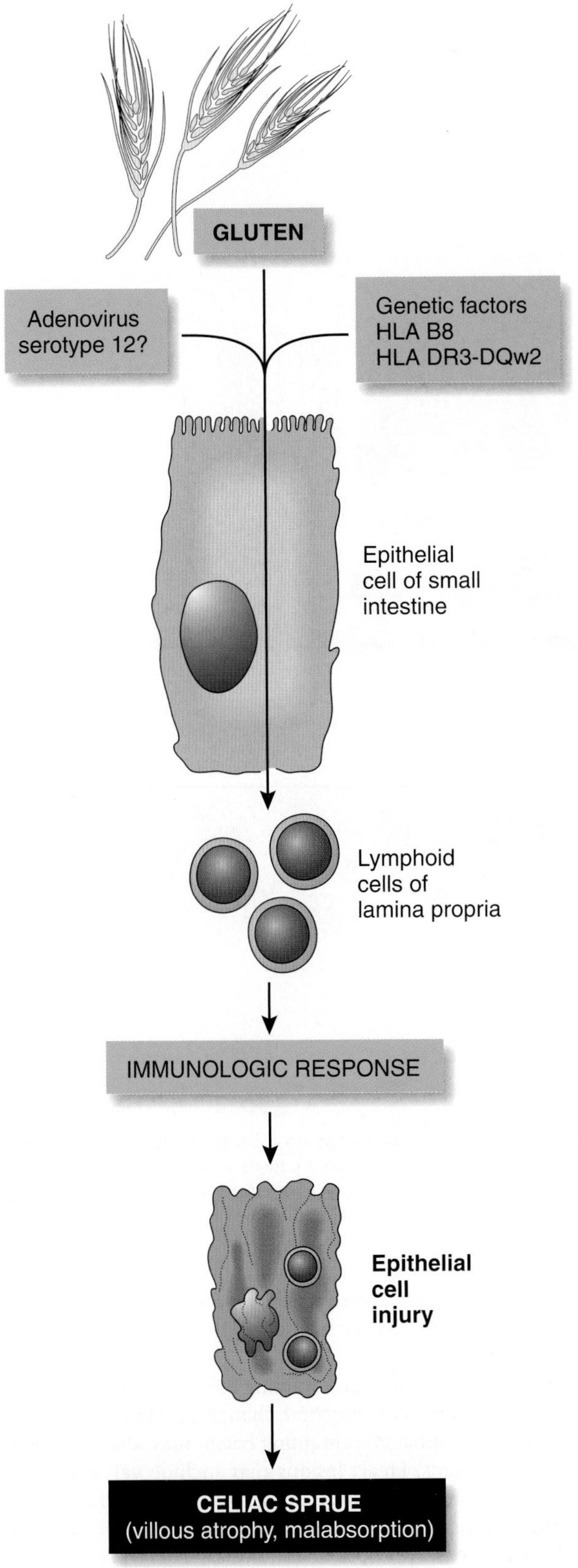

FIGURE 13-31. **Hypothetical mechanisms in the pathogenesis of celiac disease.** HLA = human leukocyte antigen.

The total mucosal thickness may not be decreased, because lengthening of the crypts compensates for villous shortening. The absorptive cells are flattened and more basophilic than normal, and the basal polarity of their nuclei is lost. Lymphocytes and plasma cells in the lamina propria are markedly increased. Most of the plasma cells produce IgA (as in the normal small bowel). Polymorphonuclear leukocytes and eosinophils may also be increased in the epithelium and lamina propria.

CLINICAL FEATURES: *Fully developed celiac disease is characterized by generalized malabsorption.* Not infrequently, overt signs of malabsorption in children are lacking, and the disease is suspected only because of growth retardation. In adults, iron deficiency anemia resistant to oral therapy is often the clue to celiac disease. The symptoms and signs of generalized malabsorption are often initially manifested in older children, adolescents, and adults. With the application of IgA anti-endomysial and IgA anti-tissue transglutaminase antibodies, it has become evident that celiac disease is more common than previously thought.

The systemic manifestations of celiac disease are related to the various deficiency states that result from generalized malabsorption. Late complications in some cases include ulcerative jejunitis and small bowel T-cell lymphoma. Adenocarcinoma of the small bowel and carcinoma of the oropharynx and esophagus also occur and an increased risk for colorectal carcinoma is reported. Other extraintestinal manifestations include follicular keratosis, peripheral neuropathy, and infertility. Treatment with a strict gluten-free diet is usually followed by a complete and prolonged clinical and histopathologic remission. Some patients have refractory sprue and respond only to corticosteroids.

Collagenous sprue *refers to a rare disorder characterized by the deposition of collagen in the lamina propria of the small bowel.* The disorder initially mimics celiac disease but does not respond to removal of gluten from the diet. The prognosis in collagenous sprue is grave: all reported patients have died of the disease.

Whipple Disease Is a Rare Infection of the Small Bowel

Malabsorption is the most prominent feature of Whipple disease. White men in their 30s and 40s are most affected. The disease is systemic, and other clinical findings include fever, increased skin pigmentation, anemia, lymphadenopathy, arthritis, pericarditis, pleurisy, endocarditis, and central nervous system involvement.

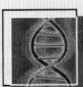

PATHOGENESIS: *Whipple disease typically shows infiltration of the small bowel mucosa by macrophages packed with small, rod-shaped bacilli.* The causative organism is one of the actinomycetes, *Tropheryma whippelii.* Interestingly, *T. whippelii* is distantly related to mycobacteria such as *Mycobacterium avium-intracellulare* and *Mycobacterium paratuberculosis,* both of which have been associated with illnesses resembling Whipple disease. The results of several studies suggest that host susceptibility factors, possibly defective T-lymphocyte function, may be important in predisposing to the disease. Macrophages from patients with Whipple disease exhibit decreased ability to degrade intracellular microorganisms. Circulating cells expressing CD11b, a cell-adhesion and complement-receptor molecule on macrophages, are reduced. CD11b is involved in activating macrophages to kill intracellular pathogens. Dramatic clinical remissions occur with antibiotic therapy.

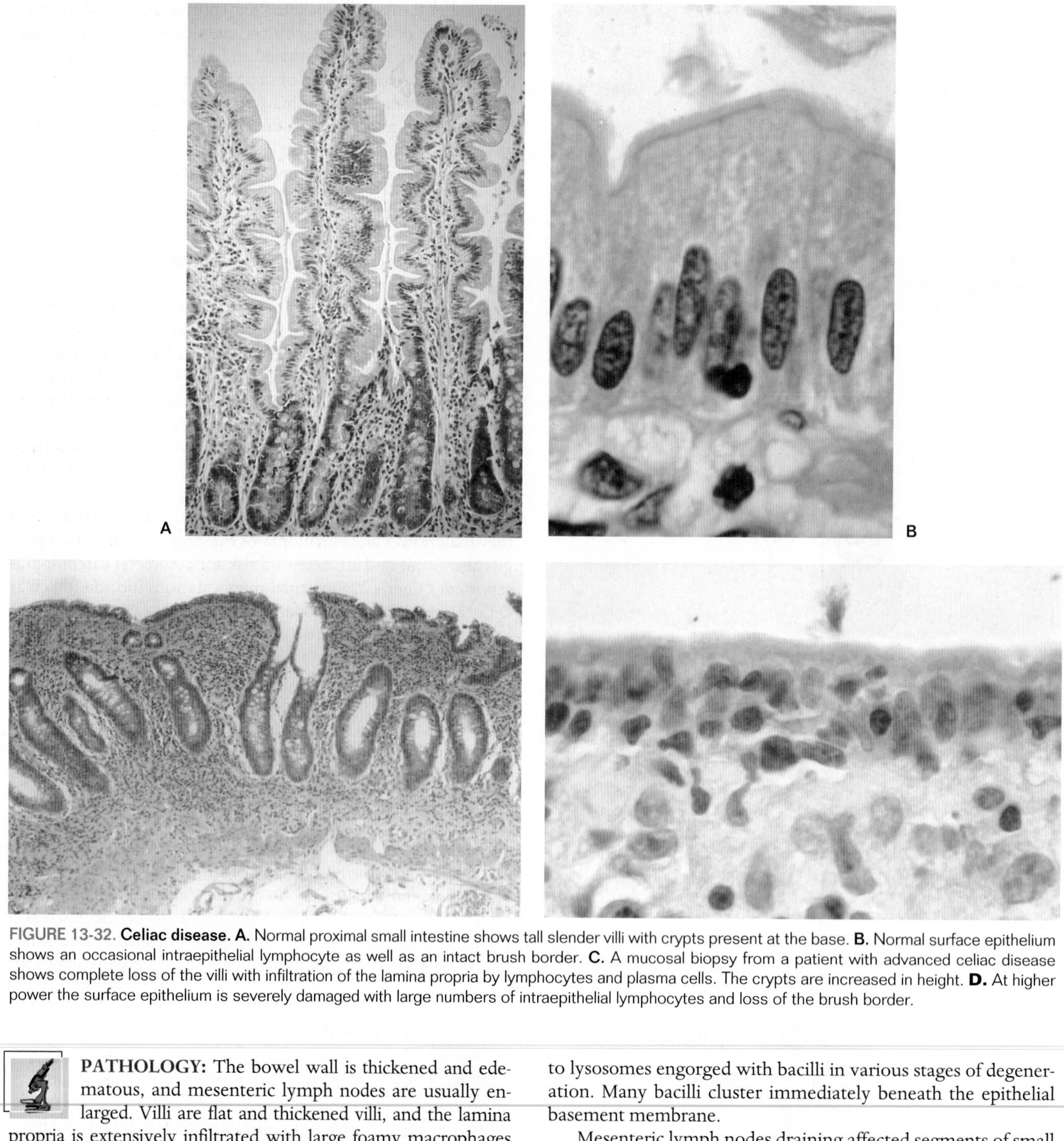

FIGURE 13-32. **Celiac disease. A.** Normal proximal small intestine shows tall slender villi with crypts present at the base. **B.** Normal surface epithelium shows an occasional intraepithelial lymphocyte as well as an intact brush border. **C.** A mucosal biopsy from a patient with advanced celiac disease shows complete loss of the villi with infiltration of the lamina propria by lymphocytes and plasma cells. The crypts are increased in height. **D.** At higher power the surface epithelium is severely damaged with large numbers of intraepithelial lymphocytes and loss of the brush border.

PATHOLOGY: The bowel wall is thickened and edematous, and mesenteric lymph nodes are usually enlarged. Villi are flat and thickened villi, and the lamina propria is extensively infiltrated with large foamy macrophages (Fig. 13-33A) whose *cytoplasm is filled with large glycoprotein granules that stain strongly with periodic acid–Schiff (PAS)* (see Fig. 13-33B). The other normal cellular components of the lamina propria (i.e., plasma cells and lymphocytes) are depleted. The lymphatic vessels in the mucosa and submucosa are dilated and large lipid droplets abound within lymphatics and in extracellular spaces, a finding that suggests lymphatic obstruction. In contrast to the striking distortion of the villous architecture, epithelial cells show only patchy abnormalities, including attenuation of microvilli and accumulation of lipid droplets within the cytoplasm.

Electron-microscopic examination reveals numerous small bacilli within macrophages and free in the lamina propria (see Fig. 13-33C). The PAS-positive granules seen by light microscopy correspond to lysosomes engorged with bacilli in various stages of degeneration. Many bacilli cluster immediately beneath the epithelial basement membrane.

Mesenteric lymph nodes draining affected segments of small bowel reveal similar microscopic changes. A characteristic infiltration by macrophages containing bacilli may also be found in most other organs. Heart lesions may include valvular vegetations which contain bacilli-laden macrophages, sometimes with superimposed streptococcal endocarditis. Treatment of Whipple disease is with appropriate antibiotics.

Abetalipoproteinemia Involves Failure to Make Apoprotein B

Abetalipoproteinemia is inherited as an autosomal recessive disease. The missing apoprotein B is a constituent of the membrane coat of low-density lipoproteins. Small intestinal absorptive cells that lack

A B C

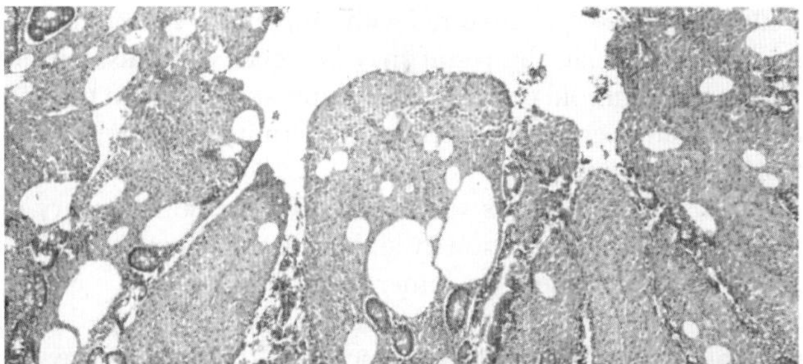

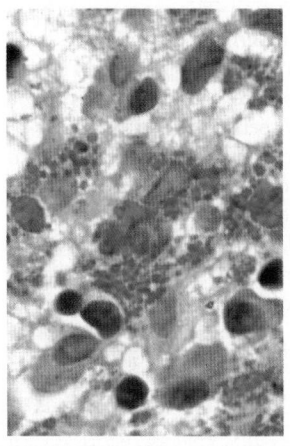

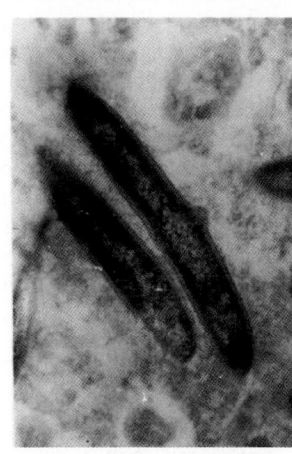

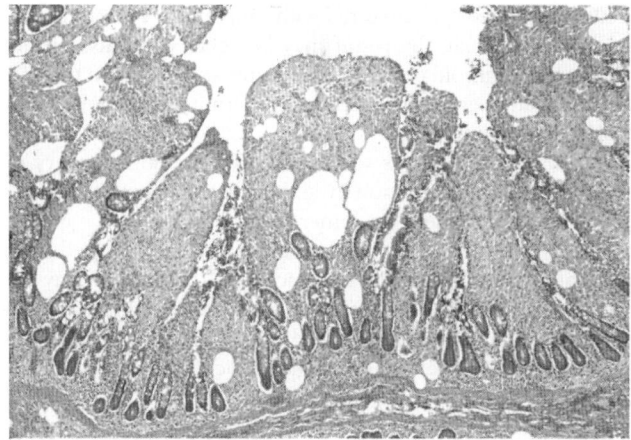

FIGURE 13-33. **Whipple disease. A.** A photomicrograph of a section of jejunal mucosa shows distortion of the villi. The lamina propria is packed with large, pale-staining macrophages. Dilated mucosal lymphatics are prominent. **B.** A periodic acid–Schiff (PAS) reaction shows numerous macrophages filled with cytoplasmic granular material. **C.** An electron micrograph shows small bacilli in a macrophage.

apoprotein B do not assemble chylomicrons, an essential component of lipid transport out of the cell. This leads to acanthocytosis in erythrocytes and selective demyelinization, particularly of the posterior columns in the central nervous system. Typical neurologic manifestations are loss of deep tendon reflexes, sensory ataxia, and a mild form of retinitis pigmentosa. The serum shows a total absence of chylomicrons, very-low-density lipoproteins and low-density lipoproteins. In addition, serum levels of cholesterol and triglycerides are low and serum lipids are mostly carried within high-density lipoprotein particles.

Microscopically, the villi, lamina propria, and submucosa appear normal. The epithelial cells contain lipid vacuoles, but no lipid is seen in intestinal lymphatics. This lipid probably represents triglyceride that has been assembled within the cell but cannot be transported into the basolateral intercellular space because of the lack of apoprotein B.

Malabsorption in abetalipoproteinemia is partially reversed by ingestion of medium-chain (rather than the usual long-chain) triglycerides; these lipids are transported through the absorptive cells without an apoprotein coat.

Hypogammaglobulinemia May Lead to Malabsorption

The small intestine in hypogammaglobulinemia contains few or no plasma cells in the lamina propria, and often displays nodular lymphoid hyperplasia. Occasionally, there is a flat mucosa, similar to the lesion of celiac sprue; in this case, the disorder is termed **hypogammaglobulinemic sprue.**

Most hypogammaglobulinemic patients with malabsorption have small intestinal infection with *Giardia lamblia.* Treatment with metronidazole is followed by improved intestinal absorption.

Congenital Lymphangiectasia Is a Generalized Malformation That Causes Malabsorption

Congenital lymphangiectasia is a poorly understood disease that usually begins in childhood. In addition to steatorrhea caused by impaired transport of chylomicrons by intestinal lymphatics, these patients have **protein-losing enteropathy,** i.e., excessive loss of plasma proteins into the gut. A syndrome of intestinal lymphangiectasia and peripheral lymphedema is known as **Milroy disease.**

Other important features of congenital lymphangiectasia are lymphopenia and impaired cell-mediated immunity, caused by loss of small lymphocytes into the bowel lumen. Chylous ascites (milky, lipid-containing peritoneal fluid), due to leakage of lymph from the mesenteric or serosal lymphatic vessels into the peritoneal cavity may occur.

Grossly, lesions of congenital lymphangiectasia are opalescent white spots which microscopically are **dilated lymphatics (lacteals)** in the lamina propria. The submucosal lymphatics also tend to be dilated. The epithelium is normal, but the villi may be blunted or even absent in areas overlying severe lymphatic dilation.

Acquired intestinal lymphangiectasia, with all or some of the clinical features described above, may be a secondary manifestation of small intestinal or retroperitoneal lymphoma, other retroperitoneal tumors, tuberculosis, sarcoidosis, chronic pancreatitis, and retroperitoneal fibrosis.

Tropical Sprue Is a Disease of Unknown Etiology That Causes Folate Deficiency

Tropical sprue is endemic in certain tropical areas and is characterized by progressively severe malabsorption and nutritional deficiency. Cure, or at least amelioration of symptoms, usually follows treatment with oral tetracycline and folic acid. The cause of tropical sprue is not known. Some studies suggest that **long-standing contamination of the bowel with bacteria,** perhaps toxigenic strains of *E. coli,* may be important and that the resultant **folate deficiency** may play a role in perpetuating the intestinal lesion.

The histologic findings are variable, ranging from mild widening and blunting of villi to a completely flat mucosa similar to that seen in celiac sprue. The morphologic injury in the epithelium and the inflammation of the lamina propria usually parallel the severity of the alterations in the villi.

Typically, steatorrhea, anemia, and weight loss are followed by progressively severe manifestations of folic acid and vitamin B_{12} deficiencies, and hypoalbuminemia. Laboratory findings include increased fecal fat, impaired D-xylose absorption, megaloblastic anemia, and decreased disaccharidase activity in the intestinal mucosa.

Radiation Enteritis Results From Abdominal Radiotherapy

Transient damage to the small intestinal mucosa is seen. Anorexia, abdominal cramps, and changes in bowel habits occur frequently during abdominal radiation treatments, and laboratory studies in such patients indicate malabsorption of bile salts and disaccharides. Transient histologic changes include shortening of small bowel villi, increased cellularity in the lamina propria, and submucosal edema.

Occasionally, subacute or chronic radiation damage occurs, especially if (1) the radiation dose is very high, (2) segments of small bowel become fixed as a result of postoperative or inflammatory adhesions, (3) the bowel's blood supply is impaired, or (4) radiation is combined with chemotherapeutic agents that may augment radiation damage.

The major histologic features of subacute and chronic radiation damage to the small intestine are similar to those elsewhere in the gastrointestinal tract and include (1) mucosal ulceration, (2) swelling and detachment of endothelial cells of small arterioles in the submucosa, (3) obliteration by fibrin plugs of arteriolar lumina, and (4) large foam cells beneath the intima. Thickening and fibrosis of the submucosa ensue, together with signs of progressive ischemia, to produce stricture.

Mechanical Obstruction

Mechanical obstruction to the passage of intestinal contents can be caused by (1) a luminal mass, (2) an intrinsic lesion of the bowel wall, or (3) extrinsic compression.

INTUSSUSCEPTION: In this form of intraluminal small bowel obstruction a segment of bowel (intussusceptum) protrudes distally into a surrounding outer portion (intussuscipiens) (Fig. 13-34). Intussesception usually occurs in infants or young children, in whom it occurs without a known cause. In adults, the leading point of an intussusception is usually a lesion in the bowel wall, such as Meckel diverticulum or a tumor. Once the leading point is entrapped in the intussuscipiens, peristalsis drives the intussusceptum forward. In addition to acute intestinal obstruction, intussusception compresses the blood supply to the intussusceptum, which may become infarcted. If the obstruction is not relieved spontaneously, treatment requires surgery.

VOLVULUS: This is a cause of an acute abdomen and is an example of intestinal obstruction in which a segment of gut twists on its mesentery, kinking the bowel and usually interrupting its blood supply. Volvulus virtually always indicates an underlying congenital abnormality. Malrotation of the bowel permits undue mobility of the bowel loops and predisposes to **midgut volvulus.** When the cecum or right colon is invested with a mesentery rather than being retroperitoneal, the result may be **cecal volvulus.** An unusually long sigmoid colon, which occurs sometimes in patients with idiopathic chronic constipation, permits the development of **sigmoid volvulus.**

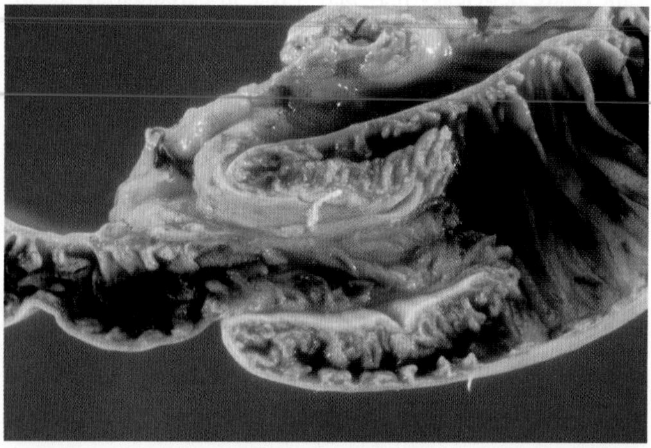

FIGURE 13-34. **Intussusception.** A cross section through the area of the obstruction shows "telescoped" small intestine surrounded by dilated small intestine.

ADHESIONS: Fibrous scars caused by previous surgery or peritonitis cause obstruction by kinking or angulating the bowel or directly compressing the lumen.

HERNIAS: Loops of small bowel may be incarcerated in an inguinal or femoral hernia, in which case, the lumen may become obstructed and the vascular supply compromised. Similarly, portions of the bowel may be trapped internally by hernias that represent congenital or surgically acquired defects in the mesentery.

PSEUDO-OBSTRUCTION: Patients who have signs and symptoms of intestinal obstruction but who lack overt mechanical causes are said to have pseudo-obstruction. The process may be familial or sporadic. There may be an underlying myopathy or a neuropathy, but in many cases no anatomic lesion is found. The myopathies feature fibrosis around muscle cells in the lamina propria. Neuronal inclusions are occasionally seen in the neuropathies.

A particularly common form of psuedo-obstruction is limited to the colon in which no morphologic lesion is usually demonstrable, referred to as severe idiopathic constipation. Pseudo-obstruction may be secondary to intestinal involvement by diseases such as scleroderma, amyloidosis, hypothroidism, or adverse drug effect. Such cases are often referred to as secondary pseudo-obstruction.

Neoplasms

Less than 5% of all gastrointestinal tumors arise in the small intestine.

Benign Tumors Include Adenomas, Peutz-Jeghers Polyps, and Stromal Tumors

Adenomas

Small bowel adenomas resemble those of the colon. Depending on the predominant component, adenomatous polyps of the small intestine may be tubular, villous, or tubulovillous. Villous adenoma is rare in the small intestine, usually occurring in the duodenum, especially the periampullary region. Adenomas, especially the villous type, may undergo malignant transformation. Benign adenomas are frequently asymptomatic, but bleeding and intussusception are occasional complications.

Peutz–Jeghers Syndrome

Peutz–Jeghers syndrome is an autosomal dominant hereditary disorder characterized by intestinal hamartomatous polyps and mucocutaneous melanin pigmentation, which is particularly evident on the face, buccal mucosa, hands, feet, and perianal and genital areas. Except for the buccal pigmentation, the frecklelike macular lesions usually fade at puberty. The polyps occur mostly in the proximal small intestine but are sometimes seen in the stomach and the colon. Patients usually have symptoms of obstruction or intussusception; in as many as one fourth of cases, however, the diagnosis is suggested by pigmentation in an otherwise asymptomatic person.

Peutz-Jeghers syndrome is associated with inactivating mutations of a gene (*LKB1*) on chromosome 19p that encodes a protein kinase. Carriers of the defective gene are also at increased risk for cancers of the breast, pancreas, testis, and ovary.

Peutz-Jeghers polyps are hamartomas, with branching networks of smooth muscle fibers continuous with the muscularis mucosae supports the glandular epithelium of the polyp (Fig. 13-35). Peutz-Jeghers polyps are generally considered benign, but 3% of patients develop adenocarcinoma, although not necessarily in the hamartomatous polyps.

Gastrointestinal Stromal Tumors

GISTs occur throughout the small intestine but most often in the jejunum. They grow as intramural masses covered by intact mucosa and are similar to those in other locations. Intestinal obstruction is uncommon, but volvulus may be a complication. Small intestinal GIST tumors are more likely to behave aggressively than their gastric counterparts.

Malignant Tumors of the Small Bowel are Uncommon

Adenocarcinoma

EPIDEMIOLOGY: Although small intestinal adenocarcinomas are a minute proportion of all gastrointestinal tumors, they account for half of all malignant small bowel tumors. Most are located in the duodenum and jejunum. The majority occur in middle-aged persons, and there is a moderate male predominance. Interestingly, the geographic variation in the incidence of small bowel adenocarcinoma correlates with that of colon cancer but not with that of stomach cancer.

Crohn disease of the small bowel is a risk factor for adenocarcinoma. For such patients, the mean age for developing adenocarcinoma is 10 years younger than the average. Such cancers tend to occur in the same area as the inflammatory lesions, namely the ileum. Familial adenomatous polyposis, HNPCC syndrome (Lynch syndrome), and celiac disease are additional risk factors.

PATHOLOGY AND CLINICAL FEATURES: Adenocarcinoma of the small intestine may be polypoid or ulcerative or simply annular and stenosing. In addition to causing intestinal obstruction directly, a polypoid tumor may be the lead point of an intussusception. Adenocarcinomas originate from crypt epithelium, rather than the villi and, therefore, resemble colorectal cancers.

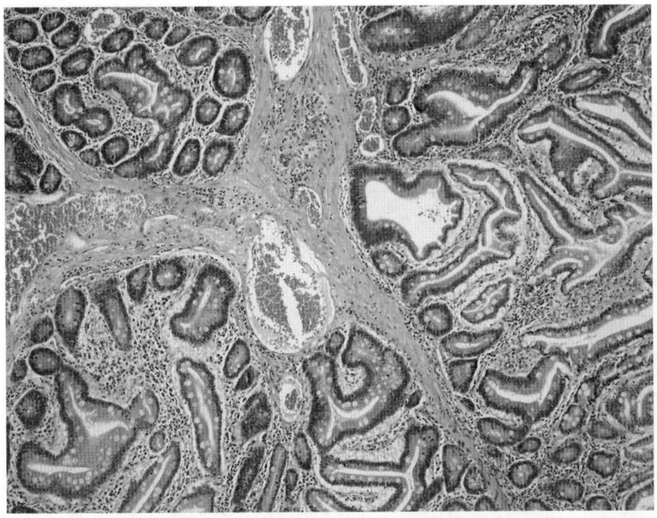

FIGURE 13-35. **Peutz-Jegher polyps.** The intestinal epithelium has peculiar shapes but unremarkable nuclear and cytoplasmic features. Arborizing large bundles of smooth muscle are characteristic.

The symptoms of small bowel adenocarcinoma commonly relate to progressive intestinal obstruction. Occult bleeding is common and often leads to iron-deficiency anemia. If adenocarcinoma of the duodenum involves the papilla of Vater, it is termed **ampullary carcinoma.** This tumor causes obstructive jaundice or pancreatitis. By the time the patient becomes symptomatic, most adenocarcinomas have metastasized to local lymph nodes and overall 5-year survival is less than 20%. This neoplasm is the second most common cause of death in patients with familial adenomatous polyposis.

Primary Intestinal Lymphoma

Primary lymphoma originates in nodules of lymphoid tissue normally present in the mucosa and superficial submucosa, termed mucosa-associated lymphoid tissue (MALT). Lymphoma is the second most common malignant tumor of the small intestine in industrialized countries, where it accounts for about 15% of small bowel cancers.

Another type of primary lymphoma comprises more than two-thirds of all cancers of the small intestine in less developed countries. The latter variety of intestinal lymphoma was originally described in Mediterranean populations, but it is now clear that it is distributed throughout the poorer parts of the world. These two types of lymphoma have distinct epidemiologic, clinical, and pathologic features and are respectively termed, **Western type** and **Mediterranean lymphoma.**

The cause of primary lymphoma of the small bowel is unknown, but association with celiac disease is well documented, occurring in as many as one tenth of patients with primary lymphoma. The persistent activation of lymphocytes in the bowel is felt to predispose to subsequent development of T-cell lymphoma. However, while a gluten-free diet usually improves the inflammatory component of the enteropathy, T-cell lymphoma can still occur.

The risk of intestinal lymphoma is also increased in conditions that favor development of nodal lymphoma, particularly immunodeficiency following treatment with immunosuppressive drugs.

MEDITERRANEAN LYMPHOMA: Mediterranean lymphoma typically occurs in poor countries in young men of low socioeconomic status; it is therefore thought by some to have an environmental cause. This neoplasm is associated with **α-heavy chain disease,** a proliferative disorder of intestinal B lymphocytes that secrete the heavy chain of IgA without light chains. Mediterranean lymphoma and α—chain disease are believed to be the same disorder, termed **immunoproliferative small intestinal disease.**

Mediterranean intestinal lymphoma predominantly involves the duodenum and proximal jejunum. A long segment of small intestine, or even the entire small bowel, is characteristically affected. Typically a diffuse infiltrate of plasmacytoid lymphocytes or plasma cells is seen in the mucosa and submucosa (Fig. 13-36). Lymphomatous infiltration of the mucosa leads to mucosal atrophy and severe malabsorption.

WESTERN-TYPE INTESTINAL LYMPHOMA: This disorder usually affects adults older than 40 and children younger than 10. It is most common in the ileum, where it is seen as (1) a fungating mass that projects into the lumen, (2) an elevated ulcerated lesion, (3) a diffuse segmental thickening of the bowel wall, or (4) plaquelike mucosal nodules. As a result, intestinal

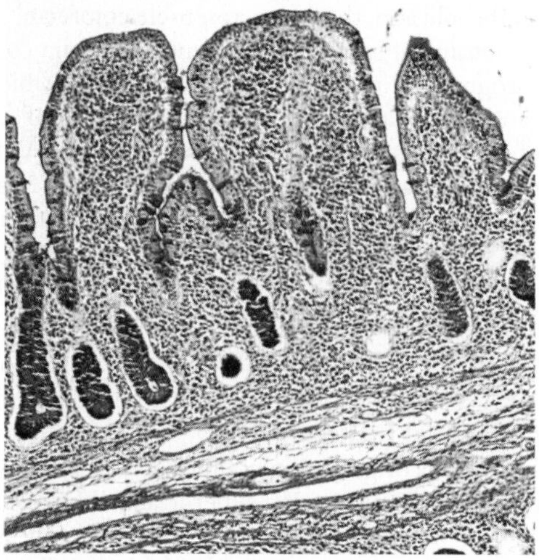

FIGURE 13-36. **Mediterranean intestinal lymphoma.** The villi are short and blunted, and the lamina propria is filled with lymphoid cells.

obstruction, intussusception, and perforation are important complications. Occult bleeding is common, although massive acute hemorrhage may also occur. Microscopically, all varieties of malignant lymphoma are encountered. Those associated with celiac disease tend to be T-cell lymphomas. When extraintestinal spread is present, the 5-year survival rate is less than 10%.

Chronic abdominal pain, diarrhea, and clubbing of fingers are the most frequent clinical signs of intestinal lymphoma. Diarrhea and weight loss reflect the underlying malabsorption. Patients with Mediterranean lymphoma tend to survive longer than those with the Western type of lymphoma.

Carcinoid Tumor (Neuroendocrine Tumors)

The term *carcinoid tumor* has been largely replaced by the term **neuroendocrine tumors** (NETs). These tumors are all considered malignant, but usually with low metastatic potential. The gut is the most common site for NETs (the bronchus is the next most common site). The site of origin is a major determinant of behavior. Other important considerations include size, depth of invasion, hormonal responsiveness, and presence or absence of function.

The appendix is the most common gastrointestinal site of origin, followed by the rectum. Tumors of these sites are usually small and rarely aggressive. The next most common site is ileum, where they are often multiple, and more aggressive. *NETs account for about 20% of all small intestinal malignancies.* They are also seen in association with the multiple endocrine neoplasia (MEN) syndromes, usually type I.

PATHOLOGY: Macroscopically, small carcinoid tumors present as submucosal nodules covered by intact mucosa. Large carcinoids may grow in a polypoid, intramural, or annular pattern (Fig. 13-37A) and often undergo secondary ulceration. The cut surface is firm and white to yellow. As they enlarge, carcinoid tumors invade the muscular coat and penetrate the serosa, often causing a conspicuous desmoplastic reaction. This fibrosis is responsible for peritoneal adhesions and kinking of the bowel, which may lead to intestinal obstruction.

Microscopically, these neoplasms appear as nests, cords and rosettes of uniform small, round cells (see Fig. 13-37B). Occasional glandlike structures are also seen. Nuclei are remarkably regular and mitoses are rare. Abundant eosinophilic cytoplasm contains cytoplasmic granules, which by electron microscopy are typically of the neurosecretory type. Goblet cell carcinoids or adenocarcinoid tumors have glandular differentiation. These tumors have a higher rate of aggressive behavior than do typical carcinoids.

NETs metastasize first to regional lymph nodes. Subsequently, hematogenous spread produces metastases at distant sites, particularly the liver.

CLINICAL FEATURES: Carcinoid syndrome is a unique but uncommon clinical condition caused by release of a variety of active tumor products that marks a small percentage of carcinoid tumors. Most NETs are to some extent functional, but this syndrome mainly occurs in patients with extensive hepatic metastases. *Classic symptoms include diarrhea (often the most distressing symptom), episodic flushing, bronchospasm, cyanosis, telangiectasia, and skin lesions.* Half of patients also have right-sided cardiac valvular disease. Diarrhea is thought to be caused by serotonin.

After its release into the blood, serotonin is metabolized to 5-hydroxyindoleacetic acid (5-HIAA) by monoamine oxidase either in the tumor or in other tissues. Urine 5-HIAA is a diagnostic test

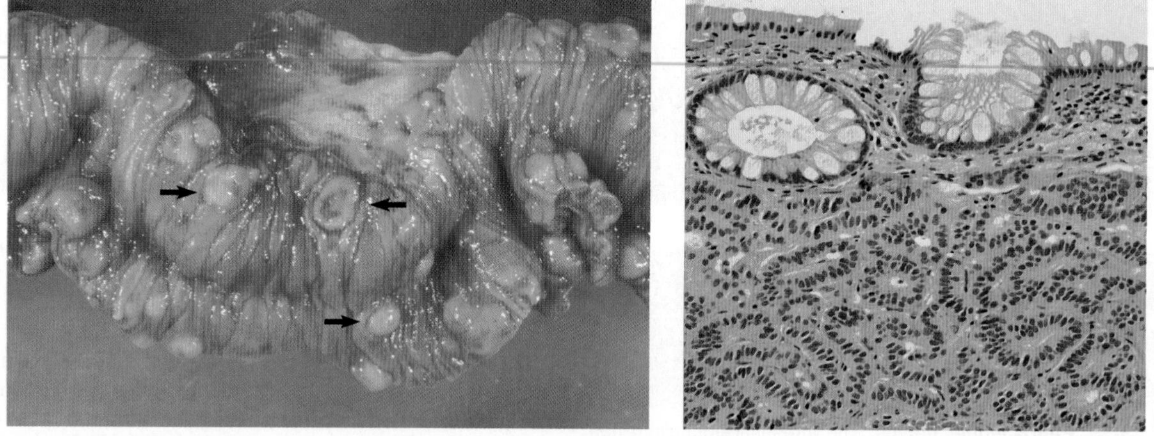

FIGURE 13-37. **Neuroendocrine tumor of small intestine. A.** A resected segment of distal ileum shows multiple neuroendocrine tumors (arrows). **B.** A photomicrograph of the lesion in *A* demonstrates cords of uniform small, round cells.

for the carcinoid syndrome. Whereas liver, lung, and brain all have high levels of activity of monoamine oxidase and (presumably) of enzymes that inactivate other tumor secretions, the right side of the heart is exposed to the full effects of tumor products that released into the vena cava from hepatic metastases. As a result, endocardial fibrosis occurs, probably as a reaction to endothelial damage. Fibrous plaques form on the tricuspid and pulmonic valves, the endocardium of the right-sided cardiac chambers, the vena cava, the coronary sinus, and the pulmonary artery. *Distortion of the valves leads to pulmonic stenosis and tricuspid regurgitation.*

Metastatic Tumors

The most common malignant tumors in the small intestine are metastatic. Cancer of adjacent organs (e.g., stomach, pancreas, or colon) may spread to the small intestine by direct extension. Lung and female genital organs and skin (melanomas) are the most frequent primary sites of small-intestinal metastases. Secondary involvement of the small intestine with systemic lymphoma may simulate metastatic carcinoma. Solitary, submucosal metastatic tumors may easily be mistaken for a primary cancer, and the symptoms may be indistinguishable.

Pneumatosis Cystoides Intestinalis

Pneumatosis cystoides intestinalis is an uncommon disorder in which numerous pockets of gas are found in the gut wall anywhere in the gastrointestinal tract. Most cases are associated with an underlying gastrointestinal disease, including intestinal obstruction, peptic ulcer, Crohn disease, mesenteric ischemia, volvulus, and neonatal necrotizing enterocolitis. Some are associated with chronic obstructive pulmonary disease or mechanical ventilation. Pneumatosis in adults is ordinarily benign, depending on the underlying disease. However, intestinal pneumatosis associated with neonatal necrotizing enteritis has a high mortality.

The cause of intestinal pneumatosis depends on the associated conditions. A mechanical break in mucosal continuity allows entry of air from the lumen to the submucosa. Alternatively, the gas can be a product of bacterial action, particularly in neonatal necrotizing enterocolitis. Dissection of air bubbles along the mesentery is common in patients with obstructive pulmonary disease or ventilation.

PATHOLOGY: Macroscopically, cysts appear as bubbles under the serosa of the intestine, and the bowel wall feels spongy. In some cases, air cysts are located principally in the submucosa, in which case, the cut surface of the bowel wall appears to be honeycombed. The cysts vary from a few millimeters to several centimeters in diameter. Cysts may also occur in the stomach and the mesentery. Microscopic examination reveals cystic spaces in the submucosa or beneath the serosa, which are often lined by large macrophages and multinucleated giant cells.

CLINICAL FEATURES: Many cases are found during investigation of symptoms unrelated to the pneumatosis. Some patients have episodic diarrhea. There is often blood in the stools, and rectal bleeding may be brisk. When intestinal pneumatosis is a complication of neonatal necrotizing enterocolitis, bowel perforation and peritonitis are frequent, but these complications are rare in adults.

Gas cysts may disappear spontaneously or may persist for years. Relief of symptoms may be obtained by oxygen inhalation or treatment with metronidazole.

THE LARGE INTESTINE

Anatomy

The large intestine is the portion of the gastrointestinal tract from the ileocecal valve to the anus. It is 90 to 125 cm in length in adults and includes the colon and rectum. Like the small intestine,the proximal colon is derived from embryonic midgut and supplied by the superior mesenteric artery. The distal half of the large intestine derives from embryonic hindgut, is supplied by the inferior mesenteric artery, and is mainly for storage.

MACROSCOPIC FEATURES: The large intestine is divided into six regions proceeding distally from the ileocecal valve: (1) cecum, (2) ascending colon, (3) transverse colon, (4) descending colon, (5) sigmoid colon, and (6) rectum. The bend between the ascending and transverse colon in the right upper quadrant is the **hepatic flexure,** and that between the transverse and descending segments in the left upper quadrant is the **splenic flexure.** The caliber of the lumen progressively diminishes from the cecum to the sigmoid colon.

Like the small intestine, the colon has outer longitudinal and inner circular muscle coats. However, in the colon, the longitudinal muscle has three separate bundles, the **taeniae coli.** Evaginations of the colonic wall between the taeniae, the **haustra,** appear as external sacculations. The appendices epiploicae are small serosal masses of fat, invested by peritoneum. The vermiform appendix arises at the apex of the cecum and terminates as a blind tube; it averages about 8 cm in length but occasionally measures up to 20 cm.

The ileocecal valve is a sphincter that regulates the flow of intestinal contents into the cecum. However it is an incompetent sphincter, and reflux of cecal contents into the ileum is usual. The internal sphincter of the anal canal is continuous with colonic smooth muscle. The external anal sphincter is the major mechanism by which bowel continence is maintained. It surrounds the anal canal with a layer of skeletal muscle. The mucosal surface of the large bowel has prominent folds, which are less pronounced in the rectum.

MICROSCOPIC FEATURES: Histologically, the colonic mucosal surface is flat and punctuated by numerous pits, the **crypts of Lieberkuhn.** Both are lined by tall columnar epithelium. The surface epithelium is primarily simple columnar cells with occasional goblet cells. The crypts mostly contain goblet cells, except at their bases, where a few undifferentiated cells and a variety of neuroendocrine cells are located. The basal undifferentiated cells constitute the reserve cell population of the colonic mucosa and exhibit numerous mitoses. Mucosal cells migrate from the bases of the crypts toward the luminal surface. Programmed cell death (apoptosis) and sloughing of the mucosal cells balance proliferation in maintaining the crypt epithelial cell population.

The lamina propria contains lymphocytes, plasma cells, macrophages and fibroblasts, with occasional eosinophils. Lymphoid aggregates interrupt the continuity of the muscularis mucosae and extend into the submucosa. The submucosa is similar to that in small intestine, but lymphatic channels are far less prominent. The lymphatics drain into paracolic nodes in the serosal fat, intermediate nodes along the course of the colic

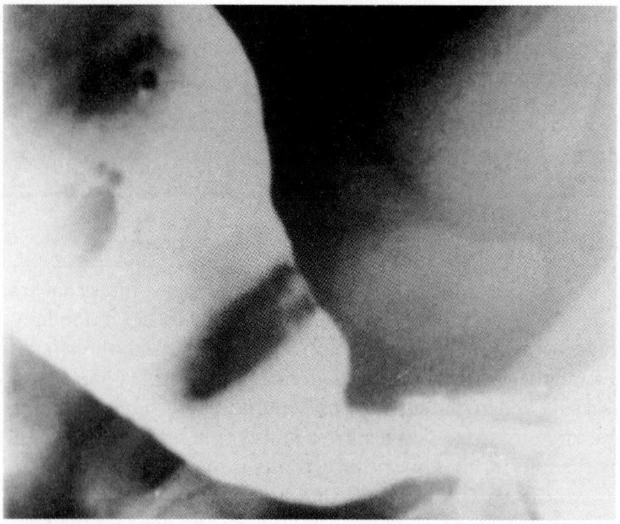

FIGURE 13-38. **Hirschsprung disease.** A contrast radiograph shows marked dilation of the rectosigmoid colon proximal to the narrowed rectum.

blood vessels and central nodes near the aorta. Parasympathetic and sympathetic innervations terminate in Meissner submucosal and Auerbach myenteric plexuses.

Congenital Disorders

Congenital Megacolon (Hirschsprung Disease) Reflects a Segmental Absence of Ganglion Cells

Hirschsprung disease is a disorder in which colon dilation (Fig. 13-38) *results from a defect in colorectal innervation: congenital absence of ganglion cells, in most cases in the wall of the rectum* (Fig. 13-39). In one fourth of cases, ganglion cells are deficient in moreproximal portions of the colon and in unusual instances, the lesion may extend as far as the small intestine. The incidence of the disorder is estimated to be 1 in 5000 live births, and 80% of patients are male.

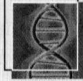

PATHOGENESIS: The pathogenesis of Hirschsprung disease can be traced to an interruption of the developmental sequence that leads to innervation of the colon. The normal caudal migration of cells from the neural crest that leads to the intramural ganglion cells is cut short. Because the internal anal sphincter is the terminus of this migration, the aganglionic segment always includes the rectum and may extend for variable distances proximally, depending on the point at which the primitive neuroblast migration halts. Given that the aganglionic rectum and occasionally the adjacent colon are permanently contracted because of the absence of relaxation stimuli, the fecal contents do not readily enter this stenotic area. The proximal bowel becomes dilated because of functional distal obstruction.

Most cases of Hirschsprung disease are sporadic, but 10% of cases are familial. Half of the familial cases and 15% of sporadic ones reflect inactivating mutations of the RET receptor tyrosine kinase gene on chromosome 10q (see MEN2 syndrome, Chapter 21). Some cases involve mutations in the endothelin-B receptor or in genes that encode ligands of the RET receptor and endothelin-B receptor.

The incidence of congenital megacolon is 10 times higher than normal in infants with **Down syndrome;** 2% of patients with Down syndrome are born with Hirschsprung disease. Although most cases are uncomplicated by other lesions, the disorder also has been reported associated with other congenital abnormalities, including anomalies of the kidneys and lower urinary tract, imperforate anus, and ventricular septal defect.

PATHOLOGY: The large intestine in Hirschsprung disease has a constricted and spastic segment that is the aganglionic zone. Proximal to this, the bowel is very dilated. The definitive diagnosis of Hirschsprung disease is made on the basis of absence of ganglion cells in a rectal biopsy specimen (see Fig. 13-39B). There is also a striking increase in nonmyelinated cholinergic nerve fibers in the submucosa and between the muscle coats (neural hyperplasia). The absence of ganglion cells leads to accumulation of acetylcholine and acetylcholinesterase. Histochemical demonstration of this enzyme, which is not visualized in normal rectal mucosa, enhances the reliability of a diagnosis based on rectal biopsy.

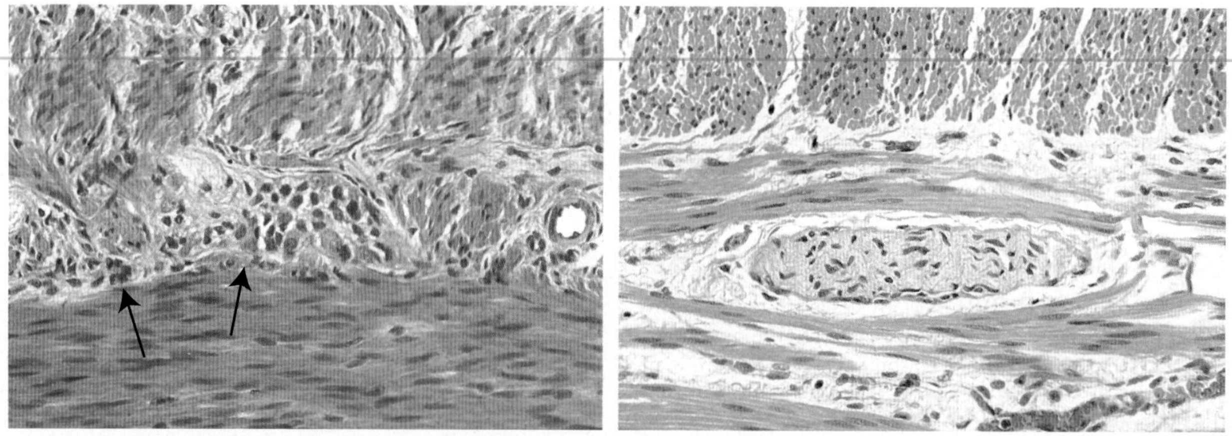

A B

FIGURE 13-39. **Hirschsprung disease. A.** A photomicrograph of ganglion cells in the wall of the rectum *(arrows)*. **B.** A rectal biopsy specimen from a patient with Hirschsprung disease shows a nonmyelinated nerve in the mesenteric plexus and an absence of ganglion cells.

Interestingly, like achalasia, which is caused by destruction of esophageal ganglion cells, Chagas disease may cause aganglionic megacolon.

CLINICAL FEATURES: Hirschsprung disease is the most common cause of congenital intestinal obstruction. The clinical signs are delayed passage of meconium by a newborn and development of vomiting in the first few days of life. In some cases, complete intestinal obstruction requires immediate surgical relief. In children who have short rectal segments lacking ganglion cells and who have only partial obstruction, constipation, abdominal distention, and recurrent fecal impactions are characteristic.

The most serious complication of congenital megacolon is an enterocolitis, in which necrosis and ulceration affect the dilated proximal segment of the colon and may extend into the small intestine. The treatment for Hirschsprung disease is surgical removal of the aganglionic segment and reconstruction.

Acquired Megacolon Often Reflects Laxative Use

Acquired megacolon sometimes occurs in children and often has a psychogenic background. It is frequently associated with chronic constipation and prolonged laxative use ("cathartic colon"). However, some cases in which ganglion cells are seen by rectal biopsy begin in infancy and are associated with fecal incontinence. The cause is not well understood, but it is thought to represent a functional abnormality of colonic motility. Acquired megacolon in adults can result from disorders that interfere with bowel innervation or smooth muscle function, such as diabetic neuropathy, parkinsonism, myotonic dystrophy, scleroderma, amyloidosis, and hypothyroidism.

Anorectal Malformations Are Common Developmental Defects

These malformations vary from minor narrowing to serious and complex defects. The lesions result from arrested development of the caudal region of the gut in the first 6 months of fetal life. These anomalies are classified based on the relation of the terminal bowel to the levator ani muscle: (1) high or supralevator deformities, in which the bowel ends above the pelvic floor; (2) intermediate deformities; and (3) low or translevator deformities, in which the bowel ends below the pelvic floor.

- **Anorectal agenesis and rectal atresia** are supralevator deformities.
- **Anal agenesis and anorectal stenosis** are classified as intermediate deformities.
- **Imperforate anus** is a low or translevator deformity in which the opening is covered by a cutaneous membrane behind which meconium is visible. **Anal stenosis** is a variant of imperforate anus.
- **Fistulas** between the malformation and the bladder, urethra, vagina, or skin may occur in all types of anorectal anomalies.

Infections of the Large Intestine

The principal infections of the colon, including tuberculosis and amebiasis, are discussed in Chapter 9 or above in the context of small intestine infectious diarrhea. Most of the remaining infectious diseases are transmitted sexually and involve the anorectal region, often in male homosexuals, including gonorrhea, syphilis, lymphogranuloma venereum, anorectal herpes, and venereal warts (condylomata acuminata). Immunosuppressed people have a high incidence of colonic infections (e.g., amebiasis and shigellosis). Bone marrow transplant recipientss often contract cytomegalovirus and herpes infection of the gastrointestinal tract.

Pseudomembranous Colitis Usually Follows Antibiotic Treatment

Pseudomembranous colitis is a generic term for an inflammatory disease of the colon that is characterized by exudative plaques on the mucosa.

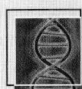

PATHOGENESIS: After the introduction of antibiotics in the early 1950s, it became clear that administration of these drugs, principally tetracycline and chloramphenicol, often led to pseudomembranous colitis. *Clostridium difficile,* which is also implicated in neonatal necrotizing enterocolitis, is the offending organism. It is not invasive, but produces toxins that damage the colonic mucosa.

Other conditions which can produce pseudomembranes include various diseases of the colon, shock, burns, uremia, and chemotherapy.

The mechanism by which *C. difficile* becomes pathogenic is not entirely clear. Alteration of fecal flora by antibiotics contributes. Only 2% to 3% of healthy adults harbor the organism, while 10% to 20% of those who were recently treated with antibiotics are infected. However, the microbe can be isolated from the stools of 95% of patients with antibiotic-associated pseudomembranous colitis.

PATHOLOGY: Macroscopically, the colon, particularly the rectosigmoid region, shows raised yellowish plaques up to 2 cm in diameter that adhere to the underlying mucosa (Fig. 13-40). The intervening mucosa appears congested and edematous but is not ulcerated. In severe cases, plaques coalesce into extensive pseudomembranes. Necrosis of the superficial epithelium is believed to be the initial pathologic event. Subsequently, crypts become disrupted and expanded by mucin and neutrophils. The pseudomembrane consists of the debris of necrotic epithelial cells, mucus, fibrin, and neutrophils. In milder cases, well formed pseudomembranes may be absent, and the pathology is more subtle, with focal damage to the surface epithelium.

When both small and large bowel are involved, the condition is referred to as **pseudomembranous enterocolitis.** Pseudomembranes occur occasionally in other enteric infections, involving *Staphylococcus aureus, Candida,* invasive bacteria, and verotoxin-producing *E. coli.* Ischemic bowel disease may also show pseudomembranes.

CLINICAL FEATURES: Antibiotic-associated infections with *C. difficile* are virtually always accompanied by diarrhea, but in most cases, the disorder does not progress to colitis. In patients with pseudomembranous colitis, fever, leukocytosis, and abdominal cramps are superimposed on the diarrhea. Before there were antibiotics, many patients with

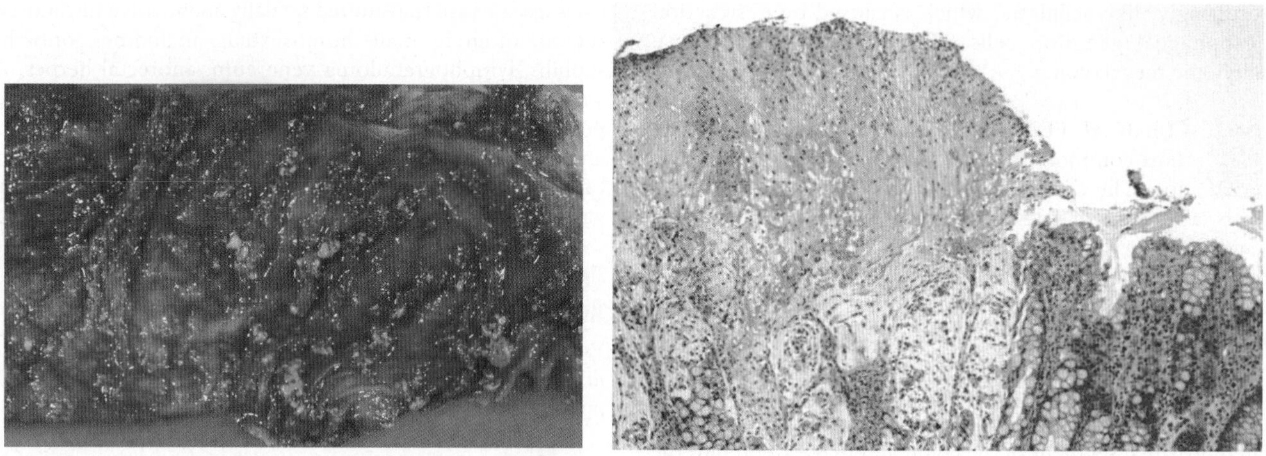

FIGURE 13-40. **Pseudomembranous colitis. A.** The colon shows variable involvement ranging from erythema to yellow-green areas of pseudomembrane. **B.** Microscopically, the pseudomembrane consists of fibrin, mucin and inflammatory cells (largely neutrophils).

this form of colitis died within hours or days from ileus and irreversible shock. Today, pseudomembranous colitis, although still serious, is usually controlled with antibiotics and supportive fluid and electrolyte therapy. Milder cases can be confused with an array of diarrheal diseases.

Neonatal Necrotizing Enterocolitis Complicates Prematurity

Necrotizing enterocolitis is one of the most common acquired surgical emergencies in newborns. It is particularly common in premature infants after oral feeding and is likely related principally to an ischemic event involving the intestinal mucosa, which is followed by bacterial colonization, usually with *C. difficile.* The lesions vary from those of typical pseudomembranous enterocolitis to gangrene and perforation of the bowel.

Diverticular Disease

Diverticular disease refers to two entities: a condition termed **diverticulosis** and an inflammatory complication called **diverticulitis.**

Diverticulosis Reflects Environmental and Structural Factors

Diverticulosis is an acquired herniation (diverticulum) of the mucosa and submucosa through the muscular layers of the colon.

EPIDEMIOLOGY: Diverticulosis shows a striking geographic variation, being common in Western societies and infrequent in Asia, Africa, and underdeveloped countries. Diverticulosis increases in frequency with age. Some 10% of persons in Western countries are afflicted.

PATHOGENESIS: The striking variation in the prevalence of diverticulosis implies that environmental factors are primarily responsible for the disease. Western populations consume a diet in which refined carbohydrates and meat have replaced crude cereal grains and it is widely assumed that the lack of indigestible fibers in some way predisposes to formation of diverticula in susceptible persons. In this respect, the larger fecal mass in those who ingest a high-fiber diet diminishes spontaneous motility and intraluminal pressure in the colon.

INCREASED INTRALUMINAL PRESSURE: According to the fiber theory, Western diets lack dietary residue, leading to sustained bowel contractions and consequently increased intraluminal pressure. Such prolonged increased pressure is believed to lead to herniation of the superficial coats of the colon through the muscular layers into the serosa.

DEFECTS IN THE WALL OF THE COLON: In addition to pressure, defects in the wall of the colon are required for the formation of a diverticulum. The circular muscle of the colon is interrupted by connective tissue clefts at the sites of penetration by the nutrient vessels that supply the submucosa and mucosa. In persons of advancing age, this connective tissue loses its resilience and, therefore, its resistance to the effects of increased intraluminal pressure. This concept is supported by the observation that persons with heritable disorders of connective tissue (e.g., Marfan syndrome, Ehlers-Danlos syndrome) acquire precocious diverticulosis, primarily of the small bowel.

PATHOLOGY: True diverticula all layers of the intestinal wall. The abnormal structures in diverticulosis are instead pseudodiverticula, in which only the mucosa and submucosa are herniated through the muscle layers. The sigmoid colon is affected in 95% of cases, but diverticulosis can affect any segment of the colon, including the cecum. Diverticula vary in number from a few to hundreds. Most appear in parallel rows between the mesenteric and lateral taeniae. They measure up to 1 cm and are connected to the intestinal lumen by necks of varying length and caliber. The muscular wall of the affected colon is consistently thickened.

Microscopically, a diverticulum characteristically is seen as a flasklike structure that extends from the lumen through the muscle layers (Fig. 13-41). Its wall is continuous with the surface mucosa and thus has an epithelium *and* a submucosa. The base of the diverticulum is formed by serosal connective tissue.

CLINICAL FEATURES: *Diverticulosis is generally asymptomatic, and 80% of affected persons remain symptom free.* Many patients complain of episodic colicky abdominal pain. Both constipation and diarrhea, sometimes

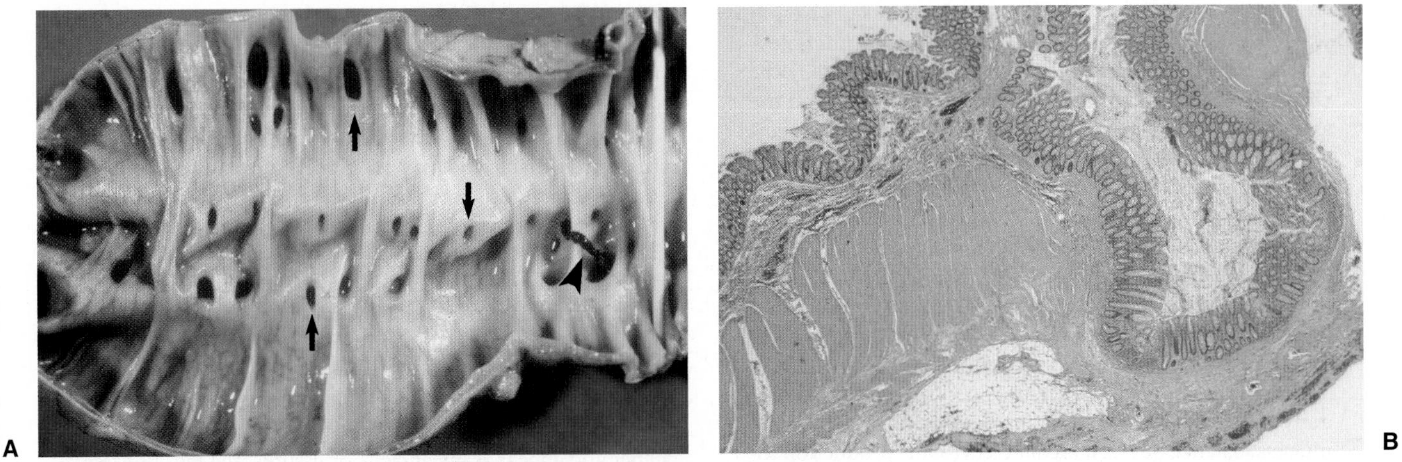

FIGURE 13-41. **Diverticulosis of the colon. A.** The colon was inflated with formalin. The mouths of numerous diverticula are seen between the taenia (arrows). There is a blood clot seen protruding from the mouth of one of the diverticula (arrowhead). This was the source of massive gastrointestinal bleeding. **B.** Sections show mucosa including mucularis mucosae which has herniated through a defect in the bowel wall producing a diverticulum.

alternating, may occur, and flatulence is common. Sudden, painless and severe bleeding from colonic diverticula is a cause of serious lower gastrointestinal hemorrhage in the elderly, occurring in as many as 5% of persons with diverticulosis. Chronic blood loss may lead to anemia.

Diverticulitis Refers to Inflammation at the Base of a Diverticulum

Diverticulitis presumably results from irritation caused by retained fecal material. In 10% to 20% of patients with diverticulosis, diverticulitis supervenes at some point.

PATHOLOGY: Diverticulitis produces inflammation of the wall of the diverticulum, an event that may lead to perforation and release of fecal bacteria into the peridiverticular tissues. The resulting abscess is usually contained by the appendices epiploicae and the pericolonic tissue. Infrequently, free perforation leads to generalized peritonitis. Fibrosis in response to repeated episodes of diverticulitis may constrict the bowel lumen, causing obstruction. Fistulas may form between the colon and adjacent organs, including the bladder, vagina, small intestine, and skin of the abdomen. Additional complications include pylephlebitis and liver abscesses.

CLINICAL FEATURES: The most common symptoms of diverticulitis, usually following microscopic or gross perforation of the diverticulum, are persistent lower abdominal pain and fever. Changes in bowel habits, ranging diarrhea to constipation, are frequent and dysuria indicates bladder irritation. Most patients have tenderness in the left lower quadrant, and a mass in that area may be palpated. Leukocytosis is the rule. Antibiotic treatment and supportive measures usually alleviate acute diverticulitis, but about 20% of patients eventually require surgical intervention.

Inflammatory Bowel Disease

Inflammatory bowel disease is a term that describes two diseases: **Crohn disease** and **ulcerative colitis.** Although these two disorders usually differ enough to be clearly distinguishable, they have certain common features. Similarities apart, Crohn disease and ulcerative colitis have different clinical courses and natural histories.

Crohn Disease Is Chronic Segmental Transmural Inflammation of the Intestine

Crohn disease occurs principally in the distal small intestine, but may involve any part of the digestive tract and even extraintestinal tissues. The colon, particularly the right colon, may be affected. Crohn disease has variously been referred to as **terminal ileitis** and **regional ileitis** when it involves mainly the ileum, and **granulomatous colitis** and **transmural colitis** when it principally affects the colon.

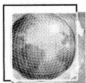

EPIDEMIOLOGY: Crohn disease is worldwide, with an annual incidence of 0.5 to 5 per 100,000. Reports from various countries indicate that the incidence has increased dramatically over the past 30 years. The disease usually appears in adolescents or young adults and is most common among persons of European origin, with a considerably higher frequency among Jews. There is a slight female predominance (1.6:1).

PATHOGENESIS: Epidemiologic studies, particularly concordance rates in twin pairs and siblings, strongly implicate a genetic predisposition to Crohn disease. A family history of inflammatory bowel disease is more common for Crohn disease than ulcerative colitis. A putative susceptibility locus for Crohn disease has been assigned to the centromeric region of chromosome 16, at least in non-Jewish patients. Other susceptibility loci may reside on chromosomes 3, 7, and 12. *NOD2* and *CARD15* mutations determine ileal disease, and the clinical pattern of Crohn disease has been linked to specific genotypes. Crohn disease has only rarely been described in both a husband and a wife, a fact that suggests that environmental factors alone do not suffice to cause the disease. Interestingly, smoking is associated with Crohn disease, but ulcerative colitis is uncommon in smokers. Several infectious agents have been suggested as possible causative agents, but definitive associations are lacking. Several studies report impaired cell-mediated immunity in patients with Crohn disease. Some investigators have suggested increased suppressor T cell activity, and others have claimed depressed phagocytic function.

The possibility that Crohn disease reflects immunologically mediated damage to the intestine is suggested by the chronic and recurrent nature of the inflammation and the association with systemic manifestations that often suggest with autoimmune diseases. Most recent immunologic studies focus on the possible role of cell-mediated cytotoxicity. Some studies support the hypothesis that cytotoxic T cells sensitized to bacterial or other antigens damage the intestinal wall. In this respect, cyclosporine, a potent inhibitor of cell-mediated immunity that is widely used to prevent rejection of transplanted organs, has been reported to ameliorate the symptoms of Crohn disease.

TNF-α production is increased in vitro in mucosal cells derived from patients with Crohn disease, as is a shift in the mucosal balance of T-cell mediated cytokine production toward TNF-α. Administration of anti–TNF-α antibodies to patients with Crohn disease provides effective short-term symptom remission.

The fecal stream appears to be of prime importance in the pathogenesis of Crohn disease, as evidenced by (1) the beneficial effects of surgical bypass, (2) the pattern of pre-anastomotic recurrence in patients with side-to-end anastomotic sites, and (3) the frequency of early inflammatory lesions (aphthoid erosions) in the epithelium in association with mucosal lymphoid tissue.

PATHOLOGY: Two major characteristics of Crohn disease differentiate it from other gastrointestinal inflammatory diseases. First, the inflammation usually involves all layers of the bowel wall and is, therefore, referred to as **transmural inflammatory disease.** Second, the involvement of the intestine is discontinuous; that is, segments of inflamed tissue are separated by apparently normal intestine.

It is convenient to classify Crohn disease into four broad macroscopic patterns, although many patients do not fit any one of them precisely. The disease involves (1) mainly the ileum and cecum in about 50% of cases, (2) only the small intestine in 15%, (3) only the colon in 20%, and (4) mainly the anorectal region in 15%. Disease of the ileum and cecum is more frequent in young persons; colitis is common in older patients. Crohn disease is occasionally seen in the duodenum and stomach as focal acute inflammation with or without granulomas. More rarely, it occurs in the esophagus and oral cavity, almost always in association with small intestinal disease. In women with anorectal Crohn disease, the inflammation may spread to involve the external genitalia.

The macroscopic and microscopic pathologies of Crohn disease are variable and may comprise almost any combination of features characteristic of the disease. Grossly, the bowel and adjacent mesentery are thickened and edematous. Mesenteric fat often wraps around the bowel ("creeping fat"). Mesenteric lymph nodes are frequently enlarged, firm, and matted together. The intestinal lumen is narrowed by edema in early cases and by a combination of edema and fibrosis in long-standing disease. Nodular swelling, fibrosis, and mucosal ulceration lead to a "cobblestone" appearance (Fig. 13-42A). In early cases, ulcers have either an aphthous or a serpiginous appearance; later they become deeper and appear as linear clefts or fissures (see Fig. 13-42B).

The cut surface of the bowel wall shows the transmural nature of the disease, with thickening, edema, and fibrosis of all layers. Involved loops of bowel are often adherent and fistulas between such segments are frequent. These fistulas, presumably a late result of the deep mural ulcers, may also penetrate from the bowel into other organs, including the bladder, uterus, vagina, and skin. Most fistulas end blindly, forming abscess cavities in the peritoneal cavity, mesentery, or retroperitoneal structures. Lesions in the distal rectum and anus may create perianal fistulas, a well-known presenting feature.

Microscopically, Crohn disease appears as a chronic inflammatory process. During early phases of the disease, the inflammation may be confined to the mucosa and submucosa. Small, superficial mucosal ulcerations (aphthous ulcers) are seen, together with mucosal and submucosal edema and an increase in the number of lymphocytes, plasma cells, and macrophages. Destruction of mucosal architecture, with regenerative changes in crypts and villous distortion, are frequent. Pyloric metaplasia and Paneth cell hyperplasia is common in the small intestine and colorectum. Later, long, deep, fissurelike ulcers are seen, and vascular hyalinization and fibrosis become apparent.

The microscopic hallmark of Crohn disease is transmural nodular lymphoid aggregates, accompanied by proliferative changes of the muscularis mucosae and nerves of submucosal and myenteric plexuses (Fig. 13-43). *Discrete, noncaseating*

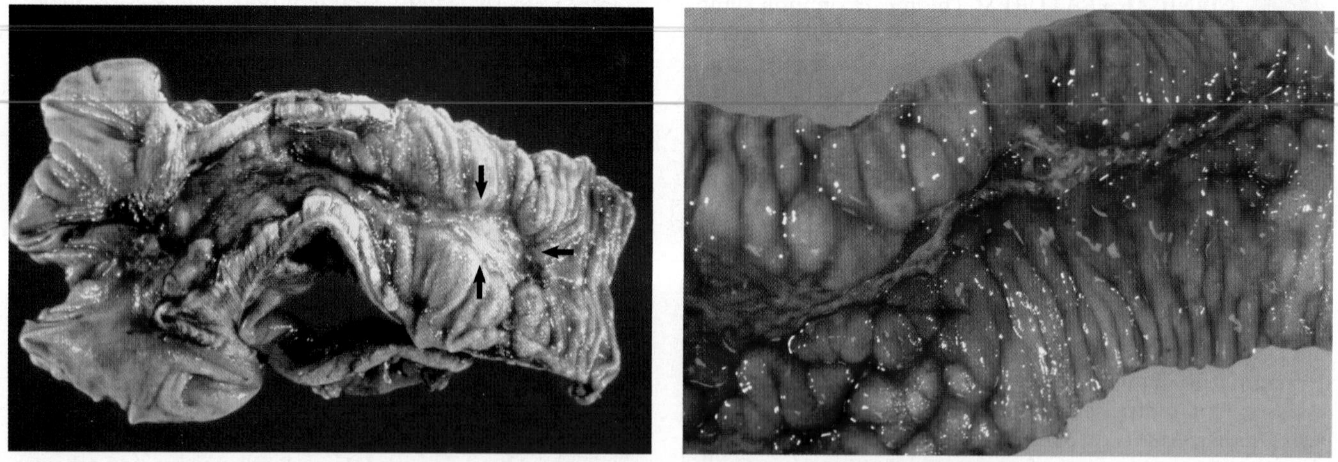

A B

FIGURE 13-42. **Crohn disease. A.** The terminal ileum shows striking thickening of the wall of the distal portion with distortion of ileocecal valve. A longitudinal ulcer is present (*arrows*). **B.** Another longitudinal ulcer is seen in this segment of ileum. The large rounded areas of edematous damaged mucosa give a "cobblestone" appearance to the involved mucosa. A portion of the mucosa to the lower right is uninvolved.

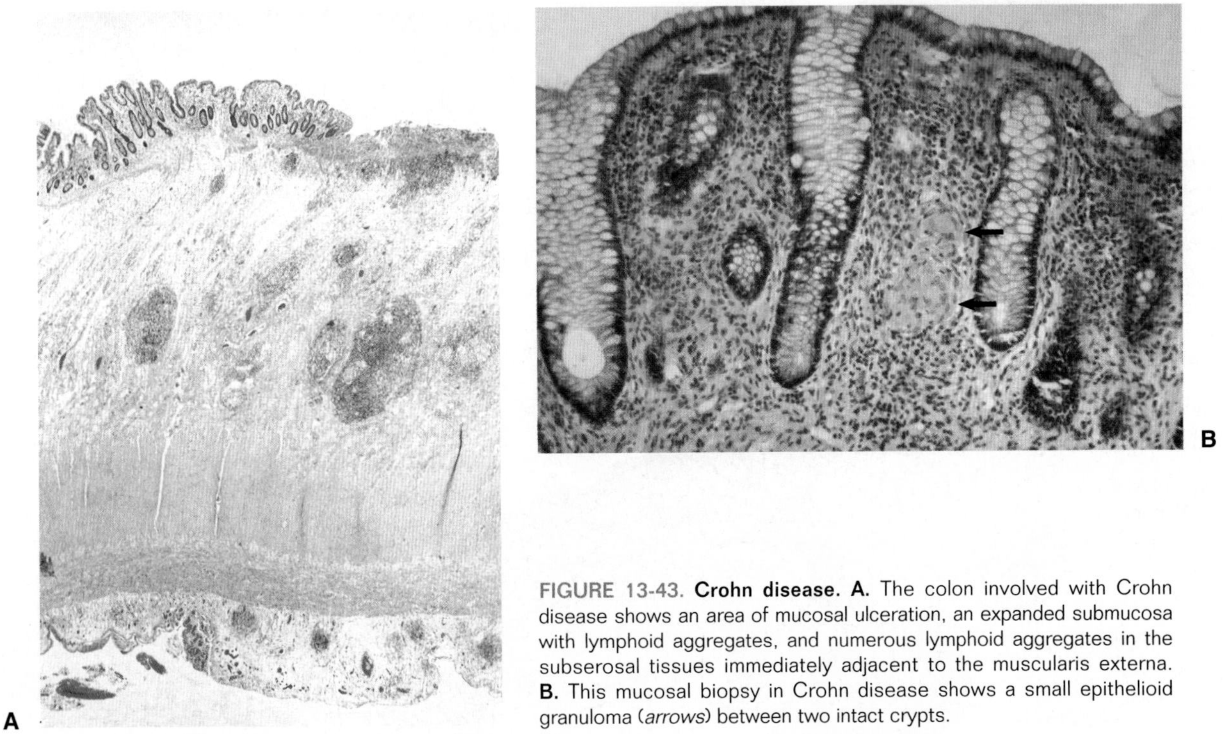

FIGURE 13-43. **Crohn disease. A.** The colon involved with Crohn disease shows an area of mucosal ulceration, an expanded submucosa with lymphoid aggregates, and numerous lymphoid aggregates in the subserosal tissues immediately adjacent to the muscularis externa. **B.** This mucosal biopsy in Crohn disease shows a small epithelioid granuloma (*arrows*) between two intact crypts.

granulomas, mostly in the submucosa, may be present. These granulomas are like those of sarcoidosis and consist of focal aggregates of epithelioid cells, vaguely limited by a rim of lymphocytes. Multinucleated giant cells may be present. The centers of the granulomas usually display hyaline material and only very rarely necrosis.

Although the presence of discrete granulomas is strong evidence in favor of Crohn disease, the absence of granulomas does not exclude the diagnosis, as less than half the cases show the typical granulomas.

The pathologic features of Crohn disease are summarized in Figure 13-44.

CLINICAL FEATURES: The clinical manifestations and natural history of Crohn disease are highly variable and relate to the anatomical sites involved by the disease. The most frequent symptoms are **abdominal pain** and **diarrhea,** which are seen in over 75% of patients, and recurrent **fever,** evident in 50%. When disease mainly involves the ileum and cecum, sudden onset may mimic appendicitis, and the diagnosis is occasionally first made at the time of abdominal surgery. If the disease predominantly involves the ileum, the major clinical features are right lower quadrant pain, intermittent diarrhea and fever, and frequently a tender mass in the right lower quadrant of the abdomen. When the small intestine is diffusely involved, **malabsorption** and malnutrition may be major features. Lipid malabsorption may also result from interruption of enterohepatic cycle of bile salts because of ileal disease. Crohn disease of the colon leads to **diarrhea** and sometimes **colonic bleeding.** In a few patients, the major site of involvement is the anorectal region and recurrent anorectal fistulas are the presenting sign.

Intestinal obstruction and **fistulas** are the most common intestinal complications of Crohn disease. Occasionally, free perforation of the bowel occurs. **Small bowel cancer** is at least threefold more common in patients with Crohn disease, and the disease also predisposes to **colorectal cancer.** When Crohn disease begins in childhood, it may lead to retardation of growth and physical development. Systemic complications also include liver disease (sclerosing cholangitis), cholelithiasis, renal oxalate stones, and amyloidosis. The most frequent extraintestinal inflammatory features are in the eye (episcleritis or uveitis), medium-sized joints (arthritis), and skin (erythema nodosum).

No cure is available. Several medications suppress the inflammatory reaction, including corticosteroids, sulfasalazine, metronidazole, 6-mercaptopurine, cyclosporine, and anti-TNF antibodies. Surgical resection of obstructed areas or of severely involved portions of intestine and drainage of abscesses caused by fistulas are required in some cases. Preanastomotic or prestomal recurrences after construction of an enterostomy is a hallmark of Crohn disease, a feature that makes clinical management difficult. The need for repeated resections can lead to short-bowel syndrome in some patients.

Ulcerative Colitis Is a Chronic Superficial Inflammation of the Colon and Rectum

Ulcerative colitis is characterized by chronic diarrhea and rectal bleeding, with a pattern of exacerbations and remissions and with the possibility of serious local and systemic complications. The disorder occurs principally, but not exclusively, in young adults.

EPIDEMIOLOGY: In Europe and North America, the incidence of ulcerative colitis is 4 to 7 per 100,000 population, and its prevalence is 40 to 80 per 100,000. It usually begins in early adult life, with peak incidence in the third decade. However, it also occurs in childhood and old age. In the United States, whites are affected more commonly than blacks.

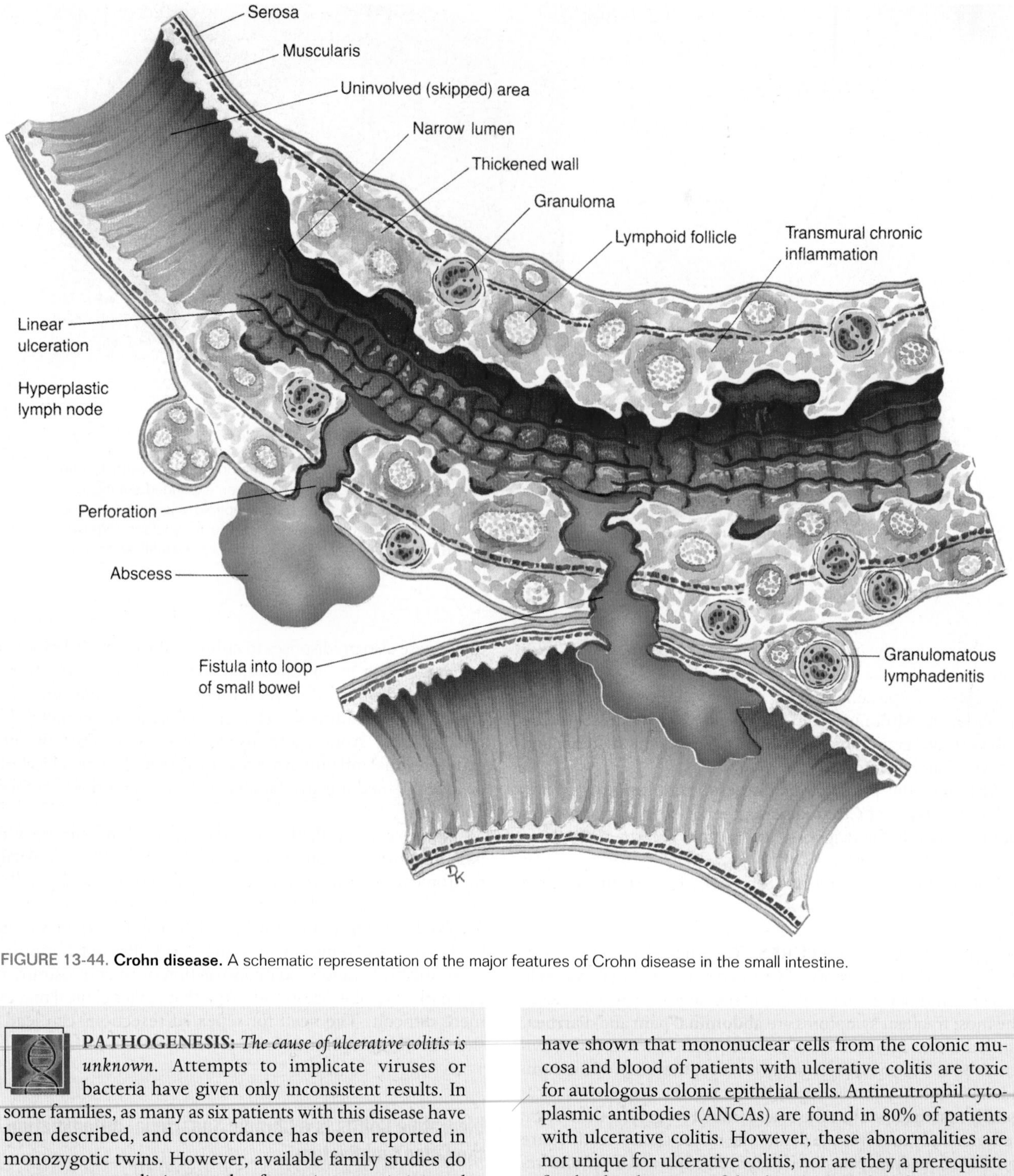

FIGURE 13-44. **Crohn disease.** A schematic representation of the major features of Crohn disease in the small intestine.

PATHOGENESIS: *The cause of ulcerative colitis is unknown.* Attempts to implicate viruses or bacteria have given only inconsistent results. In some families, as many as six patients with this disease have been described, and concordance has been reported in monozygotic twins. However, available family studies do not suggest any distinct mode of genetic transmission and studies of HLA distribution in patients with ulcerative colitis have not demonstrated a consistent pattern.

The possibility that an abnormal immune response may be involved has been studied extensively. There is abundant lymphoid tissue throughout the colon, and this disorder may have autoimmune-like concomitants, such as uveitis, erythema nodosum, and vasculitis. Several studies have demonstrated increased circulating antibodies against antigens in colonic epithelial cells and against cross-reacting antigens in enterobacteria. Furthermore, in vitro studies have shown that mononuclear cells from the colonic mucosa and blood of patients with ulcerative colitis are toxic for autologous colonic epithelial cells. Antineutrophil cytoplasmic antibodies (ANCAs) are found in 80% of patients with ulcerative colitis. However, these abnormalities are not unique for ulcerative colitis, nor are they a prerequisite for the development of the disease. It is, therefore, possible that some or all of these immune features are, the result, not the cause, of mucosal damage.

PATHOLOGY: Three major pathologic features characterize ulcerative colitis and help to differentiate it from other inflammatory conditions:

- **Ulcerative colitis is a diffuse disease.** It usually extends from the most distal part of the rectum for a variable distance proximally (Fig. 13-45). When it involves the rectum alone, it

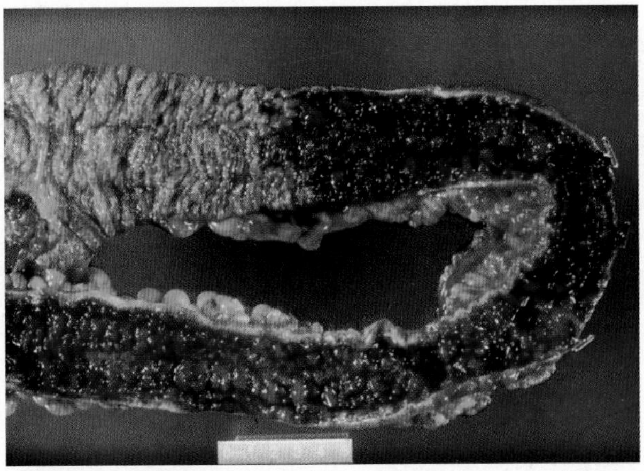

FIGURE 13-45. **Ulcerative colitis.** Prominent erythema and ulceration of the colon begin in the ascending colon and are most severe in the rectosigmoid area.

is called **ulcerative proctitis.** When the process extends toward the splenic flexure, the terms **proctosigmoiditis** and **left-sided colitis** are used. Sparing of the rectum or involvement of the right side of the colon alone is rare and suggests the possibility of another disorder, such as Crohn disease.

- **Inflammation in ulcerative colitis is generally limited to the colon and rectum.** It rarely involves the small intestine, stomach, or esophagus. If the cecum is affected, the disease ends at the ileocecal valve, although minor inflammation of the adjacent ileum is sometimes noted (backwash ileitis).
- **Ulcerative colitis is essentially a mucosal disease.** *Deeper layers are uncommonly involved,* mainly in fulminant cases, usually in association with toxic megacolon.

The following morphologic sequence may develop rapidly or over a course of years.

EARLY COLITIS: Early in the evolution of the disease, the mucosal surface is raw, red, and granular. It is frequently covered with a yellowish exudate and bleeds easily. Later small, superficial erosions or ulcers may appear. These occasionally coalesce to form irregular, shallow, ulcerated areas that appear to surround islands of intact mucosa.

The microscopic features of early ulcerative colitis correlate with colonoscopic appearances and include (1) mucosal congestion, edema, and microscopic hemorrhages; (2) a diffuse chronic inflammatory infiltrate in the lamina propria; and (3) damage and distortion of the colorectal crypts, which are often surrounded and infiltrated by neutrophils. Suppurative necrosis of the crypt epithelium gives rise to the characteristic **crypt abscess,** which appears as a dilated crypt filled with neutrophils (Fig. 13-46).

PROGRESSIVE COLITIS: As the disease continues, mucosal folds are lost (atrophy). Lateral extension and coalescence of crypt abscesses can undermine the mucosa, leaving areas of ulceration adjacent to hanging fragments of mucosa. Such mucosal excrescences are termed **inflammatory polyps** (Fig. 13-47). Tissue destruction is accompanied by manifestations of tissue repair. Granulation tissue develops in denuded areas. Importantly, the strictures characteristic of Crohn disease are absent. Microscopically, colorectal crypts may appear tortuous, branched, and shortened in the late stages and the mucosa may be diffusely atrophic.

ADVANCED COLITIS: In long-standing cases, the large bowel is often shortened, especially in the left side. Mucosal folds are indistinct and are replaced by a granular or smooth mucosal pattern. Microscopically, advanced ulcerative colitis is characterized by mucosal atrophy and a chronic inflammatory infiltrate in the mucosa and superficial submucosa. Paneth metaplasia is common.

CLINICAL FEATURES: The clinical course and manifestations are very variable. Most patients (70%) have intermittent attacks, with partial or complete remission between attacks. A small number (<10%) have a very long remission (several years) after their first attack. The remaining 20% have continuous symptoms without remission.

MILD COLITIS: Half of patients with ulcerative colitis have mild disease. Their major symptom is rectal bleeding, sometimes accompanied by tenesmus (rectal pressure and discomfort). The disease in these patients is usually limited to the rectum but may extend to the distal sigmoid colon. Extraintestinal complications are uncommon, and in most patients in this category, disease remains mild throughout their lives.

MODERATE COLITIS: About 40% of patients have moderate ulcerative colitis. They usually have recurrent episodes of loose bloody stools, crampy abdominal pain, and frequently low-grade fever, lasting days or weeks. Moderate anemia is a common result of chronic fecal blood loss.

SEVERE COLITIS: About 10% of patients have severe or fulminant ulcerative colitis, sometimes from its onset but often during a flare of activity. They may have more than 6 and sometimes more than 20, bloody bowel movements daily, often with fever and other systemic manifestations. Blood and fluid loss rapidly leads to anemia, dehydration, and electrolyte depletion. Massive hemorrhage may be life-threatening. A particularly dangerous complication is **toxic megacolon,** which is characterized by extreme dilation of the colon. Patients with this condition are at high risk for perforation of the colon. Fulminant ulcerative colitis is a medical emergency requiring immediate, intensive medical therapy, and, in some cases, prompt colectomy. About 15% of patients with fulminant ulcerative colitis die of the disease.

The medical treatment of ulcerative colitis depends on the sites involved and the severity of the inflammation. The 5-aminosalicylate–based compounds are the mainstays of treatment for patients with mild-to-moderate ulcerative colitis. Corticosteroids and immunosuppressive and immunoregulatory agents (azathioprine or mercaptopurine) are used in patients who have severe and refractory disease.

Extraintestinal Manifestations

Arthritis is seen in 25% of patients with ulcerative colitis. Eye inflammation (mostly **uveitis**) and skin lesions develop in about 10%. The most common cutaneous lesions are **erythema nodosum** and **pyoderma gangrenosum,** the latter a serious, noninfective disorder characterized by deep, purulent, necrotic ulcers in the skin.

Liver disease occurs in about 4% of patients, most commonly **primary sclerosing cholangitis.** Those with primary sclerosing cholangitis are at risk for the development of **cholangiocarcinoma.** Thromboembolic phenomena, mostly deep vein thromboses of the lower extremities, occur in 6% of ulcerative colitis patients.

The various complications of ulcerative colitis are shown in Figure 13-48.

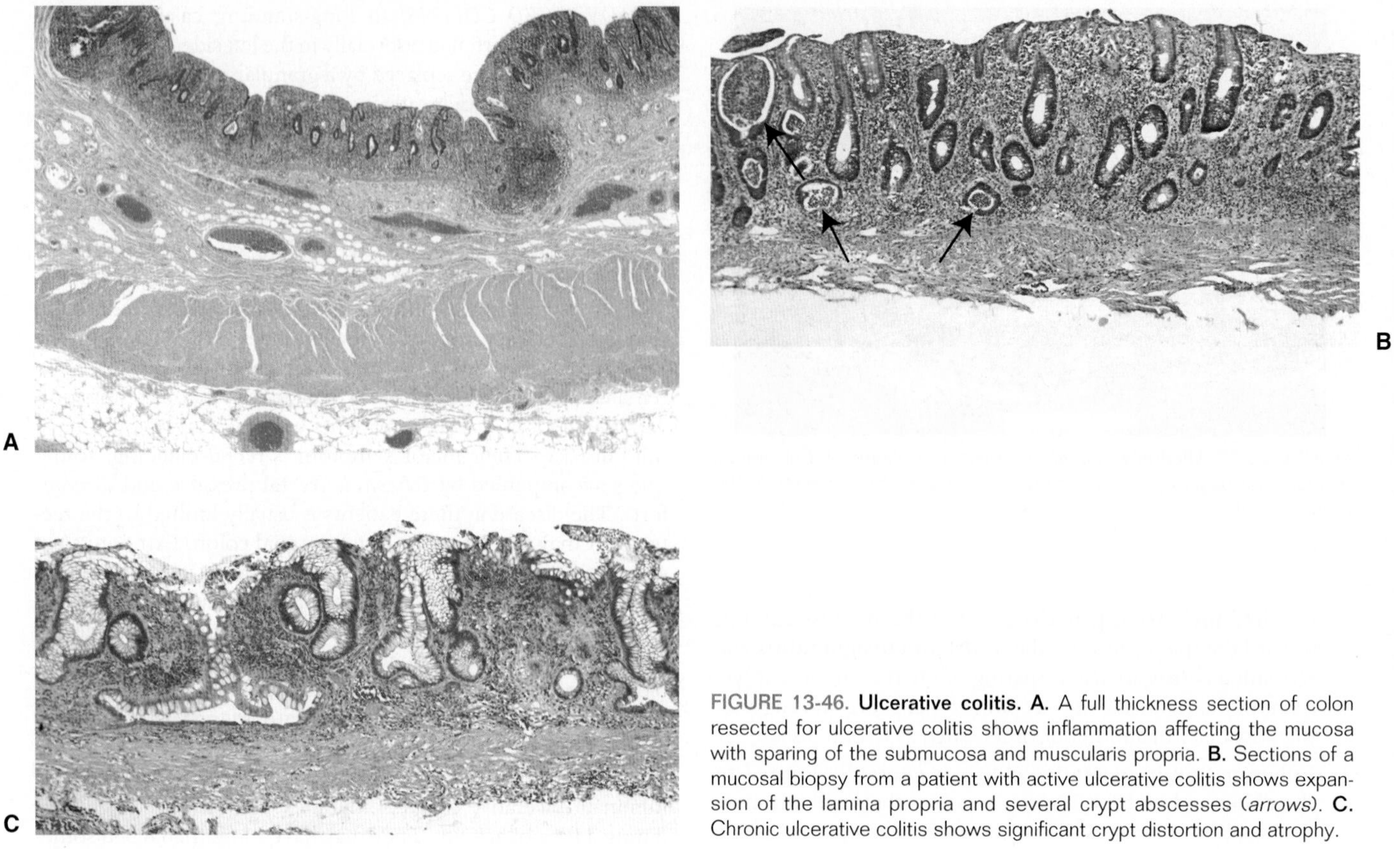

FIGURE 13-46. **Ulcerative colitis. A.** A full thickness section of colon resected for ulcerative colitis shows inflammation affecting the mucosa with sparing of the submucosa and muscularis propria. **B.** Sections of a mucosal biopsy from a patient with active ulcerative colitis shows expansion of the lamina propria and several crypt abscesses (*arrows*). **C.** Chronic ulcerative colitis shows significant crypt distortion and atrophy.

Differential Diagnosis

The most important conditions to be distinguished from ulcerative colitis are other forms of chronic colitis due to specifically treatable causes, and Crohn disease. Other conditions that should be considered in the differential diagnosis of ulcerative colitis are bacterial infections and amebic colitis, especially in areas where it is endemic. When inflammation is limited to the rectum, other infectious agents, including viruses, *Chlamydia,* fungi, and other parasites merit consideration. Proctitis due to these agents is common in male homosexuals and a variety of opportunistic infections of the bowel are encountered in patients with AIDS. Other conditions that may mimic ulcerative colitis are ischemic colitis, antibiotic-associated colitis, radiation injury, and solitary rectal ulcer syndrome.

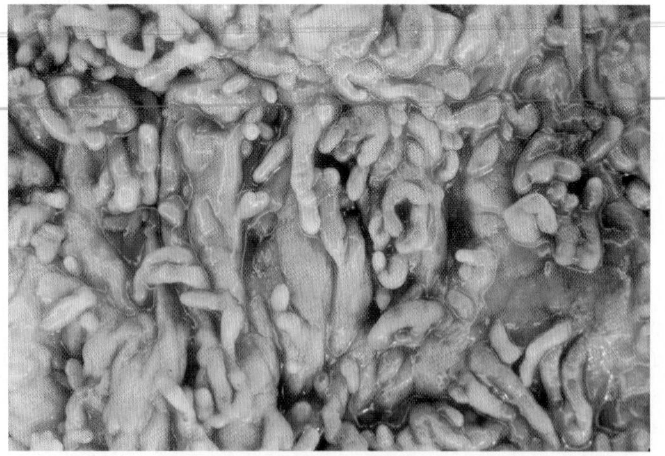

FIGURE 13-47. **Inflammatory polyps of the colon in ulcerative colitis.** Nodules of regenerative mucosa and inflammation surrounded by denuded areas provide a diffuse polypoid appearance of the mucosa.

The distinction between ulcerative colitis and Crohn colitis is based on different anatomical localization and histopathology (Table 13-1). Ulcerative colitis is a diffuse process, usually more severe distally, while Crohn colitis is patchy or segmental and often spares the rectum. The inflammation in ulcerative colitis is superficial (i.e., usually limited to the mucosa) and is characterized by an acute inflammatory infiltrate, with neutrophils and crypt abscesses. By contrast, Crohn colitis is transmural and involves all layers, with granulomas in some of the specimens.

If the disease stops at the ileocecal valve or is limited to the colon distal,ulcerative colitis is more likely. Involvement of the terminal ileum suggests Crohn colitis.

In 10% of cases, definitive discrimination is not possible. This occurs mostly in fulminant colitis; the inflammatory bowel disease is then termed **indeterminate colitis.** The distinction between ulcerative colitis and Crohn colitis is important because of (1) different surgical therapy (Crohn disease often has recurrences, so that continent ileostomy and ileoanal pouch procedures may be contraindicated), (2) a higher risk of cancer in ulcerative colitis, and (3) different medical therapy.

Ulcerative Colitis and Colorectal Cancer

Persons with long-standing ulcerative colitis have a higher risk of colorectal cancer than the general population. The risk is related to the extent of colorectal involvement and the duration of the inflammatory disease. Thus, if the entire colon is involved, the

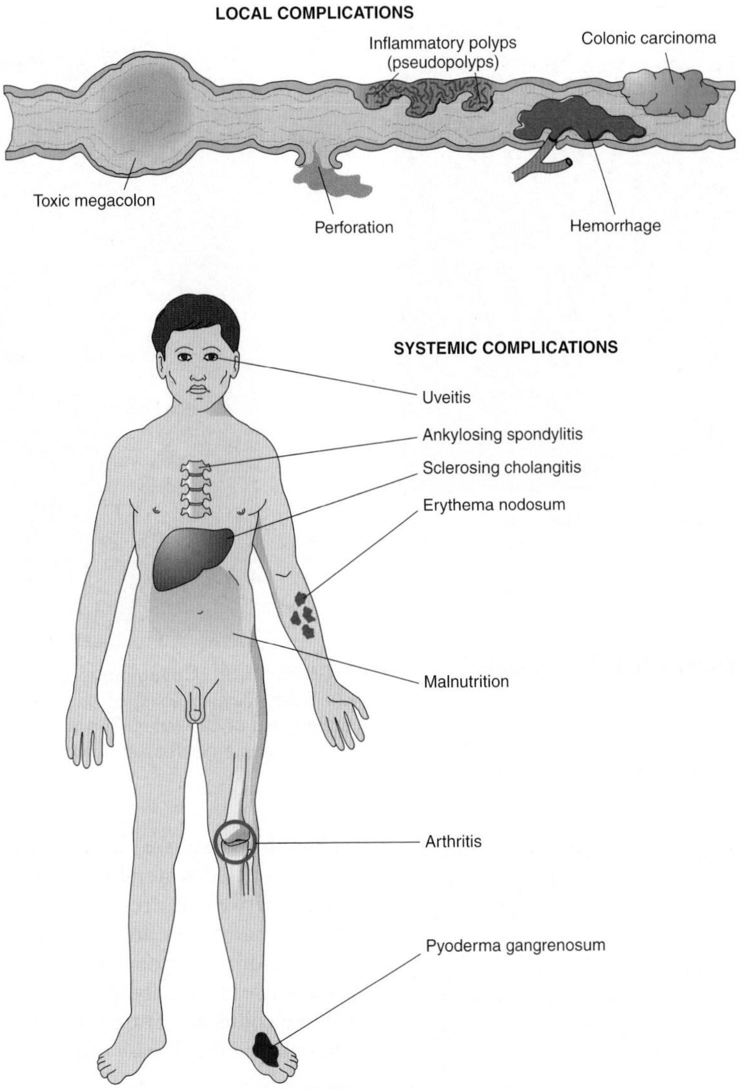

FIGURE 13-48. **Complications of ulcerative colitis.**

TABLE 13-1

Comparison of the Pathologic Features in the Colon of Crohn Disease and Ulcerative Colitis

Lesion	Crohn Disease	Ulcerative Colitis
Macroscopic		
Thickened bowel wall	Typical	Uncommon
Luminal narrowing	Typical	Uncommon
"Skip" lesions	Common	Absent
Right colon predominance	Typical	Absent
Fissures and fistulas	Common	Absent
Circumscribed ulcers	Common	Absent
Confluent linear ulcers	Common	Absent
Pseudopolyps	Absent	Common
Microscopic		
Transmural inflammation	Typical	Uncommon
Submucosal fibrosis	Typical	Absent
Fissures	Typical	Rare
Granulomas	Common	Absent
Crypt abscesses	Uncommon	Typical

risk of developing colorectal cancer is greater. If the inflammatory disease is limited to the rectum, the risk of colorectal cancer is like that of the general population. Incidence of colorectal cancer in the United States is estimated to be between 5% to 10% for each decade of pancolitis. Young age at the onset of colitis is not an independent risk factor, but since patients in whom ulcerative colitis develops at a young age have a longer duration of disease, they also have a high cumulative incidence of cancer.

Colorectal **epithelial dysplasia** is a neoplastic epithelial proliferation and precursor to colorectal carcinoma in patients with long-term ulcerative colitis (Fig. 13-49). The histopathologic criteria include (1) alteration of mucosal architecture, (2) epithelial abnormalities (hypercellularity and stratification of nuclei), and (3) epithelial dysplasia (variation in the size, shape, and staining qualities of nuclei). Dysplasia is divided into low-grade and high-grade dysplasia. High-grade epithelial dysplasia reflects a high risk for the development of colorectal cancer and when identified in a biopsy, it is a strong indication for colectomy. Routine surveillance by colonoscopic biopsy of all patients with ulcerative colitis is, therefore, recommended.

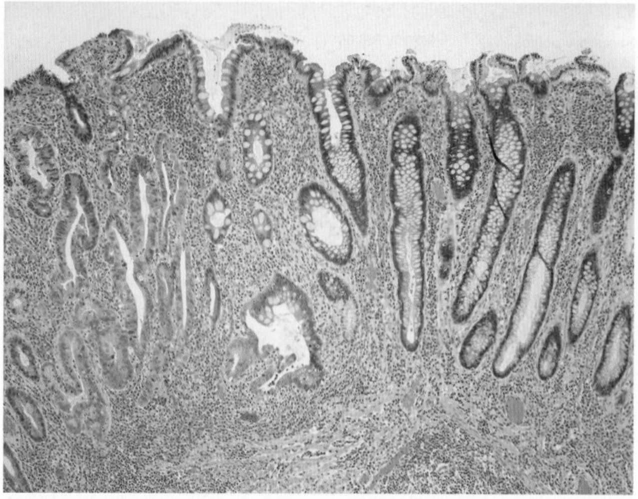

FIGURE 13-49. **Dysplasia in ulcerative colitis.** The colonic mucosa shows the chronic changes of ulcerative colitis (see Fig. 13-46). The crypts to the left are dysplastic.

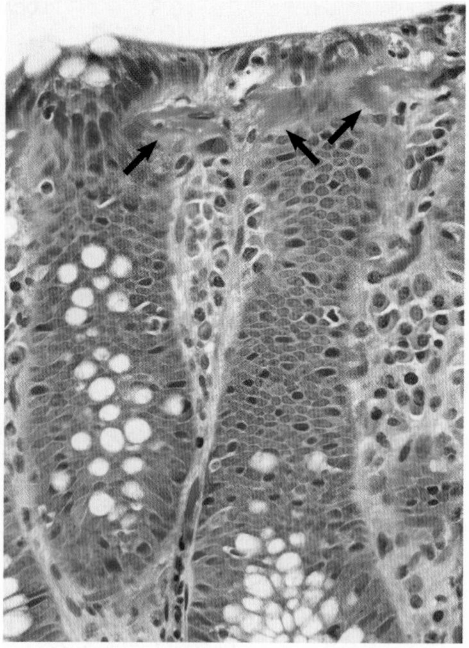

FIGURE 13-50. **Collagenous colitis.** A trichrome stainhighlights the characteristic thickening of the collagen table (blue, note *arrows*) with entrapment of capillaries. The intercryptal surface epithelium is flattened and contains an increased number of intraepithelial lymphocytes.

Collagenous Colitis and Lymphocytic Colitis Cause Chronic Diarrhea

Collagenous colitis is an inflammatory disorder of the colon characterized clinically by chronic watery diarrhea and pathologically by a thickened subepithelial collagen band. The disorder mainly afflicts middle-aged and elderly women.

The colonic mucosa appears grossly normal. The histopathologic diagnosis of collagenous colitis is made by demonstrating a chronic inflammatory cell infiltrate in the mucosa and a band of collagen immediately beneath the surface epithelium that measures up to 80 μm (Fig. 13-50). The surface epithelium shows flattened or cuboidal cells and even separation of epithelial cells from underlying structures. Intraepithelial lymphocytes are common. The lamina propria contains increased numbers of chronic inflammatory cells and neutrophils are also found in some patients. **Lymphocytic colitis** also features prominent infiltration of the damaged colonic epithelium by lymphocytes but lacks the collagen table and has an equal sex distribution. Patients with lymphocytic colitis have more than 10 lymphocytes for every 100 epithelial cells.

The etiologies of collagenous colitis and lymphocytic colitis are unknown. The fibrosis of collagenous colitis may result from persistent inflammation. Although the diseases have not been consistently linked to other systemic disorders, an autoimmune etiology also has been suggested, based on a putative association with rheumatoid arthritis and thyroid dysfunction. Compared with patients with collagenous colitis, those with lymphocytic colitis have an increased frequency of HLA-A1 and decreased HLA-A3. Many patients with these diseases have taken nonsteroidal anti-inflammatory drugs. Lymphocytic colitis is common in patients with celiac disease.

Vascular Diseases

The Colon is Subject to the Same Types of Ischemic Injury as the Small Intestine

Unlike the small bowel, extensive infarction of the colon is uncommon and chronic segmental disease is the rule. The most vulnerable areas are those between adjacent arterial distributions, so-called **watershed areas.** For example, the splenic flexure lies between the regions supplied by the superior and inferior mesenteric arteries, and the rectosigmoid area shares blood from the inferior mesenteric and internal iliac arteries. However, the rectum itself is usually spared in ischemic colitis. Most cases of ischemic colitis are caused by atherosclerosis of major intestinal arteries, and the disease usually occurs in persons older than 50.

PATHOLOGY: Some patients with symptoms and complications of bowel infarction require immediate surgical intervention. However, in most patients, the acute signs stabilize, and radiographic examination shows only the pattern associated with intramural hemorrhage and edema. On endoscopy, multiple ulcers, hemorrhagic nodular lesions, or a pseudomembrane is seen. Biopsy reveals ischemic necrosis of the bowel: mucosal ulceration, crypt abscesses, edema, and hemorrhage (Figure 13-51). Such patients may recover completely or may develop a colonic stricture, in which case, surgical removal of the obstructed segment is necessary. Segments of ischemic stricture show variable mucosal ulceration and inflammation, as well as submucosal widening by granulation tissue and fibrosis. Hemosiderin-laden macrophages may be noted, and patchy fibrosis of the muscular coats also may be present.

CLINICAL FEATURES: Ischemic disease of the rectosigmoid area typically manifests as abdominal pain, rectal bleeding, and a change in bowel habits. On clinical grounds alone, ischemic colitis often cannot be distinguished from some forms of infective colitis, ulcerative colitis, and Crohn colitis. Prognosis and treatment depend on the primary cause and extent of involvement. The goal is to improve blood supply to the colon by treating patients' overall cardiovas-

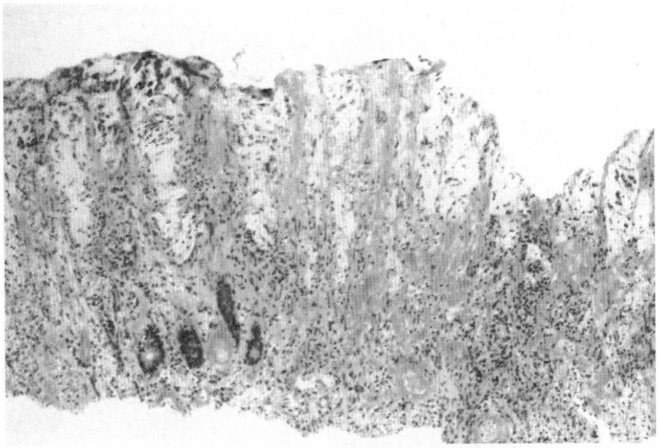

FIGURE 13-51. **Ischemic colitis.** A mucosal biopsy shows coagulative necrosis with "ghostly" outlines the preexisting crypts. Only a small portion of the base of several crypts remain.

cular status. Acute interruption of blood supply to the colon can be fatal in neonates and elderly persons.

Angiodysplasia (Vascular Ectasia) May Cause Intestinal Bleeding

Angiodysplasia (vascular ectasia) refers to localized arteriovenous malformations, mainly in the cecum and ascending colon, which produce lower intestinal bleeding. The mean age at presentation is 60 years. Younger persons preferentially exhibit lesions at other sites, including the rectum, stomach, and small bowel. Interestingly, angiodysplasia is associated with aortic valve disease in some patients. It has been suggested that it may be the result of chronic circulatory insufficiency of the intestine, intestinal muscle hypertrophy, and consequent venous obstruction. Patients typically complain of multiple bleeding episodes, although chronic occult bleeding may also occur. Radiologic studies and examination at laparotomy are usually negative. Thus, the diagnosis is difficult and often requires selective mesenteric arteriography or colonoscopy. Surgical removal of the affected segment is curative.

PATHOLOGY: The resected specimen displays small, often multiple vascular lesions, usually smaller than 0.5 cm in diameter. Microscopically, the submucosal veins and capillaries are tortuous, thin walled, and dilated. The attenuated walls of these vessels are presumably responsible for their propensity to bleed.

Hemorrhoids Tend to Bleed

Hemorrhoids are dilated venous channels of the hemorrhoidal plexuses. They result from downward displacement of the anal cushions. Internal hemorrhoids arise from the superior hemorrhoidal plexus above the pectinate line, whereas external hemorrhoids originate from the inferior hemorrhoidal plexus below that line. *Hemorrhoids are common in Western countries, to some degree afflicting at least half the population over 50 years.* Hemorrhoids are common in pregnancy, presumably because of the increased abdominal pressure.

PATHOLOGY: Microscopic examination of hemorrhoidectomy specimens discloses dilated vascular spaces with excess smooth muscle in their walls. Hemorrhage and thrombosis of varying severity are common.

CLINICAL FEATURES: The salient clinical feature of hemorrhoids is bleeding. Chronic blood loss may lead to **iron-deficiency anemia. Rectal prolapse** often develops. Prolapsed hemorrhoids may become irreducible, and lead to painful strangulated hemorrhoids. **Thrombosis** of external hemorrhoids is exquisitely painful and requires evacuation of the intravascular clot.

Radiation Enterocolitis

Radiation therapy for malignant disease of the pelvis or abdomen may be complicated by injury to the small intestine and colon.

PATHOLOGY: Clinically significant radiation colitis is most common in the rectum. The lesions produced by radiation therapy range from a reversible injury of the intestinal mucosa to chronic inflammation, ulceration, and fibrosis of the intestine. In the short term, radiation results in epithelial and endothelial damage, including decreased mitoses and, in the small bowel, villous shortening. Mucosal inflammation is conspicuous and abscesses may be seen in the colorectal crypts. Failure of epithelial renewal may lead to ulceration. Subacute changes, occurring 2 to 12 months after radiation therapy, are noted after the mucosa has healed. Damage to submucosal vessels leads to thrombosis. The submucosa becomes fibrotic and often contains bizarre fibroblasts. As a result of radiation vascular injury, progressive ischemia further damages the bowel.

Complications of radiation enterocolitis include perforation and the subsequent development of internal fistulas, hemorrhage, and stricture, occasionally severe enough to lead to intestinal obstruction.

Solitary Rectal Ulcer Syndrome

Internal mucosal prolapse of the rectum can produce mucosal changes that can be mistaken clinically and pathologically for chronic inflammatory disease or a neoplasm. The hallmark of solitary rectal ulcer syndrome is smooth muscle proliferation from the muscularis mucosae into the lamina propria. Despite the name, some patients have no ulcers, whereas others display multiple erosions, ulcers, or even polypoid lesions. Mucosal abnormalities often appear as a mass that can simulate a neoplasm. Dilated glands can be entrapped in the rectal wall, a condition termed **colitis cystica profunda.**

Polyps of the Colon and Rectum

A gastrointestinal polyp is defined as a mass that protrudes into the lumen of the gut. Polyps are subdivided according to their attachment to the bowel wall (e.g., sessile or pedunculated, with a discrete stalk), their histopathologic appearance (e.g., hyperplastic or adenomatous) and their neoplastic potential (i.e., benign or malignant). By themselves, polyps are only infrequently symptomatic and their clinical importance lies in their potential for malignant transformation.

Adenomatous Polyps Are Premalignant Lesions

Adenomatous polyps (tubular adenomas) are neoplasms that arise from the mucosal epithelium. They are composed of neoplastic epithelial cells that have migrated to the surface and have accumulated beyond the needs for replacement of the cells sloughed into the lumen.

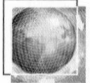

EPIDEMIOLOGY: The prevalence of adenomatous polyps of the colon is highest in industrialized countries. As in diverticular disease, the diet is the only consistent environmental difference between high-risk and low-risk populations that has been identified. In the United States, it appears that at least one adenomatous polyp is present in half of the adult population, a figure that increases to more than two thirds among persons older than 65 years. There is a modest male predominance (1.4:1) and blacks have a higher proportion of right-sided adenomas and cancers. In one-fourth of those who have at least one adenoma, two or more are present.

PATHOLOGY: *Almost half of all adenomatous polyps of the colon in the United States are located in the rectosigmoid region and can, therefore, be detected by digital examination or by sigmoidoscopy.* The remaining half are evenly distributed throughout the rest of the colon. The macroscopic appearance of an adenoma varies from a barely visible nodule or small, pedunculated adenoma to a large, sessile (flat) adenoma. Adenomas are classified by architecture into tubular, villous, and tubulovillous types. They are the usual precursor to colon carinoma, and their epithelium is often dysplastic.

TUBULAR ADENOMAS: These constitute two thirds of the benign large bowel adenomas. Tubular adenomas are typically smooth-surfaced lesions, usually less than 2 cm in diameter, which often have a stalk (Fig. 13-52). Some tubular adenomas, particularly the smaller ones, are sessile.

Microscopically, tubular adenoma has closely packed epithelial tubules, which may be uniform or irregular and excessively branched (see Fig. 13-52C). Tubules are embedded in a fibrovascular stroma similar to the normal lamina propria. Although most tubular adenomas show little epithelial dysplasia, one fifth (particularly larger tumors) may have dysplastic features, which vary from mild nuclear pleomorphism to frank invasive carcinoma (Fig. 13-53). In high-grade dysplasia, glands become crowded and highly irregular in size and shape. Papillary or cribriform (sievelike or perforated) growth patterns are common. *As long as the dysplastic focus is confined to the mucosa, the lesion is cured by resection of the polyp.*

The risk of invasive carcinoma correlates with the size of the tubular adenoma. Only 1% of tubular adenomas under 1 cm display invasive cancer at the time of resection; among those between 1 and 2 cm, 10% harbor malignancy; and among those over 2 cm, 35% are cancerous. Small flat adenomas may be missed during conventional endoscopy and have a high malignant potential.

VILLOUS ADENOMAS: These polyps constitute one tenth of colonic adenomas and are found predominantly in the rectosigmoid region. They are typically large, broad-based, elevated lesions with a shaggy, cauliflower-like surface (Fig. 13-54A), but they can be small and pedunculated. Most are over 2 cm in diameter. On occasion, they reach 10 to 15 cm across. Microscopically, villous adenomas are composed of thin, tall, fingerlike processes that superficially resemble the villi of the small intestine. They are lined externally by neoplastic epithelial cells and are supported by a core of fibrovascular connective tissue corresponding to the normal lamina propria (Fig. 13-54B).

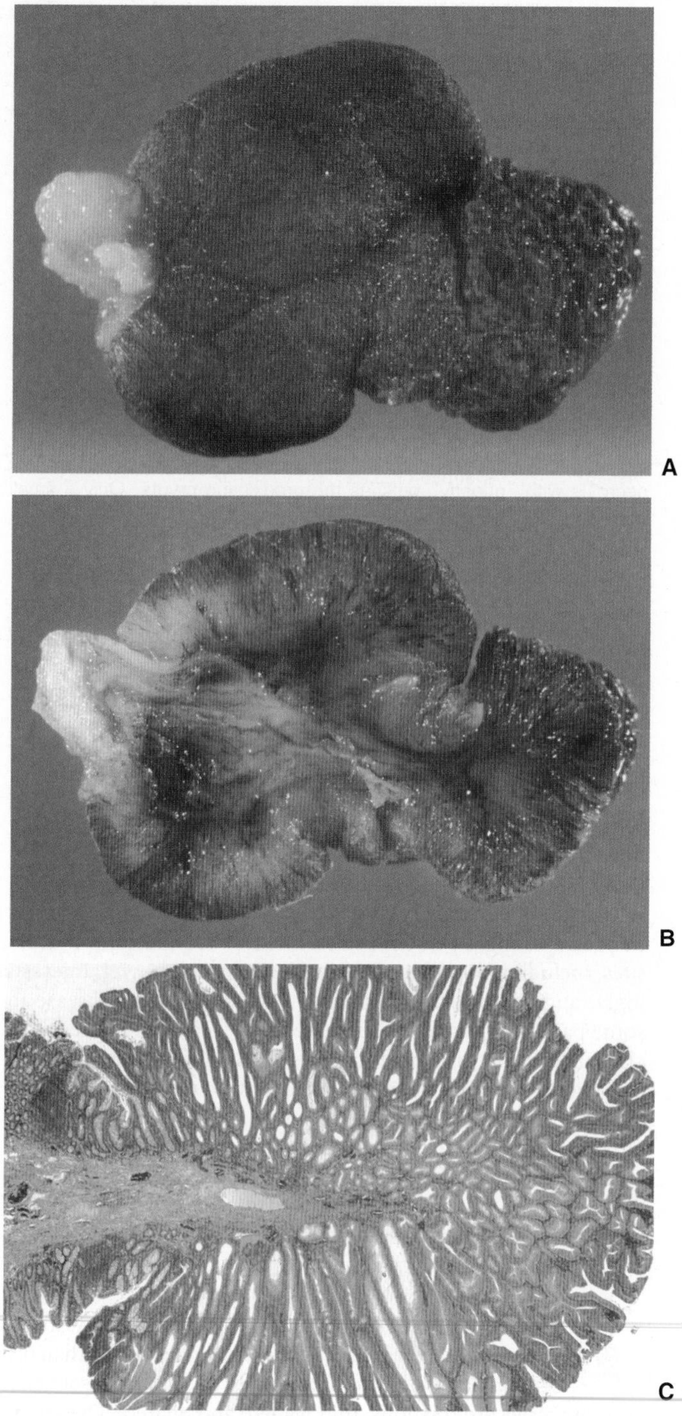

FIGURE 13-52. **Tubular adenoma of the colon. A.** The adenoma shows a characteristic stalk and bosselated surface. **B.** The bisected adenoma shows the stalk covered by the adenomatous epithelium. The ashen white color is cautery at the polypectomy resection margin from the polypectomy. **C.** Microscopically, the adenoma shows a repetitive pattern that is largely tubular. The stalk, which is in continuity with the submucosa of the colon, is not involved and is lined by normal colonic epithelium.

The histopathology of dysplasia in villous adenomas is comparable to that in tubular adenomas. *However, villous adenomas contain foci of carcinoma more often than tubular adenomas.* In polyps less than 1 cm across, the risk is 10 times higher than that for comparably sized tubular adenomas. Of greater importance is the fact that 50% of villous adenomas larger than 2 cm harbor invasive carcinoma. *Given that most villous adenomas measure more*

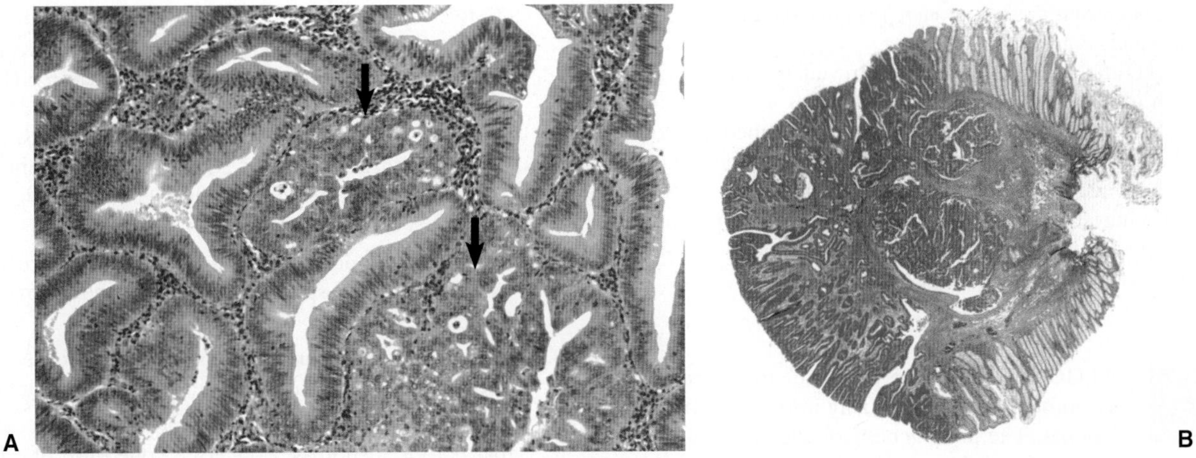

FIGURE 13-53. **Adenocarcinoma arising in a pedunculated adenomatous polyp. A.** Both low-grade dysplasia and high-grade dysplasia are present. The latter is characterized by a cribriform pattern and increased nuclear pleomorphism (*arrows*). **B.** Trichrome stain showing tumor invading the stalk (blue). Since there was a margin of resection of over 1 mm, polypectomy was sufficient therapy.

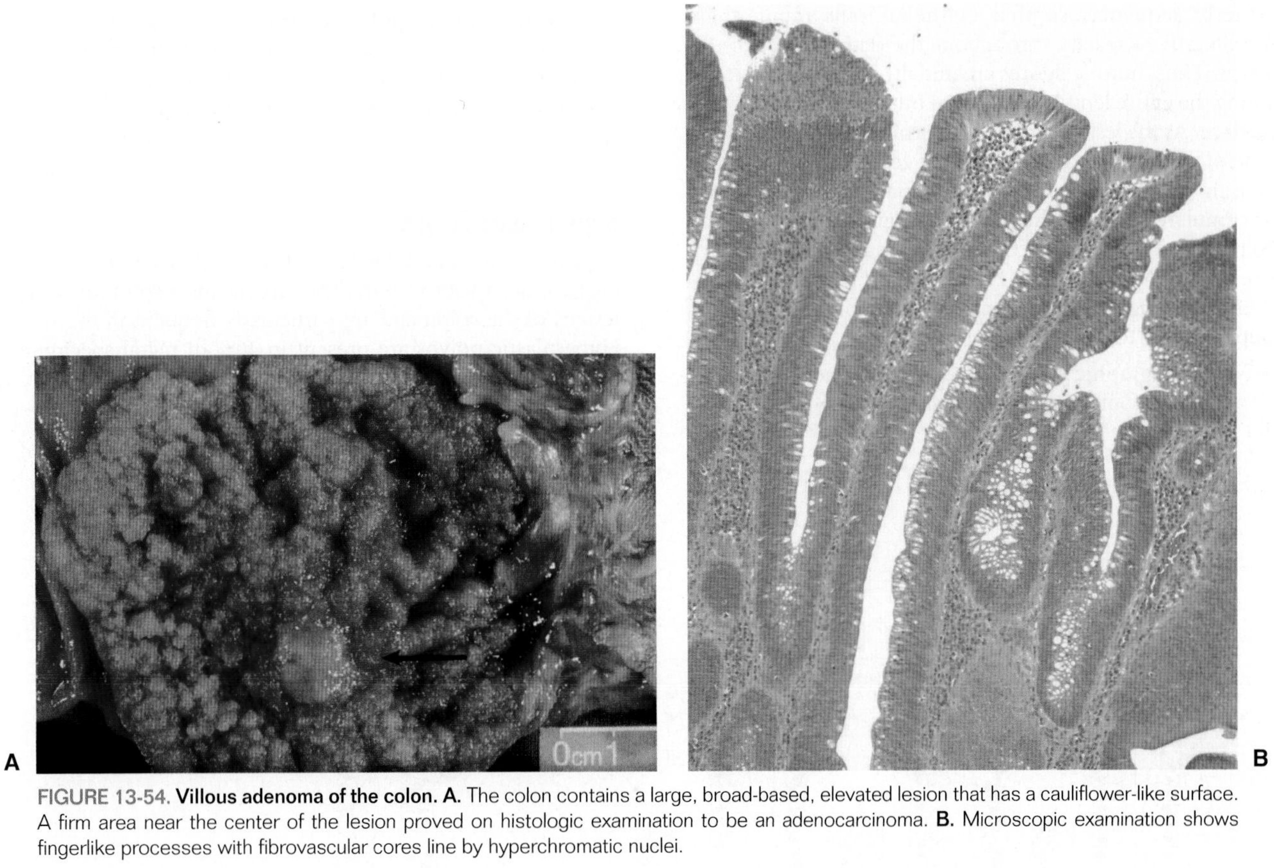

FIGURE 13-54. **Villous adenoma of the colon. A.** The colon contains a large, broad-based, elevated lesion that has a cauliflower-like surface. A firm area near the center of the lesion proved on histologic examination to be an adenocarcinoma. **B.** Microscopic examination shows fingerlike processes with fibrovascular cores line by hyperchromatic nuclei.

than 2 cm in greatest dimension, more than one third of all resected villous adenomas contain invasive cancer.

TUBULOVILLOUS ADENOMAS: Many adenomatous polyps have both tubular and villous features. Polyps with more than 25% and less than 75% villous architecture are termed tubulovillous. These adenomas tend to be intermediate in distribution and size between the tubular and villous forms, one fourth to one third being larger than 2 cm across. Tubulovillous polyps are also intermediate between tubular and villous adenomas in the risk of invasive carcinoma.

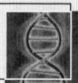

PATHOGENESIS: The precursor to colorectal carcinoma is dysplasia, usually in the form of an adenoma. The pathogenesis of adenomas of the colon and rectum involves neoplastic alteration of crypt epithelial homeostasis with (1) diminished apoptosis, (2) persistent cell replication, and (3) failure to mature and differentiate as the epithelial cells migrate toward the surface of the crypts (Fig. 13-55). Normally, DNA synthesis ceases when cells reach the upper third of the crypts, after which they mature, migrate to the surface, and become senescent. They then undergo apoptosis or are sloughed into the lumen. Adenomas represent focal disruption of this orderly sequence, so that epithelial cells retain their proliferative capacity throughout the entire depth of the crypt. Thus, mitotic figures are initially visualized not only along the entire length of the crypt but also on the mucosal surface. As the lesion evolves, cell proliferation exceeds the rate of apoptosis and sloughing and cells begin to accumulate in upper crypts and on the surface. Eventually, the accumulated cells on the mucosal surface form tubules or villous structures, in concert with stromal elements.

ADENOMATOUS POLYPS AND COLORECTAL CANCER: The origin of colon cancer in adenomatous polyps is supported by the following:

- **The geographic coincidence** in the frequencies of adenomatous polyps and colorectal cancer suggests a causal relation. In geographic regions in which there is a high risk of colorectal cancer, adenomatous polyps tend to be larger, are more often villous, and display more high-grade dysplasia than those in low-risk areas. The anatomical distributions of adenomas and carcinomas are similar, both being most frequent in the sigmoid colon in Western countries.
- **Adenomatous polyps tend to antedate colon cancer by 10 to 15 years,** suggesting that the latter follows the former.
- **Carcinomas are found in adenomas,** and some carcinomas have adenomatous remnants at their periphery.
- **An associated carcinoma** is commonly found in colons that harbor adenomas. Conversely, one third of colons resected for cancer contain an adenomatous polyp. Moreover, the presence of an adenomatous polyp in the same colon specimen resected for cancer doubles the risk that another carcinoma will develop in the remaining colon.
- **In familial adenomatosis polyposis** (see below), the innumerable adenomatous polyps are initially benign, but colorectal cancer invariably develops at a later age.

Prophylactic polypectomies have significantly reduced the risk of subsequent cancer development, a finding that provides powerful support for the concept that most colorectal cancers arise in adenomatous polyps.

Hyperplastic Polyps

Hyperplastic polyps are small, sessile mucosal excrescences that with exaggerated crypt architecture. They are the most common polypoid lesions of the colon and are particularly frequent in the rectum. Hyperplastic polyps are present in 40% of rectal specimens in persons younger than 40 and in 75% of older persons. They are more common than usual in colons with adenomatous polyps and in populations with higher rates of colorectal cancer.

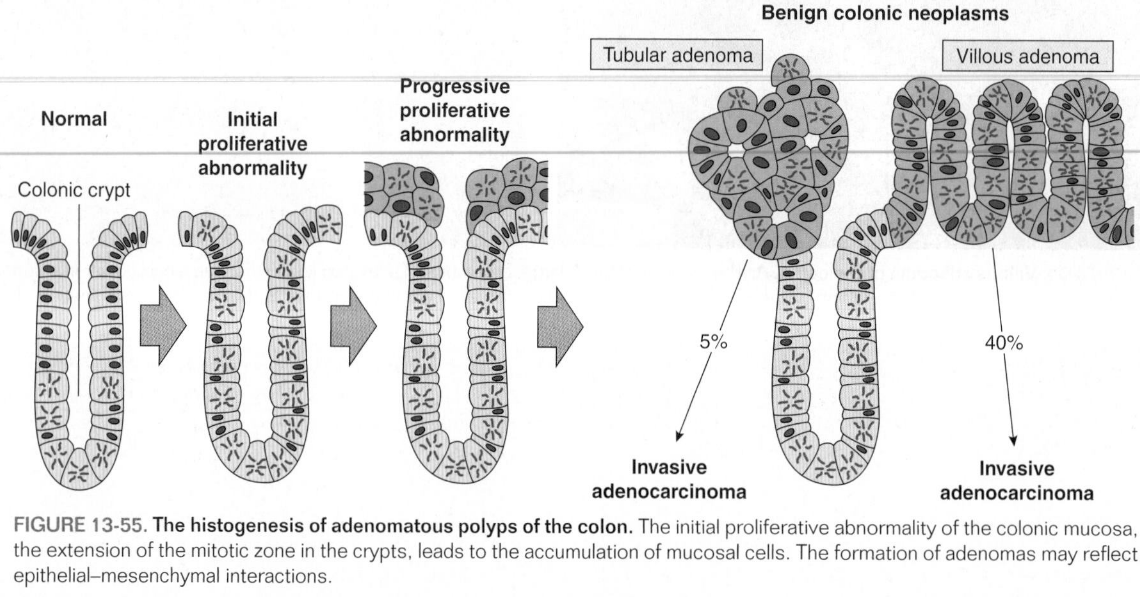

FIGURE 13-55. **The histogenesis of adenomatous polyps of the colon.** The initial proliferative abnormality of the colonic mucosa, the extension of the mitotic zone in the crypts, leads to the accumulation of mucosal cells. The formation of adenomas may reflect epithelial–mesenchymal interactions.

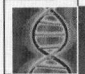

PATHOGENESIS: Hyperplastic polyps are believed to arise due to a defect in proliferation and maturation of normal mucosal epithelium. In a hyperplastic polyp, proliferation occurs at the base of the crypt, and upward migration of the cells is slowed. Thus, epithelial cells differentiate and acquire absorptive characteristics lower in the crypts. Moreover, cells persist at the surface longer do than normal cells.

PATHOLOGY: Hyperplastic polyps are small, sessile, raised mucosal nodules, up to 0.5 cm in diameter but occasionally larger. They are almost always multiple and have even been mistaken for familial adenomatous polyposis (FAP). Histologically, the crypts of hyperplastic polyps are elongated and may show cystic dilation (Fig. 13-56). The epithelium contains goblet cells and absorptive cells, with no dysplasia. The surface cells are elongated giving a tufted appearance; this accounts for the serrated contour of the glands near the surface.

There are Several Variants of Hyperplastic Polyps (Serrated Adenomas)

There is debate over current nomenclature of these variants. One form has a serrated configuration like that of hyperplastic polyps but with nuclear features of adenomas, and is termed **serrated adenoma** (Fig. 13-57A). Another type is called **sessile serrated adenoma,** and resembles classic hyperplastic polyps, but does not show adenomatous features, and often appear as a large deformed mucosal fold (Fig. 13-57B and C). Yet a third variant exhibits juxtaposed areas of hyperplastic polyp and adenoma, referred to as **mixed hyperplastic adenomatous polyps** (Fig. 13-57D). *Unlike classic hyperplastic polyps, patients with these variants have an increased risk for the development of carcinoma.* These lesions have a high incidence of microsatellite instability. The carinomas that arise from them tend to be bulky, mucinous, and right-sided.

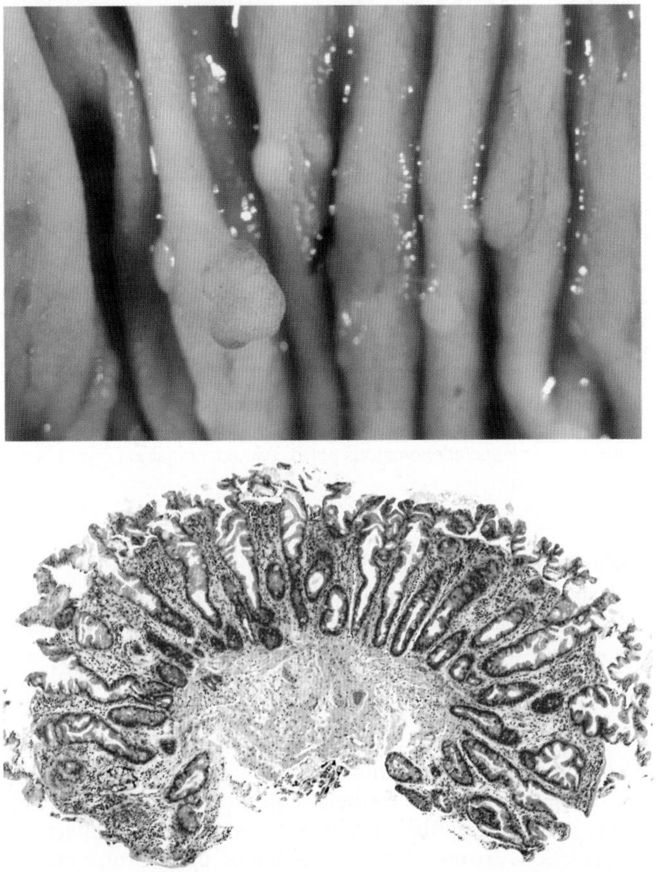

FIGURE 13-56. **Hyperplastic polyp. A.** This hyperplastic polyp is small, sessile and pale. There are smaller adjacent hyperplastic polyps. **B.** Microscopically, there is a "sawtooth" appearance to the surface.

Familial Adenomatous Polyposis (FAP) is an Autosomal Dominant Trait that Invariably Leads to Cancer

Also termed **adenomatous polyposis coli** (APC), FAP accounts for less than 1% of colorectal cancers. It is caused by a mutation of the *APC* gene on the long arm of chromosome 5 (5q21-22) (see below). Most cases are familial, but 30% to 50% reflect new mutations. FAP is characterized by hundreds to thousands of adenomas carpeting the colorectal mucosa, sometimes throughout its length, but particularly in the rectosigmoid area (Fig. 13-58). The adenomas are mostly of the tubular variety, although tubulovillous and villous adenomas are also present. Microscopic adenomas, sometimes involving a single crypt, are numerous. A few polyps are usually present by age 10, but the mean age for occurrence of symptoms is 36 years, by which time cancer is often already present. *Carcinoma of the colon and rectum is inevitable, the mean age of onset being 40 years.* Total colectomy before onset of cancer is curative, but some patients also have tubular adenomas in the small intestine and stomach that have the same malignant potential as those in the colon.

Genetic testing for FAP is available, but mutations are found in only 75% of familial cases. Subtypes of FAP include:

- **Attenuated FAP:** In this condition adenomas in the colon number less than 100.
- **Gardner syndrome:** This variant features extracolonic lesions including osteomas of the skull, mandible, and long bones; epidermoid cysts; desmoid tumors; and congential hypertrophy of the retinal pigment epithelium. *APC* gene mutations do not predict this phenotype.
- **Turcot syndrome:** This rare disorder combines FAP with malignant tumors of the central nervous system. Many cases, especially those with medulloblastoma, are due to germline mutation of the *APC* gene. Some cases, especially those with glioblastoma multiforme, are part of the spectrum of the HNPCC syndrome (see below).

Non-neoplastic Polyps Are Acquired Lesions

Non-neoplastic polyps are entirely different entities and are grouped together solely because of their gross appearance as raised lesions of the colonic mucosa.

Juvenile Polyps (Retention Polyps)

Juvenile polyps are hamartomatous proliferations of the colonic mucosa. They are most common in children younger than 10 years, although one third occur in adults.

PATHOLOGY: Juvenile polyps are single or (rarely) multiple. They mostly occur in the rectum, but may be seen anywhere in the small or large bowel. Grossly,

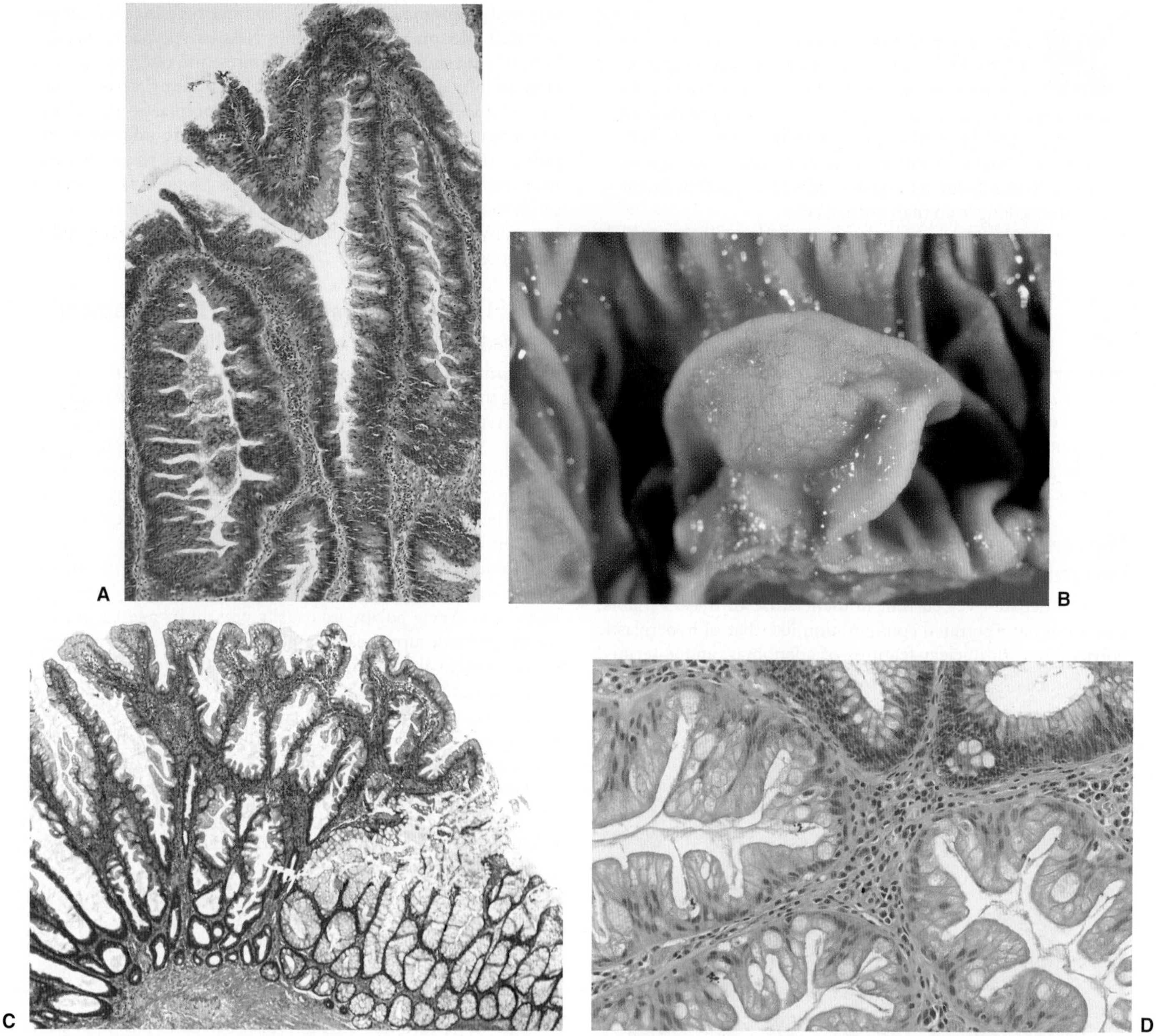

FIGURE 13-57. **Variants of hyperplastic polyps. A.** Serrated adenoma. The epithelium shows contours typical of hyperplastic polyp with adenomatous nuclear features. **B.** Sessile serrated adenoma. A polypoid lesion appears to be an enlarged flattened fold. **C.** Microscopically, sessile serrated adenoma features irregular, asymmetric crypts that are often dilated by mucin. **D.** Mixed hyperplastic adenomatous polyp. Two adenomatous crypts in the upper right contrast with the three hyperplastic crypts.

most are pedunculated lesions up to 2 cm in diameter. They have smooth, rounded surfaces, unlike fissured surfaces of adenomatous polyps. Microscopically, dilated and cystic epithelial tubules filled with mucus (hence the name "retention polyp") are embedded in a fibrovascular lamina propria (Fig. 13-59). Surface epithelial erosion is common, and reactive epithelial proliferation is evident, but the epithelium usually lacks dysplasia.

Patients with five or more juvenile polyps, or juvenile polyps present outside the colon along with a family history of juvenile polyps have a high likelihood of the syndrome of familial juvenile polyposis. These patients have an increased risk for gastrointestinal carcinoma, not necessarily arising from the polyps or even the segment of the gastrointestinal tract in which they are located.

Inflammatory Polyps

Inflammatory polyps are not neoplasms but are elevated nodules of inflamed, regenerating epithelium. They are commonly found in association with ulcerative colitis and Crohn disease; they are also encountered in cases of amebic colitis and bacterial dysentery. Microscopically, inflammatory polyps are composed of a variable component of distorted and inflamed mucosal glands, often intermixed with granulation tissue.

As healing proceeds, epithelial regeneration characterized by large, basophilic epithelial cells restores mucosal architecture. These lesions are not precancerous, but occur in chronic inflammatory diseases that are associated with a high incidence of cancer (e.g., ulcerative colitis) and must thus be distinguished from adenomatous polyps.

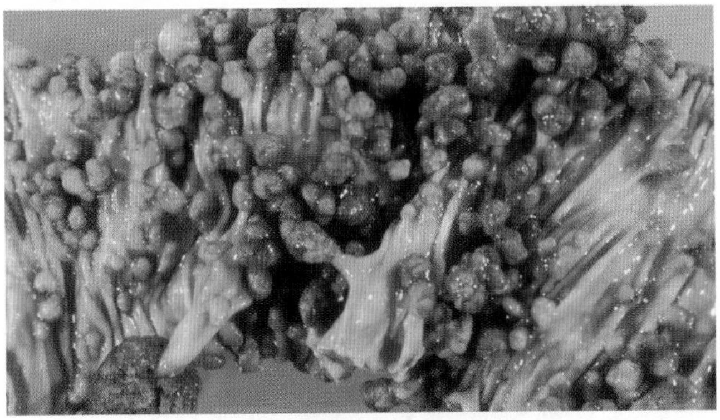

FIGURE 13-58. **Familial polyposis.** The colon containes thousands of adenomatous polyps with only several exceeding 1 cm in diameter.

Lymphoid Polyps

Lymphoid polyps are submucosal accumulations of lymphoid tissue, almost invariably in the rectum, which are seen as single, sessile nodules measuring from pinpoint size to as large as 5 cm in diameter. On occasion, multiple lesions impart a cobblestone appearance to the mucosa. Microscopically, these polyps are covered by intact mucosa and are composed of prominent lymphoid follicles with germinal centers. In this context, lymphoid tissue is normally present in the colorectal mucosa. Lymphoid polyps are more common in women than men and occur at any age, including childhood. They are benign and usually asymptomatic.

Nodular lymphoid hyperplasia is seen primarily in children or with common variable immunodeficiency syndrome, and features excessive accumulation of the normal follicular lymphoid tissue of the colon. Macroscopically, the mucosa exhibits numerous small sessile or polypoid nodules up to 0.5 cm in diameter. The microscopic appearance is similar to that of lymphoid polyps. The condition is only rarely related to malignant lymphoma, but the radiologic appearance can be mistaken for FAP.

Malignant Tumors

Adenocarcinoma of the Colon and Rectum Is an Example of Multistep Carcinogenesis

In Western societies, colorectal cancer is the most common cause of cancer deaths that are not directly attributable to tobacco use. Some 5% of Americans develop this cancer during their lifetime. Although the widely used term **colorectal** implies a common biology, the differences between cancers of the colon and rectum seem to be more fundamental than simple location. For instance, whereas colon cancer is much more common in the United States than in Japan, the incidence of rectal cancer in the two populations is nearly the same. In general, rectosigmoid carcinoma accounts for a much higher proportion of large bowel cancers in populations at high risk for this tumor (including the United States) than in low-risk populations. Moreover, colon cancer shows a slight female preponderance, whereas rectal cancer is somewhat more common in men. The proportion of cancers in the distal colorectum has been declining in recent decades.

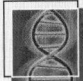

PATHOGENESIS: Most cancers of the colon and rectum arise in adenomatous polyps and so factors associated with the development of such polyps are relevant to the genesis of colorectal cancer. The importance of environmental factors in the pathogenesis of colorectal cancer is emphasized by the high incidence of the disease in industrialized countries and among emigrants from low-risk to high-risk regions.

DIETARY FIBER: A diet low in indigestible fiber and high in animal fat has been implicated in the etiology of other colonic diseases, including diverticulosis and appendicitis. Such a diet is associated with slower transit of fecal contents through the colon, and some suggest that this permits longer exposure of the mucosa to possibly toxic substances in the stools. It has also been suggested that fiber may bind potential mutagens and dilute their concentration by increasing stool bulk. However, more recent analyses and clinical trials of diets high in fiber have cast doubt on such an explanation.

DIETARY FAT: Consumption of animal fats is paralleled by increased colorectal cancer. Moreover, certain ethnic groups in the United States that consume diets lower in animal fat have a lower incidence of colorectal cancer. Ingestion of fat elicits bile secretion into the intestine, and some bile acids may augment the tumorigenicity of experimental intestinal carcinogens. In this context, cholecystectomy, which increases the colonic content of secondary bile acids, has been claimed in some studies (although not in others) to be associated with an increased risk of right-sided colon cancer.

ANAEROBIC BACTERIA: The feces of persons in high-risk populations have a higher content of anaerobic bacteria than do those in low-risk populations. Some of these bacteria, particularly *Bacteroides* species, can convert bile salts into compounds that are potentially mutagenic. Repopulation of the colon with *Lactobacillus* protects experimental animals against chemically induced colon cancer.

OTHER DIETARY FACTORS: A low prevalence of colorectal cancer has been correlated with high levels of selenium in the soil and plants in certain geographic areas. In this context, the endogenous antioxidant, glutathione peroxidase, is a selenium-containing enzyme. Exogenous antioxidants (e.g., butylated hydroxytoluene and vitamin E) and a reducing agent such as ascorbic acid have protected experimental animals from colonic cancer. Diets rich in cruciferous vegetables (e.g., cauliflower, Brussels sprouts, and cabbage) and those that provide vitamin A may be associated with a lower incidence of colorectal cancer.

Molecular Genetics of Colorectal Cancer

In 85% of cases of colorectal carcinoma, it has been estimated that at least 8 to 10 mutational events must accumulate before an invasive cancer with metastatic potential develops. This process is initiated in histologically normal mucosa, proceeds through an adenomatous precursor stage, and ends as invasive adenocarcinoma.

The most important mutational events are illustrated in Figure 13-60 and involve:

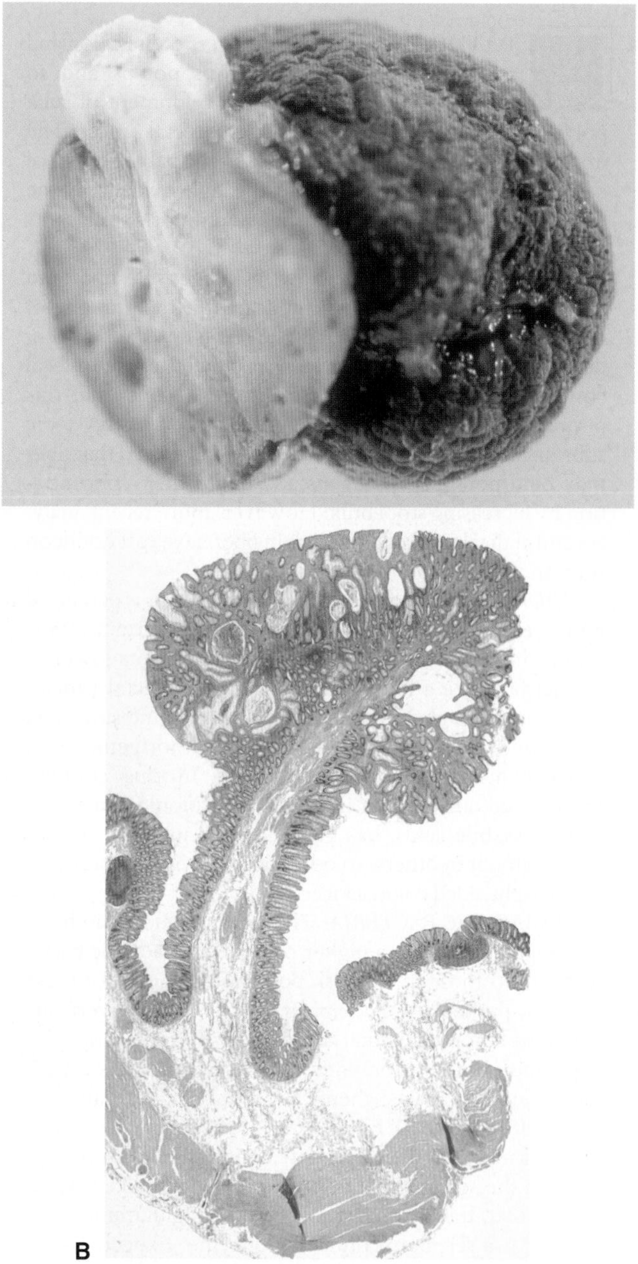

FIGURE 13-59. **Juvenile polyp. A.** The resected specimen shows a rounded surface which is dark because of hemorrhage and ulceration. The cut surface (left) is cystic. **B.** Microscopically, the polyp displays cystically dilated glands.

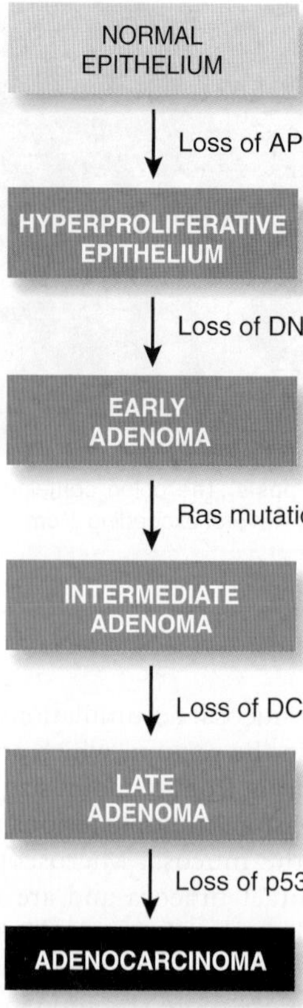

FIGURE 13-60. Model of some of the genetic alterations involved in colonic carcinogenesis following the tumor suppressor pathway. APC = adenomatous polyposis coli; DCC = "deleted in colon cancer."

- ***APC* gene:** As noted above, germline mutations in *APC* (adenomatous polyposis coli), a putative tumor-suppressor gene, lead to familial adenomatous polyposis. In most sporadic colorectal cancers the same gene is mutated. Some tumors with normal *APC* have mutations in the β-catenin gene, whose product binds to the *APC* protein. A specific *APC* mutation (T→A, 1307) is found in 6% of Ashkenazi Jews and seems to render surrounding regions of the gene susceptible to inactivating frame-shift mutations. *APC* mutations are seen in normal colonic mucosa preceding development of sporadic adenomas. These data suggest an important role for *APC* in the early development of most colorectal neoplasms.
- ***Ras* oncogene:** Activating mutations of the *ras* protooncogene occur early in tubular adenomas of the colon.
- ***DCC* gene:** A putative tumor-suppressor gene, *DCC* ("deleted in colon cancer") is located on chromosome 18 and is often missing in colorectal cancers.
- ***p53* tumor-suppressor gene:** In the most common type of adenocarcinoma of the colon, mutation of *p53* participates in the transition from adenoma to carcinoma and is a late event in the carcinogenic pathway.

In 15% of colorectal cancers, DNA mismatch repair (MMR) is impaired, leading to deficient repair of spontaneous replication errors, particularly in simple repetitive sequences (microsatellites). MMR deficiencies can occur through two mechanisms in a hereditary form (HNPCC, Lynch syndrome), a germline mutation in one of the MMR genes is followed by a somatic mutation of the other allele ("second hit") later in life. In a sporadic form, hypermethylation of the MMR promoter, *MLH1,* inactivates transcription of the gene.

Risk Factors

AGE: Increasing age is probably the single most important risk factor for colorectal cancer in the general population. Risk is low before age 40. It increases steadily to age 50, after which it doubles with each decade.

PRIOR COLORECTAL CANCER: Patients with a prior colorectal cancer are at increased risk for a subsequent tumor. In fact, 5% to 10% of patients treated for colorectal cancer subsequently develop a second colorectal malignancy. Moreover, 2% to 5% of those with a new colorectal cancer harbor a second (synchronous) colorectal primary cancer.

ULCERATIVE COLITIS AND CROHN DISEASE: These chronic inflammatory diseases increase the risk of colorectal cancer in proportion to their duration and extent of involvement within the large bowel.

GENETIC FACTORS: Colorectal cancer is increased in frequency among relatives of patients with the disease, a finding that suggests a genetic contribution to tumorigenesis. Persons with two or more first- or second-degree relatives with colorectal cancer constitute 20% of all patients with this tumor. Some 5% to 10% of all colorectal cancers are inherited as autosomal dominant traits. A history of cancer at other sites, particularly breast or genital cancer in women, is associated with a higher than normal frequency of colorectal cancer.

DIET: As previously noted, prospective studies involving large populations in various countries have reported that the daily consumption of red meat and animal fat leads to a higher risk of colorectal cancer than that in persons who eat little or no meat.

PATHOLOGY: Grossly colorectal cancers resemble adenocarcinomas elsewhere in the gut. *They tend to be polypoid and ulcerating or infiltrative and may be annular and constrictive* (Fig. 13-61A). Polypoid cancers are more common in the right colon, particularly in the cecum, where the large caliber of the colon allows unimpeded intraluminal growth. Annular constricting tumors are more common in the distal colon. Ulceration of tumors, irrespective of growth pattern, is common.

The vast majority of colorectal cancers are adenocarcinomas (see Fig. 13-61B) that are microscopically similar to their counterparts in other parts of the digestive tract. Some 10% to 15% secrete large quantities of mucin; these are called **mucinous** adenocarcinomas. The degree of differentiation influences the prognosis; better-differentiated tumors tend to have a more favorable outlook.

Colorectal cancer spreads by direct extension or vascular invasion. The former is commonly seen in resected specimens. The connective tissues of the serosa offer little resistance to tumor spread, and cancer cells are often found in the fat and serosa at some distance from the primary tumor. The peritoneum is occasionally involved, in which case, there may be multiple deposits throughout the abdomen.

Colorectal cancer invades lymphatic channels and initially involves the lymph nodes immediately underlying the tumor. Venous invasion leads to blood-borne metastases, which involve the liver in most patients with metastatic disease. The prognosis of colorectal cancer is more closely related to tumor extension through the large bowel wall than to its size or histopathological characteristics.

Current staging of colorectal carcinomas uses TNM classification (tumor, lymph nodes, metastasis). In this system T1 tumor invades the submucosa; T2 tumor infiltrates into, but not through, the muscularis propria; T3 tumor invades into the subserosal tissue; and T4 tumors penetrate the serosa or involve adjacent organs. N refers to presence or absence of nodal metastases, and M to the presence or absence of extranodal metastases.

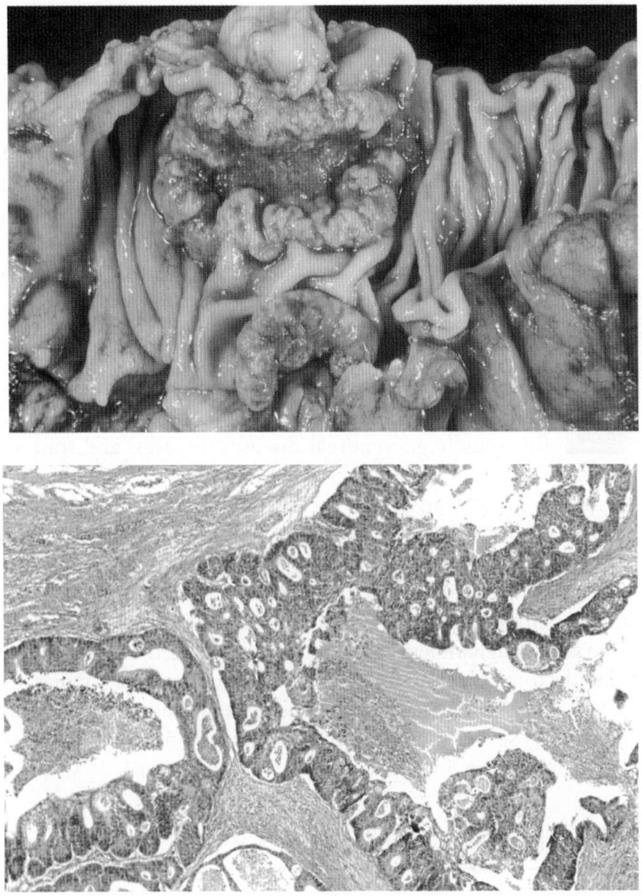

A

B

FIGURE 13-61. **Adenocarcinoma of the colon. A.** A resected colon shows an ulcerated mass with enlarged, firm, rolled borders. **B.** Microscopically, this colon adenocarcinoma consists of moderately differentiated glands with a prominent cribriform pattern and frequent central necrosis.

CLINICAL FEATURES: Initially, colorectal cancer is clinically silent. As the tumor grows, the most common sign is **occult blood in the feces** when the tumor is in the proximal portions of the colon. Both occult blood and **bright red blood** in the feces may occur if a lesion is in the distal colorectum.

Cancers on the left side of the colon, where the caliber of the lumen is small and the fecal contents more solid, often constrict the lumen, producing **obstructive symptoms.** These are manifested as changes in bowel habits and abdominal pain. Occasionally, colorectal cancer **perforates** early and induces peritonitis. By contrast, on the right side of the colon, particularly in the cecum, the colon lumen is large and fecal contents are liquid, tumors can grow to large size without causing symptoms of obstruction. In this situation, chronic asymptomatic bleeding may cause **iron-deficiency anemia,** which is often the first indication of colorectal cancer. When a tumor has extended beyond the confines of the colorectum, it may produce enterocutaneous and rectovaginal **fistulas,** tumor masses in the abdominal wall, bladder symptoms, and sciatic nerve pain. Spread within the abdomen may cause **small intestinal obstruction** and malignant **ascites.**

A positive test result for fecal occult blood predicts the presence of a cancer or an adenoma in 50% of cases. Periodic fiberoptic colonoscopy and testing for occult blood in feces improves the prognosis of colorectal cancer, because these methods can often detect the disease at an early stage.

The only curative treatment for colorectal cancer is surgery. Small polyps are easily removed endoscopically; large lesions require segmental resection. Tumors close to the anal verge

TABLE 13-2

Hereditary Nonpolyposis Colorectal Cancer (HNPCC)

Amsterdam criteria
At least three relatives must have histologically verified colorectal cancer.
One must be a first-degree relative of the other two
At least two successive generations must be affected
At least one of the relatives with colorectal cancer must have received the diagnosis before the age of 50 years
Familial adenomatous polyposis must have been excluded
Bethesda guidelines
Amsterdam I criteria met
Individuals with more than one HNPCC
Colorectal cancer (CRC) and first-degree relative with CRC/HNPCC, one cancer younger than 45 years or one adenoma younger than 40
CRC/endometrial cancer younger than age 45
Right-sided CRC, undifferentiated, younger than 45
Signet-ring CRC younger than 45
Adenomas younger than 40 years

often necessitate abdominal–perineal resection and colostomy, although newer surgical techniques may allow sphincter preservation. In rectal cancers, use of adjuvant chemotherapy and radiotherapy before surgery improves the prognosis.

Hereditary Nonpolyposis Colorectal Cancer Syndrome

HNPCC, or Warthin-Lynch syndrome is an autosomal dominant inherited disease that accounts for 3% to 5% of all colorectal cancers. It is characterized by (1) onset of colorectal cancer at a young age (Table 13-2); (2) few adenomas (hence "nonpolyposis"); (3) a high frequency of carcinomas proximal to the splenic flexure (70%); (4) multiple synchronous or metachronous colorectal cancers; and (5) extracolonic cancers, including endometrial and ovarian cancers, adenocarcinomas of the stomach, small intestine, and hepatobiliary tract, as well as transitional cell carcinomas of the renal pelvis and ureter. Patients with HNPCC may also have sebaceous adenomas and carcinomas and multiple keratoacanthomas. Histologically, HNPCC-related colorectal cancers are characterized by a high frequency of mucinous, signet ring cell and solid (medullary) carcinomas, and frequent intratumoral lymphocytes.

PATHOGENESIS: HNPCC is caused by germline mutations in a DNA mismatch repair gene. In most cases, *hMSH2* (human MutS homolog 2) on chromosome 2p and *hMLH1* (human MutL homolog 1) on chromosome 3p are affected. A smaller number of cases are caused by mutations in *hMSH6* (human MutS homolog 6) and *hPMS2* (human postmeiotic segregation 2) on chromosomes 2p and 7p, respectively. In patients with HNPCC there is a germline mutation in one allele of one of the mismatch repair genes, and the second allele is deleted in a somatic "second hit." The result is that spontaneous replication errors are not repaired effectively. This leads to widespread genomic instability, particularly in simple repetitive sequences (microsatellites), which are particularly prone to replication errors. Thus, genes that regulate growth and differentiation, and other mismatch repair genes, are disabled by unrepaired mutations.

Mismatch repair deficiency can be assessed by testing for microsatellite instability and loss of immunohistochemical expression of mismatch repair proteins in a tumor. If suspicion of HNPCC persists, mutation analysis of mismatch repair genes is available.

Carcinoid Tumors (Neuroendocrine Tumors)

Colorectal carcinoid tumors behave like similar tumors of the small intestine. Half of carcinoid tumors of the colorectum have metastasized at the time they are discovered.

Large Bowel Lymphoma is Usually B-cell Lymphoma

Primary lymphoma of the colorectum is uncommon. It may be seen as (1) segmental involvement of the mucosa, (2) diffuse polypoid lesions, or (3) a mass extending beyond the confines of the colorectum. Presenting symptoms are similar to those of other primary intestinal cancers, but the diffuse polypoid form may resemble inflammatory polyps or adenomatous polyps. Most large bowel lymphomas are derived from B cells.

Cancers of the Anal Canal Are Epidermoid Carcinomas

Carcinomas of the anal canal, which constitute 2% of cancers of the large bowel, may arise at or above the dentate line. These tumors occur in both sexes, but are more common in women and in blacks.

PATHOLOGY: Anal cancers have various histologic patterns, such as squamous, basaloid (cloacogenic) or mucoepidermoid, but the different tumor types exhibit similar clinical behavior and so are all classed as **epidermoid carcinomas. Bowen disease of the anus** is squamous carcinoma in situ, while **extramammary Paget disease** at this site reflects intraepithelial adenocarcinoma (either primary of the mucosa or metastatic). Carcinoma of the anus penetrates directly into surrounding tissues, including internal and external sphincters, perianal soft tissues, prostate, and vagina.

CLINICAL FEATURES: Infection with human papilloma virus (HPV) and chronic inflammatory disease of the anus (e.g., venereal disease), fissures, and trauma predispose to anal cancer. Factors associated with genital carcinoma (cancer of the penis, scrotum, cervix or vulva), poor hygiene, indiscriminate sexual practices, and genital warts also contribute to the development of anal cancer.

The usual symptoms of anal cancers include bleeding, pain, and an anal or rectal mass. Often a tumor is not clinically recognized as a malignant lesion and may be discovered only in a hemorrhoidectomy specimen. Combined chemotherapy and radiation therapy is the customary treatment, although abdominal–perineal resection is sometimes carried out. More than half of patients survive for at least 5 years.

Miscellaneous Disorders

Endometriosis Involves the Colon and Rectum in 15% to 20% of Cases

Colorectal endometriosis is mostly asymptomatic and discovered only incidentally during laparotomy for other reasons. When symptoms do occur (abdominal pain, constipation, and even intestinal obstruction), they may be mistaken for those of colorectal cancer. **Endometriomas** are seen as indurated tumors of up to 5 cm in diameter in the serosa and muscularis propria of the bowel, although they may penetrate the submucosa. As a result of repeated hemorrhage, the lesions are surrounded by reactive fibrosis.

Melanosis Coli is Usually the Result of Chronic Use of Anthracene Laxatives

The cathartics include cascara sagrada, rhubarb, senna, and aloe, and the finding can indicate surreptitious laxative abuse. In melanosis coli the mucosa is dark brown. Despite the name, the pigment is lipofuscin-like, and is unrelated to melanin. Microscopically, macrophages in the lamina propria contain brown pigment granules. The pigment is lysosomal and is derived from the breakdown of cellular membranes.

Gastrointestinal Infections Are Common Complications of AIDS

The AIDS epidemic has resulted in numerous gastrointestinal infections previously considered rare. Most patients with AIDS (50%–90%) have chronic diarrhea. Virtually all forms of infectious agents–including bacteria, fungi, protozoa, and viruses–afflict patients with AIDS (Table 13-3).

Kaposi sarcoma of the gut is found almost exclusively in patients with AIDS. One third to one half of AIDS patients with cutaneous Kaposi sarcoma show digestive tract involvement. In most patients, intestinal Kaposi sarcoma does not lead to symptoms, although gastrointestinal bleeding, obstruction, and malabsorption have been reported.

A common presentation of lymphoma complicating AIDS is involvement of the gastrointestinal tract. Any portion may be affected. The histologic appearance and prognosis of these tumors in AIDS patients are similar to those elsewhere.

TABLE 13-3

Gastrointestinal Pathogens Associated with AIDS

Bacteria	
	Mycobacterium avium-intracellulare
	Shigella
	Salmonella
	Clostridium difficile
Viruses	
	Cytomegalovirus
	Herpes simplex
Fungi	
	Candida
	Aspergillus
Protozoa	
	Cryptospordium
	Toxoplasma
	Giardia
	Entameba histolytica
	Microsporidia
	Isopora belli
Helminths	
	Strongyloides
	Enterobius

THE APPENDIX

Anatomy

The vermiform appendix, which is usually 8 to 10 cm in length, typically has a retrocecal attachment to the cecum, but its tip is generally not fixed and can therefore move freely. It is invested with a mesentery, the **mesoappendix.** The wall of the appendix is composed of the same layers as the rest of the intestine. The most prominent microscopic feature is the predominance of submucosal lymphoid tissue, which develops in early infancy, reaches its largest size during adolescence and then progressively atrophies.

Appendicitis

Acute appendicitis is an inflammatory disease of the wall of the vermiform appendix that leads to transmural inflammation and perforation and peritonitis. This condition is by far the most common disease of the appendix and is the most frequent cause of an abdominal emergency. Although incidence peaks in the second and third decades, acute appendicitis may occur in persons of any age.

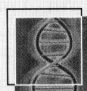

PATHOGENESIS: *Acute appendicitis relates to obstruction of its orifice, with secondary distention of the lumen and bacterial invasion of the wall.* Mechanical obstruction by fecaliths or solid fecal material in the cecum is found in one third of cases. Occasionally tumors, parasites such as *Enterobius vermicularis* or foreign bodies are incriminated. Lymphoid hyperplasia due to bacterial or viral infection (e.g., by *Salmonella* or measles) may obstruct the lumen and lead to appendicitis. *However, no obstruction is demonstrated in up to half of patients with appendicitis,* and the factor that precipitates the disease in these patients is unknown.

As secretions distend an obstructed appendix, intraluminal pressure increases and eventually exceeds the venous pressure. This causes venous stasis and ischemia,and leads to mucosal ulceration and invasion by intestinal bacteria. Neutrophil accumulation produces microabscesses. Interestingly, appendectomy protects against development of ulcerative colitis but not Crohn disease.

PATHOLOGY: The appendix is congested, tense, and covered by a fibrinous exudate. Its lumen often contains purulent material. A fecalith may be evident (Fig. 13-62). Microscopically, early cases show mucosal microabscesses and a purulent exudate in the lumen. As infection progresses, the entire wall becomes infiltrated with neutrophils, which eventually reach the serosa. Perforation of the wall releases the luminal contents into the peritoneal cavity.

The complications of appendicitis are principally related to perforation, which occurs in one third of children and young adults. Almost all children under 2 years have a perforated appendix at the time of operation, as do three fourths of patients over 60.

- **Periappendiceal abscesses** are common, although abscesses may develop anywhere in the abdominal cavity.

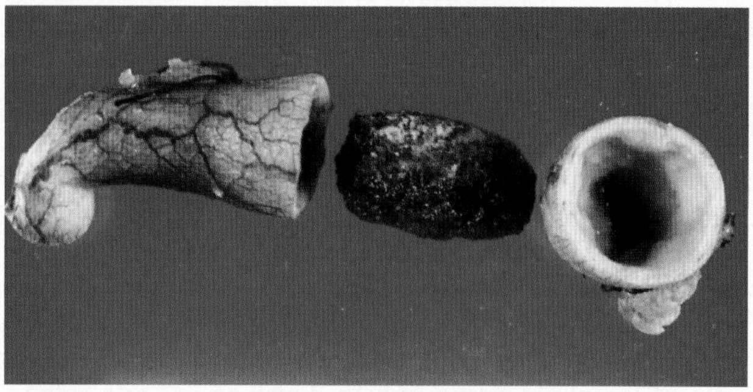

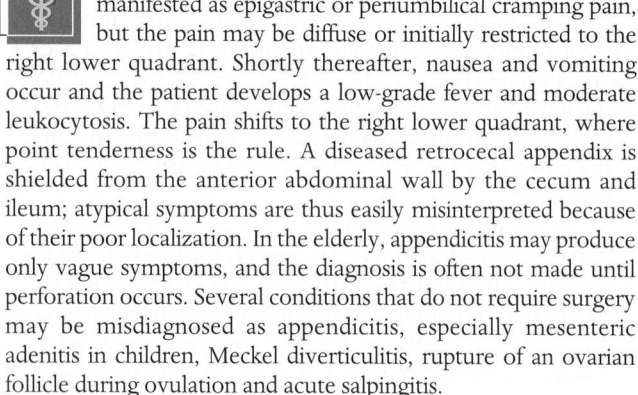

FIGURE 13-62. **Acute appendicitis.** The lumen of this acutely inflamed appendix is dilated and contains a large fecalith.

- **Fistulous tracts** may appear between the perforated appendix and adjacent structures, including the small and large bowel, bladder, vagina, or abdominal wall.
- **Pylephlebitis** (thrombophlebitis of the intrahepatic portal vein radicals) and **secondary hepatic abscesses** may occur, because venous blood from the appendix drains into the superior mesenteric vein.
- **Diffuse peritonitis and septicemia** are dangerous sequelae.
- **Wound infection** is the most common complication of acute appendicitis after surgery; it occurs in one fourth of patients with perforation and in one third of those who develop a periappendiceal abscess.

CLINICAL FEATURES: Acute appendicitis is typically manifested as epigastric or periumbilical cramping pain, but the pain may be diffuse or initially restricted to the right lower quadrant. Shortly thereafter, nausea and vomiting occur and the patient develops a low-grade fever and moderate leukocytosis. The pain shifts to the right lower quadrant, where point tenderness is the rule. A diseased retrocecal appendix is shielded from the anterior abdominal wall by the cecum and ileum; atypical symptoms are thus easily misinterpreted because of their poor localization. In the elderly, appendicitis may produce only vague symptoms, and the diagnosis is often not made until perforation occurs. Several conditions that do not require surgery may be misdiagnosed as appendicitis, especially mesenteric adenitis in children, Meckel diverticulitis, rupture of an ovarian follicle during ovulation and acute salpingitis.

Treatment is surgical in the vast majority of cases. As perforation carries a much higher risk of death than does laparoscopic surgery, early surgical intervention is warranted, even if the diagnosis of acute appendicitis is not entirely secure.

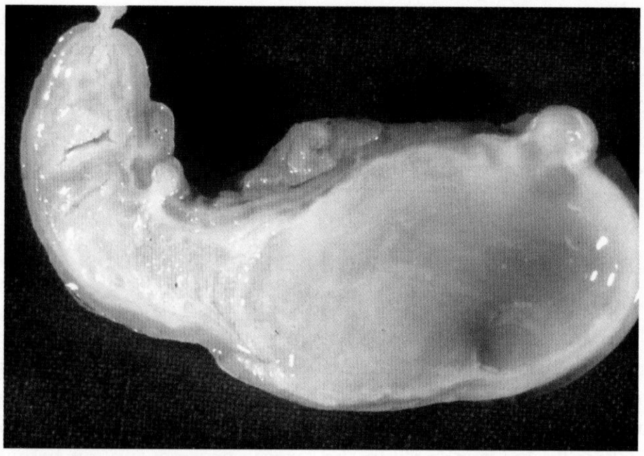

FIGURE 13-63. **Mucocele of the appendix.** The appendix is conspicuously dilated by mucinous material secreted by a cystadenoma.

Mucocele

Mucocele refers to a dilated mucus-filled appendix. The pathogenesis may be neoplastic or non-neoplastic. In the non-neoplastic variety chronic obstruction leads to retention of mucus in the appendiceal lumen.

Most mucoceles are associated with neoplastic epithelium. In the presence of a **mucinous cystadenoma** (Fig. 13-63) or a **mucinous cystadenocarcinoma,** the dilated appendix is lined by a villous adenomatous mucosa. Cystadenocarcinoma exhibits infiltrating neoplastic glands into the wall of the appendix.

A mucocele may become secondarily infected and rupture, discharging mucin and debris into the peritoneum. This material may be mistaken at laparotomy for peritoneal tumor implants. However, when a mucocele results from mucus secretion by a cystadenoma or cystadenocarcinoma of the appendix, perforation may lead to seeding of the peritoneum by mucus-secreting tumor cells, a condition known as **pseudomyxoma peritonei.** In less than one third of cases, pseudomyxoma peritonei is caused by disease of the appendix; in half, it originates from ovarian mucinous cystadenocarcinoma.

Neoplasms

Carcinoid tumors of the appendix are common, and are unlikely to metastasize unless they are over 1.5 cm, which is very rare.

Figure 13-64 through Figure 13-67 summarize the causes of gastrointestinal bleeding and obstruction and the major benign and malignant tumors of the gastrointestinal tract.

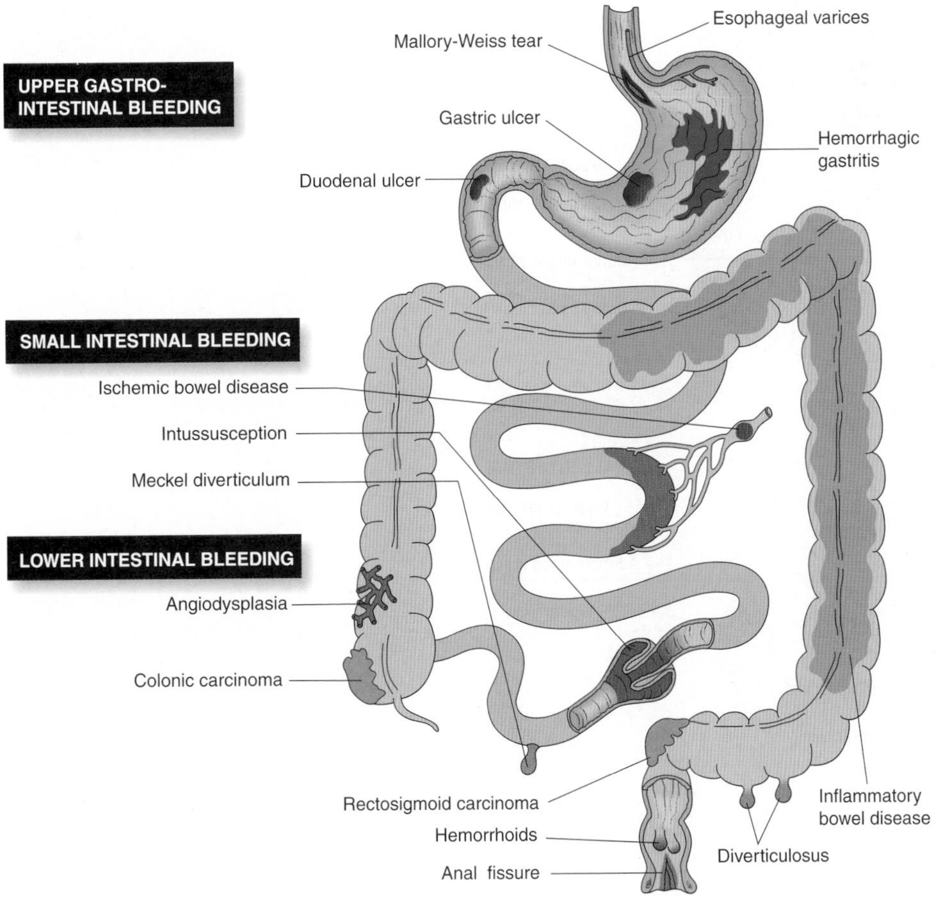

FIGURE 13-64. **Causes of gastrointestinal bleeding.**

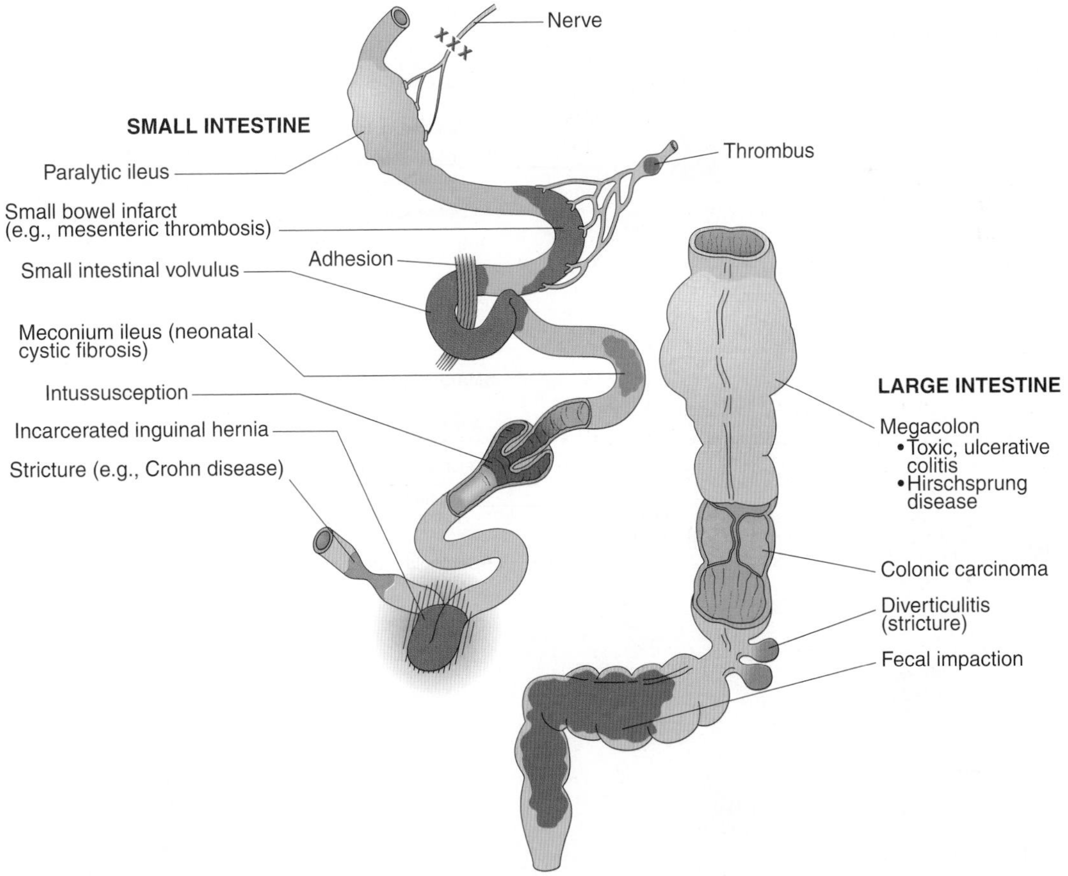

FIGURE 13-65. **Causes of gastrointestinal obstruction.**

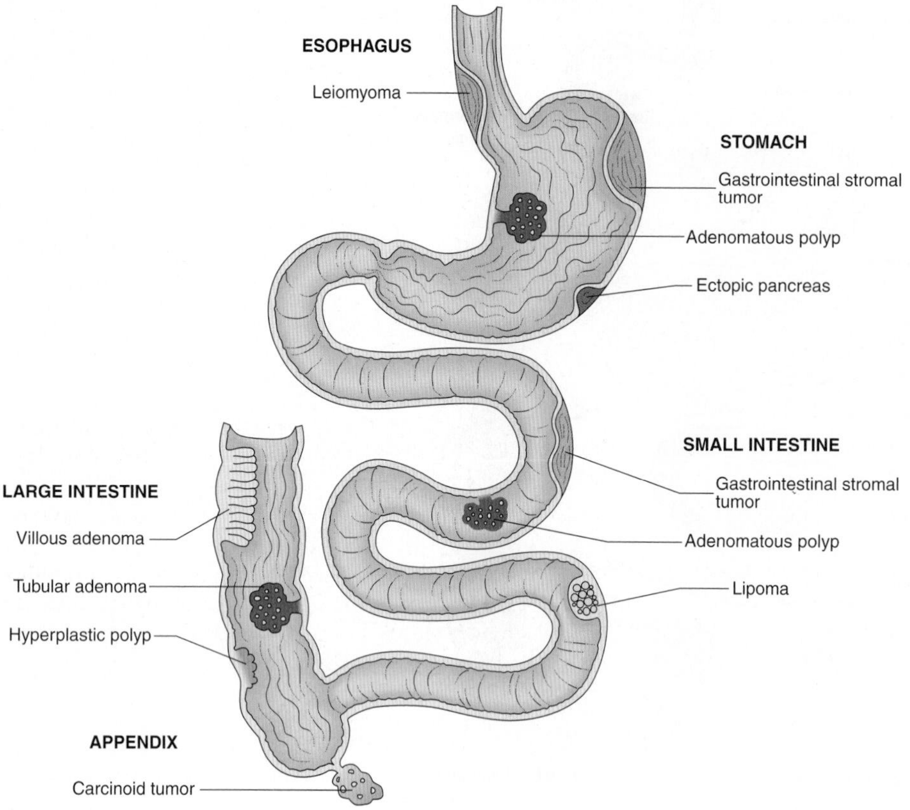

FIGURE 13-66. **Major benign tumors of the gastrointestinal tract.**

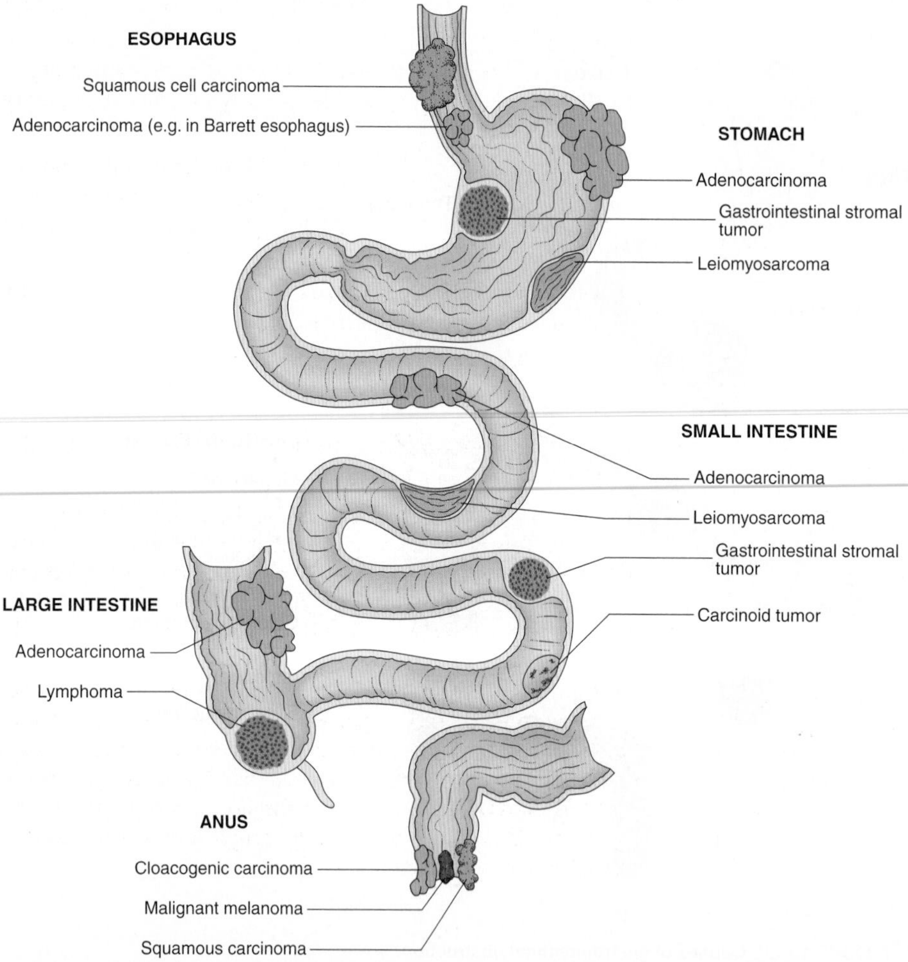

FIGURE 13-67. **Major malignant tumors of the gastrointestinal tract.**

THE PERITONEUM

The peritoneum is the mesothelial lining of the abdominal cavity and its viscera. The visceral peritoneum invests the gastrointestinal tract from stomach to rectum and encircles the liver. The parietal peritoneum lines the abdominal wall and retroperitoneal space. The omentum, which has a double layer of peritoneum, encloses blood vessels and a variable amount of fat.

Peritonitis

Bacterial Peritonitis Is Usually Caused by Intestinal Organisms

PATHOGENESIS:

PERFORATION: The most common cause of bacterial peritonitis is perforation of an abdominal viscus, as in an inflamed appendix, peptic ulcer, or colonic diverticulum. Peritonitis results in an acute abdomen, in which severe abdominal pain and tenderness predominate. Nausea, vomiting, and a high fever are usual, and in severe cases, generalized peritonitis, paralytic ileus, and septic shock ensue. Often the perforation becomes "walled off," in which case a peritoneal abscess results.

The bacteria released into the peritoneal cavity from the gastrointestinal tract vary according to the site of perforation and the duration of the peritonitis. Commonly, several aerobic and anaerobic species are cultured, including *E. coli, Bacteroides* species, various *Streptococcus* species, and *Clostridium*. Despite antibiotic treatment, surgical drainage and débridement and supportive measures, generalized peritonitis still carries substantial mortality and is especially dangerous in the elderly.

PERITONEAL DIALYSIS: Chronic peritoneal dialysis is today a frequent cause of bacterial peritonitis, owing to contamination of instruments or dialysate. The clinical course is usually milder than that noted with a perforated viscus and the offending organisms are mostly *Staphylococcus* and *Streptococcus* species. One fourth of cases of peritonitis associated with chronic dialysis are aseptic; they are presumably caused by some chemical in the dialysate to which the peritoneum is sensitive.

SPONTANEOUS BACTERIAL PERITONITIS: This term refers to a peritoneal infection lacking a clear precipitating circumstance, such as a perforated viscus. *The most common cause of spontaneous bacterial peritonitis in adults is cirrhosis complicated by portal hypertension and ascites.* The pathogenesis appears to involve movement of enteric organisms, mainly gram-negative bacilli, from the gut to mesenteric lymph nodes. Seeding of ascitic fluid then ensues, with depressed phagocytic activity and low antibacterial activity in ascitic fluid.

Spontaneous bacterial peritonitis in children can be a complication of the **nephrotic syndrome,** in part because ascites is more common in nephrotic children than in adults. Most cases of spontaneous peritonitis in children are caused by gram-negative organisms, usually derived from urinary tract infections. The disease causes symptoms of an acute abdomen and ordinarily leads to surgical intervention, unless the child is known to have the nephrotic syndrome. Even with antibiotic treatment, mortality is 5% to 10%.

TUBERCULOUS PERITONITIS: This infection is rarely seen in industrialized countries today, but occasionally complicates tuberculosis in developing countries. Many patients with tuberculous peritonitis do not have apparent pulmonary or miliary tuberculosis, an observation that suggests activation of latent tuberculous foci in the peritoneum derived from previous hematogenous dissemination.

PATHOLOGY: Grossly, bacterial peritonitis resembles purulent infection elsewhere. A fibrinopurulent exudate covers the surface of the intestines, and on organization, fibrinous and fibrous adhesions form between loops of bowel, which become joined to each other. Such adhesions may eventually be lysed, or they may lead to **volvulus** and **intestinal obstruction.** Bacterial salpingitis, usually gonococcal, may lead to pelvic peritonitis and adhesions, which define **pelvic inflammatory disease.**

Chemical Peritonitis Usually Results from Endogenous Sources

- **Bile peritonitis** is caused by escape of bile into the peritoneum, usually from a perforated gallbladder but sometimes from a needle biopsy of the liver. This abrupt insult may lead to shock.
- **Hydrochloric acid or hemorrhage** from a perforated peptic ulcer of the stomach or duodenum may elicit an inflammatory reaction in the peritoneum.
- **Acute pancreatitis** causes release and activation of potent lipolytic and proteolytic enzymes that produce severe peritonitis and fat necrosis. Shock is common and may be lethal unless adequately treated.
- **Foreign materials** introduced by surgery (e.g., talc) or by trauma are unusual causes of chemical peritonitis.
- **Leakage of urine** can produce ascites.

Familial Paroxysmal Polyserositis (Familial Mediterranean Fever) Leads to Peritonitis and Amyloidosis

Familial Mediterranean fever (FMF) is an inherited autosomal recessive disorder that features recurrent episodes of aseptic peritonitis with fever and abdominal pain. It is caused by mutations in a gene on the short arm of chromosome 16. FMF initially presents as peritonitis in half of cases, as arthritis in one-fourth, and as pleuritis in 5% of patients. However, almost all affected persons eventually manifest peritonitis, and more than half develop arthritis and pleuritis at some time. The disease predominates in Sephardic Jews and other Mediterranean populations, such as Armenians, Turks, and Arabs. The pathogenesis of FMF remains obscure, but in the absence of complications, the prognosis is good. Unfortunately, **amyloidosis** is a frequent complication (see Chapter 23).

Retroperitoneal Fibrosis

Idiopathic retroperitoneal fibrosis, an uncommon fibrosing condition of the abdomen, becomes symptomatic when it causes obstruction of the ureters. Although no cause is discernible in most cases, it has been linked to treatment of migraine headaches with methysergide. A similar idiopathic fibrosis also has been described in the mediastinum and may affect the mesentery, causing secondary intestinal obstruction.

Neoplasms of the Peritoneum

Mesenteric and Omental Cysts are Usually of Lymphatic Origin

They may also derive from other embryonic tissues. Usually a slowly enlarging, painless mass is discovered in a child older than 10 years. The cyst may come to medical attention because of rupture, bleeding, torsion or intestinal obstruction. Surgical excision is curative.

Mesotheliomas are the Most Common Primary Peritoneal Tumor

One fourth of all mesotheliomas arise in the peritoneum. *Like pleural mesotheliomas, most of these malignant tumors are associated with exposure to asbestos.* The pathologic characteristics of peritoneal mesotheliomas are identical to those of their pleural counterparts (see Chapter 12).

Primary Peritoneal Carcinoma Resembles Ovarian Carcinoma

Primary peritoneal carcinoma presents as tumor masses involving the omentum and peritoneum. It is morphologically identical to ovarian serous carcinoma of the ovary, except that the ovaries are normal.

Metastatic Carcinoma is the Most Common Malignancy of the Peritoneum

Ovarian, gastric, and pancreatic carcinomas are particularly likely to seed the peritoneum, but any intra-abdominal carcinoma can spread to the peritoneum.

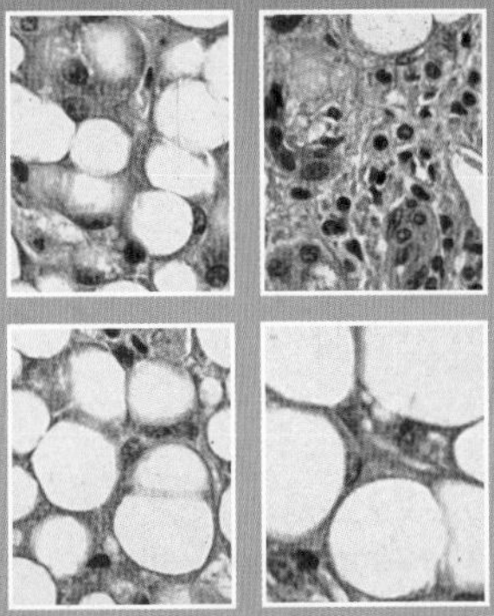

14 The Liver and Biliary System

Raphael Rubin
Emanuel Rubin

THE LIVER

Anatomy

The liver arises from the embryonic foregut as an entodermal bud that differentiates into the hepatic diverticulum. Strands of entodermal cells mingle with proliferating mesenchymal cells to form all the structures of the adult liver, the gallbladder, and the extrahepatic biliary ducts.

The liver weigh about 1500 g in the average adult man. Situated in the right upper quadrant of the abdomen immediately below the diaphragm, it consists of two lobes, a larger **right lobe** and a smaller **left lobe,** which meet at the level of the gallbladder bed. Inferiorly, the right lobe exhibits lesser segments, the **caudate** and **quadrate lobes.** The **gallbladder** is located inferiorly in a fossa of the right hepatic lobe and normally extends slightly beyond the inferior margin of the liver.

The liver has a dual blood supply consisting of (1) **the hepatic artery,** a branch of the celiac axis; and (2) **the portal vein,** formed by the convergence of the splenic and superior mesenteric veins. **The hepatic veins** empty into the inferior vena cava, which is partly surrounded by the posterior surface of the liver. The hepatic lymphatics drain principally into lymph nodes of the porta hepatis and the celiac axis.

The common hepatic duct, formed by the union of the right and left hepatic ducts, receives the cystic duct from the gallbladder to form the common bile duct. The common bile duct joins with the pancreatic duct just before emptying into the duodenum. It terminates in the ampulla of Vater, where its lumen is guarded by the sphincter of Oddi.

The Liver Lobule Is the Basic Unit of the Liver

The liver lobule is a polyhedral structure (Fig. 14-1 and Fig. 14-2), classically depicted as a hexagon. **Portal triads** (or portal tracts), found peripherally at the angles of the polygon, are so named because they contain intrahepatic branches of the (1) **bile ducts,** (2) **hepatic artery,** and (3) **portal vein.** The collagenous portal tracts are surrounded by an adjacent circumferential layer of hepatocytes called **the limiting plate**. As its name implies, the **central vein** (also known as the **terminal hepatic venule**) resides in the center of the lobule. Radiating from it are **one-cell-thick plates of hepatocytes,** which extend to the perimeter of the lobule, where they are continuous with the plates of other lobules. Between the plates of hepatocytes are the **hepatic sinusoids,** which are lined by endothelial cells, Kupffer cells, and stellate cells.

The large blood vessels that enter the liver at the porta hepatis eventually divide into the small interlobular branches of the hepatic artery and portal vein in the portal triads. From the portal triads, the interlobular vessels distribute blood to the hepatic sinusoids, where it flows centripetally into the central vein. The central veins coalesce to form sublobular veins, which eventually merge into the hepatic veins.

Bile flows in a direction opposite to that of the blood. Bile is secreted by hepatocytes into the bile canaliculi, formed by the apposed lateral surfaces of contiguous hepatocytes. Contraction of the bile canaliculus, mediated by the pericanalicular cytoskeleton of the hepatocytes, propels the bile toward the portal tract.

From the canaliculi, the bile flows into the bile ductules (canals of Hering or cholangioles) at the border of the portal tract

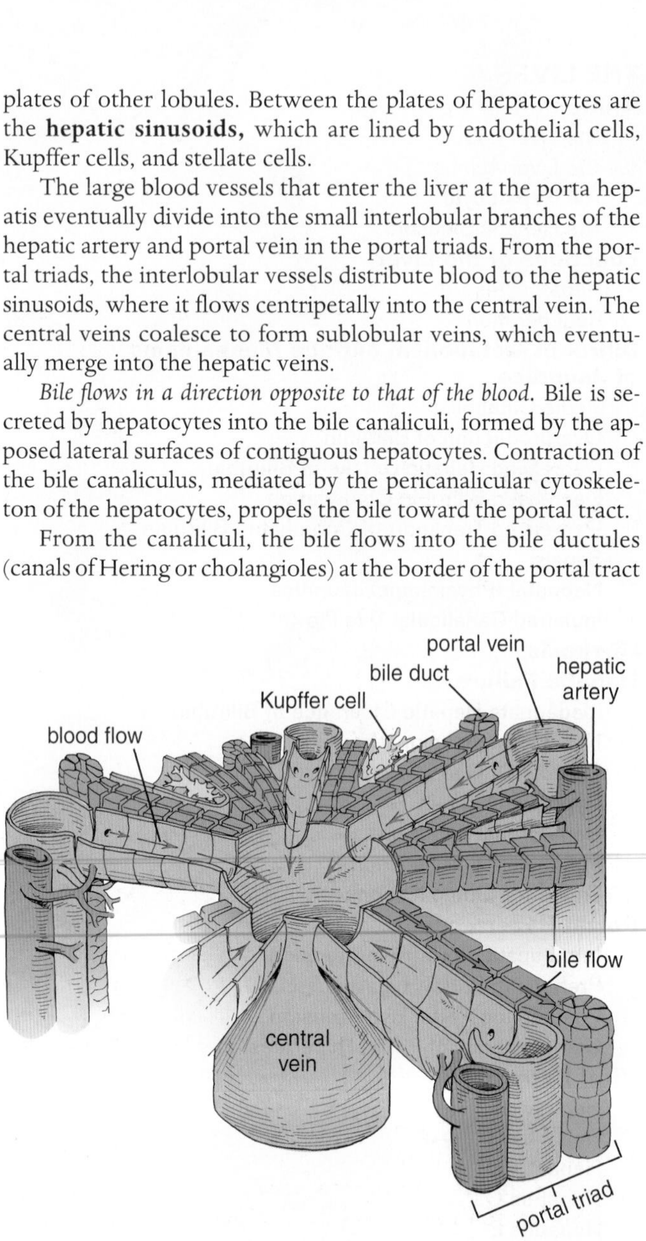

FIGURE 14-1. **Microanatomy of the liver.** The classic lobule is composed of portal triads, hepatic sinuses, terminal hepatic venule (centeral vein), and asociated plates of hepatocytes. *Red arrows* indicate the direction of sinusoidal blood flow. *Green arrows* show the direction of bile flow. (Used with permission from Ross & Pawlina, p 18.)

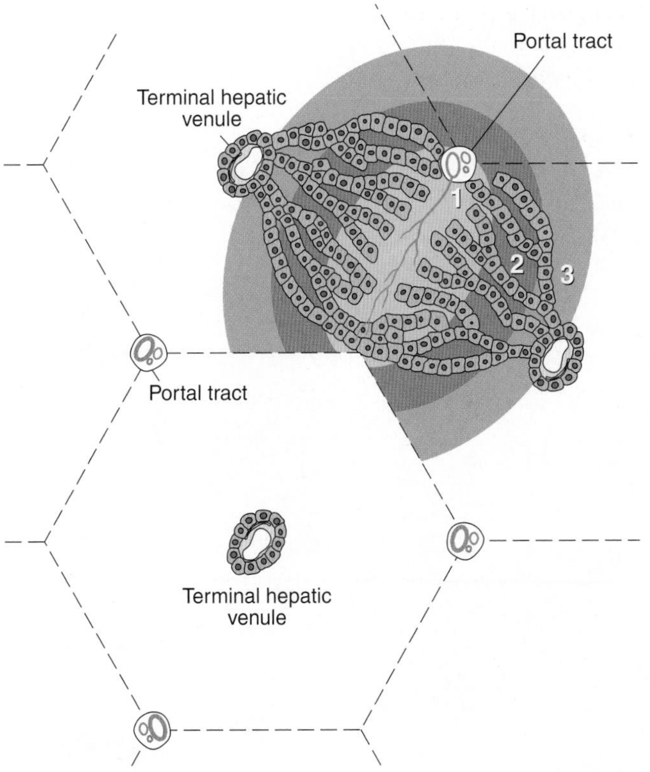

FIGURE 14-2. **Morphologic and functional concepts of the liver lobule.** In the classic *morphologic* liver lobule, the periphery of the hexagonal lobule is anchored in the portal tracts, and the terminal hepatic venule is in the center. The *functional* liver lobule is an acinus derived from the gradients of oxygen and nutrients in the sinusoidal blood. In this scheme, the portal tract, with the richest content of oxygen and nutrients, is in the center (zone 1). The region most distant from the portal tract (zone 3) is poor in oxygen and nutrients and surrounds the terminal hepatic venule.

and then enters a branch of the intrahepatic bile ducts. Within each lobe of the liver, smaller bile ducts progressively merge, eventually forming the right and left hepatic ducts.

The Liver Acinus Is the Functional Interpretation of the Lobule

The classic lobule described above is depicted as arranged around the central vein simply because of the histologic appearance of the liver. *However, from a functional point of view, the lobule can be thought of as an acinus with its center in the portal tract* (see Fig. 14-2). Such a concept takes into account the functional gradients that exist within the lobule. Concentrations of oxygen, nutrients, and hormones in the blood are highest at the portal tracts and decline progressively as the blood courses through the sinusoids to the central vein. This functional heterogeneity of the liver lobule can be expressed in terms of concentric functional zones around portal tracts. **Zone 1,** the most highly oxygenated zone, encircles the portal tracts, whereas **zone 3,** which surrounds the central veins, is oxygen poor. The intermediate or midlobular area is referred to as **zone 2.** Differences in hepatocytes are not restricted to blood flow. The acinus is also heterogeneous with respect to metabolism, independent of oxygenation. In particular, toxic injury is often prominent in zone 3, owing to enrichment in hepatocyte enzymes involved in drug detoxification and biotransformation. For convenience, pathologic changes in the liver are usually designated in relation to the classic histologic lobule. For example, centrilobular necrosis refers to a lesion around the central veins, whereas periportal fibrosis is seen at the periphery of the classic lobule.

The Hepatocyte Performs the Major Functions of the Liver

Although 60% of the total cell population of the liver consists of hepatocytes, these cells account for 90% of the volume of the liver. The hepatocyte, roughly 30 μm across, has three specialized surfaces: sinusoidal, lateral, and canalicular. Each cell has two sinusoidal surfaces, which exhibit numerous slender microvilli. The sinusoidal surface is separated from the endothelial cells that line the sinusoids by the **space of Disse** (Fig. 14-3). The canalicular surfaces of adjacent hepatocytes form the **bile canaliculus,** a collecting structure that is actually an intercellular space without a separate and distinct wall. The canalicular surface displays microvilli extending into the lumen. A tight junctional complex between adjacent hepatocytes prevents leakage of bile from the canaliculus. The lateral, or intercellular, surfaces of adjacent hepatocytes are in close contact and contain gap junctions.

The centrally placed, spherical nucleus of the hepatocyte exhibits one or more nucleoli. The nuclei vary in size in ratios of 2 (diploid), 4 (tetraploid), and 8 (octaploid), with most being diploid. The cytoplasm is rich in organelles and shows prominent rough and smooth endoplasmic reticulum, Golgi complexes, mitochondria, lysosomes, and peroxisomes. In addition, in the fed state, abundant glycogen and occasional fat droplets are evident.

The Hepatic Sinusoid Is the Channel through Which Blood Traverses the Liver

The sinusoids contain three cell types: endothelial, Kupffer, and stellate cells.

ENDOTHELIAL CELLS: The hepatic sinusoid is lined by a sheet of endothelial cells, which are penetrated by numerous holes called **fenestrae** (see Fig. 14-3). Unlike their counterparts in other tissues, adjacent endothelial cells do not form junctions, and there are many gaps between them. The result is a sievelike structure that affords free communication between the sinusoidal lumen and the space of Disse. Free access of sinusoidal plasma to the hepatocyte is further facilitated by the absence of a basement membrane between the endothelial cells and liver cells.

KUPFFER CELLS: The phagocytic Kupffer cells are located either in the gaps between adjacent endothelial cells or on their surfaces (see Fig. 14-1). Kupffer cells belong to the monocyte/macrophage system derived from the bone marrow. For that reason, after liver transplantation, the Kupffer cell population eventually originates from the recipient rather than the donor. Like other macrophages, they provide a first line of defense against infection and circulating toxic molecules (e.g., endotoxin). Activated Kupffer cells also release a variety of cytokines, including tumor necrosis factor (TNF), interleukins (IL), interferons, and transforming growth factors (TGFs) α and β.

STELLATE CELLS: Beneath the endothelial cells in the space of Disse are found occasional stellate cells (also known as Ito cells), which have specialized storage capacities. These cells contain fat, vitamin A, and other lipid-soluble vitamins. The stellate cell also secretes extracellular matrix components, including various collagens, laminin, and proteoglycans. In a number of

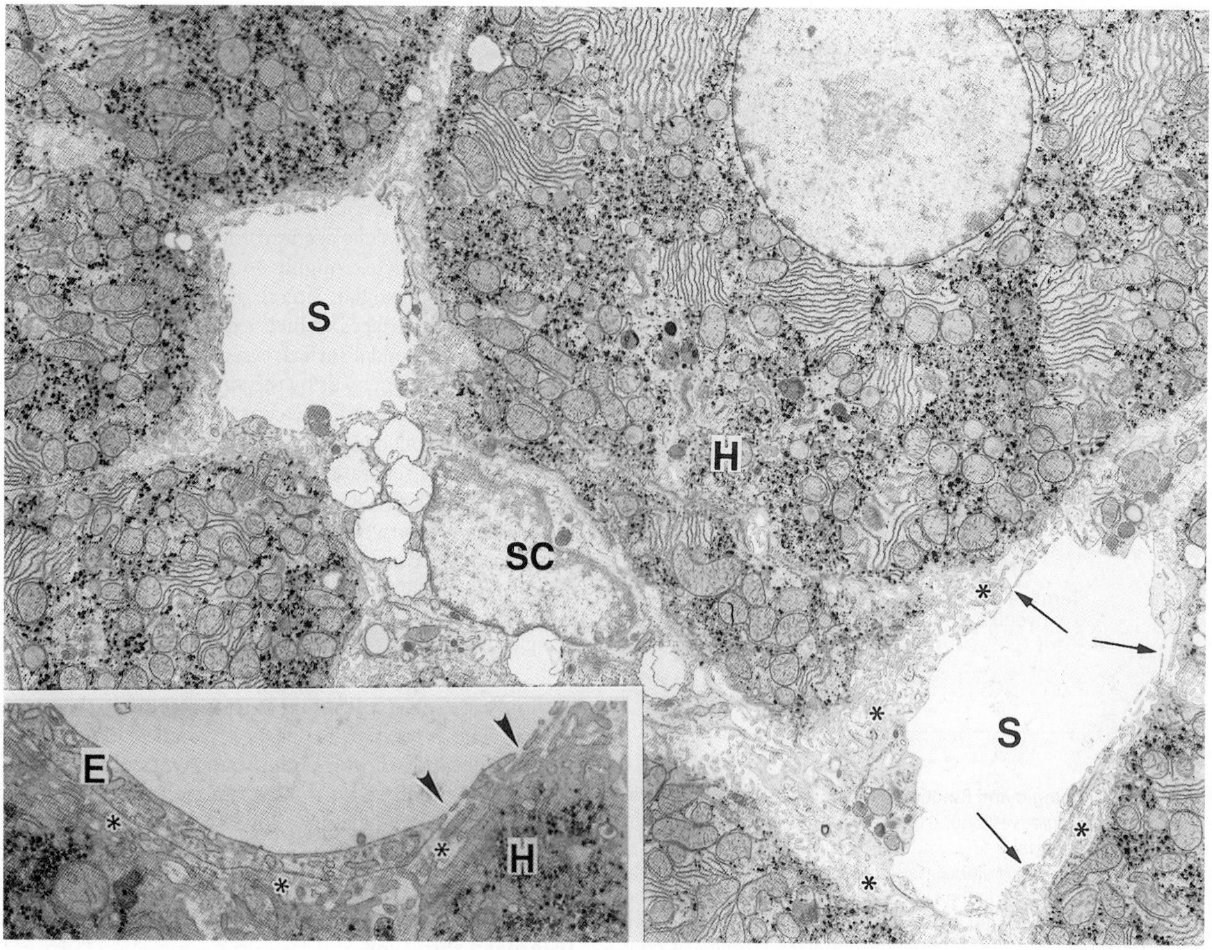

FIGURE 14-3. **Hepatic sinusoids and space of Disse.** An electron micrograph illustrates the relationship between hepatocytes, sinusoids, the space of Disse, and hepatic stellate cells (Ito cells, fat-storing cells). *H,* hepatocyte; *S,* sinusoid; *SC,* stellate cell; *arrow,* endothelial cell; *asterisk,* space of Disse. The *inset* illustrates the relationship between hepatocytes *(H)* and endothelial cells *(E)*. The *arrowheads* indicate fenestrae in the endothelial cells; the *asterisks* are in the space of Disse.

pathologic states, these matrix constituents are formed in great excess, leading to the hepatic fibrosis characteristic of cirrhosis.

The most abundant extracellular matrix component in the space of Disse is fibronectin. Occasional bundles of type I collagen fibers provide the scaffold of the liver lobule. There is no continuous basement membrane barrier between the plasma and the surface of the hepatocyte, although by light microscopy, reticulin stains impart the false impression of a continuous membrane.

FUNCTIONS OF THE LIVER

The Hepatocyte Subserves Myriad Functions

The functions served by the hepatocyte can be broadly categorized as metabolic, synthetic, storage, catabolic, and excretory.

METABOLIC FUNCTIONS: The liver is the central organ of **glucose homeostasis** and responds rapidly to fluctuations in the concentration of blood glucose. In the fed state, excess blood glucose is shunted to the liver to be stored as glycogen; in the fasting state, the liver maintains blood glucose levels by glycogenolysis and gluconeogenesis. For **gluconeogenesis,** the liver uses amino acids, lactate, and glycerol. The nitrogenous portion of amino acids is converted to urea. Free fatty acids are taken up by the liver, where they are oxidized to produce energy. Alternatively, they are converted to triglycerides, and secreted in the form of **lipoproteins** to be used elsewhere.

SYNTHETIC FUNCTIONS: Most serum proteins, with the major exception of the immunoglobulins, are synthesized in the liver. **Albumin** is the principal source of plasma oncotic pressure, and its decrease in chronic liver disease contributes to the development of edema and ascites. Blood coagulation depends on the continuous production of **clotting factors,** most of which, including prothrombin and fibrinogen, are synthesized by hepatocytes. Liver failure is thus characterized by a severe and often life-threatening bleeding diathesis. Endothelial cells of the liver manufacture **factor VIII,** and hemophilia is ameliorated by liver transplantation. **Complement** and other acute-phase reactants are also secreted by the liver, as are numerous specific binding proteins—for example, the **binding proteins** for iron, copper, and vitamin A.

STORAGE FUNCTIONS: The liver is an important storage site for glycogen, triglycerides, iron, copper, and lipid-soluble vitamins. Severe liver disease can result from excessive storage—for instance, abnormal glycogen in type IV glycogenosis and excess iron in hemochromatosis.

CATABOLIC FUNCTIONS: Endogenous substances, including hormones and serum proteins, are catabolized by the liver to maintain a balance between their production and their elimination. Thus, in chronic liver disease, impaired catabolism of estrogens contributes to feminization in men. The liver is also the principal site for the **detoxification of foreign compounds** (xenobiotics), such as drugs, industrial chemicals, environmental contaminants, and perhaps products of bacterial metabolism in the intestine. Removal of ammonia, a product of amino acid metabolism, occurs principally in the liver. Serum ammonia increases in liver failure and is used as a marker for this condition.

EXCRETORY FUNCTIONS: The principal excretory product of the liver is **bile,** an aqueous mixture of conjugated bilirubin, bile acids, phospholipids, cholesterol, and electrolytes. Bile not only provides a repository for the products of heme catabolism but is also vital for fat absorption in the small intestine. Bile also contains immunoglobulin A (IgA), which is involved in an enterohepatic circulation. Normal bile formation is critical for elimination of environmental toxins, carcinogens, and drugs and their metabolites.

Regeneration Is a Unique Characteristic of the Liver

Liver size is normally maintained within narrow limits relative to body size. When liver tissue is damaged (e.g., after a mechanical, toxic, or viral challenge that has caused a substantial loss of functional tissue), recovery occurs by regrowth of the undamaged tissue in a process called **liver regeneration**. The parenchymal cells in the liver, which normally are in a fully differentiated, quiescent state (G_0), reenter the cell cycle and go through one or more synchronized rounds of replication to recover the original size of the tissue. Uniquely, this process takes place while maintaining the differentiated functions of the liver. Little is known about the factors that guide this part of the process or how the liver recognizes the recovery of its normal size and architecture. *Conditions that interfere with the regenerative process may result in permanent liver dysfunction and lead to fibrosis and cirrhosis.*

Several phases can be distinguished in liver regeneration:

- **Priming:** Liver tissue has to recognize that damage has occurred and that the remaining functional parenchymal cells must make the transition from the quiescent G_0 state to the G_1 phase of the cell cycle. This phase is often referred to as "priming." It is associated with the expression of immediate-early genes, many of which are transcription factors required for the expression of cell cycle proteins. The priming phase depends on the release of different cytokines, notably TNF-α and IL-6.
- **Progression to mitosis:** The second phase involves progression through the G_1 phase of the cell cycle and transition into S phase, where DNA synthesis occurs. This sequence is followed by the G_2 phase and M phase, where cell division takes place. A number of growth factors promote this part of the process, including hepatocyte growth factor, also known as scatter factor (HGF/SF), epidermal growth factor (EGF), TGF-α, and several others. Several growth factors (e.g. HGF, IL-6) promote hepatoprotection and survival in various models of liver injury. After completion of one or two rounds of cell division (depending on need), the cells revert to the quiescent state and resume normal function.
- **Nonparenchymal cells:** The third phase of liver regeneration involves the replication of nonparenchymal cells (sinusoidal endothelial cells, Kupffer cells, stellate cells, and biliary epithelial cells) and the remodeling of the tissue architecture, with recovery of the original structure of liver cell plates. Hepatic progenitor cells ("oval cells") that exist within the terminal branches of the bile ductules and canals of Hering contribute to ductular proliferation after hepatic necrosis. However, controversy remains over the importance of these cells to hepatic regeneration, as well as the potential contribution of bone marrow-derived stem cells (see Chapter 3).

Bilirubin Metabolism and the Mechanisms of Jaundice

Bilirubin Is the End Product of Heme Catabolism

Bilirubin has no known physiologic function, although a role as an antioxidant has been suggested. *Up to 85% of bilirubin is derived from senescent erythrocytes, which are removed from the circulation by mononuclear phagocytes of the spleen, bone marrow, and liver.* The remaining bilirubin arises from the degradation of heme produced from other sources, the most important of which is the premature breakdown of hemoglobin in developing erythroid cells in the bone marrow.

After release of bilirubin into the circulation, it is bound to albumin for transport to the liver. Albumin in the circulation and the extracellular space constitutes a large binding reservoir for bilirubin and ensures a low extracellular concentration of free (unbound) bilirubin. Free bilirubin, unlike that bound to albumin or conjugated with glucuronic acid, is toxic to the brain in newborns and in high concentrations causes irreversible brain injury, termed **kernicterus.**

The transfer of bilirubin from the blood to the bile involves four steps:

1. **Uptake:** On reaching the sinusoidal plasma membrane of the hepatocyte, the albumin–bilirubin complex is dissociated, and bilirubin is transported across the plasma membrane. This transport system has the characteristics of a carrier-mediated process and likely involves specific recognition of bilirubin by a plasma membrane receptor.
2. **Binding:** Within the hepatocyte, bilirubin is bound to a group of cytosolic proteins known collectively as **glutathione-S-transferases** (also termed ligandin).
3. **Conjugation:** For its excretion, bilirubin must be converted to a water-soluble compound by complexing with glucuronic acid. Bilirubin is transferred to the endoplasmic reticulum, which contains the uridine diphosphate-glucuronyl transferase (UGT) system responsible for the conjugation of bilirubin with glucuronic acid. This reaction forms water-soluble bilirubin diglucuronide and a small amount (<10%) of the monoglucuronide.
4. **Excretion:** Conjugated bilirubin diffuses through the cytosol to the bile canaliculus, where it is excreted into the bile by an energy-dependent carrier-mediated process, which is the rate-limiting step for overall transhepatic transport of bilirubin.

After its excretion into the small intestine in bile, conjugated bilirubin is not absorbed and remains intact until it reaches the distal small bowel and colon, where it is hydrolyzed by the bacterial flora to free bilirubin. In turn, free bilirubin (now unconjugated) is reduced to a mixture of pyrroles, known collectively as **urobilinogen**. Most of the urobilinogen is excreted in the feces,

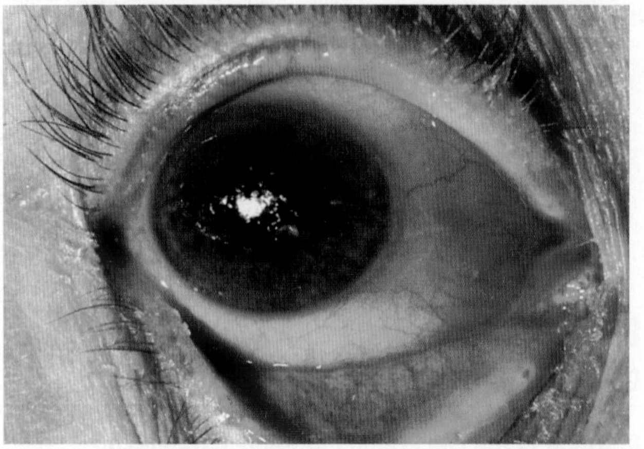

FIGURE 14-4. **Jaundice.** A patient in hepatic failure displays a yellow sclera.

but a small proportion is absorbed in the terminal ileum and colon, returned to the liver, and reexcreted into the bile. Bile acids are also reabsorbed in the terminal ileum and salvaged by the liver. Collectively, the reabsorption of bile constituents is referred to as the **enterohepatic circulation of bile**. Some urobilinogen escapes reabsorption by the liver and reaches the systemic circulation, after which it is excreted in the urine.

- **Hyperbilirubinemia** refers to an increased concentration of bilirubin in the blood (>1.0 mg/dL).
- **Jaundice** or **icterus** describes yellow skin and sclerae (Fig. 14-4), whose color becomes apparent when the circulating bilirubin concentration exceeds 2.0 to 2.5 mg/dL.
- **Cholestasis** is the presence of plugs of inspissated bile in dilated bile canaliculi and visible bile pigment in hepatocytes.
- **Cholestatic jaundice** is characterized by histologic cholestasis and hyperbilirubinemia.

As shown in Figure 14-5, many conditions are associated with hyperbilirubinemia.

Overproduction of bilirubin, interference with hepatic uptake or intracellular metabolism of bilirubin, and impairment of bile excretion are all causes of jaundice.

Overproduction of Bilirubin Can Lead to Unconjugated Hyperbilirubinemia

An increased production of bilirubin results from increased destruction of erythrocytes (i.e., hemolytic anemia) or ineffective erythropoiesis ***(dyserythropoiesis)***. In unusual circumstances, the breakdown of erythrocytes in a large hematoma (e.g., after trauma) may also provide excess bilirubin.

In the adult, even severe hemolytic anemia does not produce a sustained rise in serum bilirubin concentration beyond 4.0 mg/dL, provided that hepatic bilirubin clearance remains normal. However, the combination of prolonged hemolysis, as in sickle cell anemia, and intrinsic liver disease, such as viral hepatitis, leads to extraordinarily high levels of circulating bilirubin (up to 100 mg/dL) and pronounced jaundice.

The hyperbilirubinemia of uncomplicated hemolytic disease principally involves unconjugated bilirubin, whereas in parenchymal liver disease, both conjugated and unconjugated bilirubin participate. Although the unconjugated hyperbilirubinemia of hemolytic disease is of little clinical significance in the adult, in the newborn it may be catastrophic. Hemolytic disease of the newborn may result in concentrations of unconjugated bilirubin high enough to cause kernicterus (see Chapter 6). Kernicterus has generally been associated with bilirubin concentrations over 20 mg/dL, but subtle psychomotor retardation may follow considerably lower bilirubin concentrations.

In disorders characterized by ineffective erythropoiesis (e.g., megaloblastic and sideroblastic anemias), the fraction of bilirubin derived from the bone marrow may be increased to the point that hyperbilirubinemia develops. A rare hereditary disease of unknown etiology, "primary shunt hyperbilirubinemia" or "idiopathic dyserythropoietic jaundice," is characterized by massive overproduction of bilirubin in the bone marrow and is associated with chronic unconjugated hyperbilirubinemia.

Decreased Hepatic Uptake of Bilirubin Is a Common Cause of Jaundice

Hyperbilirubinemia can result from impaired hepatic uptake of unconjugated bilirubin. Such a situation occurs in generalized liver cell injury, exemplified by viral hepatitis. Certain drugs (e.g., rifampin and probenecid) interfere with the net uptake of bilirubin by the liver cell and may produce a mild unconjugated hyperbilirubinemia.

Decreased Bilirubin Conjugation Occurs in a Number of Hereditary Syndromes

Crigler-Najjar Syndrome

Crigler-Najjar syndrome type I is a rare, recessively inherited malady characterized by chronic, severe, unconjugated hyperbilirubinemia, owing to the complete absence of hepatic UGT activity. A variety of mutations in the *UGT* gene lead to the synthesis of a completely inactive enzyme. As a result, treatment with phenobarbital, an inducer of microsomal enzymes (including UGT), is without effect.

The bile in this condition is colorless and contains no conjugated bilirubin and no more than trace amounts of unconjugated bilirubin. *The morphologic appearance of the liver is normal.* In the era before liver transplantation, infants with Crigler-Najjar syndrome type I invariably developed bilirubin encephalopathy and usually died in the first year of life. However, current therapy with ultraviolet light succeeds in keeping many such patients alive well into adolescence.

Crigler-Najjar syndrome type II is similar to but less severe than type I and manifests only a partial decrease in the activity of UGT. Almost all patients with type II syndrome develop normally, but neurologic changes resembling kernicterus are observed in some.

Gilbert Syndrome

Gilbert syndrome is an inherited, mild, chronic unconjugated hyperbilirubinemia (<6 mg/dL) that is caused by ***impaired clearance of bilirubin*** *in the absence of any detectable functional or structural liver disease.* The syndrome runs in families, and both autosomal dominant and recessive patterns of inheritance have been suggested, although the latter is favored today. Mutations in the promotor region of the *UGT* gene lead to reduced transcription of the gene and, consequently, inadequate synthesis of the enzyme. In a few patients with a normal *UGT* gene promotor region, missense mutations of the coding region have been described. Factors that elevate serum bilirubin concentrations in normal persons, such as fasting or an intercurrent illness, pro-

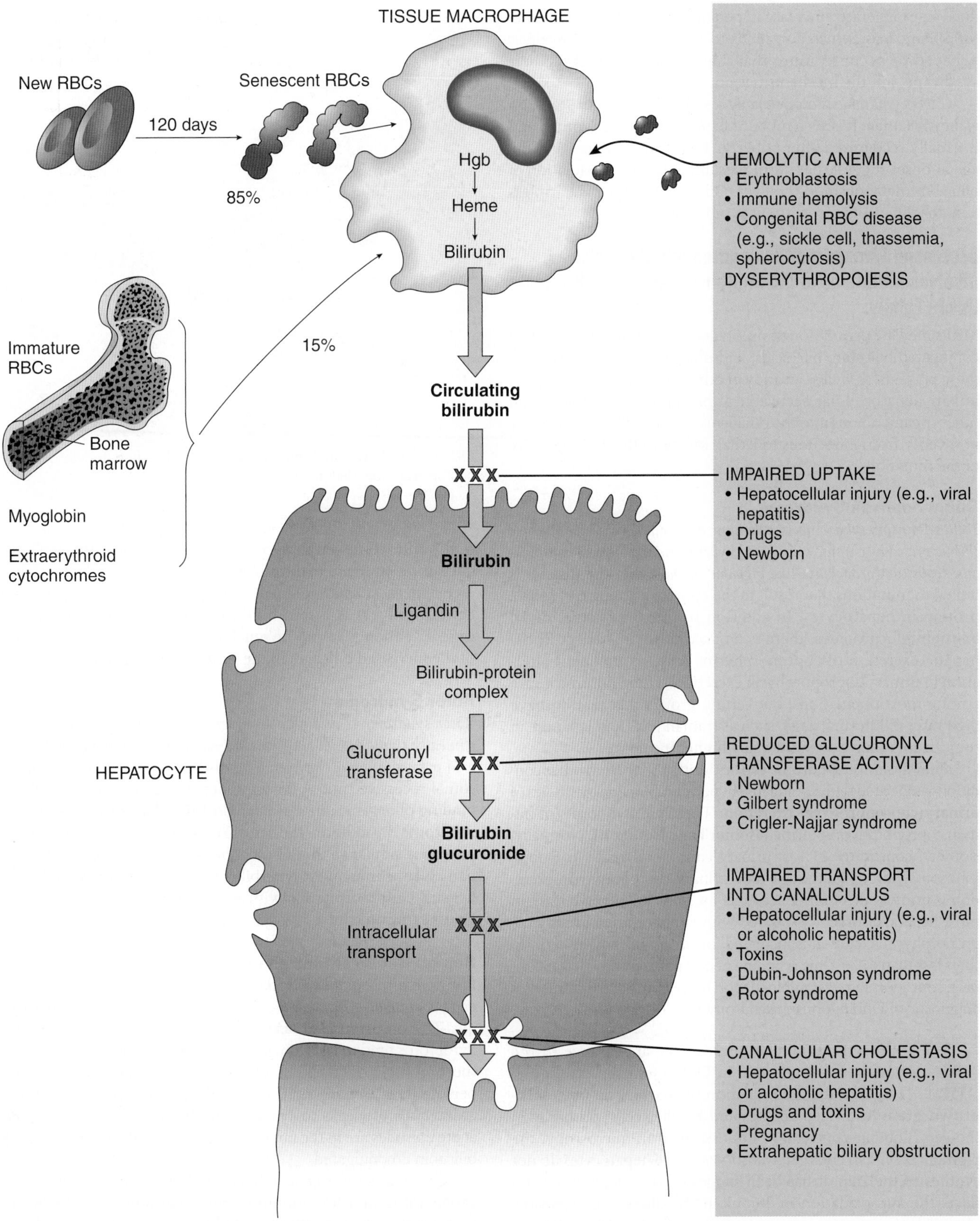

FIGURE 14-5. **Mechanisms of hyperbilirubinemia at the level of the hepatocyte.** Bilirubin is derived principally from the senescence of circulating red blood cells (RBCs), with a smaller contribution from the degradation of erythropoietic elements in the bone marrow, myoglobin, and extraerythroid cytochromes. Hyperbilirubinemia and jaundice results from overproduction of bilirubin (hemolytic anemia), dyserythropoiesis, impaired bilirubin uptake, or defects in its hepatic metabolism. The locations of specific blocks in the metabolic pathway of bilirubin in the hepatocyte are illustrated. Hgb = hemoglobin.

duce an exaggerated increase in persons with Gilbert syndrome. Mild hemolysis, which also tends to increase bilirubin levels, is believed to occur in more than half of persons with Gilbert syndrome, but the mechanism is unclear.

Gilbert syndrome is exceptionally common, occurring in 3% to 7% of the population. It is seen more often in men than in women and is usually recognized after puberty. The sex differences and the age at onset suggest that hormones influence the modulation of bilirubin metabolism in the liver. Gilbert syndrome is harmless and, for the most part, without symptoms.

Decreased Transport of Conjugated Bilirubin Often Involves Mutations in the Multidrug Resistance Protein (MRP) Family

MRPs mediate organic ion transport across membranes, including conjugated bilirubin, bile acids, and phospholipids. Mutations in these proteins, as well as an array of other canalicular transporters, impair hepatocellular secretion of bilirubin glucuronides and other organic anions into the canalicular lumen. The diseases vary in severity from innocuous to lethal, owing to the heterogeneity of the mutations.

Dubin-Johnson Syndrome

Dubin-Johnson syndrome is a benign autosomal recessive disease characterized by chronic conjugated hyperbilirubinemia and conspicuous deposition of melanin-like pigment in the liver. The disease is linked to mutations that result in the complete absence of MRP2 protein in hepatocytes. In addition to impaired secretion of bilirubin glucuronides, there is an accompanying defect in the hepatic excretion of coproporphyrins and a consequent alteration in urinary coproporphyrin excretion. The syndrome is rare among most populations, but certain groups that tend to have high rates of intermarriage, such as Iranian Jews and Japanese in remote areas, have a considerably higher incidence.

Dubin-Johnson syndrome can be distinguished from other conditions associated with conjugated hyperbilirubinemia by studies of **urinary coproporphyrin excretion.** There are two forms of human coproporphyrins, termed **isomer I** and **isomer III.** Normally, isomer I constitutes 25% of urinary coproporphyrins. In Dubin-Johnson syndrome, although total urinary coproporphyrin excretion is normal, this isomer accounts for fully 80%. By contrast, in most hepatic disorders associated with jaundice, total urinary coproporphyrin excretion is increased, but coproporphyrin I constitutes less than 65%. Thus, a finding of normal excretion of total urinary coproporphyrins combined with more than 80% as isomer I is diagnostic of Dubin-Johnson syndrome

PATHOLOGY: The microscopic appearance of the liver is entirely normal in Dubin-Johnson syndrome, except for the accumulation of coarse, iron-free, **dark-brown granules** in hepatocytes and Kupffer cells, primarily in the centrilobular zone (Fig. 14-6). By electron microscopy, the pigment is seen in enlarged lysosomes. Since hepatocytes do not synthesize melanin, it has been suggested that the pigment reflects the autooxidation of anionic metabolites (e.g., tyrosine, phenylalanine, tryptophan) and possibly of epinephrine. The accumulation of this intracellular pigment is reflected in a grossly pigmented, or "black," liver.

CLINICAL FEATURES: Except for mild intermittent jaundice, most patients with Dubin-Johnson syndrome do not complain of any symptoms, although vague nonspecific complaints are common. Half of those affected have dark urine. In women, the disease may be discovered when jaundice appears during pregnancy or as a result of the use of oral contraceptives. The serum bilirubin value varies from 2 to 5 mg/dL, although it may be much higher transiently. About 60% of the increased bilirubin in the serum is conjugated.

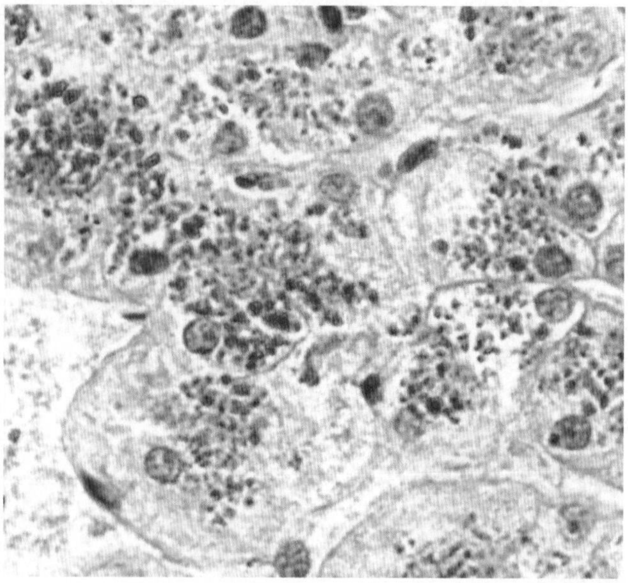

FIGURE 14-6. **Dubin-Johnson syndrome.** The hepatocytes contain coarse, iron-free, dark-brown granules.

Rotor Syndrome

Rotor syndrome is a familial conjugated hyperbilirubinemia that is clinically similar to Dubin-Johnson syndrome but without the associated pigmentation of the liver. The disease is inherited as an autosomal recessive trait. A defect in hepatic uptake or intracellular binding of organic ions has been postulated as the basis of Rotor syndrome. In addition, the pattern of urinary coproporphyrin excretion is similar to that of most hepatobiliary disorders accompanied by conjugated hyperbilirubinemia (i.e., increased total urinary coproporphyrins with 65% of isomer I). Patients with Rotor syndrome have few symptoms and lead normal lives.

Benign Recurrent Intrahepatic Cholestasis

Benign recurrent intrahepatic cholestasis is characterized by self-limited, periodic episodes of intrahepatic cholestasis preceded by malaise and itching. The occurrence of familial cases suggests a genetic origin. Symptoms tend to last from several weeks to several months. The mean number of attacks in a lifetime is 3 to 5, but some affected persons have as many as 10 attacks. Recurrences have been noted at intervals of weeks to years. Serum bilirubin levels during the acute episodes are in the range of 10 to 20 mg/dL, and most of the bilirubin is conjugated.

The liver shows centrilobular cholestasis (bile plugs in bile canaliculi) and a few mononuclear inflammatory cells in the portal tracts. All the structural and functional alterations disappear during remissions, and no permanent sequelae have been reported.

Progressive Familial Intrahepatic Cholestasis

Progressive Familial Intrahepatic Cholestasis (PFIC) *is a heterogeneous group of uncommon, inherited, autosomal recessive disorders of infancy or early childhood in which intrahepatic cholestasis progresses relentlessly to cirrhosis.* The first reported cases were descendents of an Amish man, Jacob Byler (Byler syndrome), but PFIC is not limited to that ethnic group. These disorders have been linked to mutations in several proteins, including FIC1, an aminophospholipid transporter, bile salt transporters, and MRPs. There is an associated high incidence of retinitis pigmentosa, and the children are often mentally retarded. Most affected children die within the first 2 years of life.

Intrahepatic Cholestasis of Pregnancy

Intrahepatic cholestasis of pregnancy is a disorder characterized by pruritus and cholestatic jaundice that usually occurs in the last trimester of each pregnancy and promptly disappears after delivery. Half of the patients have other family members who have experienced jaundice during pregnancy or after the use of oral contraceptives; the remainder are sporadic. In some familial cases, mutations in the MRP protein genes have been described. The increase in gonadal and placental hormones during pregnancy is likely responsible for the cholestasis in susceptible women. Maternal health is unaffected by this disease, but the effects on the fetus are often grave and include fetal distress, stillbirth, prematurity, and an increased risk of intracranial hemorrhage during delivery. The liver of the mother exhibits no specific changes other than centrilobular cholestasis.

Sepsis Can Cause Jaundice

Severe conjugated hyperbilirubinemia may be associated with septicemia involving both gram-positive and gram-negative bacteria, although the latter infection is more common. In these situations, the serum alkaline phosphatase activity and cholesterol levels are usually low, suggesting the possibility of an isolated defect in the excretion of conjugated bilirubin. In jaundice associated with sepsis, the histologic changes in the liver are nonspecific and include mild canalicular cholestasis and slight fat accumulation. The portal tracts may contain excess inflammatory cells, and varying degrees of proliferation of bile ductules may be seen. Occasionally, dilated ductules are filled with inspissated bile.

Neonatal (Physiologic) Jaundice Occurs in Most Newborns

Infants who exhibit hyperbilirubinemia in the absence of any specific disorder are said to suffer from physiologic jaundice.

Transhepatic clearance of bilirubin in the fetus is negligible; hepatic uptake, conjugation, and biliary excretion are all much lower than in children and adults. Hepatic UGT activity is less than 1% of that in adults, and ligandin levels are low. Nevertheless, fetal bilirubin levels remain low because bilirubin traverses the placenta, after which it is conjugated and excreted by the maternal liver.

The liver of the newborn assumes the responsibility for bilirubin clearance before its conjugating and excretory capacities are fully developed. Moreover, the demands on the liver in the newborn are actually increased because of augmented destruction of circulating erythrocytes during this period. *As a consequence, 70% of normal newborns exhibit transient unconjugated hyperbilirubinemia.* This physiologic jaundice is more pronounced in premature infants, both because the hepatic clearance of bilirubin is less developed and because the turnover of erythrocytes is more pronounced than in the term infant. The hepatic bilirubin-conjugating capacity reaches adult levels about 2 weeks after birth; the ligandin level takes somewhat longer to reach adult values. As a result of this hepatic maturation, serum bilirubin levels rapidly decline to adult values shortly after birth. Absorption of light by unconjugated bilirubin generates water-soluble bilirubin isomers. Thus, phototherapy is now routinely used to treat neonatal jaundice.

In cases of maternal–fetal blood group incompatibilities that lead to erythroblastosis fetalis (see Chapter 6), a striking overproduction of bilirubin in the fetus results from immune-mediated hemolysis. However, although newborns with erythroblastosis fetalis display increased bilirubin levels in cord blood, jaundice becomes severe only after birth, because maternal metabolism of bilirubin no longer compensates for the immaturity of the neonatal liver.

Impaired Canalicular Bile Flow Accompanied by Visible Biliary Pigment (Cholestasis) Reflects Either Extrahepatic or Intrahepatic Biliary Obstruction

Functionally, cholestasis represents decreased bile flow through the canaliculus and reduced secretion of water, bilirubin, and bile acids by the hepatocyte. The clinical diagnosis is based on the accumulation in the blood of materials normally transferred to the bile, including bilirubin, cholesterol, and bile acids, and the presence in the blood of elevated activities of certain enzymes, typically alkaline phosphatase. Cholestasis may be produced by intrinsic liver disease, in which case the term **intrahepatic cholestasis** is used (see Fig. 14-5), or by obstruction of the large bile ducts, a condition known as **extrahepatic cholestasis**. In any event, cholestasis is caused by a defect in the transport of bile across the canalicular membrane.

The inability to excrete bile acids into the canaliculus results in elevated serum and hepatocellular bile acid concentrations. These hydrophobic molecules have potent hepatotoxic properties, and much of the hepatic injury and progression to cirrhosis associated with cholestasis is due to the accumulation of bile acids within hepatocytes. Bile acids induce injury by their detergent action and by direct activation of apoptotic pathways. Elevated serum bile acid concentrations is the likely cause of severe itching (**pruritis**).

The extrahepatic biliary system may be obstructed by a number of lesions. These include gallstones passing through the cystic duct to lodge in the common bile duct, cancer of the bile duct or surrounding tissues (pancreas or ampulla of Vater), external compression by enlarged neoplastic lymph nodes in the porta hepatis (as in Hodgkin disease), benign strictures (postoperative scarring or primary sclerosing cholangitis), and congenital biliary atresia (Fig. 14-7).

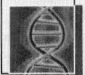

PATHOGENESIS: The secretion of bile into the canaliculus and its passage into the biliary collecting system are active processes that depend on a number of factors, including (1) the functional and structural characteristics of the canalicular microvilli, (2) the permeability of the canalicular plasma membrane, (3) the intracellular contractile system surrounding the canaliculus (microfilaments, microtubules), and (4) the interaction of bile acids with the secretory apparatus.

The biochemical basis of cholestasis is not entirely clear, but a number of abnormalities in the formation and movement of bile have been described. In the case of extrahepatic biliary obstruction, the effects clearly begin with increased pressure in the bile ducts. However, in the early stages, the biochemical and morphologic events at the canalicular level are similar to those that occur with intra-

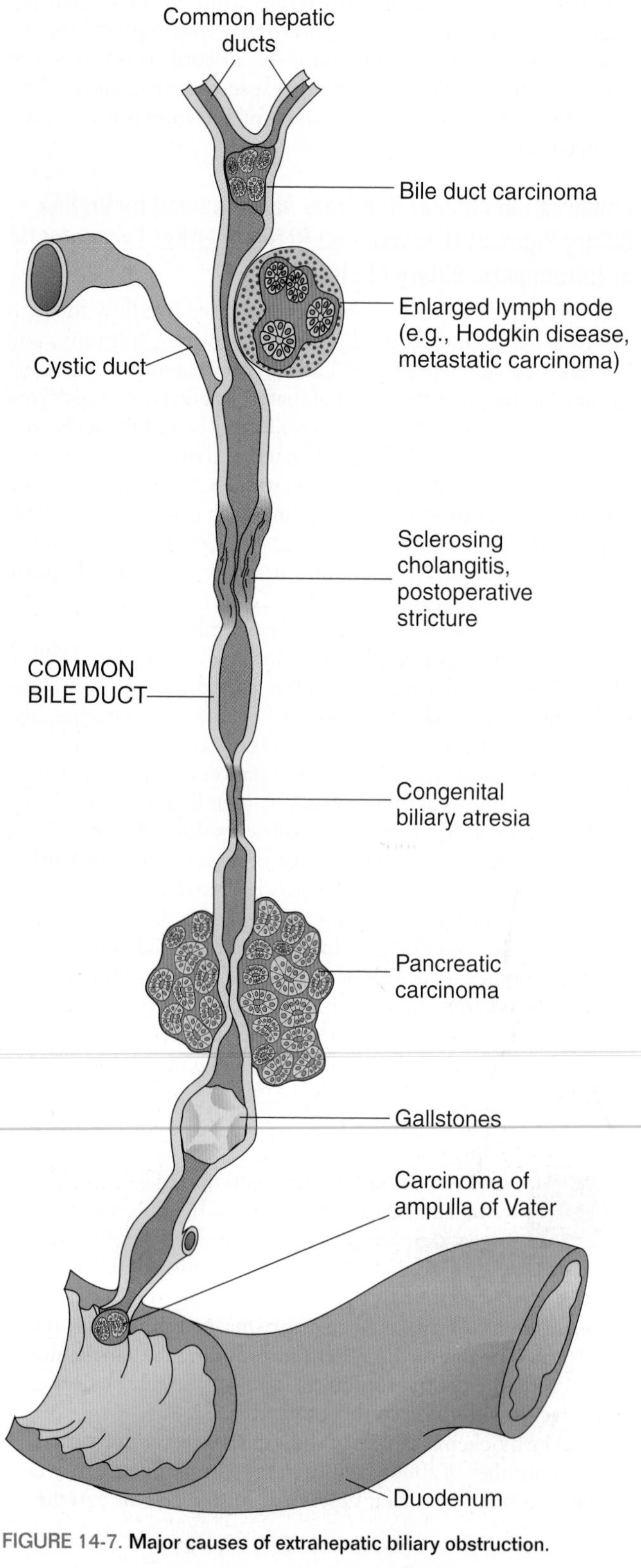

FIGURE 14-7. **Major causes of extrahepatic biliary obstruction.**

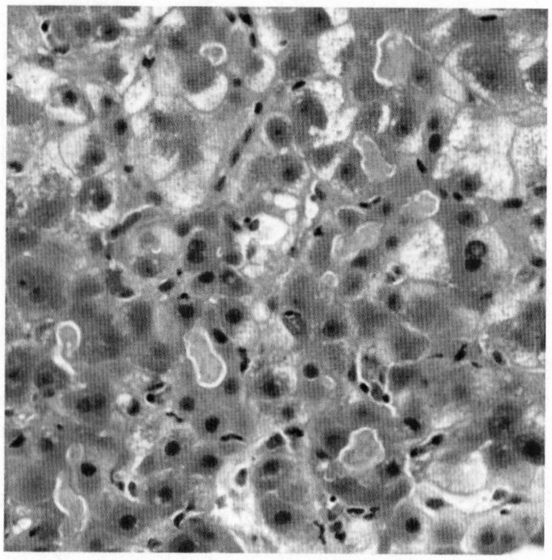

FIGURE 14-8. **Bile stasis.** A photomicrograph of the liver shows prominent bile plugs in dilated bile canaliculi.

hepatic cholestasis, including *a centrilobular predilection for the appearance of canalicular bile plugs* (Fig. 14-8).

The invariable presence of bile constituents in the blood of persons with cholestasis implies regurgitation of conjugated bilirubin from the hepatocyte into the bloodstream. The hepatic clearance of unconjugated bilirubin in cholestasis is normal. Even in the presence of complete bile duct obstruction, the serum bilirubin level rises only as high as 30 to 35 mg/dL because renal excretion of bilirubin prevents further accumulation.

Both intrahepatic and extrahepatic cholestasis are characterized initially by a preferential localization of visible bile pigment in the centrilobular zone. Fluid secretion into the canalicular bile is divided into two components: one dependent on the secretion of bile acids and the other independent of bile acid secretion. Since the periportal hepatocytes secrete most of the bile acids, the fluid content in the periportal zone of the canaliculus exceeds that in the central zone, a condition that tends to keep bilirubin in solution. Moreover, the bile acids themselves, which act as detergents in the intestine, also solubilize aggregates of bilirubin in the periportal areas. To the above factors is added the higher activity of microsomal mixed-function oxidases in the central zone, which predisposes central hepatocytes to injury by a variety of drugs and toxins. Such an effect may favor the deposition of bile in the centrilobular areas in cholestatic disorders.

Several mechanisms of cholestasis have been proposed:

DAMAGE TO THE CANALICULAR PLASMA MEMBRANE: The canalicular plasma membrane is the site of sodium (and therefore fluid) secretion into the bile. In addition, this membrane participates in the secretion of bile acids and bilirubin. The secretion of fluid is under the control of the Na^+/K^+-ATPase of the canalicular membrane. Alterations in the canalicular membrane by a number of drugs and other agents capable of perturbing its structure inhibit Na^+/K^+-ATPase, decrease bile flow, or produce morphologic alterations.

ALTERATION IN THE CONTRACTILE PROPERTIES OF THE CANALICULUS: Bile is propelled along the canaliculus by a peristalsis-like contractile activity of the hepatocytes. Agents that interact with the pericanalicular actin microfilaments (e.g., cytochalasin, phalloidin) inhibit this peristalsis and may cause cholestasis.

ALTERATIONS IN THE PERMEABILITY OF THE CANALICULAR MEMBRANE: It has been suggested that certain agents that produce cholestasis, including estrogens and taurolithocholate, permit back-diffusion of bile components by making the canalicular membrane more permeable, or "leaky."

PATHOLOGY: *The morphologic hallmark of cholestasis is the presence of brownish bile pigment within dilated canaliculi and in hepatocytes* (see Fig. 14-8). The canaliculus is enlarged. By electron microscopy, the microvilli are blunted and fewer in number or even absent. Bile stasis in the hepatocyte is reflected in the presence of large, bile-laden lysosomes.

When cholestasis persists, secondary morphologic abnormalities develop. Scattered necrotic hepatocytes probably reflect a toxic effect of excess intracellular bile. Within the sinusoids, the macrophages and Kupffer cells contain bile pigment and cellular debris. *Whereas early cholestasis is restricted almost exclusively to the central zone, chronic cholestasis is also marked by the appearance of bile plugs in the periphery of the lobule.*

In extrahepatic biliary obstruction, the liver is swollen and bile stained. In prolonged obstruction, the bile becomes almost colorless ("white bile") because of the suppression of bilirubin secretion, although the liver remains green. Initially, centrilobular cholestasis is accompanied by edema of the portal tracts. As obstruction proceeds, mononuclear inflammatory cells infiltrate the portal tracts. Tortuous and distended bile ductules, characterized by a high cuboidal epithelium, proliferate (Fig. 14-9). Damaged hepatocytes containing large amounts of bile manifest (1) hydropic swelling, (2) diffuse impregnation with bile pigment, and (3) a reticulated appearance. This triad is termed **feathery degeneration** (Fig. 14-10). The cholestasis eventually extends to the periphery of the lobule. Dilated bile ducts may rupture, promoting the formation of **bile lakes** (Fig. 14-11), which appear as focal, golden-yellow deposits that are surrounded by degenerating hepatocytes. Infection of the obstructed biliary passages often leads to a superimposed suppurative cholangitis, intraluminal pus, and even intrahepatic

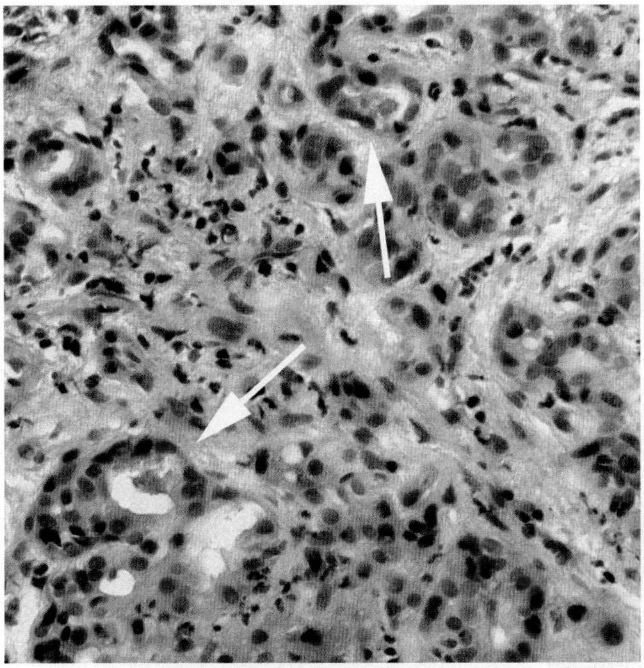

FIGURE 14-9. **Extrahepatic biliary obstruction.** A portal tract is expanded by proliferated bile ducts and acute and chronic inflammation. Several ducts are plugged with bile *(arrows)*.

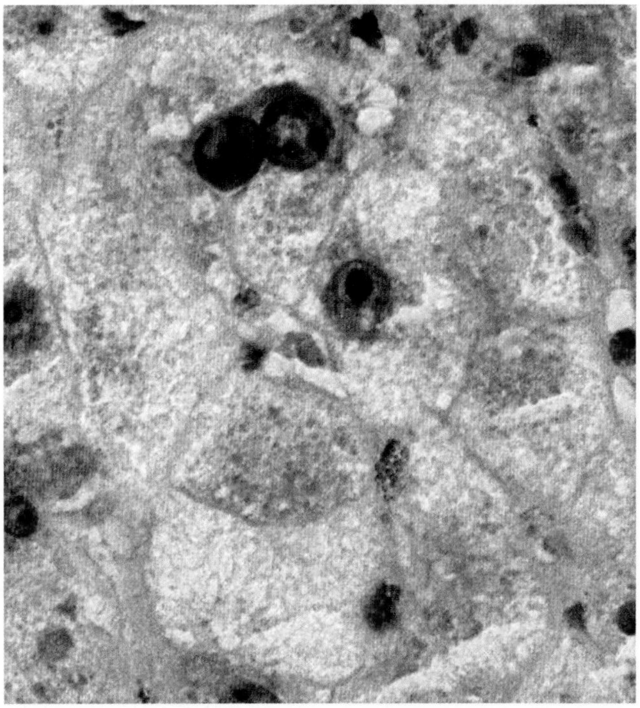

FIGURE 14-10. **Cholestasis.** Hepatocytes are swollen and bile stained (feathery degeneration)

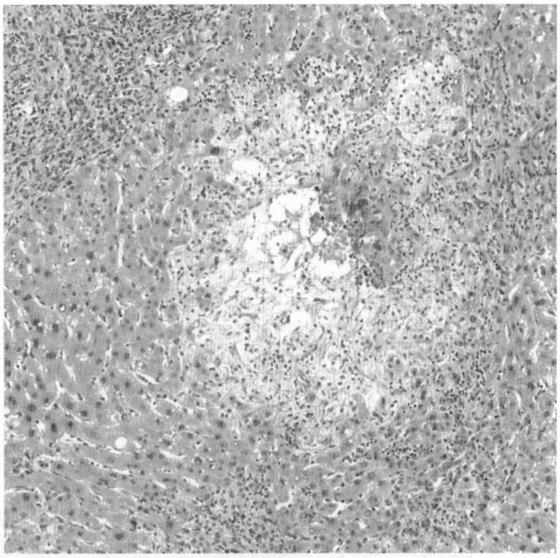

FIGURE 14-11. **Bile infarct (bile lake).** A photomicrograph of the liver in a patient with extrahepatic biliary obstruction shows an area of necrosis and the accumulation of extravasated bile.

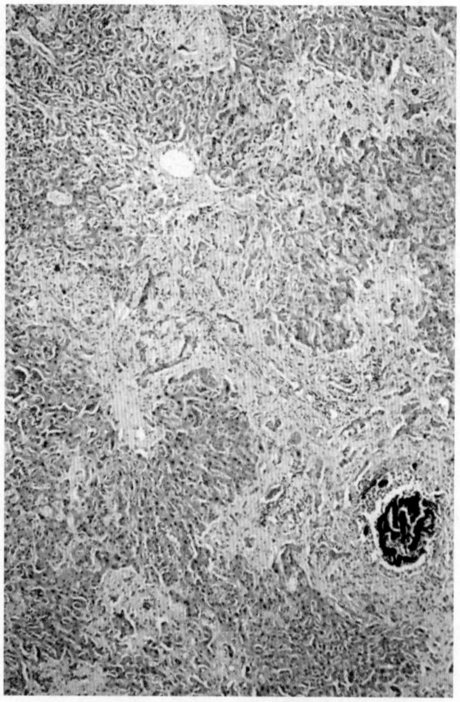

FIGURE 14-12. **Secondary biliary cirrhosis.** A photomicrograph of the liver from a patient with a carcinoma of the pancreas that obstructed the common bile duct. Irregular fibrous septa extend from an enlarged portal tract *(lower right)* containing a dilated interlobular bile duct that encloses a dense biliary concretion. Numerous proliferated bile ductules are seen within the septa.

abscesses. Within bile ducts and proliferated ductules, biliary concretions may be conspicuous.

With time, the portal tracts become enlarged and fibrotic (Fig. 14-12). In untreated extrahepatic biliary obstruction, septa eventually extend between the portal tracts of contiguous lobules to form **micronodular cirrhosis** (discussed below).

CLINICAL FEATURES: Cholestasis usually presents with jaundice, irrespective of its underlying cause. **Pruritis** (itching) is common, and can be severe and intractable. It may be caused by deposition of bile acids within the skin, but other components of bile may be play a role. Choesterol accumulates in the skin in the form of **xanthomas. Malabsorption** may develop in cases of protacted cholestastis (see Chapter 13).

Cirrhosis

Cirrhosis, the end stage of chronic liver disease, is defined as the destruction of the normal liver architecture by fibrous septa that encompass regenerative nodules of hepatocytes. This morphologic pattern invariably results from persistent liver cell necrosis. Advanced cases of cirrhosis all tend to have a similar appearance, and often the cause can no longer be ascertained by morphologic examination alone. During earlier stages, on the other hand, the characteristic features of the inciting pathogenic insult may be evident. For example, fat and Mallory bodies are typical of alcoholic liver injury, whereas chronic inflammation and periportal necrosis define chronic hepatitis.

The number of terms applied to the different forms of cirrhosis rivals the number of causative agents incriminated in chronic liver disease. Out of this apparent complexity, we can extract a simple spectrum of nodular patterns. At one end of this spectrum, usually in the early evolution of cirrhosis, is the **micronodular** type, characterized by small, uniform nodules separated by thin fibrous septa (discussed below). At the other end of the spectrum, ordinarily late in the course of the disease, is **macronodular cirrhosis**. This pattern consists of grossly visible, coarse, irregular nodules, which are mirrored histo-

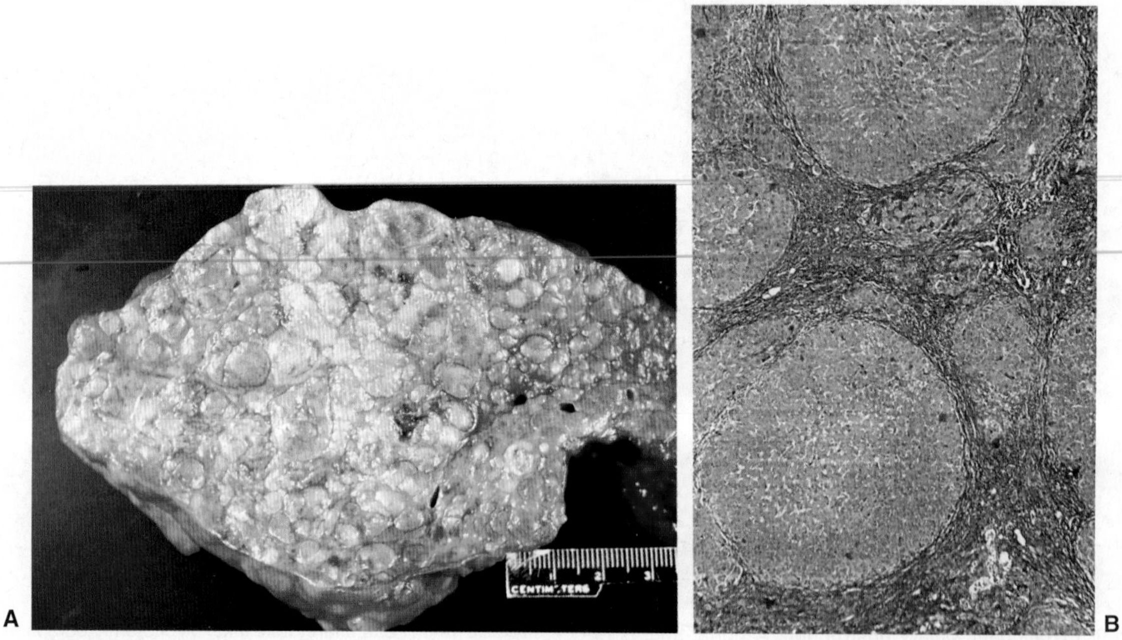

FIGURE 14-13. **Macronodular cirrhosis. A.** The liver is misshapen, and the cut surface reveals irregular nodules and connective tissue septa of varying width. **B.** A photomicrograph shows nodules of varying size and irregular fibrous septa.

logically by large nodules of varying size and shape that are encircled by bands of connective tissue (Fig. 14-13). These collagenous septa also vary conspicuously in width. Between these two extremes are many cases that show features of both types.

Historically, cirrhosis has been considered an irreversible condition. Recent observations suggest that collagen resorption and hepatic remodeling can occur over years to decades, assuming that the underlying cause of cirrhosis has abated. However, despite functional and structural improvement in the cirrhotic liver, it is unlikely that complete regression ever occurs.

MICRONODULAR CIRRHOSIS: This form of liver disease was previously termed **Laennec cirrhosis**, which honors the early 19th century French physician who provided the first accurate description of this disease (Laennec also invented the stethoscope). Micronodular cirrhosis exhibits nodules scarcely larger than a lobule, measuring less than 3 mm in diameter. The micronodules show no landmarks of lobular architecture in the form of portal tracts or central venules. The connective tissue septa separating the nodules are usually thin, but irregular focal collapse of parenchyma may lead to the presence of wider septa. In active stages of the cirrhotic process, numerous mononuclear inflammatory cells and proliferated bile ductules inhabit the septa. *The prototype of micronodular cirrhosis is alcoholic cirrhosis, but this pattern may also be observed in cirrhosis of many other causes.*

MACRONODULAR CIRRHOSIS: Macronodular cirrhosis is classically associated with chronic hepatitis. It also occasionally results from submassive confluent necrosis (see below), in which case the liver may be grossly misshapen. The connective tissue septa in macronodular cirrhosis are characteristically broad and contain elements of preexisting portal tracts, mononuclear inflammatory cells, and proliferated bile ductules. *Micronodular cirrhosis can be converted into a macronodular pattern by continued regeneration and expansion of existing nodules.* This is particularly true of alcoholics who are persuaded to abstain from drinking.

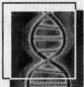

PATHOGENESIS: The diseases associated with cirrhosis are listed in Table 14-1. They have little in common except that they are all accompanied by persistent liver cell necrosis. Most cases of cirrhosis are attributable to alcoholism and chronic viral hepatitis. Despite advances in diagnostic modalities, some 15% of cases are of unknown origin and are classified as **cryptogenic cirrhosis.** Recent evidence suggests that nonalcoholic steatohepatitis accounts for a significant proportion of cryptogenic cirrhosis (see below).

Hepatic Failure

Hepatic failure is the clinical syndrome that occurs when the mass of liver cells or their function is inadequate to sustain the vital activities of the liver. Liver failure may develop acutely, most commonly as a result of viral hepatitis or toxic liver injury. By contrast, chronic liver diseases, such as chronic viral hepatitis or cirrhosis, may lead to an insidious onset of hepatic failure. The consequences of acute and chronic hepatic failure are depicted in Figure 14-14, which deals

TABLE 14-1

Major Causes of Cirrhosis

Alcoholic liver disease	
Nonalcoholic fatty liver disease	
Chronic hepatitis	
Chronic viral hepatitis	
Autoimmune hepatitis	
Drugs	
Biliary disease	
Extrahepatic biliary obstruction	
Primary biliary cirrhosis	
Sclerosing cholangitis	
Metabolic disease	
Hemochromatosis	Glycogen storage disease
Wilson disease	Hereditary fructose intolerance
α_1-Antitrypsin deficiency	Hereditary storage diseases
Tyrosinemia	Galactosemia
Cryptogenic	

with the complications of cirrhosis, the most common cause of hepatic failure. Although advances in supportive care have improved survival in acute hepatic failure, the mortality rate for this condition remains above 50%.

Inadequate Clearance of Bilirubin by the Liver Causes Jaundice

Hyperbilirubinemia associated with hepatic failure is for the most part conjugated, although the level of unconjugated bilirubin also tends to increase. On occasion, increased erythrocyte turnover may add to unconjugated hyperbilirubinemia, thereby aggravating the jaundice.

Hepatic Encephalopathy Refers to Neurologic Signs and Symptoms of Liver Failure

Hepatic encephalopathy progresses according to the following stages:

- **Stage I:** Sleep disturbance, irritability, and personality changes
- **Stage II:** Lethargy and disorientation
- **Stage III:** Deep somnolence
- **Stage IV:** Coma

This sequence may occur over a period of many months or may evolve rapidly in days or weeks in cases of fulminant hepatic failure. Associated neurologic symptoms include (1) a flapping tremor of the hands, called **asterixis**, and hyperactive reflexes in the earlier stages; (2) extensor toe responses later; and (3) a decerebrate posture in the terminal stages. Whereas intensive supportive measures may be adequate therapy in the early stages of hepatic encephalopathy, patients with stages III and IV encephalopathy are usually salvaged only by liver transplantation.

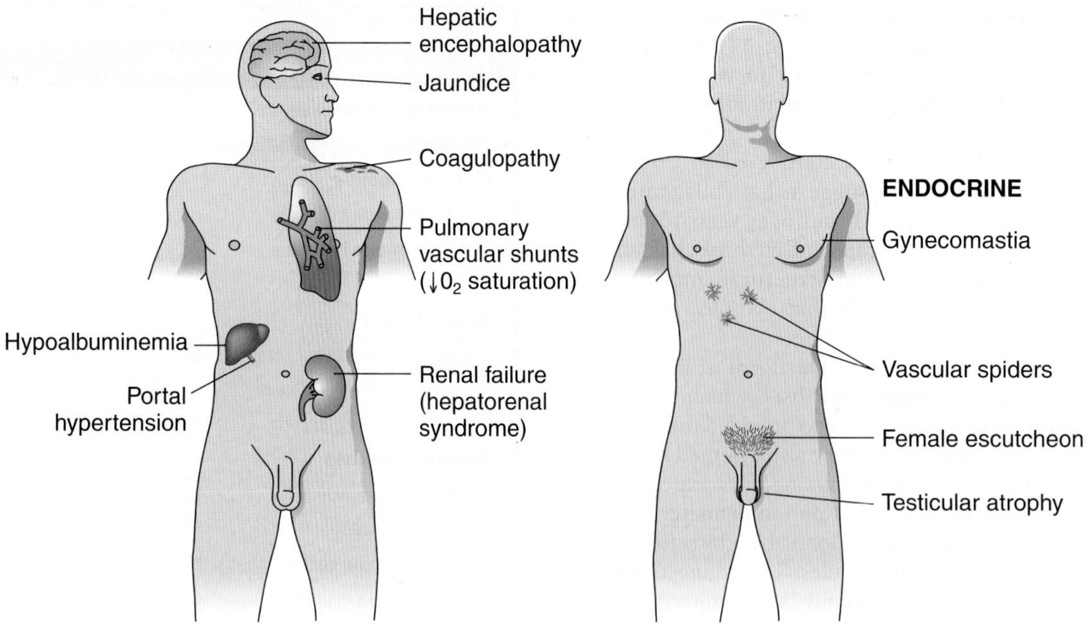

FIGURE 14-14. **Complications of cirrhosis and hepatic failure.**

PATHOGENESIS: The pathogenesis of hepatic encephalopathy remains elusive, and no single factor has been proved to account for the clinical syndrome. It is probable that the condition is caused in part by injurious compounds absorbed from the intestine that have escaped hepatic detoxification, because of either hepatocyte dysfunction or the existence of structural or functional vascular shunts. The latter mechanism is particularly evident after the surgical construction of a portal–systemic anastomosis (portal vein to inferior vena cava or its equivalent) for the relief of portal hypertension (see below), which accounts for the synonym **portasystemic encephalopathy**.

AMMONIA: Levels of ammonia are usually increased in the blood and brain of patients with hepatic encephalopathy. Most of the body's ammonia is of dietary origin and is derived from ingestion of ammonia in foods, digestion of proteins in the small intestine, and bacterial catabolism of dietary protein and urea secreted into the intestine. The brain detoxifies ammonia by synthesizing glutamate and glutamine, and excess levels of these molecules may alter neurotransmission and brain osmolality. However, the correlation between the increased concentration of blood ammonia and the severity of hepatic encephalopathy is inexact, and the neurotoxic effect of ammonia remains unexplained.

GABA: Neural inhibition, mediated by the γ-aminobutyric acid (GABA)–benzodiazepine receptor complex, is accentuated in hepatic encephalopathy by increased levels of benzodiazepine-like molecules.

OTHER SUBSTANCES: A number of other compounds have been suggested as contributing to the pathogenesis of hepatic encephalopathy. Among these are **mercaptans,** which result from the breakdown of sulfur-containing amino acids in the colon. The characteristic breath odor of patients with hepatic failure, termed **fetor hepaticus**, reflects the presence of mercaptans in saliva. Another hypothesis for the pathogenesis of hepatic encephalopathy holds that increased blood levels of aromatic amino acids, typical of hepatic failure, lead to decreased synthesis of normal neurotransmitters such as norepinephrine and augmented production of **false neurotransmitters** (e.g., octopamine). A toxic effect of **phenols** and **short-chain fatty acids** on the brain has also been postulated. Finally, there is experimental evidence for a disturbance in the blood–brain barrier in hepatic failure.

PATHOLOGY: In patients who have died with chronic liver disease and hepatic coma, the most striking changes are found in the astrocytes, termed **Alzheimer type II astrocytes**. These brain cells are increased in number and size and show swelling, nuclear enlargement, and nuclear inclusions. The deep layers of the cerebral cortex and subcortical white matter, the basal ganglia, and the cerebellum exhibit laminar necrosis and a spongiform appearance.

In patients with acute hepatic failure, **cerebral edema** is the major cause of death, occurring in more than half the cases, often in conjunction with uncal and cerebellar herniation. This edema is not simply a terminal event but is rather a specific lesion associated with hepatic coma, although the precise mechanism is obscure.

Defects Of Coagulation Often Cause Bleeding

Reduced hepatic synthesis of coagulation factors and thrombocytopenia are the principal causes for the impaired hemostasis in liver failure. Decreased production of clotting factors (fibrinogen; prothrombin; and factors V, VII, IX, and X) reflects the generalized impairment of protein synthesis by the liver.

Thrombocytopenia ($<$80,000/μL) occurs commonly in hepatic failure and is accompanied by qualitative abnormalities in platelet function. Thrombocytopenia may result from (1) hypersplenism, (2) bone marrow depression, or (3) the consumption of circulating platelets by intravascular coagulation.

Disseminated intravascular coagulation (DIC) occurs frequently in liver failure. Intravascular coagulation may be stimulated by necrosis of liver cells, activation of factor XII

(Hageman factor) by endotoxin, or inadequate hepatic clearance of activated clotting factors from the circulation.

Hypoalbuminemia Complicates Hepatic Failure

A decreased level of circulating albumin is secondary to impaired hepatic synthesis of albumin and is an important factor in the pathogenesis of the edema that often complicates chronic liver disease.

Hepatorenal Syndrome Refers to Renal Failure Secondary to Hepatic Failure

Hepatorenal syndrome is characterized by the features of renal hypoperfusion, namely, oliguria, azotemia, and increased plasma creatinine levels. The syndrome usually occurs in the setting of cirrhosis and indicates a poor prognosis. Curiously, the kidneys clearly maintain the ability to function normally. Kidneys from patients who have died of the hepatorenal syndrome function well when transplanted into recipients with chronic renal failure. Conversely, in patients with the hepatorenal syndrome, liver transplantation can restore renal function.

PATHOGENESIS: *The major determinant of the hepatorenal syndrome is decreased renal blood flow and a consequent reduction in glomerular filtration rate.* A reduction in the effective circulating blood volume leads to compensatory renal vasoconstriction. The resulting decrease in renal perfusion and the shunting of blood from the cortex to the medulla cause reduced glomerular filtration. Vasoactive substances produced by the failing liver or inadequately cleared by it seem to contribute to the renal hemodynamic changes. In any event, the hepatorenal syndrome is caused by inadequate perfusion of the kidneys when local vasodilation can no longer counteract the effects of vasoconstriction.

PATHOLOGY: At autopsy, jaundiced patients with the hepatorenal syndrome show bile staining of renal tubular cells and bile casts in the lumina, so-called *biliary nephrosis*. However, these morphologic alterations are not believed to contribute to renal dysfunction.

Pulmonary Complications Are Frequent in Cirrhosis

Decreased arterial oxygen saturation may be severe enough to result in cyanosis. Arteriovenous shunts in the lungs of patients with cirrhosis shift the hemoglobin dissociation curve to the right (reduced affinity for oxygen). In addition, ventilatory and perfusion deficits may play a role. Arterial desaturation is responsible for the clubbing of the fingers occasionally encountered in chronic liver disease.

Endocrine Complications Are Associated with Cirrhosis

It is important to distinguish between the direct effects of alcohol abuse, a common cause of liver disease, and changes that are better attributed to hepatic dysfunction. Chronic liver failure in men leads to feminization, characterized by **gynecomastia**, a female body habitus, and a female distribution of pubic hair (female escutcheon). In addition, vascular manifestations of **hyperestrogenism** are common and include **spider angiomas** in the territory drained by the superior vena cava (upper trunk and face) and **palmar erythema** (see Fig. 14-14).

Feminization is attributed to reduced hepatic catabolism of estrogens and weak androgens. The weak androgens (androstenedione and dehydroepiandrosterone) are converted to estrogenic compounds in peripheral tissues, thereby adding to the burden of circulating estrogens. Moreover, extrahepatic portal–systemic shunts secondary to portal hypertension in cirrhosis permit these hormones to bypass the liver.

Men who suffer from alcoholic liver disease are more likely to be feminized than those with liver disease from other causes, and the feminization is usually more severe. In addition, chronic alcoholics also suffer hypogonadism, manifested by testicular atrophy, impotence, and loss of libido. Alcoholic women also exhibit gonadal failure, presenting as oligomenorrhea, amenorrhea, infertility, ovarian atrophy, and loss of secondary sex characteristics. These effects on gonadal function in both sexes reflect a direct toxic action of alcohol independent of chronic liver disease.

Portal Hypertension

Portal hypertension is defined as a sustained increase in portal venous pressure and results from obstruction to blood flow somewhere in the portal circuit. Arising at the junction of the superior mesenteric vein with the splenic vein, the portal vein carries the major venous drainage from the gastrointestinal tract, the pancreas, and the spleen into the liver. It delivers two thirds of the hepatic blood flow but accounts for less than half of the total oxygen supply, the remainder being supplied by the hepatic artery. Normal pressure in the portal vein is only 7 to 14 cm H_2O (5–10 mm Hg), and a pressure greater than 30 cm H_2O defines portal hypertension. *The major complications of increased portal pressure and the opening of collateral channels are bleeding from gastroesophageal varices, ascites, and splenomegaly.*

For the sake of convenience, obstruction to the flow of portal blood can be pictured as (1) **prehepatic**, occurring before the blood enters the liver; (2) **intrahepatic,** occurring during transit through the portal tracts and lobules; and (3) **posthepatic**, occurring after exit of the blood from the lobules (Fig. 14-15).

Intrahepatic Portal Hypertension Is Usually Caused by Cirrhosis

Regenerative nodules in the cirrhotic liver impinge on the hepatic veins, thereby obstructing blood flow distal to the lobules. The small portal veins and venules are trapped, narrowed, and often obliterated by scarring of the portal tracts. Moreover, blood flow through the hepatic artery is increased and small arteriovenous communications become functional. In this way, portal hypertension due to obstruction of blood flow distal to the sinusoid is augmented by increased arterial blood flow. In addition, increased splanchnic arterial blood flow, whose cause is unclear, is an important factor in the maintenance of portal hypertension. Intrahepatic vasoconstriction in cirrhosis may further exacerbate portal hypertension. Central vein sclerosis and sinusoidal fibrosis also contribute to the development of portal hypertension in alcoholic liver disease. In fact, portal hypertension can result from alcoholic central sclerosis alone, even in cases that do not progress to cirrhosis.

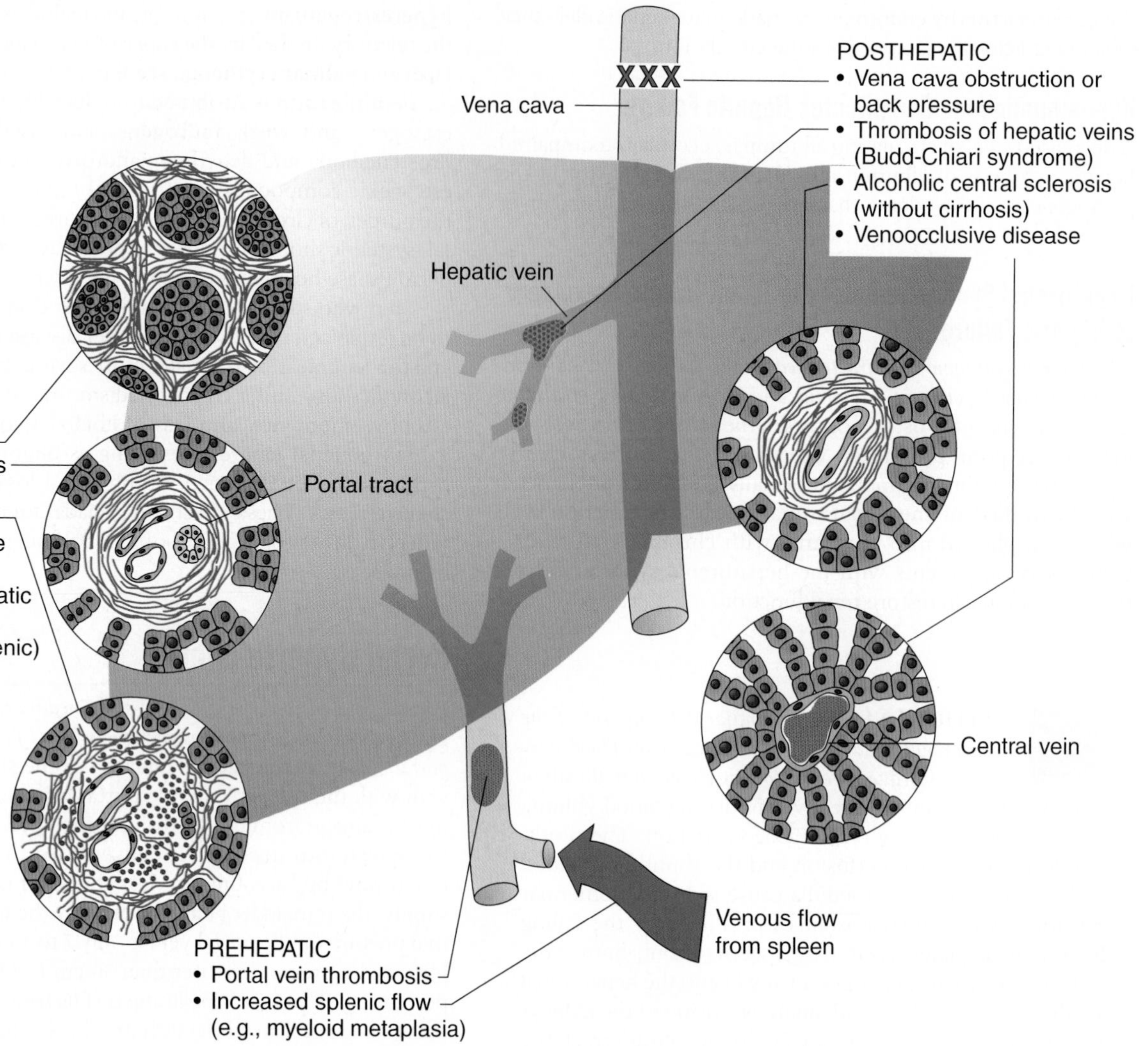

FIGURE 14-15. **Causes of portal hypertension.**

Worldwide, ***hepatic schistosomiasis*** *(Schistoma mansoni and Schistoma japonicum) is a major cause of intrahepatic portal hypertension.* The ova released from the intestinal veins traverse the portal system and lodge in the intrahepatic portal venules, where they elicit a granulomatous reaction that heals by scarring. Because the obstruction within the liver occurs predominantly before the portal blood enters the hepatic sinusoids, hepatic schistosomiasis is functionally similar to prehepatic portal hypertension. Thus, hepatic function is well maintained, but the intrahepatic presinusoidal vascular obstruction leads to severe portal hypertension.

Idiopathic portal hypertension refers to occasional cases of intrahepatic portal hypertension with splenomegaly that occur in the absence of any demonstrable intrahepatic or extrahepatic disease. In some countries (England, Japan), idiopathic portal hypertension accounts for 15% to 35% of all cases that require surgery to decompress the portal circulation.

Intrahepatic portal hypertension can be caused by other conditions that interfere with the flow of blood through the liver, including (1) cystic disease of the liver (see Chapter 16, which includes a discussion of cystic disease of the kidney), (2) partial nodular transformation of the liver in the region of the porta hepatis, and (3) nodular regenerative hyperplasia (small regenerative nodules without fibrosis that compress the intervening hepatic parenchyma).

Prehepatic Portal Hypertension Is Often Caused by Portal Vein Thrombosis

Portal vein thrombosis occurs most commonly in the setting of cirrhosis. Other causes of portal vein thrombosis include tumors, infections, hypercoagulability states, pancreatitis, and surgical trauma. Some cases are of unknown etiology. Primary hepatocellular carcinoma characteristically invades branches of the portal vein and occasionally occludes the main portal vein. When the portal vein is obstructed by a septic thrombus, bacteria may seed the intrahepatic branches of the portal vein (suppurative pylephlebitis) and cause multiple hepatic abscesses.

Occlusion of the portal vein may be manifested in the neonatal period or in early childhood. In some cases, umbilical sepsis is an important cause, but other local and systemic infections may also play a role. Sometimes the thrombosed portal or splenic vein is replaced by a fibrous cord or interlacing vascular channels, a condition termed **cavernous transformation.**

The liver normally offers little resistance to the outflow of blood through the sinusoids and can, therefore, accommodate substantial increases in blood flow without a secondary increase in pressure. However, under some uncommon circumstances, increased portal venous blood flow can result in prehepatic portal hypertension. An arteriovenous fistula (i.e., an abnormal communication between an artery and the portal vein) may lead to prehepatic portal hypertension. It generally arises from trauma or rupture of an aneurysm of the splenic or hepatic artery. Such a fistula may also be found in association with hereditary hemorrhagic telangiectasia (Osler-Weber-Rendu syndrome). Portal hypertension also occasionally occurs in patients with splenomegaly from a variety of causes, including polycythemia vera, myeloid metaplasia, and chronic myelogenous leukemia. In cirrhosis, the accompanying splenomegaly may further aggravate portal hypertension.

Posthepatic Portal Hypertension Refers to Obstruction to Blood Flow beyond the Liver Lobules

Budd-Chiari syndrome is a congestive disease of the liver caused by occlusion of the hepatic veins and their tributaries.

PATHOGENESIS: The principal cause of the Budd-Chiari syndrome is thrombosis of the hepatic veins, in association with such diverse conditions as polycythemia vera (10%–40% of cases) and other myeloproliferative disorders, hypercoagulable states associated with malignant tumors, the use of oral contraceptives, pregnancy, bacterial infections, paroxysmal nocturnal hemoglobinuria, metastatic and primary tumors in the liver, and surgical trauma. In 20% of cases, no specific cause is evident. Thrombosis is most common in the large hepatic veins close to their exit from the liver and in the intrahepatic portion of the inferior vena cava. In parts of Africa and the Orient, membranous webs of unknown cause, presumably congenital, compromise the vena cava above the orifices of the hepatic veins and commonly cause the Budd-Chiari syndrome. Increased back-pressure in the venous system caused by severe congestive heart failure, tricuspid stenosis or regurgitation, or constrictive pericarditis may mimic the Budd-Chiari syndrome.

Hepatic veno-occlusive disease is a variant of the Budd-Chiari syndrome and is caused by occlusion of the central venules and small branches of the hepatic veins. Most commonly, this disorder is traced to the ingestion of toxic pyrrolizidine alkaloids present in plants of the *Crotalaria* and *Senecio* genera, which are used in the formulation of "bush teas" in primitive societies. It is also seen in patients treated with certain antineoplastic chemotherapeutic agents, and after hepatic irradiation. Veno-occlusive disease also occurs in association with bone marrow transplantation, possibly as a manifestation of graft-versus-host disease.

PATHOLOGY: In the acute stage of **hepatic vein thrombosis**, the liver is swollen and tense, and the cut surface exhibits a mottled appearance and oozes blood (Fig. 14-16A). In the chronic stage, the cut surface is paler, and the liver is firm, owing to an increase in connective tissue. Microscopically, the hepatic veins display thrombi in varying stages of evolution, from recent clots to well-organized thrombi that have been canalized.

In the acute stage of both the Budd-Chiari syndrome and veno-occlusive disease, the sinusoids of the central zone are dilated and packed with erythrocytes. The liver cell plates are compressed, and there is necrosis of centrilobular hepatocytes (see Fig. 14-16B). In long-standing venous congestion, fibrosis of the central zone radiating into the more peripheral portions of the lobules is conspicuous. The sinusoids are dilated, and the central to midzonal hepatocytes show pressure atrophy. Eventually, connective tissue septa link adjacent central zones to form nodules with a single portal tract in the center, a process known as reverse lobulation. The fibrosis is usually not severe enough to justify a label of cirrhosis.

A

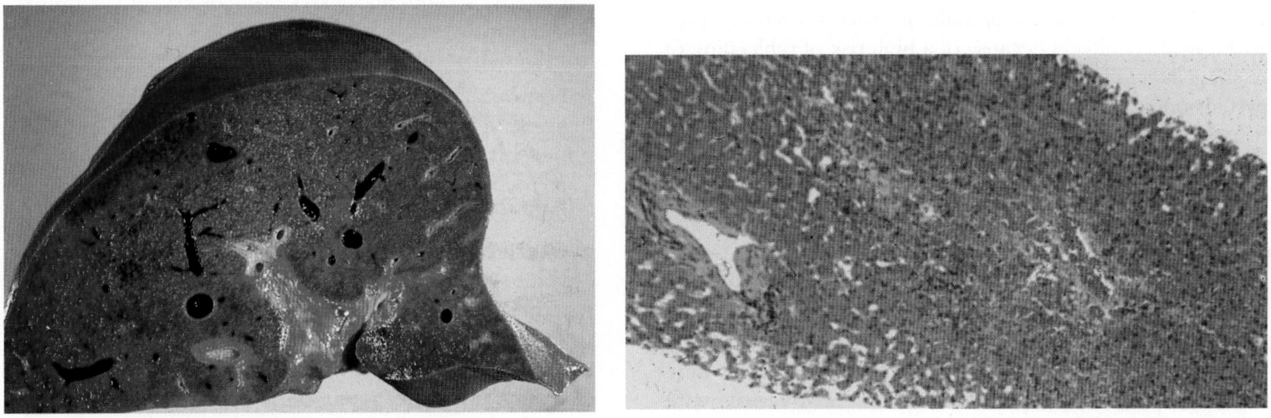

B

FIGURE 14-16. **Budd-Chiari syndrome. A.** The cut surface of the liver from a patient who died from Budd-Chiari syndrome shows thrombosis of the hepatic veins and diffuse congestion of the parenchyma. **B.** A needle biopsy of the liver from a patient with acute Budd-Chiari syndrome reveals centrilobular necrosis and hemorrhage.

CLINICAL FEATURES: *Complete thrombosis of the hepatic veins presents as an acute illness characterized by abdominal pain, enlargement of the liver, ascites, and mild jaundice.* Acute hepatic failure and death often occur rapidly. The more usual course, in which the obstruction of the hepatic venous circulation is incomplete, is marked by similar symptoms but may pursue a protracted course over periods ranging from a month to a few years. More than 90% of patients with Budd-Chiari syndrome develop ascites, usually severe, and splenomegaly is seen in over 30%. Typically, the serum bilirubin and aminotransferase activities increase only modestly. Most patients eventually die in hepatic failure or from the complications of portal hypertension. Liver transplantation has been successful in curing the disease.

Portal Hypertension Leads to Systemic Complications

Esophageal Varices

Esophageal varices represent the most important complication of portal hypertension and arise from the opening of portal–systemic collaterals as an adaptation to decompress the portal venous system. One of the most common causes of death in patients with cirrhosis and other disorders associated with portal hypertension is exsanguinating upper gastrointestinal tract hemorrhage from **bleeding esophageal varices.**

PATHOGENESIS: The collaterals of most clinical significance are located in the submucosa of the lower esophagus and upper stomach and are the result of communications between the portal vein and the gastric coronary vein. Because of the increased blood flow and higher pressure that follow the opening of these collaterals, the submucosal veins in the vicinity of the esophagogastric junction become dilated and protrude into the lumen (see Chapter 13). There is no simple correlation between portal venous pressure and the risk of variceal bleeding, although the risk does rise with increasing size of the varices.

CLINICAL FEATURES: The prognosis in patients with bleeding esophageal varices is poor, and the acute mortality may be as high as 40%. In patients with cirrhosis who survive an initial episode of variceal bleeding, long-term survival is unlikely because of a high risk of rebleeding or worsening liver failure. By contrast, patients in whom the portal hypertension is caused by a presinusoidal block, such as hepatic schistosomiasis, have a much better prognosis than those with cirrhosis because of the absence of underlying liver dysfunction. Importantly, death associated with bleeding esophageal varices is frequently not attributable directly to exsanguination and shock. Rather it is the result of hepatic failure precipitated by stress, ischemic necrosis of the liver, and the encephalopathy caused by the acute nitrogenous load imposed by blood in the intestinal tract.

Acute variceal hemorrhage may be treated by direct tamponade with an inflatable balloon, injection of varices with sclerosing agents through an endoscope, endoscopic variceal ligation, or intravenous administration of vasopressin to reduce splanchnic blood flow and portal venous pressure. For patients with repeated episodes of variceal bleeding in whom sclerotherapy has failed, permanent decompression of the portal circulation can be achieved by surgically constructed portasystemic shunts. These procedures divert blood from the high-pressure portal circulation to the lower-pressure systemic venous circulation. Intrahepatic portasystemic shunts can also be constructed by invasive angiography, in which a catheter in a hepatic vein is thrust through hepatic parenchyma into a dilated branch of the portal vein (transjugular intrahepatic portasystemic shunt [TIPS]). In some cases, liver transplantation is an alternative to shunt surgery.

The back-pressure in the portal vein is also transmitted to its tributaries, including the inferior hemorrhoidal veins, which become dilated and tortuous (**anorectal varices**). Collateral veins radiating about the umbilicus produce a pattern known as **caput medusae.**

Splenomegaly

The spleen in portal hypertension enlarges progressively and often gives rise to the syndrome of **hypersplenism**—that is, a decrease in the life span of all of the formed elements of the blood and, therefore, a reduction in their circulating numbers (pancytopenia). Hypersplenism is attributed to an increased rate of removal of erythrocytes, leukocytes, and platelets because of the prolonged transit time through the hyperplastic spleen.

On gross examination, the spleen is firm and enlarged, up to 1000 g, and its cut surface is uniformly deep red, with an inapparent white pulp. Microscopically, the splenic sinusoids are dilated, and their walls are thickened by fibrous tissue and lined by hyperplastic endothelial cells and macrophages. Focal hemorrhages lead to the formation of fibrotic, iron-laden nodules, known as **Gamna-Gandy bodies.**

Ascites

Ascites refers to the accumulation of fluid in the peritoneal cavity. It often accompanies portal hypertension, and the amount of fluid may be so great (frequently many liters) that it not only distends the abdomen but also interferes with breathing. The onset of ascites in cirrhosis is associated with a poor prognosis.

PATHOGENESIS: The retention of sodium and water in cirrhosis is clearly important in the pathogenesis of ascites. The mechanisms for altered sodium and water homeostasis in cirrhosis remain controversial, but three major hypotheses can be considered:

- **Hypovolemia:** It was initially held that increased pressure in the portal system caused sodium and water transudation into the abdominal cavity. The resulting hypovolemia was postulated to stimulate increased retention of renal sodium and water (Fig. 14-17).
- **Overflow:** Subsequently, it was shown that the total blood volume in cirrhotic patients with ascites actually increases rather than decreases. In fact, expansion of blood volume and sodium and water retention by the kidney precede the formation of ascites. These findings suggest that renal sodium and water retention in decompensated cirrhosis results from an alteration in volume regulation that is not secondary to decreased intravascular volume.

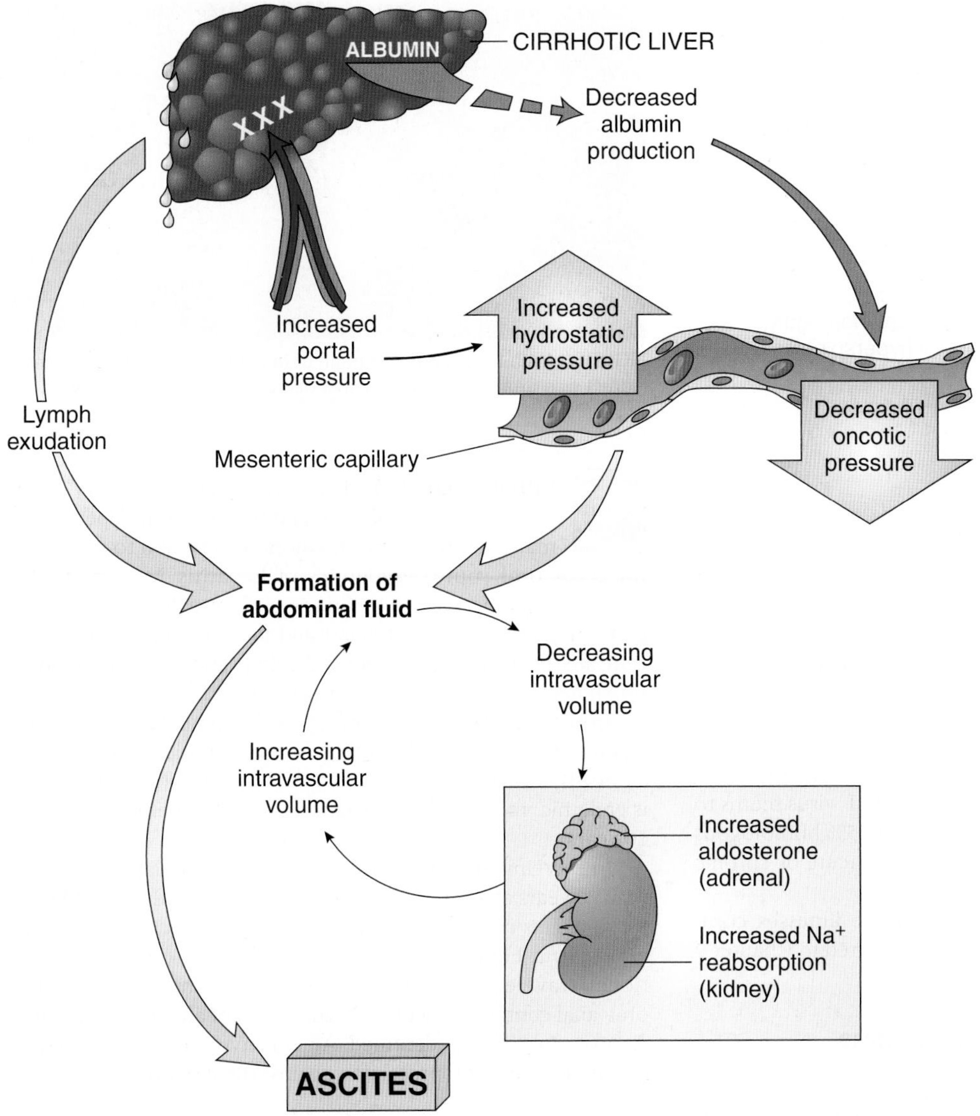

FIGURE 14-17. **Pathogenesis of ascites.** In addition to the other factors depicted, the traditional concept holds that renal retention of sodium is a response to a decreased "effective" blood volume. An alternative view (overflow hypothesis) considers the increased renal reabsorption of sodium to be a primary effect of cirrhosis that precedes the formation of ascites. Peripheral vasodilation should also considered.

- **Vasodilation:** It has been proposed that peripheral arterial vasodilation is an initiating event in the renal retention of sodium and water in cirrhosis. Vasodilation results in a decreased effective arterial blood volume, owing to the diversion of blood to the periphery. This process serves as a potent stimulus for the renal retention of sodium and water.

Other factors contribute to the formation of ascites in cirrhosis. Portal hypertension increases the hydrostatic pressure in the mesenteric capillaries. At the same time, the low serum albumin characteristic of cirrhosis is associated with decreased plasma oncotic pressure. As in the formation of peripheral edema (see Chapter 7), the resulting imbalance in Starling forces leads to transudation of fluid into the peritoneal cavity. Finally, the rate of formation of hepatic lymph exceeds the capacity of the lymphatics to remove it, and the liver "weeps" lymph into the abdomen.

Spontaneous Bacterial Peritonitis

Spontaneous bacterial peritonitis is an important complication in patients with both cirrhosis and ascites. The infection is extremely dangerous and carries a very high mortality, even when treated with antibiotics. Presumably, the ascitic fluid is seeded with bacteria from the blood or lymph or by the passage of bacteria through the bowel wall. Typically, the leukocyte count in the ascitic fluid of spontaneous bacterial peritonitis is greater than 500/μL, and more than half are neutrophils.

The complications of portal hypertension are summarized in Figure 14-18.

Viral Hepatitis

Viral hepatitis is an infection of hepatocytes that produces necrosis and inflammation of the liver. The disease has been recognized as "epidemic jaundice" for millennia. Worldwide, over 500 million people are infected with hepatotropic viruses and are at considerable risk for the development of hepatocellular carcinoma. Many viruses and other infectious agents can produce hepatitis and jaundice (Table 14-2), but in the industrialized world, more than

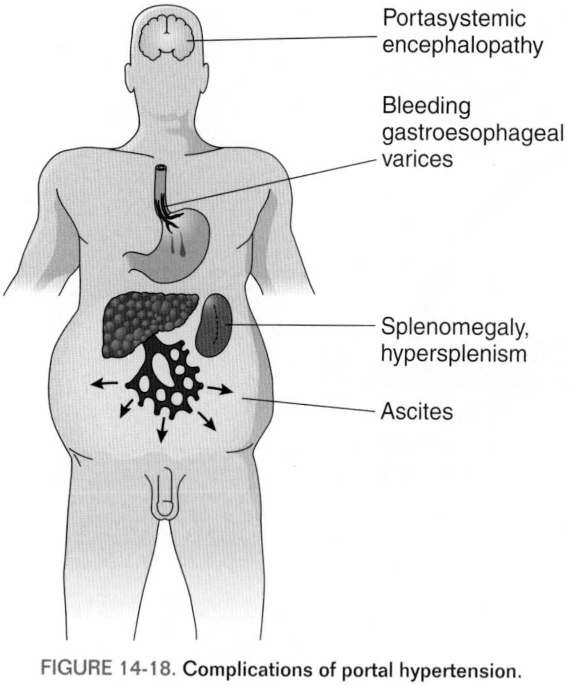

FIGURE 14-18. **Complications of portal hypertension.**

95% of cases of viral hepatitis involve a limited number of hepatotropic viruses, named from A to G. Hepatitis F virus seems to be a variant of hepatitis B. Hepatitis G virus is 25% homologous with hepatitis C virus, but it does not lead to acute or chronic hepatitis.

The following discussion emphasizes the illnesses commonly termed *viral hepatitis*. The reader is referred to Chapter 9 for consideration of the other agents.

Hepatitis A Virus Is the Most Common Cause of Acute Hepatitis

Hepatitis A virus (HAV) is a small RNA-containing enterovirus of the picornavirus group (which includes the polio virus) (Fig. 14-19). The hepatocyte is the principal site of viral replication, although gastrointestinal epithelial cells may also be infected. Shedding of progeny virus into the bile accounts for its appearance in the feces. HAV is not directly cytopathic, and hepatic injury has been attributed to an immunologic reaction to virally infected hepatocytes.

TABLE 14–2

Infectious Agents That Cause Hepatitis

Hepatitis A virus (HAV)	Herpes simplex virus
Hepatitis B virus (HBV)	Cytomegalovirus
Hepatitis C virus (HCV)	Enteroviruses other than HAV
Hepatitis E virus	
Yellow fever virus	Leptospires (leptospirosis)
Epstein-Barr virus (infectious mononucleosis)	*Entamoeba histolytica* (amebic hepatitis)
Lassa, Marburg, and Ebola viruses	

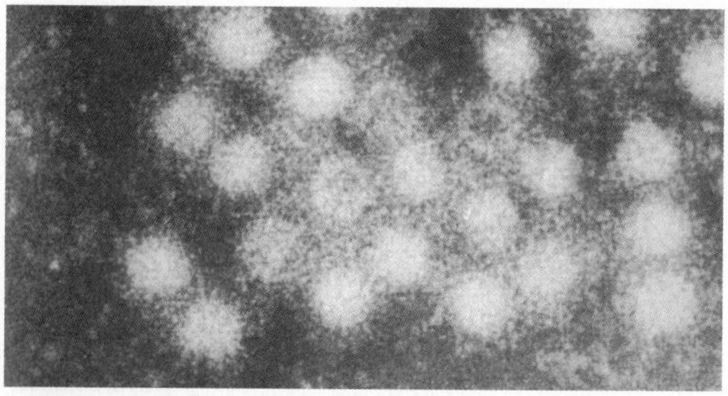

FIGURE 14-19. **Electron micrograph of hepatitis A virus (HAV).** A fecal extract was treated with convalescent serum containing anti-HAV.

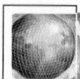

EPIDEMIOLOGY: The only reservoir for HAV is the acutely infected person, and transmission depends primarily on serial transmission from person to person by the fecal–oral route. Epidemics of hepatitis A occur under crowded and unsanitary conditions, such as exist in warfare, or by fecal contamination of water and food. Edible shellfish concentrate the virus in contaminated waters and may lead to infection if eaten after being inadequately cooked.

In the industrialized countries, which have low rates of infection, most cases of hepatitis A are seen in older children and adults. By contrast, in less-developed regions, where the disease is endemic, most of the population is infected before the age of 10 years.

In the United States, about 10% of the population younger than 20 years of age have serologic evidence of previous HAV infection. *This circumstance indicates that most infections with HAV are anicteric.* Hepatitis A is common in day care centers, international travelers, and male homosexuals, the last reflecting oral–anal contact. However, in about half of all cases of hepatitis A, no source can be identified. An effective vaccine for hepatitis A confers long-term protection against the disease.

CLINICAL FEATURES: Following an incubation period of 3 to 6 weeks (with a mean of about 4 weeks), persons infected with HAV develop nonspecific symptoms, including fever, malaise, and anorexia. Concomitantly, liver injury is evidenced by a rise in serum aminotransferase activity (Fig. 14-20). As the activities of aminotransferases begin to decline, usually 5 to 10 days later, jaundice may appear. It remains evident for an average of 10 days but may persist for more than a month. In most cases, the elevated levels of aminotransferases return to normal by the time jaundice has disappeared. *Hepatitis A never pursues a chronic course. There is no carrier state, and infection provides lifelong immunity.* Moreover, virtually all patients recover without hepatic encephalopathy, and fatal fulminant hepatitis occurs only rarely.

HAV can be detected in the liver about 2 weeks after infection. It reaches a maximum in another 2 weeks, and it disappears shortly thereafter (see Fig. 14-20). Fecal shedding of HAV follows its appearance in the liver by about a week and lasts for only a brief time. The period of viremia is also short, occurring early in the course of the disease.

The first detectable antibody response to HAV infection is the appearance of IgM anti-HAV in the blood during the acute illness (see Fig. 14-20). The antibody titer begins to fall within a few weeks and generally disappears by 3 to 5 months. IgG anti-HAV

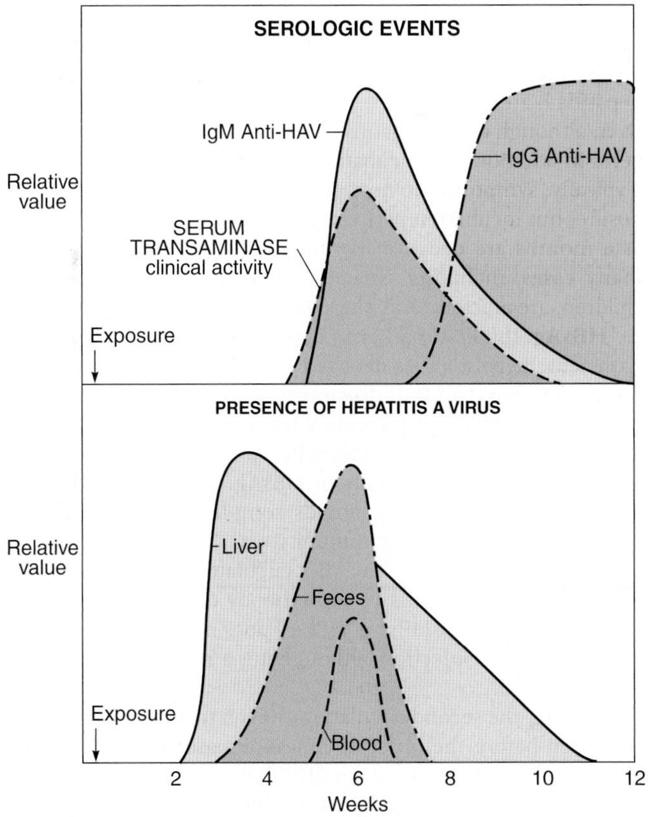

FIGURE 14-20. **Typical serologic events associated with hepatitis A (HAV).**

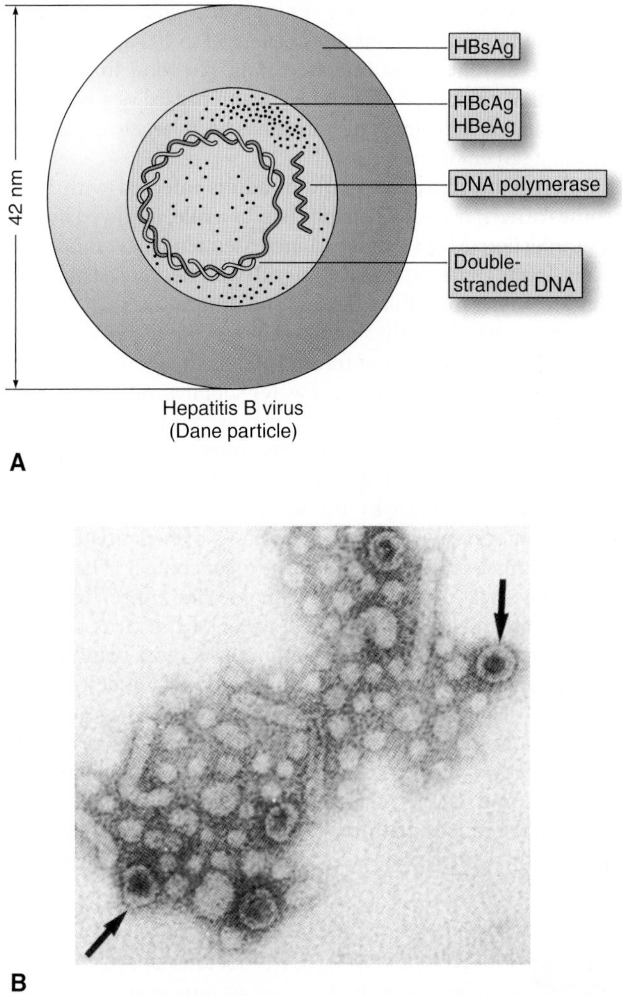

FIGURE 14-21. **Hepatitis B virus. A.** Schematic representation of the hepatitis B virus (HBV) and serum particles associated with HBV infection. (Antigens (Ag) for hepatitis B are indicated by their letters: c = core, e, and s = surface.) **B.** Electron micrograph of particles from centrifuged serum in a case of hepatitis. Rodlike and spherical particles containing HBsAg are evident. The complete virion, composed of the viral core and its surrounding envelope, is represented by Dane particles *(arrows)*.

is detected as the patient recovers; it maintains peak levels after the IgM antibody has disappeared and persists for life. Finding IgM anti-HAV in the serum of a patient with acute hepatitis confirms HAV as the cause.

Hepatitis B Virus Is a Major Cause of Acute and Chronic Liver Disease

Hepatitis B virus (HBV) is a hepatotropic DNA virus that was the first of the so-called hepadnaviruses. The genomes of the hepadnaviruses are among the smallest of all known viruses. The DNA of HBV is predominantly double-stranded and consists of one long circular strand containing the entire genome, and a shorter complementary strand that varies from 50% to 85% of the length of the longer strand (Fig. 14-21). The HBV genome contains four genes:

- **Core *(C)* gene:** The core of the virus contains the **core antigen (HBcAg)** and the **e antigen (HBeAg),** both products of the *C* gene. The *C* gene includes two consecutive open reading frames, the precore and core regions. Transcription of the core frame alone yields HBcAg, whereas HBeAg is derived from the proteolysis of the translation product of the entire *C* gene.
- **Surface gene:** The core of HBV is enclosed in a coat that expresses an antigen termed **hepatitis B surface antigen (HBsAg).** The surface coat is synthesized by the infected hepatocyte independently from the viral core and is secreted into the blood in vast amounts. This material is visualized by electron microscopy in centrifuged serum as two distinct particles (see Fig. 14-21), one a 22-nm sphere and the other a tubular structure 22 nm in diameter and 40 to 400 nm in length. HBsAg particles are immunogenic but not infectious. The intact and infectious virus is also found in the same preparations as a 42-nm sphere *(Dane particle)* that contains viral DNA.
- **Polymerase gene:** The *P* gene encodes the DNA polymerase.
- ***X* gene:** The small X protein activates viral transcription and probably plays a role in the pathogenesis of hepatocellular carcinoma associated with chronic HBV infection.

EPIDEMIOLOGY: It is estimated that there are about 200 million chronic carriers of HBV in the world, constituting an enormous reservoir of infection. Depending on the incidence of primary infection with HBV, the carrier rates vary from as low as 0.3% (United States and western Europe) to 20% (Southeast Asia, sub-Saharan Africa, and Oceania). In the latter populations, an important avenue by which the high carrier rate is sustained is vertical transmission of the virus from a carrier mother to her newborn.

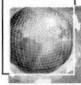

In the United States, it is estimated that there are between 500,000 and 1.5 million chronic HBV carriers, and 200,000 to 300,000 persons are newly infected with HBV annually. Of these new cases, only one-fourth are clinically recognized because of jaundice. Fulminant hepatitis B results in 250 to 300 deaths a year. Before the advent of routine screening of blood for HBsAg, chronic HBV carriers posed a public health hazard as a source of post-transfusion hepatitis. This threat has been largely eliminated by routine screening for HBsAg.

Whereas no more than 10% of adults infected with HBV become carriers, neonatal hepatitis B is, as a rule, followed by persistent infection. Males exhibit an increased tendency to become carriers. In the United States, chronic HBV carriers are particularly common among male homosexuals and drug addicts.

Humans are the only significant reservoir of HBV. Unlike hepatitis A, hepatitis B is not transmitted by the fecal–oral route, nor does it contaminate food and water supplies. *Although HBsAg is found in most secretions, infectious virus has been demonstrated only in blood, saliva, and semen.* Historically, transmission of hepatitis B was believed to be limited to direct transfer of blood products, either by transfusion or by the use of contaminated needles. However, it is now clear that most cases of hepatitis B result from transmission associated with intimate contact. The routes by which contact-transmission occurs are not entirely defined, but it seems probable that direct transfer of the virus through breaks in the skin or mucous membranes is most common. In this respect anal sexual contact is an important mode of transmission.

Synthetic vaccines for hepatitis B, composed of recombinant HbsAg or its immunogenic epitopes, are highly effective and confer lifelong immunity. In some regions where hepatitis B is endemic, its use has significantly reduced the prevalence of the disease. It is now routine in the United States to administer the vaccine to infants.

PATHOGENESIS: HBV is not directly cytopathic, as reflected in the fact that asymptomatic chronic carriers of the virus maintain a large burden of infectious virus in the liver for years without functional or biochemical evidence of liver cell injury. Cytotoxic ($CD8^+$) T lymphocytes (CTLs) directed against multiple HBV epitopes are the major mediators of the destruction of hepatocytes and consequent clinical liver disease. In conjunction with human leukocyte antigen (HLA) class I molecules, the target viral antigens are expressed on the surface of infected hepatocytes. In that location, they are recognized by $CD8^+$ CTLs, which in turn kill the infected hepatocytes.

The infectivity of blood from patients with chronic hepatitis B tends to decline with the duration of the disease. This is due in large measure to a decline in episomal (extrachromosomal) replication of infectious virions. Although the intact viral genome is not integrated into the host DNA, genomic fragments are progressively integrated, after which they produce a variety of viral antigens. Thus, despite declining infectivity of the blood, chronic hepatitis tends to persist.

CLINICAL FEATURES: There are three well-recognized clinical courses associated with HBV infection (Fig. 14-22):

- Acute hepatitis
- Fulminant hepatitis
- Chronic hepatitis

ACUTE HEPATITIS B: Most patients have acute, self-limited hepatitis similar to that produced by HAV, in which complete recovery and lifelong immunity are the rule. The symptoms of hepatitis B are, for the most part, also similar to those of hepatitis A, although acute hepatitis B tends to be somewhat more severe. In addition, the incubation period is considerably longer. Typically, symptoms do not appear until 2 to 3 months after exposure, but incubation periods of less than 6 weeks and as long as 6 months are occasionally encountered. As in hepatitis A, many cases, including virtually all infections in infants and children, are anicteric and, therefore, not clinically apparent.

HBsAg, the first marker to appear in the serum of patients with acute hepatitis B, is detected 1 week to 2 months after exposure (see Fig. 14-22). It disappears from the blood during the convalescent phase in patients who recover rapidly from the acute hepatitis. Simultaneously with, or shortly after, the disappearance of HBsAg, antibody to HBsAg (anti-HBs) is found in the blood. Its appearance heralds complete recovery, and its presence provides lifelong immunity.

HBcAg (core antigen) does not circulate in the serum of persons with acute hepatitis B, but antibody to HBcAg (anti-HBc) appears shortly after HBsAg. HBcAg does not clear the virus or protect against reinfection, although it is a marker of a previous HBV infection.

HBeAg, the second circulating antigen to appear in hepatitis B, is seen before the onset of clinical disease and after the appearance of HBsAg. It generally disappears within about 2 weeks, while HBsAg is still present. *The presence of HBeAg in the serum correlates with a period of intense viral replication and, hence, maximal infectivity of the patient.* Anti-HBe appears shortly after the disappearance of the antigen and is detectable for up to 2 or more years after resolution of the hepatitis. A minor subset of patients who seroconvert to anti-HBe antibody and lose serum HBeAg have persistent HBV replication. The HBV virus in these cases are replication-competent but are unable to produce HbeAg owing to mutations either in the precore region ('precore mutants') or the basic core promoter region of the HBV genome. Hepatitis is particularly severe in patients infected with precore HBV mutants, and progression to cirrhosis and hepatocellular carcinoma is accelerated in comparison to wild-type virus infection.

FULMINANT HEPATITIS B: More often than hepatitis A, but still only rarely, acute hepatitis B pursues a fulminant course, characterized by massive liver cell necrosis, hepatic failure, and a high mortality.

CHRONIC HEPATITIS B: Chronic hepatitis refers to the presence of necrosis and inflammation in the liver for more than 6 months. In 5% to 10% of patients with hepatitis B, HBs antigenemia does not resolve, in which case the infection persists, and the disease progresses to chronic hepatitis B. For reasons unknown, 90% of patients with chronic hepatitis B are male.

Patients with chronic hepatitis B do not have detectable anti-HBs in the blood. Some chronic HBV carriers manifest circulating HBsAg–anti-HBs complexes; although the patients produce antibody, the level is inadequate to clear the virus from the circulation. These immune complexes cause a variety of **extrahepatic** ailments, including a serum sickness-like syndrome (fever, rash, urticaria, acute arthritis), polyarteritis, glomerulonephritis, and cryoglobulinemia. In fact, one third to one half of patients with polyarteritis nodosa are carriers of HBV. Some chronic carriers who were initially negative for anti-HBs eventually develop measurable antibody (often after many years), clear the virus, and are restored to full health. Others (no more than 3% of all

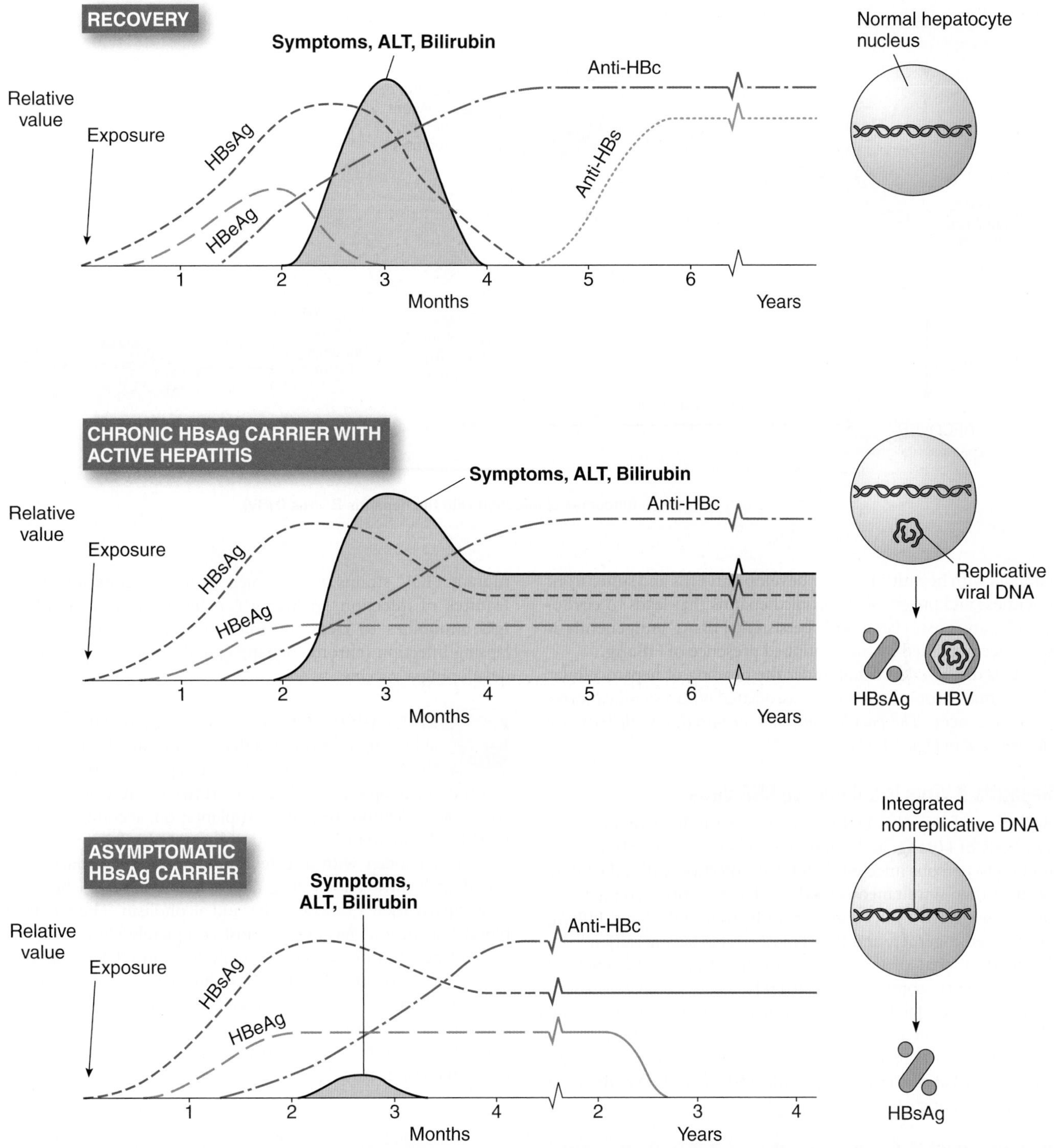

FIGURE 14-22. **Typical serologic events in three distinct outcomes of hepatitis B.** *(Top panel)* In most cases, the appearance of antibody to HBsAg (anti-HBs) ensures complete recovery. Viral DNA disappears from the nucleus of the hepatocyte. *(Middle panel)* In about 10% of cases of hepatitis B, HBs antigenemia is sustained for longer than 6 months, owing to the absence of anti-HBs. Patients in whom viral replication remains active, as evidenced by sustained high levels of HBeAg in the blood, develop active hepatitis. In such cases, the viral genome persists in the nucleus but is not integrated into host DNA. *(Lower panel)* Patients in whom active viral replication ceases or is attenuated, as reflected in the disappearance of HBeAg from the blood, become asymptomatic carriers. In these individuals, fragments of the hepatitis B virus (HBV) genome are integrated into the host DNA, but episomal DNA is absent.

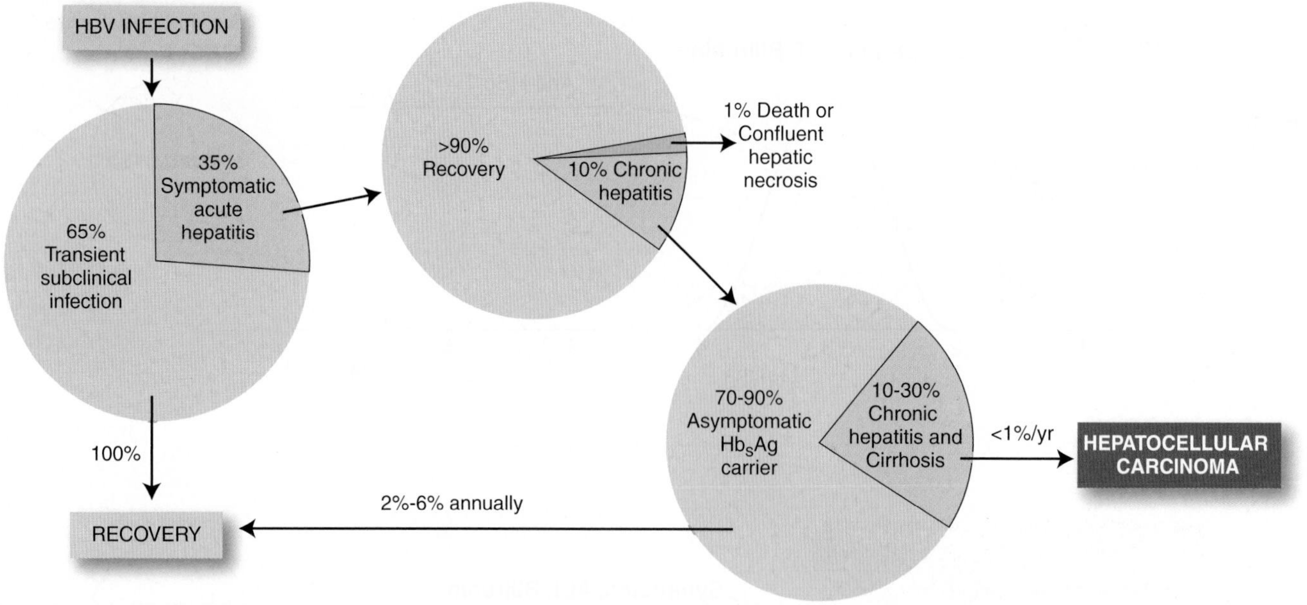

FIGURE 14-23. **Possible outcomes of infection with the hepatitis B virus (HBV).**

patients with hepatitis B) never develop anti-HBs and suffer from relentless and progressive chronic hepatitis that leads to cirrhosis. Hepatitis associated with persistent HBsAg antigenemia is often accompanied by the continued presence of HBeAg.

As is discussed in detail under the heading of hepatocellular carcinoma, chronic hepatitis B is associated with a significant risk of liver cancer. *The possible outcomes of infection with HBV are summarized in Figure 14-23.*

Hepatitis D Virus Is a Defective RNA Virus

Assembly of hepatitis D virus (HDV) in the liver requires the synthesis of HBsAg, and, therefore, infection with this agent is limited to persons infected with HBV. Infection with HDV may occur either simultaneously with HBV infection (coinfection) or following HBV infection (superinfection). HDV and HBsAg are cleared together, and the clinical course is generally no different from that of the usual acute hepatitis B. However, in some patients, coinfection with HDV leads to severe, fulminant, and often fatal hepatitis, particularly in intravenous drug abusers. *Superinfection of an HBV carrier with HDV typically increases the severity of an existing chronic hepatitis.* In fact, 70% to 80% of HBsAg carriers superinfected with HDV develop chronic hepatitis.

Hepatitis C Virus Is a Common Cause of Chronic Hepatitis and Cirrhosis

Hepatitis C virus (HCV) is classified as a flavivirus and contains a single strand of RNA. The genome consists of a single open reading frame that encodes a polyprotein of about 3000 amino acids. The transcript is cleaved into single proteins, including three structural proteins (one core and two envelope proteins) and four nonstructural proteins. The virus is genetically unstable, which leads to multiple genotypes and subtypes. Six different but related HCV genotypes are recognized, types 1, 2, and 3 being the most common (72% in the United States and Western Europe). Genotypes 2 and 3 are more responsive to antiviral therapy than is type 1. In an individual patient, many mutant HCV strains arise, which likely accounts for several features of infection, including (1) the inability of anti-HCV IgG antibodies to clear the infection; (2) persistent and relapsing infection (chronic hepatitis); and (3) lack of progress in developing a vaccine.

EPIDEMIOLOGY: The prevalence of HCV is variable, ranging from less than 1% in Canada and 1.8% in the United States, to 22% in Egypt. It is estimated that 200 million people are infected worldwide. HCV is the most common indication for liver transplantation, accounting for up to 50% of patients on the waiting list. HCV infection is transmitted by contact with infected blood and is particularly associated with intravenous drug abuse, high-risk sexual behavior (particularly male homosexuals), and alcoholism. The risk from blood transfusions has been almost completely eliminated owing to screening of the blood supply for anti-HCV antibodies. Vertical transmission of HCV from an infected mother to her newborn baby is infrequent (about 5%), although it is more common in the case of women infected with human immunodeficiency virus (HIV). A minority of cases occur in the absence of known risk factors.

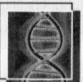

PATHOGENESIS: HCV is not directly cytopathic, as evidenced by the fact that many chronic carriers of the virus often have no evidence of liver cell injury. Despite active humoral and cellular immune responses directed against all viral proteins, most patients display persistent viremia. Liver cell injury has been attributed to cytotoxic T cell responses to virally infected hepatocytes. The mechanisms by which HCV persists has not been clarified. In addition to mutational escape (see above), defects in HCV-specific cellular immunity have been described.

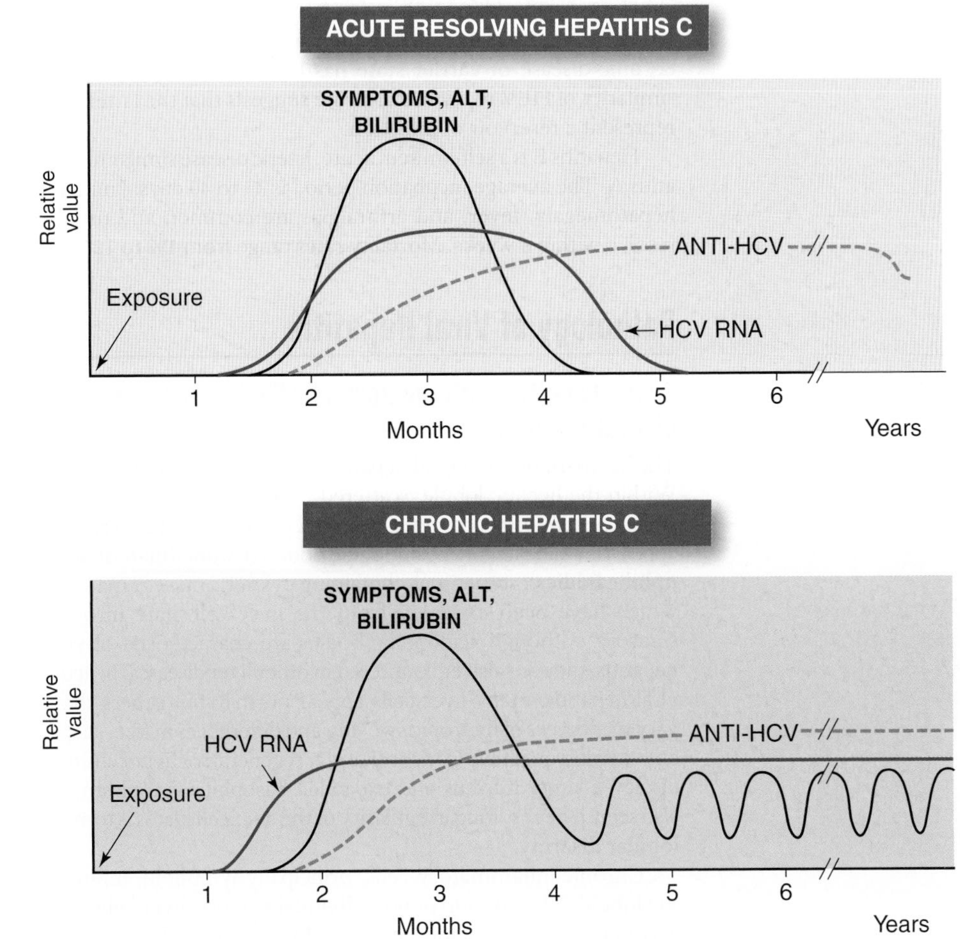

FIGURE 14-24. **Clinical course of hepatitis C.** Typical serologic events in two distinct outcomes. *(Top panel)* About 20% of the patients with acute hepatitis C have a self-limited infection that resolves in a few months. Anti-HCV appears at the end of the clinical course and persists. *(Bottom panel)* The remaining patients with hepatitis C develop chronic illness, with exacerbations and remissions of clinical symptoms. The development of anti-HCV does not affect the clinical outcome. Chronic hepatitis often eventuates in cirrhosis. ALT = alanine aminotransferase.

CLINICAL FEATURES: The incubation period of hepatitis C is similar to that of hepatitis B. Elevated serum aminotransferase activities (Fig. 14-24) are usually detected within 1 to 3 months of exposure to the virus (range, 2–26 weeks). The presence of HCV RNA in the serum can be detected by polymerase chain reaction (PCR) within 2 weeks of infection. Anti-HCV antibodies are usually detectable 7 to 8 weeks after HCV infection and persist during the chronic phase of infection. The clinical course of acute hepatitis C is surprisingly mild and is only very rarely complicated by fulminant hepatitis. In fact, only 10% of patients become jaundiced in the acute phase.

The major consequences of infection with HCV relate to chronic disease (Fig. 14-25). Despite complete recovery from clinical and biochemical acute liver disease, the probability of persistent HCV infection and chronic hepatitis is at least 80% and may be higher. Moreover, chronic hepatitis ensues in 50% to 70% of infected persons. Clinical morbidity in most patients remains mild for at least 10 years, and in many cases for 20 or more years. Importantly, some 20% of patients with chronic hepatitis C eventually develop cirrhosis. *In patients with well-established cirrhosis, up to 5% a year develop primary hepatocellular carcinoma.*

Liver disease in patients with chronic HCV infection tends to be more severe in the face of concurrent hepatitis B, alcoholic liver disease, hemochromatosis, and α_1-antitrypsin deficiency. Interestingly, a quarter of patients with advanced alcoholic liver disease have antibodies to HCV, although the rates vary in different geographical areas. Alcohol consumption has also been shown to worsen the course of chronic hepatitis C. The relationship is unexplained, and the possibility that HCV actually accounts for a proportion of cases otherwise classified as alcoholic cirrhosis is intriguing. Chronic HCV infection is also an important risk factor for the development of hepatocellular carcinoma, a topic discussed below.

Extrahepatic manifestations of hepatitis C are well recognized. Chronic HCV infection has been associated with essential mixed cryoglobulinemia, membranoproliferative glomerulonephritis, porphyria cutanea tarda, and sicca syndrome. A higher incidence of lymphoma has also been described in patients with chronic hepatitis C.

Treatment with α-interferon and antiviral agents has been beneficial in many patients with chronic hepatitis C.

Table 14-3 compares the major features of the common forms of viral hepatitis.

Hepatitis E Virus Is a Major Cause of Epidemics of Hepatitis in Underdeveloped Countries

Hepatitis E virus (HEV) is an enteric RNA virus transmitted by the fecal–oral route. It accounts for more than half of cases of acute viral hepatitis in young to middle-aged persons in poor regions of the world. Large outbreaks have been reported in India, Nepal, Burma, Pakistan, the former Soviet Union, Africa, and Mexico. Most of these epidemics have followed heavy rains in areas with inadequate sewage disposal. Similar to hepatitis A, clinical illness from hepatitis E is far more common in adults than in children, suggesting that infection in the latter is often

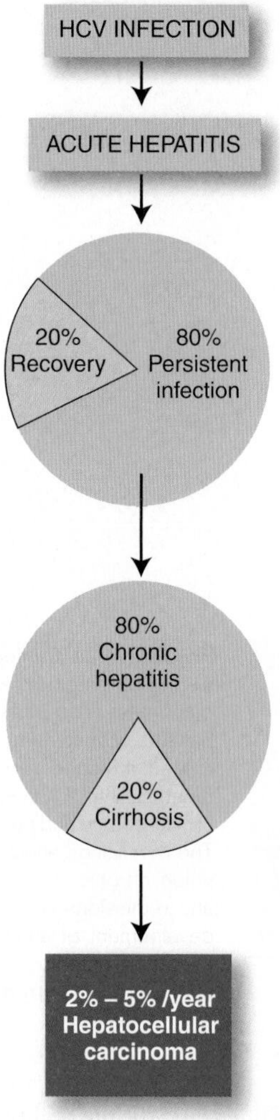

FIGURE 14-25. **Possible outcomes of infection with the hepatitis C virus (HCV).**

subclinical. The disease is especially dangerous in pregnant women, with mortality rates as high as 20% to 40% reported. No chronic disease or carrier state has been identified. The close similarity of HEV to a virus in swine suggests that the latter may represent a reservoir of infection.

Hepatitis E is a self-limited, acute, icteric disease similar to hepatitis A. The average incubation period is 35 to 40 days. Jaundice, hepatomegaly, fever, and arthralgias are common and usually resolve within 6 weeks. Mortality rates range from 1% to 12%.

Pathology of Viral Hepatitis

Acute Hepatitis Is Morphologically Similar in All Forms of Viral Hepatitis

The hallmark of acute viral hepatitis is liver cell death (Fig. 14-26). Within the hepatic lobule, scattered necrosis of single cells or of small clusters of hepatocytes is seen. A few apoptotic liver cells appear as small, deeply eosinophilic bodies (**Councilman or acidophilic bodies**), sometimes containing pyknotic nuclear material, which have been extruded from the liver cell plate into the sinusoid. Although acidophilic bodies are characteristic of viral hepatitis, they are also encountered in other liver diseases. In acute viral hepatitis, many liver cells appear normal, but others show varying degrees of hydropic swelling and differences in size, shape, and staining qualities. Concomitantly, regenerative liver cells that display a larger nucleus and expanded basophilic cytoplasm are also seen. The resulting irregularity of the liver cell plates is termed **lobular disarray**.

Chronic inflammatory cells, principally lymphoid, infiltrate the lobule diffusely, surround individual necrotic liver cells, and accumulate in areas of focal necrosis. In addition to the lymphoid cells, macrophages may be prominent, and eosinophils and polymorphonuclear leukocytes are not uncommon. Characteristically, lymphoid cells infiltrate between the wall of the central vein and the liver cell plates, an appearance termed **central phlebitis**. Swelling and proliferation of the endothelial cells of

TABLE 14-3

Comparative Features of the Common Forms of Viral Hepatitis

	Hepatitis A	Hepatitis B	Hepatitis C
Genome	RNA	DNA	RNA
Incubation period	3–6 weeks	6 weeks–6 months	7–8 weeks
Transmission	Oral	Parenteral	Parenteral
Blood	No	Yes	Yes
Feces	Yes	No	No
Vertical	No	Yes	5%
Fulminant hepatic necrosis	Very rare	Yes	Rare
Chronic hepatitis	No	10%	80%
Carrier state	No	Yes	Yes
Liver cancer	No	Yes	Yes

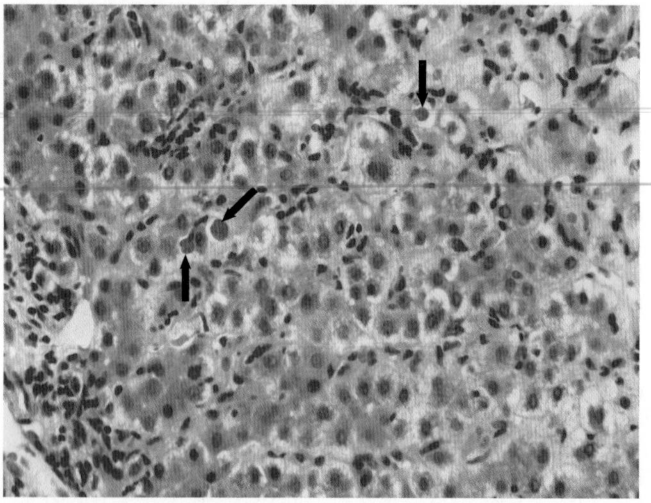

FIGURE 14-26. **Acute viral hepatitis.** A photomicrograph shows disarray of liver cell plates, swollen (ballooned) hepatocytes, and an infiltrate of lymphocytes and scattered mononuclear inflammatory cells. The remnants of necrotic hepatocytes have been extruded into the sinusoids, where they appear as acidophilic, or Councilman, bodies *(arrows)*.

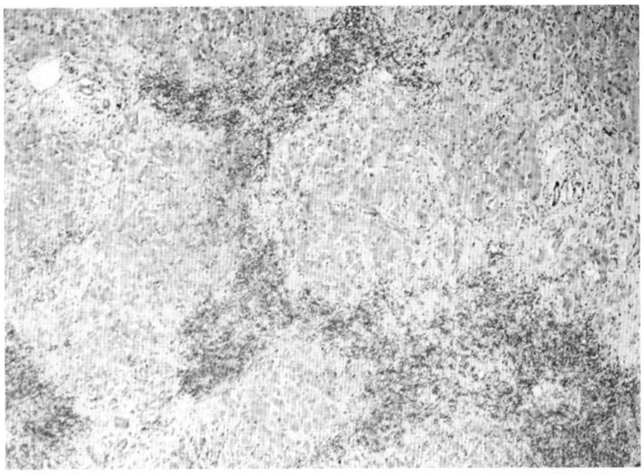

FIGURE 14-27. **Confluent hepatic necrosis.** Hemorrhagic zones of necrosis bridge adjacent portal tracts (bridging necrosis).

the central vein (**endophlebitis**) often develop. The Kupffer cells are enlarged, project into the lumen of the sinusoid, and contain lipofuscin pigment and phagocytosed debris. Cholestasis is common and when severe is termed **cholestatic hepatitis**. In this situation, many liver cells are arranged around a lumen, thereby presenting an acinar or glandular appearance. The lumen of such an "acinus" may contain a large bile plug.

Chronic inflammatory cells accumulate within the portal tracts and mirror the distribution of those in the lobule. Occasionally, aggregates of lymphoid cells within the portal tracts assume a follicular form, particularly in hepatitis C. The limiting plate of hepatocytes around the portal tracts is usually intact. The portal tracts commonly exhibit only a few proliferated bile ductules, although occasionally this phenomenon may be more conspicuous. All of the pathologic changes are gradually reversed during recovery, and the normal hepatic architecture is completely restored.

Confluent Hepatic Necrosis Affects Whole Regions of the Lobule

*The term **confluent hepatic necrosis** refers to particularly severe variants of acute viral hepatitis, which are characterized by the death of numerous hepatocytes in a geographical distribution and, in extreme cases, by the death of almost all the liver cells (massive hepatic necrosis).* The most common cause is acute hepatitis B, and only rarely does confluent hepatic necrosis result from infection with other hepatotropic viruses. Importantly, the lesions are not confined to viral hepatitis but may also be encountered after exposure to a variety of hepatotoxic agents and in autoimmune hepatitis (see below). *In contrast to the most common forms of acute viral hepatitis, in which the necrosis of hepatocytes appears to be random and patchy, confluent hepatic necrosis typically affects whole regions of the lobule.* The lesions of confluent hepatic necrosis, in order of increasing severity, are bridging necrosis, submassive necrosis, and massive necrosis.

BRIDGING NECROSIS: At the milder end of the spectrum of lesions that constitute confluent hepatic necrosis are bands of necrosis (bridging necrosis) that stretch between adjacent portal tracts, between adjacent central veins, and between portal tracts and central veins (Fig. 14-27). The death of adjacent plates of hepatocytes results in the collapse of the collagenous stroma to form bands of connective tissue, best visualized with a reticulin stain. When such bands encircle an area of liver cells, a nodular pattern, similar to that seen in cirrhosis, may be apparent.

SUBMASSIVE CONFLUENT NECROSIS: This form of acute hepatitis defines an even more severe injury involving necrosis of entire lobules or groups of adjacent lobules. Clinically, these patients manifest severe hepatitis, which may rapidly proceed to hepatic failure, in which case the disease is classed clinically as **fulminant hepatitis**.

MASSIVE HEPATIC NECROSIS (ACUTE YELLOW ATROPHY): Although uncommon, massive hepatic necrosis is the most feared variant of acute viral hepatitis, because it is a form of fulminant hepatitis that is almost invariably fatal. Grossly, the liver is shrunken to as little as 500 g (one third of normal weight). The capsule is wrinkled, and the mottled, red-tan parenchyma is soft and flabby. Microscopic examination reveals that virtually all the hepatocytes are dead (Fig. 14-28), and the hepatic lobule is represented only by the collagenous framework, which in many areas has collapsed. Macrophages, erythrocytes, and necrotic debris fill the sinusoids. For unknown reasons, the massive necrosis does not elicit a vigorous inflammatory response in either the parenchyma or the portal tracts.

A

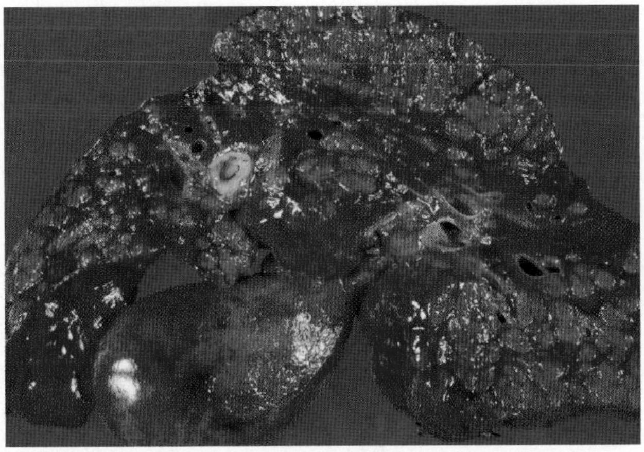

B

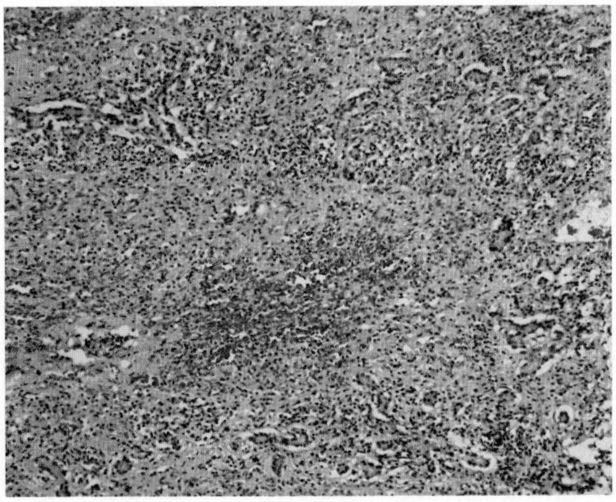

FIGURE 14-28. **Massive hepatic necrosis. A.** The liver is soft and reduced in size (note size of gallbladder) and shows a mottled, irregularly hemorrhagic cut surface. The surviving parenchyma appears as tan nodules. **B.** A photomicrograph shows the loss of most of the hepatocytes. Necrotic lobules are hemorrhagic, and the reticulin framework has collapsed. A sparse chronic inflammatory infiltrate is present within the lobules and portal tracts. The portal tracts are expanded and contain proliferated bile ducts.

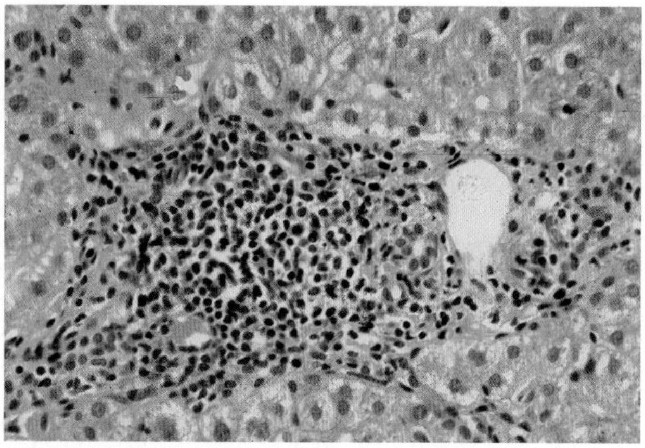

FIGURE 14-29. **Mild chronic hepatitis.** A photomicrograph shows a portal tract infiltrated by mononuclear inflammatory cells. The lobular parenchyma is intact.

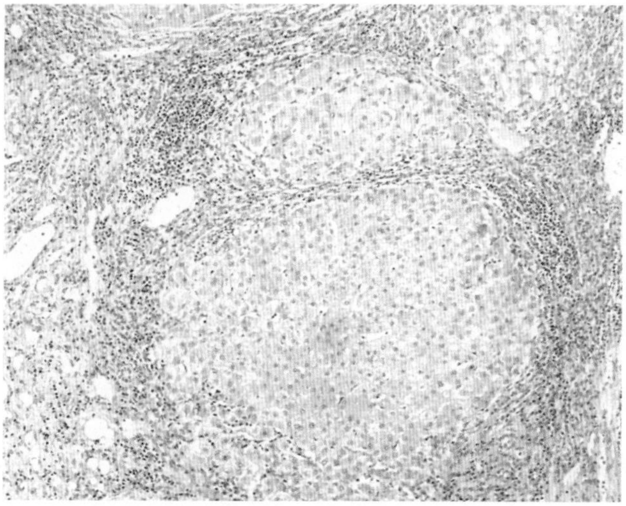

FIGURE 14-31. **Chronic hepatitis with cirrhosis.** A photomicrograph of the liver from a patient with long-standing chronic hepatitis B shows hepatocellular nodules and chronically inflamed fibrous septa.

Liver transplantation is a mainstay of therapy for severe forms of confluent hepatic necrosis.

Chronic Hepatitis Is a Complication of Hepatitis B and C, As Well As a Number of Metabolic and Immune Disorders

The morphologic spectrum of chronic hepatitis ranges from mild, portal inflammation with little or no evidence of liver cell necrosis (Fig. 14-29) to a widespread inflammatory, necrotizing, and fibrosing condition that often eventuates in cirrhosis (Fig. 14-30 and Fig.14-31).

PIECEMEAL NECROSIS: This lesion is essentially periportal and refers to focal destruction of the limiting plate of hepatocytes. A periportal chronic inflammatory infiltrate creates an irregular border between the portal tracts and the lobular parenchyma (see Fig. 14-30).

PORTAL TRACT LESIONS: Chronic hepatitis is characterized by variable infiltration of the portal tracts by lymphocytes, plasma cells, and macrophages (see Fig. 14-29 and Fig. 14-30).

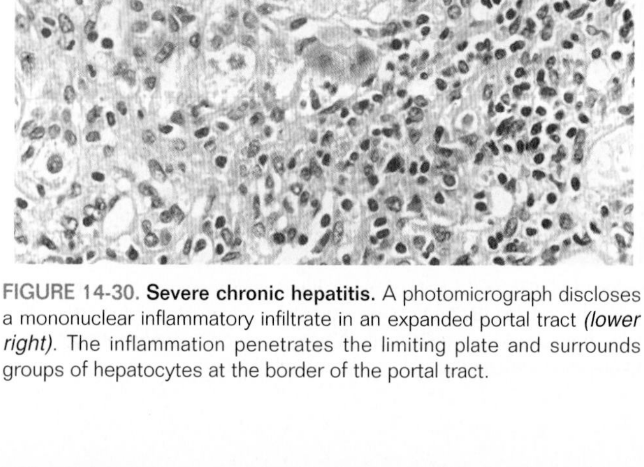

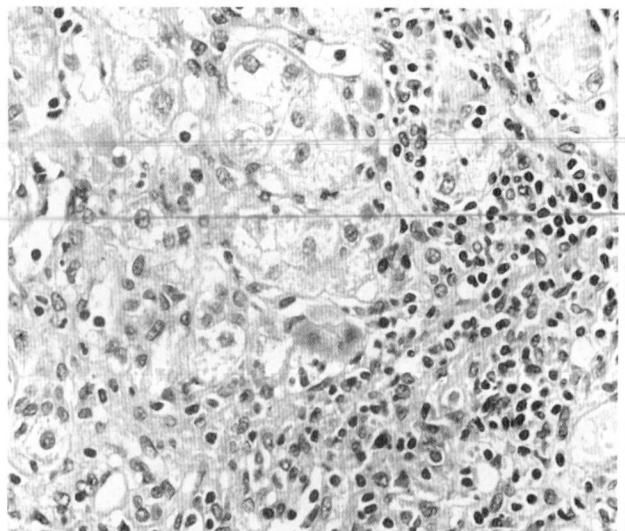

FIGURE 14-30. **Severe chronic hepatitis.** A photomicrograph discloses a mononuclear inflammatory infiltrate in an expanded portal tract *(lower right)*. The inflammation penetrates the limiting plate and surrounds groups of hepatocytes at the border of the portal tract.

The expanded portal tracts often display mild-to-severe proliferation of bile ductules, which represents a nonspecific response to chronic liver injury. In the case of chronic hepatitis C, lymphoid aggregates or follicles with reactive centers are often present.

INTRALOBULAR LESIONS: Focal necrosis and inflammation within the parenchyma are typical of chronic hepatitis. Scattered acidophilic bodies are common, and enlarged Kupffer cells are seen within the sinusoids. The liver in chronic hepatitis B often exhibits scattered hepatocytes with a large granular cytoplasm containing abundant HBsAg (**ground-glass hepatocytes**) (Fig. 14-32).

PERIPORTAL FIBROSIS: The progressive erosion of the periportal hepatocytes by piecemeal necrosis leads to the deposition of collagen, which gives the portal tract a stellate (star-shaped) appearance. With time, the fibrosis may extend to adjacent portal tracts or into the lobule itself toward the central vein, ultimately developing into cirrhosis.

Autoimmune Hepatitis

Autoimmune hepatitis is a severe type of chronic hepatitis of unknown cause that is associated with circulating autoantibodies and high levels of serum immunoglobulins. The disorder occurs predominantly among young women, but up to one third of patients are men, and the disease may appear at any age. In the United States, autoimmune hepatitis affects up to 200,000 persons and accounts for 6% of liver transplants.

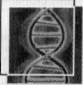

PATHOGENESIS: Two distinct types of autoimmune hepatitis have been identified.

- **Type I** autoimmune hepatitis is the most common form of the disease (80% of cases) and features antinuclear and anti-smooth muscle antibodies. Some 70% of cases occur in women younger than 40 years of age, among whom a third have other autoimmune diseases, including thyroiditis, rheumatoid arthritis, and ulcerative colitis.

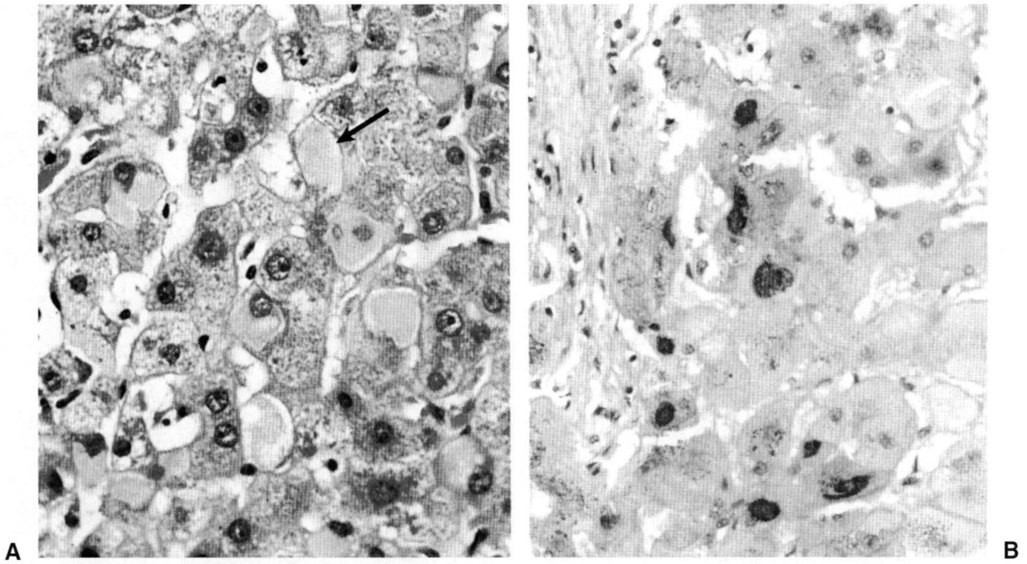

FIGURE 14-32. **"Ground-glass" hepatocytes. A.** A photomicrograph of liver from a patient with chronic hepatitis B shows scattered hepatocytes *(arrow)* with an abundant granular cytoplasm containing HBsAg. **B.** The same specimen has been stained for HBsAg by the immunoperoxidase method. The abundant cytoplasmic HBsAg appears brown.

Importantly, a quarter of patients with type I autoimmune hepatitis present with cirrhosis, indicating that the disease usually has a prolonged asymptomatic course. Antibodies against numerous cytosolic enzymes have been described, but the asialoglycoprotein receptor on the hepatocyte surface is the leading candidate target for antibody-dependent cell-mediated cytotoxicity. Susceptibility to type I autoimmune hepatitis resides mainly within the HLA-*DRB1* gene. A minority of patients present with a poorly characterized "overlap syndrome" which features mixed clinical and histologic features of autoimmune hepatitis and either primary biliary cirrhosis or primary sclerosing cholangitis.

- **Type II** autoimmune hepatitis occurs principally in children aged 2 to 14 years and is recognized by the presence of antibody to liver and kidney microsomes (anti-LKM). However, the target autoantigen is a P450-type drug-metabolizing enzyme (CYP 2D6). These patients often suffer from other autoimmune diseases, especially type I diabetes and thyroiditis. The genetic background for this type of autoimmune hepatitis is less well defined than is that for type I.

PATHOLOGY: In general, the histologic appearance of autoimmune hepatitis resembles that of chronic viral hepatitis, although lobular inflammation and necrosis tends to be more pronounced. An inflammatory infiltrate rich in plasma cells is an important diagnostic feature.

CLINICAL FEATURES: In most patients, the disease begins insidiously. Eventually, serum aminotransferase levels become conspicuously elevated, and liver failure may ensue. A fulminant presentation is occasionally observed. In many patients, autoimmune hepatitis progresses to cirrhosis. Pronounced hyperglobulinemia is characteristic of the disease.

In contrast to viral hepatitis, autoimmune hepatitis usually responds to therapy with corticosteroids, particularly when combined with immunosuppressive drugs. Liver transplantation is an option for patients whose disease progresses to end-stage cirrhosis. Recurrence of autoimmune hepatitis occurs in up to 20% of patients after liver transplantation.

Alcoholic Liver Disease

The deleterious effects of excess alcohol (ethanol, ethyl alcohol) consumption have been recognized since the early days of recorded history. The prophet Isaiah warned, "Woe to him that is mighty to drink wine." Although early investigators confused alcoholic liver injury with the effects of malnutrition, ethanol per se is today recognized as a hepatotoxin that acts both directly and indirectly.

EPIDEMIOLOGY: *The prevalence of cirrhosis is highest in those countries with the highest per capita consumption of alcohol.* This relationship is valid regardless of the specific nature of the preferred beverage (e.g., wine in France, beer in Australia, and spirits in Scandinavia). Although only a minority of chronic alcoholics develop cirrhosis, a dose–response relationship between the lifetime dose of alcohol (duration of exposure and the daily amount of alcohol consumed) and the appearance of cirrhosis has been established.

It is estimated that some 10% of the adult male population in the United States abuse alcohol, and this figure is considerably higher in many other countries. *About 15% of alcoholics can be expected to develop cirrhosis, and many of these persons die in hepatic failure or from the extrahepatic complications of cirrhosis.* In fact, in many urban areas of the United States with high alcoholism rates, cirrhosis of the liver is the third or fourth leading cause of death in men younger than 45 years of age.

The amount of alcohol required to produce chronic liver disease varies widely, depending on body size, age, sex, and ethnicity, but the lower range seems to be about 80 g/day (8 ounces

[240 mL] of 86 proof [43%] whiskey, two bottles of wine, or six 12-ounce bottles of beer). In general, more than 10 years of alcoholism are required to produce cirrhosis, although a few cirrhotic patients give shorter histories of heavy alcohol use.

The epidemiology of alcoholic liver disease has recently been complicated by the discovery of its association with hepatotropic viruses. The prevalence of serum HBV markers is two- to fourfold higher in alcoholics than in corresponding control populations. The prevalence of anti-HCV antibodies is up to 10% among alcoholics and is considerably higher among alcoholics with chronic liver disease. The significance of these data with respect to the epidemiology of alcoholic cirrhosis deserves further study.

The Metabolism of Ethanol Occurs Primarily in the Liver

Ethanol is rapidly absorbed from the stomach and is eventually distributed in body water space. Almost all of the ethanol consumed is metabolized by the liver to acetaldehyde and acetate. Between 5% and 10% is excreted unchanged, principally in the urine and expired breath. The principal route of ethanol oxidation in the liver is through cytosolic **alcohol dehydrogenase** (**ADH**). A minor metabolic pathway is a **microsomal ethanol-oxidizing system** in the smooth endoplasmic reticulum, which is a mixed-function oxidase. In contrast to most drugs, the clearance of alcohol from the body is linear—that is, a fixed quantity is metabolized per unit time. A rough guide for the average man is 7 to 10 g of alcohol eliminated per hour. However, chronic alcoholics metabolize ethanol at a substantially higher rate, provided that they do not suffer from active liver disease.

A Spectrum of Liver Diseases Is Produced by Alcohol Consumption

Alcoholic liver disease spans three major morphologic and clinical entities: **fatty liver, acute alcoholic hepatitis,** and **cirrhosis**. Although these lesions usually occur sequentially, they may coexist in any combination and may actually be independent entities.

Fatty Liver and Associated Lesions

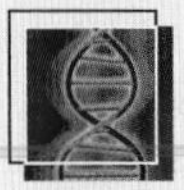

PATHOGENESIS: Virtually all chronic alcoholics accumulate fat in hepatocytes (**steatosis**). The pathogenesis of fatty liver is not precisely understood, and the relative contributions of different pathways may vary, depending on the amount of alcohol consumed, dietary lipid content, body stores of fat, hormonal status, and other variables. Nevertheless, the accumulation of fat clearly depends on the intake of ethanol, since it is fully and rapidly reversible on discontinuation of alcohol ingestion.

Dietary fat, in the form of chylomicrons and free fatty acids, is transported to the liver, where it is taken up by the hepatocytes. Triglycerides are then hydrolyzed to free fatty acids. These, in turn, undergo β-oxidation in the mitochondria or are converted to triglycerides in the endoplasmic reticulum. The newly synthesized triglycerides are secreted in the form of lipoproteins or are retained for storage.

Most of the fat deposited in the liver after chronic alcohol consumption is derived from the diet. Ethanol increases lipolysis and thus the delivery of free fatty acids to the liver. Within the hepatocyte, ethanol (1) increases fatty acid synthesis, (2) decreases mitochondrial oxidation of fatty acids, (3) increases the production of triglycerides, and (4) impairs the release of lipoproteins. Collectively, these metabolic consequences produce a fatty liver.

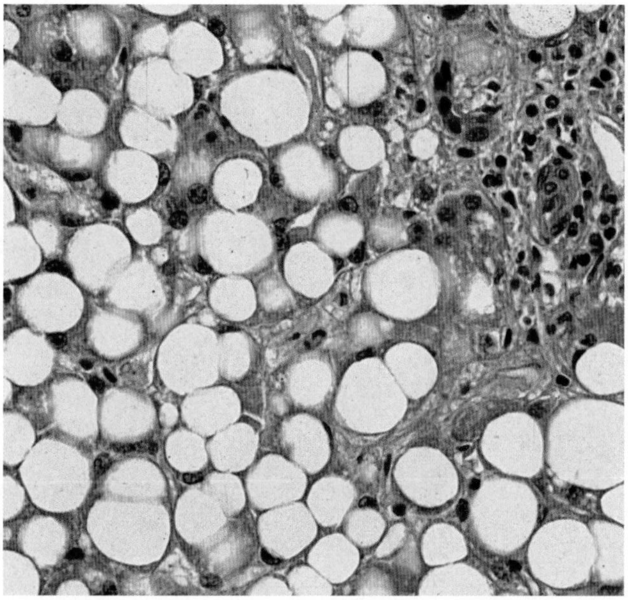

FIGURE 14-33. **Alcoholic fatty liver.** A photomicrograph shows the cytoplasm of almost all the hepatocytes distended by fat that displaces the nucleus to the periphery.

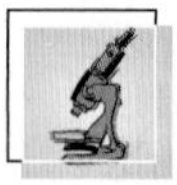

PATHOLOGY: In the alcoholic, the liver becomes yellow and enlarged, sometimes massively, to as much as three times the normal weight. The increased weight does not reflect fat accumulation alone, since protein and water content also increase. Microscopically, the extent of visible fat accumulation varies from minute droplets scattered in the cytoplasm of a few hepatocytes to distention of the entire cytoplasm of most cells by coalesced droplets (Fig. 14-33). In the latter situation, the liver cell is scarcely recognizable as such and bears a resemblance to an adipocyte, the cytoplasm being represented by a distended clear area, and the nucleus flattened and displaced to the periphery of the cell.

The ultrastructural appearance of the hepatocyte in alcohol-induced fatty liver reflects the cytotoxicity of ethanol rather than an effect of the fat per se. The mitochondria are enlarged, with occasional bizarre giant forms. The smooth endoplasmic reticulum exhibits hyperplasia resembling that produced by other inducers of microsomal drug-metabolizing enzymes.

The ultrastructural changes in mitochondria and endo-lplasmic reticulum produced by chronic ethanol ingestion are paralleled by functional alterations. Hepatic mitochondria show decreased rates of substrate oxidation (e.g., of fatty acids) and impaired formation of adenosine triphosphate (ATP). Hyperplasia of the smooth endoplasmic reticulum is accompanied by an increase in the activity of the cytochrome P450-dependent mixed-function oxidases. Not only is the microsomal ethanol-oxidizing system induced, but the metabolism of a variety of drugs is also enhanced. *The increased microsomal function also augments the metabolism of hepatic toxins, thereby exaggerating the danger produced by agents such as acetaminophen.* In contrast to chronic alcohol consumption, which promotes microsomal functions, the presence of ethanol after acute alcohol ingestion inhibits the activity of mixed-function oxidases and acutely reduces the rate of clearance of drugs from the body.

CLINICAL FEATURES: Patients with uncomplicated alcoholic fatty liver have surprisingly few symptoms of liver disease. Despite the striking morphologic change in the liver, alcoholic fatty liver is a fully reversible lesion and does not by itself progress to more severe disease, notably cirrhosis. A fatty liver, although characteristic of alcoholism, is not restricted to that condition but is also noted in nonalcoholic fatty liver disease (see below), in kwashiorkor, and following prolonged administration of corticosteroids.

Alcoholic Hepatitis

Alcoholic hepatitis is an acute necrotizing lesion characterized by (1) necrosis of hepatocytes, predominantly in the central zone; (2) cytoplasmic hyaline inclusions within hepatocytes; (3) a neutrophilic inflammatory response, and (4) perivenular fibrosis (Fig. 14-34). The pathogenesis of alcoholic hepatitis is mysterious. Alcoholics may have mild fatty liver for many years and, without any change in drinking habits, suddenly develop acute alcoholic hepatitis.

PATHOLOGY: In the typical case of acute alcoholic hepatitis, the hepatic architecture is basically intact, with a normal relation of portal tracts to central venules. The hepatocytes show variable hydropic swelling, which gives them a heterogeneous appearance. Isolated necrotic liver cells or clusters of them exhibit pyknotic nuclei and karyorrhexis. Scattered hepatocytes contain **Mallory bodies (alcoholic hyalin)** (see Fig. 14-34). These cytoplasmic inclusions, which are more common in visibly damaged, swollen hepatocytes, are visualized as irregular skeins of eosinophilic material or as solid eosinophilic masses, often in a perinuclear location. Ultrastructurally, they are composed of aggregates of intermediate (cytokeratin) filaments. The damaged, ballooned hepatocytes, particularly those containing Mallory bodies, are surrounded by neutrophils, although a more diffuse, intralobular inflammatory infiltrate is also present. Cholestasis, varying from mild to severe, is present in as many as one third of cases. Alcoholic hepatitis is usually superimposed on an existing fatty liver, although there is no evidence that fat accumulation predisposes or contributes to the development of alcoholic hepatitis.

A

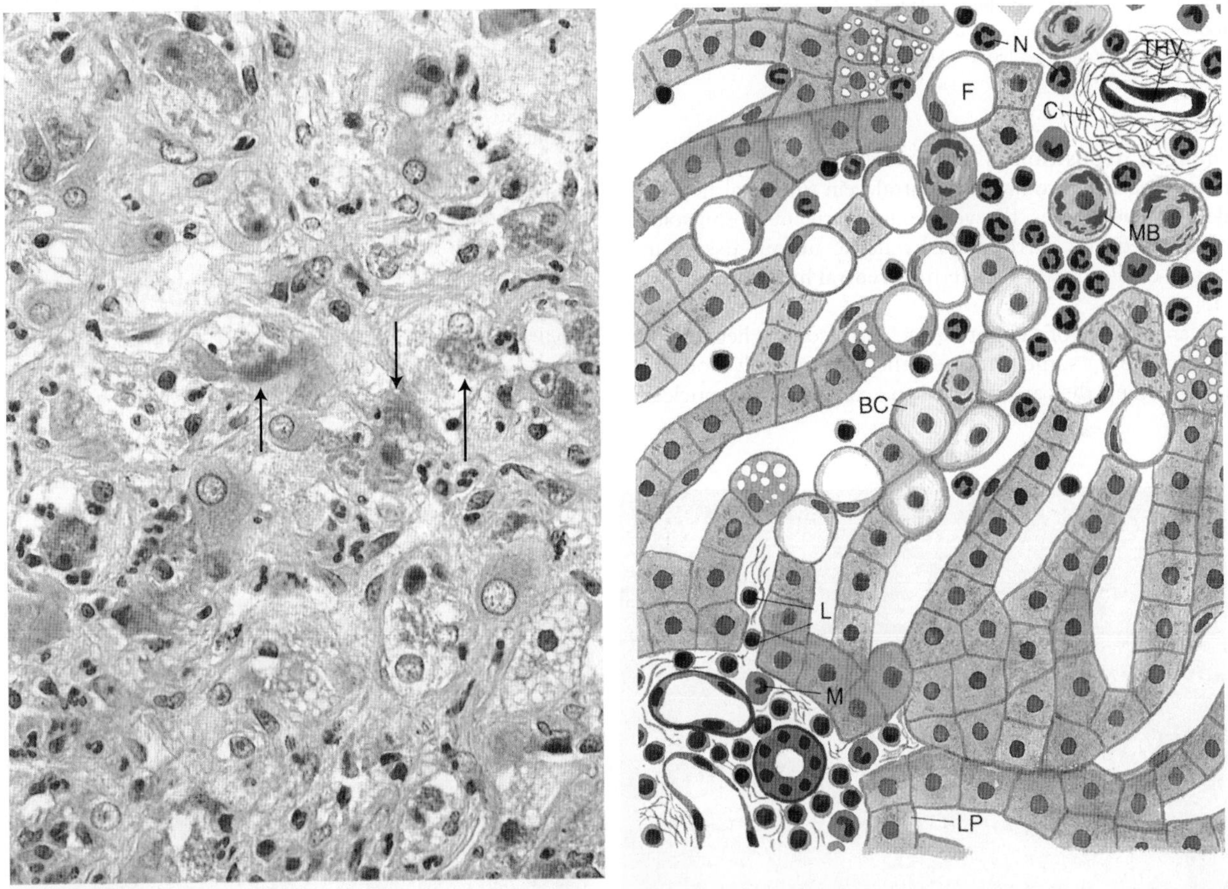

B

FIGURE 14-34. **Alcoholic hepatitis. A**. A photomicrograph shows necrosis and degeneration of hepatocytes; Mallory bodies (eosinophilic inclusions) in the cytoplasm of injured hepatocytes *(arrows)*; and infiltration by neutrophils. **B**. Schematic representation of the major pathologic features of alcoholic hepatitis. The lesions are predominantly centrilobular and include necrosis and loss of hepatocytes, ballooned cells *(BC)*, and Mallory bodies *(MB)* in the cytoplasm of damaged hepatocytes. The inflammatory infiltrate consists predominantly of neutrophils *(N)*, although a few lymphocytes *(L)* and macrophages *(M)* are also present. The central vein, or terminal hepatic venule *(THV)*, is encased in connective tissue *(C)* (central sclerosis). Fat-laden hepatocytes *(F)* are evident in the lobule. The portal tract displays moderate chronic inflammation, and the limiting plate *(LP)* is focally breached.

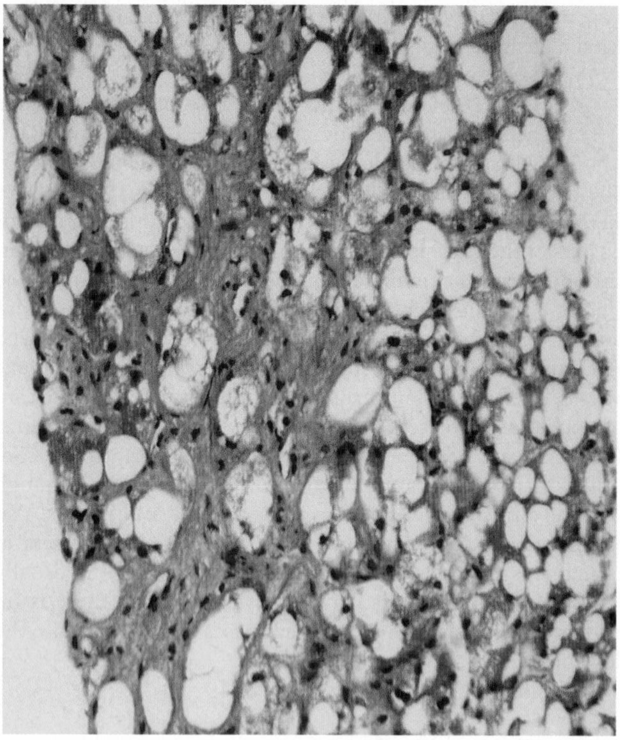

FIGURE 14-35. **Central hyaline sclerosis.** This photomicrograph (trichrome stain) from the liver of a patient with alcoholic liver disease shows the central terminal venule to be obliterated by fibrous tissue (blue).

Collagen deposition is a constant feature of alcoholic hepatitis, especially around the central vein (terminal hepatic venule). In severe cases, the venule and perivenular sinusoids are obliterated and surrounded by dense fibrous tissue, in which case the lesion has been termed **central hyaline sclerosis** (Fig. 14-35).

The appearance of the portal tracts in alcoholic hepatitis is highly variable. In some instances, they are virtually normal, whereas in others they are enlarged and contain a mononuclear infiltrate and proliferated bile ductules. The altered portal tracts often display spurs of fibrous tissue that penetrate the lobules.

CLINICAL FEATURES: Alcoholic hepatitis features malaise and anorexia, fever, right upper quadrant abdominal pain, and jaundice. A mild leukocytosis is common. The serum aminotransferase activities, particularly that of aspartate aminotransferase, are moderately elevated, but not to the levels often noted in viral hepatitis. Serum alkaline phosphatase activity is usually increased. In severe cases, the prothrombin time may be prolonged, a situation associated with an ominous prognosis.

The prognosis in patients with alcoholic hepatitis correlates with the severity of the liver cell injury. In some patients, the disease rapidly progresses to hepatic failure and death. The mortality in the acute stage of alcoholic hepatitis is about 10%. Among those who abstain from alcohol after recovery from acute alcoholic hepatitis, most recover. However, of those who continue to drink, up to 70% may ultimately develop cirrhosis. No specific treatment for acute alcoholic hepatitis is available, although corticosteroids and dietary supplementation may improve short-term survival.

Alcoholic Cirrhosis

In about 15% of alcoholics, hepatocellular necrosis, fibrosis, and regeneration eventually lead to the formation of fibrous septa surrounding hepatocellular nodules, the two features that define cirrhosis (Fig. 14-36). The other lesions of alcoholic liver disease—namely, fatty liver and acute or persistent alcoholic hepatitis—are often seen in conjunction with cirrhosis. The prognosis in cases of established alcoholic cirrhosis is considerably better in those who abstain from alcohol abuse. Nevertheless, many patients progress to end-stage liver disease, and alcoholic liver disease is a common indication for liver transplantation.

Nonalcoholic Fatty Liver Disease

Nonalcoholic fatty liver disease (NAFLD) is so named because of its close resemblance to alcoholic liver disease. It represents a spectrum of liver injuries that initially display simple steatosis, with or without

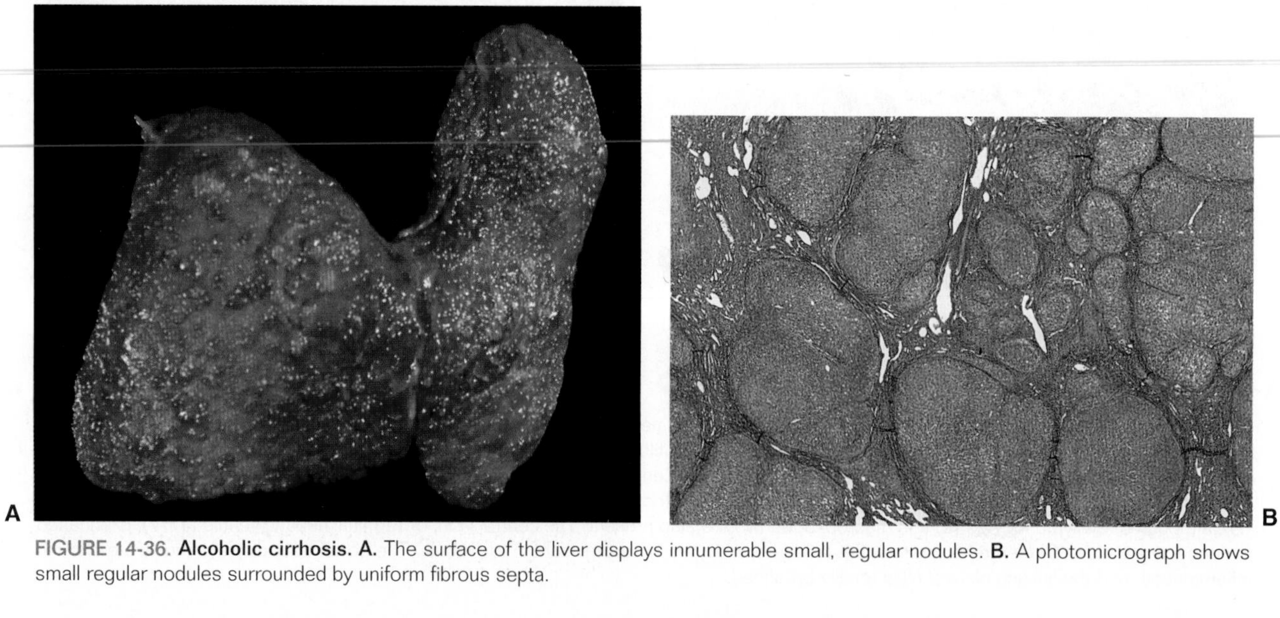

FIGURE 14-36. **Alcoholic cirrhosis. A.** The surface of the liver displays innumerable small, regular nodules. **B.** A photomicrograph shows small regular nodules surrounded by uniform fibrous septa.

associated hepatitis (nonalcoholic steatohepatitis [NASH]), and progress to bridging fibrosis and cirrhosis. Risk factors for NAFLD include obesity, type 2 diabetes mellitus, and hyperlipidemia. Importantly, approximately half of persons with both severe obesity and diabetes have NASH, and as many as a fifth of this population seems to develop cirrhosis.

Histologic features of NAFLD overlap with alcoholic liver disease and include steatosis, lobular and portal inflammation, hepatocyte necrosis, Mallory's hyaline, and fibrosis. As in alcoholic liver disease, centrilobular fibrosis is commonly observed. With the development of cirrhosis, steatosis often disappears. *Thus, NAFLD is the likely cause of many cases of so-called cryptogenic cirrhosis.* The pathogenesis of NAFLD is obscure, although insulin resistance, increased hepatic mitochondrial oxidation of free fatty acids, increased oxidative stress, and lipid peroxidation have been proposed as etiologic factors.

Progression to cirrhosis in NAFLD is often insidious, and many patients remain asymptomatic, with only moderate increases in serum liver enzymes. Weight loss tends to improve NAFLD, but no drug therapy is effective.

Primary Biliary Cirrhosis

Primary biliary cirrhosis (PBC) is a chronic progressive cholestatic liver disease characterized by destruction of the intrahepatic bile ducts (nonsuppurative destructive cholangitis). The loss of bile ducts leads to impaired bile secretion, cholestasis, and hepatic damage. PBC occurs principally in middle-aged women (10:1 female predominance). The use of the term *cirrhosis* in this context is somewhat misleading, in that cirrhosis is actually a late complication of the disease.

PBC accounts for up to 2% of deaths from cirrhosis. Cases are sporadic, although several familial clusters of the disease have been reported. The prevalence in families of patients with PBC is considerably higher than that in the general population, suggesting a hereditary predisposition.

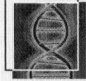

PATHOGENESIS: *PBC is associated with many immunologic abnormalities and is, therefore, widely held to be an autoimmune disease.* Most (85%) patients with primary biliary cirrhosis have at least one other disease usually classed as autoimmune, and almost half (40%) have two or more such ailments. Among these disorders are chronic thyroiditis, rheumatoid arthritis, scleroderma, Sjögren syndrome, and systemic lupus erythematosus. Molecular mimicry to certain bacteria and environmental agents has been proposed as a mechanism for the initiation of of autoimmunity in PBC, but definitive evidence is lacking.

Both humoral and cellular immunity appear to be altered. Serum immunoglobulin levels are increased, especially the level of IgM. *More than 95% of patients have circulating antimitochondrial antibodies, a finding commonly used in the diagnosis of PBC.* These autoantibodies recognize epitopes associated with the mitochondrial pyruvate dehydrogenase complex. Despite the specificity of the antimitochondrial antibodies, they have no inhibitory effect on mitochondrial function and play no known role in the pathogenesis or progression of the disease. Other circulating autoantibodies are antinuclear, antithyroid, antiplatelet, anti-acetylcholine receptor, and antiribonucleoprotein antibodies. The complement system is also chronically activated.

The cells surrounding and infiltrating the sites of bile duct damage are predominantly suppressor/cytotoxic ($CD8^+$) lymphocytes, suggesting that they mediate the destruction of the ductal epithelium.

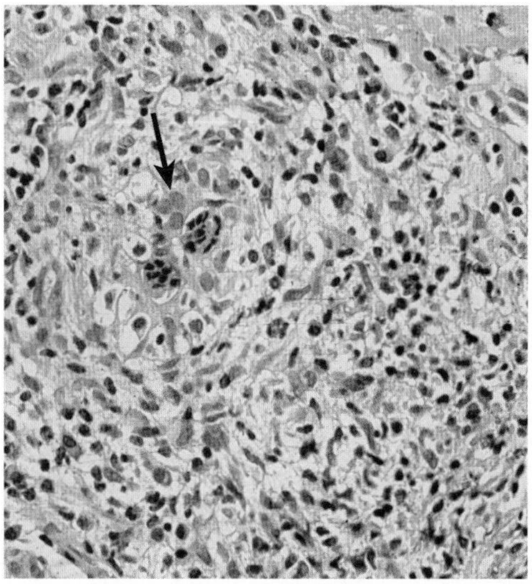

FIGURE 14-37. **Primary biliary cirrhosis (PBC), stage 1.** A photomicrograph shows a portal tract expanded by an inflammatory infiltrate consisting of lymphocytes, plasma cells, and macrophages. A bile duct *(arrow)* is damaged by the inflammation.

PATHOLOGY: The pathological stages in the evolution of PBC are characterized by ductal lesions, scarring, and cirrhosis.

STAGE I: THE DUCT LESION. Early PBC features a unique lesion, namely a **chronic destructive cholangitis** affecting the intrahepatic small and medium-sized bile ducts (Fig. 14-37). The injury to the bile ducts is segmental and therefore appears focal in histologic sections. The bile ducts are surrounded principally by lymphocytes, but plasma cells and macrophages are also seen. Characteristically, the bile duct epithelium is irregular and hyperplastic, with stratification of epithelial cells and occasional papillary ingrowths. In some portal tracts, lymphoid follicles, occasionally containing germinal centers, are conspicuous. Discrete epithelioid granulomas often occur in the portal tracts and may impinge on the bile ducts. In stage I PBC, the lobular parenchyma tends to be normal.

STAGE II: SCARRING. As a result of the destructive inflammatory process characteristic of stage I PBC, the small bile ducts virtually disappear, and scarring of medium-sized bile ducts is common. Proliferation of bile ductules within the portal tracts is usual and may be florid. Collagenous septa extend from the portal tracts into the lobular parenchyma and begin to encircle some lobules. Cholestasis, when present, may be severe and is located at the periphery of the portal tracts.

STAGE III: CIRRHOSIS. The end-stage of PBC is cirrhosis, characterized by a dark green bile-stained liver that exhibits fine nodularity. Microscopically, small bile ducts are scarce and medium-sized ducts are conspicuously fewer in number. There is little inflammation within either the fibrous septa or the parenchymal nodules.

CLINICAL FEATURES: *Women, usually between 30 and 65 years of age, constitute some 90% to 95% of those afflicted with PBC.* A substantial proportion of patients with PBC have no symptoms during the early stages of the disease. Fatigue and pruritus are the most common initial symptoms. Some remain asymptomatic and appear to have an excellent prognosis; others ultimately develop advanced cirrhosis and its complications.

In a typical case of PBC, high serum alkaline phosphatase activity is accompanied by a normal or only slightly elevated serum bilirubin level. The patient often suffers from severe pruritus. As the disease advances, most patients have a progressive increase in serum bilirubin level. Serum aminotransferase activities are only moderately elevated. The serum cholesterol level increases strikingly, and an abnormal lipoprotein (lipoprotein-X) appears that is found in many forms of chronic cholestasis. Cholesterol-laden macrophages accumulate in the subcutaneous tissues, where they appear as localized lesions termed **xanthomas.** The impairment in the excretion of bile into the intestine often leads to severe **steatorrhea,** owing to fat malabsorption. Because of associated malabsorption of vitamin D and calcium, **osteomalacia** and **osteoporosis** are important complications of PBC. About one third of patients develop gallstones. Patients who eventually develop cirrhosis die in hepatic failure or of the complications of portal hypertension.

PBC generally pursues an indolent course, which may be as long as 20 to 30 years. Liver transplantation is highly effective in end-stage PBC.

Primary Sclerosing Cholangitis

Primary sclerosing cholangitis (PSC) is a chronic cholestatic liver disease of unknown cause, in which an inflammatory and fibrosing process narrows and eventually obstructs the intrahepatic and extrahepatic bile ducts. Up to 70% of patients are men with a mean age of 40 years, and a prevalence of 14 cases per 100,000 population. Progressive biliary obstruction typically leads to persistent obstructive jaundice and eventually to secondary biliary cirrhosis.

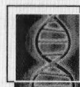

PATHOGENESIS: *Although the cause of PSC is unknown, two thirds of patients also have ulcerative colitis.* A few cases have been described in patients with Crohn disease of the colon. PSC has also been reported in association with retroperitoneal fibrosis, lymphoma, and the fibrosing variant of chronic thyroiditis (Riedel struma). In one fourth of cases, no associated disease is discerned. Increased colonic permeability to bacteria associated with ulcerative colitis has been proposed as a source of antigen in the pathogenesis of PSC. However, this hypothesis remains unproved.

Genetic and immunologic factors contribute to the pathogenesis of PSC. The disease occasionally occurs in families and shows an association with certain HLA haplotypes, including HLA B8 and DR3. Hypergammaglobulinemia is common, as are circulating antineutrophil cytoplasmic antibodies (perinuclear or P-ANCAs), immune complexes in the serum, and activation of the complement system by the classic pathway. The portal tracts exhibit an increased number of T cells.

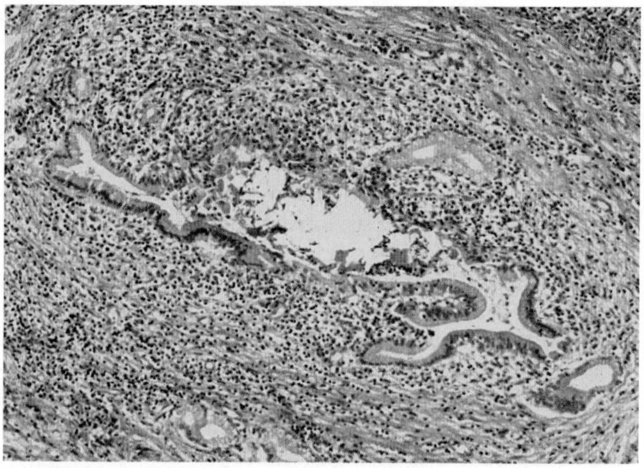

FIGURE 14-38. **Primary sclerosing cholangitis.** A photomicrograph of a liver removed for hepatic transplantation shows an edematous, fibrotic, and inflamed portal tract. Inflammatory debris is present within the lumen of the bile duct.

PATHOLOGY: The liver disease associated with PSC can be divided into three histologic stages:

- **Stage I:** The initial lesion is periductal inflammation and fibrosis in the portal tracts (Fig. 14-38).
- **Stage II:** Many bile ducts become obliterated, and fibrous septa extend into the parenchyma.
- **Stage III:** Secondary biliary cirrhosis eventually develops.

Similar inflammatory and fibrotic changes may be seen in the large intrahepatic and extrahepatic bile ducts, where they lead to obstruction of the lumen and true extrahepatic biliary obstruction. Since the disease tends to be segmental, a characteristic beaded appearance of the intrahepatic biliary tree is noted by contrast radiography. The same inflammatory process affects the wall of the gallbladder. A subset of patients with typical clinical features of PSC have normal-appearing bile ducts on cholangiography, in which case the condition is termed "small duct PSC."

CLINICAL FEATURES: PSC has a poor prognosis: the mean survival after the appearance of symptoms is 6 years. *Cholangiocarcinoma has been reported to develop in up to 20% of patients with PSC.* Liver transplantation is curative, but recurrence of PSC is not uncommon.

Iron-Overload Syndromes

A number of conditions are characterized by the excessive accumulation of iron in the body (siderosis). Iron overload is divided into two major categories based on the etiology of the increased body iron. **Hereditary hemochromatosis** (HH) is caused by a common genetic alteration in the control of the intestinal absorption of iron. **Secondary iron overload** is a condition that (1) complicates certain hematologic disorders; (2) is associated with parenteral iron overload, in which the iron is obtained from multiple blood transfusions or the parenteral administration of iron itself; or (3) is caused by an enormous dietary intake of iron.

The body of a normal man contains 3 to 4 g of iron, two thirds of which is present in hemoglobin, myoglobin, and iron-containing enzymes. The remainder is represented by storage iron, which exists in two forms, soluble ferritin and insoluble hemosiderin. **Ferritin,** the primary iron storage protein, is present in the cytoplasm of all cells and, in small amounts, in the circulation. **Hemosiderin** is a product of the degradation of ferritin but, unlike the latter, is visualized by light microscopy as golden-yellow granules that stain with the Prussian blue reaction. The liver is an important organ for the storage of iron, although a comparable amount of storage iron exists in the bone marrow.

The absorption of iron from the gastrointestinal tract is controlled by the need to maintain appropriate iron stores. Thus, in the face of iron deficiency, small-intestinal absorption of iron increases. When body stores of iron are adequate, iron absorption is relatively constant. The obligatory daily iron loss through the urine and desquamated cells of the gut and skin is about 1 mg in men. Women suffer extra losses during menstruation and pregnancy. The possible range of daily iron absorption is from less than 0.5 mg in persons with a normal iron balance to an upper limit of 4 mg in those with iron deficiency. Dietary ascorbate is important in iron absorption because ferric iron in the diet is reduced by ascorbic acid to ferrous iron, the form in which it can be absorbed by the small intestine. The absence of dietary vitamin C significantly decreases the amount of iron that can be absorbed.

Hereditary Hemochromatosis Is a Common Disorder of Iron Metabolism

HH is characterized by excessive iron absorption and the toxic accumulation of iron in parenchymal cells, particularly of the liver, heart, and pancreas. In this disease, 20 to 40 g of iron (i.e., up to 10 times the normal content) accumulates in the body. The excess iron in HH is located exclusively within the storage compartment, and thus iron stores are increased up to 50 times normal. *The clinical hallmarks of advanced HH are cirrhosis, diabetes, skin pigmentation, and cardiac failure* (Fig. 14-39). The disease is most often manifested clinically in patients age 40 to 60, and men are afflicted 10 times as often as women. This striking male predilection may be attributed to the increased loss of iron in women during the reproductive years. However, given sufficient time to absorb additional iron, postmenopausal women also seem to be at risk for the development of hemochromatosis. Since maximum daily iron absorption is about 4 mg, hemochromatosis clearly takes years to develop.

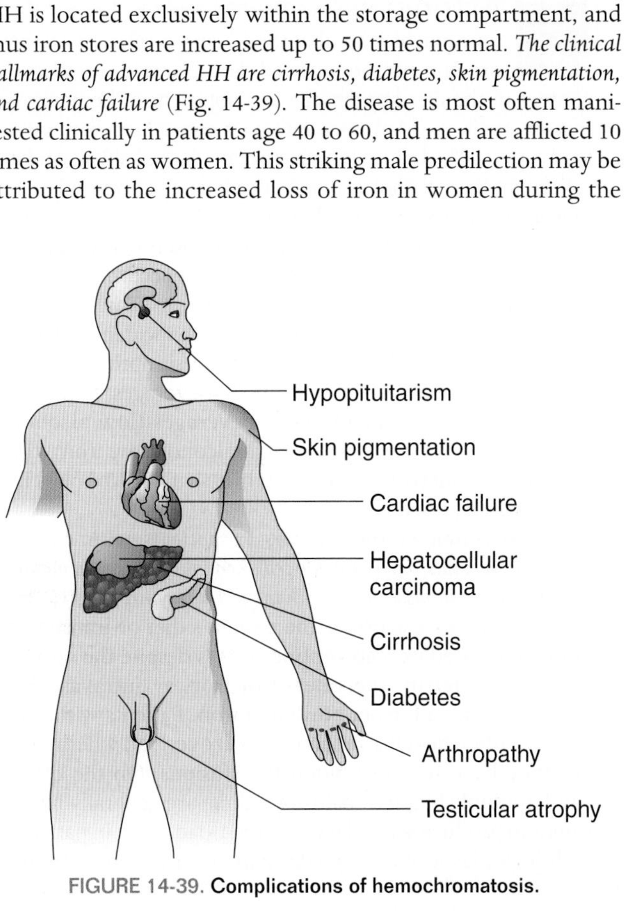

FIGURE 14-39. **Complications of hemochromatosis.**

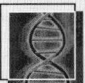

PATHOGENESIS: HH is inherited as an **autosomal recessive** disorder, in which increased intestinal absorption of iron leads to its deposition in many organs. Lesser degrees of iron overload are often found in relatives of those with the disease.

The gene involved in HH, known as *HFe,* is located on the short arm of chromosome 6 and encodes a transmembrane protein that is similar to MHC class-1 molecules. Mutations in other genes that control iron metabolism less commonly lead to iron overload and syndromes similar to hemochromatosis. The most common form of HH reflects a homozygous mutation (C282Y) in the *HFe* gene. In populations of European descent, the heterozygous frequency is about 10%, and 1 of 200 to 400 persons is homozygous. Interestingly, some persons who are homozygous for the mutation do not have the HH phenotype and do not exhibit iron overload. Thus, only 1 in 400 persons develops clinically apparent hemochromatosis.

The iron content of the body is regulated by intestinal iron absorption. A divalent metal transporter (DMT-1) on the luminal surface of mucosal cells in the duodenum binds dietary ferrous iron and transfers it to the intracellular compartment, from which it is absorbed into the circulation. In the blood, most of the iron is bound to transferrin, but a lesser amount circulates bound to another protein(s). Iron is then transferred to all cells of the body through the transferrin receptor and, to a lesser extent, by the uptake of non–transferrin-bound iron. The HFe protein associates with the transferrin receptor and influences intracellular iron delivery to the cytoplasm, although the precise effect remains controversial. *A current hypothesis holds that the mutant HFe protein, including that of the duodenal enterocytes, cannot promote iron uptake. As a result, duodenal crypt cells sense an iron deficiency and upregulate DMT-1 expression, which then* ***increases absorption of dietary iron.*** The accelerated transfer of iron across the mucosal cell leads to an increased concentration of non–transferrin-bound iron in the blood and its subsequent accumulation in parenchymal organs.

A competing hypothesis invokes a role for the novel protein **hepcidin,** which is thought to down-regulate iron release by enterocytes and macrophages. Hepcidin levels are depressed in persons with HFe-related disease and in Hfe-knockout mice. However, the relationship between HFe activity and hepcidin expression, as well as the specific role of hepcidin in HH, has not been clarified.

As noted in Chapter 1, iron is an essential factor in cellular injury mediated by activated oxygen species. The presence of excess iron in cells probably renders them more susceptible to oxidative injury.

PATHOLOGY: HH is characterized pathologically by the accumulation of very large amounts of iron in the parenchymal cells of a variety of organs and tissues.

LIVER: The liver is always affected in HH, containing more than 0.5 g iron per 100 g wet weight in the late stages. The liver is

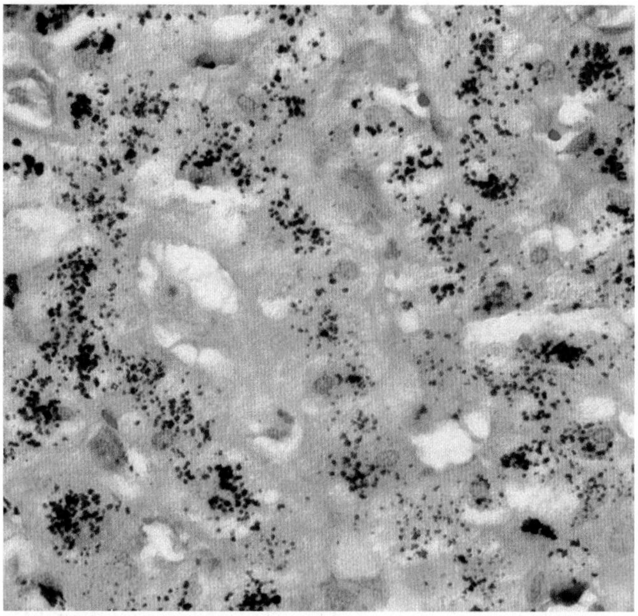

FIGURE 14-40. **Hemochromatosis.** Prussian blue stain demonstrates considerable iron in hepatocytes.

enlarged and reddish brown and exhibits micronodular cirrhosis. The hepatocytes and bile duct epithelium are filled with iron granules (Fig. 14-40). The excess cellular iron is stored predominantly in lysosomes in the ferric form. Late in the disease, many Kupffer cells contain large deposits of iron derived from the phagocytosis of necrotic hepatocytes. Within the fibrous septa, iron is conspicuous in proliferated bile ductules and macrophages. Eventually, as in micronodular cirrhosis of other causes, the pattern is transformed to that of a macronodular cirrhosis.

SKIN: The skin in patients with HH is typically pigmented, but only half of patients exhibit increased iron deposition in the skin. Most patients display increased melanin in the basal melanocytes.

PANCREAS: Diabetes is a common complication of HH, and results from the deposition of iron in the pancreas. Grossly, the organ appears rust-colored and fibrotic. Both exocrine and endocrine cells contain excess iron, and there is degeneration of acinar cells and a reduction in the number of islets of Langerhans. The combination of pigmented skin and glucose intolerance in patients with HH is referred to as **bronze diabetes.**

HEART: Congestive heart failure is a common cause of death in patients with HH. The myocardial fibers contain iron pigment, which is more extensive in the ventricles than in the atria. Necrosis of cardiac myocytes and accompanying interstitial fibrosis are common.

ENDOCRINE SYSTEM: Numerous endocrine glands are involved in HH, including the pituitary, adrenal, thyroid, and parathyroid glands. However, tissue damage is not a usual feature in these organs, except for the pituitary, in which the release of gonadotropins is impaired. As a result, testicular atrophy is seen in a fourth of male patients, even without iron deposition in the testes. The disturbance in the pituitary–gonadal axis is characterized by loss of libido and amenorrhea in women and impotence and sparse body hair in men.

JOINTS: Arthropathy, most severe in the fingers and hands, occurs in about half of patients with HH. When arthritis affects the larger joints, such as the knee, it may be severe enough to be disabling.

CLINICAL FEATURES: Symptomatic organ involvement generally starts in midlife. The liver disease in HH generally pursues an indolent and prolonged course, but among untreated patients, a fourth eventually die in hepatic coma or from gastrointestinal hemorrhage. *Hepatocellular carcinoma is a significant late complication of HH-induced cirrhosis.* In fact, among patients with cirrhosis, the 10-year cumulative probability of developing liver cancer is as high as 30%. By contrast, noncirrhotic patients with HH treated by phlebotomy are not at increased risk of hepatocellular carcinoma.

The normal value for plasma iron is 80 to 100 g/dL, and transferrin is ordinarily about one-third saturated. In patients with HH, the serum iron concentration is more than doubled, and transferrin is entirely saturated. The concentration of ferritin in the blood, which parallels the amount of storage iron, is greatly increased in HH.

The treatment of HH is based on the removal of iron from the body, most effectively by repeated phlebotomy. Weekly phlebotomies for 2 to 3 years can remove 20 to 40 g of iron, after which phlebotomies every 2 to 3 months maintain iron balance. The beneficial effect of repeated phlebotomies is impressive. In homozygotes who have neither cirrhosis nor diabetes, iron depletion results in a life expectancy identical to that of the general population. By contrast, the 10-year survival of untreated patients with HH is a mere 6%.

Secondary Iron Overload Syndromes Occur in Persons Who Do Not Carry the Gene for HH

PATHOGENESIS: Within certain limits, the amount of iron absorbed bears a relation to the amount of iron ingested. For example, a low iron content in the diet renders the development of hemochromatosis unlikely. Many patients with secondary iron overload (up to 40%) have a long history of alcohol abuse, and it is thought that alcohol may enhance both the accumulation of iron and its associated cell injury.

An interesting example of secondary hemochromatosis is presented by the well-recognized iron accumulation in blacks of sub-Saharan Africa, commonly misnamed "Bantu siderosis." These populations show a high incidence of iron overload, presumably because of the consumption of large amounts of iron-containing alcoholic beverages. With the replacement of "home-brewed" beverages (low alcohol, high iron) by Western spirits (high alcohol, low iron), the incidence of siderosis has fallen while that of alcoholic cirrhosis has increased.

Massive iron overload occurs in patients with certain hemolytic anemias, such as sickle cell anemia, thalassemia major, and other anemias associated with ineffective erythropoiesis. The source of the excess iron is the patient's diet or transfused blood. Increased iron absorption occurs despite the saturation of transferrin; the release of iron by intravascular hemolysis adds a further burden of iron. Patients with thalassemia often develop secondary iron overload whether or not they have received blood transfusions. On the other hand, multiple blood transfusions alone are generally insufficient to produce secondary iron overload, even in patients with hypoplastic anemia given many transfusions (250 mg

TABLE 14-4

Causes of Iron Overload

Increased iron absorption	
	Hereditary hemochromatosis
	Chronic liver disease
	Iron-loading anemias
	Porphyria cutanea tarda
	Congenital diseases (e.g., atransferrinemia)
	Dietary iron overload (Bantu siderosis)
	Excess medicinal iron
Parenteral iron overload	
	Multiple blood transfusions
	Injectable medicinal iron

iron/500 mL unit of blood). In these patients, iron is concentrated principally in mononuclear phagocytes, and cirrhosis is rare.

The causes of iron overload are summarized in Table 14-4.

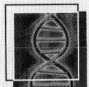

PATHOLOGY: Cirrhosis with secondary iron overload shows varying degrees of iron accumulation, but iron deposition in the liver is generally less extensive than that in HH and is often restricted to the periphery of the nodules. Transfusional and other types of siderosis are characterized by the uniform, initial deposition of iron in Kupffer cells, with eventual spillover into the hepatocytes.

Heritable Disorders Associated With Cirrhosis

Wilson Disease (Hepatolenticular Degeneration) Is a Rare Disorder of Copper Metabolism

Wilson disease (WD) is an autosomal recessive malady in which excess copper may be deposited in the liver and brain. The carrier rate is 1 in 100, and the incidence of clinical disease is 1 in 30,000 live births. The mutated gene has a worldwide distribution.

PATHOGENESIS: The intake of copper in the diet usually exceeds requirements, and the liver clears excess copper via excretion into the bile. In addition to biliary secretion, copper is normally bound to ceruloplasmin in the hepatocyte, and the complex is secreted into the blood. The gene for WD, namely *ATP7B*, codes for an ATP-dependent transmembrane cation channel that transports copper within the hepatocytes before it is excreted. *Mutations in the WD gene renders copper transport ineffective, and both biliary excretion of copper and its incorporation into ceruloplasmin are deficient.* Some 200 different mutations in the WD gene on chromosome 13 have been described. In European and North American populations, a single mutation, His1069Gln, accounts for 70% of WD, whereas this mutation is rare in India and Asia. Most patients are compound heterozygotes, possessing alleles with two different mutations.

Wilson disease is characterized by a striking reduction in the serum levels of ceruloplasmin. However, this deficiency is thought to be secondary to hepatic copper overload. After excess copper leads to the death of hepatocytes, copper is released into the blood and subsequently deposits in extrahepatic tissues. The primacy of the liver as the seat of WD is attested to by its cure with liver transplantation.

The mechanism by which excess copper injures cells remains elusive. Like iron, copper can catalyze the formation of potent oxidizing species from superoxide anions and hydrogen peroxide produced by normal oxygen metabolism. In this regard, copper can replace iron in the Fenton reaction, in which ferrous iron and hydrogen peroxide generate hydroxyl radicals (see Chapter 1).

PATHOLOGY: *Liver disease in WD progresses from mild to severe chronic hepatitis. Cirrhosis may develop rapidly, even in childhood.* The periportal hepatocytes often contain Mallory's hyaline, and cholestasis is not infrequent. Mitochondrial abnormalities are observed by electron microscopy. An initial micronodular cirrhosis eventually assumes a macronodular pattern. Chemical measurement of liver copper in unfixed tissue from livers of patients with WD reveals more than 250 μg of copper per gram of dry weight.

In the brain, the corpus striatum and occasionally the subthalamic nuclei may display a reddish brown discoloration. The central white matter of the cerebral or cerebellar hemispheres may manifest spongy softening or cavitation, in which case the overlying cortex is atrophic. Astrocytes proliferate in the putamen, and the number of neurons is decreased.

CLINICAL FEATURES: Half of patients with WD display some symptoms by adolescence. The remainder usually become ill in their early adult years, but later presentations can occur. The presenting symptoms are referable to chronic liver disease in about half of patients, one third initially present with neurologic complaints, and about one tenth are seen because of psychiatric manifestations.

LIVER: The liver disease begins insidiously with nonspecific symptoms and may progress to chronic liver disease indistinguishable from that of other forms of chronic hepatitis. Eventually, chronic hepatitis and cirrhosis result in jaundice, portal hypertension, and hepatic failure. Unlike hemochromatosis, WD is not associated with an increased risk of primary hepatocellular carcinoma.

BRAIN: The neurologic disease begins with mild incoordination and tremors. In untreated patients, dysarthria and dysphagia appear, and in late stages, disabling dystonia and spasticity occur.

EYE: Ophthalmic manifestations invariably accompany the neurologic disease. **Kayser-Fleischer ring** is a golden-brown, bilateral discoloration of the cornea that encircles the periphery of the iris and obscures its muscular pattern (Fig. 14-41). It represents a deposition of copper in Descemet membrane. In some patients, Kayser-Fleischer rings are accompanied by "sunflower cataracts," which are green disks of copper deposition in the anterior capsule of the lens.

BONES: Skeletal lesions are commonly found on radiographic examination. They include osteomalacia, osteoporosis, spontaneous fractures, and various arthropathies.

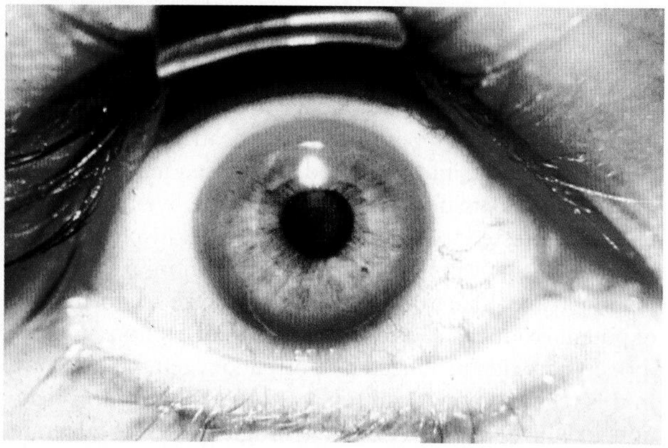

FIGURE 14-41. **Kayser-Fleischer ring.** The deposition of copper in Descemet membrane is reflected in a peripheral brown color, which obstructs the view of the underlying iris.

KIDNEY: Renal glomerular and tubular dysfunction, manifested by proteinuria, lowered glomerular filtration, aminoaciduria, and phosphaturia, is common in WD. These abnormalities are secondary to copper deposition in the renal tubules.

BLOOD: Transient acute hemolytic episodes, presumably related to a sudden release of free copper from the liver, occur in as many as 15% of patients with WD.

Treatment of WD not only prevents the accumulation of tissue copper but also extracts copper that has already been deposited. Trientine, and D-Penicillamine, copper-chelating agents, augment the excretion of copper in the urine. Both central nervous system dysfunction and the symptoms of liver disease are often reversed by treatment. (D-Penicillamine is not recommended as a first treatment for patients presenting with neurologic symptoms; but if necessary, add vitamin B_6 to prevent the deficiency of this vitamin.) In addition, tetrathiomolybdate is still in the experimental stage in the United States and Canada. As the blood copper levels drop, zinc maintenance may be added.

For presymptomatic patients, maintenance treatment is with zinc, that blocks the intestinal absorption of copper. Liver transplantation is curative for WD.

Cystic Fibrosis May Cause Biliary Obstruction

Biliary obstruction results from the accumulation of tenacious mucous plugs in the intrahepatic biliary tree and may present in the first few weeks of life. Recovery typically occurs in 1 to 6 months, although some infants die in hepatic failure. *In children who survive to adolescence, clinically symptomatic liver disease develops in some 15%, and secondary biliary cirrhosis is found in 10% of patients who survive beyond the age of 25 years.*

α_1-Antitrypsin (α_1-AT) Deficiency Leads to Cirrhosis

α_1-AT deficiency is inherited as an autosomal recessive trait and was initially described as a cause of emphysema (see Chapter 12). Thereafter, cases of liver disease without pulmonary involvement were described, and disease of both organs has also been recognized. In infants and children, α_1-AT deficiency is the most common genetic cause of liver disease and the most frequent genetic disease for which liver transplantation is indicated. Although the disorder is found in 1 of 2000 live births, only 10% to 15% of those affected develop liver injury.

PATHOGENESIS: α_1-AT is synthesized in the liver, and both the pulmonary and hepatic disorders result from a defect in the secretion of a mutant variant by the liver. The α_1-AT gene locus is termed *Pi*, and over 75 isoforms have been identified. The two most frequent types are designated PiS and PiZ. The substitution of a lysine for a glutamate in the PiZ variant (95% of all cases) causes the retention of mutant protein within the lumen of the endoplasmic reticulum, where it folds abnormally as an insoluble aggregate, thereby damaging that cell.

PATHOLOGY: *The characteristic feature in the liver of patients with α_1-AT deficiency is the presence of faintly eosinophilic,* periodic acid–Schiff *(PAS)-positive cytoplasmic droplets* (Fig. 14-42). Electron microscopy visualizes these inclusions as amorphous material within dilated cisternae of the endoplasmic reticulum. The disease often terminates in cirrhosis.

α_1-AT deficiency is a cause of hepatitis in the newborn (see below). *Micronodular cirrhosis develops by the age of 2 to 3 years in these children and may ultimately become macronodular.*

CLINICAL FEATURES: The clinical expression of liver disease in α_1-AT deficiency is highly variable, ranging from a rapidly fatal neonatal hepatitis to an absence of any hepatic dysfunction. *Of those infants with the ZZ genotype—that is, those who are susceptible to the development of clinical disease—10% develop neonatal cholestatic jaundice (conjugated hyperbilirubinemia).* In fact, α_1-AT accounts for up to 30% of all cases of neonatal conjugated hyperbilirubinemia. Most infants recover within 6 months, but 10% to 20% develop permanent liver disease. Children with cirrhosis usually die before the age of 10 years from hepatic failure or other complications of α_1-AT deficiency. However, liver transplantation is curative.

Some patients are asymptomatic until early adulthood, when they may present with symptoms of cirrhosis as the initial complaint. *The cirrhosis of α_1-AT deficiency is complicated by a high incidence of hepatocellular carcinoma.*

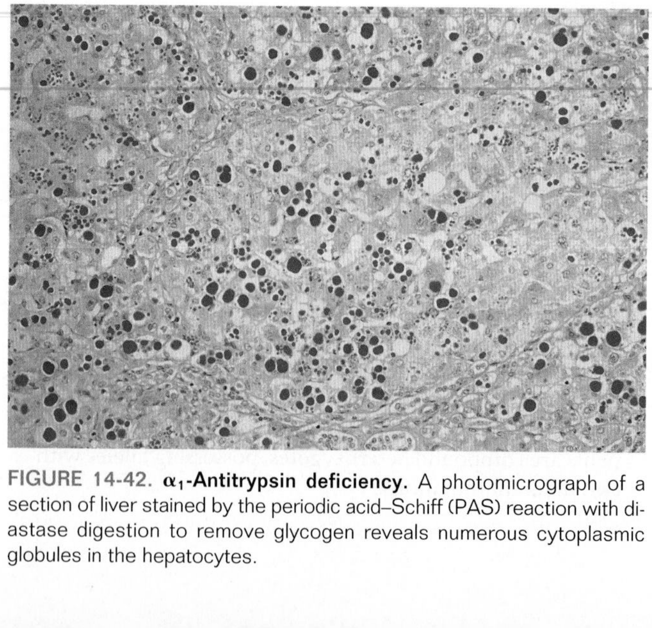

FIGURE 14-42. **α_1-Antitrypsin deficiency.** A photomicrograph of a section of liver stained by the periodic acid–Schiff (PAS) reaction with diastase digestion to remove glycogen reveals numerous cytoplasmic globules in the hepatocytes.

Inborn Errors of Carbohydrate Metabolism Affect the Liver

Glycogen Storage Diseases

The biochemical basis of the glycogen storage diseases is discussed in Chapter 6. *Only glycogenosis type IV (brancher deficiency, Andersen disease) is usually complicated by cirrhosis.* A slowly developing cirrhosis may occur in glycogenosis type III (debrancher deficiency, Cori disease) but is not inevitable. Glycogenosis type I (glucose-6-phosphatase deficiency, von Gierke disease) is associated with striking hepatomegaly, and type II (acid-glucosidase deficiency, Pompe disease) features mild hepatomegaly. Neither type I nor type II is complicated by cirrhosis.

GLYCOGENOSIS TYPE I: The hepatocytes are distended by large amounts of glycogen, which appears pale in sections stained with hematoxylin and eosin and red with PAS. Fat accumulation varies from mild to severe, but fibrosis is usually absent. Hepatic adenomas often develop in adolescence but regress with dietary therapy.

GLYCOGENOSIS TYPE III: Infants with this malady show severe hepatomegaly, and the liver morphologically resembles that seen in type I. Fat is less conspicuous, but fibrosis is present and may progress to cirrhosis.

GLYCOGENOSIS TYPE IV: Infants present with severe hepatomegaly and usually die of cirrhosis by the age of 4 years. Sharply circumscribed, PAS-positive inclusions are present in enlarged hepatocytes. By electron microscopy these inclusions consist of fibrillar material that represents abnormal glycogen. Deposits of mutant glycogen are also found in the heart, skeletal muscle, and brain. Liver transplantation is curative for glycogenosis type IV.

Galactosemia

Galactosemia, inherited as an autosomal recessive trait, is caused by a deficiency of galactose-1-phosphate uridyl transferase, the enzyme that catalyzes the second step in the conversion of galactose to glucose. As a result of this metabolic defect, galactose and its metabolites accumulate in the liver and other organs. Infants with this disorder who are fed milk rapidly develop **hepatosplenomegaly, jaundice,** and **hypoglycemia.** Cataracts and mental retardation are common.

Microscopically, within 2 weeks of birth the liver shows extensive and uniform fat accumulation and striking proliferation of bile ductules in and around the portal tracts. Cholestasis is often present in canaliculi and bile ductules. Bile plugs fill many of these pseudoacini. *At about 6 weeks of age, fibrosis begins to extend from the portal tracts into the lobule and within 6 months progresses to cirrhosis.* Institution of a galactose-free diet ameliorates the disease and reverses many of the morphologic alterations.

Hereditary Fructose Intolerance

Hereditary fructose intolerance is an autosomal recessive disease caused by a deficiency of fructose-1-phosphate aldolase. When fructose is fed early in infancy, hepatomegaly, jaundice, and ascites develop. However, the feeding of fructose after the age of 6 months results in far less severe disease, and the only clinical impairment is spontaneous hypoglycemia. Infants who suffer from liver disease show many of the changes of neonatal hepatitis. Fat accumulation may be marked, in which case the appearance resembles that of galactosemia. Progressive fibrosis culminates in cirrhosis.

Tyrosinemia

Tyrosinemia is an autosomal recessive trait that interferes with the catabolism of tyrosine to fumarate and acetoacetate. The biochemical defect is a deficiency of fumarylacetoacetate hydrolase (FAH) in the liver caused by more than 30 mutations in the *FAH* gene. Damage to the liver and kidney is caused by the accumulation of succinyl acetone and succinyl acetoacetate, both of which are potent electrophiles that can react with the sulfhydryl groups of glutathione and proteins.

Acute tyrosinemia, which begins within a few weeks or months of birth, is characterized by hepatosplenomegaly and is associated with liver failure and death, usually before the age of 12 months. The appearance of the liver is remarkably similar to that in galactosemia, including progression to cirrhosis.

Chronic tyrosinemia begins in the first year of life and is characterized by growth retardation, renal disease, and hepatic failure. Death usually supervenes before the age of 10 years. *The incidence of hepatocellular carcinoma associated with chronic tyrosinemia is extraordinarily high.* Tyrosinemia is treated by liver transplantation.

Miscellaneous Inherited Causes of Cirrhosis

A number of inborn errors of metabolism have been associated with cirrhosis, including storage diseases, such as Gaucher disease, Niemann-Pick disease, mucopolysaccharidoses, neonatal adrenoleukodystrophy, Wolman disease, and Zellweger syndrome.

Indian Childhood Cirrhosis

Indian childhood cirrhosis (ICC) is a fatal disorder largely restricted to preschool children on the Indian subcontinent. Similar cases have occasionally been described elsewhere. The disorder affects predominantly boys between the ages of 1 and 4 years from middle-class Hindu families. The liver displays micronodular cirrhosis and abundant Mallory bodies, similar to alcoholic liver disease.

The etiology and pathogenesis of ICC are not well understood. Familial cases have been reported, but no hereditary pattern has been established. Interestingly, children with this disease display a marked excess of copper and copper-binding protein in the liver, but the significance of these findings remains obscure.

Toxic Liver Injury

Acute, chemically induced hepatic injury spans the entire spectrum of liver disease, from transient cholestasis to fulminant hepatitis to cirrhosis. Chronic toxic injury to the liver is equally diverse; at one extreme is a mild chronic hepatitis and at the other, active cirrhosis. Although hepatic injury caused by drugs accounts for less than 5% of all cases of jaundice, it constitutes up to 25% of cases of fulminant hepatic failure.

Some hepatotoxic chemicals invariably produce liver cell necrosis—that is, their action is entirely **predictable**. Among such agents are substances as diverse as yellow phosphorus, the organic solvent carbon tetrachloride, the mushroom poison phalloidin, and the analgesic acetaminophen. The defining characteristics of the liver injury produced by predictable hepatotoxins are as follows:

- The agent, in sufficiently high doses, always produces liver cell necrosis
- The extent of hepatic injury is dose-dependent
- These compounds produce the same lesions in different animal species
- The liver necrosis is characteristically zonal—often, but not exclusively, centrilobular

- The period between administration of the toxin and the development of liver cell necrosis is brief

Chapter 1 includes a discussion of the possible mechanisms by which these toxins produce liver necrosis. Briefly, toxic liver necrosis is, in most cases, a consequence of the metabolism of the compound by the mixed-function oxidase system of the liver, by which activated oxygen species and reactive metabolites are produced. The rate of drug metabolism is influenced by many factors, including age, sex, nutritional status, interactions with other drugs, and prior induction of hepatic drug-metabolizing activity.

In contrast to the aforementioned classic poisons, most reactions to therapeutic drugs are ***unpredictable*** *and seem to represent idiosyncratic events or manifestations of unusual sensitivity to a dose-related side effect.* Sensitive persons may be predisposed to idiosyncratic reactions either because they possess metabolic pathways different from those of the general population or because they are particularly susceptible to a uniform pharmacologic effect of the drug other than the desired therapeutic response.

Genetic variations in systems of biotransformation and in the production or detoxification of reactive metabolites may determine the toxicity of some drugs. An immunologic reaction to drugs, their metabolites, or modified liver cells has not been ruled out. Drugs that are principally cholestatic do not necessarily depend on metabolism for their action.

With these considerations in mind, we shall discuss toxic liver injury in terms of the morphologic patterns of the resulting reaction.

Zonal Hepatocellular Necrosis Is Caused by the Metabolites of Drugs and Chemicals

The centrilobular localization of necrosis presumably reflects the greater activity of drug-metabolizing enzymes in the central zones. Examples of agents that produce such injury agents are carbon tetrachloride, acetaminophen (Fig. 14-43), and the toxins of the mushroom *Amanita phalloides*. In the affected zones, hepatocytes show coagulative necrosis, hydropic swelling, and variable amounts of fat. Inflammation tends to be sparse. If the dose of the hepatotoxin is sufficiently large, necrosis may extend to involve the entire lobule, leaving only a thin rim of viable hepatocytes surrounding the portal tracts. Patients either die in acute hepatic failure or recover without sequelae.

The chronic administration of hepatotoxins that cause zonal necrosis, exemplified by carbon tetrachloride, produces cirrhosis in experimental animals. However, this is generally not a problem in humans; once the acute toxic injury has been recognized, measures are usually taken to preclude reexposure to the offending agent.

Fatty Liver Is a Response to a Variety of Hepatotoxins

The accumulation of triglycerides within the hepatocytes (i.e., hepatic steatosis or fatty liver) generally occurs in a predictable fashion. Although substantial overlap may exist, two morphologic patterns occur, namely macrovesicular and microvesicular steatosis.

Macrovesicular Steatosis

In macrovesicular steatosis, light microscopy shows the cytoplasm of the liver cell to be occupied by fat, seen as a large clear area that distends the cell and displaces the nucleus to the periphery. In addition to its association with chronic ethanol ingestion, macrovesicular fat results from the experimental administration of, or accidental exposure to, such direct hepatotoxins as carbon tetrachloride and the poisonous constituents of certain mushrooms. Moreover, corticosteroids and some antimetabolites, such as methotrexate, may cause macrovesicular steatosis. There is no reason to believe that the presence of fat per se is injurious to the hepatocyte. Rather, its accumulation reflects the underlying liver cell damage.

A puzzling variant of toxic macrovesicular steatosis that resembles alcoholic hepatitis, termed **steatohepatitis**, occurs after the administration of certain drugs (e.g., amiodarone in the treatment of arrhythmias).

Microvesicular Steatosis

In contrast to macrovesicular steatosis, which by itself tends to be clinically inconsequential, microvesicular fatty liver is commonly associated with severe, and sometimes fatal, liver disease. Small fat vacuoles are dispersed throughout the cytoplasm of hepatocytes, and the nucleus retains its central position (Fig. 14-44). Again, it is not the presence of fat but the underlying metabolic defects that produce the liver dysfunction.

REYE SYNDROME: This rare acute disease of children is characterized by microvesicular steatosis, hepatic failure, and encephalopathy. Cerebral edema and fat accumulation are reported in the brain. The symptoms usually begin after a febrile illness, commonly influenza or varicella infection, and are claimed to correlate

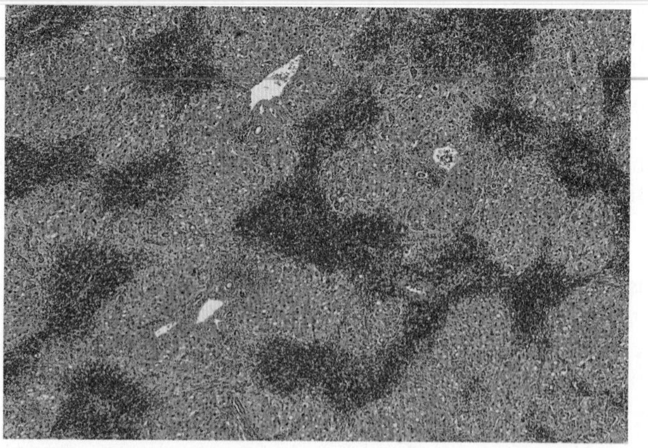

FIGURE 14-43. **Toxic centrilobular necrosis.** The autopsy specimen in a case of acetaminophen overdose discloses prominent hemorrhagic necrosis of the centrilobular zones of all liver lobules.

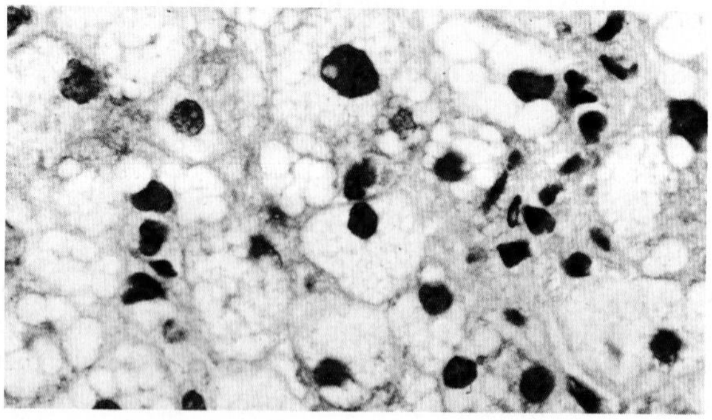

FIGURE 14-44. **Microvesicular fatty liver.** A liver biopsy specimen in a case of Reye syndrome shows small-droplet fat in hepatocytes and centrally located nuclei.

with the administration of aspirin. Clearly, Reye syndrome is more complex than simple aspirin toxicity, because the doses of aspirin consumed were far too small to produce liver injury. In any event, with the decline in the use of aspirin in children and possibly a reduced incidence of influenza, Reye syndrome is now distinctly uncommon.

FATTY LIVER OF PREGNANCY: Microsteatosis, not infrequently associated with hepatic failure, may occur during pregnancy and ordinarily improves on delivery. Women who have suffered fatty liver of pregnancy may complete subsequent pregnancies without untoward effects.

PHOSPHOLIPIDOSIS: Triglycerides are not the only lipids that can accumulate in the liver in response to toxic injury. Phospholipidosis, which resembles certain heritable disorders of lipid metabolism (e.g., Niemann-Pick and Tay-Sachs disease), occurs after the administration of drugs such as amiodarone. By light microscopy, both hepatocytes and Kupffer cells are enlarged and show a foamy cytoplasm.

Acute Intrahepatic Cholestasis Is a Frequent Manifestation of Drug-Induced Liver Disease

Histologically, the lesions may range from bland centrilobular cholestasis with virtually no hepatocellular necrosis or inflammation to panlobular cholestasis with scattered foci of hepatocellular necrosis. Drugs incriminated in this type of liver injury include anabolic steroids and tranquilizing agents. Except for mild jaundice, pruritus, and an elevated serum alkaline phosphatase level, the patients feel well.

Lesions Resembling Viral Hepatitis Are Unpredictable

All the features of acute viral hepatitis occasionally occur after administration of a variety of drugs. Historically, the most widely appreciated examples are the inhalation anesthetic halothane, the antituberculosis agent isoniazid, and the antihypertensive drug methyldopa. Although the incidence of these viral hepatitis like reactions is low, they are far more dangerous than viral hepatitis itself, causing more severe disease and a much higher mortality rate. The entire range of acute liver injury, from mild anicteric hepatitis to rapidly fatal massive hepatic necrosis, is encountered.

Chronic Hepatitis Can Follow the Persistent Intake of Hepatotoxic Drugs

Like chronic hepatitis caused by persistent viral infection, drug-induced chronic hepatitis may progress to cirrhosis, albeit rarely. On discontinuation of drug administration, the lesion usually resolves, although this may require many months. In patients who have progressed to cirrhosis, the scarring remains, but the inflammatory and necrotizing activity is halted. Among the drugs incriminated in the production of chronic hepatitis are the antituberculosis drug isoniazid and certain sulfonamides.

Granulomatous Hepatitis is a Rare Reaction to Drugs

Noncaseating "sarcoid-like" granulomas may appear in the portal tracts and the lobular parenchyma after the intake of some drugs. The liver damage is transient and does not lead to chronic lesions. Among the many drugs that have been associated with granulomatous hepatitis are the anti-inflammatory agent phenylbutazone, the antiarrhythmic drug quinidine, and allopurinol, used in the treatment of gout.

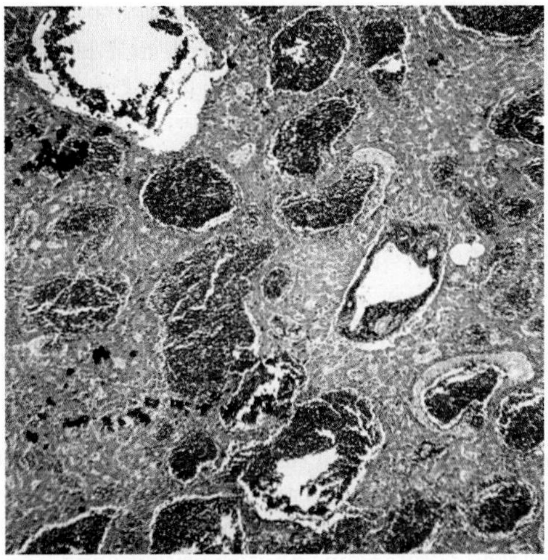

FIGURE 14-45. **Peliosis hepatis.** The liver contains numerous large, irregular, blood-filled spaces.

Vascular Lesions May Complicate Hormone Therapy

Occlusion of the hepatic veins (**Budd-Chiari syndrome**) (see Fig. 14-16) has been reported to follow the use of oral contraceptive agents, presumably reflecting the general hypercoagulable state associated with the use of these steroids.

***Peliosis hepatis** is a peculiar hepatic lesion, characterized by cystic, blood-filled cavities that are not lined by endothelial cells* (Fig. 14-45). Anabolic sex steroids, contraceptive steroids, and the antiestrogen compound tamoxifen sometimes produce this lesion.

Neoplastic Lesions Are Rare Reactions to Drugs

Hepatic adenomas are uncommon benign tumors that arise after the use of oral contraceptives and (uncommonly) of anabolic steroids (see below). **Hemangiosarcomas** of the liver appeared many years after the intravenous administration of thorium dioxide (Thorotrast), a radioactive compound used in the past to visualize the liver. This particulate isotope is engulfed by Kupffer cells, where it remains inert indefinitely, emits local radiant energy, and thereby produces neoplastic transformation. Chronic exposure to inorganic arsenic, usually in the form of insecticides, and the inhalation of vinyl chloride in an industrial setting have also been linked to the development of hemangiosarcoma of the liver.

The Porphyrias

The porphyrias comprise both acquired and inherited conditions; they are caused by deficiencies in the pathway of heme biosynthesis and are characterized by the accumulation of porphyrin intermediates (see Chapter 20). The porphyrias are divided into two types—hepatic and erythropoietic porphyrias—based on the location of defective heme metabolism and the accumulation of porphyrins and their precursors. The molecular genetics of the porphyrias is heterogeneous, with unique mutations usually occurring within individual families.

The hepatic porphyrias are inherited as autosomal dominant traits and are often precipitated by the administration of drugs, sex hormones, starvation, hepatitis C, HIV infection, and alcohol consumption. The liver in hepatic porphyrias variably displays steatosis, hemosiderosis, fibrosis, and cirrhosis. Needle-shaped cytoplasmic inclusions may be present.

ACUTE INTERMITTENT PORPHYRIA: This malady is the most common genetic porphyria and reflects a deficiency of porphobilinogen deaminase activity in the liver. However, only 10% of gene carriers suffer clinical symptoms, which generally affect young adults. Colicky abdominal pain and neuropsychiatric symptoms predominate.

PORPHYRIA CUTANEA TARDA: This chronic hepatic porphyria is the most frequent porphyria and is either acquired or inherited as an autosomal dominant trait. It reflects deficient uroporphyrinogen decarboxylase activity in the liver. The typical patient is middle-aged or elderly, displays cutaneous photosensitivity, and suffers from liver disease with hepatic iron overload.

Other inherited porphyrias, termed **erythropoietic porphyrias** and **congenital erythropoietic porphyria**, are caused by enzyme deficiencies in cells of erythrocytic lineage. They are characterized by cutaneous photosensitivity and occasionally liver disease.

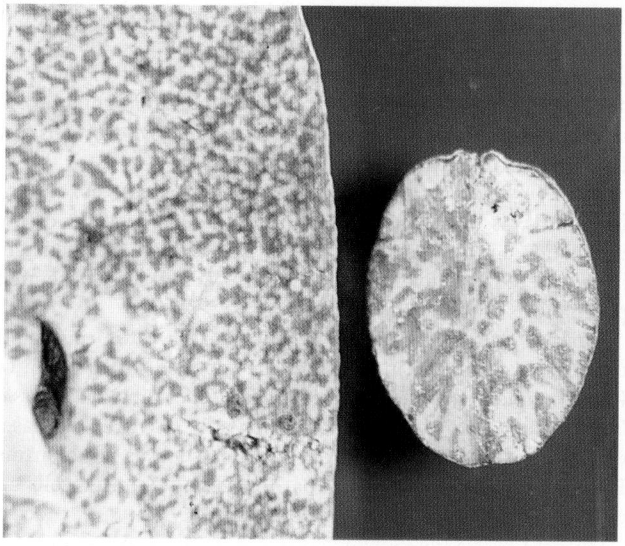

FIGURE 14-46. **Chronic passive congestion of the liver.** The surface of this fixed liver exhibits an accentuated lobular pattern, an appearance resembling that of a nutmeg *(right)*.

Vascular Disorders

Congestive Heart Failure Is the Major Cause of Liver Congestion

Acute Passive Congestion

At autopsy, it is common for the liver to be acutely congested, presumably because of a failing heart in the agonal period. On cut section, the liver is diffusely speckled with small red foci. Microscopically, they represent centrilobular zones with dilated and congested sinusoids and terminal venules. These changes are not clinically significant.

Chronic Passive Congestion

In the face of persistent congestive heart failure, the pressure in the peripheral venous circulation increases, thereby impeding venous outflow from liver and producing chronic passive congestion of that organ. The chronically congested liver is often reduced in size. The cut surface exhibits an accentuated lobular pattern, with a mottled appearance of alternating light and dark areas (Fig. 14-46), termed **nutmeg liver**. In severe cases, the centrilobular terminal venules and adjacent sinusoids are markedly dilated and filled with erythrocytes, and the liver cell plates in this zone are thinned by pressure atrophy.

In cases of particularly severe and long-standing **right-sided heart failure** (e.g., tricuspid valvular disease or constrictive pericarditis), chronic passive congestion progresses to varying degrees of hepatic fibrosis. Delicate fibrous strands envelop terminal venules, and septa radiate from the centrilobular zones. Fibrous septa may link adjacent central veins, thereby producing a "reverse lobulation." Pressure atrophy of the centrilobular hepatocytes remains prominent. The older term "cardiac cirrhosis" is inappropriate, since the complete septa and regenerative nodules of true cirrhosis are rarely encountered.

Chronic passive congestion of the liver is of more pathologic than clinical interest, since the condition has little effect on hepatic function. Features of portal hypertension, including splenomegaly and ascites, sometimes accompany chronic passive congestion of the liver.

Shock Results in Decreased Perfusion of the Liver

Shock from any cause often leads to ischemic necrosis of the centrilobular hepatocytes. The centrilobular zone, referred to as zone 3 in the functional concept of the hepatic acinus (see Fig. 14-2), is most distal to the blood supply from the portal tracts and is the area most vulnerable to ischemic insults. Microscopically, coagulative necrosis of centrilobular hepatocytes is accompanied by frank hemorrhage.

Infarction of the Liver Is Uncommon Because of Its Dual Blood Supply and the Anastomotic Structure of the Hepatic Sinusoids

Acute occlusion of the hepatic artery or its branches is unusual but can occur as a result of embolism, polyarteritis nodosa, or accidental ligation during surgery. Under such circumstances, irregular pale areas, often surrounded by a hyperemic zone, reflect the underlying ischemic necrosis.

Acute occlusion of intrahepatic branches of the portal vein, generally in the presence of elevated hepatic venous pressure, classically produces the **Zahn infarct,** a dark-red, triangular area with its base on the surface of the liver. Microscopically only dilation and congestion of the sinusoids are noted. Thus, the traditional term "infarct" is actually a misnomer.

Bacterial Infections

Bacterial infections are uncommon causes of liver disease in the industrialized countries and are for the most part complications of infections elsewhere. The characteristic reactions in the liver are granulomas, abscesses, and diffuse inflammation. Infections associated with granulomatous inflammation elsewhere (e.g., tuberculosis, tularemia, and brucellosis) also cause granulomatous hepatitis.

Pyogenic liver abscesses are produced by staphylococci, streptococci, and gram-negative enterobacteria. The morphologic appearance of a pyogenic abscess in the liver is similar to

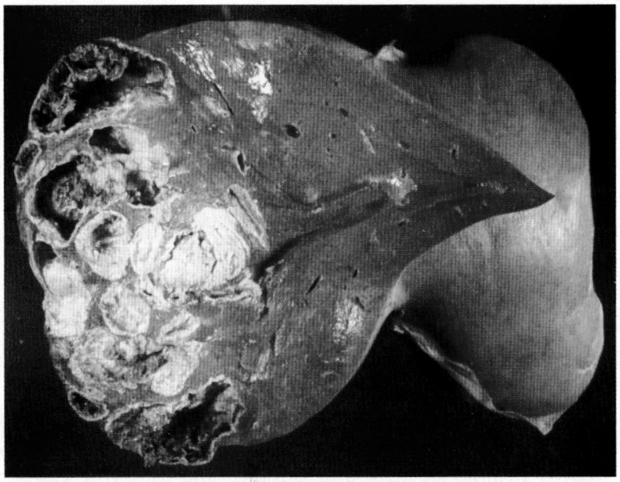

FIGURE 14-47. **Pylephlebitic abscesses of the liver.** The cut surface of the liver shows large, confluent, irregular abscess cavities.

that in other sites. Anaerobic inhabitants of the gastrointestinal tract, particularly *Bacteroides* species and microaerophilic streptococci, are common causes of liver abscesses. Organisms reach the liver in arterial or portal blood or through the biliary tract. In cases of septicemia, the liver is seeded with organisms from distant sites through the arterial blood.

Pylephlebitic abscesses (Fig. 14-47) result from intra-abdominal suppuration, as in peritonitis or diverticulitis, with the organisms being transmitted to the liver in portal blood. At one time, pylephlebitis was the most common cause of hepatic abscesses, but the control of abdominal sepsis with antibiotics has rendered this route of infection uncommon.

Cholangitic abscesses in the liver are today the most common form of hepatic abscess in Western countries. Biliary obstruction from any cause is often complicated by bacterial infection of the biliary tree, termed **ascending cholangitis.** The retrograde biliary dissemination of organisms (usually *Escherichia coli*) then leads to the formation of cholangitic abscesses.

Hepatic abscesses are more commonly located in the right lobe of the liver. Diffuse inflammation of the liver from bacterial infection is distinctly uncommon today but may be encountered in various septicemic states, particularly in immunocompromised patients. In about half of all cases of hepatic abscess, the source of infection cannot be demonstrated.

CLINICAL FEATURES: A patient with a hepatic abscess typically presents with high fever, rapid weight loss, right upper quadrant abdominal pain, and hepatomegaly. Jaundice occurs in a fourth of cases, but the serum alkaline phosphatase level is almost always elevated. Solitary abscesses are treated with surgical drainage and antibiotics, but multiple abscesses present a difficult therapeutic problem. The complications of hepatic abscess relate principally to rupture and direct spread of the infection. Pleuropulmonary fistulas, from the rupture of an abscess through the diaphragm, and peritonitis, from leakage into the abdominal cavity, occur. The dissemination of organisms in the blood may lead to septicemia and metastatic abscesses in other parts of the body. The mortality from hepatic abscess, even in treated cases, remains high, ranging from 40% to 80%.

Parasitic Infestations

Parasitic infestations of the liver are a serious public health problem worldwide, although they are uncommon in industrialized countries. These diseases are discussed in Chapter 9. Here we summarize the major parasitic diseases that affect the liver.

Protozoal Diseases Frequently Involve the Liver

AMEBIASIS: In the United States, the carrier rate for *Entamoeba histolytica* is probably less than 5%, but a prevalence of up to 35% has been reported in homosexual men. Amebiasis of the liver, the most common extraintestinal complication, leads to amebic abscesses, which are multiple in about half of cases (Fig. 14-48).

On gross examination, an amebic abscess typically ranges from 8 to 12 cm in diameter, appears well circumscribed, and contains thick, dark material that has been likened to anchovy paste or chocolate. Microscopically, the trophozoites can usually be visualized in the periphery of the necrotic debris.

The symptoms associated with amebic abscesses are similar to those that characterize pyogenic abscesses. With appropriate treatment (tissue amebicides), the abscess may heal and leave only residual scar tissue. Surgical drainage of large abscesses is important. If an amebic abscess continues to grow, it may rupture into the peritoneal cavity, where it produces peritonitis, a complication associated with a mortality rate as high as 40%. The amebae may also invade the blood, in which case abscesses of the brain and lung may ensue.

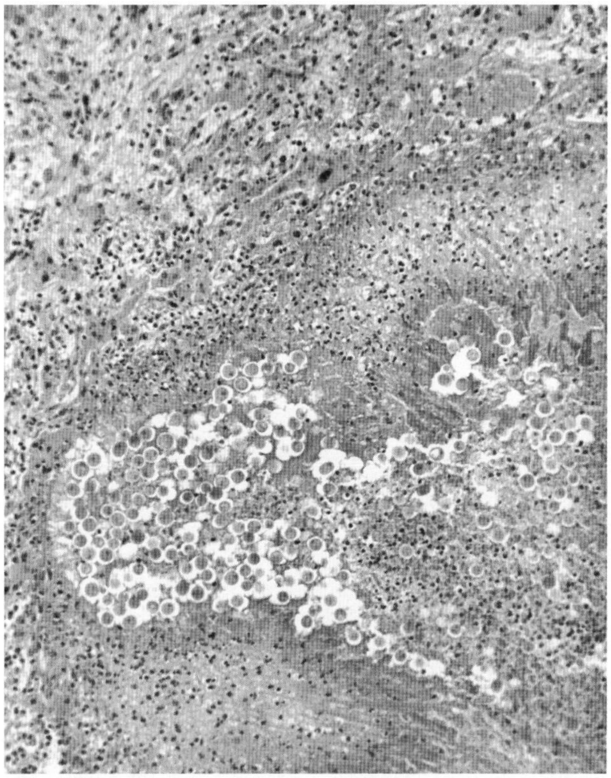

FIGURE 14-48. **Amebic abscess of the liver.** A photomicrograph of the margin of an amebic abscess shows fibroblastic proliferation surrounding the cavity and amebic trophozoites in the lumen.

MALARIA: Hepatic involvement in malaria is a frequent cause of hepatomegaly in endemic areas. It reflects Kupffer cell hypertrophy and hyperplasia secondary to phagocytosis of the debris resulting from the rupture of parasitized erythrocytes. This hepatic involvement does not give rise to significant hepatic dysfunction.

VISCERAL LEISHMANIASIS (KALA-AZAR): As in malaria, the hepatomegaly of chronic visceral leishmaniasis reflects hyperplasia of mononuclear phagocytes in the liver. In contrast to malaria, however, the Kupffer cells ingest the parasitic organisms themselves, which appear as **Donovan bodies**. Clinically, there is little evidence of hepatic dysfunction.

Helminthic Diseases Are Problems of Underdeveloped Areas

Diseases caused by helminths are described in Chapter 9, and **hepatic schistosomiasis** is discussed above in the context of portal hypertension.

ASCARIASIS: From the duodenum, the worms of *Ascaris lumbricoides* gain access to the biliary tree, where they may produce acute biliary colic. When the worms lodge in the intrahepatic biliary passages, their disintegration results in the liberation of innumerable eggs, which precipitates severe, suppurative cholangitis. The resulting cholangitic abscesses may rupture into the peritoneal cavity or into the pleural space. Spread of the infection into the hepatic or portal veins causes pylephlebitis, a highly dangerous complication. At autopsy, the liver is enlarged and numerous irregular cavities contain foul-smelling material in which the remnants of degenerated parasites are found.

LIVER FLUKES: The major parasitic flukes that involve the human liver are *Clonorchis sinensis* and *Fasciola hepatica*. Humans are the definitive host for *C. sinensis*, whereas sheep and cattle are the principal reservoir of *F. hepatica*. Both parasites lodge in the intrahepatic biliary tree, where they provoke hyperplasia of the biliary epithelium, particularly severe in clonorchiasis (Fig. 14-49). In severe infestation with *C. sinensis*, the accumulation of material from degenerated worms, parasite eggs, and viscid mucus (secreted by metaplastic goblet cells in the biliary epithelium) obstructs intrahepatic bile flow and leads to intrahepatic pigment gallstones. Secondary infection of the bile with *E. coli* causes cholangitis and cholangitic abscesses, which are common causes of surgical emergencies in some Asian countries. *Biliary infestation with C. sinensis is an etiologic factor in the development of cholangiocarcinoma.*

ECHINOCOCCOSIS (CYSTIC HYDATID DISEASE): Infection with the tapeworms of the genus *Echinococcus,* principally *Echinococcus granulosus,* is an important zoonosis that involves the human liver. Echinococcal cysts expand slowly and produce symptoms only after many years. Within the liver, the cyst behaves as a space-occupying lesion; systemic manifestations reflect toxic or allergic reactions to the absorption of constituents of the organisms.

Leptospirosis (Weil Disease) Is an Accidental Infection from a Zoonosis

Leptospira spirochetes infect many animal species. Despite the animal reservoir of leptospira, fewer than one fifth of patients who contract leptospirosis give a history of direct contact with animals. **Weil syndrome** refers to leptospirosis complicated by prolonged fever and jaundice and in severe cases by azotemia, hemorrhages, and altered consciousness. Weil syndrome occurs in only 1% to 6% of all cases of leptospirosis. The morphologic alterations of the liver in fatal cases are nonspecific and include focal necrosis, enlarged Kupffer cells, and centrilobular cholestasis. The organisms are generally not demonstrable in the liver.

Hepatic Lesions of Syphilis Were Common but Are Now Rare

Congenital syphilis causes neonatal hepatitis, which results in diffuse fibrosis in the portal tracts and around individual liver cells or groups of hepatocytes. **Tertiary syphilis** is characterized by hepatic gummas (i.e., focal lesions resembling granulomas), which heal with dense scars. Retraction produces deep clefts and a gross pseudolobation of the liver, termed **hepar lobatum,** a condition that should not be confused with cirrhosis.

Cholestatic Syndromes of Infancy

Diseases characterized by prolonged cholestasis and jaundice in infants represent either diseases primarily affecting the hepatocytes or obstruction of the biliary system.

Neonatal Hepatitis Is an Entity of Multiple Causes

Neonatal hepatitis features prolonged cholestasis, morphologic evidence of liver cell injury, and inflammation.

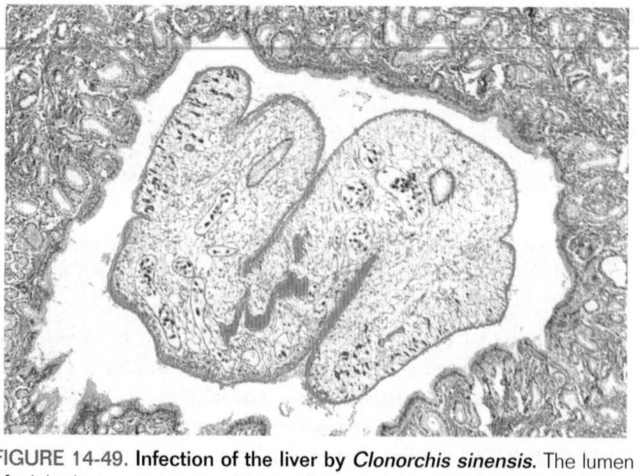

FIGURE 14-49. **Infection of the liver by *Clonorchis sinensis*.** The lumen of a bile duct contains an adult liver fluke, and the mucosa is hyperplastic.

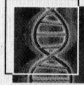

PATHOGENESIS: In about half of all cases of neonatal hepatitis, the cause is discernible (Table 14-5), and about 30% of cases are assigned to α_1-antitrypsin deficiency alone. Most of the other cases with known causes can be attributed to viral hepatitis B and infectious agents such as those of the TORCH group (toxoplasmosis, "other", rubella, cytomegalovirus, and herpes simplex). A few cases represent hepatic injury associated with metabolic defects, for instance, galactosemia or fructose intolerance. Occasional cases of neonatal hepatitis are seen in association with Down syndrome and other chromosomal disorders. The remaining half of all cases of neonatal hepatitis are of unexplained etiology.

TABLE 14–5

Causes of Neonatal Hepatitis

Idiopathic
Idiopathic neonatal hepatitis
Prolonged intrahepatic cholestasis
Arteriohepatic dysplasia (Alagille syndrome)
Paucity of intrahepatic bile ducts not associated with specific syndromes
Zellweger syndrome (cerebrohepatorenal syndrome)
Byler disease
Mechanical obstruction of the intrahepatic bile ducts
Congenital hepatic fibrosis
Caroli disease (cystic dilation of intrahepatic ducts)
Metabolic disorders
Defects of carbohydrate metabolism
Galactosemia
Hereditary fructose intolerance
Glycogenosis type IV
Defects in lipid metabolism
Gaucher disease
Niemann-Pick disease
Wolman disease
Tyrosinemia (defect of amino acid metabolism)
α_1-Antitrypsin deficiency
Cystic fibrosis
Parenteral nutrition
Hepatitis
Hepatitis B
TORCH agents (toxoplasmosis, "other", rubella, cytomegalovirus, and herpes simplex)
Varicella
Syphillis
ECHO viruses
Neonatal sepsis
Chromosomal abnormalities
Down syndrome
Trisomy 18
Extrahepatic biliary obstruction

PATHOLOGY: The characteristic hepatic lesion of neonatal hepatitis is giant cell transformation of hepatocytes, hence the former term **giant cell hepatitis** (Fig. 14-50). The giant cells contain as many as 40 nuclei and may appear detached from other cells in the liver plate. The pale, distended cytoplasm contains large amounts of glycogen and iron. The number of giant cells decreases with time, and they are rare in children older than 1 year of age. Bile pigment is often prominent within canaliculi and hepatocytes. Ballooned hepatocytes, acinar transformation of hepatocytes, and acidophilic bodies are also typical of neonatal hepatitis. Extramedullary hematopoiesis is often conspicuous. Chronic inflammatory infiltrates are seen in the portal tracts as well as in the lobular parenchyma. Pericellular fibrosis around degenerating hepatocytes, singly or in groups, is common, and fibrous tissue septa extend from the portal tracts.

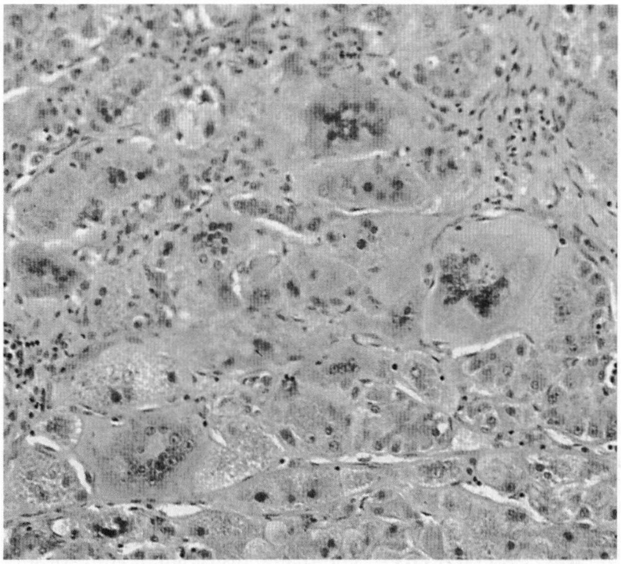

FIGURE 14-50. **Neonatal hepatitis.** A photomicrograph shows multinucleated giant hepatocytes, liver cell injury, and a mild chronic inflammatory infiltrate.

Biliary Atresia Refers to the Lack of a Lumen in the Biliary Tree

Both extrahepatic and intrahepatic biliary atresias are often associated with the morphologic features of neonatal hepatitis.

Extrahepatic Biliary Atresia

Extrahepatic biliary atresia (EXBA) *is a cholestatic disease characterized by obliteration of the lumen of all or part of the biliary tree external to the liver, not associated with calculi, neoplasm or rupture.* It accounts for almost half of all cases of persistent cholestasis in the neonatal period and occurs in 1 of 800 to 18,00 live births. Biliary atresia is the most common indication for liver transplantation in children. EXBA is thought to represent the end result of heterogeneous conditions during gestational and perinatal development. Congenital anomalies are present in 20% of cases, including abnormalities of the heart, intestine, and spleen. Other instances of extrahepatic biliary obstruction are associated with known causes of neonatal hepatitis, such as chromosomal abnormalities (trisomies) and a number of viral infections. Cholangiograms in EXBA fail to demonstrate flow into the duodenum or liver, depending on the site of the affected segment of the biliary tract.

PATHOLOGY: EXBA may involve all the extrahepatic bile ducts or may be restricted to segments of the proximal or distal biliary tree. The gallbladder is often atretic. At one extreme, acute and chronic periluminal inflammation is prominent. Epithelial necrosis is evident, and cellular debris is found in the obstructed or narrow lumen. At the other extreme, the original lumen is completely replaced by mature connective tissue, and little or no inflammation is present. Histologically, cholestasis and periportal bile ductular proliferation in the liver are evident. A minority of cases display multinucleated giant hepatocytes, identical to those seen in neonatal hepatitis. Although the intrahepatic bile ducts may initially appear normal, they are gradually obliterated with the persistence of cholestasis. Eventually, secondary biliary cirrhosis supervenes.

Intrahepatic Biliary Atresia

Intrahepatic biliary atresia refers to a paucity of bile ducts within the liver. The disorder occurs under three different circumstances:

- In association with known causes of neonatal hepatitis (e.g., α_1-AT deficiency, various chromosomal anomalies, and metabolic derangements)
- **Alagille syndrome** (syndromic bile duct paucity), an autosomal dominant disease, also characterized by congenital abnormalities of the heart, eye, skeleton, kidneys, and central nervous system, which involves mutations in the Notch signaling pathway
- Unassociated with other conditions (idiopathic

Many observations support the concept that neonatal hepatitis, intrahepatic biliary atresia, EXBA, and possibly choledochal cyst all result from a common inflammatory process ("infantile obstructive cholangiopathy").

PATHOLOGY: The major histologic feature of intrahepatic biliary atresia is a scarcity of bile ducts in the liver. Cholestasis, giant cell transformation, and bile ductular proliferation are usual. However, cirrhosis is uncommon.

CLINICAL FEATURES: Most patients who have uncomplicated neonatal hepatitis recover without sequelae. Intrahepatic biliary atresia associated with neonatal hepatitis carries a grave prognosis, given that many of these children progress to biliary cirrhosis. By contrast, the outlook in Alagille syndrome is good. Uncorrected EXBA invariably results in progressive secondary biliary cirrhosis and is incompatible with survival. Although surgical correction has been successful in some anatomically favorable cases, most cases of both extrahepatic and intrahepatic biliary atresia are cured only by liver transplantation.

Benign Tumors and Tumor-Like Lesions

Hepatic Adenomas Are Benign Tumors of Hepatocytes That Occur Principally in Women

Hepatic adenomas were exceedingly rare before the availability of oral contraceptives, but since their introduction, many such neoplasms have been reported. The incidence has been reduced by the use of newer combinations of estrogen and progesterone.

PATHOLOGY: Hepatic adenomas usually occur as solitary, sharply demarcated masses, up to 40 cm in diameter and 3 kg in weight (Fig. 14-51). In a fourth of cases, multiple smaller adenomas are present. On gross examination, the tumor is encapsulated and paler than the surrounding parenchyma. Microscopically, the neoplastic hepatocytes resemble their normal counterparts, except that they are not arranged in a lobular architecture (see Fig. 14-51). Portal tracts and central venules are absent. The cells making up the adenoma may be very large and eosinophilic or filled with glycogen, which makes the cytoplasm appear clear. The tumor is circumscribed by a fibrous capsule of variable thickness, and the adjacent hepatocytes appear compressed. Large, thick-walled arteries are often seen in the vicinity of the capsule, and arteries and veins traverse the tumor.

CLINICAL FEATURES: *In about one third of patients with hepatic adenomas (particularly in pregnant women who have used oral contraceptives), the tumors bleed into the peritoneal cavity and require treatment as a surgical emergency.* Even large adenomas have been reported to disappear after discontinuation of oral contraceptive use. A few adenomas are encountered in men, and they have occasionally been reported in association with the use of anabolic steroids.

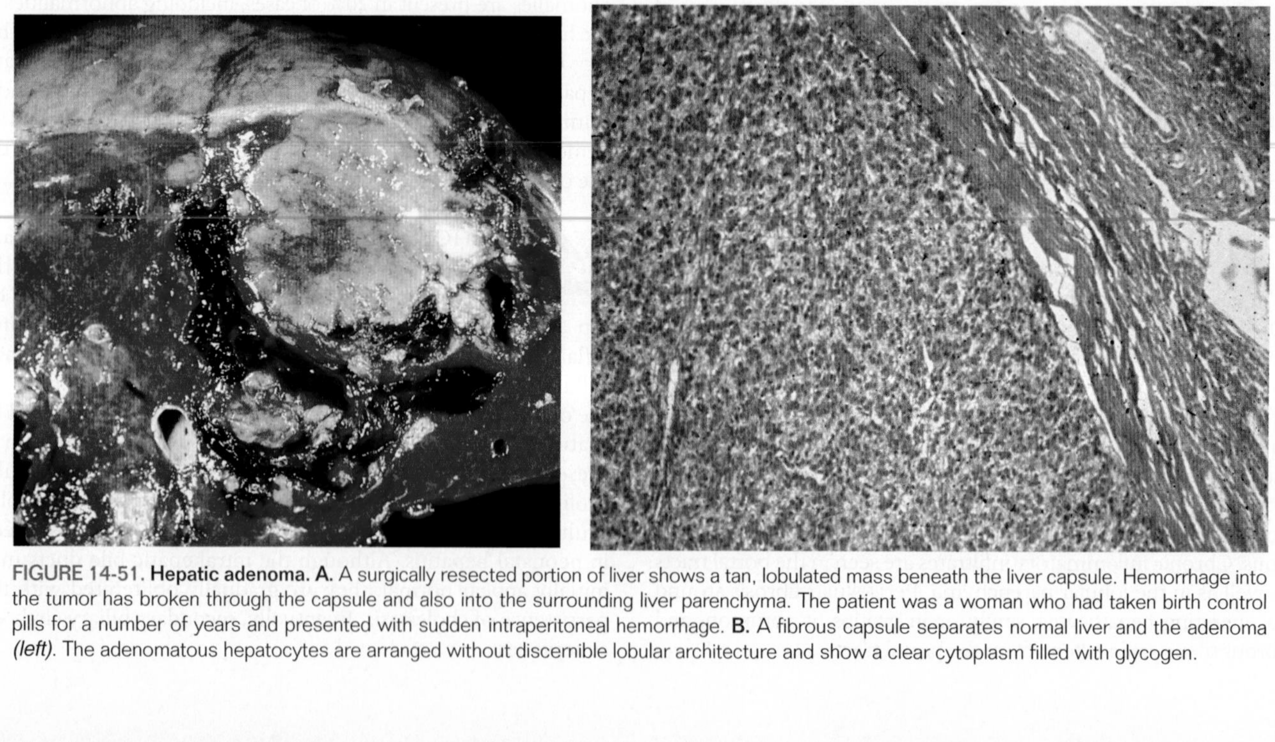

A B

FIGURE 14-51. **Hepatic adenoma. A.** A surgically resected portion of liver shows a tan, lobulated mass beneath the liver capsule. Hemorrhage into the tumor has broken through the capsule and also into the surrounding liver parenchyma. The patient was a woman who had taken birth control pills for a number of years and presented with sudden intraperitoneal hemorrhage. **B.** A fibrous capsule separates normal liver and the adenoma *(left)*. The adenomatous hepatocytes are arranged without discernible lobular architecture and show a clear cytoplasm filled with glycogen.

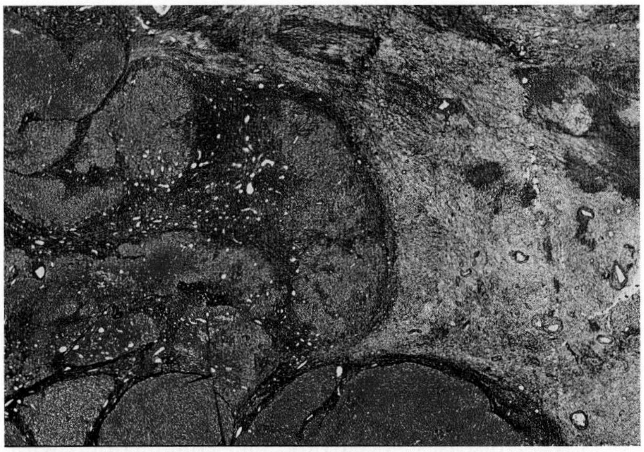

FIGURE 14-52. **Focal nodular hyperplasia.** A photomicrograph of a surgically resected mass from the liver shows a vascular central scar and irregular fibrous septa dissecting hepatic parenchyma, accounting for the resemblance to cirrhosis.

Focal Nodular Hyperplasia Is a Nodular Lesion That Resembles Cirrhosis

The lesion of focal nodular hyperplasia varies from 5 to 15 cm in diameter and weighs as much as 700 g. On occasion, it protrudes from the surface of the liver, and it may even be pedunculated. The cut surface exhibits a characteristic central scar from which fibrous septa radiate. The division of the mass by multiple fibrous septa accounts for the older term "focal cirrhosis." Microscopically, hepatocytic nodules are circumscribed by fibrous septa (Fig. 14-52), which contain numerous tortuous bile ducts and mononuclear inflammatory cells. Within the nodules, lobular architecture is absent. The lesion exhibits large arteries and veins in the septa, but hemorrhage is uncommon.

Focal nodular hyperplasia occurs in both sexes and at all ages but most often in young women. It is not a neoplasm and is not associated with the use of oral contraceptives.

Nodular Regenerative Hyperplasia (Nodular Transformation of the Liver, Partial Nodular Transformation) Causes Portal Hypertension

Nodular regenerative hyperplasia is characterized by small, hyperplastic nodules without fibrosis in an otherwise normal liver. The lesion may be partial and located predominantly in the perihilar region or may be diffuse throughout the liver. The nodules are composed of liver cells arranged in plates that are two and three cells thick, which compress the surrounding parenchyma.

The clinical importance of nodular regenerative hyperplasia relates to its association with portal hypertension, which accounts for the older term **noncirrhotic portal hypertension.** The etiology is unknown, but it has been reported in association with the use of oral contraceptives or anabolic steroids, extrahepatic infections, neoplasms, chronic inflammatory disorders, and autoimmune diseases. Nodular regenerative hyperplasia is not preneoplastic.

Hepatic Hemangiomas Are the Most Common Tumors of the Liver

Benign hemangiomas in the liver occur at all ages and in both sexes and are found in up to 7% of autopsy specimens. They are ordinarily small and asymptomatic, although larger tumors have been reported to cause abdominal symptoms and even hemorrhage into the peritoneal cavity. Grossly, the tumor is usually solitary and less than 5 cm in diameter, but multiple hemangiomas and giant forms have been described. Microscopically, the tumor is similar to cavernous hemangiomas found elsewhere.

Infantile hemangioendothelioma, a rare cellular tumor that appears during the first 2 years of life (and sometimes at birth), contains arteriovenous shunts that may be large enough to cause congestive heart failure. Malignant transformation has been reported in a few cases.

Cystic Disease of the Liver Represents a Spectrum of Lesions

BILE DUCT MICROHAMARTOMAS (vON MEYENBURG COMPLEXES): These clinically inapparent lesions consist of anomalous, small cystic bile ducts embedded in a fibrous stroma. They are usually multiple and vary from barely visible grayish white foci to nodules 1 cm in diameter. Microscopically, the cysts are lined by bile duct epithelium and sometimes contain inspissated bile.

SOLITARY AND MULTIPLE SIMPLE CYSTS: Simple cysts of the liver are lined by cuboidal to columnar epithelium and are occasionally associated with adult polycystic disease of the kidney (see Chapter 16). They are not infrequently seen in livers that contain von Meyenburg complexes.

CONGENITAL HEPATIC FIBROSIS: This recessively inherited disorder is marked by enlarged portal tracts that exhibit extensive fibrosis and numerous bile ductules. It is seen predominantly in children and adolescents. The bile ductules may be so dilated that they resemble microcysts, but even in these cases, they retain their communication with the biliary system. Regenerative nodules are absent, an appearance that distinguishes this condition from cirrhosis. The origin of the lesion is unknown, but it has been postulated that it may result from abnormal differentiation of primitive duct structures. *The principal complication of congenital hepatic fibrosis is severe portal hypertension with recurrent bleeding from esophageal varices.* **Infantile polycystic disease** of the liver resembles congenital hepatic fibrosis and is also inherited as an autosomal recessive trait.

Malignant Tumors of the Liver

Hepatocellular Carcinoma (HCC) Is a Malignant Tumor That Derives from Hepatocytes or Their Precursors

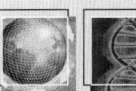

EPIDEMIOLOGY AND PATHOGENESIS: HCC is probably the most common malignant tumor of humans. It occurs in all parts of the world, but its incidence shows a striking geographical variability. In Western industrialized countries, the tumor is uncommon, although the incidence of HCC has nearly doubled in the last 20 years; in sub-Saharan Africa, Southeast Asia, and Japan, the rates are up to 50 times greater. For example, in Mozambique, which seems to have the highest incidence in the world, two thirds of all cancers in men and one third in women are HCC. The incidence of HCC in the United States is expected to rise owing to the increased prevalence of HCV infection.

HEPATITIS B: There is a strong association between HBV infection and HCC. More than 85% of cases of HCC occur in countries with a high prevalence of chronic HBV infection. Most patients have chronic HBV infection for many years, the disease often being transmitted from an infected mother to her newborn child perinatally. Persistent HBV infection is indeed dangerous, since such persons are estimated to have as much as a 200-fold increased risk of developing HCC. One fourth of those with chronic hepatitis B acquired at or near birth ultimately develop HCC. The risk of HCC in men who are positive for HBsAg and HBeAg is about four times as great as in those who are positive only for HBsAg. Most (>80%) cases of HCC associated with HBV infection occur in patients with cirrhosis, although numerous instances are reported in noncirrhotic chronic hepatitis B.

It has been traditionally held that the repeated cycles of liver cell regeneration in chronic hepatitis provides the soil for emergence of a neoplastic clone (see Chapter 5). However, a significant proportion of HBV-associated HCCs develop in patients without cirrhosis. *The genome of HBV is integrated into the host DNA of both the nonneoplastic liver cells and the tumor cells.* The *X* gene of HBV encodes a viral protein (HBxAg) that inactivates tumor suppressor proteins and transactivates certain oncogenes. Additionally, HBV integration by itself may have oncogenic effects. The worldwide use of a vaccine for HBV should significantly decrease the prevalence of HCC in the future.

HEPATITIS C: Although hepatitis C has a lower global prevalence than hepatitis B, the former is associated with most cases of HCC in Europe and North America and has overtaken hepatitis B as a cause of HCC in Japan. In the United States, HCV infection is present in about 50% of HCC. As in hepatitis B, most patients with HCV who develop HCC have underlying cirrhosis. The cumulative rate for HCC in persons with HCV-induced cirrhosis is as high as 70% after 15 years.

The risk of liver cancer in persons who are infected with both HCV and HBV is three times higher than with either alone. The mechanism by which HCV leads to HCC is not understood, but experimental evidence suggests an important role for the interaction of HCV core protein with a variety of cellular proteins.

OTHER CAUSES OF HCC: **Alcoholic cirrhosis** predisposes to HCC, but the risk is not large, and the mechanism is unknown. The strength of this correlation is difficult to estimate owing to high incidence of infection with HBV and HCV in patients with alcoholic cirrhosis. Alcoholics with chronic hepatitis C have as much as a two-fold increased risk for HCC as compared with the risk in HCV infection alone.

Liver diseases occurring in conjunction with **hemochromatosis** and **α_1-AT deficiency** carry a substantial risk of HCC; about 10% of patients with hemochromatosis may be expected to develop the tumor. On the other hand, the incidence of HCC is not increased in patients with "autoimmune" chronic hepatitis and cirrhosis, Wilson disease, and PBC. As in the case of HBV-associated HCC arising in noncirrhotic livers, these observations cast further doubt on the hypothesis that cirrhosis by itself causes neoplastic transformation of hepatocytes.

Aflatoxin B_1, a fungal contaminant of many foods, particularly in less-developed countries, produces HCC in a number of mammalian species. The incidence of liver cancer in humans has also been roughly correlated with the content of aflatoxin in the diet. Studies in China have reported that the presence of urinary metabolites of aflatoxin B_1 is associated with a threefold increased risk of HCC, and the combination of these metabolites with HBV is synergistic, increasing the risk of HCC 60-fold.

Analyses of DNA from HCC in Africa and China, two areas with a high incidence of this cancer, revealed that as many as half of the samples had mutations in the *p53* gene. Interestingly, most of these mutations were G-to-T substitutions in one particular codon (249), a change known to be produced experimentally by aflatoxin B_1.

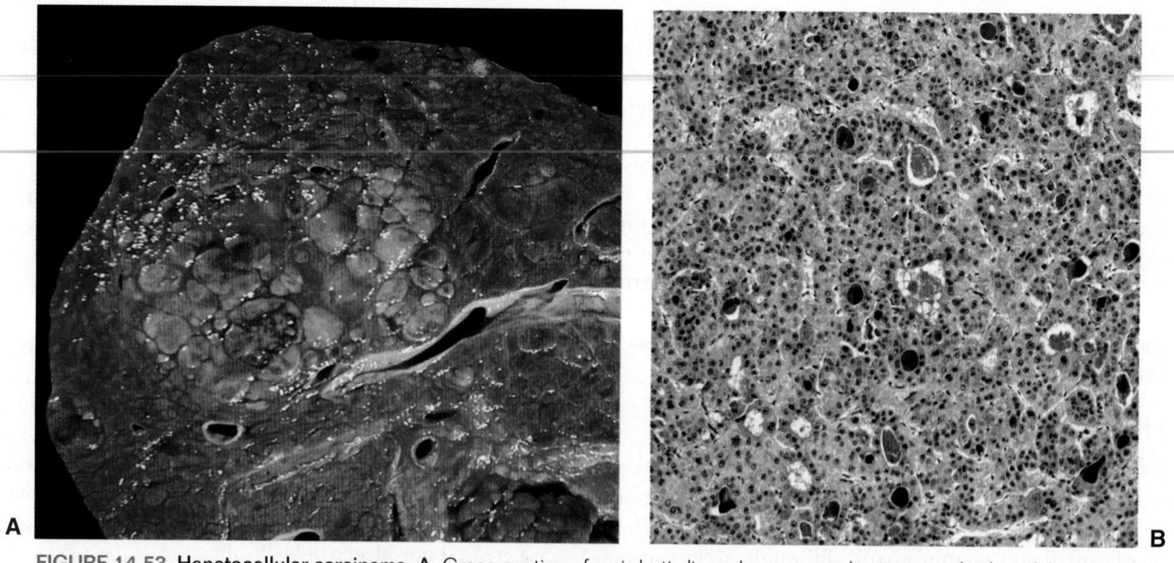

FIGURE 14-53. **Hepatocellular carcinoma. A.** Cross-section of a cirrhotic liver shows a poorly circumscribed, nodular area of yellow, partially hemorrhagic hepatocellular carcinoma. **B.** A photomicrograph of the tumor shows a trabecular pattern of malignant hepatocytes. Many cells are arranged in an acinar pattern and surround concretions of inspissated bile.

PATHOLOGY: HCCs appear grossly as soft, hemorrhagic tan masses in the liver (Fig. 14-53). Occasionally, a green color is present, indicating bile staining. In some cases, a large solitary tumor occupies a portion of the liver; in other cases, many smaller tumors are found. Multiple lesions may indicate a multicentric origin of the tumor, although intrahepatic metastases from a single HCC cannot be excluded. The tumor has a tendency to grow into portal veins and may extend into the vena cava and even the right atrium through the hepatic veins. Metastases occur widely, but the most common sites are the lungs and portal lymph nodes.

The histologic spectrum of HCC is variable, ranging from a well-differentiated tumor difficult to distinguish from normal liver to an anaplastic or undifferentiated appearance. A number of histologic patterns are recognized, but no prognostic significance can be attributed to any of them. Most HCCs exhibit a "trabecular pattern," that is, the tumor cells are arranged in trabeculae or plates that resemble the normal liver. The plates are separated by endothelium-lined sinusoids. A second histologic variant is termed the "pseudoglandular (adenoid, acinar) pattern" (see Fig. 14-53B). In this variety, malignant hepatocytes are arranged around a lumen and thus resemble glands. The lumina may contain bile. The acini formed by the tumor cells are not true glands, and the lesion should not be confused with adenocarcinoma.

***Fibrolamellar HCC** is an uncommon variant that has a distinctive histologic appearance and arises in an apparently normal liver, principally in adolescents and young adults.* The tumor is composed of large, eosinophilic, neoplastic hepatocytes arranged in clusters and surrounded by delicate collagen fibers (Fig. 14-54). The prognosis is considered more favorable than in most cases of HCC, although recent data have called this into question.

CLINICAL FEATURES: HCC usually presents as a painful and enlarging mass in the liver. The prognosis is dismal, and patients die of malignant cachexia, rupture of the tumor with catastrophic bleeding into the peritoneal cavity, or complications of cirrhosis.

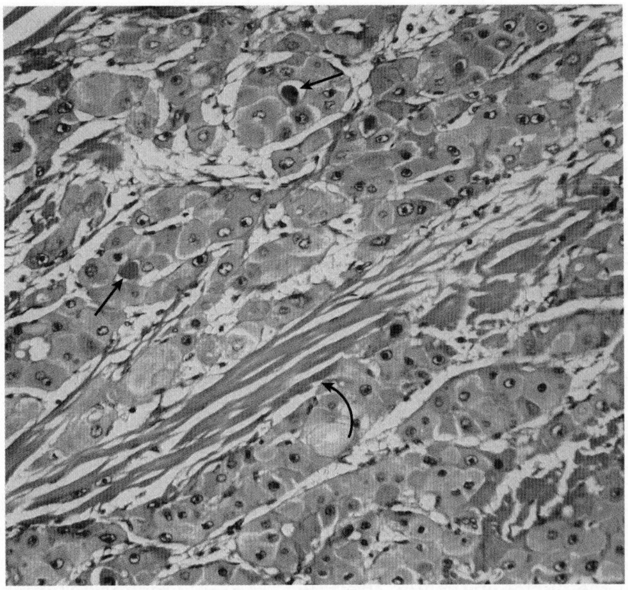

FIGURE 14-54. **Fibrolamellar hepatocellular carcinoma.** Eosinophilic tumor cells show a lamellar pattern. A fibrous band (curved arrow) traverses the tumor. Bile casts (straight arrows) are seen within neoplastic acini.

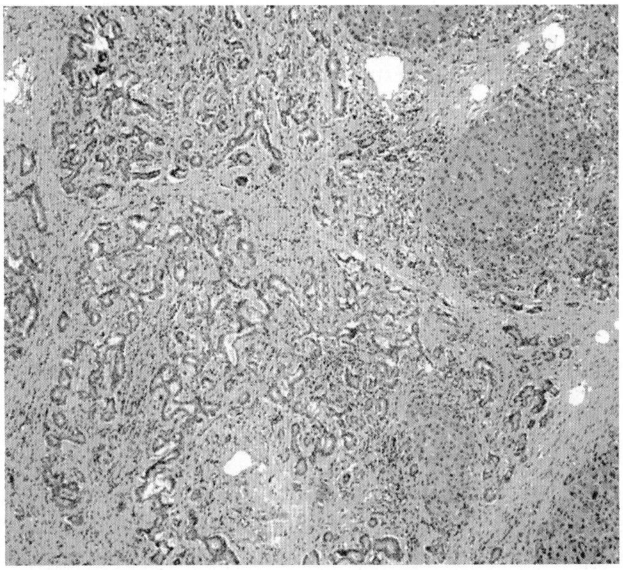

FIGURE 14-55. **Cholangiocarcinoma.** Well-differentiated neoplastic glands are embedded in a dense fibrous stroma.

HCC may be associated with a variety of paraneoplastic manifestations (e.g., polycythemia, hypoglycemia, hypercalcemia) as a result of hormone production by the tumor. α-Fetoprotein levels are often elevated in HCC (and may also be encountered in other neoplastic and non-neoplastic liver diseases and in some extrahepatic disorders).

In the cases of small tumors confined to one hepatic lobe, segmental resections of the liver have been successful in curing HCC in as many as half of patients. Hepatic transplantation has been used for larger tumors with disappointing results.

Cholangiocarcinoma (Bile Duct Carcinoma) Arises from Biliary Epithelium

Cholangiocarcinoma originates anywhere in the biliary tree, from the large intrahepatic bile ducts at the porta hepatis to the smallest bile ductules at the periphery of the hepatic lobule. The tumor occurs predominantly in older persons of both sexes, with an average age at presentation of 60 years. This cancer is particularly frequent in the parts of Asia in which the liver fluke *(Clonorchis sinensis)* is endemic, although cholangiocarcinoma is encountered in all parts of the world. A strong association exists between PSC and cholangiocarcionoma. A quarter of livers with PSC explanted at the time of transplantation have cholangiocarcinoma. Choledochal cysts and Caroli disease are additional risk factors for cholangiocarcinoma.

PATHOLOGY: Peripheral cholangiocarcinomas are composed of small cuboidal cells arranged in a ductular or glandular configuration (Fig. 14-55). Characteristically, they show substantial fibrosis, and on liver biopsy, they may be confused with metastatic scirrhous carcinoma of the breast or pancreas. A combined form of HCC and peripheral cholangiocarcinoma has been labeled **cholangiohepatocellular carcinoma.**

Hilar cholangiocarcinomas are extrahepatic lesions that arise at the convergence of the right and left hepatic ducts. They present in three histologic patterns: (1) a small sclerosing tumor that obliterates the duct, (2) a tumor that spreads within the wall of the duct, and (3) a rare intraductal papillary variant. They produce symptoms of extrahepatic biliary obstruction.

Cholangiocarcinomas show less tendency to invade the portal and hepatic veins than do HCCs. They metastasize to a wide range of extrahepatic sites and show a greater predilection for the portal lymph nodes than do HCCs. Liver transplantation has been attempted in patients with cholangiocarcinoma but is rarely successful in eradicating the tumor. The finding of cholangiocarcionma in livers explanted for PSC carries a dismal prognosis.

Hepatoblastoma Is a Rare Malignant Tumor of Children

Hepatoblastoma is usually discovered at birth or before the age of 3 years.

PATHOLOGY: Hepatoblastoma presents as a partially necrotic and hemorrhagic circumscribed mass up to 25 cm in diameter. Microscopically, cells of epithelial and mesenchymal appearance are seen, but occasionally the latter are missing. The epithelial component of hepatoblastoma includes cells resembling embryonal and fetal cells. The "embryonal" cells are small and fusiform and are arranged in ribbons or rosettes. The "fetal" cells more closely resemble hepatocytes, contain glycogen and fat, and are arranged in trabeculae with intervening sinusoids. Foci of squamous epithelium are occasionally encountered. The mesenchymal elements include those often present in teratomas, including connective tissue, cartilage, and osteoid.

CLINICAL FEATURES: Attention is called to the presence of a hepatoblastoma by enlargement of the abdomen, vomiting, and failure to thrive. The serum α-fetoprotein level is almost invariably elevated, and occasionally secretion of ectopic gonadotropin leads to sexual precocity. Some of these children also exhibit congenital anomalies, including cardiac and renal malformations, hemihypertrophy, and macroglossia. Untreated hepatoblastomas are fatal, but liver transplantation or surgical resection by partial hepatectomy has been curative in many instances.

Hemangiosarcoma May Result from Exposure to Chemicals

Hemangiosarcoma is the only significant sarcoma of the liver. As noted above, this malignant vascular tumor may result from exposure to thorium dioxide, vinyl chloride, or inorganic arsenic. Hemangiosarcoma of the liver is now distinctly uncommon.

PATHOLOGY: On gross examination, hemangiosarcoma is characteristically multicentric, presenting as multiple hemorrhagic nodules that may coalesce. Microscopic examination reveals spindle-shaped, neoplastic, endothelial cells that line the sinusoids and compress the liver cell plates. The neoplasm may form cavernous blood spaces and solid masses of neoplastic cells. Widespread metastases are usual.

CLINICAL FEATURES: Patients with hemangiosarcoma of the liver present with hepatomegaly, jaundice, and ascites. Hematologic abnormalities, including pancytopenia and hemolytic anemia, are often prominent and in many cases reflect splenomegaly from noncirrhotic portal hypertension. The tumor may rupture and bleed vigorously into the abdominal cavity. The prognosis is poor.

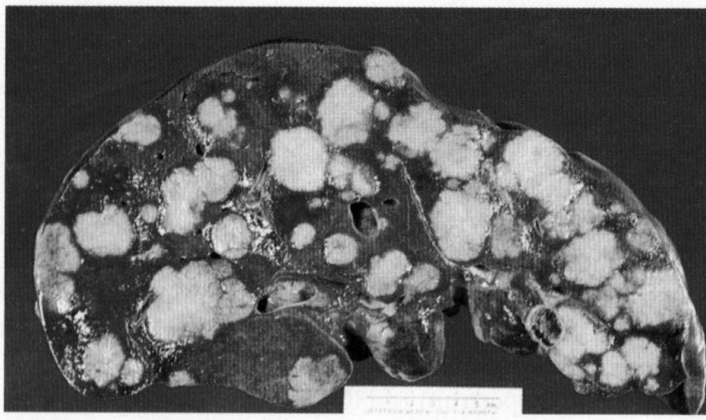

FIGURE 14-56. **Metastatic carcinoma in the liver.** The cut surface of the liver shows many firm, pale masses of metastatic colon cancer.

Metastatic Cancer Is the Most Common Malignant Tumor of the Liver

The liver is involved in a third of all metastatic cancers, including half of those of the gastrointestinal tract, breast, and lung. Other tumors that characteristically metastasize to the liver are pancreatic carcinoma and malignant melanoma, although virtually any cancer may find its way to the liver.

PATHOLOGY: The liver may show only a single nodule of tumor or may be virtually replaced by metastases (Fig. 14-56), and liver weights of 5 kg or more are not uncommon. *In fact, liver metastases are the most common cause of massive hepatomegaly.* Metastatic carcinomas are often seen on the surface of the liver as umbilicated masses, a reflection of central necrosis and hemorrhage. The metastatic deposits tend to be histologically similar to the primary tumor, but on occasion are so undifferentiated that the primary site cannot be determined.

CLINICAL FEATURES: Weight loss is a common early finding in cases of metastatic cancer in the liver. Portal hypertension with splenomegaly, ascites, and gastrointestinal bleeding may occur. Obstruction of the major bile ducts or replacement of most of the liver parenchyma leads to jaundice. If the patient lives long enough, hepatic failure may ensue. Often the first indication of a metastatic tumor is an unexplained increase in the serum alkaline phosphatase level. Most patients die within a year of the diagnosis of liver metastases. However, surgical resection of a solitary metastasis to the liver has often resulted in cures.

Liver Transplantation

The increasing availability of hepatic transplantation and the accompanying problems related to allograft rejection have focused attention on the morphologic criteria by which the outcome can be assessed and therapy recommended. Despite immunosuppressive therapy, some patients subjected to hepatic transplantation develop graft rejection.

PATHOLOGY: Acute rejection features distortion of the bile ducts by a portal inflammatory infiltrate, atypism of bile duct epithelial cells, and often inflammation of the ductal epithelium itself (Fig. 14-57). Lymphocytes often adhere to the endothelium of terminal venules and small branches of the portal veins, with or without subendothelial inflammation (endotheliatitis).

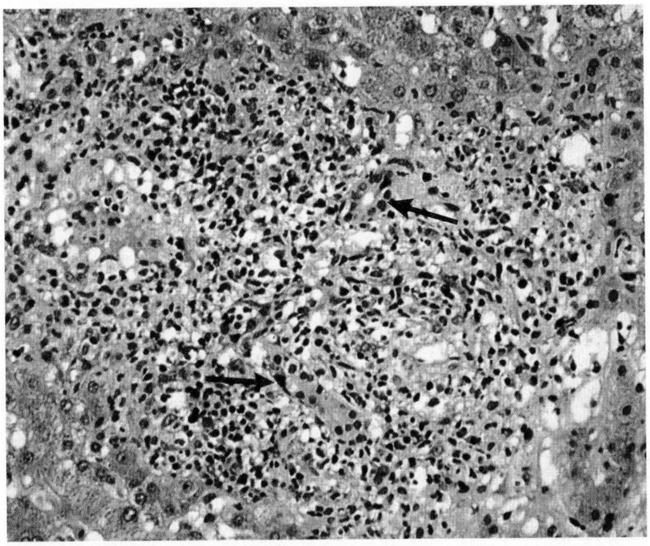

FIGURE 14-57. **Acute rejection of a liver transplant.** A portal tract is expanded by a polymorphous inflammatory infiltrate consisting of large and small lymphocytes, plasma cells, macrophages, and neutrophils. The bile ducts *(arrows)* are damaged.

Allograft rejection persisting for more than 2 months generally exhibits damage to interlobular bile ducts. As the lesion progresses, these small bile ducts are destroyed, and persistent cholestasis ensues. The end stage of this process is referred to as **vanishing bile duct syndrome**. Subintimal foam cells, intimal sclerosis, and myointimal hyperplasia may narrow or occlude these arteries (Fig. 14-58).

THE GALLBLADDER AND EXTRAHEPATIC BILE DUCTS

Anatomy

The gallbladder originates from the same foregut diverticulum that gives rise to the liver. It is a thin elongated sac about 8 cm long and about 50 mL in volume that occupies a fossa on the inferior surface of the liver between the right and the quadrate lobes. The primary function of the gallbladder is the storage, concentration, and release of bile. The cystic duct, which drains the gallbladder into the hepatic duct, is about 3 cm long. Dilute bile from the hepatic duct passes into the gallbladder through the cystic duct, where it is concentrated and subsequently discharged into the common bile duct.

The wall of the gallbladder is composed of a mucous membrane, a muscularis, and an adventitia and is covered by a reflection of the visceral peritoneum. The mucosa is thrown into folds and consists of a columnar epithelium and a lamina propria of loose connective tissue. Dipping into the wall of the gallbladder are mucosal diverticula (**Rokitansky-Aschoff sinuses).**

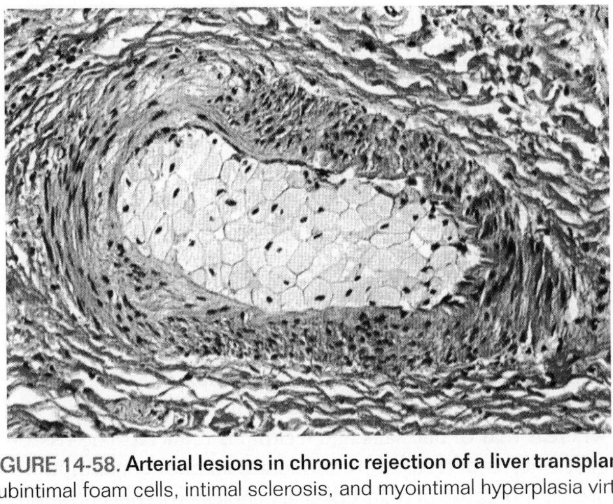

FIGURE 14-58. **Arterial lesions in chronic rejection of a liver transplant.** Subintimal foam cells, intimal sclerosis, and myointimal hyperplasia virtually obliterate the lumen of a hepatic artery.

Congenital Anomalies

Developmental anomalies of the gallbladder are rare and of little clinical significance except for the surgeon. Anomalies of the bile duct include **duplication** and **accessory bile ducts**. Congenital dilations of the bile duct are termed **choledochal cyst** (85% of all cases), **choledochal diverticulum**, and **choledochocele** (Fig. 14-59). Multiple cysts may occur as segmental dilations in the entire extrahepatic biliary tree. Similar multiple dilations in the intrahepatic portion of the biliary tree, termed **Caroli disease**, predispose to bacterial cholangitis. It has been suggested that choledochal cysts form part of the same complex as neonatal hepatitis and biliary atresia.

Cholelithiasis

Cholelithiasis is defined as the presence of stones within the lumen of the gallbladder or in the extrahepatic biliary tree. Three fourths of gallstones in the industrialized countries consist primarily of cholesterol, and the remainder are composed of calcium biliru-

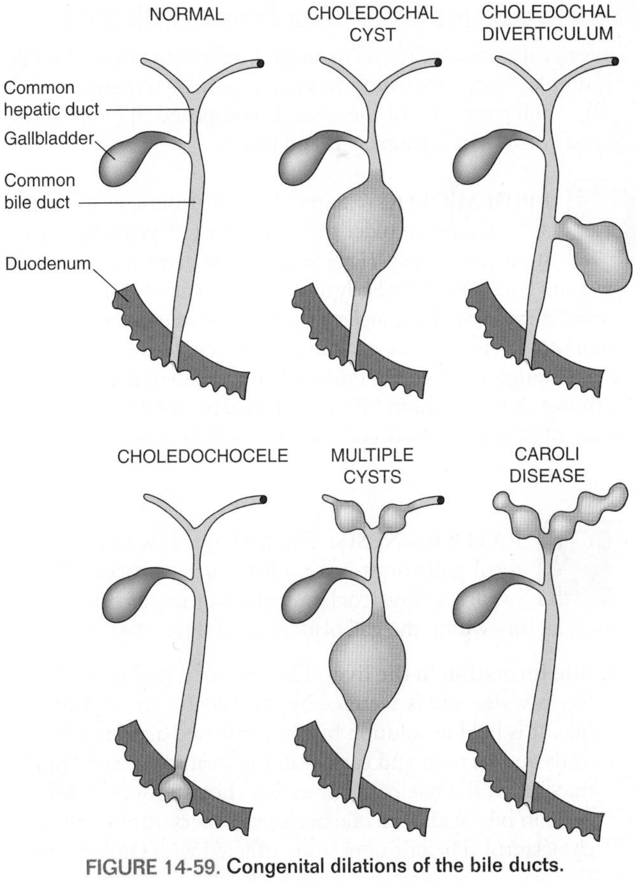

FIGURE 14-59. **Congenital dilations of the bile ducts.**

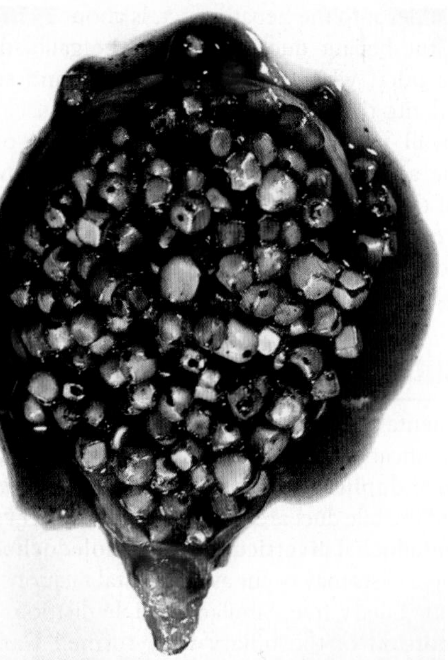

FIGURE 14-60. **Cholesterol gallstones.** The gallbladder has been opened to reveal numerous yellow cholesterol gallstones.

binate and other calcium salts (pigment gallstones). However, pigment stones predominate in the tropics and the Orient. Most gallstones are not radiopaque, but they are readily visualized by ultrasound examination. Although gallstones are frequently asymptomatic, they often cause mild-to-severe pain (**biliary colic**) as a result of impaction in the cystic duct or (less frequently) in the common bile duct.

Cholesterol Stones Are the Most Common Gallstones

Cholesterol stones are round or faceted, yellow to tan, and single or multiple. They vary from 1 to 4 cm in greatest dimension (Fig. 14-60). Well over 50% of the stone is composed of cholesterol; the rest consists of calcium salts and mucin.

EPIDEMIOLOGY: Some 20% of American men and 35% of women older than the age of 75 years have gallstones at autopsy. *However, during their reproductive period, women are three times more likely to develop cholesterol gallstones than are men, the incidence being higher in users of oral contraceptives and in women with several pregnancies.* Interestingly, cholesterol gallstones are exceedingly common in Pima Indian women of the American Southwest, among whom 75% are affected by age 25 and 90% by the age of 60 years. This occurrence may reflect genetic factors.

PATHOGENESIS: The pathogenesis of cholesterol gallstones is a multifactorial process that involves physicochemical qualities of bile and local factors within the gall bladder itself (Fig. 14-61):

- **Bile formation in the liver.** Cholesterol is highly insoluble in water and is secreted by the hepatocytes into the bile. It is held in solution by the combined action of bile acids and lecithin and carried in the form of mixed lipid micelles. If the bile contains excess cholesterol or is deficient in bile acids, the bile becomes supersaturated with cholesterol. The bile of persons afflicted with cholesterol gallstones has more cholesterol and less bile salts as it leaves the liver than that of normal persons, and the supersaturated cholesterol precipitates as solid crystals and forms stones (lithogenic bile). In obese persons, cholesterol secretion by the liver is augmented, further adding to the supersaturation of the bile with cholesterol.
- **Local factors in the gallbladder.** Bile in the gallbladder from patients with gallstones crystallizes more easily than normal. Pronucleating biliary proteins and hypersecretion of gallbladder mucus accelerate the rate of cholesterol precipitation from gallbladder bile.
- **Gallbladder motility.** Impaired gallbladder motor function leads to bile stasis and permits the formation of biliary sludge, which then progresses to macroscopic stones.

The higher prevalence of gallstones in premenopausal women has been attributed to the fact that estrogens stimulate the formation of lithogenic bile by the liver. Estrogens increase the hepatic secretion of cholesterol and decrease the secretion of bile acids. These effects are augmented during pregnancy because the gallbladder empties more slowly in the last trimester, thereby causing stasis and increasing the opportunity for precipitation of cholesterol crystals. Indeed, progesterone, the predominant hormone of pregnancy, inhibits the discharge of bile from the gallbladder. These mechanisms are also invoked to explain the increased incidence of gallstones in users of oral contraceptives.

Other major risk factors for the development of cholesterol gallstones can be divided into those that relate to increased biliary cholesterol secretion, those that contribute to decreased secretion of bile salts and lecithin, and those that reflect a combination of the two.

Risk factors associated with **increased biliary cholesterol secretion** include the following:

- Increasing age
- Obesity
- Membership in certain ethnic groups (e.g., Chilean women, some northern European groups)
- Familial predisposition
- Diet high in calories and cholesterol
- Certain metabolic abnormalities associated with high blood cholesterol levels (e.g., diabetes, some genetic hyperlipoproteinemias, and PBC)

There is a linear correlation between the magnitude of obesity and the risk of symptomatic gallstones, reaching a value as high as five times the risk in nonobese persons. Hepatic cholesterol synthesis is stimulated by insulin, and the increased biliary excretion of cholesterol associated with obesity may relate to the hyperinsulinism that accompanies increased body fat.

Decreased secretion of bile salts and lecithin occurs in nonobese whites who develop gallstones. Gastrointestinal absorptive disorders that interfere with the enterohepatic circulation of bile acids (e.g., pancreatic insufficiency secondary to cystic fibrosis and Crohn disease) also decrease secretion of bile acids and favor gallstone formation.

In American Pima Indians and in people who take certain drugs (e.g., clofibrate), cholesterol synthesis increases, whereas that of bile salts and lecithin is reduced. The risk of gallstones is decreased by moderate alcohol consumption, probably because of reduced biliary cholesterol concentration.

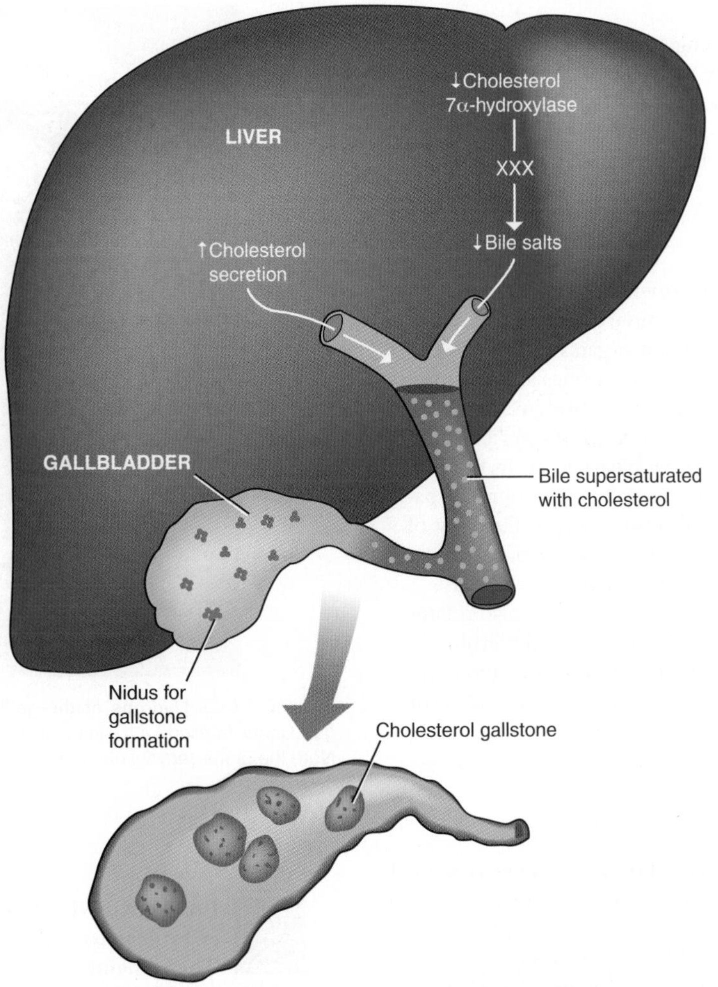

FIGURE 14-61. **Pathogenesis of cholesterol gallstones.**

Pigment Stones Are Classed As Black or Brown Stones

Black Pigment Stones

Black pigment stones are irregular and measure less than 1 cm across. On cross-section, the surface appears glassy (Fig. 14-62). Black stones contain calcium bilirubinate, bilirubin polymers, calcium salts, and mucin.

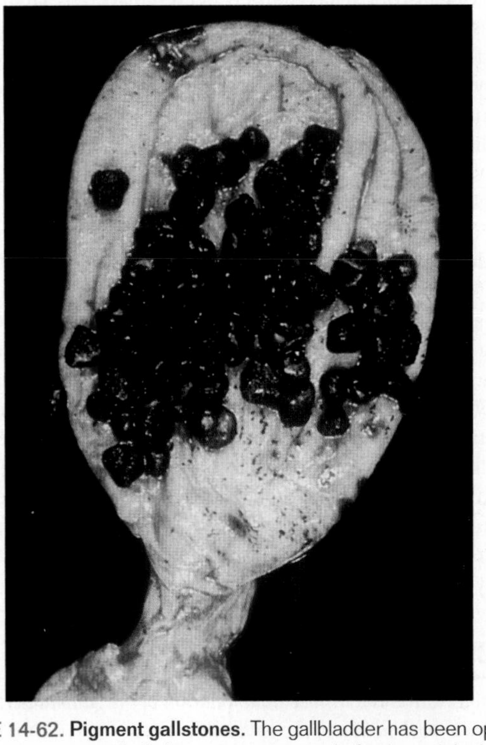

FIGURE 14-62. **Pigment gallstones.** The gallbladder has been opened to reveal numerous small, dark stones composed of calcium bilirubinate.

PATHOGENESIS: The incidence of black stones is increased in older or undernourished persons, but no correlations with gender, ethnicity, or obesity have been made. Chronic hemolysis, such as occurs with sickle cell anemia and thalassemia, predisposes to the development of black pigment stones. Cirrhosis, either because it leads to increased hemolysis or because of damage to liver cells, is also associated with a high incidence of black stones. However, in most instances, no predisposing cause for the formation of black pigment stones is evident.

Unconjugated bilirubin is insoluble in bile and is usually present in only trace amounts. When increased amounts are secreted by the hepatocyte, the unconjugated bilirubin precipitates as calcium bilirubinate, probably around a nidus of mucinous glycoproteins. For unexplained reasons, patients without known predisposing factors who develop black pigment stones have increased concentrations of unconjugated bilirubin in the bile.

Brown Pigment Stones

Brown pigment stones are spongy and laminated and contain principally calcium bilirubinate mixed with cholesterol and calcium soaps of fatty acids. In contrast to the other types of gallstones, brown pigment stones are found more frequently in the intrahepatic and extrahepatic bile ducts than in the gallbladder.

PATHOGENESIS: Brown stones are almost always associated with bacterial cholangitis, in which *E. coli* is the predominant organism. Rare or uncommon in Western countries, brown stones are not infrequent in Asia, where they are almost entirely restricted to persons infested with *Ascaris lumbricoides* or *Clonorchis sinensis,* helminths that may invade the biliary tract. In the rare cases in Western countries, brown stones are found in patients with chronic mechanical obstruction to the flow of bile, as in sclerosing cholangitis or the presence of a catheter in the common bile duct after common bile duct surgery.

The pathogenesis of brown pigment stones also relates to an increased concentration of unconjugated bilirubin in the bile. Conjugated bilirubin is hydrolyzed to unconjugated bilirubin by the action of bacterial β-glucuronidase or other hydrolytic enzymes.

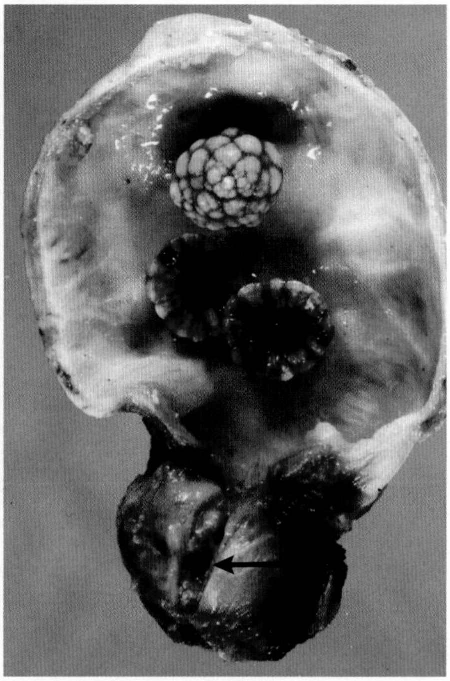

FIGURE 14-63. **Hydrops of the gallbladder.** The lumen of the dilated gallbladder is filled with clear mucus and contains cholesterol stones. Note the stone *(arrow)* obstructing the cystic duct.

CLINICAL FEATURES OF GALLSTONES Gallstones may remain "silent" in the gallbladder for many years, and few patients ever die of cholelithiasis itself. The 15-year cumulative probability that asymptomatic stones will lead to biliary pain or other complications is less than 20%. Medical treatment of gallstones, including the oral administration of bile acids, and extracorporeal lithotripsy (ultrasonic disruption of gallstones) have largely been replaced by laparoscopic cholecystectomy.

Most of the complications of cholelithiasis relate to the obstruction of the cystic duct or common bile duct by gallstones. Passage of a stone into the cystic duct often, but not invariably, causes severe biliary colic and may lead to acute cholecystitis. Repeated episodes of acute cholecystitis then produce chronic cholecystitis. The latter condition can also result from the presence of stones alone. Gallstones may pass into the common duct (**choledocholithiasis**), where they may lead to obstructive jaundice, cholangitis, and pancreatitis. In fact, in populations in whom alcoholism is not a factor, gallstones are the most common cause of acute pancreatitis. Passage of a large gallstone into the small intestine has been known to cause intestinal obstruction, a condition called **gallstone ileus**. In obstruction of the cystic duct, with or without acute cholecystitis, the bile in the gallbladder is reabsorbed, to be replaced by a clear mucinous fluid secreted by the gallbladder epithelium. The term **hydrops of the gallbladder (mucocele)** (Fig. 14-63) is applied to the distended and palpable gallbladder, which may become secondarily infected.

Acute Cholecystitis

Acute cholecystitis is a diffuse inflammation of the gallbladder, usually secondary to obstruction of the gallbladder outlet.

PATHOGENESIS: *Some 90% of cases of acute cholecystitis are associated with the presence of gallstones.* The remaining cases (**acalculous cholecystitis**) occur in conjunction with sepsis, severe trauma, infection of the gallbladder with *Salmonella typhosa,* and polyarteritis nodosa. Bacterial infection is usually secondary to biliary obstruction, rather than a primary event.

It has been theorized that obstruction of the cystic duct by a gallstone leads to the release of phospholipase from the epithelium of the gallbladder. In turn, this enzyme may hydrolyze lecithin and release lysolecithin, a membrane-active toxin. At the same time, disruption of the mucous coat of the epithelium renders the mucosal cells vulnerable to damage by the detergent action of concentrated bile salts. Bile supersaturated with cholesterol may be toxic to the epithelium.

PATHOLOGY: The external surface of the gallbladder in acute cholecystitis is congested and layered with a fibrinous exudate. The wall is remarkably thickened by edema, and opening the viscus reveals a fiery red or purple mucosa. Gallstones are usually found within the lumen, and a stone is often seen obstructing the cystic duct. On rare occasions, when obstruction of the cystic duct is complete and bacteria have invaded the gallbladder, the cavity may be distended by cloudy, purulent fluid, a condition termed **empyema of the gallbladder.**

Microscopically, edema and hemorrhage in the wall are striking, with accompanying acute and chronic inflammation (Fig. 14-64). Secondary bacterial infection may lead to suppuration in the gallbladder wall. The mucosa shows focal ulcerations

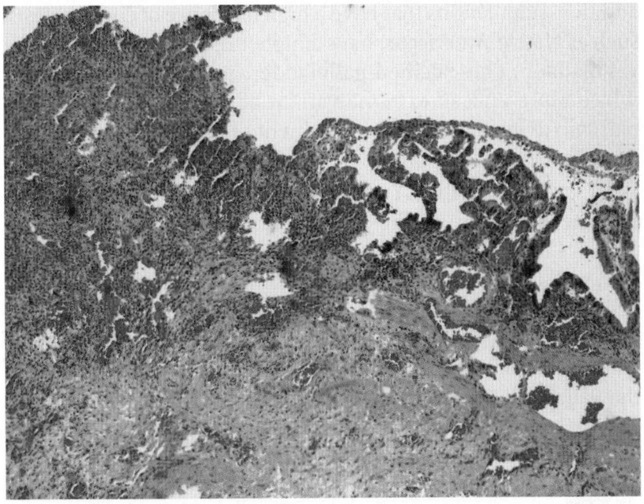

FIGURE 14-64. **Acute cholecystitis.** A photomicrograph of a gallbladder removed from a patient with acute cholecystitis demonstrates ulceration of the mucosa, edema, and acute and chronic inflammation.

or, in severe cases, widespread necrosis, in which case the term **gangrenous cholecystitis** is applied.

Perforation is a feared complication in severe cases and may occur after secondary bacterial infection, most commonly of the fundus. Discharge of bile into the abdominal cavity results in **bile peritonitis**. More commonly, the contents of the perforated gallbladder are localized by inflammatory adhesions, a lesion known as a **pericholecystic abscess.** The gallbladder contents may also erode into the small or large intestine, creating a **cholecystenteric fistula.**

CLINICAL FEATURES: The initial symptom of acute cholecystitis is abdominal pain in the right upper quadrant, and most patients have already experienced episodes of biliary colic. Mild jaundice, caused by stones in, or edema of, the common bile duct, is evident in 20% of patients. In most cases, the acute illness subsides within a week, but persistent pain, fever, leukocytosis, and shaking chills indicate progression of the acute cholecystitis and the need for cholecystectomy. As the inflammatory process resolves, the gallbladder wall becomes fibrotic and the mucosa heals. However, the function of the gallbladder usually remains impaired.

Chronic Cholecystitis

Chronic cholecystitis, the most common disease of the gallbladder, is a persistent inflammation of the gallbladder wall that is almost invariably associated with gallstones. Chronic cholecystitis may also result from repeated attacks of acute cholecystitis. In the latter case, the pathogenesis probably relates to chronic irritation and chemical injury to the gallbladder epithelium.

PATHOLOGY: Grossly, the wall of the chronically inflamed gallbladder is thickened and firm (Fig. 14-65A), and the serosal surface may show fibrous adhesions to surrounding structures as a result of previous episodes of acute cholecystitis. Gallstones are usually found within the lumen, and the bile often contains gravel or sludge (i.e., fine precipitates of calculous material). The bile is infected with coliform organisms in about half of cases. The mucosa may be focally ulcerated and atrophic or may appear intact. Microscopically, the wall is fibrotic and often penetrated by sinuses of Rokitansky-Aschoff (see Fig. 14-65B). Chronic inflammation of variable degree may be seen in all layers. In long-standing chronic cholecystitis, the wall of the gallbladder may become calcified (**porcelain gallbladder**).

CLINICAL FEATURES: Many patients with chronic cholecystitis complain of nonspecific abdominal symptoms, although it is not at all clear that these are

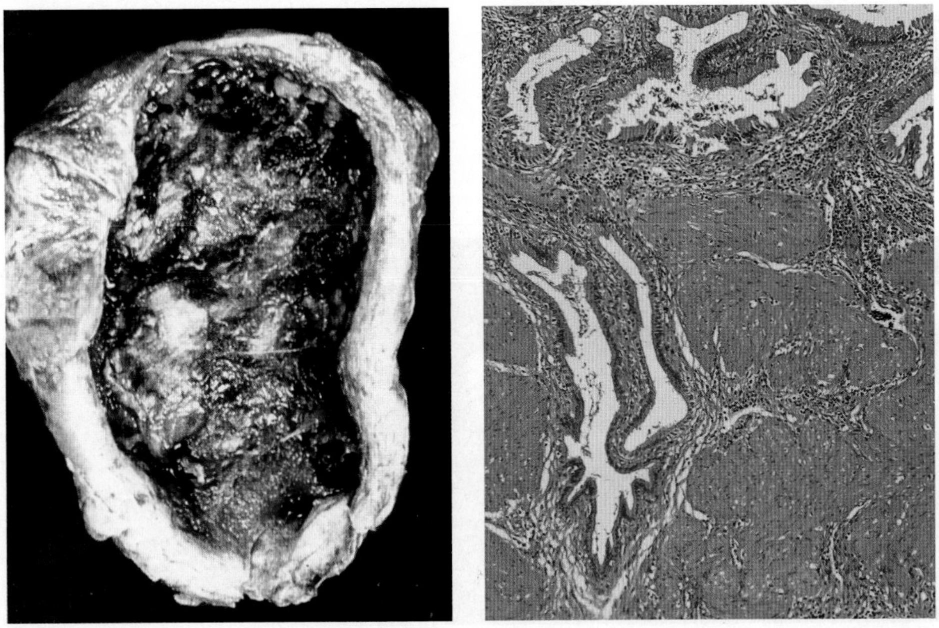

A B

FIGURE 14-65. **Chronic cholecystitis. A.** The gallbladder is thickened and fibrotic, and the lumen contains several gallstones. **B.** A photomicrograph of (A) shows chronic inflammation of the gallbladder and a sinus of Rokitansky-Aschoff extending into the muscularis.

necessarily related to the gallbladder disease. On the other hand, pain in the right hypochondrium is typical and often episodic. The diagnosis is best made by ultrasound examination, which demonstrates gallstones in a thick, contracted gallbladder. Cholecystectomy is the definitive treatment.

Cholesterolosis

Cholesterolosis of the gallbladder is defined as the accumulation of cholesterol-laden macrophages within the submucosa. It is a common incidental finding at autopsy but is not ordinarily associated with symptoms. Cholesterolosis is often associated with the presence of bile supersaturated with cholesterol. Grossly, the appearance of scattered, yellow mucosal flecks accounts for the term "strawberry gallbladder." Microscopically, the mucosal folds are swollen with large, foamy macrophages, in which a small nucleus is displaced to the periphery.

Tumors

Benign Tumors of the Gallbladder and Extrahepatic Biliary Ducts Are Rare

Papillomas are the most common benign tumors of the gallbladder and may be single or multiple. In three fourths of cases, they are associated with gallstones. The combination of smooth muscle proliferation and an adenoma has been termed **adenomyoma**. Fibromas, lipomas, leiomyomas, and myxomas have also been recorded. The bile ducts are affected by the same benign tumors that occur in the gallbladder. Such tumors are clinically more important because they may obstruct biliary flow and cause jaundice.

Adenocarcinoma Is the Most Common Tumor of the Gallbladder

Adenocarcinoma of the gallbladder is not rare, being incidentally found in 2% of patients who undergo gallbladder surgery. *Because this cancer is usually associated with cholelithiasis and chronic cholecystitis, it is considerably more common in women than in men.* In addition, populations that have a high incidence of cholelithiasis, such as Native Americans, have a higher risk of carcinoma of the gallbladder. The calcified gallbladder (porcelain gallbladder), which represents an extreme variant of chronic cholecystitis, is particularly prone to the development of gallbladder cancer.

PATHOLOGY: Gallbladder carcinoma may occur anywhere in the gallbladder but most frequently appears in the fundus. The tumor is characteristically an infiltrative, well-differentiated adenocarcinoma (Fig. 14-66). It is usually desmoplastic, and thus the wall of the gallbladder becomes thickened and leathery. Anaplastic, giant cell, and spindle cell forms of gallbladder carcinoma are reported. The rich lymphatic plexus of the gallbladder provides the most common route of metastasis, although vascular dissemination and direct spread into the liver and contiguous structures occur.

CLINICAL FEATURES: The symptoms produced by carcinoma of the gallbladder are similar to those encountered with gallstone disease. However, by the time the tumor becomes symptomatic, it is almost invariably incurable, the 5-year survival rate being less than 3%. For practical purposes, surgical cure is obtained only in patients who undergo cholecystectomy for gallbladder disease in whom the cancer is an incidental finding.

Carcinoma of the Bile Duct and the Ampulla of Vater Present As Obstructive Jaundice

Cancer of the extrahepatic bile ducts (extrahepatic cholangiocarcinoma; see above) is almost always adenocarcinoma. It may occur anywhere along the length of the bile duct, including the location where the right and left hepatic ducts join to form the common hepatic duct.

The tumor is less common than gallbladder cancer, and the female predominance of gallbladder cancer is not evident. Gallstones are frequently found in those affected, and there is an association with inflammatory disease of the colon. The tumor has also been reported to arise in choledochal cysts and in Caroli disease. In the Orient, bile duct carcinoma is associated with biliary

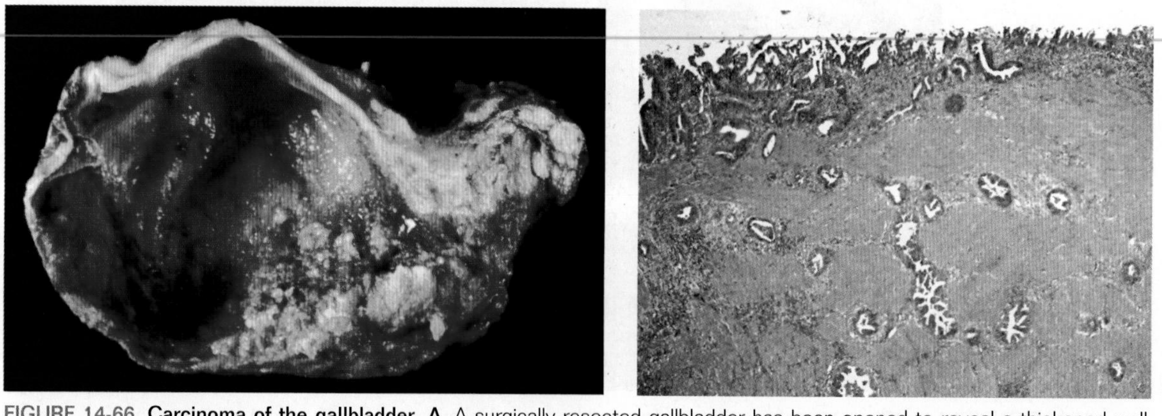

A B

FIGURE 14-66. **Carcinoma of the gallbladder. A.** A surgically resected gallbladder has been opened to reveal a thickened wall infiltrated by adenocarcinoma, which also demonstrates exophytic growth into the lumen. **B.** The gallbladder wall is infiltrated by a moderately differentiated adenocarcinoma, which has stimulated a desmoplastic response.

infestation by the fluke *Clonorchis sinensis*. As in carcinoma of the gallbladder, growth may be endophytic (into the lumen) or diffusely infiltrative. The prognosis is poor, but because symptoms arise early in the course of the disease, the outcome is somewhat better than that of gallbladder carcinoma.

Adenocarcinoma of the ampulla of Vater may also obstruct the bile duct. The initial symptom is again obstructive jaundice, although a few patients present with pancreatitis. In contrast to bile duct carcinoma, surgical treatment of cancer of the ampulla of Vater leads to a 35% 5-year survival rate.

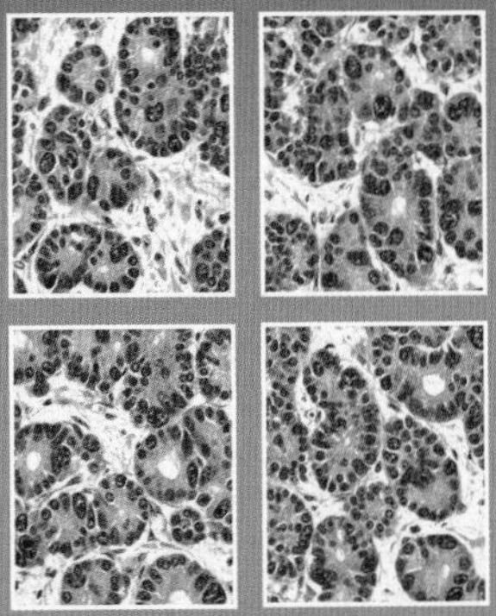

15 The Pancreas

Gregory Y. Lauwers
Mari Mino-Kenudson
Raphael Rubin

Anatomy And Physiology

Pancreatic development begins at 4 weeks as two endodermal outpouchings on the dorsal and ventral sides of the embryonic duodenal tube. The duct systems of the two embryonic pancreatic anlagen merge at 7 weeks, giving rise to a main pancreatic duct (**duct of Wirsung**). A remnant of the dorsal duct anlage commonly persists as the **duct of Santorini.** The ducts branch into elongate ductules, which arborize to form a complex ductal system. Acinar cells arise from the ductules and acquire their distinctive zymogen granules. Islet cells are also derived from larger ducts and acquire small, dense, secretory granules characteristic of the endocrine pancreas.

The pancreas is a mixed exocrine/endocrine gland that lies transversely in the upper abdomen, cradled between the loop of the duodenum and the hilum of the spleen. It is retroperitoneal, behind the lesser omental sac and the stomach. This location renders it largely inaccessible to physical examination. The adult pancreas is 10 to 15 cm long and weighs 60 to 150 g. It is divided into three anatomical subdivisions: (1) **the head** lies in the concavity of the duodenum and extends to the superior mesenteric vessels immediately behind the organ, (2) **the body** includes most of the gland, and (3) a tapered **tail** ends at the hilum of the spleen.

Exocrine pancreatic secretions drain into the duct of Wirsung, which usually empties into the common bile duct immediately proximal to the ampulla of Vater. The common channel that carries bile and pancreatic secretions into the duodenum is invested with a circular complex of smooth muscle fibers that condense into the sphincter of Oddi as they pass through the duodenal wall. The accessory duct of Santorini opens in the minor papilla.

Exocrine tissue makes up 80% to 85% of the pancreas and consists of secretory cells organized as acini that connect with ductules. Pancreatic acini are composed of a single layer of pyramidal cells, whose basophilic cytoplasm is filled with acidophilic zymogen granules. By electron microscopy, acinar cells exhibit conspicuous rough endoplasmic reticulum, a prominent Golgi apparatus, and numerous electron-dense zymogen granules in the apex of the cell. *Acinar cells synthesize some 20 different digestive enzymes, mostly in the form of inactive proenzymes.* These are secreted and activated in the intestine after neural and hormonal stimulation, and include trypsin, chymotrypsin, carboxypeptidase, phospholipase, and elastase. Amylase and lipase are secreted in their active forms. The daily secretion of 1.5 to 3 liters of pancreatic juice attests to the remarkable synthetic and secretory capacity of the exocrine pancreas.

The endocrine pancreas is organized into islets distributed throughout the organ but comprising only 1% to 2% of the total pancreatic mass. Islets contain several cell types, each of which synthesizes one or more hormones, including insulin and glucagon, among others, which are secreted directly into the blood (see below). The major endocrine disease of the pancreas, diabetes mellitus, is discussed in Chapter 22.

Congenital Anomalies

Developmental defects of the pancreas are rarely of clinical significance.

PANCREAS DIVISUM: Pancreas divisum, the most common congenital anomaly, results from failure of the two pancreatic rudiments to fuse, leading to the formation of two separate glands, each with its own duct draining into the duodenum. Consequently, the main pancreatic anlage is drained by the canal of Santorini. Chronic pancreatitis develops in up to 25% of persons with pancreas divisum.

HETEROTOPIC PANCREAS: In this anomaly, there is pancreatic tissue outside its normal location, most commonly localized in the wall of the duodenum, stomach, and jejunum. It is an incidental finding in 2% to 15% of autopsies. The heterotopic tissue contains most or all components of normal pancreas, namely, acini, ducts, and islets. Malignant transformation has been rarely reported.

ANNULAR PANCREAS: In this uncommon condition, the pancreatic head surrounds the second portion of the duodenum; encirclement may be complete or partial. Such infants frequently have other congenital anomalies, including trisomy 21 (Down syndrome). Annular pancreas may be associated with duodenal atresia, an anomaly that requires surgery immediately after birth. About half of patients with annular pancreas do not require surgery in early life but develop symptoms at 60 or 70 years of age.

CYSTS: True cysts of the pancreas are believed to arise from faulty development of pancreatic ducts. There is an association with other anatomic anomalies, including renal tubular dysplasia, anorectal malformations, polydactyly, and thoracic dystrophy.

PARTIAL AND COMPLETE PANCREATIC AGENESIS: Homozygous germline mutations of the homeodomain transcription factor IPF1 (PDX1) have been reported in these rare conditions.

Acute Pancreatitis

Pancreatitis is an inflammatory condition of the exocrine pancreas that results from injury to acinar cells. The devastation of acute pancreatitis was justly described by Lord Moynihan in 1925 as the "most terrible of all calamities [of] the abdominal viscera. The suddenness of its onset, the illimitable agony which accompanies it and the mortality attendant upon it render it a formidable disease." For unknown reasons, the incidence of acute pancreatitis has increased ten-fold in the past few decades.

Pancreatitis presents in a variety of clinical forms. At one end of the spectrum is a mild, self-limited disease, with acute inflammation and stromal edema, and little or no acinar cell necrosis. At the other extreme is a severe, sometimes fatal, acute hemorrhagic pancreatitis with massive necrosis. Repeated episodes of acute pancreatitis may lead to chronic pancreatitis, which is characterized by recurrent attacks of severe abdominal pain and progressive fibrosis, ultimately leading to pancreatic insufficiency. However, no acute episodes are recognized clinically in about half of the cases of chronic pancreatitis.

Interstitial or **edematous pancreatitis** is a mild and presumably reversible form of acute pancreatitis. An infiltrate of polymorphonuclear leukocytes and edema of the connective tissue between lobules of acinar cells constitute the initial lesion. There is no necrosis or hemorrhage. It is usually well-managed medically.

Acute hemorrhagic pancreatitis usually occurs in middle age, with a peak incidence at 60 years. Alcoholism (more commonly in men) or chronic biliary disease (more often in women) account for over 80% of cases. Acute pancreatitis erupts abruptly, usually after a heavy meal or excessive alcohol intake, and is associated with high morbidity and mortality.

PATHOGENESIS: Acinar cell injury and duct obstruction are the major causes of acute pancreatitis. These processes lead to inappropriate extracellular leakage of activated digestive enzymes and consequent autodigestion of pancreatic and extrapancreatic tissues. A number of factors have been implicated in acute pancreatitis.

ACTIVATED PANCREATIC ENZYMES: Acinar cells are shielded from the potentially destructive action of their digestive enzymes (proteases, nucleases, amylase, lipase, and phospholipase A) by three mechanisms.

1. Various enzymes are physically isolated from cytoplasmic components by an intricate, intracellular, cavitary system of endoplasmic reticulum, Golgi complex, and zymogen granule membranes.
2. Many of the digestive enzymes are synthesized as inactive forms (e.g., chymotrypsinogen, proelastase, prophospholipase, and trypsinogen).
3. Specific enzyme inhibitors tend to protect the pancreas.

Trypsin activation is central to the pathogenesis of acute pancreatitis. By itself, trypsin does not produce cell necrosis, but it activates other pancreatic proenzymes, including prophospholipase A_2 and proelastase. Under the appropriate circumstances, phospholipase A_2 attacks membrane phospholipids (yielding lysolecithin) to cause necrosis, and elastase digests blood vessel walls, causing hemorrhage. Liberation of pancreatic lipase into the interstitium contributes to fat necrosis. *Inappropriate activation of pancreatic proenzymes occurs in all forms of pancreatitis.*

SECRETION AGAINST OBSTRUCTION: Most enzymes secreted by acinar cells are discharged into the ductal system and enter the duodenum. A small amount diffuses back into periductular extracellular fluid and eventually into plasma. Any condition that narrows the lumina of pancreatic ducts or impairs the easy outflow of exocrine secretions can raise intraductal pressure and exacerbate back-diffusion across the ducts. This phenomenon is suspected to cause inappropriate activation of digestive proenzymes. Heavy meals may lead to release of pancreatic secretagogues, and so augment production of pancreatic enzymes.

Gallstones can cause pancreatic duct obstruction. Some 45% of all patients with acute pancreatitis also have cholelithiasis. *About 5% of patients with gallstones develop acute pancreatitis and the risk of developing acute pancreatitis in patients with gallstones is 25 times higher than in the general population.* Also, unless gallstones are eliminated after the first attack, recurrent acute pancreatitis occurs in half the cases. However, fewer than 5% of patients with acute pancreatitis have impacted stones at the ampulla of Vater, and the reason for the association between pancreatitis and cholelithiasis remains obscure. Neither ligation of the pancreatic duct nor its occlusion by tumor causes acute pancreatitis. It has been suggested that the reflux of bile or duodenal contents into the pancreatic duct may lead to pancreatitis, but there is little evidence to support this theory.

Anatomic anomalies (e.g., pancreas divisum) and **neoplasms** (ampullary and pancreatic neoplasms) can also lead to acute pancreatitis

PROTEASE INHIBITORS: The various inhibitors of proteolytic enzymes present in many body fluids and tissues constitute a defense against inappropriate activation of pancreatic proenzymes. Four potent protease inhibitors have been identified in human plasma: α_1-antitrypsin, α_2-macroglobulin, C_1 esterase inhibitor and pancreatic secretory trypsin inhibitor. Despite the variety of trypsin inhibitors in different body compartments, the protection they render is clearly incomplete. Since trypsin activates other pancreatic proenzymes, its incomplete inhibition in pancreatic juice poses a hazard.

ETHANOL: *Chronic alcohol abuse accounts for one third of cases of acute pancreatitis, although only 5% of chronic alcoholics develop this complication.* Ethanol is well recognized as a chemical toxin, but a significant injurious effect on pancreatic acinar or duct cells has yet to be demonstrated. Ethanol consumption may adversely affect the pancreas by causing spasm or acute edema of the sphincter of Oddi, especially after an alcoholic binge. It also stimulates secretion from the small intestine, which triggers the exocrine pancreas to release pancreatic juice. When these effects occur together (enhanced secretion into an obstructed duct), the results may be disastrous.

OTHER CAUSES OF PANCREATITIS: Other rare causes of acute pancreatitis are:

- **Viruses,** such as mumps, coxsackievirus, and cytomegalovirus can cause pancreatitis. The incidence of acute pancreatitis is particularly high in patients with acquired immunodeficiency syndrome (AIDS) owing to human immunodeficiency virus (HIV) itself, or, most commonly, cytomegalovirus infection.
- **Therapeutic drugs,** of which more than 85 have been reported to cause acute pancreatitis. These include immunosuppressive drugs (e.g., azathioprine), antineoplastic agents, estrogens, sulfonamides, and diuretics. The mechanisms of pancreatic injury by these compounds are unclear.
- **Blunt trauma** to the upper abdomen can cause contusive injury to the pancreas, with leakage of digestive enzymes into the pancreas and peripancreatic tissues. Patients undergoing endoscopic retrograde cholangiopancreatography (ERCP) occasionally develop acute pancreatitis.
- **Acute ischemia** due to shock, vasculitis, and thrombosis may injure the pancreas.
- **Hyperlipidemia** can induce acute pancreatitis. The mechanism is thought to involve hydrolysis of triglycerides in the extracellular space by inappropriate leakage of lipase by pancreatic cells. Released free fatty acids are cytotoxic.
- **Hypercalcemia,** regardless of cause, is associated with acute pancreatitis. **Obesity** is a risk factor for pancreatitis, especially for severe disease. Obese persons have increased deposition of peripancreatic fat, which may predispose them to more extensive fat necrosis after local release of pancreatic lipase.
- **Idiopathic pancreatitis** is still the third most common form of the disease, accounting for 10% to 20% of all cases.
- **Parasites** (e.g., *Ascariasis*), bacteria (e.g., *Mycoplasma* species), and **pregnancy** are rare causes of acute pancreatitis.

Factors involved in the pathogenesis of acute hemorrhagic pancreatitis are shown in Figure 15-1.

PATHOLOGY: In acute hemorrhagic pancreatitis, the pancreas is initially edematous and hyperemic. Within a day, pale, gray foci appear, rapidly becoming friable and hemorrhagic (Fig. 15-2A). *In severe cases, these foci enlarge and become so numerous that most of the pancreas is converted into a large retroperitoneal hematoma, in which pancreatic tissue is barely recognizable.* Yellow-white areas of fat necrosis appear around the pancreas, including the adjacent mesentery (see Fig. 15-2B). These nodules of necrotic fat have a pasty consistency that becomes firmer and chalklike as more calcium and magnesium soaps are produced. Saponification reflects the interaction of cations with free fatty acids released by the action of activated lipase on triglycerides in fat cells. As a result, the level of blood calcium may be depressed, sometimes to the point of causing neuromuscular irritability.

The most prominent microscopic findings in acute pancreatitis are acinar cell necrosis, intense acute inflammation and foci of necrotic fat cells (Fig. 15-3). Necrosis is usually patchy, rarely involving the entire gland. Irregular fibrosis of the pancreas and occasionally calcification are the residuals of healed acute pancreatitis.

PANCREATIC PSEUDOCYST: As many as half of patients who survive acute pancreatitis are at risk for development of pancreatic pseudocysts (Fig. 15-4). These are delimited by connective tissue and contain degraded blood, debris of necrotic pancreatic tissue, and fluid rich in pancreatic enzymes. Pseudocysts may enlarge to compress and even obstruct the duodenum. They may become secondarily infected and form an abscess. Rupture of a pseudocyst is a rare complication that leads to a chemical or septic peritonitis or both.

CLINICAL FEATURES: Patients with acute pancreatitis present with severe epigastric pain that is referred to the upper back and is accompanied by nausea and vomiting. Catastrophic peripheral vascular collapse and shock may ensue within hours. If shock is sustained and profound, adult respiratory distress syndrome and acute renal failure may occur within the first week. Early in the disease, pancreatic digestive enzymes are released from injured acinar cells into the blood and the abdominal cavity. *Elevated serum amylase and lipase within 24 to 72 hours is diagnostic for acute pancreatitis.* The necrotic pancreas becomes infected with gram-negative bacteria from the intestinal tract in half of cases of acute pancreatitis, which greatly increases mortality.

Chronic Pancreatitis

Chronic pancreatitis is the progressive destruction of pancreatic parenchyma with irregular fibrosis and chronic inflammation. Since the original description of the disease and its association with stones two centuries ago, the pathogenesis, clinical course and treatment of chronic pancreatitis remain enigmatic. Clinically, it manifests as recurrent or persisting abdominal pain or simply as evidence of pancreatic exocrine or endocrine insufficiency.

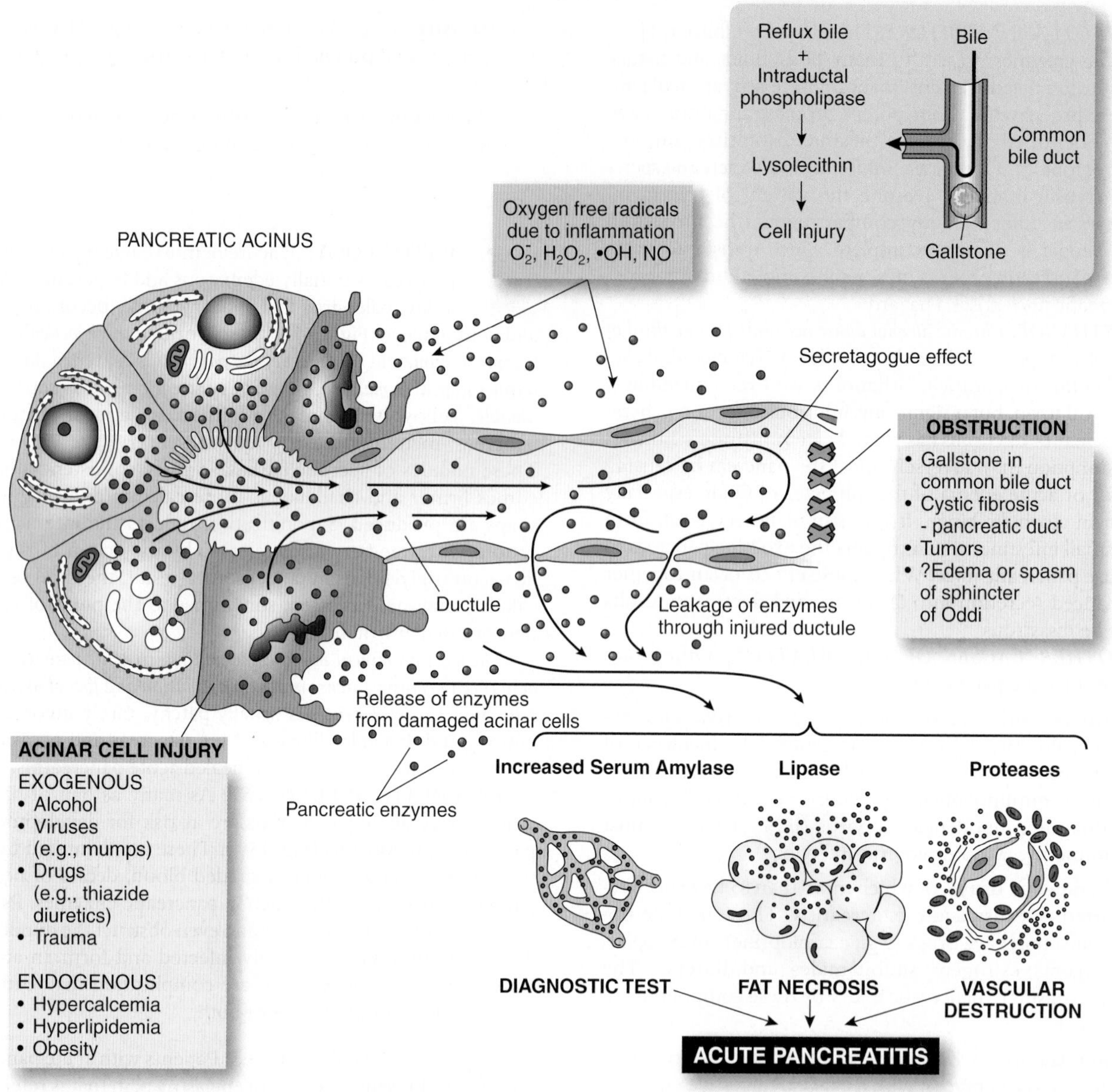

FIGURE 15-1. **The pathogenesis of acute pancreatitis.** Injury to the ductules or the acinar cells leads to the release of pancreatic enzymes. Lipase and proteases destroy tissue, thereby causing acute pancreatitis. The release of amylase is the basis of a test for acute pancreatitis. H_2O_2 = hydrogen peroxide; NO• = nitric acid; O_2^- = superoxide ion; •OH = hydroxyl radical.

PATHOGENESIS: Most factors that cause acute pancreatitis also cause chronic pancreatitis. The fact that chronic pancreatitis is often characterized by intermittent "acute" attacks followed by periods of quiescence suggests that it may evolve from repeated bouts of acute pancreatitis, followed by scarring. However, about half of patients present without a history of acute episodes, and the pathogenesis of these cases of chronic pancreatitis may relate to persistent necrosis and insidious scarring, similar to the progression of cirrhosis of the liver.

- **Alcoholism** of long standing is the major cause of chronic pancreatitis, being responsible for two thirds of adult cases. In almost half of alcoholics who had no symptoms of chronic pancreatitis during life, autopsy reveals evidence of this disease. A comparable proportion of asymptomatic alcoholics manifest abnormal results for pancreatic exocrine function tests. The role of alcohol is undisputed, but the mechanism by which it causes chronic pancreatitis is still debated.
- The earliest morphologic abnormality in alcoholic chronic pancreatitis is precipitation of protein plugs in the ducts, which serve as niduses for subsequent calculi that obstruct the ductal system. Alcohol is a pancreatic secretagogue, so early chronic pancreatitis features hypersecretion of enzyme proteins by acinar cells, without concomitantly increased fluid. As a result, protein plugs precipitate in the small branches of the pancreatic ducts. These deposits, initially include degenerating cells within a reticular framework, then enlarge to form laminar aggregates through accretion of amorphous material. Intra-

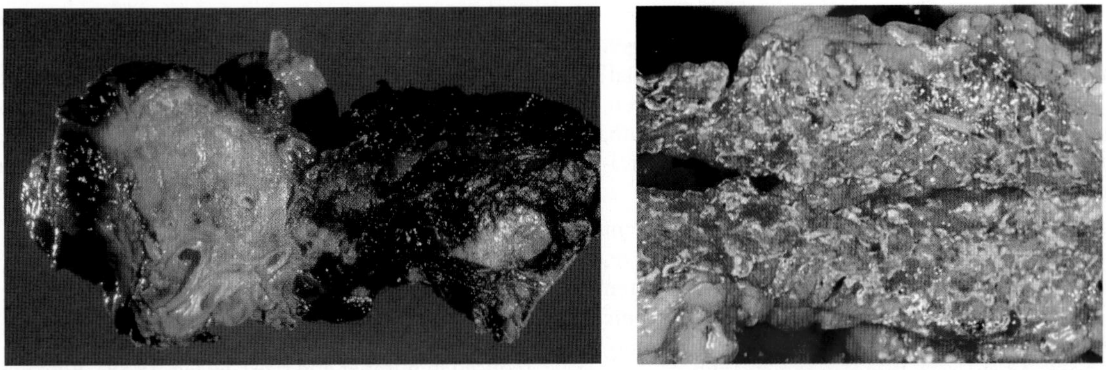

FIGURE 15-2. **Acute hemorrhagic pancreatitis. A.** Large areas of the pancreas are intensely hemorrhagic. **B.** The cut surface of the pancreas in a less severe case of acute pancreatitis, and at a somewhat later stage than in (*A*), shows numerous yellow-white foci of fat necrosis.

ductal stones then form when calcium carbonate is precipitated in the plugs.

- **Obstruction of the pancreatic duct** by pancreas divisum or mechanical blockage by cancer or by inspissated mucus in cystic fibrosis (CF) leads to chronic pancreatitis. However, obstruction by gallstones does not seem to lead to chronic pancreatitis, and cholecystectomy does not alter the course of the disease.
- **Chronic injury to acinar cells** (e.g., in hemochromatosis) is associated with pancreatic fibrosis and atrophy.
- **Chronic renal failure** is linked to increased incidence of acute and chronic pancreatitis.
- **Autoimmune chronic pancreatitis** (also termed **lymphoplasmacytic sclerosing pancreatitis**) frequently occurs in association with autoimmune disorders such as Sjögren syndrome, primary sclerosing cholangitis, primary biliary cirrhosis, retroperitoneal fibrosis, and inflammatory bowel disease (ulcerative colitis and Crohn disease). The disorder affects both sexes, often in early adulthood. Symptoms vary from abdominal discomfort to painless jaundice. Imaging studies can be particularly worrisome, ranging from a mass-like lesion (mimicking an adenocarcinoma) to irregular beading of the pancreatic duct. Microscopically, a lymphoplasmacytic infiltrate targets duct epithelium, acini and veins (venulitis), and there is diffuse fibrous replacement of the pancreatic parenchyma.

  The pathogenesis of autoimmune pancreatitis is unclear. Serum immunoglobulin (Ig)G4 is often elevated and IgG4-positive plasma cells are present in the parenchyma. Immunoglobulin deposits within basement membranes have been described. Autoimmune etiology is further suggested by hypergammaglobulinemia and serum autoantibodies, including antinuclear antibody (ANA), rheumatoid factor, anti-lactoferrin, and anti-carbonic anhydrase.

- **Cystic fibrosis** (see Chapter 16) is briefly reviewed here because it may manifests as chronic pancreatitis. In a pancreas of a patient with CF, intraductal secretions are abnormally viscid, accounting for the older name, **mucoviscidosis**. Plugs of inspissated mucus obstruct cystically distended pancreatic ducts, leading to chronic pancreati-

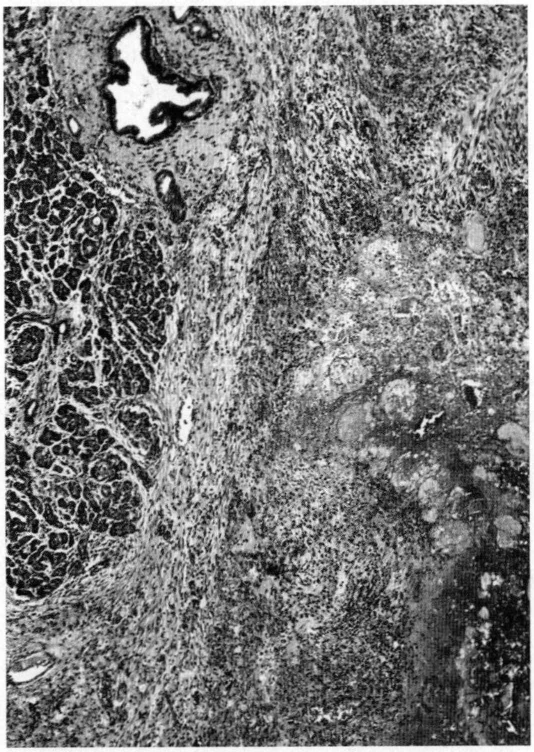

FIGURE 15-3. **Acute hemorrhagic pancreatitis.** A photomicrograph of the pancreas shows areas of acinar cell necrosis, hemorrhage, and fat necrosis (*lower right*). An intact lobule is seen on the left.

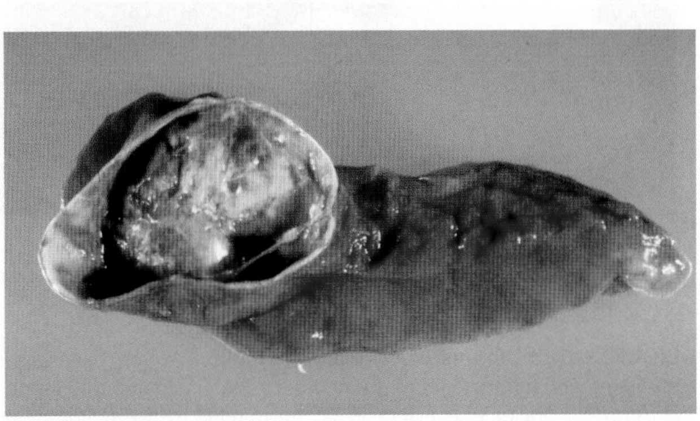

FIGURE 15-4. **Pancreatic pseudocyst.** A cystic cavity arises from the head of the pancreas.

tis and exocrine pancreatic insufficiency. In its late stages, the entire parenchyma is replaced by adipose tissue. Malabsorption this is a common feature of CF in children, who may have bulky, fatty stools (steatorrhea). Death, however, usually results from the pulmonary complications of the disease.

- **Hereditary pancreatitis** is a rare autosomal dominant disease with 80% penetrance. It is characterized by recurring episodes of severe abdominal pain that often manifests in childhood. Point mutations in the **cationic trypsinogen gene (protease serine 1,** ***PRSS1;*** chromosome 7_q) and in the **serine protease inhibitor gene** (*SPINK 1*) have been associated with the disease. Most forms of hereditary pancreatitis are caused by one of three point mutations in the **cationic trypsinogen** gene. One mutation affects a trypsin sensitive hydrolysis site in the chain linking the two globular domains of the trypsin molecule, thereby eliminating an important fail safe mechanism against trypsin autoactivation. Failure to inactivate trypsin allows its activation within the pancreas, leading to autodigestion and pancreatitis. Another mutation may affect intracellular trypsinogen transport.

  Hereditary pancreatitis is occasionally accompanied by aminoaciduria, although the two conditions are not necessarily linked etiologically. Some patients exhibit hypercalcemia secondary to parathyroid hyperplasia or adenomas. *About 40% of patients with hereditary pancreatitis subsequently develop pancreatic ductal adenocarcinoma.* The clinicopathologic features of hereditary pancreatitis are indistinguishable from those of other forms of chronic pancreatitis, including ductal stones and the late complications.

- **Idiopathic chronic pancreatitis** has a bimodal distribution: a juvenile form with a mean age of 25 years; and a second form that occurs in older patients with a peak at age 60. Mutations in the cystic fibrosis transmembrane conductance regulator *(CFTR)* gene are seen in 10% to 30% of patients with idiopathic chronic pancreatitis. Somatic mutations in the gene for pancreatic secretory trypsin inhibitor *(SPINK1)* have also been associated with chronic pancreatitis.

PATHOLOGY: By the time chronic pancreatitis is clinically evident, it is usually well advanced. Chronic calcifying pancreatitis is the most common type of the disease and is associated with chronic alcoholism in over 90% of cases. The pancreas can be affected in a focal, segmental, or diffuse manner. The parenchyma is firm, and the cut surface lacks the usual lobular appearance (Fig. 15-5A). The main pancreatic duct and its tributaries are commonly dilated, owing to obstruction by thick proteinaceous plugs, intraductal stones or strictures. Pseudocysts or abscess formation are common.

Microscopically, large regions of the pancreas show irregular areas of fibrosis, and exocrine and endocrine elements are reduced in number and size (see Fig. 15-5B). Remaining islets of Langerhans are embedded in the sclerotic tissue, and may appear fused and enlarged. The islets eventually disappear. Fibrotic areas contain activated fibroblasts, adjacent to which are infiltrates of lymphocytes, plasma cells, and macrophages, particularly around surviving pancreatic lobules. Pancreatic ducts of all sizes contain variably calcified proteinaceous material, a finding more commonly associated with alcoholism. Ductal epithelium may be atrophic or hyperplastic, and may show squamous metaplasia.

CLINICAL FEATURES: Half of patients with chronic pancreatitis suffer from repeated episodes of acute pancreatitis. One third of cases are characterized by the gradual onset of continuous or intermittent pain, without any acute attacks (Fig. 15-6). In a few patients, chronic pancreatitis is initially painless but presents with diabetes or malabsorption. Once pancreatic calcifications are visible radiologically, most patients have developed diabetes, malabsorption, or both. Conspicuous weight loss is common, and unrelenting epigastric pain, radiating to the back, may cripple the patient. The mortality rate is 3% to 4% per year, and approaches 50% within 20 to 25 years. One fifth of patients die of complications associated with attacks of acute pancreatitis. The other deaths are from other causes, particularly alcohol-related disorders.

Pancreatic Cystic Neoplasms

Liberal use of abdominal imaging has led to increased recognition of cystic pancreatic neoplasms.

SEROUS CYSTADENOMA: Serous cystic neoplasm is a benign tumor composed of cystic structures uniformly lined by

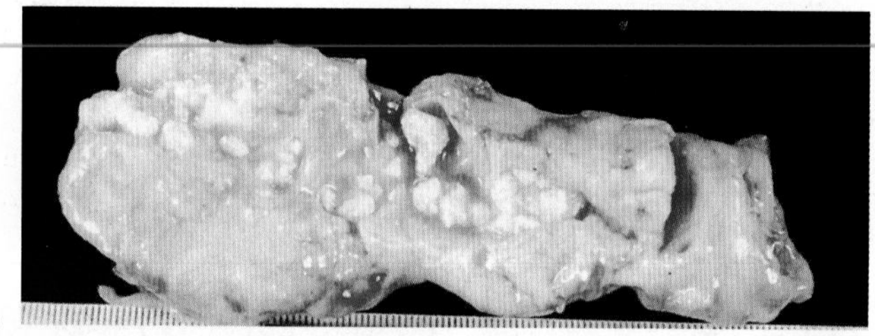

A

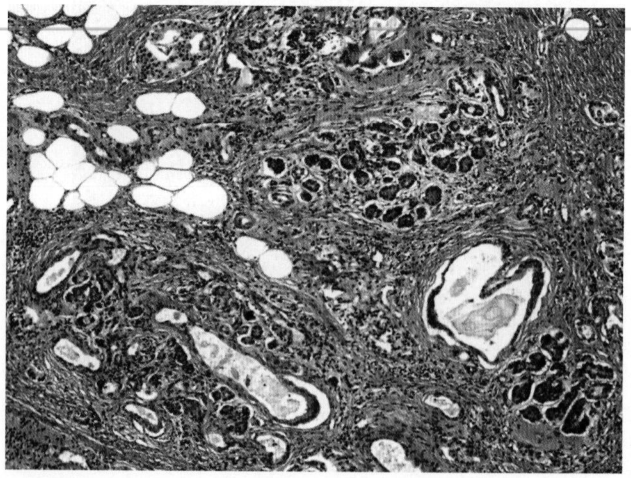

B

FIGURE 15-5. **Chronic calcifying pancreatitis. A.** The pancreas is shrunken and fibrotic, and the dilated duct contains numerous stones. **B.** Atrophic lobules of acinar cells are surrounded by dense fibrous tissue infiltrated by lymphocytes. The pancreatic ducts are dilated and contain inspissated proteinaceous material.

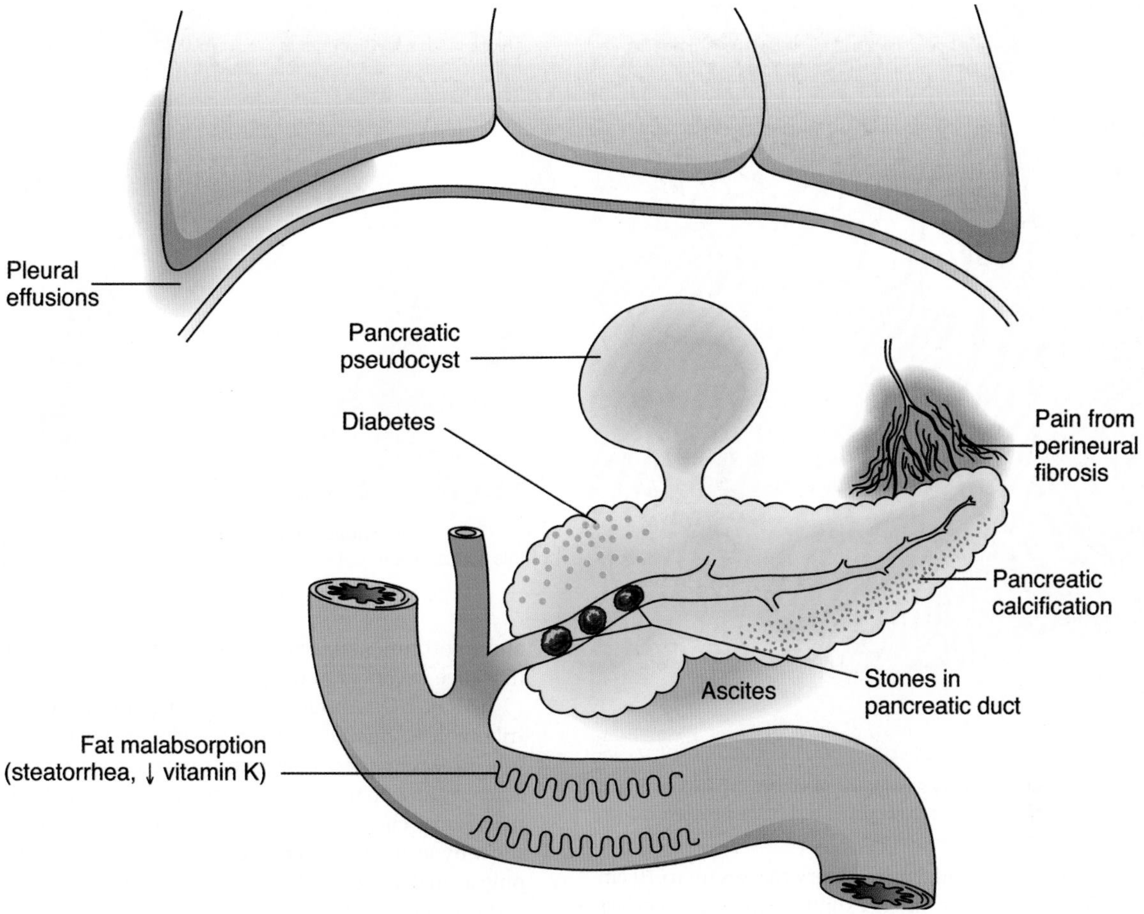

FIGURE 15-6. **Complications of chronic pancreatitis.**

glycogen-rich cuboidal epithelium (Fig.15-7). It usually occurs in the pancreatic body or tail. The tumor occurs in adults, with a 3:1 female predominance, and patients with von Hippel-Lindau syndrome are at increased risk for its development. Serous cystadenomas range from 1 to 25 cm in diameter. Most patients present with nonspecific symptoms related to local mass effects, but about a third are asymptomatic. There is often a large, stellate central scar, sometimes with microcalcifications giving a "sunburst" pattern on imaging studies.

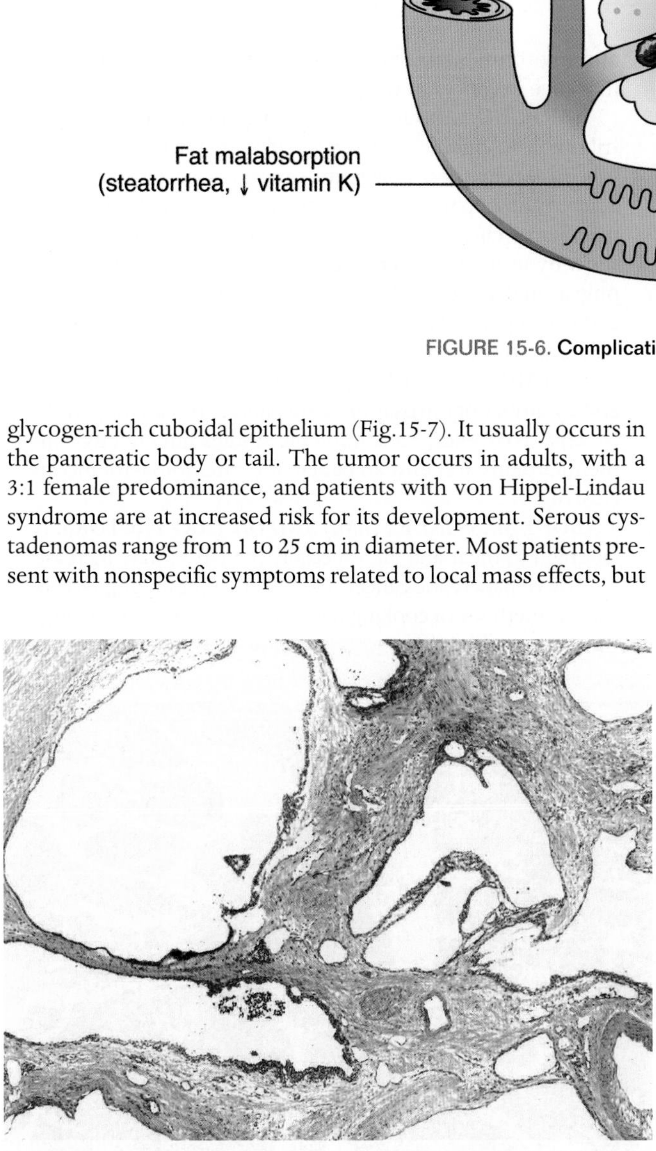

FIGURE 15-7. **Serous cystadenoma.** Cysts are embedded in a dense, fibrous stroma. The epithelial lining is composed of a single layer of glycogen-rich cells.

INTRADUCTAL PAPILLARY MUCINOUS NEOPLASM: Intraductal papillary mucin-producing neoplasms (IPMNs) are composed of papillary proliferations of neoplastic mucin-secreting cells that arise in the main pancreatic duct or its major branches (Fig. 15-8). IPMNs are usually diagnosed in late adulthood. Most IPMNs arise in the head of the pancreas. Duct involvement may be unifocal, multifocal, or diffuse. IPMNs measure up to 10 cm. The distended duct(s) are usually filled by viscous, yellow mucus. IPMNs exhibit a varying degrees of epithelial atypia, and are classified accordingly: benign (adenoma), borderline, and malignant (either invasive or noninvasive). A focus of invasive adenocarcinoma is found in up to one third of cases.

PANCREATIC MUCINOUS CYSTIC NEOPLASM: Mucinous cystic neoplasm (MCN) is a uni- or multilocular tumor composed of tall or cuboidal mucin-secreting epithelium supported by a cellular ovarian-type stroma (Fig. 15-9). MCN occurs almost exclusively in adult women. Tumors may reach 10 cm in diameter and do not communicate with the pancreatic duct system. MCNs have a predilection for the body and tail of the pancreas. The prognosis of MCN (noninvasive) is excellent if it is completely removed

SOLID PSEUDOPAPILLARY NEOPLASM: Solid pseudopapillary neoplasm (SPN) occurs almost exclusively in adolescent girls and young women. It is composed of monomorphic cells forming loose solid sheets and pseudopapillary structures (Fig.

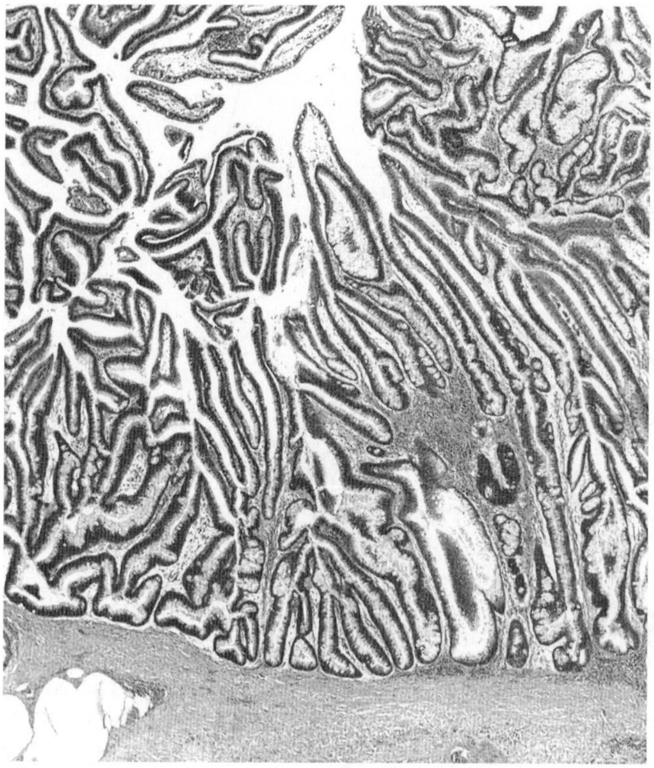

FIGURE 15-8. **Intraductal papillary mucinous neoplasm.** An exuberant papillary proliferation of tall mucin-secreting epithelium fills the pancreatic duct.

15-10). SPN presents as round, large solitary masses up to 10 cm in diameter. The cut surface often exhibits extensive necrosis and hemorrhage with cystic spaces filled with necrotic debris. In some cases, the tumor may be entirely hemorrhagic and cystic, mimicking a pseudocyst. SPN is generally considered a benign neoplasm with an excellent prognosis following resection. However, aggressive tumor behavior can occur.

Pancreatic Cancer

In the United States, pancreatic carcinoma is the fourth most common cause of cancer death in men, and the fifth in women. The prognosis is dismal: the 5-year survival is only 5%. The incidence of pancreatic cancer seems to be increasing in all countries studied, and has tripled in the United States over the past 50 years. Ductal adenocarcinoma accounts for 90% of all pancreatic cancers.

EPIDEMIOLOGY: Pancreatic cancer is seen worldwide. The highest incidence (twice that in the United States) is among male Maoris, Polynesian aborigines of New Zealand and female natives of Hawaii. It shows a significant male predominance (up to 3:1) in younger age groups but almost equal sex distribution in old age. In the United States, it is more common in Native Americans and blacks, in whom the incidence is approximately 50% higher than in whites. Pancreatic carcinoma is a disease of late life, with the greatest incidence in persons older than 60 years of age, although its appearance as early as the third decade is not rare.

PATHOGENESIS: The factors involved in the development of pancreatic cancer are obscure. Epidemiologic studies have implicated both host and environmental factors as being of possible etiologic significance in cancer of the pancreas.

SMOKING: About 25% of pancreatic cancers are attributable to cigarette smoking, and there is a two- to threefold increased risk of pancreatic cancer in cigarette smokers. There is an apparent dose–response relationship, with the number of cigarettes smoked per day, and smokers often show hyperplastic pancreatic ducts at autopsy. However, as only a small fraction of smokers develop pancreatic cancer, additional genetic and environmental factors are undoubtedly important.

CHEMICAL CARCINOGENS: Polycyclic hydrocarbons and a number of nitrosamines are pancreatic carcinogens in rodents. However, epidemiologic studies linking environmental toxins and human pancreatic carcinoma are inconclusive.

BODY MASS INDEX (BMI) AND DIETARY FACTORS: A diet high in meat and fat, especially the latter, may increase the risk of pancreatic cancer. However, confounding factors such as methods of cooking (i.e., frying, boiling, barbecuing)

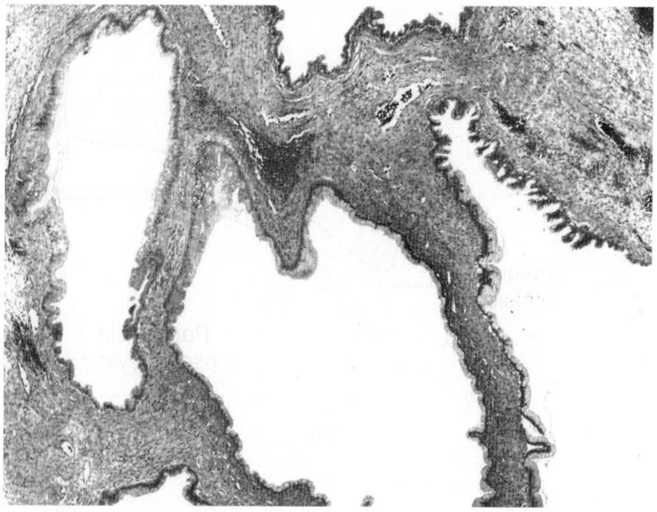

FIGURE 15-9. **Mucinous cystic neoplasm.** A mucin-rich epithelial lining of this cystic lesion rests on an ovarian type stroma.

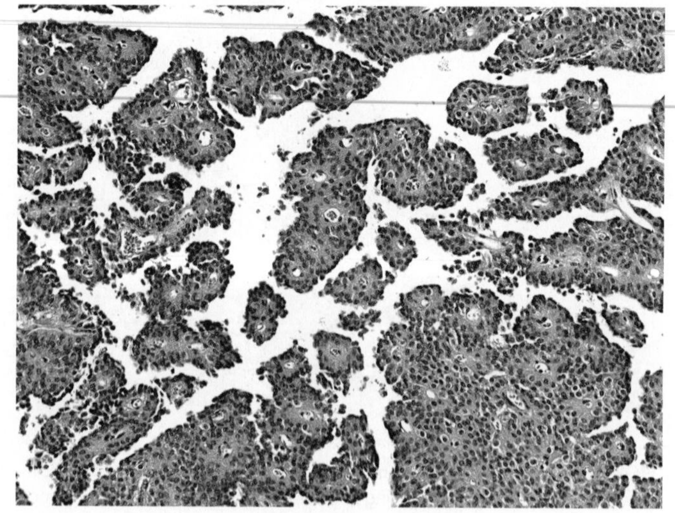

FIGURE 15-10. **Solid pseudopapillary neoplasm.** The tumor is composed of pseudopapillae with vascular cores.

may play a role. A positive association between BMI and pancreatic cancer is reported.

DIABETES MELLITUS: Diabetics are at increased risk for carcinoma of the pancreas. Up to 80% of patients with pancreatic cancer have evidence of diabetes mellitus at the time of cancer diagnosis. Patients with diabetes mellitus for 5or more years have double the risk for pancreatic cancer. In some patients, diabetes may be caused by pancreatic cancer, rather than the reverse. However, prospective studies of people with abnormal glucose tolerance document the subsequent increased incidence of pancreatic cancer.

CHRONIC PANCREATITIS: Chronic pancreatitis is a risk factor for pancreatic adenocarcinoma, although it accounts for few cases. As chronic pancreatitis may occasionally be mild and clinically silent, its role in the development of pancreatic carcinoma may be underestimated.

ADDITIONAL FACTORS: Aspirin, nonsteroidal anti-inflammatory drugs, coffee, and alcohol have been reported to increase risk of pancreatic cancer. However, the evidence is tenuous.

MOLECULAR GENETICS: Pancreatic duct cancers exhibit a number of genetic alterations. A tumor progression model based upon specific gene mutations has been proposed, which is supported by the finding of preneoplastic duct epithelial lesions, termed **pancreatic intraductal neoplasia** (PanIN). An early event is mutational activation of K-*ras* (G→A transition in the second position of codon 12), which is observed in up to 95% of pancreatic carcinomas. Mutational inactivation or deletion of tumor suppressor genes appear later in the sequence of tumor progression, including *p53* (50%), *p16 (MST1)* (85%), and *DPC-4* (deleted in pancreatic cancer, locus 4) (55%). Interestingly, deletions in chromosome 18 are present in 90% of pancreatic cancers. Although *DPC-4* is located on chromosome 18, only half of all pancreatic cancers show loss or inactivation of this gene, suggesting that another nearby tumor suppressor gene contributes to the development of the remaining 40%. Overactivity or inappropriate expression of several growth factors and their receptors has been described, including epidermal growth factor (EGF) and its receptor, transforming growth factor-β (TGF-β), and fibroblast growth factor (FGF) and its receptor. Up to 10% of pancreatic carcinomas have inactivating mutations of *BRCA2*.Several familial cancer syndromes have a strong risk for the development of pancreatic carcinoma (Table 15-1; also see Chapter 5).

PATHOLOGY: Carcinoma arises anywhere in the pancreas, the most frequent focus being in the head (60%), followed by the body (10%), and tail (5%). The pancreas is diffusely involved in the remaining 25%. Carcinomas of the head of the pancreas may cause biliary obstruction and jaundice by compressing the ampulla of Vater and common bile duct. They thus tend to be smaller at diagnosis than those of the body and tail and show more limited spread to regional lymph nodes and distant sites.

On gross examination, pancreatic carcinoma is a firm, gray, poorly demarcated, multinodular mass (Fig. 15-11), often embedded in a dense connective tissue stroma. Tumors of the head of the pancreas may invade the common duct and duodenal wall. They may also obstruct the duct of Wirsung and cause atrophy of the body and tail.

Microscopically, more than 75% of pancreatic cancers are well-differentiated **ductal adenocarcinomas**, secrete mucin, and are associated with collagen deposition. The remaining 25% of cancers that originate from pancreatic ducts and ductules are colloid carcinoma, medullary carcinoma, adenosquamous carcinoma, undifferentiated carcinoma, and osteoclastic giant cell carcinoma.

Pancreatic cancer metastasizes most commonly to regional lymph nodes and liver. Other frequent metastatic locations include peritoneum, lungs, adrenals, and bones. Direct extension into neighboring organs (e.g., the stomach and duodenum) occasionally occurs. Perineural infiltration by tumor is characteristic of pancreatic cancer and accounts for the early and persistent pain of this disease.

CLINICAL FEATURES: Patients with pancreatic carcinoma present with anorexia, conspicuous weight loss and a gnawing pain in the epigastrium, which often radiates to the back. *Jaundice is seen in about half of all patients with cancer localized to the head of the pancreas,* but in less than 10% of tumors of the body or tail. Serum levels of cancer antigen (CA)19-9, a Lewis blood group antigen, are usually increased. Early diagnosis of pancreatic cancer is unusual because the tumor is not ordinarily symptomatic until it is well advanced. Most have already metastasized at the time of diagnosis, and curative surgery is uncommon. Progressive deterioration almost invariably ensues, with intractable pain, cachexia, and death. Half of patients die within 6 months of diagnosis, and the overall 5-year survival rate is less than 5%.

Courvoisier sign is acute, painless gallbladder dilation accompanied by jaundice, owing to common bile duct obstruction by tumor. In about one third of patients it may be the first sign of pancreatic cancer but it does not identify potentially curable tumors.

TABLE 15–1

Familial Cancer Syndromes and Relative Risk for Pancreatic Cancer

Syndrome	Chromosome	Gene Mutation	Relative Risk of Pancreatic Cancer
Peutz-Jegher syndrome	19p13	*STK11/LKB1*	132-fold
Hereditary pancreatitis	7q35	*PRSS1*	50- to 80-fold
Familial atypical multiple mole melanoma syndrome (FAMM)	9p21	*P16 (CDKN2A)*	9- to 38-fold
Hereditary breast-ovarian cancer syndrome (HBOC)	13q12–13	*BRCA2*	3.5- to 10-fold
Hereditary nonpolyposis cancer syndrome (HNPCC)	3p21, 2p22	*hMLH1, hMSH2*	Unknown

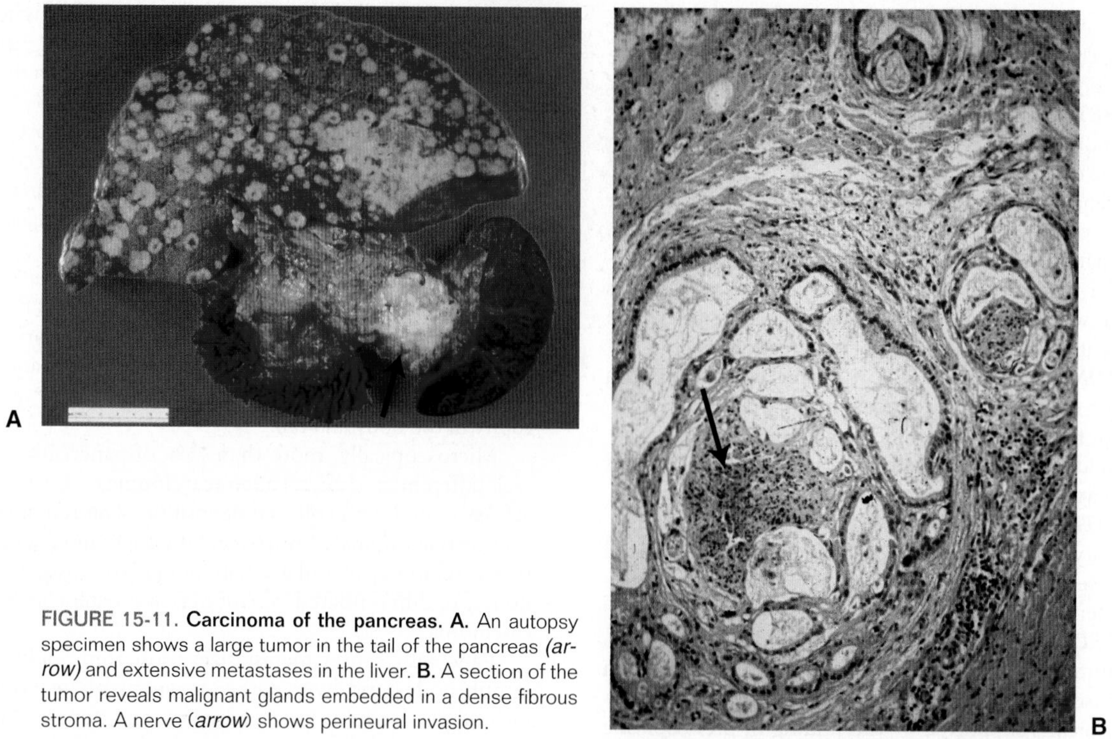

FIGURE 15-11. **Carcinoma of the pancreas. A.** An autopsy specimen shows a large tumor in the tail of the pancreas *(arrow)* and extensive metastases in the liver. **B.** A section of the tumor reveals malignant glands embedded in a dense fibrous stroma. A nerve *(arrow)* shows perineural invasion.

Migratory thrombophlebitis (deep venous thrombosis) develops in 10% of patients with pancreatic cancer, especially when the tumor involves the body and tail of the pancreas. It is not uncommon for migratory thrombophlebitis, also known as **Trousseau syndrome**, to be the first evidence of an underlying pancreatic malignancy, although it may be seen with other cancers as well. Unexplained thrombophlebitis in an otherwise healthy person demands a careful search for occult malignancy. Thrombi develop in multiple veins, including the deep veins of the legs, the subclavian vein, the inferior and superior mesenteric veins, and even the vena cava. Portal vein thrombosis may also occur, occasionally as the presenting event. The mechanisms responsible for the hypercoagulable state that leads to migratory thrombophlebitis are not completely understood, but the following facts are known: (1) a serine protease synthesized and released by malignant tumor cells directly activates plasma factor X; (2) tumor cells spontaneously shed plasma membrane vesicles, which exhibit procoagulant activity; and (3) intracellular tissue thromboplastin is released from necrotic tumor.

The complications of pancreatic ductal carcinoma are shown in (Figure 15-12).

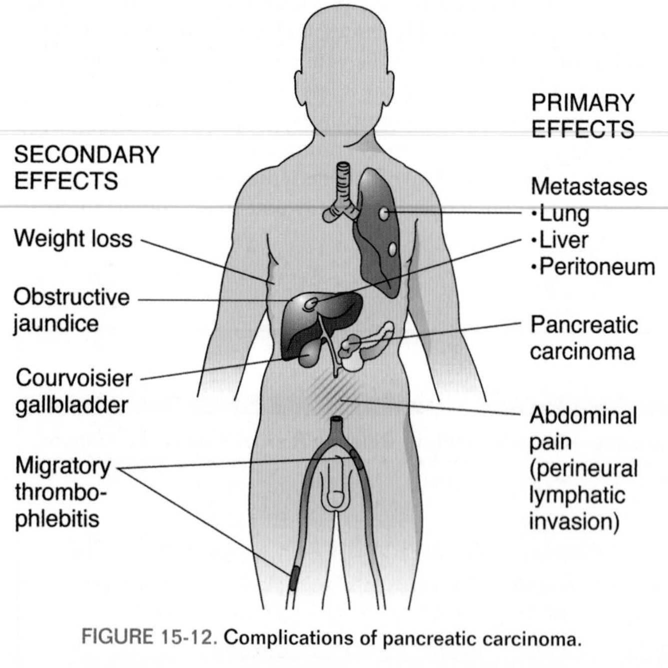

FIGURE 15-12. **Complications of pancreatic carcinoma.**

Acinar Cell Carcinoma Is an Uncommon Tumor of Older Adults

Acinar cell carcinomas are usually large and tend to metastasize to regional lymph nodes and liver and more distantly to the lungs and other body sites.(Fig. 15-13) The tumors are usually detected in the seventh decade. Some patients develop a curious syndrome

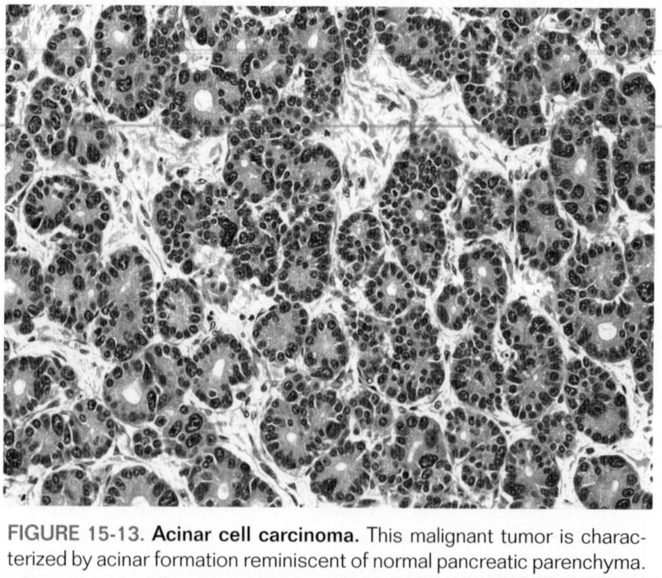

FIGURE 15-13. **Acinar cell carcinoma.** This malignant tumor is characterized by acinar formation reminiscent of normal pancreatic parenchyma.

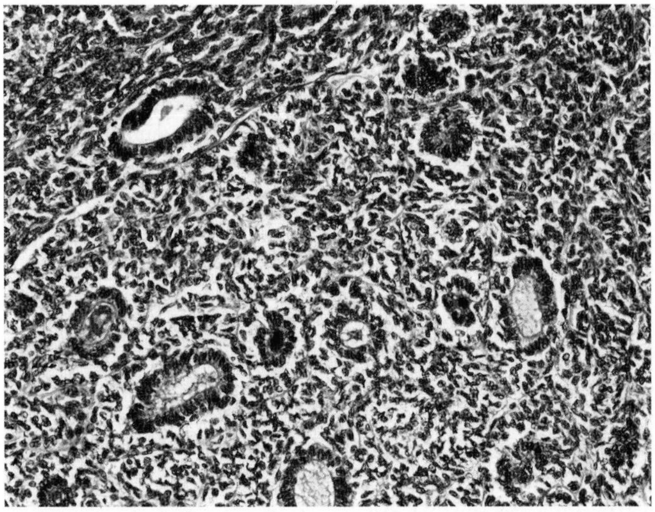

FIGURE 15-14. **Pancreatoblastoma.** There are sarcomatoid features and scattered acinar structures.

of fat necrosis in subcutaneous tissues and bone marrow, polyarthralgia, and occasional constipation. The resemblance of this complication to the extrapancreatic manifestations of acute pancreatitis suggests that it is attributable to hypersecretion of pancreatic enzymes into serum (e.g., lipase). The clinical course is less rapidly fatal than ductal adenocarcinoma.

Pancreatoblastoma is a Tumor of Childhood

Usually detected in the first decade of life, pancreatoblastoma is a solitary lobulated neoplasm of the head of the pancreas. The tumor may occur in the setting of Beckwith-Wiedemann syndrome. Serum α-fetoprotein may be elevated. Microscopically, the tumor is composed of polygonal cells arrayed in nests and less commonly acinar structures, with interspersed squamoid islands (Fig. 15-14). Lymph node or hepatic metastases occur in a third of patients, and are associated with a poor prognosis. Surgery and chemotherapy can be curative in patients without metastatic disease.

The Endocrine Pancreas

The Islets of Langerhans Form the Endocrine Pancreas

These islets are scattered throughout the pancreas and consist of richly vascularized globular masses of large epithelioid cells. Six distinct cell types are correlated with specific hormones (Table 15-2).

TABLE 15-2

Secretory Products of Islet Cells and Their Physiological Actions

Cell	Secretory Product	Physiological Actions
Alpha	Glucagon	Catabolic, stimulates glycogenolysis and gluconeogenesis, raises blood glucose
Beta	Insulin	Anabolic, stimulates glycogenesis, lipogenesis, and protein synthesis, lowers blood glucose
Delta		Inhibits secretion of alpha, beta, D_1, and acinar cells
D	Somatostatin	
D_1	Vasoactive intestinal polypeptide (VIP)	Same as glucagon; also regulates tone and motility of GI tract and activates cAMP of intestinal epithelium
PP	Human pancreatic polypeptide (hpp)	Stimulates gastric enzyme secretion, inhibits intestinal motility and bile secretion
EC	Serotonin, substance P (motilin)	Induces vasodilation, increases vascular permeability, stimulates motility of gastric muscle and tone of lower 1esophageal sphincter

- **Alpha cells** synthesize glucagon and are located in the outer rim of the islets. They constitute 15% to 20% of the total islet cell population (Fig. 15-15A). Glucagon induces glycogenolysis and gluconeogenesis in the liver, thereby raising blood glucose. Its secretion is stimulated by hypoglycemia and by ingestion of a low-carbohydrate, high-protein meal. By virtue of these responses, glucagon, together with insulin, serves to maintain fuel homeostasis.
- **Beta cells** are 60% to 70% of all islet cells, and produce insulin (see Fig. 15-15B). By electron microscopy, cellular insulin is resolved into characteristic polygonal and rhomboidal crystals enclosed in secretory vesicles. The major obligatory stimulus for insulin secretion is the binding of glucose to receptors on the beta cell surface.

A 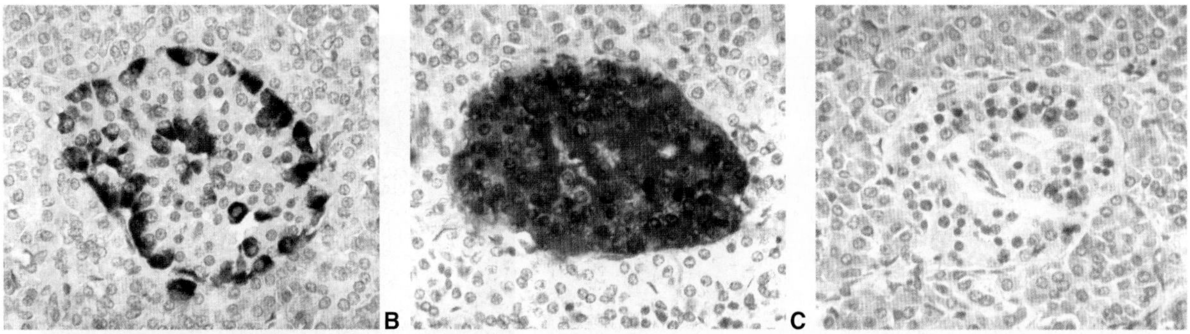 B C

FIGURE 15-15. **Localization of hormones of the pancreatic islet by specific antibodies.** The immunoperoxidase technique reveals (**A**) glucagon in alpha cells at the periphery of the islet, (**B**) insulin in beta cells distributed throughout the islet, and (**C**) somatostatin in sparsely distributed delta cells.

- **Delta cells** are subdivided into D and D_1 types, which secrete somatostatin and vasoactive intestinal polypeptide (VIP), respectively. They are fewer in number and slightly larger than alpha cells and, like them, tend to be at the periphery of the islets (see Fig. 15-15C). Delta cells are situated between the alpha and beta cells, so that the three cell types are often contiguous. Pancreatic somatostatin is identical to hypothalamic somatostatin. It inhibits pituitary release of growth hormone, secretion by alpha, beta, and D_1 cells, acinar cells of the exocrine pancreas, and certain hormone-secreting cells in the gastrointestinal tract. Coupled with the topographic cell–cell relations noted above, these hormonal interactions suggest that somatostatin plays a regulatory role in glucose homeostasis.
- **D_1 cells** are smaller than the other islet cell types and are rare in normal human islets. Their hormone, VIP, has also been localized in ganglion cells and nerve fibers of pancreas, gut, and brain. Like glucagon, VIP induces glycogenolysis and hyperglycemia and regulates ion and water secretion by epithelial cells of the gastrointestinal tract.
- **Pancreatic polypeptide-secreting cells** are located primarily in the islets of the head of the pancreas. They synthesize a polypeptide that appears to have variable and opposed functions, including stimulation secretion of enzymes from the gastric mucosa and inhibiting a number of functions, such as smooth muscle contraction in intestine and gallbladder, production of gastric acid and secretion by the exocrine pancreas and biliary system.
- **Enterochromaffin cells** occur, rarely, in islets the head of the pancreas. They synthesize serotonin and **motilin,** a peptide that stimulates gastric smooth muscle motility and increases sphincter tone at the gastroesophageal junction.

Pancreatic Endocrine Tumors (PETs) Comprise About 10% of Pancreatic Neoplasms

Most are nonfunctional and are discovered as incidental findings at autopsy. The tumors are usually composed of monotonous sheets of small round cells with uniform nuclei and infrequent mitoses. By electron microscopy, the cells contain neurosecretory granules, and often display clear vesicles that correspond to neuronal synaptic vesicles.

PETs often invade and metastasize, but it is difficult to distinguish between benign and malignant PETs on the basis of histology alone. Hormone secretion by PETs results in distinctive clinical syndromes. Functional islet cell tumors may occur alone or as part of the multiple endocrine neoplasia syndrome type I (MEN I).

The molecular pathogenesis of sporadic PETs is not well established. The most common chromosomal anomaly is allelic loss of 11q which includes the *MEN-1* locus. Somatic mutations of the *MEN-1* gene have been identified in about a third of sporadic or nonfamilial PETs. Allelic loss of the *VHL* gene is frequent.

Insulinomas (Beta Cell Tumors) Are the Most Common Islet Cell Neoplasms

***Insulinomas (beta cell tumors)** (75% of islet cell neoplasms) may release enough insulin to induce severe hypoglycemia.* Neoplastic beta cells, unlike their normal counterparts, are not regulated by blood glucose level and continue to secrete insulin autonomously, even when blood glucose is very low. Insulinomas and other islet cell neoplasms occur both sporadically and in the context of the MEN I syndrome (see Chapter 21).

PATHOLOGY: *Most insulinomas are benign lesions in the body or tail of the pancreas* (Fig. 15-16). They are generally less than 3 cm in diameter and occasionally as small as 1 mm. Most (90%) are solitary and can be surgically excised. Only a minority (5% to 15%) show malignant behavior. Histologically, insulinoma cells resemble normal beta cells but are dispersed in trabecular or solid patterns (Fig. 15-17). The tumor often elicits a desmoplastic reaction, and amyloid (derived from a peptide hormone secreted with insulin and termed **amylin**) may be found in the stroma. Electron microscopy shows pleomorphic, paracrystalline granules surrounded by a clear halo, an appearance typical of insulin stored in normal beta cells. A reliable distinction between benign and malignant insulinomas is difficult on histologic grounds and in most cases awaits the appearance or absence of metastases. However, tumor size (3 cm or larger), high mitotic rate, and marked nuclear atypia generally are associated with aggressive behavior.

CLINICAL FEATURES: Low blood sugar produces a syndrome of sweating, nervousness and hunger, which may progress to confusion, lethargy, and coma. Symptoms can be relieved by eating, so patients with insulinomas are often overweight. The diagnosis is frequently delayed by abnormal behavior that causes some patients to seek psychiatric care. Most cases are characterized by only a mild hypoglycemia, and in some, the tumor is not functional at all. The diagnosis is established by demonstrating high levels of insulin in the blood and the tumor cells (see Fig. 15-17B).

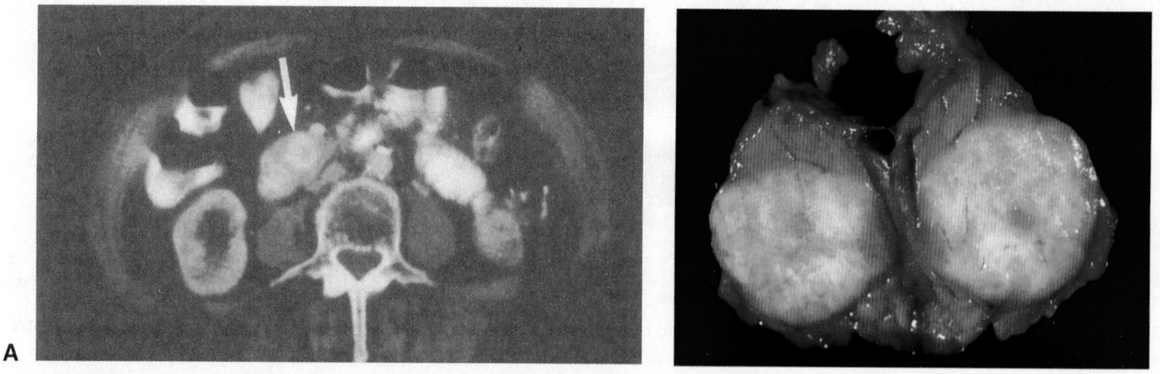

FIGURE 15-16. **Insulinoma. A.** A computed tomography (CT) scan of the abdomen shows a solitary insulinoma *(arrow)*. **B.** An insulinoma is embedded in tan, lobular pancreatic tissue.

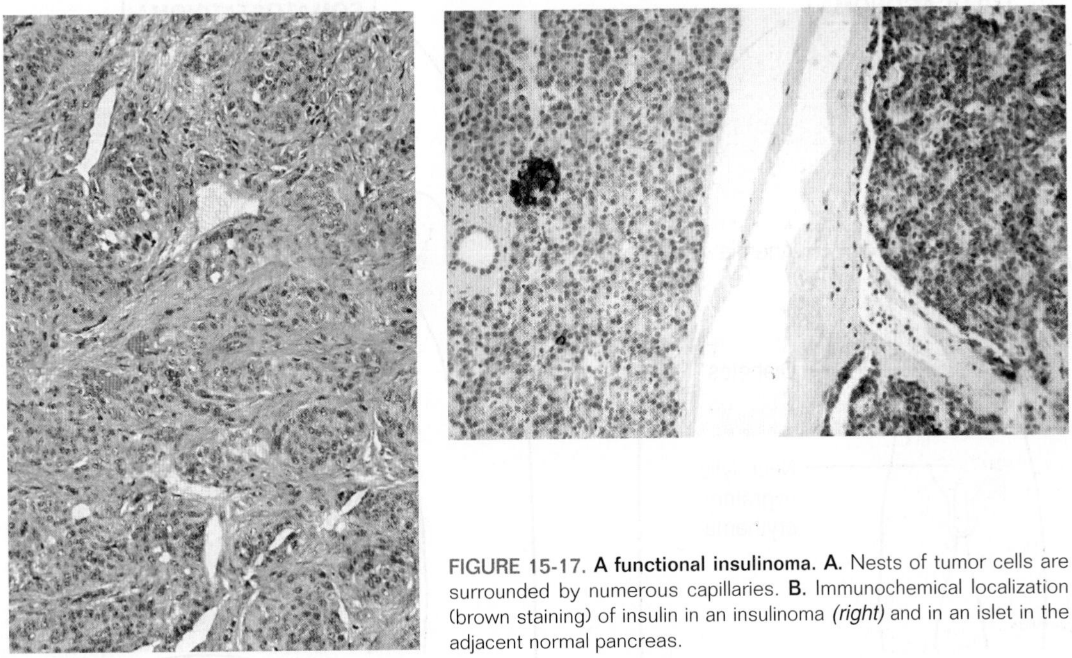

FIGURE 15-17. **A functional insulinoma. A.** Nests of tumor cells are surrounded by numerous capillaries. **B.** Immunochemical localization (brown staining) of insulin in an insulinoma *(right)* and in an islet in the adjacent normal pancreas.

Pancreatic Gastrinomas (Zollinger-Ellison Syndrome) Induce Gastric Acid Secretion

Pancreatic gastrinoma is an islet cell tumor consisting of so-called G cells, which produce gastrin, a potent hormonal stimulus for gastric acid secretion. The location of this tumor in the pancreas is curious, because gastrin-containing cells do not normally occur in the islets. By electron microscopy, tumor cells strongly resemble the gastrin-secreting cells of the duodenal mucosa. The pancreatic tumor is believed to arise from multipotent primitive endocrine cells that have undergone inappropriate differentiation to form G cells in the islets. Pancreatic gastrinoma causes **Zollinger-Ellison syndrome,** a disorder characterized by (1) intractable gastric hypersecretion, (2) severe peptic ulceration of the duodenum and jejunum, and (3) high blood gastrin levels.

Among islet cell tumors, pancreatic gastrinomas are second in frequency only to insulinomas, accounting for one fourth of islet cell tumors. They are most common between the ages of 30 and 50, with a slight male predominance. Fifteen percent of patients with Zollinger-Ellison syndrome have gastrinomas outside the pancreas, particularly in duodenum. *Most gastrinomas are malignant (70% to 90%).* The tumor may be solitary or multiple, the latter usually in the context of MEN I. Histologically, gastrinomas are remarkably similar to intestinal carcinoid tumors. Metastases to regional lymph nodes and the liver are often functional.

Glucagonomas (Alpha Cell Tumors)

Alpha cell tumors (glucagonomas) are associated with a syndrome of (1) mild diabetes; (2) a necrotizing, migratory, erythematous rash; (3) anemia; (4) venous thromboses; and (5) severe infections. They are rare (1% of functional islet cell tumors) and occur between the ages of 40 and 70 years, with a slight female predominance. Two-thirds of symptomatic glucagonomas are malignant.

Functional glucagonomas are usually large and invade surrounding structures. Microscopically, they show trabecular and solid patterns like insulinomas. By immunochemistry, tumor cells contain glucagon, and electron microscopy shows characteristic alpha cell granules (Fig. 15-18). In patients with alpha cell tumors, plasma glucagon levels are elevated up to 30 times above normal. In addition to hyperglycemia, fasting plasma amino acid levels are decreased to as low as 20% of normal.

Somatostinomas (Delta Cell Tumors)

Somatostatinomas are rare and produce a syndrome consisting of mild diabetes, gallstones, steatorrhea, and hypochlorhydria. These effects result from the inhibitory actions of somatostatin on other cells of the pancreatic islets and on neuroendocrine cells of the gastrointestinal tract. Consequently, levels of insulin and glucagon in blood are low. In addition to producing somatostatin, some delta cell tumors also secrete calcitonin or adrenocorticotropic hormone (ACTH). The tumors are usually solitary. Most are malignant, with metastases already present at the time of diagnosis.

VIPomas (D1 Tumors)

Verner-Morrison syndrome is caused by elevated levels of VIP and is characterized by explosive and profuse watery diarrhea, accompanied

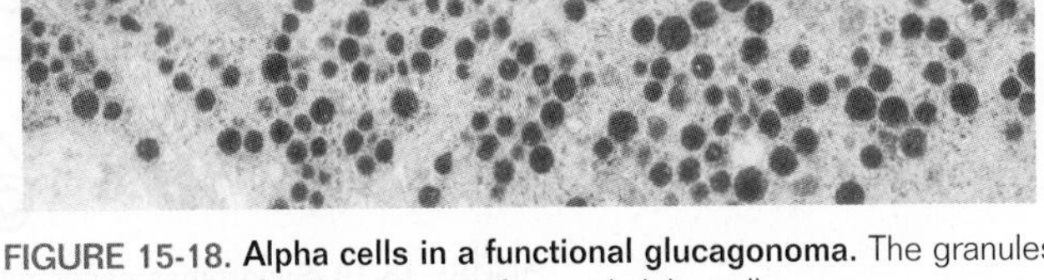

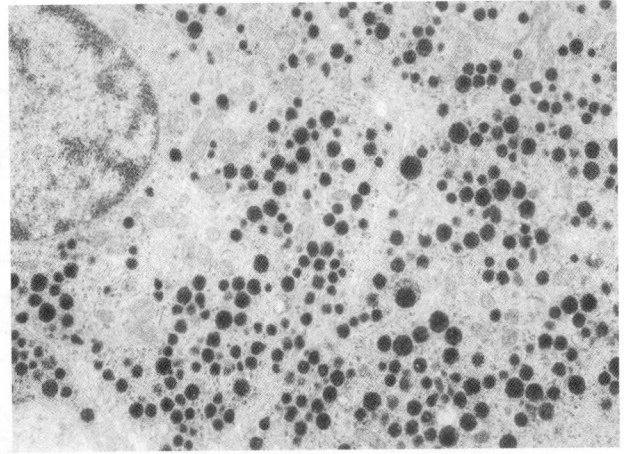

FIGURE 15-18. **Alpha cells in a functional glucagonoma.** The granules are indistinguishable from those of normal alpha cells.

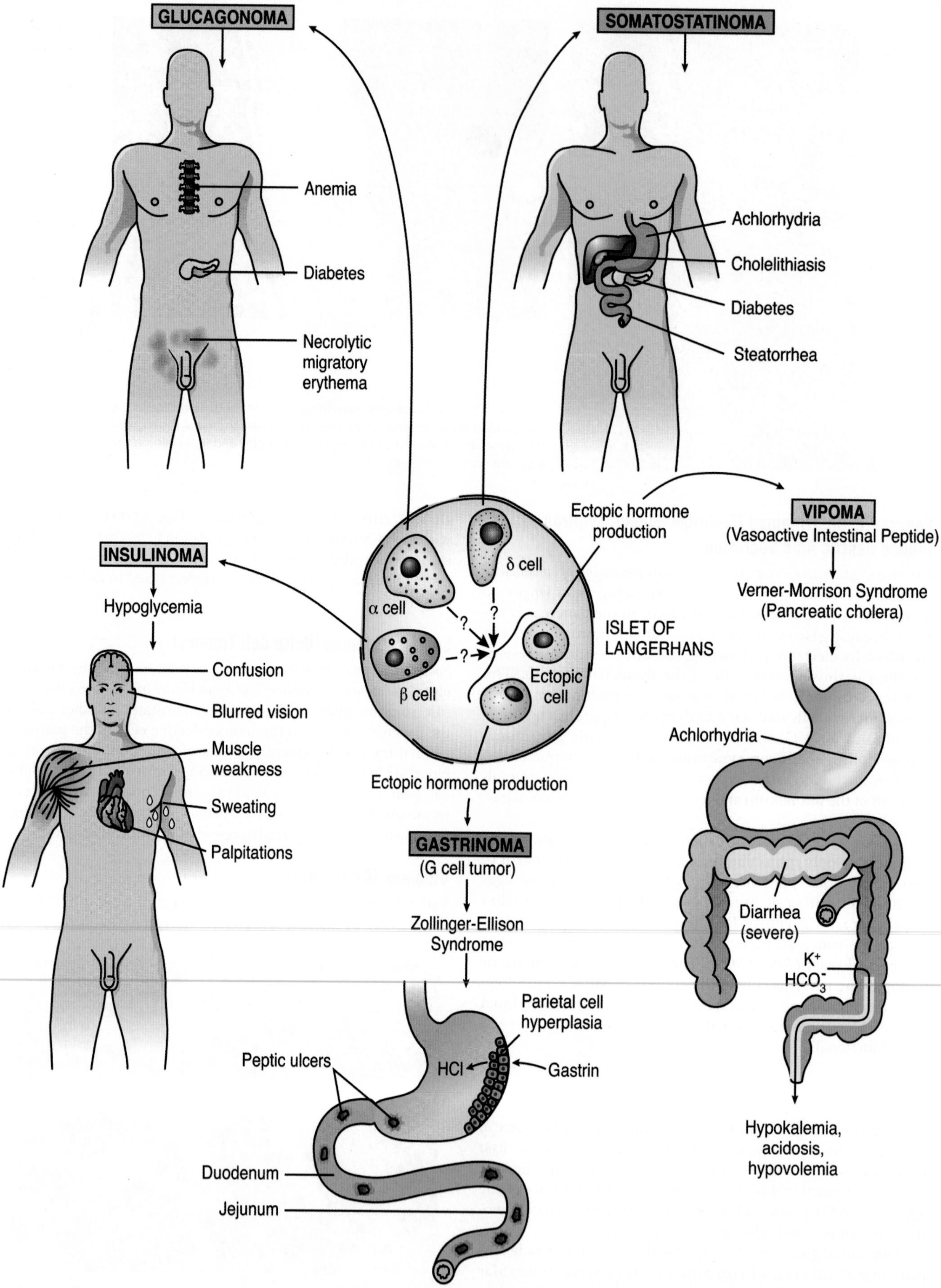

FIGURE 15-19. Syndromes associated with islet cell tumors of the pancreas.

by hypokalemia and hypochlorhydria. The disorder has also been referred to as **pancreatic cholera**. VIPomas are rare tumors (less than 5% of all islet tumors), are usually large and solitary, and in most cases are malignant.

High levels of circulating VIP and severe diarrhea have also been encountered in patients with a variety of nonpancreatic neoplasms containing different types of neuroendocrine cells (e.g., ganglioneuroma, pheochromocytoma of the adrenal medulla, medullary thyroid carcinoma, and bronchogenic carcinoma). In some patients, MEN I causes Verner-Morrison syndrome.

Pancreatic Polypeptide-Secreting Tumors Are Asymptomatic

No clinical syndrome occurs despite the fact that pancreatic polypeptide-secreting tumors secrete high levels of pancreatic polypeptide in the blood. The tumors are usually single and benign, although a few have metastasized to the liver. In addition to their own specific hormones, other islet cell tumors may secrete pancreatic polypeptide.

Enterochromaffin Cell (Carcinoid) Tumors Produce Serotonin

Carcinoid tumors of the pancreas are rare malignancies that resemble intestinal carcinoids and contain enterochromaffin cells. When confined to the pancreas, they may induce an atypical carcinoid syndrome, with a severe facial flush, hypotension, periorbital edema, and lacrimation. Carcinoid tumors that have metastasized to the liver cause the classic carcinoid syndrome (see Chapter 13).

The syndromes and complications of the major types of islet cell tumors are summarized in Figure 15-19.

Multiple Endocrine Neoplasia Syndrome Type I (MEN I) Is an Infrequent Familial Disorder

MEN I is characterized by multiple adenomas of the pituitary, parathyroids, and endocrine pancreas. It is frequently associated with the Zollinger-Ellison syndrome, in which case gastrin-secreting islet cell tumors are present. PETs occur in more than 60% of patients with MEN-1. The MEN syndromes are described in detail in Chapter 21.

Ectopic Hormone Syndromes May Be Caused by Islet Cell Tumors

Islet cell tumors may secrete a variety of normal hormones that are not ordinarily produced in the pancreas (ectopic hormones), including ACTH, parathyroid hormone, calcitonin, and vasopressin. These ectopic hormones may be produced either alone or in combination with normally occurring pancreatic hormones. Endocrine tumors of the pancreas account for 10% of paraneoplastic Cushing syndrome, in this respect being second only to small cell carcinoma of the lung.

16

The Kidney

J. Charles Jennette

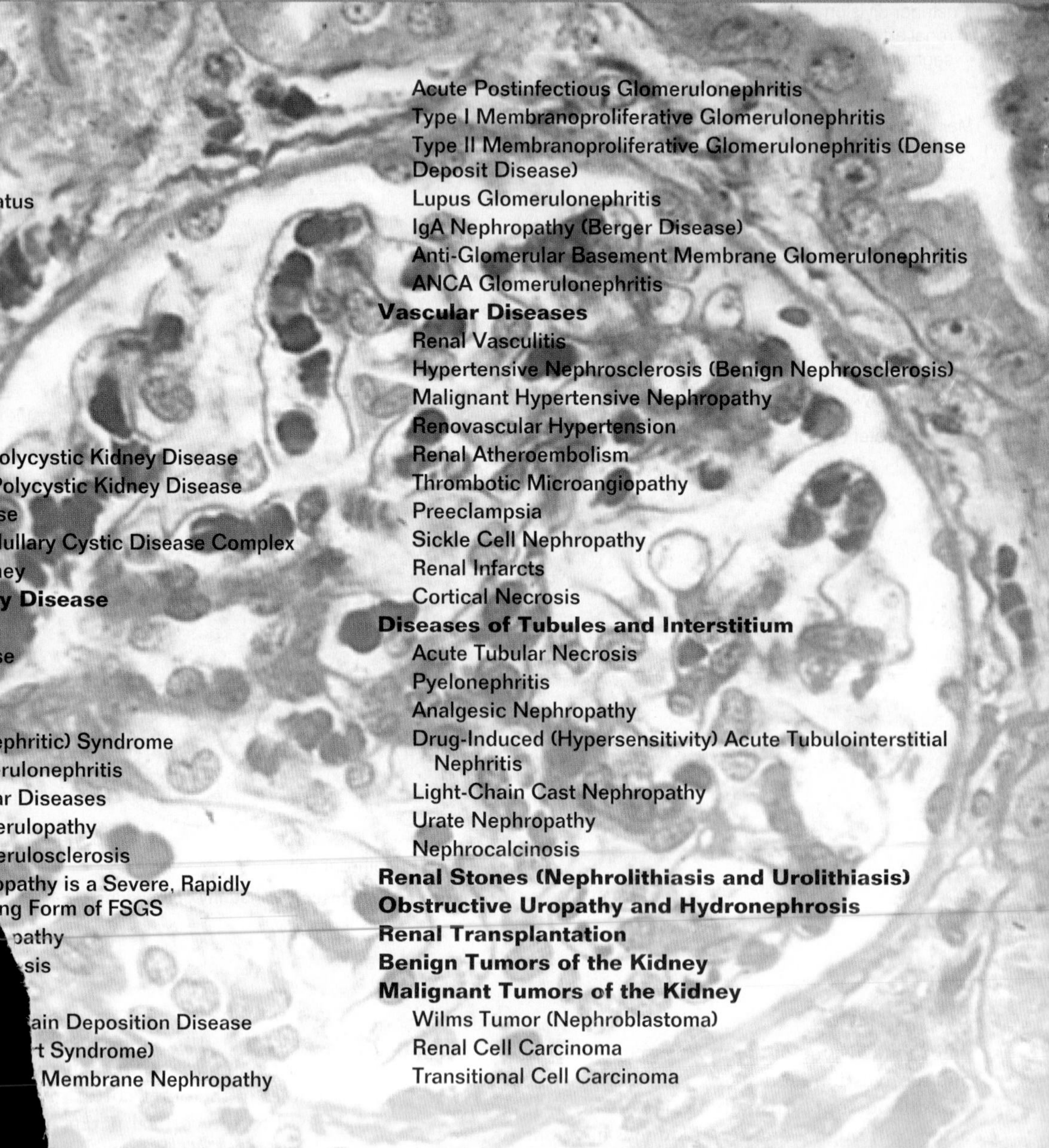

naped organs located on both in the retroperitoneal space. are approximately 11 cm long, kidney consists of an outer . 16-1). When a kidney is bisected, the medulla has approximately 12 pyramids, with their bases at the corticomedullary junction. Each medullary pyramid and the overlying cortex constitute a renal lobe. A pyramid has an inner and an outer zone. The inner zone, the **papilla,** empties into a calyx, which is a funnel-shaped structure that conducts urine into the renal pelvis. The pelvis in turn empties into the ureter.

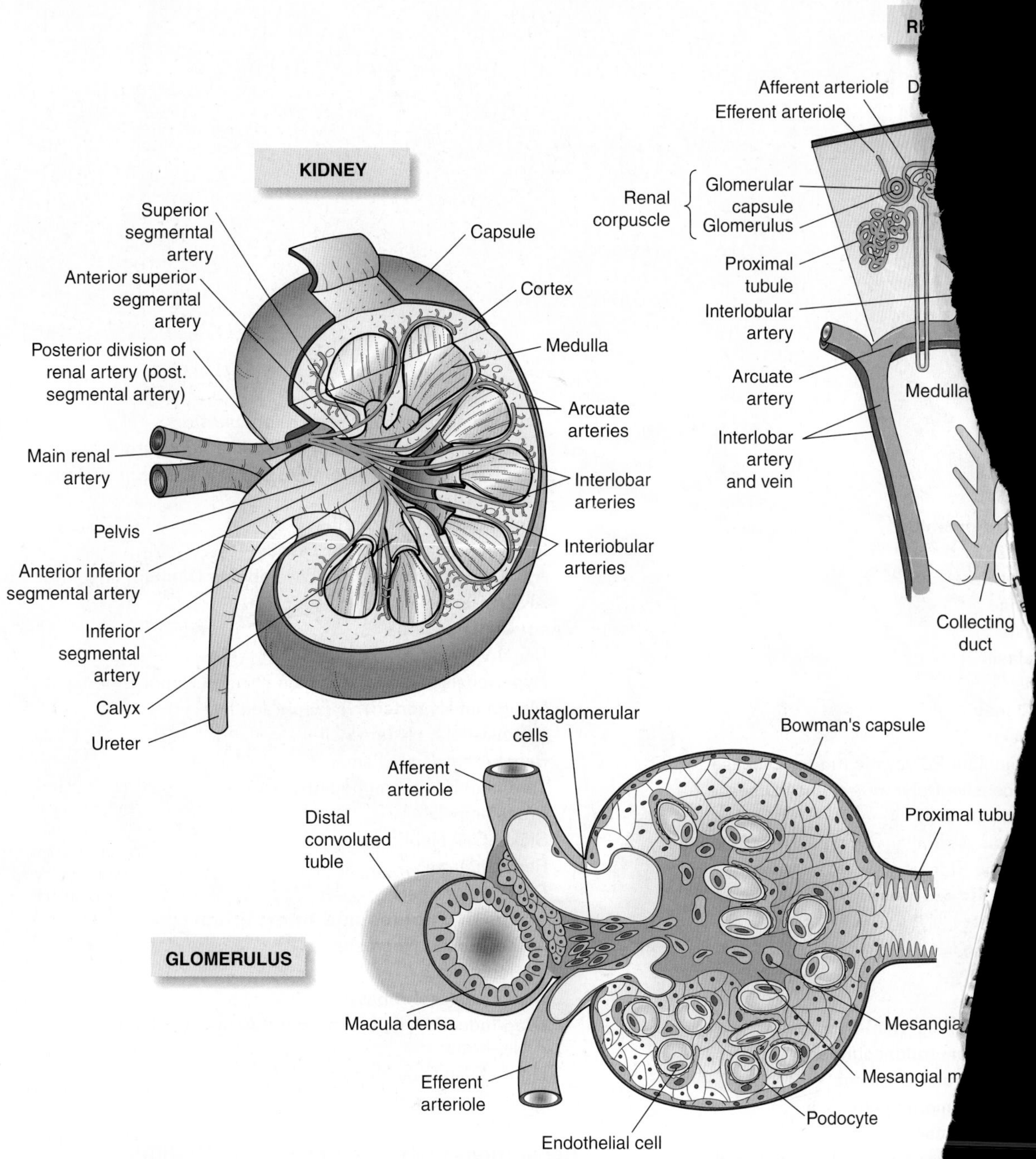

FIGURE 16-1. **The gross and microscopic anatomy of the kidney.**

Blood Vessels

The kidney is one of the most vascularized organs in the body and receives about one fifth to one fourth of the cardiac output. The blood supply usually derives from a single main renal artery, although a quarter of kidneys have one or more accessory renal arteries. Before entering the renal parenchyma, the main renal artery divides into anterior and posterior branches, which in turn give rise to the interlobar arteries (see Fig. 16-1). The latter branch into the arcuate arteries, which course parallel to the renal surface near the junction of the medulla and the cortex. The interlobular arteries arise from the arcuate arteries and extend toward the renal surface. The interlobular arteries

give off the afferent arterioles, e
glomerulus. After emerging fro
arteriole branches into capillari
terioles in the outer cortex giv
blood to the cortical parench
glomeruli in the deep cortex,
vessels that extend into the m
peritubular vessels, namely, th

The Glomerulus is the Rena

The nephron is the architec
cludes the glomerulus and its

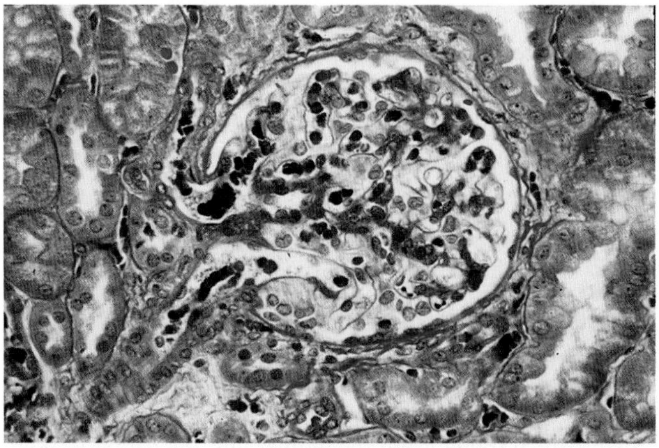

FIGURE 16-2. **Normal glomerulus, light microscopy.** The Masson trichrome stain shows a glomerular tuft with delicate blue capillary wall basement membranes, small amounts of blue matrix surrounding mesangial cells, and the hilum on the left. The afferent arteriole enters below and the efferent arteriole exits above.

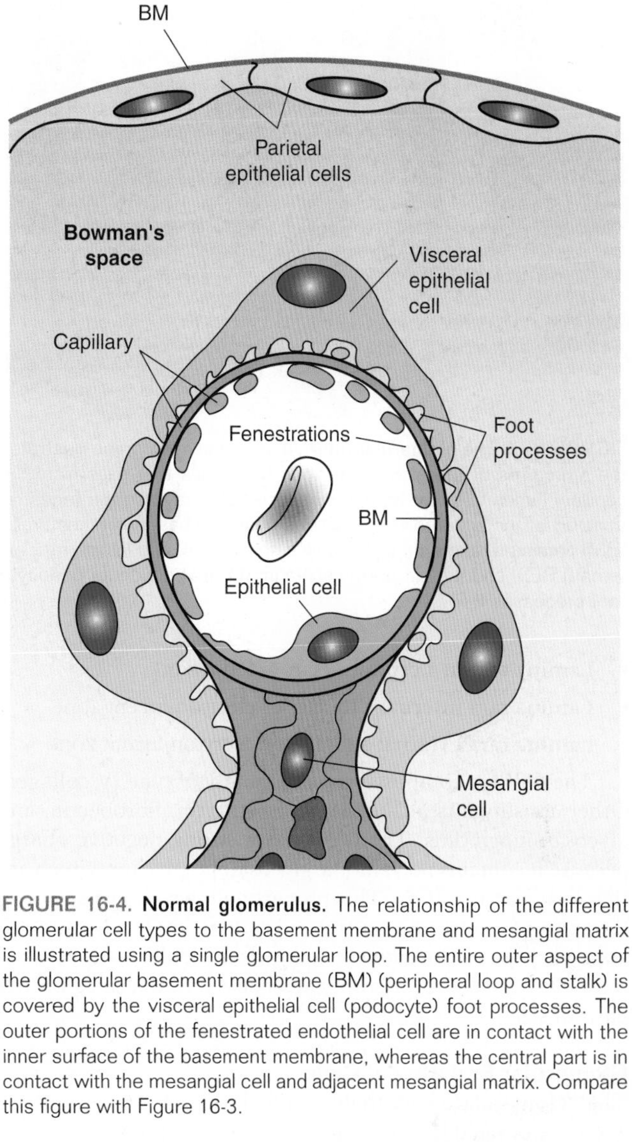

FIGURE 16-4. **Normal glomerulus.** The relationship of the different glomerular cell types to the basement membrane and mesangial matrix is illustrated using a single glomerular loop. The entire outer aspect of the glomerular basement membrane (BM) (peripheral loop and stalk) is covered by the visceral epithelial cell (podocyte) foot processes. The outer portions of the fenestrated endothelial cell are in contact with the inner surface of the basement membrane, whereas the central part is in contact with the mesangial cell and adjacent mesangial matrix. Compare this figure with Figure 16-3.

the common collecting system (see Fig. 16-1). The glomerulus is a specialized network of capillaries covered by epithelial cells and supported by modified smooth muscle cells called **mesangial cells** (see Fig. 16-1 and Fig. 16-2, Fig. 16-3, and Fig. 16-4). As it enters the glomerulus the afferent arteriole branches into capillaries, which form the convoluted glomerular tuft and eventually coalesce into the efferent arteriole that exits the glomerulus. The glomerular capillaries are lined by fenestrated endothelial cells lying on a basement membrane. The outer surface of this basement membrane is covered by specialized epithelial cells called **podocytes** or **visceral epithelial cells.** Podocytes line the glomerular side of Bowman's space, whereas the parietal epithelial cells line Bowman's capsule on the opposite side.

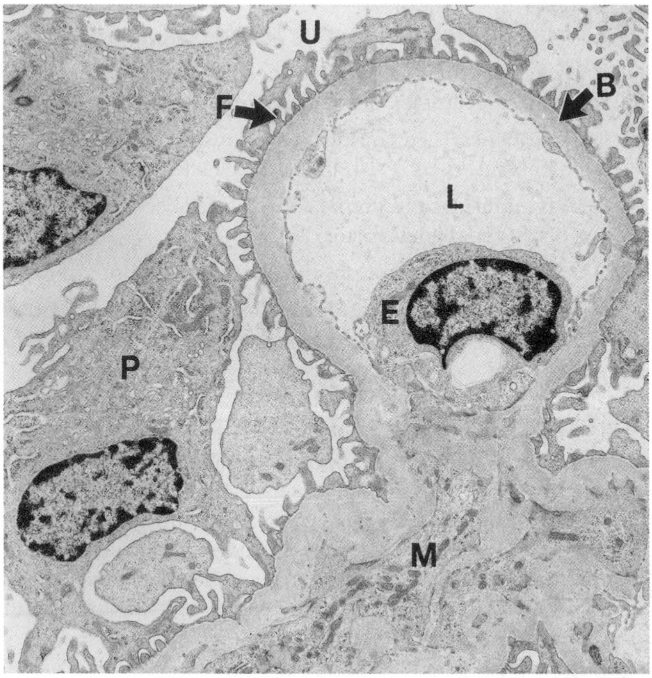

FIGURE 16-3. **Normal glomerulus.** In this electron micrograph of a single capillary loop and adjacent mesangium, the capillary wall portion of the lumen (L) is lined by a thin layer of fenestrated endothelial cytoplasm that extends out from the endothelial cell body (E). The endothelial cell body is in direct contact with the mesangium, which includes the mesangial cell (M) and adjacent matrix. The outer aspect of the basement membrane (B) is covered by foot processes (F) from the podocyte (P) that line the urinary space (U). Compare this figure with Figure 16-4.

Glomerular Basement Membrane

The glomerular basement membrane (GBM) (see Fig. 16-3 and Fig 16-4, and Fig 16-5) lies between the endothelial cells and the podocytes in peripheral capillary walls and between the mesangium and the podocytes. Thus, the GBM does not completely surround each capillary lumen but rather splays out over the mesangium as the paramesangial GBM. Thus a potential pathway exists for substances in the blood to enter the mesangium without crossing the GBM.

Although morphologically similar to many other basement membranes, the GBM is functionally and chemically distinct. Ultrastructurally, it is approximately 350 nm thick and has three definable layers (see Fig. 16-5):

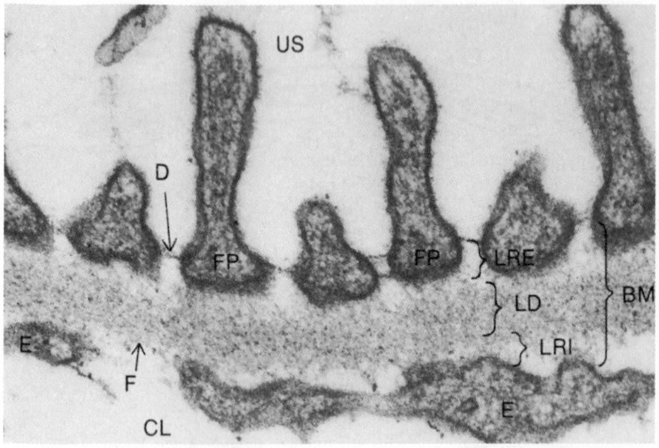

FIGURE 16-5. **The glomerular filter.** An electron micrograph illustrates the structures of the glomerular filter. Molecules that pass from the capillary lumen (CL) to the urinary space (US) traverse the fenestrations (F) of the endothelial cell (E), the trilaminar basement membrane (BM) (lamina rara interna [LRI], lamina densa [LD], and lamina rara externa [LRE]), and the slit pore diaphragm (D) that connects podocyte foot processes (FP).

- **Lamina densa:** a central electron-dense zone
- **Lamina rara interna:** a thin inner electron-lucent zone
- **Lamina rara externa:** a thin outer electron-lucent zone

The GBM is composed predominantly of type IV collagen. Other constituents include laminin, entactin, fibronectin, and glycosaminoglycans. The GBM has a strong negative charge because it contains polyanionic glycosaminoglycans, which are rich in heparan sulfate. This property allows charge-selective filtration of electrically neutral and cationic molecules and relative exclusion of negatively charged molecules such as albumin. The GBM also discriminates between molecules on the basis of size.

Glomerular Endothelial Cells

The glomerular endothelial cell layer is 50 nm thick and is fenestrated by numerous 60- to 100-nm pores (Fig. 16-5). These pores are not a major filtration barrier to plasma constituents. Endothelial surface membrane proteins (e.g., adhesion molecules) and endothelial secretory products (e.g., prostaglandins and nitric oxide), play important roles in the pathogenesis of inflammatory and thrombotic glomerular diseases.

Podocytes

Podocytes rest on the outer aspect of the GBM. They send cytoplasmic projections, termed **foot processes,** onto the lamina rara externa of the GBM (see Fig. 16-5). Between adjacent foot processes is a thin membrane called the **filtration slit diaphragm,** which is a modified adherens junction. The podocytes are the major size-selective glomerular filtration barrier, whereas the GBM is the major charge-selective barrier. Genetic abnormalities in the proteins that compose the slit diaphragm, such as **nephrin** and **podocin,** can result in abnormal protein loss into the urine (proteinuria).

ngium

ngium is a cellular and matrix network that supports lus. Mesangial cells are modified smooth muscle he center of the glomerular tuft between capil- tant functions of the mesangium are

- Mechanical support for the glomerulus
- Endocytosis and processing of plasma proteins, including immune complexes
- Maintenance of basement membrane and matrix elements
- Modulation of glomerular filtration by the contractility of mesangial cells
- Generation of molecular mediators (e.g., prostaglandins and cytokines)

The Tubules Comprise Most of the Nephron

The major segments of the tubule that arises from each glomerulus are the proximal tubule, loop of Henle, and distal tubule, which empties into the collecting duct. At the origin of the proximal tubule from the glomerulus, the flat parietal epithelium abruptly transforms into tall columnar cells of the **proximal tubule,** which have numerous tall microvilli that form a brush border. The initial segment is the proximal tubule is very tortuous and thus is called the **proximal convoluted tubule.** As it descends into the medulla, the proximal tubule straightens into the thick **descending limb of the loop of Henle.** Further into the medulla, the thick descending limb thins into the **thin limb of the loop of Henle,** which eventually loops back toward the cortex. As it approaches the cortex, the thin limb becomes the **thick ascending limb,** which returns to the glomerulus from which the tubule arose and contributes to the juxtaglomerular apparatus of that glomerulus. It then becomes the **distal convoluted tubule.** Several distal tubules unite to form a **collecting duct,** which ultimately empties into the ducts of Bellini, the structures that discharge urine through the papillae into the calyces.

The Juxtaglomerular Apparatus Secretes Hormones

The juxtaglomerular apparatus, located at the hilus of the glomerulus, is a complex that consists of:

- **Macula densa,** a region of the thick ascending limb of the loop of Henle that has closely packed nuclei
- **Extraglomerular mesangial cells,** located between the macula densa and the hilar arterioles
- **Terminal afferent arteriole and proximal efferent arteriole**

The wall of the afferent arteriole contains characteristic granular cells involved in the synthesis and secretion of renin and angiotensin.

The Interstitium Offers Structural Support

The renal interstitium is composed of interstitial cells that resemble fibroblasts and surrounding collagenous matrix. The interstitium occupies only 10% of cortical volume but constitutes 20% to 30% of medullary volume. In addition to structural support, interstitial cells have homeostatic secretory functions. For example, some cortical interstitial cells secrete erythropoietin and some medullary cells elaborate prostaglandins.

Congenital Anomalies

Potter Sequence Results from Insufficient Amniotic Fluid

Potter sequence (oligohydramnios sequence) is the syndrome of pathologic abnormalities that are caused by markedly reduced intrauterine urine production (also see Chapter 6). Reduced urine production results in less amniotic fluid (oligohydramnios). The amniotic fluid normally cushions the fetus. With less fluid, the fetus is compressed by the uterus; this causes low-set ears, small receding chin, beaklike nose, and abnormally bent lower extremities. The most life-threatening component of Potter sequence is pulmonary hypoplasia, which is caused by inadequate maturational stimuli from amniotic fluid and by compression of the chest wall by the uterus. Because even neonates can be dialyzed, severe respiratory insufficiency secondary to Potter sequence (rather than renal insufficiency) may be the cause of death in infants with severe congenital renal anomalies.

Renal Agenesis Is the Complete Absence of Renal Tissue

Most infants born with bilateral renal agenesis are stillborn and have Potter sequence. Bilateral agenesis is often associated with other congenital anomalies, especially elsewhere in the urinary tract or lower extremities. Unilateral renal agenesis is not a serious matter if there are no associated anomalies, because the contralateral kidney undergoes sufficient hypertrophy to maintain normal renal function. Later in life, however, there is an increased risk for developing progressive glomerular sclerosis (secondary focal segmental glomerulosclerosis [FSGS]) because of overwork of the nephron.

Renal Hypoplasia Refers to a Congenital Reduction in Renal Mass

The kidney shows no histologic malformation and is formed by six or fewer renal lobes (medullary pyramids with overlying cortex). Renal hypoplasia must be differentiated from small kidneys secondary to atrophy or scarring. A frequent variant of hypoplasia features enlargement of the too few glomeruli and thus is termed **oligomeganephronia.**

Ectopic Kidney Is an Abnormal Location of the Organ

The misplaced kidney is usually in the pelvis. Most commonly, this condition results from failure of the fetal kidney to migrate from the pelvis to the flank. Renal ectopia may involve only one kidney or it may be bilateral. In **simple ectopia,** the ureters drain into the appropriate side of the bladder. In **crossed ectopia,** the ectopic kidney is on the same side as its normal mate, and the ectopic ureter crosses the midline and drains into the contralateral side of the bladder.

Horseshoe Kidney Is a Single, Large, Midline Organ

The infant is born with fused kidneys, usually at the lower poles (Fig. 16-6). This anomaly usually has no clinical consequences but does increase the risk for obstruction and pyelonephritis because the ureters must cross over the junction between the two kidneys when the organ is fused at the lower pole.

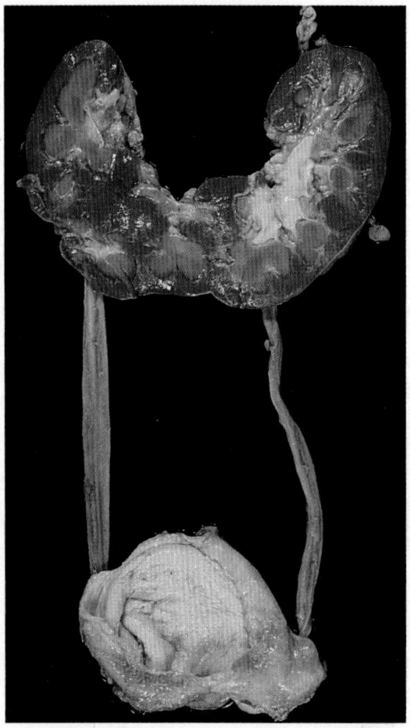

FIGURE 16-6. **Horseshoe kidney.** The kidneys are fused at the lower pole.

Renal Dysplasia Is a Developmental Disorder

Renal dysplasia is characterized by undifferentiated tubular structures surrounded by primitive mesenchyme, sometimes with heterotopic tissue such as cartilage. Cysts often form from the abnormal tubules.

PATHOGENESIS: Renal dysplasia results from an abnormality in metanephric differentiation. There are multiple genetic and somatic causes. Some familial forms of dysplasia probably result from abnormal differential signals that affect the inductive interactions between the ureteric bud and the metanephric blastema. Many forms of dysplasia are accompanied by other urinary tract abnormalities, especially ones that cause obstruction of urine flow. This association suggests that an obstruction to the flow of urine in utero can cause dysplasia. Frequent associated anomalies include:

- Ureteral agenesis
- Ureteral atresia
- Ureteropelvic junction obstruction
- Ureterovesical stenosis or posterior urethral valves

PATHOLOGY: The histologic hallmark of renal dysplasia is undifferentiated tubules and ducts lined by cuboidal or columnar epithelium. These structures are surrounded by mantles of undifferentiated mesenchyme that sometimes contain smooth muscle and islands of cartilage (Fig. 16-7). Rudimentary glomeruli may be present, and the tubules and ducts may be cystically dilated. Renal dysplasia can be unilateral or bilateral, and the involved kidney can be abnormally large or very small.

- **Aplastic renal dysplasia** results in very small misshapen dysplastic kidneys, which may be difficult to identify by gross examination.
- **Multicystic renal dysplasia** is usually unilateral and is characterized by renal enlargement by multiple cysts, ranging from microscopic to several centimeters in diameter. The kidney does not have the usual kidney shape, but is rather an irregular mass of cysts (Fig. 16-8).
- **Diffuse cystic renal dysplasia** features more uniformly size cysts and preservation of a kidney shape.

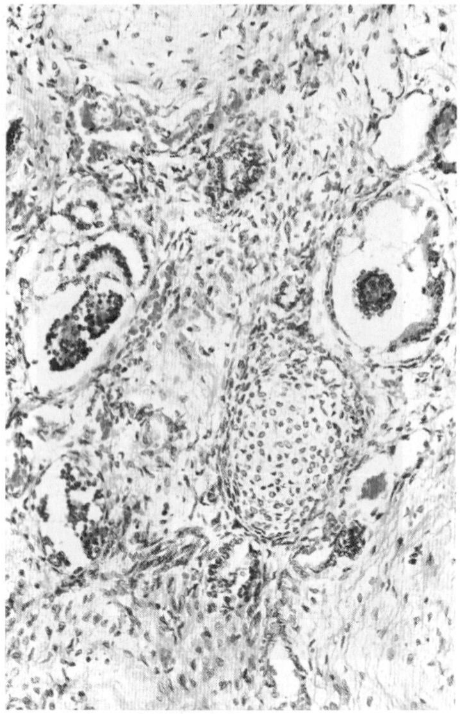

FIGURE 16-7. **Renal dysplasia.** Immature glomeruli, tubules, and cartilage are surrounded by loose, undifferentiated mesenchymal tissue.

- **Obstructive renal dysplasia** is focal or diffuse, unilateral or bilateral dysplasia caused by an overt intrauterine obstruction to urine flow, such as posterior urethral valves or ureteropelvic junction stenosis.

CLINICAL FEATURES: In most patients with multicystic renal dysplasia, a palpable flank mass is discovered shortly after birth, although small multicystic kidneys may not become apparent until many years later. *Unilateral multicystic renal dysplasia is the most common cause of an abdominal mass in newborns.* Unilateral dysplasia is adequately treated by removing the affected kidney. Bilateral aplastic dysplasia and diffuse cystic dysplasia cause oligohydramnios and the resultant Potter sequence and life-threatening pulmonary hypoplasia. Aplastic renal dysplasia and diffuse cystic dysplasia are more often hereditary than multicystic dysplasia, especially if they are associated with multiple anomalies in other organs, as in Meckel-Gruber syndrome.

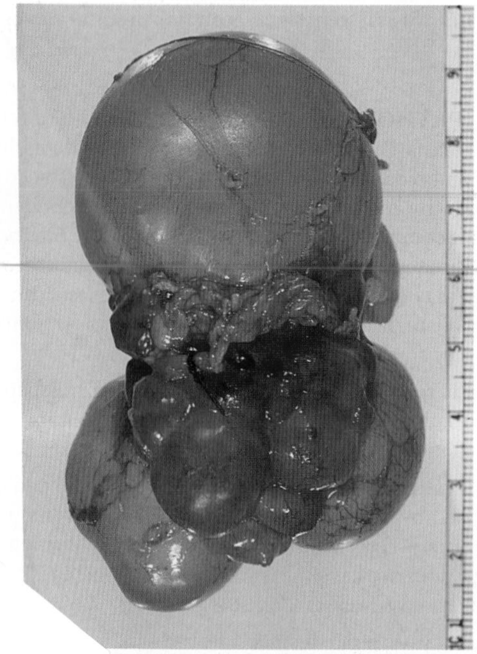

.lticystic renal dysplasia. An irregular mass of variably
ꜱ not have a reniform shape.

Autosomal Dominant Polycystic Kidney Disease (ADPKD) Features Enlarged, Multicystic Kidneys

ADPKD is the most common of a group of congenital diseases that are characterized by numerous cysts within the renal parenchyma (Fig. 16-9). It affects 1:400 to 1:1000 persons in the United States. Half of all patients with this disease eventually develop end-stage renal failure. ADPKD is responsible for 5% of all cases of renal disease that require dialysis or transplantation. Only diabetes and hypertension cause more end-stage renal disease than does ADPKD.

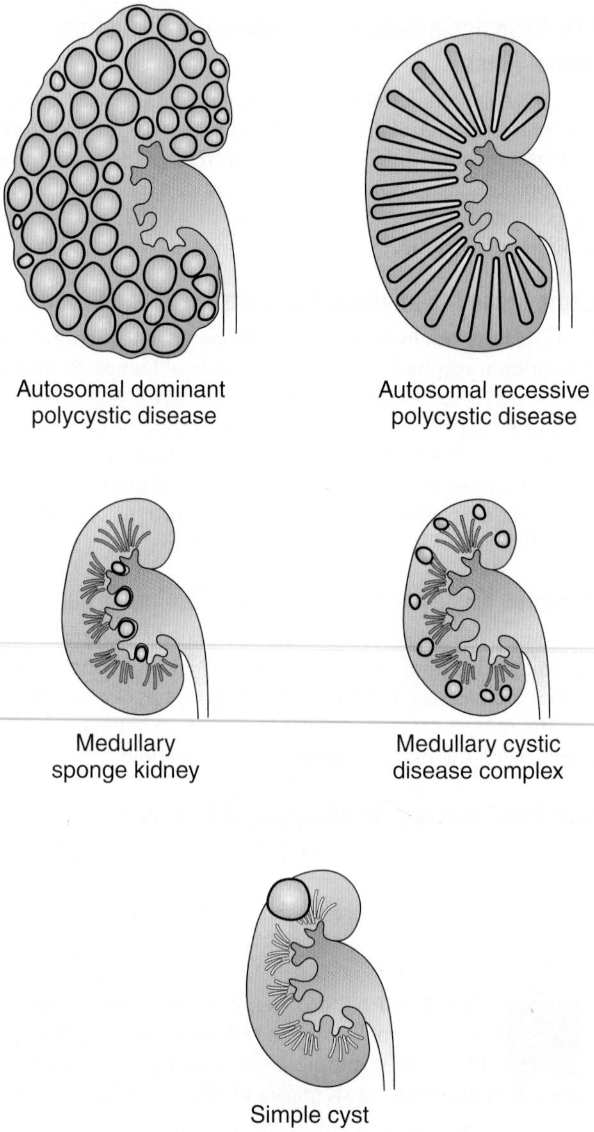

FIGURE 16-9. **Cystic diseases of the kidney.**

PATHOGENESIS: Some 85% of ADPKD is caused by mutations in the polycystic kidney disease 1 gene *(PKD1) and* 15% by mutations in *PKD2*. The products of these genes, polycystin-1 and polycystin-2, are in the primary cilia of tubular epithelial cells. These cilia sense urine flow and regulate tubule growth. Defects in these proteins disrupt calcium signaling from cilia that normally inhibits renal tubule growth.

Although the precise pathogenesis of ADPKD remains unclear, it is held that cysts arise in segments of renal tubules from a few cells that proliferate abnormally. The wall of the tubule becomes covered by an undifferentiated epithelium composed of cells with a high nucleus-to-cytoplasm ratio and only few microvilli. Concomitantly, a defective basement membrane immediately underlying the abnormal epithelium allows dilation of the affected tubule portion. Cyst fluid is initially derived from the glomerular filtrate, but eventually most of the cysts become disconnected from the tubules, in which case the fluid accumulates by transepithelial secretion. Historically, end-stage renal disease in ADPKD has been attributed to the pressure exerted by the dilating cysts on the surrounding normal parenchyma. However, it is now appreciated that cysts originate in less than 2% of nephrons, and that factors other than crowding of normal tissue by the expanding cysts likely contribute to the loss of functioning renal tissue. Apoptotic loss of renal tubules and accumulation of inflammatory mediators have been incriminated in the destruction of normal renal mass.

PATHOLOGY: The kidneys in ADPKD are markedly enlarged bilaterally, each weighing as much as 4500 g (Fig. 16-10). The external contours of the kidneys are distorted by numerous cysts, as large as 5 cm in diameter, which are filled with a straw-colored fluid. Microscopically, the cysts are lined by a cuboidal and columnar epithelium. They arise from virtually any point along the nephron, including glomeruli, proximal tubules, distal tubules, and collecting ducts. Areas of normal renal parenchyma are found between the cysts.

One third of patients with ADPKD also have **hepatic cysts,** whose lining resembles bile duct epithelium. Cysts occur in the spleen in 10% of patients and in the pancreas in 5%. One fifth of patients have an associated **cerebral aneurysm,** and intracranial hemorrhage is the cause of death in 15% of patients with ADPKD. Interestingly, many patients with ADPKD also develop colonic diverticula.

CLINICAL FEATURES: Most patients with ADPKD do not develop clinical manifestations until the fourth decade of life, which is why this condition was once called *adult* polycystic kidney disease. A small minority of patients develop symptoms during childhood, and rare ones are symptomatic at birth. Symptoms include a sense of heaviness in the loins, bilateral flank and abdominal masses, and passage of blood clots in the urine. Azotemia (elevated blood urea nitrogen) is common, and in half of patients progresses to uremia (clinical renal failure) over a period of several years.

Autosomal Recessive Polycystic Kidney Disease (ARPKD) Occurs in Infants

ARPKD is characterized by cystic transformation of collecting ducts. It is rare compared with ADPKD, occurring in about 1 in 10,000 to 50,000 live births. Seventy-five percent of these infants die in the perinatal period, often because of pulmonary hypoplasia caused by oligohydramnios (Potter sequence) and by the large size of the kidneys, which impairs expansion of the lungs. Exceptional cases of ARPKD manifest in older children and adults. ARPKD is caused by mutations in the *PKHD1* gene. The gene product, **fibrocystin,** is found in kidney, liver, and pancreas, and appears to be involved in regulation of cell proliferation and adhesion. Mutations of *PKHD1* also result in ARPKD, pancreatic cysts, and hepatic biliary dysgenesis and fibrosis.

PATHOLOGY: In contrast to ADPKD, the external kidney surface in the infantile disorder is smooth. The disease is invariably bilateral. The kidneys are often so large that delivery of the infant is impeded. The cysts are fusiform dilations of cortical and medullary collecting ducts and have a striking radial arrangement perpendicular to the renal capsule (Fig. 16-11). Interstitial fibrosis and tubular atrophy are common, particularly in children whose disease presents at an

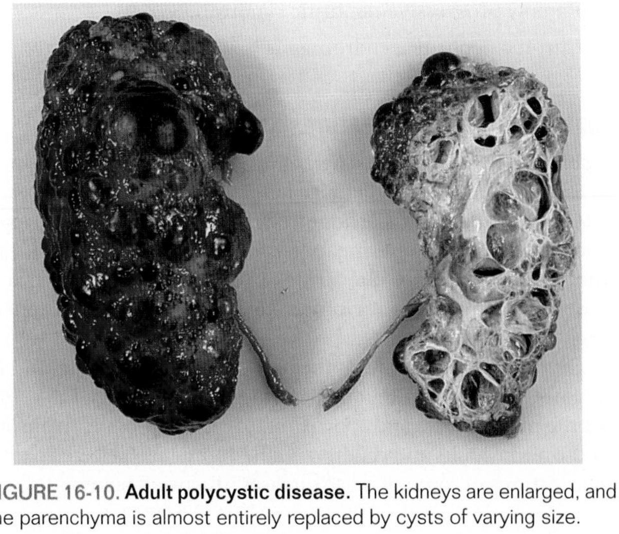

FIGURE 16-10. **Adult polycystic disease.** The kidneys are enlarged, and the parenchyma is almost entirely replaced by cysts of varying size.

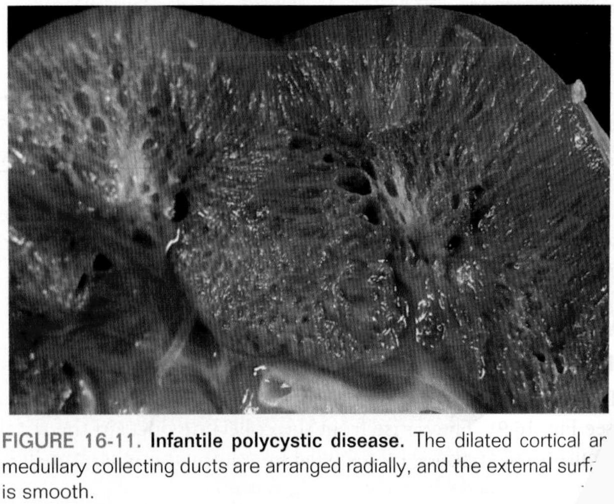

FIGURE 16-11. **Infantile polycystic disease.** The dilated cortical ar medullary collecting ducts are arranged radially, and the external surf. is smooth.

older age. As in ADPKD, the calyceal system in ARPKD is normal. The liver usually is affected by **congenital hepatic fibrosis,** which exhibits fibrous expansion of portal tracts with bile duct proliferation (see Chapter 14).

In Glomerulocystic Disease Bowman's Capsule is Dilated in Many Glomeruli

The disorder occurs as an isolated process or as a component of other cystic disease, such as ADPKD, nephronophthisis–medullary cystic disease complex, and diffuse cystic dysplasia. Thus, there are multiple causes for glomerulocystic disease. One form is autosomal dominant, caused by mutations in the gene for hepatocyte nuclear factor-1 beta (HNF-1β).

PATHOLOGY: Kidneys with primary glomerulocystic disease may be large or small. The cut surface reveals numerous small round cysts rarely more than 1 cm in diameter. Light microscopy shows dilation of Bowman's capsule in many glomeruli. The residual glomerular tuft is often distorted or appears immature.

In Nephronophthisis–Medullary Cystic Disease Complex Kidneys Show Tubulointerstitial Injury and Medullary Cysts

Nephronophthisis–medullary cystic disease complex comprises a group of autosomal recessive and autosomal dominant diseases. The pathogenesis may involve a developmental defect in tubular basement membranes.

PATHOLOGY: The kidneys are small and when sectioned often display multiple, variably sized cysts (up to 1 cm) at the corticomedullary junction (see Fig. 16-9). The cysts arise from the distal portions of the nephron. Atrophic tubules with markedly thickened and laminated basement membranes and loss of tubules out of proportion to the glomerular loss are early histologic features of the disease. Eventually, corticomedullary cysts may develop, and the remainder of the parenchyma becomes increasingly atrophic. Secondary glomerular sclerosis, interstitial fibrosis, and nonspecific inflammatory infiltrates dominate the late histologic picture.

CLINICAL FEATURES: Medullary cystic disease complex accounts for 10% to 25% of renal failure in childhood. Patients present initially with deteriorating tubular function, such as impaired concentrating ability and sodium wasting, manifested as polyuria, polydipsia, and enuresis (bed wetting). Progressive azotemia and renal failure follow, usually within 5 years of the onset of symptoms. Nephronophthisis is an autosomal recessive disease with onset in childhood and adolescence that often progresses to end-stage renal disease by 25 years of age. Defects in different genes determine onset in infancy (*NPHP2*), childhood (*NPHP1 and 4*), or adolescence (*NPHP3*). Medullary cystic disease is autosomal dominant with defects in the *MCKD1* or *2* genes, has onset of symptoms in adolescence, and usually does not cause renal failure until the third decade.

edullary Sponge Kidney Is Distinguished by Cysts Papillae

v cysts are multiple and small (<5 mm in diameter) They arise from the collecting ducts in the renal e lined by cuboidal or columnar epithelium. The disease is bilateral in 75% of patients. A few familial cases have been described.

Medullary sponge kidney is asymptomatic in young adults. Symptomatic cases are usually discovered between the ages of 30 and 60, when affected people complain of flank pain, dysuria, hematuria or "gravel" in the urine caused by stone formation in the cysts. Although the disease itself does not pose a threat to health, the cysts may predispose to secondary pyelonephritis.

Acquired Cystic Kidney Disease

Simple Renal Cysts Are Seen in Half of People over 50 Years Old

These cysts are usually incidental findings at autopsy and rarely clinically symptomatic unless they are very large. These fluid-filled cysts may be solitary or multiple and are usually located in the outer cortex, where they bulge the capsule. Simple cysts less commonly occur in the medulla. Microscopically, they are lined by a flat epithelium.

Long-Term Dialysis Leads to Acquired Cystic Disease

This disorder is characterized by multiple cortical and medullary cysts that form in the kidneys of patients with end-stage renal disease who are maintained on dialysis. After 5 years of dialysis, over 75% of patients acquire bilateral cystic kidneys. The cysts are initially lined by flat-to-cuboidal epithelium, but hyperplastic and neoplastic epithelial proliferation may develop.

Glomerular Diseases

A extensive variety of renal disorders are caused by injury to the glomerulus. A glomerular disease may be the only major site of disease (primary glomerular disease; e.g., immunoglobulin [Ig]A nephropathy) or may be a component of a disease that affects multiple organs (secondary glomerular disease; e.g., lupus glomerulonephritis). The signs and symptoms of glomerular disease fall into one of the following categories:

- Asymptomatic proteinuria
- Nephrotic syndrome
- Asymptomatic hematuria
- Acute nephritic syndrome
- Rapidly progressive nephritic syndrome
- Chronic nephritic syndrome

Nephrotic Syndrome Features Severe Proteinuria

Nephrotic syndrome is characterized by heavy proteinuria (>3.5 g of protein/24 hours), hypoalbuminemia, edema, hyperlipidemia, and lipiduria. The major pathogenetic abnormality is increased glomerular capillary permeability, allowing protein to be lost from the plasma into the urine (proteinuria). Proteinuria is caused by many different glomerular diseases and by a variety of mechanisms.

Severe proteinuria causes the nephrotic syndrome (Fig. 16-12), but lower levels of proteinuria may be asymptomatic. Table 16-1 lists the major causes and approximate frequency of the nephrotic syndrome in adults and children. Table 16-2 details selected pathologic features of some of these diseases (discussed below).

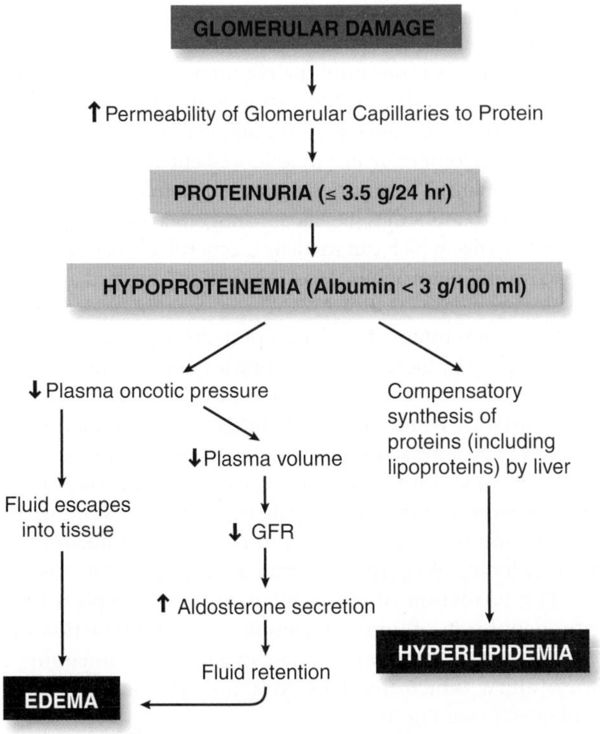

FIGURE 16-12. **Pathophysiology of the nephrotic syndrome.** (GFR = glomerular filtration rate).

Important differences exist in the rates of specific glomerular diseases that produce nephrotic syndrome in adults versus those in children. For example, minimal-change glomerulopathy is responsible for most (70%) cases of nephrotic syndrome in children but only 15% in adults. The primary glomerular diseases most often responsible for nephrotic syndrome in adults are membranous glomerulopathy and FSGS.Membranous glomerulopathy is the most frequent cause in Caucasians and Asians, whereas FSGS is the most common etiology in American blacks. The incidence of FSGS has been increasing over the past decade. Systemic diseases that involve the kidney, such as diabetes, amyloidosis, and systemic lupus erythematosus (SLE), are responsible for many cases of nephrotic syndrome in adults. Membranoproliferative glomerulonephritis is a much more frequent reason for nephrotic syndrome in underdeveloped countries that have a high prevalence of chronic infectious diseases.

TABLE 16-1

Frequency of Causes for the Nephrotic Syndrome Induced by Primary Glomerular Diseases in Children and Adults

Cause	Children (%)	Adults (%)
Minimal-change glomerulopathy	75	15
Membranous glomerulopathy	5	30
Focal segmental glomerulosclerosis	10	30
Type I membranoproliferative glomerulonephritis	5	5
Other glomerular diseases*	5	20

* Includes many forms of mesangioproliferative and proliferative glomerulonephritis, such as immunoglobulin (Ig)A nephropathy, which often also cause nephritic features.

Nephritic (Glomerulonephritic) Syndrome Is an Inflammatory Disease

Nephritic syndrome is characterized by hematuria (either microscopic or visible grossly), variable degrees of proteinuria, and decreased glomerular filtration rate. It results in elevated blood urea nitrogen and serum creatinine, oliguria, salt and water retention, edema, and hypertension. Glomerular diseases associated with the nephritic syndrome are caused by inflammatory changes in glomeruli, such as infiltration by leukocytes, hyperplasia of glomerular cells, and, in severe lesions, necrosis. Sufficient injury to glomerular capillaries results in spillage of protein and blood cells into the urine (proteinuria and hematuria). The inflammatory damage may also impair glomerular flow and filtration, resulting in renal insufficiency, fluid retention, and hypertension. Nephritic manifestations may (1) develop rapidly and result in reversible renal insufficiency (acute glomerulonephritis); (2) progress rapidly, with renal failure that resolves only with aggressive treatment (rapidly progressive glomerulonephritis); or (3) persist continuously or intermittently for years and proceed slowly to renal failure (chronic glomerulonephritis).

As shown in Table 16-3, some glomerular diseases tend to cause the nephrotic syndrome, whereas others lead to the nephritic syndrome. However, with the possible exception of minimal-change glomerulopathy (which almost always causes the nephrotic syndrome), all glomerular diseases occasionally

TABLE 16-2

Pathologic Features of Important Causes of the Nephrotic Syndrome

	Minimal change glomerulopathy	Focal segmental glomerulosclerosis	Membranous glomerulopathy	Membranoproliferative glomerulonephritis
Light microscopy	No lesion	Focal and segmental glomerular condsolidation	Diffuse global capillary wall thickening	Capillary wall thickening and endocapillary hypercellularity
Immuno-fluorescence microscopy	No immune deposits	No immune deposits	Diffuse capillary wall immunoglobulin	Diffuse capillary wall complement
Electron microscopy	No immune deposits	No immune deposits	Diffuse subepithelial dense deposits	Subendothelial (type I) or intramembranous (type II) dense deposits

TABLE 16-3

Tendencies of Glomerular Diseases to Manifest Nephrotic and Nephritic Features

Disease	Nephrotic	Nephritic
Minimal-change glomerulopathy	++++	–
Membranous glomerulopathy	+++	++
Focal segmental glomerulosclerosis	+++	++
Mesangioproliferative glomerulonephritis*	++	++
Membranoproliferative glomerulonephritis	++	++
Proliferative glomerulonephritis *	+	+++
Crescentic glomerulonephritis *	+	++++

*These histologic phenotypes can be caused by many categories of glomerular disease, including immunoglobulin (Ig)A nephropathy, postinfectious glomerulonephritis, lupus glomerulonephritis, antineutrophil cytoplasmic autoantibody glomerulonephritis, and antiglomerular basement membrane glomerulonephritis.

produce mixed nephritic and nephrotic manifestations that confound clinical diagnosis. *Renal biopsy evaluation is the only means of definitive diagnosis for glomerular diseases, although clinical and laboratory data may provide presumptive evidence for a specific disease.*

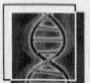

PATHOGENESIS: Glomerulonephritis is frequently caused by immunologic mechanisms. Both antibody-mediated and cell-mediated types of immunity play roles in the production of glomerular inflammation. However, three mechanisms of antibody-induced inflammation have been incriminated as the major pathogenetic processes in most forms of glomerulonephritis (Fig. 16-13):

- In situ immune complex formation
- Deposition of circulating immune complexes
- Antineutrophil cytoplasmic autoantibodies (ANCAs)

Immune complex formation in situ involves binding of circulating antibodies to intrinsic antigens or foreign antigens within glomeruli. For example, anti-GBM autoantibodies bind to a very specific epitope on the alpha 4 chain of type IV collagen in GBMs. The resultant immune complexes in the glomerular capillary walls attract leukocytes and activate complement and other humoral inflammatory mediator systems, resulting in inflammatory injury.

Circulating immune complexes may deposit in glomeruli and incite inflammation like that produced by immune complex formation in situ. For example, antigens released into the circulation by bacterial or viral infection can bind to circulating antibodies to produce immune complexes. If these complexes escape phagocytosis, they can de-…it in glomeruli and incite inflammation.

…unofluorescence microscopy using anti-human an-…cts the glomerular localization of immune complexes. Anti-GBM antibodies produce linear staining of GBMs, whereas other immune complexes produce granular staining in capillary walls, mesangium, or both.

ANCAs cause a severe glomerulonephritis that exhibits little or no glomerular immunofluorescent staining for immunoglobulins. These patients have a high frequency of circulating autoantibodies specific for antigens in the cytoplasm of neutrophils, which can mediate glomerular inflammation by activating neutrophils. Most ANCAs are directed against myeloperoxidase (MPO-ANCA) or proteinase-3 (PR3-ANCA). Even minor stimulation of neutrophils and monocytes, such as by increased circulating levels of cytokines during viral infection, causes them to express MPO and PR3 on their surfaces, where these autoantigens can interact with ANCAs. This interaction leads to neutrophil activation and results in adhesion to endothelial cells in the microvasculature, especially glomerular capillaries. In that location they release injurious products that promote vascular inflammation, including glomerulonephritis, arteritis, and venulitis.

The formation of glomerular immune complexes in situ, deposition of immune complexes, and interaction of ANCA with leukocytes all initiate of glomerular inflammatory injury, which involves attraction and activation of leukocytes (see Fig. 16-13).

PATHOLOGY: Many specific glomerular diseases have distinctive pathologic features, as well as different natural histories and appropriate treatments. *Accurate pathologic diagnosis of glomerular diseases requires evaluation of renal tissue by light, immunofluorescence, and electron microscopy, together with integration of the findings with clinical information.* Table 16-4 lists pathologic features that are useful for diagnosing glomerular diseases. Table 16-2 summarizes the pathologic features of important causes for the nephrotic syndrome. The algorithm in Figure 16-14 shows how pathologic and clinical data are integrated to diagnose specific glomerular diseases.

In general, the pathologic features that indicate acute inflammation, such as endocapillary and extracapillary hypercellularity, leukocyte infiltration and necrosis, are more common in disorders that have predominantly nephritic features than in those with nephrotic attributes. **Glomerular crescent formation** (extracapillary proliferation) correlates with a more rapidly progressive course. Crescent formation is not specific for a particular cause of glomerular inflammation. It is rather a marker for severe injury that has resulted in extensive rupture of capillary walls, which allows inflammatory mediators to enter Bowman's space, where they stimulate macrophage infiltration and epithelial proliferation.

Minimal-Change Glomerulopathy Causes Nephrotic Syndrome

Pathologically, the disease is characterized by effacement of podocyte foot processes.

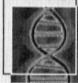

PATHOGENESIS: The pathogenesis of minimal-change glomerulopathy is unknown. Involvement of the immune system has been postulated because the disease frequently enters remission when treated

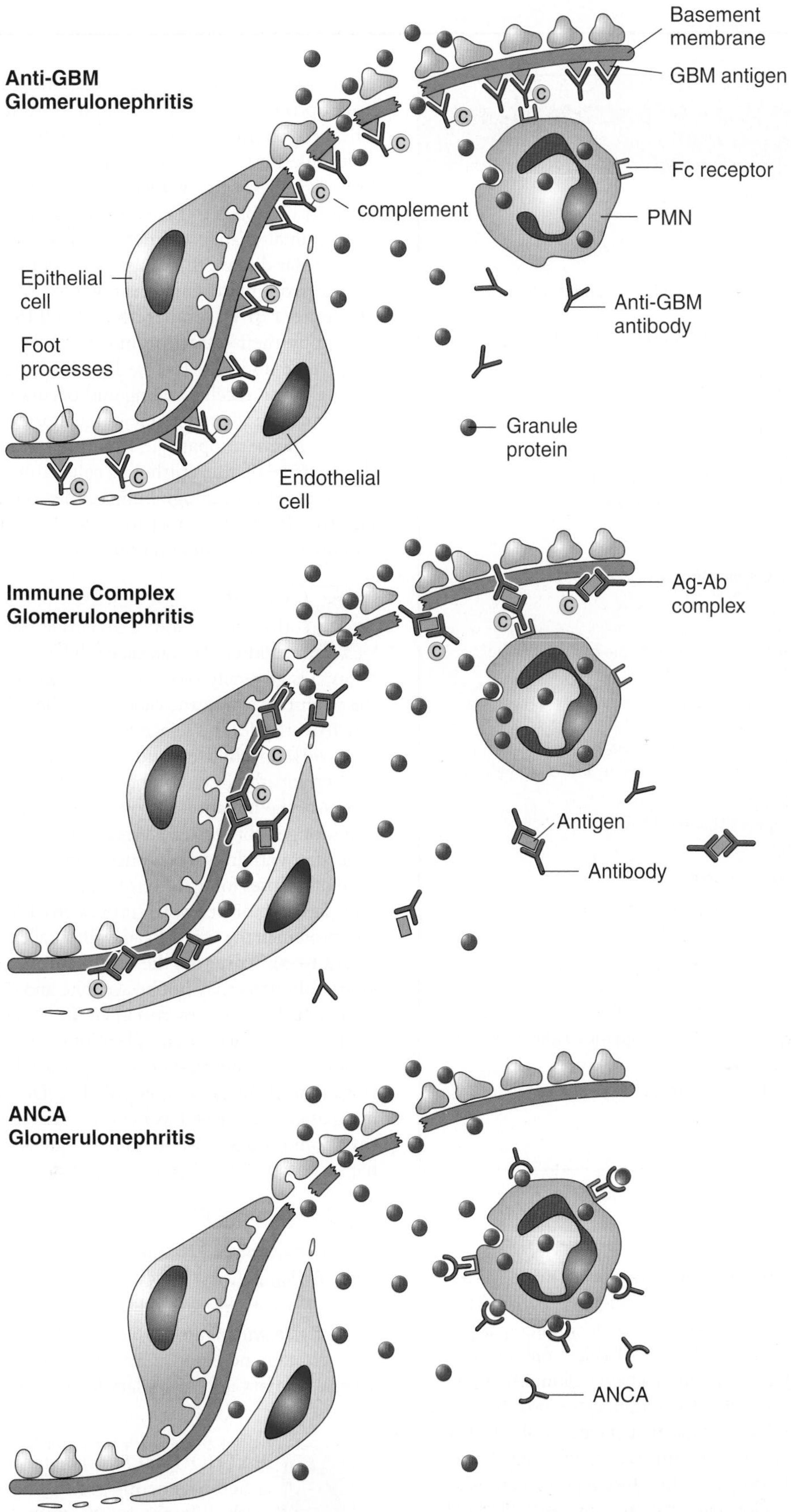

FIGURE 16-13. **Antibody-mediated glomerulonephritis. (Top panel):** Anti-glomerular basement membrane (GBM) antibodies cause glomerulonephritis by binding in situ to basement membrane antigens. This activates complement and recruits inflammatory cells. PMN = polymorphonuclear neutrophil. **(Middle panel):** Immune complexes that deposit from the circulation also activate complement and recruit inflammatory cells. Ag-Ab complex = antigen-antibody complex. **(Bottom panel):** Antineutrophil cytoplasmic antibodies (ANCA) cause inflammation by activating leukocytes by direct binding of the antibodies to the leukocytes and by Fc receptor engagement of ANCA bound to antigen.

TABLE 16–4

Diagnostic Features of Glomerular Diseases

I. Light microscopic features

A. Increased cellularity
- Infiltration by leukocytes (e.g., neutrophils, monocytes, macrophages)
- Proliferation of "endocapillary" cells (i.e., endothelial and mesangial cells)
- Proliferation of "extracapillary" cells (i.e., epithelial cells) (crescent formation)

B. Increased extracellular material
- Localization of immune complexes
- Thickening or replication of glomerular basement membrane (GBM)
- Increases in collagenous matrix (sclerosis)
- Insudation of plasma proteins (hyalinosis)
- Fibrinoid necrosis
- Deposition of amyloid

II. Immunofluorescence features

A. Linear staining of GBM
- Anti-GBM antibodies
- Multiple plasma proteins (e.g., in diabetic glomerulosclerosis)
- Monoclonal light chains

B. Granular immune complex staining
- Mesangium (e.g., IgA nephropathy)
- Capillary wall (e.g., membranous glomerulopathy)
- Mesangium and capillary wall (e.g., lupus glomerulonephritis)

C. Irregular (fluffy) staining
- Monoclonal light chains (AL amyloidosis)
- AA protein (AA amyloidosis)

III. Electron microscopic features

A. Electron-dense immune complex deposits
- Mesangial (e.g., IgA nephropathy)
- Subendothelial (e.g., lupus glomerulonephritis)
- Subepithelial (e.g., membranous glomerulopathy)

B. GBM thickening (e.g., diabetic glomerulosclerosis)

C. GBM replication (e.g., membranoproliferative glomerulonephritis)

D. Collagenous matrix expansion (e.g., focal segmental glomerulosclerosis)

E. Fibrillary deposits (e.g., amyloidosis)

IgA = immunoglobulin A

with corticosteroids and because it may occur in association with an allergic disease or a lymphoid neoplasm. The occasional association with Hodgkin disease (a condition associated with T cell dysfunction) and with T cell lymphomas has led to the speculation that minimal-change glomerulopathy may be caused by a disorder of T lymphocytes, possibly production by T cells of a cytokine that increases glomerular permeability. The heavy proteinuria of minimal-change glomerulopathy is accompanied by a loss of polyanionic sites on the GBM, which allows anionic proteins, particularly albumin, to pass more easily through the GBM.

PATHOLOGY: *The light microscopic appearance of glomeruli in minimal-change glomerulopathy is essentially normal* (Fig. 16-15). Electron microscopy shows diffuse obliteration of podocyte foot processes. Loss of protein in the urine leads to hypoalbuminemia, and compensatory increase in lipoprotein secretion by the liver results in hyperlipidemia. The loss of lipoproteins through the glomeruli causes lipid accumulation in the proximal tubular cells, which is reflected histologically as glassy (hyaline) droplets in tubular epithelial cytoplasm. Droplets in the tubular epithelial cells are not specific for minimal-change glomerulopathy but are produced by any glomerular disease that causes the nephrotic syndrome.

Electron microscopic examination of glomeruli reveals total **effacement of visceral epithelial cell foot processes,** an effect caused by their retraction into the parent epithelial cell bodies (Fig. 16-16 and Fig. 16-17). This retraction presumably results from extensive cell swelling and occurs in virtually all cases of proteinuria in the nephrotic range; it is not specific for minimal-change glomerulopathy. Numerous microvilli protrude from the surface of the epithelial cells. Immunofluorescence microscopy for immunoglobulins and complement are most often negative, but there is occasional weak mesangial staining for IgM and the complement component C3.

CLINICAL FEATURES: Minimal-change glomerulopathy causes 90% of nephrotic syndrome cases in young children, 50% in older children, and 15% in adults. Proteinuria is generally more selective (albumin > globulins) than in the nephrotic syndrome caused by other diseases, but there is too much overlap for this selectivity to be used as a diagnostic criterion. Over 90% of children and fewer adults with minimal-change glomerulopathy have complete remission of proteinuria within 8 weeks of the initiation of corticosteroid therapy. Adults often require longer corticosteroid treatment to induce remission. However, after withdrawal of corticosteroids, most patients suffer intermittent relapses for up to 10 years. A small subgroup of patients has only partial remission with corticosteroid therapy and continues to lose protein in the urine. In an even smaller group that is totally resistant to corticosteroid therapy, the diagnosis of minimal-change glomerulopathy may not be accurate and FSGS that was not sampled in the initial biopsy specimen may be present.

In the absence of complications, the long-term outlook for patients with minimal-change glomerulopathy is no different from that of the general population. Development of azotemia in a patient diagnosed as having minimal-change glomerulopathy should suggest an incorrect diagnosis, usually FSGS or perhaps a complication such as drug-induced interstitial nephritis.

Focal Segmental Glomerulosclerosis is a Feature of Multiple Disease Processes

FSGS is characterized by glomerular consolidation that affects some (focal), but not all, glomeruli and initially involves only part of an affected glomerular tuft (segmental). The consolidated segments often contain increased collagenous matrix (sclerosis). There are several primary and secondary forms of FSGS.

PATHOGENESIS: The term **FSGS** is applied to a heterogeneous group of glomerular diseases with different causes, pathologies, responses to treatment, and outcomes. FSGS occurs as an idiopathic (primary) process or secondary to a number of conditions (Table 16-5). It is likely that multiple factors can lead to a final common pathway of injury. Pathologic features and genetic evidence suggest that injury to podocytes may be common to all types of FSGS.

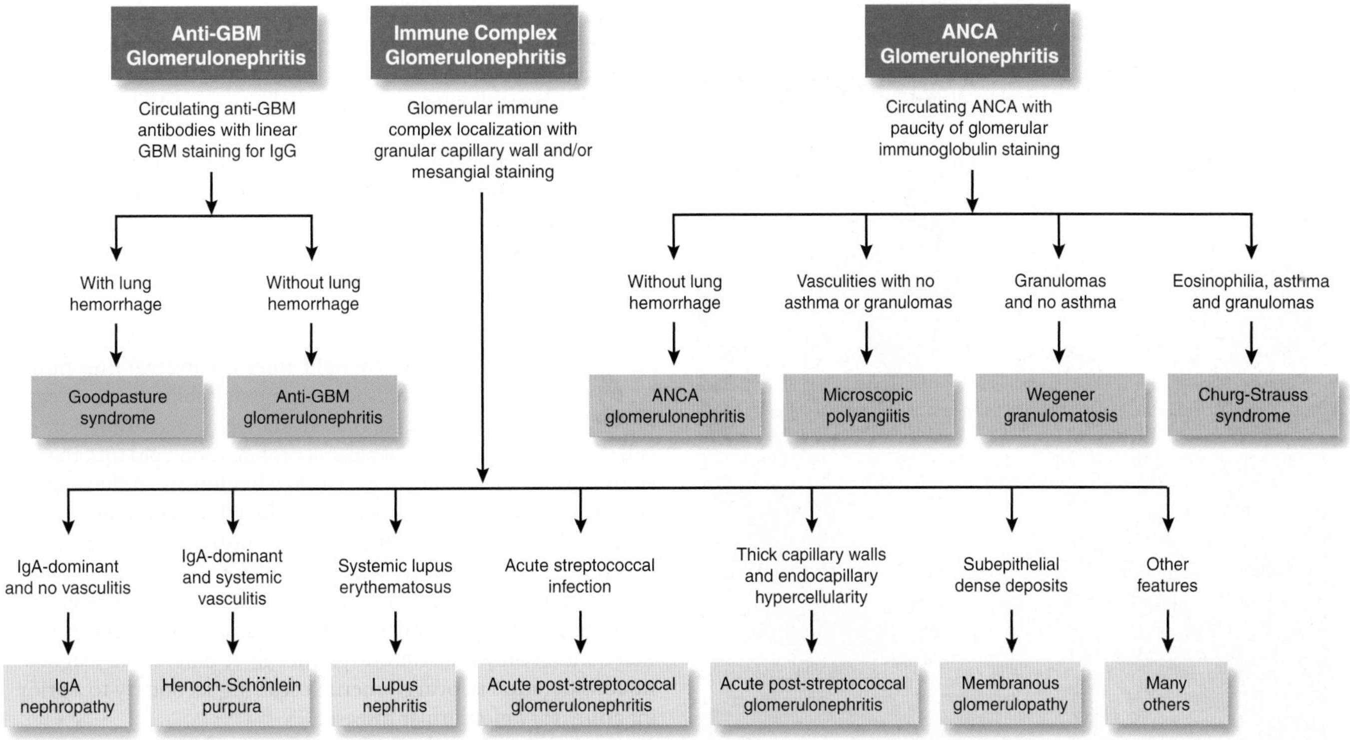

FIGURE 16-14. **Algorithm demonstrating the integration of pathologic findings with clinical data to make a diagnosis of a specific form of primary or secondary glomerulonephritis.** Note that an important initial categorization is as anti-glomerular basement membrane (GBM), immune complex, or antineutrophil cytoplasmic autoantibody (ANCA) glomerulonephritis. Once this determination is made, more specific diagnoses depend on additional clinical or pathologic observations.

Several hereditary forms of FSGS have been traced to genetic abnormalities in podocyte proteins, for example, podocin, α-actinin-4, and transient receptor potential cation channel 6 (TRPC6). This supports the hypothesis that injury to, or dysfunction of, podocytes causes FSGS.

Congenital (e.g., unilateral agenesis) and acquired (e.g., reflux nephropathy) reductions in renal mass place adaptive stress on the reduced number of nephrons. In turn this strain appears to cause FSGS as a consequence of overwork, with increased glomerular capillary pressure and filtration, and glomerular enlargement. A normal amount of renal tissue can also be stressed by excessive body mass (obesity), resulting in FSGS. Reduced oxygen in the blood (e.g., as caused by

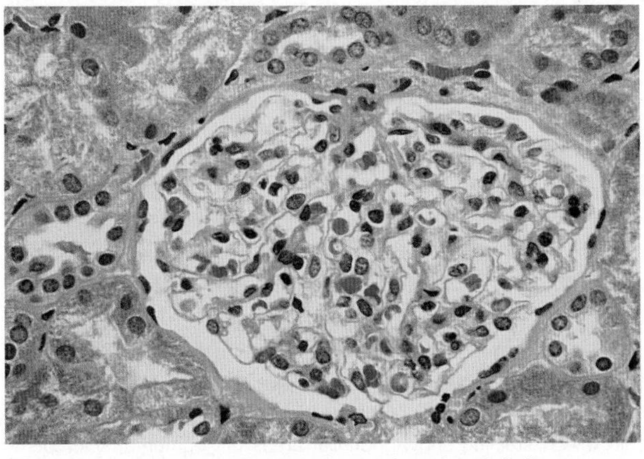

FIGURE 16-15. **Minimal-change glomerulopathy.** A light micrograph shows no abnormality.

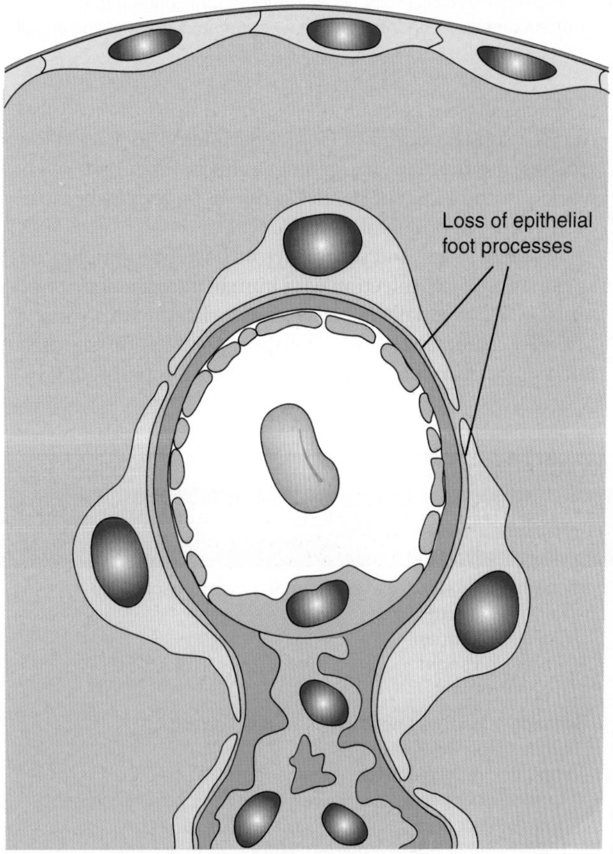

FIGURE 16-16. **Minimal-change glomerulopathy.** This condition is characterized predominantly by epithelial cell changes, particularly the effacement of the foot processes. All other glomerular structures appear intact.

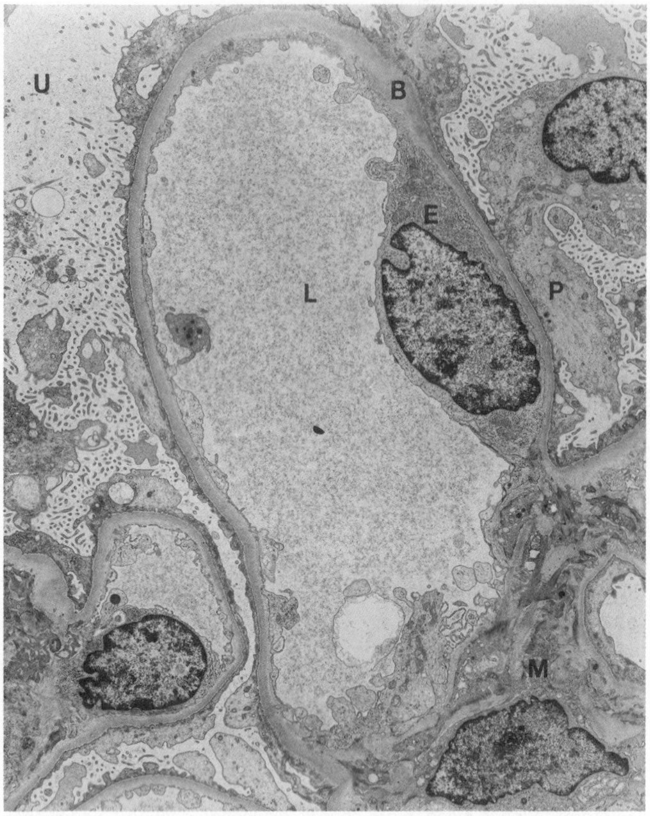

FIGURE 16-17. **Minimal-change glomerulopathy.** In this electron micrograph, the podocyte (P) displays extensive effacement of foot processes and numerous microvilli projecting into the urinary space (U). (B = basement membrane; E = endothelial cell; L = lumen; M = mesangial cell).

sickle cell disease or cyanotic congenital heart disease) also causes a similar pattern of glomerular injury. In all of these settings, glomerular enlargement reflects functional overwork, which places substantial stress on podocytes because of their limited proliferative capacity.

Viruses, drugs, and serum factors have been implicated as causes of FSGS. Infection with human immunodeficiency virus (HIV), especially in blacks, is associated with a variant of FSGS characterized by a collapsing pattern of sclerosis. Such an appearance may also occur in idiopathic FSGS.

TABLE 16-5

Categories of Focal Segmental Glomerulosclerosis

Idiopathic (primary) focal segmental glomerulosclerosis
Perihilar variant
Collapsing variant
Tip lesion variant
Cellular variant
Secondary focal segmental glomerulosclerosis
Obesity (perihilar variant)
Reduced renal mass (perihilar variant)
Cyanotic congenital heart disease (usually perihilar variant)
Sickle cell nephropathy (usually perihilar variant)
ʻuman immunodeficiency virus (collapsing variant)
ʻdronate (collapsing variant)
ous drug abuse (usually collapsing variant)

There is speculation that collapsing FSGS is caused by viral infection of podocytes. Pamidronate, a drug used to treat osteolytic bone disease in patients with cancer, causes collapsing FSGS in some patients. This drug probably causes FSGS by injuring podocytes. A serum permeability factor has been detected in some patients with FSGS, which suggests a systemic cause for the glomerular injury. This is further supported by the recurrence of FSGS in renal transplants, especially in patients who have the permeability factor.

PATHOLOGY: By light microscopy, varying numbers of glomeruli show segmental obliteration of capillary loops by increased matrix or accumulation of cells, or both. Insudation of plasma proteins and lipid into the lesions causes a glassy appearance, called **hyalinosis.** Adhesions to Bowman's capsule occur adjacent to the sclerotic lesions. Uninvolved glomeruli may appear entirely normal, although mild mesangial hypercellularity is occasionally present. Because uninvolved glomeruli usually appear normal, FSGS can be mistaken for minimal-change glomerulopathy in small biopsy specimens that contain only nonsclerotic glomeruli. A differential diagnostic consideration is focal glomerular scarring secondary to a prior inflammatory glomerular disease.

Several histologic variants of segmental glomerulosclerosis have been recognized. In some patients, especially those with reduced renal mass or obesity, the sclerosis has a predilection for *perihilar* segments within glomeruli and for glomeruli in the deep cortex (juxtamedullary glomeruli) (Fig. 16-18). A *collapsing* pattern of sclerosis with hypertrophied and hyperplastic podocytes adjacent to sclerotic segments is typical of HIV-associated nephropathy and also occurs with intravenous drug abuse and pamidronate-induced disease and as an idiopathic process. This collapsing variant has a poor prognosis, and half of patients reach end-stage disease within 2 years. Sclerosis confined to the glomerular segment adjacent to the origin of the proximal tubule has been designated **tip lesion** and is most frequent in older patients with marked proteinuria. A **cellular variant** of FSGS has prominent lipid-laden cells within the sites of glomerular consolidation.

By electron microscopy, FSGS exhibits diffuse effacement of epithelial cell foot processes, with occasional focal detachment or loss of podocytes from the GBM. Increased matrix material,

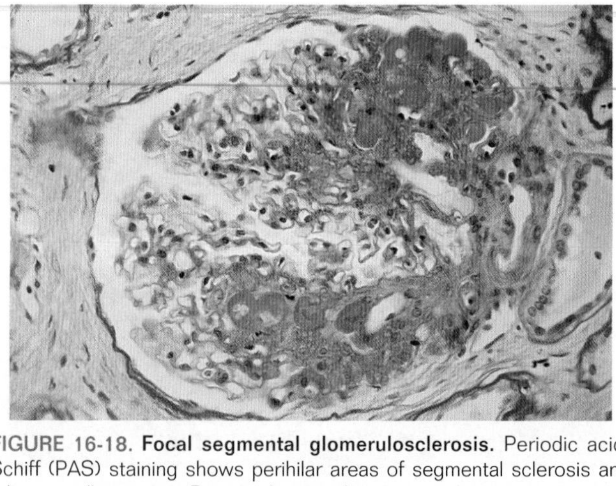

FIGURE 16-18. **Focal segmental glomerulosclerosis.** Periodic acid-Schiff (PAS) staining shows perihilar areas of segmental sclerosis and adjacent adhesions to Bowman's capsule.

folding and thickening of the basement membranes, and capillary collapse are present in sclerotic segments. Accumulation of electron-dense material in sclerotic segments represents insudative trapping of plasma proteins, which corresponds to the hyalinosis seen by light microscopy. Immune complexes are absent.

Immunofluorescence microscopy demonstrates trapping of IgM and C3 in the segmental areas of sclerosis and hyalinosis. IgG, C4, and C1q are less frequently found in sclerotic segments. Nonsclerotic segments have no staining or only trace mesangial staining, usually for IgM and C3.

CLINICAL FEATURES: FSGS is the cause of 30% of nephrotic syndrome in adults and 10% in children. It is more common in blacks than in whites and is the leading cause of nephrotic syndrome in American blacks. Its frequency has been increasing over the past few decades for unknown reasons. Clinical presentations and outcomes vary among the different patterns of injury. The most common clinical presentation is an insidious onset of asymptomatic proteinuria, which frequently progresses to the nephrotic syndrome. Many patients are hypertensive. Microscopic hematuria is frequent.

Most persons with FSGS show persistent proteinuria and progressive decline in renal function. Many progress to end-stage renal disease after 5 to 20 years. Some, but not all, patients appear to improve with corticosteroid therapy. Although renal transplantation is the preferred treatment for end-stage renal disease, FSGS recurs in half of transplanted kidneys.

Patients with FSGS secondary to obesity or reduced renal mass usually have a more indolent course that benefits from treatment with angiotensin-converting enzyme (ACE) inhibitors. Patients with the tip lesion variant often present with severe nephrotic syndrome but respond better to corticosteroids than those with other forms of FSGS. HIV-associated and idiopathic collapsing FSGS have the worst prognoses and typically manifest with severe nephrotic syndrome and renal failure, often progressing to end-stage renal disease within a year.

HIV-Associated Nephropathy is a Severe, Rapidly Progressive Collapsing Form of FSGS

PATHOGENESIS: The occurrence of nephropathy in patients with HIV infection has raised the possibility that it is caused by the virus within the renal parenchyma. A different hypothesis proposes that the nephropathy is caused by another virus that has infected the kidney of an immunocompromised person.

PATHOLOGY: HIV-associated nephropathy has a distinctive collapsing pattern of focal sclerosis that may be segmental or global (Fig. 16-19). Sclerotic segments display collapse of capillaries, frequently with adjacent swollen podocytes that contain numerous protein droplets. In addition to the glomerular injury, interstitial fibrosis and infiltration by mononuclear leukocytes are frequent. Tubular epithelial atrophy and degeneration are conspicuous, and cystically dilated tubules contain proteinaceous casts. By electron microscopy, numerous tubuloreticular inclusions are seen in endothelial cells, similar to those in lupus nephritis.

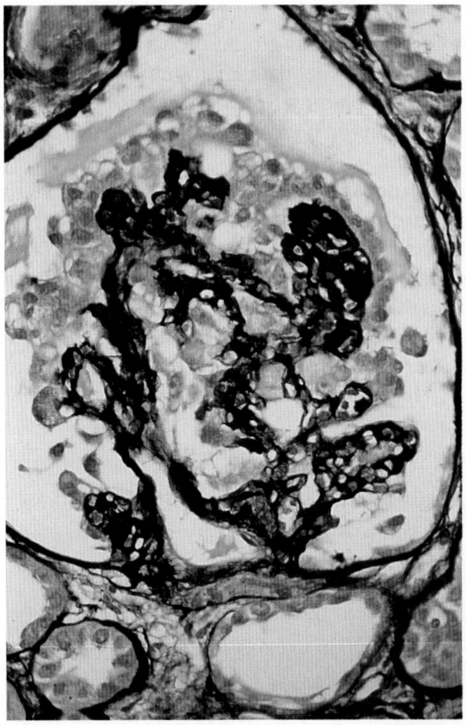

FIGURE 16-19. **Human immunodeficiency virus (HIV)-associated nephropathy.** Silver staining shows a collapsing pattern of focal segmental glomerulosclerosis (FSGS), with collapse of glomerular capillaries, increased matrix material (sclerosis), and hypertrophy of podocytes.

CLINICAL FEATURES: Some 10% of HIV-positive patients, of whom over 90% are black, develop nephropathy. Idiopathic collapsing FSGS also occurs predominantly in blacks. The disease presents with severe proteinuria (>10 g/day) and renal insufficiency. Patients typically progress to end-stage renal disease in less than a year.

Membranous Glomerulopathy Is an Immune Complex Disease

Membranous glomerulopathy is a frequent cause of the nephrotic syndrome in adults. It is caused by accumulation of immune complexes in the subepithelial zone of glomerular capillaries.

PATHOGENESIS: Immune complexes localize in the **subepithelial zone** (between the visceral epithelial cell and the GBM) as a result of immune complex formation in situ or deposition of circulating immune complexes. Formation in situ is the favored hypothesis because of the resemblance between membranous glomerulopathy and the experimental animal disease called *Heymann nephritis*. In the latter, rats are immunized with a renal epithelial antigen and develop autoantibodies. The antibodies cross GBMs and bind to antigens on podocytes. Resultant immune complexes are shed into the adjacent subepithelial zone and produce membranous glomerulopathy. An analogous pathogenesis is postulated for human idiopathic membranous glomerulopathy, and is supported by rare examples of neonatal membranous glomerulopathy caused by transplacental passage of antibodies that react with alloantigens on neonatal podocytes that are not shared by the mother.

Membranous glomerulopathy is also induced in animals by chronic injection of foreign proteins. This procedure results in the formation of circulating immune complexes and, in some circumstances, free antigens and antibodies that can form immune complexes in situ. The result is a chronic serum sickness model, which may be analogous to certain forms of secondary membranous glomerulopathy. The following are general causes of membranous glomerulopathy:

- Idiopathic (primary) membranous glomerulopathy
- Secondary membranous glomerulopathy
  - Autoimmune disease (SLE)
  - Infectious disease (hepatitis B)
  - Therapeutic agents (penicillamine)
  - Neoplasms (lung cancer)

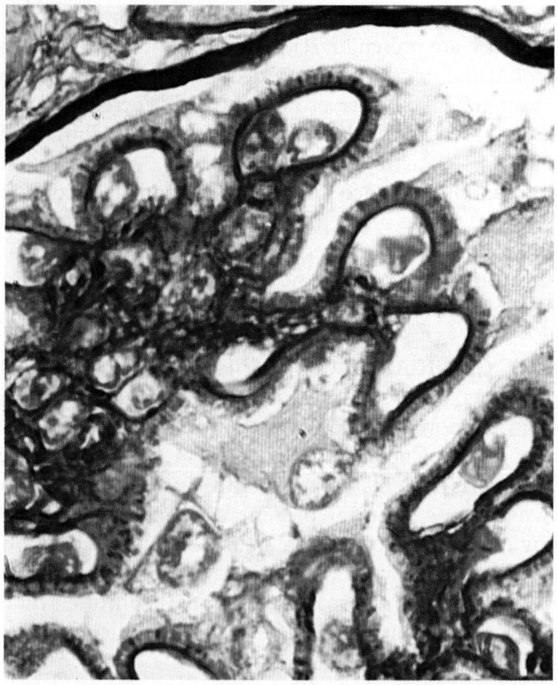

FIGURE 16-21. **Membranous glomerulopathy.** Silver staining reveals multiple "spikes" diffusely distributed in the glomerular capillary basement membranes. This pattern corresponds to the stage II lesion illustrated in Figure 16-23. The appearance is produced by the deposition of silver-positive basement membrane material around silver-negative immune complex deposits.

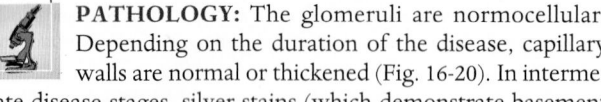

PATHOLOGY: The glomeruli are normocellular. Depending on the duration of the disease, capillary walls are normal or thickened (Fig. 16-20). In intermediate disease stages, silver stains (which demonstrate basement membrane material) reveal multiple projections or "spikes" of argyrophilic material on the epithelial surface of the basement membrane (Fig. 16-21). Such spikes are projections of basement membrane material deposited around the subepithelial immune complexes, which do not stain with silver. As disease progresses, capillary lumina are narrowed, and glomerular sclerosis eventually ensues. Advanced lesions of membranous glomerulopathy cannot be distinguished from those in other forms of chronic glomerular disease. Atrophy of tubules and interstitial fibrosis parallel the degree of glomerular sclerosis.

By electron microscopy, immune complexes appear in capillary walls as electron-dense deposits (Fig. 16-22 and Fig.16-23).

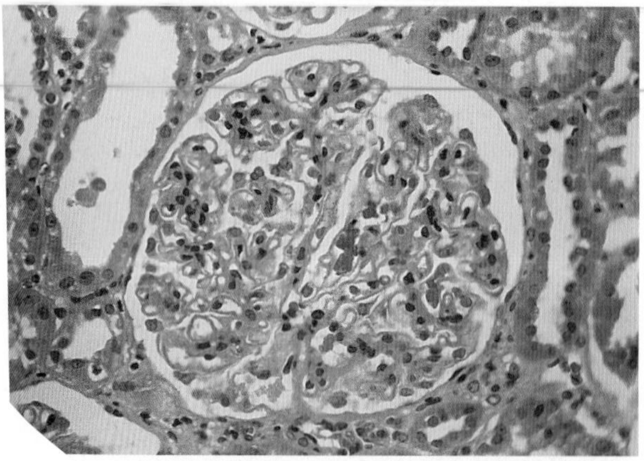

20. **Membranous glomerulopathy.** The glomerulus is slightly ... ows diffuse thickening of the capillary walls. There is no

The progressive ultrastructural alterations that are induced by the subepithelial immune complexes are divided into stages:

- **Stage I:** Subepithelial dense deposits without adjacent projections of GBM material
- **Stage II:** Projections of GBM material around these dense deposits (see Fig. 16-23)
- **Stage III:** Enclosure of the dense deposits within GBM material
- **Stage IV:** Rarefaction of the deposits within a thickened GBM

Mesangial electron-dense deposits are rare in idiopathic membranous glomerulopathy but common in secondary membranous glomerulopathy (e.g., as in lupus erythematosus). This difference may reflect the fact that idiopathic disease is caused by antigens present only in the subepithelial zone (as in Heymann nephritis), whereas the secondary type is produced by circulating antigens.

Immunofluorescence microscopy reveals diffuse granular staining of capillary walls for IgG and C3 (Fig. 16-24). There is intense staining for terminal complement components, including the membrane attack complex, which participate in the induction of glomerular injury.

CLINICAL FEATURES: Membranous glomerulopathy is the most frequent primary glomerular cause of the nephrotic syndrome in white and Asian adults in the United States (the most common secondary glomerular cause is diabetic glomerulosclerosis). The course of membranous

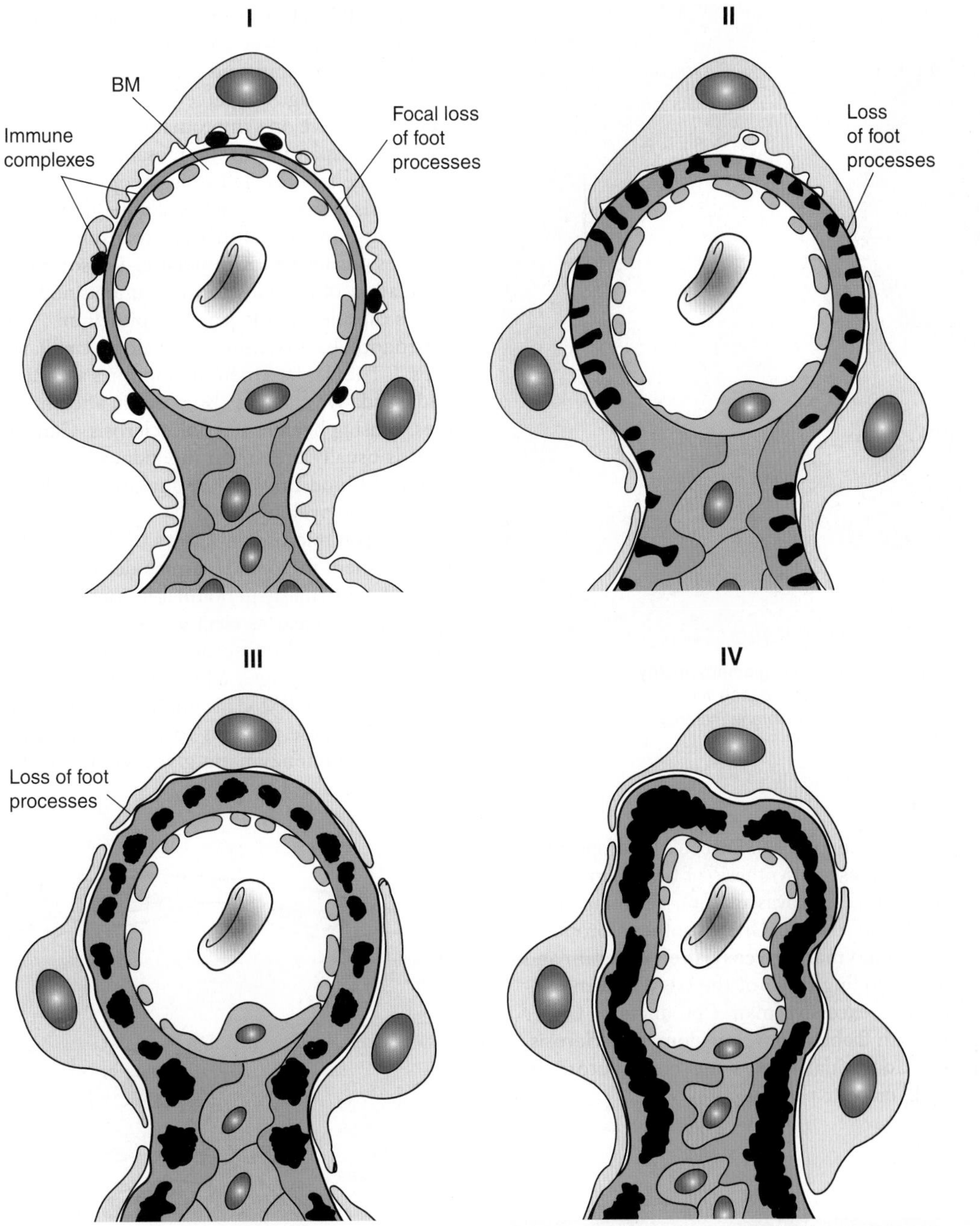

FIGURE 16-22. **Membranous glomerulopathy.** This disease is caused by the subepithelial accumulation of immune complexes and the accompanying changes in the basement membrane (BM). Stage I exhibits scattered subepithelial deposits. The outer contour of the basement membrane remains smooth. Stage II disease has projections (spikes) of basement membrane material adjacent to the deposits. In stage III disease, newly formed basement membrane has surrounded the deposits. With stage IV disease, the immune-complex deposits lose their electron density, resulting in an irregularly thickened basement membrane with irregular electron-lucent areas.

glomerulopathy is highly variable. Approximately 25% of patients have spontaneous remission within 20 years, 50% have persistent proteinuria and stable or only partial loss of renal function, and 25% develop renal failure. Treatment of idiopathic membranous glomerulopathy is controversial. Patients with progressive renal failure are treated with corticosteroids or immunosuppressive drugs, or both. The prognosis is better in children because of a higher rate of permanent spontaneous remission.

Diabetic Glomerulosclerosis Results in Proteinuria and Progressive Renal Failure

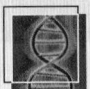

PATHOGENESIS: Glomerulosclerosis is a part of the diabetic vasculopathy that involves small vessels throughout the body in patients with

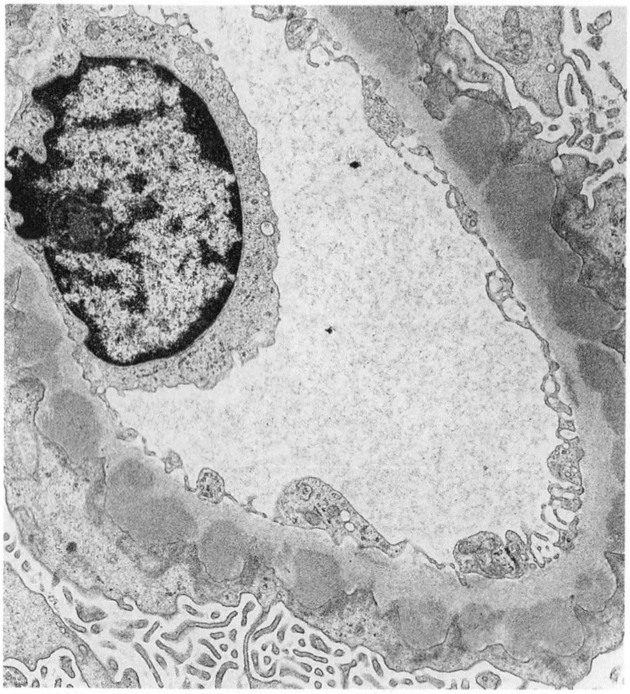

FIGURE 16-23. **Stage II membranous glomerulopathy.** An electron micrograph shows deposits of electron-dense material, with intervening delicate projections of basement membrane material.

diabetes mellitus (see Chapter 22). Diabetes is complicated by a generalized increase in synthesis of basement membrane material by the microvasculature, resulting from the abnormal metabolic state. One hypothesis proposes that abnormal **nonenzymatic glycosylation** of serum and matrix proteins, including those of the GBM and mesangial matrix, induces excessive matrix production. Under half of patients with diabetes develop glomerulosclerosis, suggesting that additional factors are contributory in some, but not all, diabetic patients.

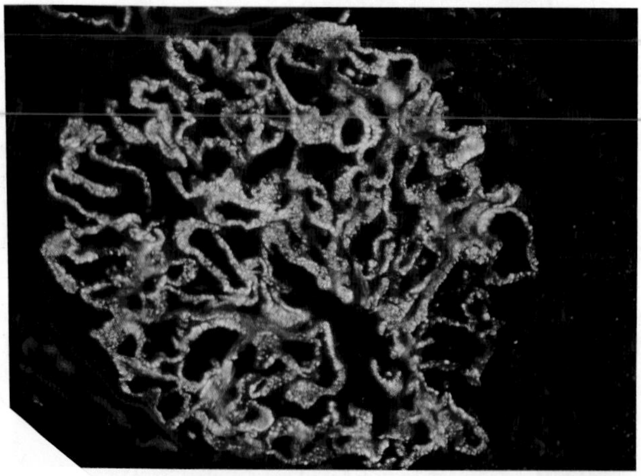

24. **Membranous glomerulopathy.** Immunofluorescence ws granular deposits of IgG outlining the glomerular

PATHOLOGY: The earliest lesions of diabetic glomerulosclerosis are glomerular enlargement, GBM thickening, and mesangial matrix expansion (Fig. 16-25). Mild mesangial hypercellularity may also be present. In patients who develop symptomatic disease, GBM thickening, and especially expansion of the mesangial matrix result in changes that can be seen by light microscopy. Overt diabetic glomerulosclerosis is characterized by diffuse global thickening of GBMs and diffuse mesangial matrix expansion, accompanied by sclerotic lesions termed **Kimmelstiel-Wilson nodules** (Fig. 16-26). Insudation of proteins forms rounded nodules between Bowman's capsule and the parietal epithelium ("capsular drops") or subendothelial accumulations along capillary loops ("hyaline caps"). Tubular basement membranes are thickened. Sclerosing and insudative changes also occur in afferent and efferent arterioles, causing hyaline arteriolosclerosis. Generalized arteriosclerosis is usually present in the kidney. Vascular narrowing and reduced blood flow to the medulla predisposes to papillary necrosis and pyelonephritis.

Electron microscopy shows up to 5- to 10-fold widening of the basement membrane lamina densa. Mesangial matrix is increased, particularly in nodular lesions (Fig. 16-27). The insudative lesions appear as electron-dense masses that contain lipid debris. Immunofluorescence microscopy demonstrates diffuse linear trapping of IgG, albumin, fibrinogen, and other plasma proteins in the GBM. This finding reflects nonimmunologic adsorption of these proteins to the thickened GBM, possibly as a result of nonenzymatic glycosylation of GBM and plasma proteins.

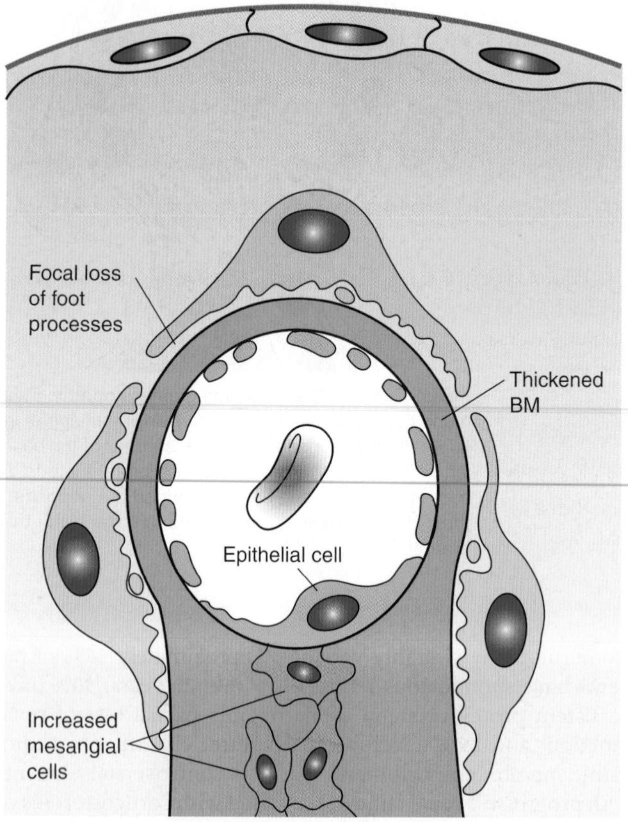

FIGURE 16-25. **Diabetic glomerulosclerosis.** The lamina densa of the glomerular basement membrane (BM) is thickened, and there is an increase in mesangial matrix material.

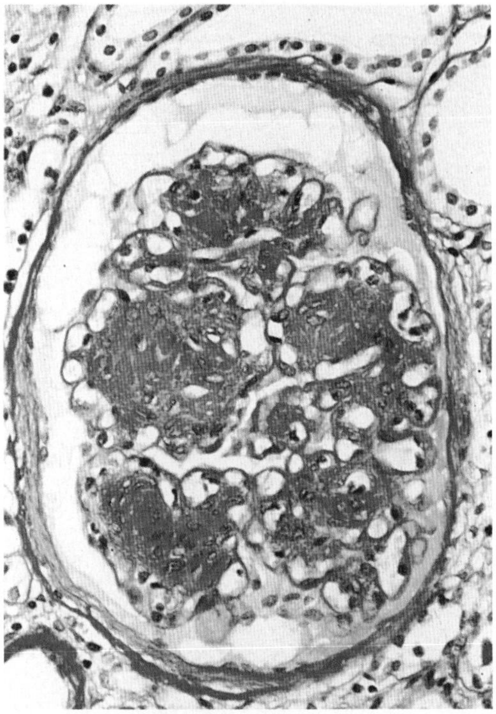

FIGURE 16-26. **Diabetic glomerulosclerosis.** Periodic acid-Schiff (PAS) staining reveals a prominent increase in the mesangial matrix, forming several nodular lesions. Dilation of glomerular capillaries is evident, and some capillary basement membranes are thickened.

CLINICAL FEATURES: Diabetic glomerulosclerosis is the leading cause of end-stage renal disease in the United States, accounting for a third of all patients with chronic renal failure. It occurs in type 1 and type 2 diabetes mellitus. The earliest manifestation is micro-albuminuria (slightly increased proteinuria). Overt proteinuria occurs between 10 and 15 years after the onset of diabetes and often becomes severe enough to cause the nephrotic syndrome. In time, diabetic glomerulosclerosis progresses to renal failure. Strict control of blood glucose reduces the incidence of diabetic glomerulosclerosis and retards progression once it develops. Control of hypertension and dietary protein restriction also slow progression of the disease.

Amyloidosis Leads to Nephrotic Syndrome and Renal Failure

Renal disease is a frequent complication of AA and AL amyloidosis (see Chapter 23).

PATHOGENESIS: Amyloid may be formed from a number of different polypeptides. In each case, the amyloid has the same histologic and ultrastructural appearance, and immunohistochemical tests are required to differentiate between the different forms. **AA amyloid** is derived from serum amyloid A protein (SAA), which increases markedly during inflammatory processes. Thus, deposition of AA amyloid is often associated with chronic inflammatory disorders (e.g., rheumatoid arthritis, chronic tuberculosis, and familial Mediterranean fever). AL amyloid is derived from λ or, less often, κ immunoglobulin light chains produced by a neoplastic clone of B cells or plasma cells. Thus, it frequently is associated with, or is a harbinger of, multiple myeloma.

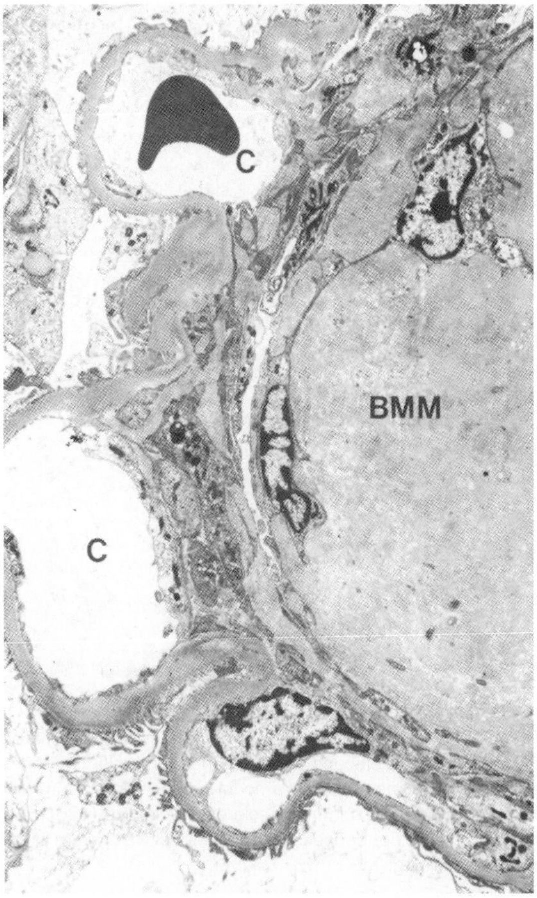

FIGURE 16-27. **Advanced diabetic glomerulosclerosis.** An electron micrograph shows a nodular aggregate of basement membrane-like material (BMM). The peripheral capillary (C) demonstrates diffuse basement membrane widening but a normal texture.

PATHOLOGY: Histologically, amyloid is an eosinophilic, amorphous material (Fig. 16-28) that has a characteristic apple-green color in sections stained with Congo red and examined by polarized light microscopy (Fig. 16-29). Acidophilic deposits initially are most apparent in the mesangium but later extend into capillary walls and may obliterate capillary lumens (see Fig. 16-28 and Fig. 16-30). Glomerular structure is completely obliterated in advanced amyloidosis, and glomeruli appear as large eosinophilic spheres.

Amyloid is composed of nonbranching fibrils, approximately 10 nm in diameter. These fibrils are most prominent in the mesangium, but often extend into capillary walls, especially in advanced cases (see Fig. 16-30 and Fig. 16-31). The epithelial foot processes overlying the GBM are effaced.

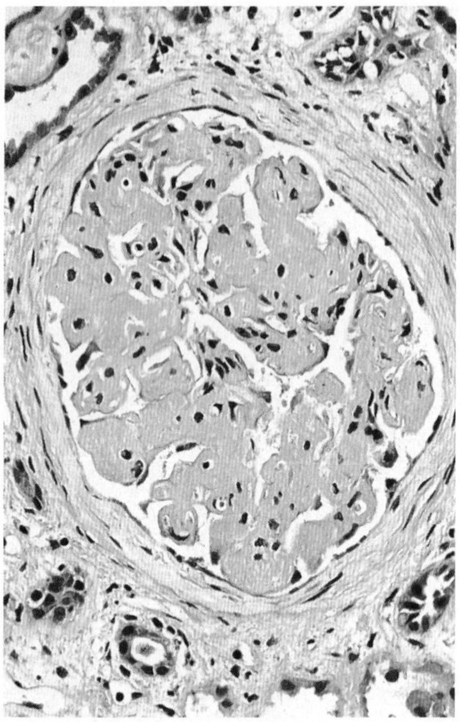

FIGURE 16-28. **Amyloid nephropathy.** Amorphous acellular material expands the mesangial areas and obstructs the glomerular capillaries. The deposits of amyloid may take on a nodular appearance, somewhat resembling those of diabetic glomerulosclerosis (see Fig. 16-26). However, amyloid deposits are not periodic acid-Schiff–positive and are identifiable by Congo red staining.

CLINICAL FEATURES: Renal involvement is prominent in most cases of systemic AL and AA amyloidosis. Proteinuria is often the initial manifestation. Proteinuria is nonselective (i.e., both albumin and globulins appear in the urine) and produces nephrotic syndrome in 60% of patients. Eventually, severe infiltration of the glomeruli and blood vessels by amyloid results in renal failure. AL amyloidosis is treated with chemotherapy analogous to that used for multiple myeloma. AA amyloidosis, especially when caused by familial Mediterranean fever, is ameliorated by colchicine therapy.

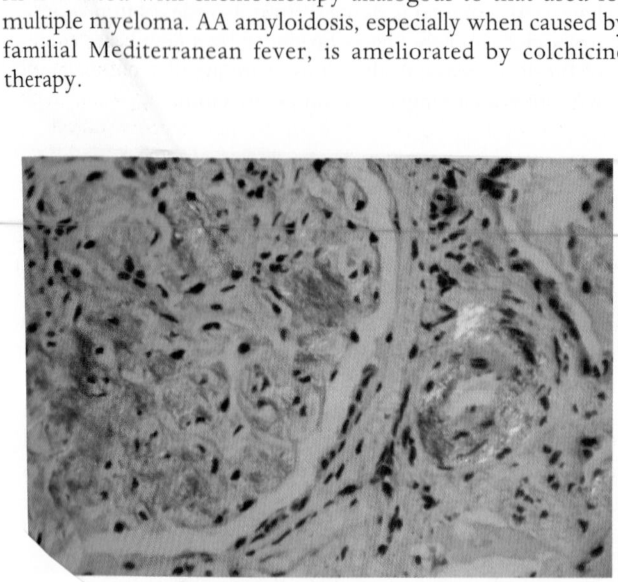

-29. **Amyloid nephropathy.** In a section stained with Congo
ned under polarized light, the amyloid deposits in the
the adjacent arteriole show a characteristic apple-green

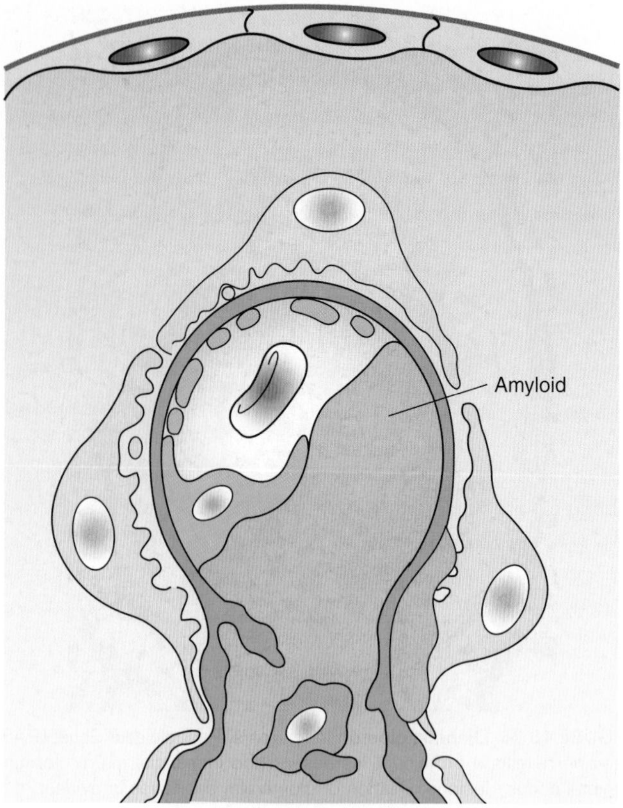

FIGURE 16-30. **Amyloid nephropathy.** This disorder is initially associated with the accumulation of characteristic fibrillar deposits in the mesangium. These inert masses, which are fibrillar by electron microscopy, extend along the inner surface of the basement membrane, frequently obstructing the capillary lumen. Focal extension of amyloid through the basement membrane may elevate the epithelial cell, in which case irregular spikes are seen along the outer surface of the basement membrane.

Light Chain and Heavy Chain Deposition Disease Occur in B-Cell Neoplasia

Both light chain and heavy chain deposition diseases reflect deposition of monoclonal immunoglobulin light chains in GBMs, glomerular mesangial matrix, and tubular basement membranes. The underlying B cell neoplasm may be occult or there may be overt multiple myeloma or lymphoma. The most common offender in light chain disease is κ light chains. The immunoglobulin heavy chains that cause this pattern of injury have deleted domains, so they resemble light chains. Monoclonal immunoglobulin deposition stimulates increased matrix production in basement membranes, causing thickening of glomerular and tubular basement membranes. Nodular expansion of mesangial regions resembles diabetic glomerulosclerosis. Importantly, the increased extracellular material does not stain with Congo red. Electron microscopy reveals a uniform, finely granular, electron-dense material along the glomerular and tubular basement membranes and within the mesangial matrix. Amyloid fibrils are not present. Immunofluorescence microscopy demonstrates linear staining for monoclonal immunoglobulin chains along the involved basement membranes. Light chain and heavy chain deposition disease usually manifest clinically as nephrotic syndrome and renal failure.

Hereditary Nephritis (Alport Syndrome) Reflects Abnormal Type IV Collagen in GBMs

Hereditary nephritis is a proliferative and sclerosing glomerular disease, often accompanied by defects of the ears or the eyes. It is caused

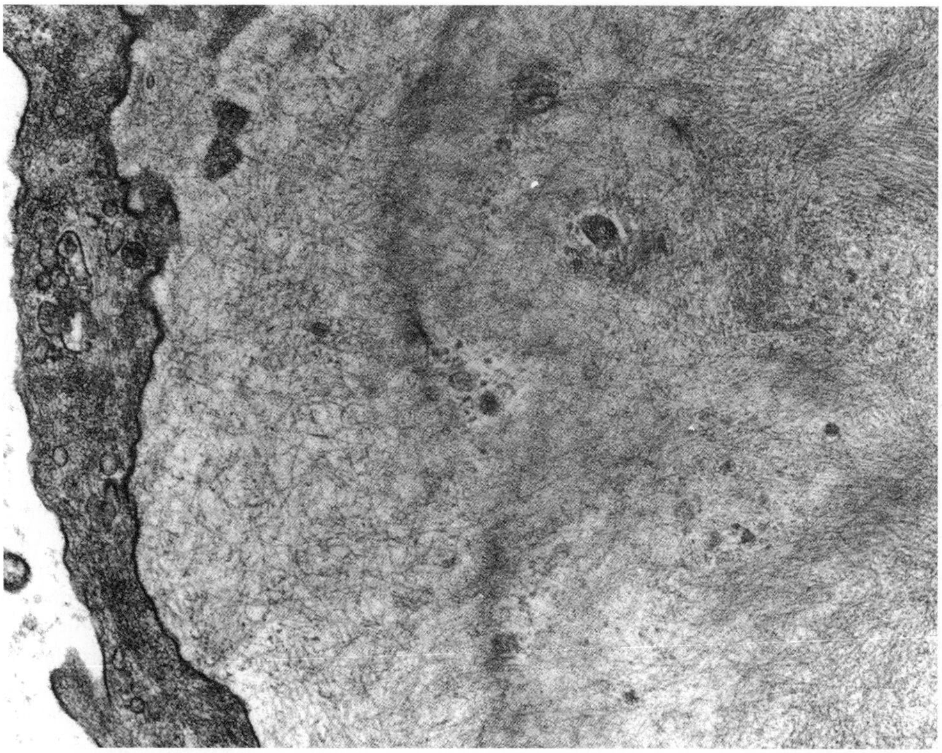

FIGURE 16-31. **Amyloid nephropathy.** Deposits of fibrils (10 nm diameter) in a glomerulus adjacent to podocyte cytoplasm with effaced foot processes.

by mutations in type IV collagen. In Alport syndrome hereditray nephritis is accompanied by a hearing deficit.

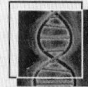

PATHOGENESIS: A variety of genetic mutations cause molecular defects in the GBM that produce the renal lesions of hereditary nephritis. The most common defect accounting for 85% of hereditary nephritis is X-linked and is caused by a mutation in the gene for the $\alpha 5$ chain of type IV collagen (*COL4A5* gene). A deletion at the 5′ end of *COL4A5* that extends into the *COL4A6* gene, which codes for the $\alpha 6$ chain of type IV collagen, causes hereditary nephritis and multiple leiomyomas in the gastrointestinal and genital tracts. An autosomal recessive form of hereditary nephritis is caused by mutations in *COL4A3* and *COL4A4*.

Because of disturbed basement membrane structure in hereditary nephritis, serum from patients with anti-GBM disease (e.g., Goodpasture syndrome) fails to react with GBMs from patients with hereditary nephritis. Conversely, patients with hereditary nephritis who have renal transplants are at risk for developing antibodies to allograft GBMs, although this rarely causes significant disease.

PATHOLOGY: Early glomerular lesions of hereditary nephritisshow mild mesangial hypercellularity and matrix expansion. Renal disease progression is associated with increasing focal and eventually diffuse glomerular sclerosis. Advanced glomerular lesions are accompanied by tubular atrophy, interstitial fibrosis, and the presence of foam cells in the tubules and interstitium. The most diagnostic morphologic lesion is seen only by electron microscopy as an irregularly thickened GBM with splitting of the lamina densa into interlacing lamellae that surround electron-lucent areas (Fig. 16-32).

CLINICAL FEATURES: Males with X-linked hereditary nephritis develop microscopic hematuria early in childhood and usually develop proteinuria,, and progressive renal failure during the second to fourth decades of life. Females with X-linked disease generally have a milder form, the slower progression of which varies substantially among patients possibly related to the degree of random inactivation (lionization) of the mutated X chromosome. Autosomal recessive hereditary nephritis resembles X-linked disease except that affects males and females equally. Autosomal dominant hereditary nephritis with progressive renal failure is rare and difficult to distinguish from severe thin basement membrane disease (see below). Sensorineural, high frequency hearing loss affects approximately 50% of males with X-linked disease and a higher proportion of males and females with autosomal disease. A quarter to a third of patients have ocular defects, most often involving the lens.

Thin Glomerular Basement Membrane Nephropathy Is a Benign Cause of Hematuria

Thin basement membrane nephropathy, also termed **benign familial hematuria,** *is a common hereditary GBM disorder that typically manifests as asymptomatic microscopic hematuria, and occasionally with intermittent gross hematuria.* This disease and IgA nephropathy are the two major diagnostic considerations in patients with asymptomatic glomerular hematuria. Patients with thin basemer membrane nephropathy usually do not develop renal failure

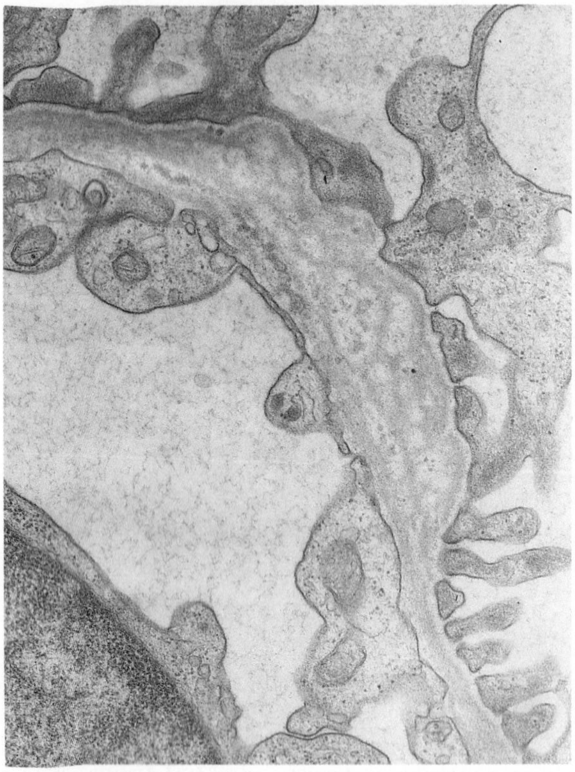

FIGURE 16-32. **Hereditary nephritis (Alport syndrome).** The lamina densa of the glomerular basement membrane is laminated rather than forming a single dense band (compare this electron micrograph with Fig. 16-5).

substantial proteinuria. By light microscopy, glomeruli are unremarkable. Electron microscopy reveals a reduced thickness of the GBM (150 to 300 nm, compared with the normal 350 to 450 nm). The most common mode of inheritance is autosomal dominant. Heterozygous mutations in the *COL4A3* and *COL4A4* genes lead to thin basement membrane disease, and homozygous ones to Alport syndrome.

Acute Postinfectious Glomerulonephritis Is an Immune Complex Disease of Childhood

Acute postinfectious glomerulonephritis usually occurs after infection with group A (β-hemolytic) streptococci and is caused by deposition of immune complexes in glomeruli.

PATHOGENESIS: *Acute postinfectious glomerulonephritis is most often caused by certain nephritogenic strains of* group A (β-hemolytic) streptococci. Occasional examples are caused by staphylococcal infection (e.g., acute staphylococcal endocarditis, staphylococcal abscess) and rare cases result from viral (e.g., hepatitis B) or parasitic (e.g., malaria) infections. The exact mechanism by which infection causes the characteristic inflammatory changes in the glomeruli is not completely understood. Similarities to experimental acute serum sickness suggest that postinfectious glomerulonephritis is caused by glomerular localization of immune complexes composed of antibody plus bacterial antigens. Both poststreptococcal glomerulonephritis in patients and acute serum sickness caused by injecting foreign proteins into animals have a latent period of 9 to 14 days between the time of exposure to a new antigen and the occurrence of glomerulonephritis. The granular immunofluorescence pattern of immune-complex staining and the ultrastructural appearance of dense deposits are similar in the human and experimental diseases. Immune complexes could localize in glomeruli by deposition from the circulation or formation in situ as bacterial antigens trapped in the glomeruli bind circulating antibodies. The specific nephritogenic streptococcal antigens have not been conclusively identified. Candidates include streptokinase, endostreptosin, and streptococcal erythrogenic toxin B, which can activate complement even in the absence of antibodies.

Immune complexes within glomeruli initiate inflammation by activating complement, as well as other humoral and cellular inflammatory mediators. Complement activation is so extensive that over 90% of patients develop hypocomplementemia. The inflammatory mediators attract and activate neutrophils and monocytes and stimulate mesangial and endothelial cell proliferation. These effects result in marked glomerular hypercellularity, which defines acute diffuse proliferative glomerulonephritis.

PATHOLOGY: The acute phase of postinfectious glomerulonephritis is characterized by diffuse glomerular enlargement and hypercellularity (Fig. 16-33). Hypercellularity reflects proliferation of both endothelial and mesangial cells (Fig. 16-34) and infiltration by neutrophils and monocytes. Crescents are uncommon. Interstitial edema and mild infiltration of mononuclear leukocytes occur in parallel with the glomerular changes.

The acute phase begins 1 or 2 weeks after the onset of the nephritogenic infection and resolves in over 90% of patients after several weeks. Neutrophils and endothelial hypercellularity disappear first. Mesangial hypercellularity and matrix expansion remain, but all histologic changes resolve completely in most patients after several months.

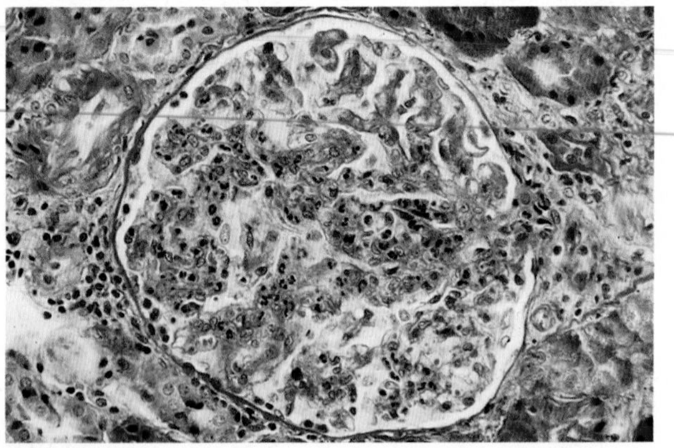

FIGURE 16-33. **Acute poststreptococcal glomerulonephritis.** The glomerulus of a patient who developed glomerulonephritis after a streptococcal infection contains numerous neutrophils (Masson trichrome stain).

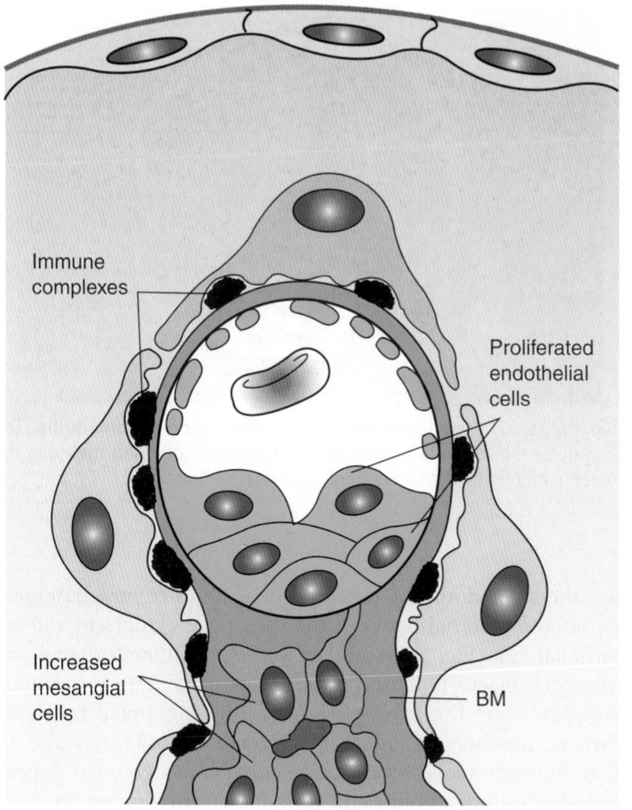

FIGURE 16-34. **Postinfectious glomerulonephritis.** Accumulation of numerous subepithelial immune complexes as humplike structures is a characteristic feature. Less prominent subendothelial immune complexes are associated with endothelial cell proliferation and are related to increased capillary permeability and narrowing of the lumen. Frequently, proliferation of mesangial cells and a thickened mesangial matrix (BM) result in widening of the stalk and conspicuous trapping of immune complexes.

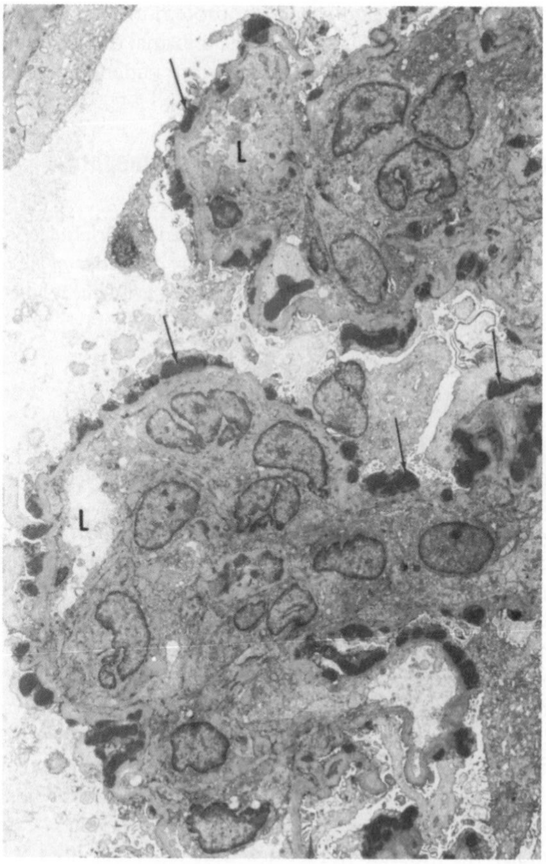

FIGURE 16-35. **Acute postinfectious glomerulonephritis.** An electron micrograph demonstrates numerous subepithelial humps *(arrows)*. The capillary lumina (L) are markedly narrowed.

The most distinctive ultrastructural features of acute postinfectious glomerulonephritis are **subepithelial dense deposits** that are shaped like **"humps"** (see Fig. 16-34 and Fig. 16-35). These deposits are invariably accompanied by mesangial and subendothelial deposits, which may be more difficult to find but are probably more important in pathogenesis because of their proximity to the inflammatory mediator systems in the blood. The variably sized, dome-shaped humps are situated on the epithelial side of the basement membrane. They are not as diffusely distributed as the deposits of membranous glomerulopathy (compare Figs. 16-22 and 16-34). In the first few weeks of disease, immunofluorescence microscopy typically reveals granular deposits corresponding to IgG and C3 along the basement membrane, in locations corresponding to the humps. Later in the disease, C3 is present without IgG, possibly because immune complexes containing IgG no longer accumulate in the glomeruli after the infection clears (Fig. 16-36).

CLINICAL FEATURES: Acute poststreptococcal glomerulonephritis is less common than in the past, but remains one of the most common childhood renal diseases. The primary infection involves the pharynx (pharyngitis) or, in hot and humid environments, the skin (pyoderma). In recent years, the proportion of cases following staphylococcal infection has been increasing. Because organisms may not be recoverable at the time of the nephritis, diagnosis depends on serologic evidence of a rise in antibody titers to streptococcal products. The nephritic syndrome begins abruptly with oliguria, hematuria, facial edema, and hypertension. Serum C3 levels are lower during the acute syndrome, but return to normal within 1 to 2 weeks. Overt nephritis resolves after several weeks,

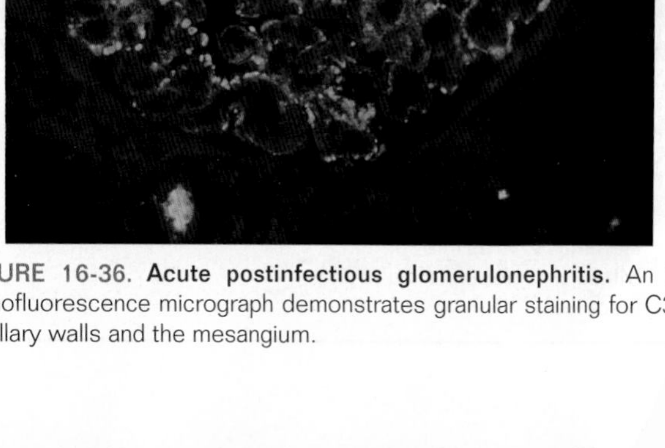

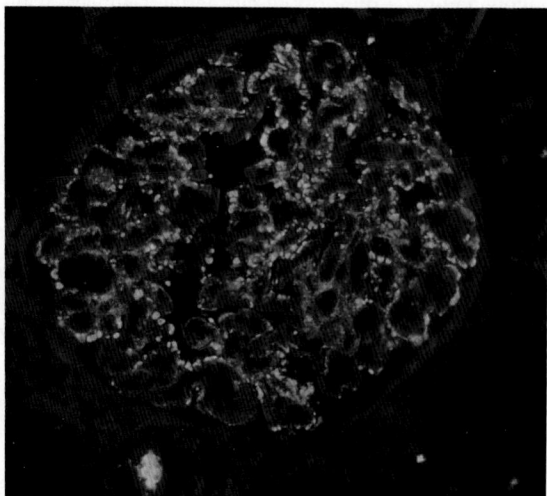

FIGURE 16-36. **Acute postinfectious glomerulonephritis.** An immunofluorescence micrograph demonstrates granular staining for C3 in capillary walls and the mesangium.

although hematuria and especially proteinuria may persist for several months. A few patients have abnormal urinary sediment for years after the acute episode, and rare patients (particularly adults) develop progressive renal failure.

Type I Membranoproliferative Glomerulonephritis Is a Chronic Immune-Complex Disease

Type I membranoproliferative glomerulonephritis is characterized by hypercellularity and capillary wall thickening; deposition of mesangial and subendothelial immune complexes causes mesangial proliferation and extension into the subendothelial zone.

PATHOGENESIS: Type I membranoproliferative glomerulonephritis, also called **mesangiocapillary glomerulonephritis,** is caused by localization of immune complexes to mesangium and the subendothelial zone of capillary walls. In most patients, the origin of nephritogenic antigen is unknown, but some have associated conditions that are the apparent source of the antigen (Table 16-6).

Elimination of the associated condition, such as bacterial endocarditis or osteomyelitis, leads to resolution of the glomerulonephritis, which supports a causal relationship between the two. Unlike the agents that cause acute postinfectious glomerulonephritis, those that are responsible for type I membranoproliferative glomerulonephritis cause persistent, indolent infections that are associated with chronic antigenemia. This condition leads to chronic localization of immune complexes in glomeruli and resultant hypercellularity and matrix remodeling.

PATHOLOGY: Glomeruli in type I membranoproliferative glomerulonephritis are diffusely enlarged, with conspicuous mesangial cell proliferation. The resulting lobular distortion ("hypersegmentation") of the glomeruli (Fig. 16-37) has in the past been termed **lobular glomerulonephritis.** Among these patients, 20% will have crescents, usually involving only a minority of glomeruli. Capillary walls are thickened, and silver stains show a doubling or complex replication of GBMs.

Electron microscopy shows that the capillary wall thickening and replication of GBMs are a consequence of the marked mesangial expansion, with extension of mesangial cytoplasm into the subendothelial zone and deposition of new basement membrane material between the mesangial cytoplasm and endothelial cell (Fig. 16-38 and Fig. 16-39). Subendothelial and mesangial electron-dense deposits, corresponding to immune complexes, are the likely stimuli for the mesangial response. Variable numbers of subepithelial dense deposits may also be seen. Immunofluorescence microscopy shows granular deposition of immunoglobulins and complement in glomerular capillary loops and mesangium (Fig. 16-40).

TABLE 16-6

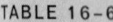

Classification of Type I Membranoproliferative Glomerulonephritis

Primary (idiopathic)
Secondary
Subacute bacterial endocarditis
Infected ventriculoatrial shunt
Osteomyelitis
Hepatitis C virus infection
Mixed cryoglobulinemia
Neoplasia

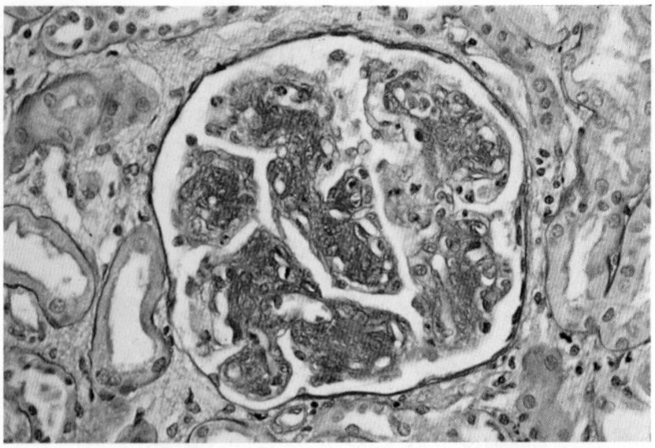

FIGURE 16-37. **Type I membranoproliferative glomerulonephritis.** The glomerular lobulation is accentuated. Increased cells and matrix in the mesangium and thickening of capillary walls are noted.

CLINICAL FEATURES: It can occur at any age, but type I membranoproliferative glomerulonephritis is most frequent in older children and young adults. It may manifest as either nephrotic or nephritic syndrome or a combination of both. Type I disease accounts for 5% of nephrotic syndrome in children and adults in United States. It is much more common in underdeveloped countries that have a high prevalence of chronic infections. Patients often have low levels of C3. Acute postinfectious glomerulonephritis and lupus glomerulonephritis, both of which can cause nephritis with hypocomplementemia, are in the differential diagnosis. Type I membranoproliferative glomerulonephritis is usually a persistent but slowly progressive disease. Half of patients reach end-stage renal disease after 10 years.

Type II Membranoproliferative Glomerulonephritis (Dense Deposit Disease) Features Complement Deposition

Type II membranoproliferative glomerulonephritis is characterized by a pathognomonic electron-dense transformation of GBMs and extensive complement deposition.

PATHOGENESIS: Although the cause of the extensive localization of complement in the GBMs and mesangial matrix in this disease suggests that complement activation is a major mediator of the structural and functional abnormalities, the basis for complement deposition is unknown. The virtual absence of immunoglobulin in glomeruli probably excludes immune complex involvement. Deficiency of, and mutations in, alternative pathway complement regulatory factors (e.g., factor H) are associated with type II membranoproliferative glomerulonephritis, suggesting that dysregulation of the alternative pathway may be involved in disease induction. Most patients have a serum IgG autoantibody, termed **C3 nephritic factor,** which stabilizes the activated C3 convertase enzyme (C3bBb) of the alternative complement activation pathway. The result is prolongation of C3 cleaving activity. A similar C3 nephritic factor is also present in a minority of patients with type I membranoproliferative glomerulonephritis and lupus nephritis. The role of this factor, if any, in type II membranoproliferative glomerulonephritis is unclear. However, type II membranoproliferative glomerulonephritis often recurs in renal transplants, suggesting that glomerular injury is mediated through some unknown humoral factor.

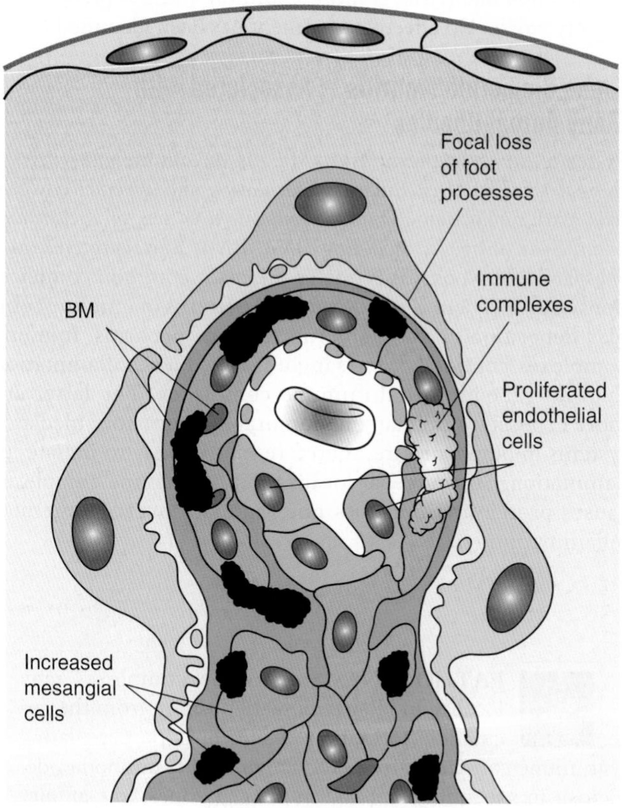

FIGURE 16-38. **Membranoproliferative glomerulonephritis, type I.** In this disease, the glomeruli are enlarged. Hypercellular tufts and narrowing or obstruction of the capillary lumen are seen. Large subendothelial deposits of immune complexes extend along the inner border of the basement membrane. The mesangial cells proliferate and migrate peripherally into the capillary. Basement membrane (BM) material accumulates in a linear fashion parallel to the basement membrane in a subendothelial position. The interposition of mesangial cells and basement membrane between the endothelial cells and the original basement membrane creates a double-contour effect. The accumulation of mesangial cells and stroma in the tufts narrows the capillary lumen. The proliferation of mesangial cells and the accumulation of basement membrane material also widen the mesangium. The entire process leads progressively to lobulation of the glomerulus. Note the proliferation of endothelial cells and focal effacement of foot processes.

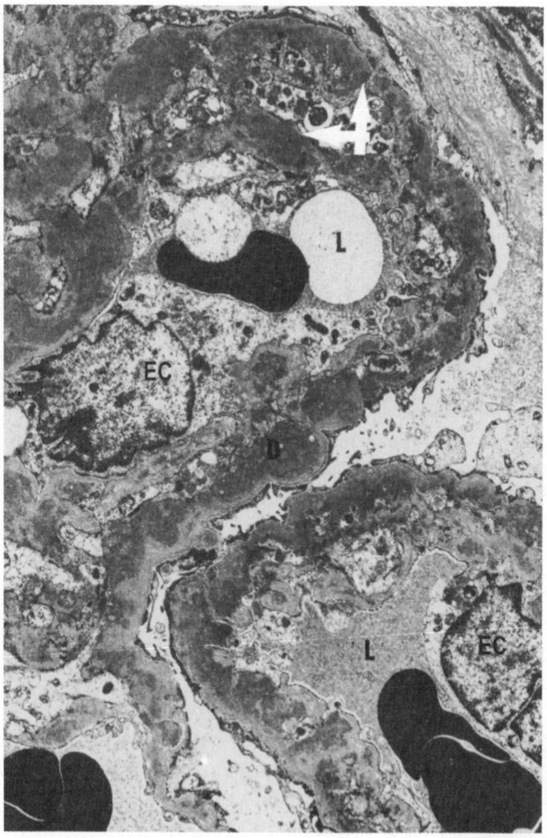

FIGURE 16-39. **Type I membranoproliferative glomerulonephritis.** An electron micrograph demonstrates a double-contour basement membrane *(arrow),* with mesangial interposition and prominent subendothelial deposits. EC = endothelial cell; L = capillary lumen.

PATHOLOGY: The histologic appearance of type II membranoproliferative glomerulonephritis may be similar to that of type I, with capillary wall thickening and hypercellularity (Fig. 16-41). However, many patients have less-pronounced or absent hypercellularity, which makes the term "proliferative" problematic. The distinctive ribbonlike zone of increased density in the center of a thickened GBM and in the mesangial matrix (Fig. 16-42), justifies the alternative name **dense deposit disease.** Areas of density may also be found

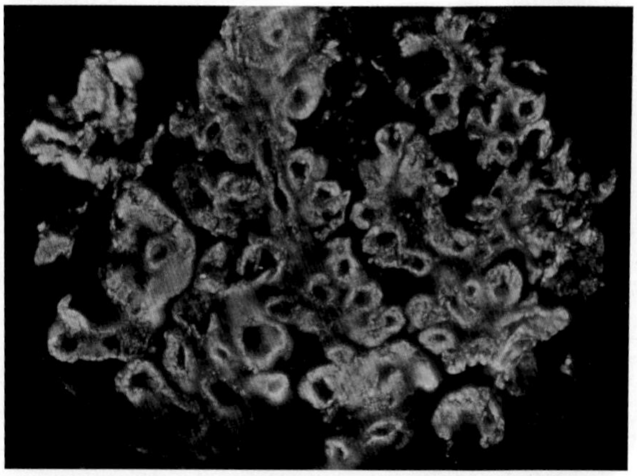

FIGURE 16-40. **Type I membranoproliferative glomerulonephritis.** An immunofluorescence micrograph demonstrates granular to bandlike staining for C3 in the capillary walls and mesangium.

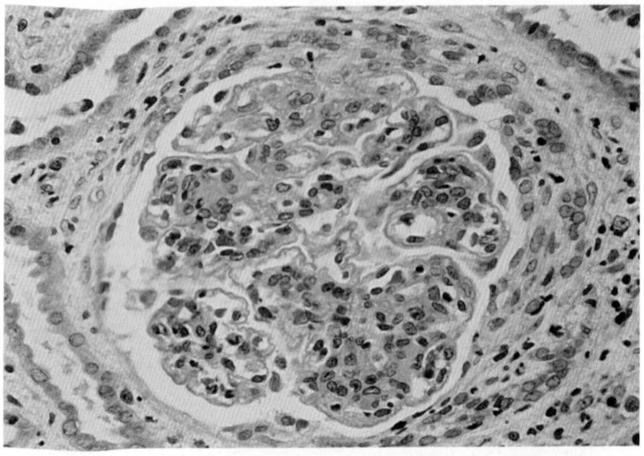

FIGURE 16-41. **Type II membranoproliferative glomerulonephritis (dense deposit disease).** Capillary wall thickening, hypercellularity, and a small crescent are evident.

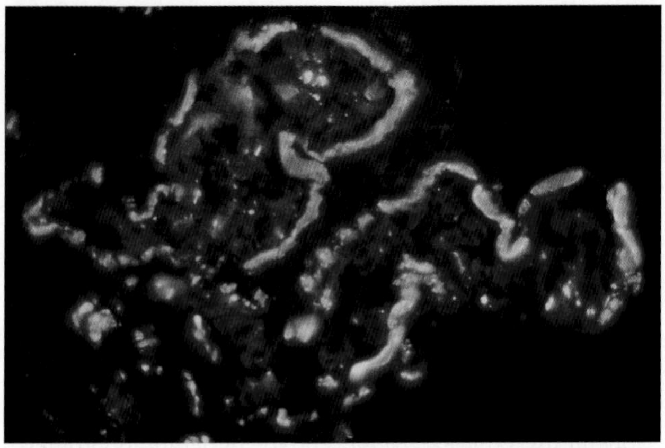

FIGURE 16-43. **Type II membranoproliferative glomerulonephritis (dense deposit disease).** An immunofluorescence micrograph demonstrates bands of capillary wall staining and coarsely granular mesangial staining for C3.

in the membranes of peritubular capillaries and in the elastic laminae of arterioles. Immunofluorescence microscopy shows linear staining of capillary walls for C3, with little or no staining for immunoglobulins (Fig. 16-43).

CLINICAL FEATURES: Type II membranoproliferative glomerulonephritis is rare. It resembles type I disease in clinical presentation and course, save that hypocomplementemia is more common and the prognosis is slightly worse. No effective treatment has been identified.

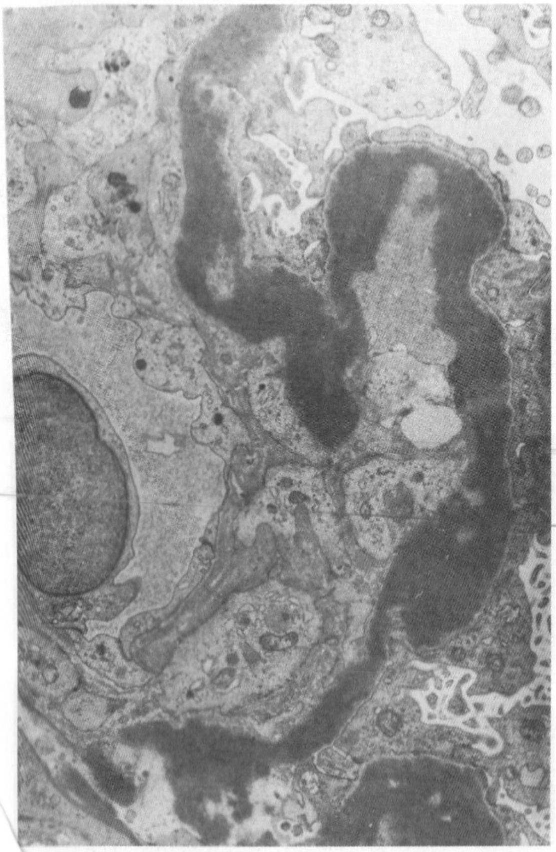

'E 16-42. **Type II membranoproliferative glomerulonephritis 'eposit disease).** An electron micrograph demonstrates thicken- 'asement membrane and intramembranous dense deposits.

Lupus Glomerulonephritis Is Associated with Many Autoantibodies

Systemic lupus erythematosus (SLE) is an autoimmune disease characterized by a generalized dysregulation and hyperactivity of B cells, with production of autoantibodies to a variety of nuclear and nonnuclear antigens, including DNA, RNA, nucleoproteins, and phospholipids. Nephritis is one of the most common complications of SLE. There is a wide range of patterns of immune complex deposition in the glomeruli of lupus nephritis. Immune complexes confined to mesangium cause less inflammation than do subendothelial immune complexes. The latter are more exposed to cellular and humoral inflammatory mediator systems in blood and are, therefore, more likely to initiate inflammation. Subepithelial localization of immune complexes causes proteinuria but does not stimulate overt glomerular inflammation.

PATHOGENESIS: Immune complexes may localize in glomeruli by deposition from the circulation, formation in situ, or both. Circulating immune complexes formed by high-avidity antibodies deposit in subendothelial and mesangial zones; low-affinity antibodies form immune complexes in situ in the subepithelial zone. Formation of immune complexes in situ may involve antigens such as DNA, which have been planted on GBMs or mesangial matrix by charge interactions. Glomerular immune complexes activate complement and initiate inflammatory injury. Complement activation in the kidneys and elsewhere often results in hypocomplementemia. Immune complexes also localize in the renal interstitium, walls of interstitial vessels, and tubular basement membranes. These complexes may be involved in the tubulointerstitial inflammation seen in patients with lupus nephritis.

PATHOLOGY: The pathologic and clinical manifestations of lupus nephritis are highly variable because of variable patterns of immune complex accumulation in different patients (Table 16-7) and in the same patient over time.

- **Class I (minimal mesangial lupus nephritis):** Immune complexes are confined to mesangium and cause no changes by light microscopy.
- **Class II (mesangial proliferative lupus nephritis):** Immune complexes are confined to mesangium and cause varying degrees of mesangial hypercellularity and matrix expansion (Fig. 16-44).
- **Class III (focal proliferative lupus nephritis):** Immune complex accumulation in the subendothelial zone, which is always accompanied by mesangial immune complexes, stimulates inflammation with proliferation of mesangial and endothelial cells, and the influx of neutrophils and monocytes. This overt glomerular inflammation is termed **focal proliferative lupus glomerulonephritis** if it involves less than 50% of glomeruli.
- **Class IV (diffuse proliferative lupus nephritis):** This type is similar to class III but involves more than 50% of glomeruli. Glomerular involvement may be predominantly global (IV-G) or predominantly segmental (IV-S).
- **Class V (membarnous lupus nephritis):** Immune complexes are mostly in the subepithelial zone. Some patients have a background of class V injury and a concurrent class III, or IV injury. Even pure class V lupus nephritis has mesangial immune complexes that can be detected by electron microscopy.
- **Class VI (advanced sclerosing lupus nephritis):** Advanced chronic disease.

Electron microscopy demonstrates the varied locations of immune-complex dense deposits in mesangial, subendothelial, and subepithelial locations. Class I and II lesions primarily have mesangial deposits. Classes III and IV have mesangial and subendothelial deposits and usually scattered subepithelial deposits (Fig. 16-45). Class V lesions have numerous subepithelial dense deposits. The dense deposits of lupus glomerulonephritis occasionally have a patterned appearance, like a fingerprint. Some 80% of specimens have **tubuloreticular inclusions** in endothelial cells. Lupus nephritis and HIV-associated nephropathy are the only renal diseases with a high frequency of these structures.

By immunofluorescence, the subepithelial complexes are granular and the subendothelial deposits appear granular or bandlike (Fig. 16-46). The immune complexes often stain most intensely for IgG, but IgA and IgM are also almost always present, as are C3, C1q, and other complement components. Granular staining along tubular basement membranes and interstitial vessels is present in over 50% of patients.

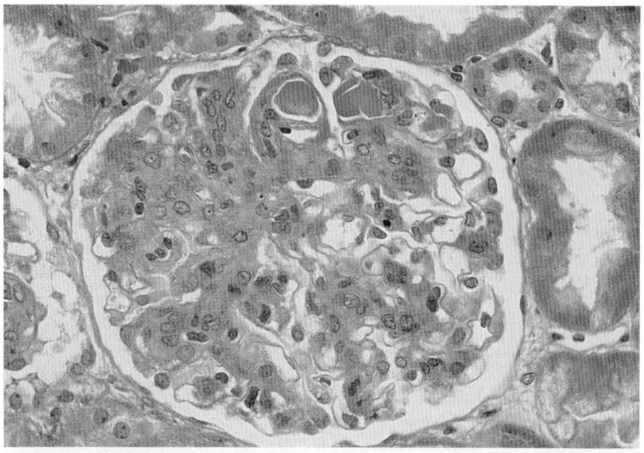

FIGURE 16-44. **Proliferative lupus glomerulonephritis.** Segmental endocapillary hypercellularity and thickening of capillary walls are present.

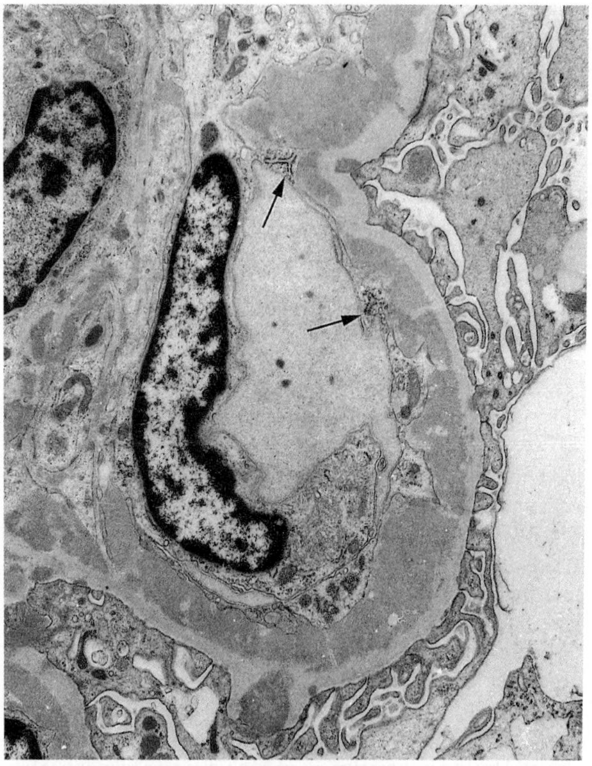

FIGURE 16-45. **Diffuse proliferative lupus glomerulonephritis.** An electron micrograph reveals large subendothelial and mesangial dense deposits and a few subepithelial deposits. Endothelial tubuloreticular inclusions *(arrows)* are present.

TABLE 16-7

Pathologic and Clinical Features of Lupus Nephritis

Location of Immune Class	Clinical Complexes	Manifestations
I: No lesion by light microscopy	Mesangial	Mild hematuria and proteinuria
II: Mesangial proliferative	Mesangial	Mild hematuria and proteinuria
III: Focal proliferative	Mesangial and subendothelial	Moderate nephritis
IV: Diffuse proliferative	Mesangial and subendothelial	Severe nephritis
V: Membranous	Subepithelial	Nephrotic syndrome
VI: Chronic	Variable	Chronic renal failure

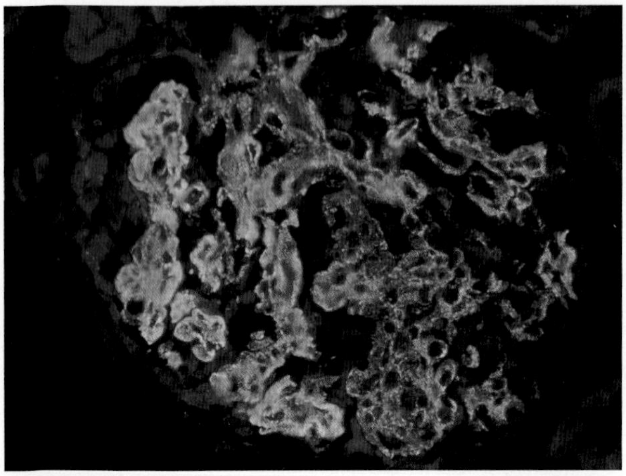

FIGURE 16-46. **Diffuse proliferative lupus glomerulonephritis.** An immunofluorescence micrograph demonstrates segmental staining for immunoglobulin G in the capillary walls and mesangium.

CLINICAL FEATURES: Seventy percent of all patients with SLE develop renal disease, which is the major cause for morbidity and mortality in many patients. The disease is most common in black women. As noted in Table 16-7, the clinical manifestations and prognosis of renal dysfunction are varied and depend on the pathologic nature of the underlying renal disease. *Renal biopsy specimens from patients with lupus are used to assess disease category, activity, and chronicity, rather than merely to make a diagnosis of lupus glomerulonephritis.* Class III and class IV lupus nephritis have the poorest prognosis and are treated most aggressively, usually with high doses of corticosteroids and other immunosuppressive drugs. Over time, sometimes prompted by treatment, there can be transitions from one type of lupus nephritis to another, with the expected changes in clinical manifestations. Currently, less than 25% of patients with class IV disease reach end-stage renal failure within 5 years.

IgA Nephropathy (Berger Disease) Is Caused by Immune Complexes of IgA

PATHOGENESIS: Although deposition of IgA-dominant immune complexes is the cause of IgA nephropathy, the constituent antigens and mechanism of accumulation (deposition versus formation in situ) are not known. Patients with IgA nephropathy often have elevated blood levels of IgA, and circulating IgA-containing immune complexes have been detected. *Exacerbations of IgA nephropathy are often initiated by respiratory or gastrointestinal infections.* A leading hypothesis proposes that mucosal exposure to viral, bacterial, or dietary antigens stimulates a nephritogenic, IgA-dominant, immune response that results in the glomerular immune complex accumulation. Possible involvement of dietary antigens is supported by an association in a small number of cases between IgA nephropathy and gluten-sensitive enteropa-[illegible]hy, and by the improvement in both diseases when dietary [illegible]n is eliminated. There is evidence for major histocom-[illegible] complex (MHC)–linked susceptibility to IgA nephropathy, possibly mediated via dysregulation of IgA immune responses. Abnormal glycosylation of the hinge region of IgA appears to be an important predisposing factor in many patients with IgA nephropathy.

IgA-containing immune complexes within the mesangium most likely activate the alternative complement pathway. This concept is supported by the demonstration of C3 and properdin, but not C1q and C4, in the IgA deposits.

PATHOLOGY: Immunofluorescence microscopy is essential for diagnosis of IgA nephropathy. The diagnostic finding is mesangial staining for IgA more intense than, or equivalent to, staining for IgG or IgM (Fig. 16-47). This is almost always accompanied by staining for C3. IgA deposition in the glomerular capillary wall (in addition to the mesangium) may be present in more severe cases and suggests a less favorable prognosis.

Depending on the severity and duration of glomerular inflammation, IgA nephropathy manifests a continuum of histologic appearances, ranging from (1) no discernible light microscopic changes, to (2) focal or diffuse mesangial hypercellularity, to (3) focal or diffuse proliferative glomerulonephritis (Fig. 16-48) to (4) chronic sclerosing glomerulonephritis. At the time of initial diagnosis, focal proliferative glomerulonephritis is the most frequent manifestation. Crescent formation is uncommon, except in unusually severe cases. This spectrum of pathologic changes is analogous to that seen with lupus nephritis but tends to be less severe.

Ultrastructural examination reveals mesangial electron-dense deposits (Fig. 16-49 and Fig. 16-50). A minority of patients, usually those with severe disease, have dense deposits in the capillary walls.

CLINICAL FEATURES: IgA nephropathy (Berger disease) is the most common form of glomerulonephritis in the world. It accounts for 10% of cases in the United States, 20% in Europe, and 40% in Asia. IgA nephropathy has a high frequency in Native Americans and is rare in blacks. It is most common in young men, with a peak age

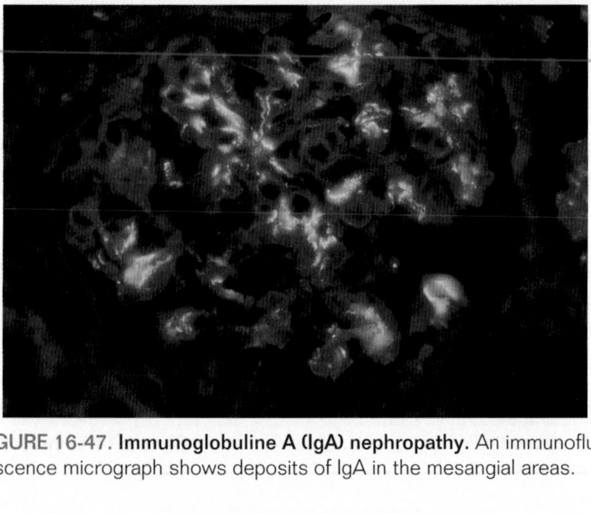

FIGURE 16-47. **Immunoglobuline A (IgA) nephropathy.** An immunofluorescence micrograph shows deposits of IgA in the mesangial areas.

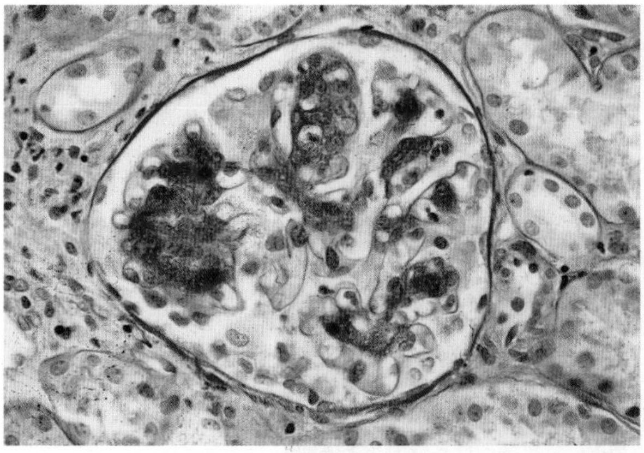

FIGURE 16-48. **Immunoglobulin A nephropathy.** Segmental mesangial hypercellularity and matrix expansion caused by the mesangial immune deposits. (periodic acid-Schiff stain)

of 15 to 30 years at diagnosis. The clinical presentations are varied, which reflects the varied pathologic severity: 40% of patients have asymptomatic microscopic hematuria, 40% have intermittent gross hematuria, 10% have nephrotic syndrome, and 10% have renal failure. The disease rarely resolves completely but may follow an episodic course, with exacerbations often occurring at the time of an upper respiratory tract infection. IgA nephropathy has a slowly progressive course, with 20% of patients reaching end-stage renal failure after 10 years. When these patients are treated by renal transplantation, IgA deposits

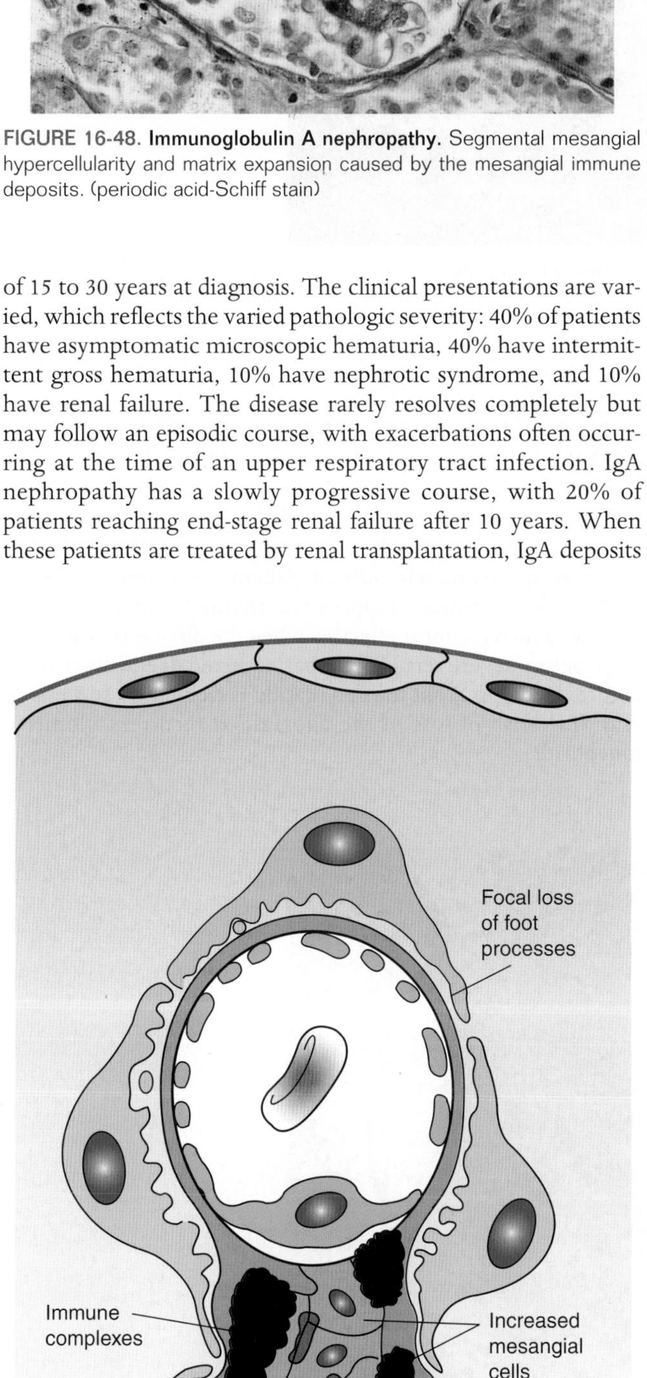

FIGURE 16-49. **Immunoglobulin A (IgA) nephropathy.** Significant accumulation of IgA is seen in the mesangium, most commonly, between the mesangial cells and the basement membrane.

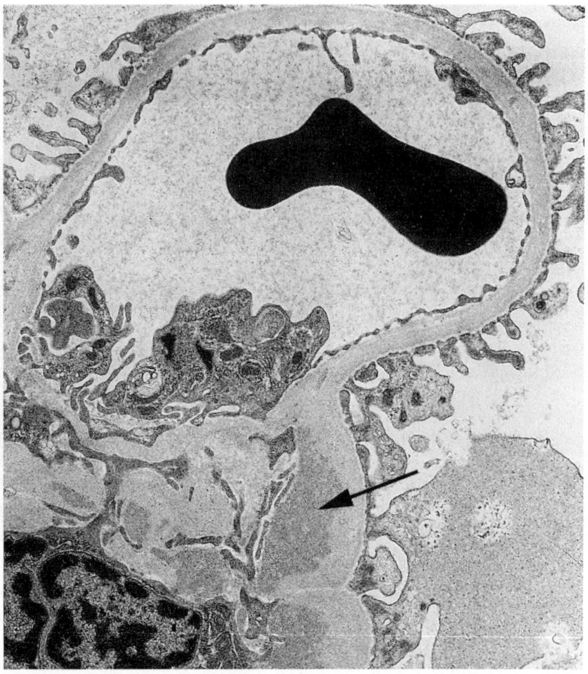

FIGURE 16-50. **Immunoglobulin A nephropathy.** An electron micrograph demonstrates prominent dense deposits in the mesangial matrix.

frequently recur in the allograft, although graft function is usually not impaired.

Anti-Glomerular Basement Membrane Glomerulonephritis Is Often Associated with Pulmonary Hemorrhage

Anti-GBM antibody glomerulonephritis is an uncommon but aggressive form of glomerulonephritis that occurs as a renal-limited disease or combined with pulmonary hemorrhage (Goodpasture syndrome).

PATHOGENESIS: *Anti-GBM glomerulonephritis is mediated by an autoimmune response against a component of the GBM within the globular noncollagenous domain of type IV collagen.* The specific epitope is on the α3 chain. Because the target antigen is also expressed on pulmonary alveolar capillary basement membranes, half of patients also have pulmonary hemorrhages and hemoptysis, sometimes severe enough to be life-threatening. If both lungs and kidneys are involved, the eponym **Goodpasture syndrome** is used (see Fig. 16-14). Anti-GBM antibodies, anti-GBM T cells, or both may mediate the injury. The antibodies bind the autoantigens in situ. Resultant immune complexes could initiate acute inflammation by activating mediator systems, such as complement. Experimental observations suggest that T cells with specificity for GBM antigens may mediate the vascular injury. Genetic susceptibility to anti-GBM disease is associated with human leukocyte antigen *(HLA)-DR2* genes. Disease onset often follows viral upper respiratory tract infections, and pulmonary involement appears to require synergistic injurious agents, such as cigarette smoke.

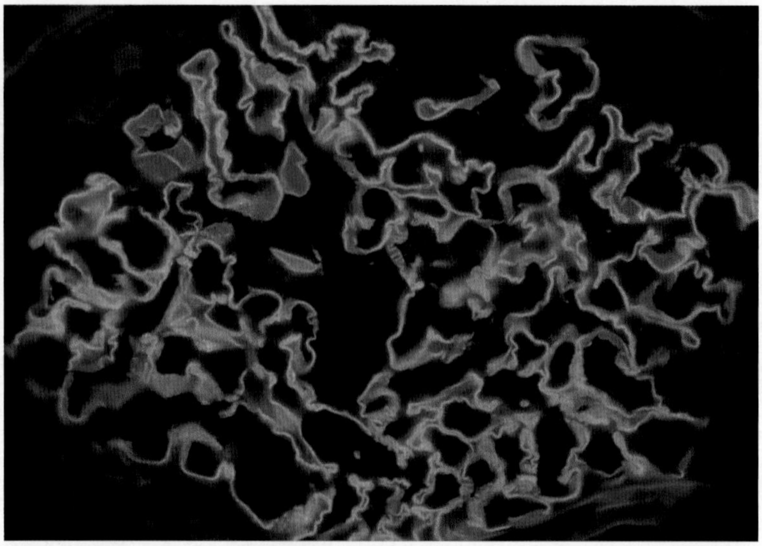

FIGURE 16-51. **Anti-glomerular basement membrane (GBM) glomerulonephritis.** Linear immunofluorescence for immunoglobulin G is seen along the GBM. Contrast this linear pattern of staining with the granular pattern of immunofluorescence typical for most types of immune complex deposition within capillary walls (see Fig. 16-36).

PATHOLOGY: *The pathologic hallmark of anti-GBM glomerulonephritis is diffuse linear staining of GBMs for IgG, which indicates autoantibodies bound to the basement membrane* (Fig. 16-51). Linear staining for IgG, however, is not entirely specific. For example, nonimmunologic binding of IgG to basement membranes occurs in diabetic glomerulosclerosis. *Over 90% of patients with anti-GBM glomerulonephritis have glomerular crescents* (**crescentic glomerulonephritis**) (Fig. 16-52 and Fig. 16-53), *usually involving over 50% of glomeruli.* Focal glomerular fibrinoid necrosis is common. Involved lungs exhibit marked intraalveolar hemorrhage. Electron microscopy shows focal breaks in GBMs, but no immune-complex-type electron-dense deposits.

CLINICAL FEATURES: Anti-GBM glomerulonephritis typically presents with rapidly progressive renal failure and nephritic signs and symptoms. It accounts for 10% to 20% of rapidly progressive (crescentic) glomerulonephritis (Table 16-8). Serum anti-GBM antibodies occur in approximately 90% of patients. Treatment consists of high-dose immunosuppressive therapy and plasma exchange, which are most effective when the disease is in an early stage before severe renal failure has occurred. If end-stage renal failure develops, renal transplantation is frequently successful, with little risk of loss of the allograft to recurrent glomerulonephritis.

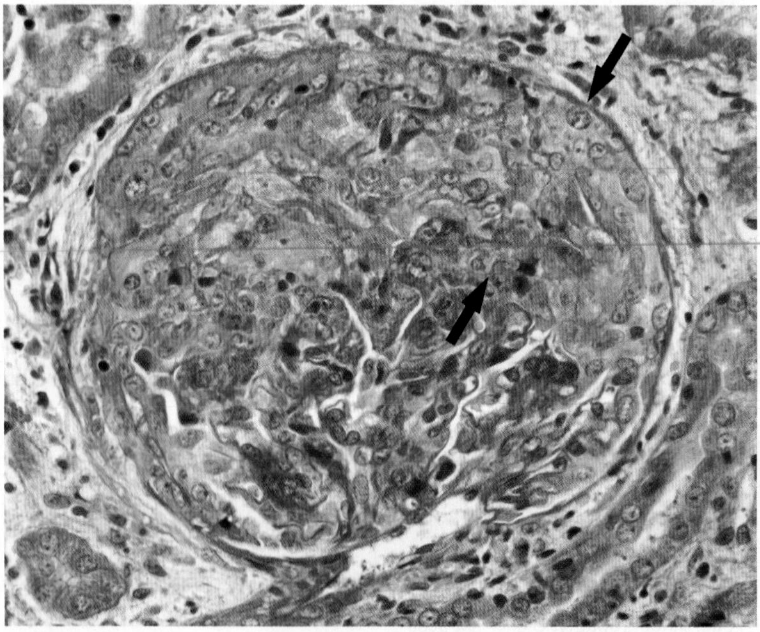

'GURE 16-52. **Crescentic anti-glomerular basement membrane glomerulonephritis.** Bowman's space is filled by a cellular cent (between arrows). The injured glomerular tuft is at the bottom. (Masson trichrome stain).

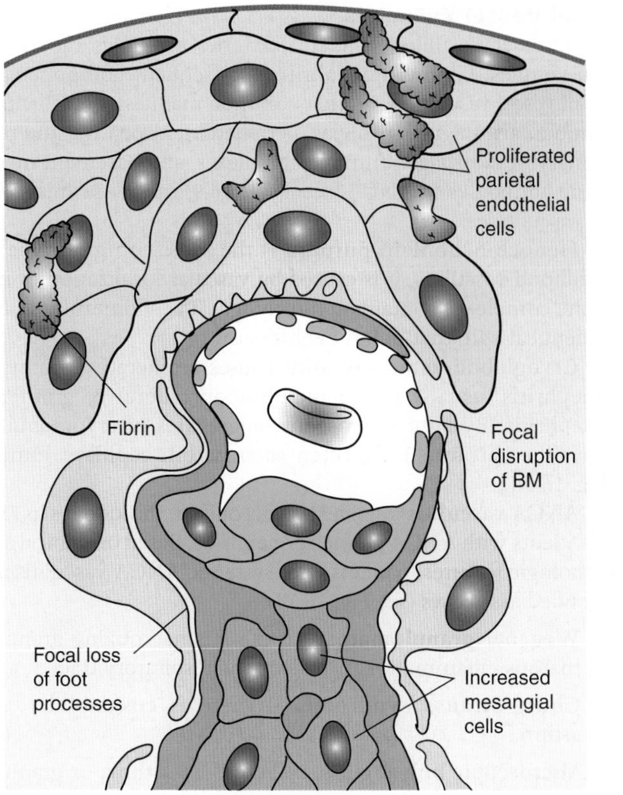

FIGURE 16-53. **Crescentic (rapidly progressive) glomerulonephritis.** A variety of different pathogenic mechanisms cause crescent formation by disrupting glomerular capillary walls. This allows plasma constituents into Bowman's space, including coagulation factors and inflammatory mediators. Fibrin forms, and there is proliferation of parietal epithelial cells and influx of macrophages, resulting in crescent formation.

ANCA Glomerulonephritis Features Neutrophil-Induced Injury

ANCA glomerulonephritis is an aggressive, neutrophil-mediated disease that is characterized by glomerular necrosis and crescents.

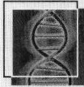

PATHOGENESIS: ANCA glomerulonephritis was once called *idiopathic crescentic glomerulonephritis* because immunofluorescence microscopy did not demonstrate evidence of glomerular deposition of anti-GBM antibodies or immune complexes. The discovery that 90% of patients with this pattern of glomerular injury have circulating ANCAs led to the demonstration that these autoantibodies cause the disease. *ANCAs are specific for proteins in the cytoplasm of neutrophils and monocytes, usually MPO-ANCA or PR3-ANCA.* These autoantibodies activate neutrophils and cause them to adhere to endothelial cells, release toxic oxygen metabolites, degranulate, and kill the endothelial cells. Transplacental transfer of MPO-ANCA can cause neonatal glomerulonephritis and pulmonary hemorrhage, which supports the pathogenic potential of ANCA.

PATHOLOGY: Over 90% of patients with ANCA glomerulonephritis have focal glomerular necrosis (Fig. 16-54) and crescent formation (Fig. 16-55). In many

TABLE 16-8

Frequency (%) of Immunopathologic Categories of Crescentic Glomerulonephritis* in Different Age Groups

Category	Age (years) <20	20–64	>65
Antiglomerular basement membrane	10	10	10
Immune complex	55	40	10
Antineutrophil cytoplasmic autoantibody (ANCA)	30	45	75
No evidence for the three categories above	5	5	5

* Glomerulonephritis with crescents in >50% of glomeruli.

patients, over 50% of glomeruli exhibit crescents. Nonnecrotic segments may appear normal or have slight neutrophil infiltration or mild endocapillary hypercellularity. Immunofluorescence microscopy demonstrates an absence or paucity of staining for immunoglobulins and complement, which distinguishes ANCA glomerulonephritis from anti-GBM glomerulonephritis and immune-complex glomerulonephritis. A minority of patients with crescentic glomerulonephritis have serologic and pathologic evidence for overlapping expression of ANCA glomerulonephritis with anti-GBM glomerulonephritis or immune-complex glomerulonephritis. Electron microscopy demonstrates no immune-complex-type dense deposits in ANCA glomerulonephritis.

CLINICAL FEATURES: The most common clinical presentation for ANCA glomerulonephritis is rapidly progressive renal failure, with nephritic signs and symptoms. The disease accounts for 75% of rapidly progressive (crescentic) glomerulonephritis in patients over 60 years old, 45% in middle-aged adults and 30% in young adults and children (see Table 16-8). *Three quarters of patients with ANCA glomerulonephritis have systemic small vessel vasculitis (see below), which has many manifestations, including pulmonary hemorrhage.* ANCA glomerulonephritis with pulmonary vasculitis is actually a much

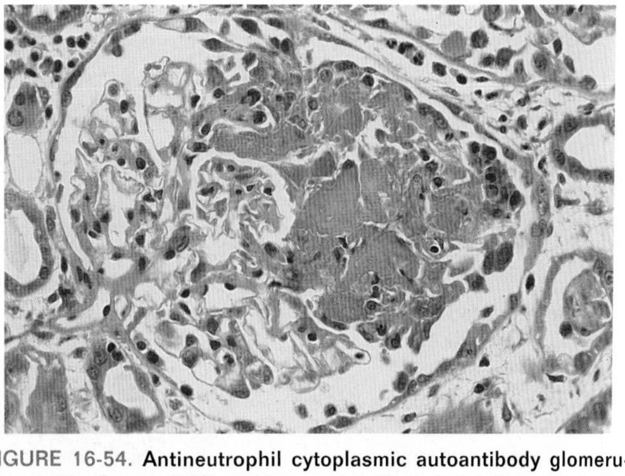

FIGURE 16-54. **Antineutrophil cytoplasmic autoantibody glomerulonephritis.** Segmental fibrinoid necrosis is illustrated. In time, this lesion stimulates crescent formation.

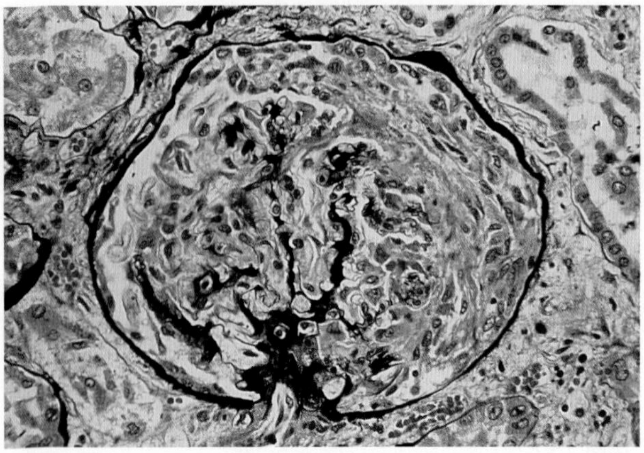

FIGURE 16-55. **Antineutrophil cytoplasmic autoantibody glomerulonephritis.** Silver staining shows focal disruption of glomerular basement membranes and crescent formation within Bowman's space.

more frequent cause of **pulmonary–renal vasculitic syndrome** than is Goodpasture syndrome. Without treatment, over 80% of patients with ANCA glomerulonephritis develop end-stage renal disease within 5 years. Immunosuppressive therapy decreases the development of end-stage disease at 5 years to less than 25%. Once remission of disease is induced with high-dose immunosuppressive treatment, patients are at risk for recurrent disease. ANCA glomerulonephritis recurs in 15% of patients who receive renal transplants.

Vascular Diseases

Renal Vasculitis May Affect Vessels of All Sizes

The kidney is involved in many types of systemic vasculitis (Table 16-9). *In a sense, glomerulonephritis is a local form of vasculitis that affects glomerular capillaries.* The glomeruli may be the only site of vascular inflammation or the renal disease may be a component of a systemic vasculitis.

Small Vessel Vasculitis

Small vessel vasculitis affects small arteries, arterioles, capillaries, and venules. Glomerulonephritis is a frequent component of small vessel vasculitides. Other common manifestations include purpura, arthralgias, myalgias, peripheral neuropathy, and pulmonary hemorrhage. Immune complexes, anti-basement membrane antibodies or ANCA (see Table 16-9) can cause small vessel vasculitides.

Henoch-Schönlein purpura is the most common type of childhood vasculitis. It is caused by vascular localization of immune complexes containing mostly IgA. The glomerular lesion is identical with that of IgA nephropathy.

Cryoglobulinemic vasculitis causes proliferative glomerulonephritis, usually type I membranoproliferative glomerulonephritis. By light microscopy, aggregates of cryoglobulins ("hyaline thrombi") are often seen within capillary lumina (Fig. 16-56).

ANCA vasculitis involves vessels outside the kidneys in 75% of patients with ANCA glomerulonephritis. Based on clinical and pathologic features, patients with systemic ANCA vasculitis are classified as follows (see Fig. 16-14):

- **Wegener granulomatosis,** if there is necrotizing granulomatous inflammation, usually in the respiratory tract
- **Churg-Strauss syndrome,** if there is eosinophilia and asthma
- **Microscopic polyangiitis,** if there is no asthma or granulomatous inflammation

In addition to causing necrotizing and crescentic glomerulonephritis, the ANCA vasculitides often display necrotizing inflammation in other renal vessels, such as arteries (Fig. 16-57), arterioles, and medullary peritubular capillaries.

Medium-Sized Vessel Vasculitis

Medium-sized vessel vasculitides affect arteries, but not arterioles, capillaries, or venules (see Chapter 10). **Polyarteritis nodosa,** which occurs mainly in adults, and **Kawasaki disease,** which principally afflicts young children, are rare causes of renal dysfunction. These diseases are characterized by necrotizing

TABLE 16-9

Types of Vasculitis That Involve the Kidneys

Type of Vasculitis	Major Target Vessels in Kidney	Major Renal Manifestations
Small-vessel vasculitis		
Immune-complex vasculitis		
Henoch-Schönlein purpura	Glomeruli	Nephritis
Cryoglobulinemic vasculitis	Glomeruli	Nephritis
Anti-GBM vasculitis		
Goodpasture syndrome	Glomeruli	Nephritis
ANCA-vasculitis		
Wegener granulomatosis	Glomeruli, arterioles, interlobular arteries	Nephritis
Microscopic polyangiitis	Glomeruli, arterioles, interlobular arteries	Nephritis
Churg-Strauss syndrome	Glomeruli, arterioles, interlobular arteries	Nephritis
Medium-sized-vessel vasculitis		
Polyarteritis nodosa	Interlobar and arcuate arteries	Infarcts and hemorrhage
Kawasaki disease	Interlobar and arcuate arteries	Infarcts and hemorrhage
Large-vessel vasculitis		
Giant cell arteritis	Main renal artery	Renovascular hypertension
Takayasu arteritis	Main renal artery	Renovascular hypertension

..utrophil cytoplasmic autoantibody; GBM= glomerular basement membrane.

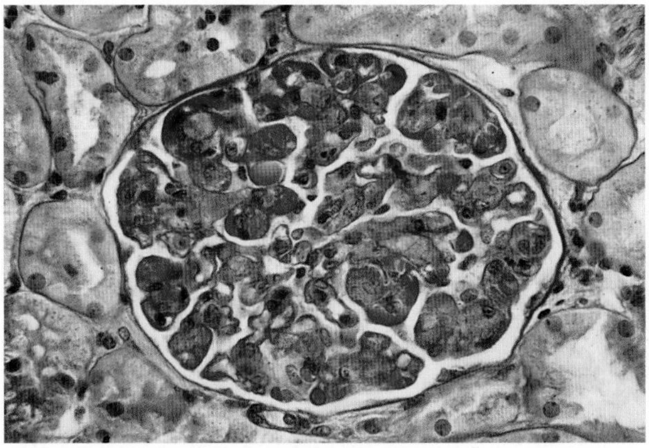

FIGURE 16-56. **Cryoglobulinemic glomerulonephritis.** The pattern of glomerular inflammation is similar to that of type I membranoproliferative glomerulonephritis. However, as in this specimen, there typically are conspicuous glassy aggregates ("hyaline thrombi") in the capillary lumina and subendothelial spaces. These are not true thrombi but rather are large aggregates of cryoglobulins. (periodic acid-Schiff stain)

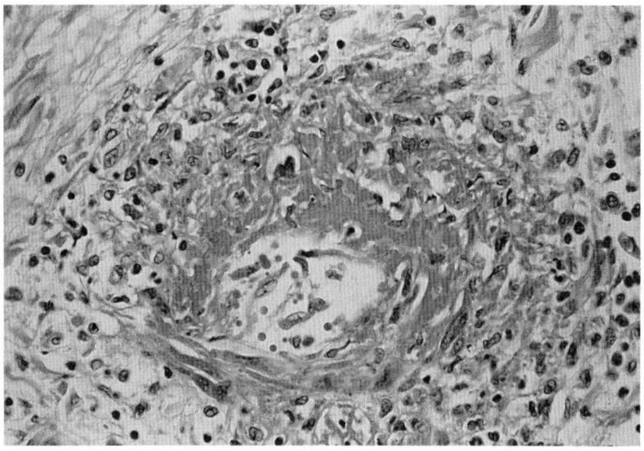

FIGURE 16-57. **Antineutrophil cytoplasmic autoantibody necrotizing arteritis.** Fibrinoid necrosis and inflammation involve an interlobular artery in the renal cortex.

arteritis, which can involve renal arteries and lead to pseudoaneurysm formation and renal thrombosis, infarction, and hemorrhage.

Large Vessel Vasculitis

Large vessel vasculitides, such as **giant cell arteritis** and **Takayasu arteritis,** affect the aorta and its major branches. These disorders may cause renovascular hypertension by involving the main renal arteries or the aorta at the origin of the renal arteries (see Chapter 10). Narrowing or obstruction of these vessels results in renal ischemia, which stimulates increased renin production and consequent hypertension (see Table 16-9).

Hypertensive Nephrosclerosis (Benign Nephrosclerosis) Leads to Obliteration of Glomeruli

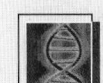

PATHOGENESIS: Sustained systolic pressures over 140 mm Hg and diastolic pressures over 90 mm are generally considered to represent hypertension (see Chapter 10). Mild-to-moderate hypertension causes typical hypertensive nephrosclerosis and thus is not truly benign. In fact hypertensive nephrosclerosis is identified in approximately 15% of patients with "benign hypertension." Changes similar to those in hypertensive nephrosclerosis occasionally occur in older individuals who have never had hypertension, and are attributed to aging itself.

PATHOLOGY: The kidneys are smaller than normal (atrophic) and are usually affected bilaterally. The cortical surfaces have a fine granularity (Fig. 16-58), but coarser scars are occasionally present. On cut section, the cortex is thinned. Microscopically, many glomeruli appear normal; others show varying degrees of ischemic change. Initially, glomerular capillaries are thickened because of thickening, wrinkling, and collapse of GBMs. Cells of the glomerular tuft are progressively lost, and collagen and matrix material are deposited within Bowman space. Eventually, the glomerular tuft is obliterated by a dense, eosinophilic globular mass within a scar, all inside Bowman's capsule. Tubular atrophy, a consequence of glomerular obsolescence, is associated with interstitial fibrosis and infiltration by chronic inflammatory cells. Globally sclerotic glomeruli and surrounding atrophic tubules are often clustered in focal subcapsular zones, with adjacent areas of preserved glomeruli and tubules (Fig. 16-59), an effect that is the basis for the granular surfaces of nephrosclerotic kidneys.

The pattern of change in the renal blood vessels depends on the size of the vessel. Arteries down to the size of the arcuate arteries have fibrotic thickening of the intima, with replication of the elastica-like lamina and partial replacement of the muscularis with fibrous tissue. Interlobular arteries and arterioles may develop medial hyperplasia. Arterioles exhibit concentric hyaline thickening of the wall, often with the loss of smooth muscle cells

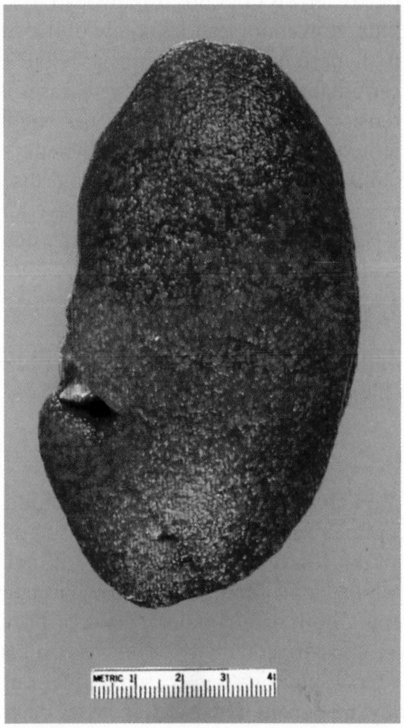

FIGURE 16-58. **Hypertensive nephrosclerosis.** The kidney is reduced in size, and the cortical surface exhibits fine granularity.

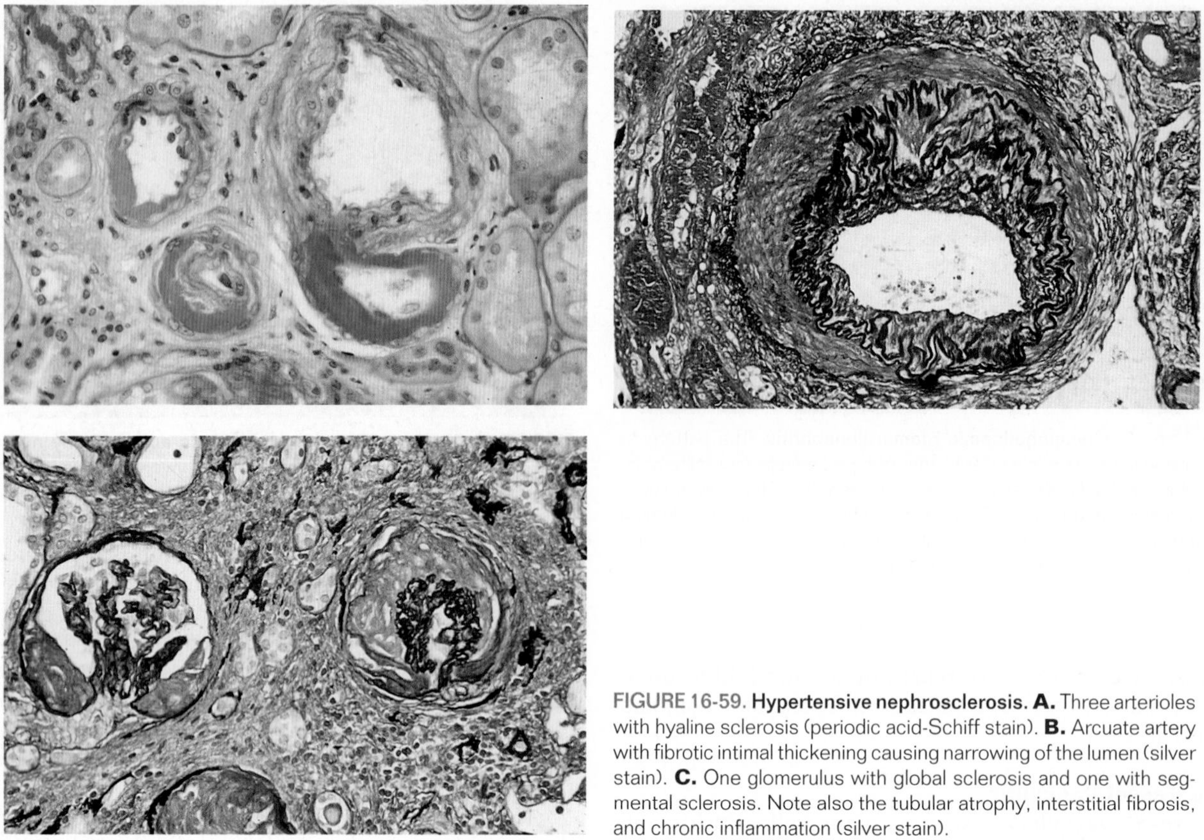

FIGURE 16-59. **Hypertensive nephrosclerosis. A.** Three arterioles with hyaline sclerosis (periodic acid-Schiff stain). **B.** Arcuate artery with fibrotic intimal thickening causing narrowing of the lumen (silver stain). **C.** One glomerulus with global sclerosis and one with segmental sclerosis. Note also the tubular atrophy, interstitial fibrosis, and chronic inflammation (silver stain).

or their displacement to the periphery. This arteriolar change is termed **hyaline arteriolosclerosis.**

CLINICAL FEATURES: Although hypertensive nephrosclerosis does not usually lead to significant renal function abnormalities, a few of the many persons with "benign" hypertension develop progressive renal failure, which may terminate in end-stage renal disease. Because "benign" hypertension is so prevalent, even the small proportion of these patients who develop renal insufficiency amounts to one third of all patients with end-stage renal disease. Benign nephrosclerosis is most prevalent and aggressive among blacks. *In fact, among blacks in the United States, hypertension without any evidence of a malignant phase is the leading cause of end-stage renal disease.*

Malignant Hypertensive Nephropathy Is a Potentially Fatal Renal Disease

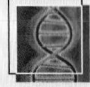

PATHOGENESIS: No specific blood pressure defines malignant hypertension, but diastolic pressures over 130 mm Hg, retinal vascular changes, papilledema, and renal functional impairment are usual criteria. About half of patients have prior histories of benign hypertension, and many others have a background of chronic renal injury caused by many different diseases. ...asionally, malignant hypertension arises de novo in ap...ly healthy persons, particularly young black men.

The pathogenesis of the vascular injury in patients with malignant hypertension is not completely elucidated. One hypothesis proposes that extremely high blood pressures, combined with microvascular vasoconstriction, cause injury to endothelium as the blood slams into the narrowed small vessels. At sites of vascular injury, plasma constituents leak into injured walls of arterioles (resulting in fibrinoid necrosis), into intima of arteries (causing edematous intimal thickening), and into the subendothelial zone of glomerular capillaries (leading to glomerular consolidation). At these sites of vascular injury, thrombosis can result in focal renal cortical necrosis (infarcts).

PATHOLOGY: The size of the kidneys in malignant hypertensive nephropathy varies from small to enlarged, depending on the duration of preexisting benign hypertension. The cut surface is mottled red and yellow and occasionally exhibits small cortical infarcts. Microscopically, malignant hypertensive nephropathy is often superimposed on a background of hypertensive nephrosclerosis, with edematous (myxoid, mucoid) intimal expansion in arteries and fibrinoid necrosis of arterioles. Variable glomerular changes range from capillary congestion to consolidation to necrosis (Fig. 16-60). Severe cases show thrombosis and focal ischemic cortical necrosis (infarction). Electron microscopy demonstrates electron-lucent expansion of the subendothelial zone in glomeruli. Immunofluorescence microscopy documents focal insudation of plasma proteins into injured vessel walls. These pathologic changes are

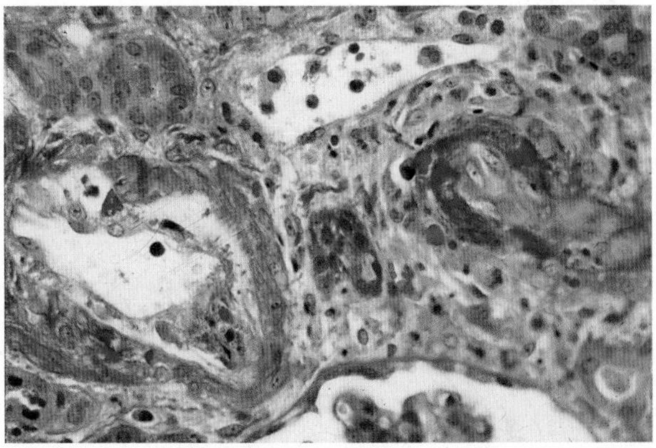

FIGURE 16-60. **Malignant hypertensive nephropathy.** Red fibrinoid necrosis in the wall of the arteriole on the right and clear edematous expansion in the intima of the interlobular artery on the left from a patient with malignant hypertension (Masson trichrome stain).

identical to those observed in other forms of thrombotic microangiopathy (see below).

CLINICAL FEATURES: Malignant hypertension occurs more often in men than in women, typically around the age of 40 years. Patients suffer headache, dizziness, and visual disturbances and may develop overt encephalopathy. Hematuria and proteinuria are frequent. Progressive deterioration of renal function develops if the malignant hypertension persists. Aggressive antihypertensive therapy often controls the disease.

Renovascular Hypertension Follows Narrowing of a Renal Artery

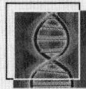

PATHOGENESIS: Stenosis or total occlusion of a main renal artery produces hypertension that is potentially curable by reconstitution of the arterial lumen. Harry Goldblatt carried out the initial experiments that led to the understanding of this syndrome in rats more than a half century ago, and since that time, the kidney deprived of vascular supply has been known as the **Goldblatt kidney.** In patients with renal artery stenosis, hypertension reflects increased production of renin, angiotensin II, and aldosterone. Renal vein renin from the ischemic kidney is elevated, whereas it is normal in the contralateral kidney. Most (95%) cases are caused by atherosclerosis, which explains why this disorder is twice as common in men as in women and is seen primarily in older age groups (average age, 55 years). Fibromuscular dysplasia and vasculitis are less common causes overall but are the most frequent causes in children.

PATHOLOGY: No matter what the cause of renal artery stenosis, the kidney parenchymal changes are the same. The size of the involved kidney is reduced. Glomeruli appear normal are closer to each other than normal, because the intervening tubules show marked ischemic atrophy without extensive interstitial fibrosis. Many glomeruli lose their attachment to the proximal tubule. The juxtaglomerular apparatus is prominent and reveals hyperplasia and increased granularity.

When vascular stenosis is caused by atherosclerosis, atherosclerotic plaques impinge on the aortic ostium or narrow the renal artery lumen, more frequently on the left than on the right. Occasionally, an atherosclerotic aneurysm of the abdominal aorta compromises the origin of the renal arteries. Takayasu arteritis and giant cell arteritis cause renal artery stenosis by producing inflammatory and sclerotic thickening of the artery wall with resultant narrowing of the lumen.

Fibromuscular dysplasia is characterized by fibrous and muscular stenosis of the renal artery. There are several patterns of renal artery involvement. The major categories are intimal fibroplasia, medial fibroplasia, perimedial fibroplasia, and periarterial fibroplasia. As the names imply, these disorders affect different layers of the artery, from the intima to the adventitia. Medial fibroplasia is the most common and accounts for two thirds of all fibromuscular dysplasia. This process creates areas of medial thickening alternating with areas of atrophy, produces a "string of beads" pattern in angiograms.

CLINICAL FEATURES: Renovascular hypertension is characterized by mild-to-moderate blood pressure elevations. A bruit may be heard over the renal artery. The diagnosis requires some type of imaging, such as angiography. In over half of patients, surgical revascularization, angioplasty, or nephrectomy cures hypertension. When there is long-standing renovascular hypertension, the uninvolved kidney may become damaged by hypertensive nephrosclerosis.

Renal Atheroembolism May Complicate Aortic Atherosclerosis

In patients with severe aortic atherosclerosis, embolization of atheromatous debris into the renal arteries and vascular tree as far as glomerular capillaries may cause acute renal failure. Atheroembolization may be spontaneous or initiated by trauma, such as angiographic procedures. **Cholesterol clefts** are observed within vessel lumina (Fig. 16-61). Early lesions are surrounded by atheromatous material or thrombus. They may later elicit a foreign body reaction and may stimulate fibrosis in the adjacent vessel wall.

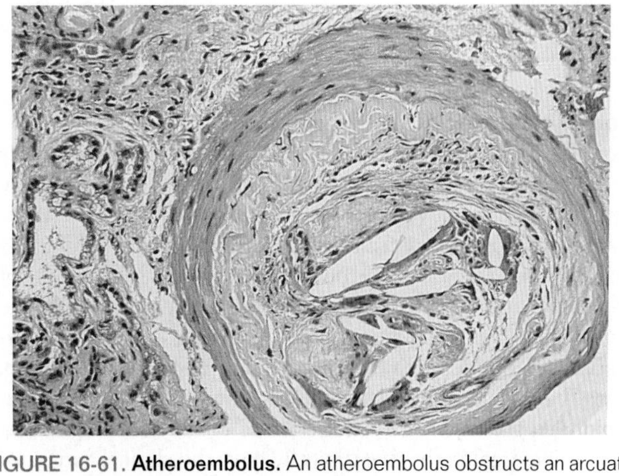

FIGURE 16-61. **Atheroembolus.** An atheroembolus obstructs an arcuate artery. Note the cholesterol clefts.

Thrombotic Microangiopathy Refers to Systemic Diseases with Similar Renal Lesions

PATHOGENESIS: Thrombotic microangiopathy has a variety of causes, all of which cause endothelial damage that initiates a final common pathway of vascular changes. A leading theory holds that endothelial damage allows plasma constituents to enter the intima of arteries, walls of arterioles, and the subendothelial zone of glomerular capillaries, resulting in narrowing of vessel lumina and ischemia. The injured endothelial surfaces promote thrombosis, which worsens ischemia and may cause focal ischemic necrosis. The passage of blood through the injured vessels leads to a nonimmune (Coombs negative) hemolytic anemia, characterized by misshapen and disrupted erythrocytes (schistocytes) and thrombocytopenia. This hematologic syndrome is termed **microangiopathic hemolytic anemia.** The kidneys are ubiquitous targets of thrombotic microangiopathies, but other organs may also be injured.

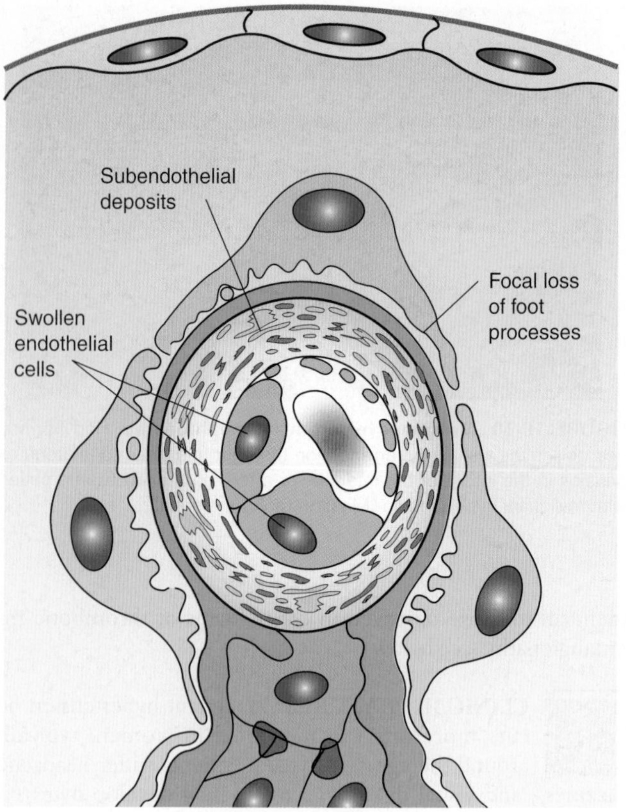

FIGURE 16-62. **Hemolytic–uremic syndrome.** A wide band of subendothelial electron-lucent material causes narrowing of the capillary lumen. Endothelial cell swelling also contributes to narrowing of the lumen.

PATHOLOGY: The renal pathologic changes are comparable to those in malignant hypertensive nephropathy, which is a form of thrombotic microangiopathy. The basic renal lesions are

- Arteriolar fibrinoid necrosis
- Arterial edematous intimal expansion
- Glomerular consolidation, necrosis, or congestion
- Vascular thrombosis

Electron microscopy of glomeruli demonstrates electron-lucent expansion of the subendothelial zone (Fig. 16-62 and Fig. 16-63), which results from insudation of plasma proteins under injured endothelial cells. Immunofluorescence microscopy reveals the accumulation of fibrin and insudation of plasma proteins in injured vessel walls.

CLINICAL FEATURES: Various clinical presentations and causes allow recognition of different categories of thrombotic microangiopathy. The various clinical disorders share microangiopathic hemolytic anemia, thrombocytopenia, hypertension, and renal failure, although these features are expressed to different degrees.

Hemolytic–Uremic Syndrome

Hemolytic–uremic syndrome (HUS) features microangiopathic hemolytic anemia and acute renal failure, with little or no evidence for significant vascular disease outside the kidneys. *HUS is the most common cause of acute renal failure in children.* Major causes for HUS are Shiga toxin-producing strains of *Escherichia coli,* which are ingested in contaminated food such as poorly cooked hamburger. The toxin injures endothelial cells, setting in motion a sequence of events that produces thrombotic microangiopa-
v. These patients present with hemorrhagic diarrhea and
'ly progressive renal failure. Some of the causes of throm-
-roangiopathy that typically have the clinical and patho-
-res of HUS are listed in Table 16-10.

Thrombotic Thrombocytopenic Purpura

Thrombotic thrombocytopenic purpura (TTP) displays systemic microvascular thrombosis and is characterized clinically by thrombocytopenia, purpura, fever, and changes in mental status. Unlike HUS, renal involvement is often absent or less

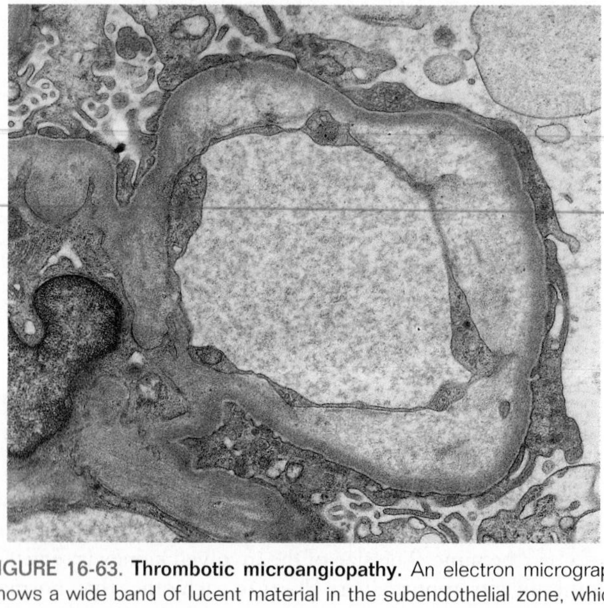

FIGURE 16-63. **Thrombotic microangiopathy.** An electron micrograph shows a wide band of lucent material in the subendothelial zone, which causes marked narrowing of the lumen.

TABLE 16–10

Causes of Thrombotic Microangiopathy
Infections
Escherichia coli
Shigella spp.
Pseudomonas spp.
Drugs
Mitomycin
Cisplatin
Cyclosporin
Tacrolimus
Autoimmune diseases
Systemic sclerosis (scleroderma)
Systemic lupus erythematosus
Antiphospholipid antibody syndrome
Malignant hypertension
Pregnancy and postpartum factors

important than other organ disease. Bleeding, caused by the consumptive thrombocytopenia, is also more severe in TTP than it is in HUS. At least in some patients, TTP involves a genetic or acquired deficiency in the activity of a protease that cleaves multimers of von Willebrand factor. The large uncleaved multimers promote platelet aggregation and microvascular thrombosis.

Preeclampsia is Characterized by Hypertension, Proteinuria, and Edema in the Third Trimester of Pregnancy

When these features are complicated by convulsions, the term **eclampsia** *is applied* (see Chapter 18). The kidney is by definition involved in preeclampsia. Glomeruli are uniformly enlarged and endothelial cells are swollen, an appearance that results in an apparently bloodless glomerular tuft (Fig. 16-64 and Fig. 16-65). By electron microscopy, the swollen endothelial contain large, irregular vacuoles. Vacuoles are also present in podocytes. Mild and moderate disease can be controlled with bed rest and antihypertensive agents. Severe cases may require induction of delivery. Hypertension and proteinuria typically disappear 1 to 2 weeks after delivery.

Sickle Cell Nephropathy Is the Most Common Organ Manifestation of Sickle Cell Disease

The interstitial tissue in which the vasa recta course is hypertonic and has a low oxygen tension. As a result, in patients with sickle cell disease erythrocytes in the vasa recta tend to sickle and occlude the lumen. Infarcts in the medulla and papilla ensue, sometimes severe enough to cause papillary necrosis. Ischemic scarring of the medulla leads to focal tubular loss and atrophy. Glomeruli are conspicuously congested with sickle cells. FSGS or, less often, membranoproliferative glomerulonephritis occurs in a minority of patients and may cause the nephrotic syndrome.

Renal Infarcts Usually Result from Embolization

Renal infarcts are, for the most part, caused by arterial obstruction, and most represent embolization to interlobar or arcuate arteries.

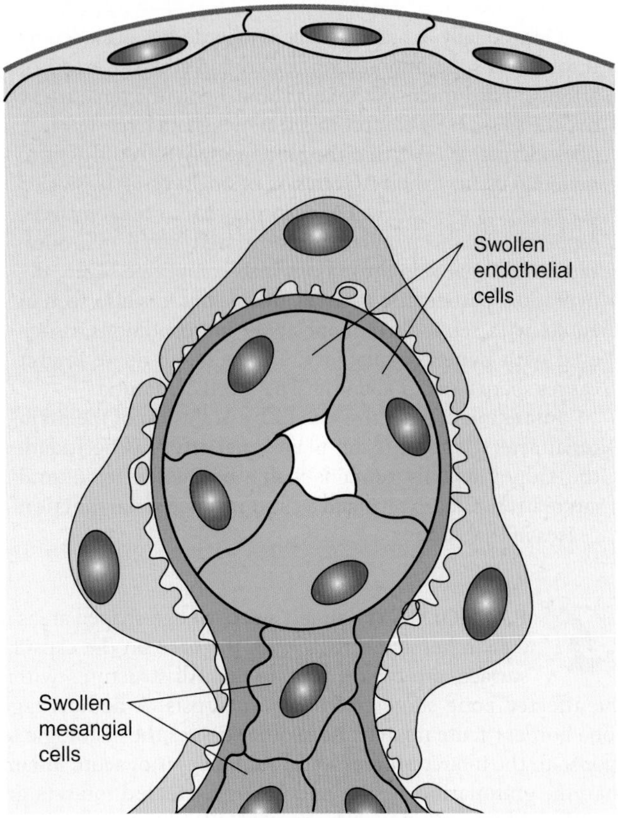

FIGURE 16-64. **Preeclamptic nephropathy.** Preeclamptic nephropathy, or pregnancy-induced nephropathy, exhibits marked swelling of endothelial cells with narrowing of the lumina. Both endothelial and mesangial cells are enlarged and have multiple vacuoles and vesicular structures.

PATHOGENESIS: The size of the infarct varies with the size of the occluded vessel. Common sources of emboli include:

- **Mural thrombi** overlying myocardial infarcts or caused by atrial fibrillation
- **Infected valves** in bacterial endocarditis
- **Complicated atherosclerotic plaques** in the aorta

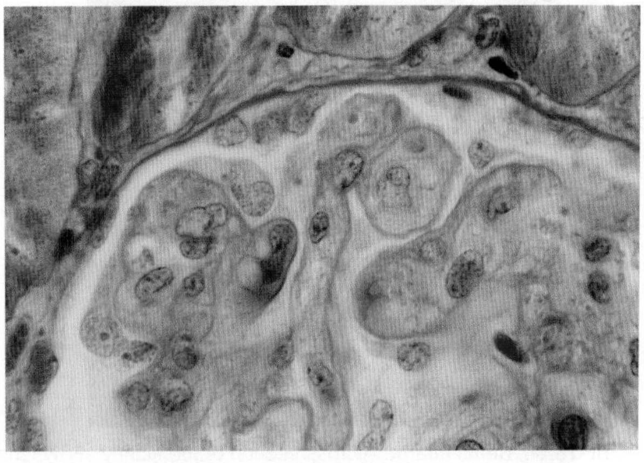

FIGURE 16-65. **Preeclampsia.** Capillary lumens are obliterated by swollen endothelial cells (Masson trichrome stain).

Occasionally, a branch of the renal artery is occluded by thrombosis superimposed on underlying atherosclerosis or arteritis. The lumens of the small branches of the renal artery may be so severely compromised in malignant hypertension, scleroderma or HUS that the blood supply is insufficient to maintain tissue viability. Occlusion of small vessels by sickled erythrocytes in sickle cell anemia may cause renal infarcts, especially in the papillae. Hemorrhagic renal infarction caused by renal vein thrombosis may complicate severe dehydration, particularly in small infants, but it is also seen in adults with septic thrombophlebitis and conditions associated with hypercoagulability. Typically, an acute infarct causes sharp flank or abdominal pain and hematuria.

Infarction of an entire kidney by occlusion of the main renal artery is rare. If the main renal artery is occluded, the kidney usually remains viable because of collateral circulation. Clearly, in such a circumstance renal function ceases in that kidney.

PATHOLOGY: Variably sized, wedge-shaped areas of pale ischemic necrosis, with the base on the capsular surface, are typical (Fig. 16-66). All structures within the affected zone show coagulative necrosis. A hemorrhagic zone borders acute infarcts. As in other tissues,the histologic response to the infarct progresses through phases of acute inflammation, granulation tissue, and fibrosis. Healed infarcts are sharply circumscribed and depressed cortical scars containing ghosts of obliterated glomeruli, atrophic tubules, interstitial fibrosis, and a mild chronic inflammatory infiltrate. Dystrophic calcification is occasionally encountered in old infarcts. At the margins of a healed infarct, the viable tissue resembles that seen in chronic ischemia, with tubular atrophy, interstitial fibrosis and infiltration by chronic inflammatory cells.

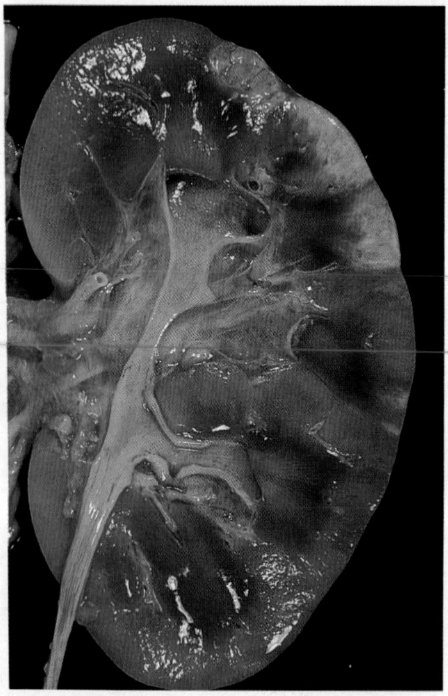

‑ 16-66. **Renal infarct.** A cross-section of the kidney shows mul- ...f infarction characterized by marked pallor, which extends to ...r surface.

Cortical Necrosis Is Secondary Severe Ischemia and Spares the Medulla

Cortica necrosis affects part or all of the renal cortex. The term **infarct** is used when there is one area (or a few areas) of necrosis caused by occlusion of arteries, whereas **cortical necrosis** implies more-widespread ischemic necrosis.

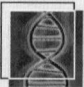

PATHOGENESIS: Historically, the most common cause for renal cortical necrosis was premature separation of the placenta (abruptio placentae), in the third trimester of pregnancy. Renal cortical necrosis can complicate any clinical condition associated with hypovolemic or endotoxic shock. Since all forms of shock are associated with acute tubular necrosis (ATN), it is not surprising that there is an overlap between that condition and cortical necrosis, both clinically and pathologically.

Vasa recta that supply arterial blood to the medulla arise from juxtamedullary efferent arterioles, proximal to vessels supplying the outer cortex. Thus, occlusion of outer cortical vessels, for example by vasospasm, thrombi, or thrombotic microangiopathy, leads to cortical necrosis and sparing of the medulla. Experimentally, vasoconstrictors such as vasopressin and serotonin produce cortical necrosis. The experimental Schwartzman phenomenon, which is characterized by disseminated intravascular coagulation with widespread fibrin thrombi, also results in cortical necrosis.

PATHOLOGY: The extent of cortical necrosis varies from patchy to confluent (Fig. 16-67). In the most severely involved areas, all parenchymal elements exhibit coagulative necrosis. The proximal convoluted tubules are invariably necrotic, as are most of the distal tubules. In the adjacent viable portions of the cortex, the glomeruli and distal convoluted tubules are usually unaffected, but many of the proximal convoluted tubules have features of ischemic injury, such as epithelial flattening or necrosis.

With extensive necrosis, the cortex has a marked pallor. The cortex is diffusely necrotic, except for thin rims of viable tissue immediately beneath the capsule and at the corticomedullary junction, which are supplied by capsular and medullary collateral blood vessels, respectively. Patients who survive cortical necrosis may develop striking dystrophic calcification of the necrotic areas.

CLINICAL FEATURES: Severe cortical necrosis manifests as acute renal failure, which initially may be indistinguishable from that produced by ATN. However, the former is more often irreversible. A renal arteriogram or biopsy may be required for diagnosis. Recovery is determined by the extent of the disease, but there is a significant incidence of hypertension among survivors.

Diseases of Tubules and Interstitium

Acute Tubular Necrosis (ATN) Causes Acute Renal Failure

ATN is a severe, but potentially reversible, renal failure due to impairment of tubular epithelial function caused by ischemia or toxic injury.

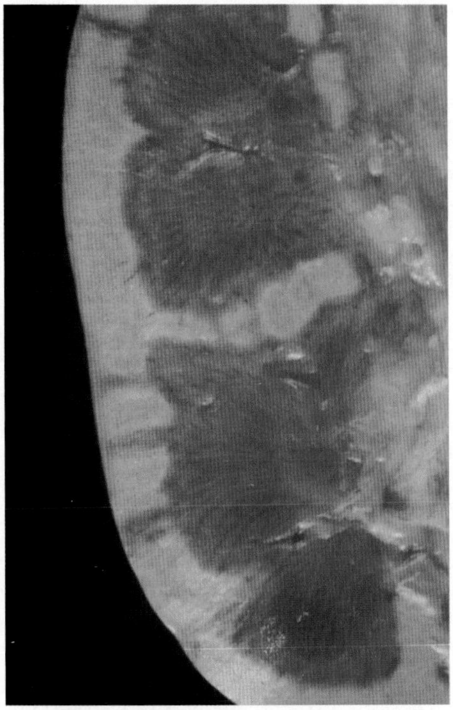

FIGURE 16-67. **Renal cortical necrosis.** The cortex of the kidney is pale yellow and soft owing to diffuse cortical necrosis.

Because necrosis often is not a prominent feature of ATN, this process also is called acute renal injury (ARI).

PATHOGENESIS: Some causes of ATN are listed in Table 16-11.

Ischemic ATN results from reduced renal perfusion, usually associated with hypotension. Tubular epithelial cells, with their high rate of energy-consuming metabolic activity and numerous organelles, are particularly sensitive to hypoxia and anoxia, which cause rapid depletion of intracellular adenosine triphostphate (ATP) in tubular epithelium. Tubular epithelial cells may be simplified (flattened) but not necrotic in some patients with typical clinical ATN.

Nephrotoxic ATN is caused by chemically induced injury to epithelial cells. Tubular epithelial cells are preferred targets for certain toxins because they absorb and concentrate toxins. The high rate of energy consumption by epithelial cells also makes them susceptible to injury by toxins that perturb oxidative or other metabolic pathways. Hemoglobin and myoglobin can be considered endogenous toxins that can induce ATN (**pigment nephropathy**) when they are present in the urine in high concentrations.

The pathophysiology of ATN appears to involve some or all of the following perturbations (Fig. 16-68), various combinations of which result in a reduced glomerular filtration rate and tubular epithelial dysfunction:

- Intrarenal vasoconstriction
- Alteration of arteriolar tone by tubuloglomerular feedback
- Decreased glomerular hydrostatic pressure
- Decreased glomerular capillary permeability (K_f)
- Tubular obstruction by cellular debris, with increased hydrostatic pressure
- Backleakage of glomerular filtrate into the interstitium through damaged tubular epithelium

TABLE 16-11

Causes of Acute Tubular Necrosis

Ischemia	
	Massive hemorrhage
	Septic shock
	Severe burns
	Dehydration
	Prolonged diarrhea
	Congestive heart failure
	Volume redistribution (e.g., pancreatitis, peritonitis)
Nephrotoxins	
	Antibiotics (e.g., aminoglycosides, amphotericin B)
	Radiographic contrast agents
	Heavy metals (e.g., mercury, lead, cisplatin)
	Organic solvents (e.g., ethylene glycol, carbon tetrachloride)
	Poisons (e.g., paraquat)
Heme proteins	
	Myoglobin (from rhabdomyolysis, e.g., with crush injury)
	Hemoglobin (from hemolysis, e.g., with transfusion reaction)

PATHOLOGY: **Ischemic ATN** is characterized by swollen kidneys that have a pale cortex and a congested medulla. No pathologic changes are seen in glomeruli or blood vessels. Tubular injury is focal and is most pronounced in the proximal tubules and the thick limbs of the loop of Henle in the outer medulla. The proximal tubules display focal flattening of the epithelium, with dilation of the lumina and loss of the brush border (epithelial simplification). This results in part from sloughing of the apical cytoplasm, which appears in the distal tubular lumina and urine as brown granular casts. The color reflects renal cytochrome pigments. Electron microscopy confirms the loss of the proximal tubular brush border and also demonstrates decreased infoldings at the basolateral membrane of proximal tubular epithelial cells. A characteristic feature of ischemic ATN is the absence of widespread necrosis of tubular epithelial cells, although simplification may be prominent. Instead, "necrosis" is more subtle and is reflected in individual necrotic cells within some proximal or distal tubules. These single necrotic cells as well as a few viable cells are shed into the tubular lumen, with resulting focal denudation of tubular basement membrane (Fig 16-69). Interstitial edema is common. The vasa recta of the outer medulla are congested and frequently contain nucleated cells, which are predominantly mononuclear leukocytes.

Toxic ATN shows more-extensive necrosis of tubular epithelium than is usually caused by ischemic ATN (compare Fig. 16-69 and Fig.16-70). In most cases, however, the necrosis is limited to certain tubular segments that are most sensitive to the particular toxin. The most common site of injury is the proximal tubule. ATN due to hemoglobin or myoglobin also has many red-brown tubular casts that are colored by heme pigments.

During the recovery phase of ATN, the tubular epithelium regenerates, with mitoses, increased size of cells and nuclei, and

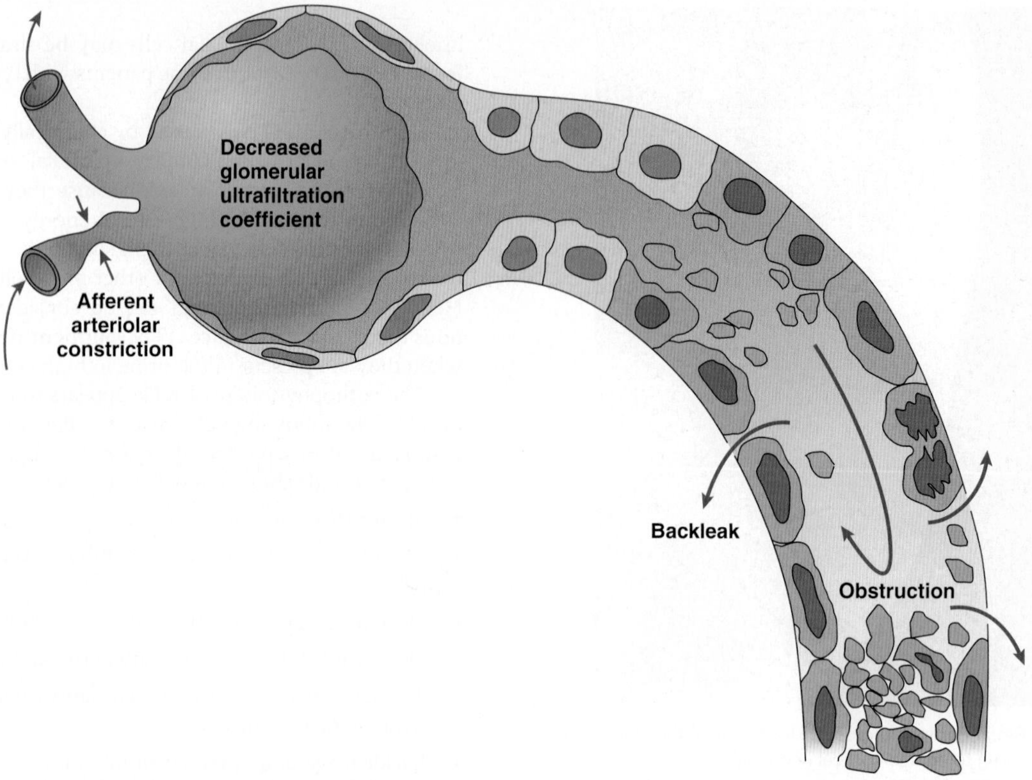

FIGURE 16-68. **Pathogenesis of acute tubular necrosis.** Sloughing and necrosis of epithelial cells result in cast formation. The presence of casts leads to obstruction and increased intraluminal pressure, which reduces glomerular filtration. Afferent arteriolar vasoconstriction, caused in part by tubuloglomerular feedback, results in decreased glomerular capillary filtration pressure. Tubular injury and increased intraluminal pressure cause fluid backleakage from the lumen into the interstitium.

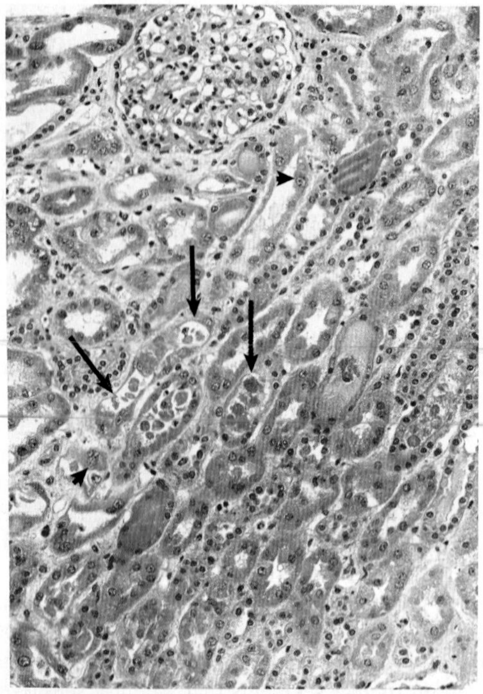

FIGURE 16-69. **Ischemic acute tubular necrosis.** Necrosis of individual tubular epithelial cells is evident both from focal denudation of the tubular basement membrane *(arrows)* and from the individual necrotic epithelial cells present in some tubular lumina. Some enlarged, regenerative epithelial cells are also present *(arrowheads)*. Note the lack of interstitial inflammation.

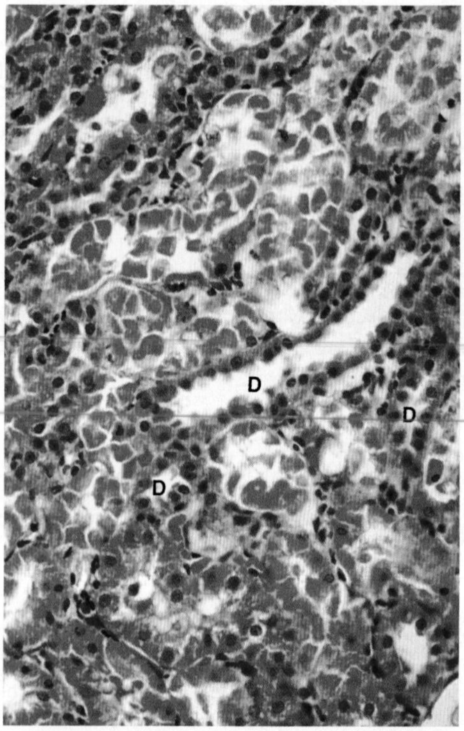

FIGURE 16-70. **Toxic acute tubular necrosis due to mercury poisoning.** There is widespread necrosis of proximal tubular epithelial cells, with sparing of distal and collecting tubules (D). Interstitial inflammation is minimal.

cell crowding. Survivors eventually display complete restoration of normal renal architecture.

CLINICAL FEATURES: ***ATN is the leading cause of acute renal failure.*** It manifests as a rapidly rising serum creatinine level, usually associated with decreased urine output (oliguria). ATN less commonly induces nonoliguric acute renal failure. Urinalysis demonstrates degenerating epithelial cells and **"dirty brown" granular casts** (acute renal failure casts) with cellular debris rich in cytochrome pigments. Urinalysis is useful in differentiating among the three major intrinsic renal diseases that cause acute renal failure (Table 16-12).

The duration of renal failure in patients with ATN depends on many factors, especially the nature and reversibility of the cause. Many patients, at least transiently, develop uremia (azotemia, fluid retention, metabolic acidosis, hyperkalemia) and may require dialysis. If the cause is immediately removed after the initiation of the injury, renal function often recovers within 1 to 2 weeks, although it may be delayed for months. Increased urine output and a fall in serum creatinine herald the recovery phase.

Pyelonephritis Refers to Bacterial Infection of the Kidney

Acute Pyelonephritis

PATHOGENESIS: Gram-negative bacteria from the feces, most commonly *E. coli,* cause 80% of acute pyelonephritis. Infection reaches the kidney by ascending through the urinary tract, a process that depends on several factors:

- Bacterial urinary infection
- Reflux of infected urine up the ureters into the renal pelvis and calyces
- Bacterial entry through the papillae into the renal parenchyma

Bladder infection precedes acute pyelonephritis. Bladder infection is more common in females because of a short urethra, lack of antibacterial prostatic secretions, and facilitation of bacterial migration by sexual intercourse. The normal urethral commensal flora are replaced by fecal organisms in some women who are unusually vulnerable to recurrent attacks of urinary tract infection. This change in flora may reflect poor hygiene, hormonal effects and genetic predisposition (e.g., increased numbers of receptors for *E. coli* on urothelial cells).

TABLE 16-12

Urinalysis in Acute Renal Failure

Causes of Acute Renal Failure	Urinalysis Findings
Acute tubular necrosis	Dirty brown casts and epithelial cells
Acute glomerulonephritis	Red blood cell casts and proteinuria
Acute tubulointerstitial nephritis	White blood cell casts and pyuria

Asymptomatic bacteriuria occurs in 10% of pregnant women, one-fourth of whom develop acute pyelonephritis. This increase in acute pyelonephritis in pregnancy can also be attributed to an increased residual urine volume. Under the influence of high levels of progesterone, bladder musculature becomes flaccid and does not expel urine with its customary efficiency.

During micturition, the bladder normally empties all but 2 to 3 mL of residual urine. The subsequent addition of sterile urine from the kidneys dilutes any bacteria that may have found their way into the bladder. Under some circumstances, the residual urine volume is increased, for example, in prostatic obstruction or in an atonic bladder caused by neurogenic disorders such as paraplegia or diabetic neuropathy. As a result, the bladder contents are not sufficiently diluted with sterile urine from the kidneys to prevent bacterial accumulation. Diabetic glycosuria also predisposes to infection by providing a rich medium for bacterial growth.

Bacteria in bladder urine usually do not gain access to the kidneys. The ureter commonly inserts into the bladder wall at a steep angle (Fig. 16-71) and in its most distal portion courses parallel to the bladder wall between the mucosa and muscularis. The intravesicular pressure produced by micturition occludes the distal ureteral lumen, preventing urinary reflux. In many persons who are particularly susceptible to pyelonephritis, an abnormally short passage of the ureter within the bladder wall is associated with an angle of insertion that is more perpendicular to the mucosal surface of the bladder. Thus, on micturition, rather than occluding the lumen, intravesicular pressure forces urine into the patent ureter. This reflux is powerful enough to force the urine into the renal pelvis and calyces.

Even when present in the calyces, bacteria are not necessarily carried into the renal parenchyma by the reflux pressure. The simple papillae of the central calyces are convex and do not readily admit reflux urine (see Fig. 16-71). By contrast, the concave shapes of peripheral compound papillae allow easier access to the collecting system. However, if the pressure is prolonged, as in obstructive uropathy, even simple papillae are eventually vulnerable to the retrograde entry of urine. From the collecting tubules, bacteria gain access to the interstitial tissue and other tubules of the kidney.

In addition to ascending through urine, bacteria and other pathogens can gain access to renal parenchyma through blood. For example, gram-positive organisms, such as staphylococci, can disseminate from an infected valve in bacterial endocarditis and establish a focus of infection in the kidney. The kidney is commonly involved in miliary tuberculosis. Fungi, such as *Aspergillus,* can seed the kidney in an immunocompromised host. Hematogenous infections of the kidney preferentially affect the cortex.

PATHOLOGY: The kidneys of acute pyelonephritis have small white abscesses on the subcapsular surface and on cut surfaces. Pelvic and calyceal urothelium may be hyperemic and covered by purulent exudate. *Acute pyelonephritis is often focal, and much of the kidney may appear normal.* Most infections involve only a few papillary systems. Microscopically, the parenchyma, particularly the cortex, typically shows extensive focal destruction by the inflammatory process, although vessels and glomeruli often are preferentially pre-

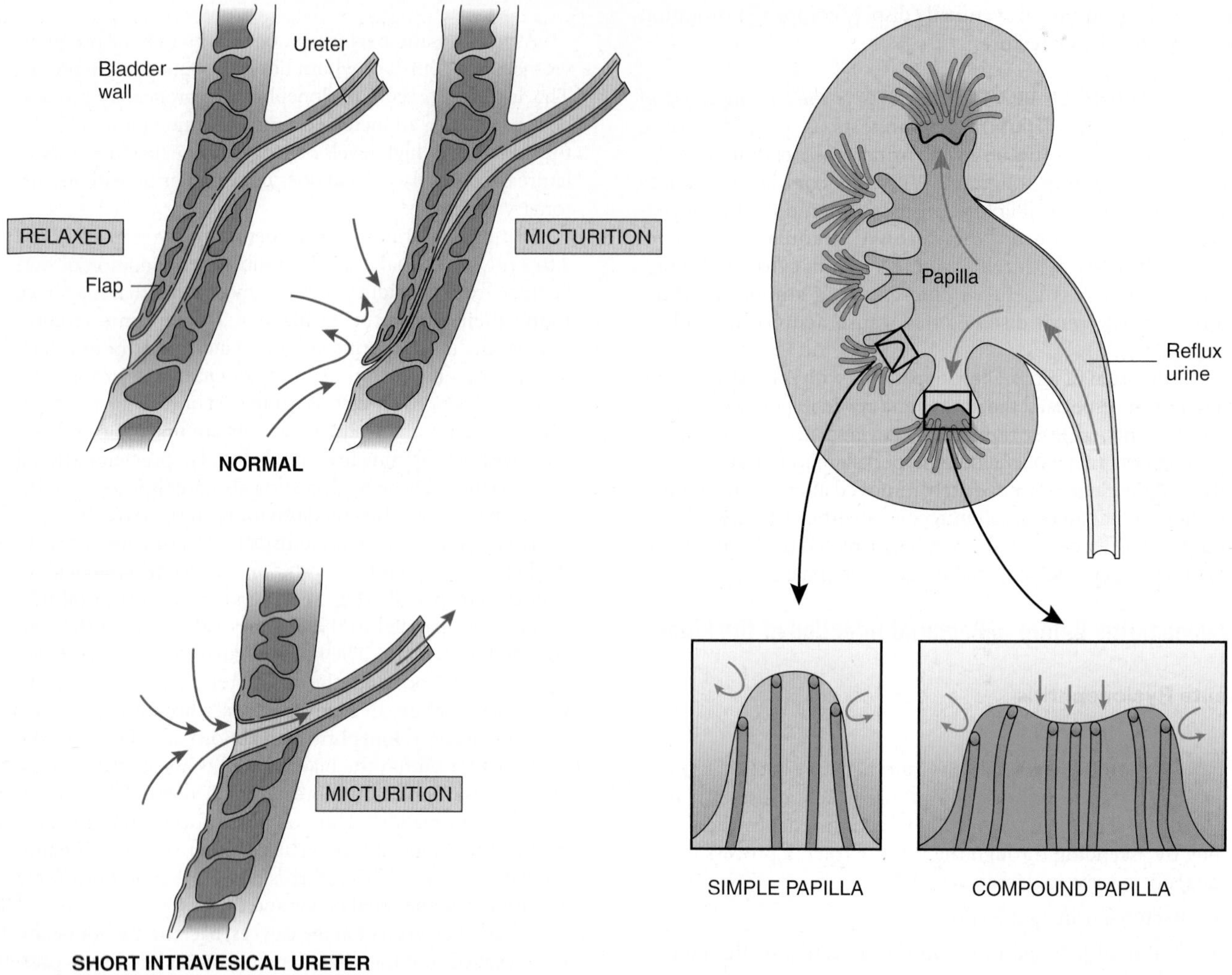

FIGURE 16-71. **Anatomical features of the bladder and kidney in pyelonephritis caused by ureterovesical reflux.** In the normal bladder, the distal portion of the intravesical ureter courses between the mucosa and the muscularis, forming a mucosal flap. On micturition, the elevated intravesicular pressure compresses the flap against the bladder wall, thereby occluding the lumen. Persons with a congenitally short intravesical ureter have no mucosal flap, because the angle of entry of the ureter into the bladder approaches a right angle. Thus, micturition forces urine into the ureter. In the renal pelvis, simple papillae of the central calyces are convex and do not readily allow reflux of urine. By contrast, the peripheral compound papillae are concave and permit entry of refluxed urine.

served. Inflammatory infiltrates mainly contain neutrophils, which often fill tubules and especially collecting ducts (Fig. 16-72). In severe cases of acute pyelonephritis, necrosis of the papillary tips may occur (Fig. 16-73) or infection may extend beyond the renal capsule, to cause a perinephric abscess.

CLINICAL FEATURES: Symptoms of acute pyelonephritis include fever, chills, sweats, malaise, flank pain, and costovertebral angle tenderness. Leukocytosis with neutrophilia is common. Differentiating upper from lower urinary tract infection is often clinically difficult, but the finding of **leukocyte casts** in the urine supports a diagnosis of pyelonephritis.

Chronic Pyelonephritis

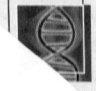

PATHOGENESIS: Chronic pyelonephritis is caused by recurrent and persistent bacterial infection secondary to urinary tract obstruction, urine reflux, or both (Fig. 16-74). Whether urine reflux without infection can produce pathologic changes identical to chronic pyelonephritis is controversial.

In chronic pyelonephritis caused by reflux or obstruction, the medullary tissue and overlying cortex are preferentially injured by recurrent acute and chronic inflammation. Progressive atrophy and scarring ensue, with resultant contraction of the involved papillary tip (or sloughing if there is papillary necrosis) and thinning of the overlying cortex. *This process results in the distinctive gross appearance of a broad depressed area of cortical fibrosis and atrophy overlying a dilated calyx* (**caliectasis**) (Fig. 16-75).

PATHOLOGY: The microscopic appearance of chronic pyelonephritis is nonspecific. Many diseases that cause chronic injury to the tubulointerstitial compartment induce chronic interstitial inflammation, interstitial fibrosis and tubular atrophy. Thus, chronic pyelonephritis is one

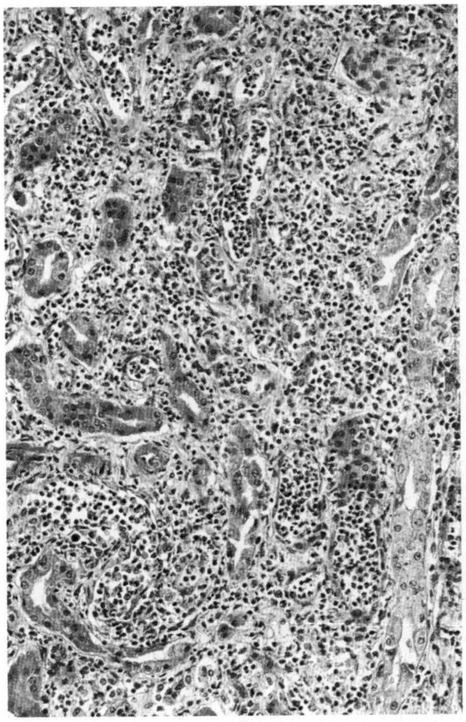

FIGURE 16-72. **Acute pyelonephritis.** An extensive infiltrate of neutrophils is present in the collecting tubules and interstitial tissue.

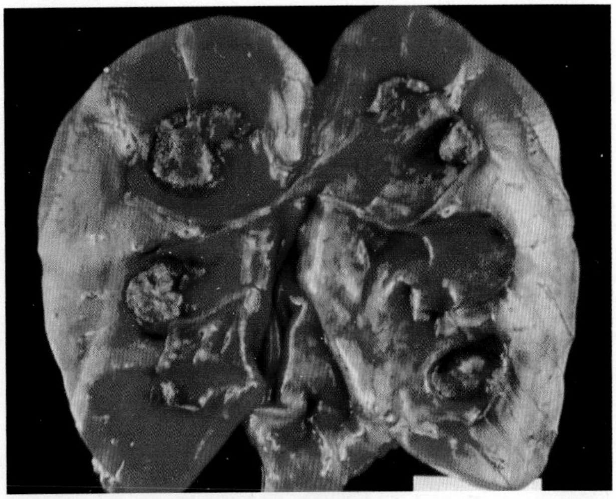

FIGURE 16-73. **Papillary necrosis.** The bisected kidney shows a dilated renal pelvis and dilated calyces secondary to urinary tract obstruction. The papillae are all necrotic and appear as sharply demarcated, ragged, yellowish areas.

of many causes of the pattern of injury termed **chronic tubulointerstitial nephritis.** The gross appearance of chronic pyelonephritis is more distinctive. Only chronic pyelonephritis and analgesic nephropathy produce a combination of caliectasis with overlying corticomedullary scarring. In obstructive uropathy, all of the calyces and the renal pelvis are dilated, and the parenchyma is uniformly thinned (see Fig. 16-75). In cases associated with vesicoureteral reflux, the calyces at the poles of the kidney are preferentially expanded and are associated with overlying discrete, coarse scars that cause indentation of the renal surface. Microscopically, the scars have atrophic dilated tubules surrounded by interstitial fibrosis and infiltrates of chronic inflammatory cells (Fig. 16-76). The most characteristic (but not specific) tubular change is severe epithalial atrophy, with diffuse, eosinophilic, hyaline casts. Such tubules, which are "pinched-off" spherical segments, resemble colloid-containing thyroid follicles, a pattern called "thyroidization." This appearance results from the breakup of tubules, with residual segments forming spherules. Glomeruli may be completely uninvolved,

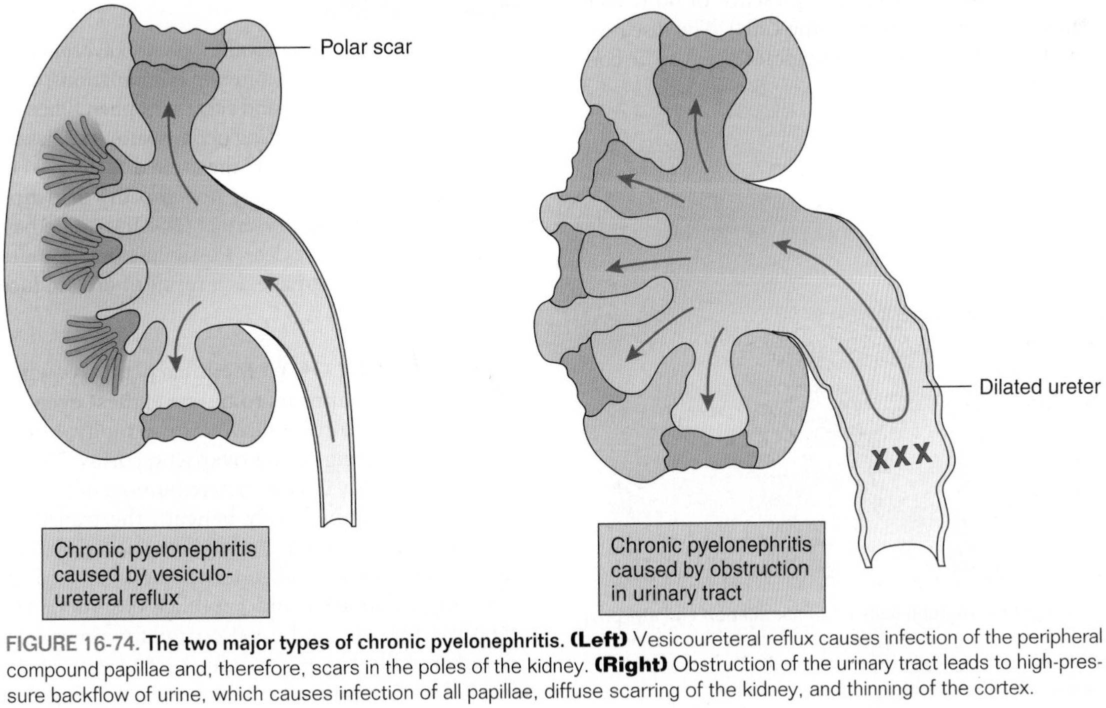

FIGURE 16-74. **The two major types of chronic pyelonephritis. (Left)** Vesicoureteral reflux causes infection of the peripheral compound papillae and, therefore, scars in the poles of the kidney. **(Right)** Obstruction of the urinary tract leads to high-pressure backflow of urine, which causes infection of all papillae, diffuse scarring of the kidney, and thinning of the cortex.

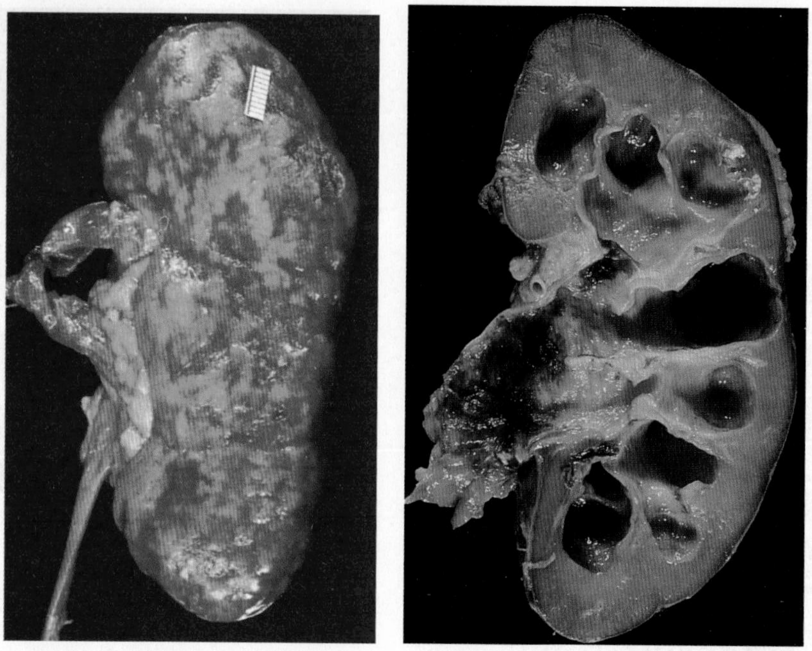

A B

FIGURE 16-75. **Chronic pyelonephritis. A.** The cortical surface contains many irregular, depressed scars (reddish areas). **B.** There is marked dilation of calyces (caliectasis) caused by inflammatory destruction of papillae, with atrophy and scarring of the overlying cortex.

show periglomerular fibrosis or be sclerotic. The loss of most functioning nephrons may induce secondary focal segmental glomerulosclerosis. Fibrosis of the walls of arteries and arterioles is common. There is marked scarring and chronic inflammation of the calyceal mucosa.

Xanthogranulomatous pyelonephritis is an uncommon form of chronic pyelonephritis that is often caused by a variety of pathogens including *Proteus, E. coli, Klebsiella,* and *Preudomonas.* The name derives from the yellow gross appearance of the nodular renal lesions, which results from the presence of numerous lipid-laden foamy macrophages (**xanthoma cells**). The disease is usually unilateral. The clinical and pathologic features can be confused with renal cell carcinoma (RCC).

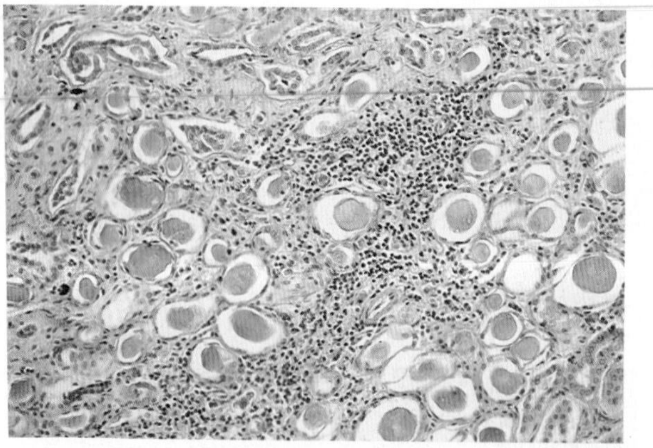

'GURE 16-76. **A light micrograph shows tubular dilation and atrophy,** ...many tubules containing eosinophilic hyaline casts resembling the ...f thyroid follicles (so-called thyroidization). The interstitium is ...d contains a chronic inflammatory cell infiltrate.

CLINICAL FEATURES: Most patients with chronic pyelonephritis have episodic symptoms of urinary tract infection or acute pyelonephritis, such as recurrent fever and flank pain. Some patients have a silent course until end-stage renal disease develops. Urinalysis shows leukocytes, and imaging studies reveal caliectasis and cortical scarring.

Analgesic Nephropathy Results from Chronic Overdosage of Drugs

Patients with analgesic nephropathy typically have consumed more than 2 kg of analgesic compounds, often in combinations, such as aspirin and phenacetin, or aspirin and acetaminophen. Phenacetin carries the greatest risk for developing nephropathy and has been banned in many countries, including the United States. Acetaminophen poses a higher risk for inducing nephropathy than aspirin or nonsteroidal anti-inflammatory drugs (NSAIDs). The basis for analgesic nephropathy is not clear. Possibilities include direct nephrotoxicity or ischemic damage as a result of drug-induced vascular changes or both.

PATHOLOGY: Medullary injury with papillary necrosis appears to be the earliest event in analgesic nephropathy, followed by atrophy, chronic inflammation, and scarring of the overlying cortex. The earliest histologic abnormality is a distinctive homogeneous thickening of capillary walls immediately beneath the transitional epithelium of the urinary tract. Early parenchymal changes are confined to the papillae and inner medulla, and consist of focal thickening of tubular and capillary basement membranes, interstitial fibrosis, and focal coagulative necrosis. Necrotic areas eventually become confluent and extend to the corticomedullary junction, after which the collecting ducts become involved. Few inflammatory cells are found around the necrotic foci. Eventually, the entire papilla becomes necrotic (**papillary necrosis**), often remaining in place as a structureless mass. Dystrophic calcification of such necrotic papillae is common. Papillae may have incomplete detachment at the demarcation zone or be completely sloughed. There is secondary tubular atrophy, interstitial fibrosis, and chronic inflammation in the overlying cortex.

CLINICAL FEATURES: Signs and symptoms occur only in the late stages of analgesic nephropathy and include an inability to concentrate the urine, distal tubular acidosis, hematuria, hypertension, and anemia. Sloughing of necrotic papillary tips into the renal pelvis may result in colic as they pass through the ureters. Progressive renal failure often develops and may lead to end-stage renal disease.

Drug-Induced (Hypersensitivity) Acute Tubulointerstitial Nephritis Is a Cell-Mediated Immune Response

PATHOGENESIS: Acute drug-induced tubulointerstitial nephritis is characterized histologically by infiltrates of activated T lymphocytes and eosinophils, a pattern that indicates a type IV cell-mediated immune reaction. The immunogen could be the drug itself, the drug bound to certain tissue components, a drug metabolite, or a tissue component altered in response to the drug. Drugs most commonly implicated include nonsteroidal antiinflammatory drugs, diuretics and certain antibiotics, especially β-lactam antibiotics, such as synthetic penicillins and cephalosporins.

PATHOLOGY: Microscopically, there is patchy infiltration of cortex and (to a much lesser extent) medulla by lymphocytes and a small number of eosinophils (5% to 10% of the total leukocytes in the tissue) (Fig. 16-77). The eosinophils tend to be concentrated in small foci and may be seen within tubular lumina and in the urine. Neutrophils are rare, and their presence should raise suspicion of pyelonephritis or hematogenous bacterial infection. Foci of granulomatous inflammation may be present, especially in the later phase of the disease. Proximal and distal tubules are focally invaded by white blood cells ("tubulitis"). Glomeruli and vessels are not inflamed, although some instances of drug-induced tubulointerstitial nephritis, usually caused by NSAIDs, are accompanied by minimal-change glomerulopathy.

CLINICAL FEATURES: Acute tubulointerstitial nephritis usually manifests as acute renal failure, typically about 2 weeks after drug administration is started. The urine contains erythrocytes, leukocytes (including eosinophils), and sometimes leukocyte casts. Tubular defects are common, including sodium wasting, glucosuria, aminoaciduria, and renal tubular acidosis. Systemic allergic symptoms such as fever and rash may also be present. Most patients recover fully within several weeks or months if the drug is discontinued.

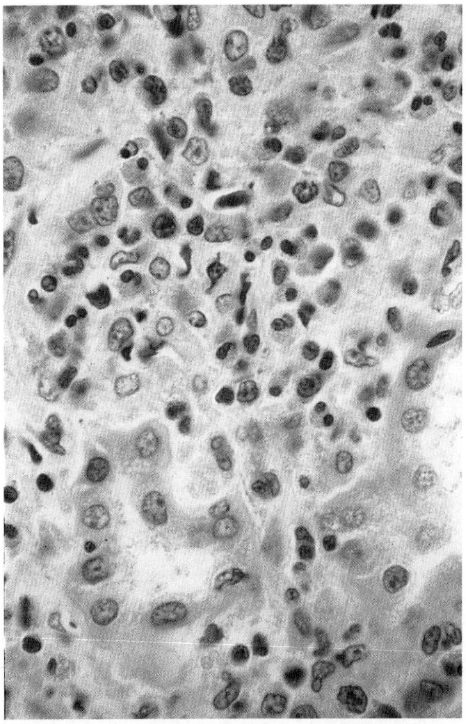

FIGURE 16-77. **Hypersensitivity tubulointerstitial nephritis.** There is interstitial edema and infiltration by mononuclear leukocytes, with admixed eosinophils.

Light-Chain Cast Nephropathy May Complicate Multiple Myeloma

Light-chain cast nephropathy is renal injury caused by monoclonal immunoglobulin light chains in the urine, which produce tubular epithelial injury and numerous tubular casts.

PATHOGENESIS: As discussed above, multiple myeloma may produce AL amyloidosis, light-chain deposition disease, heavy-chain deposition disease, and light-chain cast nephropathy. The latter is the most common form of renal disease associated with multiple myeloma, and is caused by glomerular filtering of circulating light chains. At the acidic pH typical of urine, the light chains bind to Tamm-Horsfall glycoproteins, which are secreted by distal tubular epithelial cells, and form casts. Renal dysfunction results from the toxic effects of free light chains on tubular epithelial cells and obstruction from the casts. The molecular structure of light chains determines whether they will induce disease by causing light-chain cast nephropathy, AL amyloidosis, or light-chain deposition disease. Occasional patients show several of these renal diseases.

PATHOLOGY: The characteristic tubular lesion exhibits numerous dense, hyaline casts in the distal tubules and collecting ducts (Fig. 16-78). These casts are brightly eosinophilic and glassy (hyaline) and often have fractures and angular borders. They may have a crystalline appearance. Casts may elicit foreign body reactions, with macrophages

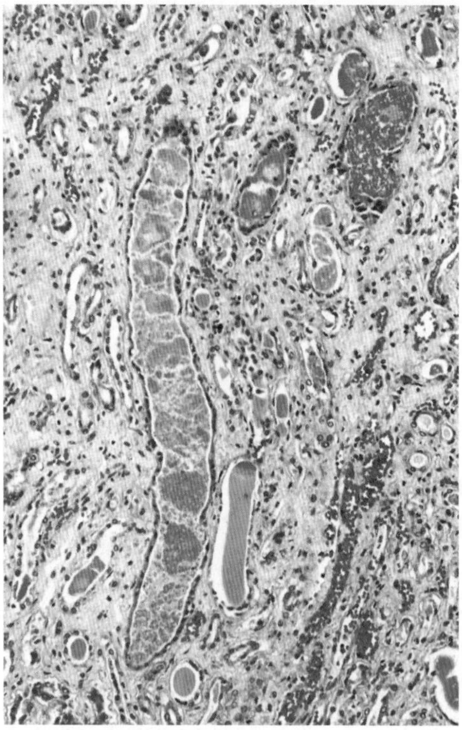

FIGURE 16-78. **Light-chain cast nephropathy.** A light micrograph shows numerous casts within tubular lumina.

and multinucleated giant cells. Interstitial chronic inflammatory infiltrates, as well as interstitial edema, typically accompany the tubular lesions. More chronic lesions show interstitial fibrosis and tubular atrophy. Focal calcium deposits (**nephrocalcinosis**) are also frequently noted in the fibrotic interstitium of the tubules. Immunostaining shows that the casts contain light chains and Tamm-Horsfall proteins.

CLINICAL FEATURES: Light-chain cast nephropathy may manifest as either acute or chronic renal failure. Proteinuria is usually present, although not necessarily in the nephrotic range, and most often consists predominantly of immunoglobulin light chains. If a patient has nephrotic-range proteinuria with multiple myeloma, AL amyloidosis or light-chain deposition disease is more likely than light-chain cast nephropathy.

Urate Nephropathy Displays Urate Crystals in the Tubules and Interstitium

Any condition with elevated blood levels of uric acid may cause urate nephropathy. The classic chronic disease in this category is primary gout (see Chapter 26).

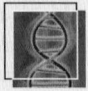

PATHOGENESIS: **Chronic urate nephropathy** caused by gout is characterized by tubular and interstitial deposition of crystalline monosodium urate. **Acute urate nephropathy** can be caused by increased cell turnover (e.g., leukemia or polycythemia). For example, chemotherapy for malignant neoplasms results in a sudden increase in blood uric acid because of the massive necrosis of cancer cells (**tumor lysis syndrome**). Hepatic catabolism of large amounts of purines released from the DNA of necrotic cells leads to hyperuricemia. Acute renal failure reflects the obstruction of the collecting ducts by precipitated crystals of uric acid, a result of increased concentrations of uric acid in the acidic pH of the urine. Conditions that interfere with excretion of uric acid can also result in hyperuricemia, e.g., chronic intake of certain diuretics. Chronic lead intoxication interferes with uric acid secretion by proximal tubules and leads to **saturnine gout.**

PATHOLOGY: In acute urate nephropathy, the precipitated uric acid in the collecting ducts is seen grossly as yellow streaks in the papillae. Histologically, the tubular deposits appear amorphous, but in frozen sections, birefringent crystals are apparent (Fig. 16-79). The tubules proximal to the obstruction are dilated. Penetration of collecting ducts by uric acid crystals may provoke a foreign-body giant cell reaction.

The basic disease process of chronic urate nephropathy is similar to that of the acute form, but the prolonged course results in more substantial deposition of urate crystals in the interstitium, interstitial fibrosis and cortical atrophy. The most diagnostic feature is the **gouty tophus,** a focal accumulation of urate crystals surrounded by inflammatory cells, which may appear granulomatous and include multinucleated giant cells. Uric acid stones account for one tenth of all cases of urolithiasis and occur in 20% of patients with chronic gout and 40% of those with acute hyperuricemia.

CLINICAL FEATURES: Acute urate nephropathy manifests as acute renal failure, whereas chronic urate nephropathy causes chronic renal tubular defects. Although histologic renal lesions are found in most persons with

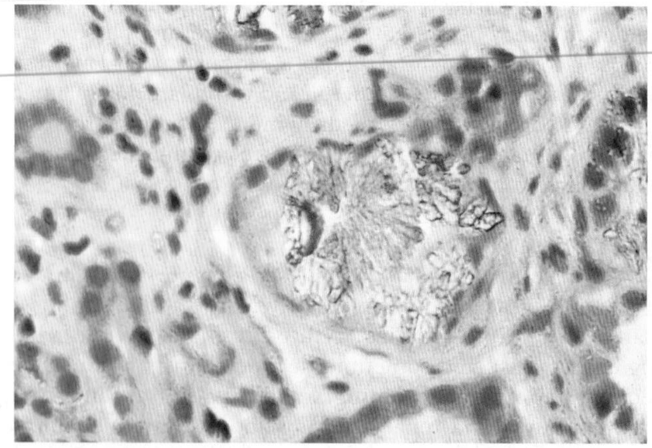

FIGURE 16-79. **Urate nephropathy.** A frozen section demonstrates tubular deposits of uric acid crystals.

chronic gout, fewer than half show significant compromise of renal function.

Nephrocalcinosis Is Deposition of Calcium in the Renal Parenchyma

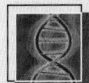

PATHOGENESIS: Hypercalciuria may result in nephrocalcinosis (Table 16-13), formation of calcium-containing stones (**nephrolithiasis**) or both. Nephrocalcinosis may cause abnormal renal function, especially tubular defects such as impaired concentrating ability, salt wasting, and renal tubular acidosis. When nephrocalcinosis is caused by hypercalcemia, it is categorized as **metastatic calcification,** in contrast to calcification at sites of renal parenchymal injury (e.g., infarcts or cortical necrosis), which is representative of **dystrophic calcification.**

PATHOLOGY: At autopsy, 20% of kidneys have small calcium deposits that have no functional significance or recognized association with hypercalcemia. In patients with nephrocalcinosis caused by hypercalcemia, the extent of calcification varies from microscopic deposits to marked calcium accumulation visible grossly and radiologically. In the presence of severe hypercalcemia (e.g., caused by primary hyperparathyroidism), gross examination characteristically reveals wedge-shaped scars interspersed with relatively normal renal tissue. These scars reflect parenchymal atrophy and interstitial fibrosis caused by the calcification. Histologically, there is striking calcification of renal tubular basement membranes, particularly in the proximal convoluted tubules. The interstitial tissue also contains calcium deposits. Such deposits also accumulate in the cytoplasm of tubular epithelial cells, which eventually degenerate and are sloughed into the lumina to aggregate as calcified casts. Scattered glomeruli show calcification of Bowman's capsule. The walls of intrarenal arteries may also be calcified. Calcium deposits are deeply basophilic with hematoxylin; with the more specific von Kossa stain, they are black. By electron microscopy, the mitochondria of renal tubular epithelial cells contain abundant calcium deposits.

TABLE 16-13

Causes of Hypercalcemia That Lead to Nephrocalcinosis

Increased resorption of calcium from bone
Renal osteodystrophy
Primary hyperparathyroidism
Neoplasms producing parathormone or parathormone-like protein
Osteolytic neoplasms and metastases
Increased intestinal absorption of calcium
Idiopathic hypercalcenia
Vitamin D excess
Milk-alkali syndrome
Sarcoidosis

Renal Stones (Nephrolithiasis and Urolithiasis)

*Nephrolithiasis and urolithiasis are stones within the collecting system of the kidney **(nephrolithiasis)** or elsewhere in the collecting system of the urinary tract **(urolithiasis)**.* Renal pelvis and calyces are common sites for calculi to form and accumulate. Stones vary in composition, depending on individual factors, geography, metabolic alterations, and the presence of infection. For unknown reasons, renal stones are more common in men than in women. They vary in size from gravel ($<$1 mm in diameter) to large stones that dilate the entire renal pelvis. Kidney stones may be well tolerated, but in some cases, they lead to severe hydronephrosis and pyelonephritis. Moreover, they can erode the mucosa and cause hematuria. Passage of a stone into the ureter causes excruciating flank pain, termed **renal colic.** Until recently, most kidney stones required surgical removal, but ultrasonic disintegration (lithotripsy) and endoscopic removal are now effective.

In most cases, the presence of a urinary stone is associated with an increased blood level and urinary excretion of its principal component. This is the case with uric acid and cystine stones. However, in many patients with calcium stones, hypercalciuria occurs in the absence of hypercalcemia. Mixed uric acid and calcium stones are common in the presence of increased uric acid excretion, because urate crystals act as a nidus around which calcium salts precipitate.

- **Calcium stones:** Most (75%) kidney stones contain calcium complexed with oxalate or phosphate or a mixture of these anions. Calcium oxalate is more common in the United States, whereas in England, calcium phosphate predominates. A calcium oxalate stone is hard and occasionally dark, because it is covered by hemorrhage from the mucosa of the renal pelvis injured by the sharp calcium oxalate crystals. Calcium phosphate stones tend to be softer and paler.
- **Infection stones:** Some 15% of stones are caused by infection. In the presence of urea-splitting bacteria, usually *Proteus* or *Providencia* species, the resulting alkaline urine favors precipitation of magnesium ammonium phosphate (**struvite**) and calcium phosphate (**apatite**). These stones vary from hard to soft and friable. Infection stones occasionally fill the pelvis and calyces to form a cast of these spaces, referred to as a **staghorn calculus** (Fig. 16-80). Infection stones are the most troublesome as they cause frequent complications, such as intractable urinary tract infection, pain, bleeding, perinephric abscess, and urosepsis.
- **Uric acid stones:** These stones occur in 25% of patients with hyperuricemia and gout, but most patients with uric acid stones do not have either condition (**idiopathic urate lithiasis**). The stones are smooth, hard, and yellow and are usually less than 2 cm in diameter. Importantly, in contrast to calcium-containing stones, pure uric acid stones are radiolucent.
- **Cystine stones:** These stones account for only 1% of stones overall but represent a significant proportion of childhood calculi and occur exclusively with hereditary cystinuria. Although the stones are composed entirely of cystine, they may be enveloped by a layer of calcium phosphate.

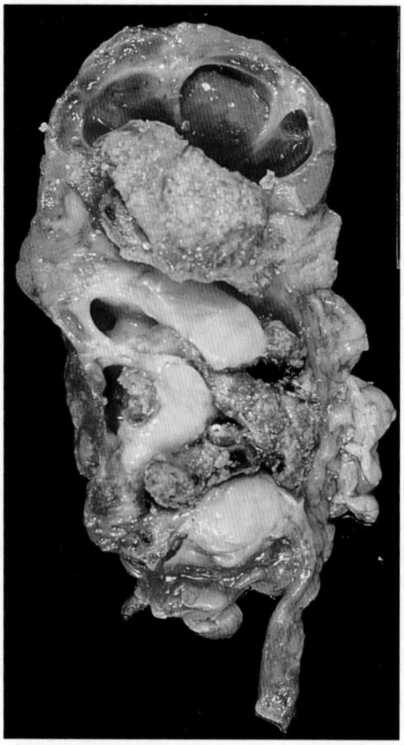

FIGURE 16-80. **Staghorn calculi.** The kidney shows hydronephrosis and stones that are casts of the dilated calyces.

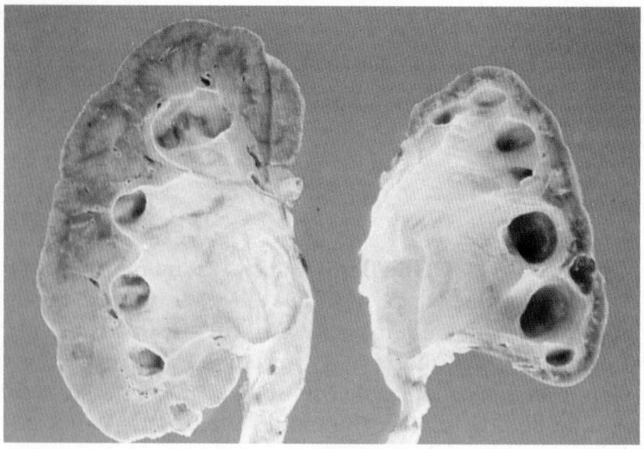

FIGURE 16-81. **Hydronephrosis.** Bilateral urinary tract obstruction has led to conspicuous dilation of the ureters, pelves, and calyces. The kidney on the right shows severe parenchymal atrophy.

Obstructive Uropathy and Hydronephrosis

Obstructive uropathy is caused by structural or functional abnormalities in the urinary tract that impede urine flow, which may cause renal dysfunction (obstructive nephropathy) and dilation of the collecting system (hydronephrosis). The causes of urinary tract obstruction are discussed in detail in Chapter 17.

PATHOLOGY: The most prominent microscopic finding in early hydronephrosis is dilation of the collecting ducts, followed by dilation of proximal and distal convoluted tubules. Eventually, the proximal tubules become widely dilated, and loss of tubules is common. Glomeruli are usually spared. Grossly, progressive dilation of the renal pelvis and calyces occurs, and atrophy of the renal parenchyma ensues (Fig. 16-81). In the presence of hydronephrosis, the kidney is more susceptible to pyelonephritis, which causes additional injury.

CLINICAL FEATURES: Bilateral acute urinary tract obstruction causes acute renal failure (**postrenal acute renal failure**). Unilateral obstruction is frequently asymptomatic. Because many causes of acute obstruction are reversible, prompt recognition is important. Left untreated, an obstructed kidney undergoes atrophy. In the case of bilateral obstruction, chronic renal failure ensues.

Renal Transplantation

Renal transplantation is the treatment of choice for most patients with end-stage renal disease. The major obstacle is immunologic rejection, but recurrence of the disease that destroyed the native kidneys and nephrotoxicity from immunosuppressive drugs also injure the renal allograft. Table 16-14 lists distinct, but often coexisting, patterns of humoral and cellular renal allograft rejection.

ABO blood group antigens and **HLAs** are the two principal targets of immune attack against a transplanted kidney. Incompatible ABO blood group antigens, expressed on endothelial cells and erythrocytes, are absolute barriers to a successful transplant. ABO-incompatible grafts encounter preformed, circulating antibodies that bind to endothelial cells and cause immediate (hyperacute) rejection. *The more commonly encountered (and more gradual) patterns of acute and chronic rejection are caused primarily by donor–recipient differences in HLAs (MHC antigens), which are encoded by several closely related loci on chromosome 6 and expressed on most cell membranes.* Sensitization of kidney allograft recipients to HLAs produces both cell-mediated and antibody-mediated reactions (Chapter 4). Renal allograft rejection can be classified on the basis of the clinical course, pathological features, and presumed pathogenesis, as shown in Table 16-14. However, more than one type of rejection can involve the allograft at the same time.

HYPERACUTE HUMORAL REJECTION: Hyperacute rejection is rare because of current compatibility testing; it occurs in

TABLE 16-14

Categories of Renal Allograft Rejection

Category	Most Characteristic Lesion
Hyperacute humoral rejection	Neutrophils, hemorrhage and necrosis
Acute cellular rejection	
Acute tubulointerstitial rejection	Tubulitis (mononuclear leukocytes in tubules)
Acute cellular vascular rejection	Endarteritis (mononuclear leukocytes in intima)
Acute humoral rejection	
Acute humoral capillary rejection	Neutrophils and C4d in capillaries
Acute necrotizing vascular rejection	Arterial fibrinoid necrosis
Chronic rejection	Arterial intimal fibrosis, cortical atrophy

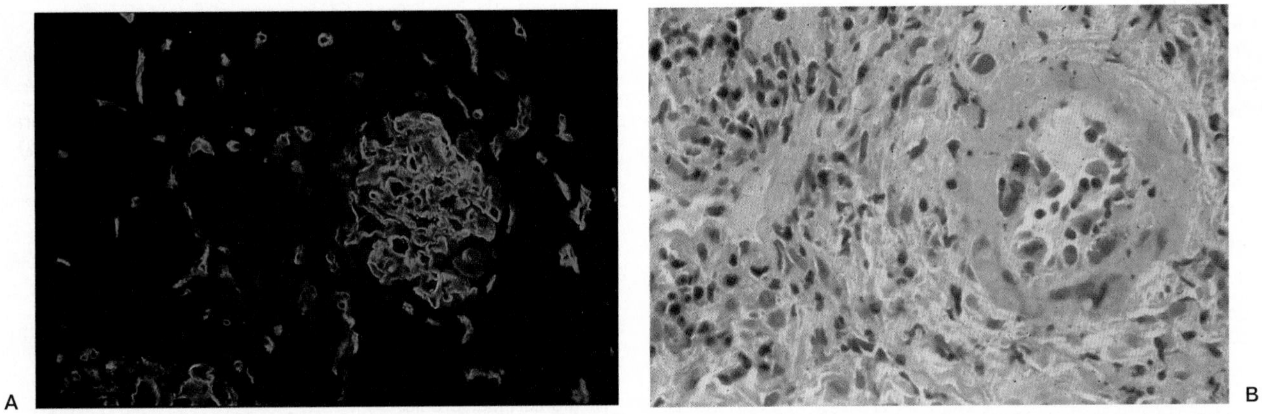

FIGURE 16-82. **Acute humoral allograft rejection. A.** Staining of peritubular and glomerular capillaries with a fluoresceinated anti-C4d antibody showing evidence of complement activation by antibodies directed against donor antigens on endothelial cells. **B.** Acute humoral necrotizing acute vasculitis in an interlobular artery with extensive fibrinoid necrosis of the muscularis. The vascular and interstitial infiltrates of mononuclear leukocytes indicate concurrent acute cellular rejection.

less than 0.5% of allografts. When recipient blood containing antibodies to major alloantigens (usually ABO or class I HLAs) begins flowing through allograft vessels, these antibodies immediately bind endothelial cells and causes prompt and irreversible injury in minutes, which may become apparent intraoperatively by mottling, cyanosis, and poor tissue turgor of the graft. Antibody binding to endothelial alloantigens induces complement activation, which attracts neutrophils. The cytotoxic effects of complement and neutrophil activation cause endothelial cell swelling, vacuolization, and lysis. The accumulation of neutrophils in glomerular capillaries is a sign of impending rejection. Endothelial cell changes are followed by platelet thrombi and later by fibrin thrombi. Interstitial edema, hemorrhage, and cortical necrosis develop over the following 12 to 24 hours.

ACUTE HUMORAL REJECTION: The most common type of acute humoral rejection is directed primarily at capillaries and may cause only subtle or no pathologic changes by light microscopy. The most common feature is increased neutrophils in peritubular and glomerular capillaries and in tubules. The most consistent finding is localization of complement activation products, especially C4d, in the walls of peritubular and glomerular capillaries (Fig. 16-82A). The most severe, but least common, pattern of acute humoral rejection is characterized by **necrotizing arteritis** with fibrinoid necrosis involving the media (see Fig. 16-82B). It occurs in less than 1% of allografts in patients whose immunosuppression includes a calcineurin inhibitor, although it occurred in 5% of renal allografts prior to the introduction of this therapy. Once necrotizing arteritis develops, the chances of graft survival for 1 year are less than 30%, even with aggressive immunosuppression.

ACUTE CELLULAR REJECTION: This is the most common form of acute rejection, and is characterized by infiltration of the interstitium, tubules, arteries, arterioles, or glomeruli by T lymphocytes and macrophages. Nuclei of infiltrating lymphocytes vary in size and shape because the cells are at various stages of activation. Occasional cells are completely transformed into immunoblasts. Interstitial infiltrates are typically patchy rather than diffuse. Involvement of tubules (**tubulitis**) is manifested by lymphocytes crossing tubular basement membranes and lying between tubular epithelial cells (see Fig. 16-83A). Arterial involvement by cellular rejection leads to penetration of T lymphocytes and monocytes across the endothelium, resulting in an expanded intima filled with mononuclear leukocytes (**intimal arteritis, or endarteritis**) (see Fig. 16-83B). Arterioles are

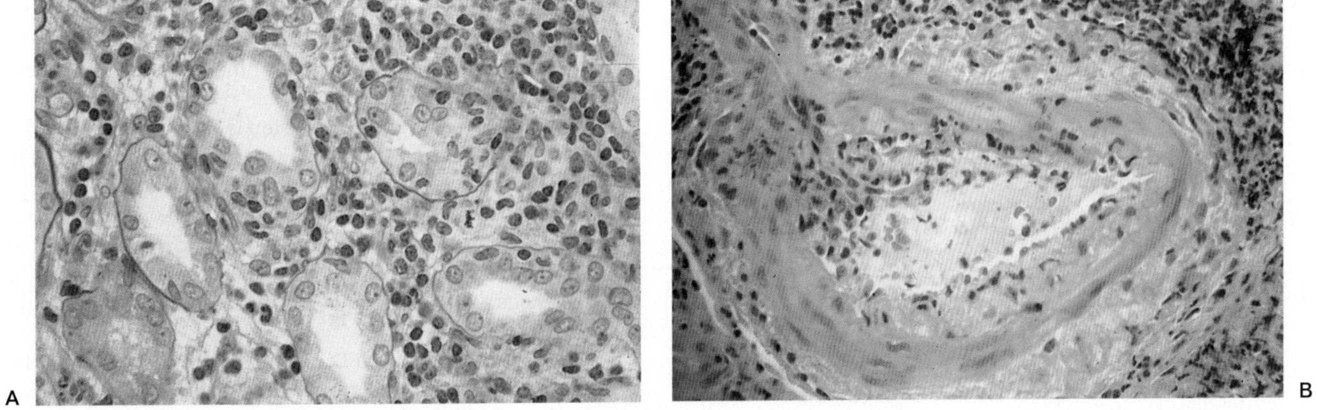

FIGURE 16-83. **Acute cellular allograft rejection. A.** Acute tubulointerstitial cellular rejection with tubulitis indicated by the lymphocytes on the epithelial side of the basement membrane (period acid–Schiff stain). **B.** Acute cellular vascular rejection with endarteritis indicated by the mononuclear leukocytes infiltrating into the intima of an arcuate artery.

TABLE 16-15

Histological Features of Chronic Renal Allograft Rejection

Fibrotic intimal thickening of arteries
Tubular atrophy
Interstitial fibrosis
Interstitial mononuclear leukocytes
Glomerular capillary wall thickening and mesangial expansion
Glomerular sclerosis

occasionally involved by similar infiltration. Glomerular infiltration by mononuclear leukocytes with obliteration of capillary lumens (**acute transplant glomerulopathy**) is an uncommon manifestation of acute cellular rejection. Renal transplants found to have tubulitis without endarteritis have an 80% chance for 1-year graft survival, compared with 60% for allografts with endarteritis.

CHRONIC REJECTION: Pathologic changes attributed to chronic rejection are listed in Table 16-15.

The arterial changes of chronic rejection affect a wide spectrum of vessels, ranging from small arteries to the main renal artery. There is prominent initial widening, caused by stromal cell proliferation and matrix deposition (Fig. 16-84). Mononuclear leukocytes within the vessel wall are much less prominent than with active intimal arteritis. Foam cells may be conspicuous and the internal elastic lamina may be interrupted. Peritubular capillaries demonstrate thickening and replication of basement membranes. Tubular atrophy and interstitial fibrosis may be

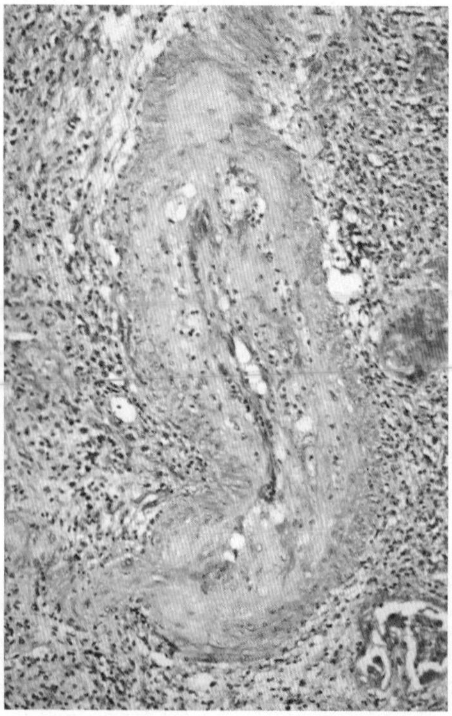

FIGURE 16-84. **Chronic allograft rejection.** The lumen of this medium-sized artery is occluded by a thickened and fibrotic intima, which contains a few inflammatory cells.

TABLE 16-16

Recurrence of Disease in Renal Allografts

Disease	Recurrence Rate (%)	Rate of Graft Loss (%)
Type II membranoproliferative glomerulonephritis	>90	15
Diabetic glomerulosclerosis	>90	<5
IgA nephropathy	40	<10
Focal segmental glomerulosclerosis	35	30
Type I membranoproliferative glomerulonephritis	30	<10
Membranous glomerulopathy	20	<5
ANCA glomerulonephritis	15	<5
Anti-GBM glomerulonephritis	5	<5
Lupus glomerulonephritis	5	<5

ANCA = antineutrophil cytoplasmic autoantibody; GBM = glomerular basement membrane; Ig = immunoglobulin.

caused at least in part by ischemia secondary to narrowing of arteries and peritubular capillaries. Tubulointerstitial injury may also result from indolent tubulitis. Glomerular involvement (**chronic transplant glomerulopathy**) manifests as thickening of capillary walls and mesangial widening. Electron microscopy shows electron-lucent expansion of the subendothelial zone and occasional mesangial interposition and replication of basement membranes. The arterial, peritubular capillary, and glomerular injury all may result from persistent, low-level, immune injury to the vascular endothelium.

RECURRENCE OF KIDNEY DISEASE: The same disease that led to renal failure in native kidneys can recur in a renal transplant. The frequency and significance of recurrence vary among different types of glomerular disease (Table 16-16).

NEPHROTOXICITY OF CYCLOSPORINE AND TACROLIMUS (FK506): The calcineurin inhibitors, cyclosporine and tacrolimus, are immunosuppressive drugs that have dramatically improved the survival of not only kidney allografts, but also other allografts (e.g., liver, heart, lungs). Unfortunately, both drugs injure kidney allografts, as well as the native kidneys of patients who are receiving immunosuppressive treatment for other reasons. The toxicity can cause acute or chronic renal failure.

The most characteristic renal lesion is an **arteriolopathy** that begins with smooth muscle cell degeneration and necrosis. The destroyed arteriolar muscle cells are replaced by acidophilic hyaline material (Fig. 16-85). In fulminant cases, vascular lesions take on the appearance of a full-blown thrombotic microangiopathy, with circumferential fibrinoid necrosis of arterioles. In chronic toxicity there are zones of interstitial fibrosis and tubular atrophy ("striped fibrosis").

BK POLYOMAVIRUS INFECTION: Reactivation of latent BK virus infection in a transplant can be caused by immunosuppression, and can result in acute tubular injury and tubulointerstitial nephritis. Intranuclear viral inclusions in tubular cells raise this possibility, which can be confirmed by immuohistochemistry.

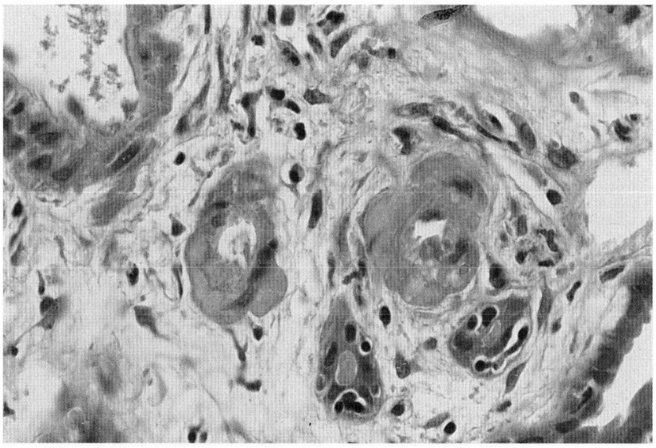

FIGURE 16-85. **Cyclosporine nephrotoxicity and arteriolopathy.** Marked destructive hyalinosis of arterioles is present.

Benign Tumors of the Kidney

RENAL ADENOMA: Whether any renal epithelial cell neoplasm should be designated an **adenoma,** a term that signifies no malignant potential, is controversial. Tumor size has been used to separate adenomas from carcinomas, but this is problematic because all carcinomas begin as small lesions. Renal epithelial neoplasms less than 3 cm in diameter rarely metastasize, but "rarely" is not "never." Neoplasms with cells that resemble clear cell, chromophobe, or collecting duct RCCs should not be designated adenomas even if they are small. Neoplasms under 5 mm with papillary or tubulopapillary growth patterns can be considered adenomas. Renal adenomas increase in frequency with age, and are found at autopsy in 40% of patients over 70.

RENAL ONCOCYTOMA: This tumor has plump cells with abundant, finely granular, acidophilic cytoplasm and round nuclei without atypia. Electron microscopy demonstrates numerous mitochondria as the basis for the distinctive appearance of the cytoplasm. Grossly, oncocytomas have a characteristic mahogany-brown color, caused by the lipochrome pigments in the mitochondria. These tumors rarely metastasize.

MEDULLARY FIBROMA: Medullary fibromas (renomedullary interstitial cell tumors) are typically small (<0.5 cm in diameter), pale gray, well-circumscribed tumors that are usually located in the midportion of the medullary pyramid. Histologically, the neoplasms are composed of small stellate to polygonal cells lying in a loose stroma. Renal medullary fibromas can be identified in half of all adult autopsies.

ANGIOMYOLIPOMA: These lesions exhibit an admixture of well-differentiated adipose tissue, smooth muscle, and thick-walled vessels. Grossly, the tumors are yellow and bosselated and may resemble RCC. However, they are always well encapsulated and lack areas of necrosis. *Angiomyolipomas have a strong association with tuberous sclerosis.* Fully 80% of patients with tuberous sclerosis have angiomyolipomas, although less than 50% of patients with angiomyolipomas have tuberous sclerosis.

MESOBLASTIC NEPHROMA: Mesoblastic nephromas are congenital benign neoplasms or hamartomas that are usually recognized during the first 3 months of life and must be differentiated from Wilms tumor. The lesions range from less than 1 cm in diameter to over 15 cm. Histologically, they are composed of spindle cells of fibroblastic or myofibroblastic lineage. Characteristically, tumor margins are irregular, with bands of cells interdigitating with adjacent parenchyma. If some of these tongues of tumor tissue are left behind after surgical resection, local recurrence is possible.

Malignant Tumors of the Kidney

Wilms Tumor (Nephroblastoma) Is Composed of Embryonal Elements

Wilms tumor is a malignant neoplasm of embryonal nephrogenic elements composed of mixtures of blastemal, stromal, and epithelial tissue. It is the most frequent abdominal solid tumor in children, with a prevalence of 1 in 10,000.

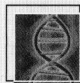

PATHOGENESIS: In most (90%) cases the Wilms tumor is sporadic and unilateral. In 5% of cases, however, it arises in the context of three different congenital syndromes, all of which include increased risk for development of this cancer at an early age and often bilaterally:

- **WAGR syndrome**—for *W*ilms tumor, *a*niridia, *g*enitourinary anomalies, mental *r*etardation
- **Denys-Drash syndrome (DDS)**—Wilms tumor, intersexual disorders, glomerulopathy
- **Beckwith-Wiedemann syndrome (BWS)**—Wilms tumor, overgrowth ranging from gigantism to hemihypertrophy, visceromegaly, and macroglossia

Some 6% of cases of Wilms tumor are familial, have an early onset and are bilateral but are not associated with any other syndrome.

Two decades ago, karyotypic analysis of children with WAGR syndrome revealed a deletion in the short arm of one copy of chromosome 11 (11p13). The WAGR deletion affects contiguous genes, including *PAX6,* the aniridia gene, and ***WT1*, the Wilms tumor gene.** Loss or mutation of one *WT1* allele leads to genitourinary anomalies, whereas a defect in *PAX6* is responsible for aniridia. One third of children with WAGR syndrome eventually develop Wilms tumor. The presence of a germline mutation in one *WT1* allele and loss of heterozygosity at this locus in the tumors of WAGR syndrome imply that a second mutation in the normal *WT1* allele is responsible for the appearance of Wilms tumor (similar to the pathogenesis of hereditary retinoblastoma; see Chapter 5). In contrast to deletions in WAGR syndrome, specific mutations of the *WT1* gene characterize DDS. The fact that the phenotype of DDS is far more severe than that of WAGR syndrome suggests that mutated *WT1* is actually a dominant negative mutation.

WT1 is a tumor-suppressor protein that regulates transcription of several other genes, including insulin-like growth factor-II (IGF-II) and platelet-derived growth factor (PDGF). WT1 protein also forms a complex with the p53 protein. *Whereas Wilms tumors arising in the context of WAGR syndrome all display defects of WT1, less than 10% of sporadic tumors exhibit such abnormalities.* Thus, it is believed that other genes play a more critical role than does *WT1* in the genesis of sporadic Wilms tumors.

A second gene for susceptibility to Wilms tumor *(WT2)* was discovered in sporadic tumors that showed loss of heterozygosity (LOH) on chromosome 11 (11p15), a site distinct from, but close to, the *WT1* gene. *WT2* is also linked to BWS. Interestingly, in LOH at the *WT2* locus in sporadic Wilms tumors, the allele lost is invariably the maternal one. Importantly, some patients with BWS show germline duplication of the paternal *WT2* allele, and others have inherited both apparently normal copies of this gene from the father and none from the mother *(paternal uniparental isodisomy). WT2* may normally be expressed only by the paternal allele *(genomic imprinting),* so that overexpression of *WT2* may be responsible for the overgrowth characteristic of BWS. Since the *IGF-II* gene has also been mapped to chromosome 11p15 and is also paternally imprinted, it is possible that increased dosage of *IGF-II* might contribute both to BWS and to tumorigenesis. Another possibility is that *WT2* is expressed only by the maternal allele acting as a tumor suppressor. Thus, loss of the maternal allele would contribute to tumorigenesis.

Nephrogenic rests (small foci of persistent primitive blastemal cells) are found in the kidneys of all children with syndromic Wilms tumors and in one third of sporadic cases. Given that such rests in the nontumorous kidney contain the same somatic mutations in *WT1* as are present in the tumors, it is thought that these rests represent clonal precursor lesions that are at least one step along the pathway to tumor formation.

PATHOLOGY: Wilms tumor tends to be large when detected, with a bulging, pale tan, cut surface enclosed within a thin rim of renal cortex and capsule (Fig. 16-86). Histologically, the tumor is composed of elements that resemble normal fetal tissue (Fig. 16-87), including (1) metanephric blastema, (2) immature stroma (mesenchymal tissue) and (3) immature epithelial elements.

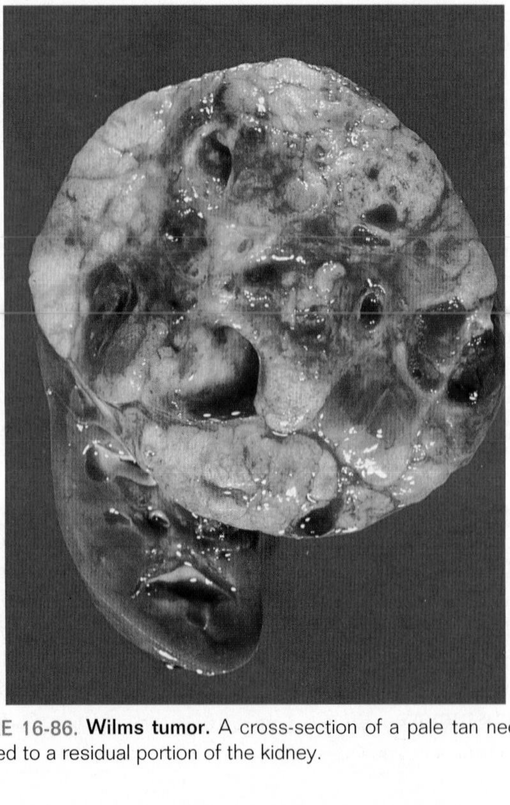

FIGURE 16-86. **Wilms tumor.** A cross-section of a pale tan neoplasm attached to a residual portion of the kidney.

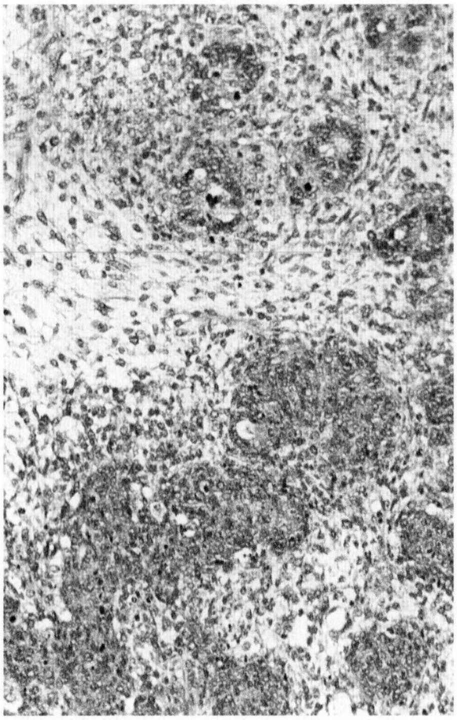

FIGURE 16-87. **Wilms tumor (nephroblastoma).** This photomicrograph of the tumor shows highly cellular areas composed of undifferentiated blastema, loose stroma containing undifferentiated mesenchymal cells, and immature tubules.

Although most Wilms tumors contain all three elements in varying proportions, occasionally they contain only two elements or even only one. The component corresponding to blastema is composed of small ovoid cells with scanty cytoplasm, growing in nests and trabeculae. The epithelial component appears as small tubular structures. In some cases, structures resembling immature glomeruli are found. The stroma between the other elements is composed of spindle cells, which are mostly undifferentiated but occasionally display smooth muscle or fibroblast differentiation. Skeletal muscle is the most common heterotopic stromal element, although bone, cartilage, fat, or neural tissue may rarely be encountered.

CLINICAL FEATURES: Wilms tumor usually presents between 1 and 3 years of age, and 98% occur before 10 years of age. The few familial cases usually exhibit autosomal dominant inheritance. Only 5% of sporadic cases are bilateral, contrasted with 20% of familial cases. Most often, the diagnosis is made after recognition of an abdominal mass. Additional manifestations include abdominal pain, intestinal obstruction, hypertension, hematuria, and symptoms of traumatic tumor rupture.

A number of histologic and clinical parameters have been used with varying success to predict the behavior of Wilms tumor. Patients younger than 2 years of age tend to have a better prognosis. Invasion of the tumor beyond the renal capsule, noted at the time of surgery, is a negative prognostic indicator. Anaplasia (nuclear enlargement, hyperchromasia, and atypical mitotic figures) also indicates a poorer prognosis. Anaplasia is more common in older patients, a feature that contributes to the overall worse prognosis in these cases. Chemotherapy and radiation therapy, combined with surgical resection, have dramatically improved the outlook of patients with this tumor, and many centers now report an overall long-term survival rate of 90%.

Renal Cell Carcinoma Is the Most Common Primary Cancer of the Kidney

RCC is a malignant neoplasm of renal tubular or ductal epithelial cells. It accounts for 80% of all renal cancers and more than 30,000 cases a year in the United States.

PATHOGENESIS: Most cases of RCC are sporadic, but about 5% are inherited. Hereditary RCC occurs in the context of three distinct syndromes:

- **Autosomal dominant RCC,** in which a clear cell tumor is the primary manifestation and occurs in half of the persons at risk
- **von Hippel-Lindau (VHL) disease,** an autosomal dominant cancer syndrome, characterized by cerebellar hemangioblastomas, retinal angiomas, clear cell RCC (40% of all cases of VHL disease), pheochromocytoma, and cysts in various organs
- **Hereditary papillary RCC**

All forms of hereditary RCC tend to be multifocal and bilateral, and appear at a younger age than sporadic RCC. It is estimated that some 5% of cases of RCC are hereditary, and a family history of RCC places a person at a four- to five-fold increased risk for this malignancy.

In genetic studies a variety of translocations involving a breakpoint on chromosome 3 have been recognized in autosomal dominant RCC. Studies of patients with sporadic RCC have demonstrated deletions and LOH in the short arm of chromosome 3 (3p) in the tumor tissue. Finally, the *VHL* gene is localized to 3p. *VHL* is a tumor-suppressor gene. *Loss of one allele of the VHL gene occurs in virtually all (98%) sporadic clear cell RCC, and mutations in the gene are found in more than half of these tumors.* Thus, the evidence strongly suggests that loss of the tumor suppressive function of *VHL* is an important event in the genesis of clear cell RCC.

Unlike clear cell RCC, hereditary papillary RCC shows no association with the *VHL* gene. Trisomies of chromosomes 7, 16, and 17 and loss of the Y chromosome have been demonstrated in many cases. Mutations in the c-*met* protooncogene *(MET)* are implicated in the development of hereditary papillary RCC.

Tobacco, whether smoked or chewed, is associated with increased risk of RCC: one third of these tumors are linked to tobacco use. Both inherited and acquired cystic diseases of the kidney may be complicated by development of RCC, especially papillary RCC. The cancer has also been tied to analgesic nephropathy.

TABLE 16-17

Categories of Renal Cell Carcinoma

Category	Frequency (%)
Clear cell type	70–80
Papillary type	10–15
Chromophobe type	5
Collecting duct type	1

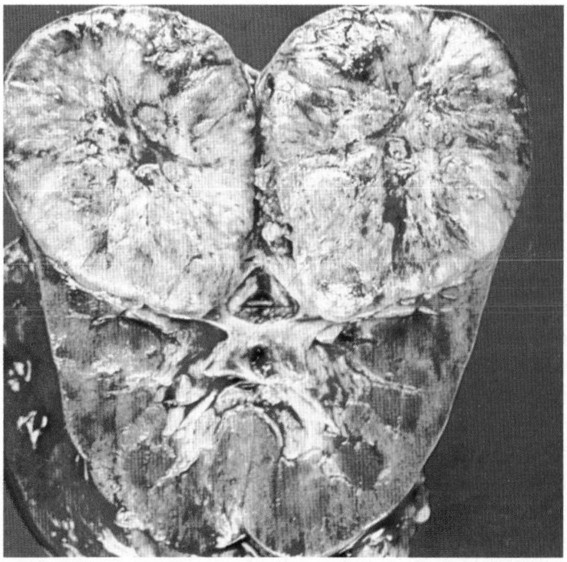

FIGURE 16-88. **Clear cell renal cell carcinoma.** The kidney contains a large irregular neoplasm with a variegated cut surface. Yellow areas correspond to lipid-containing cells.

PATHOLOGY: There are pathologic variants of RCC that reflect differences in histogenesis and predict different outcomes. The various histologic categories are shown in Table 16-17.

Clear cell RCC is the most common type and arises from proximal tubular epithelial cells. It is typically yellow-orange and often shows conspicuous focal hemorrhage and necrosis (Fig. 16-88). The tumors are solid or focally cystic. The clear cytoplasm of the neoplastic cells (Fig. 16-89) reflects the removal of abundant cytoplasmic lipids and glycogen by the water and solvents used to prepare the tissue. The cells are often arranged in round or elongated collections demarcated by a network of delicate vessels, and little cellular or nuclear pleomorphism is present.

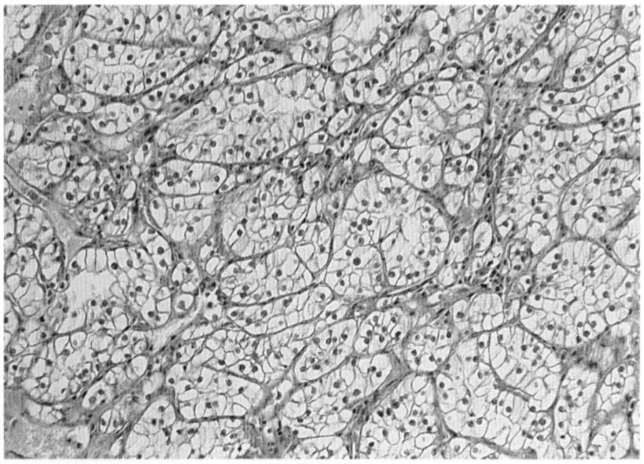

FIGURE 16-89. **Clear cell renal cell carcinoma.** Photomicrograph showing islands of neoplastic cells with abundant clear cytoplasm.

Papillary RCC is characterized by neoplastic cells arranged on fibrovascular stalks. Type 1 papillary RCC has small cells and type 2 has large cells. Type 2 papillary RCC is more aggressive with a worse prognosis. The cytoplasm may be eosinophilic or basophilic. These tumors arise from proximal tubular epithelial cells.

Chromophobe RCC shows a mixture of acidophilic granular cells and pale transparent cells with prominent cell borders, which impart a plant cell-like appearance. The cytoplasm contains numerous vesicles filled with a distinctive mucopolysaccharide that can be stained with the Hale colloidal iron technique. In the pale cells, these vesicles displace other organelles to the periphery, causing a central cytoplasmic pallor. Chromophobe RCC appears to arise from the intercalated cells of renal collecting ducts.

Collecting duct RCC is a rare variety that arises from medullary collecting ducts but may extend into the cortex. Histologically, it is composed of tubular and papillary structures lined by a single layer of cuboidal cells that may have a hobnail appearance. Renal medullary carcinomas are a variant of collecting duct carcinomas that develop almost exclusively in African Americans with sickle cell trait or disease.

"Sarcomatoid" changes may occur in any variant of RCC and portends a worse clinical outcome. The recommended histologic grading system for RCC is the Fuhrman system:

- **Grade I:** Nuclei round, uniform, 10 μm; nucleoli inconspicuous or absent
- **Grade II:** Nuclei irregular, 15 μm; nucleoli evident
- **Grade III:** Nuclei very irregular, 20 μm; nucleoli large and prominent
- **Grade IV:** Nuclei bizarre and multilobated, 20 μm or more; nucleoli prominent

CLINICAL FEATURES: The incidence of RCC peaks in the sixth decade. RCC is twice as frequent in men as in women. *The classic clinical triad of hematuria, flank pain, and a palpable abdominal mass occurs in less than 10% of patients. Hematuria is the single most common presenting sign.* Known in clinical medicine as one of the "great mimics," RCC is a potential source of ectopic hormone production and is frequently associated with fever and paraneoplastic syndromes. For example, secretion of a parathormone-like substance leads to hyperparathyroidism; production of erythropoietin causes erythrocytosis; release of renin results in hypertension. Often a patient with RCC initially presents with symptoms due to a metastasis. For instance, a sudden convulsion, or a cough in a previously healthy person leads to discovery of an unsuspected tumor in the brain or lung, which proves on further examination to be RCC.

The prognosis for RCC is influenced by many factors, including tumor size, extent of invasion and metastasis, histologic type, and nuclear grade. Few patients with prominent sarcomatoid features survive for more than 1 year. By contrast, 1-year overall survival after nephrectomy for clear cell RCC is 50%. The papillary and chromophobe types have a better prognosis than the clear cell type. Tumor stage (a measure of invasion and metastasis) is the most important prognostic factor. The 5-year survival is 90% if the RCC has not extended beyond the renal capsule; survival drops to 30% if there are distant metastases. The tumor spreads most frequently to the lungs and bones.

Transitional Cell Carcinoma

Between 5% and 10% of primary neoplasms of the kidney are transitional cell carcinomas of the renal pelvis or calyces (see Chapter 17). These are morphologically identical to the more common transitional cell carcinomas of the urinary bladder and are associated with them in half of cases. Less than 5% of transitional cell carcinomas occur in the collecting system proximal to the bladder.

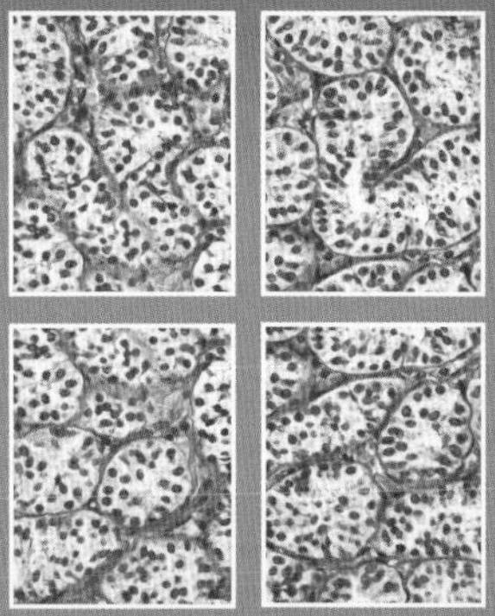

17 The Lower Urinary Tract and Male Reproductive System

Ivan Damjanov

ANATOMY AND EMBRYOLOGY

Lower Urinary Tract

The ureters, urinary bladder, and the urethra—also known as the lower urinary tract—form the outflow part of the urinary system (Fig. 17-1). In males, the lower urinary tract is closely related to the reproductive system.

The Urinary Bladder is in the Retroperitoneal Space of the Lower Abdomen

In males, the urinary bladder is anterior to the rectum and superior to the prostate. In females, it is anterior to the lower uterine corpus and anterior vaginal fornix.

The urinary bladder can be subdivided anatomically into several parts: apex (dome), midportion, and base, the last comprising the trigone and bladder neck. The apex is located behind the margin of the symphysis pubis and is linked in the

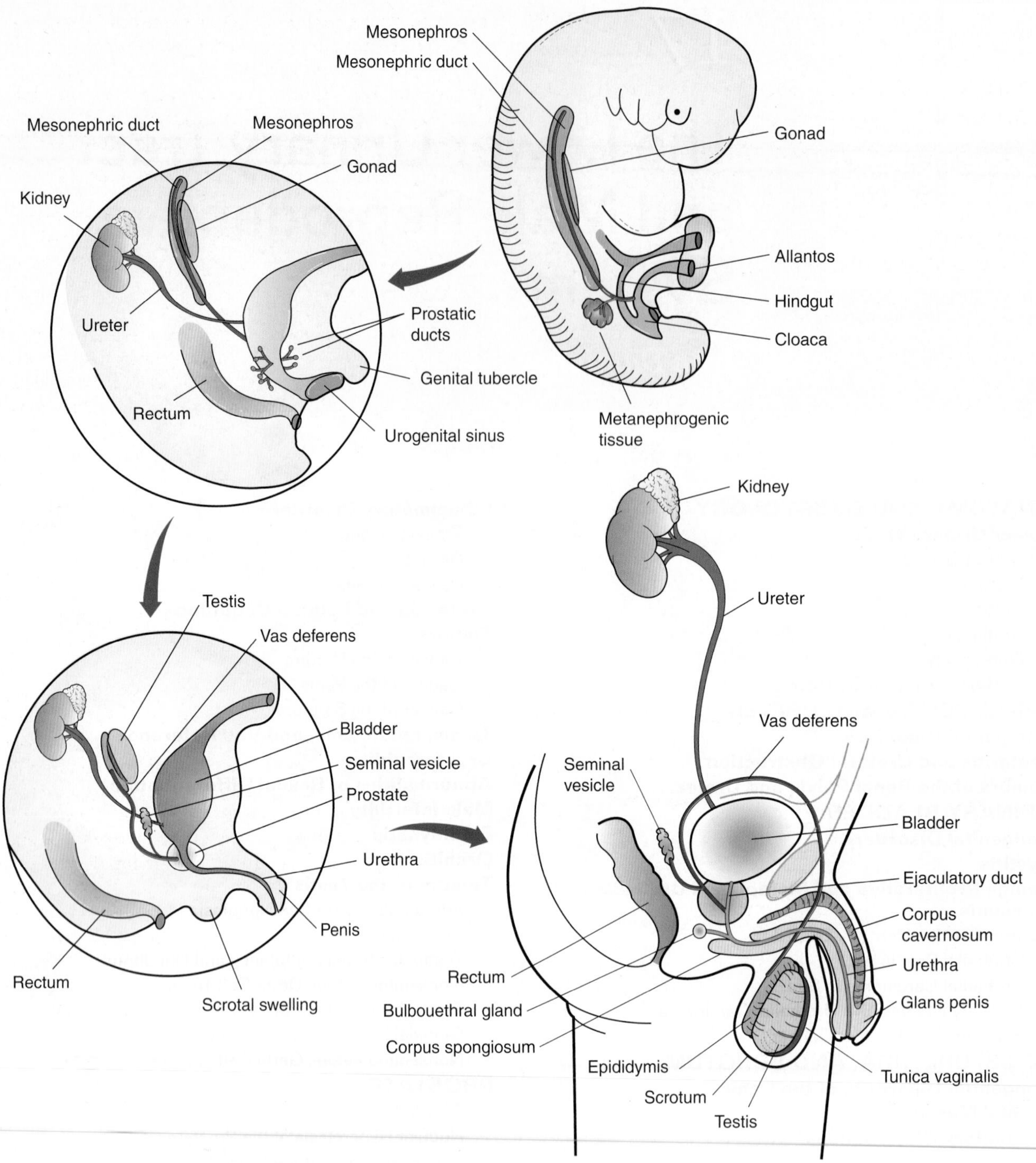

FIGURE 17-1. **Embryologic development of the urinary tract and male reproductive system.**

midline to the umbilicus by the umbilical ligament, a fibrous strand representing the involuted fetal **urachus**. The bladder neck in males rests on the upper surface of the prostate, where the smooth muscle fibers of the two organs intertwine. Inside the bladder, the posterior aspect of the base of the bladder has a triangular shape and is called the **trigone,** a region that is devoid of mucosal folds and appears flattened. Superiorly, the trigone is bound by a muscular ridge joining the laterally placed orifices of the ureters. The inferior tip of the trigone is formed by the funnel-shaped internal orifice of the urethra.

The Ureters are in the Posterior Retroperitoneal Space, Lateral to the Vertebrae

The ureters are paired organs linking each renal pelvis with the bladder. The lowermost part of the ureters is embedded in the wall of the urinary bladder, which forms the ureterovesical valves.

These valves allow urine to pass downward from the ureters into the urinary bladder but not in the opposite direction.

The Urethra is the Terminal Conduit of the Urinary Outflow Tract

The male urethra, on average 20 cm long, is divided into (1) prostatic urethra, extending through the prostate; (2) membranous urethra, penetrating through the pelvic floor; and (3) spongy or penile urethra, occupying the central portion of the penis. The prostatic urethra contains the ostia of ejaculatory and prostatic ducts. The posterior part of penile urethra, also termed **bulbous urethra**, receives secretions from the mucous bulbourethral (Cowper) glands. The penile urethra terminates in the fossa navicularis, immediately proximal to the external orifice, or meatus, located on the tip of the penis.

The female urethra is shorter, measuring only 3 to 4 cm in length. It extends from its internal orifice at the urinary bladder to its external orifice in the vulva, immediately below the clitoris. The wall of the female urethra also contains mucous glands.

Transitional Epithelium (Urothelium) Lines the Ureters, Bladder, and Posterior Urethra

The terminal urethra is lined by squamous epithelium. The urothelium consists of three epithelial zones. The basal layer lies on a basement membrane and contains cells that can divide and replace damaged superficial cells. Superficial to the basal layer are 3 to 4 layers of polygonal cells, the intermediate zone. Both the basal and the polygonal cells can flatten when the bladder dilates. The superficial layer of the urothelium consists of "umbrella cells," which are resistant to the urine that constantly bathes them.

Under the epithelium lies the lamina propria, composed principally of loose connective tissue and blood vessels. The muscularis mucosae is incomplete and poorly developed. The lamina propria is externally surrounded by a thick muscle layer that is covered by adventitia. Since the bladder, ureters, and urethra are retroperitoneal, they do not have an external serosa. Only part the bladder dome has serosa.

The Lower Urinary Tract Develops Mostly from the Cloaca

The cloaca is a fetal structure that is partitioned early in ontogenesis into an anterior part, the urogenital sinus, and the posterior part, which is the primordium of the rectum (see Fig. 17-1). The urogenital sinus is the anlage of the urinary bladder, the proximal urethra, and the urachus, a temporary fetal structure connecting the urinary tract with the umbilicus. The caudal urogenital sinus makes contact with an invagination of the urogenital membrane, thereby forming the urethra. The urachus gradually involutes into the umbilical ligament. The fetal urinary bladder forms symmetrical lateral outpouchings that grow cranially as ureteric buds. When these epithelial buds reach the nephrogenic zone, they induce formation of the metanephros, the kidney primordium.

Male Reproductive System

The male reproductive system includes the testis, epididymis, ductus (vas) deferens, seminal vesicles, prostate, and penis (see Fig. 17-1). The adult testes are in the scrotum and measure 4 × 3 × 3 cm. The epididymis lies along the lateral–posterior aspect of the testis, and extends into the ductus deferens. The testis is invested with the **tunica vaginalis,** a layer of mesothelial cells that covers the outer fibrous capsule of the testis, the **tunica albuginea.** This capsule has internal septal ramifications that divide the testis into about 250 lobules. Each lobule consists of coiled seminiferous tubules and loose interstitial tissue containing blood vessels and Leydig interstitial cells.

Arterial supply to the testis is via testicular arteries, which originate from the abdominal aorta. The right internal spermatic vein empties into the vena cava, while the left drains into the ipsilateral renal vein. This anatomical difference has several clinical implications discussed below.

Seminiferous tubules are the principal functional unit of the testis. They contain seminiferous epithelium and Sertoli cells, which provide support to **spermatogenesis**. **Sertoli cells** also secrete **inhibin**, which provides feedback information to the pituitary, thereby regulating the secretion of **gonadotropins**, i.e., follicle-stimulating hormone (FSH) and luteinizing hormone (LH). The interstitial spaces of the testis contain **Leydig cells,** the primary source of testosterone.

In prepubertal testes the seminiferous tubules contain two cell types: **germ cells** at the stage of spermatogonia and **Sertoli cells.** At puberty, LH stimulates Leydig cells to produce testosterone and initiate spermatogenesis, and FSH acts on both germ cells and Sertoli cells to support spermatogenesis.

Hormonal stimuli lead to an increased number of germ cells, primarily **spermatogonia,** which also begin differentiating into primary **spermatocytes.** Meiotic division of primary spermatocytes produces **secondary spermatocytes,** which contain a haploid number (23) of chromosomes. Secondary spermatocytes mature to **spermatids,** and the latter to **spermatozoa,** which are discharged through the channels of rete testis into the epididymal ducts. In the **epididymis,** spermatozoa are admixed with fluid secreted by epididymal lining cells and are carried through the **vas deferens,** which empties its contents into the urethra. The final semen to be ejaculated through the penile urethra is a mixture of spermatozoa in the epididymal secretions and fluids produced by the **accessory glands,** namely, the seminal vesicles, prostate, Cowper bulbourethral glands, and urethral glands.

The prostate is the largest and the most important accessory gland. It is in the pelvis, in contact with the posterior and inferior external layers of the urinary bladder, close to the rectum. Anatomically, the prostate has five parts: anterior, middle, posterior, and two lateral lobes. Microscopically it is a tubuloalveolar gland with a rich fibromuscular stroma. It develops under the influence of testosterone, which is essential for maintaining its production of seminal fluid.

The **testes** develop from the **genital ridges,** which form on the posterior surface of the celomic cavity. These ridges are populated by migratory **primordial germ cells** (formed initially in the yolk sac) that enter the fetal body through the midline, then migrate laterally into the right and left genital ridges. Complex interactions of germ cells and stromal cells in the genital ridges lead to formation of the fetal testes, which are on the posterior wall of the midabdomen. At the same time, the testes connect with the future epididymis and vas deferens, which develop from the **wolffian ducts.** At that point the testes begin their gradual descent into the inguinal canal, to the scrotum.

The scrotum and penis develop simultaneously with the testes but from another anlage that corresponds mostly to the

genital tubercle and partly to the anterior **urogenital sinus.** These primordia of the external genital organs are at first identical in both sexes. In a male fetus testosterone drives their development into penis, penile urethra, and scrotum; in a female they become clitoris, labia minora, and labia majora.

RENAL PELVIS AND URETER

Congenital Disorders

Developmental anomalies of the renal pelvis and ureters are found in 2% to 3% of all persons. They do not usually cause clinical problems, but on occasion may predispose to obstruction and urinary tract infections. The most important developmental anomalies include agenesis, ectopia, duplications, obstructions, and dilations (Fig. 17-2).

AGENESIS OF THE RENAL PELVIS AND URETERS: This rare anomaly is always associated with agenesis of the corresponding kidney. Unilateral agenesis is usually asymptomatic. Bilateral agenesis of ureters and kidneys, a feature of **Potter syndrome**, is incompatible with life (see Chapter 16).

ECTOPIC URETERS: Ureteric buds may develop at the wrong anatomical site during embryogenesis. The lower orifices of ectopic ureters can be found in many anomalous places, such as midportion of the urinary bladder, seminal vesicles, urethra, or vas deferens.

DUPLICATIONS: Single or multiple ureteric buds may be duplicated on the side of the fetal urinary bladder. These duplications may be unilateral or bilateral, complete or partial. Usually there are two parallel ureters, each with its own renal pelvis and separate vesical orifice. **Bifid ureters** (subdivided by a septum), **bifurcate ureters,** and many variations of this anomaly can be encountered, but most are not clinically significance.

URETERAL OBSTRUCTION: Obstructions can be traced to congenital **atresia** or abnormal **ureteral valves**. However, congenital **obstruction of the ureteropelvic junction,** the most common form of hydronephrosis in infants and children, cannot be explained in those terms. It is thought to be related to abnormal layering of smooth muscle cells and/or fibrosis replacing the smooth muscle cells at the ureteropelvic junction. Urinary obstruction in these children is usually unilateral, but is bilateral in 20% of cases. This form of hydronephrosis is often associated with other urinary tract anomalies and, in some cases, with agenesis of the contralateral kidney.

DILATIONS OF THE RENAL PELVIS OR URETERS: can be localized in the form of **diverticula** or generalized. Dilation of the entire ureter, **congenital megaureter**, may be unilateral or bilateral. The pathogenesis of congenital megaureters is mostly unknown. The ureters are tortuous and lack peristalsis. Resulting stagnation of urine (**hydroureter**) is typically associated with progressive hydronephrosis, ultimately leading to renal failure.

Ureteritis And Ureteral Obstruction

Ureteritis is an inflammation of the ureters. It is a complication of descending infections of kidneys or ascending infections if there is vesicoureteric reflux. Ureteritis is often associated with ureteral obstruction, which may be either intrinsic or extrinsic (Fig. 17-3).

Intrinsic causes of ureteral obstruction include calculi, intraluminal blood clots, fibroepithelial polyps, inflammatory strictures, amyloidosis, and tumors of the ureter.

Extrinsic causes of ureteral obstruction include aberrant renal vessels to the lower pole of the kidney that cross the ureter, endometriosis, and tumors in adjacent lymph nodes. In addition, the pregnant uterus can compress the ureters.

Ureteral obstruction may also result from diseases that involve urinary bladder, prostate, and urethra, e.g., bladder cancer in the vicinity of the ureteral orifice or bladder neck, neurogenic bladder, and prostatic hyperplasia. Proximal causes of ureteral obstruction tend to be unilateral, whereas more distal ones, such as prostatic hyperplasia, lead to bilateral hydronephrosis, with the possibility of renal failure in untreated cases.

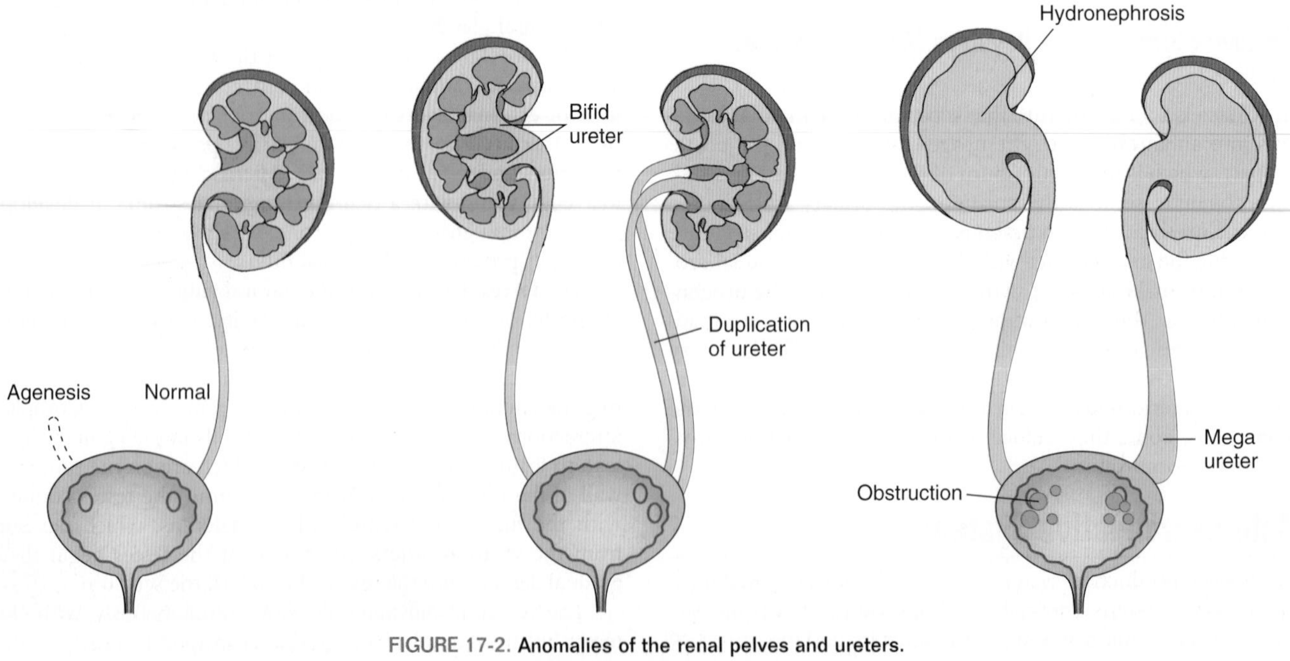

FIGURE 17-2. **Anomalies of the renal pelves and ureters.**

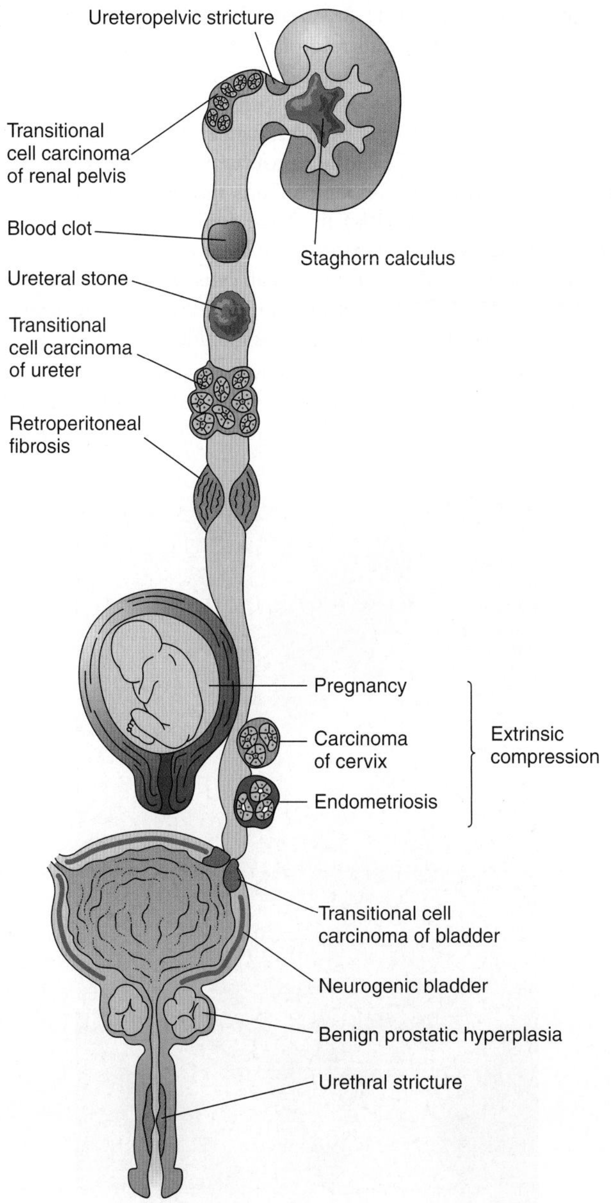

FIGURE 17-3. **Most common causes of ureteral obstruction.**

Idiopathic retroperitoneal fibrosis is a rare cause of ureteral obstruction, characterized by dense fibrosis of retroperitoneal soft tissues and a modest, nonspecific, chronic inflammatory reaction. The etiology is unknown, although use of certain drugs (methysergide, β-adrenergic blockers) and autoimmunity have been proposed as causes. On occasion, idiopathic retroperitoneal fibrosis is accompanied by inflammatory fibrosis in other areas, including Riedel struma (thyroid), sclerosing cholangitis (liver) and mediastinal fibrosis. The disease may respond to treatment with corticosteroids and immunosuppressive agents.

Tumors Of The Renal Pelvis And Ureter

Tumors of the renal pelvis and ureter resemble those of urinary bladder except that they are much less common. Histologically, most (>90%) are **transitional cell carcinomas.** The etiologic factors associated with epithelial tumors of the renal pelvis and ureter are similar to those observed in bladder cancer, suggesting a "field effect" in which the entire urothelial mucosa represents a continuous "target organ." Five percent of urothelial tumors originate in the renal pelvis and ureters.

Patients most frequently present in their sixth and seventh decades with hematuria (80%) and flank pain (25%). Transitional cell carcinoma of ureter or renal pelvis requires radical nephroureterectomy. The entire ureter must be removed because of the high frequency of concurrent and subsequent transitional cell carcinomas. The prognosis is related to the tumor stage at the time of diagnosis.

URINARY BLADDER

Congenital Disorders

Congenital malformations of the urinary bladder include (1) bladder exstrophy, (2) diverticula, (3) urachal remnants, and (4) congenital vesicoureteral valve incompetence.

EXSTROPHY OF THE BLADDER: This developmental abnormality is characterized by absence of the anterior bladder wall and part of the anterior abdominal wall. The estimated frequency is 1 per 50,000 births. In some male infants it is associated with **epispadias** (i.e., incomplete formation of the penile urethra).

Exstrophy of the bladder results from incomplete resorption of the anterior cloacal membrane. In normal embryogenesis this membrane is replaced by smooth muscle, but if it persists, it forms the anterior vesical wall. Since the membrane is thin, it ultimately ruptures, leaving a large defect that is accompanied by defective closure of the anterior muscular wall of the abdominal cavity. These two defects expose the posterior bladder wall to the exterior and transform the bladder into a cuplike organ that cannot hold urine (Fig. 17-4). The posterior wall of the bladder exposed to mechanical injury undergoes squamous or glandular metaplasia and is prone to frequent infection. Although exstrophy can be surgically repaired, the metaplastic mucosa has an increased risk of malignant transformation. In fact, the incidence of bladder cancer is increased in persons who have lived for 50 to 60 years after surgical repair of exstrophy.

DIVERTICULA: These saclike outpouchings of bladder wall are related to incomplete formation of the muscular layers. They can be soli-

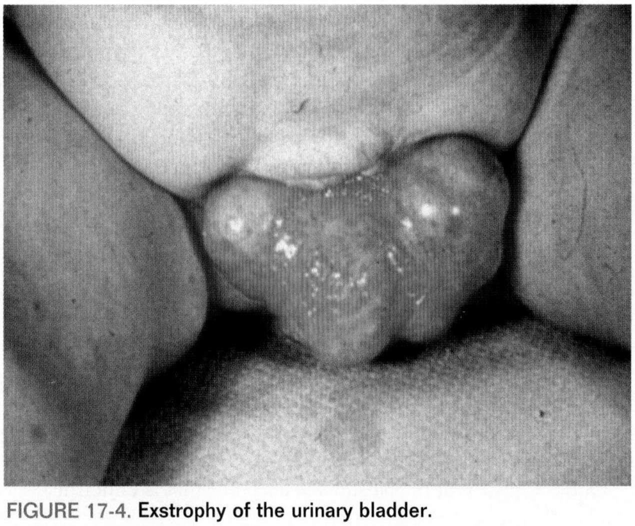

FIGURE 17-4. **Exstrophy of the urinary bladder.**

tary or multiple. Urine retained inside such diverticula is commonly infected, a complication that may lead to the urinary stone formation. Congenital diverticula must be distinguished from **acquired vesical diverticula** which typically occur in long-standing urinary tract obstruction caused by prostatic hyperplasia.

URACHAL REMNANTS: The urachus (i.e., the fetal allantoic stalk connecting the urinary bladder and umbilicus) may fail to involute completely. If it remains patent throughout, it forms a **vesical–umbilical fistula**. Incomplete regression of the urinary end, midportion, or umbilical end of the urachus results in an **urachal diverticulum, umbilical– urachal sinus**, or **urachal cyst**, respectively. The columnar epithelium of the urachal remnants may give rise to **adenocarcinoma**. Urachal remnants are the site of only 0.2% of the bladder cancers, they represent one third of bladder adenocarcinomas.

CONGENITAL INCOMPETENCE OF THE VESICOURETERAL VALVE: This anomaly results from an abnormal junction between the ureters and the urinary bladder. The ureters normally enter the wall of the bladder obliquely and have a long intravesical portion. The muscle layer of the urinary bladder serves as a sphincter that prevents backflow of urine into normal ureters during micturition. By contrast, ureters that enter the bladder perpendicularly have a short intravesical segment, which does not adequately prevent urine backflow during micturition. **Vesicoureteric reflux** (VUR) is more common in young girls than boys and is often familial. In 75% of cases, VUR is asymptomatic, but it may lead to reflux pyelonephritis. Congenital VUR is distinguished from the acquired form that occurs during pregnancy or in conditions associated with bladder hypertrophy.

Cystitis

Cystitis is inflammation of the bladder. It may be acute or chronic. It is the most common urinary tract infection and is often seen as a nosocomial infection in hospitalized patients.

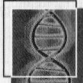

PATHOGENESIS: In most cases cystitis is secondary to infection of the lower urinary tract. Factors related to bladder infection include the age and sex of the patient, presence of bladder calculi, bladder outlet obstruction, diabetes mellitus, immunodeficiency, prior instrumentation or catheterization, radiation therapy, and chemotherapy. The risk of cystitis is increased in females because of a short urethra, especially during pregnancy. Bladder outlet obstruction secondary to prostatic hyperplasia predisposes men to cystitis. Introduction of pathogens into the bladder may also occur during instrumentation (cystoscopy) and is particularly common in patients in whom indwelling catheters remain for prolonged periods.

Coliform bacteria are the most common cause of cystitis, mostly *Escherichia coli, Proteus vulgaris, Pseudomonas aeruginosa,* and *Enterobacter* spp. Tuberculosis of the bladder is almost always secondary to renal tuberculosis. Fungal cystitis may be seen in immunosuppressed patients. Gas-forming bacilli, usually in persons with diabetes, may produce characteristic interstitial bubbles in the lamina propria of the urinary bladder (**emphysematous cystitis).** Virtually unknown in the Western world, schistosomiasis as a cause of cystitis is common in North Africa and the Middle East, where *Schistosoma haematobium* is endemic.

PATHOLOGY: Stromal edema, hemorrhage and a neutrophilic infiltrate of variable intensity are typical of acute cystitis (Fig. 17-5). Lack of resolution of the inflammatory reaction is associated with the hallmarks of chronic inflammation, including a predominance of lymphocytes (Fig. 17-6) and fibrosis of the lamina propria. Occasionally, the mucosa of the inflamed bladder contains numerous lymphocytic follicles (**follicular cystitis**) or dense infiltrates of eosinophils (**eosinophilic cystitis**). **Granulomatous cystitis** is a feature of tuberculosis. Ova of *S. hematobium* can cause simultaneous granulomatous reactions and eosinophilic infiltrates. The specific pathological forms of chronic cystitis include:

- **Hemorrhagic cystitis:** Focal petechial mucosal hemorrhages are often seen in acute bacterial cystitis. Bleeding

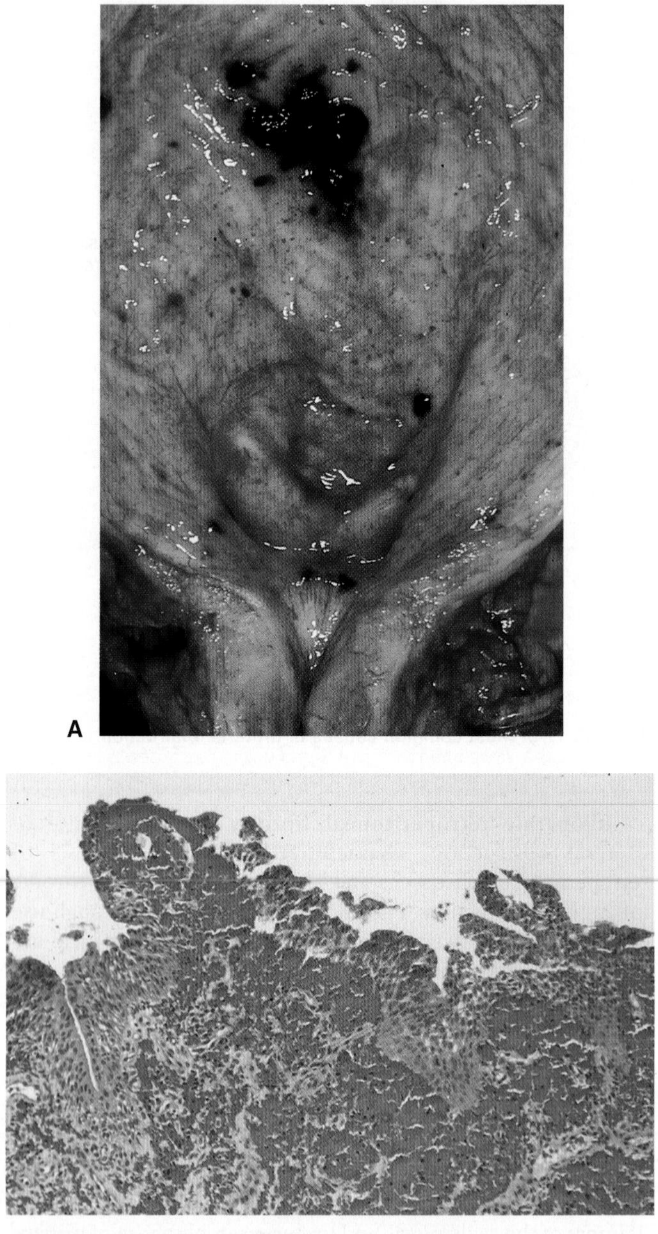

FIGURE 17-5. **Acute hemorrhagic cystitis.** The patient died 2 days after surgery, and the cystitis was obviously caused by an indwelling catheter. **A.** Several foci of hemorrhage are seen on the hyperemic bladder mucosa. **B.** Microscopic foci of mucosal hemorrhage.

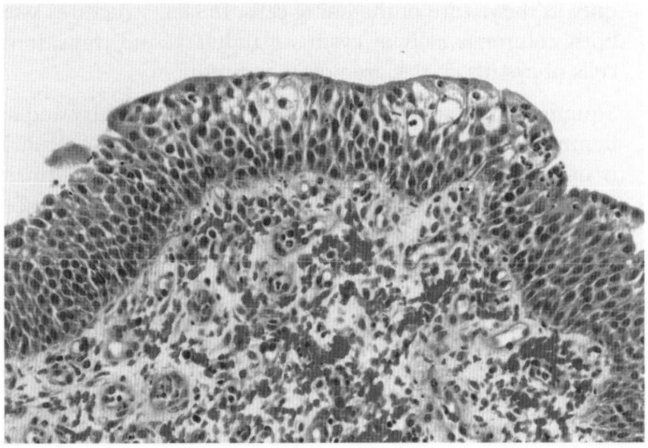

FIGURE 17-6. **Chronic cystitis.** A nonspecific inflammatory infiltrate composed of lymphocytes and plasma cells is present in the edematous lamina propria.

diatheses (e.g., leukemia or treatment with cytotoxic drugs) and disseminated intravascular coagulation often cause extensive hemorrhagic cystitis.

- **Ulcerative cystitis:** Chronic irritation, caused for example by indwelling catheters or traumatic cystoscopy, may lead to ulceration and focal mucosal hemorrhage. **Solitary mucosal ulcer** is also found in interstitial cystitis (see below).
- **Suppurative cystitis:** Pus may cover the bladder mucosa, fill the lumen, or permeate the wall. Suppurative cystitis may develop during local infection, but more often it is a complication of sepsis, pyelonephritis, or purulent infections secondary to bladder surgery.
- **Pseudomembranous cystitis:** Pseudomembranes (i.e., shaggy layers of necrotic, gray or yellow material) sometimes cover the mucosa of the urinary bladder. They can be removed to expose the underlying hemorrhagic ulcerated mucosa. Typically, pseudomembranous cystitis is a complication of infection that follows treatment with cytotoxic drugs, usually cyclophosphamide. Pseudomembranes consist of cell detritus, fibrin, inflammatory cells, and blood.
- **Calcific cystitis:** This form of chronic inflammation is typically found in schistosomiasis. Calcification of ova produces encrustations of the bladder wall similar to grains of sand. These grains gradually coalesce and transform the entire urinary bladder into a calcified rigid vessel.

CLINICAL FEATURES: Virtually all patients with acute or chronic cystitis complain of excessive urinary frequency, painful urination (**dysuria**), and lower abdominal or pelvic discomfort. Examination of urine usually reveals inflammatory cells and the causative agent can be identified by urine culture. Most cases of cystitis respond well to treatment with antimicrobial agents.

CHRONIC INTERSTITIAL CYSTITIS: This disorder of unknown cause typically affects middle-aged women and features transmural inflammation of the bladder wall, which is occasionally associated with mucosal ulceration ***(Hunner ulcer)*** (Fig. 17-7). Chronic inflammation, including increased numbers of mast cells, and fibrosis are commonly observed in the mucosa and muscularis. A Hunner ulcer displays an intense acute inflammatory reaction.

The most common symptoms of chronic interstitial cystitis are long-standing suprapubic pain, frequency, and urgency, with or without hematuria. At cystoscopy, mucosal edema, focal petechiae, and irregular hemorrhagic areas are characteristic, most often in the dome and posterior wall. Urine cultures are usually negative. The disease is typically persistent and refractory to all forms of therapy

MALAKOPLAKIA (from the Greek, malakos, *soft; plax, plaque): An uncommon inflammatory disorder of unknown etiology, malakoplakia is identified by the accumulation of characteristic macrophages.* The disorder, originally described in the bladder, has since been seen in numerous other sites, both within and outside the urinary tract. Malakoplakia is found in all age groups, the peak frequency being in the fifth to seventh decades. There is a marked female preponderance, regardless of the site.

Malakoplakia is often associated with urinary tract infection by *E. coli,* although a direct causal relationship is dubious. A clinical background of immunosuppression, chronic infections or cancer is common.

PATHOLOGY: Malakoplakia is characterized by soft, yellow plaques on the mucosal surface of the bladder (Fig. 17-8). Histologically, the most striking feature is a chronic inflammatory cell infiltrate composed predominantly of large macrophages with abundant, eosinophilic cytoplasm containing periodic acid–Schiff (PAS)-positive granules (von Hansemann cells). Some of these macrophages exhibit laminated, basophilic calcospherites, termed **Michaelis-Gutmann bodies**. Ultrastructurally, these granules are engorged lysosomes that contain fragments of bacteria, suggesting that malakoplakia may reflect an acquired defect in lysosomal degradation. The Michaelis-Gutmann bodies result from calcium salt deposition in these enlarged lysosomes.

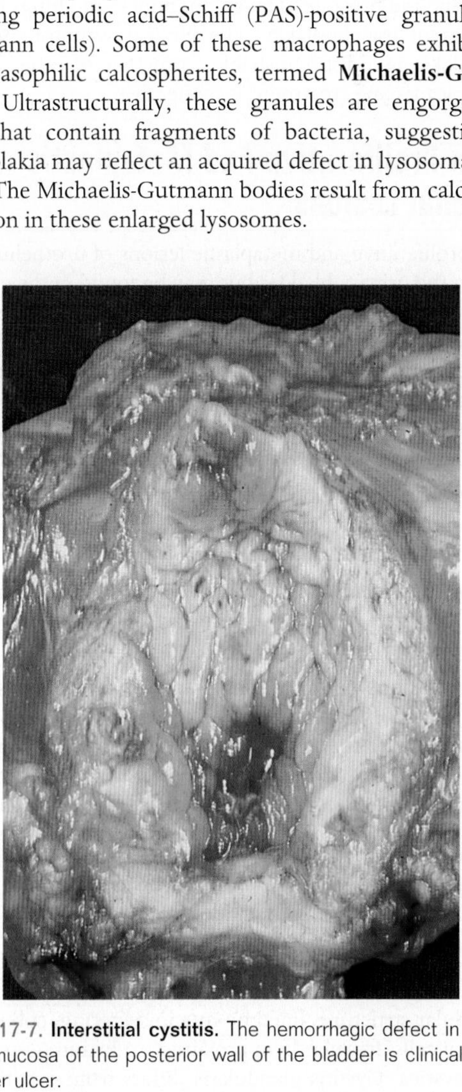

FIGURE 17-7. **Interstitial cystitis.** The hemorrhagic defect in the edematous mucosa of the posterior wall of the bladder is clinically known as Hunner ulcer.

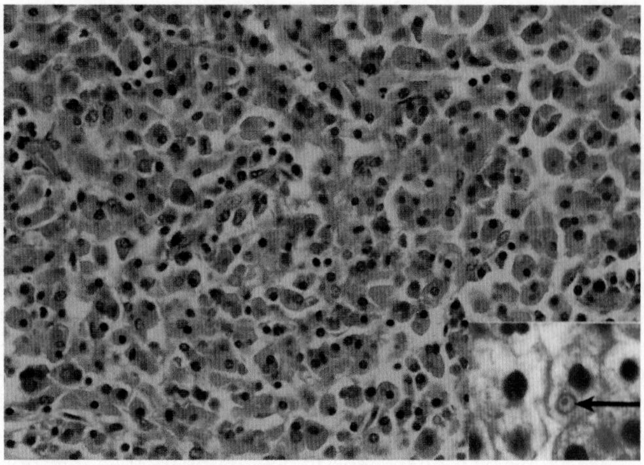

FIGURE 17-8. **Malakoplakia.** Inflammatory cells are composed principally of macrophages, with fewer lymphocytes. *(inset)* A Michaelis-Gutmann body (*arrow*) is seen at high magnification.

The urinary bladder is the most common site of malakoplakia, with half of cases occurring in this organ. This enigmatic disorder has also been reported in other regions of the genitourinary system, including the kidney, renal pelvis, ureter, testis, epididymis, and prostate. The colon, bones, and lungs have also been sites of malakoplakia. The clinical symptomatology of malakoplakia is indistinguishable from that of other forms of chronic cystitis and treatment is ineffective.

Benign Proliferative And Metaplastic Urothelial Lesions

Benign proliferative and metaplastic lesions of urothelium occur mostly in the urinary bladder but may be found in the entire urinary tract. These nonneoplastic lesions are characterized by hyperplasia or by combined hyperplasia and metaplasia (Fig. 17-9). They are found mostly in association with chronic inflammation caused by urinary tract infections, calculi, neurogenic bladder, and (rarely) bladder exstrophy. They are also occasionally observed in the absence of any preexisting inflammatory condition.

- **Brunn buds** are bulbous invaginations of the surface urothelium into the lamina propria. They are found in over 85% of bladders and are considered normal variants of the urothelium.
- **Brunn nests** are similar to Brunn buds, but the urothelial cells have detached from the surface and are seen within the lamina propria.
- **Cystic lesions of the urinary bladder** (**cystitis cystica**) appear as fluid- filled grouped cysts. Similar cysts can be seen in the urethra or the ureter (**urethritis cystica, ureteritis cystica**) (Fig. 17-10). Cystitis cystica is common, being found histologically in 60% of otherwise normal bladders. These cysts may become large enough to be apparent on cystoscopy. Histologically, all these lesions correspond to cystic Brunn nests and are lined by normal transitional epithelium. Eosinophilic, proteinaceous material may be present within the cyst lumina.
- **Cystitis glandularis** is a mucosal lesion characterized by glandular structures lined by mucin-secreting, columnar epithelial cells, frequently in proximity to Brunn nests and cystitis cystica. Cystitis glandularis differs from cystitis cystica only in the nature of the lining cells. In fact, structures with both columnar cells of cystitis glandularis and transitional cells of cystitis cystica are not uncommon.
- **Squamous metaplasia** is a reaction to chronic injury and inflammation, particularly when it is associated with calculi. It is now apparent that squamous metaplasia of the urinary tract, presumably associated with infections, is considerably more common than previously appreciated and is present in as many as 50% of normal adult women and 10% of men.
- **Nephrogenic metaplasia** is a lesion caused by transformation of transitional epithelium into epithelium resembling renal tubules. It is most common in the urinary bladder but is seen less often in urethra and ureter. Numerous small tubules clustered in the lamina propria produce a papillary exophytic nodule. The histogenesis is unsettled, but in some cases, the lesions seem to result from implants of detached renal tubular cells carried downstream by urine. The lesion may produce tumorlike protrusions in the urinary bladder. These may obstruct the ureters, in which case they require surgical treatment.

CLINICAL FEATURES: Proliferative and metaplastic urothelial lesions are of limited clinical significance, save that such lesions should not be confused with cancer. However, patients with these changes are at greater risk for urothelial bladder carcinoma and, in the case of cystitis glandularis, of adenocarcinoma as well. Yet there is no evidence to suggest that these lesions themselves are preneoplastic. Rather, the persistence of the injury that leads to the proliferative and metaplastic urothelial lesions is more likely the important factor in the pathogenesis of bladder cancer.

Tumors Of The Urinary Bladder

The most important facts about bladder cancer are as follows:

- The urinary bladder is the most common site of urinary tract tumors.
- Most bladder tumors occur in older patients (median age 65 years) and are rare under the age of 50 years.
- Tumors are more common in men than in women.
- Most tumors are microscopically classified as urothelial (transitional cell) neoplasms. Squamous cell carcinomas, adenocarcinomas, neuroendocrine carcinomas, and sarcomas are rare.
- Most tumors are malignant, but their aggressiveness and prognosis vary, depending on the clinical stage and microscopic grade and type of each tumor.
- Tumors are often multifocal and can occur in any part of the urinary tract lined by transitional epithelium, from the renal pelvis to the posterior urethra.
- Surgical treatment is often followed by tumor recurrence.

EPIDEMIOLOGY: Some 50,000 new cases of bladder cancer are diagnosed every year in the United States, accounting for 3% to 5% of all cancer-related deaths. Bladder cancer shows significant geographic and sex differences throughout the world. The highest frequencies are among urban whites in the United States and western Europe, whereas a low prevalence obtains in Japan and among American blacks.

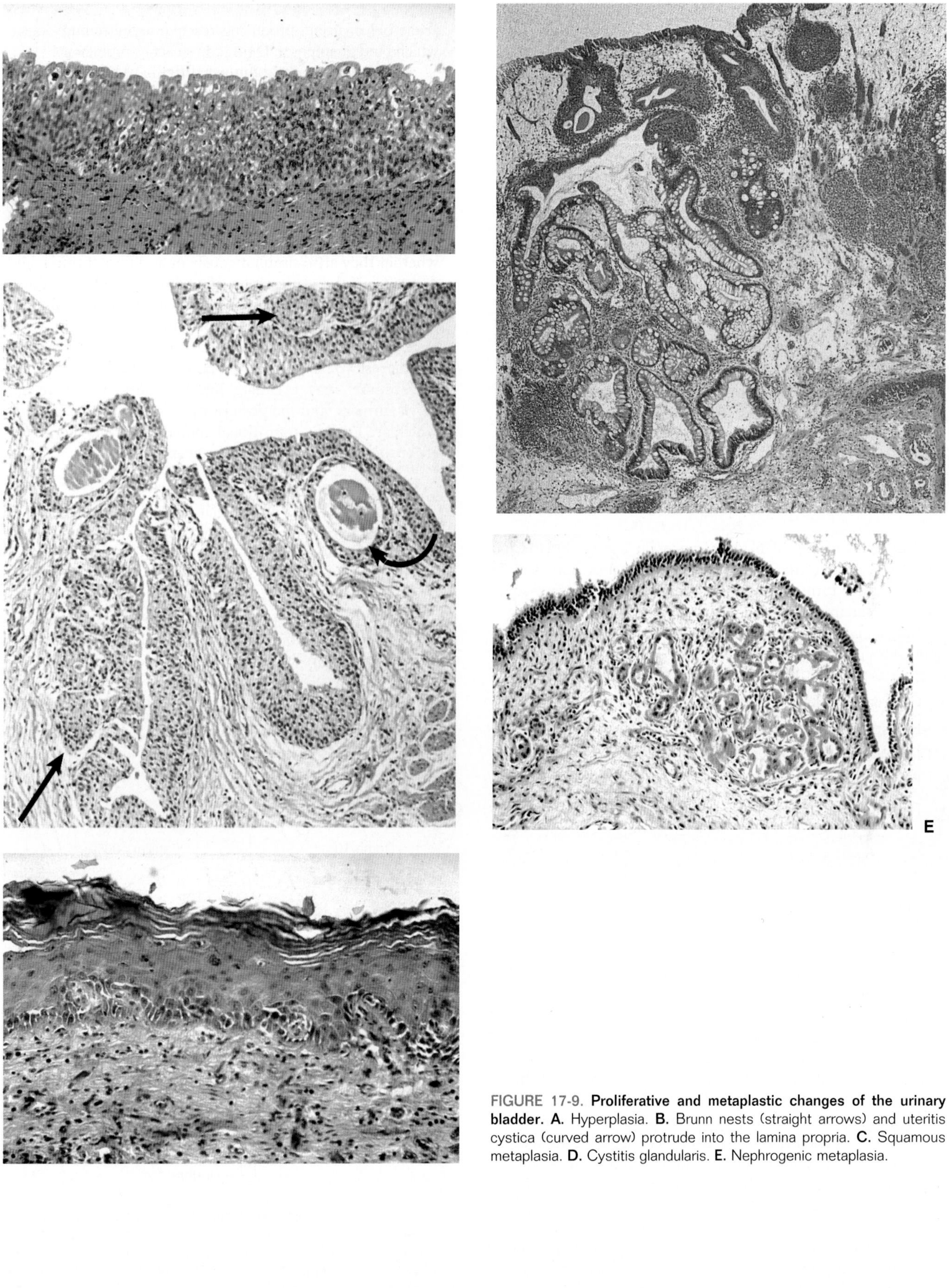

FIGURE 17-9. **Proliferative and metaplastic changes of the urinary bladder. A.** Hyperplasia. **B.** Brunn nests (straight arrows) and ureteritis cystica (curved arrow) protrude into the lamina propria. **C.** Squamous metaplasia. **D.** Cystitis glandularis. **E.** Nephrogenic metaplasia.

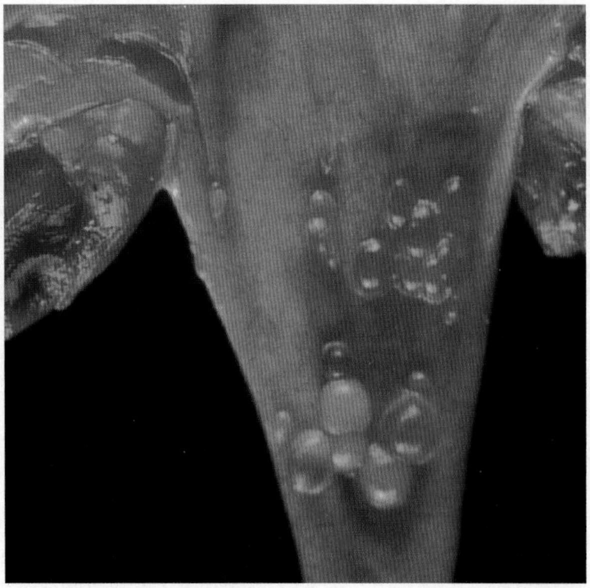

FIGURE 17-10. **Ureteritis cystica.** The mucosa of the proximal ureter exhibits small cystic structures.

A high incidence of bladder cancer in Egypt, Sudan, and other African countries is due to endemic schistosomiasis. In 70% of cases, tumors complicating schistosomiasis are squamous cell carcinomas.

Bladder cancer may be encountered at any age, but most patients (80%) are 50 to 80 years old. Men are affected three times as often as women. The most important risk factors are:

- Cigarette smoking (four-fold increased risk)
- Industrial exposure to azo dyes
- Infection with *S. haematobium*
- Drugs, such as cyclophosphamide and analgesics
- Radiation therapy (cervical, prostate, or rectal cancer)

PATHOGENESIS: The association of bladder cancer with occupational exposure to certain organic chemicals among workers in the German aniline dye industry was described in 1895 and was subsequently confirmed in similar workers in the United States. This was one of the first occupational cancers known. Later, increased risk of bladder cancer was noted in the leather, rubber, paint, and organic chemical industries. Improved industrial hygiene has reduced this risk. *Today, polycyclic hydrocarbons from cigarette smoke are the most important risk factor for urinary bladder carcinoma.*

A role for chemicals in bladder cancer has been strengthened by the demonstration that administration of β-naphthylamine, to which the dye industry workers were exposed, produces bladder cancer in dogs. The metabolism of naphthylamines explains their organ specificity. Arylamines are conjugated with glucuronic acid in the liver, after which the conjugates are excreted in the urine. In the bladder, β-glucuronidase hydrolyzes the glucuronic acid conjugate at the acidic pH of urine, producing reactive arylnitrenium ions, which bind guanines in DNA, and so act as mutagens.

Specific cytogenetic abnormalities have been observed in 50% of bladder cancers. These include most often deletion of chromosome 9 or its short or long arm (9p- or 9q-) and deletions of 11p, 13p, 14q, or 17p. Chromosomal deletions in 9p, which contains the **tumor-suppressor gene *p16***, are the only consistent finding in low grade papillary tumors and flat carcinomas in situ. Deletions in 17p, the site of the ***p53* gene**, are often found in invasive bladder cancers.

There is evidence that multiple bladder tumors, whether they arise simultaneously or at different times, all derive from the same **clone of neoplastic cells** and thus represent seeding of additional sites within the vesical mucosa from a single original tumor. Tumor multiplicity was once regarded as a "**field effect**" on a urothelial mucosa "not at rest." This theory is supported by the fact that identical tumors may originate simultaneously in the renal pelvis, ureters, and the posterior part of the urethra, all of which are lined by transitional epithelium. Thus the "field effect theory" cannot be dismissed entirely.

PATHOLOGY: Epithelial tumors, most of which are urothelial carcinomas, constitute more than 98% of all primary bladder tumors. Neoplastic transitional cell epithelial lesions arising from the bladder mucosa comprise a spectrum that at one end includes benign papillomas and low-grade exophytic papillary carcinomas and at the other, invasive transitional cell carcinomas and highly malignant tumors (Fig. 17-11). Other tumors listed in Table 17-1 are less common.

Urothelial (Transitional Cell) Papilloma Is a Benign Lesion

Urothelial papilloma of the urinary bladder is uncommon and is often encountered incidentally or after painless hematuria.

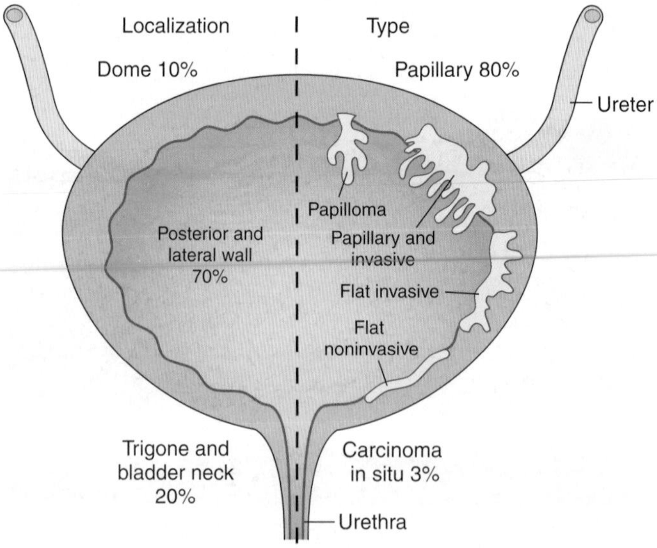

FIGURE 17-11. **Urothelial neoplasms.** Most tumors occur in the urinary bladder and are classified histologically as urothelial (transitional cell) carcinomas (TCCs). Ureters and the posterior urethra are also lined by transitional epithelium and can give rise to TCC. TCCs can be flat, papillary, papillary and invasive, or simply invasive. Benign transitional cell papillomas are rare.

TABLE 17-1

Tumors of Urinary Bladder

Urothelial cell papilloma Exophytic papilloma Inverted papilloma
Urothelial carcinoma in situ
Papillary urothelial carcinoma, low grade or high grade
Squamous cell carcinoma
Adenocarcinoma
Neuroendocrine (small cell) carcinoma
Carcinosarcoma
Sarcoma

Papillomas make up 2% to 3% of bladder epithelial tumors and occur most frequently in men above the age of 50 years. Two forms are classical exophytic papilloma and inverted papilloma.

Exophytic papilloma features papillary fronds lined by transitional epithelium that is virtually indistinguishable from normal urothelium. Tumors that meet this criterion are uncommon, and have only recently been accepted as papillomas rather than low-grade urothelial carcinomas. On cystoscopy, most patients show single lesions, 2 to 5 cm in diameter, although multiple papillomas are not unusual. Recurrent exophytic papillomas are common (70%), and invasive carcinoma develops in 7% of patients.

Transitional cell papillomas are not malignant, but they arise in a mucosa that is not at rest. Evolving tumors may be seen on repeated examinations for years. In most cases, "recurrences" represent new tumors that develop elsewhere in the urinary bladder.

Inverted papillomas are rare and typically present as nodular mucosal lesions in the urinary bladder, usually in the trigone area. They have also been observed in renal pelvis, ureter, and urethra. Inverted papillomas are covered by normal urothelium, from which cords of transitional epithelium descend into the lamina propria. These lesions are more frequent in men, with a peak incidence in the sixth and seventh decades. Hematuria of recent onset is the usual clinical presentation.

Urothelial Carcinoma in Situ Is Confined to Flat Urothelium

The term ***carcinoma in situ*** *is reserved for full-thickness, malignant changes confined to flat urothelium in nonpapillary bladder mucosa.* The lesion is characterized by a urothelium of variable thickness that shows cellular atypia of the entire mucosa, from the basal layer to the surface (Fig. 17-12). Atypia features nuclear changes, including enlargement, hyperchromatism, irregular shape, prominent nucleoli, and coarse chromatin. Occasional multinucleated cells are present. A disorganized appearance reflecting variation in nuclear polarity is a constant feature.

In one third of cases, carcinoma in situ of the bladder is associated with subsequent invasive carcinoma. In turn, most invasive transitional cell carcinomas arise from carcinoma in situ rather than from papillary transitional cell cancers. Confined to the mucosal surface, the in situ lesion appears most often as multiple, red, velvety, flat patches topographically close to exophytic papillary transitional cell carcinoma (see below). Concurrent involvement with in situ cancer elsewhere in the bladder or in the ureters, urethra, and prostatic ducts is common. Carcinoma in

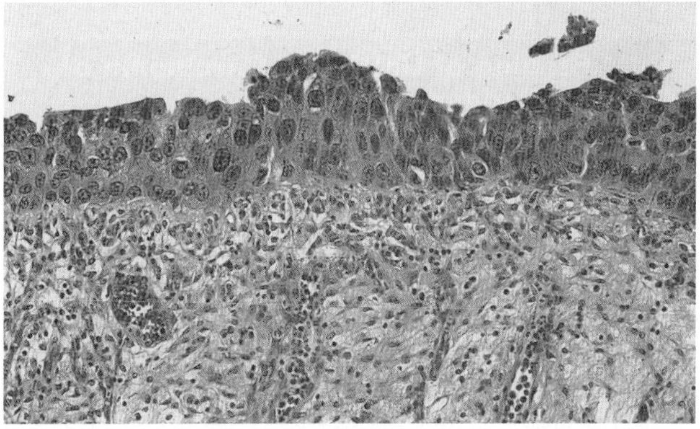

FIGURE 17-12. **Urothelial carcinoma in situ.** The urothelial mucosa shows nuclear pleomorphism and lack of polarity from the basal layer to the surface, without evidence of maturation.

situ is often multifocal at the time of discovery, or similar lesions may develop shortly thereafter. When confined to the bladder, transitional cell carcinoma in situ is currently treated with intravesical chemotherapy agents or Bacille Calmette-Guérin (BCG). Patients are followed closely. Radical surgery is performed only when repeat biopsy indicates progression (bladder wall invasion or prostate involvement). However, a growing respect for the aggressiveness of bladder carcinoma in situ has prompted some to advocate radical cystectomy for such lesions.

Urothelial Carcinoma Ranges from Superficial Papillary to Deeply Invasive

Bladder cancers vary from exophytic, without invasion to flat and deeply penetrating.

PATHOLOGY: Papillary cancer arises most frequently from the lateral or posterior bladder walls. At cystoscopy, tumors may be small, delicate, low-grade papillary lesions limited to the mucosal surface or larger, higher-grade, solid invasive masses that are often ulcerated (Fig. 17-13). Papillary and exophytic cancers tend to be better differentiated; infiltrating tumors are usually more anaplastic.

Bladder cancers are staged according to the TNM classification system (Table 17-2; Fig. 17-14). In order of decreasing frequency, metastases of bladder cancer occur in regional and periaortic lymph nodes, liver, lung, and bone.

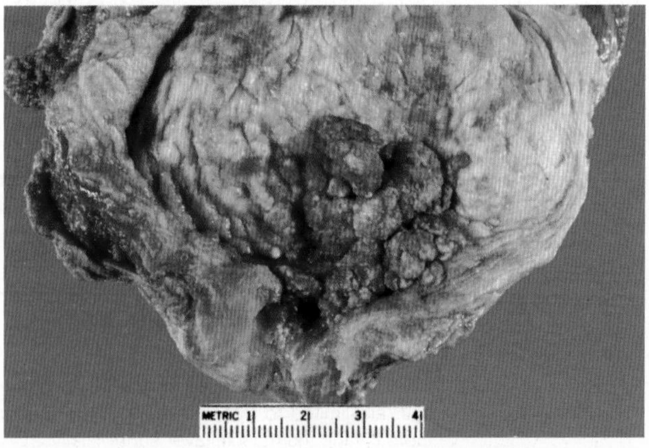

FIGURE 17-13. **Urothelial carcinoma of the urinary bladder.** A large exophytic tumor is situated above the bladder neck.

TABLE 17-2

TNM Staging of Urothelial Carcinoma of Urinary Bladder

T—Primary tumor	
T0	No grossly visible tumor
Ta	Noninvasive papillary carcinoma
Tis	Carcinoma in situ
T1	Invasion of the lamina propria
T2	Invasion of the muscularis propria
T2a	Superficial invasion of the muscularis (inner half)
T2b	Invasion of deep muscle (outer half)
T3	Invasion of the perivesical tissue
T4	Extravesical spread into adjacent organs or distant metastases
N—Regional lymph nodes	
N0	No lymph node involvement
N1	Single lymph node metastasis
N2, N3	More lymph nodes involved
M—Distant metastases	
M0	No metastases
M1	Distant metastases

Histologically, these carcinomas are classified as low grade papillary urothelial carcinomas or high grade papillary urothelial carcinomas. (Fig. 17-15A–D):

- **Low grade papillary urothelial carcinoma:** Papillary projections are lined by neoplastic transitional epithelium with minimal architectural and cytologic atypia. The cells are moderately hyperchromatic with minimal nuclear pleomorphism and mitotic activity. Papillae are long and delicate and fusion of papillae is focal and limited. In about 10% of cases there is invasion of the lamina propria or into the muscle layer of the bladder (muscularis propria).
- **High grade papillary urothelial carcinoma:** These tumors show significant nuclear hyperchromasia and pleomorphism. The epithelium is disorganized and there are mitoses in all layers. Approximately 80% of all high grade tumors show invasion into the lamina propria, and less often into the muscularis propria or through the entire thickness of the bladder wall.

A small minority of urothelial tumors are histologically intermediate between benign papillomas and low grade papillary urothelial carcinomas. Such lesions are classified as potentially malignant and are termed **papillary urothelial neoplasms of low malignant potential** (PUNLMP). These are usually larger than papillomas but do not show the architectural and cytologic atypia of low grade carcinomas. Like low grade carcinoma, PUNLMP may recur or in some instances progress to a higher grade tumor.

CLINICAL FEATURES: Urothelial carcinoma of the bladder typically manifests as sudden **hematuria** and less frequently as **dysuria.** Cystoscopy reveals single or multiple tumors. At the time of initial presentation, 85% of tumors are confined to the urinary bladder, and 15% have regional or distant metastases. Papillary lesions limited to the mucosa (stage T0) or lamina propria (stage T1) are commonly treated conservatively by transurethral resection. Radical cystectomy is done for patients whose tumors show muscle invasion, and occasionally for advanced-stage tumors.

The probability of tumor extension and subsequent recurrence correlates with a number of factors:

- Large size
- High stage
- High grade
- Presence of multiple tumors
- Vascular or lymphatic invasion
- Urothelial dysplasia (including carcinoma in situ) at other sites in the bladder

The estimated 5-year survival of patients with T0 and T1 tumors is 80%, T2 60%, T3 30% to 50%, and T4 less than 20%. Noninvasive or superficially invasive transitional cell tumors are

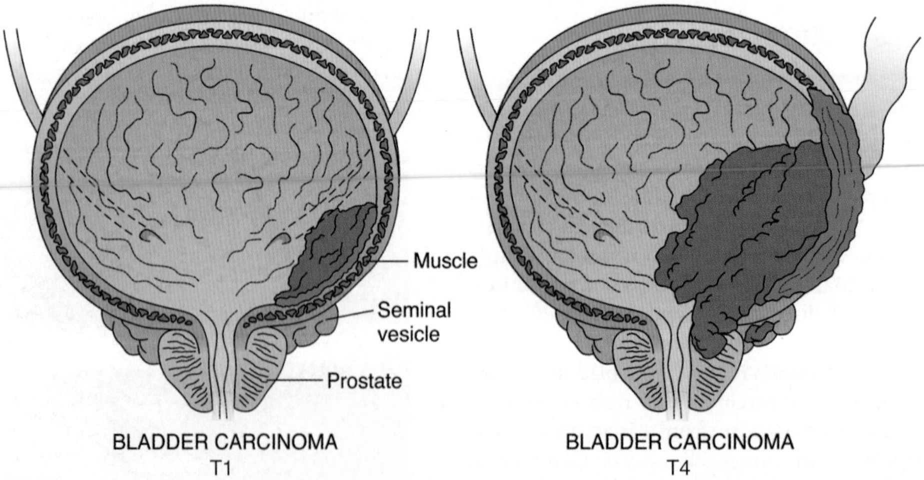

FIGURE 17-14. **Staging of urothelial carcinoma of the urinary bladder.** Stage T0 tumors (carcinoma in situ) are limited to the epithelium of the mucosa. T1 tumors show invasion of the lamina propria. T2 tumors invade the muscle layer superficially. T3 tumors invade the perivesical tissue. T4 tumors invade into the adjacent organs or show local and distant metastases. (See Table 17-2 for classification of urothelial carcinoma.)

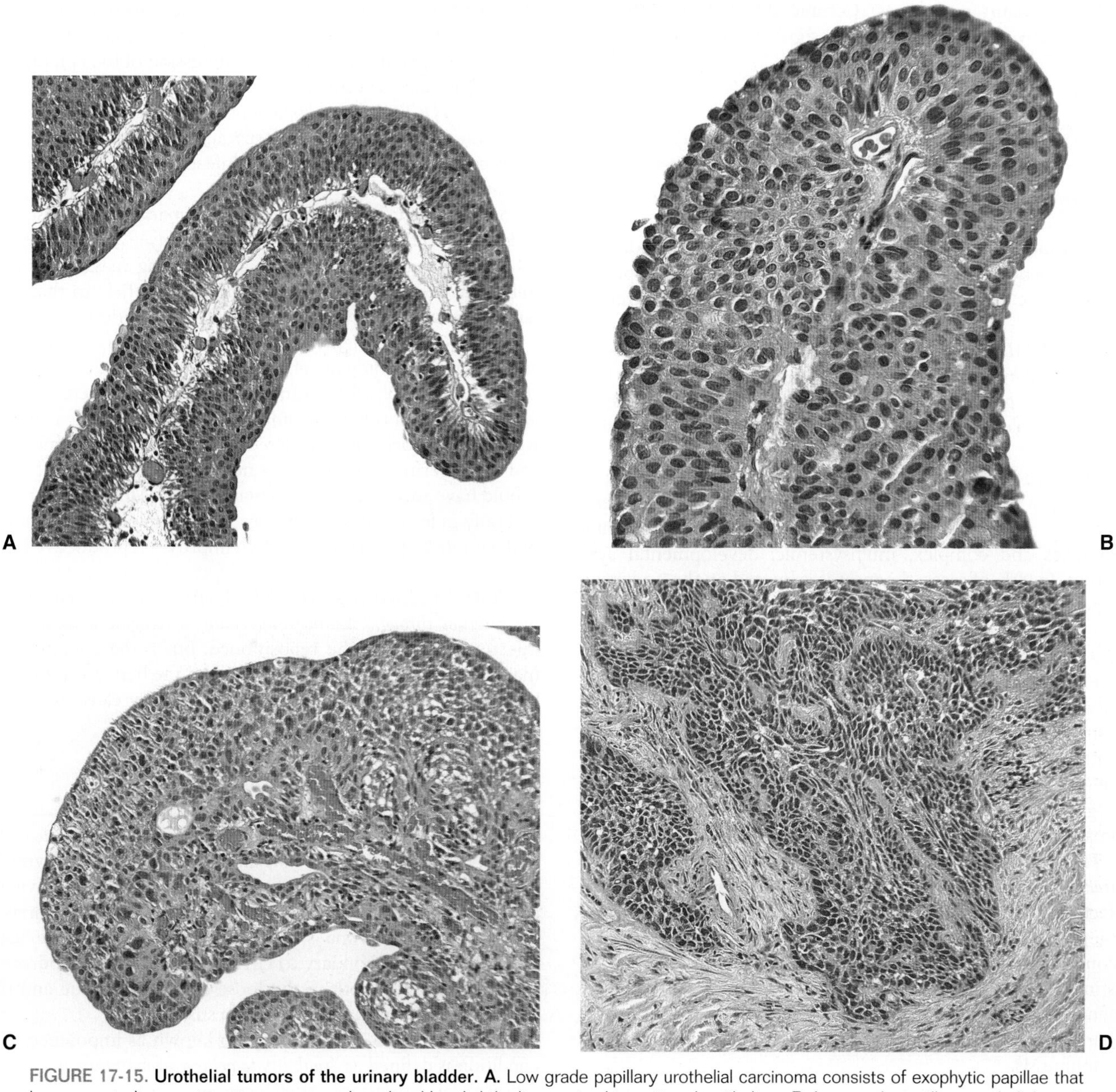

FIGURE 17-15. **Urothelial tumors of the urinary bladder. A.** Low grade papillary urothelial carcinoma consists of exophytic papillae that have a central connective tissue core and are lined by slightly disorganized transitional epithelium. **B.** Low grade papillary urothelial carcinoma at higher magnification shows mild architectural and cytologic atypia. **C.** High grade papillary urothelial carcinoma shows prominent architectural disorganization of the epithelium which contains cells with pleomorphic hyperchromatic nuclei. **D.** Invasive high grade papillary urothelial carcinoma consists of irregular nests of hyperchromatic cells invading into the muscularis.

treated conservatively, even though as many as 30% of such tumors may eventually exhibit extension. Tumor invasion into the muscle layer and beyond worsens the prognosis. However, recent advances in chemotherapy have significantly improved treatment outcome. The most common causes of death are uremia (from obstruction of the urinary outflow tract) and carcinomatosis.

Nonurothelial Forms of Bladder Cancer are Rare

Squamous cell carcinoma of the bladder develops in foci of squamous metaplasia, usually due to schistosomiasis. Virtually all patients with this tumor demonstrate bladder wall invasion at the time of initial presentation and thus have a poor prognosis.

Adenocarcinoma accounts for only 1% of all malignant tumors of the bladder. It originates from foci of cystitis glandularis or intestinal metaplasia or from remnants of urachal epithelium in the bladder dome. Most bladder adenocarcinomas are deeply invasive at the time of initial presentation and are not curable.

Neuroendocrine carcinoma, resembling small cell lung carcinoma, is sometimes seen in the urinary bladder. The tumor is highly malignant and has a poor prognosis.

Rhabdomyosarcoma, typically of the embryonal type, manifests most commonly in children as **sarcoma botryoides** (i.e., edematous, mucosal, polypoid masses that have been likened to a cluster of grapes). Combined treatment with radiation therapy and chemotherapy has greatly increased survival rates.

PENIS, URETHRA, AND SCROTUM

Congenital Disorders Of The Penis

Developmental anomalies of the penis include rare conditions such as agenesis, occasional abnormalities such as hypoplasia, and the more frequent anomalies that involve the penile urethra and prepuce.

HYPOSPADIAS: This term refers to a congenital anomaly in which the urethra opens on the underside (ventral) of the penis, so that the meatus is proximal to its normal glandular location. It results from incomplete closure of the urethral folds of the urogenital sinus.

Hypospadias has a frequency of 1 in 350 male neonates. Most cases are sporadic but a familial occurrence has been noted. It also shows an association with other urogenital anomalies and complex, multisystemic, developmental syndromes. In 90% of cases, the meatus is located on the underside of the glans or the corona. Less often it is found along the midshaft of the penis, in the scrotum, and even in the perineum. Surgical repair is usually uncomplicated.

EPISPADIAS: In this rare congenital anomaly the urethra opens on the upper side (dorsal) of the penis. In the most common form of epispadias, the entire penile urethra is open along the entire shaft. Severe epispadias may be associated with bladder exstrophy (see Fig. 17-4). In its mildest form, the defect is limited to the glandular urethra. Surgical treatment of epispadias is more complicated than that of hypospadias.

PHIMOSIS: The orifice of the prepuce may be too narrow to allow retraction over the glans penis. Phimosis predisposes the penis to infections. If a narrow prepuce is forcefully retracted, it may strangulate the glans and impede the outflow of venous blood, a condition termed **paraphimosis**. Congenital phimosis must be distinguished from acquired phimosis, which is usually a consequence of recurrent infections or trauma of the prepuce in uncircumcised men. Circumcision cures both phimosis and paraphimosis.

Scrotal Masses

Scrotal masses and conditions that lead to scrotal swelling or enlargement often reflect abnormalities of testicular, epididymal, and scrotal development. Clinical problems related to these pathologic conditions are most often encountered in children but may be found in adults (Figure 17-16A–D).

HYDROCELE: This term refers to a collection of serous fluid in the scrotal sac between the two layers of the tunica vaginalis. The cavity is lined by mesothelium. Hydrocele may be congenital or acquired.

Congenital hydrocele reflects a patent processus vaginalis testis or its incomplete obliteration. It is the most common cause of scrotal swelling in infants and is often associated with inguinal hernia.

Acquired hydrocele in adults is secondary to some other disease affecting the scrotum, such as infection, tumor, or trauma. The cause cannot be found. The diagnosis is made by ultrasound or by transluminating the fluid in the cavity. Hydrocele is a benign condition that disappears once the causal disease has been eliminated. However, long-standing hydrocele may cause testicular atrophy or compression of the epididymis, or the fluid may become infected and lead to **periorchitis.**

HEMATOCELE: An accumulation of blood between the layers of tunica vaginalis may develop after trauma or hemorrhage into a hydrocele. Testicular tumors and infections may also lead to a hematocele.

SPERMATOCELE: This mass is a cyst formed from protrusions of widened efferent ducts of the rete testis or epididymis. It manifests as a hilar paratesticular nodule or a fluctuating mass filled with milky fluid. The cyst is lined by cuboidal epithelium that contains spermatozoa in various stages of degeneration.

VARICOCELE: Dilation of testicular veins appears as a nodularity on the lateral side of the scrotum. Most are asymptomatic and are discovered during physical examination of infertile men. Massive varicocele is mentioned in clinical texts as resembling a "bag of worms." Varicocele is considered a common cause of infertility and oligospermia, although it is not clear why dilation of veins should have such effects. Testicular atrophy is found only rarely and only in long-standing disease. Surgical resection by ligation of the internal spermatic vein often improves reproductive function.

SCROTAL INGUINAL HERNIA: Protrusion of the intestines into the scrotum through the inguinal canal is recognized as a mass. Intestinal loops may be repositioned, but if the condition remains untreated, adhesions develop and the hernia can only be repaired surgically. Long-standing hernia may cause testicular atrophy.

Circulatory Disturbances

SCROTAL EDEMA: Lymph or serous fluid may accumulate in the scrotum due to obstruction of lymphatic or venous drainage. **Lymphedema** from lymphatic obstruction can be caused by pelvic or abdominal tumors, surgical scars, or infections such as filariasis. **Transudation** of plasma is common in patients who have heart failure, anasarca secondary to cirrhosis or nephrotic syndrome. Fluid accumulates both in the loose connective tissue and the cavity lined by the tunica vaginalis testis.

ERECTILE DYSFUNCTION: Also known as impotence, this condition is defined as *"inability to achieve or maintain an erection sufficient for satisfactory sexual performance."* Its prevalence increases with age, from 20% at the age of 40 years to 50% by the age of 70 years.

Erection requires adequate filling of the penile corpora cavernosa and spongiosa with blood. The tumescence of the penis is the end result of a complex interaction of mental, neural, hormonal, and vascular factors. Filling of these vascular spaces depends on nitric oxide (NO•)-mediated relaxation of vascular smooth muscle cells in the erectile cylinders. Since NO• release is related to cyclic guanosine 3′,5′-monophosphate (cGMP), drugs that inhibit the phosphodiesterase that degrades cGMP (e.g., sildenafil [Viagra], vardenafil hydrochloride [Levitra], tadalafil [Cialis]) are used to treat erectile dysfunction. Disorders associated with erectile dysfunction are listed in Table 17-3.

PRIAPISM: Continuous penile erection unrelated to sexual excitation is painful. Most often the cause of priapism is unknown and its treatment is ineffective. Secondary priapism may be a complication of several diseases, including (1) pelvic diseases that impede outflow of blood from the penis (e.g., pelvic tumors or hematomas, thrombosis of pelvic veins, infections); (2) hemato-

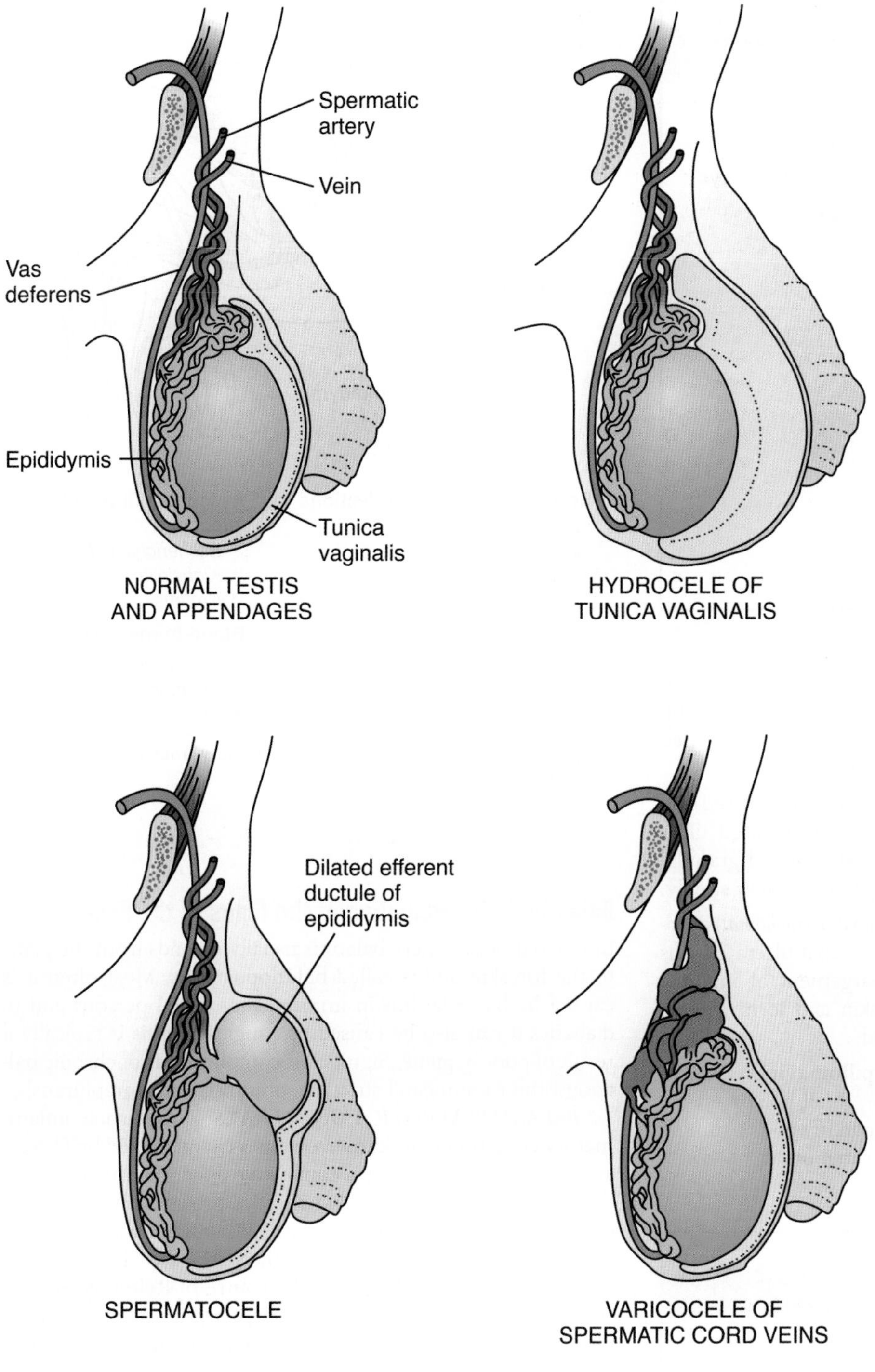

FIGURE 17-16. **Scrotal masses. A.** Normal testis. **B.** Hydrocele. **C.** Spermatocele. **D.** Varicocele.

logic disorders (e.g., sickle cell anemia, polycythemia vera, leukemia); and (3) brain and spinal cord diseases (e.g., tumors, syphilis).

Inflammatory Disorders

The most important inflammatory conditions affecting the penis are (1) sexually transmitted diseases (STDs); (2) nonspecific infections; (3) diseases of unknown etiology, such as balanitis xerotica obliterans; (4) dermatoses; and 5) dermatitis involving the shaft of the penis and scrotum (Table 17-4).

Sexually Transmitted Diseases Cause Discrete Penile Lesions

Sexually transmitted diseases (STDs) are reviewed here briefly in the context of other infections of the lower urinary tracts (Fig. 17-17) (for more detail, see Chapter 9).

- **Genital herpes** (herpes simplex virus [HSV]-2) is the most common STD affecting the glans. It manifests typically as grouped vesicles that ulcerate and transform into crusts.
- **Syphilis** *(Treponema pallidum)* manifests as a solitary, soft ulcer (**chancre**).

TABLE 17-3

Erectile Dysfunctions

Neuropsychiatric
Psychiatric disorders (e.g., depression)
Spinal cord injury
Nerve injury during surgery (e.g. pelvic or perineal surgery)
Endocrine
Hypogonadism
Pituitary diseases (e.g., hyperprolactinemia)
Hypothyroidism, Cushing syndrome, Addison disease
Vascular
Diabetic microangiopathy
Hypertension
Atherosclerosis
Drugs
Antihypertensives
Psychotropic drugs
Estrogens, anticancer drugs, etc.
Idiopathic
"Performance anxiety"
Age-related "impotence"

- **Chancroid** (*Haemophilus ducreyi*) manifests as a papule that transforms into a pustule and finally ulcerates. Shallow ulcers on the glans or the skin of the shaft are often associated with painful suppurative inguinal lymphadenitis.
- **Granuloma inguinale,** a tropical disease caused by *Calymmatobacterium granulomatis,* appears as a raised ulcer with a copious chronic inflammatory exudate and granulation tissue. Such ulcers tend to enlarge and heal very slowly.
- **Lymphogranuloma venereum** *(Chlamydia trachomatis)* appears as a small, often innocuous, vesicle that ulcerates. It is typically accompanied by tender enlargement of inguinal lymph nodes, which adhere to the skin and form sinuses draining pus and serosanguineous fluid.
- **Condylomata acuminata (human papillomavirus)** are flat-topped warts on the shaft (Fig. 17-18), small polyps on the glans and urethral meatus, or larger cauliflower-like tumors that may be confused with verrucous carcinoma.

TABLE 17-4

Inflammatory Lesions of the Penis

Sexually transmitted diseases
Herpes genitalis
Syphilis
Chancroid
Granuloma inguinale
Lymphogranuloma venereum
Human papillomavirus infections
Nonspecific infectious balanoposthitis
Bacterial, fungal, viral
Diseases of unknown etiology
Balanitis xerotica obliterans
Circinate balanitis
Plasma cell balanitis (Zoon balanitis)
Peyronie disease
Dermatitis involving the shaft of the penis and scrotum
Infectious (bacterial, viral, fungal)
Noninfectious (e.g., lichen planus, bullous skin diseases)

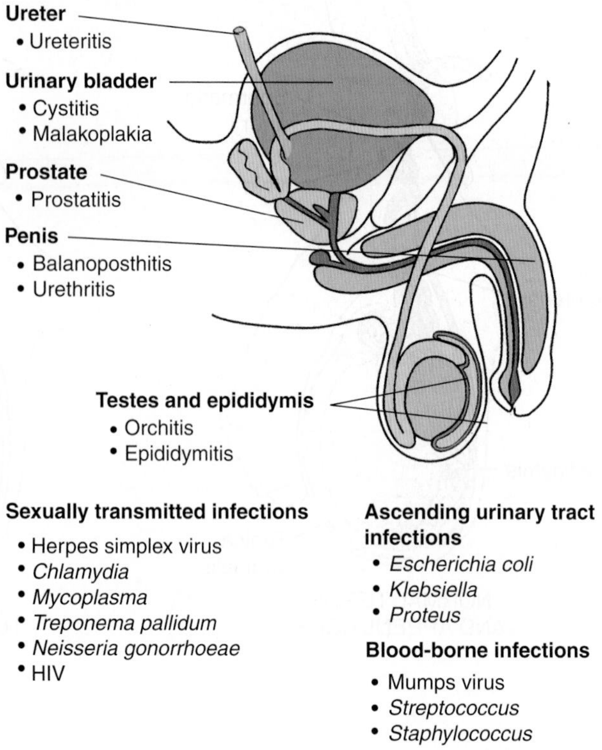

FIGURE 17-17. **Infections of the lower urinary tract and male reproductive system.**

Balanitis Is Inflammation of the Glans of the Penis

In uncircumcised men, balanitis usually extends from the glans to the foreskin and is called **balanoposthitis**. Most often it is caused by bacteria, but in immunosuppressed persons and in diabetics it can also be caused by fungi. Balanitis is typically a result of poor hygiene. Significant complications of chronic balanoposthitis are meatal stricture, phimosis, and paraphimosis.

BALANITIS XEROTICA OBLITERANS: This chronic inflammatory condition of unknown origin is characterized by fibrosis and sclerosis of subepithelial connective tissue. The affected portion of the glans is white and indurated. Fibrosis may constrict the urethral meatus or cause phimosis. This condition is equivalent to lichen sclerosus et atrophicus of the vulva (see Chapter 18).

CIRCINATE BALANITIS: In the course of **Reiter syndrome** (see below), the glans may show circular, linear or confluent, plaquelike discolorations, occasionally associated with superficial ulcerations.

PLASMA CELL BALANITIS: Also known as **Zoon balanitis,** this disease of unknown origin causes macular discoloration or painless papules on the glans. Histologically, the connective tissue shows infiltrates of plasma cells and lymphocytes and the overlying epithelium is thickened. The disease is chronic but innocuous.

DERMATOSES: Many inflammatory skin diseases may involve the penis. Such conditions are discussed in Chapter 24.

Peyronie Disease Is a Fibrous Induration of the Penis

Peyronie disease is a malady of unknown etiology characterized by focal, asymmetric fibrosis of the penile shaft. Penile curvature (penile strabismus) results, accompanied by pain during erection. The typical case is an ill-defined induration of the penile shaft in a

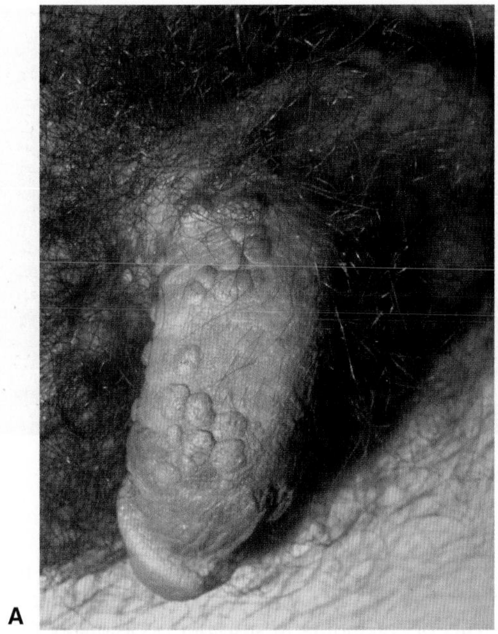

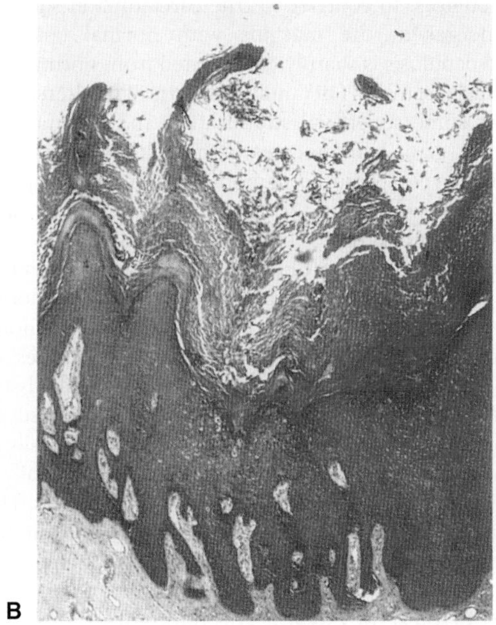

FIGURE 17-18. **Condylomata acuminata of the penis. A.** Raised, circumscribed lesions are seen on the shaft of the penis. **B.** Section of a lesion shows epidermal hyperkeratosis, parakeratosis, acanthosis, and papillomatosis.

young or middle-aged man, with no change in the overlying skin. On microscopic examination, dense fibrosis is associated with sparse, nonspecific, chronic inflammatory infiltration. Collagen focally replaces muscle in the septum of the corpus cavernosum.

Peyronie disease affects 1% of men over the age of 40, but in most instances, it is mild and does not interfere with sexual function. Severe penile curvature may be so incapacitating as to require surgery, although the outcome is not always satisfactory.

Urethritis And Related Conditions

Urethritis is inflammation of the urethra. It may be either acute or chronic.

SEXUALLY TRANSMITTED URETHRITIS: Urethritis is the most common manifestation of STDs in men, in whom it typically presents with urethral discharge. Women rarely notice distinct urethral discharge and usually complain of vaginal discharge.

Gonococcal and nongonococcal urethritis have an acute onset and are related to recent sexual intercourse. The infection manifests with a typically purulent and greenish yellow urethral discharge. Symptoms include pain or tingling at the meatus of the urethra and pain on micturition (**dysuria**). Redness and swelling of the meatus are usually seen in both sexes. Acute gonococcal and nongonococcal urethritis can both become chronic.

The diagnosis is made by identifying the causative agent. In gonococcal urethritis the discharge contains *Neisseria gonorrhoeae,* which can be identified microscopically in smears of urethral exudates. Nongonococcal urethritis is mostly caused by *Chlamydia trachomatis* or *Ureaplasma urealyticum* but may be related to a variety of other pathogens.

NONSPECIFIC INFECTIOUS URETHRITIS: Uropathogens such as E. coli and Pseudomonas can cause urethritis. Typically infection is associated with cystitis but may be related to other diseases (e.g., prostatic hyperplasia or urinary stones). In men, infectious urethritis may be the only sign of prostatitis; in women, it may be a complication of vaginitis and vulvitis. In hospitalized patients it commonly follows cystoscopy and other urologic procedures and is almost inevitable in patients with indwelling urethral catheters.

Nonspecific infectious urethritis manifests clinically with urgency and a burning sensation during urination. Usually there is no discharge, although men can express some milky fluid by "stripping" or "milking" the urethra.

URETHRAL CARUNCLES: Polypoid inflammatory lesions near the female urethral meatus produce pain and bleeding. They occur exclusively in women, mostly after menopause. The etiology and pathogenesis are unclear; prolapse of the urethral mucosa and associated chronic inflammation have been suggested as the cause.

Urethral caruncle presents as an exophytic, often ulcerated, polypoid mass, 1 to 2 cm in diameter, at or near the urethral meatus. Microscopically, it exhibits acutely and chronically inflamed granulation tissue and ulceration and hyperplasia of transitional cell or squamous epithelium. Although complex patterns of papillomatosis and occasional dysplastic epithelium may give this inflammatory lesion a superficial resemblance to carcinoma, it does not lead to cancer. Treatment is surgical excision.

REITER SYNDROME: This condition is a triad of ***urethritis, conjunctivitis, and arthritis*** *of weight-bearing joints (e.g., knee, sacroiliac and vertebral joints).* Other clinical findings encountered in variable proportions are circinate balanitis, cervicitis, and skin eruptions. Reiter syndrome tends to affect young adults with human leukocyte antigen (HLA)-B27 haplotype. Symptoms usually appear a few weeks after chlamydial urethritis or enteric infection with such pathogens as *Shigella, Salmonella, or Campylobacter.* It is thus thought to represent an inappropriate immune reaction to unknown microbial antigen(s). Symptoms usually disappear spontaneously over 3 to 6 months, but arthritis recurs in half of patients.

Tumors

Cancer Of The Urethra Arises From Squamous Or Transitional Epithelium

Urethral carcinoma is an uncommon tumor usually found in elderly women. Some penile cancers arise in the terminal part of the penile urethra.

PATHOLOGY: Most urethral cancers are squamous cell carcinomas originating in the distal urethra. Urothelial carcinoma similar to that in the bladder arises in the proximal urethra.

CLINICAL FEATURES: Urethral cancer is most frequently observed in the sixth and seventh decades. Patients present with urethral bleeding and dysuria. Despite the accessible location and associated symptoms, most tumors have spread to adjacent tissues or regional lymph nodes at the time of presentation. Radical surgery is the main therapy.

Cancer of the Penis Occurs Mostly in Uncircumcised Men

Cancer of the penis originates from the squamous mucosa of the glans and contiguous urethral meatus or the prepuce and skin covering the penile shaft.

EPIDEMIOLOGY: In the United States, invasive squamous cell carcinoma of the penis is an uncommon tumor. It accounts for less than 0.5% of all cancers in men. The average age of patients is 60 years. Penile cancer is much more common in less-developed countries: in some parts of Africa and Asia it constitutes 10% of male cancers. Since it is virtually unknown in men circumcised at birth, these geographic variations have been attributed to differences in the frequency of circumcision.

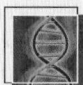

PATHOGENESIS: No single agent has been identified as the cause of penile cancer. Current interest centers on the possible influence of accumulated keratin debris and inflammatory exudate (**smegma**) that accumulate beneath the prepuce. Most patients with cancer of the penis have had phimosis since an early age, suggesting that prolonged contact between smegma and the penile epithelium may play a role. Human papillomavirus (HPV) types 16 and 18 have also been suggested as factors in the pathogenesis of penile cancer.

PATHOLOGY: Penile carcinoma occurs in a preinvasive form (carcinoma in situ) and an invasive variety.

SQUAMOUS CELL CARCINOMA IN SITU: Historically, carcinoma in situ of the penis was described in two forms: Bowen disease and erythroplasia of Queyrat.

Bowen disease appears as a sharply demarcated, erythematous or grayish white plaque on the shaft. **Erythroplasia of Queyrat** manifests as solitary or multiple, shiny, soft, erythematous plaques on the glans and foreskin.

Both of these conditions appear microscopically as **squamous cell carcinoma in situ** similar to that in other sites. The lesions show cytologic atypia of the keratinocytes of all layers of the epidermis, with parakeratosis or hyperkeratosis; papillomatosis with broad epidermal papillae; and thinning of the granular layer. By definition, the atypical keratinocytes do not invade the underlying dermis. Chronic inflammation may be present in the subjacent dermis. The frequency of progression to invasive squamous cell carcinoma remains unsettled but is estimated to be less than 10% of cases.

Bowenoid papulosis of the penis is caused by HPV and affects young, sexually active men. In contrast to the solitary lesion of Bowen disease, bowenoid papulosis appears as multiple brownish or violaceous papules. Microscopically, it resembles other variants of carcinoma in situ, but occasionally there are some differences. In contrast to true carcinoma in situ, which slowly merges at the margins with normal epithelium, bowenoid papulosis is sharply demarcated from normal epidermis and thus resembles HPV-induced warts. The altered epidermis shows some superficial stratification and maturation and may contain giant keratinocytes with multinucleated atypical nuclei. HPV type 16 can be demonstrated in 80% of patients. Virtually all lesions of bowenoid papulosis regress spontaneously and do not progress to invasive carcinoma.

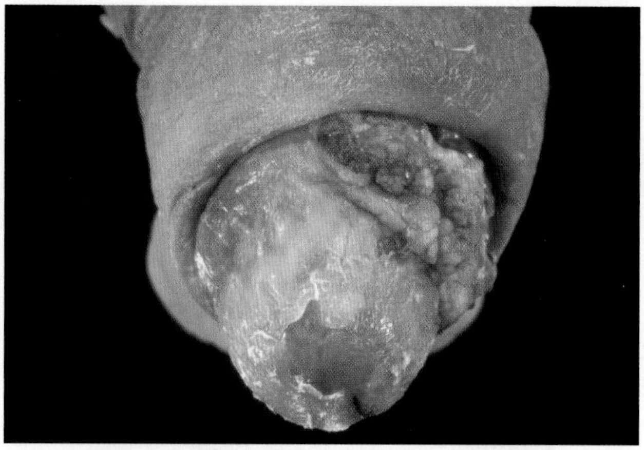

FIGURE 17-19. **Carcinoma of the penis.** This verrucous carcinoma arises on the glans and appears as an exophytic mass.

INVASIVE SQUAMOUS CELL CARCINOMA: The tumor presents as (1) an ulcer; (2) indurated crater; (3) friable hemorrhagic mass; or (4) exophytic, fungating, papillary tumor. Squamous cell carcinoma usually involves the glans or prepuce and less commonly the penile shaft. Extensive destruction of penile tissue, including the urethral meatus, is observed in neglected cases. Microscopically, it is typically a well-differentiated, focally keratinizing, squamous cell carcinoma. Invasive tumors usually have a dense, chronic inflammatory cell infiltrate in the dermis. The adjacent epidermis often shows dysplastic changes. The tumor may invade deeply along the penile shaft and spread to inguinal lymph nodes, then to iliac nodes and ultimately distant organs.

VERRUCOUS CARCINOMA: This tumor deserves to be separated from other penile cancers because it is a cytologically benign but clinically malignant exophytic squamous cell carcinoma (Fig. 17-19). It is grossly and cytologically similar to **condyloma acuminatum**, but unlike the latter, it shows local invasion. This low-grade squamous cell carcinoma usually does not metastasize and surgical removal is curative.

CLINICAL FEATURES: Most squamous cell cancers are confined to the penis at the time of initial presentation, but occult metastases to inguinal lymph nodes are not uncommon. Conversely, half of patients with enlarged regional lymph nodes do not have nodal metastases, but only reactive changes due to tumor-associated inflammation.

Survival of patients with penile cancer is related to clinical stage and, to a lesser degree, the histologic grade of the tumor. Amputation of the penis is usually necessary. Patients with superficially invasive cancer have 90% 5-year survival; inguinal lymph node metastases reduce 5-year survival to 20% to 50%, depending on the extent of spread.

Cancer of the Scrotum Was First Identified n Chimney Sweeps

In 1775 Sir Percival Pott identified scrotal cancer as an occupational disease of chimney sweeps, thereby introducing the idea of chemical carcinogenesis (see Chapters 5, 8). Pott implicated constant exposure to soot as the causative agent, but later investigators incriminated a large variety of industrial chemicals in the pathogenesis of this tumor. Industrial hygiene has improved so that scrotal cancer is today distinctly uncommon.

Squamous cell carcinoma of the scrotum typically affects older men and mostly in their sixth and seventh decades. At initial presentation, many patients show invasion of the scrotal contents and metastases to regional nodes. Therapy is surgical excision.

TESTIS, EPIDIDYMIS, AND VAS DEFERENS

Cryptorchidism

Cryptorchidism, clinically known as **undescended testis,** *is a congenital abnormality in which one or both testes are not found in their normal position in the scrotum.* It is the most common urologic condition requiring surgical treatment in infants. In 5% of male infants born at term and 30% of those born prematurely, the testes are not in the scrotum or are easily retracted. In the large majority of these infants, testes descend into the scrotum during the first year of life. Accordingly, the prevalence of cryptorchidism from the end of the first year of life into adulthood is in range of 1%. Cryptorchidism is usually unilateral but is bilateral in 30% of affected men.

PATHOGENESIS: The causes of testicular maldescent are usually unknown, but theoretically the condition could be related to (1) developmental disorders of the gonad, (2) endocrine factors, or (3) mechanical factors that prevent passage of the fetal testis through the inguinal canal. It is usually an isolated developmental disorder, but may rarely be associated with other congenital anomalies.

PATHOLOGY: Testicular descent may be arrested at any point from the abdominal cavity to the upper scrotum (Fig. 17-20). Cryptorchid testes are classified by their location as **abdominal, inguinal, or upper scrotal.** Rarely, the testes are located in unusual locations, such as perineum or calf.

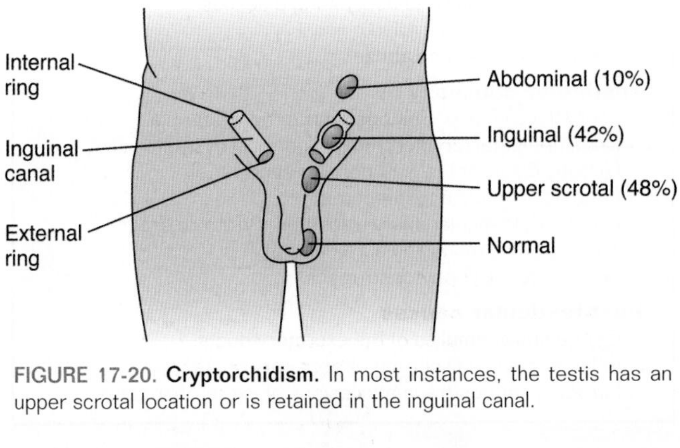

FIGURE 17-20. **Cryptorchidism.** In most instances, the testis has an upper scrotal location or is retained in the inguinal canal.

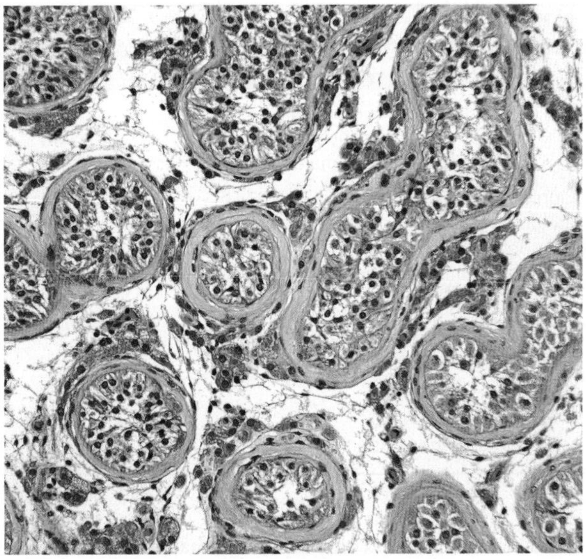

FIGURE 17-21. **Cryptorchidism.** This testis removed from a postpubertal man shows markedly thickened hyalinized basement membrane of seminiferous tubules, which show no signs of spermatogenesis.

Cryptorchid testes are smaller than normal even at an early age, and the difference between the affected and the normal testis becomes more prominent with age. Such testes appear firm, owing to parenchymal fibrosis.

The histology of cryptorchid testes varies with age. In infancy and early childhood the seminiferous tubules in the affected testes are smaller and have fewer germ cells than normal. Postpubertal testes also contain fewer germ cells than normal and spermatogenesis is limited to a minority of tubules. Hyaline thickening of tubular basement membranes and prominent stromal fibrosis are observed (Fig. 17-21). Eventually, tubules become devoid of spermatogenic cells and are entirely hyalinized. **Orchiopexy** (surgical placement of a testis into the scrotum) performed either in childhood or after puberty does not prevent the loss of seminiferous epithelium and tubules; both the untreated and the repositioned testes show no signs of spermatogenesis in half of the cases. A few adult cryptorchid testes (2%) contain atypical germ cells corresponding to carcinoma in situ.

CLINICAL FEATURES: The clinical significance of undescended testes is not related to the abnormal position of the gonad per se (patients are asymptomatic) but to an increased incidence of **infertility** and **germ cell neoplasia.** All men with bilateral cryptorchid testes have **azoospermia** and are infertile. Unilateral cryptorchidism is associated with **oligospermia**, defined as a sperm count below 20 million/mL, in 40% of cases. Although oligospermia is a cause of reduced fertility, most men with one normal testis have a reasonable chance of fathering a child. Orchiopexy done in childhood or after puberty has no effect on the sperm count. Most urologists recommend orchiopexy between the ages of 6 months and 1 year, but it is not clear whether this treatment improves the eventual sperm count.

Cryptorchidism is associated with a 20- to 40-fold greater than normal risk for testicular cancer. Conversely, 10% of patients with germ cell neoplasia have cryptorchid testes. Intra-abdominal testes are at higher risk than those retained in the inguinal canal; in turn, inguinal testes are at higher risk than those high in the scrotum. The contralateral, normally descended testis is also at risk, but the inci-

TABLE 17-5 Disorders of Sexual Differentiation
Sex chromosomal abnormalities
Klinefelter syndrome and its variants
Turner syndrome 46,XX males
Single gene defects
Adrenogenital syndromes
Androgen insensitivity syndromes
Müllerian inhibitory substance deficiency
Prenatal hormonal effects
Exogenous hormones during pregnancy
Maternal hormone-producing tumors
Idiopathic conditions
Hermaphroditism
Gonadal dysgenesis

dence of cancer in there is only four times that in normal men. Unfortunately, orchiopexy does not reduce cancer risk.

Abnormalities Of Sexual Differentiation

Disorders of gonadogenesis and the formation of external genital organs, as well as development of secondary sex characteristics, can pertain to:

- Genetic sex; the presence or absence of X and Y chromosomes
- Gonadal sex; the presence or absence of testes or ovaries
- Genital sex; the appearance of external genital organs
- Psychosocial sexual orientation

Various conditions are listed in Table 17-5. Some of these, such as Klinefelter and Turner syndromes, are discussed in Chapter 6.

HERMAPHRODITISM: *This rare developmental disorder is characterized by ambiguous genitalia in a person who has both male and female gonads.* Gonads may become ovotestes (combination of ovary and testis) or one gonad may be testis and the other ovary. Half of these patients have a female karyotype (46,XX). The others are genetic males (46,XY) or mosaics or have a missing sex chromosome(45,X).

FEMALE PSEUDOHERMAPHRODITISM: *Virilization of external genitalia may occur in genetic females (46,XX) who have normal ovaries and internal female genital organs.* The vulva may show fusion into scrotal folds. Clitoromegaly is usually associated. This phenotype is most often seen in the adrenogenital syndrome caused by 21-hydroxylase deficiency (see Chapter 21). Lack of this enzyme leads to excess androgen production in the adrenal gland during fetal life, and the ambiguous genitalia are seen at birth. Excess androgens in a pregnant woman can have the same effects on the external genitalia of the baby.

A 46,XX karyotype is found in 1 of 25 patients with classical signs of Klinefelter syndrome. These **46,XX males** carry on one of the X chromosomes the locus for the sex-determining region of chromosome Y (SRY). It is not known how this translocation occurs, but it is probably related to the crossover that occurs during male meiosis.

MALE PSEUDOHERMAPHRODITISM: *A spectrum of congenital disorders affects genetically male persons who have a normal 46,XY karyotype.* The gonads are cryptorchid testes, but external genitalia appear feminine or ambiguously female with signs of virilization. Male pseudohermaphroditism occurs most often in **androgen insensitivity syndromes** due to a congenital deficiency of the androgen receptor, also known as **testicular feminization syndrome.**

Male Infertility

Infertility is empirically defined as inability to conceive after 1 year of coital activity with the same sexual partner without contraception. Some 15% of couples are childless in the United States, but the true prevalence of infertility is difficult to assess because it is confounded by various cultural and social determinants. The causes of infertility can be found in the male partner in 20% of cases, in the female in 40%, and in both partners in 20%. In the remaining 20% of infertile couples, a cause cannot be identified. The causes of male infertility are listed in Table 17-6 and illustrated in Figure 17-22.

Supratesticular causes of infertility are factors that influence or regulate hormonal and metabolic aspects of spermatogenesis. The best examples are injuries of the hypothalamic–pituitary area. Infertility can result from transection of the pituitary stalk, destruction of the hypothalamus by a brain tumor, or pressure on the pituitary by a craniopharyngioma. A pituitary tumor secreting prolactin (prolactinoma) may act as a mass lesion that destroys the gonadotropin-secreting pituitary cells or compresses the pituitary stalk. It also secretes prolactin, which suppresses spermatogenesis.

Testicular infertility, the most common variety of male infertility, is related to pathologic changes in the testis. A male infertility (andrologic) work-up includes urological examination, sonography, semen analysis, hormonal studies, and in some cases testicular biopsy.

Post-testicular infertility refers to blockage of the excretory ducts through which sperm reach the urethra. Chronic infections of the epididymis or vas deferens are often responsible. Previous trauma or congenital atresia are the causes.

TABLE 17-6 Causes of Male Infertility
Supratesticular causes
Disorders of the hypothalamic-pituitary-gonadal axis
Endocrine disease of the adrenal, thyroid; diabetes
Metabolic disorders
Major organ diseases (e.g., renal, hepatic, cardiopulmonary diseases)
Chronic infectious and debilitating diseases (e.g., tuberculosis, AIDS)
Drugs and substance abuse
Testicular causes
Idiopathic: hypospermatogenesis or azoospermia
Developmental (cryptorchidism, gonadal dysgenesis)
Genetic disorders (e.g. Klinefelter syndrome)
Orchitis (immune and infectious)
Iatrogenic testicular injury (radiation, cytotoxic drugs)
Trauma of the testis and surgical injury
Environmental (? phytoestrogens)
Post-testicular causes
Congenital anomalies of the excretory ducts
Inflammation and scarring of excretory ducts
Iatrogenic or posttraumatic lesions of excretory ducts

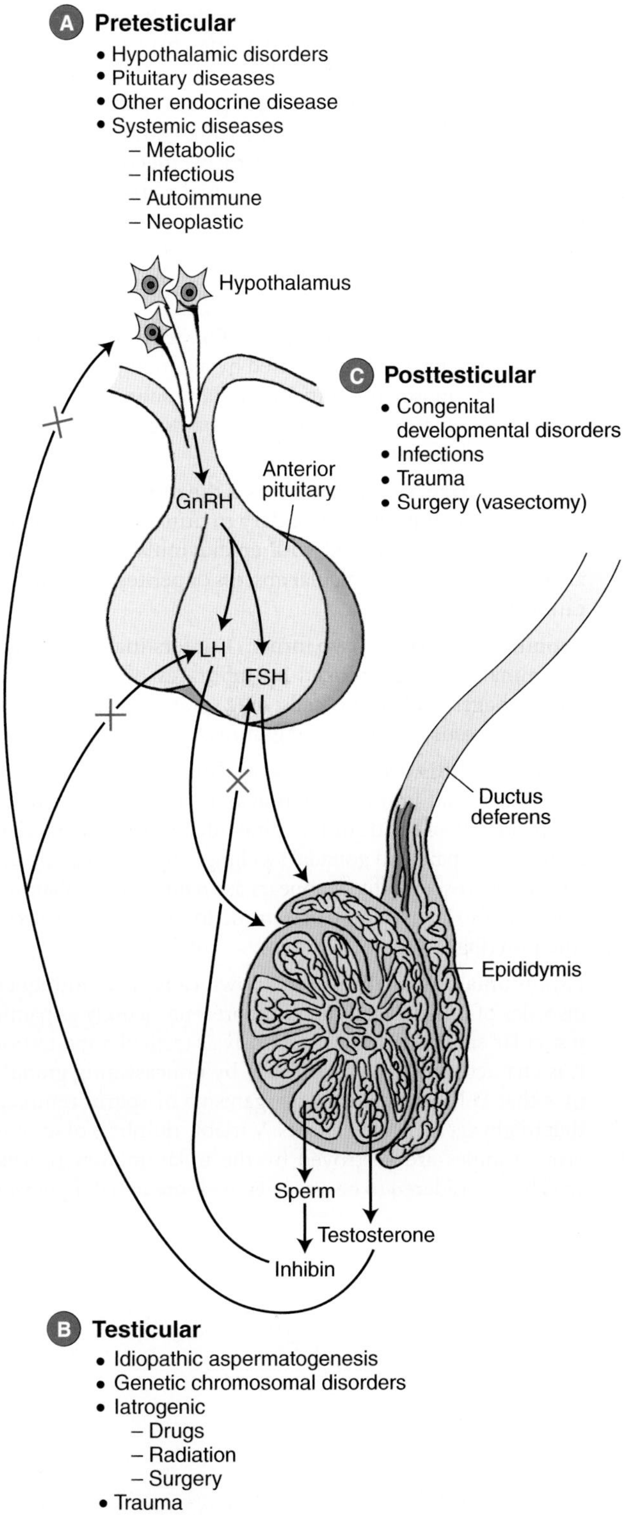

FIGURE 17-22. **Causes of male infertility. A.** Pre-testicular infertility. FSH = follicle-stimulating hormone; LH = luteinizing hormone; GnRH = gonadotropin-releasing hormone. **B.** Testicular infertility. **C.** Post-testicular (obstructive) infertility.

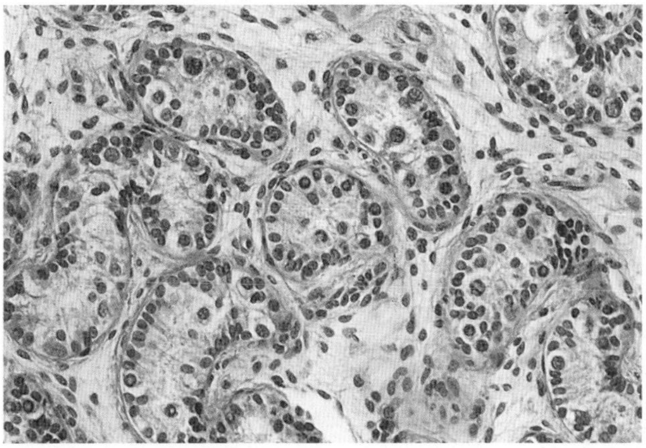

FIGURE 17-23. **Hypogonadotropic hypogonadism.** The testis of this 25-year-old man is composed of immature seminiferous tubules similar to those seen in prepubertal boys.

PATHOLOGY: Morphologic alterations in the testicular biopsy that may identify the cause of infertility include:

- **Immaturity of the seminiferous tubules** is typically found in hypogonadotropic hypogonadism caused by pituitary or hypothalamic diseases (Fig. 17-23). Seminiferous tubules show no signs of spermatogenic differentiation and resemble those of prepubertal testes.
- **Decreased spermatogenesis (hypospermatogenesis)** occurs in several systemic and endocrine diseases, including malnutrition and acquired immunodeficiency syndrome (AIDS). Hypospermatogenesis is also found in cryptorchid testes and following vasectomy.
- **Germ cell maturation arrest** is usually idiopathic. It can occur at the level of spermatogonia, spermatocytes, or spermatids.
- **Germ cell aplasia** ("Sertoli cells only" syndrome) is mostly idiopathic (Fig. 17-24). An underlying genetic mutation has been identified in some patients. It can be seen in drug-induced and toxic injury of the seminiferous epithelium.
- **Orchitis** is caused by viruses (e.g., mumps) or autoimmune diseases.
- **Peritubular and tubular fibrosis** may be related to congenital disorders such as cryptorchidism or to previous infection, ischemia, or radiation (Fig. 17-25).

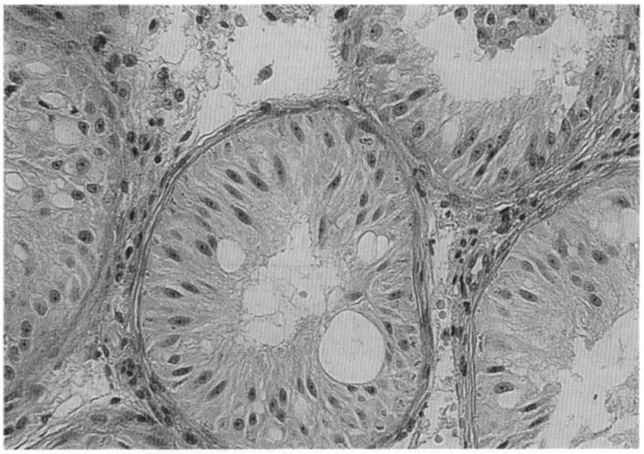

FIGURE 17-24. **Germ cell aplasia–Sertoli cell only syndrome.** The seminiferous tubules are lined by Sertoli cells and do not contain germ cells.

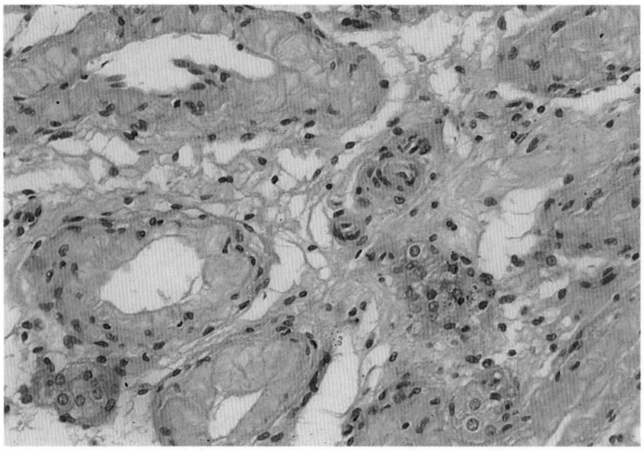

FIGURE 17-25. **Postirradiation tubular atrophy of the testis.** Seminiferous tubules are hyalinized, and there is no evidence of spermatogenesis.

Epididymitis

Epididymitis is acute or chronic inflammation of the epididymis, usually caused by bacteria.

Bacterial epididymitis in young men most often occurs in an acute form as a complication of gonorrhea or as a sexually acquired infection with *Chlamydia*. It is characterized by suppurative inflammation (Fig. 17-26). In older men, *E. coli* from associated urinary tract infections is the most common causative agent. Patients present with intrascrotal pain and tenderness, with or without associated fever. Epididymitis of recent origin shows the usual hallmarks of acute inflammation. Persistent chronic epididymitis is associated with accumulation of plasma cells, macrophages, and lymphocytes and, ultimately, with fibrotic obstruction of infected ducts. Gonorrheal epididymitis is a common cause of male infertility.

Tuberculous epididymitis is now infrequent and is usually associated with previously established pulmonary and renal tuberculosis. The infection is manifested clinically by a palpable enlargement of the epididymis and beading of the vas deferens. Microscopically, the nodules consist of confluent caseating granulomas.

Spermatic granulomas result from an intense inflammatory response to sperm present in the interstitium of the epididymis.

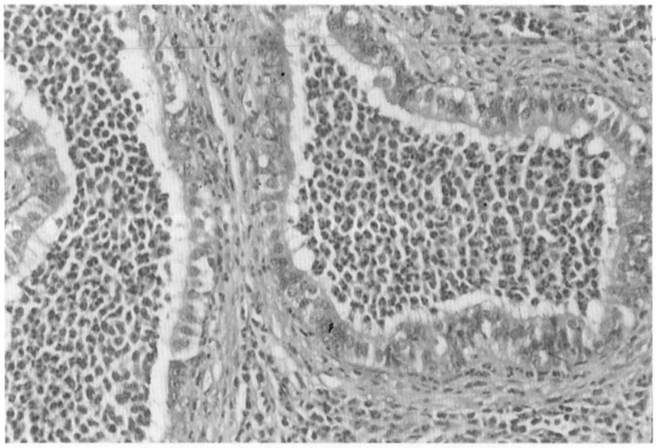

FIGURE 17-26. **Bacterial epididymitis.** The epididymal ducts contain numerous polymorphonuclear leukocytes.

The reason for sperm extravasation is often obscure, but traumatic rupture of the epididymal ducts may play a role. Patients present with scrotal pain and swelling, frequently lasting weeks or months. Microscopically, the epididymis displays a mixed inflammatory cell infiltrate with numerous extravasated sperm fragments and phagocytosis of sperm by macrophages. Ultimately, inflammation results in interstitial fibrosis, ductal obstruction, and infertility.

Orchitis

Orchitis is acute or chronic inflammation of the testis. It may be part of epididymo-orchitis, usually caused by ascending infection, or it may occur as an isolated testicular inflammation. It is usually secondary to hematogenous spread of pathogens or is an immune-mediated disease.

- **Gram-negative bacterial orchitis** is the most common form of the disease. It is often secondary to urinary tract infection, and is typically associated with epididymitis. Infection may also manifest as intratesticular abscess or peritesticular suppuration and fibrosis.
- **Syphilitic orchitis** has two forms: (1) interstitial perivascular inflammation, characterized by infiltrates of lymphocytes, macrophages, and plasma cells; or (2) granulomatous inflammation of testis in the form of gummas.
- **Mumps orchitis** occurs in 20% of adult males with mumps, but widespread immunization against mumps has reduced the incidence of the disorder. Viral infection is characterized by testicular pain and gonadal swelling, most commonly unilateral. Microscopically, it appears as an interstitial inflammation that also leads to destruction and loss of seminiferous epithelium (Fig. 17-27).
- **Granulomatous orchitis** of unknown cause is an infrequent disorder of middle-aged men that presents acutely as painful testicular enlargement or insidiously as testicular induration. It is characterized microscopically by noncaseating granulomas that fail to reveal either organisms or sperm remnants that might act as inciting agents. Variable numbers of seminiferous tubules are destroyed by the inflammatory process, which is considered to be a type IV (cell-mediated) hypersensitivity reaction.

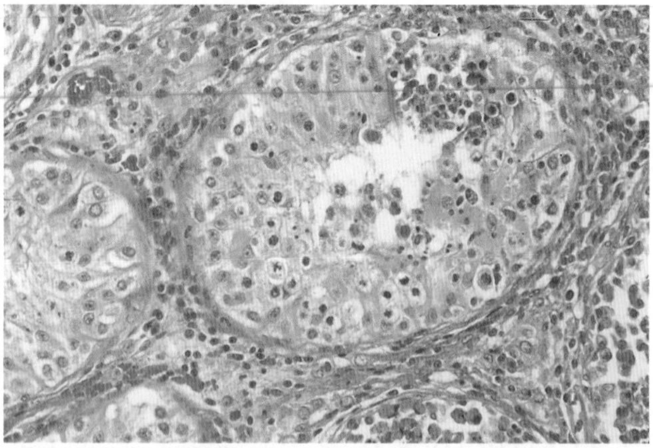

FIGURE 17-27. **Viral orchitis.** The interstitial spaces are infiltrated with mononuclear cells that spill focally into the lumen of seminiferous tubules. Note that the inflammation has interrupted normal spermatogenesis and that the seminiferous tubules do not contain sperm.

- **Malakoplakia** of the testis has the same microscopic features and presumably the same histogenesis as malakoplakia elsewhere.

Tumors Of The Testis

Tumors of the testis account for less than 1% of all malignancies in adult males. More than 90% of these tumors are characterized by:

- Diagnosis between 25 and 45 years of age.
- Germ cell origin
- Malignancy
- Curable by a combination of surgery and chemotherapy
- Cytogenetic marker, namely isochromosome p12
- Metastasize first to periaortic abdominal lymph nodes
- Most (65%) testicular tumors release markers detectable in the blood.

PATHOGENESIS: The etiology of testicular tumors is unknown. There is a geographic variation in the incidence of testicular cancer. Incidence is highest in Denmark, Sweden, and Norway, but is low in Finland and southern European countries. The tumors are five times more common among Americans of European descent than those of African heritage. Familial occurrence of testicular cancer in brothers or sons and fathers are on record but are rare and provide no support for a genetic theory of tumorigenesis. The only consistent cytogenetic abnormality is an additional fragment of chromosome 12 (isochromosome p12). As discussed previously, the only documented risk factors for testicular tumors are **cryptorchidism and gonadal dysgenesis**.

Malignant transformation of germ cells may occur during fetal development and involve (1) migrating primordial germ cells, (2) fetal germ cells interacting with stromal cells in the genital ridge, or (3) early fetal spermatogonia. Since germ cell tumors rarely occur before puberty, some investigators believe that malignant transformation occurs in the peripubertal period and involves spermatogonia that are stimulated hormonally to proliferate and differentiate into spermatocytes. There is disagreement as to the initial events in testicular neoplasia, a consensus holds that germ cell tumors progress through two pathways (Fig. 17-28). Most commonly, a carcinoma in situ stage, also known as **intratubular testicular germ cell neoplasia** (ITGCN), precedes and progresses to invasive carcinoma (see below). This pathway accounts for most adult germ cell tumors, although ITGCN is not found in spermatocytic seminomas, teratomas of prepubertal testes, or yolk sac tumors of infancy, which develop directly from germ cells without an in situ phase. It is possible that some migratory primordial germ cells have not found their way into the seminiferous tubules during fetal testicular organogenesis and that such "misplaced" cells become progenitors of yolk sac tumors and teratomas. Such germ cells can also give rise to extragonadal germ cell tumors in the retroperitoneum, sacral region, anterior mediastinum, and the area of the pineal.

TABLE 17-7

Testicular Tumors

Germ cell tumors – 90%	
Seminoma (40%)	
Nonseminomatous germ cell tumors	
Embryonal carcinoma (5%)	
Teratocarcinoma (35%)	
Choriocarcinoma (<1%)	
Mixed germ cell tumors (15%)	
Teratoma (1%)	
Spermatocytic seminoma (1%)	
Yolk sac tumor of infancy (2%)	
Sex cord cell tumors – 5%	
Leydig cell tumors (60%)	
Sertoli cell tumors	
Metastases – 5%	

PATHOLOGY: Testicular tumors are classified histogenetically on the basis of their cell of origin into several groups (Table 17-7).

Tumor cells of ITGCN resemble spermatogonia or fetal germ cells but have much larger polyploid nuclei (Fig.17-29). Like fetal germ cells, these cells express placental-like alkaline phosphatase on their surface. In infertile men with a history of cryptorchid testes, ITGCN can persist unchanged for 5 to 10 years, after which the neoplastic cells acquire invasive properties, penetrate through the tubular basement membrane, and give rise to infiltrating malignant tumors.

The malignant cells that retain the phenotypic features of spermatogonia give rise to **seminomas.** Alternatively, the neoplastic germ cells can differentiate into malignant embryonic cells (**embryonal carcinoma**) by a process that resembles **parthenogenetic activation** of oocytes in the female gonads of amphibians and reptiles.

In some cases, embryonal carcinoma cells proliferate in an undifferentiated form. In others, they differentiate into the three embryonic germ layers (ectoderm, mesoderm, endoderm) or extraembryonic tissues that form the fetal membranes and the placenta. Further differentiation of germ layer cells leads to formation of various somatic tissues. Ectoderm differentiates into skin, central nervous system, retinal pigment, and other related tissues. Mesoderm gives rise to smooth and striated muscle, cartilage, bone, and so forth. Endoderm forms intestinal tissue, bronchial epithelium, salivary glands, and so forth. The extraembryonic derivatives of embryonal carcinoma cells give rise to chorionic epithelium (cytotrophoblast and syncytiotrophoblast) and yolk sac-like epithelium. These complex tumors composed of malignant undifferentiated embryonal carcinoma cells and their somatic and extraembryonic derivatives are called **teratocarcinomas** or **malignant teratomas**. When embryonal carcinoma cells proliferate without further differentiating and exhibit a single histologic pattern, the tumor is labeled **embryonal carcinoma.** In rare instances, extraembryonic components of teratocarcinomas overgrow and destroy all other components. Such tumors are composed of a single tumor type and are classified as **yolk sac carcinoma** or **choriocarcinoma.**

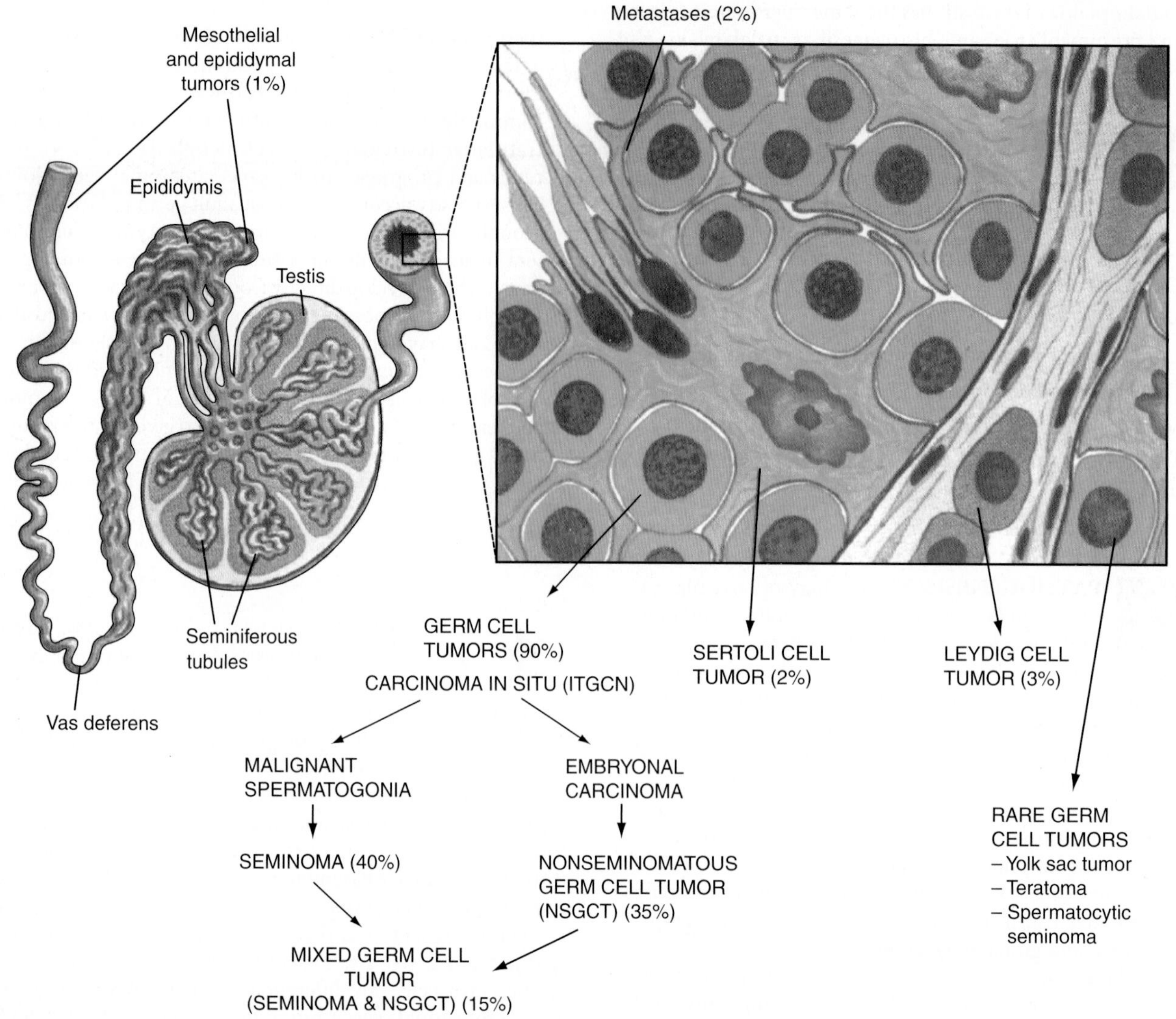

FIGURE 17-28. **Tumors of the testis, epididymis, and related structures.** Most testicular tumors originate from germ cells and are preceded by a carcinoma in situ stage known as intratubular germ cell neoplasia (ITGCN). Germ cell tumors of adult testis can be classified as seminomas (40%) or nonseminomatous germ cell tumors (NSGCTs) (35%). In 15% of cases seminomatous elements are intermixed with NSGCT, forming mixed germ cell tumors. Some germ cell tumors (yolk sac tumor of childhood, childhood teratomas, and spermatocytic seminomas) develop without passing through a preinvasive ITGCN stage. Tumors originating from sex cord stromal cells (Leydig and Sertoli cell tumors), epididymal tumors, tumors of the mesothelial lining of the tunica vaginalis (adenomatoid tumors), and metastases are rare.

For clinical purposes, all germ cell tumors with embryonal carcinoma as their malignant stem cells are termed **nonseminomatous germ cell tumors (NSGCTs),** to distinguish them from seminomas. Pure yolk sac carcinomas of the adult testis and choriocarcinomas are also included in this group because it is assumed that these tumors must contain a few embryonal carcinoma cells that are not readily recognizable.

In 15% of cases, germ cell tumors contain both seminoma and nonseminomatous elements. Such **mixed germ cell tumors** are treated clinically as nonseminomatous neoplasms.

Intratubular Germ Cell Neoplasia Refers to Testicular Carcinoma in Situ

ITGCN represents a preinvasive form of germ cell tumors.

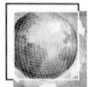

EPIDEMIOLOGY: ITGCN can be seen as (1) an isolated focal histologic change in 2% of cryptorchid testes or testicular biopsies performed for infertility, (2) widespread carcinoma in situ adjacent to almost all invasive germ, and (3) lesions in 5% of contralateral testes in patients who had an orchiectomy for a testicular germ cell tumor.

PATHOLOGY: ITGCN involves testes in a patchy manner, usually affecting less than 10% to 30% of the tubules. Seminiferous tubules harboring ITGCN have thick basement membranes and no sperm. The normal germ cells are replaced by neoplastic germ cells that are broadly attached to the basal lamina (see Fig. 17-29). The neoplastic cells appear larger than normal spermatogonia. Their nuclei are large, have finely dispersed chromatin, and display prominent nucleoli. The nuclei are centrally located and surrounded by abundant, clear cytoplasm that contains large amounts of glycogen. The nuclear DNA content is increased, suggesting that the cells are triploid. The plasma membrane is distinct and stains with antibodies to **placental alkaline phosphatase** (PLAP).

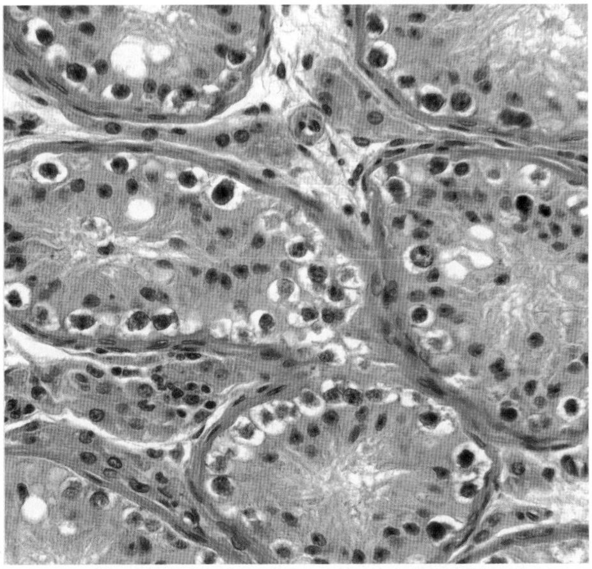

FIGURE 17-29. **Intratubular germ cell neoplasia (ITGCN).** The seminiferous tubules show no signs of spermatogenesis but instead contain large atypical cells corresponding to intratubular carcinoma in situ.

CLINICAL FEATURES: ITGCN is a precursor of invasive carcinoma that develops at an unpredictable pace. Half of men with ITGCN will develop invasive cancer within 5 years and 70% in 7 years. Microscopic diagnosis of ITGCN on testicular biopsy is an indication for prophylactic orchiectomy.

Seminoma Contains Monomorphous Cells That Resemble Spermatogonia

EPIDEMIOLOGY: Seminoma, the most common testicular cancer, accounts for 40% of all germ cells tumors. Peak incidence is between 30 to 40 years. Seminomas are never found in prepubertal children, except in those who have dysgenetic gonads.

PATHOLOGY: On gross examination, the tumors are solid, rubbery-firm, bosselated masses. Tumor tissue is usually sharply demarcated from normal testicular tissue, which may be compressed, atrophic, and fibrotic. On cross section the tumors appear lobulated and homogeneously tan or grayish yellow (Fig. 17-30). Areas of necrosis or hemorrhage are usually inconspicuous but may be seen in larger tumors.

Microscopically, seminoma is equivalent to **ovarian dysgerminoma**. The tumor features a single population of uniform polygonal cells with centrally located vesicular nuclei. The ample cytoplasm may appear pale and eosinophilic or clear in standard histologic sections because it contains large amounts of glycogen and some lipid. Tumor cells are arranged as nests or sheets separated by fibrous septa infiltrated with lymphocytes, plasma cells, and macrophages. Occasionally, the septa contain granulomas with giant cells. Tumor cells invade the testicular parenchyma but also spread through the seminiferous tubules and into rete testis. Invasion of the epididymis is seen later in the disease, usually before spread to abdominal lymph nodes.

Seminoma cells resemble immature spermatogonia. Like fetal spermatogonia and primordial germ cells in the fetus, they express PLAP on the plasma membrane. PLAP is shed into the blood in small amounts but cannot be used for diagnostic purposes.

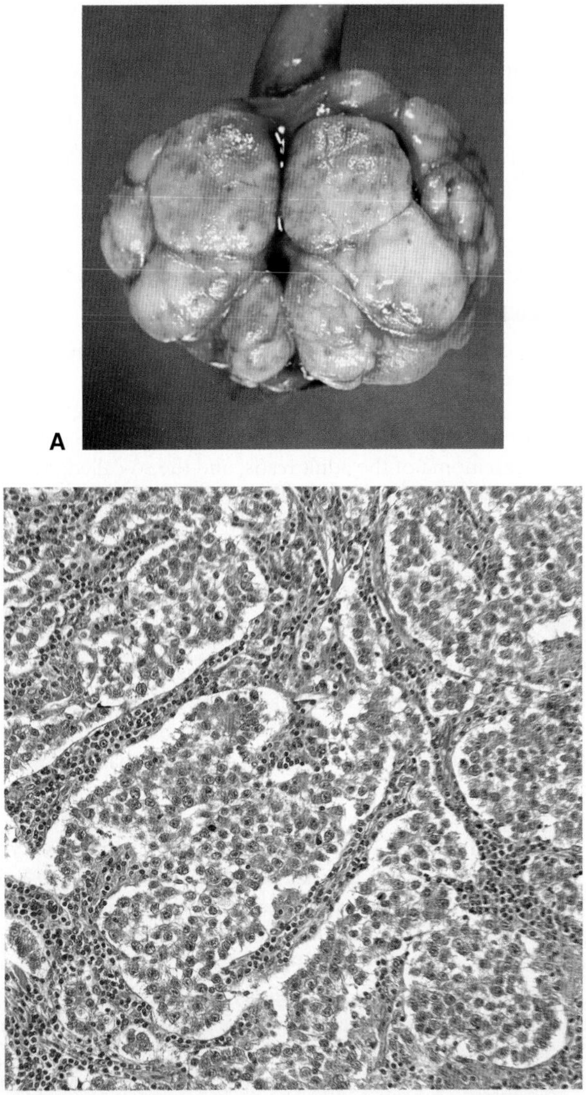

FIGURE 17-30. **Seminoma. A.** The cut surface of this nodular tumor is tan and bulging, suggesting that the tumor is firm and rubbery. **B.** Groups of tumor cells are surrounded by fibrous septa infiltrated with lymphocytes. Tumor cells have vesicular nuclei which are much larger than the small round nuclei of the lymphocytes.

Pathologists recognize two subtypes of seminoma: (1) **seminoma with syncytiotrophoblastic giant cells** and (2) **anaplastic seminoma**. The first subgroup includes 20% of tumors that contain syncytiotrophoblastic cells. These multinucleated giant cells are best demonstrated with antibodies to human chorionic gonadotropin (hCG). Although they secrete hCG, blood hCG levels are usually below detectable limits. Some 5% of seminomas show brisk mitotic activity and nuclear pleomorphism and are classified as anaplastic seminoma. There are no clinical differences between classical seminomas and these two microscopic tumor variants.

CLINICAL FEATURES: Seminoma manifests as a progressively growing scrotal mass and is usually diagnosed while it can still be cured by orchiectomy, with or without abdominal lymph node dissection. Seminomas are highly radiosensitive, and radiotherapy plays an important role in treating tumors that cannot be cured by surgery alone. Those in advanced stages of dissemination are treated with additional chemotherapy. *The cure rate for all histologic types of seminoma is over 90%.*

Spermatocytic seminoma is a rare tumor unrelated to classical seminoma. These are benign tumors of men over 40 years of age. They are not associated with ITGCN and do not elicit a lymphocytic reaction. Spermatocytic seminomas contain three cell types: large, small, and intermediate cells. Orchiectomy is curative.

Nonseminomatous Germ Cell Tumors Are Derived from Embryonal Cells

NSGCTs of the testis include several pathologic entities, two of which account for most of the cases: (1) pure embryonal carcinomas; and (2) teratocarcinomas, also known as **malignant teratomas** or **mixed germ cell tumors**. Pure choriocarcinoma, pure yolk sac carcinoma of the adult testis, and the so-called growing benign teratoma are rare NSGCTs. Mixed germ cell tumors are NSGCTs combined with seminomas.

EPIDEMIOLOGY: NSGCTs constitute 55% of all testicular germ cell tumors. Teratocarcinomas account for two thirds of all NSGCTs, followed by mixed germ cell tumors and pure embryonal carcinomas. All other tumors of this group are extremely rare. Like seminomas, NSGCTs have peak incidence in the 25- to 40-year-old age group. At diagnosis, these patients are usually somewhat younger than those with seminomas.

PATHOLOGY: Nonseminomatous tumors vary in size and shape, and may be solid or partially cystic. Solid areas vary in color from white to yellow to red, indicating that they are composed of viable tumor cells, foci of necrosis and hemorrhage, respectively (Fig. 17-31).

The histology of NSGCTs is highly variable. Pure embryonal carcinomas are composed exclusively of undifferentiated embryonal carcinoma cells similar to cells from preimplantation-stage embryos (Fig. 17-32). Because the tumor cells have little cytoplasm, their hyperchromatic, disproportionately large nuclei seem to overlap. Embryonal carcinoma cells may be arranged as broad solid sheets, cords, glandlike tubules and acini, and sometimes even line papillary structures. Numerous mitoses and apoptotic cells are characteristic. Antibodies to keratins are used to distinguish keratin-rich embryonal carcinoma from seminoma, lymphoma, sarcoma, and melanoma, which lack keratin. Embryonal carcinoma invades the testis, epididymis, and blood vessels and metastasizes to abdominal lymph nodes, lungs, and other organs.

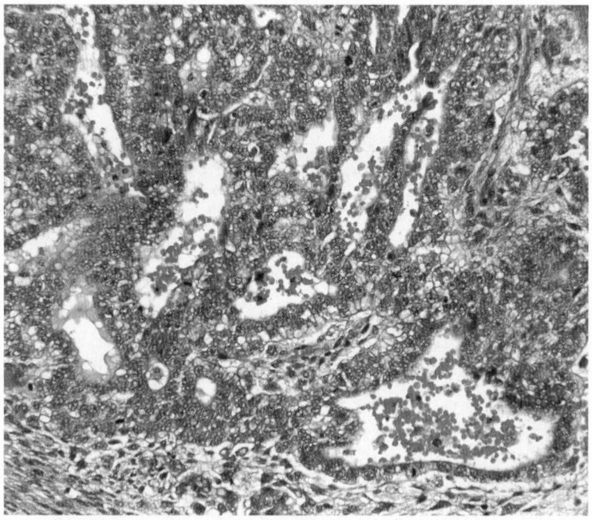

FIGURE 17-32. **Embryonal carcinoma component of a NSGCT.** Because these undifferentiated cells have scant cytoplasm, their hyperchromatic nuclei impart a bluish color to the tumor. The nuclei appear crowded and seem to overlap each other. The cells form cords and sheets surrounding dilated vascular channels filled with red blood cells.

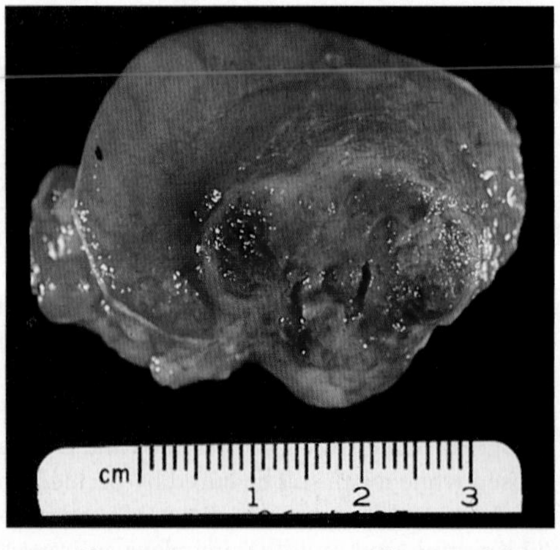

FIGURE 17-31. **Nonseminomatous germ cell tumor of the testis.** The cut surface of this small testicular tumor shows considerable heterogeneity, varying in color from white to dark red.

Embryonal carcinoma cells are the stem cells of **teratocarcinomas** (malignant teratomas), which feature differentiated somatic elements (i.e., tissues that are normally found in various organs, and extraembryonic elements, including yolk sac cells and trophoblastic cells). Microscopically, such nonseminomatous tumors thus reveal foci of embryonal carcinoma and a variety of other tissues (Fig. 17-33). For example, a tumor might be composed of embryonal carcinoma yolk sac components and trophoblastic components corresponding to choriocarcinoma. A similar tumor that also contains seminoma cells would, however, be called **mixed germ cell tumor**. In most tumors, malignancy resides in embryonal carcinoma cells. Interestingly, when these cells metastasize, they can differentiate into somatic or extraembryonic tissues, in which case the metastatic tumor can resemble the original one.

NSGCTs can give rise to clones of highly malignant cytotrophoblastic and syncytiotrophoblastic cells that overgrow other elements. Tumors composed exclusively of malignant chorionic epithelium are termed **choriocarcinomas**. Likewise, clones of malignant yolk sac epithelium produce **yolk sac carcinoma.**

Some histologically benign teratomas of postpubertal young men may have a malignant clinical course, even though they appear to be only mature, nonproliferating somatic tissues, without embryonal elements (Fig.17-34). In some instances it is assumed that the tumor was actually a teratocarcinoma in which almost all embryonal cells have differentiated into mature somatic tissues but that a few remaining malignant cells were undetected by the pathologist or had metastasized before resection. These tumors are clinically known as the **growing teratoma syndrome.** In other cases, teratoma tissues remain undifferentiated and resemble embryonic organs or embryonic tumors such as neuroblastoma. These **immature teratomas** are also potentially malignant tumors.

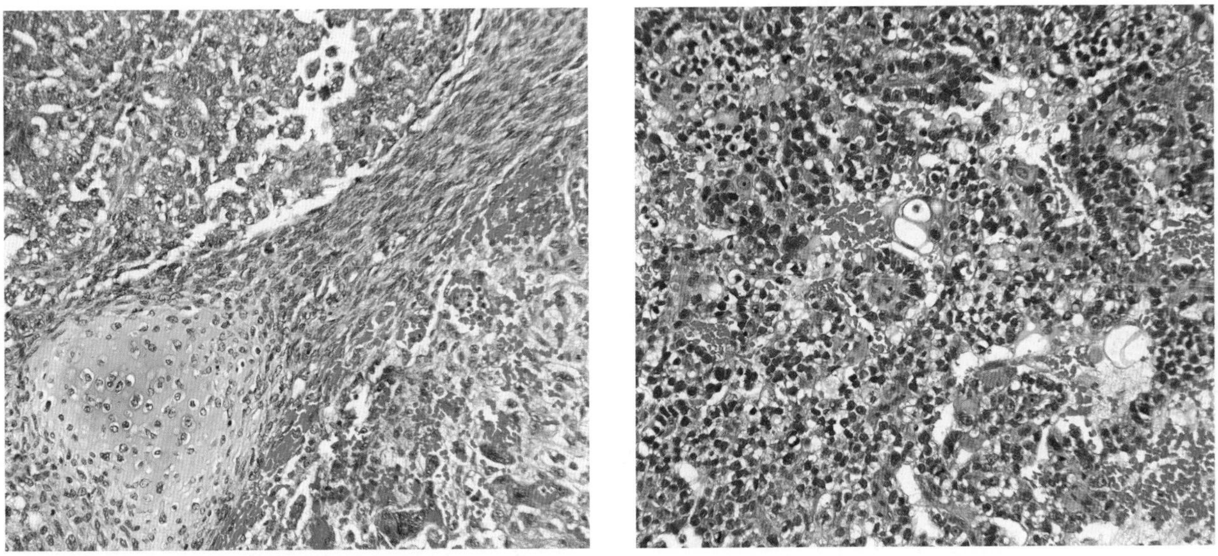

A B

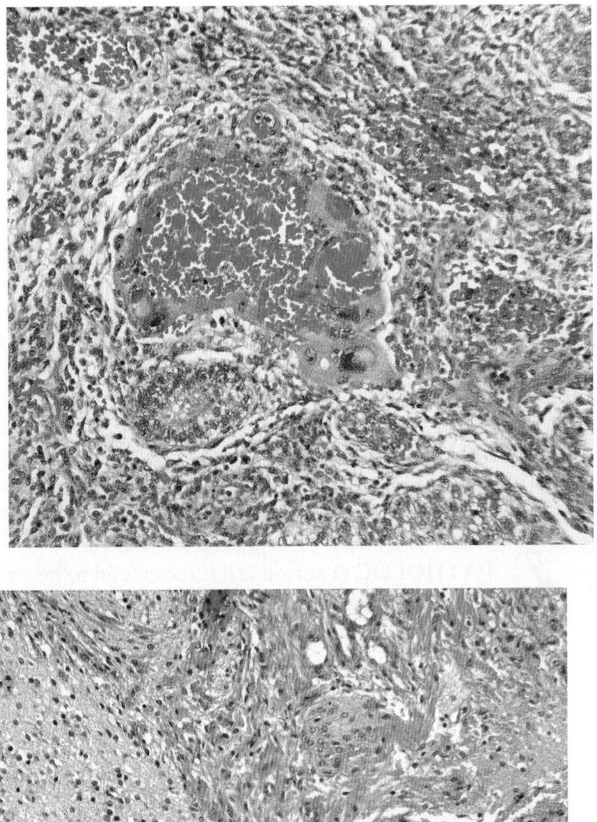

C

FIGURE 17-33. **Nonseminomatous germ cell tumor (NSGCT). A.** Somatic tissue of this tumor includes well-differentiated cartilage and nondescript connective tissue separating the embryonal carcinoma *(upper left corner)* from the hemorrhagic choriocarcinoma *(right lower corner)*. **B.** Yolk sac component consists of interlacing cord of epithelial cells surrounded by loose stroma resembling the early yolk sac. **C.** Choriocarcinoma component of the NSGCT consists of multinucleated syncytiotrophoblastic giant cells and mononuclear cytotrophoblastic cells. Invasive growth of trophoblasts is usually associated with hemor-

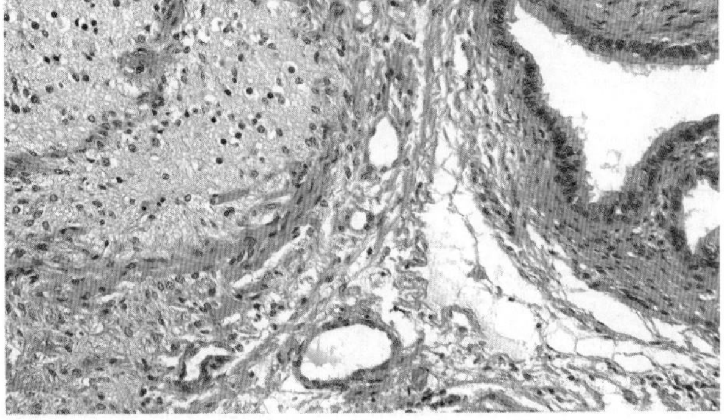

FIGURE 17-34. **Teratoma.** The tumor consists of neural tissue (*left*) connective tissue and smooth muscle cells (midportion) and glands lined by columnar epithelium (*right side of the picture*).

CLINICAL FEATURES: Most NSGCTs manifest as testicular masses. They tend to grow faster than seminomas and metastasize more readily and more widely. Hence, in some NSGCTs metastases may be the first sign of the neoplastic disease.

In contrast to seminomas, NSGCTs often contain yolk sac components and syncytiotrophoblastic cells. Yolk sac cells secrete α-fetoprotein (AFP), a fetal plasma protein that is not normally found in the blood. Syncytiotrophoblastic cells release hCG, a hormone of pregnancy, that is also not found in males. *Elevated serum AFP or hCG are found in 70% of patients harboring NSGCTs and are thus reliable tumor markers.* These antigens are most useful in postoperative follow-up of patients who have been treated for NSGCT. Persistently elevated AFP and/or hCG indicate that a patient is not tumor free. Patients whose initially high levels of AFP and hCG normalize after treatment but subsequently rise again have metastases.

Treatment of NSGCT includes orchiectomy to remove the primary tumor, then platinum-based chemotherapy, and, if indicated, surgical dissection of abdominal lymph nodes. Chemotherapy usually eliminates metastatic embryonal carcinoma cells, but differentiated tissues originating from them are resistant. Such tissues do not grow and are not likely to endanger

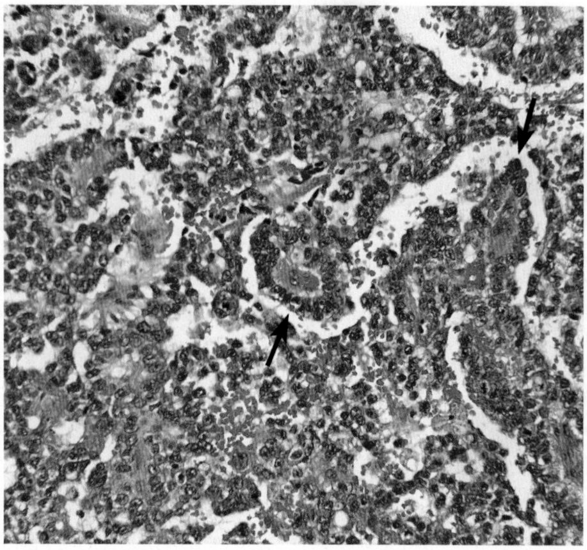

FIGURE 17-35. **Yolk sac tumor.** This childhood tumor is composed of interlacing strands of epithelial cells surrounded by loose connective stroma. The glomeruloid structures (Schiller-Duval bodies) are marked by arrows.

the patient. Nevertheless, it is better to remove any residual neoplasia than to take a chance that a few malignant tumor cells might be hiding in the residuals tumors. Only 3 decades ago, patients with NSGCTs had only a 35% chance for 5-year survival. *By contrast, complete cures are now recorded in over 90% of cases.*

Testicular Tumors are Rare in Prepubertal Boys

In the first 4 years of life, most testicular neoplasms are yolk sac tumors. Benign teratomas are the most common testicular tumor in the age group between 4 and 12 years.

YOLK SAC TUMORS: These neoplasms are composed of cells arranged into structures reminiscent of parts of fetal yolk sac. The diagnosis is based on recognizing multiple microscopic tumor patterns and the so-called glomeruloid **Schiller-Duval bodies** (Fig. 17-35). The histology of neonatal tumors are similar to those of the yolk sac elements in NSGCTs. Yolk sac tumors of infancy and early childhood are considered malignant, but timely orchiectomy and removal of the tumor cures over 95% of patients.

TERATOMAS: These tumors of prepubertal testes are benign and are composed of mature somatic tissues. Orchiectomy, and even testis-sparing surgery, are curative.

Gonadal Stromal/Sex Cord Tumors are Composed of Cells That Resemble Sertoli or Leydig Cells

Gonadal stroma/sex cord tumors constitute 5% of all testicular tumors.

LEYDIG CELL TUMORS: Rare neoplasms are composed of cells resembling interstitial (Leydig) cells of the testis. They can be hormonally active and secrete androgens, estrogens, or both. Leydig cell tumors can occur at any age, with two distinct peaks, one in childhood and one in adults from the third to the sixth decade.

PATHOLOGY: Leydig cell tumors are well circumscribed, and some appear encapsulated. They vary from 1 to 10 cm in diameter. The cut surface is yellow to brown, and larger tumors have fibrous trabeculae, giving them a lobular appearance. Leydig cell tumors are composed of uniform cells with round nuclei and

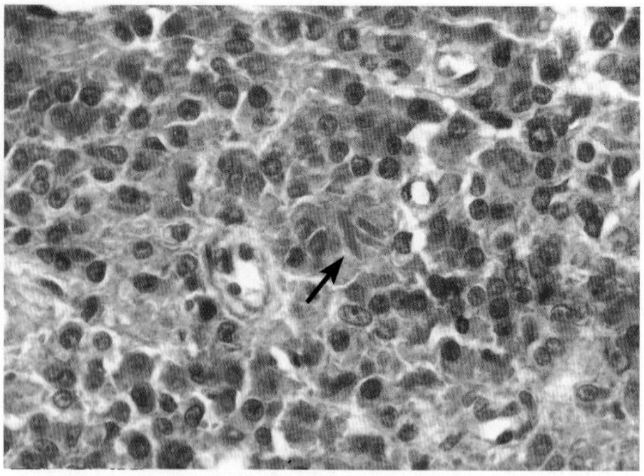

FIGURE 17-36. **Leydig cell tumor.** The tumor cells have uniform round nuclei and well-developed eosinophilic cytoplasm. Three cytoplasmic Reinke crystals are seen in the center of the field *(arrow)*.

well-developed eosinophilic or vacuolated cytoplasm (Fig. 17-36). **Reinke crystals**—rectangular, eosinophilic, cytoplasmic inclusions—are typically found in normal Leydig cells and are present in 30% of tumors. Although most (90%) of Leydig cell tumors are benign (only 10% are malignant), it is difficult to predict biological behavior on histologic grounds.

CLINICAL FEATURES: The androgenic effects of testicular Leydig cell tumors in prepubertal boys lead to precocious physical and sexual development. By contrast, feminization and gynecomastia are observed in some adults with this tumor. Either estrogen or testosterone levels may be elevated, but there is no characteristic pattern. All Leydig cell tumors in children and almost all tumors in adults are cured by orchiectomy.

SERTOLI CELL TUMORS: Some testicular sex cord stromal cell tumors are composed of neoplastic Sertoli cells. Most (90%) tumors are benign and produce few if any hormonal symptoms.

PATHOLOGY: Sertoli cell tumors tend to be small (1 to 3 cm), solid, well-circumscribed, yellow–gray nodules. Microscopically, they contain columnar tumor cells arranged into tubules or cords in a fibrous trabecular framework (Fig. 17-37). The rare malignant variant exhibits greater cel-

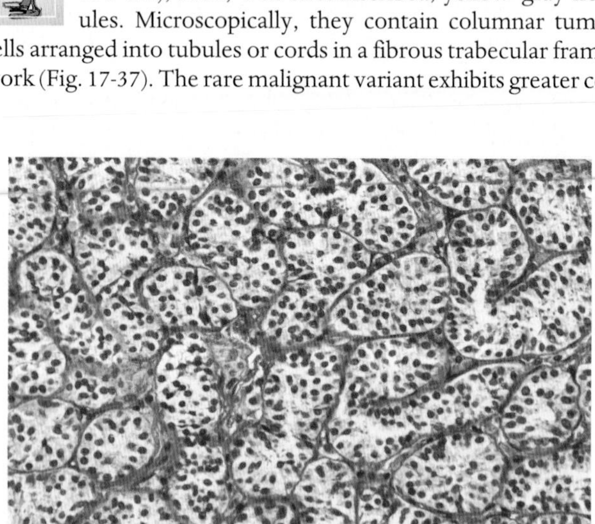

FIGURE 17-37. **Sertoli cell tumor.** The neoplastic cells are arranged in tubules surrounded by a basement membrane. These structures are reminiscent of seminiferous tubules devoid of germ cells.

lular pleomorphism, areas of necrosis, and little tendency to form cords and tubules. Most patients with Sertoli cell tumors are under 40 years of age and come to medical attention because of a scrotal mass. Endocrine effects are uncommon and, if present, are vague. Orchiectomy is curative.

Metastatic Tumors to Testis

METASTASES: Involvement of the testis with metastases accounts for 5% of all testicular tumors. Most of these spread from primary cancers of the prostate, large intestine, or bladder.

MALIGNANT LYMPHOMA: This cancer is the most common neoplasm in the testes of men older than 60 years. It usually occurs in the context of systemic disease, but a few cases of primary lymphoma of the testis have been reported. Most but not all patients with lymphomatous involvement of the testis have a poor prognosis.

ADENOMATOID TUMOR: Adenomatoid tumor ***(benign mesothelioma)*** *is a benign tumor that originates from the mesothelial layer of the testicular tunica vaginalis.* These neoplasms are usually seen in the upper pole of the epididymis, with fewer cases involving the tunica vaginalis or spermatic cord. They are well-demarcated tan nodules that vary from a few millimeters to 2 cm, but may rarely reach 6 cm in size.

PROSTATE

Prostatitis

Prostatitis is inflammation of the prostate. It can occur in acute and chronic forms. It is usually caused by coliform uropathogens, but often the cause cannot be determined.

ACUTE PROSTATITIS: Typically a complication of other urinary tract infections, acute prostatitis results from reflux of infected urine into the prostate. An acute inflammatory infiltrate is seen in prostatic acini and stroma. The disorder causes intense discomfort on urination and is often associated with fever, chills, and perineal pain. Most patients respond well to standard antibiotic treatment.

CHRONIC BACTERIAL PROSTATITIS: This infection of longer duration that may or may not be preceded by an episode of acute prostatitis. Most patients with chronic prostatitis complain of dysuria and burning at the urethral meatus. Suprapubic, perineal, and low back pain, or discomfort and nocturia may be also present. The urine usually contains bacteria. In addition to reflux of urine, factors such as prostatic calculi and local prostatic duct obstruction may contribute to development of chronic bacterial prostatitis. Microscopically, infiltrates of lymphocytes, plasma cells, and macrophages are the rule. Prolonged antibiotic therapy is often, but not necessarily, curative.

NONBACTERIAL PROSTATITIS: There exists a form of chronic prostatitis in which no causative organism is identified. It is the most common form of inflammation in prostatic biopsy or prostatectomy specimens or at autopsy. Nonbacterial prostatitis typically affects men older than 50 years of age, but has been seen at virtually all ages. It has been hypothesized that some cases may be due to *Chlamydia trachomatis, Mycoplasma, Ureaplasma. urealyticum,* and *Trichomonas vaginalis*. However, in practice it is a diagnosis of exclusion. The most common histologic pattern consists of dilated glands filled with neutrophils and foamy macrophages and surrounded by chronic inflammatory cells. The condition may be asymptomatic or cause symptoms similar to those in chronic bacterial prostatitis. The diagnosis requires fractionated collection of urine combined with transrectal prostatic massage. In most cases no specific therapy is available.

GRANULOMATOUS PROSTATITIS: This chronic inflammation is characterized by the presence of granulomas. In most cases, the cause cannot be established. Rarely, granulomatous prostatitis can be traced to specific causative agents, including *Mycobacterium tuberculosis* or such fungal pathogens as *Histoplasma capsulatum*. A granulomatous lesion resembling rheumatoid nodules has been recognized and related to previous transurethral resection of a portion of the prostate. The symptoms of chronic granulomatous prostatitis are vague and the diagnosis is made histologically. Caseating or noncaseating granulomas are associated with localized destruction of prostatic ducts and acini and, in later stages, with fibrosis.

CLINICAL FEATURES: As indicated above, the symptoms of chronic prostatitis are highly variable and treatment may be quite frustrating. Most importantly, chronic prostatitis may cause elevated serum prostate-specific antigen (PSA), raising the specter of prostatic malignancy. The diagnosis is thus often made by biopsy done to exclude carcinoma.

Nodular Hyperplasia Of The Prostate

Nodular prostatic hyperplasia, also termed ***benign prostatic hyperplasia*** *(BPH), is a common disorder characterized clinically by enlargement of the prostate and urinary outflow tract obstruction, and pathologically by proliferation of glands and stroma.*

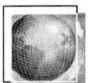

EPIDEMIOLOGY: BPH is most frequent in western Europe and the United States and least common in Asia. The prevalence of the disorder in the United States is higher among blacks than among whites. Clinical prostatism (i.e., BPH severe enough to interfere with urination) peaks in the seventh decade. However, the prevalence of BPH is far greater at autopsy than is suggested by clinically apparent prostatism. In fact, 75% of men 80 years of age or older have some degree of prostatic hyperplasia. The disorder is rarely observed in men younger than 40.

PATHOGENESIS: The earliest histogenetic events in BPH are still not understood. Although noted previously, prepubertal castration prevents the subsequent development of BPH, exogenous testosterone has no effect on either the histologic appearance of the hyperplastic nodules or the areas of the prostate that show senile atrophy. Advancing age is associated with a comparable reduction in circulating testosterone in men with and without BPH. Moreover, no change in serum dihydrotestosterone (DHT) is observed in men with BPH, although the ratio of circulating testosterone to DHT may be abnormally low. Interestingly, changes resembling BPH have been produced in dogs by administration of DHT; drugs that block 5α-reductase (e.g., finasteride) reduce the size of the prostate in men with BPH.

PATHOLOGY: Early nodular hyperplasia begins in the submucosa of the proximal urethra (**the transitional zone**). The enlarging nodules compress the centrally located urethral lumen and the more peripherally located normal prostate (Fig. 17-38). In well-developed BPH, the normal gland is actually limited to an attenuated rim of tissue beneath the capsule. On cut section, an individual nodule is clearly demarcated by an enveloping fibrous pseudocapsule (Fig. 17-39). Focal hemorrhage and infarction may be present, especially in larger nodules. On occasion, there are small stones within dilated hyperplastic acini.

Histologically, BPH features proliferation of epithelial cells of acini and ductules, smooth muscle cells and stromal fibroblasts, all in variable proportions. Accordingly, five types of nodules have been described: (1) stromal (fibrous), (2) fibromuscular, (3) muscular, (4) fibroadenomatous and (6) fibromyoadenomatous, the most common type.

In the typical fibromyoadenomatous nodule, variably sized hyperplastic prostatic acini are randomly scattered throughout the stroma of the nodule. The epithelial (adenomatous) component is composed of a double layer of cells, with tall columnar cells overlying the basal layer (see Fig. 17-39B). Papillary hyperplasia of glandular epithelium is characteristic. Hyperplastic nodules often contain chronic inflammatory cells, and corpora amylacea (eosinophilic laminated concretions) are frequently seen within the acini. The glands of the uninvolved peripheral region of the prostate are frequently atrophic and compressed by the expanding nodules. The stroma of each type of nodule differs in composition, but elastic fibers are always absent. Immunoperoxidase staining of hyperplastic epithelium is consistently positive for PSA and prostatic acid phosphatase.

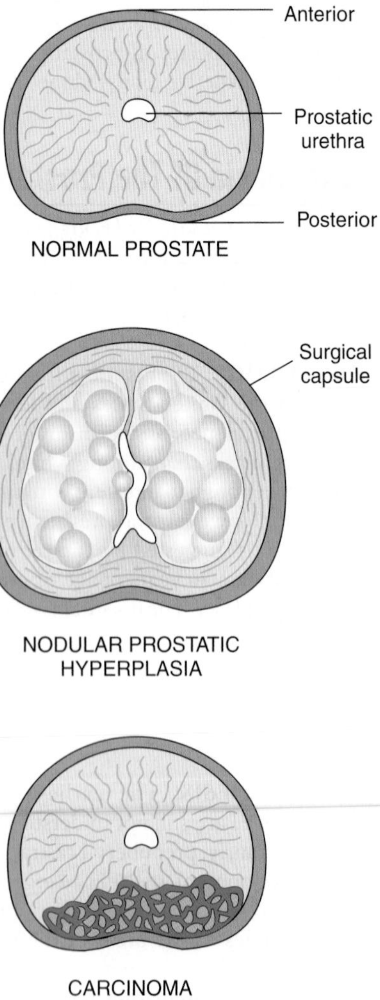

FIGURE 17-38. **Normal prostate, nodular hyperplasia, and adenocarcinoma.** In prostatic hyperplasia, which involves predominantly the periurethral part of the gland, the nodules compress and distort the urethra. The expansion of the central prostatic glands leads to compression of the peripheral parts and fibrosis, resulting in the formation of so-called surgical capsule. Prostatic carcinoma usually arises from the peripheral glands, and compression of the urethra is a late clinical event.

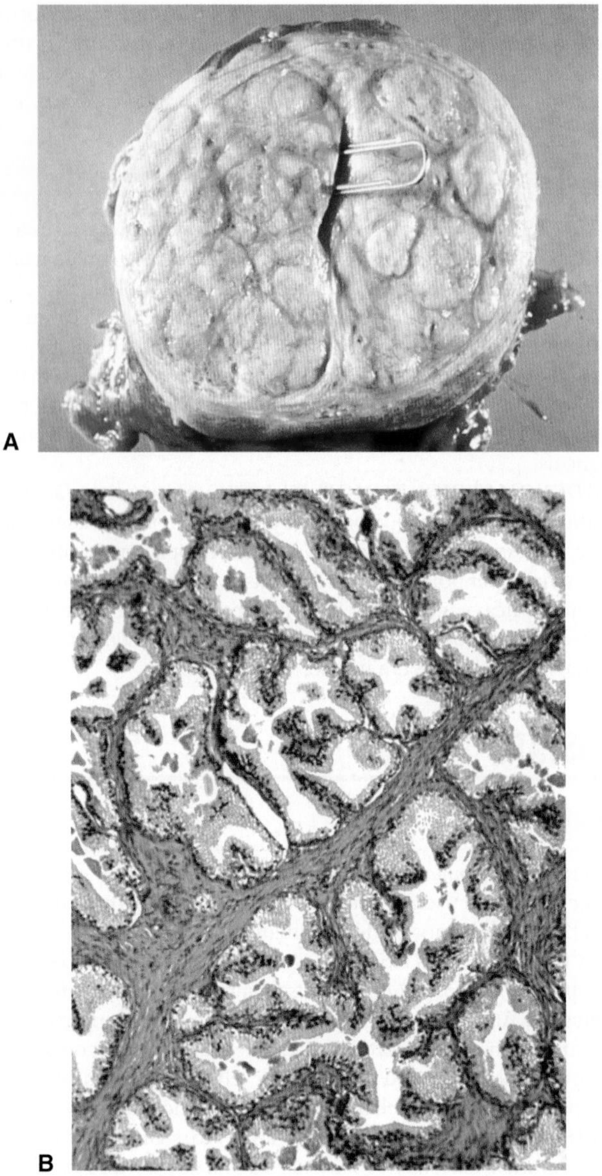

FIGURE 17-39. **Nodular hyperplasia of the prostate. A.** The cut surface of a prostate enlarged by nodular hyperplasia shows numerous well-circumscribed nodules of prostatic tissue. The prostatic urethra *(paper clip)* has been compressed to a narrow slit. **B.** The columnar epithelium lining the acini is composed of two cell layers: polarized clear cuboidal cells lining the acinar lumen and flattened basal cells interposed between the cuboidal acinar cells and the stroma. Hyperplastic cells line papillary projections protruding into the lumina of the acini.

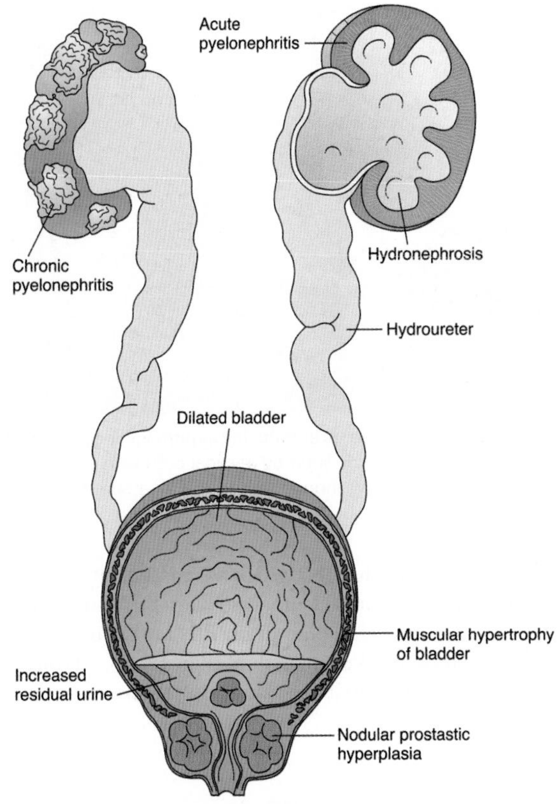

FIGURE 17-40. **Complications of nodular prostatic hyperplasia.**

Nonspecific prostatitis is frequently seen in specimens with nodular hyperplasia. There is a dense intraglandular and periglandular infiltrate of lymphocytes, plasma cells, and macrophages, often with acute inflammatory cells and focal gland destruction. Focal infarcts of varying age are observed in 20% of cases. Squamous metaplasia of ductal epithelium at the periphery of infarcts is typical. In 10% of surgical specimens submitted with preoperative diagnoses of BPH contain incidental foci of prostatic adenocarcinoma.

CLINICAL FEATURES: The clinical symptoms of nodular hyperplasia result from compression of the prostatic urethra and consequent bladder outlet obstruction (Fig. 17-40). A history of decreased vigor of the urinary stream and increasing urinary frequency is typical. Rectal examination reveals a firm, enlarged, nodular prostate. If the duration of severe obstruction is prolonged, back-pressure results in hydroureter, hydronephrosis, and ultimately renal failure and death.

The classic treatment of BPH was surgical. Transurethral prostate resection or, less commonly, suprapubic enucleation of the hyperplastic tissue alleviated the symptoms of prostatism. Both procedures remove the central hyperplastic nodules, leaving behind the more peripheral (subcapsular) prostatic glandular tissue. Currently, drugs that inhibit 5α-reductase are usually used to decrease prostate size. α-Adrenergic blockers reduce muscular tone in the prostate and ameliorate the symptoms of urinary obstruction.

In Situ And Invasive Adenocarcinoma Of The Prostate

EPIDEMIOLOGY: *In 1990, prostatic adenocarcinoma became the cancer most frequently diagnosed in American men, surpassing lung cancer for the first time.* An estimated 220,000 new cases are diagnosed yearly in the United States. Approximately 30,000 American men die annually of this malignancy, a figure that is still far lower than the mortality from lung cancer. Prostate cancer is largely a disease of elderly men and of all patients with this diagnosis, 75% are 60 to 80 years of age. Patients under 50 years of age constitute less than 1% of cases. At the age of 50, the estimated lifetime probability of developing clinically apparent prostatic carcinoma is 10% for American men.

Autopsy studies have shown that the true frequency of prostatic carcinoma is considerably higher than its clinical incidence. Most cases (70% to 90%) are incidental microscopic findings at autopsy or are discovered in a specimen resected for prostatic hyperplasia. The prevalence of prostatic carcinoma at autopsy increases with age, from under 10% in men 40 to 50 years of age to over 70% in those older than 80.

There is considerable geographic variation in the age-related death rates for adenocarcinoma of the prostate throughout the world, the highest being in the United States and the Scandinavian countries, and the lowest in Mexico, Greece, and Japan. Most western European countries have intermediate rates. American blacks, who exhibit a rate twice as high as white Americans, have the highest prostate carcinoma death rates in the world. Migrant studies have shown that in the United States, descendants of Polish and Japanese immigrants have a higher incidence of prostatic carcinoma than men in their original countries. Similarly, mortality from prostatic carcinoma among black American men exceeds that among blacks in Africa.

In addition to geographic, racial, and age differences, heredity, and possibly diet, influence the risk of prostate cancer. One tenth of cases are familial, with a significantly increased risk in persons whose first-degree relatives are afflicted with prostate cancer. There is some evidence that dietary fat content may increase the risk of prostate cancer, but further studies are required to confirm this relationship.

PATHOGENESIS: The cause of prostatic adenocarcinoma is unknown, but the principal focus of research interest is endocrine influences. Androgenic control of normal prostatic growth and the responsiveness of prostate cancer to castration and exogenous estrogens support a role for male hormones. However, patients with prostate cancer do not typically have higher levels of serum androgens. Elevated urinary estrone-to-testosterone ratios have been reported. However, rats have developed the tumor after prolonged administration of testosterone.

There is no evidence that prostatic adenocarcinoma originates from hyperplastic nodules. Current attention addresses intraductal dysplastic foci termed **prostatic intraepithelial neoplasia** *(PIN). PIN refers to resident prostatic ducts lined by cytologically atypical luminal cells and concomitant decrease in basal cells. Substantial evidence now supports the contention that PIN lesions are premalignant changes that progress to prostatic adenocar-*

cinoma. Such lesions precede invasive cancer by two decades, and their severity increases with increasing age.

Morphologic evidence linking PIN to invasive prostate cancer includes (1) both lesions are mainly peripheral, (2) cytological similarity of high-grade PIN to invasive cancer, and (3) close topographical proximity of high-grade PIN to invasive cancer. Finally, PIN lesions are more frequent in prostates harboring cancer than in those without tumors. Certain markers are similar in high-grade PIN and invasive cancer (e.g., aneuploidy, tumor growth factor [TGF]-α, type IV collagenase, and expression of *bcl*-2 and c-*erb*-2 oncogenes).

High-grade PIN is an important marker for carcinoma when identified in needle biopsies. Many patients with only high-grade PIN on initial biopsy have invasive carcinoma in subsequent follow-up biopsies performed within weeks to months.

PATHOLOGY: Adenocarcinomas, which account for the vast majority of all primary prostatic tumors, are commonly multicentric and located in the peripheral zones in over 70% of cases. The cut surface of the prostate shows irregular, yellow–white, indurated subcapsular nodules.

RELATIONSHIP OF PIN FOCI TO FOCI OF CARCINOMA: Notably, in the vicinity of most invasive carcinomas, one may identify lesions of **high-grade PIN,** which microscopically are dilated branching glands with intraluminal papillary projections lined by atypical cells. The nuclei of high-grade PIN are enlarged, contain nucleoli, and show marked crowding (Fig. 17-41). Atypical cells within PIN-affected ducts may also show a flat or a cribriform growth pattern.

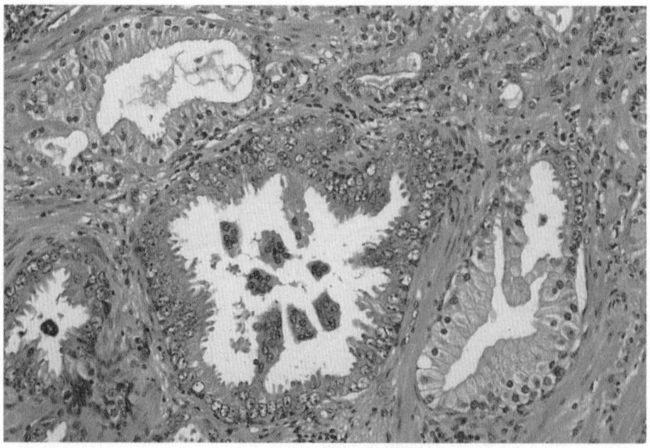

FIGURE 17-41. **High-grade prostatic intraepithelial neoplasia (PIN).** The large duct in the center is lined by atypical cells with enlarged nuclei and prominent nucleoli. Two normal ducts are located adjacent to the neoplastic one.

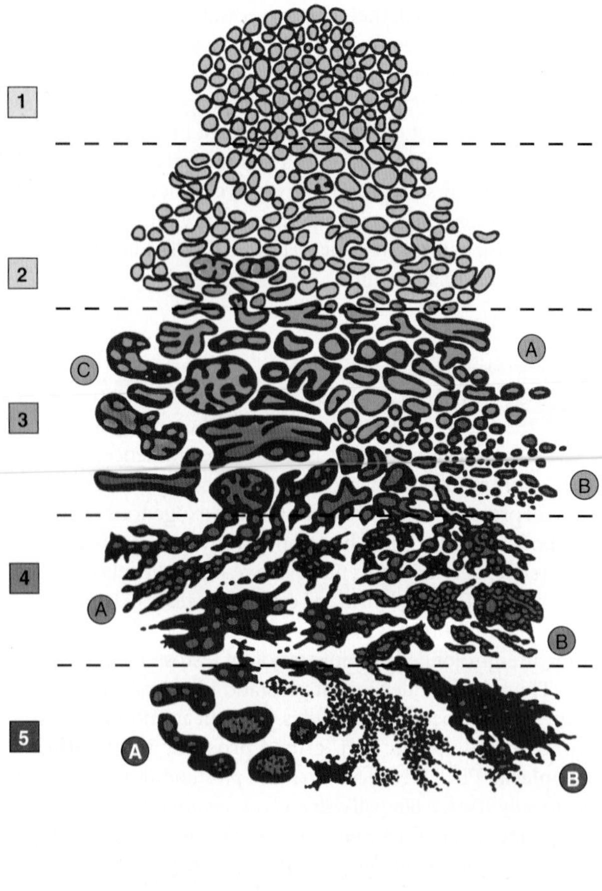

GLANDS

Differentiation	Distribution
1 'Round,' lined by single layer of cuboidal cells	Close packed in rounded masses; definite edge
2 More variable in size and shape	Separated up to one gland diameter; 'loose' edge
3a Irregular shape; medium to large size	Irregularly spaced apart; poorly defined 'edge'; surround normal strucutres
3b Small to minute glands, not fused or 'chained'	Very irregular spacing and distribution; no 'edge'; surround normal structures
3c Masses of cribriform or papillary epithelium with smooth outer surfaces	
4a Ragged masses of fused glandular epithelium; bare tumor cells in stroma	Ragged infiltrating masses that overrun normal structures; No smooth surfaces against stroma
4b Same as 4a; large clear cells	
5a Smooth, cribriform to solid masses; often central necrosis 'comedocarcinoma'	Ragged infiltrating masses that infiltrate stromal fibers
5b Anaplastic carcinoma with vacuoles and glands that suggest adenocarcinoma	

FIGURE 17-42. **Prostate carcinoma. Gleason grading system.**

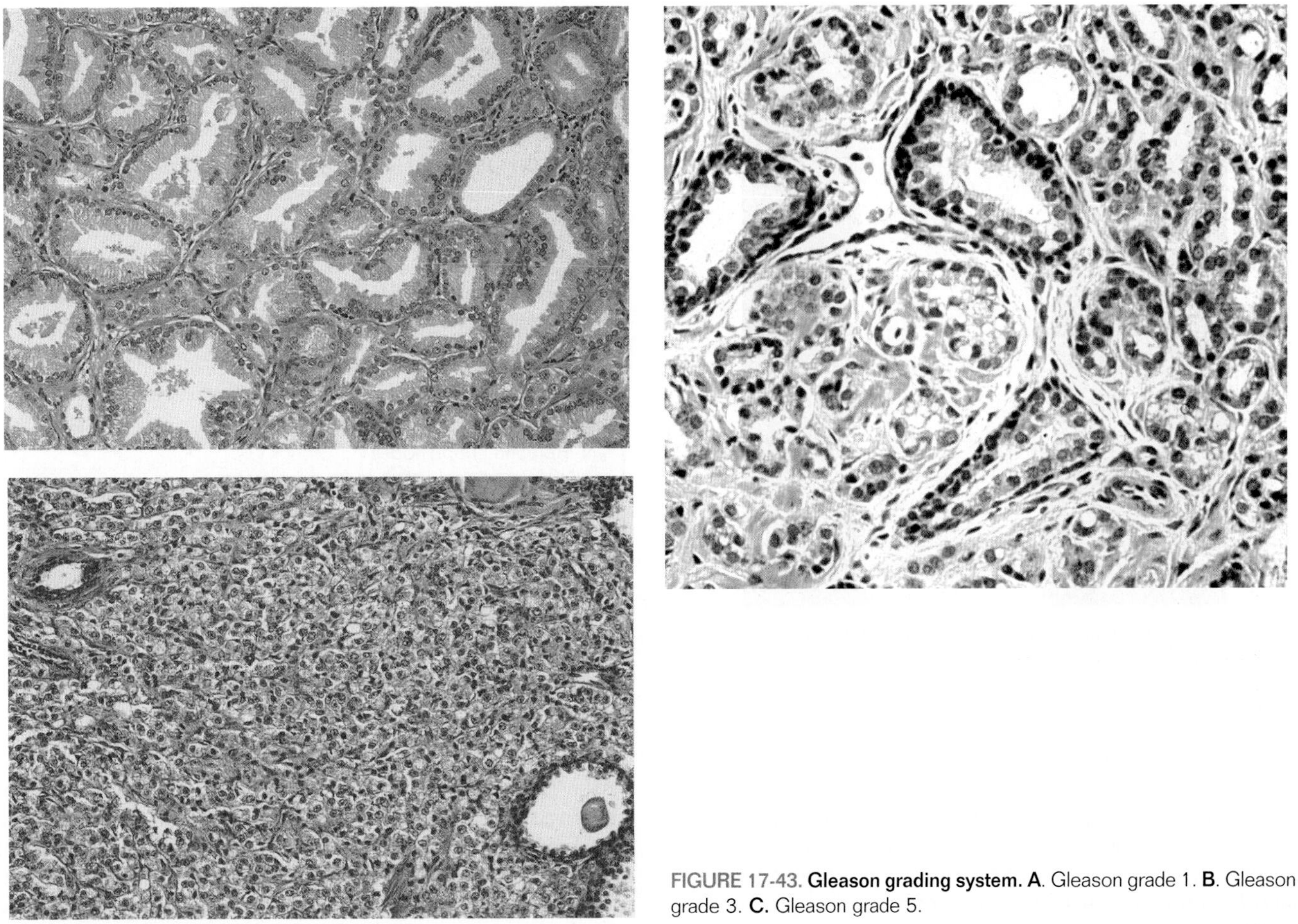

A B C

FIGURE 17-43. **Gleason grading system. A**. Gleason grade 1. **B**. Gleason grade 3. **C**. Gleason grade 5.

HISTOLOGIC FEATURES OF INVASIVE CARCINOMA: Most prostatic adenocarcinomas are of acinar origin and feature small to medium-sized glands that lack organization and infiltrate the stroma. Well-differentiated tumors show uniform medium-sized or small glands (Fig. 17-42) that are lined by a single layer of uniform neoplastic epithelial cells. *In fact, a single layer of cuboidal cells lining neoplastic acini is the most frequently used criterion to diagnose prostatic adenocarcinoma.* Progressive loss of differentiation of prostatic adenocarcinomas is characterized by:

- Increasing variability of gland size and configuration
- Papillary and cribriform patterns
- Rudimentary (or no) gland formation, with only solid cords of infiltrating tumor cells. Uncommonly, a prostate cancer is composed of small undifferentiated cells growing individually or in sheets, without evidence of any structural organization.

CYTOLOGIC FEATURES: The prominence of pleomorphic and hyperchromatic nuclei is highly variable. One or two conspicuous nucleoli in a background of chromatin clumped near the nuclear membrane is the most frequent nuclear feature. The cytoplasm stains slightly eosinophilic or may be so vacuolated that it simulates the clear cells of renal cell carcinoma. Cell borders are distinct in better-differentiated tumors, but are not well demarcated in the more poorly differentiated ones.

GRADING: Prostatic adenocarcinoma is most commonly classified according to the **Gleason grading system** (see Figs. 17-42 and Fig. 17-43), which is based on five histologic patterns of tumor gland formation and infiltration. Recognizing the high frequency of mixed tumor patterns, the Gleason score is the sum of the grades (1 through 5) attributed to the most prominent pattern and that of the minority pattern. The best-differentiated tumors have a Gleason score of 2 (1 + 1), while very poorly differentiated cancers have scores of 10 (5 + 5). Most tumors score 4 to 7 (2 + 2, to 3 + 4 or 4 + 3). When combined with the tumor stage, the Gleason grading system has prognostic value: lower scores correlate with better prognoses.

INVASION AND METASTASIS: The high frequency of invasion of the prostatic capsule by adenocarcinoma relates to the subcapsular location of the tumor. Perineural tumor invasion within the prostate and adjacent tissues is usual. Since peripheral nerves are devoid of perineural lymphatic channels, this mode of invasion represents contiguous spread of the tumor along a tissue space that offers the plane of least resistance.

The seminal vesicles are almost always involved by direct extension of prostate cancer. Invasion of the urinary bladder is less common until late in the clinical course. The earliest metastases occur in the obturator lymph node, with subsequent dissemination to iliac and periaortic lymph nodes. Metastases to the lung reflect further lymphatic spread through the thoracic duct and through dissemination from the prostatic venous plexus to the inferior vena cava. Bony metastases, particularly to the vertebral column (Fig. 17-44), ribs and pelvic bones, are painful and present a thorny clinical problem.

CLINICAL FEATURES: One tenth of all cases of prostate cancer are initially discovered in the fragments of tissue obtained at the time of transurethral resection

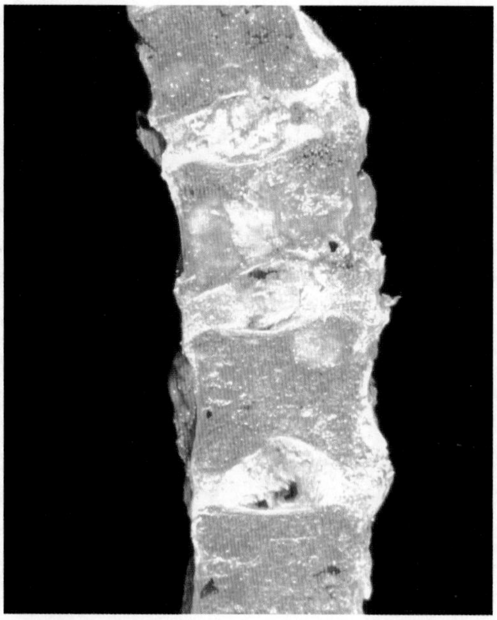

FIGURE 17-44. **Prostatic carcinoma metastatic to the spine.** The vertebral bodies contain several nodular osteoblastic metastases.

TABLE 17-8

TNM Staging of Prostatic Carcinoma

T-Primary tumor
T1 No clinically detectable tumor
T1a Histologic tumor found in 5% or less of tissue examined
T1b Histologic tumor found in more than 5% of tissue examined
T2 Tumor confined to the prostate
T2a Tumor in one lobe only
T2b Tumor in both lobes
T3 Tumor extends through the capsule
T3a Extracapsular extension only
T3b Tumor extends into seminal vesicles
T4 Tumor invades adjacent structures other than seminal vesicles
N-Regional lymph nodes
N0 No regional lymph node involvement
N1 Regional lymph node metastases present
M-Distant metastases
M0 No distant metastases
M1 Distant metastases present

for prostatic hyperplasia. The current widespread screening programs for prostate cancer that use digital rectal examination in combination with serum PSA detect this malignancy in most cases. Patients with elevated serum PSA are further evaluated by needle biopsies. *Preoperative PSA levels are correlated with cancer volume.* Uncommonly, patients with prostate cancer present with bladder outlet obstruction or symptoms referable to metastatic tumor.

The principles of clinical staging of prostate cancer are shown in Figure 17-45 and Table 17-8. At the time of initial presentation, 10% of prostate cancers are stage T1. In patients with tumors clinically judged to be localized to the prostate (stage T2), 60% show microscopic evidence of capsular penetration or seminal vesicle invasion (stage T3). Metastases are observed in lymph nodes, bones, lung and liver, in order of decreasing frequency. Widespread tumor dissemination (carcinomatosis), frequently with terminal pneumonia or sepsis, is the most common cause of death.

The immunohistochemical demonstration of PSA on biopsy specimens of metastatic sites has proved valuable in identifying the prostate as the primary site of the tumor. A new marker for prostate carcinoma, α-methylacyl-CoA racemase (AMCAR) is

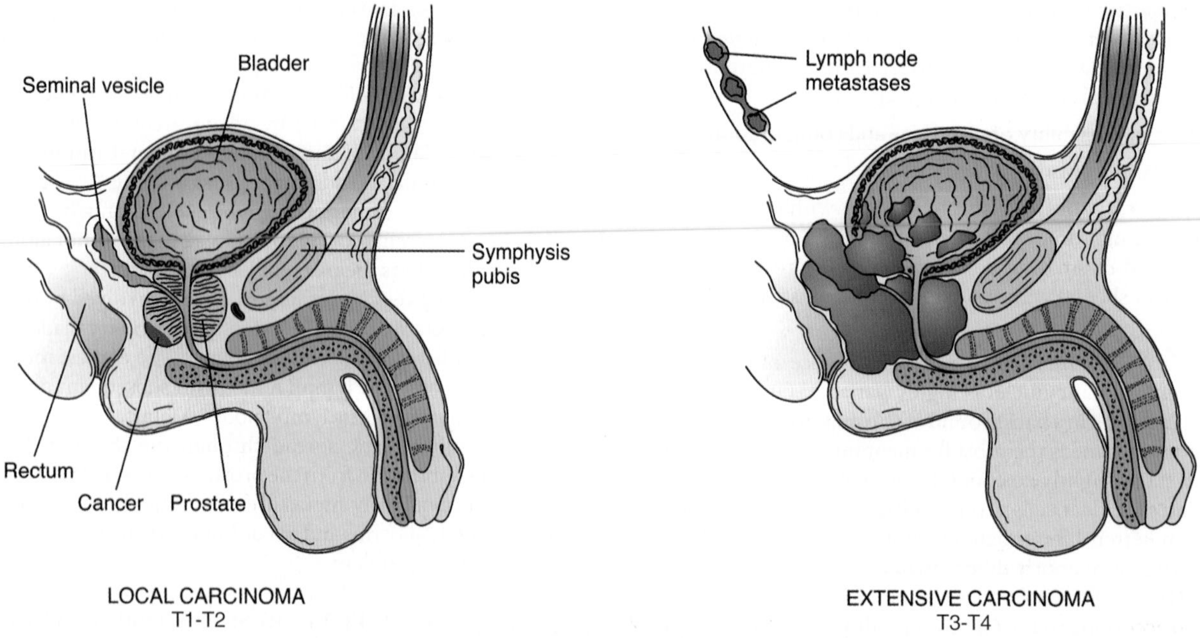

FIGURE 17-45. **Tumor, Node, Metastasis (TNM) staging of prostatic carcinoma.**

also useful for identifying prostatic adenocarcinoma inside the gland as well as in metastatic sites. PSA is also detectable in the serum of patients with prostate cancer. Serum PSA is a useful screening test for the disease and an indicator of response to treatment. Serum prostatic alkaline phosphatase (PSAP) levels are elevated in patients with osteoblastic bony metastases.

Therapy for prostate cancer depends on the stage of the tumor. Patients with stage T1 and T2 cancers are treated by radical prostatectomy or radiation therapy. In stage T3 tumors, radiation therapy is the treatment of choice, acknowledging that half of these patients have occult pelvic lymph node metastases (and possibly further systemic dissemination), which cannot be cured by surgical means.

For patients whose tumors progress clinically and for all patients judged to have regional or distant metastases at initial presentation, the principal form of therapy is hormonal. This treatment involves orchiectomy or administration of pituitary LH or LH-releasing hormone (LHRH) antagonists. In either case, the goal is androgen deprivation.

The 5-year survival rates depend on stage and Gleason grade (see Fig. 17-42). Using only the staging data, survival is: stages T1 and T2, 90%; stage T3, 40%; and stage T4, 10%.

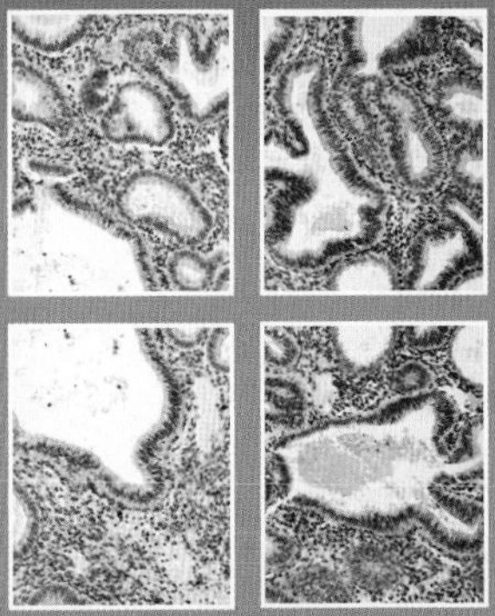

18

The Female Reproductive System

Stanley J. Robboy
Maria J. Merino
George L. Mutter

Embryology

The gonadal anlage, which forms as a swelling of the embryonic urogenital ridge, is initially in an indifferent state. Both sex chromosomes and autosomal chromosomes in gonadal stromal cells determine whether it will differentiate into testis or ovary. If the gonadal stroma is male, a gene on the Y chromosome (testis-determining gene) interacts with somatic components in the primitive gonad to initiate development of seminiferous tubules. An ovary develops if the gonadal stroma is female and there is no stimulus to form a testis. The ovary is derived from mesoderm, except for the germ cells, which are endodermal. By about the 40th day, the ovaries and testes are histologically distinct.

The **wolffian (mesonephric) ducts** begin their development at about day 25, regardless of the embryo's sex. If stimulated by testosterone (secreted by Leydig cells starting at about day 70), the ducts differentiate into vas deferens, epididymis, and seminal vesicle. If not stimulated by day 84, the ducts regress and remain as vestigial rests in the female. They may form cysts in the cervix or vagina (**mesonephric cyst**).

The **müllerian (paramesonephric) ducts** comprise the anlage of the fallopian tubes, uterus, and vaginal wall. They appear at about day 37 as funnel-shaped openings of celomic epithelium. These develop into paired, undifferentiated tubes, using the wolffian ducts as "guide wires" to reach the region of the future hymen. If the wolffian duct is absent, as in renal agenesis, the vagina and cervix are almost always abnormal or absent. At day 54, the müllerian ducts fuse to become a straight uterovaginal canal.

A central tenet of genital tract development in both sexes is that müllerian tubes will develop along female lines unless specifically impeded by embryonic testicular factors. In males, Sertoli cells in developing testes produce **antimullerian hormone**, also called **müllerian-inhibiting substance**, a protein that causes müllerian ducts to regress.

Development of external genitalia into a masculine form depends on local conversion of testosterone to dihydrotestosterone. Without dihydrotestosterone (i.e., relative estrogen excess), the results is persistence of female external genitalia. The genital tubercle develops into clitoris, genital folds into labia minora, and genital swellings into labia majora. The basic architecture of the female genital tract is completed by day 120.

Genital Infections

Genital Infections Are Commonly Sexually Transmitted

Infectious diseases of the female genital tract are common and are caused by many pathogenic organisms (Table 18-1), which are also discussed in Chapter 9. Most of the important infectious diseases affecting the female genital tract are sexually transmitted.

Bacterial Infections

Gonorrhea

Gonorrhea is caused by *Neisseria gonorrhoeae,* a fastidious, gram-negative diplococcus. A million cases of gonorrhea occur yearly in the United States. The infection is a frequent cause of acute salpingitis and pelvic inflammatory disease (PID) (Fig. 18-1).

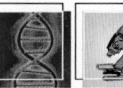

PATHOGENESIS AND PATHOLOGY: The organisms ascend through the cervix and the endometrial cavity, where they cause acute endometritis. The bacteria then attach to mucosal cells in the fallopian tube and elicit an acute inflammatory reaction, which is confined to the mucosal surface (**acute salpingitis**). From the tubal lumen, the infection spreads to involve ovary, sometimes resulting in a **tuboovarian abscess**. It may also involve pelvic and abdominal cavities, with formation of subdiaphragmatic and pelvic abscesses.

Systemic complications of gonorrhea include septicemia and septic arthritis. The organisms induce a purulent inflammatory reaction at all sites of infection. Resolution is rarely complete, and dense fibrous adhesions remain. The healing process distorts and destroys the plicae of the fallopian tube, often leading to sterility.

Syphilis

Syphilis (see Chapter 9) is caused by *Treponema pallidum,* a thin, motile, spiral-shaped bacterium, called a spirochete. It is acquired as a result of sexual contact with an infected person, or transplacental spread (congenital syphilis). *T. pallidum* penetrates small cuts in the skin or normal mucosal membranes. Untreated syphilis is a chronic infection that may wax and wane, progressing through primary, secondary, and tertiary stages.

- In the **primary stage** the **chancre** usually appears after an incubation period of about 3 weeks, be it on the penis, vulva,

TABLE 18–1

Infectious Diseases of the Female Genital Tract

Organism	Disease	Diagnostic Feature
Sexually Transmitted Diseases		
Gram-negative rods and cocci		
Calymmatobacterium granulomatis	Granuloma inguinale	Donovan body
Gardnerella vaginalis	*Gardnerella* infection	Clue cell
Haemophilus ducreyi	Chancroid (soft chancre)	
Neisseria gonorrhoeae	Gonorrhea	Gram-negative diplococcus
Spirochetes		
Treponema pallidum	Syphilis	Spirochete
Mycoplasmas		
Mycoplasma hominis	Nonspecific vaginitis	
Ureaplasma urealyticum	Nonspecific vaginitis	
Rickettsiae		
Chlamydia trachomatis type D-K	Various forms of PID	
Chlamydia trachomatis type L_{1-3}	Lymphogranuloma venereum	
Viruses		
Human papillomavirus (HPV)	Condyloma acuminatum/planum	Koilocyte
	Neoplastic potential	
Types 6, 11, 40, 42, 43, 44, 57	Low risk	
Types 16, 18, 31, 33, 35, 39, 45, 51, 52, 56, 58, 66	High risk	
Herpes simplex, type 2	Herpes genitalis	Multinucleated giant cell with intranuclear homogenization and inclusion bodies
Cytomegalovirus (CMV)	Cytomegalic inclusion disease	Bulbous intranuclear inclusion body
Molluscum contagiosum	Molluscum infection	Molluscum body
Protozoa		
Trichomonas vaginalis	Trichomoniasis	Trichomonad
Selected Nonsexually Transmitted Diseases		
Actinomyces and related organisms		
Actinomyces israelii	PID (one of many organisms)	Sulphur granules
Mycobacterium tuberculosis	Tuberculosis	Necrotizing granulomas
Fungi		
Candida albicans	Candidiasis	*Candida* species

PID = pelvic inflammatory disease.

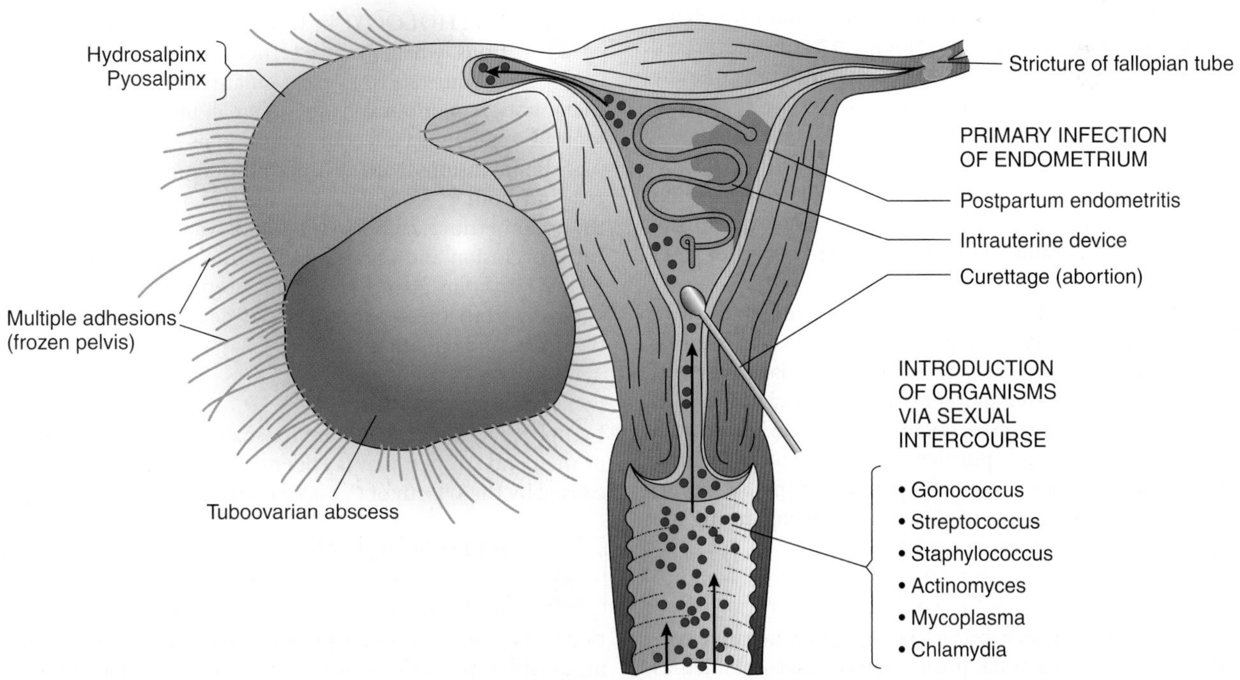

FIGURE 18-1. **Pelvic inflammatory disease.**

tongue, or other portals of bacterial entry. The chancre manifests as a painless, indurated papule, 1 cm to several centimeters in diameter. It is surrounded by an inflammatory cuff that breaks down to form an ulcer. The lesion may persist for 2 to 6 weeks. It then heals spontaneously.

- The **secondary stage** appears after a latent period of several weeks to months. Common features include low-grade fever, headache, malaise, lymphadenopathy, and highly contagious syphilitic lesions called **condylomata lata** (syphilitic warts). The secondary infectious lesions heal after 2 to 6 weeks and symptoms disappear spontaneously.
- The **tertiary stage** develops any time thereafter and may be complicated by severe damage to the cardiovascular and nervous systems.

PATHOLOGY: The hallmark of syphilis in biopsy specimens is a dense inflammatory infiltrate with lymphocytes and plasma cells, particularly adjacent to blood vessels, and prominent endothelial swelling. Silver impregnation techniques (Warthin-Starry stain or its modifications) help demonstrate the spirochetes. The more advanced stages of disease show greater obliterative endarteritis and subsequent tissue destruction.

Granuloma Inguinale

Granuloma inguinale is caused by *Calymmatobacterium granulomatis,* a sexually transmitted, gram-negative, encapsulated rod. The disease occurs with equal frequency in women and men.

PATHOLOGY: The primary lesion begins as a painless, ulcerated nodule involving genital, inguinal, or perianal skin. The organisms invade through skin abrasions and spread locally by direct extension, destroying skin and underlying tissues. Extensive local spread and lymphatic permeation occur later. Vacuolated macrophages teem with characteristic intracellular bacteria (**Donovan bodies**). The organism, best seen with the Wright stain, resembles a closed safety pin. Hyperplasia of the squamous epithelium overlying an involved area may be exuberant enough to be misinterpreted as a squamous cell carcinoma. Relapses after antibiotic therapy are common.

Chancroid

Chancroid, also called **soft chancre**, is caused by *Haemophilus ducreyi,* a gram-negative bacillus. This disease is rare in the United States but is common in underdeveloped countries.

PATHOLOGY: Single or sometimes multiple small, vesiculopustular lesions appear on cervix, vagina, vulva, or perianal region usually 3 to 5 days after sexual contact with an infected partner. Histologic examination at this stage reveals granulomatous inflammation. The lesion often ruptures to form a painful, purulent ulcer that bleeds easily. There may be associated inguinal lymphadenopathy, fever, chills, and malaise. A major complication is scarring during the healing phase, which may cause urethral stenosis.

Gardnerella

Sexual transmission of *Gardnerella vaginalis,* a gram-negative coccobacillus, causes a substantial proportion of cases classified as nonspecific vaginitis. Biopsies usually are normal because the organism does not penetrate the mucosa or elicit an inflammatory reaction. Diagnosis is best established by identifying organisms in a wet mount specimen of a vaginal discharge or a Papanicolaou-stained smear (Pap smear). The **clue cell** is pathognomonic and shows squamous cells covered by coccobacilli. Other aids to diagnosis are a thin, homogeneous, milklike vaginal discharge; vaginal pH above 4.5; and a fishy odor when the discharge is alkalinized with 10% potassium hydroxide.

Mycoplasma

Mycoplasmas (see Chapter 9) are minute pleomorphic organisms that resemble the so-called L bacterial forms but differ by having no cell wall. They are common commensals of the oropharyngeal and urogenital tracts. Colonization of the lower genital tract by mycoplasmas occurs through sexual contact. *Ureaplasma urealyticum* can be isolated from the lower genital tract in 40% of healthy women and may cause infertility, adverse effects on pregnancy, and perinatal infections. *Mycoplasma hominis,* found in the lower genital tract of 5% of healthy women, is responsible for a small proportion of cases of symptomatic cervicitis and vaginitis. *M. hominis* is frequently cultivated in association with *G. vaginalis* or *Trichomonas vaginalis* infection. Although the role of mycoplasma in genital tract infection is not completely understood, the organisms are encountered in PID, acute salpingitis, spontaneous abortion, and puerperal fever. Affected tissue is usually unremarkable histologically.

Chlamydia Infections

Chlamydia trachomatis is a common, venereally transmitted organism, which is a gram-negative obligate, intracellular rickettsia. Fifteen serotypes are known. Infection with *C. trachomatis* results in a variety of disorders in women, men, and infants. This organism has been found in the genital tract of about 8% of asymptomatic women and 20% of women presenting with symptoms of lower genital tract infection. Chlamydia is easily confused with gonorrhea, as the symptoms of both diseases are similar.

PATHOLOGY: In the more common genital infections, which involve serotypes D through K, the cervical mucosa is severely inflamed and endocervical and metaplastic squamous cells reveal small inclusion bodies. Cytologically, chlamydia infection manifests as perinuclear intracytoplasmic inclusions with distinct borders and intracytoplasmic **coccoid bodies**. Complications include ascending infection of the endometrium, fallopian tube, and ovary, which may result in tubal occlusion and infertility. Chlamydia also gives rise to infected Bartholin glands and acute urethritis. Infants delivered vaginally from infected mothers may develop conjunctivitis, otitis media, and pneumonia.

Lymphogranuloma Venereum

Lymphogranuloma venereum is a sexually transmitted infection of men and women that is endemic in tropical countries and is caused by the L form of *C. trachomatis,* serotypes L1 through L3.

PATHOLOGY: After a few days to a month, a small painless vesicle forms at the site of inoculation. It heals rapidly and in many instances is not even noticed. The second stage presents with bilaterally enlarged inguinal lymph nodes that may rupture and form suppurative fistulas. Inguinal nodes in men and perirectal nodes in women become matted and painful. In some untreated patients, a third stage appears after a latency of several years. This chronic phase shows scarring, which causes lymphatic obstruction and resulting genital elephantiasis and rectal strictures. In the second and third stages, infected tissues contain necrotizing granulomas, neutrophilic infiltrates and, occasionally, inclusion bodies within macrophages.

Viral Infections

Human Papillomavirus

Human papillomavirus (HPV) is a DNA virus that infects a number of skin and mucosal surfaces to produce wartlike lesions, referred to as **verrucae** and **condylomata**. Over 100 HPV serotypes are known, one-third of which cause genital tract lesions. The median time from infection to first detection of HPV is 3 months. In the United States, as many as two thirds of graduating college women have genital HPV infections, which result from sexual contact with an infected person. Even in women who have had only one sexual partner, by 3 years after first intercourse, the risk of acquiring cervical HPV was 50% in one study. Approximately 20 million people are currently infected with HPV in this country. HPV types 6 and 11 are detected in over 80% of the macroscopically visible condylomata.

Several strains of HPV are the major etiologic factors for squamous cell cancer in the female lower genital tract. Types 16, 18, 31, and 45 are the most common serotypes linked to intraepithelial neoplasia and invasive cancer (see the section on cervix below).

Most cases of HPV are diagnosed by cervical Pap smear. Recent tests can directly assay for HPV DNA. Current treatment for HPV infection is inadequate, but most spontaneously dissappear. The FDA approved a vaccine in 2006 against HPV.

Condyloma Acuminatum

Condyloma acuminatum is caused by HPV infection. It is a benign, exophytic, papillomatous lesion on the skin or mucous membranes of the lower female genital tract, which is often visible to the naked eye, but sometimes requires colposcopy to be seen.

PATHOLOGY: Condylomata acuminata occur on the vulva, perianal region, perineum, vagina, and cervix. They may also involve the urethra, bladder, and rectum. Condylomata grow as papules, plaques, or nodules and eventually as spiked or cauliflower-like excrescences (Fig. 18-2A). Microscopy reveals striking papillomatous proliferation of squamous epithelium. A characteristic finding is the **koilocyte** (from the Greek *koilos,* hollow), an epithelial cell with a perinuclear halo and a wrinkled nucleus that contains HPV particles (see Fig. 18-2B). The virus DNA typically remains episomal and replicates within the cell. The large numbers of particles cause extensive cytoplasmic destruction, creating the koilocyte (see Fig. 18-2C).

Herpesvirus

Herpes simplex type 2 is a double-stranded DNA virus that is a common cause of sexually transmitted genital infections. After an incubation period of 1 to 3 weeks, small vesicles develop on the vulva and erode into painful ulcers. Similar lesions occur in the vagina and cervix. Epithelial cells adjacent to intraepithelial vesicles show ballooning degeneration and many contain large nuclei with eosinophilic inclusions.

Genital herpes tends to become latent, at which times the virus remains in the sacral ganglia. If the virus reactivates in pregnancy, the newborn may acquire fatal herpes infection during passage through the birth canal. For this reason, active herpetic lesions in the vagina at the time of delivery are an indication for Cesarean section.

Cytomegalovirus

Cytomegalovirus (CMV) is a double-stranded DNA virus of the Herpesvirus family. It is ubiquitous: more than 80% of persons over the age of 35 have antibodies to it. Several lines of evidence suggest that many cases are sexually transmitted: (1) the seroprevalence of CMV has risen in young adults, (2) the virus is recovered more frequently from cervical secretions and semen than from any other body sites, and (3) viral titers in semen are 100,000 times higher than those in urine. Nevertheless, CMV only rarely causes genital infections in women. Infection in the endometrium may result in spontaneous abortion or infection of the newborn. Infected cells exhibit characteristic large, eosinophilic, intranuclear inclusions and, occasionally, cytoplasmic inclusions.

Molluscum Contagiosum

Molluscum contagiosum (see Chapter 24) is a highly contagious double-stranded DNA poxvirus. Infection leads to multiple smooth, gray-white nodules that are centrally umbilicated and exude a cheesy material. The lesions occur predominantly in the genital region but may be found elsewhere on the body. Characteristic large, cytoplasmic viral inclusions (**molluscum bodies**) are found in infected epithelial cells. Most lesions regress spontaneously, but untreated ones may persist for years.

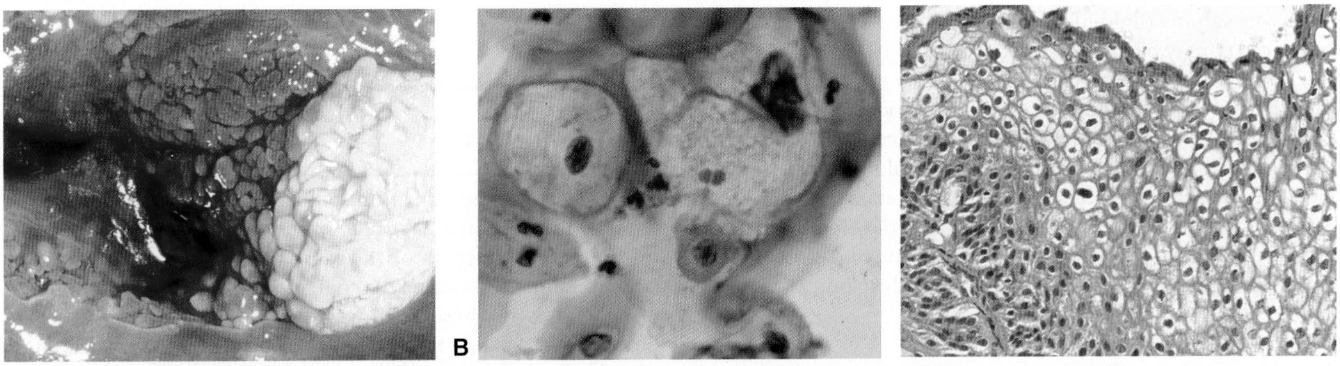

A B C

FIGURE 18-2. **Human papillomavirus-induced condylomatous infections. A.** Condyloma acuminatum on the cervix, visible with the naked eye as cauliflower-like excrescences. **B.** A cervical smear contains characteristic koilocytes, with a perinuclear halo and a wrinkled nucleus that contains viral particles. **C.** Biopsy of the condyloma shows koilocytes with perinuclear halos but lacking nuclear atypia.

Trichomoniasis

T. vaginalis is a large, pear-shaped, flagellated protozoan that commonly causes vaginitis. The disease is sexually transmitted, and 25% of infected women are asymptomatic carriers. Infection manifests as a heavy, yellow-gray, thick, foamy discharge accompanied by severe itching, dyspareunia (painful intercourse), and dysuria (painful urination). The diagnosis is confirmed by a wet mount preparation in which the motile trichomonads are seen. The organisms are also demonstrated in Pap smears.

Pelvic Inflammatory Disease

PID describes an infection of pelvic organs that follows extension of any of a variety of microorganisms beyond the uterine corpus (see Fig. 18-1). Ascent of the infection results in bilateral acute salpingitis, pyosalpinx, and tuboovarian abscesses. *N. gonorrhoeae* and chlamydia are the principal organisms causing PID, but most infections are polymicrobial. The incidence of PID is far greater in sexually promiscuous women than in those who are monogamous. Occasionally, PID is a sequel to postpartum endometritis or a complication of endometrial curettage.

Patients with PID typically present with lower abdominal pain. Examination reveals bilateral adnexal tenderness and marked discomfort when the cervix is manipulated (chandelier sign). Complications of PID include (1) rupture of a tuboovarian abscess, which may result in life-threatening peritonitis; (2) infertility from scarring of the healed tubal plicae; (3) increased rates of ectopic pregnancy; and (4) intestinal obstruction from fibrous bands and adhesions.

Some Genital Infections Are Not Transmitted Sexually

Tuberculosis

Mycobacterium tuberculosis may infect any segment of the female genital tract. Genital tuberculosis is found in 1% of infertile women in the United States and in more than 10% of such women in less-developed countries. Identification of acid-fast-bacilli (AFB) confirms the diagnosis.

PATHOLOGY:

TUBERCULOUS SALPINGITIS: Inflammation of the fallopian tube is the initial lesion in most cases of tuberculous genital infection. The mycobacteria usually reach the tube by hematogenous dissemination from lung. Tuberculous salpingitis results in fibrinous adhesions and scarring of the fallopian tube. In turn, these complications lead to multiple functional abnormalities (e.g., infertility, ectopic gestation, pelvic pain). The tubes may become nodular and mimic salpingitis isthmica nodosa. **Pyosalpinx** (fallopian tube distended with pus) and **hydrosalpinx** (fluid-filled tube) are late sequelae, and the adjacent ovary may become infected.

TUBERCULOUS ENDOMETRITIS: This condition complicates half of cases of tubal tubercular infection. Noncaseating, poorly formed granulomas with rare giant cells are typical. In other areas afflicted with this infection, granulomas have time to develop caseous necrosis and characteristic Langhans giant cells. By contrast, tuberculous granulomas that develop in the endometrium are no more than one cycle old, owing to menstrual shedding, and thus are at an earlier stage of development.

Candidiasis

Ten percent of women are asymptomatic carriers of fungi in vulva and vagina, *Candida albicans* being the most common offender. However, only 2% of women present with clinically apparent candidal vulvovaginitis. Pregnant women are considerably more susceptible, and 10% of such women are symptomatic. Diabetes mellitus and use of oral contraceptives also promote vaginal candidiasis. Infection manifests as vulvar itching and a white discharge. Clinical examination reveals firmly adherent, small white plaques on mucous membranes ("thrush"). Biopsy shows submucosal edema and chronic inflammation. The fungi do not penetrate epithelium, and the white patches correspond to foci of desquamated, necrotic epithelial cells, cellular debris, bacterial flora, candidal spores, and pseudohyphae. If untreated, infection waxes, wanes and frequently disappears following delivery. Characteristic spores and pseudohyphae in a wet mount preparation or with a Pap stain are diagnostic.

Actinomycosis

Genital tract actinomycosis is uncommon but is increasingly reported in association with use of intrauterine devices (IUDs). *Actinomyces israelii,* the causative organism, is a gram-positive rod found in 4% of normal genital tracts. It is believed to enter the uterine cavity by way of the tail of the IUD. It ascends to infect the fallopian tube, ovary, and broad ligaments and forms a tuboovarian abscess. Suppurating lesions display drainage tracts that contain dense microcolonies of organisms ("sulfur granules"). Actinomycosis results in extensive fibrosis and scarring of the female genital tract.

Toxic Shock Syndrome Is Associated with Vaginal Staphylococcal Infection

Toxic shock syndrome is an acute, sometimes fatal disorder characterized by fever, shock and a desquamative erythematous rash. In addition, vomiting, diarrhea, myalgias, neurologic signs, and thrombocytopenia are common. Certain strains of *Staphylococcus aureus* release an exotoxin called **toxic shock syndrome toxin-1**. This toxin exerts its own effects and alters the function of mononuclear phagocytes, thus impairing clearance of other potentially toxic substances, such as endotoxin. In addition to the pathologic alterations characteristic of shock, the lesions of disseminated intravascular coagulation are usually prominent. The disease was first recognized when long-acting tampons were first introduced, providing sufficient time for the staphylococcal organisms to proliferate. The contraceptive "sponge" was also associated. The occurrence of toxic shock syndrome has decreased markedly since recognition of the role of tampons in promoting colonization of the vagina by *S. aureus*.

VULVA

Anatomy

The vulva comprises the mons pubis, labia majora and minora, clitoris, and vestibule. With the onset of puberty, the mons pubis and lateral borders of the labia majora acquire increased subcutaneous fat and grow coarse hair. Sebaceous and apocrine glands in these regions develop concomitantly. The paired external openings of the paraurethral glands (**Skene glands**) flank the urethral meatus. **Bartholin glands**, located immediately posterolateral to the introitus, are branching, mucus- secreting, tubuloalveolar glands drained by a short duct lined by transitional epithelium. In addition, microscopic mucous glands are scattered throughout the area bounded by the labia minora. The inguinal and femoral lymph nodes provide the primary lymph drainage routes, except for the clitoris (the homologue of the penis), which shares the lymphatic drainage of the urethra.

Developmental Anomalies and Cysts

ECTOPIC BREAST TISSUE: Small, isolated nodules of ectopic breast tissue may extend in the "milk line" to the vulva and enlarge during pregnancy.

BARTHOLIN GLAND CYST: The paired Bartholin glands produce a clear mucoid secretion that continuously lubricates the vestibular surface. The ducts are prone to obstruction and consequent cyst formation (Fig. 18-3). In turn, cyst infection leads to abscess formation. Bartholin gland abscess was formerly associated with gonorrhea, but staphylococci, chlamydia, and anaerobes are now more frequently the cause. Treatment consists of incision, drainage, marsupialization, and appropriate antibiotics.

FOLLICULAR CYSTS: The follicular cyst recapitulates the most distal portion of the hair follicle. Also termed **epithelial inclusion cysts** or **keratinous cysts**, follicular cysts frequently appear on the vulva, especially the labia majora. They contain a white cheesy material and typically are lined by stratified squamous epithelium.

MUCINOUS CYSTS: Mucinous glands of the vulva, a normal but generally unrecognized finding, occasionally become obstructed and subsequently cystic. Mucinous columnar cells line the cyst and may become infected.

Dermatoses

Acute Dermatitis of the Vulva Appears as Reddened Vesiculated Skin

PATHOLOGY: As vesicles (Fig. 18-4) rupture onto the surface, the fluid forms a crust on the skin surface. Histologically, the epidermis shows a range of inflammatory cells and spongiotic areas form spongiotic vesicles that rupture to produce the exudative lesions. The dermis shows a perivascular lymphocytic infiltrate and edema, manifested by separation of collagen fibers. Telangiectatic lymphatics and dilated capillaries are typical.

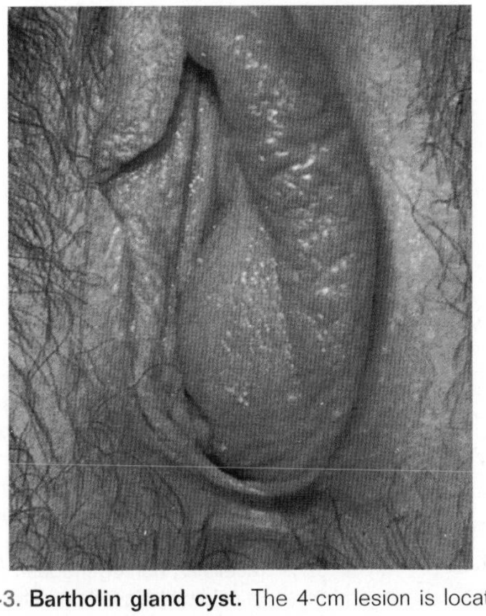

FIGURE 18-3. **Bartholin gland cyst.** The 4-cm lesion is located to the right of and posterior to the vaginal introitus.

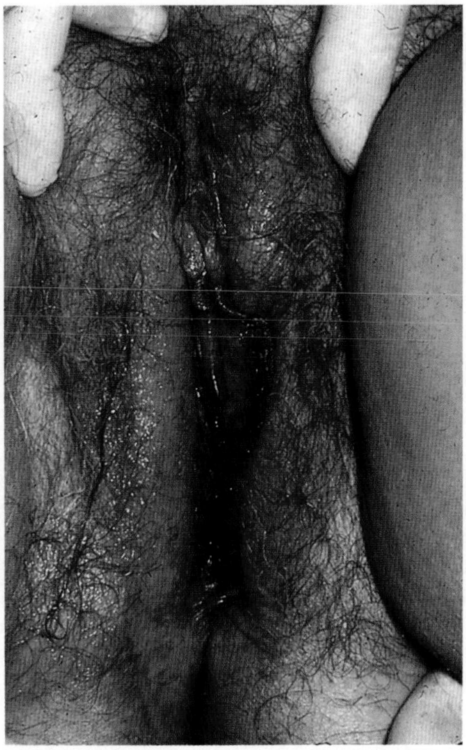

FIGURE 18-4. **Vulvar acute dermatitis (eczema).** Erythema and edema are present, with linear excoriations due to scratching.

The most common endogenous types of acute dermatitis are atopic (hypersensitivity) dermatitis and seborrheic dermatitis, seen as a scaly macular eruption. Dermatitis with an exogenous cause that manifests as acute or chronic dermatitis includes irritant dermatitis (urine on the vulvar skin) and contact allergic dermatitis (a type 4 delayed hypersensitivity reaction).

Chronic Dermatitis, or Lichen Simplex Chronicus is the End Stage of Many Vulvar Inflammatory Diseases

Vulvar chronic dermatitis (Fig. 18-5) follows many diseases that are clinically pruritic and thus subject to repeated scratching in their active phase. It may also occur in other disorders such as lichen planus, psoriasis, and lichen sclerosus. The skin is thickened with exaggerated skin markings ("lichenification") and white, due to marked hyperkeratosis. Scaling is generally present, and excoriations due to recent scratching can often be seen.

LICHEN SCLEROSUS: Lichen sclerosus is an inflammatory disease of the vulva associated with autoimmune disorders such as vitiligo, pernicious anemia, and thyroiditis.

PATHOLOGY: The condition is represented by white plaques, atrophic skin, a parchmentlike or crinkled appearance, and, occasionally, marked contracture of the vulvar tissues (Fig. 18-6A). Histological findings include hyperkeratosis, loss of rete ridges, epithelial thinning with flattening of rete pegs, cytoplasmic vacuolation of the basal layer and a homogeneous, acellular zone in the upper dermis (see Fig. 18-6B). A band of chronic inflammatory cells consisting

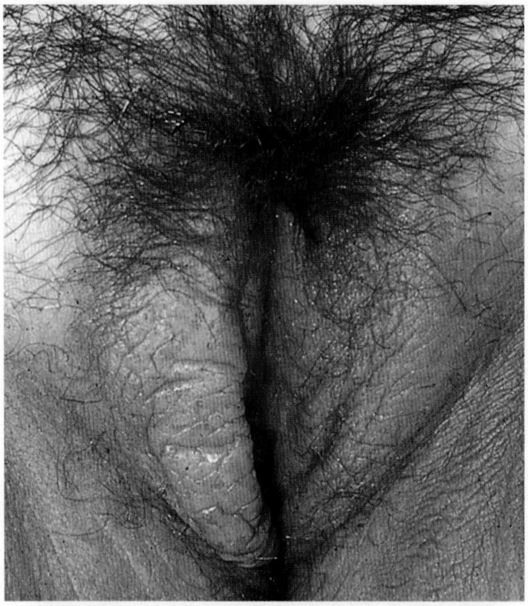

FIGURE 18-5. **Lichen simplex chronicus of the right labium majus.** There is thickening and accentuation of skin markings, with surface excoriation due to recent scratching.

of lymphocytes with few plasma cells typically lies beneath this layer. Itching is the most common symptom. Dyspareunia is frequent. The disease develops insidiously and is progressive. Women with symptomatic lichen sclerosus have a 15% chance of developing squamous cell carcinoma.

Benign Tumors

HIDRADENOMA: This benign tumor of apocrine sweat gland origin appears chiefly in the labia majora as a sharply circumscribed nodule, rarely larger than 1 cm. Microscopically, it is composed of papillary tubules and acini lined by two layers of cells: an inner layer of apocrine columnar cells and an outer one of myoepithelial cells.

SYRINGOMA: An adenoma of eccrine glands, syringoma manifests as a flesh-colored papule within the dermis of labia majora. This asymptomatic tumor is composed of a proliferation of small ducts embedded in a dense fibrous and sclerotic stroma. The walls of the ducts have two layers of cells: an inner layer of serous cells and an outer one of myoepithelial cells. The lumen contains eosinophilic material or amorphous debri.

CONNECTIVE TISSUE TUMORS: **Senile hemangiomas** (cherry hemangiomas) are small, purple skin papules, which on surface trauma may bleed. **Pyogenic granuloma,** previously thought to be a reaction to superficial wound infection, is a variant of hemangioma. Secondary infection occurs, as the surface of the lesion is fragile and easily traumatized. Soft tissue tumors found elsewhere in the body also occur in the vulva, including granular cell tumor, leiomyoma, fibroma, lipoma, and histiocytoma.

PIGMENTED VULVAR LESIONS: **Lentigo** presents as small macules. It occurs in about 10% of women. **Nevi** and **seborrheic keratosis** can also occur in this area.

Malignant Tumors and Premalignant Conditions

Vulvar Intraepithelial Neoplasia (VIN) Is a Precursor of Invasive Cancer

VIN reflects a spectrum of neoplastic changes that range from minimal cellular atypia to the most marked cellular changes short of invasive cancer. Since 1980, there has been a 5- to 10-fold increase in the frequency of VIN and a 10-fold increase in the number of women with the disease under 40 years of age. Younger women also increasingly develop an undifferentiated form of VIN, sometimes called **warty** or **basaloid dysplasia**, which typically displays HPV 16. A second form of VIN, found more often in older women, is more differentiated. If left untreated, some of these women develop invasive squamous cell carcinoma after 6 to 7 years. *Thus, like comparable lesions in the cervix (cervical intraepithelial neoplasia, CIN), VIN is a precursor of vulvar squamous cell carcinoma, of which at least 30% to 40% are*

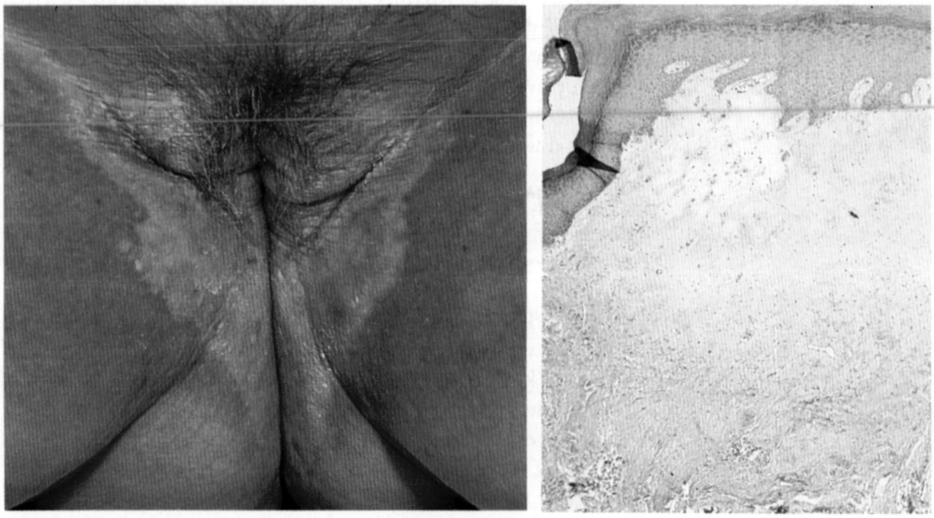

A B

FIGURE 18-6. **Lichen sclerosus of vulva. A.** The sharply demarcated white lesion affects the vulva and perineum. **B.** The epidermis is thin and exhibits hyperkeratosis and a lack of the normal rete pattern. The dermis displays an acellular, homogeneous zone overlying a mild chronic inflammatory infiltrate.

caused by ***HPV***. Clinically, most patients present with vulvar itching, burning, and raised well-defined skin lesions of variable sizes, which may be pink, red, brown, or white.

PATHOLOGY: The lesions of VIN may be single or multiple, and macular, papular, or plaquelike. Microscopically, the grades are labeled VIN I, II, and III, corresponding to mild, moderate, and severe dysplasia, respectively. Grade III also includes squamous cell carcinoma in situ (CIS). The criteria used in establishing the grade of VIN include (1) nuclear size and atypia, (2) number and degree of atypical mitoses, and (3) loss of cytoplasmic differentiation toward the epithelial surface. In the undifferentiated form seen in younger women, the entire epithelium consists of cells with highly atypical nuclei and negligible cytoplasm. Mitoses, including many atypical forms, are frequent. The more differentiated form in older women shows atypia confined to the basal or parabasal walls, with keratin pearls in the rete pegs. This type is more frequently associated with invasive carcinoma but less commonly with HPV infection. **Bowen disease**, a term still common in the dermatologic literature, is a synonym for VIN III. Lesions associated with oncogenic HPV types generally are reactive for p16.

VIN, even if locally excised, often recurs (25%), in which case it may progress to invasive squamous cell carcinoma (6%). Women with VIN may have squamous neoplasms similar to VIN elsewhere in the lower genital tract.

Squamous Cell Carcinoma Follows VIN

Squamous cell carcinoma of the vulva (Fig. 18-7) is the end result of a multistep process that begins with VIN. This tumor accounts for 3% of all genital cancers in women and is the most common cancer of the vulva (86%). In the past, it mainly affected older women, but like VIN it now occurs with increasing frequency in younger women. Two thirds of larger tumors are exophytic; the others are ulcerative and endophytic. Pruritus of long duration is commonly the first symptom. Ulceration, bleeding, and secondary infection may develop. The tumors grow slowly, then extend to the contiguous skin, vagina, and rectum. They metastasize to superficial inguinal and then deep inguinal, femoral, and pelvic lymph nodes.

Staging for vulvar cancer uses 2 cm in greatest dimension as the critical size to differentiate stage I and stage II lesions (Table 18-2). In one series, each centimeter of tumor size increases risk of death by 50%. In addition to increased size, factors affecting survival include tumor grade, and the presence and location of lymph node metastases. Better differentiated tumors have a higher mean survival, approaching 90% when nodes are uninvolved. Two thirds of women with inguinal node metastases survive for at least 5 years, but only a fourth of those with pelvic node metastases live that long.

TABLE 18-2

Clinical Staging of Carcinoma of Vulva

Stage	Description
0	Carcinoma in situ
I	Tumor ≤ 2 cm, confined to vulva
Ia	Stromal invasion ≤1 mm
Ib	Stromal invasion >1 mm
II	Tumor >2 cm confined to vulva
III	Tumor of any size extending to the lower urethra, vagina, or anus; or ulilateral regional lymph node metastasis
IV	Tumor extension
IVa	Mucosa of bladder or rectum; bone or upper urethra; or bilateral regional lymph nodes
IVb	Distant metastases, including pelvic lymph nodes

A 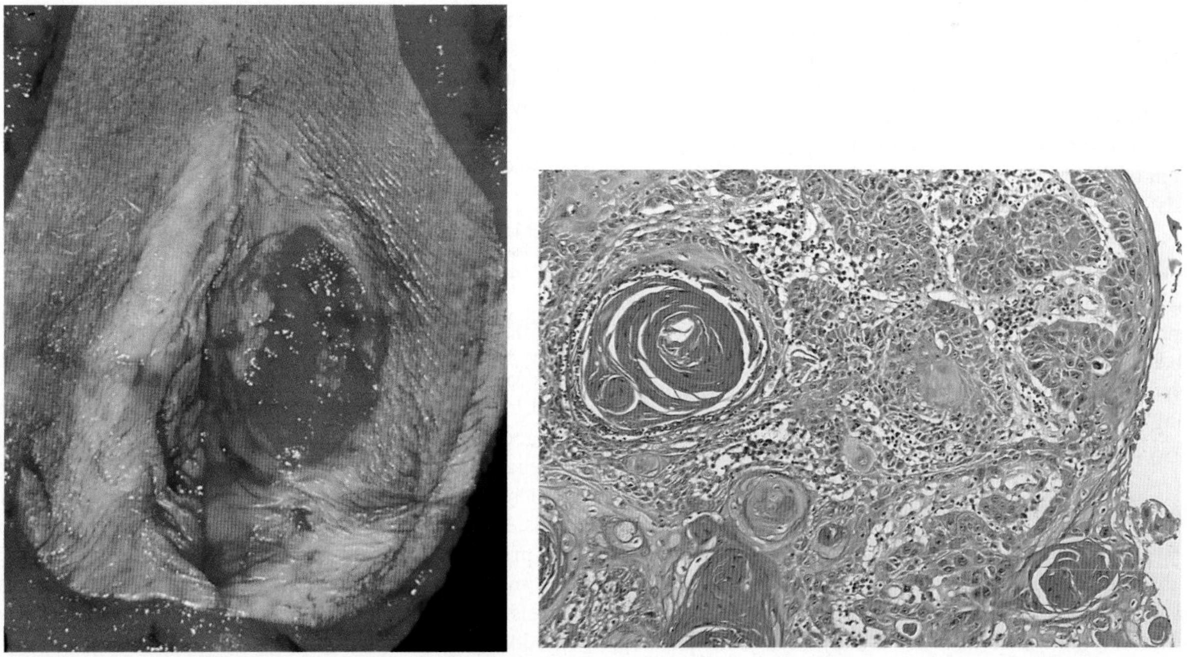 B

FIGURE 18-7. **Squamous cell carcinoma of vulva. A.** The tumor is situated in an extensive area of lichen sclerosus *(white)*. **B.** Small nests of neoplastic squamous cells, some with keratin pearls, are evident in this well-differentiated tumor

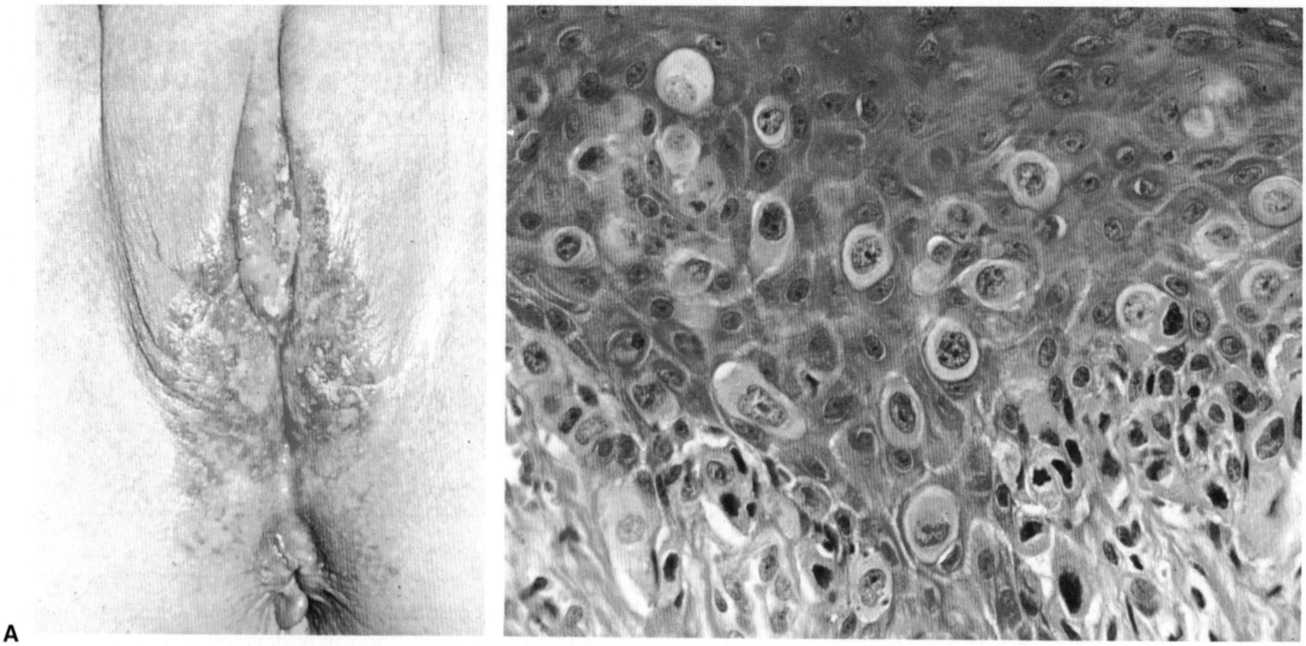

A B

FIGURE 18-8. **Paget disease of the vulva. A.** The lesion is red, moist, and sharply demarcated. **B.** Individual Paget cells, characterized by an abundant pale cytoplasm, infiltrate the epithelium and are interspersed among normal keratinocytes.

Prognosis correlates with stage of disease and lymph node status. The number of inguinal lymph nodes with metastases is the most important single factor. The prognosis of patients with vulvar cancer is generally good with an overall 5-year survival of 70%.

Verrucous Carcinoma

Verrucous carcinoma of the vulva is a distinct variety of squamous cell carcinoma that manifests as a large fungating mass resembling a giant condyloma acuminatum. HPV, usually type 6 or 11, is commonly identified. The tumor is very well differentiated, being composed of large nests of squamous cells with abundant cytoplasm and small, bland nuclei. Squamous pearls are common, and mitoses are rare. The tumor "invades" with broad tongues, and the stromal interface frequently exhibits a heavy infiltrate of lymphocytes and plasma cells. Verrucous carcinoma rarely metastasizes. Wide local surgical excision is the treatment of choice, but other forms of therapy (cryosurgery and retinoids) have been used successfully.

Malignant Melanoma

Although uncommon, malignant melanoma is the second most frequent cancer of the vulva (5%). It occurs in the sixth and seventh decades but occasionally is found in younger women. The tumor has biological and microscopic characteristics of melanoma occurring elsewhere in the body. It is highly aggressive, and the prognosis is poor.

Extramammary Paget Disease Exhibits Intraepithelial Cells with Copious Pale Cytoplasm

Paget disease of the vulva is named after similar-appearing tumors in the nipple and extramammary sites, such as the axilla and perianal region. The disorder usually occurs on the labia majora in older women. Women with Paget disease of the vulva complain of pruritus or a burning sensation for many years.

PATHOLOGY: The lesion of Paget disease is large, red, moist, and sharply demarcated. The exact origin of the diagnostic cells (Paget cells) is controversial; they are thought to arise in the epidermis or epidermally-derived adnexal structures. Paget cells have pale, vacuolated cytoplasm (Fig. 18-8) with abundant glycosaminoglycans; it stains with periodic acid–Schiff (PAS) and mucicarmine and expresses carcinoembryonic antigen (CEA). They appear as large single cells or, less often, as clusters of cells that lack intercellular bridges and are usually confined to the epidermis.

Intraepidermal Paget disease may have been present for many years and is often far more extensive throughout the epidermis than preoperative biopsies indicate. In contrast to Paget disease of the breast, which is almost always associated with underlying duct carcinoma, extramammary Paget disease is only rarely associated with carcinoma of the skin adnexa. Metastases rarely occur, so treatment requires only wide local excision or simple vulvectomy.

VAGINA

Anatomy

The vagina extends from the uterus to the vestibule of the vulva and is lined by hormone-responsive squamous epithelium. Estrogens stimulate proliferation and maturation of vaginal epithelial cells. Maturation is marked by accumulation of glycogen, which imparts a clear appearance to the cytoplasm of epithelial cells. By contrast, maturation of vaginal epithelium is inhibited by progesterone. As a result, during the secretory phase of the menstrual cycle or during pregnancy—when progesterone levels are high—intermediate cells, rather than superficial ones, predominate in vaginal smears.

Lymph drains through the lateral perivaginal plexus. Lymphatics from the vaginal vault and upper vagina communicate with branches from the cervix to drain into pelvic and then para-aortic nodes. The lower vagina also drains to inguinal and femoral nodes.

Nonneoplastic Conditions and Benign Tumors

Congenital Anomalies of the Vagina Are Rare

Congenital absence of the vagina is generally associated with anomalies of the uterus and urinary tract. If there is a functional uterus, absence of a vagina may lead to accumulation of menstrual blood in the uterus.

Septate vagina results from failure of embryonic müllerian ducts to fuse properly, and the resulting median wall does not resorb.

Vaginal atresia and imperforate hymen prevent transformation of the vaginal embryonic lining from a müllerian to a squamous epithelium, an effect that is a cause of vaginal adenosis.

Atrophic Vaginitis Results From Diminished Estrogenic Stimulation

Atrophic vaginitis is thinning and atrophy of the vaginal epithelium. The thinned epithelium in an estrogen-deficient woman is a poor barrier to infections or abrasions. Atrophic vaginitis occurs most commonly in postmenopausal women in whom estrogen levels are low. Dyspareunia and vaginal spotting are common symptoms.

Vaginal Adenosis Occurs in Females Exposed to Diethylstilbestrol (DES) in Utero

Vaginal adenosis is the failure of the glandular epithelium that normally lines the embryonic vagina to be replaced during fetal life by squamous epithelium. The use of DES to prevent miscarriages in women who were prone to repetitive abortions led, in the 1970s, to a substantial increase in the incidence of this disorder in young daughters of women who had received DES during pregnancy. At the 10th week of gestation, the upgrowth of a squamous epithelium derived from the urogenital sinus replaces the glandular (müllerian) epithelium lining the vagina and exocervix. DES exposure at any time during this critical window, which lasts until about the 18th week, arrests the transformation process. Hence, some glandular tissue (i.e., adenosis) remains.

Adenosis manifests as red, granular patches on the vaginal mucosa, which microscopically are comprised of mucinous columnar cells (resembling those lining the endocervix) and ciliated cells (similar to those lining the endometrium and fallopian tubes). Many of these lesions have disappeared as the young women have grown older. Rare cases of **clear cell adenocarcinoma** of the vagina have also occurred in the daughters of women treated with DES. Clear cell adenocarcinomas are almost invariably curable when they are small and asymptomatic, but in more advanced stages, they may spread by hematogenous or lymphatic routes.

Fibroepithelial Polyp

Vaginal polyps are uncommon benign growths composed of a connective tissue core and an outer lining of vaginal squamous epithelium. They are usually single, gray-white, and less than 1 cm in diameter. Simple excision is usually curative.

Benign Mesenchymal Tumors

Most benign tumors in the vagina resemble those in other parts of the female genital tract and include leiomyomas, rhabdomyomas, and neurofibromas. These are solid submucosal tumors usually less than 2 cm in diameter.

Malignant Tumors

Primary malignant tumors of the vagina are uncommon, constituting about 2% of all genital tract tumors. Most (80%) vaginal malignancies represent secondary spread. The most common symptoms are a vaginal discharge and bleeding during coitus, but advanced tumors may cause pelvic or abdominal pain and edema of the legs. Tumors confined to the vagina are usually treated by radical hysterectomy and vaginectomy.

Squamous Cell Carcinoma Accounts for over 90% of Primary Vaginal Malignancies

It is generally a disease of older women, with a peak incidence between the ages of 60 and 70. It appears most commonly in the anterior wall of the upper third of the vagina, where it usually manifests as an exophytic mass. **Vaginal intraepithelial neoplasia** (VAIN), a term replacing both "vaginal dysplasia" and "carcinoma in situ," frequently precedes invasive carcinoma. Not infrequently, squamous cell carcinoma of the vagina develops some years after cervical or vulvar carcinoma, a sequence that supports the concept of a carcinogenic field effect in the lower genital tract related to HPV infection.

Since most preinvasive and early invasive cancers are clinically silent, the routine use of vaginal cytology remains the most effective method to detect squamous cell carcinoma of the vagina. The prognosis is related to the spread of the tumor at the time of its discovery (Table 18-3). The 5-year survival rate for tumors confined to the vagina (stage I) is 80%, whereas it is only 20% for those with extensive spread (stages III/IV).

Embryonal Rhabdomyosarcoma (Sarcoma Botryoides) Is a Malignant Childhood Tumor

Embryonal rhabdomyosarcoma is a rare vaginal tumor that appears as confluent polypoid masses resembling a bunch of grapes, hence the name sarcoma botryoides *(from the Greek* botrys, *grapes)* (Fig. 18-9). It occurs almost exclusively in girls under 4 years of age. The tumor arises in the lamina propria of the vagina and

TABLE 18-3

Clinical Staging of Carcinoma of Vagina

Stage	Description
0	Carcinoma in situ
I	Limited to vaginal wall
II	Involves subvaginal tissue, but does not extend to pelvic wall
III	Extends to pelvic wall
IV	Extends beyond true pelvis or involves mucosa of bladder or rectum
IVa	Spread to adjacent organs
IVb	Spread to distant organs

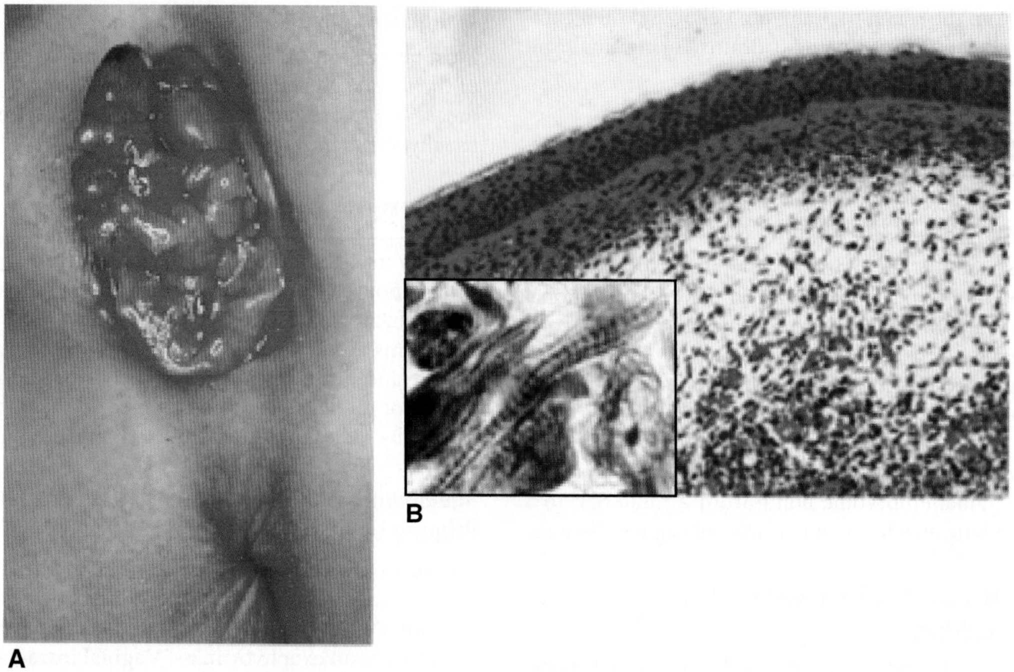

FIGURE 18-9. **Embryonal rhabdomyosarcoma (sarcoma botryoides) of vagina. A.** The grapelike tumor protrudes through the introitus. **B.** A section of the tumor shows a dense layer of neoplastic stroma termed the ***cambium layer*** (c) beneath the surface epithelium of the vagina. A loose neoplastic stroma is present beneath the cambium layer. The tumor contains rhabdomyoblasts characterized by cross striations (PTAH stain) ***(inset)***.

consists of primitive spindle rhabdomyoblasts, some of which display cross striations. Myofibrils composed of myosin and actin are often demonstrable. A dense zone of round rhabdomyoblasts (the cambium layer) is present beneath the vaginal epithelium. Deep to this layer the stroma is myxomatous and shows fewer neoplastic rhabdomyoblasts.The tumor is usually detected because of spotting on the child's diaper. Tumors under 3 cm in greatest dimension tend to be localized and may be cured by wide excision and chemotherapy. Larger tumors are likely to have invaded adjacent structures, metastasized to regional lymph nodes and spread hematogenously to distant sites. Even in advanced cases, half of patients survive with radical surgery and chemotherapy.

CERVIX

Anatomy

The cervix (from the Latin *collare,* neck) is the inferior portion of the uterus that connects the corpus to the vagina (Fig. 18-10). Its

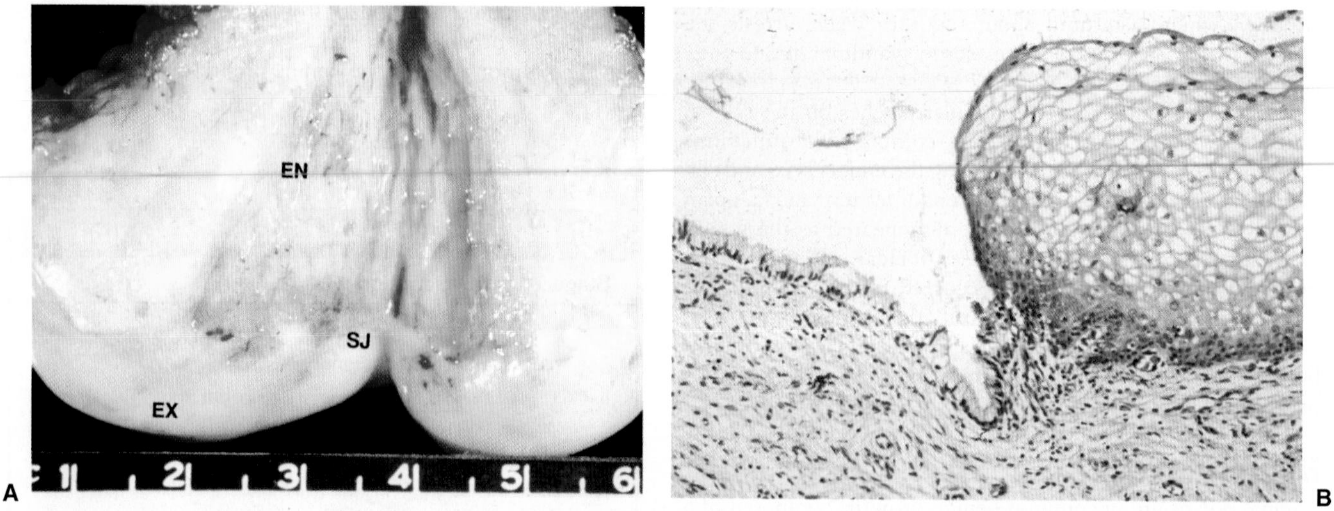

FIGURE 18-10. **Anatomy of the cervix. A.** The cervix has been opened to show the endocervix (EN), squamocolumnar junction (SJ), and exocervix (EX). The thick layer of squamous cells covering the exocervix accounts for its white color. **B.** A microscopic view of the squamocolumnar junction. The endocervix is lined by a single layer of columnar mucus-producing cells that abruptly meets the exocervix lined by mature squamous cells. ***Note:*** In specimens in which the squamocolumnar junction is on the ectocervix or in the endocervical canal, the region between it and the external os is called the ***transformation zone*** (see Fig. 18-11).

exposed portion (also termed the **exocervix**, **ectocervix** or **portio vaginalis**) protrudes into the upper vagina and is covered by glycogen-rich squamous epithelium. The **endocervix** is the canal that leads to the endometrial cavity. It is lined by longitudinal mucosal ridges made of fibrovascular cores lined by a single layer of mucinous columnar cells. Occasionally, the outlet of the endocervical glands becomes blocked. As a result, mucin is retained and produces macroscopically visible cystic dilations of these glands, termed **nabothian cysts**. The external os is the *macroscopically* visible junction between the exocervix and endocervix. The squamocolumnar junction is the *microscopic* anatomical junction of the squamous and mucinous columnar epithelia. The area between the endocervix and endometrial cavity is called the **isthmus** or **lower uterine segment**.

The exocervix remodels continuously throughout life. During embryonic development, the upward migration of squamous cells meets the columnar epithelium of the endocervix to form the initial squamocolumnar junction (Fig. 18-11). In some young women, this "original" squamocolumnar junction is located at the internal os. In most young women, however, the columnar epithelium extends onto the exocervix, in which case the squamocolumnar junction is also located on the exocervix. In the latter situation, the areas of the exocervix lined by columnar epithelium are referred to as **endocervical ectropion** and appear by colposcopic examination as reddish discolorations. With

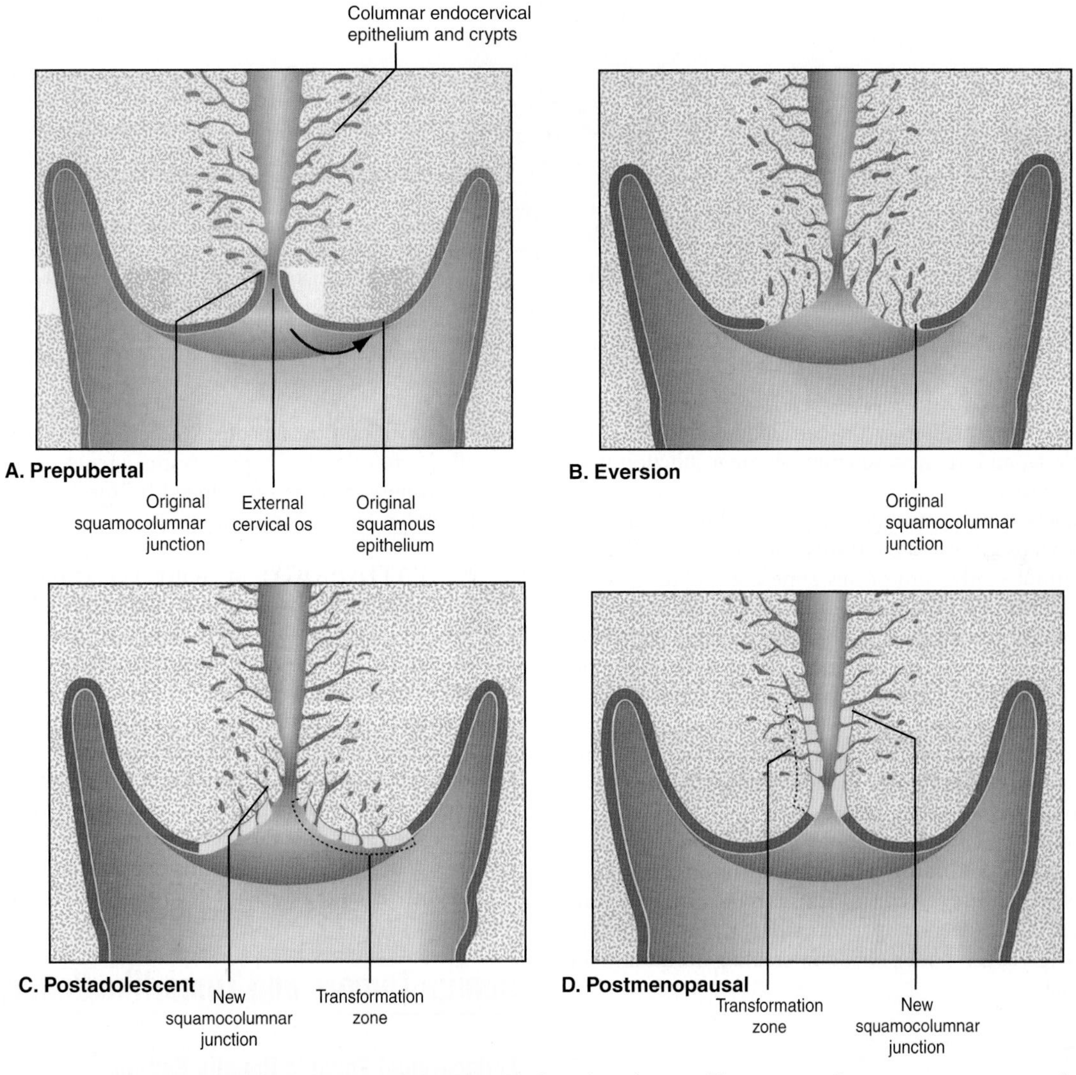

FIGURE 18-11. **The transformation zone of the cervix. A.** Prepubertal cervix. The squamocolumnar junction is situated at the external cervical os. The leaders show the direction of the movement that takes place as a result of the increase in bulk of the cervix during adolescence. **B.** The process of eversion. On completion, endocervical columnar tissue lies on the vaginal surface of the cervix and is exposed to the vaginal environment. **C.** Postadolescent cervix. The acidity of the vaginal environmental is one of the factors that encourage squamous metaplastic change, replacing the exposed columnar epithelium with squamous epithelium. **D.** Postmenopausal cervix. At this time, cervical inversion occurs. This phenomenon is the reverse of eversion, which was so important in adolescence. The transformation zone is now drawn into the cervical canal, often making it inaccessible to colposcopic examination.

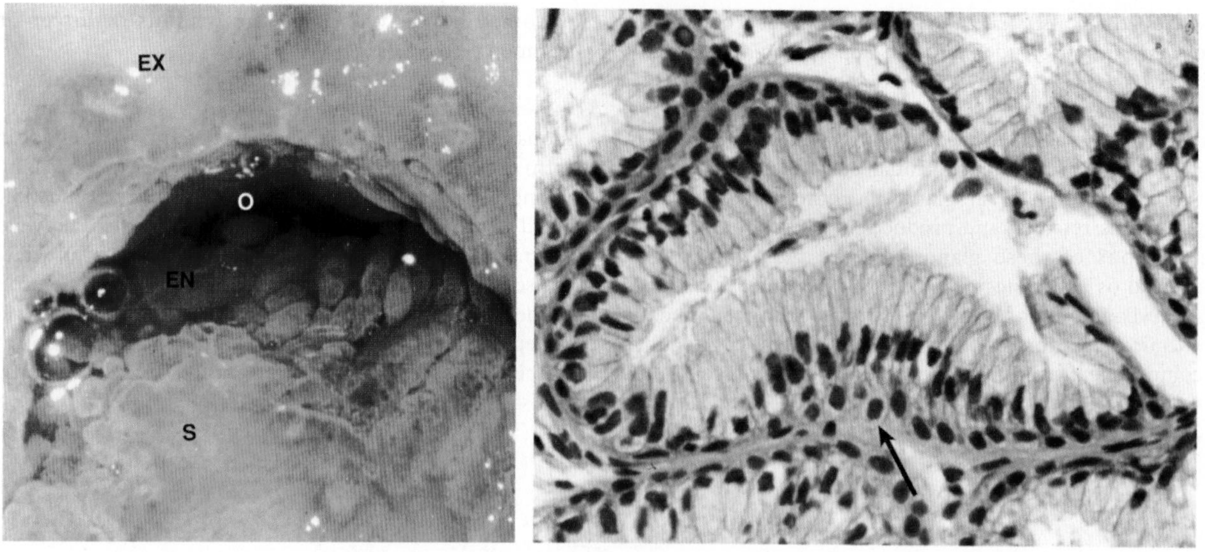

A B

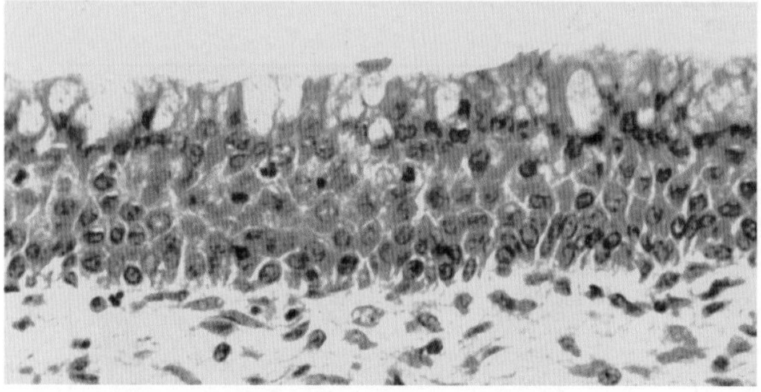

C

FIGURE 18-12. **Squamous metaplasia in the transformation zone. A.** In this colposcopic view of the cervix, a white area of metaplastic squamous epithelium (S) is situated between the exocervix (EX) and the mucinous endocervix (EN), which terminates at the internal os (O). **B.** In the early stages of squamous metaplasia of the transformation zone, the reserve cells, which normally constitute a single layer, begin to proliferate *(arrow)*. **C.** At a later stage, the proliferating reserve cells displace the glandular epithelium. As a final step, the metaplastic cells mature into glycogen-rich squamous cells, resembling those in Figure 18-10B.

age, the columnar epithelium of the ectropion undergoes squamous metaplasia, and the new squamocolumnar junction is located at the internal os.

The area between the most distal squamocolumnar junction and the external os is termed the **transformation zone**.The immature squamous epithelium of this zone displays progressive nuclear maturation and increasing amounts of glycogen-free cytoplasm toward the surface. Colposcopy reveals the development of a thin white membrane, which eventually becomes thicker and whiter as the squamous epithelium matures (Figs. 18-11 and 18-12). Subsequently, the cells accumulate glycogen and are indistinguishable from normal squamous epithelium lining the exocervix. The transformation zone is the site of cervical squamous carcinoma (see below).

Examination of the transformation zone by iodine staining is the basis of the **Schiller iodine test**. If the squamous cells lining the exocervix are mature (glycogen rich), as is normal, they stain with iodine and the exocervix appears mahogany brown. If they are immature (glycogen poor), no iodine staining occurs and the exocervix is pale.

Cervicitis

Inflammation of the cervix is common and is related to constant exposure to bacterial flora in the vagina. Acute and chronic cervicitis result from infection with many microorganisms, particularly endogenous vaginal aerobes and anaerobes, *Streptococcus, Staphylococcus, and Enterococcus.* Other specific organisms include *Chlamydia trachomatis, Neisseria gonorrhoeae, and* occasionally herpes simplex, type 2. Some agents are sexually transmitted; others may be introduced by foreign bodies, such as residual fragments of tampons and pessaries.

PATHOLOGY: In **acute cervicitis,** the cervix is grossly red, swollen, and edematous, with copious pus "dripping" from the external os. Microscopically, the tissues exhibit an extensive infiltrate of polymorphonuclear leukocytes and stromal edema.

In **chronic cervicitis,** which is more common, the cervical mucosa is hyperemic (Fig. 18-13), and there may be true epithelial erosions. Microscopically, the stroma is infiltrated by mononuclear cells, principally lymphocytes and plasma cells. Metaplastic squamous epithelium of the transformation zone may extend into endocervical glands, forming clusters of squamous epithelium with slightly enlarged nuclei, which must be differentiated from carcinoma.

Benign Tumors and Tumorlike Conditions

Endocervical Polyp is Usually Benign

Endocervical polyps are the most common cervical growths (Fig. 18-14). They appear as single smooth or lobulated masses, usually under 3 cm in greatest dimension. They typically manifest as vaginal bleeding or discharge. The lining epithelium is mucinous, with varying degrees of squamous metaplasia, but

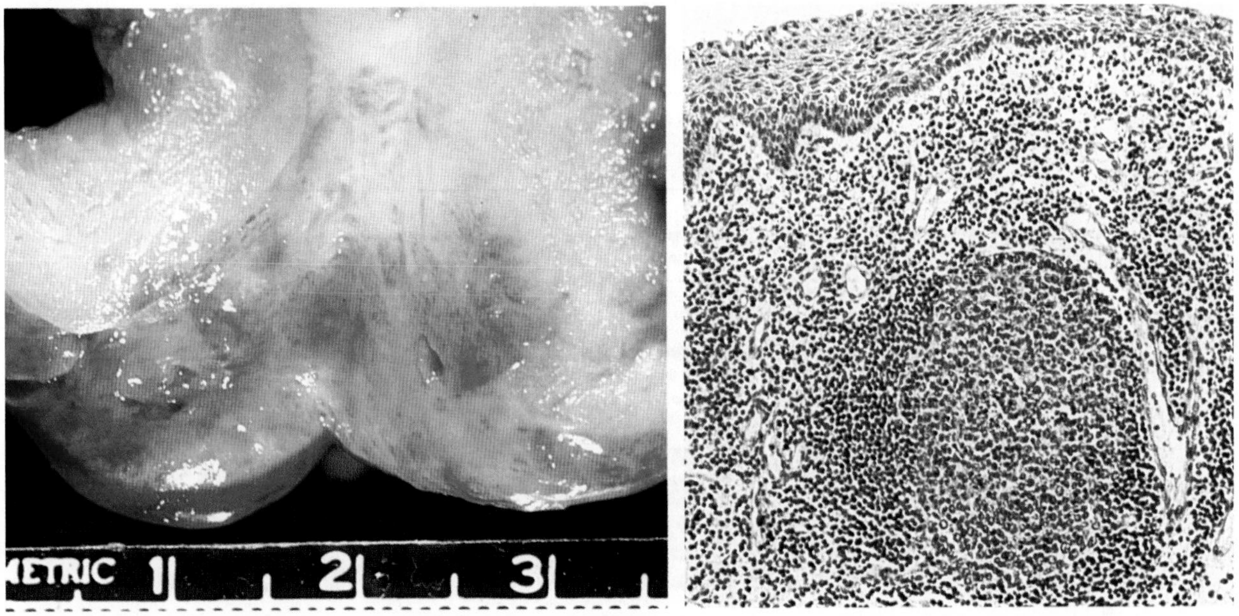

A B

FIGURE 18-13. **Chronic cervicitis. A.** The cervix has been opened to reveal the reddened exocervix. **B.** Microscopic examination discloses chronic inflammation and the formation of a lymphoid follicle.

may feature erosions and granulation tissue in women with symptoms. Simple excision or curettage is curative. Cancer rarely arises in an endocervical polyp (0.2% of cases).

Microglandular Hyperplasia Reflects Progestational Stimulation

Microglandular hyperplasia of the cervix is a benign condition showing closely packed vacuolated glands that lack an intervening stroma and display a neutrophilic infiltrate. Microscopically, glands vary in size and are lined by a flattened-to-cuboidal epithelium. (Fig. 18-15). The nuclei are uniform, and mitotic figures are rare. Squamous metaplasia and reserve cell hyperplasia are common. It should not be confused with well-differentiated adenocarcinoma. Microglandular hyperplasia is usually asymptomatic and is typically associated with progestin stimulation. It usually occurs during pregnancy, in the postpartum period and in women taking oral contraceptives.

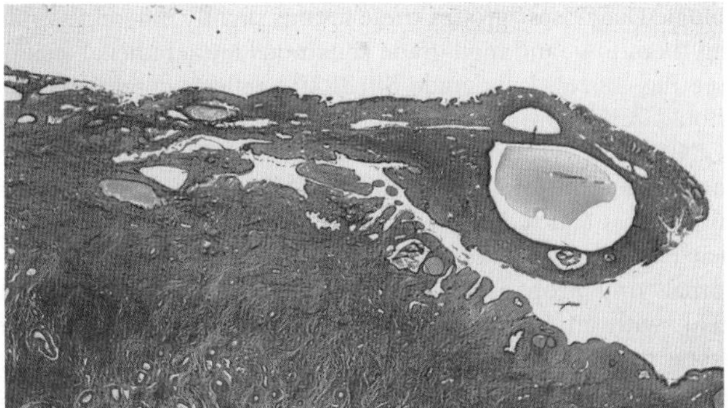

FIGURE 18-14. **Endocervical polyp.** An epithelial lining covers a fibrovascular core.

Leiomyoma

Leiomyomas of the cervix can bleed or prolapse into the endocervical canal, leading to uterine contractions and pain resembling the early phases of labor. The appearance is similar to that of uterine leiomyomas (see below).

Squamous Cell Neoplasia

Fifty years ago, cervical cancer was the leading cause of cancer death in American women. The introduction and widespread use of cytologic screening have decreased cervical carcinoma by 50% to 85% in Western countries. It is the sixth most common female cancer in the United States, and the mortality rate has fallen by 70%. However, worldwide, cervical cancer remains the second most common cancer in women.

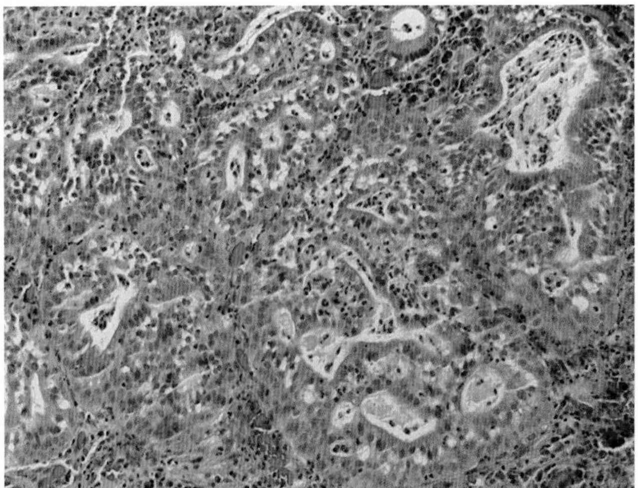

FIGURE 18-15. **Microglandular hyperplasia.** Proliferated glands are admixed with a neutrophilic infiltrate.

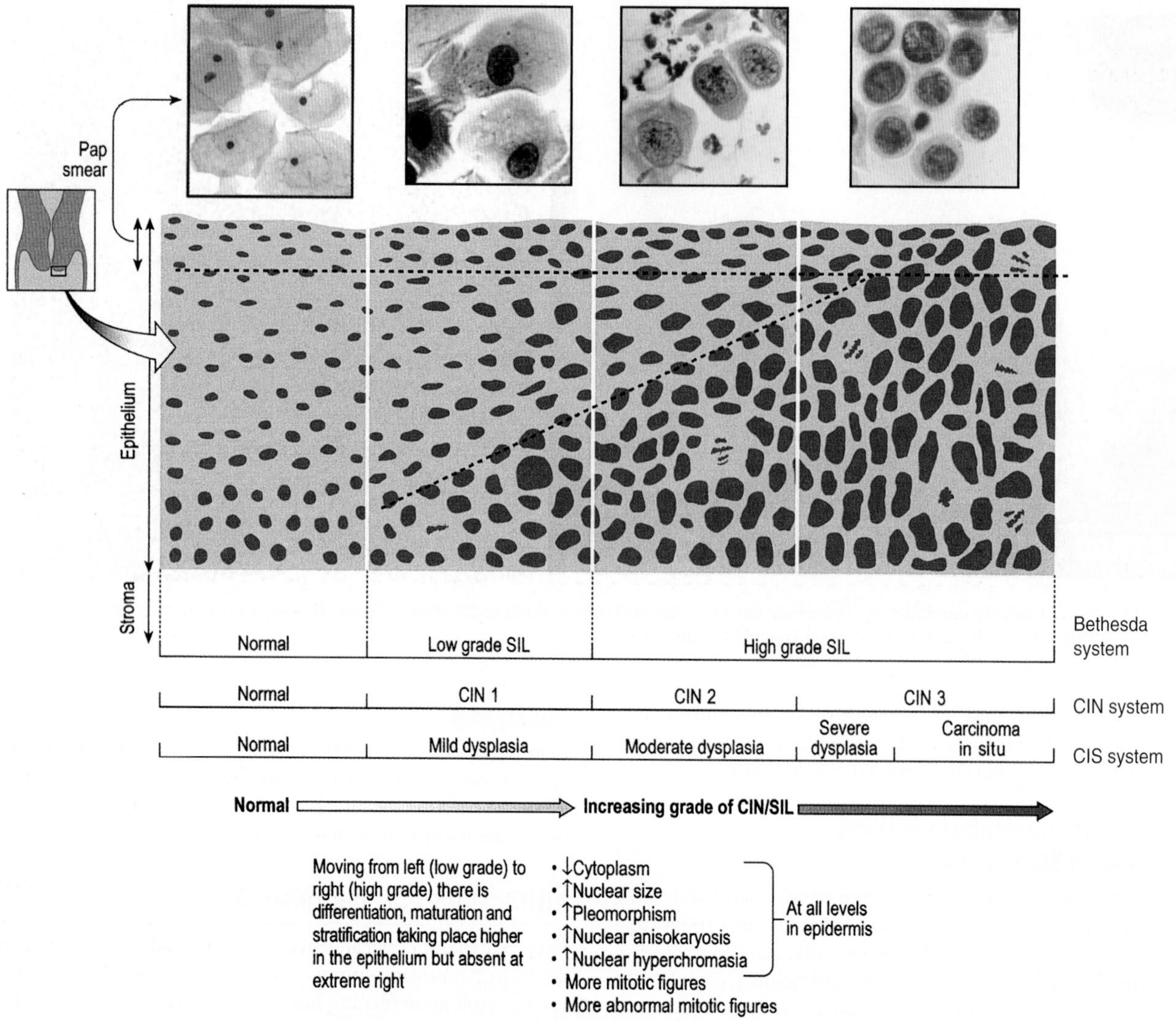

FIGURE 18-16. **Interrelations of naming systems in premalignant cervical disease.** This complex chart integrates multiple aspects of the disease complex. It lists the qualitative and quantitative features that become increasingly abnormal as the premalignant disease advances in severity. It also illustrates the changes in progressively more abnormal disease states and provides translation nomenclature for the dysplasia/carcinoma in situ (CIS) system, cervical intraepithelial neoplasia (CIN) system, and Bethesda system. Finally, the scheme illustrates the corresponding cytologic smear resulting from exfoliation of the most superficial cells, indicating that even in the mildest disease state, abnormal cells reach the surface and are shed. SIL = squamous intraepithelial lesion.

Cervical Intraepithelial Neoplasia Is the Precursor of Invasive Cancer

CIN is defined as a spectrum of intraepithelial changes that begins with minimal atypia and progresses through stages of more-marked intraepithelial abnormalities to invasive squamous cell carcinoma (Fig. 18-16). **CIN, dysplasia, CIS, and squamous intraepithelial lesion (SIL)** are commonly used interchangeably.

Dysplasia in the cervical epithelium carries a risk for ***malignant transformation*** (Fig. 18-16 and Fig. 18-17). The concept of CIN emphasizes that dysplasia and carcinoma in situ are points on a disease spectrum rather than separate entities.

The grades of CIN are as follows:

- CIN-1: mild dysplasia
- CIN-2: moderate dysplasia
- CIN-3: severe dysplasia and CIS

The "Bethesda System for Reporting Cervical/Vaginal Cytologic Diagnoses" groups these lesions slightly differently, calling them low- and high-grade squamous intraepithelial lesions (see Fig. 18-16). Low-grade SIL (LSIL) reflects conditions that should rarely progress in severity and commonly disappear (CIN-1, mild dysplasia). High-grade SIL (HSIL) corresponds to more severe histologic lesions (CIN-2 and CIN-3), which tend to progress and require treatment. There is accumulating evidence that early phases of infection by all HPV types show episomal viral propagation throughout a polyclonal epithelial field, with an LSIL cytology. Oncogenic types of HPV are prone to monoclonal outgrowth of those cells that undergo genomic integration of virus and elaboration of transforming viral proteins (e6/e7) with progression to HSIL. Lesions associated with nononcogenic types often progress no further than LSIL and then disappear.

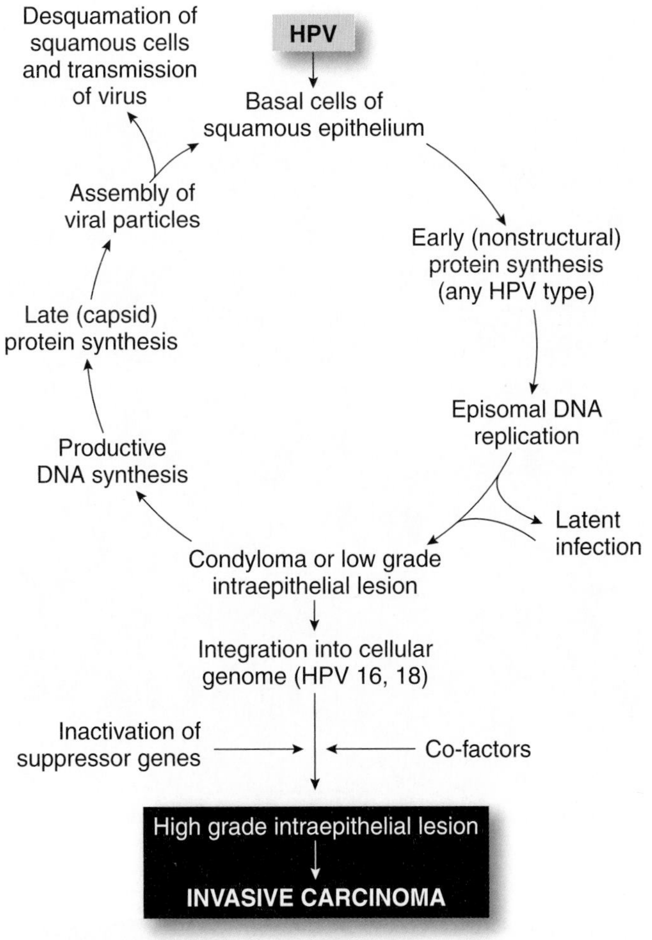

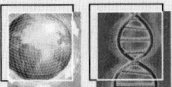

FIGURE 18-17. **Role of human papillomavirus (HPV) in the pathogenesis of cervical neoplasia.**

EPIDEMIOLOGY AND PATHOGENESIS: Epidemiologic features of CIN and invasive cancer are similar. Cervical cancer usually manifests between the ages of 40 and 60 years (mean 54), but CIN generally occurs under the age of 40. *The critical factor is HPV infection, which correlates with multiple sexual partners and early age at first coitus.* Thus CIN is essentially a **sexually transmitted disease.** Smoking seems to increase the incidence of cancer of the cervix, but the mechanism is obscure.

HPV infection leads to CIN and cervical cancer (see Fig. 18-17). Low-grade CIN is an example of a permissive infection, in which HPV is episomal and freely replicates, thereby causing cell death. Massive numbers of viral copies must accumulate in the cell cytoplasm before it can be seen microscopically as a **koilocyte**.

In most cases of higher-grade CIN, viral integration into the cell genome occurs. Proteins encoded by *E6* and *E7* genes of HPV 16 bind and inactivate p53 and Rb proteins, respectively, thereby vitiating their tumor suppressor functions (see Chapter 5).

After HPV integrates into host DNA, the viral capsid becomes superfluous. As a result, copies of the whole virus do not accumulate and koilocytes are absent in many cases of high-grade dysplasia and all invasive cancers.

Some 85% of low-grade CIN lesions harbor low-risk HPV. Many genital warts (condylomata acuminata) on the cervix contain HPV 6 or 11, which are regarded as low-risk HPV types. By contrast, cells in high-grade CIN usually contain HPV types 16, 18, 31, 33, 35, 39, 45, 51, 52, 56, 58, 59, and 68. **HPV types 16 and 18** are found in 70% of invasive cancers, and the other high-risk types account for another 25%.

Hormonally induced eversion of the cervix and an acidic vaginal environment encourage the development of the transformation zone. Under physiologic conditions, benign squamous metaplasia is the eventual outcome. In the presence of HPV or other carcinogenic agents, the benign metaplastic process is diverted into a malignant transformation, resulting first in increasingly severe CIN and then, in an unknown proportion of women, progressing to invasive squamous cell carcinoma.

There is uncertainty concerning how far along the process metaplastic squamous cells remain susceptible to carcinogenesis. Cells at the early reserve cell hyperplasia stage are usually considered to be at greatest risk and mature metaplastic squamous epithelium at no risk. The potential for cellular transformation between these two extremes is unknown. Local and systemic immune defenses are probably important in counteracting the changes generated by the carcinogenic agents.

PATHOLOGY: CIN is nearly always a disease of metaplastic squamous epithelium in the transformation zone or the endocervix. *Practically, the extent of the transformation zone determines the distribution of CIN, and hence cervical cancer, on the exposed portion of the cervix.*

The normal process by which cervical squamous epithelium matures is disturbed in CIN, as evidenced morphologically by changes in cellularity, differentiation, polarity, nuclear features, and mitotic activity. In CIN-1 (mild dysplasia), the most pronounced changes are seen in the basal third of the epithelium. However, abnormal cells are present throughout the entire thickness of the epithelium. Substantial cytoplasmic differentiation proceeds as abnormal cells migrate through the upper two thirds of the epithelium, but the nuclei in the upper levels are still morphologically abnormal. Thus, the sloughed cells can be detected as abnormal in Papsmears. In CIN-2 (moderate dysplasia), most of the cellular abnormalities are in the lower and middle thirds of the epithelium. Cytodifferentiation occurs in cells in the upper third, but it is less than in CIN-1.

CIN-3 is synonymous with severe dysplasia and CIS. In severe dysplasia, the cells in the superficial (upper) epithelium disclose some, albeit minimal, differentiation, whereas CIS shows none at all. The sequence of histologic changes from CIN-1 to CIN-3 is illustrated in Figure 18-18. Dysplasia and CIS can often be detected on colposcopic examination by signs associated with their altered vasculature and epithelial changes. Mosaicism (irregular surface resembling inlaid woodwork) (Fig. 18-19) (dots differentiated from surrounding tissue surface by color and texture) are the two patterns most often found in high-grade CIN. The oncogenic process is more common on the anterior than the posterior cervical lip, and often extends to involve the endocervical glands.

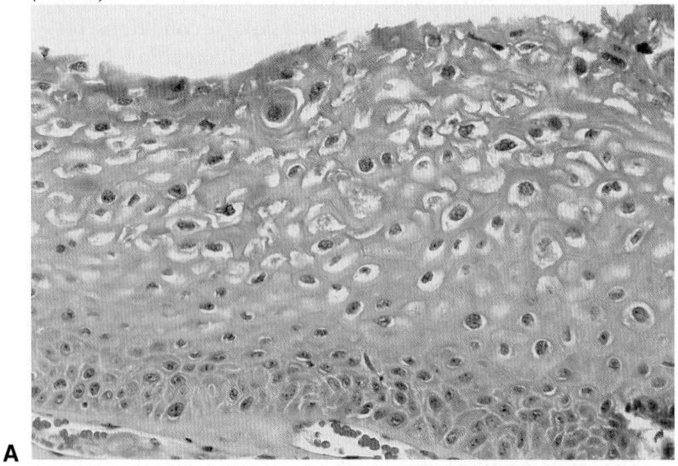
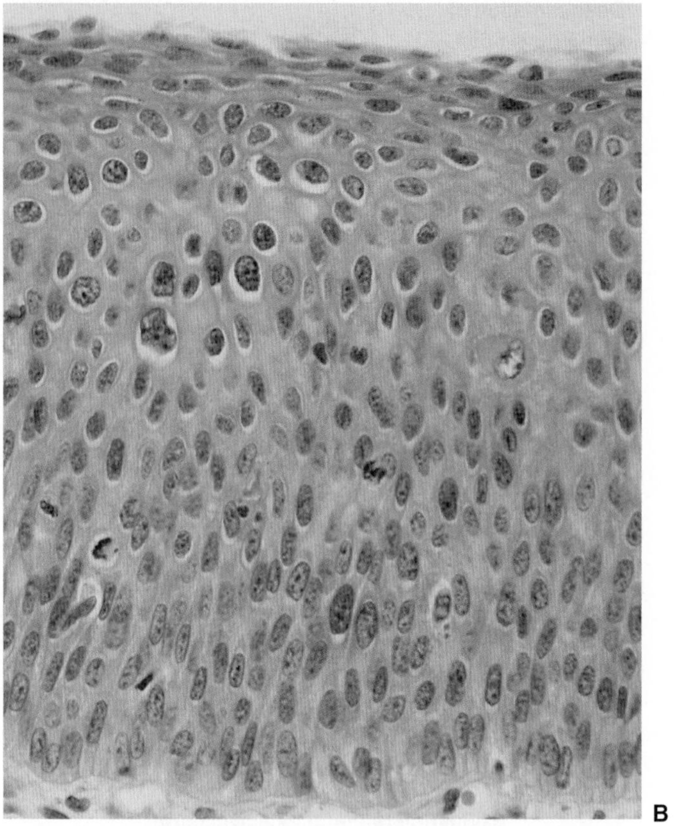
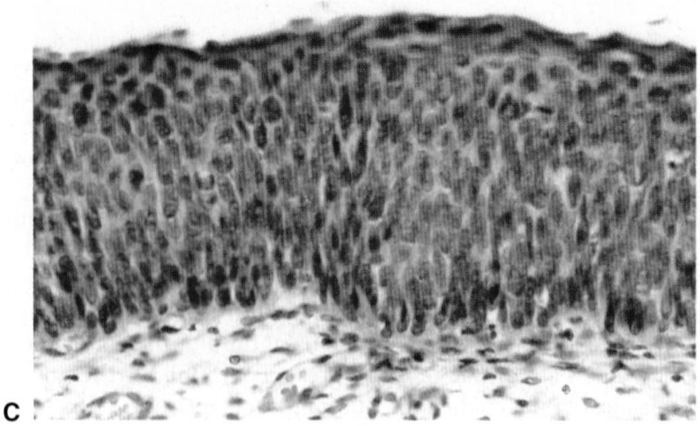
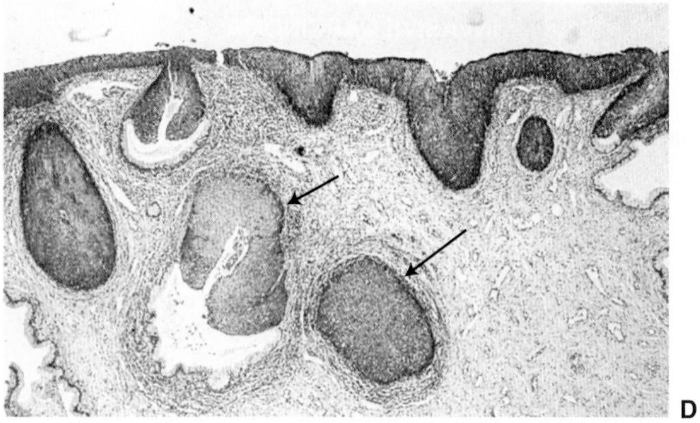

FIGURE 18-18. **Cervical intraepithelial neoplasia (CIN). A.** CIN-1: The cervical epithelium shows pronounced cellular atypia in the basal third. Some cells in the upper two thirds of the epithelium have abnormal nuclei, but all show cytoplasmic differentiation. **B.** CIN-2 to CIN-3: The lower two thirds of the epithelium displays pronounced cell atypia. Although cytodifferentiation occurs in the upper third of the epithelium, it is less pronounced than in CIN-1. **C.** CIN-3 (carcinoma in situ, CIS): Neoplastic cells are present throughout the entire epithelium. **D.** CIN-3: CIS partially or completely replaces the columnar epithelium of the endocervical glands *(arrows)*.

The mean age at which women develop CIN is 24 to 27 years for CIN-1 and CIN-2, and 35 to 42 for CIN-3. Based on morphologic criteria, half of cases of CIN-1 regress, 10% progress to CIN-3, and less than 2% become invasive cancer. The frequency is much greater and the time required much shorter for progression to CIS for initially higher grades of CIN. The average time for all grades of dysplasia to progress to carcinoma in situ is about 10 years. *At least 20% of cases of CIN-3 progress to invasive carcinoma within that time.*

CLINICAL FEATURES: When CIN is discovered, colposcopic examination in combination with a Schiller test is important to delineate the extent of the lesion and to indicate areas to be biopsied. Diagnostic endocervical curettage is also useful for determining the extent of endocervical involvement. Women with CIN-1 are often followed conservatively (i.e., repeated Papsmears plus close 1follow-up), although some gynecologists now advocate local ablative treatment. High-grade lesions are treated according to the extent of disease. LEEP (loop electrosurgical excision procedure), which can be performed on an outpatient basis, is commonly used. In certain situations, cervical conization (removal of a cone of tissue around the external os), cryosurgery, and (rarely) hysterectomy are done. Follow-up smears and clinical examinations should continue for life, since vaginal or vulvar squamous cancer may develop later.

Microinvasive Squamous Cell Carcinoma Is the Earliest Stage (Ia) of Invasive Cervical Cancer

Microinvasive cancer features neoplastic cells that invade the stroma minimally (Fig. 18-20). About 7% of specimens removed for CIS show foci of microinvasive cancer. Small clusters of cells or solid lesions in the stroma have the following characteristics (see Table 18-4):

- Invasion to a depth of less than 3 mm (stage 1a1) or 5 mm (stage 1a2) below the basement membrane.
- 7 mm maximum lateral extension.

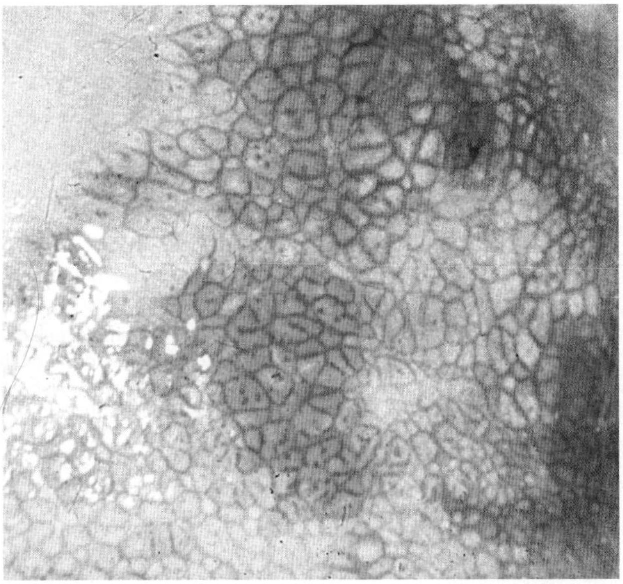

FIGURE 18-19. **Dysplasia of the cervix.** Examination with the colposcope discloses a mosaic pattern resembling inlaid woodwork.

Most American gynecological oncologists further limit the definition of microinvasive carcinoma to:

- Lack of vascular invasion
- No lymph node metastases

Lymph node metastases are encountered in only 3% to 5% of stage 1a2 microinvasive carcinomas. Conization or simple hysterectomy generally suffices to cure microinvasive cancers less than 3 mm deep.

Invasive Squamous Cell Carcinoma Is Still Common Worldwide

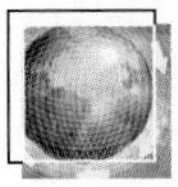

EPIDEMIOLOGY: Squamous cell carcinoma is by far the most common type of cervical cancer. Even in the United States (Table 18-5), it still accounts for some 13,000 new cases annually, which is less than the incidence of either endometrial or ovarian cancer. However, in underdeveloped areas, where cytologic screening is less available, squamous cell cancer of the cervix is still a major cause of cancer death. A **cervical cancer vaccine** has recently been approved, which in clinical trials decreased risk of cervical cancer by 97%. Vaccinated women developed neither HPV-associated pre-cancer nor invasive cervical cancer.

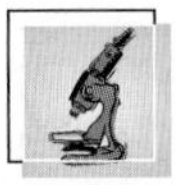

PATHOLOGY: Early stages of cervical cancer often manifest as poorly defined, granular, eroded lesions or nodular and exophytic masses (Fig. 18-21A). If it is predominantly within the endocervical canal, it may appear as an endophytic mass, infiltrating stroma and causing diffuse enlargement and hardening of the cervix (barrel-shaped cervix). On

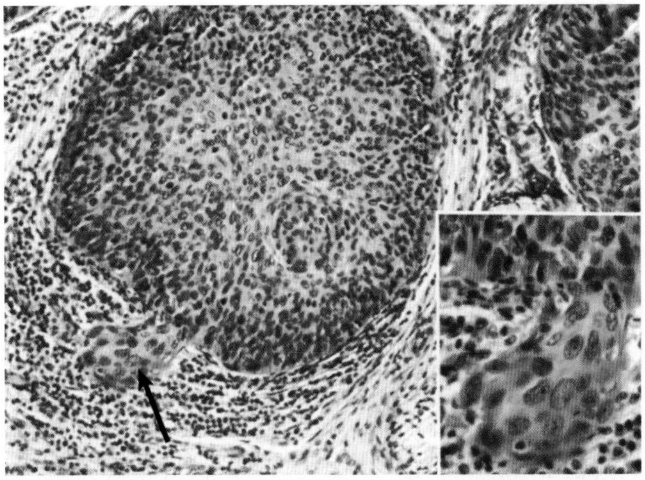

FIGURE 18-20. **Microinvasive squamous cell carcinoma.** Section of the cervix shows that carcinoma in situ in an endocervical gland has broken through the basement membrane *(arrow)* to invade the stroma. *(Inset)* A higher-power view of the microinvasive focus.

TABLE 18-4

Clinical Staging of Cervical Cancer (FIGO)

Stage	Description
0	Carcinoma in situ (cervical intraepithelial neoplasia III)
I	Carcinoma confined to cervix (extension to corpus disregarded)
Ia	Invasive cancer identified *only* microscopically. Maximum depth, 5.0 mm; maximum width, 7.0 mm.
1a1	Depth = 3.0 mm
1a2	Depth >3.0 mm
Ib	Any cancer *grossly* visible
1b1	Clinical size = 4.0 cm
1b2	Clinical size >4.0 cm
II	Carcinoma extending beyond cervix, but not to lateral pelvic wall; involvement of vagina limited to upper two thirds
IIa	Paracervical extension not suspected
IIb	Paracervical extension suspected
III	Invasive carcinoma extending to lateral pelvic wall or lower one third of vagina
IIIa	No extension to pelvic wall
IIIb	Extension to pelvic wall, hydronephrosis, or nonfunctioning kidney
IV	Extended spread involving
IVa	Mucosa of urinary bladder or rectum
IVb	Tissues beyond true pelvis

TABLE 18-5

Incidence of Gynecological Cancer in the United States [2004]

	New Cases		Death	
	Cases	%*	Cases	%*
Endometrium	40,320	6	7090	3
Ovary	25,580	4	16,090	6
Cervix, invasive	10,520	3	3900	2
Vulva, invasive	3970	<1	850	
Vagina, invasive	1000	<1		
Other	2000	<1		

* % = percentage of all cases of cancer in females.
Carcinoma in situ of cervix >50,000 new case/year.

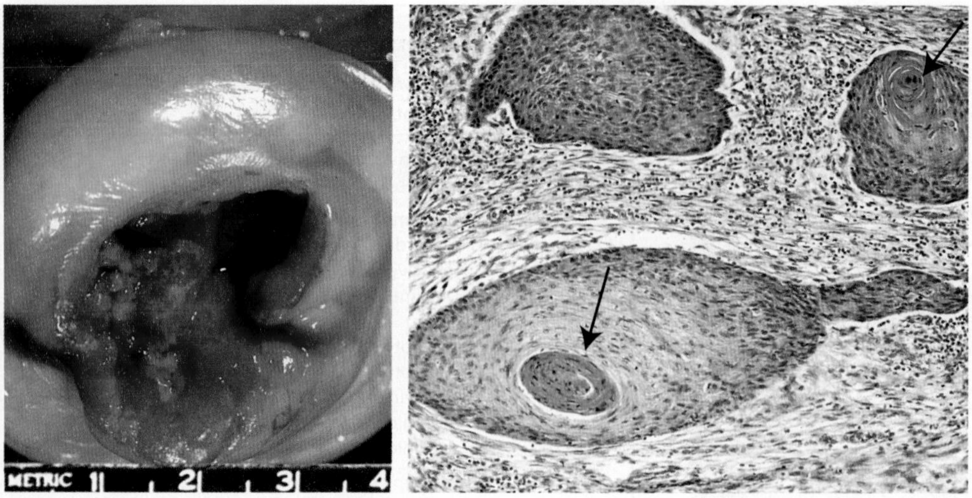

A B

FIGURE 18-21. **Squamous cell cancer. A.** The cervix is distorted by the presence of an exophytic, ulcerated squamous cell carcinoma. **B.** The keratinizing pattern of the tumor is manifested as whorls of keratinized cells ("keratin pearls") *(arrows).*

microscopic examination, most tumors display a nonkeratinizing pattern characterized by solid nests of large malignant squamous cells, with no more than individual cell keratinization. Most of the remaining cancers exhibit nests of keratinized cells organized in concentric whorls, so-called keratin pearls (see Fig. 18-21B).

The least common pattern of squamous cell cancer is small cell carcinoma, which is the most aggressive cancer of the cervix and has the worst prognosis. It consists of infiltrating masses of small, cohesive, nonkeratinized, malignant cells.

Cervical cancer spreads by direct extension and through lymphatic vessels (Fig. 18-22) and only rarely by the hematogenous route. Local extension into surrounding tissues (parametrium) results in **ureteral compression** (stage IIIb, see Table 18-4); the corresponding clinical complications are hydroureter, hydronephrosis, as well as renal failure, the most common cause of death (50% of patients). Bladder and rectal involvement (stage IVa) may lead to fistula formation. Metastases to regional lymph nodes involve paracervical, hypogastric, and external iliac nodes. Overall, the cancer's growth and spread are relatively slow, since the average age for patients with stage 0 tumor (CIN-III) is 35 to 40 years; for stage 1A, 43 years and for stage IV, 57 years.

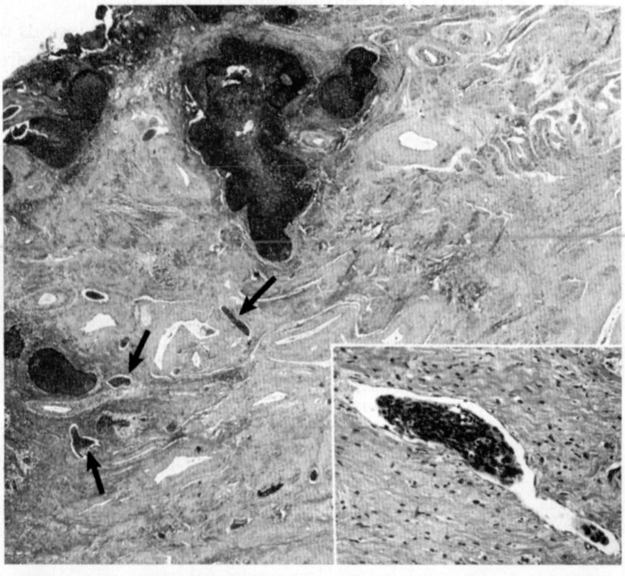

FIGURE 18-22. **Squamous cell cancer of the cervix with lymphatic invasion.** Low magnification shows a squamous cell carcinoma that has invaded the stroma and permeated the lymphatics *(arrows). (Inset)* A high-power view of lymphatic invasion.

CLINICAL FEATURES: In the earliest stages of cervical cancer, patients complain most often of vaginal bleeding after intercourse or douching. With more advanced tumors, symptoms are referable to the route and degree of spread. The Pap smear remains the most reliable screening test for detecting cervical cancer. A newer assay for squamous cell carcinoma antigen (SCC-Ag) on Pap smear is positive in one third of cases of stage I tumor and in over half of higher-stage cases.

The clinical stage of cervical cancer is the best prognostic index of survival (see Table 18-4). Overall 5-year survival is 60%, and for each stage it is as follows: I, 90%; II, 75%; III, 35%; and IV, 10%. About 15% of patients develop recurrences on the vaginal wall, bladder, pelvis, or rectum within 2 years of therapy. Radical hysterectomy is favored for localized tumor, especially in younger women; radiation therapy or combinations of the two are used for more advanced tumors.

Endocervical Adenocarcinoma Accounts for 20% of Malignant Cervical Tumors

Increased incidence of cervical adenocarcinoma has been reported recently, with a mean age at presentation of 56 years. Most tumors are of the endocervical cell (mucinous) type, but the various subtypes have little importance for overall survival. Adenocarcinoma shares epidemiologic factors with squamous cell carcinoma of the cervix and spreads similarly. The tumors are often associated with adenocarcinoma in situ and are frequently infected with HPV types 16 and 18.

PATHOLOGY

ADENOCARCINOMA IN SITU: This lesion, also called **cervical glandular intraepithelial neoplasia (CGIN)**, generally arises in the region of the squamocolumnar junction and extends into the endocervical canal. It displays tall columnar cells with eosinophilic or mucinous cytoplasm, sometimes resembling goblet cells. The pattern of spread and involvement of endocervical glands resemble those of CIN. Adenocarcinoma in situ typically is an intraepithelial proliferation. Normal endocervical gland architecture is maintained. The cells show slight enlargement, atypical hyperchromatic nuclei, increased nuclear-to-cytoplasmic ratio, and variable numbers of mitoses. Abrupt transitions help distinguish neoplastic from neighboring normal endocervical cells. Associated high-grade squamous cell CIN occurs in 40% of cases of adenocarcinoma in situ.

INVASIVE ADENOCARCINOMA: This tumor typically manifests as a fungating polypoid or papillary mass. Microscopically, exophytic tumors often have a papillary pattern, whereas endophytic ones display tubular or glandular patterns. Poorly differentiated tumors are predominantly composed of solid sheets of cells.

Adenocarcinoma of the endocervix spreads by local invasion and lymphatic metastases, but overall survival is somewhat worse than that for squamous carcinoma. The tumor is treated similarly to squamous carcinoma.

UTERUS

Anatomy

The uterine corpus (body) is smaller than the cervix at birth and during childhood, but increases rapidly in size after puberty. The endometrium is composed of glands and stroma. It is thin at birth, when it consists of a continuous surface of cuboidal epithelium that dips to line a few sparse tubular glands. After puberty, it thickens. The superficial two-thirds, the "zona functionalis," respond to hormones and is shed with each menstrual phase. The deepest third, the basal layer, is the germinative portion and with each cycle regenerates a new functional zone.

The endometrium is supplied by arcuate arteries that traverse the outer myometrium and give off two sets of vessels, one to the myometrium and the other, the radial arteries, to the endometrium. In turn, the radial arteries branch into two types of vessels. The basal arteries supply the basal endometrium and the spiral arteries nourish the superficial two thirds.

The Menstrual Cycle

The normal endometrium undergoes a series of sequential changes that support the growth of implanted fertilized ova (zygotes) (Fig. 18-23). If conception does not occur, the endometrium is shed, then regenerated to support a fertilized ovum in the next cycle.

PROLIFERATIVE PHASE: During the first 14 days of the menstrual cycle, the endometrium is under estrogenic stimulation. The functional zone exhibits tubular to coiled glands, which are evenly distributed and supported by a cellular,

Day of Cycle		Before 14	15–16	17	18	19–22	23	24–25	26–27	28+
Post-ovulatory day			1–2	3	4	5–8	9	10–11	12–13	14+
Cycle phases		Proliferative	Interval	Early secretory		Mid-secretory			Late secretory	Menstrual
Key feature		Mitoses	Mitoses and subnuclear vacuoles	Maximum subnuclear vacuoles	Subnuclear vacuoles present	Stromal edema	Focal decidua around spiral arteries	Patchy decidua	Extensive decidua	Stromal crumbling
Microscopic features of functional zone	Stroma	Loose stroma. Mitoses	Same as proliferative	Loose stroma. Scanty mitoses	Loose stroma	Stromal edema	Focal decidua around spiral arteries. Edema prominent	Decidua throughout stroma. Some edema	Extensive decidua. Prominent granulated lymphocytes	Stromal crumbling. Hemorrhage
	Glands	Straight to tightly coiled tubules. Mitoses	Some subnuclear vacuoles, otherwise as proliferative	Extensive subnuclear vacuoles	Dilated glands. Some subnuclear vacuoles	Dilated glands with irregular outline. Luminal secretion		`Saw tooth' glands	Prominent 'saw tooth' glands	Disrupted glands. Secretory exhaustion. Regenerating epithelium
Appearances		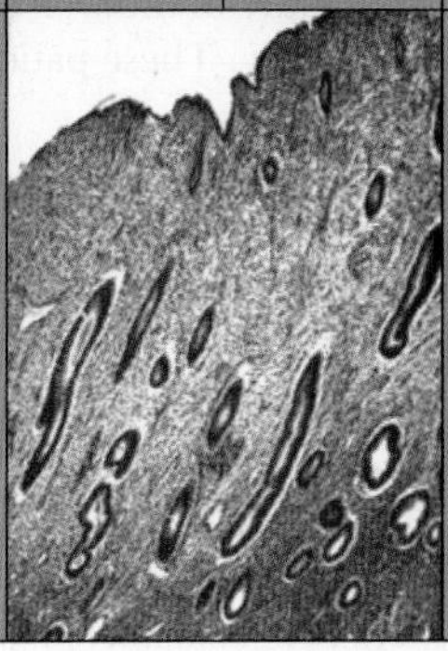 A				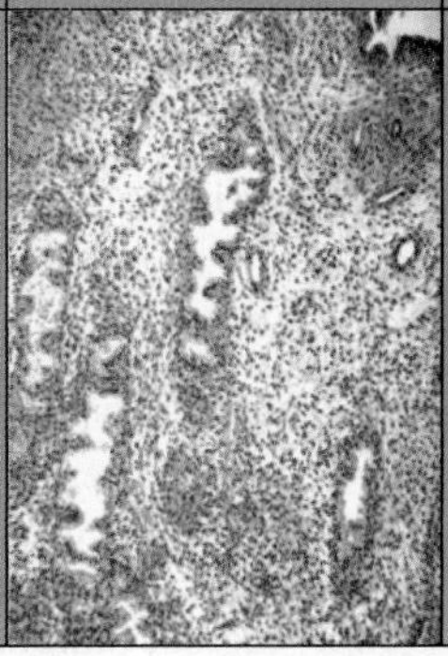 B			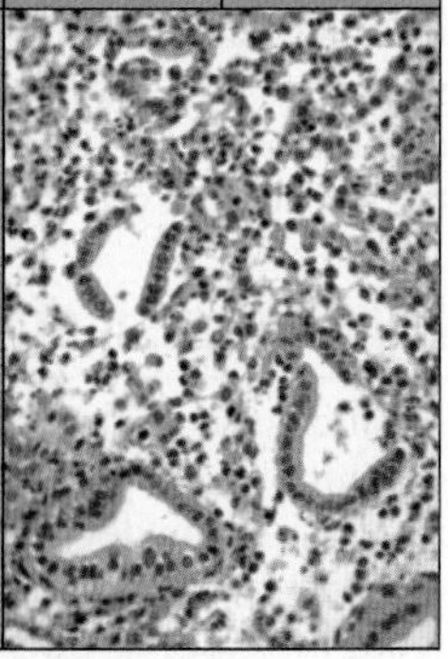 C	

FIGURE 18-23. **Main histologic features of the endometrial phases of the normal menstrual cycle. A.** Proliferative phase. Straight tubular glands are embedded in a cellular monomorphic stroma. **B.** Secretory phase, day 24. Dilated tortuous glands with serrated borders are situated in a predecidual stroma. **C.** Menstrual endometrium. Fragmented glands, dissolution of the stroma, and numerous neutrophils are evident.

monomorphic stroma (see Fig. 18-23A). Early during the proliferative phase, the glands are narrow, but as proliferation progresses, they coil more and increase slightly in caliber. The columnar cells lining the tubules increase from one layer in thickness to a pseudostratified epithelium that is mitotically active. The glands produce a watery alkaline secretion that facilitates the passage of sperm through the endometrial cavity into the fallopian tubes. The stroma is also mitotically active. Spiral arteries are narrow and mostly inconspicuous.

SECRETORY PHASE: Ovulation occurs about 14 days after the last menstrual period. Afterwards, the graafian follicle that has discharged its ovum becomes a corpus luteum. The granulosa cells of the corpus luteum begin to secrete progesterone, the hormone that transforms the endometrium from a proliferative into a secretory state.

- **Days 17 to 19 (postovulatory days 3–5):** Endometrial glands enlarge, dilate, and become more coiled. The lining cells develop abundant and prominent, glycogen-rich, subnuclear vacuoles (day 17). Over the next several days, the glandular cells produce copious secretions that can support a zygote while it develops early chorionic villi capable of invading the endometrium.
- **Days 20 to 22 (postovulatory days 6–8):** The endometrium displays prominent glandular secretions and stromal edema. The glands dilate and are more tortuous.
- **Day 23 (postovulatory day 9):** The stromal cells enlarge and exhibit large, round, vesicular nuclei and abundant eosinophilic cytoplasm. These cells, which normally appear first about the spiral arterioles, are the precursors of the decidual cells of pregnancy and are referred to as "predecidual."
- **Day 27 (postovulatory day 13):** The full thickness of the stroma is now predecidualized and prepared for menstruation. The tubular glands continue to dilate and develop serrated (saw-toothed) borders.

MENSTRUAL PHASE: In the absence of pregnancy, i.e., without a blastocyst to elaborate human chorionic gonadotropin (hCG), granulosa and thecal cells of the corpus luteum degenerate. As the corpus luteum degenerates, progesterone levels fall, the endometrium becomes desiccated, the spiral arteries collapse, and the stroma disintegrates. Menses commence on day 28, last 3 to 7 days, and result in a flow of about 35 mL of blood. The denuded surface is reepithelialized by extension of the residual glandular epithelium.

ATROPHIC ENDOMETRIUM: After menopause, the number of glands and quantity of stroma progressively decrease. Remaining glands often are oriented parallel to the surface and the stroma contains abundant collagen. The glands of the atrophic endometrium are often conspicuously dilated, an appearance termed **senile cystic atrophy of the endometrium.**

Endometrium of Pregnancy

Maintenance of the corpus luteum of pregnancy depends on continuous stimulation by hCG secreted by placental trophoblast of the developing embryo. The trophoblast begins to develop about day 23. Under the influence of hCG, the corpus luteum increases its output of progesterone, thereby stimulating secretion of fluid by endometrial glands. The hypersecretory endometrium of pregnancy shows widely dilated glands lined by cells with abundant glycogen. These features can persist for up to 8 weeks after delivery.

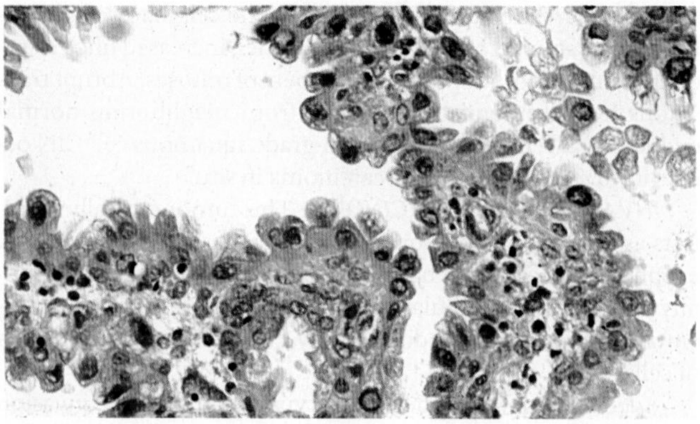

FIGURE 18-24. **Arias-Stella reaction of pregnancy associated with human chorionic gonadotropin (hCG) stimulation.** A section of endometrium shows enlarged, bulbous nuclei that protrude into the gland lumen.

The hypersecretory response may become exaggerated with intrauterine pregnancy, ectopic pregnancy, or trophoblastic disease. In this circumstance, the nuclei of the glandular cells become enlarged, bulbous, and polyploid, because the DNA has replicated, but the cells have not divided. The nuclei protrude beyond the apparent cellular cytoplasmic limits into the gland lumen, an appearance referred to as the **Arias-Stella phenomenon** (Fig. 18-24). Enlarged nuclei are polyploid, not to be confused with aneuploidy, a condition sometimes seen in adenocarcinoma.

Congenital Anomalies

Congenital anomalies of the uterus are rare.

- **Congenital absence of the uterus (agenesis)** reflects failure of the müllerian ducts to develop. Since elongation of the müllerian ducts during embryonic life depends on the presence of the wolffian ducts as guides, uterine agenesis is almost always accompanied by other anomalies of the urogenital tract as well as an absent vagina and fallopian tubes.
- **Uterus didelphys** refers to a double uterus, due to failure of the two müllerian ducts to fuse in early embryonic life. A double vagina commonly accompanies this anomaly.
- **Uterus duplex bicornis** is a uterus with a common fused wall between two distinct endometrial cavities. The common wall between the apposed müllerian ducts fails to degenerate to form a single uterine cavity.
- **Uterus septus** is a single uterus with a partial remaining septum, owing to failure of the wall of the fused müllerian ducts to resorb completely. These patients have increased risk for habitual abortion.
- **Bicornuate uterus** refers to a uterus with two cornua (horns) and a common cervix. Didelphic and bicornuate uterine fusion defects lead to a small increase in the incidence of premature birth.

Endometritis

Endometritis, or an inflamed endometrium, is a diagnosis based on the finding of an abnormal inflammatory infiltrate in the endometrium. It must be distinguished from the normal presence of polymorphonuclear leukocytes during menstruation and a mild lymphocytic infiltrate at other times. The findings in most cases of endometritis are nonspecific and rarely point to a specific cause.

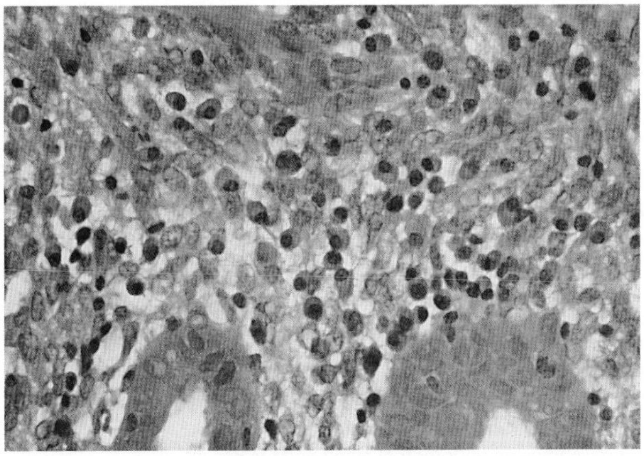

FIGURE 18-25. **Chronic endometritis.** The inflammatory infiltrate is composed largely of lymphocytes and plasma cells.

ACUTE ENDOMETRITIS: This condition is defined as the abnormal presence of polymorphonuclear leukocytes in the endometrium. Most cases result from an ascending infection from the cervix, e.g., after the usually impervious cervical barrier is compromised by abortion, delivery, or medical instrumentation. Curettage is diagnostic and often curative, because it removes necrotic tissue that has served as the nidus of the ongoing infection. Nowadays, the condition is of little significance, although it was quite dangerous before antibiotics.

CHRONIC ENDOMETRITIS: Although lymphocytes and lymphoid follicles are occasionally scattered in a normal endometrium, plasma cells in the endometrium are diagnostic of chronic endometritis (Fig. 18-25). The disorder is associated with IUDs, PID, and retained products of conception after an abortion or delivery. Without a culture, the pathologic findings alone do not distinguish between infective and noninfective causes. Patients usually complain of bleeding, pelvic pain, or both. The condition is generally self-limited.

PYOMETRA: Defined as pus in the endometrial cavity, pyometra is associated with gross anatomic defects such as fistulous tracts between bowel and uterine cavity, bulky or perforating malignancies, or cervical stenosis. Long-standing pyometra may rarely be associated with development of endometrial squamous cell cancer.

Traumatic Lesions

INTRAUTERINE DEVICE: IUDs predispose bearers to (1) increased menstrual flow, (2) uterine perforation, and (3) spontaneous abortion if conception occurs with the IUD in place. However, IUD use reduces endometrial cancer risk by half. Much of the adverse publicity about IUDs relates to early devices, and only 1% of women who desire contraception now use an IUD.

INTRAUTERINE ADHESIONS (ASHERMAN SYNDROME): Intrauterine fibrous adhesions sometimes develop after a uterus has been curetted, particularly for postpartum complications or therapeutic abortion. These bands traverse, but do not necessarily obliterate, the endometrial cavity. Additional complications include amenorrhea or, in the event of a subsequent pregnancy, increased abortion rates, preterm labor and placenta accreta.

Adenomyosis

Adenomyosis is the presence of endometrial glands and stroma within the myometrium. The most clinically significant correlation between symptoms of pain, dysmenorrhea, or menorrhagia and pathologic finding of adenomyosis occurs if the glands are located at least 1 mm or more beneath the endometrial myometrial junction. Adenomyosis is more likely to be symptomatic the more deeply it penetrates the myometrium. Pain occurs as foci of adenomyosis enlarge when blood is entrapped during menses. One fifth of all uteri removed at surgery show some adenomyosis.

PATHOLOGY: The uterus may be enlarged. The myometrium discloses small, soft, tan areas, some of which are cystic (Fig. 18-26). Microscopic examination reveals glands lined by mildly proliferative to inactive endometrium and surrounded by endometrial stroma with varying degrees of fibrosis. Secretory changes are rare, except during pregnancy and in patients treated with progestins. Sometimes the uterus is enlarged by smooth muscle that hypertrophies about adenomyotic foci. Over time, the uterus may also become enlarged from cyclic bleeding into these foci. Varying degrees of glandular hyperplasia may be seen, and occasionally hyperplastic surface endometrium extends into the foci of adenomyosis.

CLINICAL FEATURES: Many patients with adenomyosis are asymptomatic, but varying degrees of pelvic pain, dysfunctional uterine bleeding, dysmenorrhea, and dyspareunia are common. These symptoms appear in parous women of reproductive age and regress after menopause. The cause of adenomyosis remains unknown.

Hormonal Effects

Contraceptive Steroids Prevent Pregnancy and Many Gynecological Cancers

Oral contraceptive agents induce a number of endometrial changes that reflect the types, potencies, and dosages of estrogens and progestins used in these formulations. Combined preparations generally contain potent progestins and weak estrogens. The pseudodecidual change, therefore, appears early and overshadows the weak glandular growth. Over time (i.e., after a number of cycles), endometrial glands atrophy. More recently developed contraceptive combinations contain lower doses of hormones and correspondingly elicit less change. *Women who use contraceptive steroids that include progestational agents have significantly lower rates of endometrial and ovarian cancer, reflecting the growth-inhibiting properties of progesterone, and in the ovary, a reduction in the number of ovulations.*

Dysfunctional Uterine Bleeding Occurs During or Between Menstrual Periods

In dysfunctional bleeding, the cause lies outside the uterus. It is one of the most common gynecological disorders of women of reproductive age but is still poorly understood. Most cases are related to an endocrine disturbance that involves an aspect of the hypothalamic–pituitary–ovarian axis (Table 18-6). Ovarian dysfunction is usual, especially in the presence of anovulation.

Some causes of menstrual irregularity are intrinsic to the uterus and are not considered dysfunctional. These include (1) growths (e.g., carcinoma, endometrial intraepithelial neoplasia [EIN], submucous leiomyomata. and polyps), (2) inflammation

A

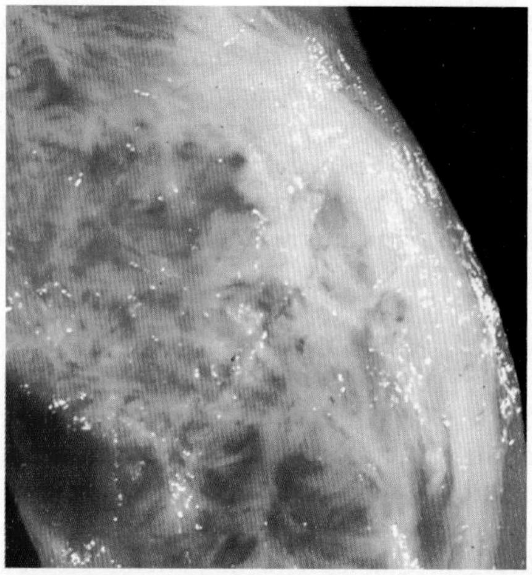

B

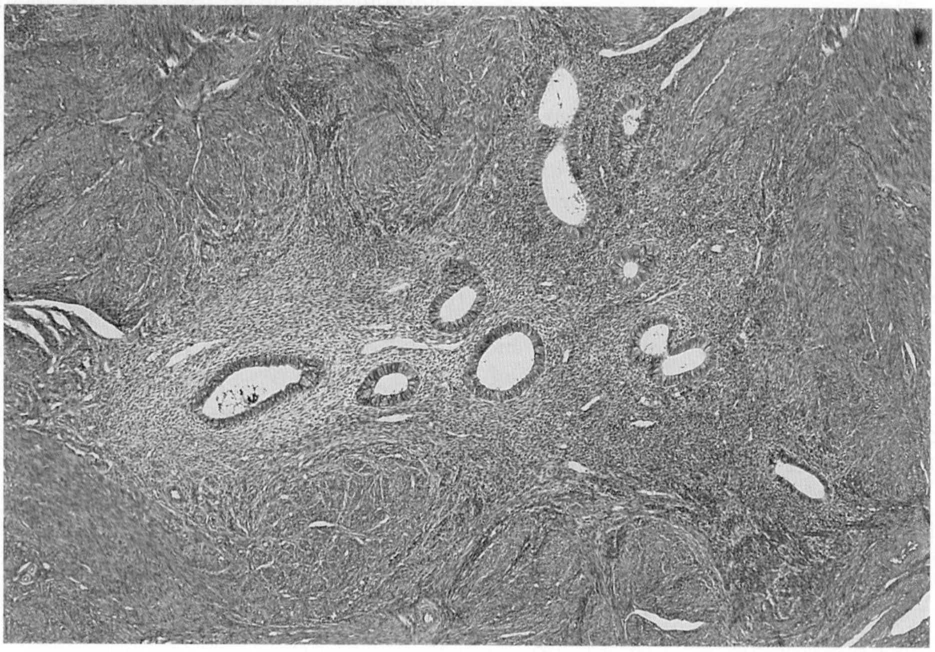

FIGURE 18-26. **Adenomyosis. A.** The cut surface of the uterus reveals small, red areas corresponding to endometrial glands in the myometrium. **B.** A microscopic view shows an endometrial gland and stroma in the myometrium.

(e.g., endometritis), (3) pregnancy (e.g., complications of intrauterine or ectopic pregnancy). and (4) the effects of IUDs (see Table 18-6).

Anovulatory Bleeding Is the Most Common Form of Dysfunctional Bleeding

Anovulotory bleeding is a complex syndrome of many causes that manifests as the absence of ovulation during the reproductive years. It is most often noted at either end of reproductive life (i.e., menarche and menopause).

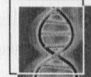

PATHOGENESIS AND PATHOLOGY: In an anovulatory cycle, failure of ovulation leads to excessive and prolonged estrogen stimulation, without a postovulatory rise in progesterone. The result is that the endometrium remains in a proliferative state but exhibits a disordered and fragmented appearance. In the absence of adequate progesterone, the spiral arteries of the endometrium do not develop normally. When the estrogen level falls, "breakthrough bleeding" occurs. Since estrogen maintains the stromal fluid turgescence that supports the endometrial blood vessels, a drop in estrogen level causes stromal fluid loss and hence loss of support for endometrial blood vessels. Subsequent compression of the poorly developed spiral arteries leads in turn to stasis, thrombosis, infarction, and hemorrhage. Bleeding also occurs if the endometrium continues to proliferate should estrogen levels remain unchanged. In this case, the proliferative endometrium is inadequately nourished and withdrawal bleeding ensues.

Microscopically, the glands in anovulatory bleeding are frequently disordered and appear crowded because of severe stromal necrosis and collapse of the proliferative endometrium. Fragments of menstrual-type endometrium are also present.

TABLE 18-6

Causes of Abnormal Uterine Bleeding (Including Uterine and Extrauterine Causes)

Newborn	Maternal estrogen
Childhood	Iatrogenic (trauma, foreign body, infection of vagina) Vaginal neoplasms (sarcoma botryoides) Ovarian tumors (functional)
Adolescence	Hypothalamic immaturity Psychogenic and nutritional problems Inadequate luteal function
Reproductive age	Anovulatory Central: psychogenic, stress Systemic: nutritional and endocrine disease Gonadal: functional tumors End-organ: benign endometrial hyperplasia Pregnancy: ectopic, retained placenta, abortion, mole Ovulatory Organic: neoplasia, infections (PID), leiomyomas Polymenorrhea: short follicular or luteal phases Iatrogenic: anticoagulants, IUD Irregular shedding
Menopause	Carcinoma, EIN, benign hyperplasias, polyps, leiomyomata
Postmenopause	Carcinoma, EIN, polyps, leiomyomata

EIN = endometrial intraepithelial neoplasia; IUD = intrauterine device; PID = pelvic inflammatory disease.

Luteal Phase Defect Is Caused by Inadequate Progesterone

Luteal phase defect results in an abnormally short menstrual cycle: menses occur 6 to 9 days after the surge of luteinizing hormone (LH) associated with ovulation. A luteal phase defect occurs when a corpus luteum develops improperly or regresses prematurely. The disorder is primarily of interest in infertility investigations and occasionally in analysis of abnormal uterine bleeding. Luteal phase defects are responsible for 3% of cases of infertility. The diagnosis is confirmed by endometrial biopsy showing an endometrium more than 2 days out of synchrony with the chronological day of the menstrual cycle.

Tumors

Endometrial Polyp Is a Benign Stromal Neoplasm in the Endometrial Cavity

Endometrial polyps occur most commonly in the perimenopausal period. They do not occur before menarche. Polyps arise as monoclonal outgrowths of endometrial stromal cells genetically altered by chromosomal translocation, with secondary induction of polyclonal glandular elements. The stroma and glands of endometrial polyps have diminished hormonal responsiveness and do not slough during menstruation.

PATHOLOGY: Most endometrial polyps arise in the fundus (Fig. 18-27), although they may originate anywhere within the endometrial cavity. They vary from several millimeters to growths filling the entire endometrial cavity. Most are solitary but 20% are multiple. Microscopically, the core of a polyp is composed of (1) endometrial glands, which often are cystically dilated and hyperplastic; (2) a fibrous endometrial stroma; and (3) thick-walled, coiled, dilated blood vessels, derived from a straight artery that normally would

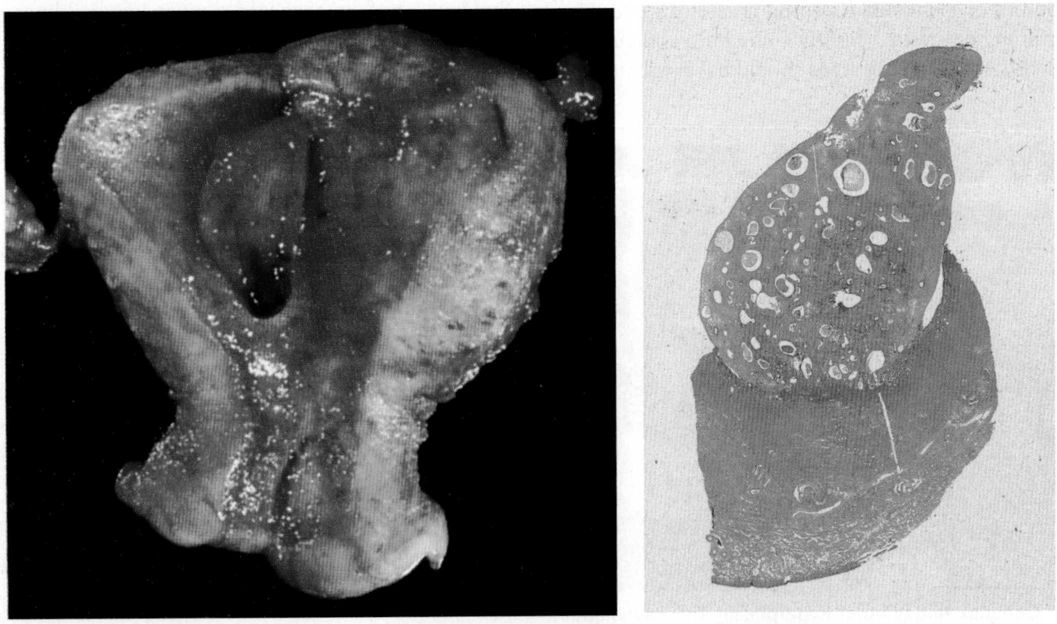

A B

FIGURE 18-27. **Endometrial polyp. A.** A single polyp extends into the endometrial cavity. The necrotic tip is responsible for clinical bleeding. **B.** On microscopic section, a polyp exhibits slightly dilated endometrial glands embedded in a markedly fibrous stroma.

have supplied the basal zone of the endometrium. A mantle of endometrial epithelium covers the polyp. The glandular epithelium uncommonly is at the same stage of the cycle as that of the adjacent, normal endometrium.

CLINICAL FEATURES: Endometrial polyps typically present with intermenstrual bleeding, owing to surface ulceration or hemorrhagic infarction. Since bleeding in an older woman may be due to endometrial cancer, this sign must be thoroughly evaluated. Endometrial polyps are not ordinarily precancerous, but up to 0.5% harbor adenocarcinoma.

Benign Endometrial Hyperplasia Is Caused by Excess Estrogenic Stimulation

Benign endometrial hyperplasia refers to a spectrum of endometrial-wide changes resulting from abnormal estrogenic stimulation, exhibiting randomly distributed architectural and cytologic changes. Estrogenic stimulation of the endometrium beyond the 2-week interval of a normal proliferative menstrual cycle causes progressive changes that have been associated with a 2- to 10-fold increased risk of endometrial cancer. Risk has been defined by epidemiologic clinical outcome studies using historical information of estrogen dose and duration over time. Aside from women with co-existing EIN (see below), it is not possible on histopathologic grounds to stratify cancer risk within this group of patients by a single histologic examination. Endometrial histopathology does vary greatly, however, as a function of the sequence and tempo of hormonal stimulation amongst women with benign endometrial hyperplasia. The earliest changes are isolated cystic expansion of scattered proliferative glands without a substantial change in gland density, often designated "persistent proliferative" or "disordered proliferative" endometrium. Morphologic transition to benign endometrial hyperplasia is gradual and arbitrarily defined, but can be said to occur when gland density becomes irregular throughout, with some regions having more glands than stroma.

PATHOLOGY: Benign endometrial hyperplasia affects the entire endometrial compartment, where remodeling of glands and stroma creates an irregular density of commingled cystic, slightly branching and tubular glands (Fig. 18-28). At least some areas should have a gland area that exceeds the stromal area, but the cytology of the crowded foci is representative of that seen elsewhere. As long as circulating estrogens persist, glands are proliferative and, if ciliation occurs, suggest scattered tubal differentiation.

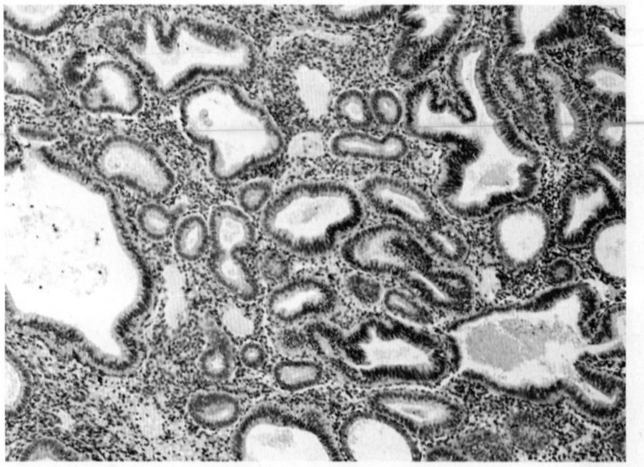

FIGURE 18-28. **Complex endometrial hyperplasia.** The endometrial glands, which are in the proliferative phase, are closey packed and display moderate architectural disarrrry (budding and branching). No cytologic atypia is present.

There are now two classifications of endometrial hyperplasia. An older classification centers on the presence of cytologic atypia and abnormal glandular architecture. *Cytologic atypia is the most important prognostic feature.*

- **Simple hyperplasia:** This proliferative lesion shows minimal glandular complexity and crowding and no cytologic atypia. The epithelial lining is usually one cell layer thick and the stroma between the glands is abundant. One percent of cases of simple endometrial hyperplasia progress to adenocarcinoma.
- **Complex hyperplasia:** This variant exhibits marked glandular complexity and crowding but no cytologic atypia (see Figure 18-28). Glands are increased in number and may vary in size. The stroma between the glands is scanty. Three percent develop adenocarcinoma.
- **Atypical hyperplasia:** This lesion shows cytologic atypia and marked glandular crowding, often as back-to-back glands. Glands may show complex architecture, with an intraluminal papillary arrangement or the appearance of budding glands in the stroma (Fig. 18-29). Epithelial cells are enlarged and hyperchromatic, with prominent nucleoli and increased nuclear-to-cytoplasmic ratios. One fourth of these cases progress to adenocarcinoma, which is almost always of the endometrioid type.

With increasing estrogen exposure, stromal breakdown and resultant gland collapse occur, often accompanied by fibrin vascular thrombi. Although prototypically an estrogenic lesion, architectural and metaplastic changes which persist after gradual weaning from a hyperestrogenic state can be construed as manifestations of benign endometrial hyperplasia in which proliferative activity is weak or absent. Stromal predecidualization caused by superimposed progestin therapy or delayed ovulation may develop between irregular glands of benign hyperplasia. Sudden loss of estrogen leads to massive shedding with attendant heavy menses.

CLINICAL FEATURES: Benign endometrial hyperplasia may result from anovulatory cycles, polycystic ovary syndrome, an estrogen-producing tumor, therapeutic administration of estrogens, or obesity. In such cases, therapy aimed at the primary cause may alleviate estrogenic stimulation. Treatment with large doses of progestins can produce temporary symptomatic relief or objective remission, depending on persistence of the underlying hormonal condition. Short term risk for endometrial cancer remains low for women with benign endometrial hyperplasia, providing the endometrium is well sampled, and no EIN is seen. Longer term risks of refractory benign endometrial hyperplasia are best assessed by repeat evaluation.

Endometrial Intraepithelial Neoplasia (EIN) and Adenocarcinoma Are Separate from Benign Endometrial Hyperplasia

Any classification of endometrial proliferations must incorporate our increasing understanding of molecular biology and biological behavior. Pathologic nomenclature is thus continually evolving.

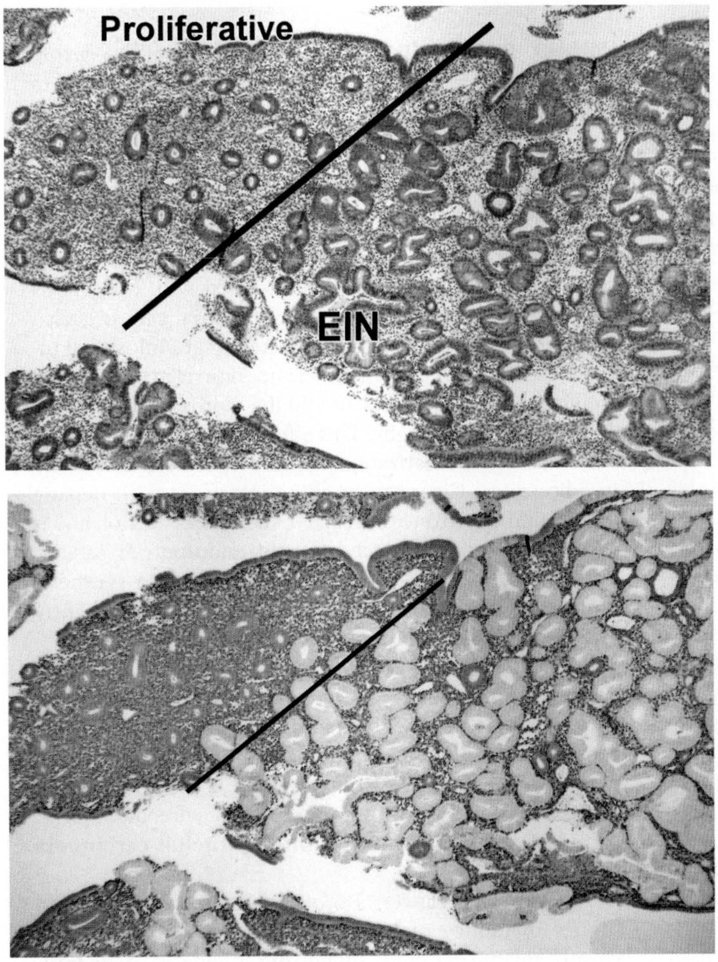

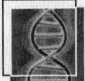

FIGURE 18-29. **Endometrial intraepithelial neoplasia (EIN).** **A.** Tight clusters of cytologically altered neoplastic endometrial glands with abundant cytoplasm and rounded nuclei *(right)* are offset from the background endometrium *(left)* in this geographic focus of EIN. Measurement across the perimeter of this aggregate of individual tubular glands exceeds 1 mm, and features of adenocarcinoma such as cribriform, mazelike, or solid architecture are lacking. **B.** Glands affected by EIN show loss of PTEN expression by immunohistochemistry (loss of brown staining).

The more classical categorization presented above may therefore be supplanted or supplemented by groupings that better account for known molecular and biological parameters. Thus, endometrial hyperplasias of the several types mentioned above may be considered endometrial in situ neoplasia (EIN). *In this paradigm, EIN are recognized as monoclonal neoplastic growths of genetically altered cells having a greatly increased clinical risk of clinical conversion to the endometrioid type of endometrial adenocarcinoma.* Benign endometrial hyperplasia, by contrast, is intrinsically normal endometrium displaying global morphologic changes due to the extrinsic influence of unopposed estrogens. EIN and benign endometrial hyperplasia coexist in many individual patients and are discretely different histologies. Systemic hormonal factors are relevant to both diseases, as they can act as positive or negative selection factors for mutated cells within an EIN lesion.

Endometrial Intraepithelial Neoplasia

EIN is monoclonal neoplastic proliferation prone to malignant transformation. It shows a continuity of acquired genetic markers upon transformation into a malignant phase.

PATHOGENESIS: EIN lesions are aggregates of neoplastic endometrial glands with altered cytology and architecture that offset them from the background from which they sprang. Unlike benign endometrial hyperplasia, which involves all the endometrium at inception, EIN lesions begin locally and only later overrun the endometrial compartment. The PTEN tumor suppressor gene, which is hormonally regulated in normal endometrium, is an informative biomarker for endometrial carcinogenesis. Loss of PTEN function occurs clonally in two-thirds of EIN lesions, and an increased fraction in subsequent endometrial carcinomas. Additional evidence that PTEN is important in this context comes from heterozygous PTEN knockout mice, which uniformly develop an "endometrial hyperplasia" that evolves to carcinoma in one fifth of animals. Cancers that develop in women with EIN are usually endometrioid adenocarcinoma. Commonly, there is a relationship to estrogen exposure.

PATHOLOGY: At emergence, EIN lesions have a geographic epicenter that extends centripetally by interposition of neoplastic glands between normal glands. They are composed of tight aggregates of individually recognizable glands that as a group differ cytologically from the background endometrium, have a gland area that exceeds that of stroma, and measure more than 1mm in dimension in a single fragment. Unlike the diffuse architectural and randomly dispersed cytologic changes associated with unopposed estrogen, EIN originates as a focus of cytologically altered glands, only later becoming more diffuse. When correlated with the older hyperplasia classification system, 5% of simple hyperplasias, 44% of complex hyperplasias, and 79% of atypical hyperplasias were rediagnosed as EIN (see Fig. 18-29). Malignant transformation of EIN is evident when the glands develop solid, cribriform, or mazelike patterns characteristic of adenocarcinoma.

CLINICAL FEATURES: Women newly diagnosed with EIN have a 39% chance of having endometrial cancer diagnosed within 1 year, indicating that in most cases the cancer was already present at the time of the initial biopsy. This also explains the clinical adage, "not cancer but better out," as patients with a diagnosis of "atypical hyperplasia" in the older World Health Organization (WHO) classification system often had cancer if the uterus was removed immediately. Excluding women with concurrent cancer (i.e., only looking at those with a cancer-free interval of 1 year), EIN-positive patients have a 45-fold increased risk of developing of endometrial cancer.

Exclusion of coexisting carcinoma, and prevention of future cancer are the goals of clinical management. Hysterectomy fulfills both objectives, and is usually considered the therapy of choice if a woman has decided not to have any more children. There is clinical interest, however, in the alternative of hormonal therapy with progestins for women who wish to retain fertility or who are poor surgical risks.

Endometrial Adenocarcinoma

EPIDEMIOLOGY: Endometrial carcinoma is the fourth most frequent cancer in American women and the most common gynecological cancer (see Table 18-5). It can be divided into (1) endometrioid cancers, which are associated with EIN precursors, prior estrogen exposure, and a slow clinical course; and (2) nonendometrioid types which emerge without warning generally in older women and have much higher fatality rates. Endometrial carcinoma was responsible for an estimated 6000 deaths in the United States in 2002 (7% of all cancers in women). The incidence of this cancer was stable between 1950 and 1970, but then increased by 40% by 1975. The rise was attributed to the practice of prescribing estrogens for easing the symptoms of menopause. By 1985, rates had returned nearly to 1950 levels, a trend that correlated with use of lower doses of estrogen, incorporation of progestins (estrogen antagonists) into estrogen replacement regimens, and increased surveillance of women treated with estrogens.

The occurrence of endometrial cancer varies with age. The incidence is 12 cases per 100,000 women at age 40, but is sevenfold higher in 60-year-olds. Three quarters of women with endometrial cancer are postmenopausal. The median age at diagnosis is 63.

PATHOGENESIS: *The major form of endometrial cancer, endometrioid adenocarcinoma, is linked to prolonged estrogenic stimulation of the endometrium and defects in the PTEN tumor suppressor pathway.* In addition to treatment with exogenous estrogens, the most common risk factors are obesity, diabetes, nulliparity, early menarche, and late menopause. Each risk factor points to relative hyperestrinism. Women with ovarian agenesis do not develop endometrial cancer unless treated with exogenous estrogens. A high frequency of endometrial cancer is also found in women with estrogen-secreting granulosa cell tumors. Incidence of endometrial cancer correlates with body weight: the risk increases 10-fold if a woman is more than 23 kg (50 lb) overweight. This effect of obesity is related to the enhanced aromatization of androstenedione to estrone in adipocytes. Cigarette smoking interferes with hepatic conversion of estrone to its active metabolite estriol, and is associated with a reduced risk of endometrial cancer. Treatment of breast cancer with tamoxifen, a synthetic antiestrogen that also has agonist activity, may slightly increase the risk of endometrial cancer.

Nonendometrioid cancers, especially **serous and clear cell adenocarcinoma**, are unrelated to estrogen exposure and usually occur in women in their 60s and 70s. The adjacent endometrium is usually atrophic, a sign of estrogen deficiency. These tumors frequently have p53 gene mutations. Occasionally, the tumor may show a precursor form, termed **serous endometrial intraepithelial carcinoma** (see below).

Endometrial cancer also occurs in association with a higher incidence of both breast and ovarian cancer in closely related women, suggesting a genetic predisposition. It is also the most common extracolonic cancer in women with hereditary nonpolyposis colon cancer syndrome, a defect in DNA mismatch repair that is also associated with breast and ovarian cancers.

PATHOLOGY: Endometrial cancer grows in a diffuse or exophytic pattern (Fig. 18-30). Regardless of its site of origin, the tumor often tends to involve multiple areas. Large tumors are usually hemorrhagic and necrotic.

ENDOMETRIOID ADENOCARCINOMA OF THE ENDOMETRIUM: This type of endometrial cancer is composed entirely of glandular cells and is the most common histologic variant (60%). The FIGO system divides this tumor into three grades on the basis of the ratio of glandular to solid elements, the latter signifying poorer differentiation (Table 18-7; Fig. 18-31).

- **Grade 1:** Well differentiated; composed almost exclusively of neoplastic glands, with only minimal (<5%) solid areas.
- **Grade 2:** Moderately differentiated; formed partly of glandular elements and partly (<50%) of solid tumor.
- **Grade 3:** Poorly differentiated; shows large (>50%) areas of solid tumor.

The nuclei of endometrial adenocarcinoma range from bland to markedly pleomorphic, usually showing prominent nucleoli. Mitotic figures are abundant, and may be abnormal in less differentiated tumors. Tumor cells that grow in solid sheets generally are poorly differentiated.

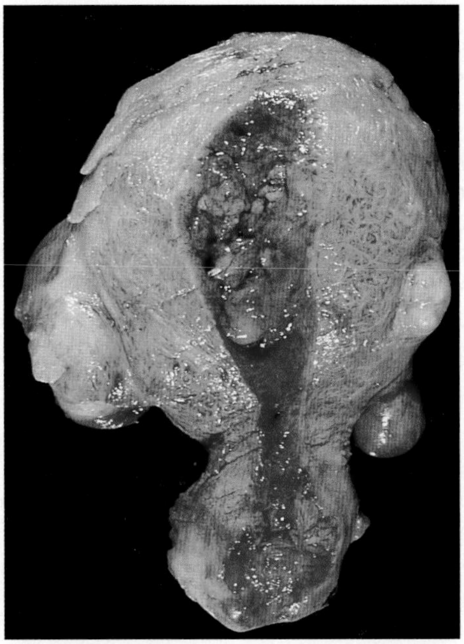

FIGURE 18-30. **Adenocarcinoma of the endometrium.** The uterus has been opened to reveal a partially necrotic, polypoid endometrial cancer.

TABLE 18-7

Surgical Staging and Histopathologic Grading of Endometrial Cancer

Stage		Description
O		Atypical hyperplasia or carcinoma in situ
I		Confined to corpus
	Ia	Confined to endometrium
	Ib	Invades <1/2 myometrium
	Ic	Invades >1/2 myometrium
II		Involves cervix
	IIa	Endocervical glandular involvement only (i.e., in situ in glands)
	IIb	Cervical stromal invasion
III		Extends beyond uterus but not outside true pelvis
	IIIa	Involves serosa or adnexa, or has positive peritoneal cytology
IV		Extends beyond true pelvis or involves the mucosa of bladder or rectum
	IVa	Spread to adjacent organs
	IVb	Spread to distant organs

Grading (FIGO) of glandular tissue: G1 = <5% solid (highly differentiated); G2 = 5%–50% solid (differentiated with partly solid areas); G3 = >50% solid (predominantly solid or entirely undifferentiated).

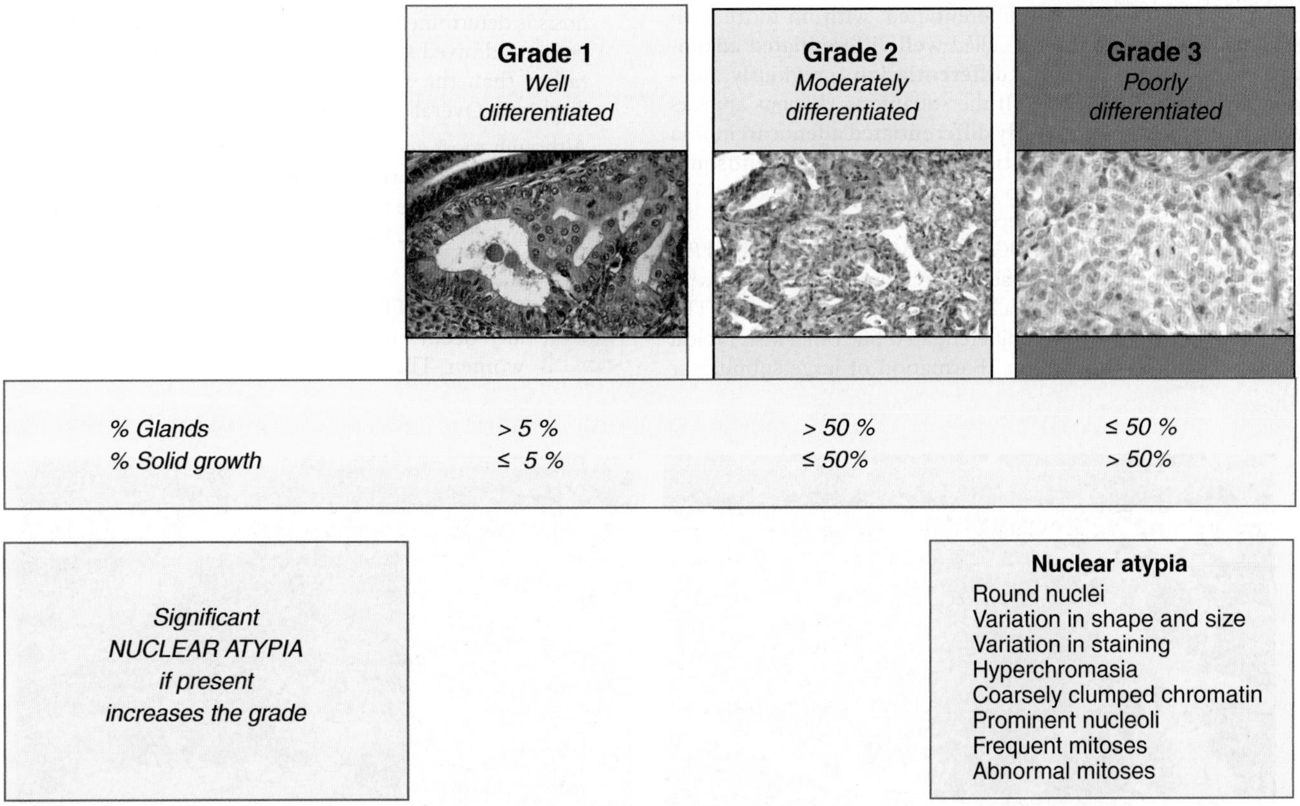

FIGURE 18-31. **Grading of endometrial adenocarcinoma.** The grade depends primarily on the architectural pattern, but significant nuclear atypia changes a grade 1 tumor to grade 2, and a grade 2 tumor to grade 3. Nuclear atypia is characterized by round nuclei; variation in shape, size, and staining; hyperchromasia; coarsely clumped chromating; prominent nucleoli; and frequent and abnormal mitoses. Significant nuclear atypia if present increases the tumor grade.

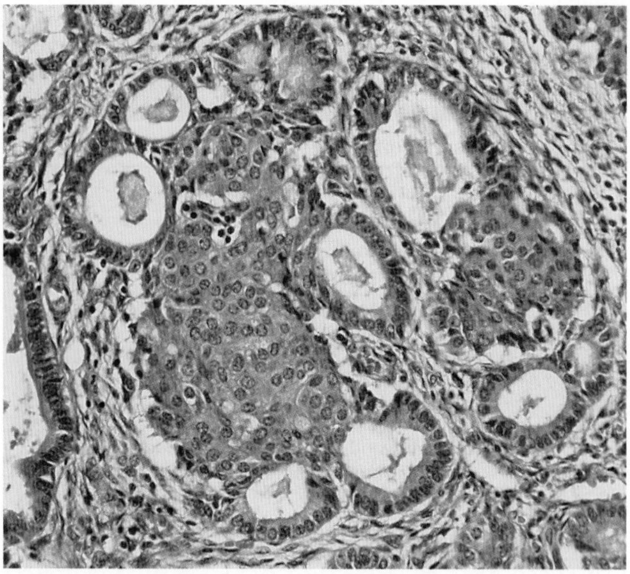

FIGURE 18-32. **Squamous differentiation in endometrioid adenocarcinoma of the endometrium.** The well-differentiated squamous cells show minimal atypia. The pattern has been called adenoacanthoma when the squamous cells form squamous morules and nest among glands.

ENDOMETRIOID ADENOCARCINOMA, WITH SQUAMOUS DIFFERENTIATION: One third of all endometrial carcinomas contain squamous cells in addition to glandular elements. If the squamous element is well differentiated, with no more than minimal atypia, the tumor is called **well-differentiated adenocarcinoma with squamous differentiation** (previously, **adenoacanthoma**) (Fig. 18-32). If the squamous element appears malignant, the tumor is **poorly differentiated adenocarcinoma with squamous differentiation** (also known as **adenosquamous carcinoma**). These two variants represent 22% and 7% of all endometrial cancers, respectively.

ENDOMETRIOID ADENOCARCINOMA, SECRETORY TYPE: Is a variant of endometrioid adenocarcinoma having cells with subnuclear vacuolization, usually in premenopausal women. The tumor is an extremely well differentiated but otherwise typical endometrial adenocarcinoma. Formation of large subnuclear vacuoles of glycogen in some cases is dependant on progesterone stimulation in as much as it may be present in only one of several serial specimens. Secretory carcinoma has the most favorable outcome of any adenocarcinoma, presumably because the cells are well differentiated

OTHER TYPES (NONENDOMETRIOID) OF ENDOMETRIAL CARCINOMA: Nonendometrioid types of endometrial carcinoma are less common, and unassociated with estrogen exposure. Because they tend to be aggressive as a group, histologic grading is not of clinical value.

- **Serous adenocarcinoma** histologically resembles serous adenocarcinoma of the ovary (Fig. 18-33A). It also behaves more like an ovarian carcinoma than an endometrial tumor, often showing transtubal spread to celomic spread. An in situ form has been termed "serous endometrial intraepithelial carcinoma" (serous EIC), not to be confused with EIN, described earlier. Patients with this type of tumor need to be staged and treated as if they had ovarian cancer.
- **Clear cell adenocarcinoma** is a tumor of elderly women. It is composed of large cells with abundant cytoplasmic glycogen ("clear cells") or of cells with bulbous nuclei that line glandular lumina ("hobnail cells") (see Fig. 18-33B). Serous and clear cell carcinomas are associated with adverse outcomes.
- **Carcinosarcoma (malignant mixed mesodermal tumor):** In this highly malignant tumor, pleomorphic **epithelial** components are intermingled with cells that show **mesenchymal** differentiation. These mixed neoplasms are derived from a common clone believed to be of epithelial origin. The prognosis is determined by the presence of a mesenchymal component admixed with the malignant epithelial component, rather than the specific type of mesenchymal histology displayed. Overall 5-year survival is 25%.

Although most endometrial carcinomas arise in the uterine corpus, a small proportion originate in the lower uterine segment (isthmus). These tumors often occur in women under the age of 50 and are often high grade and deeply invasive.

CLINICAL FEATURES: Endometrial carcinoma usually occurs in perimenopausal or postmenopausal women. The chief complaint is commonly abnormal

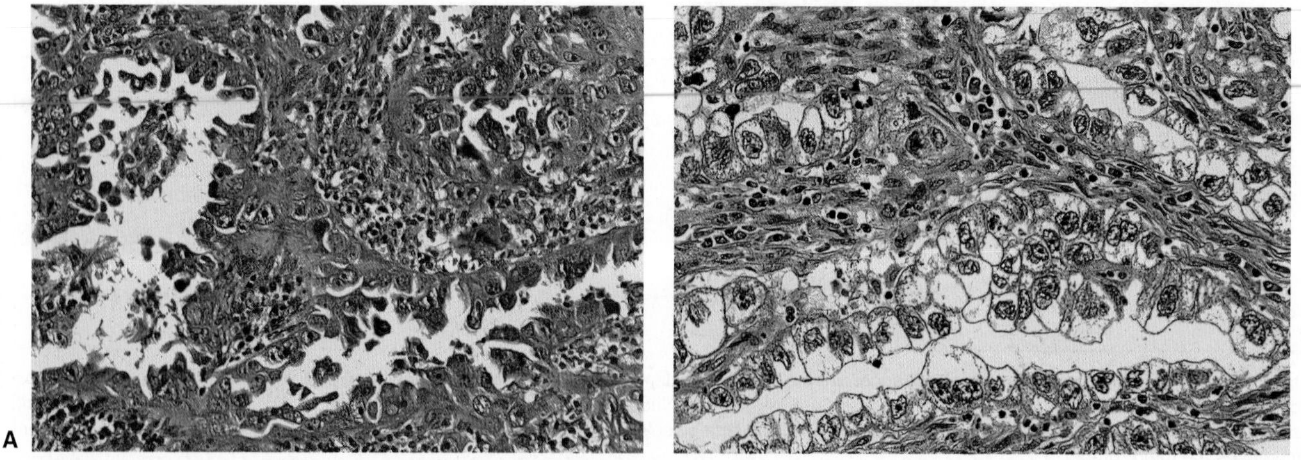

FIGURE 18-33. **Nonendometrioid types of endometrial adenocarcinoma. A.** Serous adenocarcinoma. Large cells with bulbous, pleomorphic nuclei grow in a papillary configuration. **B.** Clear cell adenocarcinoma. The clear appearance of the cytoplasm is due to the dissolution of glycogen when the specimen was processed for microscopic examination. Hobnail cells with bulbous nuclei line glandular lumina.

uterine bleeding, especially if the tumor is in its early stages of growth (i.e., confined to the endometrium). Unfortunately, cervicovaginal cytological screening is unsuitable for early detection of endometrial cancer. Fractional curettage is needed to assess spread to the cervix, whereas peritoneal washing detects tubal reflux and abdominal contamination. Transvaginal ultrasonography is a valuable diagnostic modality; endometrium more than 5 mm thick is considered highly suspicious. Unlike cervical cancer, endometrial cancer may spread directly to paraaortic lymph nodes, thereby skipping pelvic nodes. Patients with advanced cancers may also develop pulmonary metastases (40% of cases with metastases).

Women with well-differentiated cancers confined to the endometrium are usually treated by simple hysterectomy. Postoperative radiation is considered if (1) the tumor is poorly differentiated or nonendometrioid in type, (2) myometrium is deeply invaded, (3) the cervix is involved, or (4) lymph nodes contain metastases.

Survival in endometrial carcinoma is related to multiple factors, including (1) stage and grade; (2) age; and (3) other measurable risk factors, such as progesterone receptor activity, depth of myometrial invasion, extent of lymphovascular invasion, and results of peritoneal washings. High levels of estrogen and progesterone receptors in the tumor and low levels of proliferative activity correlate with a better prognosis. Actuarial survival of all patients with endometrial cancer following treatment is 80% after the second year, decreasing to 65% after 10 years. Tumors that have penetrated the myometrium or invaded lymphatics are more likely to have spread beyond the uterus. Endometrial cancers involving the cervix have a poorer prognosis. Those that extend outside the uterus have the worst outlook (Table 18-8).

TABLE 18-8

Stage, Grade, and Survival for Endometrial Cancer

	5-Year Survival (%)		
Stage	**G-1***	**G-2**	**G-3**
I	90	69	52
II	80	42	12
III, IV	25	33	17

* G = FIGO grade.

Endometrial Stromal Tumors Account for Fewer Than 2% of All Uterine Cancers

Some endometrial stromal tumors are pure sarcomas; others exhibit intimate admixtures of sarcomatous (stromal) and epithelial elements. The nomenclature of these tumor types, the spectrum of their histologic components and the correlation of each tumor type with its potential for malignant behavior are presented in Table 18-9.

Endometrial Stromal Sarcoma

Pure stromal tumors are divided into two major categories, based on whether the tumor margin is expansile or infiltrating. Expansile lesions that do not invade are **benign stromal nodules**, which have little clinical significance. Tumors with infiltrating margins are termed **stromal sarcomas**.

PATHOLOGY: Endometrial stromal sarcomas may be polypoid and fill the endometrial cavity, or they may diffusely invade the myometrium. Large masses of spindle cells with scant cytoplasm dissect the myometrium and invade vascular channels. The neoplastic cells resemble endometrial stromal cells in the proliferative phase. A feature characteristic of all endometrial stromal tumors is a rich vascular supporting framework, with the neoplastic cells concentrically arranged around blood vessels (Fig. 18-34). Nuclear atypism may be minimal to severe and mitotic activity may be restrained. Expression of CD-10 and estrogen and progesterone receptors helps confirm the diagnosis. Higher-grade sarcomas originating in the endometrium lose all antigenic and

TABLE 18-9

Nomenclature of Uterine Tumors

Tumor	Epithelium	Stroma	Clinical Behavior
Epithelium and Stroma			
Endometrial polyp	Polyclonal benign	Neoplastic	Benign
Benign endometrial hyperplasia	Polyclonal		Benign
Endometrial intraepithelial neoplasia	Neoplastic	–	Premalignant
Endometrial adenocarcinoma	Neoplastic	–	Malignant
Endometrial stromal nodule	–	Neoplastic	Benign
Endometrial stromal sarcoma		Neoplastic	Low-grade malignant
Undifferentiated sarcoma	–	Neoplastic	Malignant
Adenosarcoma	Neoplastic	Neoplastic	Low-grade malignant
Carcinosarcoma	Neoplastic	Neoplastic, transformed epithelial cells	Malignant
Smooth Muscle			
Leiomyoma	–	Neoplastic	Benign
Cellular leiomyoma	–	Neoplastic	Benign
Intravenous leiomyomatosis	–	Neoplastic	Locally aggressive
Leiomyosarcoma	–	Neoplastic	Malignant

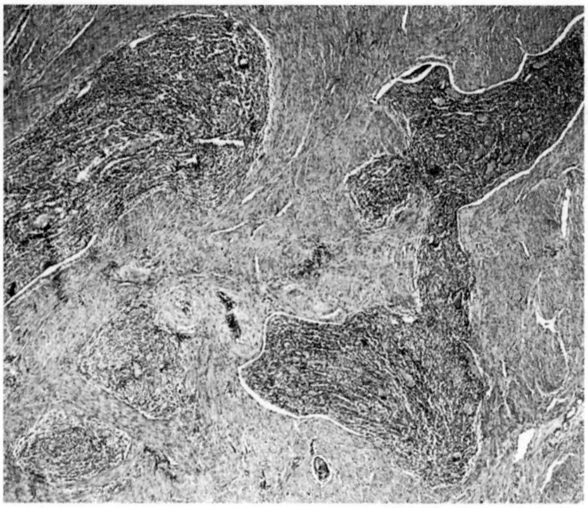

FIGURE 18-34. **Endometrial stromal sarcoma, low grade.** The myometrium is irregularly invaded by the tumor, which displays a rich vascular network.

morphologic resemblance to endometrial stroma and are thus designated as **undifferentiated endometrial sarcoma.**

CLINICAL FEATURES: Many years may elapse before recurrent endometrial stromal sarcoma becomes clinically evident, and metastases may occur even if the tumor was confined to the uterus at initial surgery. Recurrences usually involve the pelvis initially, to be followed by pulmonary metastases. Prolonged survival and even cure are feasible, despite metastases. By contrast, undifferentiated endometrial sarcomas recur early, generally with widespread metastases, even if there had been little myometrial invasion. Endometrial stromal sarcomas can be successfully treated with surgery and progestin therapy, with an expectation of 90% survival 10 years after diagnosis.

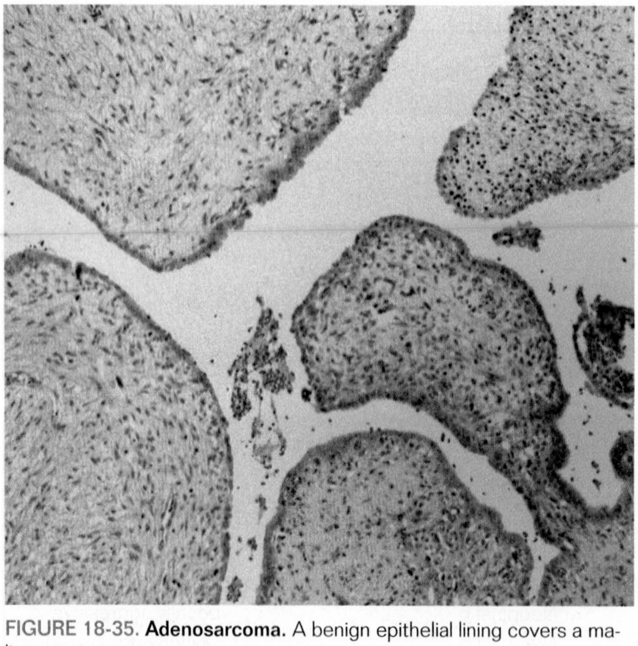

FIGURE 18-35. **Adenosarcoma.** A benign epithelial lining covers a malignant stroma.

UTERINE ADENOSARCOMA

Uterine (müllerian) adenosarcoma is a distinctive low-grade tumor that combines benign glandular epithelium and malignant stroma (Fig. 18-35). It should be distinguished from carcinosarcoma, which has both malignant epithelial and stromal elements and is highly aggressive.

Adenosarcoma typically presents as a polypoid mass within the endometrial cavity. The glandular epithelium resembles proliferative phase endometrial glands, but occasionally squamous epithelium and mucinous-type epithelium are seen. The stroma is cellular, may exhibit mitotic activity, is often densest about the glandular epithelium (periglandular cuffing) and resembles endometrial stromal cells in the proliferative phase of the cycle. One fourth of patients with adenosarcoma eventually succumb to local recurrence or metastatic spread.

Leiomyoma Is the Most Common Tumor of the Female Genital Tract

Leiomyoma, a benign tumor of smooth muscle origin, is colloquially known as a "myoma" or "fibroid." If minute tumors are included, leiomyomas occur in 75% of women over 30 years of age. They are rare before age 20, and most regress after menopause. Although often multiple, each leiomyoma is monoclonal (see Chapter 5). Estrogen promotes their growth, although it does not initiate them.

PATHOLOGY: Grossly, leiomyomas are firm, pale gray, whorled, and without encapsulation (Fig. 18-36 and Fig.18-37). They range from 1 mm to more than 30 cm in diameter. The cut surface bulges and borders are smooth and distinct from neighboring myometrium. Most

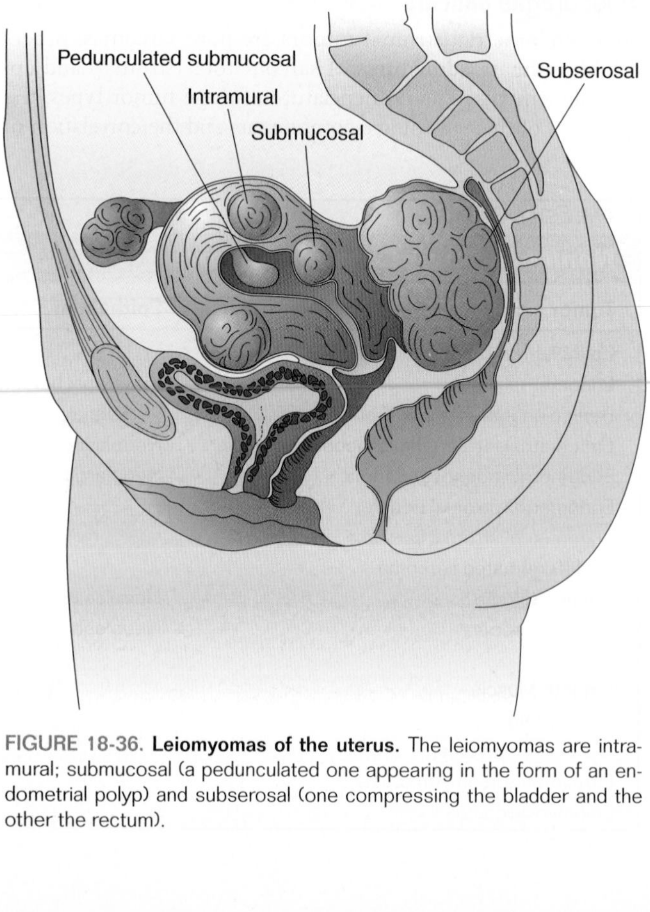

FIGURE 18-36. **Leiomyomas of the uterus.** The leiomyomas are intramural; submucosal (a pedunculated one appearing in the form of an endometrial polyp) and subserosal (one compressing the bladder and the other the rectum).

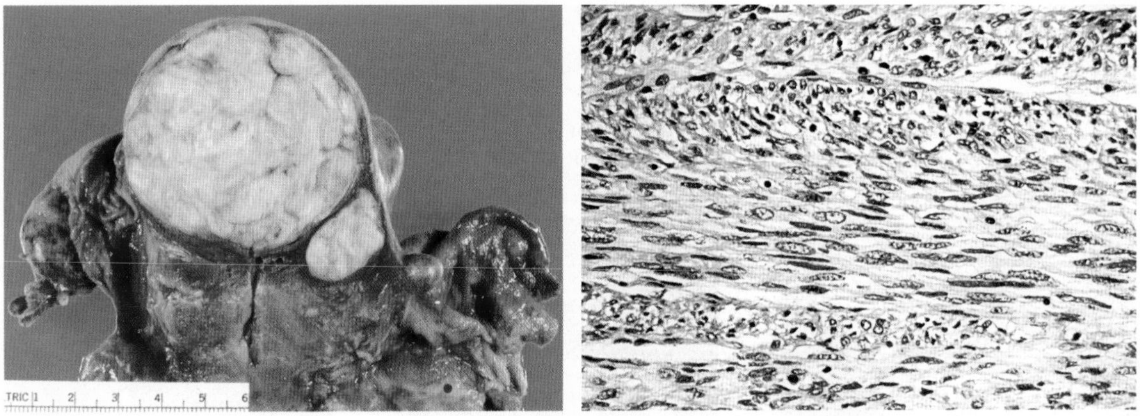

A B

FIGURE 18-37. **Leiomyoma of the uterus. A.** A bisected uterus displays a prominent, sharply circumscribed, fleshy tumor. **B.** Microscopically, smooth muscle cells intertwine in bundles, some of which are cut longitudinally (elongated nuclei) and others transversely.

leiomyomas are intramural, but some are submucosal, subserosal or pedunculated. Many, especially larger ones, show areas of degenerative hyalinization that are sharply demarcated from adjacent normal myometrium. Leiomyomas that display low mitotic activity (=4 mitoses per 10 high-power fields [HPFs]), lack nuclear atypia and geographical necrosis, and have little or no malignant potential. "**Mitotically active leiomyoma,**" a condition usually benign, is a leiomyoma that shows brisk mitotic activity but is relatively small, is sharply demarcated from the adjacent normal myometrium and lacks both geographical necrosis and significant cellular atypia.

Microscopically leiomyomas exhibit interlacing fascicles of uniform spindle cells, in which nuclei are elongated and have blunt ends (see Fig. 18-37B). The cytoplasm is abundant, eosinophilic, and fibrillar. The myocytes of leiomyomas and adjacent myometrium are cytologically identical, but leiomyomas are easily distinguished by their circumscription, nodularity, and denser cellularity.

CLINICAL FEATURES: Submucosal leiomyomas may cause bleeding due to ulceration of the thinned, overlying endometrium. Some submucosal leiomyomas become pedunculated and protrude through the cervical os, eliciting cramping pains. Many intramural leiomyomas are symptomatic because of sheer bulk, and large ones may interfere with bowel or bladder function or cause dystocia in labor. Pedunculated leiomyomas on the uterine serosa may interfere with the function of neighboring viscera. Leiomyomas may also infarct and become painful if they undergo torsion.

Leiomyomas usually grow slowly, but occasionally enlarge rapidly during pregnancy. Large symptomatic leiomyomas are removed by myomectomy or hysterectomy. Ablation by arterial thrombosis has also been used recently.

Intravenous Leiomyomatosis Does Not Metastasize

Intravenous leiomyomatosis is a rare condition that features growth of benign smooth muscle within uterine and pelvic veins. The condition may originate from vascular invasion by a preexisting uterine leiomyoma or growth of venous smooth muscle. It may be evident at surgery as wormlike extensions near the external uterine surface or as projections into uterine veins in the broad ligament. Although they may grow extensively inside blood vessels, these neoplasms do not metastasize. Rare fatalities have resulted from direct extension of leiomyomatous tissues within pelvic veins into the inferior vena cava and right atrium. Treatment consists of total abdominal hysterectomy.

Leiomyosarcoma Is Very Rare in Comparison to Leiomyoma

Leiomyosarcoma is a malignancy of smooth muscle origin whose incidence is only 1/1000 that of its benign counterpart. It accounts for 2% of uterine malignancies. Its pathogenesis is uncertain, but at least some appear to arise from within leiomyomas. Women with leiomyosarcomas are on average more than a decade older (age above 50) than those with leiomyomas, and the malignant tumors are larger (10 to 15 cm vs. 3 to 5 cm).

PATHOLOGY: Leiomyosarcoma should be suspected if an apparent leiomyoma is soft, shows areas of necrosis on gross examination, has irregular borders (invasion into neighboring myometrium), or does not bulge above the surface when cut (Fig. 18-38). Mitotic activity, cellular atypia, and geographical necrosis are the best diagnostic criteria. There is usually a sharp transition from viable tumor to large zones of necrosis, with an intervening rim of partially viable tumor cells. Blood vessels, if present, may be surrounded by a thin rim of viable tumor cells. The following are evidence that a smooth muscle tumor is a leiomyosarcoma: (1) Presence of geographic necrosis; (2) 10 or more mitoses per 10 HPFs, provided the tumor is more than about 5 cm in diameter; (3) 5 or more mitoses per 10 HPFs, with geographical necrosis and diffuse cytoplasmic/nuclear atypia; and (4) myxoid and epithelioid smooth muscle tumors with 5 or more mitoses per 10 HPFs. Size is an important: tumors under 5 cm in diameter almost never recur.

Most leiomyosarcomas are large and are advanced when detected. They thus are usually fatal despite combinations of surgery, radiation therapy, and chemotherapy. Nearly half of recurrences first present in the lung, and 5-year survival is about 20%.

FALLOPIAN TUBE

Anatomy

The fallopian tubes extend from the uterine fundus to the ovaries. An interstitial portion, termed the **isthmus**, lies within the cornua

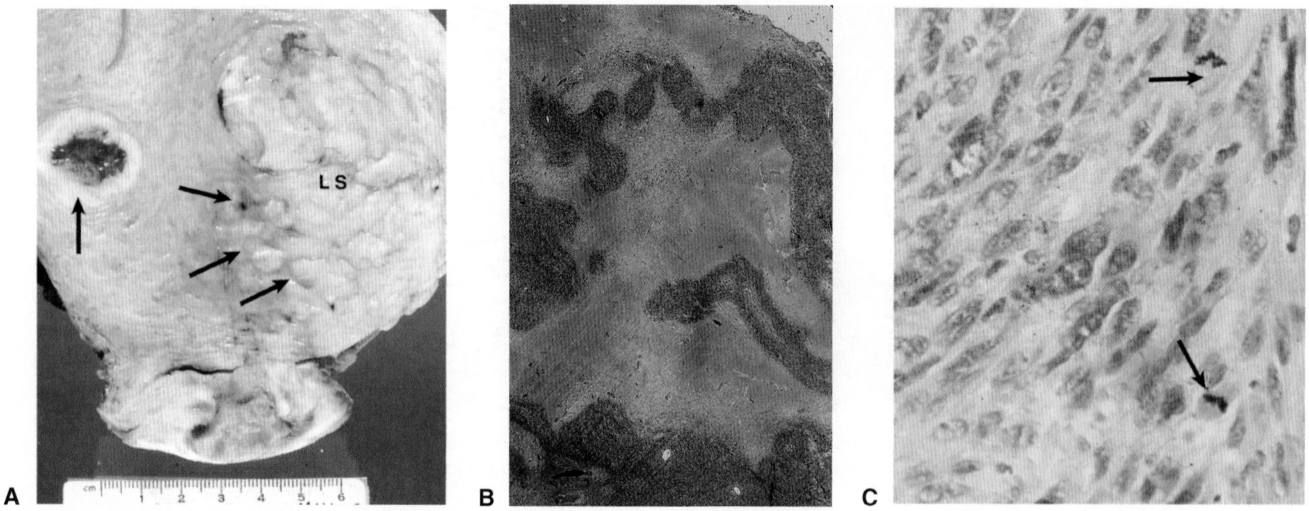

FIGURE 18-38. **Leiomyosarcoma of the uterus. A.** The uterus has been opened to reveal a large, soft leiomyosarcoma (LS) that has irregular borders *(horizontal arrows)* and invades the surrounding myometrium. By comparison, a small, firm leiomyoma *(vertical arrow)* with a hemorrhagic center is sharply demarcated. **B.** At low magnification, areas of necrosis are sharply demarcated from the viable tumor. **C.** The malignant cells are moderately disorganized in arrangement, they are irregular in shape, and display numerous mitoses *(arrows)*.

of the uterus and connects the uterine cavity with the straight portion of the tube. As the tube extends to the ovary, it increases in diameter to form the **ampulla**, which merges with the **infundibulum**. The fimbriated end opens like the bell of a trumpet and has many fingerlike extensions that envelop the ovary. The lining cells are ciliated and are important in transport of ova.

Salpingitis

Salpingitis is inflammation of the fallopian tubes, typically due to infections ascending from the lower genital tract. The most common causative organisms are *Neisseria gonorrhoeae, Escherichia coli, Chlamydia, and Mycoplasma.* Infection is typically polymicrobial. Acute episodes of salpingitis (particularly those associated with chlamydial infection) may be asymptomatic. A fallopian tube damaged by prior infection is particularly susceptible to reinfection. In most cases, chronic salpingitis develops only after repeated episodes of acute salpingitis.

PATHOLOGY AND CLINICAL FEATURES: In acute salpingitis, microscopic examination reveals marked infiltration by polymorphonuclear leukocytes, pronounced edema and congestion of the mucosal folds (plicae). The inflammatory infiltrate in chronic salpingitis consists of lymphocytes and plasma cells; edema, and congestion tend to be minimal. In late stages, the fallopian tube may seal and become distended with pus (**pyosalpinx**) or a transudate (**hydrosalpinx**).

The fallopian tube allows ascending microorganisms from the lower genital tract to reach the peritoneal cavity, leading to peritonitis and PID. Fibrinous adhesions between the fallopian tube serosa and surrounding peritoneal surfaces organize into thin fibrous adhesions ("violin string" adhesions). The adjacent ovary may also be involved, sometimes giving rise to a **tuboovarian abscess**.

Complications also ensue from damage to the fallopian tube itself. Destruction of the epithelium or deposition of fibrin on the mucosa results in formation of fibrin bridges, which cause the plicae to adhere to one another. In severe chronic salpingitis, adhesions are dense and form a blunted, clubbed end of the tube. The consequence of the blocked lumen may be hydrosalpinx or pyosalpinx. The damage wrought by chronic salpingitis may impair general tubal motility and passage of sperm, in which case **infertility** results. Chronic salpingitis is a common cause of **ectopic pregnancy**, since adherent mucosal plicae create pockets in which ova are entrapped.

Ectopic Pregnancy

Ectopic pregnancy means implantation of a fertilized ovum outside the endometrium. The frequency of ectopic pregnancy in the United States has increased threefold, to 1.5% of live births, during the past two decades, although mortality has sharply declined. *Over 95% of ectopic pregnancies occur in the fallopian tube, mostly in the distal and middle thirds.*

PATHOLOGY: Ectopic pregnancy results when passage of the conceptus along the fallopian tube is impeded, for example, by mucosal adhesions or abnormal tubal motility secondary to inflammatory disease or endometriosis. The trophoblast readily penetrates the mucosa and muscular tubal wall. Thus, ectopic pregnancy resembles placenta increta or placenta percreta of the uterus (see below). Blood from the implantation site in the tube enters the peritoneal cavity, causing abdominal pain. In addition, ectopic pregnancy is often associated with anomalous uterine bleeding after a period of amenorrhea, and Arias-Stella cells in the endometrium. The thin tubal wall usually ruptures by the 12th week of gestation. *Tubal rupture is life-threatening because it can result in rapid exsanguination.*

Rupture of the tube's interstitial portion produces greater intra-abdominal hemorrhage than rupture in other locations because vasculature there is richer and rupture occurs later in gestation. In the isthmus, the tube ruptures early (within the first 6 weeks), because its thick muscular wall does not allow much distention. Tubal pregnancies in the ampulla tend to be of longer duration, since the distensible tubal wall can accommodate a growing pregnancy for a longer time.

Ectopic pregnancy must be treated promptly with surgical or chemotherapeutic intervention. Administration of methotrexate terminates ectopic pregnancy, and is used when the conceptus is smaller than 4 cm.

Fallopian Tumors

Tumors of the fallopian tube are rare. The most common is the small, circumscribed **adenomatoid tumor**, which is of mesothelial origin. It arises in the mesosalpinx and shows benign mesothelial cells that line slitlike spaces.

Fallopian tube involvement by metastases or implants from adjacent ovarian and uterine neoplasms far exceeds the frequency of the rare primary cancer. Most primary malignancies are adenocarcinomas, with peak incidence among 50- to 60-year-olds. The tumor is bilateral in 25% of cases. Prognosis is poor, as the disease is almost always detected at a late stage. Fallopian tube cancer is treated similar to ovarian cancer.

OVARY

Anatomy and Embryology

The ovaries are paired organs that flank the uterus. They are attached to the posterior surface of the broad ligament in a shallow peritoneal fossa between the external iliac vessels and the ureter. Each ovary consists of (1) an epithelial surface, (2) a mesenchymal stroma containing steroid-producing cells, and (3) germ cells. It has an outer cortex and inner medulla.

Ovaries appear early in fetal life as swellings of the genital ridges. At the 19th day of gestation, germ cells migrate from the primitive yolk sac to the gonads and multiply by mitotic division. By the 40th day, ovaries and testes are histologically distinct. Towards the third trimester of fetal life, germ cells stop multiplying and instead continue to develop by meiosis. Of 1 million primordial follicles present at birth, only 70% remain by puberty and fewer than 15% persist to age 25 years. Only some 450 ova are actually shed during a woman's 35-year reproductive lifetime.

The ovarian cortex mesenchyme consists of spindle-shaped, fibroblast-like cells. These give rise to the granulosa and theca cells, which form a functional unit about each ovum (theca interna and theca externa). The complex of the germ cell and supporting granulosa cells is known first as a **primordial follicle**. During the reproductive period, a dominant follicle develops every month into a **graafian follicle**, which then ruptures during ovulation. Ovulation itself is often associated with mild cramping pain which, if severe, is called **mittelschmerz** (i.e., midcycle pain). It is frequently confused with appendicitis. Following ovulation the follicle granulosa cells luteinize, a change characterized by hypertrophy and lipid accumulation. At that time they secrete progesterone in addition to estrogens. The collapsed follicle turns bright yellow and becomes the **corpus luteum** (yellow body).

The cells of ovarian stromal origin include hilus cells and those resembling luteinized cells of the theca interna, both of which respond to pituitary hormones. These specialized cells synthesize and secrete both androgens and estrogens, which stimulate proliferation in end organs, (e.g., uterus). They inhibit hypothalamic function by negative feedback loops.

Cystic Lesions of the Ovaries

Cysts are the most common cause of enlarged ovaries. Cysts arising from the invaginated surface epithelium (serous cysts) are quite common. Almost all of the rest derive from ovarian follicles.

Follicle Cysts Tend to be Asymptomatic

Follicle cysts are thin-walled, fluid-filled structures lined internally by granulosa cells and externally by theca interna cells. They occur at any age up to menopause, are unilocular and may be single or multiple, unilateral or bilateral. These cysts arise from ovarian follicles and are probably related to abnormalities in pituitary gonadotropin release.

PATHOLOGY: Follicle cysts rarely exceed 5 cm greatest dimension. In an unstimulated state, the granulosa cells of the cyst have uniform, round nuclei and little cytoplasm. Thecal cells are small and spindle-shaped. Occasionally, the layers may be luteinized, in which case the lumen contains fluid high in estrogen or progesterone. If the cyst persists, hormonal output can cause precocious puberty in a child and menstrual irregularities in an adult. The only significant complication is mild intraperitoneal bleeding (Fig. 18-39).

Corpus Luteum Cyst Can Bleed

A corpus luteum cyst results from delayed resolution of a corpus luteum's central cavity. Continued progesterone synthesis by the luteal cyst leads to menstrual irregularities. Rupture of a cyst can cause mild hemorrhage into the abdominal cavity. A corpus luteum cyst is typically unilocular, 3 to 5 cm in size, and possessed of a yellow wall. The contents of the cyst vary from serosanguineous fluid to clotted blood. Microscopic examination shows numerous large, luteinized granulosa cells. The condition is self-limited.

Theca Lutein Cysts Relate to High Gonadotropin Levels

Theca lutein cysts are also known as hyperreactio luteinalis and are commonly multiple and bilateral. They are associated with high levels of circulating gonadotropin (e.g., in pregnancy, hydatidiform

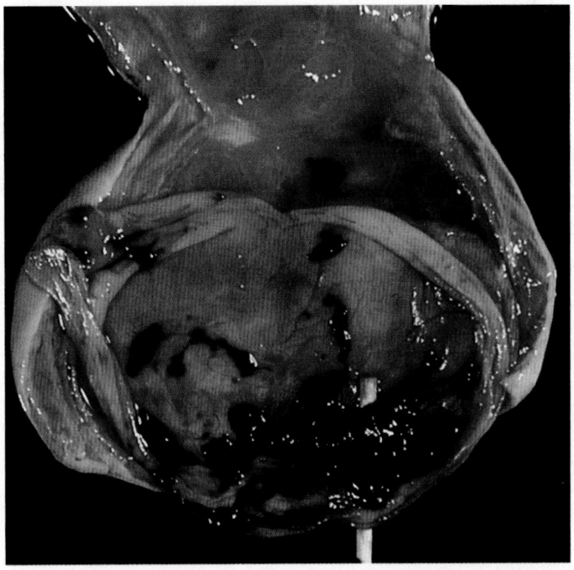

FIGURE 18-39. **Follicle cyst of the ovary.** The rupture of this thin-walled follicular cyst (dowel stick) led to intraabdominal hemorrhage.

mole, choriocarcinoma, and exogenous gonadotropin therapy) or physical impediments (dense adhesions, cortical fibrosis) to ovulation. The excessive gonadotropin levels lead to exaggerated stimulation of the theca interna and extensive cyst formation.

PATHOLOGY: Multiple thin-walled cysts filled with clear fluid replace both ovaries. Microscopically, cysts show a markedly luteinized layer of theca interna. Ovarian parenchyma shows edema and foci of luteinized stromal cells. Intra-abdominal hemorrhage secondary to torsion or rupture of the cyst may require surgical intervention.

Polycystic Ovary Syndrome

Polycystic ovary syndrome, known as ***Stein-Leventhal syndrome,*** *describes (1) clinical manifestations related to the secretion of excess androgenic hormones, (2) persistent anovulation, and (3) ovaries containing many small subcapsular cysts.* It was described initially as a syndrome of **secondary amenorrhea, hirsutism, and obesity.** However, clinical presentations are now known to be far more variable and include amenorrheic women who appear otherwise normal and, even rarely, have ovaries lacking polycystic features. *This condition a common cause of infertility: up to 7% of women experience polycystic ovary syndrome.*

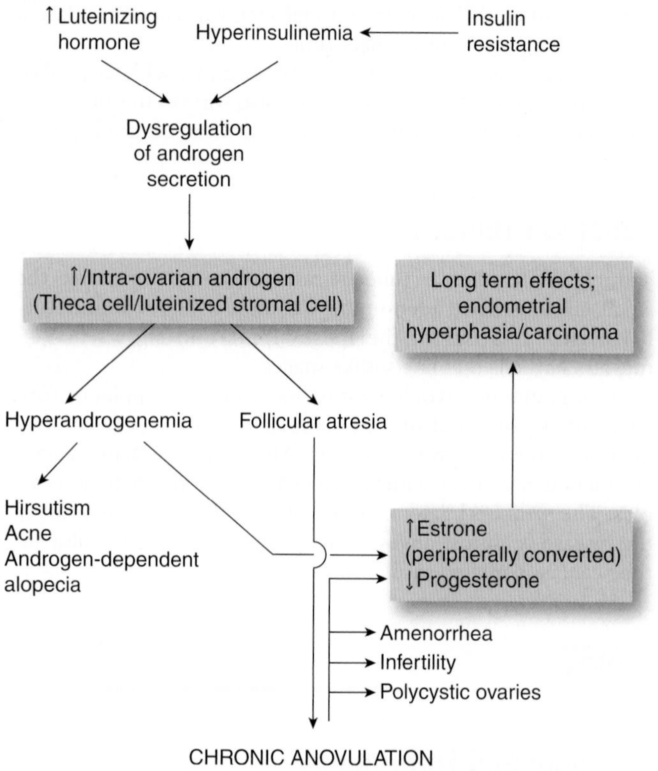

FIGURE 18-40. **Pathogenesis of the polycystic ovary syndrome.**

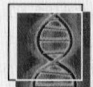

PATHOGENESIS: Polycystic ovary syndrome is a state of functional ovarian hyperandrogenism with elevated levels of LH, although increased LH is probably a result, rather than a cause, of ovarian dysfunction (Fig. 18-40).

1. The central abnormality is thought to be increased ovarian production of androgens, although adrenal hypersecretion of androgens may also be present. The rate-limiting enzyme in biosynthesis of androgens, namely, cytochrome P450$_{c17\alpha}$ (17α-hydroxylase), which is expressed in both the ovary and the adrenal gland, is abnormally regulated.
2. Excess ovarian androgens act locally to cause (a) premature follicular atresia, (b) multiple follicular cysts, and (c) a persistent anovulatory state. Impaired follicular maturation causes decreased secretion of progesterone. Peripherally, hyperandrogenism leads to hirsutism, acne, and male-pattern (androgen-dependent) alopecia. These patients may have high serum concentrations of androgenic hormones, such as testosterone, androstenedione, and dehydroepiandrosterone sulfate. But there are individual variations and some patients have normal androgen levels.
3. Excess androgens are converted to estrogens in peripheral adipose tissue, which effect is exaggerated by obesity. Acyclical estrogen production and progesterone deficiency increase pituitary secretion of LH.
4. Women with polycystic ovary syndrome exhibit marked peripheral insulin resistance, out of proportion to the degree of obesity. The mechanism appears to involve a post–insulin- receptor defect, possibly related to decreased expression of a glucose transporter.

In any event, the resulting hyperinsulinemia seems to contribute to increased ovarian hypersecretion of androgens and direct stimulation of pituitary LH production.

PATHOLOGY: On gross examination, both ovaries are enlarged. The surface is smooth, reflecting the absence of ovulation. On cut section, the cortex is thickened and discloses numerous theca-lutein type cysts, typically 2 to 8 mm in diameter, arranged peripherally around a dense core of stroma or scattered throughout an increased amount of stroma (Fig. 18-41). Microscopically, the following features are present: (1) numerous follicles in early stages of development; (2) follicular atresia; (3) increased stroma, occasionally with luteinized cells (hyperthecosis); and (4) morphologic signs of an absence of ovulation (thick, smooth capsule, and absence of corpora lutea and corpora albicantiae). Many subcapsular cysts show thick zones of theca interna, in which some cells may be luteinized.

CLINICAL FEATURES: In the United States, 15% of married couples cannot conceive. Nearly three-quarters of those with anovulatory infertility have polycystic ovary syndrome. Patients are typically in their 20s and tell of early obesity, menstrual problems, and hirsutism. Half of women with polycystic ovary syndrome are amenorrheic and most others have irregular menstrual periods. Only 75% of affected women are actually infertile, indicating that some do occasionally ovulate. Unopposed acyclic estrogen activity increases incidence of endometrial hyperplasia and adenocarcinoma.

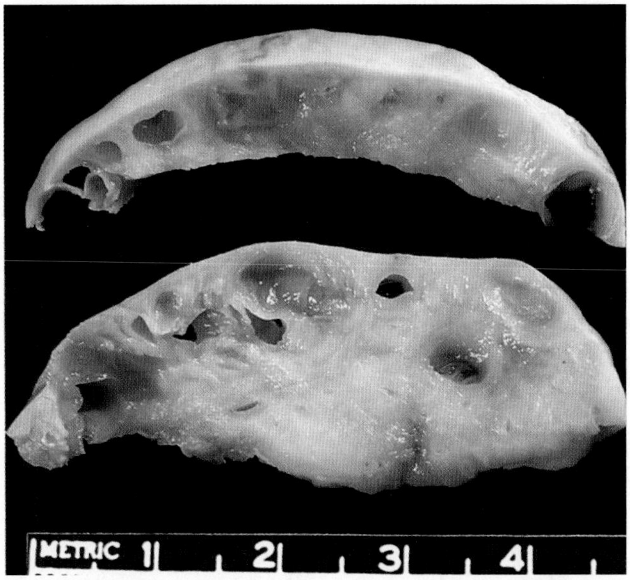

FIGURE 18-41. **Polycystic disease of the ovary.** Cut sections of an ovary show numerous cysts embedded in a sclerotic stroma.

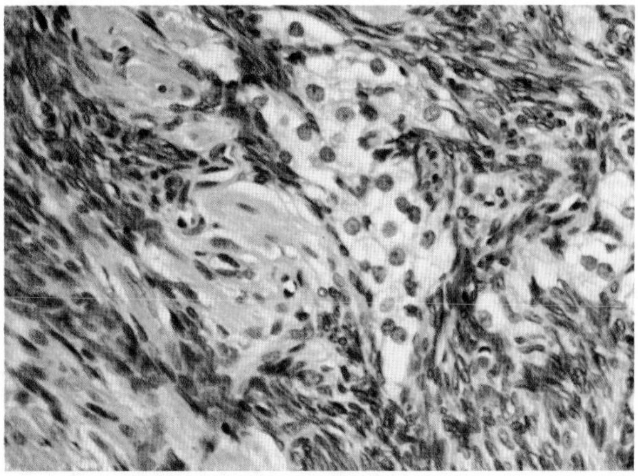

FIGURE 18-42. **Hyperthecosis of the ovary.** Nests of luteinized (lipid-rich) stromal cells are present.

Treatment of polycystic ovary syndrome encompasses two common problems in reproductive endocrinology—hirsutism and anovulation. Therapy is mostly hormonal and is directed towards interrupting the constant excess of androgens. Wedge resection of the ovary has provided temporary remission of the syndrome, but is rarely used today.

Stromal Hyperthecosis

Stromal hyperthecosis is focal luteinization of ovarian stromal cells. These stromal cells are often functional and cause **virilization.** The condition is most common in postmenopausal women and, in a microscopic form, is found in one third of postmenopausal ovaries.

PATHOLOGY: In women in whom stromal hyperthecosis is detected clinically, usually on the basis of masculinizing signs, both ovaries may be enlarged, sometimes up to 8 cm in greatest dimension. The ovarian serosa is smooth, and the cut surface is homogeneous, firm and brown to yellow. Microscopically, single nests or nodules of luteinized stromal cells are present in the cortex or medulla (Fig. 18-42). The cytoplasm of these cells is deeply eosinophilic and often vacuolated. The luteinized cells have a central large nucleus with a prominent nucleolus, a feature shared with all hormonally active stromal cells in the ovary.

Ovarian Tumors

Ovarian cancer is the second most frequent gynecological malignancy after endometrial cancer. In the United States it carries a higher mortality rate than all other female genital cancers combined (see Table 18-5). Unfortunately, this cancer is difficult to detect early in its evolution when it is still curable. More than three-fourths of patients already have extragonadal tumor spread to the pelvis or abdomen at the time of diagnosis. Approximately 26,000 new cases of ovarian cancer are diagnosed each year in the United States and more than 16,000 women die from the disease (see Table 18-5). The lifetime risk of developing ovarian cancer is 2%. These tumors predominate in women older than 60 years, but may occur in younger women with family history of the disease.

There are more than 25 major types of ovarian neoplasms. With variants and rare entities, they number over 100. The most common malignancy, serous adenocarcinoma (also termed **serous cystadenocarcinoma**), occurs in 1% to 2% of women.

The broad range of histologic features in these tumors reflects the diverse anatomical structure of the ovary itself. The classification of ovarian tumors identifies them by the tissue of origin (Fig. 18-43). Most frequently encountered tumors arise from surface epithelium and are termed **common epithelial tumors**. Other important groups include germ cell tumors, sex cord/stromal tumors, steroid cell tumors, and tumors metastatic to the ovary. About one sixth of ovarian tumors are of a mixed type.

Epithelial Tumors Account for over 90% of Ovarian Cancers

Tumors of common epithelial origin can be broadly classified as (1) benign, (2) of borderline malignancy (also called **atypical proliferating** or **low malignant potential**), and (3) malignant.

EPIDEMIOLOGY: Epidemiologic studies suggest that common epithelial neoplasms are related to repeated disruption and repair of the epithelial surface, which is part of cyclic ovulation. Thus, tumors most commonly afflict women who are nulliparous and, conversely, occur least often in women in whom ovulation has been suppressed (e.g., by pregnancy or oral contraceptives). Irritants, such as powder used for feminine hygiene, have also been implicated, since they may be transported up the reproductive tract and reach the ovaries.

A family history of ovarian carcinoma is occasionally elicited. Women with a first-degree relative with ovarian cancer have a 3.5-fold increased risk of developing the same disease. Women with a history of ovarian carcinoma are also at greater risk for breast cancer and vice versa. A gene implicated in many hereditary breast cancers, *BRCA-1* (17q12-q23), has been incriminated in familial ovarian cancers as well. As for endometrial carcinoma, women who suffer from hereditary nonpolyposis colon cancer (HNCC) are also at greater risk for ovarian cancer.

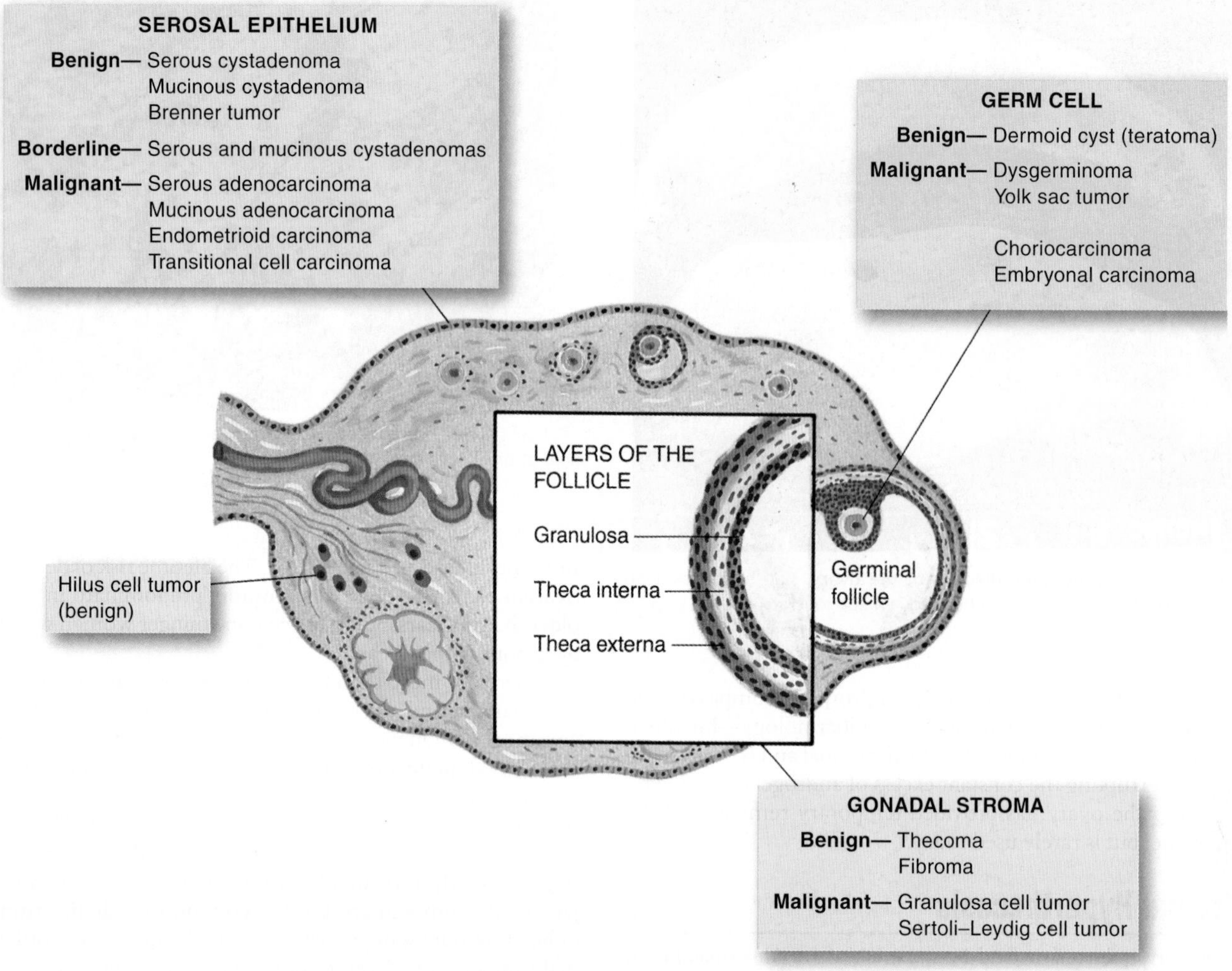

FIGURE 18-43. **Classification of ovarian neoplasms based on cell of origin.**

Women who bear *BRCA-1* tend to develop ovarian cancer much earlier than those who have sporadic ovarian cancer, but their prognosis is considerably better. Ovaries that are clinically normal in a woman who is a *BRCA-1* heterozygote rarely show any evidence of premalignant alterations, suggesting that prophylactic oophorectomy may not be warranted in such women.

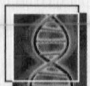

PATHOGENESIS: Most common epithelial tumors, especially serous carcinomas, arise from the ovarian surface epithelium or serosa. A few, especially Brenner tumor, arise elsewhere in the ovary. During embryonic life, the celomic cavity is lined by a mesothelium, parts of which become specialized to form the serosal epithelium covering the gonadal ridge. The same mesothelial lining gives rise to müllerian ducts, from which fallopian tubes, uterus, and vagina arise (Fig. 18-44).

As the ovary develops, the surface epithelium may extend into the ovarian stroma to form glands and cysts. In some cases, these inclusions become neoplastic and exhibit a variety of müllerian-type differentiations (Fig. 18-45).

PATHOLOGY: In order of decreasing frequency, the **common epithelial tumors** are:

- **Serous tumors** that resemble the epithelium of the fallopian tube
- **Mucinous tumors** that mimic the mucosa of the endocervix
- **Endometrioid tumors** that are similar to the glands of the endometrium
- **Clear cell tumors** that display glycogen-rich cells that resemble endometrial glands in pregnancy
- **Transitional cell tumors** that resemble the mucosa of the bladder
- **Mixed**

Cystadenomas

Benign common epithelial tumors are almost always serous or mucinous adenomas and generally arise in women between 20 and 60 years old. The neoplasms are frequently large, often 15 to 30 cm in diameter. Some, particularly the mucinous variety, reach massive proportions, exceeding 50 cm in diameter, in which case they may mimic the appearance of a term pregnancy. Benign epithelial tumors are typically cystic, hence the term **cystadenoma**.

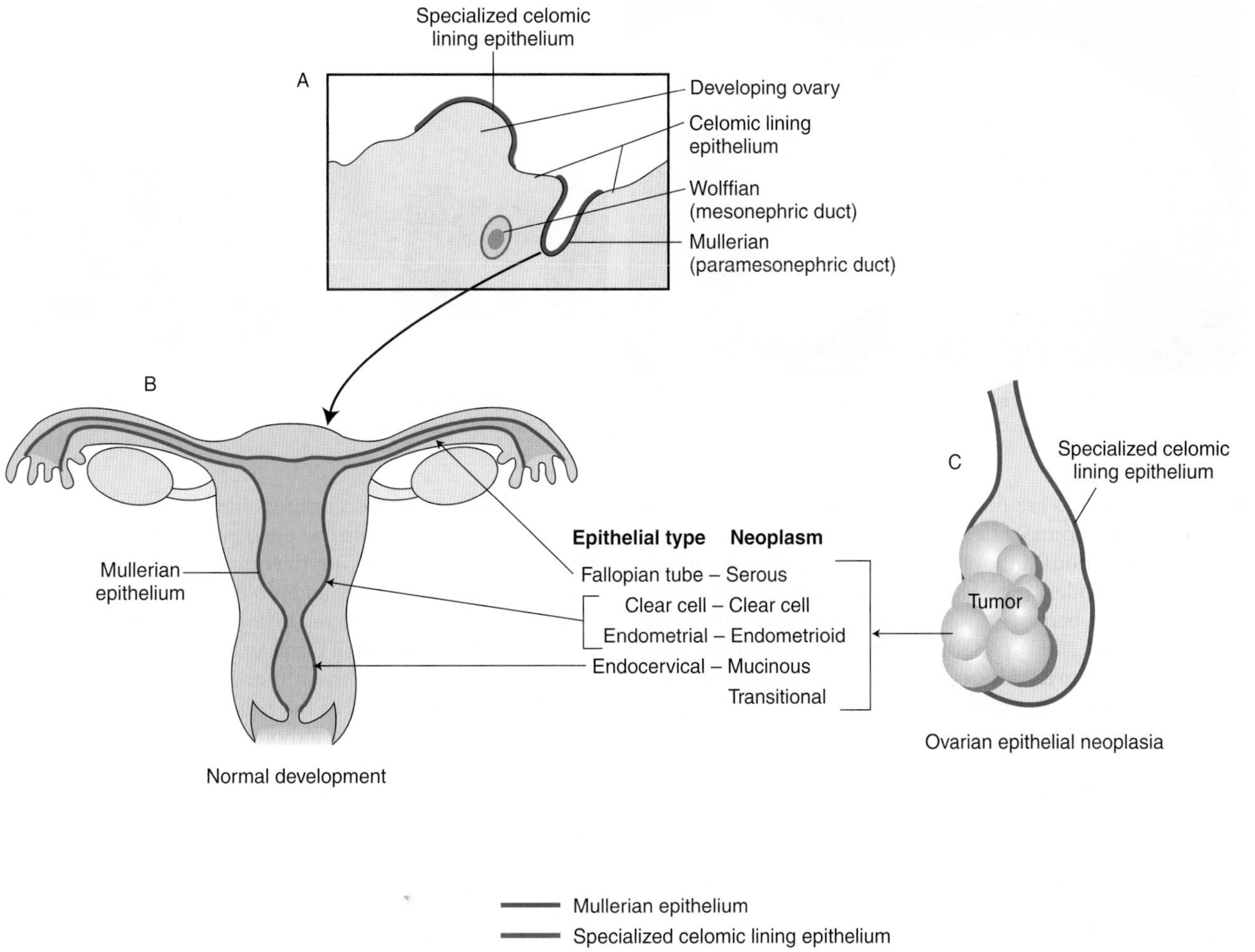

FIGURE 18-44. **The müllerian relations of epithelial/stromal tumors of the ovaries.**

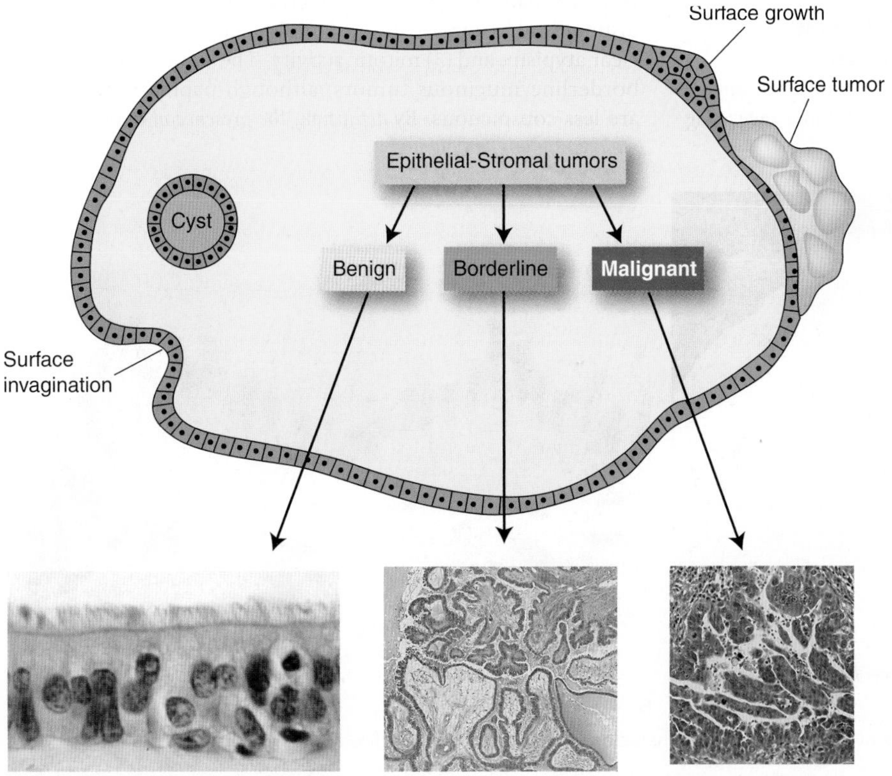

FIGURE 18-45. **Histogenesis of ovarian epithelial-stromal tumors.**

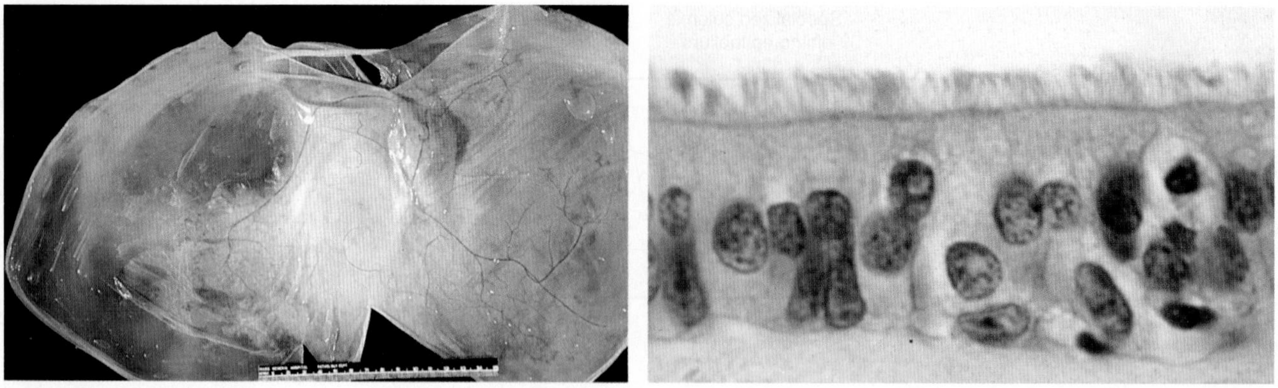

A B

FIGURE 18-46. **Serous cystadenoma of the ovary.** The fluid has been removed from this huge unilocular serous cystadenoma. The wall is thin and translucent. On microscopic examination, the cyst is lined by a single layer of ciliated tubal-type epithelium.

Serous cystadenomas are more commonly bilateral (15%) than mucinous cystadenomas and tend to be unilocular (Fig. 18-46). By contrast, **mucinous tumors** characteristically show hundreds of small cysts (locules) (Fig. 18-47). As opposed to their malignant counterparts, benign ovarian epithelial tumors tend to have thin walls and lack solid areas. Microscopically, one layer of tall columnar epithelium lines the cysts. Papillae, when present, consist of a fibrovascular core covered by a single layer of tall columnar epithelium identical to that of the cyst lining.

Transitional Cell Tumor (Brenner Tumor)

The typical Brenner tumor is benign and occurs at all ages, with half of cases presenting in women over the age of 50. Size varies from a microscopic focus to masses as large as 8 cm or more in diameter. Histologically, it Brenner tumors show solid nests of transitional-like (urothelium-like) cells encased in a dense, fibrous stroma (Fig. 18-48). The most superficial epithelial cells may exhibit mucinous differentiation.

Borderline Tumors (Tumors of Low Malignant Potential) or Atypical Proliferative Tumors

"Borderline tumors" comprise a well-defined group of ovarian tumors that share an excellent prognosis, despite histologic features suggesting cancer. They generally occur in women between the ages of 20 and 40 years but may also be encountered in older women. In terms of biological behavior, the tumor is "of low malignant potential," but show atypical and proliferative morphology. Chromosomal abnormalities found in borderline tumors are different from those in the common forms of cancer. A surgical cure is almost always possible if the tumor is confined to the ovaries. Even when it has spread to the pelvis or abdomen, 80% of patients are alive after 5 years, although there is a significant rate of late recurrence. The tumors rarely recur beyond 10 years.

Serous tumors of borderline malignancy are more commonly bilateral (34%) than mucinous ones (6%) or other types. The tumors vary in size, although mucinous ones are sometimes gigantic (100+ kg). In serous tumors of borderline malignancy, papillary projections, ranging from fine and exuberant to grape-like clusters arising from the cyst wall, are common (Fig. 18-49). The presence of ovarian surface excrescences does not seem to predict progression of disease. Microscopically, these structures resemble papillary fronds in benign cystadenomas, but they are distinguished from them by (1) epithelial stratification, (2) nuclear atypism, and (3) mitotic activity. The same criteria apply to borderline mucinous tumors, although papillary projections are less conspicuous. *By definition, the presence of more than focal*

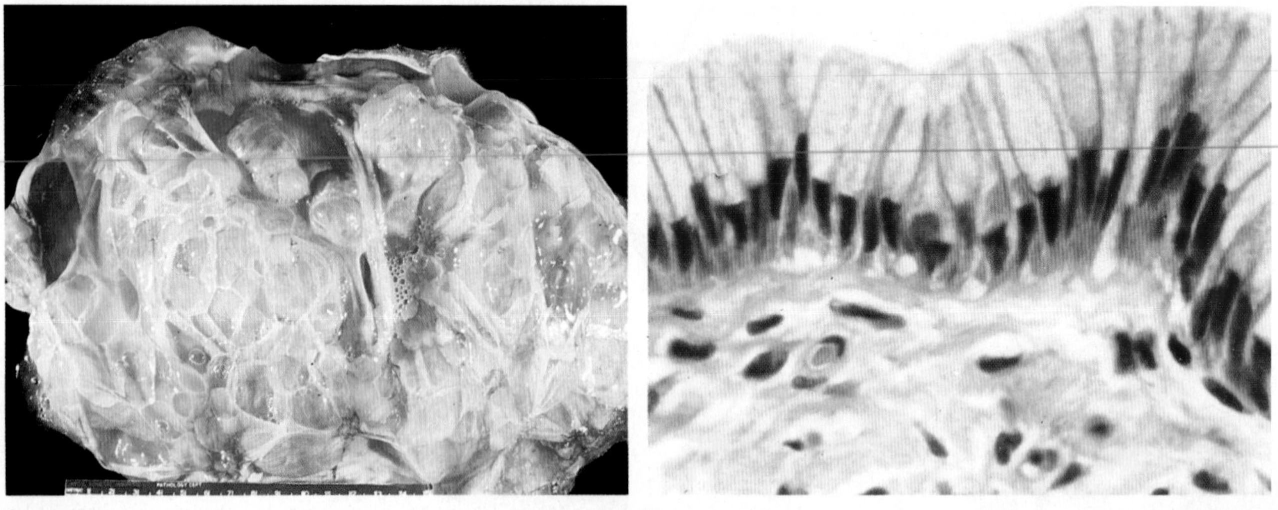

A B

FIGURE 18-47. **Mucinous cystadenoma of the ovary. A.** The tumor is characterized by numerous cysts filled with thick, viscous fluid. **B.** A single layer of mucinous epithelial cells lines the cyst.

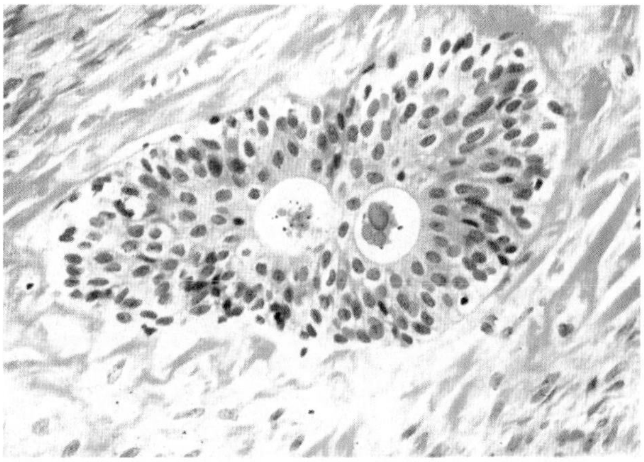

FIGURE 18-48. **Brenner tumor.** A nest of transitional-like cells is embedded in a dense, fibrous stroma.

microinvasion (i.e., discrete nests of epithelial cells that invade less than 3 mm into the ovarian stoma) identifies a tumor as frankly malignant, rather than borderline. However, borderline tumors with lymph node metastases or implants in the peritoneum, whether noninvasive or invasive, are still considered "borderline," reflecting that this category is well defined and carries a prognosis far better than the usual adenocarcinoma.

Malignant Epithelial Tumors

Malignant epithelial tumors of ovary are most common between the ages of 40 and 60, and are rare under the age of 35. By the time an ovarian cancer has reached 10 to 15 cm, it has often spread beyond the ovary and seeded the peritoneum.

SEROUS ADENOCARCINOMA: This tumor (commonly called "cystadenocarcinoma") is the most common malignancy of the ovary, accounting for a third of all ovarian cancers. Since tumors of advanced stage are bilateral more than twice as often as those of low stage, it seems that the cancer commonly spreads to the other ovary by implantation. In fact two thirds of serous cancers with extragonadal spread are bilateral. On gross examination, serous tumors tend to be uniform throughout, and are usually uniloculated or pauciloculated, with soft, delicate papillae lining the entire surface. Solid areas, often with necrosis and hemorrhage, are common (Fig. 18-50).

Microscopically, serous adenocarcinomas vary from well differentiated to poorly differentiated. In the latter, the papillary pattern may be inconspicuous, with most areas composed of solid sheets of malignant cells. Stromal and capsular invasion by the tumor cells is evident. Laminated calcified concretions, referred to as *psammoma bodies,* are present in a third of cases (see Fig. 18-50C).

MUCINOUS ADENOCARCINOMA: Mucinous cystadenocarcinoma constitutes about 10% of ovarian cancers. When confined to the ovary, one-sixth of cases are bilateral. Mucinous cancers are typically multilocular, with hundreds to thousands of small cysts. Primary ovarian mucinous tumors often contain some solid areas or others with papillary projections. The cystic areas typically appear as benign or borderline tumors and clearly malignant features are found only in the solid regions. Microscopically, the same mucinous tumor may display a full range of appearances from well to poorly differentiated. Well-differentiated mucinous tumors contain neoplastic glands lined by tall columnar, mucin-producing cells, usually with some solid or cribriform areas (Fig. 18-51). Poorly differentiated mucinous adenocarcinomas exhibit irregular nests and cords of tumor cells and numerous mitoses. Stromal invasion is the rule, and infiltration of the serosa is common. Mucinous ovarian carcinomas that lack benign or borderline components are often metastases from gastrointestinal primary sites such as appendix or colon.

ENDOMETRIOID ADENOCARCINOMA: Endometrioid adenocarcinoma histologically resembles its endometrial counterpart, may include areas of squamous differentiation and is second only to serous adenocarcinoma in frequency, accounting for 20% of all ovarian cancers. The tumor occurs most commonly after menopause. In contrast to serous and mucinous neoplasms, most endometrioid tumors are malignant. Up to one half of these cancers are bilateral.

On gross examination, endometrioid carcinomas vary in size from 2 cm to more than 30 cm. Most are largely solid and exhibit necrotic areas, although they may be cystic. Microscopically, they are graded according to the same scheme used for

A

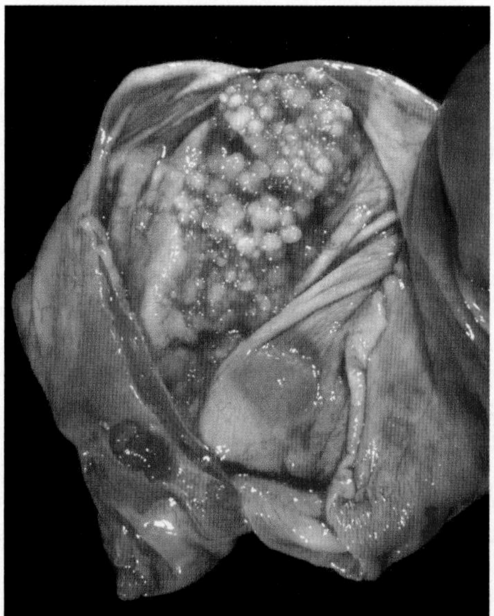

B

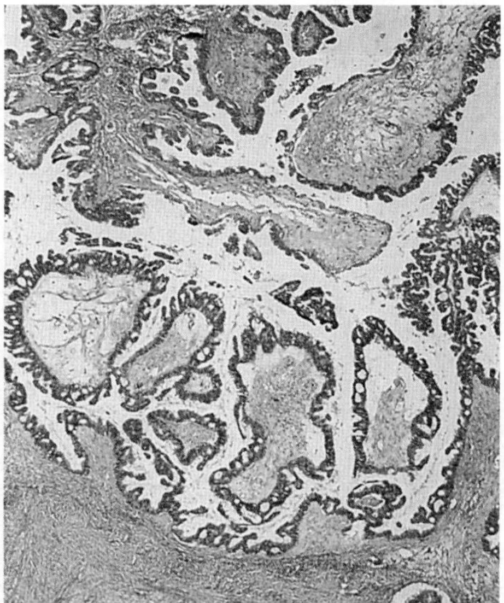

FIGURE 18-49. **Serous ovarian tumor of borderline malignancy. A.** Papillary excrescences project from the cyst wall. **B.** A microscopic view demonstrates the papillary structure of the tumor.

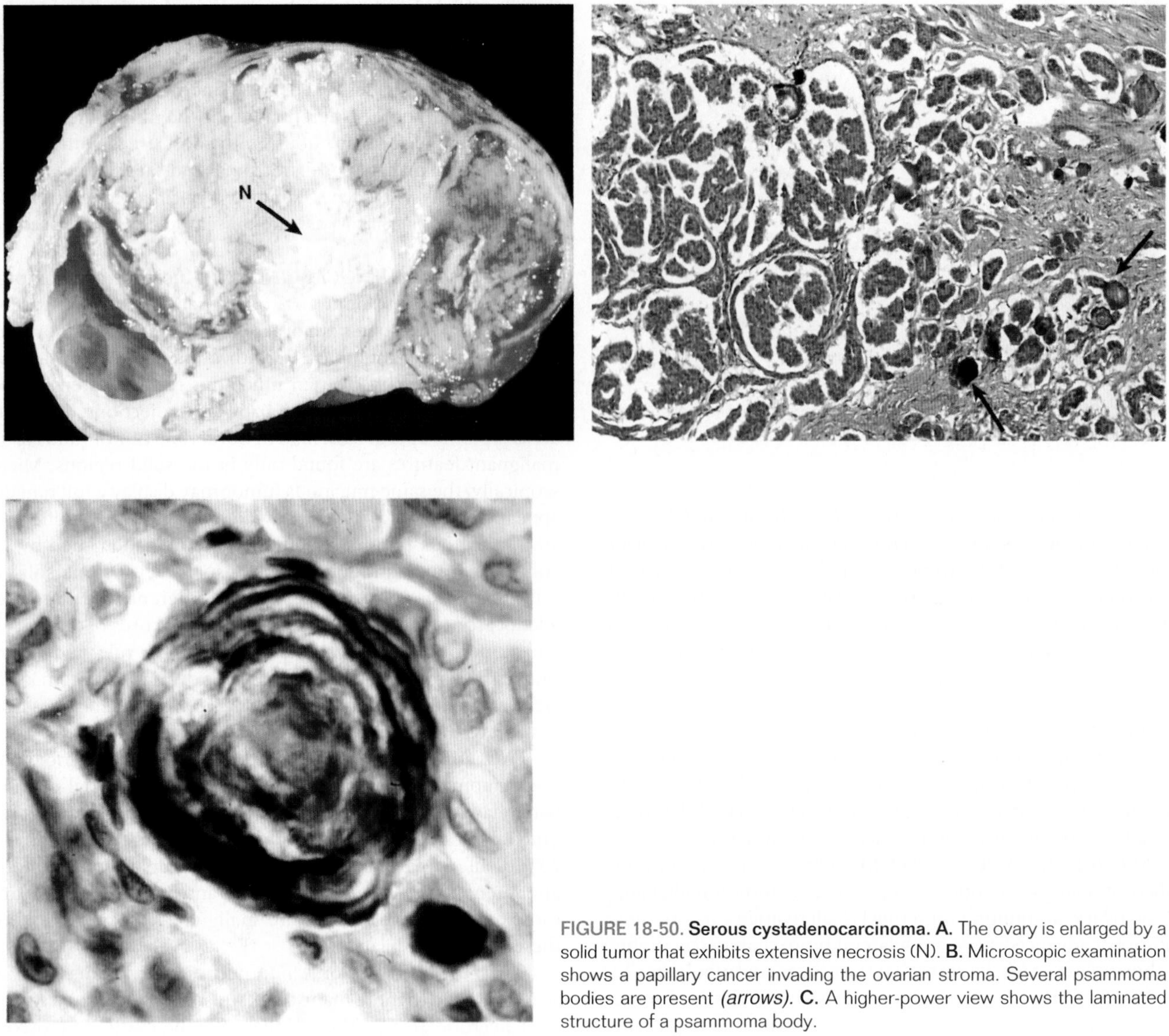

A B C

FIGURE 18-50. **Serous cystadenocarcinoma. A.** The ovary is enlarged by a solid tumor that exhibits extensive necrosis (N). **B.** Microscopic examination shows a papillary cancer invading the ovarian stroma. Several psammoma bodies are present *(arrows).* **C.** A higher-power view shows the laminated structure of a psammoma body.

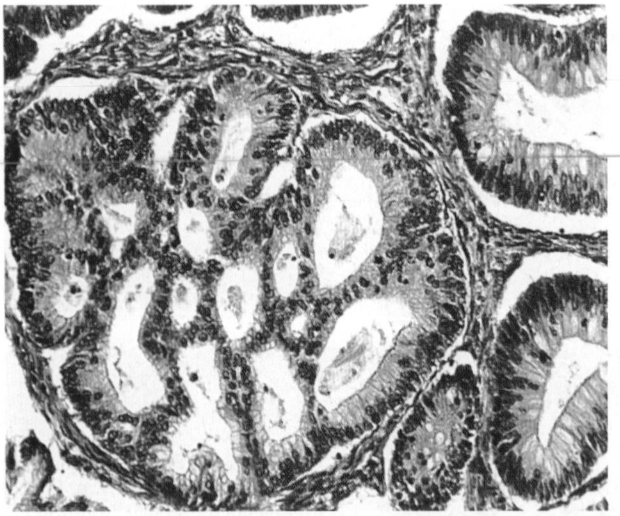

FIGURE 18-51. **Mucinous cystadenocarcinoma.** The malignant glands are arranged in a cribriform pattern and are composed of mucin-producing columnar cells.

endometrial adenocarcinomas. Many patients with endometrioid carcinoma of the ovary also harbor an endometrial cancer, the rates in various series ranging from 15% to 50%. Strong evidence suggests that coexisting ovarian and endometrial cancers most frequently arise independently, but some are metastases from one or the other. The 5-year survival exceeds 85% in such synchronous tumors. As with all malignant epithelial tumors of the ovary, prognosis depends on the stage at which it presents.

CLEAR CELL ADENOCARCINOMA: This ovarian cancer, which is closely related to endometrioid adenocarcinoma, often occurs in association with endometriosis. It constitutes 5% to 10% of all ovarian cancers usually occurring after menopause. The size ranges from 2 to 30 cm in diameter, and 40% are bilateral. Most of these tumors are partially cystic and exhibit necrosis and hemorrhage in the solid areas.

Microscopically, clear cell ovarian adenocarcinoma displays sheets or tubules of malignant cells with clear cytoplasm. In its tubular form, malignant cells often display bulbous nuclei that protrude into the lumen of the tubule ("hobnail cell"; see Fig. 18-33B), an appearance similar to the Arias-Stella reaction in gestational endometrium (see Fig. 18-24). The microscopic appearance of clear cell adenocarcinoma resembles that of its counterpart in the vagina. The clinical course parallels that of endometrioid carcinoma.

CLINICAL FEATURES: Most ovarian tumors do not secrete hormones. However, an antibody to the cancer antigen, CA-125, in the serum detects about half of the epithelial tumors that are confined to the ovary and about 90% that have already spread. The specificity of this test is 90%; the sensitivity is 75%.

Ovarian masses rarely cause symptoms until they are large. When they distend the abdomen, they cause pain, pelvic pressure, or compression of regional organs. By the time ovarian cancers are diagnosed, many have metastasized (implanted) to the surfaces of the pelvis, abdominal organs, or bladder. Evaluation of a patient with an ovarian cancer of epithelial origin requires an intimate knowledge of staging, grading and routes of tumor spread. For example, ovarian tumors have a tendency to implant in the peritoneal cavity on the diaphragm, paracolic gutters, and omentum. Lymphatic dissemination carries malignant cells preferentially to paraaortic lymph nodes near the origin of the renal arteries and to a lesser extent to external iliac (pelvic) or inguinal lymph nodes. In addition to specific symptoms, metastatic cancers are associated with ascites, weakness, weight loss, and cachexia.

Survival for patients with malignant ovarian tumors is generally poor. The single most important prognostic index is the surgical stage of the tumor at the time it is detected (Table 18-10). Overall, 5-year survival is only 35%, because more than half of tumors have spread to the abdominal cavity (stage 3) or elsewhere by the time they are discovered. Prognostic indices for epithelial tumors also include grade, histologic type, and the size of the residual neoplasm.

The cornerstone to managing ovarian cancer is surgery, which removes the primary tumor, establishes the diagnosis, and assesses the extent of spread. At laparotomy, the surgeon must examine the peritoneal surfaces, omentum, liver, subdiaphragmatic recesses, and all abdominal regions, so as to remove as much of the metastatic tumor as possible. Adjuvant chemotherapy is used to treat distant occult sites of tumor spread.

At some time after the initial operation, another exploratory laparotomy (second-look laparotomy) has been used to assess the effectiveness of therapy. However, even when no residual disease is apparent, one third of older patients eventually develop recurrences. Risk factors for recurrence include (1) high stage, (2) high grade, and (3) more than 2 cm of residual disease remaining after the primary operation.

Germ Cell Tumors Tend to Be Benign in Adults and Malignant in Children

Tumors derived from germ cells constitute a fourth of all ovarian tumors. In adult women, germ cell tumors are virtually all benign (mature cystic teratoma, dermoid cyst), whereas in children and young adults, they are largely cancerous. In children, germ cell tumors are the most common ovarian cancer (60%); they are rare after menopause.

The neoplastic germ cell may follow one of several lines of differentiation, giving rise to tumors analogous to those found in the male testis (Fig. 18-52).

- **Dysgerminoma** is composed of neoplastic germ cells, resembling oogonia of the fetal ovary.
- **Teratoma** differentiates toward somatic (embryonic or adult) tissues.

TABLE 18-10

Clinical Staging of Ovarian Cancer

Stage	Description
I	Limited to ovaries; capsule intact; no tumor on the external surface
Ia	Limited to one ovary; ascitic fluid, if present, lacks malignant cells
Ib	Limited to both ovaries; capsule intact; no tumor on the external surface; ascitic fluid, if present, lacks malignant cells
Ic	Any of above, but with ascites or positive peritoneal washings
II	With pelvic extension
IIa	Extension or metastases to uterus or tubes
IIb	Extension to other pelvic tissues
IIc	Any of above, but with ascites or positive peritoneal washings
III	With intraperitoneal metastases outside the pelvis, or positive retroperitoneal nodes, or both. Tumor limited to true pelvis with histologically proven malignant extension to small bowel or omentum.
IIIa	Microscopic seeding on abdominal-peritoneal surface
IIIb	Implants =2 cm on abdominal peritoneal surface
IIIc	Implants >2 cm on abdominal peritoneal surface
IV	With distant metastases. If pleural effusion present, positive cytology required. Liver metastases must be parenchymal.

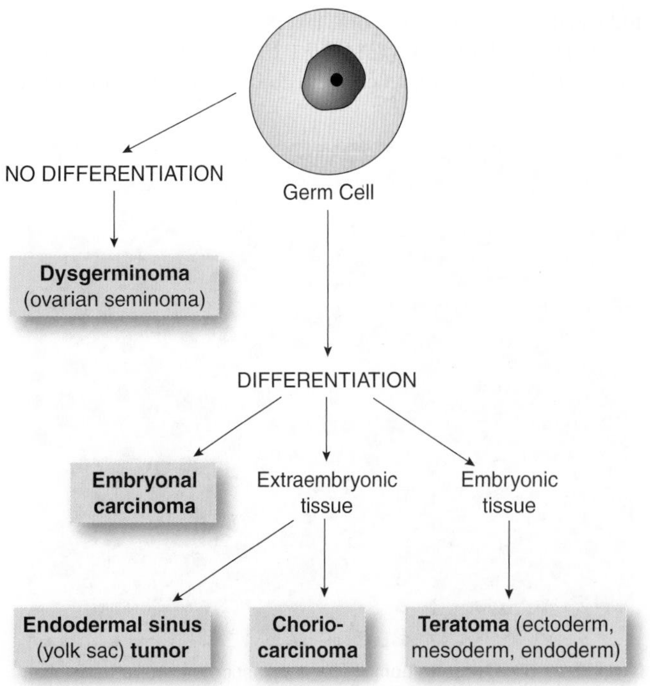

FIGURE 18-52. **Classification of germ cell tumors of the ovary.**

- **Yolk sac tumor** differentiates toward extraembryonic tissue and resembles the placental mesenchyme or its precursors.
- **Choriocarcinoma** features cells similar to those covering the placental villi.

Germ cell tumors in infants tend to be solid and immature (e.g., yolk sac tumor and immature teratoma). Tumors in young adults show greater differentiation, as in mature cystic teratoma. Malignant germ cell tumors in women older than 40 years of age usually result from transformation of one of the components of a benign cystic teratoma.

Malignant germ cell tumors tend to be highly aggressive. At one time, solid germ cell tumors of the ovary were uniformly fatal, but with the advent of chemotherapy, survival rates for many exceed 80%.

Dysgerminoma

Dysgerminoma is the ovarian counterpart of testicular seminoma, and is composed of primordial germ cells. It accounts for less than 2% of all ovarian cancers, but constitutes 10% of these malignancies in women younger than 20 years. Most patients are between 10 and 30. The tumors are bilateral in about 15% of cases.

PATHOLOGY: Grossly, dysgerminomas are often large and firm and have a bosselated external surface. The cut surface is soft and fleshy. Microscopic examination reveals large nests of monotonously uniform tumor cells, which have a clear glycogen-filled cytoplasm and irregularly flattened central nuclei (Fig. 18-53). Fibrous septa containing lymphocytes traverse the tumor.

Dysgerminoma is treated surgically, and 5-year survival for patients with stage I tumor approaches 100%. Because the tumor is highly radiosensitive and also responsive to chemotherapy, 5-year survival rates even for higher-stage tumors still exceed 80%.

Teratoma

Teratoma is a tumor of germ cell origin that differentiates toward somatic structures. Most teratomas contain tissues from at least two and usually all three, embryonic layers.

MATURE TERATOMA (MATURE CYSTIC TERATOMA, DERMOID CYST): This benign neoplasm accounts for one fourth of all ovarian tumors with a peak incidence in the third decade. Mature teratomas develop by parthenogenesis. Haploid (postmeiotic) germ cells endoreduplicate to give rise to diploid genetically female tumor cells (46,XX).

PATHOLOGY: Mature teratomas are cystic and more than 90% contain skin, sebaceous glands and hair follicles (Fig. 18-54). Half exhibit smooth muscle, sweat glands, cartilage, bone, teeth, and respiratory tract epithelium. Tissues such as gut, thyroid, and brain are seen less frequently. When present, nodular foci in the cyst wall ("mammary tubercles" or "Rokitansky nodules") contain tissue elements of all three germ cell layers: (1) ectoderm (e.g., skin and glia), (2) mesoderm (e.g., smooth muscle or cartilage), and (3) endoderm (e.g., respiratory epithelium).

Struma ovarii refers to a cystic lesion composed predominantly of thyroid tissue (5% to 20% of mature cystic teratomas). Rare cases of hyperthyroidism have been associated with struma ovarii.

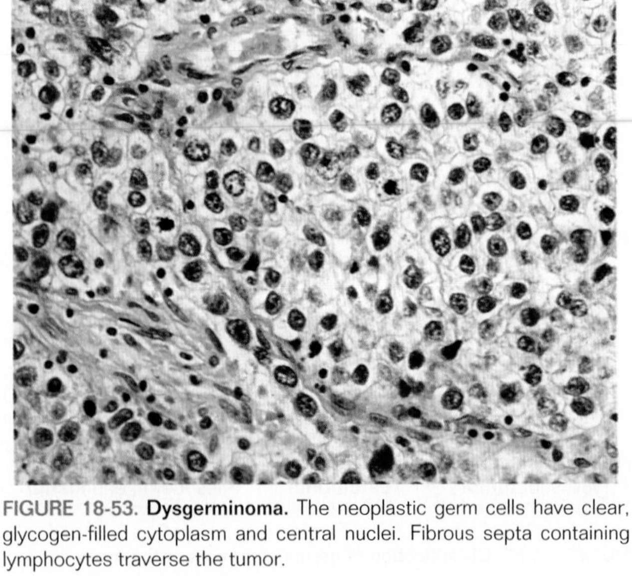

FIGURE 18-53. **Dysgerminoma.** The neoplastic germ cells have clear, glycogen-filled cytoplasm and central nuclei. Fibrous septa containing lymphocytes traverse the tumor.

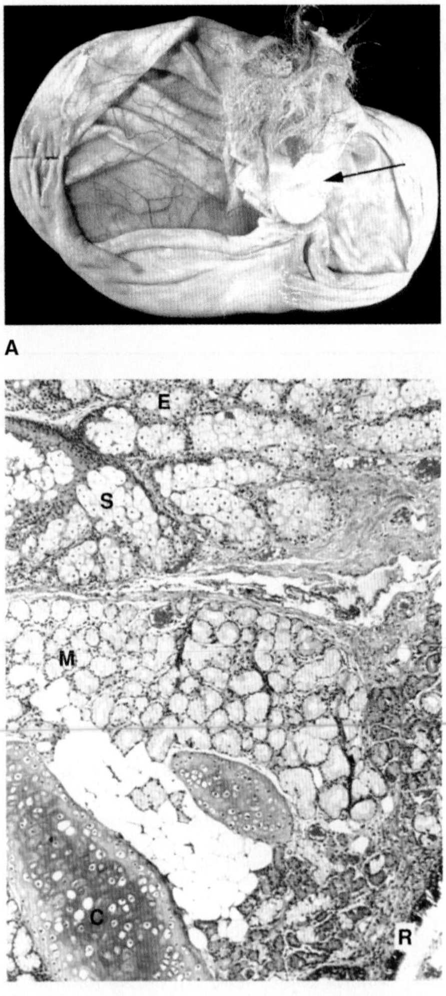

FIGURE 18-54. **Mature cystic teratoma of the ovary. A.** A mature cystic teratoma has been opened to reveal a solid knob *(arrow)* from which hair projects. **B.** A photomicrograph of the solid knob shows epidermal and respiratory components. Tissue resembling the skin exhibits an epidermis (E) with underlying sebaceous glands (S). The respiratory tissue consists of mucous glands (M), cartilage (C), and respiratory epithelium (R).

Very few (1%) of dermoid cysts become malignant. These cancers usually occur in older women and correspond to the tumors that arise in other differentiated tissues of the body. Three fourths of all cancers that arise in dermoid cysts are squamous cell carcinomas. The remainder includes carcinoid tumor, basal cell carcinoma, thyroid cancer, adenocarcinoma, and others. In rare cases, derivatives of gut may be functional and produce carcinoid syndrome. The prognosis of patients with malignant transformation of mature cystic teratoma is related largely to stage of the cancer.

IMMATURE TERATOMA: Immature teratomas of the ovary are composed of elements derived from the three germ layers. However, unlike mature cystic teratoma, the immature variety contains embryonal tissues. Immature teratoma accounts for 20% of malignant tumors at all sites in women under the age of 20 and becomes progressively less common in older women.

PATHOLOGY: Immature teratoma is predominantly solid and lobulated, with numerous small cysts. Solid areas may contain grossly recognizable immature bone and cartilage. Microscopically, multiple tumor components are usually found, including those differentiating toward nerve (neuroepithelial rosettes and immature glia) (Fig. 18-55), glands and other structures found in mature cystic teratomas. Grading is based on the amount of immature tissue present. Metastases of immature teratomas are composed of embryonal, usually stromal, tissues. By contrast, rare metastases of mature cystic teratomas, resemble epithelial adult-type malignancies.

Survival correlates with tumor grade. Well-differentiated immature teratomas generally have a favorable outcome, but high-grade tumors (predominantly embryonal tissue) have a poor prognosis.

Yolk Sac Tumor

Yolk sac tumor is a highly malignant tumor of women under the age of 30 that histologically resembles the mesenchyme of the primitive yolk sac. It is the second most common malignant germ cell tumor and is almost always unilateral.

PATHOLOGY: Typically, the neoplasm is large and displays extensive necrosis and hemorrhage. Microscopic examination reveals multiple patterns. The most common appearance is a reticular, honeycombed structure of communicating spaces lined by primitive cells. **Schiller-Duval bodies** (Fig. 18-56), which resemble the endodermal sinus of the rodent placenta, are found sparingly in a few tumors, but are characteristic. They consist of papillae that protrude into a space lined by tumor cells, resembling the glomerular Bowman space. The papillae are covered by a mantle of embryonal cells and contain a fibrovascular core and a central blood vessel.

Yolk sac tumor should not be confused with embryonal cell carcinoma, which is common in the testis. The former secretes α-fetoprotein, which can be demonstrated histochemically within eosinophilic droplets. Detection of αfetoprotein in the blood is useful for diagnosis and for monitoring the effectiveness of therapy. Previously nearly always fatal, with chemotherapy 5-year survival for stage I yolk sac tumors exceeds 80%.

Choriocarcinoma

Choriocarcinoma of the ovary is a rare tumor that mimics the epithelial covering of placental villi, namely, cytotrophoblast and syncytiotrophoblast. Derivation from ovarian germ cells is assumed if the tumor arises before puberty or in combination with another germ cell tumor. In women of reproductive age, however, ovarian choriocarcinoma may also be a metastasis from an intrauterine gestational tumor. Choriocarcinoma of germ cell origin manifests in young girls as precocious sexual development, menstrual irregularities, or rapid breast enlargement.

PATHOLOGY: Choriocarcinoma is unilateral, solid, and widely hemorrhagic. Microscopically, it shows a mixture of malignant cytotrophoblast and syncytiotrophoblast (see placenta, choriocarcinoma, below). The syncytial cells secrete hCG, which accounts for the frequent finding of a positive pregnancy test result. Bilateral theca lutein cysts, a result of hCG stimulation, may also be found.

Serial serum hCG determinations are useful both for diagnosis and follow-up. The tumor is highly aggressive but responds to chemotherapy.

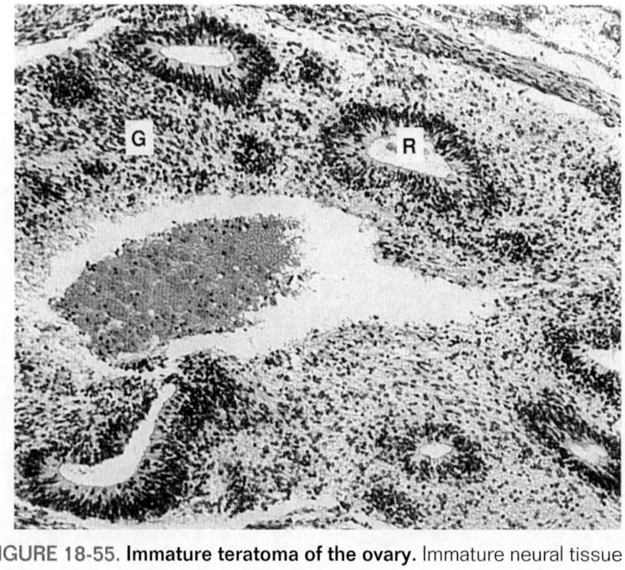

FIGURE 18-55. **Immature teratoma of the ovary.** Immature neural tissue exhibits rosettes (R) with multilayered nuclei. Embryonal glia (G) display densely packed, atypical nuclei.

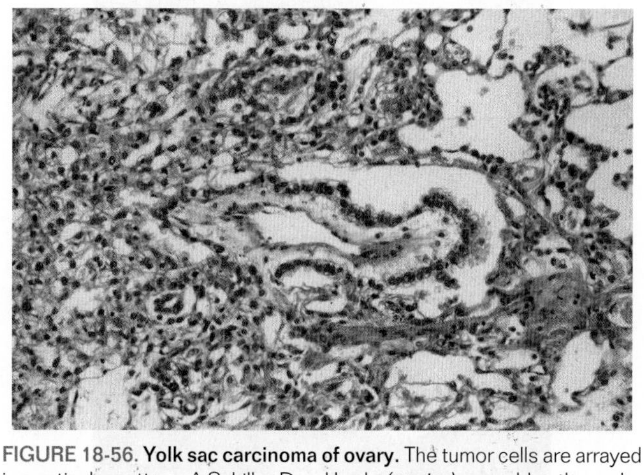

FIGURE 18-56. **Yolk sac carcinoma of ovary.** The tumor cells are arrayed in a reticular pattern. A Schiller-Duval body *(center)* resembles the endodermal sinuses of the rodent placenta and consists of a papilla protruding into a space lined by tumor cells.

Gonadoblastoma

Gonadoblastoma is a rare ovarian tumor that is distinctive because of its association with various types of gonadal dysgenesis, especially in women who bear a Y chromosome. It occurs in phenotypic women under 30 years of age, although 20% are found in phenotypic men with cryptorchidism, hypospadias, and female internal sex organs. Most affected women are virilized and suffer from primary amenorrhea and developmental abnormalities of the genitalia. Microscopically, cellular nests show a mixture of germ cells and sex cord derivatives that resemble immature Sertoli and granulosa cells, which is why some consider the tumor to be an in situ form of germinoma. In half of cases, gonadoblastoma is overgrown by dysgerminoma. The gonadoblastoma itself does not metastasize, but its overgrowths do.

Sex Cord/Stromal Tumors Are Clinically Functional

Tumors of sex cord and stroma originate from either primitive sex cords or from mesenchymal stroma of the developing gonad. They account for 10% of ovarian tumors. They range from benign to low-grade malignant and may differentiate toward female (granulosa and theca cells) or male (Sertoli and Leydig cells) structures.

Fibroma

Fibromas account for 75% of all stromal tumors and 7% of all ovarian tumors. They occur at all ages, with a peak in the perimenopausal period, and are virtually always benign.

PATHOLOGY: Tumors are solid, firm and white (Fig. 18-57). Microscopically, the cells resemble the stroma of the normal ovarian cortex, being well-differentiated spindle cells, and variable amounts of collagen. Half of the larger tumors are associated with ascites and, rarely, with ascites and pleural effusions (**Meigs syndrome**).

Thecoma

Thecomas are functional ovarian tumors that arise in postmenopausal women and are almost always benign. They are closely related to fibromas, but additionally contain varying amounts of steroidogenic cells that in many cases produce estrogens or androgen.

PATHOLOGY: Thecomas are solid tumors, mostly 5 to 10 cm in diameter. The cut section is yellow, due to the many lipid-laden theca cells. Microscopically, the cells are large and oblong to round, with a vacuolated cytoplasm that contains lipid (Fig. 18-58). Bands of hyalinized collagen separate nests of theca cells.

Because of estrogen output by the tumor, thecomas in premenopausal women commonly cause irregularity in menstrual cycles and breast enlargement. Endometrial hyperplasia and cancer are well-recognized complications.

Granulosa Cell Tumor

Granulosa cell tumor is the prototypical functional neoplasm of the ovary associated with estrogen secretion. This tumor should be considered malignant because of its potential for local spread and the rare occurrence of distant metastases.

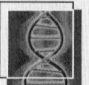

PATHOGENESIS: Most granulosa cell tumors occur after menopause (adult form), and are unusual before puberty. The juvenile form occurs in children and young women and has distinct clinical and pathologic features (hyperestrinism and precocious puberty. In contrast to common epithelial tumors, in which repeated ovulation is a contributing factor, experimental evidence suggests that development of granulosa cell tumors is linked to loss of oocytes. Oocytes appear to regulate granulosa cells, and tumorigenesis occurs when follicles are disorganized or atretic.

PATHOLOGY: Adult-type granulosa cell tumors, like most ovarian tumors, are large and focally cystic to solid. The cut surface shows yellow areas, representing lipid-laden luteinized granulosa cells, and white zones of stroma and focal hemorrhages (Fig. 18-59). Microscopically, granulosa cell tumors display an array of growth patterns: (1) diffuse (sarcomatoid), (2) insular (islands of cells), or (3) trabecular (anastomotic bands of granulosa cells). Haphazard orientation of nuclei about a central degenerative space (**Call-Exner bodies**) results in

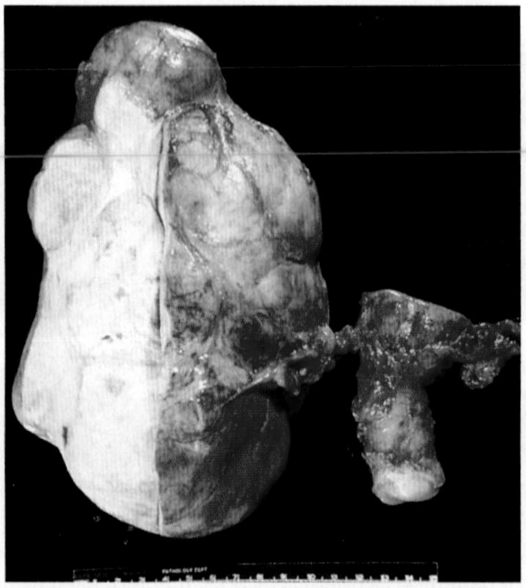

FIGURE 18-57. **Fibroma of ovary.** The ovary is conspicuously enlarged by a firm, white, bosselated tumor.

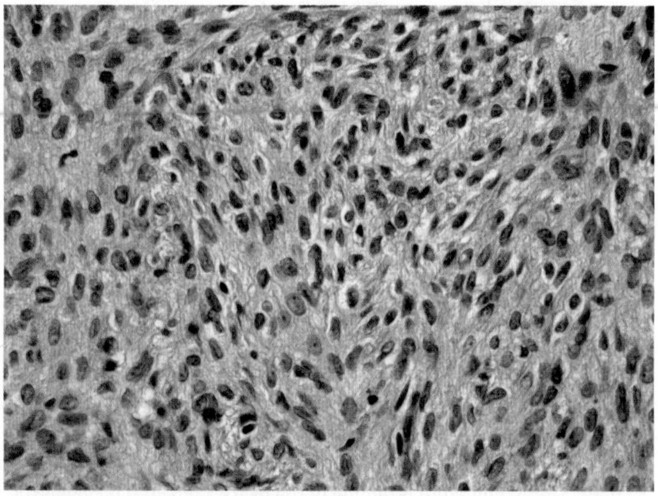

FIGURE 18-58. **Thecoma of ovary.** Oblong cells are invested by collagen. The cytoplasm contains lipid.

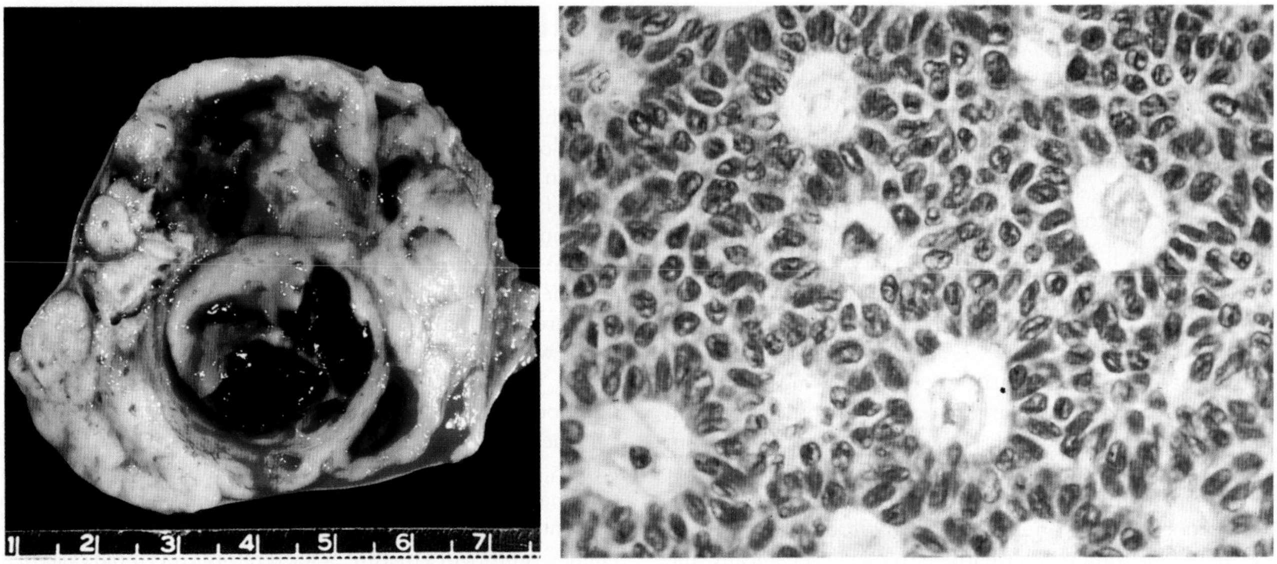

A B

FIGURE 18-59. **Granulosa cell tumor of the ovary. A.** Cross-section of the enlarged ovary shows a variegated solid tumor with focal hemorrhages. The yellow areas represent collections of lipid-laden luteinized granulosa cells. **B.** The orientation of tumor cells about central spaces results in the characteristic follicular pattern (Call-Exner bodies).

a characteristic follicular pattern (see Fig. 18-59B). Tumor cells are typically spindle-shaped and commonly have a cleaved, elongated nucleus (coffee bean appearance). They secrete **inhibin,** a protein that suppresses pituitary release of follicle-stimulating hormone (FSH). Granulosa cell tumors can also express **calretinin**, a primarily neuronal protein, which suggests a possible neural differentiation or derivation for these neoplasms.

CLINICAL FEATURES: *Three fourths of granulosa cell tumors secrete estrogens.* Thus, benign endometrial hyperplasia is a common presenting sign. It predisposes to EIN or endometrial adenocarcinoma if the functioning granulosa cell tumor remains undetected. When detected clinically, 90% of granulosa cell tumors are confined to the ovary (stage I). These patients have a greater than 90% 10-year survival. Tumors that have extended into pelvis and lower abdomen have a poorer prognosis. Late recurrence after surgical removal is not uncommon after 5 to 10 years and is usually fatal.

Sertoli-Leydig Cell Tumors

Ovarian Sertoli-Leydig cell tumor (arrhenoblastoma or androblastoma) is a rare mesenchymal neoplasm of low malignant potential that resembles the embryonic testis. It is the prototypical androgen-secreting ovarian tumor. The tumor cells typically secrete weak androgens (dehydroepiandrosterone), which accounts for the large tumor size that is required to achieve masculinizing signs. Sertoli-Leydig cell tumors occur at all ages but are most common in young women of childbearing age.

PATHOLOGY: Sertoli-Leydig cell tumors are unilateral, most measuring between 5 and 15 cm in diameter. They tend to be lobulated, solid, and brown to yellow. Microscopically, they vary from well differentiated to poorly differentiated and some exhibit heterologous elements (e.g., mucinous glands and, rarely, even cartilage). The most characteristic features are large Leydig cells, which have abundant eosinophilic cytoplasm and a central round to oval nucleus with a prominent nucleolus. The tumor cells are embedded in a sarcomatoid stroma (Fig. 18-60). The stroma in some areas often differentiates into immature solid tubules of embryonic Sertoli cells.

CLINICAL FEATURES: Nearly half of all patients with Sertoli-Leydig cell tumors exhibit androgenic effects (i.e., signs of virilization: hirsutism, male escutcheon, enlarged clitoris, and deepened voice). The initial signs are often defeminization, manifested as breast atrophy, amenorrhea, and loss of hip fat. Once the tumor is removed, these signs disappear or at least lessen. Well-differentiated tumors are virtually always cured by surgical resection, but poorly differentiated ones may metastasize.

Steroid Cell Tumor

Steroid cell tumors of ovary, also called **lipid cell** and **lipoid cell tumors**, are composed of cells that resemble lutein cells, Leydig cells, and adrenal cortical cells. Most steroid cell tumors are

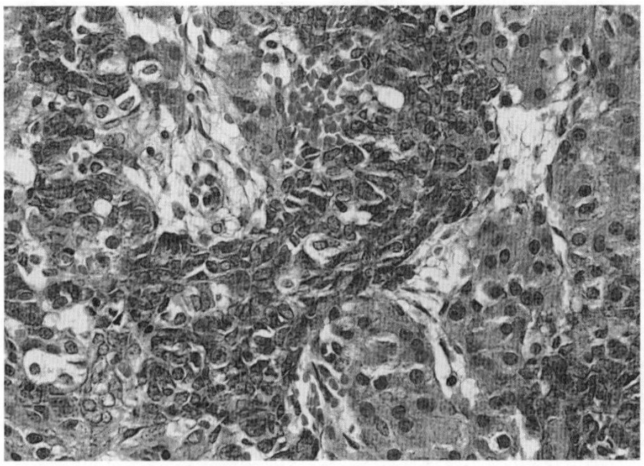

FIGURE 18-60. **Sertoli-Leydig cell tumor.** Immature solid tubules of embryonic Sertoli cells are adjacent to clusters of Leydig cells that exhibit abundant eosinophilic cytoplasm.

hormonally active, usually with androgenic manifestations. Some secrete testosterone; others synthesize weaker androgens. **Hilus cell tumor** is a specialized form of steroid cell tumor that is typically a benign neoplasm composed of Leydig cells. It arises in the hilus of the ovary, usually after menopause and secretes testosterone–the most potent of the common androgens. As a result, masculinizing signs are frequent (75%), despite the typically small size of the tumor. Most hilus cell tumors contain "crystalloids of Reinke" (rodlike cytoplasmic structures).

Tumors Metastatic to the Ovary May Mimic a Primary Tumor

About 3% of ovarian cancers arise elsewhere, the most common primary sites being breast, large intestine, endometrium, and stomach, in descending order. These tumors vary in size from microscopic lesions to large masses. Metastases from the breast are in most cases microscopic and are found in 10% of ovaries removed prophylactically in cases of advanced breast cancer. Of those metastatic tumors large enough to manifest clinically, the colon is the most frequent site of origin. Commonly, the tumor cells stimulate the ovarian stroma to differentiate into hormonally active cells (luteinized stromal cells), thereby inducing androgenic and sometimes estrogenic symptoms.

***Krukenberg tumors** are ovarian metastases in which the tumor appears as nests of mucin-filled "signet-ring" cells within a cellular stroma derived from the ovary* (Fig. 18-61). The stomach is the primary site in 75% of cases and most of the other Krukenberg tumors are from the colon.

Bilateral ovarian involvement and multinodularity are important clues to the diagnosis of metastatic carcinoma. Both ovaries are grossly involved in 75% of cases. In metastatic disease that is clinically unilateral, the seemingly normal ovary may also contain surface implants or minute foci of tumor within the parenchyma. Thus, when metastasis to one ovary is documented, the surgeon must remove the other as well. It may be possible to differentiate based on the fact that ovarian tumors are positive for cytokeratin 7 while gastrointestinal tumors express cytokeratin 20.

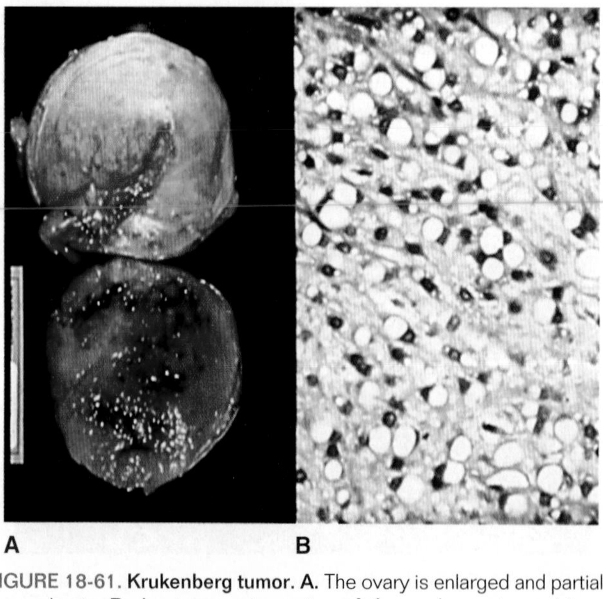

FIGURE 18-61. **Krukenberg tumor. A.** The ovary is enlarged and partially hemorrhagic. **B.** A microscopic section of *A* reveals mucinous (signet-ring) cells infiltrating the ovary.

PERITONEUM

The peritoneum is a nearly continuous membrane that lines the peritoneal cavity and separates the viscera from the abdominal wall The peritoneal cavity in men is a closed system. In women, it is an "open system" interrupted in the pelvis by the fallopian tubes. The fallopian tubes provide a final conduit for transmission of pathogens and chemicals from the genital tract to the peritoneal cavity.

The cells that line the peritoneal cavity and those that form the serosa of the ovary are both of celomic epithelial origin. Thus, whether tumors and tumorlike lesions of peritoneum and ovary (i.e., müllerian epithelial lesions) are the same entity in both locations remains an open question.

The peritoneum is the site of a wide range of inflammatory lesions, including granulomatous peritonitis as a response to suture materials, surgical glove powder, contrast media; intestinal contents following perforation (e.g., in Crohn disease or diverticulitis); rupture of a mature cystic teratoma (dermoid cyst) of the ovary; and of course, tuberculosis. It is also the site of reactive mesothelial proliferation, which occurs with the slightest irritation. Peritonitis is discussed in Chapter 13.

Endometriosis

Endometriosis is the presence of benign endometrial glands and stroma outside the uterus. It afflicts 5% to 10% of women of reproductive age and regresses after natural or artificial menopause. The mean age at diagnosis is the late 20s to early 30s, although it may appear any time after menarche. Sites most frequently involved are the ovaries (>60%), other uterine adnexae (uterine ligaments, rectovaginal septum, pouch of Douglas) and the pelvic peritoneum covering the uterus, fallopian tubes, rectosigmoid colon, and bladder (Fig. 18-62). Endometriosis can be even more widespread and occasionally affects the cervix, vagina, perineum, bladder, and umbilicus. Even pelvic lymph nodes may contain foci of endometriosis. On rare occasions, distant areas such as lungs, pleura, small bowel, kidneys, and bones contain lesions.

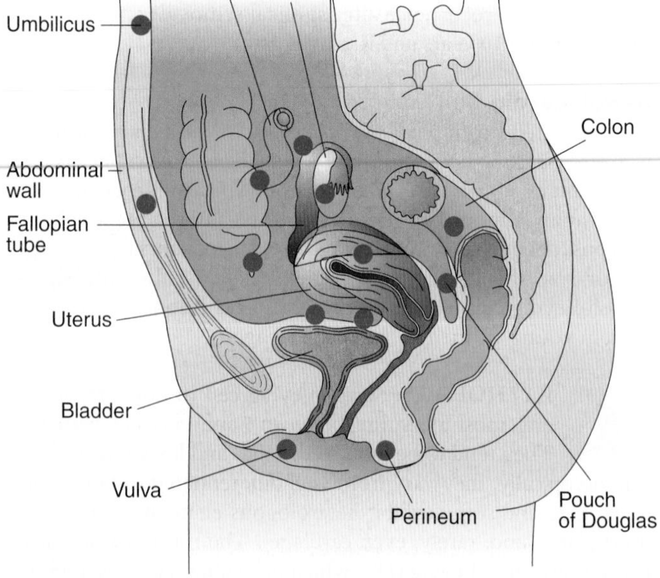

FIGURE 18-62. **Sites of endometriosis**

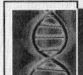

PATHOGENESIS: There are three theories to explain the histogenesis of endometriosis. They are not necessarily mutually exclusive, and may be effective to varying degrees in different individuals and sites.

1. **Transplantation** of endometrial fragments to ectopic sites
2. **Metaplasia** of the multipotential celomic peritoneum
3. **Induction** of undifferentiated mesenchyme in ectopic sites to form lesions after exposure to substances released from shed endometrium.

TRANSPLANTATION: The most widely accepted theory holds that foci of menstrual endometrium reflux through the fallopian tubes and implant at ectopic sites. In this context, retrograde menstruation through the fallopian tubes occurs in 90% of women. An extension of the transplantation theory is lymphatic and hematogenous dissemination, which would explain endometriosis at such distant sites as the lungs and kidneys. The observation that pulmonary endometriosis occurs almost exclusively in women who have been had uterine surgery supports this contention. The presence of endometriosis in lymph nodes is consistent with similar lymphatic dissemination.

CELOMIC METAPLASIA: The metaplastic theory proposes that endometriosis arises in the pelvis and elsewhere by endometrial metaplasia of peritoneal serosa or serosa-like structures. According to this concept, pelvic peritoneum can potentially differentiate, if appropriately stimulated, into any type of müllerian epithelium.

INDUCTION THEORY: This concept suggests that a substance secreted by the endometrium induces development of endometrial epithelium and stroma in ectopic sites.

PATHOLOGY: On gross examination, the lesions of endometriosis vary in color. Yellow-red stains, when confined to the serosa, reflect breakdown of blood products and often are the earliest detectable lesions. Red lesions also reflect an early form of the disease, in which foci of endometriosis are actively growing. Pathologists usually see black lesions in operative specimens, which show some degree of resolution. Such foci on the ovary and peritoneal surfaces, termed "mulberry" nodules, are 1 to 5 mm in diameter. With repeated cycles, hemorrhage and the onset of fibrosis, the affected surface may show scarring and take on a grossly brown discoloration ("powder burns"). Over time, fibrous adhesions may become more pronounced. Sometimes, scarring leads to complications, such as intestinal obstruction. In the ovaries, repeated hemorrhage may cause endometriotic foci to form cysts up to 15 cm in diameter, which contain inspissated, chocolate-colored material ("chocolate cysts").

Microscopically, endometriosis shows ectopic endometrial glands and stroma (Fig. 18-63). Occasionally, healed foci of endometriosis may consist only of fibrous tissue and hemosiderin-laden macrophages, features that by themselves are not diagnostic. Demonstration of CD-10 expression can be diagnostic.

CLINICAL FEATURES: The signs and symptoms of endometriosis depend on the location of the implants. The most common complaint is dysmenorrhea, due to implants on the uterosacral ligaments. These lesions swell immediately before or during menstruation, producing pelvic pain. In fact, half of all women with dysmenorrhea have endometriosis. Dyspareunia and cyclical abdominal pain may be troublesome.

Infertility is the primary complaint in a third of women with endometriosis (Fig. 18-64). The hormonal milieu in a woman who does not achieve pregnancy encourages development of endometriosis. In turn, once endometriosis develops, it contributes to the infertile state and a vicious circle is established. Conversely, pregnancy often has a beneficial effect on the disease. With conservative surgery to restore pelvic anatomy, many women who suffer from endometriosis may eventually become pregnant.

Malignancy occurs in about 1% to 2% of cases of endometriosis. Clear cell and endometrioid tumors are the most frequent forms. Adenosarcoma, although rare, is the most common sarcoma.

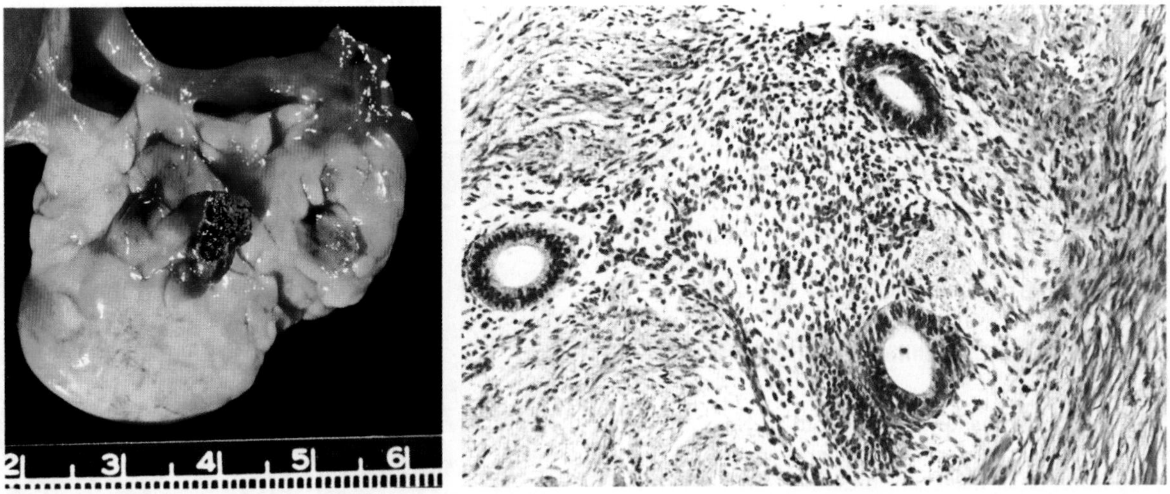

A B

FIGURE 18-63. **Endometriosis. A.** Implants of endometriosis on the ovary appear as red-blue nodules. **B.** A microscopic section shows endometrial glands and stroma in the ovary.

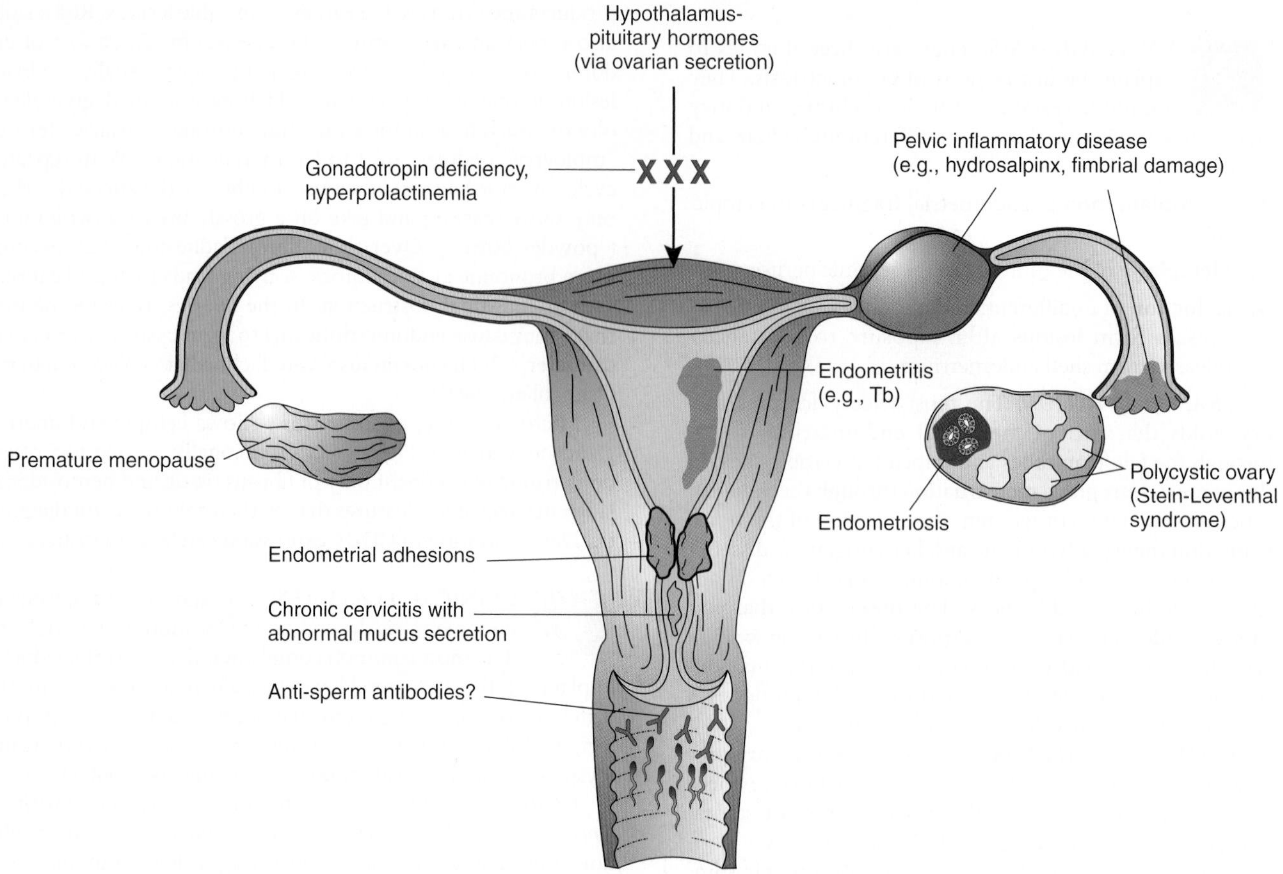

FIGURE 18-64. **Causes of acquired infertility.** Tb = Tuberculosis

Mesothelial Tumors

Tumors of mesothelial origin range from neoplastic but benign to multicentric and aggressive malignancies.

Adenomatoid Tumor Is a Benign Mesothelial Neoplasm

Adenomatoid tumor is encountered in the fallopian tube and in the subserosal tissue of the uterine corpus near the fallopian tube. It is seldom found elsewhere in the peritoneum.

Well-Differentiated Papillary Mesotheliomas are Benign

Well-differentiated papillary mesotheliomas are rare tumors of women of reproductive age. They are typically asymptomatic and are usually found incidentally at operation. The tumors are typically solitary, small, broad-based, wartlike polypoid, or nodular excrescences. Microscopically, thick papillae are covered by a single layer of small cuboidal cells with bland nuclei (Fig. 18-65). These lesions often resemble serous epithelial tumors, but the two are treated differently.

Diffuse Malignant Mesothelioma Is an Invariably Fatal Peritoneal Tumor

Diffuse malignant mesotheliomas arise from the mesothelium of the peritoneum. They are rare in women and constitute only a small proportion of all malignant mesotheliomas, which are mostly pleural. These tumors need to be distinguished from serous adenocarcinomas, including those arising from the peritoneal surface itself and those metastatic from ovary, because survival rates of mesothelioma are so poor and treatment differs from that of serous adenocarcinoma. Most patients are middle-aged or postmenopausal. Clinical manifestations are nonspecific and include ascites, abdominal discomfort, digestive disturbances, and weight loss. Although asbestos exposure is uncommon in women with peritoneal mesothelioma compared to pleural tumors, as many as 2 million fibers per gram of wet weight have been reported in some tumors.

PATHOLOGY: Diffuse malignant mesothelioma extensively involves and thickens the peritoneum and serosa of the various abdominal and pelvic organs. On

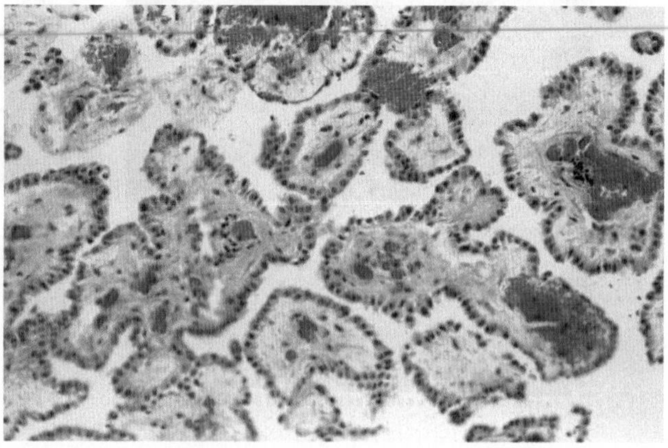

FIGURE 18-65. **Well-differentiated peritoneal mesothelioma.** Cuboidal epithelium lines papillae.

microscopic examination, it has a tubulopapillary to solid pattern. Unlike pleural mesothelioma, the sarcomatoid type is rare. The epithelial variant displays polygonal or cuboidal neoplastic cells with abundant cytoplasm. Calretinin, thrombomodulin, cytokeratin 5/6, and HBME-1 are markers of malignant mesothelioma, whereas CA-125, CEA, and estrogen and progesterone receptors (ER & PR) are markers of ovarian epithelial tumors. No effective treatment is available.

Serous Tumors (Primary and Metastatic)

Unlike the ovary, which features a wide range of tumors, serous tumors are virtually the only type found in the peritoneum. Mucinous tumors in the peritoneum are metastases from a primary neoplasm in the appendix or ovary.

Serous Tumor of Borderline Malignancy Resembles the Ovarian Neoplasm

Most serous borderline tumors in the peritoneum are metastases from the ovary, but some may be primary in the peritoneum. In the latter case, serous peritoneal tumors without evidence of invasion usually are benign; those that are invasive carry a worse prognosis.

PATHOLOGY: Whether it is in the ovary or the peritoneum, a serous tumor of borderline malignancy is characterized by papillary processes, small clusters of cells, cell stratification, detached cellular clusters, nuclear atypia, and mitotic activity in the absence of invasion. Grossly, implants appear as fine granularities or small nodules. Microscopic examination discloses clusters of blunt papillae or glandular structures, often with complex cellular tufts (Fig. 18-66). Psammoma bodies are common and may fill the core of the papillae. Mild-to-severe cytologic atypia with some stratification is common but is substantially less than that seen in adenocarcinoma.

Serous Adenocarcinoma Occurs in Women With Normal Ovaries

The frequency of serous adenocarcinoma arising de novo in the peritoneum is estimated as 10% of its counterpart in the ovary. The mean age of women with this tumor is 50 to 65 years. The diagnosis of a primary peritoneal tumor requires demonstration of normal ovaries. Abdominal pain and ascites are frequent presentations. Like ovarian cancer, serous adenocarcinoma primary in the peritoneum may have a familial basis and can metastasize to distant locations.

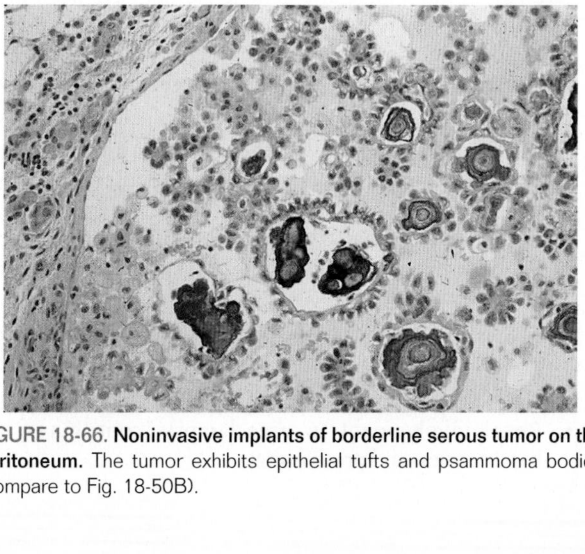

FIGURE 18-66. **Noninvasive implants of borderline serous tumor on the peritoneum.** The tumor exhibits epithelial tufts and psammoma bodies (compare to Fig. 18-50B).

Pseudomyxoma Peritonei

Pseudomyxoma peritonei *refers to the accumulation of jellylike mucus in the pelvic or peritoneal cavity.* Although historically interpreted as stage 3 spread from mucinous ovarian tumors, it is now recognized that many if not most of the tumors are actually mucus-producing adenocarcinomas of the appendix.

PATHOLOGY: The condition may be extensive and appear as semisolid gelatin covering all abdominal structures, or there may be little more than a slightly thickened gelatinous coat over a focal area of bowel or omentum. The appendix will commonly be enlarged or adherent to omentum that is covered with the gelatinous material. Microscopically, the gelatin discloses strips of extremely well differentiated, intestinal-type, mucinous epithelium (Fig. 18-67). If only isolated foci are present, the epithelium may be so well differentiated that it resembles a simple mucinous adenoma. Occasionally, cribriform patterns or other histologic features of malignancy, such as signet-ring cells, warrant a diagnosis of adenocarcinoma.

Low-grade tumors are usually treated for cure, which consists of aggressive surgical debulking and intraperitoneal chemotherapy. The 5-year survival is under 50%.

PLACENTA AND GESTATIONAL DISEASE

Development

The fertilized ovum implants in the endometrium about 5 days after ovulation. The blastocyst gives rise to three layers of trophoblast:

- **The cytotrophoblast** constitutes the germinative layer of the placenta and is devoid of hormones. The cells are small and mononuclear.
- **The syncytiotrophoblast,** the most differentiated form of trophoblast, is composed of large multinucleated cells. These cells contain numerous hormones, among them hCG and human placental lactogen (hPL).

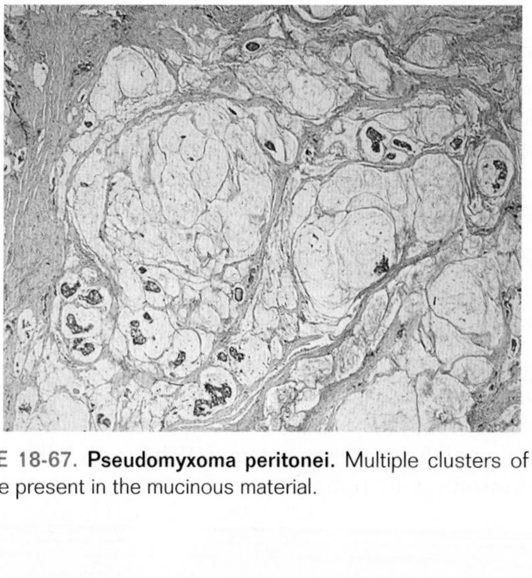

FIGURE 18-67. **Pseudomyxoma peritonei.** Multiple clusters of tumor cells are present in the mucinous material.

- **The intermediate trophoblastic cells** are a transitional form between cytotrophoblasts and syncytiotrophoblasts. These are mononuclear cells but have an eosinophilic cytoplasm closely resembling syncytiotrophoblast. Intermediate cells contain mainly hPL and small quantities of hCG.

The trophoblast: (1) fosters implantation of the blastocyst, (2) develops the uteroplacental circulation, and (3) synthesizes hormones.

Chorionic villi develop on day 21 from the primary villous stems that extend into the intervillous space. By the fourth month of gestation, a definitive placenta develops and no further anatomical alterations occur, although growth continues until parturition.

Anatomy

The placenta contains some 200 subunits called **lobules**. Primary stem villi originate from the chorionic plate and branch into secondary and then tertiary stem villi. The lobules form from the tertiary stem villi, which course through the intervillous space toward the basal plate. There they insert and reenter the intervillous space, dividing into a complex terminal villous network. Fetal blood enters the placenta through two umbilical arteries that spiral around the umbilical vein. Each artery supplies half of the placenta.

The terminal villus is the placenta's functional unit. It consists of an inner layer of cytotrophoblast (**Langhans cells**), a middle layer of intermediate trophoblast and an outer layer of syncytiotrophoblast. The villous stroma is loose mesenchyme containing macrophages (**Hofbauer cells**). In the second trimester, villi become smaller and more numerous, cytotrophoblastic cells and intermediate trophoblast become less prominent and the syncytiotrophoblast attenuates. Villous capillaries grow larger and more numerous and remain mainly within the centers of villi. This process continues until term.

In the third trimester, syncytiotrophoblastic nuclei aggregate to form multinuclear protrusions, **syncytial knots**. In other areas along the villous surface, syncytium between the knots becomes markedly attenuated. At these points, the trophoblastic cytoplasm comes into direct contact with the endothelium of the fetal capillaries to form the **vasculosyncytial membrane**. These specialized zones facilitate gas and nutrient transfer across the placenta. Nonmembranous areas play a role in hormone synthesis.

Infections

Chorioamnionitis Results from Ascending Infection

Chorioamnionitis is inflammation of the amnion and chorion, and the extraplacental membranes. Infectious organisms ascend from the maternal birth canal, commonly owing to premature rupture of the membranes. The inflammatory process affects primarily the membranes (chorioamnionitis) rather than the chorionic villi.

PATHOLOGY: The amniotic fluid is usually cloudy. Membrane walls are slightly opaque, malodorous, and edematous. Microscopically, they show a neutrophilic infiltrate, often with fibrin deposition. With more-extensive spread, the umbilical cord may become infected (**funisitis**) and may exhibit vasculitis of one or more umbilical vessels or inflammation of the cord mesenchyme (**Wharton's jelly**). Generally, chorionic villi remain free of inflammatory infiltrate. Microorganisms isolated from placentas with chorioamnionitis, in descending frequency, are genital mycoplasmas (*Ureaplasma urealyticum, Mysoplasma hominis)* anaerobic organisms of the *Bacteroides* group and aerobes (group *B* streptococci, *E. coli and Gardnerella vaginalis)*.

CLINICAL FEATURES: Acute chorioamnionitis is found in 10% of placentas and is associated with preterm labor, fetal and neonatal infections, and intrauterine hypoxia. The risks of chorioamnionitis to the fetus include (1) pneumonia after inhalation of infected amniotic fluid; (2) skin or eye infections from direct contact with organisms in the fluid, and (3) neonatal gastritis, enteritis, or peritonitis from ingestion of infected fluid. Major risks to the mother are intrapartum fever, postpartum endometritis, and pelvic sepsis with venous thrombosis.

Villitis May Reflect Hematogenous Infection

Infection of chorionic villi results from endometritis or transplacental passage of organisms delivered by way of the maternal circulation. The process is frequently focal. Although the infection cannot be demonstrated in most cases, the microorganisms include (1) bacteria (*Listeria, Treponoma pallidum, Mycobacterium tuberculosis, Mycoplasma* sp., *Chlamydia* sp.), (2) viruses (rubella, CMV, herpes), (3) parasites and protozoa (*Toxoplasma* sp.), and (4) fungi (*Candida* sp.). The most important consequence of hematogenous placental infection is establishment of an inflammatory focus that can then secondarily infect the fetus. Approximately 30% of the villi must be destroyed before perinatal mortality significantly increases.

Preeclampsia and Eclampsia

The hypertensive disorders of pregnancy—preeclampsia and eclampsia—define a syndrome of hypertension, proteinuria, and edema, and, most severely, convulsions. Preeclampsia occurs in 6% of pregnant women in their last trimester, especially with the first child. The disorder becomes **eclampsia** if convulsive seizures appear. (An archaic term, toxemia of pregnancy, is a misnomer and is rarely used any more.)

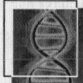

PATHOGENESIS: The pathogenesis of preeclampsia and eclampsia is still not resolved. Immunologic and genetic factors have been invoked as well as altered vascular reactivity, endothelial injury, and coagulation abnormalities (Fig. 18-68). Regardless of the precise cause, certain features are characteristic:

- Preeclampsia occurs with hydatidiform mole (see below), which suggests that the trophoblast is the most likely responsible tissue and that preeclampsia is a trophoblastic disease. Even though the hemodynamic, renal, and endothelial systems are essential for this disorder to develop, preeclampsia is not a primary disease in any of these systems.
- Maternal blood flow to the placenta is markedly reduced because the normal changes in the maternal spiral arteries of the placental bed do not take place.
- Renal involvement in preeclampsia contributes to hypertension and proteinuria.

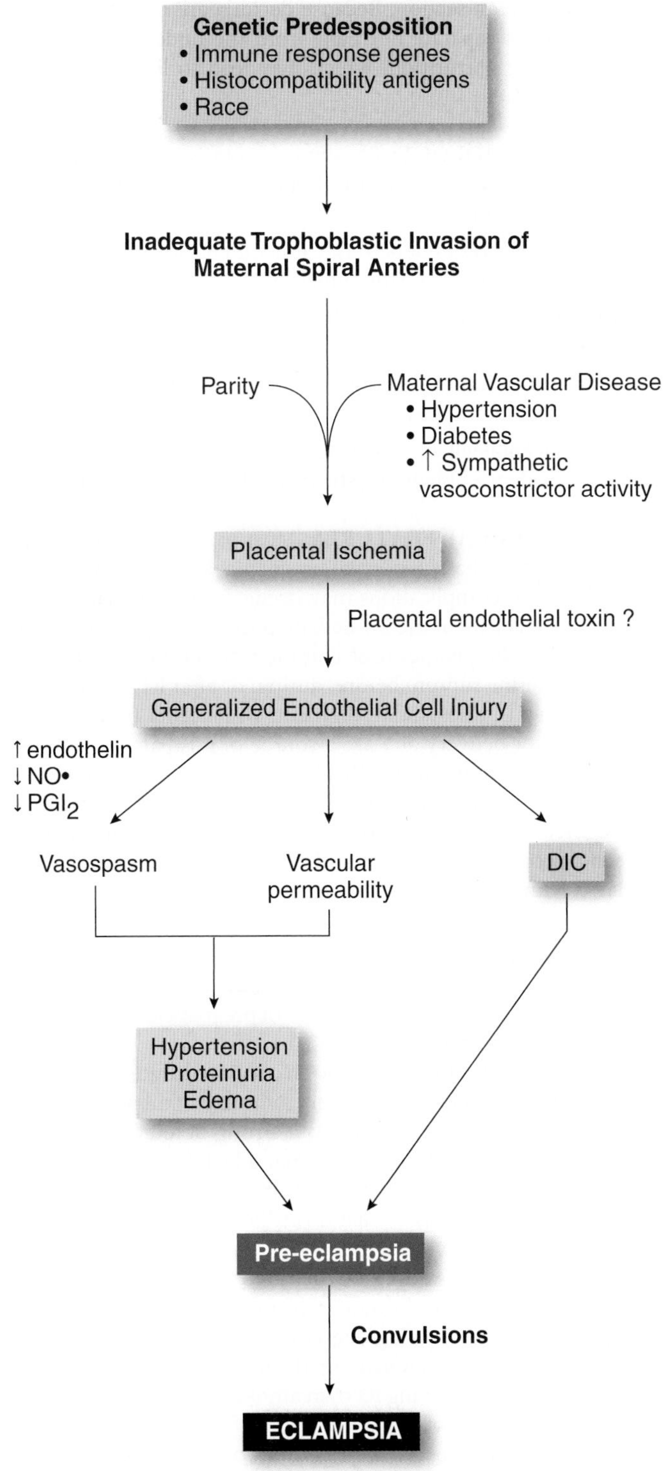

FIGURE 18-68. **Pathogenesis of preeclampsia and eclampsia.** NO• = nitric oxide; PGI_2 = prostacyclin.

- Disseminated intravascular coagulation is a prominent feature of preeclampsia, manifested as fibrin thrombi in the liver, brain, and kidneys. Treatment with antiplatelet agents, particularly low dose aspirin, ameliorates or prevents it.
- The risk of preeclampsia in the first pregnancy is manyfold higher than in subsequent pregnancies. Incidence is also increased in women whose current pregnancy was conceived with a different partner than the first pregnancy and in women with a history of using barrier contraception. These findings suggest that previous antigen exposure may protect against the disease.
- Eclampsia is a cerebrovascular disorder characterized by seizures, worsening hypertension, and cerebral edema. It is often the first sign of preeclampsia but does not necessarily evolve from it.

The pathologic changes in the placenta reflect reduced maternal blood flow to the uteroplacental unit. *The key factor in preeclampsia resides in the spiral arteries of the uteroplacental bed, which never fully dilate.* These arteries are smaller than normal and retain their musculoelastic wall, which is ordinarily attenuated by infiltrative trophoblasts. Normally, extravillous trophoblast invades these arteries and destroys their vascular tone. As a result, vessels become dilated passive conduits of blood from the mother to the fetoplacental unit. In preeclampsia, up to half of spiral arteries escape invasion by endovascular trophoblastic tissue and thus never dilate. There is an inappropriate immune response between the trophoblastic tissue and the musculoelastic tissue of the spiral artery that prevents appropriate invasion by trophoblast. There are also data to suggest that cytotrophoblastic cells do not differentiate properly and do not express the appropriate adhesion molecules that allow vascular invasion.

In women with preeclampsia, the spiral arteries commonly exhibit **acute atherosis**, namely fibrinoid necrosis with accumulation of lipid-laden macrophages. Thrombosis of these vessels is frequent and results in focal placental infarctions. The combination of vasoconstriction and structural changes in the spiral arteries contributes to inadequate blood flow and placental ischemia.

PATHOLOGY: The placenta and maternal organs of women with preeclampsia show conspicuous changes. Extensive placental infarction is seen in nearly one third of women with severe preeclampsia, although it is often negligible in mild preeclampsia. Retroplacental hemorrhage occurs in 15% of patients. Microscopically, chorionic villi show signs of underperfusion. The cytotrophoblastic cells lining them are hyperplastic, and the basement membrane is thickened.

Kidneys always show glomerular changes. Glomeruli are enlarged and endothelial cells are swollen. Fibrin is present between the endothelial cells and the glomerular capillary basement membrane. Mesangial cell hyperplasia is the rule. The changes in the maternal kidneys are reversible with therapy or after delivery.

Fatal cases of eclampsia often show cerebral hemorrhages, ranging from petechiae to large hematomas.

CLINICAL FEATURES: Preeclampsia usually begins insidiously after the 20th week of pregnancy with (1) excessive weight gain occasioned by fluid retention, (2) increased maternal blood pressure, and (3) proteinuria. As the preeclampsia progresses from mild to severe, diastolic pressure persistently exceeds 110 mm Hg, proteinuria is greater than 3 g/day, and renal function declines. Disseminated intravascular coagulation often supervenes. Preeclampsia is treated with antihypertensive and antiplatelet drugs, but definitive therapy requires removing the placenta, hopefully by normal delivery. Eclampsia is treated with magnesium sulfate, which reduces cerebrovascular tone.

Retroplacental Hematoma

Retroplacental hematoma is defined as blood between the basal plate of the placenta and the uterine wall. Retroplacental hematoma is one of the most common causes of perinatal mortality, accounting for 8% of perinatal deaths. The source of the hemorrhage is usually a ruptured maternal artery or premature separation of the placenta. In one third of cases, a retroplacental hematoma occurs without clinical hemorrhage (**abruptio placenta**). The reverse is also true. About half of cases of retroplacental hematoma are associated with maternal smoking, advanced maternal age, acute chorioamnionitis, and cocaine abuse.

PATHOLOGY: The hematomas may be small or may occupy the entire maternal surface of the placenta. Recent hematomas are soft, red, and easily detached from the maternal surface. Older ones are firm, brown, and more adherent to the placental surface. Adverse perinatal outcome associated with retroplacental hematoma relates to its size and the severity of accompanying disorders, particularly preeclampsia, systemic lupus erythematosus, and placental infarction.

Placenta Accreta

Placenta accreta is abnormal adherence of part or all of the placenta to the underlying uterine wall (Fig. 18-69). A deficiency of decidua at the implantation site may result from implantation of the placenta close to or over the cervix (**placenta previa**). A similar situation may arise when implantation occurs on scars from a previous cesarean section. Because decidua are absent, the placenta does not separate normally from the underlying uterine wall following parturition, which may lead to life-threatening bleeding.

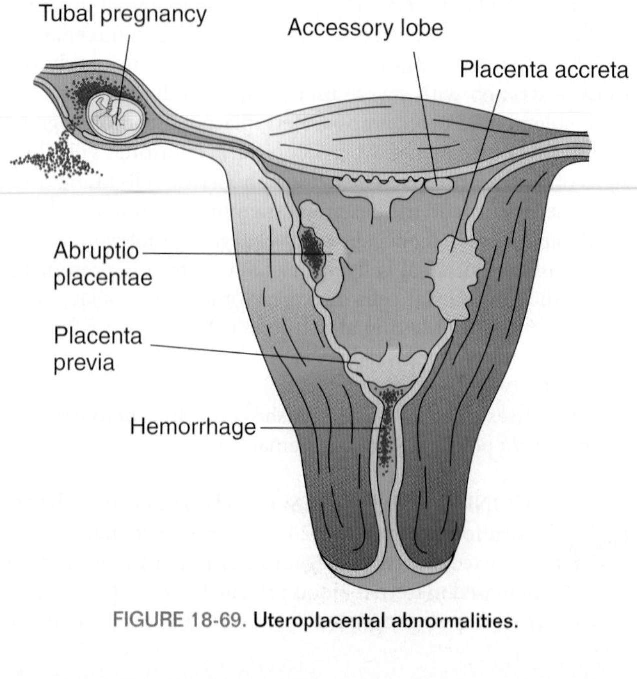

FIGURE 18-69. **Uteroplacental abnormalities.**

PATHOLOGY: Placenta accreta is subclassified according to the depth of villous invasion into the myometrium:

- **Placenta accreta** refers to the attachment of villi to the myometrium without further invasion.
- **Placenta increta** defines villi invading the underlying myometrium.
- **Placenta percreta** describes villi penetrating the full thickness of the uterine wall.

The placental villi in these placental disorders are normal and show no evidence of hyperplastic trophoblastic proliferation.

CLINICAL FEATURES: Most patients with placenta accreta have a normal pregnancy and delivery. However, complications may occur during pregnancy, delivery, or especially in the immediate postpartum period. Third trimester bleeding is the most common presenting sign before delivery. Uterine rupture before, during, or after labor occurs in 15% of patients. Substantial fragments of placenta may remain adherent after delivery and are a source of postpartum hemorrhage. The bleeding can be difficult to control and often requires emergency hysterectomy. Attempts to remove attached placental fragments can cause hemorrhage and even uterine inversion. Placenta accreta is a serious complication of pregnancy and is associated with a maternal death rate of 2%.

Multiple Gestations

Twinning occurs in slightly under 1% of pregnancies and may be dizygotic or monozygotic (Fig. 18-70).

DIZYGOTIC TWINS: Fertilization of two separate ova results in twins that are genetically different, whether of the same or opposite sex. Dizygotic twinning has a strong hereditary component, which is confined to the maternal side. Dizygotic twinning and multiple gestations are more common in women who have used hormones to induce ovulation artificially or who have been impregnated after in vitro fertilization.

Separate placentas develop when two fertilized ova implant apart from one another. If they implant nearby each other, the two placentas show varying degrees of fusion, and may appear as one. When the ova implant apart, there are discrete conceptuses, each placenta having its own amniotic sac. When the placentas fuse, microscopic examination of the membranes between the two fetuses shows two amnions and two chorions (diamnionic, dichorionic gestation).

MONOZYGOTIC TWINS: Early division of a single fertilized ovum results in twins that are genetically identical and therefore of the same sex. If a single fertilized ovum divides within 2 days of fertilization, before the trophoblast has differentiated, two separate embryos develop, each with its own placenta and amniotic sac (dichorionic, diamniotic twinning). Hence, dichorionic placentas may be either monozygotic or dizygotic, whereas monochorionic placentas are always monozygous. If division occurs between the 3rd and 8th days after conception, the trophoblast (but not the amniotic cavity) has already differentiated. A single placenta with two amniotic sacs develops (monochorionic,

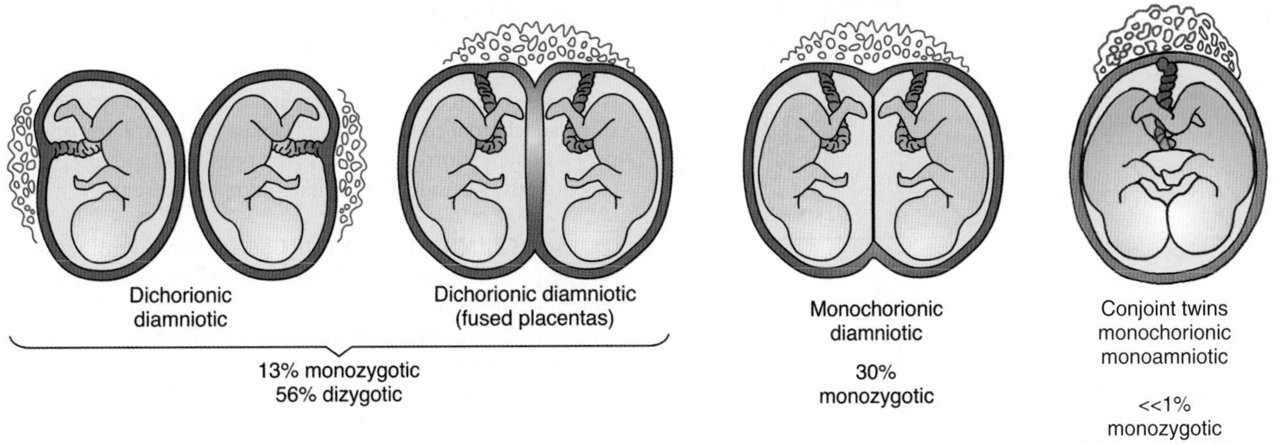

FIGURE 18-70. **Placental structure in twin pregnancies.** The percentages in the figure refer to the proportion of total twin pregnancies (100%) accounted for by each variant.

diamniotic twinning). A monochorionic, monoamniotic placenta is formed if division occurs between the 8th and 13th day after conception, because the amniotic cavity has already developed. Incomplete separation of monozygous twins results in conjoint (formerly Siamese) fetuses within a monoamniotic monochorionic placenta. The mechanisms by which triplet, etc., pregnancies arise may include one or more of the above.

Spontaneous Abortion

A pregnancy that terminates before the fetus is capable of extrauterine life, currently about the 22nd week of gestation, is called a spontaneous abortion. Some 15% of recognized pregnancies abort spontaneously, and an additional 30% of women abort without being aware that pregnancy has occurred. ***Thus, about 45% of pregnancies end in spontaneous abortion.***

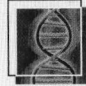

PATHOGENESIS: The principal factors responsible for abortion are maternal and fetal and include:

- Infection early in pregnancy
- Mechanical factors (e.g., submucous uterine leiomyoma or cervical incompetence)
- Endocrine factors (e.g., inadequate progesterone production)
- Immunologic factors
- Fetal congenital abnormalities (e.g., neural tube defects)
- Chromosomal abnormalities

PATHOLOGY: Pathologic examination of the abortus and placenta is often difficult because the aborted tissue is often fragmented and/or macerated by the time the pathologist receives it. Fetal products, if identified, should be examined for changes suggesting chromosomal anomalies. An empty gestational sac with hydropic swelling of the chorionic villi (blighted ovum) suggests early demise of the fetus. Microscopically, chorionic villi in spontaneous abortions may appear normal for gestational age or show intravillous fibrosis or hydropic change.

Gestational Trophoblastic Disease

The term **gestational trophoblastic disease** is a spectrum of disorders with abnormal trophoblast proliferation and maturation, as well as neoplasms derived from trophoblast (Fig. 18-71).

Complete Hydatidiform Mole Does Not Contain an Embryo

Complete hydatidiform mole is a placenta with grossly swollen chorionic villi, resembling bunches of grapes, and showing varying degrees of trophoblastic proliferation. Villi are enlarged, often exceeding 5 mm in diameter (Fig. 18-72).

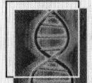

PATHOGENESIS: Complete mole results from fertilization of an empty ovum that lacks functional maternal DNA. Most commonly, a haploid (23,X) set of paternal chromosomes introduced by monospermy duplicates to 46,XX, but dispermic 46,XX and 46,XY moles also occur. The characteristic feature is complete lack of maternal chromosomes. Paternally imprinted genes such as *p57* which are normally expressed only from the maternal allele are not expressed in villous trophoblast of androgenetic derived complete moles. Since the embryo dies at a very early stage, before placental circulation has developed, few chorionic villi develop blood vessels and fetal parts are absent.

RISK FACTORS: The risk of hydatidiform mole relates to maternal age and has two peaks. Girls younger than 15 years of age have a 20-fold higher risk than women between 20 and 35. Risk increases progressively for women over 40. In fact, women older than 50 years of age have 200 times the risk of those between 20 and 40. Ethnic background and obstetric history also influence the risk of developing hydatidiform mole. Incidence is many-fold higher in Asian women than among white women. In Taiwan the risk is 25 times that in the United States. Women with a prior hydatidiform mole have a 20-fold greater risk of a subsequent molar pregnancy than the general population.

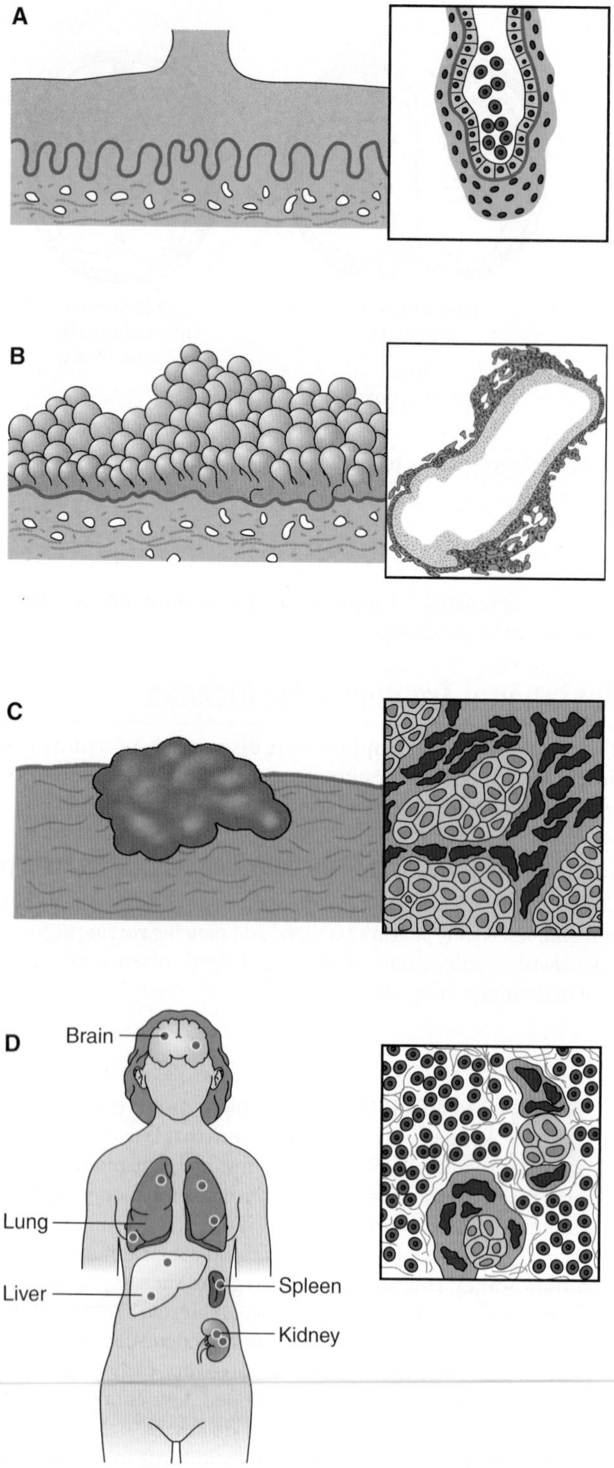

FIGURE 18-71. **Proliferative disorders of the trophoblast. A.** Normal chorionic villus of 8-week fetus, with blood vessel containing nucleated red blood cells. **B.** Complete hydatidiform mole with hydropic villi (also see Fig. 18-72). The villi are enlarged by an edematous stroma devoid of blood vessels. The trophoblastic epithelium is hyperplastic and exhibits variable atypia. **C.** Choriocarcinoma that has arisen in a molar pregnancy invades the myometrium and consists of admixed syncytiotrophoblastic and cytotrophoblastic elements. **D.** Common sites of metastasis from choriocarcinoma.

PATHOLOGY: Molar tissue is voluminous and consists of macroscopically visible villi that are obviously swollen. Microscopically, many individual villi have cisternae, which are central, acellular, fluid-filled spaces devoid of mesenchymal cells. The trophoblast is hyperplastic and composed of syncytiotrophoblast, cytotrophoblast and intermediate trophoblast. Considerable cellular atypia is present.

CLINICAL FEATURES: Patients with complete moles commonly present between the 11th and 25th weeks of pregnancy and complain of excessive uterine enlargement and often abnormal uterine bleeding. Passage of tissue fragments, which appear as small grapelike masses, is common. The serum hCG concentration is markedly elevated, and serial determinations disclose rapidly increasing levels.

Complications of complete mole include uterine hemorrhage, disseminated intravascular coagulation, uterine perforation, trophoblastic embolism, and infection. *The most important complication is the development of choriocarcinoma, which occurs in about 2% of patients after the mole has been evacuated.*

Treatment consists of suction curettage of the uterus and subsequent monitoring of serum hCG levels. As many as 20% of patients require adjuvant chemotherapy for persistent disease, as judged by stable or rising hCG levels. The presence of aneuploidy in the molar tissue may help to identify patients who will require adjuvant treatment. With such management, survival approaches 100%.

Partial Hydatidiform Mole Features Triploid Cells

Partial hydatidiform mole is a distinct form of mole that almost never evolves into choriocarcinoma (see Table 18-11). Partial hydatidiform moles have 69 chromosomes (triploidy), of which one haploid set is maternal and two paternal in origin. This abnormal chromosomal complement results from fertilization of a normal ovum (23,X) by two normal spermatozoa, each carrying 23 chromosomes, or a single spermatozoon that has not undergone meiotic reduction and bears 46 chromosomes. The fetus associated with a partial mole usually dies after 10 weeks' gestation, and the mole is aborted shortly thereafter. In contrast to a complete mole, fetal parts may be present.

PATHOLOGY: Partial moles have two populations of chorionic villi. Some are normal; others are enlarged by hydropic swelling and show central cavitation, resulting from tangential histologic sections of invaginated surface epithelium ("fjord-like") (Fig. 18-73). Trophoblastic proliferation is focal and less pronounced than in complete mole. Blood vessels are typically found within chorionic villi and contain fetal (nucleated) erythrocytes.

Invasive Hydatidiform Mole Penetrates the Underlying Myometrium

PATHOLOGY: Villi of a hydatidiform mole may extend only superficially into the myometrium or may invade the uterus and even the broad ligament. The mole tends to enter dilated venous channels in the myometrium, and a third of them spread to distant sites, mostly the lungs. Unlike choriocarcinoma (see below), distant deposits of an invasive mole do not penetrate beyond the confines of the blood vessels in which they are lodged, and death from such spread is unusual.

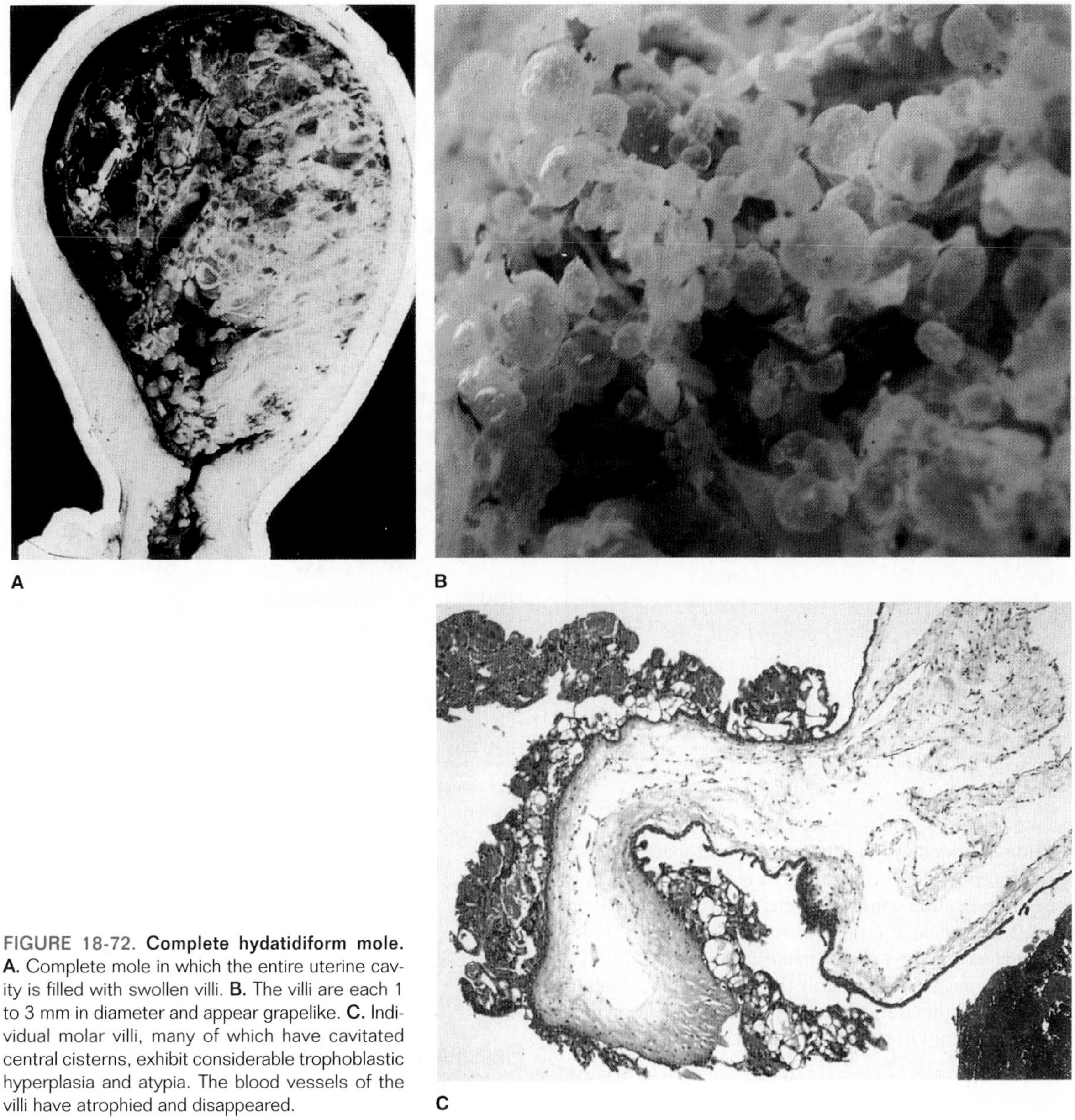

A B C

FIGURE 18-72. **Complete hydatidiform mole.** **A.** Complete mole in which the entire uterine cavity is filled with swollen villi. **B.** The villi are each 1 to 3 mm in diameter and appear grapelike. **C.** Individual molar villi, many of which have cavitated central cisterns, exhibit considerable trophoblastic hyperplasia and atypia. The blood vessels of the villi have atrophied and disappeared.

The clinical distinction between invasive mole and choriocarcinoma is often difficult.

Histologically, invasive moles show less hydropic change than complete moles. Trophoblastic proliferation is usually prominent. Uterine perforation is a major complication, but occurs in only a minority of cases. Theca lutein cysts, which may occur with any form of trophoblastic disease as a result of hCG stimulation, are prominent with invasive moles.

Choriocarcinoma Is a Tumor Allograft in the Host Mother

Gestational choriocarcinoma is a malignant tumor derived from trophoblast.

EPIDEMIOLOGY: Choriocarcinoma occurs in 1 in 30,000 pregnancies in the United States; in eastern Asia, the frequency is far greater. The incidence seems related to abnormalities of pregnancy. Thus, it occurs in 1 of 160,000 normal gestations, 1 of 15,000 spontaneous abortions, 1 of 5000 ectopic pregnancies, and 1 of 40 complete molar pregnancies. In whites, 25% of choriocarcinomas arise from term deliveries, 25% from spontaneous abortions, and 50% from complete hydatidiform moles. Although the risk that a complete hydatidiform mole will transform into choriocarcinoma is only 2%, it is still several orders of magnitude higher than if the pregnancy were normal.

PATHOLOGY: The uterine lesions of choriocarcinoma range from microscopic foci to huge necrotic and hemorrhagic tumors. Viable tumor is usually confined to the rim of the neoplasm because, unlike most other cancers, choriocarcinoma lacks an intrinsic tumor vasculature. Histologically, the tumor contains a dimorphic population of cytotrophoblast and syncytiotrophoblast, with varying degrees of intermediate trophoblast (Fig. 18-74). The tumor resembles the trophoblast in early implanting blastocyst. Rims of syncytiotrophoblast surround central cores of cytotrophoblast, in ad-

TABLE 18-11

Comparative Features of Complete and Partial Hydatidiform Mole

Features	Complete Mole	Partial Mole
Karyotype	46,XX	47,XXY or 47,XXX
Parental origin of haploid genome sets	Both paternal	1 maternal, 2 paternal
Preoperative diagnosis	Mole	Missed abortion
Marked vaginal bleeding	3+	1 +
Uterus	Large	Small
Serum hCG	High	Less elevated
Hydropic villi	All	Some
Trophoblastic proliferation	Diffuse	Focal
Atypia	Diffuse	Minimal
hCG in tissue	3+	1+
Embryo present	No	Some
Blood vessels	No	Common
Nucleated erythrocytes	No	Sometimes
Persists after initial therapy	20%	7%
Choriocarcinoma	2% after mole	No choriocarcinoma

hCG = human chorionic gonadotropin.

dition to being arranged around maternal blood spaces, which resemble the intervillous space of normal placentation. hCG is localized to the syncytiotrophoblastic element. *By definition, tumors containing any villous structures, even if metastatic, are considered hydatidiform mole and not choriocarcinoma.*

Choriocarcinoma invades primarily through venous sinuses in the myometrium. It metastasizes widely by the hematogenous route, especially to lungs (over 90%), brain, gastrointestinal tract, liver and vagina (Table 18-12).

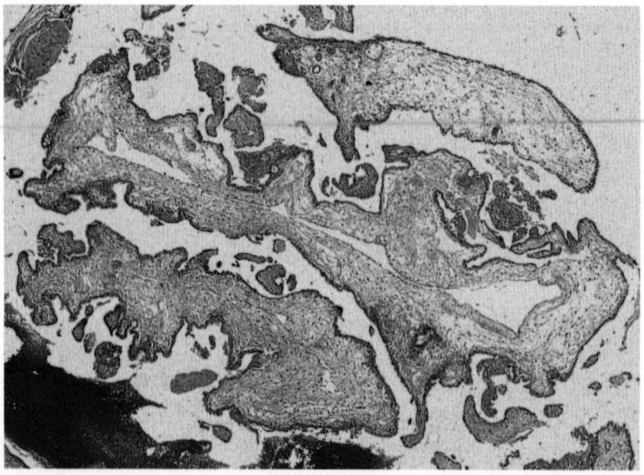

FIGURE 18-73. **Partial hydatidiform mole.** Two populations of chorionic villi are evident. Some are normal; others are conspicuously swollen. Trophoblastic proliferation is focal and less conspicuous than in a complete mole.

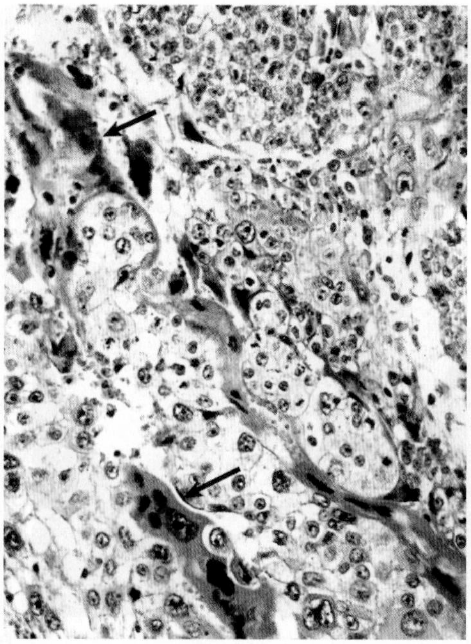

FIGURE 18-74. **Choriocarcinoma.** Malignant cytotrophoblast and syncytiotrophoblast *(arrows)* are present.

CLINICAL FEATURES: Abnormal uterine bleeding is the most frequent initial indication that heralds choriocarcinoma. Occasionally, the first sign relates to metastases to lungs or brain. In some cases, it may only become evident 10 or more years after the last pregnancy.

With currently available chemotherapy, recognition of risk factors (high hCG levels and prolonged interval since antecedent pregnancy), and early treatment, most patients are cured. Survival rates exceed 70% for tumors that have metastasized and virtually 100% remission is expected if a tumor is localized. Serial serum hCG levels monitor the effectiveness of treatment.

Placental Site Trophoblastic Tumor Outcomes are Unpredictable

Placental site trophoblastic tumor, the least common of the various forms of trophoblastic disease, is composed predominantly of intermediate trophoblastic cells.

TABLE 18-12

Clinical Staging of Gestational Trophoblastic Tumors

I	Confined to the uterus
Ia	0 risk factors
Ib	1 risk factor
Ic	2 risk factors
II	Extends outside of the uterus but limited to genital structures
III	Extends to lungs
IV	All other metastatic sites

Risk factors affecting stage include (1) human chorinonic gonadotropin (hCG) > 100,000 mIU/mL, and (2) duration of disease >6 months from termination of antecedent pregnancy.

PATHOLOGY: The gross appearance of placental site trophoblastic tumor is more variable than that of choriocarcinoma. Often, the myometrium shows an ill-defined, yellowish tumor mass that does not display conspicuous hemorrhage. The degree of myometrial invasion varies. Microscopically, the pattern of infiltration resembles that of normal trophoblast in the placental bed. Since intermediate trophoblast in the normal developing pregnancy functions to anchor the pregnancy into the superficial myometrium, the microscopic appearance of the tumor is typically that of an exaggerated placental site. Mononuclear and multinuclear trophoblast may be present as single cells or as cords, islands, and sheets of cells interspersed among myometrial cells. Neither necrosis nor chorionic villi is present. Placental site trophoblastic tumor is also distinguished from choriocarcinoma by its monomorphic (intermediate) trophoblastic proliferation, contrasted with the dimorphic pattern of trophoblast in choriocarcinoma. Most trophoblastic cells are positive for hPL, but a few express hCG.

CLINICAL FEATURES: The age and parity of patients with placental site trophoblastic tumor resemble those of patients with choriocarcinoma. Half of patients with placental site trophoblastic tumor report amenorrhea, whereas vaginal bleeding usually occurs with choriocarcinoma. Compared with patients with choriocarcinoma, many fewer women with this tumor have had a preceding molar pregnancy (5% vs. 50%).

Placental site trophoblastic tumor must be excised completely (hysterectomy) to prevent local recurrence, and sometimes metastasizes and may prove fatal. Large tumors and mitotic index of more than 5 mitoses/10 HPFs are associated with worse prognosis. Because of the short half-life of hPL, serum levels of hCG are more useful in monitoring response to treatment. Generally, conservative management suffices. If hCG persists, even at low levels, or mitotic count is elevated, aggressive treatment with hysterectomy or chemotherapy is indicated.

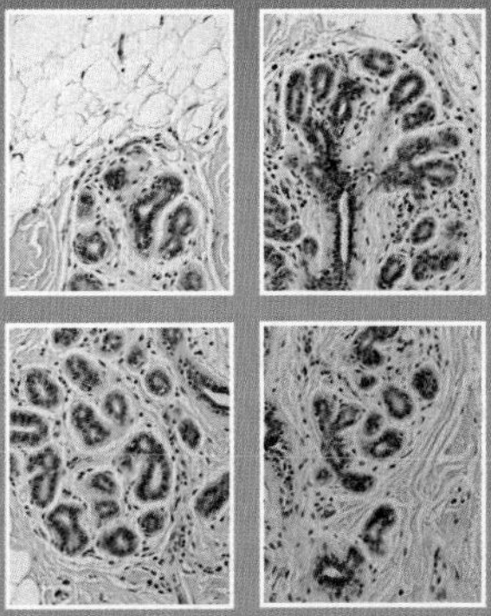

19

The Breast

Ann D. Thor
Adeboye O. Osunkoya

Anatomy and Development

The human breast is first recognizable at about 6 weeks of embryonic development, as ectodermal, ridge-like bilateral thickenings. By the ninth week of gestation, solid epithelial cords grow from the epidermal layer into the underlying mesenchyme. These solid cellular invaginations eventually form branching primary mammary ducts with lumens. Breast development is rudimentary at birth, although in both male and female neonates the breast bud is responsive to maternal hormones and may be prominent. With age the ducts elongate and branch, a process that accelerates in females at puberty. Under the influence of cyclic estrogen and progesterone the terminal end buds and connective tissue stroma proliferate, differentiate, and remodel to form the adult mammary glands.

Extending posteriorly from the nipple, the large and medium sized ducts, glandular structures, and surrounding stroma form approximately 20 interconnected lobes. Within a single lobe the small ducts branch and terminate in glands known as **terminal duct lobular units** (TDLUs). The TDLUs consist of (1) the terminal ductules, whose epithelium differentiates into the secretory "acini" of the pregnant or lactating breast; (2) the intralobular collecting duct; and (3) the specialized intralobular stroma (Fig. 19-1). Each of the lobes drains into its own lactiferous duct, which opens onto the surface of the nipple.

The parenchyma of the female breast consists of the ducts and lobules, interlobular fibrous tissue, and abundant adipose tissue. The amount of adipose tissue varies considerably, depending on the age and general habitus of the woman. Adolescent women typically have dense fibrous breasts whereas postmenopausal women generally have predominantly fatty breasts. Women of reproductive age typically have variable patterns of stromal fibrosis, which is typically influenced by steroid hormone levels, age, and other biologic factors.

The nipple consists predominantly of dense fibrous tissue mixed with fascicles of smooth muscle. The latter component gives the nipple its erectile capability and contributes to expression of milk. The skin immediately surrounding the nipple, the areola, is more heavily pigmented than the surrounding skin of the breast and becomes even more so during pregnancy. In this area the skin has pilosebaceous units, and it is one of the few areas of the body that contains apocrine as well as eccrine sweat glands.

The breast is richly vascularized and contains lymphatic channels that directly communicate with the lower pectoralis axillary nodes (75%) as well as mediastinal (parasternal) lymph nodes (25%, typically the medial breast). *This rich vascularity and*

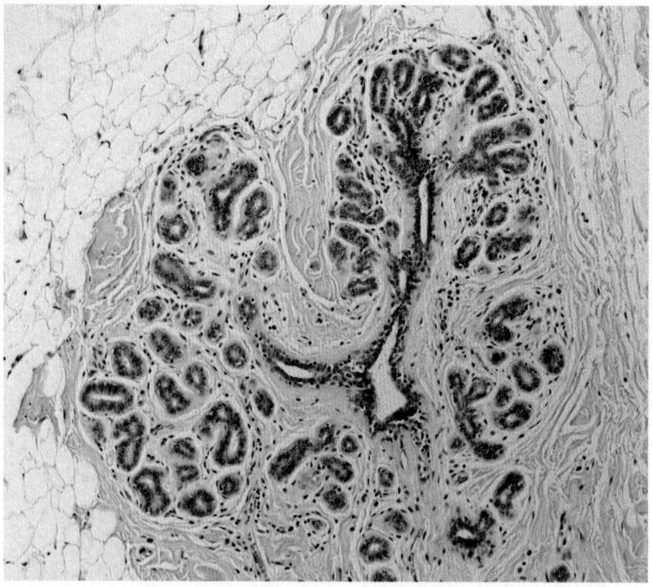

FIGURE 19-1. **Terminal duct lobular units are the functional units of the breast.**

lymphatic drainage may facilitate metastatic spread of breast cancers when they occur.

Hormonal Control of Development and Function

With the onset of menarche and the attendant increase in estrogen and progesterone, the TDLUs develop more fully and the epithelial cells differentiate (Fig. 19-2A and B). The TDLUs are dynamic structures that undergo marked cellular alterations, not only at the time of pregnancy but also, to a lesser degree, during the regular menstrual cycles. These cyclical changes include proliferation and programmed cell death (apoptosis) of epithelium as well as changes in the intralobular stromal components.

The TDLUs are responsible for breast secretory activity that occurs during lactation (see Fig. 19-2C). The female breast and endometrium are governed by many of the same hormones. The endometrium shows mitotic activity during the first half of the menstrual cycle, but the breast epithelium proliferates most during the second half of the menstrual cycle. The early mutational events that may eventually lead to breast cancer may take place during this part. There are several critical hormonal phases that influence both benign and malignant breast gland activity.

- **Follicular phase** of the menstrual cycle: During the first half, or follicular phase, of the cycle, terminal ducts are few and lined by a simple, two-cell layer of epithelium surrounded by a layer of myoepithelial cells.

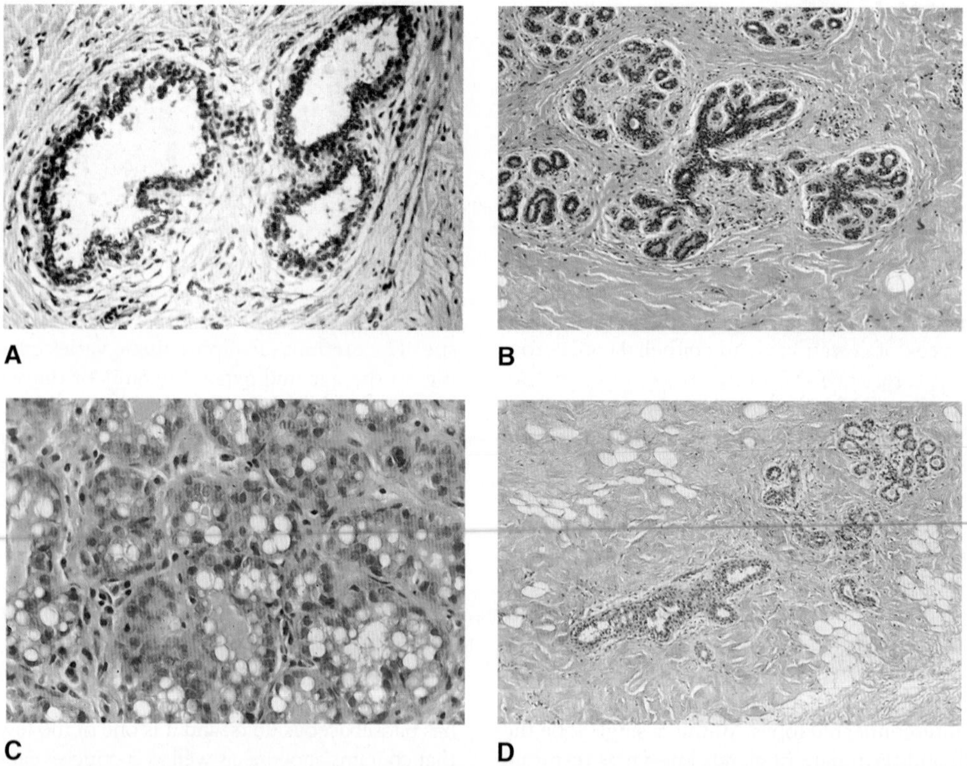

FIGURE 19-2. **Normal breast architecture at various ages. A.** Adolescent breast. Large and intermediate-size ducts are seen within a dense fibrous stroma. No lobular units are present. **B.** Postpubertal breast. The terminal duct lobular unit consists of small ductules arrayed around an intralobular duct. The two-cell-layered epithelium shows no secretory or mitotic activity. The intralobular stroma is dense and confluent with the interlobular stroma. **C.** Lactating breast. The terminal duct lobular units are conspicuously enlarged, with inapparent interlobular and intralobular stroma. The individual terminal ducts, now termed acini, show prominent epithelial secretory activity (cytoplasmic vacuolization). The acinar lumina contain secretory material. **D.** Postmenopausal breast. The terminal duct lobular units are absent. The remaining intermediate ducts and larger ducts are commonly dilated. There is little interlobular fibrous connective tissue, and much of the breast is composed of fat.

- **Luteal phase:** After ovulation, enhanced mitotic activity in the terminal duct epithelium results in a conspicuous increase in the number of terminal ducts within a lobule. Simultaneously, the basal layer of epithelial cells becomes vacuolated. The intralobular stroma becomes edematous and distinct from the dense fibrous tissue that surrounds each lobule. Clinically, women perceive progressive fullness and tenderness of the breast during the luteal phase of the menstrual cycle.
- **Menses:** With the onset of menstruation, as levels of estrogen and progesterone fall, apoptotic cell death increases in the terminal duct epithelium. Progressive lymphocyte infiltration occurs in the intralobular stroma. By the end of menses, TDLUs regress to their state during the follicular phase.
- **Pregnancy:** In pregnancy, there is a pronounced hormonally induced increase in the number of terminal ducts. The lobular epithelium is increased to such a point that it is the major component of the breast tissue.
- **Lactation:** During lactation, epithelial cells become vacuolated, and ductal lumina are distended with secretions (see Fig. 19-2C). When lactation ceases, lobular units involute and revert to their former state.
- **Postmenopause:** After menopause, TDLUs atrophy, but large and intermediate duct systems remain, and minor cystic dilation of residual ducts is common, accompanied by a concomitant loss of the dense, interlobular, fibrous connective tissue. Consequently, the percentage of the breast that is adipose tissue increases. By 80 years of age, 80% of women have predominantly fatty breasts although cuffs of dense fibrous tissue may persist around the remaining ducts (see Fig. 19-2D).
- **The male breast:** Until puberty the male breast develops similarly to the female breast. At puberty, further development is arrested. Thus, the adult male breast consists of large to intermediate-sized ducts resembling those of the immature female breasts.

Congenital Anomalies

It is common for a tail of breast tissue to extend into the lower axilla. Uncommonly, breast or nipple tissue may be present elsewhere along the original embryonic breast ridge (milk line). Thus, accessory breast tissue may be found along the anterior trunk, superior or inferior to the main breast, all the way to the inguinal area, and even occasionally into the vulva. Breast cancer may rarely arise from such an accessory gland. The most frequent variant of the normal breast is **inversion of the nipple**. This is of clinical significance, because it may cause difficulty in nursing. Secondary nipple inversion may be caused by traction from an underlying carcinoma.

Juvenile Hypertrophy

Neonatal breast hypertrophy occurs in both male and female newborns, in response to maternal hormones. It regresses with age and does not require clinical treatment.

Juvenile (pubertal) hypertrophy may be bilateral or unilateral and occurs in either girls or boys. Unless there is an underlying hormonal abnormality, juvenile breast hypertrophy usually regresses spontaneously.

PATHOLOGY: Morphologically, the fibrous stroma expands and ducts increase in number. Duct epithelium becomes hyperplastic and branching structures more exaggerated. Since lobules are not yet formed, they do not participate in this process.

SECONDARY HYPERTROPHY: Secondary hypertrophy of the breast may occur owing to abnormally high hormone levels, such as those induced by a functioning ovarian, adrenocortical, or pituitary tumor.

Gynecomastia

Gynecomastia refers to an enlargement of the adult male breast. It is typically bilateral, and is usually caused by hormones or certain medications, and is morphologically similar to juvenile hypertrophy of the female breast (Fig. 19-3). Unilateral or focal male breast enlargement is not gynecomastia and is usually cause for a biopsy.

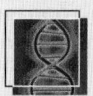

PATHOGENESIS: Gynecomastia is caused by an absolute increase in circulating estrogens or by a relative increase in the estrogen/androgen ratio, most commonly due to: (1) intake of exogenous estrogens or estrogen-like agents (e.g., digitalis, opiates); (2) hormone-secreting adrenal or testicular tumors; (3) paraneoplastic production of gonadotropins by cancers of the liver, lung, and other organs; and (4) metabolic disorders such as liver disease and hyperthyroidism that lead to increased conversion of androstenedione into estrogen. Low levels of androgen may also enhance estrogenic activity due to modification of the estrogen/androgen ratio and may reflect inadequate testicular secretion of testosterone (Klinefelter syndrome, castration, orchitis, atrophy) or androgen insensitivity (testicular feminization). There is no evidence that gynecomastia is associated with an increased risk of cancer in males.

Acute Mastitis

Acute mastitis is an emergent clinical condition resulting from a bacterial infection of the breast. Acute mastitis may be seen at any age, but most frequently presents in the postpartum or lactating breast. Patients with acute mastitis may present with localized symptoms including pain, swelling, or redness. Sys-

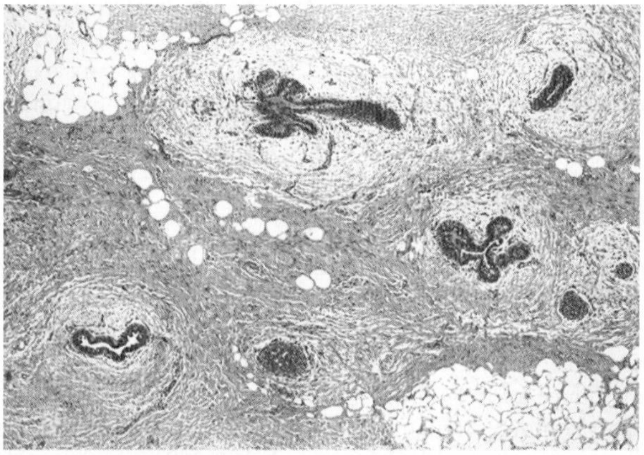

FIGURE 19-3. **Gynecomastia.** There is proliferation of branching, intermediate-sized ducts. The ductal epithelium is hyperplastic, and mitoses are present. A concomitant increase in the surrounding fibrous tissue causes a palpable mass.

temic symptoms may include fever or malaise. Acute mastitis is most often secondary to obstruction of the duct system by inspissated secretions, with stasis and a secondary bacterial infection. The most common organisms isolated are *Staphylococcus* and *Streptococcus*. Acute bacterial mastitis may resolve with aggressive mechanical suction to empty the breast of milk and by the administration of antibiotics. Untreated or unresponsive infections may progress to abscess formation and or systemic bacterial infection. A firm, walled-off, nontender abscess or chronic, localized scar may be mistaken for cancer on physical exam.

Duct Ectasia

Duct ectasia refers to the presence of dilated large and intermediate breast ducts containing pasty, inspissated material, with accompanying periductal inflammation and fibrosis. It is common in elderly women, in whom it affects the large collecting ducts immediately under the areola. Morphologically, involved ducts are dilated and contain acellular debris and foamy macrophages. These dilated ducts may rupture. The release of grumous material incites in surrounding stroma a sterile but substantial chronic inflammatory response, often with foreign body granulomas. By virtue of its firmness, duct ectasia may be difficult to distinguish from carcinoma clinically and so may be subjected to biopsy.

Fat Necrosis

Fat necrosis is a distinct clinical and histologic entity, resulting in either a localized or more diffuse mass lesion of the breast. A history of trauma can often be elicited. Trauma may induce tissue damage, the release of fat and blood, and subsequent inflammation. Clinically, pain, swelling, redness, discoloration, and/or a mass lesion may suggest cancer.

PATHOLOGY: Initially, the lesion consists of necrosis of adipocytes and hemorrhage, after which inflammatory cells phagocytize the lipid debris. Macrophages may produce a granulomatous inflammatory response. Fibro-blastic proliferation and collagen deposition during healing may lead to fibrous scar tissue (fibrosis) that extends into the adjacent breast or dermis (overlying skin). As a result, an irregular, fixed, hard mass may ensue and clinically resemble breast cancer. **Dystrophic calcification**, a common feature of breast cancer, may also be detected radiographically in areas of ancient fat necrosis. Thus, significant fat necrosis may also be detected radiographically in areas of ancient fat necrosis, and may require biopsy to establish its benign character.

Granulomatous Mastitis

Granulomatous mastitis is an uncommon inflammatory lesion. It is associated with intra-mammary foreign material, often implanted or injected to modify the shape or size of the breast. These may include silicone or other foreign substances, which may induce a foreign body giant cell or granulomatous inflammatory response. Implants are often surrounded by formation of a fibrous pseudocapsule due to the chronic inflammation at their periphery. The use of saline, rather than silicone implants, has significantly reduced implant-associated granulomatous mastitis. Granulomatous breast inflammation secondary to mycobacterial or fungal infections is much less common.

Fibrocystic Change

Fibrocystic change is a constellation of morphologic features characterized by (1) cystic dilation of terminal ducts, (2) a relative increase in fibrous stroma, and (3) variable proliferation of terminal duct epithelial elements. It is most often diagnosed in women from their late 20s to the time of menopause. Some fibrocystic change occurs in 75% of adult women in the United States. Symptomatic fibrocystic change, in which large, clinically detectable cysts are formed may be seen in 10% of women between 35 and 55 years old. The frequency of fibrocystic change decreases after menopause.

Fibrocystic change with giant cysts and proliferative epithelial lesions is more common in populations that have an increased risk of breast cancer, but progression to carcinoma has not been documented. Florid proliferative lesions are designated **proliferative** fibrocystic change. Fibrocystic change without epithelial proliferation (**nonproliferative** fibrocystic change) does not involve increased risk of breast cancer.

PATHOLOGY: The morphologic hallmarks of nonproliferative fibrocystic change are an increase in dense, fibrous stroma and some cystic dilation of the terminal ducts (Fig. 19-4B and C). Fibrocystic change always occurs in multiple areas of both breasts, although involvement may vary from one area to another. Most often, cystic changes are minor and do not cause discrete masses. However, a dominant cyst or aggregate of fibrous connective tissue containing smaller cysts may appear to be a discrete "mass," and be cause for biopsy to exclude the possibility of cancer.

The large cysts, up to 5 cm in diameter, often contain dark, thin fluid that imparts a blue color to the unopened cysts—the so-called *blue-domed cysts of Bloodgood* see Fig. 19-4B). Aspiration of a large cyst will usually cause it to collapse and the mass to disappear.

On microscopic examination, the epithelium lining the cysts varies from columnar to flattened or may even be entirely absent. **Apocrine metaplasia** frequently is seen in nonproliferative fibrocystic change (see Fig. 19-4D). The metaplastic cells are larger and more eosinophilic than the usual duct lining cells and resemble apocrine sweat gland epithelium.

Proliferative fibrocystic change refers to several forms of epithelial proliferation that occur in the background of nonproliferative fibrocystic change. The most common proliferative change is an increase in the number of cells or layers lining the dilated terminal ducts, termed **ductal epithelial hyperplasia** (see Fig. 19-4E). Epithelial proliferation can at times become exuberant and widespread forming intraductal epithelial papillary structures with central fibrovascular cores (**papillomatosis**).

Proliferative (hyperplastic) lesions may also demonstrate cytologic atypia. These atypical lesions are subclassified by the degree of microscopic atypia and the extent of breast involvement (see below).

Proliferative fibrocystic change increases the risk of cancer.

- **Nonproliferative fibrocystic change** does not confer an increased risk for the development of invasive breast cancer.

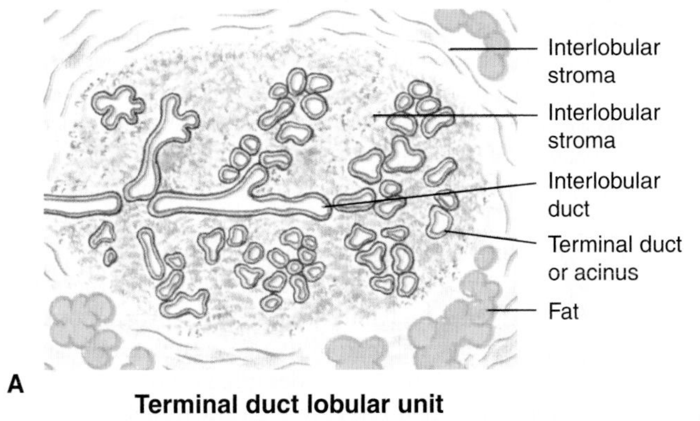

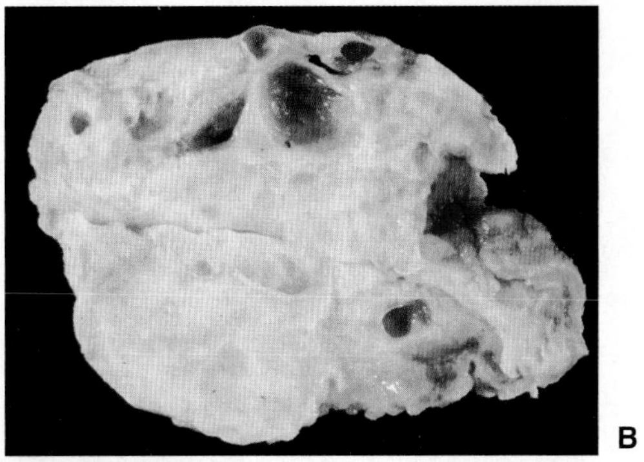

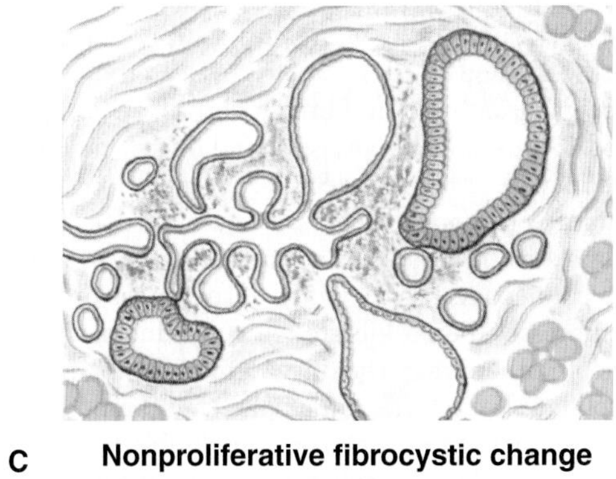

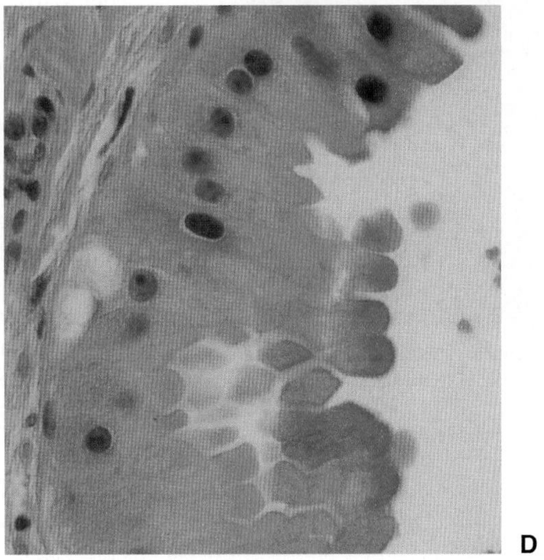

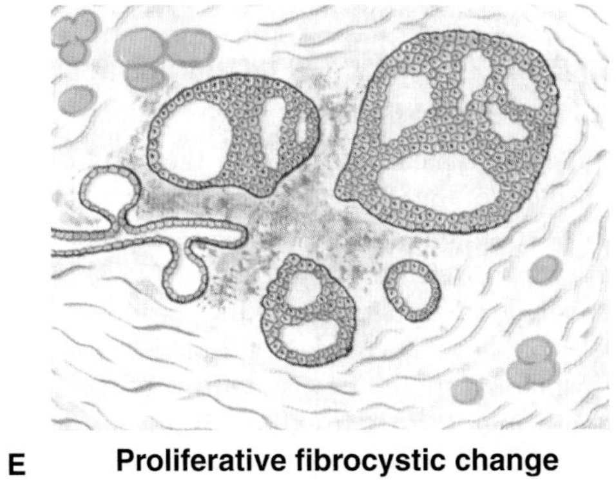

FIGURE 19-4. **Fibrocystic change. A**. Normal terminal lobular unit. **B**. Surgical specimen: Cysts of various sizes are dispersed in dense, fibrous connective tissue. Some of the cysts are large and contain old blood-tinged proteinaceous debris. **C.** Nonproliferative fibrocystic change combines cystic dilation of the terminal ducts with varying degrees of apocrine metaplasia of the epithelium and increased fibrous stroma. **D.** Apocrine metaplasia: Epithelial cells have apocrine features with eosinophilic cytoplasm. **E.** Proliferative fibrocystic change: Terminal duct dilation and intraductal epithelial hyperplasia are present.

- **Proliferative, nonatypical fibrocystic change** is associated with a minimal increased risk for the development of invasive cancer (1.5- to 2-fold).
- **Atypical hyperplasia** with fibrocystic change (atypical proliferative fibrocystic change) is associated with a 4- to 5-fold increased risk for developing invasive cancer compared to the general population. This risk increases further if there is a strong family history of the disease.
- **Proliferative lesions** increase the risk of subsequent cancer equally in both breasts.

The risk of breast cancer associated with proliferative fibrocystic change increases with the level and extent of atypia, age, and family history of breast cancer. Women at high risk may reduce their chances of developing breast cancer by chemical or surgical castration and anti-estrogenic agents (e.g., tamoxifen). Exogenous hormones (e.g., estrogens) may increase the risk of breast cancer, particularly in postmenopausal women or women at high risk for breast cancer, although the extent to which this might occur is controversial.

Sclerosing Adenosis is a Less Common Variant of Proliferative Fibrocystic Change

Sclerosing adenosis is characterized by proliferation of small ducts and myoepithelial cells with surrounding stromal fibrosis (Fig. 19-5). Sclerosing adenosis is almost always associated with other forms of proliferative fibrocystic change. On mammogram, these lesions often demonstrate microcalcifications in patterns that resemble those seen in malignancies and may be difficult to distinguish clinically from carcinoma. Sclerosing adenosis may also present a diagnostic challenge for the pathologist. Microscopically, lobular units may be deformed and enlarged, forming a mass of epithelial and stromal elements (see Fig. 19-5), which can be difficult ot distinguish from invasive carcinoma.

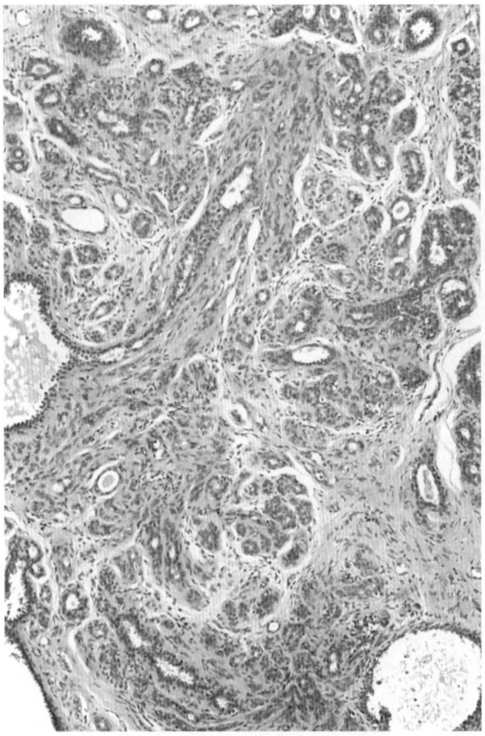

FIGURE 19-5. **Sclerosing adenosis.** This lesion is characterized by the proliferation of small, abortive, ductlike structures and myoepithelial cells expands and distorts the lobule in which it arises. The lesion is well circumscribed, in contrast to a cancerous lesion.

Benign Tumors

Fibroadenoma is the Most Common Benign Neoplasm of the Breast

These benign neoplasms are composed of epithelial and stromal elements that originate from the TDLU. Fibroadenomas are usually solitary masses, although some women develop more than one during their lifetime. They are most often diagnosed in women between the ages of 20 and 35. Fibroadenomas commonly enlarge more rapidly during pregnancy (i.e., they are hormone-responsive) and cease to grow after menopause. A causal relationship between hormones and the development of fibroadenomas has not been established.

The rarer **juvenile fibroadenoma** arises in adolescence and may grow rapidly. Some fibroadenomas are associated with an increase in breast cancer risk, including a complex fibroadenoma, fibroadenoma with adjacent proliferative disease, or fibroadenoma in patients with a first-degree family history of breast cancer.

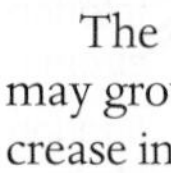

PATHOLOGY: Fibroadenomas vary in size, from a microscopic, incidental lesion to a large tumor most often 2 to 4 cm. in diameter. Fibroadenomas are rubbery tumors that are sharply demarcated from the surrounding breast. These lesions can be identified on mammography or by palpation. Fibroadenomas are typically mobile and may be tender, particularly during the mid-to-late menstrual cycle. The cut surface appears glistening, gray-white and sharply demarcated from adjacent breast (Fig. 19-6A).

On microscopic examination, fibroadenomas are composed of a mixture of fibrous connective tissue and ducts (see Fig. 19-6B). The ducts may be either simple and round or elongate and branching, and are dispersed within a characteristic fibrous stroma that varies from loose and myxomatous to hyalinized collagen. This connective tissue, which forms most of the tumor, often compresses the proliferated ducts, reducing them to curvilinear slits. In other areas, the ducts remain patent because the stroma proliferates circumferentially around them. The appearance of the epithelium ranges from the double layer of epithelium of normal lobules to varying degrees of hyperplasia.

Intraductal papillomas occur in the lactiferous ducts of middle-aged and older women.

Intraductal papillomas typically arise from the surface of the large, subareolar ducts of middle aged and older women. **Intraductal papillomas** are often associated with a serous or bloody nipple discharge, which typically brings the patient to her physician for clinical evaluation. A solitary intraductal papilloma is not a premalignant lesion, nor is it a marker of risk for breast cancer. An intraductal papilloma should be distinguished from papillomatosis, the latter being a form of multifocal epithelial hyperplasia that occurs in the peripheral ducts and is a component of proliferative fibrocystic change.

A

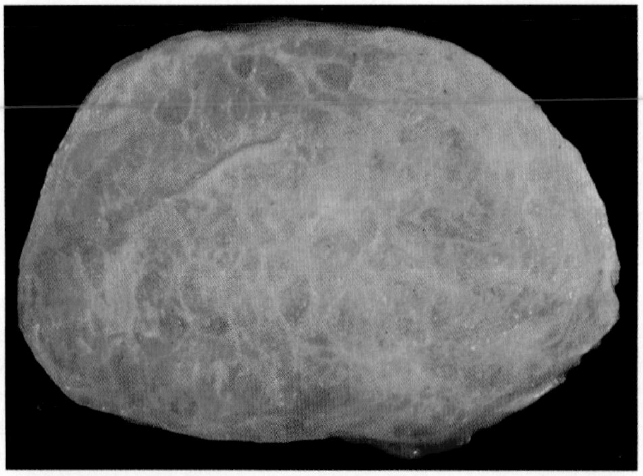

B

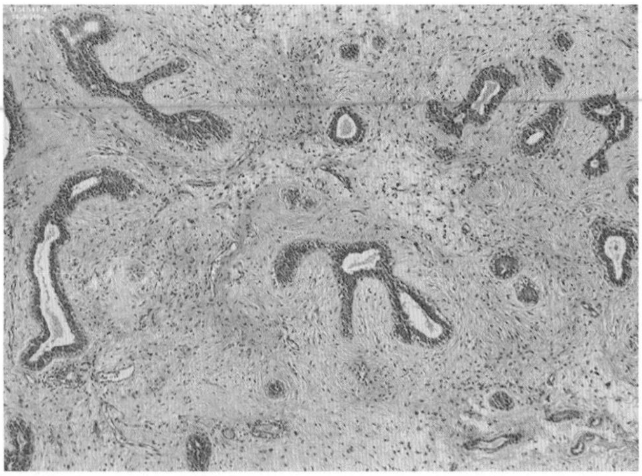

FIGURE 19-6. **Fibroadenoma. A.** Surgical specimen. This well-circumscribed tumor was easily enucleated from the surrounding tissue. The cut surface is characteristically glistening tannish-white and has a septate appearance. **B.** Microscopic section. Elongated epithelial duct structures are situated within a loose, myxoid stroma.

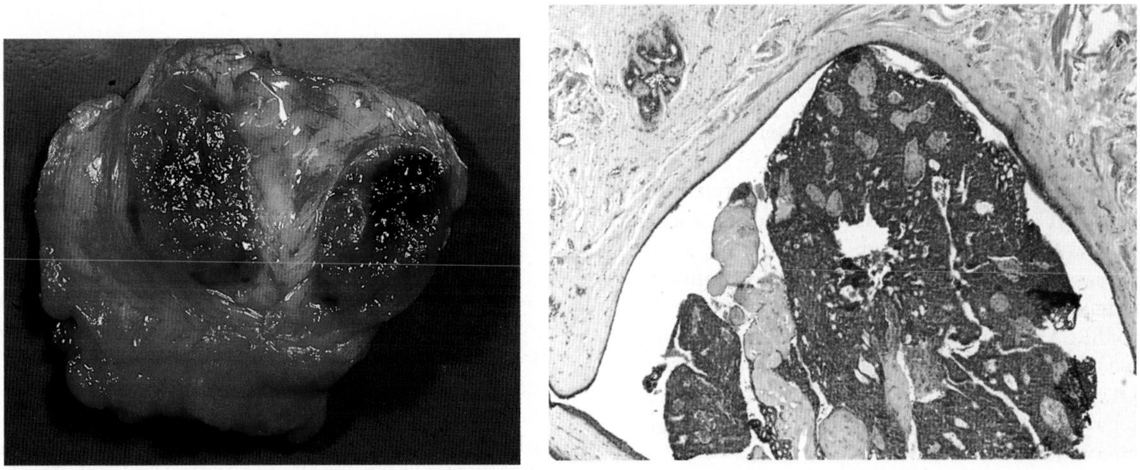

A B

FIGURE 19-7. **Intraductal papilloma. A.** A large papillary mass is seen within dilated ducts. **B.** A photomicrograph shows a benign papillary growth in a subareolar duct.

PATHOLOGY: Intraductal papilloma (Fig. 19-7A and B) is a single tumor, usually a few millimeters in diameter, which is attached to the wall of the duct by a fibrovascular stalk. The papillomatous portion consists of a double layer of epithelial cells, an outer one of cuboidal or columnar cells and an inner layer of more-rounded myoepithelial cells.

Carcinoma of the Breast

Breast cancer is the most common malignancy of women in the United States, and the mortality from this disease among women is second only to that of lung cancer.

EPIDEMIOLOGY: The incidence of breast cancer has slowly increased over the past 50 years. Currently, one in nine American women may be expected to develop breast cancer, of whom one-third will die of the disease. In Western industrialized countries with high rates of breast cancer, the incidence of this tumor continues to increase throughout life, albeit at a slower rate in elderly women. In populations at low risk for breast cancer, the incidence reaches a plateau prior to menopause and then does not increase further. Breast cancer is uncommon before the age of 35 years.

Breast cancer is 4 to 5 times more frequent in Western industrialized countries than in less-developed countries and in Native Americans in the United States. Furthermore, the risk of breast cancer in daughters and granddaughters of women who migrate to the United States from countries where breast cancer incidence is low (e.g., Japan), increases to approach that in white American women. It has been suggested that diet, in particular dietary fat, may in part explain differences in the geographical distribution ofbreast cancer, but this concept remains controversial.

Breast cancer is uncommon but may occur in women before the age of 35 years. Breast cancer in young women under 40 is more often associated with inherited, genetic defects. Breast cancer rarely develops in men, although when it occurs it may be equally if not more deadly. Patients with mutations in both BRCA2 genes develop a Fanconi anemia-like disease (see Chapter 20)

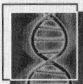

PATHOGENESIS: The pathogenesis of breast cancer is poorly understood, but epidemiologic, molecular, and genetic studies outline complex risk factors. Breast cancers also exhibit diversity in histopathology, molecular features, and overall patient outcomes. Hence, the disease can be viewed as a multifaceted and complex epithelial malignancy.

Approximately 5% of Breast Cancers are Thought to Reflect a Hereditary Predisposition

The strongest association with an increased risk for breast cancer is a family history, specifically breast cancer in first-degree relatives (mother, sister, daughter). The risk is greater when the relative is afflicted at a young age or with bilateral breast cancer. A woman who has two sisters with breast cancer, one of whom had bilateral tumors, or a mother and sister who show the same pattern, has a greater than 25% chance of developing breast cancer by age 70.

The ***BRCA1* gene** (breast cancer 1), a tumor suppressor gene located on chromosome 17 (17q21), has been implicated in the pathogenesis of hereditary breast and ovarian cancers. Mutations in this tumor-suppressor gene are thought to be carried by 1 in 200 to 400 people in the United States. Germline point mutations and deletions in *BRCA1* confer a 60% to 85% lifetime risk for breast cancer, with over half of the tumors developing before 50 years of age. Inherited *BRCA1* mutations are involved in , <2% of cases of breast cancer discovered after 70 years of age, but 30% of women in whom the tumor is detected before the age of 45 carry these mutations. It is currently suspected that mutated *BRCA1* is responsible for 20% of all cases of **inherited** breast cancer (about 3% of all breast cancers). Somatic mutations in *BRCA1* are infrequently detected in **sporadic** (nonfamilial) breast cancers. The *BRCA1* protein is involved in double strand DNA break repair, ubiquitination (see Chapter 1), transcriptional regulation and heterochromatin formation (see Chapter 5).

Women with *BRCA1* mutations are also at greater lifetime risk of ovarian cancer, which has been estimated to range from 15% to 40%. There is some evidence that persons with mutations in this gene may also be at increased risk of prostate and colon cancers.

The ***BRCA2* gene**, located on chromosome 13q12, has been incriminated in approximately 20% of hereditary breast cancers. Women with one copy of a mutated BRCA2 gene have a 30% to 40% lifetime chance of developing breast cancers. Like patients with *BRCA1*, these women have increased risk of ovarian cancer. *BRCA2* mutations also put male carriers at increased risk of breast cancer. Mutations of *BRCA2* are particularly common amongst Ashkenazi Jewish women. *BRCA2* protein is closely related to the FANCD1 protein and is important in DNA double strand break repair and, in association with RAD1, homologous recombination.

For both *BRCA1* and *BRCA2*, specific germ line mutations and disease patterns vary among families. If a founder mutation can be defined, family members can be screened for that specific mutation rather than a more complex molecular analysis. The ***p53* gene** is mutated in the Li-Fraumeni syndrome (see Chapter 5). This rare familial cancer syndrome features tumors of the brain and adrenals in children and breast cancer in young women. It is estimated that germline (inherited) mutations in p53 account for 1% of breast cancers among women in whom the tumor is detected before the age of 40 years. However, almost all (90%) women with Li-Fraumeni syndrome who survive childhood cancers will develop breast cancer. Somatic *p53* mutations are common in sporadic breast cancers.

Most Breast Cancers are Not Associated with Heritable Factors

HORMONAL STATUS: A link between breast cancer and the hormonal status of women is strongly suggested by the conspicuous association between the incidence of this tumor and the age of menarche, menopause, and first pregnancy. *Early menarche, late menopause, and older age at first-term pregnancy all increase the risk of breast cancer.* Nulliparous women, or those who become pregnant for the first time after age 35, have a twofold to threefold higher risk of breast cancer than women whose first pregnancy occurred before age 25. Oophorectomy before age 35, but not afterwards, dramatically lowers the risk of breast cancer. Oral contraceptive agents have not been associated with increased risk of breast cancer, in contrast with peri- and postmenopausal hormone supplementation, which confer a slightly higher probability of breast cancer.

RADIATION: The female breast is susceptible to radiation- induced neoplasia. The risk of breast cancer was increased in atomic bomb survivors, women irradiated for postpartum mastitis, Hodgkin disease, and so forth. The increased risk of breast cancer is highest when exposure occurs in children and adolescents. Therapeutic radiation after the age of 40 is not known to increase the incidence of breast cancer. Modern mammographic techniques use extremely low doses of radiation that do not pose a hazard.

PREVIOUS CANCER OF THE BREAST: Women who have previously had breast cancer have at least a 10-fold increased risk of developing a second primary breast cancer, in the same or the contralateral breast. Hormonal treatment by anti-estrogenic agents decreases the risk of a second primary cancer of the breast.

PATHOLOGY: Breast cancers are almost entirely adenocarcinomas derived from progenitor cells of the glandular epithelium. They are classified based on a combination of histologic pattern and cytologic characteristics. Breast cancers are subdivided into **in situ** (not invasive through the basement membrane of the gland) and **invasive** forms. Further subclassification into ductal, lobular, or specialized subtypes is based upon the microscopic appearance of the cancer cells, phenotypic profiling and other clinical and pathologic data.

Carcinoma In Situ of the Breast is Often a Preinvasive Lesion

The term **carcinoma in situ** *refers to the presence of apparently malignant epithelial cells that have not penetrated the basement membrane.* The name *carcinoma in situ* implies that these lesions are obligate precursors of invasive carcinoma, and histologically, the various subtypes of carcinoma *in situ* do have invasive counterparts. However, only 20% to 30% of women with biopsy-proven ductal carcinoma in situ (DCIS), but who received no further therapy, subsequently developed invasive cancer. The likelihood of an invasive cancer arising after the diagnosis of *in situ* carcinoma varies with the histologic subtype, grade, and extent of their *in situ* disease. A strong family history for breast cancer further elevates the risk for breast cancer in women with *in situ* disease.

The recognition and subsequent incidence of DCIS has risen significantly in the last three decades, with the advent of mammography. Intraductal carcinomas arise within TDLUs: dysplastic cells replace normal or hyperplastic cells and tend to spread by lumenal extension. The growth pattern and cytologic appearances of *in situ* carcinomas are used to divide these lesions into low, moderate, and high grade. Low- and moderate-grade lesions show little cell proliferation or necrosis. High-grade lesions have pronounced cytologic atypia, rapidly proliferating cells and necrosis.

DCIS-COMEDO (HIGH-GRADE) SUBTYPE: This subtype is composed of very large, pleomorphic epithelial cells with abundant cytoplasm, irregular nuclei, and often prominent, heterogeneous nucleoli. Cancer cells grow rapidly within ducts and frequently demonstrate intraductal necrosis (Fig. 19-8). Grossly, a high-grade in situ carcinoma often shows distended duct-like structures containing white, necrotic material resembling comedos (hence the term **comedocarcinoma**). The cellular necrotic debris often undergoes dystrophic calcification, resulting in multiple, microscopic calcified bodies, which can be visualized on a mammogram. These microcalcifications may assume a linear, branching appearance due to their intraductal location (see Fig. 19-8A). Even though the malignant cells do not invade through the basement membrane, this form of carcinoma in situ may incite a periductular chronic inflammatory response and the formation of new vessels in a periductular distribution (see Fig. 19-8B and C). The cancer may extend within the duct system beyond the clinically detectable tumor growth. The consequent difficulties in obtaining complete excision of the primary tumor frequently necessitates mastectomy rather than "lumpectomy."

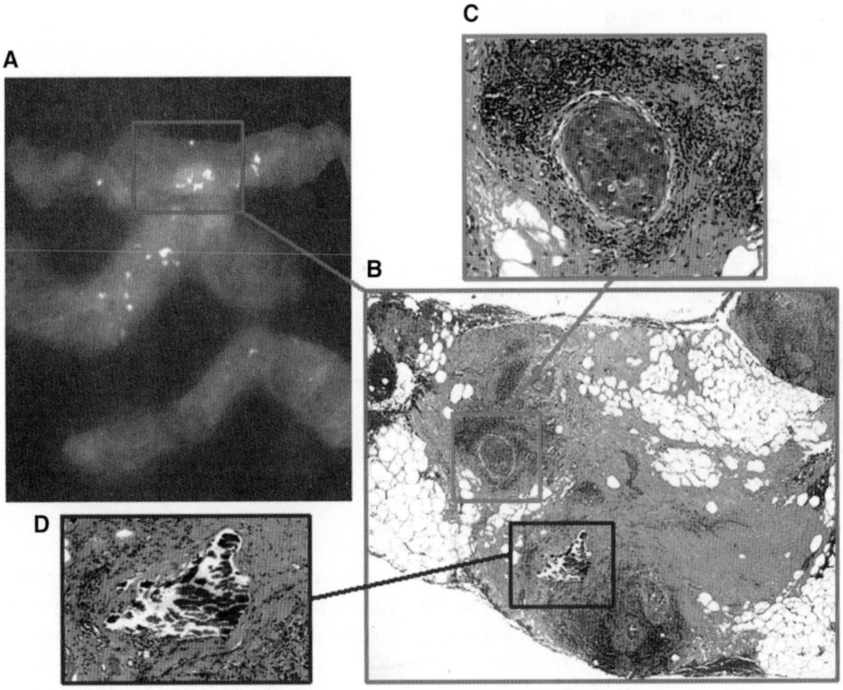

FIGURE 19-8. **Ductal carcinoma in situ. A.** Specimen radiograph of core biopsy shows linear and punctate atypical calcifications that are highly suspicious for cancer. **B.** Low-power photomicrograph showing high grade in situ ductal carcinoma. **C.** High power image of a duct expanded by in situ ductal carcinoma. **D.** High power photomicrograph of tissue calcification.

DCIS-NONCOMEDO (LOW-TO MODERATE-GRADE SUBTYPES): This tumor has multiple architectural patterns, which are often intermixed and exhibit a spectrum of cytologic atypia. The patterns are classified as micropapillary, cribriform (Fig. 19-9), and solid. The tumor cells and nuclei are smaller and more regular than those of the comedo type. Noncomedo intraductal carcinoma in situ is less likely than the comedo type to incite a desmoplastic response in the surrounding tissue. Necrosis is minimal or absent.

DCIS, treated only by biopsy, carries a 30% risk of developing invasive carcinoma in the same breast over the ensuing 20 years. The risk of cancer in the contralateral breast is also increased, but not to the same degree as with lobular carcinoma in situ (LCIS, see below). The chance of local recurrence as either *in situ* or invasive cancer is substantially greater for the comedo than noncomedo subtypes.

Data from prospective clinical trials indicate that hormone therapy reduces the risk of recurrence or progression in patients with DCIS whose tumors express the estrogen or progesterone receptor. In all, the critical prognostic factors for patients with DCIS include the size of the lesion, histopathologic subtype and grade, completeness of excision, and hormone receptor status. Each of these factors must be carefully evaluated to optimize the treatment for each patient.

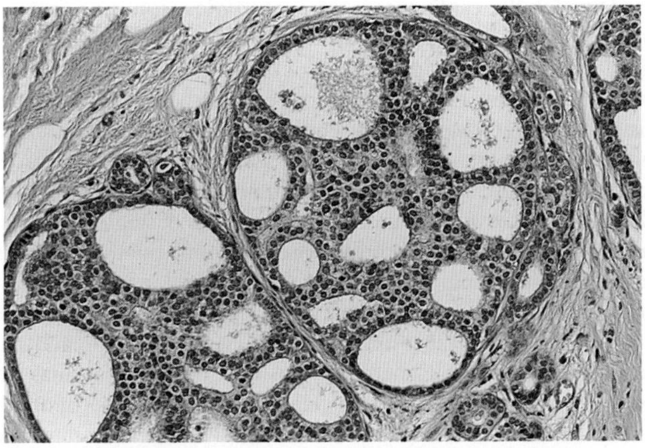

FIGURE 19-9. **Ductal carcinoma in situ-noncomedo type.** A cribriform arrangement of tumor cells is evident.

LOBULAR CARCINOMA IN SITU: LCIS, the second most common subtype of in situ breast carcinoma, also arises in TDLU. In this tumor cells tend to be smaller and more monotonous than in DCIS, with round, regular nuclei and minute nucleoli (Fig. 19-10). The malignant cells appear as solid clusters that pack and distend the terminal ducts, but not to the extent of DCIS. A more aggressive form of LCIS with larger, pleomorphic higher grade cells is known as **pleomorphic LCIS**. LCIS may also have duct microcalcifications that are detectable radiographically. The lesion does not usually incite dense fibrosis and chronic inflammation so characteristic of DCIS and so is less likely to cause a detectable mass. LCIS is often an "incidental" finding in a biopsy that was prompted by benign changes.

Lobular carcinoma is associated with truncating mutations of the E-cadherin gene. This gene encodes a transmembrane glycoprotein that functions as an adhesion molecule. E-cadherin is typically expressed by both benign breast epithelium and ductal cancers. Thus, a lack of E-cadherin expression can be used to confirm the lobular nature of neoplastic cells.

As with DCIS, 20% to 30% of women with LCIS receiving no further treatment after biopsy will develop invasive cancer within 20 years. About half of these invasive cancers will arise in the contralateral breast and may be either lobular or ductal cancers. Thus, LCIS, more than DCIS, is a harbinger of increased risk of subsequent invasive cancer in both breasts.

PAPILLARY CARCINOMA IN SITU: Papillary carcinoma in situ is much less common than either ductal or lobular carcinoma in situ. This neoplasm originates in the larger branches of the ductal system. The tumor is usually well differentiated and exhibits a papillary configuration. The neoplastic cells are typi-

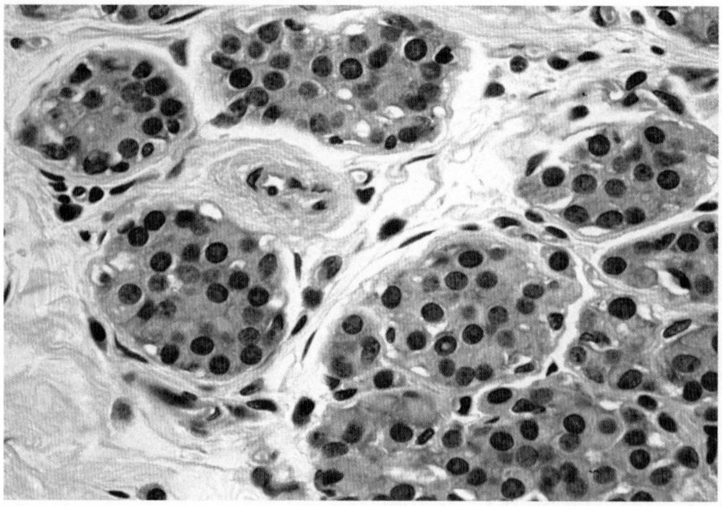

FIGURE 19-10. **Lobular carcinoma in situ.** The lumina of the terminal duct lobular units are distended by tumor cells, which exhibit round nuclei and small nucleoli. The cancer cells in the lobular form of carcinoma in situ are smaller and have less cytoplasm than those in the ductal type.

cally small and regular, making it difficult in some cases to distinguish from a benign intraductal papilloma. Papillary carcinoma in situ does not carry an increased risk of developing invasive cancer if it is completely resected.

Invasive Breast Carcinoma Exhibits Multiple Histological Types

Invasive carcinoma of the breast exhibits a morphologic spectrum, with different subtypes being associated with varying prognosis (Table 19-1).

Invasive Ductal Carcinoma

Invasive (or infiltrating) ductal carcinoma is the most common histologic type of breast cancer. Invasion is defined by the presence of tumor cells outside of the duct-lobular units and extending into breast stroma. Invasion of the stroma by malignant cells typically incites a pronounced fibroblastic proliferation (**desmoplasia**). This stromal reaction may lead to a firm, palpable mass, which may modify the contour of the breast or be visible as a dense mass lesion by mammography or ultrasonography (Fig. 19-11A). Invasive breast cancers are variably associated with calcifications. Early invasive breast cancers are typically asymptomatic, whereas later stage presentations may include large ulcerating masses, deformation of the breast, or symptoms associated with regional or distant metastases.

TABLE 19–1

Frequency of Histologic Subtypes of Invasive Breast Cancer

Subtype	Frequency (%)
Invasive ductal carcinoma	
Pure	55
Mixed with other types (including lobular)	25
Invasive lobular carcinoma (pure)	10
Medullary carcinoma (pure)	<5
Mucinous carcinoma (pure)	2
Other pure types	2
Other mixed types	1

On gross examination, the tumor is typically firm and shows irregular margins. The cut surface is pale gray and gritty and flecked with yellow, chalky streaks (see Fig. 19-11B). Microscopically, invasive ductal cancer is characterized by irregular nests and cords (tubules) of cytologically aberrant epithelial cells outside of the ductal-lobular units and located haphazardly within the stroma (see Fig. 19-11C).

Invasive ductal carcinomas are graded histologically on the basis of their similarity to benign breast glands. Well-differentiated (or low grade) cancers form abortive glands, whereas less-differentiated (higher grade) cancers may show solid sheets or individually invasive neoplastic cells. Higher grade tumors generally have abundant molecular alterations, grow the most rapidly, and may display extensive necrosis and/or apoptosis.

Paget Disease

Paget's disease is an uncommon variant of ductal carcinoma, either in situ or invasive, that extends to involve the epidermis of the nipple and areola (Fig. 19-12A). This condition usually comes to medical attention because of an eczematous change in the skin of the nipple and areola. Microscopically, large cells with clear cytoplasm (**Paget cells**) are found singly or in groups within the epidermis (see Fig. 19-12B). The prognosis of Paget disease is related to that of the underlying ductal cancer.

Invasive Lobular Carcinoma

Invasive lobular carcinoma is the second most common form of invasive breast cancer. The incidence of invasive lobular carcinoma has increased significantly since the mid-1980s, mostly in peri- and postmenopausal women. Because the amount of fibrosis is variable, the clinical presentation of invasive lobular carcinoma varies from a discrete firm mass, similar to ductal carcinoma, to a more subtle, diffuse, indurated area. Microscopically, the classic invasive lobular carcinoma consists of single strands of malignant cells infiltrating between stromal fibers, a feature termed Indian filing (Fig. 19-13A). Occasionally, a more solid or trabecular growth pattern is observed. The small, regular cells are cytologically identical to those in LCIS (see Fig. 19-10), and mitotic activity is rare. Generally, invasive lobular carcinomas express molecular markers associated with higher degrees of differentiation and are less aggressive than invasive ductal carcinomas.

Variants of classical lobular carcinoma display an overall growth pattern that is identical to that of the ordinary invasive

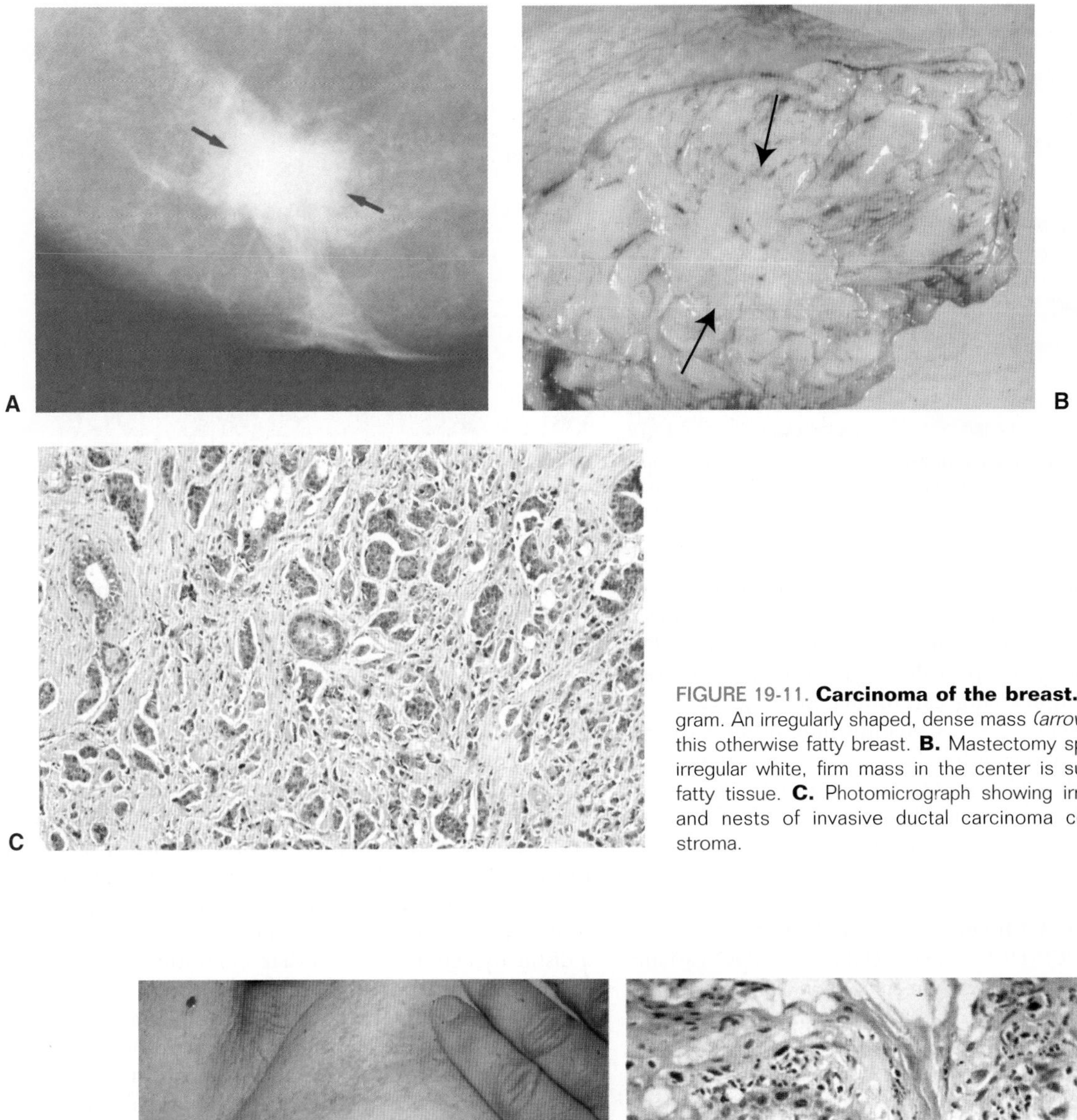

FIGURE 19-11. **Carcinoma of the breast. A.** Mammogram. An irregularly shaped, dense mass (*arrows*) is seen in this otherwise fatty breast. **B.** Mastectomy specimen. The irregular white, firm mass in the center is surrounded by fatty tissue. **C.** Photomicrograph showing irregular cords and nests of invasive ductal carcinoma cells invading stroma.

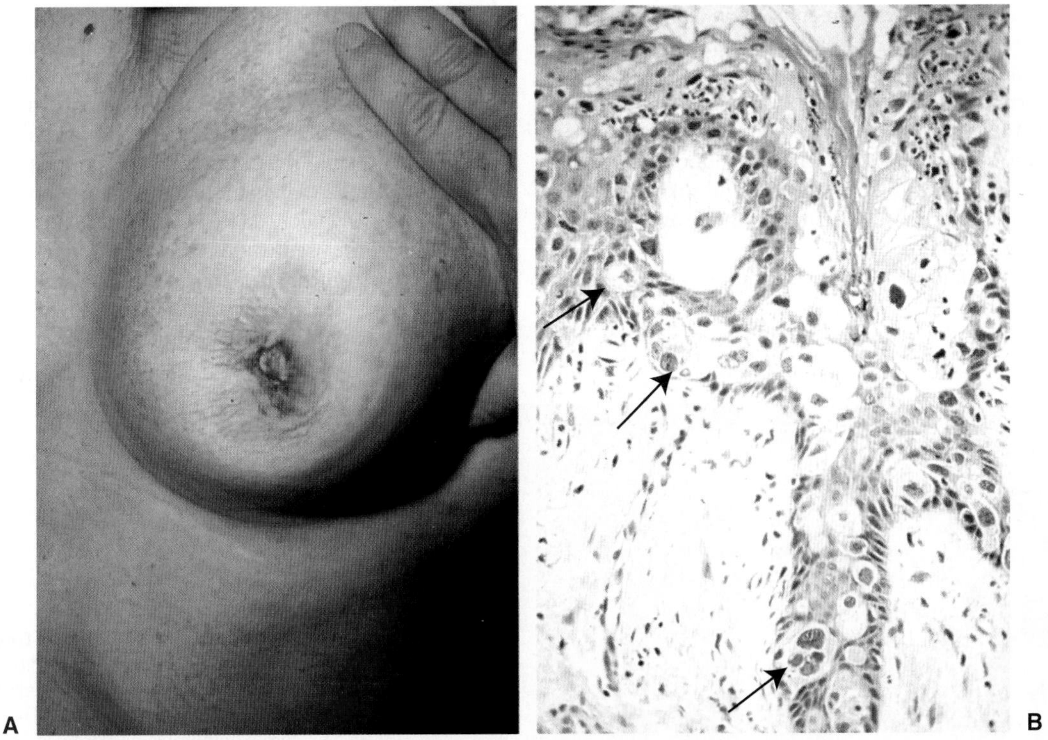

FIGURE 19-12. **Paget disease of the nipple. A**. An erythematous, scaly, and weeping "eczema" involves the nipple. **B**. The epidermis contains clusters of ductal type carcinoma cells that are larger and have more abundant pale cytoplasm (*arrows*) than surrounding keratinocytes.

A 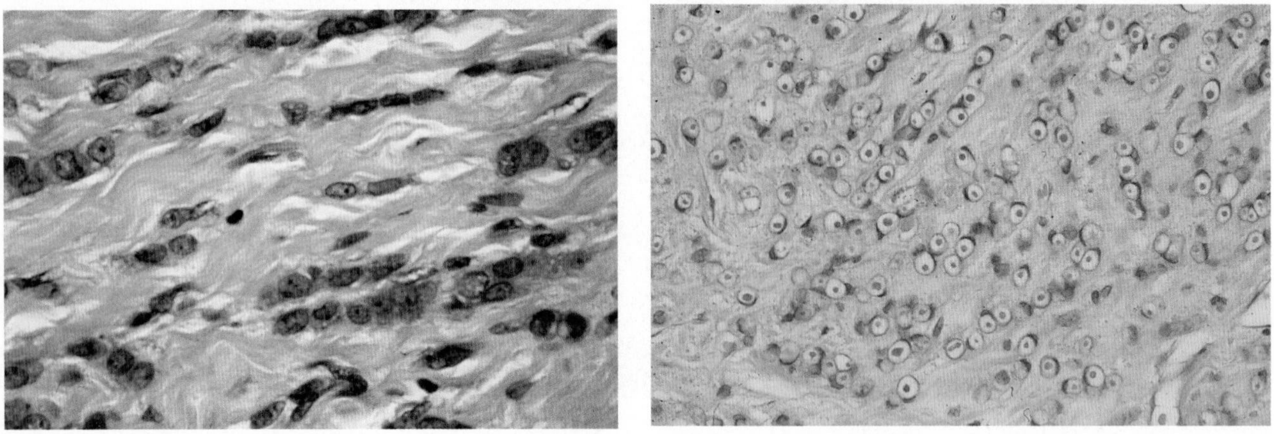 B

FIGURE 19-13. **Lobular carcinoma. A.** Invasive lobular carcinoma. In contrast to invasive ductal carcinoma, the cells of lobular carcinoma tend to form single strands that invade between collagen fibers in a single pattern. The tumor cells are similar to those seen in lobular carcinoma in situ. **B.** Signet ring carcinoma. The tumor cells contain large amounts of clear mucin.

lobular carcinoma. However, the nuclear characteristics are different. In one form, the small, regular tumor cells possess intracellular mucin. The mucin commonly compresses the nucleus to one side, giving the cell a "signet ring" appearance, hence the term **signet ring carcinoma** (see Fig. 19-13B). Another variant referred to as **pleomorphic lobular carcinoma** maintains the usual lobular growth pattern, but has more marked nuclear pleomorphism, and is more aggressive than most lobular carcinomas. *Twenty-five percent of invasive carcinomas have features of both ductal and lobular carcinoma (see Table 19-1).*

Uncommon Types Of Invasive Breast Cancer

COLLOID (MUCINOUS) CARCINOMA: This IDC variant tends to occur in older women. On cut section, colloid carcinomas have a glistening surface and mucoid consistency. Microscopically, they are comprised of small clusters of epithelial cells, occasionally forming glands, floating in pools of extracellular mucin (Fig. 19-14A). In its pure form, colloid carcinoma has a considerably better prognosis than infiltrating ductal or lobular carcinoma. When colloid differentiation is admixed with the more typical infiltrating ductal carcinoma, the prognosis is determined by the ductal component.

TUBULAR CARCINOMA: Invasive tubular carcinoma is a very well differentiated invasive ductal carcinoma that forms small ducts that invade stroma in a haphazard pattern. The individual cancer cells are typically small and mimic benign epithelium. The prognosis of pure tubular carcinoma is excellent; it is virtually always cured by excision. The incidence of regional or distant metastasis is very low with this histologic subtype.

MEDULLARY CARCINOMA: Medullary cancers present as a circumscribed, rapidly growing mass that usually lacks calcifications. Medullary carcinoma has a distinctive gross appearance, being well-circumscribed, fleshy, and pale gray. Microscopically, it is composed of sheets of highly pleomorphic cancer cells with a distinct, rounded border and surrounded by a chronic inflammatory infiltrate (see Fig. 19-14B). In spite of its highly malignant appearance, medullary carcinoma has a distinctly better prognosis than infiltrating ductal or lobular carcinomas.

METAPLASTIC CARCINOMA: This is a rare invasive variant of invasive ductal carcinoma in which the malignant cells show metaplastic changes (differentiation towards another type of epithelium or mesenchymal tissue). Such tumors may show areas of malignant squamous, fibrous, cartilaginous, or bony tissue, admixed with the malignant glandular component.

INFLAMMATORY CARCINOMA: This is a clinical, not a pathologic term used to describe a particular clinical presentation of breast cancer. It features swollen, erythematous breast tissue, and accentuation of skin structures owing to dermal plugging of lymphatic vessels by tumor cells. The lymphatics may be

A,B 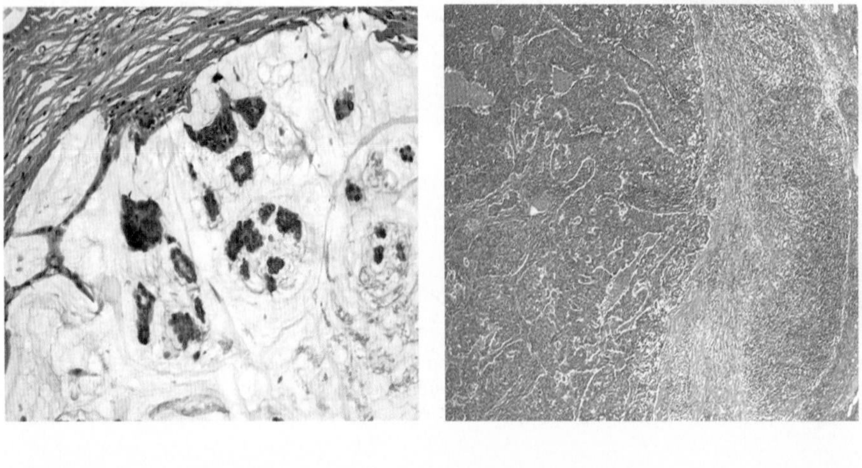

FIGURE 19-14. **A. Colloid (mucinous) carcinoma.** Clusters of malignant cells float in large pools of extracellular mucin. **B. Medullary carcinoma.** The malignant cells are pleomorphic and grow in solid sheets, forming a blunt margin. There is no gland formation. Numerous mitoses are present. The tumor is surrounded by a dense lymphocytic infiltrate.

so involved that skin drainage is blocked, causing lymphedema and thickening of the skin, so called Peau d'orange. The prominent lymphatic involvement signifies extensive lymph node and other metastases: the prognosis of inflammatory carcinoma is not good.

Breast Cancer Usually Metastasizes First to Regional Lymph Nodes

Breast cancer spreads regionally by direct extension (e.g., to chest wall) or via lymphatic channels (to regional lymph nodes, including the axillary, internal mammary, and supraclavicular nodes). Small or low grade invasive breast cancers may be localized to the breast and may be curable by complete surgical excision alone. *The axillary lymph nodes are the most common site of regional metastases.* Breast cancer patients are typically stratified into node "negative" or node "positive" based on an axillary lymph node excision. The most proximate lymph node, the "'sentinel node," is identified by prior instillation of dye or radioactive material within the breast, and is assumed to be the initial site of nodal metastasis. Further axillary lymph node dissection is performed if the sentinal node contains metastatic tumor. Prognosis is a function of the extent of lymph node metastasis.

The most common sites of distant metastases are the lung and pleura, liver, bone, adrenals, skin, and brain. Metastases commonly present as painful pathologic bone fractures. The presence of distant metastases portends poor prognosis. Unlike many tumors, breast cancers may recur and metastasize decades after a primary tumor was removed (see Chapter 5).

Key Factors Influencing Breast Cancer Prognosis Include the Extent of Metastases, Histologic Grade, and Molecular Markers of Differentiation

Breast cancer survival is strongly influenced by the stage of the tumor:

- **Stage 0:** In situ carcinoma (DCIS or LCIS)
- **Stage I:** Early invasive cancer. The tumor is <2 cm in diameter AND there are no lymph node metastases.
- **Stage II:** Tumor size >2 cm and/or (for tumors <5 cm) metastases are detected that are confined to local lymph nodes
- **Stage III:** Locally advanced cancer. Metastatic tumor has spread beyond the confines of lymph nodes into soft tissues
- **Stage IV:** Cancer has metastasized to other organs or other parts of the body.

Fortunately, with growing public awareness of breast cancer and the expanding use of screening mammography, more than half of breast cancers currently diagnosed in the United States are stage I.

Histologic Grade

In addition to the histologic subtype and stage of the cancer, the histologic grade of the primary tumor is also a useful prognostic indicator. The histologic grade includes (1) the degree of glandular differentiation, (2) the degree of nuclear atypia, and (3) the mitotic index.

Estrogen and Progesterone Receptors

Steroid receptor proteins are expressed by benign breast epithelial cells and over half of breast cancers. The receptors can bind their respective ligands (estrogen, progesterone) and induce cell growth. Women whose cancers express hormone receptors are typically older and have lower grade tumors and a better prognosis. The presence of these receptors also portends a greater probability of response to anti-estrogenic therapy or oophorectomy. These anti-estrogenic strategies may be equally effective as chemotherapy in some women, whereas with more aggressive cancers combinations of chemotherapy and anti-estrogenic therapy may also be used.

Proliferative Capacity and Ploidy

In general, increased proliferative capacity is associated with a poorer prognosis. Several methods are used to evaluate the proliferative capacity of breast cancers, including (1) mitotic index, as judged by histologic evaluation; (2) estimation of the proportion of cells in the S phase of the cell cycle by flow cytometry; and (3) immunohistochemical staining for nuclear proteins expressed in cells that are actively proliferating (Ki67 or mib1 antigens). When proliferative capacity is evaluated by flow cytometry, cell cycle analysis can also detect the presence of aneuploid cell populations. Aneuploidy, which is found in two thirds of breast cancers, is also associated with a poorer prognosis.

HER2 (erbB-2) Oncogene Alterations

Overexpression of *HER2/neu* is identified in 10% to 35% of primary breast tumors and is mostly attributable to gene amplification. Amplification or overexpression of *HER2/neu* has also been described in cancers of the lung, ovary, and stomach. Overexpression can be determined by immunohistologic detection of the c-erbB2 protein on the cell membrane (19-15A) or by analysis of the *HER2/neu* gene using fluorescent in situ hybridization (FISH) (see Fig. 19-15B). Patients whose tumors demonstrate *HER2* gene amplification benefit from therapy with a monoclonal antibody that selectively binds to the extracellular domain of the protein.

Other Potential Prognostic Factors Related to Invasion and Metastasis

A number of enzymes, cell adhesion molecules, and angiogenic markers have been reported to bear some relationship to breast cancer metastasis and recurrence. These include stromelysin, urokinase-plasminogen activator, laminin receptor, and high vascular density. However, these markers have demonstrated only limited predictive power, and their significance remains to be established. Recent studies have reported that the "gene expression signature" of a tumor can be a significant predictor of survival in breast cancer. Microarray analysis of candidate genes encoding tumor suppressor proteins, growth factors, and hormonal receptors, together with genes expressed primarily by B and T cells of infiltrating lymphocytes, have permitted the separation of patients with stage I and stage II disease into either good or poor prognostic groups, regardless of the lymph node status of the patient.

Improved Therapies Have Led to Substantially Better Survival in Breast Cancer

One of the most significant advancements in the treatment of this cancer was the shift from the disfiguring radical mastectomy (en bloc removal of the breast, all axillary lymph nodes, and underlying chest wall muscles) to the modified radical mastectomy. For most patients, even more limited surgical

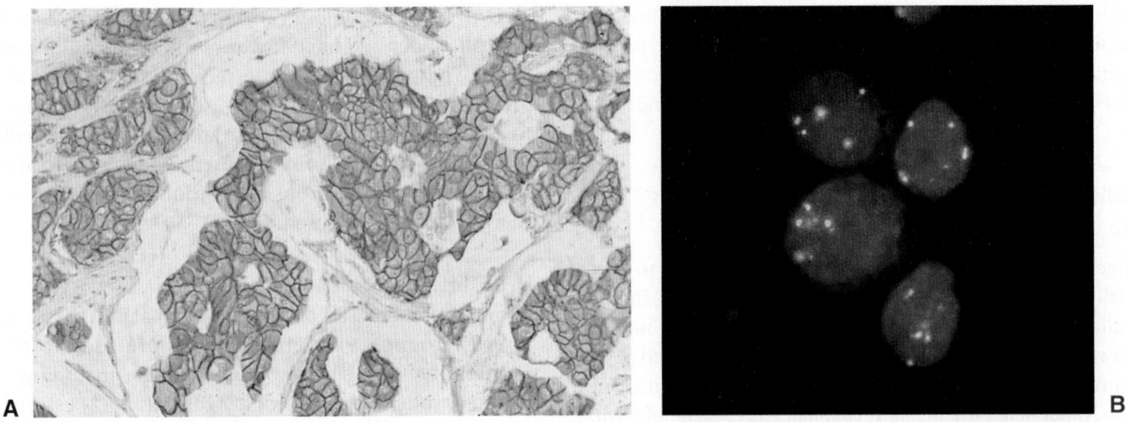

FIGURE 19-15. ***HER2/neu* abnormalities in a breast cancer. A.** Immunoperoxide staining of an invasive ductal carcinoma shows over expression of the *HER2* (erbB-2) protein. **B.** Fluorescence in situ hybridization (FISH) methodology identifies the gene copies of *HER2* (erbB-2) in cancer cells. The *HER2* probe is red, and a normal cell should have 2 copies. More than 2 copies indicates *HER2* gene amplification. The green probe identifies the centromeric region of chromosome 17.

approaches have supplanted modified radical mastectomy, including lumpectomy, quadrantectomy, and sentinel node or limited axillary lymph node dissection. In selected patients with bulky disease, tumors can be pretreated with neoadjuvant therapy, making the patient eligible for more limited surgical approaches.

Hormonal therapy, chemotherapy, and radiation therapy have become increasingly important partners in the limited-surgery approach. In general, patients with the greatest risk for mortality stand to gain the most from hormonal treatment and/or chemotherapy. Clinical studies have shown that the benefit of routinely adding chemotherapy to surgery in the treatment of all stage I patients is marginal and not without morbidity. Thus, there is an impetus to identify specific subsets of women who might particularly benefit from chemotherapy in addition to surgery.

Targeted molecular therapy has emerged as an important tool in controlling breast cancer. Notably, a monoclonal antibody that binds the extracellular portion of the *HER-2* (erbB-2) transmembrane protein and blocks downstream signal activation has been used effectively to treat cancers in which overexpression of *HER-2* is detected.

Early Detection of Breast Cancer has Greatly Enhanced Survival

Regular self- and physician-examination of the breasts, adherence to recommended guidelines for screening mammograms, and periodic physician checkups have been estimated to decrease mortality from breast cancer by about 30%. Women with strong risk factors are likely to benefit the most from vigilant screening. Preventive agents are increasingly given to women in the significant risk category to reduce their lifetime incidence of invasive breast cancer.

There is a significant difference in survival between women with stage 0 or I disease and those with axillary node metastases (stage II). Thus, 5-year survival with stage 0 or I breast cancer approaches 100%. For stage II, the comparable statistic is 80% to 90%, depending on the number of lymph nodes involved. Within stage II disease, survival decreases as the number of involved axillary nodes increases. Women with advanced local or regional disease (stage III) can be palliated but usually not cured. The prognosis for women with distant metastases (stage IV) is poor in terms of survival, but palliative treatment may significantly prolong life.

Cancer of the Male Breast is Distinctly Uncommon

Cancer in the male breast accounts for less than 1% of all cases of breast cancer. As in women, the most common subtype is infiltrating ductal carcinoma. Because there is less fat in the male breast, these tumors more often invade the musculature of the chest wall. For cancers of the same stage, however, the prognosis for males is similar to that of the female. Predisposing factors for the development of breast cancer in men are largely unknown. Mutations of the *BRCA2* gene have been associated with an increased risk of male breast cancers.

Phyllodes Tumor

Phyllodes tumor of the breast is a proliferation of stromal elements accompanied by a benign growth of ductal structures (Fig. 19-16). These tumors usually occur in women between 30 and 70 years of age, with a peak in the fifth decade. The original term for this tumor, **cystosarcoma phyllodes**, implies malignant behavior, although only a minority of these tumors are capable of invasion and metastasis. Thus, current terminology refers to **phyllodes tumor**, with the additional designation of benign or malignant.

PATHOLOGY: Phyllodes tumors resemble fibroadenomas in their overall architecture and the presence of glandular and stromal elements. Like fibroadenoma, benign phyllodes tumor is sharply circumscribed, and the cut surface is firm, glistening, and grayish white. Benign and malignant phyllodes tumor are similar in gross appearance. Average sizes today are ~5 cm in diameter.

Microscopically, the stroma of a benign phyllodes tumor is hypercellular and has mitotic activity. Differentiation from fibroadenoma is by the histologic and cytologic characteristics of

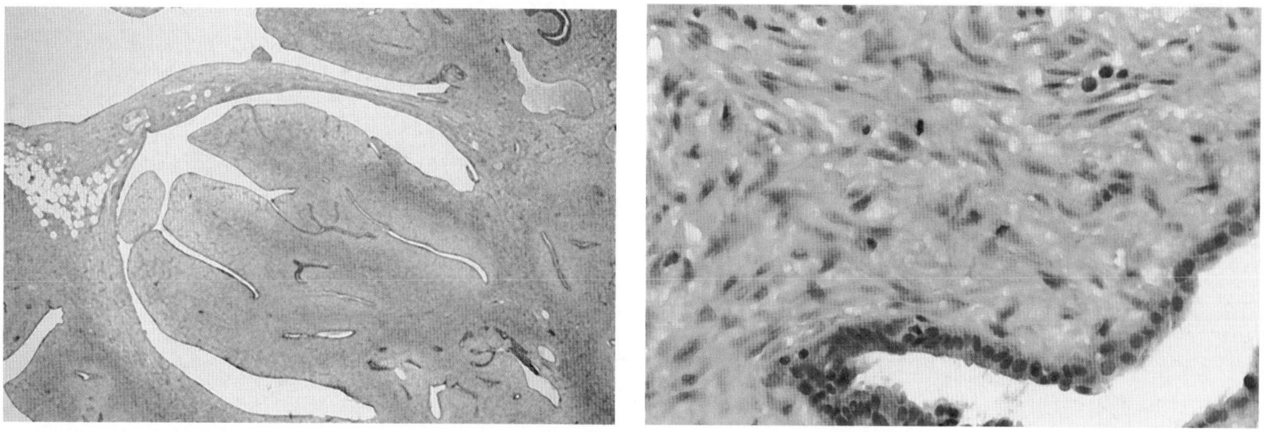

FIGURE 19-16. **Phyllodes tumor: A.** A polypoid tumor with a leaflike pattern expands a duct. **B.** The stromal component adjacent to ductal epithelium is similar to a fibroadenoma, but is more cellular. The residual ductal structure is benign.

the stromal component. By the same token, it is the appearance of the stromal component that distinguishes malignant phyllodes tumors: these have an obviously sarcomatous stroma with abundant mitotic activity, and the stromal component is increased out of proportion to the benign duct elements. They are usually poorly circumscribed and locally invasive. Malignant tumors may exhibit various sarcomatous tissue types, such as malignant fibrous histiocytoma, chondrosarcoma, and osteosarcoma.

CLINICAL FEATURES: Benign phyllodes tumors are adequately treated by local excision. The initial treatment of a malignant phyllodes tumor is wide excision if the tumor is small or a simple mastectomy if the tumor is large. An axillary lymph node dissection is not indicated. Malignant phyllodes tumors tend to recur locally, and 15% eventually metastasize to both distant sites and axillary lymph nodes.

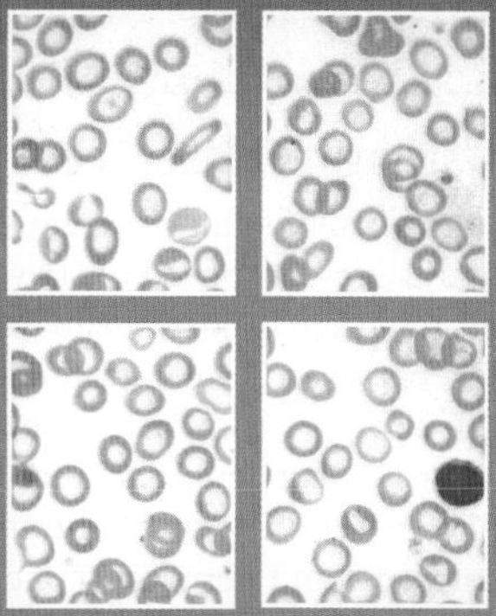

20 Hematopathology

Roland Schwarting
Steven McKenzie
Raphael Rubin

BONE AND NORMAL MYELOPOIETIC CELLS

Embryology

Hematopoiesis, or blood cell formation, first occurs in the fetal yolk sac. Erythrocyte formation shifts after the third week of embryogenesis to liver and spleen, where the cells contain fetal hemoglobins rather than embryonic hemoglobins produced during the yolk sac phase. At term, erythropoiesis in the liver and spleen has ceased, and marrow erythropoiesis has become fully established.

From birth until 4 years of age, all bone cavities are densely packed with hematopoietic tissue. Thereafter, the size of the bone cavities outgrows the volume required for hematopoiesis. By adulthood, fat occupies most of the available space. The marrow in the axial skeleton continues to be active and full of "red marrow" until old age, when resorption of cancellous bone enlarges marrow cavities and leads to further replacement by fat.

Local expansion of red (cellular) marrow and reactivation of peripheral yellow marrow allow the hematopoietic system to meet demands for increased blood cell formation. Reactivation of hepatic and splenic hematopoiesis rarely occurs during adult life. *The finding of significant extramedullary hematopoiesis in soft tissue sites usually suggests a clonal (malignant) disorder, rather than a reactive one.*

Bone Marrow

Hematopoietic Cells Derive From Multipotent Stem Cells

Bone marrow consists of a complex network of solid cords separated by sinusoids (Fig. 20-1). The cords are composed of stromal and hematopoietic cells, knitted together by extracellular matrix. The semipermeable barrier between sinusoids and cords consists of an endothelial cell layer, a thin basement membrane, and an outer interrupted layer of reticular adventitial cells. These reticular cells branch extensively throughout the cords and provide a scaffold for stromal and hematopoietic cells. Other stromal cells include macrophages, endothelial cells, lymphocytes, and fibroblasts.

Within the cords are islands of erythroblasts, usually located in concentric rings around a macrophage (inappropriately termed a **"nurse cell"**), which stores excess iron. These islands lie close to sinusoid walls, as do megakaryocytes. Granulocyte precursors are located deeper in the cords.

STEM CELLS: These undifferentiated cells are a self-perpetuating pool, in which differentiation and exit are balanced by self-renewal (Fig. 20-2). Stem cells are small mononuclear cells that are difficult to identify by observation by observation. They are semidormant (noncycling) that undergo differentiation to progenitor cells of specific cell lines as needed. When marrow elements are injected into irradiated mice, stem cells form visible colonies in the spleen (**colony-forming unit, spleen; CFU-S**). In

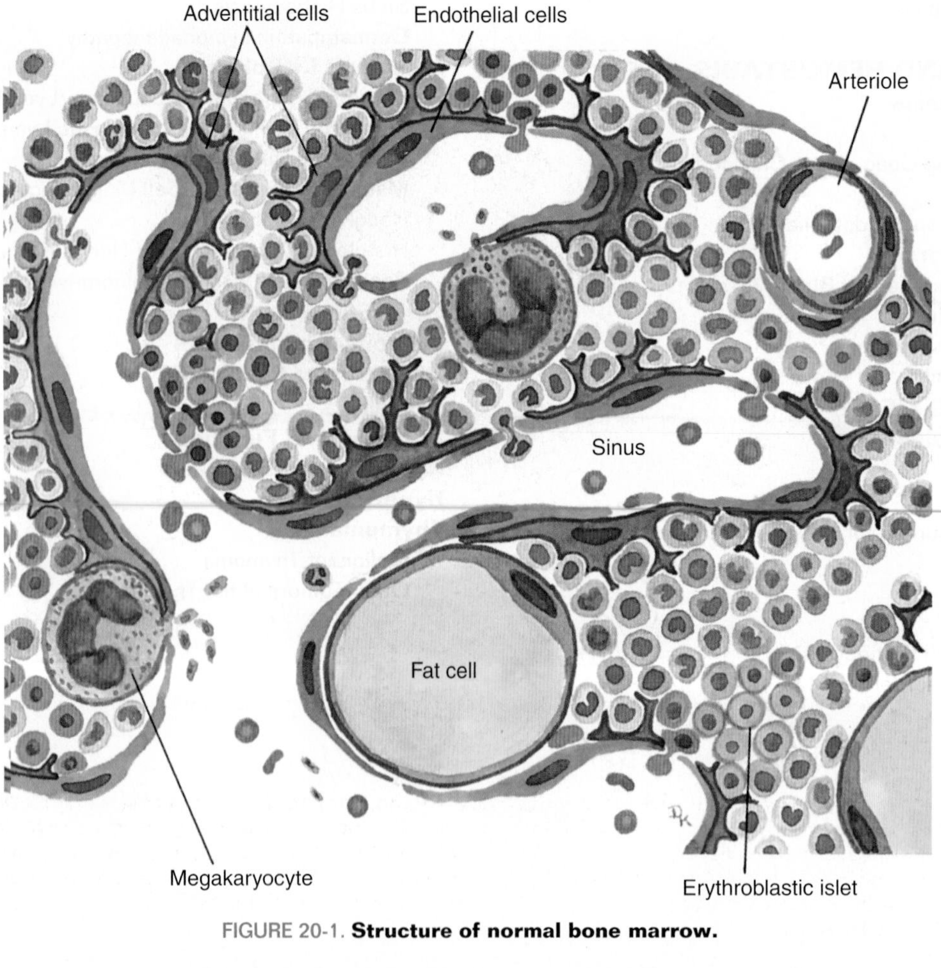

FIGURE 20-1. **Structure of normal bone marrow.**

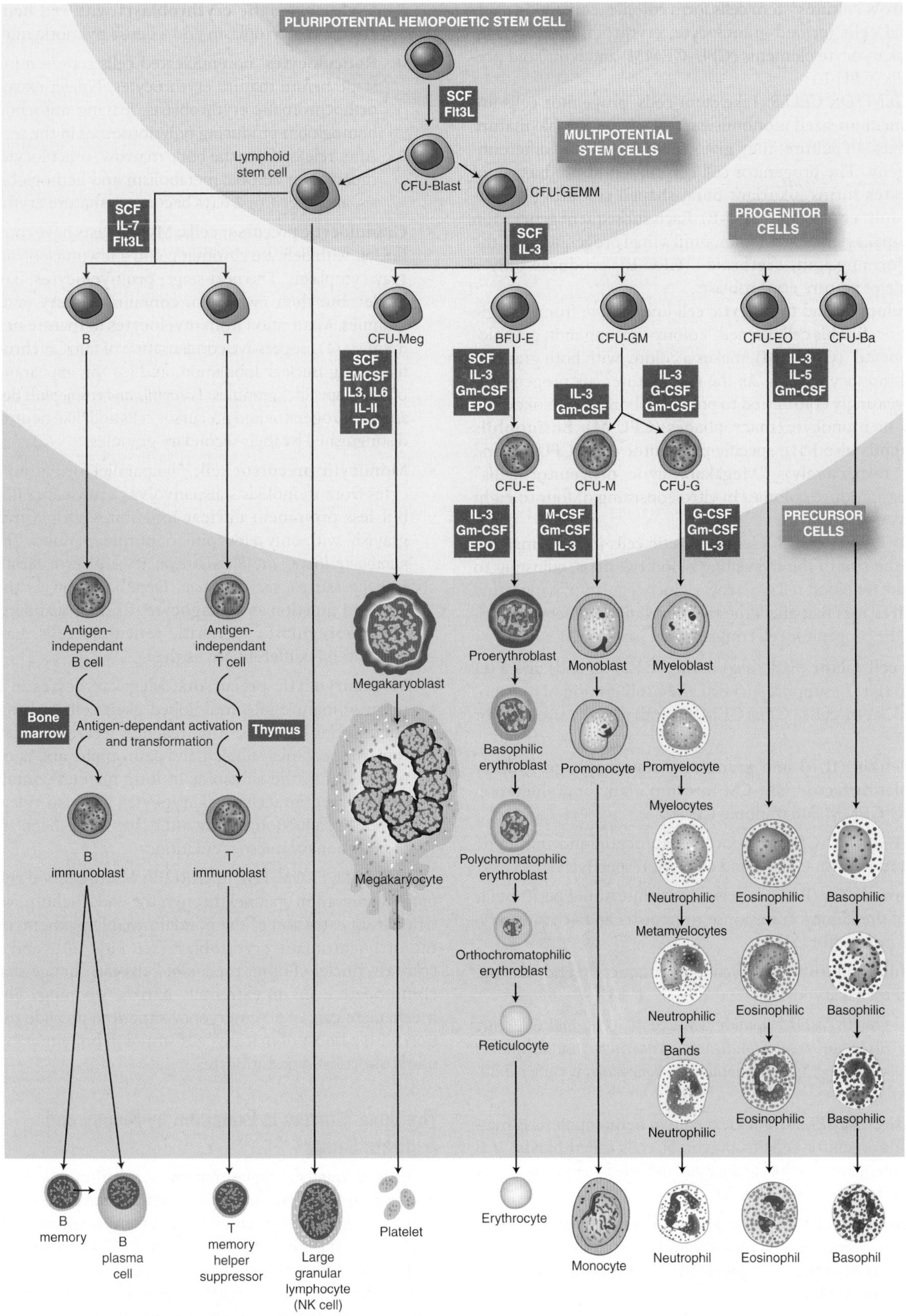

FIGURE 20-2. **Cellular differentiation and maturation of the lymphoid and myeloid components of the hematopoietic system.** Only the precursor cells (blasts and maturing cells) are identifiable by light microscopic evaluation of the bone marrow. BFU = burst-forming unit; CFU = colony-forming unit [Ba = basophils; E = erythroid; Eo = eosinophils; G= polymorphonuclear leukocytes; GM = granulocyte-monocyte; M= monocyte/macrophages; Meg = megakaryocytic]; EPO = erythropoietin; GM-CSF = granulocyte-macrophage colony stimulating factor; IL = interleukin; NK = natural killer; SCF = stem cell facor; TPO = thrombopoietin.

bone marrow cultures, stem cells form colonies containing **multipotential cells** termed granulocyte, erythroid, macrophage, and megakaryocyte elements (**CFU-GEMM**) and lymphoid precursor cells (**CFU-L**) .

PROGENITOR CELLS: Like stem cells, progenitor cells are small to medium-sized mononuclear cells that resemble mature lymphocytes. In culture, they give rise to colonies of differentiated progeny. The progenitor cell committed to production of **erythrocytes** forms luxuriant burst-shaped colonies ("**burst-forming unit, erythroid**" (**BFU-E**). Each subsequent generation of BFU-E makes smaller colonies, until a final progenitor cell, the "colony-forming unit, erythroid" (**CFU-E**), produces only a small clone of mature erythroblasts.

Granulocytic and **monocytic** cell lines derive from a single progenitor cell. This cell, named "colony-forming unit, granulocyte-monocyte" (**CFU-GM**), makes a colony with both granulocytic and monocytic cells. As the cell matures, its progeny become increasingly committed to polymorphonuclear leukocytes (**CFU-G**) or monocyte/macrophages (**CFU-M**). **Eosinophils** and **basophils** also have specific progenitor cells (**CFU-Eo** and **CFU-Ba**, respectively). "Megakaryocytic progenitor cells" (**CFU-Meg**) produce colonies in vitro consisting of four to eight megakaryocytes.

GROWTH FACTORS: Hematopoietic cells in bone marrow maintain the size of the circulating blood cell mass, adjusting to compensate for blood cell senescence. Such regulation is mediated by growth factors that affect the rate of cellular proliferation, primarily in the progenitor cell compartment (see Fig. 20-2).

- **Stem cell factor** (SCF; also named c-KIT ligand) and **Flt3 ligand** (Flt3L) support survival and proliferation of pluripotential stem cells, CFU-GEMM, and various progenitor cells.
- **Interleukin (IL)-3** and **granulocyte-macrophage -colony stimulating factor (GM-CSF)** are important for proliferation of CFU-GEMM and multiple CFUs.
- **G-CSF and M-CSF** promote granulocytic and moncytic maturation from CFU-G and CFU-M, respectively.
- **Erythropoietin (EPO)** is released by interstitial peritubular cells of the kidney in response to hypoxia and activates erythroid progenitor cells.
- **Thrombopoietin (TPO)** facilitates production and maturation of megakaryocytes.

Several growth factors, notably GM-CSF, G-CSF, and EPO, are widely used to treat conditions requiring stimulation of hematopoiesis (e.g., postchemotherapy, bone marrow transplantation, renal failure; see below).

PRECURSOR CELLS: The next step in hematopoiesis is maturation of progenitor cells to precursor cells called **blasts**. *It is only at the precursor stage and beyond that the cells are morphologically recognizable in terms of their lineage.*

- **Erythroid precursor cells**: The **proerythroblast** is a large cell with intense blue cytoplasm and a round homogeneous nucleus, containing a few nucleoli. The proerythroblast matures sequentially:

  1. **Basophilic erythroblasts** without nucleoli.
  2. **Polychromatic erythroblasts** with grayish cytoplasm (due to hemoglobin synthesis) and a nucleus with coarsely clumped chromatin.
  3. **Orthochromatic erythroblasts** with red hemoglobin-containing cytoplasm and a dense pyknotic nucleus.
  4. **Reticulocytes**, non-nucleated cells representing the last stage before mature erythrocytes. Nuclei extruded from orthochromatic erythroblasts, leaving mitochondria and hemoglobin-producing polyribosomes in the reticulocyte. After release from the bone marrow, reticulocytes lose the capacity for aerobic metabolism and hemoglobin synthesis, and after 1 or 2 days becomes a mature erythrocyte.

- **Granulocytic precursor cells: Myeloblasts** have round to oval nuclei, with delicate chromatin and a few nucleoli and a blue-gray cytoplasm. The next stage, **promyelocytes**, have similar nuclei, but their cytoplasm contains primary (azurophilic) granules. Maturation from **myelocytes** to mature **neutrophils** involves (1) progressive condensation of nuclear chromatin, (2) increasing nuclear lobulation, and (3) the appearance of secondary (specific) granules. *Basophils and eosinophils* derive from specific progenitor and precursor cells and, like neutrophils, are distinguished by their secondary granules.
- **Monocytic precursor cell:** The parallel formation of monocytes from monoblasts also involves a nuclear condensation, but less prominent nuclear lobation. Cytoplasm becomes grayish, with only a few pink or purple granules. *Then, after a monocyte leaves the bloodstream it becomes a member of the mononuclear phagocyte system.* Depending on its tissue location and function as a **phagocyte** (fixed or wandering) or an **immunoregulator** (dendritic reticulum cells, Langerhans cells), it may differentiate further.
- **Megakaryocytic precursors:** Megakaryocytes in the bone marrow mature into multilobed giant cells by a number of endomitotic divisions. After reaching a certain ploidy, the cytoplasm becomes stippled and azurophilic and is eventually released into the sinusoids in long platelet-containing ribbons. Some intact megakaryocytes are also released, and platelet production occurs after they have been trapped in the pulmonary microcirculation.

RELEASE FROM THE MARROW: Mature blood cells form a narrow migration channel through the endothelium, which participates in extrusion of the nondeformable pyknotic nucleus of the orthochromatic erythroblast (see Figs. 20-1 and 20-2). By contrast, nuclei of other precursor cells can change shape to accommodate even an extremely narrow opening. The release mechanism can, in an emergency situation, provide the circulation with a boost of mature cells stored in bone marrow, particularly short-lived granulocytes.

The Bone Marrow Is Examined by Biopsy and Aspirate Smear

Cellular elements of bone marrow are commonly evaluated by needle biopsy and marrow aspiration from the posterior iliac crest. Marrow can also be obtained in infants from anterior tibia and in adults from the sternum. Examination of biopsy sections allows evaluation of the amount of hematopoietic elements and marrow architecture (Fig. 20-3A), whereas specific precursor cells are identified in smears of the aspirate (see Fig. 20-3B). In a normal adult, about half of the biopsy surface area is fat cells and half is active hematopoietic tissue. The proportion of hematopoietic cells is called the **cellularity**. Cellularity is high in children and lower in the elderly.

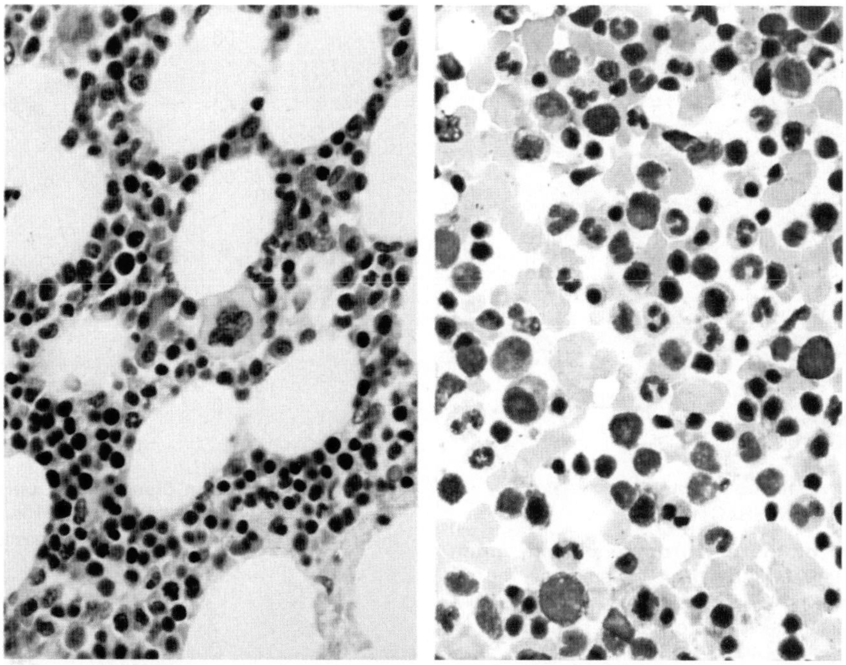

FIGURE 20-3. **Normal bone marrow. A.** A photomicrograph of a tissue section shows the normal relationship (1:1) of cellular elements to fat, a normal myeloid-to-erythroid ratio, and a megakaryocyte in the center. **B.** A smear of the bone marrow aspirate from the same patient demonstrates normal hematopoietic elements and varying stages of differentiation.

Normal proportions of granulocytic precursors (myeloid cells) and erythroblastic precursors (erythroid cells), or the **myeloid-to-erythroid (M:E) ratio,** vary from 2:1 and 5:1 (Table 20-1). Blast cells are few, and the most mature cells are plentiful. Changes in this distribution are designated as a "**left shift**" (toward immaturity) or a "**right shift**" (toward maturity). There are usually 2 to 5 megakaryocytes per high-power field. Normal bone marrow contains fewer than 3% plasma cells, up to 20% lymphocytes, and only rare mast cells and macrophages.

Evaluation of bone marrow iron stores uses Prussian blue stain, which highlights blue hemosiderin granules in macrophages and in the interstitium. Minute hemosiderin granules are found in the cytoplasm of 10% of erythroid precursors (**sideroblasts**).

TABLE 20-1

Normal Adult Bone Marrow (Age 18–70 Years)

Fat: cell ratio, 50:50 ± 15%
Myeloid-to-erythroid ratio, 2:1 to 5:1
Cell distribution (% surface area) Fat cells, 35%–65% Erythroid series, 10%–20% Granulocytic (myeloid) series, 40%–65%
Megakaryocytes, 2–5/high-power field
Plasma cells, <3% of nucleated cells
Lymphocytes, <20% of nucleated cells
No fibrosis

RED BLOOD CELLS

Normal Structure and Function

Red blood cells (RBCs), or erythrocytes, transport oxygen to tissues. Mature erythrocytes are nonnucleated 7- to 8-μm biconcave disks, similar in size to the nucleus of a small lymphocyte (Fig. 20-4). On Wright-stained blood smears, they are round with reddish, eosinophilic cytoplasm. The red color is imparted by hemoglobin, their main cytoplasmic component. Because of their biconcave disk shape, RBCs display an area of central pallor approximately 1/3 the diameter of the cell. Erythrocytes are released from the

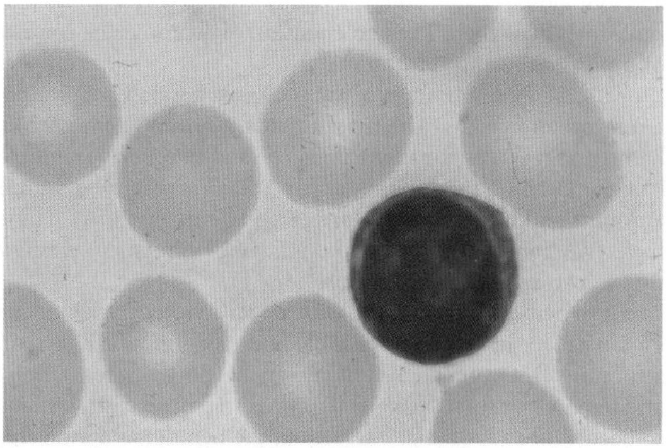

FIGURE 20-4. **Normal red blood cells** are approximately the same size as the nucleus of a lymphocyte.

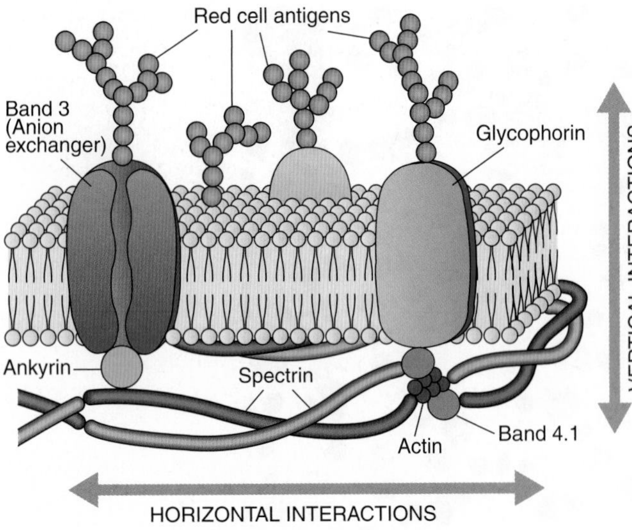

FIGURE 20-5. **Structure of the erythrocyte plasma membrane.** The membrane is stabilized by a number of interactions. The two vertical ones are spectrin-ankyrin–band 3 and spectrin-protein 4.1– glycophorin. The two horizontal interactions are spectrin heterodimer assembly and spectrin-actin–protein 4.1.

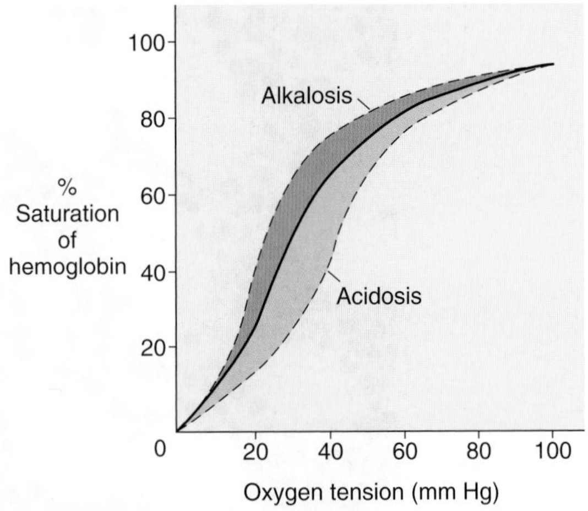

FIGURE 20-6. **Oxygen dissociation curve of hemoglobin.** With decreasing pH (acidosis) the oxygen affinity declines (shifts right); with increasing pH (alkalosis) the affinity increases (shifts left).

marrow as reticulocytes, which are larger and have more diffusely basophilic gray cytoplasm than mature RBCs. Reticulocyte polychromatophilia is due to their higher content of ribosomes, since these cells still synthesize hemoglobin.

RBC membranes are attached to an underlying cytoskeletal network (Fig. 20-5). Transmembrane proteins that act as receptors, channels, and anchors for other membrane components, and the underlying cytoskeleton are inserted into the lipid bilayer. *Addition of carbohydrate groups to some membrane proteins leads to formation of different red cell antigen groups.* The erythrocyte cytoskeleton contains interconnected spectrin dimers and other stabilizing proteins (ankyrin, actin, band 4.1), which allows for the inherent deformability of RBCs. *Changes in this membrane-cytoskeletal unit lead to increased cell rigidity and premature destruction of circulating erythrocytes.*

Hemoglobin accounts for the oxygen-carrying capacity of RBCs. Each hemoglobin molecule contains four heme groups and four globin chains, and, when fully saturated, transports four molecules of oxygen. The heme portion of the molecule consists of a porphyrin ring (protoporphyrin IX), with one ferrous ion (Fe^{2+}). The globin portion of the molecule has pairs of two different protein chains. The most abundant normal hemoglobin, hemoglobin A, contains two alpha (α) and two beta (β) globin chains. Other hemoglobins are normally present in minor amounts and include hemoglobin F and hemoglobin A_2. These have two gamma (γ) and two delta (δ) globin chains, respectively, instead of β globin chains.

Each heme group interacts with a hydrophobic pocket of one globin chain, and the entire molecule has a globular tertiary structure. Deoxygenated hemoglobin has low oxygen affinity and requires increased oxygen tension for heme–oxygen binding to occur. After this initial interaction, the hemoglobin molecule undergoes a conformational change that facilitates subsequent oxygen binding to the 3 remaining heme groups. The progressive increase in oxygen affinity is reflected in the sigmoid shape of the oxygen dissociation curve (Fig. 20-6). The slope of the oxygen dissociation curve can be shifted to the right by acidosis or increased 2,3-diphosphoglycerate (2,3-DPG) (a product of an alternate pathway of glycolysis), thus enhancing tissue oxygen delivery. Alkalosis shifts the curve to the left, and results in increased oxygen binding.

The average life span of the erythrocyte in the blood is 120 days. Changes in membrane proteins and phospholipids appear in aged red cells and are likely signals for erythrocyte removal by mononuclear phagocytes.

The erythroid component of the blood is best analyzed by a complete blood count (CBC) plus microscopic examination of a blood smear (Table 20-2). The CBC measures hemoglobin (Hgb), red blood cell (RBC) count, and mean corpuscular volume (MCV). From these values, additional parameters can be calculated including **hematocrit** (Hct = MCV × RBC), **mean corpuscular hemoglobin** (MCH = Hgb/RBC), and **mean corpuscular hemoglobin concentration** (MCHC = Hgb/Hct). The degree of variation in RBC size or red cell distribution width (RDW) is also derived. Reticulocytes can be accurately quantitated using supravital dyes which stain their cytoplasmic ribosome aggregates.

Anemia

Anemia is a reduction in circulating erythrocyte mass. A diagnosis of anemia is made by demonstrating a reduction in hemoglobin, hematocrit, or RBC count. Anemia leads to decreased oxygen transport by the blood and ultimately tissue hypoxia.

Anemias are Classified by Morphology or Pathophysiology

Anemias are classified by morphology or pathophysiology.

Morphologic classification of anemia is based on erythrocyte appearance, as determined by automated blood counters and microscopic evaluation of a blood smear. RBC size (gener-

TABLE 20-2

Complete Blood Count (CBC): Normal Adult Values

Erythrocytes	
Hemoglobin	Male, 14–18 g/dL Female, 12–16 g/dL
Hematocrit	Male, 40%–54% Female, 35%–47%
Red blood cell (RBC) count	Male, 4.5–6 × $10^6/\mu L$ Female, 4–5.5 × $10^6/\mu L$
Reticulocytes	0.5%–2.5%
Indices	
Mean corpuscular volume	82–100 μm^3
Mean corpuscular hemoglobin	27–34 pg
Mean corpuscular hemoglobin concentration	32%–36%

Leukocytes

	Absolute Count/μL	Differential Count (%)
White blood cells (WBC)	4000–11,000	
Neutrophil granulocytes	1800–7000	50–60
Neutrophil bands	0–700	2–4
Lymphocytes	1500–4000	30–40
Monocytes	0–800	1–9
Basophils	0–200	0–1
Eosinophils	0–450	0–3

Platelets

Quantitative normal value: 150,000–400,000/μL

Qualitative estimation on smear: Number of platelets/oil immersion field × 10,000 = estimated platelet count

Normal ratio of RBC to platelets = 15:1 to 20:1

TABLE 20-3

Morphologic Classification of Anemia

Macrocytic

Megaloblastic	Hypothyroidism
Alcohol use	Reticulocytosis
Liver disease	Primary bone marrow disease

Microcytic

Iron deficiency
Thalassemias
Sideroblastic

Normocytic

Anemia of chronic disease/inflammation
Anemia of renal disease
Acute blood loss

ally measured by analyzers), is reflected in the MCV, which allows division of anemias into three groups: (1) **microcytic** (decreased MCV), (2) **normocytic,** and (3) **macrocytic** (increased MCV) (Table 20-3). Blood smear analyis may show abnormally shaped RBCs (**poikilocytes**) which can be seen in a wide variety of anemias. The particular type of poikilocyte can aid in diagnosis (Fig. 20-7).

Pathophysiologic classification of anemia includes 4 major groups (Table 20-4):

1. **Acute blood loss**
2. **Decreased production** of red cells by the bone marrow, either by **stem cell and progenitor-cell defects**
3. **Ineffective hematopoiesis** with reduced release of erythrocytes from marrow
4. **Increased destruction** of RBCs after release from the bone marrow, either **intracorpuscular** or **extracorpuscular**

Anemias associated with increased destruction of red cells are usually characterized by increased numbers of circulating reticulocytes (**reticulocytosis**)which allows distinction from other groups.

CLINICAL FEATURES: In the face of anemia, the body has several compensatory mechanisms, to enhance oxygen delivery to tissues.

- Increased cardiac output
- Increased respiratory rate
- Shunting of blood flow to provide increased tissue perfusion of vital organs
- Decreased hemoglobin–oxygen affinity
- Increased marrow erythrocyte production due to EPO stimulation

Clinical signs and symptoms (tachycardia, shortness of breath, and systolic murmurs) may develop secondary to these compensatory processes. If anemia is sufficiently severe (i.e., hemoglobin levels below 7 g/dL), tissue hypoxia is uncompensated and additional clinical findings may include easy fatigability, faintness, angina and dyspnea on exertion.

Acute Blood Loss Leads to Normocytic Normochromic Anemia

Acute anemia reflects the loss of blood from the intravascular compartment.

PATHOLOGY AND CLINICAL FEATURES: Initial manifestations of acute blood loss reflect volume depletion and decreased tissue perfusion. Since whole blood is lost, the severity of the anemia may not be appreciated initially. Within 24 to 48 hours after significant hemorrhage, however, fluid is mobilized from extravascular locations into the intravascular space to restore overall blood volume. This is when the extent of the anemia becomes apparent, since red cell replacement is not as rapid. If the underlying bleeding is stopped, EPO-driven bone marrow erythroid hyperplasia will gradually correct the anemia. Examination of blood smear reveals no specific red cell abnormalities, but polychromasia is seen during the recovery phase.

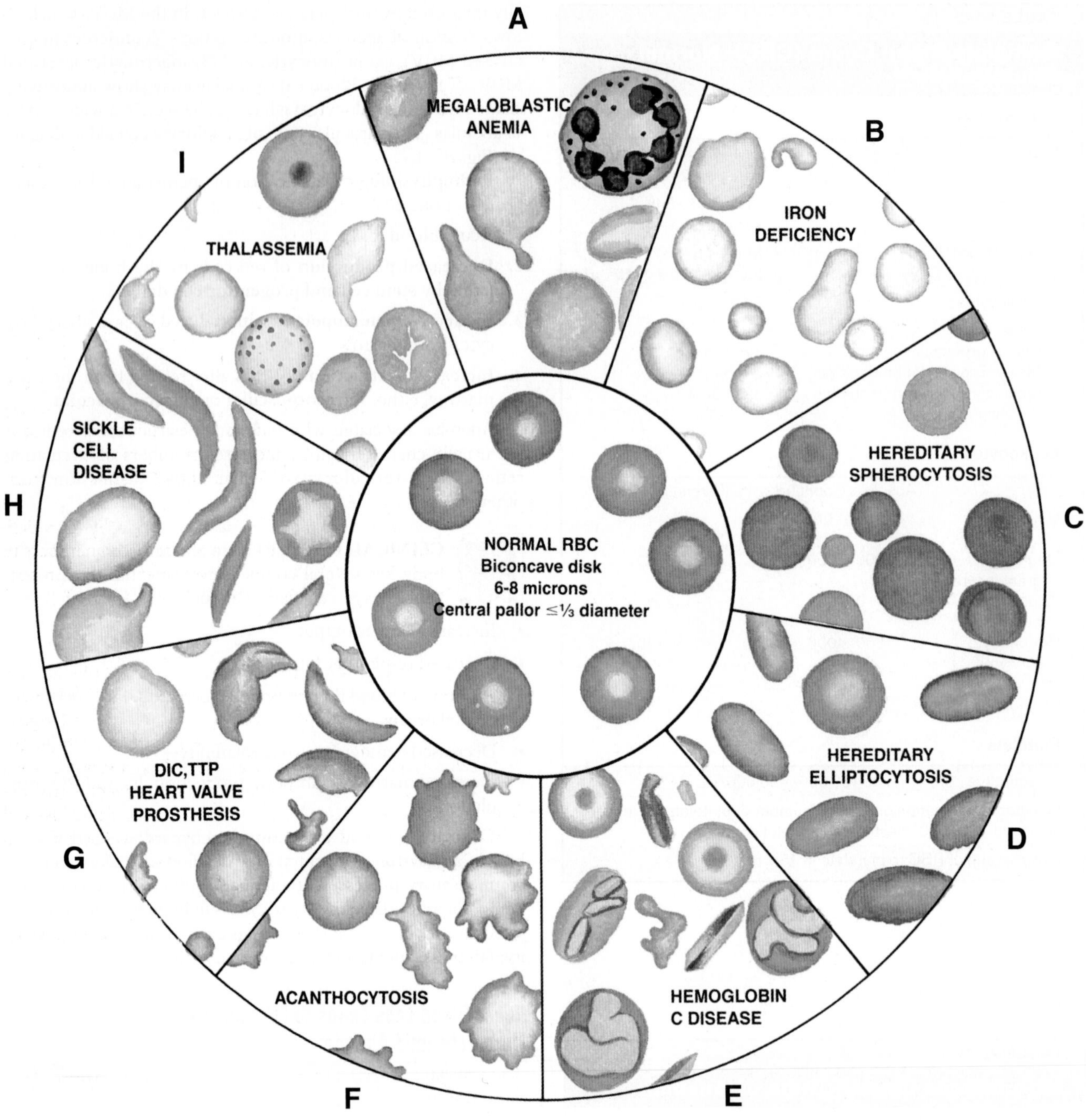

FIGURE 20-7. **Anemias.** The pathophysiology of characteristic morphologic features of various anemias are shown. The morphology of normal erythrocytes is contrasted in the central circle.

A. Megaloblastic anemia **(disturbance in DNA synthesis):** Oval macrocytes, teardrop poikilocytosis, and hypersegmented neutrophils
B. Iron deficiency **(disturbance in hemoglobin synthesis; lack of iron):** Hypochromic, microcytic erythrocytes
C. Hereditary spherocytosis **(membrane defect):** Spherocytes
D. Hereditary elliptocytosis **(membrane defect):** Elliptocytes
E. Hemoglobin C disease **(abnormal globin chain):** Target cells, rhomboid crystals
F. Acanthocytosis **(membrane lipid defect, e.g., abetalipoprotenemia):** Irregular spiculation
G. Disseminated intravascular coagulation (DIC), thrombocytic thrombocytopenic purpura (TTP), heart valve prosthesis sequela **(mechanical damage to erythrocytes):** Schistocytes
H. Sickle cell disease **(abnormal globin chain):** Sickle cells
I. Thalassemia **(disturbance in hemoglobin synthesis):** Hypochromic, microcytic erythrocytes, poikilocytosis, basophilic stipling

TABLE 20–4

Pathophysiologic Classification of Anemia

Acute blood loss	
Decreased Production	
Stem Cell and Progenitor Cell Defects	
Iron deficiency	Leukemia
Anemia of chronic disease	Myelodysplastic syndromes
Aplastic anemia	Marrow infiltratio n
Pure red cell aplasia	Lead poisoning
Paroxysmal nocturnal hemoglobinuria	Anemia of renal disease
Ineffective hematopoiesis	
Megaloblastic anemia	Thallasemia
Increased Destruction	
Intracorpuscular	
Membrane defect	Hemoglobinopathies
Enzyme defect	
Extracorpuscular	
Immunologic	
Autoimmune	Alloimmune
Nonimmunologic	
Mechanical	Infectious
Hypersplenism	Chemical

Decreased Red Blood Cell Production Often Reflects Impaired Erythrocyte Precursor Development

Iron Deficiency Anemia

Iron deficiency interferes with normal heme (hemoglobin) synthesis and leads to impaired erythropoiesis and anemia. Iron deficiency is the most common cause of anemia worldwide.

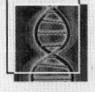

PATHOGENESIS: The normal Western adult diet contains about 20 mg of iron, 1 to 2 mg of which is absorbed by the duodenum and proximal jejunum (see Chapter 14). The rate of iron absorption is regulated by normal losses, but with anemia (especially in cases of ineffective erythropoiesis) intestinal absorption is increased and may ultimately lead to iron overload. About 85% of absorbed iron is transported by a carrier protein, transferrin, to be incorporated into developing red cells through specific transferrin receptors on their surface. As senescent red cells are removed from circulation, hemoglobin is broken down into component parts and iron is recycled. Excess iron is stored as **hemosiderin** and as **ferritin**. Hemosiderin is large aggregates of iron with a disorganized structure, while ferritin is complexed with protein (apoferritin) and appears highly organized.

Many underlying conditions give rise to iron deficiency. In infants and children, dietary iron may be inadequate for growth and development. Iron also increases during pregnancy and lactation. In adults, iron deficiency typically results from chronic blood loss or, less commonly, intravascular hemolysis. One milligram of iron is contained in 2 mL of whole blood lost from the body. In women of reproductive age, gynecologic blood loss (menstruation, parturition, vaginal bleeding) is most common. In postmenopausal women and men, unexplained iron deficiency should prompt study of the gastrointestinal tract for tumors or vascular lesions, as this is the most common site of chronic blood loss.

PATHOLOGY: Iron deficiency anemia is characterized by a microcytic, hypochromic anemia (Fig. 20-8). Variation in erythrocyte size and shape (**anisopoikilocytosis**) is reflected in an increased RDW, which is a measure of **anisocytosis**. **Ovalocytes** may be found, some of which are very thin and are designated **pencil cells**. Because of the production defect in the marrow, there is no associated reticulocytosis. The bone marrow displays erythroid hyperplasia. Prussian blue staining shows no stored iron.

Serum iron and ferritin levels are decreased by iron deficiency, while total iron-binding capacity is increased (due to increased serum transferrin level). As a result, the percent saturation of transferrin is conspicuously lowered (often less than 5%).

CLINICAL FEATURES: The symptoms of iron deficiency are those of anemia in general. With advanced disease, a smooth and glistening tongue (**atrophic glossitis**) and inflammation at the corners of the mouth (**angular stomatitis**) may be encountered, as well as a spoon-shaped deformity of the fingernails (**koilonychia**)**.** Treatment of iron deficiency involves correcting the source of chronic blood loss and oral iron supplementation. Parenteral iron is available for patients who are not compliant.

Anemia of Chronic Disease

Anemia of chronic disease arises in association with chronic inflammatory and malignant conditions.

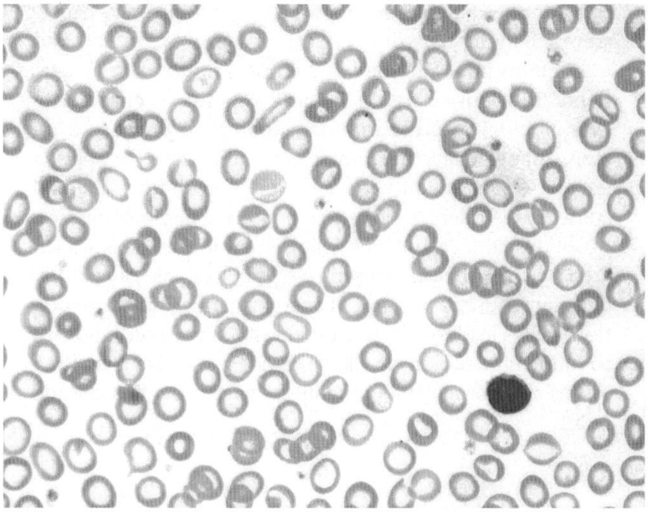

FIGURE 20-8. **Microcytic hypochromic anemia caused by iron deficiency.** Red blood cells are significantly smaller than the nucleus of a lymphocyte.

PATHOGENESIS: Chronic disease causes ineffective use of iron from macrophage stores in bone marrow, resulting in a functional iron deficiency, although iron stores are normal or even increased. Other factors that may contribute to anemia are decreased erythrocyte life span, blunted renal EPO responses to tissue hypoxia and impaired bone marrow response to erythropoietin. Inflammatory cytokines (lactoferrin, IL-1, tumor necrosis factor-α [TNF-α], and interferon) may interfere with iron mobilization.

PATHOLOGY: The anemia of chronic disease is mild to moderate; red cells are often microcytic but can be normocytic. Prussian blue staining shows normal or increased iron storage. Serum iron levels tend to be reduced. However, unlike iron deficiency anemia, total iron binding capacity also tends to be decreased (as is serum albumin). Successful treatment of the underlying disease restores normal hemoglobin levels.

Aplastic Anemia

Aplastic anemia is a disorder of pluripotential stem cells that leads to bone marrow failure. The disorder features hypocellular bone marrow and pancytopenia (decreased circulating levels of all formed elements in the blood).

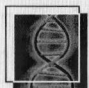

PATHOGENESIS: Aplastic anemia results from injury to bone marrow stem cells. Most cases are idiopathic, and no specific initiating etiology can be identified (Table 20-5). There are two main mechanisms of stem cell injury. The first is a predictable, dose-dependent, toxic injury, typified by exposure to certain chemotherapeutic drugs, chemicals, and ionizing radiation. The other is idiosyncratic, dose-independent, immunologic injury, as seen in idiopathic cases or after certain drug exposures or viral infections. Rarely aplastic anemia (e.g., Fanconi anemia) may be inherited. Depending on its cause, stem cell injury may or may not be reversible.

The immune etiology of stem cell injury in some patients is supported by the clinical response to antithymocyte globulin or other immunosuppressive agents. An intrinsic abnormality of stem cells in other cases of aplastic anemia is suggested by the subsequent evolution of clonal stem cell disorders (paroxysmal nocturnal hemoglobinuria, myelodysplasia, acute leukemia). Aplastic anemia is associated with **Fanconi anemia** (see below) is caused by germline mutations in *FAC* (Fanconi anemia complementation) genes lead to chromosomal instability upon exposure to ionizing radiation or alkylating agents. Aplastic aneima in this syndrome usually manifests within the first decade of life.

TABLE 20-5

Etiology of Aplastic Anemia

Idiopathic (⅔ of cases)
Ionizing radiation
Drugs
Chemotherapeutic agents Chloramphenicol Anticonvulsants Nonsteroidal antiinflammatory agents Gold
Chemicals
Benzene
Viruses
Hepatitis C virus (HCV) Epstein-Barr virus (EBV) Human immunodeficiency virus (HIV) Parvovirus B19
Hereditary
Fanconi anemia

PATHOLOGY: The bone marrow in aplastic anemia shows variably reduced cellularity, depending on the clinical stage of the disease. Myeloid, erythroid, and megakaryocytic lineage cells are fewer, with a relative increase in marrow lymphocytes and plasma cells. As bone marrow cellularity decreases, there is a corresponding increase in fat (Fig. 20-9). Anemia, leukopenia (mainly granulocytopenia), and thrombocytopenia characterize aplastic anemia. Despite elevated EPO levels, reticulocytosis is not present, which underscores the underlying stem cell defect.

CLINICAL FEATURES: Patients with aplastic anemia present with signs and symptoms attributable to pancytopenia, namely: weakness, fatigue, infection, and bleeding. For untreated aplastic anemia, the prognosis is grim, with a 3- to 6-month median survival. Only 20% survive over 1 year. Immunosuppressive therapy often leads to transient remissions and bone marrow or stem cell transplantation may be curative.

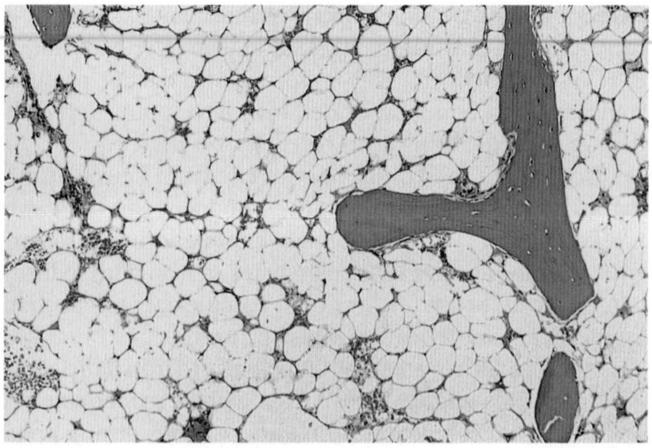

FIGURE 20-9. **Aplastic anemia.** The bone marrow consists largely of fat cells and lacks normal hematopoietic activity.

Pure Red Cell Aplasia

Pure red cell aplasia (PRCA) is selective suppression of committed erythroid precursors in the bone marrow. White blood cells and platelets are unaffected.

PATHOGENESIS: PRCA most often results from immune suppression of red cell production. the stimulus for which is unknown. On occasion, it is secondary to viral infection (parvovirus B19) or thymic lesions (e.g., thymoma, thymic hyperplasia). The P antigen system on the red cell membrane is a receptor for parvovirus and explains the restricted infection of erythroid precursors by this agent.

Diamond-Blackfan syndrome is a heritable type of PRCA that appears in the first year of life and is associated with defective erythroid precursors that show a diminished response to erythropoietin and decreased erythroid burst and colony- forming capacities.

PATHOLOGY: In PRCA, overall marrow cellularity is normal, but there is a selective absence of erythroid precursors. Erythroid precursors are completely absent or are arrested at the erythroblast stage. In cases secondary to parvovirus B19, intranuclear viral inclusions in proerythroblasts can be observed. Myeloid and megakaryocytic precursors are adequate in number and show normal maturation.

Patients with PRCA develop moderate to severe anemia, often with macrocytic indices. Despite increased EPO, there is no accompanying reticulocytosis.

CLINICAL FEATURES: Acquired PRCA manifests as an acute self-limited illness or a chronic relapsing process. **Acute self-limited PRCA** is often due to parvovirus B19. This condition may not be clinically apparent unless the patient suffers from an underlying chronic hemolytic anemia (e.g., hereditary spherocytosis, sickle cell anemia). Such cases may be complicated by a so-called aplastic crisis, i.e., sudden worsening of anemia. Immunocompromised patients cannot clear parvovirus infection and anemia may be prolonged. **Chronic relapsing PRCA** may be idiopathic, or associated with an underlying thymic lesion. In these cases, thymectomy may correct the anemia.

Anemia of Renal Disease

Anemia of chronic renal insufficiency reflects decreased production of EPO.

PATHOGENESIS: Renal disease of varying causes is associated with decreased production of EPO and subsequent development of anemia. The severity of anemia is proportional to the underlying degree of renal insufficiency. Administration of recombinant EPO is the treatment of choice. A "uremic toxin," which suppresses erythroid precursors, plus a minor hemolytic component, have been suggested (but not proven) as contributing to the anemia of chronic renal disease.

PATHOLOGY: The anemia of chronic renal disease is normocytic and normochromic. In some cases, erythrocytes with scalloped cell membranes can be seen (Burr cells). If renal insufficiency is secondary to malignant hypertension, red cell fragmentation with formation of schistocytes may be observed.

Anemia Associated with Marrow Infiltration (Myelophthisic Anemia)

Myelophthisic anemia is a hypoproliferative anemia associated with infiltration of bone marrow by a variety of processes.

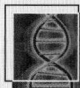

PATHOGENESIS: Any infiltrative process—e.g., myelofibrosis, hematologic malignancies, metastatic carcinoma, or granulomatous disease—may replace normal hematopoietic elements and cause anemia (and often leukopenia and thrombocytopenia). In an attempt to maintain blood cell production, extramedullary hematopoiesis may develop, mostly in the spleen and liver.

PATHOLOGY: Bone marrow infiltration causes moderate to severe normocytic anemia, with anisopoikilocytosis and teardrop cells. Circulating immature granulocytes and nucleated erythrocytes (**leukoerythroblastosis**) are frequently seen.

Anemia of Lead Poisoning

Lead poisoning results in anemia by interfering with several enzymes involved in heme synthesis (see Chapter 8).

In Ineffective Red Cell Production There are Fewer Circulating Erythrocytes

Various anemias reflect abnormal erythrocyte production due to ineffective hematopoesis. In contrast with stem cell or precursor cell disorders, the bone marrow erythrocyte precursor pool is expanded. Thus, sufficient erythrocyte precurosors are are formed in the bone marrow, but erythrocytes do not enter the circulation.

Megaloblastic Anemias

Megaloblastic anemias are caused by impaired DNA synthesis, usually because of either vitamin B_{12} or folic acid deficiency.

PATHOGENESIS: Impaired DNA synthesis results in abnormal nuclear development, which in turn leads to ineffective erythrocyte maturation and anemia. Certain chemotherapeutic agents (methotrexate, hydroxyurea) or antiretroviral drugs (5-azacytidine) may also cause megaloblastic anemia. Less commonly, inherited defects in purine or pyrimidine metabolism may be involved.

Folate and B_{12} are critical for normal DNA synthesis. Tetrahydrofolate is converted from methyl tetrahydrofolate by methyltranferase and vitamin B_{12}, which serves as a

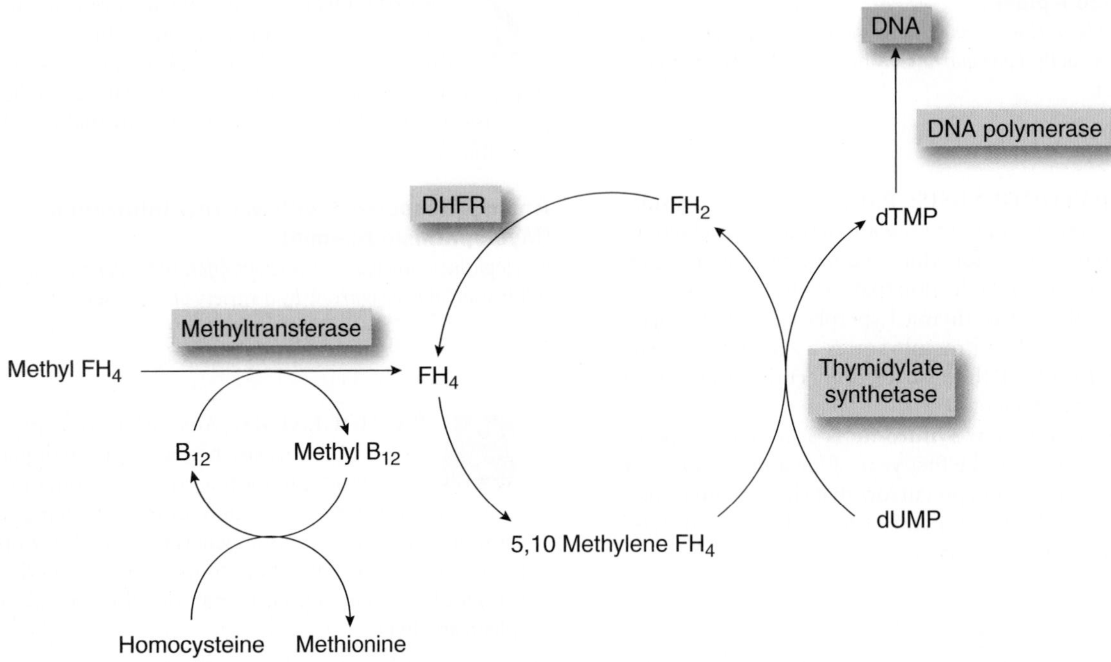

FIGURE 20-10. **Relationship of folic acid to vitamin B_{12}.** A 1-carbon transfer mediated by folic acid, methylates dUMP to dTMP, which is then used for the synthesis of DNA. To enter this cycle, folate (methyl FH_4) is demethylated to FH_4, vitamin B_{12} acting as the cofactor. Thus, both vitamin B_{12} and folic acid deficiencies lead to impaired DNA synthesis and megaloblastic anemia. FH_4 = tetrahydrofolate; dUMP = deoxyuridine monophosphate; dTMP = deoxythymidine monophosphate; FH_2 = dihydrofolate; DHFR = dihydrofolate reductase.

cofactor. Vitamin B_{12} is also required for converting homocysteine to methionine. Using tetrahydrofolate as a cofactor, thymidylate synthetase converts uridylate to thymidylate (Fig. 20-10). Dihydrofolate reductase restores tetrahydrofolate.

In the face of defective DNA synthesis, nuclear development is impaired, whereas cytoplasm matures normally. This situation, termed **nuclear to cytoplasmic asynchrony**, results in formation of large nucleated erythrocyte precursors (**megaloblasts**). Since megaloblast precursors do not mature enough to be released into the blood, they undergo intramedullary destruction. Released erythrocytes are macrocytic.

Vitamin B_{12} (cyanocobalamin) is found in a variety of animal food sources and is synthesized by intestinal microorganisms. Proper vitamin B_{12} absorption requires its binding to intrinsic factor, which protects vitamin B_{12} from degradation by intestinal enzymes (Fig. 20-11). Intrinsic factor is produced, along with hydrochloric acid, by gastric parietal cells. Vitamin B_{12} is absorbed in the distal ileum via specific receptors. In the blood, vitamin B_{12} is transported by a group of proteins called **transcobalamins**, of which transcobalamin II is the most important. The daily usage of vitamin B_{12} is 1 μg. Therefore, normal body stores of 1000 to 5000 μg provide several years of reserve.

Vitamin B_{12} deficiency arises from diverse causes. Inadequate dietary intake of vitamin B_{12} is rare and is usually encountered only in strict vegetarians (vegans). *Most commonly, lack of intrinsic factor leads to impaired absorption of vitamin B_{12}.* Intrinsic factor may be deficient as a result of previous gastric surgery in which the parietal cell mass of the stomach has been removed.

Pernicious anemia is an autoimmune disorder: patients develop antibodies against parietal cells and intrinsic factor. Anti-parietal cell antibodies also lead to atrophic gastritis with achlorhydria. Primary intestinal disorders (inflammatory bowel disease) or previous intestinal surgery (ileal bypass) can impair vitamin B_{12} absorption. Microbiologic competition, e.g., from bacterial overgrowth of a blind loop or infestation by a fish tapeworm, *Diphyllobothrium latum*, may lead to vitamin B_{12} deficiency.

Folic acid is present in leafy vegetables, in meat, and eggs. Dietary folic acid exists in a polyglutamate form but is deconjugated to monoglutamates in the intestines and primarily absorbed in the jejunum. Folate is then reduced and methylated to 5-methyl tetrahydrofolate, which is transported in the blood by folate-binding protein. The daily requirement for foliate is about 50 μg. Body stores of folate average 2000 to 5000 μg, providing a few months reserve before signs of deficiency develop.

The most common cause of folic acid deficiency is inadequate dietary intake. This occurs most often in patients with poorly balanced diets (alcoholics, recluses). Demand for folic acid is increased in pregnancy, lactation, periods of rapid growth, and chronic hemolytic processes; deficiency may result unless folate supplementation is provided. Primary intestinal diseases (inflammatory bowel disease, sprue) may interfere with absorption of folic acid. Various medications can also impair folic acid absorption (phenytoin) or metabolism (methotrexate).

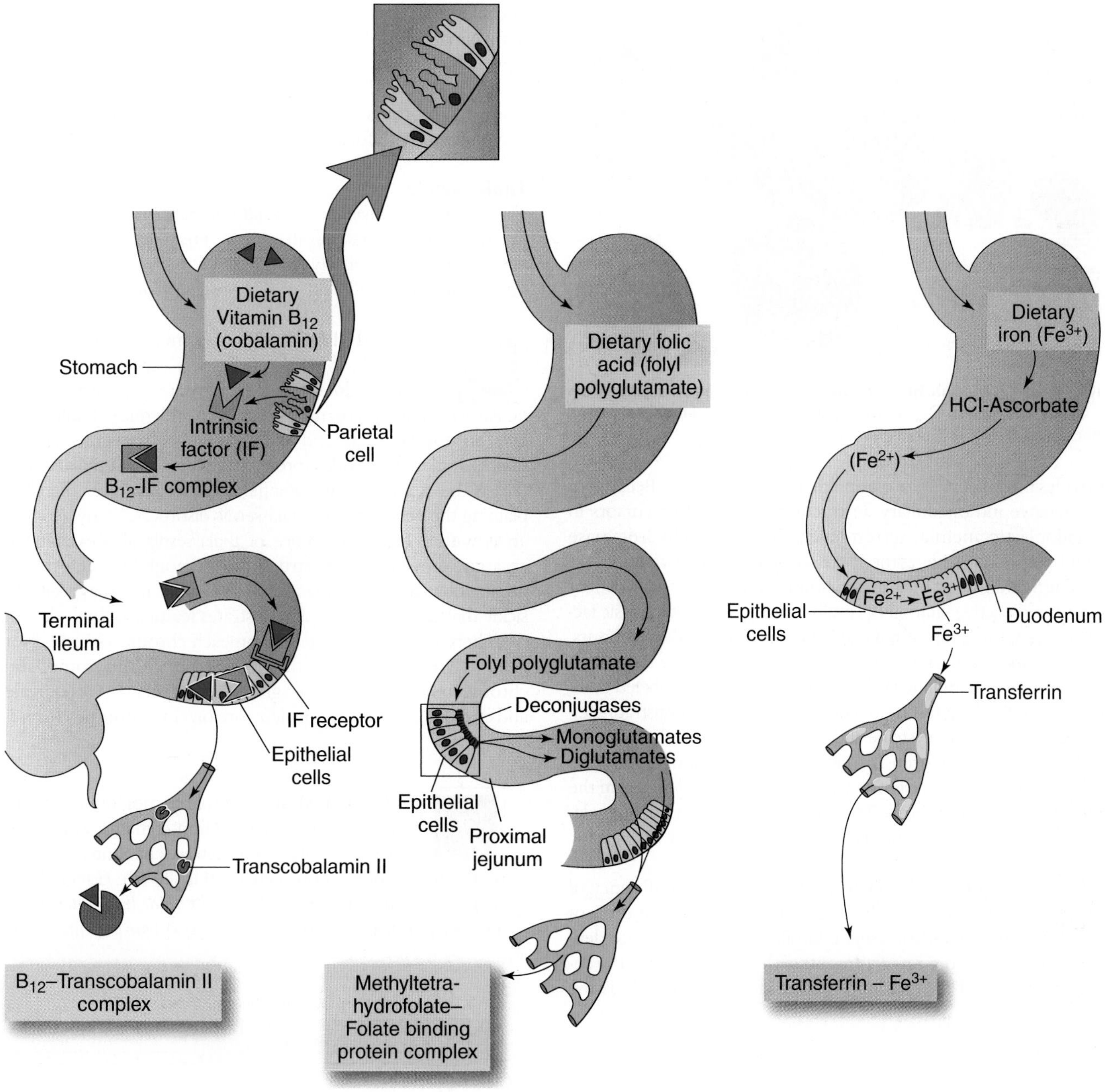

FIGURE 20-11. **Absorption of vitamin B_{12}, folic acid, and iron.** Absorption of vitamin B_{12} requires initial complexing with intrinsic factor (IF), which is produced by the parietal cells of the gastric mucosa. Absorption then occurs in the terminal ileum, where there are receptors for the IF–B_{12} complex. Dietary folic acid is conjugated by conjugase enzymes to polyglutamate. Absorption occurs in the jejunum following deconjugation in the intestinal lumen. Reduction and methylation result in the generation of methyl tetrahydrofolate, which is then transported by folate-binding protein. Dietary ferric iron (Fe^{3+}) is reduced to ferrous iron (Fe^{2+}) in the stomach and absorbed principally in the duodenum. Iron is transported by transferrin in the circulation.

PATHOLOGY: The hematologic manifestations, in bone marrow and blood, are identical for either folic acid or vitamin B_{12} deficiency. Although the bone marrow tends to be hypercellular, the blood demonstrates pancytopenia because of **ineffective hematopoiesis**. Megaloblastic maturation, characterized by cellular enlargement with asynchronous maturation between the nucleus and cytoplasm (Fig. 20-12), is noted in bone marrow precursors from all lineages.

The degree of anemia varies but may be severe. Erythrocytes are macrocytic and may be oval (oval macrocytes). Anisopoikilocytosis is usually prominent and teardrop cells may be seen. Circulating neutrophils often show nuclear hypersegmentation (more than five lobes) (Fig. 20-13). No increase in reticulocytes occurs.

The distinction between folic acid and vitamin B_{12} deficiency can usually be established by measuring serum levels of these compounds. Occasionally, specific measurement of red cell folate

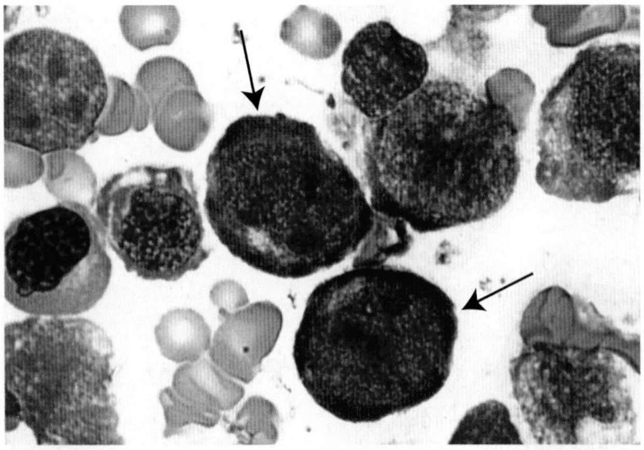

FIGURE 20-12. **Megaloblastic anemia.** A bone marrow aspirate from a patient with vitamin B_{12} deficiency (pernicious anemia) shows prominent megaloblastic erythroid precursors (*arrows*).

provides more useful information than serum analyses. Because of the massive intramedullary destruction of red cell precursors in megaloblastic anemia, serum levels of lactate dehydrogenase (LDH), especially isoenzyme 1, are conspicuously elevated.

The **Schilling test** measures vitamin B_{12} absorption. The patient is given radioactive vitamin B_{12} orally, with or without intrinsic factor. Urinary excretion of radioactivity is measured over 24 hours, Based on the result, the cause of the deficiency can be suggested. However, owing to difficulties in working with rad-iolabeled compounds the Schilling test is not commonly used. Demonstrating elevated levels of homocysteine and methyl ma-lonic acid may prove useful in cases of vitamin B_{12} deficiency. Circulating antibodies against gastric parietal cells or intrinsic factor can be detected in the setting of pernicious anemia. The former antibody is more often detected; the latter is more specific for pernicious anemia.

CLINICAL FEATURES: Whether due to deficiency of vitamin B_{12} or folic acid, the clinical presentation of megaloblastic anemia is similar. In general, folate deficiency develops more rapidly (months) than does vitamin B_{12} deficiency (years). The most important difference clinically is the neurologic symptoms with vitamin B_{12} deficiency, secondary to demyelination of the posterior and lateral columns of the spinal cord, which may cause both sensory and motor deficiencies (see Chapter 28). Without appropriate and prompt therapy, neurologic symptoms may be irreversible. Such findings are not encountered with folate deficiency.

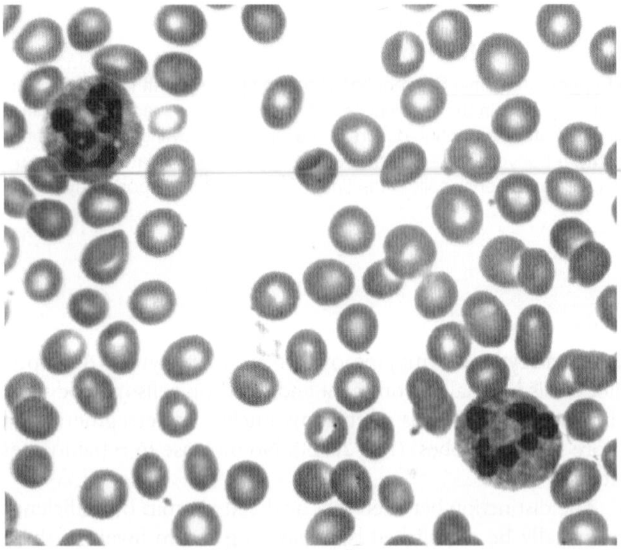

FIGURE 20-13. **Hypersegmented granulocytes in a patient with vitamin B_{12} deficiency.**

Thalassemia

Thalassemias are anemias that result from defective globin chains. Ineffective hematopoeisis results from precipitation of abnormal hemoglobins within newly formed RBCs and increased erythrocyte fragility, features that lead to erythrocyte destruction in the marrow.

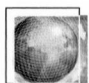

EPIDEMIOLOGY: Thalassemia is most common around the Mediterranean Sea, especially in Italy and Greece. It does, however, have a wide distribution, particularly in areas where malaria has been endemic (Middle East, India, Southeast Asia, and China). A heterozygous state for thalassemia may provide a protective effect against malaria and increase the reproductive potential of heterozygotes, thereby explaining the persistence of thalassemic disorders. Many geographic areas with a higher incidence of thalassemia also exhibit an increased prevalence of structural hemoglobin defects (e.g., hemoglobin S). This situation leads double heterozygosity (e.g., sickle thalassemia), which demonstrates features of both disorders.

There are 4 α genes, paired on each chromosome 16. Non-α genes, two γ, one δ, and one β gene per chromosome, are on chromosome 11. Embryonic globin genes zeta (ζ) (α equivalent) and epsilon (ϵ) (non-α equivalent) are on chromosomes 16 and 11.

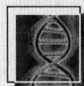

PATHOGENESIS: Normal hemoglobin contains 4 globin chains: 2 α and 2 non-α chains. Three normal variants of hemoglobin are encountered, based on the nature of the non-α chains (Fig. 20-14). *Hemoglobin A ($\alpha_2\beta_2$) accounts for 95% to 98% of the total in adults; minor amounts of hemoglobin F ($\alpha_2\gamma_2$) and A_2 ($\alpha_2\delta_2$) are present.*

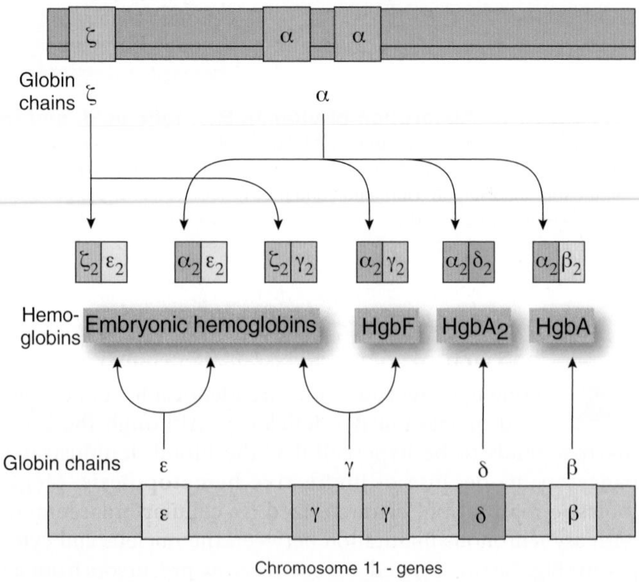

FIGURE 20-14. **Assembly of subunit chains to form different hemoglobins Hgb.**

Thalassemias are generally classified according to the affected globin chain. The two most clinically significant forms involve deficits of α and β chains. Thalassemias involving γ and δ globin chain synthesis have also been described but are not common.

β Thalassemia

PATHOGENESIS: β Thalassemias are a heterogeneous group of disorders that are most often caused by point mutations in the β globin gene. Mutations may be in the gene's promoter region, a splice site or other coding regions, or may lead to creation of an inappropriate stop codon. The result is that transcription of the gene is entirely (β^o) or partly (β^+) suppressed. Occasionally, a mutation may also affect the adjacent δ globin gene, leading to a β-δ thalassemia.

PATHOLOGY AND CLINICAL FEATURES: Homozygous β thalassemia (Cooley anemia) is characterized by moderate-to-severe, microcytic and hypochromic anemia (Fig. 20-15). There is a marked excess of α chains, which form unstable tetramers (α_4) that precipitate in the cytoplasm of developing erythroid precursors. In the β^o type, fetal hemoglobin accounts for most of the hemoglobin, although increased levels (5%–8%) of hemoglobin A_2 are also present. In the case of $\beta+$ type, some hemoglobin A may be detected (depending on the nature of the underlying defect) and hemoglobin A_2 is mildly increased. A modest increase in hemoglobin A_2 is characteristic of all forms of β thalassemia, as δ globin genes are upregulated.

In addition to microcytosis and hypochromia, blood smears demonstrate striking anisopoikilocytosis (uneven size and shape) with target cells, basophilic stippling and circulating normoblasts (especially after splenectomy). The increased oxygen affinity of hemoglobin F plus the underlying anemia impair oxygen delivery and lead to increased EPO. The latter causes marked bone marrow erythroid hyperplasia. The marrow space is expanded, causing facial and cranial bone deformities. Extramedullary hematopoiesis contributes to hepatosplenomegaly and formation of soft tissue masses.

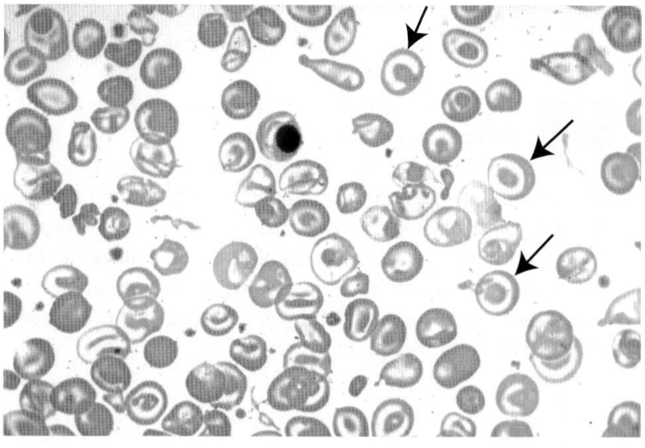

FIGURE 20-15. **Thalassemia.** The peripheral blood erythrocytes are hypochromic and microcytic and show anisocytosis, poikilocytosis, and target cells (*arrows*).

Excess erythropoiesis leads to increased iron absorption, which, together with repeated transfusions, creates iron overload. Excess iron deposition in tissues is a major cause of morbidity and mortality in thalassemic patients and often requires aggressive chelation therapy.

Heterozygous β thalassemia is associated with microcytosis and hypochromia. The degree of microcytosis is disproportionate to the severity of the anemia, which is generally mild. There is often an accompanying erythrocytosis (increased RBC count) but minimal anisocytosis (normal RDW). Target cells, basophilic stippling, and a mild increase in hemoglobin A_2 are present. Most patients are entirely asymptomatic.

α Thalassemia

PATHOGENESIS: Unlike β thalassemias, α thalassemias are most frequently due to gene deletions. More syndromes are clinically observed because of the potential number (up to four) of α globin genes that may be affected. α Thalassemia is associated with excess β or γ chains, which can then form the tetrameric hemoglobin H (β_4) and hemoglobin Bart (γ_4). Hemoglobins H and Bart are both unstable and precipitate in the cytoplasm, forming Heinz bodies, but to a lesser degree than α_4 tetramers. Further, they have high oxygen affinities and cause decreased tissue oxygen delivery. The relative amount of these tetrameric hemoglobins depends on the number of α genes involved and the patient's age. Because of the underlying impairment in hemoglobin synthesis, circulating red cells usually are microcytic and hypochromic.

PATHOLOGY AND CLINICAL FEATURES:

- **Silent carrier α thalassemia** (one gene affected) is difficult to diagnose, because patients' only hematologic abnormalitiy is small amounts of hemoglobin Bart, detectable only in infancy. There is no anemia, and patients are asymptomatic. α **Thalassemia trait** (two genes affected) is associated with a mild microcytic anemia. Like heterozygous β thalassemia, the degree of microcytosis is disproportionately low compared to the degree of anemia. Hemoglobin A_2 is not increased, allowing distinction between α and β thalassemia traits. Up to 5% hemoglobin Bart can be seen during infancy.

  Two different genotypes are possible in heterozygous α thalassemia. There may be a single gene deleted from each chromosome 16, or alternatively, both genes may be deleted from the same chromosome 16. The former scenario is more common in persons of Mediterranean and African descent; the latter is more frequent in Southeast Asia. Clinically, both genotypes present similarly, but homozygous α thalassemia (see below) can only develop if both genes are deleted from the same chromosome.

- **Hemoglobin H disease** (3 genes affected) is associated with moderate microcytic anemia. Increased hemoglobin Bart (up to 25% in infancy) and variable levels of hemoglobin H can be detected. Both hemoglobins H and Bart can be recognized by hemoglobin electrophoresis, since they migrate faster than hemoglobin A. Precipitated hemoglobin H (Heinz bodies) can also be demonstrated by supravital staining of a blood smear.

- **Homozygous** (four genes affected) α **thalassemia,** also termed α hydrops fetalis, is incompatible with life. Affected infants die in utero or shortly after birth with severe anemia, marked anisopoikilocytosis and large amounts of hemoglobin Bart. Severe impairment in tissue oxygen delivery is associated with heart failure and generalized edema. Massive hepatosplenomegaly is secondary to extramedullary hematopoiesis.

Hemolytic Anemias Feature Increased Red Cell Destruction

Premature elimination of circulating erythrocytes is called **hemolysis.** The resulting anemias are **hemolytic anemias**. These anemias are classified by the site of red cell destruction. In **extravascular hemolysis** the monocyte/macrophage system in the spleen and, to a lesser extent, the liver are involved. In **intravascular hemolysis**, erythrocytes are destroyed in the circulation.

Hemolytic anemias are characterized by a compensatory increase in red cell production and release. In the blood this manifests as polychromasia of red cells due to increased reticulocytes. Other laboratory findings commonly associated with hemolysis include increased LDH (particularly isoenzyme 1) and unconjugated (indirect) bilirubin, decreased haptoglobin, free (extracellular) hemoglobin in the blood and urine, increased urobilinogen, and urine hemosiderin.

Erythrocyte Membrane Defects

Erythrocyte membranes are normally remarkably flexible, and can deform to allow red cells to circulate unimpaired through the microcirculation and splenic vasculature. The red cell membrane consists of a lipid bilayer attached to an underlying cytoskeleton (see Fig. 20-5). The main component of the cytoskeleton is spectrin, a dimer of α and β subunits. Ankyrin (band 2.1) anchors spectrin to transmembrane proteins (band 3, anion exchanger proteins), whereas spectrin is bound to actin and glycophorin by protein 4.1. *Alterations in any portion of the red cell membrane can reduce the normal plasticity and render erythrocytes susceptible to hemolysis.*

Hereditary Spherocytosis

Hereditary spherocytosis (HS) is a heterogeneous group of inherited disorders of RBC cytoskeletons, characterized by a deficiency of spectrin or another cytoskeletal component (ankyrin, protein 4.2, band 3).

PATHOGENESIS: The deficiency of a cytoskeletal protein in HS leads to a **"vertical"** defect in the red cell membrane, with uncoupling of the lipid bilayer from the underlying cytoskeleton. The result is progressive loss of membrane surface area and **spherocyte** formation. These abnormal red cells are more rigid and cannot easily traverse the spleen. While circulating through the spleen, spherocytes become "conditioned" and lose additional surface membrane before they ultimately succumb to extravascular hemolysis. Most forms of HS are inherited as autosomal dominant traits and the rare recessive cases all involve the α subunit of spectrin.

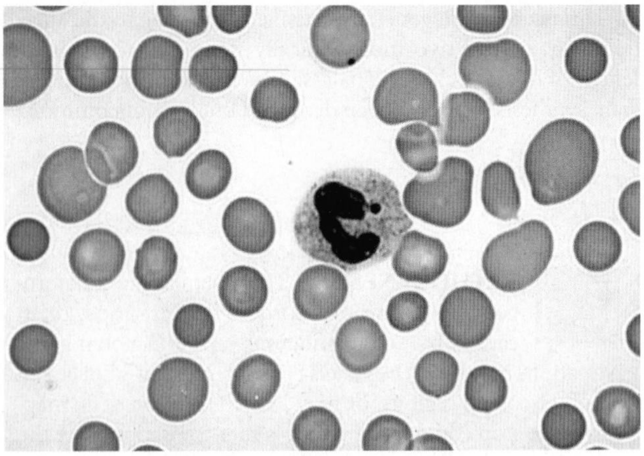

FIGURE 20-16. **Hereditary spherocytosis.** The peripheral blood smear shows many erythrocytes with decreased diameter, intense staining, and no central pallor (spherocytes).

PATHOLOGY: Most patients with HS have a moderate normocytic anemia. Conspicuous spherocytes that appear hyperchromic (no central pallor) are typical, along with polychromasia and reticulocytosis (Fig. 20-16). The bone marrow shows erythroid hyperplasia.

Spherocytes show greater **osmotic fragility** than normal erythrocytes. Laboratory findings typical of hemolysis (decreased haptoglobin, increased indirect bilirubin, increased LDH) are often present.

CLINICAL FEATURES: Most patients have splenomegaly due to chronic extravascular hemolysis. They may appear jaundiced, and up to 50% develop cholelithiasis, with pigmented (bilirubin) gallstones. Despite chronic hemolysis, transfusion is generally not required. An exception is a sudden decline in hemoglobin and reticulocytes, which heralds an aplastic crisis (usually due to infection by parvovirus B19). Anemia may also become more severe in so-called hemolytic crisis, during which there is a transient acceleration of the hemolysis. Patients with HS can be managed effectively by splenectomy, although spherocytes still persist in the circulation.

Hereditary Elliptocytosis

Hereditary elliptocytosis (HE) is a heterogeneous group of inherited disorders involving the erythrocyte cytoskeleton.

PATHOGENESIS: HE features a ***"horizontal"*** abnormality within the cytoskeleton. More commonly described variants of HE include defects in self-assembly of spectrin, spectrin–ankyrin binding, protein 4.1, and glycophorin C. Regardless of the underlying molecular abnormality, most circulating red cells are elliptical or oval. They still have an area of central pallor, since there is no loss of the lipid bilayer (as seen in HS). Most forms of HE are autosomal dominant.

PATHOLOGY AND CLINICAL FEATURES: HE usually manifests with only mild normocytic anemia. Many patients are asymptomatic.

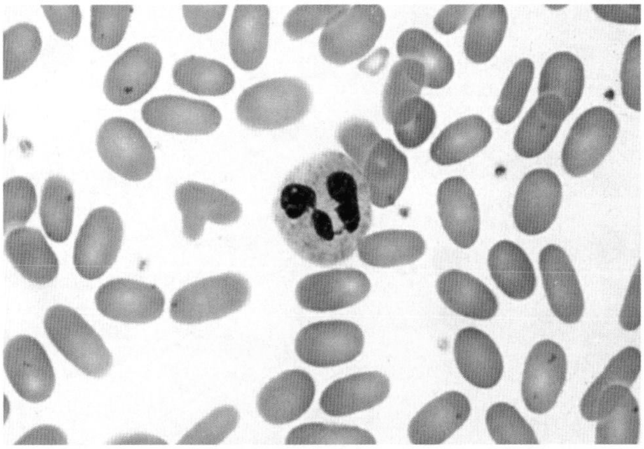

FIGURE 20-17. **Hereditary elliptocytosis.** A smear of peripheral blood reveals that virtually all of the erythrocytes are elliptical.

Blood smears show numerous elliptocytes with only minimal reticulocytosis (Fig. 20-17). Generally, less hemolysis and subsequent anemia are seen than are seen with HS. Occasional patients with more severe hemolysis may require splenectomy.

Acanthocytosis

Acanthocytosis results from a defect within the lipid bilayer of the red cell membrane and features spiny projections of the surface, which may be associated with hemolysis.

PATHOGENESIS: The most common cause is chronic liver disease, in which increased free cholesterol is deposited within cell membranes. Acanthocytes are also a prominent feature in cases of abetalipoproteinemia, an autosomal recessive disorder associated with lipid membrane abnormalities (see Chapter 13).

PATHOLOGY AND CLINICAL FEATURES: Abnormalities in the lipid membrane cause erythrocytes to become deformed and develop irregular spiny surface projections and centrally dense cytoplasm (no central pallor) (Fig. 20-18). These red cells are called **acanthocytes** (spur cells). They should be distinguished from burr cells (crenated cells, echinocytes), which have more uniform cell membrane scalloping and maintain an area of central pallor. Hemolysis and anemia in acanthocytosis are mild.

Enzyme Defects

Energy generation within erythrocytes occurs primarily by glycolysis. Inherited defects of enzymes in the glycolytic pathway can predispose circulating red cells to hemolysis. The most common enzyme defect involves glucose-6-phosphate dehydrogenase (G6PD), which catalyzes conversion of glucose-6-phosphate to 6-phosphogluconate. Deficiencies of other glycolytic enzymes are rare and autosomal recessive. Among these, pyruvate kinase deficiency is the most common. Clinically, these defects cause variable degrees of anemia and are designated **hereditary nonspherocytic anemias.**

G6PD deficiency *is an X-linked disorder in which abnormal red cell sensitivity to oxidative stress manifests as hemolytic anemia.*

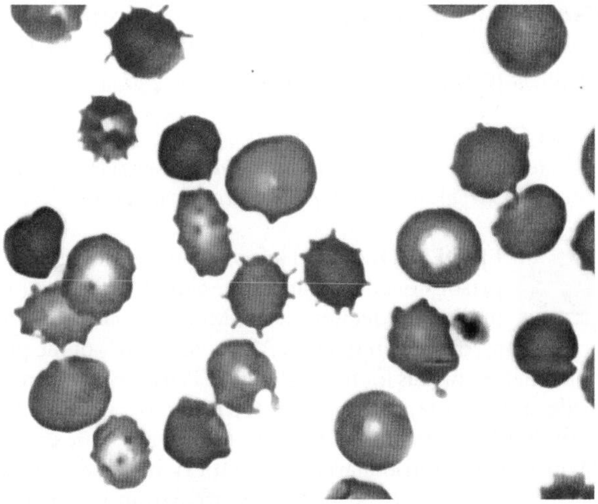

FIGURE 20-18. **Acanthocytes.** The red cells lack central pallor and display spikes on the surface.

G6PD deficiency has a variable worldwide distribution, with highest prevalence in areas where malaria is historically endemic, notably Africa and the Mediterranean region. Various mutations have been identified. G6PD mutations appear to provide some protective effect against malaria.

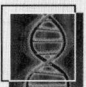

PATHOGENESIS: Because G6PD helps to recycle reduced glutathione, red cells deficient in this enzyme are susceptible to oxidative stress (e.g., infections, drugs, or fava bean ingestion [favism]). Oxidation of hemoglobin leads to formation of methemoglobin, in which $Fe2^{+}$ ions are converted to ferric (Fe^{3+}) ions. Methemoglobin cannot transport oxygen, is unstable and precipitates in the cytoplasm as Heinz bodies. Precipitated methemoglobin increases cell rigidity and leads to hemolysis.

PATHOLOGY: In quiescent periods, erythrocytes in G6PD deficiency appear normal. However, in a hemolytic episode precipitated by oxidative stress, Heinz bodies can be demonstrated by supravital staining. After passage through the spleen, circulating red cells may have part of their membrane removed, forming so-called **bite cells**.

CLINICAL FEATURES: Full expression of G6PD deficiency is seen only in males, with females being asymptomatic carriers. The A–variant of G6PD is seen in 10% to 15% of American blacks and is associated with reduced enzyme activity (10% of normal) because of instability of the molecule. In affected patients, exposure to oxidant drugs, such as the antimalarial agent primaquine, may result in hemolysis. In the Mediterranean type of G6PD mutation, enzyme activity is absent and, therefore, exposure to oxidant stress, causes more sustained and severe hemolysis. Potentially lethal hemolysis may follow ingestion of fava beans (**favism**) in susceptible patients.

Hemoglobinopathies

Most clinically relevant hemoglobinopathies are caused by point mutations in the β globin chain gene.

Sickle Cell Disease

In sickle cell disease, an abnormal hemoglobin, hemoglobin S, transforms the erythrocyte into a sickle shape upon deoxygenation.

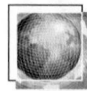

EPIDEMIOLOGY: Hemoglobin S is most common in persons of African ancestry, although the gene is also present in Mediterranean, Middle Eastern, and Indian populations. In some regions of Africa, up to 40% of the population is heterozygous for hemoglobin S. Ten percent of American blacks are heterozygous and 1 in 650 is homozygous. Heterozygosity for hemoglobin S is thought to provide some protection against falciparum malaria. Infected erythrocytes selectively sickle and are removed from the circulation by splenic and hepatic macrophages, effectively destroying the parasite.

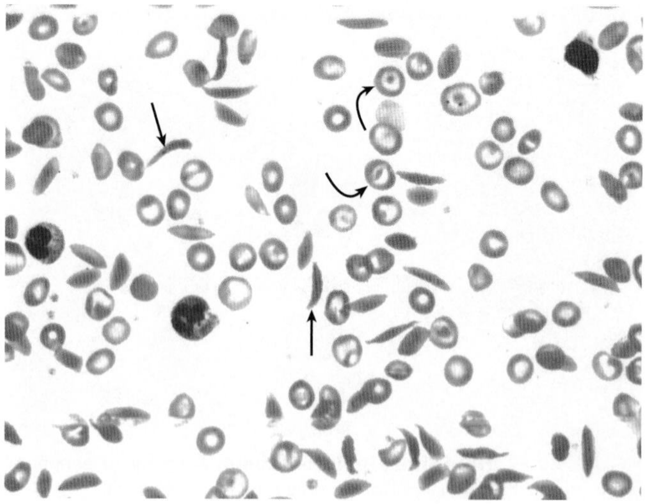

FIGURE 20-19. **Sickle cell anemia.** Sickled cells (*straight arrows*) and target cells (*curved arrows*) are evident.

PATHOGENESIS: In hemoglobin S a point mutation in the gene for the β globin chain gene substitutes valine for glutamic acid at the sixth amino acid. This single change generates in a structurally abnormal molecule that polymerizes under conditions of deoxygenation. Polymerization of hemoglobin S transforms the cytoplasm into a rigid filamentous gel and leads to the formation of less deformable sickled erythrocytes.

The rigidity of sickled erythrocytes results in obstruction of the microcirculation, with subsequent tissue hypoxia and ischemic injury in many organs. The inflexible nature of sickle cells also renders them susceptible to destruction (hemolysis) during circulation through the spleen. Thus, the two primary manifestations of sickle cell disease are recurrent ischemic events and chronic extravascular hemolytic anemia.

Erythrocyte sickling is initially reversible with reoxygenation, but after several cycles of sickling and unsickling, the process becomes irreversible. Sickled erythrocytes also have changes in the phospholipids of the membrane, and so adhere more strongly to endothelial cells, which further impairs capillary blood flow.

People who are homozygous for hemoglobin S show the full clinical presentation of sickle cell disease. A sickling disorder is also observed in patients who are doubly heterozygous for two β chain mutations (e.g. hemoglobin SC disease, sickle/β-thalassemia). Heterozygotes for hemoglobin S (sickle cell trait), however, do not develop red cell sickling, because their hemoglobin A prevents hemoglobin S polymerization. Hemoglobin F also interferes with hemoglobin S polymerization and patients who are homozygous for hemoglobin S and have increased levels of hemoglobin F have a milder form of disease.

PATHOLOGY: Homozygous patients (hemoglobin SS) have severe normocytic or macrocytic anemia. The macrocytosis can be attributed to increased numbers of reticulocytes, secondary to chronic hemolysis. Blood smear examination reveals marked anisopoikilocytosis and polychromasia. Classic sickle cells and target cells, as well as a variety of other abnormally shaped erythrocytes, are observed (Fig. 20-19). Howell-Jolly bodies, representing nuclear remnants, are seen in most patients beyond childhood and reflect hyposplenism caused by ischemic loss of splenic tissue.

Electrophoretic analysis shows that and hemoglobin S accounts for 80% to 95% of the total hemoglobin and hemoglobin A is absent. Hemoglobins F and A_2 account for remaining hemoglobin.

CLINICAL FEATURES: Infants with SS hemoglobin are asymptomatic for their first 8 to 10 weeks of life, because they have high levels of hemoglobin F. Clinical symptoms first appear in children when synthesis of γ globin chains declines. This event is somewhat delayed in homozygous S patients. Although patients suffer from lifelong hemolysis, adaptation occurs over time and most may not require regular transfusions. Instead, the clinical picture is dominated by sequelae of repeated **vasoocclusive disease**. In an attempt to minimize these complications by decreasing the amount of hemoglobin S in circulation, a chronic exchange transfusion program may become necessary. Sickle cell anemia is a systemic disorder and is eventually responsible for impaired function in most organ systems and tissues (Fig. 20-20).

Patients with sickle cell disease develop episodic painful crises, the number of which varies. Capillary occlusion leads to ischemia and hypoxic cell injury, which cause severe pain, especially in the chest, abdomen and bones. Painful crises can be triggered by various stimuli (e.g. underlying infection, acidosis, or dehydration).

APLASTIC CRISIS: In aplastic crisis, the bone marrow fails to compensate for the high level of red cell loss. Hemoglobin levels drop rapidly and there is no reticulocyte response. Parvovirus B19 is the most frequent cause of an aplastic crisis, although other viral and bacterial infections may also cause transient bone marrow suppression.

SEQUESTRATION CRISIS: In this case, sudden pooling of erythrocytes, especially in the spleen, results in a decreased circulating blood volume and low hemoglobin levels. The etiology is not well understood, but it most frequently develops in young children, who still have a functioning spleen. This complication

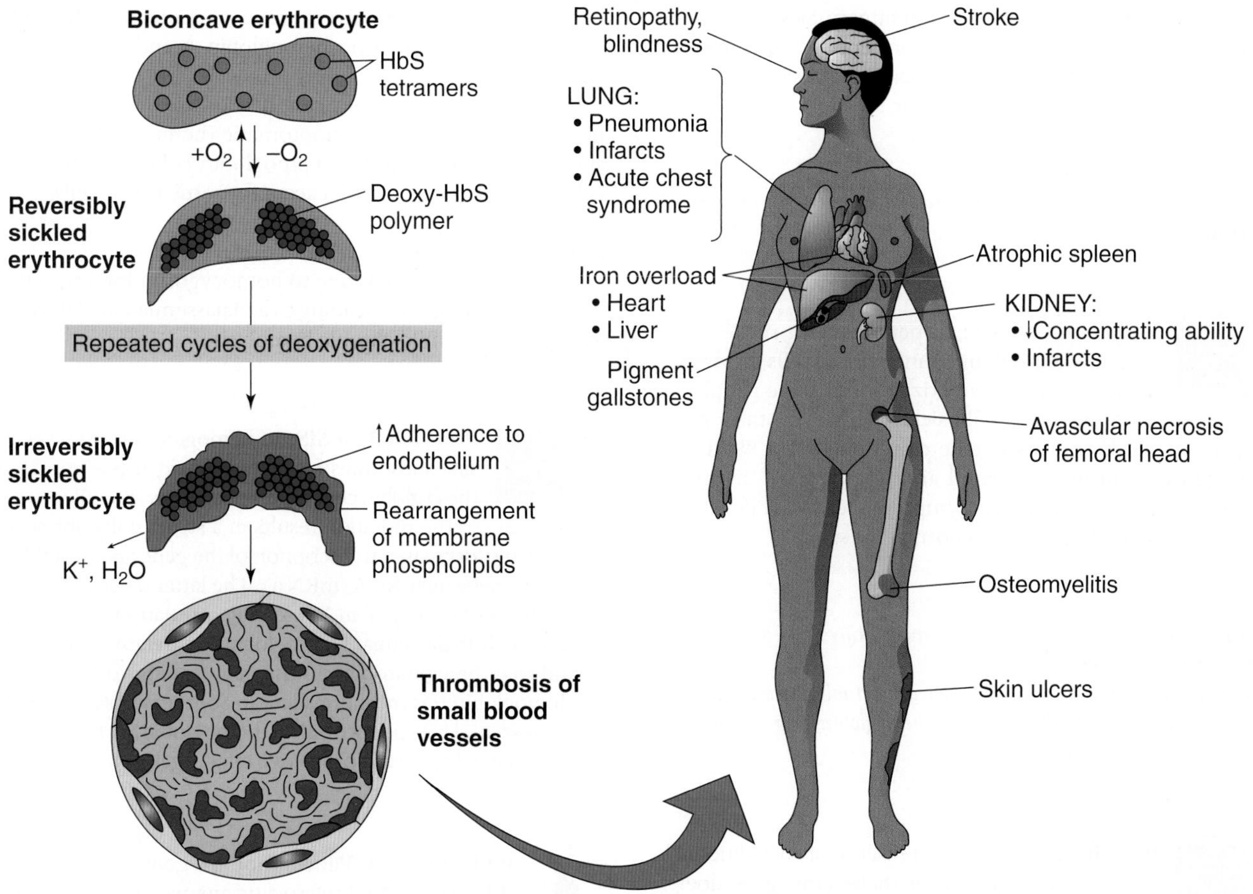

FIGURE 20-20. **Pathogenesis of the vascular complications of sickle cell anemia.** Substitution of valine for glutamic acid leads to an alteration in the surface charge of the hemoglobin molecule. Upon deoxygenation ($-O_2$), sickle hemoglobin (HbS) tetramers aggregate to form poorly soluble polymers. The erythrocyte change shape from a biconcave disk to a sickle form with the polymerization of HbS. This process is initially reversible upon reoxygenation ($+O_2$), but with repeated cycles of deoxygenation and reoxygenation, the erythrocytes become irreversibly sickled. Irreversibly sickled cells display a rearrangement of phospholipids between the outer and inner monolayers of the cell membrane, in particular an increase in aminophospholipids in the outer leaflet. Potassium (K^+) and water (H_2O) are lost from the cells. The erythrocytes are no longer deformable and are more adherent to endothelial cells, properties that predispose to thrombosis of small blood vessels. The resulting vascular occlusions lead to widespread ischemic complications.

is followed by hypovolemic shock and is the most frequent cause of death early in life.

- **Heart:** Chronic demand for increased cardiac output may lead to cardiomegaly and congestive heart failure. In addition, obstruction of coronary microcirculation may cause myocardial ischemia. Myocyte function may also be impaired by excess iron deposition, due to the chronic hemolysis and repeated transfusions.
- **Lungs:** Up to one-third of patients with sickle cell anemia show a rapid decrease in respiratory function, associated with pulmonary infiltrates on chest x-ray. This **acute chest syndrome** may be fatal. Pulmonary infarction may occur, and sickle cell patients are more susceptible to a variety of pulmonary infections.
- **Spleen:** Although splenomegaly is often found in childhood, repeated splenic infarction leads to a functional autosplenectomy. In most adults, only a small fibrous remnant of the spleen remains. The asplenic state renders the patient prone to infections with encapsulated bacteria, especially pneumococcus.
- **Brain:** Patients with sickle cell anemia develop neurologic complications related to vascular obstruction, including transient ischemic attacks, overt strokes, and cerebral hemorrhages. Occlusion of retinal microvasculature may lead to retinal hemorrhage and detachment, proliferative retinopathy, and blindness.
- **Kidney:** Sickling commonly occurs in the renal medulla because of the hypoxic, acidotic, and hypertonic environment that normally exists there. Complications include inability to form concentrated urine, renal infarcts, and papillary necrosis. Male patients may develop priapism, which, if not treated promptly, may lead to permanent erectile dysfunction.
- **Liver:** As in any form of chronic hemolytic anemia, patients with sickle cell anemia have increased levels of unconjugated (indirect) bilirubin, which predisposes to development of pigmented bilirubin gallstones. Cholelithiasis may lead to cholecystitis, which then may require cholecystectomy. Hepatomegaly and increased hepatic iron deposition are also seen.
- **Extremities:** Cutaneous ulcers over the lower extremities, especially near the ankles, are common and reflect obstruction of dermal capillaries. "Hand–foot syndrome," with self-limited swelling of the hands and feet, may develop in children because of underlying bone infarcts. A vascular necrosis of the

femoral head requires corrective hip surgery. Sickle cell disease is also associated with increased incidence of osteomyelitis, particularly with *Salmonella typhimurium,* possibly related to the underlying impairment in splenic function.

Sickle Cell Trait

Heterozygosity for the hemoglobin S mutation is referred to as ***sickle cell trait.***

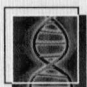

PATHOGENESIS: In persons with sickle cell trait, the hemoglobin A in their red cells prevents hemoglobin S polymerization, so these people's erythrocytes do not normally sickle. However, their red cells may sickle under extreme conditions (e.g., flight at high altitude in unpressurized aircraft, deep sea diving). Heterozygotes are clinically asymptomatic, do not develop hemolytic anemia and have a normal life span.

Double Heterozygosity for Hemoglobin S and Other Hemoglobinopathies

Some patients with a sickling disorder are actually heterozygous for both hemoglobin S and other abnormal hemoglobins (e.g., hemoglobin C or D) or for thalassemia.

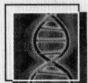

PATHOGENESIS: The presence of an additional abnormal hemoglobin or thalassemic gene does not prevent polymerization of hemoglobin S, and the clinical expression and severity of disease may be affected. Doubly heterozygous individuals may have less frequent crises, higher baseline hemoglobin values, microcytic red cell indices, or persistent splenomegaly into adult life.

Hemoglobin C Disease

Hemoglobin C disease results from homozygous inheritance of a structurally abnormal hemoglobin, which leads to increased erythrocyte rigidity and mild chronic hemolysis.

PATHOGENESIS: In hemoglobin C involves lysine replaces glutamic acid at the sixth amino acid of β globin. Hemoglobin C precipitates in erythrocyte cytoplasm and leads to cellular dehydration and decreased deformability. Upon passage through the spleen, the abnormal red cells are removed from the circulation, causing mild anemia and splenomegaly. Given that hemoglobin C has reduced oxygen affinity, tissue oxygen delivery is increased, which lessens the severity of disease. Hemoglobin C is mosty found in the same populations as hemoglobin S, although its incidence is less.

PATHOLOGY: Homozygosity for hemoglobin C disease (CC) causes a mild normocytic anemia. Hemoglobin may be unevenly distributed within red cells and dense, rhomboidal crystals (representing precipitated hemoglobin C) are present in some erythrocytes. Hemoglobin electrophoresis reveals no hemoglobin A and more than 90% hemoglobin C.

Two to 3% of American blacks are heterozygous for hemoglobin C and are asymptomatic (hemoglobin C trait). In such people, about 40% of hemoglobin is hemoglobin C. Red cell morphology is normal, except for some target cells.

Hemoglobin E Disease

Hemoglobin E disease is due to homozygosity for a structurally abnormal hemoglobin, leading to a thalassemia-like defect that is associated with mild chronic hemolysis.

PATHOGENESIS: In hemoglobin E involves lysine substitutes for glutamic acid at position 26 of the β globin chain. This position is at a splice site in the gene, so the mutation results in a structurally abnormal molecule, decreased transcription of the gene and unstable β globin messenger RNA (mRNA). The latter defects diminish synthesis of hemoglobin E, creating a situation akin to that seen with thalassemia. Hemoglobin E is relatively unstable and may precipitate within the cell, leading to hemolysis. Hemoglobin E is most prevalent in Southeast Asia and globally is second in incidence only to hemoglobin S. Hemoglobin E is believed to exert a protective effect against malaria.

PATHOLOGY: Patients homozygous for hemoglobin E (EE) have a mild microcytic anemia. MCV is decreased and there is often erythrocytosis because of the thalassemia-like component. Blood smear examination reveals microcytic, hypochromic red cells, and target cells. More than 90% of hemoglobin is hemoglobin E.

Other Hemoglobinopathies

Several hundred additional hemoglobin variants have been described that result from mutations in α or β globin genes. These mutations may lead to structural abnormalities or to a functional derangement of the hemoglobin molecule.

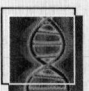

PATHOGENESIS: Some mutations alter the tertiary structure of hemoglobin, leading to its destabilization and precipitation in the cytoplasm. As a group, these hemoglobins are referred to as **unstable hemoglobins** and are often named after the geographic location in which they were first discovered (e.g., hemoglobin Köln). Unstable hemoglobins precipitate and form Heinz bodies within the erythrocytes that can be shown with supravital staining. Heinz bodies bind to cell membranes, increasing their rigidity and leading to mild chronic hemolysis. Patients may suffer jaundice and splenomegaly.

Other hemoglobin mutations cause **abnormal oxygen affinity. Increased oxygen affinity** leads to decreased tissue oxygen delivery. Resulting hypoxia leads to increased EPO production and erythroid hyperplasia in the bone marrow. This in turn causes erythrocytosis. Patients are mostly asymptomatic, but in some cases they may have symptoms related to hyperviscosity. Abnormal hemoglobins with **decreased oxygen affinity** readily release oxygen at the tissue level. EPO levels are low, and most patients have mild anemia. Because of increased of deoxyhemoglobin, patients appear cyanotic.

Immune Hemolytic Anemias

In immune hemolytic anemias, red cell destruction (hemolysis) is caused by antibodies against antigens at the erythrocyte surface. The red cells themselves are intrinsically normal but are targets for an immune-mediated attack. Immune hemolytic anemia can develop secondary to either auto- or alloantibodies, and the site of hemolysis may be extravascular or intravascular.

Autoimmune Hemolytic Anemia

Autoimmune hemolytic anemia (AIHA) features autoantibodies against red cells. Autoantibodies can be classified as either warm or cold antibodies.

Warm Antibody AIHA

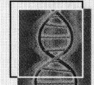

PATHOGENESIS: Warm autoantibodies have optimal reactivity at 37°C (98.6°F) and account for 80% of all cases of AIHA. They are usually IgG and are usually directed against erythrocyte Rh determinants. They do not bind complement, so extravascular hemolysis occurs, primarily in the spleen. Splenic macrophages have Fc receptors that recognize erythrocyte-bound warm antibodies and remove segments of the membrane with attached antibody. Progressive loss of membrane leads to formation of spherocytes, which ultimately undergo hemolysis.

Warm antibody AIHA affects women more often than men, and half of cases are idiopathic. In remaining cases, warm antibody reflects an underlying condition, such as infection, collagen vascular disease, lymphoproliferative disorders, and drug reactions.

Drug-induced warm antibodies may arise by several different mechanisms. In the **hapten** mechanism, a drug such as penicillin binds to erythrocyte surfaces. With this modification, the red cell-drug complex elicit antibodies, some of which react with the erythrocyte itself. In the **immune complex** mechanism, a drug such as quinidine reacts with specific circulating antibody to form immune complexes, which are then bound to red cell membranes. In the **autoantibody** mechanism, a drug (e.g., α-methyldopa) leads to the formation of antibodies that cross-react with red cell membrane components. In both hapten and immune-complex models, the drug is required for hemolysis, whereas in the autoantibody model, hemolysis occurs in the absence of the initiating drug.

PATHOLOGY AND CLINICAL FEATURES: Warm antibody AIHA is associated with normocytic or occasionally macrocytic anemia, with spherocytes, and polychromasia. The direct antiglobulin (Coombs) test is usually positive and is useful in distinguishing immune from nonimmune spherocytosis. In the direct Coombs test, the patient's red cells are incubated with anti-human globulin serum. Agglutination indicates antibody is present on the cell surface. Warm antibody AIHA is treated with corticosteroids or other immunosuppressive agents. Refractory cases may require splenectomy or transfusions.

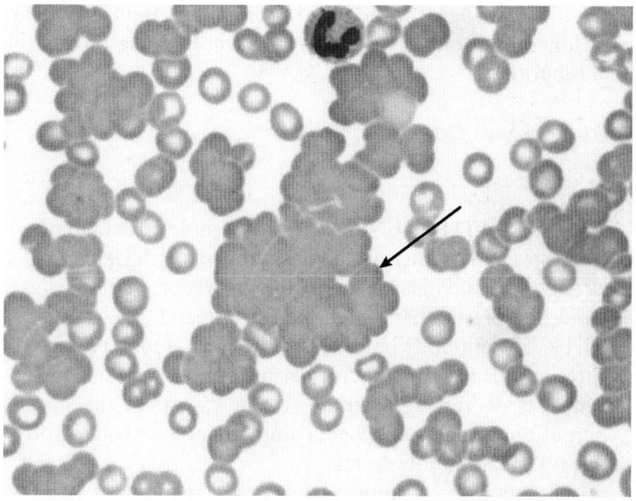

FIGURE 20-21. **Clumped red cells *(arrow)* caused by cold agglutinins.**

Cold Antibody AIHA

Cold antibodies have maximal reactivity at 4°C (39.2°F). Some 20% of cases of AIHA are caused by cold IgM or IgG antibodies, which occur as cold agglutinins or hemolysins.

PATHOGENESIS: Cold agglutinins are mostly IgM directed against the I/i antigen system on red cells. At cooler temperatures in the peripheral circulation, these antibodies bind and agglutinate red cells (Fig. 20-21), and fix complement. Upon rewarming in the central circulation, the antibody dissociates from the erythrocyte surface, leaving unactivated complement attached. These complement-coated red cells may undergo extravascular hemolysis in the liver, because Kupffer cells have more complement receptors than do splenic macrophages. Occasionally, the thermal amplitude of a cold agglutinin is high enough for the antibody to remain attached; complement becomes activated and intravascular hemolysis occurs. Cold agglutinins may be idiopathic or develop secondary to an underlying condition, mostly infections (Epstein-Barr virus [EBV], *Mycoplasma*) or lymphoproliferative disorders.

PATHOLOGY AND CLINICAL FEATURES: Cold agglutinins often are activated upon cooling of blood to room temperature, and erythrocyte agglutination in vitro can be noted on blood smears (see Fig. 20-21). Agglutination leads to falsely low RBCs and Hct and falsely elevated MCV and MCHC. Warming a blood sample to 37°C (98.6°F) prior to analysis corrects the spurious results. The direct Coombs test is positive but usually only for the presence of complement on red cells. Significant hemolysis is uncommon with cold agglutinins and patients are more likely to develop peripheral vascular symptoms (Raynaud phenomenon) upon cold exposure, because of red cell agglutination.

Cold Hemolysin Disease

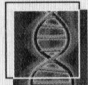

PATHOGENESIS: Cold hemolysins (Donath-Landsteiner antibodies) are usually IgGs and directed against the P antigen system on red cells. Cold hemolysins have biphasic activity and rarely cause AIHA. The antibody binds to erythrocytes at low temperatures and fixes complement. Because the antibody is IgG, red cells do not agglutinate. Upon warming, the cold hemolysin remains attached, complement is activated and intravascular hemolysis occurs.

The clinical syndrome related to cold hemolysins is designated **paroxysmal cold hemoglobinuria (PCH)**. PCH most often follows a viral illness. Immunosuppressive therapy and splenectomy are usually ineffective and supportive therapy is required.

PATHOLOGY: Patients with PCH may develop severe anemia, decreased haptoglobin levels, and hemoglobinuria secondary to intravascular hemolysis. The direct Coombs test is positive for complement but may be negative for IgG, since cold hemolysins may readily dissociate from red cells in vitro.

Hemolytic Transfusion Reactions

An **immediate hemolytic transfusion** reaction occurs when grossly incompatible blood is administered to a patient with preformed alloantibodies, usually because of a clerical error. Massive hemolysis of the transfused blood may be associated with severe complications, including hypotension, renal failure, and even death. *Hemolytic transufion reaction and hemolytic disease in the newborn (see below) are examples of* ***alloimmune hemolytic anemia****, which refers to the destruction of fetal red cells by alloantibodies.*

Delayed hemolytic transfusion reactions usually involve antibodies to minor red cell antigens. Following initial exposure to such antigens, antibody levels rise, but then may decline to the point where they are undetectable in routine pretransfusion screening tests. Subsequent re-exposure to the offending antigen elicits an anamnestic antibody response, with hemolysis occurring several days later. Delayed hemolytic transfusion reactions are usually less severe than immediate reactions and may be clinically undetectable. In both types of hemolytic transfusion reactions, the direct antiglobulin test is positive.

Hemolytic Disease of the Newborn

Hemolytic disease of the newborn (HDN) reflects incompatibility of blood types between a mother and her developing fetus; the mother lacks an antigen that is expressed by the fetus. Maternal IgG alloantibodies can then cross the placenta and cause hemolysis of fetal erythrocytes and erythroblastosis detectable in peripheral blood smears (Fig. 20-22). Most commonly, HDN antibodies react to ABO or Rh antigens.

With ABO-type HDN, the mother is type O and the fetus is usually type A. Naturally occurring maternal anti-A antibodies cause hemolysis in the fetus. No prior exposure through pregnancy or transfusion is required for hemolysis to develop. The anemia associated with ABO incompatibility is usually mild. Affected babies develop hyperbilirubinemia, spherocytosis, and a positive direct antiglobulin test.

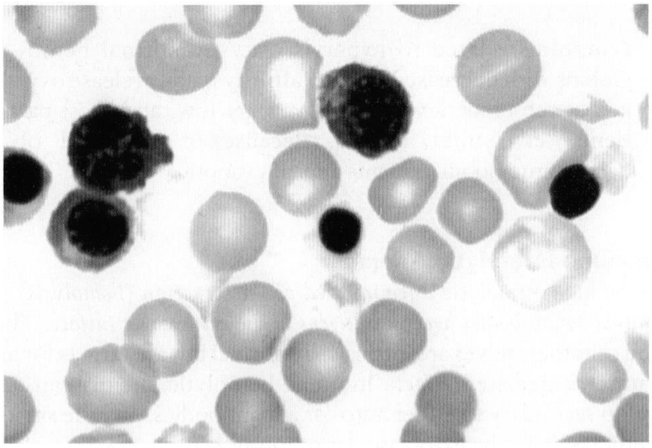

FIGURE 20-22. **Hemolytic disease of the newborn.** The peripheral blood contains numerous erythroid precursors (erythroblasts), which are normally confined to the bone marrow.

With Rh-type HDN, the mother is Rh-negative and the fetus is Rh-positive. The D antigen is most frequently involved, although minor Rh antigens can also cause disease. Prior maternal exposure reflects previous pregnancy or transfusion. The severity of the disease varies, but hemolysis in Rh incompatibility is generally more significant than in ABO-type HDN. Severely affected fetuses may develop **hydrops fetalis**, characterized by heart failure, generalized edema, and intrauterine death (see Chapter 6). Fortunately, today most cases of D-related HDN are preventable by passive immunization of Rh-negative mothers during pregnancy with injections of Rh immune globulin. Laboratory findings are similar to those described above for ABO HDN.

Mechanical Red Cell Fragmentation Syndromes

In red cell fragmentation syndromes intrinsically normal erythrocytes are subjected to mechanical disruption as they circulate in the blood (intravascular hemolysis).

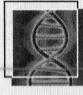

PATHOGENESIS: *These disorders are classified as macroangiopathic (large vessels) or microangiopathic (capillaries), according to the site of hemolysis.* Mechanical fragmentation of red cells is due to alteration of the endothelial surface of blood vessels or disturbances in blood flow patterns that lead to turbulence and increased shear stress.

Macroangiopathic hemolytic anemia most often reflects direct red cell trauma from an abnormal vascular surface (e.g., prosthetic heart valve, synthetic vascular graft).

Microangiopathic hemolytic anemia (see Fig. 20-7) more frequently results from abnormalities in the microcirculation that cause turbulent blood flow patterns. Classic examples of microangiopathic hemolysis are disseminated intravascular coagulation (DIC) and thrombotic thrombocytopenic purpura (TTP), both of which feature

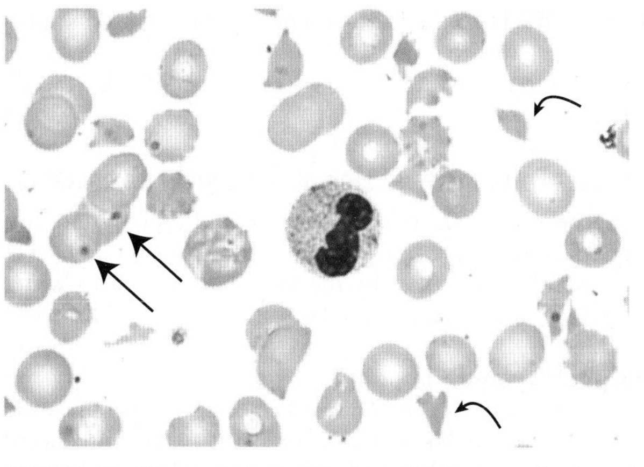

FIGURE 20-23. **Microangiopathic hemolytic anemia.** Irregular, fragmented erythrocytes (schistocytes, *curved arrows)* are seen in the blood smear of a patient with disseminated intravascular coagulation. Howell-Jolly bodies are also present (*straight arrows*).

generalized capillary thrombosis (see below). Long distance running or walking ("march hemoglobinuria") or prolonged vigorous exercise can cause repetitive trauma to red cells and lead to hemolysis. Alterations in blood flow, as are encountered in malignant hypertension or vasculitis syndromes, may also lead to mechanical fragmentation of erythrocytes.

PATHOLOGY: Laboratory findings are similar in macro- and microangiopathic hemolytic anemias. Anemia is mild to moderate and an appropriate reticulocyte response is seen. Blood smears show fragmented erythrocytes (schistocytes) and polychromasia (Fig. 20-23). Abnormalities in coagulation and thrombocytopenia characterize DIC, whereas thrombocytopenia alone is seen in cases of TTP (see below).

Paroxysmal Nocturnal Hemoglobinuria

Paroxysmal nocturnal hemoglobinuria (PNH) is an acquired clonal stem cell disorder characterized by episodic intravascular hemolytic anemia due to increased sensitivity of erythrocytes to complement-mediated lysis.

PATHOGENESIS: The underlying defect in cases of PNH involves somatic mutation of the *phosphatidylinositol glycan-class A (PIG-A)* gene, on the short arm of the X chromosome (Xp22.1) in hematopoietic stem cells. Mutation of the *PIG-A* gene leads to disrupted synthesis of glycosyl phosphatidylinositol (GPI), which normally anchors many proteins (e.g., cluster designation [CD]14, CD16, CD55, CD59) to red cell membranes. Consequent loss of **decay acceleration factor** (CD55) and more importantly **membrane inhibitor of reactive lysis** (CD59) from erythrocyte surfaces renders the cells susceptible to complement-mediated hemolysis. Leukocytes and platelets derived from the abnormal stem cells also show loss of GPI-linked membrane proteins.

PNH may develop as a primary disorder or evolve from preexisting aplastic anemia. Because the defect is clonal it may progress to myelodysplasia or overt acute leukemia. Some patients exhibit several abnormal clonal erythrocyte populations, with varying susceptibility to complement.

PATHOLOGY: During hemolytic episodes, patients develop varyingly severe normocytic or macrocytic anemia, with an appropriate reticulocyte response. Because the hemolysis is intravascular, hemoglobinuria is present, and iron deficiency may develop over time from recurrent iron loss in the urine. Traditionally, increased lysis of patient red cells when incubated with sugar (sucrose hemolysis test) or acidified serum (Ham test) suggest PNH. Both manipulations enhance complement binding to red cells. Today, PNH is diagnosed by demonstrating loss of GPI-anchored proteins on blood cells by flow cytometry. Leukopenia and thrombocytopenia are frequently detected, and sensitivity to complement may lead to inappropriate platelet activation.

CLINICAL FEATURES: Patients develop intermittent intravascular hemolysis, although it is nocturnal in only a minority of cases. Venous and arterial thrombosis, notably Budd-Chiari syndrome (hepatic vein thrombosis), are increased in PNH due to complement-mediated platelet activation. Thrombocytopenia may lead to bleeding. Treatment is supportive; bone marrow transplantation is curative.

Hypersplenism

A mild hemolytic anemia may develop in patients with hypersplenism and congestive splenomegaly.

PATHOGENESIS: Splenomegaly causes pooling of blood and delayed transit of blood cells through the splenic circulation. Prolonged exposure of red cells to splenic macrophages may lead to their premature destruction.

PATHOLOGY AND CLINICAL FEATURES: The anemia of hypersplenism shows no specific morphologic features. Leukopenia and thrombocytopenia are often encountered, but these are due to sequestration of these elements within the enlarged spleen, not destruction. Bone marrow examination shows compensatory hyperplasia of all cell lines.

Other Hemolytic Anemias

Severe thermal burns lead to intravascular hemolysis of erythrocytes. Normal red cells undergo membrane disruption and fragmentation when exposed to temperatures over 49°C (120.2°F). Blood smears reveal numerous schistocytes and microspherocytes, as well as polychromasia. The direct Coombs test is negative.

Several infectious microorganisms specifically parasitize erythrocytes and can cause significant hemolysis. All species of *Plasmodium* have an intraerythrocytic life cycle, which upon completion results in lysis of the red cell (see Chapter 9). Infected red cells are also removed from circulation by splenic macrophages. *Babesiosis,* found in more temperate climates (northeastern United States), is also associated with hemolysis after the intraerythrocytic life cycle is over. In both cases, blood smears reveal the parasites within red cells.

Polycythemia

Polycythemia (erythrocytosis) refers to an increase in the RBC mass.

PATHOGENESIS: Polycythemia can be arbitrarily defined as a Hct greater than 54% in men and 47% in women. At Hcts above 50%, blood viscosity increases exponentially, and cardiac function and peripheral blood flow may be impaired. With a Hct above 60%, blood flow may be so compromised as to lead to tissue hypoxia.

Polycythemia can be further divided on the basis of overall red cell mass into relative and absolute categories.

- **Relative polycythemia**, characteristic of dehydration, is characterized by decreased plasma volume with a normal red cell mass.
- **Gaisbock syndrome (spurious polycythemia)** is seen in middle-aged, overweight, hypertensive smokers and is due to a combination of plasma volume depletion and increased red cell production. Nicotine in cigarettes is a diuretic and leads to reduction in plasma volume, while increased carbon monoxide levels cause hypoxia and a compensatory increase in erythropoiesis.
- **Absolute polycythemia** is a true increase in red cell mass and can be subclassified as primary and secondary.
  - **Primary polycythemia**, or **polycythemia vera (PV),** is an autonomous, EPO-independent, proliferation of erythroid cells that due to an acquired, clonal, hematopoietic stem cell disorder. PV is considered to be a chronic myeloproliferative disorder, and is discussed below.
  - **Secondary polycythemia** arises from EPO-dependent stimulation of erythropoiesis, usually as a compensatory response to general tissue hypoxia. Causes of tissue hypoxia, include chronic lung disease, cigarette smoking, residence at high altitudes, a right-to-left shunt in the heart, and the presence of an abnormal hemoglobin with high oxygen affinity.

    Secondary polycythemia can also occur under certain circumstances unrelated to generalized tissue hypoxia. Neoplasms may produce ectopic EPO as a paraneoplastic syndrome, particularly renal cell carcinoma, hepatocellular carcinoma, cerebellar hemangioblastoma, and uterine leiomyoma. Some non-neoplastic conditions of the kidney may cause secondary polycythemia. Renal cysts or hydronephrosis may exert direct pressure on the kidney, thereby leading to localized hypoxia and increased EPO production.

PLATELETS AND HEMOSTASIS

Normal Hemostasis

Platelets, endothelium, and coagulation factors participate in hemostasis. Hemostasis is normally achieved by clot formation. Initially, platelets **adhere** to the vascular endothelium and subsequently form **aggregates** that are stabilized by fibrin after the coagulation cascade is activated. Clots can be dissolved by the **fibrinolytic system**.

Platelets Form the First Line of Defense in Hemostasis

Hematopoietic stem cells proliferate and differentiate in the bone marrow to form megakaryocytes, under the influence of **TPO**, which is produced by the liver. Each megakaryocyte releases 1000 to 4000 anucleate platelets.

Morphology and Function

At rest, platelets are small discoid cells, 2 to 3 μm in diameter (Fig. 20-24) that circulate freely for about 10 days at concentrations between 150,000 and 400,000/μL. On Wright-stained smears they are pale blue with faint pink granules. By electron microscopy, they contain mitochondria, glycogen particles, dense granules, and α granules. Dense granules contain various nucleotides, including the potent aggregating molecule adenosine diphosphate (ADP). α Granules contain many polypeptides, including adhesive proteins like fibrinogen, von Willebrand factor (vWF), fibronectin, and thrombospondin, as well as the chemokines platelet factor 4 and neutrophil-activating peptide 2.

When vascular endothelium is disrupted, platelets respond by creating a platelet plug to minimize bleeding. Platelets are particularly important in sealing damaged blood vessels that are subjected to high shear rate, such as arteries and arterioles. In certain diseases, platelets respond to activated leukocytes and endothelial cells (see Chapter 2).

Platelet Activation

There are multiple sequential steps in the platelets activation that follows blood vessel injury and loss of an intact endothelial cell layer (see Fig. 20-24).

1. **Platelet adhesion** to subendothelial matrix proteins, such as collagen and vWF, by specific platelet surface glycoprotein receptors. GP Ib/IX binds vWF and GP Ia/IIa and GPVI bind collagen.
2. **Shape change,** from discoid to spherical to stellate
3. **Secretion of platelet granule contents,** including ADP, epinephrine, calcium, vWF, and platelet-derived growth factor (PDGF)
4. **Thromboxane A_2** generation by cyclooxygenase 1
5. **Membrane changes** expose P-selectin and procoagulant anionic phospholipids such as phosphatidylserine
6. **Aggregation of platelets** through fibrinogen receptor GP IIb/IIIa cross-linking

Each of these functional steps has specific consequences. Initial adhesion signals further activation. Secreted granule contents and thromboxane A_2 provide positive feedback to activate additional platelets via their surface receptors. The stellate shape projects the procoagulant membrane surface and activated GP IIb/IIIa/fibrinogen to the site of interaction with coagulation factors and other platelets, respectively. *Thus the surface of activated platelets is an optimal environment for propagating assembly of the coagulation-factor complex, including the prothrombinase complex. The resulting thrombin has many consequences, particularly further platelet activation.* Finally, P-selectin participates in binding leukocytes and localizing them to participate in healing, together with substances secreted by platelets such as PDGF. *As a result of*

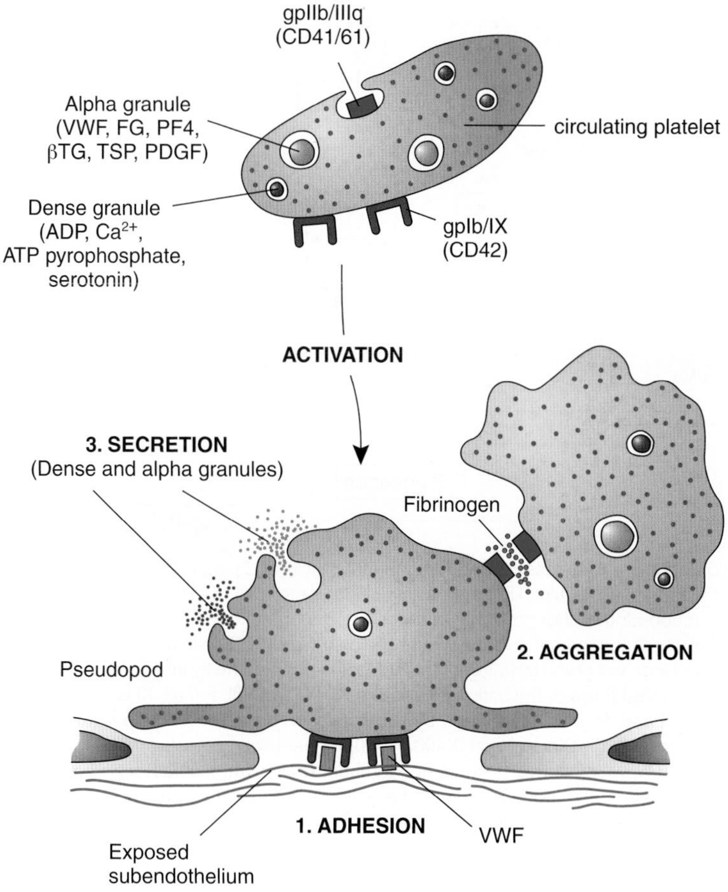

FIGURE 20-24. **Platelet activation involves three overlapping mechanisms.** ***(1)*** Adhesion to the exposed subendothelium is mediated by the binding of von Willebrand factor (vWF) to gpIb/IX (CD42) and is the initiation signal for activation. ***(2)*** Exposure of gpIIb/IIIa (CD41/61) to the fibrinogen (FG) receptor on the platelet surface allows for platelet aggregation. ***(3)*** At the same time, platelets secrete their granule contents, which facilitates further activation. α-Granules contain vWF, fibrinogen, platelet factor 4 (PF4), thromboglobulin (TG), thrombospondin (TSP), and platelet-derived growth factor (PDGF).

these concerted steps, activated platelets form a strong primary plug and then an aggregate within a platelet–fibrin meshwork, which stops bleeding and initiates healing.

Activation of the Coagulation Cascade Completes Blood Clot Formation

Platelets and leukocytes circulate in an inactive state. Similarly, coagulation factors are present as inactive zymogen forms. Aactivation of platelets and coagulation factors is concerted and highly constrained in space and time, to limit dissemination of clots through the circulation. The localization of coagulation-factor complexes to activated surfaces of blood cells, especially platelets, accelerates activation of coagulation factors, and avoids the many anticoagulant factors in plasma.

Activation of the coagulation cascade by damaged tissue culminates in conversion of prothrombin (factor II) to thrombin (factor IIa), and generation of fibrin from fibrinogen (Fig. 20-25). Thrombin has additional roles, namely: (1) activation of platelets and (2) feedback activation of factors that sustain the coagulation response (see Chapter 10).

There are three essential procoagulant complexes and one anticoagulant complex (Fig. 20-25 and Fig. 20-26). *As a general rule, each active enzyme in the cascade is assisted by a cofactor and localized to a phospholipid surface (PL).*

PROCOAGULANT PATHWAYS. Factor Xa, together with its cofactor Va (Xa/Va complex) cleaves factor II (prothrombin) to IIa (thrombin). There are two complexes that activate factor X, the so-called Xase complexes.

1. The complex of **tissue factor** (**TF**) **and factor VIIa** initiats coagulation. Its activation is controlled by exposure to subendothelial cells or activated monocytes and endothelial cells. Microparticles derived from activated leukocytes and endothelial cells contribute to a pool of circulating TF that participates in hemostasis and thrombosis. TF/VIIa/PL initiates factor X activation but is then rapidly shut off by **TF pathway inhibitor** (**TFPI**) (also see Fig. 20-26). The TF/VIIa/PL complex also cleaves and thus activates a small amount of factor IX.
2. The **IXa/VIIIa/PL complex** also initiates factor X activation, with ongoing activation of factor IX by XIa.

Note that thrombin activates the Xase complexes by activating factors XI, VIII, and V. *In summary, the three procoagulant complexes are the prothrombinase complex, Xa/Va/PL and the two Xase complexes, TF/VIIa/PL and IXa/VIIIa/PL.*

ANTICOAGULANT PATHWAYS. An anticoagulant complex activates protein C (see Fig. 20-26). The **protein $\mathbf{C_{ase}}$ complex** is composed of thrombin and thrombomodulin in the endothelial cell plasma membrane. Endothelial protein C receptor also participates in forming this cell surface complex. Activated Protein C, with its cofactor Protein S, inactivates the key cofactors VIIIa and Va, thus limiting further generation of Xa and IIa (see Chapter 10).

Antithrombin inhibits thrombin activity. Antithrombin also cleaves activated factors IXa, Xa, XIa, and XIIa. In vivo this effect is accentuated by heparan sulfate proteoglycans and, most dramatically, by therapeutic administration of heparin.

Thrombolysis Is Mediated by Plasminogen Activation

After a thrombus is firmly established, its further growth is curtailed by removal of platelet-activating factors and coagulation proteins. Endothelial cells near the thrombus produce

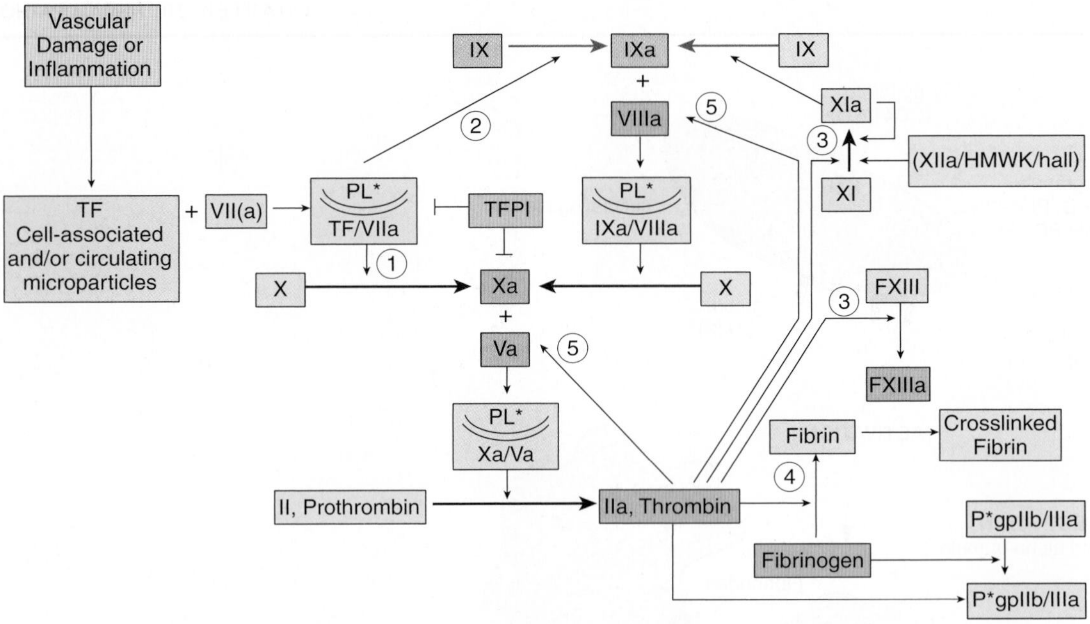

FIGURE 20-25. **Hemostasis and thrombosis.** Following injury to a vessel, rupture of an atherosclerotic plaque, or the presence of major inflammation, coagulation is initiated when tissue factor (TF) binds to circulating factor VII, a small proportion of which is activated (VIIa). TF is located on cells (subendothelial or activated endothelial cells or leukocytes) or circulating microparticles. The TF/VIIa complex is activated by localizing to an activated phospholipid surface (PL*) such as that provided by activated platelets. TF/VIIa activates factor X to form Xa *(1)* and IX to form IXa *(2)*. However, TF pathway inhibitor (TFPI) inhibits both *(1)* and *(2)*. Sustained amplification is achieved through the actions of factors XI, IX, and VIII. Factor XI is activated through the small amount of initial thrombin formed and, to a limited extent, by autoactivation or factor XIIa. Cofactors V and VIII, when activated by thrombin, form complexes with X (Xa/Va) and IX (IXa/VIIIa), respectively, on activated PL surfaces. Note the central and multiple roles for thrombin *(4)*, which converts fibrinogen to fibrin, *(5)* activates cofactors V and VIII, *(3)* activates factors XI and XIII, and activates platelets. Fibrinogen binds to the gpIIb/IIIa integrin receptor on activated platelets (P*). Note the extensive control in time and space of these concerted surface reactions. The combined result is the platelet–fibrin thrombus.

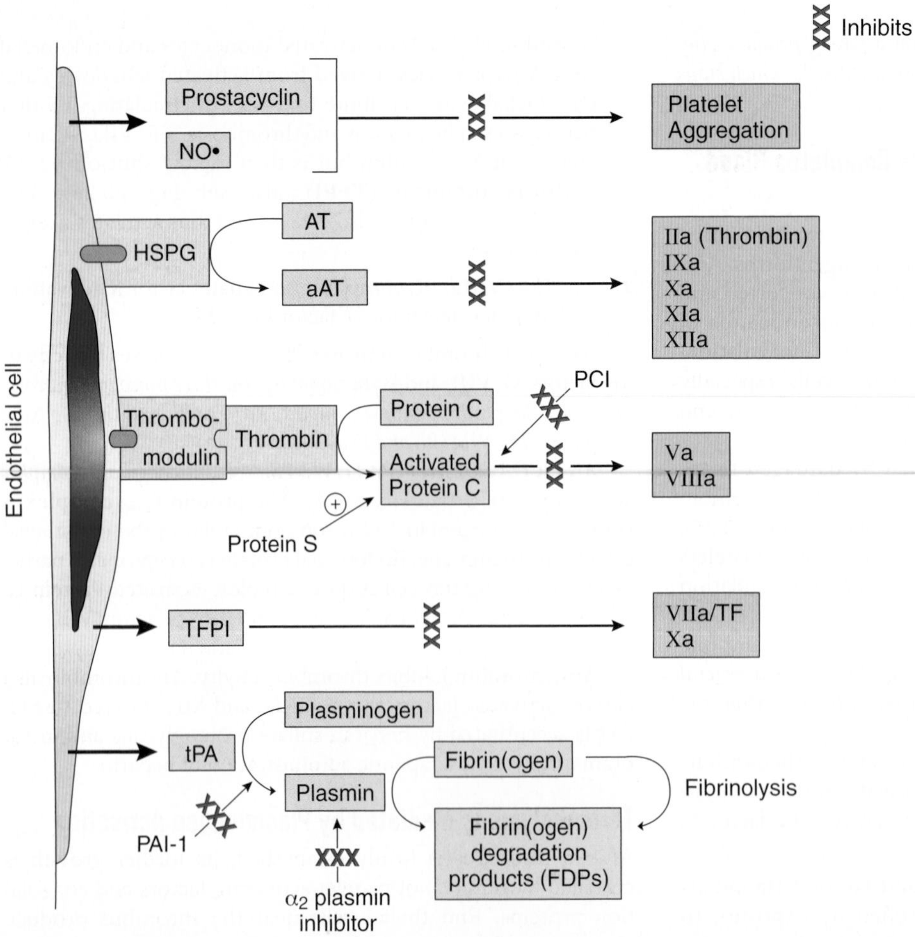

FIGURE 20-26. **The role of endothelium in anticoagulation,** platelet inhibition, and thrombolysis. The endothelial cell plays a central role in the inhibition of various components of the clotting mechanism. Heparan sulfate proteoglycan potentiates the activation of antithrombin (AT) 15-fold. Thrombomodulin stimulates the activation of protein C by thrombin 30-fold. NO• = nitric oxide; HSPG = heparan sulfate proteoglycan; PCI = protein C inhibitor; tPA= tissue plasminogen activator; PAI-I = plasminogen activator inhibitor-I.

plasminogen activators, which activate circulating plasminogen to plasmin and initiate thrombolysis (also known as **fibrinolysis**). There are two major plasminogen activators, **tissue plasminogen activator** (t-PA) and **urokinase-type plasminogen activator** (u-PA). Plasminogen cleavage to plasmin and plasmin action are tightly regulated by several naturally occurring inhibitors, including plasminogen activator inhibitor-I (PAI-I), antiplasmin, and thrombin-activatable fibrinolysis inhibitor (TAFI). Together, the protease plasmin and the activity of macrophages dissolve the thrombus. Plasmin targets specific sites in the fibrin meshwork for degradation, helping to localize its activity to sites where it is needed (see Chapter 10).

Thrombolysis is also coincident with the start of wound repair (see Chapter 7). The latter involves migration and proliferation of fibroblasts and endothelial cells, secretion of new extracellular matrix, and restoration of blood vessel patency. Angiogenesis (i.e., new blood vessels budding from existing ones) occurs in the setting of tissue ischemia or damage. Many products of coagulation and fibrinolysis pathways are potent angiogenic agents.

Blood Vessels and Endothelial Cells Interact with Platelets

The above discussion highlights the many roles of endothelial cells in regulating platelets and coagulation (see Fig. 20-26). Endothelial cells rest on a matrix that contains collagens, elastin, laminin, fibronectin, vWF, and other structural and adhesive proteins. The subendothelial cells are a potent source of TF. When exposed, the matrix of the intima is intensely thrombogenic. Its adhesive proteins bind corresponding platelet membrane glycoprotein receptors and cause them to adhere to the exposed matrix. TF binds circulating activated factor VIIa to activate factors X and IX (see Fig. 20-25).

The endothelium provides smooth, nonthrombogenic surface. The synthesis of anticoagulant molecules on the endothelium prevents unstimulated platelets from adhering to, or penetrating, the endothelial barrier. Endothelial cells also synthesize the potent vasodilator prostacyclin, which inhibits platelet function. Nitric oxide exerts similar effects. These actions keep the blood fluid until injury to the endothelium exposes subendothelial tissue (see Chapters 2 and 10).

Hemostatic Disorders

Defects of the system for maintaining fluid blood passage through intact vessels fall into two categories: **hemostatic** disorders and **thrombotic** disorders. *Failure of the hemostatic system to restore the integrity of an injured vessel causes **bleeding**. Inability to maintain the fluidity of blood results in **thrombosis**.*

The clinical manifestations of hemorrhage associated with disorders of each component of the hemostatic system tend to be distinctive (Table 20-6). Platelet abnormalities result in both petechiae and purpuric hemorrhages in the skin and mucous membranes. Deficiencies of coagulation factors lead to hemorrhage into muscles, viscera, and joint spaces. Disorders of the blood vessels usually cause purpura.

Hemostatic Disorders of Blood Vessels Reflect Dysfunction of Vascular or Extravascular Tissues

Dysfunction of the extravascular or vascular tissues may cause hemorrhages ranging from cosmetic blemishes to life-threatening blood loss.

TABLE 20-6

Principal Causes of Bleeding

Vascular disorders
Senile purpura
Purpura simplex
Glucocorticoid excess
Dysproteinemias
Allergic (Henoch-Schönlein) purpura
Hereditary hemorrhagic telangiectasia
Platelet abnormalities
Thrombocytopenia (see Table 20-7)
Qualitative disorders
Inherited
Glycoprotein IIb/IIIa deficiency (Glanzmann thrombasthenia)
Glycoprotein Ib/IX/V deficiency (Bernard-Soulier syndrome)
Storage pool diseases (α and δ)
Abnormal arachidonic acid metabolism
Acquired
Uremia
Drugs
Cardiopulmonary bypass
Myeloproliferative disorders
Liver disease
Coagulation factor deficiencies
Inherited
von Willebrand disease
Hemophilia A
Hemophilia B
Acquired
Vitamin K deficiency/antagonism
Liver disease
Disseminated intravascular coagulation

Extravascular Dysfunction

SENILE PURPURA: The most common disorder in extravascular dysfunction, senile purpura, is age-related atrophy of supporting connective tissues. Senile purpura is associated with superficial, sharply demarcated, persistent purpuric spots on the forearms and other sun-exposed areas.

PURPURA SIMPLEX: A similar type of purpura occurs principally in women during menses. Purpura simplex occurs in the deep dermis and resolves quickly.

SCURVY: Collagen synthesis is disturbed in vitamin C deficiency, and purpura is a common manifestation (see Chapter 8). Perifollicular hemorrhages are characteristic.

Vascular Dysfunction

Deposition of immunoglobulin fragments in vessel walls may occur in **amyloidosis** (see Chapter 23), **cryoglobulinemia, and other paraproteinemias** and can cause vessel wall weakness and purpura. Certain types of **arteritis** also injure the vessel wall and may lead to hemorrhage (see Chapter 10).

Hereditary Hemorrhagic Telangiectasia (Rendu-Osler-Weber Syndrome)

Hereditary hemorrhagic telangiectasia is an autosomal dominant disorder of blood vessel walls (venules and capillaries) that results in tortuous, dilated vessels (telangiectasias). The underlying defect is dilation and thinning of vessel walls, due to inadequate elastic tissue and smooth muscle. At first, telangiectasias are punctate reddish spots on the lips and nose, up to 0.5 cm in diameter. They can remain as telangiectasias or progress to arteriovenous malformations or aneurysmal dilations throughout the body.

CLINICAL FEATURES: Patients with hereditary hemorrhagic telangiectasia have recurrent hemorrhages, which may occur spontaneously or following trivial trauma, and anemia. Although bleeding may occur at the site of any lesion, over 80% of patients have recurrent epistaxis beginning at an early age. Later in life, gastrointestinal hemorrhage may be the dominant symptom. Arteriovenous fistulas in the lung, brain, and retina may be troublesome and lead to hemorrhage or clinically significant shunting of blood. Recurrent bleeding may limit a patient's activities, but death from exsanguination is rare.

Allergic Purpura (Henoch-Schönlein Purpura)

Allergic purpura is a vascular disease that results from immunological damage to blood vessel walls (see Chapter 16). In children, it often follows viral infections and is self-limited. In adults, it is associated with exposure to a variety of drugs and may be chronic.

PATHOLOGY: Histologically, Henoch-Schönlein purpura is characterized by **leukocytoclastic vasculitis**, with perivascular infiltration of neutrophils and eosinophils, fibrinoid necrosis of vessel walls, and platelet plugs in vascular lumens. IgA and complement complexes circulate in the blood and are often seen in vessel walls. Purpuric spots are often accompanied by raised urticarial lesions. Intestinal cramps and bleeding indicate gastrointestinal involvement. If kidneys are affected, renal failure may ensue.

The Most Common Platelet Disorders Impair Hemostasis

Patients may have a history of easy bruising or life-threatening bleeding. Bleeding can occur in any damaged vascular bed, but a particular pattern of mucocutaneous bleeding, including gingival bleeding, epistaxis, and menorrhagia, is common. More severe manifestations are bleeding into the gastrointestinal tract, genitourinary tract, and brain. Petechiae, which are characteristic of platelet disorders, are nonblanching red lesions less than 2 mm in size. They usually occur in lower extremities, in dependent regions of the body, on the buccal mucosal and soft palate and at pressure points (waistband, wristwatch band). Petechiae may also occur in vascular disorders. *Platelet disorders reflect:*

1. Decreased production
2. Increased destruction
3. Impaired function

Thrombocytopenia

Thrombocytopenia is defined as platelet counts under 150,000/μL. The lower the platelet count, the greater the risk of traumatic and perioperative bleeding. Patients with fewer than 10,000 platelets/μL are at increased risk of spontaneous hemorrhage (Table 20-7).

Decreased platelet production *is caused by bone marrow infiltration with leukemic cells or metastatic cancer, which impair megakaryopoiesis.* Ineffective megakaryopoiesis in myelodysplasia also results in thrombocytopenia. Bone marrow failure in patients with aplastic anemia or who received radiotherapy or chemotherapy produces pancytopenia, including thrombocytopenia. Certain viral infections such as cytomegalovirus or any megaloblastic anemia may cause severe thrombocytopenia.

TABLE 20-7

Principal Causes of Thrombocytopenia

Decreased production
Aplastic anemia Bone marrow infiltration (neoplastic, fibrosis) Bone marrow suppression by drugs or radiation
Ineffective production
Megaloblastic anemia Myelodysplasias
Increased destruction
Immunologic (idiopathic, HIV, drugs, alloimmune, posttransfusion purpura, neonatal) Nonimmunologic (DIC, TTP, HUS, vascular malformations, drugs)
Increased sequestration
Splenomegaly
Dilutional
Blood and plasma transfusions

DIC = disseminated intravascular coagulation; HIV = human immunodeficiency virus; HUS = hemolytic-uremic syndrome; TTP = thrombocytic thrombocytopenic purpura.

May-Hegglin anomaly is a hereditary defect in megakaryocyte maturation in which thrombocytopenia is associated with circulating giant platelets and blue cytoplasmic inclusions within neutrophils (Döhle bodies). The disorder is one of the constellation of MYH9 syndromes. These are giant platelet syndromes caused by mutations in the *myosin heavy chain 9* gene.

Increased platelet destruction may reflect immune-mediated damage and removal of circulating platelets, as in idiopathic thrombocytopenic purpura and drug-induced thrombocytopenia. Alternatively, intravascular platelet aggregation may produce thrombocytopenia (e.g., in TTP).

Idiopathic (Immune) Thrombocytopenic Purpura

Idiopathic thrombocytopenic purpura (ITP) is a decrease in blood platelets caused by antibodies against platelet or megakaryocytic antigens. It is, thus, more appropriately called *immune thrombocytopenic purpura.* ITP occurs in two forms: an acute, self-limited, hemorrhagic syndrome in children; and a chronic bleeding disorder in adolescents and adults.

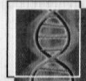

PATHOGENESIS: Like autoimmune hemolytic anemia, ITP reflects antibody-mediated destruction of platelets or their precursors. In most patients, these autoantibodies are of the IgG class, but IgM antiplatelet antibodies also occur.

Acute ITP typically appears in children of either sex after a viral illness and is likely caused by virus-induced changes in platelet antigens that elicit autoantibodies. Complement bound at the surface causes platelets to be lysed in the blood or phagocytosed and destroyed by splenic and hepatic macrophages.

Chronic ITP occurs mainly in adults (male to female ratio of 1:2.6) and may be associated with collagen vascular diseases (e.g., systemic lupus erythematosus) or a malignant lymphoproliferative disease, especially chronic lymphocytic leukemia. It is also common in people infected with human immunodeficiency virus (HIV). The extent of thrombocytopenia in ITP is determined by the balance between: (1) levels of antiplatelet antibodies; (2) the degree of inhibition of platelet production in the bone marrow, as some antibodies may bind to megakaryocytes; and (3) expression of Fc and complement receptors on the surface of macrophages. This expression is upregulated in infection and pregnancy but is ameliorated by certain drugs, for example, corticosteroids, danazol, and intravenous gamma globulin, all of which are used to treat ITP.

PATHOLOGY: In acute ITP, the platelet count is typically less than 20,000/μL. In chronic adult ITP, platelet counts vary from a few thousand to 100,000/μL. Peripheral blood smears show numerous large platelets, which reflect accelerated release of young platelets by bone marrow actively engaged in platelet production. Accordingly, bone marrow examination reveals compensatory increases in megakaryocytes (Fig. 20-27). IgG is detected on the platelets in more than 80% of patients with chronic ITP and in half of these, increased platelet-associated C3 can be demonstrated.

CLINICAL FEATURES: Children with acute ITP experience sudden onset of petechiae and purpura but are otherwise asymptomatic. Spontaneous recovery occurs within 6 months in over 80% of cases. The major threat (<1% of cases) is intracranial hemorrhage. Treatment is rarely necessary, but with serious disease, corticosteroids and intravenous immunoglobulin may be needed. Glucocorticoids decrease production of antiplatelet antibodies and down-regulate macrophage Fc receptors. γ-Globulin interferes with clearance of IgG-coated platelets from the circulation via multiple mechanisms.

Chronic ITP in adults manifests as bleeding episodes, such as epistaxis, menorrhagia or ecchymoses. Life-threatening hemorrhages are uncommon. Occasionally, asymptomatic persons are discovered to have thrombocytopenia on a routine blood cell count. Most adults with chronic ITP improve when given corticosteroids and intravenous γ-globulin. Danazol (a synthetic anabolic steroid) acts similarly to glucocorticoids. In 70% of patients who do not respond adequately to drug therapy within 2 to 3 months, splenectomy produces complete or partial remission.

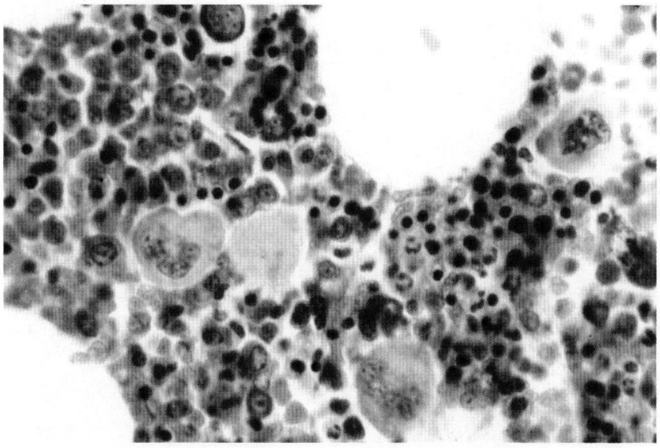

FIGURE 20-27. **Idiopathic thrombocytopenic purpura.** A section of the bone marrow reveals increased megakaryocytes.

Drug-Induced Thrombocytopenia

Many drugs are known to cause immune-mediated platelet destruction: quinine, quinidine, heparin, sulfonamides, gold salts, antibiotics, sedatives, tranquilizers, and anticonvulsants. The drug often forms a complex with a platelet-related protein to make a neoepitope that elicits antibody production. By contrast, chemotherapeutic agents, ethanol, and thiazides cause thrombocytopenia by suppression of platelet production.

In **heparin-induced thrombocytopenia,** 25% of patients experience a mild, transient thrombocytopenia within the first 2 to 5 days of treatment initiation. However, 1% to 3% develop profound consumptive thrombocytopenia after 7 to 10 days of heparin therapy. These patients are predisposed to arterial and venous thromboembolic events that may be lethal. The diagnosis of heparin-induced thrombocytopenia is supported by demonstrating antibodies to the complex of heparin and platelet factor 4.

Pregnancy-Associated Thrombocytopenia

Minimal thrombocytopenia occurs frequently during the third trimester of pregnancy, due to dilution of platelets. Since platelet count are usually above 100,000/μL, no special management is needed. Conversely, preeclampsia/eclampsia syndromes can result in maternal thrombocytopenia. A related condition is called **HELLP** (hemolysis, elevated liver enzyme tests and low platelets). The latter two syndromes can be life-threatening.

Neonatal Thrombocytopenia

Neonatal thrombocytopenias are either *inherited* or *acquired.*

Inherited causes associated with increased platelet destruction include **Wiskott-Aldrich syndrome** (WAS), which is caused by a defect in the *WASP* gene on the X-chromosome. Affected boys have small platelets, eczema and immunodeficiency (see Chapter 4). A variant of WAS is **X-linked thrombocytopenia**, which displays defects in the same gene but features only thrombocytopenia. Inherited causes associated with poor production include amegakaryocytic thrombocytopenia, thrombocytopenia-absent radius syndrome, Fanconi anemia, and other genetic defects in platelet development. Thrombocytopenia can also be seen in infants with trisomy 13, 18, or 21.

Fanconi anemia is a genetic bone marrow failure disorder manifesting often with thrombocytopenia and RBC macrocytosis. There is a high incidence of associated congenital anomalies, such as skin hypopigmentation and hyperpigmentation, short stature, microcephaly, microphthalmia, and radial/thumb abnormalities. Defects in a family of genes responsible for Fanconi anemia have been identified.

Neonatal alloimmune thrombocytopenia (NAIT) is due to increased destruction of platelets, caused by alloimmunization to HPA-1a and other platelet-specific antigens that occur during pregnancy. The mechanism for alloimmunization in this condition is similar to Rh alloimmunization in that the fetus is HPA-1a positive, whereas the mother is negative. In NAIT, the fetus or neonate but not the mother is thrombocytopenic. NAIT predisposes to fetal and neonatal intracranial hemorrhage.

Nonimmune causes of thrombocytopenia in the neonate are similar to those in adults, with additional considerations such as birth asphyxia, hypoxic injury, sepsis and DIC, necrotizing enterocolitis, hemangiomas, and thrombosis.

Post-Transfusion Purpura

After a transfusion, HPA-1–negative persons may develop alloantibodies to HPA-1–positive platelets. Newly infused HPA-1–positive platelets are destroyed by these antibodies. Curiously, the patient's own HPA-1–negative platelets are also destroyed, perhaps related to the passive acquisition of the antigen by these platelets or the development of immune complexes. In any event, a self-limited thrombocytopenia occurs about a week after the transfusion.

Thrombotic Thrombocytopenic Purpura

TTP is a rare syndrome featuring thrombocytopenia, microangiopathic hemolytic anemia, neurologic symptoms, fever, and renal impairment. Platelet aggregation leads to widespread microvascular deposition of platelets as characteristic hyaline thrombi.

PATHOGENESIS: The pathogenesis of TTP is obscure, but the most tenable hypothesis holds that it results from the introduction of one or more platelet-aggregating substances into the circulation. The theory that has received the most attention is the cross-linking of platelets by inappropriate vWF multimers from injured endothelial cells. vWF monomers are normally assembled into multimeric molecules of varying size (up to millions of daltons) within endothelial cells and released locally in response to endothelial stimulation (see below). *For unknown reasons, in TTP, unusually large multimers of vWF are present in the plasma, where they are thought to mediate intravascular platelet aggregation.* A protease that cleaves vWF (ADAMTS13) is genetically absent or defective in familial TTP, and is inactivated by autoantibodies in sporadic TTP. Plasma infusion is most effective in familial forms of TTP and plasma exchange is preferred in acquired types.

Although most cases arise in otherwise normal persons, TTP may also complicate autoimmune collagen vascular disorders (systemic lupus erythematosus, rheumatoid arthritis, Sjögren syndrome) and drug-induced hypersensitivity reactions. It has also been triggered by infections, cancer chemotherapy, bone marrow transplantation, and pregnancy. Occurrence of TTP in siblings suggests a hereditary predisposition.

PATHOLOGY: The morphologic hallmark of TTP is the deposition of PAS-positive hyaline microthrombi in arterioles and capillaries throughout the body, mainly in the heart, brain, and kidneys (Fig. 20-28). These microthrombi contain platelet aggregates, fibrin, and a few erythrocytes and leukocytes. Unlike immune-mediated vasculitis there is no inflammation in TTP, Fragmented erythrocytes (schistocytes) are always evident in peripheral blood smears (Fig. 20-29), as are numerous reticulocytes.

A

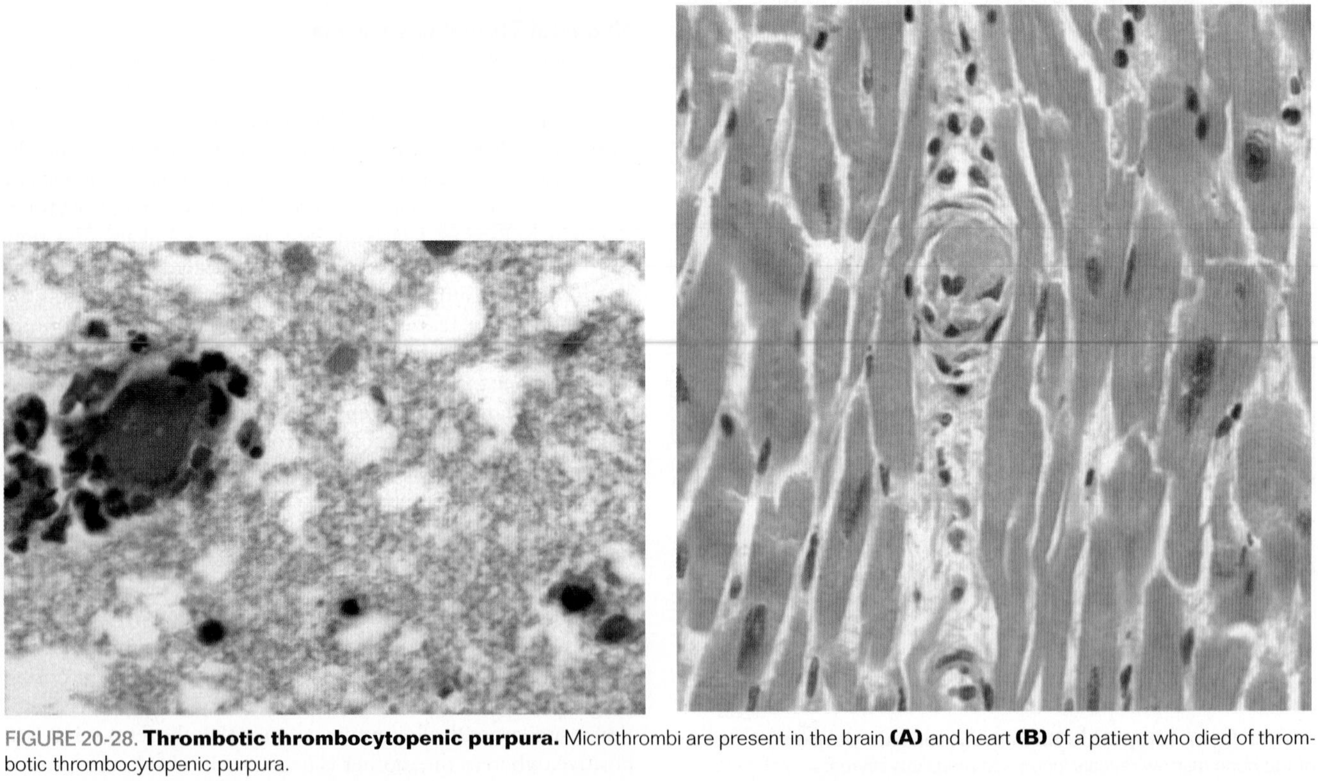

B

FIGURE 20-28. **Thrombotic thrombocytopenic purpura.** Microthrombi are present in the brain **(A)** and heart **(B)** of a patient who died of thrombotic thrombocytopenic purpura.

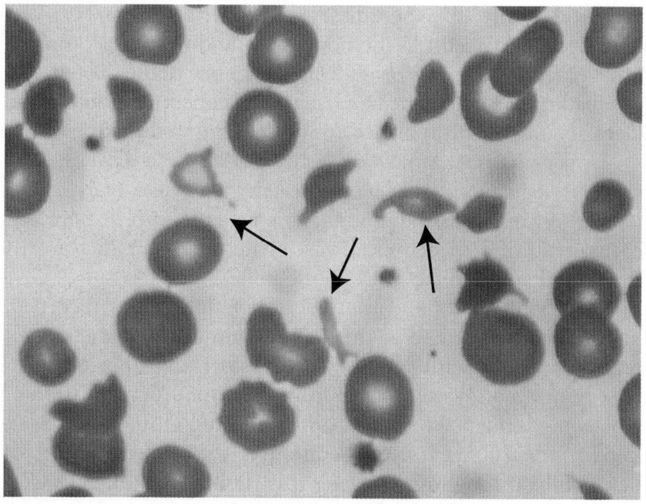

FIGURE 20-29. **Microangiopathic hemolytic anemia.** Numerous schistocytes (arrows) are present in a patient with thrombotic thrombocytopenic purpura.

CLINICAL FEATURES: TTP occurs at virtually any age, but is most common in women in the fourth and fifth decades. It may be chronic and recurrent for years or, more frequently, occurs as an acute, fulminant disease that is often fatal. Most patients present with neurologic symptoms, including seizures, focal weakness, aphasia, and alterations in the state of consciousness. Widespread purpura is often present and vaginal bleeding may occur in women. Anemia is a constant feature, hemoglobin levels are often below 6 g/dL. Jaundice due to hemolysis may be severe. Renal dysfunction is often prominent, half of patients being azotemic.

More than half of patients with TTP have platelet counts below 20,000/μL. Despite the presence of aggregated platelets, activation of the coagulation cascade does not occur. Consequently, the prothrombin time (PT), partial thromboplastin time (PTT), and fibrinogen concentration remain normal, distinguishing this syndrome from DIC (see below). Acute TTP was formerly fatal, but the cure rate is approximately 80% with plasma infusion and plasmapheresis.

Hemolytic–Uremic Syndrome

Hemolytic–uremic syndrome (HUS) resembles TTP and its adult form is a variant of the latter. Classic HUS occurs in children, usually after an acute enteric infection. It seems to be a result of glomerular endothelial cell injury produced by verotoxins elaborated, usually by *Escherichia coli* or *Shigella dysenteriae* (see Chapter 16). In HUS, aggregated platelet thrombi are found primarily in the renal microvasculature. Kidney failure, rather than neurologic abnormalities, is the main clinical feature. Adult HUS is not related to enteric infection, and the pathogenesis of the endothelial injury is unknown.

Splenic Sequestration of Platelets

Many patients with splenomegaly, irrespective of the cause, show **hypersplenism**, a syndrome that includes sequestration of platelets in the spleen. One third of platelets are normally stored temporarily in the spleen, but in massive splenomegaly, up to 90% of the total platelet pool may be captured in that organ. Interestingly, the platelet life span is normal or only slightly reduced. Thrombocytopenia associated with hypersplenism is rarely severe and by itself does not produce a hemorrhagic diathesis.

Other Causes of Thrombocytopenia

Vascular malformations, including hemangiomas and arteriovenous malformations, can cause thrombocytopenia. In hemangiomas, consumption of platelets has been called the **Kasabach-Merritt syndrome**. Platelet loss occurs in patients who have massive hemorrhage, such as in bleeding from a peptic ulcer or during surgery with heavy blood loss. Transfused blood does not contain viable platelets because it is stored at 4°C (39.2°F) before administration. Thus, thrombocytopenia in transfused patients is due to platelet loss and dilution. Platelet transfusion may be used to prevent development of thrombocytopenia.

Hereditary Disorders of Platelets

Bernard-Soulier Syndrome (Giant Platelet Syndrome)

Bernard-Soulier Syndrome is an autosomal recessive trait in which platelets have a quantitative or qualitative defect in the membrane glycoprotein complex (GPIb/IX [CD42] and sometimes GPV) that serves as a receptor for vWF. The complex plays a prominent role in the adhesion of normal platelets to vWF in injured subendothelial tissues. The platelets in Bernard-Soulier syndrome vary widely in size and shape, and the diagnosis is suggested by the presence of thrombocytopenia and giant platelets on the blood smear. Bernard-Soulier syndrome manifests in infancy or childhood with a bleeding pattern characteristic of abnormal platelet function: ecchymoses, epistaxis, and gingival bleeding. At a later age, traumatic hemorrhage, gastrointestinal bleeding, and menorrhagia occur. Many patients have only a mild bleeding disorder but others suffer more severe hemorrhage requiring frequent platelet transfusions and may even be fatal.

Glanzmann Thrombasthenia

Glanzmann thrombasthenia is an autosomal recessive defect in platelet aggregation caused by a quantitative or qualitative abnormality in the glycoprotein complex IIb/IIIa (CD41/61). In normal platelets, this complex is activated during platelet adhesion and serves as a receptor for fibrinogen and vWF, mediating platelet aggregation and the generation of a solid plug. The IIb/IIIa complex is also linked to the platelet cytoskeleton, and transmits the force of contraction to adherent fibrin, a mechanism that promotes clot retraction. In Glanzmann thrombasthenia the lack of aggregation and clot retraction impairs hemostasis and causes bleeding, despite a normal platelet count.

The disease becomes clinically apparent shortly after birth when an infant has mucocutaneous or gingival hemorrhage, epistaxis, or bleeding after circumcision. Later, patients may suffer unexpected hemorrhage after trauma or surgery. Disease severity varies, and only a few patients experience life-threatening hemorrhage. Platelet transfusions correct the condition temporarily.

Alpha Storage Pool Disease (Grey Platelet Syndrome)

A rare inherited malady, alpha storage pool disease is characterized by the absence of morphologically recognizable α granules in platelets. The defect resides in abnormal granule membranes. Thrombocytopenia is common; platelets are large and pale. The bleeding diathesis tends to be mild.

Delta Storage Pool Disease

This heterogeneous malady affects the dense granules of platelets. It is sometimes associated with other multisystem hereditary disorders, including Chediak-Higashi syndrome or Hermansky-Pudlak syndrome (a type of oculocutaneous albinism; see Chapter 6). Bleeding manifestations are mild to moderate.

Acquired Qualitative Disorders of Platelets

A variety of acquired disorders may adversely affect platelet function (see Table 20-7).

- **Drugs:** Various drugs can impair platelet function. Aspirin irreversibly acetylates cyclooxygenase, primarily COX-1 and thus blocks production of platelet thromboxane A_2, which is important in platelet aggregation. Platelets cannot synthesize cyclooxygenase, so the aspirin effect lasts for the life span of platelets (7 to 10 days). Nonsteroidal analgesics, such as indomethacin or ibuprofen, impair platelet function, but as their inhibition of cyclooxygenase is reversible, their effect on platelets is short. Antibiotics, particularly β-lactams (penicillin and cephalosporins), can cause platelet dysfunction. Ticlopidine, which is used to suppress platelet function in patients with thromboembolic disease, causes marked impairment of platelet function and even TTP.
- **Renal failure:** End-stage kidney disease is often accompanied by a qualitative platelet defect that results in a prolonged bleeding time and a tendency towards hemorrhage. The platelet abnormality is heterogeneous and is aggravated by uremic anemia. Restoring a normal hematocrit by administering EPO may restore bleeding time to normal without affecting the azotemia.
- **Cardiopulmonary bypass:** Platelet dysfunction due to platelet activation and fragmentation occurs in the extracorporeal circuit during bypass surgery.
- **Hematologic malignancies:** In chronic myeloproliferative disorders and myelodysplastic syndromes, platelet dysfunction is due to intrinsic platelet defects. In dysproteinemias, platelets are impaired because they are coated with plasma paraprotein.

Thrombocytosis

Reactive Thrombocytosis

An increase in platelet counts occurs in association with: (1) iron deficiency anemia, especially in children; (2) splenectomy; (3) cancer; and (4) chronic inflammatory disorders. Reactive thrombocytosis is rarely symptomatic, but it has been associated with thrombotic episodes, especially in patients bedridden after splenectomy.

Clonal Thrombocytosis

Patients with chronic myeloproliferative syndromes such as PV and essential thrombocythemia have a malignant proliferation of megakaryocytes (see below). Resulting increases in circulating platelets may lead to episodes of thrombosis or bleeding (see below).

Coagulopathies Are Caused by Deficient or Abnormal Coagulation Factors

Quantitative and qualitative disorders of all of coagulation factors have been identified. These conditions may be hereditary or acquired. Only the hereditary deficiencies of factor VIII (hemophilia A), factor IX (hemophilia B), and vWF are common. Most of these disorders result from deficiency of the protein factor, leading to inadequate hemostasis and concomitant bleeding. Occasionally the protein factor is present but dysfunctional.

Hemophilia is an X-linked recessive disorder of blood clotting that results in spontaneous bleeding, particularly into joints, muscles, and internal organs. Classic hemophilia is actually two distinct diseases, resulting from mutations in the genes for factor VIII (hemophilia A) and factor IX (hemophilia B).

Hemophilia is one of the oldest genetic diseases recorded, having been described in the Talmud almost 2000 years ago: male infants of Jewish families with a history of fatal bleeding after circumcision were excused from this ritual. Transmission of a bleeding tendency to boys from unaffected mothers has been known for 200 years. Subsequently, the dissemination of hemophilia throughout Europe's royal families by Queen Victoria's daughters highlighted this disease. The gene for factor VIII was cloned in 1984, allowing investigation of the molecular basis of hemophilia A.

Hemophilia A (Factor VIII Deficiency)

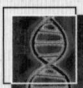

PATHOGENESIS: *Hemophilia A is the most common sex-linked inherited bleeding disorder (1 per 5000 to 10,000 males).* Causative mutations in the very large factor VIII gene at the tip of the long arm of the X chromosome (Xq28) include deletions, inversions, point mutations, and insertions. Each family with a history of hemophilia actually harbors a different mutation (private mutant allele). In half of cases hemophilia A can be traced through many generations, but in the other half, de novo mutations arise within two generations of the index case. In most of these de novo mutations, an origin in the mother, maternal grandfather, or maternal grandmother has been identified.

CLINICAL FEATURES: Patients with hemophilia A have mild, moderate, or severe bleeding tendencies. In most, the severity of the illness parallels the activity of factor VIII in the blood. Half of patients have virtually no factor VIII activity and often suffer spontaneous bleeding. A third of patients, who have up to 10 units of factor VIII per deciliter, bleed spontaneously only occasionally, but often do so after minor trauma. One fifth have more than 10 U/dL and bleed only after significant trauma or surgery.

The most frequent complication of hemophilia A is a deforming arthritis caused by repeated bleeding into many joints. Although uncommon, bleeding into the brain was formerly the most common cause of death. Hematuria, intestinal obstruction, and respiratory obstruction may all occur with bleeding into the respective organs.

Treatment with factor VIII to maintain levels of this clotting factor generally control the bleeding diathesis. Unfortunately, many of these patients developed acquired immunodeficiency syndrome (AIDS) and viral hepatitis from contamination of pooled factor VIII preparations. These complications have been virtually eliminated by screening blood donors and heat treatment of purified factor VIII to inactivate HIV. The availability of human recombinant factor VIII now avoids these infectious complications. Screening to detect female carriers and prenatal diagnosis using DNA markers are highly accurate.

Hemophilia B

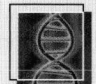

PATHOGENESIS: *Hemophilia B is an X-linked heritable disorder of factor IX deficiency.* At 1 in 20,000 male births, hemophilia B is four times less common than hemophilia A and accounts for 15% of all cases of hemophilia. Factor IX is a vitamin K-dependent protein that is made in the liver. Many different mutations, from single base substitutions to gross deletions, have been linked to hemophilia B.

CLINICAL FEATURES: The bleeding manifestations in hemophilia B, are like those of hemophilia A. Treatment relies on infusion of purified or recombinant protein.

von Willebrand Disease

von Willebrand disease (vWD) is a heterogeneous complex of hereditary bleeding disorders related to deficiency or abnormality of vWF. Over 20 distinct subtypes are known. A simplified classification (see below) recognizes three major categories. Variable expression of vWF (especially type I) confounds estimates of prevalence, although some hold that vWD is the most common inherited coagulopathy (1%–2% of the population).

vWF is an adhesive molecule produced by endothelial cells and megakaryocytes as a 250-kd monomer that polymerizes to multimers with molecular weights in the millions. It is stored in cytoplasmic Weibel-Palade bodies of endothelial cells from which it is released into subendothelial tissues and plasma. After endothelial injury, subendothelial vWF binds to platelet glycoprotein receptors (GPIb/IX or CD42), promoting platelet adherence and sealing the endothelial injury (Fig. 20-30). vWF can also bind to GPIIb/IIIa (CD41/61) to promote platelet aggregation. In plasma, it binds to and protects factor VIII; its absence is always associated with impaired factor VIII activity.

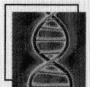

PATHOGENESIS: vWD is an autosomal disease, affecting men and women. The *vWF* gene on chromosome 12 is large and complex (180 kb with 52 exons). Three types of the disease are recognized, each of which is heterogeneous:

- **TYPE I** vWD: These variants constitute 75% of all cases of vWD and are inherited as autosomal dominant traits with variable penetrance. Type I vWD is a **quantitative**

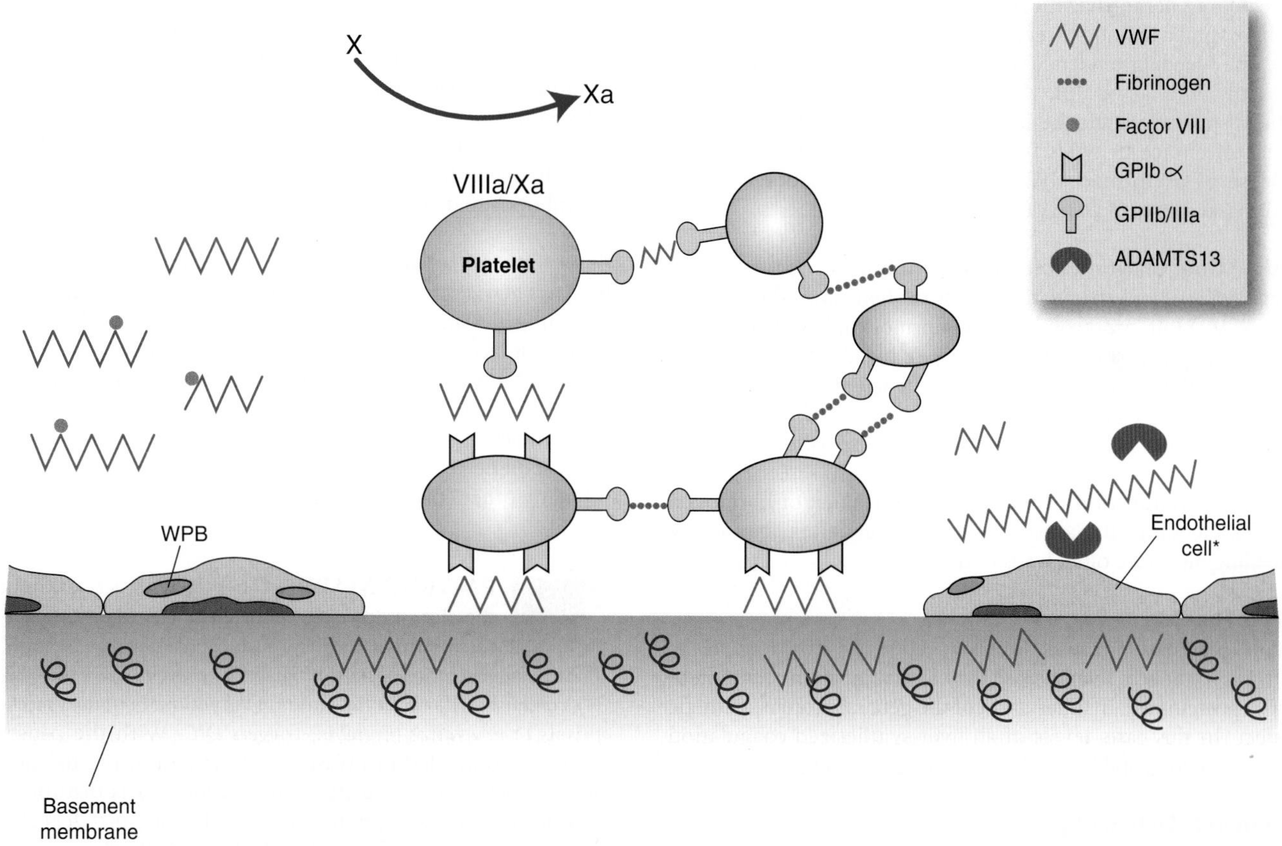

FIGURE 20-30. **von Willebrand factor.** vWF is stored in Weibel-Palade bodies (WBP) of endothelial cells, and is secreted from activated endothelial cells (*) into the subendothelial space. vWF is also secreted from platelet alpha granules. After endothelial injury, vWF binds to platelet glycoprotein receptors GPIbα and promotes platelet adherence and protects factor VIII. Released vWF stablizes platelet adehesion to the damaged vessel wall and promotes platelet-fibrin interactions. vWF also binds GPIIB/IIA on the activated platelet surface to promote platelet aggregation. ADAMTS13 is the protease that cleaves ultralarge multimers of vWF.

deficiency in vWF, in which levels of **all** multimers are reduced, though their relative concentrations remain unchanged.

- **TYPE II** vWD: **Qualitative defects in vWF** characterize type II variants, which account for 20% of vWD. In type II disease, interactions of vWF and the blood vessel wall are defective. The plasma activities of both vWF and factor VIII are low. In type IIa, higher-molecular-weight multimers are **absent** from platelets and plasma. Type IIb is caused by synthesis of an **abnormal** vWF with increased affinity for platelets, and may be associated with thrombocytopenia.
- **TYPE III** vWD: This severe form of vWD is least common and is inherited as an autosomal recessive trait. Some patients are compound heterozygotes (different mutations in the two vWF alleles). vWF activity is absent and plasma levels of factor VIII are less than 10% of normal.

CLINICAL FEATURES: Most cases of vWD are associated with only a mild bleeding diathesis, with the exception of type III. Easy bruising, epistaxis, gastrointestinal bleeding, and (in women) menorrhagia are frequent. The presenting symptom is often excessive hemorrhage after trauma or surgery. Patients with type III vWD may have life-threatening hemorrhage from the gut; hemarthroses like those in hemophilia are not infrequent.

The bleeding tendency in all forms of vWD is treated successfully with factor VIII, vWF concentrates or cryoprecipitate. The vasopressin analogue desmopressin (DDAVP) is the treatment of choice in types I and IIa vWD because it increases release of preformed VWF from endothelial storage pools. Intranasal sprays of DDAVP are now available.

Other Coagulation Factor Deficiencies

Deficiencies of all coagulation factor proteins, including factors VII, X, V, XI, II (prothrombin), and fibrinogen, have been noted in humans. As expected, the severity of bleeding usually correlates with the level of functional protein activity. Prolonged PT or PTT in patients with bleeding manifestations helps to identify a problem with coagulation factors. Factor-specific assays confirm the diagnosis. The thrombin time helps to screen for deficiency or dysfunction of fibrinogen. Deficiency of fibrinogen causes bleeding. By contrast, dysfibrinogenemia may cause bleeding but more often leads to thrombosis.

Liver Disease

Many coagulation factors are produced in the liver (e.g., II, V, VII, IX, X). Severe liver disease may cause impaired secretion of these proteins as a manifestation of the general protein synthetic defect. In this case, levels of all liver-synthesized coagulation factors are low, and both PT and PTT are prolonged.

Vitamin K Deficiency

Liver-derived coagulation factors depend on vitamin K as an essential cofactor in γ-carboxylation of glutamic acid residues to Gla residues. Only if Gla residues are present are the secreted proteins functional. By contrast, factor V is made in the liver but does not require vitamin K. Thus, in vitamin K deficiency activities of factors II, VII, IX, and X are low but factor V activity is normal. However, in severe liver disease, all of these factors have low activity.

CLINICAL FEATURES: Levels of vitamin K are physiologically low in neonates, and it is standard practice to administer vitamin K to newborns to prevent hemorrhagic disease. In adults, vitamin K deficiency may reflect inadequate dietary intake. Since bacteria in the colon produce the form of vitamin K that is best absorbed, prolonged antibiotic intake, or large colonic resections, may lead to vitamin K deficiency.

Inhibitors of Coagulation Factors

Acquired inhibitors of coagulation factors, **circulating anticoagulants**, are usually IgG autoantibodies. Most are directed against factor VIII and vWF, although rarely antibodies against most of the other coagulation factors are seen. In hereditary coagulation disorders, especially hemophilia, circulating anticoagulants arise in response to administration of plasma concentrates containing the deficient factor. Anticoagulants also develop in some patients with autoimmune disorders (e.g., systemic lupus erythematosus, rheumatoid arthritis), presumably as a result of abnormal immune regulation. Finally, acquired anticoagulants often appear in apparently normal persons.

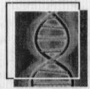

CLINICAL FEATURES: Acquired anticoagulants may be asymptomatic laboratory findings, or they may cause life-threatening hemorrhage. These autoantibodies are difficult to eliminate, but one third of patients have spontaneous remissions. Treatment includes plasma concentrates, corticosteroids, or immunosuppressive agents.

Lupus anticoagulants are antiphospholipid antibodies in patients with systemic lupus erythematosus and other autoimmune conditions or in otherwise asymptomatic persons. Bleeding is distinctly uncommon, but these patients have a hypercoagulable (thrombotic) tendency (see below).

Disseminated Intravascular Coagulation

DIC refers to widespread ischemic changes secondary to microvascular fibrin thrombi, which are accompanied by consumption of platelets and coagulation factors and a hemorrhagic diathesis. DIC is a serious, often fatal, disorder that typically occurs as a complication of massive trauma, sepsis from numerous organisms, and obstetric emergencies. It is also associated with metastatic cancer, hematopoietic malignancies, cardiovascular and liver disease, and many other conditions.

PATHOGENESIS: DIC begins with activation of the clotting cascades within the vascular compartment by tissue injury, endothelial damage or both. *Subsequent generation of substantial amounts of thrombin (Fig. 20-31), combined with the initial failure of the natural inhibitory mechanisms to neutralize thrombin, triggers DIC.* With the consequent uncontrolled intravascular coagulation, the delicate balance between coagulation and fibrinolysis is disrupted. This leads to consumption of clotting factors, platelets and fibrinogen and a consequent hemorrhagic diathesis.

Procoagulant TF is released into the circulation after injury in a variety of circumstances, including direct trauma, brain injury, and obstetric accidents (e.g., prema-

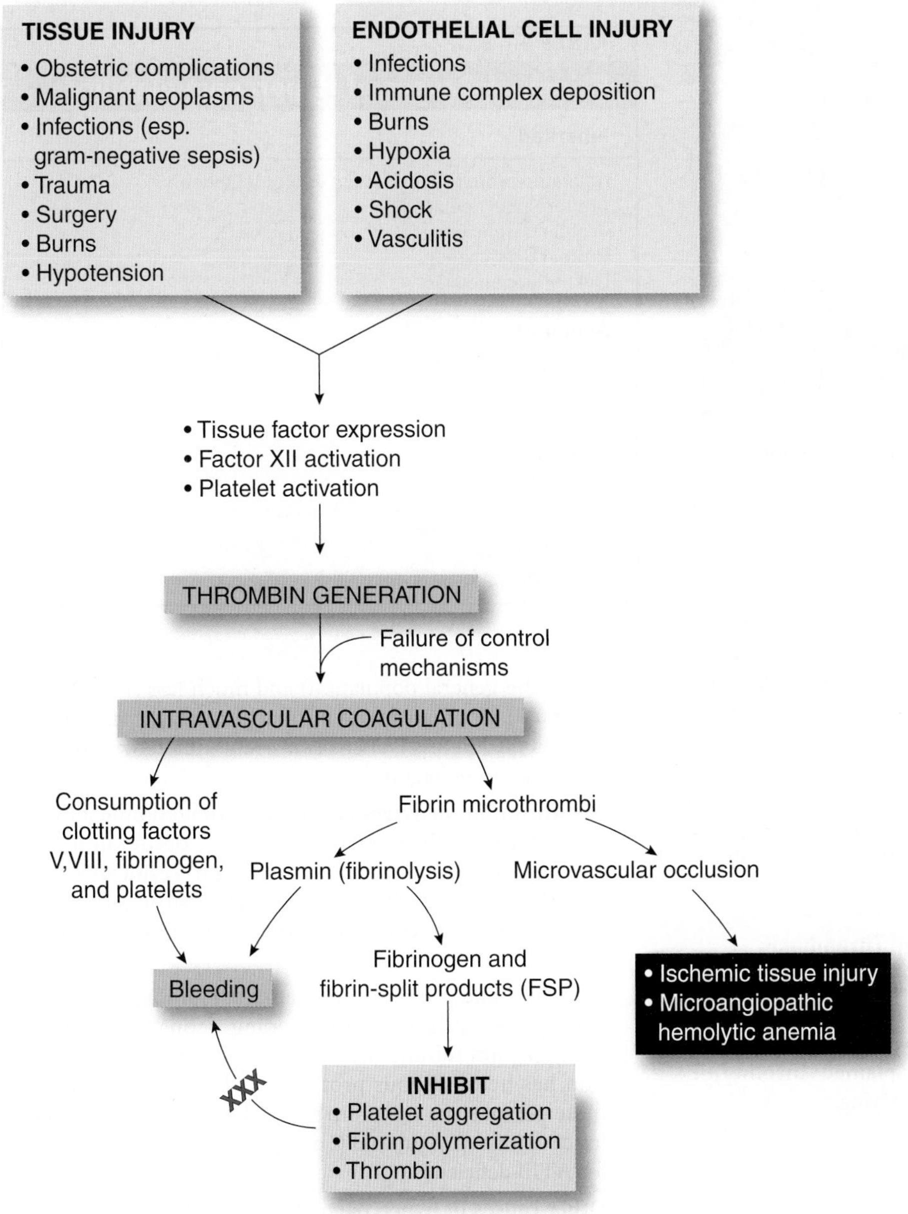

FIGURE 20-31. **The pathophysiology of disseminated intravascular coagulation (DIC).** The DIC syndrome is precipitated by tissue injury, endothelial cell injury, or a combination of the two. These injuries trigger increased expression of tissue factor on cell surfaces, and activation of clotting factors (including XII and V) and platelets. With the failure of normal control mechanisms, generation of thrombin leads to intravascular coagulation.

ture separation of the placenta) (see Chapter 18). **Bacterial endotoxin** also stimulates macrophages to release TF. **Certain tumor cells** cause DIC by releasing TF. With activation of the clotting cascade, intravascular fibrin microthrombi are deposited in the smallest blood vessels. Stimulation of the fibrinolytic system by fibrin generates fibrin split products, which possess anticoagulant properties and contribute to the bleeding diathesis.

Endothelial injury often plays an important role in the pathogenesis of DIC. The anticoagulant properties of the endothelium (see Fig. 20-26) are impaired by widely varying injuries, including (1) TNF in gram-negative sepsis; (2) other inflammatory mediators, such as activated complement, IL-1, or neutrophil proteases; (3) viral or rickettsial infections; and (4) trauma (e.g., burns). Thus, platelet aggregates form in the microvasculature.

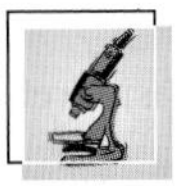

PATHOLOGY: Arterioles, capillaries, and venules throughout the body are occluded by **microthrombi** composed of fibrin and platelets (Fig. 20-32). However, owing to the enhancement of fibrinolysis, these thrombi may no longer be visualized at the time of autopsy. Microvascular obstruction is associated with widespread **ischemic changes,** particularly in the brain, kidneys, skin, lungs, and gastroinstestinal tract. These organs are also sites of bleeding, which, in the case of the brain and gut, may be fatal.

Erythrocytes become fragmented (**schistocytes**) by passage through webs of intravascular fibrin, resulting in **microangiopathic hemolytic anemia.** Consumption of activated platelets leads to **thrombocytopenia,** while **depletion of clotting factors** is reflected in prolonged PT and PTT and decreased plasma fibrinogen. Plasma fibrin split products prolong the thrombin time. Fibrinopeptide A and D-dimers are elevated (as markers of coagulation and fibrinolytic activation, respectively).

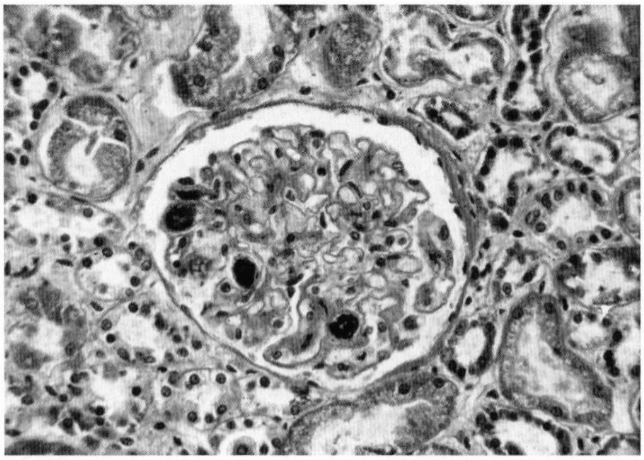

FIGURE 20-32. **Disseminated intravascular coagulation.** A section of a glomerulus stained with phosphotungstic acid hematoxylin (PTAH), which colors fibrin deep purple, demonstrates several microthrombi.

CLINICAL FEATURES: The symptoms of DIC reflect both microvascular thrombosis and a bleeding tendency. Ischemic changes in the brain lead to seizures and coma. Depending on the severity of DIC, renal symptoms range from mild azotemia to fulminant acute renal failure. Acute respiratory distress syndrome may supervene, and acute gastrointestinal ulcers may bleed. The bleeding diathesis is evidenced by cerebral hemorrhage, ecchymoses and hematuria. Patients with DIC are treated with (1) heparin anticoagulation to interrupt the cycle of intravascular coagulation and (2) replacement of platelets and clotting factors to control the bleeding.

Hypercoagulability Causes Widespread Thrombosis

Hypercoagulability is defined as an increased risk of thrombosis in circumstances that would not cause thrombosis in a normal person. Laboratory evaluation of an underlying hypercoagulable state is warranted in persons who have unexplained thrombotic episodes that show one or more of the following:

- Recurrence
- Development at a young age
- Family history of thrombotic episodes
- Thrombosis in unusual anatomical locations
- Difficulty in controlling with anticoagulants

Disorders that enhance thrombosis have been considered elsewhere (Chapters 7, 10, 11).

Hypercoagulable states are divided into inherited and acquired forms (Table 20-8).

TABLE 20-8

Principal Causes of Hypercoagualability

Inherited
Activated protein C resistance (factor V Leiden)
Antithrombin deficiency
Protein C deficiency
Protein S deficiency
Dysfibrinogenemias
Acquired
Lupus inhibitor
Malignancy
Nephrotic syndrome
Therapy
Factor concentrates
Heparin
Oral contraceptives
Hyperlipidemia
Thrombotic thrombocytopenic purpura

Inherited Hypercoagulability

Inherited hypercoagulable states are due to genetic mutations that affect one of the natural anticoagulant mechanisms. The hereditary tendency to develop thrombosis, irrespective of its origin, is referred to as **thrombophilia.**

- **Activated protein C (APC) resistance—factor V Leiden:** A point mutation in the *factor V* gene (factor V Leiden) renders it resistant to the inhibitory effect of APC. *Resistance APC action is the most common genetic disorder associated with hypercoagulability, and its prevalence in patients with venous thrombosis has been reported to be as high as 65%.* The factor V Leiden mutation is found worldwide, but more so in whites (up to 5% of the general population) and much less so in Africans (near 0%). Compared with normal persons, the risk for deep venous thrombosis is increased 7-fold in heterozygotes and 80-fold in homozygotes.
- **Antithrombin deficiency:** This autosomal dominant disorder, which has incomplete penetrance, occurs in 0.2% to 0.4% of the general population and can result in either a quantitative or a qualitative effect on antithrombin. The risk of a thrombotic event (usually venous) ranges between 20% and 80% in different families.
- **Protein C and protein S deficiencies:** Homozygous protein C deficiency causes life-threatening neonatal thrombosis with **purpura fulminans**. Up to 0.5% of the general population has heterozygous protein C deficiency, but many of these persons are symptom free. The clinical presentations for deficiencies of protein C and protein S are similar to that for ATIII deficiency.
- **Other causes of hypercoagulability:** Prothrombin also has a known genetic variant (G20210A) in the 3′ untranslated region of the mRNA that is associated with thrombosis. The mechanism is not defined but may involve excessively high prothrombin levels in persons with the variant. Unusually high levels of fibrinogen, factor VII, and factor VIII are associated with thrombosis, although the molecular basis for the elevated levels remains to be elucidated. Some dysfibrinogenemias are also associated with thrombosis.

Acquired Hypercoagulability

Venous stasis contributes to the hypercoagulability associated with prolonged immobilization and congestive cardiac failure. Increased platelet activation probably accounts for the clotting tendency in patients with myeloproliferative disorders, heparin-associated thrombocytopenia, and TTP.

Antiphospholipid Antibody Syndrome

Antibodies directed against several negatively charged phospholipids are associated with the development of antiphospholipid antibody syndrome. This disorder features (1) thromboembolic events, (2) spontaneous abortions, and (3) thrombocytopenia. Combinations of laboratory tests help to confirm the diagnosis of antiphospholipid syndrome. Antibodies (IgG primarily but not exclusively) react with proteins that bind anionic phospholipids such as phosphatidylserine (PS) or cardiolipin. These membrane lipids are only exposed when cells such as platelets are activated. Many plasma proteins and Gla-domain-containing procoagulant proteins (e.g., prothrombin) bind to PS and related anionic phospholipids. The laboratory tests are (1) detection of lupus-type anticoagulant activity, (2) anticardiolipin antibodies, and (3) antibodies to plasma protein β2-GPI. Anticardiolipin antibodies bind to β2-GPI in the presence of cardiolipin.

The antiphospholipid antibody syndrome is the leading acquired hematologic cause of thrombosis. The thrombosis in this syndrome has several proposed mechanisms, including platelet activation, endothelial cell activation, and alterations in the coagulation factor assembly on membranes. Interference with placental vascular function is the likely mechanism in recurrent fetal loss.

The lupus anticoagulant (which is not restricted to patients with systemic lupus erythematosus) is an antiphospholipid antibody that results in paradoxical prolongation of PTT in vitro (due to phospholipid inhibition) but hypercoagulability in vivo (probably through platelet activation). The latter accounts for the frequent occurrence of arterial thrombosis and is the most common of the acquired blood protein defects that cause thrombosis.

WHITE BLOOD CELLS

The reader is referred to Chapters 2-4 for discussions of white blood cell structure and function.

Nonmalignant Disorders

Neutropenia is an Absolute Neutrophil Count below 1800/μL

In most patients with neutropenia (**granulocytopenia**), the number of neutrophils is adequate to defend against microorganisms. When the number declines to 1000/μL, patients become vulnerable to microbial infections, but there is serious risk with absolute counts below 500/μL. The term **agranulocytosis** denotes virtual absence of neutrophils, caused by depletion of both the marginated pool and the bone marrow reserve.

Neutropenia reflects decreased production or increased destruction of neutrophils (Table 20-9). Most cases of neutropenia are asymptomatic and unexplained, and the term **chronic benign neutropenia** is used. In some cases, the total granulocyte pool is normal, but excessive neutrophils are stored in the marrow or marginated in blood vessels.

DECREASED PRODUCTION OF NEUTROPHILS: Radiation or chemotherapeutic drugs interfere with generation of neutrophils by generally suppressing marrow cell proliferation. Certain drugs, such as phenothiazines, phenylbutazone, antithyroid drugs, and indomethacin, can cause an **idiosyncratic** suppression of the bone marrow. Viral infection and alcohol intake may also suppress myelopoiesis. Decreased production of granulocytes is seen in a number of rare hereditary disorders, including **Kostmann syndrome** and **infantile genetic agranulocytosis.**

TABLE 20-9
Principal Causes of Neutropenia

Decreased production
Irradiation
Drug induced (long and short term)
Viral infections
Congenital
Cyclic
Ineffective production
Megaloblastic anemia
Myelodysplastic syndromes
Increased destruction
Isoimmune neonatal
Autoimmune
Idiopathic
Drug induced
Felty syndrome
Systemic lupus erythematosus
Dialysis (induced by complement activation)
Splenic sequestration
Increased margination

Ineffective myelopoiesis is involved in the neutropenia of megaloblastic anemias and myelodysplastic syndromes. In **cyclic neutropenia,** episodes recur regularly about every 21 days.

INCREASED PERIPHERAL DESTRUCTION OF GRANULOCYTES: Accelerated elimination of granulocytes is caused by:

- Increased consumption of neutrophils in overwhelming infections
- Increased sequestration in hypersplenism
- Increased destruction by antibodies

Neutropenia is a common feature in AIDS and is multifactorial. Virus-induced depression of neutrophil production is aggravated by infectious consumption of neutrophils and often by antiretroviral drugs (e.g., zidovudine).

Many drugs can lead to immunologically mediated neutrophil destruction, especially sulfonamides, phenylbutazone, and indomethacin. The toxic effect results from attachment of circulating antigen–antibody complexes to granulocyte surfaces, with subsequent complement-mediated injury.

Neutrophilia Is an Absolute Neutrophil Count above 7000/μL

Neutrophilia has many causes (Table 20-10) and reflects (1) **increased mobilization** of neutrophils from bone marrow storage, (2) **enhanced release** from the peripheral blood marginal pool, or (3) **stimulation of granulopoiesis** in the bone marrow. Increased mobilization of neutrophils from the bone marrow pool or from the peripheral marginal pool occurs in acute traumatic or infectious disorders. A mild neutrophilia occurs in 20% of women during the third trimester of pregnancy, but the mechanism is poorly defined.

LEUKEMOID REACTION: In acute infections, neutrophilia may be so pronounced that it may be mistaken for leukemia, especially chronic myeloid leukemia (CML), in which case it is termed a **leukemoid reaction.** Clues to the benign (or reac-

TABLE 20-10
Principal Causes of Neutrophilia

Infections	
Primarily bacterial	
Immunological inflammatory	
Rheumatoid arthritis Rheumatic fever	Vasculitis
Neoplasia	
Hemorrhage	
Drugs	
Glucocorticoids Colony-stimulating factors (CSFs)	Lithium
Hereditary	
CD18 deficiency	
Metabolic	
Acidosis Uremia	Gout Thyroid storm
Tissue necrosis	
Infarction Trauma	Burns

tive) nature of a leukemoid reaction include: (1) the cells in the peripheral blood are usually more mature than myelocytes; (2) leukocyte alkaline phosphatase activity is high in a leukemoid reaction, but low in CML; and (3) benign neutrophils often contain large blue cytoplasmic inclusions (**Döhle bodies**) or prominent blue-black granulation of the cytoplasm (**toxic granulation**).

Qualitative Disorders of Neutrophils Are Associated with Impaired Function

If granulocyte functionality is impaired, resistance to infection may decrease despite a normal granulocyte count. A number of rare hereditary disorders of granulocytes have been described earlier (see Chapter 2), including chronic granlomatous disease, myeloperoxidase deficiency, and Chédiak-Higashi syndrome.

Eosinophilia Occurs with Allergic Reactions and Malignancies

Eosinophils differentiate in the bone marrow under the influence of eosinophil growth factors (e.g., IL-5). They circulate briefly in the blood, then migrate preferentially to the gastrointestinal and respiratory tracts and the skin. Eosinophils respond to chemotactic substances produced by mast cells or are induced by the presence of persistent antigen–antibody complexes, such as occur in chronic parasitic, dermatologic, and allergic conditions. The principal causes of eosinophilia are listed in (Table 20-11).

TABLE 20-11
Principal Causes of Eosinophilia

Allergic disorders
Skin diseases
Parasitic (helminth) infestations
Malignant neoplasms
Hematopoietic Solid tumors
Collagen vascular disorders
Miscellaneous
Hypereosinophilic syndromes Eosinophilia–myalgia syndrome IL-2 therapy

Idiopathic hypereosinophilic syndrome refers to an increase in circulating eosinophils above 1500/μL for more than 6 months without evident underlying disease. Accumulation of eosinophils in tissue often leads to necrosis, particularly in the myocardium, where it produces endomyocardial disease (see Chapter 11). Neurologic dysfunction may also develop. Eosinophil-mediated cell injury is related to constituents of the eosinophil granules, particularly major basic protein, and cationic protein (see Chapter 2). The prognosis of untreated idiopathic hypereosinophilic syndrome is serious: only 10% of untreated patients survive 3 years. With aggressive corticosteroid therapy, 70% survive more than 5 years, even with cardiac involvement.

Basophilia Is Associated with Allergic Reactions and Myeloproliferative Diseases

The basophil, the least abundant of all leukocytes, differentiates in the bone marrow, circulates briefly in the blood, then passes to the tissues. Its relationship to mast cells is controversial. Basophil granules contain a number of preformed mediators of the inflammatory response, including histamine and chondroitin sulfate. Upon stimulation, these cells also synthesize leukotriene and other mediators. The principal causes of basophilia are listed in (Table 20-12). Basophilia is most commonly observed in immediate-type hypersensitivity reactions and in chronic myeloproliferative syndromes.

Monocytosis Is Seen in Malignant and Inflammatory Conditions

Monocytosis is defined as a peripheral blood monocyte count above 800/μL. The main causes include hematologic disorders, immunologic and inflammatory conditions, infectious diseases, and solid cancers. The former account for at least half of peripheral blood monocytoses. For example, monocytes may constitute a component of acute or CML. In such cases, they may be either morphologically normal or immature and dyspoietic cytologically. Monocytosis often occurs in neutropenic states, probably as a compensatory mechanism. Peripheral blood monocytosis may also accompany malignant lymphomas and Hodgkin lymphoma.

TABLE 20-12

Principal Causes of Basophilia
Allergic (drug, food)
Inflammation
Juvenile rheumatoid arthritis Ulcerative colitis
Infection
Viral (chickenpox, influenza) Tuberculosis
Neoplasia
Myeloproliferative syndromes Basophilic leukemia Carcinoma
Endocrine
Diabetes mellitus Myxedema Estrogen administration

Langerhans Cell Histiocytosis is Neoplastic Proliferation of Langerhans cells, That Occurs Mainly in Children

Langerhans cell histiocytosis (LCH) is a spectrum of uncommon proliferations of Langerhans cells. The diseases range from asymptomatic involvement at a single site, such as bone or lymph nodes, to an aggressive systemic multiorgan disorder.

Langerhans cells are mononuclear phagocytes derived from precursor cells in the bone marrow. They are found in the epidermis, lymph nodes, spleen, thymus, and mucosal tissues. Langerhans cells ingest, process and present antigens to T lymphocytes. In lymph nodes, Langerhans cells are termed **interdigitating reticulum cells** (IDCs).

The etiology and pathogenesis of LCH are unknown. The disease may represent an atypical immunologic reaction or an unusual manifestation of an autoimmune disorder, but the recent demonstration of the clonality of Langerhans cells in all forms of LCH suggests that it may be a neoplastic disorder. Infants, children, and young adults are most affected. The extent of disease and rate of progression correlate inversely with the age at presentation. Certain eponyms were traditionally attached to the various presentations of LCH.

- **Eosinophilic granuloma** is a localized, usually self-limited, disorder of older children (5- to10-years-old) and young adults (under 30 years). It accounts for almost 75% of all cases of LCH and afflicts males four times as frequently as females. The bones and lungs are the principal sites affected.
- **Hand-Schüller-Christian disease** is a multifocal and typically indolent disorder, usually in children 2 to 5 years of age, which represents about one-fourth of all cases of LCH. Boys and girls are affected equally. Bony lesions tend to predominate, although involvement of endocrine glands may be prominent.
- **Letterer-Siwe disease** is a rare (less than 10% of cases), acute, disseminated variant of LCH in infants and children under 2 years of age. There is no sex predominance. Skin lesions and involvement of visceral organs and the hematopoietic system are characteristic.

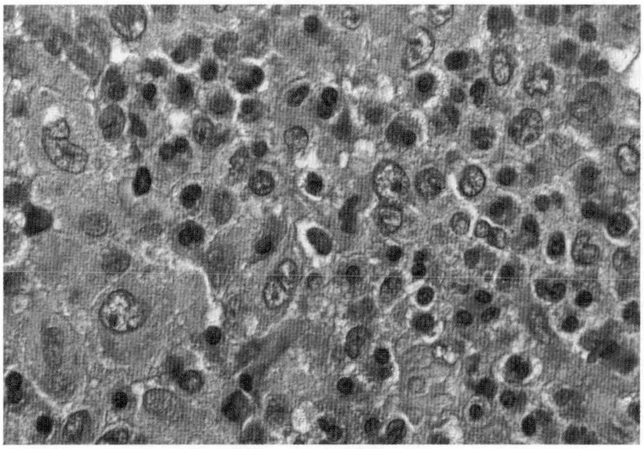

FIGURE 20-33. **Eosinophilic granuloma.** A section of an affected rib shows proliferated Langerhans cells and numerous eosinophils.

PATHOLOGY: Despite their clinical heterogeneity LCHs share common histopathological findings (Fig. 20-33). The cells that accumulate are large (15–25 μm in diameter), with round to indented nuclei, delicate vesicular chromatin, and small nucleoli. By electron microscopy, a distinctive rod-shaped or tubular cytoplasmic inclusion with a dense core and a double outer sheath, the **Birbeck granule** (Fig. 20-34), is commonly observed. Frequently, one end of the granule is bulbous, in which case it resembles a tennis racket. Characteristic immunologic cell markers identical to those of epidermal Langerhans cells include S-100 protein and CD1.

CLINICAL FEATURES: The clinical manifestations of LCH reflect the sites involved. Skin involvement, principally in the Letterer-Siwe variant, takes the form of seborrheic or eczematoid dermatitis, most prominent on the scalp, face, and trunk. Otitis media is common. Painless localized or generalized lymphadenopathy and hepatosplenomegaly are frequent. Lytic lesions of bone cause pain or tenderness to palpation. Bone manifestations of LCH are discussed in Chapter 26. Proptosis (protrusion of the eyeball) may be a complication of infiltration of the orbit. Diabetes insipidus occurs when the

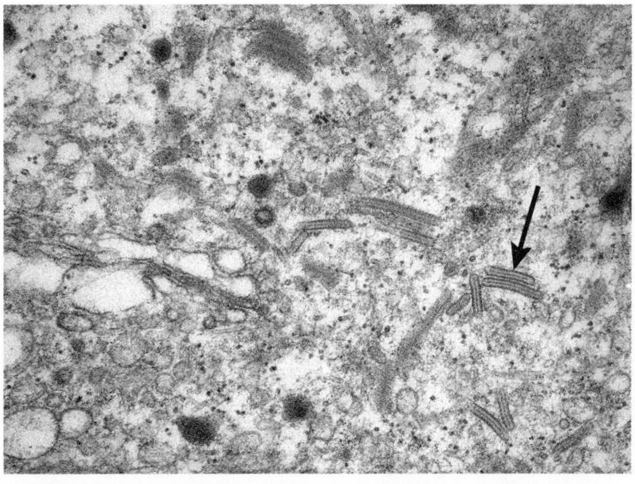

FIGURE 20-34. **Electron micrograph showing a Birbeck granule (*arrow*) in Langerhans histiocytosis.**

hypothalamic–pituitary axis is affected. *The classic triad of diabetes insipidus, proptosis, and defects in membranous bones occurs in only 15% of cases of Hand-Schüller-Christian disease.* The prognosis in LCH depends mainly on age at presentation, extent of disease and rate of progression. In general, the disorder is self-limited and benign in older persons (eosinophilic granuloma), whereas children younger than 2 years (Letterer-Siwe disease) tend to do poorly. Rarely, the clinical course is aggressive and indistinguishable from that of a malignant neoplasm.

Proliferative Disorders of Mast Cells Release Inflammatory Mediators

Mast cells derive from precursor cells in the bone marrow and are found in the connective tissues, usually in close proximity to blood vessels (see Chapter 2). Mast cell granules contain inflammatory mediators, such as histamine, heparin, eosinophil and neutrophil chemotactic factors, and certain proteases. The symptoms of mast cell proliferative diseases are due to the release of these substances and include flushing, pruritus, and hives. The secretion of heparin also causes bleeding from the nasopharynx or gastrointestinal tract. The spectrum of mast cell proliferative disorders comprises a variety of benign and malignant conditions.

MAST CELL HYPERPLASIA (REACTIVE MASTOCYTOSIS): This process occurs in immediate- and delayed-type hypersensitivity reactions and in lymph nodes that drain the sites of malignant tumors. It is also observed in Waldenström macroglobulinemia, in the bone marrow of women with postmenopausal osteoporosis, in myelodysplastic syndromes, and after chemotherapy for leukemia.

LOCALIZED MASTOCYTOSIS (MASTOCYTOMA): This lesion presents either as a single, tan-brown, cutaneous nodule in newborns or as several groups of skin nodules in young children. Microscopically, a diffuse dermal infiltrate of mast cells is noted. The disorder resolves spontaneously and secondary extracutaneous involvement is rare.

URTICARIA PIGMENTOSA: This entity presents as multiple, symmetrically distributed, tan-brown, cutaneous macules or papules, most commonly in infants and young children. The skin of the trunk is predominantly affected, but any cutaneous site may be involved. Microscopically, a diffuse dermal infiltrate of mast cells is observed. Spontaneous resolution usually occurs at puberty and systemic involvement is unusual.

SYSTEMIC MASTOCYTOSIS: This rare disorder is characterized by infiltration of many organs with mast cells, including the skin, lymph nodes, spleen, liver, bones and bone marrow, and gastrointestinal tract. In most cases of systemic mastocytosis there is an activating mutation in the tyrosine kinase domain of the protooncogene *c-kit* (D816V), which underscores the neoplastic nature of this disorder. Systemic mastocytosis occurs at any age, but adults in the sixth and seventh decades of life are most commonly affected. Systemic mastocytosis may accompany urticaria pigmentosa.

PATHOLOGY: In systemic mastocytosis, the lymph nodes initially show perifollicular and perivascular infiltration by mast cells. The spleen exhibits nodular aggregates of mast cells with accompanying dense fibrosis in the red pulp, particularly in relation to the fibrous trabeculae and the capsule. In the liver, the portal triads are first involved. Involvement of the bone marrow may be peritrabecular, perivascular, or diffuse (Fig. 20-35) and there is often accompanying fibrosis.

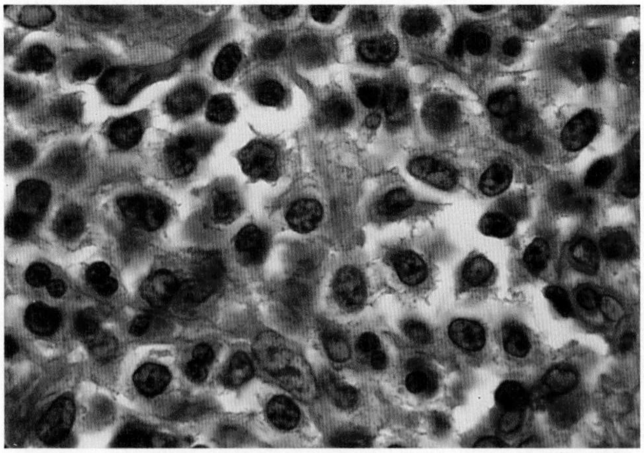

FIGURE 20-35. **Mastocytosis.** A section of lymph node shows effacement of the normal architecture by sheets of mast cells. The centrally situated nuclei are round to elongated, and occasionally indented. The cytoplasm is pale pink and finely granular.

CLINICAL FEATURES: Patients with systemic mastocytosis suffer symptoms related to the overproduction of a number of mediators normally produced by mast cells and basophils, including histamine, prostaglandin D_2 and thromboxane B_2. Most experience gastrointestinal pain and diarrhea. Anaphylactic episodes–with pruritus, flushing, and asthmatic symptoms–are common. Extensive mast cell infiltration of the bone marrow leads to secondary anemia, leukopenia, and thrombocytopenia. Systemic mastocytosis follows a chronic, indolent course, with about half of patients surviving for 5 years. Symptomatic relief is obtained, at least partially, with H1- and H2-receptor antagonists. There is no effective therapy for the underlying disease process.

MAST CELL LEUKEMIA: This complication develops in 15% of cases of systemic mastocytosis. The circulating cells exhibit the typical cytological features of mast cells or of less-differentiated variants. The leukocyte count may be markedly increased.

Leukemias and Myelodysplastic Syndromes

Malignant leukocytes originate from either myeloid cells or lymphoid cells. Malignant proliferations of myeloid cells are derived from bone marrow cells and manifest as ***myelodysplastic syndromes, chronic myeloproliferative diseases,*** *or* ***acute myelogenous leukemias****. By contrast, malignant lymphocytes can arise in any compartment that contains lymphoid cells.* The World Health Organization (WHO) classification is based upon conventional morphologic criteria, cytogenetics, molecular abnormalities, and immunophenotype. The WHO has recently added **neutrophilic leukemia and chronic eosinophilic leukemia** to the list of myeloproliferative disorders. The reader is referred to other sources for discussion of these rare entities.

Chronic Myeloproliferative Diseases Are Clonal Stem Cell Disorders

Chronic myeloproliferative diseases involve increased proliferation of one or more myeloid lineages (granulocytes, erythrocytes, or megakaryocytes). Four types are usually distinguished: **chronic myelogenous leukemia, polycythemia vera, chronic idiopathic myelofibrosis, and essential thrombocythemia** (Table 20-13).

TABLE 20–13

Chronic Myeloproliferative Syndromes

	Chronic Myelogenous Leukemia	Polycythemia Vera	Chronic Idiopathic Myelofibrosis	Essential Thrombocythemia
Clinical Features				
Peak age range (years)	25–60	40–60	50–70	50–70
Splenomegaly	90%	75%	100%	30% (slight)
Hepatomegaly	50%	40%	80%	40% (slight)
Acute leukemic conversion	80%	5%–10%	5%–10%	2%–5%
Median survival (years)	3–4	13	5	>10
Bone Marrow				
Histopathology	Panhyperplasia (predominantly granulocytic)	Panhyperplasia (predominantly erythroid)	Panhyperplasia with fibrosis	Large megakaryocytes in clusters
M:E ratio	10:1 to 50:1	≤2:1	2:1 to 5:1	2:1 to 5:1
Fibrosis	<10%	15%–20%	90%–100%	<5%
Laboratory Findings				
Hemoglobin	Mild anemia	>20 g/dL	Mild anemia	Mild anemia
RBC morphology	Slight aniso- and poikilocytosis	Slight aniso- and poikilocytosis	Immature erythrocytes and marked aniso- and poikilocytosis	Hypochromic microcytes
Granulocytes	Moderate to markedly increased with spectrum of maturation	Normal to mildly increased; may show a few immature forms	Normal to moderately increased; some immature WBC	Normal to slightly increased
Platelets	Normal to moderately increased	Normal to moderately increased	Increased to decreased	Markedly increased with abnormal forms
Genetics	Philadelphia chromosome: *BCR/ABL* gene rearrangement	JAK2 activating mutation	JAK2 activating mutation	JAK2 activating mutation

M:E ratio = ratio of myeloid-to-erythroid.

Chronic myeloproliferative diseases typically affect adults between 40 and 80 years old. They are relatively uncommon, with a yearly incidence of 5 to 10 cases per 100,000. The cause is usually unknown, although radiation or benzene exposure have sometimes been implicated. Characteristic oncogene mutations and translocations occur in certain myeloproliferative syndromes (see below).

Chronic Myelogenous Leukemia

CML is derived from an abnormal pluripotent bone marrow stem cell and results in prominent neutrophilic leukocytosis over the full range of myeloid maturation. A **Philadelphia chromosome**, or molecular demonstration of the ***BCR/ABL*** **fusion gene**, is required to establish the diagnosis. CML is the most common myeloproliferative disease and accounts for 15% to 20% of all cases of leukemia.

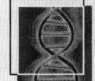

PATHOGENESIS: The cause in most cases of CML is unknown. Radiation exposure and myelotoxic agents such as benzene have been implicated in a small number of cases. Leukemic cells represent transformed pluripotent stem cells with predominantly granulocytic differentiation. In 95% of CML cases, the Philadelphia chromosome, which results from t(9:22)(q34:q11) translocation, can be shown by conventional cytogenetics and fluorescence in situ hybridization (FISH) (Fig. 20-36). The Philadelphia chromosome itself is a derived (shortened) chromosome 22 [DER(22q)]. The *BCR* (break point cluster region) gene on chromosome 22 is fused to the *ABL* gene on chromosome 9. A small number of cases involve additional chromosomal abnormalities or cryptic translocation of 9q34 and 22q11 that cannot be identified by conventional cytogenetics. In these cases, the *BCR/ABL* fusion gene is detected by FISH (see Fig. 20-36B), polymerase chain reaction (PCR) or molecular techniques, which show a fused *BCR/ABL* gene or fusion transcripts on chromosome 22.

The BCR/ABL *gene encodes a fusion protein, p210, which is a constitutively activated tyrosine kinase.* Much less commonly, *BCR/ABL* fusion genes result from breakage in the minor break point cluster region and yield a fusion protein termed p190. P190 is most common in **Philadelphia chromosome-positive acute lymphoblastic leukemia**. Acquisition of additional chromosomal abnormalities (e.g., second Philadelphia chromosome or trisomy 8) indicates a more aggressive clinical course.

PATHOLOGY: CML may present in **chronic**, **accelerated**, or **blast phases**.

- **Chronic phase of CML** features conspicuous leukocytosis, consisting mainly of maturing neutrophils. By definition, blasts are less than 10% of cicrulating leukocytes. Basophilia and eosinophilia are frequent. The platelet count is typically increased and may exceed $10^6/\mu L$. Bone marrow biopsy shows hypercellularity, with total effacement of the marrow space by

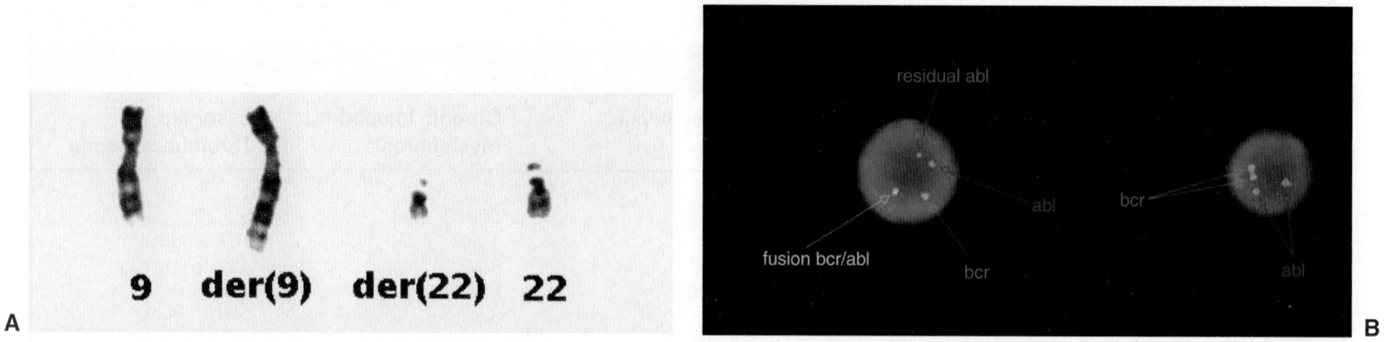

FIGURE 20-36. **Chronic myelogenous leukemia. A.** The Philadelphia chromosome der(22) is shown. **B.** Fluorescence in situ hybridization (FISH) in a patient with t(9;22) (Philadelphia chromosome) positive chronic myeloid leukemia. Right image: A normal cell contains two separate bcr (chromosome 22) and abl (chromosome 9) genes; Left image: A leukemic cell with a fusion bcr/abl signal, residual abl signal, and two normal abl and bcr signals derived from normal chromosomes 9 and 22, respectively.

predominantly myeloid cells and their precursors (Fig. 20-37). Megakaryocytes often form clusters and show abnormal morphologic features, including micromegakaryocytes and hypolobation of nuclei.

- **Accelerated phase of CML** often follows the chronic phase and may be associated with (1) 10% to 20% blasts in the blood or bone marrow, (2) more than 20% blood basophils, (3) persistent thrombocytopenia or thrombocytosis unresponsive to therapy, (4) splenomegaly, (5) increasing white blood cell count unresponsive to therapy, and (6) additional chromosomal abnormalities.
- **Blast phase of CML** is the ultimate outcome and features (1) at least 20% blasts in the bone marrow, (2) extramedullary proliferation of blasts (skin, lymph nodes, spleen, bone, brain), and (3) clusters of blasts in the bone marrow biopsy. Blast phase heralds a poor prognosis. In most cases (70%), the leukemic cells in blast phase exhibit morphology and immunophenotype of myeloid lineage; in 30%, they resemble lymphoblasts, usually with a B cell precursor immunophenotype (expressing CD10, CD19, CD34, and terminal deoxynucleotidyl transferase [TdT]).

CLINICAL FEATURES: Peak incidence is in the fifth and sixth decades, with a slight male predominance. Patients with CML report fatigue, anorexia, weight loss, and vague abdominal discomfort owing to hepatosplenomegaly. Acute left upper quandrant pain is often a symptom of splenic infarction. There is mild to moderate anemia. Peripheral granulocytes are markedly increased with a full maturation range. Clinical deterioration often heralds blast phase.

CML is a paradigm for a malignancy with a well-defined cytogenetic abnormality that can be targeted by specific drug therapy. The drug imatinib, blocks the adenosine triphosphate (ATP)-binding site on the *BCR/ABL* tyrosine kinase, thereby inactivating it. A high level of sustained remissions has been achieved with imatinib, but disease control appears to require continued treatment with the drug. Allogeneic bone marrow transplantation is also used with curative intent in patients with CML.

Polycythemia Vera

PV is a myeloproliferative disease arising from a clonal hematopoietic stem cell and resulting in uncontrolled production of RBCs. The increase in erythrocytes in PV is autonomous and is not regulated by EPO. As several benign conditions resemble PV clinically, the WHO established diagnostic criteria for polycythemia. Major criteria include: (1) Increased RBC mass (hemoglobin >18.5 g/dL in men and >16.5 g/dL in women); (2) No elevation of EPO level; (3) No cause of secondary

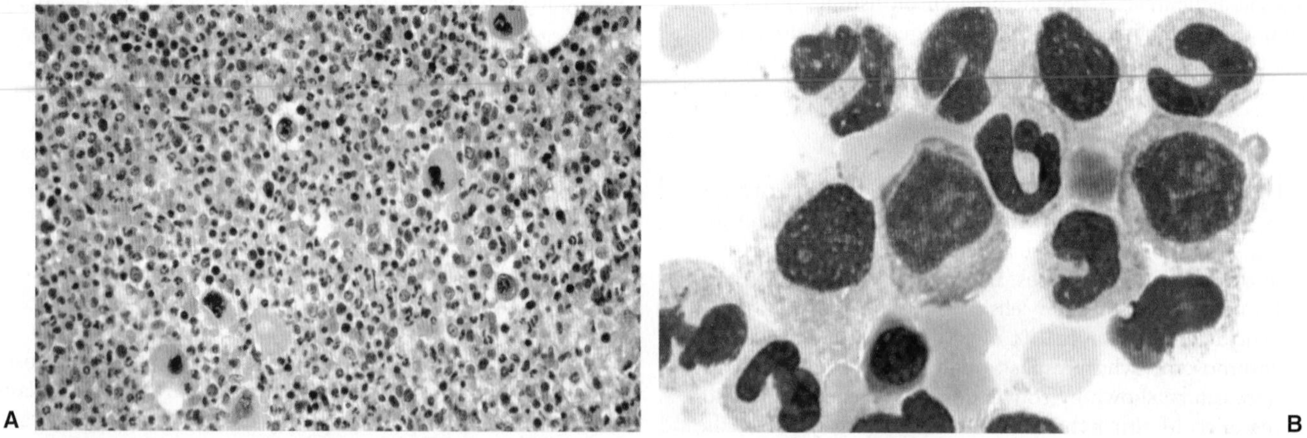

FIGURE 20-37. **Chronic myelogenous leukemia. A.** The bone marrow is conspicuously hypercellular, owing to an increase in granulocyte precursors, mature granulocytes, and megakaryocytes. **B.** A smear of the bone marrow aspirate from the same patient reveals numerous granulocytes at various stages of development.

erythrocytosis; (4) Splenomegaly; (5) Demonstration of a clonal genetic abnormality other than the Philadelphia chromosome; and (6) Erythroid colony formation in vitro in the absence of growth factor stimulation.

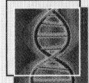

PATHOGENESIS: PV derives from malignant transformation of a single hematopoietic stem cell with primary commitment to the erythroid lineage. Proliferation of the neoplastic clone occurs mainly in the bone marrow but may involve such extramedullary sites as the spleen, lymph nodes, and liver (**myeloid metaplasia**).

The neoplastic erythroid progenitor cells of PV are sensitive to EPO like their normal counterparts. In semisolid culture media, they form luxuriant clusters of erythroid cells (BFU-E) when exposed to EPO. However, at the more mature colony-forming stage (CFU-E), the neoplastic cells form erythroid colonies in semisolid culture media even without erythropoietin stimulation. These autonomous erythroid colonies, "endogenous CFU-E," and are characteristic of PV throughout the disease. By contrast, CFU-E formation in normal erythroid progenitor cells requires added EPO ("exogenous CFU-E"). Autonomous proliferation of the more mature cells confers a proliferative advantage to neoplastic clones, since the increased erythrocyte mass suppresses normal EPO secretion and the function of the remaining normal progenitors. Serum EPO levels are thus either normal or low in PV, unlike secondary (functional) erythrocytosis, in which EPO levels are increased. No specific recurrent genetic defect has been identified in PV, although some cytogenetic abnormalities have been described.

Recent studies show a close association between an activating mutation in the cytoplasmic protein-tyrosine kinase Janus kinase 2 (JAK2; V617F) and bcr/abl-negative myeloproliferative diseases, including PV, essential thrombocythemia, and myelofibrosis. The JAK2 family of transcription factors plays a critical role in cytokine signaling in normal hematopoietic cells primarily by activating signal transducers and activators of transcription (STAT) proteins. In vitro studies indicate that the activating JAK2 mutation confers a proliferative and survival advantage to hematopoietic precursors. Patients with the JAK2 mutation have a longer duration of disease and a higher risk for bleeding complications and fibrosis.

PATHOLOGY: *The bone marrow in PV is hypercellular, with hyperplasia of all elements* (see Table 20-13). Unlike CML, erythroid precursor cells predominate, and the myeloid-to-erythroid ratio is less than 2:1. Erythroid maturation is normal (normoblastic). The granulocyte series also shows normal maturation. Megakaryocytes are typically increased in number and size and tend to cluster. In 90% of cases, marrow stainable iron is decreased or absent. A mild-to-moderate increase in reticulin is common, and 10% of cases progress to severe collagenous fibrosis.

The spleen is typically enlarged, with prominent accumulation of erythrocytes in the red pulp cords and sinuses. There may be myeloid metaplasia, characterized by erythroid precursor cells, immature granulocytes, and megakaryocytes. Myeloid metaplasia is also common in the liver and lymph nodes.

The peripheral blood smear reveals normal erythrocytes, although hypochromia and microcytosis are seen if there is iron deficiency. Iron deficiency anemia is common in PV, largely because storage iron is diverted to the increased red cell mass.

Blood hemoglobin concentration may exceed 20 g/dL, and the Hct surpasses 60% (see Table 20-13). In the blood smear, formed elements are usually increased. A mild-to-moderate leukocytosis of 10,000 to 25,000/μL occurs initially in two thirds of cases. A mild-to-moderate thrombocytosis (400,000–800,000 platelets/μL) occurs initially in half of cases, often withabnormal morphologic features. Hyperuricemia and secondary gout may be present and are related to rapid cell turnover.

CLINICAL FEATURES: In North America, 8 to 10 cases of PV per million are seen annually. The mean age at diagnosis is 60 years. Onset tends to be insidious, and symptoms are generally nonspecific, typically relating to the increased erythrocyte mass. Plethora and splenomegaly are early findings. Headache, dizziness, and visual problems result from vascular disturbances in the brain and retina. Angina pectoris, secondary to slowing of coronary artery blood flow, and intermittent claudication caused by sluggish peripheral blood flow in the lower extremities may be observed. Gastric or duodenal ulcers may result from circulatory problems in the gastrointestinal tract and possibly (in part) from histamine release by basophils. Major thrombotic complications occur in a third of cases, including stroke and myocardial infarction.

The clinical course of PV tends to proceed as a series of phases. In the **proliferative phase,** there is erythroid proliferation and an increased erythrocyte mass. In one third of patients, the disease progresses to other stages. In 10% of cases of polycythemia overall, excessive proliferation of erythroid cells ceases, resulting in stable or decreased erythrocyte mass (**spent phase**). Another 10% of cases progress to myelofibrosis, like that in other chronic myeloproliferative syndromes (**postpolycythemic myelofibrosis with myeloid metaplasia**). **Acute myelogenous leukemia** occurs in 5% to 10% of cases of PV, and may be due in part to treatment with ^{32}P or alkylating agents.

Median survival with PV is 13 years. The most common causes of death are those associated with old age. Specific causes of death related to the disease itself include thrombosis, hemorrhage, acute myeloid leukemia (AML), and the spent phase. Therapeutic reduction of erythrocyte mass, by repeated phlebotomy or chemotherapy, is effective management in most cases.

Chronic Idiopathic Myelofibrosis

Chronic idiopathic myelofibrosis is a clonal myeloproliferative disease in which marrow fibrosis is accompanied by prominent megakaryopoiesis and granulopoiesis.

PATHOGENESIS: As in other types of myeloproliferative disease, exposure to benzene or radiation has occasionally been implicated in chronic idiopathic myelofibrosis. The malignant megakaryocytes produce PDGF and TGF-β, both of which are powerful fibroblast mitogens. Ultimately, the entire marrow space is displaced by connective tissue, although fibroblasts are not part of the clonal stem cell disorder. In the fibrotic phase, malignant stem cells enter the circulation and give rise to extramedullary hematopoiesis at multiple anatomic sites. No genetic defect has been identified.

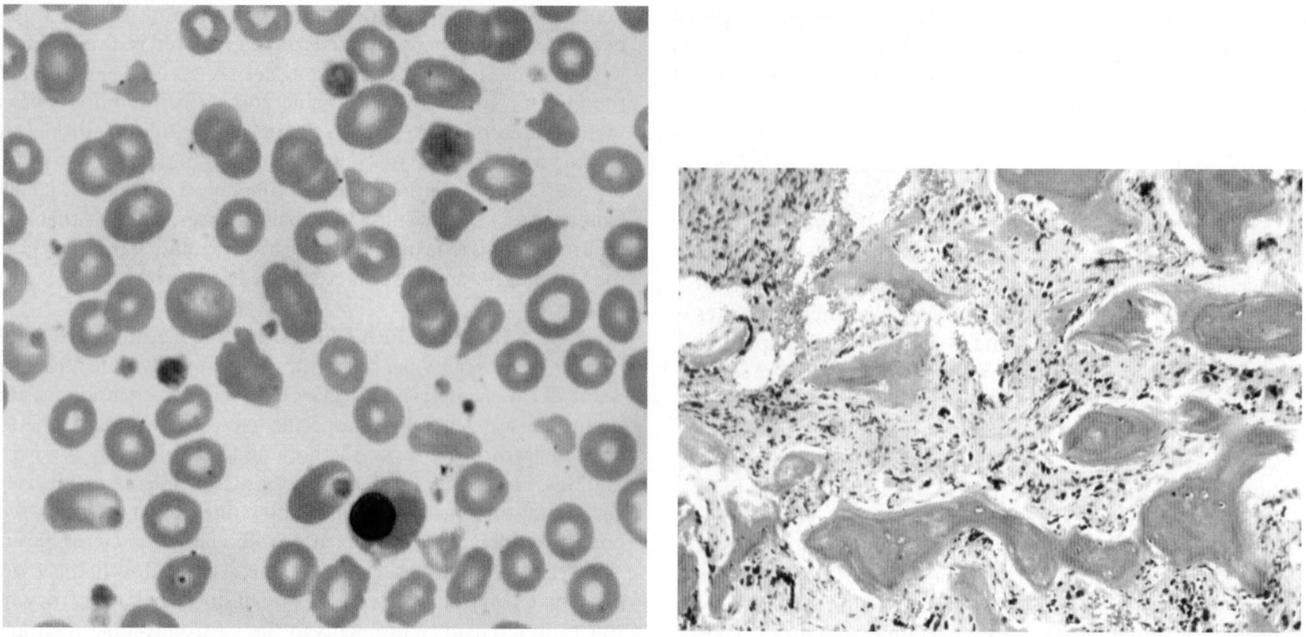

A B

FIGURE 20-38. **Chronic idiopathic myelofibrosis. A.** Peripheral smear shows anisocytosis, poikilocytosis with teardrop forms, and nucleated erythrocytes. Giant platelets are also present. **B.** A section of bone marrow shows collagenous fibrosis, osteosclerosis, and numerous abnormal megakaryocytes.

PATHOLOGY: Most patients are diagnosed at the fibrotic stage, but 25% are first detected in a cellular phase. The **prefibrotic, cellular stage** features a hypercellular bone marrow, with predominant neutrophilic and megakaryocytic proliferation. The megakaryocytes are clustered and atypically lobated. In the **fibrotic stage,** the blood shows either leukopenia or marked leukocytosis, and myeloid precursors and nucleated RBCs (leukoerythroblastosis) are usually present. The red cells exhibit poikilocytosis and teardrop forms (Fig. 20-38A). Conspicuous reticulin or collagen fibrosis in the marrow defines this stage (see Fig. 20-38B). As in the cellular phase, many atypical megakaryocytes are present. Extramedullary hematopoiesis leads to splenomegaly, hepatomegaly, and lymphadenopathy, and may be seen in other organs.

CLINICAL FEATURES: The annual incidence of idiopathic myelofibrosis is estimated at 0.5 to 1.5 per 100,000. It is a disease of the elderly, with a peak incidence in the 7th decade. A quarter of patients with idiopathic myelofibrosis are asymptomatic at diagnosis, the disease being detected by splenomegaly on physical examination or by demonstration of teardrop red cells or thrombocytosis. Early clinical symptoms are nonspecific and include fatigue, low-grade fever, night sweats, and weight loss. Platelet function may be impaired and associated with either increased platelet aggregation and thrombosis or decreased platelet aggregation with a bleeding diathesis. Transformation to AML occurs in 15% of cases. (See Table 20-13.)

Essential Thrombocythemia

Essential thrombocythemia is an uncommon neoplastic disorder of hematopoietic stem cells, characterized by uncontrolled proliferation of megakaryocytes. A marked increase in circulating platelets ($>600{,}000/\mu L$) is accompanied by recurrent episodes of thrombosis and hemorrhage. The disease affects middle-aged persons, with a slight male predominance (see Table 20-13).

PATHOGENESIS: Essential thrombocythemia is a clonal disorder believed to derive from malignant transformation of a single hematopoietic stem cell with principal, but not exclusive, commitment to megakaryocytic lineage. The disease features marked proliferation of megakaryocytes, with up to a 15-fold or greater increase in platelet production. Chromosomal abnormalities are identified in fewer than 25% of patients.

PATHOLOGY: Abnormalities of platelet function are common in primary thrombocythemia. Recurrent episodes of thrombosis in arteries or veins are attributed to severe thrombocytosis and hemorrhage reflects defects in platelet function. Thromboses in the spleen, with subsequent infarctions, may result in splenic atrophy. Iron deficiency anemia follows hemorrhage from gastrointestinal or urogenital tracts. The bone marrow is markedly hypercellular, with decreased fat cells and increased megakaryocytes (Fig. 20-39), which form cohesive clusters or sheets. Reticulin fibers in the marrow are increased in one-third of cases, but overt fibrosis is rare. Iron stores are normal or low.

The spleen is mildly enlarged in half the cases of primary thrombocythemia. Microscopically, myeloid metaplasia is common. Myeloid metaplasia of hepatic sinusoids and lymph nodes is occasionally observed.

The diagnosis of essential thrombocythemia is one of exclusion. Other chronic myeloproliferative diseases must be excluded before this dignosis is established.

CLINICAL FEATURES: The clinical course of primary thrombocythemia is protracted, with a median survival of over 10 years. In untreated cases, thrombosis of large arteries and veins is common, especially in the legs,

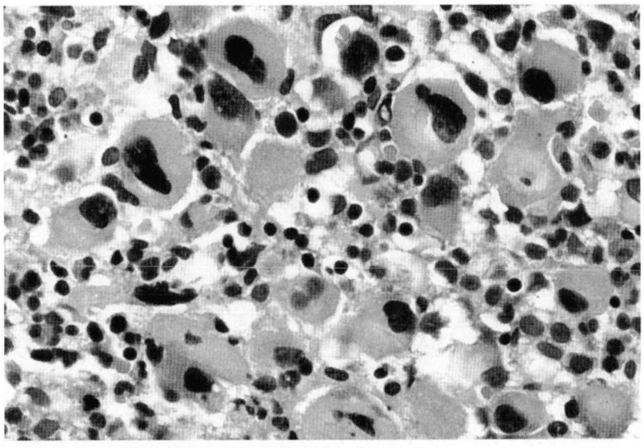

FIGURE 20-39. **Essential thrombocythemia.** A section of bone marrow exhibits a conspicuous increase in the number of megakaryocytes, which display atypical features and hypolobated forms.

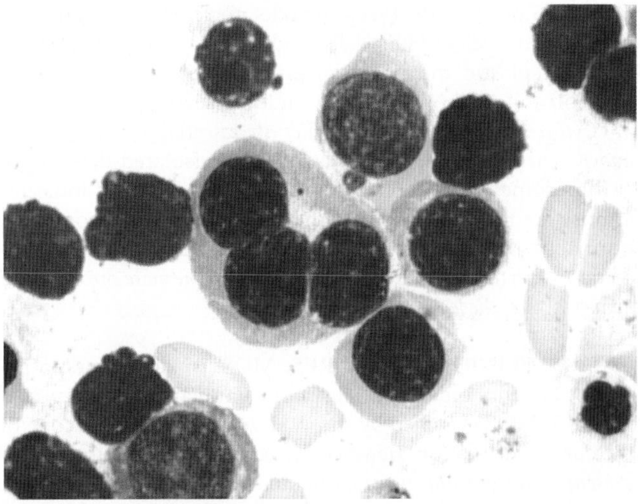

FIGURE 20-40. **Myelodysplastic syndrome.** Dysplastic, multinucleated, megaloblastoid erythroid precursors are shown.

heart, intestine, and kidneys. Hemorrhage is usually mild and not life-threatening. AML supervenes in up to 5% of cases. The disease is treated with plateletpheresis and myelosuppressive chemotherapy.

Myelodysplastic Syndromes (MDS) Are Clonal Disorders That Cause Ineffective Hematopoiesis

Dysplastic morphology in one or more hematopoietic lineages is characteristic of MDS. The disease is most common in the elderly. There is a discrepancy between the paucity of peripheral blood elements and the marked hyperplasia seen in the bone marrow. This is due to ineffective hematopoiesis and increased apoptosis in the marrow. The WHO classifies several subtypes of MDS. *However, all types manifest refractory anemia or other cytopenias.* Unlike myeloproliferative diseases, MDS displays neither leukocytosis nor thrombocytosis. MDS also must be distinguished from AML, which exhibits at least 20% blasts in the bone marrow. Because MDS frequently converts to AML, it is also referred to as **preleukemic syndrome**.

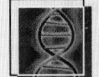

PATHOGENESIS: MDS may be either primary (de novo) or secondary (therapy-related). Patients with secondary myelodysplasia usually have a history of chemotherapy, especially alkylating agents or radiation therapy. Other risk factors for MDS include viruses, benzene exposure, cigarette smoking, and Fanconi anemia.

PATHOLOGY: The morphologic classification of MDS is based upon the presence of abnormally shaped hematopoietic cells and the proportion of myeloblasts. Dysplastic features may be present in one or more hematopoietic lineages. They are most frequent in erythroid precursors, which show megaloblastoid changes, multinucleation, nuclear budding, bridging between nuclei, and karyorrhexis (Fig. 20-40). Erythroid precursors with iron-laden mitochondria around the nuclei (**ringed sideroblasts**) are common (Fig. 20-41A).

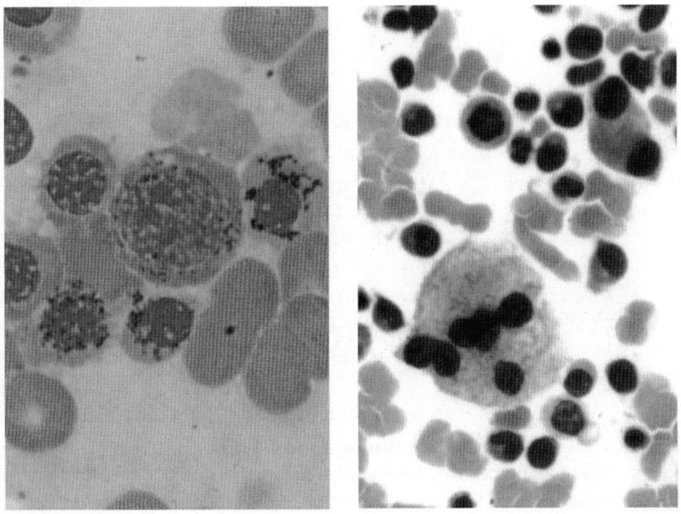

A,B

FIGURE 20-41. **Myelodysplastic syndrome. A**. Smear of a bone marrow aspirate stained with Prussian blue shows an erythroid precursor cell containing iron-laden mitochondria that encircle the nuclei (ringed sideroblast). **B.** Dysplastic megakaryocyte with nuclear separation.

Dysgranulopoietic features include nuclear hyposegmentation (pseudo-Pelger-Huët cells) and cytoplasmic hypogranulation. Dysplastic megakaryocytes may be mononuclear or hypolobated, or show nuclear separation (see Fig. 20-41B).

Cytogenetic and molecular studies are essential for the diagnosis and prognosis of myelodysplastic syndromes. Isolated deletion of chromosome 5 (5q-) occurs primarily in women and indicates a more favorable prognosis. Other favorable chromosomal abnormalities are −y and 20q-. By contrast, deletion of chromosome 7 (7q-) has an unfavorable prognosis. *The more chromosomal abnormalities, the less favorable is the outcome.*

CLINICAL FEATURES: MDS usually occurs in patients older than 60 years. The various subtypes of MDS classified by the WHO are beyond the scope of the current discussion. *However, as a general common feature, MDS presents with anemia, neutropenia and thrombocytopenia,* which commonly leads to infection and bleeding. Up to 40% of patients with MDS progress to AML and the higher the proportion of blasts in the bone marrow, the greater is the risk.

Acute Myeloid Leukemia is a Clonal Proliferation of Myeloblasts in the Marrow with their Subsequent Appearance in Blood and Tissues

According to the WHO classification, a diagnosis of AML requires more than 20% blasts in the bone marrow. If less than 20% blasts are present, the process should be designated **refractory anemia with excess blasts**. These blasts should have cytochemical and immunophenotypic characteristics of myeloid cells. AML is classified into four types (Table 20-14):

1. **AML with recurrent genetic abnormalities**
2. **AML evolving from multilineage dysplasia**
3. **AML therapy-related**
4. **AML not otherwise categorized**

Of all acute leukemias, 70% are myeloid leukemias. The rest are lymphoblastic leukemias (discussed below under lymphoid malignancies). Most cases of AML occur in adults, with a median age of 60 years at onset.

PATHOGENESIS: Most cases of AML are of unknown etiology, but in a few instances a causal relationship between radiation, cytotoxic chemotherapy, or benzene exposure has been documented. An increase in AML was noted after the detonation of atomic bombs in Hiroshima and Nagasaki (see Chapter 8). Cigarette smoking doubles the risk for AML.

PATHOLOGY: Malignant myeloblasts of AML are detectable in the bone marrow and, in most instances, in the blood. Typically, the malignant cells pack the bone marrow and displace normal hematopoietic cells (Fig. 20-42). Myeloblasts are medium-sized to large cells with round or slightly irregular nuclei. Depending on the AML subtype, Auer rods may be present in the cytoplasm (Fig. 20-43). These inclusions are specific for the myeloid lineage and preclude a diagnosis of lymphoblastic leukemia.

TABLE 20-14

WHO Classification of Acute Myeloid Leukemia (AML)

Acute myeloid leukemia with recurrent genetic abnormalities
AML with t(8;21)(q22;q22);(AML1/ETO) AML with abnormal bone marrow eosinophils inv(16)(p13q22) or t(16;16)(p13;q22);(CBFβ/MY<H1>1) Acute promyelocytic leukemia (AML with t(15;17)(q22;q12)(PML/RARα) and variants (**M3**) AML with 11q23 (MML) abnormalities
Acute myeloid leukemia with multilineage dysplasia
Following a myelodysplastic syndrome or myelodysplastic syndrome/myeloproliferative disorder Without antecedent myelodysplastic syndrome
Acute myeloid leukemia and myelodysplastic syndromes, therapy-related
Alkylating agent related Topoisomerase type II inhibitor related (some may be lymphoid) Other types
Acute myeloid leukemia not otherwise categorized
AML minimally differentiated (**M0**) AML without maturation (**M1**) AML with maturation (**M2**) AML (**M4**) Acute monoblastic and monocytic leukemia (**M5**) Acute erythroid leukemia (**M6**) Acute megakaryoblastic leukemia (**M7**)

MML = myelomonocytic leukemia; PML = promyelocytic leukemia; RAR = retinoic acid receptor; WHO = World Health Organization.

Immunophenotyping by flow cytometry and cytogenetic studies is essential for correct classification of AML. Myeloid antigens frequently expressed include CD13, CD15, CD33, CD34, and CD117. AML with megakaryoblastic differentiation may show the platelet/megakaryocyte markers CD41 and CD61 (platelet GPIIb/IIIa complex).

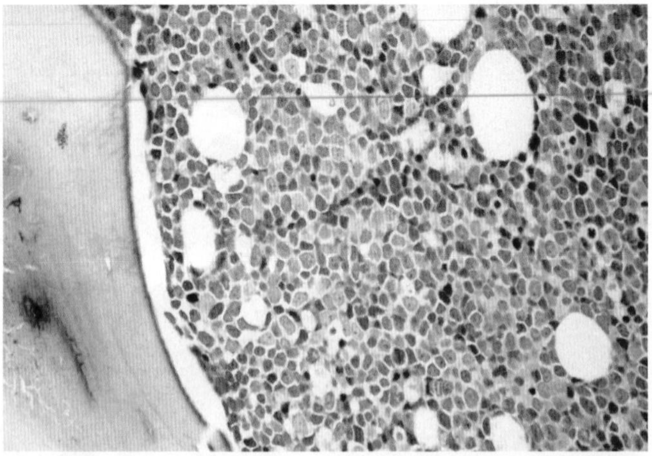

FIGURE 20-42. **Acute myelogenous leukemia.** A bone marrow section is hypercellular, owing to effacement of the normal architecture by myeloblasts.

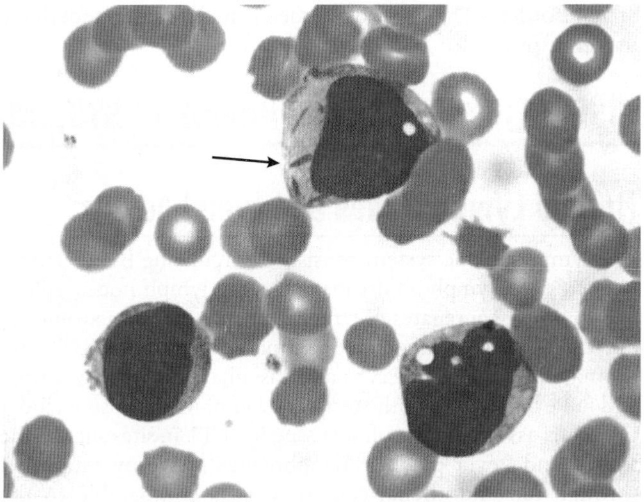

FIGURE 20-43. **Acute promyelocytic leukemia.** Auer rods are prominent (*arrow*).

Important cytochemical markers include myeloperoxidase, Sudan black and nonspecific esterase (NSE). Myeloperoxidase and Sudan black decorate myeloid cells and their precursors with increased staining intensity in more mature forms. NSE labels monoblasts and promonocytes and is a marker for AML with monocytoid differentiation.

CLINICAL FEATURES: *The major problems associated with AML reflect the progressive accumulation in the marrow of immature myeloid cells that lack the potential for further differentiation and maturation.* Whereas leukemic myeloblasts replicate at a slower rate than do normal hematopoietic precursor cells, the frequency of spontaneous cell death is also less than normal. The expanded pool of abnormal leukemic blasts encroaches on the marrow and suppresses normal hematopoiesis. *Thus, the major clinical problems in AML are granulocytopenia, thrombocytopenia, and anemia.* Infections, particularly with opportunisitic organisms (e.g., fungi), are common, as are cutaneous bleeding (petechiae and ecchymoses) and serosal hemorrahges over viscera. Untreated AML carries a dismal prognosis. Chemotherapy leads to remission in over 50% of patients, but overall 5-year survival is less than 30%. Bone marrow transplantation is a common mode of treatment for high-risk forms of AML, and for AML in relapse.

Selected AML subtypes are considered:

ACUTE PROMYELOCYTIC LEUKEMIA (APL): Categorized under "acute leukemia with recurrent genetic abnormalities," APL is defined by a chromosomal translocation involving the PML1 *gene and the retinoic acid receptor (RAR) gene.* Promyelocytic leukemia (PML) mainly affects middle-aged patients and accounts for 5% to 10% of all cases of AML. *APL is a paradigm for a molecularly defined disease in which the underlying genetic defect determines the type of treatment.* The underlying genetic defect in APL is a translocation involving the *PML* gene on chromosome 15 and the *RARα* gene on chromosome 17. The resulting *PML/RARα* fusion gene encodes a functional retinoic acid receptor. The receptor can be targeted by all-*trans*-retinoic acid (ATRA), which mediates maturation of the tumor cells. The bone marrow is packed with tumor cells that have promyelocytic morphologic features. Auer rods may be abundant (see Fig. 20-43). Leukemic cells are strongly reactive for myeloperoxidase or Sudan black. *Patients with APL frequently present with DIC.* Senescent leukemic cells degranulate and activate the coagulation cascade. Treatment with ATRA induces maturation of the tumor cells and prevents both degranulation and DIC.

THERAPY-INDUCED AML AND MYELODYSPLASTIC SYNDROMES: Treatment of solid tumors with chemotherapy or radiation therapy can induce later hematopoietic cancers. Secondary AML is often associated with monocytoid morphology and immunophenotype. The most common therapy-induced secondary malignancies are MDS and AML. Alkylating agents and topoisomerase II inhibitors (epipodophylotoxins) most often give rise to AML. AML or MDS after treatment with alkylating agents or radiation have a median latency of approximately 6 years, whereas AML after treatment with topoisomerase II inhibitor occurs on average 3 years after treatment.

ACUTE MYELOID LEUKEMIA, NOT OTHERWISE CATEGORIZED: This set of leukemias was organized according to the French-American-British (FAB) classification. The WHO classification incorporates the FAB scheme (Fig. 20-44):

- **M0—AML, minimally differentiated:** The leukemic cells are immature myeloblasts with no defining morphologic criteria of the myeloid lineage Immunophenotyping by flow cytometry establishes the myeloid nature of the tumor cells. The prognosis is unfavorable.

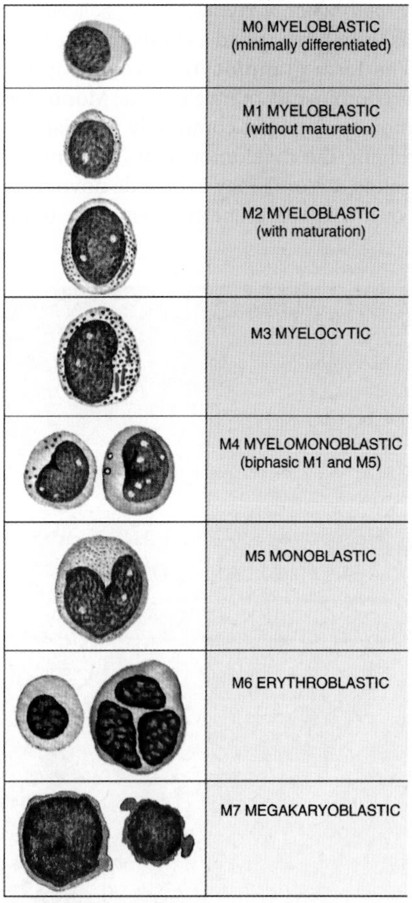

FIGURE 20-44. **Morphology of acute myeloid leukemia** (AML) in the traditional French-American-British (FAB) classification, now within the framework of the World Health Organization (WHO) classification "AML-not otherwise categorized."

- **M1—AML without maturation:** Less than 10% of the myeloid cells are promyelocytes or more mature myeloid cells. The disease occurs most often in middle-aged persons.
- **M2—AML with maturation:** More than 10% maturing myeloid cells (promyelocytes and later) are present.
- **M3—APL:** Classified under AML with genetic abnormalities, see above.
- **M4—Acute myelomonocytic leukemia (AMML):** Some 20% to 80% of tumor cells show monocytoid features. AMML accounts for 20% of all AMLs.
- **M5—Acute monoblastic/monocytic leukemia (AMoL):** At least 80% of the myeloid cells have monocytoid differentiation. AMoL constitutes 5 to 8% of all cases of AML and is seen in younger patients.
- **M6—Acute erythroid leukemia:** Acute erythroid leukemias feature prominent erythropoietic proliferation; over 50% of nucleated cells in the bone marrow are erythroid precursors. At least 20% of the remaining cells are myeloblasts. A rare, more chronic, form of this disease displays pure erythroblasts and is referred to as **erythremic myelosis** or **di Guglielmo syndrome.**
- **M7—Acute megakaryoblastic leukemia (AMegL):** At least 50% of the blasts show a megakaryocytic immunophenotype.

A tumor of myeloblasts or monoblasts can occur that differs from the AML types listed above. **Myeloid sarcoma** *is an extramedullary solid tumor of myeloblasts or monoblasts* (Fig. 20-45). This entity is sometimes called a **chloroma** because of its greenish color. The term **granulocytic sarcoma** applies to lesions composed predominantly of myeloblasts. **Monoblastic sarcoma** is less common, and is most commonly associated with translocations involving the myelomonocytic leukemia (MML) gene (11q23). Myeloid sarcoma may evolve de novo or in association with AML, or it may represent the blast phase in myeloproliferative disorders. The prognosis is determined by the underlying leukemic process.

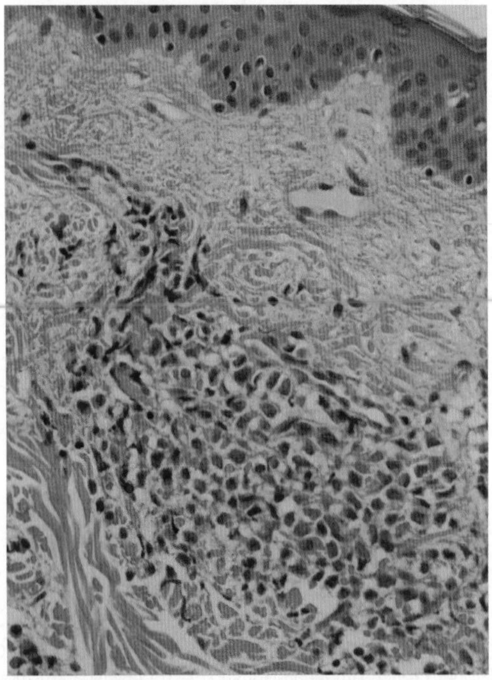

FIGURE 20-45. **Myeloid sarcoma.** The skin from a patient with acute monoblastic leukemia (leukemia cutis) shows neoplastic myeloid cells.

DISORDERS OF THE LYMPHOPOIETIC SYSTEM

Normal Lymph Nodes and Lymphocytes

The lymphopoietic system consists of circulating B and T lymphocytes and lymphoid organs, including lymph nodes, spleen and thymus. Aggregates of lymphoid tissue in the gastrointestinal tract, mucosa-associated lymphoid tissue (MALT), are prominent in the oropharynx and nasopharynx (Waldeyer ring) and in Peyer patches of the terminal ileum. MALT also includes bronchus-associated lymphoid tissue (BALT). In sites such as the tonsils and Peyer patches, lymphocytes arrive by migration through tall endothelial cells of vessels comparable to the postcapillary venules of the lymph nodes. (MALT) plays an important role in immunologic protection of the host in areas vulnerable to potential invaders. IgA secretion is a prominent component of this protective function.

Lymphocytes are derived from bone marrow stem cells (see Fig. 20-2). Lymphocytes that differentiate and mature in the thymus are **T cells***;* those that develop in the bone marrow are **B cells**. Lymphocyte development is associated with sequential gain and loss of several cytoplasmic and surface antigens. *The pattern of expression of these antigens identifies the character of the cells or the maturation stage of a neoplastic clone (discussed below).* The reader is referred to Chapter 4 for a detailed discussion of T and B lymphocyte development and function.

LYMPH NODES: Lymph nodes consist of organized collections of lymphoid tissue located along lymphatic vessels. Typically grayish white and ovoid or bean-shaped, they are 2 mm to 2 cm in diameter. A fibrous capsule and radiating trabeculae provide a supporting structure and a delicate reticular network contributes internal support. Lymph nodes exhibit an outer cortex and an inner medulla (Fig. 20-46).

Lymph or interstitial fluid enters the nodes through afferent lymphatics in the convexity of the cortex. It percolates first through the subcapsular sinuses, then the radial sinuses and exits through efferent lymphatics. The sinuses are lined by mononuclear phagocytes. The arrangement of the sinuses maximizes exposure of foreign antigens in lymph to macrophages and immunoreactive B cells and T cells.

The **cortex** contains defined B cell and T cell domains. Circulating B and T lymphocytes enter lymph nodes by migrating through the tall endothelial cells of the postcapillary venules in the **paracortex**. T lymphocytes tend to remain in the paracortex; B lymphocytes home to the **germinal centers**.

The B-cell–dependent cortex consists of two types of follicles. Immunologically inactive follicles are termed **primary follicles,** which consist of cohesive aggregates of small, normal-appearing lymphocytes; active follicles that contain germinal centers are referred to as **secondary follicles**. Germinal centers contain large lymphocytes (**centroblasts**) and small lymphocytes with cleaved nuclei (**centrocytes**). There are also scattered macrophages that contain phagocytized nuclear and cytoplasmic debris ("tingible body" macrophages).

In lymphoid tissue outside of germinal centers, B cells are more regular and have round-to-oval hyperchromatic nuclei and blue-purple cytoplasm. Immunoblast-like cells with prominent blue-purple cytoplasm are **plasmacytoid immunoblasts**.

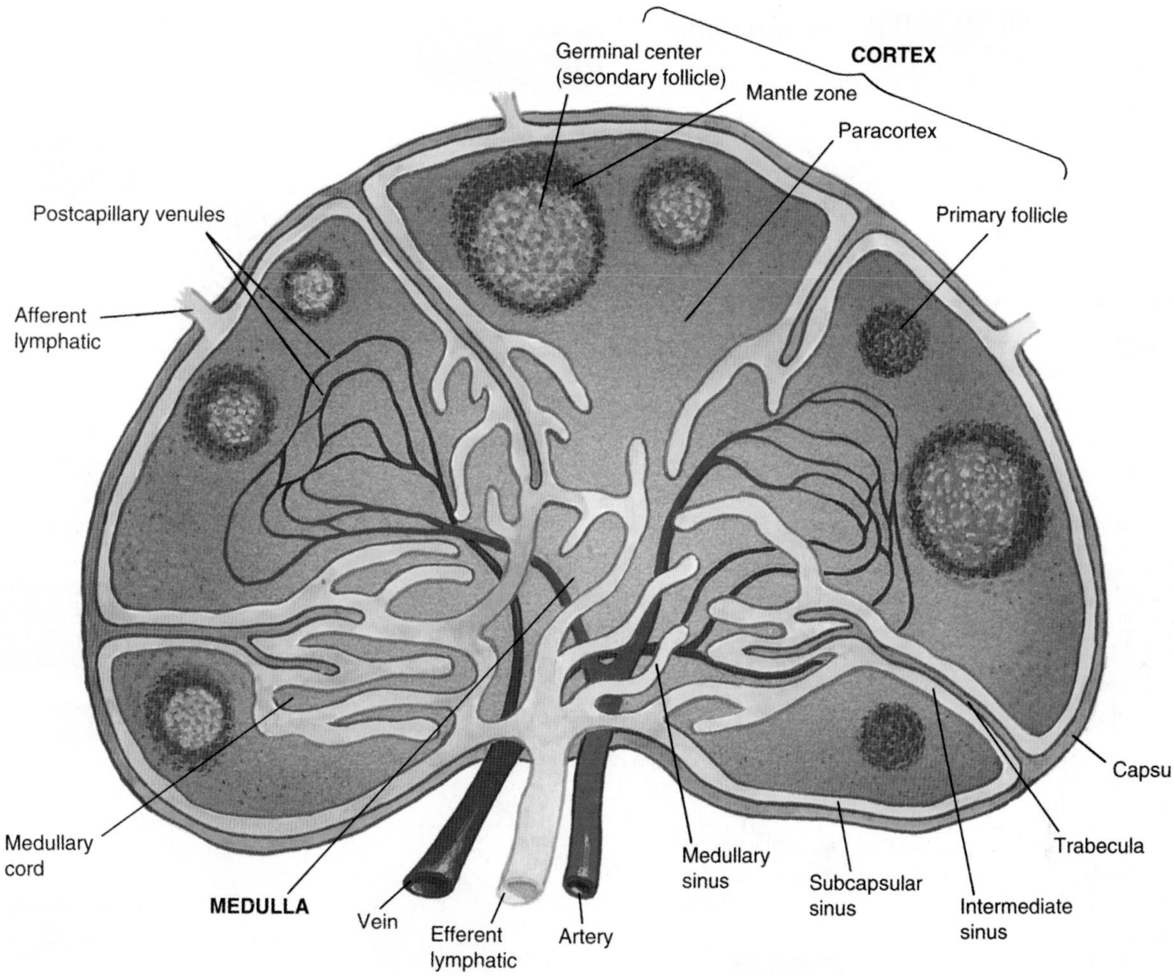

FIGURE 20-46. **Structure of a normal lymph node.**

Follicular dendritic cells (**FDCs**) are stellate cells with long cytoplasmic processes. They present antigens to follicular B cells. Macrophages and, to a lesser extent, dendritic cells provide growth factors for activated B cells.

The T cell-dependent paracortex, also known as the deep cortex, is between the B cell follicles and deep to them. In addition to T lymphocytes, scattered macrophages and IDCs are found in the paracortex. IDCs process and present antigens to T lymphocytes.

B LYMPHOCYTE DEVELOPMENT: **Precursors** of B cells acquire their repertoire of cytoplasmic and cell surface antigens in the bone marrow (Fig. 20-47). The earliest B cell antigens are **CD19**, CALLA (common acute leukemia/lymphoma antigen, **CD10**) on the cell membrane, and the nuclear antigen TdT.

As B lymphocytes mature, the genes for immunoglobulin heavy chains are rearranged in preparation for the synthesis of IgM molecules. In precursor B cells, IgM is expressed in the cytoplasm. After activation and clonal expansion in germinal centers, B lymphocytes migrate to the B cell-dependent medullary cords of the lymph nodes to become Ig-secreting plasma cells or to exit lymph nodes as memory B lymphocytes.

Mature B cells express ***surface*** *pan B cell antigens CD19, CD20, CD22, plus Ig heavy and light chains.* When activated by antigen and stimulated by an appropriate T helper cell, B cells develop into plasma cells that synthesize and export immunoglobulins. At this stage, they no longer display heavy or light Ig chains on the surface membrane.

Terminally differentiated, effector B lymphocytes are recognized as **plasma cells** in both smears and tissue sections. Plasma cells have eccentric nuclei with clumped chromatin marginated at the nuclear membrane, traditionally described as "clockface chromatin." The abundant blue-purple cytoplasm of plasma cells often displays a clear paranuclear clear zone representing the Golgi complex.

T LYMPHOCYTES: The lymphocytic stem cells that migrate to the thymus are exposed to a number of thymic hormones that first induce expression of CD2 surface receptors that bind sheep erythrocytes (Fig. 20-48). At this point, recombination of the T cell receptor genes leads to generation of diversity in T cell receptors, each of which recognizes a single antigen. The T cell receptor on the membrane associates with a **CD3** molecule; *CD2 and CD3 antigens define the cells as T cells.* Other antigens appear, such as **CD5** and particularly **CD4** (**helper**) or **CD8** (**suppressor**). The cells then migrate from the thymus to lymph nodes, spleen, and peripheral blood.

When exposed to antigens specific for their receptors, CD4+ cells become activated. These antigens are peptide fragments derived from partial digestion of proteins by macrophages or antigen-presenting cells. When such antigens are presented in association with class 2 human leukocyte antigen (HLA)

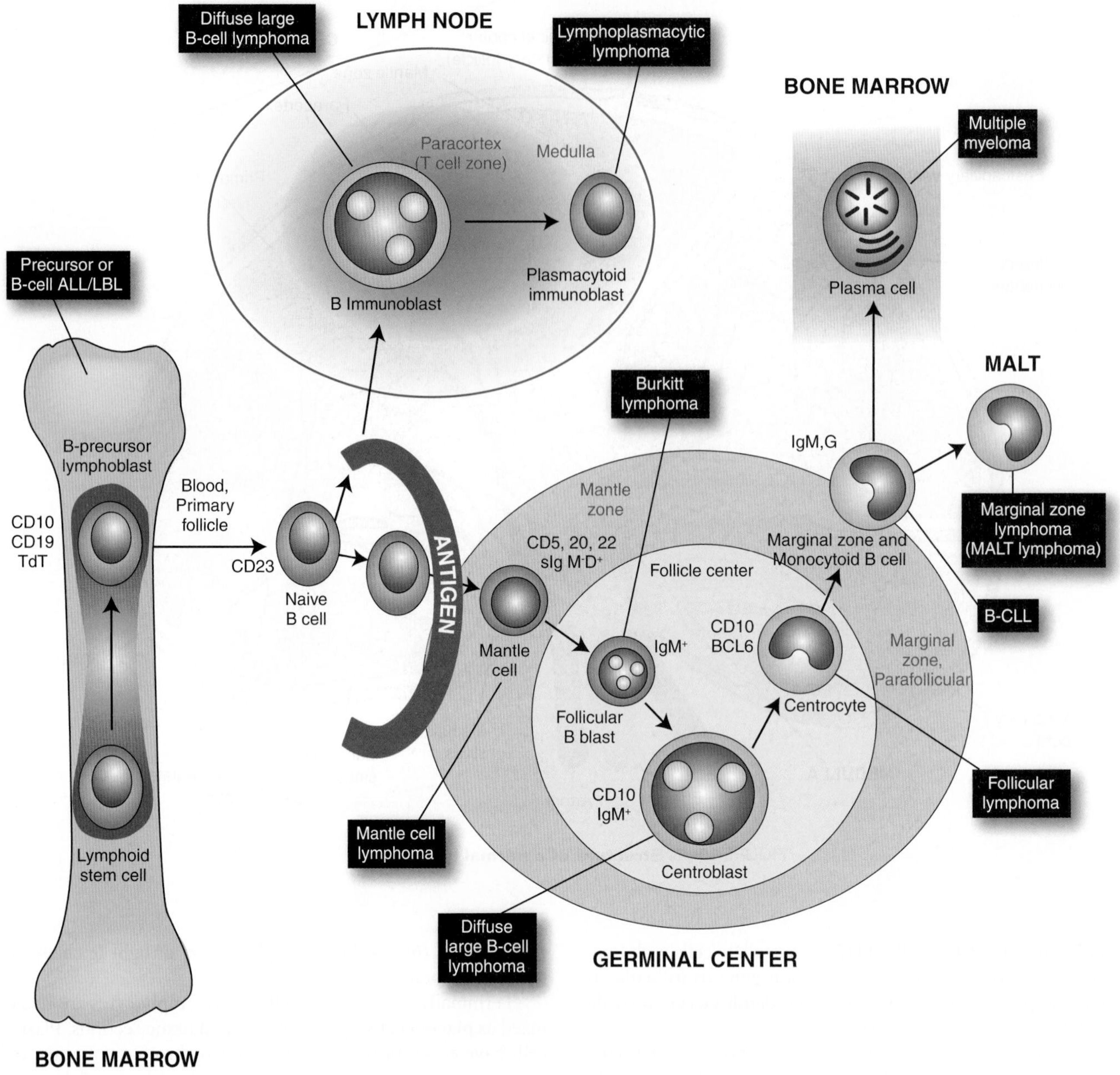

FIGURE 20-47. **Pathway of B cell differentiation and corresponding B-cell lymphomas.** Following the precursor status, B cells mature into naive B lymphocytes. The germinal-center response represents an important turntable for immunoglobulin variable region gene mutations, Ig heavy-chain switch, and differentiation into plasma cells and memory cells. Cluster designation (CD) markers are shown. B immunoblasts and plasmacytoid immunoblasts reside in the T-cell-rich paracortex and medulla, respectively. Marginal zone B cells home to mucosa-associated lymphoid tissue (MALT) sites and bone marrow. Neoplastic transformation occurs at all phases of B-cell differentiation. ALL/LBL = acute lymphoblastic leukemia/lymphoma; B-CLL= B-cell chronic lymphocytic leukemia; Ig = immunoglobulin.

molecules, CD4+ cells become activated, release mitogenic growth factors (IL-1 and IL-2) and develop into helper/inducer cells. In turn these T cells interact with B lymphocytes that express the same antigenic specificity, prompting the latter to proliferate and inducing them to differentiate to plasma cells.

CD8+ cells are activated when their receptors recognize peptides presented in association with a class I HLA antigen, after which they become suppressor/cytotoxic cells. *CD8+ cells limit expansion of activated B cells and stop their immune response.*

A subpopulation of T lymphocytes activated by antigenic peptides becomes **cytotoxic lymphocytes (killer cells)**, which eliminate foreign cells or viruses bearing the recognized antigen.

NATURAL KILLER (NK) AND CYTOTOXIC CELLS: a small proportion of lymphocytes express neither B nor T cell differentiation antigens. They may act as cytotoxic or **natural killer cells** (NK cells), which do not require antigenic recognition for their function. NK cells are large lymphocytes with granular cytoplasm (large granular lymphocytes) (Fig. 20-49). These cells are usually CD56+, CD3−, and CD8−, but are heterogeneous with respect to other cell membrane antigens.

Lymphocytes exhibit a heterogeneous morphologic appearance. Small to medium-sized lymphocytes may be primitive, antigen-independent B and T cells, or antigen-dependent, committed cells that have not been reexposed to the specific sensitizing

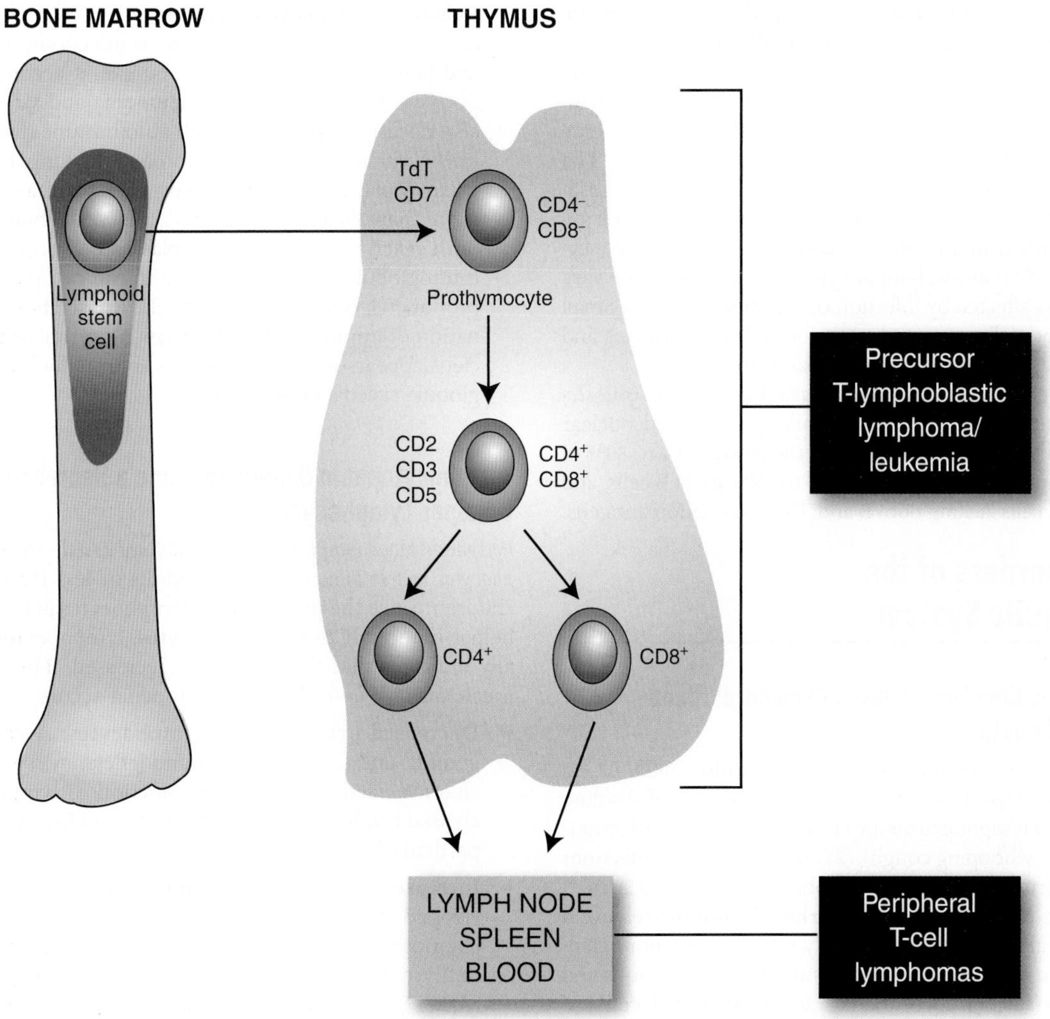

FIGURE 20-48. **Pathways of T-cell development and corresponding lymphomas.** CD = cluster designation; TdT = terminal deoxynucleotidyl transferase.

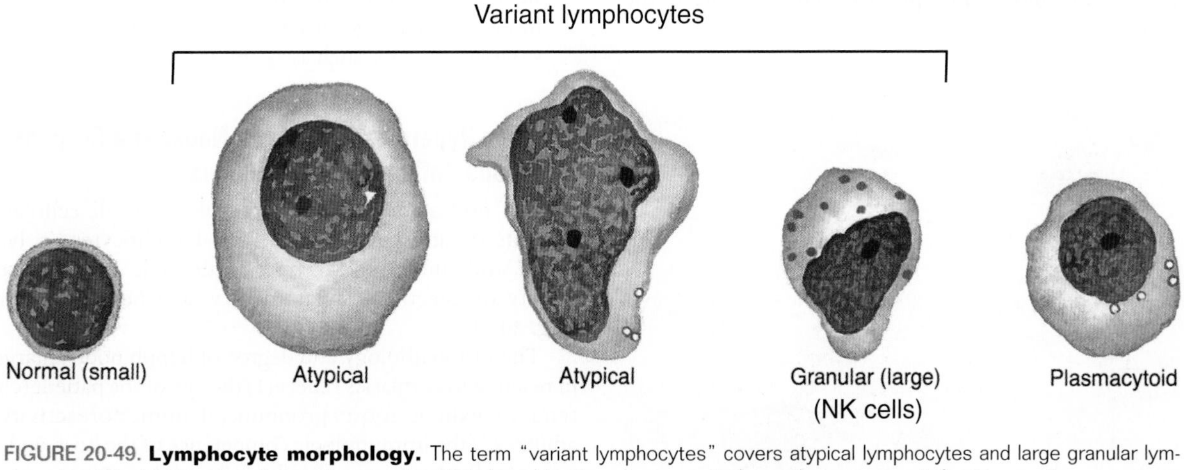

FIGURE 20-49. **Lymphocyte morphology.** The term "variant lymphocytes" covers atypical lymphocytes and large granular lymphocytes. *Atypical lymphocytes* are large and exhibit deep blue to pale gray cytoplasm; they are seen in benign reactive processes. *Large granular lymphocytes* are medium-to-large lymphoid cells with some pink cytoplasmic granules. They are suppressor T lymphocytes, some with natural killer (NK) function, and may be increased in benign or malignant disorders. *Plasmacytoid lymphocytes* have abundant blue cytoplasm and are seen in some reactive disorders.

antigen. *When activated by antigen, both B and T cells develop into large, protein-synthesizing cells, called* **immunoblasts** (see Fig. 20-46 and Fig. 20-49). In peripheral blood smears, transformed cytotoxic T cells are called variant lymphocytes (sometimes "atypical lymphocytes"). Variant lymphocytes tend to have abundant blue-gray cytoplasm and multiple nucleoli on Wright-Giemsa staining. The same cells in tissue sections stained with hematoxylin and eosin have round to oval nuclei, one to several eosinophilic nucleoli apposed to the nuclear membrane and abundant clear to purple cytoplasm. For these reasons, lymphocyte size and appearance vary widely in tissues affected by infection or immune reactions. Small lymphocytes, partially activated (transformed) lymphocytes and large activated lymphocytes (immunoblasts) are all seen.

T lymphocytes are usually indistinguishable from B cells in tissue sections. Infrequently, they show an irregularly contoured nuclear membrane and pale, clear cytoplasm. In the blood, 60% to 80% of circulating lymphocytes are T cells, 10% to 15% are of B cells, and the rest are NK cells lacking both B and T differentiation antigens.

Benign Disorders of the Lymphopoietic System

Lymphocytosis Denotes Elevated Peripheral Blood Lymphocyte Counts

The upper limits of normal are 4000/μL in adults, 7000/μL in children, and 9000/μL in infants. The principal causes of absolute peripheral blood lymphocytosis are (1) acute infections (infectious mononucleosis, whooping cough), (2) chronic bacterial infections (tuberculosis, brucellosis), and (3) lymphoproliferative diseases.

In addition to lymphocytosis, **variant lymphocytes** are a hallmark of viral infections, particularly infectious mononucleosis and some immunologic disorders, such as drug reactions and serum sickness (see Fig. 20-49 and Fig. 20-50). Most such cells are of the T cell lineage (CD8+ cytotoxic/suppressor cells).

Plasmacytosis Is Most Common in End-Stage Multiple Myeloma

- **Peripheral blood plasmacytosis:** An increase in plasma cells in the blood is uncommon. The most frequent cause is **plasma cell neoplasia (multiple myeloma)**, usually in the terminal stages of the disease.

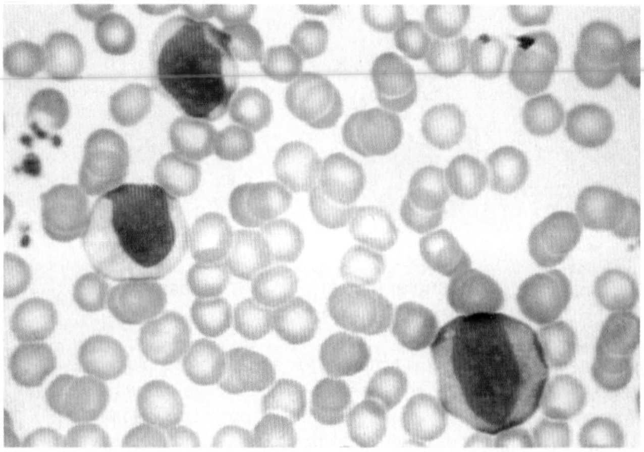

FIGURE 20-50. **Infectious mononucleosis.** Atypical lymphocytes are characteristic.

- **Reactive bone marrow plasmacytosis:** An increase in plasma cells in the marrow occurs various infectious, inflammatory, and neoplastic disorders. For example, it accompanies infections as diverse as bronchopneumonia and viral hepatitis. It also occurs in association with autoimmune diseases and epithelial cancers, such as carcinoma of the lung. Reactive bone marrow plasmacytosis is present when plasma cells constitute more than 3% of the nucleated cells in the bone marrow. In both reactive and neoplastic plasma cell proliferations, immunoglobulin may accumulate in the cytoplasm to form a prominent eosinophilic globule, the **Russell body**. The invagination of immunoglobulin-containing cytoplasm into the nucleus appears in cross section as an intranuclear eosinophilic globule called a **Dutcher body**.

Lymphocytopenia Usually Reflects a Decrease in T-Helper Lymphocytes

Peripheral blood lymphocytopenia is defined as a decrease in blood lymphocytes to less than 1500/μL in adults or less than 3000/μL in children. Since the predominant lymphocytes in the blood are T helper-inducer (CD4+) lymphocytes, lymphocytopenia generally indicates that these cells are decreased. There are several mechanisms by which lymphocytopenia occurs:

- **Decreased production of lymphocytes:** A variety of congenital and acquired immunodeficiency syndromes are characterized by reduced production of lymphocytes. Decreased production of T cells occurs in Hodgkin lymphoma, particularly in advanced stages.
- **Increased destruction of lymphocytes:** Lymphocytes are destroyed by medical treatments, such as x-irradiation; chemotherapy for malignant tumors; and administration of antilymphocyte globulin, adrenocorticotropic hormone (ACTH), or corticosteroids. Some viral infections, particularly AIDS, are characterized by destruction of T cells.
- **Loss of lymphocytes:** Intestinal disorders that are associated with damage to lymphatics result in the loss of lymph and its lymphocytes into the intestinal lumen. These include protein-losing enteropathies, Whipple disease, and disorders associated with increased central venous pressure (e.g., right-sided heart failure and chronic constrictive pericarditis). Immunologic damage to lymphocytes may occur in collagen vascular diseases, such as systemic lupus erythematosus.

Reactive Hyperplasia of Lymph Nodes Is a Response to Infections, Inflammation or Tumors

Lymph nodes may exhibit hyperplasia of all cellular components or any combination of B lymphocytes, T lymphocytes, and mononuclear phagocytic cells in response to a variety of infectious, inflammatory, and neoplastic disorders (Fig. 20-51).

The histopathology and degree of lymph node enlargement in reactive hyperplasias reflect (1) the age of the patient (children tend to exhibit more pronounced immunoreactivity than adults), (2) the immunologic competence of the host, and (3) the type of infectious agent or inflammatory disorder.

Acute suppurative or necrotizing lymphadenitis occurs in lymph nodes that drain a site of acute bacterial infection. Suppurative lymph nodes enlarge rapidly because of edema and hyperemia and are tender, due to distention of the capsule.

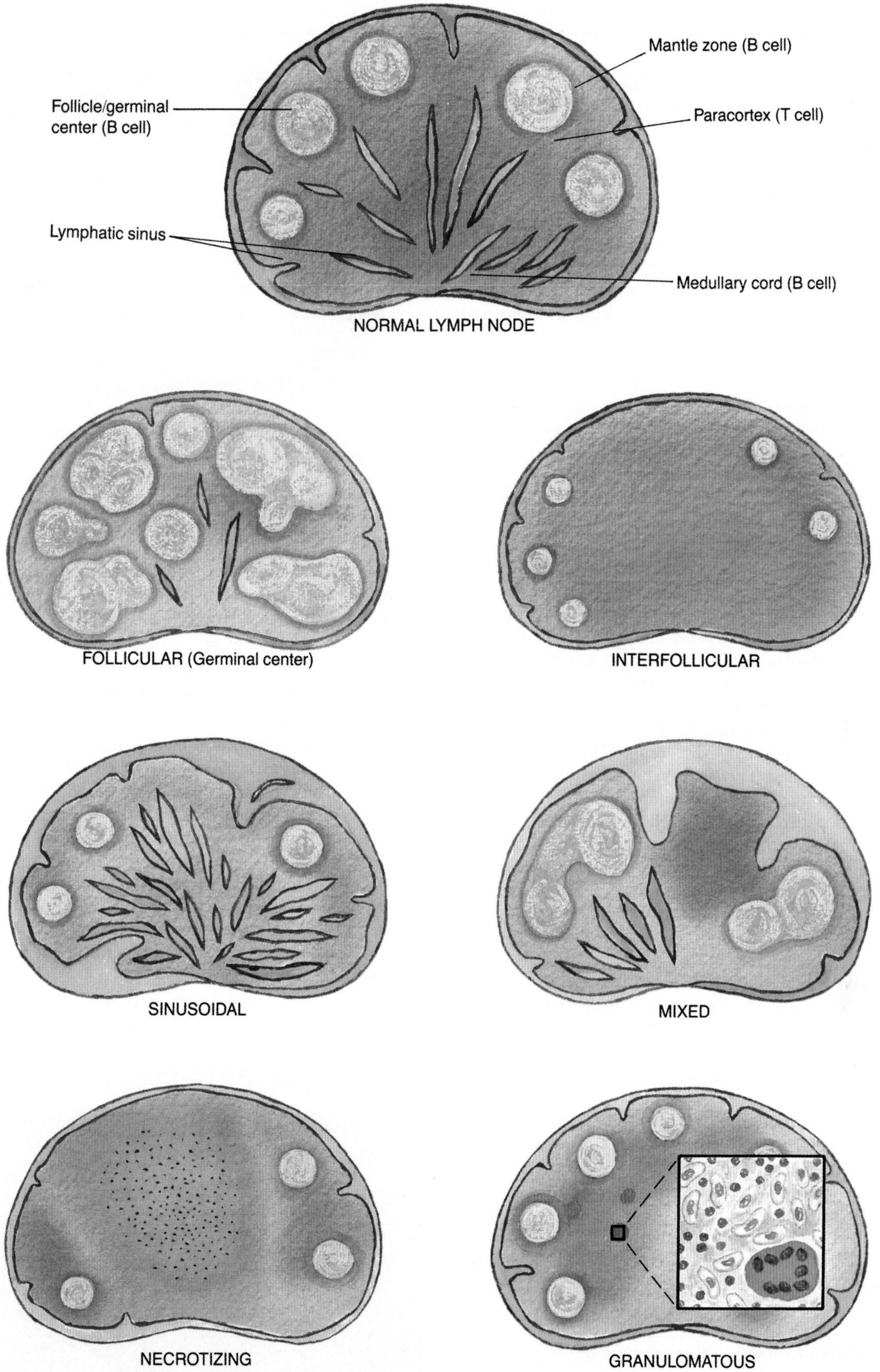

FIGURE 20-51. **Lymph nodes.** Patterns of benign reactive hyperplasia are contrasted with the structure of a normal lymph node. *Follicular hyperplasia* with prominent enlarged and irregular benign follicles, is characteristic of B cell immunoreactivity. *Interfollicular hyperplasia* is typical of T cell immunoreactivity. The *sinusoidal pattern* with expansion of sinuses by benign macrophages is seen in reactive proliferations of the mononuclear–phagocyte system. Mixed patterns of follicular, interfollicular, and sinusoidal hyperplasia are common in a variety of complex immune reactions. In *necrotizing lymphadenitis,* variable necrosis of the lymph node architecture with residual cell debris is present. In *granulomatous inflammation,* cohesive clusters of macrophages and occasional multinucleated giant cells are characteristic.

Microscopically, infiltration of lymph node sinuses and stroma by polymorphonuclear leukocytes and prominent follicular hyperplasia are noted.

The anatomical site of lymphadenopathy often provides a clue to its cause. For example, posterior auricular lymph nodes are commonly enlarged in rubella infection; occipital lymph nodes in scalp infections; posterior cervical lymph nodes in toxoplasmosis; axillary lymph nodes in infections of the arms or chest wall; and inguinal lymph nodes in venereal infections and infections of the legs. Generalized lymphadenopathy may occur in systemic infections, hyperthyroidism, drug reactions and collagen vascular diseases.

Follicular Hyperplasia

Hyperplasia of secondary follicles (germinal centers) and plasmacytosis of medullary cords indicate B lymphocyte immunoreactivity.

In **nonspecific reactive follicular hyperplasia,** a benign condition, prominent hyperplastic follicles occur principally in the cortex of the lymph node (see Fig. 20-51). Follicles are round or irregular and may be confluent. The activated B cells in the follicles range from small cells with irregular, cleaved nuclei to large immunoblasts. Numerous mitotic figures reflect the rapid proliferation of activated B lymphocytes. Scattered benign macrophages, with abundant pale cytoplasm containing pyknotic nuclear and cytoplasmic debris, impart the characteristic "starry sky" pattern of benign follicles. A well-defined mantle of normal small B lymphocytes surrounds the follicles, sharply separating them from the interfollicular regions.

The cause of nonspecific reactive follicular hyperplasia is frequently not known, although a viral, drug, or inflammatory etiology is often suspected. The clinical course features rapid and complete resolution of the lymphadenopathy.

Lymphadenopathy, either localized or generalized, is common in rheumatoid arthritis. Follicular hyperplasia is also encountered in AIDS. Additionally, the lymph nodes in AIDS show a high incidence of superimposed malignant neoplasms, including diffuse B-cell lymphomas, Burkitt lymphoma, Hodgkin lymphoma, and Kaposi sarcoma.

Interfollicular Hyperplasia

Hyperplasia of the deep cortex or paracortex (interfollicular or diffuse hyperplasia) is characteristic of T lymphocyte immunoreactivity.

Reactive nonspecific interfollicular hyperplasia (see Fig. 20-51 and Fig. 20-52) is most commonly due to viral infections or to immunologic reactions. Although the precise cause is often not determined, the condition resolves promptly. Interfollicular lymph node hyperplasia is a common finding in viral diseases, including infectious mononucleosis, varicella-herpes zoster infection, measles, and cytomegalovirus lymphadenitis.

Systemic lupus erythematosus is often associated with lymphadenopathy characterized by interfollicular hyperplasia with prominent immunoblasts and plasma cells and focal-to-massive necrosis. Arteriolitis, with fibrinoid necrosis of vessel walls, is frequently observed.

Mixed Patterns of Reactive Hyperplasia of Lymph Nodes

Some infectious diseases are associated with mixed patterns of lymph node hyperplasia, in which several different features are prominent. For example, in **toxoplasmosis** one sees prominent follicular hyperplasia and small collections of epithelioid macrophages in interfollicular regions (see Fig. 20-51 and Fig. 20-53). **Cat-scratch disease** elicits follicular hyperplasia and suppurative granulomas. Lymphadenitis caused by **lymphogranuloma venereum** and **tularemia** (see Chapter 9) is indistinguishable from cat-scratch disease.

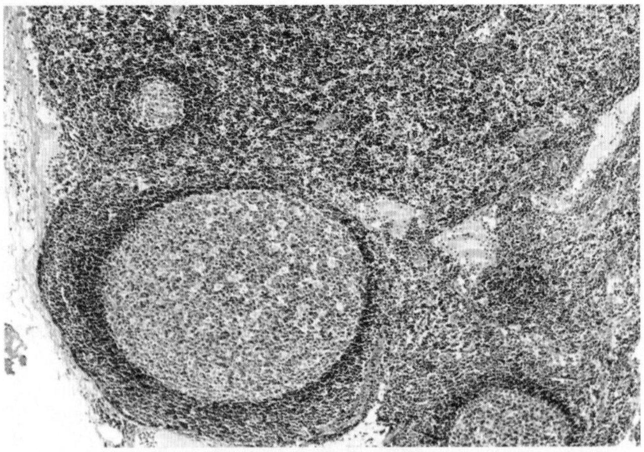

FIGURE 20-52. **Lymph node with reactive follicular hyperplasia.** A section of a hyperplastic lymph node shows prominent follicles (germinal centers) containing numerous macrophages with pale cytoplasm.

Sinus Histiocytosis Represents an Increase in Macrophages

Sinus histiocytosis is an increase in tissue macrophages (histiocytes) of the subcapsular and trabecular sinuses of the lymph nodes (see Fig. 20-51). Sinus histiocytes are derived from blood monocytes. Sinus histiocytosis is common in lymph nodes draining sites of cancer and, less often, inflammatory and infectious foci. The nature of the phagocytic debris in the cytoplasm of the macrophages helps identify the origin of the sinus histiocytosis. For example, anthracotic pigment is frequently seen in macrophages of mediastinal lymph nodes that exhibit sinus histocytosis. Macrophages containing erythrocytes and hemosiderin pigment occur with autoimmune hemolytic anemia.

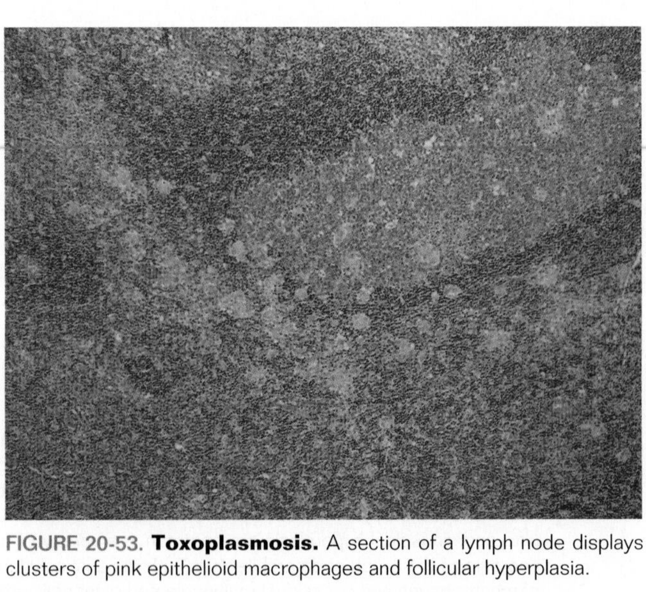

FIGURE 20-53. **Toxoplasmosis.** A section of a lymph node displays clusters of pink epithelioid macrophages and follicular hyperplasia.

Dermatopathic Lymphadenopathy Features Paracortical T cell Proliferation

***Dermatopathic lymphadenopathy** refers to specific reactive changes in lymph nodes that are caused by a variety of chronic dermatoses.* This reaction is due to drainage of lipid, melanin, and hemosiderin from the affected skin to the regional lymph nodes. The lymph nodes demonstrate an immunologic reaction to antigenic material draining from the skin, which accumulates principally in paracortical macrophages. The paracortex is expanded by a heterogeneous cell population that consists principally of macrophages whose cytoplasm contains lipid or granular, brown, melanin pigment

Malignant Lymphomas

Lymphomas are malignant proliferations of lymphocytes or lymphoblasts. B-cell and T-cell lymphomas are further categorized as derived from immature (precursor) cells or from mature (peripheral) effector cells.

Malignant lymphomas are the most heterogeneous group of human tumors (Table 20-15 and Table 20-16, and see Figs. 20-47 and 20-48). The current WHO classification of lymphomas is based upon their normal cellular counterparts and has helped to clarify an otherwise bewildering topic. Lynphomas may represent (1) **immature or mature lymphocytes,** (2) **B cells or T cells,** and (3) **lymphocytes homing to different anatomic sites**. Malignant lymphomas also exhibit characteristic immunophenotypic, cytogenetic, and molecular abnormalities. Indeed, the pathologic diagnosis of lymphomas is usually dependent upon clinical, histologic, and molecular features.

The WHO classification distinguishes between **Hodgkin lymphoma** and **non-Hodgkin lymphoma**, the latter being further divided into **B cell and T cell lymphomas**. As a general principle, the B-cell and T-cell lymphomas derive from their corresponding cell during differentiation and maturation, with corresponding immunophenotypic expression (see Fig. 20-47 and Fig. 20-48). This classification does not always distinguish between lymphoma and leukemia. For example, no distinction in principle is made between chronic lymphocytic leukemia (CLL) and small lymphocytic lymphoma (SLL).

TABLE 20-15

WHO Histological Classification of B-cell Neoplasms

Precursor B-cell neoplasm
Precursor B lymphoblastic leukemia/lymphoma
Mature B-cell neoplasms
Chronic lymphocytic leukemia/small lymphocytic lymphoma
B cell prolymphocytic leukemia
Lymphoplasmacytic lymphoma
Splenic marginal zone lymphoma
Hairy cell leukemia
Plasma cell myeloma
Monoclonal gammopathy of undetermined significance (MGUS)
Solitary plasmacytoma of bone
Extraosseous plasmacytoma
Primary amyloidosis
Heavy-chain diseases
Extranodal marginal zone B-cell lymphoma of mucosa-associated lymphoid tissue (MALT lymphoma)
Nodal marginal zone B-cell lymphoma
Follicular lymphoma
Mantle cell lymphoma
Mediastinal (thymic) large B-cell lymphoma
Intravascular large B-cell lymphoma
Primary effusion lymphoma
Burkitt lymphoma/leukemia

WHO = World Health Organization.

TABLE 20-16

WHO Histologic Classification of T cell and NK-Cell Neoplasms

Precursor T-cell neoplasm
Precursor T-lymphoblastic leukemia/lymphoma
Mature T-cell neoplasms
Leukemic/disseminated
T cell prolymphocytic leukemia
T cell large granular lymphocytic leukemia
Aggressive NK-cell leukemia
Adult T cell leukemia/lymphoma
Cutaneous
Mycosis fungoides
Sézary syndrome
Primary cutaneous anaplastic lymphoma
Large cell lymphoma
Lymphomatoid papulosis
Other extranodal
Extranodal NK/T-cell lymphoma, nasal type
Enteropathy-type T-cell lymphoma
Hepatosplenic T-cell lymphoma
Subcutaneous panniculitis-like T-cell lymphoma
Nodal
Angioimmunoblastic T-cell lymphoma
Peripheral T-cell lymphoma, unspecified
Anaplastic large cell lymphoma
Neoplasm of uncertain lineage and stage of differentiation
Blastic NK cell lymphoma

NK = natural killer; WHO = World Health Organization.

B-Acute Lymphoblastic Leukemia/Lymphoma (B-ALL/LBL) is a Malignancy of Precursor Lymphocytes

Immature (precursor) B-lymphoblasts are the malignant cells in B-ALL/LBL and represent the most common childhood leukemia. Most precursor B-cell malignancies involve primarily bone marrow and peripheral blood, and are termed **B lymphoblastic leukemia**. However, nodal involvement can occur, in which case the disease is referred to as **B lymphoblastic lymphoma**.

EPIDEMIOLOGY: Most childhood leukemias are acute lymphoblastic leukemias of B-cell type (B-ALL). Some 75% of cases occur in children under the age of 6. Almost all precursor B-cell malignancies are predominantly leukemic. Lymphoblastic lymphoma is uncommon.

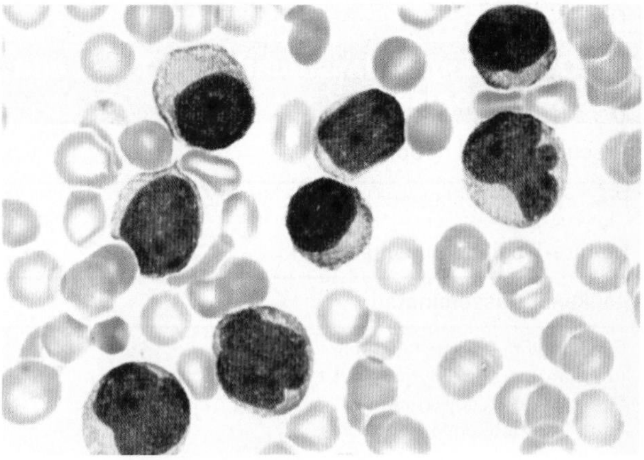

FIGURE 20-54. **Acute lymphoblastic leukemia.** The lymphoblasts in peripheral blood contain irregular and indented nuclei with prominent nucleoli and a moderate amount of cytoplasm.

PATHOLOGY: Malignant lymphoblasts comprise at least 20% of bone marrow cellularity, and are small to medium-sized cells with an increased nuclear-to-cytoplasmic ratio, delicate chromatin and inconspicuous nucleoli (Fig. 20-54). The immunophenotypes of B-ALL reflect different stages of B cell maturation (see Fig. 20-47). The earliest antigens that indicate B cell differentiation are CD10, CD19, and TdT. *B-cell tumors that express cell surface Ig are not considered precursor leukemias.*

Cytogenetic abnormalities are involved. B-ALL features numerical aberrations and chromosomal translocations, including the Philadelphia chromosome. In childhood ALL, a BCR/ABL fusion protein, P190, is produced, in contrast to the *CML* fusion protein (P210) that is seen in half of adult cases of ALL or CML. Progenitor B-ALL may present with t(4;11) involving the *MLL* gene at 11q23. About 25% of childhood pre-B-ALL patients are positive for t(1;19), which involves *PBX/E2A*.

CLINICAL FEATURES: The leukemic cells of B-ALL displace normal marrow elements, resulting in anemia, thrombocytopenia and neutropenia. Organomegaly and central nervous system involvement are common. The rapidly growing tumor cells in the marrow cause bone pain and arthralgias. In general, childhood B-ALL treated with chemotherapy has an excellent prognosis, with complete remission rates of better than 90%. However, very young age (less than 1 year), t(9;22), t(1;19) and t(4;11) are bad prognostic indicators. B-ALL also has a poor prognosis in patients over age 12. All translocations involving the *MLL* gene at 11q23 are associated with a poor prognosis irrespective of age.

Precursor T cells Compose Most Lymphoblastic Lymphomas

Precursor T acute lymphoblastic leukemia (T-ALL) and T lymphoblastic lymphoma (T LBL) are immature T-cell neoplasms. Whether the terms **leukemia** or **lymphoma** apply is often arbitrary, and the considerations are similar to those described for B-ALL.

EPIDEMIOLOGY: Only 15% of childhood ALL originates from T-cells. In adults, the percentage of T-lymphoblastic leukemia is higher. Lymphoblastic lymphoma, a tumor mass consisting of precursor lymphocytes, is 90% of T cell origin.

PATHOLOGY: The morphologic appearance of T lymphoblasts is like that of B lymphoblasts (see Fig. 20-54). Expression of antigens in T-ALL reflects normal T cell differentiation and maturation in the bone marrow and thymus (see Fig. 20-48). The earliest T cell antigen is CD7, followed by CD2 and CD5. During thymic differentiation, T cells become positive for CD1a and cytoplasmic CD3 (cCD3), CD4, and CD8. The immunophenotypes in T-ALL reflect that sequence of antigen expression. As with B-ALL, T-ALL is positive for TdT.

The genes encoding the four T cell receptor chains (α, β, γ, δ chains) often participate in chromosomal translocations with transcription factor genes such as *MYC, TAL1, RBTN1, RBTN2, and HOX11*. Juxtaposition of the T cell receptor loci to one of the transcription partner genes often results in disturbed regulation of transcription.

CLINICAL FEATURES: Blood and bone marrow are most commonly involved in T-ALL. The leukemia frequently infiltrates peripheral lymph nodes, brain, gonads, spleen, and liver. Precursor T cell malignancies that originate from thymic T cells most often present as a mediastinal mass. Like B-ALL, T-ALL has a poor prognosis after childhood.

Mature (Peripheral) B cell Lymphomas Are the Most Common Type in the Western World

Mature B cell malignancies are derived from clonal proliferation of peripheral B cells. As B cells go through multiple steps of differentiation and maturation from naïve B cells to mature plasma cells, lymphomas may arise at every step of the way (see Fig. 20-47).

EPIDEMIOLOGY: The incidence of malignant lymphomas in the United States is 15 per 100,000 annually. B-cell neoplasms by far outnumber T cell malignancies, particularly in the Western world. *The most common B-cell lymphomas are follicular lymphoma (22.1%) and diffuse large cell lymphoma (30.6%)* (Table 20-17). Except for mediastinal B cell and Burkitt lymphoma, most mature B-cell lymphomas occur in the 6th and 7th decades. Peripheral B-cell lymphomas are distinctly uncommon in children with save for Burkitt lymphoma and large cell B-cell lymphoma.

PATHOGENESIS: Most peripheral B-cell lymphomas occur without apparent cause. However, impairment of the immune system and certain infectious agents may give rise to malignant lymphomas (Table 20-18). Immunodeficiency caused by HIV infection and therapeutic immunosuppression in allograft recipients favor development of large B-cell lymphoma or Burkitt lymphoma. Low-grade malignant B-cell lymphomas can develop in patients with certain types of autoimmune disease,. For example, patients with **Sjögren disease** or **Hashimoto thyroiditis** (see Chapter 21) may develop extranodal marginal zone lymphoma (MALT lymphoma). EBV is linked to endemic Burkitt lymphoma and HIV-associated lymphomas. Other viruses that predispose to B cell malignancies include **human herpesvirus 8** (HHV-8) in primary effusion lymphoma and **hepatitis C virus** in lymphoplasmacytic lymphoma associated with type 2 cryoglobulinemia. MALT lymphoma is frequently associated with *Helicobacter pylori* infection of the stomach (see Chapter 13) and often regresses upon antibiotic treatment.

As discussed earlier, lymphomas are currently classified according to their respective normal lymphocytes during development and differentiation (see Fig. 20-47). After the precursor stage, B cells undergo immunoglobulin *VDJ* gene arrangements and mature to surface IgM- and IgD-positive naïve B cells that often express CD5. These cells give rise to **mantle cell lymphoma**. Large activated B cells (**centroblasts**) home to germinal centers where centroblasts mature into smaller cells with cleaved nuclei (**centrocytes**). Centroblasts and centrocytes lack the apoptosis inhibitor BCL-2; they express *BCL6* and *CD10*. **Follicular lymphomas** are derived from germinal center B cells and consist of a mixture of centroblasts and centrocytes. **Burkitt lymphoma** and some large **B-cell lymphomas** are also derived from germinal center lymphocytes.

Late-stage memory B cells reside in the marginal zone, the outermost compartment of the lymph follicle. Variants of **marginal zone lymphomas** include **splenic marginal zone lymphoma** and **MALT lymphomas** of the stomach and other mucosal surfaces. In addition, late-stage memory B cells give rise to **CLL/SLL.** Ultimately, some B cells differentiate into plasma cells. These cells are the only B cells that secrete immunoglobulins, although they lack immunoglobulin expression on the cell surface. Plasma cells home to bone marrow, where they may give rise to **multiple myeloma**.

TABLE 20-17

Frequency of B- and T/NK-Cell Lymphomas

Diagnosis	% of Total Cases
Diffuse large B-cell lymphoma	30.6
Follicular lymphoma	22.1
MALT lymphoma	7.6
Mature T-cell lymphomas (except ALCL)	7.6
Chronic lymphocytic leukemia/small lymphocytic lymphoma	6.7
Mantle cell lymphoma	6.0
Mediastinal large B-cell lymphoma	2.4
Anaplastic large cell lymphoma	2.4
Burkitt lymphoma	2.5
Nodal marginal zone lymphoma	1.8
Precursor T-lymphoblastic lymphoma	1.7
Lymphoplasmacytic lymphoma	1.2
Other types	7.4

ALCL = anaplastic large cell lymphoma; MALT = mucosa-associated lymphoid tissue; NK = natural killer.

TABLE 20-18

Disorders with Increased Risk of Secondary Malignant Lymphoma

Sjögren syndrome
Hashimoto thyroiditis
Renal and cardiac transplant recipients
Acquired immunodeficiency syndrome (AIDS)
EBV infection
HHV-8 infection
Helicobacter pylori-positive gastritis
Hepatitis C
Congenital immune deficiency syndromes Chediak-Higashi Wiskott-Aldrich Ataxia telangiectasia IgA deficiency Severe combined immune deficiency
α Heavy-chain disease
Celiac disease
Hodgkin lymphoma (post-treatment)

EBV = Epstein-Barr virus; HHV = human herpesvirus; Ig = immunoglobulin

CLINICAL FEATURES: Indolent lymphomas are distinguished from **aggressive** B-cell lymphomas. Typical indolent lymphomas are B-CLL and follicular lymphoma; aggressive B-cell lymphomas tend to be large B-cell lymphoma and Burkitt lymphoma. Ironically, although indolent lymphomas follow a prolonged clinical course, they are usually incurable. By contrast, aggressive lymphomas progress rapidly, but many of them are curable. Not all malignant lymphomas fall unequivocally into either category. MALT lymphomas, for example, are indolent lymphomas that can sometimes be cured by local irradiation or antibiotic treatment in some cases of gastric MALT lymphoma.

Our discussion of B-cell lymphomas follows the development of B cells outlined in Figure. 20-47.

Mantle Cell Lymphoma

Mantle cell lymphoma is a B-cell neoplasm of small to medium-sized lymphocytes with irregular nuclear features.

EPIDEMIOLOGY: Mantle cell lymphomas constitute fewer than 10% of malignant lymphomas. They do not occur in children, but affect older persons, with a median age of 60 years. Men are more likely to be affected than women.

PATHOLOGY: Small to medium-sized lymphocytes with irregular nuclear features diffusely infiltrate lymph nodes. In one variant, an expanded (malignant) follicular mantle is wrapped around (benign) germinal centers (**mantle zone lymphoma**). In another, more aggressive variant, the tumor cells appear larger and more immature (**blastoid mantle cell lymphoma**). The spleen, bone marrow, and gastrointestinal tract may be involved. In the gastrointestinal tract, mantle cell lymphoma produces nodular alterations of the mucosal surface, termed **lymphomatous polyposis**.

Mantle cell lymphoma has a B cell immunophenotype and the tumor cells express CD5 but are negative for CD23 and CD10. Tumor cells express nuclear BCL-1 protein and cyclin D1 (Fig. 20-55).

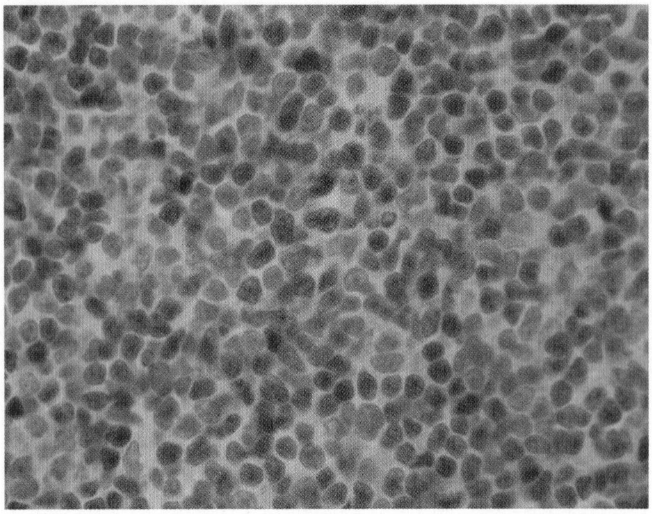

FIGURE 20-55. **Mantle cell lymphoma.** A nuclear stain for BCL-1 is positive.

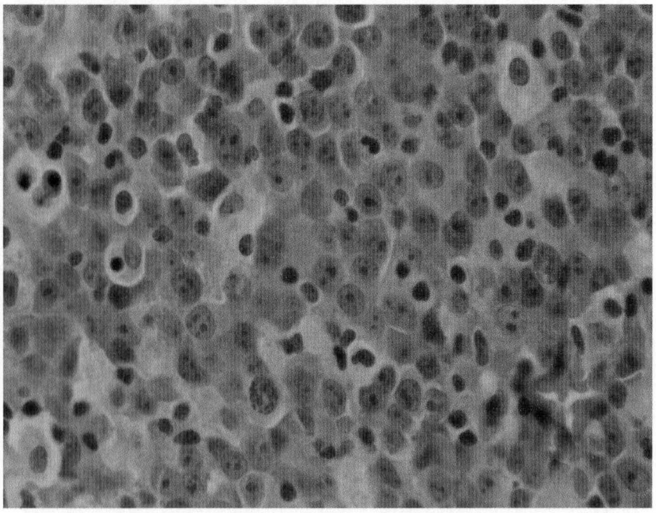

FIGURE 20-56. **Diffuse large B-cell lymphoma.** Tumor cells show prominent nucleoli.

Variable-region genes are normally not mutated, indicating derivation from a pre-germinal center B cell. The most important cytogenetic abnormality is t(11:14)(q13:q32), which involves the *cyclin D1 (BCL-1, PRAD1)* gene on chromosome 11 and the *IgH* gene on chromosome 14. Cyclin D1 exerts cell cycle control at the transition from G1 to S by complexing with Cdk 4/6. This event results in phosphorylation of Rb and subsequent activation of transcription factors (see Chapter 5). In many cases, abnormalities of the *ATM* (ataxia telangiectasia mutated) gene have been described.

CLINICAL FEATURES: Mantle cell lymphoma progresses relentlessly and half of patients do not survive 3 years.

Diffuse Large B-cell lymphoma

Diffuse large B-cell lymphoma (DLBCL) are a heterogeneous group of aggressive, potentially curable B-cell neoplasms. The disease occurs in all age groups but is most prevalent between the ages of 60 and 70 years. The cause of DLBCL is unknown, but it may be seen in association with EBV and HIV infections.

PATHOLOGY: DLBCL may involve lymph nodes or extranodal sites. The tumor cells resemble **immunoblasts** or **centroblasts** (Fig. 20-56) or appear as anaplastic bizarre cells with marked nuclear irregularities. Immunoblasts are large B cells (see Fig. 20-47) whose nuclei exhibit prominent central nucleoli.

The tumor cells of DLBCL express various B cell antigens. As in FL, clonal *BCL2* gene rearrangements are often seen, indicating a potential germinal center origin in some cases. DLBCL associated with immunodeficiency is usually positive for EBV.

CLINICAL FEATURES: Rapidly evolving, multifocal, nodal and extranodal tumor manifestations are typically seen at the time of presentation. DLBCL is potentially curable, but a high proliferation rate indicates an adverse prognosis.

Burkitt Lymphoma

Burkitt lymphoma (BL), one of the most rapidly growing malignancies, is defined by a chromosomal translocation involving 8q24, which harbors the *MYC* oncogene (see Chapter 5).

EPIDEMIOLOGY: Endemic BL is the most common childhood malignancy in Central Africa, with peak incidence at ages 3 to 7. **Sporadic BL** affects mainly children and young adults in the Western world, where it accounts for 1 to 2% of all lymphomas. As in endemic BL, males are more often affected than females. **Immunodeficiency-associated BL** mainly occurs in HIV-infected persons.

PATHOGENESIS: EBV is present in virtually all cases of endemic BL, but is seen in less than 30% of sporadic types. EBV-positive sporadic BL is associated with low socioeconomic status. Many patients experience a prodromal stage of polyclonal B cell activation caused by bacterial, viral, or parasitic infections (malaria) (see Chapter 5).

PATHOLOGY: BL typically produces extranodal tumors rather than lymphadenopathy. All types of this lymphoma have a high risk for central nervous system involvement. The classic presentation for endemic BL is a destructive tumor in the jaws or other facial bones (Fig. 20-57A). Patients with sporadic BL typically present with abdominal masses. All types may involve ovaries, kidneys, and breast. Patients with sizable bulky tumors sometimes present with Burkitt leukemia and extensive bone marrow involvement.

Microscopically, BL cells are medium-sized and lack significant cytologic atypia. Tissue sections reveal a high number of mitotic figures, which attests to the extremely high proliferation rate in this tumor. The cellular debris of apoptotic tumor cells is cleared by macrophages, whose scattered appearance is termed "starry sky macrophage" (see Fig. 20-57B). Aspirate smears stained with Wright-Giemsa demonstrate numerous lipid vacuoles in the deeply basophilic cytoplasm of the tumor cells.

Burkitt cells express surface IgM and are positive for common B cell antigens (CD19, CD20, CD22). They mark for CD10 and BCL-6 and are thus thought to be of germinal center origin.

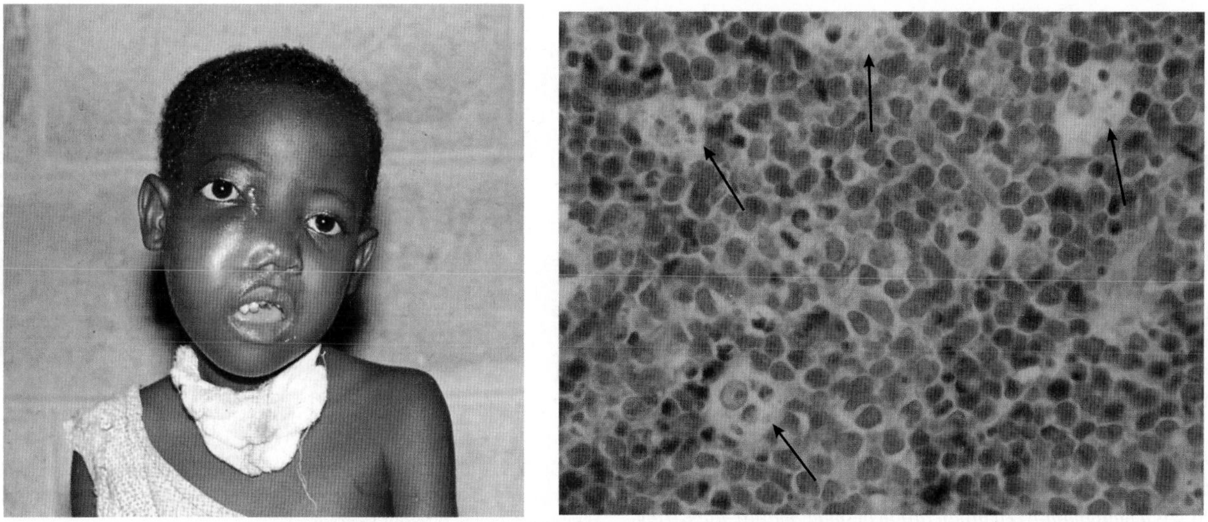

A B

FIGURE 20-57. **Burkitt lymphoma. A.** A tumor of the jaw distorts the child's face. **B.** Lymph node is effaced by neoplastic lymphocytes with several starry sky macrophages (*arrows*).

Clonal *IgH* gene arrangement can be shown for heavy- and light-chain genes. Heavy-chain genes and *MYC* genes participate in t(8;14). In endemic cases, the breakpoint on chromosome 14 occurs in the heavy chain joining region, as seen in early B cells. In sporadic BL, the translocation occurs in the Ig switch region, which is more characteristic of mature B lymphocytes. In these cases, expression of *MYC* gene driven by the Ig heavy-chain promoter leads to uncontrolled tumor cell growth (see Chapter 5).

CLINICAL FEATURES: Most patients present with bulky extranodal tumors that emerge in a short time and respond to aggressive chemotherapy. Both endemic and sporadic BL are curable in up to 90% of patients.

Follicular Lymphoma

Follicular lymphoma (FL) is the malignant counterpart of lymphocytes derived from follicle centers. Follicle (germinal) centers consist of large round cells (centroblasts) and smaller cells with irregular or cleaved nuclei (centrocytes). *Unlike any other type of lymphoma, FL mimics an entire functional unit of lymphocytes, including their ancillary cells. The opposite of FL is diffuse lymphoma.*

EPIDEMIOLOGY: FL is a particularly common neoplasm in the United States, where it constitutes 35% of all adult malignant lymphomas. The disease shows a peak incidence at 60 years of age and is somewhat more common in women than in men.

PATHOLOGY: FL (Fig. 20-58) predominantly involves lymph nodes and resembles benign follicular hyperplasia. However, FL is distinguished from the latter by extracapsular invasion into perinodal fat, among other considerations. FL may transform into a more aggressive diffuse lymphoma consisting of a mixture of centroblasts and centrocytes. Depending on the percentage of centroblasts, FL is divided into three grades. The more centroblasts present, the higher the grade.

FL usually displays surface Ig and is light-chain restricted. The tumor cells are positive for most B cell antigens and CD10 but negative for CD5. *In contrast to benign germinal center B lymphocytes, FL expresses BCL-2 protein* (Fig. 20-59).

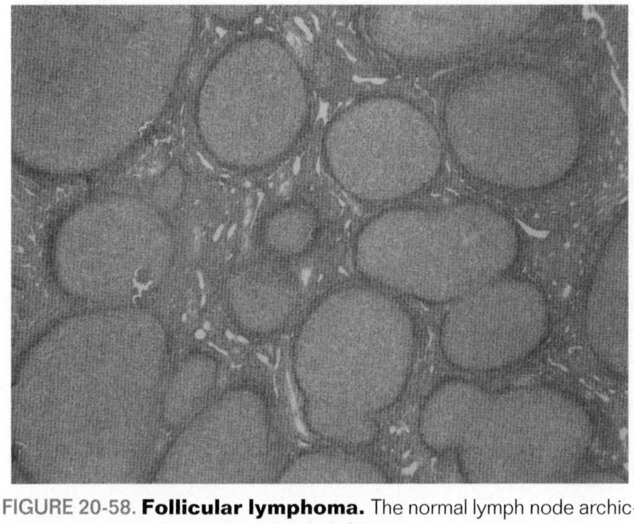

FIGURE 20-58. **Follicular lymphoma.** The normal lymph node architecture is replaced by malignant lymph follicles.

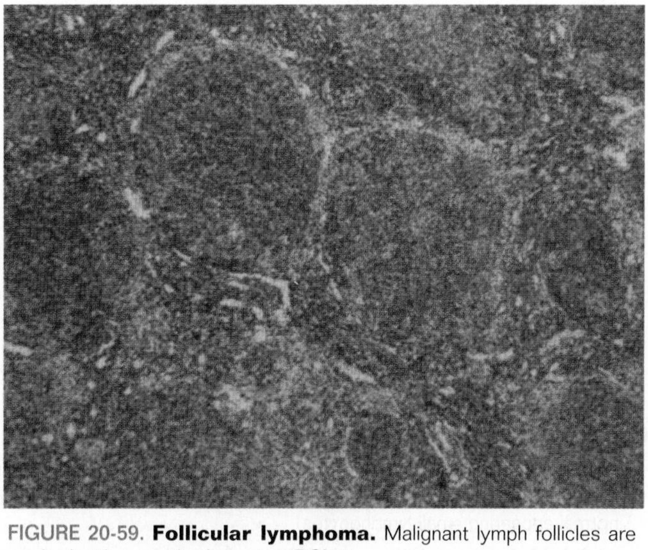

FIGURE 20-59. **Follicular lymphoma.** Malignant lymph follicles are marked with an antibody against BCL-2 .

The most common cytogenetic translocation is t(14:18)(q32:q21), with *IgH* and *BCL-2* as partner genes. BCL-2 protein is an apoptosis inhibitor located in the mitochondrial membrane. Clonal rearrangement of the *BCL-6* oncogene is common.

CLINICAL FEATURES: FL predominantly affects lymph nodes. Other sites of involvement include spleen, bone marrow, peripheral blood, head and neck region, gastrointestinal tract, soft tissue, and skin. Most patients have advanced disease at presentation. Low-grade FL is indolent, but usually incurable, whereas grade 3 FL is more aggressive but is potentially curable. The prognosis worsens with the number of genetic abnormalities. One third of patients progress to (diffuse) large B-cell lymphoma.

Chronic Lymphocytic Leukemia/Small Lymphocytic Lymphoma

CLL/SLL is a malignant B cell proliferation of small, mature-appearing, lymphocytes and a variable number of larger cells (prolymphocytes and paraimmunoblasts). A diagnosis of CLL is made if bone marrow and peripheral blood are primarily involved. If tumor cells predominantly give rise to lymphadenopathy or solid tumor masses, the term **small lymphocytic lymphoma** is more appropriate.

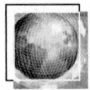

EPIDEMIOLOGY: CLL/SLL is a typical indolent malignant lymphoma of the elderly (median age 65) and accounts for 7% of malignant lymphomas.

PATHOLOGY: Lymph nodes infiltrated by CLL show complete effacement of architecture by small lymphocytes (Fig. 20-60). In the spleen, the white pulp is expanded, although tumor cells may also extend into the red pulp. Bone marrow involvement ranges from complete effacement of the marrow space to more patchy distribution. In peripheral blood smears (Fig. 20-61), some leukemic lymphocytes are destroyed and show ill-defined nuclear remnants ("smudge" cells). A variable number of larger cells with prominent nucleoli (prolymphocytes) can be seen. An increasing number of prolymphocytes may indicate a more aggressive course. Transformation of CLL/SLL into diffuse large cell lymphoma is labeled **Richter syndrome**, which is characterized by sheets of large lymphocytes (centroblasts or immunoblasts).

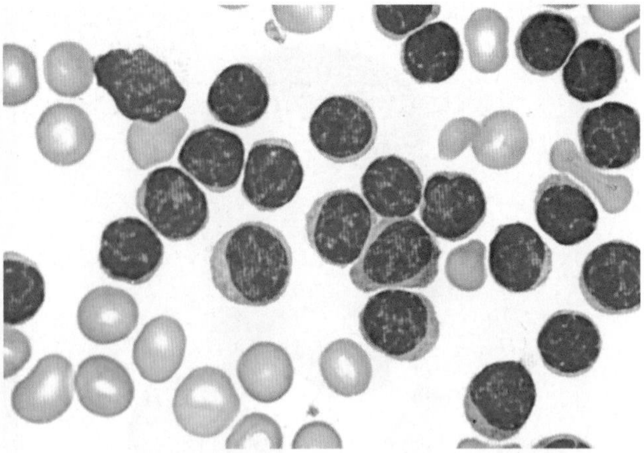

FIGURE 20-61. **Chronic lymphocytic leukemia.** A smear of peripheral blood exhibits numerous small-to-medium sized lymphocytes. A smudge cell is present (*arrow*).

SLL/CLL features a mature B cell population that expresses CD19, CD20, CD22, and CD79. Half of cases of B-CLL have not undergone somatic mutations in variable-region genes and thus reflect the genotype of naïve B cells. The other half have undergone *VH* gene mutations and resemble post-germinal center B cells.

CLINICAL FEATURES: The diagnosis of CLL is established by demonstrating a sustained peripheral blood lymphocytosis, generally more than 15,000/μL and a bone marrow lymphocytosis exceeding 40% of marrow cells. If the blood lymphocyte count is between 5,000 and 15,000/μL, a finding of monoclonality (light-chain restriction or clonal rearrangement of a light-chain gene) confirms the diagnosis of B-CLL.

The erythrocyte and platelet counts are initially normal, but with advanced disease, severe anemia, thrombocytopenia and neutropenia develop. A positive Coombs test is observed at some time in up to 20% of cases.

Immunologic deficiencies, mainly of B cells but also of T cells, are common. The cause of B cell dysfunction is not known, but hypogammaglobulinemia occurs in 50% to 75% of cases at

A

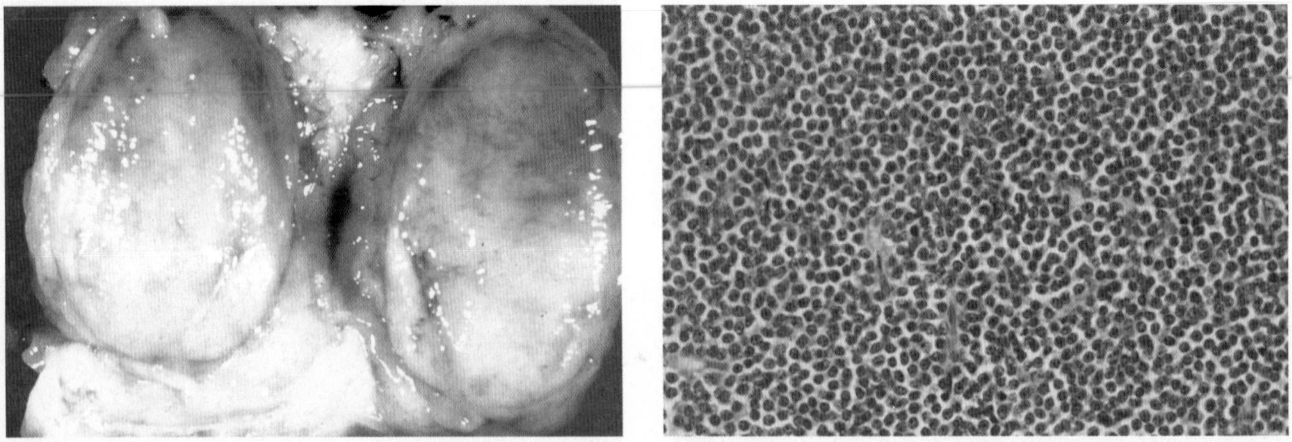

B

FIGURE 20-60. **Small lymphocytic lymphoma/leukemia. A.** A bisected, enlarged lymph node shows the characteristic uniform, glistening, gray color that imparts a fish-flesh appearance. **B.** On microscopic examination, the lymph nodal architecture is replaced by a diffuse infiltration of normal-appearing small lymphocytes.

some time in the disease. The degree of hypogammaglobulinemia generally correlates with disease stage and is responsible for infectious complications. Patients with B-CLL also have increased peripheral blood T cells (>3,000/μL). There is an increase in CD8+ T cells and a corresponding decrease in CD4+ cells, with a resulting decrease in the CD4+/CD8+ cell ratio. The T cells often show impaired delayed-type hypersensitivity in vitro, which also contributes to the increased risk of infection.

The overall mean survival in B-CLL is 6 years. Initially, most patients with B-CLL are asymptomatic and the diagnosis is suggested by finding lymphadenopathy and splenomegaly in a routine physical examination or lymphocytosis on a blood cell count. The subsequent clinical course is highly variable. In some cases, the disease progresses rapidly and patients die within 2 to 3 years. Other patients remain asymptomatic for 10 to 20 years. The most common complications are bacterial infections and, less frequently, fungal and viral ones. Coombs-positive, autoimmune hemolytic anemia, and hemorrhagic episodes secondary to thrombocytopenia are often observed.

Conversion to prolymphocytic leukemia occurs in 10% of cases of B-CLL and is characterized by a marked elevation in the blood lymphocyte count, 15% to 50% prolymphocytes, and increasing splenomegaly. Prolymphocytic conversion indicates a more aggressive clinical course, and a mean survival of less than 2 years.

Richter syndrome, a large cell lymphoma, is superimposed in 5% of cases of B-CLL. Patients with this complication present with a rapid onset of fever, abdominal pain and progressive lymphadenopathy and hepatosplenomegaly. Prominent enlargement of retroperitoneal lymph nodes and neoplastic involvement of the gastrointestinal tract are common. Richter syndrome is aggressive and refractory to therapy, with a mean survival of 2 months.

Asymptomatic patients with B-CLL who have stable lymphocyte counts are ordinarily not treated. More-advanced disease is treated with chemotherapeutic agents and antilymphocyte antibody. Splenectomy or splenic irradiation may be needed to manage refractory hypersplenism.

Extranodal Marginal-Zone B-cell lymphoma of Mucosa-Associated Lymphoid Tissue

MALT lymphomas are indolent, malignant T lymphocyte proliferations of small to medium-sized lymphocytes, with frequent monocytoid features and variable admixtures of plasma cells. The malignant T cells appear to originate from marginal-zone B cells.

EPIDEMIOLOGY: MALT lymphomas constitute 5% to 10% of all B-cell lymphomas, with a mean incidence at age 60 years. *Most primary gastric lymphomas are MALT lymphomas.*

PATHOGENESIS: MALT lymphomas occur either in glandular organs or along mucosal surfaces. They commonly arise in the context of chronic inflammatory processes or autoimmune disease. The prototypical infection-driven MALT lymphoma is gastric lymphoma associated with *H. pylori* gastritis. Examples of MALT lymphomas in autoimmune diseases include salivary gland lymphoma in Sjögren syndrome and thyroid lymphoma associated with Hashimoto thyroiditis.

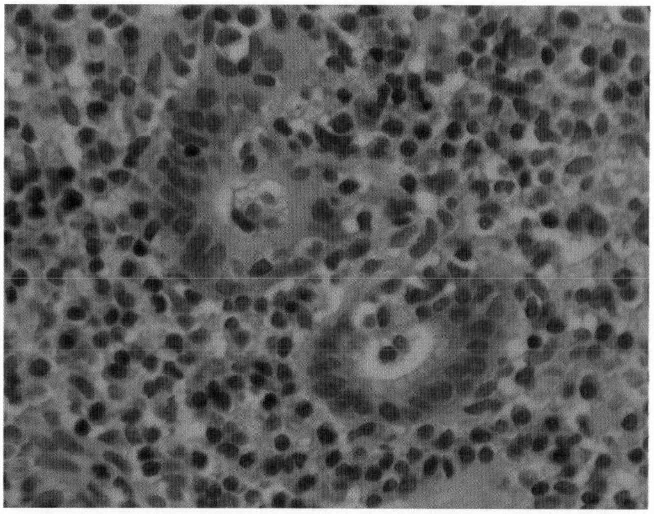

FIGURE 20-62. **Mucosa-associated lymphoid tissue (MALT) lymphoma.** Lymphoepithelial lesions of the stomach are present.

PATHOLOGY: Early-stage MALT lymphomas present microscopically with expanded marginal zone lymphocytes around reactive B cell follicles. The spectrum of malignant T lymphocytes ranges from small lymphocytes to medium-sized, monocytoid lymphocytes with more abundant cytoplasm, and a variable admixture of clonal plasma cells. The tumor cells invade glandular epithelium or epithelia of mucosal surfaces, where they form **lymphoepithelial lesions** (Fig. 20-62). Immunoproliferative small intestinal disease, also termed **α-chain disease** or **Mediterranean lymphoma**, is a subtype of MALT lymphoma that produces α heavy chains. Occasionally, transformation of (indolent) MALT lymphoma into large cell B-cell lymphoma occurs.

There is no specific immunophenotype of MALT lymphoma. Most tumor cells express IgM and show light chain restriction. MALT lymphomas express B cell-associated antigens and are negative for CD5 and CD23, which distinguishes them from B-CLL/SLL and mantle cell lymphoma. They are also negative for CD10, which differentiates them from follicular lymphoma.

MALT lymphoma typically shows somatic mutation of variable region genes and is believed to derive from memory B cells. The most common cytogenetic abnormalities are trisomy 3 and t(11:18), the latter involving the apoptosis inhibitor gene *API2* and a novel gene termed *MLT*. In cases with subtle lymphocytic infiltrates in the gastric mucosa, demonstration of clonal *IgH* gene rearrangement helps to establish the diagnosis.

CLINICAL FEATURES: Most MALT lymphomas involve the stomach or other mucosal sites, including the respiratory tract. They may also be seen in the head and neck region, ocular adnexal sites, skin, thyroid, and breast. MALT lymphomas remain localized for prolonged periods and tend to follow an indolent clinical course. MALT lymphomas involving the parotid are sensitive to radiation therapy; gastric MALT lymphomas secondary to *H. pylori* infection respond to antibiotic therapy.

Lymphoplasmacytic Lymphoma/Waldenström Macroglobulinemia

Lymphoplasmacytic lymphoma (LPL)/Waldenström disease is a neoplastic proliferation of small lymphocytes and a variable number of

IgM-secreting plasma cells of the same malignant clone. Waldenström disease is not a variant of multiple myeloma, but rather an indolent malignant lymphoma that mainly affects the elderly.

PATHOLOGY: Waldenström disease, or LPL, primarily involves the bone marrow, but can also be seen in lymph nodes, spleen and peripheral blood. In lymph nodes, LPL shows an interfollicular lymphocytic infiltrate with plasma cells. The leukemic bone marrow infiltrates are similar to those in CLL, although there may be more plasma cells. Transformation from LPL into a large cell lymphoma may occur.

LPL expresses common B cell antigens and CD5 and CD23 are negative. The most common translocation is t(9;14). As in other lymphomas with plasma cell differentiation, rearrangement of the *PAX-5* gene, which encodes B cell-specific activator protein (BSAP), is common.

CLINICAL FEATURES: Eighty percent of patients present with a monoclonal IgM spike on serum electrophoresis (>3 g/dL). Many of their clinical symptoms result from hyperviscosity. Sludging and rouleaux formation of RBCs in the microvascular system may lead to visual disturbances and stroke. Complications of hyperviscosity are treated with plasmapheresis. Excess serum IgM may bind to clotting factors, platelets, and fibrin and so cause a coagulopathy. The clinical outcome of the disease is comparable to that of other indolent lymphomas such as B-CLL.

Plasma Cell Neoplasia

Plasma cell neoplasia is a group of related malignant disorders of terminally differentiated B lymphocytes (plasma cells).

- **Plasma cell myeloma or multiple myeloma** (90% of cases) is characterized by bone marrow multifocal infiltration by malignant plasma cells. There are typically multiple destructive (lytic) lesions or diffuse demineralization of bone.
- **Solitary osseous myeloma** (5% of cases) is a single destructive lesion of bone.
- **Extramedullary plasmacytoma** (5% of cases) presents as a soft tissue mass, most frequently in the upper respiratory tract.

In most cases of plasma cell neoplasia, the tumor cells secrete a homogeneous, complete or partial, immunoglobulin molecule, an **M-component** or **paraprotein**. Based on the type of M-component, multiple myeloma can be divided into several types:

- **IgG, IgA, IgD, IgE, and IgM types**
- **Light-chain disease,** in which only κ or λ light chains are synthesized
- **Biclonal multiple myeloma,** with two distinct M-components (rare)
- **Nonsecretory myeloma,** displaying no secreted M-component (1%)

EPIDEMIOLOGY: Plasma cell neoplasia comprises 10% of all hematologic malignancies. About 7500 cases are reported annually in the United States, for an overall incidence of 3 per 100,000 population. The disorder is more than twice as common in blacks (8 per 100,000 population) than in whites. The frequency of plasma cell neoplasia increases with age, the mean age at diagnosis of multiple myeloma being 65 years and that of solitary osseous myeloma and extramedullary plasmacytoma a decade earlier. Plasma cell neoplasia is distinctly uncommon before age 40. There is a slight male predominance, the male-to-female ratio being 1.5:1.

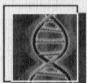

PATHOGENESIS: Several risk factors for plasma cell neoplasia have been identified.

- A **genetic predisposition** is suggested by an increased incidence of multiple myeloma in first-degree relatives of patients with plasma cell neoplasia and the higher frequency of multiple myeloma in blacks.
- **Ionizing radiation** has been incriminated in the etiology of plasma cell neoplasia. Long-term survivors of the bombing of Hiroshima and Nagasaki had a 5-fold increased incidence of multiple myeloma.
- **Chronic antigenic stimulation** may constitute a risk factor. Some cases of multiple myeloma have been associated with chronic infections, such as HIV and chronic osteomyelitis and with chronic inflammatory disorders (e.g., rheumatoid arthritis). A two-hit hypothesis is proposed by which (1) antigenic stimulation leads to reactive, polyclonal proliferation of B lymphocytes; and (2) a subsequent mutagenic event establishes a single malignant clone.

PATHOLOGY: On gross examination, the osseous and extraosseous plasma cell tumors are variably red, tan, or gray and have a consistency that ranges from fleshy to gelatinous (Fig. 20-63). The bony lesions are well demarcated from the surrounding normal tissue. The cortical bone may be destroyed, with direct tumor extension into surrounding soft tissues. In multiple myeloma, moderate enlargement of the lymph nodes, spleen, and liver is occasionally observed, although the gross appearance of these organs is not distinctive. The kidneys are often contracted in size.

- **Bone marrow:** The microscopic hallmark of multiple myeloma in bone marrow is diffuse sheets or nodular aggregates of plasma cells. Ultimately, normal hematopoietic tissues and fat cells are replaced by neoplastic plasma cells. In marrow aspirates, neoplastic plasma cells usually exceed 30% of all cells. The malignant cells may appear normal, but more often they show atypical features including: (1) prominent nucleoli; (2) irregular chromatin distribution; (3) binucleation and bizarre multinucleation; and (4) nuclear–cytoplasmic asynchrony, with immature nuclei and mature cytoplasm (Fig. 20-64). Plasmablasts–with large central nuclei, finely dispersed chromatin, prominent nucleoli, and scant blue cytoplasm–may be seen and in some cases are the predominant cell type.
- Cytoplasmic and nuclear inclusions, representing immunoglobulin accumulation, may be observed in neoplastic plasma cells. **Russell bodies** are globular, eosinophilic, refractile, cytoplasmic inclusions and **Dutcher bodies** are similar nuclear invaginations. Precipitates of crystalline immunoglobulin may also be observed in the cytoplasm.

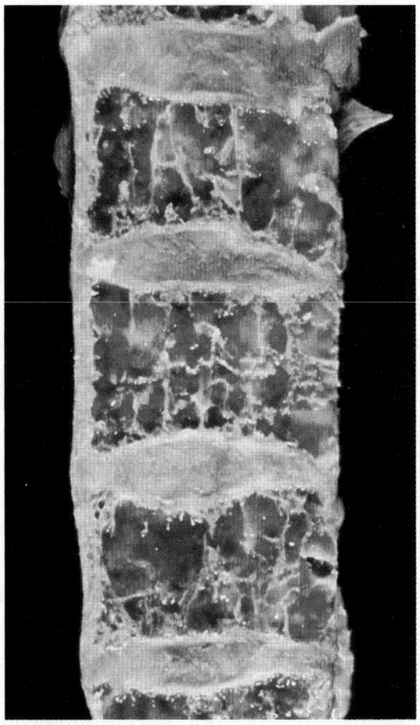

FIGURE 20-63. **Multiple myeloma.** Multiple lytic bone lesions are present in the vertebra.

- **Kidneys:** Renal abnormalities is seen in over half of cases (see Chapter 16).
- **Light-chain cast nephropathy** is a characteristic finding and is due to precipitation in the distal convoluted and collecting tubules of finely granular or lamellar protein casts made of light chains and other proteins (see Chapter 16). Secondary injury to tubules by the protein casts leads to tubular epithelial cell atrophy or hyperplasia, with formation of epithelial cell syncytia. Destruction of tubular basement membranes induces renal tubulointerstitial inflammation and secondary interstitial fibrosis.
- **Glomerulopathy** is a consequence of diffuse deposition of M-component in renal glomeruli, tubular basement membranes, and vasculature. The glomerulopathy is characterized by proliferation of mesangial cells and increased mesangial matrix. Additionally, there may be damage to both renal tubules and blood vessels.

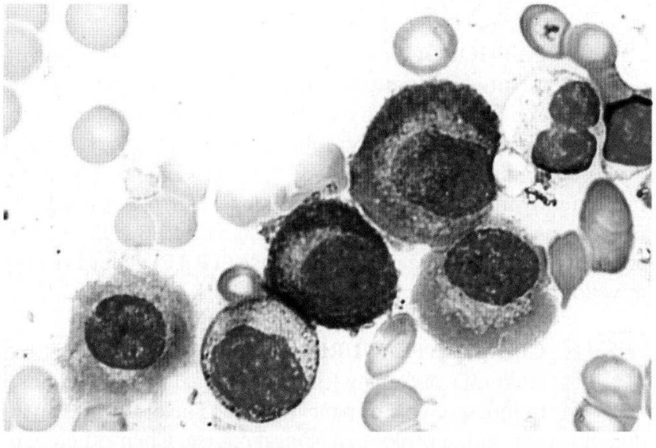

FIGURE 20-64. **Multiple myeloma.** A smear of a bone marrow aspirate shows a cluster of three neoplastic plasma cells.

- **Additional renal findings** in multiple myeloma include deposition of (1) amyloid in glomeruli and blood vessels, (2) calcium (nephrocalcinosis), and (3) uric acid crystals (urate nephropathy). Acute and chronic pyelonephritis may be seen. Focal or (rarely) massive tumor cell infiltration may be seen in the interstitium.
- **Lymph nodes:** Lymph nodes may be infiltrated by neoplastic plasma cells, initially in the B cell-dependent medullary cords. This process may progress to a total obliteration of the normal nodal architecture.
- **Spleen and liver:** The spleen shows variable infiltration of the red pulp cords and sinuses. In the liver, the portal triads may contain plasma cells, and in the case of a leukemic distribution, they are identified in the hepatic sinusoids.
- **Immunophenotypes:** In most cases the monoclonal paraprotein is IgG or IgA. Rarely, IgD or IgE is secreted. In 85% of cases, complete immunoglobulin is secreted, but in 15%, only light chains are produced (**light chain disease**). Except for CD79A, many cell surface antigens characteristic of mature B cells are absent in plasma cells.
- **Genotypes:** Clonal rearrangement for IgH can be shown by molecular studies. Numerous chromosomal abnormalities are associated with multiple myeloma, including monosomy or partial deletion of chromosome 13 in 25% of cases. As in mantle cell lymphoma, t(11;14) gene rearrangement of the *BCL-1* gene locus may occur. Similar to other clonal plasma cell proliferations, *PAX-5* abnormalities on chromosome 9 have been described. Deletions of 30q14 and 17p13 (loss of *p53*) are associated with a poorer prognosis.

CLINICAL FEATURES: Lytic lesions of the skull and other flat bones, including the spine and ribs, are characteristic (but not diagnostic) radiographic findings.

The most important disorder to consider in the differential diagnosis of multiple myeloma is the more common **monoclonal gammopathy of unknown significance (MGUS)** (Fig. 20-65), or **benign essential gammopathy.** The former term is preferred as the disorder is not necessarily benign. Of patients with MGUS, about 2% per year progress to a B-cell neoplasm (lymphoplasmacytic disorder or multiple myeloma). The strong link between MGUS and multiple myeloma suggests that a first oncogenic event produces MGUS and a second event results in multiple myeloma.

Common initial laboratory findings in multiple myeloma include normocytic, normochromic anemia, hypercalcemia, and hyperuricemia. A sharp peak or spike representing the M-component is observed with serum or urine protein electrophoresis. Immunochemistry using antibodies against Ig heavy and light chain allows better characterization of the abnormal protein. The erythrocyte sedimentation rate is elevated, owing to the M-component. On peripheral blood smears, erythrocytes may appear stacked and clumped (rouleaux formation), which is also due to the M-component.

The type of M-component determines the course of the disease and its prognosis.

- **IgG myeloma** is "typical" myeloma. Mean survival is 3 to 4 years. Infectious complications are common.
- **IgA myeloma** causes serum hyperviscosity because IgA tends to form dimers.
- **IgD myeloma** is an aggressive clinical disorder that tends to occur in middle-aged men. Mean survival is 1 year.

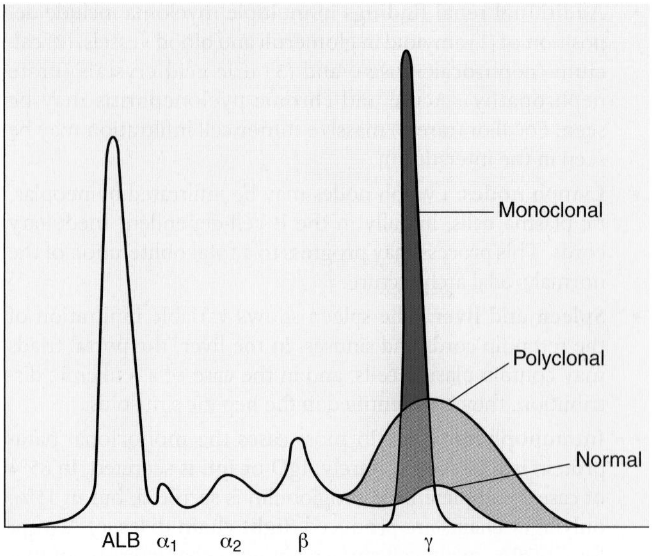

FIGURE 20-65. **Abnormal serum protein electrophoretic patterns contrasted with a normal pattern.** Polyclonal hypergammaglobulinemia, characteristic of benign reactive processes, shows a broad-based increase in immunoglobulins, owing to immunoglobulin secretion by a myriad of reactive plasma cells. Monoclonal gammopathy of unknown significance (MGUS) or plasma cell neoplasia shows a narrow peak, or spike, owing to the homogeneity of the immunoglobulin molecules secreted by a single clone of aberrant plasma cells. ALB = albumin.

- **IgE myeloma** is an uncommon and aggressive clinical disorder that also tends to occur in young adult men.
- **Light-chain disease** is an aggressive variant in which only κ or λ light chains are made. κ chain disease is twice as common as λ chain disease, reflecting the normal ratio of κ and λ light chains in plasma cells. The serum protein pattern is normal until secondary renal disease prevents glomerular filtration of light chains.

Multiple myeloma typically presents with bone pain, mostly involving vertebrae and ribs. Symptoms of anemia, hypercalcemia, and renal insufficiency are common. Amyloidosis of light-chain origin (principally λ) occurs in 15% of cases, and hyperviscosity syndrome is seen in less than 5%. There is a "primary" distribution of amyloid, with deposition in such sites as the tongue, gastrointestinal tract, and heart.

Bone destruction in multiple myeloma is due to both progressive tumor growth and secretion of osteoclast-activating factor by malignant plasma cells. Osteoclasts may also be activated by IL-6, whose activity is increased in patients with multiple myeloma. Common complications of bone destruction include vertebral collapse and pathologic fractures of long bones. Additionally, calcium released from the injured bone may precipitate in the kidneys and cause renal damage (nephrocalcinosis).

The hyperviscosity syndrome (see macroglobulinemia) is particularly common in IgG and IgA myelomas, but far less than in macroglobulinemia. Neurologic abnormalities and spontaneous bleeding episodes are observed.

Some M-components are cryoglobulins, i.e., proteins that precipitate in the cold. As a result, blood flow to distal extremities may be impaired, leading to acrocyanosis and Raynaud phenomenon.

Coagulation abnormalities are caused by (1) complexes between M-components and coagulation factors, (2) coprecipitation of M-component cryoglobulins with coagulation complexes, and (3) coating of platelets by the M-component.

Monoclonal light chains are present in the urine (Bence-Jones protein) in up to 75% of cases of multiple myeloma and in a minority of solitary osseous myelomas and extramedullary plasmacytomas. The neoplastic clone of plasma cells may secrete excess light chains, owing to unbalanced synthesis of heavy and light chains. The light chains are rapidly filtered through by glomeruli and appear in the urine as Bence-Jones protein.

Humoral immune deficiency, with decreased levels of normal serum Ig, is characteristic of multiple myeloma. This defect is due to (1) suppression of normal B lymphocytes by the neoplastic clone and (2) increased catabolism of normal IgG. Consequently, patients with multiple myeloma are susceptible to a variety of infectious complications, particularly pneumonia and pyelonephritis.

Multiple myeloma is an incurable disease, with a mean survival of 6 months in untreated patients and 3 years with chemotherapy. The clinical course tends to be biphasic. An initial chronic stable stage is followed by an aggressive or accelerated preterminal phase. Death is usually due to infection or renal failure. The disease may be complicated by superimposed MDS or AML, usually attributed to the leukemogenic effects of alkylating agent therapy. After treatment, the risk of AML occurring in 5 years is 14% and in 10 years, 20%.

Solitary osseous myeloma presents as a single lytic skeletal lesion, most commonly involving the ribs, vertebrae, or pelvic bones. The natural history of solitary osseous myeloma is progression to multiple myeloma (70%), local extension or recurrence (15%), or extension to a distant skeletal site (15%). Overall 10-year survival is 20%. Solitary osseous myeloma is treated with irradiation.

Extramedullary plasmacytomas occur in the upper respiratory tract in 80% of cases, including nasal sinuses, nasopharynx, and tonsils. The rest occur in other soft tissue sites, such as lungs, breast, and lymph nodes. Extramedullary plasmacytoma is eradicated by surgery or local irradiation. In 20% of cases progression to multiple myeloma occurs.

Hairy Cell Leukemia

Hairy cell leukemia is a clonal B cell proliferation of small to medium-sized lymphocytes with abundant cytoplasm and hairlike cell membrane protrusions. The malignant cell is postulated to arise from a post-germinal center stage peripheral B cell. Hairy cell leukemia is rare and affects mainly middle-aged to elderly men, with a male-to-female ratio of 5:1.

PATHOLOGY: Hairy cell leukemia exhibits subtle interstitial infiltrates that do not disturb normal marrow architecture. Hairy cells have more-abundant cytoplasm than normal small lymphocytes, which lends them a "fried egg" appearance (Fig. 20-66). Both liver and spleen are prominently involved. *The normal cellular counterpart of hairy cells is not known.* These cells express all established B cell antigens and **tartrate-resistant acid phosphatase (TRAP).** They are negative for CD5, CD10, and CD23.

CLINICAL FEATURES: Most patients with hairy cell leukemia present with splenomegaly and peripheral monocytopenia or pancytopenia. The disorder is an indolent tumor with a prolonged clinical course. Chemotherapeutic drugs that specifically target low-grade malignant lymphomas,

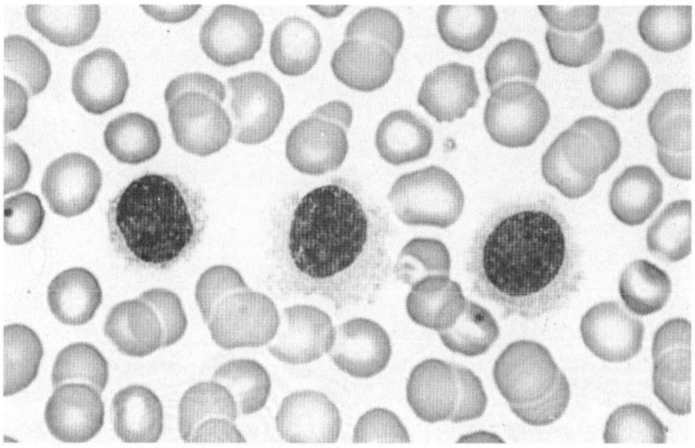

FIGURE 20-66. **Hairy cell leukemia.** Hairy cells with fine, irregular cytoplasmic projections are seen in the peripheral blood.

such as deoxycoformycin or 2-chlorodeoxyadenosine (2-CDA), can achieve long-term remissions.

Mature T-cell and NK-Cell Lymphomas Have a Poor Prognosis

Mature (peripheral) T cell and NK-cell malignancies originate from postthymic T cells (see Fig. 20-48).

EPIDEMIOLOGY: Worldwide, T cell malignancies account for 12% of non-Hodgkin lymphomas. T cell and NK-cell lymphomas are more common in Asia than in the Western world. In Japan, many T cell malignancies is attributed to infection with human T cell leukemia virus (HTLV-1) (see Chapter 5).

PATHOLOGY: The immunophenotype of mature T cell malignancies is uniformly characterized by expression of α,β or γ,δ pairs of T cell receptors, both of which are linked to CD3. By definition, NK cells lack complete T cell receptor gene expression, but are positive for the intracellular ϵ chain of CD3. γ,δ T cells constitute less than 5% of the T cell repertoire and are mainly found in association with epithelial surfaces and within the splenic red pulp. These T cells do not express CD4, CD8 and CD5, whereas α,β T cells are (CD4+) helper or CD8+ (cytotoxic).

NK cells express CD2, CD7, and CD8. NK and cytotoxic T-cell malignancies both demonstrate the granule-associated proteins **perforin, granzyme B and T cell intracellular antigen (TIA-1).**

CLINICAL FEATURES: T cell and NK-cell tumors are clinically grouped into leukemic or nodal, extranodal, and cutaneous malignancies. *These neoplasms and NK cell lymphomas are generally more aggressive than most B cell malignancies and Hodgkin lymphoma.* They are treated with standard chemotherapy for B-cell lymphomas. Many T-cell neoplasms respond poorly to treatment: overall 5-year survival is 20% to 30%.

Adult T-cell Leukemia/Lymphoma

Adult T-cell leukemia/lymphoma (ATLL) is caused by HTLV-1.

EPIDEMIOLOGY: Geographically, ATLL parallels the endemic prevalence of HTLV-1 infection in Japan, the Caribbean basin, and Central Africa. Only 2% of people who harbor the virus develop ATLL.

PATHOLOGY: ATLL is caused by gene activation mediated through HTLV-1 viral protein P40 tax. The leukemic cells in ATLL are markedly atypical and contain multilobulated nuclei (**flower cells**). Peripheral blood, bone marrow, and skin are common sites of involvement.

T cells in ATLL express CD2, CD3, and CD5. Most patients have a helper T cell (CD4+) immunophenotype.

Tumor cells show a clonal T cell receptor gene rearrangement pattern and are positive for clonally integrated HTLV-1. The normal counterpart of ATLL is a mature, activated, CD4+ T cell.

CLINICAL FEATURES: ATLL is a systemic disease with multiorgan manifestations and peripheral leukocytosis. Acute, smoldering, and chronic variants are recognized. Hypercalcemia, with or without lytic bone lesions, is typical. The skin is the most important extranodal site of involvement. Acute ATLL has a poor prognosis. Death frequently occurs from infectious complications, like those seen in HIV-infected patients. Chronic and smoldering forms have a somewhat better prognosis.

Mycosis Fungoides and Sézary Syndrome

Mycosis fungoides (MF) is a cutaneous T-cell lymphoma with epidermal tropism.

EPIDEMIOLOGY: The disease occurs mainly in adults and the elderly. Men are more affected than women.

PATHOLOGY: MF displays lymphocytic infiltrates at the dermal–epidermal junction, epidermis, and, in some cases, intraepidermal nests of tumor cells (Pautrier microabscesses) (see Chapter 24).

Most tumors show a mature T helper cell immunophenotype (CD2+, CD3+, CD5+, CD4+, CD8$^-$ and TCRα,β+). As with other peripheral T-cell lymphomas, CD7 is often absent. Clonal T cell receptor gene rearrangements are common, which helps to distinguish subtle cases of mycosis fungoides from inflammatory infiltrates.

CLINICAL FEATURES: MF is an indolent lymphoma.

- The **premycotic or eczematous stage** lasts some years and is difficult to distinguish from many benign chronic dermatoses. A skin biopsy specimen is not diagnostic of lymphoma and shows a nonspecific perivascular and periadnexal lymphocytic infiltration with accompanying eosinophils and plasma cells.
- The **plaque stage** follows the premycotic stage. It is characterized by well-demarcated, raised cutaneous plaques. Definitive diagnosis of MF can usually be made in this stage. There is a dense subepidermal bandlike infiltrate of lymphoid cells, with irregular nuclear contours and a spectrum of cell sizes. Distinctive medium-to-large lymphoid cells with hyperchromatic nuclei and cerebriform nuclear contours, **mycosis cells**, are typical. Pautrier microabscesses in intraepidermal clear spaces are observed often.
- The **tumor stage** features raised cutaneous tumors, mostly on the face and in body folds, which frequently ulcerate and

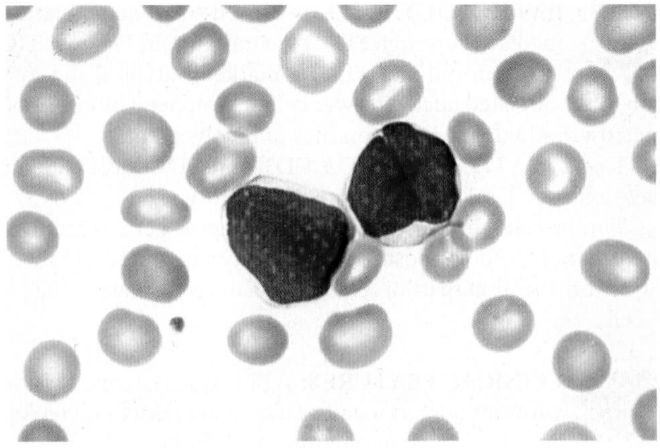

FIGURE 20-67. **Sézary cells.** Two circulating, neoplastic, T-helper cells with irregular nuclei and a thin rim of cytoplasm are seen.

become secondarily infected. The name **mycosis fungoides** derives from the raised, fungating, mushroomlike appearance of these tumors. Extracutaneous involvement, particularly of lymph nodes, spleen, liver, bone marrow, and lungs, is common.

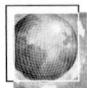

PATHOLOGY: Spread of MF to other organs, including lung, spleen, liver, and peripheral blood, is termed **Sézary syndrome.** Sézary syndrome arises after extensive cutaneous lesions have existed for a long time. Small (**Lutzner**) cells or large (**Sézary**) tumor cells are found in the peripheral blood (Fig. 20-67).

Anaplastic Large Cell Lymphoma

Anaplastic large cell lymphoma (ALCL) is characterized by large atypical tumor cells that universally express the activation marker CD30. Most cases are characterized by t(2;5) involving the **nucleophosmin** *(NPM)* and **anaplastic lymphoma kinase** *(ALK)* genes. NPM is a nuclear transfer protein and ALK is a transmembranous tyrosine kinase receptor of the insulin receptor superfamily. The fusion protein resulting from this translocation is silent in normal lymphocytes, but is upregulated in ALCL.

EPIDEMIOLOGY: ALCL has a bimodal age distribution; one peak occurs in young adulthood and a second in older persons. Many cases occur in children.

PATHOLOGY: ALCL cells are highly irregular (Fig. 20-68) with kidney- or horseshoe-shaped nuclei. Expression of T cell markers varies, but most cases express cytotoxic granule-associated proteins, granzyme B, TIA-1, and perforin.

CLINICAL FEATURES: Both nodal and extranodal sites are commonly involved. Many patients have fever. In the spectrum of T cell malignancies, ALK-positive ALCL has a favorable prognosis, with a median 5-year survival of 80%; the outlook for ALK-negative patients is worse.

Angioimmunoblastic T-cell Lymphoma (AILT)

AILT presents with generalized lymphadenopathy. T cell zones are expanded by a polymorphic T lymphoid infiltrate and proliferation of high endothelial venules. EBV can be seen in atypical B cells, but for the most part not in the malignant T cells.

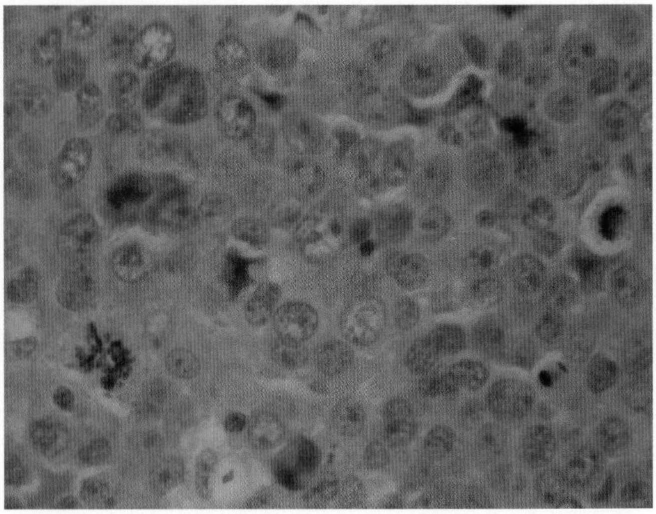

FIGURE 20-68. **Anaplastic large cell lymphoma.** Nuclei are large and highly irregular.

CLINICAL FEATURES: Most patients with AILT present with generalized lymphadenopathy, hepatosplenomegaly, bone marrow involvement, hypergammaglobulinemia, and serosal effusions. Other laboratory findings include cold hemagglutinins, hemolytic anemia, circulating immune complexes, and positive rheumatoid factor. AILT is an aggressive lymphoma: median survival is under 3 years.

Hodgkin Lymphoma (HL) Features Hodgkin Cells and Reed-Sternberg Cells Against an Inflammatory Background

Large atypical mononuclear or multinucleated tumor cells termed **Hodgkin and Reed- Sternberg cells** *are the diagnostic hallmark of Hodgkin lymphoma* (Fig. 20-69). Hodgkin disease was first recognized by Thomas Hodgkin of Guy's Hospital, London, in 1832. The first descriptions of the distinctive malignant cell were by Sternberg in 1898 and Reed in 1902. *Most cases of HL are clonal neoplasms of B lymphocytes.* However, its unique clinicopathologic features warrant its recognition as a distinctive malignancy.

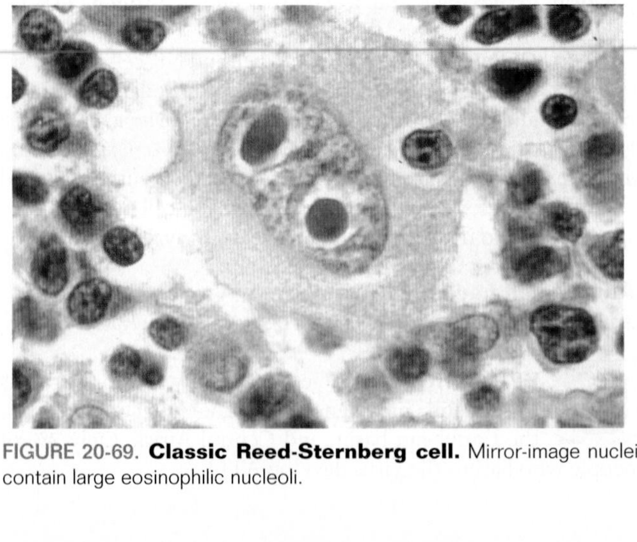

FIGURE 20-69. **Classic Reed-Sternberg cell.** Mirror-image nuclei contain large eosinophilic nucleoli.

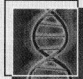

EPIDEMIOLOGY AND PATHOGENESIS: *HL is the most common malignancy of Americans between the ages of 10 and 30 years.* Some 8000 cases are reported annually in the United States, for an incidence of 3 per 100,000 population. It is somewhat more common in men than in women (4:2.5) and in whites than in blacks (3.5:2). There is a distinctive bimodal age distribution in developed countries, with a peak in the late 20s, a decrease in frequency in the fourth and fifth decades and a gradually increasing incidence after age 50.

Epidemiologic patterns in HL suggest that early and increased exposure to an unidentified agent of low oncogenic potential may be important in its development. In underdeveloped countries and less advanced regions of developed countries, HL is less common, but there is an increased frequency in children. There is also a different distribution of HL subtypes in different areas. Compared to affluent societies, less-developed regions show an increased frequency of the more aggressive "mixed cellularity" and "lymphocyte depletion" subtypes. In developed countries, less aggressive variants (nodular sclerosis and lymphocyte predominant) are more common in young adults from small families with few neighborhood playmates during childhood.

These patterns suggest that early exposure to an unidentified etiologic agent may predispose children to aggressive HL. According to this theory, delayed exposure results in a predisposition to indolent HL in young adults. This scheme does not explain whether the increasing incidence of HL after age 50 reflects exposure to the same hypothetical etiologic agent or has a different cause.

The **geographic variation** in HL incidence, and some clinicopathologic features that simulate an infectious process, suggest a viral etiology, but proof is still lacking. The possibility of horizontal transmission (i.e., by interpersonal contact) of an infectious agent has been suggested by several self-limited "mini-epidemics" of HL in children. However, such apparent case clustering is predictable on statistical grounds and has not been confirmed by broader epidemiologic studies. A possible relationship between HL and infection with EBV has been suggested. Young adults who have had EBV infection (infectious mononucleosis) have a threefold increased risk of developing HL and the EBV genome is frequently identified in the Reed-Sternberg cell (Fig. 20-70).

Genetic factors may play a role. The frequency of certain HLA subtypes, particularly HLA-B18, is higher in patients with HL. Moreover, there is a 7-fold increased risk of HL in siblings of patients with this disorder and a 100-fold increased risk when the sibling is a monozygotic twin.

Immune status seems to be a factor in at least some cases of HL. HL is more frequent in patients with compromised immunity or with autoimmune diseases, such as rheumatoid arthritis. In fact, in patients with ataxia–telangiectasia (A-T) (see later), who have a 100-fold increased incidence of cancer, 7% of the malignancies are HL.

Historically, the pathogenesis of HL has been difficult to study, in part because of the inability to define the lineage and clonality of Reed-Sternberg cells, which frequently constitute less than 1% of the total cell population. In fact, a salient feature of HL is the predominance in tumor tissue of reactive benign tissue components. Recent studies have indicated that in most patients with HL, EBV is present in Reed-Sternberg cells (see Fig. 20-70). EBV antigens can be demonstrated in situ in the tumor cells by immunohistochemistry or in situ hybridization. Mixed-cellularity HL is associated with EBV in 70% to 80% of cases, but in less than 40% of those of the nodular sclerosing type.

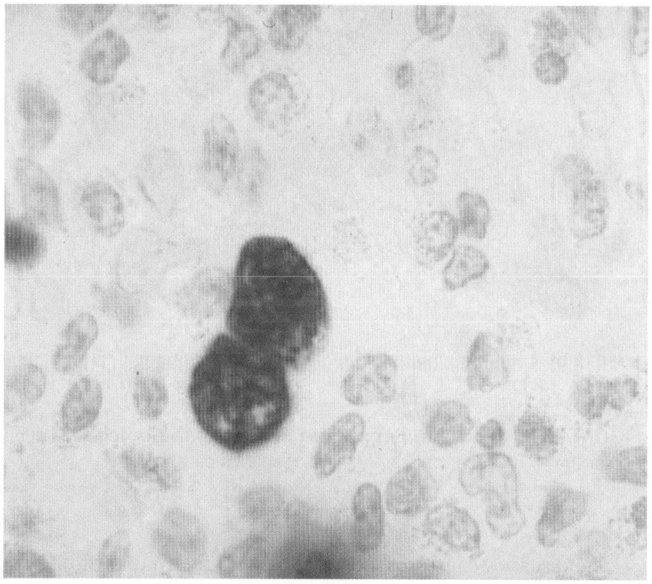

FIGURE 20-70. **EBV genome in a Reed-Sternberg cell.** EBV-RNA is visualized as red by in situ hybridization.

PATHOLOGY: Most patients with HL present with lymphadenopathy. After an initial diagnosis of HL, a comprehensive clinical and radiographic evaluation is commonly used to establish the extent, or stage, of disease. Abdominal exploratory surgery (staging laparotomy) may be performed to search for abdominal involvement. Bone marrow is also examined.

- **Lymph nodes:** On clinical examination, lymph nodes involved by HL are typically firm or rubbery, but they may be soft. If tumor tissue extends beyond the confines of individual lymph nodes, groups of nodes may be matted together.
- **Spleen:** The spleen is involved in one-third of cases of HL at the time of diagnosis and in most patients at autopsy. HL occurs first in T-cell-dependent, periarteriolar lymphoid sheaths of the white pulp or in the marginal zone between the white pulp and the red pulp. As the disease progresses, single or multiple discrete tumor nodules or confluent multinodular tumor masses in the spleen are common (Fig. 20-71). The prognosis in HL is adversely affected by multiple discrete tumor nodules in the spleen.
- **Liver:** At autopsy, the liver is involved with HL in two thirds of patients with residual disease, although it is unusual at the time of presentation.
- **Bone marrow:** The bone marrow is only rarely involved initially. Early changes in the bone marrow are discrete foci of fibrotic tumor, without destruction of bony trabeculae. As

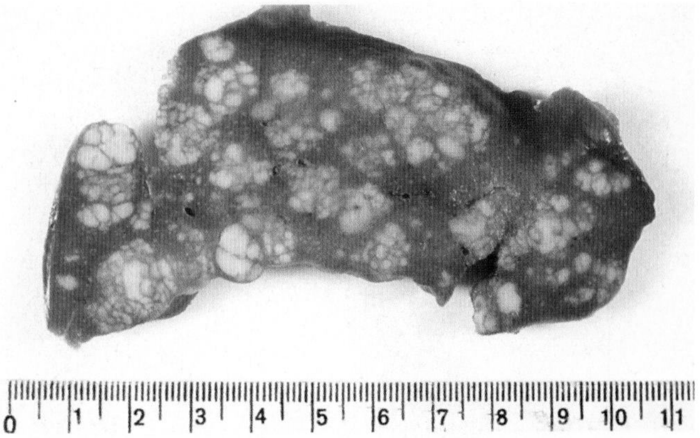

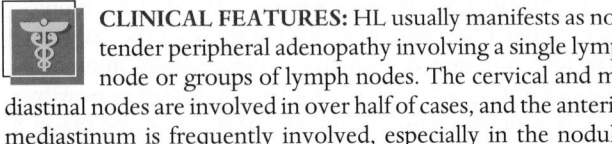

FIGURE 20-71. **Hodgkin lymphoma involving the spleen.** Multinodular tumor masses replace the normal splenic parenchyma.

the disease progresses, destruction of bone may produce an osteolytic appearance on radiologic examination.

- **Other systems:** Pulmonary involvement is seen at autopsy in over half of patients with residual disease and epidural spread of HL from paravertebral nodes through intervertebral foramina is a frequent neurological complication.

CLINICAL FEATURES: HL usually manifests as nontender peripheral adenopathy involving a single lymph node or groups of lymph nodes. The cervical and mediastinal nodes are involved in over half of cases, and the anterior mediastinum is frequently involved, especially in the nodular sclerosis type. Less commonly, axillary, inguinal, and retroperitoneal lymph nodes are initially enlarged. Peripheral lymph node groups, such as antecubital, popliteal, and mesenteric lymph nodes, tend to be spared.

Initially, HL spreads predictably between contiguous lymph node groups via efferent lymphatics. As the disease progresses, spread is kess predictable, owing to vascular invasion and hematogenous dissemination.

Constitutional ("B") symptoms are found in 40% of HL patients. These include low-grade fever, which is occasionally cyclical (Pel-Ebstein fever), night sweats, and weight loss exceeding 10% of body weight. Pruritus may occur as the disease progresses. For unknown reasons, drinking alcohol induces pain at involved sites in 10% of patients.

Deficient T lymphocyte function is characteristic of HL. Subtle defects of delayed-type hypersensitivity, which can be detected in most patients even at the time of initial diagnosis, tend to become more pronounced as the disease progresses. Anergy to skin test antigens is often noted early in HL. Such immune dysfunction is exacerbated by the immunosuppressive effects of therapy. An absolute lymphocytopenia ($<$1500 per μL) is seen in half of cases, most often in advanced HL. Humoral immunity is usually intact until late in the course of the disease.

The prognosis in HL depends mainly on the patient's age and the anatomic extent of the disease, i.e., the stage. A better prognosis is associated with (1) younger age, (2) lower clinical stage (localized disease), and (3) absence of B signs and symptoms. The comprehensive Ann Arbor staging system (Table 20-19), which is based on clinical evaluation and pathologic findings from staging laparotomy, is used to assign stage.

TABLE 20–19

Ann Arbor Staging System for Hodgkin Disease

Stage I A or B*	I	Involvement of a single lymph node region or
	I_E	A single extralymphatic organ or site
Stage II A or B	II	Involvement or two or more lymph node regions on the same side of the diaphragm or
	II_E	with localized contiguous involvement of an extra-lymphatic organ site
Stage III A or B	III	Involvement of lymph node regions on both sides of the diaphragm or
	III_E	with localized contiguous involvement of an extra-lymphatic organ or site or
	III_S	with involvement of spleen or
	III_{ES}	both extralymphatic organ or site and spleen involvement
Stage IV A or B	IV	Diffuse or disseminated involvement of one or more extralymphatic organs with or without associated lymph node involvement

*A = asymptomatic; B = presence of constitutional symptoms (fever, night sweats, and weight loss exceeding 10% of baseline body weight in preceding 6 months).

Complications of HL include compromise of vital organs by progressive tumor growth and secondary infections, owing to both the primary defect in delayed type hypersensitivity and the immunosuppressive effects of therapy. Development of second malignancies after therapy is of special concern, since more than 15% of treated patients may eventually suffer this complication. AML develops in 5% of patients and aggressive large cell lymphomas occur somewhat less frequently.

Histologic Classification of Hodgkin Lymphoma

Two major types of HL are distinguished, **nodular lymphocyte-predominant HL** (NLPHL) and **classical** HL (CHL).

Nodular Lymphocyte-Predominant Hodgkin Lymphoma

NLPHL features Reed-Sternberg cell variants called "popcorn" or L&H (lymphohistocytic) cells. NLPHL represents only a small proportion of all cases of HL.

NLPHL is a neoplasm of B lymphocyte origin. The Reed-Sternberg cells of this variant express specific B cell lineage antigens and surface Ig, and lack the CD15 and CD30, which are usually but not always found on Reed-Sternberg cells of the other subtypes of HL. Nevertheless classical HL are also considered to be B lymphocyte neoplasms.

Expression of BSAP in the vast majority of cases favors this interpretation. The *PAX5* gene encodes BSAP, a B cell-specific transcription factor. Clonal *IgH* gene rearrangement is almost always seen in the tumor cells. The rearranged *IgG* genes are positive for mutations in the variable region of IgG heavy chain, indicating that they are most likely of germinal center B cell origin. In a few cases, the normal counterpart appears to be a postthymic T cell.

NLPHL is the most indolent type. Adult men under 35 years of age are most often affected (male-to-female ratio, 4:1). At the time of diagnosis, disease is usually localized (stage I), with the high cervical, axillary, or inguinal lymph nodes most commonly involved. B signs and symptoms are present in only 20% of cases. Visceral involvement is uncommon. Unlike classical types of HL, NLPHL tends to skip anatomical lymph node regions. Mediastinal involvement is rare. The overall survival is excellent, with more than 80% 10-year survival at stages I and II. However, lymphocyte-predominant HL has a high recurrence rate.

PATHOLOGY: The tumor completely effaces lymph node architecture in a vaguely nodular pattern. The usual inflammatory background of eosinophils and plasma cells is missing. The immunophenotype of Reed-Sternberg cells in NLPHL is different from that in classical HL (see above). Genotypically, the tumor cells resemble germinal center B cells. The tumor cells in NLPHL are negative for EBV.

Classical Hodgkin Lymphoma

CHL is characterized by clonal proliferation of typical mononuclear Hodgkin cells and multinucleated Reed-Sternberg cells (HRS cells), with invariable expression of CD30 (Fig. 20-72). A variable inflammatory background of lymphocytes, eosinophils, macrophages, neutrophils, plasma cells, fibroblasts, and collagenous tissue determines the morphologic appearance. Four different types of CHL are defined: lymphocyte-rich, nodular-sclerosis, mixed-cellularity, and lymphocyte-depleted variants.

PATHOLOGY: Typical mononuclear or multinucleated Reed-Sternberg cells with large nucleoli are immersed in a rich inflammatory background. Occasionally, HRS cells undergo apoptosis, resulting in ghost cells with condensed cytoplasm and pyknotic nuclei (mummified cells). In nodular sclerosis, **lacunar cells** result from a retraction artifact in formaldehyde-fixed tissue. *Expression of the lymphocytic activation antigen CD30 unites the different types of CHL.*

HRS cells produce several cytokines that elicit characteristic tissue effects. Eosinophils are attracted by the combined effects of IL-5 and eotaxin and IL-6 can attract plasma cells. TGF-β activates fibroblasts and may account for nodular fibrosis. Other growth factors and cytokines made by HRS cells include IL 2, 7, 9, 10, and 13.

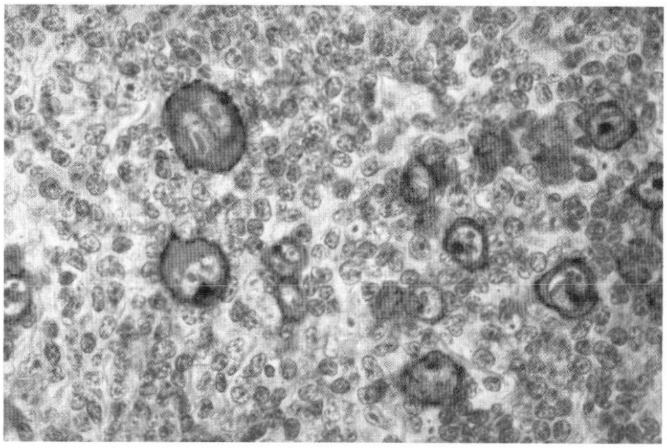

FIGURE 20-72. **Reed-Sternberg and Hodgkin cells.** The cells are positive for CD30 (immunohistochemistry)

Nodular-Sclerosis Hodgkin Lymphoma (NSHL)

NSHL features nodular architecture in which lymphoid tissue is surrounded by fibrosis (Fig. 20-73). Classical HRS cells with lacunar variants are typical. NSHL accounts for 70% of CHL, with most cases occurring between the ages of 20 and 30 years. Mediastinal involvement is most common in this type of HL.

NSHL is the most common form of HL and is often found in adolescent and young adult women, ages 15 to 35 years. It tends to manifest as lower cervical, supraclavicular, and mediastinal adenopathy (stage II). B symptoms (see Table 20-19) occur in up to 40% of patients. The prognosis is good, with a cure rate of 80% to 85%. Untreated, NSHL is fatal, with a 10-year survival rate of only 1%. With irradiation and chemotherapy, a 70% cure rate can be achieved.

Mixed-Cellularity Hodgkin Lymphoma (MCHL)

MCHL contains HRS cells against a mixed inflammatory background of eosinophils, neutrophils, macrophages and plasma cells (Fig. 20-74). The histology is like that of the nodular-sclerosis variety, but collagen bands are missing. MCHL is the most frequent HL subtype in HIV-1-infected patients and shows the highest association with EBV (see Fig. 20-70). Mediastinal involvement is uncommon.

A 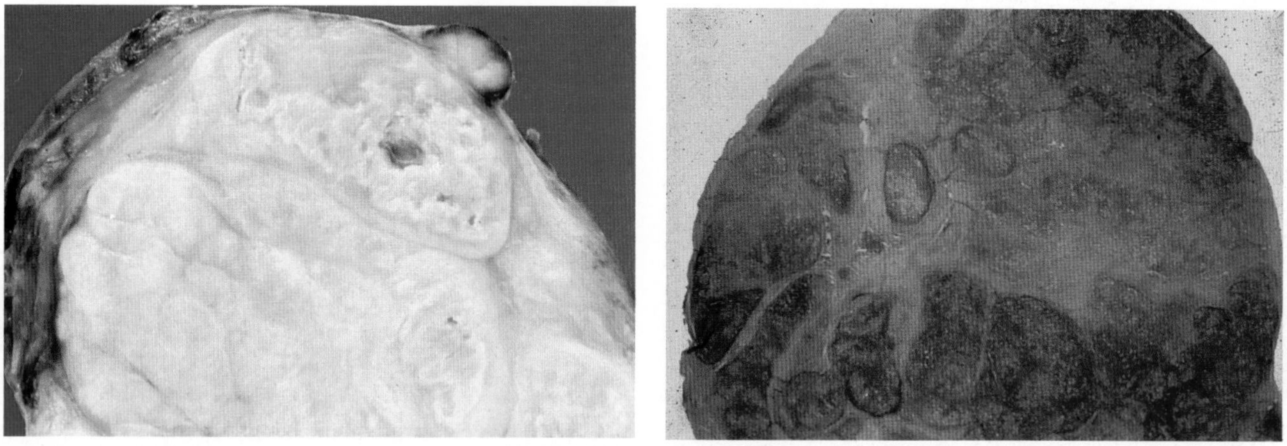 B

FIGURE 20-73. **Hodgkin lymphoma; nodular sclerosis. A.** A cut section of matted lymph nodes shows broad bands of fibrosis that divide the parenchyma into distinct nodules. Several foci of necrosis are evident. **B.** A low-power photomicrograph demonstrates broad bands of fibrosis.

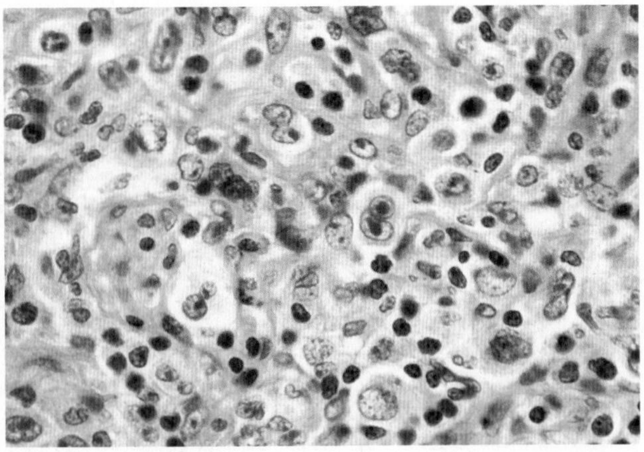

FIGURE 20-74. **Hodgkin lymphoma; mixed cellularity.** A photomicrograph of a lymph node shows classic, binucleated, and mononuclear Reed-Sternberg cells; lymphocytes; and mild diffuse fibrosis.

People of age may be affected, but MCHL is most common in the fourth and fifth decades. The left cervical lymph nodes are the most common site of initial involvement. However, after staging, most patients are found to have stage II or III disease. A minority have visceral involvement (stage IV). B signs and symptoms are present in half of the cases of MCHL. The prognosis is intermediate, with a cure rate of 75%.

Lymphocyte-Rich Hodgkin Lymphoma (LRHL)

LRHL has recently been added to the list of Hodgkin lymphomas. It is characterized by classical HRS cells in an abundant background of small lymphocytes. Mixed inflammatory cells and collagen bands are missing.

Lymphocyte-Depleted Hodgkin Lymphoma (LDHL)

LDHL is the least common type of CHL. Histologically, it shows a predominance of tumor cells and a marked absence of background lymphocytes (Fig. 20-75). LDHL is frequently associated with HIV infection. Without treatment, this type of HL has the worst prognosis. Advanced stage and B symptoms are seen in more than 70% of patients and most are positive for EBV.

LDHL is the most clinically aggressive type. Middle-aged to elderly men are most commonly affected. Advanced clinical stage (III–IV) and B signs and symptoms are present in two thirds of patients. Those with the diffuse fibrosis subtype of LDHL commonly present with fever of undetermined origin, pancytopenia, and wasting. There is usually no peripheral or mediastinal adenopathy. However, retroperitoneal adenopathy is frequently prominent and involvement of the spleen, liver, and bone marrow is common. Profound immunodeficiency develops and death commonly results from inanition or secondary infections. The reticular subtype of LDHL is characterized by bulky peripheral adenopathy, which is most frequent above the diaphragm. Patients usually die because of tumor progression. The overall cure rate in both types of LDHL is 40% to 50%.

Post-transplant Lymphoproliferative Disorder (PTLD) Is Often Associated with EBV Infection

PTLD results from immunosuppression. In most cases, the disease is an EBV-driven, monoclonal, lymphocyte proliferation with variable morphology.

EPIDEMIOLOGY: The incidence of PTLD parallels the extent of immunosuppression. Liver transplant recipients have a higher incidence of PTLD than do kidney transplant patients (5% vs. 1%). Recipients of matched bone marrow allografts show a low incidence of PTLD (1%), whereas unmatched recipients have a much higher incidence, owing to higher levels of immunosuppression.

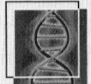

PATHOGENESIS: Most cases are caused by EBV (Fig. 20-76), with an average latency period of less than 1 year. However, EBV-negative cases may evolve more than 5 years after transplantation. In solid organ recipients, ***host*** lymphocytes become infected with EBV, but in bone marrow allograft recipients, PTLD is caused by infected ***donor*** lymphocytes.

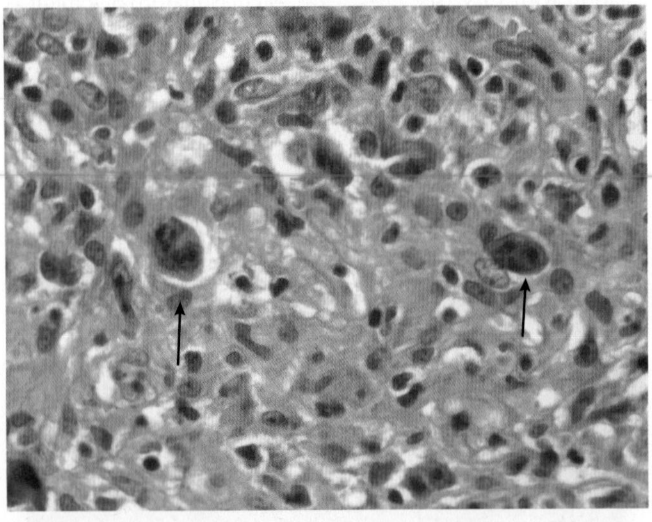

A

FIGURE 20-75. **Hodkgin lymphoma; lymphocyte-depleted type.** Two tumor cells are seen (*arrows*). The number of reactive lymphocytes in the fibrotic background is markedly reduced.

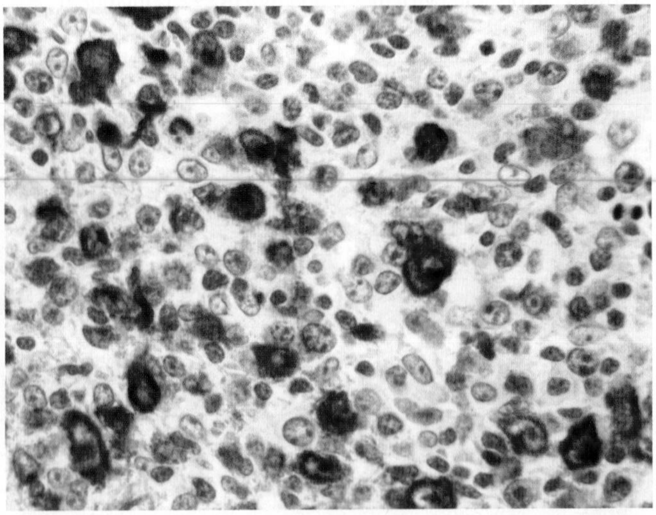

B

FIGURE 20-76. **Posttransplant lymphoproliferative disorder (PTLD).** Atypical lymphocytes are positive for latent membrane protein (LMP) of Epstein-Barr virus.

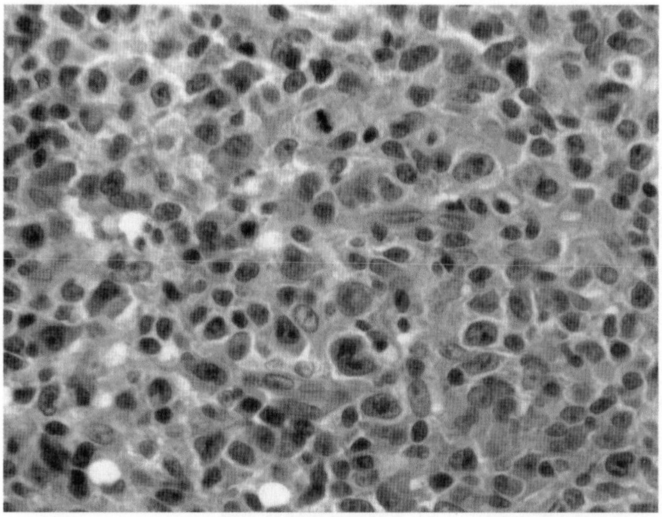

FIGURE 20-77. **Post-transplant lymphoproliferative disorder (PTLD).** Highly atypical lymphocytes are shown.

PATHOLOGY: Early lymph node lesions of PTLD are characterized by increased plasma cells or an appearance similar to that of **infectious mononucleosis.** Lymphocyte and plasma cell proliferation at this stage is not clonal.

Polymorphic PTLD is the next step in the evolution of the disease and features a mixture of immunoblasts, plasma cells, and medium-sized lymphocytes in lymph nodes or other organs (Fig. 20-77). B cells that demonstrate the full range of maturation and have numerous mitotic figures infiltrate the tissue. In spite of the polymorphic appearance of the lymphocytes, PCR almost always shows clonal *IgH* gene arrangements. Some patients may spontaneously regress if immunosuppressive therapy is reduced.

PTLD eventually acquires a **monomorphic** appearance indistinguishable from that of malignant lymphoma. Histologic types include diffuse large B-cell lymphoma, BL, HL, plasma cell myeloma or, rarely, T-cell lymphoma.

CLINICAL FEATURES: In PTLD, neoplastic lymphocytes can be seen at any nodal or extranodal site. Solid organ recipients treated with azathioprine present with PTLD after an average latency period of 48 months, whereas those given cyclosporine develop the disease within 15 months. PTLD in bone marrow allograft recipients occurs within the first 6 months. EBV-positive cases occur much earlier than EBV-negative ones. Early PTLD has an excellent prognosis and may regress at a decreased level of immunosuppression. Late-stage PTLD, with full-blown malignant lymphoma, has a mortality rate of 70%. Treatment with an anti-CD20 antibody (rituximab) has been successful in eliminating clonal B cell proliferations.

SPLEEN

Anatomy and Function

The spleen is a lymphoid organ that also serves as a versatile filter for abnormal or senescent cells. Its normal weight is 100 to 170 g; it is normally not palpable on clinical examination. The spleen's supporting structure consists of a fibrous capsule, radiating fibrous trabeculae, and a delicate stromal framework of reticulum fibers. The splenic artery enters at the hilum and branches into trabecular arteries, following the course of the fibrous trabeculae.

The white pulp: Leaving the trabeculae, central arteries become ensheathed by lymphocytes, which constitute the white pulp. The white pulp is further subdivided into a T cell domain, located in the periarteriolar lymphoid sheath; and a B cell domain that comprises the follicles and perifollicular mantle zone (Fig. 20-78). Like the lymph nodes, the follicles are either inactive or activated, the latter being associated with germinal-center formation. Arising from the central artery, follicular arteries enter the B cell follicles and terminate in the marginal sinus at the junction between the white and red pulp. Circulating lymphocytes exit the vascular system from the marginal sinus and travel to their respective B cell and T cell domains. Lymphocytes leave the white pulp and enter the red pulp by way of the same marginal sinuses.

The red pulp: this region comprises a network of stromal cords and vascular sinuses. Most of the blood from the penicilliary arteries empties directly into the sinuses (closed circulation), with subsequent drainage to the trabecular veins and ultimately to the splenic vein. A small fraction (5%–10%) is diverted into the splenic cords (open circulation) and slowly percolates through a meshwork studded with phagocytic macrophages. The blood then reenters the sinusoids through narrow slits composed of longitudinally oriented, slender endothelial cells and radially oriented ring fibers.

In the splenic cords, erythrocytes are subjected to the sustained scrutiny of mononuclear phagocytes and must be deformable to traverse the narrow interstices between the lining endothelial cells. The erythrocytes must also be able to withstand the hypoxia, hypoglycemia, and acidosis that are characteristic of the stromal cord microenvironment. Most normal erythroid cells survive, as do granulocytes and platelets. They ultimately enter the trabecular veins and leave the hilum by way of the splenic vein.

As part of the peripheral lymphoid system, effector B and T lymphocytes of the white pulp perform an immunologic function for the circulatory system comparable to the immunologic function of the lymph nodes. The white pulp is (1) the source of protection from blood-borne infection, (2) a major locale for the synthesis of opsonizing IgM antibody, and (3) a site of production of lymphocytes and plasma cells.

The red pulp is primarily a filter designed to screen and eliminate defective or foreign cells. Senescent and damaged erythrocytes are recognized and phagocytosed by splenic macrophages. The spleen ordinarily accounts for the removal of about half of aged erythrocytes, the remainder being destroyed in the liver, bone marrow, and other components of the mononuclear phagocyte system. Following phagocytosis and breakdown of erythrocytes, the iron is first stored as hemosiderin in macrophages. It is then released, bound to transferrin, and transported to the bone marrow for reuse in erythropoiesis. Abnormal erythrocyte inclusions, such as Howell-Jolly bodies (remnants of nuclear DNA), Heinz bodies (denatured hemoglobin), and siderotic granules (iron), are recognized and removed (pitted) by macrophages, without destroying the erythrocyte.

Some membrane lipids of maturing erythrocytes are removed in the red pulp. In the absence of this function, such as after splenectomy, there may be excess erythrocyte membrane in relation to hemoglobin content, which leads to central pooling of hemoglobin and a "target cell" appearance.

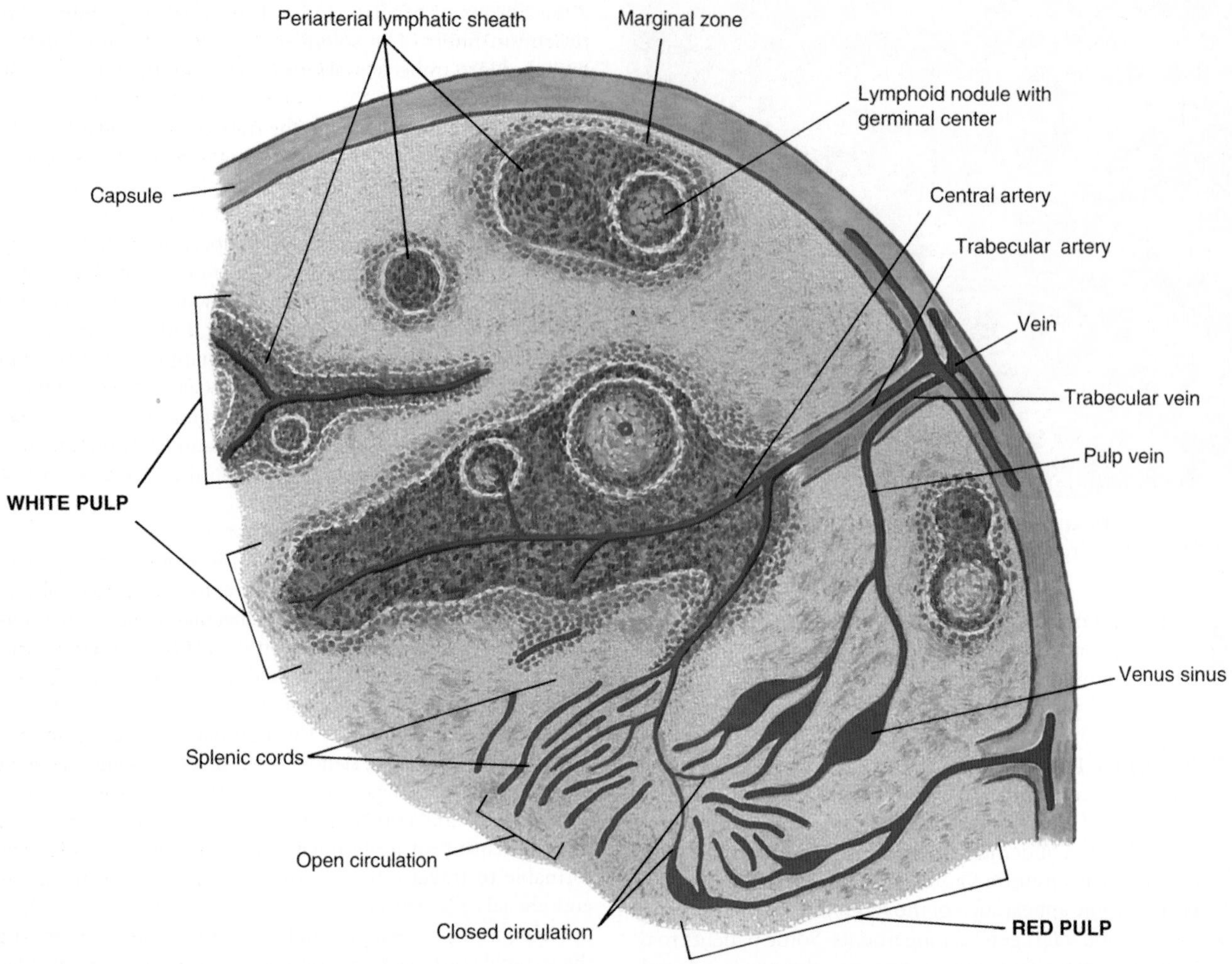

FIGURE 20-78. **Structure of the normal spleen.**

One third of the blood platelet pool and a small fraction of granulocytes are normally sequestered in the spleen without causing any damage to the cells. By contrast, there is no significant splenic sequestration of erythrocytes and splenectomy is followed only by an increase in platelet and granulocyte counts.

Disorders of the Spleen

Hypersplenism is a functional disorder, which, as noted above (see hemolytic anemia), is characterized by anemia, leukopenia, thrombocytopenia, and compensatory bone marrow hyperplasia. Hyposplenism is a situation in which normal splenic functions are reduced by disease or are absent after splenectomy. Impaired filtering leads to increased risk of severe bacteremia and mild leukocytosis and thrombocytosis. Nuclear remnants and Howell-Jolly bodies are found in many of the circulating erythrocytes.

Congenital absence of the spleen (asplenia) is rare and is often seen with other congenital anomalies. **Acquired asplenia** is most common in young adults with sickle cell anemia. Multiple infarctions eventually result in atrophy and hyposplenism. The infarctions are often painful, owing to the complication of fibrinous perisplenitis. As the result of the absence of splenic sequestration of erythrocytes, with consequent lack of removal of excess membrane and intracellular debris, many erythrocytes become targeT cells and contain nuclear remnants, Howell-Jolly bodies, or even intact nuclei.

Accessory spleens occur in 10% of normal persons, may be up to several centimeters in diameter and are most frequently found in the tail of the pancreas or in the gastrosplenic ligament. After splenectomy, accessory spleens may increase considerably in size, but they rarely become large enough to restore the functions of the lost spleen.

The spleen is a prominent member of the lymphopoietic and mononuclear phagocyte systems and **splenomegaly** is common in a variety of unrelated diseases (Table 20-20).

Reactive Splenomegaly

Reactive splenic hyperplasia occurs in a number of acute and chronic inflammatory conditions. It is probably caused by phagocytosis of blood-borne bacteria, which leads to release of growth factors and other products of the inflammatory response. The spleen is moderately enlarged (up to 400 g) and macrophages and neutrophils abound in the red pulp. Mild hyperplasia of the lymphoid white pulp is common.

In **acute and chronic parasitemias,** the red pulp may be engorged with parasites and their breakdown products. The spleen is often massively enlarged in chronic malaria (up to 10 kg). It shows fibrous thickening of the capsule and trabeculae, with a slate gray to black coloration of the pulp, due to phagocytosed malarial pigment (hematin).

In **chronic immunologic inflammatory disorders,** splenomegaly is caused by hyperplasia of the white pulp. Ger-

TABLE 20-20
Principal Causes of Splenomegaly

Infections
Acute Subacute Chronic
Immunologic inflammatory disorders
Felty syndrome Lupus erythematosus Sarcoidosis Amyloidosis Thyroiditis
Hemolytic anemias
Immune thrombocytopenia
Splenic vein hypertension
Cirrhosis Splenic or portal vein thrombosis or stenosis Right-sided cardiac failure
Primary or metastatic neoplasm
Leukemia Lymphoma Hodgkin disease Myeloproliferative syndromes Sarcoma Carcinoma
Storage diseases
Gaucher Niemann-Pick Mucopolysaccharidoses

minal centers are prominent, as in rheumatoid arthritis; and the red pulp displays an associated increase in mononuclear phagocytes, immunoblasts, plasma cells, and eosinophils.

Systemic lupus erythematosus is characterized by fibrinoid necrosis of capsular and trabecular collagen and concentric, or "onion skin," thickening of the penicilliary arteries and central arterioles of the white pulp.

In **infectious mononucleosis,** transformed lymphocytes (immunoblasts) prominently infiltrate the red pulp, whereas the white pulp may no longer be evident. Infiltration of the capsular and trabecular systems and of blood vessels by lymphoid elements weakens the supporting structure of the spleen and accounts for **traumatic splenic rupture** in infectious mononucleosis.

Congestive Splenomegaly

Chronic passive congestion of the spleen causes splenomegaly and hypersplenism. This is most common in patients with portal hypertension due to cirrhosis, thrombosis of the portal or splenic veins, or right-sided heart failure.

PATHOLOGY: The spleen is modestly enlarged (300–700 g) and has a thickened, fibrotic capsule. Focal accentuation of the capsular fibrosis leads to a "sugar-coated" appearance. The cut surface is firm, and the color varies from pink to deep red, depending on the extent of fibrosis. Microscopically, the red pulp initially shows dilated sinuses and an increased number of macrophages. Later, the parenchyma becomes fibrotic, and the red pulp is hypocellular. Foci of old hemorrhages persist as **Gamna-Gandy bodies,** which are fibrotic nodules containing iron and calcium salts encrusted on collagenous and elastic fibers. The white pulp tends to be atrophic.

Infiltrative Splenomegaly

The spleen may be enlarged by an increase in cellularity or by deposition of extracellular material, as in amyloidosis. Splenic macrophages accumulate in chronic infections, hemolytic anemias, and a variety of storage diseases, Gaucher disease being the prototype (see Chapter 6). A variety of neoplastic and reactive bone marrow disorders are accompanied by extramedullary hematopoiesis and a corresponding increase in the size of the spleen. Splenomegaly is also caused by infiltration of malignant cells in hematologic proliferative disorders, such as leukemias and lymphomas.

Splenomegaly Due to Cysts and Tumors

Splenic cysts are rare, and the most common are actually pseudocysts. The latter are lined by a fibrous wall and are the residue of previous hemorrhage or infarction. **Hydatid cysts** are encountered in areas endemic for *Echinococcus granulosus* (see Chapter 9).

Primary splenic tumors are also distinctly uncommon. The most common primary benign tumors of the spleen are hemangiomas and lymphangiomas. Usually of the cavernous type, they contain large endothelial-lined spaces and vary from minute foci to lesions that occupy most of the spleen. The spaces in hemangiomas are occupied by erythrocytes, and in lymphangiomas by lymph.

Malignant tumors, such as malignant lymphomas or HL, are usually not primary in the spleen but rather part of a generalized disease. **Splenic hemangiosarcoma** is a rare, highly malignant neoplasm of vascular endothelial cells that tends to metastasize to the liver by way of the portal drainage.

Despite its large blood supply and filtering function, the spleen is only rarely involved by metastatic tumors. The microenvironment, with its abundance of macrophages and lymphocytes, is apparently not favorable for tumor growth. Metastatic tumors are usually observed only late in the course of a widely metastasizing neoplasm.

THYMUS

Theories underlying the historical categorization of the thymus as an endocrine organ have long been discredited. Nevertheless, we know that the thymus elaborates a number of factors (thymic hormones) that play a key role in the maturation of the immune system and the development of immune tolerance. On this basis, we discuss certain entities associated with thymus abnormalities in this chapter.

Anatomy and Function

The thymus derives embryologically from the third pair of pharyngeal pouches, with an inconstant contribution from the fourth pair. The organ is irregularly pyramidal, with its base located inferiorly and its two lobes fused in the midline. Its fibrous capsule extends into the parenchyma, forming septa that delimit lobules. The thymus is largest in relation to total body size and weight at birth, when it averages about 15 g. It continues to grow until puberty, and then may weigh 30 to 40 g.

Microscopically, the lobules display an outer cortex and an inner medulla. The cortex consists of densely packed lymphocytes, which in this location are termed **thymocytes**. Thymocytes are admixed with a few epithelial and mesenchymal cells. The medulla contains many more epithelial cells and fewer thymocytes. **Hassall corpuscles** are medullary structures that are focally keratinized, concentric aggregates of epithelial cells characteristic of the thymus.

The thymus is the key site for T lymphocyte differentiation (see Chapter 4). It also has a small population of neuroendocrine cells, which may explain the occurrence of neuroendocrine tumors in this organ. The thymus also exhibits a complement of myoid cells, which resemble striated muscle cells but are nevertheless regarded as epithelial cells. Myoid cells may play a role in the autoimmune pathogenesis of myasthenia gravis.

Beginning at puberty, the thymus starts to involute and continues to diminish in size into adulthood. Initially, cortical thymocytes are decreased relative to epithelial cells. Eventually, the thymus consists of islands of epithelial cells depleted of lymphocytes and aggregates of Hassall corpuscles separated by adipose tissue.

Agenesis and Dysplasia

Alterations in the thymus vary from complete absence (**agenesis**) or severe **hypoplasia** to a situation in which the thymus is small but exhibits a normal architecture. Some small glands exhibit **thymic dysplasia**, characterized by an absence of thymocytes, few if any Hassall corpuscles and only epithelial components. Various developmental abnormalities are associated with immune deficiencies (see Chapter 4) and hematologic disorders.

- **Severe combined immunodeficiency (SCID)** represents a group of genetically distinct syndromes all characterized by defects of both T and B lymphocytes and associated with severe thymic dysplasia. Both X-linked and autosomal recessive modes of inheritance have been observed. SCID can be caused by mutations in at least 10 different genes. The most common form is the X-linked type, caused by mutations in *IL-2RG*, a cytokine-receptor gene. Common autosomal recessive inherited forms include the adenosine deaminase deficiency and IL-7Ra.
- **Chromosome 22q11.2 deletion syndrome (DiGeorge, velocardiofacial, Shprintzen, conotruncal anomaly face, and Cayler syndromes)** is a spectrum of overlapping conditions caused by 22q11.2 deletions. It is one of the most common genetic syndromes associated with variable clinical manifestations (180 at least). Patients with DiGeorge syndrome have a failure in development of the third and fourth branchial pouches, resulting in agenesis or hypoplasia of the thymus and parathyroid glands, congenital heart defects, dysmorphic facies, and a variety of other congenital anomalies. As a result, patients have hypocalcemia and a deficiency of cellular immunity, with a particular susceptibility to *Candida* infection. Recent reports indicate that patients with 22q11.2 deletion syndrome are also at increased risk for psychotic illnesses. Endocrine abnormalities include hypocalcemia, thyroid dysfunction, and short stature. The diagnosis, suspected on clinical grounds, can be readily established by FISH analysis.
- **Nezelof syndrome** is characterized by lymphopenia, hypoplastic lymphoid tissue, abnormal thymus architecture, and abnormal T cell function. It is like DiGeorge syndrome save for the lack of parathyroid and cardiac involvement.
- **Wiskott-Aldrich syndrome (WAS)** is an X-linked, recessive immunodeficiency caused by mutations in the gene encoding WAS protein and characterized by a hypoplastic thymus, recurrent infections, eczema, and thrombocytopenia (see Chapter 4). Patients have increased susceptibility to lymphoid malignancies and autoimmune disorders.
- **Reticular dysgenesis (RD)** is a very rare, severe form of immune deficiency characterized by a vestigial thymus and developmental failure of bone marrow stem cells, resulting in lymphopenia, granulocytopenia, and death in utero or in the neonatal period. The primary defect that disturbs the differentiation of the myeloid and lymphoid cell precursors is currently unknown.
- **Swiss-type hypogammaglobulinemia** is an autosomal recessive disorder featuring severe thymic hypoplasia or dysplasia. Infants with this condition have no lymphocytes or Hassall corpuscles in the thymus and die within a few years from a variety of infections. The anomaly represents a failure of the thymic anlage in the neck to descend into the mediastinum.
- **Ataxia telangiectasia (A-T)** is an autosomal recessive cerebellar ataxia associated with immunodeficiency, telangiectasia, increased sensitivity to ionizing radiation, and frequent occurrence of lymphoma. The involuted thymus lacks epithelial differentiation and Hassall corpuscles. Classic A-T results from two-truncating ATM mutations that cause complete loss of ATM protein kinase.

Hyperplasia

Thymic hyperplasia denotes the presence of lymphoid follicles in the thymus irrespective of the size of the gland (Fig. 20-79). The total weight of the thymus is usually within the normal range, although it may be increased. The follicles contain germinal centers and are composed largely of B lymphocytes that contain IgM and IgD. The follicles tend to occupy and distort the medullary zones.

The best known association of thymic hyperplasia is with **myasthenia gravis** (see Chapter 27), in which two-thirds of patients exhibit this thymic abnormality. Interestingly, thymic epithelial and myoid cells contain nicotinic acetylcholine receptor protein, suggesting a potential source for the development of antibodies directed against this receptor. Thymic follicular hyperplasia may also be found in other diseases in which autoimmunity is believed to play a role, including Graves disease, Addison disease, systemic lupus erythematosus, scleroderma, and rheumatoid arthritis.

Thymoma

Thymoma is a neoplasm of thymic epithelial cells. This tumor almost always occurs in adult life and most (80%) are benign.

PATHOLOGY: Most thymomas are in the anterosuperior mediastinum, although a few have been described in other locations where thymic tissue is found, including the neck, middle and posterior mediastinum, and pul-

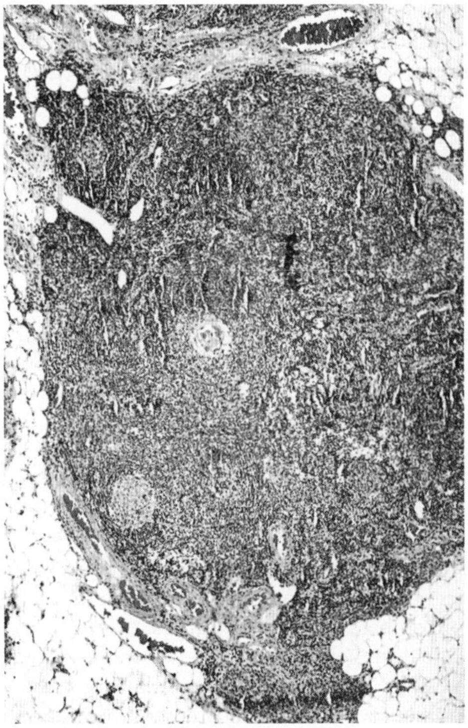

FIGURE 20-79. **Thymic hyperplasia.** This thymus removed from a patient with myasthenia gravis shows lymphoid follicles with germinal centers.

monary hilus. Benign thymomas are irregularly shaped masses that range from a few centimeters to 15 cm or more in greatest dimension. They are encapsulated, firm and gray to yellow tumors that are divided into lobules by fibrous septa (Fig. 20-80). Large tumors show foci of hemorrhage, necrosis, and cystic degeneration. In some instances, the entire thymoma becomes cystic and multiple sections are required to identify the true nature of the lesion.

On microscopic examination, thymomas consist of a mixture of neoplastic epithelial cells and non-tumorous lymphocytes. The proportions of these elements vary in individual cases and even among different lobules. The epithelial cells are plump or spindle-shaped and have vesicular nuclei. In cases in which epithelial cells predominate, they may exhibit an organoid differentiation, including perivascular spaces containing lymphocytes and macrophages, tumor cell rosettes and whorls suggesting abortive Hassall corpuscle formation.

MYASTHENIA GRAVIS: Fifteen percent of patients with myasthenia gravis have thymoma. Conversely, one-third to one-half of patients with thymoma develop myasthenia gravis. The occurrence of thymoma in persons with myasthenia gravis is more common in men over 50.

When thymoma is associated with myasthenic symptoms, the epithelial cells are of the plump, rather than spindle cell, variety. Antigens related to the nicotinic acetylcholine receptor have also been detected in thymomas. Thymic hyperplasia is almost always present in the nontumorous thymic tissue and lymphoid follicles may even be present in the thymoma itself.

OTHER ASSOCIATED DISEASES: Thymoma is also associated with many other immune disorders. More than 10% of patients have hypogammaglobulinemia and 5% have erythroid hypoplasia. In contrast to the situation with myasthenia gravis, the epithelial component of the thymoma is spindle shaped in these cases. Other associated diseases include myocarditis, dermatomyositis, rheumatoid arthritis, lupus erythematosus, scleroderma, and Sjögren syndrome. Certain malignant tumors have also been associated with thymoma, including T-cell leukemia-lymphoma and multiple myeloma.

Malignant Thymoma Invades Locally and May Metastasize

One-fourth of thymomas are not encapsulated and exhibit malignant features.

PATHOLOGY: **Type I malignant thymoma** is the most common cancer of the thymus and is virtually indistinguishable histologically from encapsulated, benign thymoma. However, it penetrates the capsule; implants on pleural or pericardial surfaces; and metastasizes to lymph nodes, lung, liver, and bone.

Type II malignant thymoma is a very uncommon, invasive tumor, that is also termed **thymic carcinoma**. Its morphology is highly variable and takes the form of squamous cell carcinoma, lymphoepithelioma-like carcinoma (identical to that found in the oropharynx; see Chapter 25), a sarcomatoid variant (carci-

A

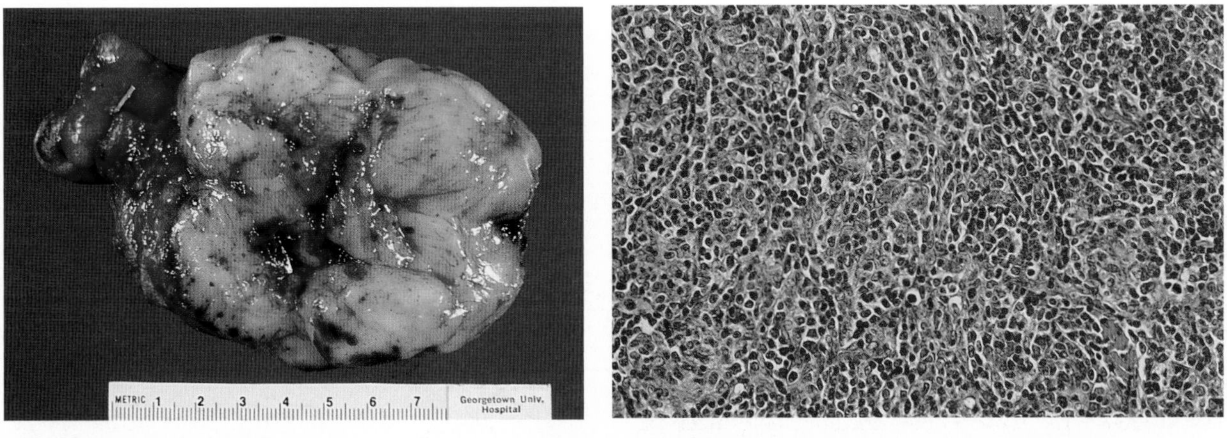

B

FIGURE 20-80. **Thymoma. A**. The tumor in cross section is whitish and has a bulging surface with areas of hemorrhage. Note the attached portion of normal thymus. **B.** Microscopically, the tumor consists of a mixture of neoplastic epithelial cells and nontumorous lymphocytes.

nosarcoma) and a number of other rare patterns. These variants share a distinct epithelial appearance and a mediastinal tumor that lacks this feature is probably not a thymic carcinoma.

CLINICAL FEATURES: Malignant thymoma is treated by surgical excision and radiation therapy. Chemotherapy is added in cases with distant metastases. The prognosis for benign thymoma is excellent and the presence or absence of myasthenic symptoms has little prognostic value. For type I malignant thymomas, prognosis correlates with the extent of disease. Most patients with type II thymomas die within 5 years of diagnosis.

Other Tumors of the Thymus Are Uncommon

NEUROENDOCRINE TUMORS: Several neuroendocrine tumors, which are similar in appearance and natural history to comparable tumors elsewhere, arise in the thymus. These include carcinoids (typical and atypical) and carcinomas (small and large cell). Neuroendocrine tumors are immunoreactive for cytokeratins (AE1/AE3, CAM5.2) and endocrine markers (synaptophysinn, cromogranin, NSE). ACTH may be produced in such tumors that cause Cushing syndrome. Interestingly, nuclear expression of TTF-1 is reportedly negative in many thymic neuroendocrine tumors.

CARCINOID: Thymic carcinoid tumors are malignant and tend to invade locally and metastasize widely, although if well-circumscribed they may be cured by local excision. Interestingly, one third of these patients show Cushing syndrome, but carcinoid syndrome is exceedingly rare. Thymic carcinoid tumors occur both sporadically, in familial forms and may also arise in the context of multiple endocrine neoplasia (MEN)-1 and -2A. Association with neurofibromatosis type I is also described. Most thymic carcinoids are atypical (intermediate category) with frequent mitoses and/or necrosis.

SMALL CELL CARCINOMA: Small cell carcinomas (SCCs), indistinguishable from those in the lung, may also arise in the thymus. Thymic SCCs may be admixed with squamous cell carcinomas.

GERM CELL TUMORS: Thymic germ cell tumors account for 20% of all mediastinal tumors. It is felt that these arise from cells left behind when germ cells migrate during embryogenesis. The histologies of mediastinal germ cell tumors are like those in the gonads (see Chapters 17 and 18). Mature cystic teratoma is most common. Seminoma, embryonal carcinoma, endodermal sinus tumor, teratocarcinoma, immature teratoma, and choriocarcinoma all occur; and mixed germ cell tumors are common. Mediastinal germ cell tumors may on occasion contain a somatic-type malignant component of sarcoma, carcinoma, or hematologic malignancies. Save for mature cystic teratoma, which affects both sexes equally, the other tumors occur mostly in males and thymic seminoma arises only in men. Prognosis is like that of comparable gonadal tumors, except for mediastinal nonseminomatous germ cell tumors, are more aggressive.

Other lesions include benign and malignant stromal tumors. **Thymolipoma** is a benign, well-circumscribed mass composed of mature adipose tissue and unremarkable thymic parenchyma. **Thymic stromal sarcomas** are low-grade malignant mesenchymal tumors with variable morphology, but frequently of liposarcomatous nature.

Nonneoplastic masses include thymic, mesothelial, and enteric-type cysts.

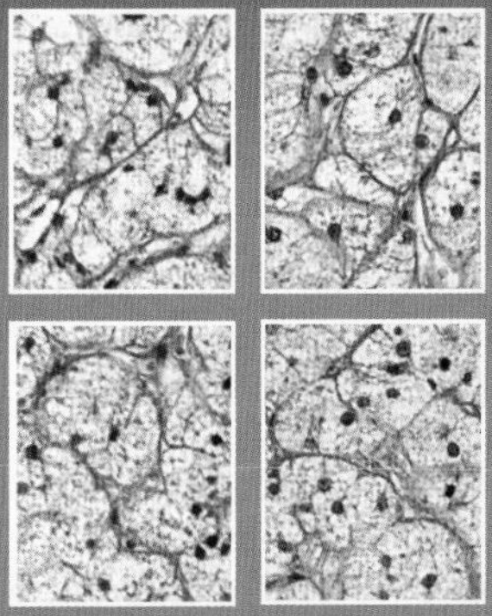

21

The Endocrine System

Maria Merino
Martha Quezado
Emanuel Rubin
Raphael Rubin

The main function of the endocrine system is communication. Although there is some overlap between nervous and endocrine systems in the soluble mediators they use and the functions they serve, the key element of the endocrine system is its ability to communicate at a distance using soluble mediators, hormones.

The term **hormone** (from the Greek, *horman,* "set in motion") applies to chemicals secreted by "ductless" (i.e., endocrine) glands into the circulation, which carries it to the target organ. Many hormones, such as thyroid hormone, corticosteroids, and pituitary hormones, fit this definition. By contrast, some traditionally recognized hormones, such as catecholamines, are produced in a variety of sites and act either locally or through the circulation. Other mediators function only in restricted circulation compartments, e.g., hypothalamic hormones only act on the pituitary and reach it via portal tributaries without entering the systemic circulation. Finally, many hormones exert their effects in the same tissues in which they are formed, such as müllerian-inhibiting substance. These diverse forms of chemically mediated cell-to-cell communication are summarized in Figure 21-1.

To qualify as a hormone, a chemical messenger must bind to a receptor, either on the surface of the cell or within it. Hormones act either on the final effector target or on other glands that in turn produce another hormone. For instance, thyroid hormone acts directly on many types of peripheral cells, whereas thyroid-stimulating hormone (TSH) is released by the pituitary and thereafter promotes thyroid hormone secretion by the thyroid gland. Diseases of the endocrine system may lead to excessive or insufficient production of hormones. In addition, insensitivity of target tissues leads to effects similar to those associated with underproduction of hormones.

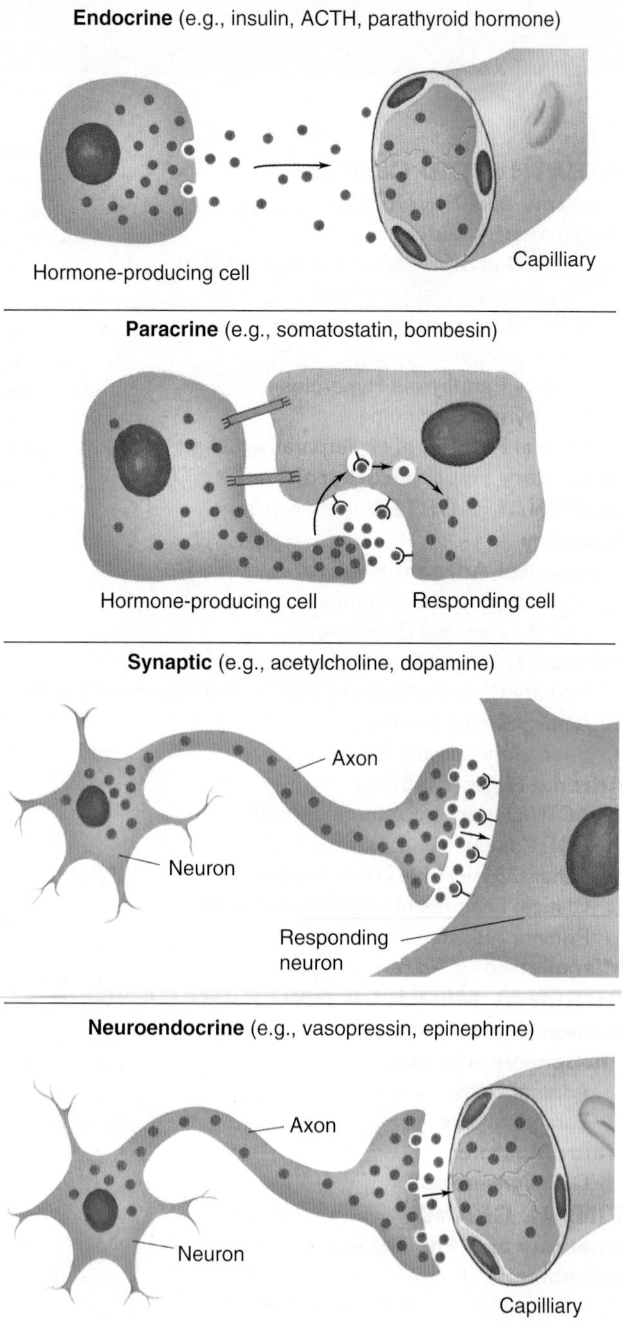

FIGURE 21-1. **Mechanisms of chemically mediated cell-to-cell communication.** Biological messages may be transmitted by mechanisms other than the classic endocrine pathway via the circulation. These include paracrine, synaptic, and neuroendocrine modes of communication.

PITUITARY GLAND

Anatomy

The pituitary gland, also termed the **hypophysis,** sits in the sella turcica, located within the sphenoid bone at the base of the brain. It has two lobes: the **adenohypophysis** or anterior lobe, which comprises 80% of the gland and is populated by epithelial cells and the posterior lobe or **neurohypophysis**, which is a neural structure (Fig. 21-2). The adult human gland is approximately 1.3 × 0.9 × 0.6 cm and weighs 0.6 g. It is near the optic chiasm and cranial nerves III, IV, V, and VI; thus, pituitary tumors may cause partial blindness or various cranial nerve palsies.

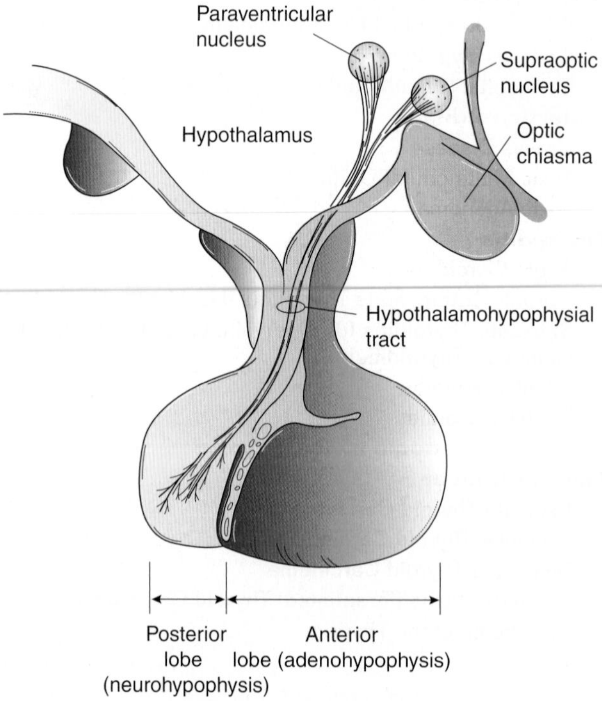

FIGURE 21-2. **The pituitary gland.**

The two lobes of the pituitary are anatomically distinct and derived from different embryologic anlagen. The anterior lobe develops from Rathke's pouch, an endodermal evagination from the developing oral cavity. Along its migration tract, this craniopharyngeal duct may leave intrasphenoidal squamous epithelial rests that may later give rise to tumors known as **craniopharyngiomas**. The neurohypophysis (posterior lobe) begins as a downward projection of the brain and remains connected to the hypothalamus by the hypophyseal stalk. Flanked on either side by the anterior and posterior lobes is the vestigial intermediate lobe, composed of a few cystic cavities lined by cuboidal or columnar epithelium.

The pituitary has a dual circulation, composed of a complex portal system that originates from the hypothalamus, and by a separate arterial and venous blood supply. The hypophysial portal system transports stimulatory and inhibitory hypothalamic-releasing hormones to the anterior pituitary. The venous drainage of the pituitary follows the cavernous sinus to both inferior petrosal sinuses.

Axons and unmyelinated nerve fibers from the hypothalamus proceed along the pituitary stalk to the neurohypophysis and are the nerve supply of the posterior lobe. An important function of these nerves is to regulate secretion of arginine vasopressin (**antidiuretic hormone** [ADH]) and **oxytocin**, which are made in the hypothalamus, stored in the posterior lobe, and later released into the systemic circulation.

Microscopically, the constituent cells of the anterior pituitary are arranged in cords or nests within a highly vascular stroma. On the basis of staining with hematoxylin and eosin (H&E), these cells were classically divided into two groups of equal number: stainable and unstainable cells, the latter termed **chromophobe** cells. The cytoplasmic granules of the stainable cells appeared acidophilic (eosinophilic) (40%) and basophilic (10%). *However, the tinctorial properties of the granules are unrelated to their function, and the histologic classification has been replaced by one that defines cells according to the hormone secreted.* The cellular localization of specific pituitary hormones is determined by immunohistochemical staining methods (Fig. 21-3). The hormone-producing cells in the anterior pituitary are:

- **Corticotrophs:** These basophilic cells secrete proopiomelanocortin (POMC) and its derivatives including adrenocorticotropic hormone (ACTH, corticotropin), which controls adrenal secretion of corticosteroids, melanocyte-stimulating hormone (MSH), lipotropic hormone (LPH), and endorphins. Pituitary corticotrophs, when subjected to glucocorticoid excess, may exhibit a morphologic alteration, the so called Crooke's hyaline change. Basophilic corticotrophs of the **pars intermedia** may cluster and spread deep into the posterior lobe, a phenomenon called "basophil invasion."
- **Lactotrophs:** These acidophilic cells secrete prolactin, which is essential for lactation in addition to numerous other metabolic activities.
- **Somatotrophs:** These acidophilic cells elaborate growth hormone and constitute half of all hormone-producing cells of the adenohypophysis.
- **Thyrotrophs:** TSH is produced by pale basophilic or amphophilic cells, which constitute only 5% of the cells of the anterior lobe.
- **Gonadotrophs:** Follicle-stimulating hormone (FSH) and luteinizing hormone (LH) are secreted by the same basophilic cell. FSH stimulates Graafian follicle formation in the ovary. LH induces ovulation and formation of corpora lutea in the ovary.

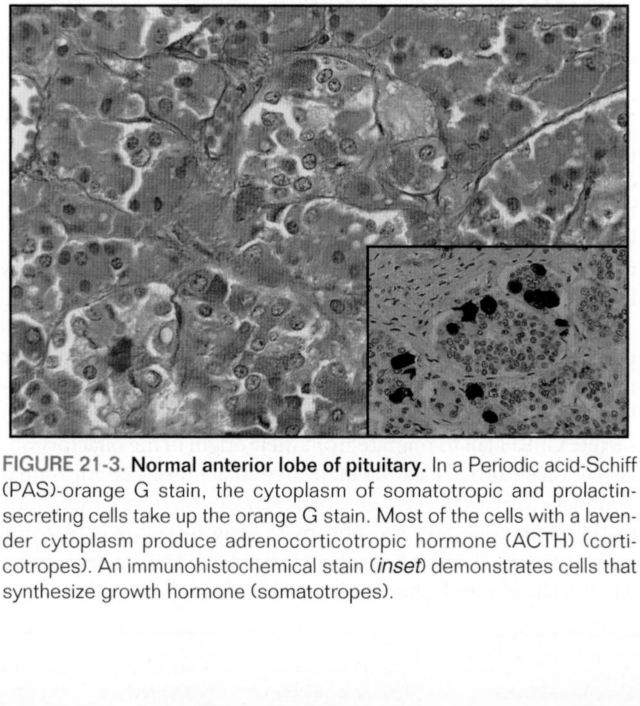

FIGURE 21-3. **Normal anterior lobe of pituitary.** In a Periodic acid-Schiff (PAS)-orange G stain, the cytoplasm of somatotropic and prolactin-secreting cells take up the orange G stain. Most of the cells with a lavender cytoplasm produce adrenocorticotropic hormone (ACTH) (corticotropes). An immunohistochemical stain (*inset*) demonstrates cells that synthesize growth hormone (somatotropes).

Histologically, the posterior lobe of the pituitary is composed of pituicytes, a modified glial cell without secretory function, axon terminals, and unmyelinated nerve fibers containing ADH and oxytocin. Both of these hormones are formed in nerve cell bodies in the hypothalamus and transported along axons to the neurohypophysis. ADH promotes water resorption from the distal renal tubules; oxytocin stimulates the pregnant uterus to contract at term and also stimulates cells around the mammary lactiferous ducts.

Hypopituitarism

Hypopituitarism refers to deficient secretion of one or more of the pituitary hormones. It has many causes and various clinical presentations. Most commonly, only one or a few pituitary hormones are deficient. Occasionally, total failure of pituitary function, **panhypopituitarism,** occurs. The effects of hypopituitarism vary with (1) the extent of the loss, (2) specific hormones involved, and (3) age of the patient. In general, symptoms relate to deficient function of the thyroid and adrenal glands and the reproductive system. In children, growth retardation and delayed puberty are additional problems.

PITUITARY TUMORS: Over half of all hypopituitarism in adults is caused by pituitary tumors, usually adenomas. The tumor itself may be functional, but symptoms of hypopituitarism often result from compression of adjacent tissue by the mass.

SHEEHAN SYNDROME: In this condition, panhypopituitarism is caused by ischemic necrosis of the gland, often due to severe hypotension from postpartum hemorrhage. It may be rarely encountered without massive bleeding or after normal delivery. The pituitary is particularly vulnerable during pregnancy, because of a reduction in blood flow associated with its enlargement at this time. Agalactia, amenorrhea, hypothyroidism, and adrenocortical insufficiency are important consequences (Fig. 21-4). Sheehan syndrome has become rare.

PITUITARY APOPLEXY: Hemorrhage and/or infarction can occur in a normal pituitary, but at least half of cases occur in association with endocrinologically inactive adenomas. On occasion, pituitary apoplexy leads to hypopituitarism.

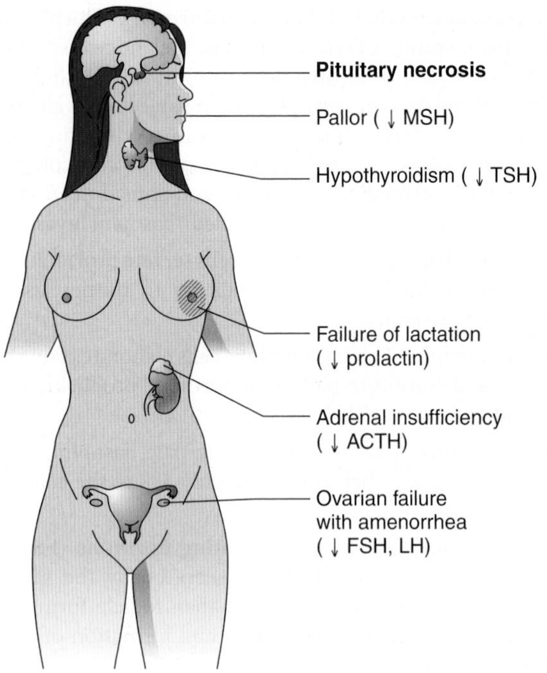

FIGURE 21-4. **Major clinical manifestations of panhypopituitarism.** ACTH = adrenocorticotropic hormone; FSH = follicle-stimulating hormone; LH = luteinizing hormone; MSH = melanocyte-stimulating hormone; TSH = thyroid-stimulating hormone.

IATROGENIC HYPOPITUITARISM: Radiation damage to the hypothalamic-pituitary axis or neurosurgical procedures frequently cause neuroendocrine abnormalities, including hypopituitarism.

TRAUMA: Traumatic brain injury is associated with significant risk to the pituitary gland, with potential development of diabetes, hypopituitarism and other endocrinopathies.

INFILTRATIVE DISEASES: Bacterial and viral infections may lead to inflammation, which can damage the gland. Involvement of the hypothalamic-pituitary axis in Langerhans' cell histiocytosis (see Chapter 20) results in endocrine abnormalities including diabetes insipidus in 5% to 50% of patients and panhypopituitarism in 5% to 20%. Panhypopituitarism may occur in hemochromatosis (see Chapter 14), owing to iron deposition in the pituitary.

GENETIC ABNORMALITIES OF PITUITARY DEVELOPMENT: Congenital growth hormone deficiency constitutes a unique group of disorders. It may occur in isolation, in the so-called **isolated growth hormone deficiency** (IGHD), or in association with other anterior and posterior pituitary hormone deficiencies. Four types of familial and sporadic IGHD have been described. Inheritance can be autosomal recessive (AR), autosomal dominant (AD), or X-linked recessive. Inherited IGHD is linked to mutations, including deletions, amino acid substitutions, and splice site mutations, in the genes for **human growth hormone** (GH) or the growth hormone-releasing hormone (GHRH) receptor. Recombinant GH is the treatment of choice for children with this disorder.

Several mutations targeting transcription factors during embryogenesis have been identified:

- **Pit-1:** Pit-1 is a POU homeodomain transcription factor important for the development of somatotrophs, lactotrophs, and thyrotrophs. It is encoded by the *POU1F1* gene on human chromosome 3p11. Mutations in this gene appear to cause combined pituitary hormone deficiency (CPHD) with low levels or absence of GH, prolactin (PRL), and TSH.
- **PROP1 (5q):** Prop 1 is a pituitary specific paired-like homeodomain transcription factor. Mutations of PROP1 inactivate LH, FSH, GH, PRL, and TSH.
- **HESX1 (3p21):** This gene is a member of the paired-like class of homeobox genes important for development of the optic nerve and the pituitary. Its expression begins before that of other developmental genes. Mutations of *HESX1* gene are seen in patients with septo-optic dysplasia, a rare congenital anomaly characterized by midline forebrain abnormalities, optic nerve hypoplasia, and hypopituitarism. Endocrinopathies are characterized by growth hormone deficiency followed by TSH and ACTH deficiency.
- **PITX2:** This gene is expressed in the fetal pituitary, and in most cells of the adult gland. Mutations are associated with **Rieger syndrome,** an AD condition with variable phenotypic expression including pituitary abnormalities.
- **LX3/LX4:** These genes belong to the LIM family of homeobox genes that are expressed early in Rathke's pouch. *LHX3* is localized to chromosome 9q and mutations are associated with GH, TSH, LH, FSH, and PRL deficiencies. Rarely, mutation of the *LX4* gene may present as GH, TSH, and ACTH deficiency.

GROWTH HORMONE INSENSITIVITY (LARON SYNDROME): Laron dwarfism is a rare, AR form of short stature due to extreme resistance to GH due to abnormalities in growth hormone receptor (GHR). Clinically, these dwarfs tend to be obese and have high levels of serum GH and low concentrations of insulin-like growth factor-I (IGF-I). This condition is seen predominantly in people of Mediterranean origin, especially Sephardic Jews. Interestingly, the same lesion is responsible for the dwarfism of African pygmies.

Laron syndrome is caused by more than 30 *GHR* mutations, all of which involve the extracellular domain of the receptor. Clinical presentation is heterogeneous, and most cases are unique to particular families or geographic areas. Since GH exerts its effects by promoting IGF-I secretion, IGF-I is effective replacement therapy for Laron syndrome, mimicking most effects ascribed to GH itself.

ISOLATED GONADOTROPIN DEFICIENCY (KALLMANN SYNDROME): Kallmann syndrome is characterized by hypogonadotropic hypogonadism (due to gonadotropin-releasing hormone [GnRH] deficiency) and anosmia (absent sense of smell). Cleft lip/palate and other anomalies may also be present. Kallmann syndrome is usually diagnosed at puberty because of a delay in the appearance of secondary sex characteristics. Kallmann syndrome is likely to be three to five times more common in males than females (1:8,000). Most cases are sporadic, although familial forms have been described, some being X-linked and others AD or AR. The X-linked Kallman syndrome (KAL1) is associated with mutations of the *KAL1* gene (Xp23.3), which encodes an extracellular matrix component with putative antiprotease activity and cell adhesion function. As a result of this mutation, neurons destined to secrete GnRH fail to migrate from their origin in the olfactory anlage to their normal location in the hypothalamus. The autosomal dominant form of the disease (KAL2) is associated with mutations of the gene encoding the fibroblast growth factor receptor 1 (8p11). A third form of Kallman syndrome (KAL3) appears to be AR, but the affected gene is not yet identified.

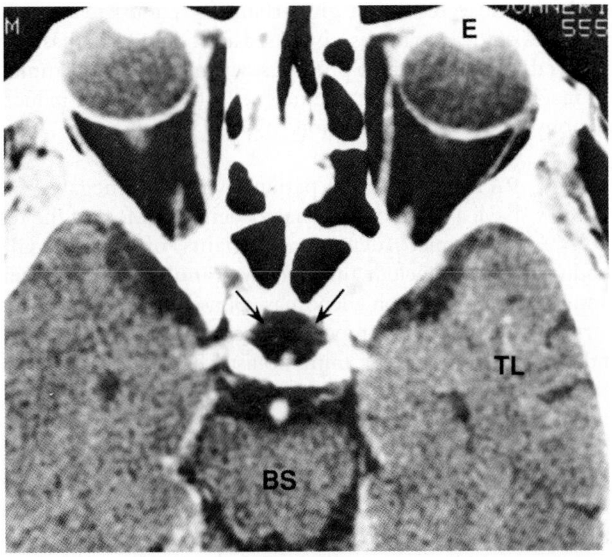

FIGURE 21-5. **Empty sella syndrome.** A computed tomography (CT) scan of the cranium in an axial section demonstrates an empty sella turcica *(arrows)*. *BS*, brainstem. *E*, eye; *TL*, temporal lobe.

EMPTY SELLA SYNDROME: This is primarily a radiologic term that describes an enlarged sella containing a thin, flattened pituitary at the base (Fig. 21-5). It is secondary to a congenitally defective or absent diaphragma sella, which permits transmission of cerebrospinal fluid pressure into the sella. Empty sella syndrome can cause various degrees of pituitary dysfunction and endocrine abnormalities. It has been linked to both pituitary and nonpituitary causes. Endocrine disturbances include hyperprolactinemia, oligomenorrhea or amenorrhea, frank hypopituitarism, acromegaly, diabetes insipidus, and Cushing syndrome.

Pituitary Adenomas

Pituitary adenomas are benign neoplasms of the anterior lobe of the pituitary and are often associated with excess secretion of pituitary hormones and corresponding endocrine hyperfunction (Table 21-1). They occur in both sexes, are more common in adults, comprising only 2% of all adenomas in children. **PRL-producing adenomas** are the most common hormone-secreting tumors of all adults and children. **Gonadotroph adenomas** are more common in the elderly. Small, apparently **nonfunctioning pituitary adenomas** are found incidentally in as many as 27% of adult autopsies.

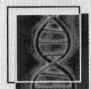

PATHOGENESIS: The etiology of pituitary adenomas is still obscure, but it is clear that its pathogenesis is related to hormonal and genetic factors. Rarely, they occur in the context of multiple endocrine neoplasia (MEN) type 1, a hereditary disposition to the formation of pituitary adenomas, parathyroid hyperplasia or adenoma and islet cell adenomas of the pancreas (see Chapter 15). There is no evidence that mutations of the MEN1 gene are involved in sporadic pituitary tumorigenesis. Acquired activating mutations in the stimulatory subunit of the G_s protein that activates adenylyl cyclase have been reported in 40% of growth hormone-secreting pituitary adenomas. More specifically, elevation of intracellular cyclic adenosine monophosphate (cAMP) levels is thought to stimulate hypersecretion of GH and cell proliferation. Some human pituitary tumors express a kinase-containing variant of fibroblast growth factor/receptor (FGFR4), which causes pituitary tumor formation in transgenic mice. Mutations or overexpression of a number of regulatory genes have been described in a number of pituitary adenomas, including *cyclin D_1, CREB, ras,* and *pituitary tumor transforming* gene.

TABLE 21-1

Frequency of Adenomas of the Anterior Pituitary

Cell Type	Hormone	Frequency (%)
Lactotrope	Prolactin	26
Null cell	None	17
Corticotrope	ACTH (corticotropin)	15
Somatotrope	Growth hormone	14
Plurihormonal	Multiple	13
Gonadotrope	FSH, LH	8
Oncocytoma	None	6
Thyrotrope	TSH	1

ACTH = adrenocorticotropic hormone; FSH = follicle-stimulating hormone; LH = luteinizing hormone; TSH = thyroid-stimulating hormone.

PATHOLOGY: Pituitary adenomas were traditionally classified as either acidophil, basophil, or chromophobe adenomas depending on how constituent cells stained. Acidophil adenomas were associated with overproduction of GH, basophil adenomas with excess secretion of ACTH, and chromophobe adenomas with no endocrine hyperfunction. Since H&E staining properties of the tumor cells does not correlate with the type of hormone secreted, pituitary adenomas are now classified according to the hormone(s) they produce. The 2004 World Health Organization (WHO) classification of pituitary lesions takes in account histologic, histochemical, immunohistochemical, and electron microscopic features.

Pituitary adenomas range from small lesions that do not enlarge the gland to expansive tumors that erode the sella turcica and impinge on adjacent cranial structures (Fig. 21-6). In general, adenomas under 10 mm are referred to as **microadenomas;** larger tumors are **macroadenomas**. Microadenomas are not symptomatic until they secrete hormones. Macroadenomas tend to cause local compressive symptoms, by virtue of their size, and systemic manifestations, as a result of overproduction of hormones.

CLINICAL FEATURES: Pituitary macroadenomas exert a mass effect by impinging on the optic chiasm, causing severe headaches, bitemporal hemianopsia and loss of central vision. Oculomotor palsies occur when a tumor invades the cavernous sinuses. Large adenomas may invade the hypothalamus; interfere with normal hypothalamic input to

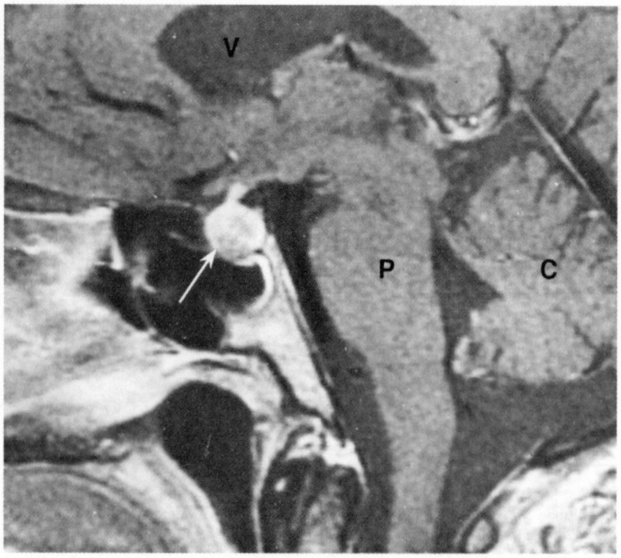

FIGURE 21-6. **Pituitary adenoma.** A magnetic resonance sagittal view of the brain shows a distinct pituitary tumor *(arrow)*. *C*, cerebellum. *P*, pons; *V*, lateral ventricle;

the pituitary; and lead to loss of temperature regulation, hyperphagia, and hormonal syndromes.

Hyperprolactinemia is the Most Common Endocrinopathy Caused by Pituitary Adenomas

Almost half of all pituitary microadenomas contain PRL, but many fewer appear to secrete this hormone. PRL-producing tumors are most often symptomatic in young women, but more than half of all macroadenomas that elaborate PRL are found in men. This difference in sex distribution is related to the more frequent occurrence of endocrine symptoms in women. The true incidence in unselected autopsies is similar in both sexes. In general, larger adenomas secrete more PRL.

PATHOLOGY: Lactotroph adenomas tend to be chromophobic and contain spheroid nuclei with a prominent nucleolus. Endocrine amyloid (see Chapter 23) and psammoma bodies (calcospherites) are seen but are not pathognomonic. Lactotroph adenomas stain for PRL in a dot-like "Golgi pattern" by immunohistochemistry.

CLINICAL FEATURES: In women, functional lactotroph adenomas lead to amenorrhea, galactorrhea, and infertility. The consistently elevated blood PRL levels inhibit the surge of pituitary LH necessary for ovulation. Men tend to suffer from decreased libido and impotence. Functional lactotroph microadenomas are successfully treated with dopamine agonists (bromocriptine) to inhibit PRL secretion, whereas macroadenomas may require surgery or radiation therapy. Excess PRL secretion may be caused by factors other than pituitary adenomas, including pregnancy, lactation, administration of certain drugs, or pressure on the hypothalamus by other tumors.

Somatotrope Adenomas Secrete Growth Hormone

Dramatic changes result from excess secretion of GH. A somatotroph adenoma that arises in a child or adolescent before epiphyses close results in **gigantism**. By contrast, after the epiphyses of the long bones have fused and adult height has been achieved, the same tumor produces **acromegaly**. Most tumors are macroadenomas and cause mass effects and tumor-induced adenohypophyseal hypofunction.

PATHOLOGY: In patients with acromegaly, 75% have a somatotroph macroadenoma. Most of the rest have microadenomas. Variants of isolated GH-producing tumors include the **densely granulated** and **sparsely granulated** somatotroph adenomas. Densely granulated somatotroph adenomas are composed of acidophilic cells (Fig. 21-7) and exhibit strong, diffuse immunohistochemical reactivity for GH. Acidophilic somatotroph adenomas usually grow slowly and remain within the sella. Sparsely granulated adenomas are composed of chromophobe cells which show characteristic spheroid cytoplasmic inclusions known as "fibrous bodies" that are comprised of keratin intermediate filaments, especially keratin 8. The chromophobic variant is typically faster growing and invasive, and microscopically manifests cellular and nuclear pleomorphism.

In **mixed somatotroph-lactotroph adenomas** the two cell types elaborate GH and PRL, respectively. **Mammosomatotroph adenomas** are monomorphous with a single cell type expressing both GH and PRL. **Acidophil stem cell adenomas** are monomorphous, slightly acidophilic tumors with nuclear pleomorphism and large cytoplasmic vacuoles. Key features include giant mitochondria, keratin 8-positive fibrous bodies, and misplaced exocytosis. This subtype is clinically more aggressive.

CLINICAL FEATURES: Acromegaly is uncommon, with an annual incidence of three cases per million. Over many years, patients with acromegaly gradually develop coarse facial features (Fig. 21-8), with overgrowth of the mandible (prognathism) and maxilla, increased space between upper incisor teeth, and a thickened nose. Hands and feet are often enlarged and hat size increases.

Acromegaly has serious complications. Cardiovascular, cerebrovascular, and respiratory deaths are increased. Most acromegalics have neurologic and musculoskeletal symptoms, including headaches, paresthesias, arthralgias, and muscle weakness. One-third have hypertension, and even half of normotensive acromegalics have increased left ventricular mass and are at risk

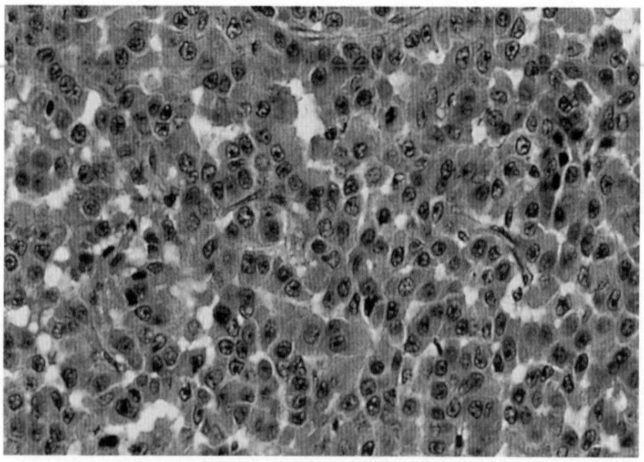

FIGURE 21-7. **Pituitary somatotrope adenoma from a man with acromegaly.** The tumor cells are arranged in thin cords and ribbons.

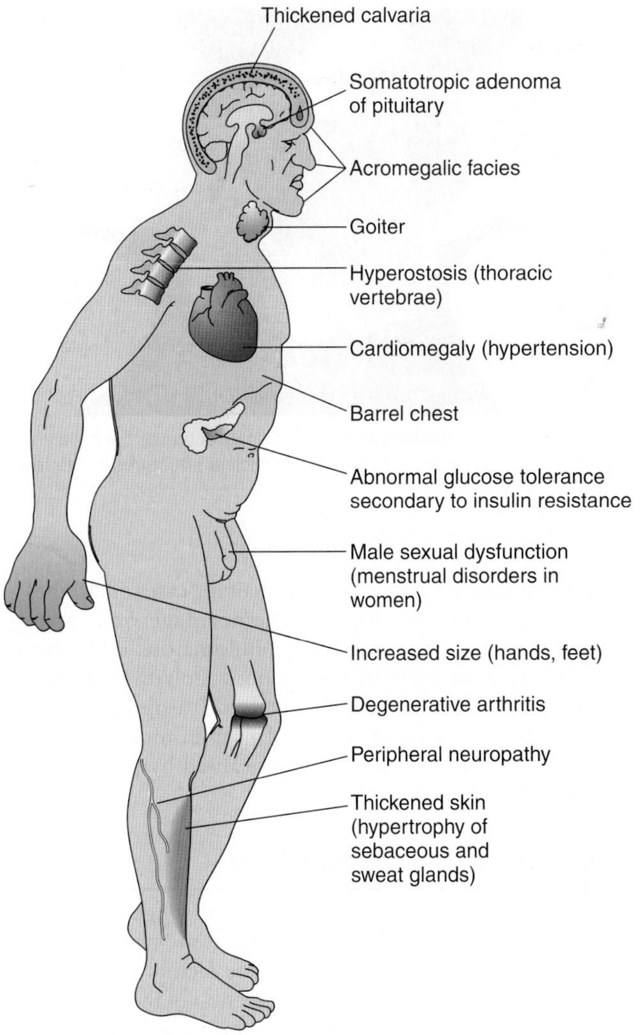

FIGURE 21-8. **Clinical manifestations of acromegaly.**

for congestive heart failure. Visceral hypertrophy is common. Diabetes occurs in as many as 20%, and hypercalciuria and renal stones are present in another fifth of patients. In half of patients with acromegaly, hyperprolactinemia is severe enough to be symptomatic (see above).

Treatment for somatotroph adenomas is usually trans-sphenoidal hypophysectomy, after which circulating GH levels may decline to normal levels within hours. Radiation therapy is an alternative when surgery is contraindicated. A long-acting analogue of somatostatin, an antagonist of GH, is a useful therapeutic adjunct.

Corticotrope Adenomas Produce ACTH

ACTH excess induces adrenal cortical hypersecretion to produce **Cushing disease** (see below). In most cases, the tumor is a microadenoma that is intensely basophilic and periodic acid–Schiff (PAS)-positive. Immunohistochemistry demonstrates ACTH and related peptides, such as endorphins and lipotropin. A few functional corticotroph adenomas are chromophobic and more aggressive than their basophilic counterparts.

By electron microscopy, basophilic adenomas contain numerous secretory granules and perinuclear bundles of fine, keratin-positive, intermediate filaments (type I filaments). These filaments may be abundant enough to be visible by light microscopy as **Crooke hyalinization**, a change related to the suppression of ACTH secretion by high levels of circulating cortisol. **Crooke's adenomas** represent ACTH-producing tumors with massive cell hyaline deposition.

Gonadotrope Adenoma Secretes LH and FSH

Most of these tumors are macroadenomas, hormonally inactive, and are detected either incidentally or due to compressive effects. Clinical presentations include headache, visual disturbance, and hypopituitarism.

In general, gonadotrope adenomas are chromophobic and PAS-negative. Tumor cells are strongly immunopositive for FSH, LH, or both. Treatment is surgical resection.

Thyrotrope Adenomas Produce TSH

Thyrotrope adenomas are the rarest of all pituitary adenomas, and come to medical attention when there are symptoms of hyperthyroidism, goiter, or apituitary mass lesion. Circulating levels of TSH and thyroid hormone are usually elevated, a situation unique to this tumor. Thyrotroph adenomas are chromophobic, with polyhedral or columnar cells forming collars around blood vessels. They stain for α and β-TSH. By electron microscopy, secretory granules are often arranged in a single row immediately beneath the plasma membrane.

In patients with long-standing hypothyroidism, hyperplasia of pituitary thyrotrophs (thyroid deficiency cells) is a well-described entity and is presumably secondary to inadequate feedback inhibition by thyroid hormones.

Nonfunctional Pituitary Adenomas Do Not Cause Endocrinopathies

One-quarter of pituitary tumors removed surgically do not secrete excess hormones. They are slowly growing macroadenomas diagnosed in older persons due to mass effect.

Null cell adenomas are usually chromophobic, PAS-negative, and exhibit a pseudo-papillary growth pattern. By immunochemistry, tumor cells are negative for all anterior pituitary hormones or display a few immunoreactive cells. They are typically immunoreactive for chromogranin A and synaptophysin.

Oncocytoma is a variant of nonfunctional null cell adenoma characterized by enlarged, eosinophilic and often granular cells. By electron microscopy, the neoplastic cells are packed with mitochondria but are otherwise similar to other null cell adenomas.

Silent adenomas are distinguished from other nonfunctional pituitary adenomas by a well-differentiated ultrastructural appearance, and in many cases, immunoreactivity for ACTH and other hormones.

PLURIHORMONAL ADENOMAS: These unusual adenomas produce a variety of pituitary hormones. The most frequent combinations include GH, PRL, and one or more glycoprotein hormone subunits. The aggressive subtype 3 has a unique ultrastructural profile and expresses PRL and TSH staining.

PITUITARY CARCINOMAS: Distinction of pituitary adenoma from carcinoma based on morphology is not possible. Pituitary carcinoma implies the existence of cerebrospinal and/or systemic metastases. When functional, pituitary carcinomas primarily secrete PRL or ACTH.

Posterior Pituitary

Central diabetes insipidus (Fig. 21-9) is the only significant disease associated with the posterior pituitary. It is characterized by an inability to concentrate urine and consequent chronic water diuresis (polyuria), thirst, and polydipsia caused by deficiency of ADH (vasopressin). ADH is secreted by the posterior pituitary under the influence of the hypothalamus. One third of cases of central diabetes insipidus are of unknown etiology or can be attributed to sporadic or familial mutations in the vasopressin–neurophysin II gene. Currently, more than 35 mutations have been linked to familial neurohypophysial diabetes insipidus. Mutations or deletions in the vasopressin V2-receptor (Xq28) and the vasopressin-sensitive aquaporin-2 water channel genes have also been described in the context of **nephrogenic diabetes insipidus.**

One fourth of cases of central diabetes insipidus are associated with brain tumors, particularly **craniopharyngioma** (Fig. 21-10). This tumor arises above the sella turcica from remnants of Rathke pouch and invades and compresses adjacent tissues (see Chapter 28). Trauma and hypophysectomy for anterior pituitary tumors account for most remaining cases of diabetes insipidus. Uncommonly, localized hemorrhage or infarction, Langerhans cell histiocytosis or granulomatous infiltrates involve the posterior pituitary stalk or body. Polyuria may be controlled by powdered posterior pituitary or vasopressin given as snuff. Ectopic secretion of ADH and a syndrome of inappropriate ADH secretion (SIADH) may be caused by paraneoplastic secretion of ADH by tumor cells.

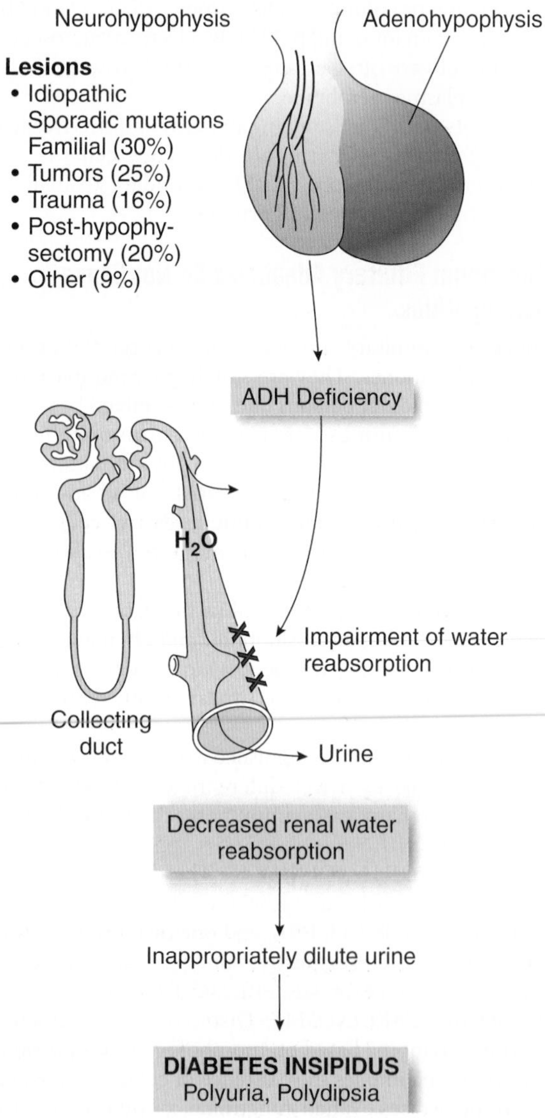

FIGURE 21-9. **Mechanism of diabetes insipidus.**

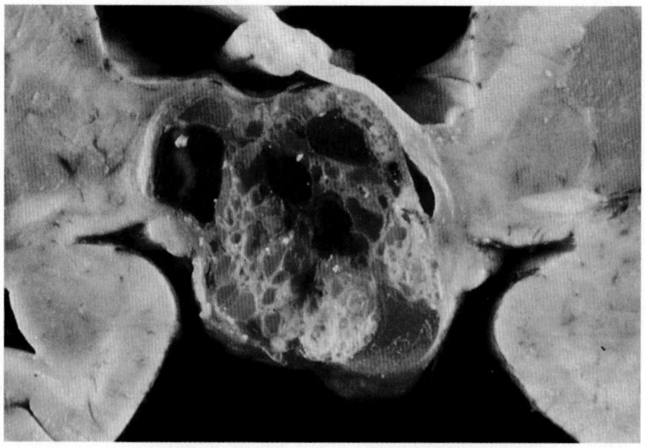

FIGURE 21-10. **Craniopharyngioma.** Coronal section of the brain shows a large, cystic tumor mass replacing the midline structures in the region of the hypothalamus.

Hypothalamic–Pituitary Axis

The hypothalamus, pituitary stalk, and pituitary gland constitute an anatomically and functionally integrated "neuroendocrine system." Hypothalamic neurons secrete factors that stimulate the anterior pituitary (Table 21-2). Secretion of these hypothalamic factors is, in turn, antagonized by hormones secreted by the peripheral target organs, thereby completing the feedback loop. Specific hypothalamic inhibitory hormones have also been identified. For example, dopamine inhibits pituitary PRL secretion.

The hypothalamus may be damaged by a variety of primary and metastatic tumors, viral infections and granulomatous inflammations, as well as several degenerative and hereditary disorders. In many instances, hypothalamic dysfunction occurs without an identifiable anatomical abnormality. Diverse conditions result from disturbances of hypothalamic function and include, among others, hypogonadism, precocious puberty, amenorrhea, and eating disorders (obesity or anorexia). Some pituitary disorders characterized by increased or decreased hormone secretion have their origin in hypothalamic dysfunction. A detailed description of the hypothalamic syndromes is beyond the scope of this chapter, and the reader is referred to additional sources under "Suggested Reading."

THYROID GLAND

Anatomy

The thyroid is one of the largest endocrine organs. It forms early in fetal life and can be recognized as early as 24 days of development. The primitive thyroid descends to its eventual location in the lower anterior neck by elongation of its tubular attachment to

TABLE 21-2
Hormones of the Hypothalamic-Pituitary-Target Gland Axis

Hypothalamus	Pituitary	Target Gland	Peripheral Inhibitory Hormone
CRH	ACTH	Adrenal	Corticosteroids
TRH	TSH	Thyroid	T_3, T_4
GHRH	Growth hormone	Varied	IGF-I
Somatostatin	Growth hormone	Varied	IGF-I
LHRH	LH FSH	Gonads Gonads	Estradiol, testosterone Inhibin, estradiol, testosterone
Dopamine	Prolactin	Breast	Unknown

CRH = corticotropin (ACTH)-releasing hormone; GHRH = growth hormone-releasing hormone; IGF-I = insulin-like growth factor-I; LHRH = luteinizing hormone-releasing hormone; T_3 = triiodothyronine; T_4 = tetraiodothyronine (thyroxine); TRH = thyrotropin-releasing hormone.

the tongue, the thyroglossal duct, which then atrophies around the seventh week of life. The adult thyroid has two lobes connected by an isthmus, and is situated below the thyroid cartilage anterior to the trachea. Each lobe is about 4 cm in greatest dimension. The entire gland weighs 25 to 35 g. The cut surface has a glistening, light brown, lobulated appearance. In its early development, the gland contains cords of cells that will give origin to the follicles or acini which constitute the functional unit of the thyroid gland. Follicles average about 200 μm in diameter and are formed by a single row of cuboidal cells surrounded by a delicate basement membrane. Approximately 20 to 40 follicles comprise a thyroid lobule, supplied by a lobular artery and sustained by a diffuse mesh of fibrous stroma, lymphatics, and connective tissue. The follicles eventually become filled by an eosinophilic, proteinaceous material called **colloid.** This substance represents secreted thyroglobulin, from which active thyroid hormones are released.

In addition to follicular epithelial cells, the thyroid also contains **parafollicular** or **C cells**, in the lateral aspects of the upper portion of both thyroid lobes and in close proximity with the follicles. C cells produce calcitonin, a calcium-lowering hormone. C cells are difficult to identify using routine stains, but they are readily seen by immunostaining for calcitonin. They also express neuroendocrine markers.

Thyroid Function

The main function of the thyroid gland is to make the thyroid hormones triiodothyronine (T_3) and tetraiodothyronine (thyroxine, T_4). T_4 is principally a prohormone; the major effector of thyroid function is T_3. These molecules are formed by iodination of tyrosines in thyroglobulin by the follicular cells. Iodinated thyroglobulin is then secreted into the lumen of the follicle. Alone among endocrine glands, the thyroid can store a large amount of preformed hormone.

On demand, thyroglobulin is reabsorbed by follicular cells. T_4 and T_3 are then liberated by proteolytic cleavage and released into the blood. Most secreted hormone is T_4, which is de-iodinated in peripheral tissues to its more active form, T_3. Thyroid hormones in the blood are both free and bound to thyronine-binding globulin (TBG). Peripheral cells take up only free hormone, which binds to nuclear receptors and initiates specific protein synthesis.

Thyroid hormone affects almost all organs. It stimulates basal metabolic rate and metabolism of carbohydrates, lipids, and proteins. It increases body heat and hepatic glucose production by increasing gluconeogenesis and glycogenolysis. It promotes synthesis of many structural proteins, enzymes, and other hormones. Glucose use, fatty acid synthesis in the liver, and adipose tissue lipolysis are all increased. In general, thyroid hormone upregulates the body's overall metabolic activities, both anabolic and catabolic.

Thyroid structure and function are governed principally by pituitary TSH. In turn, thyroid hormone suppresses TSH secretion, to complete a feedback loop. Maintenance of normal thyroid hormone production depends on an adequate dietary supply of iodine.

Congenital Anomalies

THYROID AGENESIS: Complete absence of thyroid tissue (athyrosis) is a rare congenital abnormality, usually not discovered until several weeks after birth because of maternal thyroid hormone supplies the fetus through the placenta.

ECTOPIC THYROID: Thyroid tissue can be found outside the thyroid gland in a variety of locations as a result of abnormal migration during development These tissues are functionally normal and capable of producing thyroid hormone. Malignant tumors can develop from the displaced thyroid tissue.

LATERAL ABERRANT THYROID: This term describes the presence of thyroid tissue located lateral to the jugular veins. Ectopic thyroid tissue may occur in lymph nodes and soft tissue adjacent to the normal gland. The origin of lateral aberrant thyroid is controversial. Some hold that all of these cases actually represent well-differentiated metastases from an occult thyroid cancer, while others see them as embryonal rests lateral to the thyroid. If the aberrant thyroid tissue is histologically malignant (see below) then the lesion should be considered a metastasis.

LINGUAL THYROID: If the thyroid fails to descend during embryogenesis, it remains at its origin as a nodule at the base of the tongue. This happens more in females and usually is found because of difficulty in swallowing, speaking, or breathing. Removal may result in total hypothyroidism. These tissues resemble normal thyroid histologically.

HETEROTOPIC THYROID TISSUE: Nests of thyroid tissue may be found anywhere along the pathway of its descent into the lower neck. Thyroid tissue is also occasionally encountered in the pericardium or mediastinum.

THYROGLOSSAL DUCT CYST: Failure of a thyroglossal duct to involute completely can result in a cystic, fluid-filled remnant anywhere along the route of the duct. This condition affects patients in all age groups. It presents as cystic masses of variable size (1 to 4 cm) often in the middle of the neck and attached to the hyoid bone or soft tissues. The cysts can be lined by squamous or respiratory-type epithelium, and contain variable amounts of thyroid tissue. Malignant tumors can develop in the cysts, usually papillary carcinoma. Surgical excision is curative.

Nontoxic Goiter

Goiter refers to thyroid gland enlargement, either nodular or diffuse. It is classified according to its function.

Nontoxic goiter *(from the Latin,* guttur, *"throat"), also termed simple, colloid, or multinodular goiter, is enlargement of the thyroid without functional, inflammatory, or neoplastic alterations.* Thus, patients with nontoxic goiter are euthyroid and do not suffer from any form of thyroiditis (see below). The disease is far more common in women than in men (8:1). Diffuse goiter is frequent in adolescence and during pregnancy, whereas the multinodular type usually occurs in persons older than 50 years.

PATHOGENESIS: In nontoxic goiter, the capacity of the thyroid to produce thyroid hormone is impaired. Resulting increased secretion of TSH leads to enlargement of the gland, which maintains the euthyroid state. The etiology of the decrease in thyroid hormone production is unknown.

Simple nodular thyroid enlargement tends to be familial, suggesting a genetic factor in the disorder. Indeed, mutations in the thyroglobulin gene have been detected in a number of families affected by simple goiter. Goiters can develop in patients receiving a variety of medications such as sulfonamides or having an excess of iodine intake.

PATHOLOGY: Nontoxic goiters range from double the size of a normal gland (40 g) to massive thyroid weighing hundreds of grams (Fig. 21-11).

Diffuse nontoxic goiter characterizes the early stages of the disease. The gland is diffusely enlarged and microscopically exhibits hypertrophy and hyperplasia of the follicular epithelial cells. On occasion, the epithelium is papillary. At this stage, the amount of colloid in the follicles is decreased.

Multinodular nontoxic goiter reflects more chronic disease. The enlarged gland becomes increasingly nodular, and the cut surface is typically studded with numerous irregular nodules. When these nodules contain large amounts of colloid, the thyroid tends to be soft, glistening, and reddish. Microscopically, nodules vary considerably in size and shape. Some are distended with colloid; others are collapsed. Large colloid-containing follicles may fuse to form even larger "colloid cysts." Lining epithelial cells are flat to cuboidal and are occasionally arrayed as papillae that project into the follicular lumen. Hemosiderin deposition and cholesterol granulomas

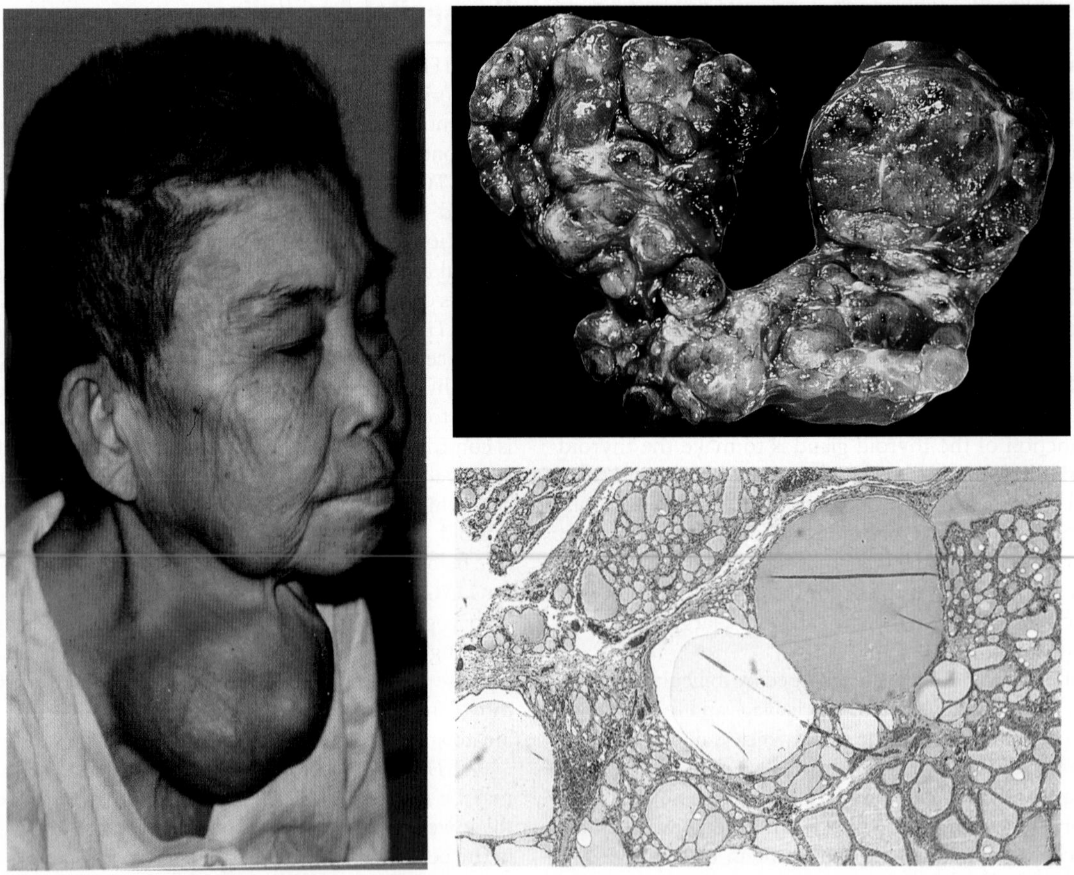

A B C

FIGURE 21-11. Nontoxic goiter. A. In a middle-aged woman with nontoxic goiter, the thyroid has enlarged to produce a conspicuous neck mass. **B.** Coronal section of the enlarged thyroid gland shows numerous irregular nodules, some with cystic degeneration and old hemorrhage. **C.** Microscopic view of one of the macroscopic nodules shows marked variation in the size of the follicles.

are evidence of old hemorrhage. The individual follicles or groups of follicles are separated by dense fibrosis and dystrophic calcifications. Hemorrhage and chronic inflammation are common.

CLINICAL FEATURES: Patients with nontoxic goiter are typically asymptomatic and come to medical attention because of a mass in the neck. Large goiters may cause dysphagia or inspiratory stridor by compressing the esophagus or trachea. Pressure on neck veins leads to venous congestion of the head and face. Hoarseness may result from recurrent laryngeal nerve compression. Occasionally, hemorrhage into a nodule or cyst leads to local pain. Blood concentrations of T_4, T_3, and (usually) TSH are normal.

Nontoxic goiter is most commonly treated with thyroid hormone to reduce TSH levels and, thus, the stimulation to thyroid growth. In older patients with low TSH levels, further suppression by exogenous thyroid hormone may be ineffective, and radioactive iodine therapy is indicated. Surgery is ordinarily contraindicated, but may be necessary if local obstructive symptoms become troublesome. Many patients with nontoxic goiter eventually develop hyperthyroidism, in which case the term **toxic multinodular goiter** is applied (see below).

Hypothyroidism

Hypothyroidism refers to the clinical manifestations of thyroid hormone deficiency. It can be the consequence of three general processes:

- **Defective thyroid hormone synthesis,** with compensatory goitrogenesis (goitrous hypothyroidism)
- **Inadequate thyroid parenchyma function,** usually due to thyroiditis, surgical resection of the gland, or therapeutic administration of radioiodine
- **Inadequate secretion of TSH** by the pituitary or of thyroid-releasing hormone (TRH) by the hypothalamus

Symptoms of hypothyroidism reflect decreased circulating thyroid hormone (Fig. 21-12). They develop insidiously. Often the first manifestations are tiredness, lethargy, sensitivity to cold, and inability to concentrate. Many organ systems are affected, but all are hypofunctional. Hypothyroidism is treated effectively with thyroid hormone.

SKIN: Alterations in the skin are almost universal in patients with clinically apparent hypothyroidism. Proteoglycans accumulate in the extracellular matrix and bind water, resulting in a peculiar form of edema termed **myxedema**. Myxedematous patients have boggy facies, puffy eyelids, edema of the hands and feet, and enlarged tongues. Thickening of the mucous membranes of the larynx causes patients to be hoarse. A pale, cool skin reflects cutaneous vasoconstriction. The skin is also dry and coarse, because sebaceous and sweat gland secretions are inadequate. Ecchymoses are common because of increased capillary fragility. Skin wounds heal slowly.

NERVOUS SYSTEM: Hypothyroidism in pregnancy has grave neurologic consequences for the fetus, expressed after birth as cretinism (see below). Hypothyroid adults are lethargic and somnolent, show memory loss and slowed mental processes. Psychiatric symptoms are prominent: paranoid ideation and depression are common. Severe agitation, **myxedema madness,** may develop. Sensory defects, including deafness and night blindness, occur. Cerebellar ataxia may appear and tendon reflexes are slow. Microscopically, the brain shows mucinous accumulations in nerve fibers and in the cerebellum.

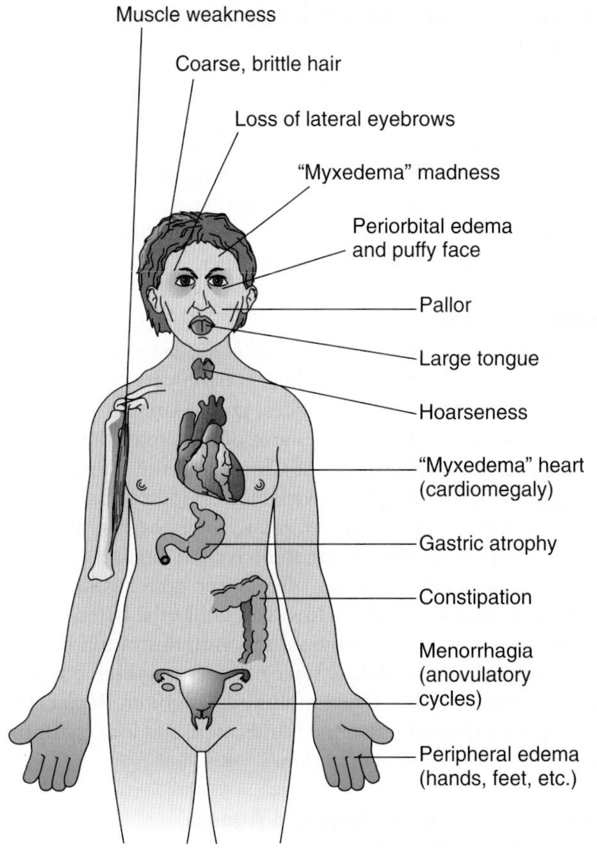

FIGURE 21-12. **Dominant clinical manifestations of hypothyroidism.**

HEART: In early hypothyroidism the heart rate and stroke volume are reduced, resulting in decreased cardiac output. In untreated hypothyroidism, so-called **myxedema heart** develops, which is characterized by a dilated heart and a pericardial effusion. On pathologic examination, the heart is flabby and microscopically shows interstitial edema and swelling of the myocytes. Coronary atherosclerosis is a common finding.

GASTROINTESTINAL TRACT: Constipation, owing to decreased peristalsis, is common, and may be severe enough to lead to fecal impaction (**myxedema megacolon).**

REPRODUCTIVE SYSTEM: Women with hypothyroidism suffer ovulatory failure, progesterone deficiency, and irregular and excessive menstrual bleeding. In men, erectile dysfunction and oligospermia are common.

Primary (Idiopathic) Hypothyroidism Is Often Autoimmune

Primary hypothyroidism is most common in the fifth and sixth decades and, like most thyroid disorders, is more common in women than in men. Three-fourths of patients have circulating antibodies to thyroid antigens, suggesting that these cases represent the end stage of autoimmune thyroiditis (see below). Nongoitrous hypothyroidism may also result from antibodies that block TSH or TSH receptor without activating the thyroid. Some cases of primary hypothyroidism are part of multiglandular autoimmune syndrome, including insulin-dependent diabetes, pernicious anemia, hypoparathyroidism, adrenal atrophy, and hypogonadism (see below).

Goitrous Hypothyroidism Reflects Inadequate Secretion of Thyroid Hormone

There are a number of conditions in which thyroid enlargement (goiter) is associated with hypothyroidism. The etiology of goitrous hypothyroidism includes iodine deficiency, antithyroid agents (drugs or dietary goitrogens), long-term iodide intake, and a number of hereditary defects in thyroid hormone synthesis. *The evolution of the pathology of goitrous hypothyroidism is similar to that described earlier for nontoxic goiter.*

Endemic Goiter

Endemic goiter is goitrous hypothyroidism due to dietary iodine deficiency in locales with a high prevalence of the disease. Salt water and seafood are rich sources of iodides, goiters are (or were) common far inland. The Great Lakes area of the United States, alpine Europe, central Africa, parts of China, and the Himalayas are such places. The widespread availability of iodized salt has eliminated endemic goiter in many areas. Nevertheless, more than 200 million persons worldwide still have the disease.

The pathologic evolution of endemic goiter is like that of nontoxic goiter (see above). However, unlike the latter, endemic goiter rarely causes hyperthyroidism. Administration of iodine may reverse the early, diffuse stage of endemic goiter, but has little effect on a fully developed multinodular goiter. Replacement therapy with thyroid hormone is indicated, and local symptoms may necessitate surgical resection.

Goiter Induced by Antithyroid Agents

A number of drugs and naturally occurring chemicals in foods suppress thyroid hormone synthesis and so are goitrogenic. Such goiters may or may not be associated with hypothyroidism. Common goitrogenic drugs include **lithium,** which is used to manage manic-depressive states, phenylbutazone, and *p*-aminosalicylic acid. Certain cruciferous vegetables (turnips, rutabaga, cassava) contain goitrogens, and their ingestion can potentiate an iodine-deficient diet to produce goitrous hypothyroidism.

Iodide-Induced Goiter

Goiter and/or hypothyroidism may occur in persons who consume large amounts of iodide, either as a medicinal component (potassium iodide-containing expectorants) or in foods particularly rich in this halide (e.g., seaweed in Japan). In most cases, iodide-induced goiter develops in the context of preexisting thyroid disease, such as thyroiditis. Women given large doses of iodine during pregnancy may deliver goitrous infants.

Congenital Hypothyroidism Is Also Termed Cretinism

Cretinism may be endemic, sporadic, or familial and is twice as frequent in girls as boys. In nonendemic regions, 90% of cases result from developmental defects of the thyroid (**thyroid dysgenesis**). The remainder principally have a variety of inherited metabolic defects, including mutations in the genes for TRH and its receptor, TSH and its receptor, sodium-iodide symporter, thyroglobulin, and thyroid oxidase.

CLINICAL FEATURES: Symptoms of congenital hypothyroidism appear in the early weeks of life. Infants are apathetic and sluggish. Their abdomens are large and often show umbilical hernias. Body temperatures are often below 35°C (95°F), and the skin is pale and cold. Refractory anemia and a dilated heart are frequent. By the age of 6 months, the clinical syndrome of congenital hypothyroidism is well developed. Mental retardation, stunted growth (owing to defective osseous maturation), and characteristic facies are evident. Serum T_4 and T_3 are low, and TSH levels are high (unless the problem relates to a lack of TSH secretion itself).

Prompt thyroid hormone replacement therapy is needed to prevent mental retardation and stunted growth. Although treatment may prevent dwarfism, its effects on mental development are more variable. Children in whom hypothyroidism is detected early with neonatal screening respond well to thyroid hormone treatment and are apparently normal mentally. Delayed treatment leads to irreversible brain damage.

***Endemic cretinism** refers to congenital hypothyroidism in areas of endemic goiter.* Both parents are usually goitrous. The disease encompasses two overlapping clinical presentations, a neurologic syndrome and a predominantly hypothyroid one.

- **Neurologic cretinism** features mental retardation, ataxia, spasticity, and deaf-mutism. In the pure form of neurologic cretinism, children may be of normal stature and virtually euthyroid. It is postulated that iodine deficiency in the first trimester of pregnancy damages the developing nervous system independently of its effect on thyroid hormone production.
- **Hypothyroid cretinism** is thought to arise from iodine deficiency in late fetal life and in the neonatal period. The clinical course in these children is similar to that of other forms of congenital hypothyroidism.

Hyperthyroidism

Hyperthyroidism refers to the clinical consequences of excessive circulating thyroid hormone. In general, signs and symptoms of hyperthyroidism reflect a hypermetabolic state of target tissues. Prolonged hypersecretion of thyroid hormone can result from (1) of abnormal thyroid stimulator (Graves disease), (2) intrinsic disease of the thyroid gland (toxic multinodular goiter or functional adenoma), and (3) excess TSH production by a pituitary adenoma (rare).

Graves Disease Is the Most Common Cause of Hyperthyroidism in Young Adults

Also known as **Basedow disease** in continental Europe, Graves disease is an autoimmune disorder characterized by diffuse goiter, hyperthyroidism, exophthalmos (Fig. 21-13), and dermopathy. It is the most prevalent autoimmune disease in the United States, affecting 0.5% to 1% of the population under 40 years of age.

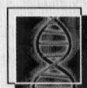

PATHOGENESIS: The etiology of Graves disease is not fully understood and seems to involve an interplay between immune mechanisms, heredity, sex, and possibly emotional factors.

IMMUNE MECHANISMS: Patients have immunoglobulin (Ig)G antibodies that bind to the TSH receptor on the plasma membrane of thyrocytes (Fig. 21-14). These antibodies act as agonists; that is, they stimulate the TSH receptor, thereby activating adenylyl cyclase and increasing thyroid hormone secretion. Under this continued stimulation, the thyroid becomes diffusely hyperplastic and excessively vascular.

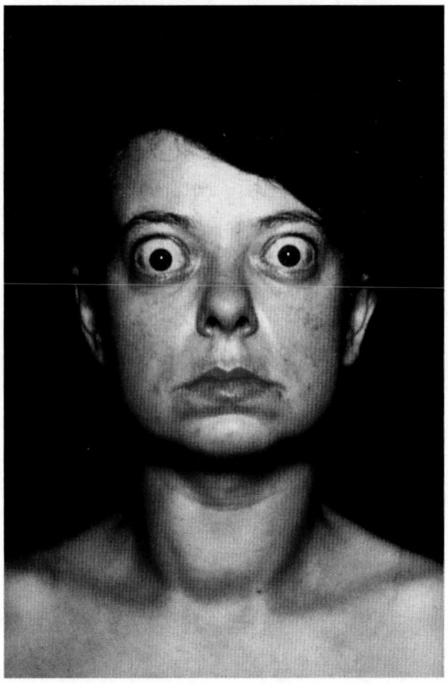

FIGURE 21-13. Graves disease. A young woman with hyperthyroidism displays a mass in the neck and exophthalmos.

Elaboration of thyroid-stimulating antibodies requires thyroid-specific helper (CD4+) T cells that recognize multiple epitopes of the TSH receptor and stimulate autoreactive B cells. These then produce thyroid-stimulating immunoglobulins. Graves autoantibodies are heterogeneous, of which those that stimulate thyroid hormone secretion represent only one component. Other antibodies seem to be cytotoxic and may account for the thyroid failure that often follows long-standing Graves disease. These include antibodies against thyroglobulin, thyroid peroxidase, and the sodium–iodide symporter, all of which may also play roles in the pathogenesis of chronic lymphocytic thyroiditis (Hashimoto disease; see below). Patients with Graves disease have decreased levels of suppressor CD8+ cells, which may play a role in the lack of immune tolerance.

GENETIC FACTORS: The strongest risk factor for Graves disease is a positive family history. No single gene is responsible or is necessary for Graves disease, and the concordance rate in monozygotic twins is only 30% to 50%, while in dizygotic twins it is merely 5%. Thus, both genetic and environmental factors are probably involved. With respect to the genetic contribution, human leukocyte antigen (HLA) class II molecules exposed on thyrocytes (e.g., HLA-DR3, HLA-DQA1) have been established as susceptibility loci, with a number of loci carrying a relative risk of Graves disease of up to 4. Graves disease is also associated with polymorphism of cytotoxic T-lymphocyte antigen-4 (CTLA-4), which indicates the importance of autoreactive T cells. Patients with Graves disease and their relatives have a considerably higher incidence of other autoimmune diseases, including pernicious anemia and Hashimoto thyroiditis. Some asymptomatic, first-degree relatives of these patients also have increased ^{131}I uptake. White patients with Graves disease more often express HLA-B8 and HLA-DR3, while Chinese patients are more likely to be positive for HLA-Bw46, and Japanese ones for HLA-Bw35.

SEX: Like other autoimmune diseases, Graves disease is far more common (7–10 times) in women than in men. Interestingly, it tends to arise during periods of hormonal imbalance, including puberty, pregnancy, and menopause. Men with Graves disease are usually older, and although the degree of thyroid hyperfunction is often greater in men than in women, symptoms tend to be less severe in men.

EMOTIONAL INFLUENCES: Endocrinologists have long observed that onset of Graves disease often follows a period of emotional stress, such as separation anxiety, death of a loved one, or near injury in an accident. Quantitative data are lacking.

SMOKING: Smoking is associated with increased risk of Graves disease, and it increases the severity of the eye disease in patients who develop ophthalmopathy.

OPHTHALMOPATHY: Although exophthalmos (protrusion of eyeballs) is a common complication of Graves disease, (see Fig. 21-13) its occurrence and severity correlate poorly with levels of thyroid hormone. It seems likely that a combination of humoral and cell-mediated immune mechanisms is involved. T lymphocytes sensitized to antigens shared by thyroid follicular cells and orbital fibroblasts (possibly TSH receptor) accumulate around the eye, where they secrete cytokines that activate fibroblasts. There is also evidence for systemic or local production of antibodies that stimulate orbital fibroblasts to proliferate and produce collagen and glycosaminoglycans.

PATHOLOGY: The thyroid in Graves disease is symmetrically enlarged, usually 35 to 100 g. Cut surfaces are firm and dark red. The tan translucence of normal thyroid, due to stored colloid, is notably absent. Microscopically, the gland is diffusely hyperplastic and highly vascular. The epithelial cells are tall and columnar and are often arranged as papillae that project into the lumen of the follicles. The colloid tends to be depleted and appears scalloped or "moth-eaten" where it abuts the epithelial cells (Fig. 21-15). Scattered B and T lymphocytes and plasma cells infiltrate the interstitial tissue and may even aggregate to form germinal follicles.

Therapy with antithyroid medication (e.g., methimazole or propylthiouracil) commonly results in increased thyroid hyperplasia and complete lack of colloid.

Exophthalmos is caused by enlargement of orbital extraocular muscles. These muscles themselves are normal, but are swollen by mucinous edema, accumulation of fibroblasts and lymphocyte infiltration. The increased orbital contents displace the eye forward (**proptosis**).

CLINICAL FEATURES: Patients with Graves disease note gradual onset of nonspecific symptoms, such as nervousness, emotional lability, tremor, weakness, and weight loss (Fig. 21-16). They are intolerant of heat, seek cooler environments, tend to sweat profusely and may report palpitations. Excess thyroid hormone reduces systemic vascular resistance, enhances cardiac contractility, and increases heart rate. In patients with preexisting heart disease, congestive heart failure may ensue. Women develop oligomenorrhea, which may progress to amenorrhea.

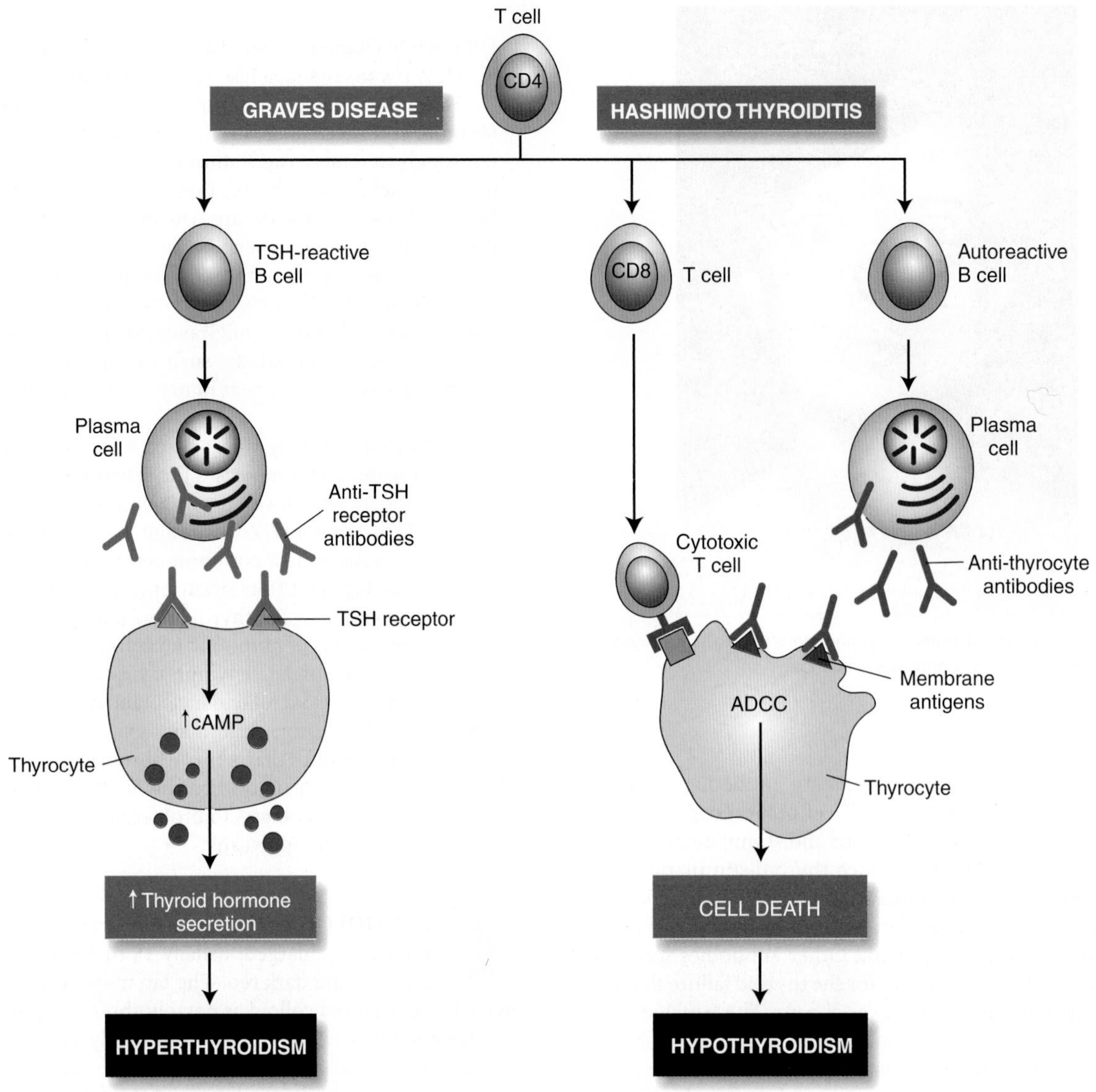

FIGURE 21-14. **Immune mechanisms of Graves disease and Hashimoto thyroiditis.** CD4+ T cells stimulate antibody production by autoreactive B cells. Anti-thyroids-stimulating hormone (TSH) receptor antibodies stimulate thyroid hormone synthesis in Graves disease. Antibodies induce thyrocyte cell death in Hashimoto thyroiditis by complement-dependent cytotoxicity and antibody-dependent cell-mediated cytotoxicity (ADDC). Thyrocyte death also results from attack by CD8+ (cytotoxic) T cells. cAMP = cyclic adenosine monophosphate

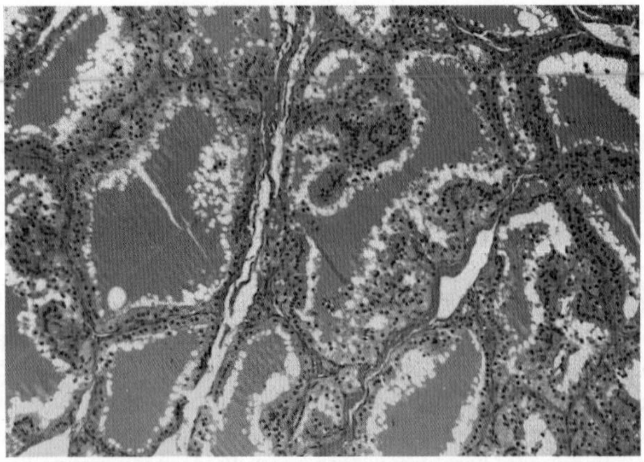

FIGURE 21-15. **Graves disease.** The follicles are lined by hyperplastic, tall columnar cells. Colloid is pink and scalloped at the periphery adjacent to the follicular cells.

Physical examination reveals a symmetrically enlarged thyroid, often with an audible bruit and a palpable thrill. Proptosis and retraction of the eyelids expose the sclera above the superior margin of the limbus. The skin is warm and moist, and some patients exhibit **Graves dermopathy**, a peculiar pretibial edema caused by accumulation of fluid and glycosaminoglycans. The diagnosis is confirmed by increased thyroid radioactive iodine uptake and elevated serum of T_4 and T_3. Serum TSH is very low.

The course of Graves disease is characterized by exacerbations and remissions. Untreated, hyperthyroidism may eventually lead to progressive thyroid failure and hypothyroidism. Treatment of the disorder depends on many individual factors and includes the use of antithyroid medication such as thioisocyanate, destruction of thyroid tissue with radioactive iodine, and adjunctive therapy with corticosteroids and adrenergic antagonists. Surgical ablation is not often done. Unfortunately, despite successful relief of hyperthyroidism, exophthalmos often persists and may even worsen.

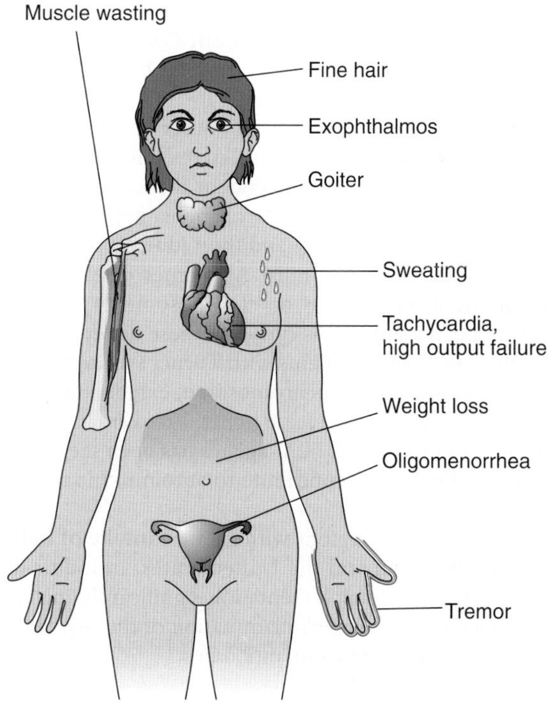

FIGURE 21-16. **Major clinical manifestations of Graves disease.**

Toxic Multinodular Goiter Results from Functional Autonomy of Thyroid Nodules

Many patients with nontoxic multinodular goiter, usually over the age of 50, eventually develop a toxic form of the disease. Like its precursor disease, toxic goiter is 10 times more frequent in women than in men.

PATHOGENESIS AND PATHOLOGY: The mechanisms by which nontoxic multinodular goiter assumes functional autonomy are not clear, but two patterns are seen. In some patients, iodine uptake is diffuse and not affected by administration of thyroid hormone. Microscopically the thyroid shows groups of small hyperplastic follicles mixed with other nodules of varying size that appear to be inactive. A second pattern is characterized by focal accumulation of radiolabeled iodine in one or more nodules. Hyperfunction of these nodules suppresses the function of the rest of the thyroid. Exogenous thyroid hormone produces no further suppression of iodine uptake, although previously inactive areas will respond to TSH by sequestering iodine. The functional nodules are clearly demarcated from the inactive areas histologically, contain large hyperplastic follicles, and thus resemble adenomas. The functional nodules do not have neoplastic characteristics, but the clinical picture is like that of a normal thyroid with a single hyperfunctioning adenoma.

CLINICAL FEATURES: Patients with toxic multinodular goiter usually have less severe symptoms of hyperthyroidism than those with Graves disease and never develop exophthalmos. Since patients with toxic goiter tend to be older, cardiac complications, including atrial fibrillation and congestive heart failure, may dominate the clinical presentation. Serum T_4 and T_3 levels are frequently only minimally elevated, and uptake of radiolabeled iodine may be normal or only slightly elevated. Radiolabeled iodine following a course of antithyroid therapy is the most common therapy.

Toxic Adenoma Is a Functional Neoplasm

Toxic adenoma is a benign, solitary, hyperfunctioning, follicular tumor in an otherwise normal thyroid. It is an infrequent cause of hyperthyroidism. Such tumors (1) display autonomous function, (2) are independent of TSH, and (3) are not suppressed if thyroid hormone is given. Hyperfunction of a toxic adenoma eventually suppresses the remainder of the thyroid, which then atrophies. Under these circumstances, a ^{131}I scintiscan shows a solitary focus of iodine uptake ("hot nodule") in a background of minimal uptake. Many, but not all, toxic adenomas exhibit a variety of somatic activating mutations of the TSH-receptor gene, leading to constitutive up-regulation of the cAMP cascade and less commonly the inositol phosphate-diacylglycerol system.

CLINICAL FEATURES: Toxic thyroid adenoma is most common in the fourth and fifth decades of life. Symptoms of hyperthyroidism usually begin when the adenoma is about 3 cm in diameter. Spontaneous necrosis and hemorrhage within an adenoma may relieve the hyperthyroidism. In this case the rest of the gland resumes its normal function, and the adenoma appears as a "cold" nodule in a scintigram, simulating thyroid cancer.

Since the normal thyroid tissue is suppressed, toxic adenoma is treated effectively with radiolabeled iodine. Large nodules may be excised surgically, especially in young patients to minimize risk of thyroid cancer that may occur many years after radiolabeled iodine administration.

Thyroiditis

Thyroiditis describes a heterogeneous group of inflammatory disorders of the thyroid gland, including those that are caused by autoimmune mechanisms and infectious agents.

Acute Thyroiditis is Caused by Bacterial or Fungal Infections

The most common causative organisms are streptococcus, staphylococcus, and pneumococcus. The disease usually develops during a systemic infection that reaches the thyroid by hematogenous spread. Patients of all ages can be affected, but children and the elderly, or immunocompromised patients, are most commonly affected.

Patients present with fever, chills, malaise, and a painful, swollen neck. Infection may involve one lobe or the entire gland. Microscopically, there is diffuse acute and chronic inflammation with focal microabscess formation. Rarely, acute thyroiditis is complicated by extension of the infection into the trachea, mediastinum, and esophagus. The prognosis is excellent when the infection is promptly treated with antibiotics.

Chronic Autoimmune Thyroiditis (Hashimoto Thyroiditis) Is the Most Common Cause of Goitrous Hypothyroidism in the United States

Hashimoto's thyroiditis (HT) occurs predominantly in women between 30 and 50 years of age, although, patients of all ages can be affected Patients present with diffuse thyroid enlargement accompanied by either mild hyperthyroidism or hypothyroidism The disease can affect several family members who often also suffer other autoimmune conditions such as lupus, Graves disease, arteritis, and scleroderma.

PATHOGENESIS: The pathogenesis of HT involves cellular and humoral immunity. The autoimmune process in HT arises from activation of CD4 (helper) T lymphocytes sensitized to thyroid antigens (see Fig. 21-14). Helper T cell activation may be initiated by viral or bacterial infection.

In turn, these CD4+ cells stimulate proliferation of autoreactive cytotoxic (CD8+) T cells, which attack thyrocytes. The activated lymphocytes secrete interferon-γ causing thyrocytes to express major histocompatability complex (MHC) class II molecules (HLA-DR, DP, DQ), thereby expanding the autoreactive T cell population. These effects account for the striking accumulation of lymphocytes in the glands of patients with autoimmune thyroiditis.

Activated CD4 cells also recruit autoreactive B cells to produce antibodies against thyroid antigens. These include antibodies against thyroid microsomal peroxidase (95%), thyroglobulin (60%), and TSH receptor. Cytotoxic antibodies that fix complement have been described in some patients, and antibody- dependent cell-mediated cytotoxicity (ADCC) may contribute to thyroid injury. Unlike the anti-TSH receptor antibodies in Graves disease, which stimulate thyroid function, antibodies in HT block TSH action. Such blocking antibodies have been described in 10% of patients with goitrous autoimmune thyroiditis and in 20% of those with end-stage atrophy of the gland. Half of all first-degree relatives of patients with this condition have anti-thyroid antibodies, which are apparently transmitted as a dominant trait. Moreover, both Graves disease and chronic autoimmune thyroiditis are described in these family members. A familial tendency for HT is further suggested by the higher prevalence of other autoimmune diseases in patients and their relatives, including MEN syndrome type 2, insulin-dependent diabetes, pernicious anemia, Addison disease, and myasthenia gravis. The high incidence of autoimmunity and thyroiditis in people with Down syndrome and familial Alzheimer disease has attracted attention to genes on chromosome 21, but none have yet been identified as causes of these disorders. Interestingly, half of adult patients with Turner syndrome, especially those with an X isochromosome, exhibit antithyroid antibodies, and a third develop hypothyroidism. Only association with HLA and CTLA-4 genes has been seen consistently, but how these contribute to autoimmune thyroiditis remains obscure.

HY is highest in regions with greatest **intake of iodine**, for example, Japan and the United States. In iodine-deficient areas, iodine supplementation significantly increases the prevalence of chronic inflammation of the thyroid and the presence of thyroid autoantibodies.

PATHOLOGY: On gross examination, the gland in patients with HT is diffusely enlarged and firm, weighing 60 to 200 g. The cut surface is pale tan and fleshy with a vaguely nodular pattern (Fig. 21-17). The capsule is intact; perithyroid tissues are not involved. Microscopically, the gland shows (1) a conspicuous infiltrate of lymphocytes and plasma cells, (2) destruction and atrophy of follicles, and (3) oxyphilic metaplasia of follicular epithelial cells (**Hürthle** or **Askanazy cells**). Lymphoid follicles, often with germinal centers, are present. The Askanazy cells are filled with mitochondria and frequently display nuclear atypia, which may be mistaken for cancer. Interstitial fibrosis is present to a varying extent and in 10% of cases is particularly conspicuous (fibrous variant). The thyroid eventually undergoes atrophy in some patients, who are left with a small, fibrotic gland infiltrated by lymphocytes. Thyroid lymphoma is a rare complication of HT.

A

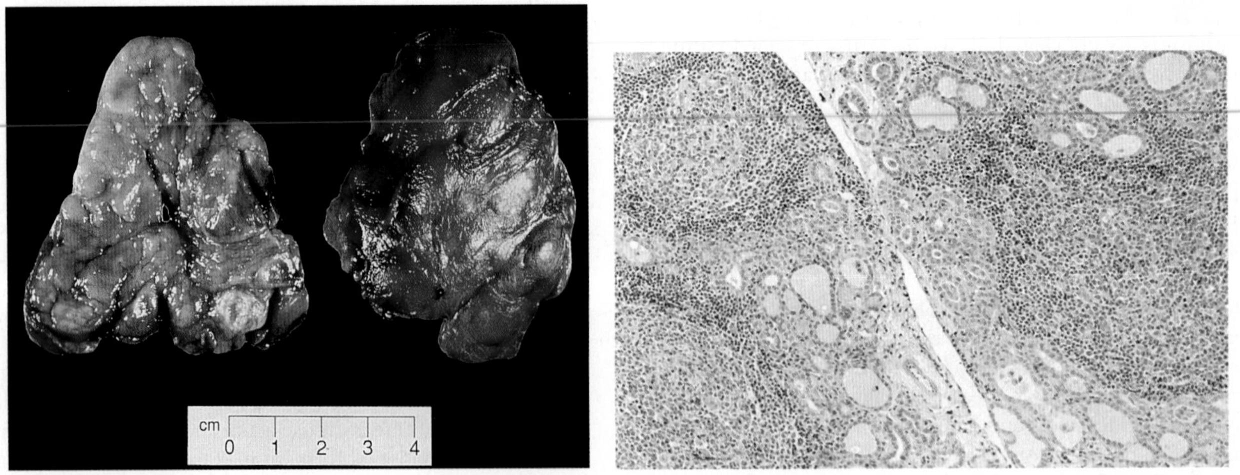

B

FIGURE 21-17. **Chronic autoimmune (Hashimoto) thyroiditis.** The thyroid gland is symmetrically enlarged and coarsely nodular. **A.** A coronal section of the right lobe shows irregular nodules and an intact capsule. **B.** A microscopic section of the thyroid reveals a conspicuous chronic inflammatory infiltrate and many atrophic thyroid follicles. The inflammatory cells form prominent lymphoid follicles with germinal centers.

CLINICAL FEATURES: HT mainly affects women between 30 and 50 years of age, although no age group is spared. Patients present with diffuse thyroid enlargement and either mild hyperthyroidism or hypothyroidism Most patients note gradual onset of a goiter, although sometimes the gland enlarges rapidly. Eventually, one-third to a half of all patients progress to an overt hypothyroid state, the risk of which is considerably greater among men than women. Rarely, hyperthyroidism may develop (**hashitoxicosis**). The diagnosis of HT is now made by the detection of circulating antithyroid antibodies (detected in 95% of patients), antithyroglobulin, and cell membrane antibodies. Such patients show low levels of T4, elevated serum thyrotropin and thyroxine index, and elevated TSH. HT may frequently co-exist with papillary cancer

Many patients require no treatment. Thyroid hormone is given to alleviate hypothyroidism and decrease the size of the gland. Surgery is reserved for patients who do not respond to suppressive hormone therapy or with troublesome pressure symptoms.

Subacute Thyroiditis (de Quervain, Granulomatous, or Giant Cell Thyroiditis) Is Caused by a Viral Infection

Subacute thyroiditis, also known as granulomatous, de Quervain, or nonsuppurative thyroiditis is an infrequent, self-limited disorder characterized by granulomatous inflammation. The disease typically occurs after upper respiratory viral infections, such as with influenza virus, adenovirus, echovirus, and coxsackievirus. Mumps virus has also been incriminated in some cases. de Quervain thyroiditis principally affects women between the ages of 30 and 50 years. The true incidence of subacute thyroiditis is unknown since many infectious thyroididites have been reported under this name.

PATHOLOGY: The thyroid is enlarged to 40 to 60 g, and its cut surface is firm and pale. Acute inflammation, often with microabscesses, is followed by a patchy infiltrate of lymphocytes, plasma cells, and macrophages throughout the thyroid. Destruction of follicles allows release of colloid, which elicits a conspicuous granulomatous reaction (Fig. 21-18). Numerous foreign body type multinucleated giant cells, often containing colloid, are present. Fibrosis of the thyroid may follow resolution of the inflammatory reaction, but the normal thyroid architecture is usually restored.

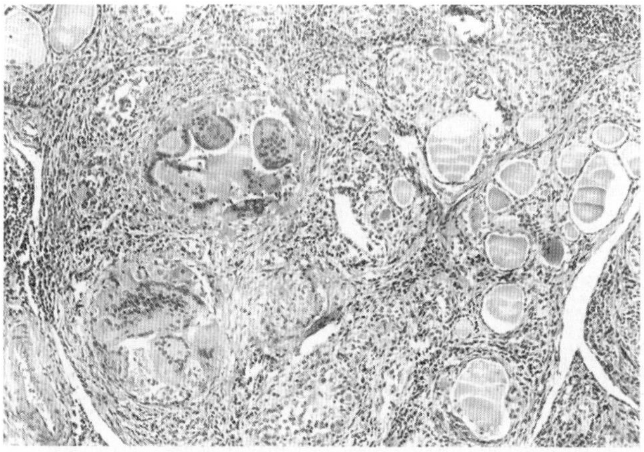

FIGURE 21-18. **Subacute thyroiditis.** The release of colloid into the interstitial tissue has elicited a prominent granulomatous reaction, with numerous foreign body giant cells.

CLINICAL FEATURES: Patients with subacute thyroiditis typically notice pain in the anterior neck, sometimes accompanied by fever, malaise, fatigue, and pain localized to the neck or radiating to the jaw. Other patients follow a mild course with only minimal symptoms. The disorder is often mistaken for a pharyngitis, because of a preceding respiratory tract infection and the presence of hoarseness and dysphagia. On physical examination, the thyroid is moderately enlarged and exquisitely tender. Subacute thyroiditis generally resolves within a few months without any clinical sequelae.

The release of preformed thyroid hormone by destruction of the follicles often elevates serum T_4 and T_3 levels, occasionally high enough to produce transient clinical hyperthyroidism. The consequent suppression of TSH leads to decreased uptake of radiolabeled iodine. This phase is followed by decreased serum T_4 and T_3 levels, but as subacute thyroiditis resolves, a euthyroid state is restored.

Silent Thyroiditis Causes Transient Hyperthyroidism

Silent thyroiditis, also termed **painless subacute thyroiditis** or **lymphocytic thyroiditis,** is characterized by painless thyroid enlargement, self-limited hyperthyroidism, destruction of gland parenchyma, and a lymphocytic infiltrate. Thus, it clinically resembles subacute thyroiditis but pathologically is more similar to HT. Importantly, silent thyroiditis differs from the latter by the lack of antithyroid antibodies or other evidence of autoimmune thyroiditis. However, association with HLA-DR3 has been reported. As in subacute thyroiditis, the hyperthyroid state reflects release of preformed thyroid hormone from the injured gland.

Silent thyroiditis predominantly affects women, often in the postpartum period. Hyperthyroidism usually persists for 2 to 4 months. Treatment is symptomatic, and most patients become euthyroid.

Riedel Thyroiditis Causes Fibrosis of the Thyroid

The "thyroiditis" in Riedel thyroiditis is something of a misnomer, as this rare disease also involves extrathyroidal soft tissues of the neck and is often associated with progressive fibrosis in other locations, including the retroperitoneum, mediastinum, and orbit. Riedel thyroiditis is mainly a disease of middle age. The female-to-male ratio is 3:1. The etiology is unknown, but it does not appear to be related to other forms of thyroiditis.

PATHOLOGY: Grossly, part or all of the thyroid is stony hard and "woody." The process is usually asymmetric and often affects only one lobe. The fibrous infiltrate extends into the thyroid gland and other tissues of the neck, including skeletal muscle and nerves, and may also surround and infiltrate lymph nodes and parathyroid glands. The surgeon may have extreme difficulty identifying a tissue plane. Microscopic examination reveals dense, hyalinized fibrous tissue and a chronic inflammatory infiltrate throughout involved portions of the thyroid (Fig. 21-19). Follicles are normal in the unaffected parts of the gland. Fibrosis surrounds and infiltrates other tissues, including skeletal muscle, nerves, fat, blood vessels, and, sometimes, the parathyroids.

CLINICAL FEATURES: Patients with Riedel thyroiditis notice gradual onset of painless goiter and present with a hard thyroid mass. They may also have

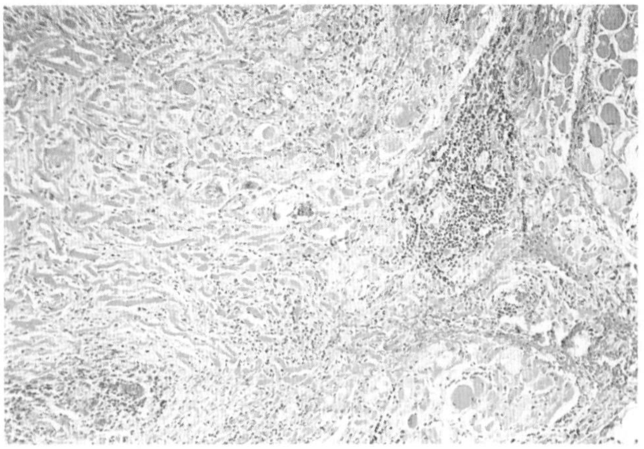

FIGURE 21-19. **Riedel thyroiditis.** The thyroid parenchyma is largely replaced by dense, hyalinized fibrous tissue and a chronic inflammatory infiltrate.

fibrosing lesions in other sites, such as the retroperitoneum, mediastinum, and retro-orbital tissues. Immunophenotyping shows a predominance of T cells with few B cells. Compression of neck organs may cause symptoms: compression of the trachea (stridor), esophagus (dysphagia), and recurrent laryngeal nerve (hoarseness). Unusual cases may involve the entire thyroid and cause hypothyroidism. Treatment is primarily surgical to relieve the compression of the local organs.

Follicular Adenoma of the Thyroid

Follicular adenoma is a benign neoplasm showing follicular differentiation. It is the most common thyroid tumor, and typically presents in euthyroid persons as a solitary "cold" nodule, i.e., a tumor that does not take up radiolabeled iodine. It is a solitary encapsulated neoplasm in which the cells are arranged in follicles resembling normal thyroid tissue or mimic stages in the embryonic development of the gland. Multiple adenomas may occur. Up to 90% of palpable, solitary follicular lesions are actually the dominant nodule in a multinodular goiter, and follicular adenomas are correspondingly infrequent. Follicular adenoma is most common in the fourth and fifth decades, with a female-to-male ratio of 7:1. The clonal origin of follicular adenomas has been established.

PATHOLOGY: Follicular adenoma is a solitary, circumscribed nodule which protrudes from the surface of the thyroid, 1 to 3 cm in diameter, surrounded completely by a thin fibrous capsule,. The tumor cut surface is soft and paler than the surrounding gland. Hemorrhage, fibrosis and cystic change are common. There are several distinctive histologic patterns (Fig. 21-20). Although these variants are of no par-

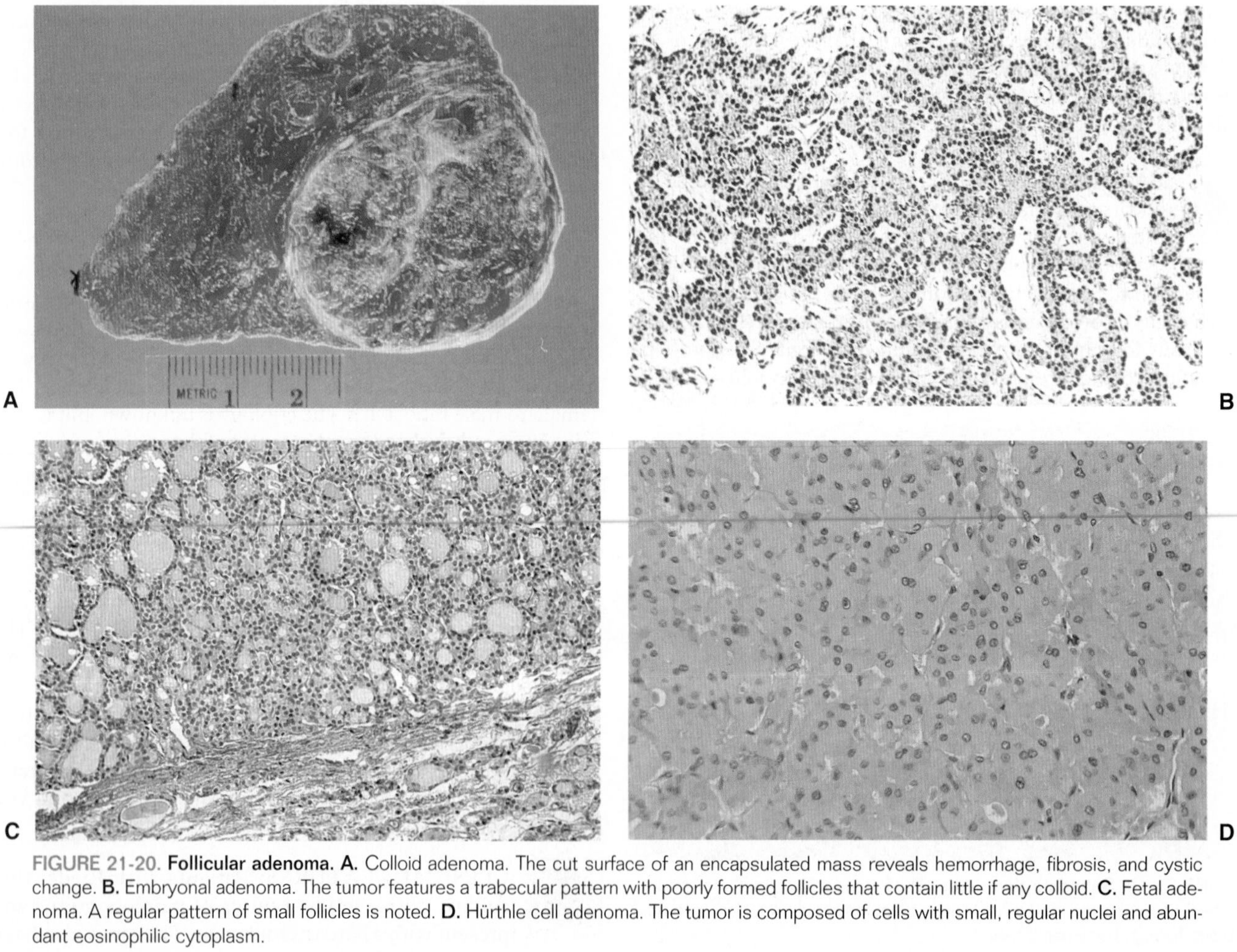

FIGURE 21-20. **Follicular adenoma. A.** Colloid adenoma. The cut surface of an encapsulated mass reveals hemorrhage, fibrosis, and cystic change. **B.** Embryonal adenoma. The tumor features a trabecular pattern with poorly formed follicles that contain little if any colloid. **C.** Fetal adenoma. A regular pattern of small follicles is noted. **D.** Hürthle cell adenoma. The tumor is composed of cells with small, regular nuclei and abundant eosinophilic cytoplasm.

ticular clinical significance, their recognition may be important in separating them from thyroid cancers.

- **Embryonal adenoma** is distinguished by a trabecular pattern in which poorly formed follicles contain little or no colloid (see Fig 21-20B).
- **Fetal adenoma** displays cells that are similar to those of embryonal adenoma but tend to be arranged in microfollicles containing little colloid (see Fig 21-20C).
- **Simple adenoma** exhibits mature follicles with a normal amount of colloid.
- **Colloid adenoma** is similar to simple adenoma except that the follicles are larger and contain more abundant colloid (see Fig 21-20A).
- **Hürthle cell adenoma** is a solid tumor characterized by oxyphil cells, small follicles, and scanty colloid (see Fig 21-20D).
- **Atypical adenoma** is a follicular tumor that with mitoses, excessive cellularity, nuclear atypism or equivocal capsular invasion, but for which a diagnosis of carcinoma cannot be established with certainty.

These benign lesions should be differentiated from follicular carcinomas which usually have thicker capsules. Careful evaluation of the capsule for capsular or vascular invasion is mandatory to make this distinction. *Malignancies can develop in association or within benign nodules.* Surgical lobectomy to remove the lesion is curative.

Papillary Hyperplastic Nodules

Papillary hyperplastic nodules occur mainly in children and young women. These solitary lesions are well-circumscribed and well encapsulated. They are composed of papillae of different sizes in which the stalk may contain small follicles. Papillae are lined by cuboidal cells with characteristic follicular nuclei, i.e., dense and dispersed chromatin. The center of nodules is often cystic and can contain colloid-like material.

Thyroid Cancer

Malignant thyroid neoplasms account for 0.4% of all cancer deaths in the United States. Approximately 10,000 new cases diagnosed each year. Mortality from thyroid cancer, however, exceeds the mortality from malignant tumors of all other endocrine organs

The difficulty of distinguishing clinically between nonneoplastic lesions, benign tumors, and thyroid cancer is a major clinical and pathologic concern. Thyroid nodules are found in 1% to 10% of the population, but malignant tumors of the thyroid account for only about 1% of all cancers. A single nodule has up to a 12% probability of being malignant, and those odds decrease significantly (3%) if a nodule is palpable.

Most cases of thyroid carcinoma occur between the third and seventh decades, but children can also be affected. Tumors occur in women 2.5 times more often than in men.

Fine-needle biopsy of thyroid nodules makes a diagnosis in most cases. Prognosis is a function of the morphology of the tumor, and may range from a virtually benign clinical course to a rapidly fatal disease. The latter outcome is fortunately uncommon.

Radioscintigraphy of the gland is helpful in diagnosing thyroid tumors, since hyperfunctioning nodules are usually benign. "Cold" or non-functioning nodules, on the other hand, although more frequently malignant, may also be benign.

Papillary Thyroid Carcinoma (PTC) Is the Most Common Thyroid Cancer

PTC accounts for up to 90% of sporadic cases of thyroid cancer in the United States. It is most frequent between the ages of 20 and 50 years, with a female-to-male ratio of 3:1. However, it may arise at any age, even in children, and it is the most common thyroid tumor type in children and young adolescents. Elderly men have a worse prognosis with this type of thyroid cancer.

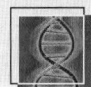

PATHOGENESIS: Although the etiology of PTC remains to be established, a number of associations have been identified.

- **Iodine excess:** PTC has been produced in animals by administering excess iodine. In endemic goiter regions, addition of iodine to the diet increased the proportion of thyroid cancers showing papillary, as compared with follicular, morphology.
- **Radiation:** External radiation to the neck of children and adults increases the incidence of later PTC. Survivors of atomic bomb explosions in Japan suffered more papillary cancers than would otherwise be expected. A substantially higher incidence of PTC has occurred in children living in contaminated areas surrounding Chernobyl, the site in Ukraine of a nuclear reactor catastrophe in 1986. On the other hand, treatment with radiolabeled iodine does not increase the risk of this tumor.
- **Genetic factors:** Epidemiologic studies have reported a 4- to 10-fold higher risk for PTC in first-degree relatives of persons with that tumor. A concordance for PTC has been described in monozygotic twins. A familial form of PTC accounts for some 5% of all cases, but the genes responsible have not been identified.
- **Somatic mutations:** The risk of PTC is higher in people with familial adenomatous polyposis. Somatic rearrangements of the *RET* protooncogene on chromosome 10 (10q11.2) are common in PTC, and 60% of such tumors in children exposed to radiation from the Chernobyl accident showed this mutation. The same mutation occurs after external radiation to the thyroid. These rearrangements cause the fusion of the tyrosine kinase domain of *RET* to various other genes, creating *RET/PTC* fusion oncogenes. Interestingly, the frequency of *RET/PTC* rearrangements in PTC varies geographically, ranging from none in Korea to 2% in Saudi Arabia, and 60% in the United States and Great Britain. Illegitimate recombination of the *NTRK1* gene on chromosome 1, which encodes the high-affinity nerve growth factor receptor *(NGFR)*, with another gene on the same chromosome *(TPM3)* has also been described in some PTCs.

PATHOLOGY: PTCs vary from microscopic lesions to tumors larger than a normal gland. Serial sections of ostensibly normal thyroids obtained at autopsy have re-

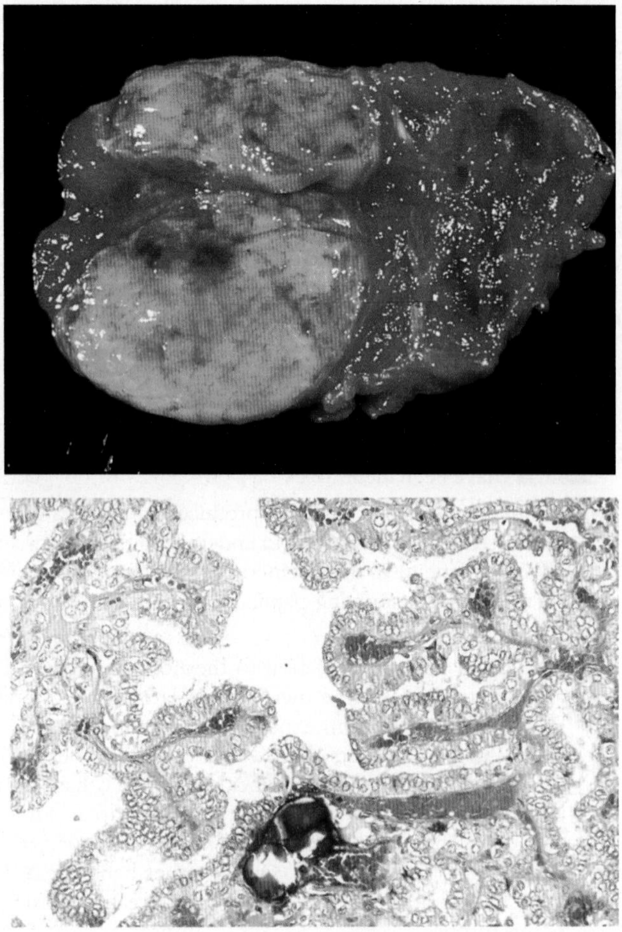

A

B

FIGURE 21-21. **Papillary carcinoma of the thyroid. A.** The cut surface of a surgically resected thyroid displays a circumscribed pale tan mass with foci of cystic change. **B.** Branching papillae are lined by neoplastic columnar epithelium with clear nuclei. A calcospherite, or psammoma body, is evident.

vealed a high proportion of papillary cancers that measure less than 1 mm across, but lymph node metastases in such cases are distinctly uncommon. Papillary cancers may be located anywhere in the gland including the isthmus. Tumors are firm, solid, white-yellowish in color, with irregular and infiltrative borders. Lesions may be multiple, and are occasionally encapsulated (Fig. 21-21A).

Microscopically, branching papillae are composed of a central fibrovascular core and a single or stratified lining of cuboidal to columnar cells (see Fig. 21-21B). Irregularly shaped or tubular neoplastic follicles are usually seen in the tumor, but the proportions of the papillary and follicular elements are highly variable. Nuclear atypism is an important diagnostic feature and includes clear (**ground-glass** or **Orphan Annie**) nuclei, eosinophilic pseudo-inclusions (which represent invaginations of the cytoplasm into the nucleus) and nuclear grooves. Many papillary cancers show dense fibrosis. Calcospherites (**psammoma bodies**) are virtually diagnostic of papillary carcinoma, being rare in other conditions, and are seen in half the cases. The stroma may be infiltrated by lymphocytes and Langerhans cells. In over three fourths of cases of PTC, careful sectioning of a resected thyroid reveals multiple microscopic foci of tumor, but it is not clear whether this represents a multifocal origin of the tumor or lymphatic spread from a solitary primary. Vascular invasion is distinctly uncommon.

PTC typically invades lymphatics and spreads to regional cervical lymph nodes. Lymph node metastases vary from microscopic foci in otherwise normal lymph nodes to large masses that dwarf the primary lesion. Direct extension of PTC into soft tissues of the neck occurs in one fourth of cases. Hematogenous metastases are less common than in other varieties of thyroid cancer, but occur occasionally, mostly to the lungs.

CLINICAL FEATURES: PTC presents as (1) a painless, palpable nodule in an otherwise normal gland; (2) a nodule with enlarged cervical lymph nodes; or (3) cervical lymphadenopathy without a palpable thyroid nodule. Tumors over 0.5 cm can be detected as cold areas in a thyroid scintiscan.

In general, the prognosis of PTC is excellent, and life expectancy for these patients differs little from that of the general population. The prognosis is more serious in patients older than 50 years, whereas in children, the outlook is good even when lung metastases are detected. PTC tends to be more aggressive in men than in women.

As a rule, the larger the primary tumor, the more aggressive it is, and direct extension into adjacent soft tissues portends a poorer prognosis. The proportion of papillary and follicular elements does not affect prognosis, but less-differentiated tumors tend to be more aggressive. The presence of metastases to cervical nodes at the time or surgery does not change the prognosis, as less than 10% of these patients die of the tumor. In fatal cases of PTC, death is caused principally by metastases to the lungs or brain or by obstruction of the trachea or esophagus.

Therapies include surgery (lobectomy or total thyroidectomy) with or without neck dissection, followed by administration of radioiodine.

Follicular Thyroid Carcinoma (FTC) Is Rarely Fatal

FTC is a purely follicular malignant tumor that contains no papillary or other elements. It comprises approximately 15% to-30% of thyroid tumors. Most patients are above 40 years of age, and the female-to-male ratio is 3:1. Incidence of follicular carcinoma is higher in endemic goiter areas among persons who do not receive iodine supplements. However, in areas where iodine is added to salt, such as the United States, FTC is uncommon, accounting for as few as 5% of all thyroid cancers.

PATHOLOGY: Follicular cancer varies in size, has a yellow-tan color and shows a thick white fibrous capsule. Areas of hemorrhage and necrosis are not uncommon as well as foci of cystic degeneration. FTCs are subdivided into minimally invasive and widely invasive variants.

Minimally invasive FTC is grossly a well-defined, encapsulated tumor. On cut section it is soft and pale tan to pink and bulges from within its capsule. Microscopically, most lesions resemble follicular adenoma, although they tend more to a microfollicular or trabecular pattern. Occasionally, hemorrhagic necrosis is seen in the center of a tumor. Mitoses are common, which distinguishes follicular cancer from benign adenoma. The principal distinction from adenoma is at the interface of the capsule and normal parenchyma. Minimally invasive cancer is diagnosed when tumor extends into, but not entirely through, the capsule.

Invasive FTC usually presents few diagnostic problems, since it extends through its capsule or shows vascular invasion

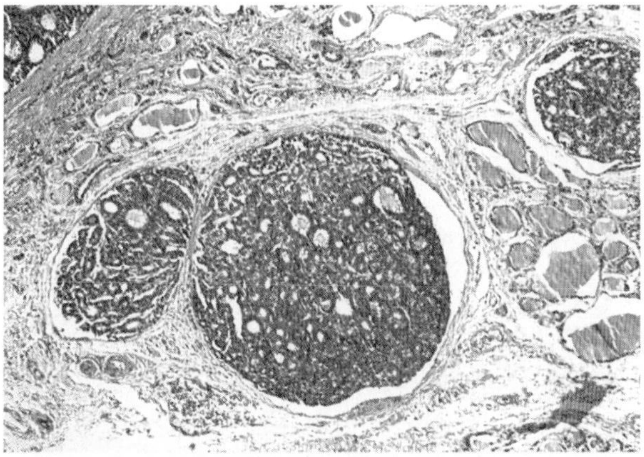

FIGURE 21-22. **Follicular carcinoma of the thyroid.** A microfollicular tumor has invaded veins in the thyroid parenchyma.

(see Fig. 21-22), often within or adjacent to the capsule. The tumor may also extend into the surrounding soft tissues.

FTC differs from PTC in that its metastases are blood-borne, not lymphatic, and are directed mainly to the bones of the shoulder and pelvic girdles, sternum, and skull.

CLINICAL FEATURES: Most follicular cancers are detected clinically as solitary palpable nodules or enlarged thyroids. However, in some cases, the presenting sign is a pathologic fracture through a bony metastasis or a pulmonary lesion. Both primary tumors and metastases take up radiolabeled iodine, although the thyroid scintiscan may indicate a cold nodule as the normal thyroid accumulates iodine more efficiently. However, the affinity for ^{131}I may be used therapeutically. Minimally invasive follicular tumors have a cure rate of at least 95%, compared with a survival of about 50% for the widely invasive form. FTC is treated with unilateral lobectomy. Metastases can be treated with radioiodine

Medullary Thyroid Carcinoma (MTC) Is Derived from C Cells of the Thyroid

These cells originate from the cells of the branchial pouches. They secrete calcitonin and other peptides such as serotonin, ACTH, and somatostatin

This tumor represents no more than 5% of all thyroid cancers. The disease occurs in sporadic and familial forms, the latter accounting for 20% of cases. Patients with the familial form of medullary carcinoma often have MEN type 2, which includes adrenal pheochromocytoma and parathyroid hyperplasia or adenoma.

Somatic mutations in the *RET* protooncogene have been detected in 25% to 70% of cases of sporadic MTC. Most of these occur at codon 918 (ATG to ACG) in the tyrosine kinase domain of the RET protein and indicate a poorer prognosis than in tumors without a *RET* mutation. *RET* is discussed more fully in the section on MEN syndromes (below).

The mean age of patients with MTC is 50 years, but familial cases appear earlier (mean age, 20 years). There is a slight female predominance (1.5:1); in familial cases, the inheritance is autosomal dominant, and the sex distribution is equal.

PATHOLOGY: On gross examination, MTC tends to arise in the superior portion of the thyroid, the region richest in C cells. In the setting of MEN type 2, tumors are often multicentric and bilateral. MTCs are not encapsulated, but are usually circumscribed. Cut surfaces are firm and grayish white. MTC histology is highly variable. Characteristically, the tumor is solid with polygonal, granular cells separated by a distinctly vascular stroma (Fig. 21-23). However, architectural patterns and appearances of the cells are highly variable. *A conspicuous feature is stromal amyloid, representing deposition of procalcitonin.* Nests of tumor cells are embedded in a hyalinized collagenous framework. Focal calcification is often present and may be extensive enough to be detected radiologically. Besides amyloid, medullary carcinoma may contain mucin, melanin, and many polypeptide hormones shown by immunohistochemistry.

By electron microscopy, the neoplastic C cells have dense-core secretory granules that stain immunohistochemically for several endocrine markers, including calcitonin, synaptophysin, chromogranin, and neuron-specific enolase. Almost all of these tumors express carcinoembryonic antigen (CEA). Many are also positive for ACTH, serotonin, substance P, glucagon, insulin, and human chorionic gonadotropin (hCG).

MTC extends by direct invasion into soft tissues and metastasizes to regional lymph nodes and to lung, liver, and bone. Sometimes, the initial presentation may be as metastatic disease. Metastases resemble primary tumors and also tend to contain amyloid.

The precursor lesion of the familial variety of MTC is C cell hyperplasia. Thus, patients with MEN types 2A and 2B (see section on adrenal medulla) who are at risk for MTC are monitored by periodic measurements of serum calcitonin, CEA and sometimes chromogranin. When these are elevated, the patient is subjected to a total thyroidectomy.

CLINICAL FEATURES: Patients with MTC often suffer symptoms related to endocrine secretion, including carcinoid syndrome (serotonin) and Cushing syndrome (ACTH). Watery diarrhea in one third of patients is caused by secretion of vasoactive intestinal peptide, prostaglandins, and several kinins. In cases of familial MTC, patients may exhibit hyperparathyroidism, episodic hypertension, and other symptoms attributable to secretion of catecholamines by pheochromocytoma.

The tumor usually presents as a firm thyroid nodule or cervical lymphadenopathy. By scintiscan, a cold nodule is characteristic. Treatment is total thyroidectomy, but tumors recur locally in one third of patients. Prognosis depends on age (younger patients and women have better prognosis), and tumor size and stage. Other prognostic parameters include: histologic type, mitotic count, necrosis and amount of calcitonin present. The 5 year survival rate is 60% to 75%.

Anaplastic (Undifferentiated) Thyroid Carcinoma Is Usually Fatal

Anaplastic thyroid cancer principally afflicts women (female-to-male ratio of 4:1) over the age of 60. The tumor constitutes 10% of thyroid cancers and is more common in areas of endemic goiter. In fact, overall, at least half of patients suffer from long-standing goiter. In addition, many patients with anaplastic carcinoma have a history of a lower-grade thyroid cancer.

A
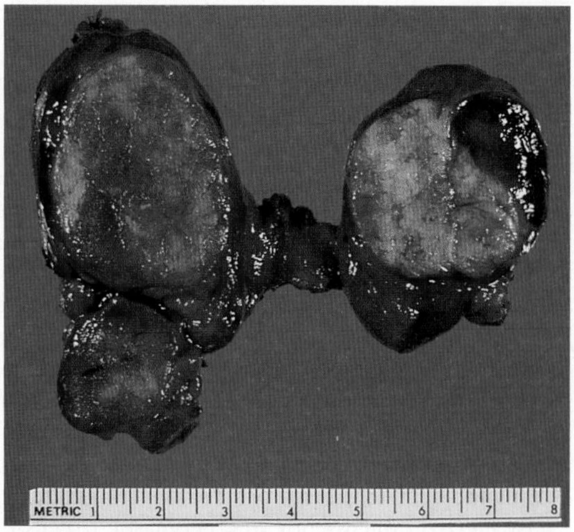

B
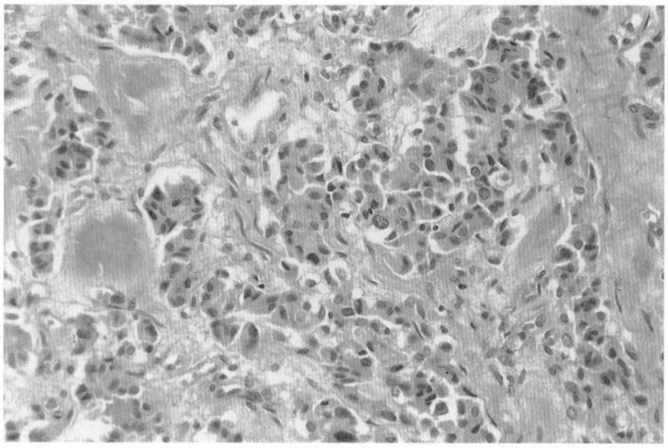

C
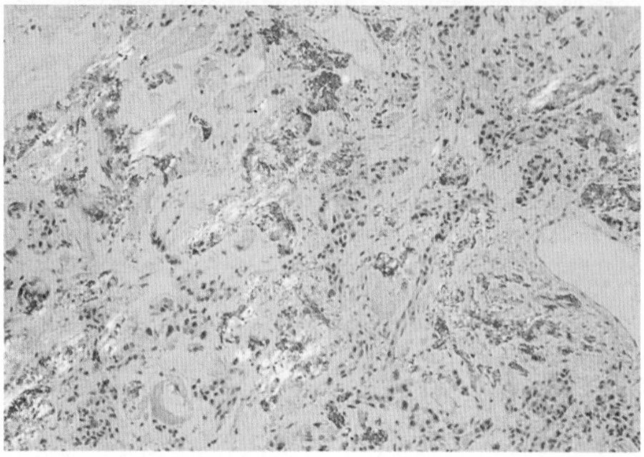

FIGURE 21-23. **Medullary thyroid carcinoma. A.** Coronal section of a total thyroid resection shows bilateral involvement by a firm, pale tumor. **B.** The tumor features nests of polygonal cells embedded in a collagenous framework. The connective tissue septa contain eosinophilic amyloid. **C.** A section stained with Congo red and viewed under polarized light demonstrates the pale green birefringence of amyloid.

Thus, it seems likely that the anaplastic variant often represents a transformation of a benign or low-grade thyroid neoplasm into a more poorly differentiated and more aggressive cancer. There is evidence that the risk of such an event is enhanced by external radiation. Mutations in the *p53* tumor suppressor gene are common in anaplastic cancers, but *RET* activation has not been observed.

PATHOLOGY: Anaplastic carcinoma of the thyroid manifests as large poorly circumscribed masses in the gland that frequently extend into the soft tissues of the neck. The cut surface is hard and grayish white. The most common histologic pattern is a sarcoma-like proliferation of bizarre spindle and giant cells, with polyploid nuclei, many mitoses, necrosis, and stromal fibrosis (Fig. 21-24). Other microscopic

A
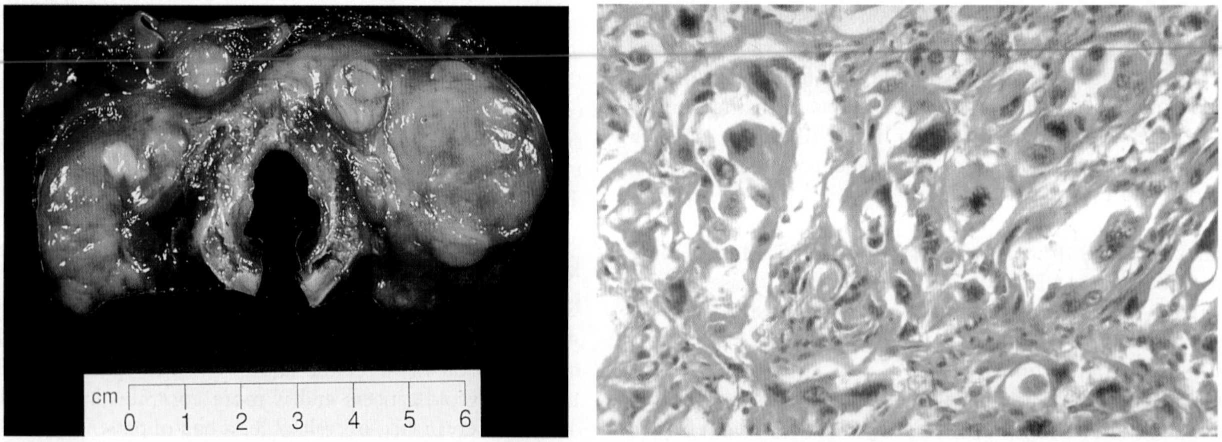

B

FIGURE 21-24. **Anaplastic carcinoma of the thyroid. A.** The tumor in transverse section partially surrounds the trachea and extends into the adjacent soft tissue. **B.** The tumor is composed of bizarre spindle and giant cells with polyploid nuclei and numerous mitoses.

patterns include distinct epithelial differentiation. The tumor tends to invade veins and arteries, often occluding the vessels and producing foci of infarction within the tumor.

CLINICAL FEATURES: Anaplastic compresses and destroys local structures. Accordingly, the tumor presents as a rapidly enlarging neck mass associated with symptoms such as dysphagia, hoarseness, dyspnea and enlargement of cervical nodes. Dysphagia and dyspnea are caused by tracheal compression or invasion. The prognosis is dismal, and widespread metastases are frequent. Less than 10% of patients survive for 5 years. Treatment with radiation and chemotherapy has had little success

Lymphomas of the Thyroid Are Largely B-Cell Tumors

Lymphoma originating in the thyroid is distinctly uncommon, accounting for 2% of all thyroid malignancies. Most if not all cases arise in the setting of chronic thyroiditis, and in regions where this disorder is frequent, up to 10% of malignant tumors of the thyroid are lymphomas. Like chronic thyroiditis, thyroid lymphoma is more common in women than in men (4:1), but the mean age at presentation (seventh decade) is older. Their histology is similar to that of lymphomas at other sites; the most common subtype is the diffuse large cell pattern.

PARATHYROID GLANDS

Anatomy and Physiology

The parathyroid glands are derivatives of branchial clefts III and IV. Most people have 4 glands, but numbers vary from 1 to 12. Normally, they are on the posterior thyroid surface, although they occasionally occur in ectopic locations such as mediastinum, pericardium, or near the recurrent laryngeal nerve.

They are the size and color of a grain of saffron-cooked rice. All glands combined weigh about 130 mg. The weight of an individual gland varies considerably, but anything in excess of 50 mg probably represents enlargement. The glands measure between 4 to 6 mm in length. Microscopically, about three fourths of the parathyroids are composed of chief cells and oxyphil cells, with the remainder being adipose tissue scattered throughout the parenchyma. The amount of fat cells vary throughout life.

Chief cells secrete parathyroid hormone (PTH). They are polyhedral cells that are characterized by a pale, eosinophilic-to-amphophilic cytoplasm with glycogen and fat droplets. Electron microscopy reveals cytoplasmic membrane-bound secretory granules. **Clear cells** are chief cells whose cytoplasm is packed with glycogen. **Oxyphil cells,** appear after puberty, are larger than chief cells and have deeply eosinophilic cytoplasm, due to numerous mitochondria. They have no secretory granules and do not secrete PTH.

The parathyroids respond to blood levels of ionized calcium and magnesium. In turn, PTH controls plasma calcium. Magnesium, a cation closely related to calcium, acts as a brake on PTH secretion. PTH is degraded in the liver and kidney.

Hypoparathyroidism

Hypoparathyroidism results from decreased secretion of PTH or end-organ insensitivity to it (pseudohypoparathyroidism) due to congenital or acquired conditions. It is clinically characterized by hypocalcemia and hyperphosphatemia.

Hypoparathyroidism is Most Often due to Surgical Removal of the Parathyroids at the Time of Thyroidectomy

The symptoms of hypoparathyroidism relate to hypocalcemia. Increased neuromuscular excitability may cause mild tingling in the hands and feet, severe muscle cramps, tetany, laryngeal stridor, and convulsions. Neuropsychiatric manifestations include depression, paranoia, and psychoses. High cerebrospinal fluid pressure and papilledema may mimic a brain tumor. Patients with all forms of hypoparathyroidism are successfully treated with vitamin D and calcium supplementation. Of patients undergoing surgery for primary hyperparathyroidism, 1% develop irreversible hypoparathyroidism. Radioactive iodine therapy can also cause hypoparathyroidism.

Familial hypoparathyroidism may be part of a polyglandular syndrome that includes adrenal insufficiency and mucocutaneous candidiasis (see below). **Familial isolated hypoparathyroidism** has variable inheritance patterns, is rare and reflects deficient PTH secretion. **Idiopathic hypoparathyroidism** is a heterogeneous group of rare disorders, sporadic and familial, that share deficient secretion of PTH. **Agenesis of the parathyroid glands** is part of the DiGeorge syndrome (see Chapter 4).

Pseudohypoparathyroidism Reflects Target Organ Insensitivity to PTH

This group of hereditary conditions is characterized by hypocalcemia, and reflects mutation of the *GNAS1* gene on the long arm of chromosome 20 that result in decreased activity of G_s, the G protein that couples hormone receptors to stimulation of adenyl cyclase. Consequently, in renal tubular epithelium production of cAMP in response to PTH is impaired, and inadequate resorption of calcium from glomerular filtrate ensues. Patients with pseudohypoparathyroidism are also often resistant to other cAMP-coupled hormones, including TSH, glucagon, FSH, and LH. These patients have a characteristic phenotype (**Albright hereditary osteodystrophy**), including short stature, obesity, mental retardation, subcutaneous calcification, and a number of congenital anomalies of bone, particularly abnormally short metacarpals and metatarsals (Fig. 21-25).

Some of those with pseudohypoparathyroidism have normal G_S activity and a normal phenotype. The basis for their resistance to PTH is unclear.

Pseudopseudohypoparathyroidism reads like a typographical error, but it refers to rare cases in which the phenotype of Albright hereditary osteodystrophy is associated with normal cAMP response to PTH. These patients also have reduced G_S activity like that reported in cases of pseudohypoparathyroidism. *GNAS1* mutations are not seen in this condition, although a candidate gene maps to a nearby region on chromosome 20.

Primary Hyperparathyroidism

Primary Hyperparathyroidism is Caused by Excessive PTH Secretion

Primary hyperparathyroidism may be caused by a parathyroid adenoma (80% to 90%), hyperplasia of all parathyroids (10% to 15%) or (rarely) parathyroid carcinoma (1% to 5%). PTH can be sporadic or part of familial syndromes such as MEN-1 and MEN-2A.

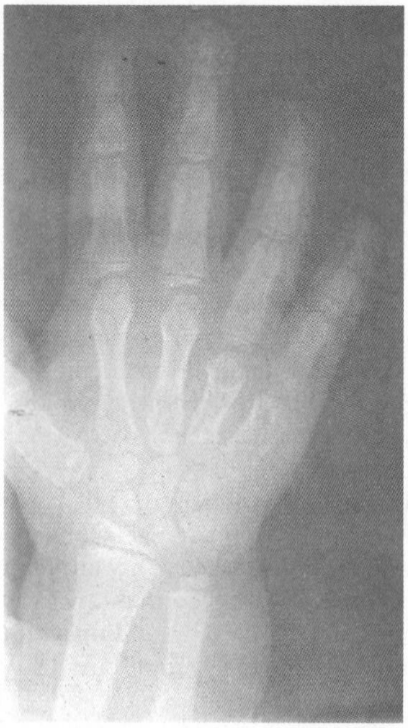

FIGURE 21-25. **Pseudohypoparathyroidism.** A radiograph of the hand reveals the characteristic shortness of the fourth and fifth metacarpal bones.

Parathyroid Adenoma Accounts for Most Cases of Hyperparathyroidism

Parathyroid adenoma is responsible for 85% of all primary hyperparathyroidism. These tumors arise sporadically or (in 20%) in the context of MEN-1 (see below). In a small minority of cases of sporadic adenoma, genetic analysis has identified rearrangement and overexpression of the cyclin D_1 *(PRAD1)* protooncogene on chromosome 11. Adenomas occur at any age but predominate after 50 years of age.

PATHOLOGY: A parathyroid adenoma is a circumscribed, reddish brown, solitary mass, measuring 1 to 3 cm in diameter, weighing 0.05 to 200g. Hemorrhagic areas are common, and cystic changes are occasionally noted. Microscopically, they show sheets of neoplastic chief cells in a rich capillary network. A rim of normal parathyroid tissue is usually evident outside the capsule and distinguishes adenomas from parathyroid hyperplasia (Fig. 21-26). The cells mostly resemble normal chief cells. Immunochemical staining for PTH documents the tumor's activity. The other three glands tend to be atrophic. Surgical resection of the tumor relieves the symptoms of hyperparathyroidism.

Primary Parathyroid Hyperplasia Causes 15% of Hyperparathyroidism

About 75% of cases occur in women. Of these, about 20% are associated with familial hyperparathyroidism or MEN syndromes (MEN types 1 and 2A). One third of sporadic primary parathyroid hyperplasia are monoclonal, suggesting a neoplastic proliferation. In such instances, both chief cell hyperplasia and multiple small adenomas are seen in the same gland. Factors associated with sporadic primary hyperparathyroidism include external radiation and lithium ingestion.

PATHOLOGY: Grossly, all four parathyroid glands are enlarged, combined weights ranging from under 1 g to 10 g. In half of patients, one gland is noticeably larger than the others, which may make the distinction from adenoma difficult. Microscopically, the normal glandular adipose tissue is replaced by hyperplastic chief cells arranged in sheets, trabecular or follicular patterns (Fig. 21-27). Scattered oxyphil

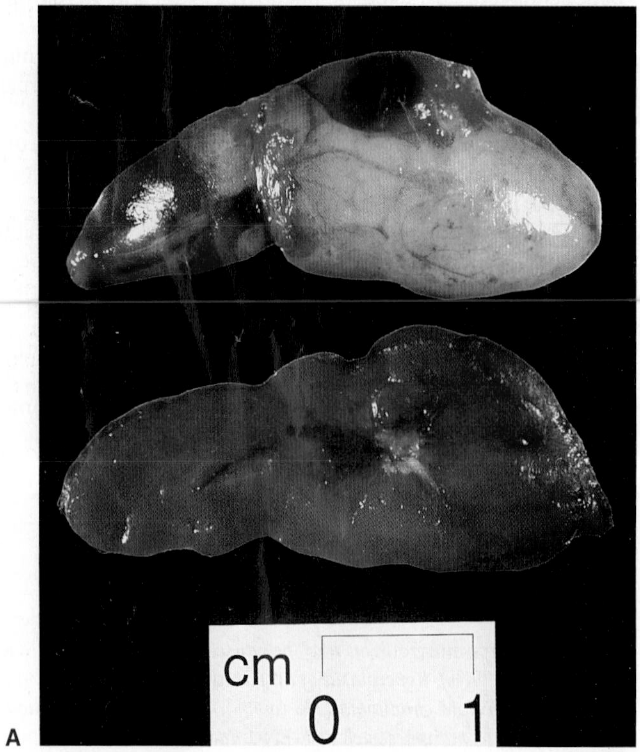

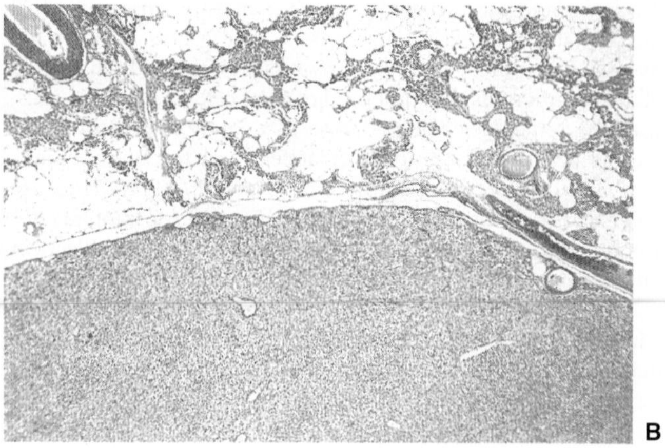

FIGURE 21-26. **Parathyroid adenoma. A.** External *(top)* and cross-section views *(bottom)* show a tan fleshy tumor. **B.** The tumor consists of sheets of neoplastic chief cells and is separated from normal parenchyma by a thin capsule.

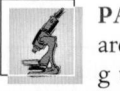

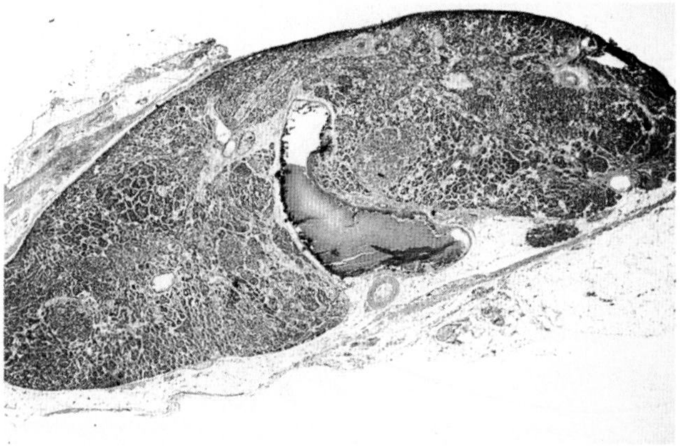

FIGURE 21-27. **Primary parathyroid hyperplasia.** The normal adipose tissue of the gland has been replaced by sheets and trabeculae of hyperplastic chief cells.

cells are common, and small foci of adipose tissue may remain. An important feature that distinguishes hyperplasia from adenoma is the lack of cellular pleomorphism in the former.

Parathyroid Carcinoma Accounts for 1% of Hyperparathyroidism

Parathyroid carcinoma is rare, occurring in both sexes principally between the ages of 30 and 60. It is usually a functioning tumor, and most patients present with symptoms of hyperparathyroidism. Similar to functioning parathyroid adenomas, overexpression of cyclin D_1 has also been described in some parathyroid carcinomas, suggesting that deregulation of this protooncogene is an important feature of parathyroid neoplasia in general. Most parathyroid carcinomas are negative for retinoblastoma protein (another cell cycle regulator); adenomas usually display normal staining. The etiology of these tumors is not known but neck radiation and hereditary syndromes with history of parathyroid adenoma are considered risks factors.

PATHOLOGY: Parathyroid carcinomas tend to be larger than adenomas, and appear as lobulated, firm, tannish, unencapsulated masses, often adherent to surrounding soft tissues. Microscopically, most show a trabecular pattern, with significant mitotic activity and thick fibrous bands. Capsular or vascular invasion is occasionally noted. Importantly, the cell atypism often seen in parathyroid adenomas is rare in carcinomas.

After surgical removal, local recurrence is common: about a third of patients develop metastases to regional lymph nodes, lungs, liver, and bone. If fatal, death is most often due to hyperparathyroidism rather than carcinomatosis. Ten year survival is approximately 50%.

Clinical Features of Hyperparathyroidism Are Highly Variable

Some patients have asymptomatic hypercalcemia, detected on routine blood analysis. Others show florid systemic, renal and skeletal disease (Fig. 21-28). Hypercalcemia and hypophosphatemia are characteristic. Excessive PTH leads to excessive loss of calcium from bones, and enhanced calcium resorption by renal tubules. Production of the activated form of vitamin D (1,25[OH]$_2$D) by renal tubules is also stimulated by PTH, increasing intestinal calcium absorption. The action of PTH on the kidney, together with hypercalcemia, leads to hypophosphatemia. Common symptoms include nausea, vomiting, fatigue, weight loss, anorexia, polyuria, and polydipsia. A neck mass is palpable in many patients. Other systems affected are:

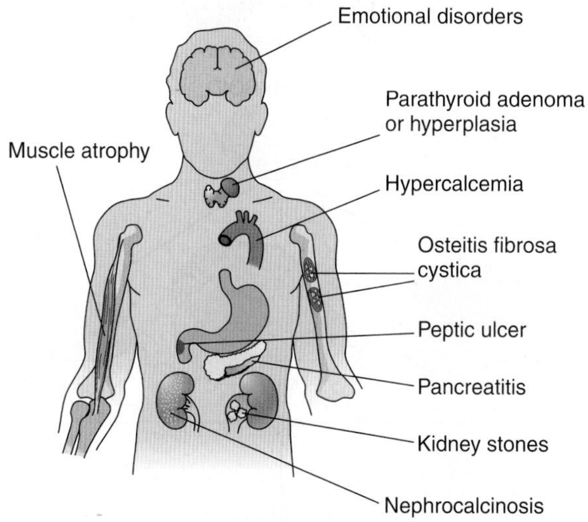

FIGURE 21-28. **Major clinical features of hyperparathyroidism.**

SKELETAL SYSTEM: The classic bone lesions of hyperparathyroidism, known as **osteitis fibrosa cystica** (see Chapter 26), are encountered in a minority of patients who follow an accelerated and serious form of the disease. Briefly, these patients present with bone pain, bone cysts, pathologic fractures, and localized bone swellings (brown tumors and epulis of the jaw). Chondrocalcinosis may be a complication of hyperparathyroidism.

KIDNEY: Ten percent of patients with primary hyperparathyroidism present with renal colic due to kidney stones. Nephrocalcinosis, observed radiologically as diffuse renal calcification, may also occur (see Chapter 16). Polyuria is caused by hypercalciuria, and leads to polydipsia.

NERVOUS SYSTEM: Psychiatric changes are common, including depression, emotional lability, poor mentation, and memory defects. Hyperactive reflexes are seen. Peripheral neuropathy with type 2 fiber atrophy of skeletal muscles leads to muscle weakness.

GASTROINTESTINAL TRACT: Peptic ulcer disease is increased in patients with hyperparathyroidism, possibly because hypercalcemia increases serum gastrin, thereby stimulating gastric acid secretion. Peptic ulcers in the context of MEN-1, which includes parathyroid hyperplasia or adenoma, may be secondary to Zollinger-Ellison syndrome (see Chapter 15). Hypercalcemia may also cause constipation and chronic pancreatitis, but the pathogenesis is not understood.

OTHER SYSTEMS: Half of patients with hyperparathyroidism are hypertensive, although the mechanism is not clear. Anemia of unknown cause is also frequent.

Secondary Hyperparathyroidism

Secondary parathyroid hyperplasia is seen mainly in patients with chronic renal failure, but it also occurs in association with vitamin D deficiency, intestinal malabsorption, Fanconi syndrome, and renal tubular acidosis (Fig. 21-29). Chronic hypocalcemia owing to renal retention of phosphate, inadequate

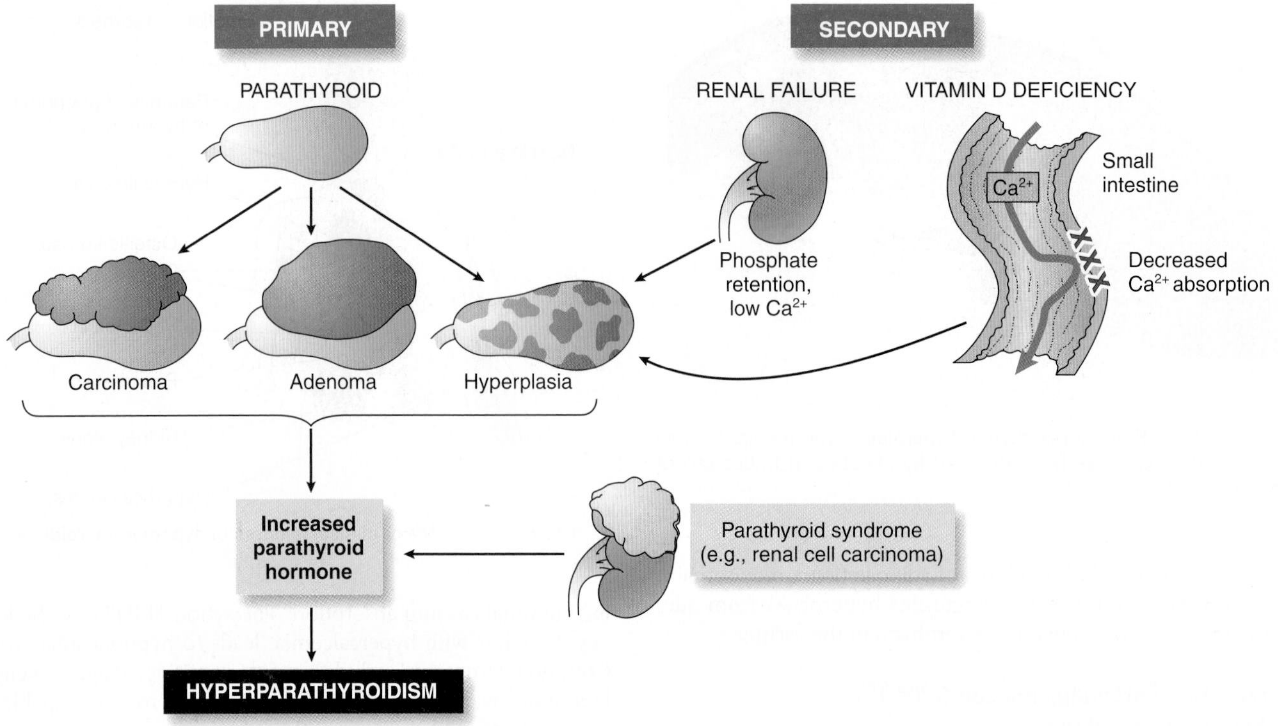

FIGURE 21-29. **Major pathogenetic pathways leading to clinical primary and secondary hyperparathyroidism.**

$1,25(OH)_2D$ production by diseased kidneys, and some skeletal resistance to PTH all lead to compensatory PTH hypersecretion. Secondary hyperplasia of all parathyroids leads to excess levels of PTH, which cause osseous manifestations of hyperparathyroidism, termed **renal osteodystrophy** (see Chapter 26). The morphology of parathyroids in secondary hyperplasia is like that in primary hyperplasia. Treatment is surgical removal of the enlarged glands with or without re-implantation.

Tertiary hyperparathyroidism is the development of autonomous parathyroid hyperplasia after long-standing hyperplasia secondary to renal failure. In these cases parathyroid hyperplasia may not regress after renal transplantation, and surgery to remove parathyroids is required. Two thirds of patients with long-standing uremia have monoclonal hyperplastic parathyroid proliferations.

ADRENAL CORTEX

Anatomy

Each adrenal gland contains two independent endocrine organs: the cortex and the medulla. Both are distinct anatomically and functionally and embryologically. The cortex arises from celomic mesenchymal cells near the urogenital ridge. The medulla is formed by neuroectodermal cells invading fetal adrenal.

Adult adrenal glands are pyramidal organs found anteriorly above each kidney. Each gland is 4 to 6 cm in greatest dimension and weighs about 4 g. Grossly, and on cut section, the cortex shows a characteristic yellow color and the medulla is paler gray-tan. Microscopically, the cortex exhibits three layers or zones.

- The **zona glomerulosa** is the outermost layer where aldosterone production is stimulated by angiotensin and potassium, and inhibited by atrial natriuretic peptide and somatostatin. The zona glomerulosa makes up 15% of the cortex and is composed of indistinct spherical nests of cells with dark-staining nuclei and a moderate number of fat droplets in the cytoplasm.
- The **zona fasciculata** comprises 75% of the cortex and is not distinctly separated from the zona glomerulosa. Radial cords of cells, each with a small nucleus and a large, foamy, clear cytoplasm, representing stored lipid, are readily appreciated.
- The **zona reticularis** is the innermost layer adjacent to the medulla. Irregular anastomosing cords are composed of compact cells with a lipid-poor, slightly granular eosinophilic cytoplasm and bland nuclei.

The cells of the fasciculata and reticularis secrete glucocorticoids under the control of ACTH. In addition, ACTH stimulates adrenal growth. These zones also produce dehydroepiandrosterone, a weak adrenal androgen.

Ectopic adrenal tissue can be present in many locations outside the gland due to migration of cells along the gonads. Common locations include the retroperitoneum, broad ligament near the ovary, near the epididymis, lung, and liver. Ectopic adrenal tissue does not contain medullary cells.

Congenital Adrenal Hyperplasia

Congenital adrenal hyperplasia (CAH) results from several autosomal recessive enzyme defects in the biosynthesis of cortisol from cholesterol (Fig. 21-30). The extent of the defects varies from mild to complete deficiencies. In general, a deficiency in corticosteroid synthesis results in the unopposed action of ACTH and hence adrenal hyperplasia. CAH occurs equally in males and females

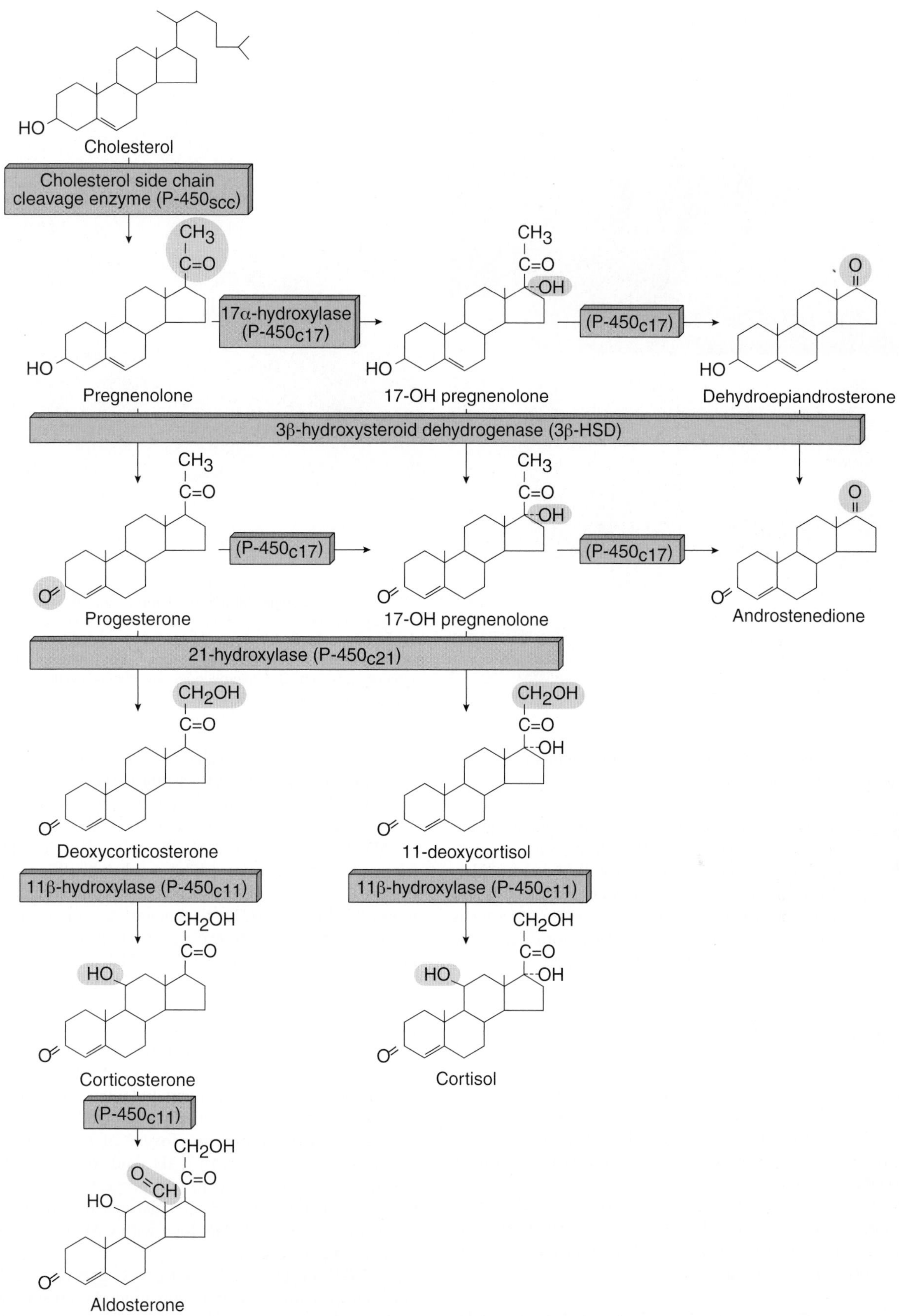

FIGURE 21-30. **Biosynthetic pathways in the synthesis of adrenal corticosteroids.**

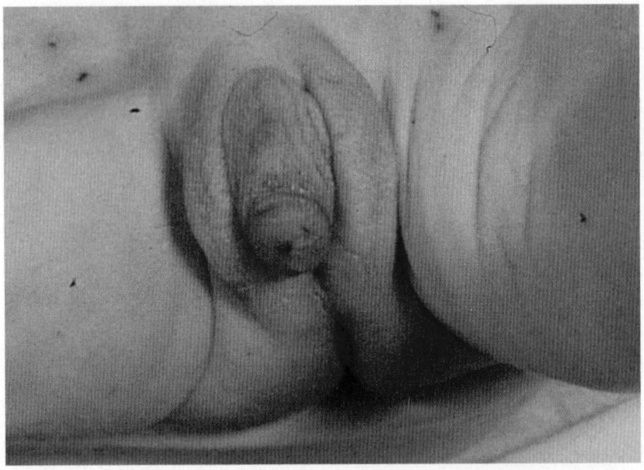

A

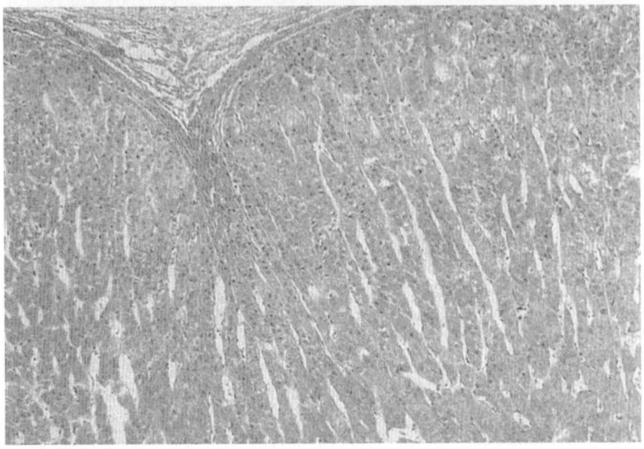

C

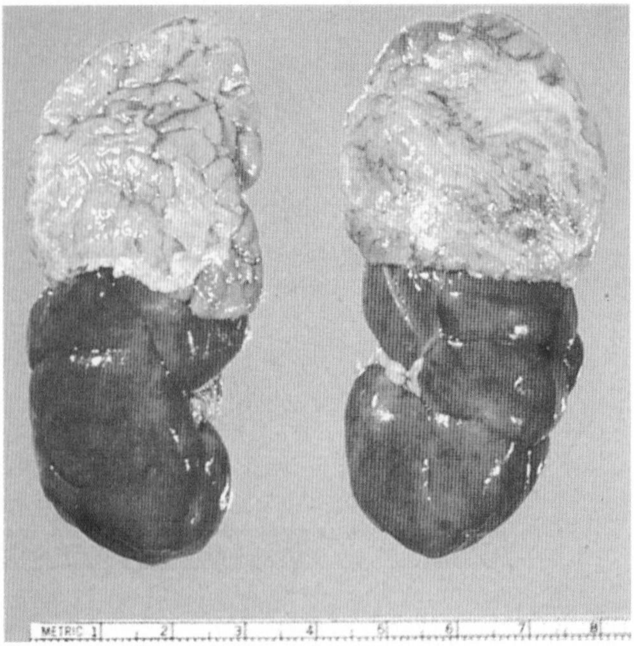

B

FIGURE 21-31. **Congenital adrenal hyperplasia. A.** A female infant is markedly virilized with hypertrophy of the clitoris and partial fusion of labioscrotal folds. **B.** A 7-week-old male died of severe salt-wasting congenital adrenal hyperplasia. At autopsy, both adrenal glands were markedly enlarged. **C.** A microscopic view shows a widened cortex containing compact eosinophilic cells.

and is the most common cause of ambiguous genitalia in newborn girls (Fig. 21-31A).

PATHOLOGY: Adrenal glands are enlarged, weighing as much as 30 g (see Fig. 21-31B). The cut surface is soft, tan to brown and either diffusely enlarged or nodular. Microscopically, the cortex is widened between the medulla and the zona glomerulosa (see Fig. 21-31C). The hyperplastic zone is filled by compact, granular, eosinophilic cells. In most cases, the zona glomerulosa is also hyperplastic, although not to the extent of the other zones, especially the zona fasciculata

21-Hydroxylase, or $P450_{C21}$ Deficiency Is the Major Cause of CAH

The gene for $P450_{C21}$ (CYP21) is linked to the *MHC* locus on the short arm of chromosome 6 (6p21.3.) and is closely associated with *HLA-B* and the *C4A* and *C4B* complement genes. The incidence of this disease varies from about 1 in 10,000 among whites to 1 in 500 in Alaskan Eskimos.

$P450_{C21}$ is a microsomal enzyme that converts 17-hydroxyprogesterone to 11-deoxycortisol. A deficiency in this enzymatic activity impairs cortisol biosynthesis, and accumulated precursors are instead converted to androgens.

CLINICAL FEATURES: Classic CAH caused by $P450_{C21}$ deficiency manifests as several genetically distinct syndromes. Two variants affect newborns. One is simple virilizing CAH; the other is a salt-wasting form that is linked to HLA-Bw47. There is also a less severe late-onset (nonclassic) variant. Mutations that result in complete inactivation of 21-hydroxylase lead to salt-wasting CAH, while those that reduce activity to 2% cause simple virilizing CAH. Late-onset CAH features intermediate values.

SIMPLE VIRILIZING CAH: Female infants exhibit pseudohermaphroditism; males exhibit no abnormalities of the sexual organs. Conversion of cortisol precursors into adrenal androgens is amplified by the ACTH-dependent increase in the size of the gland. Female newborns exposed to a large excess of adrenal androgens in utero are born with fused labia, an enlarged clitoris, and a urogenital sinus that may be mistaken for a penile urethra (see Fig. 21-21A). The sexual ambiguity may cause the infant to be mislabeled as male.

The female external genitalia are not necessarily abnormal at birth, but infant girls may develop a syndrome of androgen excess, with clitoral enlargement and pubic hair. Infant boys exhibit sexual precocity. Eventually, the high levels of adrenal androgens lead to premature closure of epiphyses and short stature. Adult women with CAH tend to be infertile because elevated levels of androgens and progestogens interfere with the hypothalamic–pituitary–gonadal axis, disturb the menstrual cycle, and inhibit ovulation. Men with CAH may be fertile, but some exhibit azoospermia.

SALT-WASTING CAH: Owing to 21-hydroxylase deficiency, aldosterone synthesis may be impaired. As a result, hypoaldosteronism develops within the first few weeks of life in two thirds of newborns with CAH, manifested as hyponatremia, hyperkalemia, dehydration, hypotension, and increased renin secretion. These effects may be rapidly fatal if the disease is untreated (see Fig. 21-31B).

Both infantile variants of CAH caused by $P450_{C21}$ deficiency are treated with glucocorticoids and mineralocorticoids to suppress ACTH and replace steroids. Reconstructive surgery may be necessary for virilized girls with ambiguous genitalia.

LATE-ONSET CAH: Patients with nonclassic variants of 21-hydroxylase deficiency show no abnormalities at birth but exhibit virilizing symptoms at puberty. In young women, late-onset CAH may be difficult to distinguish from polycystic ovary syndrome. Most young men with the disorder are asymptomatic. This form of CAH is probably more common than is classic CAH, particularly among Ashkenazi Jews, Italians, and persons from the former Yugoslavia.

11 β-Hydroxylase Deficiency Causes 5% of CAH

This disorder is distinctly uncommon in the general population, but among Jews of Iranian or Moroccan ancestry in Israel, it is the most common cause of CAH. The gene for 11 β-hydroxylase is located on chromosome 8, and thus, there is no linkage to the *HLA* locus. 11 β-Hydroxylase catalyzes terminal hydroxylation in cortisol biosynthesis. In addition to the androgenic complications of CAH, the presence of high levels of 11-deoxycortisol, a weak mineralocorticoid, often causes sodium retention and accompanying hypertension.

Rare forms of CAH have been described, including deficiencies of a variety of enzymes involved in the biosynthesis of adrenocorticosteroids. These result in variable combinations of electrolyte abnormalities and anomalies of the sex organs.

Adrenal Cortical Insufficiency

Deficient production of adrenal cortical hormones can result from (1) adrenal gland destruction, (2) pituitary or hypothalamic dysfunction with decreased ACTH production, or (3) chronic corticosteroid therapy.

Primary Chronic Adrenal Insufficiency (Addison Disease) Often Reflects an Autoimmune Destruction of the Adrenal

Addison disease is a fatal wasting disorder caused by failure of the adrenal glands to produce glucocorticoids, mineralocorticoids, and androgens. It causes weakness, weight loss, gastrointestinal symptoms, hypotension, electrolyte imbalance, and hyperpigmentation.

PATHOGENESIS: When Addison described primary adrenal insufficiency in 1855, the most common cause of the syndrome was tuberculosis of the adrenal glands. Worldwide, tuberculosis probably is still the most common cause of chronic adrenal insufficiency, but in Western societies, autoimmunity is responsible for 75% of cases. Autoimmune adrenalitis may be an isolated disorder or a part of two different polyglandular autoimmune syndromes. There is evidence that sporadic cases may in fact be a variant of type II polyglandular autoimmune syndrome (see below). Other causes of adrenal destruction include metastatic carcinoma, amyloidosis, hemorrhage, sarcoidosis, and fungal infections. In idiopathic Addison disease, the biochemical defect of adrenoleukodystrophy (see Chapter 28) is often detected. Rarely, adrenal insufficiency is due to congenital adrenal hypoplasia or familial glucocorticoid deficiency (defective ACTH receptor).

The autoimmune pathogenesis of most cases of Addison disease is supported by:

- Lymphoid infiltrates in the adrenal gland
- The presence of circulating antibodies to adrenal antigens
- Abnormalities of cellular immunity
- Associations with other autoimmune endocrinopathies
- Genetic linkage with *HLA* loci

IMMUNE MECHANISMS: Anti-adrenal antibodies that react with tissue from all three zones of the adrenal cortex have been reported in two thirds of patients with chronic adrenal insufficiency that could not be attributed to a specific cause. The major autoantigens are adrenal steroidogenic enzymes, particularly $P450_{C21}$. Autoantibodies are seen in Addison disease, but cell-mediated immunity is probably responsible for the destruction of the adrenal gland. Increased numbers of Ia+ T lymphocytes and decreased suppressor T-cell function have been detected in blood from patients with the disorder.

POLYGLANDULAR ENDOCRINOPATHIES: Half of patients with autoimmune adrenal insufficiency suffer from other autoimmune endocrine diseases. These are grouped into two polyglandular endocrine syndromes.

Type I polyglandular autoimmune syndrome is a rare autosomal recessive condition with a slight female predominance. It is seen in older children and adolescents. In addition to adrenal insufficiency, most (60%) patients also have hypoparathyroidism and chronic mucocutaneous candidiasis. Insulin-dependent diabetes (type I) is common. Premature ovarian failure, hypothyroidism, malabsorption syndromes, pernicious anemia, chronic hepatitis, alopecia totalis, and vitiligo are also encountered.

Type I polyglandular disease is prevalent among Finns and Iranian Jews. The gene associated with type I disease is *AIRE* (autoimmune regulator) on chromosome 21q22. which is expressed in thymus, lymph nodes, and fetal liver, all tissues that are involved in the maturation of the immune system and immune tolerance. Similar to the common form of autoimmune Addison disease, sera from patients with type I polyglandular disease recognize steroidogenic autoantigens and other targets.

Type II polyglandular autoimmune syndrome (Schmidt syndrome) is more common than type I and always includes adrenal insufficiency. Women are affected twice as often as men. The disorder usually manifests between 20 and 40 years of age. Half of cases are familial, but several modes of inheritance are known. HT and occasionally Graves disease occur in more than two-thirds of cases. Insulin-dependent diabetes mellitus and premature ovarian failure are common. Only rarely are other autoimmune diseases present. This condition is considered to be a polygenic disorder with linkage to HLA-DR3.

GENETIC FACTORS: Half of patients with autoimmune adrenal insufficiency as part of a polyglandular syndrome have a familial history of an autoimmune endocrinopathy. When Addison disease occurs alone, a third have an affected relative. There is a strong linkage between autoimmune adrenalitis and HLA-B8, HLA-DR3, and HLA-DR4, with the exception of cases occurring as part of polyglandular syndrome type I, which is not linked to any *HLA* alleles.

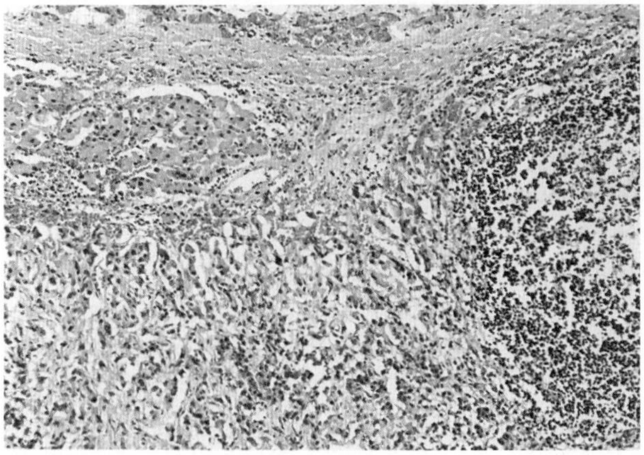

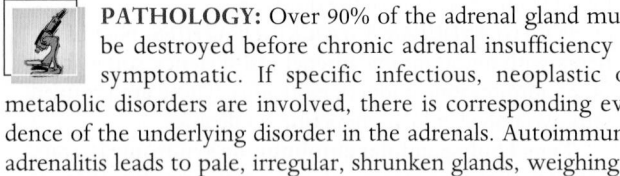

FIGURE 21-32. **Autoimmune adrenalitis.** A section of the adrenal gland from a patient with Addison disease shows chronic inflammation and fibrosis in the cortex, an island of residual atrophic cortical cells, and an intact medulla.

PATHOLOGY: Over 90% of the adrenal gland must be destroyed before chronic adrenal insufficiency is symptomatic. If specific infectious, neoplastic or metabolic disorders are involved, there is corresponding evidence of the underlying disorder in the adrenals. Autoimmune adrenalitis leads to pale, irregular, shrunken glands, weighing 2 to 3 g or less. The medulla is intact but surrounded by fibrous tissue containing small islands of atrophic cortical cells (Fig. 21-32). Depending on the stage of the disease, lymphoid infiltrates, predominantly T cells, of varying density are encountered.

CLINICAL FEATURES: Addison's original description of the clinical features of chronic adrenal insufficiency still applies for untreated cases. Patients had "general languor and debility, remarkable feebleness of the heart's action, irritability of the stomach and a peculiar change of the colour of the skin." Typically, the first symptom is insidious onset of weakness, which may become so profound that a patient is bedridden. Anorexia and weight loss are invariably present. A diffuse, tan pigmentation usually develops on the skin, and dark patches may appear on the mucous membranes. This hyperpigmentation is related to pituitary POMC stimulation of skin melanocytes. Hypotension, with blood pressures in the range of 80/50 mm Hg, is the rule. A variety of gastrointestinal symptoms, including vomiting, diarrhea, and abdominal pain, affects most patients and may be the presenting complaint. Patients with Addison disease often exhibit marked personality changes and even organic brain syndromes.

The lack of mineralocorticoid secretion, together with other metabolic derangements, leads to low serum levels of sodium and high potassium levels. The absence of glucocorticoids leads to lymphocytosis and mild eosinophilia. The diagnosis is established by measuring corticosteroid blood levels after ACTH stimulation. With glucocorticoid and mineralocorticoid replacement, patients live normal lives.

Acute Adrenal Insufficiency Is a Life-Threatening Emergency

Acute adrenal insufficiency, or adrenal crisis, reflects a sudden loss of adrenal cortical function. Symptoms are related more to mineralocorticoid deficiency than to inadequate glucocorticoids. Adrenal crisis occurs in three settings:

- Abrupt withdrawal of corticosteroid therapy in patients with adrenal atrophy that is due to long-term administration of these steroids. This is the most common cause of acute adrenal insufficiency.
- Sudden, devastating worsening of chronic adrenal insufficiency may be precipitated by the stress of infection or surgery.
- ***Waterhouse-Friderichsen syndrome*** *is acute, bilateral, hemorrhagic infarction of the adrenal cortex, most commonly secondary to meningococcus or* Pseudomonas *septicemia* (see Chapter 7). Adrenal hemorrhage in these circumstances is thought to be a local manifestation of a generalized Shwartzman reaction with disseminated intravascular coagulation. Acute adrenal insufficiency due to adrenal hemorrhage is also seen in newborns subjected to birth trauma.

CLINICAL FEATURES: The initial manifestations of adrenal crisis are usually hypotension and shock. Nonspecific symptoms commonly include weakness, vomiting, abdominal pain, and lethargy, which may progress to coma. Typically in Waterhouse-Friderichsen syndrome, a young person suddenly develops hypotension and shock, together with abdominal or back pain, fever, and purpura. Adrenal crisis is almost invariably fatal unless the patient is promptly and aggressively treated with corticosteroids and supportive measures.

Secondary Adrenal Insufficiency Reflects a Lack of ACTH

Destruction of the pituitary and consequent panhypopituitarism result in secondary adrenal insufficiency. Causes include pituitary tumors, craniopharyngioma, empty sella syndrome, and pituitary infarction. Trauma, surgery, and radiation therapy also may result in loss of pituitary function. Isolated ACTH deficiency is often associated with autoimmune endocrinopathies.

Any disorder that interferes with secretion of corticotropin (ACTH)-releasing hormone (CRH) by the hypothalamus (e.g., tumors, sarcoidosis) can result in inadequate secretion of ACTH. Secretion of glucocorticoids in response to ACTH distinguishes secondary from primary adrenal insufficiency. Pigmentary and electrolyte abnormalities are typically absent in secondary adrenal insufficiency since these processes are not regulated by ACTH.

Adrenal Hyperfunction

Excess corticosteroid secretion occurs in adrenal hyperplasia or neoplasia (Fig. 21-33). Such hyperfunction may take one of two forms, namely, **hypercortisolism** (Cushing syndrome) or **hyperaldosteronism** (Conn syndrome), disorders reflecting the two major classes of adrenal steroid hormones.

Early in the 20th century, the neurosurgeon Harvey Cushing associated "painful obesity, hypertrichosis and amenorrhea" with the presence of a pituitary tumor. The combination of pituitary hyperfunction and the signs and symptoms produced by chronic glucocorticoid excess was termed Cushing disease. It is now recognized that the constellation of clinical features caused by high glucocorticoid levels can also result from an adrenal adenoma or carcinoma, ectopic production of ACTH or CRH by a tumor or exogenous administration of corticosteroids. *Thus, hypercortisolism from any cause is now referred to as* ***Cushing syndrome,*** *and the term* ***Cushing disease*** *is reserved for excessive secretion of ACTH by pituitary corticotrope tumors.*

The most common cause of Cushing syndrome in the United States is chronic corticosteroid administration to treat immune and inflammatory

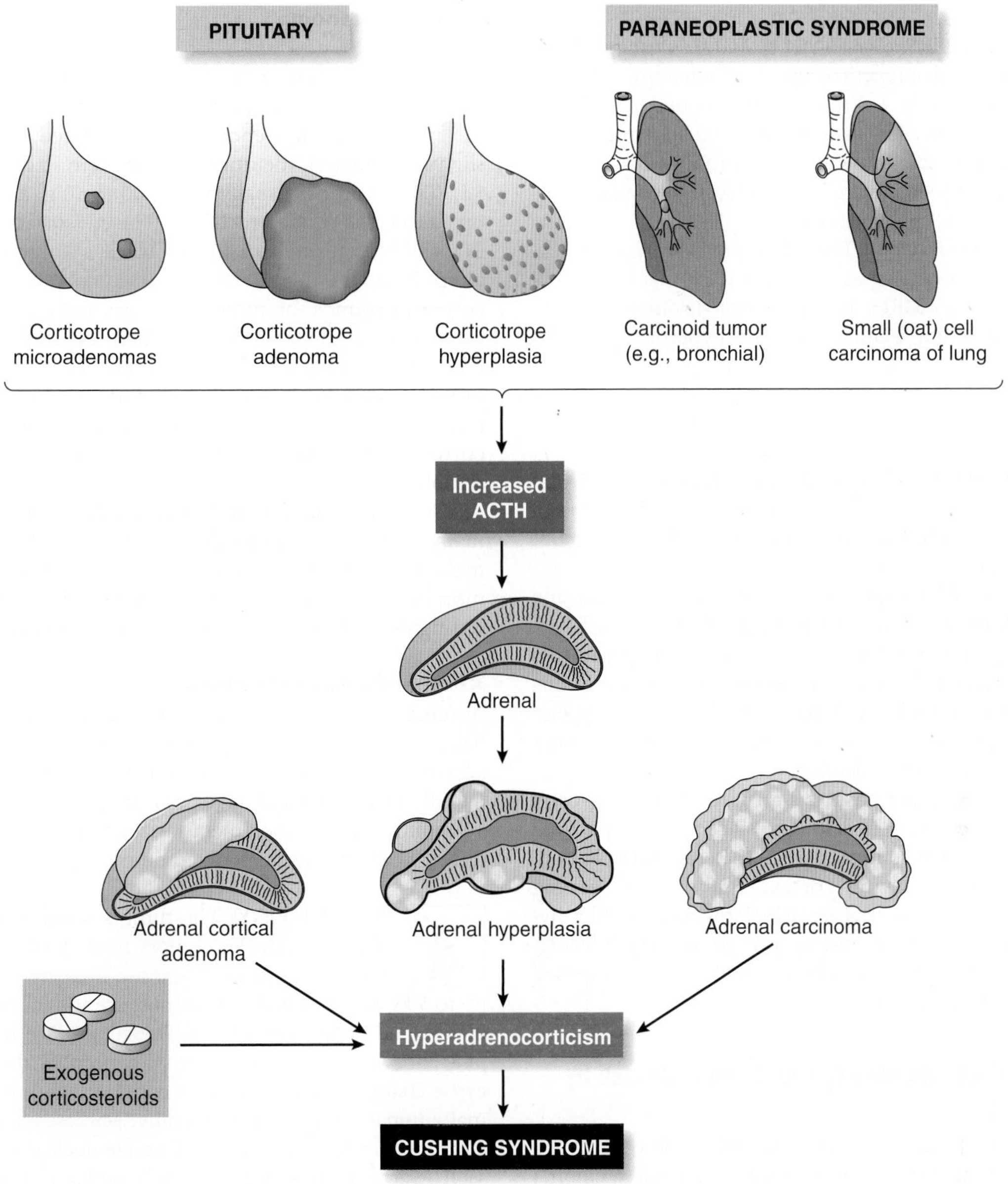

FIGURE 21-33. **The pathogenetic pathways of Cushing syndrome.** The ACTH-dependent pathway is referred to as Cushing disease. ACTH = adrenocorticotropic hormone (corticotropin).

disorders. The second most common cause is a paraneoplastic effect associated with nonpituitary cancers that inappropriately produce ACTH. Cushing disease is five times more frequent than the type of Cushing syndrome associated with adrenal tumors.

ACTH-Dependent Adrenal Hyperfunction Is of Pituitary or Ectopic Origin

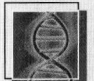

PATHOGENESIS: Women, usually 25 to 45 years old, are five times more likely than men to develop Cushing disease. Excessive secretion of ACTH leads to adrenal cortical hyperplasia. ACTH-dependent adrenal hyperfunction results from:

- Ectopic ACTH production by a nonpituitary tumor
- Primary hypersecretion of ACTH by the pituitary (Cushing disease)
- Inappropriate secretion of CRH by tumors arising outside the hypothalamus, with secondary pituitary hypersecretion of ACTH

ECTOPIC PRODUCTION OF ACTH: Inappropriate secretion of ACTH by a malignant tumor accounts for most cases of ACTH-dependent hyperadrenalism. Cancer of the lung, particularly small cell carcinoma, is responsible for more than half of the cases of ectopic ACTH syndrome. The remainder are attributable principally to carcinoids and neural crest tumors (pheochromocytoma, neuroblastoma, medullary carcinoma of the thyroid), thymoma, and islet cell adenoma of the pancreas.

PRIMARY HYPERSECRETION OF ACTH: Cushing disease usually results from corticotrope microadenomas of the pituitary, although it is occasionally secondary to a macroadenoma or, in a few patients, diffuse corticotrope hyperplasia. Whereas adenomas are clearly monoclonal, arising from a single progenitor cell, corticotrope hyperplasia is caused by chronic CRH hypersecretion.

ECTOPIC CRH PRODUCTION: Ectopic CRH syndrome is similar to ectopic ACTH syndrome, except that a malignant tumor secretes CRH. In turn, CRH stimulates pituitary ACTH secretion, leading to adrenal hyperplasia.

PATHOLOGY: Cushing disease is characterized by bilateral, diffuse (75%) or nodular (25%) hyperplasia of adrenal glands. Each gland usually weighs 8 to 10 g but occasionally as much as 20 g.

In **diffuse adrenal hyperplasia** the cortex is grossly visible and broadened, with an inner brown layer and a yellow, lipid-rich cap. Microscopically, the inner third of the cortex is composed of a compact cell layer, and the outer zone, corresponding to the zona fasciculata, displays large clear cells packed with lipid. The appearance of the zona glomerulosa varies, sometimes being prominent and at other times difficult to identify.

Nodular adrenal hyperplasia is a term reserved for grossly visible nodules up to 2.5 cm in diameter, since microscopic nodules are common in diffuse hyperplasia. Bilateral, multiple nodules compress the overlying cortex, and the intervening parenchyma exhibits diffuse hyperplasia. However, nodular hyperplasia may be asymmetric, and the two glands may differ significantly in weight. Microscopically, the nodules are composed of large, lipid-laden, clear cells.

ACTH-Independent Adrenal Hyperfunction is Caused by Adrenal Tumors

In adults, incidence of adrenal carcinoma peaks at 40 years of age and that of adenoma a decade later. In children, adrenal carcinoma accounts for one half of cases of Cushing syndrome; 15% are caused by adenoma. At all ages, the female-to-male ratio is 4:1.

Adrenal Adenoma

PATHOLOGY: Adenomas of the adrenal cortex are uncommon, provided one excludes minute nodules. A typical adenoma is encapsulated, firm, yellow, and slightly lobulated, measuring about 4 cm in diameter (Fig. 21-34). These tumors usually weigh 10 to 50 g, although weights up to 100 g have been recorded. The cut surface is mottled yellow and brown and occasionally black, owing to the deposition of lipofuscin pigment. A thin rim of compressed normal adrenal cortex surrounds the tumor. Necrosis and calcification may be present, even in small tumors. Microscopically, adenomas exhibit clear, lipid-laden (fasciculata type) cells arranged in sheets or nests, often with interspersed clusters of compact, lipid-depleted, eosinophilic (reticularis type) cells. The nontumorous cortex of the involved and contralateral gland is generally atrophic.

Nonfunctional adrenal cortical adenoma is observed in as many as 5% of adult autopsies, but less than 10% of surgically removed benign tumors of the adrenal are hormonally silent. On morphologic grounds alone, nonfunctional adenomas cannot be distinguished from their functional counterparts.

Adrenal Cortical Carcinoma

Adrenal cortical carcinoma is a rare and aggressive tumor that has an incidence of 1 case per million per year. Eighty percent of adrenal cortical carcinomas are functional. They occur more frequently in women and have poor prognosis. Median survival is 30 months. The tumor metastasizes to lung, liver, and lymph nodes. Local recurrences are common.

PATHOLOGY: The tumors weigh more than 100 g although smaller tumors have been reported due to improvement in diagnostic imaging. Tumor weights up to 5 kg are recorded. The tumors are soft, circumscribed, lobulated, and bulky (Fig. 21-35). The cut surface has a variegated pink, brown, or yellow, often with necrosis, hemorrhage and cystic change. Local invasion is common, and remnants of normal adrenal are difficult to identify. Microscopically, both clear and compact cells are present. Variable nuclear pleomorphism is seen. Mitotic figures, necrosis, and vascular invasion may or may not be apparent. In functional carcinomas, the contralateral adrenal cortex is atrophic.

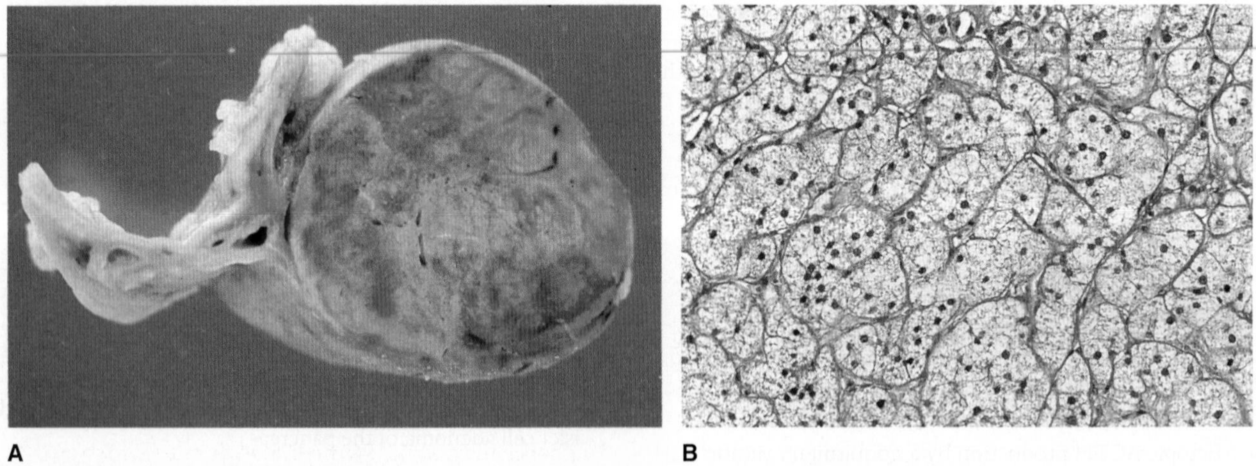

A B

FIGURE 21-34. **Adrenal adenoma. A.** The cut surface of an adrenal tumor removed from a patient with Cushing syndrome is a mottled yellow with a rim of compressed normal adrenal tissue. **B.** A microscopic view reveals nests of clear, lipid-laden cells.

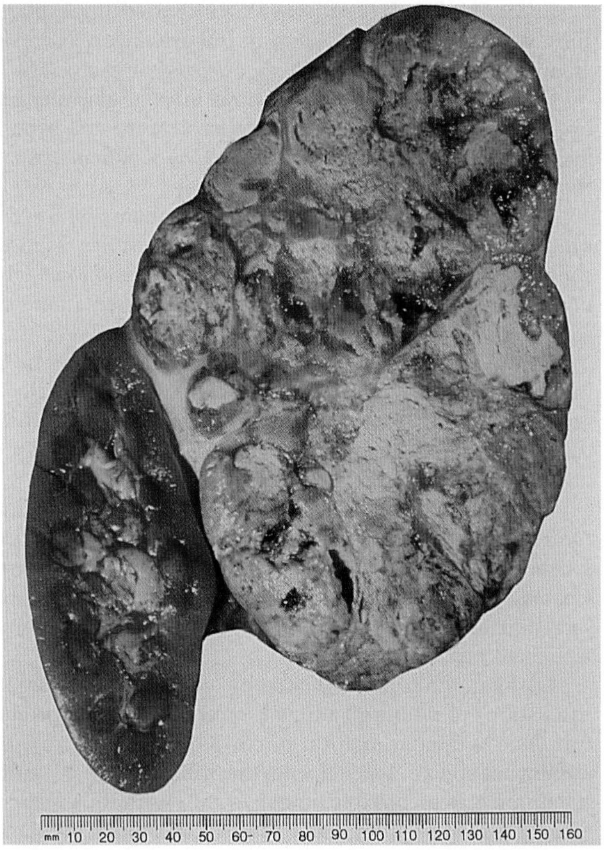

A

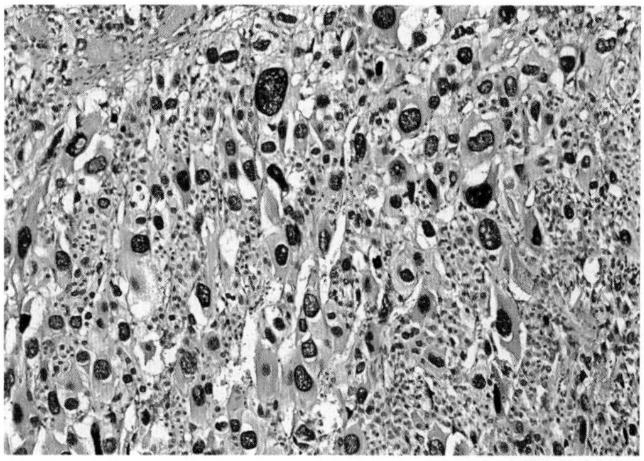

B

FIGURE 21-35. **Adrenal cortical carcinoma. A.** The bulky tumor on section is yellow to tan with areas of necrosis and cystic degeneration. **B.** A microscopic section demonstrates marked anisocytosis and nuclear pleomorphism.

Most adrenal cortical carcinomas cannot be resected completely, and even when the surgeon believes that the entire tumor has been removed, micrometastases in other organs are already present. Even with surgery, most patients survive for only 1 to 3 years.

Nonfunctional adrenal cortical carcinomas tend to be highly malignant, with weights exceeding 1 kg. They are morphologically identical to functional cancers.

Adrenal carcinomas are monoclonal, while one third of adenomas are polyclonal. Several hereditary tumor syndromes are associated with benign and malignant adrenal tumors including Li-Fraumeni syndrome, Beckwith-Wiedemann syndrome, MEN type 1, and a few other rare conditions.

Other Causes of ACTH-Independent Cushing Syndrome Include Chronic Corticosteroid Administration and Bilateral Micronodular Hyperplasia

Many immunologic and inflammatory diseases are treated with glucocorticoids, constituting by far the most common cause of Cushing syndrome. The synthetic hormones ordinarily used (e.g., dexamethasone, prednisone) have only glucocorticoid activity and few or no mineralocorticoid or androgen effects. Thus, hypertension and hirsutism, features commonly seen in Cushing syndrome due to adrenal hyperplasia or neoplasia, are usually absent in this iatrogenic disorder.

Bilateral adrenal cortical micronodular hyperplasia (Carney complex or **primary pigmented nodular adrenocortical disease)** is a rare cause of ACTH-independent Cushing syndrome, usually in children or young adults. Half have an AD disease characterized by pigmented skin lesions over much of the body, a variety of myxomas, testicular tumors, and pituitary somatotrope adenomas. The adrenals contain small, brown or black nodules, up to 0.5 cm in diameter, with large eosinophilic cells laden with lipofuscin granules. Half of patients with Carney complex carry a mutation in a tumor suppressor gene (17q22-24) that codes for a regulatory subunit of protein kinase A. Another gene in 2p16 has also been mapped to the disease.

Clinical Features of Cushing Syndrome Are Seen in Many Organs

CLINICAL FEATURES: The manifestations of Cushing syndrome (Fig. 21-36) depend on the degree and duration of excessive corticosteroid levels, as well as on the levels of adrenal androgens and mineralocorticoids.

OBESITY: Typically, the patient notes gradual onset of obesity of the face (moon face), neck (buffalo hump), trunk, and abdomen (Fig. 21-37). The extremities are characteristically unaffected or even wasted.

SKIN: The skin is atrophic. Subcutaneous fat is decreased. Enlargement of the abdomen and other areas of fat deposition stretches the thin skin and produces purplish striae, which represent venous channels that are visible through the attenuated dermis. Hyperpigmentation, similar to, but less severe than, that in Addison disease, may occur because of pituitary hypersecretion of POMC. Acanthosis nigricans is increased in frequency in Cushing syndrome.

MUSCULOSKELETAL SYSTEM: Increased bone resorption causes osteoporosis. Back pain is common, and up to a fifth of patients with Cushing syndrome have radiologic evidence of vertebral compression fractures. Fractures of ribs and occasionally long bones may occur. Proximal muscle wasting (**steroid myopathy**) causes weakness, which may be so severe that the patient cannot rise from sitting or climb a flight of stairs.

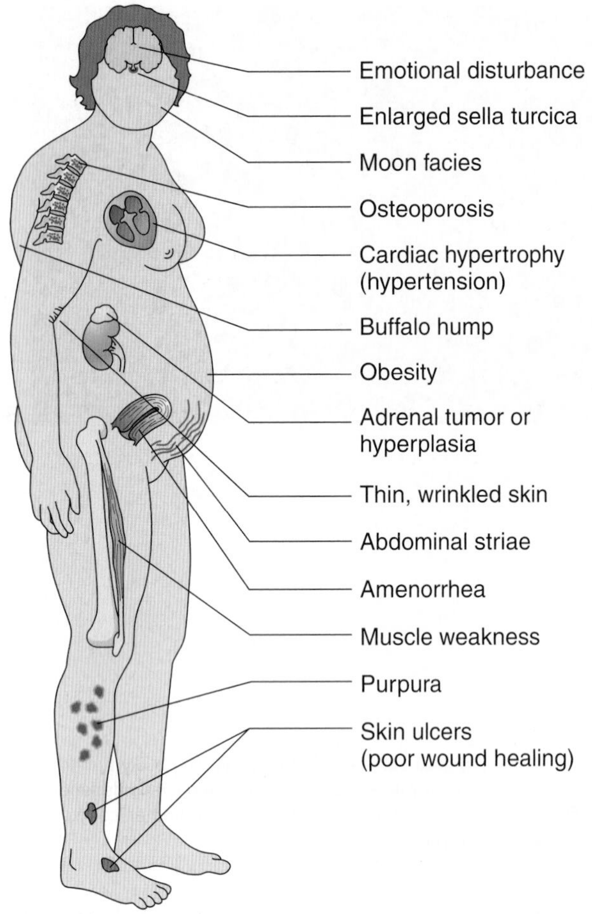

FIGURE 21-36. **Major clinical manifestations of Cushing syndrome.**

CARDIOVASCULAR SYSTEM: Hypertension is common in Cushing syndrome, often reflecting excessive mineralocorticoid activity. In older patients, congestive heart failure is a frequent sequel.

SECONDARY SEX CHARACTERISTICS: Women with Cushing syndrome tend to be virilized, with increased facial hair, thinning of scalp hair, acne, and oligomenorrhea. Excess glucocorticoid levels in men cause erectile dysfunction, and both sexes experience decreased libido.

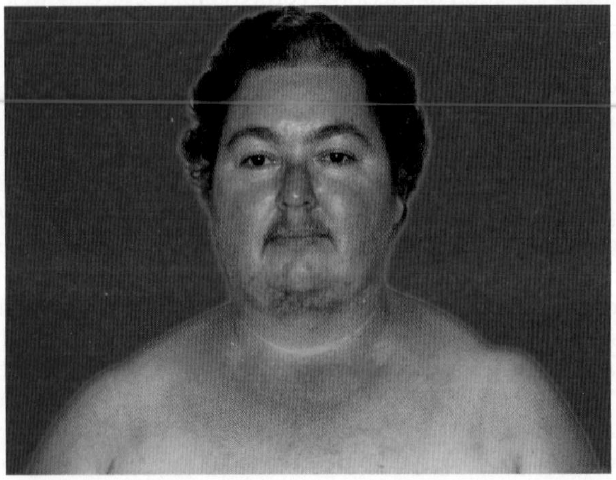

FIGURE 21-37. **Cushing syndrome.** A woman who had a pituitary adenoma that produced adrenocorticotropic hormone (ACTH) exhibits a moon face, buffalo hump, increased facial hair, and thinning of the scalp hair.

EYES: One fourth of patients have increased intraocular pressure, which may be a problem in the presence of preexisting glaucoma.

GLUCOSE INTOLERANCE: Stimulation of gluconeogenesis by glucocorticoids leads to glucose intolerance and hyperinsulinemia. Diabetes mellitus develops in 15% of patients, usually in those with a family history of diabetes.

PSYCHOLOGICAL CHANGES: Most patients with Cushing syndrome, both endogenous and iatrogenic, suffer distinct personality changes. These include irritability, emotional lability, depression, and paranoia. The disturbance in mentation may be so severe that the patient becomes suicidal.

LABORATORY FINDINGS: Half of patients exhibit an absolute lymphopenia, and one third have abnormally low eosinophil counts. Hypercalciuria is common, although serum calcium levels remain unchanged. Serum cholesterol and triglyceride levels are frequently elevated.

All forms of Cushing syndrome are characterized by increased glucocorticoid levels. The dexamethasone suppression test distinguishes ACTH-dependent and ACTH-independent forms of Cushing syndrome. Dexamethasone suppresses pituitary ACTH secretion, and hence hypercortisolism, whereas it is without effect on adrenal tumors.

Cushing syndrome is treated by (1) extirpation (surgery or irradiation) of pituitary, adrenal, or ectopic ACTH-producing tumors; (2) discontinuation of corticosteroid therapy; or (3) administration of adrenal enzyme inhibitors (e.g., aminoglutethimide, ketoconazole, metapyrone). With the exception of ectopic ACTH syndrome and adrenal carcinoma, in which patients die of cancer rather than of hypercortisolism, Cushing syndrome is highly curable.

Primary Aldosteronism (Conn Syndrome) Leads to Hypertension and Hypokalemia

Inappropriate secretion of aldosterone is caused by adrenal adenomas or hyperplasia. Aldosterone-secreting adenomas are more common in women than in men (3:1) and usually occur between the ages of 30 and 50 years.

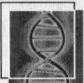

PATHOGENESIS: About 75% of causes of primary aldosteronism are caused by solitary adrenal adenomas (aldosteronoma). In a quarter of cases, adrenal hyperplasia is involved. The remainder reflect bilateral hyperplasia of the adrenal zona glomerulosa. Only a few cases of primary aldosteronism are caused by adrenal carcinomas.

Two types of familial hyperaldosteronism are defined. Type I (glucocorticoid-suppressible) is an autosomal dominant disease in which fusion of the ACTH-responsive regulatory elements of the 11β-hydroxylase gene to the aldosterone synthase gene results in a hybrid gene that is ectopically and constitutively activated in the zona fasciculata. Bilateral hyperplasia of this zone results. By suppressing ACTH release, glucocorticoids ameliorate type I disease. In contrast, type II familial hyperaldosteronism is associated with adrenal cortical adenomas and is, therefore, not suppressible by glucocorticoids.

Aldosterone hypersecretion enhances renal tubular sodium reabsorption, thus increasing body sodium. Hypertension is caused not only by retention of sodium and consequent volume expansion, but also by increased peripheral vascular resistance. Hypokalemia reflects aldosterone-induced loss of potassium in the distal renal tubule.

PATHOLOGY: Most aldosterone-secreting adenomas measure less than 3 cm in diameter, weigh less than 6 g, and are yellow. However, the size varies, and tumors up to 50 g are reported. On microscopic examination, the dominant cells are clear, lipid-rich, resembling the zona fasciculata, and arranged in cords or alveoli. Little nuclear pleomorphism is noted. In contrast to cortisol-producing adenomas, the nontumorous cortex in cases of hyperaldosteronism is not atrophic, because aldosterone does not inhibit ACTH secretion by the pituitary.

Bilateral nodular adrenal hyperplasia in Conn syndrome is characterized by yellow cortical nodules less than 2 cm in diameter. Microscopically, they are formed by clear cells that show no nuclear pleomorphism.

CLINICAL FEATURES: Most patients with primary aldosteronism are diagnosed after detection of asymptomatic diastolic hypertension. Muscle weakness and fatigue are caused by the effects of potassium depletion on skeletal muscle. Polyuria and polydipsia result from a disturbance in the concentrating ability of the kidney, probably secondary to hypokalemia. Metabolic alkalosis and an alkaline urine are common.

Primary aldosteronism that is caused by an adenoma is cured by surgical removal of the tumor. Dietary sodium restriction and treatment with the aldosterone antagonist spironolactone are also frequently effective. Bilateral adrenal hyperplasia in Conn syndrome is treated medically with aldosterone antagonists and sometimes with dexamethasone in the case of glucocorticoid-suppressible hyperaldosteronism.

Miscellaneous Adrenal Tumors

Adrenal myelolipoma is a mixture of mature adipose tissue and hematopoietic marrow and is notable for its occasional large size.

Adrenal cysts are rare, and most are actually pseudocysts that develop secondary to degenerative changes in benign adrenal tumors or resolution of hemorrhage. In some cases, they represent remnants of an underlying vascular lesion.

Metastatic cancers to adrenal glands are commonly lung or breast carcinomas, or malignant melanomas. The glands may be unilaterally or bilaterally hugely enlarged, up to 20 to 45 g. They are largely replaced by carcinoma, often with necrosis and hemorrhage. Usually, enough functional adrenal cortex remains to ensure that Addison disease does not develop, particularly in view of the limited survival of these patients.

ADRENAL MEDULLA AND PARAGANGLIA

Anatomy And Function

The adrenal medulla is entirely surrounded by the adrenal cortex and accounts for 10% of the weight of the gland. It consists of neuroendocrine cells, termed **chromaffin cells**, which are derived from primitive pheochromoblasts of the developing sympathetic nervous system (Fig. 21-38). Chromaffin cells are so named because the catecholamines in their cytoplasmic granules

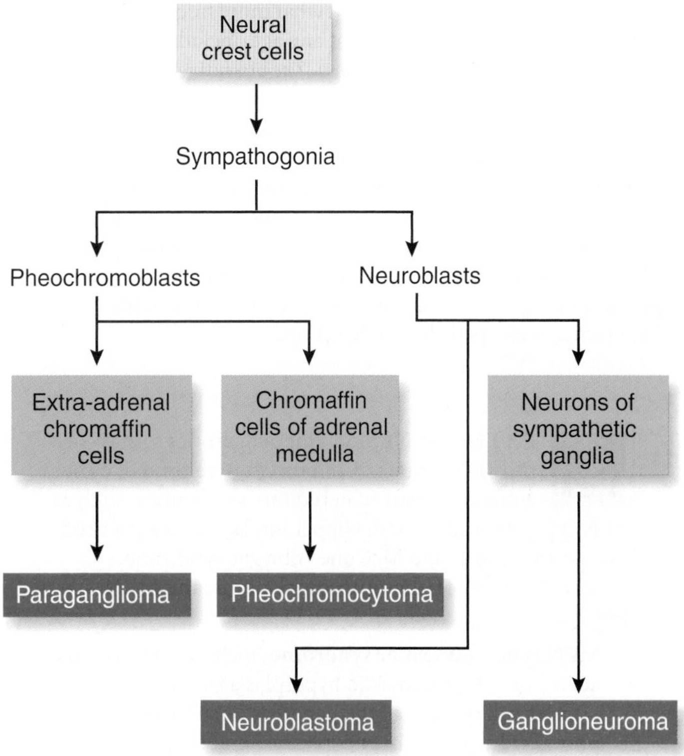

FIGURE 21-38. **Histogenesis of tumors of the adrenal medulla and extra-adrenal sympathetic nervous system.**

bind chromium salts and darken on oxidation by potassium dichromate. These cells are also present at extra-adrenal sympathetic nervous system sites, such as the preaortic sympathetic plexuses and paravertebral sympathetic chain.

Chromaffin cells appear as nests of small polyhedral cells with pale amphophilic cytoplasm and vesicular nuclei. The cells of the adrenal medulla have many electron-dense chromaffin (catecholamine-containing) granules 100 to 300 nm in diameter, resembling those of sympathetic nerve endings. Epinephrine accounts for 85% of the content of these granules, with the remainder being norepinephrine and other noncatecholamine hormones. Interspersed among the chromaffin cells are postganglionic neurons and small autonomic nerve fibers. Stored catecholamines are secreted on sympathetic stimulation as a response to stress (exercise, cold, fasting, trauma) or emotional excitation accompanying fear and anger.

The adrenal medulla is supplied by arterial and portal venous circulations that originate in the zona reticularis of the cortex. Most of the blood to the hormonally active cells of the medulla is from the portal system. The medulla is innervated from the splanchnic nerves by cholinergic preganglionic sympathetic neurons.

Pheochromocytoma

Pheochromocytomas are Rare Catecholamine-Secreting Tumors of Chromaffin Cells of the Adrenal Medulla

If pheochromocytoma arise in extra-adrenal sites, they are called **paragangliomas.** Other catecholamine-producing tumors (e.g., chemodectoma and ganglioneuroma) may also cause a syndrome similar to that associated with pheochromocytoma.

Pheochromocytomas are somewhat more frequent in women than in men. They are observed at any age, including infancy, but are uncommon after 60 years of age. *The presenting symptoms reflect sustained or episodic hypertension.* Other symptoms include pallor, anxiety, and cardiac arrhythmias. Although pheochromocytomas account for less than 0.1% of cases of hypertension, this tumor should be considered in evaluating any hypertensive patient. If detected early, pheochromocytomas are amenable to surgical resection, but when left untreated, patients can die of the complications of prolonged hypertension. Most pheochromocytomas are unexpected findings at autopsy, indicating that some curable cases of hypertension escaped clinical detection.

PATHOGENESIS: Pheochromocytomas are mostly sporadic. A minority are inherited, either alone or as part of hereditary syndromes, such as MEN types 2A and 2B, von Hippel-Lindau disease, neurofibromatosis type 1, and McCune-Albright syndrome.

The features of the autosomal dominant MEN syndromes are:

- **MEN type 1 (Wermer syndrome)** includes (1) pituitary adenoma, (2) parathyroid hyperplasia or adenoma, and (3) islet cell tumors of the pancreas (insulinoma, gastrinoma). The pancreatic neoplasms tend to be multicentric and more malignant than in sporadic cases. Two-thirds of patients have adenomas of two or more endocrine organs, and one-fifth develop tumors of three or more. Carcinoid, adrenocortical and lipoid tumors may also occur in MEN-1. Almost all people with MEN type 1 (>95%) have primary hyperparathyroidism. The disease is caused by mutation of the MEN1 tumor suppressor gene (chromosome 11q13), which encodes a protein termed **menin**. This nuclear protein is thought to interact with the transcription factor junD.
- **MEN type 2 syndromes** feature MTC in virtually all patients and pheochromocytoma in about half.

MEN-2A (SIPPLE SYNDROME): Most (95%) MEN-2 patients are classified as 2A. In addition to MTC and pheochromocytoma, a third of patients show hyperparathyroidism due to parathyroid hyperplasia or adenoma. A variety of neural crest tumors may be seen with MEN type 2A, including gliomas, glioblastomas, and meningiomas. Hirschsprung disease is also associated with MEN type 2A.

MEN-2B: This disorder resembles MEN-2A, but develops some 10 years earlier. Parathyroid disease is uncommon. The **mucosal neuroma syndrome** (ganglioneuromas of the conjunctiva, oral cavity, larynx, and gastrointestinal tract) is a feature of MEN-2B. Mucosal neuromas are always encountered, but only half of patients express the full phenotype. Many patients have a habitus similar to that in Marfan syndrome.

FAMILIAL MEDULLARY THYROID CARCINOMA: There are families who have at least four members with this tumor and no evidence of other features of MEN-2.

Adrenal medullary hyperplasia has been reported in some patients with both MEN-2A and 2B. Just as C-cell hyperplasia precedes thyroid medullary carcinomas, adrenal medullary hyperplasia is thought to antedate pheochromocytoma in these cases. Lesions are usually less than 1 cm. Grossly, an enlarged adrenal shows an expanded medulla. The chromaffin cells are larger than normal and are arranged in distinct nests or cords.

The ***RET* protooncogene** on chromosome 10q11.2 is responsible for MEN-2 syndromes. *RET* encodes a transmembrane receptor of the tyrosine kinase family. Glia-derived growth factor and neurturin are ligands for the RET receptor. Several germline, missense, and activating mutations in the cysteine-rich extracellular domain of RET have been identified in 95% of families with MEN-2A and 85% of those with familial thyroid carcinoma (Fig. 21-39).

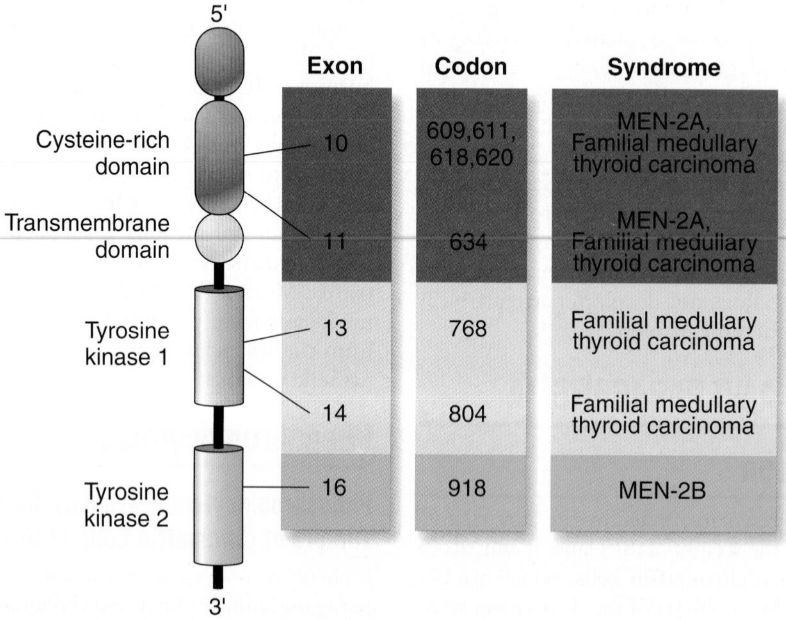

FIGURE 21-39. Representative ***RET*** protooncogene mutations in multiple endocrine neoplasia, type 2 (MEN-2).

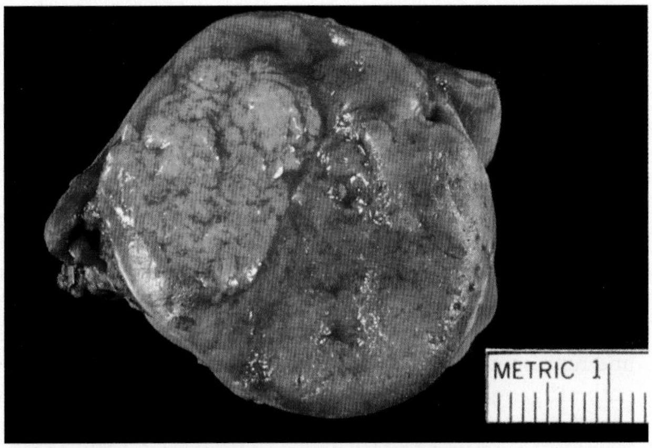

A

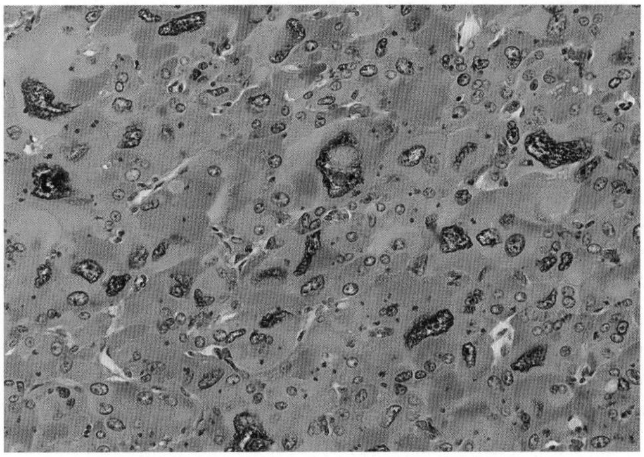

B

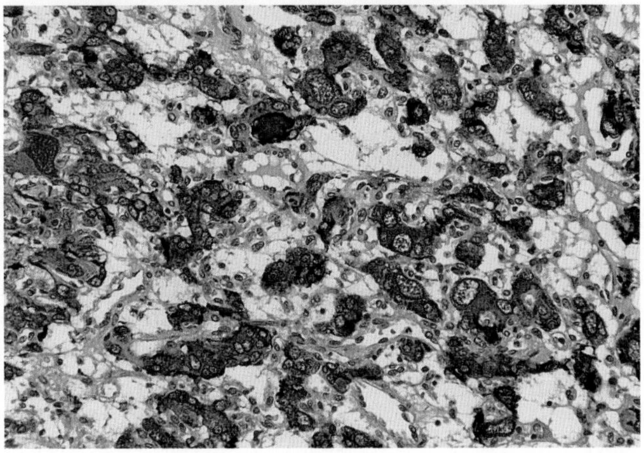

C

FIGURE 21-40. **Pheochromocytoma. A.** The cut surface of an adrenal tumor from a patient with episodic hypertension is reddish brown with a prominent area of fibrosis. Foci of hemorrhage and cystic degeneration are evident. **B.** A photomicrograph of the tumor shows polyhedral tumor cells with ample finely granular cytoplasm. Note the enlarged hyperchromatic nuclei. **C.** Many of the tumor cells show positive immunohistochemical staining for chromogranin A, a marker of neuroendocrine differentiation.

The most common mutation (codon 634) constitutively activates the receptor by promoting its dimerization, recapitulating the result of ligand binding.

A point mutation at codon 918 of the tyrosine kinase domain of *RET* is seen in 95% of patients with MEN-2B. This mutation constitutively activates the tyrosine kinase function of the receptor, and also causes it to phosphorylate substrates ordinarily preferred by other kinases (e.g., c-*src* and c-*abl*).

Identification of RET *mutations is used to confirm the diagnosis of MEN-2 and identify asymptomatic family members.* People who carry *RET* mutations are screened for thyroid cancer, pheochromocytoma, and hyperparathyroidism between 6 and 35 years of age, and are offered prophylactic thyroidectomy.

Somatic mutations in *RET* have been found in 10% to 20% of patients with sporadic pheochromocytomas. In addition, some sporadic pheochromocytomas exhibit mutations in the von Hippel-Lindau *(VHL)* and neurofibromatosis, type 1 *(NF1)* genes.

PATHOLOGY: In sporadic pheochromocytomas, 80% of tumors are unilateral, 10% are bilateral and 10% are in extraadrenal locations; 10% are malignant and 10% occur in children. By contrast, two thirds of tumors occurring in the context of MEN are bilateral. Tumors range in size from 1 cm across to large masses of more than 2 kg. Most are 5 to 6 cm in diameter and weigh 80 to 100 g.

Pheochromocytomas tend to be encapsulated, spongy, reddish masses, with prominent central scars, hemorrhage and foci of cystic degeneration (Fig. 21-40A). Their histology is highly variable. Typically, circumscribed nests (**zellballen**) of neoplastic cells are present. Tumor cells range from polyhedral to fusiform, with granular, amphophilic, or basophilic cytoplasm and vesicular nuclei. Eosinophilic globules are usually seen in the cytoplasm. Cellular pleomorphism is often prominent and may include multinucleated tumor giant cells (see Fig. 21-40B). The tumor contains numerous capillaries. Less commonly, trabecular or solid patterns are seen, with only indistinct **zellballen.**

By electron microscopy, membrane-bound, dense core granules are seen, corresponding to stored catecholamines. Immunohistochemical stains attest to the neuroendocrine nature of the tumor and show neuron-specific enolase, chromogranin (see Fig. 21-40C), and synaptophysin.

In 5% to 10% of cases, pheochromocytomas are malignant, although this figure may be higher for extra-adrenal tumors. Malignancy is only determined by a tumor's biological behavior (i.e., metastases), and cannot be determined from its histologic appearance. Both benign and malignant pheochromocytomas show mitoses, cellular pleomorphism, capsular or vascular invasion, and necrosis. Metastases are most common in the regional lymph nodes, bone, lung, and liver.

CLINICAL FEATURES: With few exceptions, the clinical features of pheochromocytomas are caused by catecholamine release by the tumor. Patients may come to medical attention because of (1) asymptomatic hypertension discovered on routine physical examination, (2) symptomatic hypertension resistant to antihypertensive therapy, (3) malignant hypertension (e.g., encephalopathy, papilledema, proteinuria), (4) myocardial infarction or aortic dissection, or (5) paroxysms of convulsions, anxiety, or hyperventilation.

Typically, episodic catecholamine release leads to a paroxysm or crisis, of up to several hours, with severe throbbing headache, sweating, palpitations, tachycardia, abdominal pain, and vomiting. Blood pressure may be elevated, often to an extreme degree. A paroxysm can be precipitated by activities that place pressure on the abdominal contents (including the tumor), such as exercise, lifting, bending or vigorous abdominal palpation. Anxiety may occur during a paroxysm, but it is not an initiating factor.

More than 90% of patients with pheochromocytoma show hypertension, which is sustained in two thirds of patients and resembles essential hypertension. In these patients, blood pressure rises to even higher levels during a paroxysm. In one third of patients, hypertension is episodic. Frequently, episodic hypertension becomes sustained, and in many untreated patients, it evolves into malignant hypertension.

There are other consequences of excess catecholamine levels. Orthostatic hypotension results from decreased plasma volume and poor postural tone. Increased basal metabolism, sweating, heat intolerance, and weight loss may mimic hyperthyroidism. Angina and myocardial infarction occur in the absence of coronary artery disease. The cardiac complications are attributed to myocardial necrosis caused by elevated catecholamine levels ***(catecholamine cardiomyopathy)***.

Pheochromocytoma is diagnosed by finding increased urinary levels of catecholamine metabolites, particularly vanillylmandelic acid (VMA), metanephrine, and unconjugated catecholamines. Treatment for pheochromocytoma is surgical removal. β-Adrenergic blocking agents are used to control hypertensive crises, and β-adrenergic receptor antagonists are helpful adjuncts.

Paraganglioma Is a Pheochromocytoma Arising at an Extra-adrenal Site

Paragangliomas arise in paraganglia in any location, including the retroperitoneum, neck, posterior mediastinum, and urinary bladder. Bladder paragangliomas may present as a peculiar syndrome of headaches and paroxysmal hypertension on urination. The tumors may also arise in the base of the skull, in the neck, in vagal or aortic bodies, or in any organ that contains paraganglionic tissue, such as the larynx and small intestine. They take origin in such paraganglia as the glomus jugulare, carotid body, and other vasoreceptor bodies. Most (90%) paragangliomas of the head and neck are benign; those in the retroperitoneum are more often malignant.

Carotid body tumor *is a prototypic paraganglioma arising at the carotid bifurcation. It forms a palpable mass in the neck.* Interestingly, carotid body tumors are 10 times more frequent in persons living at high altitude than those at sea level, suggesting that these tumors may represent a hyperplastic response to prolonged carotid body sensing of hypoxia.

Autosomal dominant transmission of paragangliomas is seen in some families, and hereditary paraganglioma was the first hereditary tumor syndrome reported to be caused by a germline mutation in a gene encoding a mitochondrial protein. Genetic linkage is traced to the *SDHD* gene (11q23), which encodes a subunit of cytochrome B that has been proposed to participate in oxygen sensing. Curiously, all affected persons, whether male or female, inherited the disease from their fathers. About 10% of these tumors can be malignant and metastasize to distant organs such as lung and bone.

Neuroblastoma

Neuroblastoma (NB) is an embryonal malignant tumor of neural crest origin that is composed of neoplastic neuroblasts and originates in the adrenal medulla, paravertebral sympathetic ganglia, and sympathetic paraganglia. Neuroblasts derive from primitive sympathogonia and represent an intermediate stage in the development of sympathetic ganglion neurons (see Fig. 21-38). *Neuroblastomas are the most common solid extracranial neoplasms of childhood, accounting for up to 10% of all childhood cancers and 15% of cancer deaths in children.* Overall incidence is 1 in 7000. The peak incidence is in the first 3 years.

NB is congenital in some cases and has even been found in premature stillborns. In fact, NB accounts for half of all cancers diagnosed in the first month of life. Occasional cases are encountered in adolescents or adults. Although the occurrence of NB is sporadic, a few instances of familial tumors are recorded. Those genetically predisposed to this disease usually have multifocal tumors at an early age and follow an AD pattern of inheritance. The short arm of chromosome 16 appears to be the affected locus. NBs may occur with neurofibromatosis type 1, Beckwith-Wiedemann syndrome, and Hirschsprung disease.

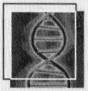

PATHOGENESIS: Embryogenesis of the adrenal medulla and presumably of other parts of the sympathetic nervous system continues during the first year of life. *Persistence and transformation of these embryonal structures may be related to the pathogenesis of NB.* The tumor is characterized by frequent deletions on chromosome 1 (1p35-36), with unbalanced translocation with 17q. Extrachromosomal double minutes and homogeneously staining regions (HSRs) are found on chromosome 2. The HSRs represent amplification of N-*myc,* which abnormality is key in determining the aggressiveness of neuroblastoma. It is thought that the locus on chromosome 1 encodes a gene that suppresses N-*myc* amplification.

PATHOLOGY: NBs can arise at any site with neural crest derived cells (i.e., from the posterior cranial fossa to the coccyx). One third of tumors are in the adrenal, another third elsewhere in the abdomen, and 20% in the posterior mediastinum.

NBs vary from minute, barely discernible nodules to tumors readily palpable through the abdominal wall. They are round, irregularly lobulated masses that may weigh 50 to 150 g or more (Fig. 21-41A). The cut surface is soft and friable, with a variegated maroon color. Areas of necrosis, hemorrhage, calcification, and cystic change are often present.

Neuroblastic tumors are classified as belonging to one of four categories:

- **Neuroblastoma** (Schwannian stroma-poor)
- **Ganglioneuroblastoma, intermixed** (Schwannian stroma-rich)

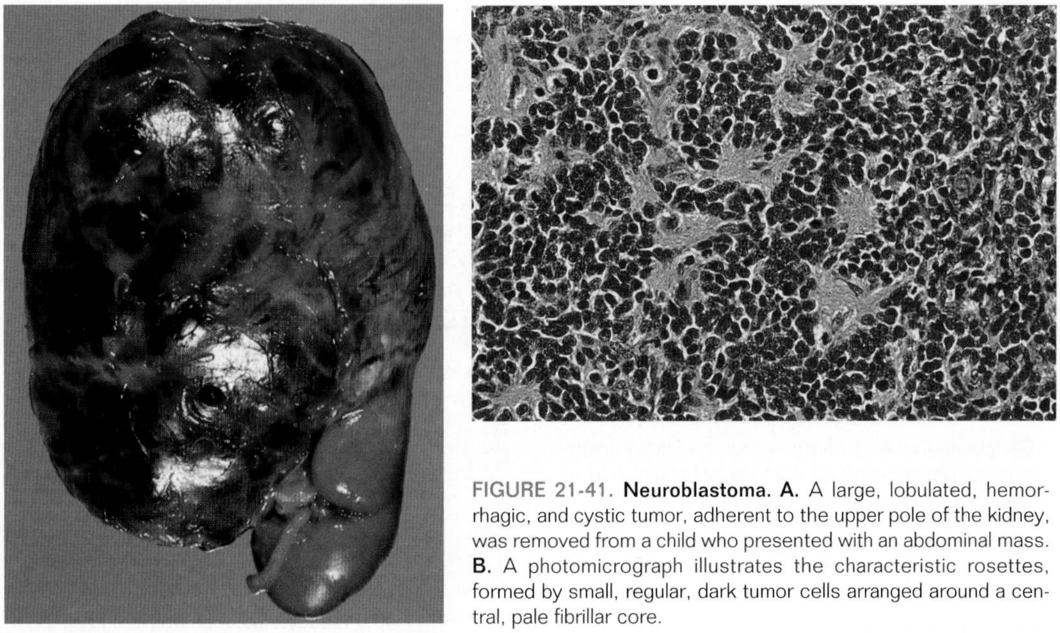

A

B

FIGURE 21-41. **Neuroblastoma. A.** A large, lobulated, hemorrhagic, and cystic tumor, adherent to the upper pole of the kidney, was removed from a child who presented with an abdominal mass. **B.** A photomicrograph illustrates the characteristic rosettes, formed by small, regular, dark tumor cells arranged around a central, pale fibrillar core.

- **Ganglioneuroma** (Schwannian stroma-dominant)
- **Ganglioneuroblastoma, nodular** (composite Schwannian stroma-rich/stroma-dominant and stroma-poor).

Each category may have one or more subtypes.

NBs are composed of dense sheets of small, round to fusiform cells with hyperchromatic nuclei and scanty cytoplasm, which are often compared with lymphocytes. Limited or no Schwannian proliferation is seen and mitoses are frequent. Characteristic Homer Wright rosettes are defined by a rim of dark tumor cells in a circumferential arrangement around a central pale fibrillar core (see Fig. 21-41B). By electron microscopy, malignant neuroblasts show peripheral dendritic processes with longitudinally oriented microtubules and neurosecretory granules and filament.

NBs readily infiltrate surrounding structures and metastasize to regional lymph nodes, liver, lungs, bones, and other sites. The tumor may differentiate into a ganglioneuroma (see below).

CLINICAL FEATURES: The presentation of NB is highly variable, a consequence of the many sites of the primary tumors and metastases. The first sign is often an enlarging abdomen in a young child. Physical examination discloses a firm, irregular, nontender mass. Hepatic metastases enlarge the liver and may cause ascites. Marked irritability may reflect pain from bony metastases. Respiratory distress accompanies large masses in the thorax, and tumors in the pelvis obstruct the bowel or ureters. Spinal cord compression may lead to gait disturbance and sphincter dysfunction. Severe diarrhea may be caused in tumors secreting vasoactive intestinal peptide. Some patients show paraneoplastic opsoclonus-myoclonus syndrome, which usually indicates an excellent prognosis, although some may develop permanent neurologic deficits.

Urinary excretion of catecholamines and their metabolites is almost invariably elevated in patients with NB. The urine contains increased amounts of **norepinephrine**, **VMA**, **homovanillic acid** (HVA), and **dopamine**.

Several factors are useful in predicting the outcome of NB:

- **Age:** Age at diagnosis is one of the most important indicators of survival. Children under 1 year have a better prognosis than do older patients with the same stage of disease. Spontaneous tumor regression is common at this age.
- **Site:** Extra-adrenal tumors tend to be better differentiated and so less aggressive.
- **Stage:** Survival is 90% in stage I (tumor confined to the organ of origin), and decreases to less than 3% in stage IV (widespread metastases). An exception is stage IVS (special), in which tumors lack the chromosomal abnormalities characteristic of neuroblastoma. Even with liver and bone marrow metastases, patients with stage IVS may experience spontaneous remissions, and have a 60% to 90% survival rate.
- **Tumor histology:** Low-grade (better differentiated) tumors have better prognoses than high-grade (undifferentiated) tumors. If **VMA/HVA ratio** is less than 1, the tumor is deficient in dopamine β-hydroxylase and likely to be more aggressive.
- **DNA ploidy**: A DNA index near-diploid/tetraploid range is unfavorable, whereas hyperdiploid or near-triploid neuroblastomas have a good prognosis. DNA ploidy has less prognostic value in patients older than 2 years of age.
- **Genomic alterations:** Amplification of N-*myc* occurs in about 20% to 25% of cases, and is associated with poor outcome. Tumors with N-*myc* amplification often have deletion of chromosome 1p (especially del 1p36.3). Allelic gain of 17q is associated with more aggressive tumors.

NBs can express 3 tyrosine kinase neurotropin receptors: TrkA, TrkB, and TrkC. High levels of *TrkA* correlate with younger age, lower stage, absence of MYCN amplification and a favorable prognosis. Conversely, TrkB expression correlates with an invasive phenotype, high-risk disease, and chemoresistance. Expression of TrkC is found in lower-stage tumors. High-

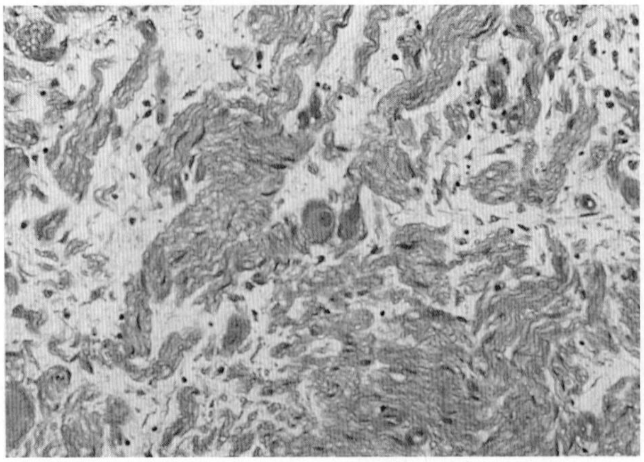

FIGURE 21-42. **Ganglioneuroma.** A photomicrograph shows mature ganglion cells interspersed among wavy spindle cells embedded in a myxoid matrix.

level expression of *EPHB6, CD44, EFNB2,* and *EFNB3* genes is associated with good clinical outcome.

Localized NBs are treated by surgical resection alone. Patients with disseminated tumor are given chemotherapy and sometimes irradiation.

Ganglioneuroma Is a Mature Variant of Neuroblastic Tumors

Ganglioneuroma, like NB, is a tumor of neural crest origin. It is seen in older children and young adults. *Ganglioneuroma is benign and arises in sympathetic ganglia, typically in the posterior mediastinum.* Up to 30% of these tumors occur in the adrenal medulla. In keeping with its degree of differentiation, ganglioneuroma does not manifest the chromosomal abnormalities characteristic of NB.

PATHOLOGY: Ganglioneuromas are well encapsulated and display a myxoid, glistening, cut surface. Microscopically, they show well-differentiated, mature ganglion cells, associated with spindle cells in a loose, abundant fibrillar stroma (Fig. 21-42). The fibrils represent neurites extending from tumor cell bodies. The cytoplasmic processes of ganglion cells contain neurosecretory granules and may form synaptic junctions. Typical neuroendocrine substances, such as neuron-specific enolase and certain peptide hormones, are readily demonstrated. As mentioned above, a NB may differentiate into a ganglioneuroma.

PINEAL GLAND

Anatomy and Function

The pineal gland is 5 to 7 mm in maximal diameter. Shaped like a minute pine cone, it is below the posterior edge of the corpus callosum and is suspended from the roof of the third ventricle over the superior colliculi. Microscopically, the gland shows a lobulated architecture compartmentalized by fibrovascular septa. It is composed of cords and clusters of large epithelial-like cells, **pinealocytes**, which have modified photosensory and neuroendocrine functions. Astrocytes comprise approximately 10% of pineal cells.

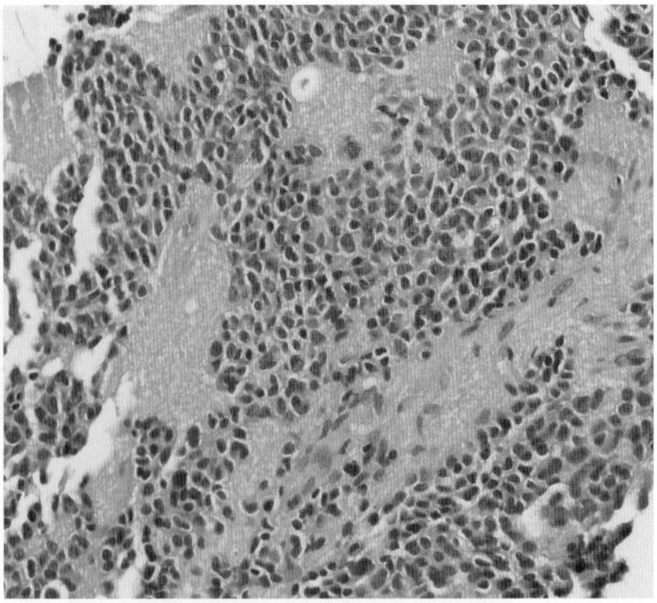

FIGURE 21-43. **Pineocytoma.** A photomicrograph shows nests of tumor cells with round nuclei and eosinophilic cytoplasm separated by connective tissue.

The pineal gland produces several neurotransmitters, among the most abundant of which is **melatonin**. Since melatonin levels are distinctly higher at night than during waking hours, it has been suggested that it may function as a sleep inducer.

Serotonin and several other peptides are also produced by the pineal. The most significant of these is arginine vasotocin, a hormone that has important antigonadotropic activity. Melatonin may act as a releasing factor for arginine vasotocin.

Beginning at about the time of puberty, calcifications (corpora arenacea or "brain sand") can be identified in autopsy specimens in the pineal gland or by various radiologic techniques. These mineralized concretions accumulate increasingly with age and is accompanied by cystic degeneration and gliosis.

Neoplasms

Tumors of the pineal gland are rare, representing less than 1% of brain tumors. They include neoplasms originating from the pineal parenchyma, presumably from the pinealocyte, neoplasms located in the pineal gland region, but not derived from the pineocyte and, rarely, metastasis from other sites.

PATHOLOGY:

- **Germ cell tumors:** These are the most frequent pineal neoplasms and are apparently derived from misplaced germ cells. Germinomas, or dysgerminomas, account for about 60% of pineal tumors and are indistinguishable from their gonadal counterparts.
- **Pineocytoma:** This benign tumor is a solid, well-circumscribed mass that replaces the pineal body. Microscopically, small tumor cells with round nuclei and eosinophilic cyto-

plasm appear as nests separated by thin strands of connective tissue (Fig. 21-43). The overall appearance is similar to that of a paraganglioma, but no neurosecretory granules are present.

- **Pineoblastoma:** This highly malignant tumor is extremely rare and occurs in young adults. Soft masses, often showing hemorrhagic and necrotic areas, invade and infiltrate the surrounding structures. Microscopically, pineoblastoma consists of small oval cells, with dark nuclei and scanty cytoplasm, resembling medulloblastoma or neuroblastoma. Mitoses are generally numerous.

CLINICAL FEATURES: Regardless of histologic type, pineal gland tumors present with signs and symptoms related to their impact on surrounding structures, including headaches and visual and behavioral disturbances. In children, these tumors are frequently associated with precocious puberty, predominantly in boys. The prognosis of pineal tumors is poor in the case of pineoblastoma but is also guarded in cases of pineocytoma. Even nonneoplastic pineal cysts pose a great threat to life because they are difficult to excise surgically.

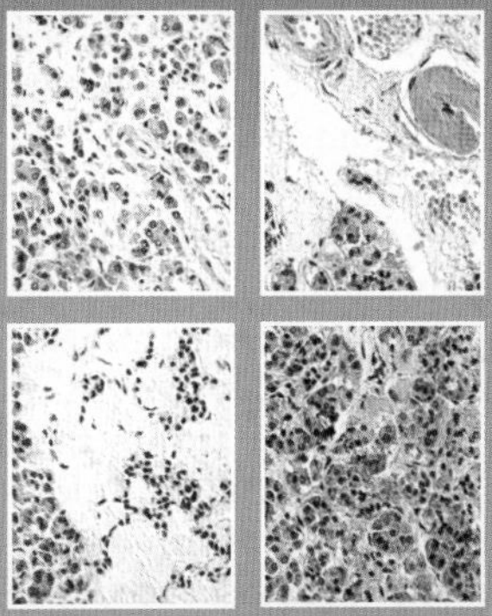

22

Obesity, Diabetes Mellitus, and Metabolic Syndrome

Barry J. Goldstein
Serge Jabbour
Kevin Furlong

Obesity

Obesity is Excessive Adipose Tissue Relative to Lean Body Mass

The standard most often used to define obesity is the body mass index (BMI):

$$\text{BMI} = [\text{weight (kg)}] \div [\text{height (m)}]^2$$

Most health organizations define a BMI between 25 and 29.9 as overweight. Someone whose BMI $\geq$ 30 is considered obese, and a BMI $>$ 40 denotes morbid obesity. These classifications are based on data from epidemiologic studies that have evaluated the relationship between BMI and mortality. Although for most people the BMI reflects body fat content, this definition is not perfect: it does not distinguish between fat mass and lean mass. Therefore, a muscular person with little body fat could be classified as obese, and a person with excess adiposity and reduced muscle mass, such as an elderly or chronically ill individual, could have a normal BMI.

Regional fat distribution is an important determinant of health risk associated with obesity. Fat depots in different parts of the body play various roles including energy metabolism, secretion of circulating proteins and metabolites into the bloodstream and the physical cushioning and protection of internal organs. Abdominal obesity (also known as central adiposity or visceral-abdominal obesity: "apple-shaped") carries a greater risk of diabetes, hypertension, heart disease, and some forms of cancer, compared to individuals with less body fat or gluteal-femoral obesity ("pear-shaped").

The BMI does not take into consideration fat distribution, so abdominal obesity is better assessed by measuring waist circumference or waist:hip ratio. Increased risk for adverse health outcomes is associated with waist circumferences $>$102cm (40 inches) or waist:hip ratios $>$ 0.9 in men, and waist circumference $>$ 88cm (35 inches) or waist:hip ratio $>$0.85 in women.

The genesis of obesity is indisputably complex but the fact remains that obesity develops because more calories are taken in than expended. This imbalance does not have to be large to have significant effects over time. For example, ingesting only 8 calories (Cal) per day more than is expended could lead to a 10-kg increase in body weight over 30 years. To understand how this occurs, some of the mechanisms that regulate energy intake and energy expenditure are reviewed.

The Brain is the Central Homeostatic Controller of Body Weight

The brain receives hormonal and neuronal signals from the periphery about the deficit or surplus of food and the rate of fuel utilization. In order to maintain homeostasis, it then coordinates a response by modulating behavioral patterns and the endocrine and autonomic nervous systems to adjust energy balance.

The ***hypothalamus*** *is the main processor of signals from the periphery and plays a crucial role in the management of energy balance.* Many hypothalamic nuclei have been reported to regulate metabolism, but the arcuate nucleus plays a central role in integrating peripheral signals. Specifically, it has two distinct populations of neurons with opposing actions on food intake. One population produces **anorexigenic** (appetite-suppressing) neuropeptides including proopiomelanocortin (POMC) and cocaine- and amphetamine-regulated transcript (CART). POMC is cleaved into α-melanocyte stimulating hormone (α-MSH), which binds MC3 and MC4 brain melanocortin receptors to decrease appetite.

The other group of neurons produces two **orexigenic** (appetite-stimulating) neuropeptides: neuropeptide Y (NPY) and agouti-related protein (AgRP). NPY is one of the most abundant neuropeptides in the mammalian brain and is a potent stimulator of feeding. It may bind any of 6 G-protein-coupled NPY receptor subtypes (Y1–Y6), but the Y1 and Y2 NPY receptors seem to be most involved with feeding. AgRP antagonizes the melanocortin receptors thereby blocking the anorexigenic effects of α-MSH, leading to increased food intake.

***Leptin** is the protein product of the ob gene and is mainly produced in adipocytes.* Its serum concentration is proportional to body fat mass and its chief physiologic role appears to be signaling the brain whether body fat stores are sufficient. POMC/CART neurons and NPY/AgRP neurons express leptin receptors and are regulated by leptin in opposite ways. Leptin directly activates (anorexigenic) POMC/CART neurons while blocking activity of (orexigenic) NPY/AgRP neurons. The result is decreased food intake. Low serum leptin levels lead to increased appetite and decreased energy expenditure. Interestingly, although blood levels of leptin are above normal in most obese individuals, this increased leptin fails to prevent excessive fat accumulation. The main role of leptin may be to protect against weight loss in times of scarcity, rather than against obesity in times of excess. Attempts to date to "treat" obesity with leptin injection have not been successful.

Endocannabinoids are recently discovered endogenous lipids that bind to cannabinoid receptors 1 and 2 (CB1, CB2). CB1 receptors are found in hypothalamic nuclei that are involved in control of energy balance and weight. CB1 receptors are also found in adipose tissue and the gastrointestinal tract. When activated, the CB1 receptor induces food intake and may play a role in the development and maintenance of obesity. A synthetic blocker of the CB1 receptor has been shown to decrease weight and improve metabolic parameters in those that are overweight or obese.

The **gastrointestinal tract** is another major player in the homeostasis of energy metabolism. It contains a diverse group of mechanoreceptors and chemosensitive receptors that relay information via vagal afferent fibers which terminate on the nucleus tractus solitarii in the brainstem. For example, activation of the vagus from gastric distension causes satiation and meal termination. Additionally, several hormones are produced by the gastrointestinal tract that signal to the central nervous system (CNS) to regulate energy intake:

- **Cholecystokinin (CCK)** is produced by gastrointestinal mucosa and is mainly concentrated in the duodenum and jejunum. It is released in response to fat and protein intake and acts on two distinct receptors. CCK stimulates release of enzymes from the pancreas and gallbladder to aid digestion, slows gastric emptying, and reduces food intake. Regulation of food intake is mediated via vagal afferent signals to the brain.
- **Peptide YY** (PYY) is secreted along the entire gastrointestinal tract, but is concentrated in the distal portion. It is present in two forms, but PYY (3–36) is the major circulating form. It is released in response to food intake and its numerous actions include delaying pancreatic and gastric secretions, gallbladder emptying, and gastric emptying. PYY (3-36) decreases appetite, duration of food intake, and total caloric intake.
- **Pancreatic polypeptide** (PP) is in the same peptide family as PYY. It is primarily produced in the pancreas, but is also found in the colon and rectum. The main stimulus to its release is food intake: it acts to reduce appetite and decrease food intake.
- **Glucagon-like-peptide-1** (GLP-1) is produced by posttranslational processing of proglucagon by the L-cells located primarily in the mucosa of the distal ileum and colon. GLP-1 decreases food intake and results in feelings of satiety. It also augments postprandial insulin secretion, decreases glucagon secretion, reduces gastric motility and inhibits gastric acid secretion. Exendin-4 is a long-acting analogue derived from the venom of the Gila monster *Heloderma suspectum* that has recently become commercially available for the treatment of type 2 diabetes mellitus (T2DM). Exendin-4 significantly lowers fasting plasma glucose, delays gastric emptying, and reduces caloric intake. Its clinical use has been associated with weight loss and it may eventually prove valuable as a potential treatment for obesity.
- **Amylin** is a peptide primarily synthesized and secreted by pancreatic β-cells, but also found in gut endocrine cells, visceral sensory neurons, and the hypothalamus. It is a potent inhibitor of gastric emptying and decreases food intake. An analogue of amylin known as pramlintide is currently available for treatment of diabetes mellitus. It is associated with weight reduction in these patients and is in clinical trials for obesity.
- **Ghrelin** is a hormone primarily produced by gastric endocrine cells, but also to a lesser extent in the duodenum, ileum, and colon. Circulating ghrelin concentrations increase during fasting, and its administration increases caloric intake. A fall in plasma ghrelin is observed following gastric bypass and this may contribute to the continued weight loss after the procedure. Conversely, patients with Prader-Willi syndrome have hyperphagia and very high plasma ghrelin levels. Moreover, serum ghrelin concentrations increase after diet-induced weight loss, which may contribute to the long-term failure of clinical weight loss programs.
- **Insulin** is well known for its role in peripheral glucose uptake, but it may also decrease food intake via insulin receptors in the arcuate nucleus of the hypothalamus. Even when blood glucose changes are taken into account, increases in peripheral insulin levels lead to hypophagia.
- **Other substances** have been found to regulate hunger, satiety, fat deposition, and so forth, in rodents, including galanin, adipocyte complement-related protein (ACRP), peroxisome proliferator-associated receptors (PPARs),and others. Known orexigenic and anorexigenic factors are illustrated in Fig. 22-1.

Energy Expenditure is Determined by a Number of Factors

Total daily energy expenditure (TEE) is comprised of three major components: (1) resting energy expenditure (REE), which is the energy expended for normal cellular and organ functioning, and is generally 70% of TEE; (2) the thermic effect of food, which is the increase in expenditure associated with digestion, and is approximately 10% of TEE; and (3) energy expended with physical activity, which includes volitional activity and nonvolitional activity (energy expended during fidgeting, maintenance of posture and spontaneous muscle contractions).

Because obesity is caused by energy intake that exceeds energy expenditure, defects in energy expenditure could be a possible mechanism for obesity. However, results from many cross-sectional studies suggest that obese individuals do not have any obvious abnormalities in the components of energy metabolism. This does not preclude possibly defective energy expenditure

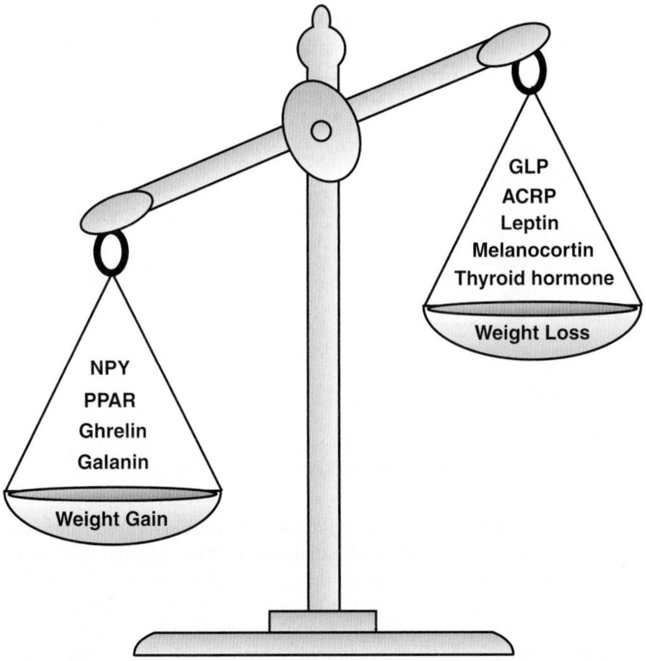

FIGURE 22-1. **The balance of chemical mediators that promote fat accumulation (weight gain) and those that promote fat loss (weight loss).** ACRP = adipocyte complement-related protein; GLP = glucagon-like peptide; NPY = neuropeptide Y; PPAR = peroxisome proliferator-activated receptor.

before they develop obesity, but this is extremely difficult to assess. Nonetheless, evidence does support a feedback control of body weight and a "fat mass set point." For example, weight gain or loss causes energy expenditure to increase or decrease, respectively, in an attempt to return to the original weight.

Furthermore, the amount of weight that is gained after overfeeding may be genetically determined, so that certain individuals tend to be more susceptible to weight gain then others. The effect of excess caloric intake has been assessed within and between twin pairs. Chronic overfeeding of 1000 Cal/day caused similar increases in weight within pairs but a large variance of weight gain between pairs. Since caloric intake was fixed and similar, weight gain differences must have been mediated by differences in energy expenditure.

EPIDEMIOLOGY: Obesity has reached epidemic proportions with a prevalence that continues to increase. Globally, one billion adults would be classified as overweight, at least 300 million of whom meet established criteria for obesity. In the United States, 35% of adults are overweight and another 30% are obese. The annual costs related to obesity have been estimated to exceed 100 billion dollars. More worrisome are the 15% of children and adolescents who are overweight or obese, one of the most rapidly increasing groups of overweight and obese people.

PATHOGENESIS: Obesity is a multifactorial condition that involves complex interaction of genetic, metabolic, physiologic, social and behavioral factors. Rarely, severe clinical obesity has monogenic causes, but most cases are due to combined effects of multiple genes, lifestyle and environmental factors.

GENETIC FACTORS: More than 250 gene markers, and chromosomal regions have been linked to human obesity in large population surveys. The clinical significance of most of these has yet to be determined, but in unusual cases, monogenic causes of obesity have been noted in humans. These rare genetic anomalies have provided a greater understanding of a few specific causes of aberrant body weight regulation in humans.

Melanocortin-4 receptor (MC4R) mutations are relatively common causes of human monogenic obesity. Mutations in MC4R are estimated to occur in approximately 5% of individuals with severe childhood-onset obesity. Patients tend to have no phenotype other than obesity. Both dominant and recessive inheritance are described.

Leptin gene mutations have been reported in a few families. Homozygotes present with hyperphagia and severe, early onset obesity. They have an increased rate of death after childhood infections and hypothalamic hypogonadism, insulin resistance and diabetes as adults. Heterozygotes have reduced circulating levels of leptin and increased body weight compared with unaffected siblings. Replacement therapy with recombinant leptin by injection is very effective in these individuals.

Leptin receptor mutations have been found in rare families with severe early-onset obesity. The phenotype is similar to that in patients with mutations in the leptin gene, except that patients with the receptor mutation have markedly elevated serum leptin levels. They also have hypogonadotropic hypogonadism, failure of pubertal development, growth delay, and secondary hypothyroidism.

Isolated cases of obesity have been linked to mutations or deficiencies in POMC/α-MSH, α-MSH, prohormone converatase 1, and hypothalamic transcription factor SIM1.

Conversely, mutations in acetylation-stimulating protein (ASP) may lead to resistance to obesity. ASP increases adipolyte triglyceride synthesis.

ENVIRONMENTAL FACTORS: The impact of sociologic and psychologic factors on development of obesity cannot be underestimated. The more that is known about the physiology of energy intake and use, the greater is its apparent complexity. The understanding gained by studies of monogenic causes of obesity notwithstanding, the vast majority of obesity is believed to be polygenic in origin and caused by complex interactions of multiple genes and the individual's environment. It is clear that there is a striking difference between the effects of individual biological mediators in rodents and in humans.

The marked increase in obesity in the last 20 years provides evidence of environmental influences in the development of obesity. Body weight control mechanisms are believed to have developed to protect against weight loss in times of scarcity, rather than obesity in times of plenty. In essence, the obese are victims of genomic evolution that provided benefit in times of food scarcity, but now leads to overweight and obesity when food calories are plentiful.

Striking examples of environmental influence on genetic predisposition include the Pima Native Americans in Arizona and the Aboriginal population of northern Australia. The Pimas are now largely sedentary and eat a diet in which 50% of energy derives from fat, as opposed to their

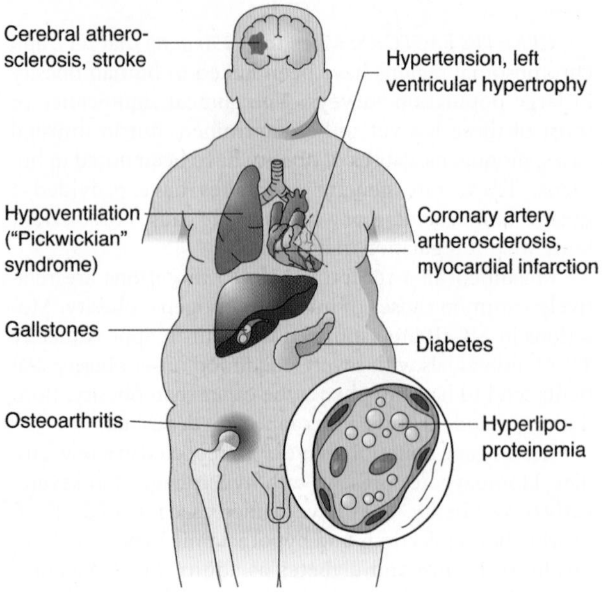

FIGURE 22-2. **Medical complications of obesity**

traditional low-fat diets. They have had dramatic increases in the incidence of obesity and diabetes. In contrast, the genetically related Pimas in the Sierra Madre Mountains of Northern Mexico are more physically active, have maintained more traditional low-fat diets, and have much lower rates of obesity and T2DM. Similarly, urbanized Aboriginal people in Australia have a high prevalence of diabetes and hypertriglyceridemia when compared with their nonurbanized counterparts. As little as a 7 week re-exposure to the traditional Aboriginal lifestyle led to weight loss; improvement in glucose tolerance and fasting glucose, insulin, and triglyceride concentrations in urbanized Aboriginal people affected with T2DM and hypertriglyceridemia.

PATHOLOGY: Many epidemiologic studies have shown that obesity and central adiposity are associated with increased mortality (Fig. 22-2). A pathologic lesion associated with these complications is hyperplasia and hypertrophy of fat cells. The excess from the imbalance between energy intake and energy expenditure is stored in adipocytes that enlarge and/or increase in number: an extremely obese adult can have four times as many adipocytes as a lean adult, each one containing twice as much lipid.

Determining how excess adiposity influences regulation of glucose and lipid metabolism and contributes to cardiovascular risk is currently an area of active research. Several hypotheses have been proposed including the portal/visceral hypothesis, secretion of circulating factors by adipose tissue, and accumulation of fat-derived molecules in metabolically active tissues including liver and skeletal muscle. The portal/visceral hypothesis proposes that increased central adiposity increases delivery of free fatty acids to the liver where they directly block insulin action. This hepatic insulin resistance has been implicated in the development of hyperglycemia in diabetes (see below).

The endocrine paradigm derives from recent research showing that adipose tissue is an active secretory organ that releases

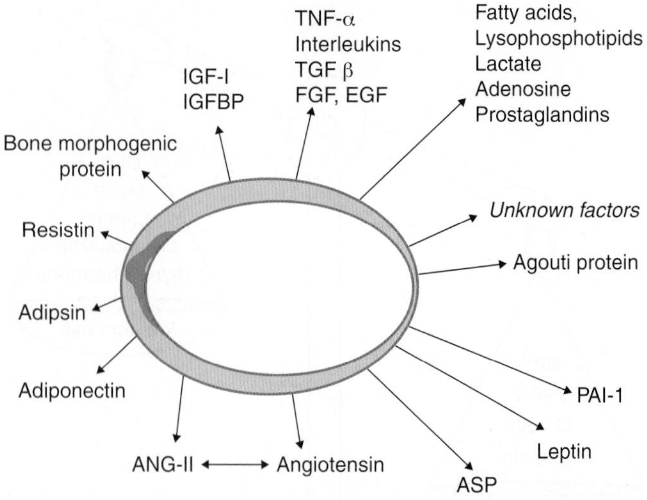

FIGURE 22-3. **Many proteins and metabolites are secreted from adipose tissue and act locally or at a distance in other organs.** They have been shown to have a strong influence on food intake, energy expenditure, insulin signaling, vascular function, and other homeostatic processes in the body. ANG-II = angiotensin II; ASP = acetylation-stimulating protein; EGF = epidermal growth factor; FGF = fibroblast growth factor; IGF= insulin-like growth factor; IGFBP = insulin-like growth factor binding protein; PAI-1 = plasminogen activator inhibitor-1; TGF = transforming growth factor; TNF = tumor necrosis factor.

many different types of factors into the blood. These substances include hormones and cytokines such as leptin, interleukin (IL)-6, angiotensin II, adiponectin, resistin, among others, which have been shown to play a critical role in development of insulin resistance in liver and skeletal muscle (Fig. 22-3). Interestingly, many of these factors are also believed to contribute to endothelial dysfunction and inflammatory changes in the vasculature that herald the onset of atherosclerosis, potentially linking adiposity with cardiovascular disease.

The ectopic fat storage hypothesis proposes that excess lipid in obesity is stored in liver, skeletal muscle, and pancreatic insulin-secreting beta cells, where it influences insulin signaling and secretion, contributing to development of T2DM. Inherited defects in mitochondrial metabolism in skeletal muscle can lead to lipid accumulation there, eventuating in insulin resistance and type 2 diabetes.

The Complications of Obesity Affect Most Organ Systems

Endocrine complications

- **T2DM.** This disorder is strongly associated with obesity: more than 80% of cases of T2DM can be attributed to obesity. The risk of diabetes increases linearly with BMI, and also with increments in abdominal fat mass, waist circumference, or waist:hip ratio at any given BMI. Conversely, weight loss and exercise decrease risk of type 2 diabetes and can prevent progression of insulin resistance to diabetes. In a large American population with impaired glucose tolerance or "pre-diabetes," simply engaging in brisk walking for 150 minutes per week and loss of 7% of body weight reduced the rate of progression of blood glucose levels to overt T2DM in 58% of subjects. Using more drastic measures for morbid obesity, weight loss occurring after gastric bypass surgery resulted in complete resolution of diabetes in 77% of patients.

- **Dyslipidemia.** Obesity is associated with several deleterious serum lipid abnormalities including elevated triglycerides, reduced high-density lipoprotein (HDL) and increased small, dense low-density lipoprotein (LDL) particles. These abnormalities are strongly associated with increased risk of cardiovascular disease, particularly in individuals with central adiposity.
- **Other**. Obesity is also associated with polycystic ovary syndrome, irregular menses, amenorrhea, infertility, and hypogonadism.

Cardiovascular complications

- **Hypertension**. Elevated blood pressure is strongly correlated with obesity, and may be related to heightened sympathetic activity. The high insulin levels that occur in obese patients with insulin resistance may enhance renal reabsorption of sodium, which contributes to hypertension. As noted above, adipose tissue also secretes substances that can cause vasoconstriction and increase blood pressure, including angiotensin II and its precursors. Obesity makes hypertension more difficult to control by interfering with the action of antihypertensive agents. Even a small reduction in weight may decrease in blood pressure in this population.
- **Coronary heart disease**. BMI has a modest and graded association with myocardial infarction, but body fat distribution, especially the waist-to-hip ratio, appears to be a stronger indicator of risk.
- **Congestive heart failure**. Obesity is associated with increased risk of heart failure owing to eccentric cardiac dilatation. Additionally, the combination of obesity and hypertension leads to ventricular wall thickening and larger heart volume. Obese patients are also at increased risk of atrial fibrillation and atrial flutter.
- **Thromboembolic disease**. The risks of deep venous thromboses and pulmonary embolism are increased in obesity. Lower extremity venous thromboembolic disease may be related to increased abdominal pressure, impaired fibrinolysis and increased circulating inflammatory mediators, particularly with abdominal obesity.

Additional complications of obesity

- **Neurologic**. Obesity increases risk of fatal and nonfatal ischemic strokes progressively as BMI increases. Obesity is also associated with increased prevalence of idiopathic intracranial hypertension. Marked weight loss in severely obese individuals can lead to a decline in intracranial pressure and resolution of symptoms.
- **Pulmonary**. Obesity can interfere mechanically with lung function. Increased weight, particularly excess abdominal obesity, depresses ventilatory drive, decreases respiratory compliance, restricts ventilation and limits ventilation of lung bases, contributing to ventilation-perfusion mismatching. Obesity is a major risk factor for development of **obstructive sleep apnea**, in which patients are prone to apnea and hypopnea during sleep. Obesity-hypoventilation syndrome is decreased ventilatory responsiveness to hypercapnia and/or hypoxia, leading to an inability to meet the increased ventilatory demands imposed by the mechanical effects of obesity. The severe form of this syndrome is termed **Pickwickian syndrome**. It is characterized by extreme obesity, irregular breathing, cyanosis, secondary polycythemia, and right ventricular dysfunction leading to fixed pulmonary hypertension.
- **Hepatobiliary**. Obese individuals, particularly females, have an increased incidence of gallstones. Interestingly, weight loss may also precipitate gallstones secondary to increased bile cholesterol supersaturation, enhanced cholesterol crystal nucleation, and decreased gallbladder contractility. A diverse array of liver abnormalities, manifested by increased liver biochemistry values, hepatomegaly and alterations in liver histology, may also complicate obesity. These represent a spectrum of disease known as **nonalcoholic fatty liver disease** (NAFLD), characterized by accumulation of fat within hepatocytes (see Chapter 14). A subset of patients with simple steatosis progress to steatohepatitis, with inflammatory changes leading to fibrosis, and potentially cirrhosis and portal hypertension.
- **Gastrointestinal**. Most large epidemiologic studies have found that gastroesophageal reflux is more common in obese persons.
- **Cancer**. Certain cancers occur with greater frequency in individuals who are obese. Thus, obese people are at increased risk for esophageal, gallbladder, pancreatic, breast, renal, uterine, cervical, and prostate cancer. Obesity also increases the likelihood of dying from cancer.
- **Musculoskeletal**. Obesity is associated with hyperuricemia and gout. Obesity increases the risk of osteoarthritis, particularly of weight-bearing joints such as the knees. However, non–weight-bearing joints can be affected, suggesting mechanisms other than increased mechanical load. Weight loss decreases the risk of osteoarthritis.
- **Skin.** Obesity can lead to stretching and thinning of the epidermis in a ribbon-like pattern called **striae. Acanthosis nigricans** is a velvety, hypertrophic, hyperpigmented alteration especially at skin fold areas (axillae, nape of the neck) in the epidermis that is believed to be a response to increased circulating insulin levels in obese individuals with insulin resistance. Excessive hair growth, **hirsutism**, can result from increased circulating levels of androgens in susceptible women.
- **Psychological and Social.** Obesity has also been associated with impaired quality of life and increased sick leave absences and disability claims.

The "Insulin Resistance/Metabolic Syndrome"

The phenomenon of insulin resistance is a common consequence of obesity, and leads to type 2 diabetes mellitus. To understand the relationship of obesity, insulin resistance. and diabetes, an understanding of insulin receptor and its function is needed.

The insulin receptor is a tetrameric glycoprotein composed of two extracellular α subunits that bind insulin and two transmembrane β subunits that contain an insulin-stimulated tyrosine kinase enzyme activity. Activation of the receptor kinase leads to tyrosine phosphorylation of several insulin receptor substrate (IRS) proteins, an event that is critical to the transmission of the insulin signal in the cell. Adaptor proteins bind to the phosphorylated sites on the IRS molecules, which activates their latent activity for downstream signaling. In turn, signaling kinases activated via phosphorylation of IRS proteins phosphorylate lipid and protein substrates, leading to the translocation of glucose transport proteins and regulation of glucose and lipid metabolism, depending

TABLE 22-1

Frequently Observed Concomitants of the Insulin Resistance/Metabolic Syndrome

Clinical Signs	
	Central (upper body) obesity with increased waist circumference
	Acanthosis nigricans (hypertrophic, hyperpigmented skin changes)
Laboratory Abnormalities	
	Elevated fasting and/or postprandial glucose
	Insulin resistance with hyperinsulinemia
	Dyslipidemia characterized by increased triglycerides and low HDL-cholesterol
	Abnormal thrombolysis
	Hyperuricemia
	Endothelial and vascular smooth muscle dysfunction
	Albuminuria
Comorbid Illnesses	
	Hypertension
	Atherosclerosis
	Hyperandrogenism with polycystic ovary syndrome

on the specific target cell type (i.e., liver, skeletal muscle, or adipose tissue). Hyperinsulinemia, secondary to insulin resistance, can down-regulate the number of insulin receptors on the plasma membrane, which may in part contribute to cellular resistance to the action of insulin.

Peripheral insulin resistance is a fundamental component in the pathogenesis of type 2 diabetes (see below). In obese persons, inhibitory mediators from adipose tissue are released (including free fatty acids and cytokines such as tumor necrosis factor (TNF)-α and adiponectin), which interfere with insulin signaling by disrupting the propagation of protein-tyrosine phosphorylation. Plasma levels of these products are strongly influenced by body fat distribution, in particular, visceral–abdominal (upper body) versus subcutaneous (hips/buttocks; lower body) adiposity. There is a higher prevalence of insulin resistance and T2DM in persons with upper body/visceral obesity. Levels of free fatty acids and TNF-α are preferentially increased in visceral adiposity. Adiponectin, which promotes insulin action on its target tissues, is reduced in visceral adiposity.

Mitochondrial abnormalities have recently been shown to be an additional mechanism in the development of T2DM (see below). In diabetic individuals who are obese, abnormal triglyceride accumulation in liver and skeletal muscle suggests a defect in mitochondrial lipid oxidation. Tissue triglyceride and acyl coenzyme A (CoA) derivatives may activate serine kinase pathways that induce insulin resistance by blocking the insulin receptor tyrosine kinase signal cascade. A genetic component for defective mitochondrial oxidative phosphorylation has been suggested.

Resistance to the action of insulin in target tissues and compensatory hyperinsulinemia are closely tied to a diverse set of cardiovascular risk factors that are prevalent in obese, sedentary persons and in patients with type 2 ("adult onset") diabetes mellitus. These risk factors, together termed the **metabolic syndrome,** include abdominal adiposity with increased waist circumference; mild hypertension (perhaps related to a failure of endothelium-dependent vascular relaxation); and a dyslipidemia, characterized by reduced HDL cholesterol, increased circulating triglycerides, and small, dense, LDL particles (Table 22-1).

DIABETES MELLITUS

Almost a century ago, the noted physician Sir William Osler defined diabetes mellitus as "a syndrome due to a disturbance in carbohydrate metabolism from various causes, in which sugar appears in the urine, associated with thirst, polyuria, wasting and imperfect oxidation of fats." Although he described

TABLE 22-2

Comparison of Type 1 and Type 2 Diabetes Mellitus

	Type 1 Diabetes	Type 2 Diabetes
Age at onset	Usually before 20	Usually after 30
Type of onset	Abrupt; symptomatic (polyuria, polydipsia, dehydration); often severe with ketoacidosis	Gradual; usually subtle; often asymptomatic
Usual body weight	Normal; recent weight loss is common	Overweight
Genetics (parents or siblings with diabetes)	<20%	>60%
Monozygotic twins	50% concordant	90% concordant
HLA associations	+	No
Antibodies to islet cell antigens (insulin, glutamic acid decarboxylase (GAD-65), IA-2)	+	No
Islet lesions	Early—inflammation Late—atrophy and fibrosis	Late-Fibrosis, amyloid
β-Cell mass	Markedly reduced	Normal or slightly reduced
Circulating insulin level	Markedly reduced	Elevated or normal
Clinical management	Insulin absolutely required	Lifestyle modification (diet, exercise); combinations of oral drugs; often insulin supplementation is needed

HLA = human leukocyte antigen; IA-2 = islet cell antigen-512 the salient clinical features of the disease, Osler also emphasized the diverse causes of diabetes.

Today, diabetes is a major health problem that affects increasing numbers of persons in the developed world. Two major forms of diabetes mellitus are recognized, distinguished by their underlying pathophysiology. **Type 1 diabetes mellitus** (**T1DM**), formerly known as **insulin-dependent** (**IDDM**) or **juvenile-onset diabetes**, is caused by autoimmune destruction of the insulin-producing β-cells in the pancreatic islets of Langerhans, and affects less than 10% of all patients with diabetes. By contrast, **type 2 diabetes mellitus**, formerly known as **non–insulin-dependent** (**NIDDM**) or **maturity-onset diabetes,** is typically associated with obesity and results from a complex interrelationship between resistance to the metabolic action of insulin in its target tissues and inadequate secretion of insulin from the pancreas (Table 22-2).

Gestational diabetes develops in a few percent of pregnant women, owing to the insulin resistance of pregnancy combined with a β-cell defect, but almost always abates following parturition. Diabetes can also occur secondary to other endocrine conditions or drug therapy, especially in patients with Cushing syndrome or during treatment with glucocorticoids. Other rare clinical syndromes are associated with abnormal glucose metabolism or overt **hyperglycemia**. Because these conditions are uncommon and have well-defined genetic etiologies that differ from the more common forms of diabetes, they will not be considered in detail.

Current criteria for the diagnosis of diabetes mellitus are based on abnormal glucose threshold levels that have been shown to be closely associated with the chronic complications of this disorder. In particular, hyperglycemia causes the "microvascular" changes of diabetic retinopathy and renal glomerular damage. In a younger patient with hyperglycemia and elevated plasma ketones or frank ketoacidosis, the diagnosis of type 1 diabetes due to absolute insulin deficiency is obvious. However, type 2 diabetes typically develops gradually over many years before it is recognized, most often in an overweight, middle-aged person with a genetic predisposition. Accepted criteria for a diagnosis of diabetes include a fasting plasma glucose level of at least 126 mg/dL or a glucose level above 200 mg/dL taken any time of day in a patient who typically experienced overt symptoms of polyuria and polydipsia. A normal fasting plasma glucose level is currently defined as <100 mg/dL; patients with fasting glucose levels of 100 to 125 mg/dL are considered to have "impaired fasting glucose," and need to be followed closely because they are at high risk of developing diabetes over time.

Type 2 Diabetes Mellitus

Type 2 diabetes mellitus (T2DM) is a heterogeneous disorder characterized by a combination of reduced tissue sensitivity to insulin and inadequate secretion of insulin from the pancreas. The disease usually develops in adults, with an increased prevalence in obese persons and in the elderly. Recently, T2DM has been appearing in increasing numbers in younger adults and adolescents, owing to worsening obesity and lack of exercise in this age group. *Hyperglycemia in T2DM is a failure of the β cells to meet an increased demand for insulin in the body.* T2DM affects more than 16 million Americans, almost half of whom are undiagnosed. Almost 10% of persons older than 65 years of age are affected, and 80% of patients with T2DM are overweight (Fig. 22-4). T2DM is most prevalent in all non-Caucasian ethnic minority groups in the United States, including African-Americans, Hispanics, Asians, and Native Americans.

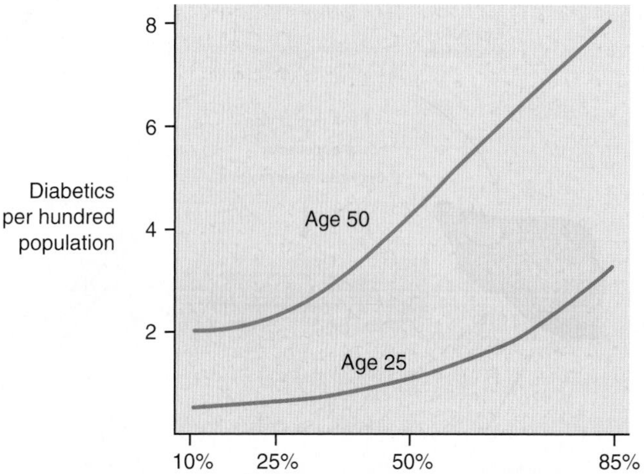

FIGURE 22-4. **Occurrence of diabetes in relation to body weight in young and older adults.** In persons over 50 years of age, the risk of diabetes increases linearly with body weight more than 25% above normal.

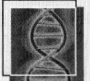

PATHOGENESIS: T2DM results from a complex interplay between underlying resistance to the action of insulin in its metabolic target tissues (liver, skeletal muscle, and adipose tissue) and reduction in glucose-stimulated insulin secretion, which fails to compensate for the increased demand for insulin. Progression to overt diabetes in susceptible populations occurs most commonly in patients exhibiting both of these defects (Fig. 22-5).

GENETIC FACTORS: Multifactorial and multigenic inheritance is a key contributor to the development of T2DM. Sixty percent of patients have either a parent or a sibling with the disease. In some populations, notably Native Americans and some indigenous populations in Pacific Island nations, adoption of a more affluent lifestyle has led to the occurrence of T2DM in 30% to 50% of the population. Among monozygotic twins, both are almost always affected. No association with genes of the major histocompatibility complex (MHC), as seen in T1DM, has been found. Despite the high familial prevalence of the disease, the inheritance pattern is complex and thought to be due to multiple interacting susceptibility genes. Constitutional factors such as obesity (which itself has strong genetic determinants), hypertension, and the amount of exercise influence the phenotypic expression of the disorder and have complicated genetic analysis.

GLUCOSE METABOLISM: In a normal person, the extracellular concentration of glucose in fed and fasting states is maintained in a tightly limited range. This rigid control is mediated by the opposing actions of insulin and glucagon. Following a carbohydrate-rich meal, absorption of glucose from the gut leads to an increase in blood glucose, which stimulates insulin secretion by the pancreatic β cells and the consequent insulin-mediated increase in glucose uptake by skeletal muscle and adipose tissue. At the same time, insulin suppresses hepatic glucose production by (1) inhibiting gluconeogenesis, (2) enhancing glycogen synthesis, (3) blocking the effects of glucagon on the liver, and (4) antagonizing the release of glucagon from the pancreas.

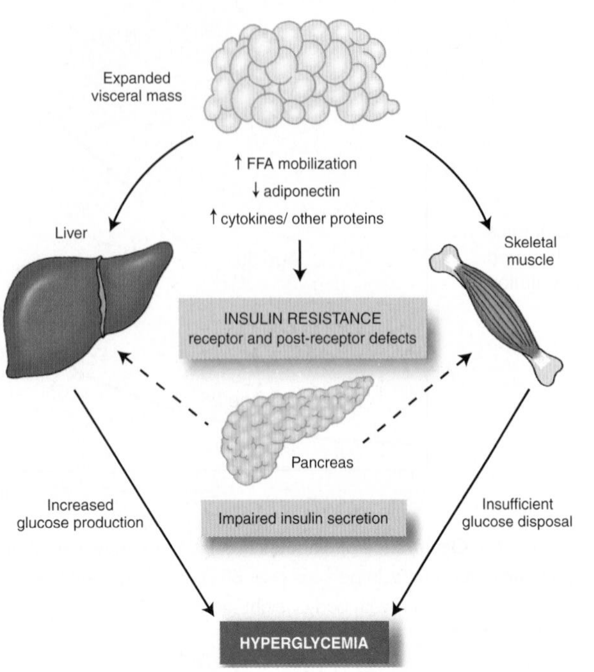

FIGURE 22-5. **Pathogenesis of obesity-related type 2 diabetes mellitus (T2DM).** The expanded visceral fat mass in upper-body obesity elaborates several factors that contribute to tissue insulin resistance. These include an increase in circulating free (nonesterified) fatty acids (FFAs) and other cytokines and proteins that inhibit insulin action, as well as a decrease in factors that enhance insulin signaling, such as adiponectin. These changes result in a block to insulin action in liver and skeletal muscle at the level of the insulin receptor and at postreceptor signaling sites, resulting in a failure of insulin to suppress hepatic glucose production and to promote glucose uptake into muscle. The resulting hyperglycemia is normally countered by increased insulin secretion by pancreatic β cells. In persons with T2DM, the combination of resistance to insulin action and a genetically determined impairment of the β-cell response to hyperglycemia results in hyperglycemia, and T2DM ensues.

β CELL FUNCTION: Persons with T2DM exhibit impaired β-cell insulin release in response to glucose stimulation, a defect that can appear early in the progression of the disease. Mild-to-moderate hyperglycemia can alter the coupling set-point between glucose levels and insulin secretion by a process known as "glucose toxicity." This functional abnormality is specific for glucose, since the β cells retain the ability to respond to other secretagogues, such as amino acids. β-cell function may also be affected by the chronically elevated plasma levels of free fatty acids that occur in obese persons.

A rare autosomal dominant form of inherited diabetes, known as **maturity-onset diabetes of the young (MODY),** has been found to be associated with a variety of gene defects that affect β-cell function, including glucokinase, an important sensor for glucose metabolism within the β cell, and several mutations in genes that control the development and function of the β-cells. Mutations in these genes, however, do not account for the typical prevalent forms of T2DM.

PATHOLOGY: A variety of microscopic lesions are found in the islets of Langerhans of many, but not all, patients with T2DM. Unlike T1DM, in T2DM there is no consistent reduction in the number of β cells, and no morphologic lesions of these cells have been found by light or electron microscopy.

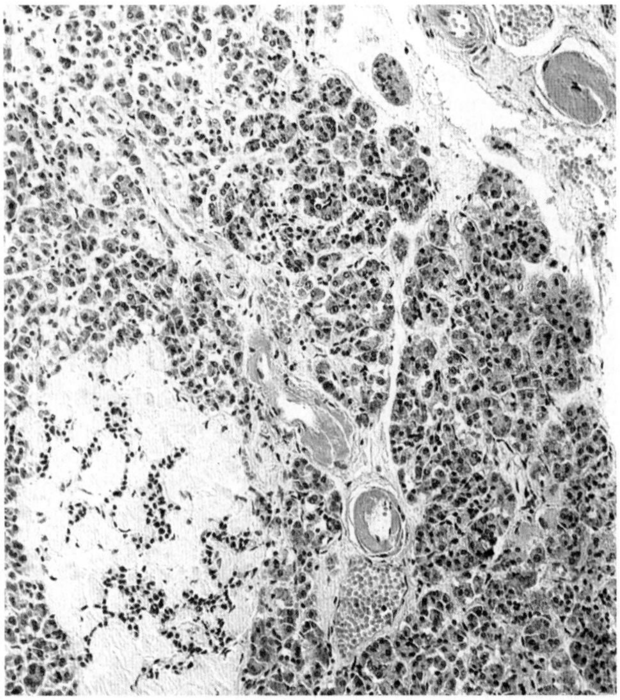

FIGURE 22-6. **Amyloidosis (hyalinization) of an islet in the pancreas of a patient with T2DM *(lower left)*.** The blood vessel adjacent to the islet shows the advanced hyaline arteriolosclerosis characteristic of diabetes.

In some islets, fibrous tissue accumulates, sometimes to such a degree that they are obliterated. Islet amyloid is often present (Fig. 22-6), particularly in patients over 60 years of age. This type of amyloid is composed of a polypeptide molecule known as **amylin**, which is secreted with insulin by the β cell. Importantly, as many as 20% of aged nondiabetic persons also have amyloid deposits in their pancreas, a finding that has been attributed to the aging process itself.

Type 1 Diabetes Mellitus

Type 1 diabetes mellitus (T1DM) is a life-long disorder of glucose homeostasis that results from the autoimmune destruction of the β cells in the islets of Langerhans. The disease is characterized by few if any functional β cells in the islets of Langerhans and extremely limited or nonexistent insulin secretion. As a result, body fat rather than glucose is preferentially metabolized as a source of energy. In turn, oxidation of fat overproduces **ketone bodies** (acetoacetic acid and β-hydroxybutyric acid), which are released into the blood from the liver and lead to metabolic ketoacidosis. Hyperglycemia results from unsuppressed hepatic glucose output and reduced glucose disposal in skeletal muscle and adipose tissue and leads to glucosuria and dehydration from loss of body water into the urine. If uncorrected, the progressive acidosis and dehydration ultimately lead to coma and death (Fig. 22-7)

EPIDEMIOLOGY: T1DM is most common among northern Europeans and their descendants and is not seen as frequently among Asians, African-Americans, or Native Americans. For example, the incidence of T1DM in

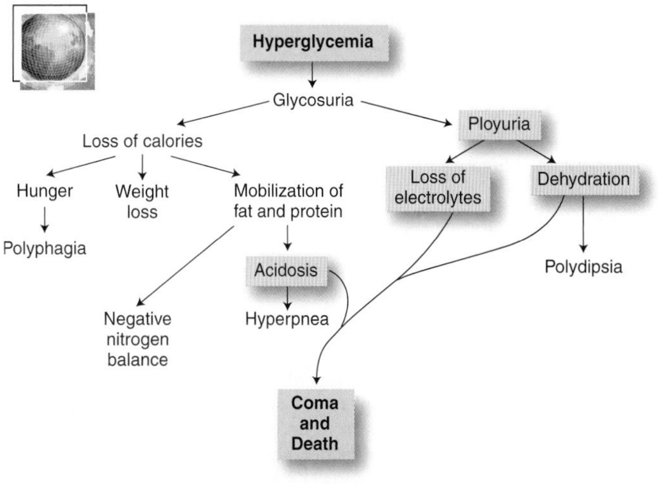

FIGURE 22-7. **Symptoms and signs of uncontrolled hyperglycemia in diabetes mellitus.**

Finland is 20 to 40 times that in Japan. Although the disorder can develop at any age, the peak age of onset coincides with puberty. Some older patients may present with autoimmune β-cell destruction that has developed slowly over many years. An increased incidence in late fall and early winter has been documented in many geographical areas.

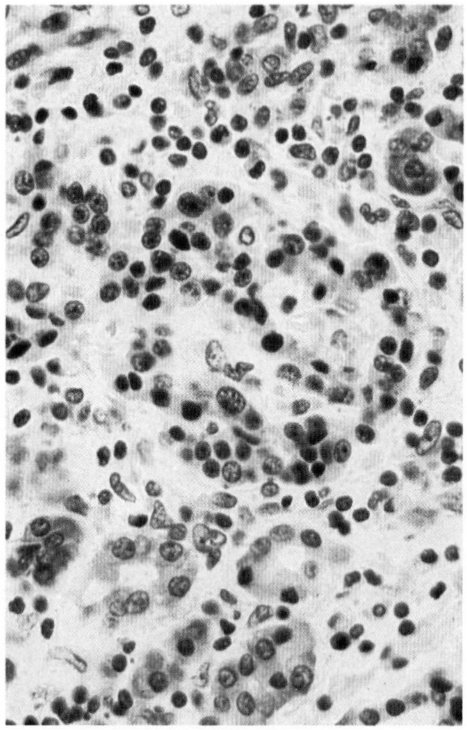

FIGURE 22-8. **Insulitis in type 1 diabetes mellitus.** A mononuclear inflammatory infiltrate is seen in and around the islet.

PATHOGENESIS: A variety of factors have been incriminated in the pathogenesis of T1DM.

GENETIC FACTORS: Fewer than 20% of those with T1DM have a parent or sibling with the disease. In identical (monozygotic) twins in which one twin is diabetic, both members of the pair are affected in less than half of cases. This lack of complete concordance suggests that environmental factors contribute in a major way to the development of the disease. However, certain genetic factors are important, especially major histocompatibility antigens. Some 95% of patients with type T1DM have either human leukocyte antigen (HLA)-DR3 or HLA-DR4, or both, compared with 20% of the general population.

There is evidence that susceptibility to T1DM is associated with the DQ locus and a single amino acid substitution at codon 57 in the DQ β-chain: 96% of patients are homozygous for this polymorphism, compared with only 19% of healthy unrelated persons. It is postulated that this mutation might modulate an autoimmune T cell response against β cells. However, 20 other, independent chromosomal regions, have thus far been associated with susceptibility to T1DM. Interestingly, the children of fathers with T1DM are three times more likely to develop the disease than are children of diabetic mothers, suggesting genetic imprinting of the paternal susceptibility gene.

AUTOIMMUNITY: The concept of an autoimmune pathogenesis for T1DM is supported by the observation that patients who die shortly after the onset of the disease often exhibit an infiltrate of mononuclear cells in and around the islets of Langerhans, termed **insulitis** (Fig. 22-8). Among the inflammatory cells, CD8+ T lymphocytes predominate, although some CD4+ cells are also present. The infiltrating inflammatory cells also elaborate cytokines, for example, IL-1, IL-6, interferon-α, and nitric oxide, which may further contribute to β cell injury.

An autoimmune origin for T1DM was initially suggested by the demonstration of circulating antibodies against components of the β cells (including insulin itself) in most newly diagnosed children with diabetes. Many patients develop islet cell antibodies months or years before insulin production decreases and clinical symptoms appear, a clinical state known as "pre-type 1 diabetes" (Fig. 22-9). However, these antibodies are regarded as a response to β-cell antigens released during destruction of β cells by cell-mediated immune mechanisms, rather than the cause of β-cell depletion. Nevertheless, detection of serum, antibodies to islet cells and certain islet antigens (glutamic acid decarboxylase [GAD]-65, islet cell antigen [ICA]-512 (IA-2), insulin, etc.) remains a useful clinical tool for differentiating between type 1 and type 2 diabetes, which does not have an autoimmune basis (see below).

Cell-mediated immune mechanisms are fundamental to the pathogenesis of T1DM, and cytotoxic T lymphocytes sensitized to β cells in T1DM persist indefinitely, possibly for a lifetime. Patients transplanted with a donor pancreas or a preparation of purified islets must be treated with immunosuppressive drugs. Ten percent of patients with T1DM manifest at least one other organ-specific autoimmune disease, including Hashimoto thyroiditis, Graves disease, myasthenia gravis, Addison disease, or pernicious anemia. Interestingly, most patients with polyendocrine immune syndromes (see Chapter 20) also possess HLA DR3 and DR4 histocompatibility antigens.

The destruction of β-cells in T1DM generally develops slowly over years, and specific stages of the disease have

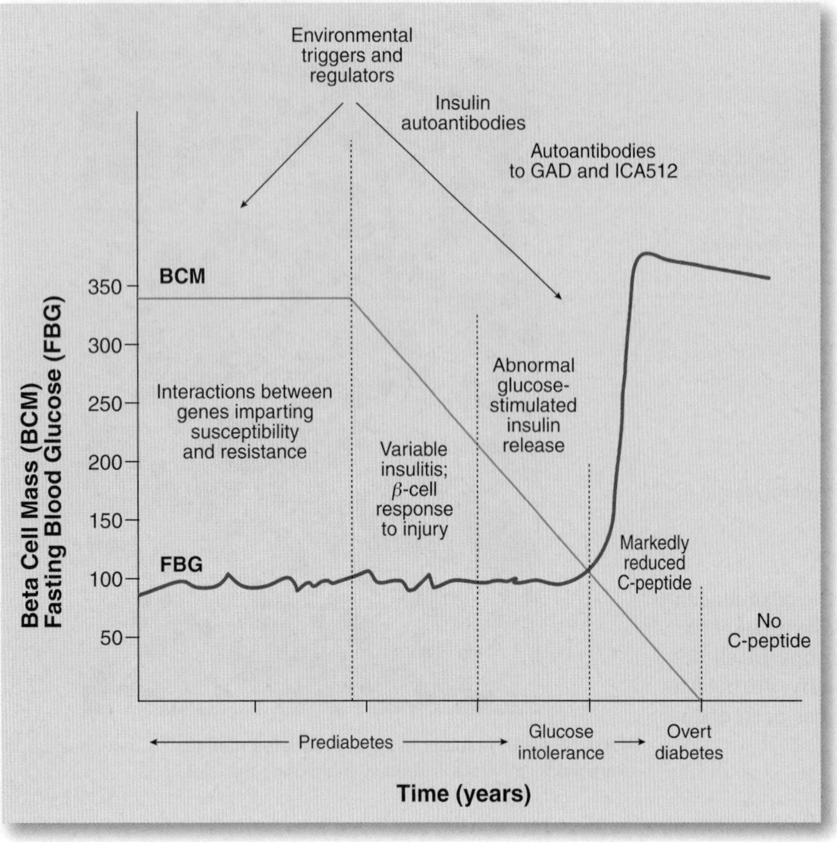

FIGURE 22-9. **Pathogenetic stages in the development of type 1 diabetes (T1DM).** The disease develops from an initial genetic susceptibility to defective recognition of β-cell epitopes and ends with essentially complete β-cell destruction in most patients. An environmental event is believed to trigger the immune attack, and persons with certain genetic markers (human leukocyte antigen [HLA]-DR3 and -DR4) are particularly susceptible to the autoimmune disease. Patients with islet cell antibodies and normal blood glucose levels are considered to have a state of "pre-diabetes." The rate of decline in β-cell mass determines the length of time between onset of β-cell destruction and eventual hyperglycemia owing to loss of >90% of functioning β cells. In the serum, autoantibodies to insulin appear early, followed by antibodies to the β-cell antigens glutamic acid decarboxylase (GAD-65) and the islet cell antigen (ICA-512).

been described (see Fig. 22-9). Clinically apparent diabetes with hyperglycemia or ketoacidosis manifests only when at least 90% of the insulin-secreting cells have been eliminated and insulin deprivation becomes severe.

ENVIRONMENTAL FACTORS: What triggers the immunologic injury to the islets of Langerhans? Viruses and chemicals have been implicated as causative factors in at least some cases of T1DM. For example, the disease occasionally develops after infection with mumps or group B coxsackie viruses. Children and young adults who were infected in utero with rubella also occasionally develop diabetes, presumably after viral injury of the fetal pancreas.

Certain viral and dietary proteins may share antigenic epitopes with human cell-surface proteins and trigger the autoreactive disease process by "molecular mimicry." For example, bovine serum albumin contains sequences similar to subunits of MHC class II proteins, and a coxsackie B virus protein has close homology to the human GAD-65 islet protein. Geographical and seasonal differences in the incidence of T1DM further suggest that environmental factors are important in its pathogenesis. The onset of T1DM in genetically identical sibs in sets of twins or triplets may also be separated by years, or not occur at all, further supporting a role for environmental factors in the clinical presentation of the disease.

PATHOLOGY: The most characteristic early lesion in the pancreas of T1DM is a lymphocytic infiltrate in the islets (insulitis), sometimes accompanied by a few macrophages and neutrophils (see Fig. 22-8). *As the disease becomes chronic, the β cells of the islets are progressively depleted; eventually insulin-producing cells are no longer discernible.* The loss of β cells results in variably sized islets, many of which appear as ribbonlike cords that are difficult to distinguish from the surrounding acinar tissue. Fibrosis of the islets is uncommon. In contrast to T2DM, deposition of amyloid in the islets of Langerhans is absent in T1DM. The exocrine pancreas in chronic T1DM often exhibits diffuse interlobular and interacinar fibrosis, accompanied by atrophy of the acinar cells.

CLINICAL FEATURES: The clinical presentation of T1DM results from the loss of insulin, which has a unique role in energy metabolism in the body. The disease classically appears with acute metabolic decompensation characterized by ketoacidosis and hyperglycemia. Depending on the degree of absolute insulin deficiency, severe ketoacidosis may be preceded by weeks to months of increased urine output (**polyuria**) and increased thirst (**polydipsia**). Excessive diuresis results from glucosuria. Weight loss in spite of increased appetite (polyphagia) is due to unregulated catabolism of body stores of fat, protein, and carbohydrate with inefficient energy use. Often the clinical onset of T1DM coincides with another acute illness, such as a febrile viral or bacterial infection.

Complications of Diabetes

The discovery of insulin early in the 20th century promised to cure diabetes, but as diabetics lived longer, it became apparent that they were subject to numerous complications. *It is now clearly estab-*

lished that the severity and chronicity of hyperglycemia in both T1DM and T2DM are the major pathogenetic factors leading to the "microvascular" complications of diabetes including retinopathy, nephropathy, and neuropathy. Thus, control of blood glucose remains the major means by which the development of microvascular diabetic complications can be minimized. It has been more difficult to demonstrate that glucose control can prevent atherosclerosis and its complications (coronary artery disease, peripheral vascular disease, and cerebrovascular disease). These "macrovascular" complications are especially common in insulin-resistant patients with T2DM, since they tend to be older and frequently harbor additional vascular risk factors.

PATHOGENESIS: A variety of biochemical mechanisms have been proposed to account for the development of pathological changes in diabetes.

EXCESSIVE REACTIVE OXYGEN SPECIES (ROS): In various cell types, hyperglycemia increases production of ROS as byproducts of mitochondrial oxidative phosphorylation. ROS are implicated in many types of cell injury (see Chapter 1).

PROTEIN GLYCOSYLATION: Glucose binds to a assortment of proteins nonenzymatically, via a process termed **glycosylation.** Glycosylation occurs roughly in proportion to the severity of hyperglycemia. Numerous cellular proteins are modified in this manner, including hemoglobin, components of the crystalline lens, and cellular basement membrane proteins. A specific fraction of the glycosylated hemoglobin in circulating red blood cells (hemoglobin A_{1c}) is measured routinely to monitor the overall degree of hyperglycemia that occurred during the preceding 6 to 8 weeks. Nonenzymatic glycosylation of hemoglobin is irreversible, so the level of hemoglobin $A_{1c,}$ serves as a maker for glycemic control, as well as ongoing hyperglycemia-related protein damage.

The initial glycosylation products (known chemically as Schiff bases) are labile and can dissociate rapidly. With time, these labile products undergo complex chemical rearrangements to form stable **advanced glycosylation products,** consisting of a glucose derivative covalently bound to the protein amino group. As a result, the structure of the protein is permanently altered and its function may be affected. For example, albumin and immunoglobulin (Ig)G do not normally bind to collagen, but they adhere to glycosylated collagen. Unstable chemical bonds in proteins containing advanced glycosylation products can lead to physical cross-linking of nearby proteins, which may contribute to the characteristic thickening of vascular basement membranes in diabetes. Importantly, unlike the initial labile glycosylation products, advanced glycosylation products can continue to cross-link proteins despite a return of blood glucose to a normal level. Thus, in a canine model of diabetic retinopathy (see below), this complication is prevented only if blood glucose is strictly controlled within 2 months of the initiation of hyperglycemia. Patients with diabetic retinopathy have higher levels of these products than do diabetics without this complication. Moreover, compounds that inhibit formation of advanced glycosylation products provide some protection against diabetic complications in experimental animals.

THE ALDOSE REDUCTASE PATHWAY: By mass action, hyperglycemia also increases uptake of glucose in tissues that do not depend on insulin. Some of the increased flux of glucose is metabolized by aldose reductase, leading to accumulation of sorbitol. This sugar alcohol has been suspected to play a role in diabetic complications in a variety of tissues, including peripheral nerves, retina, lens, and kidney. Although aldose reductase has a low affinity for glucose, it generates appreciable amounts of sorbitol in these tissues when blood glucose levels are elevated. The mechanism by which sorbitol accumulation may cause tissue injury is not fully understood. In the lens, this alcohol may simply create an osmotic gradient that causes influx of fluid and consequent swelling. Sorbitol may also be directly toxic to cells. Increased intracellular sorbitol has been linked to decreased myoinositol (a precursor of phosphoinositides), lowered activity of protein kinase C and inhibition of the plasma membrane sodium pump.

PROTEIN KINASE C (PKC) ACTIVATION: In patients with hyperglycemia, specific PKC isoforms, mainly PKC-β and PKC-δ, are activated by diacylglycerol (DAG) synthesized from glycolytic intermediates. PKC activation may lead to (1) increased production of extracellular matrix and cytokines, (2) enhanced microvascular contractility, (3) increased microvascular permeability, and (4) proliferation of endothelial and smooth muscle cells. PKC also induces activation of phospholipase A_2 and inhibits the activity of Na^+/K^+-ATPase. Inhibition of PKC-β by a selective inhibitor prevents or reverses a number of vascular abnormalities in vitro and in vivo.

Atherosclerosis is a Frequent Complication of Diabetes

Cardiovascular disease, including atherosclerotic heart disease and ischemic stroke, accounting for more than half of all deaths among adults with diabetes. The extent and severity of atherosclerotic lesions in medium-sized and large arteries are increased in patients with long-standing diabetes. Diabetes eliminates the usual protective effect of being female and coronary artery disease develops at a younger age than in nondiabetic persons. Moreover, mortality from myocardial infarction is higher in diabetics than in nondiabetic patients. As indicated above, patients with T2DM frequently exhibit multiple risk factors of the metabolic syndrome that contribute to development of atherosclerosis.

Atherosclerotic peripheral vascular disease, particularly of the lower extremities, is a common complication of diabetes. Vascular insufficiency leads to ulcers and gangrene of the toes and feet, complications that ultimately necessitate amputation. Indeed, diabetes accounts for 40% of nontraumatic limb amputations in the United States.

The mechanism whereby hyperglycemia promotes atherosclerosis is the subject of considerable study. A number of pathogenetic factors have been proposed, including glycosylated LDLs that are poorly cleared by the liver, glycosylation and cross-linking of cellular proteins (which can damage the vessel wall), a defect in lipoprotein lipase that impairs the clearance of chylomicrons and leads to postprandial hypertriglyceridemia, and accumulation of atherogenic remnant lipoprotein particles. Enhanced platelet aggregation, increased plasma fibrinogen levels, and defective endothelial production of nitric oxide with

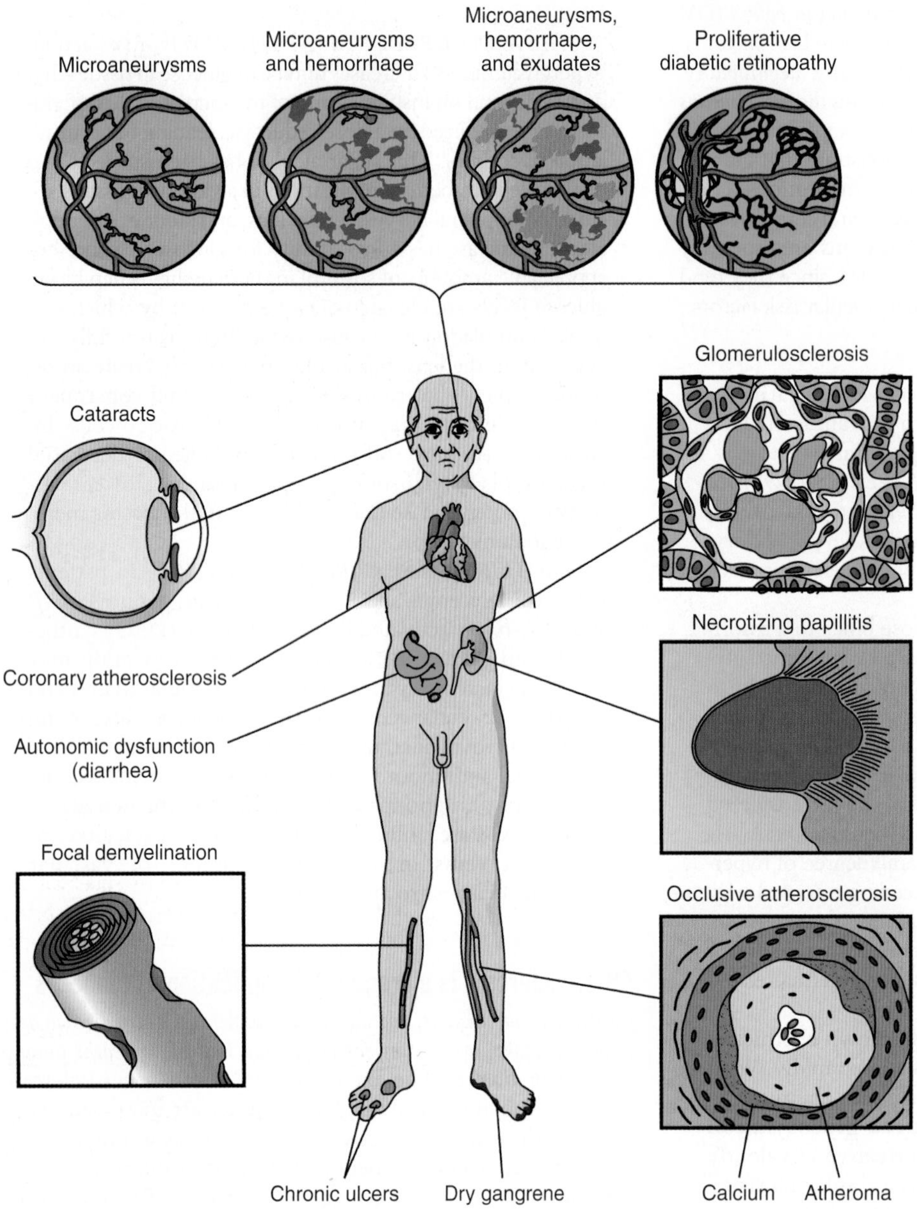

FIGURE 22-10. **Secondary complications of diabetes.** The effects of diabetes on a number of vital organs result in complications that may be incapacitating (cerebral and peripheral vascular disease), painful (neuropathy), or life-threatening (coronary artery disease, pyelonephritis with necrotizing papillitis).

impaired vasodilation of the arterial wall are also observed in patients with diabetes.

Diabetic Microvascular Disease is Responsible for Many of the Complications of Diabetes, Including Renal Failure and Blindness

Arteriolosclerosis (see Fig. 22-6) and capillary basement membrane thickening (Fig. 22-10) are characteristic vascular changes in diabetes. The frequent occurrence of hypertension contributes to the development of the arteriolar lesions. In addition, deposition of basement membrane proteins, which may also become glycosylated, increases in diabetes. Aggregation of platelets in smaller blood vessels and impaired fibrinolytic mechanisms have also been suggested as playing a role in the pathogenesis of diabetic microvascular disease.

Whatever the pathogenetic processes, the effects of microvascular disease on tissue perfusion and wound healing are profound. For example, it is believed to reduce blood flow to the heart, which is already compromised by coronary atherosclerosis. Healing of chronic ulcers that develop from trauma and infection of the feet in diabetic patients is commonly defective, in part because of microvascular disease. The major complications of diabetic microvascular disease involve the kidney and the retina.

Diabetic Nephropathy

Of patients with T1DM, 30% to 40% ultimately develop renal failure. A somewhat smaller proportion (up to 20%) of patients with T2DM are similarly affected. Conversely, since diabetes is such a common condition, diabetic nephropathy accounts for one third of all new cases of renal failure. Although some patients with T1DM die from uremia, most who develop nephropathy succumb to cardiovascular disease, the risk of which is 40 times greater in diabetics with end-stage renal disease. The prevalence of diabetic nephropathy increases with the severity and duration of the hyperglycemia. *Kidney disease due to diabetes is the most common reason for renal transplantation in adults.*

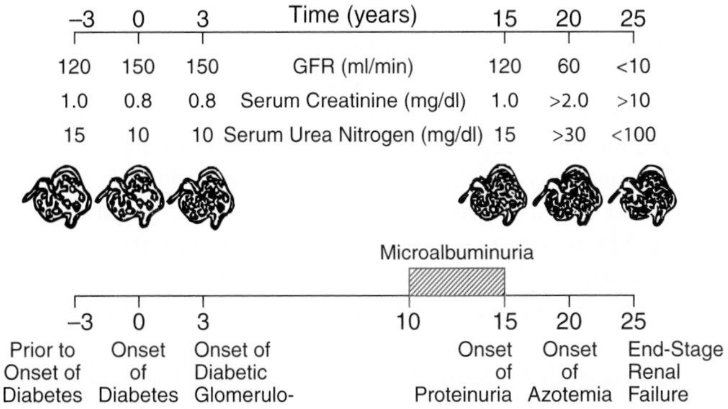

FIGURE 22-11. **Natural history of diabetic nephropathy. Initially, renal hypertrophy and hyperfiltration lead to an increase in the glomerular filtration rate (GFR).** Once the decline in renal function begins, on average at least 10 years after the onset of diabetes, leakage of a small amount of serum albumin into the urine (microalbuminuria) is the first abnormality that is easily and reliably measured. The elevation in serum creatinine and gross proteinuria occur much later.

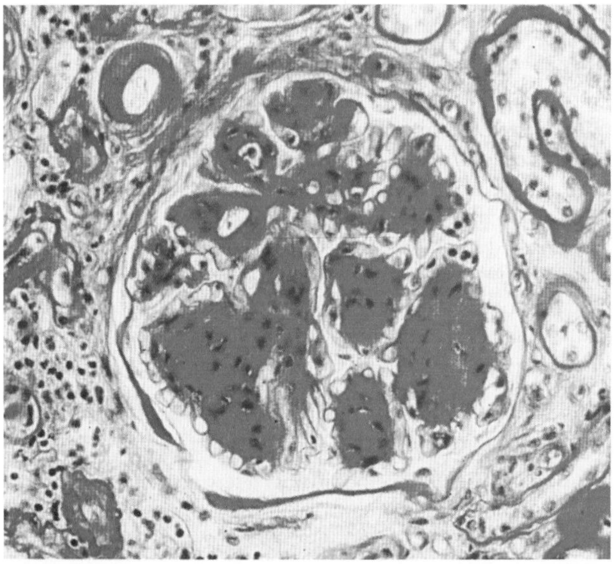

FIGURE 22-12. **Diabetic glomerulosclerosis.** A periodic acid–Schiff stain demonstrates nodular accumulations of basement membrane-like material in the glomerulus.

Initially, hyperglycemia leads to glomerular hypertension and renal hyperperfusion (Fig. 22-11). Increased glomerular pressure favors deposition of protein in the mesangium, resulting in glomerulosclerosis and, eventually, renal failure. Advanced glycosylation products and lipoprotein abnormalities may contribute to changes in the chemical composition of the glomerular basement membrane. In addition, growth factors such as transforming growth factor-β (TGF-β), induced in the kidney by hyperglycemia and its associated ROS, have been implicated in some of the cellular abnormalities in diabetic nephropathy. Regardless of the underlying mechanism, strict control of blood glucose levels and blood pressure retards development of diabetic nephropathy. Treatment with angiotensin-converting enzyme (ACE) inhibitors–which reduce systemic blood pressure, renal oxidative stress, glomerular hypertension, and renal perfusion—retards progression of diabetic nephropathy.

Eventually, the glomeruli in the diabetic kidney exhibit a unique lesion termed **Kimmelstiel-Wilson disease** or **nodular glomerulosclerosis** (see Chapter 16). Two microscopic patterns are observed. In the more common one, spherical masses of basement membrane-like material accumulate in glomerular lobules (Fig. 22-12). The other form is characterized by more diffuse, although somewhat irregular, deposition of this material throughout the glomerulus. The latter change must be differentiated from membranous nephropathy. The onset of glomerular disease is heralded clinically by the appearance in the urine of small amounts of serum albumin, termed "microalbuminuria." Proteinuria increases with time and with a progressive decline in renal function.

Diabetic Retinopathy

Diabetic retinopathy is the most important cause of blindness in the Unites States in persons under the age of 60 years. The risk is higher in T1DM than in T2DM. In fact, 10% of patients with T1DM of 30 years' duration become legally blind. Nevertheless, there are many more patients with T2DM, so these are the most numerous patients with diabetic retinopathy. Retinopathy is the most devastating ophthalmic complication of diabetes, although glaucoma, cataracts, and corneal disease are also increased. Like nephropathy, the prevalence of retinopathy in diabetes is a function of the duration and degree of glycemic control. Diabetic retinopathy is discussed in detail in Chapter 16.

Diabetic Neuropathy Affects Sensory and Autonomic Innervation

Peripheral sensory impairment and autonomic nerve dysfunction are among the most common and distressing complications of diabetes. Changes in the nerves are complex, and abnormalities in axons, the myelin sheath, and Schwann cells have all been found. Microvasculopathy involving the small blood vessels of nerves contributes to the disorder. Evidence suggests that hyperglycemia increases the perception of pain, independent of any structural lesions in the nerves.

Peripheral neuropathy is initially characterized by pain and abnormal sensations in the extremities. However, fine touch, pain detection, and proprioception are ultimately lost. As a result, diabetics tend to ignore irritation and minor trauma to feet, joints, and legs. Peripheral neuropathy can thus lead to foot ulcers, which often plague patients with severe diabetes. It also plays a role in the painless destructive joint disease that occasionally occurs.

Although autonomic nerve dysfunction is subtle, abnormalities in neurogenic regulation of cardiovascular and gastrointestinal functions frequently result in postural hypotension and problems of gut motility, such as diarrhea. Erectile dysfunction and retrograde ejaculation are common complications of autonomic dysfunction, although vascular disease is often a contributing factor. Hypotonic urinary bladder develops occasionally, results in urinary retention and predisposes to infection.

Bacterial and Fungal Infections Occur in Diabetic Patients Whose Hyperglycemia is Poorly Controlled.

Multiple abnormalities in host responses to microbial invasion have been described in such patients. Leukocyte function is compromised and immune responses are blunted. Before the use of insulin, tuberculosis and purulent infections were often life-threatening. Now, patients with well-controlled diabetes are much less susceptible to infections. However, urinary tract infections continue to be problematic because glucose in the urine provides an enriched culture medium. This is further complicated if patients have developed autonomic neuropathy leading to urinary retention from poor bladder emptying. Infection ascending from the bladder to the kidney, pyelonephritis, is thus a constant concern. Renal papillary necrosis may be a devastating complication of bladder infection.

A dreaded infectious complication of poorly controlled diabetes is mucormycosis. This often fatal fungal infection tends to originate in the nasopharynx or paranasal sinuses and spreads rapidly to the orbit and brain (see Chapter 9).

Diabetes Occurring During Pregnancy May Put both Mother and Fetus at Risk

Gestational diabetes develops in only a few percent of seemingly healthy women during pregnancy. It may continue after parturition in a small proportion of these patients. Pregnancy is a state of insulin resistance, but only pregnant women with impaired β-cell insulin secretion become diabetic. Abnormalities in the amount and timing of pancreatic insulin secretion make these women highly susceptible to overt T2DM later in life.

Poor control of gestational diabetes may lead to birth to large infants, make labor and delivery more difficult, and necessitate a cesarean section. The fetal pancreas may try to compensate for poor maternal control of diabetes during gestation. Such fetuses may develop β cell hyperplasia, which may lead to hypoglycemia at birth and the early postnatal period.

Infants of diabetic mothers have a 5% to 10% incidence of major developmental abnormalities, including anomalies of the heart and great vessels, and neural tube defects, such as anencephaly and spina bifida. The frequency of these lesions is a function of the control of maternal diabetes during early gestation.

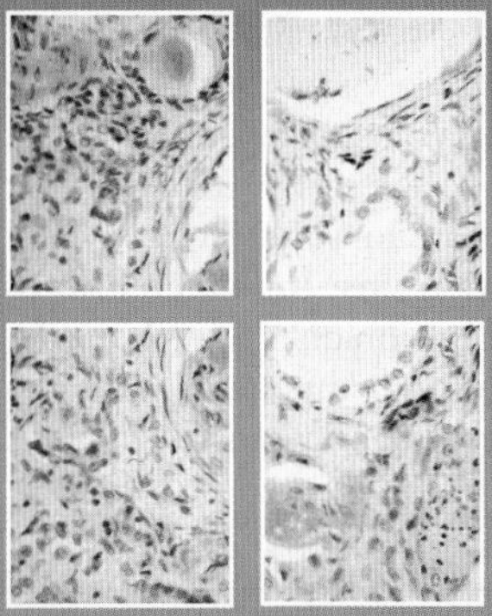

23 The Amyloidoses

Robert Kisilevsky

Constituents of Amyloid

***Amyloid** refers to a group of diverse extracellular protein deposits that have (1) common morphologic properties, (2) affinities for specific dyes, and (3) a characteristic appearance under polarized light. Although they vary in amino acid sequence, all amyloid proteins are folded in such as way as to share common ultrastructural and physical properties.*

Disorders associated with amyloid deposition have been recognized for more than 300 years, but it was not until Virchow's time in the mid-19th century that attempts were made to define the nature of the tissue deposits by their staining properties. Amyloid stained blue with acidified iodine, which was then in use for demonstrating cellulose or starch. This staining not only led to coining of the term **amyloid** (starch-like), but also deceptively intimated that it was a polysaccharide. Neither starch nor cellulose is a constituent of amyloid, and a different complex carbohydrate is responsible for the fact that it stains with iodine. Amyloid deposits are composed of two classes of constituents:

A DISEASE-SPECIFIC FIBRILLOGENIC PROTEIN: The nature of this protein varies with the underlying disease. The tertiary structure of the protein and the manner in which it interacts with other molecules are responsible for the characteristics of amyloid. *The specific fibrillogenic protein in various types of amyloid is now the determining factor in the classification of amyloid.*

A SET OF COMMON COMPONENTS FOUND IN ALL AMYLOIDS:

- The **amyloid P component** (**AP**) is a pentagonal, doughnut-shaped protein that is present in all types of amyloid. AP is identical with, and is derived from, a normal circulating serum protein, termed *serum amyloid P (SAP)*. SAP is also a structural component of normal basement membranes.
- **Other molecular building blocks of basement membranes** are present in amyloid and include laminin, collagen type IV, and the proteoglycan perlecan. The glycosaminoglycan side chain of perlecan is heparan sulfate, which is probably responsible for the iodine-staining properties of amyloid. Heparan sulfate is also crucial in altering the conformation of the disease-specific fibrillogenic proteins.
- **Apolipoprotein E** (**apoE**) is a constituent of high-density lipoproteins and normally plays a role in cholesterol transport.

Not all amyloids are the same, and the protein responsible for the fibrillary characteristics varies significantly. For example, in amyloid associated with multiple myeloma, the fibrillogenic component is a product of immunoglobulin light chains produced by myeloma cells. In amyloid associated with inflammatory diseases, the fibrillogenic component is derived from an acute phase protein that is produced by the liver and is unrelated to immunoglobulins. *In these two cases, amyloid is deposited systemically.*

In other situations, amyloid is deposited only locally. Amyloid in medullary carcinoma of the thyroid is restricted to the tumor deposits, and its fibrillogenic component is derived from a polypeptide hormone related to calcitonin. In the pancreas, amyloid located either in an islet cell tumor or in the islets in type 2 diabetes is derived from a peptide hormone secreted with insulin (amylin, or islet amyloid polypeptide [IAPP]). In Alzheimer disease, the amyloid is restricted to the brain and its blood vessels; yet it is derived from a plasma membrane protein that is found not only in the central nervous system but distributed ubiquitously in the body.

Although the nature of amyloid deposits varies widely and the conditions under which they occur are disparate, a century of usage established the term **amyloidosis** as denoting a single disease. *In current usage, however, amyloidosis refers to a group of diseases characterized by proteinaceous tissue deposits with similar morphologic, structural, and staining properties, but with variable protein composition.*

Staining Properties of Amyloid Deposits

The staining properties and general appearance of amyloid are governed primarily by the nature of its protein. Because of its compact structure, amyloid has few morphologic features visible by light microscopy. When routine stains are used, amyloid is amorphous, glassy, and almost cartilage-like. On staining with hematoxylin and eosin, amyloid stains no differently from many other proteins. However, the specific nature and underlying organization of amyloid proteins, as well as those of associated molecules (glycosaminoglycans and AP component), allow amyloid to be stained in specific ways.

CONGO RED: All amyloids stain red with the Congo red dye (Fig. 23-1A). When stained with Congo red and viewed under polarized light, amyloid deposits exhibit a red-green birefringence (see Fig. 23-1B). The fibrillary deposits organized in one plane have one color, and those organized perpendicular to that plane have the other color. *Congo red is the stain most commonly used for the diagnosis of amyloidosis.*

THIOFLAVIN T: Although not entirely specific for amyloid, staining with thioflavin T allows the amyloid to fluoresce when viewed in ultraviolet light.

ALCIAN BLUE: The presence of glycosaminoglycans in all amyloid deposits is demonstrated with a variety of Alcian blue stains, which cause the glycosaminoglycans to appear blue.

SPECIFIC ANTIBODIES: The success in isolating various amyloid proteins has led to the preparation of both polyclonal and monoclonal antibodies directed against the different proteins. In turn, immunohistochemical techniques have been devised to demonstrate the presence of AP component, as well as the specific protein present in each type of amyloid.

Structure of Amyloid

All amyloids are similar in ultrastructural appearance, regardless of which protein is responsible for the fibrillary component. By electron microscopy, groups of fibers are arranged in parallel arrays, with each group having a different orientation (see Fig. 23-2). These parallel arrays orient the specific dyes, such as Congo red, and thus give amyloid the ability to rotate polarized light, producing the classic birefringence. Although the individual fibrils vary considerably in length, all have a diameter of 7 to 13 nm. The secondary and tertiary organization of the protein that constitutes the amyloid fibril has been explored by x-ray diffraction and infrared spectroscopy. The individual protein subunits appear to be organized primarily as a **β-pleated sheet**. However, in the case of the amyloid peptide found in inflammatory diseases, there is an abundant α-helical structure as well as one segment organized into a β-pleated sheet. Similar findings have now been observed with the amyloid peptides in Alzheimer disease and in the pancreatic islets in adult-onset (type 2) diabetes. *The individually folded polypeptide subunits are stacked into fibrils.* The precise manner and mechanism by which this occurs may be different for each amyloid.

In all amyloids, the set of common components (SAP, basement membrane components, highly charged glycosaminoglycans, and apoE) are present in close association with the amyloid deposits. In at least six types of amyloid, the basement membrane form of heparan sulfate proteoglycan (perlecan) has been identified as the charged component. But, other heparan sulfate proteoglycans may play a similar role in other forms of amyloid (e.g., agrin in Alzheimer disease). The interaction of amyloid protein precursors with the common components probably changes the

A

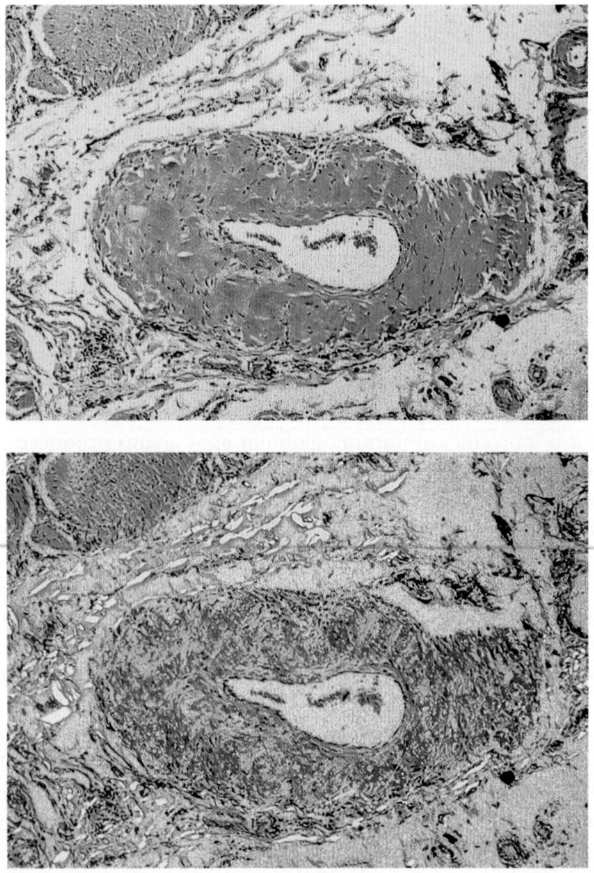

B

FIGURE 23-1. **AL amyloid** involving the wall of an artery stained with Congo red is shown under (**A**)ordinary light and (**B**) polarized light. Note the red–green birefringence of the amyloid. Collagen has a silvery appearance.

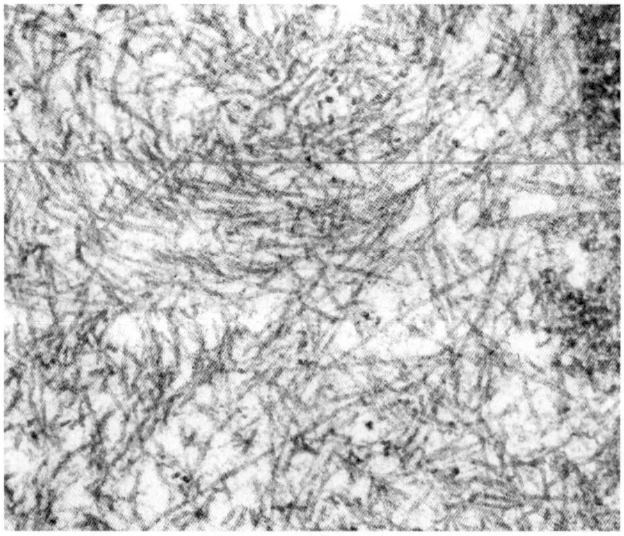

FIGURE 23-2. **Amyloid deposits in tissue.** Parallel and interlacing arrays of fibrils are evident in this electron micrograph.

conformational stability of the disease-specific protein, shifting it in favor of amyloidogenic intermediates, which in turn interact as β-pleated sheets. Thus, the basic fibril seems not to be formed simply as a result of the primary structure of the precursor or the protein fragment. *Fibril formation is most likely influenced by the manner in which the protein fragment interacts with additional components. The common secondary and tertiary organization of the proteins then results in uniform structural and staining properties.*

Definition of Amyloid

The staining and structural properties of amyloid allow a general definition, based primarily on its morphologic characteristics.

- All forms of amyloid stain positively with Congo red and show red–green birefringence when views under polarized light.
- Ultrastructurally, all forms of amyloid consist of interlacing bundles of parallel arrays of fibrils, which have a diameter of 7 to 13 nm.
- The protein in the amyloid fibrils contains a large proportion of crossed β-pleated sheet structure.

Clinical Classification of the Amyloidoses

The classification of amyloidosis has undergone a major change (Table 23-1), primarily because of the realization that the specific protein found in each type of amyloid overlaps previous groupings. Older classifications were based on the clinical presentation of the patient, and did not account for protein composition. For example, familial Mediterranean fever (FMF) and familial amyloidotic polyneuropathy were grouped together as "familial" forms of amyloid, implying incorrectly that similar processes are operative in each disease. Superficially disparate amyloids may in fact be closely related: the amyloid protein of FMF (an inherited disorder) and that deposited secondarily in a variety of inflammatory diseases are the same. Similarly, amyloid proteins in "primary" amyloidosis and that associated with a variety of plasma cell dyscrasias are identical. The amyloid of isolated cardiac amyloidosis and that of senile systemic amyloidosis are also indistinguishable. This clinically oriented categorization is not supported by current information. Although newer groupings, based on the protein type, are now coming into general use, the older classification is regrettably still used

TABLE 23-1

Classification of Human Amyloids

Amyloid Protein	Protein Precursor	Clinical Setting
AL	k or λ immunoglobulin light chain	Multiple myeloma, plasma cell dyscrasias, and primary amyloid
AH	γ immunoglobulin chain	Waldenström macroglobulinemia
Aβ2M	β2-microglobulin	Hemodialysis-related
ATTR	Transthyretin	Familial amyloidotic polyneuropathy (FAP), normal TTR in senile systemic amyloid
AA	Apo serum AA	Persistent acute inflammation; Familial Mediterranean fever; Certain malignancies
AApoAI	Apolipiprotein AI	FAP Iowa
AApoAII	ApolipoproteinAII	Familial
AApoAIV	ApolipoproteinAIV	Sporadic, age-associated
Aβ	β-protein precursor	Alzheimer disease, Down syndrome, Hereditary cerebral hemorrhage with amyloid (HCHWA) Dutch
ABri	ABriPP	Familial dementia, British
ADan	ADanPP	Familial dementia, Danish
APrP	Prion protein	CJD, scrapie, BSE, GSS, Kuru
ACys	Cystatin C	HCHWA, Icelandic
ALys	Lysozyme	Hereditary systemic amyloidosis, Ostertag-type
AFib	Fibrinogen	Hereditary renal amyloidosis
AGel	Gelsolin	Familial amyloidosis, Finnish
ACal	(Pro)calcitonin	Medullary carcinoma of the thyroid
AANF	Atrial natruretic factor	Isolated atrial amyloid
AIAPP	Islet amyloid polypeptide	Type 2 diabetes, insulinomas
AIns	Insulin	Iatrogenic
APro	Prolactin	Pituitary, age associated
AMed	Lactadherin	Senile aortic, media
AKer	Kerato-epithelin	Cornea, familial
ALac	Lactoferrin	Cornea

Apo = apolipoprotein; BSE = bovine spongiform encephalopathy; CJD = Creutzfeldt-Jakob disease; GSS = Gerstmann-Straussler-Sheinker syndrome; TTR = transthyretin.

in clinical medicine. For this reason, both classifications must be reviewed.

The older clinical classification categorizes amyloidosis as primary, secondary, familial, or isolated. Primary, secondary, and familial amyloidoses are usually, but not always, systemic diseases, in which patients frequently present with renal dysfunction or heart failure. The liver, spleen, gastrointestinal tract, tongue, and subcutaneous tissues are also frequent sites of amyloid deposition. Isolated amyloidosis is, by definition, restricted to a single organ.

Primary Amyloidosis Refers to the Presentation of Amyloid without Any Preceding Disease

In one third of these cases, primary amyloidosis is the harbinger of frank **plasma cell neoplasia**, such as multiple myeloma or other B-cell lymphomas. In this respect, primary amyloidosis forms part of the spectrum of amyloid disorders associated with B-cell dysfunction but differs from other types in that the amyloid appears before, rather than after, the overt malignancy. *Whether the amyloidosis or the B-cell neoplasm presents first, the type of amyloid protein (**AL amyloid**) is the same.*

Secondary Amyloidosis Complicates Come Chronic Inflammatory Conditions.

Secondary amyloidosis is associated with a previously existing, persistent inflammatory disorder, which may or may not have an immunologic basis. Patients with rheumatoid arthritis, ankylosing spondylitis, and occasionally systemic lupus erythematosus may develop secondary amyloidosis. Most other patients with secondary amyloidosis have long-standing inflammatory conditions (e.g., lung abscess, tuberculosis, or osteomyelitis). These disorders were the most common causes of systemic amyloidosis in the past, but the use of antibiotics and modern surgical techniques have drastically reduced the frequency of this complication.

Currently, secondary amyloidosis also occurs in persons who develop chronic skin abscesses as a result of subcutaneous self-administration of narcotics, and patients with cystic fibrosis who now live long enough with recurrent lung infections to develop amyloidosis as a complication. Secondary amyloidosis is also seen in patients with specific cancers, such as Hodgkin disease and renal cell carcinoma. The amyloid protein deposited secondary to these malignancies (**AA amyloid**) (see Table 23-1) is identical to that seen in rheumatoid arthritis, chronic infections, and FMF

Incidence of Familial Amyloidoses May Vary with Ethnicity

Several geographical populations display genetically inherited forms of amyloidosis.

FAMILIAL MEDITERRANEAN FEVER (FMF): This autosomal recessive disease is found predominantly in the Mediterranean basin among Sephardic Jews and Turks, although Armenians and Arabs may also be affected. More than 90% of the Jewish patients in Israel are of Sephardic origin. FMF is characterized by polymorphonuclear leukocyte dysfunction and recurrent episodes of serositis, including peritonitis. Since there is recurrent inflammation, the type of amyloid protein deposited (AA amyloid) (see Table 23-1) is the same as that in amyloidosis secondary to acquired inflammatory disorders. The gene for Mediterranean fever *(MEFV)* has been mapped to the short arm of chromosome 16, encoding a protein termed *pyrin* or more poetically, *marenostrin* (Latin, *Mare Nostrum*, "Our Sea," the Mediterranean). It is expressed in neutrophils and is thought to be a transcription factor that regulates other genes involved in the suppression of inflammation.

FAMILIAL AMYLOIDOTIC POLYNEUROPATHY (FAP): This is usually an autosomal dominant genetic disorder, for which at least 80 mutations have been described, scattered throughout the amyloidogenic protein (ATTR) (see Table 23-1). Each protein gives rise to a clinically distinct variant of the disease. FAP exhibits a predilection for peripheral and autonomic nerves. The most common variant is due to a methionine for valine substitution at residue 30 in **transthyretin,** the accumulation of which protein produces this form of amyloidosis. This met30val variant has been described primarily in people of Swedish, Portuguese, and Japanese origin.

HEREDITARY CONGOPHILIC ANGIOPATHY (ICELANDIC): Also termed hereditary cerebral hemorrhage with amyloid (HCHWA), this form of amyloidosis (**ACys**) (see Table 23-1) is the result of a mutation in **cystatin-c**, a protease inhibitor.

HEREDITARY CONGOPHILIC ANGIOPATHY (DUTCH): HCHWA (Dutch) is similar clinically and pathologically to the Icelandic variety but results from a mutation in the amyloid-forming segment of the **Aβ-protein precursor** of Alzheimer disease (see below). Unlike patients affected with Alzheimer disease, however, these individuals do not manifest dementia.

Isolated Amyloidosis Affects Individual Single Organs

Isolated amyloidosis has been described in the major arteries, lung, heart, and various joints and in association with endocrine tumors that secrete polypeptide hormones. In endocrine tumors, the amyloid is usually part of a hormone or a prohormone. By far, the most common organ-specific amyloids are those found in the aorta in atherosclerosis, in Alzheimer disease, and in type 2 diabetes.

Aortic Atherosclerosis and Arterial Inflammations

Amyloid has long been known to be present in the wall of the aorta at sites of atherosclerosis and in arteries with inflammation (e.g., giant cell arteritis) associated with elastic lamina. The amyloid peptide isolated in these conditions has been designated **medin**, classified as **Amed,** and shown to be a 50-residue proteolytic fragment derived from **lactadherin**. This precursor was previously described in milk fat-globule membranes and is also synthesized by smooth muscle cells of the arterial media. The function of this protein is unknown.

Alzheimer Disease

In the most common form of dementia, Alzheimer disease (see Chapter 28), **Aβ amyloid** is restricted to the brain and its vessels. The deposited protein, a 4-kilodalton peptide called the *Aβ* protein, is a fragment of a larger **Aβ-protein precursor** (**Aβ-PP**), which is a normal cell membrane constituent. The longer part of AβPP is extracellular, with the remainder traversing the cell membrane and ending in a cytoplasmic portion of approximately 100 amino acids. The Aβ protein itself is a segment of 40 to 43 amino acids that lies immediately outside and partially within the cell membrane. Aβ-PP is present not only in the cells of the central nervous system but also in most other tissues. There are at least five mRNA splicing products of the *Aβ*-PP gene, several of which have been identified in the brain, but only one of which

(Aβ-PP-695) is brain-specific. It is generally accepted, but has never been demonstrated, that the Aβ protein giving rise to Aβ amyloid is derived from a cell in the central nervous system. Since Aβ-PP is present in so many cell types, it is still possible that the source of Aβ for the vascular amyloid or the brain parenchymal amyloid in Alzheimer disease is extracerebral.

Aβ Protein is derived from Aβ-PP by a series of proteolytic steps, catalyzed by enzymes termed **secretases**. The α-secretase cuts within the Aβ-protein segment and thus precludes its involvement in producing the Aβ protein fragment. The β- and γ-secretases, respectively, cut at the amino- and carboxy-terminal ends of Aβ protein, thereby generating the 40- to 43-residue amyloidogenic fragment. Mutations adjacent to these cleavage sites (but not within Aβ protein) are associated with several familial forms of Alzheimer disease, suggesting a pathogenetic role for amyloid in these situations.

The gene for Aβ-PP is located on chromosome 21, which likely explains the observation that patients with **Down syndrome** (trisomy 21) all develop the morphologic lesions of Alzheimer disease by 35 years of age. Several other genes, in addition to Aβ-PP, have been implicated in both the pathogenesis of Alzheimer disease and the deposition of Aβ These include a locus on chromosome 19 that codes for apoE, one of the common constituents of all amyloids. The E_4 isoform of apoE is linked to Alzheimer disease. Loci on chromosomes 1 and 4, which code for two related proteins, called *presenilins,* have also been linked to Alzheimer disease. Mutations in these proteins influence γ-secretase activity and thus production and processing of Aβ protein. By itself Aβ protein in a random conformation is innocuous to neurons. However, when it is folded into aβ- sheet containing protofibrils Aβ becomes neurotoxic. There is also evidence that transforming growth factor (TGF)-β1 may contribute to amyloid deposition in Alzheimer disease through its capacity to induce amyloid-binding proteins.

Diabetes

The amyloid deposited in the islets of Langerhans in type 2 diabetes (**AIAPP**) is also derived from a larger precursor, a peptide related to a variant of calcitonin, termed **islet amyloid polypeptide** (**IAPP**), or **amylin** (see Table 23-1). Like insulin, this novel hormone is produced by the β cells of the islets and has a profound effect on glucose uptake by the liver and striated muscle cells in pharmacological doses. IAPP's physiologic function has not yet been determined. In transgenic mice that synthesize human amylin, overproduction of this protein leads to islet amyloid in the presence of a high-lipid diet. These observations imply that islet amyloid is involved in the pathogenesis of type 2 diabetes, although the subject requires further study.

Senile Cardiac Amyloidosis

Isolated amyloid deposition may occur in the heart (**ATTR**), particularly in men, after the age of 70 years. This disorder is usually asymptomatic, but occasionally, extensive deposits in the myocardium may cause heart failure. The amyloid precursor responsible is **transthyretin** (see Table 23-1).

Classification of Amyloidoses by the Type of Protein

It is now apparent that (1) specific forms of secondary amyloidosis share a common protein with primary amyloidosis, (2) FMF should be grouped with secondary forms occurring in association with inflammatory disorders and some cancers, and (3) there are isolated forms of amyloidosis that involve single-organ systems that have the same type of protein found in familial amyloidotic polyneuropathy. The presence of amyloid deposits with identical proteins in seemingly distinct clinical entities implies that common pathologic processes occur. These various amyloid proteins are designated A (amyloid), followed by a letter or abbreviation that refers to the specific origin of the protein (see Table 23-1). The most common clinically related amyloids are (1) AMed and atherosclerosis, (2) Aβ and Alzheimer disease, (3) AIAPP and type 2 diabetes, and (4) Aβ2M and chronic dialysis. The first three are covered above.

AL Amyloid Derives from Immunoglobulin Light Chains

The first amyloid protein to be isolated and sequenced was AL amyloid, which was derived from patients who had primary amyloidosis or multiple myeloma. *AL amyloid usually consists of the variable region of immunoglobulin light chains (L, light) and may be derived from either κ or λ chains.* Occasionally, the AL amyloid subunit is larger than the variable end of light chains, and may represent a complete immunoglobulin light chain. Within an individual patient, the sequence of AL amyloid protein is constant, regardless of the organ from which the amyloid is isolated. The amino acid sequence of the variable region of urinary Bence Jones protein corresponds to the patient's AL protein. Because the light chains produced by the neoplastic cells in plasma cell dyscrasias are unique to each patient, *AL amyloid isolated from different persons differs in its amino acid sequence.*

AL protein is common to primary amyloidosis and amyloidosis associated with either multiple myeloma, B-cell lymphomas, or other plasma cell dyscrasias. AL protein in isolated nodules of lung amyloid is a product of focal aggregates of plasma cells. Given that one third of patients who first present with "primary" amyloidosis subsequently develop plasma cell abnormalities or frank myeloma, "primary" amyloidosis, multiple myeloma, and immunoblastic lymphomas apparently form a spectrum of a single disorder. In some cases, the malignant disease presents first as multiple myeloma or lymphoma; in other cases, it is announced by AL deposits in various tissues.

Only some patients with multiple myeloma develop AL amyloid, probably because some κ or λ chains are more fibrillogenic than others. The mechanism by which AL amyloid is deposited is summarized in Figure 23-3.

AA Amyloid Occurs in a Variety of Chronic Inflammatory Processes

AA amyloid is common to a host of seemingly unrelated, persistent inflammatory, neoplastic, and hereditary disorders that lead to so-called secondary amyloidosis. As with AL amyloid, there is a spectrum of AA peptides of differing sizes within AA deposits. *However, in contrast to AL protein, the amino-terminal sequence of AA proteins is identical in all patients, regardless of the underlying disorder.* The intact precursor of AA is **serum amyloid A** (**SAA**). The most prevalent size is a peptide of 76 amino acids, which corresponds to the amino-terminal two-thirds of SAA. SAA is an acute phase protein, whose serum concentration increases rapidly up to 1000-fold during any inflammatory process. The amino acid sequence of SAA exhibits strong evolutionary preservation, which reflects the important role that SAA

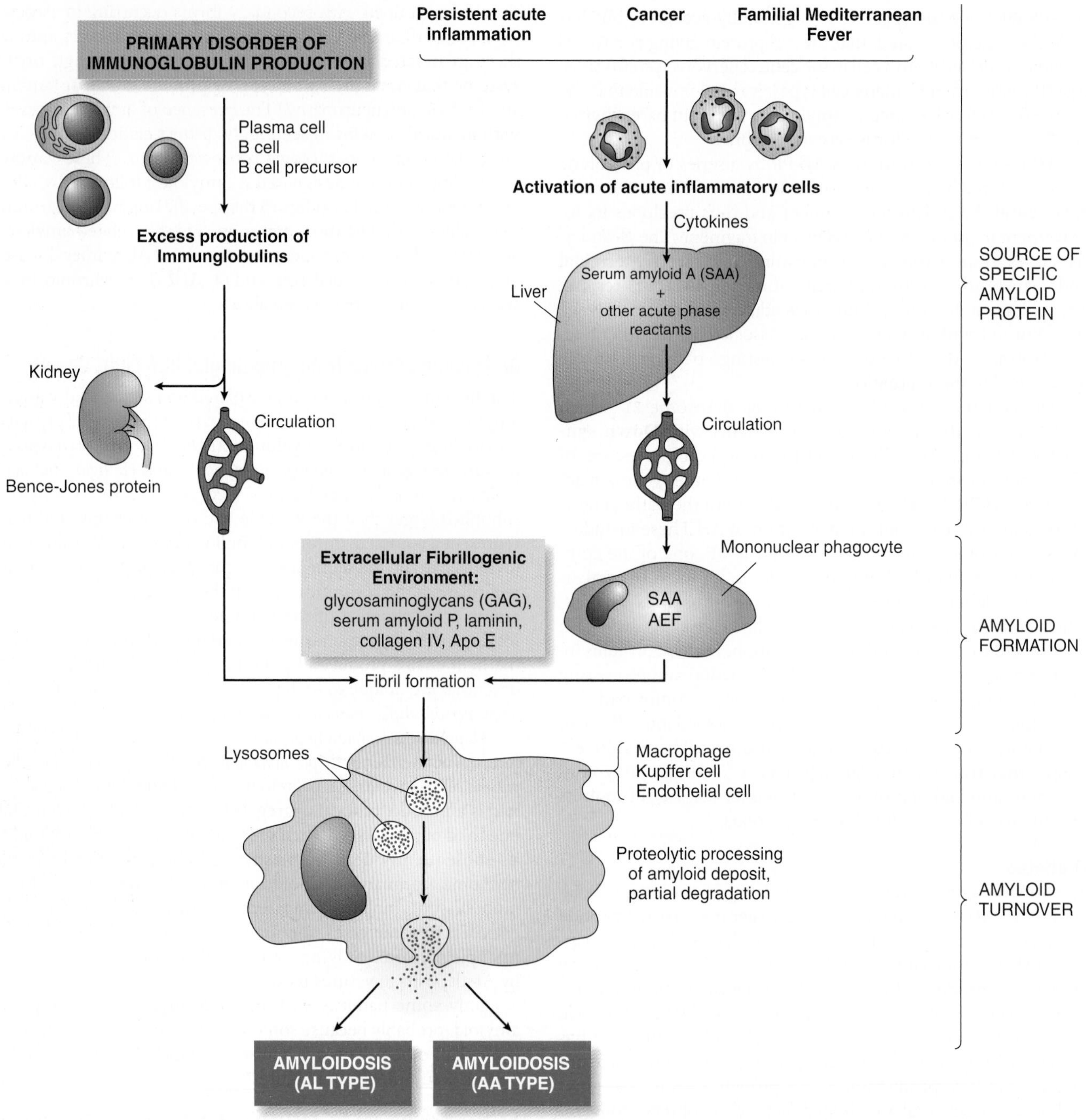

FIGURE 23-3. **The mechanisms of amyloid deposition.** For **AL amyloid**: Lymphocyte- and plasma cell-derived intact immunoglobulins light chains are amyloidogenic within a fibrillogenic environment. For **AA amyloid** deposition: A variety of diseases is associated with the activation of polymorphonuclear leukocytes and macrophages, which in turn leads to the synthesis and release of acute phase reactants by the liver, including serum amyloid A (SAA). SAA in the presence of amyloid-enhancing factor (AEF) is likely released substantially intact by macrophages. In a fibrillogenic environment the released products complex with glycosaminoglycans and serum amyloid PV (SAP). Macrophages are involved in amyloid turnover occurs by proteolytic processing.

probably plays during inflammation. In experimental animals, intact SAA is incorporated into AA fibrils, after which it undergoes postfibrillogenic proteolysis.

Circulating SAA is converted into AA (see Fig. 23-3). SAA has the characteristics of an apolipoprotein for a high-density lipoprotein (HDL); yet it is present in significant quantities only during inflammation. Denaturation of this lipoprotein, which releases a subunit termed **apoSAA**, renders it amyloidogenic. ApoSAA is synthesized primarily in the liver and binds to HDL on entering the circulation. Hepatic apoSAA messenger RNA (mRNA) synthesis is induced by interleukin (IL)-1, IL-6, and tumor necrosis factor (TNF), cytokines that are released by activated inflammatory cells at sites of inflammation. Thus, at least part of the pathway involved in AA deposition involves the normal reaction of the body to acute inflammatory stimuli. As in the case of AL amyloid, macrophages and endothelial cells are intimately related to AA amyloid deposition. Although the anatomical distribution of these cells seems to determine the localization of AA, amyloid deposition cannot be regarded as their normal activity.

Why do inflammatory and endothelial cells fail to degrade SAA completely? Persistent acute inflammation induces not only the synthesis of the amyloid precursor SAA, but also the appearance of a substance termed *amyloid enhancing factor (AEF)*. It is not clear why only a small proportion of patients with high levels of SAA develop amyloidosis. However, in experimental models, amyloid deposition does not occur without AEF, which has characteristics analogous to those of a crystallization nidus, serving as a template for AA amyloid fibril formation. When injected intravenously, AEF localizes to macrophages and endothelial cells, thereby altering their metabolic processing of SAA.

An additional element in the pathogenesis of experimental murine AA amyloid is the co-deposition of apoE and the structural constituents of basement membranes (perlecan, laminin, collagen IV, and SAP). Several amyloid precursors can directly bind to basement membrane proteins and disturb there normal binding interactions. Other evidence suggests that part of the process of amyloid formation is a derangement in basement membrane protein metabolism. Recent work with apoE and SAP "knock-out" mice has shown that the presence of these two components does not determine whether or not AA amyloid is deposited. However, in their absence, the onset of amyloidosis is delayed, and its progression is slowed considerably. These observations with apoE in mice are similar to those of apoE4 in patients with Alzheimer disease.

Thus, during inflammation, the following coincident processes are necessary for AA amyloid deposition (see Fig. 23-3):

- Generation of the amyloid precursor apoSAA.
- Generation of AEF, which in turn affects the conformation and processing of apoSAA in macrophages and endothelial cells.
- Disturbance in the metabolism of basement membrane proteins, whose components can bind to apoSAA and change its conformation.
- Presence of apoE and SAP in the progression of amyloidosis

Aβ2M Amyloid Is Associated with Renal Dialysis

The deposition of amyloid formed from β_2-microglobulin (Aβ2M) is characterized by a destructive arthropathy, owing to amyloid deposition in the major joints of patients undergoing chronic renal dialysis. Because dialysis has been in common use for only 25 to 30 years and more than 8 to 10 years are required before the manifestations of Aβ2M become apparent, the disease first appeared as a clinical entity in the early 1980s. Today 50% to75% of patients undergoing dialysis for over 10 years develop this disorder. Aβ2M amyloid is deposited in subchondral bone and periarticular tissues and the gastrointestinal tract. Blood β_2-microglobulin, the precursor pool for amyloid deposition, is markedly increased in patients with renal failure. The intact normal protein is deposited: neither altered proteolytic processing nor a mutation is involved.

APrP Amyloid Is Found in Spongiform Encephalopathies

Prion proteins (PrPs) are natural plasma membrane constituents found in a variety of cells, including the central nervous system. Their physiologic function is not yet apparent. In the vast majority of people the conformation of PrP is in a nonfibrillar, non-"infectious" state. In rare instances, a PrP protein, with or without a mutation, may experience an alteration in its conformational stability and then an altered susceptibility to proteolysis. The residual PrP, now in an altered conformation, may serve as a template for the association of additional PrP molecules and in so doing confer on them the new PrP conformation (PrPsc). Such altered PrP and its aggregates form fibrils with the characteristics of amyloid and are believed to play a role in a group of human and animal central nervous system degenerative diseases such as **kuru, Creutzfeldt-Jakob disease (CJD), Gerstmann-Straussler-Sheinker disease (GSS), scrapie, and bovine spongiform encephalopathy (BSE, mad cow disease)** (see Chapter 28). In the case of kuru and BSE, the evidence is clear that ingestion of tissue contaminated with PrPsc can induce the PrPsc conformation and the disease in recipients. Cases of CJD have been reported after surgical implantation of tissue transplants or use of pituitary extracts from infected individuals. Such clinical experience highlights the human and veterinary health issues related to transmission of PrP conformational disorders. Nevertheless, the transmissible nature of PrPsc does not involve PrPsc particle replication, but rather its ability to alter the conformation of endogenous PrP.

Deposition of ATTR Amyloid (Transthyretin Amyloid) Occurs in Several Different Types of Amyloidosis, including Familial Amyloidotic Polyneuropathy

Transthyretin (TTR) is secreted by the liver into the plasma, where it serves as a carrier of thyroid hormone and of retinal binding protein. At least 80 mutants of TTR have been described, each responsible for a clinical variant of **FAP** (see Table 23-1). The most common form of FAP is caused by a methionine for valine substitution in TTR at position 30. This mutation lowers the stability of the tetrameric native TTR, allowing the formation of a monomeric intermediate with altered conformation. There is a satisfying correlation between the mutations that give rise to the most unstable tetramers and the most severe forms of FAP. Interestingly, normal TTR is deposited in isolated cardiac amyloidosis and in a systemic form of amyloidosis associated with aging, indicating that an altered amino acid sequence is not an absolute requirement for the deposition of ATTR.

Other Amyloid Proteins May be Less Well Characterized

Other forms of amyloid are derived from normal pre-prohormones or from hormonal products secreted by endocrine tissues or tumors. Medullary thyroid carcinoma originates from thyroid C-type cells, which secrete calcitonin. Amyloid deposited in this tumor is a fragment of procalcitonin. In isolated atrial amyloid, the peptide is atrial natriuretic factor. Amyloid proteins related to keratin have been reported in the skin. In other isolated forms of human amyloidosis, e.g., amyloid in osteoarthritic joints associated with aging, the deposited materials are not yet characterized.

Conformational instability of several other proteins with amyloid-like fibril formation is believed to play a role in several other diseases (see Chapter 28). Thus, phosphorylated tau protein, complexed with heparan sulfate, has been identified as paired helical filaments in neurons of patients with Alzheimer disease. Similarly the filaments in Lewy bodies in patients with Parkinson disease are composed of α-synuclein. This protein rapidly forms such filaments *in vitro* in the presence of heparin/heparan sulfate. Finally, intranuclear protein filaments composed of long polyglutamine sequences appear to play a role in neurodegeneration in Huntington disease.

Macrophages Mediate Amyloid Turnover

Although amyloid has for decades been considered an inert stable entity once it has been deposited, recent clinical and experimental observations indicate that amyloids of various types do turnover, and can resolve with time. Examples include renal function in AA amyloid that can improve if the underlying inflammatory process responsible for AA deposition is adequately treated. Similarly AL amyloid may ameliorate if the underlying plasma cell dyscrasia is effectively treated. Neurologic improvement can occur in cases of ATTR following liver transplantation. In experimental animal models, depletion of body macrophages during the earliest phases of AA induction prevents deposition, but depletion of body macrophages following deposition enhances AA accumulation. Thus in AA amyloid, macrophages play a role both in the process of deposition and turnover of the deposits (see Fig. 23-3).

A General Scheme of Amyloidogenesis

The requirements for amyloidogenesis *in vivo* include (1) an adequate pool of an amyloidogenic protein, (2) a nidus or nucleus for fibrillogenesis, (3) conformational instability of the amyloidogenic protein (mutations, proteolysis, and protein interactions), and (4) amyloid turnover. These are schematically interrelated in Figure 23-4.

AN ADEQUATE PRECURSOR POOL: In some settings, such as ATTR associated with senile systemic or senile cardiac amyloid, the constitutive hepatic synthesis of transthyretin provides the necessary pool. In other forms of amyloid, such as AA, a physiologic response as part of inflammation leads to increased synthesis of the precursor, which inadvertently provides the necessary pool. Alternatively, mutations may alter a nonamyloidogenic protein, providing it with an amyloidogenic sequence and generating the required pool.

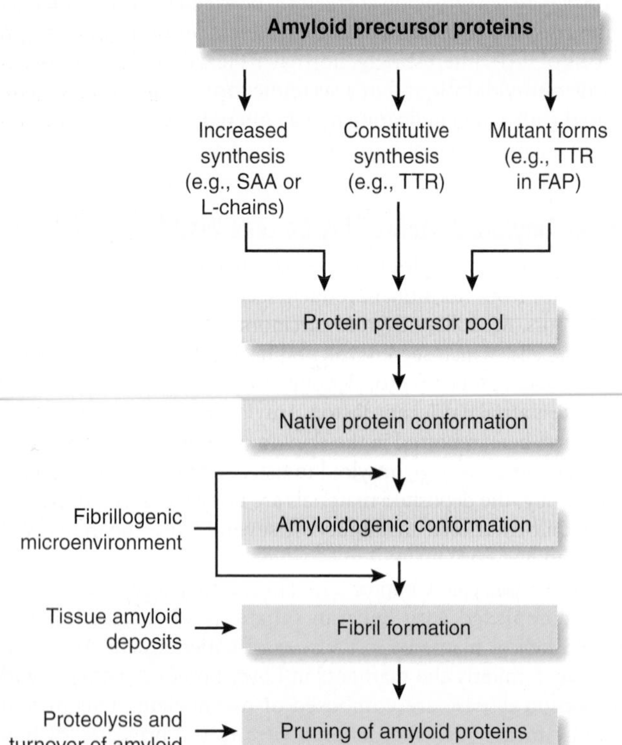

FIGURE 23-4. **General scheme for amyloidogenesis.** FAP = familial amyloidotic polyneuropathy; SAA = serum amyloid A; TTR = transthyretin.

ANATOMICAL LOCALIZATION OF AMYLOID: The physiologic function of the amyloid precursor probably determines the location of the specific form of amyloid. For instance, SAA, the precursor of AA, may target HDLs to macrophages and endothelial cells. Mishandling of SAA by such cells would set the stage for local AA deposition. Similarly, a mutation may not only provide an amyloidogenic sequence, but may also cause the protein to interact with different cells. Thus, the same protein in mutant and normal forms may be involved in amyloid at different anatomical sites. For example, normal TTR is found primarily in the heart in senile cardiac amyloidosis. Yet in FAP, the same protein in its mutant form is deposited as ATTR primarily in the peripheral nervous system.

ALTERED MICROENVIRONMENTS, FIBRILLIZATION NUCLEI AND CONFORMATIONAL INSTABILITY: An appropriate microenvironment is necessary for the precursor protein to present as amyloid. This environment likely involves changes in the metabolism of basement membrane proteins and direct molecular interactions of these proteins with the amyloidogenic protein. Examples include SAA, tau, α-synuclein, IAPP, or Aβ and their interaction with heparan sulfate. In these cases, this interaction changes the conformation of the amyloidogenic protein, thereby increasing its β-sheet content. A fibrillization nucleus may aid and abet this process by driving the equilibrium away from the native conformation in favor of the amyloid one.

PROTEOLYSIS AND TURNOVER: In some forms of amyloid, proteolysis of the precursor may be part of its processing or post-translational modification. These prefibrillogenic steps generate a normal peptide or protein, which under appropriate conditions may lead to amyloid deposition. The conversion of AβPP into Aβ in Alzheimer disease is an example. Proteolysis of amyloid precursors, which generates the varied sizes of peptides found in individual deposits, is inferred to occur at a step beyond the incorporation of the precursor into the amyloid fibrils. Proteases in various tissues process the fibrils until further degradation becomes difficult. Thus, the size of the residual amyloid peptides varies in any given deposit.

Morphologic Features of Amyloidoses

Amyloid fibrils are usually first deposited in close association with subendothelial basement membranes (Fig. 23-5). *Because amyloid accumulates along stromal networks, the deposits take on the architectural framework of the organs involved.* The morphologic differences in amyloid deposition among organs simply reflect differences between tissues in stromal organization. For example, in the medulla of the kidney, amyloid is laid down in a longitudinal fashion, parallel to the tubules and vasa recta. By contrast, in the glomerulus (Fig. 23-6), amyloid appears in a pattern determined by the lobular architecture of that structure. Splenic amyloid may be associated with either the stroma of the red pulp or that of the white pulp. On gross examination, amyloid in the red pulp imparts a diffusely pale and waxy appearance, the so-called lardaceous spleen. The cut surface of the spleen containing white pulp amyloid is different and shows multiple pale foci scattered throughout the organ, an appearance labeled *sago spleen.* Deposits in the liver follow the arteries of the portal triads or are laid down along central veins and radiate into the parenchyma along liver cell plates (Fig. 23-7).

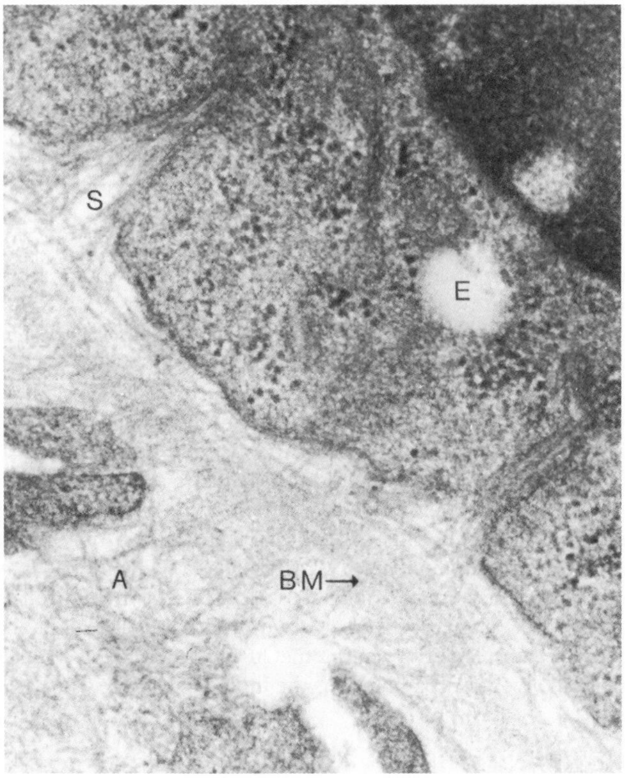

FIGURE 23-5. **Electron micrograph of glomerular amyloid** *(A)* illustrating its location relative to the basement membrane *(BM)*. Amyloid spicules *(S)* extend into the cytoplasm of the glomerular epithelial cells *(E)*.

Amyloid adds interstitial material to sites of deposition, thereby increasing the size of affected organs. This increase may be counterbalanced by the deposition of amyloid in blood vessels (Fig. 23-8), which impairs circulation and may lead to organ atrophy. Affected organs may thus increase or decrease in size. Compact amyloid deposits are essentially avascular, so the involved organs are commonly pale and firm.

Regardless of whether amyloid is laid down in a systemic or local fashion, deposits tend to occur between parenchymal cells and their blood supply, interfering with normal nutrition and gas exchange. Amyloid may eventually entrap parenchymal

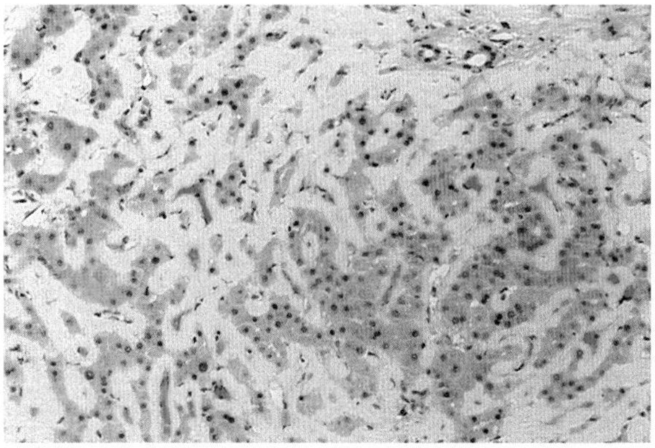

FIGURE 23-7. **Hepatic amyloidosis.** Amyloid is deposited along the sinusoids. Note the atrophic hepatocytes.

cells. Alternatively, it may have a direct toxic effect on these cells through the interaction of protofibrils and cell membranes. *In each case, amyloidosis leads to cell strangulation, atrophy, and death* (Fig. 23-9).

Clinical Features of Amyloidoses

No single set of symptoms points unequivocally to amyloidosis as a diagnosis. The symptomatology of amyloidosis is governed by both the underlying disease and the type and organ locations of the protein deposited. Amyloidosis may also be diagnosed unexpectedly in the course of evaluation for something unrelated, with no clinical manifestations referable to the amyloidosis itself. In other cases, unexplained renal and cardiac complications may be the presenting conditions.

KIDNEY: Patients with multiple myeloma, chronic longstanding inflammatory disorders, or FMF who develop nephrotic syndrome should be suspected of having amyloidosis. Proteinuria, particularly in patients with plasma cell dyscrasias, may be overlooked if the patient is already excreting a Bence Jones protein. Progressive glomerular obliteration may ultimately lead to renal failure and uremia.

HEART: Amyloid involvement of the myocardium should be suspected in systemic forms of amyloidosis in which congestive failure or cardiomegaly is associated with low voltage on the

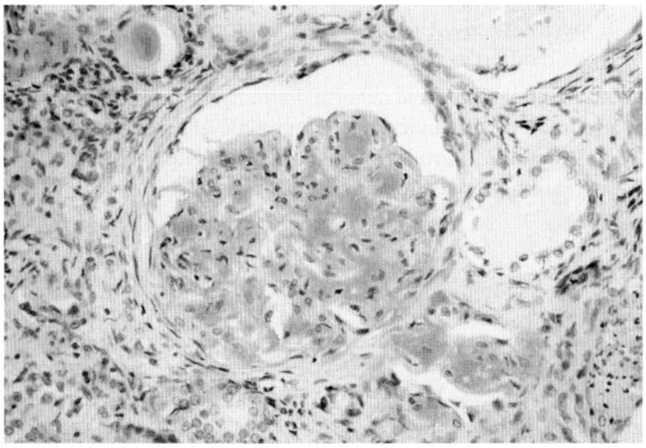

FIGURE 23-6. **Microscopic appearance of AA amyloid in a glomerulus.** Note the lobular pattern of the amyloid deposit and the involvement of the afferent arteriole.

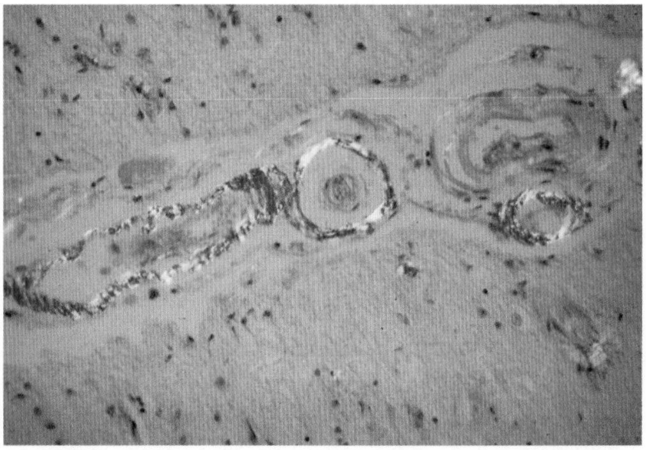

FIGURE 23-8. **Cerebrovascular amyloid in a case of Alzheimer disease.** The section was stained with Congo red and examined under polarized light.

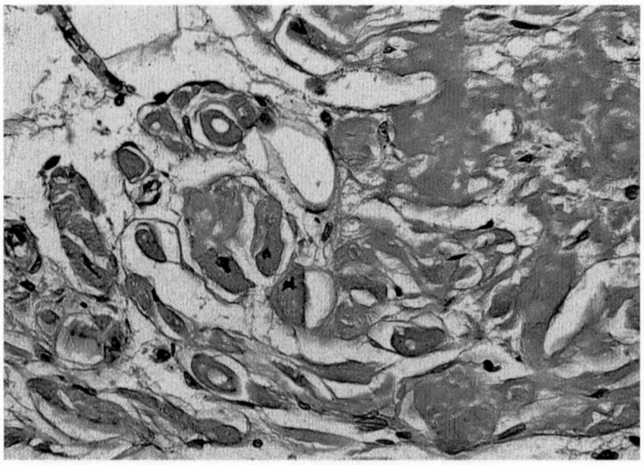

FIGURE 23-9. **Myocardial amyloid (AL type)**, showing the encroachment upon, and strangulation of, individual myocardial fibers.

electrocardiogram. Entrapment of the conduction system leads to arrhythmias, which in turn can result in sudden death. Not only does congestive failure secondary to cardiac amyloidosis respond poorly to digitalis therapy, but amyloid fibrils also sequester and concentrate digoxin, thereby precipitating digitalis toxicity and fatal arrhythmias. Amyloid deposition in the myocardium may also impair ventricular pliancy and limit filling, an effect that appears clinically as a *restrictive form of cardiomyopathy*. In some instances, cardiac amyloidosis has masqueraded as constrictive pericarditis.

GASTROINTESTINAL TRACT: The ganglia, smooth muscle, vasculature, and submucosa of the gastrointestinal tract may all be affected by amyloid. Deposits in these locations alter gastrointestinal motility and absorption. Patients complain of either constipation or diarrhea, occasionally in association with malabsorption. Enlargement of the tongue is classic, and interference with its motor function may be severe enough to affect speech and swallowing.

LIVER: The liver is frequently affected by AL, AA, and familial forms of amyloidosis. Although hepatic dysfunction is uncommon, patients may present with jaundice and even frank liver failure. Liver transplantation can be an effective treatment in some cases. Interestingly, familial met30val mutant forms of TTR amyloid largely spare the liver, but transplanted liver does not produce amyloidogenic precursor.

PERIPHERAL NERVES: The familial polyneuropathic forms of amyloid usually manifest as paresthesias, with loss in temperature and pain sensation of the extremities.

In all systemic forms of amyloidosis, the patient's course is usually unremitting and ultimately fatal. Patients with multiple myeloma and AL amyloidosis generally die within 1 to 2 years, either from the malignancy itself or from cardiac or renal complications of amyloidosis. Patients with AA amyloidosis secondary to long-standing inflammatory disease have a more protracted course, but often die, usually from cardiac or renal failure, within 5 years of diagnosis. Persons who suffer deposition of ATTR of the familial type have an extended course of 15 to 25 years. Symptoms may begin at any age but are usually postpubertal, with death most common in the fifth and sixth decades. Successful treatment of the underlying condition, such as multiple myeloma or an inflammatory disorder, may on occasion lead to resorption and resolution of amyloid deposits. These clinical observations indicate that amyloid does turn over, albeit slowly.

The diagnosis of amyloidosis, ultimately rests on histologic demonstration of amyloid deposition in biopsy specimens. Amyloid is readily demonstrated in gingival and rectal biopsy specimens and in abdominal subcutaneous fat. It is commonly visualized in renal biopsies taken as part of a general investigation of impaired renal function. The availability of antisera specific for the various amyloid proteins now allows determination of the specific forms of amyloid by immunohistochemical means, which may guide which therapy. For example, AL amyloid and TTR amyloid may be confused because of similar ages of onset. AL amyloid and its underlying malignancy is treated with chemotherapy and bone marrow transplantation. In the met30val mutant forms of TTR amyloid, liver transplantation is the therapy of choice.

Amyloid Treatment Strategies

Strategies for anti-amyloid therapy flow from the processes of amyloidogenesis outlined above.

1. *Reduction in amyloid precursor concentrations:* Since an adequate amyloid precursor pool is necessary for fibrillogenesis, attempts have been made to limit the availability of such precursors, including liver transplantation for mutant ATTR in FAP and chemotherapy and bone marrow transplantation in the treatment of multiple myeloma.
2. *Inhibition of nidus (nucleus formation):* Colchicine is the drug of choice in preventing the development of amyloidosis in patients with FMF. Experimentally, this drug acts by preventing the generation of AEF (the nidus), thereby preventing the appearance of amyloid.
3. *Inhibition of molecular interactions:* The recent recognition that amyloid fibril formation may be the product of interactions between several molecular components suggests that interfering with such interactions may inhibit amyloidogenesis. Experimentally, this approach has proved successful with several different forms of amyloid.
4. *Acceleration of amyloid removal:* Patients with AL amyloid who are treated with an iodinated analogue of doxorubicin resorb considerable amounts of their amyloid. The agent binds with high affinity to several amyloids, including AL.

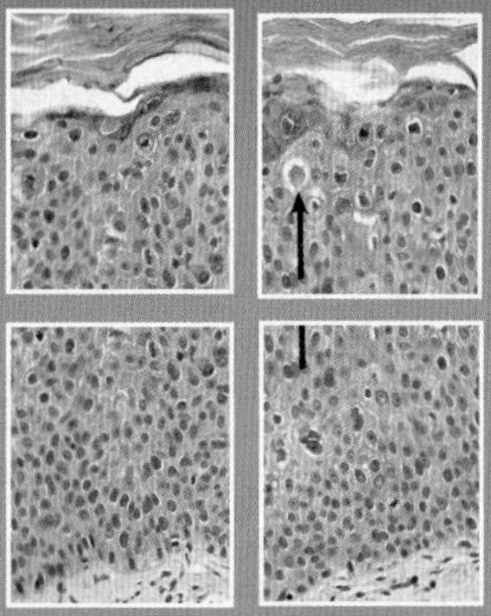

24 The Skin

Craig A. Storm
David E. Elder

The skin is an optimal organ for studying fundamental principles of pathology because lesions on its surface are readily apparent. Except for diseases of highly specialized tissues—for instance, those of the alveolus or glomerulus or the demyelinating diseases of the central nervous system—all classes of disease are seen in the skin. Some diseases, such as the blistering ones, are manifested only in the skin (except for some involvement of the mucous membranes).

Considering the imperatives of appearance in human interactions, a changed appearance of the skin may at times be the most important feature of cutaneous disease. Many cutaneous diseases have only minor symptoms, and some have no symptoms at all. Few are life-threatening, and many are self-limited. However, even self-limited, asymptomatic cutaneous diseases are often of great concern to the patient. For example, the symptoms of acne are systemically minor, but the disease can change a life. Although scalp hair is unneeded, baldness may cause considerable distress. Vitiligo, a completely asymptomatic, progressive, depigmentary disorder, may turn an otherwise normal black person into a recluse or an outcast.

Anatomy and Physiology of the Skin

The skin is a protective barrier; microorganisms find it almost impossible to penetrate the epidermis from the outside, and water loss is limited from the inside. The skin is vital in regulating temperature and protecting against ultraviolet light. A variety of sensory receptors communicate details related to the immediate environment. The skin plays a prominent role in immune regulation through skin-associated lymphoid tissues, which consist of lymphocytes and antigen-presenting cells that travel between the skin and regional lymph nodes via the lymphatics and bloodstream. Keratinocytes, Langerhans cells, mast cells, lymphocytes, and macrophages all serve functions related to immunity. Epidermal keratinocytes produce a variety of cytokines, notably interleukin (IL)-1α and IL-1β, as well as eicosanoids. This ability of keratinocytes to produce products that mediate immunity and inflammation is necessary in an organ relentlessly exposed to the external environment. Langerhans cells, the dendritic antigen-presenting cells of the skin, are bone marrow-derived, epidermal, immigrant cells. They play an important role in the development and regulation of contact hypersensitivity, allograft rejection, and graft-versus-host disease.

KERATINOCYTES: The epidermis is a multilayered sheet of keratin-producing cells. A progressive change in morphology occurs from the replicating columnar cells of the basal layer (**stratum basalis**) through the spinous layer (**stratum spinosum**) and the granular layer (**stratum granulosum**) to the nonviable flattened cells of the cornified layer (**stratum corneum**) (Fig. 24-1 and Fig. 24-2). The basal cells harbor most of the mitotic activity of the epidermis. As keratinocytes approach the superficial epidermis, they become anucleate and form flattened plates of dead cells on the skin surface (the cornified layer). Keratinocytes synthesize a sulfur-poor, filamentous protein, the **tonofibril**, which is related to the keratin molecule of the stratum corneum. Tonofibrils are composed of varying blends of acidic and basic intermediate keratin filaments, resulting in over 30 different keratins that are responsible for structures such as the stratum corneum, hair, and nails. Bundles of tonofibrils converge on, and terminate at, the plasma membrane in attachment plates called **desmosomes** (Fig. 24-3).

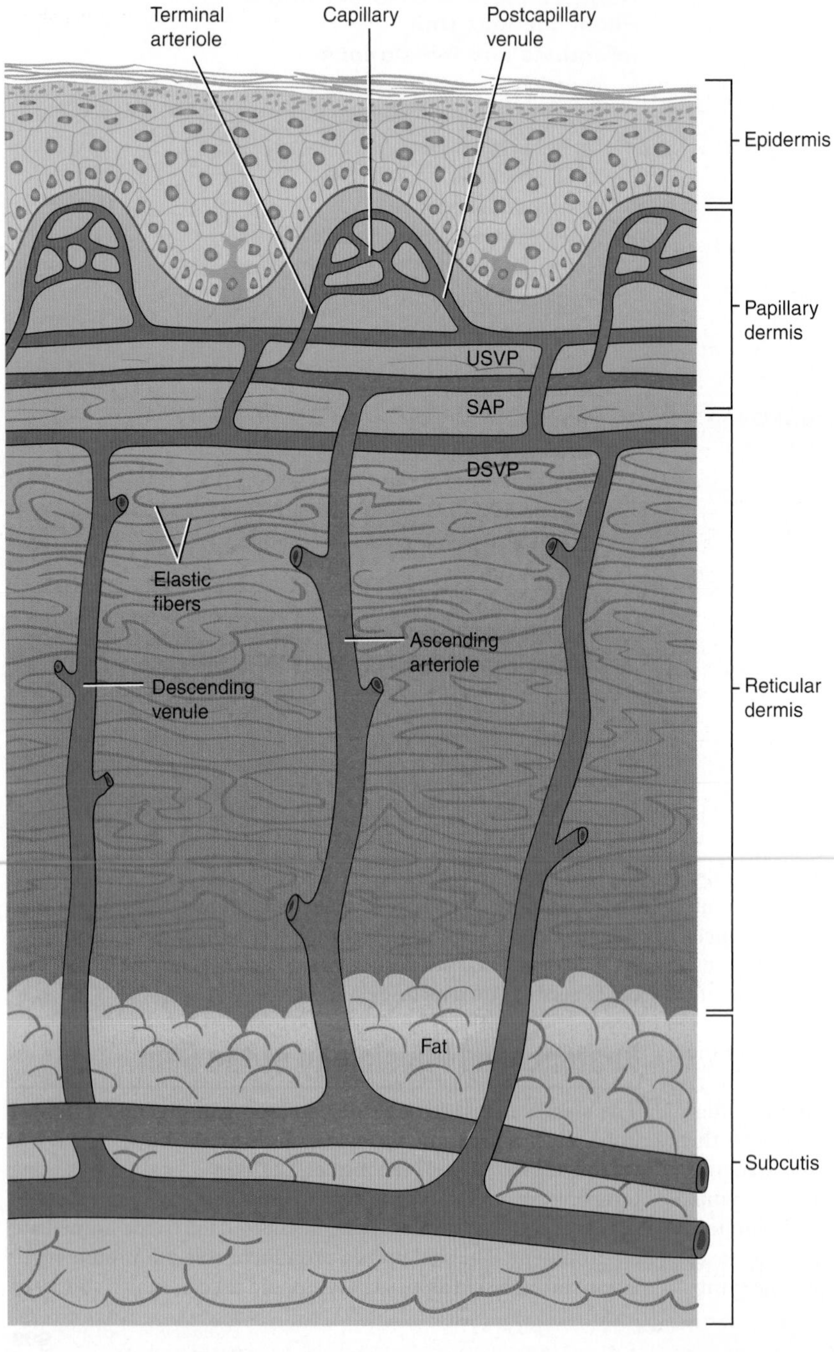

FIGURE 24-1. **The dermis and its vasculature.** The dermis is divided into two distinct anatomical regions. The papillary dermis with its vascular plexus and the epidermis usually react together in diseases that are primarily limited to the skin. The reticular dermis and the subcutis are altered in association with systemic diseases that manifest in the skin. *DSVP* = deep superficial venular plexus; *SAP* = superficial arterial plexus; *USVP* = upper superficial venular plexus.

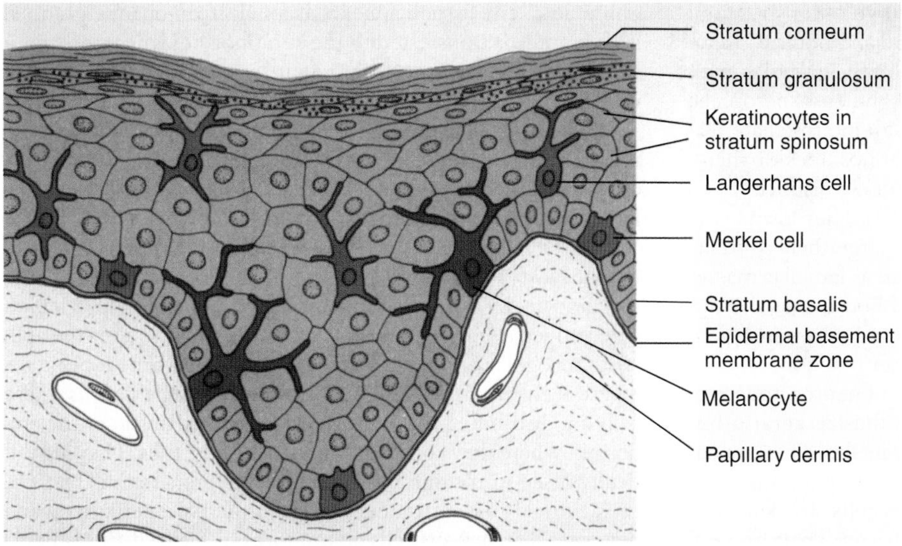

FIGURE 24-2. **Normal epidermis and the epidermal immigrant cells.** Keratinocytes form the multilayered epidermis, protecting against water loss and bacterial invasion. Melanocytes provide color as well as protection against ultraviolet radiation. Langerhans cells are among the cells responsible for the skin's function as an immunologic organ. Merkel cells may represent one of the enablers of tactile function of the skin.

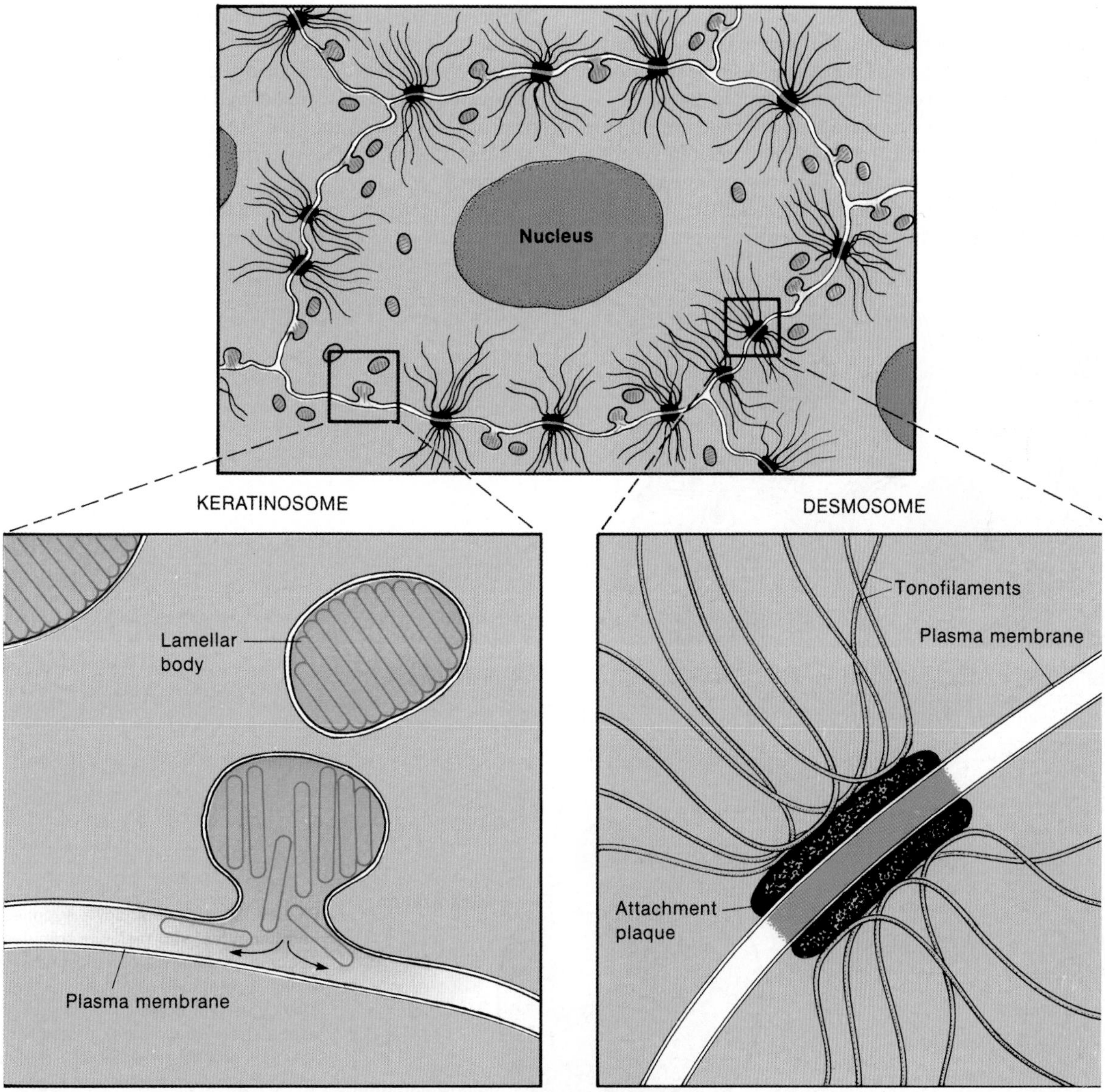

FIGURE 24-3. **The keratinocyte, keratinosome, and desmosome.** The keratinocyte cytoplasm is dominated by delicate keratin fibrils, the tonofilaments. These are part of the cytoskeleton of the cell and loop within the attachment plaque of the desmosome. The lamellar body of the keratinocyte extrudes its contents into the intercellular space. This material probably has a role in cellular cohesion.

Keratinocytes are also distinguished by two other structural products: "keratohyaline granules" and "Odland bodies." Keratohyaline granules are the defining feature of the granular layer and are composed of a histidine-rich, electron-dense, basophilic protein–profilaggrin–which is associated with intermediate filaments. Odland bodies, also known as keratinosomes or membrane-coating granules, are the only structurally distinctive, secretory product of the epidermis (see Fig. 24-3). They form in the outer spinous and granular layers and discharge their contents into the intercellular spaces, appearing there as lamellar masses parallel to the surface of the skin. Odland bodies and the discharged lamellated products are most obvious in the outer granular layer and are related to epidermal barrier function.

The epidermis harbors immigrant cells of neuroectodermal and mesenchymal origin that do not synthesize keratin but which have their own highly distinctive organelles. They appear in varying numbers and at varying levels of the epidermis. Two of these cells, **melanocytes** and **Langerhans cells**, are dendritic. The third, the **Merkel cell**, is associated with a terminal neuronal axon (see Fig. 24-2.).

MELANOCYTES: Melanocytes are dendritic cells of neural crest origin that are largely responsible for skin color. They lie in the basal layer of the epidermis and are separated from the dermis by the epidermal basement membrane zone. A single melanocyte may supply dendrites to over 30 keratinocytes (Fig. 24-4).

The **melanosome** is a cytoplasmic membrane-bound complex in which melanin is synthesized. When melanin synthesis is active, the melanosome contains filaments arranged in a parallel array along the long axis of the organelle (see Fig. 24-4). The melanosome's orderly internal structure is progressively obliterated, and it then appears as an electron-opaque granule. This granule is transferred to the keratinocyte, where it forms a supranuclear cap, protecting the nuclear material from ultraviolet light.

Skin color is largely based on the number, size, and packaging of melanosomes in keratinocytes. In hair and epidermal keratinocytes, melanins are packaged to absorb and reflect visible light, thereby forming the integumentary colors.

LANGERHANS CELLS: These cells arrive in embryonic skin in the last month of the first trimester, following the melanocytes by a month. With the arrival of these human leukocyte antigen (HLA)-DR–positive cells, the skin acquires the ability to recognize and process antigens, at which time it becomes a part of the immune system. Uncommon in the dermis, these cells are distributed throughout the nucleated layers of the epidermis, where they constitute about 4% of the cells. They are difficult to see in routine light microscopic preparations because their cytoplasm is translucent and is formed of a perikaryon and dendrites. Langerhans cells do not form specialized attachments to the apposed keratinocytes. In electron micrographs, the cytoplasm contains a moderate number of specialized organelles, the **Birbeck granules**. In two dimensions, these structures appear to be racquet-shaped, but three-dimensional reconstruction has shown them to be cup-shaped (Fig. 24-5). The function of these unique organelles that are derived from the plasma membrane is probably related to the role of Langerhans cells as antigen-presenting cells (antigenic material being internalized into Birbeck granules).

In Langerhans cell histiocytoses (see Chapter 20), Birbeck granules are attached to the plasma membrane of the proliferating

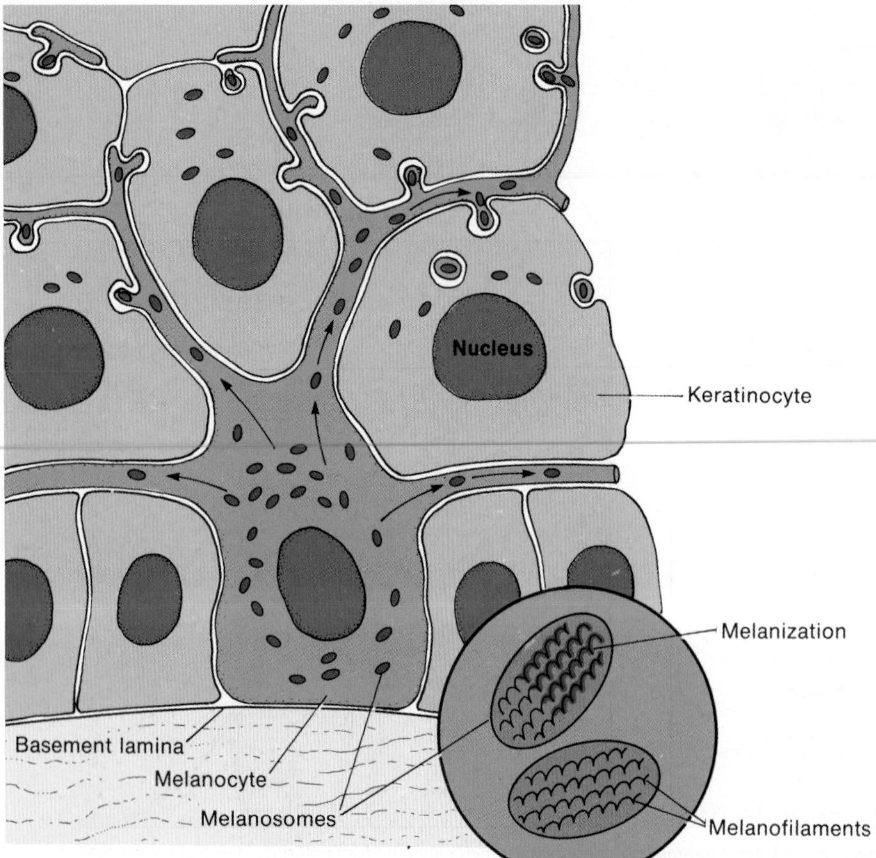

FIGURE 24-4. **A melanocyte supplies over 30 keratinocytes with melanin granules by way of complex dendritic cytoplasmic extensions.** Melanin granules are transferred to keratinocytes and come to lie in a supranuclear cap, a site indicating their protective function. Pigment granules are actually formed in the melanocytes within distinctive organelles—the melanosomes. Pigment is synthesized on small filaments within this organelle *(inset).*

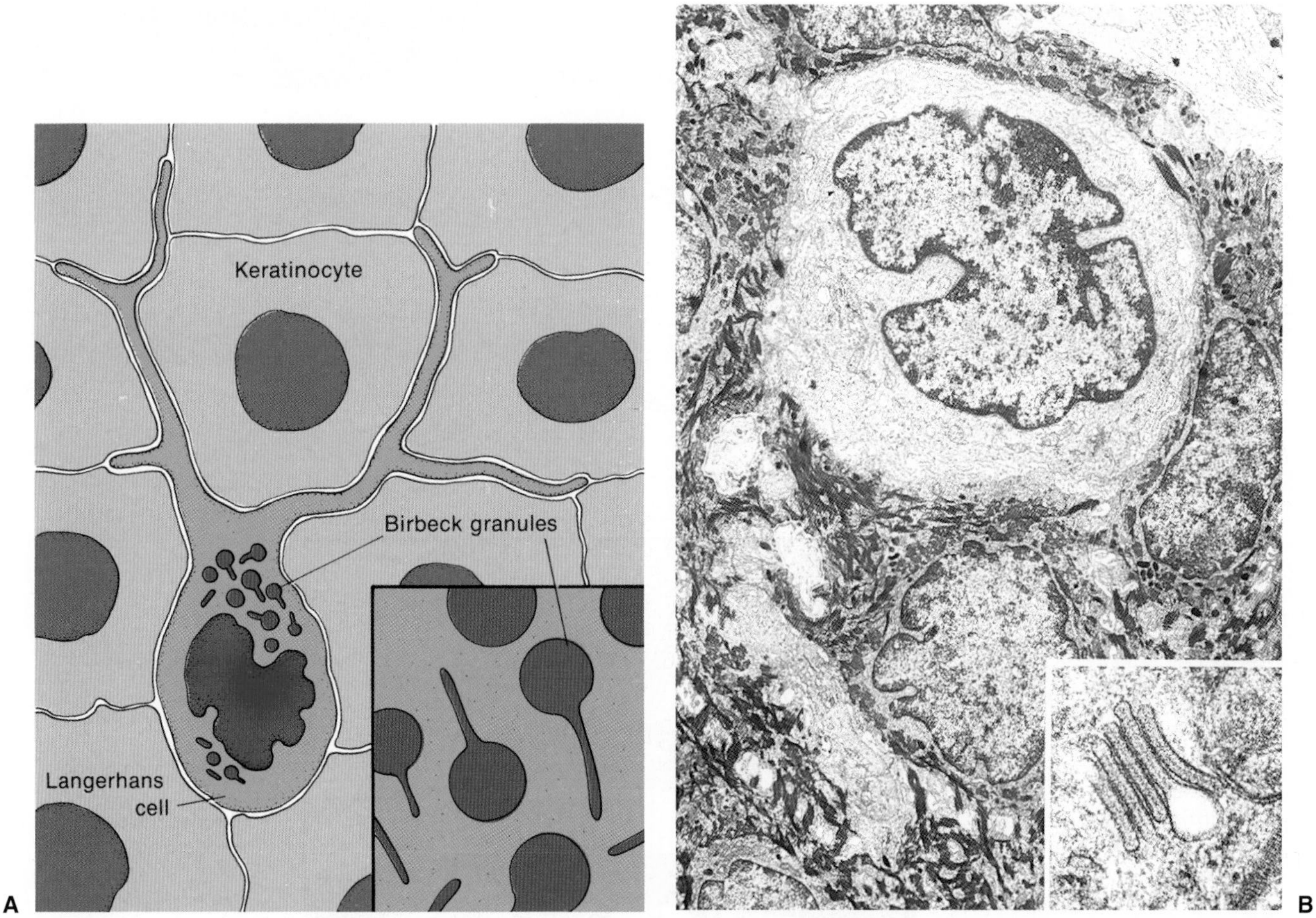

FIGURE 24-5. **The dendritic Langerhans cell can recognize and process antigens. A.** The unique racket-shaped organelles, called *Birbeck granules,* may be important in antigen presentation. **B.** An electron micrograph of a Langerhans cell shows a high-power view of the racket-shaped organelles (*inset*). The Langerhans cell body *(mid-lower portion)* is pale compared to the surrounding keratinocytes, whose cytoplasm contains electron-dense packets of tonofilaments. A dendrite is present *(upper right corner)*.

cells and are in direct communication with the extracellular space. Furthermore, they have a fuzzy coat of clathrin, a feature of "coated pits," suggesting a relationship to receptor-mediated antigen processing and recognition. Langerhans cells express major histocompatibility complex (MHC)-I, MHC-II and receptors for Fc immunoglobulin (Ig)G and Fc IgE. They are identified immunohistochemically by CD1 or, less specifically, S-100 protein.

MERKEL CELLS: Although sometimes classified as "immigrant" cells, evidence is accumulating that Merkel cells may be specialized basal keratinocytes. They form desmosomes with keratinocytes and express keratins in a fashion similar to that of keratinocytes. The cells project short, blunt cytoplasmic fingers into adjacent keratinocytes. Merkel cells do not appear in all areas of the epidermis, but are seen in special regions such as the lips, oral cavity, external root sheath of the hair follicles, and the palmar skin of the digits. They have a distinctive organelle, a membrane-bound, dense-core granule, 100 nm or wider (Fig. 24-6). Immunohistochemical and ultrastructural studies suggest that the Merkel cell has a neurosecretory function. The basal aspect of the cell is apposed to a small nerve plate, which is connected to a myelinated axon by a short, nonmyelinated axon. This complex structure may function as a tactile mechanoreceptor.

BASEMENT MEMBRANE: The basement membrane zone (BMZ) is an interface between the dermis and epidermis and is as diverse in function as it is complex in structure (Fig. 24-7). It

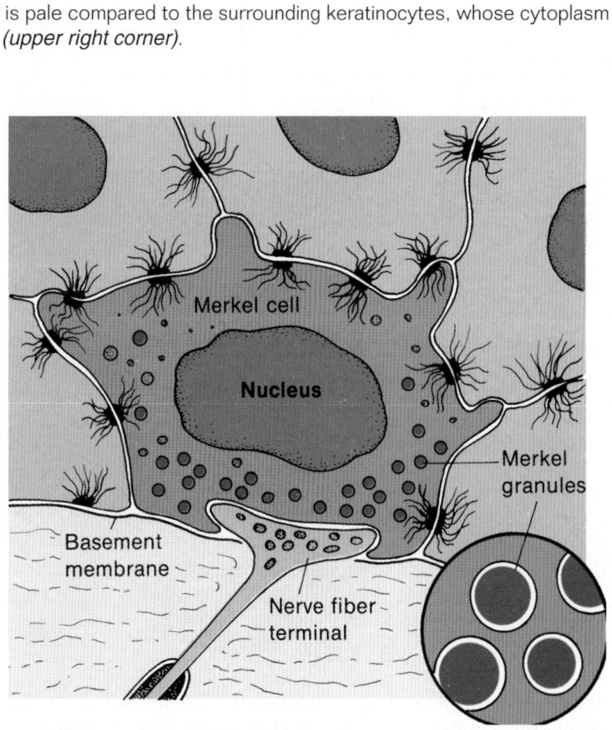

FIGURE 24-6. **The Merkel cell,** which differs from other immigrant cells, forms desmosomes with keratinocytes and is attached to a small nerve plate (nerve fiber terminal). The membrane-delimited, dense core granule is distinctive *(inset)*.

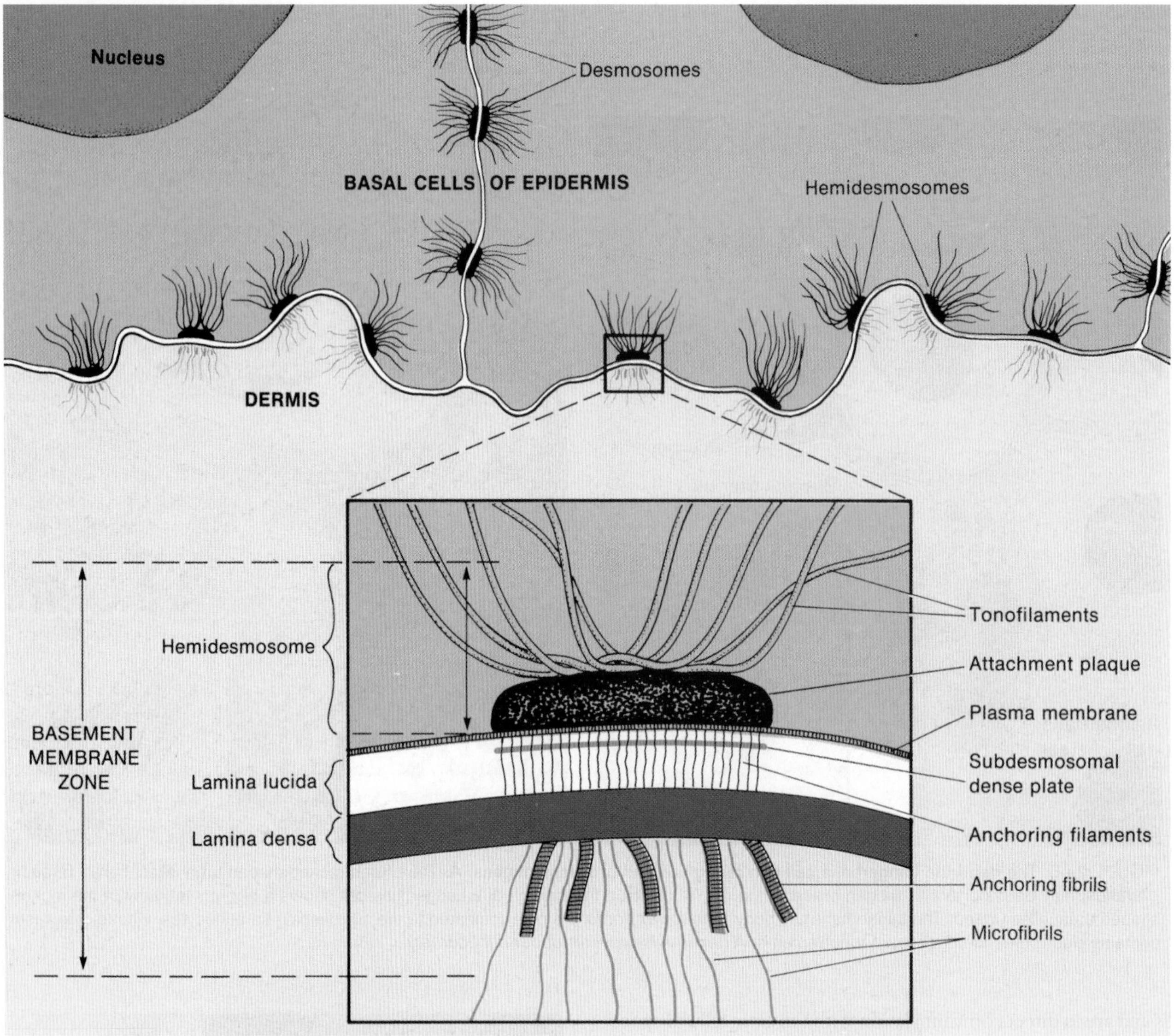

A

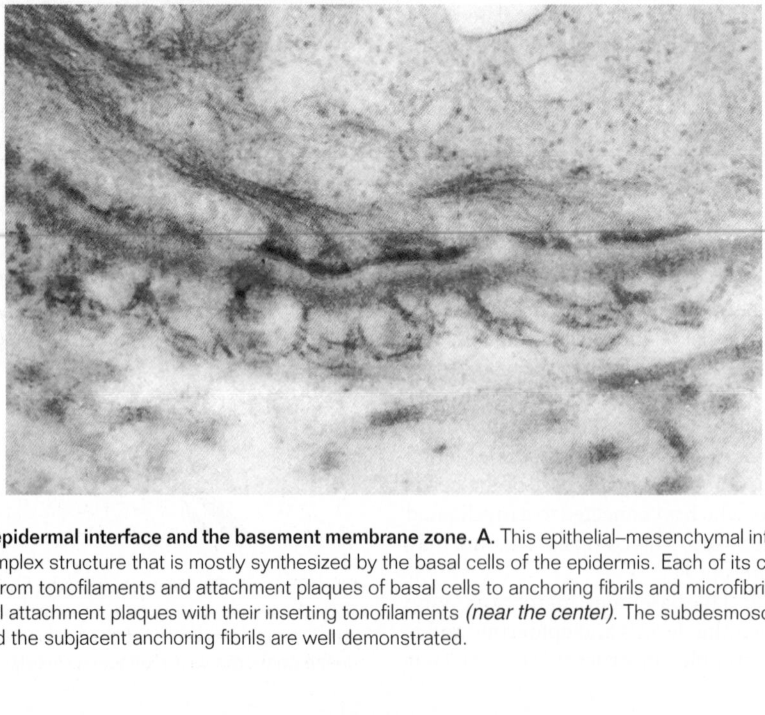

B

FIGURE 24-7. **The dermal–epidermal interface and the basement membrane zone. A.** This epithelial–mesenchymal interface is the site of the basement membrane zone, a complex structure that is mostly synthesized by the basal cells of the epidermis. Each of its complex structures is a site of change in specific disease, from tonofilaments and attachment plaques of basal cells to anchoring fibrils and microfibrils. **B.** An electron micrograph shows the hemidesmosomal attachment plaques with their inserting tonofilaments *(near the center)*. The subdesmosomal dense plates, the lamina lucida, the lamina densa, and the subjacent anchoring fibrils are well demonstrated.

is responsible for dermal–epidermal adherence and probably functions as a selective macromolecular filter. It is also a site of immunoglobulin and complement deposition in certain cutaneous diseases. Most of the structures of the BMZ are elaborated by cells of the epidermis. The basal lamina is the primary organizational feature of the BMZ and is responsible for epithelial cell polarity as well as some keratin gene expression. Ultrastructurally, the basal lamina includes:

- **Deep aspects of basal keratinocytes** including plasma membrane and tonofilaments that attach to the deep face of the hemidesmosome
- **Hemidesmosome,** with its subdesmosomal dense plate
- **Anchoring filaments** that extend from subdesmosomal dense plates across the lamina lucida and insert into the lamina densa
- **Lamina lucida,** an electron-lucent layer containing adherence proteins
- **Lamina densa,** composed principally of type IV collagen
- **Anchoring fibrils,** which are arrays of type VII collagen extending from the inner face of the lamina densa for a short distance into the papillary dermis
- **Microfibrils,** which feature delicate, long, elastic fibrils that blend with the underlying elastic fibrillary system of the skin

Certain antigenic components have been identified in the BMZ, some of which play identified roles in cutaneous disease. **Laminin** is a glycoprotein present in the lamina lucida and lamina densa of all BMZs. It assists in the organization of BMZ macromolecules and promotes cell attachment to extracellular matrix. Laminin binds to **type IV collagen**. Bullous pemphigoid (BP) antigens were identified with antibodies from patients with the blistering disorder bullous pemphigoid (discussed below). The antigens BPAG1 and BPAG2 (**type XVII collagen**) are normal constituents of the dermal–epidermal junction, but are absent in BMZs around adnexal structures and blood vessels. These BP antigens are located in the hemidesmosomes and cytoplasm of the basal keratinocytes. Type IV collagen is present in the lamina densa of all BMZs. It is the most superficial component of the complex collagen fiber network of the dermis and is important in dermal–epidermal attachment. **Type VII collagen** is present on the deep aspect of the basal lamina in anchoring fibrils. Anchoring fibril antigens (AF-1 and AF-2) reside within anchoring fibrils and possibly within the lower lamina densa.

The **dermis** is a complex organization of connective tissue deep to the BMZ and is composed predominantly of collagen, which is embedded in a ground substance rich in hyaluronic acid. The dermis consists of two zones:

PAPILLARY DERMIS: The papillary dermis is a narrow zone immediately deep to the BMZ of the epidermis. This region is pale pink with the hematoxylin and eosin stain and has little organization when viewed with the light microscope (see Figs. 24-1 and 24-2). Delicate collagen fibrils are the most apparent structures. This delicate connective tissue extends as a sheath about blood vessels, nerves, and adnexal structures. This entire network of collagen is known as the **adventitial dermis**.

The papillary dermis is generally altered in conjunction with epidermal disease and disorders affecting the superficial vascular bed. The epidermis, papillary dermis, and superficial vascular bed react jointly and influence each other in complex ways. Some primary skin diseases with few, if any, systemic manifestations, such as psoriasis and lichen planus, involve these superficial structures.

RETICULAR DERMIS: The reticular dermis is deep to the papillary dermis and contains most of the dermal collagen, which is organized into coarse bundles and associated with elastic fibers (see Fig. 24-1). The reticular dermis and subcutis (also recognized as a cutaneous structure) are less common sites of pathologic change and, when diseased, are often manifestations of systemic disease. Scleroderma (progressive systemic sclerosis) and erythema nodosum are examples.

CUTANEOUS VASCULATURE: Cutaneous circulating blood has a number of functions. The skin, via its vascular network, is important in temperature regulation. Also, many aspects of cutaneous inflammation involve the superficial cutaneous vasculature.

An ascending arteriole arises from arteries in the subcutis and directly crosses much of the reticular dermis (see Fig. 24-1). In the outer part of the reticular dermis, in conjunction with other similar ascending arteries, a superficial arteriolar plexus is formed. From this plexus a terminal arteriole extends into each dermal papilla, where an arterial capillary is formed. The arterial capillary makes a U-turn and on its descent becomes a venous capillary and a postcapillary venule. The venules then join to form a complex venular plexus in the reticular dermis, immediately deep to the papillary dermis. The venular end of this vascular structure is important in cutaneous inflammatory responses.

Cutaneous lymphatic vessels form a random network, beginning as lymphatic capillaries near the epidermis. A superficial lymphatic plexus is then formed, from which lymphatic channels drain to regional lymph nodes. Lymphatic channels are involved in drainage of tissue fluids and metastasis of cutaneous cancers, especially malignant melanoma. Cutaneous lymphatics have, at best, an incomplete basal lamina.

Mast cells are derived from the bone marrow and are normally present around dermal venules. Mast cells release of vasoactive and chemotactic substances, mediate all types of inflammation and proliferate in a spectrum of diseases **termed urticaria pigmentosa** (Fig. 24-8).

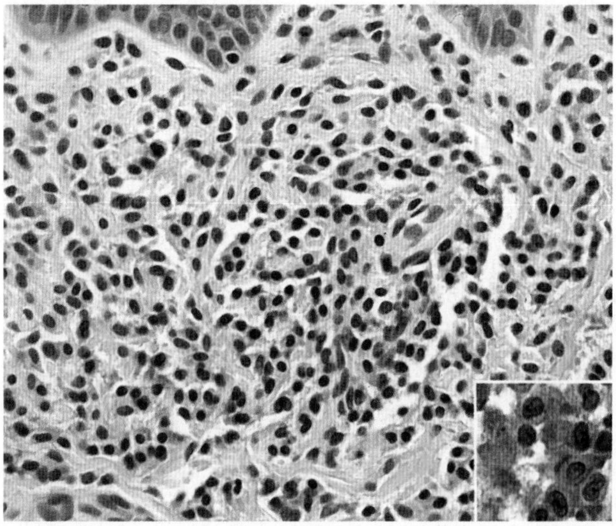

FIGURE 24-8. **Urticaria pigmentosa.** Mast cells fill and expand the papillary dermis. The cytoplasm of mast cells contains chloracetate esterase-rich granules, giving them a red hue in this Leder stain (*inset*), a useful distinguishing feature.

HAIR FOLLICLES: Hair follicles originate in the primitive epidermis and grow downward through the dermis as well as upward through the epidermis. Growing hairs of the scalp and beard have bulbs of epithelial and mesenchymal tissue firmly embedded within the subcutis. A vertical cross-section of a bulb reveals a cap of actively dividing, keratin-synthesizing cells that become arrayed in layers that join at the top of the bulb to form the cylindrical hair shaft. The differentiating hairs form the roof of the epithelial bulb and interact with an island of melanocytes that contribute melanin to the passing keratinocytes. This process results in hair color. The colored keratinocytes lose their nuclei as they form the final product, the cylindrical hair shaft. Curly hair is formed from angulated bulbs; straight hair develops from round bulbs.

THE HAIR CYCLE: Hair grows in a cyclical fashion. At any given time, 90% of hairs are normally in the **anagen**, or actively growing, phase. These have a mosaic distribution and are interspersed with hairs that show no evidence of active growth, **telogen** hairs. Hairs in the process of ceasing growth, **catagen** hairs, still have hair shafts. Catagen hairs end in the lower reticular dermis as slightly widened clublike structures, each surrounded by a rim of nucleated keratinocytes. The hair bulbs are no longer evident, and the lamina densa surrounding the catagen hair is strikingly thickened.

As the telogen phase (resting follicle) is reached, the end of the hair retreats to the level of the arrector pili muscle. The hair shaft may be missing, since it is no longer tethered at the base, leaving only a remnant of the original follicle. However, a delicate vascularized mesenchymal tract, the telogen tract, extends from the attenuated tip. At the top of this tract, the early anagen hair forms again from the follicular stem cells. With growth, it follows the delicate pathway through the reticular dermis into the panniculus, there forming a mature anagen follicle and a new hair.

ALOPECIA: Alopecia, commonly known as baldness, refers to the loss of hair. **Common alopecia**, which affects both men and women, results from a complex and poorly understood interaction of heritable and hormonal factors. Men castrated before puberty retain scalp hair and fail to grow a beard. On the other hand, the administration of testosterone to such castrated men results in growth of a beard and may lead to male-pattern baldness. Loss of scalp hair results in replacement of a large terminal hair follicle by a diminutive "vellus" hair follicle, the source of the delicate "fuzz" on the cheeks of women and the upper cheeks of men.

Growing hair is the site of active mitosis, and many systemic diseases cause cessation of mitosis in this location and subsequent alopecia. If the malady passes, mitotic activity is renewed and regrowth occurs. If a patient is subjected to a potent antimitotic regimen, such as chemotherapy for advanced cancer, hair follicles stop growth, hair is lost, and a telogen follicle follows. When therapy stops, hair cycling resumes. Almost any kind of follicular inflammation can induce the telogen phase. If fibrosis distorts the telogen tract (the regrowth pathway), permanent loss of that follicle and alopecia result.

Alopecia areata is a circumscribed area of hair loss, usually on the scalp, although other body areas may be involved. A brisk lymphocytic infiltrate is found around the hair bulb and results in formation of telogen hairs and hair loss. Alopecia areata may actually result from several diseases. This histologic pattern and the association of this phenomenon with the inheritance of HLA class II alleles (especially HLA-DQ3) has been interpreted as evidence for an autoimmune etiology. Generally, scarring does not occur, and hair may regrow normally after varying time periods.

VELLUS HAIRS: These fine hairs may play a role in touch perception in many mammals, but in humans they have no function. Microscopically, vellus hairs are diminutive anagen hairs, with a small active bulb high in the reticular dermis, together with small sebaceous glands.

SEBACEOUS FOLLICLES: These structures develop with puberty and are clinically important because they are the sites of acne. Sebaceous follicles have a minute vellus hair at the base. The central face has large sebaceous glands that dwarf the vellus hairs and fill the follicular canal with sebum.

Diseases of the Epidermis

Ichthyoses Feature Epidermal Thickening and Scales

Ichthyosiform dermatoses, many of which are heritable, are a heterogeneous group of diseases characterized by striking thickening of the stratum corneum. The term **ichthyosis** reflects the similarity of the diseased skin to coarse, fish-like scales (Fig. 24-9). Several rare ichthyoses are associated with other abnormalities such as abnormal lipid metabolism, neurologic disorders, bone diseases, and cancer.

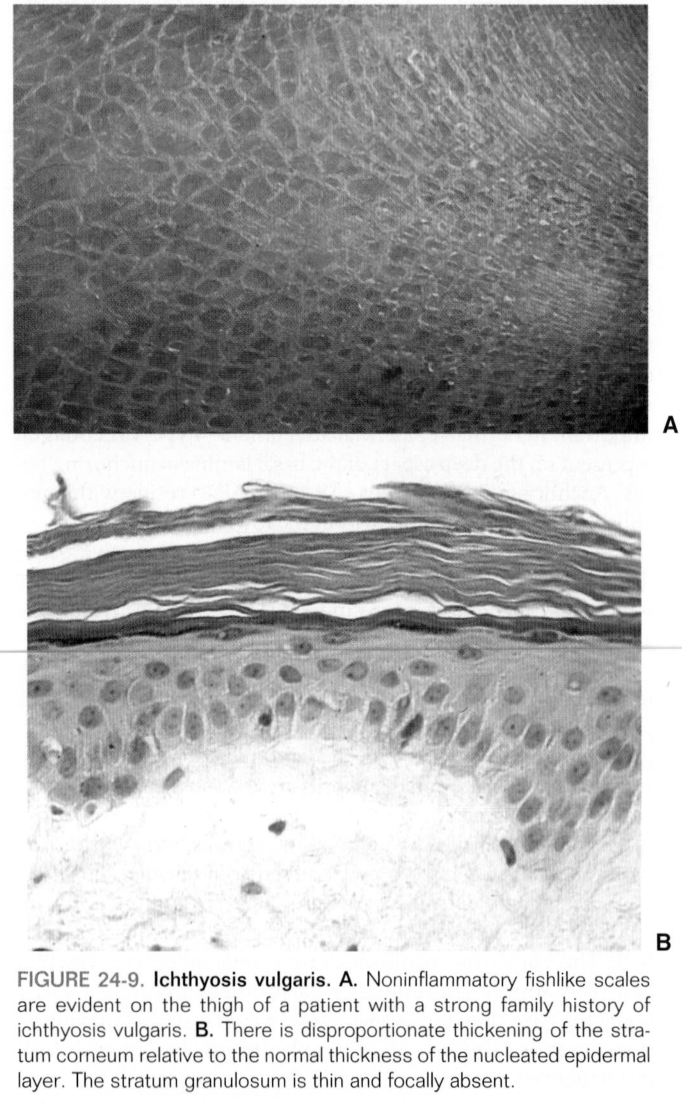

FIGURE 24-9. **Ichthyosis vulgaris. A.** Noninflammatory fishlike scales are evident on the thigh of a patient with a strong family history of ichthyosis vulgaris. **B.** There is disproportionate thickening of the stratum corneum relative to the normal thickness of the nucleated epidermal layer. The stratum granulosum is thin and focally absent.

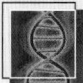

PATHOGENESIS: Three general defects are involved in the excessive epidermal cornification of the ichthyoses:

- **Increased cohesiveness** of the cells of the stratum corneum, possibly related to altered lipid metabolism
- **Abnormal keratinization,** manifested as impaired tonofilament formation and keratohyaline synthesis and as excessive cornification
- **Increased basal cell proliferation,** associated with a decrease in transit time of keratinocytes across the epidermis

PATHOLOGY: All ichthyoses (with the possible exception of lamellar ichthyosis) have a stratum corneum that is disproportionately thick in comparison with the nucleated epidermal layers. Virtually all diseases characterized by thickening of the nucleated epidermal layers also exhibit hyperkeratosis. For example, chronic scratching or rubbing of normal skin causes a thickened epidermis, hyperkeratosis, and dermal fibrosis, a condition known as lichen simplex chronicus. In this entity, the nucleated epidermis and stratum corneum may each be three times normal thickness. By contrast, in ichthyosis, the stratum corneum may be five times thicker than normal, but it overlies a disproportionately thin nucleated epidermis.

Ichthyosis Vulgaris

Ichthyosis vulgaris is an autosomal dominant disorder of keratinization characterized by hyperkeratosis and reduced or absent epidermal keratohyaline granules. Scaly skin results from increased cohesiveness of the stratum corneum. The attenuated stratum granulosum is a single layer with small, defective keratohyaline granules. *Decreased or absent synthesis of* ***profilaggrin,*** *a keratin filament "glue," is responsible for these defects.*

Ichthyosis vulgaris is the prototype of disproportionate corneal thickening. The stratum corneum is loose and has a basket-weave appearance, which differs from normal only in amount. The granular layer is greatly diminished and often appears absent (see Fig. 24-9B). Ultrastructurally, the keratohyaline granules are small and spongelike, a feature indicating defective synthesis. The basal and spinous layers appear normal. Thus, the primary defect in ichthyosis vulgaris is in the granular and cornified layers, the epidermal zones responsible for the final stage of keratinization and cornification.

CLINICAL FEATURES: Ichthyosis vulgaris is the most common of the ichthyoses and begins in early childhood. A family history of this condition is often obtained. Small white scales occur on the extensor surfaces of extremities and on the trunk and face. The disease is lifelong, but most patients can be maintained free of scales with topical treatment.

A clinical and histologic state similar to ichthyosis vulgaris is occasionally associated with other diseases or may follow the use of drugs. Lymphomas, especially Hodgkin disease; other neoplasms; systemic granulomatous disorders; and connective tissue disease may be associated with ichthyosis. Drugs may produce ichthyosis by interfering with similar pathways of lipid metabolism.

X-linked ichthyosis

This condition is a heritable epidermal disorder which in the recessive form is characterized by delayed dissolution of desmosomal disks in the stratum corneum, owing to a deficiency of steroid sulfatase. Steroid sulfatase normally degrades the Odland body product, cholesterol sulfate, which provides cellular adhesion in the lower stratum corneum. Failure of steroid sulfatase action on cholesterol sulfate leads to persistent cohesion of the stratum corneum, but in this disease the granular layer is preserved.

Epidermolytic hyperkeratosis

This congenital, autosomal dominant ichthyosis features generalized erythroderma, ichthyosiform skin and blistering. The disease results from mutations in the *K1* and *K10* keratin genes (chromosomes 12 and 17, respectively), which encode the keratins in the suprabasal epidermis. These mutations cause faulty assembly of keratin tonofilaments and impair their insertion into desmosomes. These flaws prevent normal development of the cytoskeleton, resulting in epidermal "lysis" and a tendency to form vesicles.

In epidermolytic hyperkeratosis, suprabasal keratinocytes contain thick, eosinophilic tonofilaments that whorl around the nucleus in a concentric fashion (Fig. 24-10). The cytoplasm has a clear zone (vacuolization) peripheral to the perinuclear tonofilaments, but at the periphery of the cell these filaments again become condensed. Enlarged keratohyaline granules are present. The stratum corneum is disproportionately thickened (Fig. 24-11).

CLINICAL FEATURES: Epidermolytic hyperkeratosis manifests with blistering at or shortly after birth. It may be generalized or localized to only several areas of the body. Lesions tend to appear dark and even verrucous. Other than cosmetic disfigurement, the major problem is secondary bacterial infection.

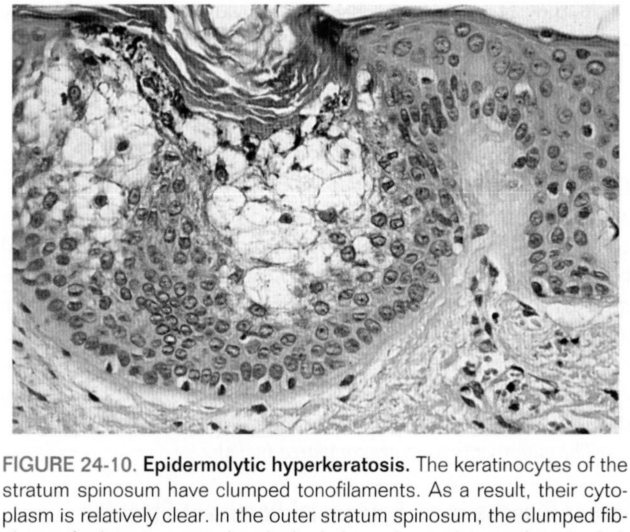

FIGURE 24-10. **Epidermolytic hyperkeratosis.** The keratinocytes of the stratum spinosum have clumped tonofilaments. As a result, their cytoplasm is relatively clear. In the outer stratum spinosum, the clumped fibrils are further compacted and whorl about the nuclei, resulting in dark cytoplasm condensed about the nuclei. These cells separate from each other to produce epidermolysis. A normal portion of epidermis is seen on the *right.*

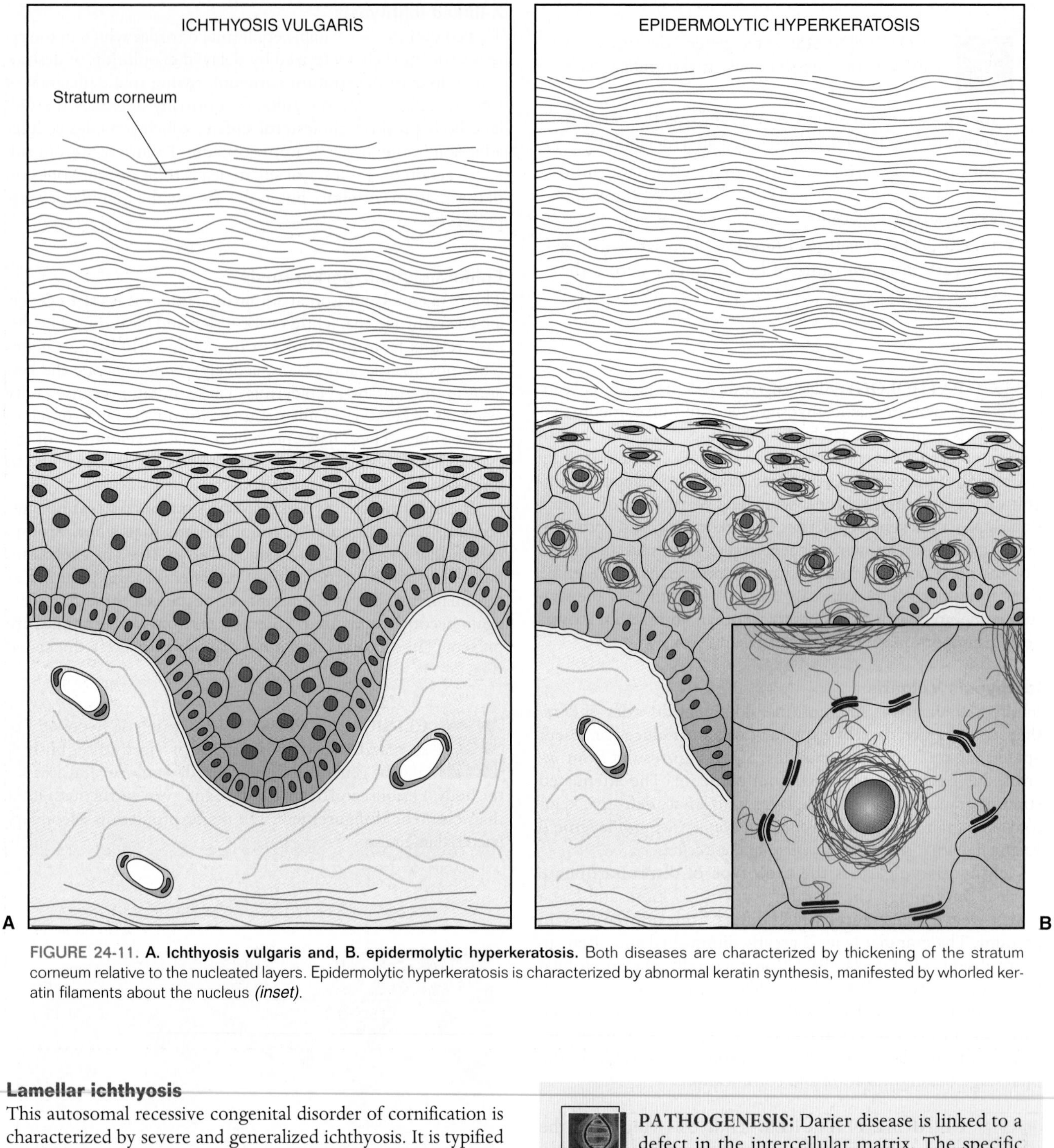

FIGURE 24-11. **A. Ichthyosis vulgaris and, B. epidermolytic hyperkeratosis.** Both diseases are characterized by thickening of the stratum corneum relative to the nucleated layers. Epidermolytic hyperkeratosis is characterized by abnormal keratin synthesis, manifested by whorled keratin filaments about the nucleus *(inset)*.

Lamellar ichthyosis

This autosomal recessive congenital disorder of cornification is characterized by severe and generalized ichthyosis. It is typified by increased cohesiveness of the stratum corneum, accompanied by numerous keratinosomes and an abnormally large amount of intercellular substance. The disease is genetically heterogeneous, but are often caused by mutations in the gene encoding transglutaminase 1 (*TGM1;* chromosome 14q11), lead to defective lamellar body secretion.

The major ichthyoses are compared in Table 24-1.

Darier Disease Is an Autosomal Dominant Disorder of Keratinization

Darier disease, also called **keratosis follicularis**, is characterized by multifocal keratoses.

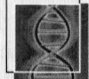

PATHOGENESIS: Darier disease is linked to a defect in the intercellular matrix. The specific gene, *ATP2A2* on chromosome 12q23-24, encodes a calcium pump of the endoplasmic reticulum, and its mutation may exert a direct effect on calcium-dependent assembly of desmosomes. The many neuropsychiatric problems among these patients may also be related to *ATP2A2* mutations.

PATHOLOGY: Microscopically, the warty papule of Darier disease has a suprabasal cleft. Above and to the side of the cleft, dyskeratotic keratinocytes with eosinophilic cytoplasm contain keratin fibrils that whorl about

TABLE 24–1

A Comparison of the Major Ichthyoses

Type of Ichthyosis	Mode of Inheritance	Present at Birth	Pathogenetic Mechanism	Histology
Ichthyosis vulgaris	Autosomal dominant	No; onset in childhood	Normal epidermal turnover Retention keratosis due to defective dissolution of adhesive mechanisms in the stratum corneum	Hyperkeratosis, loosely woven, disproportionately thick in relationship to a relatively thin stratum spinosum Thin granular layer with abnormal keratohyaline granules
Sex-linked ichthyosis	X-linked recessive	Yes; onset may be in infancy	Normal epidermal turnover Constitutional absence of steroid sulfatase and arylsulfatase-C Retention keratosis due to a failure to break down cholesterol sulfate, an important substance in stratum corneum adhesion	Compact, disproportionately thick stratum corneum. Normal granular layer. Stratum spinosum only slightly thick
Epidermolytic hyperkeratosis	Autosomal dominant	Yes	Increased germinative cell replication and decreased cellular transit time through the epidermis Defect in keratin genes *K1* and *K10*, the differentiation-specific keratins of the suprabasal epidermis	Tonofilaments aggregate at the cell periphery and have a distorted association with desmosomes, which may lead to dyshesion (acantholysis) of epidermal keratinocytes and vesicle formation; entire skin is rarely involved
Lamellar ichthyosis	Autosomal recessive	Yes	Increased number of keratinosomes and increased intercellular substance; defects in transglutaminase acylation and in lamellar body secretion	Moderate hyperkeratosis; normal or thickened granular layer

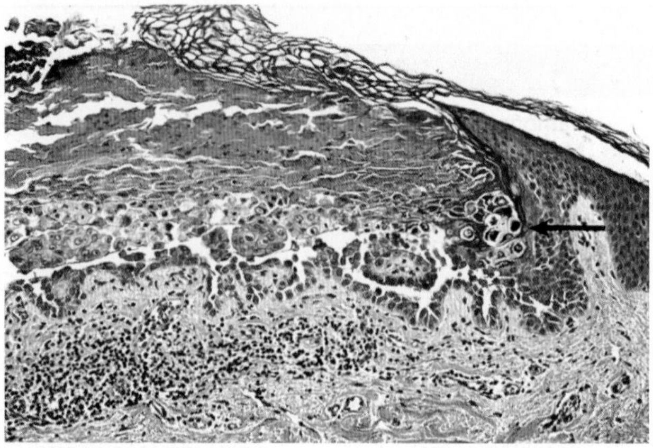

FIGURE 24-12. **Darier disease.** Virtually the entire epidermis exhibits focal acantholytic dyskeratosis. A small portion of normal epidermis is present *(right)*. In the lesion, there is a suprabasal cleft with a few dyshesive (acantholytic) keratinocytes surmounted by hyperkeratosis and parakeratosis. The cleft is not a vesicle because true vesicles contain inflammatory cells and tissue fluid. Dyskeratosis is present above the cleft.

the nucleus (Fig. 24-12). The roof of the cleft is formed by a column of compact keratotic material.

CLINICAL FEATURES: Darier disease first appears late in childhood or in adolescence as skin-colored papules that later become crusted. Affected areas have many warty elevations, 2 to 4 mm in diameter, largely on the chest, nasolabial folds, back, scalp, forehead, ears, and groin.

Psoriasis Is a Proliferative Skin Disease Characterized by Persistent Epidermal Hyperplasia

Psoriasis is a chronic, frequently familial disorder that features large, erythematous, scaly plaques, commonly on extensor cutaneous surfaces. It affects 1% to 2% of the population worldwide. It may arise at any age but shows a peak in late adolescence. Interestingly, psoriasis is not seen among Native Americans and is infrequent among Asians.

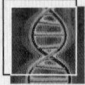

PATHOGENESIS: The pathogenesis of psoriasis is poorly understood and is likely multifactorial.

GENETIC FACTORS: Psoriasis unquestionably has a genetic component, although only one third of patients with psoriasis have a family history of the disease. The more severe the illness, the greater the likelihood of a familial background. The genetic basis for psoriasis rests on a number of observations: (1) increased incidence among relatives and offspring of patients with psoriasis; (2) 65% concordance for psoriasis in monozygotic twins; and (3) increases in certain HLA haplotypes in affected persons, especially HLA-B13, HLA-B17, HLA-Bw57, and particularly HLA-Cw6. In fact, persons with HLA-Cw6 are 10 to 15 times more likely to develop psoriasis than the general population.

ENVIRONMENTAL FACTORS: Clinical lesions may occur anywhere on the skin. In this context, a variety of stimuli, such as physical injury ("Köbner's phenomenon"), infection, certain drugs, and photosensitivity, may produce psoriatic lesions in apparently normal skin. The pathogenesis of the psoriatic plaques may be appreciated by contrasting the effect of chronic cutaneous trauma in persons with and without psoriasis. Chronic irritation of a normal person's skin—e.g., as in repeated rubbing—produces a tough, scaly, cutaneous plaque that is both clinically and histologically psoriasiform. However, the lesion disappears with cessation of the trauma. In the psoriatic patient, even less trauma produces a psoriatic plaque that may persist for years after the initial injury.

ABNORMAL CELLULAR PROLIFERATION: There is evidence to suggest that deregulation of epidermal proliferation and an abnormality in dermal microcirculation produce psoriatic lesions (Fig. 24-13). Abnormal proliferation of keratinocytes is possibly related to defective epidermal cell surface receptors. Decreased adenylyl cyclase activity in the lower proliferative compartment of the epidermis has been attributed to faulty β-adrenergic receptors. The decrease in cyclic adenosine monophosphate (cAMP) alters cutaneous responses to trauma in complex ways that are not fully understood.

Increased cAMP-regulated proteinases and augmented polyamines of low molecular weight are postulated to be associated with a growth factor-like effect. Acute inflammation follows an increase in phospholipase A_2, which enhances production of arachidonic acid. In turn, the lipo-oxygenase metabolites of arachidonic acid, notably leukotriene B_4, exert potent neutrophilic chemotactic effects.

MICROCIRCULATORY CHANGES: In psoriatic skin, the capillary loops of the dermal papillae become venular, showing multiple layers of basal lamina material, wide lumina, and "bridged" fenestrations between endothelial cells. The vascular change, which occurs in concert with a striking increase in neutrophilic chemotactic factors, leads to diapedesis of many neutrophils at the tips of dermal papillae and subsequent migration into the epidermis (the "squirting papillae") (see Fig. 24-13). This unusual pattern of neutrophilic inflammation is responsible for the dense collections of neutrophils in the stratum corneum (**Munro microabscesses**) as well as for the scattering of neutrophils throughout the epidermis (**spongiform pustules**).

IMMUNOLOGIC FACTORS: T lymphocytes may be key to the pathogenesis of psoriatic lesions. Eruption of psoriatic lesions coincides with T cell infiltration into the epidermis. By contrast, resolution of psoriatic plaques, whether spontaneous or induced by treatment, follows disappearance, or reduction in, epidermal T cells. Streptococcal superantigens reportedly induce expression of cutaneous lymphocyte antigens, which enable T cells to migrate to the skin. Finally, T lymphocytes from psoriatic patients can produce psoriasis-like plaques when transferred to nude mice.

In summary, keratinocytes of persons afflicted with psoriasis possess a genetic predisposition to hyperproliferation and altered differentiation (see Fig. 24-13). Environmental stimuli may trigger release of cytokines and growth factors by keratinocytes and other epidermal cells, and ensuing immune and inflammatory responses lead to the full development of psoriatic lesions.

PATHOLOGY: The most distinctive pathologic changes are seen at the periphery of a chronic psoriatic plaque. The epidermis is thickened and shows **hyperkeratosis** and **parakeratosis** (persistence of nuclei in the cells of the stratum corneum). Parakeratosis may be circumscribed, ellip-

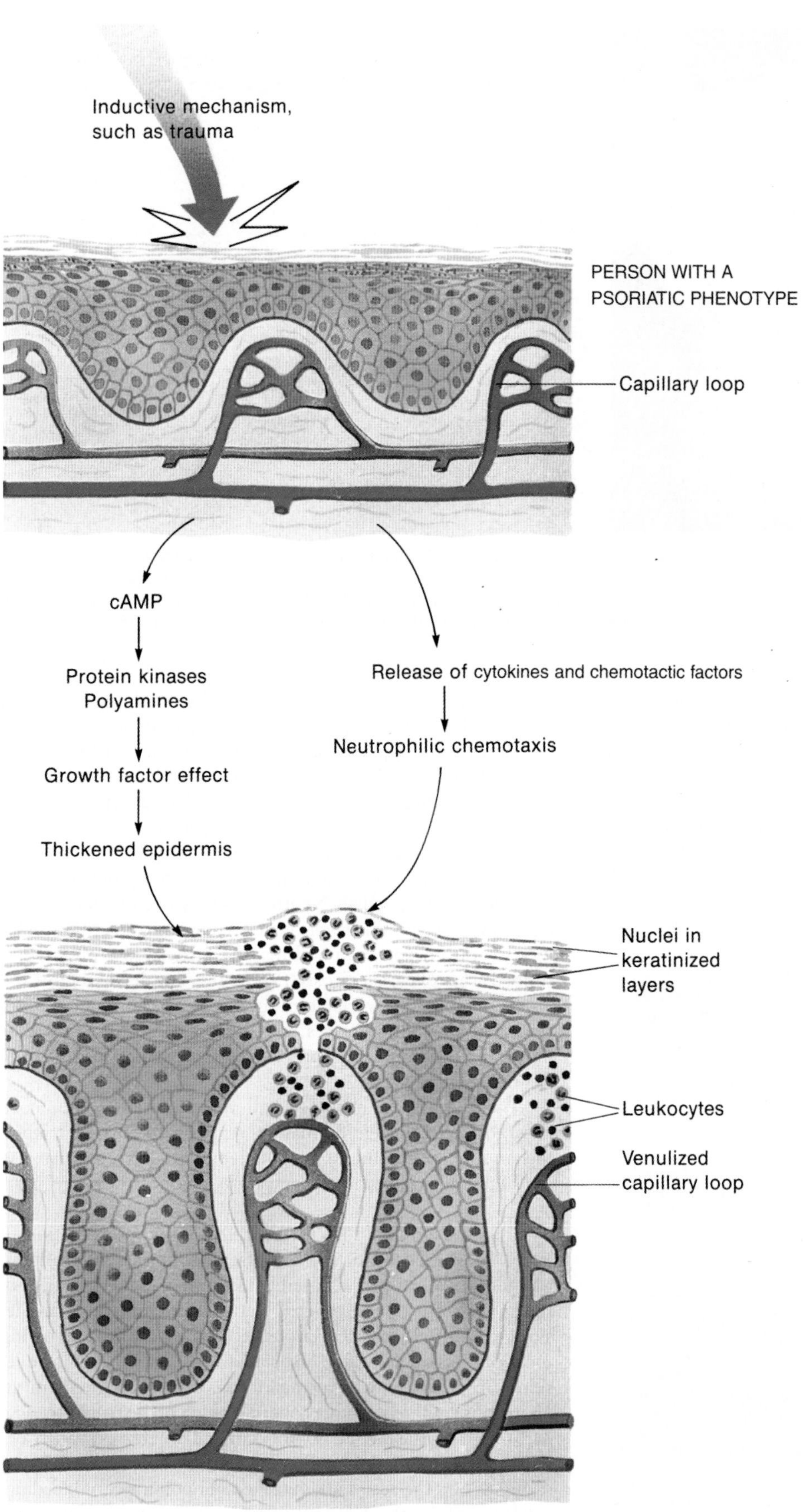

FIGURE 24-13. **Pathogenetic mechanisms in psoriasis.** The drawing depicts the deregulation of epidermal growth, venulization of the capillary loop, and a unique form of neutrophilic inflammation. The altered epidermal growth is thought to be caused by defective epidermal cell surface receptors. This results in a decrease in cyclic adenosine monophosphate (cAMP), together with the effects indicated. The decrease in cAMP is also likely to be related to the increased production of arachidonic acid, which in turn leads to activation of leukotriene B_4 (LTB-4). This potent neutrophilic chemotactic agent acts on a venulized capillary loop. Neutrophils then emerge from the tips of the capillary loop at the apex of the dermal papilla rather than from the postcapillary venule, as is the rule in most inflammatory skin diseases.

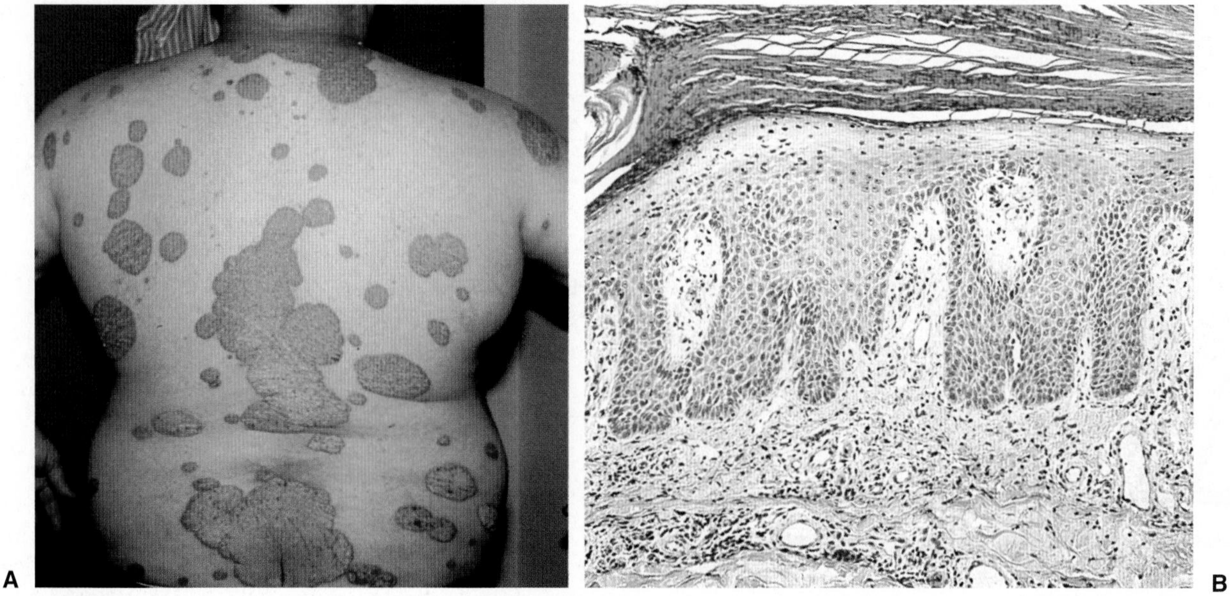

FIGURE 24-14. **Psoriasis.** This disorder is the prototype of psoriasiform epidermal hyperplasia. **A.** A patient with psoriasis shows large, confluent, sharply demarcated, erythematous plaques on the trunk. **B.** Microscopic examination of a lesion demonstrates that the rete ridges are uniformly elongated, as are the dermal papillae, giving an interlocking pattern of alternately reversed "clubs." The dermal papillae are edematous and reside beneath a thinned epidermis (suprapapillary thinning). There is striking parakeratosis, which is the scale observed clinically.

soidal foci, or it may be diffuse, in which case the granular layer is diminished or absent. The nucleated layers of the epidermis are thickened several-fold in the rete pegs and are frequently thinner over the dermal papillae (Fig. 24-14). In turn, the papillae are elongated and appear as sections of cones, with their apices toward the dermis. In chronic lesions, dermal papillae tend to appear as bulbous clubs with short handles (see Fig. 24-14 and Fig. 24-15). The rete ridges of the epidermis have a profile reciprocal to that of the dermal papillae, resulting in interlocked dermal and epidermal clubs, with alternatively reversed polarity (see Fig. 24-15). The capillaries of the papillae are dilated and tortuous. In a very early lesion, changes may be limited to capillary dilation with a few neutrophils "squirting" into the epidermis. Epidermal hyperplasia and hyperkeratosis are hallmarks of chronic lesions.

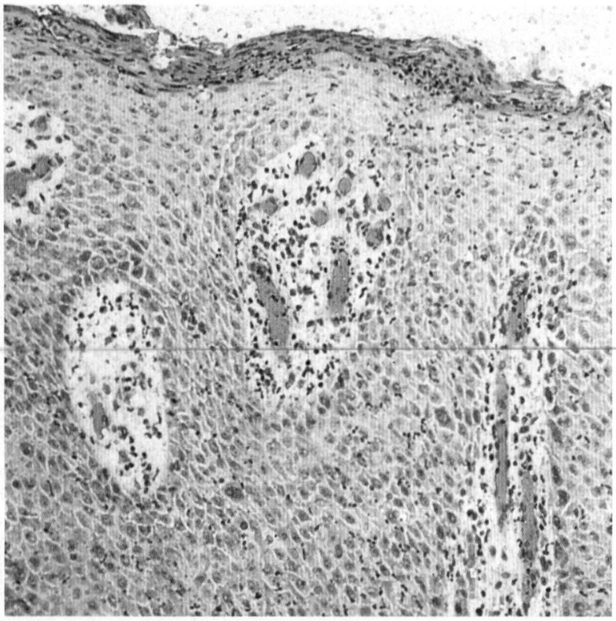

FIGURE 24-15. **Psoriasis.** The clubbed papillae contain tortuous dilated venules. The prominent venules are part of the venulization of capillaries, which may be of histogenetic importance in psoriasis. The papilla to the *right* has one cross-section of its superficial capillary venule loop, which is normal. The papilla in the *center* shows numerous cross-sections of its venule, indicating striking tortuosity.

Ultrastructurally, the capillaries are venulelike; neutrophils may emerge at their tips and migrate into the epidermis above the apices of the papillae. Neutrophils may become localized in the epidermal spinous layer or in small Munro microabscesses in the stratum corneum and may be associated with circumscribed areas of parakeratosis (Fig. 24-16). The dermis below the papillae contains a variable mononuclear inflammatory infiltrate, mostly lymphocytes, around the superficial vascular plexus. The inflammatory process does not extend into the subjacent reticular dermis.

The psoriasiform histologic pattern is common in cutaneous pathology. Seborrheic dermatitis, reaction to chronic trauma (lichen simplex chronicus) and cutaneous T-cell lymphoma (mycosis fungoides) all exhibit psoriasiform epidermal change.

CLINICAL FEATURES: The initial presentation of psoriasis is variable and disease activity is intermittent. Familial psoriasis tends to be more severe than sporadic types, but disease severity varies from annoying scaly lesions over the elbows to a serious debilitating disorder involving most of the skin and often associated with arthritis. A single lesion of psoriasis may be a small focus of scaly erythema or an enormous confluent plaque covering much of the trunk (see Fig. 24-14A). A typical plaque is 4 to 5 cm in diameter, is sharply demarcated at its margin, and is covered by a surface of silvery scales. When the scales are detached, pinpoint foci of bleeding, originating from the dilated capillaries in the dermal papillae, dot the underlying glossy erythematous surface ("Auspitz sign").

Of all patients with psoriasis, 7% develop **seronegative arthritis** (see Chapter 26). The tendency to arthropathy is linked

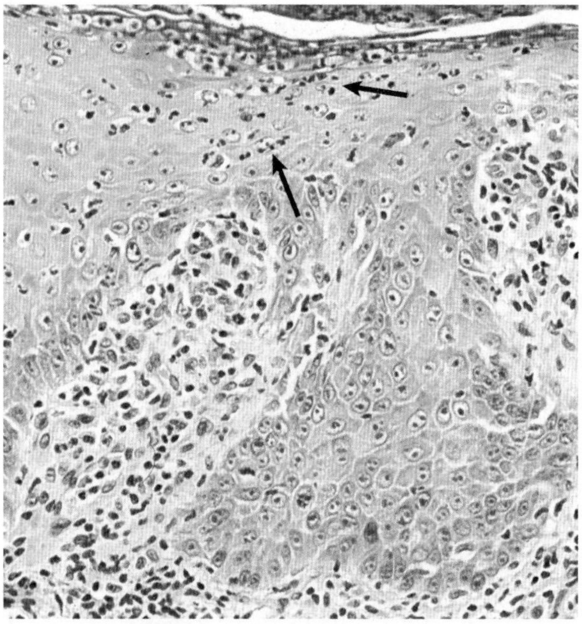

FIGURE 24-16. **Psoriasis.** Neutrophils migrate into the epidermis, emerging from the venulized capillaries at the tips of the dermal papillae. They migrate to the upper stratum spinosum and stratum corneum *(arrows)*. In some forms of psoriasis, pustules are common clinical lesions.

to several HLA haplotypes, particularly HLA-B27. Psoriatic arthritis closely resembles its rheumatoid counterpart, but it is usually milder and causes little disability.

In some variations of the disease, neutrophilic pustules dominate (**pustular psoriasis**). Severe intractable psoriasis has been observed in some patients with acquired immunodeficiency syndrome (AIDS), but the cause is not known.

Psoriasis has long been treated with coal tar or wood tar derivatives and anthralin, a strong reducing agent. Topical and systemic corticosteroids have also been used. Severe, generalized psoriasis justifies systemic treatment with methotrexate. Phototherapy ("PUVA") after administration of psoralens, an ultraviolet-absorbing compounds that bind to DNA, is often effective. More recently, synthetic vitamin A and vitamin D derivatives have been used as well.

Pemphigus Vulgaris Is a Blistering Skin Disorder Caused by Antibodies to Keratinocytes

Dyshesive disorders are cutaneous maladies in which blister formation is secondary to diminished cohesiveness of the epidermal keratinocytes. Pemphigus vulgaris (PV) (Greek, *pemphix*, "bubble"), the prototype of dyshesive diseases, is a chronic, blistering skin disorder that is most common in people between 40 and 60 years of age, but is seen in all age groups, including children. All races are susceptible, but persons of Jewish or Mediterranean heritage are at greater risk.

PATHOGENESIS: PV is an autoimmune disease: circulating IgG antibodies in patients with PV react with an epidermal surface antigen called **desmoglein 3**, a desmosomal protein. Antigen–antibody union results in dyshesion, which is augmented by release of plasminogen activator and, hence, activation of plasmin. This proteolytic enzyme acts on intercellular substance and may be the dominant factor in dyshesion. Internalization of the pemphigus antigen–antibody complex, disappearance of attachment plaques, and retraction of perinuclear tonofilaments may all act in concert with proteinases to cause dyshesion and vesiculation (Fig. 24-17).

PATHOLOGY: The blister in PV forms because of the separation of the outer epidermal layers from the basal layer. This suprabasal dyshesion results in a blister that has an intact basal layer as a floor and the remaining epidermis as a roof (Fig. 24-18). Desmoglein 3 is concentrated in the lower epidermis, explaining the location of the blister. The blister contains moderate numbers of lymphocytes, macrophages, eosinophils, and neutrophils. Distinctive, rounded keratinocytes, termed acantholytic cells, are shed into the vesicle during dyshesion. The basal cells remain adherent to the basal lamina and form a layer of "tombstone cells." Dyshesion may extend along dermal adnexa and is not always strictly suprabasal. The subjacent dermis shows a moderate infiltrate of lymphocytes, macrophages, eosinophils, and neutrophils, predominantly around the capillary venular bed.

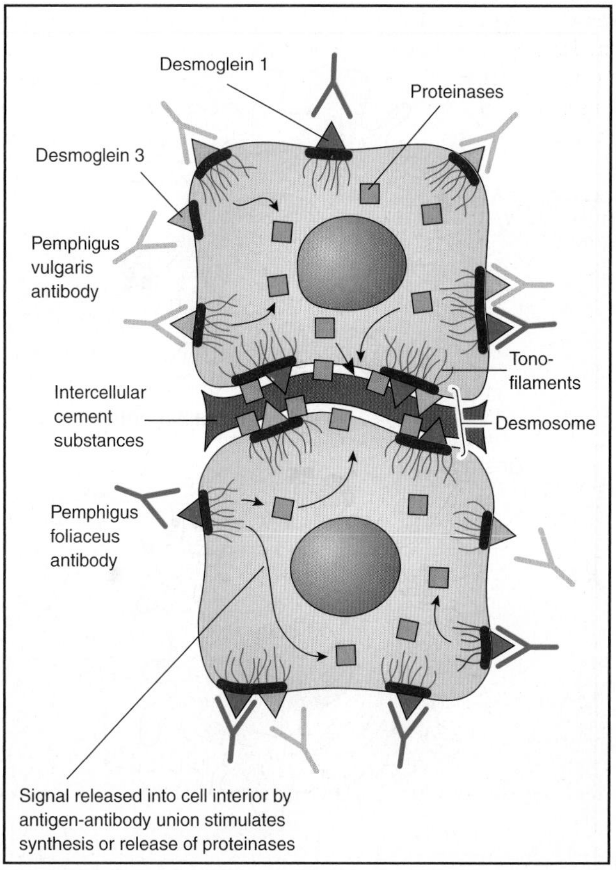

1

FIGURE 24-17. **Pemphigus vulgaris.** A pathogenetic mechanism of suprabasal dyshesion is shown. **(1)** A circulating autoantibody binds to an antigen on the outer leaflet of the plasma membrane (desmosome) of the keratinocyte, especially in the basal regions.

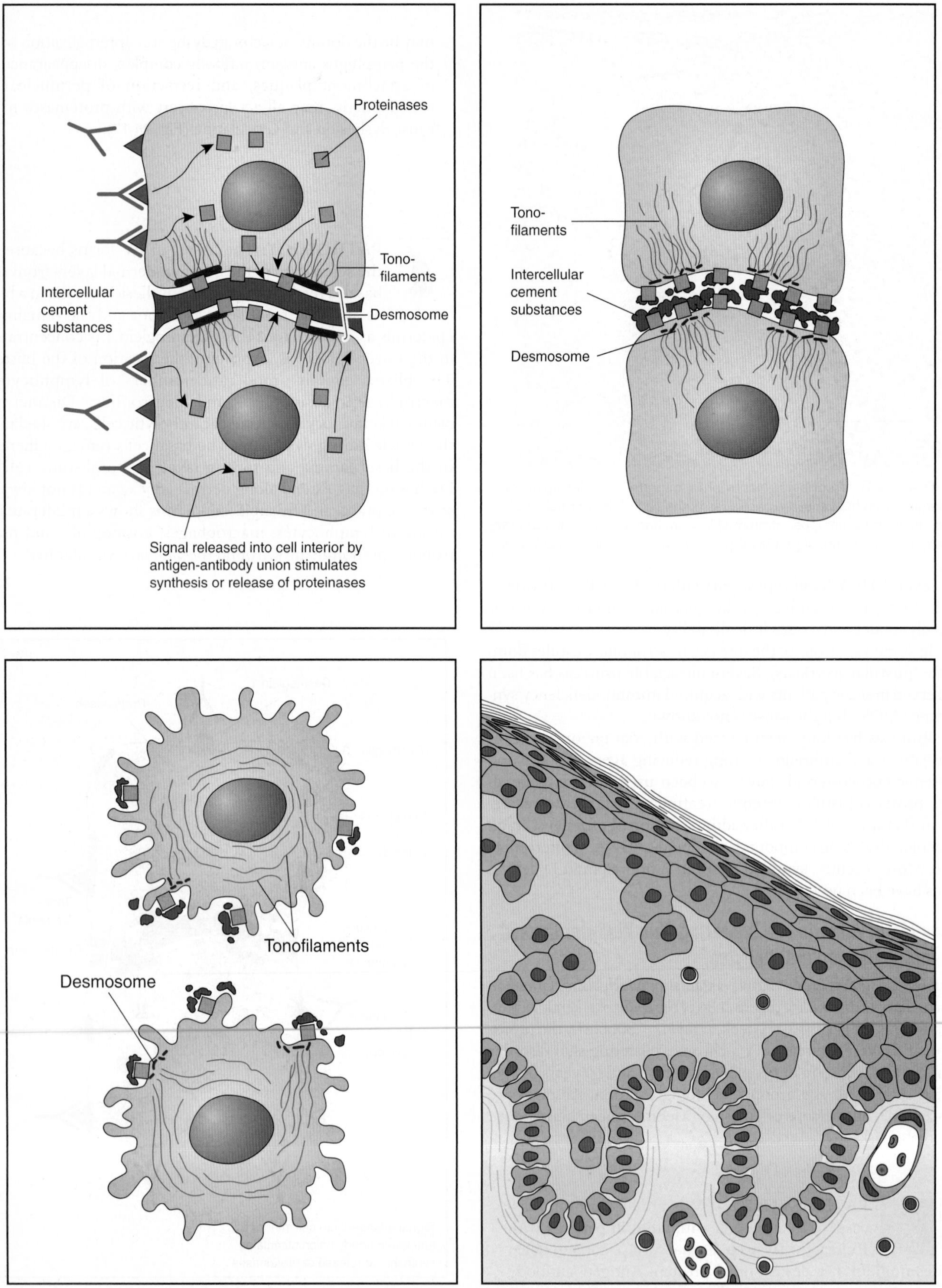

FIGURE 24-17. *(continued)* **(2)** Antigen–antibody union results in release of a proteinase (plasmin). **(3)** The proteinase interacts with intercellular cement, initiating dyshesion. **(4)** Desmosomes deteriorate, tonofilaments clump about the nucleus, the cells round up, and separation is complete. **(5)** A vesicle, which is usually suprabasal, forms. Alternatively, acantholysis may occur by direct interference with desmosomal and adherence junction attachments.

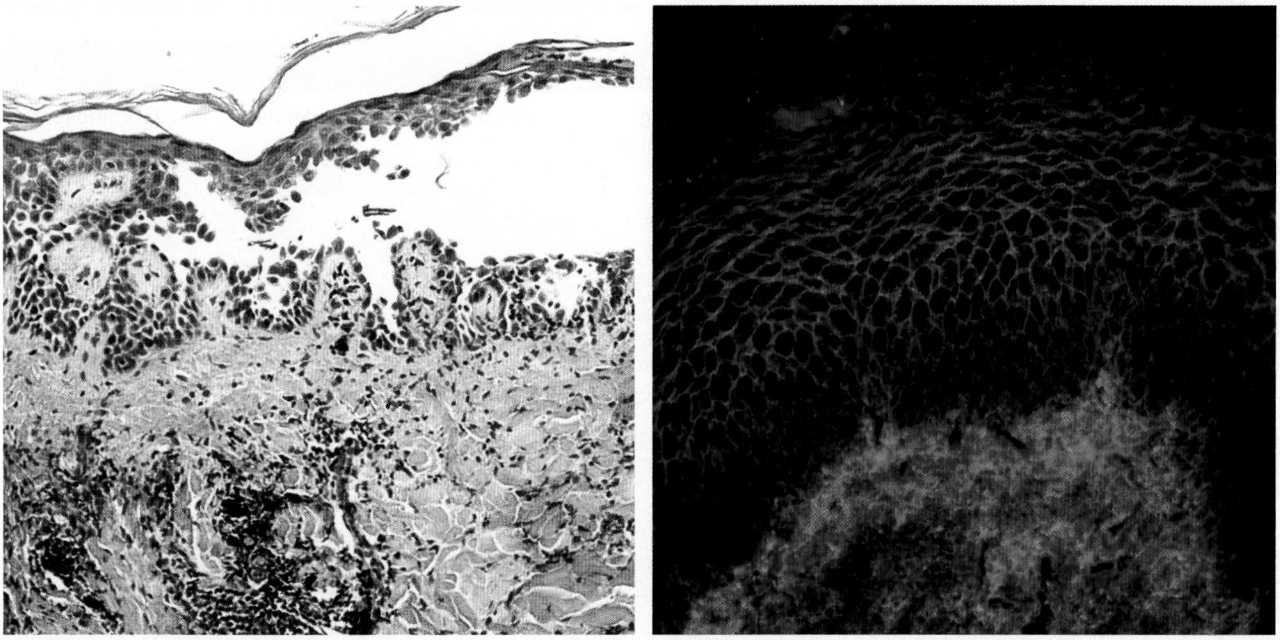

A B

FIGURE 24-18. **Pemphigus vulgaris. A.** Suprabasal dyshesion leads to an intraepidermal blister containing acantholytic keratinocytes. The basal keratinocytes are slightly separated from each other and totally separated from the stratum spinosum. The basal keratinocytes are firmly attached to the epidermal basement membrane zone. **B.** Direct immunofluorescence examination of perilesional skin reveals antibodies, usually of the immunoglobuin G (IgG) type, deposited in the intercellular substance of the epidermis, yielding a lacelike pattern outlining the keratinocytes.

CLINICAL FEATURES: The characteristic lesion of PV is a large, easily ruptured blister that leaves extensive denuded or crusted areas. Lesions are most common on the scalp and mucous membranes and in periumbilical and intertriginous areas. Without corticosteroid treatment, PV is progressive and usually fatal, and much of the skin surface may become denuded. Immunosuppressive agents are also useful for maintenance therapy. With appropriate treatment, the 10-year mortality rate for PV is less than 10%.

Other diseases caused by dyshesion that have a pathogenetic mechanism similar to PV include pemphigus foliaceus, pemphigus erythematosus, and drug-induced pemphigus (mostly associated with penicillamine and captopril). In pemphigus foliaceus antibodies to **desmoglein 1**, a desmosomal protein, cause dyshesion in the outer spinous and granular epidermal layers (in contrast with the suprabasal dyshesiveness in pemphigus vulgaris) (Fig. 24-19). Pemphigus foliaceus and pemphigus erythematosus feature dyshesion in the spinous layer. Paraneoplastic pemphigus has been described in association with cancers, usually lymphoproliferative tumors.

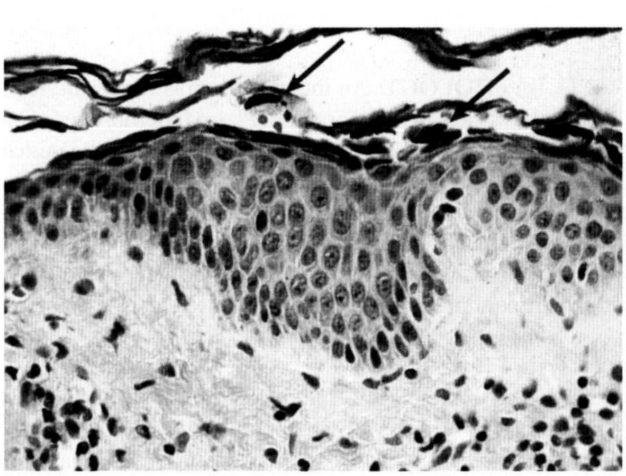

FIGURE 24-19. **Pemphigus foliaceus.** The dyshesion develops in the outer stratum spinosum and stratum granulosum. (Compare with that of pemphigus vulgaris; Fig. 24-18) Dyshesive and dyskeratotic keratinocytes of the stratum granulosum *(arrows)* are important hallmarks.

Pemphigus may be associated with other autoimmune diseases, such as myasthenia gravis and lupus erythematosus, and may also be seen with benign thymomas. Other diseases may mimic the histologic appearance of PV, namely, familial benign chronic pemphigus (Hailey-Hailey disease) and transient acantholytic dermatosis (Grover disease). However, IgG antibodies do not react with epidermal antigens in these entities.

Diseases of the Basement Membrane Zone (Dermal–Epidermal Interface)

Epidermolysis Bullosa Features Blister Formation in the Basement Membrane Zone

Epidermolysis bullosa (EB) comprises a heterogeneous group of disorders loosely bound by their hereditary nature and by a tendency to form blisters at the sites of minor trauma. The clinical spectrum ranges from a minor annoyance to a widespread, life-threatening blistering disease. *These blisters are almost always noted at birth or shortly thereafter.* The classification of these disorders is based on the site of blister formation in the BMZ (Table 24-2). The different mechanisms of blister formation underlie each of the three major categories of EB (Figure 24-20).

TABLE 24–2

Classification of Epidermolysis Bullosa (Selected Variants)

Class	Site of Blister Formation	Name of Variant	Healing Residuum	Heredity	Molecular Defect	Chromosomal Defect
Epidermolytic	Within the basal keratinocytic layer	Localized epidermolysis bullosa simplex	None	Autosomal dominant	Keratins 5 and 14	12q11–13 and 17q21
		Generalized epidermolysis bullosa simplex	None	Autosomal dominant		
Junctional	Lamina lucida	Epidermolysis bullosa letalis	None or atrophic skin	Autosomal recessive	Laminin 5	1q25–31, 1q3, and 18q11.2
					Integrins $\alpha6\beta4$	
		Generalized atrophic benign epidermolysis bullosa	Atrophic skin	Autosomal recessive	Collagen type XVII	1q32 and 10q23.4
Dermolytic	Immediately deep to the lamina densa	Dystrophic epidermolysis bullosa	Scars, nails deformed	Autosomal dominant	Collagen type VII	3p21
		Dystrophic epidermolysis bullosa	Scars, teeth, and nails deformed	Autosomal recessive		

Epidermolytic EB

This disorder, also known as **EB simplex**, is a group of autosomal dominant skin diseases in which blisters form as a result of disruption of basal keratinocytes. Epidermolytic EB has been attributed to mutations of genes encoding cytokeratin intermediate filaments, which likely provide mechanical stability to the epidermis. The blisters develop in response to minor trauma, such as merely rubbing the skin, but heal without scarring (thus, the term "simplex"). Although epidermolytic EB is cosmetically disturbing and sometimes debilitating, it is not life-threatening.

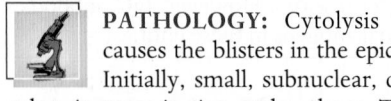

PATHOLOGY: Cytolysis of basal keratinocytes causes the blisters in the epidermolytic variety of EB. Initially, small, subnuclear, cytoplasmic vacuoles develop, increase in size, and coalesce. These vacuoles reflect abnormalities in keratins 5 and 14, which aggregate about the keratinocyte nuclei. The plasma membrane ruptures when the large vacuole reaches it, after which the cell is lysed. An intraepidermal vesicle results from lysis of several basal keratinocytes. The roof of the vesicle is an almost intact epidermis with a fragmented basal layer. The floor of the vesicle shows bits of basal cell cytoplasm attached to the lamina densa, which is seen as a well-preserved pink line at the base of the vesicle. Inflammatory cells are sparse.

Junctional EB

This type of EB is a heritable, autosomal recessive skin disease in which blisters form within the lamina lucida. The clinical expression ranges from a benign disease with no effect on life span, to a severe condition that may be fatal within the first 2 years of life.

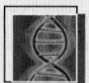

PATHOGENESIS: In the severe form, mutations in the genes for certain isoforms of laminin and the integrins have been reported. The benign form has been attributed to mutations in the gene for type XVII collagen. Both varieties heal without scarring, but there may be residual atrophy of the skin. There may also be associated abnormalities of nails and teeth.

PATHOLOGY: An intact epidermis forms the roof of the vesicle in junctional EB. Plasma membranes of basal keratinocytes are unchanged. The floor of the vesicle is an intact lamina densa, as in epidermolytic EB, but there are no attached fragments of basal cell cytoplasm. The blister, therefore, occurs within the lamina lucida. Both lesional and uninvolved skin shows fewer basal hemidesmosomes, which have poorly developed attachment plaques and subbasal dense plates.

Dermolytic EB

Also known as **dystrophic EB**, dermolytic EB is a heritable skin condition in which blisters are located immediately deep to the lamina densa. Dermolytic disease may be either dominant or recessive, the latter being more severe. In both variants, healed blisters are characterized by atrophic ("dystrophic") scarring. There may be associated abnormalities of nails and teeth.

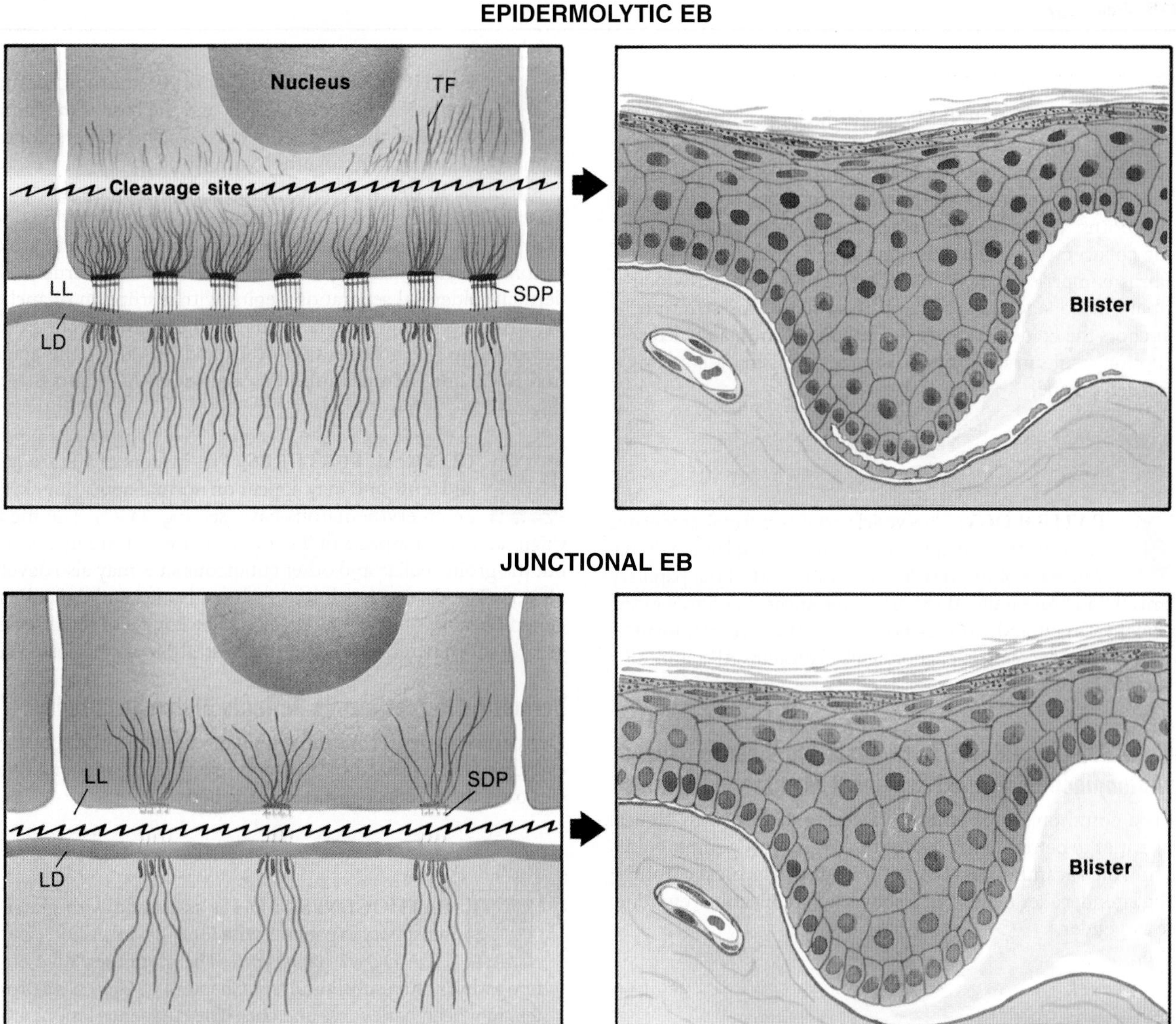

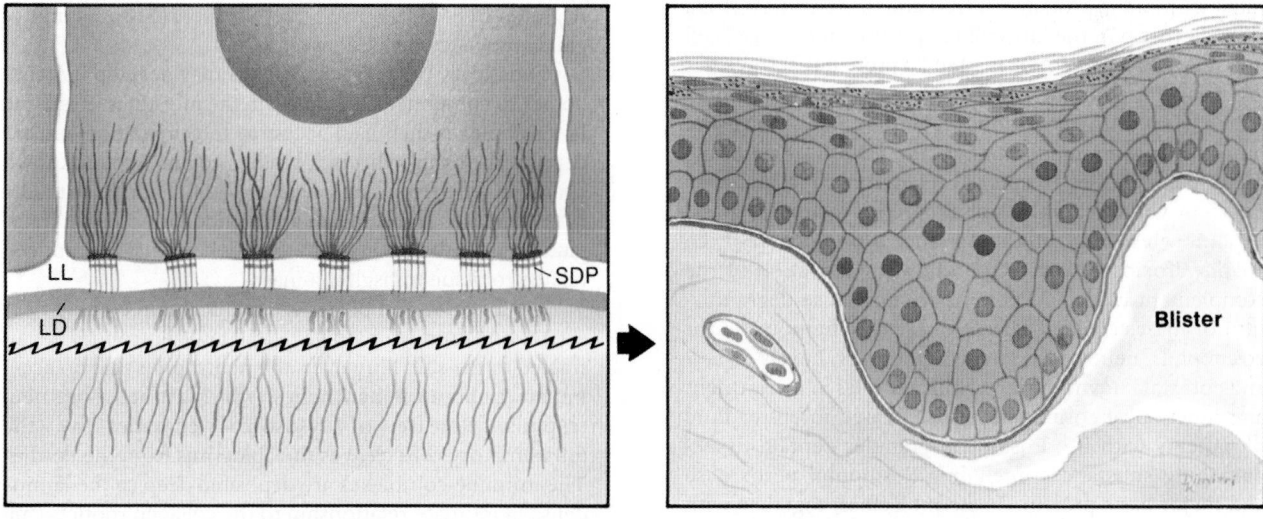

FIGURE 24-20. **Epidermolysis bullosa (EB).** Three distinct mechanisms of blister formation are shown. Electron microscopic images are diagrammed on the *left;* light microscopic images are on the *right*. Epidermolytic EB is caused by disintegration of the lowermost regions of the epidermal basal cells. The bottom portions of the basal cells cleave, and the remainder of the epidermis lifts away. Small fragments of basal cells remain attached to the basement membrane zone. Junctional EB is characterized by cleavage in the lamina lucida. Dermolytic EB is associated with rudimentary and fragmented anchoring fibrils. The entire basement membrane zone and epidermis split away from the dermis in relationship to these flawed anchoring fibrils. *LL* = lamina lucida; *LD* = lamina densa; *SDP* = subdesomosomal dense plate.

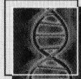

PATHOGENESIS: The development of dermolytic EB is attributed to a defect in anchoring fibrils. These fibrils are abnormally arranged and reduced in number in apparently normal skin of affected newborns. The basic defect is a mutation in the gene encoding collagen type VII on chromosome 3 (3p21). Anchoring fibrils comprise a net in the upper dermis through which fibers of collagen types I and III course. This structure anchors the epidermis to the underlying dermis, and its disruption results in subepidermal bullae arising in the sublamina densa zone.

PATHOLOGY: The vesicle roof is normal epidermis with an attached, intact lamina lucida and lamina densa. The base of the vesicle is the outer part of the papillary dermis. Ultrastructurally, there are fewer anchoring fibrils in the dominant variant and virtually no fibrils in the recessive form. A corresponding decrease in anchoring fibril proteins AF-1 and AF-2 occurs in the two variants.

Bullous Pemphigoid (BP) Is an Blistering Disease Caused by Autoanibodies Against Basement Membrane Proteins

BP is a common, autoimmune, blistering disease with clinical similarities to pemphigus vulgaris (thus, the term "pemphigoid") but in which acantholysis is absent. The disease is most common in the later decades of life, but it shows no predilection regarding race or gender.

PATHOGENESIS: Like PV, BP is an autoimmune disease, but in this case complement-fixing IgG antibodies are directed against two basement membrane proteins, BPAG1 and BPAG2. BPAG1 is a 230-kd protein in the intracellular portion of the basal cell hemidesmosome. BPAG2 is a 180-kd protein that traverses the plasma membrane and extends into the upper lamina lucida. The antigen–antibody complex may injure the basal cell plasma membrane via the C5b–C9 membrane attack complex (see Chapter 4). This damage in turn may interfere with elaboration of adherence factors by basal keratinocytes. Of greater importance is production of the anaphylatoxins C3a and C5a following activation of the complement cascade. These molecules cause degranulation of mast cells and release of factors chemotactic for eosinophils, neutrophils, and lymphocytes. Levels of IL-5 and eotaxin, known to play significant roles in recruitment and function of eosinophils, are increased in blister fluid of patients with BP. Eosinophil granules contain tissue-damaging substances, including eosinophil peroxidase and major basic protein. These molecules, together with proteases of neutrophilic and mast cell origin, cause dermal–epidermal separation within the lamina lucida (Fig. 24-21).

PATHOLOGY: The blisters of BP are subepidermal: the roof is intact epidermis and the base is the lamina densa of the BMZ (Fig. 24-22). The blisters contain numerous eosinophils, together with fibrin, lymphocytes, and neutrophils. In BP, apparently normal skin shows migration of mast cells from the venule toward the epidermis. With the onset of erythema, eosinophils appear in the upper dermis and are occasionally arranged along the epidermal BMZ. Ultrastructurally, dermal–epidermal separation begins with disruption of anchoring filaments of the lamina lucida. Immunofluorescent studies demonstrate linear deposition of C3 and IgG along the epidermal BMZ and serum antibodies against BPAG1 and BPAG2 (Fig. 24-23).

CLINICAL FEATURES: The blisters of BP are large and tense and may appear on normal-appearing skin or on an erythematous base (see Fig. 24-22). The medial thighs and flexor aspects of the forearms are commonly affected, but the groin, axillae and other cutaneous sites may also develop blisters. The disease is self-limited but chronic, and the patient's general health is usually unaffected. The course of the disease is greatly shortened by systemic administration of corticosteroids.

Dermatitis Herpetiformis Reflects Gluten Sensitivity

Dermatitis herpetiformis (DH) is an intensely pruritic cutaneous eruption characterized by urticaria-like plaques and small vesicles over the extensor surfaces of the body.

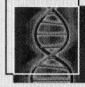

PATHOGENESIS: DH is associated with gluten sensitivity in patients with HLA-B8, HLA-DR3, and HLA-DQw2 haplotypes. The gluten-sensitive enteropathy is often subclinical (see Chapter 14). Gluten is a protein in wheat, barley, rye and oats. The cutaneous lesions are related to granular deposits of IgA at the dermal–epidermal interface, mainly at the tips of the dermal papillae. IgA immune complexes at the tips of dermal papillae are more prominent in perilesional skin than in normal-appearing skin. A gluten-free diet controls the disease; reintroduction of gluten provokes new lesions.

Genetically predisposed patients may develop IgA antibodies to components of gluten in the intestines. Resulting IgA complexes then gain access to the circulation and are deposited, possibly through binding to an as yet unknown ligand, in the dermal papillae (Fig. 24-24). Patients with DH have increased levels of IgA autoantibodies to tissue transglutaminase, suggesting that there is a dermal autoantigen related to tissue transglutaminase.

IgA immune complexes are inefficient in complement activation (alternate pathway), and few neutrophils are attracted to the site. However, the neutrophils that do accumulate elaborate leukotrienes, which attract more neutrophils. Release of lysosomal enzymes by the inflammatory cells cleaves the epidermis from the dermis. The immune complexes are deposited deep to the lamina densa in intimate relationship to the collagen rootlets (microfibrils) which, along with anchoring fibrils, are help the lamina densa attach to the subjacent papillary dermis (see Fig. 24-24).

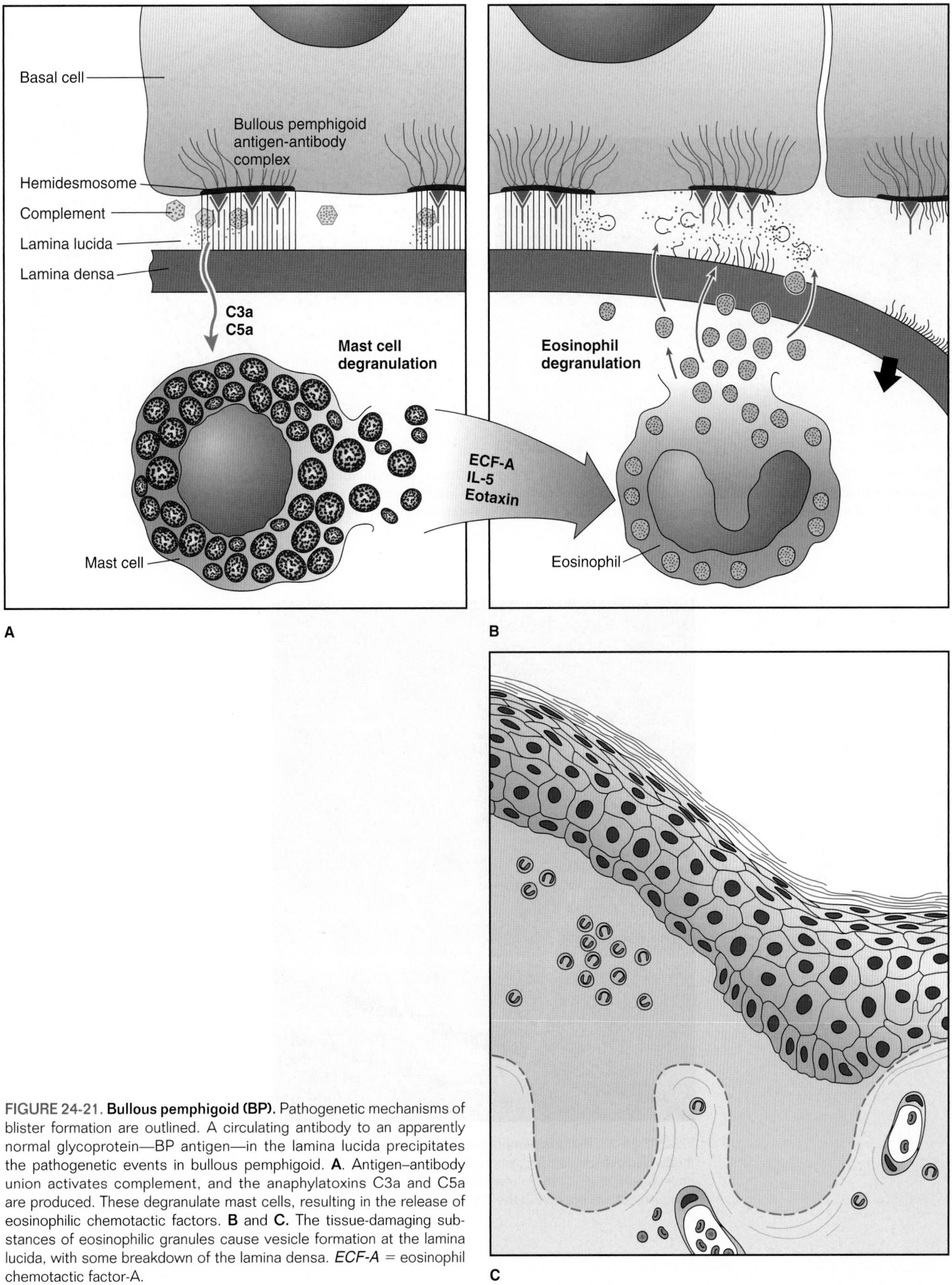

FIGURE 24-21. **Bullous pemphigoid (BP).** Pathogenetic mechanisms of blister formation are outlined. A circulating antibody to an apparently normal glycoprotein—BP antigen—in the lamina lucida precipitates the pathogenetic events in bullous pemphigoid. **A**. Antigen–antibody union activates complement, and the anaphylatoxins C3a and C5a are produced. These degranulate mast cells, resulting in the release of eosinophilic chemotactic factors. **B** and **C.** The tissue-damaging substances of eosinophilic granules cause vesicle formation at the lamina lucida, with some breakdown of the lamina densa. *ECF-A* = eosinophil chemotactic factor-A.

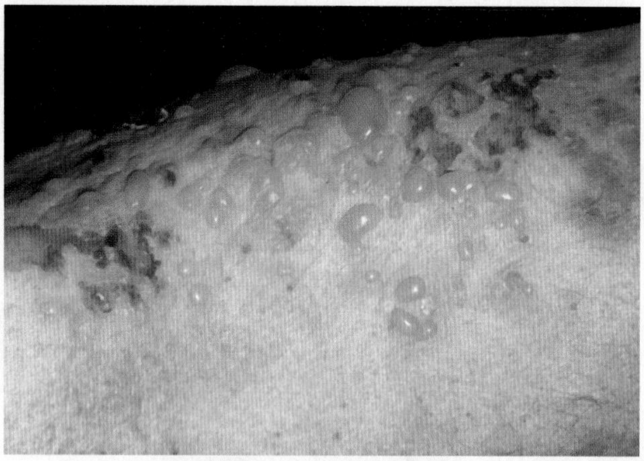
A

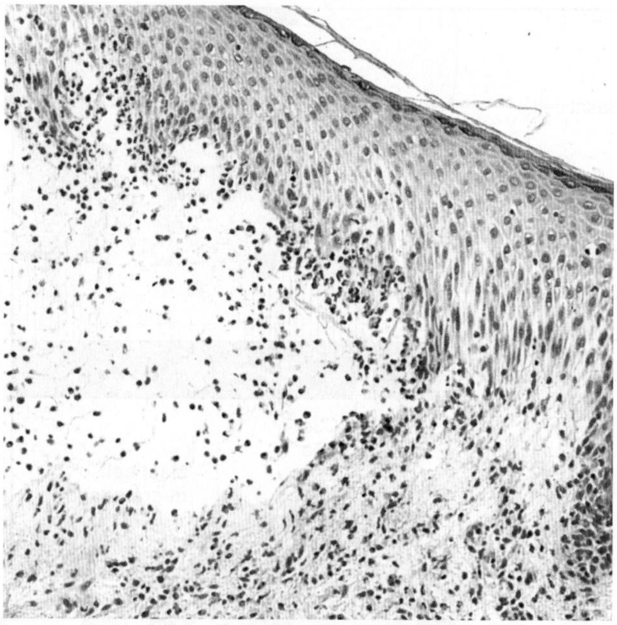
B

FIGURE 24-22. **Bullous pemphigoid. A.** The skin shows multiple tense bullae on an erythematous base and erosions, distributed primarily on the medial thighs and trunk. **B.** A subepidermal blister has an edematous papillary dermis as its base. The roof of the blister consists of the intact, entire epidermis, including the stratum basalis. Inflammatory cells, fibrin, and fluid fill the blister.

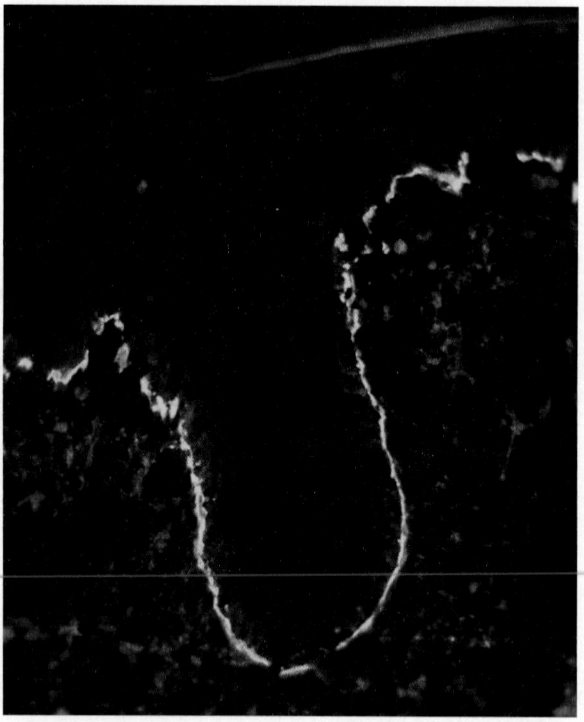

FIGURE 24-23. **Bullous pemphigoid.** Direct immunofluorescence study discloses linear deposition of IgG (and C3) along the dermal–epidermal junction. Ultrastructurally, these antibodies and complement are present in the lamina lucida.

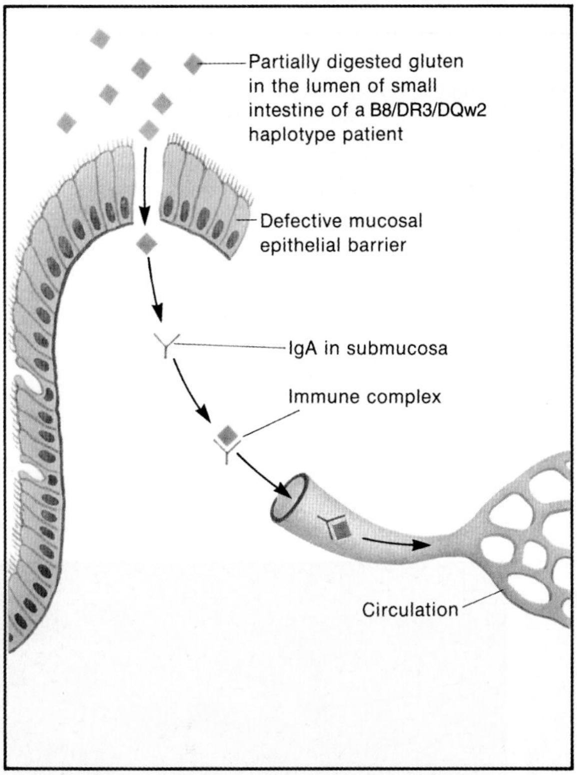

1. Formation of immune complexes in submucosa of small intestine. Passage of immune complexes into **the circulation.**

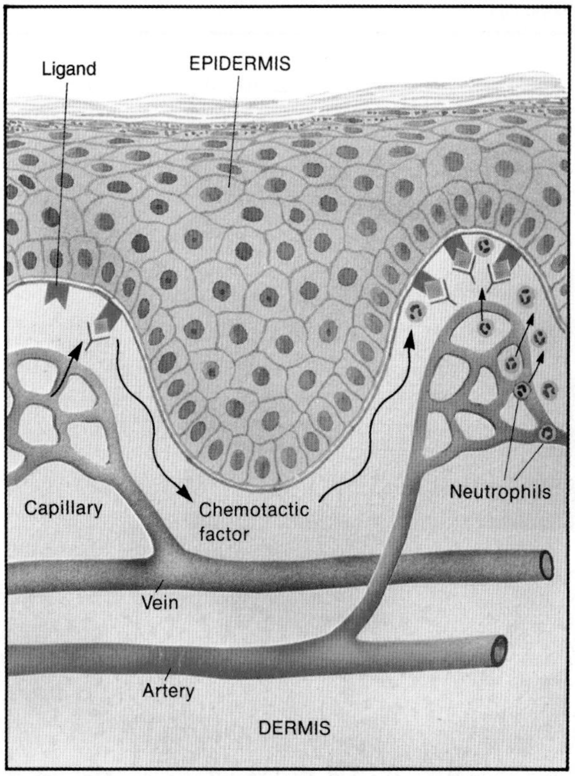

2. Ligand–immune complex union releases neutrophil chemotactic factor. Neutrophils migrate to the tips of the papillae.

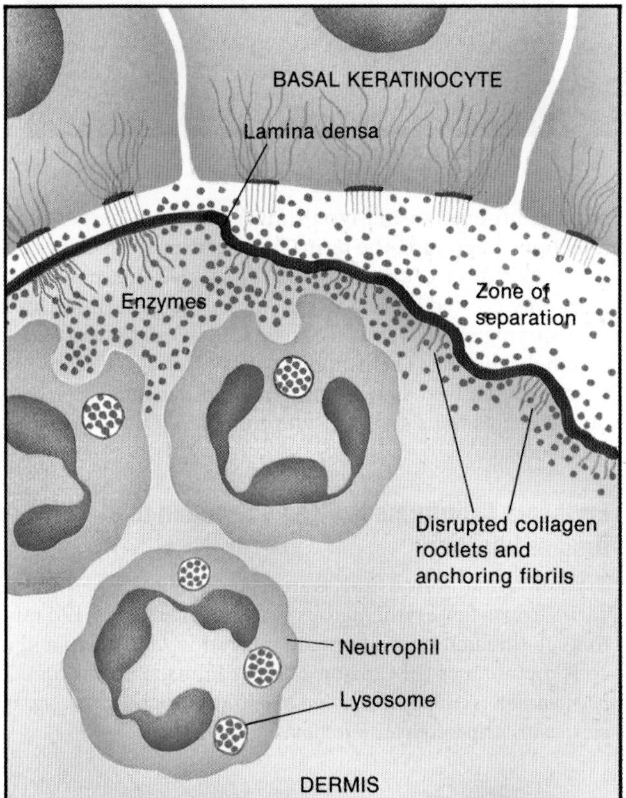

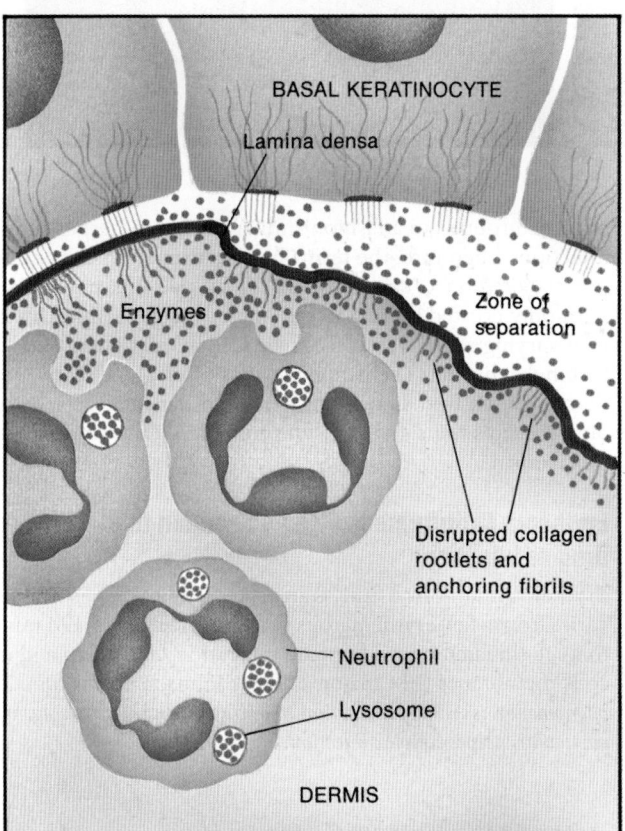

3. Dissolution of basal rootlets and anchoring fibrils by enzymes released by neutrophils. Early dermo-epidermal separation.

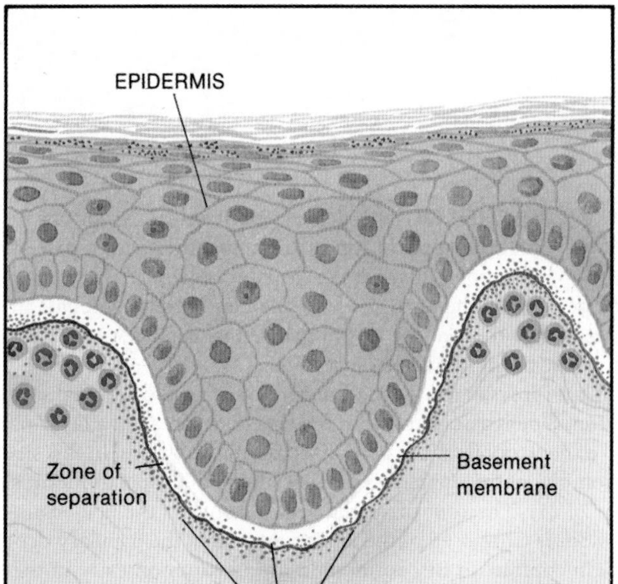

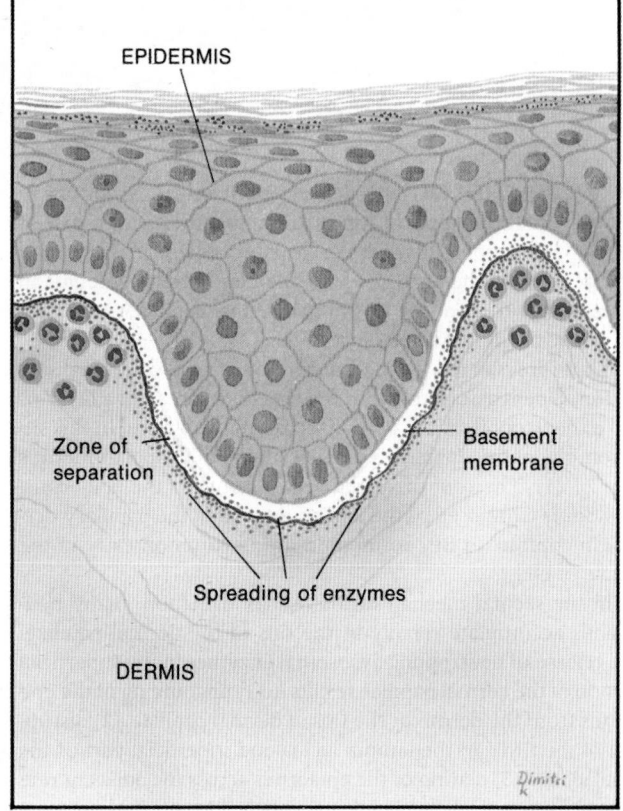

4. Concentration of neutrophils at the tips of the papillae. Spreading of enzymes along basement membrane. Lifting away of lamina densa.

FIGURE 24-24. **Dermatitis herpetiformis.** Proposed pathogenesis for cutaneous lesions. The disease is initiated in the small intestine and is likely expressed in the skin because of the presence of a ligand immediately deep to the lamina densa. IgA = immunoglobulin A.

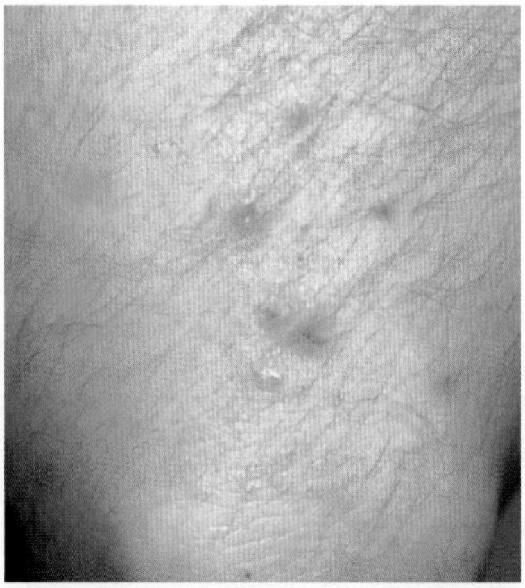

A

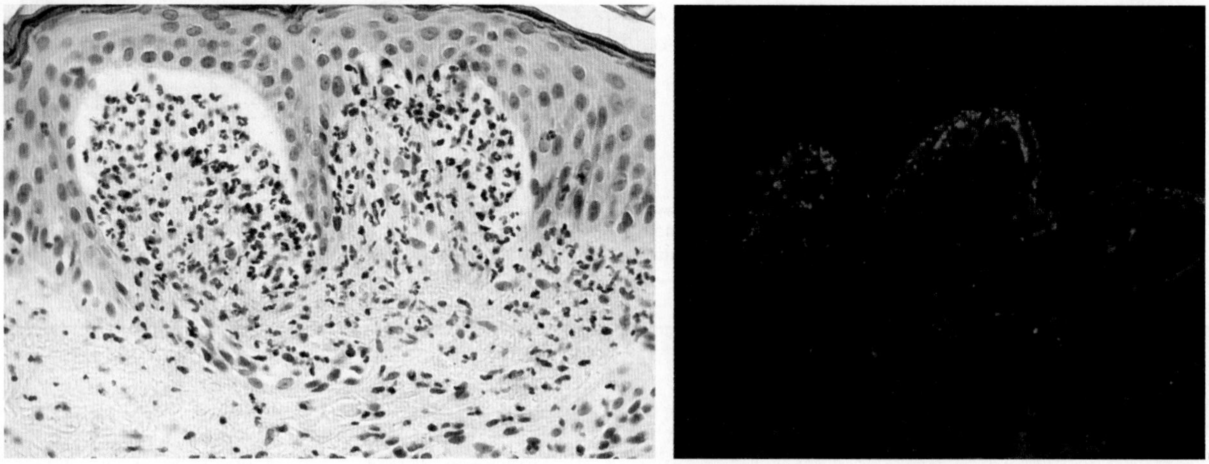

B C

FIGURE 24-25. **Dermatitis herpetiformis. A.** Pruritic, symmetric, grouped vesicles on an erythematous base are seen on the elbows and knees. **B.** Dermal papillary abscesses of neutrophils with vesicle formation at the dermal–epidermal junction are characteristic. **C.** Direct immunofluorescence reveals IgA deposited in dermal papillae in association with (but not necessarily directly upon) anchoring fibrils and elastic tissue fibers. This is the site of neutrophil infiltration and subepidermal vesicle formation.

PATHOLOGY: A delicate perivenular lymphocytic infiltrate appears appears first, together with a row of neutrophils just deep to the lamina densa in the dermal papillae. During the next 12 hours, the neutrophils aggregate in clusters of 10 to 25 at the tips of the dermal papillae to create a diagnostic histologic appearance.

There are two related mechanisms of dermal–epidermal separation. One is associated with the sheetlike spread of a layer or two of neutrophils at the dermal–epidermal interface. In this situation, the entire epidermis detaches from the papillary dermis (Fig. 24-25). The roof of such a vesicle contains the epidermis; the floor is composed of the lamina densa and the papillary dermis. In contrast to BP, eosinophils are uncommon early in the course of DH.

In the second mechanism of vesicle formation, many neutrophils accumulate rapidly in the tips of the dermal papillae. The release of neutrophilic lysosomal enzymes in the superficial portion of the dermal papillae results in (1) uncoupling of the epidermis from the dermis at the tips of dermal papillae, (2) disruption of the BMZ in the lamina lucida and superficial part of the papillae, and (3) tearing of the epidermis across the adjacent rete ridges. The roof of the resulting vesicle has alternating tears across its epidermal covering and the floor shows residual epidermal pegs alternating with the basal half of dermal papillae.

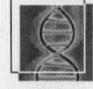

CLINICAL FEATURES: The lesions of DH are especially prominent over the elbows, knees and buttocks (see Fig. 24-25A). The intensely pruritic vesicles may become grouped in a fashion similar to that in herpes simplex infections (therefore, the term "herpetiformis") and are almost invariably rubbed until broken. Thus, patients may present with only crusted lesions and no intact vesicles. Although DH is of varying severity and characterized by remissions, it is disturbingly chronic. The healing lesions often leave scars. Other than a gluten-free diet, treatment with dapsone or sulfapyridine controls the signs and symptoms of DH by an unknown mechanism.

Erythema Multiforme Is Often a Reaction to a Drug or Infection

Erythema multiforme (EM) is an acute, self-limited disorder that varies from a few erythematous macules and blisters (EM minor) to a life-threatening, widespread ulceration of the skin and mucous membranes (EM major; Stevens-Johnson syndrome). *This phenomenon is usually a reaction to a drug or an infectious agent, in particular, herpes simplex infection.*

PATHOGENESIS: The list of agents that may provoke EM is long and includes Herpesvirus, *Mycoplasma,* and sulfonamides. However, a precipitating factor is found in only half of cases. In postherpetic EM, viral antigens, IgM, and C3 are deposited in a perivascular location and at the epidermal BMZ. The combination of infiltrating lymphocytes and antigen–antibody complexes within the lesions suggest that both humoral and cellular hypersensitivity are involved.

PATHOLOGY: The dermis in EM shows a sparse lymphocyte infiltrate about the superficial vascular bed and at the dermal–epidermal interface. The characteristic morphologic feature in the epidermis is the presence of apoptotic keratinocytes, which have a pyknotic nucleus and an eosinophilic cytoplasm. Apoptosis may be extensive and associated with a subepidermal vesicle, whose roof is an almost completely necrotic epidermis. Because of the acute onset of the disease, in most cases there is little or no change in the stratum corneum.

CLINICAL FEATURES: The characteristic "target" or "iris" lesions of EM have a central, dark red zone, occasionally with a blister, surrounded by a paler area (Fig. 24-26). In turn, the latter is encompassed by a peripheral red rim. Urticarial plaques are common. The presence of vesicles and bullae usually predicts a more severe course. EM is a common condition, with a peak incidence in the second and third decades of life. It is occasionally encountered in association with other presumably immunologic cutaneous disorders, including erythema nodosum, toxic epidermal necrolysis and necrotizing vasculitis. **Stevens-Johnson syndrome** refers to an unusually severe form of EM that involves several mucosal surfaces and internal organs and is frequently fatal.

Systemic Lupus Erythematosus Is an Immune Complex Disease

Systemic lupus erythematosus (SLE), the paradigm of an immune complex disease, is characterized by a variety of autoantibodies and other immune abnormalities (see Chapters 4 and 16). Although cutaneous involvement may be severe and cosmetically devastating, it is not life-threatening. However, the nature and pattern of immune reactants in the skin are an excellent guide to the likelihood of systemic disease.

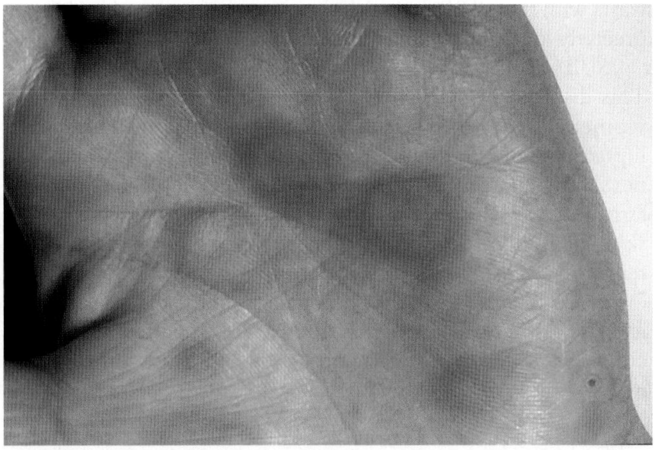

FIGURE 24-26. **Erythema multiforme.** Steroid-responsive "target" papules, characterized by central bullae with surrounding erythema, appeared after antibiotic therapy.

PATHOGENESIS: Immune complexes are not likely to be solely responsible for the cutaneous lesions of SLE. In this respect, immune complexes are present in both lesional and normal-appearing skin in SLE. Deposition of immune reactants along the epidermal BMZ (positive lupus band test) of "normal" skin is important in the diagnosis of SLE. Epidermal injury seems to be initiated by exogenous agents such as ultraviolet light and perpetuated by cell-mediated immune reactions similar to those in graft-versus-host disease. The manifestations of epidermal injury include (1) vacuolization of basal keratinocytes, hyperkeratosis, and diminished epidermal thickness; (2) release of DNA and other nuclear and cytoplasmic antigens to the circulation; and (3) deposition of DNA and other antigenic determinants in the epidermal BMZ (lamina densa and immediately subjacent dermis) (Fig. 24-27). Thus, epidermal injury, local immune-complex formation, deposition of circulating immune complexes, and lymphocyte-induced cellular injury all seem to act in concert.

The various forms of cutaneous lupus erythematosus have been classified according to their chronicity, but considerable overlap in features is possible. There is an inverse relationship between the prominence of skin lesions and the extent of systemic pathology.

CHRONIC CUTANEOUS (DISCOID) LUPUS ERYTHEMATOSUS: This form of lupus is usually limited to the skin. Disease generally manifests above the neck, on the face (especially the malar area), scalp, and ears. The lesions begin as slightly elevated violaceous papules with a rough scale of keratin. As they enlarge, they assume a disk shape, with a hyperkeratotic margin and a depigmented center. The cutaneous lesions may culminate in disfiguring scars. Elevation of circulating antinuclear antibodies (ANAs) is seen in fewer than 10% of patients.

PATHOLOGY: In discoid lupus, the nucleated epidermal layers are modestly thickened or somewhat thin. Hyperkeratosis and plugging of hair follicles are prominent features. The rete–papillae pattern of the dermal–epidermal interface is partially effaced. The basal keratinocytes are vacuolated, and eosinophilic apoptotic bodies are noted. The lamina densa is greatly thickened and reduplicated. On periodic acid-Schiff (PAS) staining, multiple layers of lamina densa extend into the subjacent dermis. The excessive quantity of lamina densa, a product of the basal keratinocytes, reflects a response of basal cells to damage. These changes all suggest that injury to basal keratinocytes is an essential pathogenetic characteristic of skin disease associated with lupus (Fig. 24-28 through Fig. 24-30).

The basal keratinocytes and BMZ contain a diffuse lymphocytic infiltrate that penetrates the basal layer focally. Deeper in the dermis, dense patches of helper and cytotoxic/suppressor T lymphocytes, often with plasma cells, are commonly found

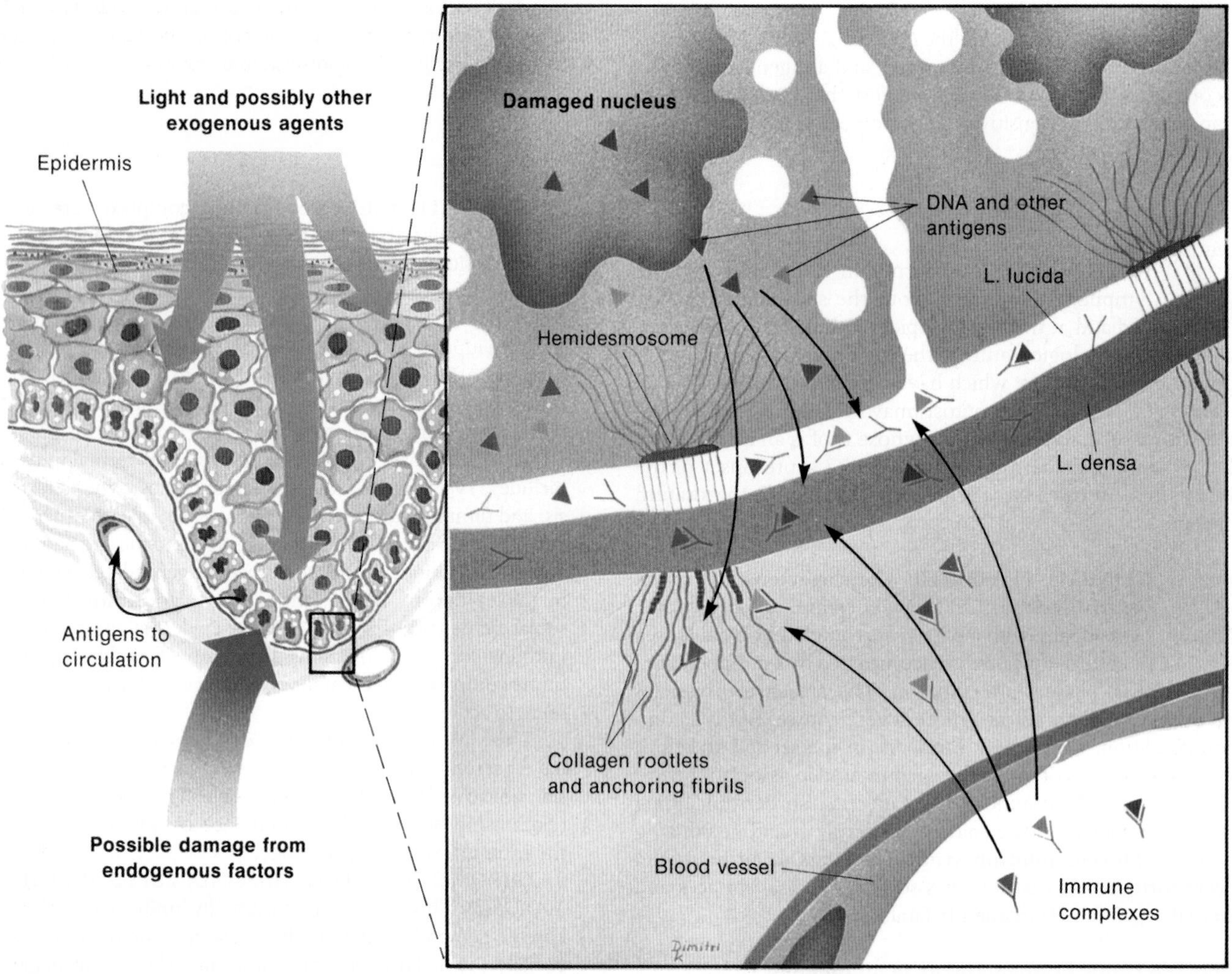

FIGURE 24-27. **Lupus erythematosus.** A cell-mediated immune reaction leads to epidermal cellular damage when initiated by light or other exogenous agents as well as endogenous ones. Such injury releases a large number of antigens, some of which may return to the skin in the form of immune complexes. Immune complexes are also formed in the skin by a reaction of local DNA with antibody that may also be deposited beneath the epidermal basement membrane zone. L. = lamina.

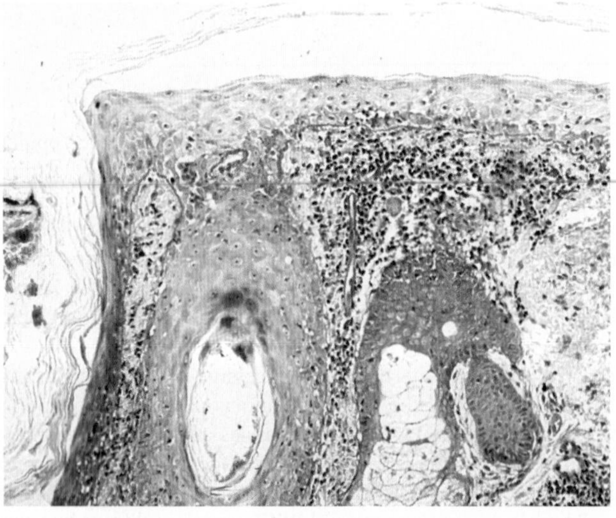

FIGURE 24-28. **Lupus erythematosus.** A variably cell-rich to cell-poor, bandlike, lymphocytic infiltrate is present in the papillary and adventitial dermis. There is epidermal atrophy arising from damage to the epidermis, which is mediated by infiltrating lymphocytes.

around skin appendages. Immune complexes are predominantly located deep to the lamina densa, but they are also seen on the lamina densa and within the lamina lucida. This pattern contrasts with that of BP, in which there are only two antigens, both precisely localized to the lamina lucida.

SUBACUTE CUTANEOUS LUPUS ERYTHEMATOSUS: This disorder primarily afflicts young and middle-aged white women. In contrast to discoid lupus, subacute cutaneous lupus may also involve the musculoskeletal system and kidneys. Initially, scaly erythematous papules develop and then enlarge into psoriasiform or annular lesions, which may fuse. The skin changes are seen in the upper chest, upper back, and extensor surfaces of the arms, a distribution indicating that light exposure plays a role in the pathogenesis of the disorder. Significant scarring does not occur. About 70% of patients have circulating anti-Ro (ss-A) antibodies, and ANA levels are elevated in 70%.

PATHOLOGY: Subacute cutaneous lupus features edema of the papillary dermis, thickening of the lamina densa and prominent vacuolar degeneration of

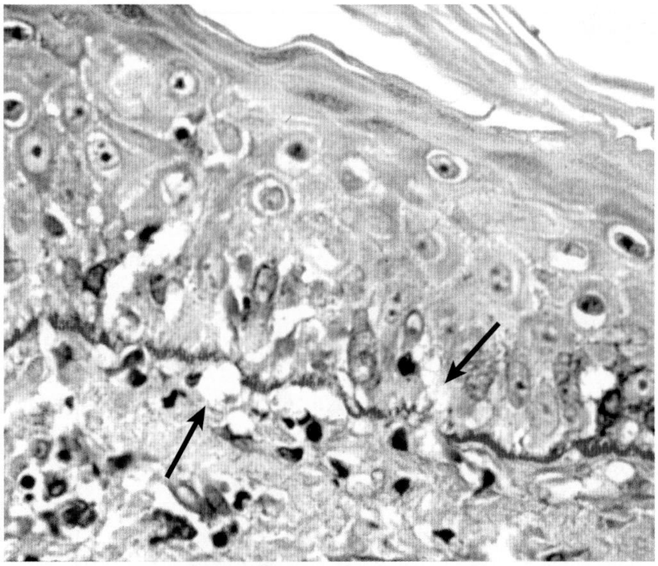

FIGURE 24-29. **Lupus erythematosus.** Basal cell necrosis with resultant basal keratinocytic migration and synthesis of new basement membrane zone leads to thickening of the epidermal basement membrane zone (BMZ), as evident in this periodic acid-Schiff (PAS) stain. Notice the vacuoles *(arrows)* on either side of the BMZ, an indicator of cellular injury.

the basilar keratinocytes. There is some lymphocytic infiltration of the BMZ, but deeper patches of lymphocytes are not observed.

ACUTE SYSTEMIC LUPUS ERYTHEMATOSUS: Over 80% of patients with SLE have acute cutaneous manifestations during their illness, in association with disease of the kidneys and joints. The rash is often the first manifestation of the disease and may precede the onset of systemic symptoms by a few months. The typical "butterfly" rash of SLE is a delicate erythema of the malar area of the face, which may pass in a few hours or a few days. Many patients exhibit a maculopapular eruption of the chest and extremities, often developing after sun exposure. Both rashes heal without scarring. Lesions indistinguishable from discoid lupus may occur. ANA levels are elevated in more than 90% of patients.

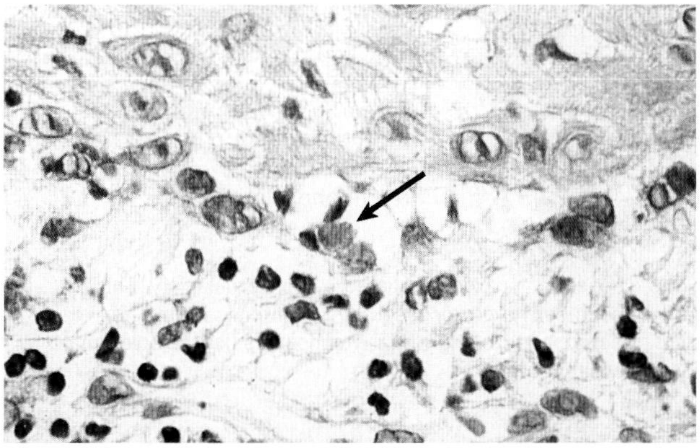

FIGURE 24-30. **Lupus erythematosus.** An active lesion shows striking basal vacuolization, with keratinocyte necrosis *(arrow)* forming a dense eosinophilic body (apoptotic/fibrillary/colloid body) that is surrounded by lymphocytes (satellitosis).

PATHOLOGY: Histologically, the earliest malar blush of acute cutaneous lupus may show only edema of the papillary dermis. More often, the changes are similar to those in the subacute form of lupus. In **bullous SLE,** blisters may occur subepidermally and beneath the lamina densa, where an autoantibody against type VII collagen, a component of anchoring fibrils, is deposited.

Lichen Planus Is a Hypersensitivity Reaction with Lymphocytic Infiltrates at the Dermal–Epidermal Junction

"Lichenoid" tissue reactions are so named because the clinical lesions resemble certain lichens that form a scaly growth on rocks or tree trunks. Histologically, a lichenoid infiltrate is characterized by a bandlike infiltrate of lymphocytes that obscures the dermal–epidermal junction. The disease is characterized by reduced epidermal turnover and subsequent hyperkeratosis without parakeratosis. Lichen planus (LP) is the prototypic disorder of this group, which includes entities such as lichen nitidus and lichenoid drug eruptions.

PATHOGENESIS: The etiology of LP is unknown. It is occasionally familial and may also accompany a variety of autoimmune disorders, such as SLE and myasthenia gravis. LP is more frequent in patients with ulcerative colitis. Drugs such as gold, chlorothiazide, and chloroquine may induce lichenoid reactions. External agents such as photographic chemicals may evoke a lichenoid response. LP-like lesions are also often observed in the later stages of chronic graft-versus-host disease. Thus, it seems that immunologic mechanisms play a role in the pathogenesis of LP (Fig. 24-31). The presence of apoptotic bodies and increased epidermal cell turnover suggest that the lesions of LP result from cell destruction and subsequent reactive epidermal proliferation. Evidence supports the notion that LP is a delayed type of hypersensitivity reaction, initiated and amplified by cytokines such as gamma interferon (IFN-γ) and IL-6, whose expression is due not only to infiltrating lymphocytes but also to stimulated keratinocytes. Association of LP with hepatitis B and C infections have been observed.

PATHOLOGY: The epidermis in LP features compact hyperkeratosis with little or no parakeratosis. The stratum granulosum is thickened, frequently in a distinctive, focal, wedge-shaped pattern, with the base of the wedge abutting the stratum corneum. The stratum spinosum is variably thickened.

The distinctive pathological changes of LP are at the dermal–epidermal interface. The basal row of cuboidal cells is replaced by flattened or polygonal keratinocytes. The undulating interface between the dermal papillae and the rounded profiles of the rete ridges is obscured by a dense infiltrate of lymphocytes and macrophages, many of the latter containing melanin pigment (melanophages) (Fig. 24-32). The lymphocytes are

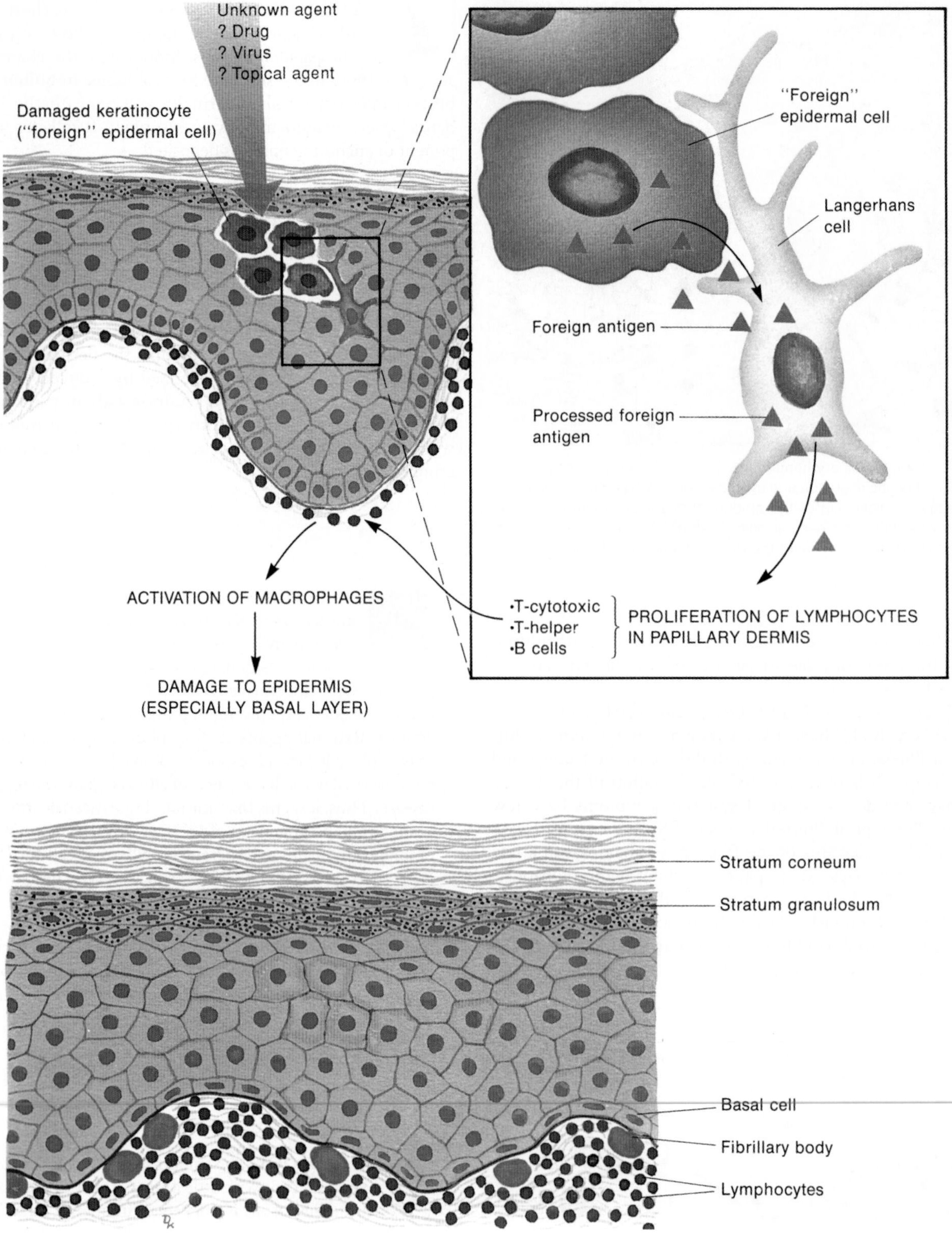

FIGURE 24-31. **Lichen planus.** Pathogenetic mechanisms are outlined. The disease is apparently initiated by epidermal injury. This injury causes some epidermal cells to be treated as "foreign." The antigens of such cells are processed by Langerhans cells. The processed antigen induces lymphocytic proliferation and macrophage activation. Macrophages, along with T lymphocytes, kill the epidermal basal cells, resulting in a reactive epidermal proliferation and the formation of fibrillary bodies.

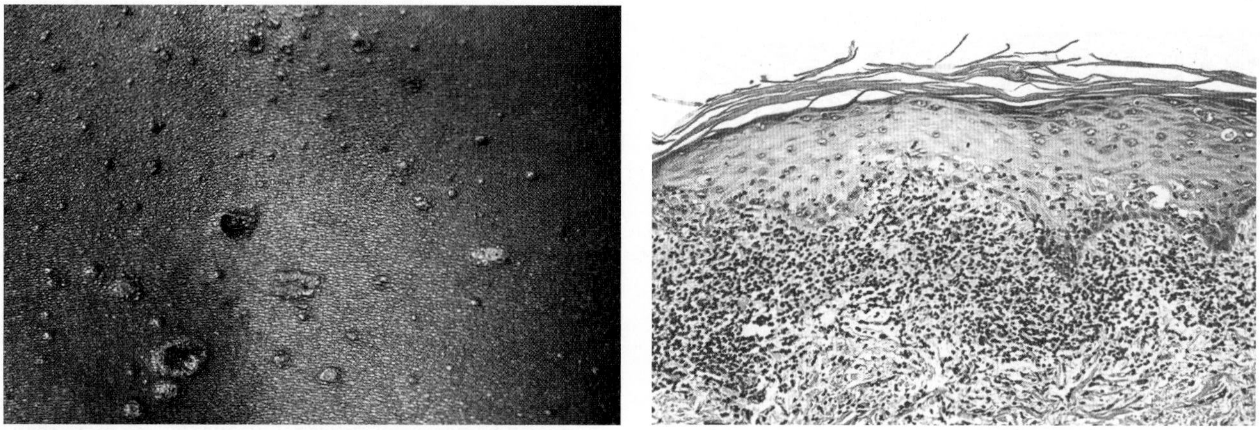

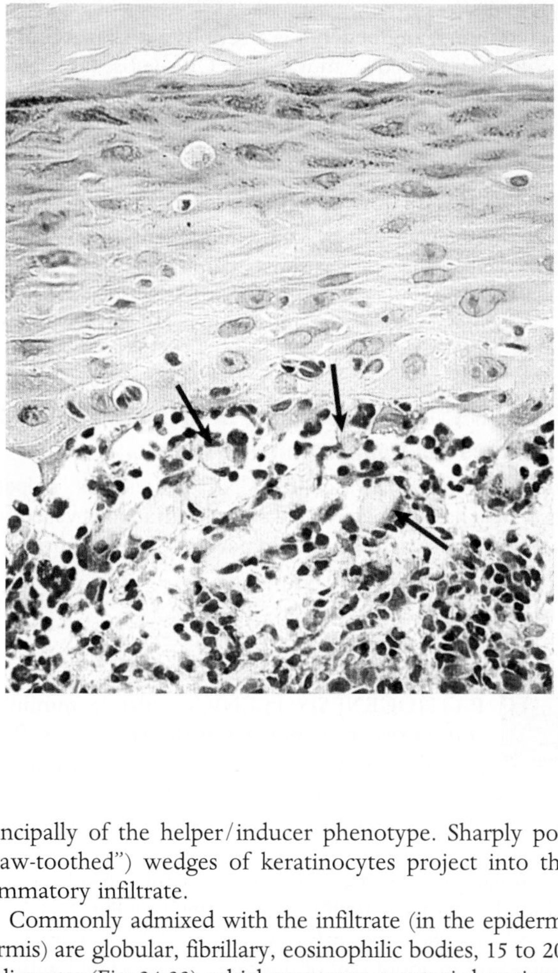

FIGURE 24-32. **Lichen planus. A.** The skin displays multiple flat-topped violaceous polygonal papules. **B.** A cell-rich, bandlike, lymphocytic infiltrate disrupts the stratum basalis. Unlike lupus erythematosus, there is usually epidermal hyperplasia, hyperkeratosis and wedgelike hypergranulosis. **C.** Hypergranulosis and loss of rete ridges are noted. The site of pathologic injury is at the dermal-epidermal junction where there is a striking infiltrate of lymphocytes, many of which surround apoptotic keratinocytes.

principally of the helper/inducer phenotype. Sharply pointed ("saw-toothed") wedges of keratinocytes project into the inflammatory infiltrate.

Commonly admixed with the infiltrate (in the epidermis or dermis) are globular, fibrillary, eosinophilic bodies, 15 to 20 μm in diameter (Fig. 24-33), which represent apoptotic keratinocytes. These structures are variably termed *apoptotic, colloid, Civatte* or *fibrillary bodies*. The fibrils within the apoptotic bodies are keratin filaments. Epidermal Langerhans cells are increased early in LP.

CLINICAL FEATURES: LP is a chronic eruption characterized by violaceous, flat-topped papules, usually on the flexor surfaces of the wrists (see Fig. 24-32A). White patches or streaks may also be present on the oral mucous membranes. In most patients, the pruritic lesions resolve in less than a year, but they may occasionally persist for longer periods.

Inflammatory Diseases of the Superficial and Deep Vascular Bed

Urticaria and Angioedema are IgE-Dependent Hypersensitivity Reactions

These reactions initiated by degranulation of mast cells sensitized to a specific antigen. **Urticaria** or hives are raised, pale, well-demarcated pruritic papules and plaques that appear and disappear within a few hours. The lesions represent edema of the superficial portion of the dermis. **Angioedema** refers to a condition in which the edema involves the deeper dermis or subcutis, resulting in an egglike swelling. Both entities have a rapid onset and range in severity from simply annoying lesions to life-threatening anaphylactic reactions. The mainstays of treatment are avoidance of the offending agent and prompt administration of antihistamines.

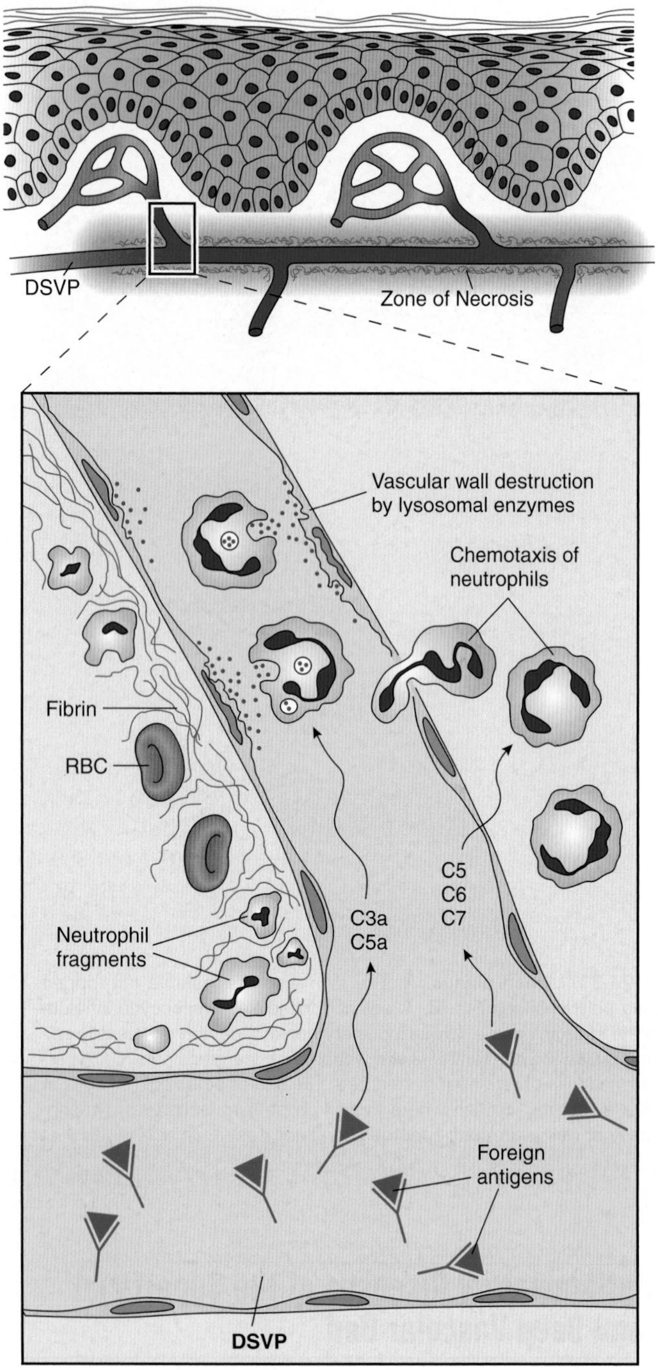

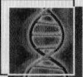

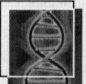

FIGURE 24-33. **Cutaneous necrotizing vasculitis.** The pathogenesis of vessel damage is depicted. The site of the vascular pathology is indicated in the *upper diagram*. Circulating immune complexes activate complement. There is neutrophilic chemotaxis *(C5a)* and neutrophilic destruction. Vascular damage occurs, with extravasation of erythrocytes, fibrin deposition, and leukocytoclasia. *RBC* = red blood cell; *DSVP* = deep superficial venular plexus.

Dermatographism is a linear hive with a rich pink flare produced by briskly stroking the skin. It is found in approximately 4% of the population and represents an exaggerated IgE-dependent response. One may write on the skin of such persons and create a hive in the form of a legible word.

PATHOGENESIS: Most cases of urticaria are IgE-dependent and reflect exaggerated venule permeability due to mast cell degranulation. An almost endless list of materials may react with IgE antibodies on the surface of the mast cell. Urticaria occur in both atopic and nonatopic persons. Atopic persons have intensely pruritic skin eruptions, a family history of similar eruptions and a personal or family history of allergies. They commonly exhibit an elevation of circulating IgE.

Initially, cutaneous venules react to degranulation of mast cells and release of their vasoactive mediators with increased permeability, resulting in rapidly forming edema. If the reaction persists, inflammatory cells are attracted to the area and a persistent urticarial plaque (lasting more than a day) results.

Hereditary angioedema is a serious autosomal dominant disorder caused by mutation of C1-esterase inhibitor.

PATHOLOGY: In urticaria, collagen fibers and fibrils are splayed apart by excess fluid. Lymphatic vessels are dilated and venules show margination of neutrophils and eosinophils. Vessels are cuffed by a few lymphocytes. Persistent urticaria shows increased lymphocytes and eosinophils, but neutrophils are sparse.

Cutaneous Necrotizing Vasculitis Is an Immune Reaction That Features Neutrophilic Inflammation

Cutaneous necrotizing vasculitis (CNV) presents as "palpable purpura," and has also been called **allergic cutaneous vasculitis, leukocytoclastic vasculitis,** and **hypersensitivity angiitis.**

PATHOGENESIS: In CNV, circulating immune complexes are deposited in the vascular walls, probably at sites of injuries, at branch points where turbulence is increased, or where the venous circulation is slowed, as in the lower extremities. The elaborated C5a complement component attracts neutrophils, which degranulate and release lysosomal enzymes, resulting in endothelial damage and fibrin deposition (see Fig. 24-33).

CNV may be either primary, without a known precipitating event in about half of the cases, or associated with a specific infectious agent (e.g., HBV or HCV). It may also be a secondary process in a variety of chronic diseases, such as rheumatoid arthritis, SLE, and ulcerative colitis. CNV may also be associated with (1) underlying malignancies such as lymphoma, (2) a drug or some other allergy, or (3) an infectious process such as Henoch-Schönlein purpura.

PATHOLOGY: The lesions of CNV show vessel walls obliterated by a neutrophilic infiltrate. The endothelial cells are difficult to visualize and vessel damage is manifested by fibrin deposition and extravasation of erythrocytes (Fig. 24-34). Many of the eutrophils are also damaged, resulting in dustlike nuclear remnants, a process known as "leukocytoclasia." The collagen fibers between affected vessels are separated by neutrophils, eosinophils, and leukocytoclastic cellular remnants, as well as the extravasated erythrocytes that account for the characteristic palpable purpura.

CLINICAL FEATURES: CNV is distinguished by 2 to 4 mm purpuric papules, which are red, palpable lesions that do not blanch under pressure (palpable purpura) (see Fig. 24-34). Multiple lesions characteristically appear in crops on the lower extremities or at sites of pressure. Lesions may be confined to the skin in an otherwise healthy person, or may involve small blood vessels in the joints, GI tract or kidney. Individual lesions persist for up to a month and then resolve, leaving hyperpigmentation or atrophic scars. Despite removal of the offending agent, episodes of CNV may recur.

Allergic Contact Dermatitis is Cell-Mediated Hypersensitivity to Exogenous Sensitizing Agents

Some of the most common sensitizing agents are members of the *Rhus* genus of plants. Some 90% of the population of the United States is sensitive to the common offenders: *Rhus radicans* (poison ivy), *Rhus diversiloba* (poison oak), and *Rhus vernix* (poison sumac). These plant dermatitides are so well known that the resultant disease is commonly labeled according to the offending plant. Patients definitively state "I have poison ivy" and go to the physician for relief, rather than for diagnosis.

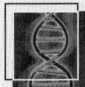

PATHOGENESIS: The offending plant contains low-molecular-weight compounds called **haptens**, in particular, oleoresins. These are not active in sensitization unless they combine with a carrier protein. This likely happens at the cell membrane of the Langerhans cell in the **sensitization phase**, a process that has been studied as a prototype of antigenic sensitization in delayed-type hypersensitivity. Formation of a hapten-carrier complex requires about 1 hour, after which it is processed as an antigen by the Langerhans cells. These cells carry the antigen through the lymphatics to regional lymph nodes and present the antigen to CD4+ T lymphocytes (Fig. 24-35). After 5 to 7 days, some clones of these T lymphocytes become sensitized to the antigen, become activated, multiply and circulate in the blood as memory cells. Some migrate to the skin, ready to react with the antigen if they encounter it. IL-1, produced by Langerhans cells, supports the proliferation of CD4+ Th1 lymphocytes, the effector cells of delayed hypersensitivity.

In the **elicitation phase**, specifically sensitized T lymphocytes in the circulation enter the skin. At the site of antigen challenge, Langerhans cells, endothelial cells, perivascular dendritic cells and monocytes process the antigen and present it to the specifically sensitized T cells, which then migrate into the epidermis. Cytokine production leads to the accumulation of more T cells and macrophages. This inflammatory infiltrate is responsible for epidermal cell injury. It is proposed that activated T cells in the skin, via IFN-α, induce apoptosis of keratinocytes by up-regulating the expression of Fas by the keratinocytes. Fas ligand enters the microenvironment after being expressed on the T cell surface.

PATHOLOGY: Allergic contact dermatitis is a model of **spongiotic dermatitis**. In the initial 24 hours following reexposure to the offending plant (elicitation phase), numerous lymphocytes and macrophages accumulate about the superficial venular bed and extend into the epidermis. The epidermal keratinocytes are partially separated by the edema fluid, creating a spongelike appearance (**spongiosis**) (Fig. 24-36). The stratum corneum contains coagulated eosinophilic fluid and plasma proteins. Later, numerous mononuclear inflammatory cells and eosinophils accumulate. Vesicles containing lymphocytes and macrophages are present, and large amounts of eosinophilic coagulated fluid accumulate in the stratum corneum.

CLINICAL FEATURES: When a person first comes into contact with poison ivy, no immediate reaction occurs. Five to 7 days after reexposure, the site of contact becomes intensely pruritic, after which erythema and small

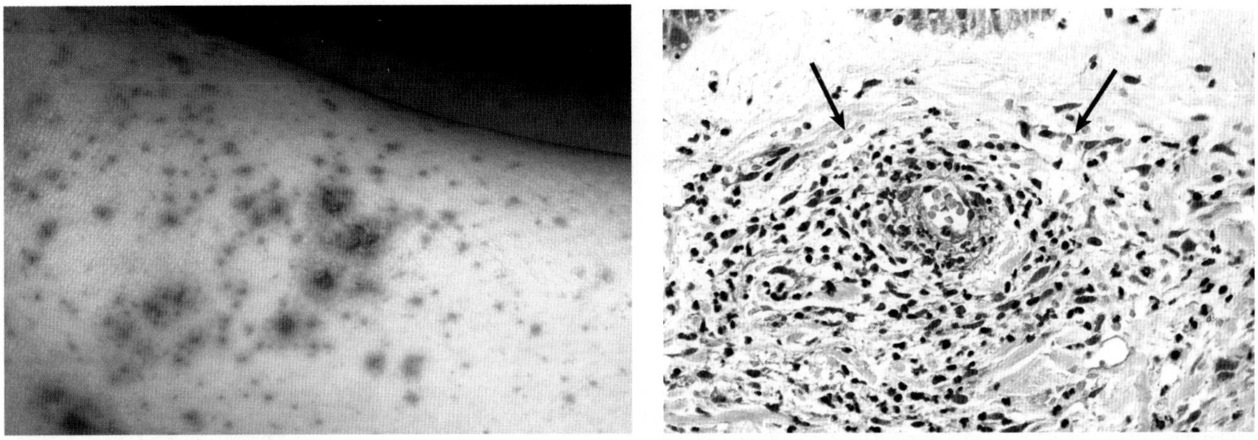

A B

FIGURE 24-34. **Cutaneous necrotizing vasculitis. A.** Palpable purpuric tender papules on the legs of a 25-year-old woman. The condition resolved after therapy for streptococcal pharyngitis. **B.** The vessel is surrounded by pink fibrin and neutrophils, many of which have disintegrated (leukocytoclasis). Extravasated red blood cells *(arrows)* and inflammation give the classic clinical appearance of "palpable purpura."

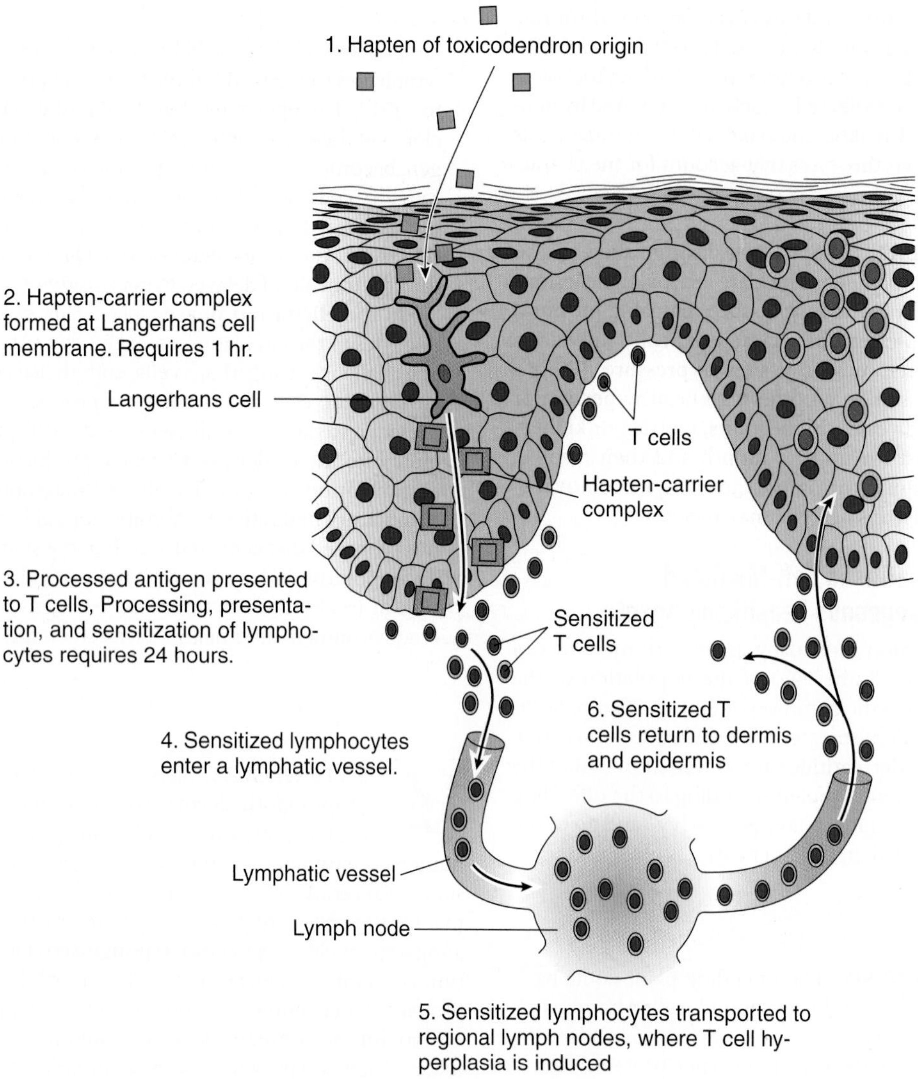
1. Hapten of toxicodendron origin
2. Hapten-carrier complex formed at Langerhans cell membrane. Requires 1 hr.
Langerhans cell
T cells
Hapten-carrier complex
3. Processed antigen presented to T cells, Processing, presentation, and sensitization of lymphocytes requires 24 hours.
Sensitized T cells
6. Sensitized T cells return to dermis and epidermis
4. Sensitized lymphocytes enter a lymphatic vessel.
Lymphatic vessel
Lymph node
5. Sensitized lymphocytes transported to regional lymph nodes, where T cell hyperplasia is induced

FIGURE 24-35. **Allergic contact dermatitis.** Pathogenetic mechanisms are shown.

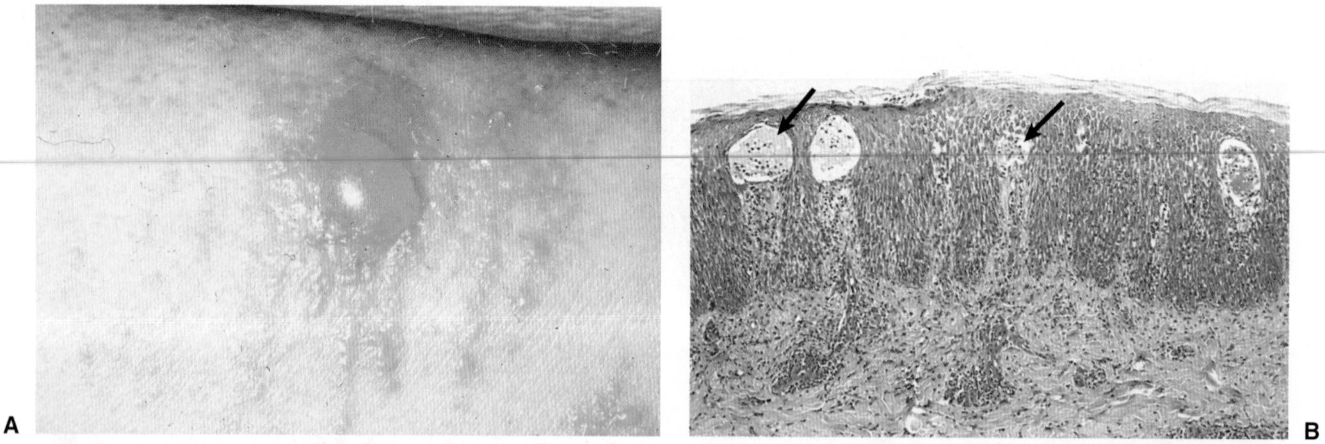
A
B

FIGURE 24-36. **Allergic contact dermatitis. A.** Vesicles and bullae developed on the volar forearm after application of perfume. **B.** Epidermal spongiosis and spongiotic vesicles *(arrows)* are present in this biopsy of "poison ivy." Infiltrating lymphocytes are apparent in the epidermis, where they effect the cell-mediated delayed hypersensitivity reaction.

vesicles rapidly develop (see Fig. 24-36). Over the next few days, the area enlarges, becomes fiery red, develops numerous vesicles and exudes a large amount of clear proteinaceous fluid. During this evolution pruritus is intense. The entire process lasts about 3 weeks. Exudation gradually subsides and the whole area is covered by an irregular crust that eventually falls off. Pruritus diminishes and healing occurs without scarring.

When a sensitized patient again comes into contact with poison ivy, the process is accelerated. Within 24 to 48 hours lesions appear, spread rapidly and produce the same clinical appearance. However, the reaction is usually more intense. Again, the lesions clear in about 3 weeks. Allergic contact dermatitis responds to topical or systemic administration of corticosteroids.

Granulomatous Dermatitis Is a Response to Indigestible Antigens

Granulomas, generally defined as localized collections of epithelioid macrophages, form in response to insoluble or slowly released antigens that produce either a focal nonallergic response or an allergic response in sensitized persons. Implicated antigens include foreign substances implanted accidentally into the skin (e.g., silicone in breast implants or endogenous antigens such as keratin). In many cases of granulomatous dermatitis, including sarcoidosis, the exact antigen is not known. Other common causes include mycobacterial and other infections (see Chapter 9) and granuloma annulare. Phagocytosis of the foreign particulate matter or processing of protein antigens is central to the activation of tissue macrophages as they become the characteristic granulomatous epithelioid cells (see Chapter 2).

Sarcoidosis May Lead to Skin Lesions

Sarcoidosis is a granulomatous disorder of unknown etiology that primarily affects the lungs but may also involve the skin, lymph nodes, spleen, eyes and other organs (see Chapter 12). Sarcoidal granulomas are the classic epithelioid cell type, without caseation necrosis (Fig. 24-37). Cutaneous manifestations of sarcoidosis are asymptomatic papules, plaques and nodules of the dermis and subcutis. Some dermal plaques may be annular, and those that involve the subcutis appear as irregular nodules. In severe cases, the cutaneous lesions are so prominent that they simulate a diffuse infiltrative neoplasm.

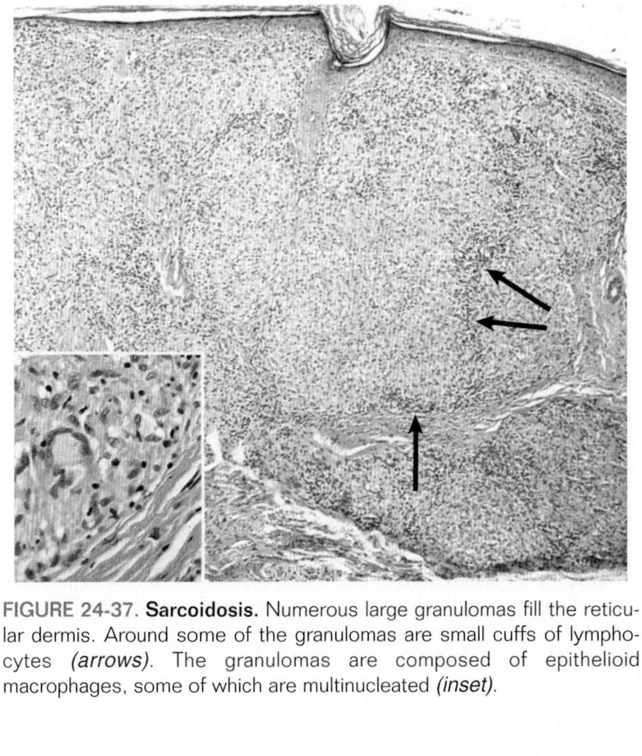

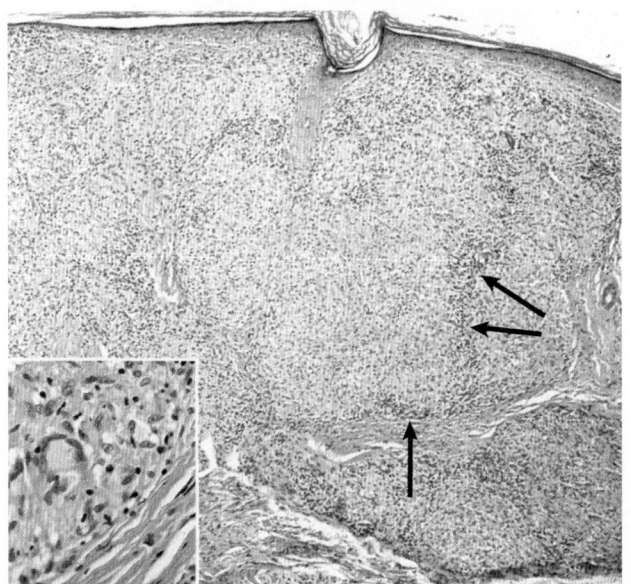

FIGURE 24-37. **Sarcoidosis.** Numerous large granulomas fill the reticular dermis. Around some of the granulomas are small cuffs of lymphocytes *(arrows)*. The granulomas are composed of epithelioid macrophages, some of which are multinucleated *(inset)*.

Granuloma Annulare Is a Reaction to an Unknown Antigen

Granuloma annulare is a benign, self-limited disorder of unknown etiology, characterized by palisading "necrobiotic" granulomas in the skin.

PATHOGENESIS: Granuloma annulare may be an immunologically mediated reaction to an unknown antigen. It can occur following insect bites, sun exposure, and viral infections. Antigenic stimuli are thought to include viral antigens, altered dermal collagen or elastic fibers or proteins in the saliva of biting arthropods. The precise type of immune reaction is unclear, but both circulating immune complexes and cell-mediated immunity may be involved. The activated macrophages may themselves contribute to the disease process by releasing lysosomal enzymes and cytokines that in turn cause focal collagen degeneration (so-called necrobiosis) characteristic of granuloma annulare.

PATHOLOGY: Well-developed lesions contain a central area of acellular degenerated collagen and mucin deposition (necrobiosis) in the superficial to mid-reticular dermis (Fig. 24-38). This central area is surrounded by palisaded macrophages, each with the long axis of the nucleus radiating outward. Occasional multinucleated cells are found along with a superficial perivascular lymphocytic infiltrate.

CLINICAL FEATURES: The most common type of granuloma annulare occurs on the dorsum of the hands and feet, primarily in children and young adults (see Fig. 24-38A). The disease features asymptomatic, skin-colored or erythematous annular plaques. About 15% of patients have disseminated granuloma annulare, with 10 or more lesions involving the trunk and neck. Granuloma annulare rarely requires treatment and usually has no medical consequences. In patients with significant cosmetic disfigurement, lesional injection of steroids is usually effective.

Scleroderma: A Disorder of the Dermal Connective Tissue

Scleroderma (Greek, *skleros*, hard) also displays variable structural and functional involvement of internal organs, including the kidneys, lungs, heart, esophagus, and small intestine. **Morphea** is similar to scleroderma, but involves only patchy, circumscribed areas of the skin. The pathogenesis and systemic manifestations of scleroderma are discussed in Chapters 4 and 16.

A
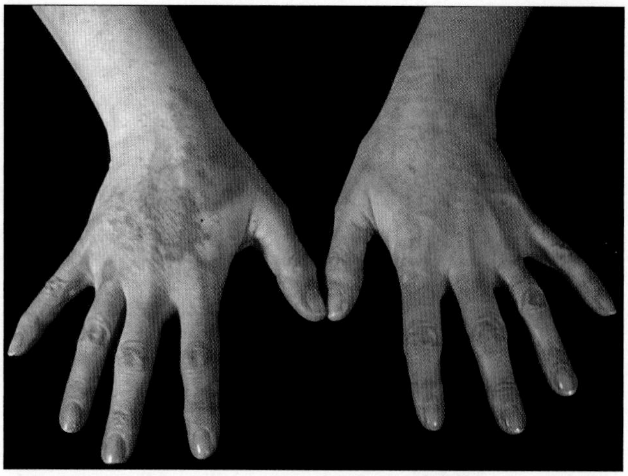

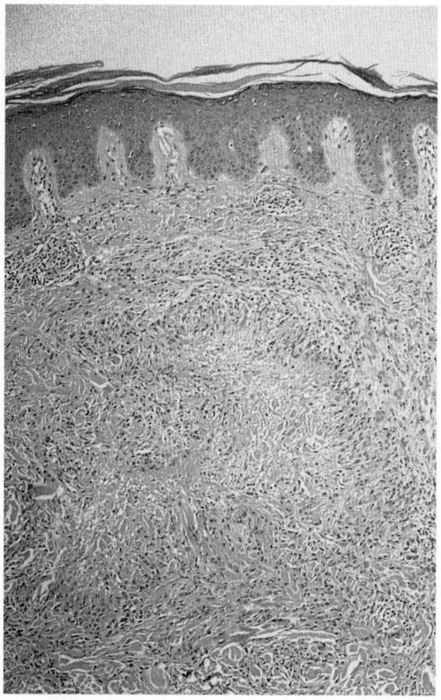
B

FIGURE 24-38. **Granuloma annulare. A.** The skin exhibits a typical annular plaque on the dorsal right hand. **B.** A central area of acellular degenerated collagen is surrounded by palisaded macrophages with the long axes of their nuclei radiating outward.

PATHOLOGY: The initial cutaneous lesions of scleroderma are in the lower reticular dermis, but eventually the entire reticular dermis and even the papillary dermis are involved. There is diminished space among collagen bundles in the reticular dermis and a tendency for the collagen bundles to be enlarged, hypocellular, and parallel to each other. A patchy lymphocytic infiltrate containing a few plasma cells is common and may also be present in the underlying subcutaneous tissue. Sweat ducts are entrapped in the thickened fibrous tissue. Normal fat around eccrine structures is lost. Hair follicles are completely obliterated (Fig. 24-39). In late stages of the disease, large areas of subcutaneous fat are replaced by newly formed collagen.

CLINICAL FEATURES: Scleroderma shows a peak incidence in persons between 30 and 50 years of age. Women are afflicted four times as often as men. Patients with early scleroderma usually present with Raynaud phenomenon (see Chapter 10) or nonpitting edema of the hands or fingers. Affected areas become hard and tense. The skin of the face becomes masklike and expressionless, and the skin around the mouth exhibits radial furrows. In late stages of the disease, the skin over large parts of the body is thickened, densely fibrotic and fixed to the underlying tissue. Prognosis is related to the extent of disease in visceral organs, particularly the lung and kidney.

Inflammatory Disorders of the Panniculus

Panniculitis denotes a heterogeneous group of diseases characterized by inflammation, mainly in the subcutis (panniculus). The various disorders gathered under the umbrella of panniculitis are classified according to their location. **Septal panniculitis** is inflammation in connective tissue septa, whereas **lobular panniculitis** denotes involvement of fat lobules. These two entities may occur with or without accompanying vasculitis.

Erythema Nodosum Is Related to Toxic and Infectious Agents

Erythema nodosum (EN) is a cutaneous disorder that manifests as self-limited, nonsuppurative, tender nodules over the extensor surfaces of the lower extremities. The disease has a peak incidence in the third decade of life and is three times more common in women than in men.

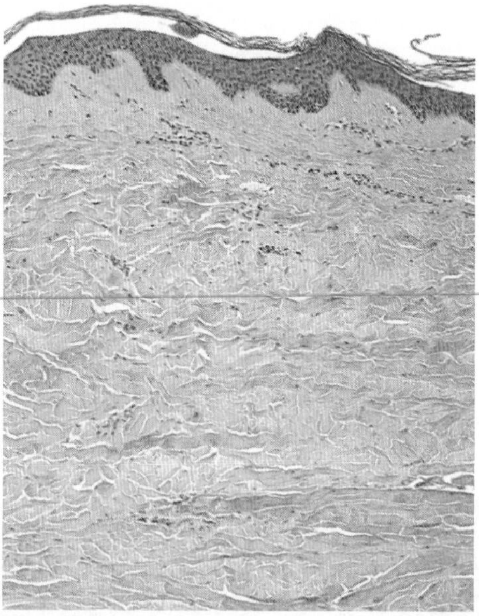

FIGURE 24-39. **Scleroderma.** The dermis is characterized by large, reticular collagen bundles that are oriented parallel to the epidermis. The large size and loss of basket-weave pattern of these collagen bundles are abnormal. No appendages are apparent because these structures have been destroyed.

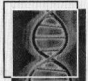

PATHOGENESIS: EN is triggered by exposure to a variety of agents, including drugs and microorganisms, and occurs in association with a number of benign and malignant systemic diseases. Common infections complicated by EN include streptococcal diseases (especially in children), tuberculosis, and *Yersinia* infection. In endemic areas deep fungal infections (blastomycosis, histoplasmosis, coccidioidomycosis) are common causes. EN also frequently occurs after acute respiratory tract infections of unknown etiology, but which are likely viral. The agents most commonly implicated in drug-induced EN are sulfonamides and oral contraceptives. Finally, Crohn disease and ulcerative colitis may be complicated by EN.

It is thought that EN represents an immunologic response to foreign antigens, although the evidence is indirect. For example, patients with tuberculosis or coccidioidomycosis do not develop EN until the skin test becomes positive, and testing with Frei antigen for lymphogranuloma venereum may itself induce EN. The early neutrophilic inflammation suggests that EN may be a response to complement activation, with resulting neutrophilic chemotaxis. Subsequent chronic inflammation, foreign body giant cells, and fibrosis are secondary to adipose tissue necrosis at the interface of septa and lobules.

PATHOLOGY: Early in the disease, EN lesions are in the fibrous septa of the subcutaneous tissue, where neutrophilic inflammation is associated with extravasation of erythrocytes. In chronic lesions, the septa are widened, with focal collections of giant cell macrophages around small areas of altered collagen, and an ill-defined lymphocytic infiltrate (Fig. 24-40). Giant cells and inflammatory cells extend into the lobule from the interface between the septum and the fat lobule. Secondary vascular involvement is occasionally noted.

CLINICAL FEATURES: EN typically manifests acutely on the anterior aspects of the lower limbs as dome-shaped, exquisitely tender, erythematous nodules. The nodules eventually become firm and less tender and disappear in 3 to 6 weeks. As some nodules heal, others arise, but all lesions resolve without residual scarring within 6 weeks.

Erythema Induratum Is Frequently Associated with Mycobaterium tuberculosis

Erythema induratum (EI) refers to chronic, recurrent subcutaneous nodules or plaques on the legs, predominantly in women. EI was traditionally considered a "tuberculid" (i.e., a hypersensitivity reaction to mycobacteria or associated antigens at a distant site). The failure of lesional tissue to yield isolates of mycobacteria in culture or in laboratory animals eventually cast doubt on this historical concept. However, subsequent investigations detected a specific *M. tuberculosis* DNA sequence in over 75% of skin biopsy specimens with EI.

PATHOLOGY: In contrast to EN, EI manifests initially as a lobular panniculitis, secondary to a vasculitis that produces ischemic necrosis of the fat lobule. The panniculus exhibits a dense, chronic inflammatory infiltrate within the lobules, which can form prominent tuberculoid granulomas or result in areas of coagulative necrosis. The lobular septa within the panniculus are relatively spared. The vascular changes are usually extensive and include (1) prominent infiltration of small and medium-sized arteries and veins by a dense lymphoid or granulomatous infiltrate; (2) endothelial swelling, which may progress to thrombosis; and (3) fibrous thickening of the intima. Extensive ischemic necrosis leads to subsequent ulceration of the overlying epidermis. Eventually, lesions heal by fibrosis.

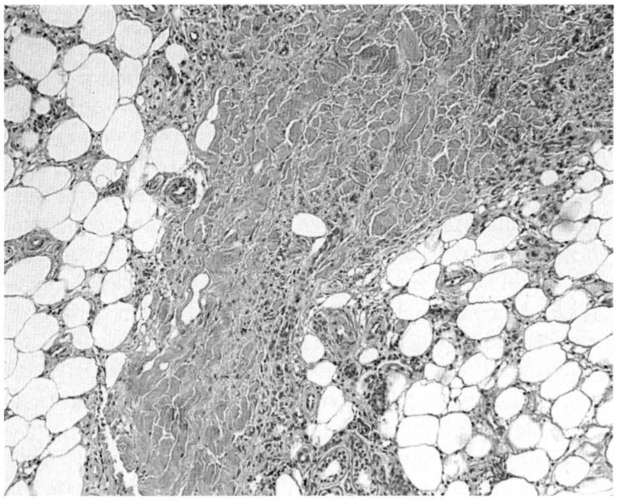

FIGURE 24-40. **Erythema nodosum.** The reticular dermis is present in *upper right.* Within the panniculus *(extending through the middle of the field)* is a widened septum. Lymphocytes and macrophages are present at its border with the adipose tissue lobules. The vessels palisading along the border of the septum are infiltrated by lymphocytes.

CLINICAL FEATURES: Patients with EI present with recurrent, tender, erythematous, subcutaneous nodules on the legs, particularly the calf. Lesions tend to ulcerate and heal with an atrophic scar. The course may last many years, and systemic steroids are usually necessary to control the disease.

Acne Vulgaris: A Disorder of the Pilosebaceous Unit

Acne vulgaris is a self-limited, inflammatory disorder of sebaceous follicles that typically afflicts adolescents, results in intermittent formation of discrete papular or pustular lesions and may lead to scarring. It is cosmetically disfiguring and often psychologically debilitating. Acne is so common that many regard it as a "rite of passage" through adolescence. In some cases, acne extends as long as the third decade.

PATHOGENESIS AND PATHOLOGY: The development of acne is related to (1) excessive hormonally induced production of sebum, (2) abnormal cornification of portions of the follicular epithelium, (3) a response to the anaerobic diphtheroid

Propionibacterium acnes, and (4) follicle rupture and subsequent inflammation. The sebaceous follicle contains a vellus hair and prominent sebaceous glands. The change in hormonal status at puberty leads to sebum production in the follicle and altered cornification in the neck of the sebaceous follicle (infundibulum), effects that lead to dilation of the follicular canal. Another round of excessive sebum production is associated with desquamation of squamous cells and accretion of keratinous debris, providing a rich environment for *P. acnes* proliferation. These combined changes produce a distended, plugged follicle, a **comedone.** Neutrophils attracted to the area by chemotactic factors released by *P. acnes,* release hydrolytic enzymes to form a follicular abscess (**pustule**). They also attack the follicle wall, thereby permitting escape of sebum, keratin, and bacteria into perifollicular tissue, where they stimulate further acute inflammation and a perifollicular abscess (Fig. 24-41). The development of an allergy to *P. acnes* intensifies the inflammatory response. Fully evolved lesions show intense neutrophilic inflammation surrounding a ruptured sebaceous follicle. In addition, numerous macrophages, lymphocytes, and foreign body giant cells accumulate in response to sebaceous follicle rupture.

CLINICAL FEATURES: Acne vulgaris features a variety of skin lesions in different stages of development, including comedones, papules, pustules, nodules, cysts, and pitted scars. Comedones, the primary noninflammatory lesions of acne, are either open (**blackheads**) or closed (**whiteheads**). More advanced inflammatory lesions vary from small, erythematous papules to large, tender, purulent nodules, and cysts.

Acne vulgaris is treated with topical cleansing and keratolytic and antibacterial agents. Severe cases are managed with topical vitamin A, systemic antibiotics, and synthetic oral retinoids (isotretinoin).

Infections and Infestations

The skin is under constant assault from countless marauders and is an effective but imperfect barrier against them: bacteria, fungi, viruses, parasites, and insects sometimes penetrate this first line of defense.

Impetigo Is an Infection by Staphylococci or Streptococci

Superficial bacterial infections of the skin, known as **impetigo**, occur mostly in children, who are often infected through minor breaks in the skin. Adults tend to contract impetigo after an underlying disease process that somehow compromises the barrier function of the skin. Honey-colored crusted erosions or ulcers, often with central healing, are present most commonly on exposed areas such as the face, hands, and extremities (Fig. 24-42). A combination of topical and systemic antimicrobial agents against staphylococci or streptococci is the mainstay of therapy. Ecthyma occurs when the organisms invade the superficial aspects of the skin to form a necrotizing ulcerated lesion in the dermis.

PATHOLOGY: Microscopically, neutrophils accumulate beneath the stratum corneum. Bacteria may be identified with special stains. Vesicles or bullae form and eventually rupture, allowing a thin, seropurulent discharge to appear. This discharge dries and forms the characteristic layers of exudate containing neutrophils and cellular debris. Reactive epidermal changes (spongiosis and elongation of the rete ridges) and superficial dermal inflammation are usually present.

Superficial Fungal Infections Are Caused by Dermatophytes

Dermatophytes are fungi that can infect nonviable keratinized epithelium, including stratum corneum, nails, and hair. They synthesize keratinases that digest keratin and provide sustenance for the organisms. Superficial fungal infections are often caused by a change in the microenvironment of the skin, which allows overgrowth of transient or resident flora. For example, use of immunosuppressive agents such as topical or systemic glucocorticoids may impair cell-mediated immune responses that normally eliminate dermatophytes. Excessive sweating or occlusion of a body part may provide an environment that "tips the balance" between fungal proliferation and elimination in favor of proliferation.

Of the 10 or so dermatophyte species that often cause human cutaneous infection, *Trichophyton rubrum* is the most common. A superficial dermatophyte infection is called a **dermatophytosis, tinea,** or **ringworm**. The tineas have distinctive clinical features depending on the site of infection. They are divided as follows: (1) **tinea capitis** (scalp; "ringworm"), (2) **tinea barbae** (beard), (3) **tinea faciei** (face), (4) **tinea corporis** (trunk, legs, arms, or neck, excluding the feet, hands, and groin), (5) **tinea manus** (hands), (6) **tinea pedis** (feet; "athlete's foot"; Fig. 24-43A), (7) **tinea cruris** (groin, pubic area, and thigh; "jock itch") and (8) **tinea unguium** (nails; "onychomycosis").

Other causes of superficial fungal infections are *Candida* species and *Malassezia furfur. Candida* species require a warm, moist environment in which to flourish, such as that found on a baby's bottom encased in a wet diaper. *M. furfur* requires a moist, lipid-rich environment. **Tinea versicolor**, caused by *M. furfur,* is more common in young adults when sebum production is greatest. Variably sized, pigmented, sharply demarcated, round or oval macules with fine scales are present, predominantly on the upper trunk.

Special stains such as PAS show budding yeast and hyphal forms in the most superficial layers of the stratum corneum. Hyperkeratosis, epidermal hyperplasia, and chronic perivascular inflammation are noted in the dermis (see Fig. 24-43B,C).

Deep Fungal Infections May Reflect Dissemination of Pulmonary Infections

Most invasive or systemic fungal infections arise from inhalation of aerosolized material contaminated with organisms such as *Histoplasma* or *Blastomyces*. A primary pulmonary infection may then spread to the skin or mucosa. Locally invasive fungal infections of the skin are rare and usually arise from traumatic implantation of organisms such as *Sporothrix* or *Fonsecaea*. An underlying immunocompromised state increases the likelihood of dissemination of fungal organisms.

Deep extension of a local cutaneous infection often results in a chancrelike lesion at the site of implantation. Intervening lymphatic vessels may become indurated and thickened. Nodules and ulcerations, especially those found bilaterally, suggest an internal source of infection.

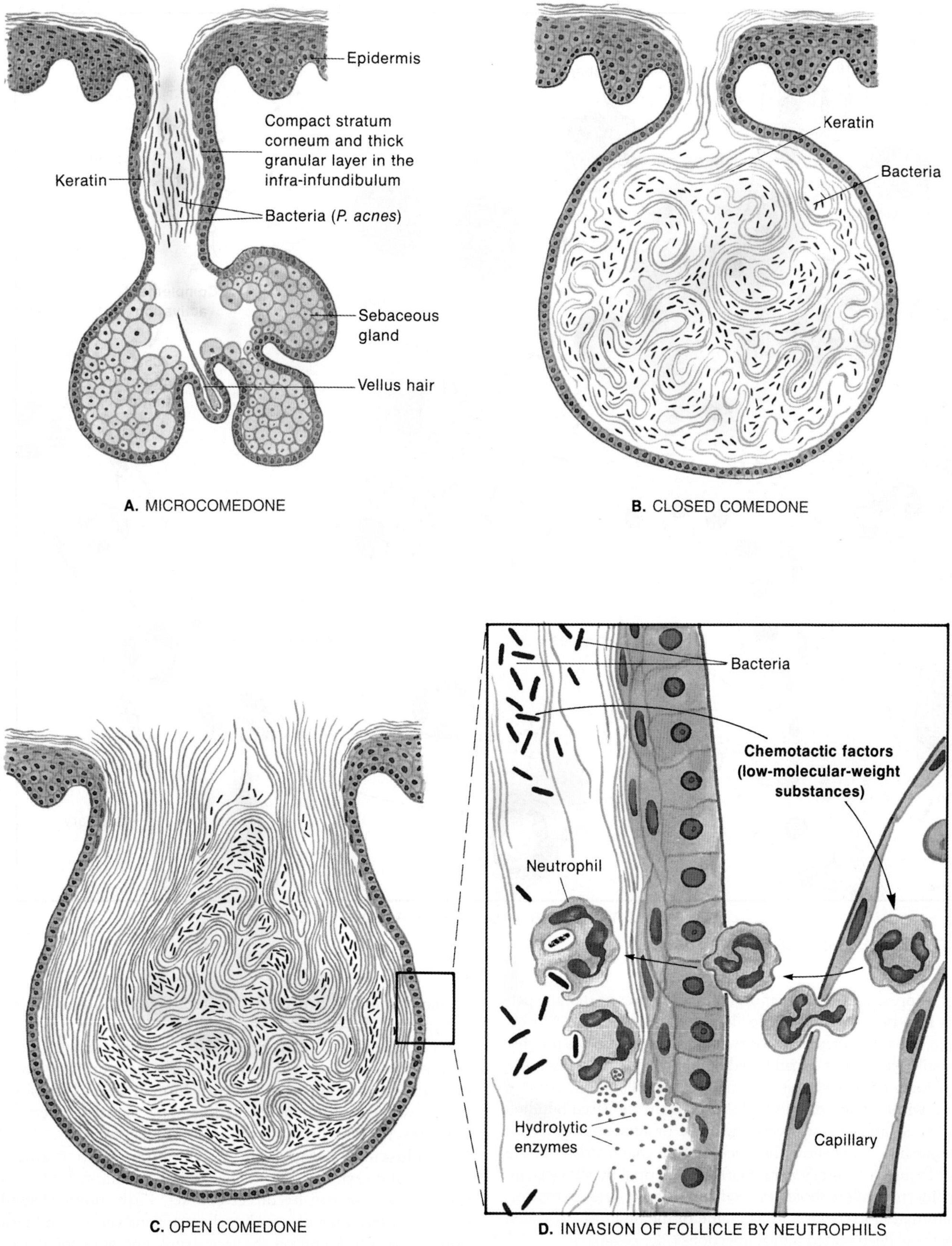

FIGURE 24-41. **Acne vulgaris.** The pathogenesis of follicular distention, rupture, and inflammation is depicted. Acne is a disease of the follicular canal of a sebaceous follicle. A compact stratum corneum and a thickened granular layer in the infrainfundibulum are the beginning of the formation of a comedone. Microcomedones (**A**), and closed (**B**) and open (**C**) comedones form. Excessive sebum secretion occurs, and the bacterium *Propionibacterium acnes* proliferates. The organism produces chemotactic factors, leading to neutrophil migration into the intact comedone. Neutrophilic enzymes are released, and the comedone ruptures, inducing a cycle of chemotaxis and intense neutrophilic inflammation (**D** and **E**).

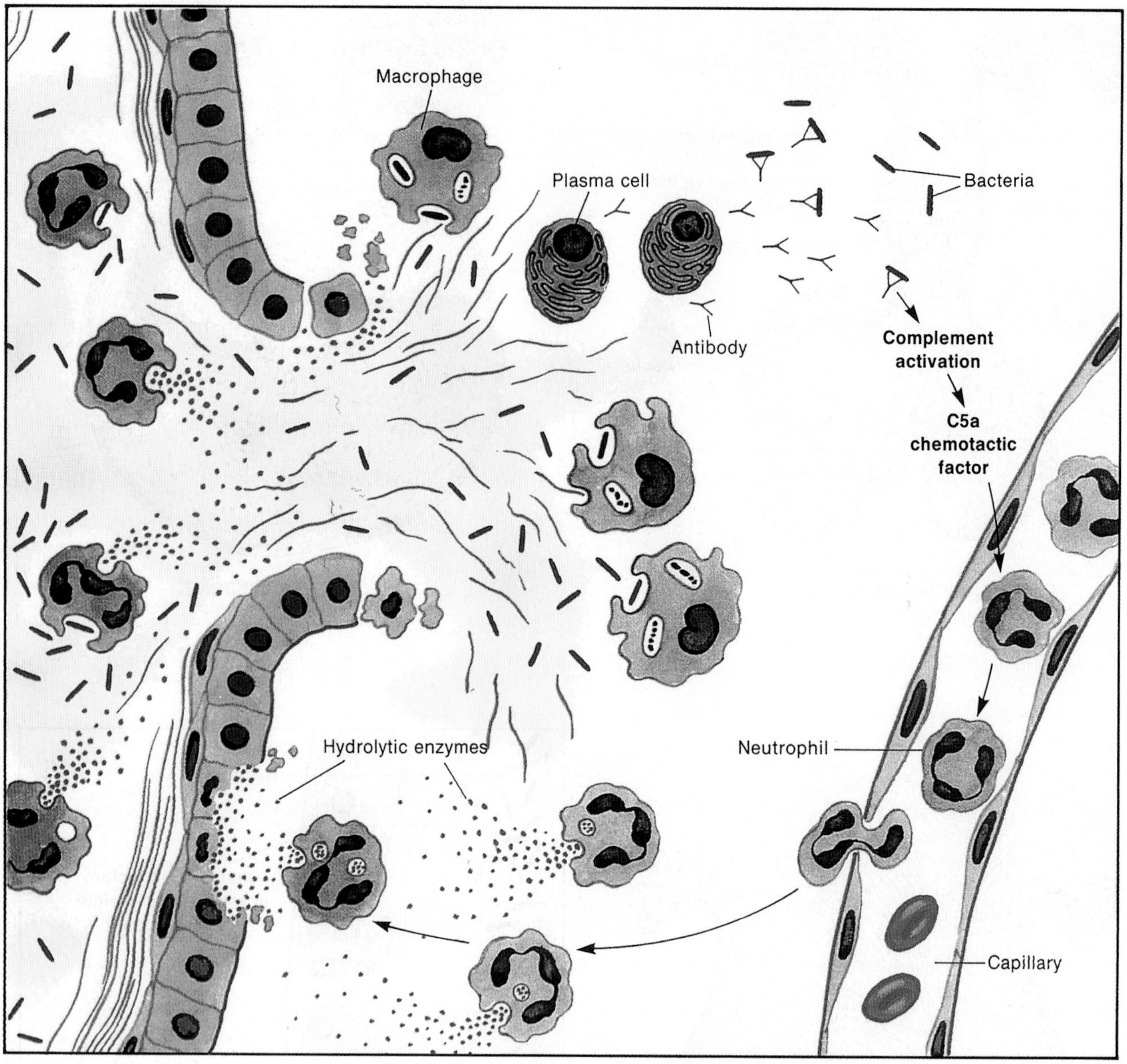

E. INFLAMMATION AND RUPTURE OF SEBACEOUS FOLLICLE

FIGURE 24-41. *(continued)*

The presence of certain morphologic features or staining patterns may provide clues to the identity of the organism. For example, the yeast form of *Blastomyces dermatitidis* displays notably refractile walls and a broad-based budding pattern, whereas the yeast form of *Histoplasma capsulatum* is much smaller, is often found within macrophages and shows a narrow-based budding pattern. Staining a smear with India ink, or a tissue biopsy with mucicarmine, may show the thick capsule characteristic of the yeast *Cryptococcus neoformans*. Marked epidermal hyperplasia, intraepidermal microabscesses, and suppurative granulomatous inflammation in the dermis are some of the findings associated with these deep-seated fungal infections (Fig. 24-44).

Viral Infections Cause a Variety of Skin Lesions

The dermatoses caused by viruses are numerous and include a wide spectrum of clinical manifestations (see Chapter 9). Some viruses, such as the poxvirus **molluscum contagiosum** or the **human papillomaviruses** (HPVs) (see below), cause transient benign epithelial proliferations that resolve spontaneously. Others (e.g., measles or *parvovirus* [erythema infectiosum]) cause febrile illnesses with self-limited cutaneous eruptions (exanthems). Primary infection by most **human herpesviruses** is often asymptomatic but results in a state of latent infection. Upon reactivation, the virus causes a vesicular eruption.

Molluscum contagiosum is a common infection among children and sexually active adults. It is a self-limited infection that is easily spread by direct contact. Firm, dome-shaped, smooth-surfaced papules with a characteristic central umbilication are usually found on the face, trunk and anogenital area. Microscopic examination shows epidermal cells containing large intracytoplasmic inclusion bodies ("molluscum bodies"), which are found within cup-shaped areas that also exhibit verrucous (papillomatous) epidermal hyperplasia. Numerous viral particles are present within these inclusion bodies (Fig. 24-45).

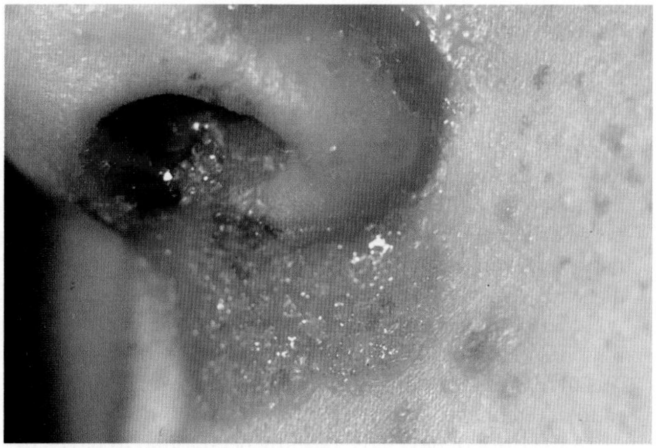

FIGURE 24-42. **Impetigo contagiosa.** Honey-colored crusts secondary to rupture of vesicopustules are seen in the nasal area of a child, an area commonly colonized by *Staphylococcus aureus.*

Arthropod Infestations Produce Pruritic Skin Lesions

Mites and lice, other insects, and spiders produce local lesions that may be intensely pruritic.

- ***Scabies*** *is* a severely pruritic, eczematous dermatitis caused by the mite *Sarcoptes scabei.* The female mite burrows beneath the stratum corneum on the fingers, wrists, trunk, and genital skin (Fig. 24-46). Intense lymphocytic and eosinophilic dermatitis is induced as a hypersensitivity reaction to the mite and its eggs and feces.
- ***Pediculosis,*** another pruritic dermatosis, may be caused by a variety of human lice. Eggs ("nits") of the lice may be found attached to hair shafts.
- **Biting insects** produce lesions that vary from small, pruritic papules to large, weeping nodules. The reaction depends on the particular arthropod species and the host immune response. For example, tick bites tend to be large, with a striking lymphocytic and eosinophilic infiltrate. Lymphoid follicles may also form. Flea bites are usually urticarial, with a scant neutrophilic infiltrate. The venoms injected by arthropods such as the brown recluse spider may lead to severe local tissue necrosis.

Primary Neoplasms of the Skin

Cutaneous tumors are a paradigm for understanding neoplasia in general. These lesions are on the body surface, where their development and evolution may be readily observed. The availability of tumor tissue from the developmentally sequential lesions has permitted the correlation of studies of tumor cells in vitro with the observed behavior of clinical lesions.

The incidence of malignant melanoma, in particular, is increasing at an alarming rate. It is estimated that over 1% of children born today will develop malignant melanoma. The

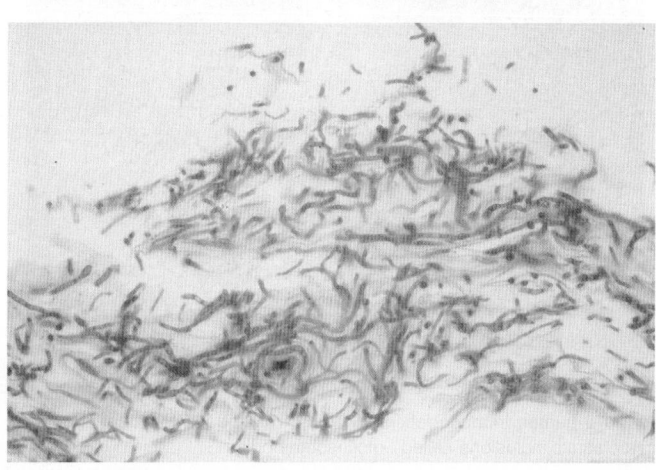

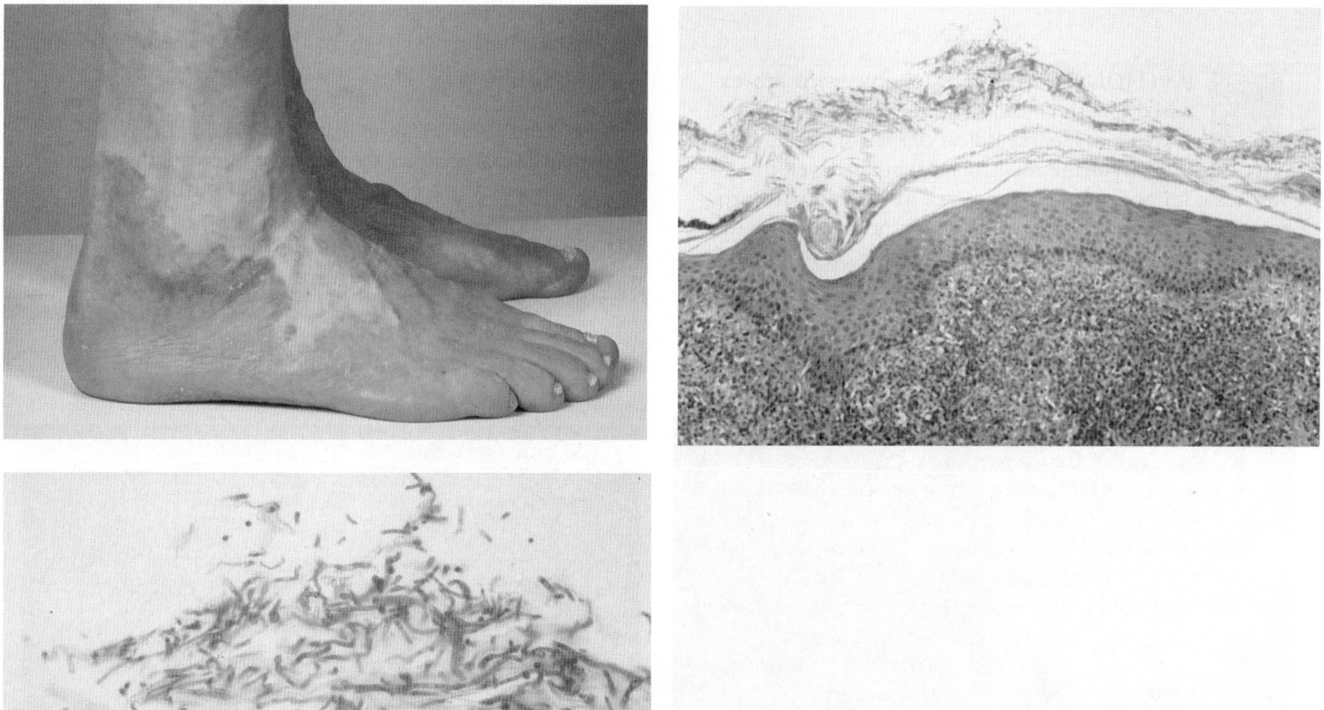

A

B

C

FIGURE 24-43. **Dermatophytosis. A.** Tinea pedis. A leading edge of scale and erythema in a moccasin distribution characterizes this infection, most commonly caused by *Trichophyton rubrum.* **B.** A dense inflammatory infiltrate is present in the epidermis and dermis and is associated with the presence of fungal hyphae in the stratum corneum. **C.** A higher power view of the fungal hyphae in the stratum corneum.

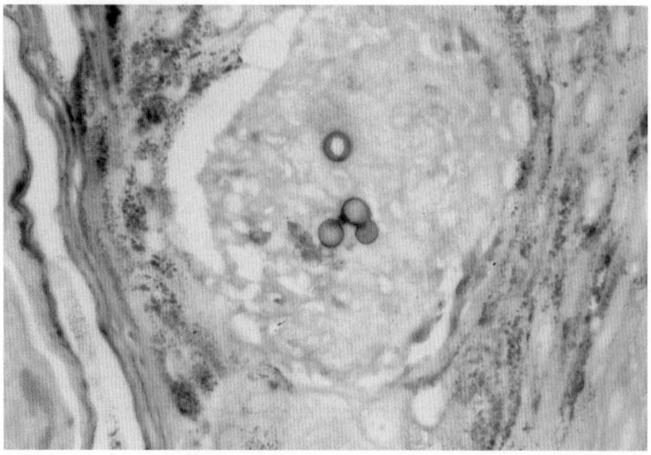

FIGURE 24-44. **Blastomycosis.** A period acid-Schiff stain highlights the organisms, which are thick-walled spores 8 to 15 microns in diameter. One of the organisms demonstrates broad-based budding.

prognosis of most melanomas is excellent if lesions are recognized and excised before entering a vertical growth phase. However, if the tumor exceeds a critical depth in the dermis, many patients will die of metastatic disease.

Common Acquired Melanocytic Nevus (Mole) Is a Localized Proliferation of Melanocytes Within the Epidermis or Dermis

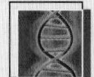

PATHOGENESIS: Most people who are exposed to a significant amount of light in the first 15 years of life, regardless of their skin color, develop 10 to 50 nevi on their skin. Black skin can develop nevi, but less commonly and they are not associated with progression to melanoma. However, if nevi are located on the palms of the hands, the soles of the feet or on the genital skin, the risk of melanoma is the same in all races. Nevi do not ordinarily develop in areas protected from light by at least two layers of clothing, such as the breasts of women. Red-haired, blue-eyed persons with milk-white skin are notable exceptions, in that they are exquisitely sensitive to light and form freckles, but they do not develop a significant number of nevi. There is an unequivocal causal relationship between ultraviolet light and melanocytic nevi (and malignant melanoma), but the relationship is complex; some people with fair skin form relatively few nevi, whereas some with dark skin develop numerous nevi. The ability to form nevi has been correlated with polymorphic variants of the melanocortin receptor and with subsequent variation in the ratio of red pheomelanin to brown eumelanin.

A majority of nevi have recently been found to have an activating mutation of the gene encoding the oncogene *B-RAF*, which can lead to growth stimulation through the mitogen-activated protein kinase (MAP-kinase) pathway. However, after an initial period of growth, nevi are stable lesions. This observation may involve the suppressor activity of p16, an inhibitor of the cyclin-mediated cell cycle mechanism encoded by the gene *CDKN2A* on chromosome 9p21, which is commonly lost in melanoma progression.

Epidemiologic studies have shown melanocytic nevi to be potential precursor lesions for melanomas. A person with 100 or more nevi that are 2 to 5 mm in greatest dimension has a threefold greater risk of developing melanoma than a person with fewer than 25 similar nevi. Patients with clinically atypical-appearing nevi or histologically proven dysplastic nevi are at even greater risk for melanoma. As nevi are very common and melanomas are rare, the risk of progression of any one nevus is small.

Melanocytic nevi begin to appear between the first and second years of life and continue to emerge for the first 2 decades of life. A nevus first appears as a small tan dot no bigger than 1 to 2 mm in diameter. During the next 3 to 4 years, the dot enlarges to become a uniform tan to brown circular or oval area. The peripheral outline usually remains regular. When it reaches 4 to 5 mm in diameter, it is flat or slightly elevated, stops enlarging peripherally and is sharply demarcated from surrounding normal skin. Over

A

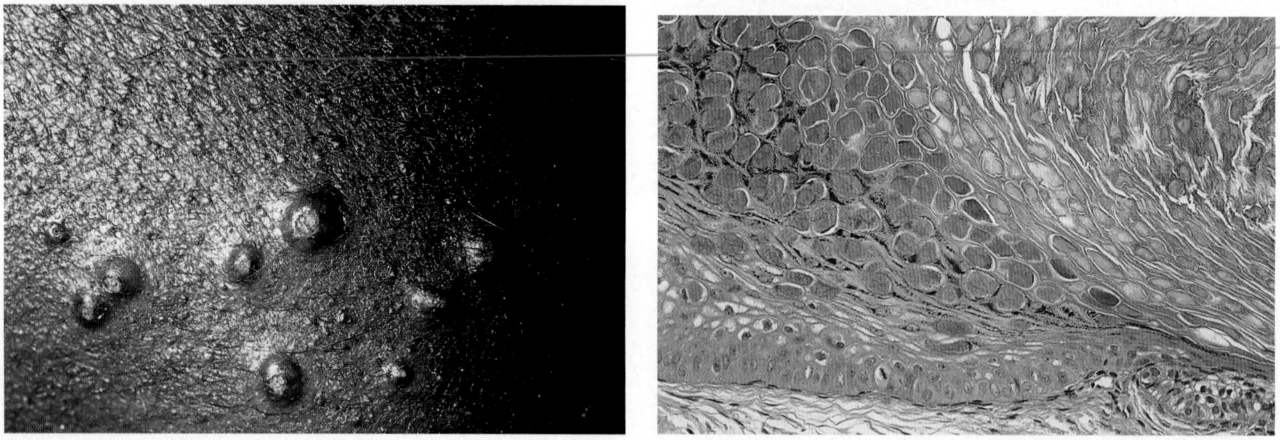

B

FIGURE 24-45. **Molluscum contagiosum. A.** Multiple umbilicated papules in a human immunodeficiency virus (HIV)-positive patient. **B.** The keratinocytes that are infected with this poxvirus show large eosinophilic cytoplasmic inclusions called "molluscum bodies."

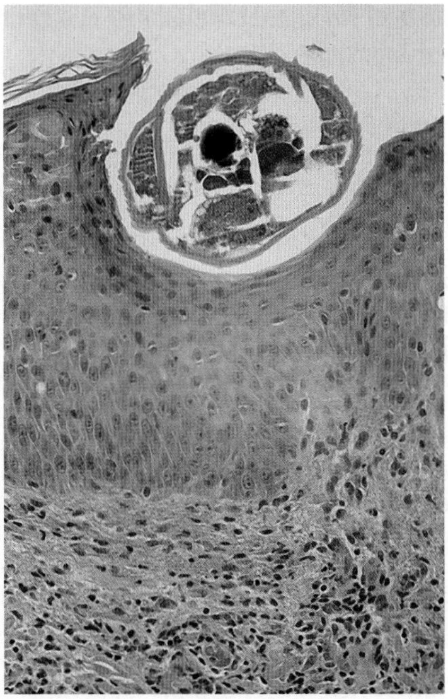

FIGURE 24-46. **Scabetic nodule.** A scabies mite is present in the stratum corneum.

the next 10 years, the lesion elevates and its color pales to the point of becoming a tan taglike protrusion. For the next decade or two, it gradually flattens and the skin may approximate a normal appearance. In most people number of nevis gradually decrease over time. Notably, many melanoma patients tend to retain increased numbers of nevi, including atypical ones, in the later decades of life.

PATHOLOGY: At the inception of a melanocytic nevus, melanocytes are increased in the basal epidermis, with subsequent hyperpigmentation. The melanocytes eventually form nests, frequently at tips of rete ridges, and then migrate into the dermis where they form small clusters. As the lesion becomes elevated, the dermal nevus cells begin to differentiate in a manner reminiscent of Schwann cells, an evolution that gradually encompasses the entire dermal component, leaving a core of delicate neuromesenchyme. The nevus may eventually flatten and possibly even disappear. The histologic classification of melanocytic nevi reflects the evolution of the lesions:

- **Junctional nevus:** Melanocytes form nests at the tips of epidermal rete ridges.
- **Compound nevus:** Nests of melanocytes are seen in the epidermis and some of the cells have migrated into the dermis (Fig. 24-47).
- **Dermal nevus:** Intraepidermal melanocytic growth has ceased (Fig. 24-48).

Dysplastic (Atypical) Nevus Is a Risk Marker for Melanoma

Some common acquired nevi do not follow the pattern of growth, differentiation, and disappearance described above. Such lesions persist and are often more than 5 mm in greatest dimension. These nevi may show foci of aberrant melanocytic growth

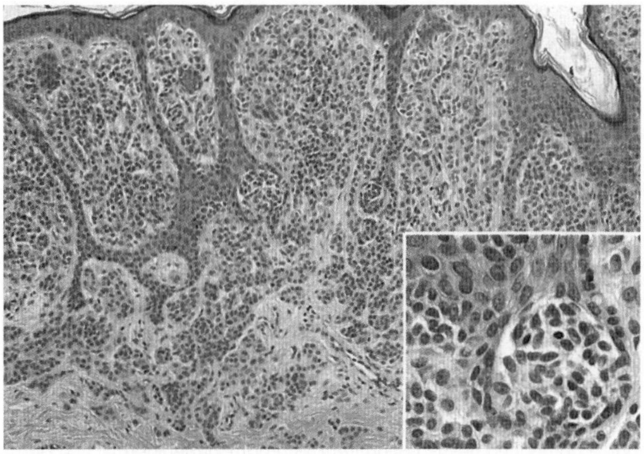

FIGURE 24-47. **Compound melanocytic nevus.** Melanocytes are present as nests within the epidermis and dermis. An intraepidermal nest of melanocytes is surrounded by keratinocytes *(inset).*

and become larger and more irregular peripherally. The irregular area is flat (macular) and extends asymmetrically from the parent nevus. Some clinically dysplastic nevi are entirely macular.

Germline mutations in the *CDKN2A* tumor-suppressor gene (also known as *p16* or *p16INK4a*), mapped to chromosome 9p21, have been found in some dysplastic nevus/melanoma patients and their family members. This gene encodes an inhibitor of cyclin-dependent kinase 4 (CDK4) that functions to suppress proliferation. Patients with dysplastic nevi are at increased risk of developing melanoma. The magnitude of this risk varies with the number of nevi, and is especially high in patients with a prior melanoma and/or a family history of melanoma. The genetic underpinnings of dysplastic nevi are not well understood, and are likely polygenic.

Melanocytic Dysplasia Features Architectural and Cytologic Atypia

Initially, the growth of melanocytes in the basal epidermis appears similar to that which occurs in the early stages of a common nevus. This area is abnormal in architectural pattern, not in cytologic features. A band of eosinophilic connective tissue ("lamellar fibroplasia") is seen around the rete ridges, which contain aberrantly growing melanocytes. These aberrant melanocytes may grow to become continuous streams of melanocytes extending from rete to rete ("bridging"). As these architectural features become more

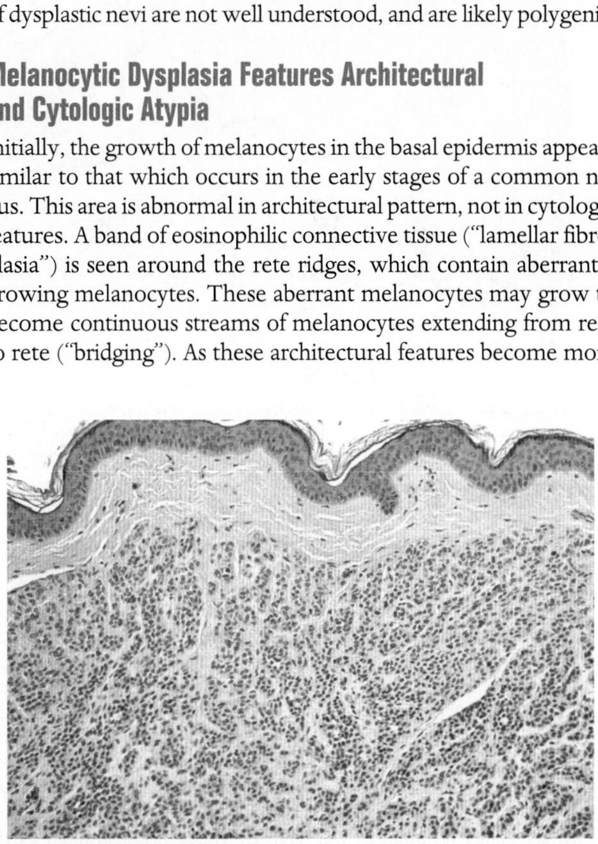

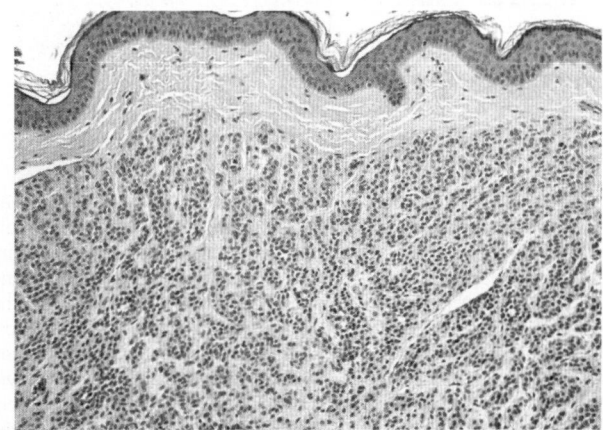

FIGURE 24-48. **Dermal melanocytic nevus.** The melanocytes are entirely confined to the dermis.

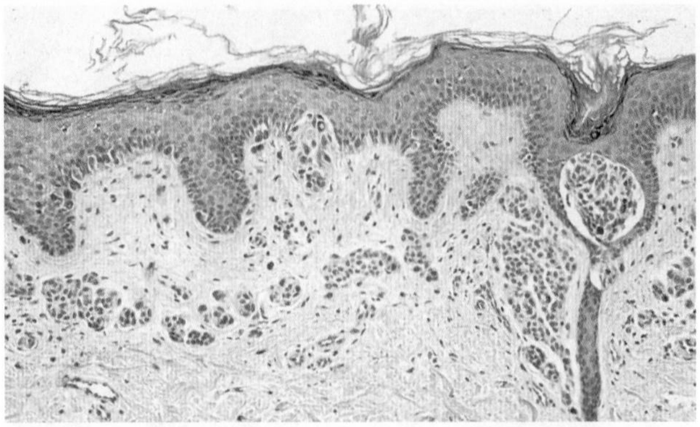

FIGURE 24-49. **Compound nevus with melanocytic dysplasia.** On the *right,* a compound nevus is apparent with both intraepidermal and dermal components. To the *left,* within the epidermis are single atypical melanocytes within the basal unit, as well as incipient lamellar fibroplasia. Dermal melanocytes are present *below.*

prominent, melanocytes with large atypical nuclei that are reminiscent of malignant cells may also appear in the areas of architectural disorder. This combination of architectural disorder and cytologic atypia constitutes a dysplastic nevus (Fig. 24-49 and Fig. 24-50). Areas of dysplasia may also be associated with a subjacent lymphocytic infiltrate. More than one third of malignant melanomas have a precursor nevus, most of which show melanocytic dysplasia. However, most dysplastic nevi are stable and will never progress to melanoma.

The Prognosis of Malignant Melanoma is a Function of the Depth of Invasion

Radial Growth Phase Melanoma

The most frequently encountered form of melanoma is the radial growth phase, also termed **superficial spreading melanoma** (Fig. 24-51).

PATHOLOGY: Large epithelioid melanocytes are dispersed in nests and as individual cells through the entire thickness of the epidermis. These melanocytes may be limited to the epidermis (**melanoma in situ**) or they may extend into the papillary dermis. In the radial growth phase, no nest has growth preference (larger size) over the other nests (Fig. 24-52), so the cells grow in all directions: upward in the epidermis, peripherally in the epidermis and downward into the dermis. Mitoses are not seen in dermal melanocytes. These lesions enlarge at the periphery, hence the term **radial.** Melanocytes of the radial growth phase are typically associated with a brisk lymphocytic response. Melanomas in the radial growth phase only rarely metastasize.

CLINICAL FEATURES: Superficial spreading melanoma (SSM) has been associated with a history of intermittent sun exposure and sunburn, and with activating mutations of the B-*raf* oncogene. Early melanomas in the radial growth phase have slightly elevated and palpable borders. The neoplasm is usually variably and haphazardly pigmented. Some parts are black or dark brown, whereas other areas may be

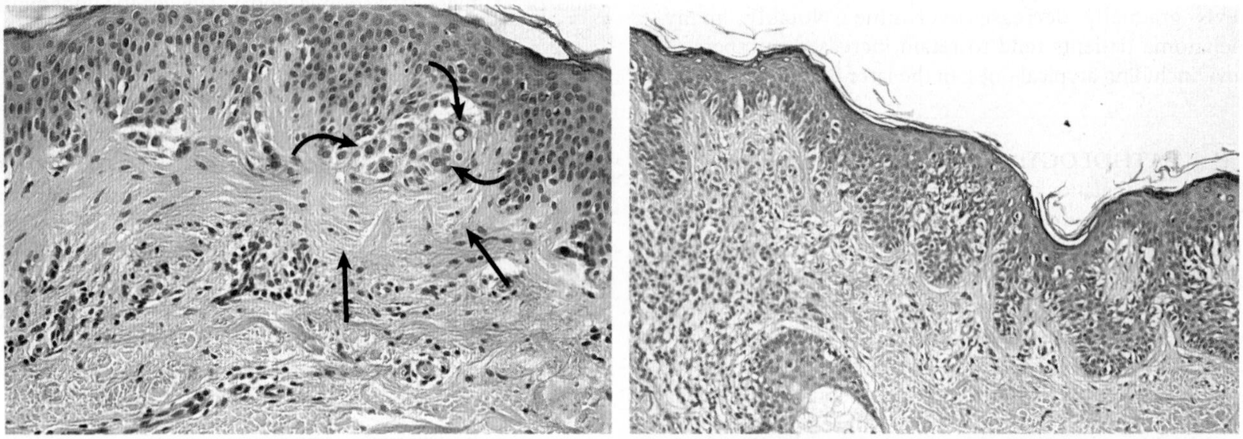

A

B

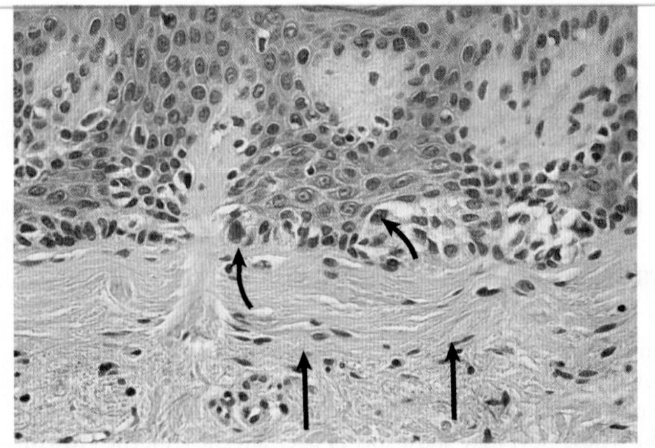

C

FIGURE 24-50. **Dysplastic nevus. A.** There is bridging of rete ridges by nests of melanocytes, melanocytes with cytological atypia *(curved arrows),* lamellar fibroplasia *(straight arrows),* and a scant perivascular lymphocytic infiltrate. **B.** To the *left* is a zone containing typical dermal nevic cells of a compound melanocytic nevus. In the epidermis on the *right* is a lentiginous proliferation of atypical melanocytes with lamellar fibroplasia. This photomicrograph is taken from the junction of the papular and macular components of this dysplastic nevus. Dysplasia usually develops in the macular portion, which takes up most of the field. **C.** These ellipsoid melanocytic nests resting above lamellar fibroplasia *(straight arrows)* exhibit large epithelioid melanocytes with atypia *(curved arrows).*

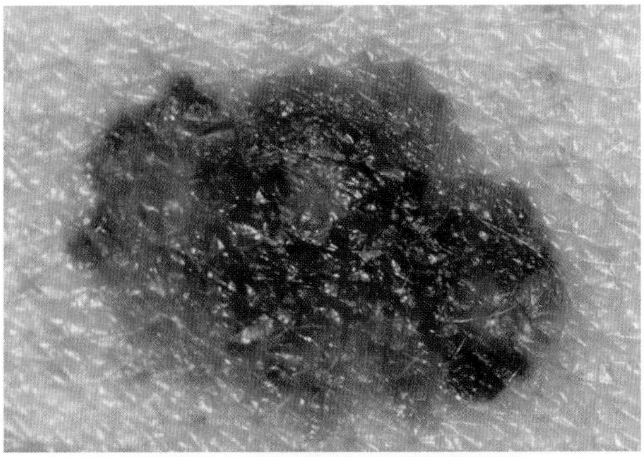

FIGURE 24-51. **The clinical appearance of the radial growth phase in malignant melanoma of the superficial spreading type.** The larger diameter is 1.8 cm.

lighter brown, possibly mixed with pink or light blue tints. The entire lesion may be purely dark brown (see Fig. 24-51). With regard to lesions that are eventually documented to be melanoma, patients frequently state that a change in a nevus occurred. Such changes can include itching, increase in size, darkening, or bleeding and oozing, though the last signs tend to appear later. Even in the absence of such observations on the part of the patient, any lesion that prompts clinical suspicion of melanoma warrants an excisional biopsy. The "ABCD rule" is a convenient mnemonic that is commonly taught to patients to help them recognize changes in nevi that should prompt them to seek medical attention: **A**symmetry of shape, **B**order irregularity, **C**olor variation, and a **D**iameter more than 6 mm. However, not all early melanomas exhibit these attributes, and any changing lesion should be evaluated for excisional biopsy.

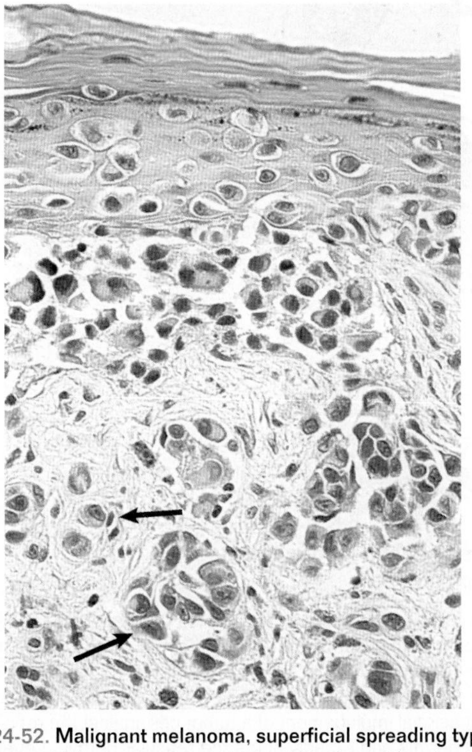

FIGURE 24-52. **Malignant melanoma, superficial spreading type, radial growth phase.** Melanocytes grow singly within the epidermis at all levels and as large, irregularly sized nests at the dermal–epidermal junction. Tumor cells are present in the papillary dermis *(arrows),* but no nest shows preferential growth over the others.

Vertical Growth Phase Melanoma

After a variable time (usually 1 to 2 years), the character of growth begins to change. Melanocytes exhibit mitotic activity and grow as spheroid nodules that expand more rapidly than the rest of the tumor in the surrounding papillary dermis (Fig. 24-53). The net direction of growth tends to be perpendicular to that of the radial growth phase, hence the term **vertical** (Fig. 24-54 through Fig. 24-56).

PATHOLOGY: The more specific characteristics of vertical growth phase are:

- The melanocytes tend to differ in appearance from those of the radial growth phase. For example, they may contain little or no pigment, whereas the cells of the radial growth phase are melanotic.
- The cellular aggregate that characterizes the vertical growth phase is larger than the clusters of melanocytes that form the intraepidermal and invasive components of the radial growth phase. The dominant site of tumor growth shifts from the epidermis to the dermis.
- Tumors that extend into the lower half of the reticular dermis are considered to be in vertical growth phase.
- The host immune response may be absent at the base of the vertical growth phase.
- Markers of cell cycle progression, such as Ki-67, increase in cells of the vertical growth phase.

Even when tumors enter vertical growth phase, they may still lack the propensity to metastasize. Thus, vertical growth phase melanomas less than 1.7 mm thick that lack mitoses and exhibit a brisk infiltrate of lymphocytes rarely metastasize. Vertical growth phase melanomas more than 3.6 mm thick, with more than 6 mitoses/mm^2, and without tumor-infiltrating lymphocytes frequently metastasize. Lesions intermediate between

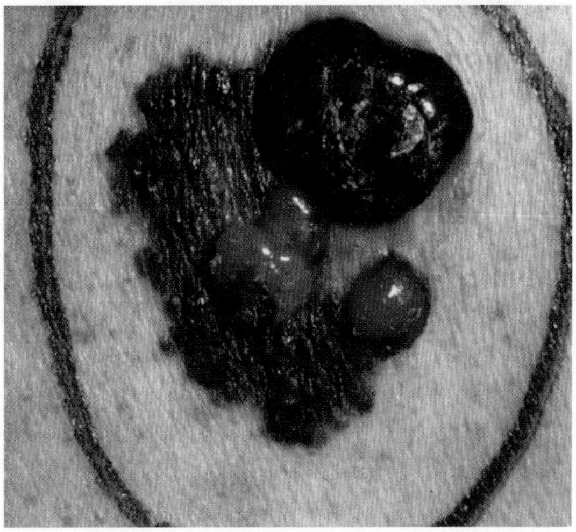

FIGURE 24-53. **Malignant melanoma.** The superficial spreading type is represented by the relatively flat, dark, brown–black portion of the tumor. Three areas in this lesion are characteristic of the vertical growth phase. All are nodular in configuration; two have a pink coloration, and the largest is a rich, ebony black.

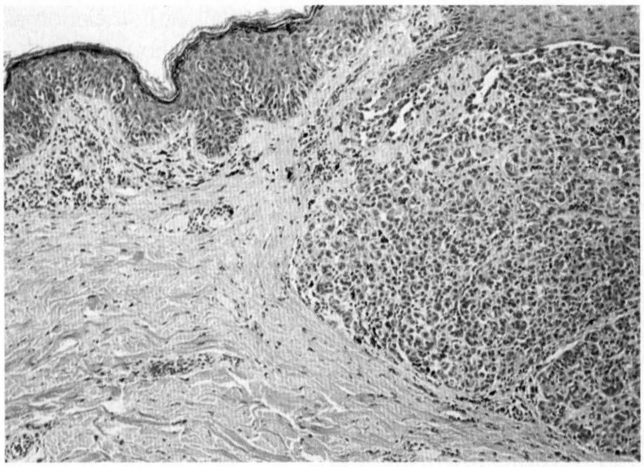

FIGURE 24-54. **Malignant melanoma, superficial spreading type, vertical growth phase.** Vertical growth is manifested by the distinct spheroid tumor nodule to the *right*. A focus of melanocytes clearly has a growth advantage (larger size) over other nests in the radial growth phase *(left)*. The nodule distorts the papillary dermal–reticular dermal junction and therefore is level III.

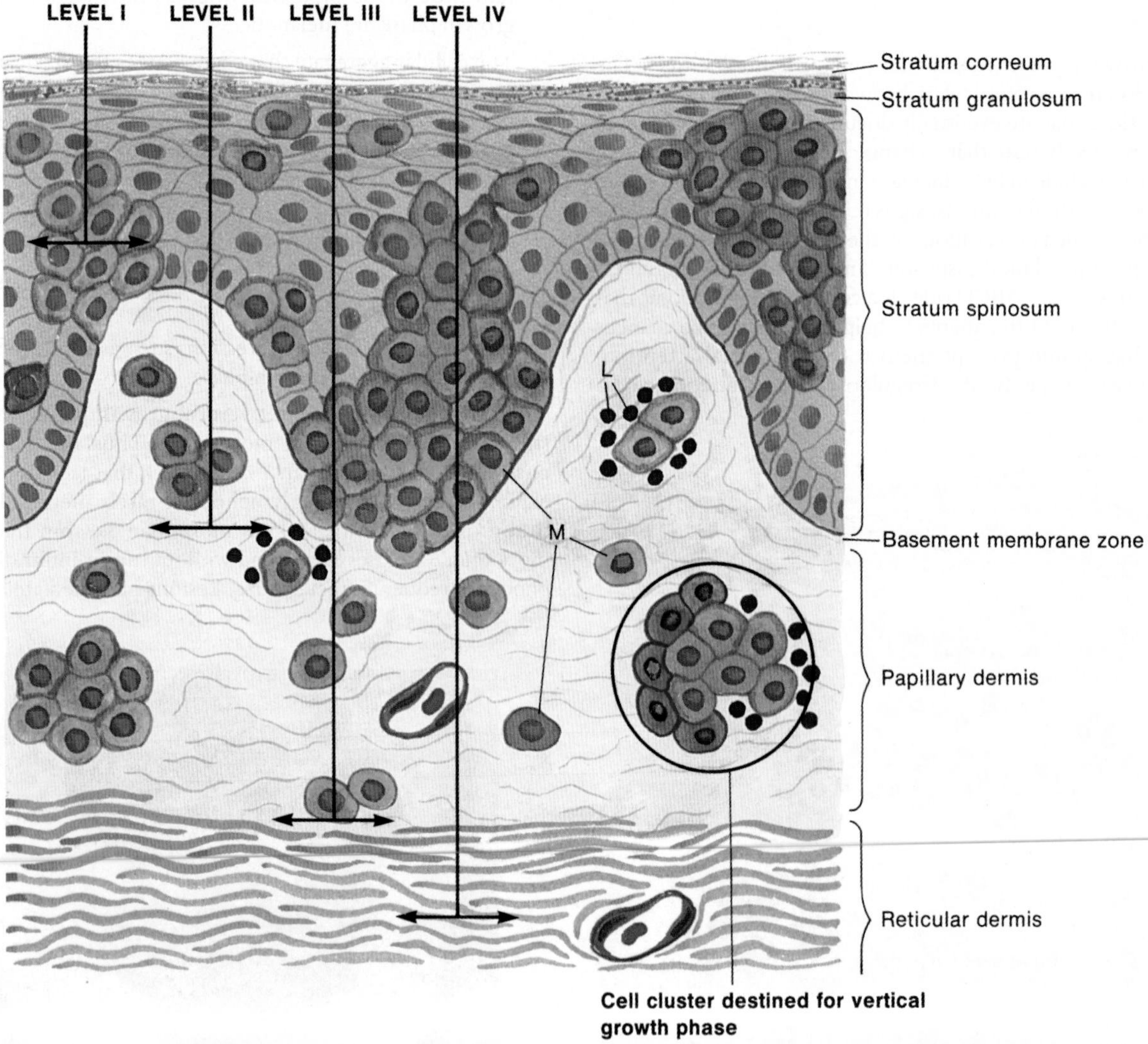

FIGURE 24-55. **Malignant melanoma.** In the radial growth phase, cells grow in the epidermis and are present in the dermis. They grow in all directions: outward, peripherally, and downward. The net direction of growth is peripheral—along the radii of an imperfect circle. Growth, as manifested by mitotic activity, is largely in the epidermis. No cells in the dermis seem to have a growth preference over others. The nest depicted here is shown as it evolves into the vertical growth phase in Figures 24-54 and 24-55. The anatomical landmarks of the levels of invasion are shown. Level III is not simply the occasional impingement of a tumor cell against the reticular dermis but indicates a collection of cells that fills and widens the papillary dermis and broadly abuts the reticular dermis. Level III invasion is usually a manifestation of the vertical growth phase. Level IV invasion should be designated only when tumor cells clearly permeate between otherwise unaltered collagen bundles of the reticular dermis.

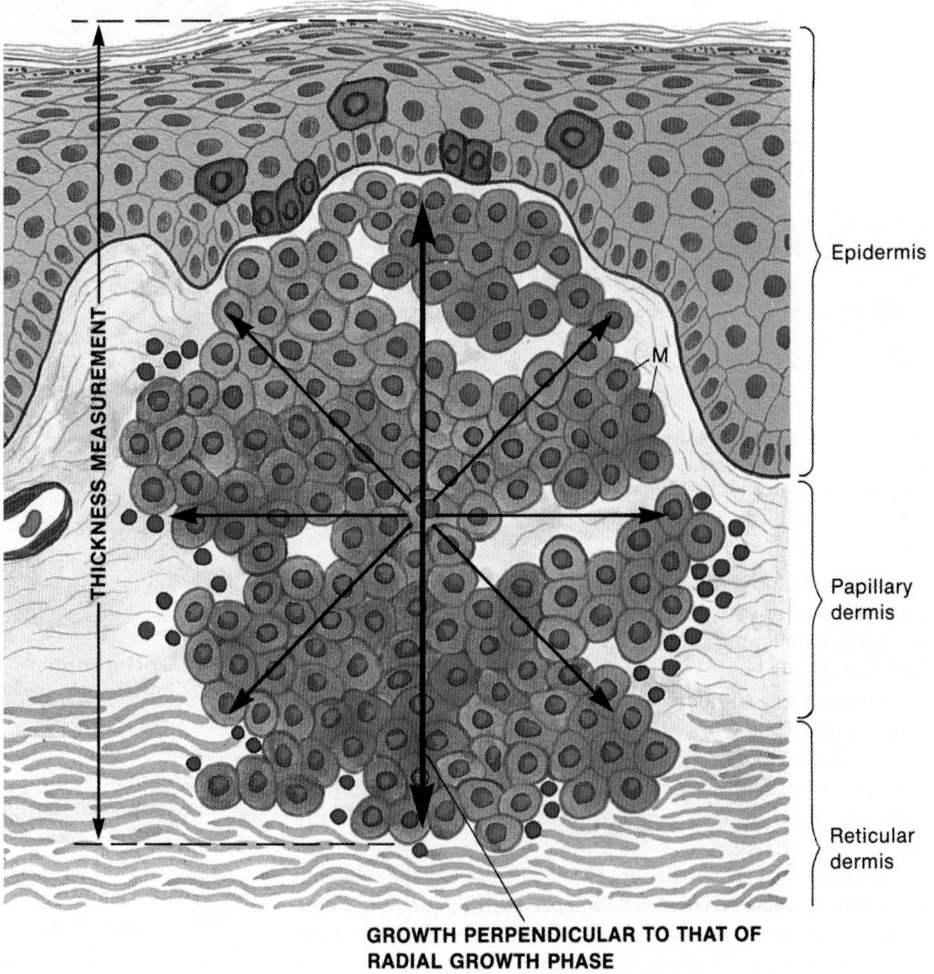

FIGURE 24-56. **Malignant melanoma.** The evolved vertical growth phase in malignant melanoma of the superficial spreading type is shown, with an indication of how thickness is measured. In this illustration, the vertical growth phase has extended into the reticular dermis. Small nodules of tumor cells that clearly have a growth preference over other tumor cells may be a manifestation of the vertical growth phase. Thickness measurements *(arrows)* are taken from the outermost granular layer across the tumor in its thick-

these extremes can be recognized and their behavior predicted through the use of prognostic models, albeit imperfectly.

Metastatic Melanoma

Metastatic melanoma arises from the melanocytes of the vertical growth phase. Initial metastases usually involve regional lymph nodes, although hematogenous spread is also possible. When the latter occurs, metastases are unusually widespread in comparison with other neoplasms; virtually any organ may be involved. Many metastatic melanomas remain dormant for long periods, only to reappear years after excision of the primary tumor.

Nodular Melanoma

Occasionally, a melanoma "bypasses" the stepwise tumor progression described above and manifests all of its malignant characteristics in the initial lesion. Nodular melanoma is an uncommon form of the tumor (10%). It appears as a circumscribed, elevated, spheroidal nodule. It does not develop through a radial growth phase but is in the vertical growth phase when initially observed (Fig. 24-57). Histologically, nodular melanoma is composed of one or more nodules of cells that grow in an expansile fashion in the dermis (Fig. 24-58 and Fig. 24-59).

Lentigo Maligna Melanoma

Lentigo maligna melanoma, also known as **Hutchinson's melanotic freckle**, is a large, pigmented macule that occurs on sun-damaged skin. It develops almost exclusively in fair-skinned, usually elderly, whites. Because it occurs on exposed body surfaces, it is probably related to chronic ultraviolet light exposure, without acute episodes of sunburn and often in outdoor workers. Lentigo maligna melanoma, like acral and mucosal melanomas (see below), is less likely than superficial spreading melanoma to be associated with mutation of B-*raf*.

PATHOLOGY: In radial growth phase, lentigo maligna melanoma (LMM) is a flat, irregular, brown- to-black patch that may cover a large part of the face or dorsal hands (Fig. 24-60). The cells of the radial growth phase

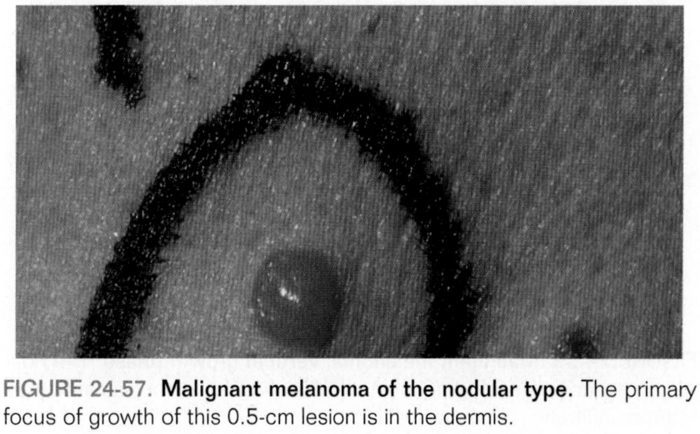

FIGURE 24-57. **Malignant melanoma of the nodular type.** The primary focus of growth of this 0.5-cm lesion is in the dermis.

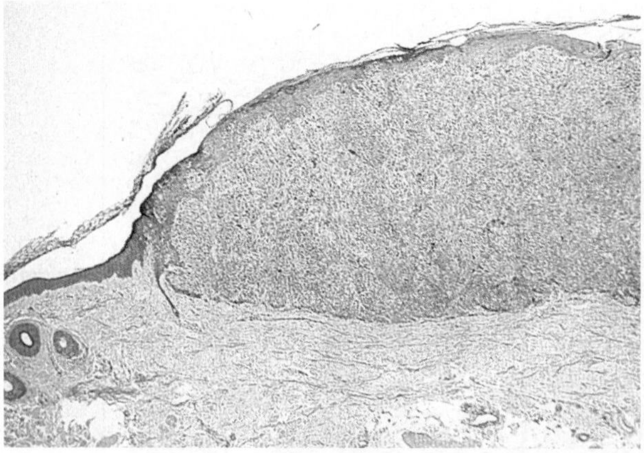

FIGURE 24-58. **Malignant melanoma, nodular type.** Intraepidermal growth is essentially absent. There is no radial growth lateral to the nodule. This tumor expands the papillary dermis and distorts the reticular dermal junction; it is therefore level III.

are predominantly in the basal layer, often forming contiguous or nearly contiguous rows of atypical single melanocytes but occasionally forming small nests that hang down into the papillary dermis (Fig. 24-61). In the radial growth phase of LMM, invasion is not as prominent or as extensive as in SSM. Cells of the radial growth phase of LMM vary in size and are usually associated with effacement of rete ridges and thinning of the epidermis. The subjacent dermis often shows a modest lymphocytic infiltrate and, with only rare exceptions, solar degeneration of the connective tissue.

In the vertical growth phase of LMM (Fig. 24-62), the cells tend to be spindle-shaped. These cells will occasionally provoke a connective tissue response to form a firm plaque (desmoplasia). Cells of the vertical growth phase may also grow along small nerves ("neurotropism").

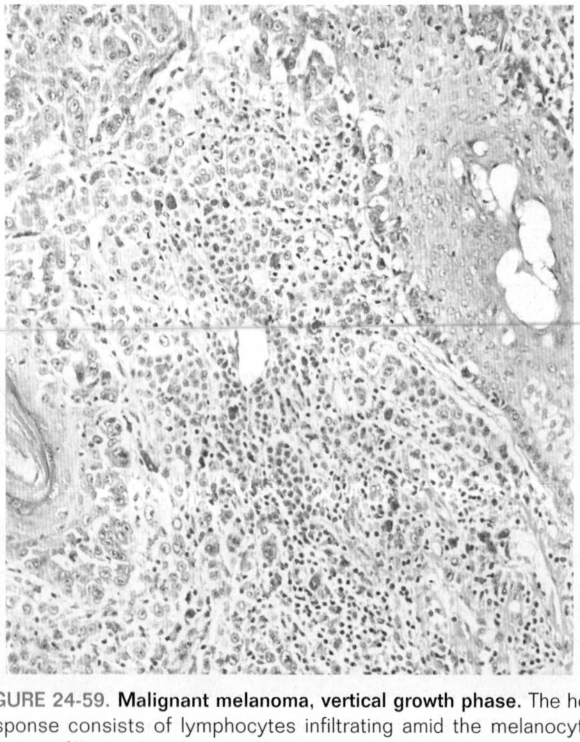

FIGURE 24-59. **Malignant melanoma, vertical growth phase.** The host response consists of lymphocytes infiltrating amid the melanocytes ("tumor-infiltrating lymphocytes").

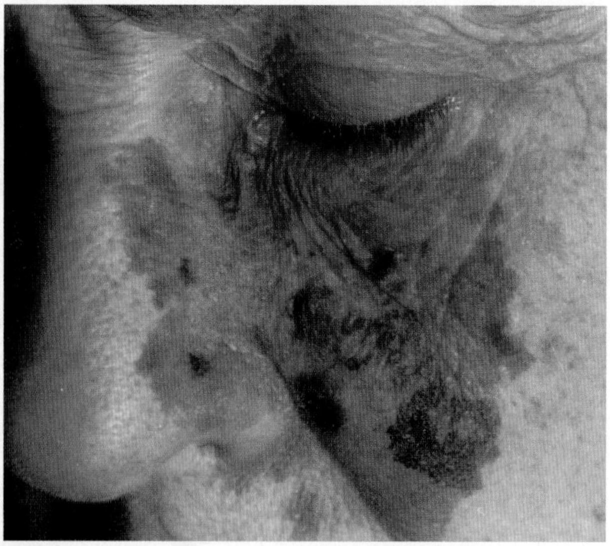

FIGURE 24-60. **Malignant melanoma of the lentigo maligna type, radial growth phase.**

Acral Lentiginous Melanoma

Acral lentiginous melanoma is the most common form of melanoma in dark-skinned people and, as the name implies, is generally limited to palms, soles, and subungual regions. A similar, though rare, tumor occurs on the mucous membranes and is called **mucosal lentiginous melanoma**.

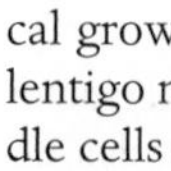

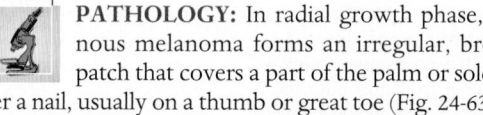

PATHOLOGY: In radial growth phase, acral lentiginous melanoma forms an irregular, brown-to-black patch that covers a part of the palm or sole or arises under a nail, usually on a thumb or great toe (Fig. 24-63). Microscopically, cells are mostly confined to the basal layer of the epidermis and maintain long dendrites (Fig. 24-64 and Fig. 24-65). A brisk lichenoid lymphocytic infiltrate is often seen.

As the vertical growth phase develops, cells may grow upward in the epidermis and become more epithelioid. The vertical growth phase (Fig. 24-66 and Fig. 24-67) is similar to that of lentigo maligna melanoma in that it commonly consists of spindle cells and occasionally includes neurotropism.

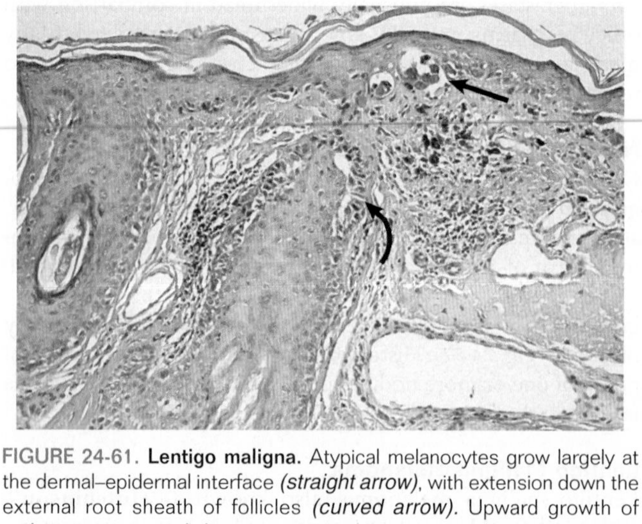

FIGURE 24-61. **Lentigo maligna.** Atypical melanocytes grow largely at the dermal–epidermal interface *(straight arrow)*, with extension down the external root sheath of follicles *(curved arrow)*. Upward growth of melanocytes is much less prominent than in intraepidermal malignant melanoma of the superficial spreading type.

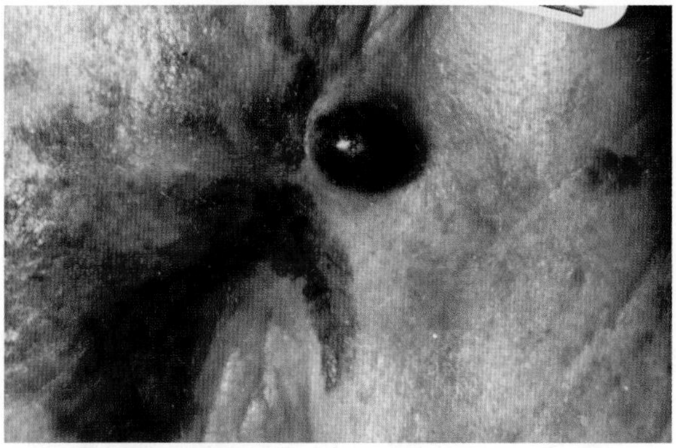

FIGURE 24-62. **Lentigo maligna.** The clinical appearance of the radial and vertical growth phase in malignant melanoma of the lentigo maligna type is shown. The lesion is 1 cm in diameter.

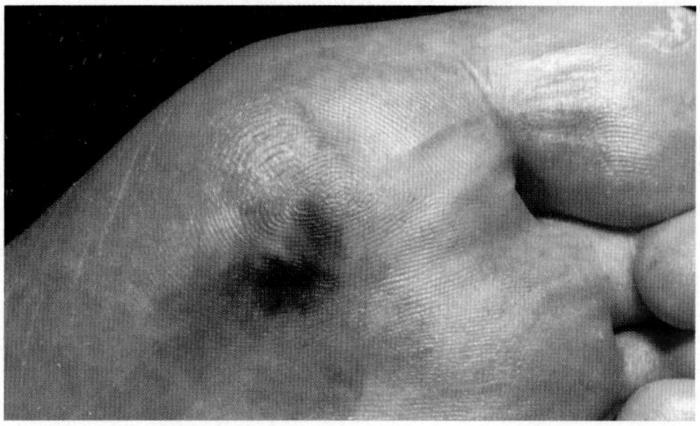

FIGURE 24-63. **Malignant melanoma, acral lentiginous type (radial growth phase).** The clinical appearance of the sole of the foot is depicted.

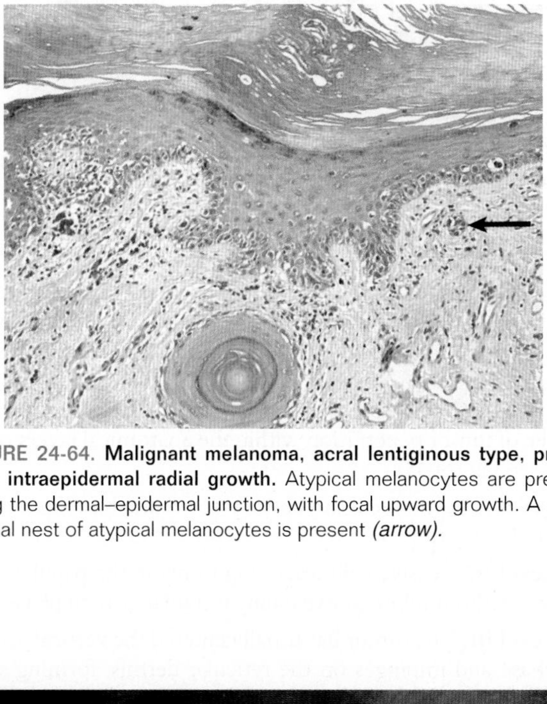

FIGURE 24-64. **Malignant melanoma, acral lentiginous type, principally intraepidermal radial growth.** Atypical melanocytes are present along the dermal–epidermal junction, with focal upward growth. A small dermal nest of atypical melanocytes is present *(arrow).*

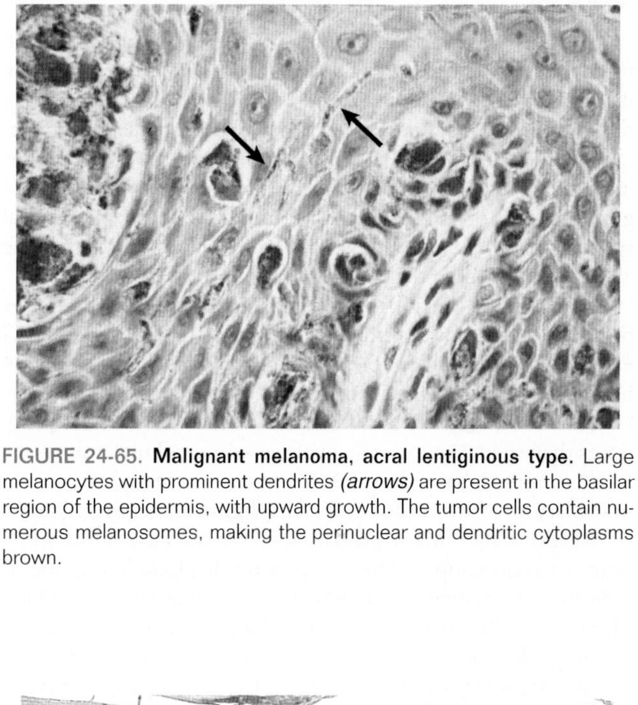

FIGURE 24-65. **Malignant melanoma, acral lentiginous type.** Large melanocytes with prominent dendrites *(arrows)* are present in the basilar region of the epidermis, with upward growth. The tumor cells contain numerous melanosomes, making the perinuclear and dendritic cytoplasms brown.

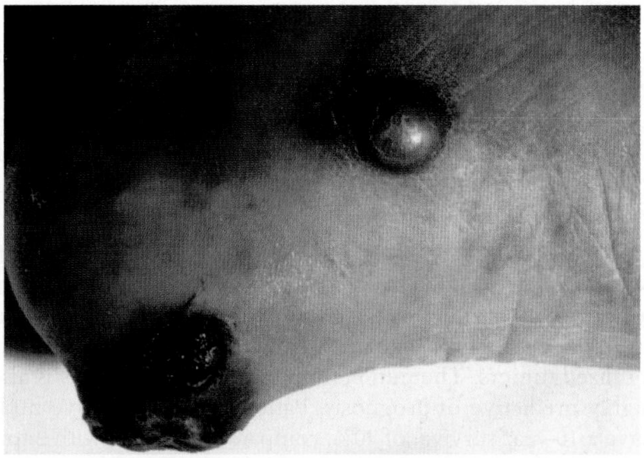

FIGURE 24-66. **Malignant melanoma, the acral lentiginous type.** The lesion on the heel is the primary tumor. The flat portion represents the radial growth phase, whereas the elevated portion indicates the vertical growth phase. The dark nodule on the instep is a metastasis.

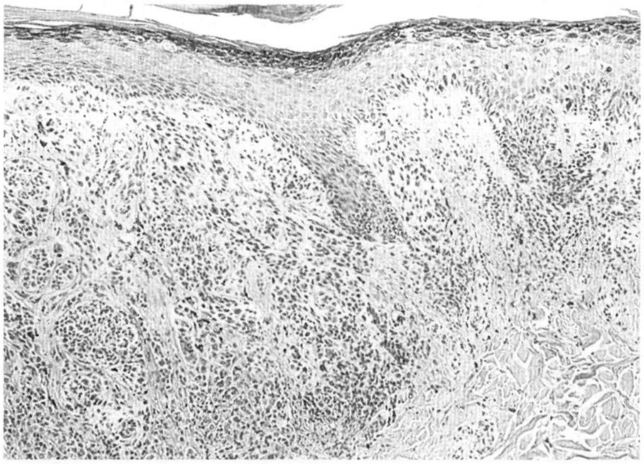

FIGURE 24-67. **Malignant melanoma, acral lentiginous type, vertical growth phase.** On the *left* is confluent growth of atypical dermal melanocytes filling and expanding the papillary dermis.

Staging and Prognosis of Melanoma

The prognosis of a patient with a melanoma in vertical growth phase is based on a number of attributes.

TUMOR THICKNESS: Tumor thickness is the strongest prognostic variable for melanomas that are apparently confined to their primary sites. The thickness of a melanoma is measured from the most superficial aspect of the stratum granulosum to the point of deepest penetration of the tumor into the dermis (see Fig. 24-56). Outcome may be predicted with some accuracy by dividing tumors into four groups without regard to the growth phase of the tumor. Prognosis up to 10 years after removal of the primary lesion may then be estimated from Table 24-3.

DERMAL MITOTIC RATE: For tumor cells in vertical growth phase, the mitotic rate is highly predictive of survival. Survival becomes progressively worse as the mitotic rate increases. The 5-year survival is 99% for patients with a mitotic rate of zero, 85% with a mitotic rate of 0.1 to 6.0/mm^2, and 68% with a mitotic rate over 6 mitoses/mm^2. Mitogenicity, or the presence of any mitoses in the dermis, has recently been identified as a risk factor for recurrence in otherwise early-stage ("thin") melanomas.

LYMPHOCYTIC RESPONSE: Interaction of lymphocytes with tumor cells in vertical growth phase is an important prognostic indicator. A cellular response is reported to be "infiltrative" when the lymphocytes actually infiltrate and disrupt the tumor, frequently forming rosettes about tumor cells (Fig. 24-68). If tumor-infiltrating lymphocytes (TILs) are present throughout the vertical growth phase or are seen across the entire base of the vertical growth phase, the infiltrate is said to be "brisk". The higher the TIL grade, the better the prognosis.

LOCATION: Melanomas on the extremities have a better prognosis than those on the head, neck, or trunk (axial). However, melanomas on the sole of the foot or the subungual region have a prognosis similar to, or worse than, axial lesions.

SEX: For every site and thickness women have better prognoses than men. For example, women with axial melanomas 0.8 to 1.7 mm thick have almost 90% 10-year survival after excision of the lesion, whereas the comparable figure in men is only 60%.

REGRESSION: Many primary melanomas show some spontaneous regression in the radial growth phase component, indicated clinically by a color change to a blue-white or white. Microscopically, such regression is characterized by a widened papillary dermis, with melanophages and a lymphocytic infiltrate. Patients whose tumors show such changes have a somewhat worse prognosis than those in whom regression is absent. It is thought that regression plays some sort of permissive role in the development of vertical growth phase.

TABLE 24-3

Tumor Thickness as Sole Predictor of Outcome 10 years after Definitive Therapy of Primary Melanoma

Thickness (mm)	Survival (%)
≤1	83–88
1.01–2	64–79
2.01–4	51–64
>4	32–54

MMP: matrix metalloproteinase
ADAM: proteins with A Disintegrin and A Metalloproteinase domain

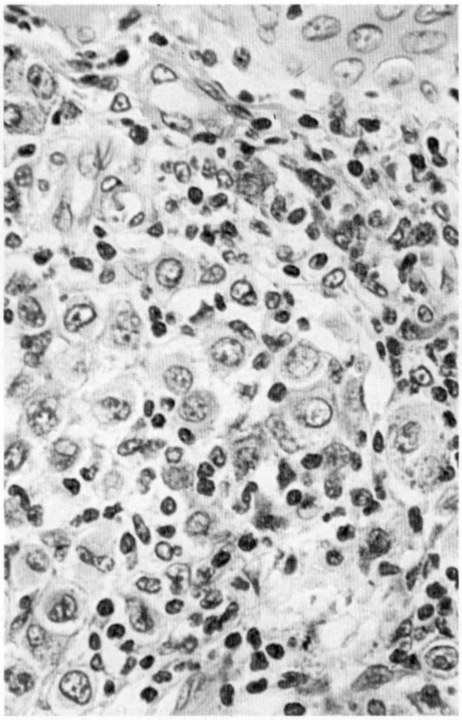

FIGURE 24-68. **Malignant melanoma, vertical growth phase.** Numerous tumor-infiltrating lymphocytes are arranged about individual tumor cells as satellites.

ULCERATION: Ulceration in a primary melanoma is associated with decreased survival. In one study, survival rates were 66% and 92% for patients with and without ulceration, respectively.

LEVELS OF INVASION: The Clark level system describes the degree of tumor penetration within the anatomical layers of the skin (see Fig. 24-55).

- **Level I:** Tumor cells are entirely above the basement membrane (in situ).
- **Level II:** Invasive cells are present only in the papillary dermis without filling or expanding it (radial growth phase).
- **Level III:** The tumor has usually entered the vertical growth phase and impinges on the reticular dermis, forming small expansile nodules that widen the papillary dermis.
- **Level IV:** Tumor cells clearly invade between the collagen bundles of the reticular dermis.
- **Level V:** The tumor extends into the subcutaneous fat. Clark levels predict the likelihood of metastasis, but not as accurately as tumor thickness. Thus, level IV invasion may predict lymph node metastases.

STAGE: The stage of the disease is perhaps the most important single factor influencing a patient's survival. Metastasis to regional lymph nodes is associated with an estimated 40% decrease in 5-year survival, compared with patients with clinically localized tumors. The number of involved lymph nodes is also highly predictive of prognosis. Patients with 1 positive node have a 10-year survival of 40%, compared with 25% with 2 to 4 nodes, and 15% with 5 or more nodes involved.

The tumor–node–metastasis (TNM) system of tumor staging incorporates features related to the primary tumor, regional lymph nodes, and soft tissues and distant metastases. The

T (primary tumor) attributes of tumor thickness, presence or absence of ulceration, and level of invasion are classified after excision of the melanoma. Numbers of lymph nodes with metastatic tumor and characterization of this tumor as micrometastasis or macrometastasis is a large part of the **N** (node) classification. **Micrometastasis** refers to nodal metastases diagnosed after sentinel or elective lymphadenectomy; **macrometastasis** refers to clinically detectable nodal metastases confirmed by therapeutic lymphadenectomy. The **M** (metastasis) properties incorporate results of evaluation for distant metastases at various anatomical sites. A TNM classification scheme based primarily on thickness, modified by ulceration, for localized primary melanomas and for the extent of regional and systemic metastatic disease, is used to determine the pathologic stage of disease, which in turn reflects the probability of survival.

The current recommendations regarding excisional removal of confirmed melanomas state that a 5-mm margin of uninvolved tissue should be obtained with in situ melanoma, a 1-cm margin with a tumor thickness of 1-mm or less, and a 2-cm margin may be considered with a tumor thickness greater than 1-mm or with Clark level IV or greater with any thickness. However many clinicians would use a 1-cm margin, at least for tumors in the lower end of these ranges, and margins are typically adjusted so as to spare important structures, such as the eyes. Sentinel lymph node sampling is generally considered with tumor thickness greater than 1 mm or with other risk factors including Clark level IV or greater or with tumorgenicity or mitogenicity, with any thickness. "Sentinel" lymph node evaluation involves biopsy of a single node that lies first in the regional node drainage pattern.

Benign Tumors of Melanocytes May Mimic Melanoma

Congenital Melanocytic Nevus

About 1% of white children are born with some form of pigmented lesion on their skin, sometimes as inconspicuous as a small patch of pale tan hyperpigmentation. Rarely, the trunk or an extremity is covered by a large pigmented patch or plaque that is cosmetically deforming ("giant hairy" or "garment" nevus). Such areas display a striking increase in intraepidermal and dermal melanocytes, which may extend deep into the subcutaneous tissue. Malignant melanoma may develop in these large congenital melanocytic nevi. Some physicians attempt to remove these large lesions, but in many instances their size makes surgical removal problematic.

Spitz Tumor

Spitz tumors (also known as spindle and epithelioid cell nevi) occur in children or adolescents and, less often, in adults. The Spitz tumor is an elevated, spheroid, pink, smooth nodule, usually on the head or neck, It grows rapidly, increasing to a diameter of 3 to 5 mm within 6 months. The lesion is composed of large spindle or epithelioid melanocytes that extend into the epidermis and into the dermis (Fig. 24-69). The cells are so atypical that an incorrect diagnosis of melanoma may be made even though melanoma is exquisitely rare in childhood. Although most Spitz tumors are benign, a few may metastasize. Therefore, the prognosis is to some extent uncertain, especially in adults.

Blue Nevus

Blue nevi appear in childhood or late adolescence as a dark blue, gray or black, firm, well-demarcated papules or nodules on the dorsum of the hands or feet or on the buttocks, scalp or face. The clinical appearance may prompt an excisional biopsy to rule out nodular melanoma. Melanin-containing melanocytes with long, thin dendrites are present in the superficial to mid-dermis, where they are often admixed with numerous melanin-containing macrophages (Fig. 24-70).

Freckle and Lentigo

Freckles, or **ephelides**, are small, brown macules that occur on sun-exposed skin, especially in people with fair skin (Fig. 24-71). They usually appear at about age 5. The pigmentation of a freckle deepens with exposure to sunlight and fades when light exposure ceases. A lentigo is a discrete, brown macule that appears at any age and on any part of the body (though a **solar lentigo**, or "liver spot," appears at an older age after long-term sun exposure) (Fig. 24-72). Unlike a freckle, the pigmentation of a lentigo does not depend on sun exposure. Freckles show hyperpigmentation of basal keratinocytes without concomitant increases in the number of melanocytes. Lentigines, on the other hand, display elongated rete ridges, increased melanin pigment

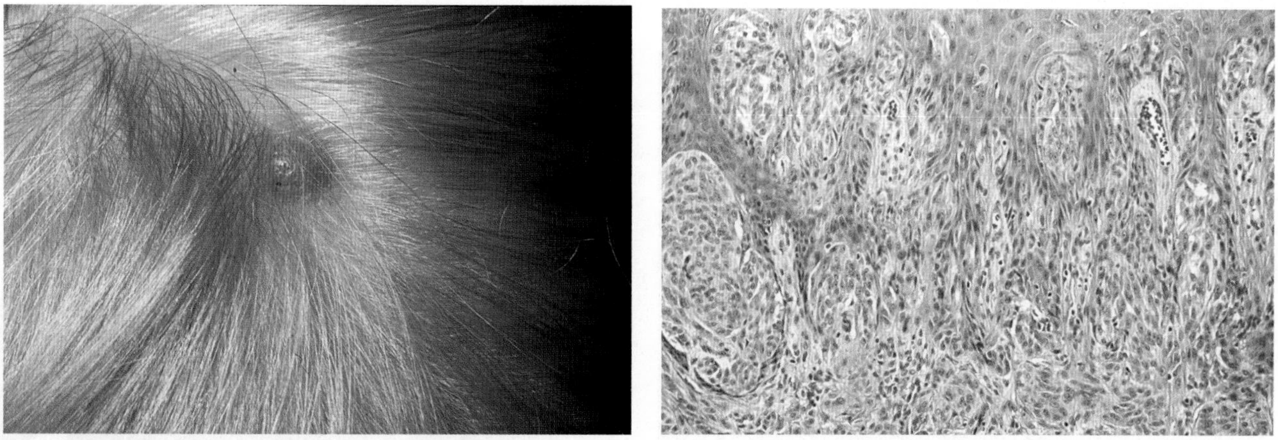

A B

FIGURE 24-69. **Spindle and epithelioid cell (Spitz) nevus. A.** A symmetric pink nodule appeared suddenly in a child but then remained stable for several weeks until it was excised. **B.** Spitz tumors are composed of large melanocytes with prominent nuclei. Within a hyperplastic epidermis, the melanocytes are disposed in large nests. Even though the cells are large and, at first glance, suggest melanoma, they are much more uniform than the cells of most malignant melanomas.

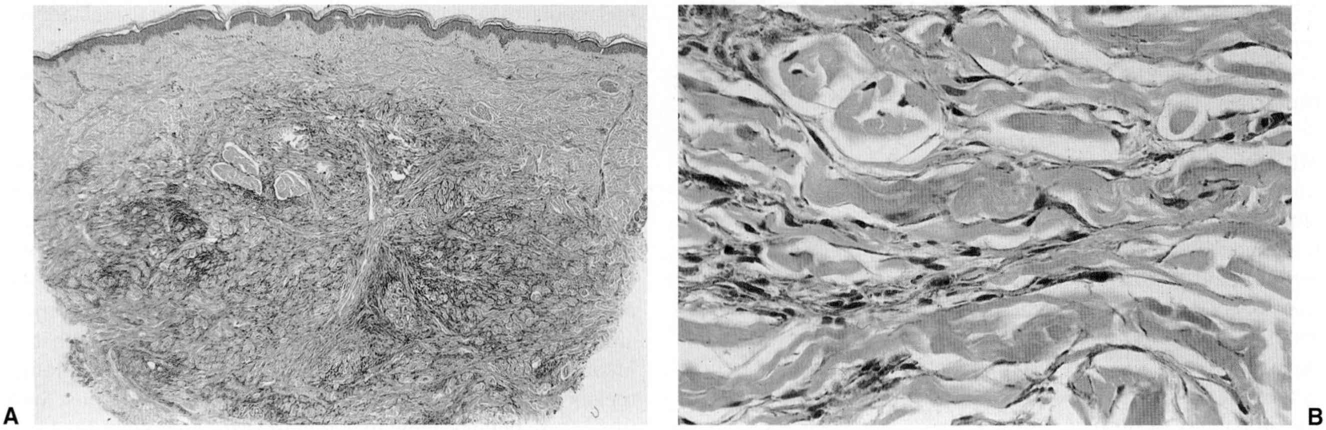

FIGURE 24-70. **Blue nevus. A.** Within the dermis there is a poorly defined but symmetric spindle cell proliferation that is dark brown. **B.** The lesion is composed of elongate cells with heavily pigmented dendrites and small bland nuclei.

in both basal keratinocytes and melanocytes and increased melanocytes. Larger lesions may need to be biopsied to rule out lentigo maligna melanoma.

Verrucae Are Warts Caused by Human Papillomavirus

Verrucae are cutaneous tumors. They are elevated, circumscribed, symmetric, epidermal proliferations that often appear papillary. *HPV is the cause of verrucae.*

PATHOLOGY:

- **Verruca vulgaris**, also known as the **common wart**, is an elevated papule with a verrucous (papillomatous) surface. They may be single or multiple and are most frequent on the dorsal surfaces of the hands or on the face. Histologically, verruca vulgaris displays hyperkeratosis and papillary epidermal hyperplasia (Fig. 24-73). **Koilocytes** (i.e., enlarged keratinocytes with a pyknotic nucleus surrounded by a halolike cleared area) are observed within the upper epidermis. Viral inclusions are difficult to identify (Fig. 24-74). HPV, especially serotypes 2 and 4, are commonly found in verruca vulgaris. There is no malignant potential.
- **Plantar warts** are benign, frequently painful, hyperkeratotic nodules on the soles of the feet. Occasionally, similar lesions appear on the palms of the hands (**palmar warts**). Histologically, plantar warts are endophytic or exophytic, papillary, squamous epithelial proliferations. The cells contain abundant cytoplasmic inclusions that are similar in appearance to the darker-staining keratohyaline granules. The nuclei of keratinocytes near the base of these warts also contain pink nuclear inclusions. HPV type 1 is the etiologic agent.
- **Verruca plana** are small flat papules that appear on the face. Microscopically, they display slight elongation of rete ridges (acanthosis), striking hypergranulosis, and superficial koilocyte formation. HPV types 3 and 10 often elicit these lesions. The lesions do not progress to cancer.
- **Condyloma acuminatum** are venereally transmitted warts usually caused by HPV serotypes 6 and 11, and occurring primarily around the genitalia. Histologically, lesions are papillary squamous proliferations. Koilocytosis and an almost continuous cap of parakeratosis are usually present. Squamous carcinomas may develop, epecially when HPV types 16 and 18 are involved (see Chapt. 18).
- **Bowenoid papulosis,** also caused by HPV types 16 and 18, is characterized by multiple hyperpigmented papules on the genitalia. Lesions may be histologically identical to squamous cell carcinoma (SCC) in situ in that they display disor-

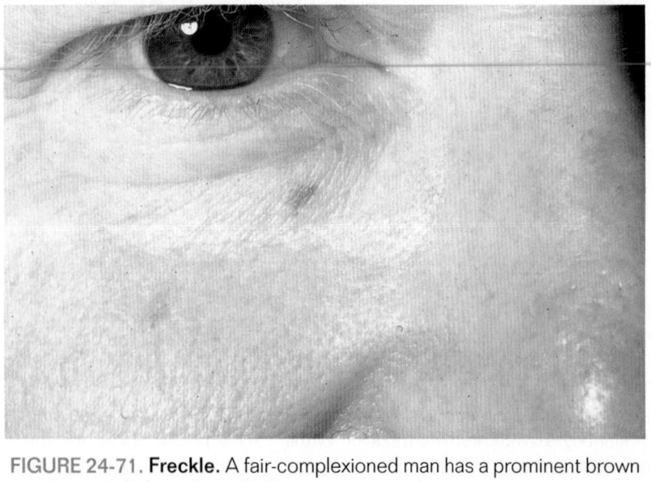

FIGURE 24-71. **Freckle.** A fair-complexioned man has a prominent brown macule that darkens in sunlight.

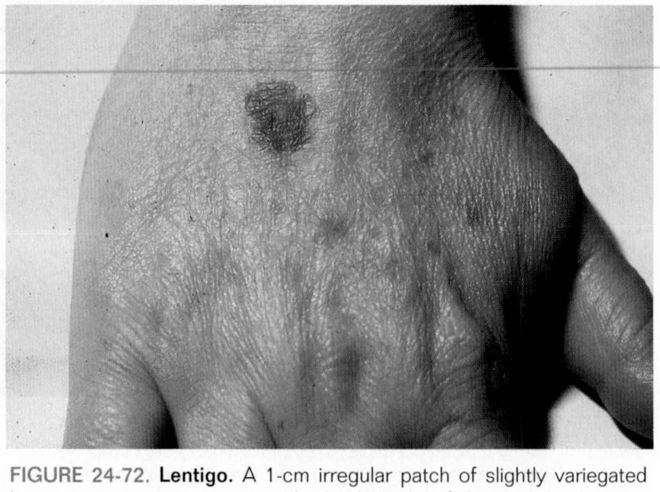

FIGURE 24-72. **Lentigo.** A 1-cm irregular patch of slightly variegated hyperpigmentation is present with a background of chronic solar damage.

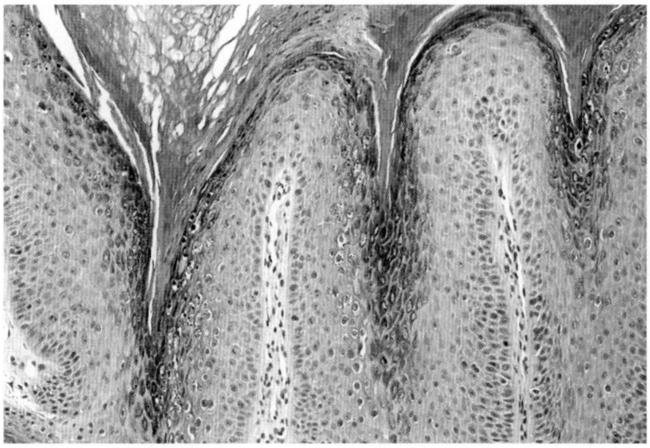

FIGURE 24-73. **Verruca vulgaris.** Verruca vulgaris is the prototype of papillary epidermal hyperplasia. Squamous epithelial-lined fronds have fibrovascular cores. The blood vessels within the cores extend close to the surface of verrucae, which makes them susceptible to traumatic hemorrhage and the resultant black "seeds" that patients observe.

dered epithelial maturation and scattered keratinocyte atypia. The lesions also exhibit parakeratosis and irregular acanthosis. Bowenoid papulosis often regresses but may progress to dysplasia or malignancy in some cases.

- **Epidermodysplasia verruciformis** is a rare autosomal recessive disease characterized by impaired cell-mediated immunity and subsequently enhanced susceptibility to HPV infection. Warts similar to those of verruca plana, with confluence into patches, are widespread. It first appears in childhood, and SCC develops in 30% to 60% of patients. HPV types 5, 8, 9, and 47 are most commonly encountered in lesions such SCCs.

Keratosis Is a Benign Horny Growth Composed of Keratinocytes

Seborrheic Keratosis

Seborrheic keratoses are scaly, frequently pigmented, elevated papules or plaques whose scales are easily rubbed off. Although they are among the most common keratoses, the etiology is unknown. The lesions generally occur in later life and tend to be familial.Clinically and

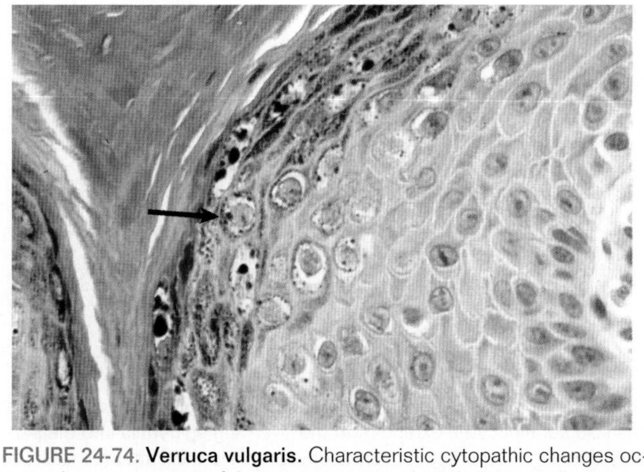

FIGURE 24-74. **Verruca vulgaris.** Characteristic cytopathic changes occur in the outer portion of the stratum spinosum and stratum granulosum, in which there is perinuclear vacuolization and prominent keratohyaline granules, with homogeneous blue inclusions *(arrow)*.

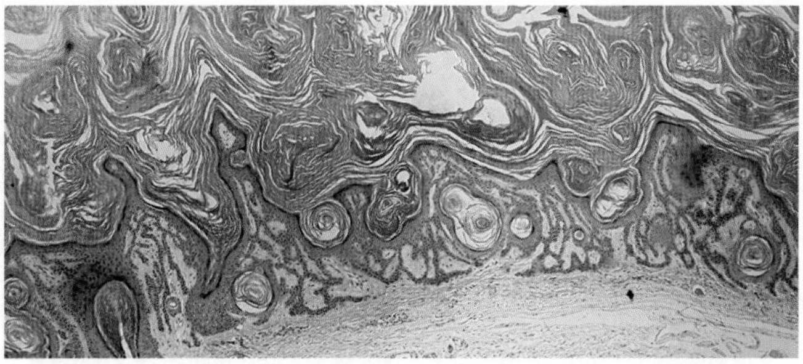

FIGURE 24-75. **Seborrheic keratosis.** Broad anastomosing cords of mature stratified squamous epithelium are associated with small keratin cysts.

microscopically, they appear "pasted on" and are composed of broad anastomosing cords of mature stratified squamous epithelium associated with small cysts of keratin (horn cysts) (Fig. 24-75). Seborrheic keratoses are innocuous but are a cosmetic nuisance. The sudden appearance of numerous seborrheic keratoses has been associated with internal malignancies ("sign of Leser-Trélat"), especially gastric adenocarcinoma.

Actinic Keratosis

Actinic keratoses ("from the sun's rays") are keratinocytic neoplasms that develop in sun-damaged skin as circumscribed keratotic patches or plaques, commonly on the backs of the hands or the face. Microscopically, the stratum corneum is no longer loose and basket-weaved but is replaced by a dense parakeratotic scale. The underlying basal keratinocytes display significant atypia (Fig. 24-76). With time, actinic keratoses may evolve into squamous cell carcinoma in situ and finally into invasive squamous cell carcinoma. However, most are stable, and many regress.

Keratoacanthoma

Keratoacanthomas are rapidly growing keratotic papules on sun-exposed skin that develop over 3 to 6 weeks into craterlike nodules. They reach a maximum diameter of 2 to 3 cm. Spontaneous regression usually follows within 6 to 12 months, leaving an atrophic scar. Some lesions may cause considerable damage before they regress, and some fail to regress. Keratoacanthomas may be considered to be variants of SCC, although this topic is controversial.

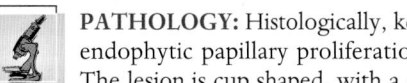

PATHOLOGY: Histologically, keratoacanthomas are endophytic papillary proliferations of keratinocytes. The lesion is cup shaped, with a central, keratin-filled umbilication and overhanging ("buttressing") edges (Fig. 24-77). At the base of the keratin, keratinocytes are large and have abundanct homogeneous, eosinophilic ("glassy") cytoplasm. At the lower aspect of the lesion, irregular tongues of squamous epithelium infiltrate the collagen of the reticular dermis. Older lesions show active fibroplasia in the dermis around these tongues. There may be focal lichenoid inflammation and the dermis may be markedly infiltrated with neutrophils, lymphocytes, and eosinophils. Microabscesses of neutrophils and entrapped dermal elastic fibers may be present within the lesion.

Basal Cell Carcinoma Is a Locally Invasive Epidermal Neoplasm

Basal cell carcinoma (BCC) is the most common malignant tumor in persons with pale skin. Although it may be locally aggressive, metastases are exceedingly rare.

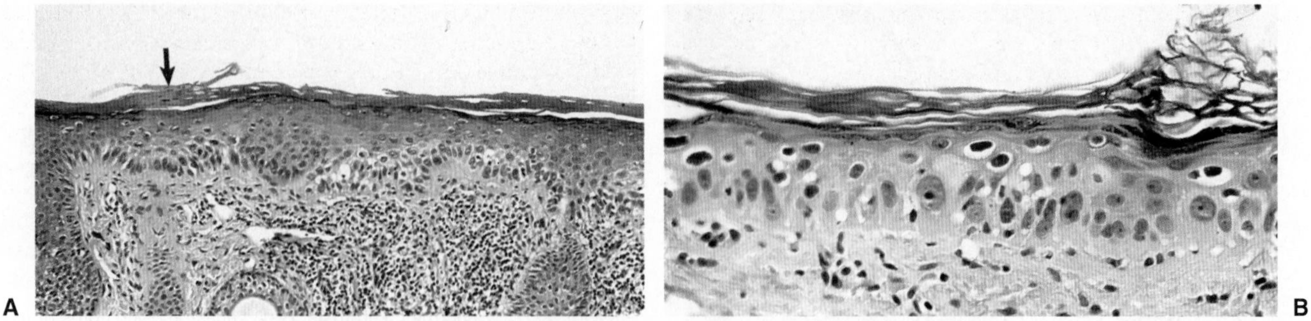

FIGURE 24-76. **Actinic keratosis. A.** A low-power view reveals cytologic atypia within the stratum basalis and lower stratum spinosum with loss of polarity. A lichenoid, bandlike, lymphocytic infiltrate is frequently present. Parakeratosis is present here only in a small focus *(arrow)*. **B.** High-power examination of an actinic keratosis reveals striking cytologic atypia of the basal keratinocytes, the hallmark of actinic keratoses.

PATHOGENESIS: BCC usually develops on sun-damaged skin of people with fair skin and freckles. However, unlike SCC, BCC also arises on areas not exposed to intense sunlight. It is unusual to find BCC on the fingers and dorsal surfaces of the hands. The tumor is thought to derive from pluripotential cells in the basal layer of the epidermis, more specifically, in the bulge region of the hair follicle.

In several heritable syndromes, BCC originates on skin that has had little light exposure. **Nevoid BCC syndrome** refers to the occurrence of multiple tumors in the context of a complex multisystem disease. The syndrome also includes pits (dyskeratoses) on the palms and soles, mandibular cysts, hypertelorism, and a predisposition to other neoplasms, including medulloblastoma. The BCCs of this syndrome appear at a young age and may number in the hundreds.

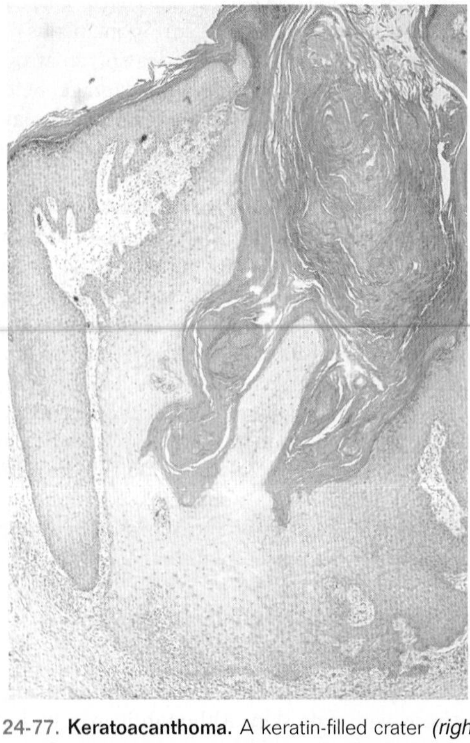

FIGURE 24-77. **Keratoacanthoma.** A keratin-filled crater *(right)* is lined by glassy proliferating keratinocytes that invade the dermis.

Germline mutations in *PTCH* tumor suppressor gene *on* chromosome 9q22, cause nevoid BCC syndrome. Somatic mutations in *PTCH* have also been implicated in up to 67% of sporadic BCC.

PATHOLOGY: BCC is composed of nests of deeply basophilic epithelial cells with narrow rims of cytoplasm that are attached to the epidermis and protrude into the subjacent papillary dermis (Fig. 24-78). The central part of each nest contains closely packed keratinocytes that are slightly smaller than the normal epidermal basal keratinocytes and show occasional apoptosis. The periphery of each nest shows an organized layer of polarized, columnar keratinocytes, with the long axis of each cell perpendicular to the surrounding BMZ ("peripheral palisading"). **Superficial, multicentric BCC** is composed of apparently isolated, but actually interconnected, nests that usually remain confined to the papillary dermis and manifest clinically as a spreading plaque. **Nodulocystic BCC** is also attached to the epidermis and exhibits the same cytologic and architectural features as the superficial type of BCC, but grows more deeply into the dermis. Usually, tumor cells of the dermal islands are associated with a mucinous ground substance and are surrounded by an array of fibroblasts and lymphocytes. The tumor nests are often separated from adjacent stroma by thin clefts ("retraction artifact"), which feature may sometimes help distinguish BCC from other adnexal neoplasms displaying

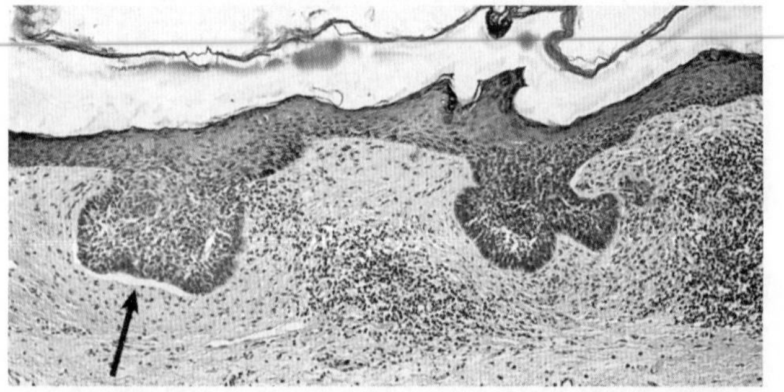

FIGURE 24-78. **Basal cell carcinoma, superficial type.** Buds of atypical basaloid keratinocytes extend from the overlying epidermis into the papillary dermis. The peripheral keratinocytes mimic the stratum basalis by palisading. The separation artifact *(arrow)* is present because of poorly formed basement membrane components and the hyaluronic acid-rich stroma that contains collagenase.

basaloid cell proliferation. BCC with particularly dense sclerotic stroma are called **morpheaform BCC** because of a clinical resemblance to lesions of localized scleroderma (also known as "morphea").

CLINICAL FEATURES: A number of common forms of BCC are recognized.

- **Pearly papule** is the prototypic nodulocystic type of lesion, so named because it resembles a 2- to 3-mm pearl (Fig. 24-79). It is covered by tightly stretched epidermis and is laced with small, delicate, branching vessels (telangiectasia).
- **Rodent ulcer** is a small crater in the center of the pearl.
- **Superficial BCC** appears as a scaly, red, sharply demarcated plaque.
- **Morpheaform BCC** is a pale, firm, scarlike tumor that is ill-defined on and especially beneath the skin surface, making it particularly difficult to eradicate.
- **Pigmented BCC** may grossly resemble malignant melanoma.

Treatment usually involves various excision or eradication procedures.

Squamous Cell Carcinoma Typically Resembles Differentiated Keratinocytes

SCC is second only to BCC in incidence and may be caused by ultraviolet light, ionizing radiation, chemical carcinogens, and HPV. SCC is most common on sun-damaged skin of fair persons with light hair and freckles, and often originates in actinic keratoses. It is exceedingly rare on normal black skin.

PATHOGENESIS: SCC has multiple causes, ultraviolet light being the most common. SCC arising in sun-damaged skin metastasizes rarely (<2%). It may also arise in chronic scarring processes such as osteomyelitis sinus tracts, burn scars, and areas of radiation dermatitis. In these settings, SCC metastasizes more often. Over 90% of SCCs, and many actinic keratoses, have mutated p53 genes.

PATHOLOGY: SCC is composed of tumor cells that mimic epidermal stratum spinosum in varying degrees, and extend into the subjacent dermis (Fig. 24-80). The edges of many tumors show changes typical of actinic keratosis, namely, a variably thickened epidermis with parakeratosis and significant atypia of the basal keratinocytes.

CLINICAL FEATURES: SCC characteristically arises in chronically sun-exposed areas such as the backs of the hands, face, lips and ears (see Fig. 24-80A). Early lesions are small, scaly or ulcerated, erythematous papules, which may be pruritic. SCCs are usually treated by electrosurgery, topical chemotherapy, excision, or radiation therapy.

Merkel Cell Carcinoma Is an Aggressive Tumor of Neurosecretory Cells That Shows Epithelial Differentiation

Merkel cell carcinoma (MCC) is typically a solitary, dome-shaped, red to violaceous nodule or indurated plaque that arises on the skin of the head and neck in elderly white patients. These are aggressive tumors that cause death in 25% to 70% of patients within 5 years.

PATHOLOGY: Most MCCs consist of large solid nests of undifferentiated cells that resemble small cell carcinoma of the lung (Fig. 24-81). At its periphery, the tumor may show a trabecular pattern. Nuclear chromatin is dense and evenly distributed, cytoplasm is scant mitotic figures and nuclear fragments are frequent. Immunostaining shows cytokeratin 20 distributed in a "perinuclear dot" cytoplasmic pattern. Tumor cells also stain positively for neuroendocrine markers such as chromogranin and synaptophysin.

Adnexal Tumors Differentiate Towards Skin Appendages

Adnexal tumors generally appear as elevated small skin nodules that often occur in people with a familial history of similar tumors. Frequently, the lesions appear at puberty. Although most are benign, malignant behavior is sometimes observed.

Cylindroma

Cylindromas are adnexal neoplasms with features of sweat gland differentiation. They may be solitary or multiple elevated

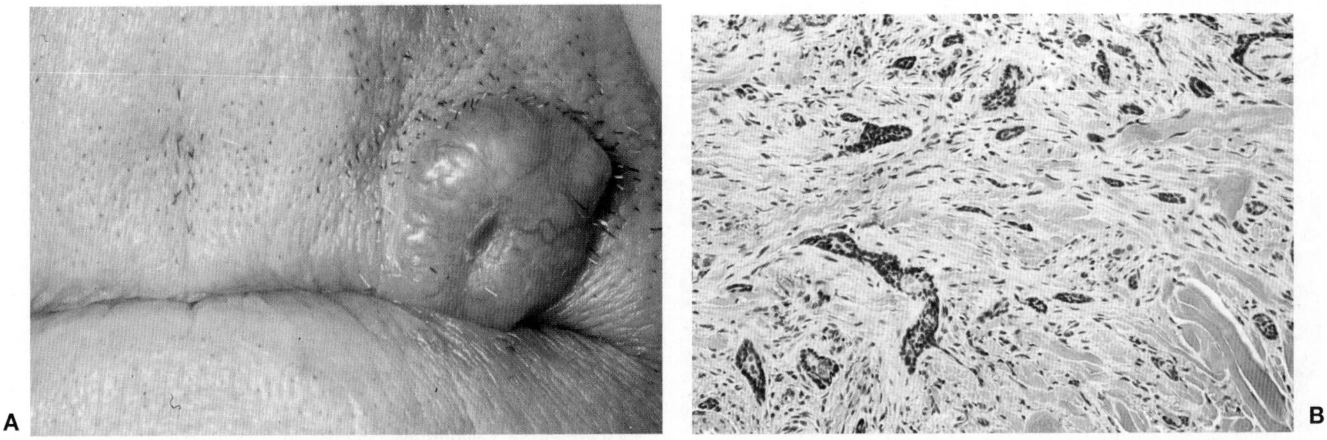

FIGURE 24-79. **Basal cell carcinoma (BCC). A.** Pearly papule: The tumor exhibits typical rolled pearly borders with telangiectases and central ulceration. **B.** Microscopic examination of morpheaform BCC shows a sclerosing and infiltrative lesion. Irregularly branching strands of tumor cells permeate the dermis, with induction of a cellular, fibroblastic, hyaluronic acid-rich stroma.

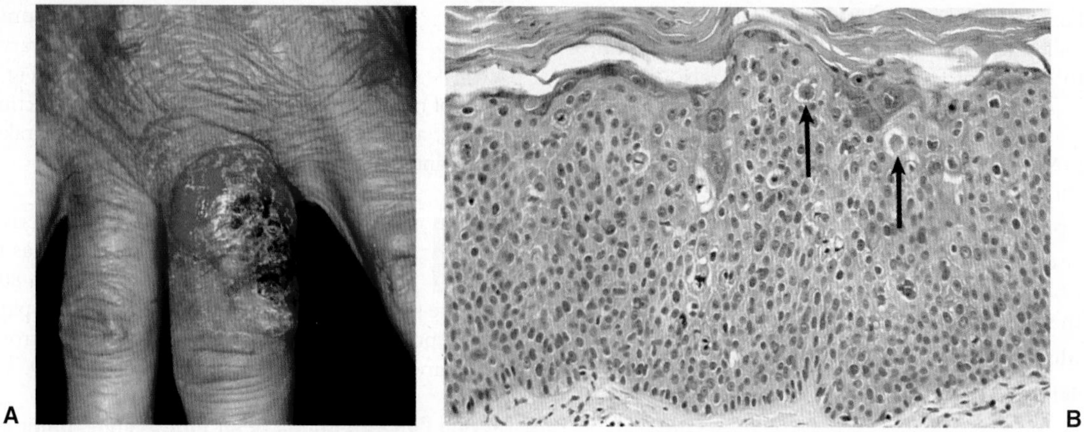

FIGURE 24-80. **Squamous cell carcinoma. A.** An ulcerated, encrusted, and infiltrating lesion is seen on the sun-exposed dorsal aspect of a finger. **B.** A microscopic view of the periphery of the lesion shows squamous cell carcinoma in situ. The entire epidermis is replaced by atypical keratinocytes. Mitoses (*curved arrow*) and multinucleation of keratinocytes are apparent, as is apoptosis *(straight arrows)*.

nodules around the scalp. An autosomal dominant, heritable variant features multiple tumors. Occasionally, cylindromas become large and cluster about the head ("turban tumors"). Microscopic examination shows sharply circumscribed nests of deeply basophilic cells surrounded by a hyalinized, thickened BMZ (Fig. 24-82).

Syringoma

Syringomas typically occur about the eyelid and upper cheek as small, elevated, flesh-colored papules. Microscopically, small ducts resembling intraepidermal portions of eccrine sweat ducts are seen (Fig. 24-83).

Poroma

Poroma is a common, solitary neoplasm histologically similar to seborrheic keratosis but with narrow ductal lumina and occasional cystic spaces (Fig. 24-84). The pattern has been interpreted as eccrine sweat gland differentiation. The tumor is a firm, raised lesion, usually less than 2 cm in diameter, that develops on the sole or sides of the foot, or on the hands or fingers. Microscopically, poromas extend from the lower portion of the epidermis into the dermis as broad, anastomosing bands of uniform, cuboidal cells. Occasional malignant lesions with ductal differentiation are termed **porocarcinomas**.

Trichoepithelioma

Trichoepithelioma is a neoplasm that differentiates toward hair structures. It is usually a solitary lesion but in "multiple trichoepithelioma syndrome" it occurs as an autosomal dominant

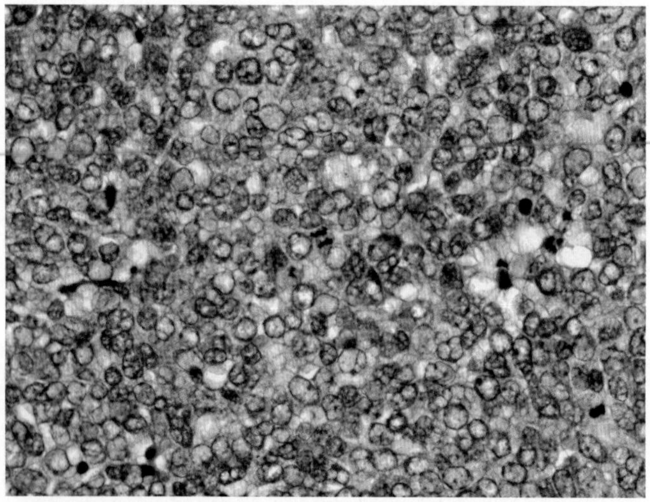

FIGURE 24-81. **Merkel cell carcinoma.** The tumor is composed of solid nests of undifferentiated cells that resemble small cell carcinoma of the lung.

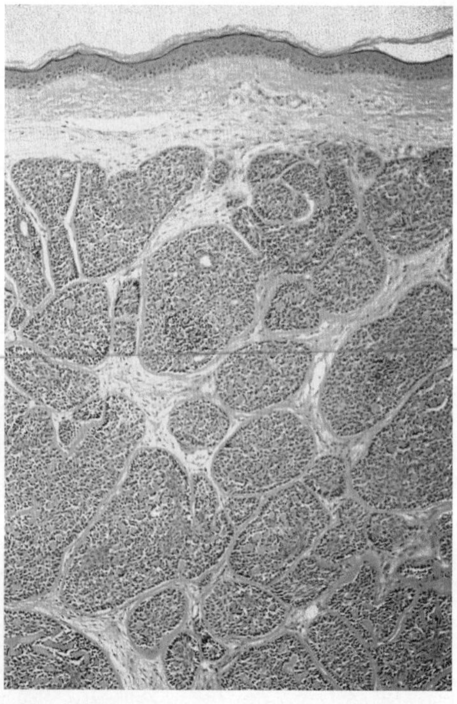

FIGURE 24-82. **Cylindroma.** Sharply circumscribed islands of basophilic epithelial cells reside in a jigsaw-puzzle-like array. Dense eosinophilic hyaline sheaths surround each island and form small circular cords within each island.

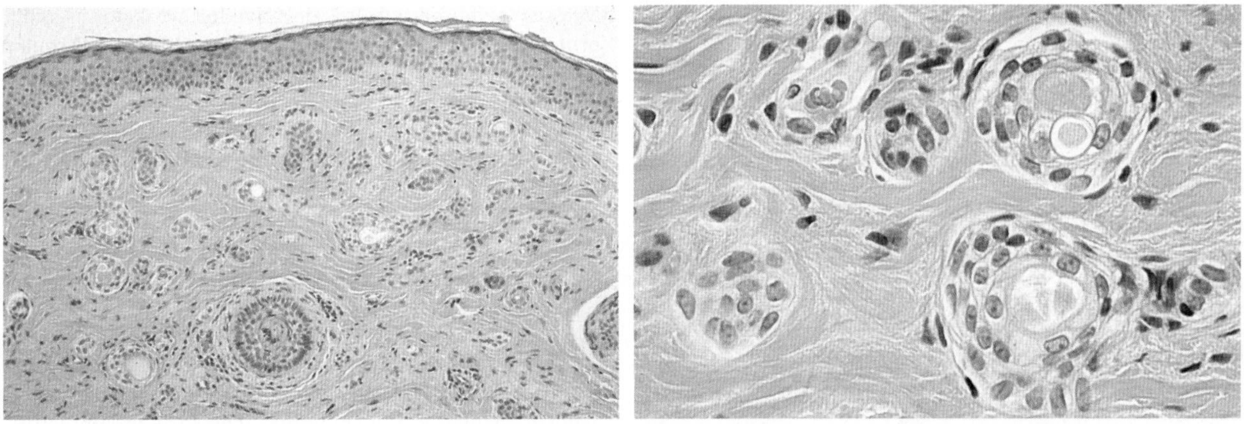

FIGURE 24-83. **Syringoma. A.** Within the upper dermis is a proliferation of epithelium-forming ducts, tubules, and solid islands amid a dense fibrous stroma. **B.** The ductal differentiation closely mimics that of the straight dermal eccrine duct, with a central lumen and cuticle formation.

trait. Lesions begin to appear at puberty, on the face, scalp, neck. and upper trunk. Microscopically, they resemble basal cell carcinomas but contain many "horn cysts": keratinized centers surrounded by basophilic epithelial cells (Fig. 24-85).

Fibrohistiocytic Tumors of the Skin Show a Varied Spectrum of Differentiation

Dermatofibroma

Dermatofibroma is a common, benign tumor of fibroblasts and macrophages. The former are the neoplastic cells. It occurs on the extremities as a dome-shaped, firm, rubbery nodule with ill-defined borders and pigmentation ranging from pink to dark brown. They are rarely more than 3 to 5 mm in diameter. Microscopically, the papillary and reticular dermis are replaced by fibrous tissue that forms ill-defined small cartwheels with small central vascular spaces (Fig. 24-86). The tumors are not well demarcated and blend with the surrounding dermis. The overlying epidermis is hyperplastic and often hyperpigmented.

Dermatofibrosarcoma Protuberans

Dermatofibrosarcoma protuberans is a slowly growing nodule or indurated plaque with intermediate malignant potential, that appears mostly on the trunk of young adults. Local recurrence after attempted complete excision is common, but metastases are rare. The most common histologic pattern is a poorly circumscribed, monotonous population of spindle cells arranged in a dense "storiform" (pinwheel-like) array (Fig. 24-87). The tumor extends into the subcutis along fat septa and interstices, creating an infiltrative, honeycomb-like pattern. Tumor cells display CD34, marker of endothelial cells, some neural tumor cells, as well as dermal fibroblast-like dendritic cells, the probable cell of origin. Positivity for CD34 may help distinguish this tumor from a dermatofibroma, which does not express this antigen.

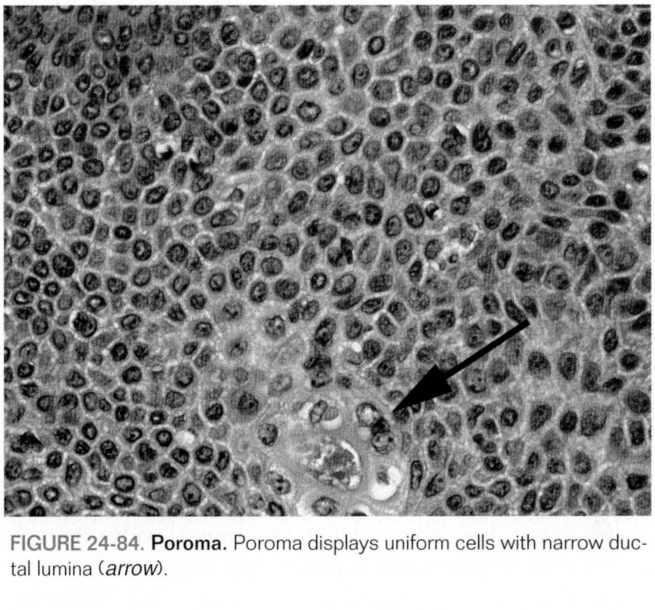

FIGURE 24-84. **Poroma.** Poroma displays uniform cells with narrow ductal lumina (*arrow*).

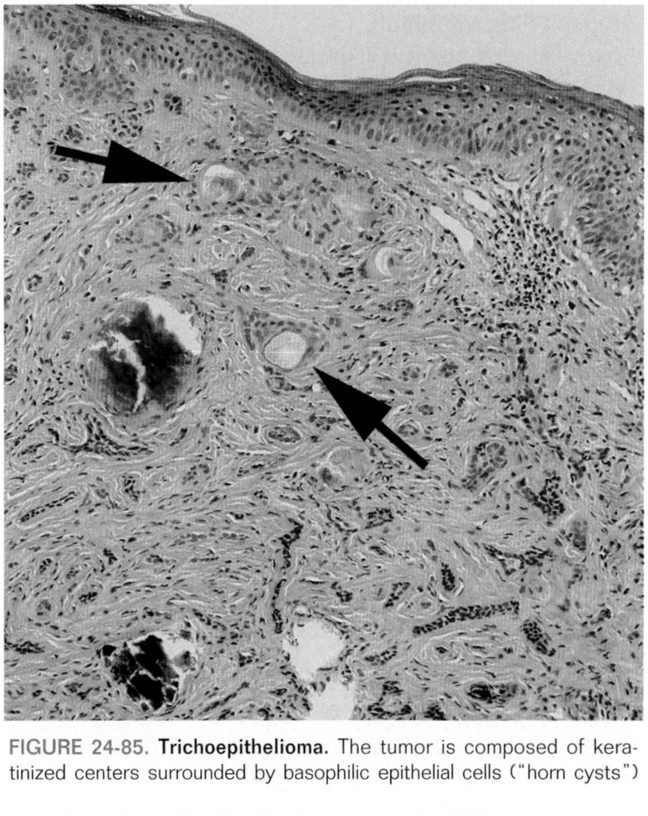

FIGURE 24-85. **Trichoepithelioma.** The tumor is composed of keratinized centers surrounded by basophilic epithelial cells ("horn cysts")

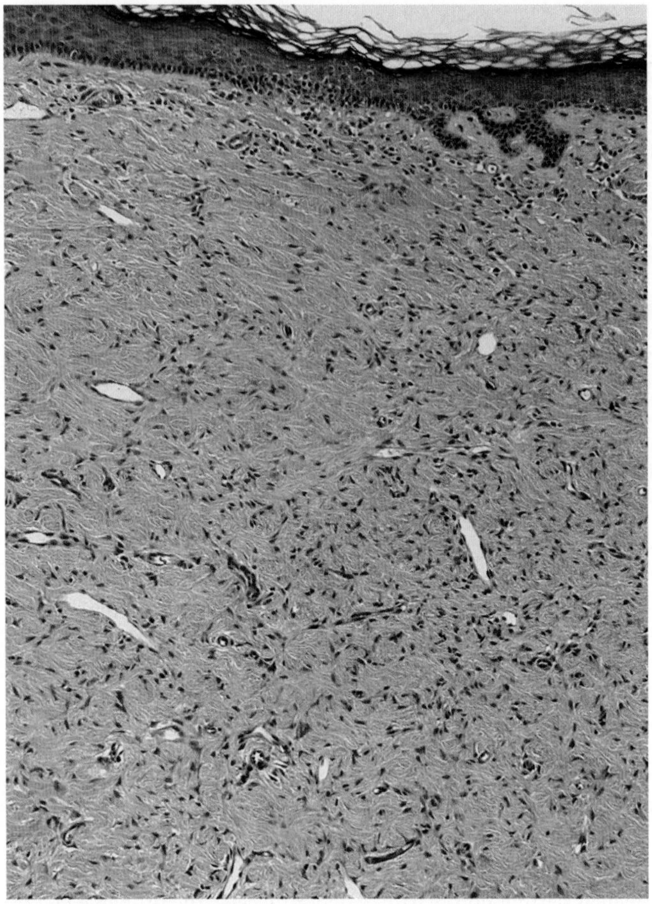

FIGURE 24-86. **Dermatofibroma.** Fibrous tissue replaces the dermis and forms poorly defined cartwheels.

Atypical Fibroxanthoma

Atypical fibroxanthoma is a low-grade malignant neoplasm that appears as a dome-shaped nodule on the sun-damaged skin of elderly persons. Microscopically, atypical spindle cells and epithelioid cells infiltrate and disrupt the dermis. Multinucleated cells, some with a finely vacuolated cytoplasm, may be prominent. Mitoses are numerous. It is negative for cytokeratins and S-100 protein, thereby differentiating it from spindle-cell squamous cell carcinoma and spindle-cell melanoma, respectively. Treatment is by excision, but local recurrence is common.

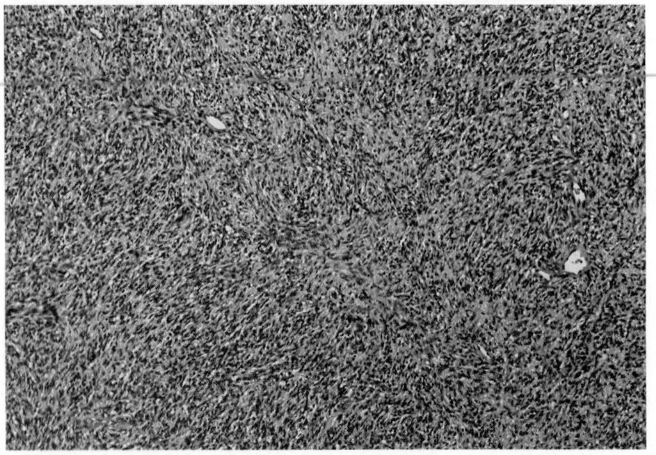

FIGURE 24-87. **Dermatofibrosarcoma protuberans.** Tumor cells form small cartwheels with central vascular spaces.

Mycosis Fungoides Is a Variant of Cutaneous T-Cell Lymphoma

The etiology of mycosis fungoides (MF) is unknown, but it is thought that malignancy of helper T cells (CD4+) may be a pathologic response to chronic exposure to an antigen.

PATHOLOGY: In the early stages of the disease, delicate, erythematous plaques appear, often by the buttocks. Microscopically, these plaques show psoriasiform changes in the epidermis. The early inflammatory cell infiltrates in the dermis are polymorphic and are often not diagnostic of MF.

Skin involvement becomes progressively more prominent and infiltrative. The most important histological feature of MF is the presence of lymphocytes in the epidermis ("epidermotropism"). In late stages, the dermal infiltrate becomes dense to the point of forming tumor nodules. Increasing numbers of atypical lymphocytes that display hyperchromatic, convoluted (cerebriform) nuclei are seen in the papillary dermis and epidermis (Fig. 24-88). Circumscribed nests of these atypical lymphocytes ("Pautrier's microabscesses") eventually appear in the epidermis. Polymerase chain reaction and Southern blotting techniques may reveal a T-cell receptor gene rearrangement, indicative of a clonal cell population.

Sézary syndrome refers to the systemic dissemination of MF. The characteristic feature is the presence of cerebriform lymphocytes in the peripheral circulation.

CLINICAL FEATURES: MF affects older age groups, has a slight male predominance and preferentially affects blacks over whites. It is classically divided into three stages: patch, plaque and tumor. In the patch stage, which may persist for months, eruptions consist of scaly, erythematous macules that may be slightly indurated. They are usually found on the lower abdomen, buttocks, and upper thighs as well as the breasts of women, and can mimic other dermatitides such as psoriasis or eczema (see Fig. 24-88A). The plaque stage lesions are more infiltrated and circumscribed. As these coalesce, involvement becomes more widespread. Large, variably shaped nodules can form on existing indurated plaques or on apparently normal skin. Spread to lymph nodes or visceral involvement portends reduced survival. Therapy includes ultraviolet light, topical nitrogen mustard, and electron beam therapy.

Human Immunodeficieny Virus (HIV) Infection is Associated with Various Skin Diseases

Kaposi Sarcoma

Kaposi sarcoma (KS) is a malignant tumor of endothelial cells. This vascular neoplasm was once seen only in older people of Mediterranean descent or in Africans. Since the advent of HIV infection, KS is most commonly seen in patients with AIDS, (see Chapters 4, 10). Human herpesvirus 8 (HHV-8) is the etiologic agent of KS.

PATHOLOGY: All cases of Kaposi sarcoma, whether associated with HIV or not, evolve through three stages: patch, plaque and nodule. In the patch

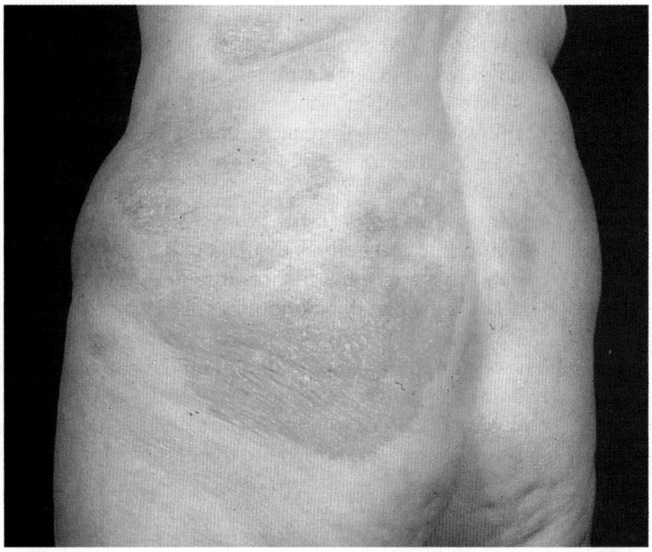
A

FIGURE 24-88. **Mycosis fungoides. A.** A 66-year-old woman presented with a 30-year history of erythematous scaly patches and plaques with telangiectases, atrophy, and pigmentation. **B.** The papillary dermis is expanded by an infiltrate of atypical lymphocytes. Lymphocytes with hyperchromatic nuclei infiltrate the thickened epidermis.

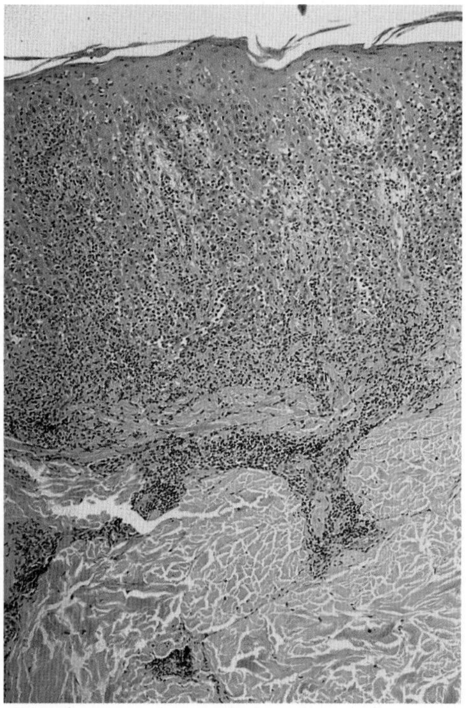
B

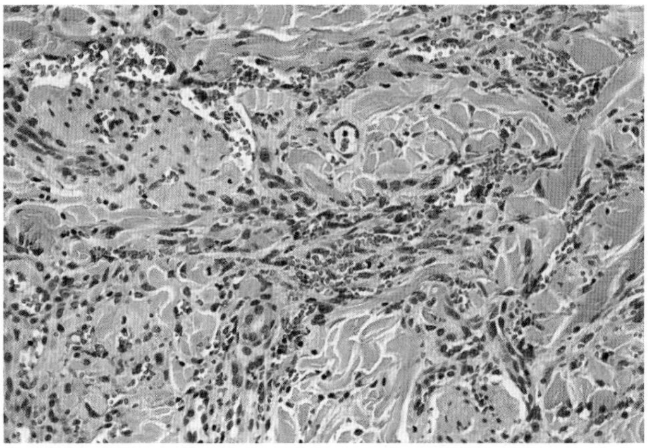

FIGURE 24-89. **Kaposi sarcoma, plaque stage.** Extending along the vascular arcades and amid reticular dermal collagen is a proliferation of endothelial cells. They form delicate vascular channels filled with red blood cells. Some endothelial cells are not canalized (have not formed lumina.)

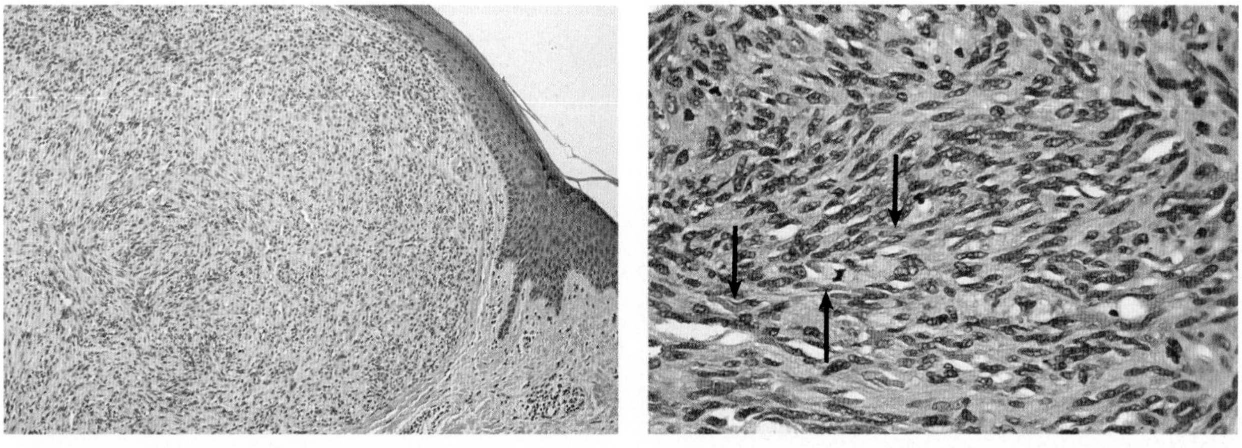
A B

FIGURE 24-90. **Kaposi sarcoma, nodule stage. A.** A large nodule is composed of proliferating endothelial cells forming fascicles and vascular spaces. **B.** A higher-power view of (A) shows cytologic atypia of the spindle cells. Red blood cells appear agglutinated *(arrows)*. The endothelial cells, in which the agglutinated red blood cells are present, form slitlike spaces.

stage, a subtle proliferation of irregular vascular channels, lined by a single layer of mildly atypical endothelial cells radiates from preexisting blood vessels and extends almost imperceptibly into the surrounding reticular dermis. Extravasated red blood cells, hemosiderin deposition and a sparse inflammatory infiltrate of lymphocytes and plasma cells are commonly observed.

In the plaque stage (Fig. 24-89), the entire reticular dermis is involved, with frequent extension into the subcutis and formation of bundles of spindle cells. In the nodule stage (Fig. 24-90), well-circumscribed dermal nodules are composed of anastomosing fascicles of spindle cells surrounding numerous slitlike spaces.

Bacillary Angiomatosis

Bacillary angiomatosis is a pseudoneoplastic proliferation of capillaries that arises in response to infection with *Bartonella* species. Patients with late-stage AIDS are at risk for infection with these organisms. The proliferative lesions appear as red-to-brown papules, often in large numbers, and may be confused with Kaposi sarcoma. Silver impregnation stains show dense masses of bacilli within the basophilic deposits. The lesions clear with antibiotic treatment.

Eosinophilic Folliculitis

Eosinophilic folliculitis (EF) is a chronic pruritic eruption of papules that are centered on hair follicles. Patients infected with HIV are a distinct population that displays EF although variants that are not related to HIV infection occur in other populations. The lesions are most often found on the trunk and proximal extremities. An infiltrate composed of lymphocytes, macrophages, and numerous eosinophils is present in the intrafollicular and perifollicular areas and around the dermal blood vessels.

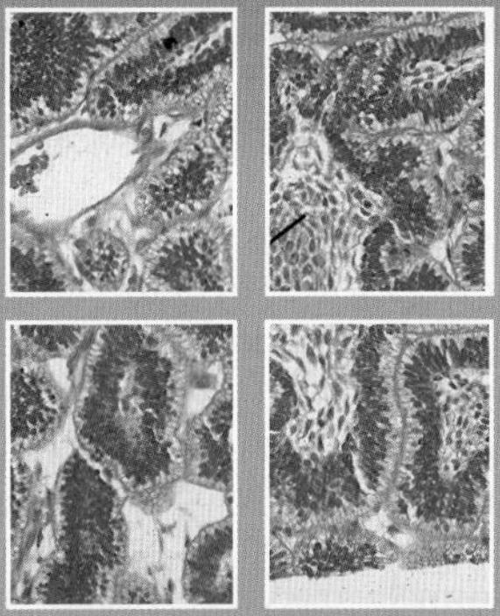

25

The Head and Neck

Bruce M. Wenig

ORAL CAVITY

The oral cavity extends from the lips to the pharynx. The anatomic borders of the oral cavity include:

- The vermilion border of the lips (anterior)
- A line drawn from the junction of the hard and soft palate to the circumvallate papillae of the tongue (posterior)
- The hard palate until its junction with the soft palate (superior)
- The anterior two-thirds of the tongue to the line of the circumvallate papillae (inferior)
- The buccal mucosa of the cheeks (lateral)

The oral mucosa consists of keratinized tissues of the attached gingiva, hard palatal mucosa, and specialized keratinized gustatory mucosa of the dorsum of the tongue. It also includes nonkeratinized mucosal surfaces of the inner lip and inner cheek, the nonattached, movable gingiva that continues into the maxillary and mandibular sulci, ventral tongue, floor of the mouth, soft palate, and tonsillar pillars.

The epithelium is three to four times the thickness of skin epidermis. Beneath the epithelium is the lamina propria of fibrous tissue and blood vessels, underneath which, in turn, is the densely fibrous periosteum of the hard palate or the alveolus of the maxilla and mandible. The term **submucosa** is sometimes loosely applied to the deep connective tissue just above the muscle layer, in which the minor salivary glands are often embedded.

Minor salivary glands, present throughout the oral cavity, appear as scattered, unencapsulated small lobules within the mucosa and submucosa. There are mucous glands in the lamina propria, particularly in the posterior hard palatal mucosa. Minor salivary glands of pure mucous type exist in the anterior ventral portion of the tongue (called Blandin, or Nunn, glands). Serous salivary glands are found near circumvallate papillae on the posterior and lateral tongue (von Ebner glands). Mixed mucoserous and mainly mucous glands predominate within the remainder of the oral cavity. Minor salivary glands are present in the retromolar mandibular ridge but the anterior hard palate and gingiva typically lack minor salivary glands.

The anterior two-thirds of the dorsum of the tongue is covered by keratinized stratified squamous epithelium that is specialized to form filiform papillae (pointed projections of keratin). Between these are the fungiform papillae, mushroom-shaped elevations of mucosa containing taste buds. Circumvallate papillae separate the anterior two-thirds from the posterior one-third, and contain taste buds at their base. The last group of papillae is the foliate papillae located in the posterior lateral tongue in a series of ridges. Each taste bud consists of a barrel-shaped collection of modified epithelial cells that extend vertically from the basal lamina to the epithelial surface, opening via a taste pore.

Developmental Anomalies

FACIAL CLEFTS: Failure of facial structures to fuse in the seventh week of embryonic life leads to formation of facial clefts, the most common of which is cleft upper lip (**harelip**). It may be unilateral or bilateral and frequently occurs in association with cleft palate (see Chapter 6).

HAMARTOMAS AND CHORISTOMAS: **Hamartomas** are non-neoplastic developmental anomalies caused by excessive growth of normal cells and/or tissue indigenous to the site. **Choristomas (heterotopias, ectopias, aberrant rests)** are non-neoplastic developmental anomalies of normal tissue that is foreign to its anatomic location. Hamartomas and choristomas are common in the oral cavity.

Fordyce granules are aggregates of sebaceous glands in the oral cavity (choristoma). They occur in 70% to 95% of the adult population, but rarely coalesce to form mass lesions.

Abnormal descent of the thyroid during development may lead to submucosal foci of **ectopic thyroid** between the tongue and suprasternal notch. The base of tongue between the foramen cecum and epiglottis is the most common location for ectopic thyroid (**lingual thyroid**). Normally placed cervical thyroid is absent in more than 75% of patients with lingual thyroid ("total migration failure"). Thus, surgical removal of a lingual thyroid can lead to hypothyroidism. Seventy percent of patients with symptomatic lingual thyroid are hypothyroid and 10% suffer from cretinism. Malignant transformation is rare but if it occurs, it will generally be papillary thyroid carcinoma.

Thyroglossal duct cysts result from persistence and cystic dilatation of the thyroglossal duct in the neck midline. The anomaly usually occurs above the thyroid isthmus but below the level of the hyoid bone. Patients are usually symptomatic before age 40. Surgery is the treatment of choice.

BRANCHIAL CLEFT CYST: Branchial cleft cysts originate from branchial arch remnants (Fig. 25-1). They occur in the lateral anterior neck or in the parotid gland, mostly in young adults, and contain thin, watery fluid, and mucoid or gelatinous material (Fig. 25-2). They are usually lined by squamous epithelium, with occasional foci of ciliated respiratory or pseudostratified columnar epithelium.

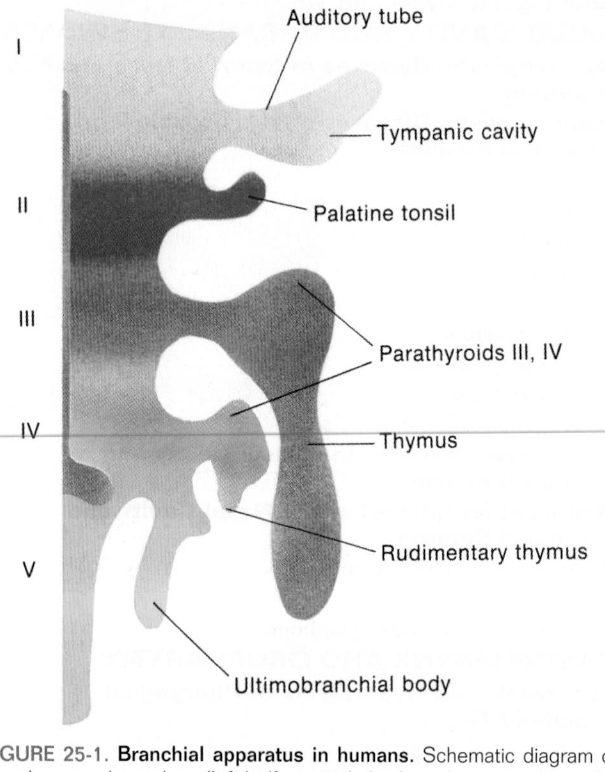

FIGURE 25-1. **Branchial apparatus in humans.** Schematic diagram of the pharyngeal pouches *(left half, ventral view)* in a human embryo of 6 weeks. Five pairs of pouches give rise to many important structures of the head, neck, and chest. A wide spectrum of congenital malformations results from abnormalities of the branchial apparatus.

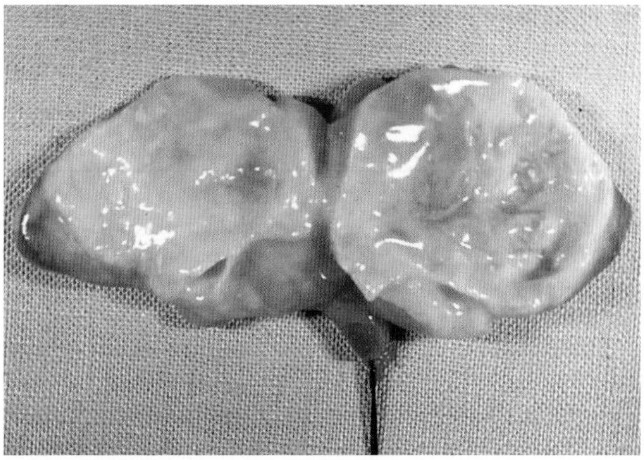

FIGURE 25-2. **Branchial cleft cyst.** Most of these cysts arise from the second branchial cleft and occur laterally in the neck. The cysts have a thin wall, contain turbid fluid, and are lined by stratified squamous or respiratory-type epithelium.

Infections of the Oral Cavity

Bacteria, spirochetes, viruses, fungi, and parasites are normal in the oral cavity, and are usually harmless. If the mucosa is injured or immunity impaired, otherwise normal oral cavity organisms can become pathogenic. (See Chapter 9 for further discussion.)

The following terms are used to describe localized inflammation of the oral cavity:

- **Cheilitis** (lips)
- **Gingivitis** (gum)
- **Glossitis** (tongue)
- **Stomatitis** (oral mucosa)

Bacterial and Fungal Infections Commonly Affect the Oral Cavity

SCARLET FEVER: Predominantly a disease of children, scarlet fever is caused by several strains of β-hemolytic streptococci (*Streptococcus pyogenes*). Damage to vascular endothelium by the erythrogenic toxin results in a rash on the skin and oral mucosa. The tongue has a white coating, through which the hyperemic fungiform papillae project as small red knobs ("strawberry tongue").

APHTHOUS STOMATITIS (CANKER SORES): Aphthous stomatitis is a common disease characterized by painful, recurrent, solitary or multiple, small ulcers of oral mucosa. The cause is unknown. Bacteria, mycoplasma, viruses, autoimmune reactions, and hypersensitivity have been implicated but are unproved. Microscopically, the lesion consists of a shallow ulcer covered by a fibrinopurulent exudate. The underlying inflammatory infiltrate is composed of mononuclear and polymorphonuclear leukocytes. The lesions heal without scar formation.

*ACUTE NECROTIZING ULCERATIVE GINGIVITIS (VINCENT ANGINA): Vincent angina is an infection by two symbiotic organisms, a fusiform bacillus and a spirochete (*Borrelia vincentii*).* The term **fusospirochetosis** is used to describe such an infection. These organisms are found in the mouths of many healthy persons, suggesting that other factors are required for development of acute necrotizing ulcerative gingivitis. The key element appears to be decreased resistance to infection due to inadequate nutrition, immunodeficiency, or poor oral hygiene. Vincent angina is characterized by punched-out erosions of the interdental papillae. The process tends to spread and eventually involve all gingival margins, which become covered by a necrotic pseudomembrane.

***Noma (cancrum oris)** is a severe fusospirochetal infection in persons who are malnourished, debilitated from infections, or weakened by blood dyscrasias. It features rapidly spreading gangrene of oral and facial tissues.* Large masses of tissue slough and leave the bones exposed, especially in children (see Chapter 9).

LUDWIG ANGINA: Ludwig angina is a rapidly spreading cellulitis, which originates in the submaxillary or sublingual space but extends locally to involve both. The responsible bacteria originate from oral flora: a variety of aerobic or anaerobic microorganisms have been implicated. This potentially life-threatening inflammatory process is uncommon in developed countries save in patients with chronic illnesses associated with immunosuppression.

Ludwig angina is most often related to dental extraction or trauma to the floor of the mouth. After extraction of a tooth, hairline fractures may occur in the lingual cortex of the mandible, providing microorganisms ready access to the submaxillary space. Infection may dissect into the parapharyngeal space along fascial planes and from there into the carotid sheath. An infected (mycotic) aneurysm of the internal carotid artery may result, erosion of which may cause massive hemorrhage. The inflammation may also dissect into the superior mediastinum, to involve the pleural space and pericardium.

DIPHTHERIA: Infection with *Corynebacterium diphtheriae* is characterized by a patchy pseudomembrane, which often begins on tonsils and pharynx but may also involve soft palate, gingiva, or buccal mucosa (see Chapter 9).

TUBERCULOSIS: Primary tuberculous lesions of the oral mucosa are rare. Most lesions are the result of pulmonary disease. The bacilli are carried in sputum and enter through small breaks in the mucosa, where they produce irregular, painful ulcers, mostly on the tongue. Biopsy reveals caseating granulomatous inflammation typical of tuberculous granulomas.

SYPHILIS: A chancre of primary syphilis may form on lips, tongue or oropharyngeal mucosa after contact with a lesion of primary or secondary syphilis (see Chapter 9). It is accompanied by a regional lymphadenitis and heals spontaneously in a few weeks. If syphilis is not treated adequately, a diffuse mucocutaneous eruption of the secondary stage develops. Lesions in the oral mucosa appear as multiple gray–white patches overlying ulcerated surfaces. They may undergo spontaneous remission but may also recur. Gummas may appear on palate and tongue after years of syphilitic infection. They are firm nodular masses that eventually ulcerate and may lead to palatal perforation.

ACTINOMYCOSIS: Actinomycetes are common inhabitants of the oral cavity of healthy persons, so that culture of the organism does not necessarily indicate infection. In the case of invasive actinomycosis, the most common offender is *Actinomyces bovis*, but *Actinomyces israelii* is sometimes encountered. The organisms produce chronic granulomatous inflammation and abscesses that drain by formation of fistulas. It is customary to distinguish cervicofacial (the most common form), pulmonary, and abdominal forms of actinomycosis according to the site of the infection. In the former, soft tissue infection may extend to adjacent bones, most commonly to mandible.

CANDIDIASIS: Also termed **thrush** or **moniliasis**, candidiasis is caused by *Candida albicans* (see Chapter 9), which is common on the surfaces of the oral cavity, gastrointestinal tract, and vagina. To cause disease, it must penetrate tissues, albeit superficially.

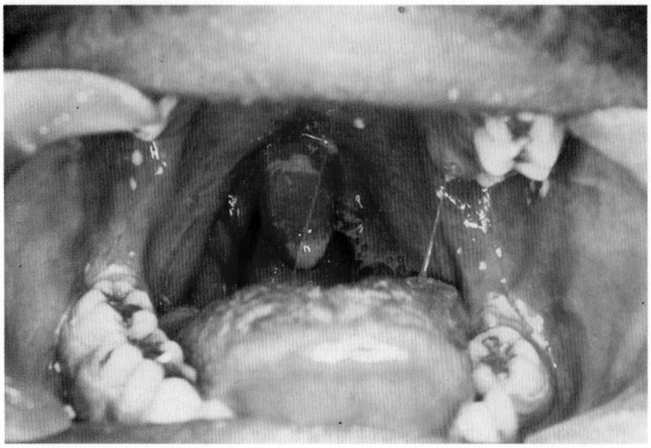

FIGURE 25-3. **Oral candidiasis.** White plaques coat mucous membranes of the oral cavity.

Oral candidiasis is mostly seen in people with compromised immune systems and in diabetics. The incidence in patients with acquired immunodeficiency syndrome (AIDS) is 40% to 90%. The lesions are white, slightly elevated, soft patches (Fig. 25-3) that consist mainly of fungal hyphae.

Viral Infections Present As Vesicular or Ulcerative Lesions

HERPES SIMPLEX VIRUS (HSV) TYPE 1: Herpes labialis (cold sores, fever blisters) and herpetic stomatitis are caused by HSV type 1 and are among the most common viral infections of lips and oral mucosa in both children and young adults. Transmission occurs by droplet infection, and the virus can be recovered from the saliva of infected persons. Disease starts with painful inflammation of the affected mucosa, followed shortly by the formation of vesicles. These vesicles rupture and form shallow, painful ulcers, ranging from punctate size to a centimeter in diameter. Microscopically, herpetic vesicle forms as a result of "ballooning degeneration" of epithelial cells. Some epithelial cells show intranuclear inclusion bodies. The ulcers heal spontaneously without scar formation.

Once HSV enters the body, it survives in a dormant state in the trigeminal ganglion. It can be reactivated to cause recurrent herpetic lesions in diverse ways, including trauma, allergy, menstruation, pregnancy, exposure to ultraviolet light, and other viral infections. Recurrent oral cavity vesicles almost invariably develop on a mucosa that is tightly bound to periosteum, for example, the hard palate.

HUMAN PAPILLOMAVIRUS (HPV) RELATED DISEASES: The HPV family of viruses (see Chapter 9) causes epithelial proliferations including papillomas (e.g., sinonasal (Schneiderian) papillomas and other mucosal papillomas of various upper aerodigestive tract sites.

EPSTEIN BARR VIRUS (EBV)-RELATED DISEASES: EBV is the cause of infectious mononucleosis, oral hairy leukoplakia and lymphoid malignancies (e.g., nasal-type natural killer (NK)/T cell lymphoma, Hodgkin lymphoma, see Chapter 20) and epithelial malignancies (e.g., nasopharyngeal-type differentiated and undifferentiated carcinomas, salivary gland undifferentiated carcinoma).

OTHER VIRAL INFECTIONS: Coxsackievirus causes **herpangina**, an acute vesicular oropharyngitis. A brief course of infection confers lasting immunity. **Cytomegalovirus** (CMV) infection typically presents with surface ulceration. Other virus infections that involve the oral mucosa include measles, rubella, chickenpox, and herpes zoster.

Benign Tumors

Benign tumors common elsewhere in the body are seen also in the oral cavity. These include pigmented nevi, fibromas, hemangiomas, lymphangiomas, and squamous papillomas. Trauma may lead to ulceration of these lesions, in which case, they may bleed or become infected.

PAPILLOMA: Squamous papilloma is a benign, exophytic epithelial neoplasm composed of branching fronds of squamous epithelium with fibrovascular cores. These are the most common benign oral cavity neoplasms, and have been associated with HPV infection. They occur mainly in the 3rd to 5th decades. The tongue, palate, buccal mucosa, tonsil, and uvula are most often involved.

BENIGN MINOR SALIVARY GLAND TUMORS: **Pleomorphic adenoma** (benign mixed tumor) is the most common oral salivary gland tumor (see below). Monomorphic adenomas such as myoepithelioma and oncocytoma occur less frequently.

Benign mesenchymal tumors may occur in the oral cavity, including hemangiomas, leiomyomas, and lipomas.

LOBULAR CAPILLARY HEMANGIOMA (PYOGENIC GRANULOMA; PREGNANCY TUMOR): Lobular capillary hemangioma is a benign polypoid form of capillary hemangioma primarily occurring on skin and mucous membranes, and are most common on gingiva. The term pyogenic granuloma is a misnomer: it is neither infectious nor granulomatous. In the oral cavity, they range from a few millimeters to a centimeter and are elevated, soft, red or purple, with smooth, lobulated, ulcerated surfaces. The lesion is characterized by submucosal vascular proliferation arranged in lobules or clusters with central capillaries and smaller ramifying tributaries (Fig. 25-4). In time, the lesions may become less vascular and may resemble a fibroma.

In pregnant women, particularly near the end of the first trimester, a gingival lesion may develop that grossly and microscopically is identical to lobular capillary hemangioma. Termed **pregnancy tumor**, it may or may not regress after delivery.

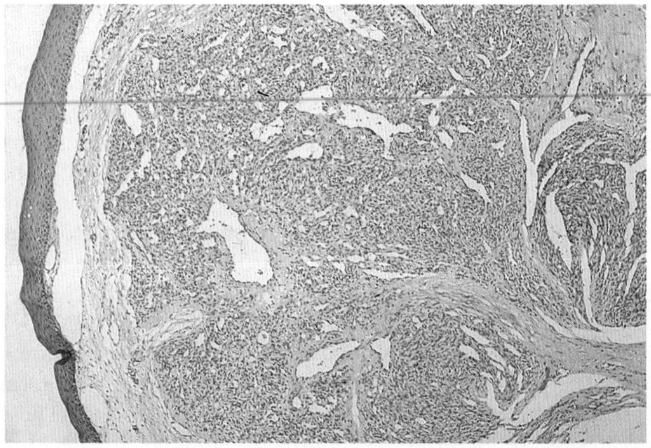

FIGURE 25-4 **Lobular capillary hemangioma (pyogenic granuloma).** Submucosal lesion characterized by the presence of cellular lobules consisting of dilated, irregularly shaped vascular spaces and surrounded by granulation tissue with a chronic inflammatory cell infiltrate.

Pre-Neoplastic or Epithelial Precursor Lesions

Premalignant lesions of the upper aerodigestive tract include leukoplakia, erythroplakia, or speckled leukoplakia, the terms reflecting the presence of a white, red, or mixed white/red lesion, respectively. ***Leukoplakia** (from the Greek,* leukos, *"white" and* plax, *"plaque") is an asymptomatic white lesion on the surface of a mucous membrane.* Some of these lesions undergo transformation to squamous cell carcinoma (SCC). The disorders occur with equal frequency in both sexes, mostly after the third decade of life. A variety of diseases appear clinically as leukoplakia, including various keratoses, hyperkeratosis, and squamous carcinoma in situ. Thus, leukoplakia is not a histologic diagnosis but rather a descriptive clinical term. Other clinical entities may also have white plaques on the oral mucosa, (e.g., candidiasis, lichen planus, psoriasis, syphilis).

The causes of leukoplakia are diverse, and include use of tobacco products, alcoholism and local irritation. The same factors also appear to be important in the etiology of oral carcinoma.

***Erythroplakia** is the red equivalent of leukoplakia.* Red areas associated with leukoplakic lesions are referred to as **speckled leukoplakia** (**erythroleukoplakia; speckled mucosa**). Erythroplakia occurs less frequently than leukoplakia. In contrast to leukoplakia, erythroplakia may represent moderate to severe dysplasia or to carcinoma. Not all red erythroplakic lesions herald dysplasia/carcinoma as many red oral mucosal lesions may be inflammatory in nature.

PATHOLOGY: Leukoplakia occurs most often on the buccal mucosa, tongue, and mouth floor. Plaques may be solitary or multiple and vary from small lesions to large patches. Erythroplakia is commonly associated with ominous histopathologic alterations, including severe dysplasia, carcinoma in situ, or invasive carcinoma. In contrast, leukoplakic lesions are not necessarily premalignant and may show a spectrum of histopathologic changes, from increased surface keratinization without dysplasia to invasive keratinizing squamous carcinoma (Fig. 25-5). Leukoplakic lesions, unlike erythroplakic ones, tend to be well defined with demarcated margins. The risk of malignant transformation in leukoplakia is 10% to 12%. Speckled leukoplakia carries an intermediate risk between "pure" leukoplakic and "pure" erythroplakic lesions for the development of a malignancy, but speckled leukoplakia should be viewed as a variant of erythroplakia.

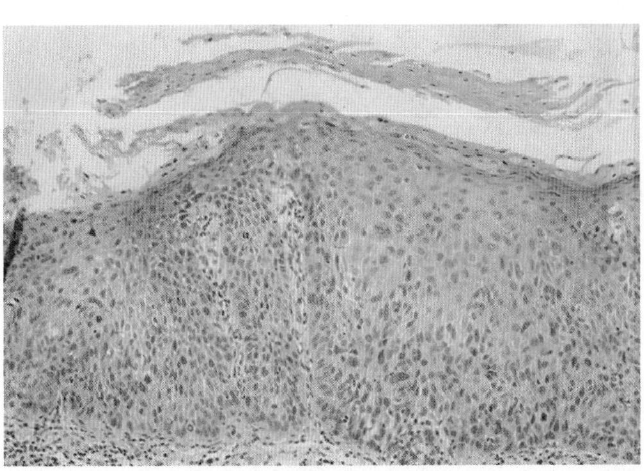

FIGURE 25-5. **Leukoplakia.** The lesion was seen as a white patch on the buccal mucosa of a heavy smoker. Histologically, epithelial hyperplasia, marked atypia, and parakeratosis are evident.

Oral hairy leukoplakia exhibits shaggy parakeratosis and edema. The EBV-infected epithelial cells have a vacuolated cytoplasm and are superficially located immediately beneath the keratin. Nuclei show dense central eosinophilic inclusions. Candidal hyphae are usually present, and concomitant HPV infection occurs in up to half of cases.

Squamous Cell Carcinoma

SCC is the most common malignant tumor of oral mucosa and may occur at any site. It most frequently involves the tongue, followed in descending order by the floor of the mouth, alveolar mucosa, palate, and buccal mucosa. The male-to-female ratio is 2:1 for the gum but 10:1 for the lip. There are substantial variations in the geographic distribution of oral cancer; for example, it is the single most common cancer of men in India.

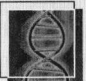

PATHOGENESIS: Predisposing factors in the pathogenesis of oral cancer include use of tobacco products, alcoholism, iron deficiency (Plummer-Vinson syndrome), physical and chemical irritants, chewing of betel nuts, ultraviolet light on the lips, and poor oral hygiene (craggy teeth and ill-fitting dentures). Not surprisingly, several of these factors also have been mentioned in connection with leukoplakia. Some SCCs of the head and neck have been associated with HPV infection, but a direct causal relationship between HPV and development of SCC is not definitively established. Multiple separate epidermoid carcinomas may be found at the same time (synchronous) or at intervals (metachronous) in the oral mucosa ("field cancerization").

PATHOLOGY: Invasive SCC of the oral cavity is similar to the same tumor in other sites and is generally preceded by carcinoma in situ. Grade I carcinoma is well differentiated and frequently keratinizing (Fig. 25-6). At the other end of the spectrum, grade IV tumors are so poorly differentiated that their origin is difficult to determine on morphologic grounds. Oral carcinoma metastasizes mainly to submandibular, superficial, and deep cervical lymph nodes. More than half of patients who die of SCC of the head and neck have distant, blood-borne metastases, most commonly in lungs, liver, and bones.

The histologic grade of SCC does not necessarily correlate with prognosis. However, tumors with broad, pushing borders, with large, cohesive cords and islands of cells, have a better prognosis than those that infiltrate in small irregular cords or single cells. These patterns of infiltration also correlate with the incidence of lymph node metastases.

Verrucous carcinoma (VC) is a highly differentiated variant of squamous cell carcinoma, which is locally destructive but do not metastasize. It generally occurs in the 6th and 7th decades of life. VCs may arise anywhere in this region but is most common on buccal mucosa, gingiva, and larynx.

VCs are usually white, warty to fungating, or exophytic, and are generally attached by a broad base (Fig. 25-7A). Microscopically, they exhibit a benign-appearing squamous epithelium (without dysplasia), marked surface keratinization, and a push-

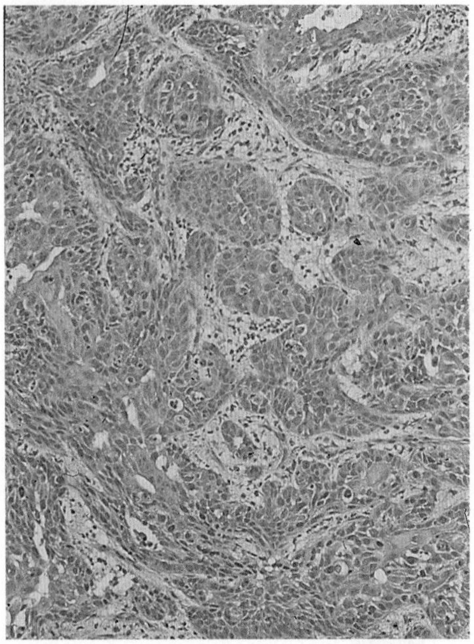

A

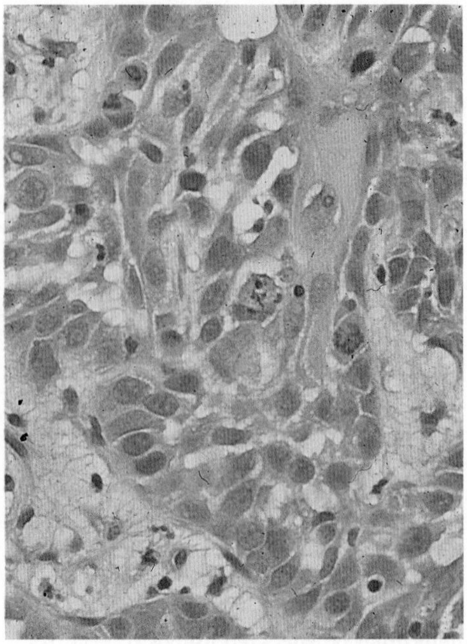

B

FIGURE 25-6. **Squamous cell carcinoma. A.** An infiltrative neoplasm is composed of cohesive nests of tumor. **B.** A less differentiated tumor displays cells with pleomorphic nuclei, prominent nucleoli, brightly eosinophilic cytoplasm indicating keratinization, and intercellular bridges connecting adjacent cells. A mitotic figure is seen (*arrow*).

ing border of bulbous rete pegs (see Fig. 25-7B). The tumor carries a good prognosis if it is completely removed.

Malignant Minor Salivary Gland Neoplasms

About 50% of intraoral minor salivary gland tumors are malignant. These include mucoepidermoid carcinoma, adenoid cystic carcinoma, and polymorphous low-grade adenocarcinoma. Some of the more common malignant major salivary gland tumors are uncommon in minor salivary gland locations (e.g., acinic cell adenocarcinoma), whereas polymorphous low-grade adenocarcinoma and clear cell carcinoma are more common in the oral cavity than in major salivary glands.

Benign Diseases of the Lips

The lips are affected by a variety of degenerative, inflammatory, and proliferative processes. Some of these, particularly those expressed in the skin and mucous membranes, are systemic; others reflect localized disease. **Mucocele** is mucous-filled cystic lesion associated with minor salivary glands that is probably caused by trauma (Fig. 25-8).

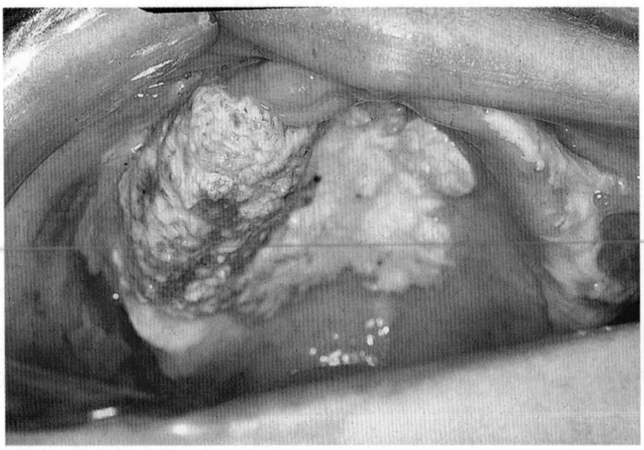

A

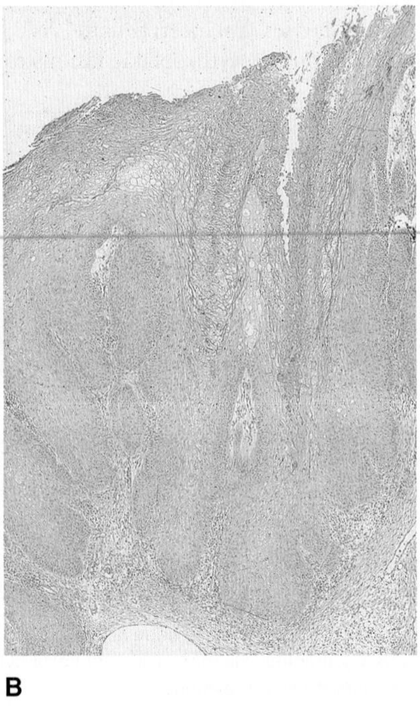

B

FIGURE 25-7. **Verrucous carcinoma. A.** The tumor is white with an exophytic appearance involving the alveolar ridge. Note the confluent flat white (leukoplakic) appearance of the palate. **B.** Microscopically, there is prominent surface keratinization ("church-spire" keratosis) composed of bland-appearing uniform squamous cells without dysplasia and broad or bulbous rete pegs with a pushing margin into the submucosa.

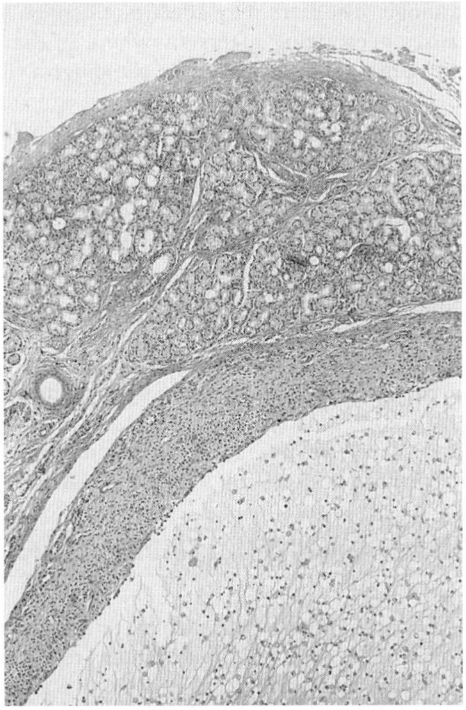

FIGURE 25-8. **Mucocele of lower lip.** This cystic lesion is associated with the minor salivary glands and is probably caused by trauma that permits escape of mucus. The cyst has a fibrous wall and is lined by granulation tissue. The lumen is filled with mucus that contains numerous macrophages.

Benign Diseases of the Tongue

MACROGLOSSIA: All components of the tongue may be involved by various localized or systemic diseases, some of which can lead to tongue enlargement. If present at birth, macroglossia is usually due to diffuse lymphangioma or hemangioma, although enlargement is rarely caused by congenital neurofibromatosis or true muscle hypertrophy. An enlarged tongue that protrudes from the mouth occurs in congenital hypothyroidism, Hurler syndrome, glycogen-storage disease type II (Pompe disease), Beckwith-Wiedemann syndrome, and Down syndrome. Acquired macroglossia is due to amyloidosis, acromegaly, and infiltration or lymphatic obstruction by tumors.

GLOSSITIS: Inflammation of the tongue can be caused by various microorganisms, physical effects, chemical agents, or systemic diseases. Some forms of glossitis are associated with vitamin deficiencies, including pernicious anemia, riboflavin deficiency, pellagra, and pyridoxine deficiency.

Dental Caries (Tooth Decay)

Caries is the most prevalent chronic disease of the calcified tissues of teeth. It affects persons of both sexes and every age group throughout the world, and its incidence has markedly increased with modern civilization.

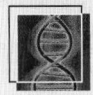

PATHOGENESIS: Dental caries results from the interactions of several factors.

BACTERIA: Dental caries is a chronic infectious disease of tooth enamel, dentin, and cementum, the organisms being part of the indigenous oral flora. Tooth surfaces are normally colonized by many microorganisms, and unless the surface is cleaned thoroughly and frequently, bacterial colonies coalesce into a soft mass known as **dental plaque**.

Carious lesions result primarily from leaching of mineral in dental tissues by acids produced from food residues by microorganisms on tooth surfaces. Numerous streptococci, lactobacilli, and actinomycetes in the oral flora have these characteristics. Indirect evidence points strongly to *Streptococcus mutans* as the primary etiologic agent that initiates caries. Organisms other than *S. mutans* may be more capable of maintaining the destructive process deeper in the enamel and dentin.

SALIVA: Saliva has a high buffering capacity that helps neutralize microbially produced acids in the mouth. In addition, it contains several bacteriostatic factors, such as lysozyme, lactoferrin, the lactoperoxidase system, and secretory immunoglobulins. **Xerostomia** (chronic dryness of the mouth from lack of saliva) results in rampant caries.

DIETARY FACTORS: One of the most important factors in caries development is a high-carbohydrate diet. The roughage in raw and unrefined foods cleanses the teeth. Additionally, roughage necessitates more mastication, which further contributes to cleansing of the teeth. By contrast, soft and refined foods tend to stick to the teeth and also require less chewing.

FLUORIDE: Fluoride protects against dental caries. It is incorporated into the crystal lattice structure of enamel, where it forms fluoroapatite, a less acid-soluble compound than the apatite of enamel. Fluoridation of drinking water in many communities led to dramatic reductions in dental caries in children whose teeth were formed while they drank fluoride-containing water.

PATHOLOGY: Caries begins with disintegration of enamel prisms after decalcification of the interprismatic substance, events that lead to accumulation of debris and microorganisms (Fig 25-9). These changes produce a small pit or fissure in the enamel. When the process reaches the

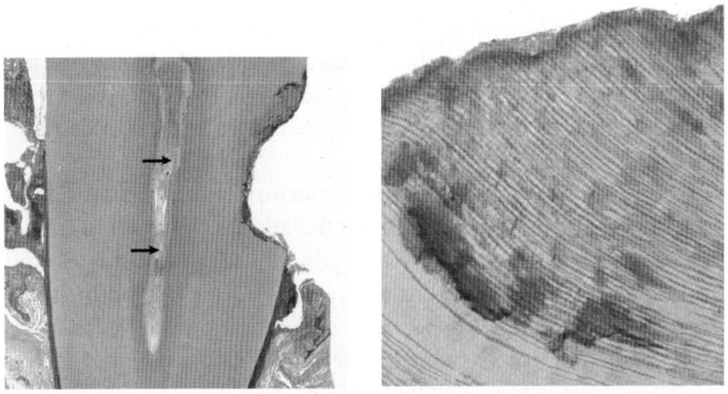

A B

FIGURE 25-9. **Dental caries. A.** A large cavity close to the gingival margin is illustrated. *Arrows,* band of secondary dentin that lines the pulp chamber. This newly formed dentin is opposite the area of tooth destruction and was produced by the stimulated odontoblasts. **B.** Deposits of debris cover the surface. Bacterial colonies *(dark purple)* have extended into dentinal canals.

dentinoenamel junction, it spreads laterally and also penetrates the dentin along the dentinal tubules. A substantial cavity then forms in the dentin, producing a flask-shaped lesion with a narrow orifice. Decalcification of dentin leads to focal coalescence of the destroyed dentinal tubules. Only when the vascular pulp of the tooth is invaded does an inflammatory reaction (**pulpitis**) appear, accompanied for the first time by pain.

Diseases of the Pulp and Periapical Tissues

The dental pulp is delicate connective tissue enclosed within the calcified walls of dentin. The pulp chamber is lined by odontoblasts and has a minute apical foramen through which blood vessels, lymphatics, and small nerves penetrate.

- **Pulpitis** results from invasion by the oral bacteria involved in dental caries. Pain in acute pulpitis reflects increased pressure in the pulp chamber, caused by edema and exudate.
- **Apical (or periapical granuloma),** the most common sequel of pulpitis, is chronically inflamed periapical granulation tissue. The inflammatory tissue gradually becomes surrounded by a fibrous capsule, and when the tooth is extracted, the encapsulated granuloma is found attached to the root.
- **Radicular cyst** (**apical periodontal cyst**) occurs when the squamous epithelium of an apical granuloma proliferates, forming a cavity or cyst.
- **Periapical abscess** may follow pulpitis.
- **Osteomyelitis** may complicate a periapical abscess, and usually cultures *Staphylococcus aureus, Staphylococcus epidermidis,* various streptococci, or mixed organisms. Infection may traverse the cortical bone and spread to various tissue spaces of head and neck, and rarely mediastinum.

Periodontal Disease

The gingiva (gum) is the part of the oral mucosa that surrounds the teeth and ends in a thin edge (free gingiva) adheres closely to the teeth. The periodontal ligament is composed of collagen fibers that hold teeth in position in the socket (alveolus) of the jawbone. These structures form the periodontium.

Periodontal disease refers to acute and chronic disorders of the soft tissues surrounding teeth, which eventually lead to the loss of supporting bone. Chronic periodontal disease typically occurs in adults with poor oral hygiene. However, many persons with apparently impeccable habits but a strong family history of periodontal disease, manifest the disorder. Chronic periodontitis causes loss of more teeth in adults than does any other disease, including caries.

Periodontal disease is caused by accumulation of bacteria under the gingiva in the periodontal pocket. As the mass of bacteria adhering to the surface of tooth (**dental plaque**) ages and mineralizes, it forms **calculus** (tartar). Adult periodontitis is mostly associated with *Bacteroides gingivalis. Bacteroides intermedius, Actinomyces* species, *Haemophilus* species, and other microorganisms may also participate.

The inflammation often starts as a marginal gingivitis, which, if untreated, progresses to chronic periodontitis. Once initiated, periodontitis continues to progress in the absence of treatment. Chronic inflammation weakens and destroys the periodontium, causing loosening and eventual loss of teeth.

Hematologic disorders may affect oral tissues. Agranulocytosis causes necrotizing ulcers anywhere in the oral and pharyngeal mucosa, but especially in the gingiva. Infectious mononucleosis often results in gingivitis and stomatitis, with exudate and ulceration. Acute and chronic leukemias of all types cause oral lesions. The most common involvement of oral tissues is seen in **acute monocytic leukemia**, in which 80% of patients exhibit gingivitis, gingival hyperplasia, petechiae, and hemorrhage. Necrosis and ulceration of the gingiva lead to severe superimposed infection, which may cause loss of teeth and alveolar bone. A hemorrhagic diathesis may be reflected in gingival hemorrhage.

Mild scurvy (vitamin C deficiency, see Chapter 8) is still encountered, particularly in poor or neglected individuals. It affects the marginal and interdental gingiva, which become swollen and bright red, and bleed and ulcerate readily. Hemorrhage into the periodontal membrane causes loosening and loss of teeth.

Odontogenic Cysts and Tumors

Odontogenic cysts include inflammatory and developmental cysts. The most common is the **radicular**, or **apical, periodontal cyst**, which involves the apex of an erupted tooth, usually after infection of the dental pulp. **Dentigerous cysts** are associated with the crown of an impacted, embedded or unerupted tooth, most often involving the mandibular and maxillary third molars. The cyst forms after the crown of the tooth has completely developed, and fluid accumulates between the crown and the overlying enamel epithelium. Dentigerous cyst may be complicated by ameloblastoma or SCC.

Ameloblastomas *are tumors of odontogenic epithelia and are the most common clinically significant odontogenic tumor.* They are slow-growing, locally invasive tumors that generally follow a benign clinical course. Most arise in the mandibular ramus or molar area, maxilla, or floor of the nasal cavity. The tumor tends to grow slowly as a central lesion of bone. Microscopically, ameloblastoma resembles the enamel organ in its various stages of differentiation, and a single tumor may show various histologic patterns. Accordingly, tumor cells resemble ameloblasts at the periphery of epithelial nests or cords, where columnar cells are oriented perpendicularly to the basement membrane (Fig. 25-10). The prognosis is favorable. Incompletely excised tumors recur, but malignant transformation does not occur.

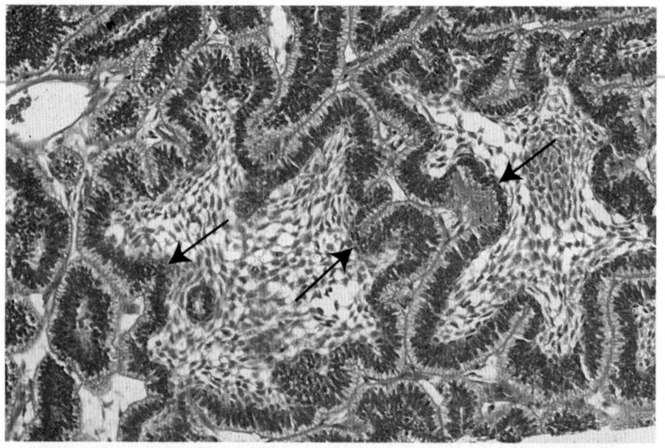

FIGURE 25-10. **Ameloblastoma.** A common histologic pattern is characterized by confluent islands of epithelium. The peripheral cells form bands that separate the tumor from the stroma *(arrows)*.

NASAL CAVITY AND PARANASAL SINUSES

The nostril apertures (**anterior nares**) lead into the nasal vestibule, a space lined by skin that contains hairs and sebaceous glands. Beyond the nares, the nasal cavity is divided by the median septum into two symmetric chambers, termed the **nasal fossae**. Each nasal fossa has an olfactory region, consisting of the superior nasal concha and the opposed part of the septum, and a respiratory region, which constitutes the rest of the cavity. On the lateral wall are the inferior, middle, and superior nasal conchae (turbinates), overhanging the corresponding nasal passages or meatuses. The paranasal sinuses are paired air spaces that communicate with the nasal cavity. The mucous membrane covering the respiratory portion of the nasal cavity has a ciliated, columnar epithelium with interspersed goblet cells.

These anatomic interrelations favor certain routes of disease spread (Fig. 25-11). Infections can spread to maxillary, ethmoid, frontal, and sphenoid sinuses, leading to intraorbital and intracranial disease. The cavernous sinus is also accessible, via the vein of Vesalius, medial to the foramen ovale.

Non-Neoplastic Diseases of External Nose and Nasal Vestibule

Virtually all diseases of the skin can occur on the external nose, including lesions due to solar damage (e.g., actinic keratosis, basal cell carcinoma, SCC, malignant melanoma). The numerous sebaceous glands of the nose are commonly involved by acne vulgaris.

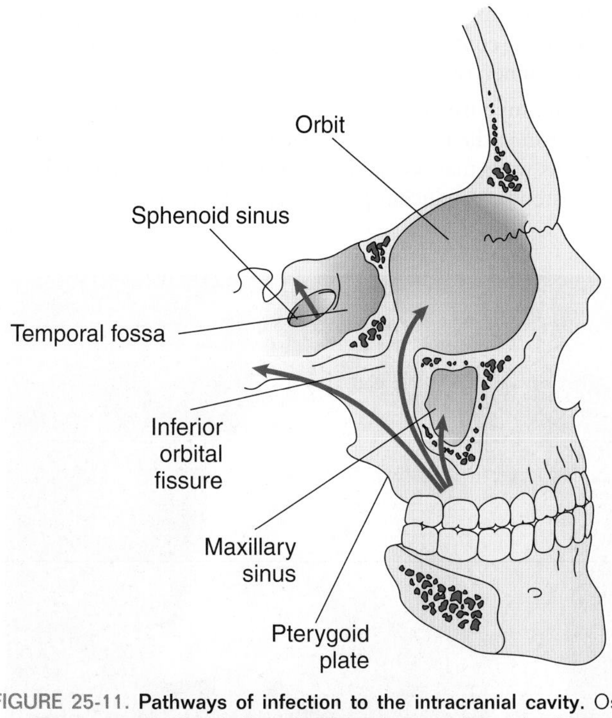

FIGURE 25-11. **Pathways of infection to the intracranial cavity.** Osseous pathways of infection from the jaws. *Arrows* indicate the direction of spread from the teeth to the maxillary sinus and through the inferior orbital fissure to the orbit. A deeper route is along the lateral pterygoid lamina up to the base of the skull, where, medial to the foramen ovale, a small aperture admits the vein of Vesalius. Through this small vein, the pterygoid plexus communicates with the cavernous sinus.

TABLE 25-1

Causes of Nasal Septum Perforation

Trauma
Specific infections (tuberculosis, syphilis, leprosy)
Wegener granulomatosis
Lupus erythematosus
Chronic exposure to dust (containing arsenic, chromium, copper, etc.)
Cocaine abuse
Malignant tumors

Rhinophyma is a protuberant bulbous mass on the nose caused by marked hyperplasia of sebaceous glands and chronic inflammation of the skin in acne rosacea.

Nosebleed (**epistaxis**) is most often caused by trauma. Other causes include hypertension, a variety of hematologic abnormalities, inflammatory conditions, and tumors of the nasal mucosa. Epistaxis frequently originates in a triangular area of the anterior nasal septum called "Little area," where the epidermis is thin. Not infrequently, numerous dilated blood vessels, or telangiectasias, are apparent. Little area is also the location of ulcers and perforations, which may be caused by various diseases or by trauma to the nasal septum (Table 25-1).

Non-Neoplastic Diseases of Nasal Cavity and Paranasal Sinuses

Rhinitis Is Usually Viral or Allergic

Rhinitis is inflammation of the mucous membranes of the nasal cavity and sinuses. The causes range from the common cold to unusual infections such as diphtheria, anthrax, and glanders.

VIRAL RHINITIS: The most common cause of acute rhinitis is viral infection, especially the common cold (**acute coryza**). The virus replicates in epithelial cells, causing the degenerating epithelial cells to be shed. The mucosa is edematous and engorged, and infiltrated by neutrophils and mononuclear cells. Clinically, mucosal swelling is manifested as nasal stuffiness. Abundant mucus secretion and increased vascular permeability lead to **rhinorrhea** (free discharge of a thin nasal mucus).

Viral rhinitis may be followed within a few days by secondary infection caused by normal nasal and pharyngeal flora. The abundant serous discharge then becomes mucopurulent, after which the surface epithelium is shed. The epithelial cells regenerate rapidly after the inflammation subsides.

ALLERGIC RHINITIS: Numerous allergens are constantly present in our environment, and sensitivity to any one of them can cause allergic rhinitis. In this condition, airborne allergenic particles (e.g., pollens, molds, animal allergens) are deposited on the nasal mucosa. Often called **hay fever**, allergic rhinitis may be acute and seasonal or chronic and perennial.

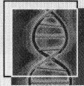

PATHOGENESIS: The few plasma cells present in the nasal mucosa normally produce immunoglobulin E (IgE). Mast cells in the nasal mucosa or free in nasal secretions also bear specific IgE directed against allergens. On contact with an allergen, mast cells release cytoplasmic granules with a variety of chemical mediators and enzymes. Some mediators are preformed and thus act rapidly (e.g., histamine); others are slowly eluted from the granule matrix (e.g., heparin or trypsin) and still others are newly synthesized (e.g., leukotrienes). Thus, an immediate, rapidly apparent reaction may give way to a prolonged inflammatory reaction as the various mediators exert their specific effects. The released mediators cause the signs and symptoms of allergic rhinitis, and many of the responses are attributable to histamine acting through its H_1 receptor.

PATHOLOGY: Increased capillary permeability mediated by vasodilator substances results in edema of the nasal mucosa, especially of the inferior turbinates. Numerous eosinophils may be seen in the nasal secretions or mucosa. The late phase of mast cell-mediated reactions is associated with persistent mucosal edema, and is seen clinically as nasal obstruction.

CHRONIC RHINITIS: Repeated bouts of acute rhinitis may lead to chronic rhinitis. A deviated nasal septum is often a contributory factor. Chronic rhinitis is characterized by nasal mucosal thickening due to persistent hyperemia, mucous gland hyperplasia, and lymphocyte and plasma cell infiltration.

Nasal Polyps Are Focal Inflammatory Swellings

Sinonasal inflammatory polyps are nonneoplastic lesions of the mucosa (Fig. 25-12). Most arise from the lateral nasal wall or ethmoid recess. They may be unilateral or bilateral, single or multiple. Symptoms include nasal obstruction, rhinorrhea, and headaches. The etiology involves multiple factors, including allergy, cystic fibrosis, infections, diabetes mellitus, and aspirin intolerance Sinonasal allergic polyps are lined externally by respiratory epithelium and contain mucous glands within a loose mucoid stroma, infiltrated by plasma cells, lymphocytes, and many eosinophils.

Sinusitis Is a Bacterial Infection

Sinusitis is inflammation of the mucous membranes of paranasal sinuses.

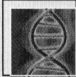

PATHOGENESIS: Any condition (inflammation, neoplasm, foreign body) that interferes with sinus drainage or aeration renders it liable to infection. If a sinus ostium is blocked, secretions or exudate accumulate behind the obstruction.

Acute sinusitis is a disorder of less than 3 weeks' duration, caused predominantly by extension of infection from the nasal mucosa. Most cases involve a rich bacterial flora, with *Haemophilus influenzae* and *Branhamella catarrhalis* most common. Maxillary sinusitis may also be caused by odontogenic infections, in which case, bacteria from the roots of the first and second molars penetrate the thin bony plate that separates them from the floor of the maxillary sinus.

Chronic sinusitis is a sequel of acute inflammation, either as a result of incomplete resolution of infection or because of recurrent acute complications. In contrast to acute sinusitis, the purulent exudate in chronic sinusitis almost always includes anaerobic bacteria.

PATHOLOGY: Acute or chronic sinusitis may be followed by a number of complications:

- **Mucocele:** *Mucocele is an accumulation of mucous secretions in a nasal sinus.* Infection of a mucocele results in a sinus filled with mucopurulent exudate, termed **pyocele**. Purulent exudate in a sinus is termed **empyema** (Fig. 25-13). Mucoceles occur most often in the anterior compartments ("cells") of frontal and ethmoid sinuses. They develop slowly and cause bone resorption by the pressure they exert. Mucoceles of anterior ethmoid or frontal sinuses may be large enough to displace the contents of the orbit and occasionally erode into the central nervous system.
- **Osteomyelitis:** Bone infection occurs when suppurative infection in the frontal sinus reaches a bone. Infection of nasal sinus walls may spread through Volkmann canals to the periosteum, producing periostitis and subperiosteal abscess.

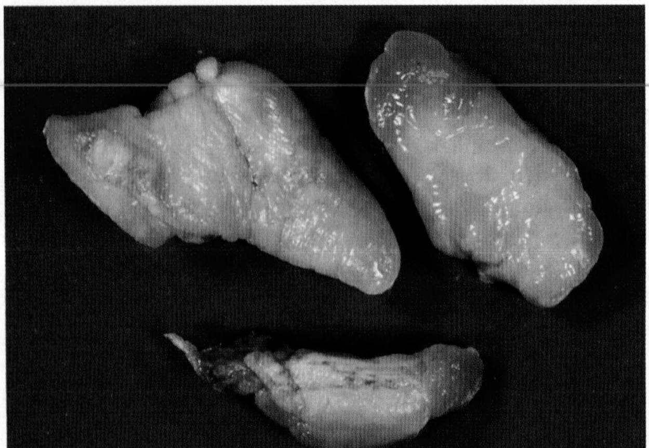

FIGURE 25-12. **Nasal polyps.** These smooth, pale, polypoid masses were removed from a patient with chronic rhinitis.

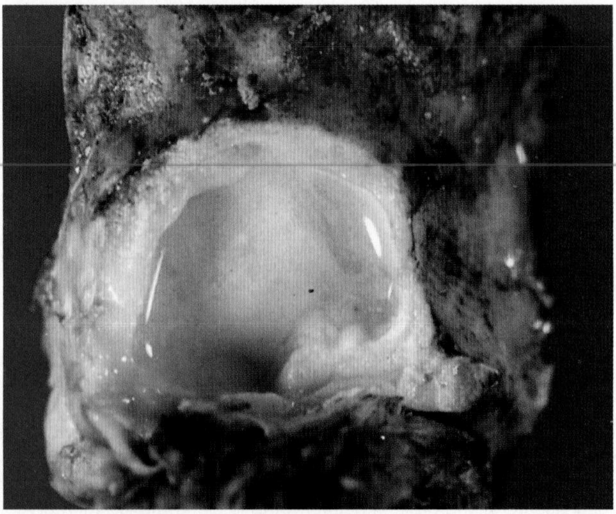

FIGURE 25-13. **Empyema of the maxillary sinus** (sagittal section). Infection followed chronic obstruction of the orifice caused by adenocarcinoma of the nasal mucosa.

If these occur on the orbital side of the bone, orbital cellulitis or an orbital abscess forms. Skin overlying the infection is often markedly edematous, and subcutaneous cellulitis or a subcutaneous abscess also may develop. Osteomyelitis also may spread rapidly between the outer and inner tables of the skull.

- **Septic thrombophlebitis:** Infection in the sinuses may penetrate the bone and spread to the frontal and diploe venous systems. Spread of septic thrombophlebitis to the cavernous venous sinus through the superior ophthalmic veins is a life-threatening complication.
- **Intracranial infections:** Spread of infection to the cranial cavity may also complicate sinusitis. Lesions include epidural, subdural, and cerebral abscesses, and purulent leptomeningitis. Such spread may occur via lymphatics and veins, and need not involve extensive destruction of bone.

Syphilis May Destroy the Nasal Bridge

Although primary chancres in the nose are rare, the mucosal lesions of secondary syphilis are common in the nose and nasopharynx. In tertiary syphilis, inflammation may involve large portions of the nasal mucosa, underlying cartilage and bone. Perichondrial or periosteal gummas may destroy nasal cartilage and bone. The nasal bridge collapses, producing so-called saddle nose. Destruction of nasal bony walls may also lead to perforation of the nasal septum, hard palate, wall of the orbit or maxillary sinus.

Leprosy Is Spread through Nasal Secretions

Mycobacterium leprae multiplies best at a lower temperatures, and so prefers infects cooler body sites, such as the nares and anterior nasal mucosa. Nasal involvement is commonly the first manifestation of leprosy. Tuberculoid and intermediate forms of leprosy account for most cases (see Chapter 9). The skin around the nares and anterior nasal mucosa shows nodules, ulceration, or perforations. Nasal involvement is important since leprosy is spread through nasal secretions that teem with bacilli.

Rhinoscleroma Is a Chronic Bacterial Infection of the Nose

*Rhinoscleroma (**scleroma**) is a chronic inflammatory process caused by a gram-negative diplobacillus,* Klebsiella rhinoscleromatis, *which usually begins in the nose and remains localized to that site, although it may extend slowly into the nasopharynx, larynx, and trachea.* Rarely, rhinoscleroma is seen in other locations, including paranasal sinuses, orbital tissues, skin, lips, oral mucosa, gastrointestinal tract, and cervical lymph nodes. Rhinoscleroma is endemic in some Mediterranean countries and in parts of Asia, Africa, and Latin America. Indigenous cases also have been recognized in the United States. It occurs in both sexes and at any age. Most patients have poor domestic and personal hygiene. Epidemiologic evidence suggests that household relationships are decisive factors in the development of this disorder.

PATHOLOGY: Infected tissues appear firm, greatly thickened, irregularly nodular, and often ulcerated. Microscopically, the granulation tissue is strikingly rich in plasma cells, lymphocytes, and foamy macrophages (Fig. 25-14). The characteristic large macrophages, referred to as *Mikulicz cells,* contain masses of phagocytosed bacilli.

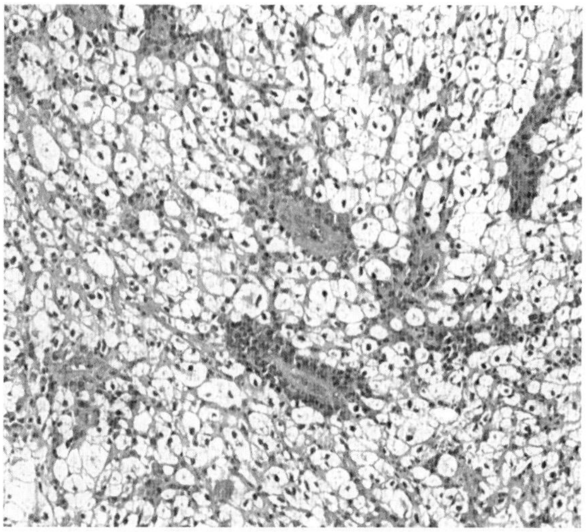

FIGURE 25-14. **Scleroma.** Granulation tissue contains numerous foamy macrophages (Mikulicz cells).

Serologic tests are valuable in establishing the diagnosis of rhinoscleroma, because specific antibodies are present in many patients. The disease is successfully treated with antibiotics.

Fungal Infections Are Usually Opportunistic

Pathogenic fungi may involve the nose and paranasal sinuses as part of cutaneous or mucocutaneous infection, particularly in a setting of immunodeficiency (see Chapter 9).

Candidiasis is the most common fungus infection of the nasal mucosa, usually accompanying oral and pharyngeal candidiasis (**thrush**). **Aspergillosis** is uncommon, and when it occurs it generally involves a paranasal sinus. The fungi may disseminate to the venous sinuses, meninges, and brain. Aspergillosis of the sinonasal tract may be noninvasive or invasive. Noninvasive types of aspergillus sinusitis include **allergic fungal sinusitis** (AFS) and **sinus mycetoma** (so-called fungus balls).

AFS is a hypersensitivity reaction to fungal antigens. It occurs in patients who are atopic or immunologically "hypercompetent." Its pathogenesis is like that of allergic bronchopulmonary aspergillosis (see Chapter 12). The disease occurs at all ages but is most common in children or young adults. It primarily involves the maxillary and ethmoid sinuses, although any sinus may be involved.

Fungus balls or **aspergillomas** occur in immunologically competent patients, usually with chronic sinus disease associated with poor drainage. In this setting, the fungus can proliferate and form a dense mass of hyphae that causes nasal obstruction. Evidence of bone destruction and ocular symptoms may be present.

Invasive fungal sinusitis usually affects immunocompromised or immunosuppressed patients. In the rare **rhinocerebral aspergillosis**, the organisms disseminate to the venous sinuses, meninges, and brain, and few patients survive.

Rhinosporidiosis of the nose is produced by the enigmatic *Rhinosporidium seeberi,* an organism whose source is unknown. It is classified among the fungi, although it has neither been grown in culture nor transmitted experimentally. The disease is endemic in Sri Lanka, and in parts of India, and Central and South America. The nasal mucosa afflicted with rhinosporidiosis contains vascular polyploid masses. Microscopically, the polyps show marked chronic inflammation and characteristic spherical 50 to 350 μm in diameter sporangia.

Leishmaniasis is also known as kala-azar

The nose is a frequent site of mucocutaneous leishmaniasis, caused by *Leishmania braziliensis* (see Chapter 9). The nasal disease, known as **espundia**, occurs in Central and South America. The initial lesion is a skin sore that heals within a few months. In some patients, mucocutaneous lesions develop in the nose or upper lip after an interval of months or years. The infection probably spreads by nasal contact with contaminated fingers. The infected mucosa has polypoid inflammatory lesions and superficial ulcers. Early in infection, many macrophages contain parasites. Later, a tuberculoid type of granulomatous response develops. Such lesions contain few recognizable parasites. Bacterial infection may supervene and lead to soft tissue destruction and collapse of the anterior cartilaginous nasal septum.

Wegener Granulomatosis May Manifest in the Nose

Wegener granulomatosis affects the lower airways (see Chapter 12).

PATHOLOGY: In its fully developed form, this rare disease involves the lungs, kidneys, and small arteries throughout the body. The sinonasal tract may be affected as part of the systemic process or disease may be localized to this region. Wegener granulomatosis often presents as septal perforation and mucosal ulceration, followed by slowly progressive destruction of the nose and paranasal sinuses, leading to a saddle nose deformity (Fig. 25-15). The resulting "runny nose," sinusitis and nosebleeds may be accompanied by constitutional symptoms, such as fever, malaise, and weight loss. Microscopically, nasal lesions reveal ischemic-type necrosis, vasculitis, mixed chronic inflammatory cell infiltrate, scattered multinucleated giant cells, and microabscesses. Well-formed granulomas are not seen. Elevated serum antineutrophil cytoplasmic antibodies (ANCAs) are associated with active disease.

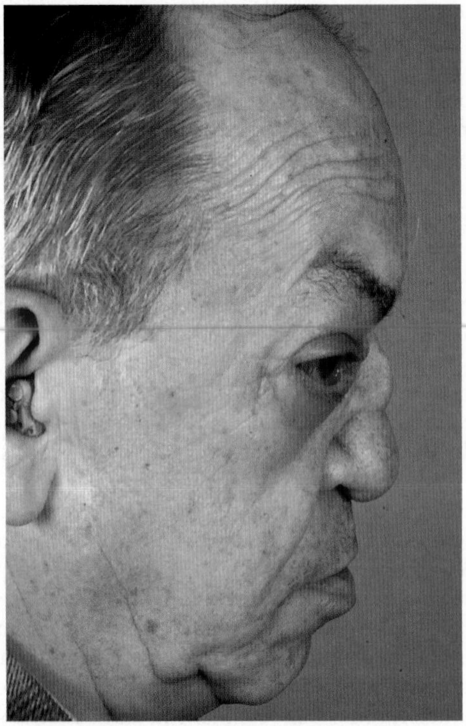

FIGURE 25-15. **Saddle nose deformity of Wegener granulomatosis.**

Benign Neoplasms of the Nasal Cavity and Paranasal Sinuses

SQUAMOUS PAPILLOMA: The most frequent benign tumor of the nasal cavity is squamous papilloma, which almost always occurs in the nasal vestibule. The lesion is often indistinguishable from a wart (verruca vulgaris).

SCHNEIDERIAN PAPILLOMAS: Schneiderian papillomas are a group of benign neoplasms composed of a squamous or columnar epithelial proliferation with associated mucous cells, and arising from the sinonasal (Schneiderian) mucosa. The ectodermally derived lining of the sinonasal tract, the Schneiderian membrane, may give rise to three morphologically distinct benign papillomas collectively called Schneiderian or sinonasal-type papillomas: **inverted**, **oncocytic** (cylindrical or columnar cell), and **fungiform** (exophytic, septal) papillomas. Collectively, Schneiderian papillomas represent less than 5% of all sinonasal tract tumors.

INVERTED PAPILLOMA: This tumor involves the lateral nasal wall and may spread into the paranasal sinuses. Inverted papillomas occur mainly in middle-aged persons. As the name implies, they show characteristic inversions of surface epithelium into the underlying stroma (Fig. 25-16). HPV types 6/11 and rarely other types (16/18, 33, 40, 57) have been found in inverted papillomas, but a cause-and-effect relationship is unproven. Although benign, these tumors may erode bone by pressure. Unless surgical resection extends beyond the boundaries of grossly visible lesions, they frequently recur. In 5% of cases, inverted papillomas give rise to SCC.

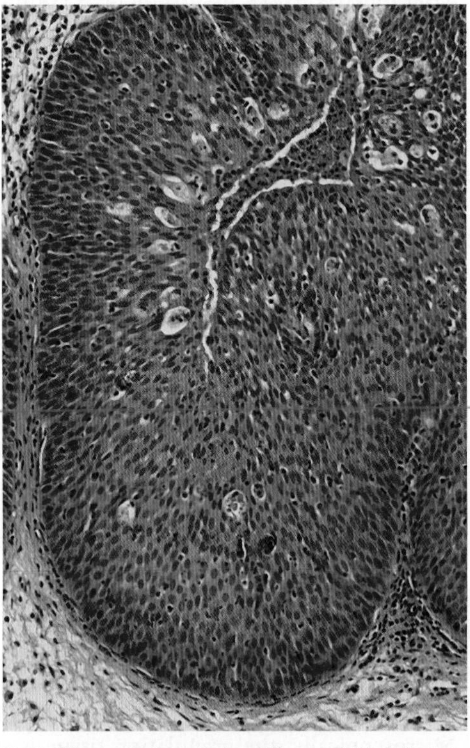

FIGURE 25-16. **Sinonasal inverted papilloma.** Epithelial nests are growing downward (inverted) into the submucosa. They are composed of a uniform cellular proliferation, which displays an inflammatory cell infiltrate and scattered microcysts.

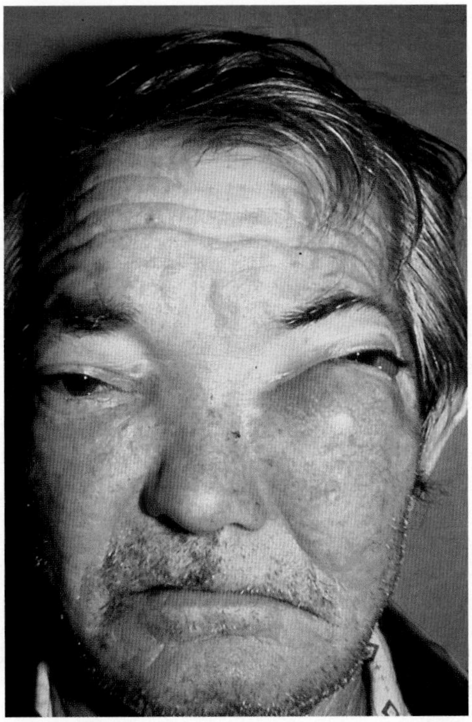

FIGURE 25-17. **Squamous cell carcinoma** of the maxillary sinus caused an obvious facial deformity, owing to invasion outside the confines of the sinus. Involvement of the orbit and facial nerve is evident. The latter is defined by drooping of the mouth to the side of the facial nerve paralysis.

Malignant Neoplasms of the Nasal Cavity and Paranasal Sinuses

Squamous Cell Carcinoma is Often Associated with Occupational Risk Factors

Over half of carcinomas of nasal cavity and paranasal sinuses originate in the antrum of the maxillary sinus, one third in the nasal cavity, 10% in the ethmoid sinus, and 1% in the sphenoid and frontal sinuses (Fig. 25-17). Most cancers of the nasal cavity and paranasal sinuses are squamous cell tumors (keratinizing and nonkeratinizing). Some 15% are adenocarcinomas, or undifferentiated carcinomas.

PATHOGENESIS: Several industrial chemicals may cause cancer of the nose and sinuses, including nickel, chromium, and aromatic hydrocarbons. Occupational settings reportedly with increased risk for cancer of the nose and sinuses (but for which a specific chemical agent is not identified) are woodworking in the furniture industry, use of cutting oils, and leather textile industries.

Tumors in nickel workers are SCCs, which usually arise from the middle turbinate, with latencies from 2 to 32 years. Tumors related to other occupational exposures are mainly adenocarcinomas and occur mostly in the maxillary and ethmoid sinuses. Because of the occupational risk factors, cancers of the nose and sinuses are far more common in men and occur after age 50 years.

Cancers of the nasal cavity and sinuses grow relentlessly and invade adjacent structures but typically do not give rise to distant metastases. Survival is usually only a few years.

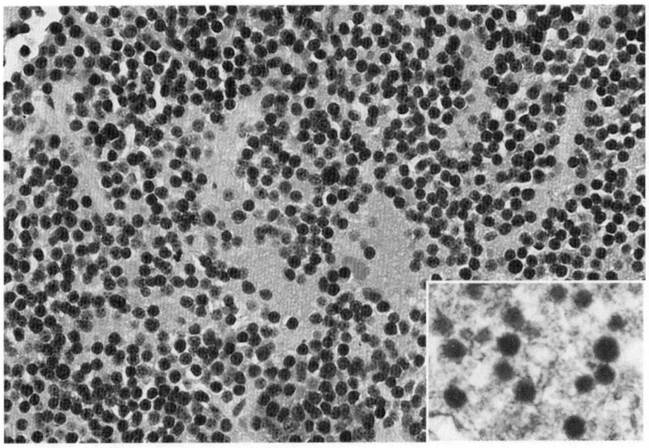

FIGURE 25-18. **Olfactory neuroblastoma.** This tumor is composed of small round cells with hyperchromatic nuclei and a background eosinophilic stroma representing neurofibrillary matrix. An electron micrograph *(inset)* shows intracytoplasmic, secretory-type, membrane-bound granules with dense cores.

Olfactory Neuroblastoma is of Neural Crest Origin

This tumor, also called **esthesioneuroblastoma**, *is an unusual malignancy of the nose.* It has a slight male predominance and occurs over a wide age range from 3 years to the ninth decade.

PATHOLOGY: This cancer arises from the olfactory mucosa that covers the superior third of the nasal septum, cribriform plate, and superior turbinate. Olfactory neuroblastoma is usually polypoid and highly vascular and displays diverse histologic patterns, depending on the amount of intercellular neurofibrillary material. Tumor cells are slightly larger than lymphocytes, exhibit round nuclei with an even distribution of chromatin and have an inconspicuous cytoplasm (Fig. 25-18). The tumor cells may form pseudorosettes (Homer Wright rosettes) or true neural rosettes (Flexner-Wintersteiner rosettes). By electron microscopy, olfactory neuroblastoma cells have intracytoplasmic secretory granules similar to those of neuroblastomas at other sites.

CLINICAL FEATURES: Olfactory neuroblastomas invade and destroy bony structures slowly, and spread readily via lymphatics to regional and distant lymph nodes. Hematogenous metastases are less frequent. The 5-year survival rate is 50%; death is usually due to invasion of the cranial cavity.

Nasal-Type Angiocentric Natural Killer/T (NK/T)-Cell Lymphoma Is an Aggressive, Highly Lethal Disease

***Nasal-type angiocentric NK/T-cell lymphoma** has supplanted previous designations of **lethal midline granuloma**, midline malignant reticulosis. and polymorphic reticulosis.* This aggressive type of lymphoma manifests as necrotizing, ulcerating mucosal lesions of the upper respiratory tract.

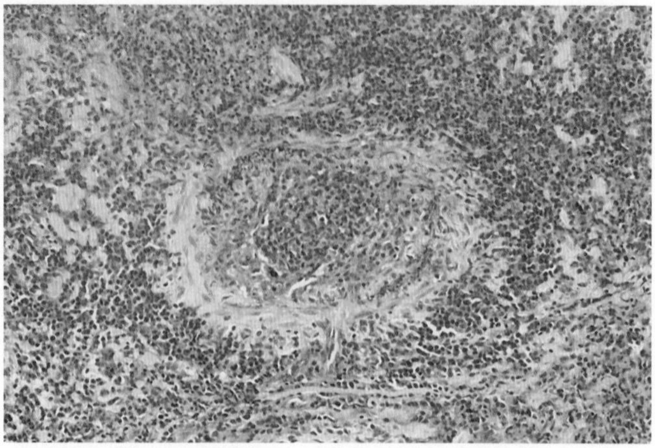

FIGURE 25-19. **Angiocentric natural killer (NK)/T cell lymphoma.** A malignant cellular infiltrate growing around and into a medium-sized blood vessel with disruption of the external elastic membrane and occlusion of the vessel lumen.

PATHOLOGY: The polymorphism of the atypical lymphocytic infiltrate is a characteristic feature that distinguishes the nasal-type NK/T-cell lymphoma from many other lymphomas. Similar necrotizing infiltrates may occur in the upper airways, lungs, and alimentary tract, but any organ can be involved. The malignant infiltrate characteristically surrounds small-to-medium-sized blood vessels (angiocentric), infiltrates through vascular walls (angioinvasive), often occludes vessel lumens like a thrombus and causes necrosis in adjacent tissues (ischemic-type) (Fig. 25-19). EBV infection is associated with this type of lymphoma.

CLINICAL FEATURES: The clinical course of nasal-type NK/T-cell lymphoma is characterized by insidious onset, with symptoms of nonspecific rhinitis or sinusitis. Gradually, the nasal mucosa becomes focally swollen and indurated and eventually ulcerated. Ulcers are covered by a black crust, under which lesions progress to erode cartilage and bone. This destruction causes defects of the nasal septum, hard palate, and nasopharynx, with serious functional consequences. The skin of the midface is often involved. The disease remains localized in half of patients, but disseminates widely in an equal proportion. Unlike Wegener granulomatosis, serum levels of ANCA are not elevated. Death is due to secondary bacterial infection, aspiration pneumonia, or hemorrhage from eroded large blood vessels.

The infiltrates of nasal-type NK/T-cell lymphoma are, at least initially, radiosensitive and remission with cytotoxic agents has also been reported.

NASOPHARYNX AND OROPHARYNX

The nasopharynx is continuous anteriorly with the nasal cavities; its roof is formed by the body of the sphenoid bone and its posterior wall is formed by the cervical vertebrae. The openings of the eustachian tubes are on the lateral walls of the nasopharynx. In the newborn it is covered by pseudostratified ciliated columnar epithelium. With advancing age, it is replaced by a stratified squamous epithelium over large areas (80%). The mucosa contains numerous mucous glands and abundant lymphoid tissue.

Waldeyer ring *is a circular band of lymphoid tissue at the opening of the oropharynx into the respiratory and digestive tracts.* The lymphoid tissue on the superior posterior wall forms the nasopharyngeal tonsils, which, when hyperplastic, are better known as **adenoids**. The palatine tonsils, situated laterally where the pharynx connects with the oral cavity, are covered by stratified squamous epithelium, which dips into the lymphoid tissue and lines the infoldings (**tonsillar crypts**). Crypts normally contain desquamated epithelium; lymphocytes; some neutrophils; and saprophytic organisms, including bacteria, *Candida,* and actinomycetes. Virulent pathogens may also be present in the pharynx of healthy persons (e.g., *Corynebacterium diphtheriae,* meningococcus).

Waldeyer ring is well developed in children and contains follicles with germinal centers. In fact, the tonsils contain the largest collection of B lymphocytes in a normal child. Pharyngeal lymphoid tissue diminishes considerably by adulthood. It gradually involutes with age, but does not totally disappear. Tonsillectomy and adenoidectomy, less widely practiced today than formerly, result in a major loss of pharyngeal lymphoid tissue. Removing tonsils and adenoids does not decrease serum immunoglobulin levels, and does not alter antibody responses to several human respiratory viruses. However, it does lead to decreased secretory IgA in the nasopharynx.

Hypoplasia and Hyperplasia of Pharyngeal Lymphoid Tissue

Bruton sex-linked agammaglobulinemia involves congenital absence of pharyngeal lymphoid tissue (see Chapter 4). This familial disease affects only male offspring, who have minimal or no lymphoid tissue in their tonsils, pharynx, and intestines (Peyer patches and appendix). They have a normally developed thymus.

Atrophy of pharyngeal lymphoid tissue is common in advanced AIDS and in chronically immunosuppressed patients. Local radiation therapy also causes marked loss of lymphoid tissue in Waldeyer ring.

Hyperplasia of nasopharyngeal lymphoid tissue follows infections or chronic irritation of the pharynx by dust, smoke, and fumes. In some primary immunodeficiencies (dysgammaglobulinemia type I or nodular lymphoid hyperplasia), the tonsils may be enlarged, presumably reflecting an adaptive response by the immune system.

Infections

Pharyngitis and tonsillitis are among the most common diseases of head and neck. Nasopharyngeal inflammation occurs mainly in children, although it is also common in adolescents and young adults. Viral or bacterial infections may be limited to the palatine tonsils, but nasopharyngeal tonsils or adjacent pharyngeal mucosa may also be involved, often as part of a general upper respiratory tract infection. In the latter case, initial infecting agents are most often viruses spread by droplet or by direct contact: usually influenza, parainfluenza, adenovirus, respiratory syncytial virus, and rhinovirus.

Streptococcus pyogenes is the most important cause of pharyngitis and tonsillitis, because of the possibility of serious suppurative and nonsuppurative sequelae. **Diphtheria** is still an important cause of pharyngitis in some countries. These infections are characterized by an exudate or, in the case of diphtheria, a pseudomembrane, on the tonsils and pharynx.

Acute tonsillitis is a bacterial infection, usually with *S. pyogenes* (group A β-hemolytic streptococci). Follicular tonsillitis is characterized by pinpoint exudates that can be extruded from the crypts.

Pseudomembranous tonsillitis refers to a necrotic mucosa covered by a coat of exudate, for instance in diphtheria or in **Vincent angina.** The latter is caused by fusiform bacilli and spirochetes that are present in the normal bacterial flora of the mouth. These organisms become pathogenic when local or systemic resistance is low (e.g., after mucosal injury or in malnutrition).

Recurrent or chronic tonsillitis is not as common as once believed, and enlarged tonsils in children do not necessarily signify chronic tonsillitis. However, repeated infections can cause enlargement of tonsils and adenoids to a degree that obstruct air passages. In children, repeated bouts of streptococcal tonsillitis may lead to rheumatic fever or glomerulonephritis, and patients may benefit from tonsillectomy.

Peritonsillar abscess (quinsy) is collection of purulent material behind the posterior capsule of the tonsil, usually due to infection with α- and β-hemolytic streptococci. Approximately one-third of patients have a prior history of tonsillitis. Untreated, peritonsillar abscesses may lead to several life-threatening situations: (1) aided by gravity, they may dissect inferiorly to the pyriform sinus, with obstruction of, or rupture into, the airway; (2) they may extend laterally into the parapharyngeal space (parapharyngeal abscess) and weaken the carotid artery wall; or (3) they may penetrate along the carotid sheath inferiorly into the mediastinum or, superiorly, to the base of the skull or cranial cavity, with disastrous consequences.

Infectious mononucleosis often presents with tonsillitis and pharyngitis, often exudative. Lymphadenopathy commonly affects posterior cervical lymph nodes. **Adenoids** represent chronic inflammatory hyperplasia of the pharyngeal lymphoid tissue. This condition is often accompanied by chronic tonsillitis or rhinitis, almost always in children. Enlarged adenoids may cause partial or complete obstruction of the eustachian tube, leading to otitis media.

Neoplasms

Nasopharyngeal Angiofibroma Is a Tumor of Adolescent Boys

Nasopharyngeal angiofibroma is an uncommon, highly vascular neoplasm of the nasopharynx, which is histologically benign but locally aggressive. Such tumors are not strictly limited to children so the older designation, "juvenile angiofibroma," is no longer recommended. As it occurs predominantly in males, the tumor is thought to be dependent on testosterone and inhibited by estrogen. There is a familial tendency to this tumor: nasopharyngeal angiofibroma is 25-times more common in patients with familial adenomatous polyposis (FAP) than an age-matched population.

PATHOLOGY: The tumor is rounded or nodular and has a sessile or pedunculated attachment to the upper posterior or lateral nasopharyngeal wall. Angiofibroma may grow into fissures and foramina of the skull or may destroy bone and spread into adjacent structures, such as the nasal cavity, paranasal sinuses, orbit, middle cranial fossa, or pterygomaxillary fossa.

Histologically, angiofibroma has vascular and stromal components (Fig. 25-20). Blood vessels vary in size and shape, and their walls characteristically lack a smooth muscle layer or show irregularly arranged smooth muscle. These vessel wall defects preclude vasoconstriction, thereby contributing to brisk bleeding after trauma. Biopsies are, therefore, dangerous and contraindicated. Although many surgeons still advocate a surgical approach, radiation therapy is also effective.

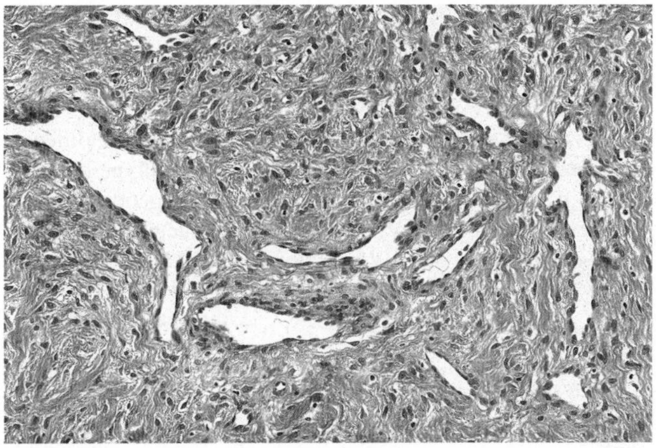

FIGURE 25-20. **Nasopharyngeal angiofibroma** is composed of slitlike vascular structures in a collagenous stroma.

The Oropharynx is a Common Site for Squamous Cell Carcinomas

These tumors tend to be less differentiated and more biologically aggressive than their counterparts in the anterior oral cavity. SCCs of the oropharynx often metastasize early because of the rich lymphatic network in this region. The primary lymphatics drain into the superior deep jugular and submandibular lymph nodes and, to a somewhat lesser degree, into the retropharyngeal lymph nodes.

Nasopharyngeal Carcinoma Is Related to EBV

Nasopharyngeal carcinoma (NPC) is a malignancy of the nasopharynx that is subclassified into keratinizing and nonkeratinizing subtypes. The latter are associated with EBV infection.

EPIDEMIOLOGY: *The undifferentiated subtype of nonkeratinizing carcinoma is particularly common in southeast Asia and parts of Africa.* By far the most common cancer of the nasopharynx, nasopharyngeal carcinoma is the most frequent of all malignant tumors in China. In Hong Kong, nasopharyngeal undifferentiated carcinoma represents 18% of all cancers, compared with 0.25% worldwide. Chinese born in the United States have about a 20-fold greater mortality from nasopharynx carcinoma than persons of other races.

PATHOGENESIS: Various environmental risk factors for nasopharyngeal carcinoma (diet, inhalation of various substances, ethnic customs) have been sought, but no association has been positively demonstrated. Recent studies point to a possible combined role for environmental and genetic factors in the pathogenesis of NPC. There is an association with the A2/sin HLA profile in the Chinese, suggesting a genetic susceptibility.

EBV is present in the tumor cells and B lymphocytes of patients with NPC. Moreover, 85% of patients also have antibodies to EBV and serum IgA anti-EBV. EBV genomes are detected in 75% to 100% of nonkeratinizing and undifferentiated types of NPC. In the keratinizing subtype detection of EBV is variable. If present, the EBV genomes are generally limited to scattered dysplastic intraepithelial cells. For more details on EBV infection and cancers, see Chapters 5 and 9.

PATHOLOGY: NPC is seen as either keratinizing (squamous cell) tumors or nonkeratinizing ones. Keratinizing tumors occur in older people and do not bear the same relation to EBV infection as do nonkeratinizing types. The latter are classified as differentiated or undifferentiated. Differentiated nonkeratinizing nasopharyngeal carcinomas display a stratified appearance and distinct cell margins. By contrast, undifferentiated tumors exhibit clusters of poorly delimited or syncytial cells bearing large oval nuclei and scant eosinophilic cytoplasm (Fig. 25-21). The undifferentiated variant often features a conspicuous lymphoid infiltrate, accounting for the obsolete (and misleading) term "lymphoepithelioma." Both subtypes are immunoreactive with cytokeratin. *The epithelial nature of this tumor is underscored by the fact that tumor cells express cytokeratin but no hematologic or lymphoid markers.*

CLINICAL FEATURES: Because of their location, most NPCs remain asymptomatic for a long time. Palpable cervical lymph node metastases are the first sign of disease in about half of cases, and even then, many patients have no complaints referable to the nasopharynx. The tumor infiltrates neighboring regions, such as the parapharyngeal space, orbit and cranial cavity, resulting in neurologic symptoms and hearing disturbances. Invasion of the base of the skull leads to involvement of cranial nerves. Neoplasms growing in the fossa of Rosenmüller and in the lateral wall of the nasopharynx produce symptoms referable to the middle ear. Obstruction of the eustachian tube is common. The rich lymphatic network draining the nasopharynx is the route of frequent and early metastases to the cervical lymph nodes.

Nasopharyngeal undifferentiated carcinoma is radiosensitive, and most patients whose tumors are restricted to the nasopharynx survive 5 or more years. Metastasis to cervical lymph nodes reduces prognosis considerably, and survival with cranial nerve involvement or distant metastasis is dismal.

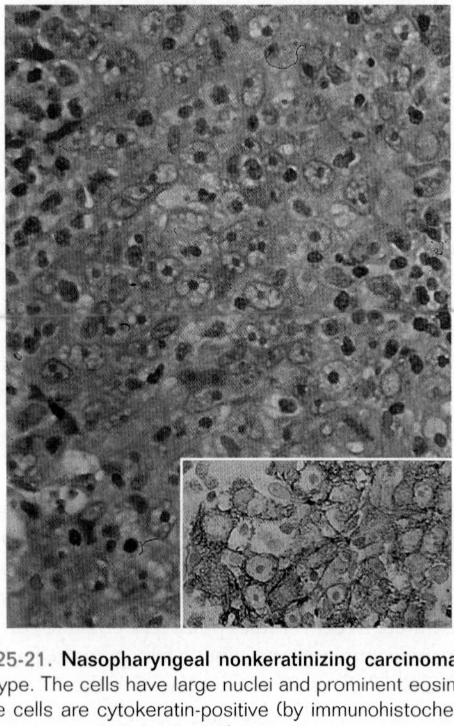

FIGURE 25-21. **Nasopharyngeal nonkeratinizing carcinoma**, undifferentiated type. The cells have large nuclei and prominent eosinophilic nucleoli. The cells are cytokeratin-positive (by immunohistochemistry; *inset*) indicating an epithelial cell proliferation.

Lymphomas of Waldeyer Ring Are Mostly Diffuse B Cell Tumors

Lymphomas comprise 5% of head and neck cancers. Waldeyer ring is by far the most common site of origin of lymphoma in this region: the palatine tonsils first, followed by the nasopharynx and the base of the tongue. Enlargement of a single tonsil in any age group, or bilateral painless tonsillar enlargement in adults, should suggest the possibility of lymphoma. In these cases, cervical lymph nodes are most often involved. Nasopharyngeal lymphomas are histologically diffuse (90%), and more than half have been classified as large cell lymphomas. In the United States and Asia, the vast majority of lymphomas of Waldeyer's ring are of B cell origin.

Plasmacytomas of the Head and Neck Comprise Three Quarters of Extramedullary Plasmacytomas

These tumors show a strong predilection for the nasopharynx, nasal cavity, and paranasal sinuses. Like extramedullary plasmacytomas in other body sites, these tumors are best considered as part of a spectrum of plasma cell disorders. The tumors may remain localized or may evolve into systemic plasma cell myeloma (see Chapter 20).

Chordomas Arise from Remnants of Embryonic Notochord

Chordoma, a malignant tumor derived from notochordal cellular remnants is uncommon in persons under 40. In one third of cases, these tumors extend into the nasopharynx. In the cranial region, they originate from the area of the sphenooccipital synchondrosis. Histologically, they exhibit large vacuolated (physaliferous) cells surrounded by abundant intercellular matrix (Fig. 25-22). Chordomas usually grow slowly, but they infiltrate bone and are ordinarily not accessible to complete surgical removal. Few patients with chordomas of the cranial region survive longer than 5 years.

Other Malignant Tumors of the Nasopharynx are Rare

They may derive from various components of mucosa or adjacent supportive soft tissues and skeleton. **Embryonal rhabdomyosarcoma** (Fig. 25-23) arises in the pharyngeal tissues of young children. This highly malignant tumor invades contiguous structures and metastasizes by both the bloodstream and lymphatics. **Kaposi sarcoma** has been reported in the nasopharyngeal mucosa of patients with AIDS.

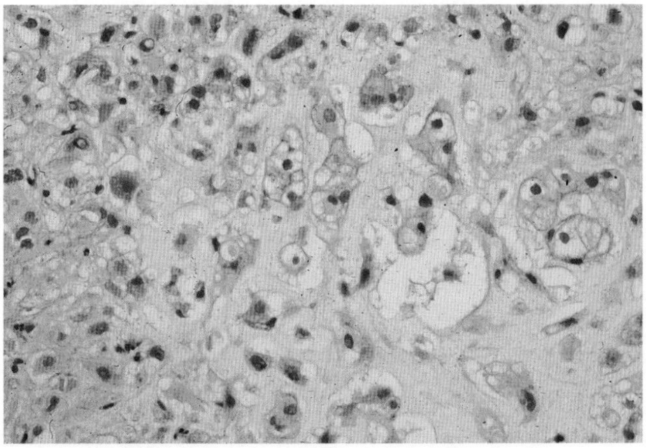

FIGURE 25-22. **Chordoma.** Large vacuolated (physaliferous) tumor cells are evident.

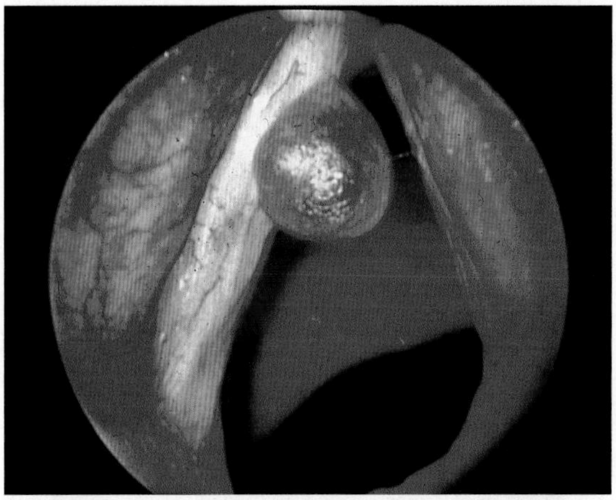

FIGURE 25-24. **Vocal cord polyp.** A solitary polypoid lesion with a glistening appearance is seen arising from the true vocal cord.

LARYNX AND HYPOPHARYNX

Infections

EPIGLOTTITIS: Inflammation of the epiglottis is a serious condition, most commonly caused by *Haemophilus influenzae*, type B. Occurring in infants and young children, this may be a life-threatening emergency. Swelling of the acutely inflamed epiglottis may obstruct airflow. Inspiratory stridor (a loud wheezing sound on inspiration) occurs and the onset of cyanosis may indicate airway obstruction so severe as to require tracheostomy.

CROUP: Croup is a laryngotracheobronchitis syndrome in young children with symptoms of inspiratory stridor, cough, and hoarseness, resulting from varying degrees of laryngeal obstruction. Croup is a complication of an upper respiratory infection, and is marked by edema of the larynx.

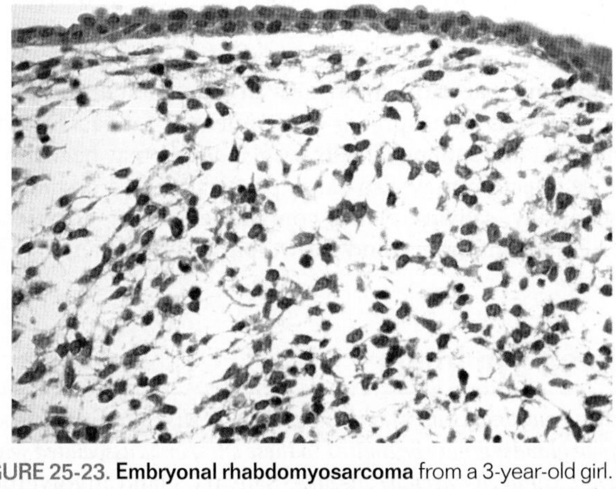

FIGURE 25-23. **Embryonal rhabdomyosarcoma** from a 3-year-old girl. This highly malignant tumor arose in the parapharyngeal space and invaded the adjacent structures. The oval or tadpole-shaped tumor cells under the epithelium have hyperchromatic, eccentric nuclei and immunohistochemical and ultrastructural features of rhabdomyoblasts.

Vocal Cord Nodule and Polyp

Vocal cord nodule/polyp is a stromal reactive process related to inflammation and/or trauma. Synonyms include screamer's, singer's, or preacher's nodules. Nodules/polyps may be seen in all age groups but are most common between the third and sixth decades (Fig. 25-24). Symptoms related to vocal cord polyps and nodules are similar and include hoarseness or voice changes ("breaking" of the voice). Lesions occur after voice abuse, infection (laryngitis), alcohol, smoking, or endocrine dysfunction (e.g., hypothyroidism). The histologic appearance varies from a myxoid, edematous, fibroblastic stroma in the early stages to a hyalinized, densely fibrotic stroma in the later stages.

Neoplasms of the Larynx

SQUAMOUS PAPILLOMA AND PAPILLOMATOSIS: Squamous papillomas of the larynx are solitary or multiple papillary growths of mature squamous cells that line the surface of fibrovascular cores. They may be multiple in children or adolescents (juvenile laryngeal papillomatosis), and may extend into the trachea and bronchi. HPV, especially types HPV-6 and HPV-11, are the principal causes. The condition may cause life-threatening respiratory obstruction and, rarely, evolve into an overt SCC, particularly in smokers or after radiation therapy. Surgical excision may not be curative, because viral infection of the mucosa is often widespread, and the tumors tend to recur over many years. Solitary laryngeal squamous papilloma occurs in adults, predominantly in men, and is usually cured surgically.

SQUAMOUS CELL CARCINOMA: Almost all laryngeal cancers are SCCs. s Virtually all of these patients are men, most of whom are cigarette smokers.

- **Glottic carcinoma** is limited to one or both true vocal cords and accounts for almost two thirds of laryngeal cancers. It is slow to metastasize to lymph nodes and has a good prognosis.
- **Supraglottic carcinoma** arises in the ventricle, false cords, or epiglottis and does not, by definition, involve the true cords. Up to one third of laryngeal carcinomas arise in this location. Nodal metastases are more common than in glottic tumors.
- **Transglottic carcinoma**, by definition, involves the true and false cords (Fig. 25-25). This uncommon tumor is

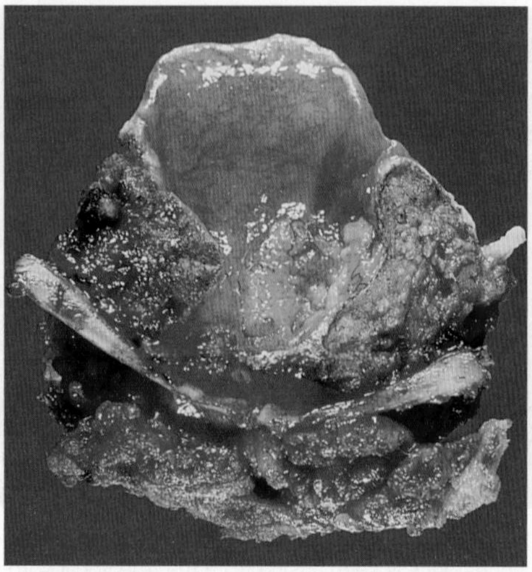

FIGURE 25-25. **Supraglottic laryngectomy specimen for squamous cell carcinoma.** The carcinoma appears as an irregular riased granular appearing area in the right supraglottic larynx.

likely to metastasize to lymph nodes and often requires total laryngectomy.

- **Infraglottic carcinoma** is an uncommon tumor located below the true cords or involving the true cords, with considerable infraglottic extension and frequent extension into the trachea. Nodal metastases are common, and total laryngectomy is generally required.

CHONDROSARCOMA: Chondrosarcoma is a rare malignant tumor of cartilage, but accounts for 75% of nonepithelial laryngeal malignancies. It also occurs in mandible, maxilla, nasal, and paranasal sinuses), and nasopharynx. Patients present with hoarseness, airway obstruction, and dyspnea.

SALIVARY GLANDS

The salivary glands develop as buds of oral ectoderm. They are tubuloalveolar structures that secrete saliva. All major salivary glands are paired organs. The parotid glands secrete serous saliva, whereas submandibular and sublingual glands produce mixed serous and mucous saliva. Minor salivary glands are widespread, being present under the mucosa of the lips, cheeks, palate, and tongue. Lymph nodes are normally embedded in the parotid gland. The intraparotid lymph nodes may be involved in a variety of inflammatory, reactive, or proliferative processes, including malignant lymphoma.

XEROSTOMIA: Xerostomia is chronic mouth dryness due to lack of saliva, and has many causes. Diseases that involve the major salivary glands and produce xerostomia include mumps, Sjögren syndrome, sarcoidosis, radiation-induced atrophy (Fig. 25-26), and drug sensitivity (antihistamines, tricyclic antidepressants, hypotensive drugs, phenothiazines).

SIALORRHEA: Increased salivary flow is associated with many conditions, including acute inflammation of the oral cavity, as in aphthous stomatitis, Parkinson disease, rabies, mental retardation, nausea, and pregnancy.

ENLARGEMENT: Unilateral enlargement of major salivary glands is usually caused by cysts, inflammation, or neoplasms. Bilateral enlargement is due to inflammation (mumps, Sjögren syndrome; see below), granulomatous disease (sarcoidosis), or diffuse neoplastic involvement (leukemia or malignant lymphoma).

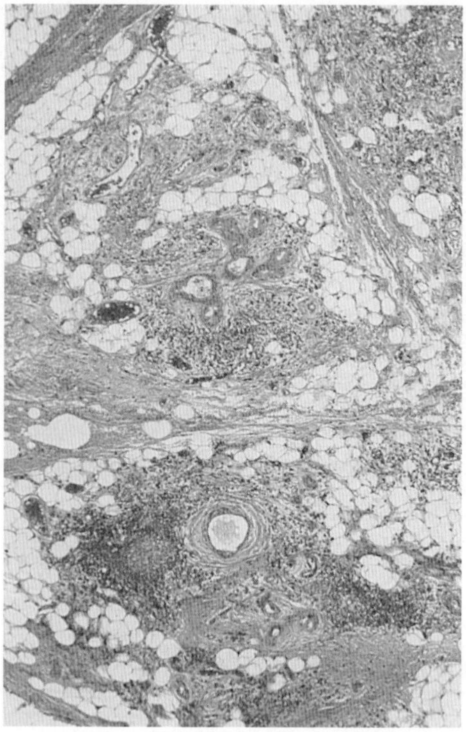

FIGURE 25-26. **Chronic sialadenitis.** Severe chronic inflammation and marked atrophy of the submandibular gland are present after irradiation of an adjacent oral cancer. The atrophic acini have been replaced by fat.

SIALOLITHIASIS: Calcific stones occur in salivary gland ducts, mostly in the submandibular gland. The most important consequence of stone formation is duct obstruction, often followed by inflammation distal to the occlusion.

PAROTITIS: Acute suppurative parotitis is caused by ascent of bacteria (usually *Staphylococcus aureus*) from the oral cavity when salivary flow is reduced. It is most often seen in debilitated or postoperative patients. Acute and chronic parotitis is often associated with stricture of salivary ducts or obstruction by stones. The stagnant secretions serve as a medium for retrograde bacterial invasion.

Epidemic parotitis (mumps) is an acute viral disease of the parotid glands that spreads with infected saliva. The submandibular and sublingual salivary glands also may be involved. Mumps infection may also cause pancreatitis and orchitis. Microscopically, salivary glands contain dense lymphocytic and macrophage infiltrates, and show epithelial degeneration and necrosis.

Sjögren Syndrome

Sjögren syndrome is a chronic inflammatory disease of salivary and lacrimal glands; it may be limited to these sites, or be associated with a systemic collagen vascular disease. Salivary gland involvement leads to xerostomia. Lacrimal gland involvement results in dry eyes (**keratoconjunctivitis sicca**). The pathogenesis and clinical features of Sjögren syndrome are discussed in Chapter 4.

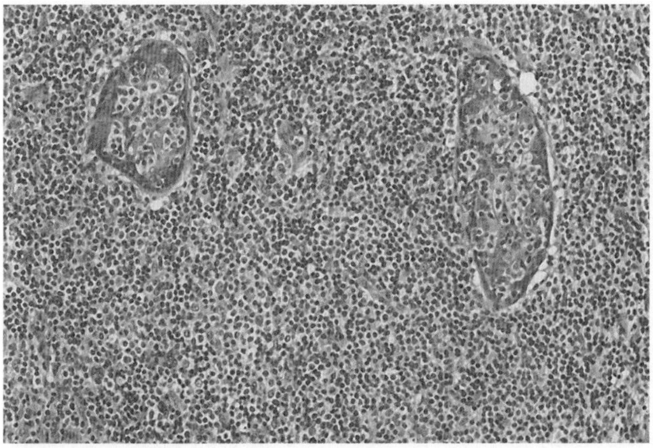

FIGURE 25-27. **Sjögren syndrome.** There is infiltration of the involved salivary gland by a mixed chronic inflammatory cell infiltrate. Extension of the infiltrate into epithelial (ductal) structures results in metaplasia and characteristic epimyoepithelial islands.

PATHOLOGY: In Sjögren syndrome parotid glands, and sometimes submandibular glands are unilaterally or bilaterally enlarged, but their lobulation is preserved. Histologically, an initial periductal chronic inflammatory infiltrate gradually extends to the acini, until the glands are completely replaced by a sea of polyclonal lymphocytes, immunoblasts, germinal centers, and plasma cells. Proliferating myoepithelial cells surround remnants of damaged ducts and form so-called epimyoepithelial islands (Fig. 25-27). The term **benign lymphoepithelial lesion** was introduced to describe these features. Similar changes can be seen in the lacrimal glands and minor salivary glands. Focal lymphocytic sialadenitis is also seen in minor salivary glands obtained by labial biopsy in most patients with Sjögren syndrome. Late in the course of the disease, affected glands become atrophic, with fibrosis and fatty infiltration of the parenchyma. The lymphoid infiltrates in Sjögren syndrome may contain monotypic cells that have restricted immunoglobulin patterns, which may not be invasive and may remain localized.

Benign Salivary Gland Neoplasms

Pleomorphic Adenoma (Mixed Tumor) is the Most Common Tumor of Salivary Glands

Pleomorphic adenoma is a benign neoplasm characterized by an admixture of epithelial and stromal elements. Two thirds of all tumors of the major salivary glands, and about half of those in the minor ones, are pleomorphic adenomas. The tumor is nine times more frequent in the parotid than in the submandibular gland and usually arises in the superficial lobe of the parotid. It occurs most often in middle-aged people and shows a female preponderance.

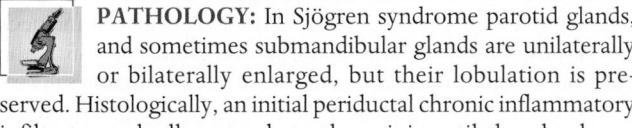

PATHOLOGY: Pleomorphic adenoma is a slowly growing, painless, movable, firm mass that has a smooth surface (Fig. 25-28). Tumors that arise deep in the parotid gland may grow between the ramus of the mandible and the styloid process and stylomandibular ligament into the parapharyngeal space, where they are seen as swellings of the lateral pharyngeal or tonsillar regions.

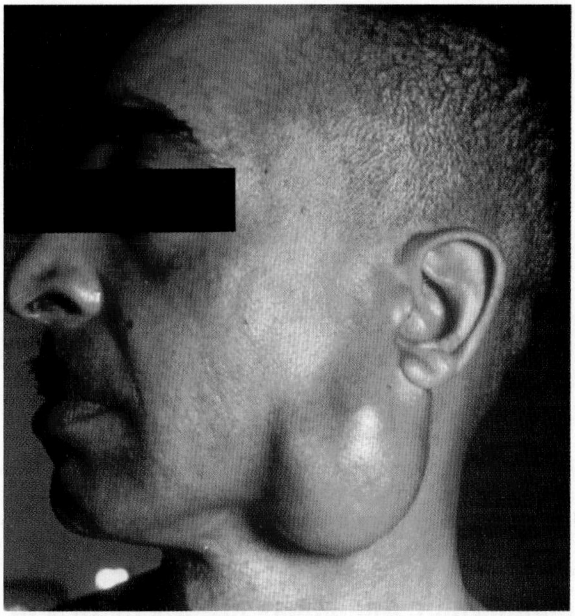

FIGURE 25-28. **Pleomorphic adenoma of the parotid.** A conspicuous tumor mass is seen at the angle of the jaw.

Microscopically, pleomorphic adenomas show epithelial tissue intermingled with myxoid, mucoid or chondroid areas (Fig. 25-29A). An older term, **mixed tumor**, reflected this mixture of epithelial and mesenchymal components. However, the neoplasm is now considered to be of epithelial origin.

The epithelial component of pleomorphic adenoma consists of ductal and myoepithelial cells. The cells lining the ducts form tubules or small cystic structures and contain clear fluid or eosinophilic, periodic acid-Schiff (PAS)-positive material. Around the ductal epithelial cells are smaller myoepithelial cells, which are the main cellular component. These cells form well-defined sheaths, cords, or nests and are often separated by a cellular ground substance that resembles cartilaginous, myxoid or mucoid material (see Fig. 25-29B).

CLINICAL FEATURES: Pleomorphic adenomas have fibrous capsules. As they grow, the surrounding fibrous tissue condenses around them. The tumors expand and tend to protrude focally into adjacent tissues, becoming nodular (see Fig. 25-28). At surgery, these tumor projections can be missed if a tumor is not carefully dissected to leave an intact capsule and an adequate margin of surrounding glandular parenchyma. Tumor implanted during surgery or tumor nodules left behind continue to grow as recurrences in the scar from the previous operation. Recurrence of pleomorphic adenomas represents local regrowth, not malignancy, and further surgery may necessitate sacrificing the facial nerve.

Rarely, carcinomas may arise in pleomorphic adenomas, **carcinoma ex pleomorphic adenoma**. In this situation a pleomorphic adenoma that has been present for many years may begin to grow rapidly or become painful. Histologic examination reveals an unequivocal carcinoma in an otherwise benign pleomorphic adenoma. These tumors are usually high-grade malignancies such as poorly differentiated adenocarcinoma and undifferentiated adenocarcinoma, but virtually any type of salivary gland malignancy may occur in this setting, including mucoepidermoid or adenoid cystic carcinomas.

A 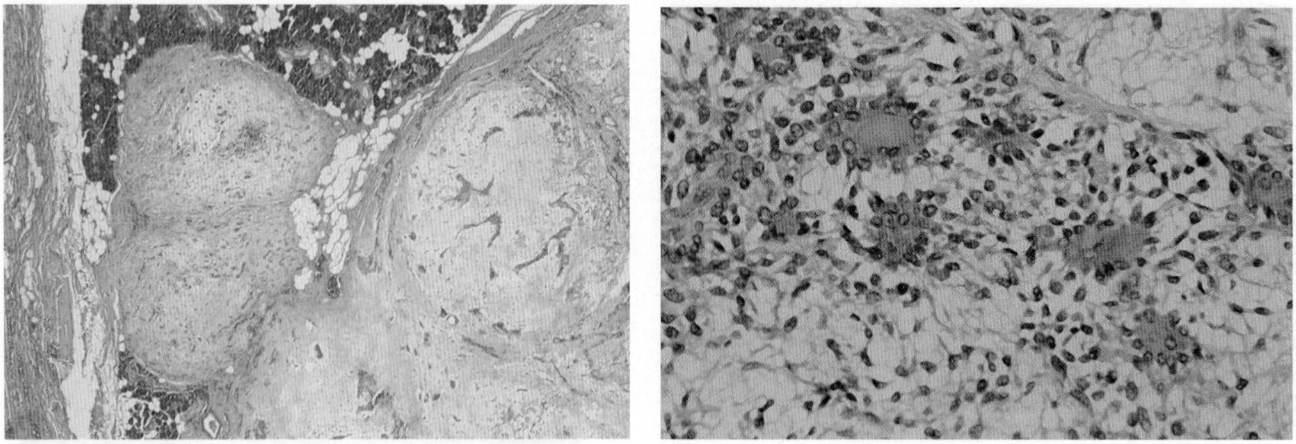 B

FIGURE 25-29. **Pleomorphic adenoma of the parotid gland. A.** The tumor contains characteristic myxoid and chondroid portions. The tumor is partly encapsulated, but a nodule protruding into the parotid gland lacks a capsule. If such nodules are not included in the resection, the tumor will recur. **B.** Cellular components of pleomorphic adenomas include an admixture of glands and myoepithelial cells within a chondromyxoid stroma.

Monomorphic Adenomas are 5% to 10% of Benign Salivary Gland Tumors

In monomorphic adenomas, the epithelium is arranged in a regular, usually glandular, pattern without a mesenchyme-like component. Monomorphic adenomas include (1) Warthin tumor (papillary cystadenoma lymphomatosum), (2) basal cell adenoma, (3) oxyphilic adenoma or oncocytoma, (4) canalicular adenoma, (5) myoepithelioma, and (6) clear cell adenoma.

Warthin Tumor

Warthin tumors are benign parotid gland neoplasms composed of cystic glandular spaces embedded in dense lymphoid tissue. This tumor is the most common monomorphic adenoma. Although the neoplasm is clearly benign, it can be bilateral (15% of cases) or multifocal within the same gland. Warthin tumor is the only tumor of salivary glands that is more common in men than in women. They generally occur after the age of 30 years, with most arising after age 50.

PATHOLOGY: Warthin tumors are composed of glandular spaces that tend to become cystic and show papillary projections. The cysts are lined by characteristic eosinophilic epithelial cells (oncocytes) and are embedded in dense lymphoid tissue with germinal centers (Fig. 25-30).

The histogenesis of this tumor has been much debated. Lymph nodes are normally found in the parotid gland and in its immediate vicinity, and usually contain a few ducts or small islands of salivary gland tissue. Warthin tumors may arise from proliferation of these salivary gland inclusions.

Oncocytoma (Oxyphil Adenoma)

Oncocytes are benign epithelial cells swollen with mitochondria, which impart a granular appearance to the cytoplasm. They are seen scattered or in small clusters among epithelial cells of various organs (e.g., thyroid and parathyroid glands). They first appear in early adulthood, and increase in number with age. Their function is unknown. Rare benign tumors composed of nests or cords of these cells occur in the parotid glands of elderly persons.

Malignant Salivary Gland Tumors

Salivary gland tumors account for about 5% of all head and neck neoplasms. Most (75%) arise in the parotid glands, 10% are in the submandibular glands, and 15% are located in minor salivary glands (mucoserous glands) of the upper aerodigestive tract. Less than 1 % occur in the sublingual glands.

Mucoepidermoid Carcinoma has Neoplastic Squamous, Glandular, and Intermediate Cells

Mucoepidermoid carcinoma is a malignant salivary gland tumor composed of a mixture of neoplastic epidermoid cells, mucus-secreting

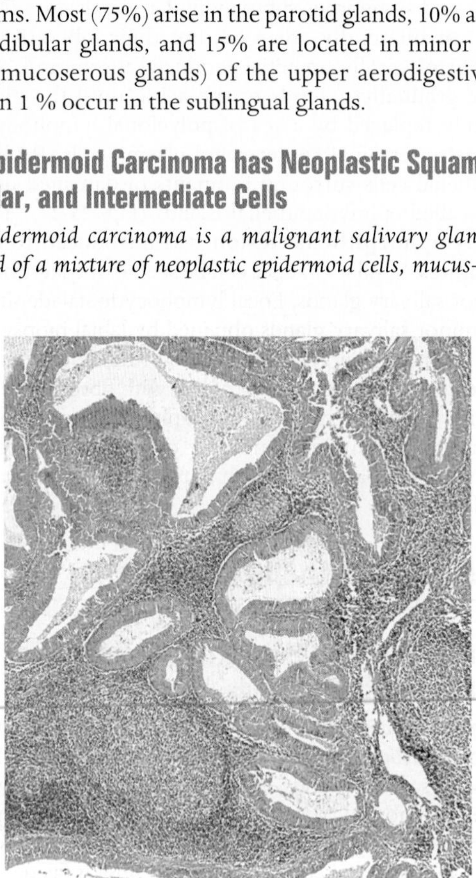

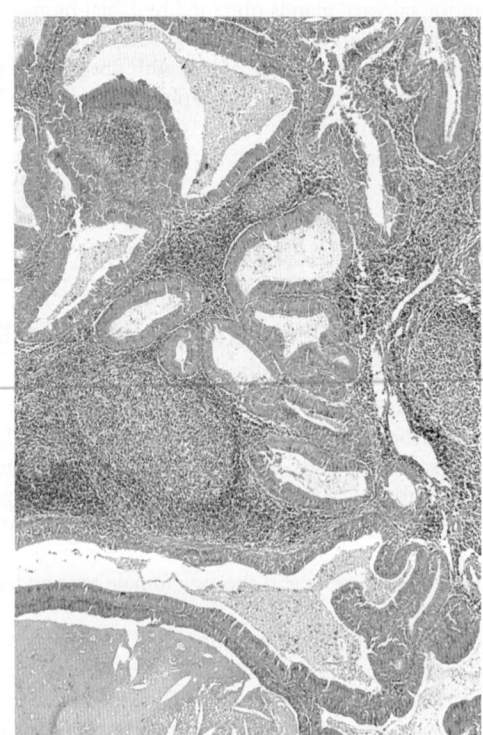

FIGURE 25-30. **Warthin tumor.** Cystic spaces and ductlike structures are lined by oncocytes. Follicular lymphoid tissue is present.

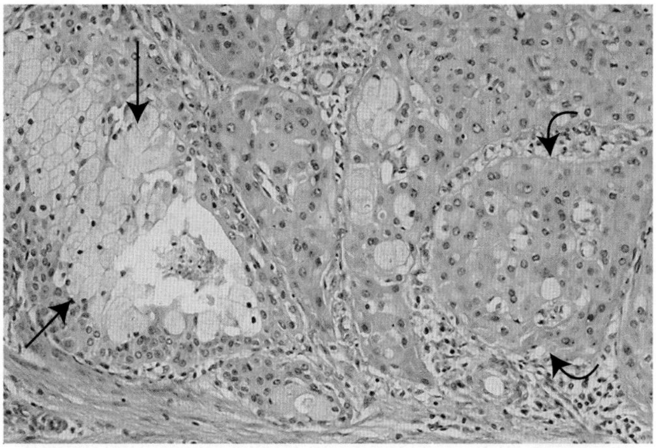

FIGURE 25-31. **Mucoepidermoid carcinoma** is characterized by an admixture of mucocytes *(straight arrows)*, epidermoid cells *(curved arrows)*, and intermediate cells. The mucocytes are clustered and have a clear cytoplasm with eccentrically situated nuclei. Epidermoid cells are squamous-like cells but lack keratinization and intercellular bridges. Intermediate cells (best seen at *lower left*) are smaller than epidermoid cells.

cells, and epithelial cells of an intermediate type. It originates from ductal epithelium, which has a considerable potential for metaplasia. This neoplasm accounts for 5% to 10% of major salivary gland tumors and 10% of those in the minor salivary glands. Within the major salivary glands, more than half of mucoepidermoid carcinomas arise in parotid gland. In minor salivary glands, they develop most frequently in the palate. Although the tumor may occur in adolescents, most arise in adults. They are more common in women.

PATHOLOGY: Mucoepidermoid carcinoma grows slowly and presents as a firm painless mass. Microscopically, low-grade (well-differentiated) tumors form irregular solid, ductlike and cystic spaces that include squamous cells, mucus-secreting cells, and intermediate cells (Fig. 25-31). Intermediate-grade tumors tend to (1) be more solid in growth, (2) contain a greater percentage of epidermoid and intermediate cells, and (3) posses fewer mucus-secreting cells. High-grade (poorly differentiated) carcinomas are a markedly pleomorphic, without evidence of differentiation save, perhaps, for scattered mucus-secreting cells.

CLINICAL FEATURES: Even low-grade (well-differentiated) mucoepidermoid carcinomas can metastasize, but 5-year survival is better than 90%, regardless of the primary site. High-grade (poorly differentiated) mucoepidermoid carcinomas have a much lower survival rate (20% to 40%).

Adenoid Cystic Carcinoma Invades Locally but Usually Recurs

Adenoid cystic carcinoma, previously termed "cylindroma," *is a slowly growing salivary gland malignancy, which is notorious for its tendency to invade locally and recur after surgical resection.* It constitutes 5% of all tumors of the major salivary glands and 20% of those of the minor salivary glands. One third of neck tumors arise in the major salivary glands and two thirds in the minor ones. They occur not only in the oral cavity but also in lacrimal glands, nasopharynx, nasal

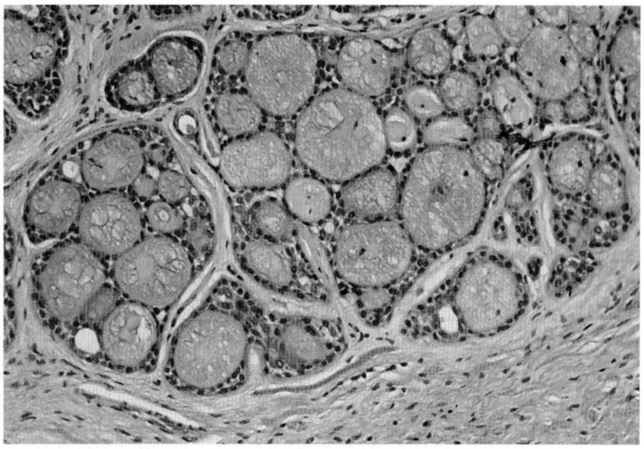

FIGURE 25-32. **Adenoid cystic carcinoma** showing cribriform growth in which cystlike spaces are filled with basophilic material. The cyst spaces are really pseudocysts surrounded by myoepithelial cells.

cavity, paranasal sinuses, and lower respiratory tract. They are most common in people 40 to 60 years of age.

PATHOLOGY: Histologically, adenoid cystic carcinomas present varying patterns. The tumor cells are small, have scant cytoplasm, and grow in solid sheets or as small groups, strands, or columns. Within these structures, the tumor cells interconnect to enclose cystic spaces, resulting in a solid, tubular or cribriform (sievelike) arrangement (Fig. 25-32). Tumor cells make a homogeneous basement membrane material that gives them the characteristic "cylindromatous" appearance.

The tumors probably originate from cells that are differentiating toward intercalated ducts and toward myoepithelium. *Adenoid cystic carcinomas tend to infiltrate perineural spaces and are often painful.* For these reasons, they are often diagnosed in an advanced stage. Although most do not metastasize for many years, they are difficult to eradicate completely, and long-term prognosis is poor.

Acinic Cell Adenocarcinoma Arises From Epithelial Secretory Cells

Acinic cell adenocarcinomas are uncommon parotid tumors (10% of all salivary gland tumors). They arise occasionally in other salivary glands and occur principally in young men between the ages of 20 and 30. They are encapsulated, round masses, usually under 3 cm across, and may sometimes be cystic. Microscopically, acinic cell adenocarcinomas are composed of uniform cells with a small central nucleus and abundant basophilic cytoplasm, similar to the secretory (acinic) cells of the normal salivary glands. The tumor may metastasize to the regional lymph nodes.

After surgical resection, most (90%) patients survive for 5 years, but local recurrence may be expected in one third of patients. Only half survive for 20 years.

THE EAR

External Ear

The outer portion of the external ear includes the auricle or pinna leading into the external auditory canal. The external auditory canal or meatus extends from the concha to its medial limit, which is the outer aspect of the tympanic membrane. The lateral portion of its wall consists of cartilage and connective tissue. The medial portion of its wall consists of bone. The tympanic membrane (ear drum) is situated obliquely at the end of the external auditory canal, sloping medially both from above downward and from behind forward. It separates the external ear from the middle ear.

Histologically, the auricle is essentially a cutaneous structure composed of keratinizing, stratified squamous epithelium with associated cutaneous adnexal structures that include hair follicles, sebaceous glands, and eccrine sweat glands. In addition to hair follicles and sebaceous glands, the outer third of the external auditory canal is noteworthy for its ceruminal glands, modified apocrine glands that replace the eccrine glands seen in the auricular dermis. Ceruminal glands produce cerumen and are arranged in clusters of cuboidal cells with eosinophilic cytoplasm often containing granular, golden-yellow pigment. These cells have secretory droplets along their luminal border. Peripheral to the secretory cells are flattened myoepithelial cells. The ducts of ceruminal glands terminate in hair follicles or on the skin. In the inner portion of the external auditory canal lack all adnexal structures. The outer surface of this airtight membrane is covered by squamous epithelium that is continuous with the skin of the external ear canal. Its inner surface is lined by the cuboidal epithelium of the middle ear. Between these two epithelial covers of the tympanic membrane is a middle layer of dense fibrous tissue.

KELOIDS: Keloids are particularly common on the ear lobes after piercing for earrings or other trauma (see Chapter 3). They are much more frequent in blacks and Asians than in whites. The lesions can attain considerable size and tend to recur. Histologically, keloids are composed of thick, hyalinized bundles of collagen in the deep dermis (see Chapter 3).

CAULIFLOWER EARS: These deformities are particularly common in wrestlers and boxers and are the result of repeated mechanical trauma to the external ear. Blows to the ears cause subperichondrial hematomas, which organize and deform the ears.

RELAPSING POLYCHONDRITIS: This rare, chronic disorder of unknown origin is characterized by intermittent inflammation that destroys the cartilage of the ears, nose, larynx, tracheobronchial tree, ribs, and joints. It may involve hyaline cartilage, elastic cartilage, or fibrocartilage.

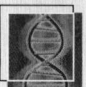

PATHOGENESIS: The cause of the cell damage is obscure, although immune mechanisms are suspected. Serum antibodies to cartilage, type II collagen, and chondroitin sulfate have been found in patients during acute attacks. Immune complexes have been demonstrated in involved cartilage. Relapsing polychondritis occurs alone or in association with one of the connective tissue diseases. Noncartilaginous tissues, such as the sclera and cardiac valves, also may be affected. Aortic involvement may lead to fatal rupture of the aorta.

PATHOLOGY: Microscopically, the perichondrium is infiltrated with lymphocytes, plasma cells and neutrophils, which also extend into the adjacent cartilage (Fig. 25-33). Chondrocytes die, and the cartilaginous matrix degenerates and fragments. Ultimately, the cartilage is destroyed and replaced by granulation tissue and fibrosis.

MALIGNANT OTITIS EXTERNA: This infection of the external auditory canal is caused by *Pseudomonas aeruginosa*. Infection

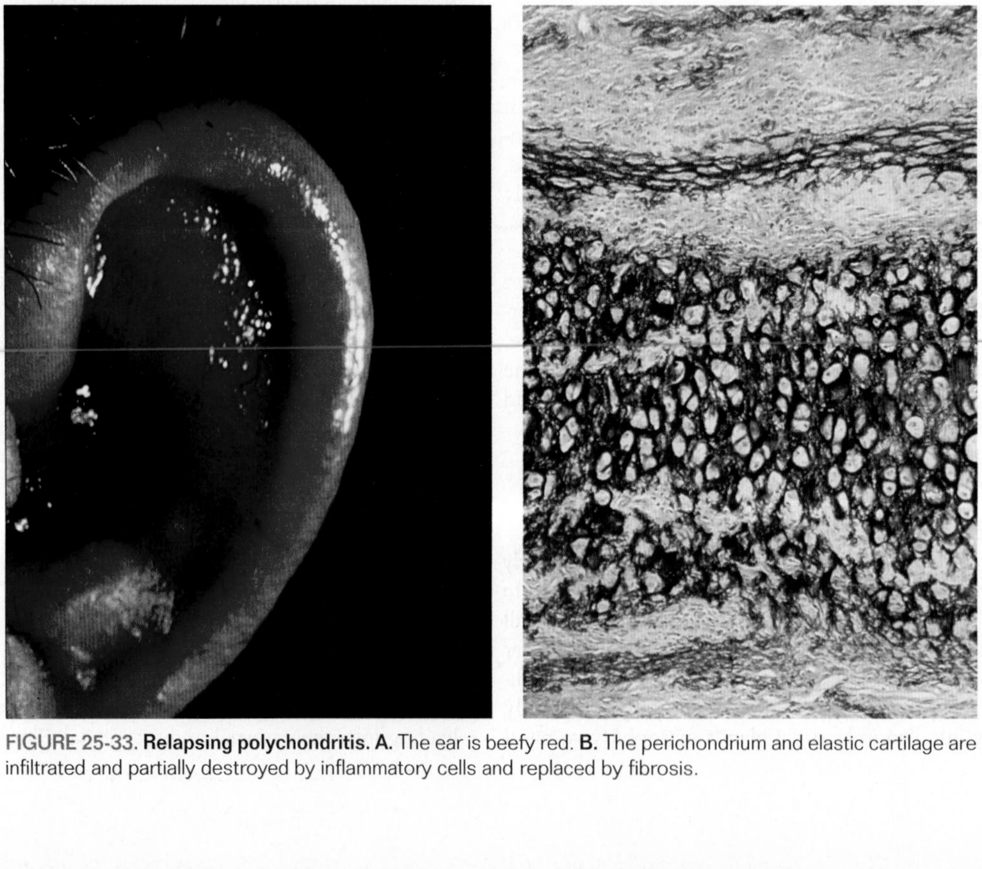

A B

FIGURE 25-33. **Relapsing polychondritis. A.** The ear is beefy red. **B.** The perichondrium and elastic cartilage are infiltrated and partially destroyed by inflammatory cells and replaced by fibrosis.

may spread through the skin and cartilage to cause mastoiditis or osteomyelitis of the skull, venous sinus thrombosis, meningitis and death. Malignant otitis externa occurs mainly in elderly diabetics but has also been reported in patients with blood dyscrasias (e.g., leukemia, granulocytopenia).

AURAL POLYPS: These benign inflammatory lesions arise from within the external ear canal or extrude into the canal from the middle ear. Aural polyps are composed of ulcerated and inflamed granulation tissue, which bleeds readily. Those arising in the middle ear result from chronic otitis media.

NEOPLASMS: Benign and malignant tumors of the external ear include the full gamut of skin related neoplasms: squamous papillomas, seborrheic keratosis, basal cell carcinoma, SCC, and benign and malignant adnexal tumors. Neoplasms arising from ceruminal glands are unique to this area. Benign tumors of these glands include ceruminoma (ceruminal gland adenoma) and salivary gland-type tumors arising from ceruminal glands (e.g., pleomorphic and monomorphic adenomas). Malignant tumors of ceruminal glands include adenocarcinoma and malignant salivary gland-type tumors (e.g., adenoid cystic carcinoma, mucoepidermoid carcinoma).

Middle Ear

The middle ear, or tympanic cavity, is an oblong space in the temporal bone lined by a mucous membrane. Together with the mastoid, it forms a closed mucosal compartment, also called the **middle ear cleft**. Most of the lateral wall consists of the tympanic membrane. Anteriorly, the eustachian tube connects the middle ear with the nasopharynx. It is an air passage that allows air pressure on both sides of the tympanic membrane to equalize. The three auditory ossicles—the malleus, incus and stapes—are a chain that connects the tympanic membrane with the oval window (on the medial wall of the tympanic cavity) and conducts sound across the middle ear. The freedom of motion of the ossicles, mainly that of the stapes in the oval window, is more important for hearing than is an intact tympanic membrane. The middle ear opens posteriorly into the mastoid antrum, a honeycomb of small, aerated, bony compartments (air cells) lined by a thin mucous membrane continuous with that of the middle ear.

Otitis Media Often Results from Obstruction of the Eustachian Tube

Otitis media is inflammation of the middle ear, and usually results from an upper respiratory tract infection that extends from the nasopharynx.

PATHOGENESIS: The infection almost invariably penetrates through the mastoid antrum into the mastoid cells. During an infection in the nasopharynx, microorganisms may reach the middle ear by ascending through the eustachian tube. Acute otitis media may be due to viral or bacterial infections or to obstruction of the eustachian tube without microorganisms. Viral otitis media may resolve without suppuration, or the middle ear may be secondarily invaded by pus-forming bacteria.

Obstruction of the eustachian tube is important in the production of middle ear effusion. When the pharyngeal end of the eustachian tube is swollen, air cannot enter the tube. Air in the middle ear is then absorbed through the mucosa, and negative pressure causes transudation of plasma and occasionally bleeding. Antibiotics usually cure or suppress the condition.

ACUTE SEROUS OTITIS MEDIA: Obstruction of the eustachian tube may result from sudden changes in atmospheric pressure (e.g., during flying in an aircraft or deep-sea diving). This effect is particularly severe if there is an upper respiratory tract infection, acute allergic reaction, or viral or bacterial infection at the orifice of the eustachian tube. Inflammation may also occur without bacterial invasion of the middle ear. More than half of children in the United States have had at least one episode of serous otitis media before their third birthday. Repeated bouts of otitis media in early childhood often contribute to unsuspected hearing loss, which is due to residual (usually sterile) fluid in the middle ear.

CHRONIC SEROUS OTITIS MEDIA: Recurrent or chronic serous effusion of the middle ear is due to the same conditions that cause acute obstruction of the eustachian tube. Carcinoma of the nasopharynx may be the cause of chronic serous otitis media in an adult and should always be suspected when a unilateral effusion occurs in the middle ear of an adult.

PATHOLOGY: In chronic serous otitis media, mucus-producing (goblet) cell metaplasia may be seen in the mucosal lining of the middle ear. If the obstruction occurs acutely, there may be accompanying hemorrhage, for example, in the mastoid cells. Extravasation of blood and degradation of erythrocytes liberate cholesterol. Cholesterol crystals stimulate a foreign-body reaction and elicit a granulation tissue response, called a **cholesterol granuloma.** Large cholesterol granulomas may destroy tissue in the mastoid or antrum. If a cholesterol granuloma is allowed to persist for many months, the granulation tissue may become fibrotic, which may eventually lead to complete obliteration of the middle ear and mastoid by fibrous tissue.

ACUTE SUPPURATIVE OTITIS MEDIA: One of the most common infections of childhood, acute suppurative otitis media, is caused by pyogenic bacteria that invade the middle ear, usually via the eustachian tube. *Streptococcus pneumoniae* (pneumococcus) is the most common causative agent in all age groups (30% to 40%). *Haemophilus influenzae* causes about 20% of cases, but is less frequent with increasing age. If a purulent exudate accumulates in the middle ear, the eardrum ruptures and the pus is discharged. In most cases, the infection is self-limited, and tends to heal even without therapy.

ACUTE MASTOIDITIS: Infection of the mastoid bone was a common complication of acute otitis media before the advent of antibiotics. It is still seen, albeit rarely, in cases of inadequately treated otitis media. Characteristically, mastoid air cells are filled with pus, and their thin osseous intercellular walls become destroyed. Extension of the infection from the mastoid to contiguous structures causes complications (Fig. 25-34).

CHRONIC SUPPURATIVE OTITIS MEDIA AND MASTOIDITIS: Neglected or recurrent infection of the middle ear and mastoid process may eventually produce chronic inflammation of the mucosa or destruction of the periosteum covering the ossicles (Fig. 25-35). Chronic otitis media is much more common in persons who had ear disease in early childhood, which may have arrested normal development of the air cells in the mastoid.

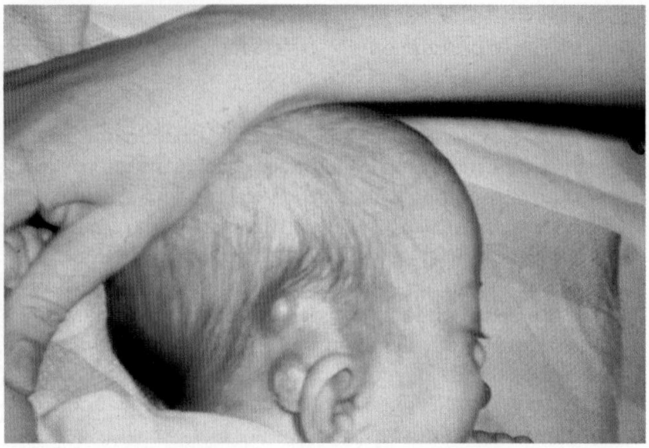

FIGURE 25-34. An unusual complication of otitis media, acute mastoiditis, appears as large bulging lesions above the child's ear.

PATHOLOGY: The inflammation tends to be insidious, persistent, and destructive. By definition, the eardrum is always perforated in chronic otitis media. Painless discharge (**otorrhea**) and varying degrees of hearing loss are constant symptoms. Exuberant granulation tissue may form polyps, which can extend through the perforated eardrum into the external ear canal.

Cholesteatoma *is a mass of accumulated keratin and squamous mucosa that results from the growth of squamous epithelium from the external ear canal thorough the perforated eardrum into the middle ear.* In that location, it continues to produce keratin. Microscopically, cholesteatomas are identical to epidermal inclusion cysts and are surrounded by granulation tissue and fibrosis. The keratin mass frequently becomes infected and shields the bacteria from antibiotics. The principal dangers of cholesteatoma arise from erosion of bone, a process that may lead to destruction of important contiguous structures (e.g., auditory ossicles, facial nerve, labyrinth).

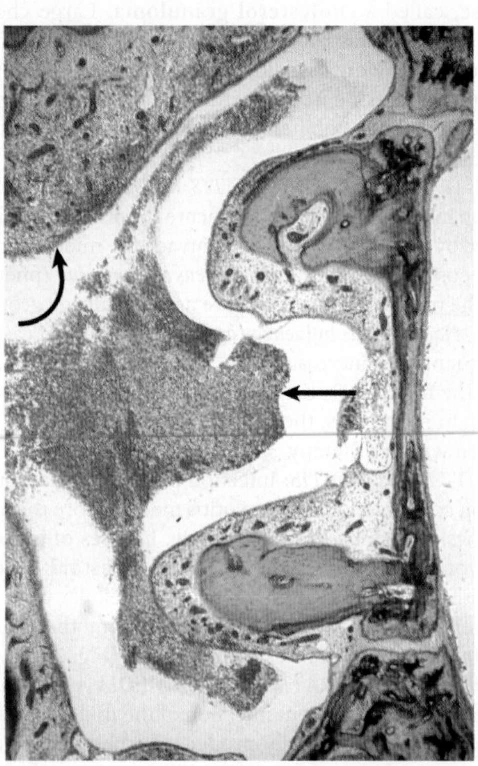

FIGURE 25-35. **Chronic suppurative otitis media.** A purulent exudate (*straight arrow*) is present in the middle ear cavity. The entire mucosa (*curved arrow*) is thickened by chronic inflammation and granulation tissue. The footplate and the crura of the stapes are at right.

COMPLICATIONS OF ACUTE AND CHRONIC OTITIS MEDIA: As a result of antibiotic treatment, complications of otitis media are now rare. However, a potential for serious, and even fatal, complications still exists with any suppurative inflammation of the middle ear. The following cranial and intracranial complications may develop:

- Destruction of the facial nerve
- Deep cervical or subperiosteal abscess, when the cortical bone of the mastoid process is eroded
- Petrositis, when the infection spreads to the petrous portion of the temporal bone through the chain of air cells
- Suppurative labyrinthitis, as a result of infection of the internal ear
- Epidural, subdural, or cerebral abscess, after extension of the infection through the inner table of the mastoid bone
- Meningitis, when the infection extends to the meninges
- Thrombophlebitis of the sigmoid sinus, which occurs when the infection spreads through the dura to the posterior cranial fossa

Jugulotympanic Paraganglioma Arises from Middle Ear Paraganglia

Jugulotympanic paraganglioma, is the most common benign tumor of the middle ear. These tumors grow slowly but, over years, may destroy the middle ear and extend into the internal ear and cranial cavity. Metastases are rare.

Histologically, middle ear paragangliomas are identical to those arising elsewhere, and show characteristic lobules of cells embedded in a richly vascular connective tissue (Fig. 25-36). The paraganglial cells are of neural crest origin and contain varying amounts of catecholamines, mostly epinephrine and norepinephrine.

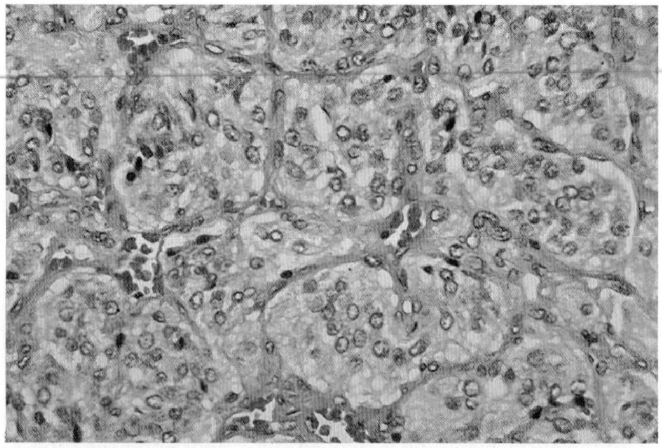

FIGURE 25-36. **Jugulotympanic paraganglioma.** Tumor cell nests are composed of cells with ill-defined cell borders and prominent eosinophilic cytoplasm (chief cells).

Internal Ear

The petrous portion of the temporal bone contains the labyrinth, which shelters the end organs for hearing (the cochlea) and equilibrium (**vestibular labyrinth**). The complex cavities of the osseous labyrinth contain the membranous labyrinth, a series of communicating membranous sacs and ducts. The osseous labyrinth is filled with a clear fluid, the perilymph. The perilymphatic system is continuous with the subarachnoid space through the cochlear aqueduct, which provides direct exchange with the cerebrospinal fluid. The membranous labyrinth contains a different fluid, the endolymph, which circulates in a closed system. Because of the lack of barriers between the cochlear and vestibular labyrinths, injury or disease of the inner ear frequently affects both hearing and equilibrium.

The **cochlea** is coiled upon itself like a snail shell and makes two and one-half turns. There are three compartments in the cochlea; two of these contain perilymph and the third (the cochlear duct) contains endolymph. The cochlear duct encompasses the end organ for hearing, the organ of Corti, which rests on the basement membrane. The organ of Corti is arranged as a spiral, with three rows of outer hair cells and a row of inner hair cells. When the hairs of these neuroepithelial cells are bent or distorted by sonic vibration, the mechanical force is converted into electrochemical impulses and interpreted in the temporal cortex as sound. The vestibular portion of the membranous labyrinth consists of the utricle, saccule, and semicircular canals. Each of these contains specialized neuroepithelium that is the end organ for equilibrium.

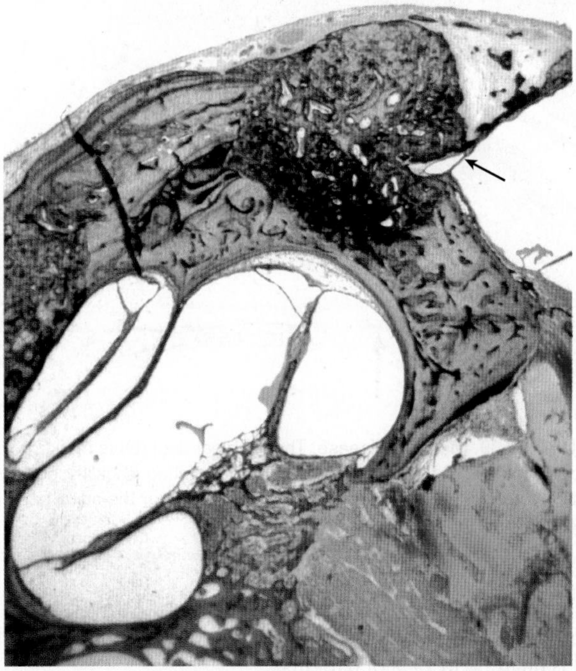

FIGURE 25-37. **Otosclerosis.** Otosclerotic foci appear as dark purple areas in the bony labyrinth. At the anterior margin of the oval window (*arrow*), otosclerosis has immobilized the footplate of the stapes by bony ankylosis.

Otosclerosis Results in Progressive Deafness

Otosclerosis is the formation of new spongy bone about the stapes and the oval window, resulting in progressive deafness. The condition is an autosomal dominant hereditary defect and is the most common cause of conductive hearing loss in young and middle-aged adults in the United States. Ten percent of white and 1% of black adult Americans have some otosclerosis, but 90% of cases are asymptomatic. The female-to-male ratio is 2:1. Both ears are usually affected. The pathogenesis of otosclerosis is obscure.

PATHOLOGY: Although any part of the petrous bone may be affected, otosclerotic bone tends to form at particular points. The most frequent site (80% to 90%) is immediately anterior to the oval window. The focus of sclerotic bone extends posteriorly and may infiltrate and replace the stapes. This process progressively immobilizes the footplate of the stapes, and the developing bony ankylosis (Fig. 25-37) is functionally manifested as a slowly progressive conductive hearing loss.

Histologically, the initial lesion of otosclerosis is resorption of bone and formation of highly cellular fibrous tissue, with wide vascular spaces and osteoclasts (Fig. 25-38). The focus of resorbed bone is later replaced by immature bone, which, with repeated remodeling, becomes mature bone.

Otosclerosis is successfully treated by surgical mobilization of the auditory ossicles.

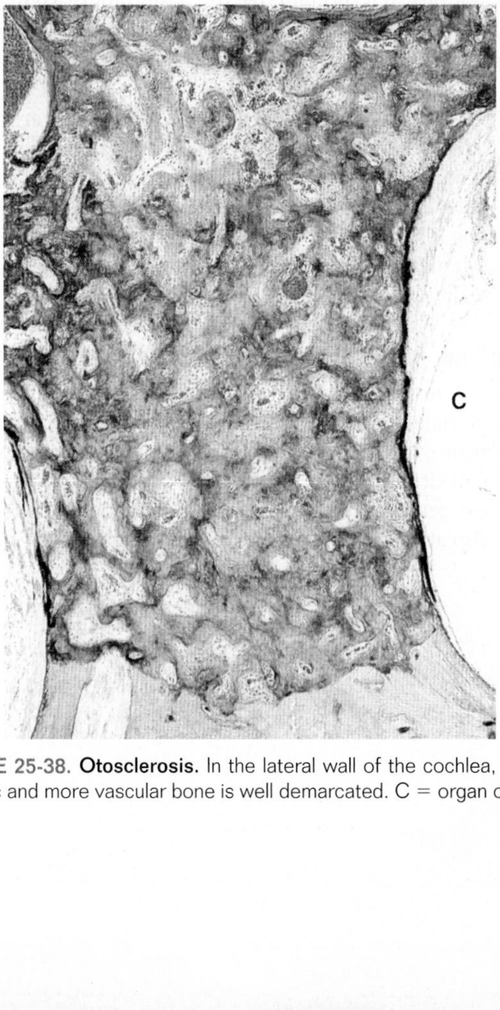

FIGURE 25-38. **Otosclerosis.** In the lateral wall of the cochlea, the basophilic and more vascular bone is well demarcated. C = organ of Corti.

Ménière Disease is the Triad of Vertigo, Sensorineural Hearing Loss and Tinnitus

A number of etiologic factors have been suggested, but the cause of **Ménière** disease is uncertain. Its pathologic correlate is hydropic distention of the endolymphatic system of the cochlea.

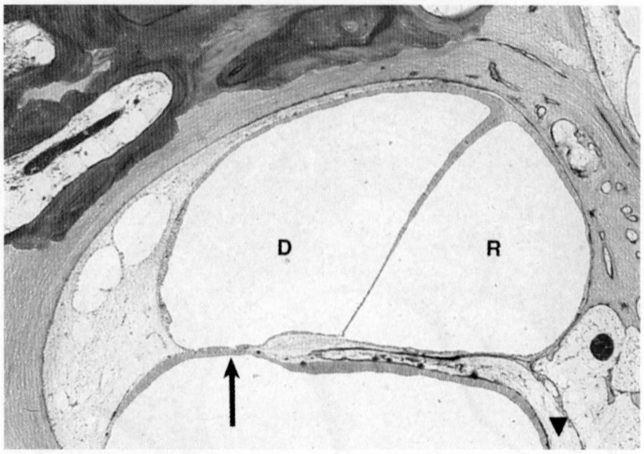

FIGURE 25-39. **Ménière disease.** The cochlear duct (D) is markedly distended, and the Reissner membrane (R) is pushed back by endolymphatic hydrops. Neither the organ of Corti *(arrow)* nor the spiral ganglion *(arrowhead)* is in its usual location.

Ménière disease is most common in the fourth and fifth decades and is bilateral in 15% of patients.

PATHOLOGY: Microscopically, the earliest change is dilatation of the cochlear duct and saccule. As the disease (**hydrops**) progresses, the entire endolymphatic system becomes dilated and the membranous wall frequently tears (Fig. 25-39). Ruptures are sometimes followed by collapse of the membranous labyrinth, but atrophy of sensory and neural structures is rare. It is thought that the symptoms of **Ménière** disease occur when endolymphatic hydrops causes rupture, and the endolymph escapes into the perilymph.

CLINICAL FEATURES: The attacks of vertigo, accompanied by often incapacitating nausea and vomiting, last less than 24 hours. Weeks or months go by before anolther episode, and in time, the remissions become longer. The hearing loss recovers between attacks but later becomes permanent. **Ménière** disease seems to be improved by a low-salt diet and use of diuretics.

Labyrinthine Toxicity is a Drug-Induced Cause of Deafness

The best known drugs that have ototoxic side effects are aminoglycoside antibiotics. These cause irreversible damage to vestibular or cochlear sensory cells. Other antibiotics, diuretics, antimalarial drugs, and salicylates may also cause transient or permanent sensorineural hearing loss. Among antineoplastic agents, cisplatin causes temporary or permanent hearing loss. The labyrinth of the embryo is especially sensitive to some drugs (congenital deafness due to thalidomide, quinine, and chloroquine).

Viral Labyrinthitis Can Result in Congenital Deafness

Viral infections are becoming increasingly recognized as causes of inner ear disorders, particularly deafness. Most cases represent invasion of the labyrinth by the virus. CMV and rubella are the best known prenatal viral infections that lead to congenital deafness through maternal-to-fetal transmission. CMV antigen has been demonstrated in the cells of the organ of Corti and neurons of the spiral ganglia.

Among postnatal viral infections mumps is the most common cause of deafness. The infection can cause rapid hearing loss, which is unilateral in 80% of cases. By contrast, prenatal infection of the labyrinth with rubella is usually bilateral, with permanent loss of cochlear and vestibular function. A number of other viruses are suspected to cause labyrinthitis, including influenza and parainfluenza viruses, EBV, herpesviruses, and adenoviruses. Temporal bone specimens of such cases reveal severe damage to the organ of Corti, with almost total loss of both inner and outer hair cells.

Acoustic Trauma

Noise-induced hearing loss is a significant health problem in industrialized countries. Occupational or recreational exposure to loud tones or noises may cause temporary or permanent loss of hearing. The earliest damage occurs in the external hair cells of the organ of Corti. Loss of sensory hairs is followed by deformation, swelling, and disintegration of the hair cells.

Tumors

SCHWANNOMA: Nearly all schwannomas in the internal auditory canal arise from the vestibular nerves. Vestibular schwannomas, which account for about 10% of all intracranial tumors, are slow growing and encapsulated. Larger tumors protrude from the internal auditory meatus into the cerebellopontine angle and may deform the brainstem and adjacent cerebellum (see Chapter. 28). Schwannomas cause slowly progressive vestibular and auditory symptoms. Neurofibromatosis, type 2, is characterized by a high incidence of bilateral vestibular schwannomas. Histologically, these tumors are indistinguishable from other vestibular schwannomas (see Chapter 28). For a more detailed discussion of acoustic neurinomas, see Chapter 28.

MENINGIOMA: Meningiomas of the cerebellopontine angle originate from the meningothelial cells in the arachnoid villi. The favored sites for these tumors are the sphenoid ridge and petrous pyramid. Meningiomas may extend into the adjacent temporal bone or dural sinuses (see Chapter 28).

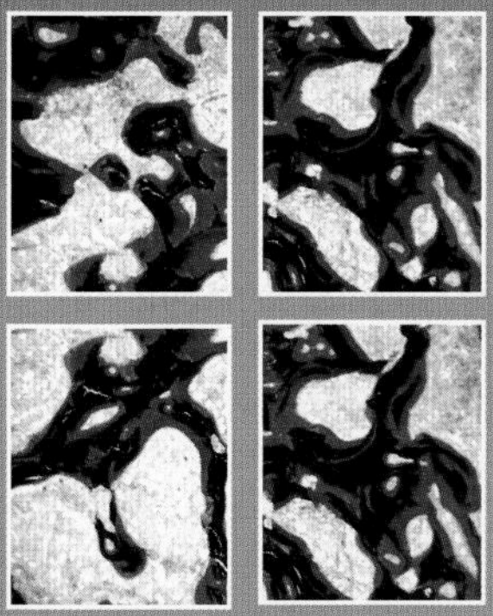

26 Bones and Joints

Benjamin L. Hoch
Michael J. Klein
Alan L. Schiller

BONES

The functions of bone are classified as mechanical, mineral storage, and hematopoietic. Mechanical functions of bone include protection for brain, spinal cord, and chest organs; rigid internal support for limbs; and deployment as lever arms in the skeletal muscle. Bone is the principal reservoir for calcium, and stores other ions such as phosphate, sodium, and magnesium. The bones also serve as hosts for hematopoietic bone marrow.

The mechanical properties of bone are related to its construction and internal architecture. Although extremely light, it has a high tensile strength. This combination of strength and light weight results from its hollow tubular shape, layering of bone tissue, and internal buttressing of the matrix.

The term **bone** can refer to both an organ and a tissue. The "organ" is composed of bone tissue, cartilage, fat, marrow elements, vessels, nerves, and fibrous tissue. Bone "tissue" is described in microscopic terms and is defined by the relation of its collagen and mineral structure to the bone cells.

Anatomy

Macroscopically two types of bone are recognized.

- **Cortical bone** is dense, compact bone, whose outer shell defines the shape of the bone. It composes 80% of the skeleton. Because of its density, its functions are mainly biomechanical.
- **Coarse cancellous bone** (also termed **spongy, trabecular, or marrow bone**) is found at the ends of long bones within the medullary canal. Cancellous bone has a high surface-to-volume ratio and contains many more bone cells per unit volume than does cortical bone. Changes in the rate of bone turnover are manifested principally in cancellous bone.

All bones contain both cancellous and cortical elements (Fig. 26-1), but their proportions differ. The body, or shaft, of a long tubular bone, such as the femur, is composed of cortical bone, and its marrow is mainly fat. Toward the ends of the femur, the cortex becomes thin and coarse cancellous bone becomes the predominant structure. By contrast, the skull is formed by outer and inner tables of compact bone, with only a small amount of cancellous bone within the marrow space, called the **diploë.**

The anatomy of bone is defined in relation to a transverse cartilage plate, which is present in the growing child. This structure is termed the **growth plate**, the **epiphyseal cartilage plate,** or **the physis** (Fig. 26-2). The terms **epiphysis**, **metaphysis,** and **diaphysis** are defined in relation to the growth plate.

- **The epiphysis** is the area of the bone that extends from the subarticular bone plate to the base of the growth plate.
- **The metaphysis** contains coarse cancellous bone, and is the region from the side of the growth plate facing away from the joint to the area where the bone develops its fluted or funnel shape. **The diaphysis** corresponds to the body or shaft of the bone and is the zone between the two metaphyses in a long tubular bone.

The metaphysis blends into the diaphysis and is the area where coarse cancellous bone dissipates. This area of bone is particularly important in hematogenous infections, tumors, and skeletal malformations.

Two additional terms are essential to an understanding of bone organization:

- **Endochondral ossification** is the process by which bone tissue replaces cartilage.
- **Intramembranous ossification** refers to the mechanism by which bone tissue supplants membranous or fibrous tissue laid down by the periosteum.

All bones are formed by at least some intramembranous ossification. Some bones (e.g., the calvaria of the skull) are forged purely by intramembranous ossification. Microscopically, it cannot be determined whether a bone resulted from replacement of cartilage or of fibrous tissue. Because bone tumors tend to recapitulate their embryologic origins, it is not surprising that cartilaginous tumors of the frontal bone have not been seen, because the calvaria of the skull do not originate from cartilage.

The Bone Marrow Resides in the Marrow Space, or Medullary Canal

The marrow space is enclosed by the cortical bone. It is supported by a delicate connective tissue framework that enmeshes the marrow cells and the blood vessels. Three types of marrow are evident to the naked eye:

- **Red marrow** corresponds to hematopoietic tissue and is found in virtually all bones at birth. At adolescence, it is confined to the axial skeleton, which includes the skull, vertebrae, sternum, ribs, scapulae, clavicles, pelvis, and proximal humerus and femur. Its presence may also be pathologic, depending on the patient's age and the site of the marrow. For example, red marrow in the femoral diaphysis of a 55-year-old man is abnormal and may reflect underlying disease, such as leukemia.

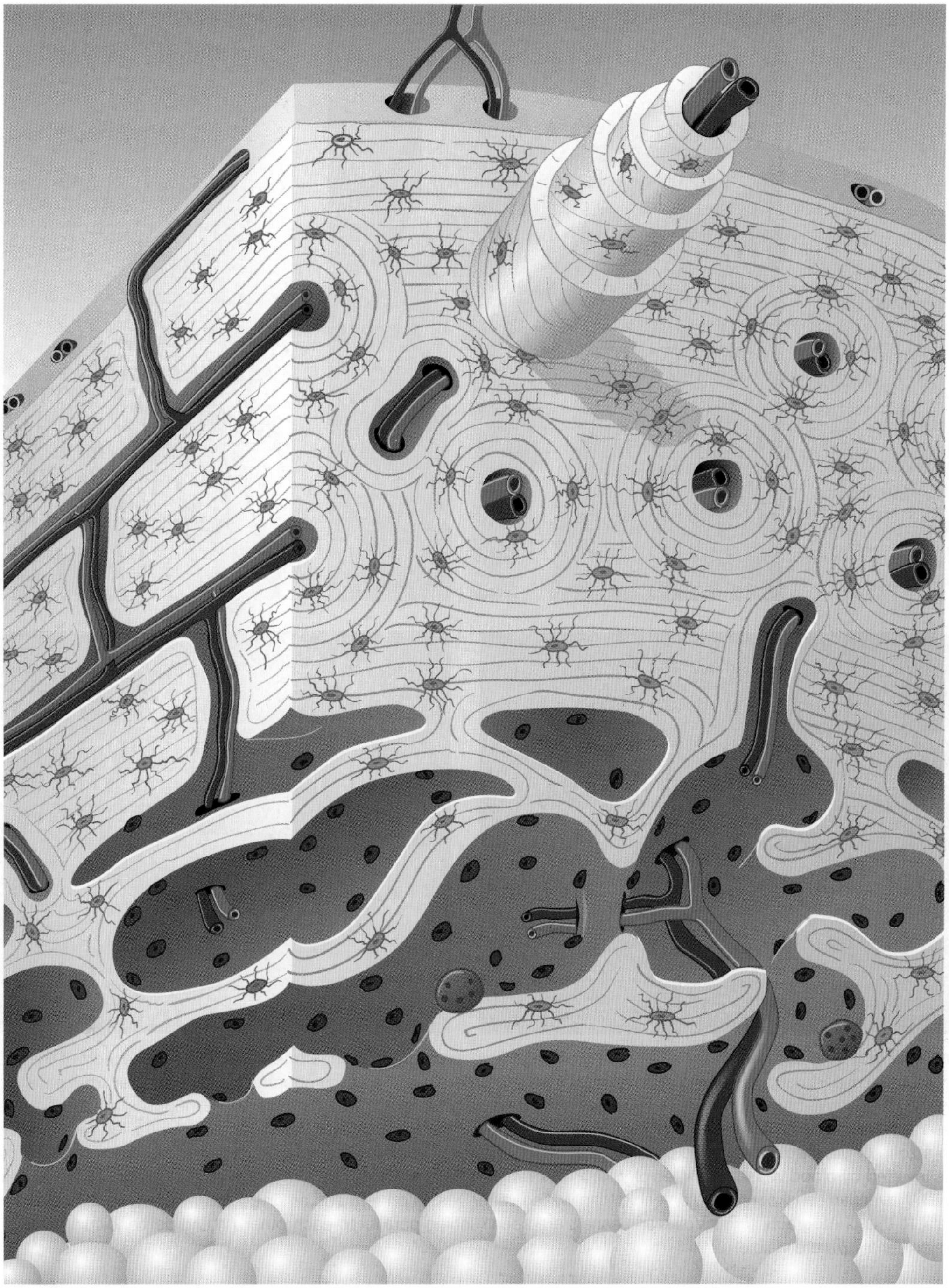

FIGURE 26-1. **Anatomy of bone.** A schematic representation of cortical and trabecular bone. The longitudinal section *(left)* shows the vasculature entering the periosteum via the periosteal perforating arteries and coursing through the bone perpendicular to the long axis in Volkmann canals. The vessels that proceed longitudinally, or parallel to the long axis, are located in haversian canals. Each artery is accompanied by a vein. Within the cortex, osteocytes reside in lacunae, and their cell processes extend into the canaliculi. The cross-sectional view *(right)* illustrates the various types of lamellar bone in the cortex. Circumferential lamellar bone is located adjacent to the periosteum and borders the marrow space. Concentric lamellar bone surrounds the central haversian canals to form an osteon. Each layer of the concentric lamellar bone displays a change in the pitch of the collagen fibers, such that each layer has a different arrangement of collagen. The interstitial lamellar bone occupies the space between osteons. The marrow space is filled with fat, and its trabecular bone is contiguous with the cortex. Multinucleated osteoclasts are present, and palisaded osteoblasts surround the bone surfaces. The perforating arteries from the periosteum and the nutrient artery from the marrow space communicate within the cortex via haversian and Volkmann canals.

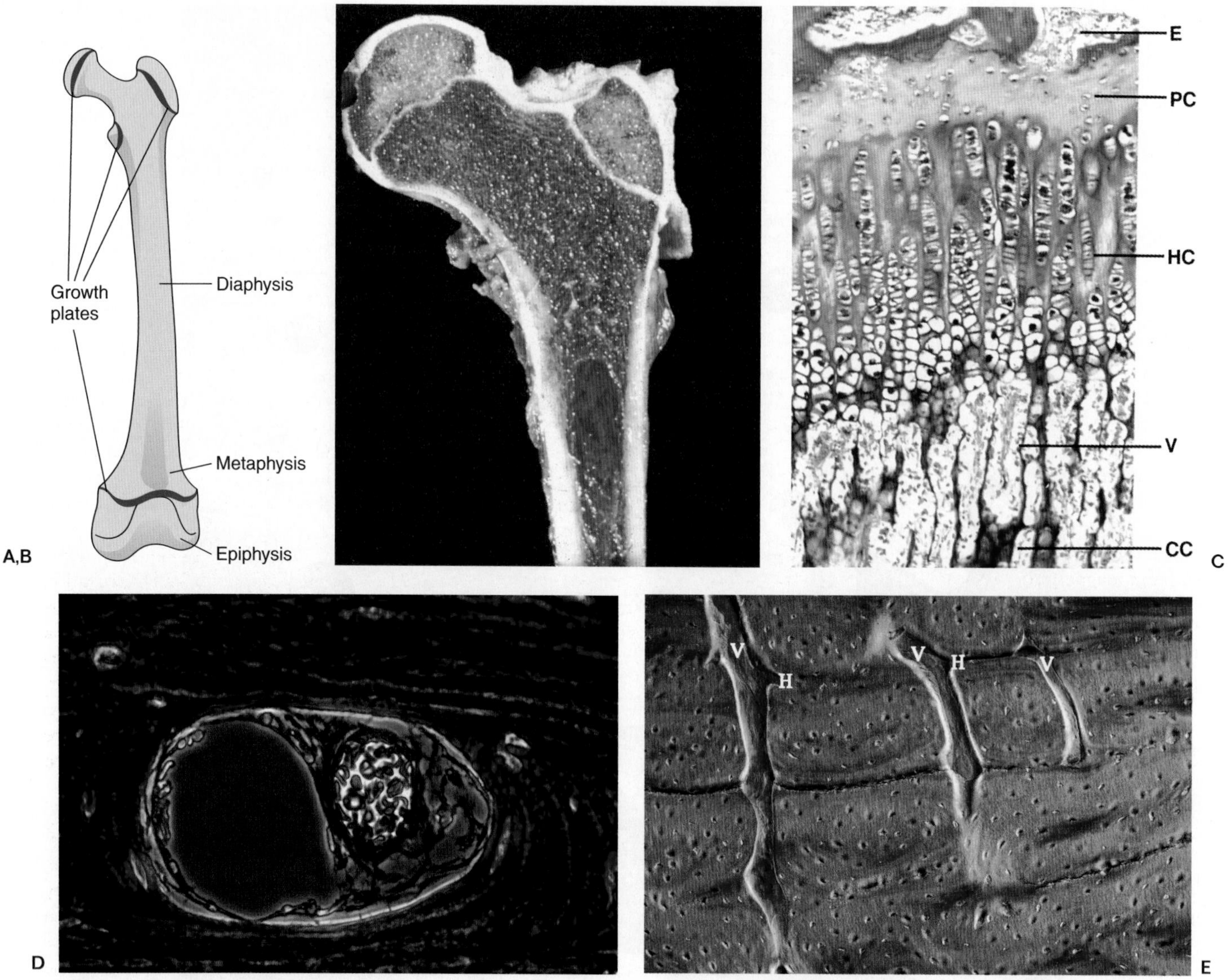

FIGURE 26-2. **Anatomy of a long bone. A.** Diagram of the femur illustrates the various compartments. **B.** Coronal section of the proximal femur illustrates the various anatomical parts of a long bone. The epiphysis of the femoral head and the apophysis of the greater trochanter are separated from the metaphysis by their respective growth plates. The cortex and the medullary cavity are well visualized. The medullary cavity contains cancellous bone until the metaphysis narrows into the diaphysis (shaft) of the bone, which is almost completely devoid of bone and filled with marrow. **C.** A section of the epiphysis with a zone of proliferating cartilage cells. Beneath this zone, the hypertrophic cartilage cells are arrayed in columns. At the *bottom,* the calcifying matrix is invaded by blood vessels. E = epiphysis; PC = proliferative cartilage; HC = hypertrophic cartilage; CC = calcified cartilage; V = vascular invasion. **D.** Haversian canal containing a venule (thin-walled wider vessel on *left*) and an arteriole (thicker-walled narrow vessel on the *right.*) **E.** Volkmann canals. In this photograph, three Volkmann canals are seen running parallel to each other *(v)* and perpendicular to the cortex. The openings of two haversian canals *(h)* are visible.

- **Yellow marrow** appears microscopically as fat tissue and is found in the limb bones. In a normally hematopoietic area, such as a vertebral body, yellow marrow is abnormal at any age.
- **Gray or white marrow** is deficient in hematopoietic elements and is often fibrotic. *It is always a pathologic tissue in a nongrowing adult bone or in areas distant from the growth plate in a child.*

Blood Supply Enters Bone Through Specialized Canals

The long tubular bones are provided with blood from two sources and contain canals to supply the tissues.

- **Nutrient arteries** enter the bone through a nutrient foramen and supply the marrow space and the internal one-third to one-half of the cortex.
- **Perforating arteries** are small straight vessels that extend inward from the periosteal arteries on the external surface of the periosteum (the fibrous capsule of the bone). The perforating arteries anastomose in the cortex with branches from the nutrient arteries coming from the marrow space.
- **Haversian canals** are spaces in cortical bone that course parallel to the long axis of the bone for a short distance and then branch and communicate with other similar canals. Each canal contains one or two blood vessels, lymphatics, and some nerve fibers.
- **Volkmann canals** are spaces within the cortex that run perpendicular to the long axis of the cortex to connect adjacent haversian canals. Volkmann canals also contain blood vessels.

Each artery has its paired vein and, perhaps, free nerve endings. Venous drainage proceeds from the cortex outwards to the periosteal veins, or inwards into the marrow space and out the nutrient veins.

Periosteum Covers All Bones and Can Form Bone

The internal layer of the periosteum, the **cambium layer**, is applied to the surface of the bone and consists of loosely arranged collagenous bundles, with spindle-shaped connective tissue cells and a network of thin elastic fibers. The outer **fibrous layer** is contiguous with soft tissue planes and fascia. It is composed of dense connective tissue containing blood vessels.

Bone Matrix Is Organic and Mineralized

Bone tissue is composed of cells (10% by weight), a mineralized phase (hydroxyapatite crystals, representing 60% of the total tissue), and an organic matrix (30%). Thus, except for its cells, bone is a biphasic structure comprising an organic and an inorganic matrix.

The **mineralized matrix** consists of poorly crystalline hydroxyapatite, $Ca_{10}(PO_4)_6(OH)_2$. Because of its net negative charge, it can neutralize substantial amounts of acid. Other important ions in bone are carbonate, citrate, fluoride, chloride, sodium, magnesium, potassium, and strontium.

The **organic matrix** consists of 88% type I collagen, 10% other proteins, and 1% to 2% lipids, and glycosaminoglycans. *Thus, type I collagen basically defines the organic matrix.* Other proteins include:

- **Osteocalcin** is produced by osteoblasts. Blood levels of this protein are a useful marker of bone formation.
- **Osteopontin** and **sialoprotein** are bone matrix proteins containing the amino acid sequence *Arg-Gly-Asp,* which is recognized by **integrins**. Thus osteopontin and bone sialoprotein probably help anchor cells to the bone matrix.

Bone Cells of Bone Maintain Its Structure

There are four types of cells in bone tissue, each of which has specific functions related to the formation, resorption, and remodeling of bone.

OSTEOPROGENITOR CELL: The osteoprogenitor cell, which ultimately differentiates into osteoblasts and osteocytes, is itself derived from a primitive stem cell. The stem cell can develop into adipocytes, myoblasts, fibroblasts, or osteoblasts. Osteoprogenitor cells are found in marrow, periosteum, and all supporting structures within the marrow cavity. They are not readily recognized by light microscopy as they are small, nonspecific, stellate, or spindle-shaped cells. In response to an appropriate signal, the osteoprogenitor gives rise to an osteoblast.

OSTEOBLAST: Osteoblasts are the protein-synthesizing cells that produce and mineralize bone tissue. They are derived from mesenchymal progenitors that also give rise to chondrocytes, myocytes, adipocytes, and fibroblasts. These large mononuclear and polygonal cells are arrayed in a line along the bone surface (Fig. 26-3A). Underlying the layer of osteoblasts is a thin, eosinophilic zone of organic bone matrix that has not yet been mineralized, termed **osteoid**. The time from the deposition of osteoid to its mineralization is known as the **mineralization lag time**. Its protein synthetic capacity is reflected in its abundant endoplasmic reticulum, prominent Golgi, and mitochondria with calcium-containing granules.Cytoplasmic processes that extend into the osteoid contact cells embedded in the matrix, called **osteocytes**. The syncytium of osteocytes and osteoblasts probably prevents bone calcium (99% of the body's calcium) from equilibrating with the general extracellular space. When an osteoblast is inactive, it flattens on the surface of bone tissue. It contains alkaline phosphatase, manufactures osteocalcin, and has parathyroid hormone (PTH) receptors. Collagenase secreted by osteoblasts may also facilitate osteoclastic activity. Finally, a number of growth factors, including transforming growth factor-β (TGF-β), insulin-like growth factor-I (IGF-I), IGF-2, platelet-derived growth factor (PDGF), interleukin-1 (IL-1), fibroblast growth factor (FGF), and tumor necrosis factor-α (TNF-α), are produced by osteoblasts and are important in regulating bone growth and differentiation.

OSTEOCYTE: The osteocyte is an osteoblast that is completely embedded in bone matrix and is isolated in a lacuna (see Fig. 26-3B). Osteocytes deposit small quantities of bone around lacunae, but with time they lose the capacity for protein synthesis. They have numerous processes that extend through bony canals, called **canaliculi** and communicate with those from other osteocytes (see Fig. 26-3C). Evidence suggests that osteocytes may be the bone cell that recognize and respond to mechanical forces.

OSTEOCLAST: Osteoclasts are the exclusive bone-resorptive cells. They are of hematopoietic origin, being members of the monocyte/macrophage family. Three major factors are required

A
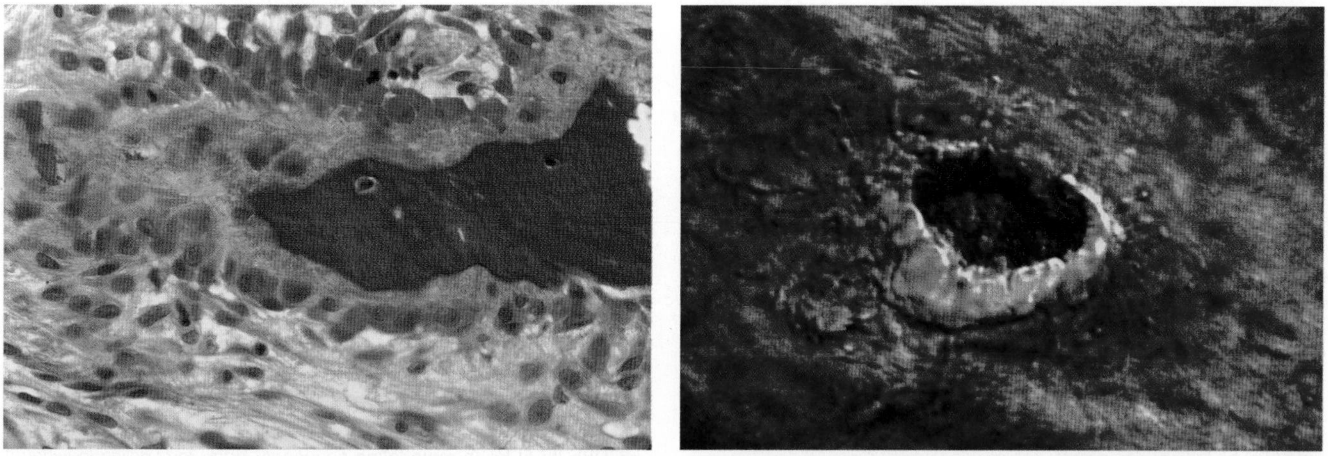
B

FIGURE 26-3. **The cells of bones. A.** A developing bone spicule demonstrates a prominent layer of plump osteoblasts lining the pink osteoid seam. The dark purple layer beneath the osteoid seam is mineralized bone. **B.** Osteocyte. Osteocytes represent trapped osteoblasts surrounded by bone matrix. The space surrounding the cell is called a *lacuna*. At this power, a few cytoplasmic extensions of the cell can be seen extending into narrow channels in the bone, called *canaliculi*.

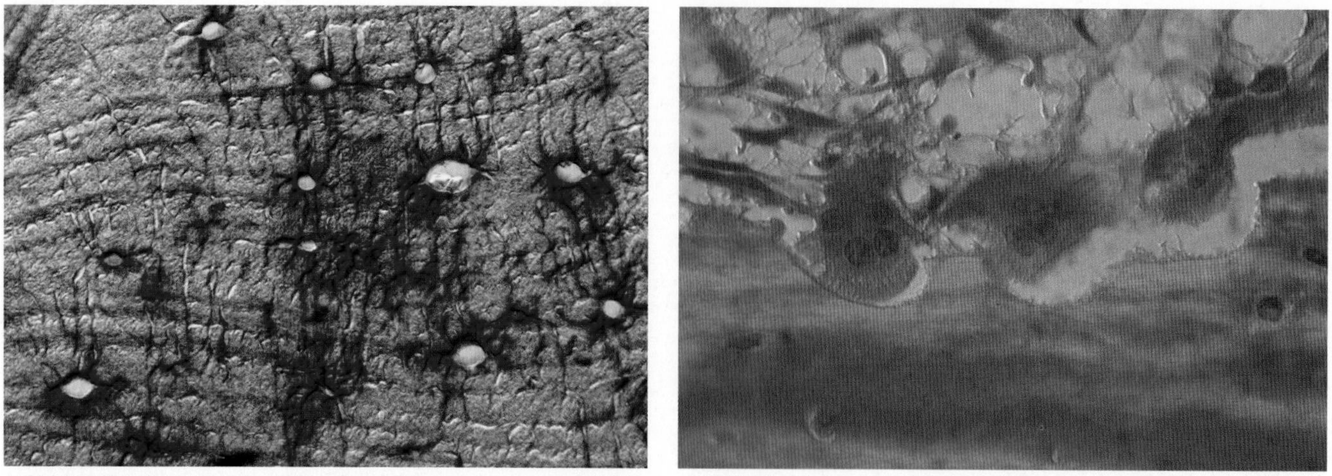
C D

FIGURE 26-3. *(continued)* **C.** The extensive intercommunication of osteocyte processes via their canalicular network in cortical bone is visible in this section. **D.** Osteoclasts. These are multinucleated giant cells found on bone surfaces within small scalloped reabsorption pits, called *Howship lacunae*.

for osteoclastogenesis: (1) TNF-related cytokine, (2) RANK ligand (RANKL; growth factor CSF-1d), (3) the activation of RANK on the surface of hematopoietic precursor cells. Binding of RANKL to RANK activates NF-*k*B signalling, which leads to increased osteoclastogenesis. Osteoclasts are multinucleated cells that contain many lysosomes and are rich in hydrolytic enzymes. They are found in small depressions, termed **Howship lacunae**, on bone surfaces (see Fig. 26-3D). By electron microscopy, they form a polarized ruffled plasmalemmal membrane (Fig. 26-4) when the cell is in contact with, and is actively degrading, bone. Osteoclastic resorption is a multistep process that involves attachment of the cell to bone by integrins. A tight gasketlike seal isolates an extracellular compartment that forms between bone and the osteoclast ruffled membrane. A proton pump then acidifies this compartment to a pH of 4.5, in effect creating a giant extracellular lysosome. This proton-rich environment mobilizes bone mineral, thereby exposing the organic bone matrix to degradation by lysosomal enzymes. Degraded fragments of bone are transported to the opposite side of the osteoclasts and then released to the extracellular space.

Although the machinery of an osteoclast is superbly suited for bone resorption, it functions only if the matrix is mineralized. *In fact, any bone that is lined by osteoid or unmineralized cartilage is protected from osteoclastic activity.* In rickets (see below), the growth plate does not calcify normally; it thus grows without osteoclastic resorption and becomes very thick.

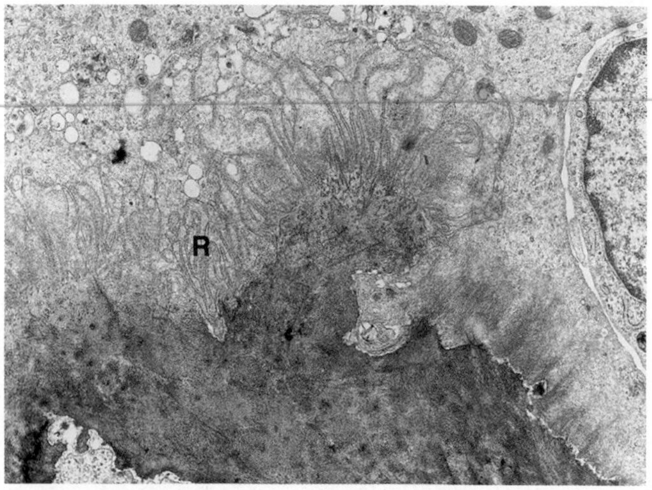

FIGURE 26-4. **Osteoclast.** An electron micrograph shows the ruffled membrane *(R)*, which consists of a complex infolding of the plasma membrane juxtaposed to bone.

Constant remodeling of bone is a normal part of skeletal maintenance (Fig. 26-5), and is initiated by activation of the cytokine receptor RANK on osteoclasts. Soluble factors released during resorption and PTH aid in recruitment of osteoblasts to the site and their activation to form new bone. *Thus, bone remodeling involves replacing old bone with newly formed bone via the functional coupling of osteoclasts and osteoblasts, termed the* ***bone remodeling unit***. Bone remodeling enables bone to adapt to mechanical stress, maintain its strength, and regulate calcium homeostasis.

There are Two Types of Bone Tissue: Lamellar Bone and Woven Bone

Both may be mineralized or unmineralized (Fig. 26-6). Unmineralized bone is called **osteoid**.

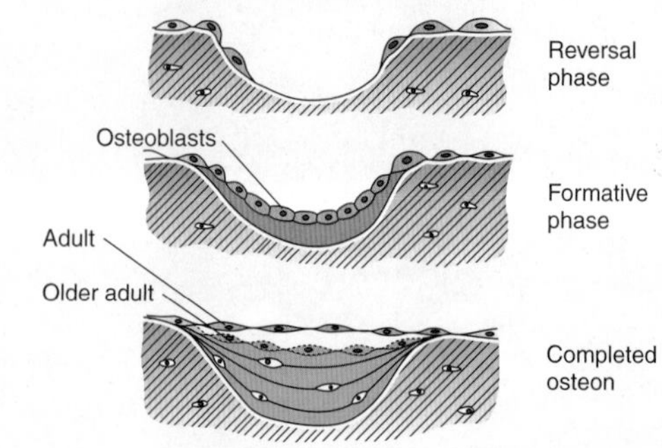

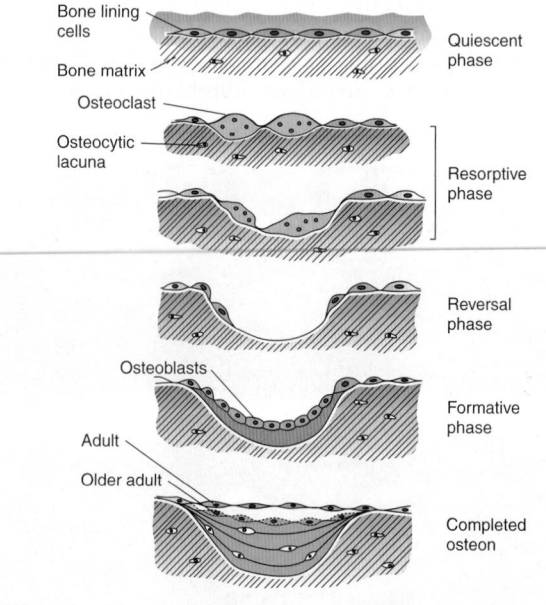

FIGURE 26-5. **Bone-remodeling sequence.** Bone remodeling is initiated by the appearance of osteoclasts on a bone surface previously lined by fusiform cells. After development of a resorption bay, osteoclasts are replaced by osteoblasts, which deposit new bone. The bone loss that attends aging (senile osteoporosis) is due to incomplete filling of resorption bays.

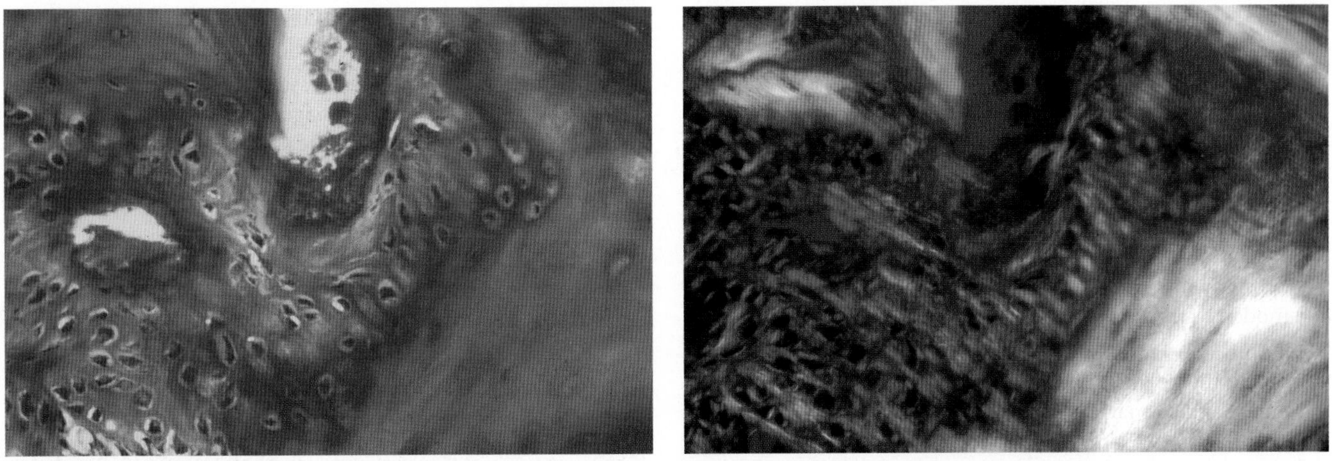

A B

FIGURE 26-6. **Woven bone. A.** In this section, the woven bone constitutes early fracture repair. Note that in the area of new bone there are many osteocytes that vary in size but are mainly large with prominent lacunae (compare with area of mature bone at *lower right*). **B.** This is the same section viewed in polarized light. Note that the collagen fibers are disposed in a pattern resembling the loose fiber pattern of coarsely woven burlap.

Lamellar Bone

Lamellar bone is made slowly and is highly organized. As the stronger bone tissue, it forms the adult skeleton. *Anything other than lamellar bone in the adult skeleton is abnormal.* Lamellar bone is defined by: (1) a parallel arrangement of type I collagen fibers, (2) few osteocytes in the matrix, and (3) uniform osteocytes in lacunae parallel to the long axis of the collagen fibers. There are 4 types of lamellar bone (Fig. 26-7).

- **Circumferential bone** forms the outer periosteal and inner endosteal lamellar envelopes of the cortex.
- **Concentric lamellar bone** is arranged around the haversian canals. In two dimensions, concentric lamellar bone and its

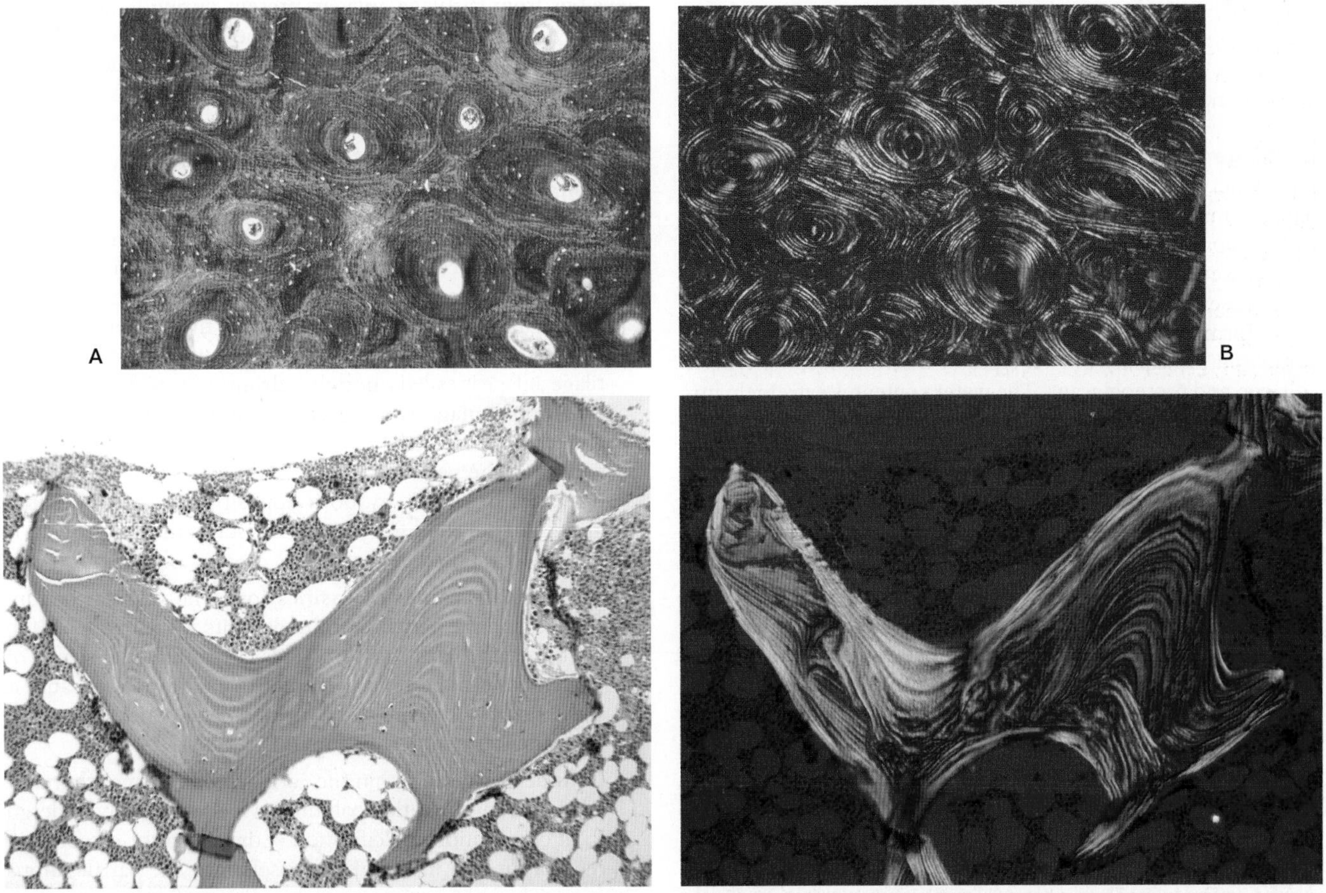

A B C D

FIGURE 26-7. **Cortical lamellar bone. A.** Lamellae of the compacta (cortex) are arranged concentrically about haversian canals. **B.** The same field in polarized light shows the alternating light and dark layered arrangement of the collagen fibers. **C.** Lamellae of the spongiosa in a single mature trabecula are shown in a bright field view. **D.** Polarized light demonstrates that the lamellae are arranged in light and dark layers, but these layers are in long plates rather than in a concentric arrangement.

haversian artery and vein constitute the **osteon** (see Fig. 26-1). In three dimensions, osteons comprise the **haversian system**. These cylinders of bone around the haversian canals run parallel to the long axis of the cortex and are the strongest bone made. The osteons form only if there is appropriate stress. Thus, a paralyzed limb has a cortex composed exclusively of poorly formed haversian systems and circumferential lamellar bone.

- **Interstitial lamellar bone** represents remnants of either circumferential or concentric lamellar bone that have been remodeled and are wedged between the osteons.
- **Trabecular lamellar bone** forms the coarse cancellous bone of the medullary cavity. It exhibits plates of lamellar bone perforated by marrow spaces.

Woven Bone

Woven bone is identified by (1) an irregular arrangement of type I collagen fibers, hence the term *woven;* (2) numerous osteocytes in the matrix, and (3) variation in osteocytesize and shape (see Fig. 26-6A and B).

Woven bone is deposited more rapidly than lamellar bone. It is haphazardly arranged and of low tensile strength, serving as a temporary scaffolding for support. It is not surprising that woven bone is found in the developing fetus, in areas surrounding tumors and infections, and as part of a healing fracture. *Its presence in the adult skeleton is always abnormal, and indicates that reactive tissue has been produced in response to some stress in the bone.*

Cartilage

In contrast to bone, cartilage does not contain blood vessels, nerves, or lymphatics. It may be focally calcified to provide some internal strength in the appropriate areas.

Cartilage Matrix

Like bone, cartilage may be viewed as an organic and inorganic biphasic material. The inorganic phase is composed of calcium hydroxyapatite crystals, equivalent to those found in bone matrix. However, the organic matrix is quite different from that of bone. Essentially, cartilage is a hyperhydrated structure, with water forming some 80% of its weight. The remaining 20% is composed principally of two types of macromolecules, type II collagen and proteoglycans. The water content is extremely important in the function of articular cartilage as it enhances the resilience and lubrication of the joint. Proteoglycans are complex macromolecules composed of a central linear protein core, to which long side arms of polysaccharides called *glycosaminoglycans* are attached. These molecules are polyanionic because of the regular presence of carboxyl groups and sulfates along the molecules. Cartilage glycosaminoglycans comprise three long-chain, unbranched, repeating, polydimeric saccharides: chondroitin-4-sulfate, chondroitin-6-sulfate, and keratan sulfate. The chondroitin sulfates are the most abundant, accounting for 55% to 90% of the cartilage matrix, depending on the age of the tissue.

Types of Cartilage

There are three types of cartilage:

- **Hyaline cartilage:** This is the prototypic cartilage, constituting the articular cartilage of joints; cartilaginous anlage of developing bones; growth plates; costochondral cartilages; cartilages of the trachea, bronchi, and larynx; and nasal cartilages. Hyaline cartilage is the most common cartilage in tumors, in fracture callus, and in areas of relative avascularity.
- **Fibrocartilage:** This tissue is essentially hyaline cartilage that contains numerous type I collagen fibers for tensile and structural strength. It is found in the annulus fibrosus of the intervertebral disk, tendinous and ligamentous insertions, menisci, the symphysis pubis, and insertions of joint capsules. Fibrocartilage may also occur in a fracture callus.
- **Elastic cartilage** is found in the epiglottis, in the arytenoid cartilages of the larynx, and in the external ear.

Chondrocytes

Chondrocytes are derived from primitive mesenchymal cells that are similar to the precursors of bone cells. The chondroblast gives rise to the chondrocyte. Activation of SOX9 transcription factor is essential for chondrocyte formation and SOX9 is expressed in cartilaginous neoplasms. As in bone, the cell that destroys calcified cartilage is the osteoclast.

Bone Formation and Growth

Bone tissue grows only by appositional growth, defined as deposition of new matrix on the surface by adjacent surface cells. By contrast, virtually all other tissues, especially cartilage, increase by interstitial cell proliferation within the matrix as well as by appositional growth.

Bone development in the fetus follows a stereotyped sequence. Most of the skeleton (except the calvaria and clavicles) develops from cartilage anlagen present during fetal development. This cartilage is eventually resorbed and replaced by bone, a process termed **endochondral ossification**. Development of bone can be illustrated by using a limb as an example.

The Process of Primary Ossification Follows a Temporal Sequence

1. **Cartilage anlage:** By 5 weeks of gestation, a thin layer of mesenchymal cells forms between the ectoderm and endoderm of the limb bud and condenses into a core of hyaline cartilage. This cartilaginous anlage is the precursor of the future long bone of that limb. The fibrous capsule of the cartilage anlage is called a **perichondrium**. The width of the cartilaginous anlage is increased by appositional growth of chondroblasts, which deposit cartilage matrix on the internal surface of the perichondrium. At the same time, the anlage increases in length by both appositional and interstitial growth of the chondrocytes. At this stage, the long "bone" is actually composed of cartilage.
2. **The primary center of ossification:** The vascular bed increases, and the perichondrium deposits woven bone on the surface of the cartilage core. This circumferential sleeve of woven bone is the primary center of ossification, because it is the first bone tissue to be formed. The perichondrium is thereafter termed **periosteum** (Fig. 26-8A).
3. **Cylinderization:** Within the cartilaginous anlage, chondrocytes form proliferating columns, which eventually undergo focal calcification. Calcification is the signal for osteoclastic resorption and invasion of vessels into the cartilaginous mass. Thus, the earliest endochondral ossification occurs after the cartilage is hollowed out from the center of the anlage. This "cavitation" of the cartilaginous core forms the

A

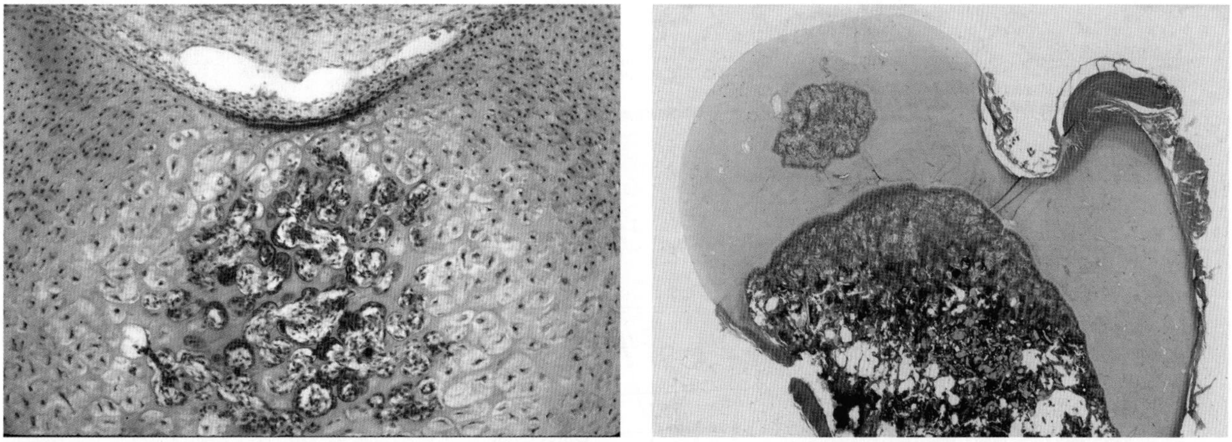

B

FIGURE 26-8. **Primary ossification. A.** This section of a short tubular bone demonstrates the first true bone tissue deposited on the outside of the midshaft of the cartilage model along with very early hollowing of the center of the cartilage model to form mixed spicules of cartilage and bone (primary spongiosa). **B.** The secondary ossification center is demonstrated in this femoral head.

future marrow space. The progressive hollowing of the diaphysis is termed **cylinderization.**

4. **Primary spongiosum:** The swollen, hypertrophied chondrocytes within the central cartilage begin to die. Capillary invasion increases. The surfaces of the calcified cartilage cores become enveloped by woven bone laid down by osteoblasts, which arrive through the pluripotential mesenchymal tissue that enters with the capillaries. This cartilaginous core, surrounded by woven bone, is called **primary spongiosum,** or **primary trabecula.** It is the first bone formed after the replacement of cartilage.

Cavitation continues along the future diaphysis toward each end of the bone. Meanwhile, the bone enlarges in width by appositional bone growth from the ever-increasing periosteal sleeve, which makes additional woven bone for the future cortex.

In Secondary Ossification, Cartilage is Stimulated and Transformed into Bone

Programmed events similar to those in the primary spongiosum take place in the cartilaginous ends of the future bone. Resting (reserve) cartilage is stimulated to become columns of proliferating cartilage, which then progress to hypertrophied chondrocytes and, eventually, calcified cartilage.

1. **The secondary center of ossification** (see Fig. 26-8B): Also termed the **epiphyseal center of ossification,** this structure is formed at the ends of the bone when cartilage is resorbed. The centrifugal enlargement of the secondary ossification is called **hemispherization** and occurs simultaneously with the longitudinal development of the marrow cavity of the diaphysis.
2. **Formation of the growth plate:** As the bony ends expand during hemispherization and cylinderization occurs in the future diaphysis, a zone of cartilage is trapped between the end of the bone and the diaphysis. This cartilage is destined to be the ***growth plate*** (Fig. 26-9A). The growth plate is a layer of modified cartilage between the diaphysis and epiphysis. Its structure is essentially unchanged from early fetal life to skeletal maturity. *The growth plate controls the longitudinal growth of bones and ultimately determines adult height.*
3. **Structure of the growth plate:** The chondrocytes of the growth plate are arranged in vertical rows, which, in three dimensions, are really helices. When viewed longitudinally, the growth plate, proceeding from epiphysis to metaphysis, is divided into zones (see Fig. 26-2B and Fig. 26-9).

- The **reserve (resting) zone** is supplied by epiphyseal arteries and has small chondrocytes and very little matrix. An additional peripheral zone, known as the **zone of Ranvier,** lies directly under the perichondrium.
- The **proliferative zone** is the next deeper zone, in which active proliferation of chondrocytes occurs both longitudinally and transversely, although the main growth thrust is longitudinal. In a very active growth plate, proliferative zones comprise over half the thickness of the growth plate.
- The **hypertrophic zone** is next, and demonstrates a substantial increase in chondrocyte size. The intercellular matrix is prominent, and a dense zone, the **territorial matrix,** surrounds chondrocytes.
- The **zone of calcification** is the cartilaginous zone closest to the metaphysis, where the matrix becomes mineralized.
- The **zone of ossification** is the area where a coating of bone is laid down on the surface of the calcified cartilage. Capillaries grow into the calcified cartilage and give access to osteoclasts, which resorb much of the calcified matrix. Residual vertical walls of calcified cartilage act as scaffolding for the deposition of bone.

The molecular mechanisms governing endochondral growth are beginning to be understood. Parathyroid hormone-related protein (PTHrP) is secreted from perichondrial cells and chondrocytes and maintains chondrocyte proliferation. PTHrP deficiency leads to severe growth retardation and distorted growth plates. The developmental regulator Indian hedgehog (Ihh) is also involved in growth plate maturation by acting in conjuction with PTHrP. A third major factor involved in growth plate regulation is FGF. FGF receptor-3 (FGFR3) is expressed on proliferating chondrocytes, and its activation leads to inhibition of growth plate proliferation. Mutations of FGFR3 lead to growth arrest (e.g., achondroplasia or other forms of dwarfism) or growth acceleration.

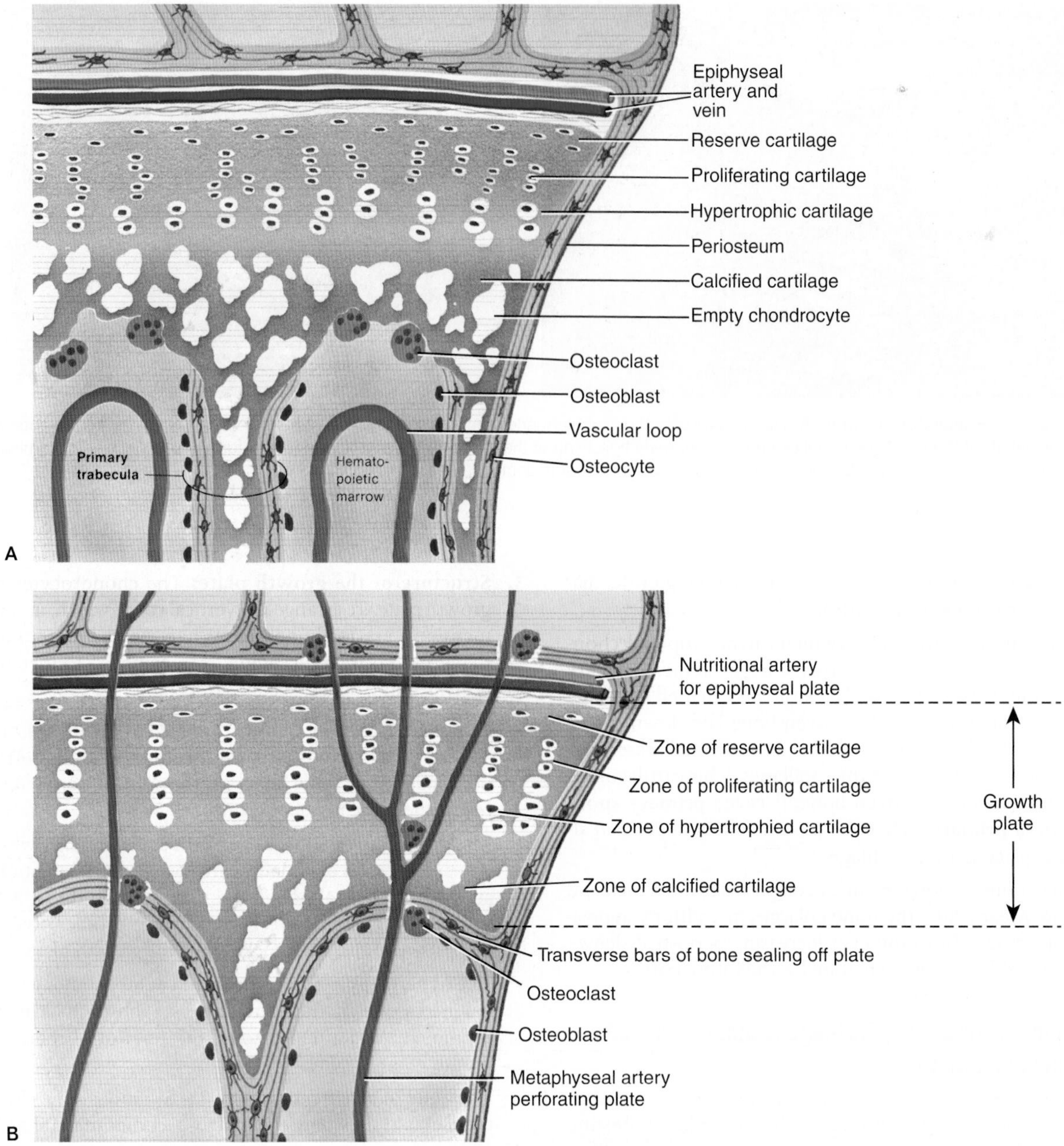

FIGURE 26-9. **Anatomy of the growth (epiphyseal) plate. A.** Normal growing epiphyseal plate. The epiphysis is separated from the epiphyseal plate by transverse plates of bone that seal the plate so that it grows only toward the metaphysis. The various zones of cartilage are illustrated. As the calcified cartilage migrates toward the metaphysis, the chondrocytes die, and the lacunae are empty. At the interface of the epiphyseal plate and the metaphysis, osteoclasts bore into the calcified cartilage, accompanied by a capillary loop from the metaphyseal vessels. Osteoblasts follow the osteoclasts and lay down osteoid on the cartilage core, thereby forming the primary spongiosum, or primary trabeculae. **B.** Normal closure. The epiphyseal cartilage has ceased to grow, and metaphyseal vessels penetrate the cartilage plate. Transverse bars of bone separate the plate from the metaphysis.

Formation of the Metaphysis is Called Funnelization

Funnelization, occurs at the ring of DeLaCroix, a periosteal cuff of bone surrounding the epiphyseal cartilage. Here a wave of periosteal osteoclasts resorbs the cortex, so that a fluted or funnel shape begins to appear. At the same time, endosteal osteoblastic bone is deposited to keep pace with, and to offset, some of the osteoclastic resorption. The net result is the funnel or fluted shape of the bone.

The Growth Plate is Normally Obliterated at a Specific Age for each Bone

Closure of the growth plate (see Fig. 26-9B) is induced by sex hormones and occurs earlier in girls than in boys. Renewal of chondrocytes slows and ultimately ceases. The entire plate is eventually replaced by bone. In some persons, a transverse bony plate representing the site of closure can be seen on X-ray.

Disorders of the Growth Plate

Cretinism Leads to Defective Cartilage Maturation

Cretinism results from maternal iodine deficiency (see Chapter 21) and has profound effects on the skeleton. Thyroid homone plays a role in regulating chondrocytes, osteoblasts, and osteoclasts through production of cytokines and other factors involved in bone development and growth. Linear growth is severely impaired in cretinism, resulting in dwarfism, with limbs disproportionately short in relation to the trunk. Delayed closure of the fontanelles of the skull causes an unusually large head. There is a delay in closure of the epiphyses, as well as radiologic stippling of these zones. Shedding of deciduous teeth and eruption of permanent teeth are retarded.

PATHOLOGY: In cretinism, chondrocytes do not follow the orderly endochondral sequence. Instead, the maturation of the hypertrophied zone is retarded, and the zone of proliferative cartilage is narrow. Endochondral ossification, therefore, does not proceed appropriately, and transverse bars of bone in the metaphysis seal off the growth plate. Although the growth plates may remain open, the failure of endochondral ossification produces severe dwarfism. The misshapen epiphyses seen on radiography reflect incomplete penetration of the secondary centers of ossification of the epiphysis.

Morquio Syndrome Features Mucopolysaccharide Deposition in Chondrocytes

Many of mucopolysaccharidoses (see Chapter 6) involve skeletal deformities, attributable to deposition of mucopolysaccharides (glycosaminoglycans) in developing bones. An example is Morquio syndrome (mucopolysaccharidosis type IV), which leads to a particularly severe form of dwarfism, in addition to dental defects, mental retardation, corneal opacities, and increased urinary excretion of keratan sulfate.

Achondroplasia Is an Inherited Dwarfism Caused by Arrest of the Growth Plate

Achondroplasia refers to a syndrome of short-limbed dwarfism and macrocephaly and represents a failure of normal epiphyseal cartilage formation. It is the most common genetic form of dwarfism (1:15,000 live births) and is inherited as an autosomal dominant trait. Most cases represent new mutations. The mean adult height in achondroplasia is 131 cm (51 inches) in men and 125 cm (49 inches) in women. Achondroplastic dwarfs have normal mentation and average life spans. However, some patients develop severe kyphoscoliosis and its complications.

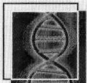

PATHOGENESIS: Achondroplasia is caused by an **activating** mutation in the FGFR3 on chromosome 16 (4p16.3). The mutation constitutively inhibits chondrocyte differentiation and proliferation, which retards growth plate development.

PATHOLOGY: The growth plate in achondroplasia is greatly thinned, and the zone of proliferative cartilage is either absent or extensively attenuated (Fig. 26-10). The zone of provisional calcification, if present, undergoes endochondral ossification, but at a greatly reduced rate. A transverse bar of bone often seals off the growth plate, thereby preventing further bone formation and causing dwarfism. Interestingly, the secondary centers of ossification and the articular cartilage are normal. Because intramembranous ossification is undisturbed, the periosteum functions normally and the bones become very short and thick. For the same reasons, the head of the dwarf appears unusually large, compared with the bones formed from the cartilage of the face. The spine is of normal length, but limbs are abnormally short.

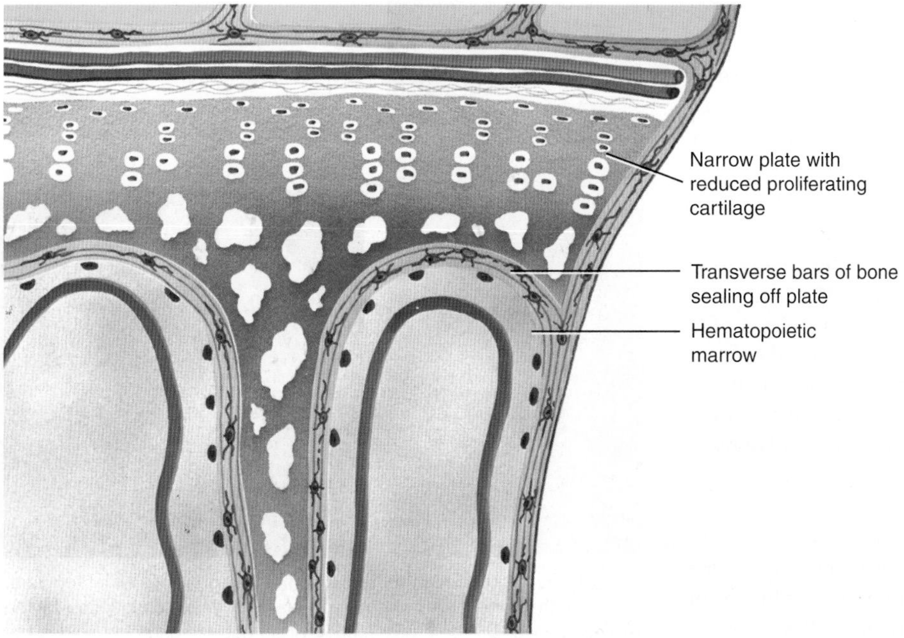

FIGURE 26-10. **The growth (epiphyseal) plate of an achondroplastic dwarf.** In achondroplasia, the epiphyseal plate is reduced in thickness, and the zones of proliferating cartilage are attenuated. Osteoclastic activity is inconspicuous, and the interface between the plate and the metaphysis is often sealed by transverse bars of bone that prevent further endochondral ossification. As a result, the bones are shortened.

Scurvy is the Disease that Results from Dietary Deficiency of Vitamin C

Today, scurvy is a rare disease (see Chapter 8).

PATHOGENESIS: Hydroxyproline and hydroxylysine are important in stabilizing the helical structure of collagen and in cross-linking the tropocollagen fibers into the proper molecular structure of collagen. Vitamin C is a cofactor in hydroxylation of proline and lysine. Wound healing and bone growth are, therefore, impaired in patients with scurvy. Furthermore, the basement membrane of capillaries is damaged by this condition and widespread capillary bleeding is common. Subperiosteal bleeding may occur, leading to joint and muscle pain.

PATHOLOGY: The skeletal changes of scurvy reflect the lack of osteoblastic function. Woven bone is not formed because osteoblasts cannot produce and normally cross-link collagen. Chondrocytes at the growth plate continue to grow. The zone of calcified cartilage may actually become more prominent, because it is more heavily calcified. Osteoclasts resorb this zone, but the primary spongiosum does not form properly, and there is irregular vascular perforation of the cartilage plate.

Asymmetric Cartilage Growth Causes Spinal Disorders and Tumors

Asymmetric cartilage growth, such as occurs in patients with knock-knees and bowed legs, develops when one part of the growth plate, either medial or lateral, grows faster than the other. Most cases are hereditary, but mechanical forces, such as trauma near the growth plate, may stimulate one side to grow faster or in an asymmetric fashion. Aside from the cosmetic appearance, these conditions may require correction to prevent future incongruity, eventual loss of articular cartilage and joint destruction.

Scoliosis and Kyphosis

Scoliosis *is an abnormal lateral curvature of the spine, usually affecting adolescent girls.* ***Kyphosis*** *refers to an abnormal anteroposterior curvature.* When both conditions are present, the term ***kyphoscoliosis*** is used.

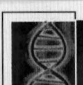

PATHOGENESIS: A vertebral body grows in length (height) from the endplates of the vertebrae, which correspond to the growth plates of long tubular bones. As in tubular bones, vertebral bodies increase in width by appositional bone growth from the periosteum. In scoliosis, for unknown reasons, one portion of the endplate grows faster than the other, producing lateral curvature of the spine.

CLINICAL FEATURES: The treatment is appropriate stress on the vertebral body through use of braces or internal fixation to straighten the spine. If kyphoscoliosis is severe, the patient may eventually develop chronic pulmonary disease, cor pulmonale, and joint problems, particularly involving the hip.

Osteochondroma

Osteochondroma is a developmental defect of the skeleton, which arises from a defect at the ring of Ranvier of the growth plate. Solitary osteochondroma is the most common form of the lesion. The tumor may have to be removed if it is cosmetically displeasing or presses upon an artery or nerve. A number of cases where the tumor increased in size have been related to pregnancy and lactation.

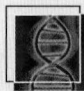

PATHOGENESIS: The ring of Ranvier guides the growth of the growth cartilage toward the metaphysis. If the ring of Ranvier is absent or defective, growth cartilage grows laterally into the soft tissue. Vessels originating in the marrow cavity of the bone extend into this cartilage mass. Continuation of this process results in a cartilage-capped, bony, stalked osteochondroma (Fig. 26-11), which is in direct continuity with the marrow cavity of the parent bone. Cytogenetic aberrations have been characterized in sporadic and hereditary osteochondromas, including chromosomes 8q24, 11p11–p13, and 19p, where the *EXT1*, *EXT2*, *EXT3* genes are located, respectively. The *EXT* genes may be involved in chondrocyte proliferation and differentiation by affecting the Indian Hedge hog-PTH-related protein (Ihh-PTHrp) pathway that is vital in the proper development of endochondral bones. *EXT* mutations inhibit chondrocyte proliferation, which may alter the direction of chondrocyte growth and lead to the development of osteochondroma.

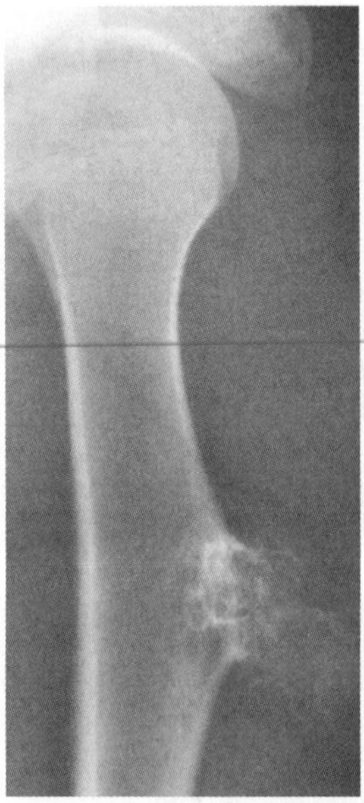
A

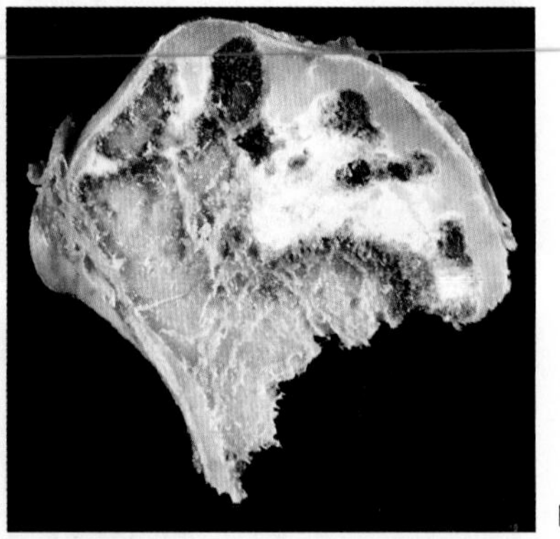
B

FIGURE 26-11. **Osteochondroma. A.** A radiograph of an osteochondroma of the humerus shows a lesion that is directly contiguous with the marrow space. **B.** The cross-section of an osteochondroma shows the cap of calcified cartilage overlying poorly organized cancellous bone.

PATHOLOGY: Osteochondromas tend to grow away from the joint. In radiographs, the cartilaginous mass is in direct continuity with the parent bone and lacks an underlying cortex. Histologically, a cartilage-capped, bony mass is surrounded by a surface fibrous membrane, which is the perichondrium. Active endochondral ossification deep to the cartilage cap allows the bony protuberance to lengthen.

HEREDITARY MULTIPLE OSTEOCHONDROMATOSIS (HMO): This inherited autosomal dominant disorder is characterized by numerous osteochondromas. HMO is one of the most common inherited musculoskeletal disorders. Loss of *EXT1* or *EXT2* gene function is the main cause of HMO. Although not as common as solitary osteochondroma, the heritable variety is not rare, with an incidence of about 1 / 50,000. It occurs predominantly in men, but because of its variable expression, a seemingly unaffected woman from an afflicted family may transmit the disorder.

PATHOLOGY: Each individual lesion in multiple osteochondromatosis is identical to a solitary osteochondroma. In severe cases of hereditary osteochondromatosis, dwarfism may result because of lateral displacement of the longitudinal growth plate by the osteochondroma. Metacarpals may be shortened and fixed pronation or supination may develop if the lesions occur in the forearm and interfere with wrist function. Further difficulties may be caused by unequal leg length and disturbed joint function because of encroaching osteochondromas. Chondrosarcoma is a rare complication.

Hemihypertrophy

Hemihypertrophy describes several conditions in which one limb's growth plate is stimulated to undergo rapid and prolonged endochondral ossification. That limb becomes much longer than the contralateral one. Infection in the metaphyseal area may stimulate the growth plate to grow rapidly. An arteriovenous malformation may also cause one growth plate to grow faster than its counterpart, as may fractures and tumors near the growth plate. In some cases, hemihypertrophy is part of an inherited syndrome. Children with isolated hemihypertrophy are at increased risk for neoplasms.

Modeling Abnormalities

Osteopetrosis Features Abnormally Dense Bone

*Osteopetrosis, also known as **marble bone disease** or **Albers–Schönberg disease**, is a heterogeneous group of rare inherited disorders characterized by increased skeletal mass due to abnormally dense bone.* The most common autosomal recessive form is a severe, sometimes fatal disease affecting infants and children. Death of infants with this severe variant is attributable to marked anemia, cranial nerve entrapment, hydrocephalus, and infection. A more benign form, transmitted as an autosomal dominant trait and seen in adulthood or adolescence, is associated with mild anemia or no symptoms at all.

PATHOGENESIS: *The sclerotic skeleton of osteopetrosis is the result of failed osteoclastic bone resorption.* The disease is caused by mutations in genes that govern osteoclast formation or function. The most common mutations cause defects in bone acidification, which is necessary for osteoclastic bone resorption. These include mutations in the *TCIRG1* gene (osteoclast proton pump; autosomal dominant), the *CLCN7* gene (osteoclast choride channel; autosomal recessive), and the **carbonic anhydrase II** gene (autosomal recessive). Other mutations that cause osteopetrosis involve transcription factors or cytokines necessary for the osteoclast differentiation.

Because osteoclast function is arrested, osteopetrosis is characterized by (1) retention of the primary spongiosum with its cartilage cores, (2) lack of funnelization of the metaphysis, and (3) a thickened cortex. The result is short, blocklike, radiodense bones, hence the term **marble bone disease** (Fig. 26-12). These bones are extremely radiopaque and weigh two to three times more than normal bone. However, they are basically weak because their structure is intrinsically disorganized and cannot remodel along lines of stress. The mineralized cartilage is also weak and friable. Thus, the bones in osteopetrosis fracture easily.

PATHOLOGY AND CLINICAL FEATURES: Grossly, bones in osteopetrosis are widened in the metaphysis and diaphysis, resulting in the characteristic "Erlenmeyer flask" deformity. Histologically, the bone tissue is extremely irregular, and almost all areas contain a cartilage core. Depending on the mutation, osteoclasts may be absent, present in normal numbers, or even abundant. In the case of osteopetrosis characterized by normal or increased numbers of osteoclasts, the molecular defect lies in a gene involved in the function of osteoclasts, rather than their formation.

Suppression of hematopoiesis in osteopetrosis is due to replacement of the marrow by sheets of abnormal osteoclasts or extensive fibrosis. Marrow suppression in patients with the malignant form of osteopetrosis may be severe enough to lead to severe anemia or pancytopenia. To compensate for loss of marrow hematopoiesis, extramedullary hematopoiesis occurs in the liver, spleen, and lymph nodes, and these structures are enlarged. Narrowing of neural foramina causes cranial nerve involvement, and subsequent strangulation of nerves leads to blindness and deafness. Osteopetrosis is treated by bone marrow transplantation, which gives rise to a new clone of functional osteoclasts.

Progressive Diaphyseal Dysplasia Features Thickened Long Bones

Progressive diaphyseal dysplasia (Camurati-Englemann disease) is an autosomal dominant disorder of children in which cylinderization does not proceed appropriately, resulting in symmetric thickening in, and increased diameter of, the diaphyses of long bones. It is due to increased bone formation linked t a mutation in the propeptide of TGF-β. The disease particularly affects the femur, tibia, fibular, radius, and ulna. Patients have pain over the affected areas, fatigue, muscle wasting, atrophy, and gait abnormalities.

Delayed Maturation of Bone

Osteogenesis Imperfecta Relates to Abnormal Type I Collagen

Osteogenesis imperfecta (OI) refers to a group of mainly autosomal dominant, heritable disorders of connective tissue, caused by mutations

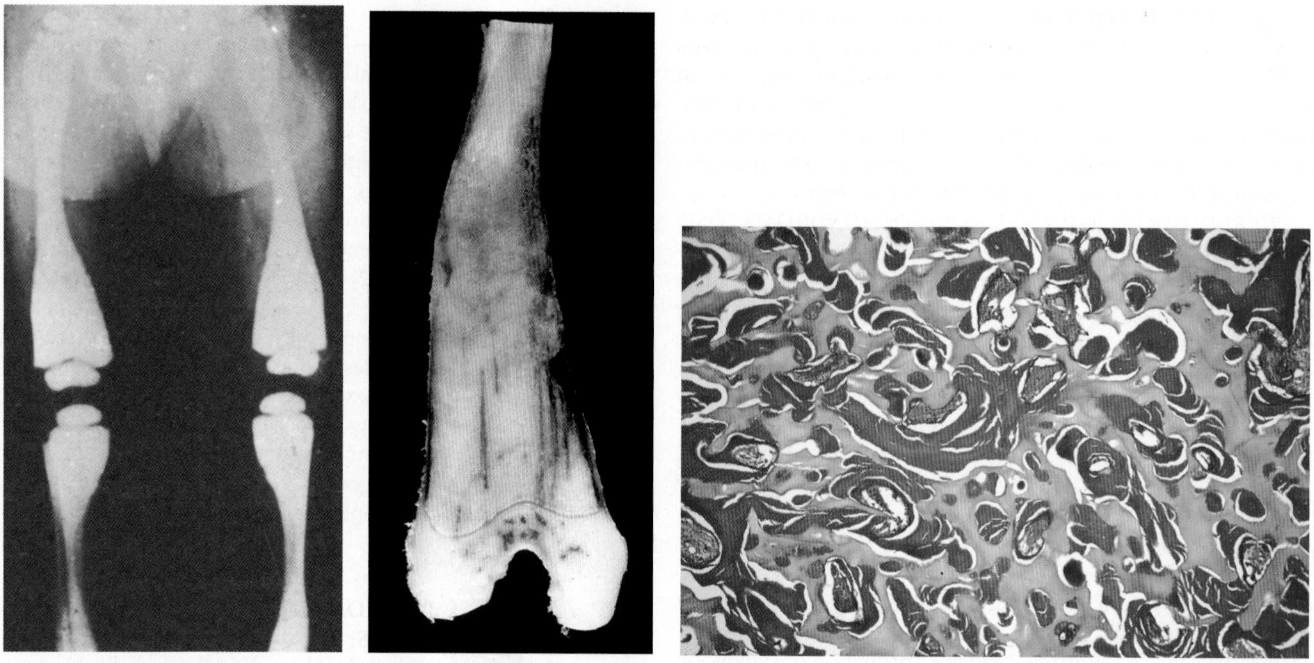

A,B C

FIGURE 26-12. **Osteopetrosis. A.** A radiograph of a child shows markedly misshapen and dense bones of the lower extremities, characteristic of "marble bone disease." **B.** A gross specimen of the femur shows obliteration of the marrow space by dense bone. **C.** A photomicrograph of the bone of a child with autosomal recessive osteopetrosis demonstrates disorganization of bony trabeculae by retention of primary spongiosa (mixed spicules) and further obliteration of the marrow space by secondary spongiosa. The result is complete disorganization of the trabeculae and absence of marrow.

in the gene for type I collagen, affecting the skeleton, joints, ears, ligaments, teeth, sclerae, and skin (see Chapter 6). There are at least four types of OI, each with a different genetic structural abnormality and clinical features.

PATHOGENESIS: The pathogenesis of OI involves mutations of *COL1A1* and *COL1A2* genes, which encode the α1 and α2 chains of type I procollagen, the major structural protein of bone. These genes are in chromosomes 17 (17q21.3–q22) and 7 (7q21.3–q22), respectively. A point mutation that affects a glycine residue in either *COL1A1* or *COL1A2* is the most typical abnormality found in OI. While *COL1A1* mutations are seen in all types of OI, mutations of *COL1A2* are found in types II, III, and IV OI. Mutations of *COL1A1* affect three-fourths of the type I collagen molecules, with half of the molecules containing one abnormal proαI chain and one quarter containing two abnormal proαI chains. By contrast, mutations in *COL1A2* affect only half of the synthesized collagen molecules. The resulting phenotype will range from mild to lethal depending on which gene is affected, the location in the collagen triple helix at which the substitution occurs and which amino acid is substitued for glycine.

Osteogenesis Imperfecta Type I

OI type I is the mildest phenotype. It is inherited as an autosomal dominant trait, characterized by multiple fractures after birth, blue sclera, and hearing abnormalities. In some patients abnormalities of the teeth are also conspicuous.

PATHOLOGY AND CLINICAL FEATURES: The initial fractures usually occur after the infant begins to sit and walk. There may be hundreds of fractures a year with minor movement or trauma. On radiologic examination, bones are extremely thin, delicate and abnormally curved (Fig. 26-13). The collagen has reduced tensile strength and bone mineralization is abnormal. The

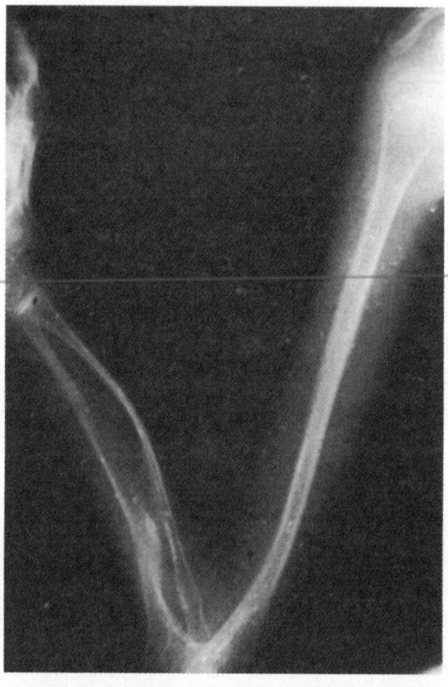

FIGURE 26-13. **Osteogenesis imperfecta.** A radiograph illustrates the markedly thin and attenuated humerus and bones of the forearm. There is a fracture callus in the proximal ulna.

combination of these abnormalities accounts for the brittleness of OI bone. In OI, insufficient bone is formed, leading to decreased cortical thickness and reduced amount of trabecular bone. When a fracture occurs, the fracture callus may be extensive enough to resemble a tumor. As the child grows, fractures tend to decrease in severity and frequency, and stature is generally unaffected.

The sclerae are very thin, with a blue color attributable to the underlying choroid. Progressive hearing loss, which develops to total deafness in adulthood, results from fusion of the auditory ossicles. The joint laxity associated with the condition eventually leads to kyphoscoliosis and flat feet. Because of hypoplasia of the dentine and pulp, the teeth are misshapen and bluish yellow.

Osteogenesis Imperfecta Type II

OI type II is a lethal, perinatal disease with an autosomal dominant inheritance pattern. Affected infants are stillborn or die within a few days, in a sense being crushed to death. They exhibit markedly short stature and severe limb deformities, and almost all of the bones sustain fractures during delivery or during uterine contractions in labor. As in OI type I, sclerae are blue.

Osteogenesis Imperfecta Type III

OI type III is the progressive, most severely deforming type of disease and is characterized by many bone fractures, growth retardation, and severe skeletal deformities. Inheritance is usually autosomal dominant, although (rarely) autosomal recessive forms are reported. Fractures are present at birth, but bones are less fragile than in the type II form. These patients eventually develop severe shortening of their stature because of progressive bone fractures and severe kyphoscoliosis. Although sclerae may be blue at birth, they become white shortly thereafter. Dental abnormalities are common.

Osteogenesis Imperfecta Type IV

OI type IV is similar to type I except that sclerae are normal. The condition is heterogeneous in presentation, and there may or may not be dental disease. In this disorder, abnormal cross-linkages of collagen result in thin, delicate, and weak collagen fibrils. This inappropriate collagen does not allow the bone cortex to mature, so that at birth the cortex of the bone resembles that of a fetus. The cortex is composed of woven bone and small areas of lamellar bone. Over a period of years, the cortex matures, but this may not occur until adolescence or even later. In any event, the frequency of fractures tends to decrease over a long period. These patients are vigorously treated with orthopedic devices, including rods inserted into the medullary cavities to prevent the dwarfing effect of multiple fractures.

Additional types of OI (types V, VI, and VII) have recently been identified from within the heterogeneous type IV group based on distinct clinical and bone histologic features.

There is no single treatment for OI. Osteoprogenitor cells for bone marrow transplantation, growth factors, bisphosphonates, and gene therapy to improve collagen synthesis have been undergoing clinical trials in an attempt to modify the course and severity of the disease. Because exuberant fracture callus occurs, it is not surprising that rare cases of OI have been interpreted as osteosarcoma.

Enchondromatosis Is Marked by Multiple Cartilaginous Tumors

*Enchondromatosis, also termed **Ollier disease** is characterized by development of numerous cartilaginous masses that lead to bony deformities.*

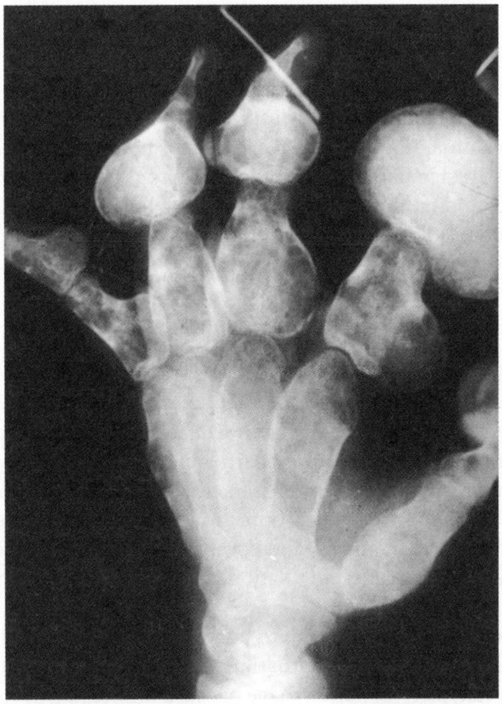

FIGURE 26-14. **Multiple enchondromatosis (Ollier disease).** A radiograph of the hand shows bulbous swellings that represent cartilage masses composed of hyaline cartilage, which is sometimes admixed with more primitive myxoid cartilage.

The condition is not strictly a disease of delayed maturation of bone, but one in which residual hyaline cartilage, anlage cartilage, or cartilage from the growth plate does not undergo endochondral ossification and remains in the bones. As a consequence, bones show multiple, tumorlike masses of abnormally arranged hyaline cartilage (enchondromas), with zones of proliferative and hypertrophied cartilage (Fig. 26-14). These tumors tend to be located in the metaphyses. As growth continues, the enchondromas settle in the diaphysis of adolescents and adults.

Enchondromatosis is asymmetric and may cause bone deformities. Whether enchondromas represent true neoplasms is debated, but they exhibit a strong tendency to undergo malignant change into chondrosarcomas in adult life. Therefore a patient with enchondromatosis who has increasing pain or an increasing abnormality at one site should be evaluated to rule out an underlying sarcoma.

Solitary enchondroma has histologic features similar to Ollier disease and principally affects the tubular bones of the hands and feet. It rarely undergoes malignant change.

Maffucci syndrome is characterized by multiple enchondromas and cavernous or spindle cell hemangiomas. It usually manifests in early childhood and may lead to significant skeletal deformities. Chondrosarcoma develops in as many as half of all patients with Maffucci syndrome. The incidence of malignant tumors in other organs is also greatly increased in patients with Mafucci syndrome.

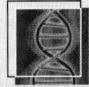

PATHOGENESIS: Most cases of enchondromatosis are sporadic, but a familial form possibly with autosomal dominant inheritance has been reported. Recent studies have disclosed mutations in the

PTHR1 gene, encoding a receptor for PTH and PTH-related protein, in some cases of enchondromatosis. The mutation results in a substitution in the receptor's extracellular domain, increasing cyclic adenosine monophosphate (cAMP) signaling. The mutant receptor may delay chondrocyte differentiation by activating Hedgehog signaling, which results in the formation of the multiple cartilaginous masses characteristic of the disease.

Fracture

The most common bone lesion is a fracture, which is defined as a discontinuity of the bone. A force perpendicular to the long axis of the bone results in a transverse fracture. A force along the long axis of the bone yields a compression fracture. Torsional force results in spiral fractures, and combined tension and compression shear forces cause angulation and displacement of the fractured ends.

A force powerful enough to fracture a bone also injures adjacent soft tissues. In this situation, there is often (1) extensive muscle necrosis; (2) hemorrhage because of shearing of capillary beds and larger vessels of the soft tissues; (3) tearing of tendinous insertions and ligamentous attachments; and (4) even nerve damage, caused by stretching or direct tearing of the nerve.

Fracture Healing is Divided into Inflammatory, Reparative, and Remodeling Phases

The duration of each phase (Fig. 26-15) depends on the patient's age, the site of fracture, the patient's overall health and nutritional status, and the extent of soft tissue injury. Local factors, such as vascular supply and mechanical forces at the site, also play a role in healing. *In the repair of a bone fracture, anything other than the formation of bone tissue at the fracture site represents incomplete healing.*

PATHOLOGY:

The Inflammatory Phase

In the first 1 to 2 days after a fracture, rupture of blood vessels in the periosteum and adjacent muscle and soft tissue leads to extensive hemorrhage. Extensive bone necrosis at the fracture site also occurs because of disruption of large vessels in the bone and interruption of cortical vessels (i.e., Volkmann and haversian canals). *Dead bone is characterized by the absence of osteocytes and empty osteocyte lacunae.*

In 2 to 5 days, the hemorrhage forms a large clot, which must be resorbed so that the fracture can heal. Neovascularization begins to occur peripheral to this blood clot. By the end of the first week, most of the clot is organized by invasion of blood vessels and early fibrosis.

The earliest bone, which is invariably woven bone, is formed after 7 days. *This corresponds to the "scar" of bone.* Because bone formation requires a good blood supply, the woven bone spicules begin to appear at the periphery of the clot. Pluripotential mesenchymal cells from the soft tissue and within the bone marrow give rise to the osteoblasts that synthesize the woven bone. In most fractures, cartilage also is formed and is eventually resorbed by endochondral ossification. Granulation tissue containing bone or cartilage is termed a **callus**. Woven bone also forms inside the marrow cavity at the periphery of the blood clot because vascular tissue is also present in this location.

The Reparative Phase

The reparative phase follows the first week after a fracture and extends for months, depending on the degree of movement and the fixation of the fracture. By this time, acute inflammation has dissipated. Pluripotential cells differentiate into fibroblasts and osteoblasts. Repair proceeds from the periphery towards the center of the fracture site and accomplishes two objectives: (1) it organizes and resorbs the blood clot; and, (2) more importantly, it furnishes neovascularization for construction of the callus, which will eventually bridge the fracture site. The events leading to repair are as follows:

1. Armies of osteoclasts within the haversian canals form **cutting cones** that bore into the cortex toward the fracture site. A new vessel accompanies the cutting cone, supplying nutrients to these cells and providing more pluripotential cells for cell renewal.
2. At the same time, the external callus, which is found on the surface of the bone and is formed from the periosteum and the soft tissue mesenchymal cells, continues to grow toward the fracture site.
3. Simultaneously, an endosteal, or internal, callus forms within the medullary cavity and grows outward toward the fracture site.
4. The cortical cutting cones reach the fracture site and the ends of the fractured bone begin to appear beveled and smooth, as the site is remodeled by osteoclasts.
5. The same is true of the endosteal surface of the cortex, as the internal callus works its way to the fracture site.
6. Where there are large areas of cartilage, new blood vessels invade the calcified cartilage, after which the endochondral sequence duplicates the normal formation of bone at the growth plate.

The Remodeling Phase

Several weeks after a fracture, the ingrowth of callus has sealed the bone ends and remodeling begins. In this phase, the bone is reorganized so that the original cortex is restored. Occasionally, the bone is strong enough to qualify as a clinically healed fracture, but biologically, the fracture may not be truly healed and may continue to undergo remodeling for years. For instance, the callus of rib fractures may remain throughout life because the continual respiratory movement of the ribs shears blood vessels and preserves extensive cartilage callus. In a child, in whom the growth plates are still open, normal modeling of growing bone overtakes the callus, so that a fracture may not be recognizable in later life. Similarly, normal modeling in a child may correct the angulation of a bone at a fracture site. If a fracture is near the growth plate, differential growth rates of the growth plate also correct the angulation. In an adult, however, because the plates are closed, angulation often requires correction with external or internal devices.

Special Considerations

There are unusual nuances to fracture healing that deserve mention.

PRIMARY HEALING: A fracture does not necessarily result in bone displacement and soft tissue injury. For example, a drill

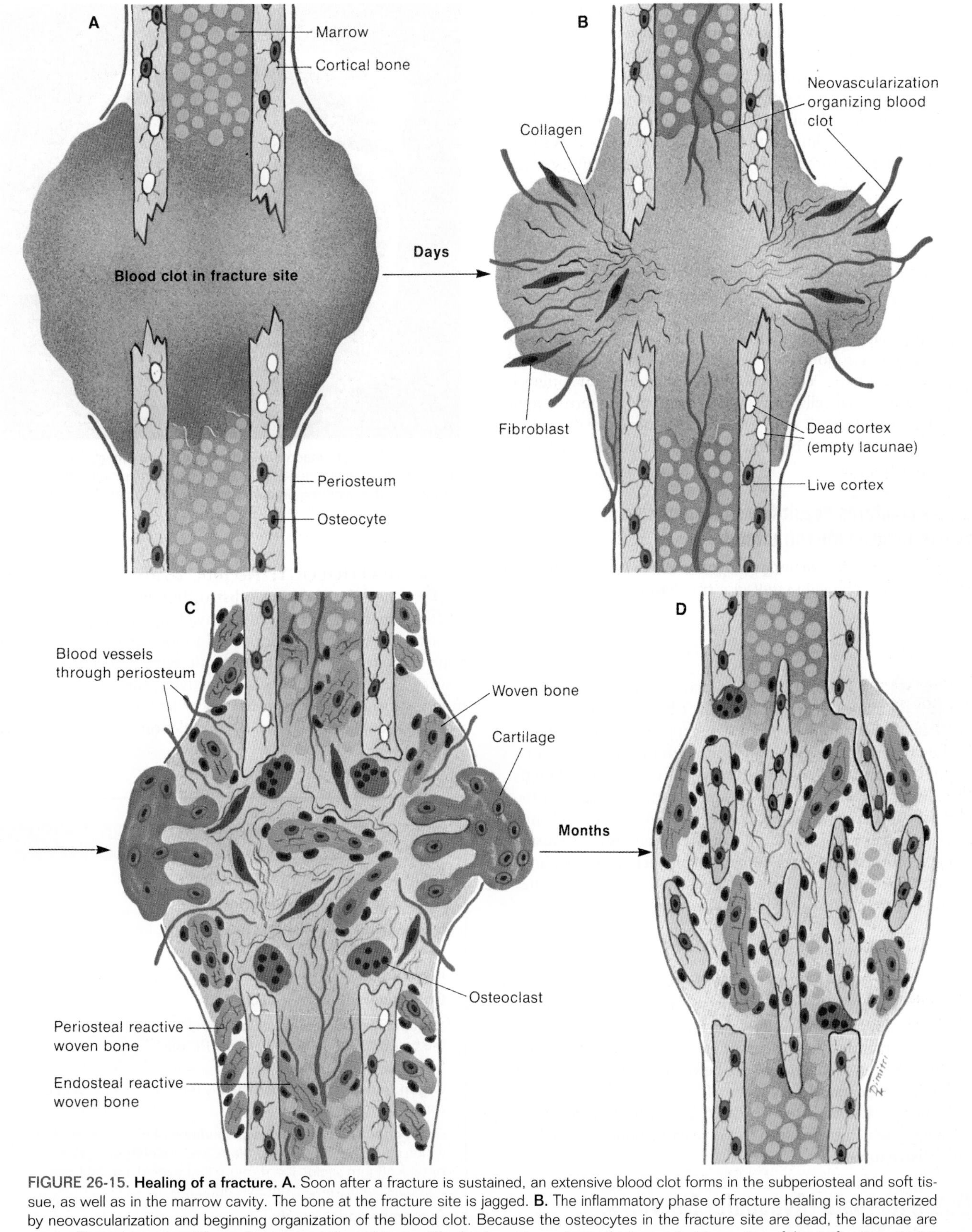

FIGURE 26-15. **Healing of a fracture. A.** Soon after a fracture is sustained, an extensive blood clot forms in the subperiosteal and soft tissue, as well as in the marrow cavity. The bone at the fracture site is jagged. **B.** The inflammatory phase of fracture healing is characterized by neovascularization and beginning organization of the blood clot. Because the osteocytes in the fracture site are dead, the lacunae are empty. The osteocytes of the cortex are necrotic well beyond the fracture site, owing to the traumatic interruption of the perforating arteries from the periosteum. **C.** The reparative phase of fracture healing is characterized by the formation of a callus of cartilage and woven bone near the fracture site. The jagged edges of the original cortex have been remodeled and eroded by osteoclasts. The marrow space has been revascularized and contains reactive woven bone, as does the periosteal area. **D.** In the remodeling phase, during which the cortex is revitalized, the reactive bone may be lamellar or woven. The new bone is organized along stress lines and mechanical forces. Extensive osteoclastic and osteoblastic cellular activity is maintained.

hole in the bone cortex or a controlled fracture, such as an osteotomy created with a fine saw during orthopedic surgery, does not displace bone. In this situation, there is almost no soft tissue reaction and callus formation because the bone is rigidly fixed. The fracture callus grows directly into the fracture site by a process called **primary healing.** This results in rapid reconstitution of the cortex, including restoration of the haversian systems. Similarly, if a fracture site is held in rigid alignment by metal screws and plates, there is also little external callus. The cortical cutting cones will then be prominent and will heal the fracture site quickly.

NONUNION: If a fracture site does not heal, the condition is termed **nonunion**. Causes of nonunion include interposition of soft tissues at the fracture site, excessive motion, infection, poor blood supply, and other factors mentioned above. Continued movement at the unhealed fracture site may also lead to **pseudoarthrosis**, a condition in which jointlike tissue is formed. Pluripotential tissue cells become histologically indistinguishable from synovial cells, secrete synovial fluid, and form a jointlike structure. In such cases, the fracture never heals and the jointlike material must be removed surgically for the fracture to heal properly.

Stress Fractures Result from Accumulation of Stress-Induced Microfractures

*In these fractures, also known as **fatigue** or **march fractures**, repeated microfractures eventually result in a true fracture through the bone cortex.*

PATHOGENESIS: A stress fracture occurs in bones in which the cortex has few osteons and forms only when stress is applied to the cortex. If the ill-prepared cortex (e.g., in the fifth metatarsal) undergoes repeated mechanical stress (e.g., from jogging, skiing, or ballet dancing), the bone produces cutting cones in an attempt to implant osteons. If the stress continues and microfractures accumulate, periosteal and endosteal calluses develop to strengthen the bone while active remodeling takes place. An actual fracture occurs as the last event if the stresses are continually applied during remodeling.

CLINICAL FEATURES: Stress fractures produce pain and swelling over the affected bone. *At the site of a future stress fracture, a callus forms before a fracture occurs.* When the actual fracture takes place, the pain becomes more severe. In the early stages of this condition, before the actual fracture, the radiologic appearance may resemble that of a tumor. A biopsy will show that the cortex is riddled with cutting cones for remodeling, which is also seen in the reactive bone at the edge of an invasive tumor.

Osteonecrosis (Avascular Necrosis, Aseptic Necrosis)

Osteonecrosis refers to the death of bone and marrow in the absence of infection (Fig. 26-16). Causes of osteonecrosis are listed in Table 26-1. Necrotic bone heals differently in the cortex and in the underlying coarse cancellous bone.

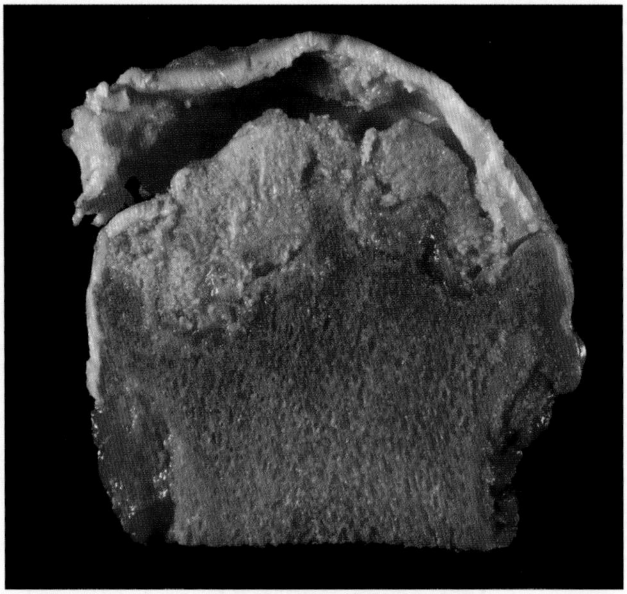

FIGURE 26-16. **Osteonecrosis of the head of the femur.** A coronal section shows a circumscribed area of subchondral infarction with partial detachment of the overlying articular cartilage and subarticular bone.

PATHOLOGY: Necrotic coarse cancellous bone heals by **creeping substitution,** in which the necrotic marrow is replaced by invading, or creeping, neovascular tissue, which provides the pluripotential cells needed for bone remodeling. Although necrotic bony trabeculae may be resorbed directly by osteoclastic activity, they are more commonly surrounded by new woven or lamellar bone generated by the osteoblastic activity of granulation tissue. Eventually,

TABLE 26-1

Causes of Osteonecrosis

Trauma, including fracture and surgery
Emboli, producing focal bone infarction
Systemic diseases, such as polycythemia, lupus erythematosus, Gaucher disease, sickle cell disease, and gout
Radiation, either internal or external
Corticosteroid administration
Specific focal bone necrosis at various sites—for instance, in the head of the femur (Legg-Calvé-Perthes disease) or in the navicular bone (Köhler disease)
Organ transplantation, particularly renal, in patients with persistent hyperparathyroidism
Osteochondritis dissecans, a condition of unknown etiology in which a piece of articular cartilage and subchondral bone breaks off into a joint. It is thought that a focal area of bone necrosis occurs and eventually detaches.
Autografts and allografts
Thrombosis of local vessels secondary to the pressure of adjacent tumors or other space-occupying lesions
Idiopathic factors, as in the high incidence of osteonecrosis of the head and the femur in alcoholics. Necrotic bone heals differently in the cortex and in the underlying coarse cancellous bone.

the sandwich composed of necrotic bone in the center and surrounding viable bone is remodeled by osteoclastic activity, and new bone is laid down through intramembranous bone formation.

Necrotic cortical bone is healed by a cutting cone. The cutting cone, as discussed above, forms by way of the preexisting vascular channels in the cortex. The appropriate signals reach this vascular channel and stimulate neovascularization by the surrounding pluripotential mesenchymal tissue. Osteoclasts make their way into the necrotic compact cortical bone, with osteoblasts trailing behind. As a result, tunnels bore their way into the necrotic cortex, leading to new bone formation. This is a slow process, and the bone is often laid down de novo as lamellar bone.

Legg-Calvé-Perthes disease is osteonecrosis in the femoral head in children; **idiopathic osteonecrosis** occurs in a similar location in adults. In both conditions, collapse of the femoral head may lead to joint incongruity and eventual severe osteoarthritis. Collapse of the subchondral bone results from several mechanisms:

- Necrotic bone may sustain stress fractures and compaction over a long period.
- The portion peripheral to the necrotic bone may undergo neovascularization. On radiologic examination, there is a lucent area surrounding the necrotic zone.
- The rigid articular cartilage and subchondral bone may actually crack as the subchondral necrotic zone collapses, producing a fracture.

A radiograph in avascular necrosis often shows the necrotic zone to be radiodense because of (1) relative osteoporosis in the surrounding viable bone compared with the unchanged necrotic bone; (2) addition of new bone through creeping substitution; (3) formation of calcium soaps, which arise as a result of the necrosis of marrow fat; and (4) actual compaction of the preexisting dead bone. Focal end-arterial vascular insufficiency may precede these events, as the necrotic zone tends to be wedge shaped.

Reactive Bone Formation

Reactive bone is intramembranous bone formed in response to stress on bone or soft tissue. Conditions such as tumors, infections, trauma, or generalized or focal disease can stimulate bone formation.

PATHOLOGY: The periosteum may respond with a so-called **sunburst** pattern (Fig. 26-17), as seen with certain tumors, or progressive layering of the periosteum, which yields an **onionskin pattern** of the cortex. The endosteal or the marrow surface may produce new bone, so that on radiologic studies, the cortex appears to be thickened, and the coarse cancellous bone appears to be denser.

Reactive bone may be either woven or lamellar, depending on the rates of deposition of the reactive bone. Around an indolent infection, as in chronic osteomyelitis, reactive bone may be laid down de novo as lamellar bone from the periosteum. In this case, the bone has time to respond to the persistent stress. Similarly, a benign tumor may cause a lamellar bone reaction. By contrast, a rapidly enlarging tumor is more likely to promote woven bone. Invariably, reactive bone is of the intramembranous type, because it is derived from the periosteum or the endosteal tissue of the marrow.

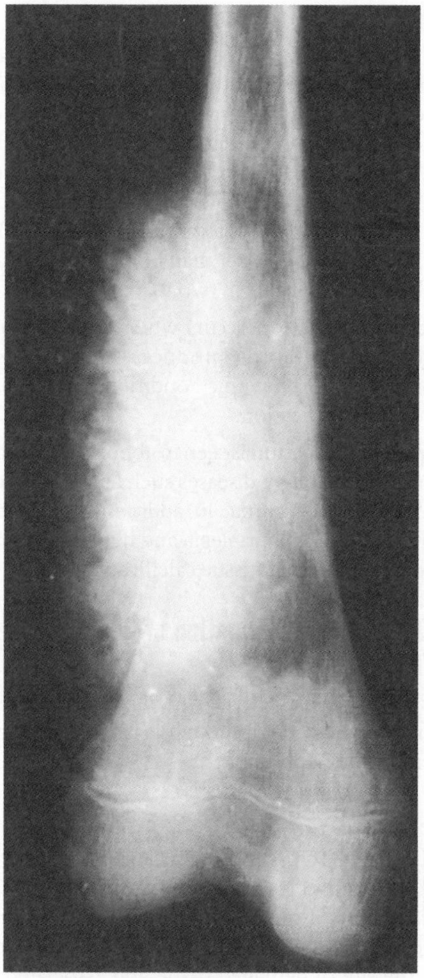

FIGURE 26-17. **Reactive bone formation.** A radiograph of a resected femur bearing an osteosarcoma shows a sunburst pattern of hyperdense new bone in the distal diaphysis and metaphysis. This radiodensity is due to woven bone produced by the sarcoma and the periosteal reaction of the host bone. The epiphyseal plate is represented as a transverse lucent line that separates the metaphysis from the epiphysis. The radiating radiodense bone extends beyond the periosteum into the soft tissues, obscuring the underlying bone architecture.

Heterotopic Ossification Is Bone Formation Outside the Skeletal System

Heterotopic ossification (**HO**) is formation of reactive bone (woven and/or lamellar) in extraskeletal sites such as the skin, subcutaneous tissue, skeletal muscle, and fibroconnective tissue around joints. HO is not associated with any metabolic diseases reflected in the fact that patients have normal serum calcium and phosphorous levels. HO occurs in five major clinical setings: genetic, post-traumatic, neurogenic, postsurgical, and as distinctive reactive lesions such as myositis ossificans. A genetic disorder know as fibrodysplasia ossificans progressiva is characterized by massive deposits of bone around multiple joints. HO may form in hematomas or skeletal muscle after trauma. Neurogenic HO occurs in muscle and periarticular fibrous tissue at multiple sites in patients with head trauma, spinal cord injury, or prolonged coma. HO can form in periarticular soft tissue following joint surgery.

Heterotopic Calcification Affects Soft Tissues

Reactive bone formation and heterotopic bone formation must be distinguished from heterotopic calcification, which is the deposition of acellular calcium salts in soft tissue. Radiologically, these entities are usually distinctive. Bone formation is characterized by a spicular or trabeculated pattern, whereas heterotopic calcification has an irregular, splotchy, amorphous appearance. Heterotopic calcification tends to occur in necrotic soft tissue or in cartilage and is usually denser than bone on radiography. Heterotopic calcification appears in two forms:

- **Metastatic calcification** occurs when there is an increase in the calcium–phosphorus product. Thus, hypercalcemic states or hyperphosphatemic conditions predispose normal soft tissues to calcification.
- **Dystrophic calcification** is seen in abnormal soft tissues such as tumors, degenerative diseases such as arteriosclerosis, and areas subjected to trauma. In addition, loss of neurologic function, as seen in quadriplegia and hemiplegia, predisposes the affected parts to soft tissue calcification.

Myositis Ossificans Is Formation of Reactive Bone in Muscle after Injury

Myositis ossificans, a distinctive form of heterotopic ossification, affects young persons and, although it is entirely benign, often mimics a malignant neoplasm.

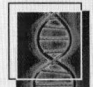

PATHOGENESIS: The lesion typically results from blunt trauma to the muscle and soft tissues, usually of the lower limb; however, some cases occur spontaneously. Peripheral neovascularization and fibrosis at the site of damaged tissue and associated hemorrhage leads in a short time to bone spicule formation. These changes are similar to those that occur at the initial hematoma in a healing fracture. Because myositis ossificans often occurs near a bone, such as the femur or tibia, on radiography it may be misdiagnosed as a malignant bone-forming tumor.

PATHOLOGY: Histologically, woven bone is formed within granulation tissue and reactive fibrous tissue (Fig. 26-18). The center of an early lesion of myositis ossificans is characterized by proliferating fibroblasts and more peripheral oseoblastic cells beginning to form woven bone. The fibroblasts are often cytologically atypical and show abundant mitoses, a histologic appearance that also resembles a malignant tumor. *The key feature that distinguishes myositis ossificans from a neoplasm is that the bone matures peripherally, whereas it is immature or not formed at all in the center of the lesion.* The phenomenon of peripheral maturity with central immaturity, the *zonation effect,* clearly indicates a reactive process. In a well-developed lesion, this phenomenon may be seen radiographically (see Fig. 26-18). A neoplasm has an opposite zonation effect: the most mature tissue of the tumor is located centrally.

The growth pattern of myositis ossificans reflects the ingrowth of neovascular tissue from the periphery into the center of the damaged area. In the late stages, the lesion may contain cartilage and even lamellar bone. Thus, in a well-developed lesion, it may mimic a sesamoid bone in the soft tissue.

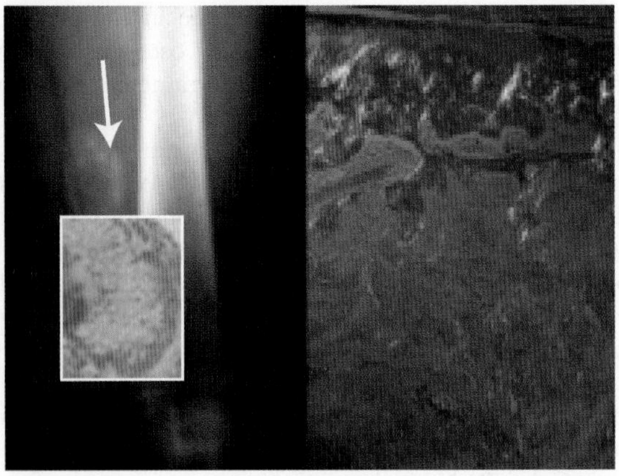

A B

FIGURE 26-18. **Myositis ossificans circumscripta. A.** Radiograph of the thigh shows a soft tissue mass (*arrow*) with a radiolucent center and ossification that becomes denser at the periphery. *Inset* demonstrates the mass at low power magnification. **B.** Higher magnification in polarized light demonstrates progression of bone formation to compacta and even the presence of a small amount of lamellar bone.

Infections

Osteomyelitis Is a Bacterial Infection of Bone and Bone Marrow

Any infectious agent may be responsible, but the term most often describes inflammation caused by bacterial infection. The most common pathogens are *Staphylococcus* species, but other organisms, such as *Escherichia coli, Neisseria gonorrhoeae, Haemophilus influenzae, and Salmonella* species, are also seen. The organisms gain entry either via the bloodstream or by direct introduction of into the bone.

Direct Penetration

Infection by direct penetration or extension of bacteria is now the most common cause of osteomyelitis in the United States. Bacterial organisms are introduced directly into bone by penetrating wounds, fractures, or surgery. Staphylococci and streptococci are still commonly incriminated, but in 25% of postoperative infections, anaerobic organisms are detected. Rarely, a gram-negative organism may seed a hip after a urological or gastrointestinal surgical procedure.

Hematogenous Osteomyelitis

Infectious organisms may reach the bone from a focus elsewhere in the body through the bloodstream. Often the focus itself, (e.g., a skin pustule or infected teeth and gums) poses little threat. Even the mere brushing of teeth may create a temporary bacteremia, which may allow organisms to reach the bone.

The most common sites affected by hematogenous osteomyelitis are the metaphyses of the long bones, such as in the knee, ankle, and hip. The infection principally affects boys aged 5 to 15 years, but it is occasionally seen in older age groups as well. Drug addicts may develop hematogenous osteomyelitis from infected needles.

PATHOGENESIS AND PATHOLOGY: Hematogenous osteomyelitis primarily affects the metaphyseal area because of the unique vascular supply in this region (Fig. 26-19). Normally, arterioles enter the calcified portion of the growth plate, form a loop, then drain into the medullary cavity without establishing a capillary bed. This loop system permits slowing and sludging of blood flow, thereby allowing bacteria time to penetrate blood vessel walls and establish infective foci within the marrow. If the organism is virulent and continues to proliferate, it creates increased pressure on the adjacent thin-walled vessels because they lie in a closed space, the marrow cavity. Such pressure further compromises the vascular supply in this region and produces bone necrosis. The necrotic areas coalesce into an avascular zone, thereby allowing further bacterial proliferation.

If infection is not contained, pus and bacteria extend into the endosteal vascular channels that supply the cortex and spread throughout the Volkmann and haversian canals of the cortex. Eventually, pus forms underneath the periosteum, shearing off the perforating arteries of the periosteum and further devitalizing the cortex. The pus flows between the periosteum and the cortex, isolating more bone from its blood supply, and may even invade the joint. Eventually, the pus penetrates the periosteum and the skin to form a draining sinus (Fig. 26-20). A sinus tract that extends from the cloaca (see below) to the skin may become epithelialized by epidermis that grows into the sinus tract. When this occurs, the sinus tract invariably remains open, continually draining pus, necrotic bone, and bacteria.

Periosteal new bone formation and reactive bone formation in the marrow tend to wall off the infection. At the same time, osteoclastic activity resorbs bone. If the infection

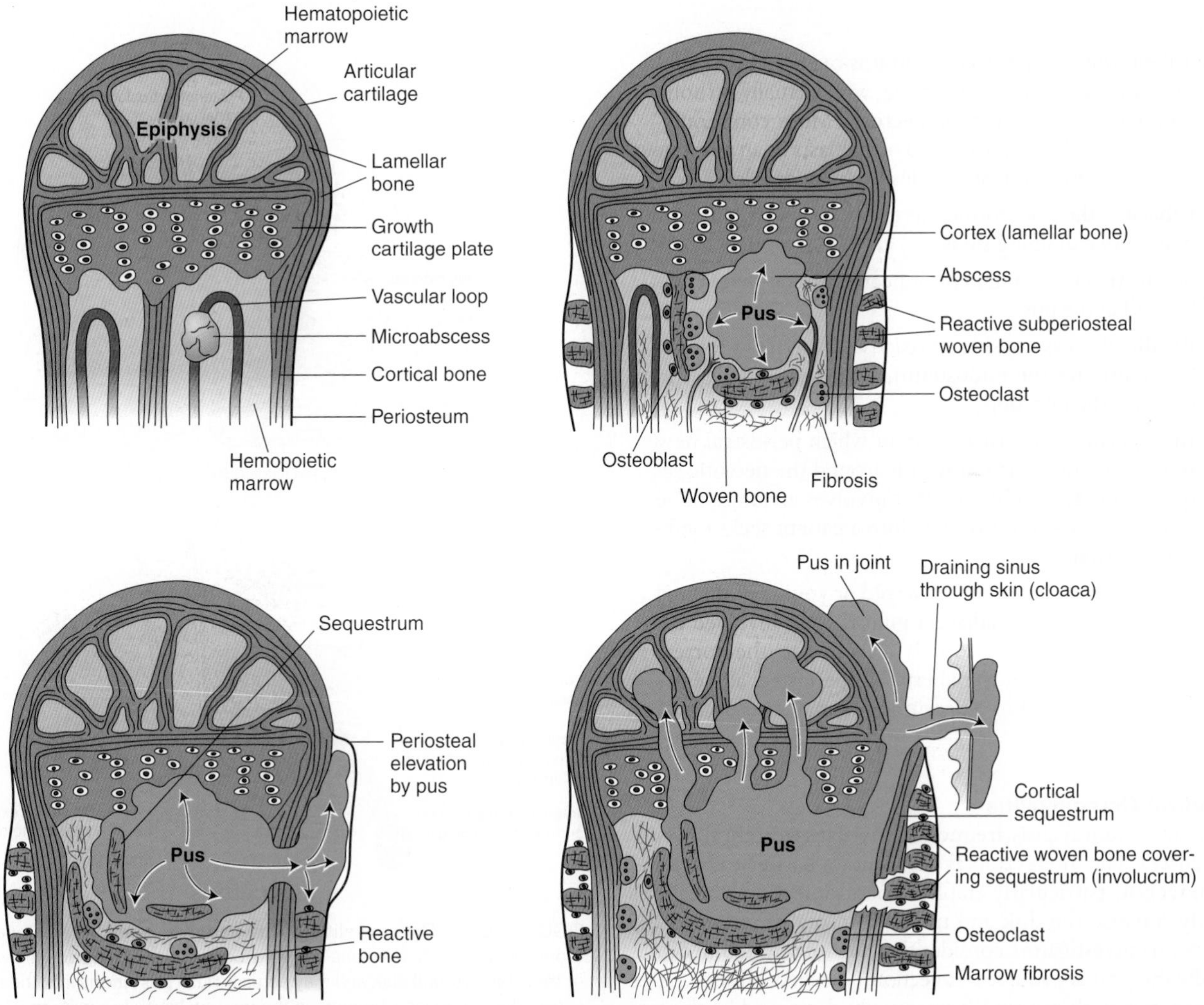

FIGURE 26-19. **Pathogenesis of hematogenous osteomyelitis. A.** The epiphysis, metaphysis, and growth plate are normal. A small, septic microabscess is forming at the capillary loop. **B.** Expansion of the septic focus stimulates resorption of adjacent bony trabeculae. Woven bone begins to surround this focus. The abscess expands into the cartilage and stimulates reactive bone formation by the periosteum. **C.** The abscess, which continues to expand through the cortex into the subperiosteal tissue, shears off the perforating arteries that supply the cortex with blood, thereby leading to necrosis of the cortex. **D.** The extension of this process into the joint space, the epiphysis, and the skin produces a draining sinus. The necrotic bone is called a ***sequestrum***. The viable bone surrounding a sequestrum is termed the ***involucrum***.

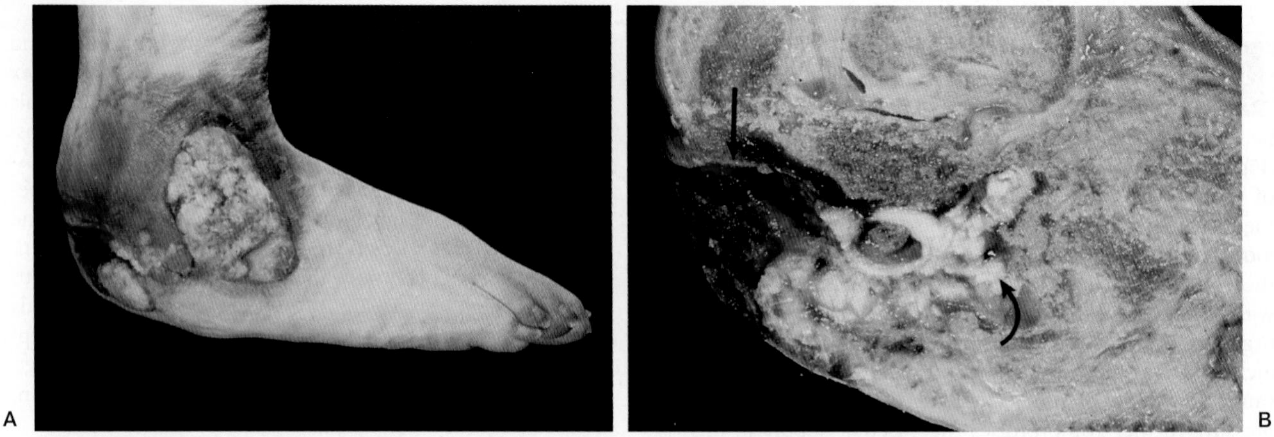

FIGURE 26-20. **Chronic osteomyelitis. A.** In this patient with chronic osteomyelitis, the skin overlying the infected bone is ulcerated and a draining sinus *(dark area)* is evident over the heel. **B.** After amputation of the foot, a sagittal section shows a draining sinus *(straight arrow)* that connects the infected bone with the surface of the ulcerated skin. The white tissue *(curved arrow)* is invasive squamous cell carcinoma, which arose in the skin.

is virulent, this attempt to contain it is overwhelmed, and the infection races through the bone, with virtually no bone formation but extensive bone necrosis. More commonly, pluripotential cells modulate into osteoblasts in an attempt to wall off the infection. Several lesions may develop:

- **Cloaca** is the hole formed in the bone during the formation of a draining sinus.
- **Sequestrum** is a fragment of necrotic bone that is embedded in the pus.
- **Brodie abscess** consists of reactive bone from the periosteum and the endosteum, which surrounds and contains the infection.
- **Involucrum** refers to a lesion in which periosteal new bone formation forms a sheath around the necrotic sequestrum. An involucrum that involves an entire bone may exist for several years before a patient seeks medical attention.

In very young children (1 year old or younger) afflicted with osteomyelitis, the adjacent joint is often involved because the periosteum is loosely attached to the cortex. From the age of 1 year to puberty, subperiosteal abscesses are common. Spread to adjacent joints may also occur in adults.

Vertebral Osteomyelitis

In adults, osteomyelitis frequently involves vertebral bodies (Fig. 26-21). The intervertebral disk is not a barrier to bacterial osteomyelitis, particularly staphylococcal infection. Infections directly traverse the disk and travel from one vertebra to the next. Some investigators consider that the intervertebral disk is actually the primary source of infection, so-called "diskitis." The disk expands with pus and is eventually destroyed as the pus bores into the adjacent vertebral bodies.

Half or more of cases of vertebral osteomyelitis are caused by *Staphylococcus aureus*. Twenty percent involve *E. coli* and other enteric organisms, many of which originate from the urinary tract. *Salmonella* species are also seen in the vertebral bodies, as

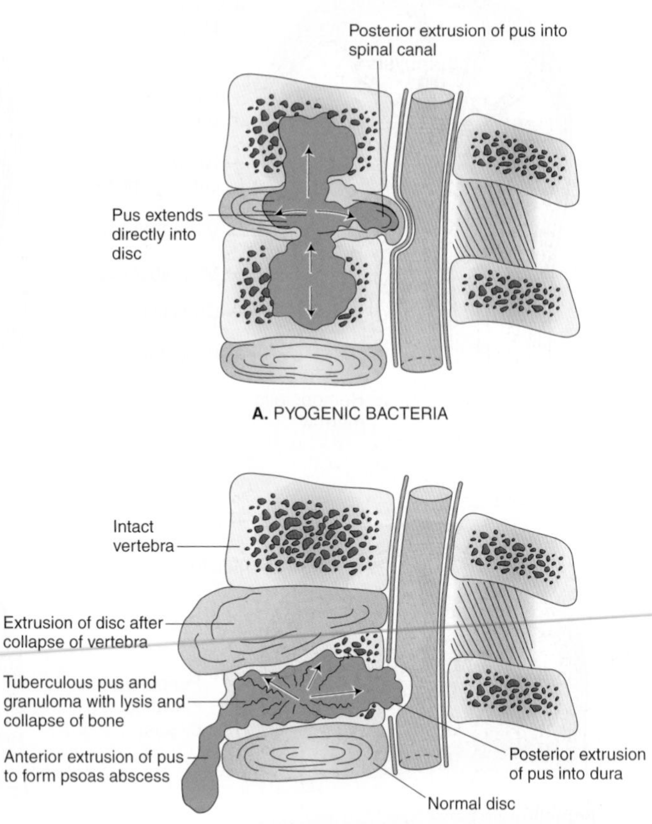

FIGURE 26-21. **Osteomyelitis of the vertebral body. A.** Bacterial osteomyelitis expands from one vertebral body to the next by direct invasion of the intervertebral disk and may actually push posteriorly into the spinal canal. The sequence of events in the marrow cavity is similar to that in a long bone. **B.** In tuberculous osteomyelitis, the bone is destroyed by resorption of bony trabeculae, which results in mechanical collapse of the vertebrae and extrusion of the intervertebral disk. Tuberculous organisms cannot penetrate the intervertebral disk directly; rather, they extend from one vertebra to the next after mechanical forces destroy and extrude the intervertebral disk.

are *Brucella* species. Predisposing factors are intravenous drug abuse, upper urinary tract infections, urological procedures, and hematogenous spread of organisms from other sites. Back pain, with point tenderness over the area of infection, is associated with low-grade fever and an increased sedimentation rate.

Occasionally, a paravertebral abscess draining the bone may "point" and emerge in the groin or elsewhere. Vertebral osteomyelitis may lead to (1) vertebral collapse with paravertebral abscesses; (2) spinal epidural abscesses, with cord compression from the abscess or from displaced fragments of the infected bone; and (3) compression fractures of the vertebral body, leading to neurologic deficits.

Complications

The complications of osteomyelitis include:

- **Septicemia:** Dissemination of organisms through the bloodstream may occur as a result of bone infection. It is unusual for osteomyelitis to result from septicemia.
- **Acute bacterial arthritis:** Joint infection is secondary to osteomyelitis at all ages, and represents a medical emergency. Direct digestion of cartilage by inflammatory cells destroys the articular cartilage and produces osteoarthritis. Rapid intervention to prevent this complication is mandatory.
- **Pathologic fractures:** Osteomyelitis may lead to fractures, which heal poorly and may require surgical drainage.
- **Squamous cell carcinoma:** This cancer develops in the bone or the sinus tract of long-standing chronic osteomyelitis, often years after the initial infection. In such cases, squamous tissue arises from the epithelialization of the sinus tract and eventually undergoes malignant transformation (see Fig. 26-20).
- **Amyloidosis:** Amyloidosis used to be a common consequence of chronic osteomyelitis, but is now only rarely seen in industrialized countries.
- **Chronic osteomyelitis:** Chronic osteomyelitis may follow acute osteomyelitis. It is difficult to treate, especially if it involves the entire bone, because necrotic bone or sequestra function as foreign bodies in avascular areas, and antibiotics do not reach the bacteria. Chronic osteomyelitis is, therefore, treated symptomatically with surgery or antibiotics for the duration of the patient's life.

CLINICAL FEATURES: Hematogenous osteomyelitis in children occurs as a sudden illness, with fever and systemic toxicity, or as a subacute illness in which local manifestations predominate. Swelling, erythema, and tenderness over the involved bone are characteristic. The leukocyte count is often conspicuously increased, but it is normal in so many cases that absence of leukocytosis does not rule out the disease.

Treatment depends on the stage of the infection. Early osteomyelitis is treated with intravenous antibiotics for 6 or more weeks. Surgery is used to drain and decompress the infection within the bone or to drain abscesses that do not respond to antibiotic therapy. In long-standing, chronic osteomyelitis, antibiotics alone are not curative, and extensive surgical débridement of necrotic bone is often required.

Tuberculosis of Bone Reflects a Primary Focus Elsewhere

Tuberculosis of bone invariably originates at other foci, usually the lungs or lymph nodes (see Chapter 9). When the bone infection is caused by the rare bovine type of tubercle bacillus, the initial focus is often in the gut or tonsils. The mycobacteria spread to the bone hematogenously, and only rarely is there direct spread from a lung or lymph node.

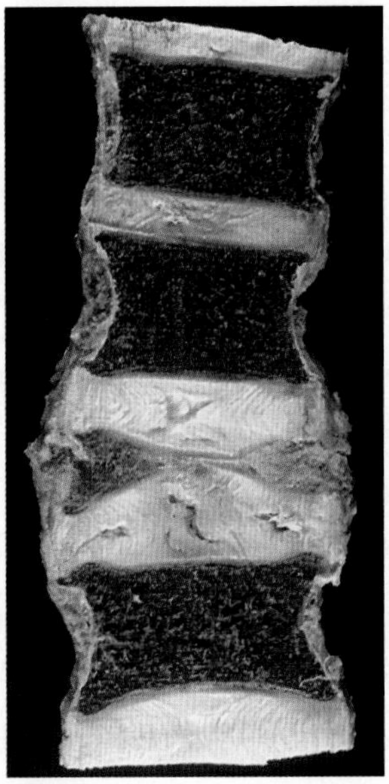

FIGURE 26-22. **Tuberculous spondylitis (Pott disease).** A vertebral body is almost completely replaced by tuberculous tissue. Note the preservation of the intervertebral disks.

Tuberculous Spondylitis (Pott Disease)

Tuberculous spondylitis, i.e., infection of the spine, is a feared complication of childhood tuberculosis. The disease affects vertebral bodies, sparing the lamina and spines and adjacent vertebrae (see Fig. 26-21 and Fig. 26-22). Thoracic vertebrae are usually affected, especially the 11th thoracic vertebra; lumbar and cervical vertebrae are less often involved. With antibiotic treatment, Pott disease is rare.

PATHOLOGY: The pathology in tuberculous spondylitis is similar to tuberculosis at other sites. The granulomas first produce caseous necrosis of the bone marrow, which leads to slow resorption of bony trabeculae and, occasionally, to cystic spaces in the bone. *Since there is little or no reactive bone formation, affected vertebrae usually collapse, leading to kyphosis and scoliosis.* The intervertebral disk is crushed and destroyed by the compression fracture, rather than by invasion of organisms. The typical hunchback of bygone days was often the victim of Pott disease.

If the infection ruptures into the soft tissue anteriorly, pus and necrotic debris drain along the spinal ligaments and form a **cold abscess**, i.e., an abscess lacking acute inflammation. A **psoas abscess**–which forms near the lower lumbar vertebrae and dissects along the pelvis, to emerge through the skin of the inguinal region as a draining sinus–may be the first manifestation of tuberculous spondylitis. Paraplegia results from vascular insufficiency of the spinal nerves, rather than from direct pressure.

Tuberculous Arthritis

Hematogenous spread of tuberculosis may bring organisms to the joint capsule, synovium, or intracapsular portion of the bone. Tuberculosis induces granulomas in synovial tissue, which then becomes edematous and papillary and may fill the entire joint space. Massive destruction of the articular cartilage results from undermining granulation tissue in the bone. The destroyed joint is replaced by bone, an effect that leads to an immovable joint (**bony ankylosis**).

Tuberculous Osteomyelitis of the Long Bones

Infection of long bones is the least common bone manifestation of tuberculosis. Tuberculosis of a long bone occurs near the joint, where it also produces arthritis. For unknown reasons, the greater trochanter of the femur is a common site for this disease.

Syphilis of Bone is Today Rare

Syphilis causes a slowly progressive, chronic, inflammatory disease of bone, characterized by granulomas, necrosis, and marked reactive bone formation. It may be acquired through sexual contact or it transplacentally, from mother to fetus (see Chapter 9). The bone changes in syphilis depend on the patient's age, endosteal and periosteal changes, and the presence or absence of gummas.

PATHOLOGY:

Congenital Syphilis

Bone involvement in congenital syphilis may appear as early as the fifth month of gestation and is fully developed at birth. Spirochetes are ubiquitous in the epiphysis and periosteum, where they produce osteochondritis (epiphysitis) and periostitis, respectively (Fig. 26-23). In severe disease, an epiphysis may become dislocated, leaving the child with a functionless limb (**pseudoparalysis of Parrot**).

The knee is most often affected by congenital syphilis. The growth plate is irregularly widened and displays a yellow discoloration. The zone of calcified cartilage is destroyed and a sea of lymphocytes, plasma cells, and spirochetes fills the marrow spaces. Because the periosteum is stimulated to produce reactive new bone, the thickness of the cortex may actually be doubled. The inflammatory infiltrate permeates the cortex through the Volkmann and haversian canals and settles in the elevated periosteum. Ultimately, as the affected bones grow they become short and deformed.

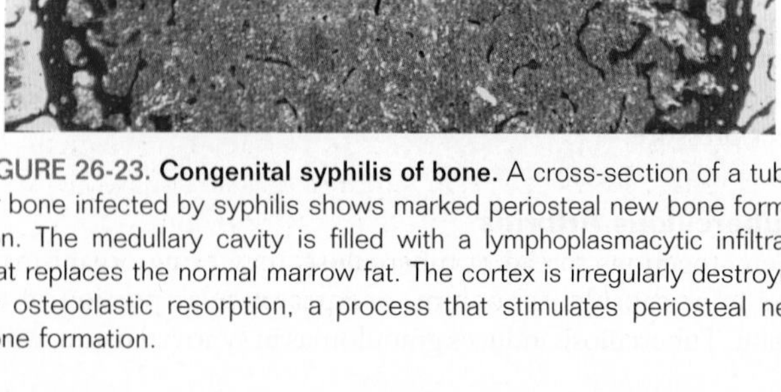

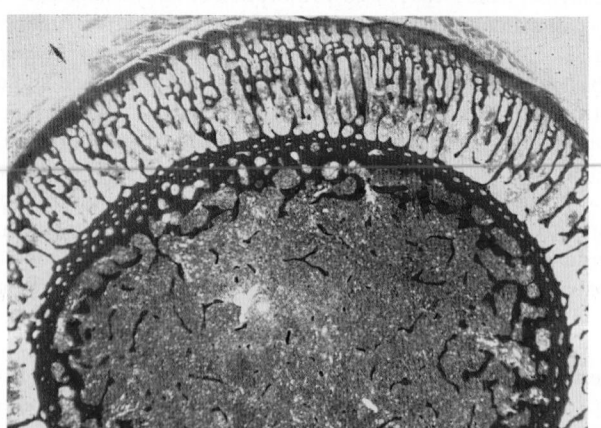

FIGURE 26-23. **Congenital syphilis of bone.** A cross-section of a tubular bone infected by syphilis shows marked periosteal new bone formation. The medullary cavity is filled with a lymphoplasmacytic infiltrate that replaces the normal marrow fat. The cortex is irregularly destroyed by osteoclastic resorption, a process that stimulates periosteal new bone formation.

Acquired Syphilis

Acquired syphilis in adults produces lesions of the bone early in the tertiary stage, 2 to 5 years after inoculation of the organisms. Periostitis is predominant because the growth plates have already closed. The bones most commonly affected are the tibia, nose, palate, and skull. Tibial lesions are marked by periostitis, with deposition of new bone on the medial and anterior aspects of the shaft, which leads to the **saber shin** deformity. The skull thickness also increases because of periosteal stimulation.

The formation of gummas is most common in tertiary syphilis. The bone adjacent to gummas is slowly replaced by fibrous marrow. Ultimately, perforations occur through the cortex. The markedly irregular, thickened periosteal surfaces, which are perforated by pits and serpiginous ulcerations, are characteristic of syphilis. Lysis and collapse of the nasal and palatal bones produce the classic **saddle nose**—perforation, destruction, and collapse of the nasal septum (see Chapter 25).

Langerhans Cell Histiocytosis

Langerhans cell histiocytosis (LCH) is a generic term (previously referred to as ***histiocytosis X****) for three entities characterized by proliferation of Langerhans cells in various tissues:* (1) **eosinophilic granuloma**, a localized form; (2) **Hand-Schüller-Christian disease,** a disseminated variant; and (3) **Letterer–Siwe disease**, a fulminant and often fatal generalized disease (see Chapter 20).

PATHOLOGY: The histologic appearance of the bones in all three variants of LCH is identical and is characterized by collections of large, phagocytic cells with pale, eosinophilic to occassionally foamy cytoplasm and convoluted or grooved nuclei (See Chapter 20). By electron microscopy these cells have the typical racquet-shaped, tubular structures, "Birbeck granules," seen in the Langerhans cells of the skin. Numerous eosinophils are located throughout the lesions, occasionally forming collections called "eosinophilic abscesses." Multinucleated **osteoclastic** giant cells are often seen, as are chronic inflammatory cells and neutrophils. Studies of X-chromosome inactivation have demonstrated that LCH is a clonal proliferative disease.

Lesions of LCH may occur anywhere in the body, including bones, skin, brain, lungs, lymph nodes, liver, and spleen. Cholesterol deposition can be prominent in histiocytic cells, but there is no defined abnormality of cholesterol metabolism, and these patients do not have hypercholesterolemia.

Radiologic findings in the bones in all three diseases are identical. The lesions may occur in the metaphysis or diaphysis of a long bone, or in a flat bone, especially in the skull (Fig. 26-24). They are punched-out lytic defects, with virtually no reactive bone. Such lesions may lead to fractures and periosteal callus formation.

Eosinophilic Granuloma Is a Self-Limited Disease

Eosinophilic granuloma, in either its solitary or multiple varieties, accounts for 70% of all cases of LCH. It is usually seen in the first two decades of life, but occasionally occurs in older persons. There are typically one or two lytic areas in bones of the axial or appendicular skeleton (see Fig. 26-24) or the vertebrae. These lesions may cause mild pain or may be incidental findings on routine chest radiographs. Foci of disease in the lower tho-

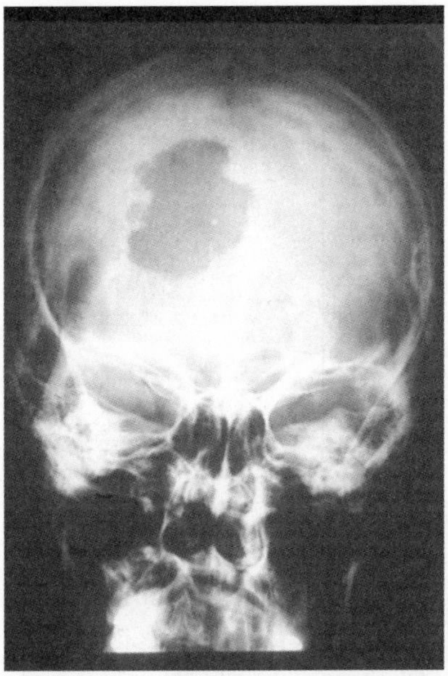

FIGURE 26-24. **Eosinophilic granuloma. A radiograph of the skull shows** a large, lytic lesion.

racic or upper lumbar vertebrae may lead to collapse and pathologic fractures. Eventual recovery is the rule.

Hand-Schüller-Christian Disease Is a Multiorgan Childhood Disease

Hand-Schüller-Christian disease occurs in children 2 to 5 years old, and is more widespread than eosinophilic granuloma. It represents some 20% of all cases of LCH. Radiolucent bony lesions characterize the disorder, most frequently in the calvaria, ribs, pelvis, and scapulae. Involvement of the jaw bone results in loss of teeth, evident radiologically as "floating teeth." Infiltratation of the retroorbital space causes exophthalmos, while infiltration of the hypothalamic stalk by Langerhans cells leads to diabetes insipidus. One-fifth of patients have lymphadenopathy and lung infiltrates.

Crusty, red, weepy skin lesions occur at the hairline and on the extensor surfaces of the extremities, abdomen, and occasionally soles of the feet. Deafness results from involvement of external auditory canal and mastoid air cells. One third of affected patients have disease in the liver and spleen, and 40% have bone lesions, half of which involve the skull. Thus, the classic triad of Hand-Schüller-Christian disease, **(1) radiolucent lesions of the skull, (2) diabetes insipidus, and (3) exophthalmos,** occurs in only one third of patients.

Letterer-Siwe Disease Is an Aggressive, Potentially Fatal, Disease of Infants

It accounts for 10% of cases of LCH. Affected children fail to thrive and become cachectic. Multiple organ involvement culminates in massive hepatosplenomegaly, lymphadenopathy, anemia, leukopenia, and thrombocytopenia. Widely scattered, seborrheic skin lesions, which are often hemorrhagic, are usual. Bone lesions are not prominent initially, but progressive marrow replacement and pulmonary infiltration occasionally cause death.

CLINICAL FEATURES: Eosinophilic granuloma is a self-limited disease, and most lesions disappear if left alone. A bone lesion may have to be curetted and packed with bone chips. Sometimes biopsy itself is enough to stimulate repair of the lytic lesion. A collapsed vertebra may actually reconstitute itself over time. Hand-Schüller-Christian disease may require radiation therapy for some bone and retroorbital lesions. Diabetes insipidus seems to be irreversible, despite irradiation of the pituitary region. Drugs such as corticosteroids, cyclophosphamide, and tumoricidal agents may also be used to treat Hand-Schüller-Christian disease. Aggressive chemotherapy for Letterer-Siwe disease may improve the prognosis.

METABOLIC BONE DISEASES

Metabolic bone diseases are defined as disorders of metabolism that result in secondary structural effects on the skeleton, including diminished bone mass due to decreased synthesis or increased destruction, reduced bone mineralization, or both. Because metabolic bone diseases are systemic, a biopsy of any bone should reveal the abnormality, even though severity may differ in various parts of the skeleton (Fig. 26-25).

Osteoporosis

Osteoporosis is a metabolic bone disease characterized by diffuse skeletal lesions in which normally mineralized bone is decreased in mass to the point that it no longer provides adequate mechanical support. Although osteoporosis reflects a number of causes, it is always characterized by loss of skeletal mass. Remaining bone has a normal ratio of mineralized to nonmineralized (i.e., osteoid) matrix. Bone loss and eventually fractures are the hallmarks of osteoporosis, regardless of the underlying causes (Fig 26-26). The etiology for bone loss is diverse but includes smoking, vitamin D deficiency, low body mass index, hypogonadism, a sedentary lifestyle, and glucocorticoid therapy.

EPIDEMIOLOGY: In normal persons of both sexes, bone mass peaks between the ages of 25 and 35 and begins to decline in the fifth or sixth decade. Bone loss with age occurs in all races, but because of higher peak bone mass, blacks are less prone to osteoporosis than are Asians and whites. Bone loss during normal aging in women has been divided into two phases: one due to menopause and one due to aging. The latter affects men as well as women. At a certain point, the loss of bone suffices to justify the label **osteoporosis** and renders weight-bearing bones susceptible to fractures. The most common fractures occur in the neck and intertrochanteric region of the femur (hip fracture, see Fig. 26-26), vertebral bodies, and distal radius (**Colles fracture**). In whites in the United States, 15% of persons have had a hip fracture by the age of 80 years and 25% by age 90. Women have twice the risk of hip fracture as men, although among blacks and some Asian populations, incidence is equal among the sexes. Compared with other osteoporotic fractures, hip fractures incur the greatest morbidity, mortality, and direct medical costs. The female predominance of 8:1 is particularly striking for vertebral fractures A subset of women in the early postmenopausal years is at particular risk of vertebral fractures, which are rare in middle-aged men. The propensity of men to sustain hip fractures as opposed to vertebral ones also reflects factors other than bone mass, such as loss of proprioception. Osteoporosis and its complications are huge public health problems that are expected to expand as life expectancy increases.

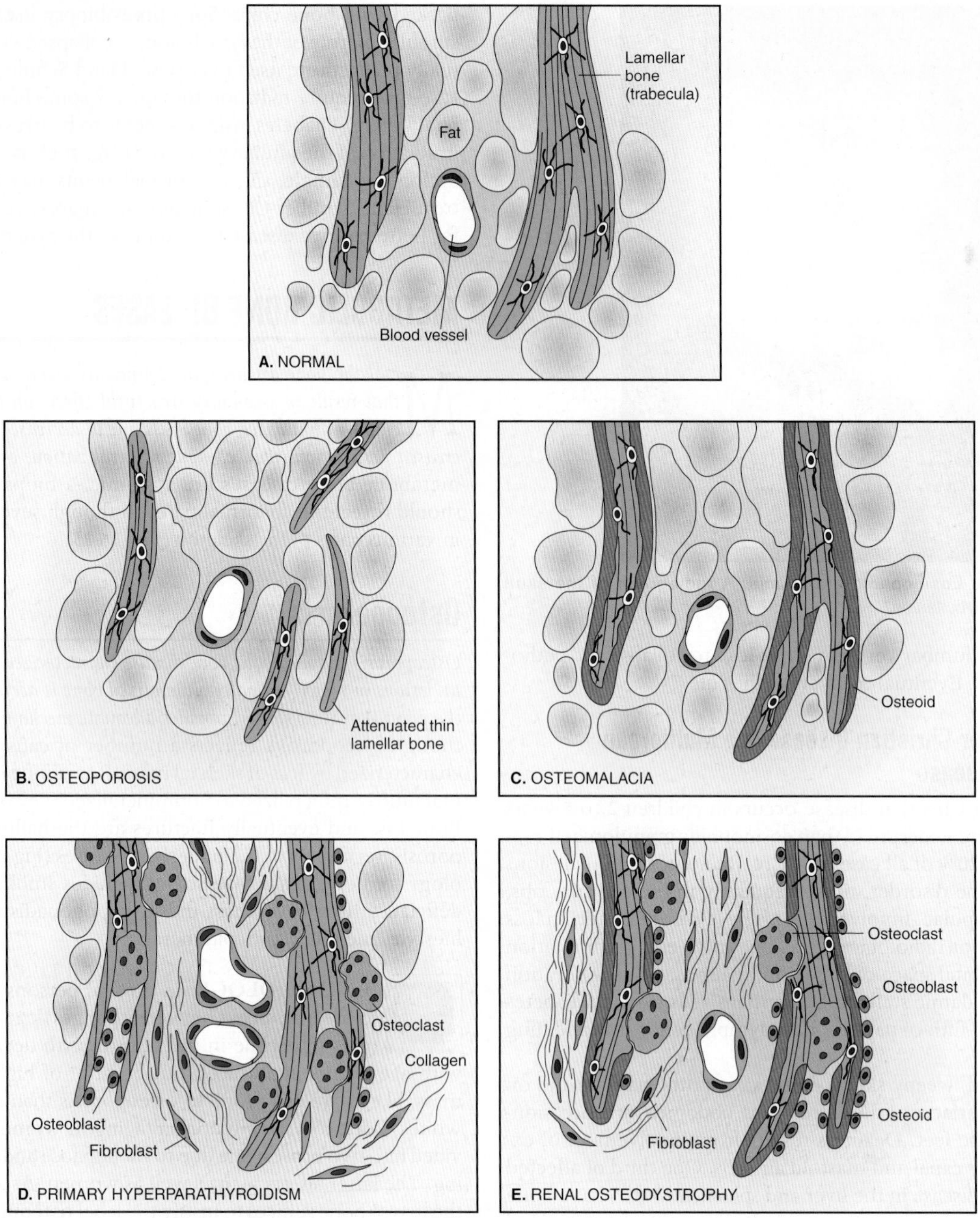

FIGURE 26-25. **Metabolic bone diseases. A.** Normal trabecular bone and fatty marrow. The trabecular bone is lamellar and contains evenly distributed osteocytes. **B.** Osteoporosis. The lamellar bone exhibits discontinuous, thin trabeculae. **C.** Osteomalacia. The trabeculae of the lamellar bone have abnormal amounts of nonmineralized bone (osteoid). These osteoid seams are thickened and cover a larger than normal area of the trabecular bone surface. **D.** Primary hyperparathyroidism. The lamellar bone trabeculae are actively resorbed by numerous osteoclasts that bore into each trabecula. The appearance of osteoclasts dissecting into the trabeculae, a process termed ***dissecting osteitis,*** is diagnostic of hyperparathyroidism. Osteoblastic activity also is pronounced. The marrow is replaced by fibrous tissue adjacent to the trabeculae. **E.** Renal osteodystrophy. The morphologic appearance is similar to that of primary hyperparathyroidism, except that prominent osteoid covers the trabeculae. Osteoclasts do not resorb osteoid, and wherever an osteoid seam is lacking, osteoclasts bore into the trabeculae. Osteoblastic activity, in association with osteoclasts, is again prominent.

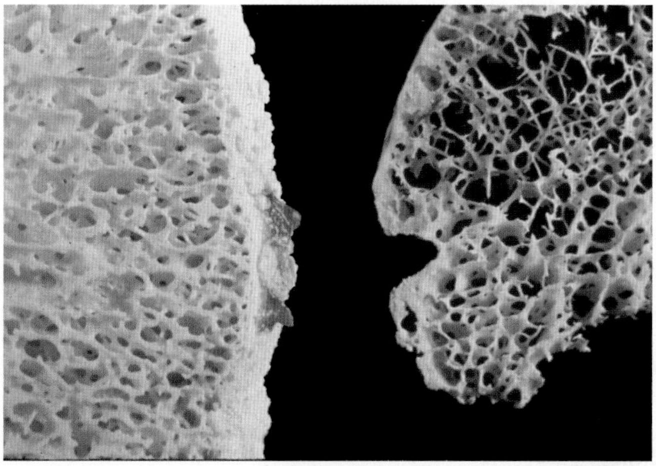

FIGURE 26-26. **Osteoporosis.** Femoral head of an 82-year-old female with osteoporosis and a femoral neck fracture *(right)* compared with a normal control cut to the same thickness *(left)*.

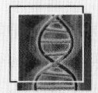

PATHOGENESIS: *Regardless of the cause of osteoporosis, it always reflects enhanced bone resorption relative to formation.* Thus this family of diseases should be viewed in the context of the remodeling cycle. Bone resorption and bone formation exist simultaneously. All osteoblasts and osteoclasts belong to a unique temporary structure, known as the **basic multicellular** (BMU or **bone remodeling unit**). The BMU is responsible for bone remodeling throughout life. Persons younger than 35 or 40 years completely replace bone resorbed during the remodeling cycle. With age, less bone is replaced in resorption bays than is removed, leading to a small deficit at each remodeling site. Given the thousands of remodeling sites in the skeleton, net bone loss, even in a short time, can be substantial.

Osteoporosis is classified as either primary or secondary. **Primary osteoporosis,** by far the more common variety, is of uncertain origin and occurs principally in postmenopausal women (type 1) and elderly persons of both sexes (type 2). **Secondary osteoporosis** is a disorder associated with a defined cause, including a variety of endocrine and genetic abnormalities.

Type 1 primary osteoporosis is due to an absolute increase in osteoclast activity. Given that osteoclasts initiate bone remodeling, the number of remodeling sites increases in this state of enhanced osteoclast formation, a phenomenon known as **increased activation frequency**.

The increased in osteoclasts in the early postmenopausal skeleton is a direct result of estrogen withdrawal. The effects of estrogen lack are not, however, targeted directly to the osteoclast, but rather to cells derived from marrow stroma, which secrete cytokines that recruit osteoclasts. These cytokines, which are believed to be estrogen sensitive, include IL-1 and IL-6, TNF, and macrophage colony-stimulating factor (M-CSF).

Type 2 primary osteoporosis, also called **senile osteoporosis**, has a more complex pathogenesis than type 1. Type 2 osteoporosis generally appears after age 70 and reflects decreased osteoblast function. Thus, although osteoclast activity is no longer increased, the number of osteoblasts and amount of bone produced per cell are insufficient to replace bone removed in the resorptive phase of the remodeling cycle.

Primary Osteoporosis Is Caused by a Number of Factors

Primary osteoporosis has been linked to a number of factors that influence peak bone mass and the rate of bone loss:

- **Genetic factors:** The development of clinically significant osteoporosis is related, in largest part, to the maximal amount of bone in a given person, referred to as the **peak bone mass.** In general, peak bone mass is greater in men than in women and in blacks than in whites or Asians. There is a higher concordance of peak bone mass in monozygotic than in dizygotic twins. Women of reproductive age whose mothers have postmenopausal osteoporosis exhibit a lower bone mineral density (BMD) than do women in the general population. BMD is the most commonly used index for defining and studying osteoporosis. Genetic factors are thought to play an important role in regulating BMD. In fact, genetic variations explain as much as 70% of the variance in BMD. Sequence variance in the vitamin D receptor (VDR), *Col1A1* collagen gene, estrogen receptor alpha (ESR1), IL-6, and low-density lipoprotein (LDL) receptor-related protein 5 (LRP5) are significantly associated with differences in BMD. Furthermore, VDR and IL-6 interact with environmental and hormonal factors (e.g., calcium intake, estrogen) to modulate BMD. Thus, environmental factors and an individual's genotype both play a role in determining peak bone mass and risk of osteoporosis.
- **Calcium intake:** The average calcium intake of postmenopausal women in the United States is below the recommended value of 800 mg/day. However, whether this apparent shorfall contributes to development of osteoporosis is controversial, in view of a number of studies to the contrary. Nevertheless, it has been recommended that both premenopausal and postmenopausal women increase the intake of calcium and vitamin D.
- **Calcium absorption and vitamin D:** Calcium absorption by the intestine decreases with age. Because calcium absorption is largely under the control of vitamin D, attention has been directed to the role of this steroid hormone in osteoporosis. Compared with controls, persons with osteoporosis have lower circulating levels of 1,25-dihydroxyvitamin D, [$1,25(OH)_2D$], the active form of vitamin D that promotes calcium absorption in the intestine. This decrease has been attributed to age-related decreases in 1α-hydroxylase activity in the kidney. This enzyme catalyzes formation of $1,25(OH)_2D$. The lower 1α- hydroxylase activity has been attributed to diminished stimulation of the enzyme by PTH, as well as an age-related decrease in responses of renal tubules to PTH. Interestingly, giving estrogens to postmenopausal women with osteoporosis increases both circulating $1,25(OH)_2D$ and calcium absorption. It has been suggested that decreased 1α-hydroxylase activity in the kidney may stimulate PTH secretion, thereby contributing to bone resorption.
- **Exercise:** Physical activity is necessary to maintain bone mass, and athletes often have increased bone mass. By contrast, immobilization of a bone (e.g., prolonged bed rest, application of a cast) leads to accelerated bone loss. As a matter of current interest, the weightlessness of space flight results in severe bone loss (33% of trabecular bone mass in 25 weeks), and vigorous exercise in this setting does not seem to increase bone mass substantially or help prevent osteoporosis.
- **Environmental factors:** Cigarette smoking in women has been correlated with increased incidence of osteoporosis. It is

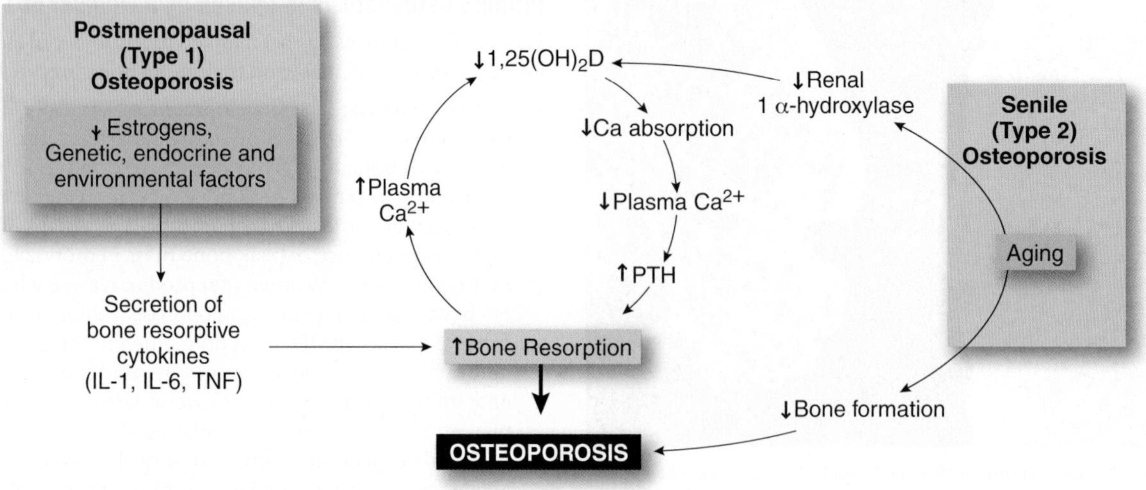

FIGURE 26-27. **Pathogenesis of primary osteoporosis.** Ca 2^+ = calcium; IL = interleukin; PTH = parathyroid hormone; TNF = tumor necrosis factor.

possible that the decreased level of active estrogens produced by smoking (see Chapter 8) is responsible for this effect.

In summary, the two major determinants of primary osteoporosis are estrogen deficiency in postmenopausal women and the aging process in both sexes. The possible mechanisms for these effects are summarized in Figure 26-27.

PATHOLOGY: The ratio of osteoid to mineralized bone is normal in persons with osteoporosis. Newer densitometric and imaging techniques, such as computerized tomography, are sufficiently sensitive and precise to detect small deficiencies of bone.

Because of the abundance of cancellous bone in the spine, osteoporotic changes are generally most conspicuous there. In vertebral body fractures caused by osteoporosis, the vertebra is deformed, with anterior wedging and collapse. If the vertebral body is not fractured, there is a general outline of both endplates, with a virtual absence of cancellous bone.

Histologically, osteoporosis is characterized by decreased thickness of the cortex and reduction in the number and size of trabeculae of the coarse cancellous bone. Whereas senile osteoporosis tends to feature reduced trabecular thickness, postmenopausal osteoporosis exhibits disrupted connections between trabeculae. The loss of trabecular connectivity, which is attended by diminished biomechanical strength and ultimately leads to fracture, is due to perforation of trabeculae by resorbing osteoclasts in remodeling sites. In histologic sections, the loss of connectivity results in the appearance of "isolated" islands of bone (see Fig. 26-25).

CLINICAL FEATURES: Postmenopausal osteoporosis is usually recognizable within 10 years after onset of the menopause, whereas senile osteoporosis generally becomes symptomatic after age 70 years. Until recently, most patients were unaware of their disease until they had a fracture of a vertebra, hip, or other bone. However, the use of sensitive screening techniques permits early diagnosis. Vertebral body compression fractures often occur after trivial trauma or may even follow lifting a heavy object. With each compression fracture, the patient becomes shorter and develops kyphosis (**dowager's hump**). Serum calcium and phosphorus levels remain normal.

Estrogen therapy is an effective, if controversial, means of preventing postmenopausal osteoporosis. Because hormone treatment carries with it slightly increased risks of breast and endometrial cancers, other bone-specific antiosteoporotic drugs have been developed. A new class of inorganic compounds, known as **bisphosphonates,** appears particularly promising. All successful antiosteoporotic agents thus far developed block or slow the rate of bone resorption but do not stimulate bone formation. Thus, the drugs may prevent disease progression but cannot cure a patient who already has osteoporosis. Dietary calcium supplementation in elderly patients reduces the risk of osteoporotic fractures by half.

Secondary Osteoporosis Reflects Extraosseous Metabolic Disorders

Osteoporosis develops in association with many other conditions. Causes of secondary osteoporosis include adverse effects of drug therapy, endocrine disorders, eating disorders, immobilization, marrow-related disorders, disorders of the gastrointestinal or biliary tracts, renal disease, and cancer.

- **Endocrine conditions:** The most common form of secondary osteoporosis is iatrogenic and results from corticosteroid administration. Bone loss may also result from an excess of endogenous glucocorticoids, as in Cushing disease. Corticosteroids inhibit osteoblastic activity, thereby reducing bone formation. They also impair vitamin D-dependent intestinal calcium absorption, an effect that leads to increased secretion of PTH and increased bone resorption.

  Estrogen is a key hormone for maintaining bone mass. Estrogen deficiency is the major cause of age-related bone loss in both sexes; estrogen deficiency or a low level of bioavailable estrogen decreases bone mass in elderly males. Its role in bone metabolism is focused on the role of proinflammatory cytokines: IL-1, IL-6, TNF-α, and RANK-L, granulocyte-macrophage colony-stimulating factor (GM-CSF), M-CSF, and prostaglandin E_2 (PGE_2). It is thought that these cytokines act upon both osteoclasts and osteoblasts via mediation by estrogen receptors.
- **Hyperparathyroidism** causes osteoclast recruitment and increased osteoclastic activity, resulting in secondary osteoporosis (see below). In both sexes, hyperparathyroidism

secondary to calcium malabsorption increases remodeling, worsening the cortical thinning and porosity, and predisposing to hip fractures.

- **Hyperthyroidism** causes accelerated turnover of bone and increases osteoclastic activity. Although thyrotoxicosis is associated with some secondary osteoporosis, bone loss is limited.
- **Hypogonadism** in both men and women is accompanied by osteoporosis. In women with primary gonadal failure (Turner syndrome) or with secondary amenorrhea as a result of pituitary disease, estrogen deficiency is likely the cause. Hypogonadal men (e.g., Klinefelter syndrome, hemochromatosis) are at risk of osteoporosis because of a deficiency of anabolic androgens. Similarly, hypogonadism contributes to bone loss in 25% of elderly males. In men, there is also evidence of decreased bone density in androgen-deprivation therapy for prostatic carcinoma.
- **Hematologic malignancies:** A variety of hematologic cancers, particularly multiple myeloma, are accompanied by significant bone loss. The malignant plasma cells of multiple myeloma secrete osteoclast-activating factor, which is presumably responsible for secondary osteoporosis. Some leukemias and lymphomas are also associated with osteoporosis. The bone loss found in systemic mastocytosis has been attributed to local release of heparin, which activates bone resorption. Even in the absence of skeletal metastases, some neoplasms are associated with severe hypercalcemia due to bone resorption. Osteoclastic activity is enhanced in these patients, owing to secretion of PTHrp by the tumor.
- **Malabsorption:** Gastrointestinal and hepatic diseases that cause malabsorption often contribute to osteoporosis, probably because of impaired absorption of calcium, phosphate, and vitamin D.
- **Alcoholism:** Chronic alcohol abuse also has been linked to development of osteoporosis. Alcohol is a direct inhibitor of osteoblasts and may also inhibit calcium absorption.

Osteomalacia and Rickets

Osteomalacia *(soft bones) is a disorder of adults characterized by inadequate mineralization of newly formed bone matrix.* ***Rickets*** *refers to a similar disorder in children, in whom the growth plates (physes) are open.* Thus children with rickets manifest defective mineralization not only of bone (osteomalacia) but also of the cartilaginous matrix of the growth plate. Diverse conditions associated with osteomalacia and rickets include abnormalities in vitamin D metabolism, phosphate deficiency states, and defects in the mineralization process itself.

Vitamin D Metabolism Influences Bone Mineralization

Vitamin D is ingested in food or synthesized in the skin from 7-dehydrocholesterol under the influence of ultraviolet light (Fig. 26-28). The vitamin is first hydroxylated in the liver to form its major circulating metabolite, 25-hydroxyvitamin D. It is then again hydroxylated in proximal renal tubules at to produce the active hormone $1,25(OH)_2D$. Exposure to sunlight provides sufficient vitamin D for bone growth and mineralization, even if there is inadequate dietary source.

Receptors for $1,25(OH)_2D$ are not only present in classic targets, such as intestine, bone, and kidney but are expressed in many cells. This steroid hormone is a general inducer of differentiation, for example, influencing maturation of hematopoietic and dermal cells, as well as many cancers. In the intestine, $1,25(OH)_2D$ stimulates calcium and phosphate absorption. It is also essential for osteoclast maturation. Although $1,25(OH)_2D$ enhances bone resorption in vitro, this effect does not occur in vivo, probably because of suppressed secretion of PTH. Regardless of mechanism, $1,25(OH)_2D$, in concert with PTH, maintain blood of calcium and phosphate at levels that are required for proper mineralization of bone. *The key determinant of the formation of $1,25(OH)_2D$ is blood calcium concentration.* Decreases in blood calcium stimulate release of PTH, which augments renal synthesis of $1,25(OH)_2D$.

Hypovitaminosis D can result from (1) inadequate exposure to sunlight, (2) deficient dietary intake, or (3) defective intestinal absorption. In addition there are hereditary and acquired disorders of vitamin D metabolism.

Dietary Deficiency of Vitamin D and Inadequate Exposure to Sunlight Cause Rickets

Rickets plagued children of the industrial cities of the United States and Europe from the 17th century through the 19th century. Of urban children in these regions 85% had rickets. These children had insufficient sun exposure, and their dietary intake of vitamin D was inadequate to avert hypovitaminosis D. Use of vitamin D-rich cod liver oil and later fortification of milk and other foods with vitamin D effectively ended widespread rickets in Western countries. However, nutritional vitamin D deficiency remains a problem elsewhere in the world, in neglected elderly persons and food faddists.

Intestinal Malabsorption Decreases the Availability of Vitamin D

In industrialized countries, diseases associated with intestinal malabsorption cause osteomalacia more often than does poor nutrition. *Intrinsic diseases of the small intestine, cholestatic disorders of the liver, biliary obstruction, and chronic pancreatic insufficiency are the most frequent causes of osteomalacia in the United States.*

Malabsorption of vitamin D and calcium complicates a number of small intestinal diseases, including celiac disease, Crohn disease, scleroderma, and the postsurgical blind-loop syndrome. In obstructive jaundice, the lack of bile salts in the intestine impairs absorption of lipids and lipid-soluble substances, among which is fat-soluble vitamin D. Furthermore, hydroxylation of vitamin D is reduced with severe liver damage. Oddly, biliary cirrhosis, a disease characterized by intestinal malabsorption and vitamin D deficiency, leads to osteoporosis rather than osteomalacia. Thus, vitamin D is essential not only for mineralization but also for the synthesis of bone collagen.

Disorders of Vitamin D Metabolism Are Inherited or Acquired

Vitamin D metabolism can be disturbed either by defective 1α-hydroxylation of vitamin D in the kidney or by insensitivity of the target organ to $1,25(OH)_2D$. Two autosomal recessive diseases associated with rickets are together known as **vitamin D-dependent rickets**.

Vitamin D-dependent rickets type I results from an inherited deficiency of renal 1α-hydroxylase activity. The clinical and biochemical changes of rickets appear during the first year of life, and these children exhibit hypocalcemia, hypophosphatemia, and high levels of serum PTH and alkaline phosphatase. The disease is controlled by the administration of $1,25(OH)_2D$.

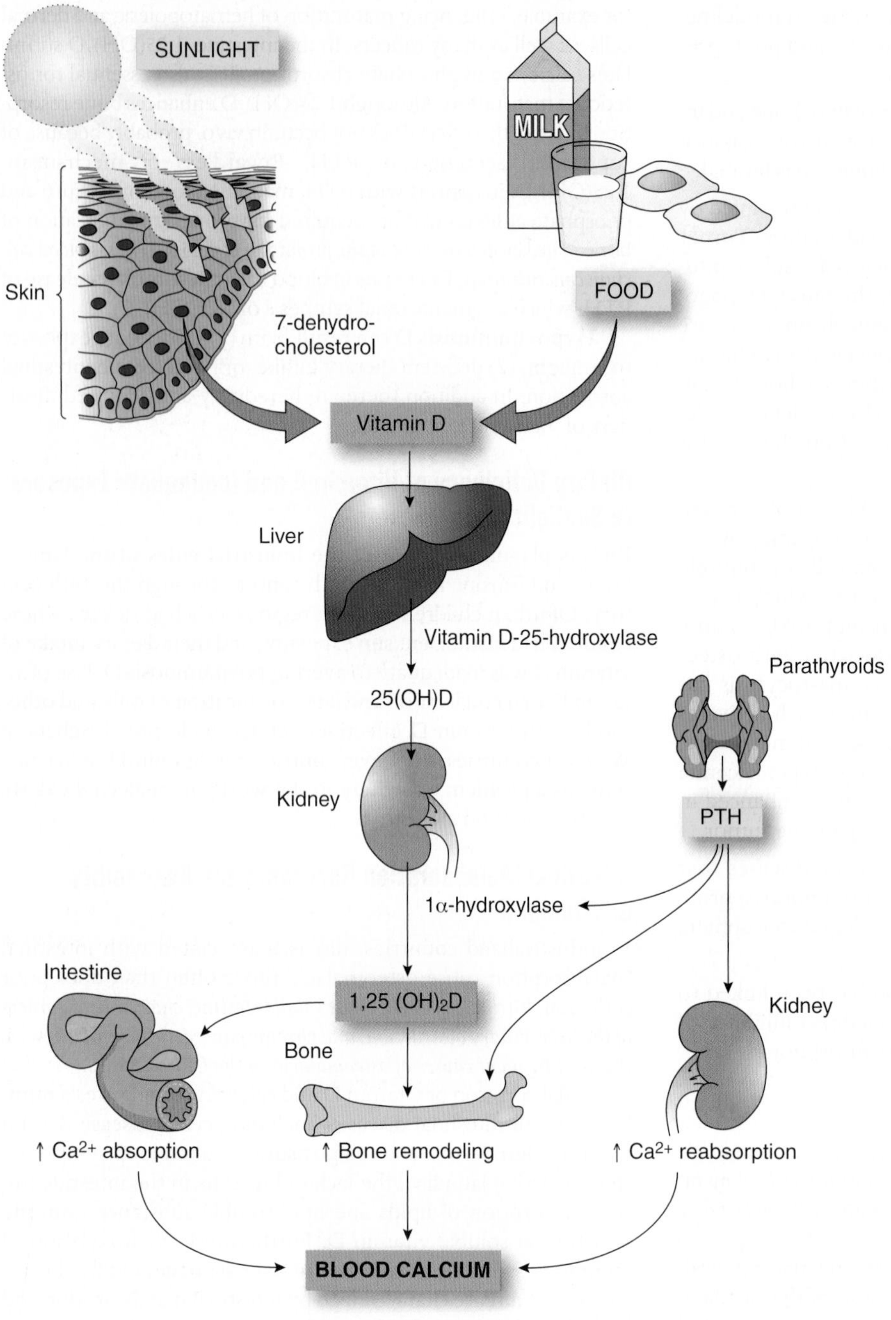

FIGURE 26-28. **Metabolism of vitamin D and the regulation of blood calcium.**

Vitamin D-dependent rickets type II involves inherited mutations of the vitamin D receptor, so that end organs are insensitive to 1,25$(OH)_2$D. The diseaes usually manifests early in life but may appear at any time up to adolescence. Serum concentrations of 1,25$(OH)_2$D are very high. Patients do not respond to 1,25$(OH)_2$D but are helped by repeated intravenous administration of calcium.

Acquired alterations in vitamin D metabolism include defective renal 1α-hydroxylation and end-organ insensitivity. Some of the causes of impaired α-hydroxylation are hypoparathyroidism, tumor-induced osteomalacia, chronic renal diseases, and osteomalacia of old age. Osteomalacia occasionally complicates the treatment of epilepsy with anticonvulsant drugs, particularly phenobarbital and phenytoin. It is believed that these drugs block the action of 1,25$(OH)_2$D on target organs.

Renal Disorders of Phosphate Metabolism Interfere with Vitamin D Metabolism

Both rickets and osteomalacia may result from impaired reabsorption of phosphate by the proximal renal tubules, with resulting hypophosphatemia.

X-LINKED HYPOPHOSPHATEMIA: This condition, also termed **vitamin D-resistant rickets** or **phosphate diabetes,** is the most common type of hereditary rickets and is inherited as a dominant trait. Mutations in the *PHEX* (phosphate-regulating) gene on the X chromosome (Xp22) impair transport of phosphate across the luminal membrane of proximal renal tubular cells. The gene product of *PHEX* is a protease that inactivates fibroblast growth factor-23 (FGF23). Increased levels of FGF23 produced renal phosphate wasting. Renal phosphate wasting is central to the disease, but osteoblast function is also impaired. In boys, florid rickets appears during childhood, but girls often suffer only hypophosphatemia. Treatment is with life-long administration of phosphate and 1,25$(OH)_2$D. Microscopically, the bones of patients with X-linked hypophosphatemia show severe osteomalacia and wide osteoid seams. They also exhibit characteristic hypomineralized areas surrounding osteocytes, known as **halos.** The presence of these structures indicates that osteocytes are responsible for the terminal mineralization of bone.

FANCONI SYNDROMES: These inborn errors of metabolism are characterized by renal wastage of phosphate, glucose, bicarbonate, and amino acids. They are all characterized by renal tubular acidosis and lead to rickets and osteomalacia. Fanconi syndromes include Wilson disease, tyrosinemia, galactosemia, glycogen-storage disease, and cystinosis. Renal tubular damage that leads to phosphate wastage may also be acquired, as in lead or mercury intoxication, amyloidosis, and Bence-Jones proteinuria.

TUMOR-ASSOCIATED OSTEOMALACIA: This disorder is a phosphate-wasting syndrome that is associated with predominantly benign and occasionally malignant tumors of soft tissue and bone. The typical laboratory features are hypophosphatemia, hyperphosphaturia, low serum concentrations of 1,25-$(OH)_2$D, and elevated serum alkaline phosphatase. Oncogenic osteomalacia mimics the clinical phenotype of X-linked hypophosphatemia and autosomally dominant hypophosphatemia. The paraneoplastic phosphaturic factors secreted by the tumor, known as **phosphatonins,** cause renal tubular phosphate wasting and prevent tubular conversion of 25-hydroxyvitamin D into 1,25$(OH)_2$D. Phosphatonins thus appear to have the same effect as inherited mutations of the PHEX gene seen in X-linked hypophosphatemia. Removal of the primary tumor is often curative. FGF23 has been implicated as a phosphatonin. Overproduction of FGF23 by tumors results in renal phosphate wasting and tumor-associated osteomalacia.

PATHOLOGY:

OSTEOMALACIA: Osteomalacia, like osteoporosis, causes an osteopenic radiologic pattern. The only findings may be vertebral compression fractures and decreased bone thickness, as in osteoporosis. However, some specific findings may be seen in osteomalacia, including the pseudofractures of **Milkman-Looser syndrome.** These are radiolucent transverse defects that are most common on the concave side of a long bone, medial side of the neck of the femur, ischial and pubic rami, ribs, and scapula.

Microscopically, defective mineralization in osteomalacia results in **exaggeration of osteoid seams,** both in thickness and in the proportion of trabecular surface covered (see Fig. 26-25 and Fig. 26-29). Osteoid seams reflect a time lag between the deposition of collagen and the appearance of the calcium salt. Although adults add 1 μm of new matrix to the surfaces of bone every day, it requires 10 days to mineralize this new bone. The normal thickness of osteoid seams, therefore, does not exceed 12 μm. Areas of pseudofracture display abundant osteoid and may function as stress points for true fractures. These areas do not evoke formation of callus and do not extend through the entire diameter of the bone.

RICKETS: Rickets is a disease of children and thus causes extensive changes at the physeal plate (Fig. 26-30), which does not become adequately mineralized. The calcified cartilage and zones of hypertrophy and proliferative cartilage continue to grow because osteoclastic activity does not resorb the cartilage growth

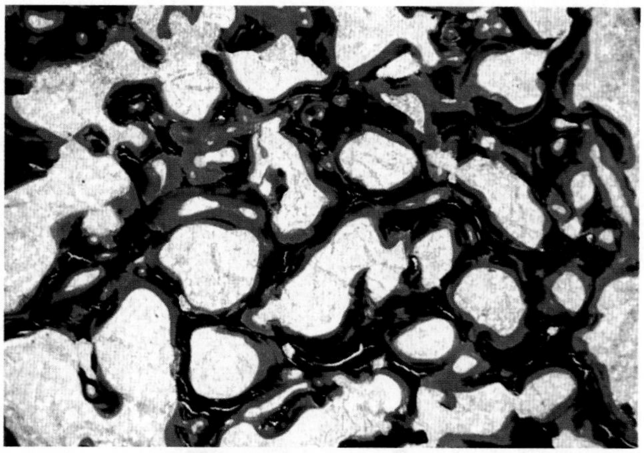

FIGURE 26-29. **Osteomalacia.** The surfaces of the bony trabeculae *(black)* are covered by a thicker than normal layer of osteoid *(red)* with the von Kossa stain, which colors calcified tissue black.

plate. As a consequence, the growth plate is conspicuously thickened, irregular, and lobulated. Endochondral ossification proceeds very slowly and preferentially at the peripheral portions of the metaphysis. The result is a flared, cup-shaped epiphysis. The largest part of the primary spongiosum is composed of lamellar or woven bone that, importantly, remains unmineralized.

Microscopically, the growth plate exhibits striking changes. The resting zone is normal, but the zones of proliferating cartilage are greatly distorted. The ordered progression of helix-forming chondrocytes is lost, and is replaced by a disorderly profusion of cells separated by small amounts of matrix. Resulting lobulated masses of proliferating and hypertrophied cartilage are associated with increasing width of the growth plate, which may be 5 to 15 times the normal width. The zone of provisional calcification is poorly defined, and only a minimal amount of primary spongiosum is formed. Masses of proliferating cartilage extend into the metaphyseal region, without any apparent vascular invasion and with little osteoclastic activity.

CLINICAL FEATURES:

OSTEOMALACIA: Clinical diagnosis of osteomalacia is often difficult. Patients have nonspecific complaints, such as muscle weakness or diffuse aches and pains. In mild forms of the disease, only slowly progressive changes in bone are seen, and many patients are totally asymptomatic for years. In advanced cases, poorly localized bone pain and tenderness are common, especially in the spine, pelvis, and proximal parts of the extremities. In such cases, the diagnosis may be made only after an acute fracture, the most common sites being the femoral neck, pubic ramus, spine, or ribs. Muscular weakness and hypotonia lead to a waddling gait in severe cases, and some patients are unable to walk.

RICKETS: Children with rickets are apathetic and irritable and have short attention spans. They are content to be sedentary, assuming a Buddha-like posture. They are short,with characteristic changes of bones and teeth. Flattening of the skull, prominent frontal bones (**frontal bossing**), and conspicuous suture lines are typical. There is delayed dentition, with severe dental caries and enamel defects. The chest has the classic **rachitic rosary** (a grossly beaded appearance of the costochondral junctions due to enlargement of the costal cartilages) and indentations of the lower ribs at the insertion of the diaphragm. **Pectus carinatum** ("pigeon breast") reflects an outward curvature of the sternum.

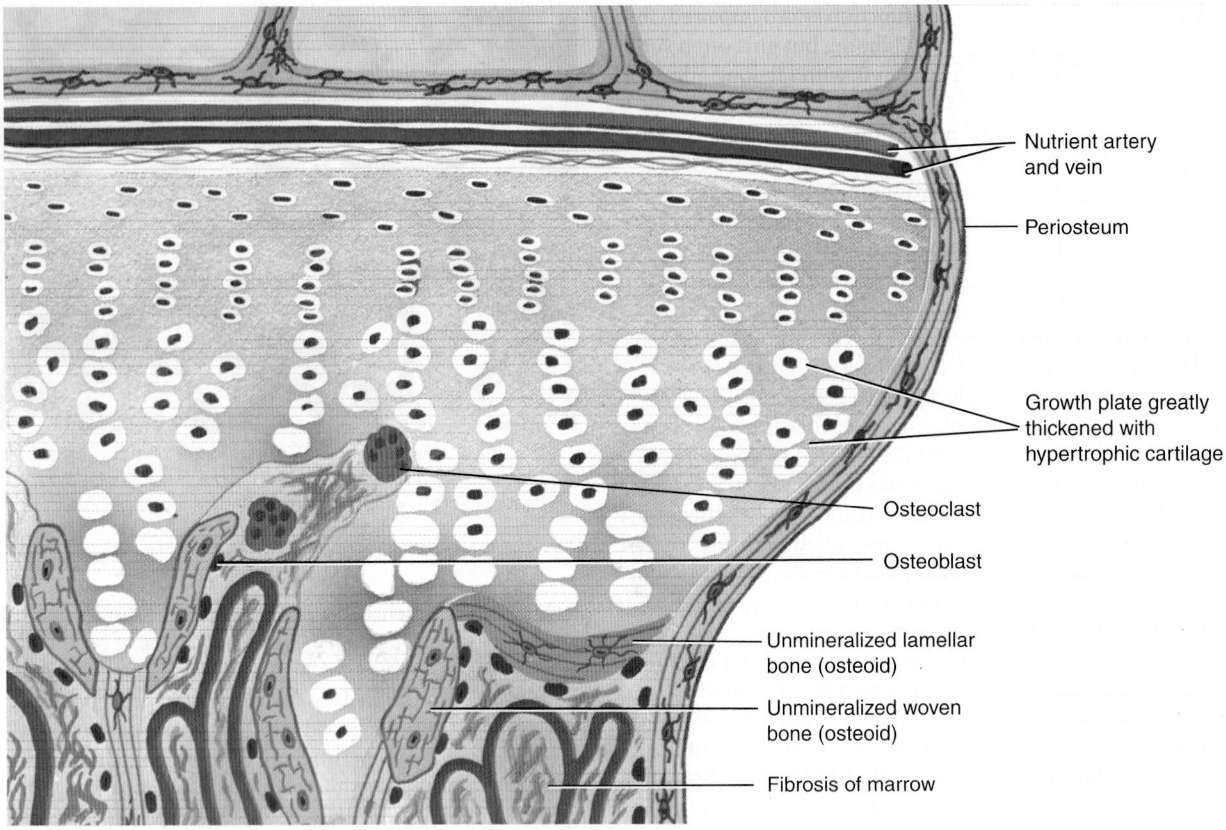

FIGURE 26-30. **The growth plate in rickets.** The growth plate is thickened and disorganized, with a large zone of hypertrophic cartilage cells. Irregular perforation of the cartilage plate by osteoclasts occurs because there is little calcified cartilage. The woven bone on the surface of some of the primary trabeculae is unmineralized and therefore easily fractured. Such microfractures often lead to hemorrhage at the interface between the plate and the metaphysis.

The overall musculature is weak, and abdominal weakness leads to a "potbelly." The limbs are shortened and deformed, with severe bowing of the arms and forearm and frequent fractures. The femoral head may dislocate from the growth plate (slipped capital femoral epiphysis).

Primary Hyperparathyroidism

Primary hyperparathyroidism is a metabolic bone disease characterized by generalized bone resorption due to inappropriate secretion of PTH. Early in the 20th century, bone disease in patients diagnosed with primary hyperparathyroidism was often advanced and crippling. Owing to screening of hospitalized patients for abnormalities of serum calcium, severe primary hyperparathyroidism is rarely encountered, and clinically significant bone disease is unusual.

The histologic changes of primary hyperparathyroidism are known as **osteitis fibrosa**. This term applies to all circumstances of markedly accelerated remodeling and may be seen in Paget disease and hyperthyroidism and even in some patients with postmenopausal osteoporosis. Almost all (90%) cases of primary hyperparathyroidism are caused by one or more parathyroid adenomas. Hyperplasia of all four glands accounts for only 10%. Rarely, hyperparathyroidism complicates a parathyroid carcinoma. Because PTH promotes phosphate excretion in the urine and stimulates osteoclastic bone resorption, low serum phosphate and high serum calcium levels are characteristic.

The effects of PTH are mediated by its effects on bone, kidney, and (indirectly) intestine.

BONE: PTH mobilizes calcium from bone, the major reservoir of calcium in the body. It increases bone resorption in the context of accelerated remodeling. Thus, enhanced bone formation is also seen in hyperparathyroidism. Depending on the relative increase in bone resorption and formation, respectively, the secretion of excess PTH may result in decreased, normal or increased bone mass.

KIDNEY: PTH stimulates reabsorption of calcium by the thick ascending and granular portions of the distal renal tubules. It also enhances phosphate excretion in proximal and distal convoluted tubules by directly inhibiting sodium-dependent phosphate transport.PTH also augments the activity of 1α-hydroxylase in the proximal tubules, thereby stimulating production of 1,25 $(OH)_2D$.

INTESTINE: PTH does not act directly on the intestine, but rather enhances intestinal calcium absorption indirectly by increasing renal synthesis of 1,25$(OH)_2D$.

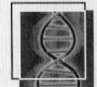

PATHOGENESIS AND PATHOLOGY: The histogenesis of osteitis fibrosa may be classified into three stages.

- **Early stage:** Initially, osteoclasts are stimulated by the increased PTH levels to resorb bone. From the subperiosteal and endosteal surfaces, osteoclasts bore their way into the cortex as cutting cones. This process is termed **dissecting osteitis** because each osteon is continually hollowed out by osteoclastic activity (see Fig. 26-25 and Fig. 26-31A). At the same time, collagen fibers are laid down in the endosteal marrow and additional osteoclasts penetrate the bone. In contrast to myelofibrosis of hematologic origin, in which fibrous tissue is randomly distributed in the marrow space, the collagen of osteitis fibrosa is deposited adjacent to trabeculae. This observation suggests that the stromal cells depositing matrix material are osteoblast precursors.

- **Osteitis fibrosa:** In the second stage, the trabecular bone is resorbed and marrow is replaced by loose fibrosis, hemosiderin-laden macrophages, areas of hemorrhage from microfractures, and reactive woven bone. These features constitute the "osteitis fibrosa" portion of the complex.
- **Osteitis fibrosa cystica:** As primary hyperparathyroidism progresses and hemorrhage continues, cystic degeneration ultimately occurs, leading to the final stage of the disease. The areas of fibrosis that contain reactive woven bone and hemosiderin-laden macrophages often display many osteoclastgiant cells. Because of its macroscopic appearance, this lesion has been termed a **brown tumor** (see Fig. 26-31B). This is not a neoplasm, but rather a repair reaction as an end stage of hyperparathyroidism.

The skeletal radiographs of most persons with primary hyperparathyroidism are normal. Some patients exhibit mottled bone cortices, with an irregular frayed surface in the outer table of the skull, tufts of the terminal digits, and shafts of the metacarpals (Fig. 26-32). A distinctive radiologic peculiarity, referred to as **subperiosteal bone resorption,** is evident in the subperiosteal outer surface of the cortex and reflects dissecting osteitis. Resorption around tooth sockets causes the lamina dura of the teeth to disappear, a well-known finding on x-ray.

A classic feature of osteitis fibrosa cystica is the presence of multiple, localized, lytic lesions, which represent hemorrhagic cysts or masses of fibrous tissue. These eccentric and well-demarcated lesions are separated from the soft tissue by a periosteal shell of bone. *The focal, tumorlike, lytic lesions always occur in the context of an abnormal skeleton produced by hyperparathyroidism.* If a single lesion is examined in isolation, it may be mistaken for a primary giant cell neoplasm of bone.

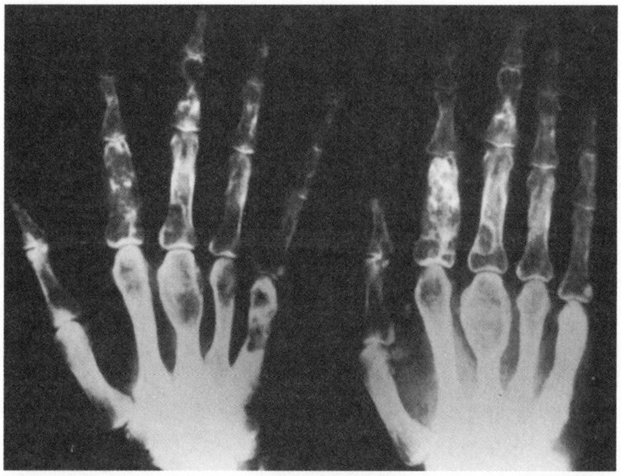

FIGURE 26-32. **Primary hyperparathyroidism.** A radiograph of the hands reveals bulbous swellings ("brown tumors") and numerous cavities, both representing bone resorption.

CLINICAL FEATURES: The symptoms of primary hyperparathyroidism are related to the abnormality of calcium homeostasis and have been summarized as **"stones, bones, moans, and groans."** The "stones" refer to kidney stones and the "bones" to the skeletal changes. The "moans" describe psychiatric depression and other abnormalities associated with hypercalcemia and the "groans" characterize the gastrointestinal irregularities associated with a high serum calcium level.

Primary hyperparathyroidism is treated with surgical removal of the parathyroid adenomas. When parathyroid hyperplasia is the cause of the disease, three and a half glands are usually removed. The remaining fragment suffices to ensure that the patient does not develop hypocalcemia. After surgery, the histologic appearance of the affected skeleton gradually normalizes.

A B

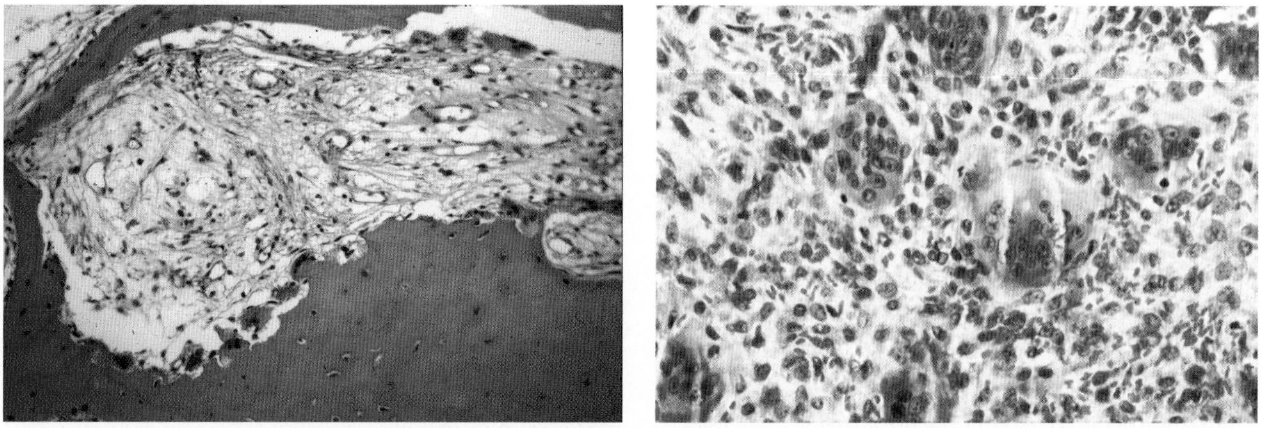

FIGURE 26-31. **Primary hyperparathyroidism. A.** Section through compact bone shows tunneling reabsorption of a haversian canal. Numerous osteoclasts and stromal fibrosis are evident. **B.** A section of tissue obtained from a "brown tumor" reveals numerous giant cells in a cellular, fibrous stroma. Scattered erythrocytes are present throughout the tissue.

A familial type of primary hyperparathyroidism is associated with mutations in the calcium-sensing receptor *(CASR)* gene, located on chromosome 3 (3q13.3).

Renal Osteodystrophy

Renal osteodystrophy is a complex metabolic bone disease that occurs in the context of chronic renal failure. Severe renal osteodystrophy is most common in patients maintained on long-term dialysis, because they live long enough to develop conspicuous bone disease.

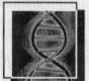

PATHOGENESIS: The pathogenesis of renal osteodystrophy is similar to that of osteomalacia, with secondary hyperparathyroidism exerting its influence by way of osteoclastic bone resorption (see Fig. 26-25). The development of renal osteodystrophy may be summarized as follows:

1. In chronic renal disease, a reduced glomerular filtration rate leads to retention of phosphate, thereby producing **hyperphosphatemia.** High serum phosphate levels drive down the serum calcium levels.
2. Tubular injury reduces 1α-hydroxylase activity, with a resulting deficiency of $1{,}25(OH)_2D$.
3. Intestinal calcium absorption is, in turn, decreased, worsening the **hypocalcemia.**
4. Hypocalcemia stimulates PTH production. In fact, most patients with end-stage renal disease have substantial hyperparathyroidism. However, PTH does not effectively promote intestinal calcium absorption or renal tubular resorption of calcium because of failure to produce adequate $1{,}25(OH)_2D$.
5. Perhaps because of hyperparathyroidism and hyperphosphatemia, a substantial proportion of patients with end-stage renal disease have increased bone mass. Renal osteosclerosis is particularly prominent in vertebrae where, owing to alternating bands of radiopaque and normally dense bone, the lesion is named **"rugger jersey spine."**

The adynamic variant of renal osteodystrophy (ARO) is characterized by arrested bone remodeling. More than 40% of adults who are treated with hemodialysis and more than 50% of those who are treated with peritoneal dialysis have bone biopsy evidence of ARO. Also, the development of adynamic bone during treatment of secondary hyperparathyroidism with large intermittent doses of calcitriol can aggravate growth retardation in prepubertal children who undergo peritoneal dialysis. Adynamic bone is characterized microscopically by an overall reduction in cellular activity in bone, with fewer osteoblasts and osteoclasts. These changes can be due to either direct inhibitory effects of systemic factors on osteoblast function or indirect changes in osteoblast activity mediated through PTH-dependent mechanisms. Old bone accumulates because it is not remodeled, thereby leading to structural compromise of the skeleton and increased tendency to fractures.

PATHOLOGY AND CLINICAL FEATURES: As a result of these effects of chronic renal failure, renal osteodystrophy is characterized by varying degrees of osteomalacia, osteitis fibrosa, osteomalacia, osteosclerosis, and adynamic bone disease (Fig. 26-33). Combinations of osteitis fibrosa and osteomalacia are particularly common. Hyperphosphatemic patients with terminal chronic renal disease may display metastatic calcification at various sites, including the eyes, skin, muscular coats of arteries and arterioles, and periarticular soft tissues.

Management of renal osteodystrophy involves not only treatment of renal failure but also control of phosphate levels by appropriate drug therapy and infusions. Occasionally, parathyroidectomy is required to control hyperparathyroidism and the administration of vitamin D may also be necessary.

Paget Disease of Bone

Paget disease is a chronic condition characterized by lesions of bone resulting from disordered remodeling, in which excessive bone resorption initially results in lytic lesions, to be followed by disorganized and excessive bone formation

EPIDEMIOLOGY: Paget disease is common and generally affects men and women older than 60 years. In predisposed populations, 3% of elderly persons manifest the disease at autopsy or on radiographic examination. The disorder has an unusual worldwide distribution, afflicting populations of the British Isles and following their migrations throughout the world. Persons of English descent living in the United States, Australia, New Zealand, and Canada have a high incidence of the disease. Northern Europeans have more Paget disease than southern Europeans. The disorder is almost nonexistent in Asia and in the indigenous populations of Africa and South America. For unknown reasons the incidence of Paget disease appears to have decreased worldwide over the last several decades.

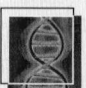

PATHOGENESIS: Sir James Paget coined the term **osteitis deformans** for this disease over a century ago, but until recently the etiology has been obscure. Paget disease resembles a metabolic disease histologically and there is a slight increase in bone turnover in affected patients, but its clinical tendency to involve one bone or only a few bones does not fulfill the definition of a metabolic disorder. A hereditary predisposition has been suggested by reports of almost 100 families in which Paget disease is generally transmitted as an autosomal dominant trait with incomplete penetrance that increases with age. There is evolving evidence that Paget disease and some related diseases are caused by mutations in genes encoding proteins in the RANK signaling pathway. Specifically, muations in *Sequestosome 1 (SQSTM1)* have been been found in familial and sporadic forms of Paget disease. The *SQSTM1* gene encodes a protein also known as p62, which may act as a scaffold protein in the RANK signaling pathway. It is currently unknown how this mutated protein leads to accelerated osteoclast activity and Paget disease. Inactivation of *SQSTM1* causes defects in RANKL-induced osteoclastogenesis indicating a significant role of p62 in osteoclast function.

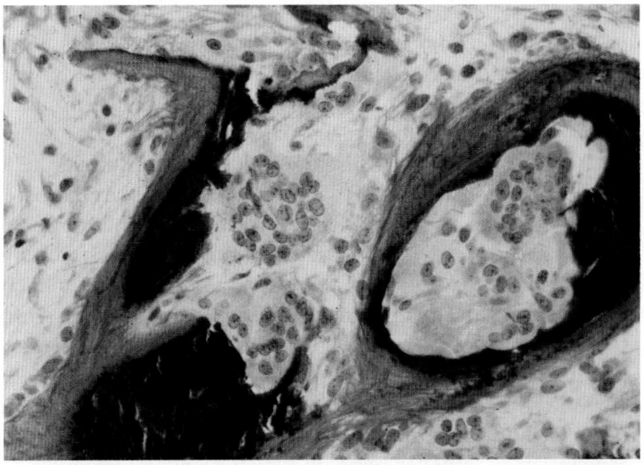
A

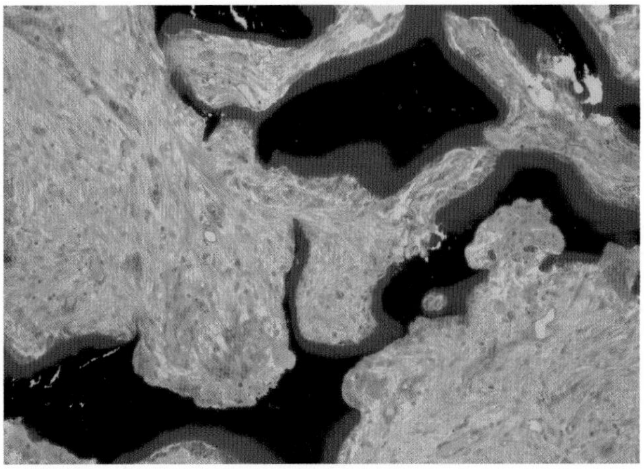
B

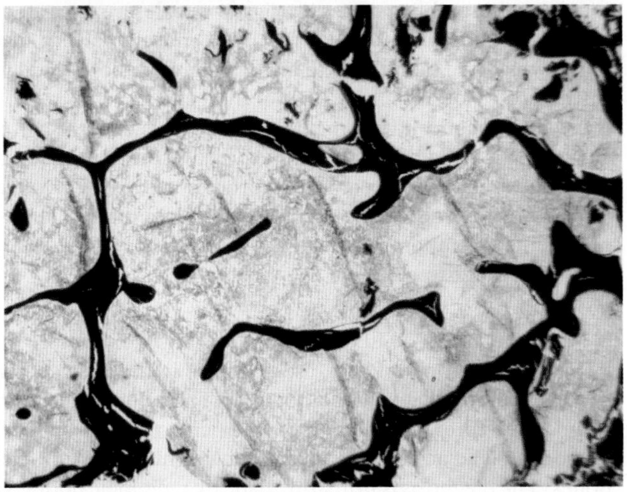
C

FIGURE 26-33. **Renal osteodystrophy. A.** Osteitis fibrosa. Several large multinucleated osteoclasts are reabsorbing these bone spicules, and the paraosseous tissue is fibrotic. Note that the osteoclastic reabsorption takes place only on the mineralized ***(blue)*** portions of the trabeculae. In this undercalcified section, the unmineralized bone (osteoid) appears ***red***. **B.** Osteomalacia. This is a Von Kossa stain prepared on an undercalcified section. The mineralized bone is ***black*** and the abundant osteoid appears ***magenta***. Osteoid is thick and lines a large proportion of the bone surfaces. Surfaces not covered by the osteoid demonstrate scalloped Howship lacunae and contain abundant osteoclasts. **C.** Adynamic bone disease in which remodeling is attenuated, with a paucity of osteoblasts, osteoclasts, and osteoid (Von Kossa stain).

Some evidence indicates that Paget disease is of viral origin. Virtually all patients exhibit nuclear inclusions consistent with the structure of a virus in osteoclasts and osteoclast precursors, which are not found in any other skeletal disease other than giant cell tumors of bone. They consist of microfilaments in a paracrystalline array and have been compared with the inclusions in the brains of patients with subacute sclerosing encephalitis (see Chapter 29). This similarity has suggested that a slow virus may be involved (Fig. 26-34). Support for this hypothesis has come from the finding that the marrow of Paget disease patients contains paramyxovirus nucleocapsid transcripts. Infection of osteoclast precursor cells with paramyxovirus can increase expression of RANK and thereby increase oseoclastic activity. In addition, paramyxoviruses stimulate osteoblasts to produce IL-6, which contributes to osteoclastogenesis. Although a viral etiology seems plausible, actual live viruses have not been isolated from Pagetic bone and it is difficult to explain monoostotic bone involvement by a systemic viral infection.

Overall, Paget disease is characterized by localized increases in osteoclast formation that leads to bone resorption and associated osteoblastic activity. The increased osteoclastogenic nature of the bone microenvironment is mediated by increases in IL-6 and the RANK signalling pathway. These are perturbed in Paget disease as a result of genetic factors such as *SQSTM1* mutations and possibly a slow virus infection that may serve as a catalyst for developing the Pagetic phenotype in genetically predisposed individuals. The result is uncoupling of the normal osteoclast/osteoblast remodeling unit.

PATHOLOGY: The lesions of Paget disease may be solitary or may occur at multiple sites. They tend to localize to the bones of the axial skeleton, including the spine, skull, and pelvis. The proximal femur and tibia may also be involved in the polyostotic form of the disease. Solitary Paget disease rarely involves the humerus, but in polyostotic disease, lesions involving this bone are common.

Paget disease is an example of bone remodeling gone awry. The disease is triphasic:

1. **"Hot" or osteoclastic resorptive stage:** Radiologically, there is a characteristic, sharply defined, flame-shaped or wedge-shaped lysis of the cortex, which may mimic a tumor (Fig 26-35A). Histologically, there is widespread osteolysis, with marrow fibrosis and dilation of marrow sinusoids.
2. **Mixed stage of osteoblastic and osteoclastic activity:** By x-ray, the bones are larger than normal. In fact, Paget disease is one of only two diseases that produce **larger than normal bones** (the other is fibrous dysplasia, discussed below). The cortex in the mixed phase is thickened, and the accentuation of the coarse cancellous bone makes the bone look heavy and enlarged (see Fig. 26-35B,C). Involvement of vertebral bodies leads to a "picture frame" appearance (see Fig. 26-35D), as cortices and endplates become greatly exaggerated compared with the coarse cancellous bone of the vertebral body. Although the bone is abnormal, the distorted, coarse cancellous bone and cortex still tend to align along stress lines. The pelvis is often thickened in the area of

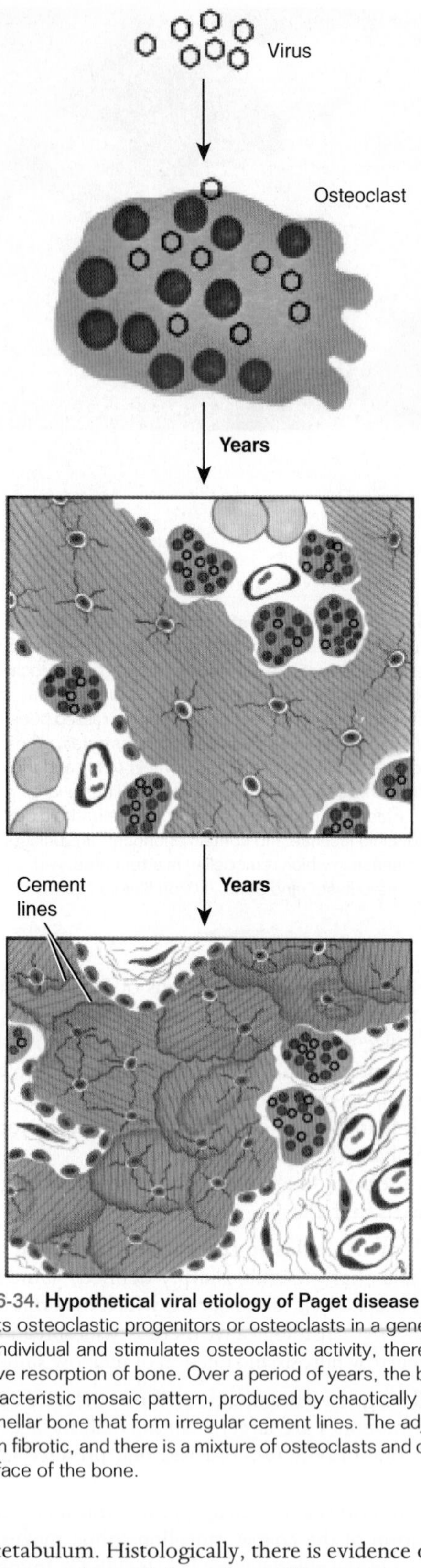

FIGURE 26-34. **Hypothetical viral etiology of Paget disease of bone.** A virus infects osteoclastic progenitors or osteoclasts in a genetically predisposed individual and stimulates osteoclastic activity, thereby leading to excessive resorption of bone. Over a period of years, the bone develops a characteristic mosaic pattern, produced by chaotically juxtaposed units of lamellar bone that form irregular cement lines. The adjacent marrow is often fibrotic, and there is a mixture of osteoclasts and osteoblasts on the surface of the bone.

the acetabulum. Histologically, there is evidence of both irregular osteoclast activity and osteoblast activity.

3. **"Cold" or burnt-out stage:** This period is characterized histologically by little cellular activity and radiologically by thickened and disordered bones.

The disease need not progress through all three stages, and in polyostotic disease, various foci may appear in different stages.

The osteoclast is the pathologic cell of Paget disease, and its appearance is characteristic. Whereas normal osteoclasts contain fewer than a dozen nuclei, those of Paget disease are huge and may have over 100 (Fig. 26-36). Nuclei may contain intranuclear inclusions that contain viruslike particles.

Because active Paget disease is a disorder of accelerated remodeling, its histologic features are those of severe osteitis fibrosa. Numerous osteoclasts, large active osteoblasts, and peritrabecular marrow fibrosis are encountered. The rapid remodeling leads to disruption of trabecular architecture. Trabeculae are characteristically distorted and irregular, with a high surface-to-volume ratio. Bone collagen is often arranged in a woven rather than lamellar pattern.

With time, the lesions of Paget disease burn out and become inactive. The diagnostic hallmark of this stage is the abnormal arrangement of lamellar bone, in which islands of irregular bone formation, resembling pieces of a jigsaw puzzle, are separated by prominent **cement lines**. The result is a **mosaic pattern** in the bone, which can be seen particularly well under polarized light. In the cortex of an affected bone, the osteons tend to be destroyed, and concentric lamellae are incomplete. Although the changes in lamellar bone are diagnostic, it is common to see woven bone as part of the pathologic process. In this situation, the woven bone is a reactive phenomenon, as in a microcallus, and represents a temporary bridge between islands of the mosaic bone of Paget disease.

CLINICAL FEATURES: The most common focal symptom of Paget disease is pain in the affected bone, although its cause is not clear. The pain may be related to microfractures, stimulation of free nerve endings by dilated blood vessels adjacent to the zbones, or weight bearing in weaker bones. The diagnosis is primarily made by radiologic findings.

SKULL: Involvement of the skull is particularly common. The skull exhibits localized lysis, generally in the frontal and parietal bones, which is termed **osteoporosis circumscripta.** Alternatively, there may be thickening of the outer and inner tables, which is most pronounced in the frontal and occipital bones. The skull becomes very heavy and may collapse over the C1 vertebra, compressing the brain and spinal cord. Hearing loss follows involvement of the ossicles and bony impingement on the eighth cranial nerve at the foramen. **Platybasia** (flattening of the base of the skull) impinges on the foramen magnum, thereby compressing the medulla and upper spinal cord.

The jaws may be grossly misshapen, and the teeth may fall out. Often, the facial bones increase in size, especially the maxillary bones, producing so-called **leontiasis ossea** (lionlike face).

PAGETIC STEAL: Occasionally, patients feel lightheaded, due to so-called pagetic steal, in which blood is shunted from the internal carotid system to the bones rather than directed to the brain.

FRACTURES AND ARTHRITIS: Bone fractures are common in Paget disease, the bones snapping transversely like a piece of chalk. Incomplete fractures without displacement are called **infractions.** Involvement of the pelvis leads to hip problems. The loss of subchondral bone compliance causes secondary osteoarthritis and destruction of the articular cartilage.

HIGH-OUTPUT CARDIAC FAILURE: With extensive Paget disease, blood flow to the bones and subcutaneous tissue increases remarkably, requiring increased cardiac output. In the presence of underlying cardiac disease, it may be severe enough to result in cardiac failure.

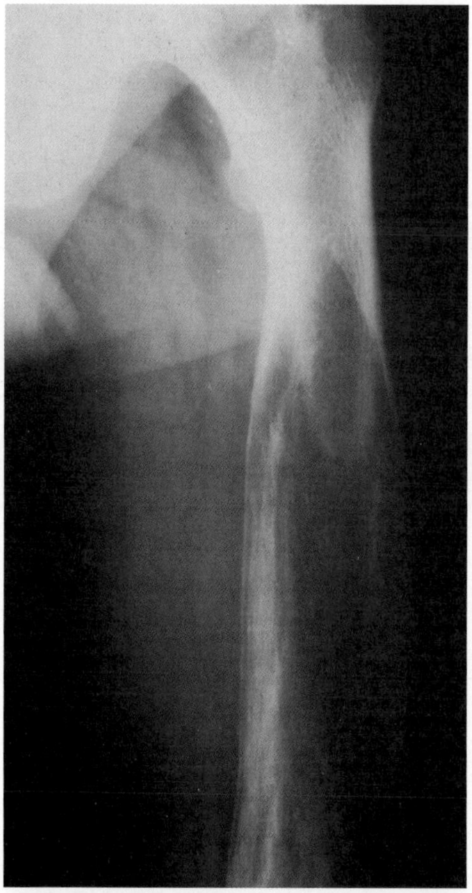
A

FIGURE 26-35. **Paget disease. A.** A radiograph of early Paget disease shows cortical dissolution, increased diameter of the diaphysis, and an advancing, wedge-shaped area of cortical reabsorption ("flame sign"). Proximal to the edge of this wedge, the femur appears entirely normal. **B.** Later Paget disease of the proximal femur and pelvis shows cortical disorganization and irregular coarse trabeculations. **C.** Gross specimen of proximal femur showing cortical thickening and coarse trabeculations of the femoral head and neck. **D.** Paget disease of the spine shows shortening and widening of the lumbar vertebral bodies. Their cortices and endplates are thickened and have a "picture-frame" appearance.

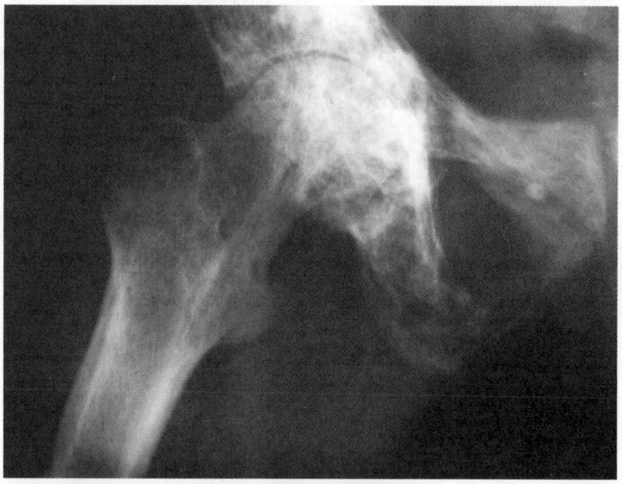
B

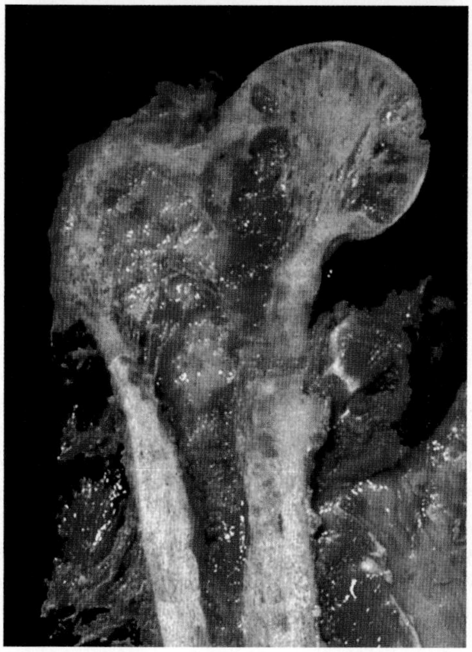
C

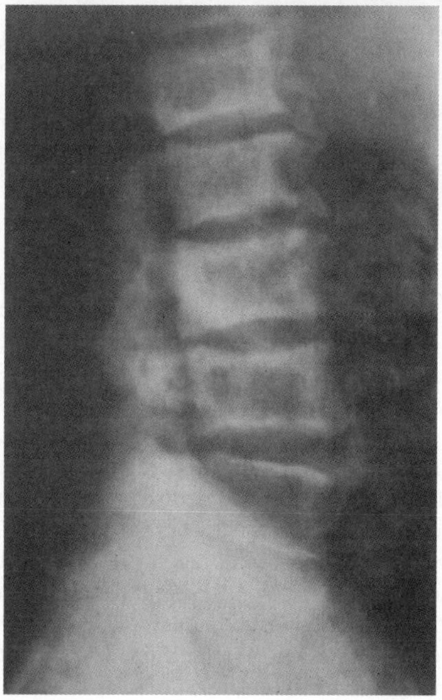
D

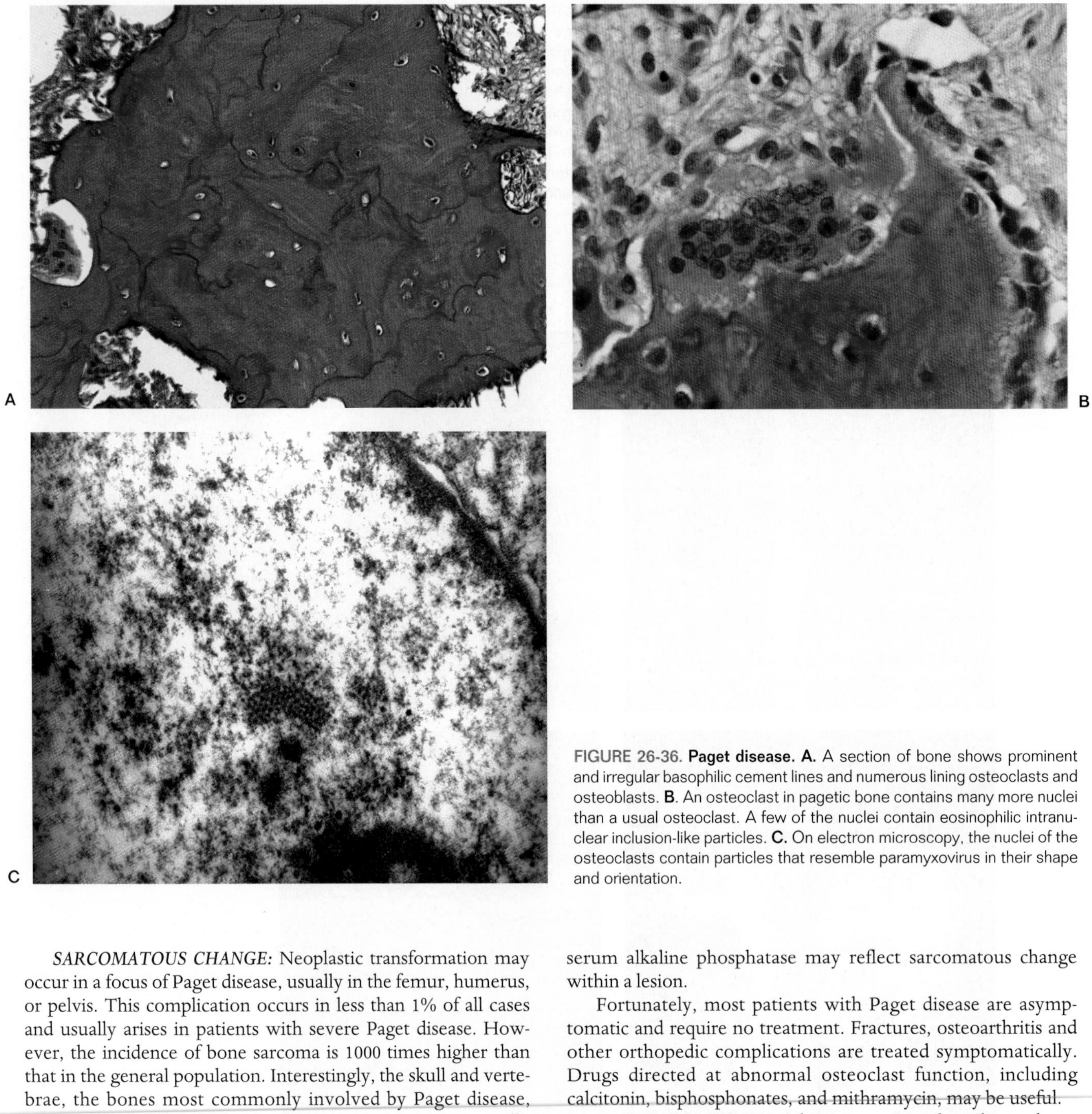

FIGURE 26-36. **Paget disease. A.** A section of bone shows prominent and irregular basophilic cement lines and numerous lining osteoclasts and osteoblasts. **B.** An osteoclast in pagetic bone contains many more nuclei than a usual osteoclast. A few of the nuclei contain eosinophilic intranuclear inclusion-like particles. **C.** On electron microscopy, the nuclei of the osteoclasts contain particles that resemble paramyxovirus in their shape and orientation.

SARCOMATOUS CHANGE: Neoplastic transformation may occur in a focus of Paget disease, usually in the femur, humerus, or pelvis. This complication occurs in less than 1% of all cases and usually arises in patients with severe Paget disease. However, the incidence of bone sarcoma is 1000 times higher than that in the general population. Interestingly, the skull and vertebrae, the bones most commonly involved by Paget disease, rarely undergo sarcomatous change. Sarcomas are usually osteogenic but may be fibrosarcoma or chondrosarcoma.

Serum calcium and phosphorus levels in Paget disease are normal, even though bone turnover increases more than 20-fold. Hypercalcemia is rare, but does occur if a patient is immobilized. The collagen structure ofbone in Paget disease is entirely normal, but because of the accelerated bone turnover, levels of collagen breakdown products (hydroxyproline and hydroxylysine) increase in the serum and urine, Hydroxyproline excretion may reach 1000 mg/day (normal, <40 mg). The serum alkaline phosphatase level is the most useful laboratory test in diagnosing Paget disease. It increases enormously and correlates with osteoblastic activity. The alkaline phosphatase levels are disproportionately high with skull involvement, but tend to be lower when only the pelvis is affected. A sudden increase in the activity of serum alkaline phosphatase may reflect sarcomatous change within a lesion.

Fortunately, most patients with Paget disease are asymptomatic and require no treatment. Fractures, osteoarthritis and other orthopedic complications are treated symptomatically. Drugs directed at abnormal osteoclast function, including calcitonin, bisphosphonates, and mithramycin, may be useful.

GIANT CELL TUMOR: This is not a neoplasm but rather a reactive phenomenon, similar to the "brown tumor" of hyperparathyroidism. Giant cell tumor is an overshoot of osteoclastic activity and an associated fibroblastic response. Radiation therapy to the giant cell tumor is curative in many cases.

Gaucher Disease

This autosomal recessive hereditary storage disease is discussed in Chapter 6. We consider here only its skeletal manisfestations. These include:

- **Failure of remodeling**. This is the most common, and least problematic, skeletal abnormality. Flaring is absent and funnelization and cylinderization are abnormal, leading to an Erlenmeyer flask shape of the distal femur and proximal tibia.

- **Crisis.** This rare, but very painful, event results from acute infarction of a large segment of bone or several bones, often after an acute viral illness. It last about 2 weeks then gradually improves.
- **Localized and diffuse bone loss.** Radiolucent lesions with overlying cortical thinning are usually asymptomatic unless a fracture occurs at the site. These lesions are packed with Gaucher cells.
- **Osteosclerotic lesions.** These reflect increased bone formation, usually in the medullary cavity of long bones and pelvis. Reactive new bone formation following osteonecrosis may be involved.
- **Corticomedullary osteonecrosis.** This disabling complication of Gaucher disease is most common in patients between 8 and 35 years old. It mostly involves femoral head or proximal humerus.
- **Pathologic fractures.** Vertebrae, long bones and even the pelvis may show spontaneous fractures.
- **Osteomyelitis and septic arthritis.** Commonly caused by coliform or anaerobic organisms, spread via bloodstream to the bones and joints of Gaucher patients is common, especially after surgery. The reason for the increased susceptibility to these infections in Gaucher disease is unknown.

Fibrous Dysplasia

Fibrous dysplasia is a developmental abnormality characterized by a disorganized mixture of fibrous and osseous elements in the medullary region of affected bones. It occurs in children or adults and may affect one (monostotic) or multiple bones (polyostotic) or other systems (McCune-Albright Syndrome).

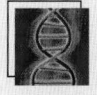

PATHOGENESIS: Activating mutations in the *GNAS1* gene encoding the α subunit of the stimulatory guanine nucleotide-binding protein ($G_S\alpha$), which is linked to adenylyl cyclase, have been described in bone cells from patients with fibrous dysplasia and McCune-Albright syndrome. The result would be constitutive activation of adenylyl cyclase and increased levels of cAMP, thereby enhancing certain functions of the affected cells (e.g., c-*fos* protooncogene, c-*jun*, IL-6, and IL-11).

PATHOLOGY AND CLINICAL FEATURES:

MONOSTOTIC FIBROUS DYSPLASIA: Monostotic fibrous dysplasia is the most common form of the disease and is most often seen in the second and third decades, with no predilection for either sex. The bones commonly involved are the proximal femur, tibia, ribs, and facial bones, although any bone may be affected. The disease may be asymptomatic or it may lead to a pathologic fracture.

POLYOSTOTIC FIBROUS DYSPLASIA: One fourth of patients with polyostotic fibrous dysplasia exhibit disease in more than half of the skeleton, including the facial bones. Symptoms usually are seen in childhood, and almost all patients have pathologic fractures, limb deformities, or limb-length discrepancies. Polyostotic fibrous dysplasia is more common in females. Sometimes the disease becomes quiescent at puberty, whereas pregnancy may stimulate the growth of lesions.

MCCUNE-ALBRIGHT SYNDROME: This condition is characterized by endocrine dysfunction, including acromegaly, Cushing syndrome, hyperthyroidism, and vitamin D-resistant rickets. The most common endocrine abnormality is precocious puberty in girls (boys rarely have McCune-Albright syndrome). As a result, premature closure of the growth plates may lead to abnormally short stature. The most common extraskeletal manifestations of McCune-Albright syndrome are characteristic skin lesions: pigmented macules ("café-au-lait" spots) with irregular ("coast of Maine") borders that do not cross the midline of the body and are usually located over the buttocks, back, and sacrum. These often overlie the skeletal lesions.

The radiographic features of fibrous dysplasia are distinctive. The bone lesion has a lucent ground-glass appearance with well-marginated borders and a thin cortex. The bone may be ballooned, deformed or enlarged, and involvement may be focal or may encompass the entire bone (Fig. 26-37A).

All forms of fibrous dysplasia have an identical histological pattern (see Fig. 26-37B,C). Benign fibroblastic tissue is arranged in a loose, whorled pattern. Irregularly arranged, purposeless spicules of woven bone that lack osteoblastic rimming are embedded in the fibrous tissue. In 10% of cases, irregular islands of hyaline cartilage are also present. Occasionally, cystic degeneration occurs, with hemosiderin-laden macrophages, hemorrhage, and osteoclasts congregated about the cyst. Rarely (<1% of cases), malignant degeneration (osteosarcoma, chondrosarcoma, or fibrosarcoma) has been reported, but most of these cases involved prior radiation therapy. Treatment of fibrous dysplasia consists of curettage, repair of fractures, and prevention of deformities.

Benign Tumors of Bone

Bone tumors of all kinds are uncommon, but are nevertheless important neoplasms because many occur in children and young persons and are potentially lethal. A primary bone tumor may arise from any of the cellular elements of bone. Most neoplasms of bone occur near the metaphyseal area, and more than 80% of primary tumors occur in the distal femur or proximal tibia (Fig. 26-38). In a growing child, these areas are characterized by conspicuous growth activity.

Osteoma Is a Benign Tumor Composed of Compact Cortical Bone

Osteoma is a benign slow-growing tumor composed of cortical type bone. These lesions can be divided into four major clinicopathologic subtypes including (1) calvarial and mandibular osteomas, (2) osteomas of the sinonasal and orbital bones, (3) bone islands occurring in medullary bone, and (4) surface osteomas of long bones. Some osteomas are likely developmental or hamartomatous in nature. However, sinonasal osteomas may be benign osteoblastic neoplasms.

Nonossifying Fibroma Is a Solitary Lesion of Childhood

Nonossifying fibroma, also termed ***fibrous cortical defect****, is a benign tumor that occurs in the metaphysis of a long bone, most commonly the tibia or femur.* It is very common and may be present in as many as 25% of all children between ages 4 and 10 years, after which it

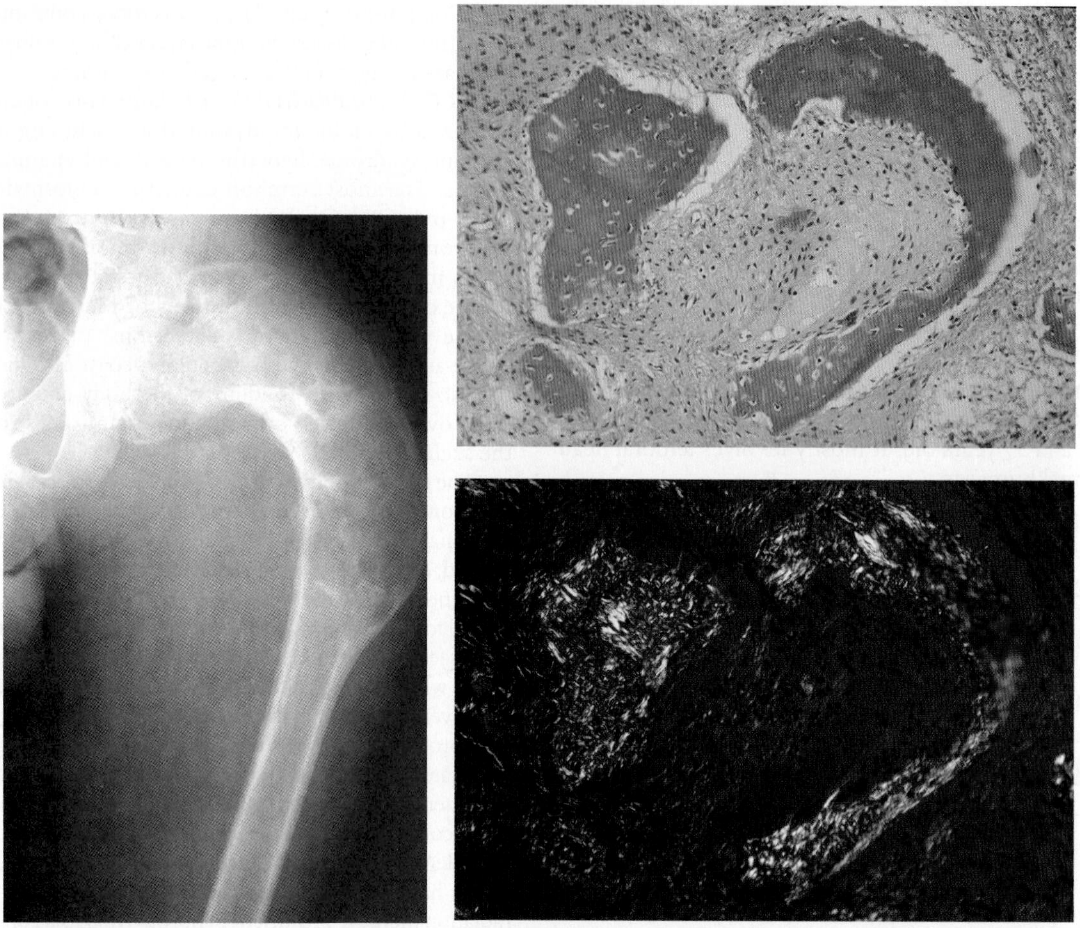

A B C

FIGURE 26-37. **Fibrous dysplasia. A.** A radiograph of the proximal femur shows a "shepherd's crook" deformity caused by fractures sustained over the years. Irregular, marginated, ground-glass lucencies are surrounded by reactive bone. The shaft has an appearance that has been likened to a soap bubble. **B.** Histologically, fibrous dysplasia consists of moderately cellular fibrous tissue in which irregular, curved spicules of woven bone develop without discernible appositional osteoblast activity. **C.** The same section in polarized light demonstrates not only that the spicules are woven, but also that their fiber pattern extends imperceptibly into the fiber pattern of the surrounding stroma.

characteristically regresses. Whether nonossifying fibroma is a neoplasm or developmental lesion remains controversial. Most cases are asymptomatic, although pain or fracture through the thin cortex overlying the lesion occasionally calls attention to the condition.

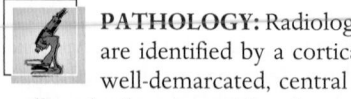

PATHOLOGY: Radiologically, nonossifying fibromas are identified by a cortical, eccentric position and by well-demarcated, central lucent zones surrounded by scalloped, sclerotic margins. On gross examination, the lesion is granular and dark red to brown. Microscopically, bland spindle cells are arranged in an interlacing, whorled pattern in which multinuclear giant cells and foamy macrophages may be seen. The rare, symptomatic, or expanded lesions are treated with curettage and bone grafting.

Solitary Bone Cyst Occurs in Children and Adolescents

Solitary, or unicameral, bone cyst is a benign, fluid-filled, unilocular, lesion. There is a male predilection (3:1). More than two thirds of all solitary bone cysts occur in the upper (proximal) humerus or femur, usually in the metaphysis adjacent to the growth plate.

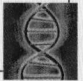

PATHOGENESIS: Solitary bone cyst seems not to be a true neoplasm but rather a disturbance of bone growth with superimposed trauma. Secondary organization of a hematoma or some abnormality of the metaphyseal vessels causes accumulation of fluid. The "tumor" then grows by expansion of the fluid cavity. The resulting pressure causes bone resorption, mediated by neighboring osteoclasts. The process is slow, so that as the endosteal surface of the cortex is resorbed, a thin periosteal shell of new bone is laid down. This sequence results in a thin, well-marginated, radiolucent bone lesion (Fig. 26-39), which is never greater in diameter than the growth plate and is particularly susceptible to pathologic fracture.

PATHOLOGY: Solitary bone cyst is not a true cyst since there is no epithelial lining, but is rather lined by fibrous tissue, a few osteoclastic giant cells, hemosiderin-laden macrophages, chronic inflammatory cells, and reactive bone. Osteoclasts are present in the advancing front of the cyst and

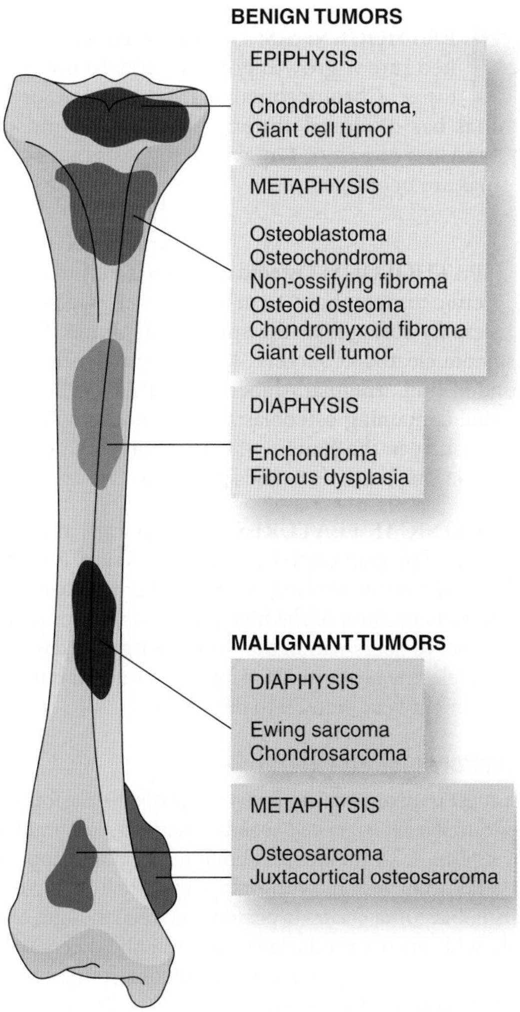

FIGURE 26-38. **Location of primary bone tumors in long tubular bones.**

allow expansion of the lesion. The cyst contains masses of amorphous proteinaceous material.

CLINICAL FEATURES: Most solitary bone cysts are entirely asymptomatic until a pathologic fracture calls attention to the lesion. Once the diagnosis is confirmed by other imaging studies and by finding clear fluid by needle aspiration, intralesional corticosteroids are administered. Curettage and deposition of bone chips are performed only when the cyst is not controlled by injection.

Aneurysmal Bone Cyst May Be Primary or Secondary

Aneurysmal bone cyst (ABC) is an uncommon, expansive lesion arising within a bone or on its surface. It occurs in children and young adults, with a peak incidence in the second decade. The lesion has been observed at every skeletal site but is most frequent in the long bones and the vertebral column.

PATHOGENESIS: The pathogenesis of ABC is controversial. Some cases represent cystic and hemorrhagic transformation of an underlying lesion, most commonly chondroblastoma, osteoblastoma, fibrous dysplasia, giant cell tumor, and osteosarcoma (termed "secondary ABC"). Other cases of ABC have no detectable associated lesion (termed "primary ABC"). Rather, primary ABC may be a true neoplasm since they are associated with a recurring chromosomal tranlocation t(16;17)(q22;p13). This translocation fuses the promoter region of the **osteoblast cadherin 11** gene (*CDH11*) on chromosome 16q22 to the coding sequence of the **ubiquitin protease** (*USP6*) gene on chromosome 17p13. USP6 *is* thought to have a role in regulating actin remodeling. However, the possible mechanism of neoplastic transformation by upregulation of USP6 has not been elucidated.

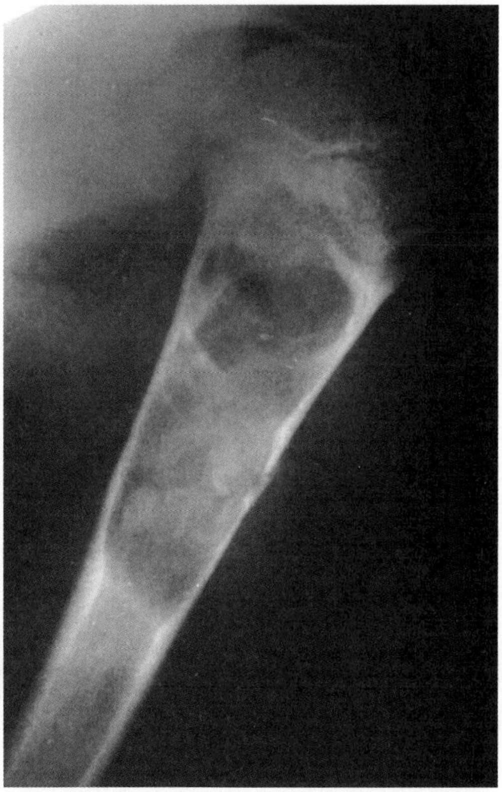

FIGURE 26-39. **Solitary bone cyst.** A radiograph of the proximal humerus of a child (note the epiphyseal plate) shows a large, well-demarcated, lytic epiphyseal and diaphyseal lesion. The cortex is thinned, but there is no cortical distortion or malformation of the shape of the bone.

PATHOLOGY: The periosteum around an aneurysmal bone cyst is ballooned but intact. In the spine, aneurysmal bone cyst may actually extend across more than one bone. By magnetic resonance imaging (MRI), fluid-fluid levels may be seen as blood cells separate from plasma. The cut surface of the lesion resembles a sponge permeated with blood and blood clots (Fig. 26-40). The walls and septa are composed of granulation tissue with multinucleated giant cells and occasional osteoid trabeculae.

CLINICAL FEATURES: Although some aneurysmal bone cysts tend to grow slowly, most expand rapidly and may be enormous. They usually manifest with

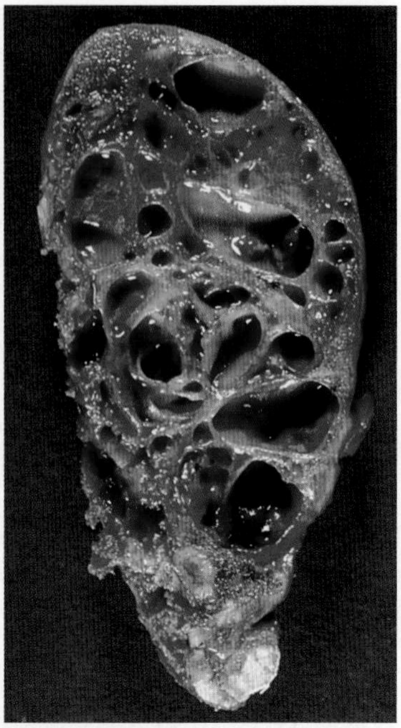

FIGURE 26-40. **Aneurysmal bone cyst.** In cross-section, the lesion consists of a spongy mass containing multiple blood-filled cysts. Some of the septa between the cysts contain bony tissue.

pain and swelling, sometimes in relation to trauma, and often develop in a short period of time. A bone cyst may "blow out," that is, rupture and produce local hemorrhage. Treatment is usually extraperiosteal excision and curettage. At surgery, incising the cyst decreases its internal pressure, causing brisk bleeding that may be difficult to control. In sites such as the vertebral column or the pelvis, selective arterial embolization has been successful.

Osteoid Osteoma Is a Benign, Painful Lesion

It composed of osseous tissue (the nidus) and surrounded by a halo of reactive bone formation. The typical patient is between 5 and 25 years old. Boys are affected more often than girls (3:1). Osteoid osteoma frequently arises in the cortex of the diaphysis of the tubular bones of the leg.

PATHOGENESIS: Osteoid osteoma have limited tumor growth potential and do not metastasize. Chromosomal analysis of a few osteoid osteomas has disclosed abnormalities of chromosome 22q13 and loss of part of 17q, which suggests that osteoid osteomas are neoplasms.

PATHOLOGY: Osteoid osteoma is a spherical, hyperemic tumor, about 1 cm in diameter, which is considerably softer than the surrounding bone (Fig. 26-41) and easily enucleated at surgery. Microscopically, the tumor is composed of thin, irregular, trabeculae within a cellular granulation tissue containing osteoblasts and osteoclasts. Trabeculae are more mature in the center, which is often partially calcified. Reactive, sclerotic bone surrounds the nidus.

CLINICAL FEATURES: Pain, typically nocturnal, is out of proportion to the size of the lesion. It is often exacerbated by drinking alcohol, and promptly relieved by aspirin, possibly because of the high prostaglandin content of the tumor and nerve fibers within the tumor. Surgical excision or radioablation (electric probe inserted into the tumor) is curative and leaves the patient very grateful to the surgeon.

Osteoblastoma Is Not Painful

Osteoblastoma is an uncommon, benign neoplasm histologically similar to osteoid osteoma but larger and not accompanied by nocturnal pain relieved by aspirin. It stimulates less bone reaction and appears as a purely radiolucent lesion, with only a thin shell of surrounding bone. Osteoblastoma occurs in persons between the ages of 10 and 35 years, with no sex predilection and mainly affects the spine and long bones. Curettage cures small osteoblastomas, but larger lesions may require wide resection.

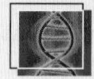

PATHOGENESIS: Several chromosomal and molecular abnormalities have been describedin oseoblastoma. However, no consistent abnormality has emerged. Aneuploid to hyperdiploid karyotypes have been demonstrated. *MDM2* gene amplification and *TP53* gene deletion implicate cell cycle abnormalities in the pathogenesis of osteoblastoma.

A

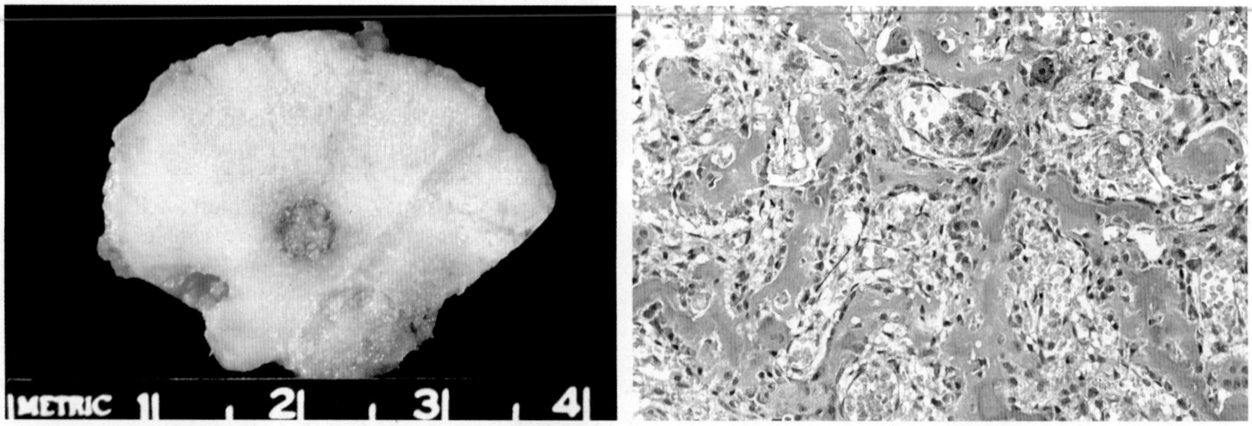

B

FIGURE 26-41. **Osteoid osteoma. A.** A gross specimen of an osteoid osteoma shows the central nidus, which is embedded in dense bone. **B.** A photomicrograph of the nidus reveals irregular trabeculae of woven bone surrounded by osteoblasts, osteoclasts, and fibrovascular marrow.

Solitary Chondroma Features Hyaline Cartilage

Solitary chondroma (enchondroma) is a benign, intraosseous tumor composed of well-differentiated hyaline cartilage. Although its neoplastic nature has been questioned, cytogenetic analyses show chromosomal abnormalities in some chondromas, suggesting that they are in fact neoplasms. The diagnosis is made at any age, and many cases are entirely asymptomatic.

PATHOLOGY: Most solitary chondromas occur in the metacarpals and phalanges of the hands, the remainder being in almost any other tubular bone. The tumor is small and grows slowly. Radiologically, it appears as a well-delimited radiolucent area, sometimes containing stippled calcifications. On gross examination, solitary chondromas have the semitranslucent appearance of hyaline cartilage, often with a few calcified areas. Microscopically, the cartilaginous tissue is well differentiated, with sparse chondrocytes. Asymptomatic chondromas are best left untreated. When pain intervenes, curettage and bone grafting are the treatment of choice.

Chondroblastoma Occurs in the Epiphyses of Long Bones

Chondroblastoma is an uncommon, benign chondrogenic tumor that favors the upper femur, tibia, and humerus. It is more common in males than in females (2:1), and 90% of cases occur in young persons between the ages of 5 and 25.

PATHOGENESIS: Genetic abnormalities suggest a neoplastic origin of chondroblastoma including aneuploidy, abnormalities involving chromosomes 5 and 8 and mutations in *TP53*.

PATHOLOGY: Chondroblastoma grows slowly, and on radiologic examination, displays an eccentric, radiolucent appearance with sharply defined borders (Fig. 26-42). On gross examination, the tumor is soft and compact with scattered gray or hemorrhagic areas. Microscopically, primitive chondroblasts are arranged as sheets of round-to-polyhedral cells that have well-defined cytoplasmic borders and large, ovoid nuclei, often with prominent nuclear grooves. The cartilage matrix is variably calcified and appears primitive. This accounts for the mottled pattern often seen in computed tomography (CT) scans.Well developed hyaline cartilage as seen in enchondroma is not found in chondroblastoma. Chondroblastoma causes bone destruction by stimulating osteoclastic resorption. In fact, these tumors may perforate the cortex, although they remain confined by the periosteum.

CLINICAL FEATURES: Because of its paraarticular location, chondroblastoma tend to cause joint pain, with mild swelling and functional limitation of joint movement. If neglected, they may rarely attain large size, destroy the epiphyseal area and invade the joint. Curettage is the treatment of choice, although in 10% of cases, the tumor recurs.

Chondromyxoid Fibroma Expresses Various Collagens

Chondromyxoid fibroma is a rare, benign cartilage-like tumor of bone that occurs in the femur or tibia of children and young adults. The tumor is also found occasionally in almost any bone.

PATHOGENESIS: Chondromyxoid fibroma is composed of tumor cells with fibroblastic or chondrocytic differentiation. Non-random clonal chromosomal rearrangement of 6q has been described. Gene expression and tumor matrix analyses have shown expression of collagens type II (chondrocytic differentiation), type I, III, and VI as well as expression of certain proteoglycans. This expression profile seems to be unique to chondromyxoid fibroma. How this expression pattern and abnormalities of chromosome 6q relate to the development of this tumor is not understood.

PATHOLOGY: Radiologically, chondromyxoid fibroma is identified as an eccentric, lucent defect with a thin scalloped border of sclerotic bone. On gross examination, the tumor is a firm, lobulated, grayish white or yellowish mass that replaces bone and thins the cortex. Microscop-

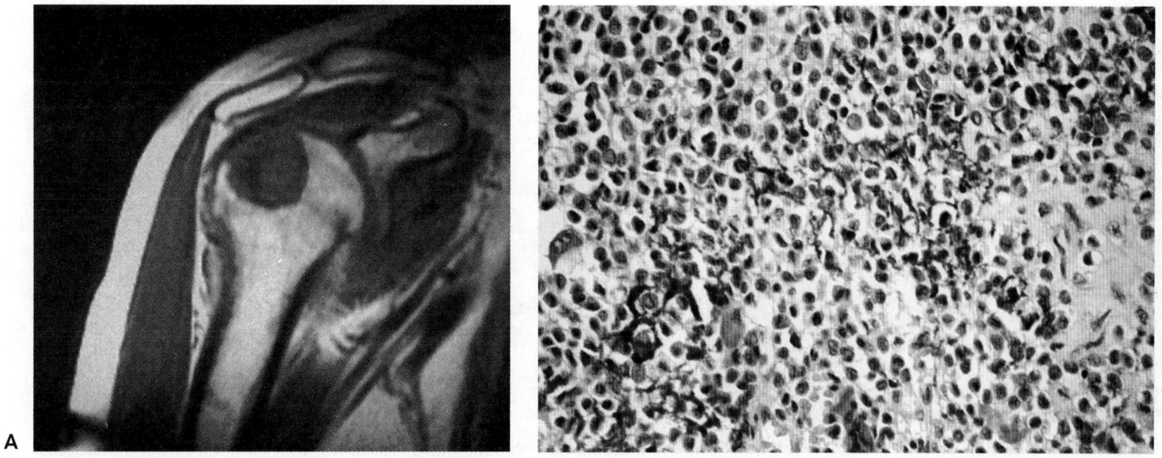

FIGURE 26-42. **Chondroblastoma. A.** A magnetic resonance image of the shoulder of a child shows a prominent lytic lesion of the head of the humerus that involves the epiphysis and extends across the epiphyseal plate. **B.** The histologic appearance of a chondroblastoma is defined by plump, round cells (chondroblasts) surrounded by a mineralized primitive chondroid matrix.

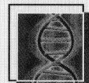

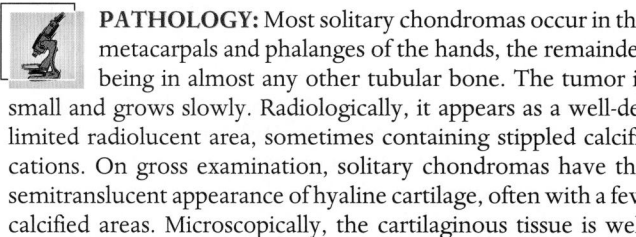

ically, sparsely cellular lobules show spindle and stellate cells and multinucleated giant cells embedded within a chondroid or myxoid matrix. The lobules are usually separated by bands of highly cellular tissue composed of plump, round, mononuclear cells, and multinucleated cells similar to those seen in chondrosarcoma. The distinct lobulation of the tumor and its characteristic sclerotic borders are important, because in some instances, the presence of large, pleomorphic cells in its chondroid matrix has led to an erroneous diagnosis of chondrosarcoma. Chondromyxoid fibroma is best treated by surgical excision because the tumor tends to recur after simple curettage.

Malignant Tumors of Bone

Osteosarcoma Is the Most Common Primary Malignant Bone Tumor

Osteosarcoma, also termed ***osteogenic sarcoma****, is a highly malignant bone tumor characterized by formation of bone tissue by tumor cells.* It represents one fifth of all bone cancers and is most frequent in adolescents between 10 and 20 years old, affecting boys more often than girls (2:1).

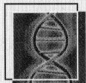

PATHOGENESIS: Osteosarcomas are associated with mutations in tumor suppressor genes: almost two thirds show mutations in the retinoblastoma *(Rb)* gene (see Chapter 5) and many also have mutations in the *p53* gene. There are also many other chromosomal and molecular abnormalities pertaining to apoptosis, replicative potential, insensitivity to growth inhibitory signals, and cell cycle regulation that contribute in some part to the development of osteosarcoma. For example, amplification of *MDM2, CDK4,* and *PRIM1* as well as overexpressin of *MET* and *FOS* have been detected in a significant proportion of cases. The tumor is more common in tall persons. Interestingly, osteosarcomas in dogs are more frequent in large breeds. When they arise in older persons, they almost always occur in the context of Paget disease or radiation exposure. For example, radium watch dial painters who wetted their brushes by licking them developed osteosarcoma many years later due to deposition of radium in their bones. Today, osteosarcoma can develop in adults and children previously subjected to external, therapeutic radiation for some other tumor such as lymphoma. Several preexisting benign bone lesions are associated with an increased risk of developing osteosarcoma, including fibrous dysplasia, osteomyelitis, and bone marrow infarcts. Although trauma may call attention to an existing osteosarcoma, there is no evidence that it ever causes the tumor.

PATHOLOGY: Osteosarcoma often arises near the knee. The lower femur (Fig. 26-43A), upper tibia, or fibula, although any metaphyseal area of a long bone may be affected. The proximal humerus is the second most common site: 75% of osteosarcomas arise adjacent to the knee or shoulder.

Radiologic evidence of bone destruction and bone formation is characteristic, the latter representing neoplastic bone. Often, the periosteum produces an incomplete rim of reactive bone adjacent to the site where it is lifted from the cortical surface by the tumor. When this appears on an x-ray as a shell of bone intersecting the cortex at one end and open at the other end, it is referred to as **Codman triangle**. A "sunburst" periosteal reaction is also often superimposed (see Fig. 26-17).

The gross appearance of the tumor is highly variable, depending on the proportions of bone, cartilage, stroma, and blood vessels. The cut surface may show any combination of hemorrhagic, cystic, soft, and bony areas. The neoplastic tissue may

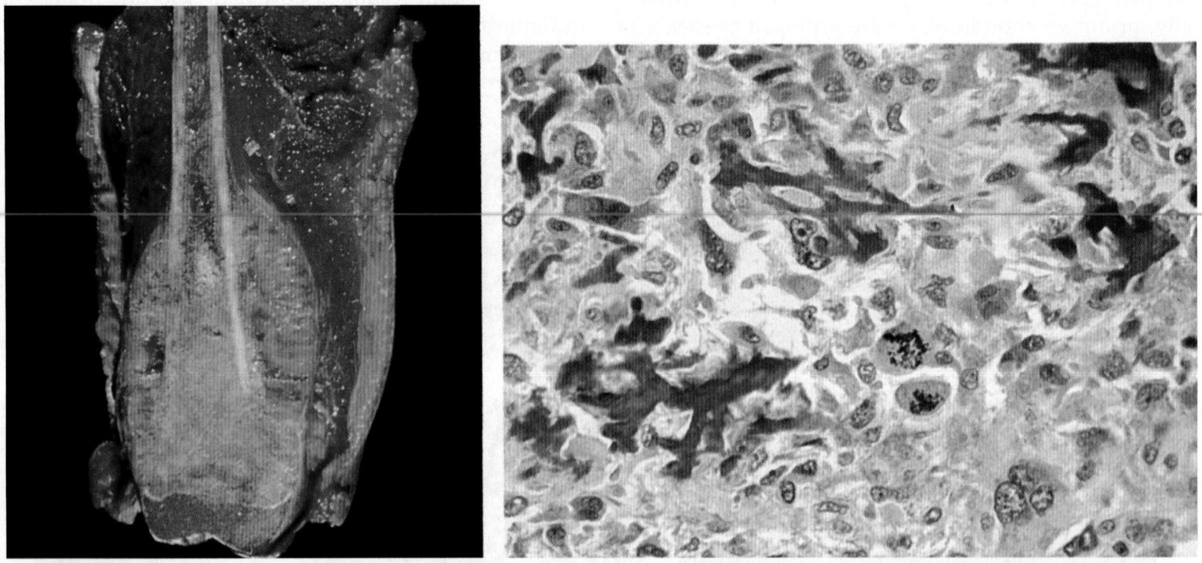

A B

FIGURE 26-43. **Osteosarcoma. A.** The distal femur contains a dense osteoblastic malignant tumor that extends through the cortex into the soft tissue and the epiphysis. **B.** A photomicrograph reveals pleomorphic malignant cells, tumor giant cells, and mitoses. The tumor produces woven bone that is focally calcified.

invade and break through the cortex, spread into the marrow cavity, elevate or perforate the periosteum, or grow into the epiphysis and even reach the joint space.

Histologic examination reveals malignant cells with osteoblastic differentiation producing woven bone (see Fig. 26-43B). The malignant cells stain prominently for alkaline phosphatase and osteonectin. The tumorous bone is laid down haphazardly and not aligned along stress lines. Often, foci of malignant cartilage cells or pleomorphic giant cells are intermixed. In areas of osteolysis, nonneoplastic osteoclasts are found at the advancing front of the tumor.

Osteosarcoma spreads through the bloodstream to the lungs. In fact, almost all patients (98%) who die of this disease have lung metastases. Less commonly, the tumor metastasizes to other bones (35%), the pleura (33%), and the heart (20%).

CLINICAL FEATURES: Osteosarcoma presents with mild or intermittent pain around the knee or other involved areas. As pain intensifies, the area becomes swollen and tender. The adjacent joint becomes functionally limited. Serum alkaline phosphatase is increased in half of patients and may decrease after amputation, only to increase again with recurrence or metastasis. Metastatic disease heralds rapid clinical deterioration and death.

Historically, osteosarcoma was treated exclusively by amputation or disarticulation of the involved limb, but the prognosis for 5-year survival did not exceed 20%. Today, standard therapy of chemotherapy and limb-sparing surgery gives 5-year disease-free rates from 60% to 80%. Resection of isolated pulmonary metastases may prolong survival.

Juxtacortical osteosarcoma is a rare variant of osteosarcoma that occurs on the periosteal surface of the bone, especially the lower posterior metaphysis of the femur (72% of cases). Unlike classic osteosarcoma, most patients are older than 25 years, and the tumor is more common in women. Juxtacortical osteosarcoma spares the deep cortex and medulla of the bone and grows external to the shaft. Usually, Codman triangle is not evident radiologically, because the periosteum is not elevated. Most juxtacortical osteosarcomas are low-grade lesions, and do not require adjunctive chemotherapy. Surgical excision is the treatment of choice. The prognosis is good, with a 5-year survival of more than 80%.

Chondrosarcoma Is a Cartilaginous Malignancy Whose Grade Determines Prognosis

Chondrosarcoma is a malignant tumor of cartilage which arise from a pre-existing cartilage rest or enchondroma. Some patients have a history of enchondromas, solitary osteochondroma, or hereditary multiple osteochondromas. Most have no known preexisting lesion. Chondrosarcoma is the second most common primary malignant bone tumor, occurring more commonly in men than in women (2:1). It is most frequently seen in the fourth to sixth decades (average age, 45 years).

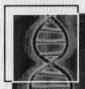

PATHOGENESIS: Numerous nonrandom chromosomal abnormalities have been discovered in chondrosarcoma. There probably is a different molecular mechanism resulting in tumor development between central chondrosarcoma and secondary peripheral chondrosarcoma (tumors arising in the cartilaginous cap of an osteochondroma) (see below). The latter may develop by upregulation of PTHrP and Bcl-2 expression in an osteochondroma along with mutations in other genes such as *TP53* and nonspecific chromosomal abnormalities. Development of central chondrosarcoma is related at least in part to abnormalities of chromosome 9p12-22 which may involve the *CDKN2A* tumor suppressor gene. The transcription factor *SOX9,* which plays a critical role in normal chondrocyte development, is expressed in chondrosarcomas.

PATHOLOGY: Chondrosarcoma occurs in three anatomical variants:

CENTRAL CHONDROSARCOMA: This form arises in the medullary cavity of pelvic bones, ribs, and long bones, although any site may be affected. Radiologically, poorly defined borders, a thickened shaft and perforation of the cortex characterize these tumors. There are usually stippled radiopacities or ringlike ossifications representing calcification or endochondral ossification in the tumor (Fig 26-44A). Although central chondrosarcoma may penetrate the cortex, extension beyond the periosteum is uncommon. On gross examination, the neoplastic cartilaginous tissue is compressed inside the bone and exhibits areas of necrosis, cystic change and hemorrhage (see Fig 26-44B). The cortex of the bone and the intertrabecular spaces of the marrow are infiltrated by the tumor.

Central chondrosarcoma begins with deep pain, which becomes more intense with time. In most cases, the tumor cannot be palpated, but in untreated cases, large masses may eventually form.

PERIPHERAL CHONDROSARCOMA: This variant is less common than the central variety of chondrosarcoma and arises outside the bone, almost always in the cartilaginous cap of an osteochondroma. It occurs after the age of 20 years and never before puberty. The most frequent location of peripheral chondrosarcoma is the pelvis, followed by the femur, vertebrae, sacrum, humerus, and other long bones. It arises only rarely distal to the knee or elbow. Radiologically, characteristic radiopacities representing calcification or ossification of the neoplastic cartilage are virtually pathognomonic for the lesion. Macroscopically, peripheral chondrosarcoma tends to be a large bosselated mass that surrounds the base of an osteochondroma and invades the bone.

Peripheral chondrosarcoma is usually seen as a slowly growing mass. Expansion of the mass causes pain and local symptoms. In the pelvis, the lumbosacral plexus may be compressed and tumors in the vertebrae may cause paraplegia.

JUXTACORTICAL CHONDROSARCOMA: This is the least common variety of chondrosarcoma and is similar to central chondrosarcoma in its predilection for middle-aged men. It tends to be situated in the metaphysis of long bones, lying on the outer surface of the cortex. Thus it is probably periosteal or parosteal in origin. Radiologically, it may be entirely translucent or focally calcified. The symptoms of juxtacortical chondrosarcoma are dominated by swelling, with little accompanying pain.

Histologically, chondrosarcomas are composed of malignant cartilage cells in various stages of maturity (see Fig. 26-44C). Occasionally, a well-differentiated chondrosarcoma is difficult to

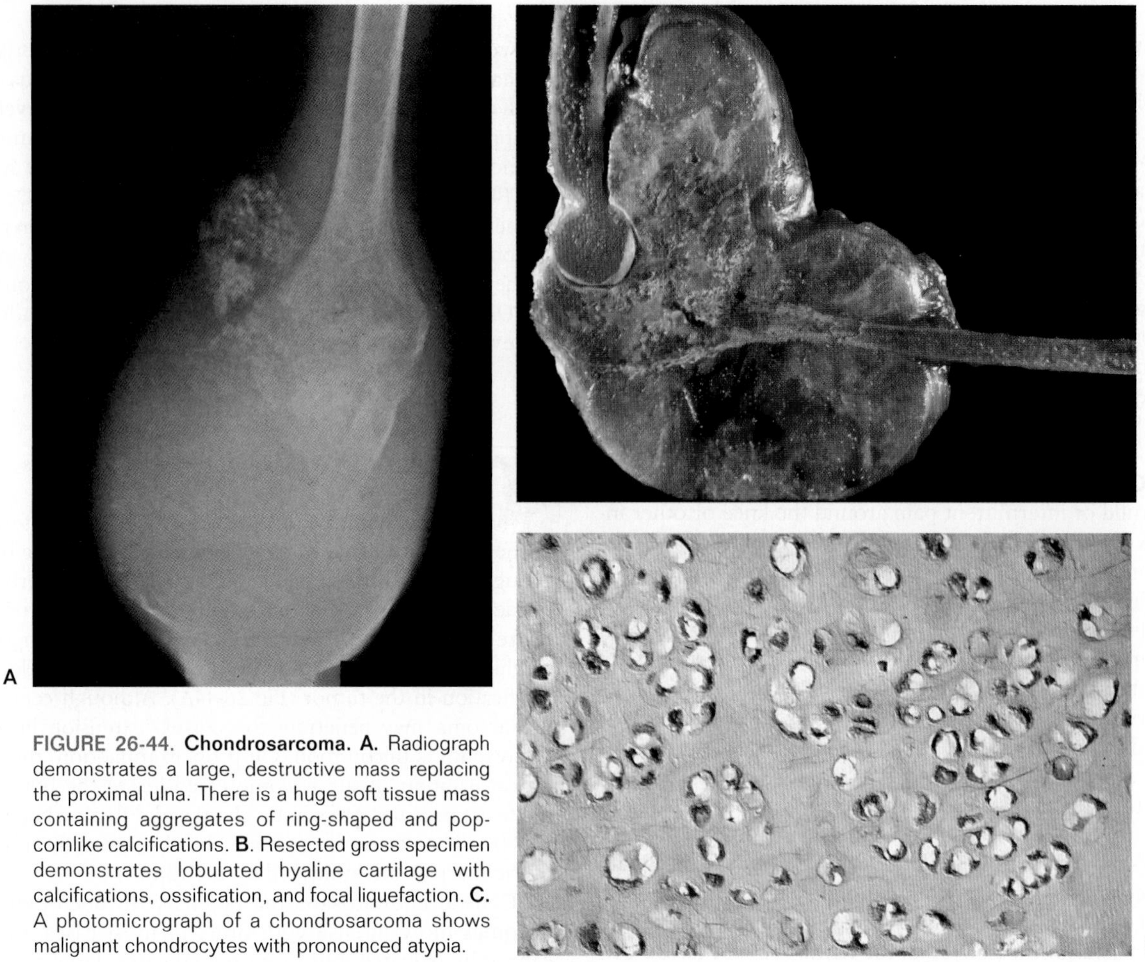

FIGURE 26-44. **Chondrosarcoma. A.** Radiograph demonstrates a large, destructive mass replacing the proximal ulna. There is a huge soft tissue mass containing aggregates of ring-shaped and popcornlike calcifications. **B.** Resected gross specimen demonstrates lobulated hyaline cartilage with calcifications, ossification, and focal liquefaction. **C.** A photomicrograph of a chondrosarcoma shows malignant chondrocytes with pronounced atypia.

distinguish from a benign tumor on cytologic grounds alone. Zones of calcification are often conspicuous and are seen radiographically as splotches or bulky masses. Chondrosarcoma expands by stimulating osteoclastic resorption of bone and often breaks through the cortex. Most chondrosarcomas grow slowly, but hematogenous metastases to the lungs are common in poorly differentiated variants.

There is a positive correlation between histologic grade, histomorphology, and the degree of karyotypic complexity. Trisomy 7 is associated with chondrosarcoma. Rearrangement of the short arm of chromosome 17 is associated with high-grade chondrosarcoma. Alterations of 12q13 are associated with tumors exhibiting myxoid features. Extraskeletal myxoid chondrosarcomas have a classical translocation (9;22)(q31;q12).

OTHER VARIANTS OF CHONDROSARCOMA: The above forms of condrosarcoma are conventional forms in that they are characterized by a hyaline cartilage matrix. Uncommon histopathologic variants of chondrosarcoma include **clear cell chondrosarcoma** which occurs almost exclusively in the proximal epiphysis of the femur or humerus and is composed of chondrocytes with abundant clear cytoplasm, areas of woven trabecular bone, and areas with a hyaline cartilage matrix. The prognosis for this tumor following complete excision is close to that of conventional low grade chondrosarcoma. **Dedifferentiated chondrosarcoma** is defined as a high grade nonchondrogenic pleomorphic sarcoma (e.g., osteosarcoma or fibrosarcoma) arising in association with a low-grade conventional chondrosarcoma or enchondroma. This tumor usually arises in flat bones of the pelvis or long bones of the extremities and has a dismal prognosis with less than 10% surviving 5 years despite surgery and chemotherapy. One other variant is known as **mesenchymal chondrosarcoma** and is histologically characterized by a two distinct components. The first is a high grade malignant small round blue cell tumor that resembles Ewing's sarcoma. Sheets of these cells are interrupted by discrete islands of malignant hyaline cartilage tumor histologically similar to conventional chondrosarcoma. The bones of the jaw and the chest wall are the most commonly affected sites. The prognosis for these tumors is poor.

CLINICAL FEATURES: Patients generally present with pain at the affected site. Chondrosarcoma is one of the few tumors in which microscopic grading has a significant prognostic value. The 5-year survival rate for low-grade conventional chondrosarcomas is 80%, for moderate-grade tumors about 50%, and for high-grade tumors only 20%. Wide excision is the usual treatment.

Giant Cell Tumor of Bone Rarely Metastasizes

Giant cell tumor (GCT) of bone is a locally aggressive, potentially malignant neoplasm characterized by the presence of osteoclastic, multinucleated, giant cells randomly and uniformly distributed in a background of proliferating mononuclear cells. It usually occurs in the third and fourth decades, has a slight predilection for women, and seems to be more common in Asia than in Western countries. GCTs in the elderly may be secondary to irradiation. Paget disease may produce a giant cell reactive lesion that closely resembles a true GCT. The neoplasms are thought to arise from primitive stromal cells that can modulate into osteoclasts.

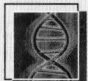

PATHOGENESIS: GCT is composed of osteoclastic giant cells and two lineages of mononuclear cells. One population of mononuclear cells is believed to be of macrophage-monocyte origin and is likely non-neoplastic. The other mononuclear cell population has chromosomal abnormalities and molecular alterations in oncogenes such as *TP53* and c-*myc*.

PATHOLOGY: In most cases (90%), GCT of bone originates at the junction between the metaphysis and the epiphysis of a long bone, with more than half being situated in the knee area (distal femur and proximal tibia; Fig. 26-45A). The lower end of the radius, humerus, and fibula are also occasionally involved. The neoplasm is often a lytic lesion that grows slowly enough to allow a periosteal reaction. Thus, radiologically, the tumor tends to be surrounded by a thin, bony shell and expands the bone. Often, it has a multiloculated or "soap bubble" appearance, representing endosteal resorption of the bone.

On gross examination, GCT is clearly circumscribed, and its cut surface is soft and light brown, without bone or calcification. Numerous hemorrhagic areas result in the appearance of a sponge full of blood. In some cases, cystic cavities and necrotic areas are present. GCT is often limited by the periosteum, although aggressive forms penetrate the cortex and the periosteum, even reaching the joint capsule and the synovial membrane.

Microscopically, GCT exhibits two types of cells (see Fig. 26-45B). The mononuclear ("stromal") cells are plump and oval, with large nuclei and scanty cytoplasm. Large osteoclastic giant cells, some with more than 100 nuclei, are scattered throughout the richly vascularized stroma. Diffuse interstitial hemorrhage is common. On low power examination, the tumor often appears as a syncytium of nuclei with poor demarcation of cytoplasmic borders and random, distribution of the giant cells. It is thought that the mononuclear cells are the neoplastic and proliferative components of GCT (mitotic activity is common in the mononuclear cells but is not observed in the giant cells). Indeed, the diagnosis of malignancy in a GCT depends upon the morphology of the mononuclear cells rather than that of the multinucleated cells.

CLINICAL FEATURES: Although the vast majority of GCTs are considered benign, but locally aggressive tumors with the potential to locally recur, all GCTs must be viewed as potentially "malignant," because rarely after simple curettage they may metastasize to distant sites, particularly the lungs. Virtually all metastases have occurred after an initial surgical intervention and have the benign histology of the primary tumor. In contrast to patients with lung metastases from other malignant bone tumors, most of these patients may enjoy an essentially normal life span, especially if the metastatic deposits are few and can be surgically removed. Thus, historical belief has been that local recurrence of the tumor reflects inadequate resection rather than biological aggressiveness, and that distant metastases may result from dislodgment of tumor fragments during surgery.

True malignancy in GCT may be occasionally observed as either a sarcomatous lesion arising in a typical GCT or as a pure sarcoma after a GCT has been curetted. Recurrence as pure sarcoma may occur spontaneously or after local radiation therapy. About 6% of GCTs demonstrate sarcomatous transformation.

GCTs manifest with pain, usually in the joint adjacent to the tumor. Microfractures and pathologic fractures are frequent, owing to thinning of the cortex. The tumor is usually treated with thorough curettage and bone grafting, although more aggressive management, including en bloc resection or even amputation, may be necessary. Local recurrence after simple curettage has been reported in one-third to one-half of cases, and 5% to 10% metastasize.

Ewing Sarcoma Is a Primitive Neuroectodermal Tumor of Childhood

Ewing sarcoma (EWS) is an uncommon malignant bone tumor composed of small, uniform, round cells. It represents only 5% of all bone tumors and is found in children and adolescents, with two thirds of cases occurring in patients younger than 20 years. Boys are affected more often than girls (2:1). EWS is very rare in African-Americans.

A

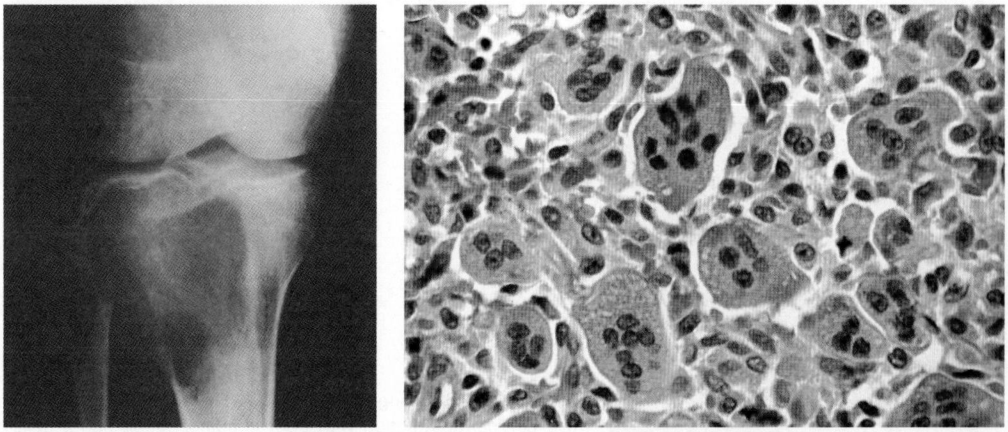

B

FIGURE 26-45. **Giant cell tumor of bone. A.** Radiograph of the proximal tibia shows an eccentric lytic lesion with virtually no new bone formation. The tumor extends to the subchondral bone plate and breaks through cortex into the soft tissue. **B.** Photomicrograph shows osteoclast-type giant cells and plump, oval, mononuclear cells. The nuclei of both types of cells are identical.

PATHOGENESIS: EWS is thought to arise from primitive marrow elements or immature mesenchymal cells. Virtually all (90%) of these tumors have a reciprocal translocation between chromosomes 11 and 22 [t(11;22)p(13;q12)], which results in the fusion of the amino terminus of the *EWS1* gene to the carboxy terminus of the *FLI-1* gene, which encodes a transcription factor. The resulting fusion protein, EWS/FLI-1, is an aberrant transcription factor whose target genes are not yet fully identified. A less common translocation t(21;22) leads to an *EWS/ERG* gene fusion and gives rise to a variant of EWS with a significantly worse prognosis.

PATHOLOGY: EWS is primarily a tumor of the long bones in childhood, especially the humerus, tibia, and femur, where it occurs as a midshaft or metaphyseal lesion. It tends to parallel the distribution of red marrow, so when it arises in the third decade or later, it affects the pelvis and spine. However, no bone is immune from involvement.

The radiographic findings are variable and depend upon the interaction of the tumor with the host bone. There is often a destructive process in which the border between normal bone and the lesion is indistinct (Fig. 26-46A). The onion-skin pattern of periosteal bone that is sometimes seen on radiologic examination represents circumferential discontinuous layers of periosteal new bone associated with a lytic lesion involving the medulla and endosteal surface of the cortex. Some patients present with fever and weakness as well as bone pain, so it is not surprising that their condition may be mistaken for osteomyelitis.

On gross examination, EWS is typically soft and grayish white, often studded by hemorrhagic foci and necrotic areas. The tumor may infiltrate the medullary spaces without destroying the bony trabeculae. It may also diffusely infiltrate the cortical bone or form nodules in which the bone is completely resorbed. In many cases, the tumor mass penetrates the periosteum and extends into the soft tissues.

Microscopically, EWS cells appear as sheets of closely packed, small, round cells with little cytoplasm, which are up to twice the size of a lymphocyte (see Fig. 26-46B). Fibrous strands separate the sheets of cells into irregular nests. There is little or no interstitial stroma, and mitoses are infrequent. In some areas, the neoplastic cells tend to form rosettes. An important diagnostic feature is the presence of substantial amounts of glycogen in the cytoplasm of the tumor cells, which is well visualized with the periodic acid-Schiff (PAS) stain (see Fig 26-46B, *inset*). EWS cells also express characteristic antigens that can be detected by immunohistochemistry, some of which are part of the translocation product (e.g., FLI-1 and CD99).

EWS metastasizes to many organs, including the lungs and brain. Other bones, especially the skull, are common sites for metastases (50% to 75% of cases).

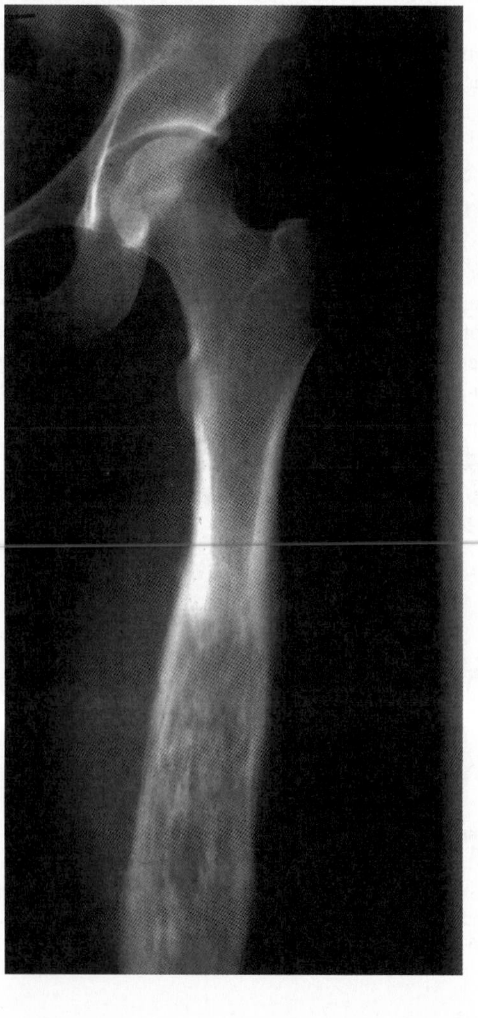

A

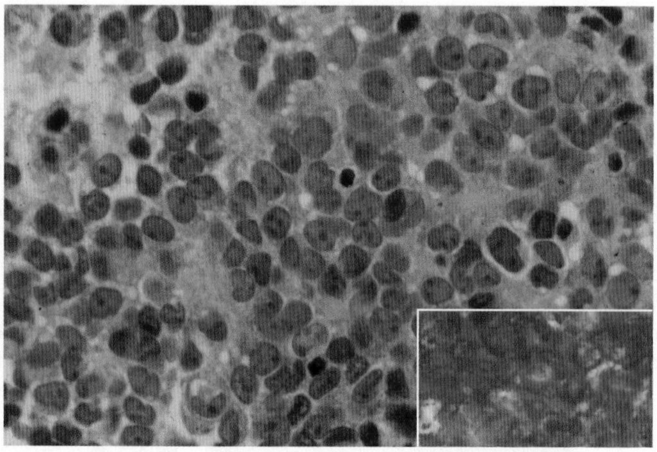

B

FIGURE 26-46. **Ewing sarcoma. A.** A clinical x-ray demonstrates expansile cortical destruction with poor circumscription and a delicate interrupted periosteal reaction. **B.** A biopsy specimen shows fairly uniform small cells with round, dark blue nuclei, paucity of mitotic activity, and poorly defined cytoplasm. A periodic acid-Schiff (PAS) stain demonstrates abundant intracellular glycogen (*inset*).

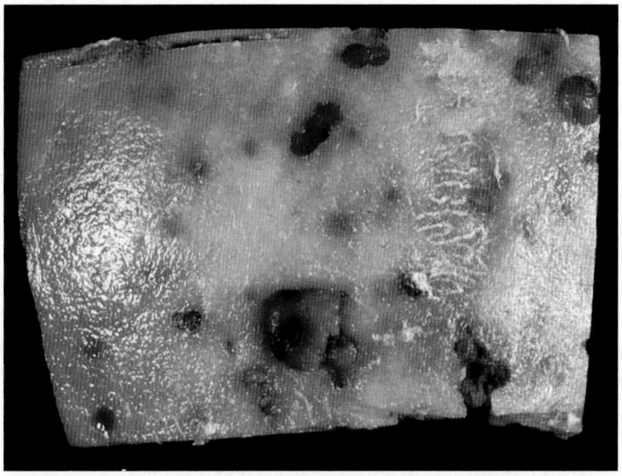

FIGURE 26-47. **Multiple myeloma.** A segment of the skull from a patient with multiple myeloma reveals numerous punched-out, lytic lesions.

CLINICAL FEATURES: EWS initially presents with mild pain, which becomes more intense and is followed by swelling of the affected area. Nonspecific symptoms, including fever and leukocytosis, commonly follow. In some cases, a soft tissue mass is encountered.

In the past, the prognosis of EWS was dismal, with 5-year survival rates of only 5% after surgery or radiation therapy. Today, with the use of chemotherapy combined with radiation and/or surgery, has now led to 5-year disease-free survivals of 60% to 75%.

Multiple Myeloma Produces Lytic Lesions

Malignant tumors of plasma cells may be either local (plasmacytoma) or diffuse (see Chapter 20). Multiple myeloma occurs mostly in older persons (average age, 65 years) and affects men twice as often as women. Because myeloma cells secrete cytokines that recruit osteoclasts, the lesions are unique in that they are almost exclusively lytic. The bones most frequently involved are the skull (Fig. 26-47), spine, ribs, pelvis, and femur. Pathologic fractures are common. On microscopic examination, sheets of plasma cells show varying degrees of maturity. Amyloid deposits, in both skeletal and extraskeletal sites, are seen in 10% of patients.

Despite irradiation and chemotherapy, the prognosis is poor (median survival is 32 months), with death is usually due to infection or kidney failure. Solitary plasmacytoma has a better prognosis, with a 60% 5-year survival.

Metastatic Tumors Are the Most Common Malignant Tumors in Bone

Most metastatic lesions to bone are carcinomas, particularly of the breast, prostate, lung, thyroid, and kidney. It is estimated that skeletal metastases are found in at least 85% of cancer cases that have run their full clinical course. The vertebral column is, by far, the most common site. Tumor cells usually arrive in the bone via the bloodstream; in the case of spinal metastases, the vertebral veins often transport them.

Some tumors (thyroid, gastrointestinal tract, kidney, neuroblastoma) produce mostly lytic lesions by stimulating osteoclasts. A few neoplasms (prostate, breast, lung, stomach) stimulate osteoblastic components to make bone (Fig. 26-48A), creating dense foci on radiographs. However, most deposits of metastatic cancer in the bones have mixtures of both lytic and blastic elements (see Fig. 26-48B).

JOINTS

A joint (or articulation) is a union between two or more bones, whose construction varies with the function of that joint. There are two types of joints: (1) **a synovial or diarthrodial joint,** which is a movable joint, such as the knee or elbow, that is lined by a synovial membrane; and (2) **a synarthrosis,** which is a joint that has little movement.

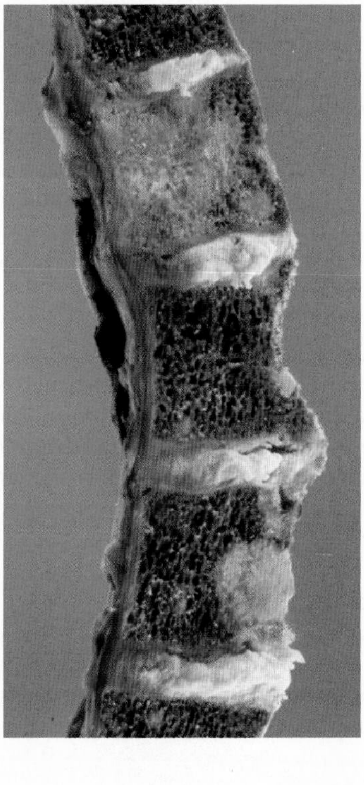

A

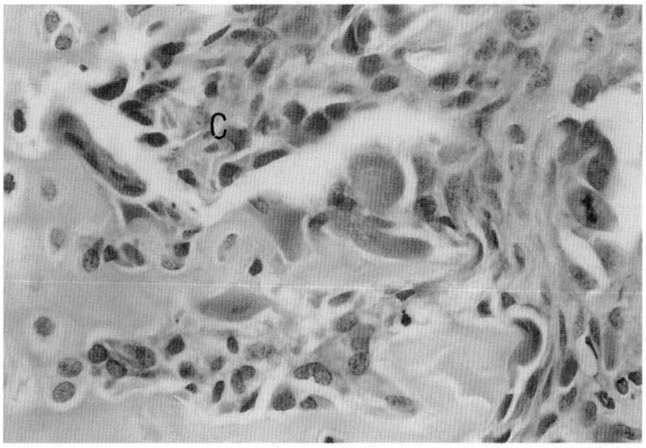

B

FIGURE 26-48. **Metastatic carcinoma to bone. A.** A section through the vertebral column reveals conspicuous tan nodules of metastatic tumor. **B.** Tumor-induce osteolysis. Breast cancer (C) metastatic to bone recruits numerous osteoclasts (*red-staining cells*), which resorb bone and lead to osteolytic lesions.

Synarthroses are further divided into four subclassifications:

- **A symphysis** is an articulation joined by fibrocartilaginous tissue and firm ligaments that allows little movement. Examples are the symphysis pubis and the ends of vertebral joints.
- **A synchondrosis** is found at the ends of bones and has articular cartilage but is not associated with synovium or a significant joint cavity, e.g., the sternal manubrial joint.
- **A syndesmosis** connects bones by fibrous tissue without any cartilaginous elements. The distal tibiofibular articulation and the cranial sutures are syndesmoses.
- **A synostosis** is a pathologic bony bridge between bones, as occurs with ankylosis of the spine.

Diseases of diarthrodial joints are among the oldest pathologic conditions known, having been found in the fossil bones of dinosaurs. One third of the population of the United States older than 50 years develop some form of clinically significant joint disease.

Classification of Synovial Joints

The synovial, or diarthrodial, joints are classified according to the type of movement they permit.

- **A uniaxial joint** allows movement around only one axis. Examples include a hinge joint such as the elbow and a pivot (rotational) joint, such as the radioulnar joint.
- **A biaxial joint** allows movement around two axes, as the condyloid joint of the wrist axis is oriented in the long diameter and the other along the short diameter of the articular surfaces. This allows four-way movement: flexion, extension, abduction, and adduction. In a saddle joint, such as the carpometacarpal joint of the thumb, joint surfaces allow movement as in a condyloid joint.
- **Polyaxial joints** permit movement in virtually any axis. In a ball-and-socket joint, such as is found in the shoulder and hip, all movements, including rotation, are possible.
- **A plane joint,** represented by the patella, allows the articular surfaces to glide over one another.

UNIT LOAD: The concept of unit load is the most important principle in understanding joint function. The unit load is the compressive force, expressed as kilograms per cubic centimeter of articular cartilage. It is fairly constant over the hip, knee and ankle (20 to 26 kg/cm^3 along the articular surfaces). Because the articular cartilage is injured if a load exceeds these values, several mechanisms protect a joint from exceeding the unit load.

Adjacent muscles are the major shock-absorbing structures that protect the joint. Deformation, even to the extent of microscopic fractures of the coarse cancellous bone, also helps protect the joint. Joint deformation allows the contact area to increase with increasing load. Diarthrodial joints may have intraarticular structures such as ligaments and menisci. Menisci hold distributed force along the articular surface and allow two planes of motion, such as flexion and rotation. However, 90% or more of energy absorption across the knee joint is by active muscle contraction and only 10% or less is by secondary mechanisms, such as by the coarse cancellous bone of the knee joint. A properly functioning joint also requires support from ligaments and tendons, periarticular connective tissues such as the joint capsule, and nerves that provide proprioception. *Thus, to protect the articular cartilage from forces that exceed the critical unit load virtually any structure is sacrificed, even to the point of a bone fracture.*

Once there is an insult to one component of the joint, the resulting dysfunction can lead to degeneration of other components of the joint. For example, knee ligament injuries sustained by athletes, such as a torn anterior cruciate ligament, can result in joint instability, which, over time, contributes to degeneration of articular cartilage due to changes in movement and load on the joint (secondary osteoarthritis).

ARTHRITIS: Arthritis is joint inflammation, usually accompanied by pain, swelling, and sometimes change in structure. Arthritis can generally be divided into two major forms: (1) **inflammatory arthritis** usually involving the synovium and mediated by inflammatory cells (e.g., rheumatoid arthritis) and (2) **noninflammatory arthritis,** as featured in primary osteoarthritis, may involve cytokines in its pathogenesis (see below).

Structures of the Synovial Joint

Movement plays a major role in the formation of a joint. Lack of movement retards joint development and may cause **arthrogryposis,** a rare but extremely crippling disease characterized by joint fusion.

Synovium

Synovial joints are partially lined on their internal aspects by the synovium. Synovial linings are not true membranes since they lack basement membranes to separate synovial lining cells from subsynovial tissue. The synovium is composed of one to three layers of lining cells, and is made up of two cell types distinguishable only by electron microscopy. **Type A cells** are macrophages with lysosomal enzymes and dense bodies. **Type B cells** secrete hyaluronic acid. Synovial cell membranes are disposed in villi and microvilli, an arrangement that creates an enormous surface area. It is estimated that the knee alone has 100 m^2 of synovial lining.

The synovium controls: (1) diffusion in and out of the joint; (2) ingestion of debris; (3) secretion of hyaluronate, immunoglobulins, and lysosomal enzymes; and (4) lubrication of the joints by secretion of glycoproteins. Synovial fluid is clear, sticky, and viscous, and is present only in small amounts, not exceeding 1 to 4 mL. It is the chief source of nourishment for chondrocytes of the articular cartilage, which lacks a blood supply. Synovial fluid is an ultrafiltrate that acts as a molecular sieve. It does not contain tissue thromboplastin and so cannot clot. α_2-Macroglobulin is absent, although it may accumulate in disease. Hyaluronate is a very large molecule. Because of it is highly charged, it has a high affinity for water.

Articular Cartilage

The hyaline cartilage that covers the articular ends of bones does not participate in endochondral ossification and is well suited for its dual role of absorbing shocks and lubricating the surfaces of movable joints. On gross examination, the articular cartilage is glistening, smooth, white, and semirigid and is generally not thicker than 6 mm.

Joint Histology

The articular surface appears smooth to the eye, but scanning electron microscopy reveals gentle waves and pits that correspond to the underlying lacunae of the surface chondrocytes. There are four zones in articular cartilage (Fig 26-49).

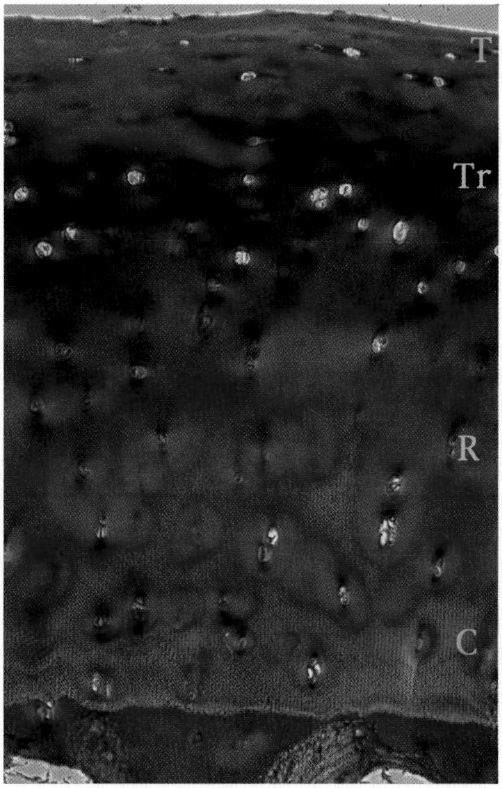

A

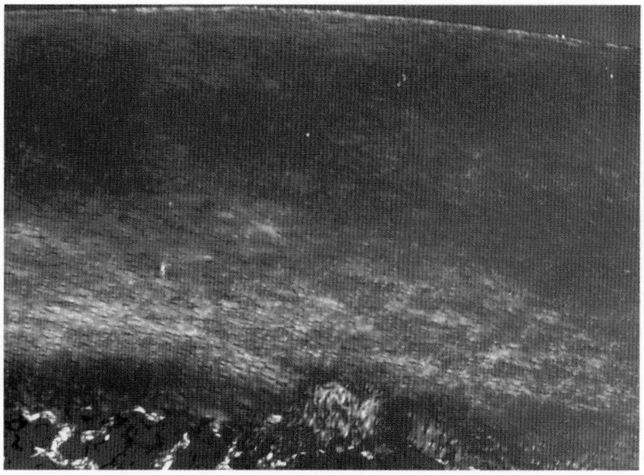

B

FIGURE 26-49. **Articular hyaline cartilage A** demonstrating tangential zone (T), transitional zone (Tr), radial zone (R), and calcified zone (C). The chondrocyte lacunae change shape in conformation with the direction of the collagen arcades in the cartilage. **B.** Articular cartilage, polarized light. The tangential and radial zones have the highest concentration of collagen fibers and appear bright yellow.

- **Tangential or gliding zone:** This is the region closest to the articular surface, where chondrocytes are elongated, flattened, and parallel to the long axis of the surface. Within this zone, a condensation of type II collagen fibers forms the so-called skin of the articular cartilage.
- **Transitional zone:** Chondrocytes in this slightly deeper zone are larger, ovoid, and more randomly distributed than those in the tangential zone. The standard hyaline cartilage matrix is present and by electron microscopy, the collagen fibers are arranged transverse to the articular surface.
- **Radial zone:** The next deeper zone is the radial zone, where chondrocytes are small and are arranged in short columns like those seen in the epiphyseal plate. In this area, collagen fibers are large and oriented perpendicular to the long axis of the articular surface.
- **Calcified zone:** Small chondrocytes and a heavily calcified matrix characterize the deepest region.

The calcified zone is separated from the radial zone by a transverse, undulating, heavily calcified "blue line" (evident on hematoxylin–eosin staining) called the **tidemark.** The tidemark is the interface between mineralized and unmineralized cartilage. Above the tidemark on the joint side, all of the cartilage is nourished by diffusion from the synovial fluid. Deep to the tidemark, the calcified cartilage is nourished by epiphyseal blood vessels.

The tidemark is the area where the cartilage cells are renewed. As a result of cell division, true articular chondrocytes migrate upward toward the joint surface. Cell division below the tidemark occurs in the calcified cartilage, if there is appropriate stimulation. For example, in acromegaly, when the epiphyseal plates have already closed, the bones may grow in minute increments, because growth hormone stimulates the calcified cartilage remnant of the epiphyseal cartilage anlage. Because the joints in acromegaly do not keep pace, joint incongruity leads to severe osteoarthritis. Deep to the calcified cartilage, the transverse bony plate, termed the **subchondral bone plate,** supports the articular cartilage. It is directly contiguous with the coarse cancellous bone of the epiphysis.

Osteoarthritis

Osteoarthritis is slowly progressive destruction of articular cartilage that affects weight-bearing joints and fingers of older persons, or the joints of younger persons subjected to trauma. Osteoarthritis is the single most common form of joint disease and the major form of noninflammatory arthritis. It is a group of conditions that have in common the mechanical destruction of a joint.

In **primary osteoarthritis**, destruction of joints to results from intrinsic defects in the joint cartilage. The prevalence and severity of primary osteoarthritis increases with age. Of 18- to 24-year-olds 4%, are affected; versus 85% of those 75 to 79 years. Before the age of 45, the disease mainly affects men. After age 55, osteoarthritis is more common in women. Many cases of primary osteoarthritis exhibit a familial clustering, suggesting a hereditary predisposition.

Primary osteoarthritis has variously been called **wear and tear arthritis** and **degenerative joint disease**. Progressive degradation of articular cartilage leads to joint narrowing, subchondral bone thickening, and eventually a nonfunctioning, painful joint. Although osteoarthritis is not primarily an inflammatory process, a mild inflammatory reaction may occur within the synovium.

Secondary osteoarthritis has a known underlying cause, including congenital or acquired incongruity of joints, trauma, crystal deposits, infection, metabolic diseases, endocrinopathies, inflammatory diseases, osteonecrosis, and hemarthrosis.

Chondromalacia is a term applied to a subcategory of osteoarthritis that affects the patellar surface of the femoral condyles of young persons and produces pain and stiffness of the knee.

PATHOGENESIS: Many factors play etiologic roles in osteoarthritis.

INCREASED UNIT LOAD: Abnormal force on the cartilage may have many causes, but is often attributable to incongruities of the joint. Thus, in congenital hip dysplasia, a fairly common abnormality, the socket of the acetabulum is shallow, covering only 30% to 40% of the femoral head (normal, 50%). Less surface is area covered by articular cartilage, which thus bears an increased load. When the critical unit load is exceeded, chondrocyte death causes degradation of articular cartilage.

RESILIENCE OF THE ARTICULAR CARTILAGE: Because articular cartilage binds extensive amounts of water, it normally has a swelling pressure of at least 3 atm. Disruption in water bonding resulting from the events discussed above leads to decreased resilience.

STIFFNESS OF SUBCHONDRAL COARSE CANCELLOUS BONE: The structure of bone adjacent to a joint is important in maintaining articular cartilage. Mechanical forces are not transferred to articular cartilage by normal stress, but rather are dissipated by microfractures of the coarse cancellous bone. Damage to the coarse cancellous bone results in an increased unit load on the cartilage because of an increase in the stiffness of subchondral bone, for example, in Paget disease.

BIOCHEMICAL ABNORMALITIES: The biochemical changes of osteoarthritis mainly involve proteoglycans. Proteoglycan content and aggregation decrease, and glycosaminoglycan chain length is reduced. Collagen fibers are thicker than normal and. the water content of osteoarthritic cartilage increases. The reduction in proteoglycans allows more water to be bound to the collagen. Thus, osteoarthritic cartilage, or any cartilage that is fibrillated, swells more than normal cartilage.

Although matrix synthesis by chondrocytes is increased early in osteoarthritis, protein synthesis eventually declines, suggesting that the cells reach a point at which they fail to respond to reparative stimuli. Similarly, chondrocytes in early osteoarthritic cartilage replicate, but cell replication diminishes with advanced disease. Acid cathepsin, which attacks the protein cores of the matrix macromolecules, increases in osteoarthritic cartilage. Collagenase is absent in normal cartilage, but is found in osteoarthritic cartilage.

GENETIC FACTORS: Studies of identical twins have demonstrated genetic contributions to the prevalence of osteoarthritis. Genetic analysis of patients with a type of familial, early-onset osteoarthritis revealed a variety of mutations in the gene for type II collagen *(COL2A1)*, the major collagen species of articular cartilage.

PATHOLOGY: Joints commonly affected by osteoarthritis are the proximal and distal interphalangeal joints of the arm, knees, and hips; and the cervical and lumbar segments of the spine. Radiologically, osteoarthritis is characterized by (1) narrowing of the joint space, which represents the loss of articular cartilage; (2) increased thickness of the subchondral bone; (3) subchondral bone cysts; and (4) large peripheral growths of bone and cartilage, called **osteophytes**. Histologic changes follow a well-described sequence.

1. First, loss of proteoglycans from the surface of the articular cartilage, is seen histologically as decreased metachromatic staining. At the same time, empty lacunae in articular cartilage indicate that chondrocytes have died (Fig. 26-50). Viable chondrocytes enlarge, aggregate into groups or clones and become surrounded by basophilic staining matrix called the **territorial matrix.**
2. Osteoarthritis may arrest at this stage for many years before progressing to the next stage, which is characterized by fibrillation (i.e., development of surface cracks parallel to the long axis of the articular surface). These fibrillations may persist for many years before further progression occurs.
3. As fibrillations propagate, synovial fluid begins to flow into the defects. The cracks are progressively oriented more vertically, parallel to the long axis of the collagen fibrils. Synovial fluid penetrates deeper into the articular cartilage along these cracks. Eventually, pieces of articular cartilage break off and lodge in the synovium, inducing inflammation and a foreign-body giant cell reaction. The result is a hyperemic and hypertrophied synovium.
4. As the crack extends down toward the tidemark and eventually crosses it, neovascularization from the epiphysis and subchondral bone extends into the area of the crack, inducing subchondral osteoclastic bone resorption. Adjacent osteoblastic activity also occurs and results in a thickening of the subchondral bone plate in the area of the crack. As neovascularization progressively extends into the area of the crack, mesenchymal cells invade and fibrocartilage forms as a poor substitute for the articular hyaline cartilage (Fig. 26-51A). These fibrocartilaginous plugs may persist, or they may be swept into the joint. The subchondral bone becomes exposed and burnished as it grinds against the opposite joint surface, which is undergoing the same process. These thick, shiny, smooth areas of subchondral bone are referred to as **eburnated** (ivorylike) bone.
5. In some areas, the eburnated bone cracks, allowing synovial fluid to extend from the joint surface into the subchondral bone marrow, where it eventually produces a **subchondral bone cyst** (see Fig. 26-51B). These cysts increase in size as synovial fluid is forced into the space but cannot exit. Eventually, osteoclasts resorb bone and osteoblasts attempt to wall off the area. The result is a subchondral bone cyst filled with synovial fluid, with a well-marginated, reactive bone wall.
6. An osteophyte develops, usually in the lateral portions of the joint, when the mesenchymal tissue of the synovium differentiates into osteoblasts and chondroblasts to form a mass of cartilage and bone. Osteophytes are pearly grayish bone nodules on the periphery of the joint surface. These osteophytes, or bony spurs, also occur at lateral edges of intervertebral disks, extending from the adjacent vertebral bodies. They produce the "lipping" pattern seen on radiologic studies as osteoarthritis of the spine. In the fingers, osteophytes at the distal interphalangeal joints are termed **Heberden nodes**.

CLINICAL FEATURES: The signs and symptoms of osteoarthritis are functions of the location of the involved joints and the severity and duration of the joint

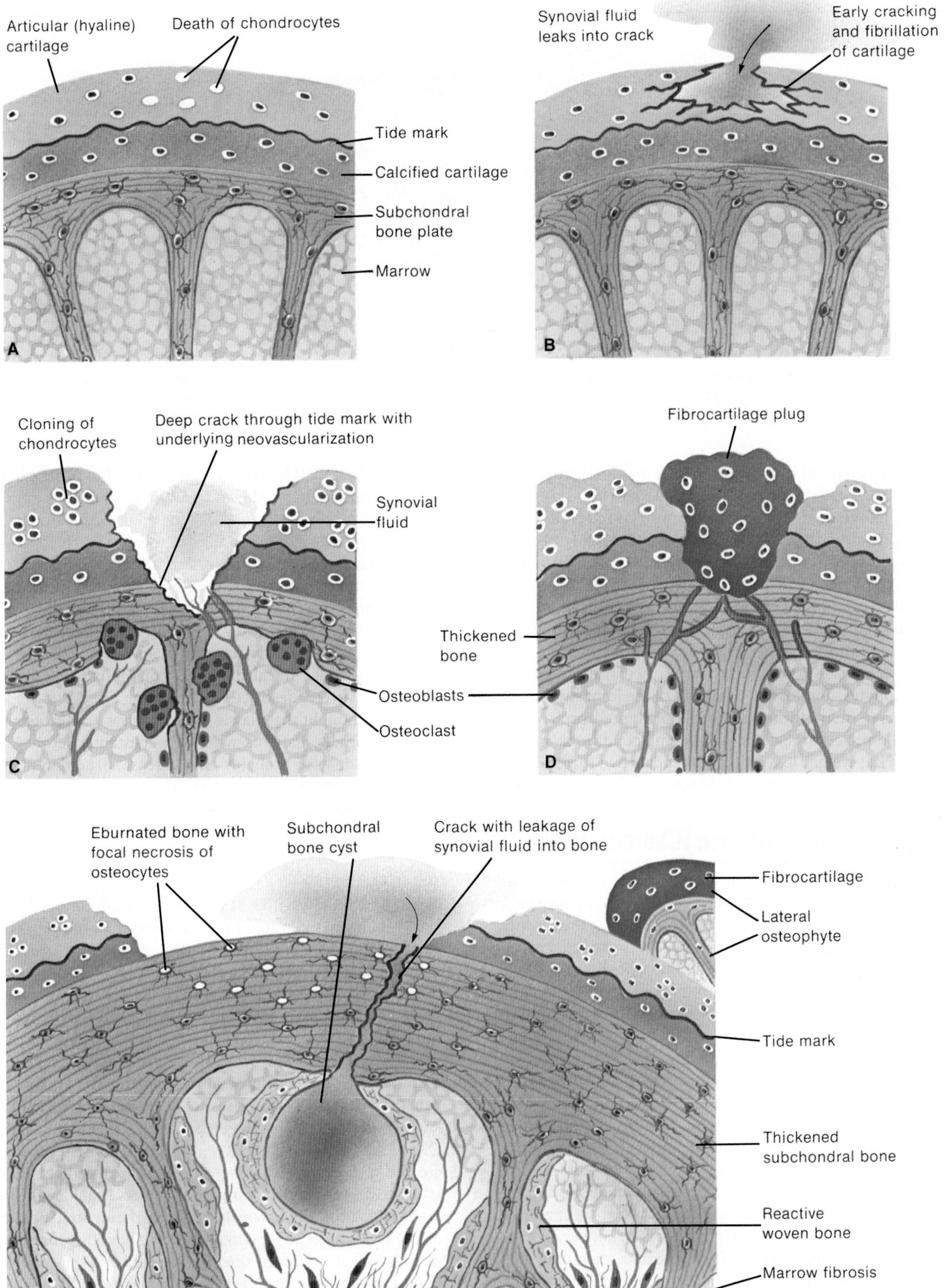

FIGURE 26-50. **Histogenesis of osteoarthritis. A and B.** The death of chondrocytes leads to a crack in the articular cartilage that is followed by an influx of synovial fluid and further loss and degeneration of cartilage. **C.** As a result of this process, cartilage is gradually worn away. Below the tidemark, new vessels grow in from the epiphysis, and fibrocartilage (**D**) is deposited. **E.** The fibrocartilage plug is not mechanically sufficient and may be worn away, thus exposing the subchondral bone plate, which becomes thickened and eburnated. If there is a crack in this region, synovial fluid leaks into the marrow space and produces a subchondral bone cyst. Focal regrowth of the articular surface leads to the formation of osteophytes.

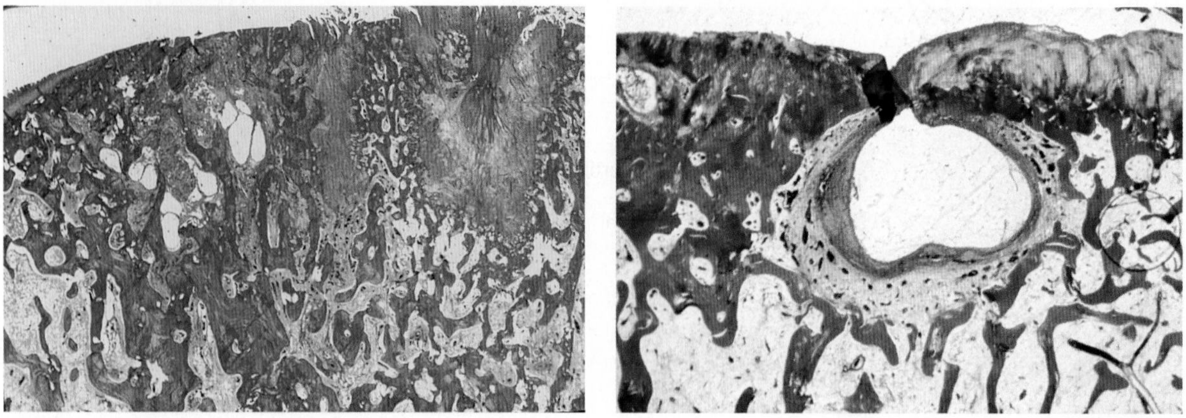

A B

FIGURE 26-51. **Osteoarthritis. A.** A femoral head with osteoarthritis shows a fibrocartilaginous plug *(far right)* extending from the marrow onto the joint surface. Eburnated bone is present over the remaining surface. **B.** A section through the articular surface of an osteoarthritic joint demonstrates focal absence of the articular cartilage, thickening of subchondral bone *(left),* and a subchondral bone cyst.

deterioration. Physical findings vary. The involved joints may be enlarged, tender, and boggy and may demonstrate crepitus. Deep, achy joint pain that follows activity and is relieved by rest is the clinical hallmark of osteoarthritis. Pain is usually a sign of significant joint destruction and arises in the periarticular structures, since articular cartilage lacks a nerve supply. Discomfort also is caused by short periods of stiffness, which is frequently experienced in the morning or after periods of minimal activity. Restricted joint motion indicates severe disease and may result from joint or muscle contractures, intraarticular loose bodies, large osteophytes, and loss of congruity of the joint surfaces.

At present osteoarthritis cannot be prevented or arrested. Therapy is directed at specific orthopedic conditions and includes exercise, weight loss, and other supportive measures. In disabling osteoarthritis, joint replacement may be necessary.

Neuropathic Joint Disease (Charcot Joint)

Neuropathic joint disease is a form of noninflammatory arthritis characterized by progressive joint destruction due to a primary neurologic disorder such as peripheral neuropathy or central motor abnormality. In the mid-19th century, Jean-Martin Charcot described destruction of knee joints in patients with syphilitic tabes dorsalis (Charcot joint). Today, the most common form of neuropathic joint disease is destruction of foot joints in people with diabetic peripheral neuropathy. Destruction of shoulder or other upper extremety joints can occur in patients with syringomelia, an abnormality affecting the cervical spinal cord.

Neuropathic joint disease can be viewed a rapid and severe form of secondary osteoarthritis in which a joint essentially fragments. Microscopically, there is marked destruction of articular cartilage and subchondral bone leading to subchondral sclerosis, cyst formation, and large amounts of cartilage and bone detritus within hyperplastic synovium. Although the pathogenesis remains uncertain, it is most likely that loss of innervation to the joint structures leads to a lack of proprioception and pain, abnormal joint mechanics and ultimately in joint destruction.

Rheumatoid Arthritis

Rheumatoid arthritis (RA) is a systemic, chronic inflammatory disease in which chronic polyarthritis involves diarthrodial joints symmetrically and bilaterally. The proximal interphalangeal and metacarpophalangeal joints, elbows, knees, ankles, and spine are most commonly affected. RA may occur at any age, but usually begins in the third or fourth decade, and prevalence increases until age 70. The disease afflicts 1% to 2% of the adult population and its incidence is greater in women than in men (3:1). The excess incidence of RA in women is firmly established before menopause, after which the frequency for men and women increases uniformly. Commonly, extremity joints are simultaneously affected, often in a symmetrically. The course of the disease varies and is often punctuated by remissions and exacerbations. The broad spectrum of clinical manifestations ranges from barely discernible to severe, destructive, mutilating disease.

It is now thought that classic RA comprises a heterogeneous group of disorders. Patients who are persistently seronegative for rheumatoid factor probably have disease of a different etiology than those who are seropositive. There are also rheumatoid-like diseases associated with underlying conditions, such as inflammatory bowel disease and cirrhosis.

PATHOGENESIS: A number of factors have been implicated in the development of RA.

GENETIC FACTORS: A contribution of hereditary factors to RA susceptibility is suggested by the increased frequency of the disease in first-degree relatives of affected persons and by the concordance for the illness in monozygotic twins (30%). In addition, it is generally agreed that certain major histocompatibility genes are expressed in a nonrandom manner in patients with RA. An important genetic locus that predisposes to RA is present in human leukocyte antigen (HLA) II genes, and a specific set of HLA-DR alleles (DR4, DR1, DR10, DR14) is consistently increased in these patients. These alleles share a pentapeptide sequence motif (shared epitope) in a hypervariable segment of the *HLA-DRB1* gene, which forms the rheumatoid pocket on the HLA molecule. It is likely that the binding properties of this pocket influence the type of peptides that can be bound by RA-associated HLA-DR molecules, thereby affecting the immune response to these peptides. Interestingly, seropositive RA (poor prognosis) is associated with a high frequency of an arginine in the shared epitope, whereas seronegative disease (good prognosis) commonly exhibits a lysine in the same position, further suggesting that the physical characteristics of the rheumatoid pocket influence the immune response in RA. Several non-HLA loci have been linked to RA, including a region of chromosome 18q21 which encodes RANK.

HUMORAL IMMUNITY: Immunologic mechanisms are important in the pathogenesis of RA. Lymphocytes and plasma cells accumulate in the synovium, where they produce immunoglobulins, mainly of the immunoglobulin (Ig)G class. In addition, immune-complex deposits are present in the articular cartilage and the synovium. Increased serum levels of IgM, IgA, and IgG are also seen.

Some 80% of patients with classic RA are positive for rheumatoid factor (RF). RF represents multiple antibodies, mostly IgM, but sometimes IgG or IgA, directed against the Fc fragment of IgG. Significant titers of RF are also found in patients with related collagen vascular diseases, such as systemic lupus erythematosus, progressive systemic sclerosis, and dermatomyositis. RF also occurs in a many nonrheumatic disorders, including pulmonary fibrosis, cirrhosis, sarcoidosis, Waldenström macroglobulinemia, tuberculosis, kala azar, lepromatous leprosy, and viral hepatitis. Even healthy elderly persons, particularly women, occasionally test positive for RF.

Although patients with classic RA may be seronegative, the presence of RF in high titer is frequently associated with severe and unremitting disease, many systemic complications and a serious prognosis. The presence of IgG RF is sometimes associated with the development of systemic complications, such as necrotizing vasculitis.

Immune complexes (IgG RF + IgG) and complement components are found in the synovium, synovial fluid, and extraarticular lesions of patients with RA. Furthermore, patients with seropositive RA have lower levels of complement in their synovial fluid than do those who are seronegative.

CELLULAR IMMUNITY: It has also been postulated that cell-mediated immunity contributes to RA. Abundant T lymphocytes in rheumatoid synovium are frequently Ia positive ("activated") and of the helper type. They are often in close contact with HLA-DR–positive cells, which are either macrophages or dendritic Ia-positive cells.

T cells may directly or indirectly interact with macrophages through production of cytokines that inhibit migration and proliferation of the latter. Such substances have been found in rheumatoid synovial fluid and in supernatants from rheumatoid tissue explants. These studies provide strong evidence that the joint destruction in RA reflects local production of cytokines, especially TNF and IL-1.

INFECTIOUS AGENTS: Infectious bacteria and viruses are not detected in joints of patients with RA, although structures resembling viruses have been reported early in the disease. Most patients with RA develop antibodies against a nuclear antigen in B cells infected with Epstein-Barr virus (EBV). This antigen, RA-associated nuclear antigen (RANA), is closely related to the nuclear antigen encoded by EBV (EBNA). Moreover, EBV is a polyclonal B-cell activator that stimulates production of RF. Interestingly, the blood of many patients with RA has increased numbers of EBV-infected B cells.

LOCAL FACTORS: Synovial cells cultured from rheumatic joints exhibit a decreased response to glucocorticoids and increased production of hyaluronate. These cells release a peptide (connective tissue-activating peptide) that may influence the function of other cells, producing increased amounts of prostaglandins, particularly PGE_2.

A hypothetical scenario consistent with the evidence presented earlier might be constructed as follows:

1. In a genetically susceptible person, an unknown agent (possibly a virus, such as EBV) infects a joint or some other tissue and stimulates antibody formation.
2. These immunoglobulins act as new antigens, triggering production of antiidiotype antibodies (RF).
3. Immune complexes containing RF are deposited in the synovium and activate complement. This increases vascular permeability and uptake of immune complexes by leukocytes, which in turn release lysosomal enzymes, activated oxygen species and other injurious products.
4. Activated macrophages in the synovium present unknown antigens to T cells, thus stimulating production of cytokines, which amplify inflammation, tissue injury, and synovial cell proliferation.

PATHOLOGY: The early synovial changes of RA are edema and accumulation of plasma cells, lymphocytes and macrophages (Fig. 26-52). Vascularity increases, with exudation of fibrin into the joint space, which may result in small fibrin nodules that float in the joint (**rice bodies).**

PANNUS FORMATION: Synovial lining cells, normally only 1 to 3 layers thick, undergo hyperplasia and form layers 8 to 10 cells deep. Multinucleated giant cells are often found among the synovial cells. *The synovial lining is thus thrown into numerous villi and frondlike folds that fill the peripheral recesses of the joint* (Fig. 26-53A). In this process the synovium creeps over the surface of the articular cartilage and adjacent structures. This inflammatory synovium, now containing mast cells, is termed a **pannus** (cloak). The pannus covers the articular cartilage and isolates it from the synovial fluid. Lymphocytes aggregate into masses and eventually develop follicular centers (*Allison–Ghormley Bodies;* see Fig. 26-53B). *The pannus erodes the articular cartilage and adjacent bone, probably through the action of collagenase produced by the pannus* (see Fig. 26-53C). Since PGE_2 and IL-1 stimulate osteoclasts and are actively produced in the rheumatoid synovium, they may mediate bone erosion.

The characteristic bone loss of RA is juxta-articular, that is, it is immediately adjacent to both sides of the joint. The pannus penetrates the subchondral bone; it may involve tendons and ligaments, leading to deformities and instabilities. Eventually, the joint is destroyed and undergoes fibrous fusion, termed ankylosis (Fig. 26-54). Long-standing cases may lead to bony bridging of the joint (**bony ankylosis**). The pannus may destroy cartilage by depriving it of nourishment; alternately, it may stimulate T lymphocytes to secrete a factor causing release of lysosomal enzymes. In turn, this process may lead to secondary osteoarthritis.

Changes in synovial fluid include a massive increase in volume, increased turbidity, and decreased viscosity. The protein content and the number of inflammatory cells in the fluid increase, correlating with the activity of the rheumatoid process. In some cases, the leukocyte count exceeds 50,000/μL, with 95% polymorphonuclear leukocytes.

RHEUMATOID NODULES: RA is a systemic disease that also involves tissues other than joints and tendons. A characteristic lesion, termed the rheumatoid nodule, is found in extra-articular locations. It has a central core of fibrinoid necrosis, which is a mixture of fibrin and other proteins, such as degraded collagen (Fig. 26-55).

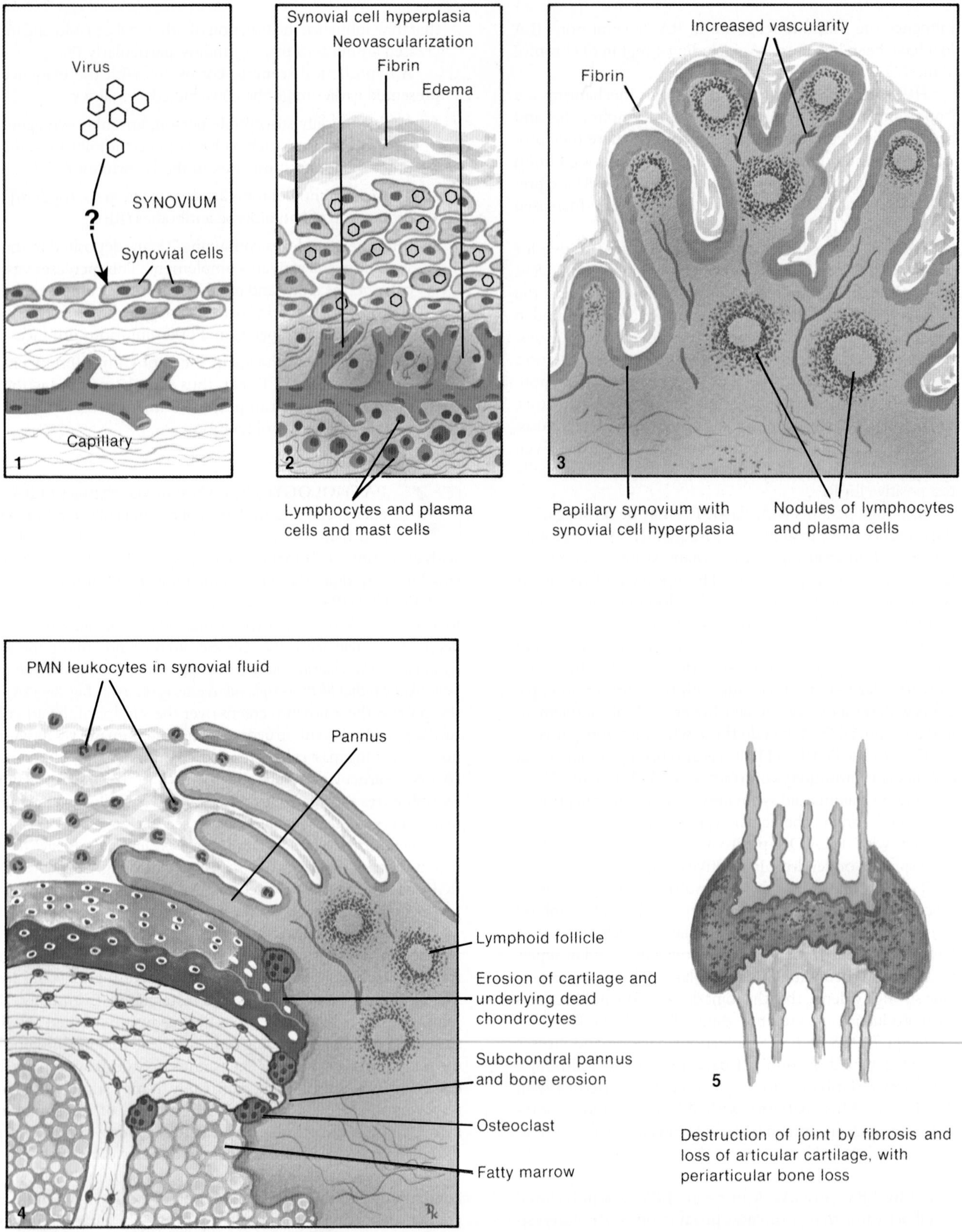

FIGURE 26-52. **Histogenesis of rheumatoid arthritis.** **1.** A virus or an unknown stress may stimulate the synovial cells to proliferate. **2.** The influx of lymphocytes, plasma cells, and mast cells, together with neovascularization and edema, leads to hypertrophy and hyperplasia of the synovium. **3.** Lymphoid nodules are prominent. **4.** Proliferating synovium extends into the joint space, burrows into the bone beneath the articular cartilage, and covers the cartilage as a pannus. The articular cartilage is eventually destroyed by direct resorption or deprivation of its nutrient synovial fluid. The synovial tissue continues to proliferate in the subchondral region, as well as in the joint. **5.** Eventually, the joint is destroyed and becomes fused, a condition termed ***ankylosis.***

A

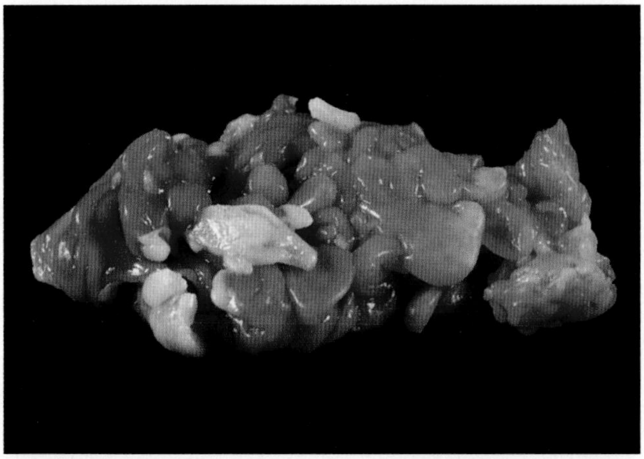

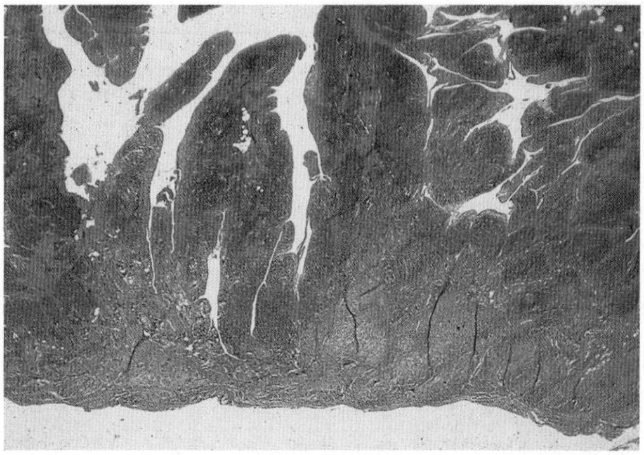

B

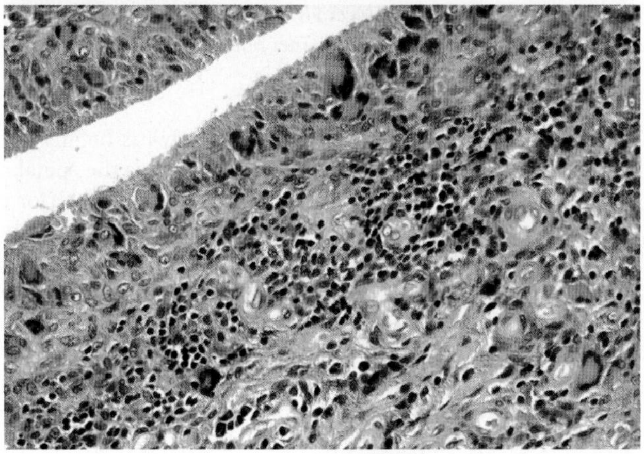

C

FIGURE 26-53. **Rheumatoid arthritis. A.** Hyperplastic synovium from a patient with rheumatoid arthritis shows numerous fingerlike projections, with focal pale areas of fibrin deposition. The brownish color of the synovium reflects hemosiderin accumulation derived from old hemorrhage. **B.** A microscopic view reveals prominent lymphoid follicles (Allison-Ghormley bodies), synovial hyperplasia and hypertrophy, villous folds, and thickening of the synovial membrane by fibrosis, and inflammation. **C.** A higher-power view of the inflamed synovium demonstrates hyperplasia and hypertrophy of the lining cells. Numerous giant cells are on and below the surface. The stroma is chronically inflamed.

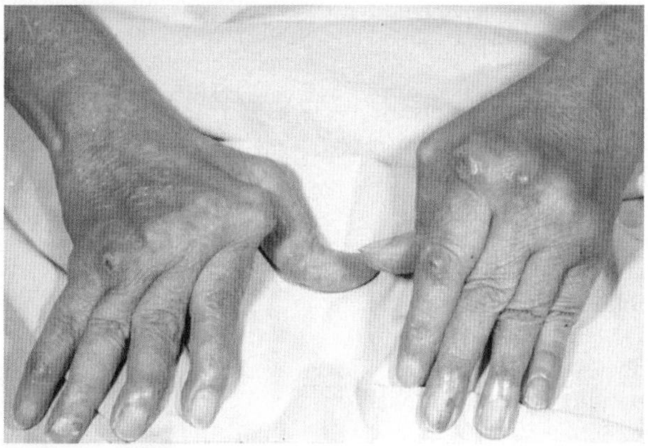

FIGURE 26-54. **Rheumatoid arthritis.** The hands of a patient with advanced arthritis show swelling of the metacarpal phalangeal joints and the classic ulnar deviation of the fingers.

A

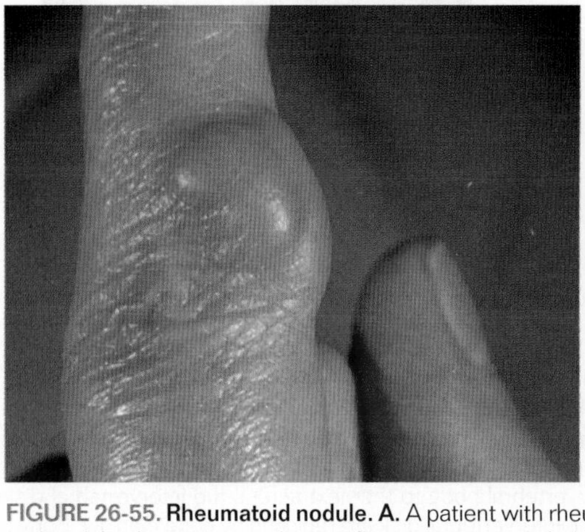

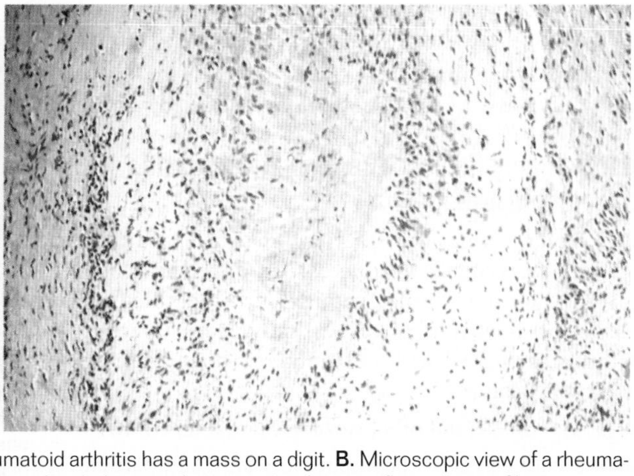

B

FIGURE 26-55. **Rheumatoid nodule. A.** A patient with rheumatoid arthritis has a mass on a digit. **B.** Microscopic view of a rheumatoid nodule shows a central area of necrosis surrounded by palisaded macrophages and a chronic inflammatory infiltrate.

A surrounding rim of macrophages is arranged in a radial, or palisading, fashion. Beyond the macrophages is a circle of lymphocytes, plasma cells, and other mononuclear cells. The overall appearance resembles a peculiar granuloma surrounding a core of fibrinoid necrosis. Rheumatoid nodules, which are usually found in areas of pressure (e.g., the skin of elbows and legs), are movable, firm, rubbery, and occasionally tender. A large nodule may ulcerate. They often recur after surgical removal.

Rheumatoid nodules may also be seen in lupus erythematous and rheumatic fever. They are sometimes found in visceral organs, such as the heart, lungs, and intestinal tract and even the dura. Nodules in the bundle of His may cause cardiac arrhythmias; in the lungs, they produce fibrosis and even respiratory failure (see Chapter 12).

RA also may be accompanied by **acute necrotizing vasculitis**, which can affect any organ.

CLINICAL FEATURES: The clinical diagnosis of RA is imprecise and is based on a number of criteria, such as the number and types of joints involved, the presence of rheumatoid nodules, and RF and radiographic features characteristic of the disease.

The onset of RA may be acute, slowly progressing, or insidious. Most patients describe slowly developing fatigue, weight loss, weakness, and vague musculoskeletal discomfort, which eventually localizes to the involved joints. Diseased joints tend to be warm, swollen, and painful. The pain is heightened by motion and is most severe after periods of disuse. Unabated disease causes progressive destruction of the joint surfaces and periarticular structures. Eventually, patients manifest severe flexion and extension deformities, associated with joint subluxation, which may terminate in joint ankylosis.

The natural history of RA is variable. In most patients, disease activity waxes and wanes. One fourth of patients seem to recover completely. Another fourth remain for many years with only slight functional impairment, whereas half have serious progressive and disabling joint disease. There is increased mortality from infection, gastrointestinal hemorrhage and perforation, vasculitis, heart and lung involvement, amyloidosis, and subluxation of the cervical spine. In fact, survival of patients with active RA is comparable to that observed in Hodgkin disease and diabetes.

Three types of drugs are used to suppress the synovial inflammation and to induce a remission:

- **Anti-inflammatory agents** include aspirin, nonsteroidal anti-inflammatory drugs (NSAIDs), phenylbutazone, glucocorticoids, and even intra-articular corticosteroid injections.
- **Remission-inducing drugs** are gold salts, penicillamine, and antimalarial drugs, such as chloroquine.
- **Immunosuppressive drugs** are used in patients with severe progressive disease who do not respond to other medications.

Spondyloarthropathy Refers to Seronegative Arthritis Mostly Linked to HLA-B27

A number of clinical entities were formerly classified as variants of RA but are now recognized to be distinct disorders. These forms of arthritis are now termed **spondyloarthropathies** and include ankylosing spondylitis, Reiter syndrome, psoriatic arthritis, and arthritis associated with inflammatory bowel disease. They share several features:

- Seronegativity for RF and other serological markers of RA
- Association with class I histocompatibility antigens, particularly HLA-B27
- Sacroiliac and vertebral involvement
- Asymmetric involvement of only few peripheral joints
- A tendency to inflammation of periarticular tendons and fascia
- Systemic involvement of other organs, especially uveitis, carditis, and aortitis
- Preferential onset in young men

Ankylosing Spondylitis

Ankylosing spondylitis is an inflammatory arthropathy of the vertebral column and sacroiliac joints. It may be accompanied by asymmetric, peripheral arthritis (30% of patients), and systemic manifestations. It is most common in young men, with peak incidence at about age 20. *Over 90% of patients have HLA-B27 (normal, 4% to 8%), although the disorder affects only 1% of persons with this haplotype.*

PATHOLOGY: Ankylosing spondylitis begins at the sacroiliac joints bilaterally, then ascends the spinal column by involving the small joints of the posterior elements of the spine. The result is ultimate destruction of these joints, after which the spine becomes fused posteriorly. The unburdened vertebral bodies become square and osteoporotic, because the main force of gravity is borne by the fused posterior elements. In such cases, the intervertebral disk undergoes ossification and may disappear. Eventually, bony fusion of the vertebral bodies ensues (Fig. 26-56).

Although a few patients with ankylosing spondylitis rapidly develop crippling spinal disease, most are able to maintain their employment and live a normal life span. However, up to 5% of patients develop AA amyloidosis and uremia and a few manifest severe cardiac involvement.

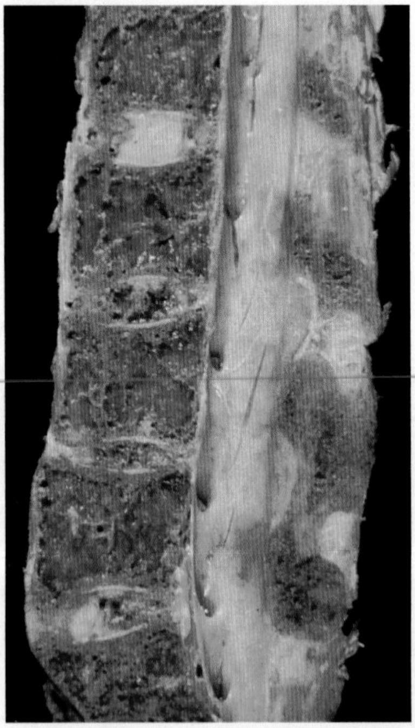

FIGURE 26-56. **Ankylosing spondylitis.** The vertebrae have been cut longitudinally. The vertebral bodies are square and have lost most of their trabecular bone, owing to osteoporosis from disuse. Bone bridges fuse one vertebral body to the next across the intervertebral disks. Portions of the intervertebral disk are replaced by bone marrow. Bony bridges also fuse the posterior elements *(ankylosis).*

Reiter Syndrome

Reiter syndrome is a triad that includes (1) seronegative polyarthritis, (2) conjunctivitis, and (3) nonspecific urethritis. It occurs almost exclusively in men and usually follows venereal exposure or an episode of bacillary dysentery. As in ankylosing spondylitis, Reiter syndrome is associated with HLA-B27 antigen in up to 90% of patients. In fact, after an attack of dysentery, 20% of HLA-B27–positive men develop Reiter syndrome.

The pathologic features of Reiter arthritis are comparable to those of RA. More than half of patients develop mucocutaneous lesions similar to those of pustular psoriasis (**keratoblennorrhagicum**) over the palms, soles, and trunk. In most patients, the disease remits within a year, but in 20%, progressive arthritis develops, including ankylosing spondylitis.

Psoriatic Arthritis

Of all patients with psoriasis, particularly in those with severe disease, 7% develop an inflammatory seronegative arthritis. HLA-B27 has been linked to psoriatic spondylitis and inflammation of distal interphalangeal joints and HLA-DR4 has been associated with a rheumatoid pattern of involvement. Joint disease is usually mild and only slowly progressive, although a mutilating form is occasionally encountered.

Enteropathic Arthritis

Ulcerative colitis and Crohn disease are accompanied by seronegative peripheral arthritis in 20% of cases and spondylitis in 10%. This form of arthritis also is seen in patients with Whipple disease and after certain bacterial infections of the gut. No particular tissue type is associated with peripheral arthritis, but most patients with ankylosing spondylitis are HLA-B27 positive. It has been proposed that HLA-B27 and proteins from enteric bacteria are structurally related in a manner that potentially affects antigen presentation to the T cell receptor. Resection of the affected bowel in ulcerative colitis relieves the arthritis, but in Crohn disease, this complication often does not resolve.

Juvenile Arthritis, Still Disease Applies to Any Inflammatory Arthritis in Children

Several different chronic arthritic conditions in children are included in this designation. In addition to RA, many children with juvenile arthritis eventually develop ankylosing spondylitis, psoriatic arthritis, and other connective tissue diseases.

- **Seropositive arthritis:** Fewer than 10% of children with arthritis are positive for RF and have a polyarticular presentation. Females predominate (80%) among children with seropositive Still disease and in most cases (75%), antinuclear antibodies are present. There is an association with HLA-D4 and more than half of the children eventually develop severe arthritis.
- **Polyarticular disease without systemic symptoms:** One fourth of juvenile arthritis patients (90% girls) have disease of several joints, are seronegative, and do not manifest systemic symptoms. Fewer than 15% of these patients eventually develop severe arthritis.
- **Polyarticular disease with systemic symptoms:** Twenty percent of children with polyarticular arthritis have prominent systemic symptoms that include high fever, rash, hepatosplenomegaly, lymphadenopathy, pleuritis, pericarditis, anemia, and leukocytosis. Most (60%) are boys who are negative for RF and one fourth of all of these children are left with severe arthritis.
- **Pauciarticular arthritis:** Children with involvement of only a few large joints, such as the knee, ankle, elbow, or hip girdle, account for half of all cases of juvenile arthritis and fall into two general groups. The larger group (80%) is mainly girls who are negative for RF but exhibit antinuclear antibodies and are positive for HLA-DR5, HLA-DRw6, or HLA-DRw8. Of these patients, one third have ocular disease characterized by chronic iridocyclitis (inflammation of the iris and ciliary body). Only a small minority of these children have residual polyarthritis or ocular damage. The smaller group of children with a pauciarticular presentation is composed almost exclusively of boys, is negative for both RF and antinuclear bodies, and is positive for HLA-B27 (75%). A few have acute iridocyclitis, which resolves spontaneously. Some of these boys subsequently develop ankylosing spondylitis.

Lyme Disease

Lyme disease usually involves the knee or other large joints and is caused by the spirochete Borrelia burgdorferi *transmitted by the Ixodes tick* (see Chapter 9). Patients generally present with joint effusion and other manifestations of Lyme disease. Although there may be a transient arthritis with acute infection, patients can develop chronic Lyme arthritis which is microscopically identical to rheumatoid arthritis..

Gout

Gout is a heterogeneous group of diseases in which the common denominator is an increased serum uric acid level and urate crystal deposition in joints and kidneys. All patients with gout have hyperuricemia, but fewer than 15% of people with hyperuricemia have gout.

Gout is characterized by acute and chronic arthritis. Gout is classified as primary and secondary, depending on the etiology of the hyperuricemia. In **primary gout** hyperuricemia occurs without any other disease, while **secondary gout** occurs in association with another illness that results in hyperuricemia. Of all cases of hyperuricemia, one third are primary and the remainder secondary.

PATHOGENESIS: Uric acid results from purine catabolism, due either to a high purine diet or increased de novo synthesis. In humans, there is a tight balance between uric acid production and tissue deposition of urates. Uric acid is only eliminated in the urine. Thus, the blood uric acid level (normal, <7.0 mg/dL in men, <6.0 in women) reflects the difference between the amount of purines ingested and synthesized, and renal excretion. Gout can result from (1) overproduction of purines, (2) increased catabolism of nucleic acids due to greater cell turnover, (3) decreased salvage of free purine bases, or (4) decreased urinary uric acid excretion (Fig. 26-57). A high dietary intake of purine-rich foods, particularly meat, by an otherwise normal person does not lead to hyperuricemia and gout.

Primary Gout Reflects Idiopathic Hyperuricemia

Most cases (85%) of idiopathic gout result from an as-yet-unexplained impairment of renal uric acid excretion. In the remain-

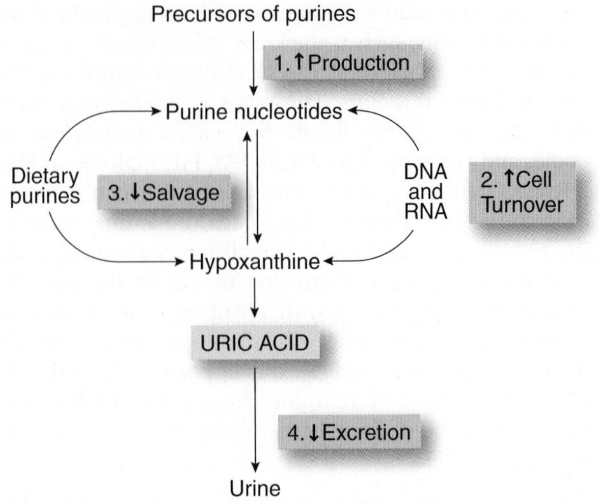

FIGURE 26-57. **Pathogenesis of hyperuricemia and gout.** Purine nucleotides are synthesized de novo from nonpurine precursors or derived from preformed purines in the diet. Purine nucleotides are catabolized to hypoxanthine or incorporated into nucleic acids. The degradation of nucleic acids and dietary purines also produces hypoxanthine. Hypoxanthine is converted to uric acid, which in turn is excreted into the urine. Hyperuricemia and gout result from (1) increased de novo purine synthesis, (2) increased cell turnover, (3) decreased salvage of dietary purines and hypoxanthine, and (4) decreased uric acid excretion by the kidneys.

der, there is a primary overproduction of uric acid, but only in a minority of cases has the underlying abnormality been identified.

A *familial tendency* to gout has been recognized since the time of Galen. Hyperuricemia is common among relatives of persons with gout. It has been proposed that primary hyperuricemia in some persons is inherited as an autosomal dominant trait with variable expression, in some as an X-linked abnormality and in others as instances of multifactorial inheritance. Precocious gout exhibits a strong familial tendency. The consensus today is that multiple genes control the level of serum uric acid.

Gout Can Be Due to Inborn Errors of Metabolism

The rate-limiting step in purine synthesis is condensation of glutamine with phosphoribosyl pyrophosphate (PP-ribose-P) to form phosphoribosylamine. Increased intracellular PP-ribose-P accelerates purine biosynthesis. PP-ribose-P, through the activity of hypoxanthine phosphoribosyl transferase (HPRT), also condenses with, and thereby salvages, purine bases (hypoxanthine and guanine) derived from the catabolism of nucleic acids. Although the specific cause of abnormally high rate of urate production is not known in most cases of primary gout, two inborn errors of metabolism are known to lead to elevated PP-ribose-P.

Lesch-Nylan syndrome represents an inherited, X-linked (Xq26–q27) deficiency of HPRT, a defect that leads to accumulation of PP-ribose-P, and in turn to enhanced purine synthesis. Children with this syndrome are clinically normal at birth but exhibit delays in development and neurologic dysfunction within the first year. Most are mentally retarded and exhibit self-mutilation. They are hyperuricemic and eventually develop gouty arthritis. In addition, obstructive nephropathy and hematologic abnormalities are often present.

Secondary Gout Often Results from DNA Turnover

A number of conditions result in hyperuricemia and secondary gout. As in primary gout, secondary hyperuricemia may reflect overproduction or decreased urinary excretion of uric acid. Increased production is most often associated with increased nucleic acid turnover, as seen in leukemias and lymphomas and after chemotherapy. Accelerated adenosine triphosphate (ATP) degradation may also lead to overproduction of uric acid and occurs in glycogen-storage diseases and tissue hypoxia. Ethanol intake leads to secondary hyperuricemia, in part owing to accelerated ATP catabolism and (to a lesser degree) decreased renal excretion of uric acid. Reduced urate excretion may result from primary renal disease. Dehydration and diuretics increase tubular reabsorption of uric acid and lead to hyperuricemia. In fact, various drugs are implicated in 20% of patients with hyperuricemia.

Saturnine gout was described in 18th century England, where this disease was prevalent among the upper classes with lead plumbing in their houses (Saturn is the symbol for lead). It is now recognized that these patients were afflicted with lead nephropathy. The Romans had a similar problem, because they drank from vessels containing lead.

EPIDEMIOLOGY: Primary gout is a disease of adult men; only 5% of cases occur in women. It is rare in children before puberty and in women during the reproductive years. The peak incidence is in the fifth decade. This sex distribution can be traced to the fact that at all ages, mean serum urate concentrations in women are lower than in men, although they increase after menopause. Many patients have a family history of gout, but environmental factors are also important. Positive correlations exist between the prevalence of hyperuricemia in a population and mean weight, protein intake, alcohol consumption, social class, and intelligence. Thus, gout is a disease that exemplifies the interplay between genetic predisposition and environmental influences.

PATHOLOGY: When sodium urate crystals precipitate from supersaturated body fluids, they absorb fibronectin, complement, and a number of other proteins on their surfaces. Neutrophils that have ingested urate crystals release activated oxygen species and lysosomal enzymes, which mediate tissue injury and promote an inflammatory response.

The presence of long, needle-shaped crystals that are negatively birefringent under polarized light is diagnostic of gout (Fig. 26-58). Monosodium urate monohydrate crystals may be found intracellularly in leukocytes of the synovial fluid. A **tophus** is an extracellular soft-tissue deposit of urate crystals surrounded by foreign-body giant cells and an associated inflammatory response of mononuclear cells. These granuloma-like areas are found in cartilage, in any of the soft tissues around joints, and even in the subchondral bone marrow adjacent to joints.

Macroscopically, any chalky white deposit on intraarticular surfaces, including articular cartilage, suggests gout. Radiologi-

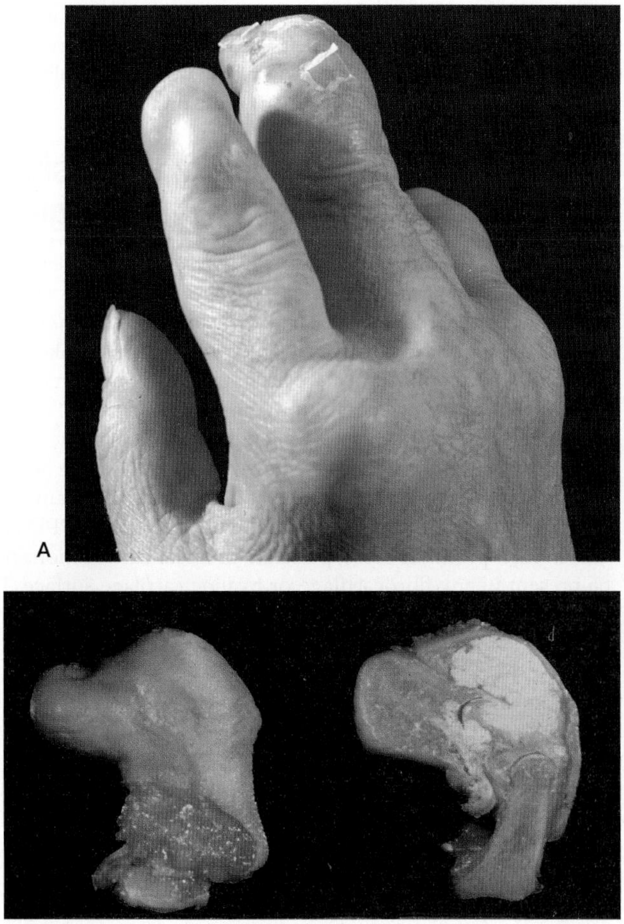

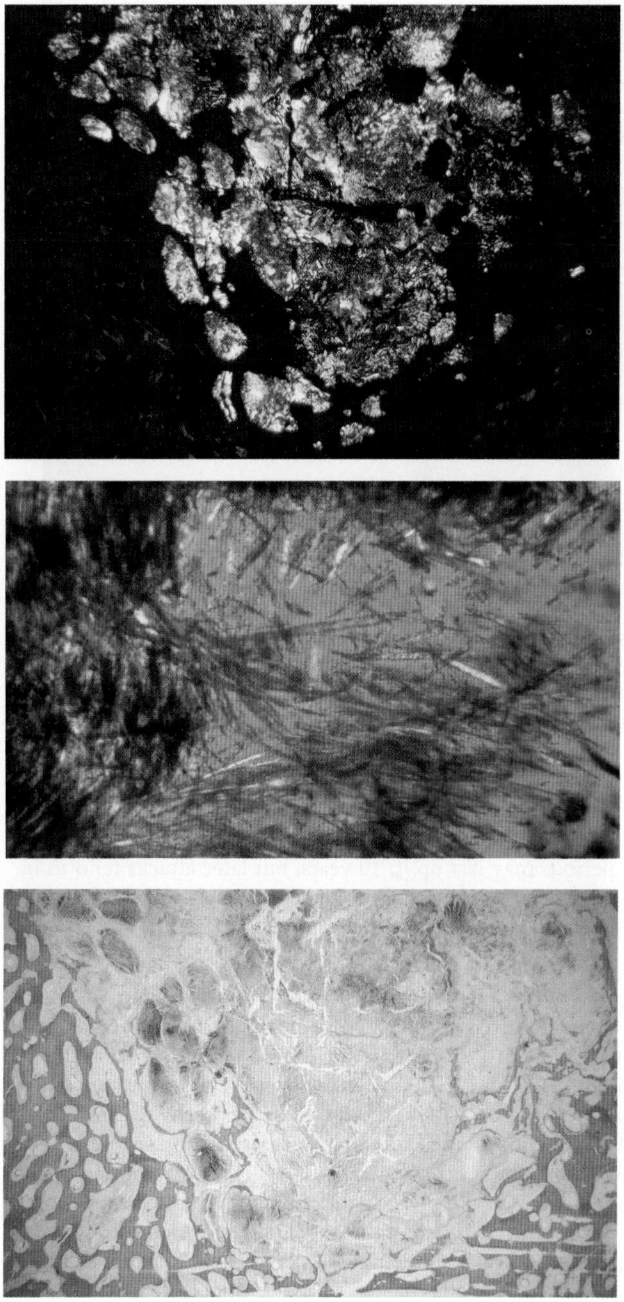

FIGURE 26-58. **Gout. A.** Gouty tophi of the hands appear as multiple rubbery nodules, one of which is ulcerated. **B.** A cross-section of a digit demonstrates a tophaceous collection of toothpaste-like urate crystals. **C.** Histologic section in bright field demonstrates brownish monosodium urate crystals within the bone. **D.** High-power micrograph in polarized light with a quartz compensator plate demonstrates negative birefringence of the crystals (those having their long axes parallel to the slow compensator axis are yellow). **E.** A section through the tophus (if usual aqueous processing is used) demonstrates a foreign body reaction around a pink, amorphous lesion from which the urate crystals have been dissolved in processing.

cally, gouty arthritis exhibits characteristic, punched-out, juxta-articular, lytic ("rat bite") lesions that are associated with only minimal reactive new bone (Fig. 26-59). In contrast to RA, there is no juxta-articular osteopenia in gout.

Renal urate deposits are between the tubules, especially at the apices of the medulla. These deposits are grossly visible as small, shiny, golden-yellow, linear streaks in the medulla.

CLINICAL FEATURES: The clinical course of gout is divided into four stages: (1) asymptomatic hyperuricemia, (2) acute gouty arthritis, (3) intercritical gout, and (4) chronic tophaceous gout. Renal stones occur in any stage except the first. In most cases, symptomatic gout appears before the renal stones, which usually require 20 to 30 years of sustained hyperuricemia.

- **Asymptomatic hyperuricemia** often precedes clinically evident gout by many years.
- **Acute gouty arthritis** was well characterized by Thomas Sydenham, who described his own disease in the 1600s. It is a painful condition that usually involves one joint, without constitutional symptoms. Later in the course of the disease, polyarticular involvement with fever is common. At least half of patients are first seen with a painful and red first metatarsophalangeal joint (great toe), designated **podagra**. Eventually, 90% of all patients have such an attack. Commonly, a gouty attack begins at night and is exquisitely painful, simulating an acute bacterial infection of the affected joint. A large meal or drinking alcoholic beverages may trigger an attack, but other specific events such as trauma, certain drugs, and surgery may also be re-

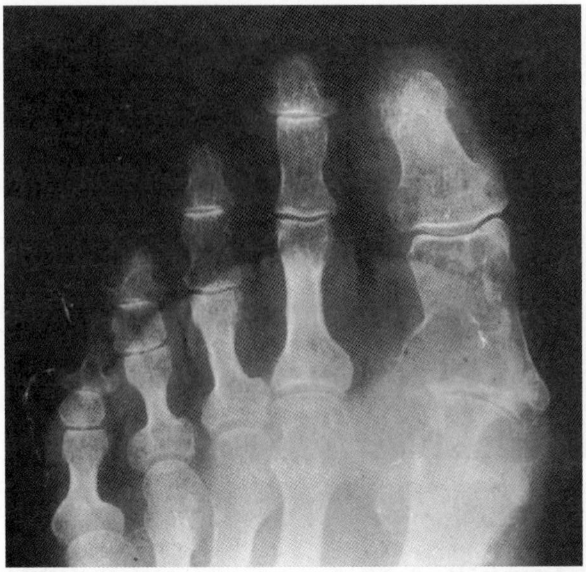

FIGURE 26-59. **Gout.** A radiograph of the first metatarsophalangeal joint shows a lytic lesion that destroys the joint space. There is an adjacent soft tissue tophus, as well as surrounding edema.

sponsible. Even when untreated, acute attacks of gout are self-limited.

- **The intercritical period** is the asymptomatic interval between the initial acute attack and subsequent episodes. These periods may last up to 10 years, but later attacks tend to be increasingly severe and prolonged and polyarticular.
- **Tophaceous gout** eventually appears in the untreated patient in the form of tophi in the cartilage, synovial membranes, tendons, and soft tissues.

Renal failure is responsible for 10% of deaths in persons with gout. One third of patients have mild albuminuria, reduced glomerular filtration, and decreased renal concentrating ability. However, the contribution of urate nephropathy to chronic renal dysfunction is unclear, and hypertension, preexisting kidney disease and the intake of analgesic drugs may be more important. In patients with severe gout caused by inherited enzyme deficiencies and in those with a precocious presentation, urate nephropathy is a prominent feature of the clinical course. **Urate stones** are 10% of all renal calculi in the United States, and up to 40% in Israel and Australia. The prevalence of urate stones correlates with the serum concentration of uric acid and affects up to 25% of gout patients. They also have an increased frequency of calcium-containing stones, in which case the uric acid may serve as a nidus for a calcium stone.

TREATMENT: Treatment of gout is designed to (1) decrease the severity of acute attacks, (2) reduce serum urate, (3) prevent future attacks, (4) promote dissolution of urate deposits, and (5) alkalinize the urine to prevent stone formation. The main drugs used to interrupt the inflammatory process, thus preventing or controlling the acute attack, are nonsteroidal anti-inflammatory agents. Colchicine has been used for hundreds of years and has been administered prophylactically during the intervals between gouty attacks to prevent recurrent episodes. Uricosuric drugs that interfere with urate reabsorption by the renal tubule are often useful.

Allopurinol is a competitive inhibitor of xanthine oxidase, the enzyme that converts xanthine and hypoxanthine to uric acid. This drug causes a prompt decrease in uricosemia and uricosuria and is used in people with renal insufficiency and those who are resistant to other uricosuric drugs. It also may be administered to patients undergoing chemotherapy for hematopoietic proliferative disorders, which increases the rate of urate production.

Calcium Pyrophosphate Dihydrate-deposition Disease (Chondrocalcinosis and Pseudogout)

Calcium pyrophosphate dihydrate (CPPD)-deposition disease refers to the accumulation of this compound in synovial membranes (pseudogout), joint cartilage (chondrocalcinosis), ligaments, and tendons. The disease can be idiopathic, associated with trauma, linked to a number of metabolic disorders, or, in rare cases, hereditary.

CPPD-deposition disease is principally a condition of old age: half of those over 85 years are afflicted. Most cases in the elderly are without symptoms. Because fully two thirds of these patients manifest preexisting joint damage, it is believed that trauma and the aging process in cartilage promote nucleation of CPPD crystals. In asymptomatic cases, punctate or linear calcifications may be present in any fibrocartilage or hyaline cartilage surface. For example, radiography of the knee may disclose linear streaks that outline the menisci.

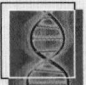

PATHOGENESIS: *The major predisposing abnormality in patients with CPPD-deposition disease is an excessive level of inorganic pyrophosphate in the synovial fluid.* This material derives from hydrolysis of nucleoside triphosphates in joint chondrocytes. Increased pyrophosphate levels in synovial fluid can result from either increased production or decreased catabolism.

CPPD deposition is commonly found in the knees after trauma and after surgical removal of the meniscus. Nucleotides releaseed after injury to articular cartilage may act as substrates for nucleotide triphosphate pyrophosphohydrolase (NTP), thereby increasing production of pyrophosphate. A number of other disorders are associated with deposition of CPPD crystals, including hyperparathyroidism, hypothyroidism, hemochromatosis, Wilson disease, and ochronosis. Iron and copper are presumed to inhibit pyrophosphatase, accounting for decreased degradation of pyrophosphate.

Mutations in the *ANKH* gene cause familial autosomal dominant CPPD chondrocalcinosis. The *ANKH* gene is thought to encode a membrane pyrophosphate transporter which inhibits mineralization of several tissues including joints, articular cartilage and tendons. Mutated ANKH elevates intracellular pyrophosphate and ruduces extracellular pyrophosphate.

Hypophosphatasia is a heritable condition in which activity of alkaline phosphatase (the enzyme that hydrolyzes pyrophosphate) in serum and tissue is deficient. As a result, pyrophosphate is not adequately metabolized and accumulates in synovial fluid.

PATHOLOGY AND CLINICAL FEATURES: A minority of patients symptomatic with CPPD-deposition disease are classified according to the nature of joint involvement.

- **Pseudogout** refers to self-limited attacks of acute arthritis lasting from 1 day to 4 weeks and involving one or two joints. Some 25% of patients with CPPD-deposition disease have an

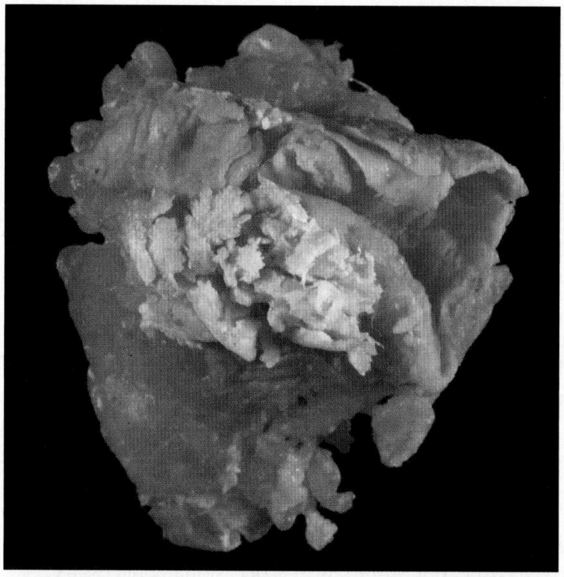

FIGURE 26-60. **Calcium pyrophosphate-deposition disease (CPPD).** Gross specimen demonstrates chalky-white calcific material.

acute onset of goutlike symptoms manifesting as inflammation and swelling of the knees, ankles, wrists, elbows, hips, or shoulders. Metatarsophalangeal joints, which are frequently affected in gout, are usually spared. The synovial fluid exhibits abundant leukocytes containing CPPD crystals.

- **Pseudorheumatoid arthritis** is a variant of CPPD-deposition disease in which multiple joints are chronically involved. The symptoms are mild and resemble those of RA.
- **Pseudoosteoarthritis** has symptoms similar to those of osteoarthritis.
- **Pseudoneurotrophic disease** is characterized by joint destruction severe enough to resemble a neurotrophic joint.

On gross examination, CPPD deposits appear as chalky white areas on the cartilaginous surfaces (Fig. 26-60). Unlike needle-shaped urate crystals, they are stubby, short and rhomboid ("coffin shaped") and have weak positive birefringence under polarized light. In contrast to urate crystals, CPPD crystals do not dissolve in water and are easily found in tissue sections. Only few mononuclear cells and macrophages surround foci of crystal deposition.

Calcium Hydroxyapatite-Deposition Disease

Calcium hydroxyapatite-deposition disease is an acute or chronic arthritis characterized by hydroxyapatite crystals within leukocytes and mononuclear cells in joint tissue and synovial fluid. Calcium hydroxyapatite (HA) is the major mineral of bone and teeth and is the compound deposited in dystrophic and metastatic calcification. HA crystals are frequently encountered in the synovial fluid of joints involved by osteoarthritis, but there is reason to believe that severe HA deposition is a distinct entity. The joints most frequently involved are the knee, shoulder, hip and fingers. Attacks may last several days.

Hemophilia, Hemochromatosis and Ochronosis

Hemophilia, hemochromatosis, and ochronosis (see Chapter 6) all produce joint disease with degradation of the matrix and destruction of the articular cartilage.

- **Hemophilia** gives rise to severe forms of arthritis because of extensive bleeding into joints (hemarthrosis), particularly the knees, elbows, ankles, shoulders, and hips. In addition to the effects within the articular cartilage matrix, synovial proliferation also simulates RA.
- **Hemochromatosis** is complicated by arthritis in half of affected patients. The hands, hips, and knees may be involved in recurrent attacks.
- **Ochronosis** is a rare, autosomal recessive disease caused by a defect in homogentisic acid oxidase. The deposition of ochronotic pigment in the cartilage of the joints, including the intravertebral disks, eventually causes them to become brittle and degenerate.

Tumors and Tumorlike Lesions of Joints

True neoplasms of the joints are rare. The most common malignant lesions of the synovium are metastatic carcinomas, particularly adenocarcinoma of the colon, breast, and lung. Lymphoproliferative diseases (e.g., leukemia) may also involve the synovium, mimicking other conditions, such as RA. It is unusual for primary malignant bone tumors to extend into the joint, although they may invade the joint capsule from the soft tissues.

Ganglion is a Small Fluid-Filled Cyst

A ganglion is a thin-walled, simple cyst containing clear mucinous fluid, which occurs most commonly on the extensor surfaces of the hands and feet, especially the wrist. The cyst arises either from the synovium or from areas of myxoid change in the connective tissue, possibly after trauma. The wall is composed of fibrous tissue. If the lesion is painful, it can be readily removed surgically, although a blow with the family Bible was the traditional treatment for a ganglion on the dorsum of the wrist.

Baker's cyst is a herniation of the synovium of the knee joint into the popliteal space. It is most often seen in association with various forms of arthritis, in which the intra-articular pressure is increased.

Synovial Chondromatosis Features Cartilage Nodules in a Joint

Synovial chondromatosis is a benign, self-limited disease in which hyaline cartilage nodules, which form in the synovium, detach from that structure and float in the synovial fluid in a manner similar to grains of sand between gears. The chronic irritation produced by these foreign bodies stimulates the synovium to secrete large amounts of synovial fluid and also causes bleeding in the synovial membrane. Synovial chondromatosis involves the large diarthrodial joints of young and middle-aged men, affecting the knee in most cases, but also the hip, elbow, shoulder, and ankle. Patients have pain, stiffness and locking of the joint, with associated bloody effusions.

Unlike cartilage that detaches from articular surface in osteoarthritis, in synovial chondromatosis fragments of hyaline cartilage are formed de novo in the synovium. They do not have a tidemark and thus differ from true articular cartilage. Occasionally, the cartilage nodules, while still residing in the synovium, undergo endochondral ossification, in which case, the disease is called **synovial osteochondromatosis**. If these nodules detach, the bony portions die, but the cartilage fragments remain viable and enlarge because they are nourished by synovial fluid. Evacuating the joint and performing a partial synovectomy treat the condition. Dysregulation of Hedgehog signaling is a factor in the development of synovial chondromatosis in animal models and suggests that this disorder is a neoplasm.

Pigmented Villonodular Synovitis Is a Benign Neoplasm of the Synovial Lining

Pigmented villonodular synovitis is characterized by exuberant proliferation of synovial lining cells with extension into the subsynovial tissue. It involves a single joint, usually in young adults, and is seen equally in males and females. The most common site (80%) is the knee, although pigmented villonodular synovitis also occurs in the hip, ankles, calcaneocuboid joint, elbow, and tendon sheaths of the fingers and toes. Several chromosomal abnormalities occur in pigmented villonodular synovitis and in localized nodular synovitis suggesting that these lesions are in fact benign neoplasms of synovium.

PATHOLOGY: The tumors arise on the synovium of tendon sheaths, bursae and diarthrodial joints. The lesions of pigmented villonodular synovitis invade the joint and erode the bone (Fig 26-61A). They may insinuate through joint capsules into soft tissue and encompass nerves and arteries, sometimes necessitating radical surgical excision. The synovium develops enlarged folds and nodular excrescences (see Fig. 26-61B). Microscopically, the tumor is composed of bland mononuclear cells with scattered multinucleated giant cells in which the nuclei are arrayed peripherally. Hemosiderin-laden macrophages reflect previous hemorrhage (see Fig. 26-61C, D).

Localized nodular synovitis is a similar condition of the knee that involves only part of the synovium rather than the entire membrane. Symptoms are limited to pain, joint locking, and joint effusions.

Localized nodular tenosynovitis, also called **giant cell tumor of the tendon sheath**, involves tendon sheaths of the hands and feet. *It is the most common soft tissue tumor of the hand.* It occurs mostly in young and middle-aged women and involves flexor surfaces of the middle or index fingers.

Treatment for all forms of pigmented villonodular synovitis is surgical. Radiation therapy produces fibrosis of the proliferating synovial tissue, but amputation is occasionally necessary.

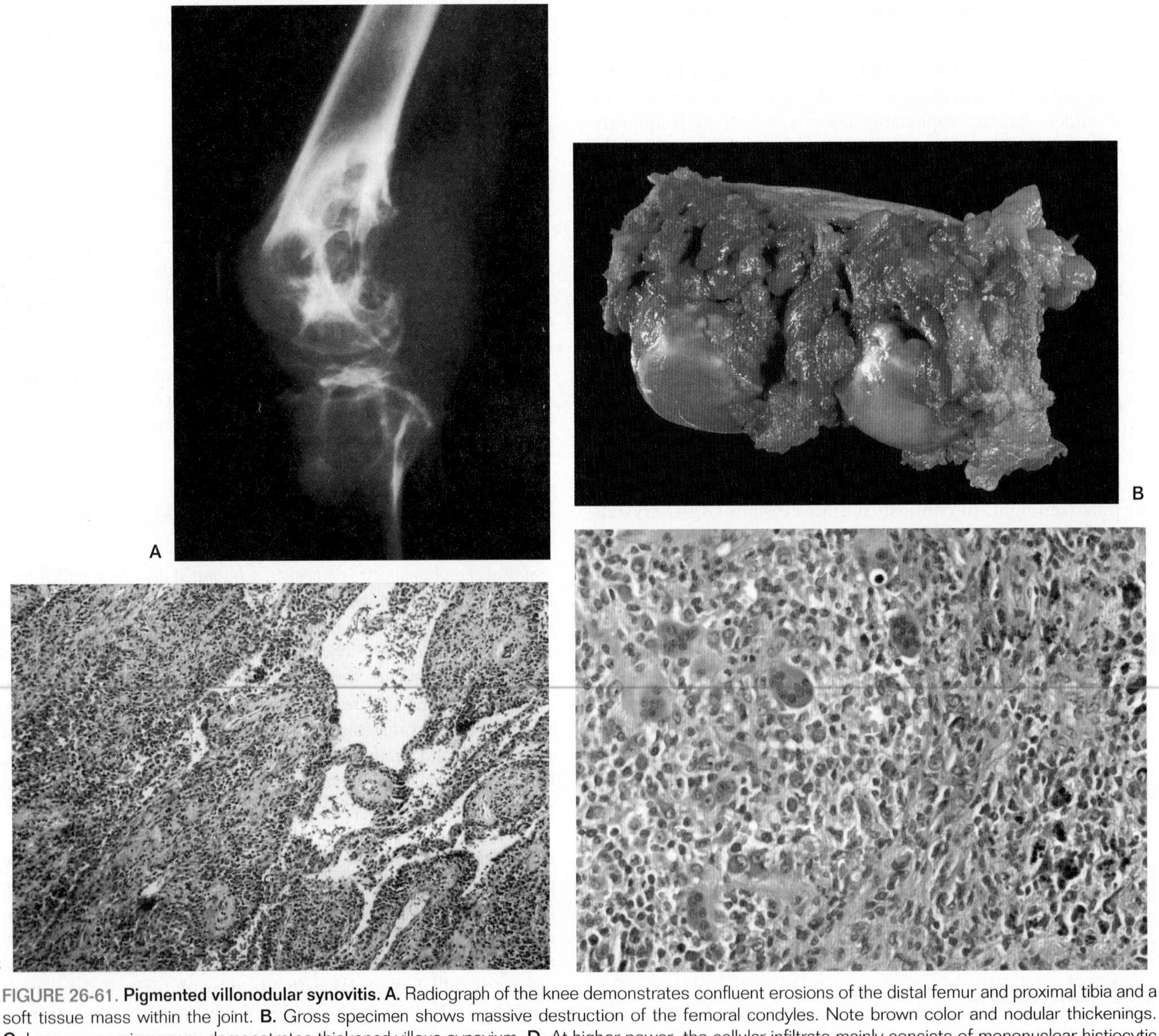

FIGURE 26-61. **Pigmented villonodular synovitis. A.** Radiograph of the knee demonstrates confluent erosions of the distal femur and proximal tibia and a soft tissue mass within the joint. **B.** Gross specimen shows massive destruction of the femoral condyles. Note brown color and nodular thickenings. **C.** Low-power microscopy demonstrates thickened villous synovium. **D.** At higher power, the cellular infiltrate mainly consists of mononuclear histiocytic synoviocytes, many of which contain brown hemosiderin pigment, and multinucleated giant cells.

SOFT TISSUE TUMORS

Soft tissue tumors are neoplasms that arise in certain extraskeletal mesodermal tissues of the body, including skeletal muscle, fat, fibrous tissue, blood vessels, and lymphatics. Tumors of peripheral nerves may be included in the category of soft tissue tumors, despite their derivation from the neuroectoderm (see Chapter 28). Soft tissue tumors are rare, accounting for less than 1% of all malignancies in the United States. Benign soft tissue neoplasms are 100 times more common than malignant ones.

Soft tissue tumors are believed to arise from multipotential mesenchymal stem cells that reside in soft tissues and are generally classified according to the phenotype they exhibit (e.g., fibroblastic, vascular, myoid). Many have characterisitic and unique chromosomal abnormalities.

In the context of soft tissue tumors, the term **benign** is somewhat relative because so-called benign tumors may invade and may recur locally (e.g., fibromatosis). Malignant soft tissue tumors (sarcomas) can metastasize, usually to the lungs. Patients generally die of metastatic disease rather than local invasion at the primary tumor site.

A group of genetic disorders associated with soft tissue tumors includes neurofibromatosis type 1, tuberous sclerosis, Osler-Weber-Rendu disease, and mesenteric fibromatosis in Gardner syndrome. Burns in childhood produce scars, which in rare instances lead to soft tissue fibroblastic tumors many years later. Radiation injury has been reported to be associated with the development of sarcomas years after exposure. There is no scientific evidence to support the association of trauma with the development of soft tissue tumors, and injury merely draws attention to a preexisting tumor.

A few important general principles relate to soft tissue tumors:

- Superficial tumors tend to be benign.
- Deep lesions are often malignant.
- Large tumors are more often malignant than small ones.
- Rapidly growing tumors are more likely to be malignant than tumors that develop slowly.
- Calcification may exist in both benign and malignant tumors.
- Benign tumors are relatively avascular, whereas most malignant ones are hypervascular.
- Some soft tissue tumors are classified on the basis of genetic or molecular findings.

Tumors and Tumorlike Conditions of Fibrous Origin

Nodular Fasciitis May Be Mistaken for Sarcoma

Nodular fasciitis is a benign but rapidly growing reactive lesion that probably results from trauma and commonly affects the superficial tissues of the forearm, trunk and back (Fig. 26-62). Most cases occur in adults and the lesion's rapid growth usually prompts a patient to seek medical attention. Histologically, nodular fasciitis may be mistaken for a sarcoma, because it is hypercellular and has abundant mitoses and numerous, pleomorphic, spindle-shaped cells. Its true nature is revealed when it is recognized that the entire "mass" is the counterpart of granulation tissue or an exuberant scar in response to trauma. Cytogenetic abnormalities involving chromosome 15 have been reported in some cases of nodular fasciitis. The affected region on chromosome 15 codes for proteins involved in tissue repair (e.g., FGF-7) and oncogenic proteins. Nodular fasciitis is self-limited and is cured by surgical excision.

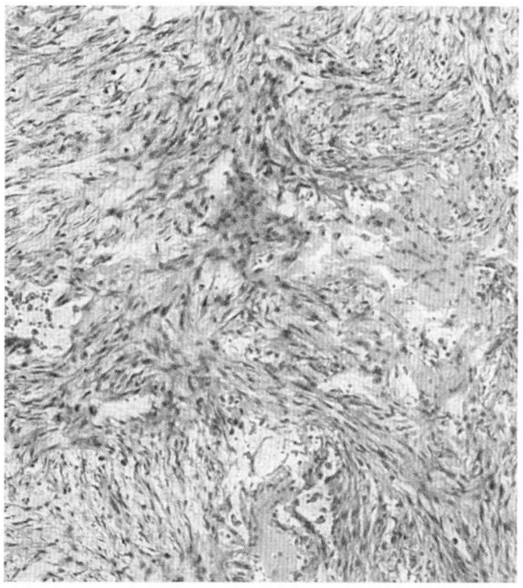

FIGURE 26-62. **Nodular fasciitis.** Swirls of tightly woven uniform spindle cells and collagen are admixed with a few lymphoid cells and vascular channels.

Fibromatosis Is a Locally Aggressive Proliferation of Fibroblasts

Fibromatosis, also known as desmoid tumor, *is a locally invasive, slowly growing, mass that may occur virtually anywhere in the body.* They do not metastasize, but are locally invasive, and surgical resection is often followed by a local recurrence. An increased incidence of fibromatosis has been reported in diabetics, alcoholics, and epileptics. Patients with familial adenomatous polyposis are also prone to developing this tumor.

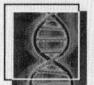

PATHOGENESIS: Inactivating mutations in the *APC* gene are found mostly in cases of fibromatosis that are associated with familial adenomatous polyposis. The APC protein binds to β-catenin, and enhances its degradation. Thus, loss of APC indirectly stabilizes β-catenin. β-catenin in turn promotes Wnt pathway signaling, which modulates develomental genes and presumably plays a role in the development of fibromatosis. Many sporadic cases of fibromatosis have activating mutations in the gene for β-catenin which. make it resistant to the inhibitory effect of APC. In short, mutations in both the *APC* and *β-catenin* genes result in persistent stabilization of β-catenin

PATHOLOGY: On gross examination, the lesions of fibromatosis tend to be large, firm, and whitish, with poorly demarcated borders and a whorled cut surface. They frequently originate in a muscular fascia. Microscopic examination reveals sheets and interdigitating fascicles of benign-appearing spindle cells (fibroblasts) with little mitotic activity.

Because microscopic tongues of tumor extend between preexisting structures, surgical "shelling out" of the lesion is followed by recurrences in half of cases. Complete surgical excision is curative.

Specific forms of fibromatosis are identified by their characteristic locations:

- **Palmar fibromatosis** (Dupuytren contracture) is the most common form of fibromatosis. It affects 1% to 2% of the general population but as many as 20% of persons older than 65 years. In half of cases, the lesion is bilateral, and in 10% of cases it is associated with fibromatosis in other locations. Fibrous nodules and cordlike bands in the palmar fascia eventually lead to flexion contractures of the fingers, particularly the fourth and fifth digits.
- **Plantar fibromatosis** is similar to palmar fibromatosis, except that it is less frequent and involves the plantar aponeurosis.
- **Penile fibromatosis** (Peyronie disease) is the least common of the localized fibromatoses and is characterized by an induration of, or mass in, the shaft of the penis, causing it to curve toward the affected side (**penile strabismus**). The lesion leads to urethral obstruction and pain on erection.

Fibrosarcoma is a Malignant Tumor of Fibroblasts

Fibrosarcoma is most common in the thigh, particularly around the knee. This tumor typically occurs in adults, although it may be seen in any age group and may even be congenital. Congenital (infantile) fibrosarcoma (CFS) has a chromosomal translocation, t(12;15)(p13;q26) that contains an *ETV6-NTRK3* fusion gene and has a poor prognosis. Fibrosarcomas arise from connective tissue, such as fascia, scar tissue, periosteum, and tendons. Macroscopically, the tumors are sharply demarcated and frequently exhibit necrosis and hemorrhage. They are characterized histologically by malignant appearing fibroblasts (Fig. 26-63), which often form densely interlacing bundles and fascicles, producing a "herringbone" pattern. There are also several morphologic variants including low grade (less aggressive) tumors. The prognosis for high-grade conventional adult fibrosarcoma is guarded; the survival at 5 years is only 40% and that at 10 years, 30%.

Pleomorphic Spindle Cell Sarcoma ("Malignant Fibrous Histiocytoma") Is the Most Common Soft Tissue Sarcoma

Malignant fibrous histiocytoma (MFH) was historically considered to be a malignant soft tissue tumor with fibroblastic and histiocytic (macrophage) differentiation. However, the term MFH now refers to a microscopic appearance that actually represents a phenotypicaly heterogeneous group of sarcomas generically termed pleomorphic spindle cell sarcomas. More recent immunohistochemical and ultrastructural studies have shown that the histologic pattern of MFH/pleomorphic spindle cell sarcoma can be seen in pleomorphic variants of liposarcoma, leiomyosarcoma, rhabdomyosarcoma, myofibroblastic sarcoma, and fibrosarcoma. Collectively, the MFH/pleomorphic spinle cell sarcoma group of tumors are the most common sarcoma in patients over the age of 40, but cases have been recorded at all ages. In half of cases, these tumors arise in the deep fascia or within skeletal muscle and have been reported in association with surgical scars and foreign bodies or after radiation treatment. In general, these tumors have complex cytogenetic abnormalities. Several oncogenes may play a role in the pathogenesis of MFH-like tumors including *SAS*, *TP53*, *RB1*, and *CDKN2A*, among others.

PATHOLOGY: Adult pleomorphic spindle cell sarcomas are usually unencapsulated gray-white or tan tumors that may have areas of hemorrhage and necrosis. Microscopically, MFH-like tumors display a highly variable morphologic pattern, with areas of spindle-shaped tumor cells arrayed in an irregularly whorled (storiform) pattern adjacent to fields with bizarre pleomorphic cells (Fig. 26-64). The spindle cells tend to be better differentiated and may resemble fibroblasts. There are occasional plump cells (histiocytes), abundant mitoses, a few xanthomatous cells, and a moderate chronic inflammatory reaction. Some tumors contain numerous tumor giant cells, which exhibit an intense eosinophilia. The extent of collagen deposition varies and sometimes dominates the microscopic pattern. A few tumors reveal a conspicuous myxoid stroma. Immunohistochemical and ultrastructural studies are generally performed to establish a specific line of differentiation (smooth muscle, skeletal muscle, fibroblast, etc.) If no such line

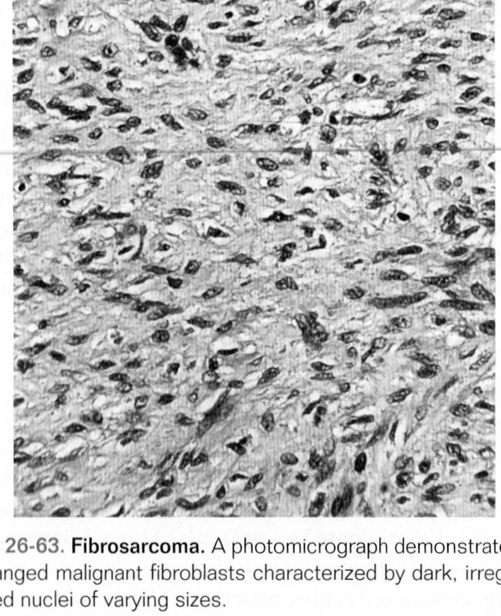

FIGURE 26-63. **Fibrosarcoma.** A photomicrograph demonstrates irregularly arranged malignant fibroblasts characterized by dark, irregular, and elongated nuclei of varying sizes.

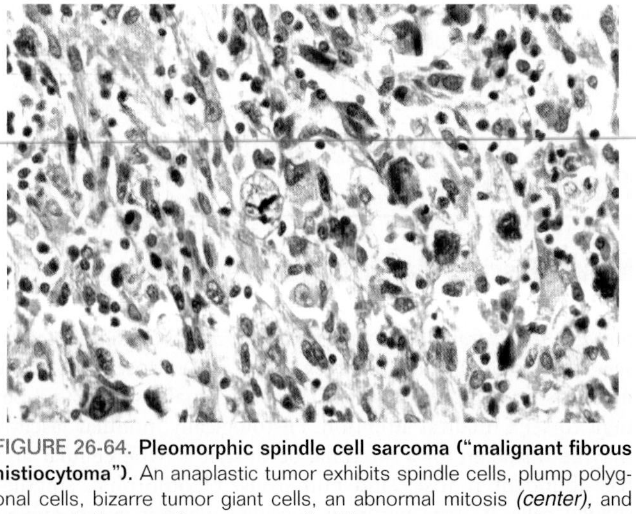

FIGURE 26-64. **Pleomorphic spindle cell sarcoma ("malignant fibrous histiocytoma").** An anaplastic tumor exhibits spindle cells, plump polygonal cells, bizarre tumor giant cells, an abnormal mitosis *(center)*, and scattered chronic inflammatory cells. This appearance can be seen in pleomorphic fibrosarcomas as well as pleomorphic sarcomas with other lines of differentiation.

of differentiation can be demonstrated, then the tumor can be considered to be an **undifferentiated pleomorphic sarcoma**.

The prognosis of adult pleomorphic spindle cell sarcomas depends on the degree of cytologic atypia, the extent of mitotic activity, and the degree of necrosis. Almost half of patients develop a local recurrence after surgery and a comparable proportion later manifest metastatic disease, particularly in the lungs. The overall 5-year survival ranges from 50% to 60%.

Radiation-induced sarcomas are a form of adult pleomorphic spindle cell sarcoma that arise in bone or soft tissue, usually 10 to 20 years after radiotherapy for a malignancy in that field. A typical story is development of osteosarcoma of a rib or vertebral body (uncommon sites for de novo osteosarcomas) after radiation to the thorax as treatment for mediastinal lymphoma or breast cancer. The incidence of postradiation sarcoma is low (<1% of irradiated patients).

Tumors of Adipose Tissue

Lipoma Closely Resembles Normal Fat

Lipoma is composed of well-differentiated adipocytes and is the most common soft tissue mass. This benign, circumscribed tumor can originate at any site in the body that contains adipose tissue. Most occur in the subcutaneous tissues of the upper half of the body, especially the trunk and neck. Lipomas are seen mainly in adults, and patients with multiple tumors often have relatives with a similar history.

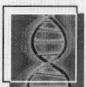

PATHOGENESIS: Numerous cytogenetic abnormalities have been documented in lipomas. In general, lipomas can be subclassified into three major groups: (1) tumors with aberrations involving 12q13–15, (2) tumors with abnormalities involving 6p21–23, and (3) tumor with loss of portions of 13q. Some tumors have the translocation t(3;12)(q27–28;q13–15) which results in the generation of a fusion gene involving the *HMGIC* gene (a member of the high mobility group of proteins) and the *LPP* gene (a member of the LIM protein family). However, the molecular pathways that are responsible for the development of lipomas are unknown. Some lipomas have no cytogenetic abnormalities and may represent localized adipocyte hyperplasia.

PATHOLOGY: On gross examination, lipomas are encapsulated, soft, yellow lesions that vary in size and may become very large. Deeper tumors are often poorly circumscribed. Histologically, a lipoma is often indistinguishable from normal adipose tissue. Lipomas are adequately treated by simple local excision.

An **angiolipoma** is a small, well-circumscribed, subcutaneous lipoma with extensive vascular proliferation usually appears shortly after puberty. Angiolipomas are often multiple and painful.

Liposarcomas are the Second most Common Sarcoma in Adults

Liposarcomas comprise 20% of all malignant soft tissue tumors. The neoplasm arises after age 50 years and is most common in the deep thigh and retroperitoneum. Liposarcomas tend to grow slowly but may become extremely large. There are several subtypes of liposarcoma including myxoid/round cell liposarcoma, well differentiated liposarcoma, and pleomorphic liposarcoma.

PATHOGENESIS: The myxoid variant of liposarcoma is another example of the growing list of human cancers that are associated with specific chromosomal translocations causing the synthesis of an abnormal fusion protein. In the case of liposarcoma, most tumors exhibit a translocation between chromosomes 12 and 16, [t(12;16)(q13;p11)], in which the *TLS/FUS* gene on chromosome 16 is fused with the *CHOP* gene on chromosome 12. The *TLS/FUS* gene product is a novel RNA-binding protein with substantial homology to the EWS protein of Ewing sarcoma, whereas the CHOP protein is a transcriptional repressor. Well differentiated liposarcomas are defined by a supernumerary circular or ring chromosome with amplification of the 12q14–15 region which includes the *MDM2* gene. MDM2 is involved in regulation of growth and survival signaling in part through inhibition of p53 (see Chapter 5).

PATHOLOGY: Liposarcomas typically measure 5 to 10 cm in diameter, although some measuring 40 cm in diameter and weighing in excess of 20 kg have been encountered. Gross appearance varies, depending on the proportions of adipose, mucinous, and fibrous tissue. Poorly differentiated liposarcomas grossly appear similar to brain tissue and display necrosis, hemorrhage, and cysts. Microscopically, myxoid/round cell liposarcoma consists of variably differentiated "signet ring" lipoblasts and variable amounts of primitive round cells embedded in a vascularized myxoid stroma (Fig. 26-65). Well-differentiated liposarcomas are often composed of large amounts of mature fat, and therefore can be confused with lipomas. Pleomorphic liposarcomas have an MFH-like histologic appearance but also contain **lipoblasts**. It is the lipoblast, a malignant appearing cell with univacuolated of multivacuolated

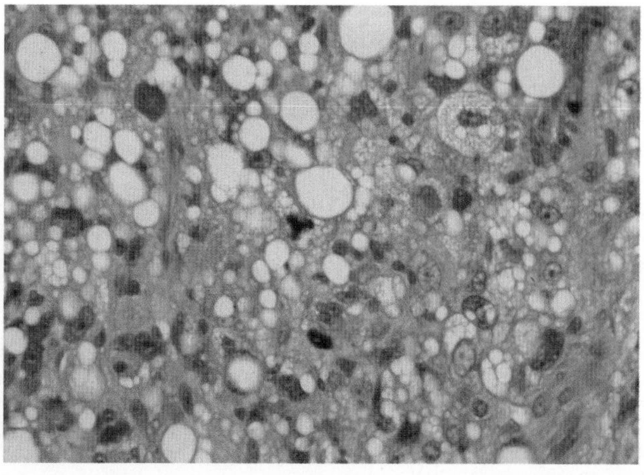

FIGURE 26-65. **Liposarcoma.** Pleomorphic cells are present, many containing lipid vacuoles that indent the nuclei or completely displace them to one side (lipoblasts).

cytoplasmic fat vesicles, that essentially defines a tumor as a liposarcoma.

Local recurrence rates and metastases after surgery are high for round cell and pleomorphic liposarcomas, and the 5-year survival for these tumors is less than 20%. By contrast, 5-year survival for patients with well-differentiated and myxoid tumors exceeds 70%.

Rhabdomyosarcoma

Rhabdomyosarcoma is a malignant tumor that displays features of striated muscle differentiation. It is uncommon in mature adults but is the most frequent soft tissue sarcoma of children and young adults. Its pathogenesis is controversial, but probably most of these tumors derive from primitive mesenchyme that has retained the capacity for skeletal muscle differentiation. Alternatively, rhabdomyosarcoma may arise from embryonal muscle tissue that is displaced into the soft tissues during embryogenesis.

PATHOLOGY: Most cases of rhabdomyosarcoma can be classified in one of four subtypes. In addition to their light microscopic features, all subtypes of rhabdomyosarcoma show immunohistochemical evidence of skeletal muscle differentiation. Tumors may express nonspecific myoid markers such as actin and desmin, or more specific markers such as the skeletal muscle specific transcription factors myogenin and MyoD1.

EMBRYONAL RHABDOMYOSARCOMA: This form is most common in children between 3 and 12 years old, and frequently involves the head and neck, genitourinary tract, and retroperitoneum. Its appearance varies from that of a highly differentiated tumor containing rhabdomyoblasts, with large eosinophilic cytoplasm and cross-striations (Fig. 26-66A), to that of a poorly differentiated neoplasm.

BOTRYOID EMBRYONAL RHABDOMYOSARCOMA: This tumor, also known as **sarcoma botryoides**, is distinguished by the formation of polypoid, grapelike tumor masses. Microscopically, the malignant cells are scattered in an abundant myxoid stroma. Botryoid foci may occur in any type of embryonal rhabdomyosarcoma, but they are most common in tumors of hollow visceral organs, including the vagina (see Chapter 18) and bladder.

ALVEOLAR RHABDOMYOSARCOMA: This neoplasm occurs less frequently than the embryonal type and principally affects persons between ages 10 and 25; rarely, it may be seen in elderly patients. It is most common in the upper and lower extremities, but it can also be distributed in the same sites as the embryonal type. Typically, club-shaped tumor cells are arranged in clumps that are outlined by fibrous septa. The loose arrangement of the cells in the center of the clusters leads to the "alveolar" pattern (see Fig. 26-66B). The tumor cells exhibit intense eosinophilia and occasional multinucleated giant cells are identified. Malignant rhabdomyoblasts, recognizable by their cross-striations, occur less commonly in the alveolar variant than in embryonal rhabdomyosarcoma, being present in only 25% of cases. Most alveolar rhabdomyosarcomas express *PAX3-FKHR* or *PAX7-FKHR* gene fusions, resulting from t(2;13)(q35;q14) or t(1;13)(p36;q14) translocations, respectively. In patients with localized tumors, the type of fusion does not correlate with the clinical outcome. However, in the presence of metastatic disease, *PAX3-FKHR*–positive tumors have a worse prognosis than do *PAX7-FKHR*–positive ones

PLEOMORPHIC RHABDOMYOSARCOMA: The least common form of rhabdomyosarcoma is found in the skeletal muscles of older persons, often in the thigh. This tumor differs from the other types of rhabdomyosarcoma in the pleomorphism of its irregularly arranged cells and can be categorized as one type of adult pleomorphic spindle cell sarcoma. Large, granular, eosinophilic rhabdomyoblasts, together with multinucleated giant cells, are common. Cross-striations are virtually nonexistent.

The historically dismal prognosis associated with most rhabdomyosarcomas has improved in the past two decades as a result of the introduction of combined therapeutic modalities, including surgery, radiation therapy, and chemotherapy. Today, more than 80% of patients with localized or regional disease are cured. Factors indicating a worse prognosis include age above 10, tumor size greater than 5 cm, alveolar and pleomorphic histologic subtypes, and advanced stage of disease.

Smooth Muscle Tumors

LEIOMYOMA: This benign soft tissue tumor usually arises in subcutaneous tissues, or from blood vessel walls. Leiomyomas are painful lesions that appear as firm, yellow, circumscribed nodules. Microscopically, intersecting fascicles of regular smooth cells are evident. Simple excision is curative.

A

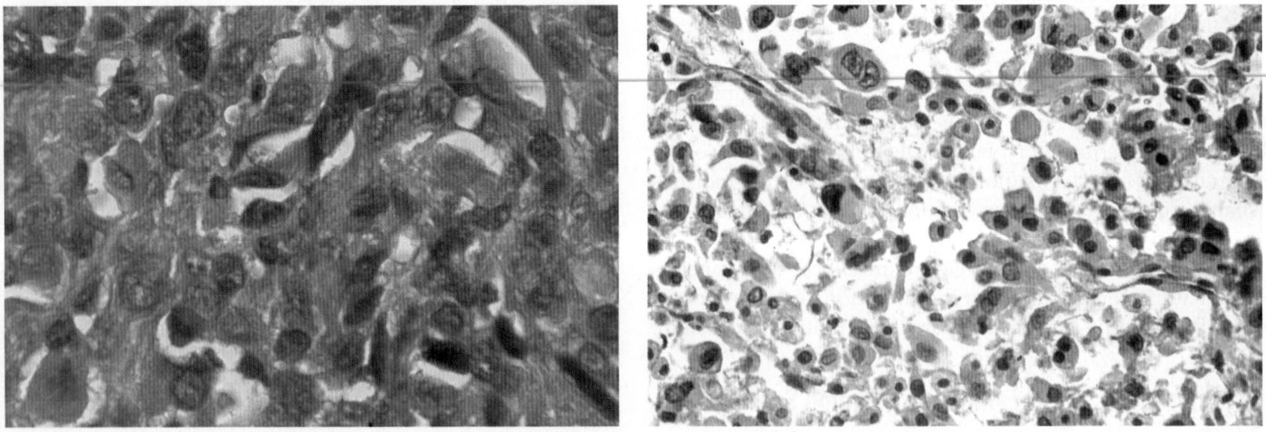

B

FIGURE 26-66. **Rhabdomyosarcoma. A.** The tumor contains polyhedral and spindle-shaped tumor cells with enlarged, hyperchromatic nuclei and deeply eosinophilic cytoplasm. A few cells have clearly visible cross striations. **B.** Alveolar rhabdomyosarcoma. The neoplastic cells are arranged in clusters that display an alveolar pattern.

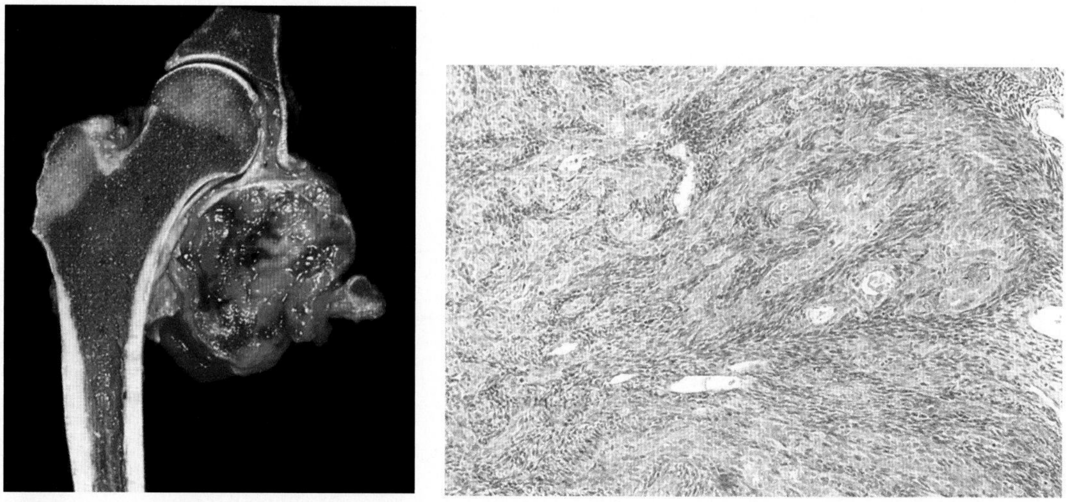

A B

FIGURE 26-67. **Synovial sarcoma. A.** Section of the upper femur and acetabulum reveals a tumor adjacent to the hip joint and the neck of the femur. **B.** A microscopic view demonstrates the biphasic appearance of a synovial sarcoma. Irregular glandular spaces are lined by plump, epithelial-like neoplastic cells. The intervening tissue contains smaller and darker staining spindle cells.

LEIOMYOSARCOMA: This malignant soft tissue neoplasm is an uncommon tumor of adults that typically arises from the wall of blood vessels in the extremities. Macroscopically, leiomyosarcomas tend to be well circumscribed, but are larger and softer than leiomyomas and often exhibit necrosis, hemorrhage, and cystic degeneration. Histologically, the tumor cells are arranged in fascicles, often with palisaded nuclei. Well-differentiated tumor cells have elongated nuclei and eosinophilic cytoplasm; poorly differentiated ones show increased cellularity and severe cytologic atypia (pleomorphic spindle cell sarcoma pattern). Leiomyosarcoma is differentiated from leiomyoma mainly by a high mitotic activity, which also indicates the prognosis. Most leiomyosarcomas eventually metastasize, although dissemination may occur as late as 15 or more years after resection of the primary tumor. Chromosomal abnormalities occur in leiomyosarcoma, but no specific alterations have been documented.

Vascular Tumors

Benign vascular tumors (hemangiomas) are among the most common soft tissue tumors and are the most frequent neoplasms of infancy and childhood. By contrast, angiosarcomas are among the rarest of soft tissue tumors, accounting for less than 1% of all sarcomas. Vascular tumors are discussed in detail in Chapter 10.

Synovial Sarcoma

Synovial sarcoma is a highly malignant soft tissue tumor that arises in the region of a joint, usually in association with tendon sheaths, bursae, and joint capsules. Fewer than 10% of synovial sarcomas are intra-articular. This tumor may also arise in other soft tissue sites as well as in other organs. Although the tumor bears a microscopic resemblance to synovium, its origin from this tissue has not been established. Thus, it is currently considerd to be a malignant soft tissue tumor with both epithelial and mesenchymal differentiation. Synovial sarcoma occurs principally in adolescents and young adults as a painful or tender mass, usually in the vicinity of a large joint, particularly the knee.

PATHOGENESIS: Synovial sarcomas display a specific, balanced chromosomal translocation involving chromosomes X and 18 [t(x;18)(p11.2;q11.2)]. This translocation results in fusion of the *SYT* (synteny) gene on chromosome 18 to the *SSX* gene (a transcriptional repressor) on the X chromosome, leading to production of a hybrid protein, SYT-SSX1 or SYT-SSX2. The **SYT-SSX2** protein is associated with a better prognosis if the disease is localized.

PATHOLOGY: On gross examination, synovial sarcomas are usually circumscribed, round or multilobular masses attached to tendons, tendon sheaths or the exterior wall of the joint capsule (Fig. 26-67A). The tumors tend to be surrounded by a glistening pseudocapsule and in many instances are cystic. They range from small nodules to masses of 15 cm or more in diameter, the average being 3 to 5 cm.

Microscopically, synovial sarcoma is classically described as having a **biphasic pattern** (see Fig. 26-67B). Fluid-filled glandular spaces lined by epithelium-like tumor cells are embedded in a sarcomatous, spindle cell background. These elements vary in proportion, distribution and cellular differentiation, with the spindle cells usually considerably more numerous than the glandular elements. If the "epithelial" component is lacking, the tumor is referred to as **monophasic synovial sarcoma**. Although monophasic synovial sarcoma resembles fibrosarcoma, its atypical spindle cells are plumper and swirled rather than being arranged in a herringbone pattern. Calcifications may be present within the tumor. Synovial sarcoma usually expresses cytokeratins or epithelial membrane antigen, further evidence of epithelial differentiation.

The recurrence rate of synovial sarcoma is high, and metastases occur in more than 60% of cases. The 5-year survival rate is about 50%, and those who die usually have extensive lung metastases.

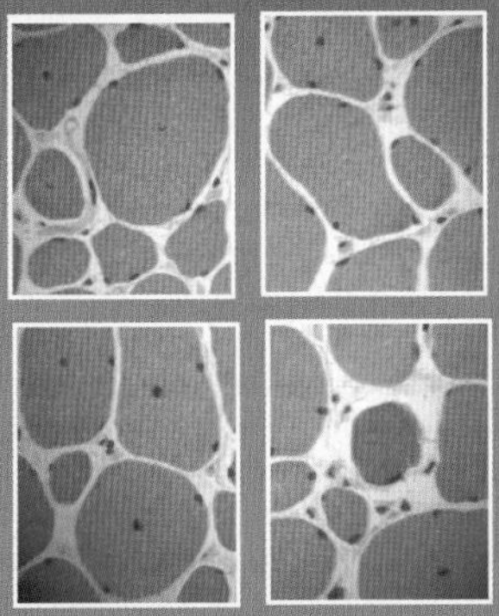

27 Skeletal Muscle

Lawrence C. Kenyon
Mark T. Curtis

Embryology and Anatomy

The myoblast is a primitive cell that fuses with other myoblasts to form a cylindrical multinucleated myotube. The periphery of the myotube rapidly accumulates myofibrils, containing myosin and actin, which become arrayed in the cross-banded pattern characteristic of striated muscle (Fig. 27-1). The myofiber has a distinctive architecture that is visualized by electron microscopy (Fig. 27-2).

The myotube matures completely when it is innervated by the terminal axon of a lower motor neuron. Before innervation, the sarcolemma of the myotube contains diffusely distributed nicotinic receptors for acetylcholine on its surface membrane. When innervation occurs, these receptors become highly concentrated at the motor endplate. Although an individual muscle fiber is innervated by only a single nerve ending, a given motor neuron innervates numerous muscle fibers. After innervation, the nuclei of each fiber move from the center to arrange themselves in a regular pattern beneath the sarcolemma (Fig. 27-3A).

The muscle fibers responsible for movement are referred to as **extrafusal fibers**, whereas those contained within stretch receptors (muscle spindle organs) are known as **intrafusal fibers.** *Most primary myopathies feature damage extrafusal fibers but not intrafusal fibers.* Thus, muscle spindle organs, which are usually inconspicuous in routine histologic preparations, become relatively more prominent as extrafusal fibers disappear.

The myofiber comprises distinct functional units. The following definitions are important for understanding muscle structure and function and the morphology of muscle dysfunction:

- **Sarcomere:** Functional unit of the myofibril that extends from one Z band to the next
- **Z band:** A distinct electron-dense band that anchors the thin actin filaments
- **I band:** Zone of the actin filaments as they extend from the Z band into the A band.
- **A band:** Structure composed of the thick myosin filaments. Actin filaments overlap myosin filaments to a variable extent, depending on the degree of muscle contraction. The thin filaments form a hexagonal array around each thick filament.
- **H zone:** Pale region in the midportion of the A band where actin filaments end
- **M line:** Zone of intermolecular bridging and thickening of myosin filaments at the midline of the A band, which forms a thin, slightly darker electron-dense band.

During contraction, actin filaments slide past myosin filaments. The sliding actin filaments advance farther into the A band, producing a shorter sarcomere length. As a result, the lengths of the I band and H zone decrease, whereas that of the A band remains nearly constant.

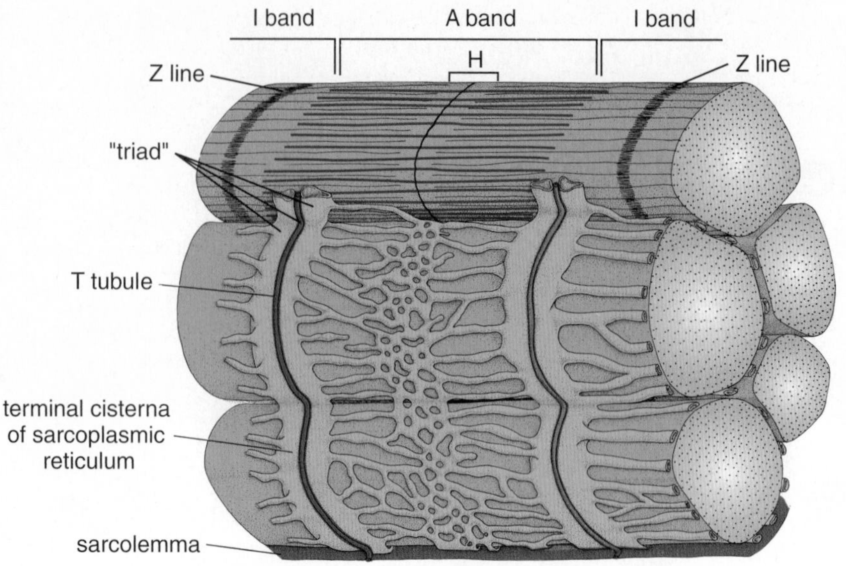

FIGURE 27-1. **Normal striated muscle.** Cross-striations of striated muscle are created by the arrangement of the myofilaments of the myofibril (compare to Fig. 27-2). The dark A band results from the thick myosin filaments and the thinner, partially overlapping actin filaments. In the middle portion of the myosin filaments where the actin does not overlap, there is a lighter band called the H zone or H band. In the middle of the H band, the center of each myosin filament thickens, forming intermolecular bridging with the adjacent myosin filament and giving rise to the M line. The finer actin filaments are anchored on the dark Z disk of the lighter I band. With contraction, the myosin filaments pull the actin filaments, causing the H zone to disappear, the A band to widen, and the I band to shrink. The mitochondria are scattered throughout the sarcoplasm among the myofibrils. The endoplasmic reticulum (sarcoplasmic reticulum) forms an extensive, complex tubular network with periodic dilations (cisternae) around each myofibril. The cisternae are closely apposed to the transverse tubules, which are derived from the cell membrane (sarcolemma) and form a transverse network, which resembles chicken wire, around each myofibril, giving extensive communication between the internal and external environments. (Used with permission from Ross. . . . p 291)

The **sarcoplasmic reticulum** surrounds each myofibril and forms an elaborate membranous network that has irregular dilations (cisternae) juxtaposed to a transverse tubular network derived from the sarcolemma (see Fig. 27-1). The **transverse tubular system** (T tubule system) is arranged across the fiber like chicken wire, each ring wrapping around an individual myofibril. This arrangement allows an electrical stimulus to proceed along the muscle fiber surface and become diffusely and rapidly internalized via the transverse tubular system. The electrical signal is translated into a chemical signal between the transverse tubule and the cisternae of the sarcoplasmic reticulum. This process releases calcium from the sarcoplasmic reticulum into the vicinity of myofibrils, where the chemical signal triggers muscle contraction.

The lower motor neuron and the fibers that it innervates are referred to as the ***motor unit***. Sizes of motor units vary. In limb muscles, a single motor unit can comprise as many as several hundred myofibers. By contrast, each motor unit of extraocular muscles may have as few as 20 myofibers. The muscles of the eye are also exceptional in that a single fiber may have more than one motor endplate.

Myofibers Are Classified as Slow Twitch or Fast Twitch

After innervation, a characteristic metabolic profile develops for different muscle fibers. In lower mammals, some muscles are deep red (type I), whereas others are pale (type II).

TYPE I FIBERS (RED, SLOW TWITCH): If a nerve stimulates a dark (red) muscle, the resulting contraction is slower and more prolonged than when a nerve excites a pale (white) muscle. For this reason, red muscles have been classified as "slow twitch." Type I fibers tend to have more mitochondria and more myoglobin, the red, oxygen-storing, pigment. The enzymes of the Krebs cycle and the carrier proteins of the electron-transport chain–mitochondrial constituents are all present in greater amounts in slow-twitch muscle than in fast-twitch muscle. The alkaline histochemical reaction for myosin ATPase gives a crisp distinction between the two fiber types. Type I fibers remain almost unstained at high (alkaline) pH, whereas type II fibers stain darkly (see Fig. 27-3B).

Functionally, type I muscles have a greater capacity for long, sustained contractions and resist fatigue. A training program that increases endurance produces little change in size of type I fibers, but conditioning of these fibers results in a proliferation of mitochondria and an expanded capacity for generating energy.

TYPE II FIBERS (WHITE, FAST TWITCH): Stimulation of type II fibers elicits faster, shorter, and more powerful contrac-

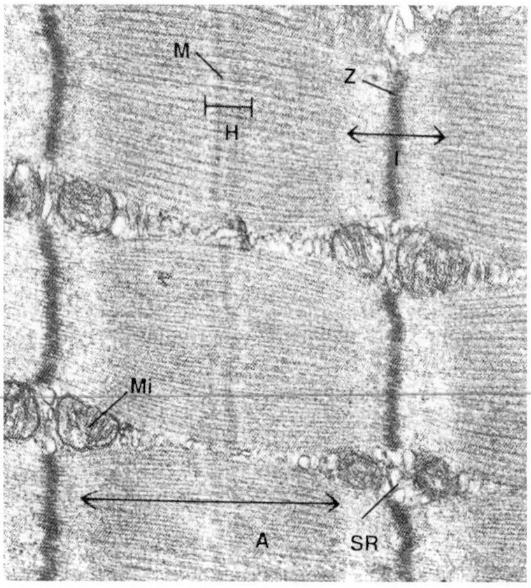

FIGURE 27-2. **Normal muscle.** This electron micrograph of the biceps muscle demonstrates the ultrastructure of the sarcomere. The thin dark band, the Z disk *(Z)*, bisects the broad, pale I band *(I)*, a zone composed of the thin actin filaments. The broad, dark band, made up of the thick myosin filaments and overlapping actin filaments, is the A band *(A)*. The middle of the A band consists of the pale H zone *(H)*, which in turn is bisected by a slightly darker M line *(M)*, representing a zone of intermolecular bridging of myosin. Small membrane-bound vesicles compose the sarcoplasmic reticulum *(SR)* and the transverse tubules. Pairs of mitochondria *(Mi)* tend to be located between myofibrils at the level of the I bands.

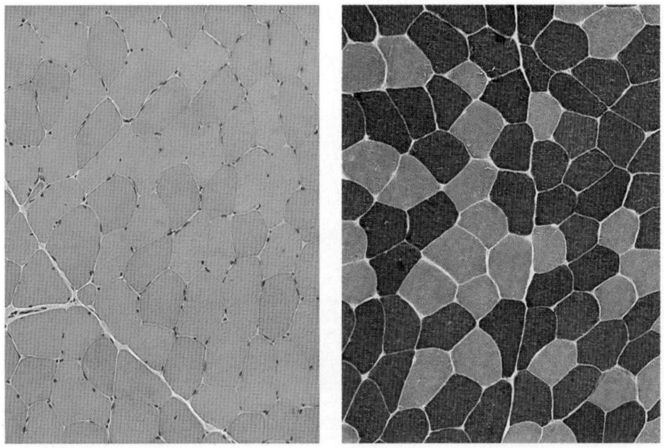

FIGURE 27-3. **Normal muscle. A.** Hematoxylin and eosin stain. In this transverse frozen section of the vastus lateralis, the polygonal myofibers are separated from each other by an indistinct, thin layer of connective tissue, the endomysium. The thicker band of connective tissue, the perimysium, demarcates a bundle or fascicle of fibers. All of the nuclei in this field are located at the periphery of the cells. Occasional nuclei are contained within satellite cells but cannot be distinguished from those of the myofibers by light microscopy. **B.** Myofibrillar (myosin) ATPase. Type I fibers are pale, at high (alkaline) pH; type II fibers are dark. Note the intermixture of fiber types.

tions than occur in type I fibers. Glycogen, phosphorylase, and other enzymes which produce energy by anaerobic glycolysis in the Embden-Meyerhof pathway are present in higher concentrations in white muscle. Type II muscle fibers are suitable for rapid contractions of brief duration and react to strength training with hypertrophy. Androgenic steroids induce type II fiber hypertrophy, and disuse of muscle results in their selective atrophy.

The lower motor neuron influences fiber type. During embryonic development of mammals, early muscle cells begin to express type-specific contractile proteins before muscle is innervated. Thus, the phenotype of a myofiber seems to be a programmed characteristic of the cell, rather than one induced by the nerve supply. However, the kind of innervation can alter the types of myofibers. For example, after denervation injury, reinnervation of a slow-twitch muscle by a nerve from a fast-twitch muscle causes the newly innervated type I fibers to assume staining characteristics of type II fibers. It is thought that the pattern or rate of discharge of the lower motor neuron plays an important role in this process. Because lower motor neurons can determine fiber type, it follows that all the muscle fibers in a given motor unit are of the same type. A cross-section of muscle stained with the alkaline ATPase reaction shows a random mixture of fiber types (see Fig. 27-3B), because motor units interdigitate extensively with each other.

In humans, no muscles are composed exclusively of one fiber type. However, the proportion of fiber types does vary from muscle to muscle. For example, the soleus muscle is composed of predominantly (≥80%) type I fibers. The pattern of fiber types in a given muscle varies between persons, a difference that is apparently genetically determined. Some evidence indicates that changing the use of a muscle over a long period through intensive training may alter the pattern of muscle fiber types.

Muscle Biopsy

Since the normal muscle pattern is more constant within a specific muscle, the same muscles are biopsied from case to case. Samples from the quadriceps femoris or biceps brachii are suitable for biopsy diagnosis in most primary muscle diseases (myopathies). Biopsy of the sural nerve and gastrocnemius muscle is often performed in patients with a suspected peripheral neuropathy. However, because some neuromuscular conditions are more focal, locations for muscle biopsies are not invariable.

Biopsy sampling from a moderately involved muscle is the most informative. Unaffected muscles may have little or no pathologic changes, whereas a severely weak muscle may be largely replaced by adipose and fibrous connective tissue (see end-stage muscle, Fig. 27-5).

Muscle is stained by a variety of histochemical reactions:

- **Nonspecific esterase:** Important for identifying denervation atrophy (see Fig. 27-22).
- **NADH-tetrazolium reductase (NADH-TR):** Type I fibers appear dark owing to abundant mitochondria (see Fig. 27-23).
- **Succinate dehydrogenase (SDH):** Sensitive histochemical index of mitochondrial proliferation caused by mutations of mitochondrial DNA (mtDNA) (see Fig. 27-20B)
- **Cytochrome C oxidase:** Fibers containing abnormal mitochondria lacking the terminal component of the electron transport chain will fail to stain (see Fig. 27-20C).
- **Alkaline phosphatase:** Regenerating fibers are selectively stained.
- **Periodic acid-Schiff (PAS):** Helpful in identification of glycogen and the diagnosis of glycogen-storage diseases.
- **Oil red orcein (Oil red O):** Marks neutral lipid and is particularly useful in evaluating lipid storage myopathies such as carnitine deficiency (see Fig. 27-19).
- **Modified Gomori trichrome stain:** Versatile stain in evaluation of myopathies.

General Pathologic Reactions

Necrosis is a common response of myofibers to injury in primary muscle diseases (**myopathies**). Widespread acute necrosis of skeletal muscle fibers (**rhabdomyolysis**) releases cytosolic proteins, including myoglobin, into the circulation, which may result in myoglobinuria and acute renal failure. In many human myopathies, necrosis occurs in a segment along the length of the fiber, leaving two intact portions that flank the site of damage (Fig. 27-4). The injury quickly elicits two responses: an influx of blood-borne macrophages into the necrotic cytoplasm and activation of the satellite cells, a population of dormant myoblasts located in close proximity to each fiber. As monocytes gradually phagocytose the necrotic debris and remove it, satellite cells proliferate and become active myoblasts. Within 2 days, they begin to fuse, to each other and to the ends of the intact fiber remnants, to form a joining multinucleated segment. This regenerating fiber is smaller in diameter than the parent fiber, and has basophilic cytoplasm and large, vesicular nuclei with prominent nucleoli.

Regeneration can restore normal structure and function of muscle fibers within a few weeks after a single episode of injury, as in the inherited disorder myophosphorylase deficiency (see below). With subacute or chronic disorders, fiber necrosis proceeds concurrently with fiber regeneration, gradually leading to atrophy of muscle fibers and fibrosis.

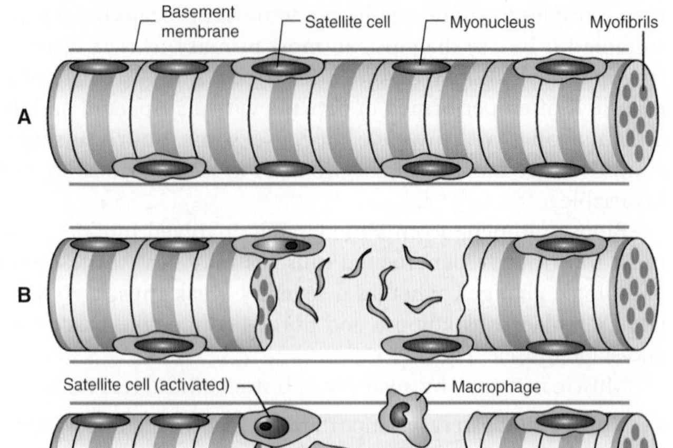

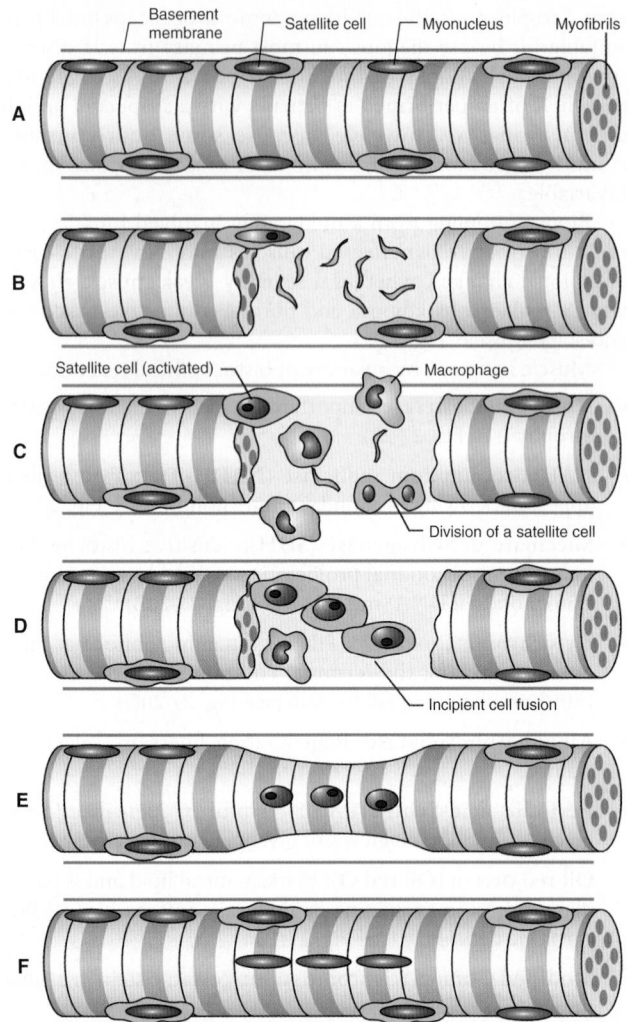

FIGURE 27-4. **Segmental necrosis and regeneration of a muscle fiber.** **A.** A normal muscle fiber contains myofibrils and subsarcolemmal nuclei and is covered by a basement membrane. Scattered satellite cells are situated on the surface of the sarcolemma, inside the basement membrane. These cells are dormant myoblasts, capable of proliferating and fusing to form differentiated fibers. They constitute 3% to 5% of the nuclei, as observed in a cross-section of skeletal muscle. **B.** In many muscle diseases (e.g., Duchenne muscular dystrophy or polymyositis), injury to the muscle fiber causes segmental necrosis with disintegration of the sarcoplasm, leaving a preserved basement membrane and nerve supply (not shown). **C.** The damaged segment attracts circulating macrophages that penetrate the basement membrane and begin to digest and engulf the sarcoplasmic contents (myophagocytosis). Regenerative processes begin with the activation and proliferation of the satellite cells, forming myoblasts within the basement membrane. Macrophages gradually leave the site of injury with their load of debris. **D.** At a later stage, the myoblasts are aligned in close proximity to each other in the center of the fiber and begin to fuse. **E.** Regeneration of the fiber segment is prominent, as indicated by the large, pale, vesicular, centrally located nuclei. **F.** The fiber is nearly normal except for a few persistent central nuclei. Eventually, the normal state (A) is restored.

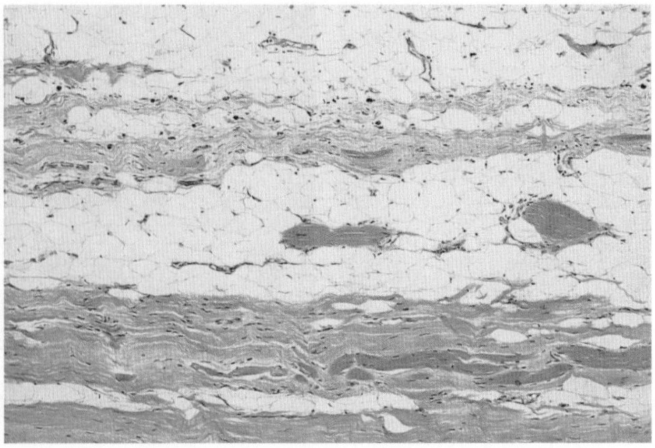

FIGURE 27-5. **End-stage neuromuscular disease.** In this section of the deltoid muscle stained by hematoxylin and eosin, skeletal muscle has been largely replaced by fibrofatty connective tissue. The few surviving muscle fibers have a deeper eosinophilia than does the abundant collagenous component.

Muscular Dystrophy

In the middle of the 19th century, physicians discovered that progressive weakness of the voluntary muscles could be caused by either a disorder of the nervous system or primary degeneration of muscles. **Muscular dystrophy** was the name applied to primary muscular degeneration. It was frequently found to be hereditary (or at least familial) and relentlessly progressive. Morphologic study of muscle tissue from these patients showed necrosis of muscle fibers, with regenerative activity, progressive fibrosis, and infiltration of the muscle with fatty tissue (Fig. 27-5). Little or no inflammation was recognized. In subsequent years, numerous variants of this type of muscle disease were described, and a classification of hereditary, progressive, noninflammatory degenerative conditions of muscle has evolved.

Duchenne and Becker Muscular Dystrophies Are Inherited Noninflammatory Myopathies

***Duchenne muscular dystrophy** is a severe, progressive, X-linked, inherited condition characterized by progressive degeneration of muscles, particularly those of the pelvic and shoulder girdles.* It is the most common noninflammatory myopathy in children. A milder form of the disease is known as **Becker muscular dystrophy** (see Chapter 6 for the molecular genetics of both diseases). The serum creatine kinase activity is greatly increased in both conditions.

PATHOGENESIS: Duchenne muscular dystrophy is caused by mutations of a large gene on the short arm of the X chromosome (Xp21). This gene codes for **dystrophin**, a 427-kd protein localized on the inner surface of the sarcolemma. Dystrophin links the subsarcolemmal cytoskeleton to the exterior of the cell through a transmembrane complex of proteins and glycoproteins that binds to laminin (Fig. 27-6). Dystrophin is absent or greatly decreased, often as a result of deletions of the gene (Fig. 27-7). Dystrophin-deficient muscle fibers thus lack the normal interaction between the sarcolemma and the extracellular matrix. This disruption may be responsible for the observed increased osmotic fragility of dystrophic muscle, excessive influx of calcium ions, and release of soluble muscle enzymes such as creatine kinase into the serum. Further evidence to support this hypothesis is the fact that a breakdown of the sarcolemma precedes muscle cell necrosis, and the basal lamina seems to separate from the sarcolemma early in the course of Duchenne muscular dystrophy.

Becker muscular dystrophy is allelic to Duchenne dystrophy. Mutated dystrophin genes produce an altered,

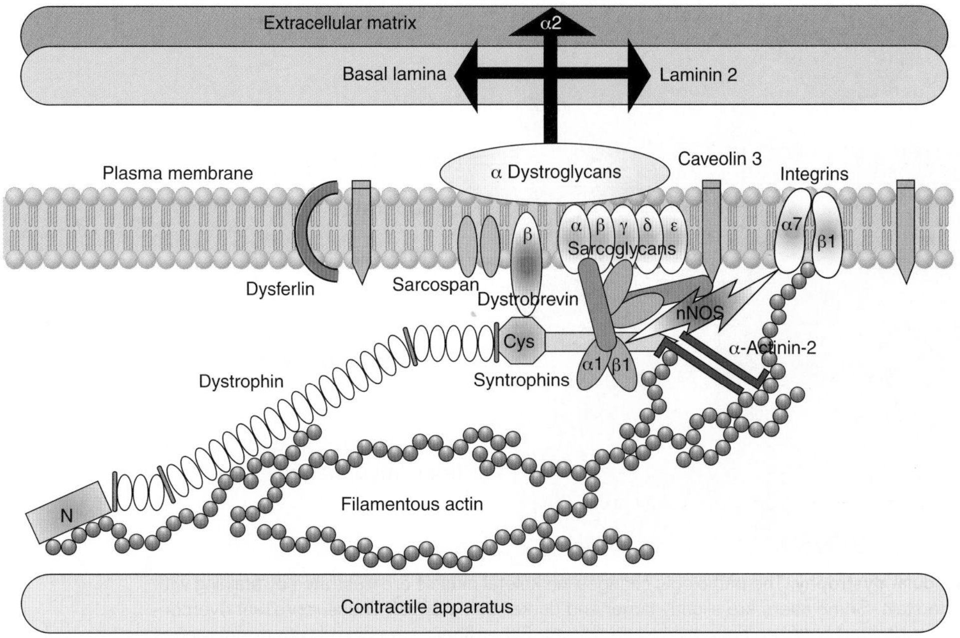

FIGURE 27-6. **Diagrammatic representation of proteins linking dystrophin to the plasma membrane and the contractile apparatus.** Several of these linking proteins are associated with known myopathies (see table 27-1)

usually truncated, protein. This mutated protein correctly localizes to the surface membrane of muscle fibers, but immunocytochemical staining is often less intense or focally absent (see Fig. 27-7). The abnormal protein apparently retains sufficient function to yield a less severe phenotype. *Other muscle diseases closely resemble Duchenne and Becker dystrophies but are inherited in a recessive autosomal fashion.* Some of these patients have mutations that affect expression of transmembrane proteins or glycoproteins and interrupt the link between the cytoskeleton and extracellular matrix (Table 27-1 and see Fig. 27-6).

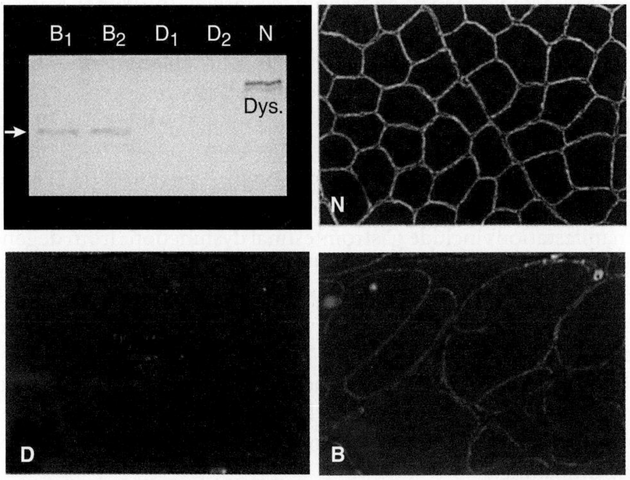

FIGURE 27-7. **Dystrophin analysis in Duchenne and Becker muscular dystrophies.** Immunofluorescence stain for dystrophin. The sections illustrate a normal subject *(N)*, a patient with Duchenne dystrophy *(D)*, and one with Becker dystrophy *(B)*. Dystrophin is normally concentrated at the surface membrane of every muscle fiber, but in Duchenne dystrophy, the protein is absent or is only barely detected in a small proportion of muscle fibers. Becker dystrophy exhibits hypertrophic muscle fibers with reduced expression of dystrophin. The immunoblot *(upper left)* of normal muscle shows a band near the top of the gel corresponding to the 427-kd protein dystrophin. Dystrophin is undetectable in Duchenne dystrophy (two patients). In Becker dystrophy, a weaker band has migrated farther down the gel relative to the normal protein, and it corresponds to a smaller, truncated protein. The combined analysis (immunolocalization and immunoblot) of the dystrophin protein is diagnostic of this group of dystrophies *(dystrophinopathies)*.

PATHOLOGY: The disease process in Duchenne dystrophy consists of (1) relentless necrosis of muscle fibers, (2) a continuous effort at repair and regeneration, and (3) progressive fibrosis. The degenerative process eventually outstrips the regenerative capacity of the muscle. As a consequence, the number of muscle fibers decreases progressively and is replaced by fibrofatty connective tissue. The end stage is characterized by almost complete loss of skeletal muscle fibers (see Fig. 27-5), but relative sparing of muscle spindle fibers (intrafusal fibers)

In the early stage of the disease, necrotic fibers and regenerating fibers tend to occur in small groups, together with scattered, large, hyalinized dark fibers. The latter are overly contracted and are thought to precede fiber necrosis (Figs. 27-8 and 27-9). Breakdown of the sarcolemma is one of the earliest

TABLE 27–1

Muscular Dystrophies and Congenital Myopathies Caused by Abnormalities in the Sarcolemma or Extracellular Matrix

Muscle Disease	Defective Proteins
Sarcoglycanopathies	Sarcoglycans α-ε (muscle fiber plasma membrane proteins)
Dysferlinopathies (Limb girdle and Miyoshi myopathy)	Dysferlin (muscle fiber plasma membrane protein)
Caveolinopathies (hereditary rippling muscle disorder, or RMD)	Caveolin-3 (muscle fiber plasma membrane protein)

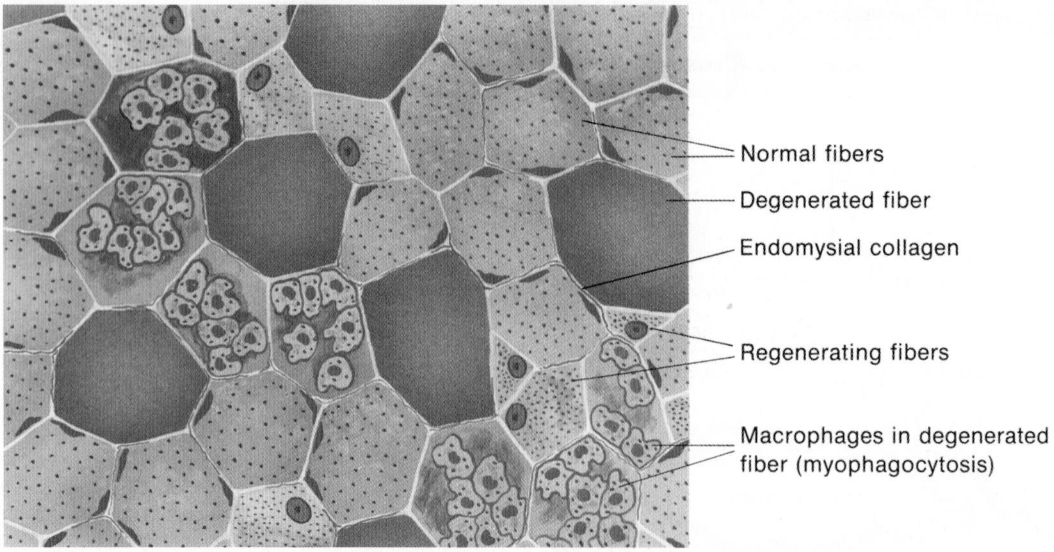

FIGURE 27-8. **Duchenne muscular dystrophy.** The pathologic changes in skeletal muscle are illustrated by staining with the modified Gomori trichrome stain. Some fibers are slightly larger and darker than normal. These represent overcontracted segments of sarcoplasm situated between degenerated segments. Other fibers are packed with macrophages (myophagocytosis), which remove degenerated sarcoplasm. Other fibers are smaller than normal and have granular sarcoplasm. These fibers have enlarged, vesicular nuclei with prominent nucleoli and represent regenerating fibers. Developing endomysial fibrosis is represented by the deposition of collagen around individual muscle fibers. The changes are those of a chronic, active noninflammatory myopathy.

ultrastructural changes. Macrophages invade necrotic fibers and reflect a scavenging function rather than an inflammatory process.

The diagnosis of Duchenne dystrophy can be established by polymerase chain reaction (PCR) analysis of genomic DNA derived from leukocytes in a blood sample. In practice, diagnosis using this method is limited to large deletions of the gene. About 30% of patients have small rearrangements or point mutations and can be evaluated by muscle biopsy, which shows little or no detectable dystrophin by immunoblot or immunocytochemistry.

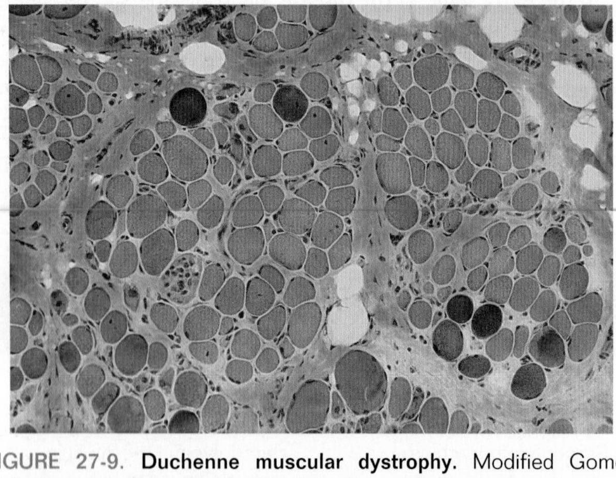

FIGURE 27-9. **Duchenne muscular dystrophy.** Modified Gomori trichrome stain. A section of vastus lateralis muscle shows necrotic muscle fibers, some of them invaded by macrophages. The endomysial septae are thickened, indicating fibrosis. Dark staining, enlarged fibers represent overly contracted fibers. Calcium influx across the defective surface membrane overwhelms mechanisms that maintain a low resting Ca^{2+} concentration and triggers excessive contraction. There is conspicuous perimysial and endomysial fibrosis.

CLINICAL FEATURES: Boys with Duchenne muscular dystrophy have markedly increased serum creatine kinase levels from birth and morphologically abnormal muscle even in utero. Clinical weakness is not detectable during the first year, but usually becomes so by the age of 3 or 4 years, mainly around pelvic and shoulder girdles (proximal muscle weakness). It is relentlessly progressive. "Pseudohypertrophy" (enlargement of a muscle due to abundant replacement of muscle fibers by fibroadipose tissue) of the calf muscles eventually develops. Patients are usually wheelchair bound by the age of 10 and bedridden by 15. Death usually results from complications of respiratory insufficiency caused by muscular weakness or cardiac arrhythmia due to myocardial involvement. Other extraskeletal manifestations include gastrointestinal dysfunction (from degeneration of smooth muscle) and intellectual impairment. Many boys affected with Duchenne dystrophy exhibit variable degrees of mental retardation, apparently due to lack of dystrophin in the central nervous system (CNS).

Occasional cases that are indistinguishable from Duchenne muscular dystrophy occur in girls. These patients represent a genetically different disease or nonrandom inactivation of the X chromosome.

CARRIER DETECTION: Because Duchenne muscular dystrophy is inherited as an X-linked recessive disease, it is passed from a mother who is a heterozygous carrier of the abnormal gene. About 30% of cases occur because of a spontaneous somatic mutation. Until recently, carriers were best detected by repeatedly measuring serum creatine kinase levels, which is moderately increased in 75% of heterozygotes. There is considerable variability in the expression of the carrier state, probably because of variations in the random inactivation of the X chromosome. Some carriers can now be detected by dystrophin immunolocalization performed on a muscle biopsy specimen. This procedure shows a characteristic mosaic pattern of deficient and normal myofibers.

Molecular probes detect more than two thirds of persons who carry large deletions.

Myotonic Dystrophy Is Characterized by Impaired Muscle Relaxation

Myotonic dystrophy, the most common form of adult muscular dystrophy, is an autosomal dominant disorder characterized by slowing muscle relaxation (myotonia) and progressive muscle weakness and wasting. Prevalence has been estimated to be as high as 14 per 100,000, although it may be higher because of the difficulty in detecting minimally affected persons. Age at onset and severity of symptoms show extreme variety. Myotonic dystrophy is classified as either adult onset and congenital.

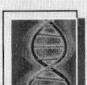

PATHOGENESIS: The gene for myotonic dystrophy has been localized to the long arm of chromosome 19 (19q13.3). Most cases seem to be descended from one original mutation, the expansion of a CTG repeat near the 3′ end of the gene. Normal persons have fewer than 30 copies of this trinucleotide repeat, whereas there may be 50 or more copies in minimally affected myotonic dystrophy patients. An interesting genetic characteristic of this disease is "anticipation" (i.e., an earlier age at onset and increasing severity of symptoms in successive generations). The number of trinucleotide repeats increases with successive generations, and the size of the repeat sequence correlates with the severity of symptoms. The gene for myotonic dystrophy encodes a novel serine–threonine protein kinase. The mechanism of injury brought about by expansion of CTG repeats in myotonic dystrophy, as in other trinucleotide repeat disorders, is not clearly understood at present (see Chapter 1).

PATHOLOGY: The pathology of adult myotonic dystrophy is highly variable, even in muscles from the same patient. Most patients display type I fiber atrophy and hypertrophy of type II fibers. Internally situated nuclei are a constant feature. The ATPase reaction shows many ring fibers, with circumferential concentration of heavily stained sarcoplasm. In these fibers, there is a circumferential orientation of the sarcomeres instead of the usual longitudinal arrangement along the fiber axis (Fig. 27-10). Necrosis and regeneration, although occasionally present, are not prominent (as they are in Duchenne muscular dystrophy).

The muscle of congenital myotonic dystrophy shows myofiber atrophy, frequent central nuclei, and failure of fiber differentiation. These pathologic features closely resemble those of the X-linked recessive type of myotubular myopathy (see below).

CLINICAL FEATURES: In addition to skeletal muscle, myotonic dystrophy affects many systems, including the heart, smooth muscle, CNS, endocrine glands, and eye. The diagnosis is based on clinical features, family history, and the characteristic electromyography, which exhibits myotonic discharges. Demonstration of an expanded trinucleotide repeat is predictive in utero and can be diagnostic in patients.

Adult myotonic dystrophy features slowly progressive muscle weakness and stiffness, principally in the distal limbs. Facial and jaw muscles are virtually always affected; ptosis can be severe. Extramuscular features of myotonic dystrophy are sometimes present and include cataracts, testicular atrophy with diminished fertility, and variable degrees of personality deterioration. A few patients exhibit involvement of smooth muscle, with disorders of the gastrointestinal tract, gallbladder, and uterus. Cardiac arrhythmias and, less commonly, cardiomyopathy have been reported.

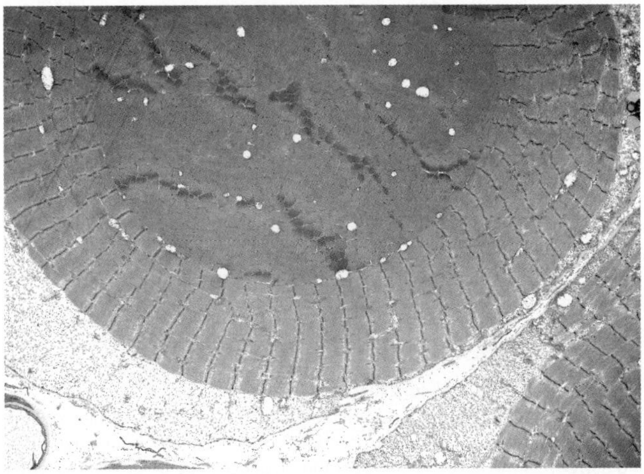

FIGURE 27-10. **Ring fiber.** Electron micrograph (magnification × 1,900). The sarcomeres are oriented perpendicular to the axis of the myofiber.

Congenital myotonic dystrophy is seen only in the offspring of women who themselves exhibit symptoms of myotonic dystrophy. The infants are born with severe muscle weakness, but myotonia is inconspicuous or absent, although it appears in later childhood. A significant number of these patients suffer mental retardation.

Congenital Myopathies

Occasionally, a newborn manifests generalized hypotonia, with decreased deep tendon reflexes and muscle bulk. Many of these children have a difficult perinatal period because of weak respiration and consequent pulmonary complications. Some have "malignant" hypotonia, which is progressive and results in death within the first 12 months of life. **Werdnig-Hoffman disease** and **infantile acid maltase deficiency (Pompe disease)** are examples.

Other hypotonic patients have a "benign" course. Although hypotonia persists throughout their lives, it shows little or no progression. Patients become ambulatory and live a normal life span, although sometimes complicated by secondary skeletal complications of the hypotonia. This group of patients is subsumed in the category of "congenital myopathies." Morphologic study of the muscle of these patients rarely reveals distinctive structural abnormalities of myofibers. Three of the most common forms of congenital myopathies are central core disease, nemaline (rod) myopathy, and central nuclear myopathy (Figs. 27-11, 27-12, and 27-13, respectively). Some generalizations can be made about these conditions. They all show congenital hypotonia, decreased deep tendon reflexes, decreased muscle bulk, and delayed motor milestones. In addition, in all three conditions the morphologic abnormality in muscle biopsies is usually limited to type I (red) fibers. Furthermore, these patients often have an abnormal predominance of type I fibers or possibly, a failure to develop type II (white) fibers. The muscle does not

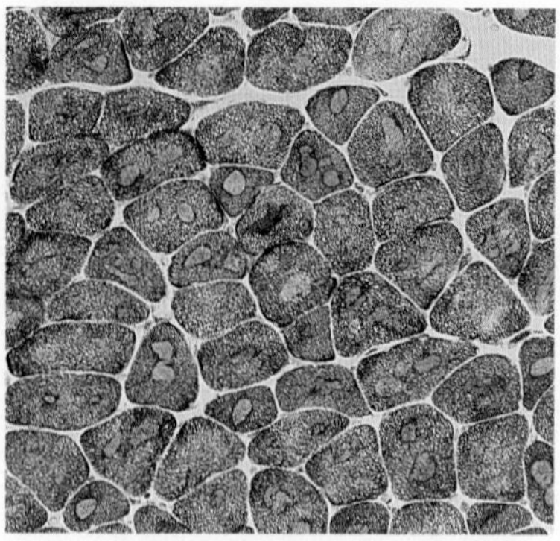

FIGURE 27-11. **Central core disease.** A section of vastus lateralis muscle stained for NADH-tetrazolium reductase shows a distinct circular zone of pallor in the center of most muscle fibers. A thin zone of excessive staining surrounds the core lesion. All of the myofibers in this case were type I, as demonstrated by the myofibrillar ATPase stain (not shown). Note the close resemblance of the core lesions to the target formations found in the muscle fibers of neurogenic disorders (see Fig. 27-23).

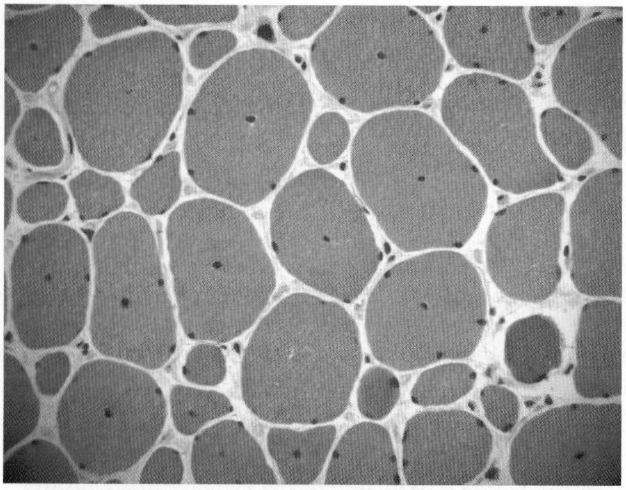

FIGURE 27-13. **Central nuclear (myotubular) myopathy.** Hematoxylin and eosin stain. Many muscle fibers contain a single central nucleus, and most of the affected muscle fibers are abnormally small. In addition, there are radiating spokes emanating from the central nuclei. These fibers resemble the late myotube stage of fetal development of skeletal muscle.

show active myofiber necrosis or fibrosis, and patients have normal serum creatine kinase.

Central Core Disease is an Autosomal Dominant Condition Characterized by Congenital Hypotonia and Proximal Muscle Weakness

Afflicted patients have decreased deep tendon reflexes and delayed motor development. The disease has been traced to a mutation on the long arm of chromosome 19 (19q13.1) that codes for the ryanodine receptor, the calcium-release channel of the sarcoplasmic reticulum. Occasional cases are sporadic or show autosomal recessive inheritance. Typical patients become ambulatory, but muscle strength remains less than normal.

PATHOLOGY: Muscle biopsy reveals striking predominance of type I fibers. Many or all of these show a central zone of degeneration with loss of NADH-TR reaction staining (Fig. 27-11). This central core abnormality extends the entire length of the fiber. The central core is difficult to see with hematoxylin and eosin staining but can often be demonstrated with the PAS reaction. By electron microscopy, the central core is characterized by a loss of mitochondria and other membranous organelles, with or without myofibril disorganization. Membranous organelles tend to condense around the margin of the central core. The periphery of the fiber is otherwise unremarkable.

The central core anomaly bears a striking resemblance to the target fibers seen in active denervating conditions (see Fig. 27-23), although there is no evidence of denervation. The motor endplates are architecturally unremarkable, and no extrajunctional nicotinic acetylcholine receptors are present in the muscle membrane.

Mutations of the ryanodine receptor gene also cause one form of **malignant hyperthermia**, a potentially fatal disorder triggered by surgical anesthesia. Both central core disease and this adverse response to anesthesia coexist in some patients.

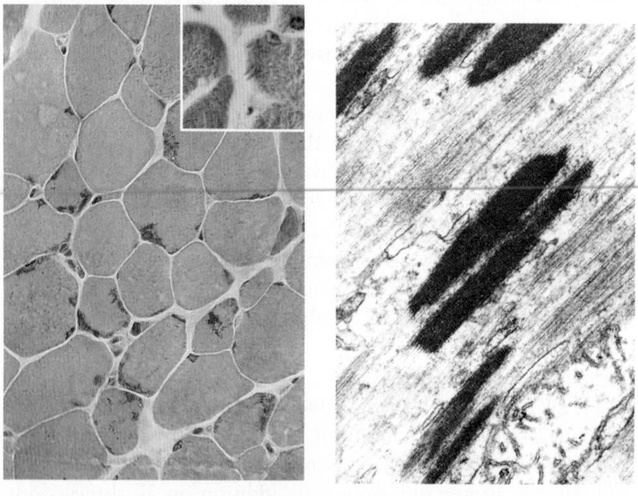

A B

FIGURE 27-12. **Rod (nemaline) myopathy. A,** Muscle fibers contain dark aggregates of rods and granules (modified Gomori trichrome stain). As shown in the inset, these rods tend to be located at the fiber periphery near nuclei. **B**. An electron micrograph of the same biopsy shows that the structures are rod-shaped and are derived from the Z-disc.

Rod (Nemaline) Myopathy Displays Inclusions That Derive from the Z Band

Rod myopathy includes a heterogeneous group of diseases that have in common the accumulation of rodlike inclusions within the sarcoplasm of skeletal muscle. The disease was initially named "nemaline" myopathy because the inclusions within the muscle fiber were interpreted as a tangled, threadlike mass. In reality, they are clusters of rod-shaped structures.

The classic congenital form of rod myopathy is characterized by congenital hypotonia, anddelayed motor milestones of variable clinical severity and secondary skeletal changes such as kyphoscoliosis. Some patients exhibit severe involvement of muscles of the face, pharynx, and neck. Later-onset (childhood and adult) forms tend to be associated with some muscle degeneration, increased serum creatine kinase levels, and a slowly progressive course. A few patients originally designated as having limb girdle muscular dystrophy have eventually been found to have rod myopathy. The etiology is unknown;

inheritance seems to be either autosomal dominant or autosomal recessive. Genes responsible for rod myopathy so far identified include slow α-tropomyosin, nebulin, skeletal muscle α-actin, β-tropomyosin, and slow troponin T. Mutations in the ryanodine receptor gene have also been associated with nemaline rod formation.

PATHOLOGY: The findings on muscle biopsy are variable predominance of type I fibers and accumulation of rod-shaped structures within their sarcoplasm. The aggregates of these inclusions are often located in subsarcolemmal regions near nuclei. They are brilliant red to dark red when stained with modified Gomori trichrome stain (see Fig. 27-12A) and may or may not be visible with hematoxylin and eosin. Ultrastructural studies demonstrate that the inclusions are indeed rod shaped and arise from the Z band, which they resemble ultrastructurally (see Fig. 27-12B).

Rods have been described in a variety of neuromuscular diseases, including denervation atrophy, muscular dystrophy, and inflammatory myopathies. Experimental tenotomy (cutting a tendon) induces formation of rods in the muscle when the nerve supply remains intact. In rod myopathy, however, the inclusions are the predominant pathologic change.

Central Nuclear Myopathy (Myotubular Myopathy) Resembles the Myotubular Stage of Embryogenesis

Central nuclear myopathy (myotubular myopathy) is a group of clinically and genetically heterogeneous inherited conditions that have in common the presence of a centrally located nucleus in skeletal muscle cells. Autosomal recessive, autosomal dominant, and X-linked recessive (Xq28) varieties have been recognized. In X-linked inheritance, newborns are strikingly weak and hypotonic, and may die of respiratory insufficiency during the neonatal period. The autosomal dominant form tends manifests later, and is associated with modestly increased serum creatine kinase. It progresses slowly and, like rod myopathy, resembles the so-called limb girdle muscular dystrophy syndrome. Some patients exhibit a striking involvement of facial and extraocular musculature.

PATHOLOGY: Biopsy specimens from patients with central nuclear myopathy are variable, but show type I fiber predominance (see Fig. 27-13). Many of these fibers are small and round, with a single central nucleus, accounting for the name of the disease. In this respect, they resemble the myotubular stage in skeletal muscle embryogenesis. This apparent immature state suggests a possible defect in the nerve supply to the muscle fiber because the lower motor neuron requires subsequent maturation of the fiber. However, studies of lower motor neurons in these patients, including motor endplates, have failed to identify any abnormality. Mutations of a gene for a tyrosine phosphatase cause the X-linked form of myotubular myopathy.

The later-onset forms of myotubular myopathy are characterized morphologically by more-mature muscle fibers, in which fibers are larger, have more numerous myofibrils, and display single central nuclei that appear more mature.

Inflammatory Myopathies

The inflammatory myopathies are a heterogeneous group of acquired disorders, all of which feature symmetric proximal muscle weakness, increased serum levels of muscle-derived enzymes, and nonsuppurative inflammation of skeletal muscle.

Inflammatory myopathies are uncommon, the annual incidence being 1 in 100,000. Dermatomyositis afflicts children and adults, whereas polymyositis almost always occurs after the age of 20 years. Both disorders are more frequent in females than males. By contrast inclusion body myositis usually occurs after age 50 years and is three times more common in men than women.

The inflammatory myopathies are thought to have an autoimmune origin because of (1) their association with other autoimmune and connective tissues diseases, (2) pathologic evidence of autoimmune mechanisms of muscle cell injury, (3) detection of autoantibodies in serum, and (4) a beneficial response to immunosuppressive agents in polymyositis and dermatomyositis (but not inclusion body myositis). No specific target autoantigens in muscle or blood vessels have been identified although antinuclear and anticytoplasmic antibodies exist in all of these diseases, with specificity to several different antigens.

The most common morphologic characteristics in the inflammatory myopathies are (1) the presence of inflammatory cells, (2) necrosis and phagocytosis of muscle fibers, (3) a mixture of regenerating and atrophic fibers, and (4) fibrosis.

CLINICAL FEATURES: All inflammatory myopathies manifest as insidious proximal and symmetric muscle weakness, gradually increasing over a period of weeks to months. Patients have problems with simple activities that require the use of proximal muscles, including lifting objects, climbing steps, or combing hair. Dysphagia and difficulty in holding up the head reflect involvement of pharyngeal and neck-flexor muscles. Some patients with inclusion body myositis have distal muscle weakness of the limbs that equals or exceeds that of proximal muscles. In advanced cases, respiratory muscles may be affected. Weakness progresses over weeks or months and leads to severe muscular wasting.

Dermatomyositis is distinguished from the other myopathies by a characteristic rash on the upper eyelids, face, trunk, and occasionally other body surfaces. It may occur alone or in association with scleroderma, mixed connective tissue disease, or other autoimmune conditions. When dermatomyositis occurs in a middle-aged man, it is associated with increased risk of epithelial cancer, most commonly lung carcinoma. Polymyositis and inclusion body myositis are not associated with malignancy.

Patients with inflammatory myopathies have increased serum creatine kinase and other muscle enzyme levels. Antinuclear and anticytoplasmic antibodies exist in all of these diseases, with specificity to several different antigens. Treatment of polymyositis and dermatomyositis with corticosteroids is usually successful, but inclusion body myositis is generally resistant to all therapy.

Polymyositis Features Direct Muscle Damage by Cytotoxic T Cells

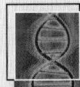

PATHOGENESIS: In polymyositis there is no evidence of microangiopathy like that found in dermatomyositis (see below). In these disorders, healthy muscle fibers are initially surrounded by CD8+ T lymphocytes (Fig. 27-14) and macrophages, after which the muscle fibers degenerate. Unlike normal muscle, muscles affected in polymyositis express major histocompatibility complex (MHC)-I antigen on the sarcolemma. Because cytotoxic

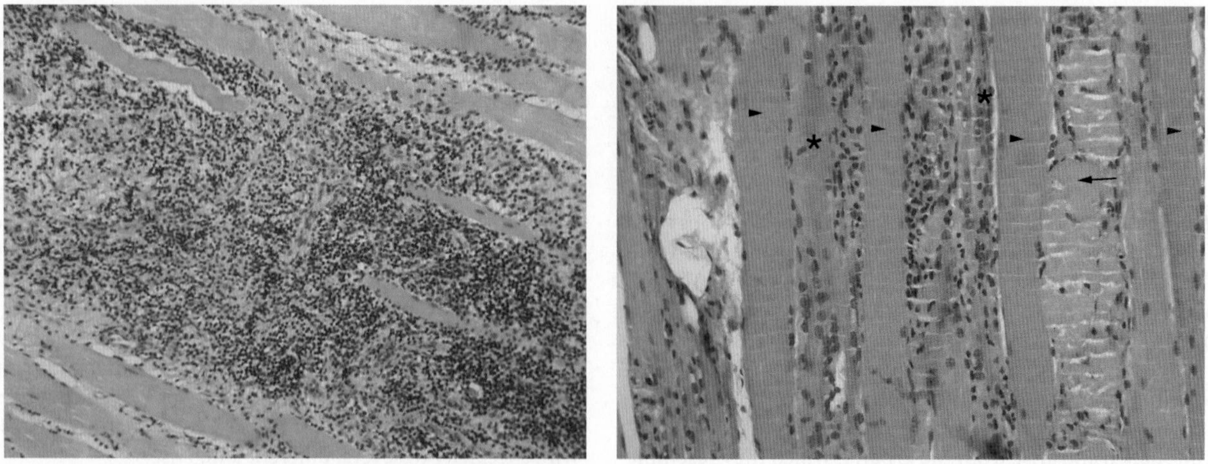

FIGURE 27-14. Polymyositis. **A.** Hematoxylin and eosin stain. A section of affected muscle shows an inflammatory myopathy. Mononuclear inflammatory cells infiltrate chiefly the endomysium. The field includes single-fiber necrosis. **B.** Region of healing inflammatory myopathy demonstrates intact fibers *(arrowheads)*, necrotic fibers *(arrow)*, and regenerating fibers characterized by enlarged nuclei and basophilic cytoplasm *(asterisk)*.

T cells attack antigenic targets in association with MHC-I molecules, these findings support an immunopathologic basis for this disorder.

The pathogenetic role of autoantibodies against nuclear antigens and cytoplasmic ribonucleoproteins in muscle injury is unknown. Polymyositis often has detectable anti-Jo-1, an antibody against histidyl-transfer RNA (tRNA) synthetase, with concomitant interstitial lung disease, Raynaud phenomenon, and nonerosive arthritis.

Viral infections may precede polymyositis, but virus cultures of muscle are negative. An inflammatory myopathy indistinguishable from polymyositis occurs in many cases of human immunodeficiency virus (HIV)-1 infection, but the role of the lentivirus is unclear.

PATHOLOGY: Inflammatory cells infiltrate connective tissue mostly within the fascicles (i.e., endomysial inflammation) and invade apparently healthy muscle fibers (see Fig. 27-14). Angiopathy is absent. Isolated degenerating or regenerating fibers are scattered throughout fascicles. Perifascicular atrophy is not present in polymyositis (see below).

Inclusion Body Myositis is Characterized by β-Amyloid Deposits

The pathologic features of inclusion body myositis resemble those of polymyositis and consist of single-fiber necrosis and regeneration with predominantly endomysial cytotoxic T cells. In addition, basophilic granular material is seen at the edge of slitlike vacuoles (rimmed vacuoles) within muscle fibers. The fibers also have small eosinophilic cytoplasmic inclusions, often near the rimmed vacuoles (Fig. 27-15A and B). The inclusions are stained by Congo red and are a form of intracellular amyloid (see Fig. 27-15C) that is immunoreactive for β-amyloid protein, the same type of amyloid present in the senile plaques of Alzheimer disease. The pathogenic significance of these inclusions is not understood. Small groups of angulated fibers are present. By electron microscopy, the granules of rimmed vacuoles contain membranous whorls. Distinctive filaments are found nearby the rimmed vacuoles (see Fig. 27-15D). The pathognomonic features of inclusion body myositis include the Congo red-positive inclusions and the characteristic filaments in the cytoplasm (or rarely in nuclei) of muscle fibers.

Dermatomyositis Is Caused by an Immune-Mediated Microangiopathy

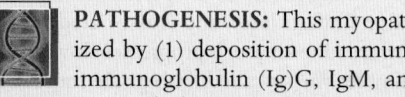

PATHOGENESIS: This myopathy is characterized by (1) deposition of immune complexes of immunoglobulin (Ig)G, IgM, and complement components, including membrane attack complement C5b-9 in the walls of capillaries and other blood vessels; (2) microangiopathy with loss of capillaries; (3) signs of injury and atrophy of myofibers; and (4) perivascular infiltrates of B cells and T cells with a predominantly CD4+-helper phenotype (Fig. 27-16). These features suggest that muscle injury in dermatomyositis occurs primarily by complement-mediated cytotoxic antibodies directed against the microvasculature of skeletal muscle tissues. In fact, complement is detectable in the capillaries before inflammation or damage to muscle fibers, and is the most specific finding of dermatomyositis. This microangiopathy is thought to lead to ischemic injury of individual muscle fibers and eventually to fiber atrophy. True infarcts may result from involvement of larger intramuscular arteries. The rash, which clinically distinguishes dermatomyositis from the other inflammatory myopathies, is presumably related to the same microangiopathy.

PATHOLOGY: Dermatomyositis features lymphoid infiltrates around blood vessels and in connective tissue of the perimysium (see Fig. 27-16). The infiltrates contain B cells and T cells, with a high ratio of CD4+ (helper) T cells to CD8+ (cytotoxic/suppressor) T cells. Immune complexes in

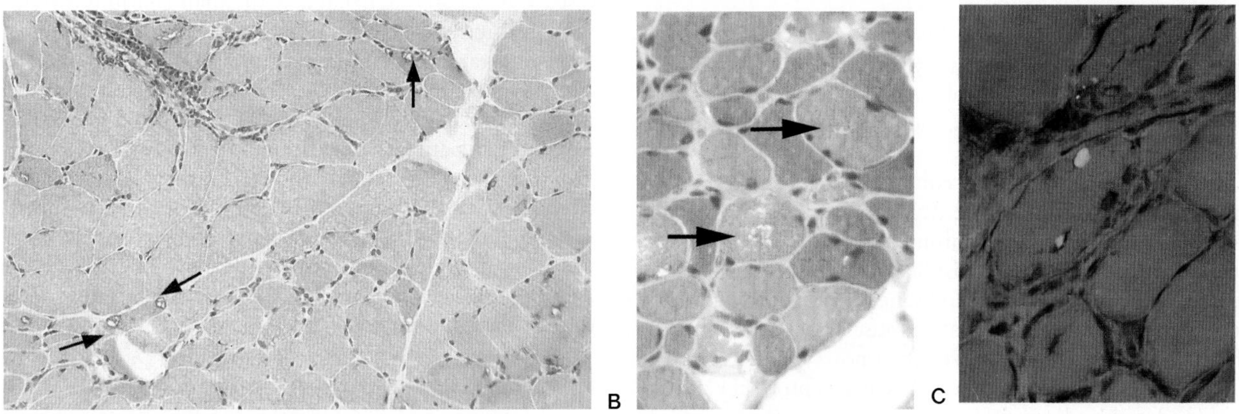

A B C

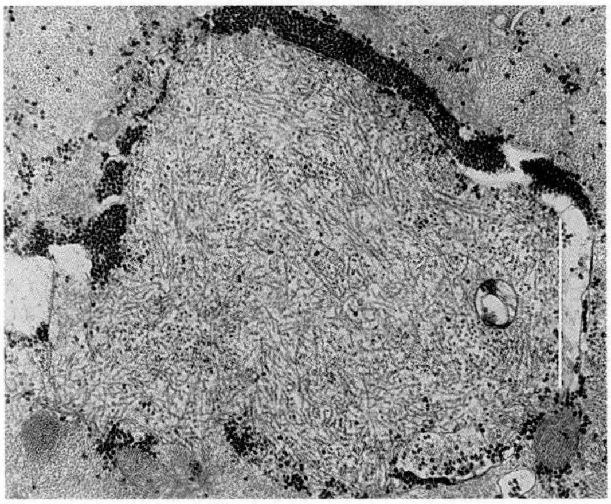

D

FIGURE 27-15. **Inclusion body myositis (IBM). A.** Hematoxylin and eosin stain. The features in IBM resemble those of polymyositis, but the muscle fibers also exhibit rimmed vacuoles *(arrows)* corresponding to enlarged lysosomes. The hyaline inclusions are sparse and difficult to visualize with this stain. **B.** Modified Gomori trichrome stain shows granular basophilic rimming of vacuoles. **C.** Congo red stain. The inclusion has weak congophilia, but the color signal is strong because it has been enhanced by fluorescence excitation. **D.** An electron micrograph shows the characteristic filaments of the amy-

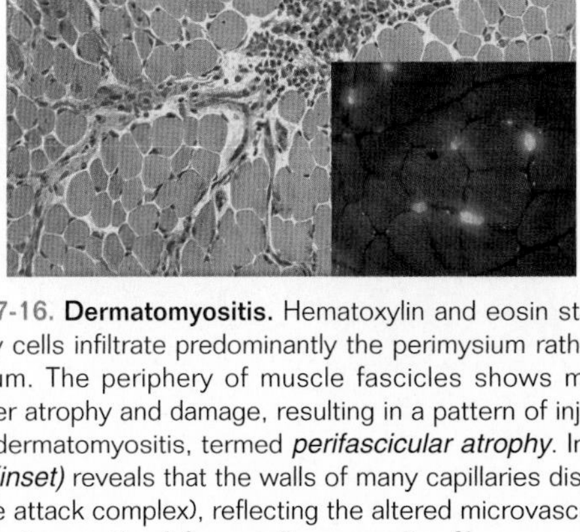

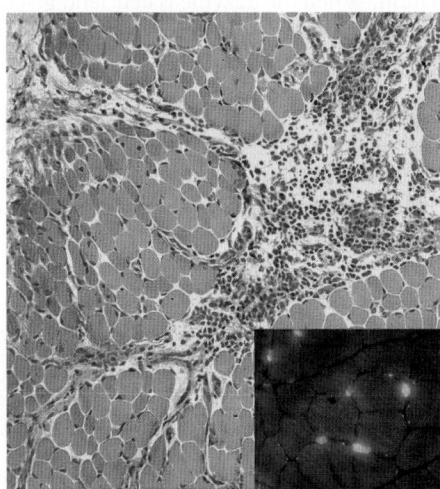

FIGURE 27-16. **Dermatomyositis.** Hematoxylin and eosin stain. The inflammatory cells infiltrate predominantly the perimysium rather than the endomysium. The periphery of muscle fascicles shows most of the muscle fiber atrophy and damage, resulting in a pattern of injury characteristic of dermatomyositis, termed *perifascicular atrophy*. Immunofluorescence *(inset)* reveals that the walls of many capillaries display C5b-9 (membrane attack complex), reflecting the altered microvasculature typical of dermatomyositis. A few small regenerating fibers are also stained by this method.

the walls of blood vessels (see Fig. 27-16, inset) are associated with microangiopathy. Intramuscular blood vessels exhibit endothelial hyperplasia, fibrin thrombi, and obliteration of capillaries. Perifascicular atrophy consists of one or more layers of atrophic fibers located at the periphery of the fascicles. The combination of perifascicular atrophy and immune complexes in capillary walls is virtually diagnostic of dermatomyositis, even in the absence of inflammation. The abnormal staining of the endomysial connective tissue with the alkaline phosphatase reaction reflects damage to the blood vessels.

Vasculitis May Occur in Skeletal Muscle as Part of Systemic Vasculitides

Vasculitis can be present in skeletal muscle in polyarteritis nodosa (PAN), Wegener granulomatosis, collagen vascular disease, and immune-mediated hypersensitivity states. In such instances, skeletal muscle may show neurogenic changes secondary to nerve damage.

Myasthenia Gravis

Myasthenia gravis is an acquired autoimmune disease characterized by abnormal muscular fatigability and caused by circulating antibodies to the acetylcholine (Ach) receptor at the myoneural junction. It occurs in all races and is twice as common in women as in men. The disease typically begins in young adults, but cases in children and the very old have also been described.

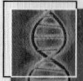

PATHOGENESIS: Myasthenia gravis is mediated by immunologic attack on the Ach receptor of the motor endplate. Antibodies attach to various receptor protein epitopes, thereby reducing the number of receptors.

This antigen–antibody complex binds complement and leads to shedding of the Ach receptor-rich terminal portions of the folds of the neuromuscular junction. The bivalent IgG antibodies also cross-link receptor proteins that remain in the postsynaptic membrane. This leads to Ach receptor endocytosis, faster than the muscle fiber can replace them. The combination of reduced postsynaptic membrane area, decreased number of Ach receptors per unit area, and widened synaptic space impairs signal transmission and causes muscle weakness and abnormal fatigability. The anti-receptor antibodies do not directly block binding of Ach to prevent neuromuscular transmission.

Up to 40% of patients with myasthenia gravis have an associated thymoma, and surgical removal of the tumor is often curative. As many as 75% of the remaining patients have thymic hyperplasia, and in such cases, thymectomy is often an effective treatment. Ach receptors have been demonstrated on the surface of some thymic cells in both thymoma and thymic hyperplasia. Thus, thymic T lymphocytes may activate B lymphocytes to produce anti-receptor antibodies.

PATHOLOGY: By light microscopy, the pathologic changes of myasthenia gravis are not impressive. At best, a muscle biopsy may reveal atrophy of type II muscle fibers and focal collections of lymphocytes within the fascicles. By electron microscopy, most muscle endplates are abnormal, even in muscles that are not weakened. There is simplification of the sarcolemmal secondary folds, breakdown and loss of the crests of the folds, and widening of the clefts.

CLINICAL FEATURES: The clinical severity of the condition is very variable, and symptoms tend to wax and wane as in other autoimmune diseases. Weakness of the extraocular muscles is typically severe and causes ptosis and diplopia. The disease may, in some cases, be confined to these muscles. More frequently, it progresses to other muscles, such as those associated with swallowing, the trunk, and extremities. Patients with myasthenia gravis also have a high incidence of other autoimmune diseases.

The overall mortality of myasthenia gravis is about 10%, often because of muscle weakness leads to respiratory insufficiency. In addition to thymectomy, corticosteroid therapy, methotrexate, and anticholinesterase drugs are used alone or in combination. Plasmapheresis reduces titers of anti-Ach receptor antibodies and can ameliorate symptoms, but such clinical improvements are short-lived.

Lambert-Eaton Syndrome

Lambert-Eaton syndrome is a paraneoplastic disorder that manifests as muscular weakness, wasting, and fatigability of proximal limbs and trunk. Also termed **myasthenic–myopathic syndrome,** the disease is usually associated with small cell lung carcinoma, though it may also occur in patients with other malignant diseases and rarely in the absence of an underlying malignancy. There is neurophysiologic evidence for a defect in Ach release at nerve terminals. This disease can be transferred to mice by IgG from human patients, and responds to corticosteroid treatment. The pathogenic IgG autoantibodies target voltage-sensitive calcium channels that are expressed in motor nerve terminals and in the cells of the lung cancer. These calcium channels, which are necessary for release of Ach, are greatly reduced in the presynaptic membrane in these patients, thereby interfering with neuromuscular transmission.

Inherited Metabolic Diseases

Skeletal muscle is dramatically affected by a variety of endocrine and metabolic diseases, such as Cushing syndrome, Addison disease, hypothyroidism, hyperthyroidism, and conditions associated with hepatic or renal failure. In the following discussion, however, primary hereditary abnormalities in the metabolism of skeletal muscle result in abnormal muscular function.

Glycogen-Storage Diseases Are Genetic Disorders That Produce Variable Effects on Muscle

Glycogen-storage diseases (glycogenoses) are autosomal recessive, inherited, metabolic disorders characterized by an inability to degrade glycogen (see Chapter 6).

Type II Glycogenosis (Acid Maltase Deficiency, *α-1,4-Glucosidase Deficiency, Pompe Disease*)

Various mutations affect muscle acid maltase activity and lead to distinctly different clinical syndromes. Acid maltase is a lysosomal enzyme that is expressed in all cells and participates in glycogen degradation. When the enzyme is deficient, glycogen is not broken down, accumulates within lysosomes, and remains membrane bound (Fig. 27-17).

PATHOLOGY: In all forms of glycogenosis due to acid maltase deficiency, the morphologic changes are distinctive and almost pathognomonic (see Fig. 27-17). In Pompe disease, muscle shows massive accumulation of

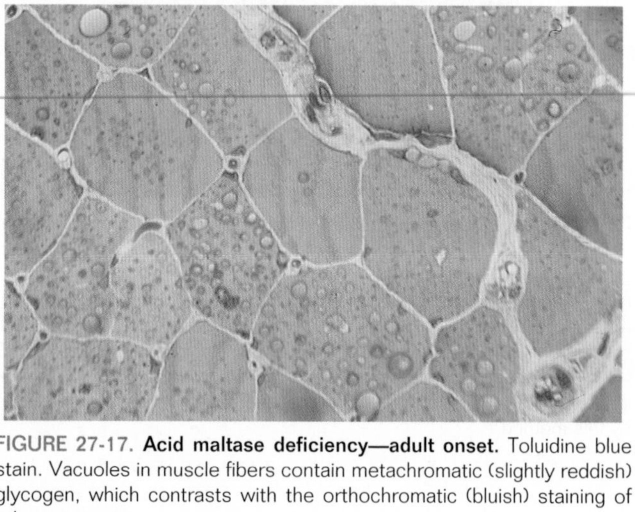

FIGURE 27-17. **Acid maltase deficiency—adult onset.** Toluidine blue stain. Vacuoles in muscle fibers contain metachromatic (slightly reddish) glycogen, which contrasts with the orthochromatic (bluish) staining of other structures.

membrane-bound glycogen and the myofilaments and other sarcoplasmic organelles disappear. Surprisingly, there is very little regeneration, and apparently inactive satellite cells are present on the surfaces of muscle fibers that have been almost completely destroyed by the disease process.

The pathologies of late infantile, juvenile, and adult-onset forms of type II glycogenosis are milder. Morphologic changes range from overt vacuolar myopathy demonstrated by routine histology to very subtle accumulation of membrane-bound glycogen particles only detectable by electron microscopy. Vacuoles observed by light microscopy are empty or contain glycogen.

CLINICAL FEATURES: Pompe disease is the most severe acid maltase deficiency. It occurs in neonates or young infants. These patients have severe hypotonia and areflexia and clinically resemble patients with Werdnig-Hoffmann disease (see below under Denervation). Sometimes patients have an enlarged tongue and cardiomegaly, and die of cardiac failure, usually within their first 2 years. Many tissues are affected, but the most significant involvement is in skeletal and cardiac muscle, the CNS, and liver. The serum creatine kinase level is slightly to moderately increased. Patients with later-onset forms of the disease have a mild, but relentlessly progressive, myopathy. Glycogen accumulates in other organs, but clinical expression of the disorder is usually limited to muscle.

Type III Glycogenosis (Debranching Enzyme Deficiency, Cori Disease, Limit Dextrinosis, Amylo-1,6-Glucosidase Deficiency)

Type III glycogenosis is a rare, autosomal recessive disease that affects children or adults. Because the debranching enzyme is absent, phosphorylase hydrolyzes the 1,4-glycosidic linkages of the terminal glucose chains of glycogen, but not beyond branch points. Hepatomegaly and growth retardation are usual. The muscle symptoms vary, and the most severe and consistent involvement is related to liver dysfunction in children.

Type V Glycogenosis (McArdle Disease, Myophosphorylase Deficiency)

Type V glycogenosis is a more common metabolic myopathy that is usually not progressive or severely debilitating. The deficient enzyme, myophosphorylase, is specific for skeletal muscle. Lacking this enzyme, skeletal muscle glycogen cannot be cleaved at 1,4-glycosidic chains to produce glucose for energy production during physical exertion. Thus, muscles cramp with exercise. Patients also cannot produce lactate during ischemic exercise, which defect is the basis for a metabolic test for the condition.

PATHOLOGY: Tissue may appear completely normal, except for the absence of phosphorylase activity. However, there is usually subtle evidence of abnormal accumulation of glycogen granules within the sarcoplasm, mainly in the subsarcolemmal area (Fig. 27-18). The specific diagnosis can be made by a histochemical reaction for myophosphorylase, but must be confirmed by biochemical assay of the muscle enzyme activity or by analysis of genomic DNA.

CLINICAL FEATURES: If patients avoid strenuous exercise, myophosphorylase deficiency does not seriously interfere with their lives. However, prolonged, vigorous exercise can lead to widespread necrosis of myofibers and release of soluble muscle proteins such as creatine kinase and myoglobin into the circulation. This event, in turn, can produce myoglobinuria and renal failure.

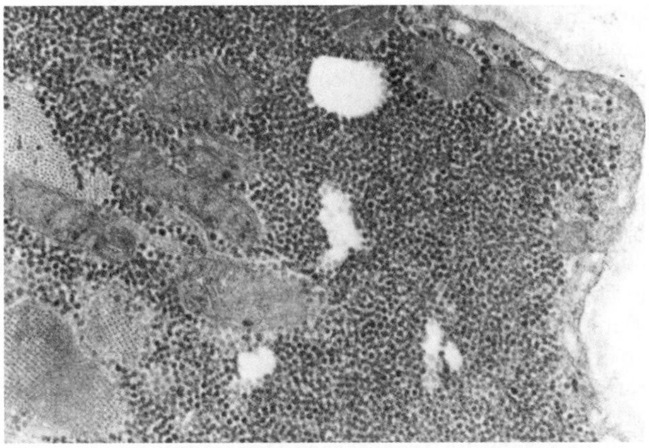

FIGURE 27-18. **McArdle disease (myophosphorylase deficiency).** An electron micrograph demonstrates an abnormal mass of glycogen particles just beneath the sarcolemma. The glycogen is not surrounded by a membrane, in contrast to the lysosomal glycogen storage of acid maltase deficiency.

Muscle biopsy should be performed several weeks after an episode of symptoms to allow regeneration of the muscle.

Type VII Glycogenosis (Phosphofructokinase Deficiency)

Phosphofructokinase (PFK) deficiency is less common than McArdle disease but causes an identical syndrome. PFK is a key enzyme in the Embden-Meyerhof pathway, which catalyzes conversion of fructose-6-phosphate to fructose-1,6-diphosphate. In muscle, this enzyme is composed of four identical subunits (M_4), whereas in erythrocytes, the tetramer contains two different subunits (the M and L subunits), each under separate genetic control. As a result, a genetic lack of the muscle subunit results in a complete absence of PFK activity in muscle, but only a 50% decrease in erythrocytes. In the latter cells, the remaining active enzyme is made up of four normal L subunits.

Patients with type VII glycogenosis often have slight anemia or low-grade hemolysis. The morphologic findings resemble those in McArdle disease, except that patients have phosphorylase activity in the muscle. By contrast, a histochemical reaction for PFK shows little or no staining for the enzyme. The diagnosis is substantiated by biochemical analysis of the enzyme activity in muscle.

Lipid Myopathies Are Caused by Defective Fat Metabolism

Occasionally, a muscle biopsy specimen from a patient with exercise intolerance or muscle weakness shows excess neutral lipids. This occurs in several metabolic disorders that affect lipid metabolism, more than a dozen of which have been identified. In brief, lipid myopathies may involve deficiencies in (1) fatty acids transport into mitochondria (carnitine-deficiency syndromes, carnitine palmityl transferase deficiency), (2) a variety of enzymes that mediate β-oxidation of fatty acids, (3) respiratory chain enzymes, and (4) triglyceride use. Only disorders involving carnitine metabolism are discussed here.

Carnitine Deficiency

Carnitine, which is synthesized in the liver and is present in large quantities in skeletal muscle, is necessary for transport of long-chain fatty acids into mitochondria. Patients with muscle carnitine deficiency, an autosomal recessive condition, have progressive proximal muscle weakness and atrophy and often show signs of denervation and peripheral neuropathy. The absence of carnitine leads to massive accumulation of lipid droplets in the sarcoplasm outside mitochondria, which is readily evident in muscle biopsies (Fig. 27-19). Sometimes oral carnitine therapy alleviates the symptoms. Carnitine deficiency in skeletal muscle also occurs as part of a systemic disorder that can affect the CNS, heart, and liver.

Carnitine Palmityl Transferase Deficiency

As in carnitine deficiency, persons with carnitine palmityl transferase deficiency cannot metabolize long-chain fatty acids because of an inability to transport these lipids into mitochondria, where they undergo β-oxidation. After prolonged exercise, these patients have muscular pain, which may progress to myoglobinuria. Prolonged fasting can produce the same symptoms. After such an episode, fibers regenerate and restore muscle structure. Biopsies are microscopically normal; the diagnosis depends on biochemical assay for carnitine palmityl transferase activity.

Mitochondrial Diseases Reflect Mutant nDNA or mtDNA

Inherited defects of mitochondrial metabolism are an uncommon but conceptually important group of disorders. Historically, diseases of muscle were recognized first and designated mitochondrial myopathies, but others affect both CNS and muscle and are known as **mitochondrial encephalomyopathies.** The nervous system, skeletal muscle, heart, kidney, and other organs can be affected in different combinations as part of a multisystem disease.

Inherited diseases of mitochondria are classified genetically into two broad groups, defects of either **nuclear DNA** (nDNA) or **mitochondrial DNA** (mtDNA). Point mutations, deletions, and duplications of mtDNA have been identified and linked to several mitochondrial encephalomyopathies. This group of syndromes is discussed here.

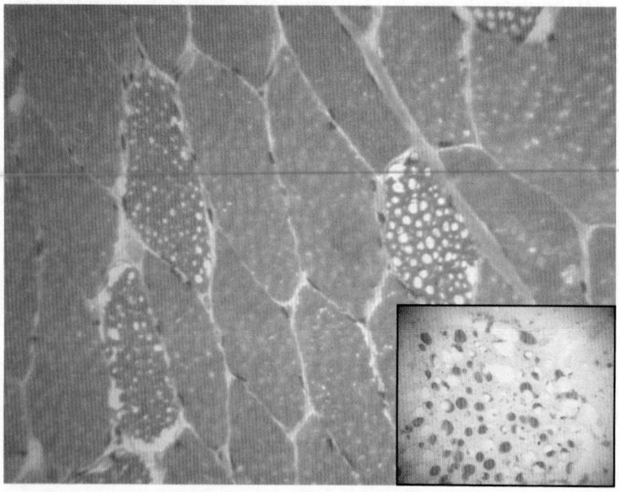

FIGURE 27-19. **Lipid storage myopathy.** Hematoxylin and eosin-stained frozen section. Numerous cytoplasmic vacuoles are present in the muscle fibers. Oil red-orcein stain *(inset)* demonstrates that the cytoplasmic vacuoles contain neutral lipid.

PATHOGENESIS: Genes for most mitochondrial proteins are in nDNA, but mtDNA encodes 13 of the approximately 80 polypeptide subunits of the respiratory chain complexes. Defects in these proteins lead to the mitochondrial encephalomyopathies.

In contrast with the Mendelian pattern of nDNA mutations, the diseases of mtDNA show maternal inheritance, because mtDNA is derived exclusively from the oocyte. The zygote and its daughter cells have many mitochondria, each of which contains several copies of the maternally derived mitochondrial genome. Mutations in mtDNA are passed on randomly to subsequent generations of cells. During growth of the fetus or later, some cells may thus contain only mutant genomes (mutant homoplasmy), whereas others will have only normal genomes (wild-type homoplasmy). Still others receive a mixed population of mutant and normal mtDNA (heteroplasmy). Clinical expression of a disease produced by a given mutation of mtDNA depends on the proportion of the total content of mitochondrial genomes that is mutant. *The fraction of mutant mtDNA must exceed a critical value for a mitochondrial disease to be symptomatic.* This threshold varies in different organs and is presumably related to cellular energy requirements.

PATHOLOGY: In skeletal muscle, the pathologic signature of a defect of mtDNA is accumulation of mitochondria, excessive numbers of which may be manifest as aggregates of reddish granular material in the sarcoplasm. This can be demonstrated by the modified Gomori trichrome stain (Fig. 27-20A). The abnormality has been termed a **ragged red fiber** because of the irregular contour of the reddish deposits at the fiber periphery. Pathogenic mutations of mtDNA in these diseases often impair the activity of complex IV (cytochrome oxidase). Three of the subunits are encoded by mtDNA, and they are required for function of the assembled electron transport carrier. Hence, histochemical stains for ragged red fibers often demonstrate deficient cytochrome oxidase activity (see Fig. 27-20C). By contrast, the ragged red fibers stain intensely for SDH (complex II), a complex that is exclusively encoded by nDNA (see Fig. 27-20B). Increased SDH, which is synthesized in the cytosol and imported into mitochondria, presumably reflects the proliferation of mitochondria. The mitochondrial defects (see Fig. 27-20D) cause atrophy of myofibers and accumulation of sarcoplasmic lipid and glycogen. Death of nerve cells and reactive astrocytosis occurs in the CNS.

CLINICAL FEATURES: Clinical manifestations of the encephalomyopathies vary, but usually begin in childhood. Some patients start with muscle weakness and then develop a brain disorder. Others present with CNS disease with or without overt muscle weakness, even though muscle biopsy indicates a mitochondrial disorder. Other organs, such as the heart, are often affected as part of a multisystem disorder.

Three neurologic syndromes have been delineated (1) **Kearns-Sayre syndrome** (progressive ophthalmoplegia, retinal pigmentary degeneration, cardiac arrhythmias, and other features), (2) **MELAS** (mitochondrial myopathy, encephalopathy, lactic

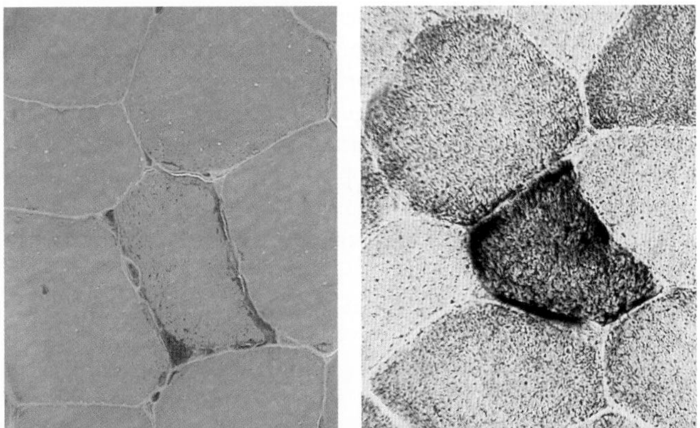

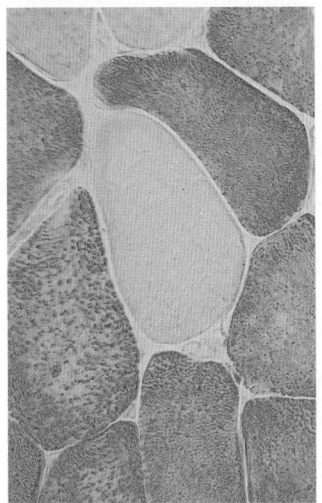

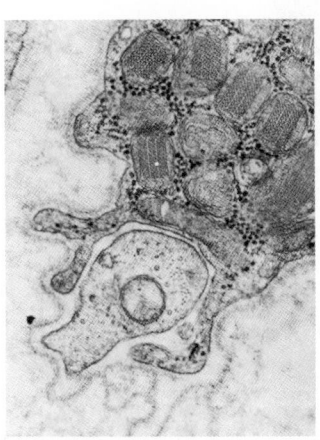

FIGURE 27-20. **Mitochondrial myopathy caused by deletions of mitochondrial DNA (mtDNA). A**. Modified Gomori trichrome. A ragged red fiber shows prominent proliferation of reddish, granular mitochondria, located chiefly in a subsarcolemmal region. **B**. Succinate dehydrogenase (SDH) stain. A ragged red fiber shows overexpression of SDH, an electron-transport carrier that is entirely encoded by nuclear DNA (nDNA). **C**. Another ragged red fiber displays lack of histochemical staining for cytochrome oxidase. Three subunits of this electron-transport carrier are coded by mtDNA, and the mutations have interfered with function in this fiber. **D**. An electron micrograph reveals mitochondria with ultrastructural abnormalities, including para-crystalline inclusions.

acidosis, and strokelike episodes), and (3) **MERRF** (myoclonic epilepsy and ragged red fibers). Most patients with Kearns-Sayre syndrome have large deletions of mtDNA that are not familial. MELAS usually involves point mutations of mitochondrial genes for certain transfer RNAs, most commonly the gene for leucine tRNA. Likewise, MERRF most commonly displays point mutations in the lysine tRNA gene, although other tRNA gene mutations may be present. As with all mitochondrial genetic disorders, these mutations show a maternal pattern of inheritance.

Myoadenylate Deaminase Deficiency Is a Frequent Cause of Mild Weakness

Adenosine monophosphate deaminase (AMP-DA) is present in large quantities in skeletal muscle, particularly in type II fibers. AMP-DA is important in regulating the purine nucleotide cycle and helps to maintain the adenosine triphosphate/adenosine diphosphate (ATP/ADP) ratio during exercise. A group of patients with mild proximal muscle weakness and exercise intolerance completely lack AMP-DA activity. It is a common, autosomal recessive condition, occurring in 1% to 2% of all muscle biopsy specimens. AMP-DA deficiency may not actually represent a separate disease: it may be a malady that is unmasked by other neuromuscular diseases.

Familial Periodic Paralysis Reflects Impaired Electrolyte Flux

Familial periodic paralysis denotes several autosomal dominant disorders characterized by episodic muscular weakness or even complete paralysis, followed by a rapid recovery. These disorders are related to abnormalities in sodium and potassium fluxes into and out of muscle cells. During an attack, the muscle fiber surface does not propagate action potentials, although delivery of calcium into the muscle fiber causes contraction. Muscle biopsies taken during an attack exhibit no detectable abnormalities of recent onset. Later, permanent mild myopathic features and sarcoplasmic vacuoles appear. These vacuoles represent dilated or remodeled sarcoplasmic reticulum and transverse tubules. In some cases, a distinct subpopulation of fibers (type IIB) contains numerous tubular aggregates derived from the tubular network of the sarcoplasmic reticulum.

There are three clinically and genetically distinct syndromes—hypokalemic, hyperkalemic, and normokalemic periodic paralysis. The hypokalemic type has been linked to mutations of the gene that encodes a voltage-gated calcium channel of skeletal muscle; the hyperkalemic and normokalemic forms reflect mutations in the *SCN4A* gene on chromosome 17q, which specifies the sodium channel.

Rhabdomyolysis

Rhabdomyolysis is the dissolution of skeletal muscle fibers and release of myoglobin into the circulation, an event that may result in myoglobinuria and acute renal failure. The disorder may be acute, subacute, or chronic. During acute rhabdomyolysis, muscles are swollen, tender, and profoundly weak.

Occasionally, an episode of rhabdomyolysis may complicate or follow influenza. Some patients develop rhabdomyolysis with apparently mild exercise and probably have some form of metabolic myopathy. After recovery, a subsequent biopsy may reveal muscle that is morphologically normal. Rhabdomyolysis also may complicate heat stroke or malignant hyperthermia after administration of an anesthetic such as halothane. Alcoholism is occasionally associated with either acute or chronic rhabdomyolysis.

Pathologic changes in rhabdomyolysis are those of an active, noninflammatory myopathy, with scattered necrosis of muscle fibers and varying degrees of degeneration and regeneration. Clusters of macrophages are seen in and around muscle fibers, but these are not accompanied by lymphocytes or inflammatory cells.

Denervation

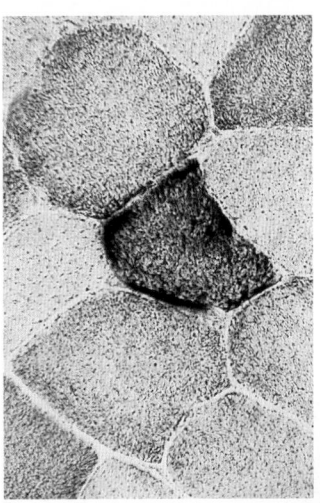

The pathology of denervation reflects lesions of the lower motor neuron. Lower motor neuron lesions can be detected by muscle biopsy, but patterns of denervation do not identify the cause of the lesion. The morphologic changes may indicate whether denervation is recent or chronic but do not, e.g., distinguish between amyotrophic lateral sclerosis, a disorder of motor neurons, and peripheral neuropathy due to diabetes mellitus. Lesions of upper motor neurons, such as occur in multiple sclerosis or stroke, lead to paralysis and atrophy, but, lower motor neurons in these conditions remain intact. Pathologic changes thus reflect nonspecific diffuse atrophy rather than denervation atrophy.

When a skeletal muscle fiber becomes separated from contact with its lower motor neuron, it invariably atrophies, owing to progressive loss of myofibrils. On cross-section, atrophic fibers have characteristic angular configurations, seemingly compressed by surrounding normal muscle fibers (Fig. 27-21). If a fiber is not reinnervated, atrophy progresses to complete loss of myofibrils, with nuclei condensing into aggregates. In the end stage, the muscle fibers disappear and are replaced chiefly by adipose tissue.

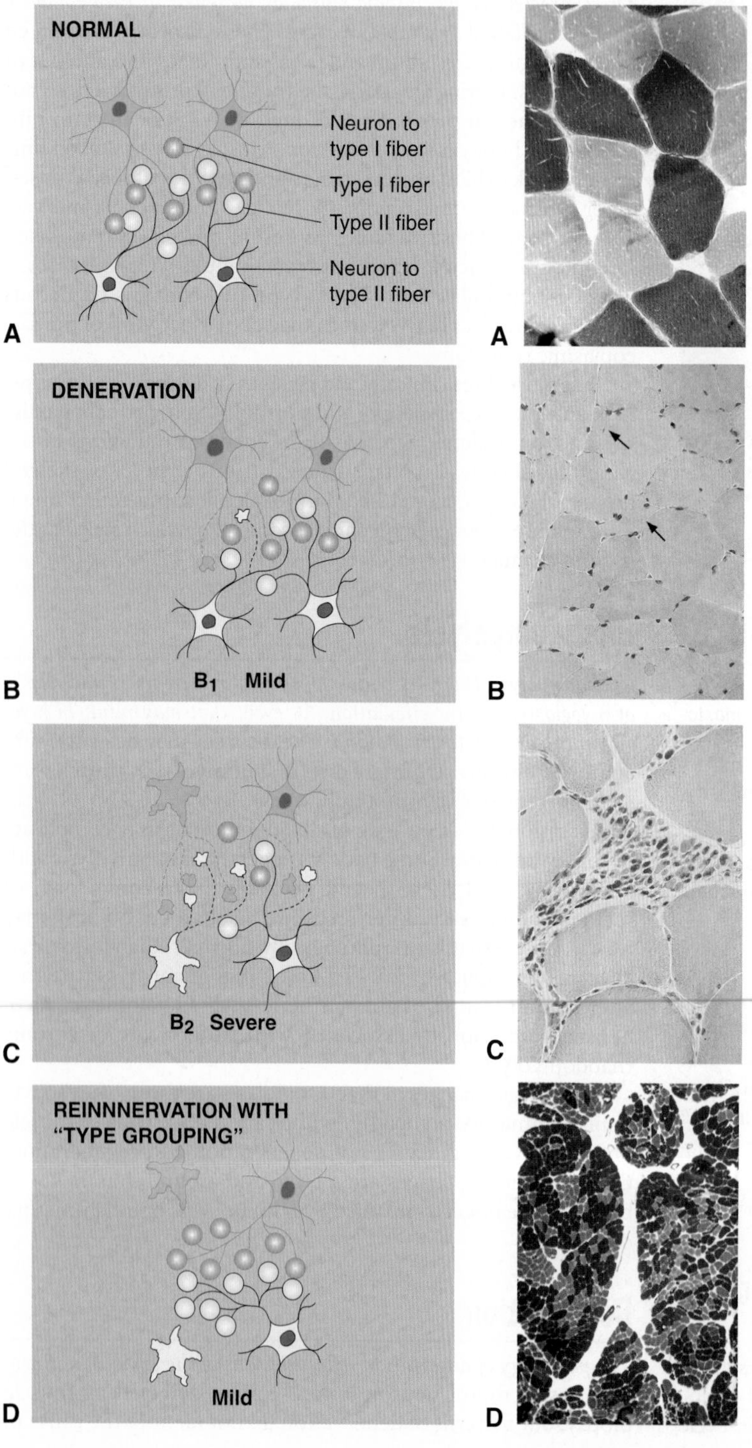

FIGURE 27-21. **Denervation/reinnervation. A.** As shown in the photomicrograph, the normal intermixed distribution of type I (*pale*) and type II (*dark*) muscle fibers is shown by staining for ATPase. In the drawing, two neurons (*red*) innervate type I muscle fibers, and two neurons (*yellow*) supply type II fibers. **B.** Denervation; hematoxylin and eosin stain. With early (mild) denervation, portions of the axonal tree degenerate, resulting in angular atrophy of scattered type I and II muscle fibers. **C.** With more advanced (severe) denervation (*B2*), entire lower motor neurons or numerous axonal processes degenerate, causing small groups of angular atrophic fibers to appear as illustrated in the photomicrograph. **D.** Reinnervation; myofibrillar ATPase. As neurons degenerate, surviving neurons sprout more nerve endings and reinnervate some of the denervated fibers. These reinnervated fibers become either type I or type II, according to the type of neuron that reinnervates them. This process results in fewer, but larger, motor units and the appearance of clusters of fibers of one type adjacent to clusters of the other type, a pattern called "type grouping." The photomicrograph demonstrates type grouping. This field would appear normal except for a few atrophic fibers if it were stained with hematoxylin and eosin.

The early phase of denervating disease is characterized by irregularly scattered, angular, atrophic fibers. As the disease progresses, these fibers are seen in groups, at first in small clusters of several fibers, and later in progressively larger groups (see Fig. 27-21B). These fibers are excessively dark when stained for nonspecific esterase (Fig. 27-22) and NADH-TR reactions, in contrast to atrophy caused by disuse or wasting. With the ATPase reaction, groups of denervated fibers are a mixture of type I and type II fibers: *denervating conditions are not selective for only one type of motor neuron.*

Another abnormality occasionally present in a denervating condition is the "target fiber" (Fig. 27-23), seen in 20% of cases. This change is apparently transient, occurring during or shortly after denervation or reinnervation and indicating that the process is active. The lesion consists of central pallor of the muscle fiber, which is surrounded by a condensed zone that in turn is surrounded by a normal zone of sarcoplasm. Target fibers are difficult to see with hematoxylin and eosin stain but are evident using NADH-TR stain, which shows greatly reduced staining in the central zone, reflecting a reduced number or absence of mitochondria.

With every episode of denervation, there is an effort at reinnervation. In a slowly progressive denervating process, reinnervation may keep pace with denervation. New sprouting nerve endings make synaptic contact with the muscle fiber at the site of the previous motor endplate. Shortly after denervation, muscle fibers becomes covered with nicotinic Ach receptors (extrajunctional receptor), as happens during the myotubular phase of embryogenesis. This denervated state induces sprouting of new nerve endings from adjacent surviving nerve. With reinnervation, the extrajunctional receptor again disappears from the sarcolemma, except at the point of synaptic contact.

In a chronic denervating condition, reinnervation of each surviving motor unit gradually becomes larger. As a specific type of lower motor neuron takes over innervation of a given field of fibers, fiber groups of one type are seen adjacent to groups of another type. This pattern, called **type grouping,** is pathognomonic of denervation followed by reinnervation (see Fig. 27-21C).

Patients with striking type grouping often have symptoms of muscle cramping in addition to progressive muscular weakness. After a single episode of denervation, such as in poliomyelitis, reinnervation often leads to a remarkable recovery of strength. Years later, a biopsy shows a conspicuous pattern of type grouping, with scattered pyknotic nuclear clumps. In such cases, there are neither angular atrophic fibers nor target fibers.

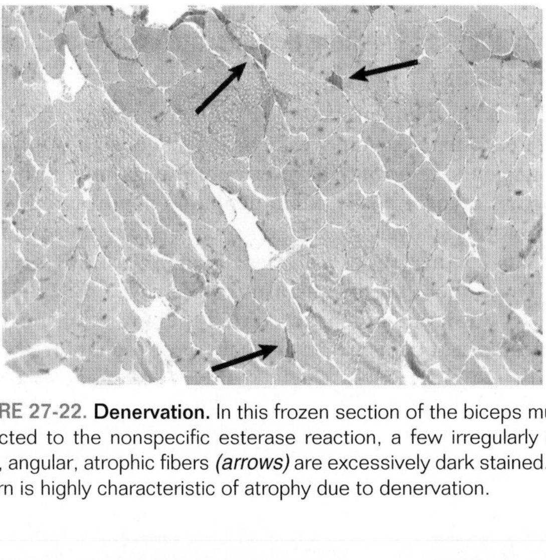

FIGURE 27-22. **Denervation.** In this frozen section of the biceps muscle subjected to the nonspecific esterase reaction, a few irregularly scattered, angular, atrophic fibers *(arrows)* are excessively dark stained. This pattern is highly characteristic of atrophy due to denervation.

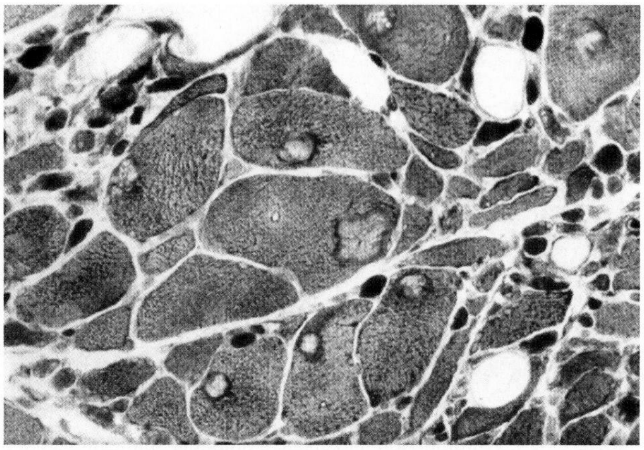

FIGURE 27-23. **Target fiber.** A cross-section of striated muscle treated with the NADH-tetrazolium reductase (NADH-TR) stain demonstrates several "target fibers," a characteristic feature of some cases of denervation. Because the enzyme reaction creates a product (formazan) that selectively fixes to membranous organelles, the centers of the target areas appear devoid of mitochondria and sarcoplasmic reticulum. The myofibrils may or may not be intact.

Occasionally, a biopsy specimen reveals abnormal prominence of one fiber type over the other, "type predominance," which may involve either type I or type II fibers. There is frequently evidence of denervation. It is possible that in type predominance, reinnervation may favor one type of lower motor neuron over another.

It is not uncommon to see occasional muscle fibers undergoing necrosis or regeneration in neuropathic conditions. In such patients, a modest increase in serum creatine kinase levels reflects muscle degeneration. This is common in slowly progressive forms of spinal muscular atrophy, e.g., Kugelberg-Welander disease and Kennedy disease.

Spinal Muscular Atrophy (SMA) Reflects Progressive Degeneration of Anterior Horn Cells

SMA is the second most common lethal autosomal recessive disorder after cystic fibrosis. Childhood SMA is classified into type I (**Werdnig-Hoffmann disease**), type II (intermediate), and type III (**Kugelberg-Welander disease**). The survival motor neuron gene (5q11.2-13.3) is absent in virtually all (99%) cases of SMA.

WERDNIG-HOFFMANN DISEASE (INFANTILE SMA): Werdnig-Hoffmann disease results in progressive and severe weakness in early infancy. Infants seldom survive beyond 1 year of life. The denervation seems to begin in utero after the establishment of motor units. The histologic pattern is virtually pathognomonic (Fig. 27-24). Groups of minute, rounded, atrophic fibers are still identifiable with the ATPase reaction as being either type I or type II. There are also fascicles of normal muscle fibers and almost invariably clusters of hypertrophied type I fibers. In addition to the absent survival motor neuron gene, a second gene (neuronal apoptosis inhibitory protein gene) has also been implicated in the pathogenesis of Werdnig-Hoffmann disease.

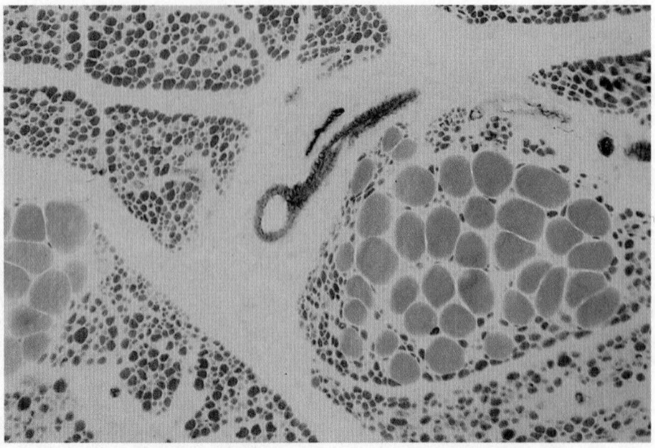

FIGURE 27-24. **Werdnig-Hoffman disease (infantile spinal muscular atrophy).** This cross-section of skeletal muscle stained for myofibrillar ATPase is derived from an infant with severe hypotonia. It shows groups of extremely atrophic, rounded type I and type II fibers and clusters of markedly hypertrophied pale type I fibers.

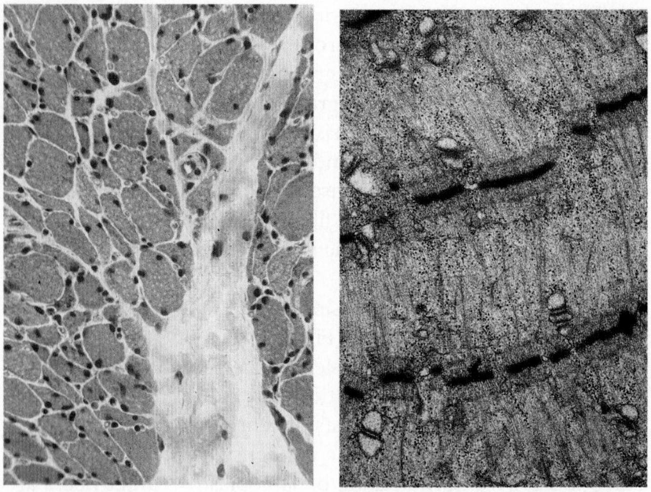

FIGURE 27-26. **Critical illness myopathy. A**. The condition frequently shows atrophic muscle with angular muscle fibers (hematoxylin and eosin). **B**. By electron microscopy, there is marked loss of thick myosin filaments, whereas α actin(thin) filaments are intact (compare to Fig. 27-2).

KUGELBERG–WELANDER DISEASE (JUVENILE SMA): This variant is a later-onset form of SMA and is not necessarily progressive. These patients had often been designated as having limb-girdle muscular dystrophy, but the electromyographic pattern of denervation helps to make the diagnosis. Muscle biopsies show type grouping and other evidence of a neurogenic disorder but can resemble a myopathy in a small sample because of coexisting necrotic fibers and regenerating fibers.

Type II Fiber Atrophy Resembles Denervation Myopathy

A commonly misinterpreted pathologic pattern in muscle biopsy specimens is atrophy resulting from disuse, wasting, upper motor neuron disease, and corticosteroid toxicity. Pathologically, this diffuse, nonspecific atrophy appears as selective angular atrophy of type II fibers. With hematoxylin and eosin stain, this pattern of atrophy may resemble that of denervation. However, in the ATPase reaction, all angular atrophic fibers are type II (Fig. 27-25), and do not stain heavily using nonspecific esterase or NADH-TR reactions. Type II atrophy is a common condition that is often related to a more chronic problem.

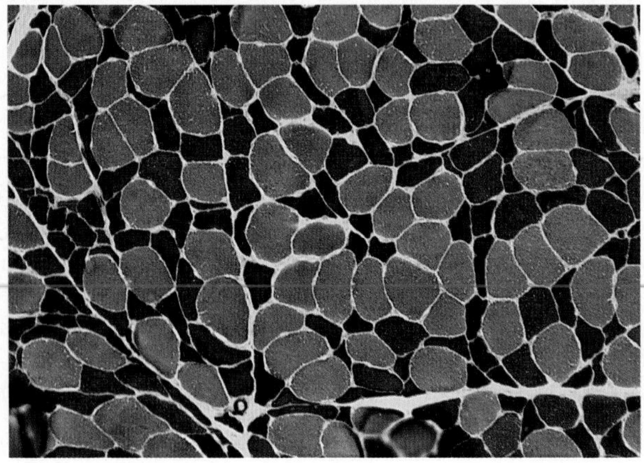

FIGURE 27-25. Type II fiber atrophy. This biopsy of the vastus lateralis muscle was taken from a 48-year-old man with proximal muscle weakness because of endogenous corticosteroid toxicity (Cushing syndrome). Virtually all of the angular atrophic fibers are type II. This form of atrophy closely mimics denervation atrophy when visualized with the hematoxylin and eosin stain.

STEROID MYOPATHY: Corticosteroid therapy can cause muscle weakness; the muscle biopsy shows type II atrophy. This pathologic feature raises an important point clinically, because patients with polymyositis are often treated with large doses of corticosteroids. If a patient's weakness worsens, the physician must decide if this development represents a relapse of polymyositis, requiring increased corticosteroids, or if it represents steroid myopathy, in which case steroid dosage should be decreased.

In weakness caused by corticosteroid toxicity, patients do not show increased serum creatine kinase level and histologically manifest selective atrophy of type II fibers, without muscle fiber degeneration and inflammation. By contrast, fiber degeneration and inflammation would be expected in recurrent polymyositis, a process that is reflected in increased serum creatine kinase activity.

Critical Illness Myopathy Is Associated with Corticosteroid Therapy

If patients on high-dose steroids and neuromuscular blocking agents experience severe weakness in spite of removal of paralyzing agents, they may have **critical illness myopathy**, also known as **myosin heavy chain depletion syndrome**. Electron microscopic analysis of skeletal muscle from these patients shows loss of thick myosin filaments from muscle fibers (Fig. 27-26). The underlying mechanism of the myosin depletion is unclear, but stopping corticosteroid therapy often results in reappearance of myosin thick filaments and resultant restoration of muscle strength.

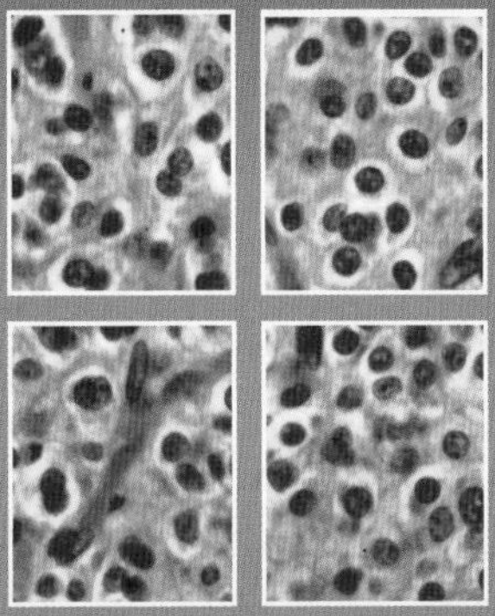

28

The Nervous System

John Q. Trojanowski
Lawrence Kenyon
(The Central Nervous System)
Thomas W. Bouldin
(The Peripheral Nervous System)

THE CENTRAL NERVOUS SYSTEM (CNS)

The nervous system is the most complex organ system in the body, and its major components (brain, spinal cord, peripheral nerves, and ganglia) are intimately interconnected to enable rapid communications. The sensory, motor, cognitive, memory, and autonomic functions of the nervous system have distinct anatomical correlates, although defects in one area may have significant effects on the functionality of other regions. Despite this intricate organization and the fact that neurons are the most asymmetric cells in the body, with extensions (e.g., axons) that extend up to meters away from the parent cell body, the nervous system is governed largely by the same principles that control the function of cells in the rest of the body.

TOPOGRAPHY: The functional properties of the nervous system are topographically localized, and neurologic diseases are also regionally distributed. The selective vulnerability of different nervous system cells and regions to disease processes is one of the most profound unresolved enigmas of neuropsychiatric illnesses. For example, Huntington disease is primarily characterized by selective degeneration of neurons in the caudate nuclei; whereas Parkinson disease targets the nigrostriatal system; and amyotrophic lateral sclerosis (ALS) singles out upper and lower motor neurons of cerebrum, brainstem, and spinal cord. Similarly, infectious diseases have distinct topographic predilections; poliomyelitis involves the anterior horn cells of the spinal cord and the motor nuclei of the brainstem, herpes simplex preferentially affects the temporal lobes, and rabies seeks out the medulla. Vascular diseases and demyelinating conditions also display regional preferences within the nervous system, and a degree of topographic predictability characterizes most brain tumors.

AGE: The nervous system is affected by neuropsychiatric disorders throughout the life span, but individual diseases commonly manifest a predilection for selected age groups. For example, inborn errors of metabolism, such as Tay-Sachs disease, the leukodystrophies, and several tumors, are encountered largely in childhood. Multiple sclerosis shows a strong preference for young adults, rarely having its onset before puberty or after the age of 40 years. Huntington disease typically strikes youthful and middle-aged adults. Parkinson disease is rarely evidenced before the later decades of life, and Alzheimer disease tends to be a malady of the aged brain.

Cells of the Nervous System

Neurons Are the Effector Cells of the Nervous System

Although mature neurons do not divide, the dogma that neurons are never generated after birth has been overturned in the past decade. However, the functional significance of the production of small numbers of new neurons in the adult brain is unknown. The nervous system indeed loses neurons with progressive aging, but these losses may not be as profound as suggested earlier.

The need for structural stability in the nervous system is counterbalanced by the need for plasticity in neuronal networks. The fact that neurons of the CNS cannot effectively regenerate axons over long distances limits the ability of the CNS to respond to many different types of injuries. Thus, an infarct that transects the internal capsule creates a permanent motor deficit because transected axons do not regenerate to reestablish lost connections. Since CNS neurons do not remyelinate efficiently after injury, a demyelinating disease like multiple sclerosis causes permanent functional deficits.

Neurons have a variety of shapes and sizes, but certain features are common to all of them. Microscopically, the centrally located, round nucleus contains a prominent nucleolus (Fig. 28-1A). The cytoplasm is abundant, and the ribosome-studded endoplasmic reticulum forms prominent basophilic granules known as Nissl bodies (see Fig. 28-1B). Some neurons, such as those in the substantia nigra or locus ceruleus, contain cytoplasmic pigment termed **neuromelanin** (Fig. 28-2).

Neurons are also highly asymmetric, with numerous branching projections (axons and dendrites) that serve to connect neurons into extended networks or functional multicellular units. Dendrites are best demonstrated by silver impregnation or antibodies to dendritic markers such as microtubule-associated protein (MAP)2. Each neuron usually gives rise to a single axon, which may extend for more than a meter to arborize in terminal synapses with the processes of other neurons or target organs such as muscle and glands. Some axons are surrounded by a myelin sheath; others are unmyelinated.

Neurons react to injury in several ways that may be reversible or culminate in cell death:

CHROMATOLYSIS: Injured neurons swell, the cytoplasm expands, and the Nissl substance disperses near the plasma membrane (Fig. 28-3). The nucleus assumes an eccentric position. This process is known as chromatolysis and is a common

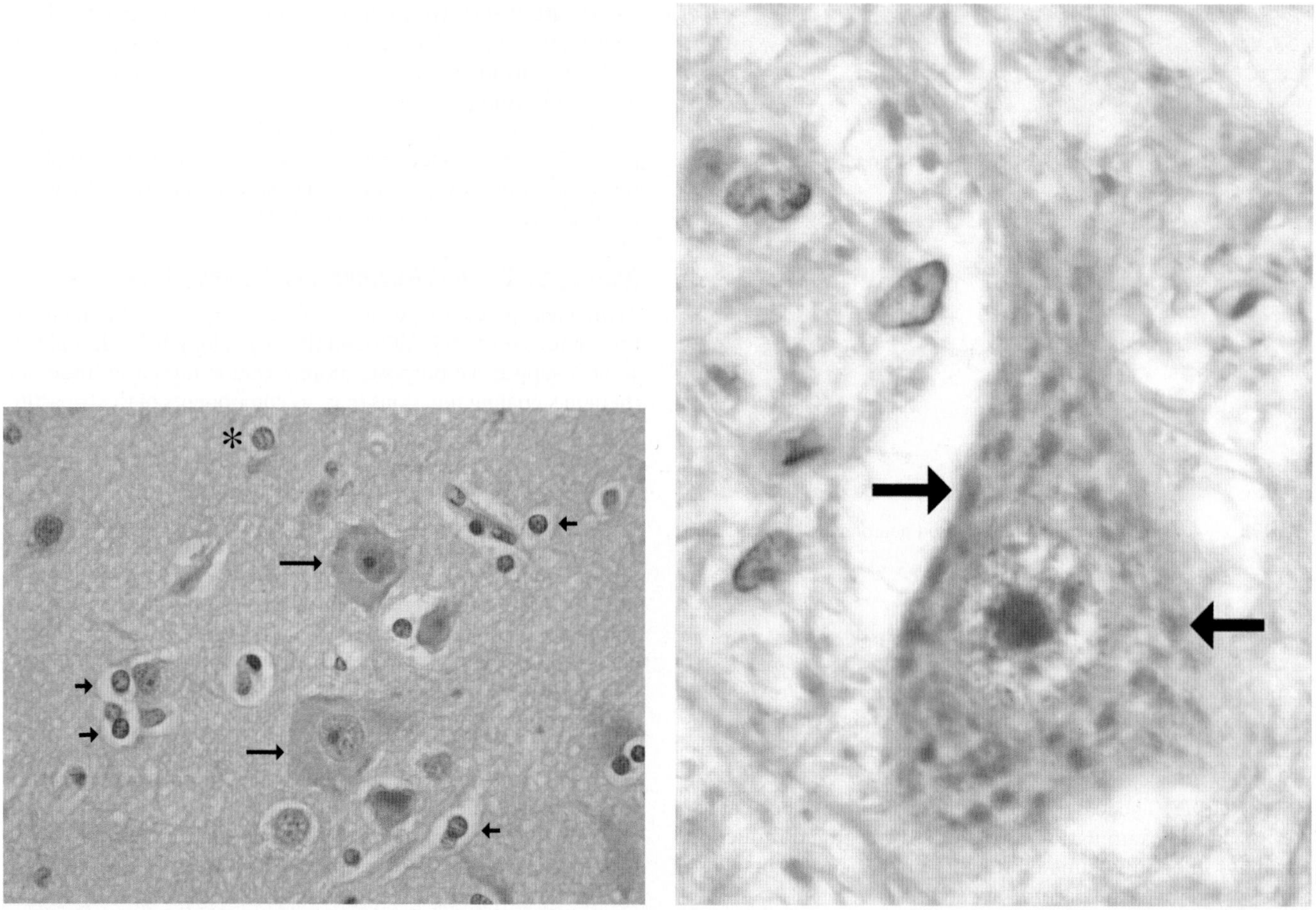

A B

FIGURE 28-1. **Brain cortex. A.** Neurons (*long arrows*) cells are typically pyramidal with a round nucleus and prominent nucleolus. Oligodendrocytes (short arrows) and astrocytes are present (asterisk). **B.** Motor neuron with abundant Nissl bodies (*arrows*). The granularity of the cytoplasm is imparted by rough endoplasmic reticulum (Nissl substance), but over 95% of the volume of large neurons is invested in its processes (axons and dendrites) that extend for very long distances (~1 m for some motor neurons), making neurons the most highly asymmetric cells in humans and other mammals.

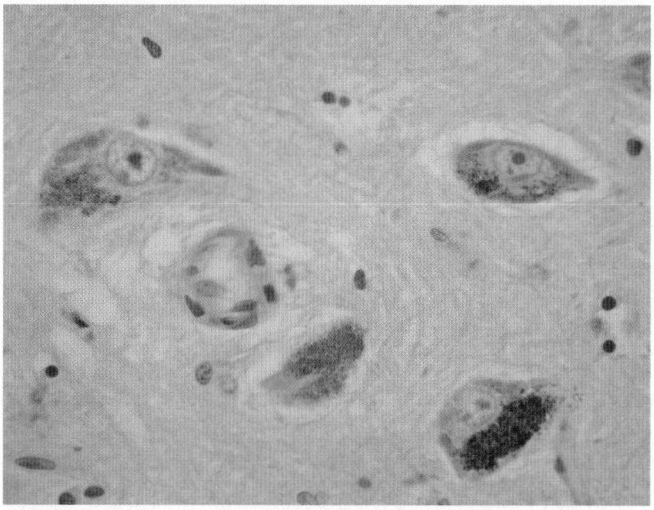

FIGURE 28-2. **Pigmented neurons.** Neurons of the substantia nigra and locus ceruleus are heavily pigmented with neuromelanin.

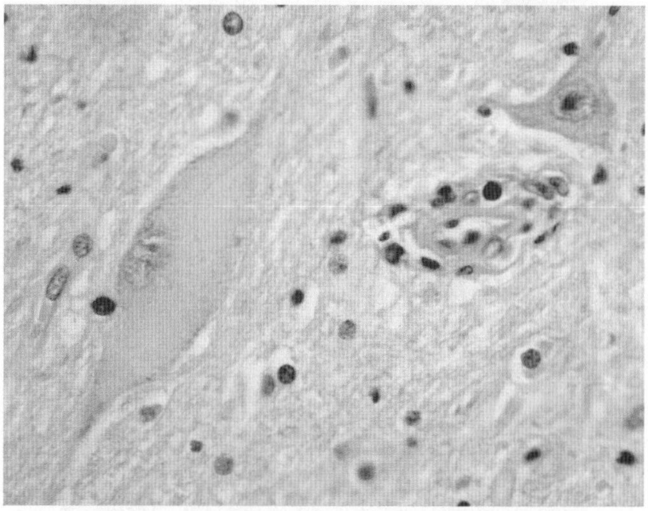

FIGURE 28-3. **Chromatolysis.** An injured neuron (*left*) appears swollen with pale cytoplasm, eccentric nucleus, and marginated Nissl substance near the plasma membrane. Compare to normal neuron at upper right.

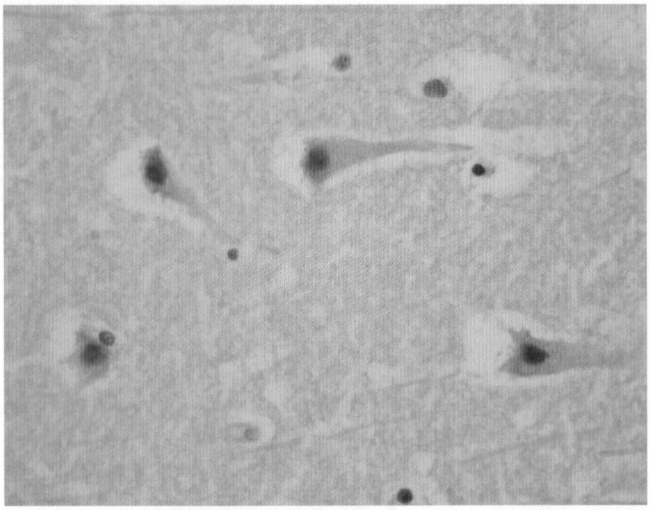

FIGURE 28-4. **Acute neuronal injury.** Injured neurons are pyknotic with hypereosinophilic cytoplasm.

response to injury (e.g., axonal transaction). It may be reversible, but it also may be a harbinger of cell death. Acutely injured neurons shrivel and become pyknotic with hypereosinophilic cytoplasm (Fig. 28-4).

ATROPHY: The loss of neurons in the brain may be appreciated on gross examination as a global or regional reduction (atrophy) in brain volume or weight. Single neurons may also atrophy or shrivel and become hyperchromatic.

NEURONOPHAGIA: Injuries that kill neurons create cellular debris and elicit phagocytosis by immune cells (i.e., brain macrophages or brain microglia). This phagocytic response is termed **neuronophagia.**

INTRANEURONAL INCLUSIONS: Diverse nuclear and cytoplasmic inclusions affect neurons, particularly in viral encephalitides and in neurodegenerative diseases characterized by intracytoplasmic amyloid deposits (see below).

Astrocytes Support Neurons and Promote Repair

Astrocytes are star-shaped glial cells that far outnumber neurons throughout the CNS. Although they have long been thought to serve a supportive purpose, more recent studies also implicate them in signaling functions (e.g., as components of the tripartite synapse) previously considered the sole domain of neurons. Astrocytes also play a prominent role in the CNS response to injury.

ANATOMY: Multiple species of CNS astrocytes have been identified, but the two best known subtypes are **fibrillary astrocytes** in white matter, and **protoplasmic astrocytes** in gray matter. By light microscopy, both types of astrocytes display a round nucleus, 7 to 10 μm in diameter, with homogeneous chromatin and scant cytoplasm (see Fig. 28-1). However, immunohistochemic stains for glial fibrillary acidic protein (GFAP) or silver impregnation reveal processes extending in all directions from the astrocyte cell body (Fig. 28-5A), some of which terminate as foot processes on blood vessels. By electron microscopy, both types of astrocytes contain a meshwork of fine glial filaments formed by polymers of GFAP.

REACTIONS: Astrocytes proliferate locally in response to injuries (e.g., trauma, abscess, tumors, infarcts, and hemorrhages). This process, referred to as **astrocytosis** or **gliosis.** Astrocytosis

A

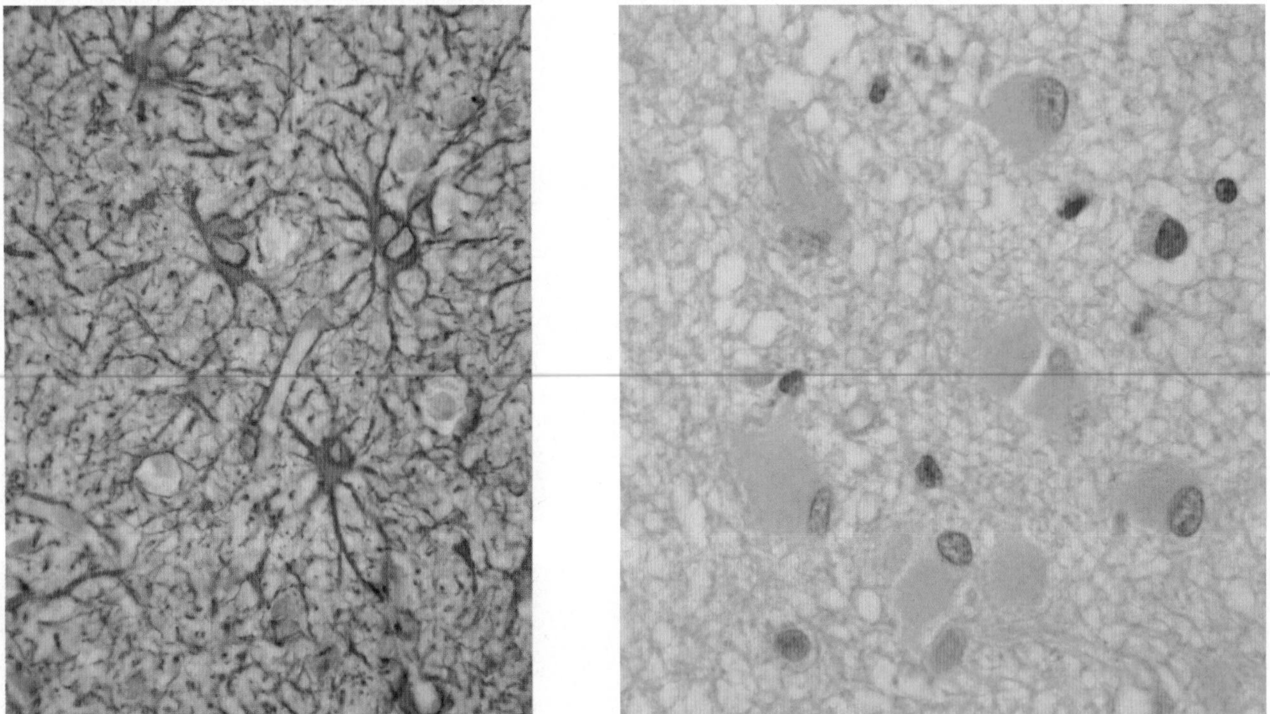

B

FIGURE 28-5. **Astrocytes. A.** The glial processes of astrocytes stain intensely for glial fibrillary acidic protein (GFAP). **B.** Hematoxylin and eosin (H&E)-stained reactive astrocytes are plump with pink cytoplasm (gemistocytic astrocytes).

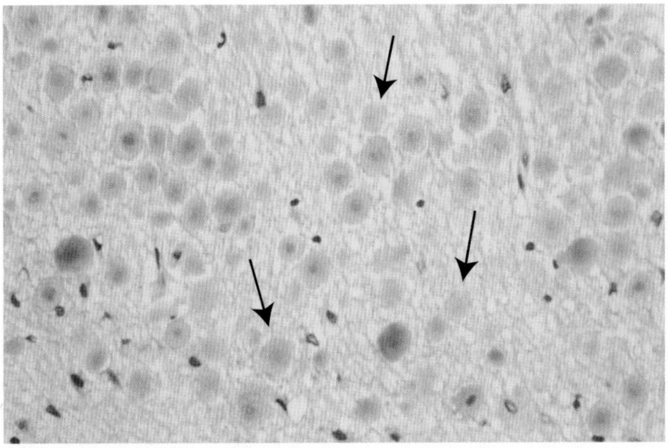

FIGURE 28-6. **Corpora amylacea.** These are amorphous, basophilic bodies *(arrows)* that accumulate in the subependymal and subpial areas of elderly persons.

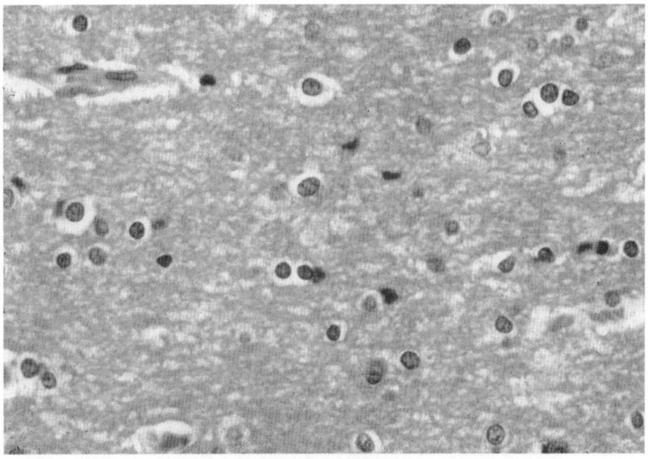

FIGURE 28-7. **Normal white matter.** The white matter contains oligodendroglia, with small nuclei and clear cytoplasm. They are often aligned along the myelinated axons.

evolves in hours to days and persists to an extent that is usually commensurate with the severity of the initiating injury. Reactive astrocytes may have plump, eosinophilic cytoplasm, termed **gemistocytic astrocytes** (see Fig. 28-5B). The consequence is a "glial scar" composed of reactive astrocytes and their processes. Astrocytes may also undergo neoplastic transformation to result in the most common primary brain tumors, namely, **gliomas** or **astrocytomas.**

Corpora amylacea are 5- to 20-nm basophilic and amorphous structures formed by aggregates of carbohydrates and proteins. These bodies accumulate with normal aging with a predilection for subpial and subependymal regions (Fig. 28-6). Although they appear extracellular by light microscopy, they evolve within processes of astrocytes.

Oligodendroglia are the Myelin-Producing Cells of the CNS

Oligodendroglia are related to astrocytes insofar as they are both of neurectodermal origin. In sections stained with hematoxylin and eosin (H&E) or Luxol fast blue, oligodendroglia have dark, round nuclei with a thin rim of cytoplasm. In the gray matter, many oligodendroglia are disposed as "satellites" around neurons, whereas oligodendrocytes in the white matter are arrayed longitudinally between myelinated fibers (Fig. 28-7). Oligodendroglia synthesize myelin during the late gestational period and through early postnatal life subsequently maintaining these lipid membranes to insulate axons and speed conduction of impulses. In diseases that affect oligodendrocytes (e.g., in multiple sclerosis and progressive multifocal leukoencephalopathy [PML]), demyelination impairs axonal function. Oligodendrogliomas are a less common type of glioma than astrocytic neoplasms.

Ependyma Regulates Fluid Transport

A single layer of ependymal cells lines the four ventricular chambers, the aqueduct of Sylvius, the central canal of the spinal cord, and the filum terminale. These cells vary from cuboidal to flat (Fig. 28-8) and modulate fluid transfer between the cerebrospinal fluid (CSF) and the CNS. During gestation, some viral infections target the ependymal cells, an event responsible in part for aqueductal stenosis and congenital hydrocephalus. Ependymomas, which result from the neoplastic transformation of ependymal cells, generally arise within a ventricle, but they also present as intramedullary tumors of the spinal cord and filum terminale.

Choroid Plexus Produces CSF

The choroid plexus is derived from the ependyma and consists of a cuboidal epithelium surrounding a fibrovascular core (see Fig. 28-8B). Tight junctions between the epithelial cells results in a

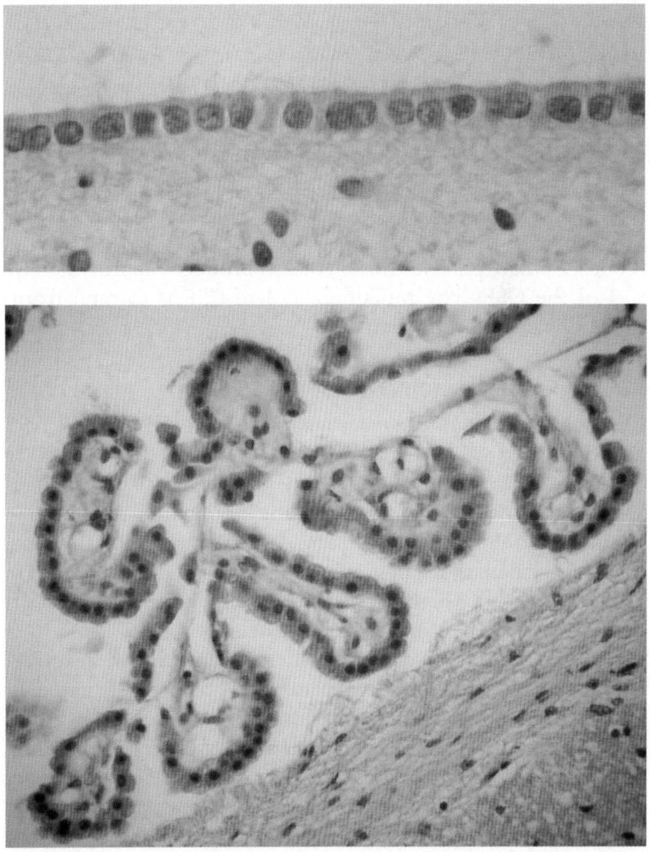

A

B

FIGURE 28-8. **Ependyma. A.** The ventricle is lined by cells of neuroglial origin that display epithelial features. **B.** Choroid plexus. A specialized structure derived from the ependyma that secretes cerebrospinal fluid.

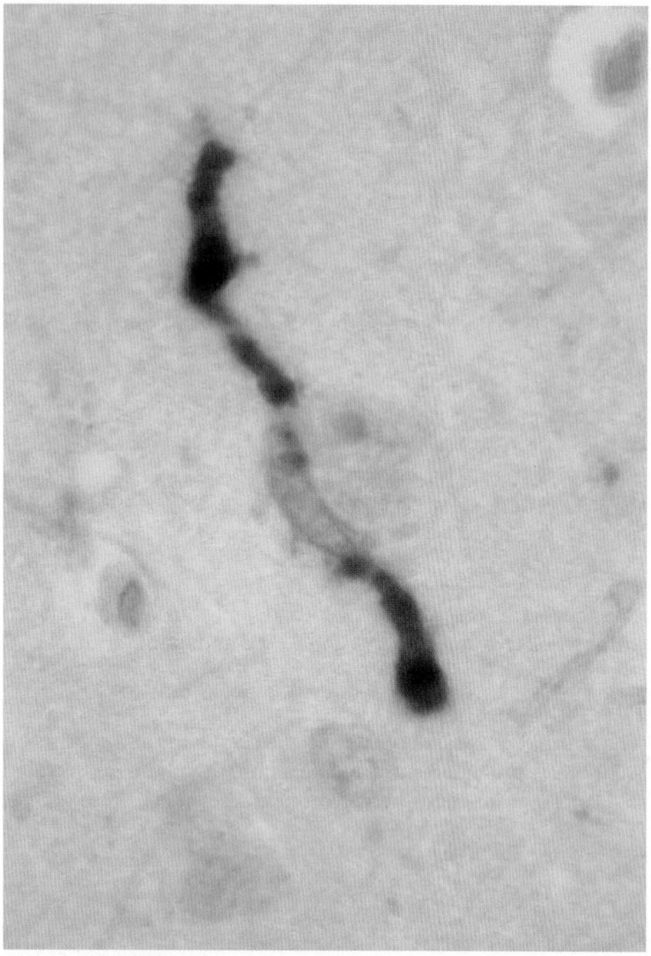

FIGURE 28-9. **Microglia.** A microglial cell stained for CD68 (lysosomal marker expressed in phagocytic cells) exhibits a rod shaped nucleus and elongated processes.

blood-CSF barrier. The choroid plexus produces approximately 2/3 of the CSF. The remaining 1/3 of CSF is formed from metabolic water production.

Microglia Are Macrophages of the CNS

Microglia are phagocytic macrophage-derived cells of the CNS, accounting for 5% of all glial cells.

ANATOMY: Resting microglia are identified in tissues stained with H&E by their hyperchromatic, elongated nuclei surrounded by a thin rim of cytoplasm. When stained with silver or for microglial markers, they appear filiform and display fine processes (Fig. 28-9). Microglia may be scattered in the neuropil or disposed around neurons or blood vessels.

REACTIONS: Microglia proliferate and show reactive changes in areas of injury. Two patterns are recognized, namely, focal microglial nodules and diffuse microgliosis. **Microglial nodules** are formed of microglia and astrocytes (Fig. 28-10), and are typical responses to viral or other infections. Some reactive microglia exhibit a prominent elongated nucleus, in which case they are referred to as **rod cells.** In response to necrosis, microglia become phagocytic, accumulate lipids and other cellular debris, and are designated **gitter cells** (Fig. 28-11). Although the embryonic derivation of microglia continues to be debated, it appears that phagocytic microglia in CNS inflammations are blood-derived monocytes.

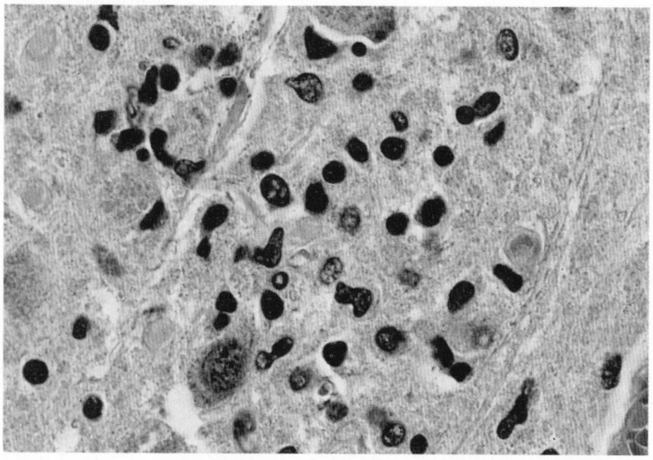

FIGURE 28-10. **Microglial nodule.** Microglia and astrocytes create cellular nodules in response to viral, protozoan, or rickettsial infections.

Congenital Malformations

The development of the CNS proceeds according to a precise schedule, and each morphologic event is the cornerstone for those that follow. For example, myelination is initiated late in embryonic development only after the neurons and oligodendroglia have differentiated and migrated to their appropriate destinations; interruption of these processes results in flawed myelination. *Thus, congenital anomalies reflect interruptions in the completion of critical developmental processes.*

Accordingly, the characteristics of a congenital malformation are defined more by the time of the insult than by the nature of the injury itself. Although specific congenital malformations may have many causes, they tend to share a common time-related target. For instance, anoxia and radiation induce anencephaly (see below) when administered to rats early in the eighth day of pregnancy but only a little later cause cleft palate.

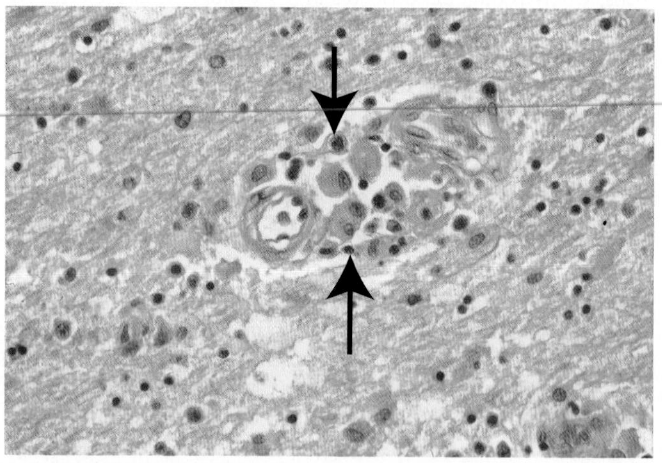

FIGURE 28-11. **Macrophages.** A cluster of pervascular macrophages (*arrows*) is seen in a patient with acquired immunodeficiency syndrome (AIDS) encephalopathy.

Neural Tube Defects (Dysraphic States) Reflect Impaired Closure of the Dorsal Aspect of the Vertebral Column

Anencephaly

Anencephaly refers to the congenital absence of all or part of the brain. Among CNS malformations, anencephaly is second in incidence to spina bifida (0.5to 2.0 per 1000 births, with a modest female predominance). Anencephalic fetuses are either stillborn or die within the first few days of life.

EPIDEMIOLOGY: Anencephaly is a typical multifactorial birth defect that exhibits a worldwide geographic variation in incidence. In the United States, the frequency of this anomaly is 0.3 per 1000 live births and stillbirths, whereas in Ireland and Wales, the frequency is 20-fold greater (5 to 6 per 1000 conceptuses). Interestingly, Irish immigrants to North America have the highest incidence of anencephaly on the continent, although it is lower (2 to 3 per 1000) than that in Ireland. The incidence of this disorder is particularly low in blacks.

PATHOGENESIS: Anencephaly is a dysraphic defect of neural tube closure (Fig. 28-12). The concurrence of anencephaly with other neural tube defects (NTDs), such as spina bifida, suggests they all may result from shared pathogenic mechanisms.

During fetal development the neural plate invaginates and is transformed into the neural tube by fusion of the posterior surfaces. The mesenchymal tissue overlying the primitive neural tube then molds the skull and the vertebral arches posterior to the spinal cord. Failure of the neural tube to close results in the lack of closure of the overlying bony structures of the cranium and an absence of the calvarium, skin, and subcutaneous tissues of this region. The exposed brain is incompletely formed or even entirely absent. In most cases, the base of the skull contains only fragments of neural and ependymal tissue and residues of the meninges. **Acrania** (complete or partial absence of the cranium) results from an injury to the fetus between the 23rd and 26th days of gestation.

Genetic factors seem to play a role in the pathogenesis of anencephaly. The anomaly is twice as common in females as in males, and it occurs with higher frequency in certain families. The risk of a second anencephalic fetus is 2% to 5%, and after two anencephalic fetuses the risk rises to 25% for each subsequent pregnancy.

Folic acid supplied in the periconceptional period lowers the incidence of NTDs. In 1998, the United States Food and Drug Administration began requiring manufacturers of enriched flour, bread, and some other products to supplement these foods with folate. This mandate has been associated with a significant decrease in the incidence of NTDs.

PATHOLOGY: The cranial vault in anencephaly is absent, and the cerebral hemispheres are a discoid mass of highly vascularized, poorly differentiated neural tissue, the so-called **cerebrovasculosa** (Fig. 28-13). This structure lies on the flattened base of the skull, behind two well-formed eyes, which mark the anterior margin of disturbed organogenesis. A well-differentiated retina attests to the preservation of the eyes, and short segments of the optic nerve extend posteriorly. The posterior aspect of the malformation forms a variable transitional zone with a recognizable midbrain, but most often the entire brainstem and cerebellum are rudimentary. The upper spinal cord is hypoplastic, and a dysraphic bony defect of the posterior spinal column (rachischisis) may involve the cervical area. Vertebral and basilar arteries usually are identifiable in a tangle of meningeal vessels

The cerebrovasculosa corresponds to the residual underdeveloped cerebral hemispheres typically containing islands of immature neural tissue. It also encloses cavities partially lined by ependyma with or without choroid plexus. However, the mass is composed predominantly of abnormal vascular channels that vary considerably in size. Beneath the cerebrovasculosa, but sharing a common origin with the brain, are cranial nerves and intraosseous ganglia.

CLINICAL FEATURES: Two thirds of anencephalic fetuses die in utero, and those that are alive at birth rarely survive for more than a week. Screening of pregnant women for serum α-fetoprotein and examination by ultrasonography allow detection of virtually all anencephalic fetuses. The use of organs from anencephalic infants for transplantation remains a thorny ethical problem.

Spina Bifida

Spina bifida is an NTD most common in the lumbosacral region. This anomaly is usually localized to the lumbar region and represents the mildest dysraphic abnormality of the CNS. Spina bifida results from an insult between the 25th and 30th days of gestation, reflecting the sequential closure of the neural tube (see Fig. 28-12). It is further classified according to the extent of the defect.

- **Spina bifida occulta:** This defect is restricted to the vertebral arches and is usually asymptomatic. It is frequently manifested externally only by a dimple or small tuft of hair.
- **Meningocele:** This condition features a more extensive bony and soft tissue defect that permits protrusion of the meninges as a fluid-filled sac. The lateral aspects of the sac are characteristically covered by skin, whereas the apex is usually ulcerated.
- **Meningomyelocele:** This term refers to a still more extensive defect that exposes the spinal canal and causes the nerve roots (particularly those of the cauda equina) to be entrapped in subcutaneous scar tissue (Fig. 28-14). Characteristically, the spinal cord appears as a flattened, ribbonlike structure.
- **Rachischisis:** In this extreme defect, the spinal column is converted into a gaping canal, often without a recognizable spinal cord (Fig. 28-15).

PATHOGENESIS: Spina bifida is induced readily in rats and chicks at the eighth to ninth gestational day by chemicals such as trypan blue or by hypervitaminosis A. It probably results from a failure of the neural tube to close, but the validity of this concept is uncertain. Maternal folic acid deficiency has been associated with an increased incidence of NTDs, and folic acid has therefore, been approved for inclusion as a food supplement in commercial flour.

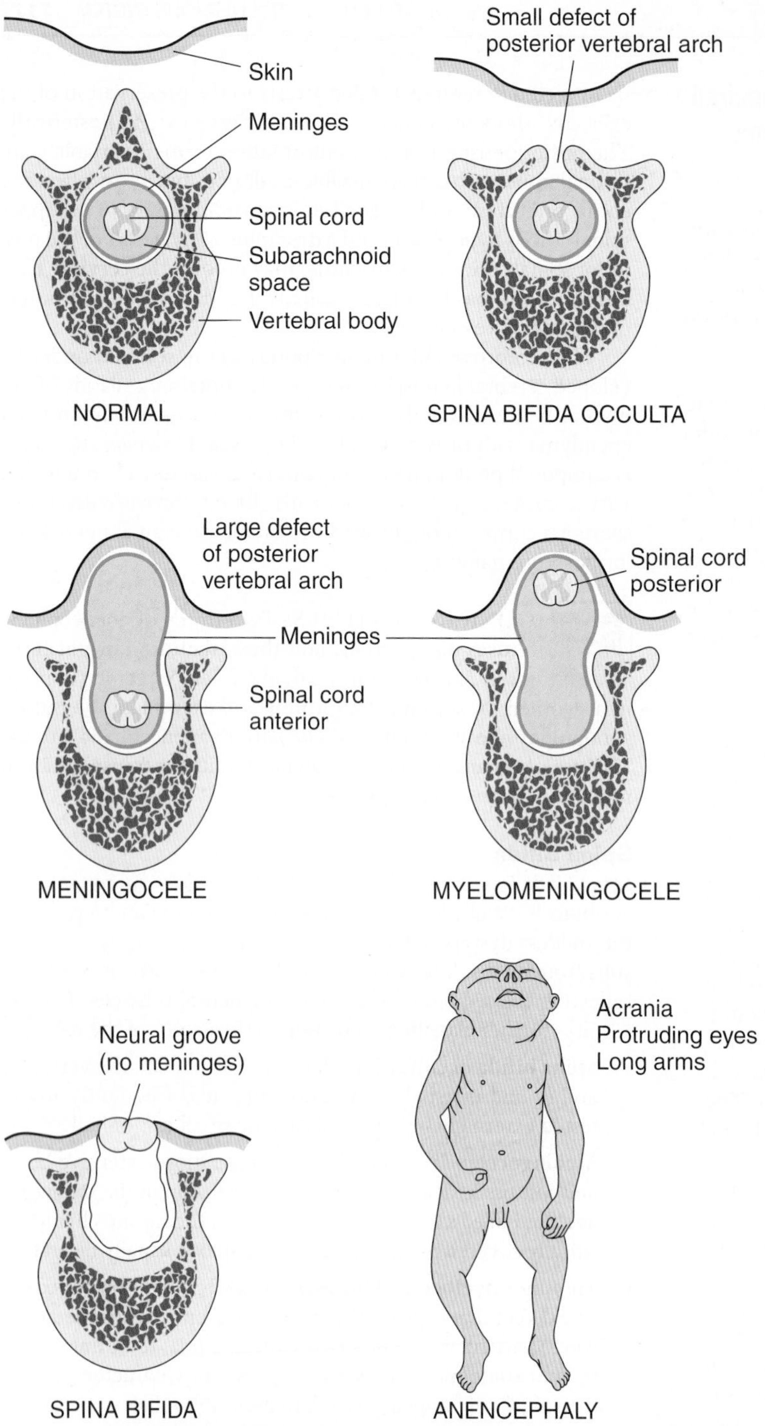

FIGURE 28-12. **Dysraphic defects of the neural tube.** Incomplete fusion of the neural tube and overlying bone, soft tissues, or skin leads to several defects, varying from mild anomalies (e.g., spina bifida occulta) to severe anomalies (e.g., anencephaly).

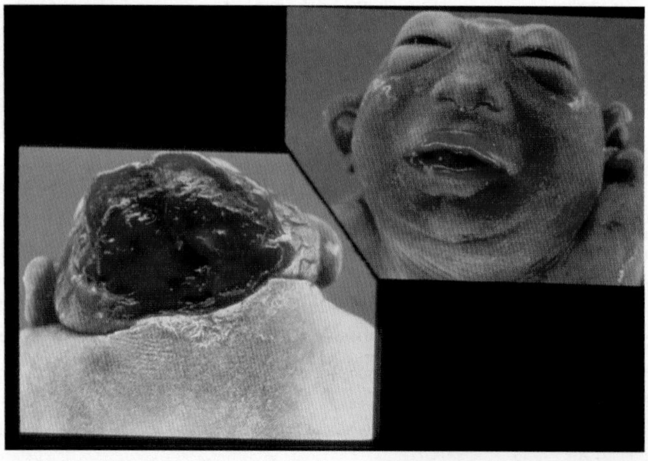

FIGURE 28-13. **Anencephaly.** The cerebral vault is absent (*upper right*), and the absence of a calvarium exposes a mass of vascularized tissue (cerebrovasculosa; *lower left*), in which there are rudimentary neuroectodermal structures. The lesion is bounded anteriorly by normally formed eyes and posteriorly by the brainstem.

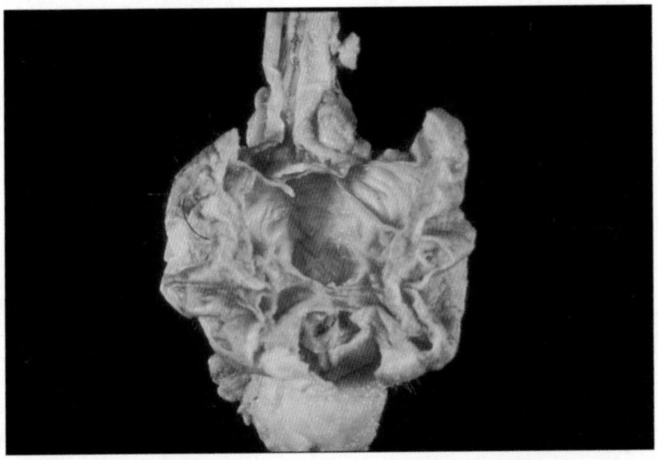

FIGURE 28-14. **Meningomyelocele.** This dysraphic defect, which is caused by lack of fusion of the spinal canal, reveals disorganized neural tissue with entrapment of nerve roots.

CLINICAL FEATURES: The spectrum of neurologic deficits in NTDs ranges from no symptoms in spina bifida occulta to lower limb paralysis, sensory loss, and incontinence with meningomyelocele. One must be aware of potential associated malformations such as Arnold-Chiari malformation, hydrocephalus, polymicrogyria, and hydromyelia of the spinal central canal (Fig. 28-16).

Malformations of the Spinal Cord are Uncommon Congenital Disorders

The spinal cord may harbor congenital malformations that are less apparent at birth than NTDs. They include rare duplications, ranging from complete (**dimyelia**) to partial duplications of spinal cord into two separate structures (**diastematomyelia**).

Hydromyelia refers to dilation of the central canal of the spinal cord (see Fig. 28-16).

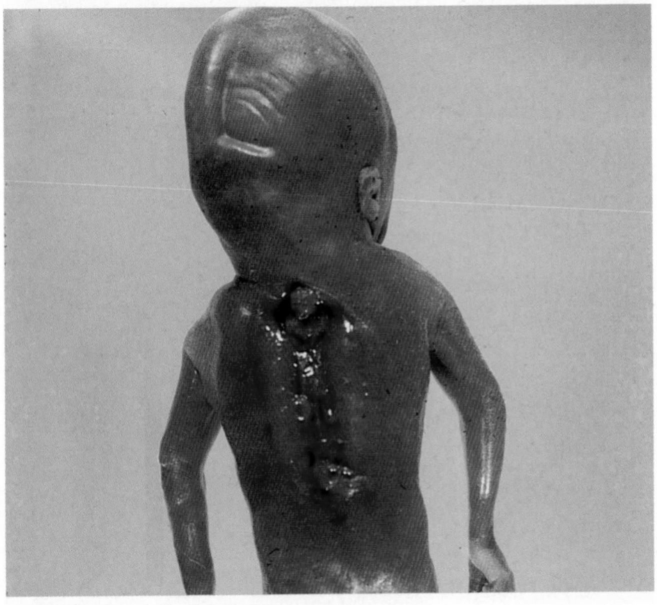

FIGURE 28-15. **Rachischisis.** A view of the vertebral column shows a bony, cutaneous defect with segmental absence of the spinal cord.

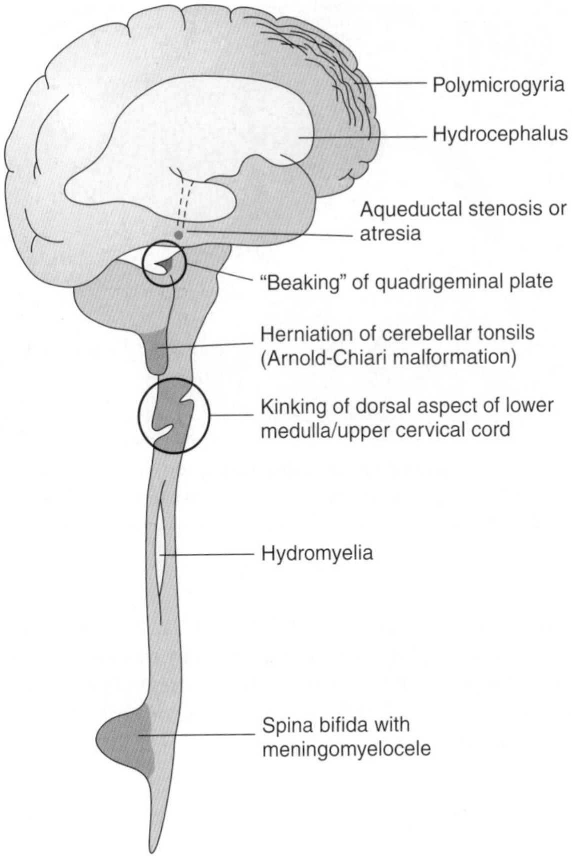

FIGURE 28-16. **Arnold-Chiari malformation and associated lesions.**

SYRINGOMYELIA: In this congenital malformation, a tubular cavitation (syrinx) extends for variable distances along the entire length of the spinal cord, which may or may not communicate with the central canal. The condition is usually encountered in adults, although many cases are thought to represent a congenital malformation. Clearly, some cases are caused by trauma, ischemia, or tumors. The syrinx is filled with a clear fluid closely resembling CSF. The symptoms of syringomyelia are related to the extent of the syrinx and its concomitant destruction of cells and fibers. Motor and sensory deficits occur at various levels, reflecting the anatomical location of the lesions in the spinal cord.

Syringobulbia is a variant of syringomyelia in which slitlike cavities are located in the medulla.

Arnold-Chiari Malformation Involves the Medulla and Cerebellum

Arnold-Chiari malformation is a condition in which the brainstem and cerebellum are compacted into a shallow, bowl-shaped posterior fossa with a low-positioned tentorium. It is often associated with syringomyelia or a lumbosacral meningomyelocele, and the symptomatology depends on the severity of the defect.

PATHOGENESIS: Arnold-Chiari malformation may result when a meningomyelocele anchors the lower end of the spinal cord and causes downward growth of the vertebral column, thereby creating traction on the medulla. However, other features of this

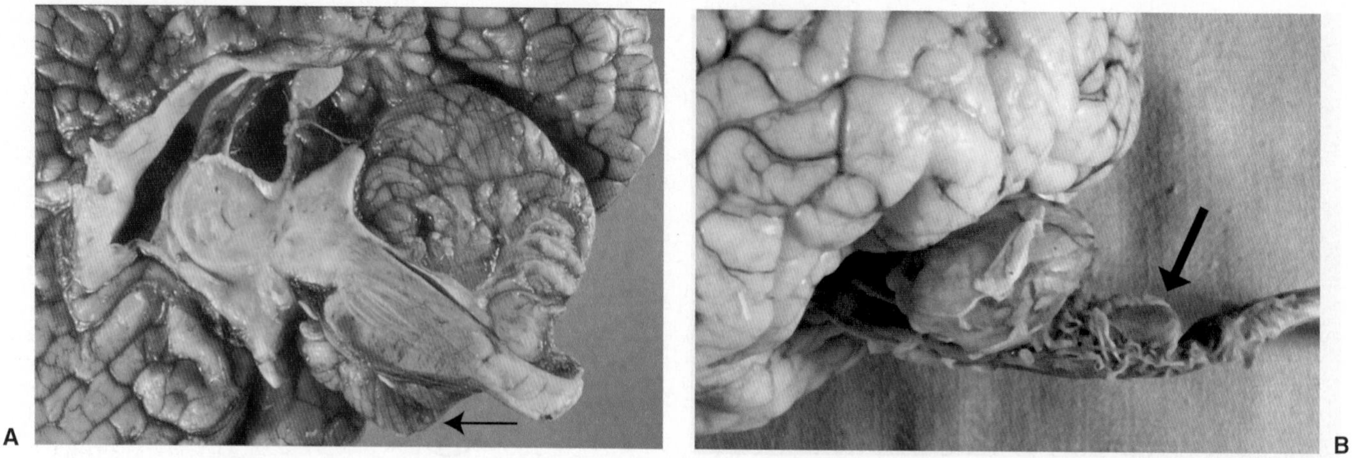

FIGURE 28-17. **Arnold-Chiari malformation. A.** The cerebellar vermis is herniated below the level of the foramen magnum *(arrow)*. The downward displacement of the dorsal portion of the cord causes the obex of the fourth ventricle to occupy a position below the foramen magnum. **B.** Herniation of the cerebellar tonsils (*arrow*) with adjacent kinking of the spinal cord.

malformation (curvature of the medulla, beaking of the quadrigeminal plate) are not explained by this mechanism. Other proposed mechanisms include increased intracranial pressure associated with hydrocephalus or limited size of the posterior fossa.

PATHOLOGY: In Arnold-Chiari malformation, the caudal aspect of the cerebellar vermis is herniated through an enlarged foramen magnum (see Fig. 28-16 and Fig. 28-17) and protrudes onto the dorsal aspect of the cervical cord, often reaching the level of C3 to C5. The herniated tissue is bound in position by thickened meninges and shows pressure atrophy (i.e., depletion of Purkinje and granular cells). The brainstem also is displaced caudally. Typically, the displacement is more exaggerated dorsally than ventrally, and landmarks such as the obex of the fourth ventricle are more caudal than ventral structures such as the inferior olive. From a lateral perspective, the lower medulla is angulated in its midsegment, thereby creating a dorsal protrusion. The foramina of Magendie and Luschka are compressed by the bony ridge of the foramen magnum. The cerebellum is flattened to a discoid contour, and the quadrigeminal plate is often deformed by a "beak-shaped" dorsal protrusion of the inferior colliculi. Hydrocephalus results from obstruction of the foramina of Magendie and Luschka.

Congenital Hydrocephalus Refers to an Excessive Amount of CSF and Ventricular Enlargement

The fluid accumulations are in varied locations and have many causes, as discussed below in the section on cerebrospinal fluid.

Congenital atresia of the aqueduct of Sylvius is the most common cause of congenital hydrocephalus (Fig. 28-18). It occurs with an incidence of 1 in 1000 live births. The brain is atrophic and features a collapsed cerebral cortex. Histologic examination of the midbrain may disclose multiple atretic channels or an aqueduct narrowed by gliosis, which may result from transplacental transmission of viruses that induce ependymitis.

Disorders of Cerebral Gyri Are Frequently Associated with Mental Retardation

Gyral malformations arise from disturbances in neuronal migration, a highly patterned event of the first trimester of embryonic development. The primitive neurons move centrifugally from the germinal epithelia to populate the cortex. The number of neurons and their positions in the cortex are determining factors in the cortical infolding that creates sulci and gyri.

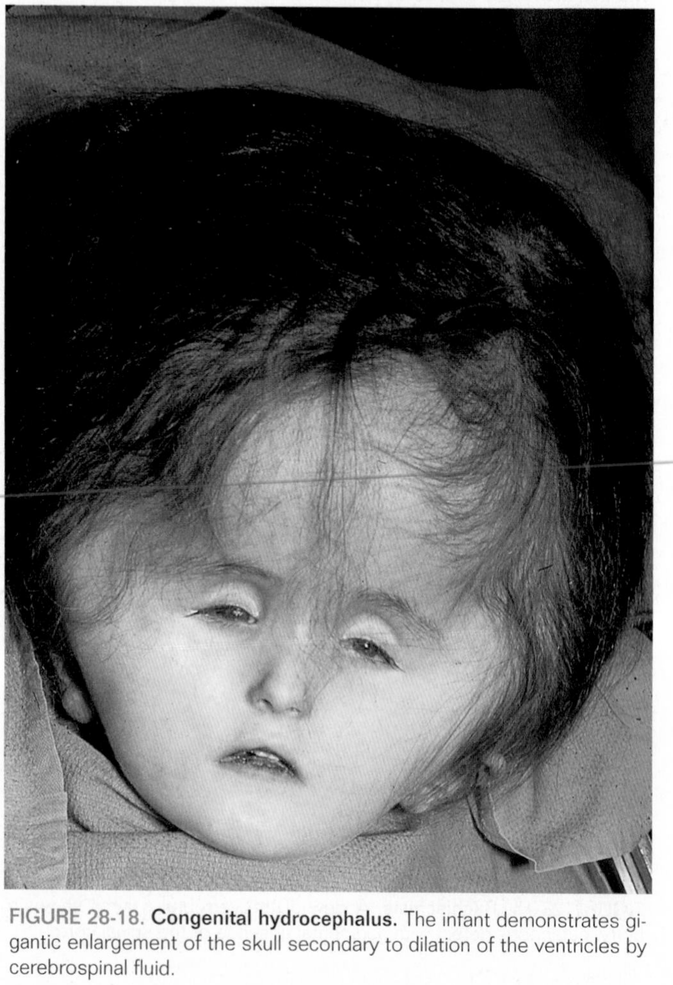

FIGURE 28-18. **Congenital hydrocephalus.** The infant demonstrates gigantic enlargement of the skull secondary to dilation of the ventricles by cerebrospinal fluid.

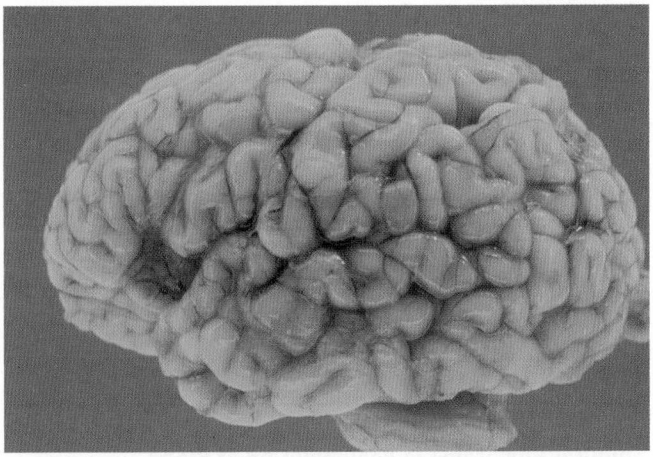

FIGURE 28-19. **Polymicrogyria.** The surface of the brain exhibits an excessive number of small, irregularly sized, randomly distributed gyral folds.

Abnormalities of the cerebral gyri, which are frequently associated with mental retardation, include a spectrum of entities exemplified by the following:

- **Polymicrogyria** refers to the presence of small and excessive gyri (Fig. 28-19).
- **Pachygyria** is a condition in which the gyri are reduced in number and unusually broad (Fig. 28-20).
- **Lissencephaly** is a congenital disorder in which the cortical surface of the cerebral hemispheres is smooth or has imperfectly formed gyri. Some 60% of patients with lissencephaly show deletions in the region of the *LIS1* gene on chromosome 17p13.3, which encodes a protein involved in cytoskeletal dynamics that plays a role in cell proliferation and motility.
- **Heterotopias** are focal disturbances in neuronal migration that lead to nodules of ectopic neurons and glia, usually in white matter. They are often associated with mental retardation and seizures and may be caused by maternal alcoholism.

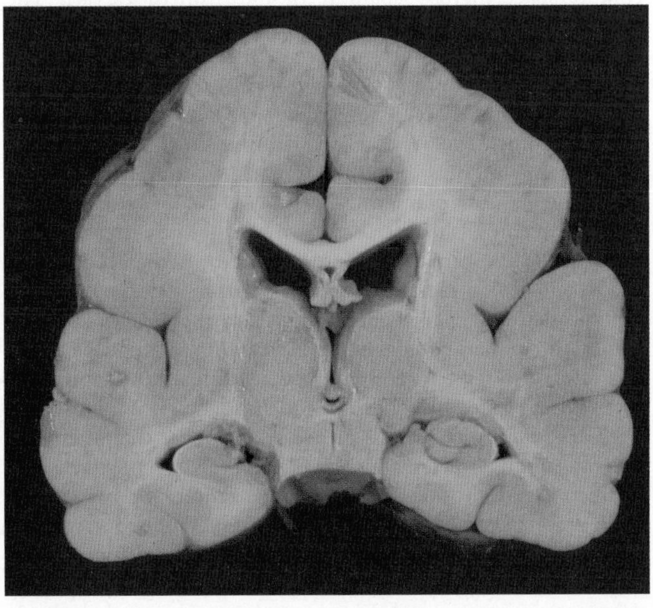

FIGURE 28-20. **Pachygyria.** A coronal section of the brain shows enlarged and thickened gyri.

Congenital Defects Are Often Associated with Chromosomal Abnormalities

Derangements of the larger autosomes, 1 through 12, are incompatible with sustained intrauterine life, and affected fetuses are spontaneously aborted. Structural and functional abnormalities attributable to gross chromosomal derangements are best exemplified by trisomies of chromosomes 13 to 15 and chromosome 21 (Down syndrome).

Down Syndrome

Down syndrome (trisomy 21) is characterized by mental retardation, distinctive facial features, and other anomalies. Although most cases reflect trisomy of chromosome 21, they rarely result from translocations or mosaicism. Down syndrome is discussed in detail in Chapter 6. The brain is moderately reduced in weight and is shortened in its anteroposterior dimension (Fig. 28-21). There is a simple gyral pattern, with disproportionately slender superior temporal gyri. The cytoarchitecture of the Down syndrome cortex closely approximates normal patterns, although patients typically develop changes of Alzheimer disease pathology (see below) by the fourth decade of life.

Trisomy 13–15

Trisomy 13-15 has an incidence of 1 per 5000 births, with a modest female predominance. The congenital deformities involve the brain, facial features, and extremities. The complex is dominated by holoprosencephaly, arrhinencephaly, microphthalmia, cyclopia, low-set ears, harelip, and cleft palate. The extremities exhibit polydactyly and "rocker bottom" feet.

HOLOPROSENCEPHALY: This term refers to a microcephalic brain in which the interhemispheric fissure is absent. The horseshoe-shaped cerebral hemispheres have fused frontal poles, across which the gyri show an irregular horizontal orientation (Fig. 28-22). A common ventricular chamber is created by lateral displacement of the posterior portions of the cerebral hemispheres. Bilobed caudate nuclei and thalami are prominent. Holoprosencephaly is rarely compatible with life beyond a few weeks or months.

ARRHINENCEPHALY: The absence of the olfactory tracts and bulbs (rhinencephalon) is associated with holoprosencephaly or occurs as a solitary malformation.

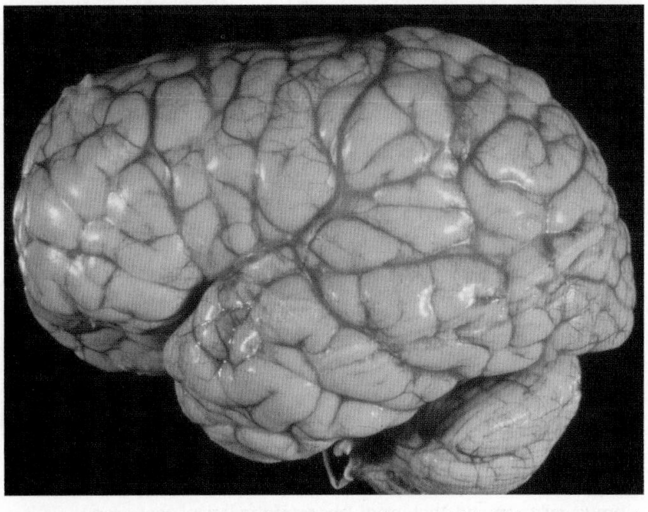

FIGURE 28-21. **Down syndrome.** Foreshortened brain with vertical occipital lobe edge and narrowed superior temporal gyrus.

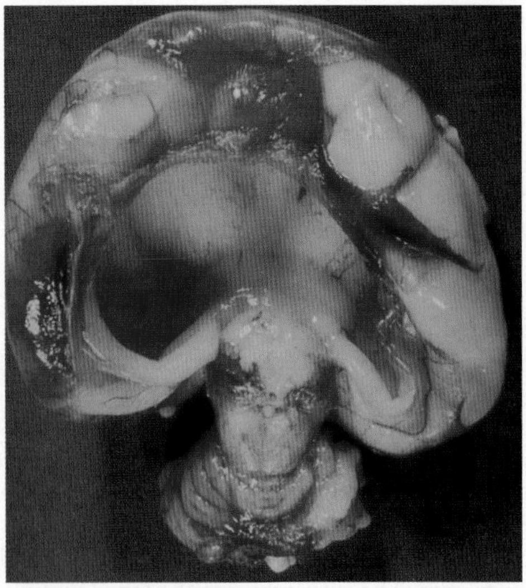

FIGURE 28-22. **Holoprosencephaly.** The brain exhibits a lack of separation of the hemispheres and a single large ventricle.

ABSENCE OF THE CORPUS CALLOSUM: This anomaly is a regular feature of holoprosencephaly, but it can also be a solitary lesion. Absence of the corpus callosum may occur without significant impairment of interhemispheric functional coordination, but it is occasionally associated with seizures. The corpus callosum physically tethers and functionally interconnects the hemispheres, and its absence (Fig. 28-23) permits the lateral ventricles to drift outward and upward, a position that is radiographically diagnostic.

Epilepsy Features Paroxysmal, Transient Disturbances (Seizures) in Brain Function

Seizures impair consciousness and cause abnormal motor activity or sensory or mental disturbances. Epilepsy has a prevalence of 6 per 1000, and newborns and infants are particularly vulnerable. Most seizures (75%) occur without a demonstrable organic lesion and are classified as idiopathic epilepsy. Most of these cases are sporadic, although hereditary forms are recognized.

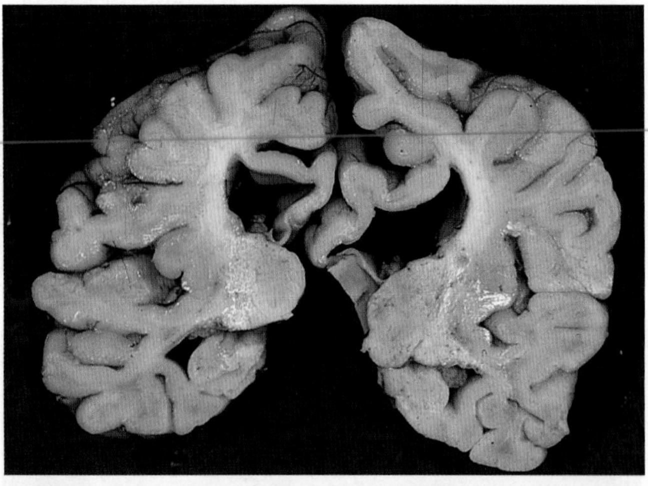

FIGURE 28-23. **Congenital absence of the corpus callosum.** A coronal section of the brain at the level of the thalamus reveals absence of the corpus callosum and "bat-wing" shape of the lateral ventricles.

PATHOLOGY: Careful studies of the brains of patients who had idiopathic epilepsy often reveal neuronal loss and reactive gliosis. The affected areas include the hippocampus, cerebellum, thalamus, and cerebral neocortex. Whether these changes are the cause of idiopathic epilepsy or result from the anoxia that occurs with generalized seizures is still debated. Heterotopias are occasionally found, and less commonly, epilepsy may be initiated by an intracranial tumor, arteriovenous malformation, or brain scar from a penetrating wound. Such lesions are more likely to cause seizures the closer they are to the motor cortex or surface of the brain.

Trauma

Epidural Hematoma Is Accumulation of Blood between the Calvaria and the Dura

Epidural hematoma usually results from a blow to the head, and unless treated promptly, is generally fatal.

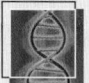

PATHOGENESIS: The intracranial dura is securely bound to the inner aspect of the calvaria and is thus analogous to the periosteum. The middle meningeal arteries occupy the space between the dura and the calvaria. They are grooved into the inner table of the bone, and their branches splay across the temporal–parietal area, generally as three major vessels. The temporal bone is one of the thinnest bones of the skull and is particularly vulnerable to fracture, so that seemingly minor trauma may fracture it and transect branches of the middle meningeal artery. The result is life-threatening epidural hemorrhage (Fig. 28-24).

PATHOLOGY AND CLINICAL COURSE: Transection of the middle meningeal artery permits the escape of arterial blood into the epidural space, thereby separating the dura from the calvaria. The hematoma enlarges relentlessly (see Fig. 28-24B). During the initial 4 to 8 hours, the intracranial events are largely asymptomatic. When the hematoma attains a volume of 30 to 50 mL, symptoms that reflect a space-occupying lesion appear. Because the supratentorial compartment has a fixed volume, the introduction of a space-occupying mass displaces an equal volume from this region. The earliest volumetric adjustments before symptoms appear are accomplished by the downward displacement of CSF through the aperture in the tentorium. If the hematoma continues to enlarge, intracranial pressure eventually exceeds the venous pressure. The large venous sinuses are then compressed, resulting in circulatory stagnation and cerebral ischemia. During this interval of global cerebral hypoxia, diffuse cortical impairment is manifested by confusion and disorientation.

The **Cushing reflex** is a protective response that augments cerebral circulation and increases cerebral oxygenation. The heart rate slows to increase ventricular filling, and myocardial contraction becomes more forceful. The blood pressure, particularly systolic pressure, increases. If bleeding continues, the hematoma can attain a size of about 60 mL within 6 to 10 hours. After compensatory mechanisms have been exhausted, the brain

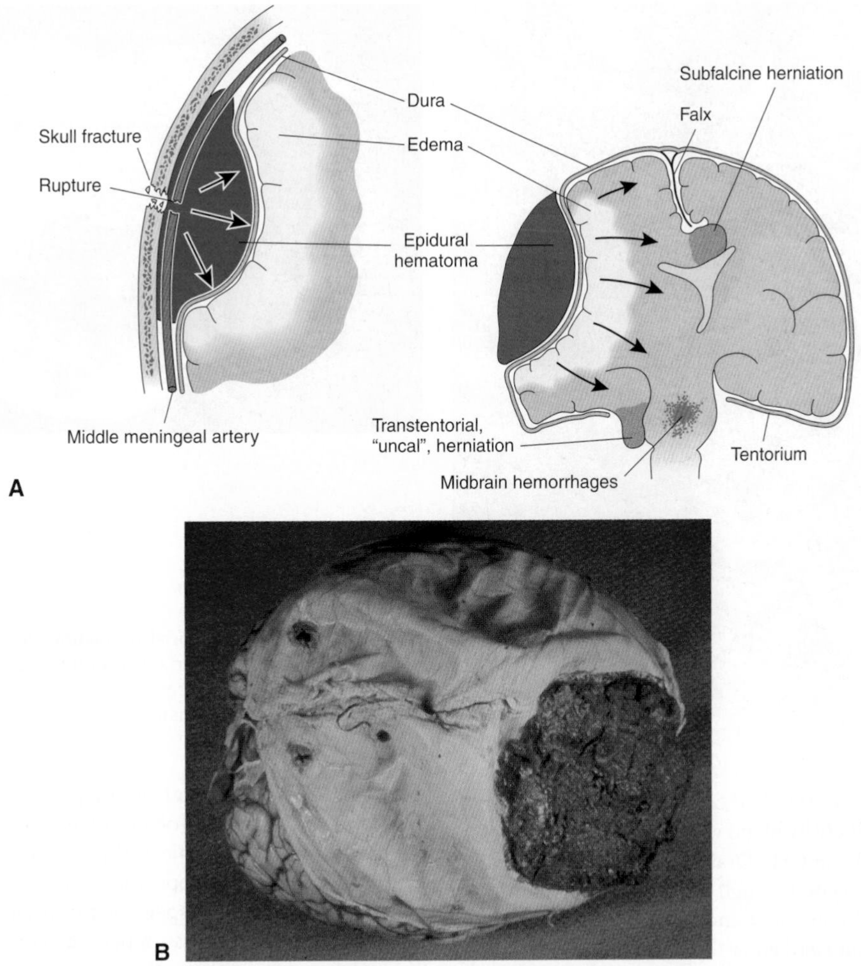

FIGURE 28-24. **Development of an epidural hematoma. A.** Transection of a branch of the middle meningeal artery by the sharp fracture initiates bleeding under arterial pressure that dissects the dura from the calvaria and produces an expanding hematoma. After an asymptomatic interval of several hours, transtentorial herniation becomes life-threatening. **B.** A discoid mass of fresh hemorrhage overlies the frontal–parietal cortex.

is shifted laterally away from the side of the lesion. The medial temporal lobe on the side of the hematoma is compressed against the midbrain to displace it downward through the opening created by the tentorium, a fatal event known as **transtentorial herniation** (Fig. 28-25). This herniation compresses the tissues of the uncus of the parahippocampal gyrus against the midbrain and also against contiguous structures, such as the cranial third nerve. Thus, the oculomotor nerve is compressed against the edge of the tentorium, causing a third-nerve palsy. The pupil, generally on the side of the lesion, becomes fixed and dilated.

The herniated uncus also compresses the vasculature of the midbrain, especially the paired mesencephalic veins (great veins of Rosenthal). Venous stagnation in the midbrain causes further hypoxia and impairs neuronal function. Damage to the reticular formation is expressed clinically as a decline in the level of consciousness. Shortly thereafter, hemorrhage (see Fig. 28-24) and necrosis of the brainstem occur, after which injury to the reticular formation becomes irreversible Death is imminent or, if the supratentorial pressure is relieved, unconsciousness is permanent. *Epidural hematomas are invariably progressive and, when not recognized and evacuated, are fatal in 24 to 48 hours.*

Concussion *is defined as the transient loss of consciousness due to trauma.* The blow to the head that causes an epidural hematoma does not necessarily have to produce a concussion. Consciousness is a positive neurologic activity that depends on the function of specific neurons, especially in the brainstem reticular formation. Concussion is exemplified in the boxing ring, as the consequence of a blow that deflects the head upward and posteriorly, often with a rotatory component. These motions impart a quick torque on the brainstem and cause functional paralysis of the neurons of the reticular formation. By contrast, a blow to the temporal–parietal area may lead to a skull fracture but does not generally cause a concussion, because lateral movement of the cerebral hemispheres is prevented by the falx.

Subdural Hematoma Reflects Torn Bridging Veins in the Subdural Space

Subdural hematoma is a significant cause of death after head injuries from falls, assaults, vehicular accidents, and sporting mishaps.

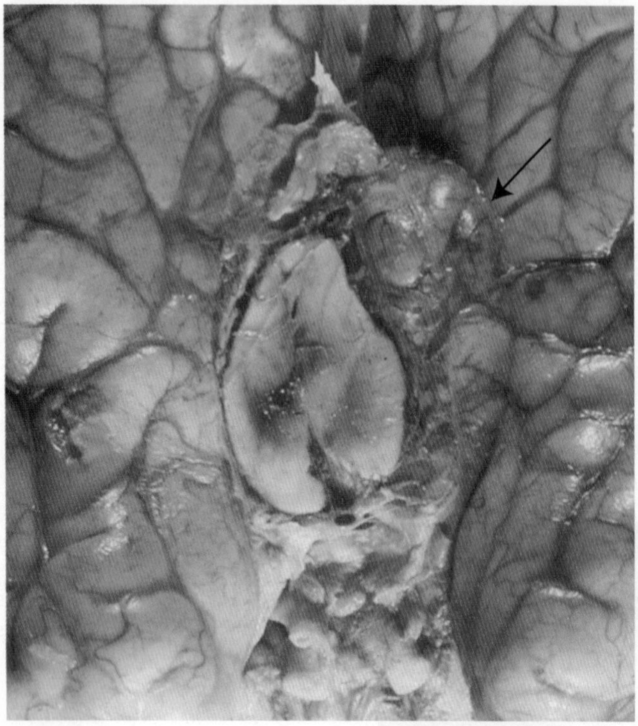

A

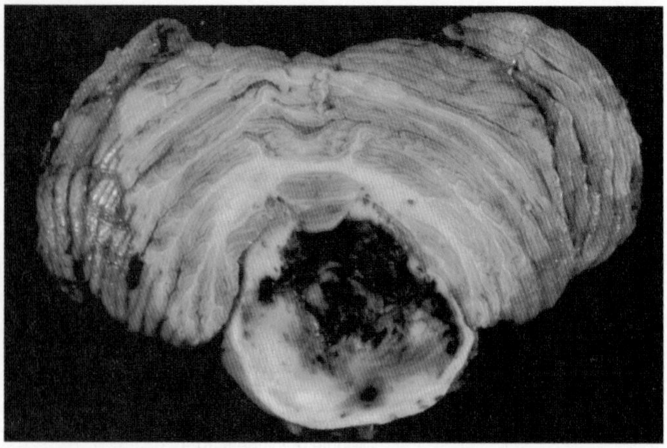

B

FIGURE 28-25. **Transtentorial herniation. A.** The uncus of the parahippocampal gyrus is herniated downward to displace the midbrain (*arrow*). **B.** Duret hemorrhages in a case of transtentorial herniation tend to be midline and to occupy the brainstem from the upper midbrain to mid-pons.

PATHOGENESIS: The cerebral hemispheres are tethered loosely by blood vessels and cranial nerves and float in the CSF. Drainage from the cerebral hemispheres flows upward through veins that cross the subarachnoid space and arachnoid and traverse the subdural space to breach the dura and enter the dural sinus.

When the frontal or occipital portion of the moving head strikes a fixed object or when the stationary head is struck by a blunt object, the cerebral hemispheres are displaced in an anteroposterior direction and hit forcefully against the inner aspect of the occipital or frontal bone. The soft cerebral tissues become compact and then recoil, producing a rippling effect through brain parenchyma. Be-

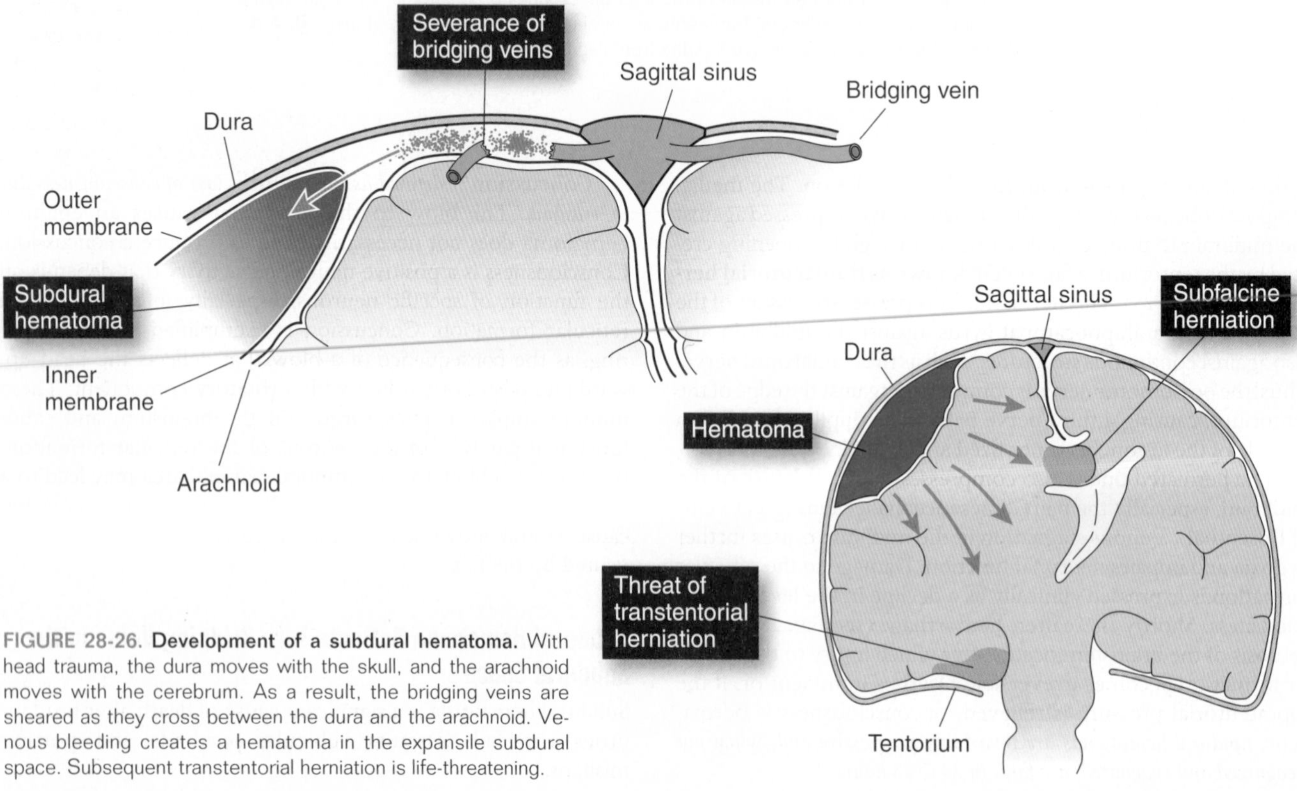

FIGURE 28-26. **Development of a subdural hematoma.** With head trauma, the dura moves with the skull, and the arachnoid moves with the cerebrum. As a result, the bridging veins are sheared as they cross between the dura and the arachnoid. Venous bleeding creates a hematoma in the expansile subdural space. Subsequent transtentorial herniation is life-threatening.

cause the dura adheres to the skull and the arachnoid is attached to the cerebrum, the disparate movement of these membranes produces a shearing effect in the subdural space, which tears the veins that pass through this compartment (see Fig. 28-26). Unlike the epidural space, the subdural space can expand. Since bleeding in this situation is from veins, it usually stops spontaneously after an accumulation of 25 to 50 mL, from a local tamponade effect. However, this also can compress severed bridging veins and cause thrombosis. Because the brain is symmetric and a force applied in the sagittal plane similarly affects both cerebral hemispheres, it is not surprising that subdural hematomas are frequently bilateral.

PATHOLOGY: A subdural hematoma, even when it is limited and too small to cause symptoms, can induce important tissue responses. Contact between the hematoma and the dura causes irritation and leads to the formation of granulation tissue over the subsequent several weeks. This process creates a membrane above the hematoma, termed the **outer membrane** (Fig. 28-27). Fibroblasts migrate from this membrane to invade the subjacent hematoma and form a fibrous membrane subjacent to the blood clot. Two weeks are required for this **inner membrane** to become visible.

A subdural hematoma, static in size and generally asymptomatic, has the potential for three routes of evolution:

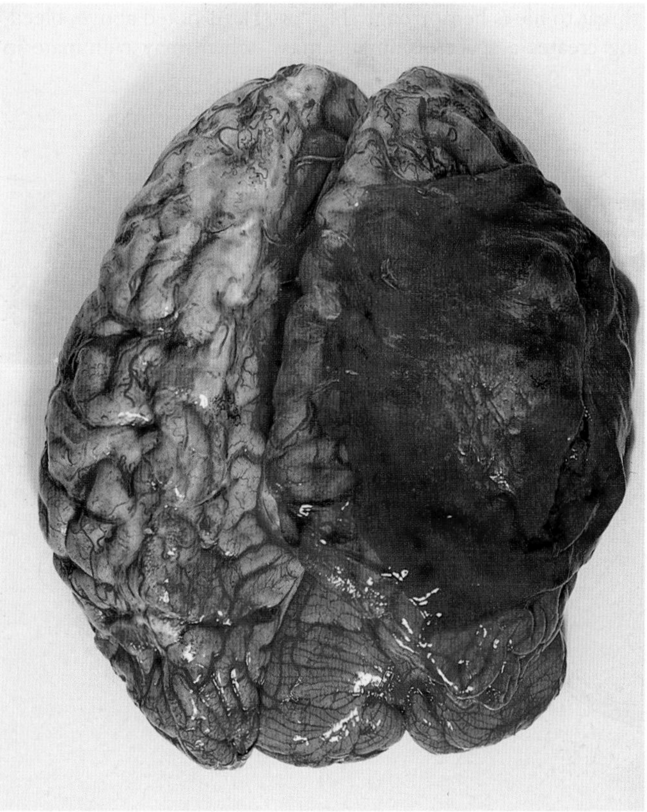

FIGURE 28-27. **Subdural hematoma.** The right hemisphere exhibits a large collection of blood in the subdural space, owing to rupture of the bridging veins.

- The hematoma may be reabsorbed and leave only a small amount of telltale hemosiderin.
- The hematoma may remain static, with the potential for calcification.
- The hematoma may enlarge.

Expansion of the hematoma, together with the onset of symptoms, commonly results from rebleeding, usually within 6 months. Since granulation tissue is vulnerable to minor trauma, even that caused by shaking the head, it can rebleed and create a new hematoma subjacent to the outer membrane. A series of events similar to those described above ensues, including formation of a second inner membrane. Such episodes of sporadic rebleeding expand the lesion periodically and at unpredictable intervals. Alternatively, it has been postulated that lysis of the original hematoma may create a hyperosmotic state that attracts fluid across the inner membrane and enlarges the lesion. If true, this process is of less consequence than rebleeding as a cause of symptoms. Remarkably, during the genesis of a subdural hematoma, the severance of the cortical bridging veins is so precisely localized to the subdural space that it compartmentalizes blood away from the CSF. *Thus, the absence of blood in the CSF does not negate the presence of a subdural hematoma.*

CLINICAL FEATURES: Subdural hematomas cause diverse clinical manifestations. Stretching of the meninges induces headaches, pressure on the motor cortex produces contralateral weakness, and focal cortical irritation can initiate seizures. Bilateral subdural hematomas may impair cognitive function and lead to a mistaken diagnosis of dementia, or rebleeding may cause a lethal transtentorial herniation.

Subarachnoid Hemorrhage Refers to Any Bleeding into the Subarachnoid Space

Subarachnoid hemorrhage (Fig. 28-28) may be seen in association with traumatic head injuries (e.g., cerebral contusion or laceration). However, it is rarely an isolated finding in the case of trauma and usually complicates hemorrhage in other parts of the brain. *Two thirds of cases of subarachnoid hemorrhages reflect the rupture of a preexisting arterial aneurysm* (see below). In 10% of cases, an arteriovenous malformation is demonstrated. The remaining

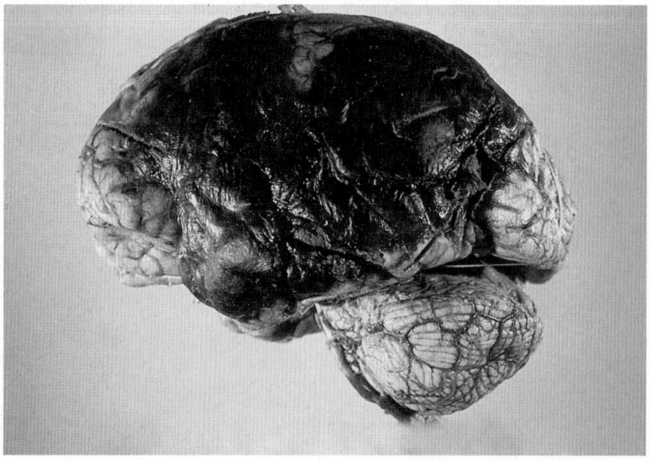

FIGURE 28-28. **Subarachnoid hemorrhage.** The subarachnoid space contains a large amount of blood secondary to rupture of an aneurysm.

instances result from a variety of conditions, including blood dyscrasias, infections, vasculitis, and tumors. Subarachnoid hemorrhage and cerebral aneurysms are discussed more fully below.

Cerebral Contusion Is a Traumatic Bruise of the Brain Surface

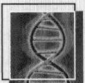

PATHOGENESIS: Like subdural hematomas, cerebral contusions generally result from anteroposterior displacements when the moving head strikes a fixed object. Anteroposterior shifts of the soft tofu-like brain renders it vulnerable to bruises or lacerations as a consequence of forces applied to the head, especially in the midsagittal plane. The severity of the contusion corresponds to the velocity of the acceleration and the abruptness of the deceleration of the head. When the contusion occurs at the point of impact, the lesion is referred to as a **coup** (from the French, "blow") injury (Fig. 28-29). If the side of the brain opposite the impact site strikes the skull, the resulting abrasions are contralateral to the point of initial contact and are termed a **contrecoup** injury.

The distant location of contrecoup lesions underscores the anatomic features that determine the nature of the injury, as illustrated by Fig. 28-29, in which the occipital bone is the site of impact. There is no injury to the subjacent cortex, but the impact causes disparate motion of the cerebrum and the skull, so that the frontal and temporal poles strike the bony surfaces of the frontal and middle fossae.

PATHOLOGY: If the force of the impact is mild, the cerebral contusion is limited to the cortex and the apex of gyri (Fig. 28-30). A greater force destroys larger expanses of cortex, creates deep cavitary lesions that extend into the white matter, or lacerates the cortex and causes hemorrhage. Together with edema, hemorrhage can create a mass lesion, which threatens life by transtentorial herniation.

Contusions are permanent. The bruised, necrotic tissue is promptly phagocytosed by macrophages and eliminated in large part via the bloodstream. Astrocytosis then leads to local scar formation, which persists as telltale evidence of a prior contusion.

The consequences of traumatic brain injury may be internal and subtle to demonstrate. The parasagittal cortex is anchored to arachnoid villi (**pacchionian granulations),** whereas the lateral aspects of the cerebrum move more freely. This anatomic feature, together with the differential density of gray and white matter, permits generation of shearing forces between different brain regions, leading to diffuse axonal shearing injuries, particularly in vehicular accidents. Shearing injuries can distort or disrupt axons, causing them to retract into "spheroids" as well as lose their myelin. This type of injury typically occurs in parasagittal white matter and may be accompanied by multiple small hemorrhages. If the injury is severe, the patient becomes comatose, although magnetic resonance imaging may show only small hemorrhages and focal edema.

Penetrating Wounds Produce Hemorrhage and Blast Effects

Penetrating objects such as bullets and knives enter the cranium and traverse the brain with variable velocities. In the absence of direct injury to the vital brain centers, the immediate threat to life is hemorrhage (Fig. 28-31). As noted above, bleeding creates a space-occupying mass, which may culminate in

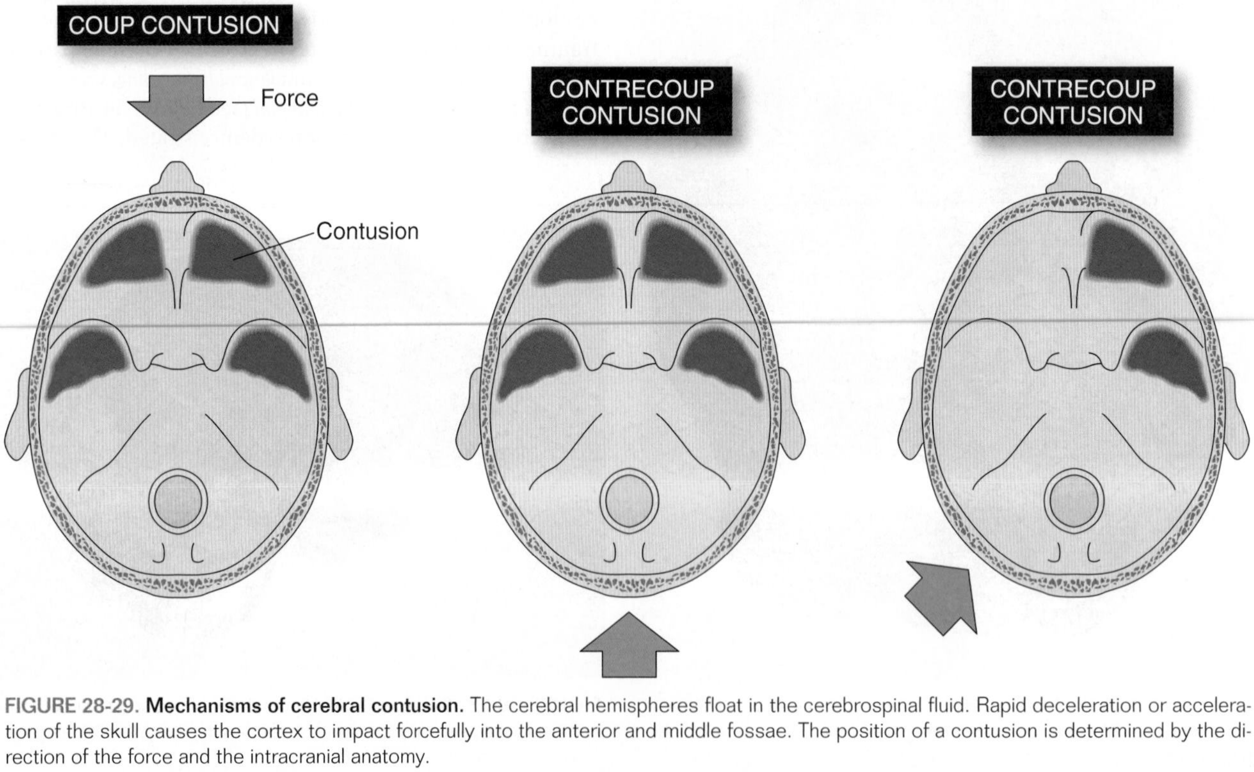

FIGURE 28-29. **Mechanisms of cerebral contusion.** The cerebral hemispheres float in the cerebrospinal fluid. Rapid deceleration or acceleration of the skull causes the cortex to impact forcefully into the anterior and middle fossae. The position of a contusion is determined by the direction of the force and the intracranial anatomy.

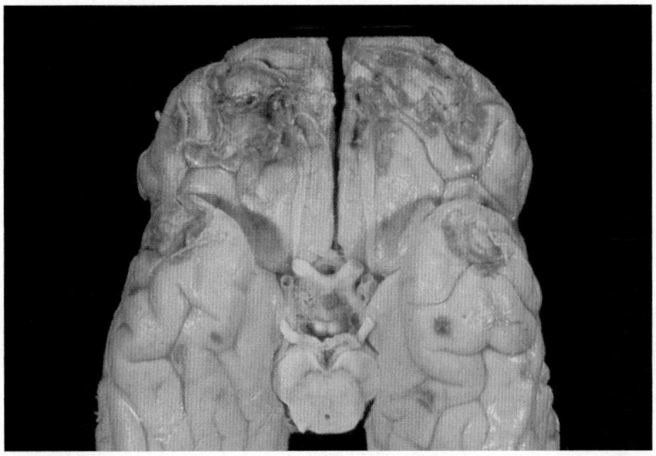

FIGURE 28-30. **Contusions of the brain.** After an automobile accident, the brain exhibits necrosis and hemorrhage involving the frontal and temporal lobes.

lethal transtentorial herniation. In the case of the cerebellum, herniation of the cerebellar tonsils into the foramen magnum is followed by compression of the medulla, thereby disabling vital cardiac and respiratory centers.

Velocity contributes a blast effect to a projectile. As a high-velocity bullet traverses the brain, it disrupts tissues by its own mass as well as by a centrifugal blast that enlarges the diameter of the cylinder of disruption. Thus, a high-velocity bullet can cause immediate death through an explosive increase in intracranial pressure. This pressure forcefully herniates the cerebellar tonsils into the foramen magnum, causing immediate death.

Seizures are a threat in healed penetrating wounds, usually occurring 6 to 12 months after the trauma. Collagenous tissue is displaced into the brain from the scalp or dura, and fibroblasts subsequently proliferate to form a dense scar. The precise mechanism by which a scar activates neurons and leads to seizures remains obscure.

Spinal Cord Injuries Often Lead to Paraplegia or Quadriplegia

Traumatic lesions of the spinal cord may result from direct injury to the cord by penetrating wounds (e.g., stab wounds, bullets) or indirect injury as a consequence of fractures or displacement of vertebrae. The spinal cord may be contused not only at the site of injury but also above and below the point of trauma. Traumatic injury may be complicated by compromise of the arterial supply to the cord, with resulting infarction.

The bodies of the vertebrae are separated by intravertebral disks and are stabilized in normal alignment by two longitudinal ligaments, as well as by the posterior bony processes. The anterior spinal ligament adheres to the ventral surface of the vertebral bodies, whereas the posterior spinal ligament is affixed to the dorsal vertebral column. As a result of extreme flexion or extension (Fig. 28-32), the angulation of the bony vertebral column brings the spinal cord forcefully into contact with bone or, alternatively, interferes with the regional circulation.

HYPEREXTENSION INJURY: When the forehead is struck from the front and driven posteriorly (e.g., as a result of diving head first into shallow water), the posterior displacement of the head (hyperextension) tears the anterior spinal ligament, thereby permitting sharp posterior angulation of the spinal canal. At the point of angulation, the posterior aspect of the spinal cord is brought into forceful and damaging contact with the posterior process of the stationary vertebral body, which lies immediately caudal to the angulation (see Fig. 28-32).

HYPERFLEXION INJURY: When the head or shoulders are struck from behind by an object of considerable weight or when this region of a falling human body (generally in a flexed position) strikes a stationary object, the head is driven forcefully forward and downward (hyperflexion). The impact forces one vertebral body down upon the underlying one. The anterior lip of the underlying vertebral body is fractured, with forward slippage and downward displacement of the overlying vertebra. This distortion of the spinal canal results in sharp forward angulation of the spinal cord. The anterior surface of the angulated cord is

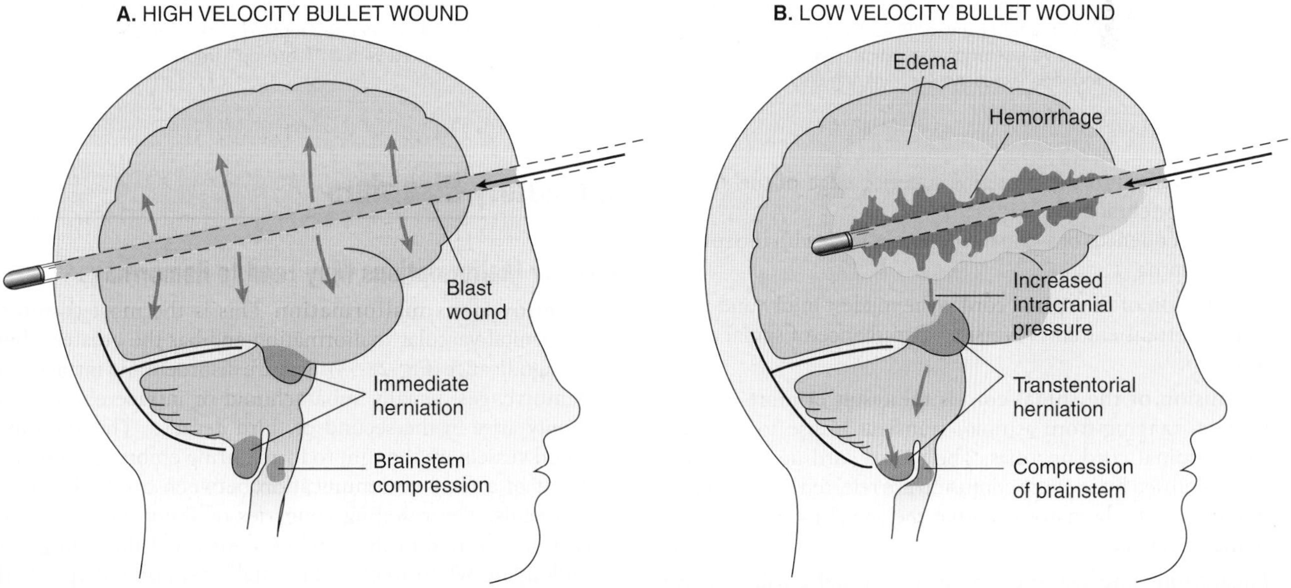

FIGURE 28-31. **Consequences of high- and low-velocity bullet wounds. A.** The "blast effect" of a high-velocity projectile causes an immediate increase in supratentorial pressure and results in death because of impaction of the cerebellum and medulla into the foramen magnum. **B.** A low-velocity projectile increases the pressure at a more gradual rate through hemorrhage and edema.

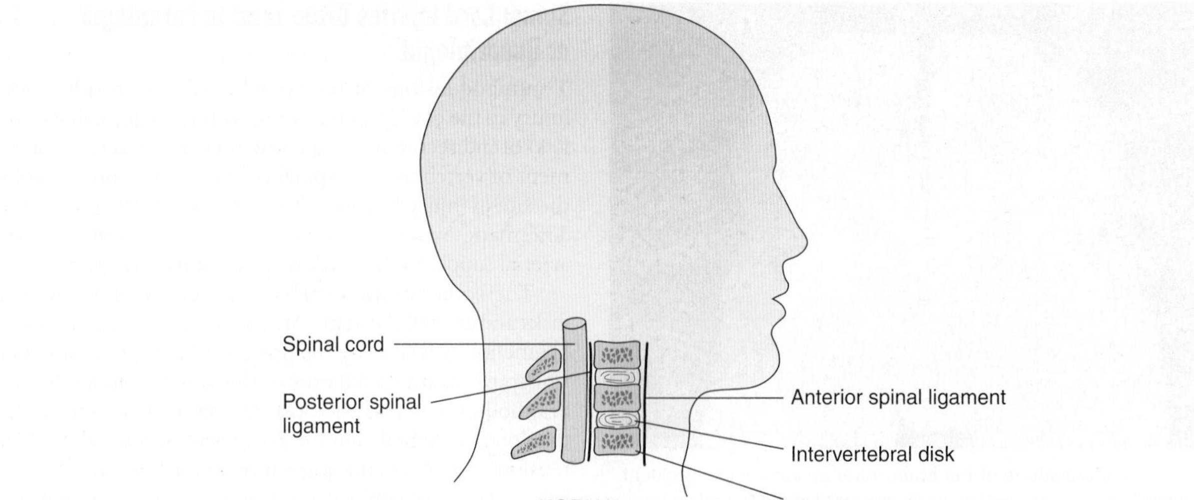

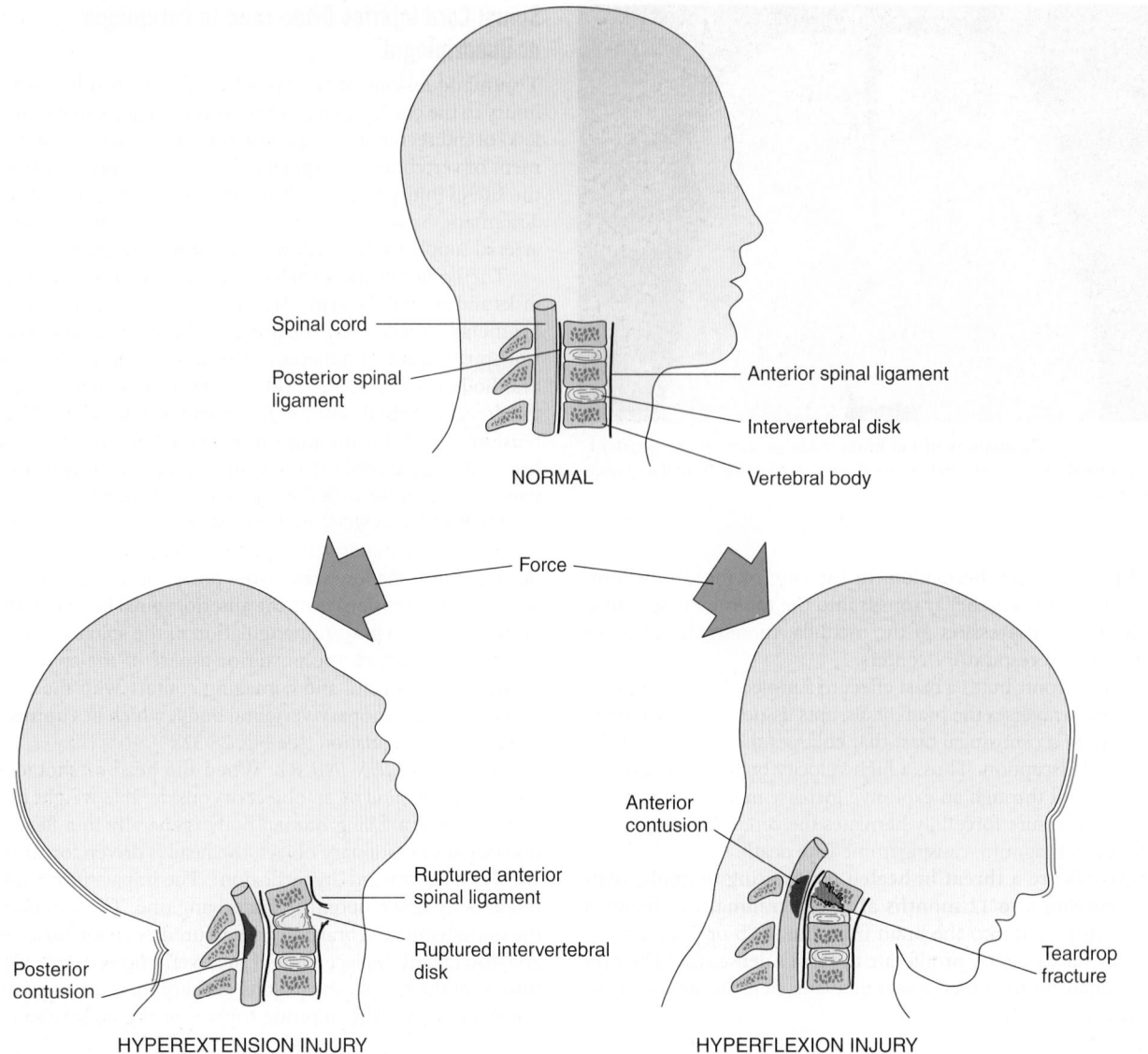

FIGURE 28-32. **Spinal injury.** Numerous different angles of force can be applied to the highly vulnerable cervical spine. Posterior (hyperextension) and anterior (hyperflexion) injuries are the most common. Hyperextension injury causes rupture of the anterior spinal ligament and excessive posterior angulation. Hyperflexion injury causes compression associated with a "teardrop" fracture of a vertebral body and produces excessive forward angulation of the cord.

driven forcefully into the posterior superior edge of the stable underlying vertebral body (see Fig. 28-32).

The consequences of a spinal cord injury vary with the severity of the trauma.

- **Concussion of the spinal cord** is the mildest injury and represents a transient and reversible disturbance of spinal cord function.
- **Contusion of the spinal cord** is the result of more severe trauma, ranging from a minor transient bruise to hemorrhagic spinal cord necrosis. The spinal cord necrosis and edema caused by a severe contusion are referred to as **myelomalacia,** and a hematoma within the spinal cord is termed **hematomyelia.**
- **Lacerations and transections of the spinal cord,** usually produced by penetrating wounds, are irreversible and result in complete loss of function. Paralysis of the lower limbs (paraplegia) or all four extremities (quadriplegia) depends on the location and extent of the injury.

Circulatory Disorders

Vascular Malformations May Lead to Hemorrhage

- **Arteriovenous malformation** This is the most common congenital vascular malformation and has the greatest clinical significance (Fig. 28-33). Seizure disorders and intracranial hemorrhages, usually subarachnoid or intracerebral, commonly arise in the second or third decades. The abnormal blood vessels are thought to form during embryogenesis as a result of a focal communication between cerebral arteries and veins. The resulting congeries of abnormal vessels are typically located in the cerebral cortex and the contiguous underlying white matter. The malformation enlarges with time and tends to involve a larger area.
- **Cavernous angioma:** This congenital anomaly is far less common than arteriovenous malformations. It is similar to cavernous angiomas elsewhere (e.g., liver) in being formed

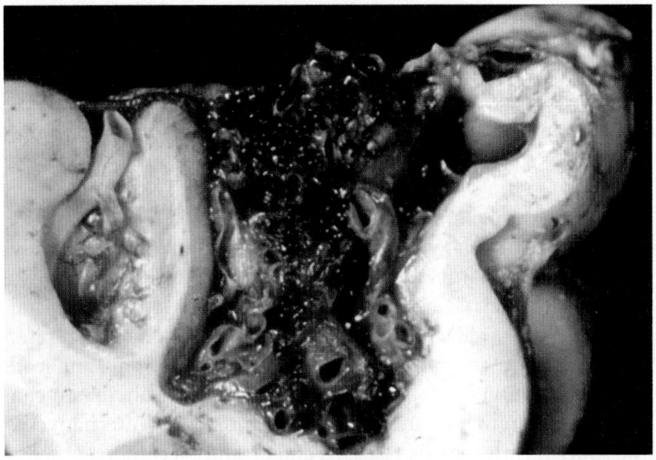

FIGURE 28-33. **Arteriovenous malformation.** A disorganized collection of arteries and veins is seen within the substance of the brain.

by large, irregular, thin-walled vascular channels. Although most cavernous angiomas are asymptomatic, they may cause intracranial bleeding, epilepsy, or focal neurologic disturbances.

- **Telangiectasia:** This focal aggregate of uniformly dilated, thin-walled small vessels with intervening neural parenchyma may initiate seizures but rarely ruptures.
- **Venous angioma:** This structure consists of a focus of a few enlarged veins and is distributed randomly in the spinal cord or brain. The lesion is generally asymptomatic, and overlaps in part with cavernous angiomas.

Cerebral Aneurysms Rupture and Lead to Fatal Hemorrhage

Intravascular pressure and weakness in arterial walls lead to the formation of cerebral aneurysms.

Berry Aneurysms

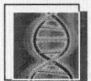

PATHOGENESIS AND PATHOLOGY: Berry (saccular) aneurysms are the consequence of arterial defects that are presumed to arise during embryogenesis when arteries bifurcate (Fig. 28-34). The muscular layer of a blood vessel that bifurcates into two branches may fail to interdigitate adequately across the branch point, thereby creating a point of congenital muscular weakness that is bridged only by endothelium, the internal elastic membrane, and a thin adventitia. Over time, the blood flow from the parent vessel exerts pressure at the point of bifurcation that expands the congenital defect. The internal elastic membrane may degenerate or fragment, after which a saccular aneurysm evolves that is precariously covered only by a layer of adventitia.

More than 90% of saccular aneurysms occur at branch points in the carotid system (Fig. 28-35). They are about equally distributed at the junction of (1) the anterior cerebral and anterior communicating arteries, (2) the internal carotid–posterior communicating–anterior cerebral–anterior choroidal arteries, and (3) the trifurcation of the middle cerebral artery. In 20% of cases, multiple berry aneurysms are present. Clinically silent berry aneurysms occur in as many as 25% of persons older than 55 years.

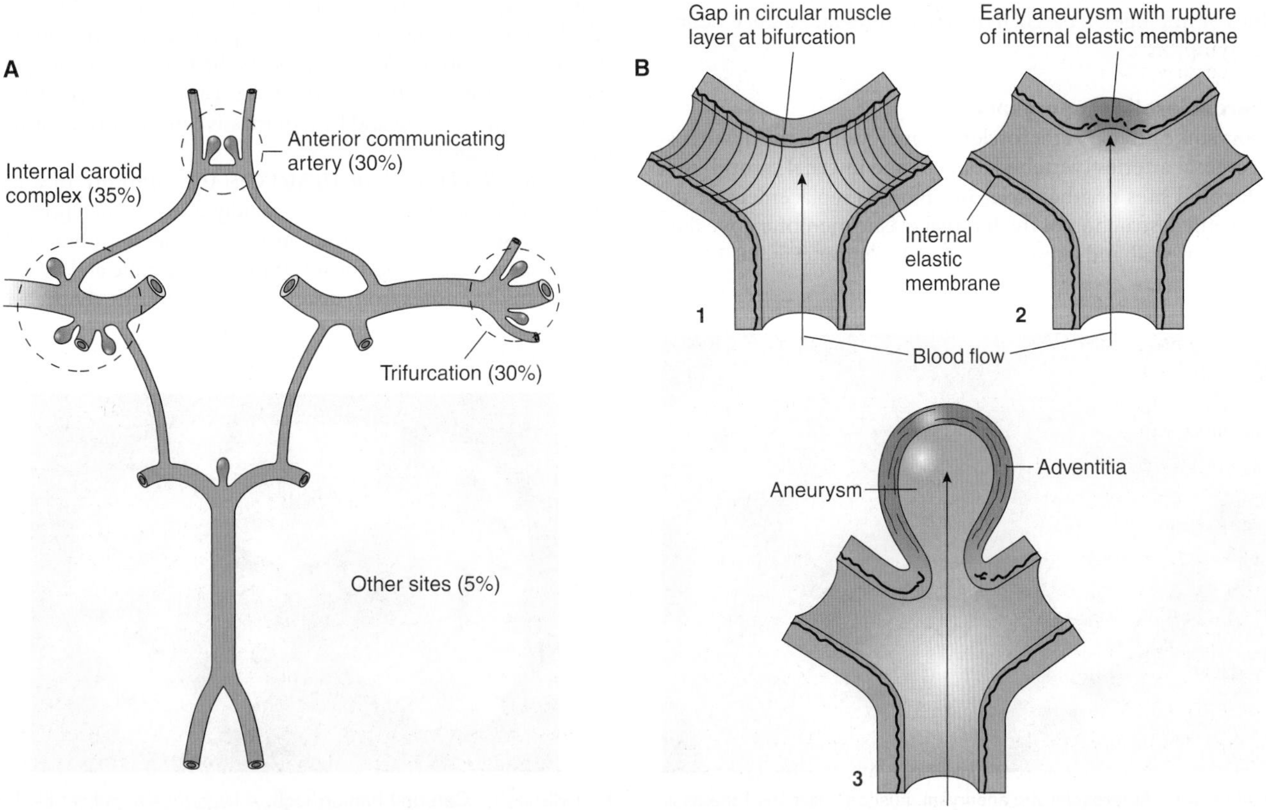

FIGURE 28-34. **Saccular aneurysm. A.** The incidence of saccular aneurysms (berry aneurysms), which preferentially involve the carotid tributaries, is shown. **B.** The lesion evolves as a result of blood acting on an early embryonic defect.

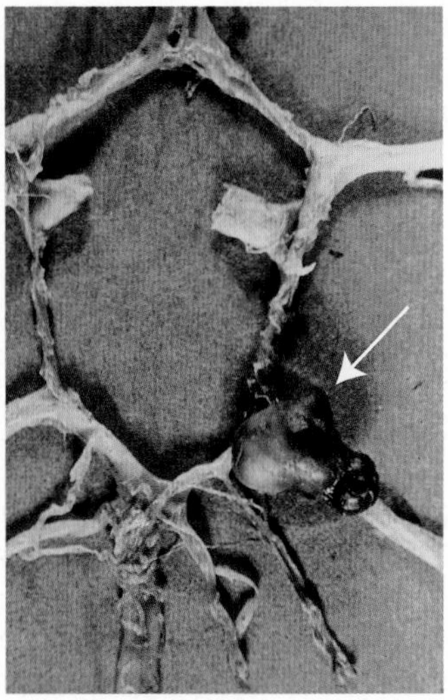

FIGURE 28-35. **Berry aneurysm.** A saccular aneurysm (*arrow*) arises from the posterior cerebral artery.

CLINICAL FEATURES: *Rupture of a berry aneurysm results in life-threatening subarachnoid hemorrhage, with a 35% mortality during the initial hemorrhage.* Rupture produces intracerebral or intraventricular hemorrhage in up to one third of patients. A sudden severe headache characteristically heralds the onset of subarachnoid hemorrhage and may be followed by coma. Patients who survive for 3 to 4 days often manifest a progressive decline in consciousness, which may be caused by arterial spasms that lead to cerebral ischemia and infarction. Survivors of the initial episode often rebleed, in which case the prognosis is worse. Enlargement of a saccular aneurysm forms a mass that may compress cranial nerves and produce palsies or impinge on parenchymal structures and induce neurologic symptoms.

Atherosclerotic Aneurysms

Aneurysms caused by atherosclerosis are localized mainly in major cerebral arteries (vertebral, basilar, and internal carotid) that are favored sites of atherosclerosis. Fibrous replacement of the media and destruction of the internal elastic membrane weaken the arterial wall and cause aneurysmal dilation (Fig. 28-36). As they enlarge, atherosclerotic aneurysms tend to be fusiform and elongate. Thus, an enlarging atherosclerotic aneurysm of the basilar artery will encroach upon the cerebellopontine angle, compress cranial nerves, and produce neurologic deficits. Atherosclerotic aneurysms rarely rupture, and the major complication is thrombosis.

Mycotic Aneurysms

Infections of arterial walls result from septic emboli that usually originate in an infected cardiac valve. The embolus flows through the carotid circulation and typically lodges in a distal branch of the middle cerebral artery, where bacteria proliferate, induce inflammation, destroy the affected arterial wall, and lead to the formation of an aneurysm. Rupture of the aneurysm can cause intracerebral or subarachnoid hemorrhage. Alternatively, microorganisms may be released and produce a cerebral abscess or meningitis.

Cerebral Hemorrhage Causes Stroke (Apoplexy)

Cerebral hemorrhages that occur without trauma (Fig. 28-37) are referred to as "spontaneous," although most are caused by a vascular anomaly (see above) or are the consequence of long-standing hypertension. **Hypertensive intracerebral hemorrhage** occurs at preferential sites, which in order of frequency are (1) the basal ganglia–thalamus (65%), (2) pons (15%), and (3) cerebellum (8%).

Hypertension compromises the integrity of cerebral arterioles by causing the deposition of lipid and hyaline material in their walls, an alteration referred to as **lipohyalinosis.** Weakening of the wall leads to the formation of **Charcot-Bouchard aneurysms,** which are located mainly along the trunk of a vessel rather than at its bifurcation.

The onset of symptoms in the case of a hypertensive cerebral hemorrhage (hemorrhagic stroke) is abrupt, and weakness usually dominates. When hemorrhage is progressive, as is common, death occurs within hours to days. As the hematoma enlarges, it may cause death by transtentorial herniation or it may rupture into a lateral ventricle and lead to massive intraventricular hemorrhage (Fig. 28-38).

INTRAVENTRICULAR HEMORRHAGE: Rupture of a cerebral blood vessel into a ventricle rapidly distends the entire ventricular system, including the fourth ventricle, with blood. The blood may emerge from the foramina of Magendie and Luschka. Death rapidly ensues from distention of the fourth ventricle and compression of vital centers in the medulla.

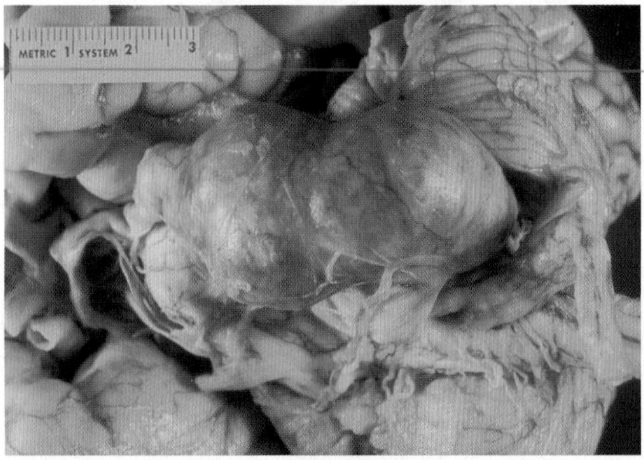

FIGURE 28-36. **Atherosclerotic aneurysm.** Fusiform dilation of the basilar artery has resulted from severe atherosclerosis.

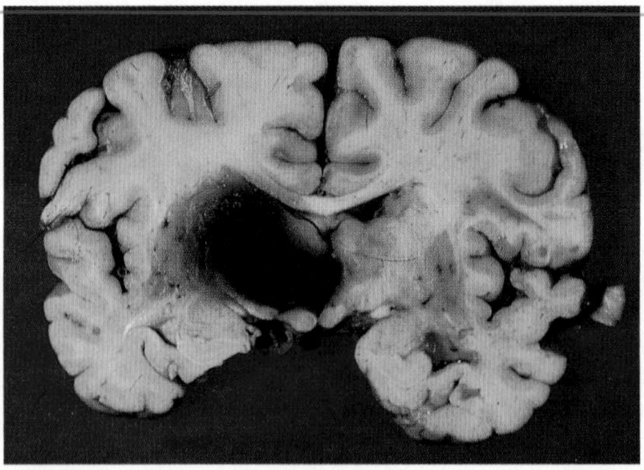

FIGURE 28-37. **Cerebral hemorrhage.** A hypertensive patient bled into the basal ganglia.

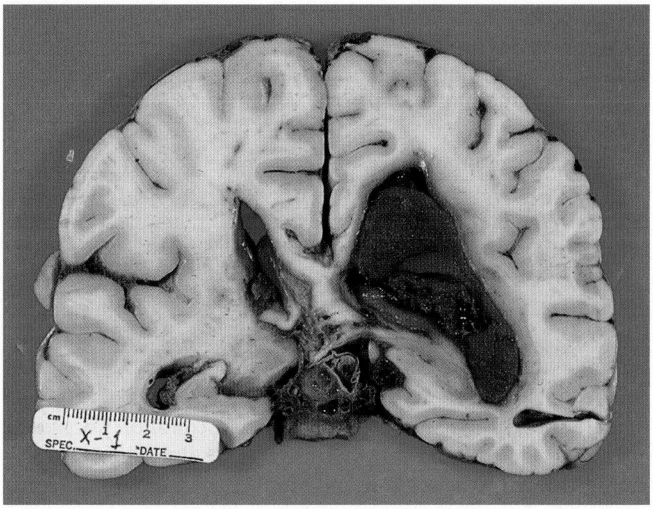

FIGURE 28-38. **Intraventricular hemorrhage.** A sagittal section of the brain shows ventricular chambers filled with blood. The patient died rapidly from compression of the brainstem by blood in the fourth ventricle.

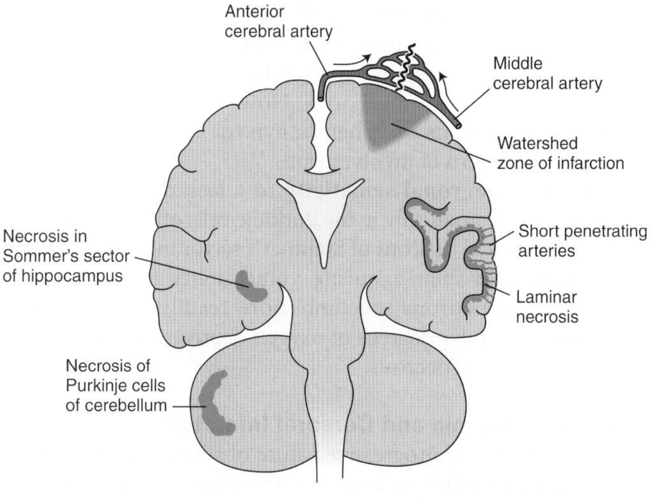

FIGURE 28-39. **Consequences of global ischemia.** A global insult induces lesions that reflect the vascular architecture (watershed infarcts, laminar necrosis) and the sensitivity of individual neuronal systems (pyramidal cells of Sommer's sector, Purkinje cells).

PONTINE HEMORRHAGE: In this catastrophic event, the loss of consciousness reflects damage to the reticular formation, an injury that overshadows all other specific cranial nerve deficits. The initial hemorrhage is generally in the midpons. With minimal enlargement, it encroaches upon vital medullary centers, commonly resulting in death before the patient arrives at the hospital.

CEREBELLAR HEMORRHAGE: Bleeding into the cerebellum causes abrupt ataxia and is accompanied by a severe occipital headache and vomiting. The expanding hematoma threatens life acutely by compressing the medulla or by producing cerebellar herniation through the foramen magnum. Surgical evacuation of the cerebellar hematoma is life-saving and may leave few serious neurologic deficits, whereas surgical intervention for cerebral hematomas generally has a very poor outcome.

Spontaneous cerebral hemorrhages due to causes other than hypertension include:

- Leakage from an arteriovenous malformation
- Erosion of a blood vessel by a primary or secondary neoplasm
- A bleeding diathesis, as exemplified by thrombocytopenic purpura
- Endothelial injury by microorganisms, notably rickettsiae
- Embolic infarction, with consequent hemorrhage into the area of necrosis

Cerebral Ischemia and Infarction Represent the Major Causes of Stroke

Inadequate perfusion of the brain results from generalized low blood flow due to extracranial events that lead to global ischemia (cardiac arrest, external hemorrhage) or from occlusive cerebrovascular disease (cerebral artery thrombosis), which produces regional ischemia and often a localized infarct. Global ischemia also results from hypoxia (near-drowning, carbon monoxide poisoning, suffocation).

Global Ischemia

The pattern of injury produced by global ischemia (or hypoxia) reflects the anatomy of the cerebral vasculature and the selective vulnerability of individual neurons to oxygen deprivation (Fig. 28-39).

WATERSHED INFARCTS: The anterior, middle, and posterior cerebral arteries perfuse partially overlapping territories, but there are no anastomoses between their terminal branches (see Fig. 28-39). For example, the anterior cerebral arteries mainly perfuse the medial aspects of both cerebral hemispheres. However, they also perfuse the parasagittal cortex by variably overlapping with the distribution of the middle cerebral arteries. Since this overlap zone is not as richly perfused as the primary territories of the anterior and middle cerebral arteries, reduced blood flow in these arteries will diminish perfusion more severely in the partial overlap zone (watershed area), thereby causing a parasagittal watershed infarct.

LAMINAR NECROSIS: This lesion also reflects the topography of the cerebral vasculature (Figs. 28-40). The cerebral cortex is perfused by short "penetrators," which originate at right angles from pial blood vessels and then penetrate gray matter,

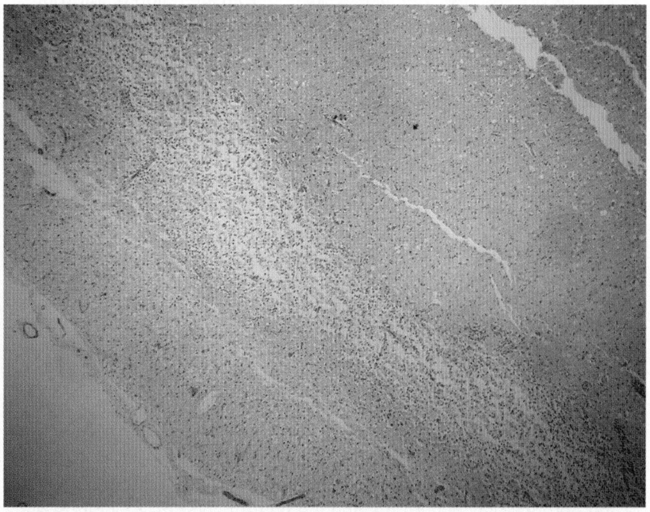

FIGURE 28-40. **Laminar necrosis.** A patient who suffered prolonged anoxia during a cardiac arrhythmia developed selective necrosis of layers in the cerebral cortex.

where they form a plexus of capillaries in cortical layers V and VI. A loss of circulatory pressure will selectively diminish perfusion of this terminal capillary plexus and cause laminar necrosis in the deeper layers of neocortex. However, the selective vulnerability of neurons to ischemia/hypoxia also contributes to this laminar pattern of involvement.

Selective neuronal sensitivity to a lack of oxygen is expressed most dramatically in the Purkinje cells of the cerebellum and the pyramidal neurons of Sommer's sector in the hippocampus. Because of their exquisite vulnerability to hypoxia/ischemia, these neurons succumb more readily than do their neighbors to similar degrees of oxygen deprivation, thereby resulting in localized necrosis.

Regional Ischemia and Cerebral Infarction

The prevalence and progressive nature of atherosclerosis are reflected in the fact that cerebrovascular occlusive disease remains a major cause of morbidity and mortality. Atherosclerosis predisposes to vascular thrombosis and embolic events, both of which result in localized ischemia and subsequent cerebral infarction (Fig. 28-41).

PATHOLOGY: Although cerebral infarcts are traditionally designated either "hemorrhagic" or "bland," these descriptors are somewhat simplistic. In general, infarcts caused by embolization are hemorrhagic, whereas those initiated by local thrombosis are ischemic (or bland). Emboli occlude vascular flow abruptly, after which the distal segments of affected blood vessels become necrotic and leak blood into the region. By contrast thrombosis progresses more slowly and gradually deprives downstream arteries of blood flow, thereby guarding against secondary hemorrhage.

An infarct of the brain acutely transforms the affected tissue into necrotic, friable debris (Fig. 28-42), which is ultimately phagocytosed and eliminated by macrophages (Fig. 28-43). Initially capillaries proliferate at the margin of the infarct, become numerous by the fifth day, and improve perfusion of the infarct penumbra. Subsequently, the necrotic area is slowly eliminated by phagocytosis to form a gliosis-lined cystic cavity. If the area of the infarction is large, the residual cyst is bridged by a cobweb of atretic blood vessels (see Fig. 28-43C). Although cerebral infarcts are examples of coagulative necrosis, large brain infarcts eventually fragment and liquefy (liquefactive necrosis).

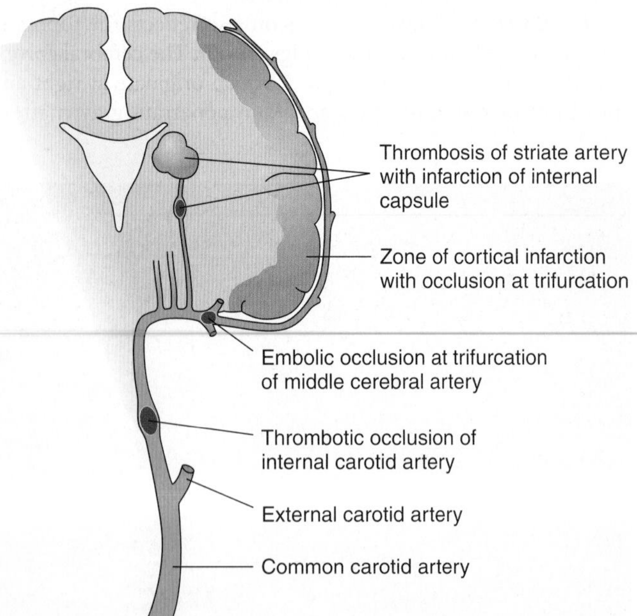

FIGURE 28-41. **Distribution of cerebral infarcts.** The normal distribution of the cerebral vasculature defines the pattern and size of infarcts and, consequently, their symptoms. Occlusion at the trifurcation causes cortical infarcts with motor and sensory loss and often aphasia. Occlusion of a striate branch transects the internal capsule and causes a motor deficit.

CLINICAL FEATURES: The diversity of the neurologic deficits caused by stroke directly reflect the consequences of occluding different cerebral vessels. For example, the lengthy and slender striate arteries, which take origin from the proximal middle cerebral artery, are commonly occluded by atherosclerosis and thrombosis. The resultant infarct often transects the internal capsule and produces hemiparesis or hemiplegia. Similarly, the trifurcation of the middle cerebral artery is a favored site for lodgment of emboli and for thrombosis secondary to atherosclerotic damage. Occlusion of the middle cerebral artery at this site deprives the parietal cortex of circulation and produces motor and sensory deficits. When the dominant hemisphere is involved, these lesions are commonly accompanied by aphasia.

Localized ischemia is associated with three distinct clinical syndromes:

- **Transient ischemic attack (TIA)** refers to focal cerebral dysfunction that lasts less than 24 hours and is often of only a few minutes' duration. Although it is followed by complete neurologic recovery, a TIA signifies an increased risk of a cerebral infarct.
- **Stroke in evolution** describes the progression of neurologic symptoms while the patient is under observation. This syndrome is uncommon and usually reflects propagation of a thrombus in the carotid or basilar arteries.
- **Completed stroke** is the term for a stable neurologic deficit resulting from a cerebral infarct.

Regional Occlusive Cerebrovascular Disease

The various occlusive cerebrovascular diseases that lead to cerebral infarcts may be classified in accord with the caliber and nature of the involved vessel.

THE LARGE EXTRACRANIAL AND INTRACRANIAL ARTERIES: These arteries are frequent sites of atherosclerosis. The most notable example is the common carotid artery, in which atherosclerotic plaques are particularly prominent at the site of its bifurcation into external and internal branches. Occlusion or stenosis of an internal carotid artery affects the ipsilateral hemisphere, but this can be offset by the variable collateral circulation through the anterior and posterior communicating arteries. *Most often, occlusion of a carotid artery produces infarcts restricted to all or some portion of the distribution of the middle cerebral artery.*

THE CIRCLE OF WILLIS: The various branches of this major vascular network of the brain may be occluded, but the consequences depend on the configuration of the circle. Thus, a large anterior communicating artery can provide collateral circulation to a frontal lobe whose arterial supply has been compromised by occlusion of the internal carotid artery. The middle cerebral artery is most often occluded by thrombosis complicating atherosclerosis in the circle of Willis. *Because the trifurcation of the middle cerebral artery is a site of a major stepdown in vascular caliber, it is the predominant site occluded by emboli, most of which emanate from the heart.*

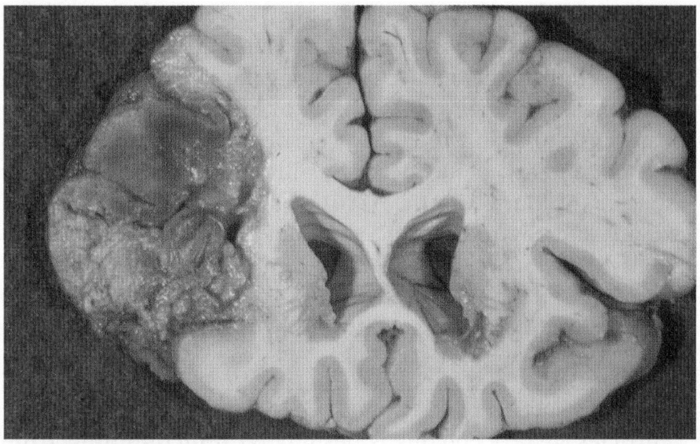
A

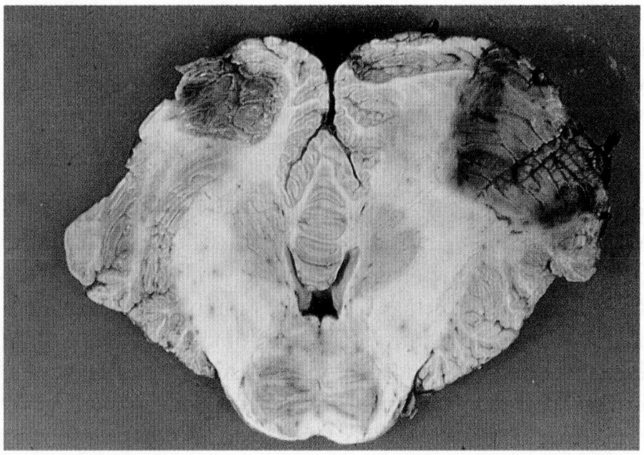
B

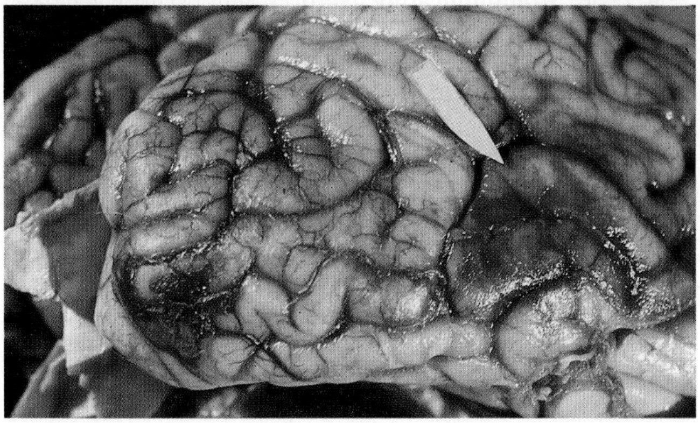
C

FIGURE 28-42. **Cerebral infarcts. A.** A coronal section of the brain of a patient who suffered thrombosis of the middle cerebral artery reveals an infarct of the left frontal lobe. **B.** Bilateral vertebral artery thrombosis resulted in infarcts of the cerebellum. **C.** Emboli from a carotid endarterectomy resulted in hemorrhagic infarcts in the territory of the middle cerebral artery (*arrow*).

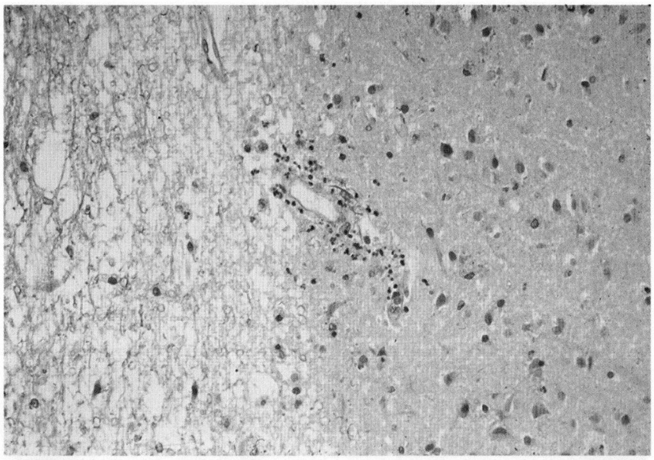
A

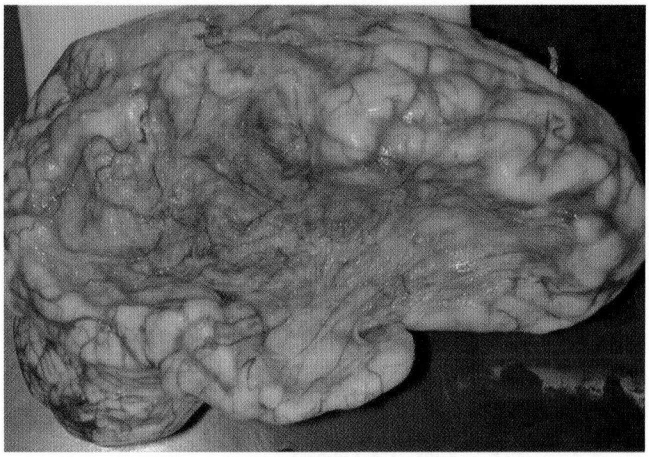
B

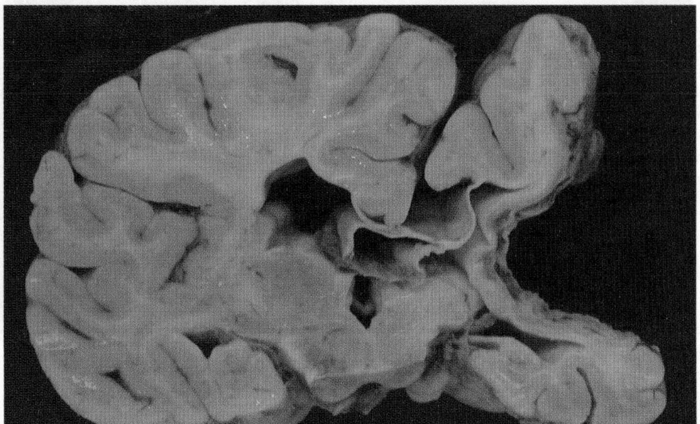
C

FIGURE 28-43. **Cerebral infarcts. A.** An 18-hour old cerebral infarct (left) shows edema, hypereosinophilic neurons, and perivascular polymorphonuclear leukocytes. **B.** Remote right middle cerebral artery infarct. **C.** Remote right middle cerebral artery infarct with complete cavitation.

THE PARENCHYMAL ARTERIES AND ARTERIOLES: These vessels rarely become atherosclerotic, but they are damaged by hypertension and become stenotic because of atherosclerosis, thereby causing small so-called **lacunar infarcts.** When multiple, these minute infarcts can impair cognition and create the entity termed **multiple infarct dementia.**

Hypertensive encephalopathy refers to the neurologic complications of malignant hypertension (see Chapter 10). As in other affected organs, hypertension can cause fibrinoid necrosis of small arteries and arterioles, as well as minute hemorrhages (petechiae). Cerebral edema may complicate the vascular pathology. Hypertensive encephalopathy usually manifests clinically as headache and vomiting that progress to coma and death. With modern antihypertensive therapy, malignant hypertension is uncommon.

THE CAPILLARY BED: Small emboli, notably those composed of fat or air, occlude capillaries.

Fat emboli, most often derived from fractured bones, are carried downstream through the cerebral vessels until the caliber of the embolus exceeds that of the blood vessel, at which point they lodge and block blood flow. The distal capillary endothelium becomes hypoxic and permeable, and petechiae develop, most commonly in the white matter.

Air emboli liberate a multitude of bubbles that further fragment as they encounter vascular bifurcations until they impede vascular flow in small blood vessels. In this situation, petechiae are less restricted to white matter than those caused by fat emboli.

THE CEREBRAL VEINS: The cerebral veins empty into large venous sinuses, the most prominent of which is the sagittal sinus because it accommodates the venous drainage from the superior portions of the cerebral hemispheres. Venous sinus thrombosis in the brain is a potentially lethal complication of the following:

- Systemic dehydration, as occurs in an infant with gastrointestinal fluid loss
- Phlebitis, caused for example by mastoiditis or bacteremia
- Obstruction by a neoplasm, notably a meningioma
- Sickle cell disease

Because venous obstruction causes stagnation upstream, abrupt thrombosis of the sagittal sinus results in bilateral hemorrhagic infarctions of the frontal lobe regions. A more indolent occlusion of the sinus (due to invasion by a meningioma) permits the recruitment of collateral circulation through the inferior sagittal sinus, which lies at the lower edge of the falx and empties into the straight sinus.

Cerebrospinal Fluid (CSF)

CSF is Produced bythe Choroid Plexus

The CSF constitutes an "accessory circulatory system" adapted to the needs of the CNS. CSF flows from its intraventricular origin to its sites of reabsorption, principally through the arachnoid villi and into the dural sinuses. The fluid transports metabolites to CNS cells, serves as a medium for clearing metabolic waste, and protects or "cushions" structures contained within it.

The volume of CSF in the adult CNS is about 150 mL. It is formed principally by the choroid plexus at a rate of approximately 500 mL/day and is reabsorbed by the arachnoid villi. A small volume of CSF also flows in the subarachnoid compartment through the Virchow-Robin spaces. With advancing age, the choroid plexus becomes fibrotic and contains cholesterol and calcium deposits, although CSF is produced throughout life.

The **choroid plexus** stretches along the roof of the third ventricle, passes through the foramina of Monro, and then angles posteriorly to span the lateral ventricles. The choroid plexus does not enter the aqueduct of Sylvius. However, the posterior aspect of the fourth ventricle is covered by choroid plexus, which extends laterally through the foramen of Luschka into the immediate subarachnoid space of the cerebellopontine angle.

Hydrocephalus Refers to Dilation of the Ventricles by Accumulated CSF

When obstruction to the flow of CSF in the brain is within the ventricles, hydrocephalus is designated **noncommunicating** (Fig. 28-44). **Communicating** hydrocephalus occurs when there is no obstruction in the ventricular system, but reabsorption of CSF by the arachnoid villi is impaired.

NONCOMMUNICATING HYDROCEPHALUS: The flow of CSF through the ventricular system may be obstructed by (1) congenital malformations, (2) neoplasms, (3) inflammation, or (4) hemorrhage. The aqueduct of Sylvius is the most common location of obstructive congenital malformations. Choroid plexus tumors and ependymomas that arise in the ventricles can obstruct CSF flow and produce hydrocephalus. Parenchymal tumors, such as gliomas, may compress the aqueduct or ventricles and thereby cause hydrocephalus. Viral ependymitis during embryogenesis may result in congenital aqueductal stenosis.

COMMUNICATING HYDROCEPHALUS: An impairment of reabsorption of CSF with resultant communicating hydrocephalus can complicate subarachnoid hemorrhage, meningitis, and the spread of tumor within the subarachnoid space.

PATHOLOGY: In hydrocephalus of all etiologies, the cerebral hemispheres are enlarged, and the ventricular system is dilated behind the point of obstruction. The external pattern of the gyri tends to be less prominent as sulci are compressed. The white matter is reduced in volume, and the basal ganglia and thalamus are attenuated.

When hydrocephalus develops *in utero* or in early life, usually because of obstruction at the aqueduct of Sylvius, the ventricles expand behind the point of obstruction, the cranial sutures separate, the head enlarges, and the cortex becomes thin. Histologic

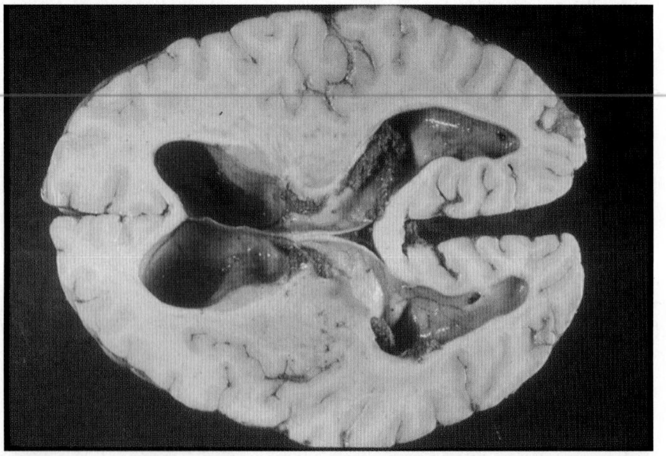

FIGURE 28-44. **Hydrocephalus.** Horizontal section of the brain from a patient who died of a brain tumor that obstructed the aqueduct of Sylvius shows marked dilation of the lateral ventricles.

examination of the obstructed aqueduct reveals multiple small, irregular, ependyma-lined canals. In some cases, a single aqueduct or a cluster of aborted canals are surrounded by gliosis, suggesting that an intrauterine viral infection caused inflammatory ependymitis. Without surgical CSF drainage or shunting, hydrocephalus is slowly progressive and lethal.

CLINICAL FEATURES: Because the infantile cranium expands easily, symptoms of increased intracranial pressure are generally absent. Convulsions are common, and optic atrophy with blindness can occur. Weakness and spasticity are frequent, but cognition may be spared, although severe ventricular dilation results in dementia. Surgical shunting of CSF controls hydrocephalus in some children.

In adults, the onset of hydrocephalus and increased intracranial pressure is heralded by headache, vomiting, and papilledema. If the obstruction is not relieved, mental deterioration ensues. Curiously, for reasons that are not known, CSF pressure is not increased in a rare dementing syndrome known as **normal pressure hydrocephalus.**

Hydrocephalus ex vacuo refers to enlargement of the ventricular system as a compensatory response to severe brain atrophy and is unrelated to obstructive lesions.

Infectious Diseases

Many organisms infect the CNS, but most localize at preferred CNS sites. For example, poliovirus targets spinal and brainstem motor neurons, herpes simplex virus localizes to the temporal lobes, PML(JC virus) preferentially involves cerebral white matter, and bacteria generally cause meningitis. Bacteria can also invade brain and result in cerebritis or brain abscess or enter the subdural space to induce subdural empyema.

Fungi such as *Cryptococcus neoformans* infect the leptomeninges, whereas *Aspergillus fumigatus* produces cerebral abscesses or leptomeningitis. *Treponema pallidum* causes syphilis by entering the CNS through the bloodstream. It can reside in the CNS for prolonged periods, where it propagates to induce distinct clinical syndromes such as dementia paralytica and tabes dorsalis. It can also invade the meninges, where it initiates fibrosis and an obliterative endarteritis, a condition termed **meningovascular syphilis.**

Rickettsial infections, such as Rocky Mountain spotted fever, target endothelial cells to produce petechiae, cerebral edema, and encephalopathy. *Toxoplasma gondii* has low virulence in healthy adults, but transplacental transmission enables infection of the fetal brain, resulting in paraventricular necrosis and calcification of the basal ganglia and thalamus. Immunocompromised adults (e.g., acquired immunodeficiency syndrome [AIDS]) may also be infected with this organism. Thus, anatomic localization, specific tissue responses, and the age and immunologic status of the patient are critical for understanding intracranial infections.

Meningitis Is a Dangerous Infection Caused by a Variety of Microorganisms

Leptomeningitis *denotes an inflammatory process localized to the pia/arachnoid* (Fig. 28-45). This compartment houses the CSF, an excellent culture medium for most microorganisms. The response of CSF to infections varies with the organism and extent of infection, including changes in its cellular, protein, sugar, and electrolyte composition and in its serological reactivity.

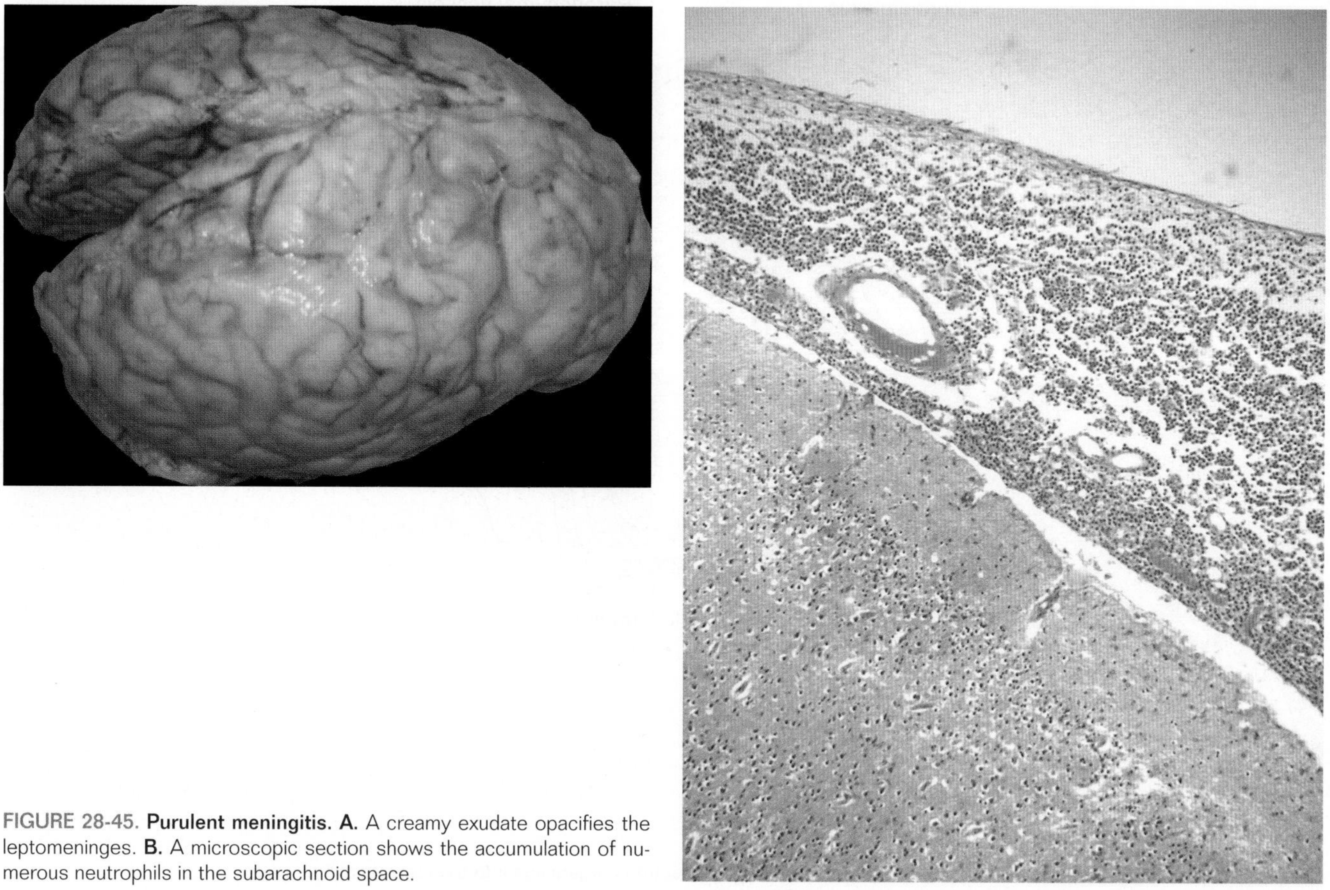

FIGURE 28-45. **Purulent meningitis. A.** A creamy exudate opacifies the leptomeninges. **B.** A microscopic section shows the accumulation of numerous neutrophils in the subarachnoid space.

***Pachymeningitis** refers to inflammation of the dura and is usually a consequence of contiguous extracranial infection such as chronic sinusitis or mastoiditis.* The dura is a substantial barrier to infection, and inflammation is usually restricted to its outer surface.

Bacterial Meningitis

With few exceptions, all forms of meningitis are initiated by microorganisms, suppurative bacteria being the principal offenders.

Suppurative Meningitis

- ***Escherichia coli:*** In the newborn, whose resistance to gram-negative bacteria has not yet fully developed, *E. coli* is the prime cause of meningitis. The transplacental transfer of maternal immunoglobulin(Ig)G imparts protection to the newborn against many bacteria. However, *E. coli* and similar gram-negative organisms require IgM for neutralization, an immunoglobulin that does not cross the placenta. Consequently, in infancy gram-negative organisms quickly produce a purulent meningitis with a high mortality.
- ***Haemophilus influenzae:*** Environmental exposure to *H. influenzae*, a gram-negative organism, is somewhat delayed, and the incidence of meningitis is maximal between 3 months and 3 years. The incidence of *H. influenza* meningitis has decreased in recent years owing to widespread vaccination against the organism.
- ***Streptococcus pneumoniae:*** The pneumococcus predominates as a cause of meningitis later in life. Patients with a history of basilar skull fracture have an unusually high incidence of pneumococcal meningitis, which often recurs after treatment.
- ***Neisseria meningitidis:*** The meningococcus resides in the nasopharynx, and airborne transmission in crowded places (e.g., schools or barracks) causes "epidemic meningitis." Initially, bacteremia causes fever, malaise, and petechial rash, but intravascular coagulopathy may cause lethal adrenal hemorrhages (**Waterhouse-Friderichsen syndrome**). Untreated meningococcal bacteremia is prone to initiate an acute fulminant meningitis.

Although organisms reach the intracranial compartment by way of the bloodstream, it is not clear how they exit (Fig. 28-46).

Because most organisms initiate a purulent or suppurative response, the presence of polymorphonuclear leukocytes in the CSF is the most definitive index of meningitis. Yet lymphocytes are the hallmark of tuberculosis and the viral meningitides, as well as of some chronic infections, such as those due to *C. neoformans*.

PATHOLOGY: Macroscopic examination reveals an exudate (leukocytes, fibrin) opacifying the arachnoid. The exudate may be mild and equivocal to the naked eye or prominent enough to obscure blood vessels. Purulent exudates are conspicuous over the cerebral hemispheres (see Fig. 28-45) but may extend to the base of the brain and from intracranial to intraspinal and subarachnoid spaces, which are in continuity. Although the pia is an effective barrier against the spread of infection, and cerebral abscesses rarely complicate meningitis, the pia forms sleeves around blood vessels that penetrate the brain (**Virchow-Robin spaces**) in continuity with the subarachnoid space.

H. influenzae elicits a dense exudate, rich in leukocytes and fibrin, that creates a barrier to antibiotics.

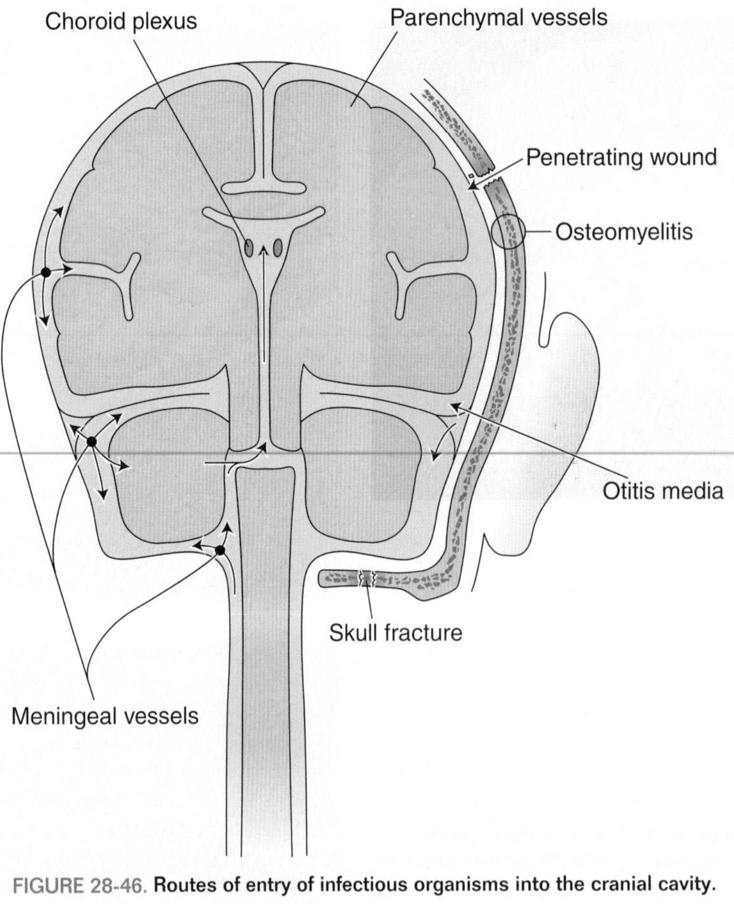

FIGURE 28-46. **Routes of entry of infectious organisms into the cranial cavity.**

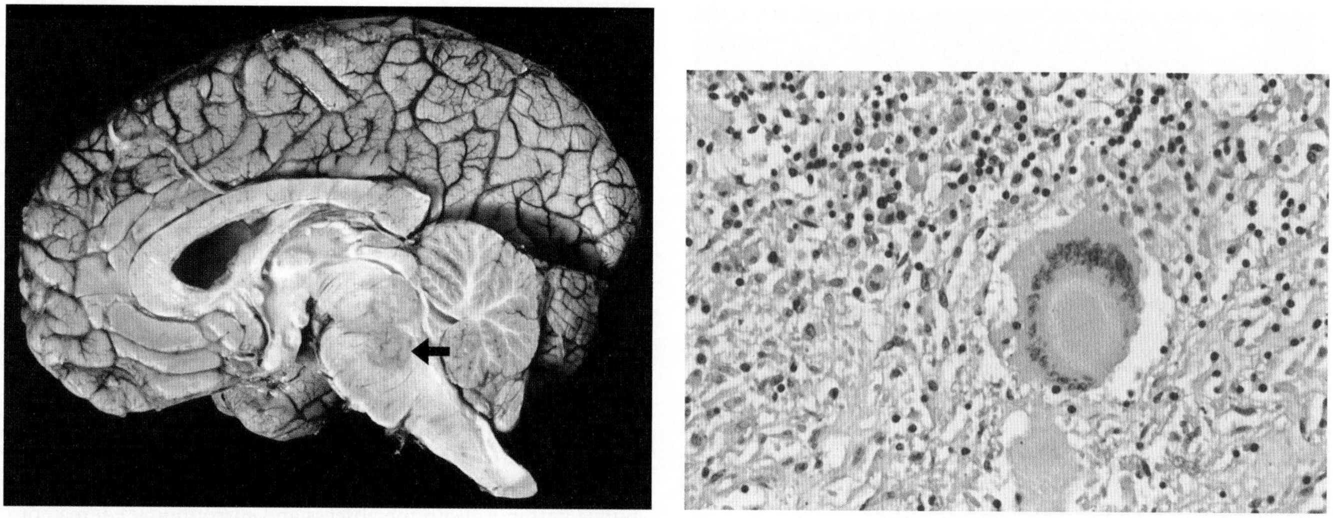

FIGURE 28-47. **Tuberculoma. A.** A focus of caseous necrosis is present in the pons and midbrain. **B.** A photomicrograph shows caseous necrosis, macrophages, and Langhans giant cells.

CLINICAL FEATURES: Suppurative meningitides share similar symptoms (albeit with a rapid or insidious onset) including headache, vomiting, fever, and convulsions (especially in children). Classic signs of meningitis include cervical rigidity, knee pain with hip flexion (Kernig sign), and knee/hip flexion when the neck is flexed (Brudzinski sign). In untreated cases, delirium gives way to coma and death.

Tuberculous Meningitis and Tuberculomas

Tuberculous granulomas in the meninges are analogous to those encountered elsewhere (Fig. 28-47). Epithelioid cells, Langhans giant cells, and lymphocytes surround areas of caseous necrosis. Inadequately treated tuberculous meningitis results in meningeal fibrosis, communicating hydrocephalus, and arteritis, the last leading to infarcts. Because tuberculous meningitis has a predilection for the base of the brain, such infarcts are often in the distribution of the striate arteries. Untreated tuberculous meningitis is fatal in 4 to 6 weeks. Parenchymal tuberculosis produces **tuberculomas** (i.e., solitary masses with central caseous necrosis surrounded by granulomatous tissue [see Fig. 28-47]).

Most cases of tuberculous meningitis follow hematogenous dissemination, although multiple portals of CNS entry are available for tubercle bacilli.

Pott disease refers to tuberculosis of the spine, in which an epidural granulomatous mass destroys the spine and causes spinal cord compression. Pott disease was formerly responsible for many so-called hunchbacks, a condition that is rare today.

Viral Meningitis

Infection of the meninges may be the most common viral disease of the CNS, but unlike bacterial meningitis, it is usually benign and leaves no sequelae. The most common causative agents are enteroviruses (e.g., coxsackievirus B, echovirus), but mumps, lymphocytic choriomeningitis, Epstein-Barr, and herpes simplex viruses are responsible for many sporadic cases.

Viral meningitis (predominantly a disease of children and young adults) is heralded by a sudden febrile illness with a severe headache. The CSF contains excess lymphocytes and a slight increase in protein but, unlike bacterial meningitis, no decrease in CSF glucose.

Cryptococcal Meningitis

Cryptococcal meningitis is an indolent infection in which the virulence of the causative agent marginally exceeds the resistance of the host. In most instances, it acts opportunistically in immunocompromised persons, but the organism on rare occasion can establish meningitis in an immunologically competent host. *Cryptococcus neoformans* customarily enters the human host by the inhalation of contaminated particulates. Birds are a major reservoir, and their inhaled excreta initiate a pneumonitis, after which the fungi enter the bloodstream and attain the intracranial compartment.

PATHOLOGY: The tissue response to *C. neoformans* in the meninges is typically sparse. The lesions are widely disseminated in the meninges, ependyma, and choroid plexus. To the naked eye, they appear as discrete white nodules, a millimeter or so in diameter. Microscopically, organisms may abound, particularly in the Virchow–Robin spaces. An occasional multinucleated giant cell, sometimes with phagocytosed organisms, is accompanied by scant epithelioid cells and a scattering of lymphocytes.

Cryptococcal organisms are encapsulated spheres, 5 to 15 μm in diameter. They have an external gelatinous capsule and reproduce by budding (Fig. 28-48). When a drop of contaminated CSF is mixed with India ink, microscopic examination shows a clear halo about the encapsulated organism. This capsule sheds specific antigens that can be detected in the CSF by the latex cryptococcal antigen test.

C. neoformans usually causes only meningitis, but rare cases of infection show collections of organisms within the brain parenchyma, forming gelatinous pseudocysts.

Amebic Meningoencephalitis

Two genera of amebae, *Naegleria* and *Acanthamoeba,* penetrate the intracranial compartment by way of the cribriform plate, via the olfactory nerves. Persons exposed to brackish water while swimming may be infected by *Naegleria,* which produces a fulminant, usually fatal, leptomeningitis. By light microscopy, the trophozoites of *Naegleria* appear similar to macrophages. Infection by *Acanthamoeba,* whose trophozoites resemble *Naegleria* (Fig. 28-49), is also fatal, but with a more protracted course.

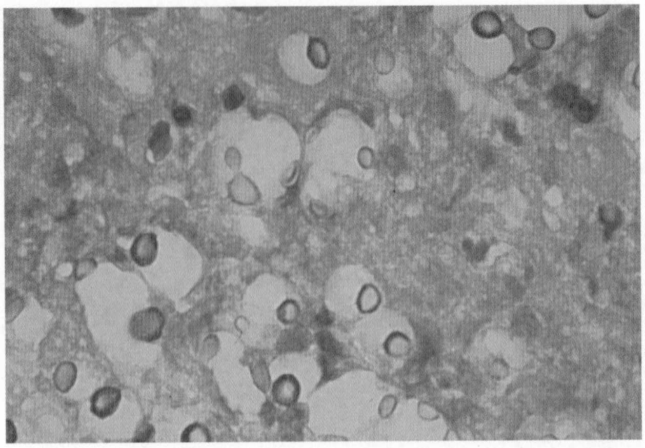

FIGURE 28-48. **Cryptococcal meningitis.** The cryptococcal organisms vary in size (5 to 15 μm in diameter) (mucicarmine stain). They reproduce by budding.

In addition to meningitis, *Acanthamoeba* produces parenchymal abscesses and a granulomatous tissue reaction. The organism has a distinctive double serrated cell wall.

Syphilitic (Luetic) Meningitis and Related Lesions

The spirochete of syphilis, *Treponema pallidum,* enters the bloodstream from the primary lesion, the chancre. The onset of secondary syphilis is marked by a maculopapular rash on the skin and mucous membranes. A few lymphocytes and plasma cells and increased protein in the CSF reflect entry of blood-borne spirochetes into the meninges. The organisms do not survive for long and the CSF reverts to normal. On occasion, however, the transient spirochete initiates a fibroblastic response in the meninges, accompanied by an obliterative endarteritis (Fig. 28-50) that induces multiple small infarcts in the cerebral cortex. Plasma cells, the hallmark of syphilis, surround the arterioles of the cerebral cortex in luetic meningovascular syphilis.

TABES DORSALIS: The initial lesion in this disorder is a variant of chronic meningitis (Fig. 28-51). The dorsal nerve roots proximal to the dorsal root ganglia are met by a conical sleeve of arachnoid filled with CSF, which can be the site of syphilitic inflammation. Fibrous tissue generated by the inflammation constricts nerve roots to cause axonal (Wallerian) degeneration. The axons that course cephalad in the posterior fasciculus do not synapse with intramedullary neurons as do all other ascending pathways in the cord. They are, rather, direct extensions of posterior root axons, so that Wallerian degeneration initiated in the dorsal spinal nerves extends into the posterior fasciculi. This is the most readily visualized morphologic lesion of tabes dorsalis and accounts for the loss of position sense in the lower extremities. The serologic reaction of the CSF generally reverts to negative before the onset of tabetic symptoms.

LUETIC DEMENTIA: T. pallidum may also lodge latently in the brain for decades. The spirochetes replicate sluggishly and escape eradication, only to cause **dementia paralytica** years after the initial infection. The morphological featur of luetic dementia include the following:

- Focal loss of cortical neurons
- Disfigurement of the topography of the residual nerve cells ("wind-blown appearance")
- Marked gliosis
- Conversion of microglia into elongated forms encrusted with iron ("rod cells")
- Nodular ependymitis

Cerebral Abscess Is a Potentially Fatal Space-Occupying Lesion

The cortex and subjacent white matter contain a rich capillary bed. It is, therefore, not surprising that blood-borne microorganisms lodge in this location, where they replicate and elicit an acute inflammatory and edematous reaction termed **cerebritis** (Fig. 28-52). Within days, liquefactive necrosis causes an expanding abscess (Fig. 28-53) and threatens life by transtentorial herniation or rupture into a ventricle.

Astrocytes predominate in cerebral repair, but fibroblasts also contribute to the formation of a capsule around abscesses. If the abscess is not drained or treated with antibiotics, pressure builds within it. Both the abscess and surrounding edema compress blood vessels, thereby disposing the affected region to ischemia. The region below an abscess also is susceptible to the growth of microorganisms that escape from the "mother" abscess, and frequently "daughter" abscesses form beneath the primary lesion. They can carry the inflammatory process to the ventricles, from which the infection can pass across the ependyma through the foramina of Magendie and Luschka and onto the meninges, with a fatal outcome.

Viral Encephalomyelitis Reflects Localization in Specific CNS Areas

The manifestations of viral infections of CNS parenchyma are heterogeneous, both clinically and pathologically (Fig. 28-54). Thus, poliomyelitis affects spinal and brainstem motor neurons, rabies localizes to the brainstem, and herpes simplex targets the temporal lobes. Subacute sclerosing panencephalitis and PML afflict the cerebral hemispheres, the former generally in childhood and the latter in immunocompromised persons. The mechanisms of viral tropism may reflect specific binding of viruses to sites on the plasma membranes of CNS cells, the ability of viruses to remain latent, or selective replication in distinct intracellular

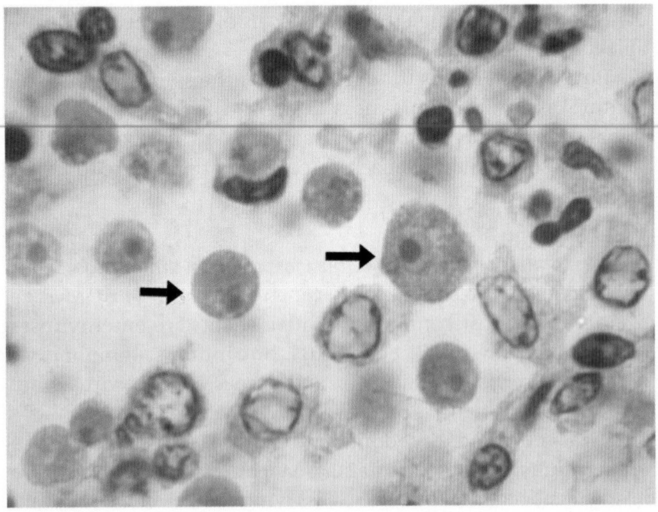

FIGURE 28-49. **Naegleria meningoencephalitis.** Amebic organisms (*arrows*) resemble macrophages but with prominent nucleoli.

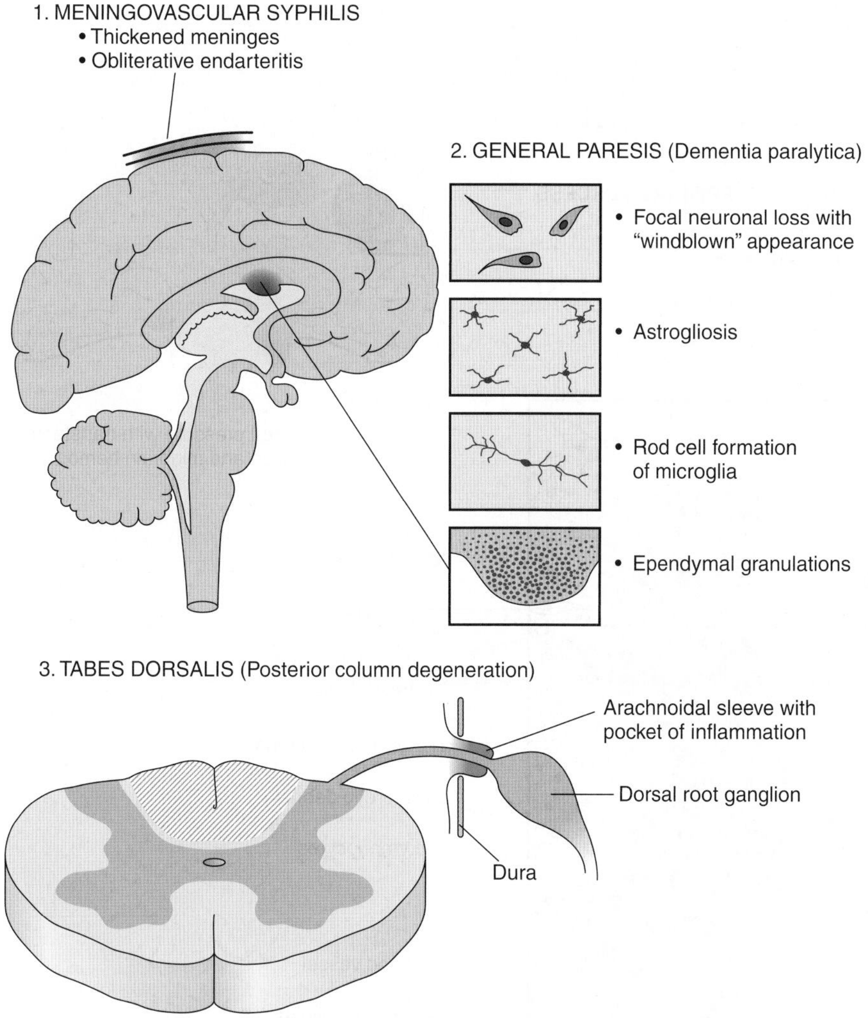

FIGURE 28-50. **Involvement of the central nervous system in syphilis.**

microenvironments. Given that axons project over long distances, viruses that enter a neuron may be transported by orthograde and retrograde axonal and dendritic transport mechanism to sites distant from their point of entry, as exemplified by rabies and herpesviruses.

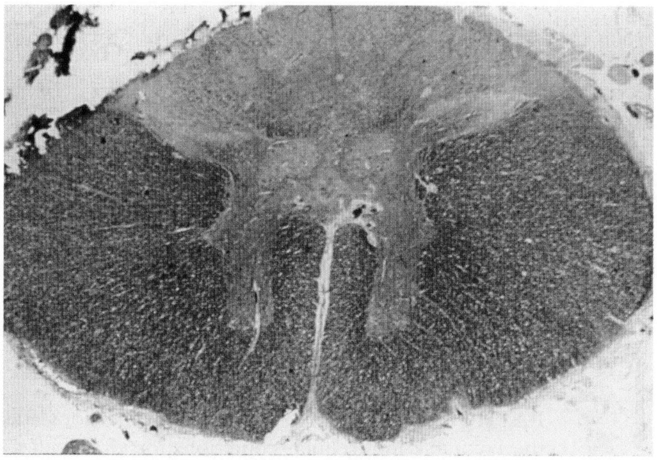

FIGURE 28-51. **Tabes dorsalis.** The spinal cord of a patient with tertiary syphilis displays posterior column degeneration (sliver impregnation stain).

PATHOLOGY: The classic hallmark of most CNS viral infections is the presence of **perivascular lymphocytes** around arteries and arterioles (Fig. 28-55), but a more diagnostic feature is the formation of viral inclusion bodies (Fig 28-56). However, inclusion bodies are not seen in all viral infections (e.g., poliomyelitis).

Viral particles also may be visualized by electron microscopy, but in situ hybridization, polymerase chain reaction (PCR), and immunohistochemistry detect viral particles most reliably and are more effective methods for the diagnosis of viral infections.

CLINICAL FEATURES: The onset of most viral encephalitides is abrupt. The more specific neurologic deficits (e.g., the paralysis of poliomyelitis or difficulty in swallowing in rabies) reflect the localization of the viral infection. Although most encephalitides run a brief course, the tempo can vary. For example, the clinical course of subacute sclerosing panencephalitis may extend over years, whereas herpes simplex virus may reside latently in the gasserian ganglion for decades and may do the same in the brain. Thus, viral infections also may be implicated in chronic cerebral disorders.

Poliomyelitis

*The term **poliomyelitis** refers to any inflammation of the gray matter of the spinal cord, but in common usage, it implies an infection by*

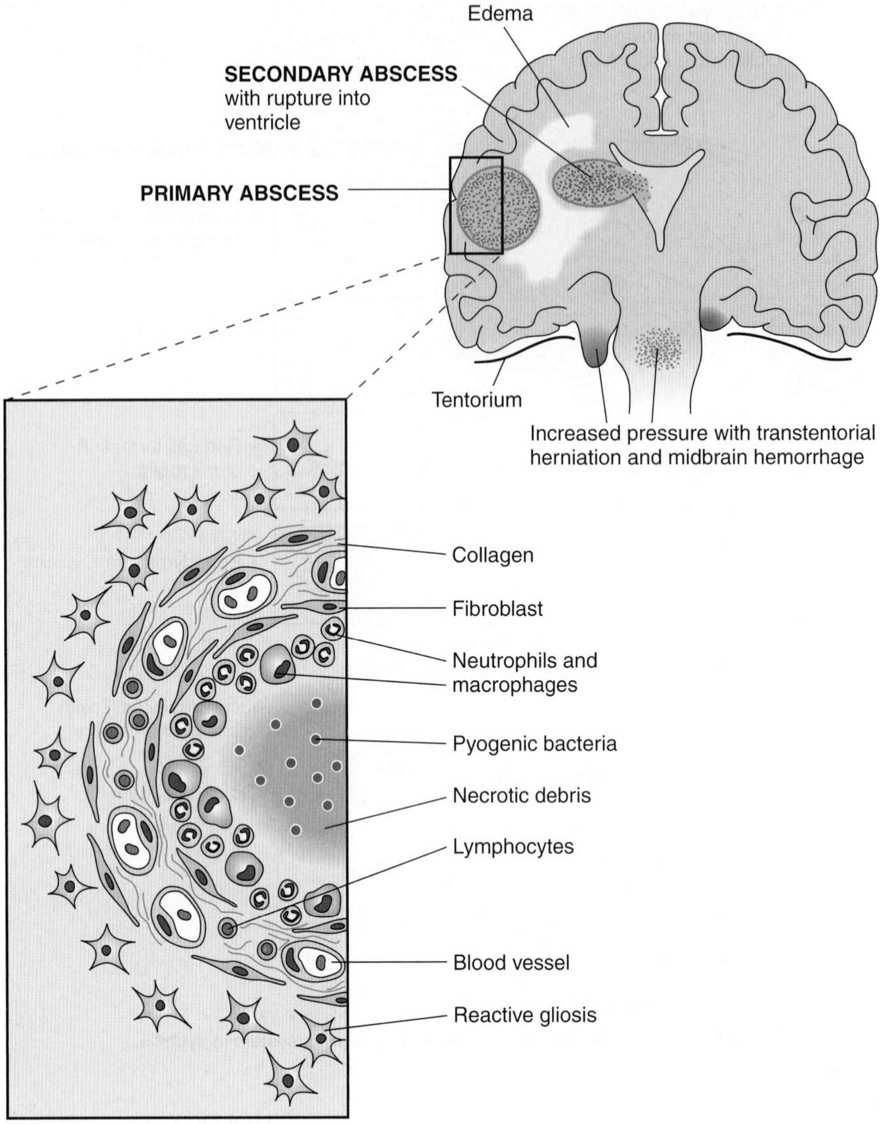

FIGURE 28-52. **Brain abscess and its complications.** A cerebral abscess may cause death through the production of secondary abscesses with intraventricular rupture; alternatively, death may result from transtentorial herniation.

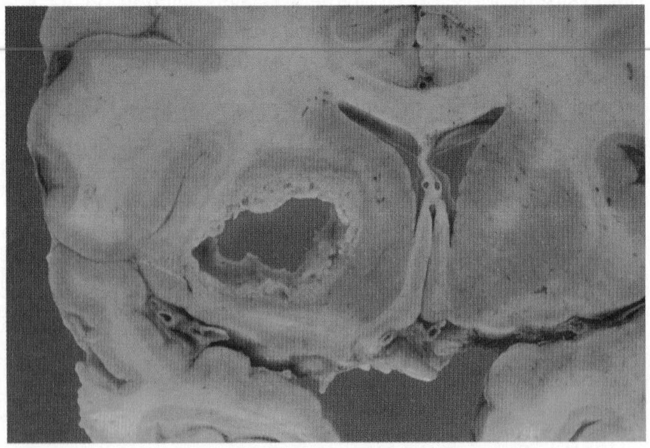

FIGURE 28-53. **Cerebral abscess.** A young man with bacterial endocarditis developed an abscess in the left basal ganglia.

poliovirus. The organism is one of the enteroviruses, which are small, nonenveloped, single-stranded, RNA viruses.

EPIDEMIOLOGY: Historical evidence suggests that poliomyelitis has occurred in epidemic form since antiquity. The medical triumph over this disease in the 20th Century depended on many years of prior research that culminated in the development of effective vaccines to prevent the disease. Persons infected with poliovirus shed large amounts of virus in their stools, and infection spreads by the fecal–oral route. The agent spreads rapidly among children in close quarters where there are opportunities for fecal–oral contact.

PATHOLOGY: Binding sites on motor neurons and the favorable intracellular conditions for viral replication permit the virus to enter these cells and replicate. The infected cells undergo chromatolysis (see Fig. 28-3), after

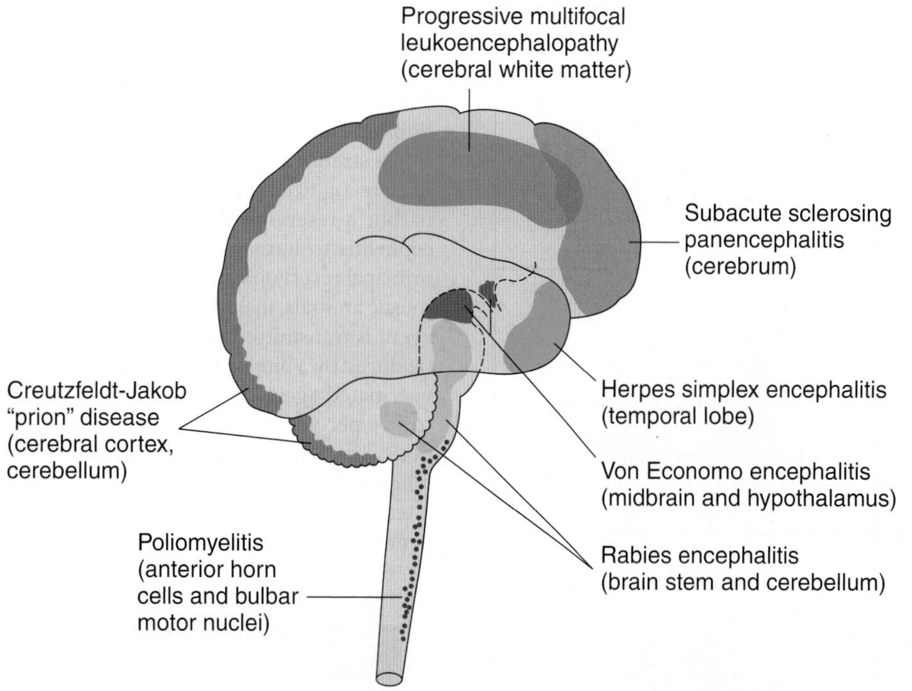

FIGURE 28-54. **Distribution of the lesions of viral encephalitides.**

which they are phagocytosed by macrophages (neuronophagia). The initial inflammatory response transiently includes polymorphonuclear leukocytes, which are followed by lymphocytes that surround blood vessels in the spinal cord and brainstem. The inflammation may also extend into the meninges. The motor cortex usually shows no inflammation but may contain "microglial nodules," (i.e., focal collections of microglia and lymphocytes) (see Fig. 28-10). Although the immunologic response of the host to poliovirus is limited, it may halt progression of clinical disease. Sections of spinal cord in cases of healed poliomyelitis show a

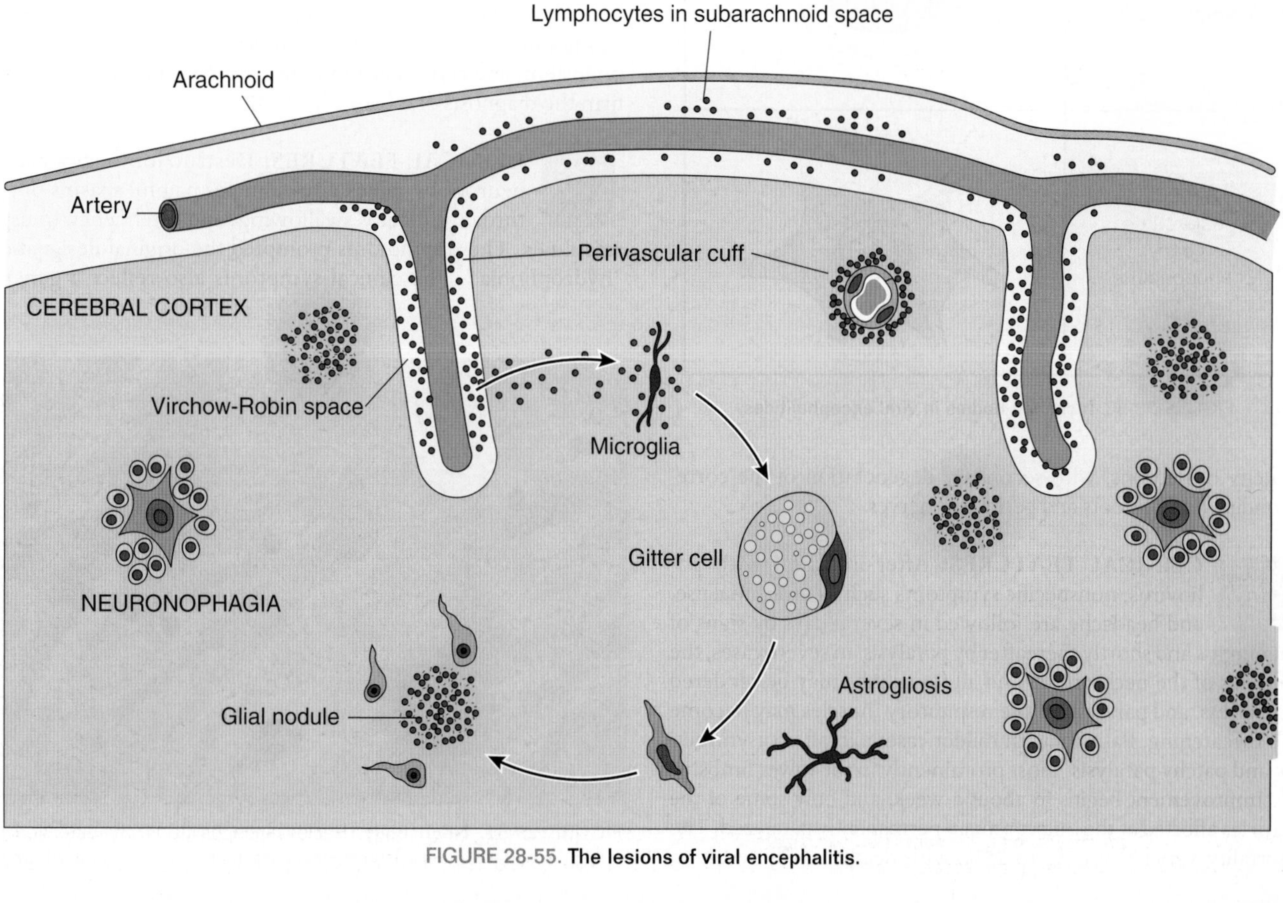

FIGURE 28-55. **The lesions of viral encephalitis.**

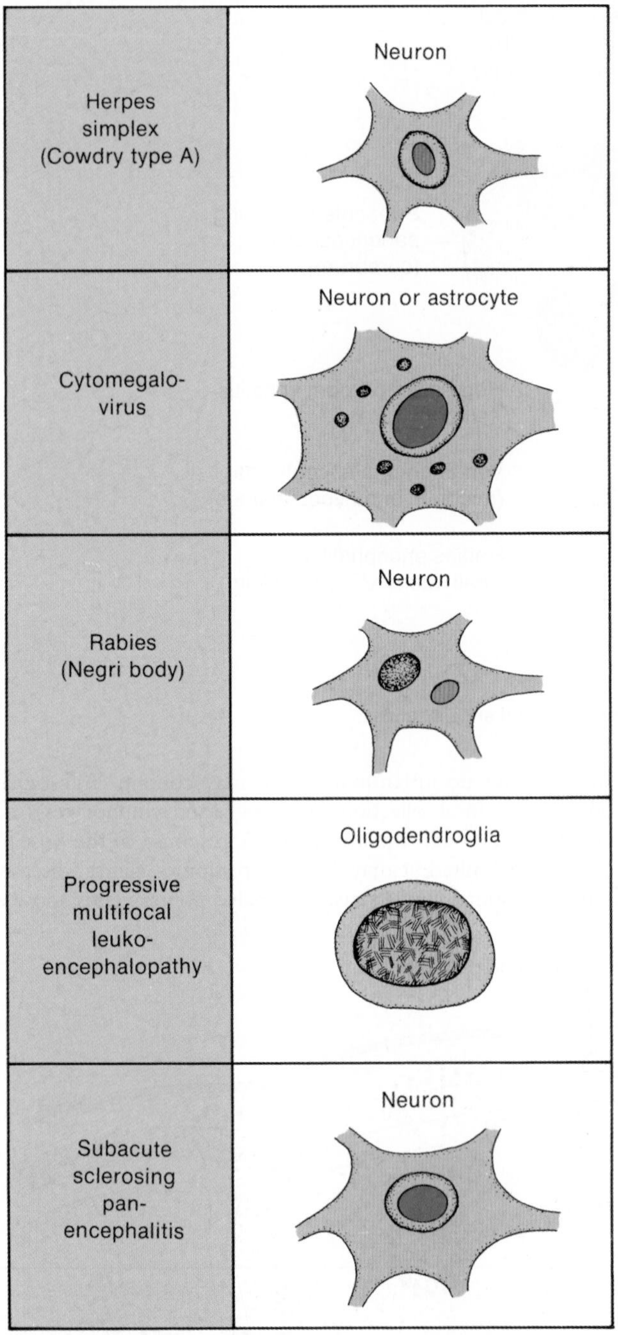

FIGURE 28-56. **Inclusion bodies in viral encephalitides.**

paucity of neurons, with secondary degeneration of the corresponding ventral roots and peripheral nerves.

CLINICAL FEATURES: After infection with poliovirus, nonspecific symptoms such as fever, malaise, and headache are followed in several days by signs of meningitis and shortly thereafter by paralysis. In severe cases, the muscles of the neck, trunk, and all four limbs may be rendered powerless, and paralysis of the respiratory muscles may become life-threatening. Patients with milder cases exhibit an asymmetric and patchy paralysis, most prominently in the lower limbs.

Improvement begins in about a week, and only some of the muscles affected at the outset remain permanently paralyzed. The mortality varies from 5% to 25%, with death usually resulting from respiratory failure. The development in the 1950s of effective vaccines against poliovirus has largely eliminated the disease.

Rabies

Rabies is an encephalitis caused by rabies virus, an enveloped, single-stranded RNA virus of the rhabdovirus group. Rabies has been recognized throughout recorded history. Lower mammals harbor a reservoir of this zoonosis and transmit the lethal encephalitis to humans. Dogs, wolves, foxes, and skunks are the principal reservoirs, but the infection also extends to bats and domestic animals, including cattle, goats, and swine. The infectious agent is transmitted to humans through contaminated saliva introduced by a bite. In the United States, where dogs are routinely vaccinated against rabies, the few human rabies infections (one to five per year) usually result from exposure to rabid wild animals. In areas of Asia, Africa, and South America, however where rabies is endemic, most human infections result from dog bites. In those areas of the world, rabies kills more than 50,000 persons annually.

PATHOGENESIS: The virus enters a peripheral nerve and is transported by retrograde axoplasmic flow to the spinal cord and brain. The latent interval varies in proportion to the distance of transport, being as short as 10 days or as long as 3 months.

PATHOLOGY: Lymphocytes aggregate about small arteries and veins in the brainstem. Scattered neurons show chromatolysis and neuronophagia, and microglial nodules develop. The inflammation is centered in the brainstem and spills into the cerebellum and hypothalamus. Eosinophilic cytoplasmic inclusion bodies in the hippocampus, brainstem, and cerebellar Purkinje cells (**Negri bodies**) can confirm the diagnosis of rabies (Fig. 28-57).

CLINICAL FEATURES: Destruction of brainstem neurons by rabies virus initiates painful spasms of the throat, difficulty swallowing, and a tendency to aspirate fluids. These symptoms prompted the original designation "hydrophobia." The clinical symptoms also reflect a general

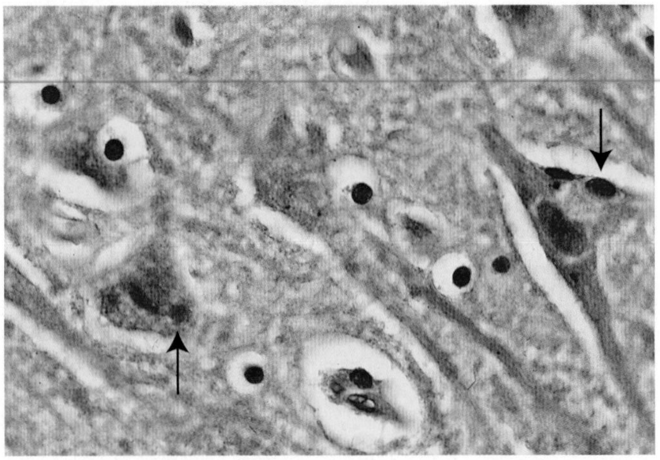

FIGURE 28-57. **Negri body.** Rabies encephalitis is characterized by round, eosinophilic cytoplasmic inclusions that resemble an erythrocyte

encephalopathy, characterized by irritability, agitation, seizures, and delirium. The CSF displays a typical viral response, including (1) a modest increase in the number of lymphocytes, (2) a moderate increase in protein content, and (3) unaltered glucose levels and CSF pressure. The illness progresses to death within one to several weeks, unless postexposure vaccination is administered in a timely manner.

Herpes Simplex Encephalitis and Related Infections

Herpesviruses include herpes simplex (types 1 and 2), varicella-zoster virus, cytomegalovirus, Epstein-Barr virus, and simian B virus.

HERPES SIMPLEX VIRUS TYPE 1 (HSV-1): HSV-1 is largely responsible for the "cold sore." The region of the vesicular lesion on the lip is innervated from the trigeminal ganglion through its mandibular nerve trunk. HSV-1 may reside latently within the trigeminal ganglion, where it proliferates during periods of stress and is transmitted centrifugally through the nerve trunk to the lip.

Herpes encephalitis is a major viral infection of the human nervous system. In adults, the encephalitis is caused principally by HSV-1 and localizes predominantly in one or both temporal lobes.

PATHOLOGY: Herpes encephalitis is a fulminant infection. The temporal lobes become swollen, hemorrhagic, and necrotic. The inflammatory exudate is predominantly lymphocytic and perivascular. The small arteries and arterioles become hemorrhagic and edematous. Intranuclear inclusions occur in both neurons and in glial cells (Fig. 28-58A). The inclusions are eosinophilic and usually surrounded by a halo. The detection of viral proteins by immunohistochemical techniques is diagnostically reliable. The diagnosis is often made by the PCR of CSF.

HERPES SIMPLEX VIRUS TYPE 2 (HSV-2): In women, HSV-2 initiates a vesicular lesion on the vulva (**genital herpes**), coupled with a latent infection in the pelvic ganglia. Newborns acquire HSV-2 from the birth canal and thereafter have an encephalitis. At this age, the neural tissues are extremely vulnerable, and the infection promptly causes extensive liquefactive necrosis in the cerebrum and cerebellum.

VARICELLA-ZOSTER VIRUS: Herpes zoster causes a disease that is anatomically analogous to the trigeminal ganglion–cold sore complex of herpes simplex. The cutaneous vesicular eruption of "shingles" occurs in the distribution of a dermatome whose dorsal root ganglion harbors the varicella-zoster virus. The infection elicits only mild inflammation and rarely spreads

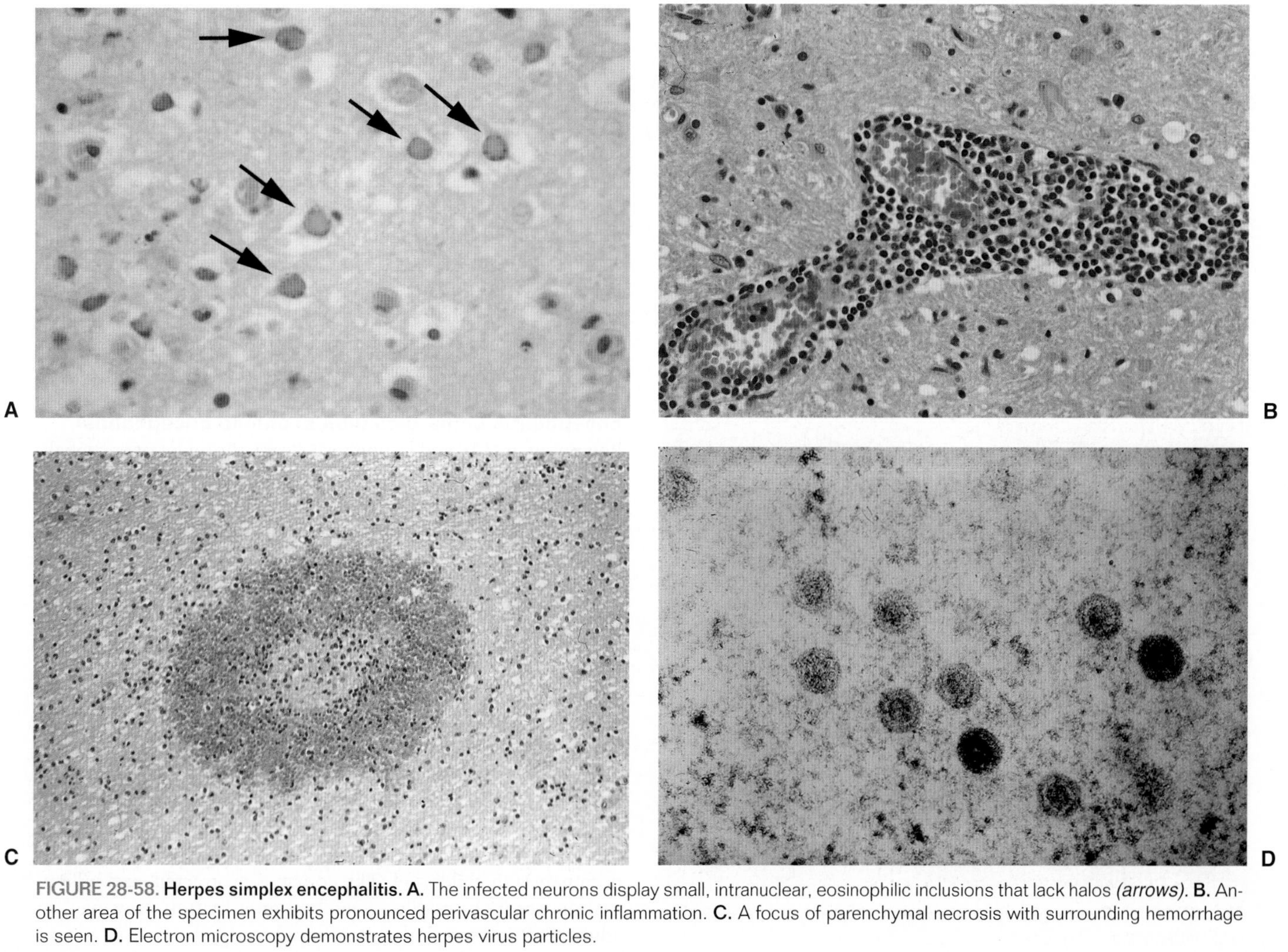

FIGURE 28-58. **Herpes simplex encephalitis. A.** The infected neurons display small, intranuclear, eosinophilic inclusions that lack halos *(arrows)*. **B.** Another area of the specimen exhibits pronounced perivascular chronic inflammation. **C.** A focus of parenchymal necrosis with surrounding hemorrhage is seen. **D.** Electron microscopy demonstrates herpes virus particles.

to the CNS. Intranuclear inclusions are indistinguishable from herpes simplex infection by morphologic appearance. Varicella-zoster is also responsible for "chicken pox" which usually causes a self-limited cutaneous viral exanthem in naïve hosts (typically children). However, the virus may also cause a fatal encephalitis. "Shingles" represents the reemergence of latent infection by the varicella-zoster virus.

CYTOMEGALOVIRUS: This agent crosses the placenta to induce encephalitis in utero. The lesions in the embryonic CNS predominate in the periventricular areas and are characterized by necrosis and calcification. Because of the proximity of these lesions to the third ventricle and the aqueduct, they are prone to induce hydrocephalus. Cytomegalovirus is one of the agents of the so-called TORCH (toxoplasmosis, other [congenital syphilis and viruses], rubella, cytomegalovirus, and herpes simplex virus) complex of newborns. In adults, cytomegalovirus initiates encephalitis in immunocompromised hosts. Eosinophilic inclusions are present in both the nucleus and cytoplasm of astrocytes and neurons. They are most conspicuous in the enlarged nucleus, where they are sharply defined and surrounded by a halo (Fig. 28-59).

Arthropod-Borne Viral Encephalitis

Arthropod-borne viruses, termed **arboviruses,** are heterogeneous and are transmitted between vertebrates by blood-sucking vectors (e.g., mosquitoes, ticks). Togaviridae and Bunyaviridae constitute most of the arboviruses that cause human encephalitis. Arbovirus infections are zoonoses of animals, and humans are infected when bitten by virus-harboring arthropods. Humans do not continue viral propagation. The various encephalitides caused by arboviruses are named principally for the location where they were first noted (Table 28-1), for example, Eastern, Western, and Venezuelan equine encephalitis; St. Louis encephalitis; Japanese B encephalitis; California encephalitis; and West Nile encephalitis.

PATHOLOGY: The response of the brain does not differentiate among the various arboviruses that cause encephalitis, and the lesions vary from mild meningitis with scattered lymphocytes to severe inflammation of gray matter, thrombosis of small blood vessels, and prominent necrosis.

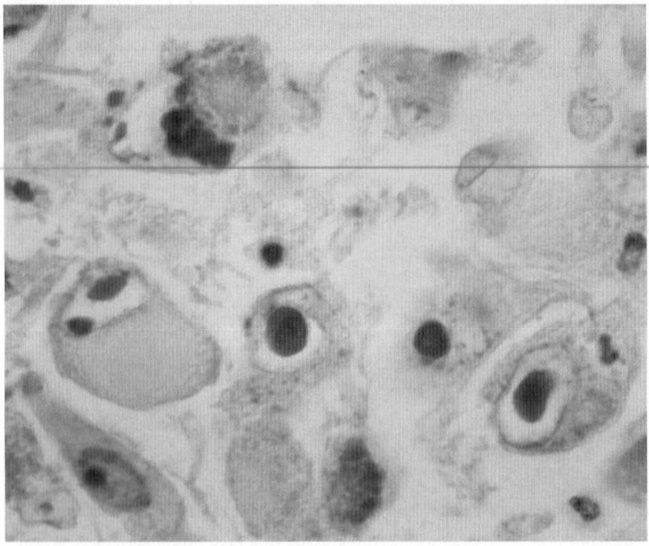

FIGURE 28-59. **Cytomegalovirus ependymitis.** Ependymal cells display large intranuclear inclusions.

TABLE 28-1

Insect-Borne Viral Encephalitis

Virus	Insect Vector	Distribution
St. Louis encephalitis	Mosquito	North and South America
Western equine encephalitis	Mosquito	North and South America
Venezuelan equine encephalitis	Mosquito	North and South America
Eastern equine encephalitis	Mosquito	North America
California encephalitis	Mosquito	North America
Murray Valley encephalitis	Mosquito	Australia, Papua New
Japanese B encephalitis	Mosquito	Eastern and south-eastern Asia
Tick-borne encephalitis	Tick	Eastern Europe, Scandinavia

No inclusions are present in the infected neurons. In necrotic foci, neuronophagia is evident, and if the patient survives, demyelination and gliosis may develop.

CLINICAL FEATURES: The arthropod-borne encephalitides share many features, but each type has a different course. For example, Eastern equine encephalitis is commonly a fulminant disease that kills in a few days, whereas Venezuelan equine encephalitis tends to be benign. Mild cases of arbovirus encephalitis may be manifested only by a mild flulike syndrome and are not diagnosed as encephalitis. In severe cases, the onset is abrupt, with high fever, headache, vomiting, and meningeal signs, followed by lethargy and coma. Most victims die within 5 days. Young children often survive but may be left with mental retardation, epilepsy, and other neurologic sequelae.

Encephalitis Lethargica (von Economo Encephalitis)

Beginning in 1916 and lasting for 5 years, the agent of encephalitis lethargica induced a severe encephalitis pandemic. Although the identity of the infectious agent is disputed, the characteristic perivascular cuffs of lymphocytes in the midbrain and hypothalamus argued for a viral cause. The dominant symptom was somnolence, which persisted for weeks. An occasional patient was left with parkinsonism (see below), but other victims developed Parkinson disease ("postencephalitic parkinsonism") a decade or so later, suggesting that subclinical injury to neurons of the substantia nigra compromised their longevity.

Subacute Sclerosing Panencephalitis

Subacute sclerosing panencephalitis (SSPE) is a chronic, lethal, viral infection of the brain caused by the measles virus. First recognized in 1933 and named "subacute inclusion-body encephalitis," its features were defined later as an encephalitis of insidious onset, predominantly in childhood. The course is protracted, and inflammation occurs primarily in cerebral gray matter. However, in adults, SSPE may follow a more rapid course.

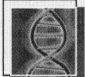

PATHOGENESIS: SSPE is a consequence of infection with the measles virus, and most patients give a history of measles in childhood. SSPE develops 6 to 8 years after the initial infection and is caused by a measles virus with defective expression of the viral M (Matrix) protein.

PATHOLOGY AND CLINICAL FEATURES: The infection is highlighted by prominent intranuclear inclusions in neurons and oligodendroglia, marked gliosis in affected gray and white matter (hence *sclerosing*), patchy loss of myelin, and ubiquitous perivascular lymphocytes and macrophages (Fig. 28-60). The intranuclear inclusions are basophilic and are rimmed by a prominent halo. In some cases, affected neurons contain neurofibrillary tangles (see below). Over a period of years, the classic disease leads insidiously to cognitive deficits, behavioral changes, motor and sensory impairments, and ultimately death. The CSF typically contains an increased titer against the measles virus.

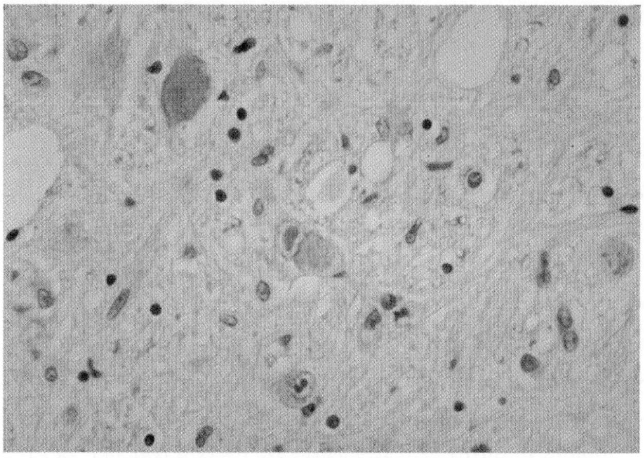

FIGURE 28-60. **Subacute sclerosing panencephalitis.** The brain shows loss of myelin and reactive gliosis.

Progressive Multifocal Leukoencephalopathy

PML is a relentlessly destructive multifocal disease caused by JC virus, which principally affects the white matter in brain. PML manifests as dementia, weakness, visual loss, and ataxia, leading to death in most patients within 6 months. The infection exemplifies the fundamental characteristics of neurotropic viruses, such as selectivity for specific cell types, notably oligodendroglia (Fig. 28-61), with demyelination caused by damage to oligodendrocytes. In contrast to many viruses, JC virus is oncogenic, at least in rodents.

JC virus is a papovavirus closely analogous to simian virus 40 (SV40 virus). Most commonly, PML is a terminal complication in immunosuppressed patients, such as those treated for cancer or lupus erythematosus, organ transplant patients, and persons

A

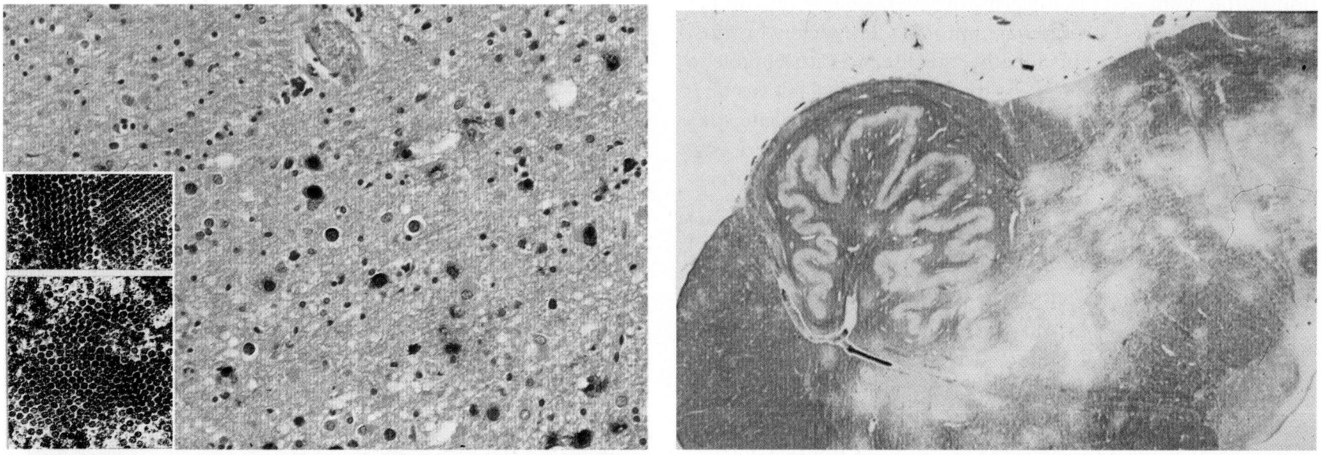

B

C

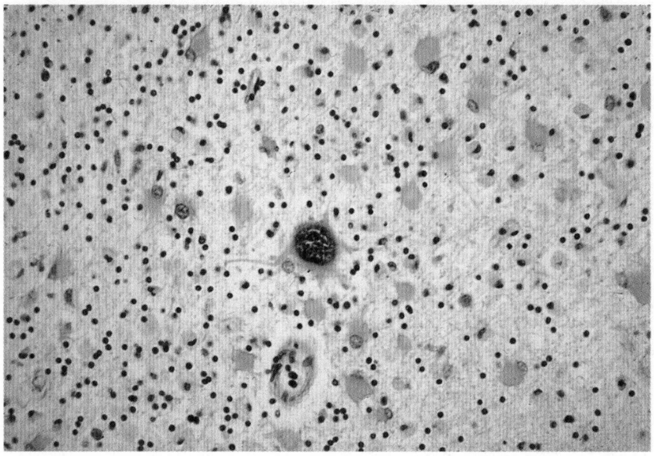

FIGURE 28-61. **Progressive multifocal leukoencephalopathy. A.** An immunohistochemical stain for JC virus demonstrates numerous infected oligodendroglia in the white matter. By electron microscopy, there are intranuclear particles (*insets*). **B.** A luxol fast blue stain of the medulla reveals severe loss of myelin. **C.** A bizarre astrocyte is present (center).

with AIDS. In fact, PML now occurs in 3% or more of AIDS patients in the United States and Europe.

PATHOLOGY: The typical lesions of PML appear as widely disseminated discrete foci of demyelination near the gray–white junction in the cerebral hemispheres and the brainstem (see Fig. 28-61B). The characteristic lesion of PML exhibits the following morphologic features:

- It is spherical, measuring several millimeters in diameter.
- A central area is largely devoid of myelin.
- Axons are retained.
- Few oligodendrocytes are seen.
- The lesion is infiltrated by macrophages, without necrosis.
- Pleomorphic bizarre astrocytes are present (see Fig. 28-61C).

A pathognomonic feature of PML is a peripheral area of demyelination that contains enlarged oligodendrocytes, with homogeneously dense, hyperchromatic, intranuclear inclusions, which lack a halo and have a ground-glass appearance. Electron microscopy discloses intranuclear, crystalline arrays of spherical virions, 35 to 40 nm in diameter (see Fig. 28-61A). The pleomorphic astrocytes appear anaplastic and contain multiple irregular nuclei, which display dense chromatin (see Fig. 28-61C). Astrocytomas have developed in some patients with PML, suggesting oncogenic potential in humans.

AIDS Encephalopathy

Many AIDS patients manifest a clinical encephalopathy and harbor brain lesions at autopsy. Some have an opportunistic infection in the brain (e.g., toxoplasmosis, cytomegalovirus, herpes simplex, PML, or a primary lymphoma). However, in most AIDS patients with encephalopathy, the disease is attributable to an active infection of the CNS by the retrovirus itself. *Dementia is the most common clinical manifestation of AIDS encephalopathy (AIDS dementia complex),* which ranges from mild to severe cognitive impairment, with paralysis and loss of sensory functions.

PATHOGENESIS: In AIDS encephalopathy macrophages and microglial cells in the CNS are productively infected by human immunodeficiency virus (HIV)-1. Although other cells, including neurons and astrocytes, may interact with the virus, they do not seem to be infected, but are injured indirectly by cytokines or other neurotoxic factors.

PATHOLOGY: On gross examination, AIDS encephalopathy is characterized by mild cerebral atrophy, with dilation of the lateral ventricles and slight prominence of the gyri and sulci. The histologic changes are usually in the subcortical gray and white matter. *The hallmark of AIDS encephalopathy is the presence of multinucleated giant cells of the monocyte/macrophage lineage associated with microglial nodules* (Fig. 28-62). In addition, myelin pallor, reflecting diffuse demyelination, intense astrogliosis, and loss of neurons are commonly found.

Vacuolar myelopathy is another disorder attributed to HIV infection, although it is less frequent than encephalopathy. It is characterized by marked vacuolation of the posterior and lateral columns, principally at the thoracic level of the spinal cord. Ataxia and spastic paraparesis dominate the clinical presentation.

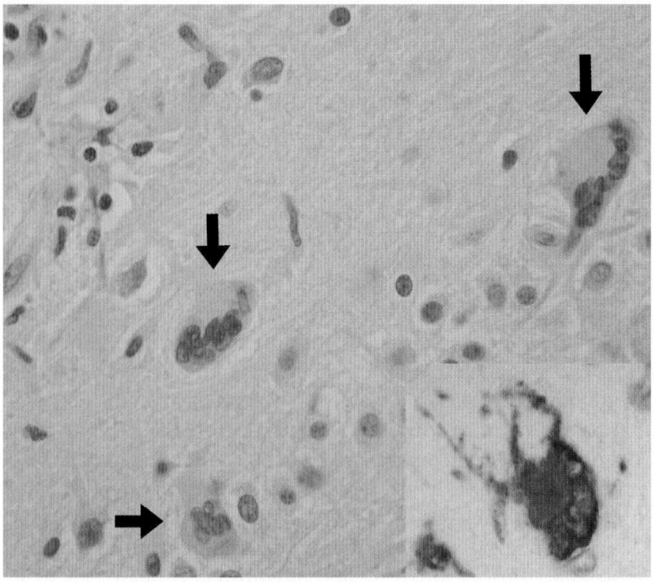

FIGURE 28-62. **Human immunodeficiency virus (HIV) encephalitis.** Multinucleated giant cells (*arrows*) often in a perivascular location are characteristic of HIV encephalitis. *Inset:* Immunohistochemical stain for HIV anti-p24.

Congenital HIV encephalopathy and myelopathy differ from the adult disease more in their intensity than in their specific attributes. Calcification of the basal ganglia and thalamus are more common in childhood infections and can be visualized radiographically.

Prion Diseases (Spongiform Encephalopathies) Are Transmissible Neurodegenerative Diseases

Prion diseases comprise a group of neurodegenerative conditions characterized clinically by slowly progressive ataxia and dementia and pathologically by accumulations of fibrillar or insoluble prion proteins, degeneration of neurons, and vacuolization termed **spongiform degeneration** (Fig. 28-63). The classic spongiform encephalopathies include several syndromes including kuru, Creutzfeldt-Jakob

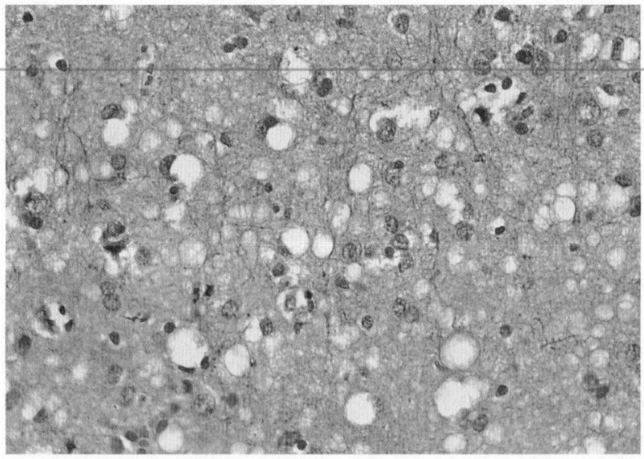

FIGURE 28-63. **Creutzfeldt-Jakob disease.** Spongiform degeneration of the gray matter is characterized by individual and clustered vacuoles, with no evidence of inflammation.

TABLE 28–2

Prion Diseases

I. Human
A. Creutzfeldt-Jakob disease (CJD) 1. Sporadic (85% of all CJD cases; incidence 1 per million worldwide) 2. Inherited mutation of the prion gene, autosomal dominant transmission (15% of all CJD cases) 3. Iatrogenic a. Hormone injection Human growth hormone (55 cases) Human pituitary gonadotropin (5 cases) b. Tissue grafts Dura mater (11 cases) Cornea (1 case) Pericardium (1 case) c. Medical devices (inadequate sterilization) Depth electrodes (2 cases) Surgical instruments (not definitely proven) 4. New variant CJD (vCJD)
B. Gerstmann-Straussler-Scheinker disease (GSS; inherited prion gene mutation, autosomal dominant transmission)
C. Fatal familial insomnia (FFI; inherited prion gene mutation, autosomal dominant transmission)
D. Kuru (confined to the Fore people of Papua New Guinea, formerly transmitted by cannibalistic ritual)
II. Animal
A. Scrapie (sheep and goats)
B. Bovine spongiform encephalopathy (BSE; "mad cow disease")
C. Transmissible mink encephalopathy
D. Feline spongiform encephalopathy
E. Captive exotic ungulate spongiform encephalopathy (nyala, gemsbok, eland, Arabian oryx, greater kudu)
F. Chronic wasting disease of deer and elk
G. Experimental transmission to many species, including primates and transgenic mice

disease (CJD), Gerstmann-Straussler-Scheinker syndrome (GSS), and fatal familial insomnia (Table 28-2). In addition, similar diseases occur in animals, including scrapie in sheep and goats, bovine spongiform encephalopathy (BSE; mad cow disease), transmissible mink encephalopathy, and chronic wasting disease in mule deer and elk.

Prion diseases encompass infectious and autosomal dominant (due to prion gene mutations) forms, but in most cases, the mode of acquisition is uncertain. In addition to their many singular clinical and molecular pathologic features, prion diseases are currently under intense scrutiny because of recent data that indicate a link between BSE ("mad cow disease") and a new variant of human CJD, namely new variant vCJD.

PATHOGENESIS: All spongiform encephalopathies are transmissible, and inadvertent human transmission of CJD has followed the administration of contaminated human pituitary growth hormone, corneal transplantation from a diseased donor, insufficiently sterilized neurosurgical instruments, and surgical implantation of contaminated dura (see Table 28-2). The infectious agent is not a conventional virus, as implied by the earlier term "slow virus" sheep scrapie, but an unprecedented protein termed the **prion (proteinaceous infectious particles).**

The human prion gene *(PRNP)* is located on the short arm of chromosome 20 and consists of a single exon encoding 254 amino acid residues. The normal prion gene product, prion protein (PrP), is a constitutively expressed cell-surface glycoprotein that is bound to the plasmalemma by a glycolipid anchor. The highest levels of PrP messenger RNA (mRNA) are found in CNS neurons, but the function of the protein is unknown. Remarkably, the normal cellular prion protein, termed *cellular PrP* or *PrP^C*, and the pathogenic (infectious) prion protein, known as scrapie PrP or PrP^{SC}, do not differ in amino acid sequence. However, they have different three-dimensional conformations and patterns of glycosylation. Specifically, PrP^C is rich in α-helix configuration, whereas the β-pleated sheet content of PrP^{SC} is predominant. This conformational change is presumed to underlie the conspicuous resistance of PrP^{SC} to proteinase digestion as well as the prion-propagation mechanism, whereby normal host PrP^C is converted to PrP^{SC}. *The newly converted proteins then change other PrP^C proteins into pathogenic PrP^{SC}. The result is an autocatalytic, exponentially expanding accrual of abnormal PrP^{SC}.* Accumulation of PrP^{SC} compromises cell function and results in neurodegeneration by mechanisms that remain to be elucidated but may be similar to those of other neurodegenerative diseases characterized by brain amyloidosis (see below).

PATHOLOGY: The cardinal morphologic features of prion diseases are neuronal degeneration and loss, gliosis, spongiform degeneration (small microcysts), and accumulations of insoluble prions with properties of amyloid (Fig. 28-64). These lesions are most prevalent in the cortical gray matter, but they also involve the deeper nuclei of the basal ganglia, hypothalamus, and cerebellum.

The various human prion diseases have distinctive features.

KURU: In 1956, a medical officer in New Guinea provided an account of kuru, a progressive, fatal neurologic disorder, in members of an isolated tribe. The disease takes its name from the word "trembling" in the language of the Fore people. The transmission of kuru was linked to ritualistic cannibalism in which women and children ate human brain.

Kuru was the first human prion disease shown to be transmissible. The disease formerly reached epidemic proportions in the Fore people but was eliminated after the cessation of cannibalism. The initial and most prominent clinical feature of kuru is ataxia of the limbs and trunk, owing to severe involvement of the cerebellum. In 70% of kuru cases, insoluble, fibrillar prion proteins accumulate extracellularly as amyloid or "kuru" plaques, and spongiform change is present in both the cerebral hemispheres and cerebellum. Late in the clinical course, some patients manifest dementia. Like all prion diseases, kuru is lethal.

CREUTZFELDT-JAKOB DISEASE (CJD): This rare, subacute encephalopathy was first fully described by Jakob in 1921. Symptoms begin insidiously, but within 6 months, the patient exhibits severe dementia and within a year is usually dead. The

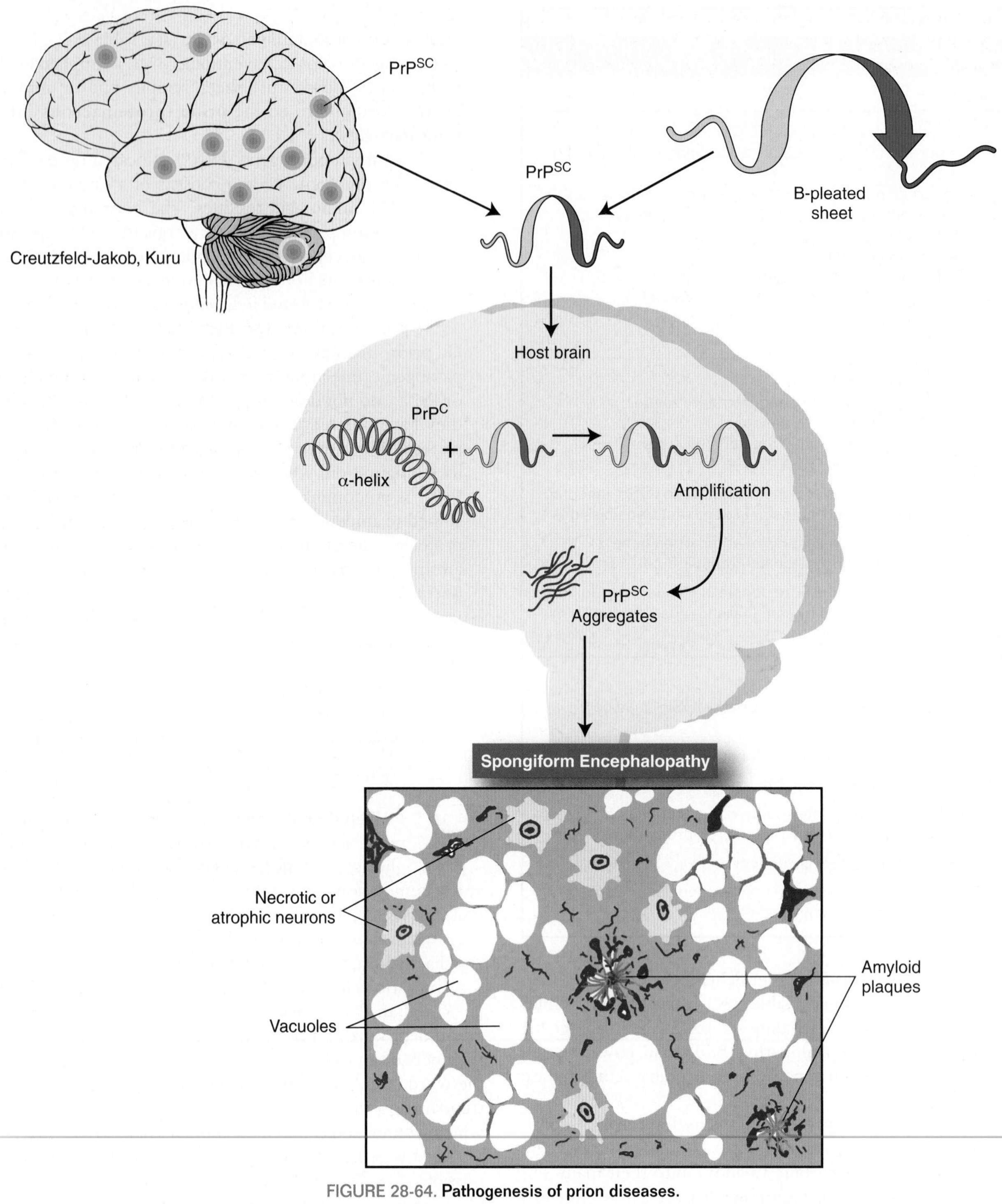

FIGURE 28-64. **Pathogenesis of prion diseases.**

involvement of the cerebellum adds ataxia to the predominant symptom of dementia and distinguishes CJD clinically from Alzheimer disease.

CJD is by far the most common form of human prion disease and can be classified into four types based on etiology:

- **Sporadic CJD:** The sporadic form occurs worldwide, with an incidence of 1 per million, and accounts for 75% of all cases of CJD. The mode of acquisition is unknown; patients do not exhibit the mutations associated with the inherited forms of CJD or other prion diseases, and there is no history of iatrogenic exposure. A normal polymorphism, which codes either for methionine (M) or valine (V), occurs at codon 129 of the prion gene. Susceptibility to all forms of CJD is influenced by this polymorphism, with a disproportionate number of patients homozygous at this locus. The frequencies for the white population are 51% M/V, 37% M/M, and 12% V/V.
- Sporadic CJD exhibits the prototypical histologic features of the spongiform encephalopathies. No host inflammatory response is seen. Clinically, sporadic CJD is characterized by the classic triad of dementia, myoclonus, and periodic spike–wave complexes in the electroencephalogram (EEG).

The dementia is rapidly progressive, with death occurring within 4 to 12 months. However, longer courses of 2 to 5 years are well documented. Some 15% of cases are first seen with ataxia similar to that of kuru, with dementia following later.

- **Inherited CJD: Familial CJD** constitutes 15% of prion diseases, with an incidence of 1 per 10 million. Several different mutations of the prion gene have been documented in various kindreds. The mutated PrP causes familial CJD, fatal familial insomnia, and Gerstmann-Straussler-Scheinker disease.

GERSTMANN-STRAUSSLER-SCHEINKER SYNDROME (GSS): This disorder was described in 1936 as a spinocerebellar ataxia with dementia. Patients exhibit progressive limb and truncal ataxia over 2 to 10 years. At autopsy, prominent prion protein amyloid or kuru-like plaques, neuron loss, and spongiform change are found in the cerebellum, cerebrum, and brainstem. Dementia is a late feature of the disease.

FATAL FAMILIAL INSOMNIA (FFI): This human prion disease is characterized by a profound disturbance of sleep–wake cycles and intractable insomnia. Dysautonomia, abnormal endocrine function, and signs of pyramidal and cerebellar dysfunction are common. Although cognitive function usually remains intact, dementia may supervene. The most conspicuous neuropathologic finding is neurodegeneration of specific thalamic nuclei. The disease has been described in several Italian families and is caused by a point mutation in codon 178 of the *PRNP* gene, leading to a substitution of aspartic acid by asparagine. Sporadic forms of FFI also occur.

- **Iatrogenic CJD:** As listed in Table 28-2, a number of iatrogenic cases of CJD have been documented, but most of the causes have been eliminated. For example, recombinant human growth hormone has supplanted human pituitary-derived preparations for therapy.
- **New variant CJD:** vCJD was identified by a surveillance program in the United Kingdom following the BSE epidemic that devastated the cattle industry between 1980 and 1996. A group of patients was identified that differed from other patients with sporadic CJD in several important characteristics, the most striking of which is age. The mean age at onset of symptoms for sporadic CJD is 65 years; it is 26 years for vCJD patients. Other differences include a longer duration of illness for vCJD (median, 12 months vs. 4 months) and an atypical clinical presentation, with vCJD patients showing various behavioral changes or sensory disturbances (dysesthesias) and none of the characteristic EEG findings of sporadic CJD. At autopsy, vCJD is characterized by prominent spongiform change in the basal ganglia and thalamus and extensive PrP plaques in the cerebrum and cerebellum. The plaques are distinctive in that they resemble those seen in kuru. Finally, brains from vCJD patients contain much more PrP than brains from sporadic CJD patients. Since physicochemical analysis revealed that the vCJD PrP^{SC} exhibits characteristics distinct from CJD PrP^{SC} but similar to the prions in BSE that were transmitted to mice and primates, BSE is likely the source of the new CJD variant.

Demyelinating Diseases

Demyelinating diseases are disorders in which the etiology relates to a selective loss of myelin. Thus, multiple sclerosis is viewed as a demyelinating disease, whereas necrosis due to infarcts or abscesses, traumatic contusions, and secondary demyelination caused by Wallerian degeneration, are not so classified.

Leukodystrophies Reflect Inherited Disturbances in the Formation and Preservation of Myelin

Metachromatic Leukodystrophy

Metachromatic leukodystrophy (MLD), the most common leukodystrophy, is an autosomal recessive disorder of myelin metabolism that is characterized by the accumulation of a cerebroside (galactosyl sulfatide) in the white matter of the brain and peripheral nerves. MLD predominates in infancy, but rare "juvenile" or "adult" cases have been described. The disorder is lethal within several years.

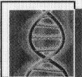

PATHOGENESIS: MLD is caused by a deficiency in the activity of arylsulfatase A, a lysosomal enzyme involved in the degradation of myelin sulfatides. Accordingly, there is progressive accumulation of sulfatides within the lysosomes of myelin-forming Schwann cells and oligodendrocytes.

PATHOLOGY: In MLD, the accumulated sulfatides form cytoplasmic spherical granules, 15 to 20 μm in diameter, which stain metachromatically with cresyl violet and toluidine blue. The brain shows diffuse myelin loss (Fig. 28-65), accumulation of metachromatic material in white

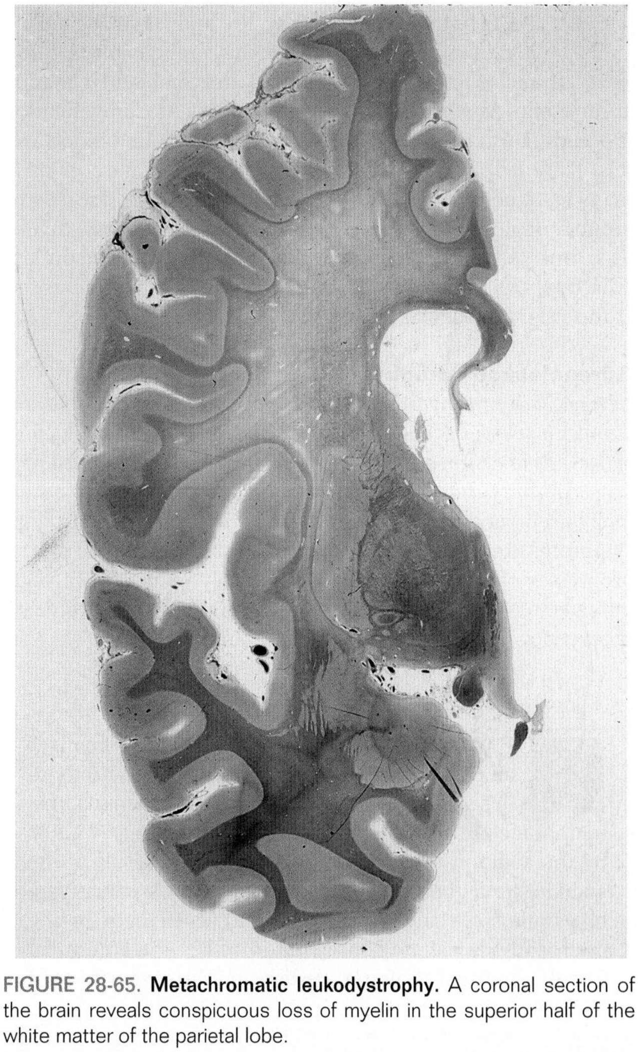

FIGURE 28-65. **Metachromatic leukodystrophy.** A coronal section of the brain reveals conspicuous loss of myelin in the superior half of the white matter of the parietal lobe.

matter, and prominent astrogliosis. Demyelination of peripheral nerves is less severe.

Krabbe Disease

Krabbe disease is a rapidly progressive, invariably fatal, autosomal recessive neurologic disorder caused by a deficiency of galactocerebroside β-galactosidase. The condition appears in young infants and is defined by the presence of perivascular aggregates of mononuclear and multinucleated "globoid cells" in the white matter, hence the alternative name **globoid cell leukodystrophy.** The globoid cells are macrophages that contain undigested galactocerebroside (galactosylceramide).

Krabbe disease appears in the early months of life and progresses to death within 1 to 2 years. Severe motor, sensory, and cognitive impairments reflect the diffuse involvement of the nervous system.

PATHOGENESIS: The brains of patients with Krabbe disease show almost complete loss of oligodendroglia and myelin. It has been hypothesized that the enzyme deficiency results in toxic, alternative metabolites that destroy oligodendroglia, thereby producing demyelination.

PATHOLOGY: At autopsy, the brain is small, and the loss of myelin is diffuse, but the cerebral cortex is normal. Marbled areas of partial and total demyelination are present. Astrogliosis is typically severe. As demyelination proceeds, clusters of globoid cells are found around blood vessels. These cells measure up to 50 μm in diameter and contain as many as 20 peripherally located nuclei. In end-stage disease, the number of globoid cells decreases, and in areas of severe myelin loss, only scattered globoid cells remain. By electron microscopy, the globoid cells contain crystalloid-like inclusions with straight or tubular profiles.

Adrenoleukodystrophy

Adrenoleukodystrophy (ALD) refers to an X-linked (Xq28), inherited disorder in which dysfunction of the adrenal cortex and demyelination of the nervous system are associated with high levels of saturated very-long-chain fatty acids (VLCFAs) in tissue and body fluids. ALD occurs in children between the ages of 3 and 10 years, and neurologic symptoms precede the signs of adrenal insufficiency. The disease progresses rapidly, and the body is quickly reduced to a vegetative state, which may persist for several years before death supervenes.

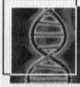

PATHOGENESIS: The cause of ALD involves an enzyme mutation that impairs the capacity to degrade VLCFAs. A defect in the peroxisomal membrane prevents the normal activation of free VLCFAs by the addition of coenzyme A (CoA). As a result of the inability to degrade VLCFAs, these fatty acids accumulate in gangliosides and myelin. Pathologic changes in the brain and adrenal are considered to reflect the accumulation of abnormal cholesterol esters and the toxic effects of VLCFAs.

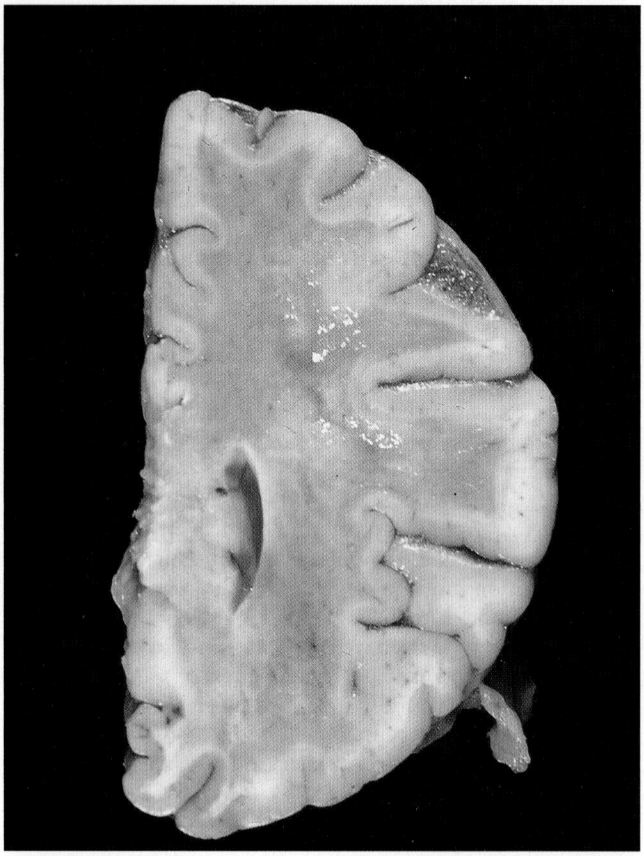

FIGURE 28-66. **Adrenoleukodystrophy.** A coronal section of the brain discloses extensive degenerative changes throughout the white matter.

PATHOLOGY: ALD is characterized in brain by confluent, bilaterally symmetric demyelination (Fig. 28-66). The most severe lesions are in the subcortical white matter of the parietooccipital region, which then extend rostrally (while sparing cortex) to result in a severe loss of myelinated axons and oligodendrocytes. Gliosis and perivascular infiltrates of mononuclear cells (mostly lymphocytes) are prominent in affected areas. Scattered macrophages contain periodic acid-Schiff (PAS)-positive and sudanophilic material. Peripheral nerves are affected, but less so than the brain. The adrenals are atrophic, and electron microscopy of cortical cells reveals pathognomonic cytoplasmic, membrane-bound, curvilinear inclusions or clefts (lamellae) containing VLCFAs. Similar inclusions occur in Schwann cells and CNS macrophages.

Alexander Disease

Alexander disease is a rare neurologic disorder of infants, children and rarely adults, that is characterized by a loss of myelin in the brain and a striking accumulation of irregular, extracellular fibers (**Rosenthal fibers;** Fig. 28-67). Clinically, children have psychomotor retardation, progressive dementia, and paralysis, and eventually die.

PATHOGENESIS: The disease is caused by mutations in the gene encoding GFAP, which leads to aggregates of fibrous structures, known as Rosenthal fibers, in astrocytes. It is not yet clear how this process impairs myelin formation and induces degeneration of oligodendrocytes and myelin.

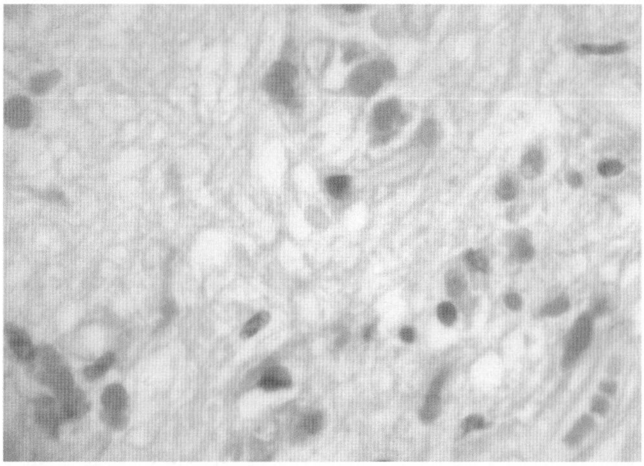

FIGURE 28-67. **Alexander disease.** The astrocytes contain deeply eosinophilic Rosenthal fibers.

PATHOLOGY: Alexander disease features the presence of abundant Rosenthal fibers (GFAP filaments with associated protein chaperones, e.g., α-B-crystallin). These irregular, beaded and fibrous lesions are deposited in the subpial regions of brain and spinal cord as well as the white matter, especially around blood vessels, where astrocyte end feet terminate. The content of myelin in the white matter is strikingly deficient. Interestingly, myelin is well preserved in the peripheral nerves, where Schwann cells express little or no GFAP.

Multiple Sclerosis Features Patches of Demyelination throughout the White Matter

Multiple sclerosis (MS) is a chronic demyelinating disease that is the most common chronic CNS disease of young adults in the United States, with a prevalence of 1 per 1000. The disorder affects sensory and motor functions and is characterized by exacerbations and remissions over many years. MS is acquired at a mean age of 30 years, with women afflicted almost twice as often as men.

PATHOGENESIS: The etiology of MS remains obscure, but experimental and clinical studies point to a genetic predisposition to MS and an immune pathogenesis. MS is principally a disease of temperate climates. Persons who emigrate before the age of 15 years from areas with a low prevalence of MS to more temperate endemic areas acquire an increased risk of developing disease, suggesting that environmental factors generate susceptibility to the disease.

GENETIC FACTORS: A genetic predisposition to MS is suggested by familial aggregation of the disease, an increased risk in second- and third-degree relatives of MS patients, and a 25% concordance for MS in monozygotic twins. Susceptibility is also linked to a number of major histocompatibility complex (MHC) alleles (e.g., HLA-DR2), thereby implying that immune mechanisms are involved in the pathogenesis. Indeed, siblings with MS may share the same T-cell receptor haplotype.

IMMUNE FACTORS: The evidence supporting a role for immune mechanisms in MS also comes from the microscopic appearance of the lesions. For example, chronic MS lesions demonstrate perivascular lymphocytes, macrophages, and numerous CD4+ (helper-inducer subset), as well as CD8+ T cells. Moreover, the CD4+ T cells isolated from the CSF of MS patients appear to be oligoclonal. Although the target antigen has not been identified, the data suggest an immune response to a specific protein of the CNS. Further support for immune mechanisms comes from the experimental production of an antigen-specific, T cell-mediated, autoimmune disease, termed **experimental allergic encephalitis (EAE).** Injection of myelin basic protein into experimental animals, including nonhuman primates, elicits a demyelinating disorder that is similar to MS, although unlike MS, EAE is a monophasic illness.

INFECTIOUS AGENTS: An assortment of viruses have been implicated in the etiology of MS, including vaccinia, mumps, rubella, herpes simplex, and measles. However, to date no direct evidence exists for the involvement of any infectious agent.

PATHOLOGY: *The demyelinated plaque is the hallmark of MS* (Fig. 28-68 and Fig. 28-69). Plaques, rarely more than 2 cm in diameter, accumulate in great numbers in the brain and spinal cord. They are discrete, with smoothly rounded contours, and are usually in white matter, although they occasionally breach the gray–white junction. The lesions exhibit a preference for the optic nerves, chiasm, and paraventricular white matter, although the CNS distribution of MS plaques is highly random. Plaques are also frequent in the spinal cord.

The evolving plaque is marked by the following morphologic hallmarks:

- Selective loss of myelin in a region of reactive axonal preservation
- A few lymphocytes that cluster about small veins and arteries
- An influx of macrophages
- Considerable edema

When neurons are within the boundaries of a plaque, the neuronal cell bodies are remarkably spared, but the same is not true of axons, which may degenerate. The number of oligodendrocytes is moderately diminished, and as the plaque ages, it becomes more discrete and less edematous. This sequence serves to emphasize the focal nature of the injury, its selectivity, and its

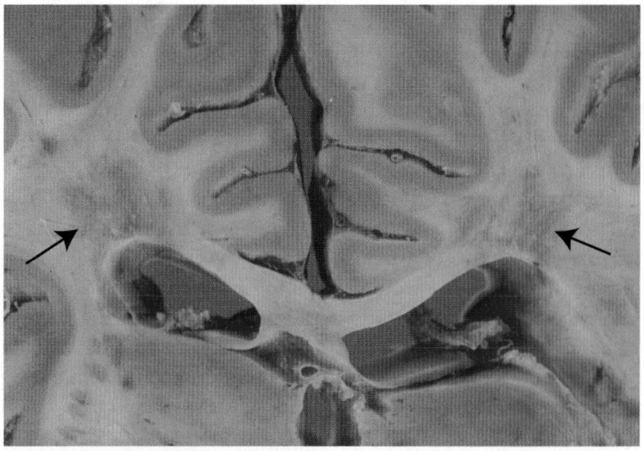

FIGURE 28-68. **Multiple sclerosis.** A coronal section of the brain shows periventricular plaques (darker areas) in the white matter (*arrows*).

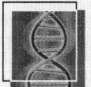

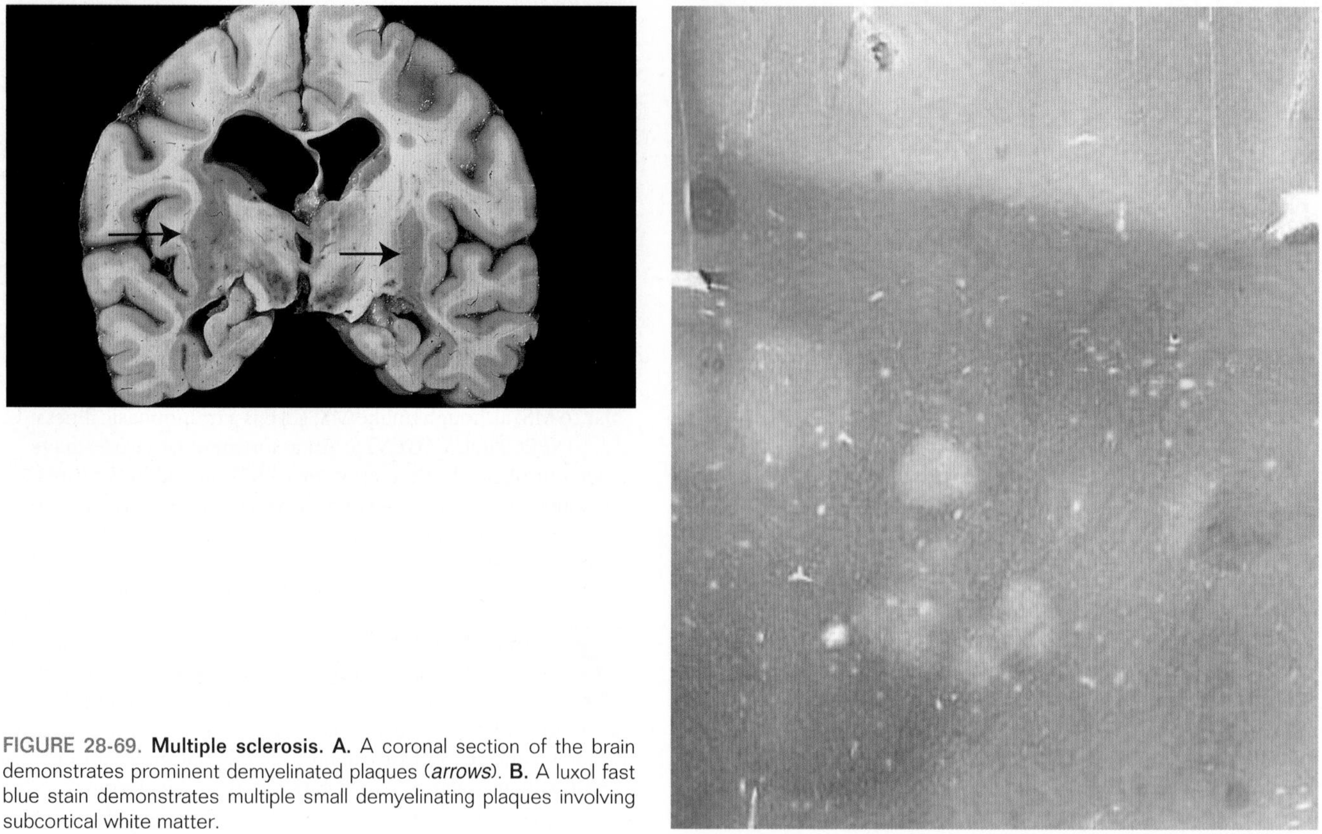
A
B

FIGURE 28-69. **Multiple sclerosis. A.** A coronal section of the brain demonstrates prominent demyelinated plaques (*arrows*). **B.** A luxol fast blue stain demonstrates multiple small demyelinating plaques involving subcortical white matter.

severity, because demyelination is total within the area of the plaque. Characteristically, axons in the plaques lose their myelin abruptly. Old MS plaques are dense and exhibit gliosis. This "scar" impairs the structural integrity of the axons.

CLINICAL FEATURES: MS usually has its onset during the third or fourth decades and is punctuated thereafter by abrupt and brief episodes of clinical progression, interspersed with periods of relative stability. However, some patients with MS suffer a relentless course without any remissions. Each exacerbation reflects the formation of additional demyelinated MS plaques. The visual system and the paraventricular areas are particularly vulnerable to the disease, whereas the peripheral nerves are uniformly spared. MS typically begins with symptoms relating to lesions in the optic nerves, brainstem, or spinal cord. Blurred vision or the loss of vision in one eye is often the presenting complaint. When the initial lesion is in the brainstem, the early symptoms are double vision and vertigo. Plaques within the spinal cord produce weakness of one or both legs and sensory symptoms in the form of numbness in the lower extremities. Many of the initial symptoms are partially reversible within a few months.

Unfortunately, in most patients with MS, the disease follows a chronic relapsing and remitting course, with development of permanent lesions. In established cases, the degree of functional impairment is highly variable, ranging from minor disability to severe incapacity, with widespread paralysis, dysarthria, severe visual defects, incontinence, and dementia. The patients usually die of respiratory paralysis or urinary tract infections while they are in terminal coma. Most patients with MS survive 20 to 30 years after the onset of symptoms. In some patients, treatment with interferon-β has been reported to be helpful.

Postinfectious and Postvaccinal Encephalomyelitis Are Immune Responses to Viral Antigens

Some viral exanthems (e.g., measles, varicella, rubella) are in rare instances followed about 3 to 21 days after the rash by an encephalomyelitis. The disease is characterized by focal perivascular demyelination and conspicuous mononuclear cell infiltrates around small to medium-sized venules in the white matter of the brain and spinal cord. This disorder is suspected to be immune-mediated, but the precise pathogenesis remains unclear.

In children, postinfectious encephalomyelitis is heralded by the sudden onset of headache, vomiting, fever, and meningeal signs. In severe cases, these symptoms may be followed by paraplegia, incontinence, and stupor, and 15% to 20% of patients die. A similar syndrome termed **postvaccinal encephalomyelitis,** may follow immunization against infectious agents (e.g., smallpox, rabies) (Fig. 28-70). The use of more-purified vaccines that are free of cross-reacting antigenic contaminants has nearly eliminated this complication.

Central Pontine Myelinolysis Occurs in Alcoholics

Central pontine myelinolysis is a rare demyelinating disorder that affects the pons. Discrete areas of selective demyelination occur in the pons (Fig. 28-71), although the lesions often are too small to have clinical manifestations and are discovered only at autopsy. In a few patients, quadriparesis, pseudobulbar palsy, or severe depression of consciousness ("pseudocoma") may occur. Central pontine myelinolysis is thought to arise from overly rapid correction of hyponatremia in alcoholics, malnourished persons, or individuals with marked electrolyte instability including persons with renal failure and liver transplant recipients.

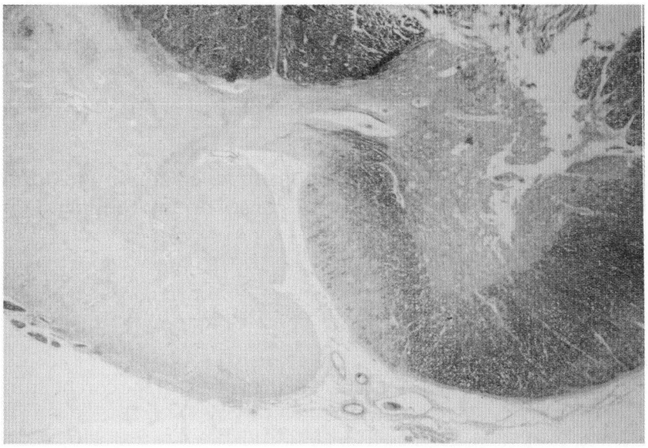

FIGURE 28-70. **Postvaccination myelitis. Luxol fast blue stain demonstrates loss of myelin in the left ventro-lateral spinal cord white matter.**

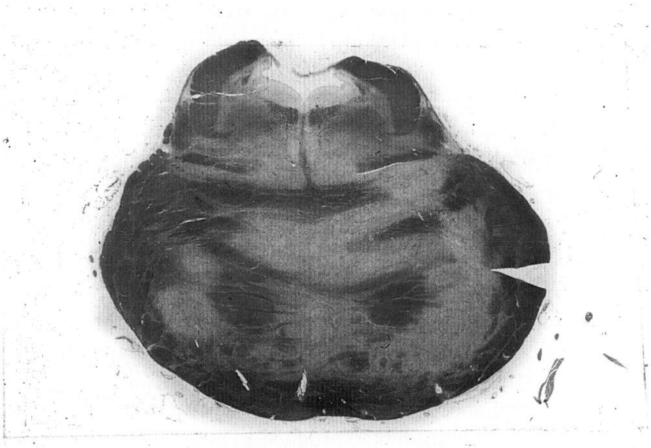

FIGURE 28-71. **Central pontine myelinolysis.** A luxol fast blue stain reveals extensive demyelination in the pons.

Neuronal Storage Diseases

Neuronal storage diseases are inherited enzyme deficiencies that result in the accumulation of normal metabolic products within lysosomes. These disorders are discussed in detail in Chapter 6, and only the highlights of the neurological manifestations are presented here.

Tay-Sachs Disease Reflects the Neuronal Accumulation of a Ganglioside

Tay-Sachs disease (amaurotic familial idiocy) is a lethal, autosomal recessive disorder caused by an inborn deficiency of hexosaminidase A, which permits the accumulation of ganglioside in CNS neurons. The disease is fatal in infancy and early childhood. Retinal involvement increases macular transparency and is responsible for a **cherry-red spot** in the macula.

The brain is the major site of storage of gangliosides, and progressively enlarges during infancy. On histologic examination, lipid droplets are seen in the cytoplasm of distended nerve cells of the CNS and peripheral nervous system (Fig. 28-72A). Electron microscopy reveals the lipid within lysosomes in the form of whorled "myelin figures" (see Fig. 28-72B). The neural tissues respond with a diffuse astrogliosis. An affected infant appears normal at birth but shows a delay in motor development by age 6 months. Thereafter, progressive deterioration leads to flaccid weakness, blindness, and severe mental impairment. Death usually supervenes before the end of the second year.

Hurler Syndrome Represents Storage of Mucopolysaccharides

Hurler syndrome is an autosomal recessive disturbance in glycosaminoglycan metabolism that results in the intraneuronal accumulation of mucopolysaccharides. The clinical variants of this syndrome are distinguished by variable involvement of visceral organs and the nervous system. The disease is typically expressed in infancy or early childhood as dwarfism, corneal opacities, skeletal deformities, and hepatosplenomegaly. The intraneuronal storage distends the cytoplasmic compartment and is accompanied by astrogliosis and progressive mental deterioration.

Gaucher Disease Features the Deposition of Glucocerebrosides

Gaucher disease is an autosomal recessive genetic disorder characterized by a deficiency of glucocerebrosidase and the accumulation of glucocerebroside, principally in macrophages. The CNS is most severely

A

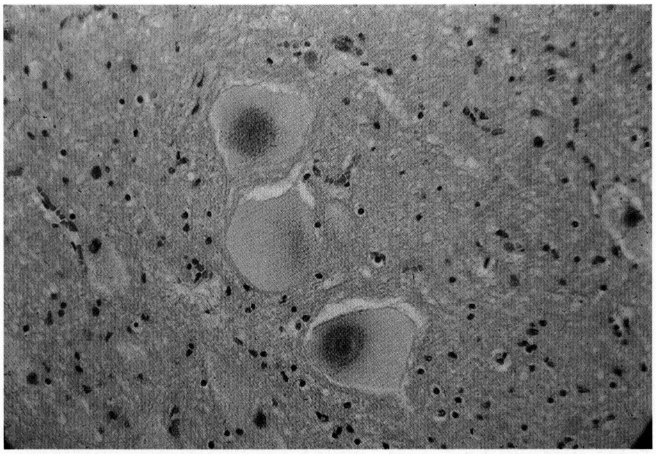

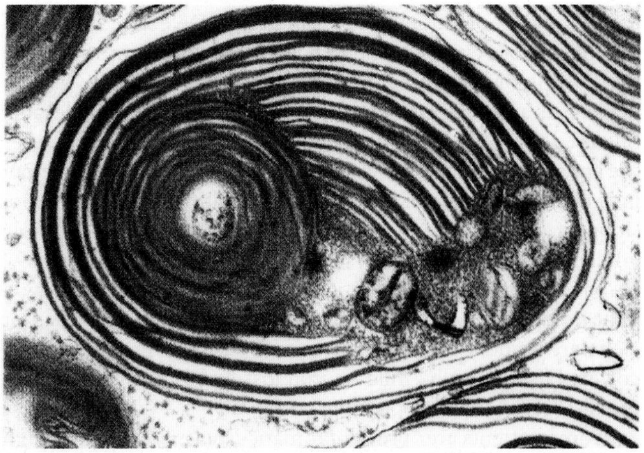

B

FIGURE 28-72. **Tay-Sachs disease. A.** The cytoplasm of neurons is distended by the accumulation of eosinophilic material. **B.** Electron microscopy reveals whorled "myelin bodies," which represent accumulated ganglioside.

involved in the infantile type (type II) of Gaucher disease. Although intraneuronal accumulation of glucocerebroside is not conspicuous, neuronal loss is severe and is accompanied by diffuse astrogliosis. These infants fail to thrive and die at an early age.

Niemann-Pick Disease Displays the Accumulation of Sphingomyelin

Niemann-Pick disease is an autosomal recessive disorder in which intraneuronal storage of sphingomyelin results from a deficiency of sphingomyelinase. The clinical symptoms occur early, and the disease is marked by failure of the infant to develop and thrive. The mononuclear phagocyte system is targeted for storage, but the nervous system may predominate symptomatically during infancy. The brain becomes atrophic and shows marked astrogliosis. Retinal degeneration may produce a cherry-red spot, similar to that in Tay-Sachs disease.

Metabolic Neuronal Diseases

Phenylketonuria Leads to Retention of Phenylalanine

Phenylketonuria (PKU) is an autosomal recessive disorder caused by a deficiency in phenylalanine hydroxylase (see Chapter 6). Phenylalanine accumulates in the blood and tissues because conversion of phenylalanine to tyrosine is blocked. The condition becomes apparent in the early months of life and leads to mental retardation, seizures, and impaired physical development. Untreated patients rarely obtain an intelligent quotient (IQ) above 50. Although there are no consistent alterations, the brain may be underweight and deficient in myelination.

Cretinism Reflects Infantile Hypothyroidism

Severe hypothyroidism in infancy, termed **cretinism,** alters the functional capacity of the CNS. The disorder is reversible by the early administration of thyroxine, but when untreated, clinical disease emerges. The brain acquires a near-normal weight, has appropriate neuronal cytoarchitecture, and is well myelinated. However, stunted growth and cognitive impairments become evident.

Wilson Disease May Exhibit Excess Copper in the Brain

Wilson disease, an autosomal recessive disease, is an inherited disorder of copper metabolism caused by mutations of the *WD* gene that affects brain and the liver; thus the synonym "hepatolenticular degeneration" (see Chapter 14). Defective biliary excretion of copper favors the deposition of copper in the brain. Symptoms of cerebral intoxication appear clinically, as evidenced in athetoid movements, usually in the second decade, but as late as the eighth (recent findings). Before, during, or after the appearance of neurologic symptoms, an insidiously developing cirrhosis of the liver may result in hepatic failure. The deposition of copper in the limbus of the cornea produces a visible golden-brown band, the **Kayser-Fleischer ring** (see Chapter 29).

Macroscopically, the lenticular nuclei of the brain show a light golden discoloration, and in 25% of cases, small cysts or clefts are evident in the putamen or in deep layers of the neocortex. Histologically, mild neuron loss and gliosis characterize the disease.

Some patients are "presymptomatic," never developing high enough levels of copper to accumulate in the brain or eyes or developing cirrhosis of the liver.

Metabolic Disorders

Alcoholism Is Associated with Several CNS Manifestations

The problems caused by alcoholism reflect poor nutrition and intoxication. Four cerebral lesions warrant consideration (Fig. 28-73):

- Wernicke syndrome
- Central pontine myelinolysis (see Fig. 28-71)
- Cortical atrophy
- Atrophy of the superior aspect of the vermis of the cerebellum

Wernicke Syndrome

Wernicke syndrome is secondary to thiamine (vitamin B_1) deficiency and is characterized clinically by the rapid onset of a disturbance in thermal regulation, altered consciousness, ophthalmoplegia, and nystagmus, and pathologically by lesions in the hypothalamus and mamillary bodies, the periaqueductal regions of the midbrain, and the tegmentum of the pons (Fig. 28-74). The syndrome arises most commonly in association with chronic alcoholism, although it may appear in patients whose nutrition is sustained by infusions that lack thiamine.

Wernicke syndrome may progress rapidly to death, but it is reversed by the administration of thiamine. In fatal cases, petechiae occur around capillaries in the mamillary bodies, hypothalamus, periaqueductal region, and the floor of the fourth ventricle. Over time, hemosiderin deposition identifies regions where petechiae occurred. Neurons and myelin are spared, but the mamillary bodies atrophy.

Wernicke-Korsakoff syndrome refers to a state of disordered recent memory often compensated for by confabulation. The histologic changes are distinguished from those of Wernicke syndrome by degeneration of neurons in the medial–dorsal nucleus of the thalamus. Thus, Wernicke syndrome and Korsakoff

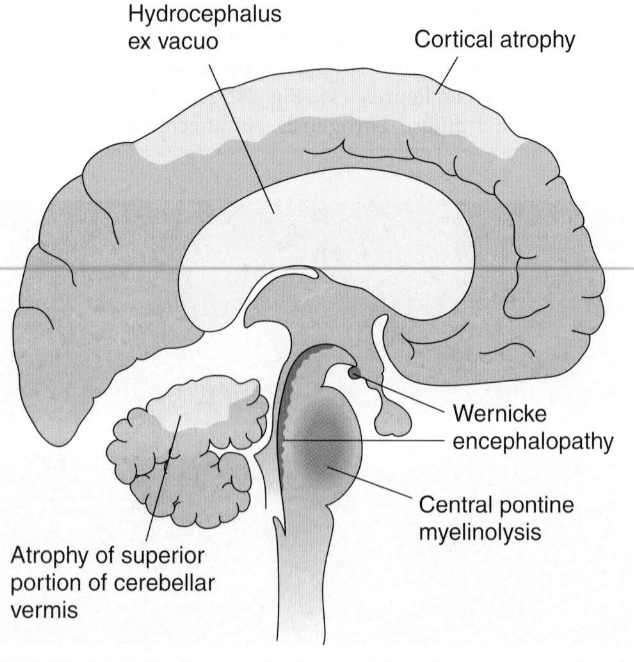

FIGURE 28-73. **Regions of the brain with lesions associated with chronic alcoholism.**

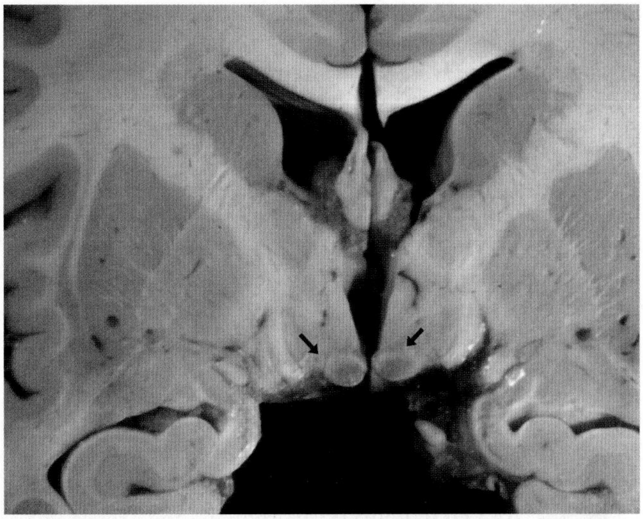

FIGURE 28-74. **Wernicke encephalopathy.** A coronal section of the brain discloses brown discoloration of the mamillary bodies (*arrows*).

psychosis occur concurrently in chronic alcoholism, but their causes may be different.

Many chronic alcoholics display cerebral atrophy, but the cause of this is not entirely clear, and the relative roles of alcohol toxicity, malnutrition, and other factors remain to be defined. Similar uncertainties prevail with regard to the atrophy of the Purkinje and granular cells of the cerebellum. These alterations are the most common corollary of chronic alcoholism and are ostensibly the cause of truncal ataxia, which persists during periods of sobriety. As noted above, central pontine myelinolysis is an iatrogenic complication caused by the rapid correction of hyponatremia.

Hepatic Encephalopathy Occurs in End-Stage Liver Disease

Hepatic encephalopathy is a common clinical expression of liver failure, manifested as delirium, seizures, and coma (see Chapter 14). In general, the clinical symptoms greatly exceed their morphologic correlates, which are restricted to the appearance of altered astroglia (termed **Alzheimer type II astrocytes**), which show enlarged nuclei and marginated chromatin, especially in the thalamus.

Subacute Combined Degeneration of the Spinal Cord Is a Complication of Pernicious Anemia

Subacute combined degeneration of the spinal cord results from a lack of vitamin B_{12} (pernicious anemia) and leads to lesions in the posterolateral portions of the spinal cord (see Chapters 14 and 20). Initially, there is symmetric myelin and axonal loss at the thoracic level of the spinal cord. Astrogliosis is mild in the acute lesions, but with time, the affected spinal cord exhibit gliosis and atrophy, especially in the posterolateral areas of the cord. A burning sensation in the soles of the feet and other paresthesias herald the onset of this rapidly progressive and poorly reversible neurologic disorder. Weakness emerges in all four limbs, followed by defective postural sensibility, incoordination, and ataxia. In addition to pernicious anemia, subacute combined degeneration may complicate a rare case of extensive gastric resection and other malabsorption syndromes. Because vitamin B_{12} is not found in plants, some extreme vegetarians who eschew all animal products, even milk and eggs, have developed subacute combined degeneration after many years on the restricted diet.

Neurodegenerative Diseases

This heterogeneous group of neurodegenerative diseases includes Parkinson disease, ALS, Huntington disease, the spinocerebellar ataxias, Alzheimer disease, and several other less common disorders. Some of these conditions primarily involve specific neuroanatomic systems (Parkinson and Huntington disease, ALS) or wider regions of the nervous system (Alzheimer disease). However, emerging data now implicate a number of different abnormal proteins that form aggregates with the properties of amyloid (congophilic and fibrillar, with a β-pleated sheet structure). The deposition of amyloid is a common factor in the onset and progression of many sporadic and hereditary neurodegenerative disorders, as summarized in Table 28-3.

For example, neurofibrillary tangles (NFTs) containing tau plus senile plaques amyloid-β (A-β) define Alzheimer disease. Lewy bodies are formed by α-synuclein fibrils and are signatures of Parkinson disease. As noted above, abnormal prions form amyloid deposits. Thus, growing evidence provides a mechanistic link

TABLE 28-3

Representative Neurodegenerative Diseases with Filamentous Amyloid Lesions

Disease	Lesion	Components	Location
Alzheimer disease	Senile plaques Neurofibrillary tangles	β-Amyloid tau	Extracellular Intracytoplasmic
Amyotrophic lateral sclerosis	Spheroids	Neurofilament subunits/superoxide dismutase (SOD-1)	Intracytoplasmic
Dementia with Lewy bodies	Lewy bodies	α-Synuclein	Intracytoplasmic
Frontotemporal dementias	Neurofibrillary tangles	tau	Intracytoplasmic
Multiple system atrophy	Glial inclusions	tau	Intracytoplasmic
Parkinson disease	Lewy bodies	α-Synuclein	Intracytoplasmic
Prion diseases	Prion deposits	Prions	Extracellular
Trinucleotide repeat diseases	Inclusions	Polyglutamine tracts	Intranuclear and cytoplasmic

between the filamentous aggregates of amyloid deposits in the CNS and the degeneration of affected brain regions in neurodegenerative disorders. Inexplicably, almost all of these neurodegenerative disorders share an enigmatic symmetry. Missense mutations in the gene encoding the disease protein cause an early onset and highly aggressive familial disorder as well as the hallmark brain lesions of the disease. However, the same brain lesions also characterize the corresponding wild-type protein in sporadic variants of these conditions. Notably, many of the familial forms of these diseases are autosomal dominant, which means that the bearer of a mutation will develop the disease if he lives to the age of disease onset, and that there are few, if any, "escapees."

It is not clear how filamentous protein aggregates cause disease. It could result from sequestration of the disease protein or other macromolecules and organelles into the aggregates, thereby rendering them unavailable to perform their normal functions. Although aggregation of the disease protein could be a protective response initially, as the aggregates enlarge, they might physically occlude axons and dendrites or block the movement of material within the cytoplasm of affected cells. In view of parallels between the brain amyloidoses in many of these neurodegenerative disorders, clarification of this mysterious symmetry in one disease could have a significant impact on understanding mechanisms underlying all of these disorders (Fig. 28-75).

Alzheimer Disease Is the Principal Cause of So-Called Senility

Alzheimer disease is an insidious and progressive neurologic disorder characterized clinically by loss of memory, cognitive impairment, and eventual dementia and pathologically by Aβ-containing senile plaques and neurofibrillary tangles formed by tau filaments. Although Alzheimer's original patients were restricted to patients younger than 65 of age and were said to suffer "presenile dementia," the term **Alzheimer disease** now refers to dementias that display characteristic pathological changes.

EPIDEMIOLOGY: Although Alzheimer disease is a worldwide disease, its distribution has been best studied in Western countries. *It is the most common cause of dementia in the elderly, accounting for more than half of all cases.* The prevalence of the condition is closely related to age. Before age 65 years, the prevalence of Alzheimer disease is at most 1% to 2%, whereas it is 40% or more after age 85 years. Women are affected twice as often as men. Most cases of Alzheimer disease are sporadic, but a familial variant is recognized.

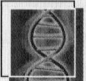

PATHOGENESIS: Although the cause of Alzheimer disease has not been fully elucidated, there have been significant advances in our understanding of the origin of both Alzheimer disease-associated amyloid and NFTs.

AMYLOID β-PROTEIN (Aβ): Increasing evidence points to the importance of the deposition of Aβ protein in the neuritic plaques of Alzheimer disease (see Chapter 23). These plaques are located in areas of the cerebral cortex that are linked to intellectual function and are a constant feature of Alzheimer disease. However, there are examples of cognitively intact elderly persons whose brains displayed

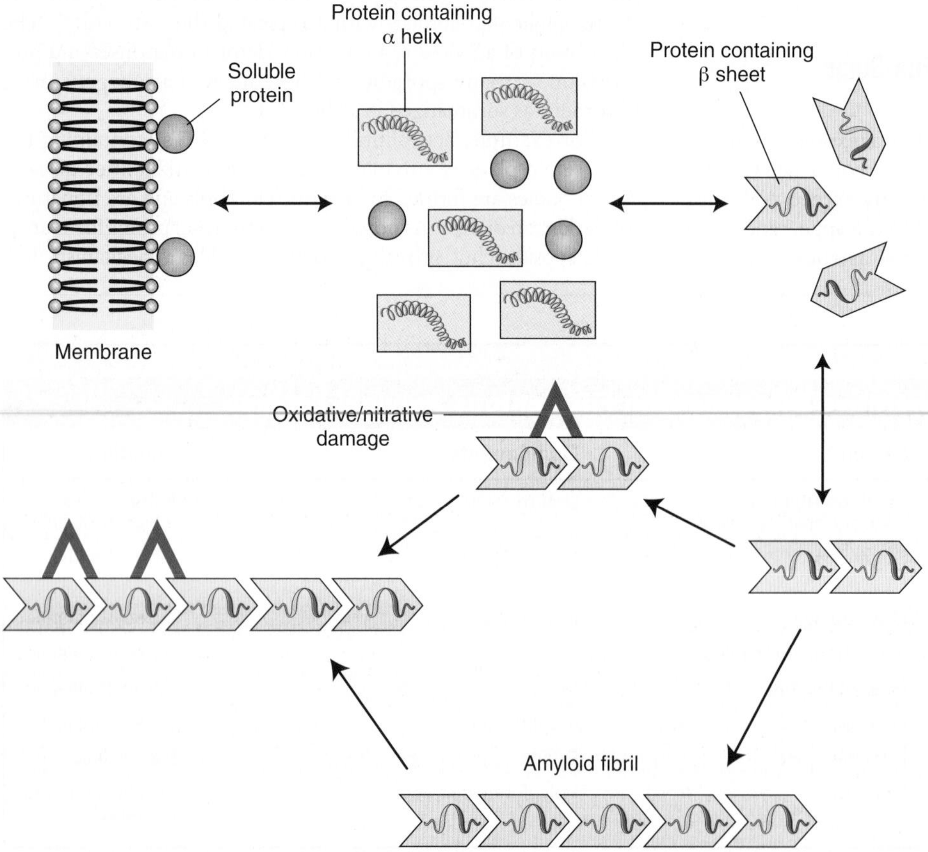

FIGURE 28-75. **Filamentous protein aggregates: Targets of novel therapies for CNS neurodegenerative diseases.** The schematic depicts the stepwise conversion of normal soluble proteins that either lack secondary structure *(orange balls)* or have an α-helical secondary structure *(blue boxes)*. They may interact normally with other structures such as organelle membranes *(box at the upper left)*. Spontaneously or due to mutations, the proteins can adopt a β-sheet structure *(unconnected arrowheads)*, which is reversible. However, if the proteins go on to form dimers, trimers, tetramers, and so forth, then they assemble into amyloid fibrils *(connected arrowheads)*. This process also may be driven by posttranslational modifications such as oxidative/nitrative damage *(red carats)*. These changes may act in several ways to promote fibrillogenesis, including cross-linking proteins or inducing conformational changes that stabilize the protein polymers into fibrils, thereby promoting formation of amyloid deposits, senile plaques, neurofibrillary tangles, Lewy bodies, glial cytoplasmic inclusions, and prion amyloid lesions.

the same burden of senile plaques as is seen in Alzheimer disease, thereby raising questions about whether or not it is the extracellular senile plaques or some intracellular process involving Aβ metabolism that compromises neuronal function in Alzheimer disease. The core of these plaques contains a distinct form of Aβ peptide, which is predominantly 42 amino acids in length. Aβ is derived by proteolysis from a much larger (695 amino acids) membrane-spanning amyloid precursor protein (APP). Full-length APP has an extracellular region, a transmembrane sequence, and a cytoplasmic domain. The region comprising Aβ serves to anchor the amino-terminal portion of APP to the membrane. The physiologic functions of APP and Aβ remain obscure.

The normal degradation of APP involves a proteolytic cleavage in the middle of the Aβ domain, with the release of a fragment extending from the middle of the Aβ domain to the amino terminus of APP. This fragment is not amyloidogenic. Proteolysis at either end of the Aβ domain then releases intact and highly amyloidogenic Aβ that accumulates in senile plaques as amyloid fibrils.

The deposition of Aβ appears to be necessary but not sufficient for the pathogenesis of Alzheimer disease because of the following considerations:

- Patients with **Down syndrome** (trisomy 21) develop the clinical and histopathologic features of Alzheimer disease, including deposition of Aβ in neuritic plaques, generally by age 40 years. The gene for APP is located on chromosome 21, and the additional dose of the gene product in trisomy 21 may predispose to precocious accumulation of Aβ.
- Some patients with the familial form of Alzheimer disease carry mutant APP genes or mutant presenilin genes. These mutations lead to increased production of Aβ, the amyloidogenic fragment of APP.
- Transgenic mice expressing mutant human APP genes develop senile plaques in the brain that are very similar to those of Alzheimer disease. However, these mice lack other critical features of Alzheimer disease such as NFTs and evidence of neurodegeneration, such as significant loss of neurons.

Neurons and glial cells are sites of APP synthesis in the brain, but Aβ also accumulates in the walls of cerebral blood vessels (Fig. 28-76).

NEUROFIBRILLARY TANGLES: NFTs are composed of paired helical filaments that consist of an abnormal form of a MAP termed **tau.** In Alzheimer disease, the phosphorylation of tau at aberrant sites results in a protein that does not associate with microtubules but instead aggregates in the form of paired helical filaments. The release of tau from microtubules deprives cells of its microtubule stabilizing effects, thereby impairing axonal transport and compromising neuronal function. Indeed, mutations in the *tau* gene on chromosome 17 cause familial frontotemporal dementia with parkinsonism. Interestingly, transgenic mouse models that over-express mutant or wild-type tau develop a neurodegenerative phenotype, with neuron loss and defective axonal transport.

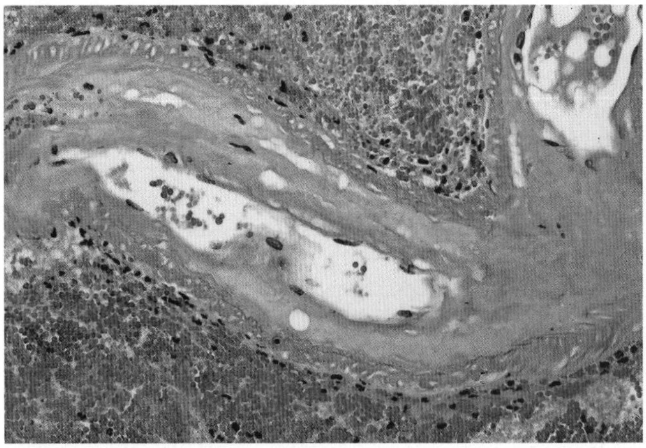

FIGURE 28-76. **Cerebral amyeloid angiopathy.** A section of cerebral cortex from a patient with Alzheimer disease demonstrates vascular deposition of amyloid (hematoxylin and eosin).

Remarkably, most cases of Alzheimer disease are also associated with abundant Lewy bodies. Thus Alzheimer disease features a "triple" brain amyloidosis, owing to accumulations of filamentous tau, Aβ, and α-synuclein.

GENETIC FACTORS: As mentioned above, mutations of the *APP* gene have been associated with certain early-onset familial variants of Alzheimer disease. Additional genetic associations (Table 28-4) involve the apolipoprotein E (apoE) genotype and the genes for PS-1 and PS-2.

APOLIPOPROTEIN E: ApoE has long been known for its role in cholesterol metabolism. Its relevance to dementia was uncovered in 1993, when it was reported that specific apoE alleles are susceptibility factors for sporadic and late-onset familial subtypes of Alzheimer disease. The human apoE gene is found on chromosome 19 (19q13.2). The

TABLE 28-4

Genetic Factors in Alzheimer Disease

Gene	Chromosome	Disease Association
Amyloid precursor protein (*APP*)	21	Mutations of the *APP* gene are associated with early-onset familial Alzheimer disease
Presenilin 1 (*PS1*)	14	Mutations of the *PS1* gene are associated with early-onset familial Alzheimer diseaseAD
Presenilin 2 (*PS2*)	1	Mutations of the *PS2* gene are associated with Volga German familial Alzheimer diseaseAD
Apolipoprotein E (*apoE*)	19	Presence of the ε4 allele is associated with increased risk and younger age of onset of both inherited and sporadic forms of late-onset Alzheimer disease

three common alleles–ϵ2, ϵ3, and ϵ4–all occur in North American apoE genotypes. An increased risk of late-onset familial and sporadic AD is associated with inheritance of the ϵ4 allele, particularly the homozygous ϵ4/ϵ4 genotype, which occurs in 2% of the population. Conversely, the ϵ2 allele may confer some protection. The age at which symptoms appear in late-onset Alzheimer disease also correlates with the ϵ4 allele; ϵ4/ϵ4 homozygotes exhibit the earliest age at onset (<70 years), whereas patients with the ϵ2 allele experience the latest onset (>90 years). The presence of the ϵ4 allele has also been correlated with an increased number of senile plaques in patients with Alzheimer disease, but the apoE genotype is not an absolute determinant of the disease and cannot be used to predict who will develop it. The mechanisms whereby these different apoE alleles influence the risk of Alzheimer disease remain poorly understood.

PRESENILIN: Two genes with significant homology are associated with different kindreds of familial Alzheimer disease. Mutations of the *PS1* gene located on chromosome 14, are associated with the most common form of autosomal dominant early-onset Alzheimer disease. The *PS2* gene resides on chromosome 1 and is associated with Alzheimer disease in Volga German pedigrees (see Table 28-4). Importantly, presenilin mutations occur in half of all inherited Alzheimer disease, compared with only a few percent for mutant *APP* genes. Both presenilin genes code for proteins characterized by multiple transmembrane domains. There is some evidence to suggest that PS1 and PS2 mutant proteins alter the processing of β-APP, thereby favoring increased production and deposition of Aβ. Cellular processing of APP releases Aβ fragments of varying lengths, but the Aβ42 variant (see above) appears to be particularly amyloidogenic. It is the Aβ molecule whose production is enhanced by mutant *PS1*.

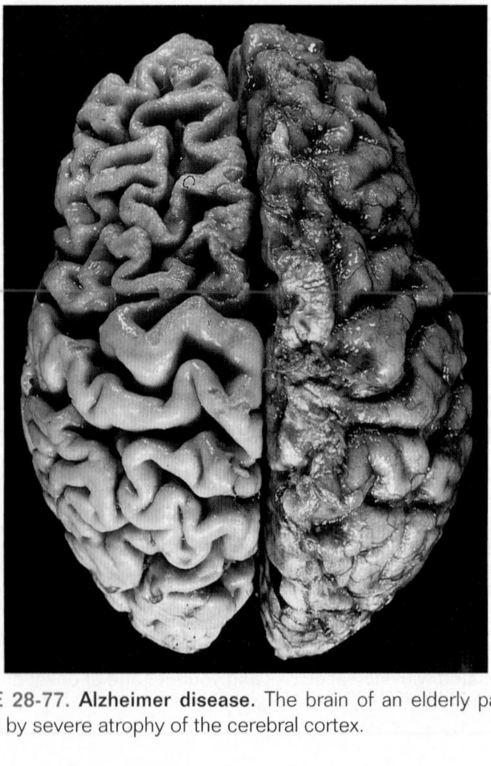

FIGURE 28-77. **Alzheimer disease.** The brain of an elderly patient is afflicted by severe atrophy of the cerebral cortex.

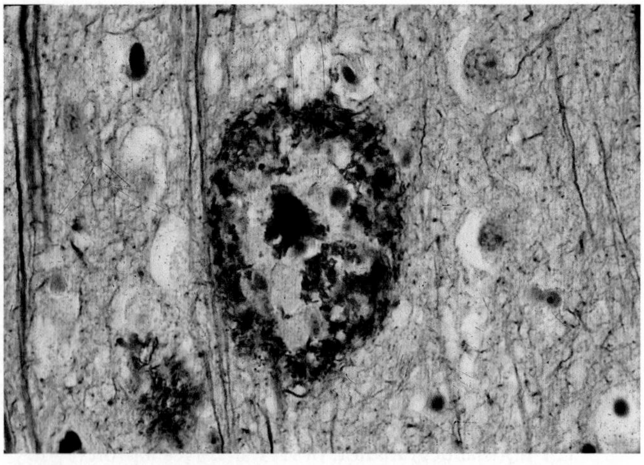

FIGURE 28-78. **Alzheimer disease.** A silver stain illustrates a senile plaque, with dystrophic neurites on the periphery and a central core of amyloid.

PATHOLOGY: During the course of Alzheimer disease, neurons are lost and gliosis occurs. The gyri narrow, the sulci widen, and cortical atrophy becomes apparent. The brain loses approximately 200 g in an interval of 3 to 8 years (Fig. 28-77). The atrophy is bilateral and symmetric and targets the frontal and hippocampal cortex.

The microscopic changes in Alzheimer disease are dominated by the presence of (1) senile plaques, (2) NFTs, and (3) neuron loss. Other lesions such as Lewy bodies and granulovacuolar degeneration are also present. Identical morphologic alterations occur in lesser intensity in the cerebrum of a large proportion of elderly persons with symptoms as minor as forgetfulness, and a prodromal phase of Alzheimer disease known as mild cognitive impairment (MCI) shows lesser changes than those in full blown Alzheimer disease.

SENILE (NEURITIC) PLAQUES: The most conspicuous histologic lesion, the senile or neuritic plaque, is a spherical deposit of Aβ several hundred μm in diameter. In end-stage disease, senile plaques converge to occupy large volumes of affected cerebral gray matter (Fig. 28-78). The plaques are positive for Congo red and thioflavin S (amyloid-binding dyes), argentophilic, and immunoreactive for Aβ at the core and periphery. They are surrounded by reactive astrocytes, microglia and tau, and display α-synuclein immunoreactive neuronal processes (dystrophic neurites).

NEUROFIBRILLARY TANGLES: Like senile plaques, abundant NFTs are required for the diagnosis of definite Alzheimer disease. These structures are formed by large intracytoplasmic masses of tau filaments (Fig. 28-79). Neuronal processes harbor more than 90% of the burden of abnormal tau. Thus, even in the absence of NFTs, a neuron could be disconnected from other neurons because of abnormal tau pathology in its processes. By light microscopy, NFTs contain irregular bundles of fibrils that are positive for Congo red and thioflavin S, argentophilic, and immunoreactive for tau. Electron microscopy reveals the tangles to be composed of paired, 10- nm thick, helical filaments. Western blots demonstrate abundant insoluble tau proteins.

NFTs also occur in neurodegenerative diseases other than Alzheimer disease, including **dementia pugilistica,** postencephalitic parkinsonism, Guam ALS/parkinsonism dementia complex, Pick disease, corticobasal degeneration, sporadic frontotemporal dementias, hereditary frontotemporal lobe dementia with parkinsonism associated with mutations on chromosome 17

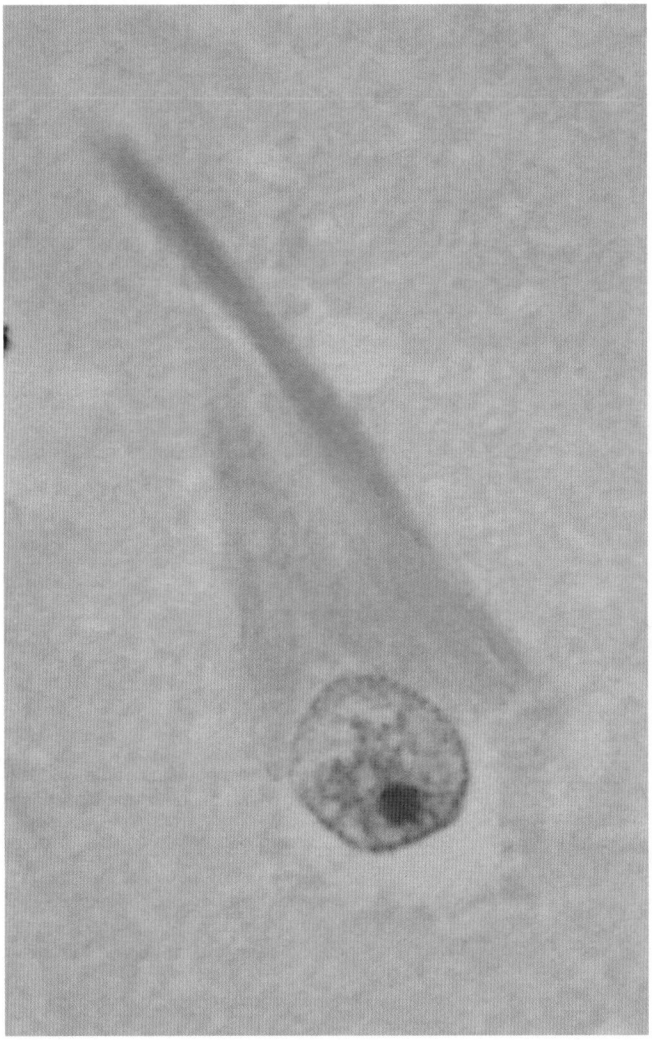
A

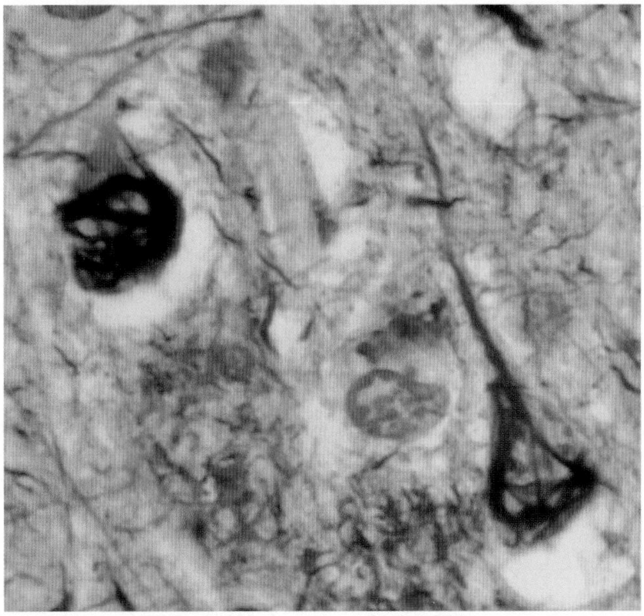
B

FIGURE 28-79. **Alzheimer disease. A.** A neuron exhibits a basophilic, cytoplasmic neurofibrillary tangle. **B.** A silver stain illustrates the intracellular structure of a neurofibrillary tangle.

(FTDP-17), and so forth. Indeed, hereditary and sporadic neurodegenerative diseases characterized by abnormal forms of tau are now classified as **taupathies,** since they may share common mechanisms of brain degeneration.

GRANULOVACUOLAR DEGENERATION: This morphological change is not diagnostic of Alzheimer disease and is largely restricted to the cytoplasm of hippocampal pyramidal cells, where it is evident as circular clear zones containing basophilic and argentophilic granules (Fig. 28-80A).

HIRANO BODIES: Like granulovacuolar degeneration, these structures are found almost exclusively in hippocampal pyramidal neurons, especially in their processes (see Fig. 28-80B). Hirano bodies are eosinophilic rods, 10 to 15 μm thick. They are not unique to Alzheimer disease but are seen in the brains of normal elderly persons and in patients with other neurologic conditions.

Proposed mechanisms underlying the development of Alzheimer disease are illustrated in Figure 28-81.

CLINICAL FEATURES: Patients with AD come to medical attention because of a gradual loss of memory and cognitive function, difficulty with language, and changes in behavior. Persons with MCI are increasingly being recognized, since they progress to full blown dementia at a rate of about 15% per year. Alzheimer disease progresses inexorably, so that previously intelligent and productive persons eventually become demented, mute, incontinent, and bedridden. Bronchopneumonia is the usual lethal outcome of Alzheimer disease.

Pick Disease

Pick disease (**lobar sclerosis**) is manifested clinically as loss of executive function followed by a dementia that can be indistinguishable from Alzheimer disease. This disorder is prototypical of frontotemporal dementias, and most cases are sporadic, although Pick disease kindreds have been described. Sporadic Pick disease becomes symptomatic in mid-adult life and progresses relentlessly to death over a period of 3 to 10 years.

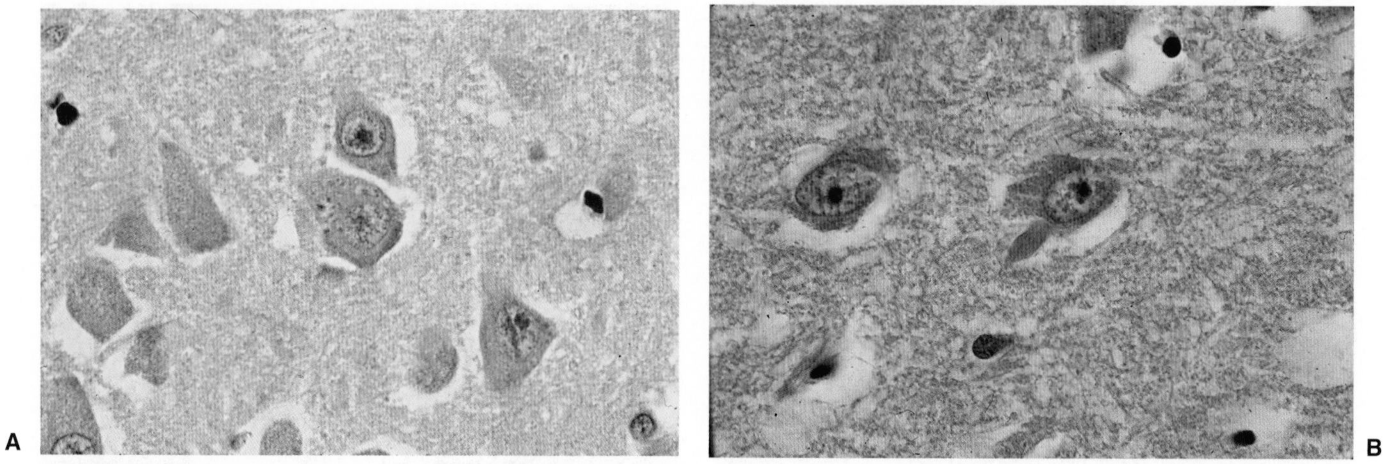

FIGURE 28-80. **Alzheimer disease. A.** Several neurons display granulovacuolar degeneration of the cytoplasm. **B.** A neuron (center) contains an eosinophilic Hirano body.

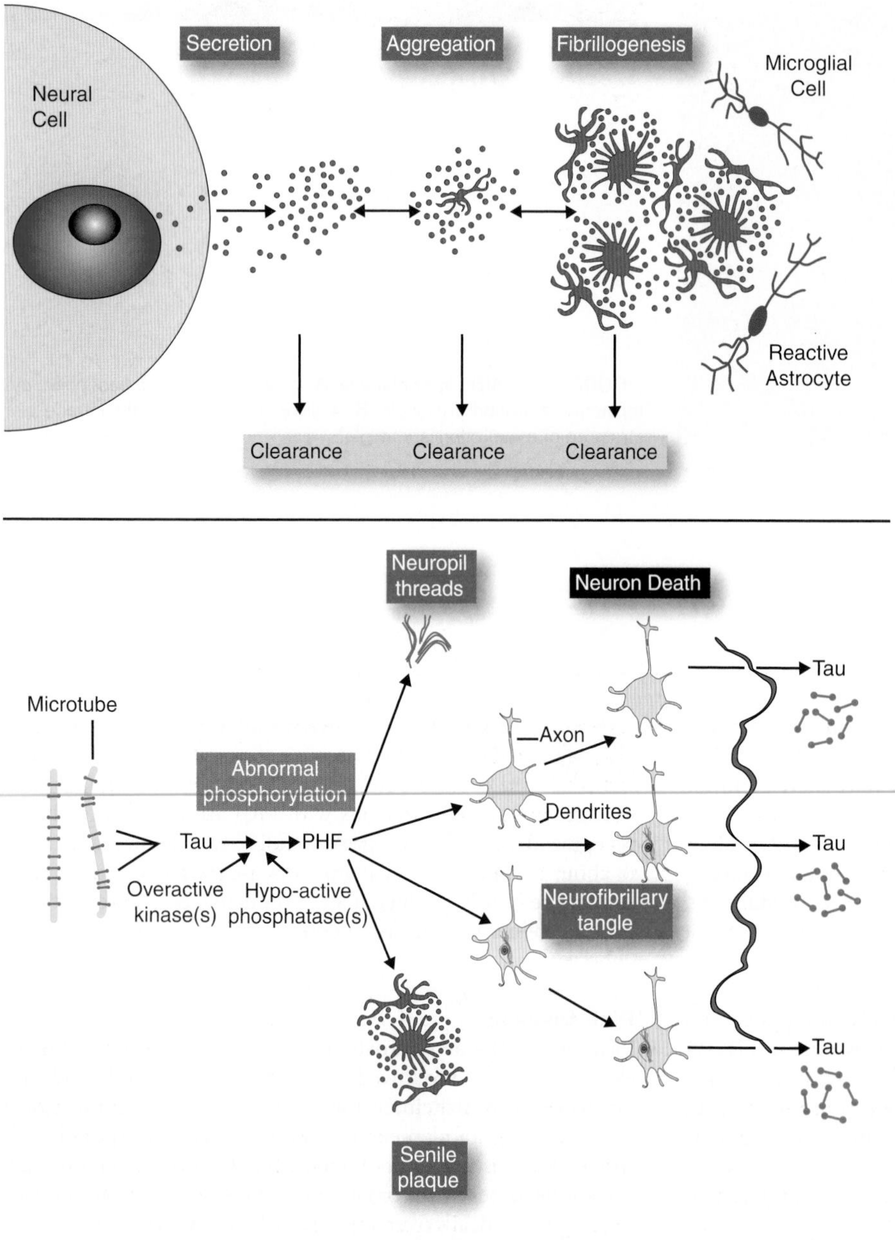

FIGURE 28-81. **Mechanisms of amyloidosis and brain degeneration in Alzheimer disease. A.** This schematic illustrates a hypothetical mechanism for the formation of senile plaques (SPs) from soluble Aβ peptides produced inside cells and secreted into the extracellular space. Amyloidogenic Aβ may encounter fibril-inducing cofactors and go on to form A fibrils to deposit in SPs *(far right)*. SPs are surrounded by reactive astrocytes and microglial cells, which secrete cytokines that may contribute to the toxicity of the SPs. These steps may be reversible. Increasing Aβ clearance or reducing its production, as well as modulating the inflammatory response, may be effective therapeutic interventions for Alzheimer disease, in combination with therapies that target brain degeneration caused by NFTs. **B.** This schematic illustrates a hypothetical mechanism leading to the conversion of normal human central nervous system (CNS) tau overlying 2 microtubules into paired helical filaments (PHFs). PHFs are generated in neuronal perikarya and their processes. Overactive kinase(s) or hypoactive phosphatase(s) may contribute to this effect. Abnormally phosphorylated tau forms PHFs in neuronal processes (neuropil threads) and neuronal perikarya (neurofibrillary tangles, NFTs). Tau in PHFs loses the ability to bind microtubules, thus causing their depolymerization, disruption of axonal transport, and degeneration of neurons. Accumulation of PHFs in neurons could exacerbate this process by physically blocking transport in neurons. The death of affected neurons would release tau and increase the levels of tau in the cerebrospinal fluid (CSF) of patients with Alzheimer disease. NFT formation may be reversible, and drugs that block NFT formation, reverse it, or stabilize microtubules may be effective therapeutic interventions for Alzheimer disease.

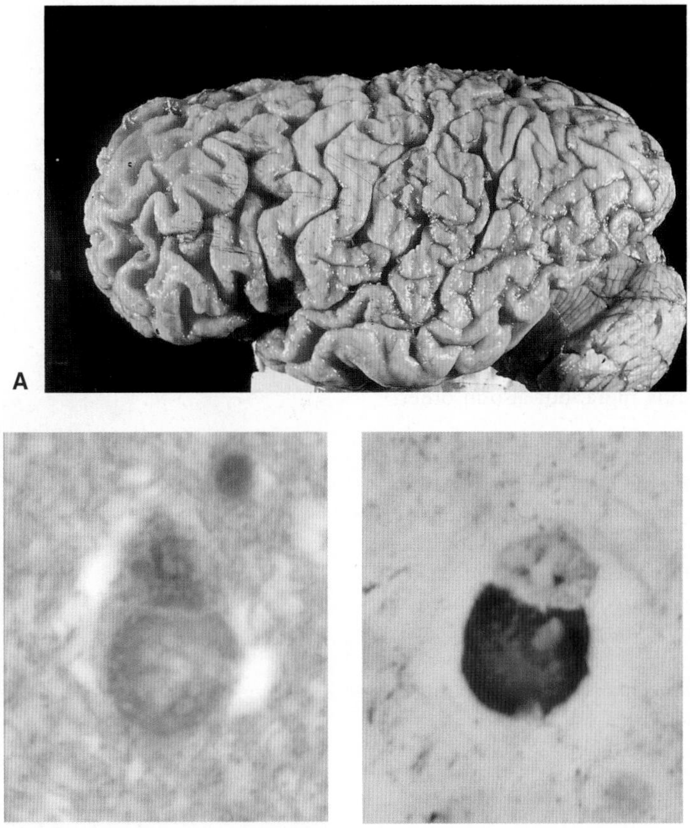

FIGURE 28-82. **Pick disease. A.** The brain demonstrates severe atrophy of the frontal lobe and the superior temporal lobe gyrus. **B.** A microscopic section of a large basophilic Pick body just below the nucleus. **C.** Silver impregnation strongly stains a Pick body.

The cortical atrophy in Pick disease is initially unilateral and localized to the frontotemporal regions, but it becomes bilateral with disease progression (Fig. 28-82). The atrophy may attain extreme proportions, so that the affected gyri are reduced to a thin edge (**knife-blade atrophy**). Histologically, the involved cortex is markedly depleted of neurons and displays conspicuous astrogliosis. Many residual neurons contain intensely argentophilic and tau immunoreactive cytoplasmic inclusions termed **Pick bodies.** By electron microscopy, these structures are formed by densely aggregated straight tau filaments.

Parkinson Disease Is a Common Movement Disorder

First described in 1817, Parkinson disease is a neurologic disorder characterized pathologically by the loss of neurons, primarily in the substantia nigra, and the accumulation of Lewy bodies, formed by filamentous α-synuclein aggregates. Clinically, Parkinson disease features tremors at rest, muscular rigidity, expressionless countenance, emotional lability, and, less commonly, cognitive impairments, including dementia late in the disease course.

EPIDEMIOLOGY: Parkinson disease typically appears in the sixth to eighth decades of life. The disease is frequent, and more than 2% of the population in North America eventually develop it. The prevalence has remained unchanged for at least the past 40 years, and no racial differences are apparent, but men are more affected than women. Although most cases are sporadic, missense mutations in the α-synuclein gene are responsible for rare cases of autosomal dominant, early-onset, familial Parkinson disease. Moreover, the demonstration that wild-type α-synuclein (a synaptic protein of unknown function) is the major building block of the aggregated filaments in Lewy bodies has led to a paradigm shift in thinking about the mechanisms underlying familial and sporadic Parkinson disease. It has also led to the recognition of a number of other diseases (e.g., multiple system atrophy, dementia with Lewy bodies, progressive autonomic failure, rapid eye movement [REM] sleep behavior disorder) that are also characterized by the accumulation of filamentous α-synuclein inclusions. These disorders are now designated α-synucleinopathies and are considered brain-specific amyloidoses. Lewy bodies and other α-synuclein inclusions share properties common to amyloid deposits within and outside the brain.

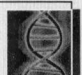

PATHOGENESIS: The vast majority of cases of Parkinson disease are idiopathic, but the disease has been recorded after viral encephalitis (von Economo encephalitis) and after intake of the toxic chemical 1-methyl-4-phenyl-1,2,3,6-tetrahydropyridine (MPTP). The substantia nigra is a component of the extrapyramidal system that relays information to the basal ganglia through dopaminergic synapses. Normal aging is associated with a loss of neurons in the substantia nigra and reduced levels of dopamine, but these features are more exaggerated in PD. Lewy bodies, composed of filamentous α-synuclein aggregates, are seen not only in neurons and their processes (Lewy neurites) in the substantia nigra, but also in other brain regions.

Accumulating evidence suggests that oxidative stress produced by the auto-oxidation of catecholamines during melanin formation injures the neurons in the substantia nigra by promoting the misfolding of α-synuclein and the formation of filamentous inclusions. A byproduct of the illicit synthesis of a meperidine analogue, MPTP, induced a Parkinson disease-like syndrome in intravenous drug users. Since MPTP inhibits mitochondrial electron transport, it may produce parkinsonism by mechanisms similar to those of naturally occurring Parkinson disease.

PATHOLOGY: Gross examination of the brain in Parkinson disease reveals a loss of pigmentation in the substantia nigra and locus ceruleus (Fig. 28-83). Other brain regions are affected to a lesser extent. On microscopic examination, pigmented neurons are scarce, and small extracellular deposits of melanin are derived from necrotic neurons. Some residual nerve cells are atrophic, and a few contain Lewy bodies, which are visualized as spherical, eosinophilic cytoplasmic inclusions (Fig. 28-84). By electron microscopy, Lewy bodies exhibit amyloid-like filaments formed by insoluble α-synuclein.

CLINICAL FEATURES: Parkinson disease is characterized by slowness of all voluntary movements and muscular rigidity throughout the entire range of movement. Most patients have a coarse tremor of the distal extremities, which is present at rest and disappears with voluntary movement. The face is expressionless (masklike), and a reduced rate of swallowing leads to drooling. There is an increased incidence of depression and dementia. In early parkinsonism, substitution therapy with levodopa is beneficial. However, this

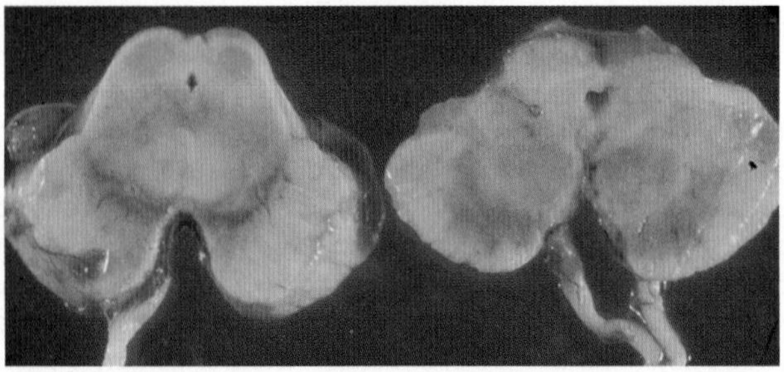

FIGURE 28-83. **Parkinson disease.** The affected substantia nigra (right) is depigmented, compared to a normal brain (left).

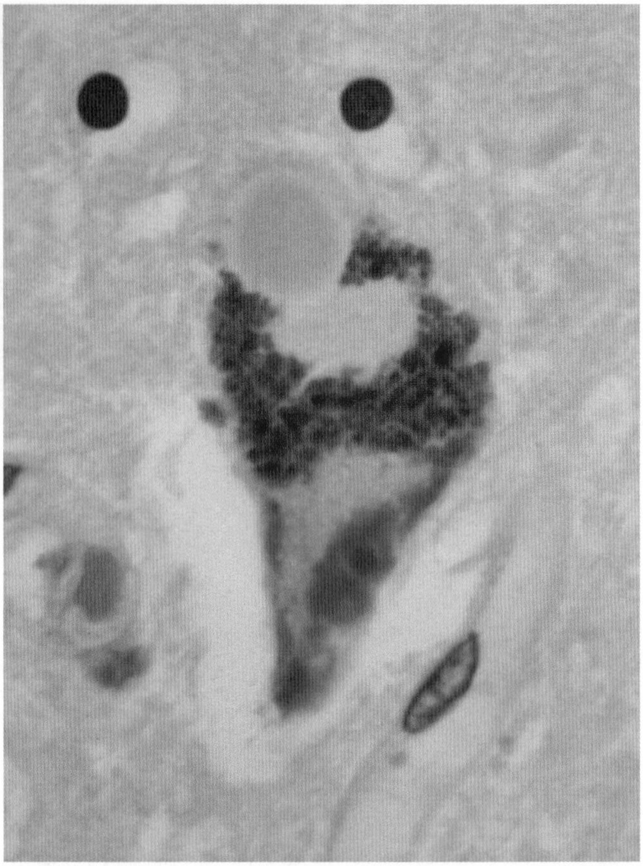

FIGURE 28-84. **Parkinson disease.** A pigmented neuron in the substantia nigra contains a Lewy body (the large eosinophilic cytoplasmic inclusion at the top with a surrounding halo).

therapy does not rectify the underlying disorder and after several years becomes ineffective. Another emerging symptomatic therapy that shows promise for the treatment of patients with Parkinson disease who no longer respond to levodopa is deep brain stimulation. Preliminary clinical trial data suggest that dopaminergic cell transplants may become viable therapies in the future.

Striatonigral degeneration is a rare disorder that mimics Parkinson disease so closely that it is rarely diagnosed during life. At autopsy, the corpus striatum (caudate and putamen) is visibly atrophied, and microscopic examination shows severe loss of neurons in this region. Less severe changes occur in the substantia nigra and locus ceruleus. This condition is also recognized with Shy-Drager disease and olivopontocerebellar atrophy as part of a syndrome complex known as **multiple system atrophy.** This syndrome is characterized by filamentous α-synuclein inclusions primarily in white matter oligodendroglia, known as glial cytoplasmic inclusions. They also occur to a lesser extent in neurons, where they exhibit the morphologic features of Lewy bodies that are similar to those in Parkinson disease.

Progressive supranuclear palsy is another unusual neurologic disorder that is clinically similar to Parkinson disease but adds a progressive paralysis of vertical eye movements. The course of the disease is relentless, with death within 5 to 10 years. The pathologic changes in the brain are more widespread than in Parkinson disease, with loss of neurons in the globus pallidus, subthalamic nucleus, red nucleus, tectum, periaqueductal gray matter, and dentate nuclei. NFTs formed by filamentous tau aggregates are noted. Thus, this disease combines clinical features of Parkinson diseasewith dementia and is a prototypical form of **neurodegenerative taupathy,** since the sole inclusions are tau-rich NFTs.

Amyotrophic Lateral Sclerosis Leads to Profound Weakness and Death

ALS is a degenerative disease of motor neurons of the brain and spinal cord that results in progressive weakness and wasting of the extremities and eventually impairment of the respiratory muscles.

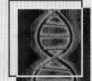

EPIDEMIOLOGY AND PATHOGENESIS: ALS is a worldwide disease with an incidence of 1 in 100,000. The frequency of the disease peaks in the fifth decade of life, and it is rare in persons younger than 35 years. There is a 1.5- to 2.0-fold excess of ALS in men. Restricted geographic areas with a particularly high incidence of ALS exist in Guam and parts of Japan and Papua New Guinea, but these cases differ from ALS in the rest of the world. Cases in the Chamorro people indigenous to Guam are characterized by abundant accumulations of tau-rich NFTs and are now classified as **neurodegenerative taupathies.** Moreover, ALS on Guam is part of a spectrum of disorders that includes dementia and parkinsonism.

Familial ALS cases, with an autosomal dominant pattern, account for 5% of all cases of ALS. The gene for familial ALS is located on chromosome 21q and has been associated with missense mutations in the gene that codes for superoxide dismutase 1 *(SOD1)*. Interestingly familial ALS caused by *SOD1* mutations is not due to deficient SOD activity. Transgenic mice that have two normal copies of the murine SOD gene but also express the human mutant SOD1 protein develop a syndrome that closely resembles ALS. This finding indicates that the mutant *SOD1* gene in ALS results in a gain of toxic function. Aggregation of SOD1 and other proteins, such as neurofilament subunits, presumably impairs the survival of motor neurons.

PATHOLOGY: ALS affects motor neurons in three locations: (1) the anterior horn cells of the spinal cord; (2) the motor nuclei of the brainstem, particularly the hypoglossal nuclei; and (2) the upper motor neurons of the cerebral cortex. The injury to the motor neurons leads to degeneration of their axons, visualized in striking alterations of the lateral pyramidal pathways in the spinal cord.

The defining histologic change in ALS is a loss of large motor neurons accompanied by mild gliosis (Fig. 28-85). This change is most evident in the anterior horns of the lumbar cord, the cervical enlargements of the spinal cord, and the hypoglossal nuclei, where neurofilaments may also aggregate in axons to form inclusions termed **spheroids.** There is also a loss of the giant pyramidal Betz cells in the motor cortex of the cerebrum. The most striking secondary change in the spinal cord is a loss of myelinated fibers in the lateral corticospinal tracts (Fig. 28-86), which imparts a pallor to these areas when they are viewed with myelin stains. The anterior nerve roots are atrophic, and the affected muscles are pale and shrunken.

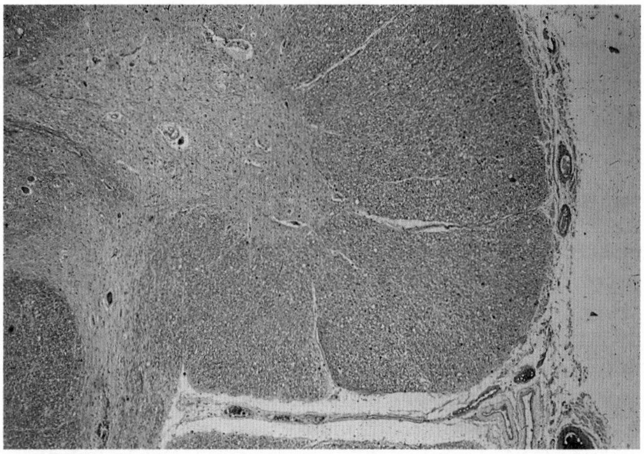

FIGURE 28-85. **Amyotrophic lateral sclerosis.** There is virtual absence of neurons in the ventral horn gray matter (Luxol fast blue stain).

CLINICAL FEATURES: ALS begins as weakness and wasting of the muscles of a hand, often accompanied by painful cramps of the muscles of the arm. Irregular rapid contractions of the muscles that do not move the limb (fasciculations) are characteristic. The disease is inexorably progressive, with increasing weakness of the limbs leading to total disability. Speech may become unintelligible, and respiratory weakness supervenes. Despite the dramatic wasting of the body, intellectual capacity tends to be preserved to the end, although a few patients with ALS also suffer dementia. The clinical course does not usually extend beyond a decade.

Trinucleotide Repeat Expansion Syndromes Comprise a Heterogeneous Group of Hereditary Neurodegenerative Diseases

A large group of neurologic diseases can now be classified on a genetic basis as trinucleotide repeat expansion syndromes. The first such disorder to be identified was fragile X syndrome in 1991, followed by spinal and bulbar muscular atrophy and myotonic dystrophy. The triplet repeat mutation disorders now include Huntington disease and Friedreich ataxia, but the number of disorders included in this category continues to expand as new mutations lead to the identification of additional variants of these diseases.

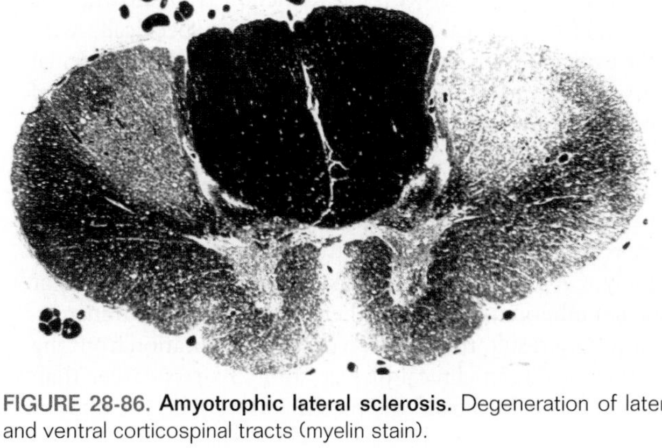

FIGURE 28-86. **Amyotrophic lateral sclerosis.** Degeneration of lateral and ventral corticospinal tracts (myelin stain).

Trinucleotide repeats are a normal feature of many genes, and expansion of the number of triplet repeats confers pathogenicity. Some triplet repeat diseases show only a small expansion compared with the normal counterpart (e.g., Huntington disease), whereas in others, the expansion is quite large (e.g., fragile X syndrome and Friedreich ataxia). This class of diseases includes examples of all forms of inheritance: X-linked, autosomal dominant, and autosomal recessive. In some of these disorders, the expansion mutation lies within the coding region of a gene segment and results in the production of an abnormal ("toxic") protein, as appears to be the case for most of the autosomal dominant CAG expansion disorders. In others, the expansion occurs in a noncoding region of the gene and presumably interferes with transcription or message processing. The resulting decreased level of protein production constitutes a loss-of-function mutation (as appears to be the case with the GAA expansion of Friedreich ataxia). Our knowledge is still nascent, but discovery of the mutations sets the stage for characterizing the normal protein function and elucidating the sequential steps in the pathogenesis of disease, which then could lead to better therapies.

Huntington Disease

Huntington disease is an autosomal dominant genetic disorder characterized by involuntary movements of all parts of the body, deterioration of cognitive function, and often severe emotional disturbance. First described by a medical student in 1872, the disorder principally affects whites of northwestern European ancestry, with an incidence of 1 in 20,000. Genealogical studies indicate that all cases of Huntington disease derive from the spread of an original focus in northern Europe; the disease is notably rare in Asia and Africa.

PATHOGENESIS: The *HD* gene is located on chromosome 4 (4p16.3) and codes for a novel protein, **huntingtin.** In 1993, it was discovered that the genetic alteration at this locus consists of expansion of a trinucleotide (CAG) repeat. The repeat is located within the coding region of the gene and results in production of an altered protein, which contains a polyglutamine tract near the N terminus. In agreement with the dominant mode of inheritance, the triplet expansion likely results in a toxic gain of function. Huntington disease is an example of a true autosomal dominant disorder, since one abnormal allele suffices to cause disease.

The huntingtin gene product is widely expressed in tissues throughout the body and in all regions of the CNS by neurons and glia. However, its function is unknown. It is thought that critical proteins may interact specifically with the expanded polyglutamine tract and become dysfunctional in affected cells. Alternatively, amyloid-like aggregates of mutant huntingtin may impede intracellular trafficking.

As with other CAG repeat expansion diseases, a strong inverse correlation is seen between the magnitude of the expansion and the age of clinical onset, and the most numerous repeats are seen in juvenile-onset cases. Interestingly, CAG length is more unstable and tends to be longer when inherited from the father than in maternal transmission. As a result, transmission of the *HD* mutation from the father results in clinical disease some 3 years earlier than when it is passed from the mother. Moreover, the ratio of children with juvenile-onset Huntington disease who inherit the expanded CAG allele from their father to those who inherit it from their mother is 10:1.

Sporadic (new mutation) cases of Huntington disease were thought to be rare, but genetic testing now reveals increasing numbers of these patients. Most new mutations arise from unstable transmission of triplet repeats from an asymptomatic parent whose alleles exhibit repeat lengths in the zone between the normal (<30) and HD (>36) ranges (referred to as "intermediate alleles").

PATHOLOGY: On gross examination of brains from patients who died of Huntington disease, the frontal cortex is symmetrically and moderately atrophic, whereas the lateral ventricles appear disproportionately enlarged, owing to the loss of the normal convex curvature of the caudate nuclei (Fig. 28-87). There is symmetric atrophy of the caudate nuclei, with lesser involvement of the putamen. Microscopically, the neuronal population of the caudate and putamen, particularly the small neurons, is greatly depleted, and there is an accompanying moderate astrogliosis. The cortical neurons are similarly, but less severely, depleted. Amyloid-like aggregates of huntingtin have been detected in neurons, especially in nuclei. Accumulations of the mutant protein also occur in neuronal processes, which could impair communication between neurons through their axons and dendrites. Biochemical assays at the termination of the disease show a marked decrease in γ-aminobutyric acid (GABA) and glutamic acid decarboxylase.

CLINICAL FEATURES: The symptoms of Huntington disease are usually first seen at about age 40 years, but 5% of persons with the disorder develop neurologic signs before 20 years of age, and a comparable proportion develop manifestations after age 60 years. Cognitive and emotional disturbances precede the onset of abnormal movements by several years in more than half of patients. Because of the prominent involvement of the extrapyramidal system, choreoathetoid movements progress to total incapacitation. Subsequent involvement of the cortex leads to a severe loss of cognitive function and intellectual deterioration, often accompanied by paranoia and delusions. The interval from the onset of symptoms to death averages 15 years.

The Inherited Spinocerebellar Ataxias

The spinocerebellar ataxias represent a heterogeneous category of disease that features (1) a broad but system-based topography, (2) a genetic

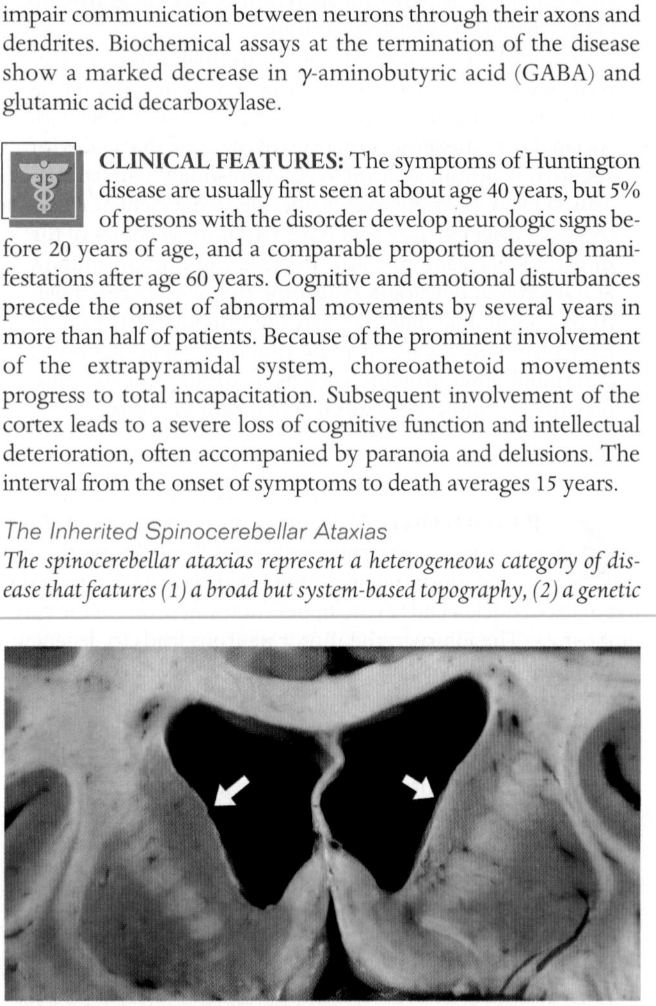

FIGURE 28-87. **Huntington disease.** There is atrophy of the caudate nuclei (*arrows*).

contribution, and (3) a precocious loss of neurons and neural tracts in the cerebellum, brainstem, and spinal cord. The symptoms reflect the topography of the lesions. Thus, ataxia and intention tremor suggest involvement of the cerebellum; rigidity and tremor reflect degeneration of the brainstem; and losses of deep tendon reflexes, vibration sense, and pain sensation are caused by disease of the spinal cord.

Because there is greater anatomic and clinical uniformity among cases from a particular family than among random cases from different families, case reports have generally focused on specific families, and the original authors' names have been appended to the different syndromes. For example, an inherited form of cerebelloolivary degeneration is designated "cerebelloolivary degeneration of Holmes," which is distinguished from the sporadic "cerebelloolivary degeneration of Marie." These cases also share many features with "olivopontocerebellar degeneration of Menzel." A similar complexity pertains to the nosology of spinal cord degeneration. This complex nosology is now being clarified by the identification of the genetic defects that cause these disorders, and many inherited ataxias, including Machado-Joseph disease and Friedreich ataxia, have been shown to be triplet repeat expansion disorders.

Friedreich Ataxia

Friedreich ataxia is the most common inherited ataxia, with a prevalence in European populations of 1 in 50,000. Although the inheritance pattern is autosomal recessive, many cases arise sporadically as new mutations without a family history. The onset of symptoms is usually before age 25 years, followed by an unremitting and progressive course of about 30 years before death. The hallmark of Friedreich ataxia is a combined ataxia of both the upper and lower limbs. Dysarthria, lower-limb areflexia, extensor plantar reflexes, and sensory loss also occur in most patients. Frequently associated systemic abnormalities are deformities of the skeletal system, (e.g., scoliosis, pes cavus), hypertrophic cardiomyopathy (which commonly causes death), and diabetes mellitus.

PATHOGENESIS: The genetic defect in Friedreich ataxia was mapped to chromosome 9 in 1988. The candidate gene *(X25)* encodes a mitochondrial protein (**frataxin**) of 210 amino acid residues, which is involved in iron transport into mitochondria. In 1996, a mutation consisting of an unstable expansion of a trinucleotide (GAA) repeat was found in the first intron of the frataxin gene (9q13.3–21.1). The recessive pattern of inheritance suggests that this expansion results in a loss of function, which is consistent with an absence of frataxin mRNA transcripts in patients with Friedreich ataxia. The expansion mutation probably interferes with transcription or RNA processing. In normal persons, the highest levels of frataxin gene expression are found in the heart and spinal cord. It is, therefore, likely that a lack of frataxin is responsible for both the neuropathologic manifestations of Friedreich ataxia and the cardiomyopathy. There is a strong inverse correlation between the size of the triplet expansion and the age of disease onset, and a direct relationship with the rate of clinical progression and the frequency of hypertrophic cardiomyopathy.

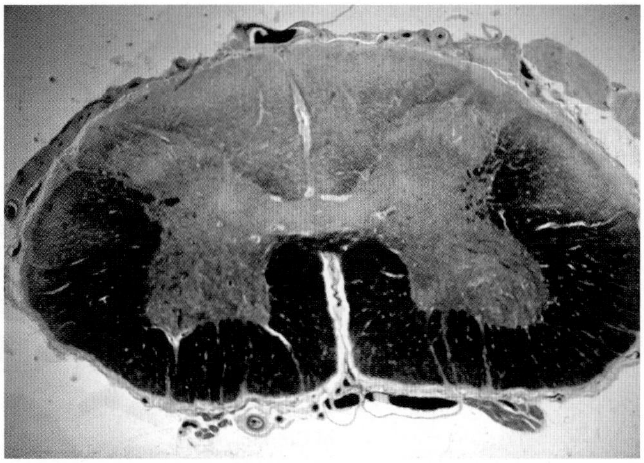

FIGURE 28-88. **Friedreich ataxia.** A section of spinal cord stained for axons (Bielchowsky stain) discloses pronounced axonal loss of the posterior columns and lateral corticospinal tracts.

The clinical spectrum of Friedreich ataxia is broader than previously thought. Many patients have sporadic ataxia, in which the typical clinical features of Friedreich ataxia are not fully expressed or in which atypical signs or symptoms are present. In such cases, identification of a GAA repeat expansion in the frataxin gene confirms the diagnosis of Friedreich ataxia. In one study, a significant proportion of patients (14%) with proven GAA expansion of the frataxin gene have an onset after 25 years of age (26 to 51), and 12% have retained lower-limb reflexes.

PATHOLOGY: The most prominent postmortem findings in Friedreich ataxia are seen in the spinal cord (Fig. 28-88). The classic lesion consists of degeneration of three major pathways: the posterior columns, corticospinal pathways, and the spinocerebellar tracts (Fig. 28-89). Posterior column degeneration accounts for the sensory loss experienced by patients with Friedreich ataxia and results from loss of the parent neuronal cell bodies, which are located in the dorsal root ganglia. In advanced cases, this degeneration can be appreciated grossly as shrinkage of the dorsal spinal roots and posterior funiculi. Similarly, atrophy of the spinocerebellar tracts, with attendant ataxia, follows neuronal degeneration in the dorsal nucleus of Clarke. The corticospinal tracts show the most pronounced degeneration more distally in the cord, with gradually less pronounced atrophy as the cord is followed proximally toward the brainstem. This process is referred to as a "dying back" phenomenon.

Tumors of the CNS

Tumors within the intracranial compartment can be classified according to five origins:

- **Neuroectoderm,** principally gliomas
- **Mesenchymal structures,** notably meningiomas and schwannomas
- **Ectopic tissues,** such as craniopharyngiomas, dermoid and epidermoid cysts, lipomas, and dysgerminomas
- **Retained embryonal structures** (e.g., paraphyseal cysts)
- **Metastases**

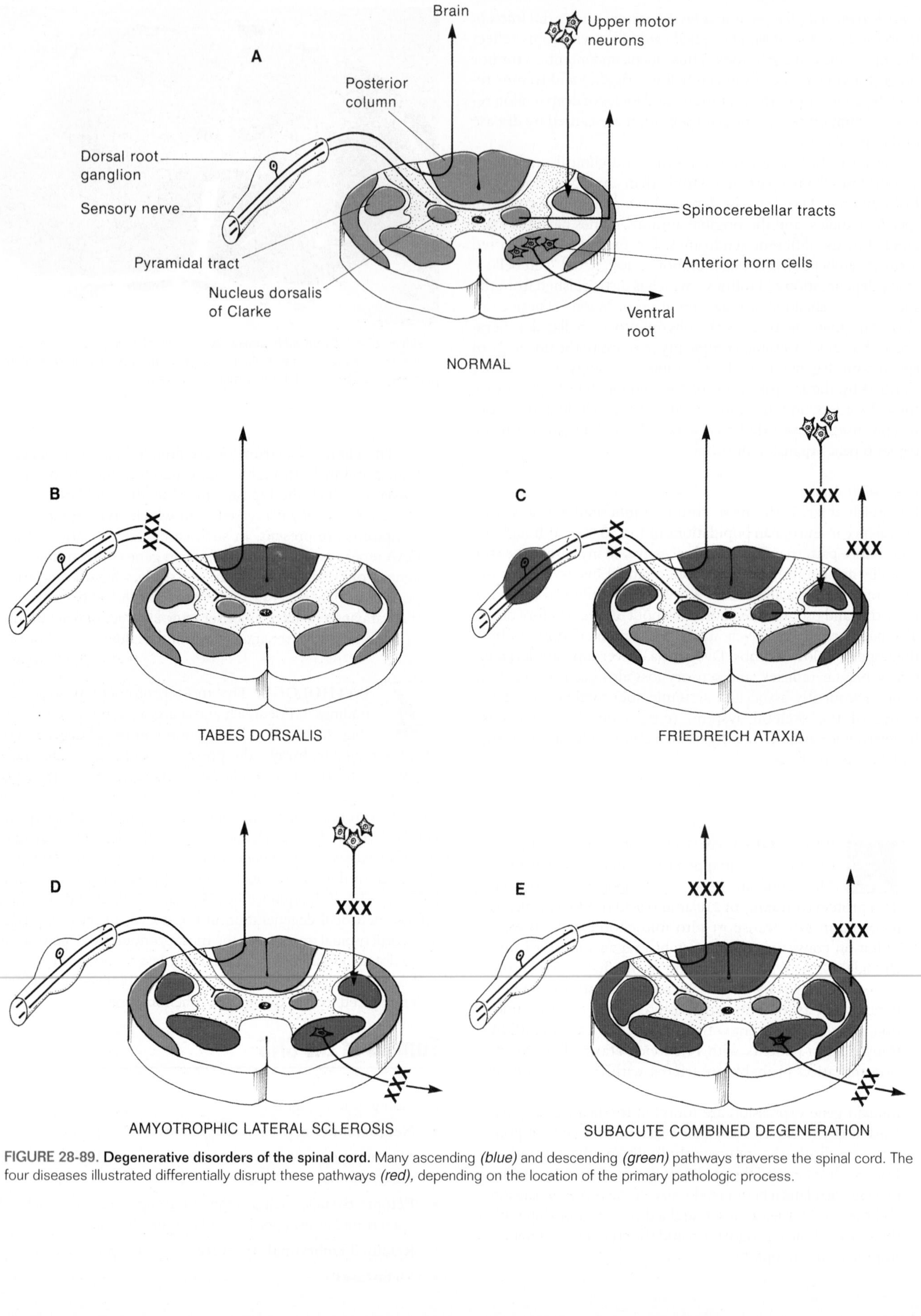

FIGURE 28-89. **Degenerative disorders of the spinal cord.** Many ascending *(blue)* and descending *(green)* pathways traverse the spinal cord. The four diseases illustrated differentially disrupt these pathways *(red)*, depending on the location of the primary pathologic process.

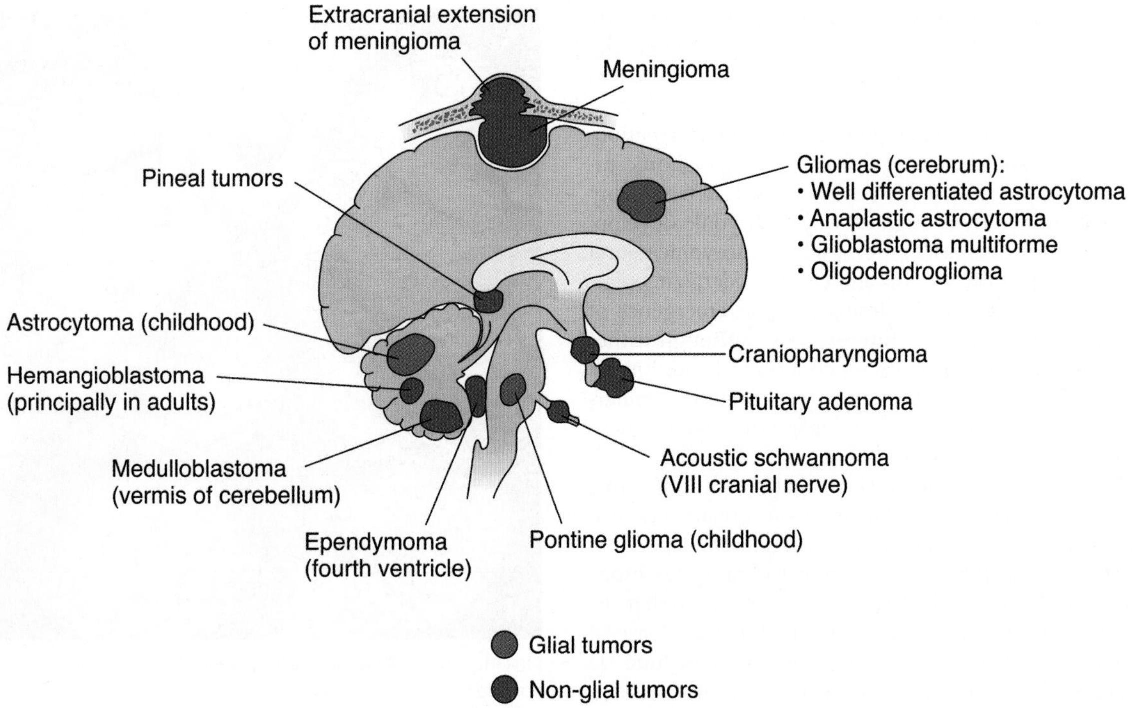

FIGURE 28-90. The distribution of common intracranial tumors.

Intracranial tumors constitute only 2% of all "aggressive" neoplasms, and most affect older persons. However the frequency of several types of brain tumors in childhood imparts clinical significance to their appearance in the young. Gliomas account for 60% of primary intracranial neoplasms, meningiomas for 20%, and all others for 20% (Fig. 28-90). Tumors of neuroectodermal origin are predominantly glial, and they are presumed to be derived from astrocytes (astrocytomas), oligodendroglia (oligodendrogliomas), or ependyma (ependymomas). Each of these tumors exhibits varying degrees of anaplasia, from well-differentiated tumors that are difficult to distinguish from normal tissue to anaplastic tumors that do not resemble CNS tissue at all.

BENIGN VERSUS MALIGNANT: The descriptive terms **benign** and **malignant** require qualification when used in reference to brain tumors, especially gliomas. For example, even a very well differentiated astrocytoma infiltrates freely through the surrounding brain tissue and has a poorly defined margin. The term **benign** may be applied to this lesion, because its growth is indolent and permits survival for 5 to 10 years. However, unlike "benign" neoplasms elsewhere, many astrocytomas are eventually fatal, owing in part to their transformation over time into more "malignant" anaplastic astrocytomas or glioblastomas and in part to encroachment upon vital centers. Unlike malignant tumors elsewhere, high-grade gliomas rarely metastasize outside the CNS.

AGE OF THE PATIENT AND LOCATION OF THE TUMOR: Most tumors in the intracranial or intraspinal compartment have predictable geographic localizations. Thus, astrocytic neoplasms occur predominantly in the cerebral hemispheres in middle life and old age, in the cerebellum and pons in childhood, and in the spinal cord in young adults. Oligodendrogliomas predominantly involve the cerebrum in adults, whereas ependymomas have their highest incidence in fourth ventricle during the first 3 decades of life, followed in frequency by intramedullary lesions that arise from the ependymal lining of the spinal canal and from the filum terminale. Inexplicably, ependymomas are least common in the lateral ventricles, which have the largest ependymal surface.

Some tumors, such as the craniopharyngiomas, medulloblastomas, and germinomas, have highly specific sites of origin. A few tumors, notably the third ventricular cyst, are rigidly restricted to a single position in the septum pellucidum, where the lesion regularly abuts against the foramen of Monro, lifts the fornix, and compresses the medial aspects of the internal capsules. Thus, the symptoms of increased intracranial pressure (hydrocephalus), personality changes, bilateral leg weakness, and urinary incontinence relate to the position of this expansible mass, which is cytologically benign but may kill by virtue of its location and surgical inaccessibility. Meningiomas arise from widely distributed arachnoidal cells but display preferred sites of origin (see below).

Within the rigidly defined volume of the intracranial compartment, a new growth compromises space. In the case of meningiomas, the mass displaces the brain, rather than infiltrating it. Glioblastoma multiforme infiltrates and destroys neural tissue. Most tumors are also associated with regional edema, which is disproportionately abundant in the immediate environs of a metastatic tumor and adds to the mass effect of the metastasis. Tumors positioned adjacent to the ventricles, particularly the fourth ventricle or the aqueduct of Sylvius, are prone to obstruct these conduits and cause hydrocephalus.

NEURONAL TUMORS: Infrequently, the neuroectoderm gives rise to a neoplasm of neuronal heritage. These tumors occur most often in childhood, and their cellular composition is usually primitive. An important example is the medulloblastoma, which arises in the cerebellum, generally in the first decade of life. This entity is usually situated in the vermis; its growth is rapid, and regional infiltration is extensive.

Although even highly anaplastic tumors rarely metastasize outside the cranial cavity, certain tumors, notably medulloblastoma and less commonly ependymoma and pineal parenchymal tumor, have a marked propensity to disseminate or "seed" by way of the CSF throughout the CNS. The implants generally involve the subarachnoid compartment over the spinal cord and cauda equina. In conformity with the principle that a cell must be capable of replication to undergo neoplastic transformation, medulloblastomas and the better-differentiated ganglionic tumors typically occur during infancy or childhood. In fact, many tumors probably have their origin during embryonic development. It is intriguing to consider that residual embryonic neural progenitor cells or stem cells of the adult brain undergo neoplastic transformation, which then culminates in the emergence of gliomas and neuronal tumors. Interestingly, although esthesioneuroblastomas of the olfactory mucosa occur in adults, the olfactory epithelium is a neural structure that retains its proliferative potential throughout adult life to replace the olfactory neurons that turn over continuously.

SYMPTOMS OF INTRACRANIAL TUMORS: An infiltrative neoplasm that destroys functional neural tissue creates a neurologic deficit, which may be sensory or motor or both, depending on the function of the affected brain region. Cognitive functions are not infrequently impaired. Alternatively, a neoplasm that "irritates" a functional area may initiate an involuntary release of neuronal activity that manifests as seizures. These include (1) motor seizures, (2) subtle visual and olfactory seizures ("uncinate fits"), and (3) seizure disorders that stem from vegetative centers of the brain. Meningiomas and the well-differentiated gliomas, such as astrocytomas, oligodendrogliomas, and gangliomas, are most likely to be associated with seizures.

The mass of a neoplasm, combined with edema or hydrocephalus, causes increased intracranial pressure, which leads to headaches and vomiting. A mass effect, if progressive, ultimately causes various herniations of neural tissue:

- **Transtentorial herniation:** The medial aspect of the parahippocampal gyrus (uncus) herniates through the tentorium, where it interferes with the circulatory dynamics of the midbrain. This effect causes a decline in the level of consciousness as a result of impaired function of the reticular formation. This herniation can compress the third nerve against the tentorium and cause a third nerve palsy, resulting in a fixed dilated pupil. Shortly thereafter, midbrain necrosis and hemorrhage lead to permanent loss of consciousness and death.
- **Foramen magnum herniation:** As a result of increased pressure in the posterior fossa, cerebellar tonsils herniate into the foramen magnum. Compression of the cardiac and respiratory centers is lethal.
- **Subfalcine herniation:** The cingulate gyrus herniates beneath the falx, which on rare occasions may result in infarction in the territories supplied by the pericallosal vessels, with weakness of, or sensory loss in, the legs.

Tumors Derived from Astrocytes Show Varying Histologic Grades

Neoplasms derived from astrocytes display a wide spectrum of differentiation, ranging from tumors whose histologic structure is remarkably similar to that of normal brain tissue to highly aggressive growths that are hardly recognizable as of glial origin. These tumors can be divided according to their increasing anaplasia into three broad categories: astrocytoma, anaplastic astrocytoma, and glioblastoma multiforme. Recognition of these glial neoplasms is facilitated by their immunopositivity for GFAP, but the abundance of GFAP diminishes with increasing malignancy.

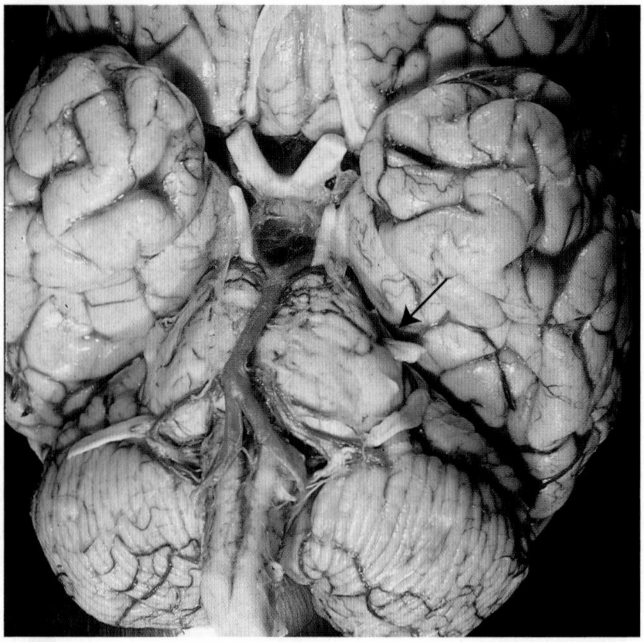

FIGURE 28-91. **Pontine astrocytoma.** A tumor markedly enlarges the pons (*arrow*).

Astrocytoma

Astrocytoma is a glioma composed of well-differentiated astrocytes. It comprises 20% of primary intracranial neoplasms. It frequents (1) the cerebral hemispheres in adults; (2) the optic nerve, walls of the third ventricle, midbrain, pons (Fig. 28-91), and cerebellum in the first two decades of life; and (3) the spinal cord, predominantly in the thoracic and cervical segments, in young adults.

PATHOLOGY: On macroscopic examination, astrocytomas are poorly demarcated and insidiously infiltrate surrounding brain. Childhood astrocytomas of the cerebellar hemispheres are frequently cystic. Astrocytomas of the cerebrum often contain microcysts, and some contain enough calcospherites to be visible radiographically. Microscopically, astrocytomas feature small glial cells with unremarkable

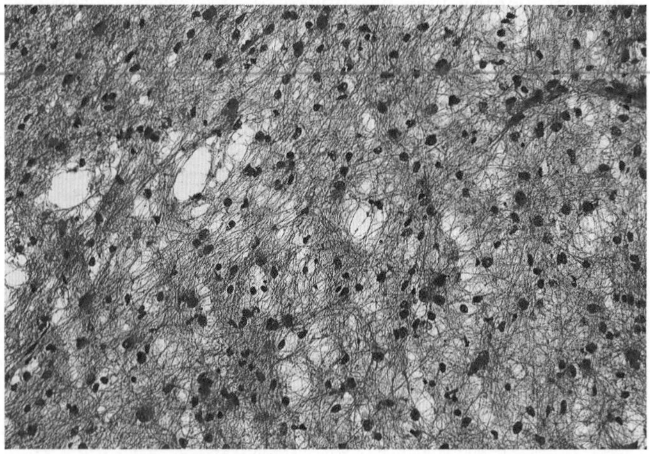

FIGURE 28-92. **Astrocytoma.** Moderately pleomorphic, neoplastic astrocytes infiltrate the white matter.

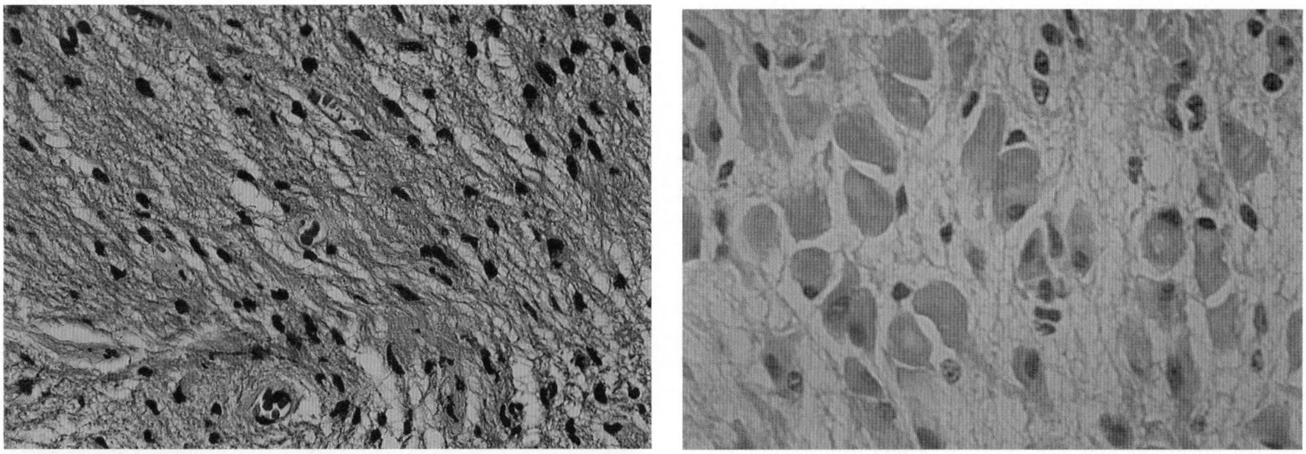

A B

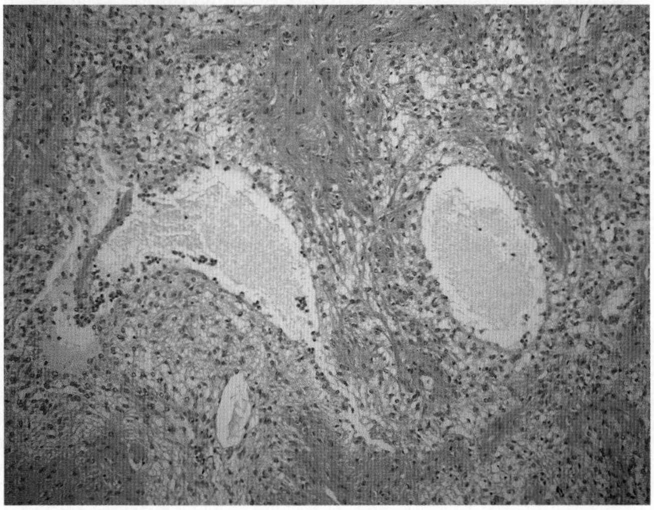

C

FIGURE 28-93. **Astrocytomas. A.** Fibrillary astrocytoma. The neoplastic astrocytes demonstrate characteristic fibrillary processes. **B.** Gemistocytic astrocytoma. Neoplastic astrocytes exhibit ample eosinophilic cytoplasm and eccentric nuclei. **C.** Pilocytic astrocytoma. A section of a cerebellar tumor reveals cystic areas containing neoplastic astrocytes against a fibrillary background.

nuclei and cytoplasmic processes (Fig. 28-92). The astrocytoma variants are:

- **Fibrillary astrocytoma:** This tumor, particularly in the cerebral hemispheres of adults, has prominent glial processes (Fig. 28-93A).
- **Gemistocytic astrocytoma:** Abundant eosinophilic cytoplasm encases the tumor cell nuclei (see Fig. 28-93B).
- **Pilocytic astrocytoma:** This neoplasm occurs in children and young adults and is characterized by abundant, hair-like glial processes. The cells typically contain Rosenthal fibers, similar to those seen in Alexander disease, albeit less abundant (see Fig. 28-93C). Pilocytic astrocytomas have an excellent prognosis with surgical excision alone resulting in long-term cure.

The life expectancy of patients with astrocytoma varies widely, but approximates 5 years. Transformation to a higher degree of anaplasia, often to glioblastoma multiforme, occurs in 10% of cases or more, in which case life expectancy is considerably shortened.

Anaplastic Astrocytoma

Anaplastic astrocytoma is distinguished from the other astrocytomas by (1) greater cellularity, (2) cellular pleomorphism, and (3) anaplasia (Fig. 28-94). The topographic distribution parallels that of astrocytoma. The growth of the tumor is rapid, and life expectancy averages 3 years.

Glioblastoma Multiforme

Glioblastoma multiforme is the extreme expression of anaplasia among the glial neoplasms and accounts for 40% of all primary intracranial tumors.

PATHOLOGY: Most glioblastomas have constituent cells with recognizable astrocytic properties, including GFAP positivity, but they display (1) marked

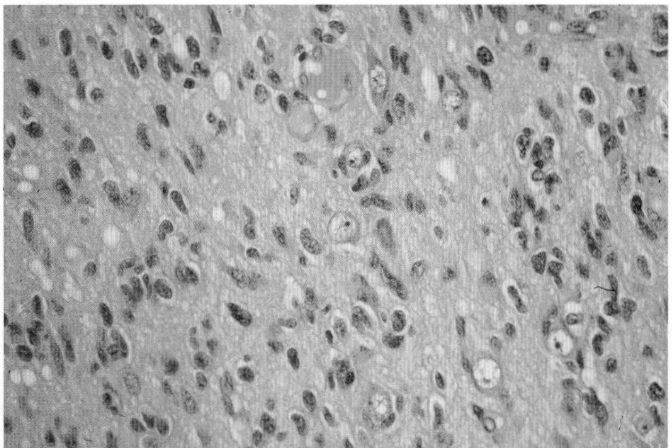

FIGURE 28-94. **Anaplastic astrocytoma.** The cerebral cortex is diffusely infiltrated by pleomorphic tumor cells.

pleomorphism, (2) frequent mitoses, (3) regional zones of necrosis, and (4) endothelial proliferation. The last feature probably reflects the release of angiogenic growth factors by these high-grade tumors. Hyperplasia of fibroblasts is also produced by glioblastomas located in or near the meninges and may actually attain malignant proportions. In such cases, the sarcomatous growth intermingles fibrosarcoma with the glioma, resulting in a **gliosarcoma.** Alternatively, the sarcomatous component may arise via de-differentiation of the glioblastoma.

Glioblastomas typically infiltrate extensively, and frequently cross the corpus callosum to result in a bilateral lesion likened to a butterfly because of its gross configuration and mottled red/yellow color (Fig. 28-95). The colors represent multiple areas of recent (red) and remote (yellow) hemorrhage. The cardinal histologic features of glioblastoma multiforme are as follows:

- **Marked cellularity,** with variable degrees of cellular pleomorphism and multinucleated cells (see Fig. 28-95)
- **Serpentine areas of necrosis** surrounded by zones of crowded tumor cells ("palisading necrosis")
- **Endothelial cell proliferation** formed by clusters of small vessels, referred to as "glomeruloid" formations

Glioblastomas predominate in the later decades of life, with twice the frequency of astrocytomas. The clinical course rarely exceeds 18 months from the time of diagnosis, regardless of therapeutic intervention.

Oligodendroglioma Arises in the White Matter and Grows Slowly

Oligodendrogliomas occur predominantly in the white matter of the cerebral hemispheres of adults.

PATHOLOGY: Histologically, the tumors have small rounded nuclei like normal oligodendrocytes (Figure 28-96), but they also exhibit increased cell density and cellular pleomorphism. Calcospherites, which on occasion are visualized radiographically, are scattered randomly throughout the lesion. The slow growth is reflected in few mitotic figures and a lack of necrosis, although markers of cell proliferation demonstrate that dividing cells are not uncommon in oligodendrogliomas.

The symptoms of oligodendroglioma are frequently ushered in by seizures. Although the lesion is infiltrative, its slow growth permits survival for 5 to 10 years.

Ependymoma Originates in the Lining of the Cavities That Contain Cerebrospinal Fluid

Ependymoma (Fig. 28-97) *is most common in the fourth ventricle, producing obstruction and resulting in hydrocephalus.* This neoplasm is

A

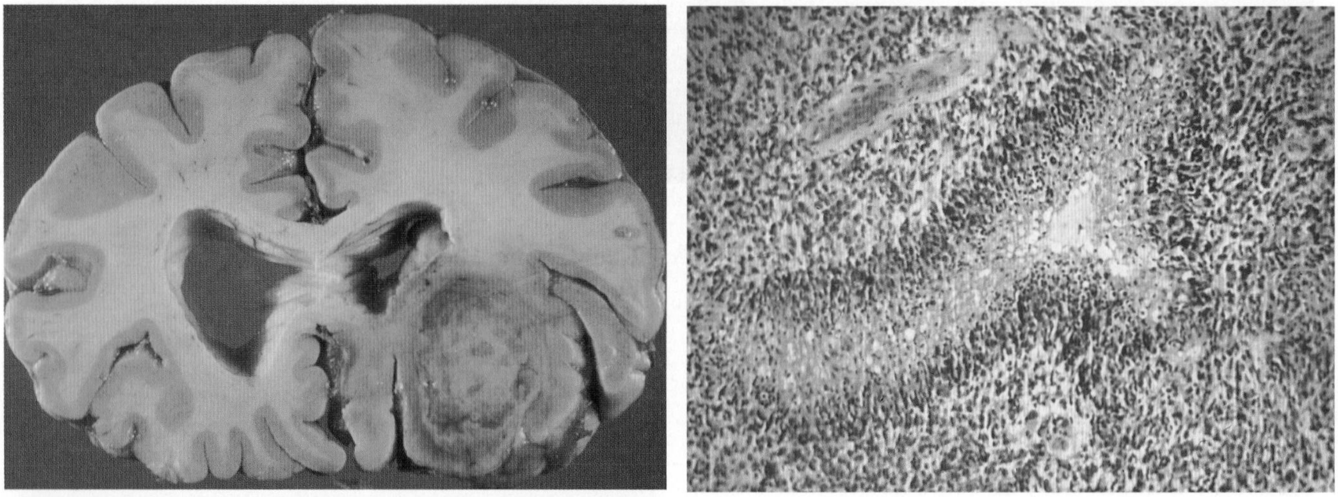

B

C

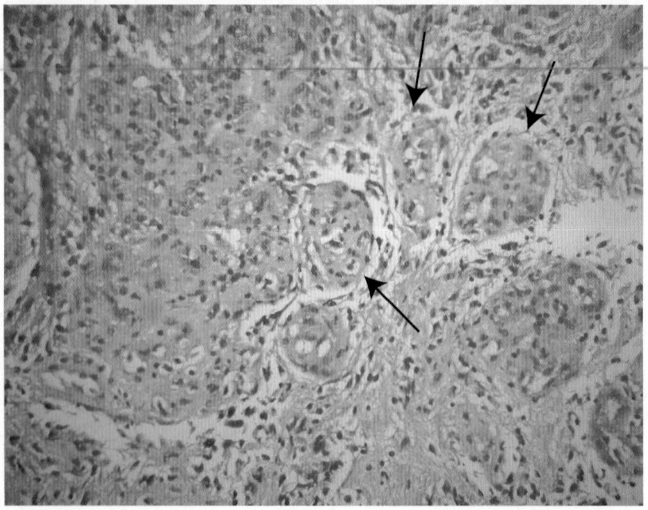

FIGURE 28-95. **Glioblastoma multiforme. A.** A coronal section of the brain shows a necrotic, hemorrhagic, expansile mass in the right hemisphere. **B.** Another area exhibits tumor necrosis, which is surrounded by pseudopalisaded tumor cells. **C.** A characteristic feature of glioblastoma multiforme is endothelial proliferation *(arrows).*

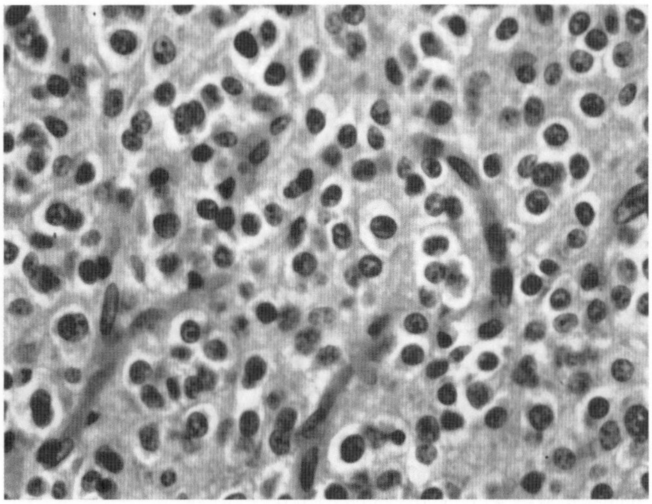

FIGURE 28-96. **Oligodendroglioma.** The tumor consists of sheets of uniform, small cells containing dark blue round nuclei (hematoxylin and eosin stain).

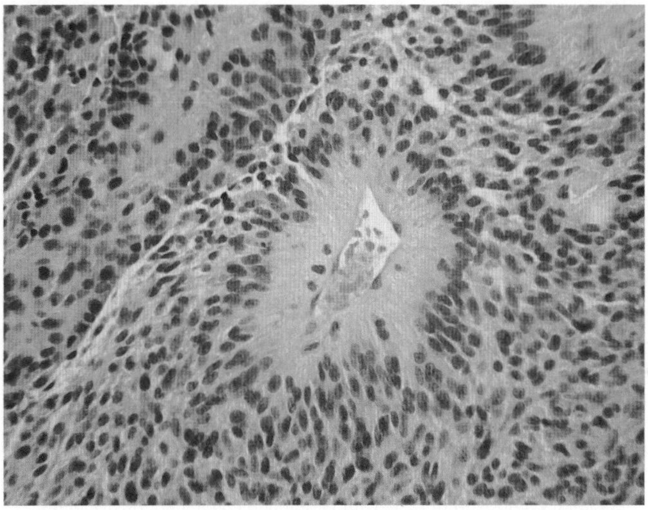

FIGURE 28-98. **Ependymoma.** A microscopic section shows a perivascular pseudorosette.

second only to astrocytoma as an intramedullary tumor of the spinal cord, where it arises from the ependymal lining of the central canal or the filum terminale. Spinal astrocytomas are most often seen at the lumbosacral level, whereas intramedullary astrocytoma, is usually located in the cervical–thoracic region. There are no specific ependymal cell markers, but loss of heterozygosity (LOH) for chromosome 22q may provide a molecular signature.

The cells of an ependymoma characteristically have an "epithelial" appearance, similar to that of normal ependymal cells. They possess ovoid nuclei, with coarse chromatin material and well-defined plasma membranes. The cells of an ependymoma form clefts or may arrange around blood vessels, creating an anuclear mantle of glial processes about the adventitia (Fig. 28-98). The tumor generally grows slowly, but it can seed the subarachnoid space.

CHOROID PLEXUS PAPILLOMA: Choroid plexus papilloma occurs most commonly in children and usually arises in the lateral or fourth ventricle. Hydrocephalus is the major complication. On gross examination, choroid plexus papilloma appears as an intraventricular papillary mass. Microscopically, it duplicates the structure of the normal choroid plexus. Transthyretin immunoreactivity is a reliable marker for these tumors. Choroid plexus papillomas can also transform into carcinomas if they are not excised.

Medulloblastoma Is a Childhood Cerebellar Tumor

Medulloblastoma, the most common intracranial neuroblastic lesion, derives from the transient, cerebellar, external granular cell layer of neuronal progenitor cells, or from their derivatives, that have migrated aberrantly into deeper regions of the cerebellar cortex. It arises exclusively in the cerebellum (Fig. 28-99) and has its highest frequency toward the end of the first decade. The tumor infiltrates aggressively and frequently disseminates through the CSF.

Medulloblastomas are characterized by cells with hyperchromatic, round-to-oval nuclei and scant cytoplasm, which often crowd together with no structural pattern (Fig. 28-100). The neuroblastic character of the cells is occasionally expressed in rosette formation, a distinctive feature of embryonic and neo-

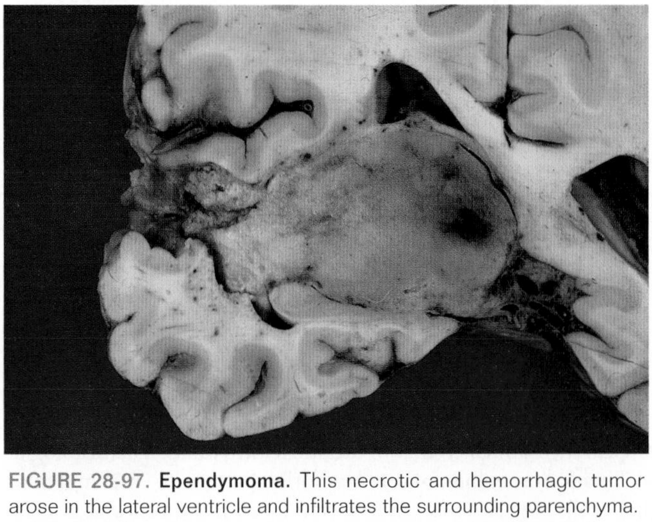

FIGURE 28-97. **Ependymoma.** This necrotic and hemorrhagic tumor arose in the lateral ventricle and infiltrates the surrounding parenchyma.

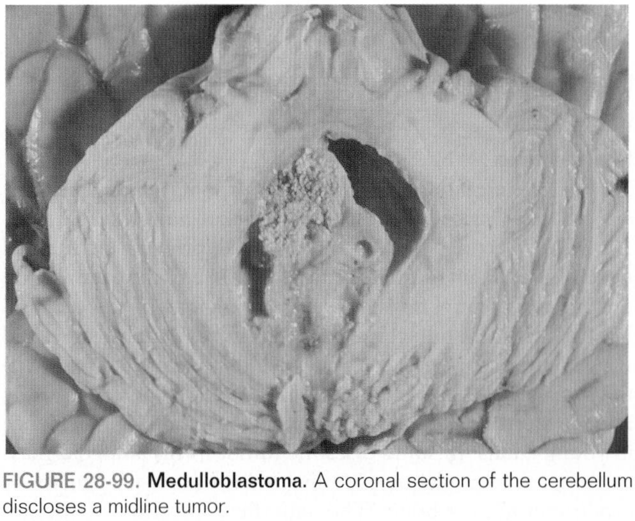

FIGURE 28-99. **Medulloblastoma.** A coronal section of the cerebellum discloses a midline tumor.

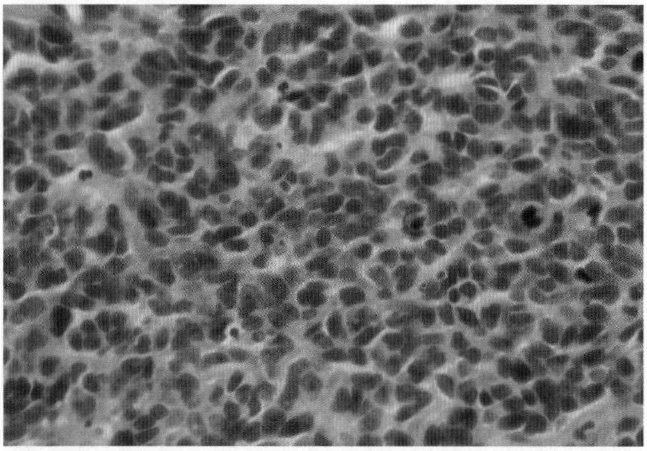

FIGURE 28-100. **Medulloblastoma.** A photomicrograph shows a cellular neoplasm composed of cells with large nuclei and scanty cytoplasm.

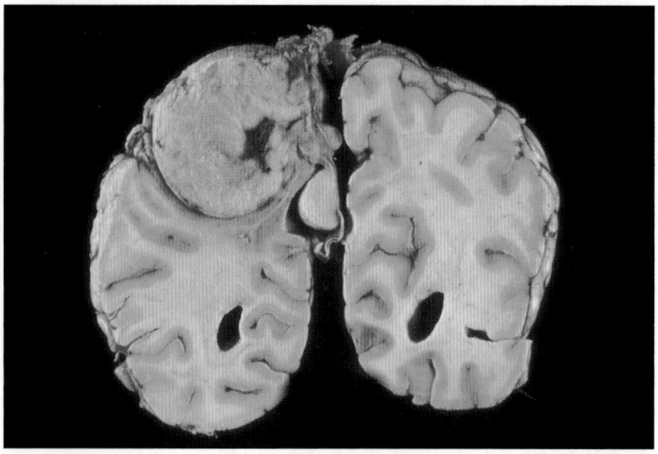

FIGURE 28-101. **Meningioma.** A coronal section of the brain shows a dural-based tumor compressing the left parietal lobe.

plastic neuroblasts. The detection of neuronal and progenitor cell markers (neurofilament proteins, synaptophysin, nestin) may be diagnostically informative in distinguishing these tumors from metastatic epithelial tumors (frequently positive for epithelial keratins), lymphomas (usually positive for leukocyte markers) or other neuroectodermal malignancies. A number of genetic abnormalities have been detected in medulloblastomas (e.g., c-*myc* and N-*myc* amplification, LOH for chromosome 17q), but none are specific.

Children with medulloblastoma are first seen with cerebellar dysfunction or hydrocephalus. Similar to embryonic neuroblasts, the tumor is highly sensitive to ionizing radiation, but unfortunately, subarachnoid dissemination is frequent. The 10-year survival rate is only 50%.

Ganglioglioma Is Composed of Mature and Immature Neurons in a Stroma of Glia

Ganglioglioma is a rare brain tumor that commonly expresses its presence in seizures during the first two decades of life. The neuronal constituents are represented by (1) small rounded nuclei of neuroblasts, (2) intermediate forms, (3) large nuclei with prominent nucleoli and the well-defined cytoplasm of neurons, and (4) the expression of multiple neuronal marker proteins. The matrix of ganglioglioma is formed by astrocytes. This tumor grows indolently and is often cured by surgical removal.

Neoplasms of Mesenchymal Origin Are External to the Brain

Meningioma

Meningiomas are intracranial tumors that arise from arachnoidal cells and produce symptoms by compressing adjacent brain tissue (Fig. 28-101). They account for almost 20% of all primary intracranial neoplasms. Meningiomas occur at almost any intracranial site but are most common in parasagittal regions of the cerebral hemispheres, the olfactory groove, and the lateral sphenoid wing. They occur with a 60:40 female-to-male incidence, but in the spinal canal, this ratio approaches 10:1. The peak frequency is in the fourth to fifth decades, but there is a significant incidence in young adults. In some cases the tumor forms a discoid mass (meningioma en plaque). Meningiomas have a propensity to erode contiguous bone. The superficial position of meningiomas, coupled with neural displacement rather than infiltration, invites total surgical excision. However, tumors at the base of the brain often invade the skull, thereby limiting complete resection and making recurrence common.

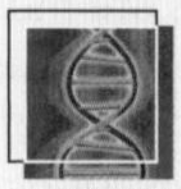

PATHOGENESIS: Meningiomas typically arise in one of three settings:

- Sporadic cases (most common)
- Iatrogenic cases caused by prior radiation therapy to the cranium
- In association with a genetic disorder, especially neurofibromatosis type 2 (NF2)

Most meningiomas arise sporadically. Many such tumors exhibit loss, partial deletion, or mutation of the *NF2* locus (22q12), suggesting that perturbations of this tumor-suppressor gene are involved not only in NF2 (see below), but also in the origin of many sporadic meningiomas (and schwannomas).

The induction of meningiomas by radiation therapy involves a latent period of a decade or more and is directly related to the radiation dosage. Low-dose scalp irradiation for tinea capitis was widely used until 1960. For these patients, the average interval between the treatment and the detection of a meningioma was 35 years. With higher radiation doses, such as those used for head and neck cancers, the interval may be as short as 5 years. Meningiomas also occur in conjunction with several genetic syndromes, most importantly NF2. An association has also been reported with basal cell nevus syndrome (Gorlin syndrome), and rare, familial, multiple meningioma syndromes have been documented.

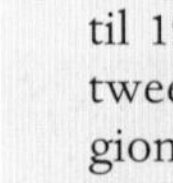

PATHOLOGY: On gross examination, most meningiomas appear as well-circumscribed, firm, bosselated masses of variable size. The cut surface presents a gray appearance similar to that of uterine leiomyomas. The histologic hallmark of meningiomas is a whorled pattern of "meningothelial" cells (Fig. 28-102), in association with psammoma bodies (laminated, spherical calcospherites). Although this morphologic

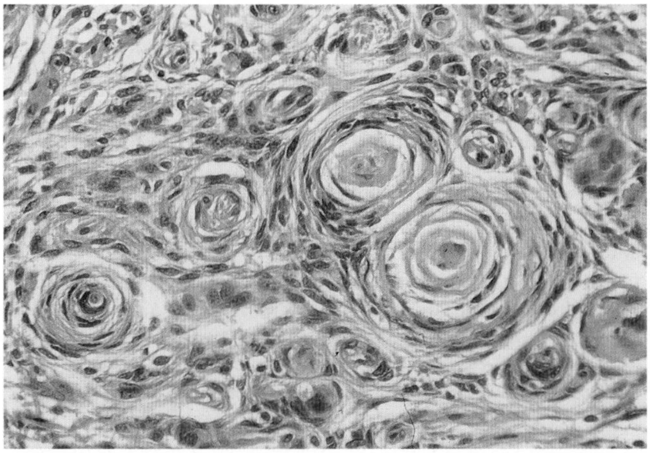

FIGURE 28-102. **Meningioma.** A microscopic section discloses a whorled arrangement of tumor cells, the so-called meningothelial appear-

appearance is distinctive, in many meningiomas it is obscured by a predominantly fibroblast-like proliferation. Some meningiomas are dominated by blood vessels (**angiomatous meningioma**); others have a papillary appearance (**papillary meningiomas**); a rare lesion features microcystic formations (**microcystic meningioma**). Many of the subtypes of meningioma do not differ significantly in their biological behavior. Meningiomas are negative for GFAP and keratins, but positive for epithelial membrane antigen.

CLINICAL FEATURES: The indolent growth of meningiomas enables them to enlarge slowly for years before becoming symptomatic, during which time they displace the brain but do not infiltrate it. Thus, seizures rather than neurologic deficits frequently characterize their clinical presentation, particularly with tumors at parasagittal sites situated over the convexity of the hemispheres. In other locations, meningiomas compress a variety of functional structures. Thus, tumors of the olfactory groove produce anosmia; those in the suprasellar region lead to visual deficits; meningiomas in the cerebellopontine angle cause cranial nerve palsies; and those in the spinal column result in dysfunction of the spinal nerve roots and spinal cord.

Because the meninges, are innervated by pain fibers, headaches are common. Penetration of the calvaria may create a tumor mass on the external surface of the skull. Meningiomas that are not completely excised tend to recur, and some may transform into malignant and invasive meningiomas, although these more aggressive variants rarely arise de novo.

Schwannoma

Schwannoma is a tumor derived from Schwann cells, which produce both collagen and myelin (see below). This tumor is also known as neurilemmoma, perineural fibroblastoma, and neurinoma. Histologically, schwannomas appear as interwoven fascicles of spindle cells. Occasionally, parallel arrays of tumor cells are noted at the ends of a fibrillar bundle and are referred to as a **Verocay body.** Fortunately, schwannomas are rarely malignant, and nuclear pleomorphism, when limited to occasional cells, does not predict accelerated growth.

Acoustic neuromas are intracranial schwannomas that are restricted to the eighth nerve. Interestingly, the tumor invariably begins at the transition from oligodendroglia to Schwann cells along CNS axons that form peripheral nerves. This junction corresponds anatomically to the position of the internal auditory meatus. Thus, acoustic neuromas may cause tinnitus and deafness as they expand the bony meatus. These schwannomas can also protrude into the cerebellopontine angle and compress other nerves.

Schwannomas also arise on spinal nerve roots. On occasion, they are entirely within the spinal canal, although at other times, they span a bony foramen, with a "dumb-bell" configuration. Together with meningiomas, schwannomas compose most intradural–extramedullary neoplasms. Tumors of Schwann cells also occur on peripheral nerves as schwannomas and neurofibromas. As mentioned above, some schwannomas exhibit deletions or mutations of the *NF2* gene.

Neoplasms Derived from Ectopic Tissues Compress Adjacent Structures

Craniopharyngioma

Craniopharyngiomas are solid and cystic lesions located above the sella turcica that arise from the epithelium of Rathke's pouch. This structure is a part of the embryonic nasopharynx that migrates cephalad and gives origin to the anterior lobe of the hypophysis (Fig. 28-103A).

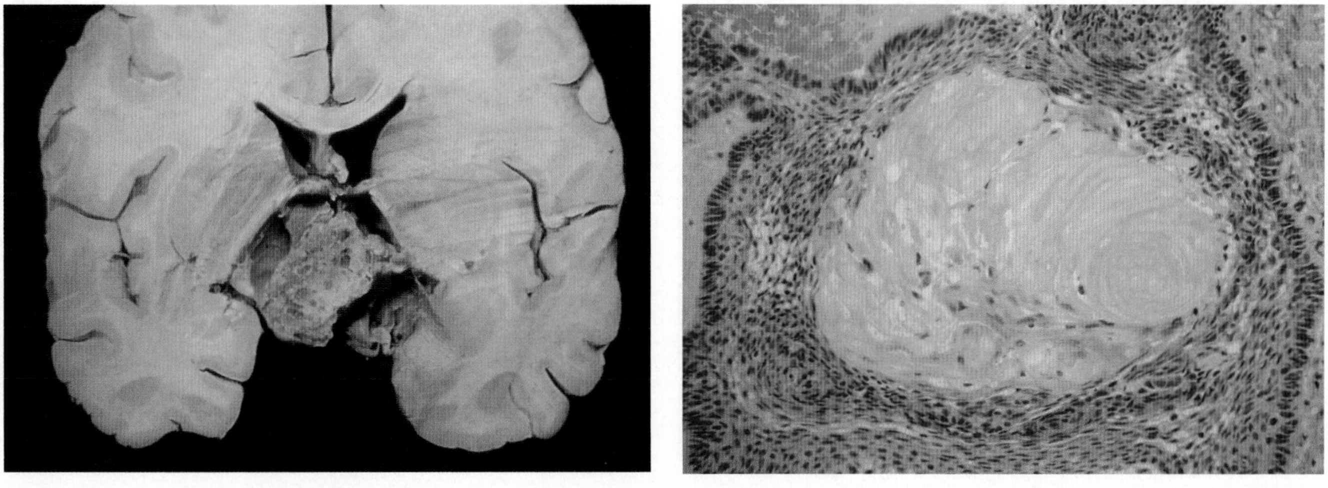

A B

FIGURE 28-103. **Craniopharyngioma. A.** A coronal section of the brain discloses a cystic mass that occupied the sella turcica. **B.** A microscopic section reveals squamous epithelium and keratin debris.

These cystic lesions are lined by squamous epithelium, and are referred to as **adamantinomatous.** Craniopharyngiomas are solid and resemble tumors of dentigerous origin such as adamantinomas and the karatinizing and calcifying odontogenic keratocyst (see Fig. 28-103B). Craniopharyngiomas generally become symptomatic in the first two decades of life, creating visual deficits and headaches. They may cause pituitary failure, including diabetes insipidus.

Dermoid and Epidermoid Cysts

Dermoid and epidermoid cysts result from misdirected embryonic development. The term **dermoid** refers to cysts lined by squamous epithelium, skin appendages, and hair. These cysts extend into bones of the skull and occasionally into the intracranial compartment. The displaced squamous cells proliferate and develop into a cyst, which fills with desquamated keratotic debris that resembles "mother of pearl." The intracranial lesions tend to occur in the posterior fossa or about the sella turcica. Although these cysts are not true neoplasms, accumulating debris causes expansion of the intracranial mass, thereby leading to symptoms.

Lipoma

Lipomas arise from rudiments of adipose tissue carried inward as the brain forms during embryogenesis. They are positioned (1) along the superior aspect of the corpus callosum, (2) the dorsum of the quadrigeminal plate (Fig. 28-104), and (3) the dorsal sagittal plane of the spinal cord near the cauda equina. Lipomas enlarge slowly, if at all, but may enmesh cranial or spinal nerves and interfere with nerve conduction. Most lipomas of the CNS are encountered incidentally at postmortem examination and histologically mimic normal adipocytes.

Tumors of Germ Cell Origin Are Similar to Gonadal Neoplasms

Neoplasms that originate from misplaced germ cells occur within the cranial cavity and, less commonly, in the spinal cord. Such tumors are almost invariably located in midline structures, especially in the area of the pineal gland, but also at sites immediately adjacent to this gland, in the cerebellopontine angle, and around the sella turcica. Intracranial germ cell tumors display a number of phenotypes that parallel gonadal neoplasms, including seminoma, choriocarcinoma, embryonal carcinoma, endodermal sinus tumor, and teratoma.

Intracranial germ cell tumors are seen primarily in young adult men, and the symptoms depend on the location of the expanding mass. Destruction of the pineal gland by a germ cell tumor may produce precocious puberty, particularly in boys. In that location it may compress the superior colliculus and restrict ocular motion. Compression of the aqueduct of Sylvius leads to hydrocephalus.

Hemangioblastoma Is a Cerebellar Tumor That Is Often Syndromic

Hemangioblastoma is a highly vascularized tumor that originates predominantly in the cerebellum (Fig. 28-105A). Although its name suggests that it arises from endothelial cells, the true cell of origin is still debated. Hemangioblastoma features endothelium-lined canals interspersed with plump cells (see Fig. 28-105B). *In 20% of cases, these cells secrete erythropoietin and induce polycythemia.* A rare hemangioblastoma arises in the spinal cord, and

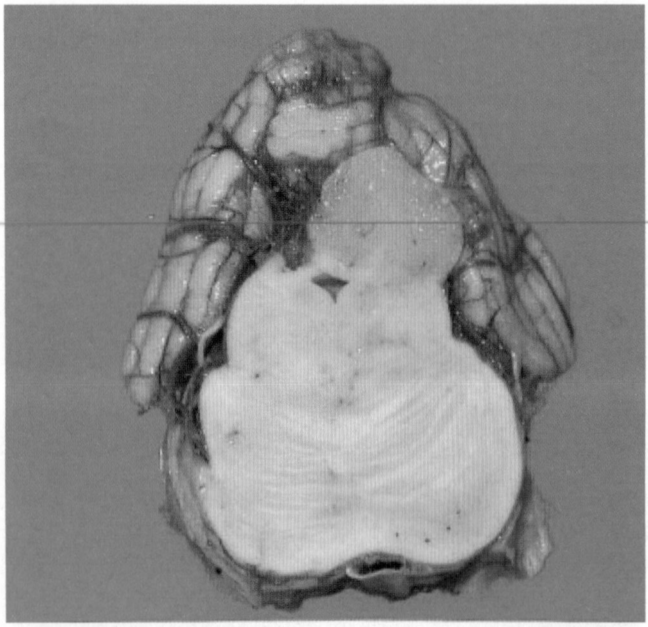

FIGURE 28-104. **Lipoma.** A fatty tumor is located superior to the pons.

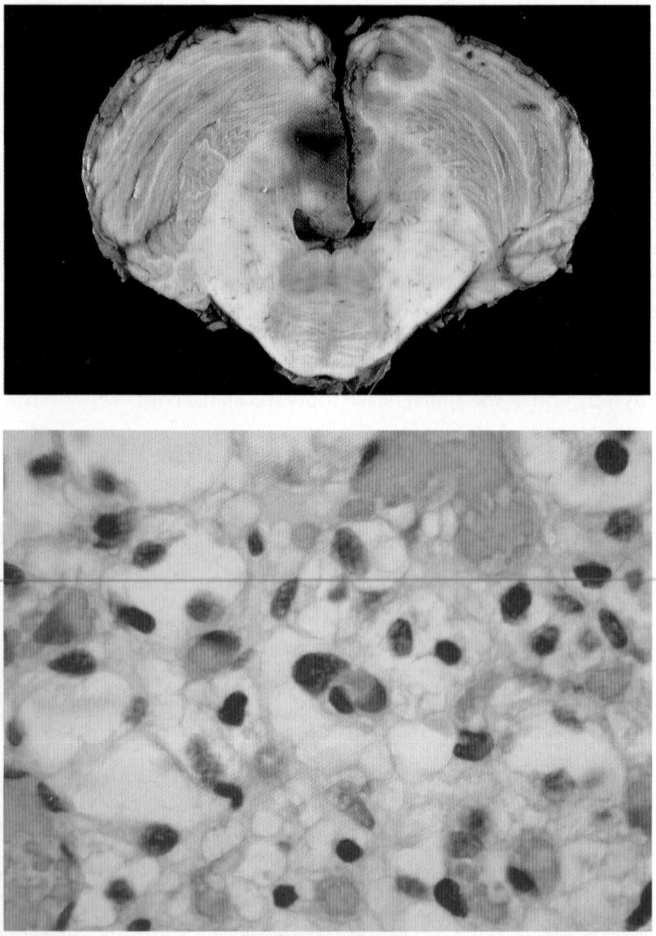

A

B

FIGURE 28-105. **Hemangioblastoma. A.** A hemorrhagic mass is located in the cerebellum. **B.** A microscopic section reveals vacuolated tumor cells and an abundant capillary network.

on occasion they originate above the tentorium. Hemangioblastoma usually becomes clinically apparent as an expanding mass between the ages of 20 and 40 years.

Lindau syndrome refers to the hereditary occurrence of a cerebellar hemangioblastoma that is not associated with other lesions.

von Hippel-Lindau syndrome is a hereditary variant in which cerebellar hemangioblastoma is associated with retinal hemangiomas and other tumors, owing to mutations in the tumor suppressor *VHL* gene (see Chapter 5).

Lymphoma Can Originate in the CNS

Lymphoma typically arises as a primary B-cell lesion in the brain in a manner analogous to its occurrence in the stomach, small bowel, or testis, but the overwhelming majority of lymphomas are metastatic to the brain from other sites. In the brain, primary lymphoma often arises deep in the cerebral hemispheres, commonly in bilateral periventricular positions. A mixture of small and large lymphocytes is angiocentric (Fig. 28-106). Lymphomas often arise in the context of immunosuppression as well as in AIDS. In some instances they have been linked etiologically to infection with Epstein-Barr virus.

Extracranial lymphomas may secondarily involve the CNS, usually late in the course of the disease. The meninges, epidural space, and nerve roots are most commonly affected.

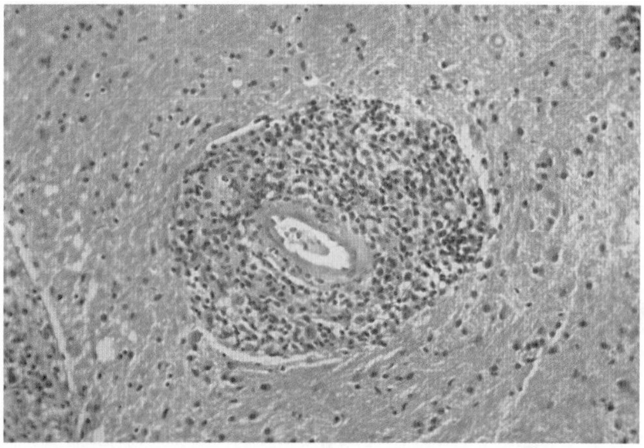

FIGURE 28-106. **Cerebral lymphoma.** A perivascular collection of neoplastic lymphocytes is present.

Metastatic Tumors Are the Most Common Intracranial Neoplasms

Metastatic tumors reach the intracranial compartment through the bloodstream, generally in patients with advanced cancer. Tumors of different organs vary in their incidence of intracranial metastases. For example, a patient with disseminated melanoma has a greater than 50% likelihood of acquiring intracranial metastases, whereas the incidence of such metastases in carcinoma of the breast and lung is 35%, and that for cancer of the kidney or colon is only 5%. Certain carcinomas, such as those of the prostate, liver, and adrenals, and sarcomas of all types rarely establish intracranial metastases. Most metastatic lesions seed to the gray–white junction, reflecting the rich capillary bed in this area. Carcinomas may spread to the calvaria and extend into the intracranial compartment.

A metastasis contrasts with a primary glioma in its discrete appearance, globoid shape, and prominent halo of edema (Fig. 28-107). Metastases to the leptomeninges permit tumor cells to grow in the CSF, suspended as if they were in tissue culture.

Colloid Cyst Exerts Pressure Effects

Colloid cysts (paraphyseal cyst, third ventricular cyst) are distinctive for their anterior, midline location in the tegmental portion of the third ventricle (Fig. 28-108). In this location, they (1) occlude the foramina of Monro, (2) elevate and compress the fornix, and (3) press on the lateral wall of the third ventricle. These effects result in hydrocephalus, alterations in personality, weakness of the lower legs, and loss of bladder control. Colloid cysts are lined by ciliated cuboidal epithelium. The lesions enlarge slowly, usually over decades, by the accumulation of desquamated and secretory products. The origin of colloid cysts remains uncertain.

A

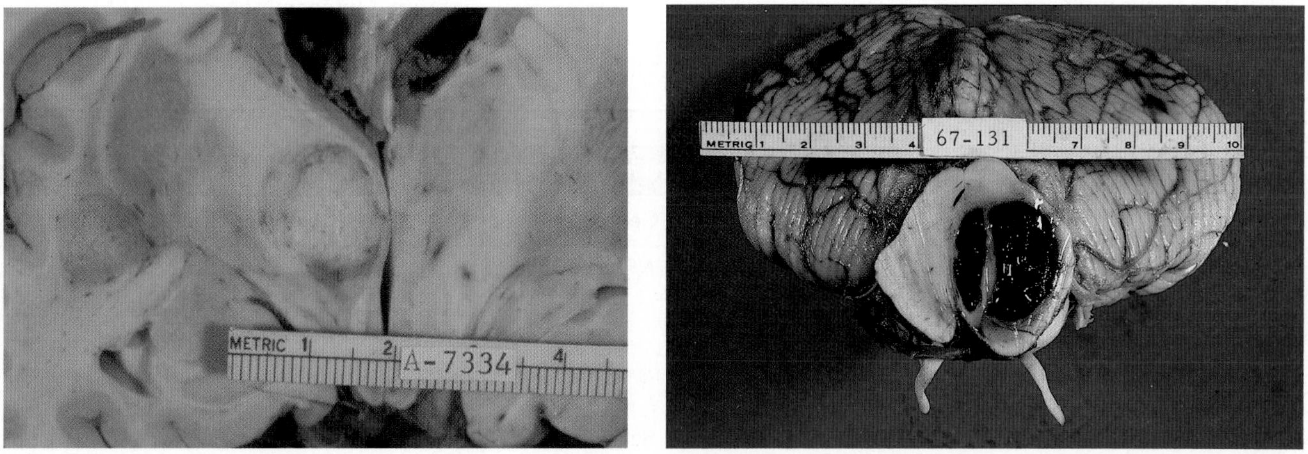

B

FIGURE 28-107. **Cerebral metastases. A.** A coronal section of the brain from a patient with disseminated adenocarcinoma of the lung shows a circumscribed tumor in the area of the left hypothalamus. **B.** A deeply pigmented tumor mass is present in the brain of a patient with metastatic malignant melanoma.

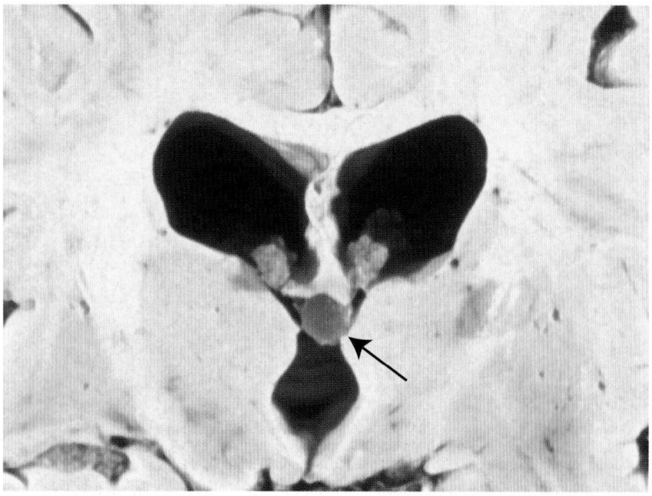

FIGURE 28-108. **Colloid cyst.** A gelatinous cystic mass (*arrow*) is present in the third ventricle.

Hereditary Intracranial Neoplasms Are Often Associated with Extracranial Tumors

A number of hereditary disorders are associated with CNS tumors, and the genetic bases of the major syndromes are listed in Table 28-5. Other inherited diseases in which neoplasms of systemic organs figure prominently include the expression of nervous system tumors. For example, malignant gliomas arise in patients with Li-Fraumeni syndrome, and medulloblastomas are associated with the gastrointestinal tumors of Turcot syndrome.

Neurofibromatosis (von Recklinghausen Disease)

NF occurs in two distinct forms, both of which are inherited as autosomal dominant traits (see Chapter 6). NF2 is usually characterized by bilateral acoustic neuromas. However, the disease can be diagnosed in patients with a unilateral eighth nerve tumor if two of the following are present: neurofibroma, meningioma, glioma, or schwannoma.

Tuberous Sclerosis (Bourneville Disease)

Tuberous sclerosis is an autosomal dominant disease characterized by hamartomas (tubers) of the brain, retina, and viscera, as well as various neoplasms. This disease reflects disordered migration and arrested maturation of the neuroectoderm, resulting in formation of "tubers" of the cerebral cortex and of subependymal giant cell astrocytomas (Fig. 28-109). The tubers are discrete cortical areas composed of bizarre cells with neuronal and glial features. The subependymal giant cell astrocytomas have been likened to "candle drippings." In addition to the intracranial lesions, the syndrome includes (1) facial angiofibromas (adenoma sebaceum), (2) cardiac rhabdomyomas, and (3) mesenchymal tumors of the kidney (angiomyolipomas). Most patients with tuberous sclerosis have seizures and are mentally retarded. Mutations in two genes have been linked to tuberous sclerosis. *TSC1* (9q34) codes for a protein termed *hamartin. TSC2* (16p13) encodes *tuberin,* a protein with homology to a GTPase-activating protein. Both genes seem to act as tumor suppressors.

Lindau Syndrome

As mentioned above, some hemangioblastomas of the cerebellum assume a hereditary pattern (Lindau syndrome). An identical tumor may occur in the retina (von Hippel-Lindau syndrome). In the latter syndrome, cysts also occur in the kidneys and pancreas.

Sturge-Weber Syndrome (Encephalofacial Angiomatosis)

Sturge-Weber syndrome is a rare, nonfamilial congenital disorder characterized by angiomas of the brain and face. The facial lesion is usually unilateral and is termed a **port wine stain (nevus flammeus).** The leptomeninges exhibit large angiomas, which in severe cases may occupy an entire hemisphere. Cerebral calcification and atrophy often underlie the intracranial angiomas (Fig. 28-110). The link between angiomas of the face and the brain has been attributed to the continuity of the embryological vascular supply of the telencephalon, the eye, and the overlying skin. In most instances, Sturge-Weber syndrome is associated with mental deficiency.

THE PERIPHERAL NERVOUS SYSTEM

Anatomy

The peripheral nervous system (PNS) is external to the brain and spinal cord and includes (1) cranial nerves, (2) dorsal and ventral spinal roots, (3) spinal nerves and their continuations, and (4) ganglia. Peripheral nerves carry somatic motor, somatic sensory, visceral sensory and autonomic fibers.

TABLE 28-5

Hereditary Syndromes Associated with Intracranial Tumors

Disease	Chromosome Locus	Gene (Protein)	Nervous System Tumor(s)
Neurofibromatosis 1	17q11	*NF1* (neurofibromin)	Neurofibroma Neurofibrosarcoma Juvenile pilocytic astrocytoma of the optic nerves ("optic glioma")
Neurofibromatosis 2	22q12	*NF2* (schwannomin/merlin)	Schwannoma Meningioma Ependymoma (spinal cord)
Tuberous sclerosis	9q34*TSC1* (hamartin)	Subependymal giant cell	
16p13.3	*TSC2* (tuberin)	Astrocytoma	
von Hippel-Lindau syndrome	3p25	*VHL*	Hemangioblastoma

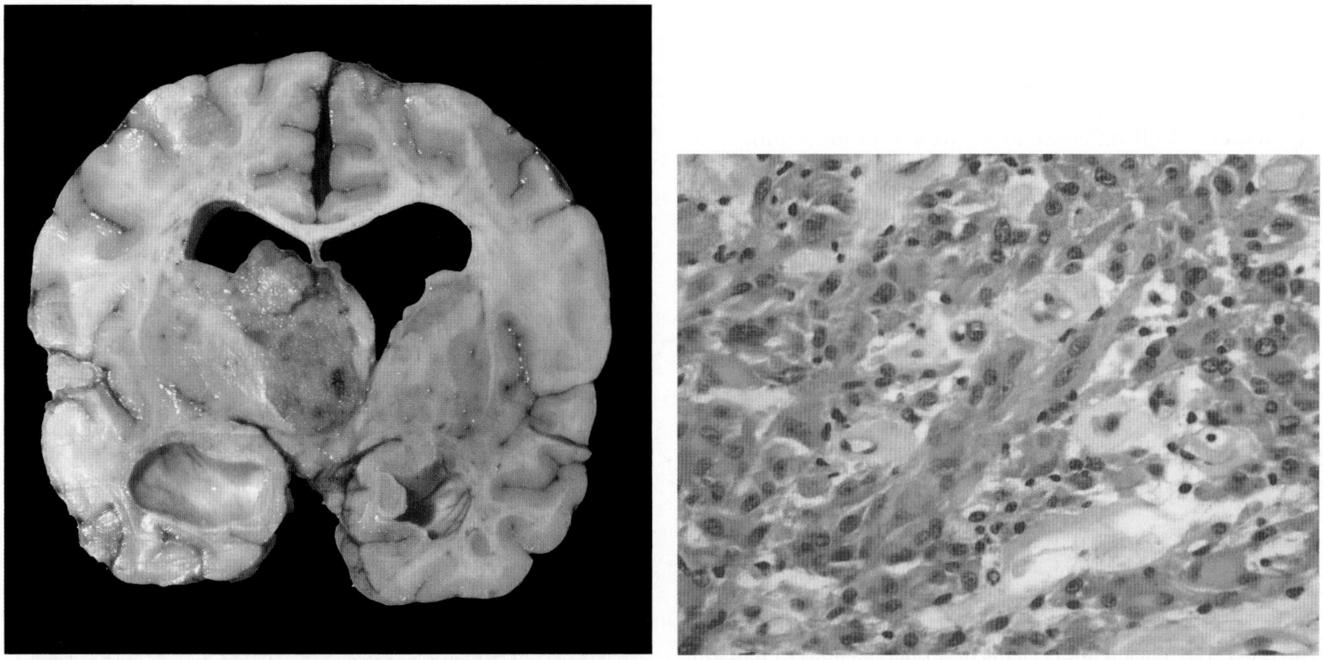

FIGURE 28-109. **Tuberous sclerosis. A.** A large subependymal giant cell astrocytoma fills much of the left lateral ventricle. **B.** Microscopic section of a subependymal giant cell astrocytoma containing large elongated cells with abundant eosinophilic cytoplasm.

Somatic motor and preganglionic autonomic fibers arise from neuronal cell bodies within the CNS. The sensory and postganglionic autonomic fibers originate from neuronal cell bodies within ganglia located on cranial nerves, dorsal roots, and autonomic nerves. The neurons and satellite cells of the ganglia and all of the Schwann cells are derived from the neural crest.

Peripheral nerves, but not their ganglia, have a blood–nerve barrier analogous to the blood–brain barrier. Endoneurial connective tissue surrounds the individual nerve fibers, which are bundled into fascicles by the **perineurial sheath.** Epineurial connective tissue binds the fascicles together and contains the nutrient arteries.

Peripheral nerve fibers are either myelinated or unmyelinated (Fig. 28-111). Myelinated fibers range from 1 to 20 μm in diameter, whereas unmyelinated ones are considerably smaller,

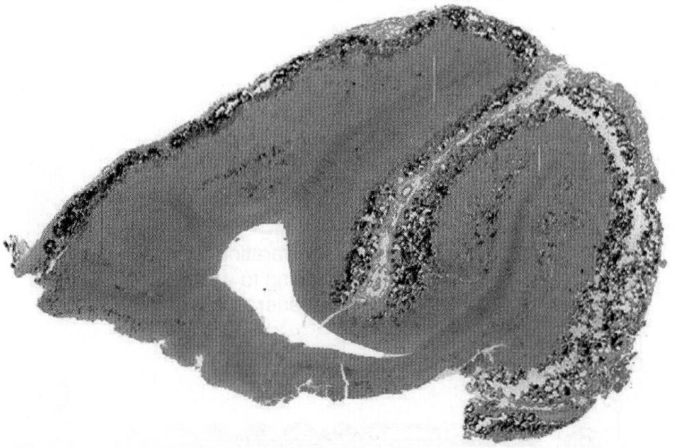

FIGURE 28-110. **Sturge-Weber Syndrome.** Portion of cerebral cortex with overlying capillary angioma involving the leptomeninges and underlying cortical calcification (purple).

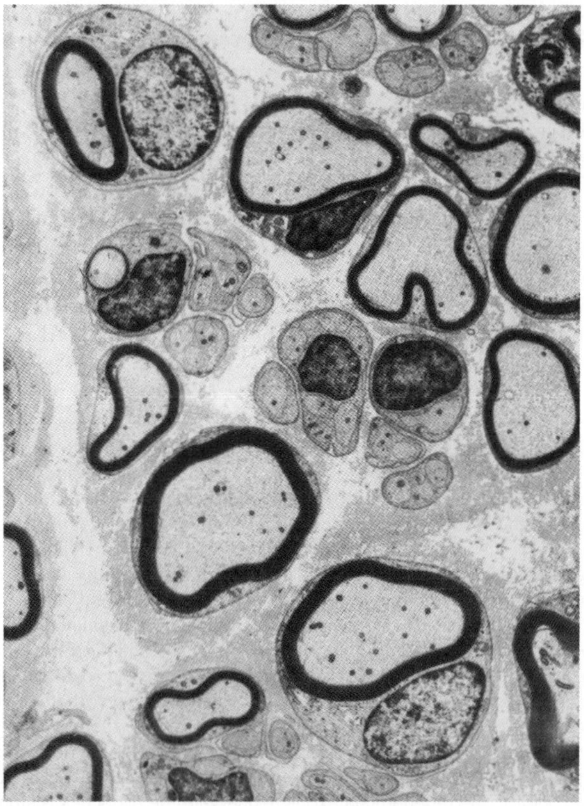

FIGURE 28-111. **Structure of peripheral nerve.** Electron micrograph of a peripheral nerve shows myelinated fibers interspersed with groups of unmyelinated fibers. Note that unlike myelinated axons, several unmyelinated axons may share a Schwann cell.

measuring 0.4 to 2.4 μm. Myelin is an elaboration of the Schwann cell plasmalemma and is necessary for saltatory nerve conduction. Schwann cells ensheathe both myelinated and unmyelinated fibers. The axon determines whether the ensheathing Schwann cell differentiates into a myelin-forming cell. Myelin-sheath thickness, internodal length (i.e., the distance between two nodes of Ranvier), and conduction velocity are proportional to the axonal diameter.

Reactions to Injury

Peripheral nerve fibers display only a limited number of reactions to injury (Fig. 28-112). The major types of nerve fiber damage are axonal degeneration and segmental demyelination. Peripheral nerve fibers differ from CNS nerve fibers in having the capacity for functionally significant axonal regeneration and remyelination.

Axonal Degeneration Is Usually Restricted to the Distal Axon

Degeneration (necrosis) of the axon occurs in many neuropathies and reflects significant injury of the neuronal cell body or its axon. Axonal degeneration is quickly followed by breakdown of the myelin sheath and Schwann cell proliferation. Myelin degradation is initiated by Schwann cells and completed by macrophages, which infiltrate the nerve within 3 days after axonal degeneration. If the degeneration is restricted to the distal axon, regenerating axons may sprout within 1 week from the intact, proximal axonal stump. There are several types of axonal degeneration.

DISTAL AXONAL DEGENERATION: In many neuropathies, axonal degeneration is initially restricted to the distal ends of the larger, longer fibers (see Fig. 28-112B). Peripheral neuropathies characterized by the selective degeneration of distal axons are known as **dying-back neuropathies** (**distal axonopathies**) and are typically seen as distal ("length-dependent" or "glove-and-stocking") neuropathies.

In distal axonal degeneration, the neuronal cell body and proximal axon remain intact. Therefore, axonal regeneration and return of nerve function may be possible if the cause of the distal axonal degeneration can be identified and removed. This must occur before the dying-back degeneration sufficiently extends centripetally to involve the proximal axon and cause death of the neuronal cell body. Recovery is also limited in some dying-back neuropathies, because the distal axonal degeneration involves not only the peripherally directed axon of the dorsal root-ganglion neuron, but also its centrally directed axon traveling in the dorsal columns of the spinal cord. These centrally directed axons, like other axons within the CNS, have little capacity for regeneration.

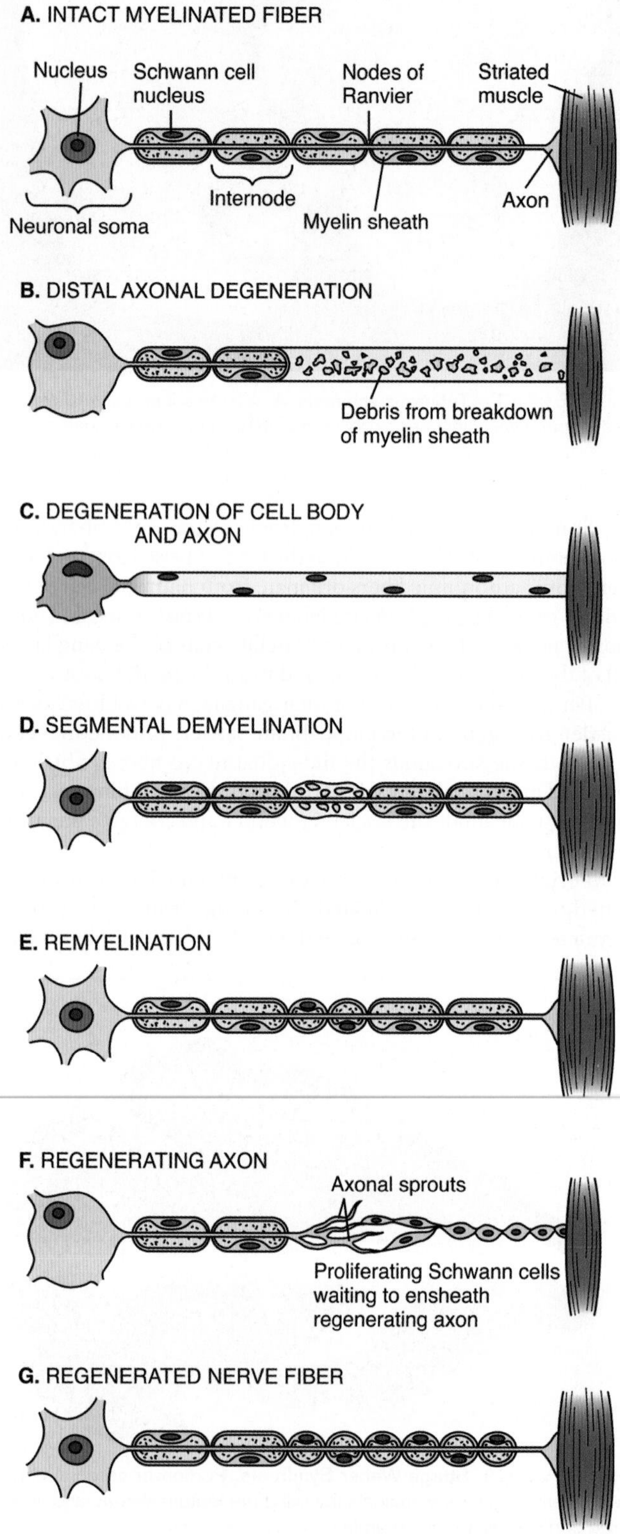

FIGURE 28-112. **Basic responses of peripheral nerve fibers to injury. A. Intact myelinated fiber.** The axon is insulated by the Schwann cell-derived myelin sheaths. **B. Distal axonal degeneration.** The distal axon has degenerated, and myelin sheaths associated with the distal axon have secondarily degenerated. The striated muscle shows denervation atrophy. **C. Degeneration of cell body and axon.** Degeneration involves the neuronal cell body and its entire axon. The myelin sheaths associated with the axon have also degenerated. **D. Segmental demyelination.** The myelin sheath associated with one Schwann cell has degenerated, leaving a segment of axon uncovered by myelin. The underlying axon remains intact. **E. Remyelination.** Proliferating Schwann cells cover the demyelinated segment of the axon and elaborate new myelin sheaths. The remyelinating Schwann cells have short internodal lengths. **F. Regenerating axon.** Regenerating axons sprout from the distal end of the disrupted axon. Ideally, the regenerating axons reinnervate the distal nerve stump, where they will be ensheathed and myelinated by Schwann cells of the distal stump. **G. Regenerated nerve fiber.** The regenerated portion of the axon is myelinated by Schwann cells with short internodal lengths. The striated muscle is reinnervated.

NEURONOPATHY: Axonal degeneration may result from death of the neuronal cell body, as occurs in an autoimmune dorsal root ganglionitis (see Fig. 28-112C). Neuropathies showing selective damage to the neuronal cell body are referred to as **neuronopathies** and are much less common than distal axonopathies. There is little potential for recovery of function in neuronopathy because death of the neuronal cell body precludes axonal regeneration.

WALLERIAN DEGENERATION: This term refers to the axonal degeneration that occurs in a nerve distal to a transection or crush of the nerve. If the transection is not too proximal, the nerve may regenerate.

Segmental Demyelination Reflects Direct Schwann Cell Injury or Underlying Axonal Abnormalities

Loss of myelin from one or more internodes (segments) along a myelinated fiber reflects Schwann cell dysfunction (see Fig. 28-112D). This condition may be caused by direct injury to the Schwann cell or myelin sheath (**primary demyelination**), or it may result from underlying axonal abnormalities (**secondary demyelination**).

Loss of the myelin sheath is not accompanied by degeneration of the underlying axon. Macrophages infiltrate the nerve and clear the myelin debris. Degeneration of the internodal myelin sheath is followed sequentially by (1) Schwann cell proliferation, (2) remyelination of the demyelinated segments, and (3) recovery of function. The remyelinated internodes have shortened internodal lengths. Repeated episodes of segmental demyelination and remyelination of peripheral nerves, as occurs in chronic demyelinating neuropathies, lead to the accumulation of supernumerary Schwann cells around axons (**onion-bulbs**) and clinically apparent nerve enlargement (**hypertrophic neuropathy;** Fig. 28-113).

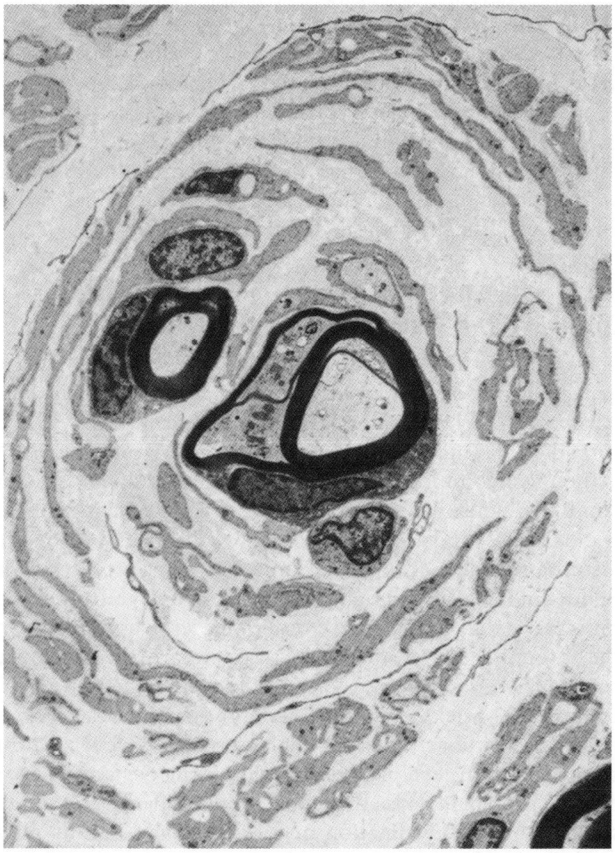

FIGURE 28-113. **Onion-bulb formation in peripheral nerve.** Electron micrograph shows multiple layers of flattened Schwann cell processes encircling two myelinated axons. Onion-bulb formations are common in the demyelinating form of Charcot-Marie-Tooth disease.

Peripheral Neuropathies

Peripheral neuropathy is a process that affects the function of one or more peripheral nerves. The disease may be restricted to the PNS, involve both the peripheral and central nervous systems, or affect multiple organ systems. Peripheral neuropathies are encountered in all age groups and may be hereditary or acquired.

The causes of peripheral neuropathy are diverse (Table 28-6). Diabetic neuropathy is the most common neuropathy in the United States. Other common causes of neuropathy include hereditary disorders, alcoholism, renal failure, neurotoxic drugs, autoimmune diseases, monoclonal gammopathy, infections, and trauma.

PATHOLOGY: The pathologic findings in most neuropathies are mainly limited to axonal degeneration, mainly segmental demyelination, or a combination of both. When axonal degeneration predominates, the neuropathy

TABLE 28-6

Etiologic Classification of Neuropathies

Immune-mediated neuropathies Guillain-Barré syndrome Acute inflammatory demyelinating polyneuropathy Acute motor axonal neuropathy Acute motor sensory axonal neuropathy Chronic inflammatory demyelinating polyneuropathy Multifocal motor neuropathy Dorsal root ganglionitis Neuropathy associated with monoclonal gammopathy Vasculitic neuropathy
Metabolic neuropathies Diabetic polyneuropathy and mononeuropathies Uremic neuropathy Critical illness polyneuropathy
Nutritional neuropathy (deficiency of vitamin B_1, B_6, B_{12}, or E)
Alcoholic neuropathy
Toxic and drug-induced neuropathies (see Table 28-7)
Amyloid neuropathy
Hereditary neuropathies (see Table 28-8 and Table 28-9)
Neuropathies associated with infections Leprosy Human immunodeficiency virus Cytomegalovirus Herpes zoster Lyme disease Diphtheria (toxin)
Paraneoplastic neuropathy
Sarcoid neuropathy
Radiation neuropathy
Traumatic neuropathy
Chronic idiopathic axonal neuropathy

is classified as an **axonal neuropathy;** when segmental demyelination predominates, the neuropathy is classified as a **demyelinating neuropathy.** *Most (80%–90%) neuropathies are axonal.* Electrophysiological studies often help to differentiate between axonal and demyelinating neuropathies. Nerve-conduction velocity is typically near normal in axonal neuropathies but conspicuously decreased in demyelinating neuropathies.

Many neuropathies do not show additional disease-specific histologic features beyond axonal loss or demyelination, so that clinicopathologic correlation is necessary to establish causation. A small number of neuropathies have disease-specific histologic features, such as necrotizing arteritis (vasculitic neuropathy), granulomatous inflammation (leprosy, sarcoid), amyloid deposits (amyloid neuropathy), abnormalities of the myelin sheath (IgM paraproteinemic neuropathy, hereditary neuropathy with liability to pressure palsies), or abnormal accumulations within Schwann cells (leukodystrophy) or axons (giant axonal neuropathy).

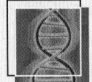

CLINICAL FEATURES: The major clinical manifestations of peripheral neuropathy are muscle weakness, muscle atrophy, altered sensation, and autonomic dysfunction. Motor, sensory, and autonomic functions may be equally or preferentially affected. Sensory abnormalities may reflect predominant involvement of large-diameter fibers (position and vibration sense) or small-diameter fibers (pain and temperature). The tempo of the neuropathy may be acute (days to weeks), subacute (weeks to months), or chronic (months to years). The disease may be localized to one nerve (**mononeuropathy**) or several nerves (**mononeuropathy multiplex**), or it may be diffuse and symmetric (**polyneuropathy**).

Diabetic Neuropathy Has Several Clinical Presentations

Peripheral neuropathy is a common complication of diabetes mellitus. The neuropathy may manifest as a distal sensorimotor polyneuropathy, autonomic neuropathy, mononeuropathy, or mononeuropathy multiplex. The mononeuropathies may involve cranial nerves (cranial neuropathy), nerve roots (radiculopathy), or proximal peripheral nerves. *Distal, predominantly sensory, polyneuropathy is the most common form of diabetic neuropathy.*

PATHOGENESIS: The pathogenesis of the nerve fiber injury in diabetes is unknown. It has long been held that the metabolic alterations of diabetes are responsible for the distal symmetric polyneuropathy, and that nerve ischemia caused by the small-vessel disease is responsible for the mononeuropathies. There is evidence, however, that local nerve ischemia may also play a significant role in the pathogenesis of the symmetric polyneuropathy.

PATHOLOGY: The distal symmetric polyneuropathy of diabetes is characterized pathologically by a mixture of axonal degeneration and segmental demyelination, with axonal degeneration predominating. The axonal loss involves fibers of all sizes, but occasionally preferentially affects the large myelinated fibers (large-fiber neuropathy) or the small myelinated fibers and unmyelinated fibers (small-fiber neuropathy). There may also be loss of neurons in the dorsal root ganglia and anterior horns, but this appears to be a consequence of centripetal progression of dying-back axonal degeneration rather than a neuronopathy.

Uremic Neuropathy May Complicate Chronic Renal Failure

Uremic neuropathy is a distal sensorimotor axonal polyneuropathy. The pathogenesis of the nerve fiber damage is not known, but the disease usually stabilizes or improves with long-term dialysis. Uremic neuropathy is characterized pathologically by both distal axonal degeneration and segmental demyelination, with axonal degeneration predominating and preferentially involving large-diameter fibers. The neuropathy resolves after renal transplantation.

Critical Illness Polyneuropathy Is Associated with Sepsis and Multiorgan Failure

Critical illness polyneuropathy is a distal axonal neuropathy that develops in severely ill patients. The pathogenesis of the condition is obscure. The acute, predominantly motor, neuropathy may first become apparent when the patient cannot be weaned from ventilatory support. A **critical illness myopathy** may also occur in these patients.

Alcoholic Neuropathy Is a Frequent Complication of Alcoholism

Alcoholic neuropathy is a distal sensorimotor axonal polyneuropathy that may be attributable to nutritional deficiencies and/or direct toxic effect of ethanol on the PNS. Peripheral nerves show loss of nerve fibers from axonal degeneration of the dying-back type.

Axonal neuropathy is also associated with a lack of vitamins B_1, B_6, B_{12}, or E but is much less common in the United States than is alcoholic neuropathy. The toxic neuropathy associated with isoniazid therapy for tuberculosis is due to the drug's interference with the metabolism of vitamin B_6.

Acute Inflammatory Demyelinating Polyneuropathy (Guillain-Barré Syndrome) Is Immune-Mediated

Acute inflammatory demyelinating polyneuropathy (AIDP) is an acquired, immune-mediated neuropathy that often follows immunization or viral, bacterial, and mycoplasmal infections. It may also be sporadic or complicate surgery, cancer, or HIV infection. AIDP is the most common cause in children and adults of the Guillain-Barré syndrome, which is acute symmetric paralysis that begins distally and ascends proximally. Sensory and autonomic disturbances may also occur. Some 5% of cases present with ophthalmoplegia, ataxia, and areflexia (**Fisher syndrome).** The muscular paralysis may cause respiratory embarrassment, and the autonomic involvement may result in cardiac arrhythmias, hypotension, or hypertension. Resolution of the neuropathy begins 2 to 4 weeks after onset, and most patients make a good recovery. Lumbar puncture characteristically reveals an increased protein level in the CSF and no pleocytosis. The increased protein level is attributable to the inflammation of the spinal roots. Demyelination may be immunologically mediated, since plasmapheresis and intravenously administered gamma globulin have proven beneficial.

AIDP may involve all levels of the PNS, including spinal roots (polyradiculoneuropathy), ganglia, craniospinal nerves, and autonomic nerves. The distribution of the lesions varies from case to case. Involved regions show endoneurial infiltrates of lymphocytes and macrophages, segmental demyelination, and relative axonal sparing. The lymphoid infiltrates are often perivascular, but there is no true vasculitis. Macrophages are frequently found adjacent to degenerating myelin sheaths and have been observed to strip off and phagocytose the superficial myelin lamellae. Such macrophage-mediated demyelination is rarely observed in other neuropathies.

Guillain-Barré syndrome may also be caused by an immune-mediated axonal neuropathy (**acute motor axonal neuropathy** or **acute motor sensory axonal neuropathy**). The axonal form of the Guillain-Barré syndrome is mainly found in China and Japan and is often associated with prior *Campylobacter jejuni* infection.

Chronic inflammatory demyelinating polyneuropathy (CIDP) is similar to AIDP but has a chronic course characterized by multiple relapses or a slow continuous progression. The nerves in CIDP may show numerous onion bulbs, owing to recurring episodes of demyelination, Schwann cell proliferation, and remyelination (see Fig. 28-112). Corticosteroid therapy is effective in CIDP but not in AIDP, suggesting that the two neuropathies have a different immune-mediated pathogenesis.

Multifocal motor neuropathy is a rare, slowly progressive, multiple mononeuropathy that may be mistaken clinically for motor neuron disease. The neuropathy may be immune-mediated. There is often an associated increased titer of anti-GM_1 antibodies. The neuropathy responds to intravenously administered gamma globulin.

Dorsal Root Ganglionitis Is an Immune-Mediated Sensory Neuronopathy

This inflammatory ganglionopathy typically manifests as a subacute or chronic sensory polyneuropathy with sensory ataxia. The pathogenesis of the neuronal degeneration is unknown. The disorder may occur in association with Sjögren syndrome and as a paraneoplastic syndrome. The paraneoplastic syndrome is frequently associated with anti-Hu antibodies (antineuronal autoantibodies). The dorsal root ganglia show infiltration by lymphocytes and loss of sensory neurons.

Vasculitic Neuropathy Causes Multiple Mononeuropathies

Necrotizing arteritis may involve the epineurial arteries of nerves as one manifestation of a more widespread, multiorgan disease, such as polyarteritis nodosa, rheumatoid arthritis, Wegener granulomatosis, Churg-Strauss syndrome, cryoglobulinemia, HIV infection, or cancer. In about a third of the cases of vasculitic neuropathy, the necrotizing arteritis appears limited to the PNS (**nonsystemic vasculitic neuropathy).** The ischemic neuropathy is characterized pathologically by axonal degeneration (Fig. 28-114).

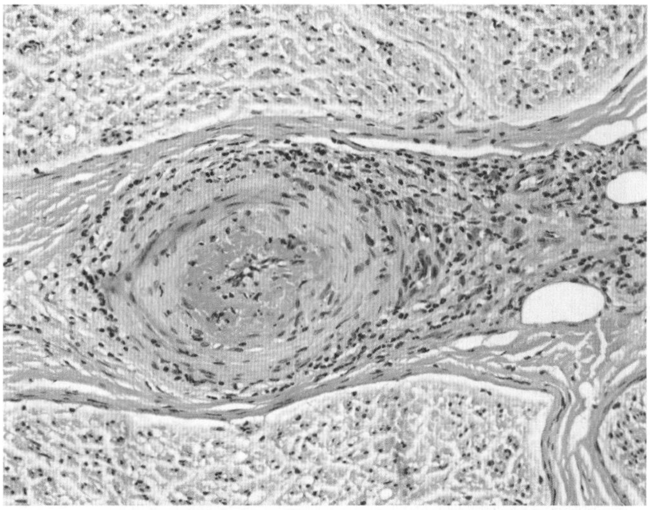

FIGURE 28-114. **Vasculitic neuropathy in a patient with polyarteritis nodosa.** Photomicrograph of a cross-section of a sural nerve reveals an inflamed epineurial artery with fibrinoid necrosis of its wall.

Neuropathies May Be Associated with Monoclonal Gammopathy

Monoclonal gammopathy may cause an amyloid neuropathy, a cryoglobulinemia-associated vasculitic neuropathy, a chronic axonal polyneuropathy, or a chronic demyelinating polyneuropathy. The monoclonal gammopathy may be of undetermined significance (MGUS) or due to a plasma cell neoplasm. The pathogenesis of the paraproteinemia-associated chronic axonal polyneuropathy is unknown. The chronic demyelinating polyneuropathy often occurs with an IgM MGUS or Waldenström macroglobulinemia, in which the paraprotein binds to myelin-associated glycoprotein (MAG), suggesting that anti-MAG antibodies are involved in the pathogenesis of demyelination. Anti-MAG antibody neuropathy is characterized by extensive segmental demyelination, a variable number of onion bulbs, axonal loss, and a distinctive widening of the myelin lamellae (Fig. 28-115). Paraproteinemic neuropathy may rarely present as the POEMS syndrome (polyneuropathy, organomegaly, endocrinopathy, monoclonal gammopathy, and skin changes).

Amyloid Neuropathy Complicates Light Chain Amyloidosis and Familial Amyloidosis

In addition to its effects on sensory and motor nerves, amyloid infiltration of the PNS often leads to prominent autonomic dysfunction. Although the disorder may be hereditary, it more commonly complicates light-chain (AL) amyloidosis associated with primary systemic amyloidosis or multiple myeloma. A point mutation in the transthyretin gene is responsible for most cases of dominantly inherited, familial amyloid polyneuropathy.

Amyloid neuropathy is characterized by the deposition of amyloid in peripheral nerves, dorsal root ganglia, and autonomic ganglia. The interstitial amyloid deposits are both endoneurial and epineurial and frequently involve blood vessel walls. Amyloid deposition is accompanied by loss of myelinated and unmyelinated fibers. Postulated mechanisms for nerve-fiber damage include direct mechanical injury of nerve fibers and ganglion cells by amyloid deposits and nerve ischemia caused by amyloid infiltration of vasa nervorum.

Carpal tunnel syndrome is a chronic entrapment neuropathy of the median nerve at the wrist and represents another complication of systemic amyloidosis. The nerve entrapment results from amyloid infiltration of the flexor retinaculum. Many other conditions, including **occupational injuries,** are also associated with carpal tunnel syndrome.

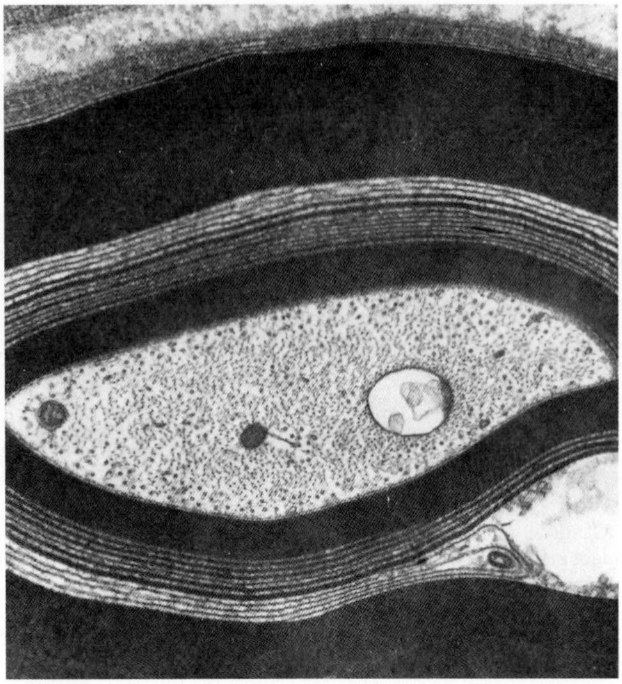

FIGURE 28-115. **Paraproteinemic neuropathy.** An electron micrograph shows a myelinated fiber with multiple, abnormally widely spaced, myelin lamellae from a patient with an immunoglobulin M (IgM) monoclonal gammopathy of unknown significance and a chronic demyelinating neuropathy.

Paraneoplastic Neuropathy Often Precedes Recognition of Underlying Cancer

Paraneoplastic diseases of the nervous system include polyneuropathy, chronic encephalomyelitis, necrotizing myelopathy, cerebellar degeneration, and the Eaton-Lambert syndrome. Several different clinicopathologic types of paraneoplastic neuropathy have been defined.

- **Paraneoplastic sensorimotor polyneuropathy:** This distal polyneuropathy is characterized by axonal degeneration and demyelination, with axonal loss predominating.
- **Paraneoplastic sensory neuronopathy:** Less commonly, paraneoplastic neuropathy may manifest as a subacute sensory neuronopathy due to a dorsal root ganglionitis. Similar histologic changes may also occur in the CNS (**paraneoplastic encephalomyelitis**). Anti-Hu antibodies are often present in these patients, and small cell carcinoma of the lung is the usual cause.
- **Inflammatory demyelinating polyneuropathy:** Acute or chronic inflammatory demyelinating polyneuropathy may be associated with cancer.
- **Paraneoplastic vasculitic neuropathy:** Vasculitic neuropathy may rarely complicate cancer.

Not all paraneoplastic neuropathies result from remote effects of the neoplasm on the nervous system. Cancer may cause neuropathy by direct compression or infiltration of nerves or nerve roots. Cancer patients may also develop chemotherapy-induced toxic neuropathy or radiation-induced neuropathy (brachial or lumbosacral plexopathy).

Toxic Neuropathy Is Often Iatrogenic

A variety of environmental agents and industrial compounds cause peripheral neuropathy (Table 28-7), but most cases of toxic neuropathy are caused by drugs. Almost all toxic neuropathies are characterized by axonal degeneration, usually of the dying-back type. Amiodarone, buckthorn toxin, and diphtheria toxin are notable for producing demyelinating neuropathies. Persons with hereditary neuropathy may be especially vulnerable to drug-induced peripheral neuropathy.

Hereditary Neuropathies Are the Most Common Form of Chronic Neuropathy in Children

Peripheral neuropathy is a manifestation of a variety of inherited diseases (Table 28-8 and Table 28–9). The neuropathy may be the sole manifestation of the hereditary disease or just one manifestation of a hereditary multisystem disease.

CHARCOT-MARIE-TOOTH DISEASE (CMT): CMT is a genetically and pathologically heterogeneous group of slowly progressive distal sensorimotor polyneuropathies that manifest in childhood or early adult life. It is the most common inherited neuropathy and among the most common inherited neurological disorders, with a prevalence of 1 in 2500. CMT may be broadly divided into demyelinating and axonal subtypes. **CMT1,** the most common subtype, has autosomal dominant inheritance and a chronic demyelinating polyneuropathy with onion bulbs and axonal loss. The less common **CMT2** subtype also shows autosomal dominant inheritance and distal axonal degeneration. X-linked (**CMTX**) and autosomal recessive (**CMT4**) subtypes have also been described. Mutations in a growing number of genes have been associated with the CMT phenotype. The majority of cases of CMT are due to mutations in three genes: peripheral

TABLE 28-7

Agents Associated with Toxic Neuropathy

Drugs	Environmental and Industrial Agents
Amiodarone	Acrylamide
Chloramphenicol	Allyl chloride
Colchicine	Arsenic
Dapsone	Buckthorn toxin
Disulfiram	Carbon disulfide
Ethambutol	Chlordecone
Gold salts	Dimethylaminopropionitrile
Isoniazid	Diphtheria toxin
Metronidazole	Ethylene oxide
Misonidazole	n-Hexane (glue sniffing)
Nitrofurantoin	Methyl n-butyl ketone
Nucleoside analogues (anti-retrovirals)	Lead
Paclitaxel (taxanes)	Mercury
Phenytoin	Methyl bromide
Platinum compounds	Organophosphates
Pyridoxine (vitamin B_6)	Polychlorinated biphenyls
Suramin	Thallium
Thalidomide	Trichloroethylene
Vincristine	Vacor

TABLE 28-8

Inherited Diseases Associated with Neuropathy

Abetalipoproteinemia
Acute intermittent porphyria
Fabry disease (α-galactosidase A deficiency)
Familial amyloid polyneuropathy (transthyretin amyloidosis)
Friedreich ataxia
Giant axonal neuropathy
Hereditary motor and sensory neuropathy (Charcot-Marie-Tooth disease)
Leukodystrophies
Refsum disease (phytanic acid storage disease)
Tangier disease

myelin protein 22 (*PMP22*), myelin protein zero (*MPZ*), and gap junction protein β 1 (*GJB1*). Classification is complex, because mutations in different genes may produce the same phenotype, and various mutations in the same gene may produce different phenotypes (see Table 28-9).

Dejerine-Sottas syndrome resembles CMT1, but is much more severe, with onset in early infancy. Peripheral nerves show a severe demyelinating neuropathy with onion bulbs and axonal loss. Several genes have been associated with this phenotype (see Table 28–9).

Hereditary neuropathy with liability to pressure palsies (HNPP) typically manifests with recurrent mononeuropathies. The nerves show demyelination, distinctive sausage-shaped thickenings (tomacula) of myelin sheaths, and axonal loss. HNPP is associated with a *PMP22* deletion.

Neuropathy Is a Complication of HIV Infection

Peripheral neuropathy is a common complaint in persons infected with HIV. The neuropathy may manifest clinically as a distal symmetric polyneuropathy, a mononeuropathy, or a lumbosacral polyradiculopathy.

- **Distal symmetrical polyneuropathy** is the most common type of neuropathy associated with HIV infection. The disorder is characterized by distal axonal degeneration and usually occurs during the later stages of AIDS. The pathogenesis of the axonal degeneration is obscure, and there is no effective therapy.
- **Inflammatory demyelinating polyneuropathy** associated with AIDS may be acute or chronic. The disorder may be immunologically mediated. It typically occurs early in the course of HIV infection, before the full onset of AIDS. The neuropathy often responds to plasmapheresis, intravenous gamma globulin, or corticosteroids.
- **Cytomegalovirus infection** of the PNS is responsible for some of the mononeuropathies and lumbosacral polyradiculopathies associated with AIDS.
- **Vasculitic neuropathy** may cause mononeuropathy and mononeuropathy multiplex in some patients with AIDS.
- **Toxic neuropathy** is caused by several drugs used in the therapy of AIDS (see Table 28-7). These antiretroviral-induced axonal neuropathies are clinically similar to AIDS-associated distal symmetrical polyneuropathy.
- **Diffuse infiltrative lymphocytosis syndrome** may be complicated by an acute or subacute axonal polyneuropathy. Peripheral nerve shows CD8-positive lymphocytic infiltrates.

Chronic Idiopathic Axonal Neuropathy

In 10% to 20% of patients with peripheral neuropathy, no cause is apparent despite careful and extensive investigation. These cryptogenic neuropathies typically occur in older patients as a chronic, distal, sensorimotor axonal polyneuropathy and have an indolent course.

Nerve Trauma

Traumatic Neuroma Is a Mass of Regenerating Axons and Scar Tissue

Traumatic neuroma forms at the end of the proximal stump of a nerve that has been disrupted physically. After transection of a peripheral nerve, regenerating axonal sprouts arise within 1 week from the distal ends of the intact axons in the proximal nerve stump. If the severed ends of the proximal and distal nerve stumps are closely

TABLE 28-9

Charcot-Marie-Tooth Disease (CMT) and Related Hereditary Motor and Sensory Neuropathies (HMSN)

Disease	Inheritance	Gene	Pathology
CMT1 (HMSN 1)	Autosomal dominant	Peripheral myelin protein 22 (PMP22), Myelin protein zero (MPZ), and others	Demyelinating neuropathy with onion bulbs; axonal loss also present
CMT2 (HMSN 2)	Autosomal dominant	Kinesin 1B (KIF1B), Neurofilament light chain (NEFL), and others	Axonal neuropathy
CMTX (HMSN X)	X-linked	Gap junction protein β1 (GJB1)	Axonal loss and myelin abnormalities
Dejerine-Sottas syndrome (congenital hypomyelinating neuropathy)	Autosomal dominant	PMP22, MPZ, *early growth response 2 (*EGR2*), and others*	Demyelinating neuropathy with onion bulbs; axonal loss also present
Hereditary neuropathy with liability to pressure palsies (HNPP)	Autosomal dominant	PMP22	Demyelinating neuropathy with tomacula

approximated, the regenerating axonal sprouts may find and reinnervate the distal stump. The regenerating axons advance in the distal stump at a rate of about 1 mm/day. However, in many instances, the severed nerve ends are not closely approximated, and there is considerable scar tissue between the proximal and distal stumps. The wide gap between the proximal and distal stumps prevents the regenerating sprouts from successfully reinnervating the distal stump. In this situation, the regenerating axons grow haphazardly into the scar tissue at the end of the proximal stump to form a painful swelling known as a **traumatic** or **amputation neuroma.**

Morton Neuroma (Plantar Interdigital Neuroma) Is a Painful Lesion of the Foot

Morton neuroma is a painful, sausage-shaped swelling of the plantar digital nerve between the second and third or third and fourth metatarsal bones. It is probably caused by repeated nerve compression. The swelling is not a true neuroma, because it results from endoneurial, perineurial, and epineurial fibrosis rather than a mass of regenerating axons. The fibrotic nerve also shows nerve fiber loss and areas of myxoid degeneration. Morton neuroma is particularly common in women who wear high heels.

Tumors

Primary tumors of the PNS are of neuronal or nerve sheath origin. The neuronal tumors (e.g., neuroblastoma and ganglioneuroma) usually arise from the adrenal medulla or sympathetic ganglia. The common nerve sheath tumors are schwannoma and neurofibroma.

Schwannoma May Arise in Any Nerve

Schwannoma is a benign, slowly growing, typically encapsulated neoplasm of Schwann cells that originates in cranial nerves, spinal roots, or peripheral nerves (Fig. 28-116A). These tumors usually are seen in adults and only very rarely undergo malignant degeneration.

VESTIBULAR SCHWANNOMA (ACOUSTIC SCHWANNOMA): Intracranial schwannomas account for 8% of all intracranial tumors. Most arise from the vestibular branch of the eighth cranial nerve within the internal auditory canal or at the meatus and cause unilateral, sensorineural hearing loss, tinnitus, and vestibular dysfunction. The slowly growing tumor enlarges the meatus, extends medially into the subarachnoid space of the cerebellopontine angle (**cerebellopontine angle tumor**), and compresses the fifth and seventh cranial nerves, brainstem, and cerebellum. The posterior fossa mass may also lead to increased intracranial pressure, hydrocephalus, and tonsillar herniation. Most vestibular schwannomas are unilateral and are not associated with NF (see chapter 6). Bilateral vestibular schwannomas are a defining feature of NF2, although sporadic schwannomas occur

INTRASPINAL AND PERIPHERAL SCHWANNOMAS: Intraspinal schwannomas are intradural, extra-axial tumors that arise most often from the dorsal (sensory) spinal roots. They produce radicular (root) pain and spinal cord compression. More peripherally located schwannomas usually arise on nerves of the head, neck, and extremities.

PATHOLOGY: Schwannomas tend to be oval and well demarcated and vary in diameter from a few millimeters to several centimeters. The nerve of origin, if large enough, may be identifiable. The cut surface is firm and tan to gray, and often shows focal hemorrhage, necrosis, xanthomatous change, and cystic degeneration. Microscopically, the proliferating Schwann cells form two distinctive histologic patterns (see Fig. 28-116B).

- **Antoni A pattern** is characterized by interwoven fascicles of spindle cells with elongated nuclei, eosinophilic cytoplasm, and indistinct cytoplasmic borders. The nuclei may palisade in areas to form structures known as **Verocay bodies.**
- **Antoni B pattern** features spindle or oval cells with indistinct cytoplasm in a loose, vacuolated background.

Degenerative changes in schwannomas are common and include collections of foam cells, recent or old hemorrhage, foci of fibrosis, and hyalinized blood vessels. Scattered atypical nuclei are frequently encountered in schwannomas, but mitotic figures are uncommon.

Neurofibroma Features Several Cell Types

Neurofibroma is a benign, slowly growing tumor of peripheral nerve composed of Schwann cells, perineurial-like cells, and fibroblasts. A distinction between neurofibroma and schwannoma is warranted because of the close association of neurofibroma with NF1 and its potential for sarcomatous degeneration to malignant peripheral nerve sheath tumor. Schwann cells may be the neoplastic cells in neurofibroma.

Neurofibromas may be solitary or multiple and may arise on any nerve. They are found in both children and adults. Most commonly, neurofibromas involve skin, major nerve plexuses, large deep nerve trunks, retroperitoneum, and gastrointestinal tract. Most **solitary cutaneous neurofibromas** occur outside the context of NF and do not have the potential for sarcomatous degeneration. The presence of multiple neurofibromas or one large plexiform neurofibroma is virtually diagnostic of NF1 and should prompt a careful search for other stigmata of the disease.

PATHOLOGY: On gross examination, a neurofibroma arising in a large nerve appears as a poorly circumscribed, fusiform enlargement. The diffuse, intrafascicular growth of tumor within multiple nerve fascicles may so enlarge the fascicles that the nerve looks like a multistranded rope (**plexiform neurofibroma**). Neurofibroma may involve long segments of the nerve, making complete surgical excision impossible. When they arise from small nerves, the nerve of origin may not be apparent. Cutaneous neurofibromas originate from dermal nerves and are seen as soft nodular or pedunculated skin tumors.

The cut surface of a neurofibroma is soft and light gray, and the greatly enlarged, individual nerve fascicles of the plexiform neurofibroma may be prominent. Microscopically, a tumor arising in a large nerve is characterized by an endoneurial proliferation of spindle cells with elongated nuclei, eosinophilic cytoplasm and indistinct cell borders (see Fig. 28-116D). The proliferating spindle cells include Schwann cells, fibroblasts, and perineurial-like cells. There are also increased numbers of mast cells. Interspersed among the spindle cells are an extracellular myxoid matrix, wavy bands of collagen and residual nerve fibers. The coursing of nerve fibers through the neurofibroma contrasts with the pattern in schwannoma, in which nerve fibers are pushed peripherally into the tumor capsule (see Fig. 28-116A and C). The neurofibromatous proliferation often extends beyond the nerve fascicle into the adjacent tissue.

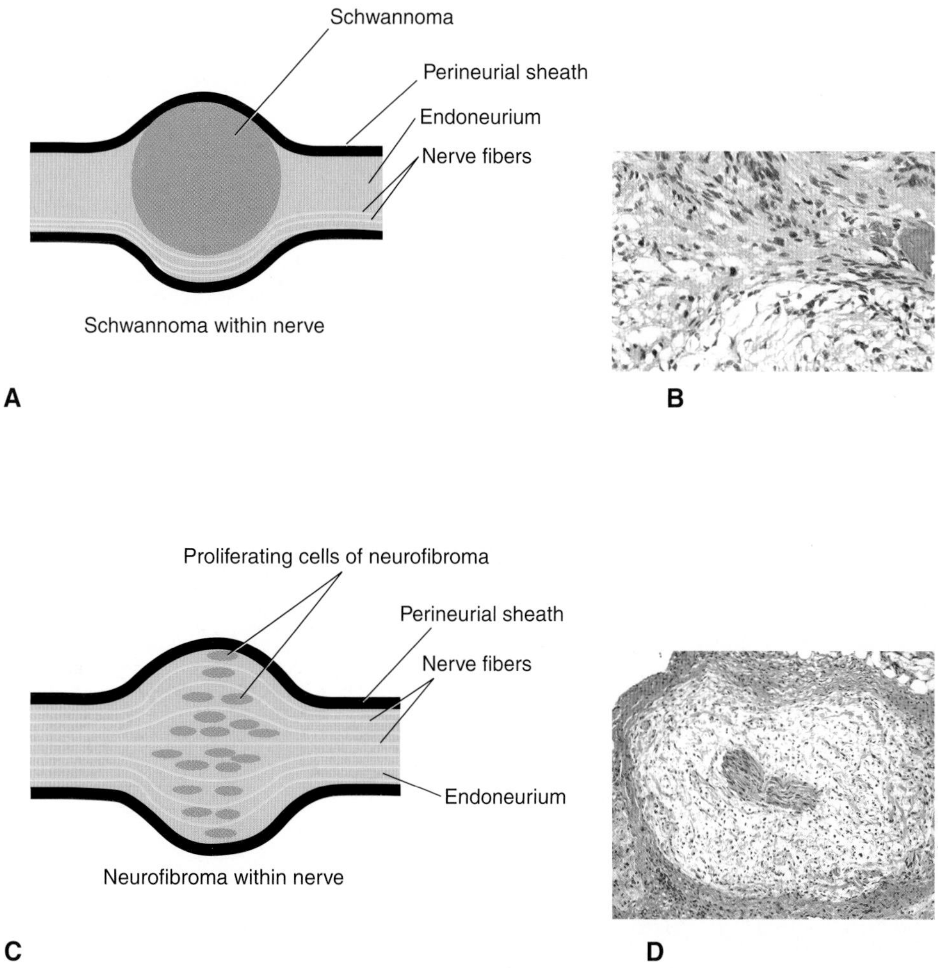

FIGURE 28-116. **Growth patterns of schwannoma and neurofibroma within peripheral nerve. A.** The cellular proliferation of the schwannoma is well-circumscribed and pushes surviving nerve fibers to the periphery of the tumor. **B.** A photomicrograph of a schwannoma shows the characteristically abrupt transition between the compact Antoni type A histologic pattern *(top)* and the spongy Antoni type B histologic pattern *(bottom)*. **C.** The cellular proliferation of the neurofibroma is interspersed among the surviving nerve fibers. **D.** Photomicrograph of neurofibroma shows that the proliferating spindle-shaped Schwann cells form small strands that course haphazardly through a myxoid matrix.

Some 5% of NF1-associated plexiform neurofibromas exhibit sarcomatous transformation to malignant peripheral nerve sheath tumor. The presence of increased cellularity and mitotic figures heralds malignant transformation.

Malignant Peripheral Nerve Sheath Tumor (Malignant Schwannoma, Neurofibrosarcoma)

Malignant peripheral nerve sheath tumor (MPNST) is a poorly differentiated, spindle cell sarcoma of peripheral nerve of uncertain histogenesis. The tumor may arise de novo or from malignant transformation of a neurofibroma. MPNST is most common in adults and typically arises in larger nerves of the trunk or proximal limbs. *About half of these sarcomas occur in patients with neurofibromatosis.* There is an increased incidence of MPNST at sites of previous irradiation.

MPNST manifests grossly as an unencapsulated, fusiform enlargement of a nerve. Microscopically, the neoplasm resembles fibrosarcoma. The tumor is prone to local recurrence and bloodborne metastases.

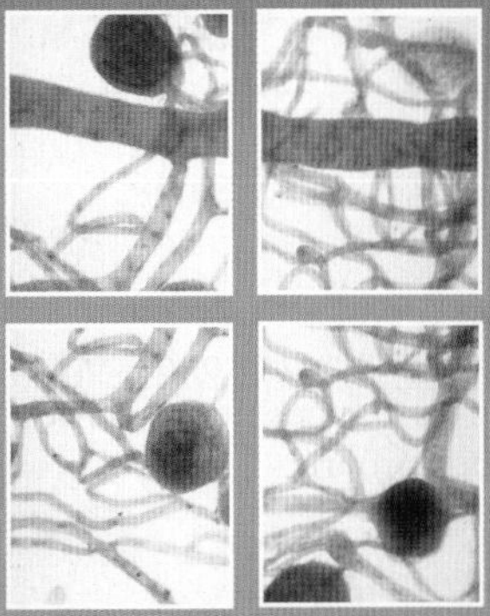

29 The Eye

Gordon K. Klintworth

Physical and Chemical Injuries

Physical trauma to the eye commonly causes ecchymosis of the highly vascular eyelids (black eye); when this occurs, other parts of the eye also may be injured. Superficial disruptions of the corneal epithelium follow traumatic abrasions, prolonged wearing of a contact lens, foreign bodies on the eye, exposure to ultraviolet light, and exposure to caustic chemicals. Blunt trauma increases intraorbital pressure momentarily, and may cause the bones in the floor of the orbit to fracture into the maxillary sinus (**blowout fracture**). The inferior rectus muscle may become entrapped in such a fracture, thereby causing the eye to sink into the orbit (**enophthalmos**).

An array of foreign materials can injure the eye. Whereas small particles often lodge in superficial ocular tissues, some penetrate into or through the eye. A foreign particle may damage the eye during entry or because of secondary infection after the introduction of microorganisms. Some foreign bodies provoke a prominent acute inflammatory or granulomatous reactions. Others, such as those containing iron, cause retinal degeneration and even discoloration of ocular tissues *(siderosis bulbi),* effects that may not be evident for several years. Other complications of ocular injuries include cataracts, retinal detachment, and glaucoma.

The eye is commonly injured by a variety of household and industrial chemicals that enter it accidentally or as a result of a malicious act. The damage created depends on the nature of the chemical.

The Eyelids

The more important conditions affecting the eyelids include:

Blepharitis is inflammation of the eyelids. It is common and sometimes produces an acute, red, tender, inflammatory mass.

Hordeolum (or sty) refers to an acute, inflammatory, focal lesion of the eyelid. Acute inflammation involving the meibomian glands is termed an **internal hordeolum,** whereas acute folliculitis of the glands of Zeis is an **external hordeolum**.

Chalazion is a granulomatous inflammation centered around the meibomian glands or the glands of Zeis. It is thought to represent a reaction to extruded lipid secretions, and usually produces painless swelling in the eyelid.

Inflammatory pseudotumor of the orbit describes an idiopathic chronic inflammatory reaction associated with a variable degree of fibrosis. It is a common cause of proptosis and partial immobility of the eyeball.

Xanthelasma refers to a yellow plaque of lipid-containing macrophages, usually involving the nasal aspect of the eyelids. It is often seen in older persons and patients with disorders of lipid metabolism (e.g., familial hypercholesterolemia, primary biliary cirrhosis).

The Orbit

Exophthalmos or Proptosis Is an Abnormal Forward Protrusion of the Eyeball

The term **exophthalmos** is used mainly when the condition is bilateral; **proptosis** refers to a unilateral protrusion of the eye. Numerous conditions cause forward protrusion of the eye. The most common cause is thyroid disease, followed by orbital dermoid cysts, and hemangiomas. Other orbital conditions can cause proptosis: various inflammatory lesions, lymphomas, developmental anomalies, vascular problems, and neoplasms all contribute cases. Proptosis also results from lesions of the paranasal sinuses and intracranial cavity.

Exophthalmos of Hyperthyroidism Continues Despite Treatment

Exophthalmos caused by Graves disease may precede or follow other manifestations of thyroid dysfunction. Exophthalmos resulting from thyroid disease usually occurs in early adult life, especially in women (female-to-male ratio, 4:1). It may be severe and progressive, particularly in middle life, when exophthalmos no longer correlates well with the state of thyroid function. Dysthyroid exophthalmos may be associated with edema of the eyelids, chemosis (conjunctival edema), and limitation of ocular motion. The pathogenesis of the exophthalmos of hyperthyroidism is discussed in Chapter 21.

CLINICAL FEATURES: Although it is usually bilateral, one eye may be involved earlier or more extensively than the other. Other ocular manifestations of hyperthyroidism include upper eyelid retraction (due to increased sympathetic tone) and a characteristic stare or apparent proptosis resulting from exposure of the conjunctiva above the corneoscleral limbus.

Complications of severe exophthalmos include several potentially blinding complications: corneal exposure with subsequent ulceration, and optic nerve compression. Paradoxically, thyroidectomy may increase the incidence and severity of exophthalmos associated with hyperthyroidism.

The Conjunctiva

Conjunctival Hemorrhage May Follow Blunt Trauma, Anoxia, or Severe Coughing

Conjunctival hemorrhages also occurs spontaneously, often first noted on arising after sleep. They do not extend into the cornea because of the barrier imposed by the close apposition of corneal epithelium to the underlying substantia propria.

Conjunctivitis May be Infectious or Allergic

Microorganisms lodging on the surface of the eye frequently cause conjunctivitis, keratitis (corneal inflammation), or a corneal ulcer. The conjunctiva, as well as other parts of the eye, may also become infected by hematogenous spread from a focus of infection elsewhere. Iatrogenic eye infections, e.g., with adenovirus, may follow ophthalmic manipulations, such as corneal grafts, intraocular implantation of lens prostheses, or use of infected eyedrops or diagnostic instruments.

At some stage in life, virtually everyone has viral or bacterial conjunctivitis. This extremely common eye disease is characterized by hyperemic conjunctival blood vessels (pink eye). The inflammatory exudate that accumulates in the conjunctival sac commonly crusts, causing the eyelids to stick together in the morning. The conjunctival discharge may be purulent, fibrinous, serous, or hemorrhagic. The inflammatory cells involved vary with the etiologic agent. As many allergens are seasonal, the allergic conjunctivitis they elicit tends to occur only at particular times of the year.

Trachoma

Trachoma is a chronic, contagious conjunctivitis caused by Chlamydia trachomatis. Different serotypes of *C. trachomatis* cause ocular, genital, and systemic infections (trachoma, inclusion conjunctivitis, and lymphogranuloma venereum) in millions of people (see Chapter 9).

EPIDEMIOLOGY: About 500 million people are afflicted by trachoma, an acute, infectious, cicatrizing keratoconjunctivitis caused by *C. trachomatis* (serotypes A, B, and C). *This infection is the most common cause of blindness in the world and is especially prevalent in Asia, the Middle East, and parts of Africa.* Trachoma is not very contagious, but overcrowding and poor hygienic conditions favor its transmission by fingers, fomites, and flies. Spontaneous healing is common in children, but in adults, the disease progresses more rapidly and rarely heals without treatment.

PATHOLOGY: Trachoma is virtually always bilateral and involves the upper half of the conjunctiva more than the lower (Fig. 29-1). The cellular infiltrate is predominantly lymphocytic, and conjunctival lymph follicles with necrotic germinal centers are characteristic. Eventually lymphocytes and blood vessels invade the superior portion of the cornea between the epithelium and Bowman's zone (**trachomatous pannus**). Scarring of the conjunctiva and eyelids distorts the eyelids. On microscopic examination, the desquamated conjunctival epithelium exhibits glycogen-rich intracytoplasmic inclusion bodies and large macrophages containing

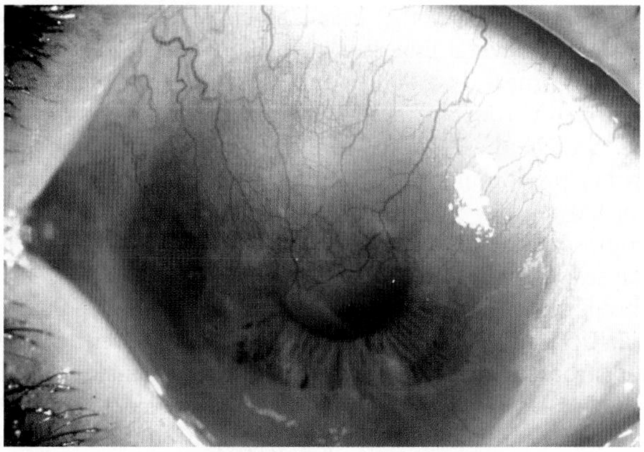

FIGURE 29-1. **Trachoma.** A clinical photograph of the cornea of a patient with severe trachoma shows extensive fibrovascular opacity (pannus) in the superior cornea.

nuclear fragments (Leber cells). Secondary bacterial infection is a common complication.

Other Chlamydial Infections

Chlamydia is responsible for a purulent conjunctivitis (**inclusion blennorrhea**) that develops in newborns, who become infected during passage through the birth canal. The infection is also acquired by swimming in nonchlorinated pools (swimming pool conjunctivitis) or from discharges of lesions of the conjunctiva, urethra, or cervix uteri.

In adults and older children, *Chlamydia* causes a chronic follicular conjunctivitis with focal lymphoid hyperplasia (**inclusion conjunctivitis**) and intracytoplasmic inclusion bodies indistinguishable from those of trachoma. In contrast to trachoma, however, the lower tarsal conjunctiva is involved. Scarring and necrosis do not develop, and keratitis is rare and mild.

Ophthalmia Neonatorum

Ophthalmia neonatorum is a severe, acute conjunctivitis with a copious purulent discharge, especially in the newborn, caused by Neisseria gonorrhoeae. The infection, which is a common cause of blindness in some parts of the world, is complicated by corneal ulceration, perforation, and scarring and panophthalmitis. Infants usually become infected while passing through the birth canal of an infected mother. Other causative organisms for ophthalmia neonatorum include other pyogenic bacteria and *C. trachomatis*. Today, newborns are usually routinely treated with 5% Betadine eye drops.

Pinguecula and Pterygium

Pinguecula *is a yellowish conjunctival lump usually located nasal to the corneoscleral limbus.* It is the most common conjunctival lump. Despite its yellowish appearance, the lesion does not contain fat; rather, it consists of sun-damaged connective tissue identical to that in similarly injured skin (actinic elastosis).

Pterygium *is a fold of vascularized conjunctiva that grows horizontally onto the cornea in the shape of an insect wing (hence the name).* It is often associated with a pinguecula and frequently recurs after excision.

The Cornea

Herpes Simplex Virus Causes Corneal Ulcerations,

Herpesvirus (HSV) has a predilection for corneal epithelium, where it causes keratitis, but it can invade corneal stroma and occasionally other ocular tissues.

PRIMARY INFECTION BY HSV TYPE 1: Subclinical or undiagnosed localized ocular lesions are caused by HSV type 1 in childhood. These infections are accompanied by regional lymphadenopathy, systemic infection, and fever. Except in newborns infected during passage through an infected mother's birth canal, HSV type 2 rarely causes ocular infection. However, when it does, it may produce widespread lesions of the cornea and retina. Most corneal lesions due to HSV are asymptomatic plaques of diseased epithelial cells that contain replicating virus. These usually heal without ulceration, but an acute unilateral follicular conjunctivitis may occur. Corneal ulcers appear after serum antibody levels increase.

REACTIVATION OF HSV INFECTION: Latent in the trigeminal ganglion, HSV may pass down the nerves and reactivate the infection. Unlike primary HSV infection, reactivation disease is characterized by corneal ulceration and a more severe inflammatory reaction. Recurrence of corneal ulcers due to HSV may be precipitated by ultraviolet light, trauma, menstruation, emotional and physical stress, exposure to light or sunlight, vaccination, and other factors.

PATHOLOGY: HSV causes multiple, minute, discrete, intraepithelial corneal ulcers (superficial punctate keratopathy). Although some of these lesions heal, others enlarge and eventually coalesce to form linear or branching fissures (dendritic ulcers, from the Greek., *dendron,* "tree"). The epithelium between the fissures desquamates, causing sharply demarcated, irregular geographical ulcers. The corneal ulcers are readily visualized after the cornea is stained with fluorescein. The affected epithelial cells, which may become multinucleated, contain eosinophilic, intranuclear inclusion bodies (Lipschütz bodies).

The lesions of the corneal stroma vary in reactivated HSV infection. Typically, a central disc-shaped corneal opacity develops beneath the epithelium, owing to edema and a minimal inflammatory cell infiltrate (**disciform keratitis**). The corneal stroma may become markedly thinned, and Descemet's membrane may bulge into it (**descemetocele**). Corneal perforation can also occur.

Onchocerciasis Leads to Blindness in Tropical Regions.

The nematode *Onchocerca volvulus,* which is transmitted by bites of infected blackflies, is by far the most important helminthic infection of the eye (see Chapter 9). *This parasite accounts for blindness in at least half a million people in regions of Africa and Latin America in which it is endemic.* Microfilaria released from fertilized adult female worms migrate into the superficial cornea, bulbar conjunctiva, aqueous humor, and other ocular tissues. The intracorneal microfilaria die and elicit an inflammatory response that leads to corneal opacification and visual impairment (**river blindness**). Less frequently, endophthalmitis, retinal lesions, and optic atrophy occur. Treatment with ivermectin is highly effective.

Arcus Lipoides is a White Arc Due to Lipid Deposition in the Peripheral Cornea

Formerly called **arcus senilis** because of its frequency in the elderly, arcus lipoides may also form an entire ring, in which case the term **annulus lipoides** is more appropriate. Although not necessarily associated with increased serum lipid levels, arcus lipoides accompanies certain disorders of lipid metabolism, and its presence alerts the perceptive clinician to the systemic disorder.

Band Keratopathy is an Opaque Horizontal Band Across the Cornea

The opacification in band keratopathy may contain calcium phosphate (calcific band keratopathy) or noncalcified protein (chronic actinic keratopathy).

In **calcific band keratopathy,** calcium phosphate deposits in a horizontal band across the superficial central cornea in conditions associated with hypercalcemia. However, the disorder most often occurs in the absence of an increased serum calcium concentration, as in chronic uveitis and other ocular disorders.

Chronic actinic keratopathy occurs worldwide but is most severe in regions in which people spend a considerable amount of time outdoors. Their unprotected eyes are exposed to excessive ultraviolet light, such as that reflected from desert, water, or snow.

Corneal Dystrophies Encompass Diverse Noninflammatory Genetic Corneal Disorders

Most corneal dystrophies are autosomal dominant or recessive, but rare cases are X-linked recessive. The corneal dystrophies have traditionally been classified according to the primary layer that is involved: (1) the outer layer composed of epithelium, basement membrane, and Bowman's layer; (2) the stroma; and (3) the endothelium and Descemet's membrane. A shortcoming of such a classification is its artificiality, because many of the conditions involve more than one layer.

EPITHELIAL DYSTROPHIES: The different epithelial dystrophies are characterized by a variety of distinct abnormalities, which include (1) microcysts or accumulations of anomalous material within the cytoplasm of the corneal epithelium, (2) defects in the epithelial basement membrane, and (3) deposition of a finely fibrillar substance in Bowman's layer. In some epithelial dystrophies, faulty desmosomes may permit the separation of adjacent epithelial cells, leading to accumulation of fluid-filled microcysts. A loss of hemidesmosomes between the epithelium and Bowman's layer leads to painful, recurrent erosions that begin in early childhood. Although there may be a slow decrease in visual acuity, epithelial dystrophies do not ordinarily cause blindness. Patients with one corneal dystrophy of the corneal epithelium *(Meesmann dystrophy)* have dominant mutations in the *KRT3* or *KRT12* genes, which encode keratin 3 and keratin 12, respectively. The mutations result in aggregations of abnormal cytokeratin filaments and severely impair cytoskeletal function in the affected cells.

STROMAL DYSTROPHIES: The stromal dystrophies are clear-cut entities in which different substances (e.g., amyloid, glycosaminoglycans, proteins, or a variety of lipids) accumulate within corneal stroma because of inherited metabolic disorders. Each stromal dystrophy causes a characteristic form of corneal opacification. The age of onset and rate of progression vary with the particular disorder. Although clinical manifestations may be limited to the cornea, other tissues are involved in some of these dystrophies. Several inherited corneal disorders, including the granular corneal dystrophies and most lattice corneal dystrophies, result from distinctly different mutations in the same gene, namely, the *TFGBI (BIGH3)* gene on chromosome 5 (5q). Another predominantly stromal corneal dystrophy (macular corneal dystrophy) results from a defect in the CHST6 gene on chromosome 16 (16q), which encodes a sulfotransferase that catalyzes sulfation of *N*-acetyl glucosamine and galactose in keratan sulfate.

ENDOTHELIAL DYSTROPHIES: Several different endothelial dystrophies are recognized, usually accompanied by abnormalities in Descemet's membrane, the basement membrane of the corneal endothelium. In one dystrophy of the corneal endothelium (Fuchs dystrophy), wartlike excrescences form on Descemet's membrane, and progressive visual loss follow corneal edema and endothelial cell degeneration. Missense mutations in *COL8A2,* the gene encoding the α_2 chain of type VIII collagen, have been identified in some patients with early-onset Fuchs dystrophy and posterior polymorphous corneal dystrophy, both of which affect the corneal endothelium and its basement membrane (Descemet's membrane).

The Lens

Cataracts are Opacifications in the Crystalline Lens.

Cataracts are a major cause of visual impairment and blindness throughout the world and are the outcome of numerous conditions.

PATHOGENESIS: Cataracts can be caused by diabetes or by deficiencies in riboflavin or tryptophan. A variety of cataracts result from genetic disorders. Others are related to the actions of toxins, drugs, or physical agents. Substances that may cause cataracts include dinitrophenol, naphthalene, ergot, phospholine iodide (topical), corticosteroids, and phenothiazines. Physical agents that cause cataracts are heat, ultraviolet light, trauma, intraocular surgery, and ultrasound.

Ocular diseases that may be complicated by cataracts include uveitis, intraocular neoplasms, glaucoma, retinitis pigmentosa, and retinal detachment. Cataracts also are associated with congenital rubella virus infection, aging, some skin diseases (atopic dermatitis, scleroderma), and various systemic diseases. A wide range of cataracts are inherited and some of them are associated with other ocular or systemic abnormalities. Cataracts can result from mutations in the heat shock transcription factor-4 *(HSF4)* gene, as well as in genes that encode specific lens proteins, including connexins, crystallins, cytoplasmic filaments, and an aquaporin. They also result from genetic mutations and chromosomal anomalies that cause numerous systemic diseases and syndromes.

PATHOLOGY: The most common cataract in the United States is associated with aging (age-related cataract). Clefts appear between the lens fibers, and degenerated lens material accumulates in these spaces (morgagnian

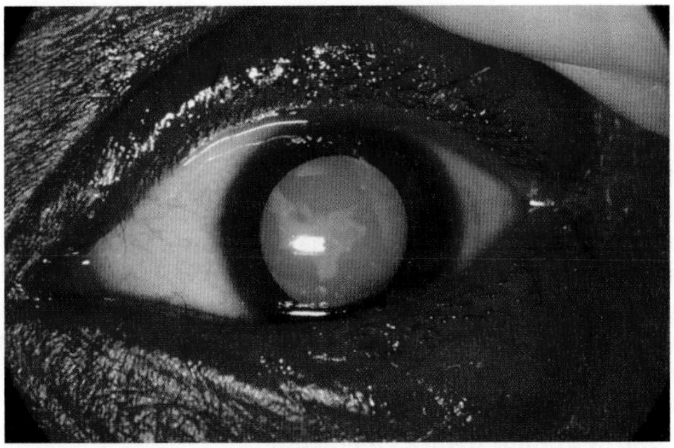

FIGURE 29-2. **Cataract.** The white appearance of the pupil in this eye is due to complete opacification of the lens ("mature cataract").

corpuscles, incipient cataract). The degenerated lens material exerts osmotic pressure, causing the damaged lens to swell by imbibing water. Such a swollen lens may obstruct the pupil and cause glaucoma (phacomorphic glaucoma).

In a mature cataract (Fig. 29-2), the entire lens degenerates, and its volume diminishes because lenticular debris escapes into the aqueous humor through a degenerated lens capsule (hypermature cataract). After becoming engulfed by macrophages, the extruded lenticular material may obstruct aqueous outflow and produce glaucoma (phacolytic glaucoma). The compressed lens fibers in the center of the lens normally harden with aging (simple nuclear sclerotic cataract) and may become brown or black. If the peripheral portion of the lens, or lens cortex, becomes liquefied (morgagnian cataract), the sclerotic nucleus may sink within the lens by gravity.

Fortunately, cataractous lenses can be surgically removed, and optical devices can be provided to permit focusing of light on the retina (spectacles, contact lenses, implantation of prosthetic lenses).

Presbyopia is a Failure of Accommodation as a Result of Aging.

With this impairment of vision, the near point of distinct vision becomes located farther from the eye. At the equator of the crystalline lens, the cuboidal subcapsular cells differentiate into elongated lens fibers throughout life. Once formed, these lens fibers persist indefinitely. Older fibers become displaced into the center of the lens, causing it to enlarge with age. After this process has occurred for many years, the lens loses its elasticity, an effect that interferes with its normal tendency to become spherical, thereby diminishing the power of accommodation. As a result, most persons after age 40 years begin to have difficulty reading and require spectacles for near vision.

Phacoanaphylactic Endophthalmitis is an Autoimmune Granulomatous Reaction to Lens Proteins.

The inflammatory lesion occurs around or within the lens (or its remains) in an eye with a traumatized or cataractous lens or after surgical removal of a cataractous lens. A similar reaction may occur spontaneously in the contralateral eye months or years later. This autoimmune reaction to unique lens proteins, which are normally sequestered from the immune system, can be provoked experimentally by immunization with autologous lens material.

The Uvea

A variety of inflammatory conditions affect the uveal tract. Inflammation of the uvea (**uveitis**) also encompasses inflammation of the iris (iritis), the ciliary body (**cyclitis**), and the iris plus the ciliary body (**iridocyclitis**). Inflammation of the iris and ciliary body typically causes a red eye, photophobia, moderate pain, blurred vision, a pericorneal halo, ciliary flush, and slight miosis. A flare is common in the anterior chamber on slit-lamp biomicroscopy, and keratic precipitates or a **hypopyon** also develop.

Posterior synechiae are adhesions that develop between the iris and the lens.

Peripheral anterior synechiae are adhesions between the peripheral iris and the anterior chamber angle. Both types of synechiae are complications of iritis and can cause glaucoma.

Sympathetic Ophthalmitis is an Autoimmune Uveitis

In sympathetic ophthalmitis, the entire uvea develops granulomatous inflammation after a latent period, in response to an injury in the other eye. Perforating ocular injury and prolapse of uveal tissue often lead to a progressive, bilateral, diffuse, granulomatous inflammation of the uvea. This uveitis develops in the originally injured eye (exciting eye) after a latent period of 4 to 8 weeks. The latent period may, however, be as short as 10 days or as long as many years. The uninjured eye (sympathizing eye) becomes affected at the same time as the injured eye, or shortly thereafter. Vitiligo and graying of the eyelashes sometimes accompanies the uveitis. Nodules containing reactive retinal pigment epithelium, macrophages, and epithelioid cells commonly appear between Bruch's membrane (lamina vitrea) and the retinal pigment epithelium (Dalen-Fuchs nodules). Experimental studies suggest that the antigen responsible for sympathetic ophthalmitis resides in the photoreceptors of the retina (arrestin).

Sarcoidosis Often Affects the Eye.

Ocular involvement occurs in one fourth to one third of patients with sarcoidosis and is frequently the initial clinical manifestation. Although any of the ocular and orbital tissues may be involved, this granulomatous disease has a predilection for the anterior segment of the eye. Ocular involvement is usually bilateral and most often takes the form of a granulomatous uveitis. Other ocular manifestations of sarcoidosis include calcific band keratopathy, cataracts, retinal vascularization, vitreous hemorrhage, and bilateral enlargement of the lacrimal and salivary glands (**Mikulicz syndrome**).

The Retina

Retinal Hemorrhage Has Different Causes

Among the causes of retinal hemorrhages are hypertension, diabetes mellitus, and central retinal vein occlusion. The appearance varies with the location. Hemorrhage in the nerve fiber layer spreads between axons and causes a flame-shaped appearance on funduscopy, whereas deep retinal hemorrhages tend to be round. When located between the retinal pigment epithelium and Bruch's membrane, blood appears as a dark mass and clinically may resemble a melanoma.

After accidental or surgical perforation of the globe, choroidal hemorrhages may detach the choroid and displace the retina, vitreous body, and lens through the wound.

Retinal Occlusive Vascular Disease Is an Important Cause of Blindness

Vascular occlusion results from thrombosis, embolism, stenosis (as in atherosclerosis), vascular compression, intravascular sludging or coagulation, or vasoconstriction (e.g., in hypertensive retinopathy or migraine). Thrombosis of ocular vessels may accompany primary disease of these vessels, as in giant cell arteritis.

Certain disorders of the heart and major vessels, such as the carotid arteries, predispose to emboli that lodge in the retina and are evident on funduscopic examination at points of vascular bifurcation. Within the optic nerve, emboli in the central retinal artery frequently lodge in the vessel where it passes though the scleral perforations (lamina cribrosa).

PATHOLOGY: The effect of vascular occlusion depends on the size of the vessel involved, the degree of resultant ischemia, and the nature of the embolus. Small emboli often do not interfere with retinal function, whereas septic emboli may cause foci of ocular infection. Retinal ischemia of any cause frequently leads to white fluffy patches that resemble cotton on ophthalmoscopic examination (**cotton-wool patches**). These round spots, which are seldom wider than the optic disc, consist of aggregates of swollen axons in the nerve-fiber layer of the retina. Affected axons contain numerous degenerated mitochondria and dense bodies related to the lysosomal system, which accumulate because of impaired axoplasmic flow. Histologically, in cross-section, individual swollen axons resemble cells (cytoid bodies). Cotton-wool spots are reversible if circulation is restored in time.

Central Retinal Artery Occlusion

Like neurons in the rest of the nervous system, those in the retina (Fig. 29-3) are extremely susceptible to hypoxia. Central retinal artery occlusion (Figs 29-4 and Fig. 29-5) may follow

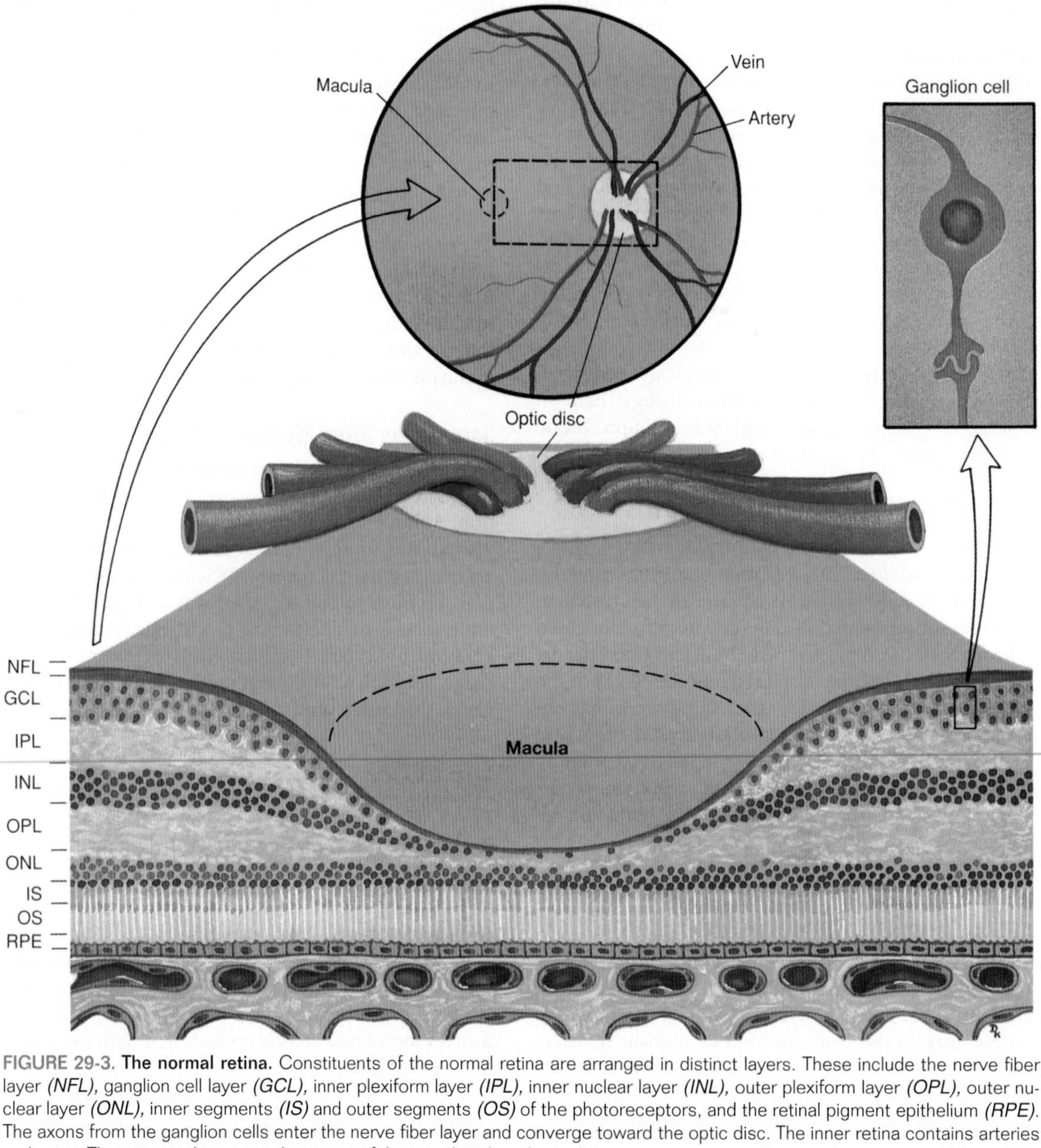

FIGURE 29-3. **The normal retina.** Constituents of the normal retina are arranged in distinct layers. These include the nerve fiber layer *(NFL)*, ganglion cell layer *(GCL)*, inner plexiform layer *(IPL)*, inner nuclear layer *(INL)*, outer plexiform layer *(OPL)*, outer nuclear layer *(ONL)*, inner segments *(IS)* and outer segments *(OS)* of the photoreceptors, and the retinal pigment epithelium *(RPE)*. The axons from the ganglion cells enter the nerve fiber layer and converge toward the optic disc. The inner retina contains arteries and veins. The retina is thinnest at the center of the macula, where bare photoreceptors rest on the retinal pigment epithelium. Only one cell thick in most of the retina, the ganglion cell layer is multilayered at the macula.

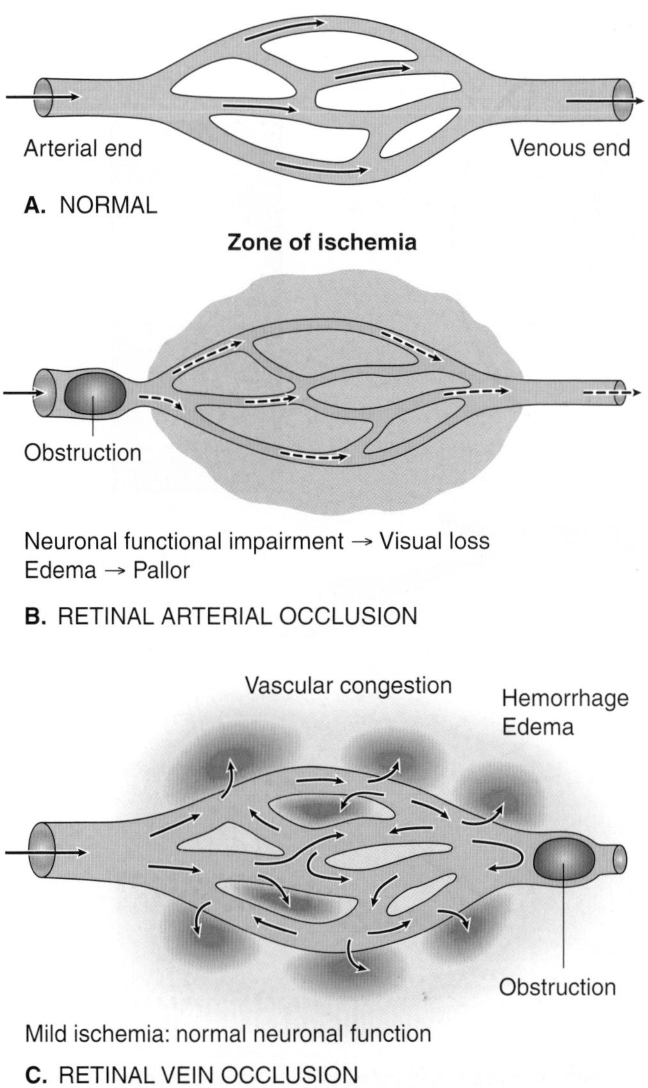

FIGURE 29-4. **Occlusion of the retinal artery and vein. A.** In the retina, as in other parts of the body, blood normally flows through a capillary network. **B.** When the retinal arteries become occluded (e.g., with an embolus) a zone of retinal ischemia ensues. This is accompanied by impaired neuronal function and visual loss, and the ischemic retina becomes pale. Because the intravascular pressure within the ischemic tissue is low, hemorrhage is inconspicuous. **C.** With retinal vein occlusion, vascular congestion, hemorrhage, and edema are prominent, whereas ischemia is mild and neuronal function remains intact.

thrombosis of the retinal artery, as in atherosclerosis or giant cell arteritis, or embolization to that vessel. Intracellular edema, manifested by retinal pallor, is prominent, especially in the macula, where ganglion cells are most numerous. The foveola, the center of the macula, stands out in sharp contrast as a prominent **cherry-red spot**, because of the underlying vascularized choroid. The lack of retinal circulation reduces retinal arterioles to delicate threads (see Fig. 29-5).

Permanent blindness follows central retinal artery obstruction, unless the ischemia is of short duration. Unilateral blurred vision, lasting a few minutes (**amaurosis fugax**), occurs with small retinal emboli.

Central Retinal Vein Occlusion

Central retinal vein occlusion results in flame-shaped hemorrhages in the nerve-fiber layer of the retina, especially around the optic disc. The hemorrhages reflect the high intravascular pressure that dilates and ruptures the veins and collateral vessels (Fig. 29-6). Edema of the optic disc and retina occurs because of an impaired absorption of interstitial fluid.

Vision is disturbed but may recover surprisingly well, considering the severity of the funduscopic changes. An intractable, closed-angle glaucoma, with severe pain and repeated hemorrhages, commonly ensues 2 to 3 months after central retinal vein occlusion (100-day glaucoma, thrombotic glaucoma, neovascular glaucoma). This distressing complication is caused by neovascularization of the iris and adhesions between the iris and the anterior chamber angle *(peripheral anterior synechiae)*.

Hypertensive Retinopathy Relates to the Severity of Hypertension

Increased blood pressure commonly affects the retina, causing changes that can readily be seen with the ophthalmoscope (Fig. 29-7 and Fig. 29-8).

PATHOLOGY: Features of hypertensive retinopathy include:

- Arteriolar narrowing
- Hemorrhages in the retinal nerve fiber layer (flame-shaped hemorrhages)
- Exudates, including some that radiate from the center of the macula (macular star)
- Fluffy white bodies in the superficial retina (cotton-wool spots)
- Microaneurysms

In the eye, arteriolosclerosis accompanies long-standing hypertension and commonly affects the retinal and choroidal vessels. Lumina of the thickened retinal arterioles become narrowed, increasingly tortuous, and of irregular caliber. At sites where the arterioles cross veins, the latter appear kinked (**arteriovenous nicking**). However, the venous diameter before the site of compression is not wider than that after it. The kinked appearance of the vein reflects sclerosis within the venous walls, because the retinal arteries and veins share a common adventitia at sites of arteriovenous crossings, rather than compression by a taut sclerotic artery.

By funduscopy, abnormal retinal arterioles appear as parallel white lines at sites of vascular crossings (**arterial sheathing**). Initially, the narrowed lumen of the retinal vessels decreases the visibility of the blood column and makes it appear orange on ophthalmoscopic examination (**copper wiring**). However, as the blood column eventually becomes completely obscured, light reflected from the sclerotic vessels appears as threads of silver wire (**silver wiring**).

Small superficial or deep retinal hemorrhages often accompany retinal arteriolosclerosis. **Malignant hypertension** is characterized by a necrotizing arteriolitis, with fibrinoid necrosis and thrombosis of the precapillary retinal arterioles.

Diabetic Retinopathy Is Primarily a Vascular Disease

The eye is frequently involved in diabetes mellitus, and ocular symptoms occur in 20% to 40% of diabetics and may even be evident at the time diabetes is diagnosed. Virtually all patients with type 1 (insulin-dependent) diabetes and many of those with type 2 (non–insulin-dependent) diabetes develop some background

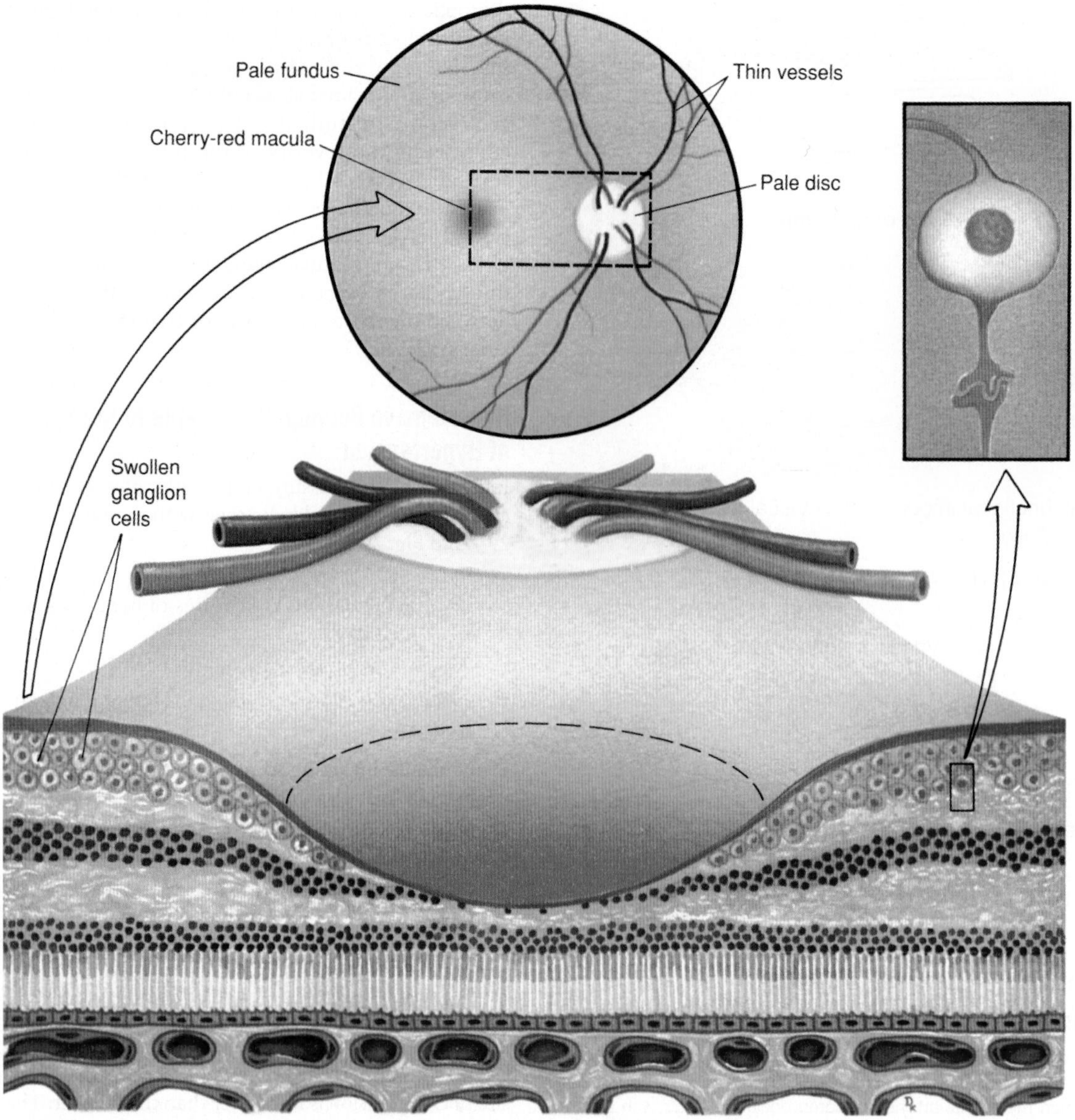

FIGURE 29-5. **Central retinal artery occlusion.** When the central retinal artery becomes occluded (e.g., with an embolus), the entire retina becomes edematous and pale. Decreased blood flow makes the retinal vessels less visible on funduscopic examination. The macula becomes cherry-red, owing to the prominent, but normal, underlying vasculature of the choroid.

retinopathy (see below) within 5 to 15 years of the onset of diabetes (Figs. 29-9 to 29-11). The more dangerous **proliferative retinopathy** does not appear until at least 10 years of diabetes, after which its incidence increases rapidly and remains high for many years. *The frequency of proliferative retinopathy correlates with the degree of glycemic control; patients whose diabetes is better controlled develop retinopathy less frequently.*

Retinal ischemia can account for most features of diabetic retinopathy, including the cotton-wool spots, capillary closure, microaneurysms, and retinal neovascularization. Ischemia results from narrowing or occlusion of retinal arterioles (as from arteriolosclerosis or platelet and lipid thrombi) or from atherosclerosis of the central retinal or ophthalmic arteries.

PATHOLOGY: The retinopathy of diabetes is characterized by background and proliferative stages.

BACKGROUND (NONPROLIFERATIVE) DIABETIC RETINOPATHY: This stage exhibits venous engorgement, small hemorrhages (dot and blot hemorrhages), capillary microaneurysms, and exudates. These lesions usually do not impair vision unless associated with macular edema. The retinopathy begins at the posterior pole but eventually may involve the entire retina.

On funduscopy, the first discernible clinical abnormality in background diabetic retinopathy is engorged retinal veins, with localized sausage-shaped distentions, coils, and loops. This is followed by small hemorrhages in the same areas, mostly in the inner nuclear and outer plexiform layers. With time, "waxy" exudates accumulate, chiefly in the vicinity of the microaneurysms. The retinopathy of elderly diabetic persons frequently displays numerous exudates (**exudative diabetic retinopathy**), which are not seen with type 1 diabetes. Because of the hyperlipoproteinemia of diabetics, the exudates are rich in lipid and thus appear yellowish (**waxy exudates**).

PROLIFERATIVE RETINOPATHY: After many years, diabetic retinopathy becomes proliferative. Delicate new blood vessels grow along with fibrous and glial tissue toward the vitreous body.

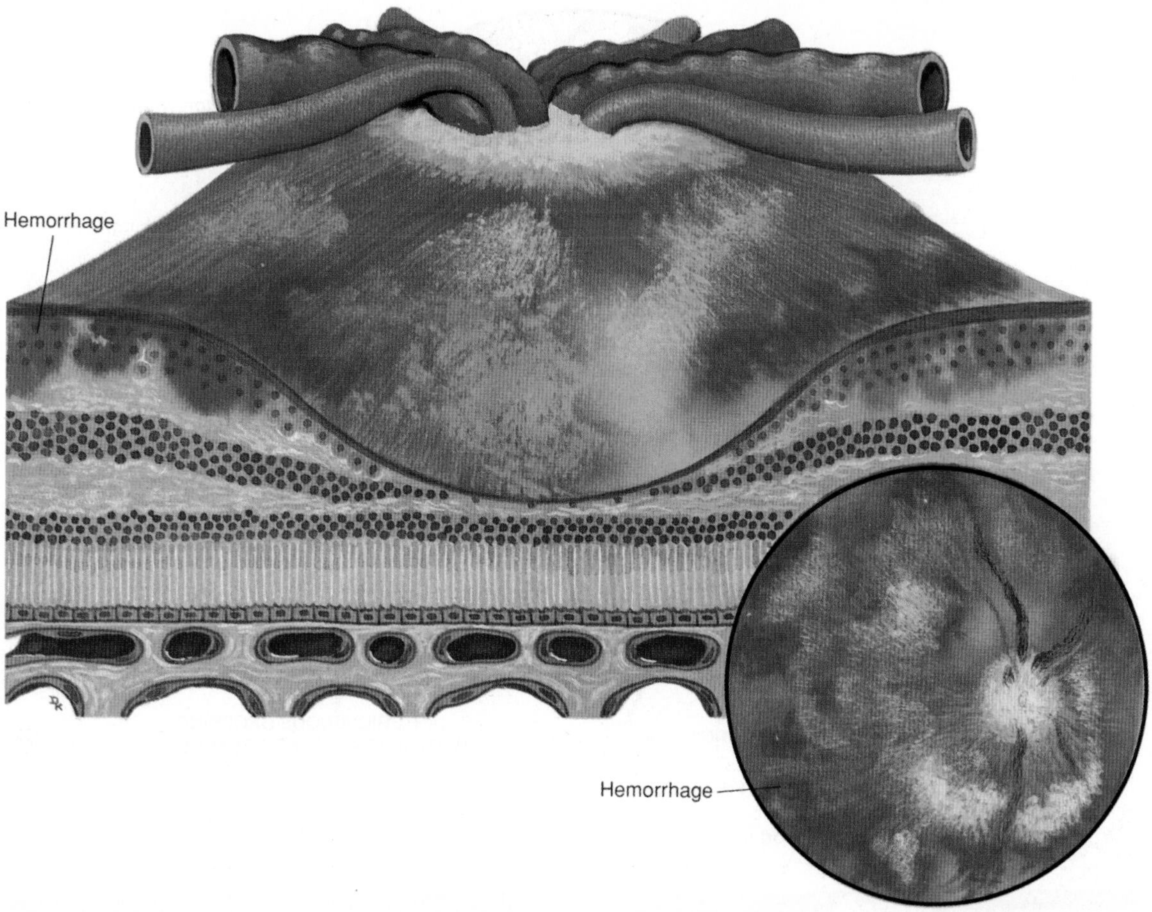

FIGURE 29-6. **Central retinal vein occlusion.** In contrast to central retinal artery occlusion, central retinal vein occlusion produces considerable vascular engorgement and retinal hemorrhage as a consequence of increased intravascular pressure.

Neovascularization of the retina is a prominent eature of diabetic retinopathy and of other conditions caused by retinal ischemia. Tortuous new vessels first appear on the surface of the retina and optic nerve head and then grow into the vitreous cavity. The newly formed friable vessels bleed easily, and resultant vitreal hemorrhages obscure vision. Neovascularization is associated with proliferation and immigration of astrocytes, which grow around the new vessels to form delicate white veils (gliosis). The proliferating fibrovascular and glial tissue contracts, often causing retinal detachment and blindness. Frequently, features of hypertensive and arteriolosclerotic retinopathy are associated with diabetic retinopathy.

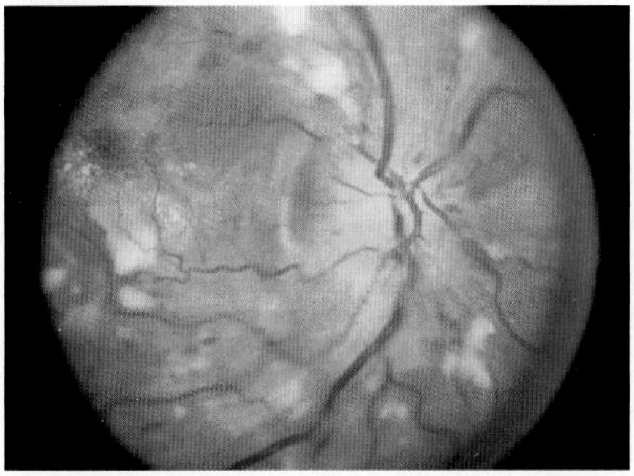

FIGURE 29-7. **Hypertensive retinopathy.** A photograph of the ocular fundus in a patient with extensive retinopathy. The optic nerve head is edematous; the retina contains numerous exudates and "cotton-wool" spots.

Diabetic retinopathy, glaucoma, and age-related maculopathy are the leading causes of irreversible blindness in the United States. Blindness in diabetic retinopathy results when the macula is involved, but it also follows vitreous hemorrhage, retinal detachment, and glaucoma. Once blindness ensues, it heralds an ominous future for the patient, because death from ischemic heart disease or renal failure often follows. In fact, the mean life expectancy in such cases is less than 6 years, and only one fifth of blind diabetics survive 10 years. Laser phototherapy and strict glycemic control early in the course of proliferative retinopathy have proved effective in controlling this complication.

Diabetic Iridopathy

In diabetics with severe retinopathy, a fibrovascular layer frequently grows along the anterior surface of the iris and in the anterior chamber angle. Because such iris neovascularization (**rubeosis iridis**) is a feature of several conditions associated with retinal ischemia, it is believed to be due to an angiogenic factor produced by the ischemic retina.

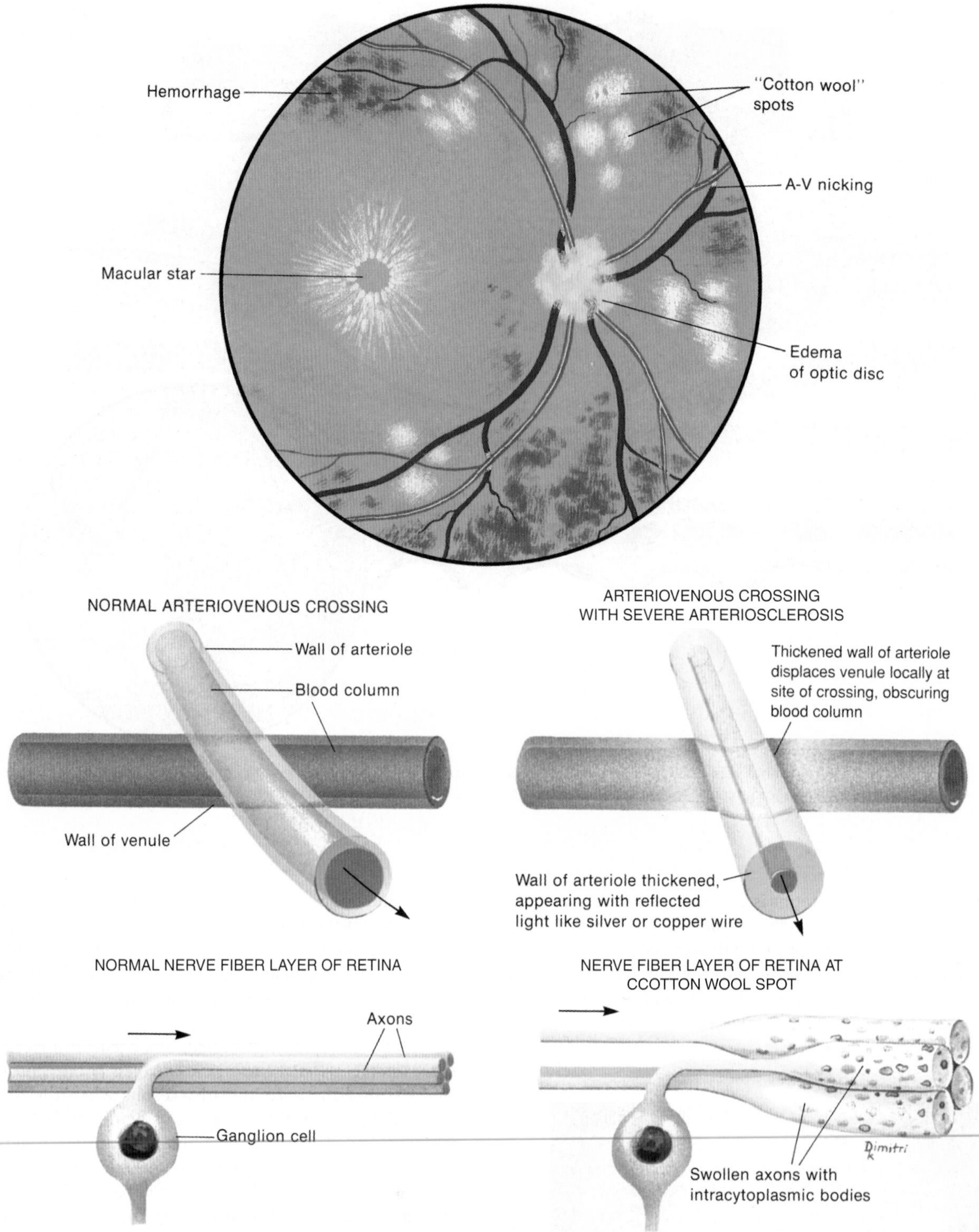

FIGURE 29-8. **Hypertensive retinopathy.** Various abnormalities develop within the retina in hypertension. The commonly associated arteriolosclerosis affects the appearance of the retinal microvasculature. Light reflected from the thickened arteriolar walls mimics silver or copper wire. Blood flow through the retinal venules is not well visualized at the sites of arteriolar–venular crossings. This effect is due to a thickening of the venular wall rather than to an impediment to blood flow caused by compression; the column of blood proximal to the compression is not wider than the part distal to the crossing. Impaired axoplasmic flow within the nerve fiber layer, caused by ischemia, results in swollen axons with cytoplasmic bodies. Such structures resemble cotton on funduscopy ("cotton-wool spots"). Hemorrhages are common in the retina, and exudates frequently form a star around the macula.

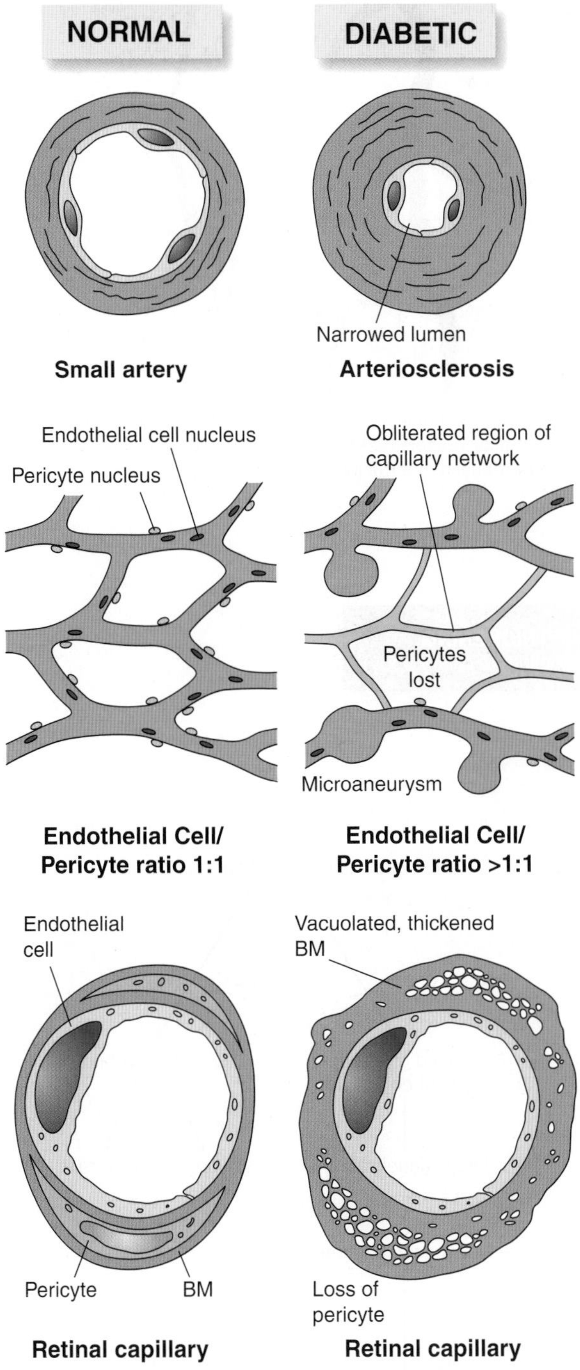

FIGURE 29-9. **Diabetic retinopathy.** In diabetic retinopathy, the microvasculature is abnormal. Arteriosclerosis narrows the lumen of the small arteries. Pericytes are lost, and the endothelial cell-to-pericyte ratio is greater than 1. Capillary microaneurysms are prominent, and portions of the capillary network become acellular and show no blood flow. The basement membrane of the retinal capillaries is thickened and vacuolated.

PATHOLOGY: A fibrovascular membrane leads to adhesions between the iris and the cornea (**peripheral anterior synechiae**) and between the iris and lens (**posterior synechiae**), while traction by the fibrovascular membrane pulls the iris pigment epithelium around the pupillary margin (**ectropion uveae**). The friable new vessels on the iris bleed easily and cause **hyphema** (hemorrhage within the anterior chamber of the eye). Neovascularization of the iris is clinically important because it frequently culminates in a blind, painful eye, owing to secondary glaucoma (**neovascular glaucoma**).

Hyperglycemia leads to glycogen storage in the pigmented epithelium of the iris, a phenomenon analogous to that produced in the renal tubules by glycosuria (Armanni-Epstein phenomenon). When tissue sections of diabetic eyes are processed in the usual manner, the pigment epithelium of the iris sometimes contains numerous vacuoles, which imparts a lacy appearance. The vacuoles result from loss of glycogen during preparation of tissue sections. Glycogen storage within the iris pigment epithelium is thought to account for the scattering of iris pigment observed clinically in diabetic patients.

Diabetic Cataracts

Patients with type 1 diabetes often develop bilateral "snowflake" cataracts, a blanket of white needle-shaped opacities in the lens immediately beneath the anterior and posterior lens capsule. The opacities coalesce within a few weeks in adolescents, and within days in children, until the whole lens becomes opaque. Snowflake cataracts can be produced experimentally in young animals and result from an osmotic effect caused by accumulation of sorbitol, the alcohol derived from glucose (see Chapter 22). The increased sorbitol content of the lens causes imbibition of water and enlargement of the lens.

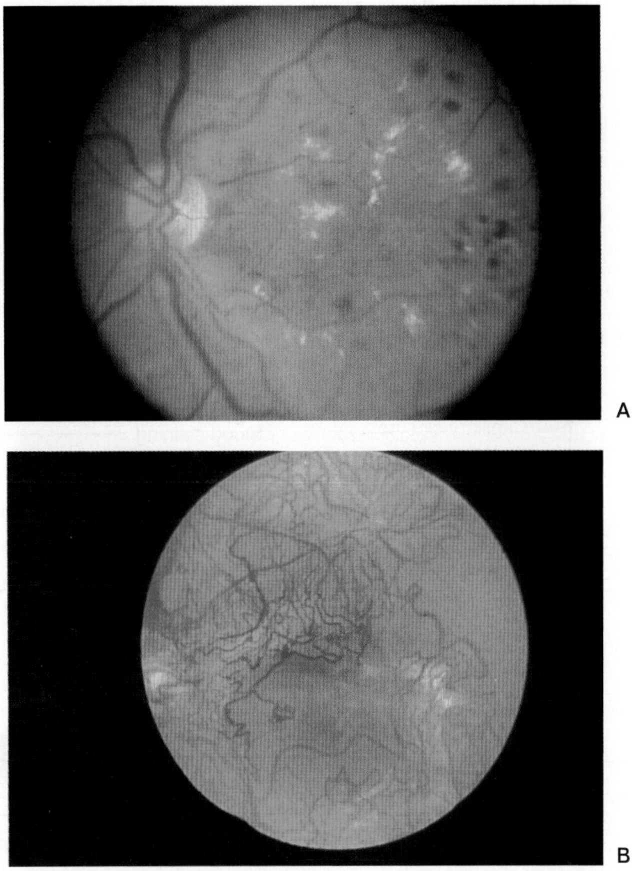

FIGURE 29-10. **Diabetic retinopathy. A.** The ocular fundus in a patient with background diabetic retinopathy. Several yellowish "hard" exudates, which are rich in lipids, are evident, together with several relatively small retinal hemorrhages. **B.** A vascular frond has extended anterior to the retina in the eye with proliferative diabetic retinopathy.

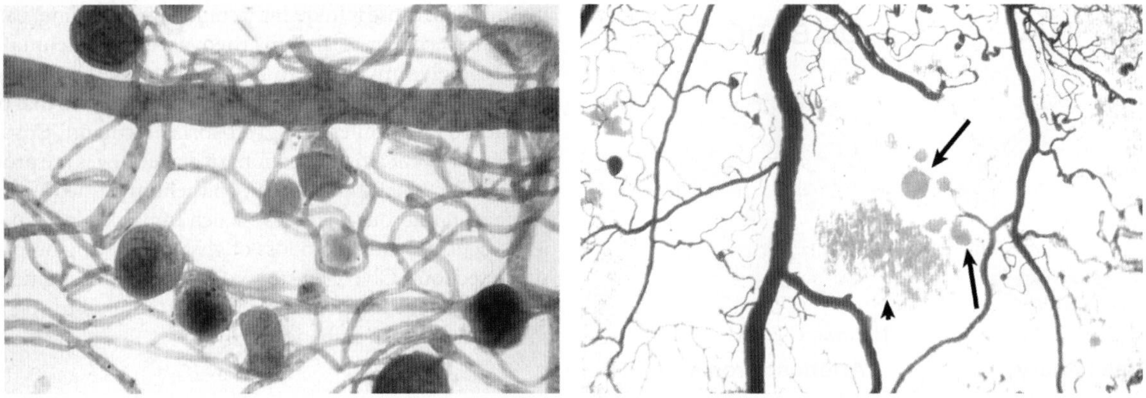

D

FIGURE 29-10. *(continued)* **C.** Numerous microaneurysms are present in this flat preparation of a diabetic retina. **D.** This flat preparation from a diabetic was stained with periodic acid–Schiff (PAS) after the retinal vessels had been perfused with India ink. Microaneurysms *(arrows)* and an exudate *(arrowhead)* are evident in a region of retinal nonperfusion.

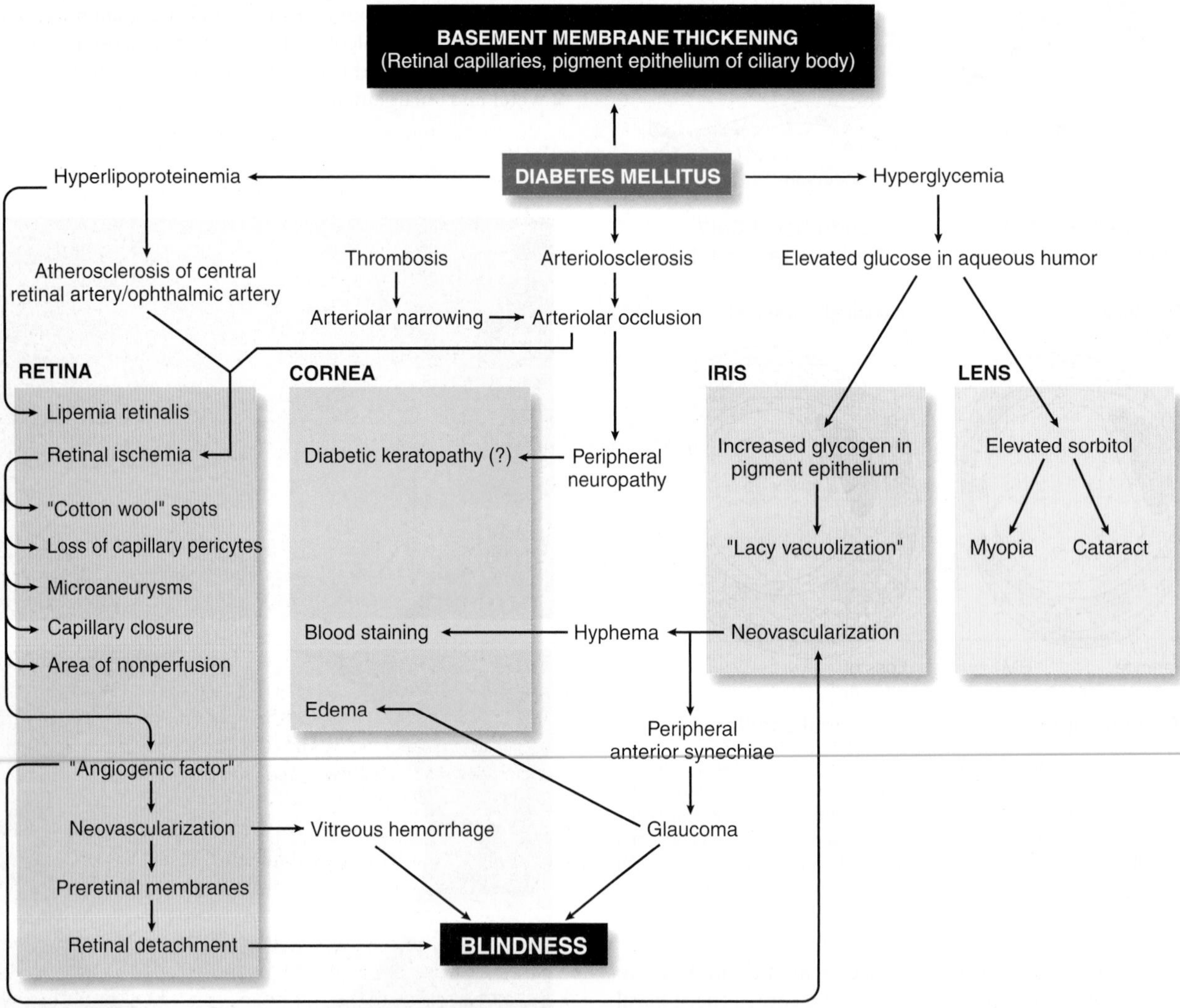

FIGURE 29-11. **Effects of diabetes on the eye.**

Age-related cataracts occur in diabetics at an earlier age than in the general population and progress more rapidly to maturity. A sudden temporary myopia, caused by increased refractive power in the lens, may be the presenting manifestation of diabetes.

Other Ophthalmic Manifestations of Diabetes

People with diabetes are at increased risk for inflammation of the anterior segment of the eye, phycomycosis (mucormycosis) of the orbit, and primary open-angle glaucoma. They are also prone to the **Argyll Robertson pupil** (unequal and irregularly shaped pupils that react to accommodation but not to light). Cranial nerve palsies occur, especially of the oculomotor nerve. Some patients with long-standing diabetes develop recurrent corneal erosions, which are thought to be due to impaired innervation of the cornea.

Retinal Detachment Separates the Sensory Retina from the Pigment Epithelium

During fetal development, the space between the sensory retina and the retinal pigment epithelium is obliterated when these two layers become apposed. However, the sensory retina readily separates from the retinal pigment epithelium when fluid (liquid vitreous, hemorrhage, or exudate) accumulates within the potential space between these structures. Such a separation is a common cause of blindness. Laser treatment has greatly improved the prognosis for patients with detached retina.

PATHOGENESIS: Factors predisposing to retinal detachment include retinal defects (due to trauma or certain retinal degenerations), vitreous traction, diminished pressure on the retina (e.g., after vitreous loss), and weakening of the fixation of the retina. The photoreceptors and retinal pigment epithelium normally function as a unit. After they separate in a retinal detachment, oxygen and nutrients that normally reach the outer retina from the choroid must diffuse across a greater distance. This situation causes the photoreceptors to degenerate, after which, cystlike extracellular spaces appear within the retina.

PATHOLOGY: Three varieties of retinal detachment are recognized—rhegmatogenous, tractional, and exudative.

RHEGMATOGENOUS RETINAL DETACHMENT: This condition is associated with a retinal tear and often with degenerative changes in the vitreous body or peripheral retina. Full-thickness holes in the retina are not complicated by retinal detachment unless liquid vitreous gains access to the potential space between the retina and the retinal pigment epithelium. Even then, some vitreoretinal traction seems to be necessary for retinal detachment to occur. Retinal detachment follows intraocular hemorrhage (e.g., after trauma) and is a potential complication of cataract extractions and several other ocular operations.

TRACTIONAL RETINAL DETACHMENT: In some instances, the retina is detached by being pulled toward the center of the eye by adherent vitreoretinal adhesions, as occurs in proliferative diabetic retinopathy, in retinopathy of prematurity, and after intraocular infection.

EXUDATIVE RETINAL DETACHMENT: Accumulation of fluid in the potential space between the sensory retina and the retinal pigment epithelium causes a detached retina in disorders such as choroiditis, choroidal hemangioma, and choroidal melanoma.

Retinitis Pigmentosa Is a Heritable Cause of Blindness

Retinitis pigmentosa (pigmentary retinopathy) is a generic term that refers to a variety of bilateral, progressive, degenerative retinopathies characterized clinically by night blindness and constriction of peripheral visual fields and pathologically by the loss of retinal photoreceptors (rods and cones) and pigment accumulation within the retina.

PATHOGENESIS: Retinitis pigmentosa is a misnomer since it does not feature inflammation of the retina. Multiple genetic disorders result in retinitis pigmentosa. Some are isolated ocular disorders, with autosomal dominant, autosomal recessive, or X-linked recessive inheritance; in others, pigmentary retinopathies are associated with neurologic and systemic disorders. At least 39 genes and loci are associated with non-syndromic retinitis pigmentosa. Some of the responsible mutated genes encode members of the rod phototransduction cascade, such as rhodopsin *(RHO)* and rod photoreceptor cyclic guanosine monophosphate (cGMP) phosphodiesterase alpha and beta subunits *(PDE6A, PDE6B)*, and peripherin. Because diverse mutations may lead to retinitis pigmentosa, a single defective protein cannot explain the death of photoreceptor cells that is characteristic of the condition. Presumably the abnormal metabolic pathways that result from all mutations ultimately converge at a final common point.

PATHOLOGY: In retinitis pigmentosa, destruction of rods and later cones is followed by migration of retinal pigment epithelial cells into the sensory retina (Fig. 29-12). Melanin appears within slender processes of spidery cells and accumulates mainly around small branching retinal blood vessels (especially in the equatorial portion of the retina), like spicules of bone. The retinal blood vessels then gradually attenuate, and the optic nerve head acquires a characteristic waxy pallor.

CLINICAL FEATURES: The clinical manifestations of retinitis pigmentosa, as well as the appearance and distribution of the retinal pigmentation, vary with the causes of the retinopathy. Half of these patients have a family history of the disease. Those with autosomal recessive and X-linked disease are more severely affected and develop night blindness and peripheral field defects in childhood. Autosomal dominant forms of retinitis pigmentosa tend to be less severe, and symptoms begin later in life. As the condition progresses, contraction of visual fields eventually leads to tunnel vision. Central vision is usually preserved until late in the course of the disease. In a few cases, the macula becomes involved, and blindness ensues.

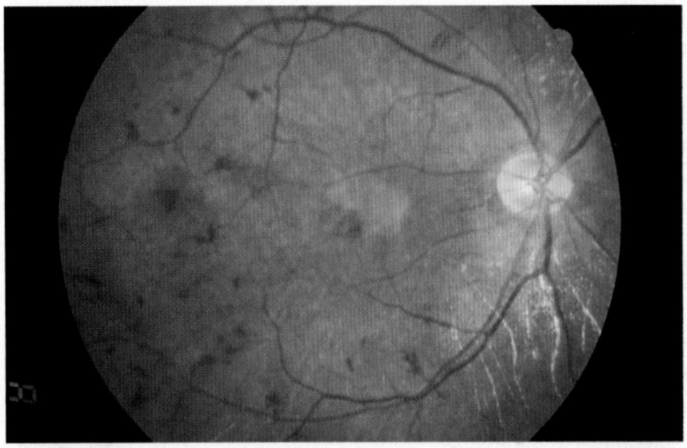

A

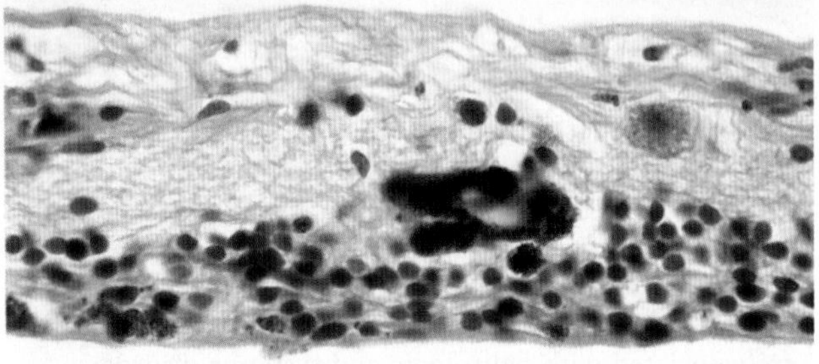

B

FIGURE 29-12. **Retinitis pigmentosa. A.** Fundus photograph of the retina of a patient with pigmentary retinopathy (retinitis pigmentosa) shows attenuated retinal vessels and foci of retinal pigmentation. **B.** Microscopic appearance of a severely degenerated retina in pigmentary retinopathy. Note the focal accumulations of pigmented cells (derived from retinal pigmented epithelium) within the retina.

Macular Degeneration Is Mostly Age-Related

The center of the macula, the foveola, is the point of greatest visual acuity. In this area, a high concentration of cones rests on the retinal pigment epithelium. Surrounding the macula, the retina has a multilayered concentration of ganglion cells. With aging, in certain drug toxicities (e.g., chloroquine), and in several inherited disorders, the macula degenerates, and central vision is impaired.

Age-related macular degeneration currently affects almost 2 million people in the United States. and is the most common cause of blindness among individuals of European descent older than age 65. Dry and wet forms of age-related macular degeneration are recognized. The wet variety of this disease is associated with subretinal fibrovascular tissue and sometimes bleeding into the subretinal space. Laser photocoagulation and other therapies are beneficial in this type of the disorder. A common missense variant of the CFH gene that encodes for complement factor H is a risk factor for about 43% of cases of age-related macular degeneration. Rare cases of age-related macular degeneration have been associated with mutations in ABCA4 (formerly called *ABCR), FBLN5,* and *FBLN6* genes. *ABCA4* encodes a rod cell protein (rim protein) thought to be a transporter involved in molecular recycling. Mutations in this gene may allow degraded material *(drusen)* to accumulate and interfere with retinal function.

Cherry-Red Spot at the Macula Describes a Bright Central Foveola

In lysosomal storage diseases, including the gangliosidoses, myriad intracytoplasmic lysosomal inclusions within the multilayered ganglion cell layer of the macula impart a striking pallor to the affected retina. As a result, the central foveola appears bright red because of the underlying choroidal vasculature (Fig. 29-13). A cherry-red spot also occurs at the macula after central retinal artery occlusion but for a different reason. Edema causes the entire retina to appear pale, which highlights the subfoveolar vascular choroid.

Angioid Streaks are Vessel-like Fractures in Bruch's Membrane

Angioid streaks are seen when the posterior segment of the eye is examined clinically. Bruch's membrane fractures spontaneously in a variety of systemic conditions, causing the characteristic irregular lines that radiate beneath the retina from the optic nerve head (angioid streaks).

Retinopathy of Prematurity Results from Oxygen Toxicity

Retinopathy of prematurity is a bilateral, iatrogenic, retinal disorder that occurs predominantly in premature infants treated with oxygen after birth. The entity was originally called *retrolental fibroplasia* because of a mass of scarred tissue behind the lens in advanced cases. More than a half-century ago, retinopathy of prematurity (Fig. 29-14) was the leading cause of blindness in infants in the United States. and many other countries. Retinopathy of prematurity is almost restricted to premature infants administered high concentrations of oxygen. In such infants, the developing retinal blood vessels become obliterated, and the peripheral retina, which is normally avascular until the end of fetal life, does not vascularize. The more mature the retina, the less the vaso-obliterative effect of hyperoxia. When the infant eventually returns to ambient air, intense proliferation of vascular endothelium and glial cells begins at the junction of the avascular and vascularized portions of the retina. This becomes apparent 5 to 10 weeks after removal of the infant from the incubator and, as in diabetic retinopathy, is thought to result from liberation of an angiogenic factor produced by the avascular and ischemic peripheral retina. This angiogenic factor is also believed to account for the neovascularization of the iris that sometimes accompanies retinopathy of prematurity. In 25% of cases, retinopathy progresses to a cicatricial phase, characterized by retinal detachment, a fibrovascular mass behind the lens (retrolental), and blindness.

The Optic Nerve

Optic Nerve Head Edema Often Reflects Increased Intracranial Pressure

Optic nerve head (optic disc) edema refers to a swelling of the optic nerve head where it enters the globe. Optic nerve head edema can result from various causes, the most important of which is increased intracranial pressure. The term **papilledema**, which is still widely used in that context, is imprecise because no optic papilla exists. Other important causes of optic nerve head edema are (1) obstruction to the venous drainage of the eye (as may occur with compressive lesions of the orbit), (2) infarction of the optic nerve (ischemic optic neuropathy), (3) inflammation of the optic nerve close to the eyeball (optic neuritis, papillitis), and (4) multiple sclerosis.

Edema of the optic nerve head is characterized clinically by a swollen optic disc that displays blurred margins and dilated vessels (Fig. 29-15). Frequently, hemorrhages (Fig. 29-16), exudates, and cotton-wool spots are seen, and concentric folds of the

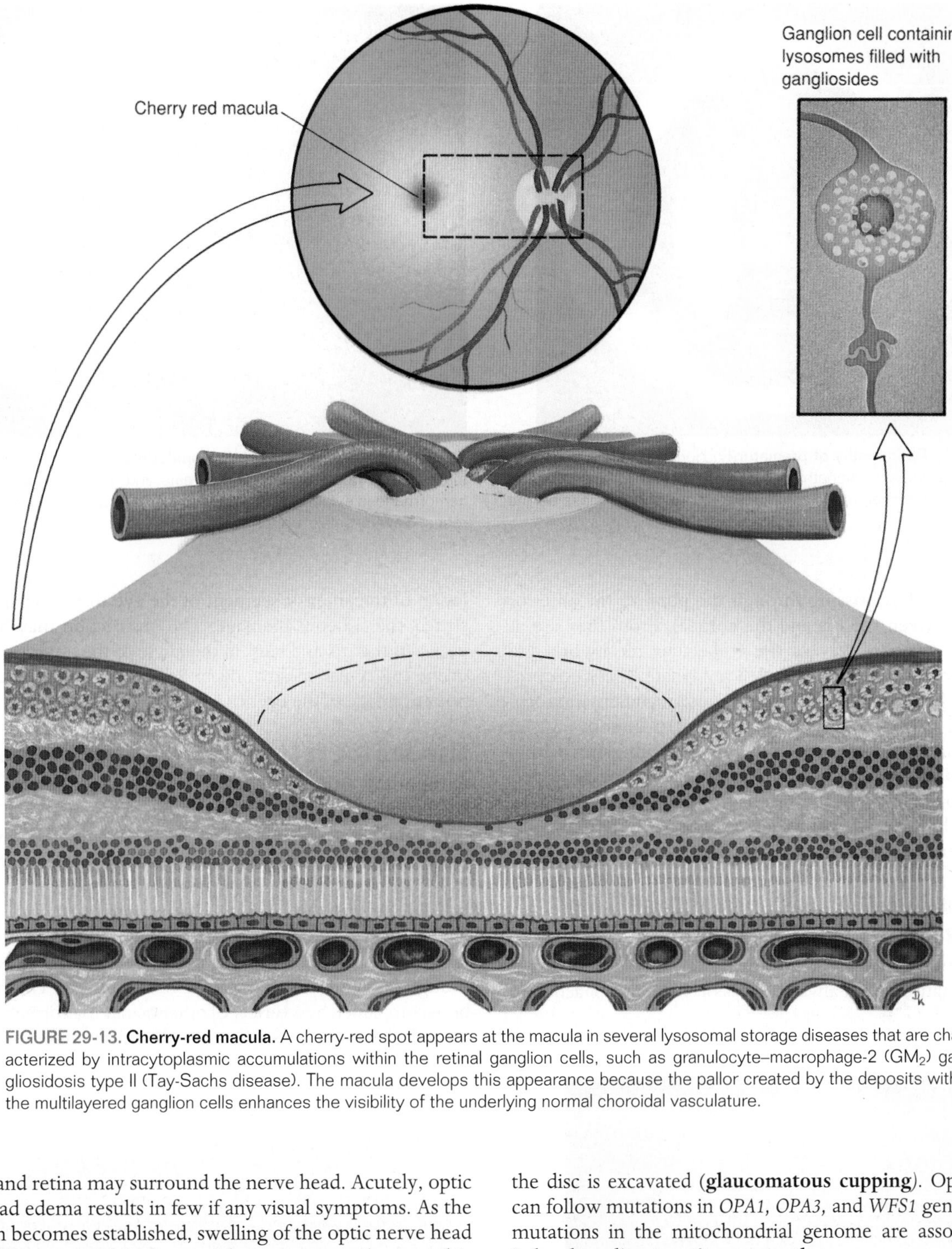

FIGURE 29-13. **Cherry-red macula.** A cherry-red spot appears at the macula in several lysosomal storage diseases that are characterized by intracytoplasmic accumulations within the retinal ganglion cells, such as granulocyte–macrophage-2 (GM_2) gangliosidosis type II (Tay-Sachs disease). The macula develops this appearance because the pallor created by the deposits within the multilayered ganglion cells enhances the visibility of the underlying normal choroidal vasculature.

choroid and retina may surround the nerve head. Acutely, optic nerve head edema results in few if any visual symptoms. As the condition becomes established, swelling of the optic nerve head enlarges the normal blind spot. After many months, atrophic changes lead to a loss of visual acuity.

Optic Atrophy is a Thinning of the Optic Nerve Caused by Loss of Axons Within its Substance

The nerve axons within the optic nerve are lost in many conditions. Possible causes include (1) long-standing edema of the optic nerve head, (2) optic neuritis, (3) optic nerve compression, (4) glaucoma, and (5) retinal degeneration. Optic atrophy also can be caused by some drugs, such as ethambutol and isoniazid. The optic nerve head is usually flat and pale in optic atrophy (Fig. 29-17), but when this disorder follows glaucoma, the disc is excavated (**glaucomatous cupping**). Optic atrophy can follow mutations in *OPA1, OPA3,* and *WFS1* genes. Multiple mutations in the mitochondrial genome are associated with **Leber hereditary optic neuropathy**.

Glaucoma

Glaucoma refers to a collection of disorders that feature an optic neuropathy accompanied by a characteristic excavation of the optic nerve head and progressive loss of visual field sensitivity. In most cases, glaucoma is produced by increased intraocular pressure (**ocular hypertension**); however, increased intraocular pressure does not necessarily cause glaucoma, and not all patients with glaucoma have elevated intraocular pressure.

After being produced by the ciliary body, the aqueous humor enters the posterior chamber (the space between the iris and

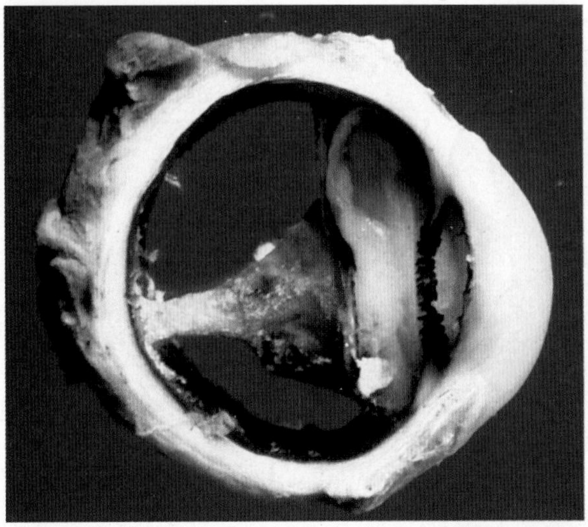

FIGURE 29-14. **Retinopathy of prematurity.** Horizontal section through an eye with advanced retinopathy of prematurity (retrolental fibroplasia) shows a totally detached retina adherent to a fibrovascular mass behind the lens.

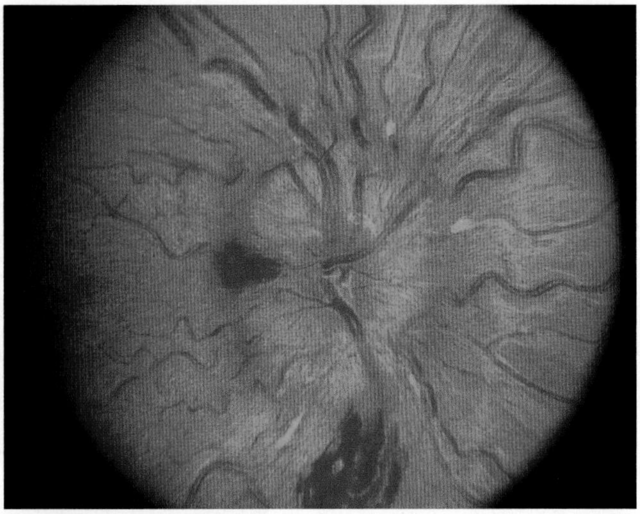

FIGURE 29-16. **Hemorrhage in papilledema.** The optic nerve head is markedly congested, with dilated veins and a blurred margin. A small hemorrhage is evident within the optic nerve head at its junction with the retina. Several small "cotton-wool" spots are present within the adjacent retina.

the zonules) before passing through the pupil to the anterior chamber (between the iris and the cornea). From that site, it drains into veins by way of the trabecular meshwork and Schlemm's canal (Fig. 29-18). A delicate balance between production and drainage of the aqueous humor maintains intraocular pressure within its physiologic range (10–20 mm Hg). In certain pathologic states, aqueous humor accumulates within the eye, and intraocular pressure increases. Temporary or permanent impairment of vision results from pressure-induced degenerative changes in the retina and optic nerve head (Fig. 29-19) and from corneal edema and opacification.

Glaucoma is Caused By an Obstruction of the Aqueous Drainage

Glaucoma, the most common cause of preventable blindness in the United States, almost always follows a congenital or acquired lesion of the anterior segment of the eye that mechanically obstructs the aqueous drainage. The obstruction may be located between the iris and lens, in the angle of the anterior chamber, in the trabecular meshwork, in Schlemm's canal, or in the venous drainage of the eye.

Glaucoma Can Be Classified into Several Different Types

Congenital Glaucoma (Infantile Glaucoma, Buphthalmos)

Congenital glaucoma is caused by obstruction to aqueous drainage by developmental anomalies. The disorder develops even though intraocular pressure may not increase until early infancy or childhood. Most cases of congenital glaucoma occur in boys (65%), and an X-linked recessive mode of inheritance is common. The developmental anomaly usually involves both eyes and, although often limited to the angle of the anterior chamber, may be accompanied by a variety of other ocular malformations. Congenital glaucoma is associated with a deep anterior chamber,

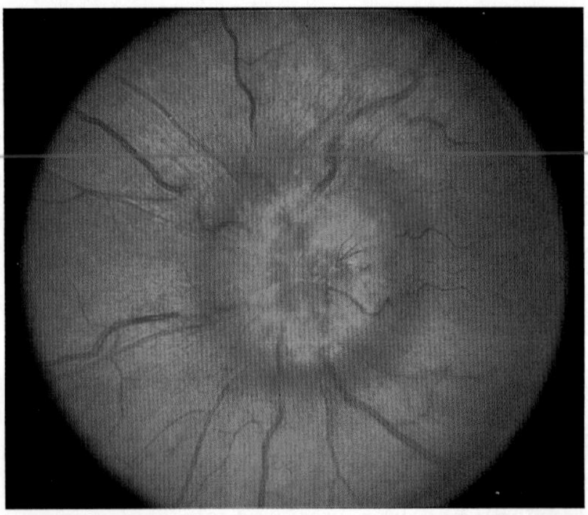

FIGURE 29-15. **Chronic papilledema.** The optic nerve head is congested and protrudes anteriorly toward the interior of the eye. It has blurred margins, and the vessels within it are poorly seen. In contrast to acute papilledema, the veins are not so congested, and hemorrhage is not a feature.

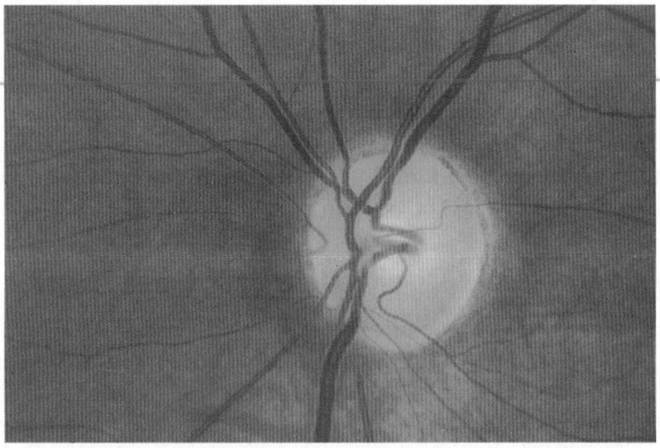

FIGURE 29-17. **Optic atrophy.** The margin of the optic nerve head is sharply demarcated from the adjacent retina. Because the myelinated axons in the optic nerve are markedly diminished, the optic nerve head appears much whiter than normal.

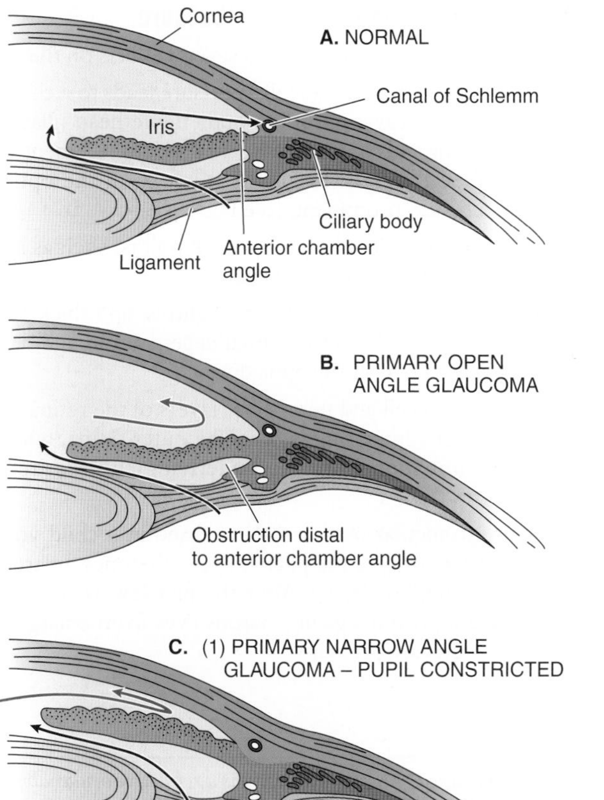

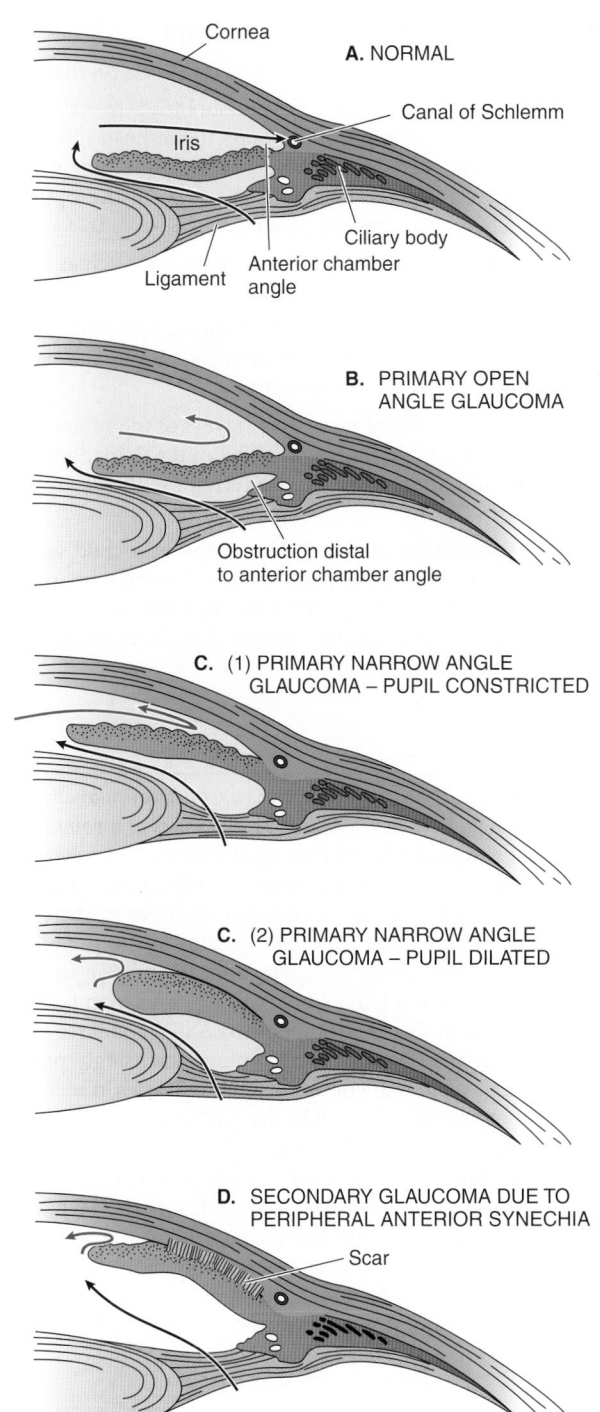

FIGURE 29-18. **Pathogenesis of glaucoma.** The anterior segment of the eye is affected differently in various forms of glaucoma. **A.** Structure of the normal eye. **B.** In primary open-angle glaucoma, the obstruction to the aqueous outflow is distal to the anterior chamber angle, and the anterior segment resembles that of the normal eye. **C.** In primary narrow-angle glaucoma, the anterior chamber angle is open, but narrower than normal when the pupil is constricted (**C1**). When the pupil becomes dilated in such an eye, the thickened iris obstructs the anterior chamber angle (**C2**), causing increased intraocular pressure. **D.** The anterior chamber angle can become obstructed by a variety of pathological processes, including an adhesion between the iris and the posterior surface of the cornea (peripheral anterior synechiae).

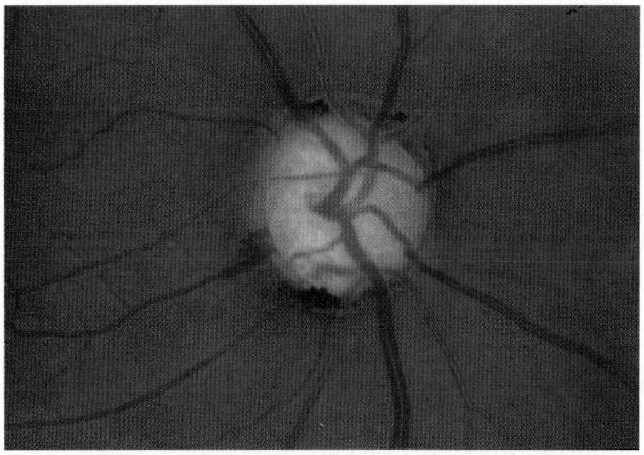

FIGURE 29-19. **Optic nerve head in glaucoma.** The anterior part of the optic nerve is depressed ("optic cupping"), and the blood vessels crossing the margin of the optic nerve head are displaced nasally. The fundus appears dark because this eye from a black patient contains numerous pigmented melanocytes in the choroid.

corneal cloudiness, sensitivity to bright lights (**photophobia**), excessive tearing, and buphthalmos. The term **buphthalmos** (from the Greek bous, "ox"; ophthalmos, "eye") describes the enlarged eyes of congenital glaucoma patients that result from expansion caused by increased intraocular pressure beneath a pliable sclera. Several genes for congenital glaucoma have been identified. Homozygous mutations in the cytochrome P4501B1 gene *(CYP1B1)* account for some cases of autosomal recessive primary infantile glaucoma. Congenital glaucoma associated with developmental anomalies of the eye (secondary congenital glaucoma) results from mutations in the fork-head transcription factor gene *(FOXC1)*, pituitary homeobox 2 gene *(PITX2)*, or paired box 6 gene *(PAX6)*.

Primary Open-Angle Glaucoma

Primary glaucoma develops in a person with no apparent underlying eye disease. The disorder is subdivided into **open-angle glaucoma,** in which the anterior chamber angle is open and appears normal, and **closed-angle glaucoma,** in which the anterior chamber is shallower than normal, and the angle is abnormally narrow (see Fig. 29-18B).

Primary open-angle glaucoma is the most frequent type of glaucoma and a major cause of blindness in the United States. It affects 1% to 3% of the population older than 40 years and occurs principally in the sixth decade. The intraocular pressure increases insidiously and asymptomatically, and although almost always bilateral, one eye may be affected more severely than the other. With time, damage to the retina and optic nerve causes an irreversible loss of peripheral vision.

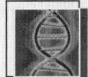

PATHOGENESIS: The angle of the anterior chamber is open and appears normal, but there is increased resistance to the outflow of the aqueous humor in the vicinity of Schlemm's canal. Persons with diabetes mellitus and myopia have increased risk of primary open-angle glaucoma.

Primary open-angle glaucoma has been mapped to several loci on many chromosomes, including chromosomes 1, 2, 3, 7, 8, 9, 10, and 20. Some cases of primary open-angle glaucoma are due to more than a dozen different mutations in the *MYOC (TGRR)* gene on chromosome 1 (1q21-q31). Primary open-angle glaucoma can occur as a manifestation of the nail–patella syndrome, in association with mutations in the Lim homeobox transcription factor *1(LMX1B)* gene. A juvenile onset primary open-angle glaucoma may result from mutations in the *CRYP1B1* gene. Susceptibility to normal tension glaucoma is associated with an intronic polymorphism of the *OPA1* gene, as well as with a mutation in the *OPTN* gene.

Primary Closed-Angle Glaucoma

Primary closed-angle glaucoma, differentiated from open-angle glaucoma above, occurs after age 40 years.

PATHOGENESIS: The disorder afflicts persons whose peripheral iris is displaced anteriorly toward the trabecular meshwork, thereby creating an abnormally narrow angle. When the pupil is constricted (miotic), the iris remains stretched so that the chamber angle is not occluded. However, when the pupil dilates (mydriasis), the iris obstructs the anterior chamber angle, thereby impairing aqueous drainage and resulting in sudden episodes of intraocular hypertension. This is accompanied by ocular pain, and halos or rings are seen around lights. In such persons, intraocular pressure may also increase if the pupil becomes blocked (e.g., by a swollen lens) and aqueous humor accumulates in the posterior chamber.

CLINICAL FEATURES: *Acute closed-angle glaucoma is an ocular emergency, and it is essential to start ocular hypotensive treatment within the first 24 to 48 hours if vision is to be maintained.* Primary closed-angle glaucoma affects both eyes, but it may become apparent in one eye 2 to 5 years before it is noted in the other. The intraocular pressure is normal between attacks, but after many episodes, adhesions form between the iris and the trabecular meshwork and cornea (peripheral anterior synechiae) and accentuate the block to the outflow of aqueous humor.

Secondary Glaucoma

The causes of secondary glaucoma are many and include inflammation, hemorrhage, neovascularization of the iris and adhesions. In secondary glaucoma, anterior chamber angles may be open or closed. Because the underlying disorder is usually limited to one eye, secondary glaucoma tends to be unilateral.

Low-Tension Glaucoma

Low-tension glaucoma refers to an entity in which the characteristic visual-field defect and all of the ophthalmoscopic features of chronic open-angle glaucoma occur without an increase in intraocular pressure. The characteristic visual-field defect and all of the ophthalmoscopic features of chronic simple (open-angle) glaucoma often occur in elderly people who do not show increased intraocular pressure. Although some eyes may be hypersensitive to normal intraocular pressure, many cases of low-tension glaucoma probably represent an infarction of the optic nerve head.

Effects of Increased Intraocular Pressure

Prolonged ocular hypertension has several effects on the eye:

- In adults, increased intraocular pressure leads to a characteristic cupped excavation of the optic nerve head (glaucomatous cupping), accompanied by a nasal displacement of the retinal blood vessels. In infants, cupping of the optic disc tends to be less prominent. (see Fig. 29-19)
- The cornea or sclera bulges at weak points, such as sites of scars in the outer coat of the eye.
- Optic atrophy, with loss of axons, gliosis, and thickening of the pial septa, follows the retinal degeneration and damage to the nerve fibers at the optic disc.
- The ganglion cell and nerve fiber layers of the retina degenerate, thereby impairing vision. The outer retina, which derives its nutrition from the underlying choroid, remains intact.
- When intraocular pressure is increased in a child younger than 3 years of age, the pliable eye sometimes enlarges extensively (buphthalmos). After the first few years of life, a rigid sclera prevents glaucomatous eyes from enlarging under the increased pressure.

Myopia

Myopia (also called "nearsightedness") is a refractive ocular abnormality in which light from the visualized object focuses at a point in front of the retina because of a longer than usual anteroposterior diameter of the eye. Myopia affects more than 70 million persons in the United States and is the most common disorder of the eye. In Asia it affects an even greater percentage of the population. Treatment requires refractive correction. In addition to glasses and contact lenses, refractive surgery using an excimer laser such as laser-assisted in situ keratomileusis (LASIK) and laser epithelial keratomileusis (LASEK) is becoming increasingly popular. Myopia usually begins in young persons and varies in severity. A mild form (stationary or simple myopia) is generally nonprogressive after cessation of body growth, whereas a genetically determined "progressive myopia" is more severe. Causes of myopia are complex, but some nonsyndromic inherited types have been mapped to 11 different loci on various chromosomes. It is a feature of several systemic diseases, including some disorders of fibrillin (Marfan syndrome), collagen (Stickler syndrome, Knobloch syndrome), and perlecan (Schwartz-Jampel syndrome type I).

Phthisis Bulbi

Phthisis bulbi refers to a nonspecific, end-stage eye that is disorganized and atrophic. This condition (Fig. 29-20) is most common after trauma to, or inflammation of, the eye. The eye is small and often extremely hard due to intraocular ossification. The choroid and ciliary body are separated from the sclera, which is thickened, wrinkled, and indented due to loss of intraocular pressure. The cornea is flattened, shrunken and opaque, intraocular contents are disorganized by diffuse scarring and detachment of the sensory retina is invariably encountered. The lens is displaced and often calcified. A typical finding in phthisis bulbi is intraocular bone formation, which seems to be derived from the hyperplastic pigment epithelium. Eyes afflicted with phthisis bulbi are often enucleated.

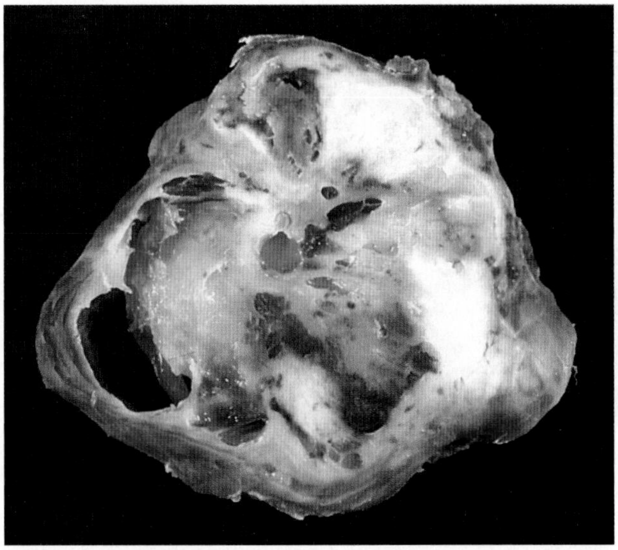

FIGURE 29-20. **Phthisis bulbi.** Section through an eye with phthisis bulbi, exemplifying the markedly disorganized nature of the intraocular contents of such atrophic disordered globes.

Ocular Neoplasms

The eye and adjacent structures contain a large number of cell types, and as one might expect, benign and malignant neoplasms arise from them. *Intraocular neoplasms arise mostly from immature retinal neurons (retinoblastoma) and uveal melanocytes (melanoma).* Although the retinal pigment epithelium often undergoes reactive proliferation, it seldom becomes neoplastic.

Malignant Melanoma Arises from Melanocytes in the Uvea

Malignant melanoma is the most common primary intraocular malignancy. It may arise from melanocytes in any part of the eye, the choroid being the most common site.

PATHOLOGY: Choroidal melanomas are mostly circumscribed and invade Bruch's membrane, causing a mushroom-shaped mass (Fig. 29-21). By contrast, some tumors are flat (diffuse melanoma) and cause a gradual deterioration of vision over many years. Some do not become apparent until extraocular dissemination has occurred. Orange lipofuscin pigment is evident over the surface of some choroidal melanomas.

Microscopically, uveal melanomas may be composed mainly of variable numbers of spindle-shaped cells without nucleoli (spindle A cells), spindle-shaped cells with prominent nucleoli (spindle B cells), and polygonal cells with distinct cell borders and prominent nucleoli (epithelioid cells). Melanomas of the ciliary body and iris may extend circumferentially around the globe (ring melanoma). Melanomas in the iris are usually diagnosed clinically 1 to 2 decades earlier than those in the choroid and ciliary body, perhaps because they are more easily seen and are often first observed by the patient.

Aside from hematogenous spread, uveal melanomas disseminate by traversing the sclera to enter the orbital tissues, usually at sites where blood vessels and nerves pass through the sclera. Lymphatic spread does not occur because the eye has no lymphatic vessels. Intraocular melanomas sometimes cause cataract, glaucoma, retinal detachment, inflammation, and even hemorrhage.

The usual treatment for most uveal melanomas is enucleation of the eye, but some are treated with other methods, such as radiotherapy or local excision. More than half of patients with uveal melanomas survive for 15 years after enucleation. Deaths have been reported within 5 years from spindle A melanomas, but tumors composed purely of epithelioid cells have the worst prognosis. Anecdotally, the diagnosis of metastatic ocular melanoma has been made intuitively by astute clinicians who discovered an enlarged liver in a patient with a "glass eye."

Retinoblastoma Originates from Immature Neurons

Retinoblastoma is the most common intraocular malignant neoplasm of childhood affecting 1:20,000 to 1:34,000 children. The tumor occurs most frequently within the first 2 years of life and may even be found at birth. Presenting signs include a white pupil (leukocoria), squint (strabismus), poor vision, spontaneous hyphema, or a red, painful eye. Secondary glaucoma is a frequent complication. Light entering the eye commonly reflects a yellowish color similar to that from the tapetum of a cat (cat's eye reflex). Most retinoblastomas occur sporadically and are unilateral. Some

A

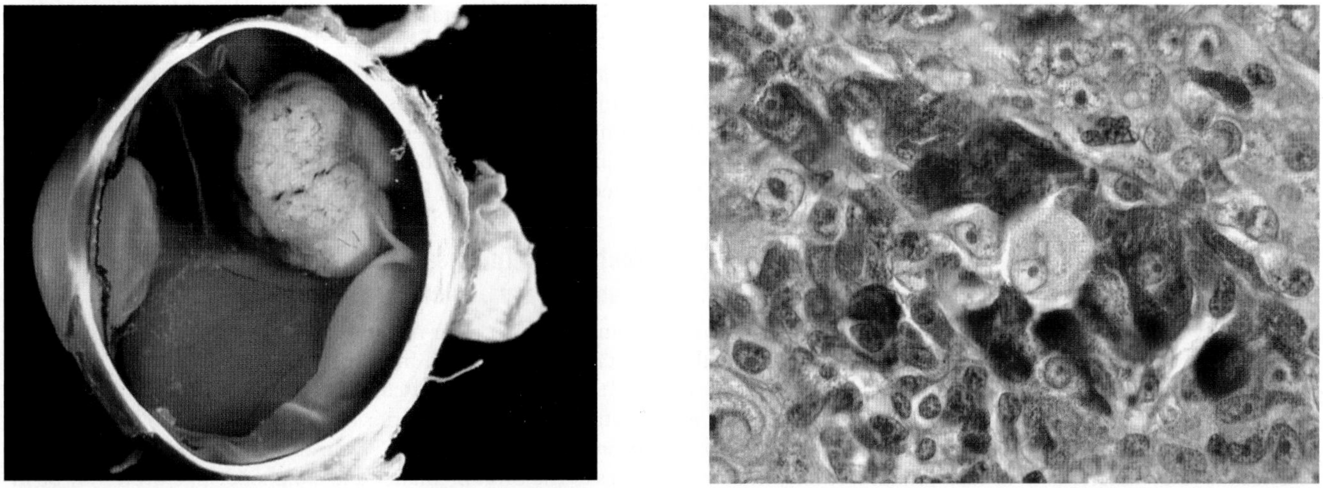

B

FIGURE 29-21. **Malignant melanoma. A.** A mushroom-shaped melanoma of the choroid is present in this eye. Choroidal melanomas commonly invade through Bruch's membrane and result in this appearance. **B.** Photomicrograph of a heavily pigmented melanoma of the choroid depicting epithelioid tumor cells with prominent nucleoli.

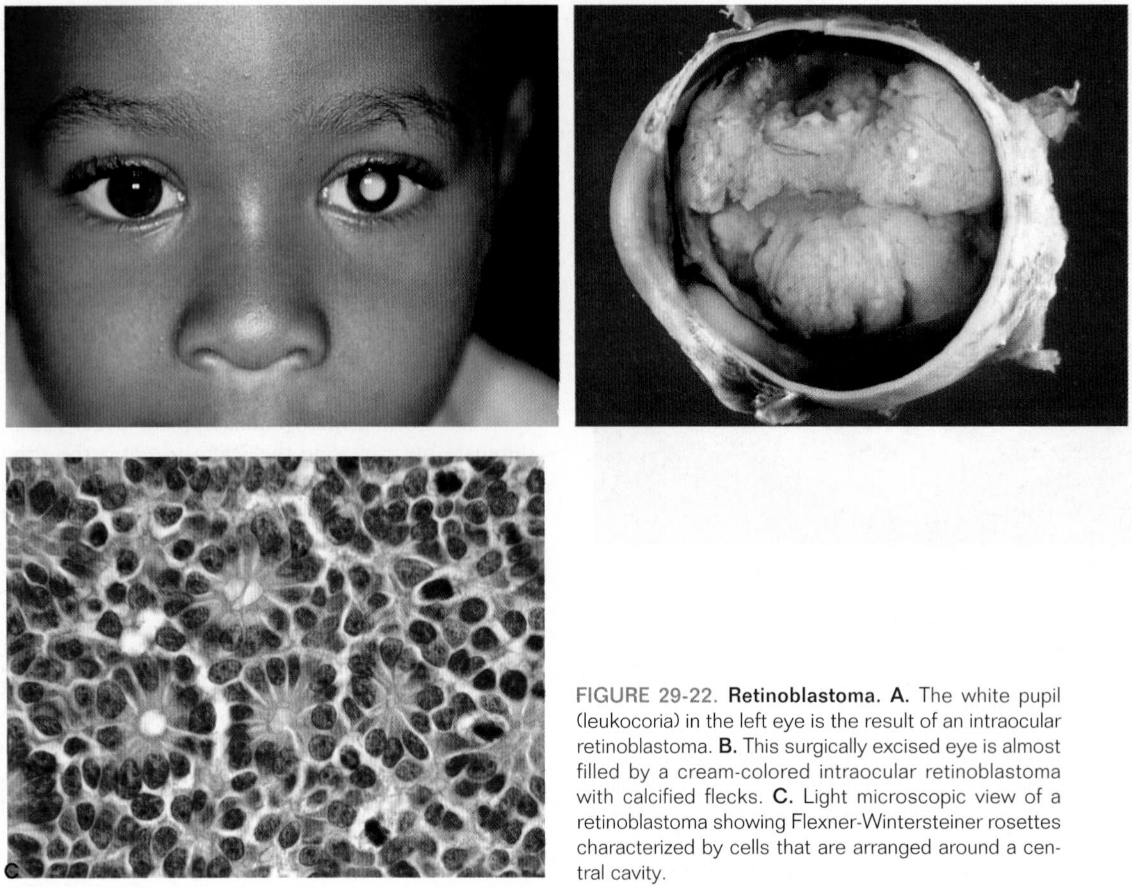

FIGURE 29-22. **Retinoblastoma. A.** The white pupil (leukocoria) in the left eye is the result of an intraocular retinoblastoma. **B.** This surgically excised eye is almost filled by a cream-colored intraocular retinoblastoma with calcified flecks. **C.** Light microscopic view of a retinoblastoma showing Flexner-Wintersteiner rosettes characterized by cells that are arranged around a central cavity.

6% to 8% of retinoblastomas are inherited. Up to 25% of sporadic retinoblastomas and most inherited retinoblastomas are bilateral.

Retinoblastomas are related to inherited or acquired deletions of, or mutations in, the retinoblastoma *(Rb)* tumor-suppressor gene, located on the long arm of chromosome 13 (13q14) (see Chapter 5).

PATHOLOGY: Some retinoblastomas grow toward the vitreous body and can be seen with an ophthalmoscope (**endophytic retinoblastoma**). Others extend between the sensory retina and the retinal pigment epithelium, thereby detaching the retina (**exophytic retinoblastoma**). A few retinoblastomas are both endophytic and exophytic. Rarely, a retinoblastoma spreads diffusely within the retina without forming an obvious mass (**diffuse retinoblastoma**). The retina often contains several distinct foci of tumor in the same eye, some of which represent a multifocal origin, whereas others are tumor implants from dissemination through the vitreous body.

Retinoblastoma is a cream-colored tumor that contains scattered, chalky white, calcified flecks within yellow necrotic zones (Fig. 29-22), which may be detected radiologically. The tumors are intensely cellular and display several morphologic patterns. In some instances, densely packed, round neoplastic cells with hyperchromatic nuclei, scant cytoplasm, and abundant mitoses are randomly distributed. In other retinoblastomas, the cells are arranged radially around a central cavity (Flexner-Wintersteiner rosettes), as they differentiate toward photoreceptors. In some cases, the cellular arrangement resembles a fleur-de-lis (fleurette). Viable tumor cells align themselves around blood vessels, and necrotic areas with calcification are seen a short distance from the vascularized regions.

Retinoblastomas disseminate by several routes. They commonly extend into the optic nerve, from where they spread intracranially. They also invade blood vessels, especially in the highly vascular choroid, before metastasizing hematogenously throughout the body. Bone marrow is a common site of blood-borne metastases, but surprisingly, the lung is rarely involved.

CLINICAL FEATURES: Retinoblastomas are almost always fatal if left untreated. However, with early diagnosis and modern therapy, survival is high (about 90%). Rarely, spontaneous regression occurs for reasons that remain unknown. Patients with inherited retinoblastomas, presumably as a consequence of the loss of *Rb* gene function, have an increased susceptibility to other malignant tumors, including osteogenic sarcoma, Ewing sarcoma, and pinealoblastoma.

Metastatic Tumors to the Eye are More Common than Primary Ocular Neoplasms

Sometimes an ocular metastasis may be the initial clinical manifestation of a cancer, but most cases are diagnosed only after death. Leukemias and cancers of the breast and lung usually metastasize to the posterior choroid and account for most cases of intraocular metastases. Neuroblastoma frequently metastasizes to the orbit in infancy and childhood. The orbit may be invaded by malignant neoplasms of the eyelid, conjunctiva, paranasal sinuses, nose, nasopharynx, and intracranial cavity.

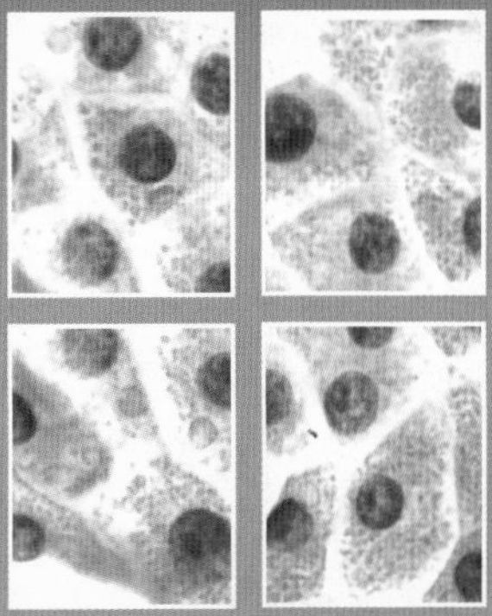

30

Cytopathology

Hormoz Ehya
Marluce Bibbo

Cytopathology refers to diagnostic techniques that are used to examine cells from various body sites to determine the cause or nature of disease. Cytologic methods date to the mid-19th century, when investigators detected abnormal cells in body fluids (e.g., urine, sputum, effusions, gastric secretions) and made sporadic attempts to collect diagnostic samples from tumors by means of a needle. In 1928, George Papanicolaou introduced a cytologic method for detection of malignant and precancerous lesions of the uterine cervix. Despite initial skepticism, cervical smear, popularly termed the **"Pap" test** became widely accepted and proved to be the most successful cancer prevention method, saving millions of lives in the past seven decades. The success of the Pap test also served as a booster to the cytologic diagnosis of cancer in other organs. In the past few decades, the applications of cytopathology have been expanded to most body sites. Exfoliated cells and cells obtained by scraping, brushing, washing, and needle aspiration are routinely evaluated by cytopathologists to determine the nature of disease and surveillance of cancer. By applying imaging techniques and **endoscopic ultrasound** (EUS) to guide in placement, the uses of fine-needle aspiration have expanded greatly. Very small lesions (a few millimeters in size) can now be targeted by EUS.

Applications of Cytopathology

Screening Is Important for Early Detection of Asymptomatic Cancer

The most important application of cytopathology in the area of cancer prevention is examination of scrapings and brushings from the uterine cervix. Widespread screening of women by Pap smears has reduced the incidence of cervical cancer in the United States and many other countries by 70%.

Early cancers can be also be detected in other organs such as bladder, stomach, lung, esophagus, endometrium, and anus. Economic considerations preclude mass screening for such tumors, but it is feasible to screen specific populations at high risk for certain malignancies such as lung cancer in uranium miners, bladder cancer in industrial workers, anal cancer in male homosexuals, and esophageal and gastric cancers in Chinese and Japanese populations, respectively.

Cytologic Methods Detect Primary and Recurrent Tumors

Cytologic evaluation with radiologic guidance is particularly important for diagnosis of tumors that may not be easily accessible or amenable to surgical treatment. Examples of such neoplasms include hepatocellular and pancreatic carcinomas with metastases and small cell lung carcinoma.

For some types of cancers, cytology is the most feasible surveillance method to detect recurrence. Thus, periodic urine cytology, usually at 3-month intervals, may be used to test for recurrence of urinary tract cancers. Cytologic methods are also used to evaluate cancer patients who develop effusions; neurologic symptoms; lymphadenopathy; or nodules in the skin, lung, or liver.

Cytologic Methods

Spontaneously Shed Cells in Body Fluids Can Be Detected

This technique is called **exfoliative cytology.** Examples of such specimens include sputum, cerebrospinal fluid, urine, effusions in body cavities (pleura, pericardium, peritoneum), nipple discharge, and vitreous and aqueous humors of the eye.

Abrasive Cytology Dislodges Cells from Body Surfaces

Abrasive methods include endoscopic brushing of mucosal surfaces of the gastrointestinal, respiratory, and urinary tracts; the balloon technique for obtaining cells from the esophagus; scraping of cutaneous or mucosal lesions to detect viral cytopathic changes; and washing (lavage) of mucosal or serosal surfaces during endoscopy or open surgery.

Fine-Needle Aspiration Cytology Samples Tumors and Cysts

Virtually any organ or tissue can be sampled by fine-needle aspiration, which uses suction under negative pressure through a thin (22–25 gauge) needle. Nodules in superficial organs such as thyroid, breast, lymph nodes, skin, and soft tissues are easily targeted. However, lesions in deep organs such as lung, mediastinum, liver, pancreas, kidney, adrenal gland, spleen, retroperitoneum, and deep lymph nodes are aspirated with guidance by fluoroscopy, computed tomography, or ultrasound. Most laboratories use a combination of Diff Quik stain for air-dried smears and Papanicolaou stain for alcohol-fixed smears for this purpose. Hematoxylin & eosin-stained sections of paraffin-embedded cell clusters and small tissue fragments allow characterization of the tumor architecture and facilitate immunocytochemical staining.

Examples of cytologic preparations from various organs are shown in Figure. 30-1 through Figure 30-13.

Morphologic Parameters In Cytological Evaluation

Specimen Cellularity Is Influenced by Various Factors

The type of tissue sampled greatly influences the cellularity of the specimen. Epithelial cells are generally detached more easily than are stromal cells or fibrous tissue. Malignant cells have lower cohesiveness than their benign counterparts and are more likely to exfoliate spontaneously or mechanically. Malignant tumors that have little connective tissue support (e.g., small cell carcinoma of the lung, lymphoma, malignant melanoma) produce more cellular samples than those with a generous fibrous stroma (e.g., scirrhous carcinoma of the breast). Carcinomas tend to exfoliate cells more readily than do sarcomas.

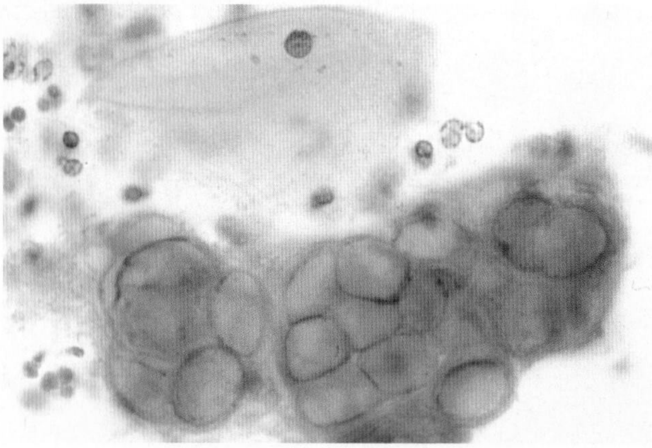

FIGURE 30-2. **Herpes simplex virus infection in a cervical smear.** Note multinucleation of squamous cells, nuclear molding, margination of the chromatin, and "ground glass" appearance of the nuclei. A normal superficial squamous cell serves for comparison.

Cell Arrangement Is an Important Cytological Parameter

The relation between cells is a helpful criterion for cytologic diagnosis. Cells may appear singly, in small groups, in monolayer sheets, or in three-dimensional clusters. Several cells may fuse, forming a large formation termed a **syncytium.** Cell clusters may form:

- **Papillary configurations** with fibrovascular cores (papillary urothelial carcinoma, papillary adenocarcinoma, malignant mesothelioma) (see Fig. 30-9A and Fig. 30-12B)
- **Glandular or tubular structures** (adenocarcinoma) (see Fig. 30-6, Fig. 30-7F, Fig. 30-8D, and Fig. 30-10B)
- **Follicles** (follicular neoplasms of the thyroid) (see Fig. 30-12A)
- **Rosettes** (neuroblastoma)
- **Pearls** (squamous cell carcinoma) (see Fig. 30-5 and Fig. 30-7E)

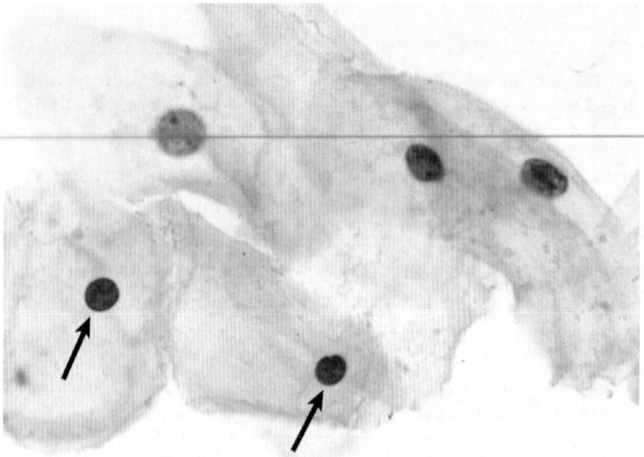

FIGURE 30-1. **Normal cervical Papanicolaou (Pap) smear.** Large squamous cells from the superficial and intermediate layers of the epithelium are illustrated. The cells have abundant cytoplasm that varies in staining from pink to blue. The nuclei are small, and the nuclear–cytoplasmic ratio is low. The most superficial cells have pyknotic nuclei *(arrows)*.

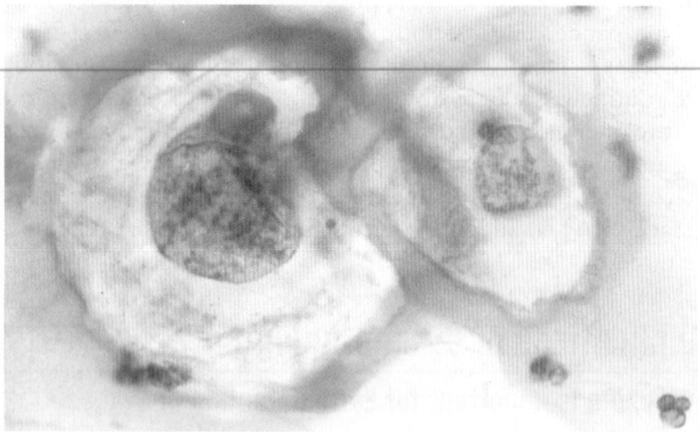

FIGURE 30-3. **Papillomavirus infection in a cervical smear.** Two superficial squamous cells exhibit koilocytotic atypia, a term that denotes the presence of sharply demarcated, large perinuclear vacuoles, combined with alterations in the chromatin pattern.

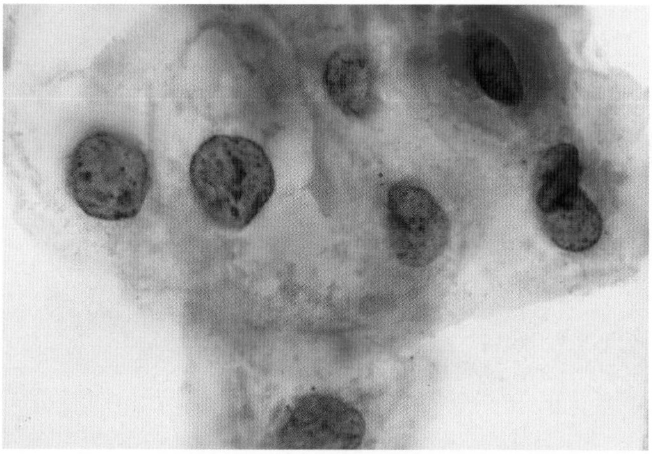

A

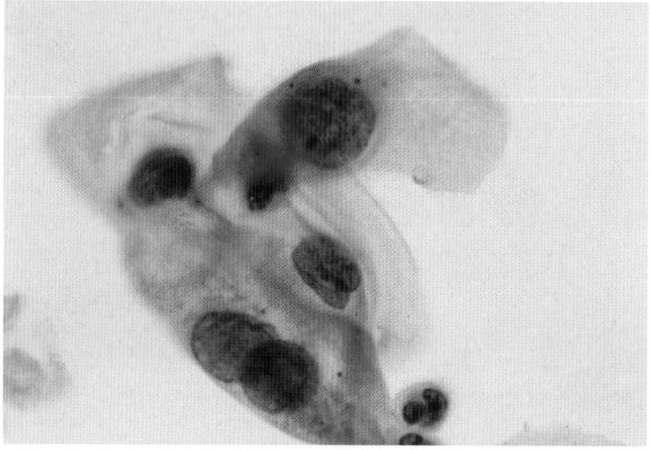

B

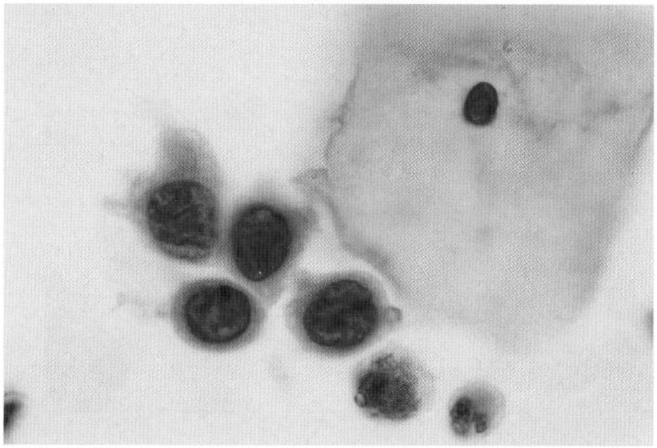

C

FIGURE 30-4. **Spectrum of squamous intraepithelial lesions (SILs) in cervical smears. A.** Low-grade SIL (mild dysplasia, cervical intraepithelial neoplasia (CIN)1). The dysplastic cells have abundant cytoplasm. The nucleus is enlarged and hyperchromatic. **B.** High-grade SIL (moderate dysplasia, CIN2). The dysplastic cells have a higher nuclear–cytoplasmic ratio than do mildly dysplastic cells. **C.** High-grade SIL (severe dysplasia, CIN3/carcinoma in situ). Multiple dysplastic squamous cells with scant cytoplasm and very high nuclear–cytoplasmic ratios are seen. Note the normal superficial squamous cell.

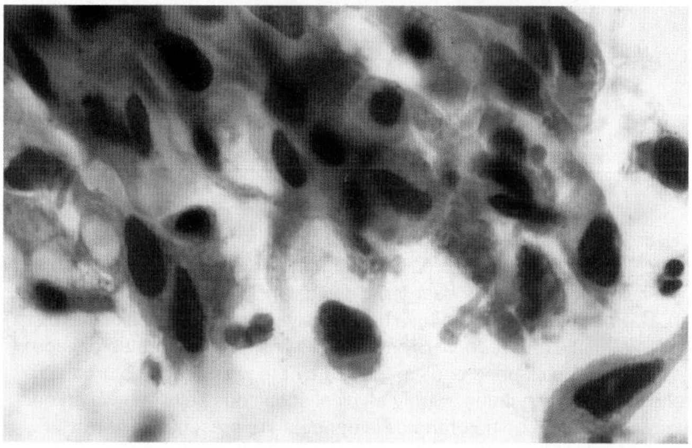

FIGURE 30-5. **Invasive squamous cell carcinoma of the cervix.** Pleomorphic elongate squamous cells, with enlarged, irregular and hyperchromatic nuclei.

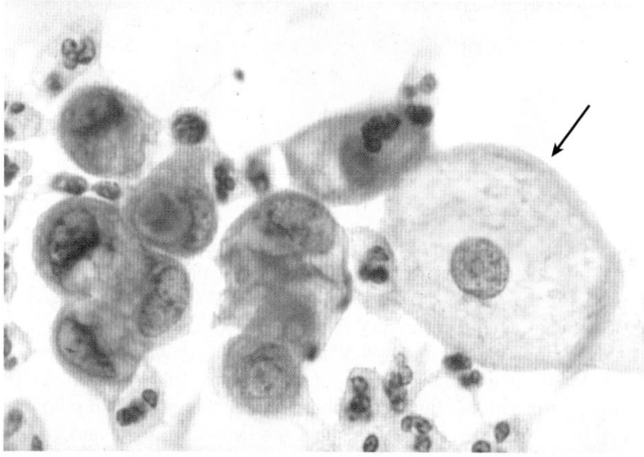

FIGURE 30-6. **Endometrial adenocarcinoma in a cervical smear.** A cluster of medium-sized malignant cells displays cytoplasmic vacuoles. The nuclei are eccentric and have irregular nuclear membranes and abnormally distributed chromatin. Note the benign squamous cell *(arrow)*.

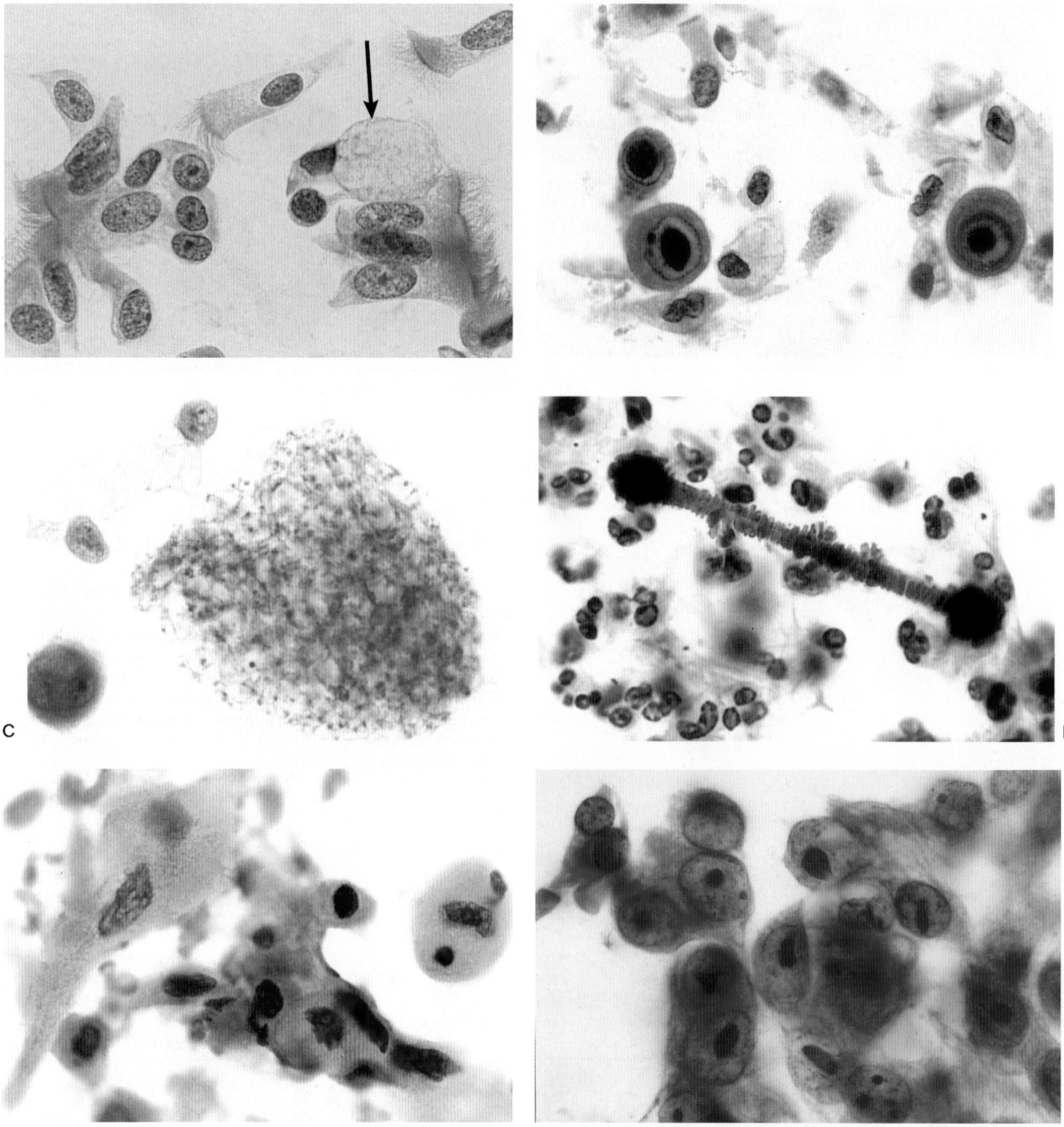

FIGURE 30-7. **Cytology of the respiratory tract. A.** Normal bronchial epithelial cells in a bronchial brush specimen. Note the ciliated columnar cells with uniform and basally located nuclei. The chromatin is finely granular and evenly dispersed; the nuclear membrane is smooth and regular. Note the goblet cell *(arrow)*. **B.** Cytomegalovirus (CMV) infection in a bronchial washing. Note the large basophilic nuclear inclusions surrounded by a halo and marginated chromatin, forming the typical target-shaped appearance. **C.** *Pneumocystis carinii* in a bronchoalveolar lavage specimen. This foamy alveolar cast composed of small cysts, each with an eccentric dot, is characteristic of *P. carinii*. Bronchial cells and an alveolar macrophage are evident. **D.** Ferruginous body in the sputum. This long, yellow, beaded structure with clubbed ends is formed by the precipitation of iron and protein complexes on asbestos fibers. **E.** Squamous cell carcinoma in a bronchial brush specimen. Highly atypical squamous cells show marked variation in size and shape. The nuclei are hyperchromatic and irregular. The orange color in some of the cells denotes the presence of keratin. **F.** Adenocarcinoma cells in bronchial brush specimen. A cluster of epithelial cells with highly atypical nuclei, prominent nucleoli, and cytoplasmic vacuoles is seen.

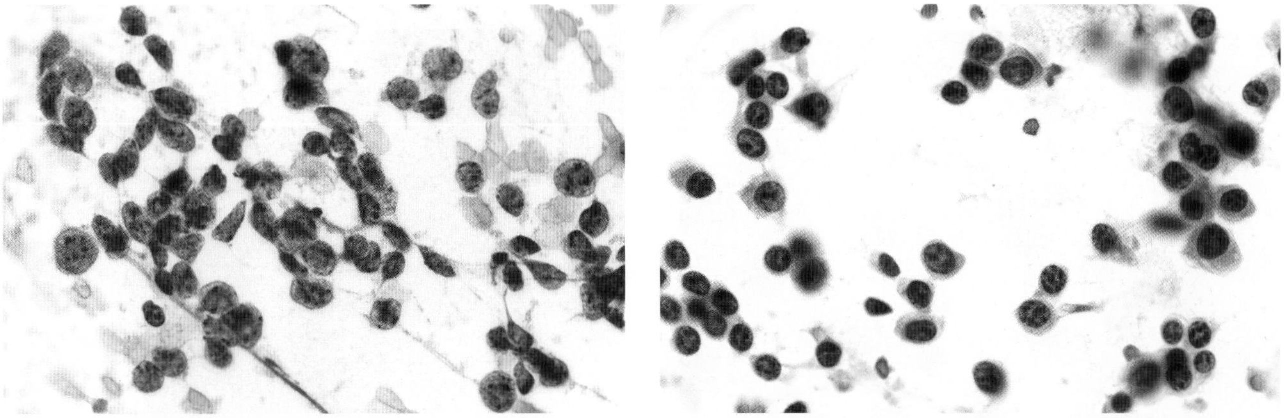

G H

FIGURE 30-7. *(continued)* **G.** Small cell carcinoma in a bronchial brush specimen. The cells are small, the cytoplasm is scanty, and the nuclei are molded where they abut adjacent ones. **H.** Carcinoid tumor in a fine-needle aspirate of the lung. These small cells are arranged in loosely cohesive sheets. They have scant cytoplasm and uniform round nuclei. The chromatin is evenly dispersed.

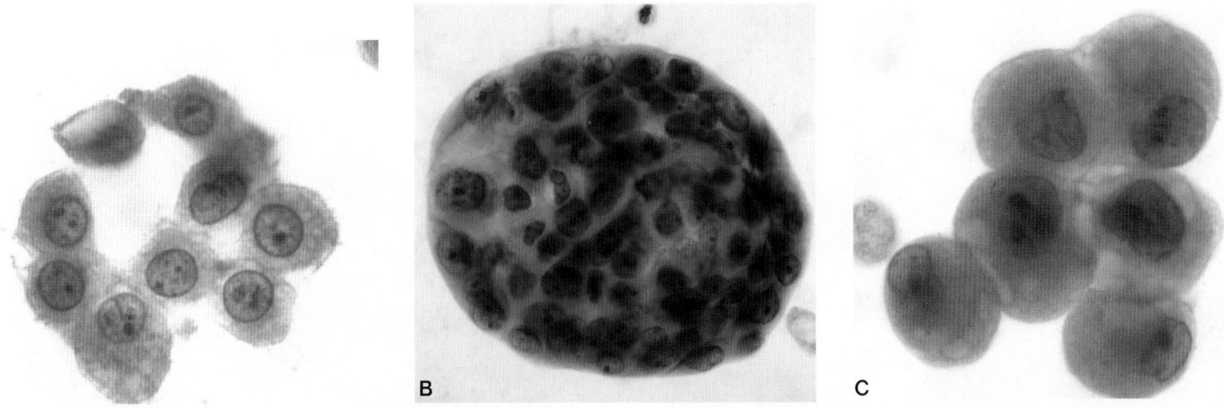

A B C

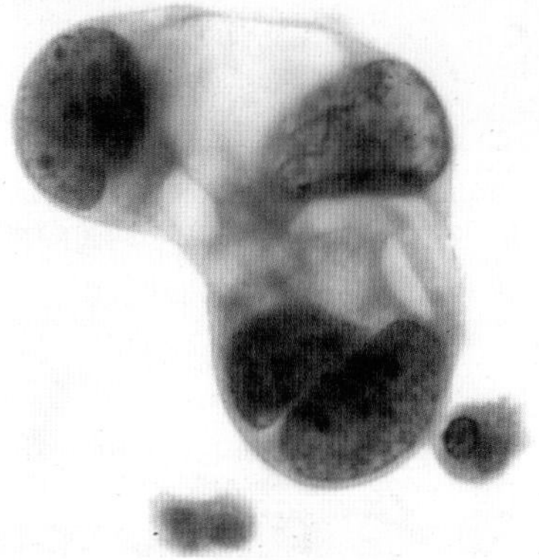

D

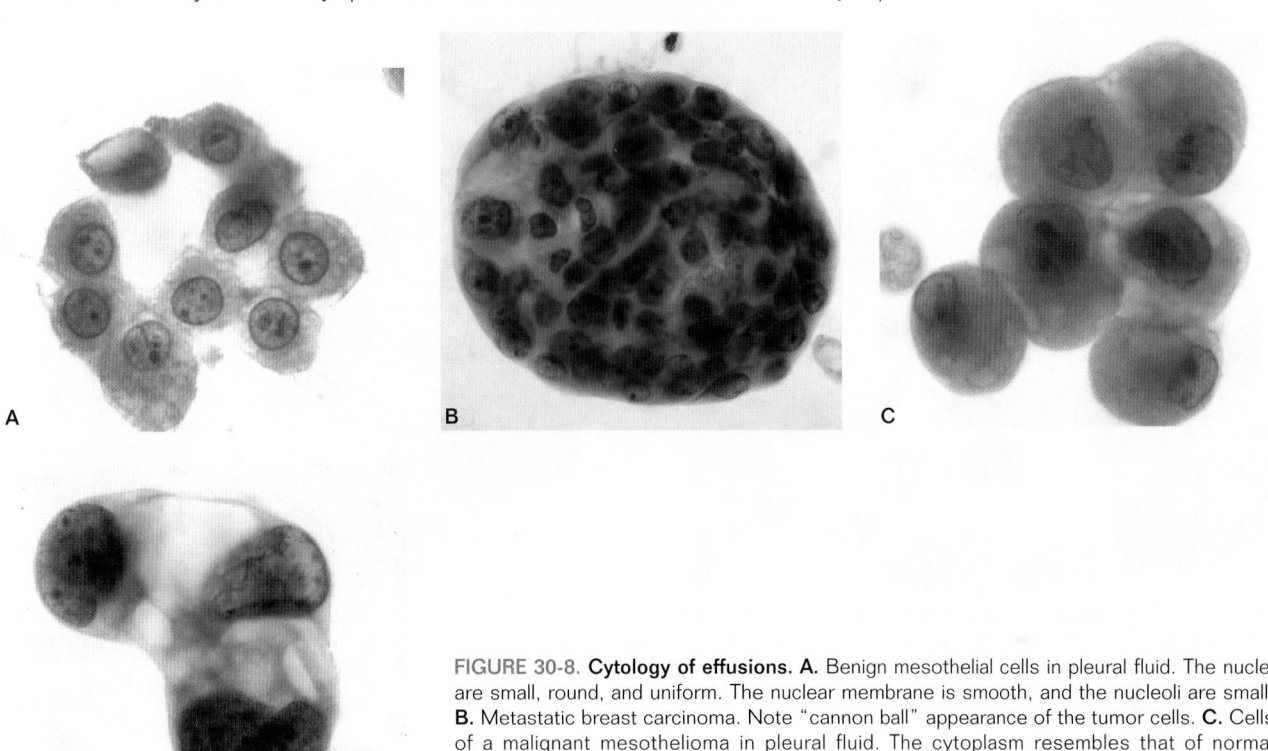

FIGURE 30-8. **Cytology of effusions. A.** Benign mesothelial cells in pleural fluid. The nuclei are small, round, and uniform. The nuclear membrane is smooth, and the nucleoli are small. **B.** Metastatic breast carcinoma. Note "cannon ball" appearance of the tumor cells. **C.** Cells of a malignant mesothelioma in pleural fluid. The cytoplasm resembles that of normal mesothelial cells, but the nuclei are large, hyperchromatic, and irregular. The chromatin is abnormally distributed, the nucleoli are prominent, and the nuclear membrane has irregular indentations. **D.** Metastatic ovarian adenocarcinoma in ascitic fluid. The nuclei exhibit malignant criteria, and the cytoplasm contains secretory vacuoles.

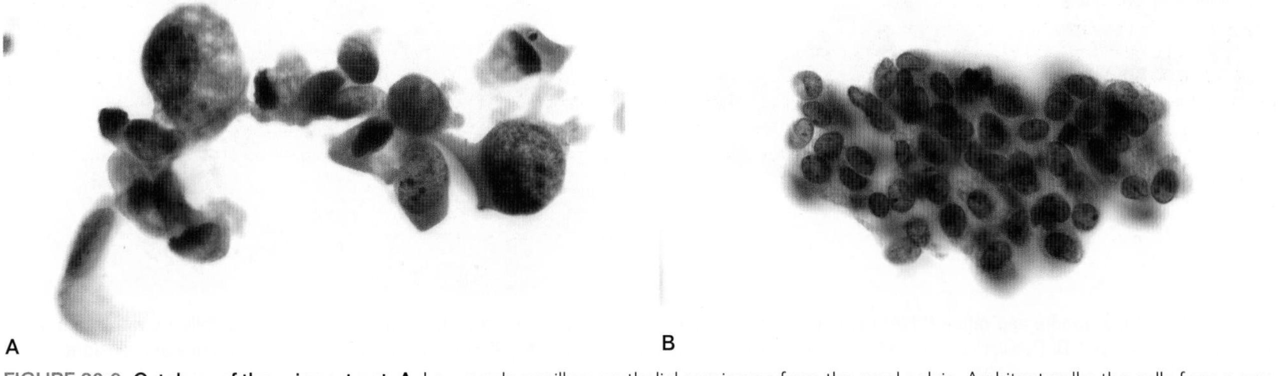

A B

FIGURE 30-9. **Cytology of the urinary tract. A.** Low-grade papillary urothelial carcinoma from the renal pelvis. Architecturally, the cells form a papillary structure, and the nuclei are crowded and hyperchromatic. **B.** High-grade urothelial carcinoma in urine. Highly pleomorphic cells with varying sized, hyperchromatic, irregular nuclei are evident.

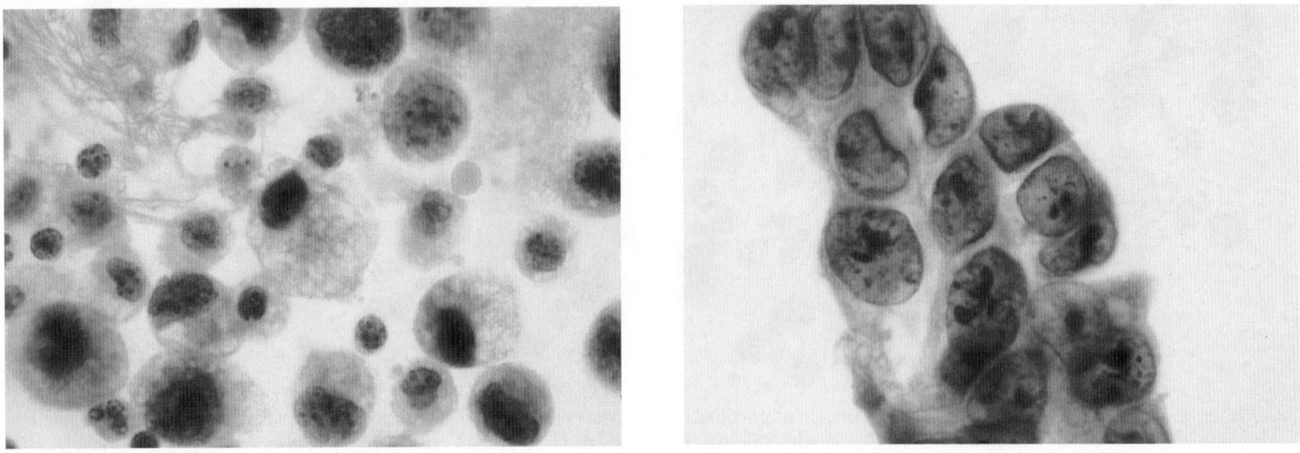

A B

FIGURE 30-10. **Cytology of the alimentary tract. A.** Gastric carcinoma in brushing specimen. Note cytoplasmic vacuoles in tumor cells. **B.** Adenocarcinoma of the colon. The malignant nuclei display variation in size and shape and prominent nucleoli.

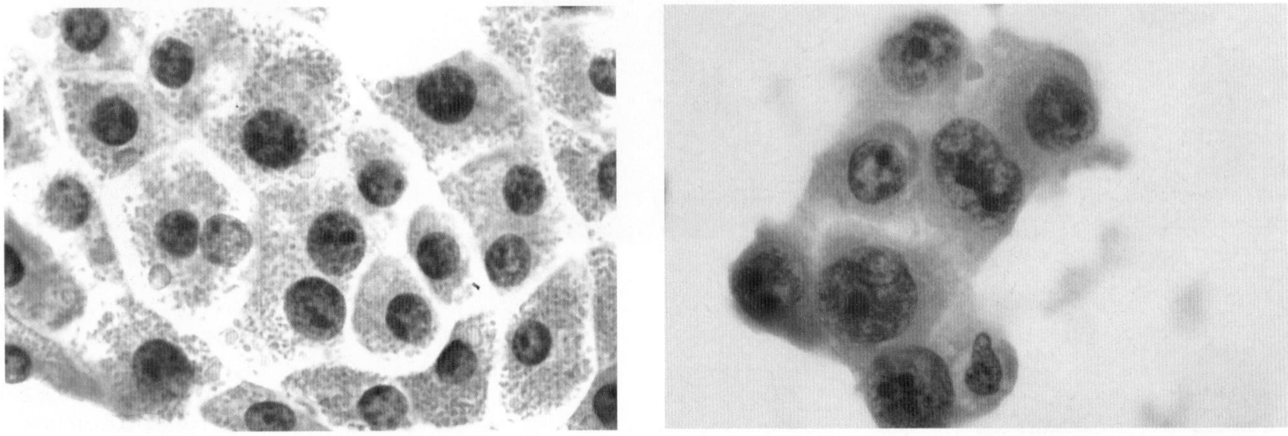

A B

FIGURE 30-11. **Fine-needle aspiration (FNA) cytology of the breast. A.** Apocrine metaplasia. These benign cells have abundant and granular cytoplasm. **B.** Mammary duct carcinoma. The cells vary in size and shape and are poorly cohesive. The nuclei are hyperchromatic, with irregular membranes and clumping of the chromatin. The nucleoli are prominent.

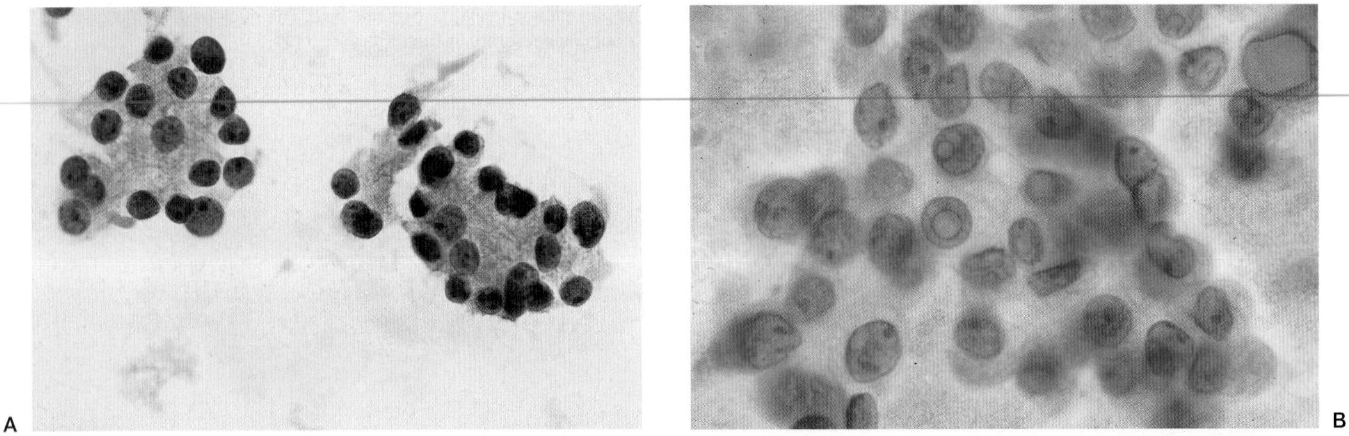

A B

FIGURE 30-12. **Fine-needle aspiration (FNA) cytology of the thyroid. A.** Follicular neoplasm. The tumor cells form small follicles with scant colloid and mild nuclear atypia. **B.** Papillary carcinoma. A papillary frond of the tumor shows nuclei with nuclear grooves and intranuclear inclusions.

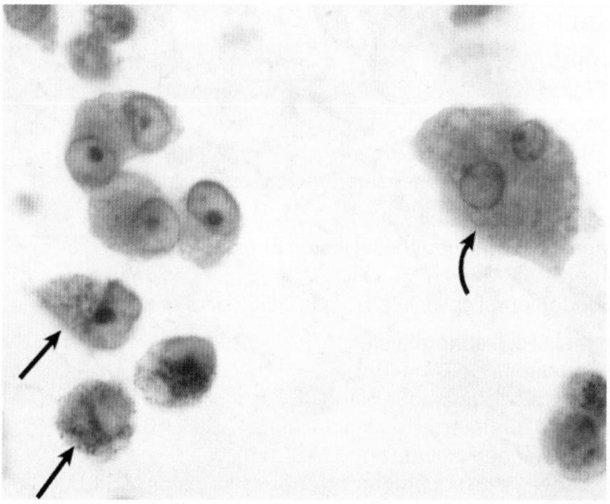

FIGURE 30-13. **Metastatic malignant melanoma in a fine-needle aspirate of the liver.** Poorly cohesive tumor cells exhibit eccentric nuclei and prominent nucleoli. The cytoplasm contains fine melanin granules *(straight arrows)*. A benign binucleated hepatocyte is evident *(curved arrow)*.

Cell Size and Shape Characteristics Help to Identify Specific Neoplasms

The size of tumor cells varies greatly depending on the type of neoplasm. Small cell carcinoma of the lung, some types of lymphoma, and many childhood tumors are composed of small cells (see Fig. 30-7G). By contrast, squamous cell carcinoma, giant cell carcinoma, pleomorphic sarcomas, some endocrine carcinomas and choriocarcinoma have very large cells. Malignant neoplasms tend to vary more in cell size than benign tumors, a feature termed **anisocytosis** (see Fig 30-7E). However, this rule does not apply to all neoplasms. Well-differentiated adenocarcinomas and low-grade urothelial carcinomas, for example, have little anisocytosis (see Fig. 30-9A). Conversely, marked anisocytosis may be seen in some benign conditions, such as lymph node hyperplasia or radiation effects. Cells are generally uniform (monomorphic) in normal tissues and benign neoplasms, whereas malignant tumors frequently exhibit significant variation in cell shape (**pleomorphism**) (see Fig. 30-5).

Cytoplasmic Features May Reveal the Tissue Origin or Etiology

The cytoplasm is evaluated for color, texture, presence of inclusions, vacuoles, pigments, and other cell products. With the Papanicolaou method, the cytoplasm assumes various shades of pink to blue; keratin stains orange (see Fig. 30-1). Cytoplasm may vary in texture from homogeneous to granular or foamy. The presence of pigments–including melanin, hemosiderin, bile, lipofuscin, and carbon particles–is helpful in identifying the cell type (see Fig. 30-13). Single or multiple cytoplasmic vacuoles indicate degenerative changes, secretory activity, or phagocytosis (see Fig. 30-8D). Viral and chlamydial infections may also produce inclusions in the cytoplasm (see Fig. 30-7B). Squamous cells infected by human papillomavirus show characteristic changes called **koilocytotic atypia**, which consists of a large perinuclear halo and nuclear abnormalities (see Fig. 30-3). Accumulation of immunoglobulin in the cytoplasm of reactive or neoplastic plasma cells forms an eosinophilic globule termed the **Russell body.** Small cytoplasmic concretions (**Michaelis-Gutmann bodies**) are seen in malakoplakia.

The Most Important Features of Malignancy Reside in the Nucleus

The size and shape of the nucleus, alterations of nuclear membrane and chromatin, prominence of the nucleolus and mitotic activity are important parameters in cytologic evaluation. Nuclei of normal cells vary little in size and shape (see Fig. 30-7A). Modest nuclear enlargement occurs in normal cells during the S phase of the cell cycle, and in reactive or regenerating cells. Malignant cells usually exhibit significant nuclear enlargement, which is frequently disproportionate to the enlargement of the cell and results in an increased nuclear-to-cytoplasmic ratio. In addition, significant variations in nuclear size (**anisokaryosis**) and shape are common in malignant neoplasms (see Fig. 30-7E). The nuclei of most cancer cells, with the exception of some well-differentiated tumors, are abnormally shaped and have an irregular contour, with protrusions, indentations, and grooves (see Fig. 30-10). Molding of the nuclei against one another is seen in some tumors (classically in small cell carcinomas), probably owing to a rapid growth rate and scanty cytoplasm (see Fig. 30-7G).

Nuclei of cancer cells are usually darker (**hyperchromatic**) than those of normal cells, and the chromatin tends to be coarser and unevenly distributed (see Fig. 30-9B). Multinucleation *per se* is not helpful in the diagnosis of malignancy, because this feature may be seen in (1) normal cells (e.g., superficial urothelial cells, osteoclasts, syncytiotrophoblast), (2) inflammatory conditions (e.g., multinucleated histiocytes in granulomas), (3) benign neoplasms (e.g., giant cell tumor of the tendon sheath), or (4) malignant neoplasms (e.g., giant cell carcinoma, malignant fibrous histiocytoma, choriocarcinoma). Cytoplasmic invagination into the nucleus, which is seen in cross-section as a pale intranuclear inclusion, may occur in some benign and malignant neoplasms and may be helpful in their classification (e.g., papillary thyroid carcinoma; see Fig. 30-12B).

The nucleoli of cancer cells, particularly in poorly differentiated tumors, are often larger and more numerous than those in their benign counterparts (see Fig.30-7F).

Although increased mitotic activity can occur in both benign and malignant tumors, cancer cells in general have a higher rate of mitosis. Additionally, the presence of abnormal mitoses (abnormal distribution of chromosomes or presence of more than two mitotic poles) is a reliable criterion for the diagnosis of malignancy.

Extracellular Material and Background Surround the Cells

The smear background is evaluated for the presence of inflammation, blood, various extracellular substances, cell products, necrotic debris, and microorganisms. The type of inflammation (acute, chronic, granulomatous) and some varieties of microorganisms–including bacteria, fungi, protozoa, and helminths–can be identified. Cell necrosis may occur in a variety of benign conditions (e.g., infections, trauma, ischemia, and irradiation) but may also be a prominent feature of many malignant neoplasms. *When present in association with malignant cells, necrosis generally indicates an invasive cancer.*

Common entities found in the smear background include:

- Mucin
- Amyloid
- Colloid
- Psammoma bodies

- Ferruginous bodies
- Curschmann spirals
- Charcot-Leyden crystals
- Renal casts
- Urinary crystals

Reporting Systems

Various methods have been used for reporting the results of cytologic tests. Most laboratories today use narrative reports for **nongynecologic** cytology, like reports used in histopathological reporting. The **Bethesda system** is the standard for **gynecologic** cytology reports. This reporting system, with revisions, has been adopted by most laboratories in the United States (Table 30-1).

Advantages of Cytopathology

Cytopathologic evaluation is invaluable from many different perspectives:

- **Less trauma** is involved sampling by cytologic techniques than by biopsy. Thus, there is less chance of hemorrhage, perforation, infection, tumor spread, or anesthetic complications.
- **A larger sampling surface** is available for cytologic methods. This is particularly important in laparoscopic and endoscopic procedures. In peritoneal washings, a very large area of the peritoneum is sampled, whereas biopsy samples are limited to a few, small, grossly visible foci. Similarly, a focus of flat *in situ* carcinoma of the bladder that may not be evident on cystoscopy is more likely to be discovered by cytologic examination of urine or bladder washings than by random biopsy sampling.
- **Tumors that are difficult to access by biopsy may be sampled by cytologic methods.** Examples include cerebrospinal fluid cytology to diagnose meningeal carcinomatosis, brushing or washing a gastrointestinal tract stricture that does not permit passage of the biopsy instrument, and fine-needle aspiration of a peripheral carcinoma of the lung that is beyond the reach of a bronchoscope.
- **Rapid diagnosis** is one of the major advantages of cytologic methods. Direct smears and fine-needle aspirates can be read within a few minutes of the collection. Fluids can be processed in less than an hour, if necessary.
- **Greater convenience** is afforded by the collection of cytologic specimens than with biopsy. In most instances, no prior preparation of the patient is necessary and the sampling is done as an office procedure. For endoscopically collected specimens, no preparations are needed beyond those required routinely for visualization.
- **An increased detection rate of malignancy** in endoscopic procedures is achieved by combining cytologic sampling (washing or brushing) with biopsy. In turn, this reduces the possibility that a repeated diagnostic procedure will be required.
- **Greater cost-effectiveness** of use of cytology for cancer detection has been amply demonstrated. Often, it eliminates needless tests, procedures, and surgical operations.

TABLE 30-1

The 2001 Bethesda System

Specimen adequacy
Satisfactory for evaluation
Unsatisfactory for evaluation . . . (specify reason)
Interpretation/result:
Negative for intraepithelial lesion or malignancy
Other
Endometrial cells (in a woman ≥40 years of age)
Epithelial cell abnormalities
Squamous Cell:
Atypical squamous cells (ASC)
Of undetermined significance (ASC-US)
Cannot exclude HSIL (ASC-H)
Low-grade squamous intraepithelial lesion (LSIL)
Encompassing: HPV/mild dysplasia/CIN1
High-grade squamous intraepithelial lesion (HSIL)
Encompassing: moderate and severe dysplasia, CIS/CIN2, and CIN3
With features suspicious for invasion (if invasion is suspected)
Squamous cell carcinoma
Glandular Cell:
Atypical
Endocervical cells (NOS or specify in comments)
Endometrial cells (NOS or specify in comments)
Glandular cells (NOS or specify in comments)
Atypical
Endocervical cells, favor neoplastic
Glandular cells, favor neoplastic
Endocervical adenocarcinoma in situ
Adenocarcinoma
Endocervical
Endometrial
Extrauterine
NOS
Other malignant neoplasms (specify)

CIN = cervical intraepithelial neoplasia; HPV = human papilloma virus; NOS = not otherwise specified

Limitations of Cytopathology

- **Classification of the type of tumor** is generally more difficult with cytologic samples than with biopsy specimens because of the small size of cytologic samples and the loss of tissue pattern. **The small size of the specimen** may preclude accurate classification of some neoplasms especially those with mixed elements, such as adenosquamous carcinoma, carcinosarcoma, or synovial sarcoma, if only one component of the tumor is sampled. In exfoliative cytology, carcinomas are more readily diagnosed than sarcomas, because epithelial neoplasms have a higher tendency to shed tumor cells.
- **The extent and depth of invasion** cannot be assessed by cytologic methods.
- **Inadequate sampling** is a major cause of false-negative diagnoses in cytology. For example, in obtaining a sample of the uterine cervix, it is critical to include the transformation zone, because most precancerous lesions of the cervix arise there. The adequacy of a sputum specimen is assessed by the presence of pulmonary macrophages, which indicates a deep cough sample.

Accuracy of Cytologic Methods

The accuracy of cytologic diagnosis depends on several factors, including the experience of the specimen collector, the sampling method, the sample adequacy, the target organ, and the expertise of the examiner. False-positive diagnoses are rarely made by experienced cytopathologists; thus, the specificity of a malignant diagnosis approaches 100%. The sensitivity of the test, however, is in the range of 80% to 90% for most specimen types. The absence of malignant cells in cytologic samples does not completely rule out the possibility of malignancy. Unless a benign cause for a lesion can be established by cytologic examination (e.g., fibroadenoma of the breast, benign cyst of the thyroid, liver abscess, granuloma of the lung), further investigation, including histologic biopsy, is warranted. The type and grade of the tumor also influence the sensitivity of cytologic diagnosis. For example, low-grade urothelial carcinomas, which by definition have little or no nuclear atypia, are difficult to detect, whereas high grade carcinomas are diagnosed with high degree of accuracy.

New Trends in Cytopathology

Liquid-based Pap test is a widely adopted technique that replaces direct smearing of collected samples. In this method, specimens from the uterine cervix or vagina are collected by means of a brush and placed in an alcohol-based solution. An automated machine is used to transfer cells from the liquid onto a glass slide and stain them by the Papanicolaou method. Additional tests for high-risk human papillomavirus and other infectious organisms can be done on the residual material.

Application of molecular tests to cytologic specimens is rapidly gaining importance as an adjunct to morphologic diagnosis. The clinical application of these methods include: (1) classifying tumors, particularly hematopoietic and mesenchymal tumors; (2) establishing clonality, particularly in the diagnosis of non-Hodgkin lymphoma); (3) identifying minimal residual disease and detecting recurrence after treatment; (4) assessing prognostic factors; and (5) providing guidance for targeted therapies.

Fluorescence in situ hybridization (FISH) and chromogenic in situ hybridization (CISH) are particularly suitable for cytologic specimens. In these methods a fluorescent or chromogen-labeled DNA probe designed for a specific chromosome, chromosomal region, or gene is used to visualize the target in cells fixed on the surface of a glass slide. These techniques allow identification of numerical abnormalities of chromosomes (gains or losses), chromosomal translocations and gene amplifications or deletions (see Chapter 5). The advantage of FISH and CISH over other molecular techniques is that the results can be easily correlated with tumor morphology.

FIGURE ACKNOWLEDGMENTS

Specific acknowledgment is made for permission to use the following material:

Chapter 1, Figure 2. Okazaki H, Scheithauer BW: Atlas of Neuropathology. New York, Gower Medical Publishing, 1988. By permission of the author.

Chapter 3, Figure 16. Okazaki H, Scheithauer BW: Atlas of Neuropathology. New York, Gower Medical Publishing, 1988. By permission of the author.

Chapter 5, Figure 5. Reprinted from Bullough PG, Vigorita VJ: Atlas of Orthopaedic Pathology. New York, Gower Medical Publishing, 1984 with permission from Elsevier.

Chapter 5, Figure 17. Reprinted from Bullough PG, Boachie-Adjei O: Atlas of Spinal Diseases. New York, Gower Medical Publishing, 1988 with permission from Elsevier.

Chapter 5, Figure 32. From US Mortality Public Use Data Tapes 1960–2002, US Mortality Volumes 1930–1959, National Center for Health Statistics, Centers for Disease Control and Prevention, 2005.

Chapter 6, Figure 30. Reprinted from Bullough PG, Vigorita VJ: Atlas of Orthopedic Pathology. New York, Gower Medical Publishing, 1988 with permission from Elsevier.

Chapter 7, Figures 3, 18, 29. Courtesy of UBC Pulmonary Registry, St. Paul's Hospital.

Chapter 7, Figures 5, 6, 12. Courtesy of Dr. Greg J. Davis, Dept. of Pathology, University of Kentucky College of Medicine.

Chapter 7, Figure 22. Courtesy of Dr. Ken Berry, Dept. of Pathology, St. Paul's Hospital.

Chapter 7, Figure 26. Courtesy of Dr. Kevin C. Kain, Centre for Travel and Tropical Medicine, Toronto General Hospital.

Chapter 7, Figure 34. Courtesy of Dr. Alex Magil, Dept. of Pathology, St. Paul's Hospital.

Chapter 8, Figure 11. Okazaki H, Scheithauer BW: Atlas of Neuropathology. New York, Gower Medical Publishing, 1988. By permission of the author.

Chapter 8, Figure 13. Reprinted from McKee PH: Pathology of the Skin. Copyright Gower Medical Publishing, 1989, with permission from Elsevier.

Chapter 9, Figures 18A, 18B, 25, 52A, 69, 80, 86, 87, 95A, and 95B. Reprinted from Farrar WE, Wood MJ, Innes JA, Tubbs H: Infectious Diseases Text and Color Atlas, 2nd ed. Copyright Gower Medical Publishing, 1992, with permission from Elsevier.

Chapter 12, Figure 40. Travis WB, Colby TV, Koss MN, Muller NL, Rosado-de-Christenson ML, and King, TE: Non-neoplastic Disorders of the Lower Respiratory Tract, Washington DC: American Registry of Pathology, 2002.

Chapter 12, Figure 55. Courtesy of the Armed Forces Institute of Pathology.

Chapter 12. The authors would like to gratefully acknowledge Dr. Anthony Gal for the contribution of Figure 70.

Chapter 13, Figures 10, 12B, 23, 26, 44, 62, 63. Reprinted from Mitros FA: Atlas of Gastrointestinal Pathology. New York, Gower Medical Publishing, 1988 with permission from Elsevier.

Chapter 13, Figure 10. Courtesy of Dr. Cecilia M. Fenoglio-Preiser.

Chapter 14, Figure 41. Yanoff M: Ocular Pathology: A Color Atlas. New York, Gower Medical Publishing, 1988.

Chapter 14, Figure 57. Thung SN, Gerber MA: Histopathology of liver transplantation. In Fabry TL, Klion FM (eds): Guide to Liver Transplantation. New York, Igaku-Shoin Medical Publishers, 1992.

Chapter 17, Figure 4 and 10. Weiss MA, Mills SE: Atlas of Genitourinary Tract Diseases. New York, Gower Medical Publishers, 1988.

Chapter 18, Figures 4, 5, 14, 25, 27, 30, 33, 38B, 45, 60, 66, 67, and 73. Reprinted with permission of Stanley J. Robboy, MD, and Gynecologic Pathology Associates, Durham and Chapel Hill, North Carolina.

Chapter 18, Figures 11, 16, 23, 26A. Robboy SJ, Anderson MC, and Russell P (eds): Pathology of the Female Reproductive Tract. London, Churchill-Livingstone, 2002, pp. 111–112, 147, 167, 140, 203, 248, 322, 354.

Chapter 18, Figures 61A and 61B. Reprinted from Woodruff JD, Parmley TH: Atlas of Gynecologic Pathology. New York, Gower Medical Publishing, 1988 with permission from Elsevier.

Chapter 21, Figure 13. Sandoz Pharmaceutical Corporation.

Chapter 22, Figure 11. Courtesy of the American Diabetes Association.

Chapter 24, Figures 9A, 22A, 25A (Courtesy W. Witmer), 26, 32A, 34A, 36A, 38A, 42, 43A, 44, 45, 46, 69A, 70, 71, 72, 79A, 88A. Elder AD, Elenitsas R, Johnson BL, et al: Synopsis and Atlas of Lever's Histopathology of the Skin. Lippincott Williams & Wilkins, Philadelphia, 1999, p 2, clin. fig. IA1; p 163, clin. fig. IVE3; p 167, clin. fig. IVE4.b; p 124, clin. fig. IIIH1.a; p 105, clin. fig. IIIF1.a; p 115, clin. fig. IIIG1.a; p 85, clin. fig. IIIB1a.a; p 219, clin. fig. VE3.a; clin. fig. IVA2.b; p 7, clin. fig. IC1; p 212, fig. VD1.d; p 51, clin. fig. IIE1.f and IIE1.1; p 226, clin. fig. VE5.f; p 283, clin. fig. VIB3.g; p 280, clin. fig. VIB3.q and VIB3.s; p 10, clin. fig. ID1.b; p 31, clin. fig. IIC1.a; clin. fig. IIF2.a; p 96, clin. fig. IIID1.d.

Chapter 26, Figures 20A, 20B, 40, 51B, 56, and 67A. Reprinted from Bullough PG: Atlas of Orthopaedic Pathology, 2nd ed. New York, Gower Medical Publishing, 1992 with permission from Elsevier.

INDEX

P

S